COMPREHENSIVE TEXTBOOK OF PSYCHIATRY/V

VOLUME 1
FIFTH EDITION

SENIOR CONTRIBUTING EDITOR

Robert Cancro, M.D., Med.D.Sc.

Professor and Chairman, Department of Psychiatry,
New York University School of Medicine
Director, Department of Psychiatry, University Hospital
of the New York University Medical Center
Director, Nathan S. Kline Institute for Psychiatric Research,
Orangeburg, New York

CONTRIBUTING EDITOR

Jack A. Grebb, M.D.

Assistant Professor of Psychiatry, New York University
School of Medicine; Assistant Attending Psychiatrist,
Bellevue Hospital; Guest Investigator,
Laboratory of Molecular and Cellular Neuroscience,
The Rockefeller University, New York, New York;
Research Scientist, Nathan S. Kline
Institute for Psychiatric Research, Orangeburg, New York

CONTRIBUTING EDITOR

Joel Yager, M.D.

Professor of Psychiatry, University of California at Los Angeles
School of Medicine; Director, Residency Education,
Neuropsychiatric Institute and Hospital
Associate Chief of Staff for Residency Education,
West Los Angeles Veterans Administration Medical Center
(Brentwood), Los Angeles, California

COMPREHENSIVE TEXTBOOK OF PSYCHIATRY/V

VOLUME 1
FIFTH EDITION

EDITORS

Harold I. Kaplan, M.D.

Professor of Psychiatry, New York University School of Medicine
Attending Psychiatrist, University Hospital of the New York University Medical Center
Attending Psychiatrist, Bellevue Hospital
New York, New York

Benjamin J. Sadock, M.D.

Professor and Vice Chairman, Department of Psychiatry,
New York University School of Medicine,
Attending Psychiatrist, University Hospital of the New York University Medical Center
Attending Psychiatrist, Bellevue Hospital
New York, New York

SANS TACHE
WILLIAMS & WILKINS
Baltimore • Hong Kong • London • Sydney

Editor: Michael G. Fisher
Associate Editor: Victoria M. Vaughn
Copy Editors: Suzanne Boyd Enright, Evelyn Tucker, Robert Whitlock, Margaret Yamashita
Design: JoAnne Janowiak
Illustration Planning: Lorraine Wrzosek
Production: Raymond E. Reter
Production Service: Rachel Hockett, Spectrum Publisher Services, Inc.
Cover Design: Dan Pfisterer
Project Editor: Lynda Abrams

The editors and the publisher of this textbook have made every effort to ensure that the drug dosage schedules herein are accurate and in accord with the standards accepted at the time of publication. Readers are advised, however, to check the product information sheet included in the package of each drug they plan to administer to be certain that changes have not been made in the recommended dose or in the indications and contraindications for administration and for adverse reactions. This recommendation is of particular importance in regard to new or infrequently used drugs.

Printed in the United States of America

First Edition 1967
Second Edition 1975
Third Edition 1980
Fourth Edition 1985

Library of Congress Cataloging in Publication Data

Main entry under title:

Comprehensive textbook of psychiatry/V.

Rev. ed. of: comprehensive textbook of psychiatry/IV. 4th ed. c1985.
Bibliography: p.
Includes index.
1. Psychiatry. I. Kaplan, Harold I. II. Sadock, Benjamin J. . III. Comprehensive textbook of psychiatry/IV. [DNLM: 1. Mental disorders. 2. Psychiatry—History. WM 100 C736]
RC454.C637 1985 616.89 83-25952

89 90 91 92
1 2 3 4 5 6 7 8 9 10

Dedicated to our wives
Nancy Barrett Kaplan
and
Virginia Alcott Sadock
without whose help and sacrifice
this textbook would not have been possible

FOREWORD

It is a curious truth that the vast majority of scientists who have ever lived are living now. This fact reveals two important facets of science: It is relatively young, and its recent growth has been exponential. Historically, there had long been a tension between scientific inquiry and theological truths. These latter truths were often revealed and not subject to rational inquiry. The church was far more powerful than science, and it held the position that if logical inquiry contradicted revealed truth, then the results of the logical inquiry were false. In this atmosphere, it was not easy for science to progress. These insights into natural science were even more pertinent to the medical sciences. Descartes made a major contribution to making a truce possible by separating the mind and the body. This partition was not only clever, but led to a marked reduction in the friction between science and theology. Medical science could focus on "mere" mechanistic questions that looked at how events transpired in the body, while the truly important questions of being, consciousness, and awareness were reserved for theology and philosophy.

For many years, this truce was an exceptionally useful one. It led to important and relatively free work in all science, with a marked reduction in church interference in scientific matters. A negative consequence of this dualism has been an arbitrary separation of mind and body in medicine, which has increasingly hampered our present understanding. The relationships among the nervous system, emotions, hormones, blood cells, immune responses, etc. are real, complex, and intimate. The organism is a whole, and our disciplinary divisions are arbitrary. While these distinctions are frequently of vital importance, they are, nevertheless, not without cost. Increasingly, the role of the nervous system and the effects of experience in all medical disorders and not merely the mental disorders can be seen.

The roots of psychiatry, as shown by this brief historical summary, are somewhat different from the roots of general medicine. The focus of psychiatry has been on the mind and its disorders. Because of its philosophical and theological origins, psychiatry frequently asked philosophical rather than biological questions. For many years, psychiatry was preoccupied with why things occurred and ignored how they occurred. This ignoring of mechanisms and search for meaning helped to obscure, rather than to enhance, the study of the problems of the human mind.

There is a second tradition in psychiatry, which was less based on observation and speculation and more on empiricism. This latter tradition has grown and in recent years has become the dominant force in American psychiatry. Sadly, the former tributaries now carry reified names, such as biological psychiatry, social psychiatry, cultural psychiatry, etc. The urgency of the need to merge these tributaries into a single psychiatry is still not sufficiently recognized. Independent of the historical antecedents, contemporary psychiatry—as also contemporary general medicine—must recognize and deal with all of the etiopathogenic forces that impinge on the individual who has become ill. Psychiatrists by the nature of the problems possessed by the patients under psychiatric care must be multidisciplinary and interdisciplinary in their perspective.

During World War II, psychiatry had been quite helpful to the armed forces. Following the war, there was an upsurge in interest in what psychiatrists could do to alleviate suffering. The period was primarily dominated in America by psychoanalytic thinking. Biological studies were going on, but they were not in the mainstream. It was not until the mid-1950s, with the introduction of pharmacologically effective compounds, that American psychiatry began to move into the pantheon of medicine.

Despite this scientific movement of the 1950s, the exuberance of the 1960s swept much of the previous rational inquiry and evolutionary growth aside. The 1960s were to bring the Age of Aquarius to mankind. If not mankind, certainly to all Americans. The goals of the French revolution were to be achieved along with peace, prosperity, and an abolishment of mental distress. It is remarkable, in retrospect, how little an understanding of human nature affected these near delusional beliefs. Senior people in American psychiatry, for example, attributed the chronicity of schizophrenia exclusively to the nature of the treatment and in no way to the nature of the disorder. All desirable outcomes were possible to those who believed. And if you did not believe, you then became part of the problem.

During this strange antirational period of massive denial and grandiose expectations, the first edition of the *Comprehensive Textbook of Psychiatry* appeared. Textbooks are written for many reasons, only a few of which are worthwhile. Personal vanity and professional visibility have driven many a person to put together a textbook that did little for the author and even less for the field. It is clear now that the driving force behind the first edition was a recognition that psychiatry was not only ready for a comprehensive textbook but in fact needed it. The field required a textbook for all the standard reasons. Very important, there was no good textbook available. Most important, psychiatry was in desperate need of a Baedeker with all of the structure and discipline it would give. The field had grown in such an extraordinary, explosive, and illogical way that it was confusing to all who looked at it. There were serious discussions about political psychiatry as if the term had some esoteric meaning. The theory of conflict resolution as a way of reducing neurotic symptoms was being generalized to the conflicts among nations. The differences between conflicting internal demands and the perfectly rational if immoral wish to exploit one's neighbor state were merely ignored. The expansionism seemed unlimited. The first edition was extremely beneficial in creating boundaries for psychiatry that were not coextensive with those of all human mental activity. This cynical sounding observation reflects quite accurately on the chaos of the field at that time, which was, in the words of Roy Grinker, going off madly in all directions simultaneously.

Textbooks always, to some degree, mirror their subject. Despite the boundaries established by the first edition, one can see in retrospect that they were still too broad. The second and third editions began to lead the specialty back to its clinical purposes and to emphasize that clinical activities had to derive from the basic sciences of psychiatry. One can also see an evolution in the second and third editions toward a more extensive scholarship. Perhaps at times defensive, the scholarship, nevertheless, reflected the growing depth and breadth of the scientific work going on. There was a necessary pruning of the excessive foliage of the Age of Aquarius and a growth of emphasis on the major mental disorders and our better understanding of them.

The fourth edition, in this writer's judgment, set a new standard. It was, in fact, a comprehensive textbook that was the equal of similar books in medicine and surgery. It was much more concise, and the scholarship, while apparent, was not ostentatious. For the first time, the textbook did not try to imply that the field was just as scientific as medicine and surgery, but merely asserted it by the quiet quality of the scholarship. One can also see in the fourth edition an increasing emphasis on the basic biological sciences that are of fundamental importance to clinical psychiatry.

Psychiatry is an application of neuroscience to the problems of particular groups of patients. This can be seen quite clearly in the fifth edition. The basic science section has been extensively redone. These changes reflect the striking developments of these past few years in neuroscience. It is remarkable to realize that it has only been four years since the fourth edition, and yet the amount of new material that is to be found in the fifth edition is truly amazing. Equally interesting is that we are getting a deeper appreciation of the role of experiential factors. People are open systems and their experiences influence their biology, just as their biology plays a role in determining their experiences. As the fourth edition previously set a new standard, so now does the fifth.

The fifth edition is a stunning accomplishment. Perhaps a more accurate name for the fifth edition would have been an integrated textbook, because, while it is comprehensive, its most striking feature is its integration. The first section on the basic sciences is literally sprinkled with clinical illustrations and applications. The clinical chapters draw heavily on the basic sciences of psychiatry in describing the diagnosis and treatment of mental disorders. This integration of basic and clinical science reflects the dramatic changes that are happening in psychiatry at a tempo whose rate is increasing exponentially. It is hard to believe that so much has changed in only four years.

The editors have invited a large number of new contributors whose efforts must be assessed by the reader. This reader believes that these changes have been salutary and that outstanding scholars and scholarship have been added. The additions are intelligible and, perhaps more importantly, interesting. If textbooks are to be read rather than collected, they must be interesting to the reader. American textbooks have long suffered from an identification with certain central European textbooks, which included such an excess of detail as to be stultifying.

The excellence of the final product reflects very positively on Harold Kaplan and Benjamin Sadock. They have worked very hard to improve the clarity and readability of the manuscripts. At times, their effort approached the heroic as particular authors defended poor prose with great zeal. This textbook has been a labor of love for Kaplan and Sadock. As in all love affairs, there is an element of irrationality. The time and effort demanded of them to make this book possible is known to only a handful of people. It is particularly known to their wives to whom the book has been traditionally dedicated (in absentia). The field owes these fine women a debt for lending us their husbands' time so unselfishly. This writer would also like to acknowledge his debt to the editors for their continued extraordinary editorial standards. Despite the harrowing pace of change, we can feel safe with Harold Kaplan and Benjamin Sadock at the controls. The *Comprehensive Textbook of Psychiatry* will continue to anticipate change and lead the field toward rational goals. It is the mission of a great textbook to educate. Any textbook will contain facts, but a great textbook must go beyond the facts. This is such a book.

Robert Cancro, Med.D.Sc.
New York University Medical Center, 1989

PREFACE

This is the fifth edition of the *Comprehensive Textbook of Psychiatry* to be published over a period of 22 years. As in previous editions, the editors have included the newest advances in the diagnosis and treatment of psychiatric disorders and have integrated those subjects with the behavioral sciences and other topics related to psychiatry. An eclectic and multidisciplinary approach has become the hallmark of this textbook through all of its editions. However, in many ways, this is a new book because of its radical departure from previous editions.

This edition contains 192 sections written by 237 contributors of whom 184 or 78 percent are new contributors who did not appear in CTP-IV. This textbook constitutes the most thorough, complete, integrated, and revised book of record of clinical psychiatry. The material is sufficiently comprehensive in scope to prepare the reader thoroughly to meet the standards of the American Board of Psychiatry and Neurology as well as the National Board of Medical Examiners.

This book forms part of a tripartite effort by the editors to provide a thorough educational system for both student and practitioner to facilitate the learning of psychiatry and to serve as a lifelong reference to the field.

At the head of this system is the *Comprehensive Textbook of Psychiatry,* which is global in depth and scope, designed for and used by psychiatrists, behavioral scientists, and all workers in the mental health field. Next is *Synopsis of Psychiatry,* a shortened, highly modified, and totally current version helpful to medical students, to psychiatric residents, and, for quick reference purposes, to the practicing psychiatrist and mental health professional. The *Study Guide and Self-Examination Review for the Synopsis of Psychiatry* consists of multiple choice questions and answers and forms the last part of the triad. That book is designed for students of psychiatry and clinical psychiatrists who require a brief review of the behavioral sciences and general psychiatry in preparation for a variety of examination situations.

Together, the three books create a multiple approach to the teaching, study, and learning of psychiatry.

CHANGES IN THIS EDITION

Format The major change is that this edition will only appear as a two-volume set since this format was preferred by most readers. Following the style of other major medical textbooks, internal citations of the literature have been eliminated. The number of references at the end of each section has been expanded from the last edition. Contributors were asked to cite 20 to 25 major books, monographs, or articles in their fields and to include very current and up-to-date references where possible. The editors asked the contributors to limit citations because of space considerations; therefore, the citation lists are not as complete as some of the contributors would have wished them to be.

Sections rewritten by new contributors Most sections were completely rewritten for this edition. They include: Perception and Cognition; Piaget's Approach to Intellectual Functioning; Learning Theory; Aggression; Anthropology and Psychiatry; Sociology and Psychiatry; Statistics and Experimental Design; Classical Psychoanalysis; Erik H. Erikson; Theories of Personality and Psychopathology: Approaches Derived from Psychology and Philosophy; The Psychiatric Interview, History, and Mental Status Examination; Medical Assessment and Laboratory Testing in Psychiatry; Clinical Manifestations of Psychiatric Disorders; Classification of Mental Disorders; Organic Mental Syndromes and Disorders; Drug Dependence: Nonnarcotics, Nicotine (Tobacco) and Caffeine; Delusional (Paranoid) Disorders; Schizoaffective Disorder, Schizophreniform Disorder, and Brief Reactive Psychosis; Atypical, Unusual, and Cultural Psychoses; Postpartum Psychotic Disorders; Somatoform Disorders; Gender Identity Disorders of Childhood, Adolescence, and Adulthood; Paraphilias; Homosexuality; Sleep Disorders; Adjustment Disorder; Impulse Control Disorder; Current Theoretical Concepts in Psychosomatic Medicine; Gastrointestional Disorders; Obesity; Respiratory Disorders; Endocrine and Metabolic Disorders; Skin Disorders; Rheumatoid Arthritis; Stress and Psychiatry; Behavior and Immunity; Psycho-oncology; Chronic Pain; Consultation-Liaison Psychiatry; Psychiatry and Surgery; Malingering; Suicide; Other Psychiatric Emergencies; Psychoanalysis and Psychoanalytic Psychotherapy; Behavior Therapy; Hypnosis; Family Therapy; Couples Therapy; Brief Dynamic and Crisis Therapy; Evaluation of Psychotherapy; Community Psychiatry; Primary, Secondary, and Tertiary Prevention of Mental Disorders; Peer Review; Legal Issues in Psychiatry; Ethics in Psychiatry; and History of Psychiatry.

Childhood disorders The chapters on child and adolescent psychiatry have been heavily rewritten. There are new discussions on the following subjects: Introduction and Overview; Normal Adolescent Development; Psychiatric Examination of the Infant, Child, and Adolescent; Pervasive Developmental Disorders; Specific Developmental Disorders of Childhood; Disruptive Behavior Disorders; Anxiety Disorders; Eating Disorders; Tic Disorders; Elimination Disorders; Other Disorders of Infancy, Childhood, and Adolescence; Child Psychiatry: Psychiatry Treatment; and Child Psychiatry: Special Areas of Interest. Almost every aspect of childhood disorders has been rewritten.

New sections **Neural sciences.** Every aspect of neuroanatomy, neurochemistry, neurophysiology, and neuroendocrinology relevant to clinical psychiatry is covered. Among these are: Introduction and Overview; Major Brain Structures; Functional Neuroanatomy; Receptors, Monoamines, and Amino Acids; Neuropeptides: Biology and Regulation; Intraneuronal Biochemical Signals; Basic Electrophysiology; Applied Electrophysiology; Basic Science of Sleep; Brain Imaging; Psychoneuroendocrinology; Neural, Endocrine, and Immune Interactions; Chronobiology; Neuronal Development and Plasticity; and Basic Molecular Genetic Neuroscience. Each subject has been covered by an outstanding worker in the field who has emphasized the application of basic science to psychiatry.

Geriatric psychiatry A major expansion of the section on geriatric psychiatry has been added to this book. This reflects the increasing importance of this subject to clinical psychiatry and the progress being made in this area. Among the sections added are: Introduction and Overview; Psychosocial Aspects of Aging; Assessment; Psychiatric Disorders of Late Life; Treatment; Psychiatric Problems of the Medically Ill Geriatric Patient; and Special Issues. Each section has been written by a leading geropsychiatric expert.

Other major changes Many other chapters have had major reorganizations with new sections and contributors. Among these are: Neurology, Schizophrenia, Mood Disorders, and Anxiety Disorders. Other new sections in this edition include: Psychiatric Rating Scales; Psychiatric Aspects of Acquired Immune Deficiency Syndrome; Psychiatry and Reproductive Medicine; Borderline Personality Disorder; Adulthood; The Economics of Psychiatry; The Chronically Mentally Ill; Graduate Psychiatric Education; and Future of Psychiatry.

Updated sections Every fifth edition contribution that was written by a previous contributor has been thoroughly updated. Each section represents the most current exposition on the subject.

DSM-III-R The psychiatric disorders discussed in this textbook are consistent with the nosology of the revised third edition of the American Psychiatric Association's *Diagnostic and Statistical Manual of Mental Disorders* (DSM-III-R), which was published in 1987.

Many of our contributors had, and still do have, distinct reservations about DSM-III-R nosology, and in several sections of this book, the reader will find those objections clearly stated. The contributors used such terms as "neurosis," "psychosis," and "psychosomatic," even though those terms are not a part of the official nosology.

A new edition of the *Manual,* DSM-IV, will appear in 1992. The editors have tried to anticipate as many of the changes as possible; for example, DSM-IV will be more consistent with the tenth revision of the World Health Organization's *International Classification of Diseases* (ICD-10). Much of the current revision of this *Classification* is described in this textbook.

The editors firmly believe that a major textbook such as the *Comprehensive Textbook of Psychiatry* must provide a forum for discussion, evaluation, criticism, and disagreement, while giving due acknowledgment to the official nomenclature. As stated in the last edition, a manual on nomenclature is just that: It is *not* a textbook.

Furthermore, the editors wish to question the timing of the publication of the various editions of DSM-III and DSM-III-R, and the aforementioned proposed publication of DSM-IV, which are occurring at such a rapid pace—1980, 1987, and 1992. Mark Zimmerman's recent article, "Why Are We Rushing to Publish DSM-IV?" which appeared in the *Archives of General Psychiatry,* in December 1988, stated that because of the large number of changes, DSM-III-R should have been labeled DSM-IV. He suggests, as do the editors of CTP, that the scheduled publication date by the APA of DSM-IV in 1992, provides insufficient time "for the accumulation of an adequate data base to guide the developers of DSM-IV." Zimmerman asks "How would the practice of psychiatry in this country have been compromised if DSM-III-R had never existed? Are the changes in DSM-IV really going to improve the practice of psychiatry in a substantial way?"

The editors of CTP strongly believe and recommend, along with Zimmerman, that revisions in DSM should follow a "restrained, sober, and deliberate pace" and that the publication date for DSM-IV be delayed. Such action would allow progress in psychiatric nosology to occur in a more timely and scientific manner and eliminate the present confusion that exists among psychiatrists as a result of the plethora of DSMs that are being published.

ACKNOWLEDGMENTS The production of this book was a major undertaking that involved the efforts of many coworkers. Lynda Abrams, M.A., Education Coordinator of the Department of Psychiatry at New York University School of Medicine, was key to the successful preparation and completion of this book. She deserves our deepest gratitude and appreciation for her skilled editing and for her prodigious work in coordinating all aspects of this textbook. She was the Project Editor and was responsible for assisting the editors in all aspects of their work. Hilary Slaven-Robinson assisted the Project Editor and was helpful throughout. She carried out her many duties with dedication and consummate skill.

Peter Kaplan, M.D., Fellow in Psychiatry at New York University School of Medicine, served as a key assistant to the editors in the preparation of this book. Not only did he represent the viewpoint of the modern-day medical student and psychiatric resident but he helped enormously in all aspects of the production of this textbook. He made particular contributions in the fields of psychopharmacology and child psychiatry, which are his areas of specialization. Rebecca Jones, M.D., Research Assistant Professor of Psychiatry at New York University School of Medicine, provided able assistance in a variety of tasks. Others who helped were Nancy B. Kaplan, James Sadock, Victoria Sadock, Amy Brown, and Phillip Kaplan, M.D.

Lissy Jarvik, M.D., Ph.D. and Gary Small, M.D. deserve special mention and acknowledgment for their leadership and prodigious effort in organizing the chapter on Geriatric Psychiatry. They suggested the areas that encompass this enormously important subspeciality of psychiatry and recommended and helped obtain contributors for this section. They also helped coordinate the integration of the various subsections in this chapter and deserve much of the credit for the content. Both the editors and the field of psychiatry owe them a debt of gratitude for their outstanding help.

We especially want to thank Virginia Alcott Sadock, M.D., Clinical Professor of Psychiatry and Director of Graduate Education in Human Sexuality at New York University School of Medicine. As in all our previous books, she has served as assistant to the editors and actively participated in every editorial decision. Her enthusiasm, sensitivity, comprehension, and depth of psychiatric knowledge were of immeasurable importance to the editors. She has ably represented not only the viewpoint of women in medicine and psychiatry but also has made many contributions to the content of this textbook. We are deeply appreciative of her outstanding help and assistance.

In the preparation of this textbook the editors have enlisted the help of two outstanding Contributing Editors, Jack Grebb, M.D., Assistant Professor of Psychiatry at New York University School of Medicine, and Joel Yager, M.D., Professor of Psychiatry at the University of California School of Medicine at Los Angeles. Dr. Grebb helped in the conceptualization and organization of the neural sciences chapter and consulted in all areas of biological and somatic psychiatry. Dr. Yager helped in consulting on various areas of clinical psychiatry.

The editors want to thank these two outstanding educators for their participation and their many contributions to the production and integration of the various contributions to this textbook.

Robert Cancro, M.D., Professor and Chairman of the Department of Psychiatry at New York University School of Medicine, participated as Senior Contributing Editor of this edition. Dr. Cancro's commitment to psychiatric education and psychiatric research is recognized throughout the world. He has been a source of great inspiration to the editors and has contributed immeasurably to this and previous editions. Dr. Cancro is renowned as a researcher, clinician, and educator. He is a much valued and highly esteemed mentor to the editors, and it is a very special privilege to work closely with him. Dr. Cancro has developed a department that represents the very best in American psychiatry. The fruitful and stimulating exchange of ideas between Dr. Cancro and the faculty, residents, medical students, and other professionals at New York University creates a unique blend of academic and clinical psychiatry for which he is responsible. Our collaboration and association with this outstanding American educator has contributed immeasurably to the new ideas and directions shaping this textbook. His role has been especially important in this edition, which reflects his breadth of knowledge, expertise in all areas of psychiatry, and dedication to the field. He is truly one of the major leaders in American psychiatry today.

Finally, we wish to express our deep appreciation to our 237 contributors, who worked with enthusiasm and who were cooperative in every aspect of this textbook.

Harold I. Kaplan, M.D.
Benjamin J. Sadock, M.D.

New York University Medical Center
New York City, 1989

CONTRIBUTORS

Gene G. Abel, M.D. Professor of Psychiatry, Emory University School of Medicine; Adjunct Professor of Psychology, Georgia State University; Medical Director, Behavioral Medicine Unit, West Paces Ferry Hospital, Atlanta, Georgia.

Paul L. Adams, M.D. Kempner Professor of Child Psychiatry, University of Texas Medical Branch at Galveston; Attending Psychiatrist, University of Texas Medical Branch and Hospital, Galveston, Texas.

Ronald D. Adelman, M.D. Assistant Professor of Medicine, State University of New York at Stony Brook School of Medicine, Stony Brook, New York; Chief, Division of Geriatrics, Winthrop University Hospital, Mineola, New York.

Anthony M. Adinolfi, Ph.D. Associate Professor of Anatomy and Cell Biology, University of California at Los Angeles School of Medicine, Los Angeles, California.

George K. Aghajanian, M.D. Professor of Psychiatry and Pharmacology, Yale University School of Medicine, New Haven, Connecticut.

W. Stewart Agras, M.D., F.R.C.P.(C) Professor of Psychiatry and Director, Behavioral Medicine Program, Stanford University School of Medicine, Stanford, California.

Huda Akil, Ph.D. Professor of Psychiatry, Research Scientist, and Director of Research, Department of Psychiatry, Mental Health Research Institute, University of Michigan Medical School, Ann Arbor, Michigan.

Hagop Souren Akiskal, M.D. Professor of Psychiatry and Director, Section of Affective Disorders, University of Tennessee, Center for the Health Sciences, College of Medicine; Special Consultant, Charter Lakeside Mood Disorders Program, Memphis, Tennessee.

George F. Alheid, Ph.D. Associate Professor of Behavioral Medicine and Psychiatry, University of Virginia School of Medicine, Charlottesville, Virginia.

Henry G. Altman, M.D. Assistant Professor of Psychiatry, Harvard Medical School; Psychiatrist, Beth Israel Hospital, Boston, Massachusetts.

Jambur Ananth, M.D., D.P.M., F.R.C.P.(C) Professor of Psychiatry, University of California at Los Angeles School of Medicine; Director of Psychopharmacology, Harbor-UCLA Medical Center, Torrance, California.

Roberta J. Apfel, M.D., M.P.H. Assistant Professor of Psychiatry, Harvard Medical School, Boston, Massachusetts; Senior Psychiatrist, Metropolitan State Hospital, Waltham, Massachusetts.

Robert F. Asarnow, Ph.D. Associate Professor of Medical Psychology, University of California at Los Angeles School of Medicine; Head, Neuropsychology Service in Child Psychiatry, Neuropsychiatric Institute and Hospital, Los Angeles, California.

Lorian Baker, Ph.D. Research Professor, Department of Child Psychiatry, University of California at Los Angeles School of Medicine, Los Angeles, California.

Jay M. Baraban, M.D., Ph.D. Assistant Professor of Neuroscience, Psychiatry, and Behavioral Sciences, Johns Hopkins University School of Medicine, Baltimore, Maryland.

Arthur J. Barsky, M.D. Associate Professor of Psychiatry, Harvard Medical School; Chief, Primary Care Psychiatry Unit, Massachusetts General Hospital, Boston, Massachusetts.

James T. Barter, M.D. Professor of Psychiatry, University of Illinois College of Medicine; Director and Attending Psychiatrist, Illinois State Psychiatric Institute; Attending Psychiatrist, University of Illinois Hospital, Chicago, Illinois.

Aaron T. Beck, M.D. University Professor of Psychiatry, University of Pennsylvania School of Medicine; Attending Psychiatrist, Hospital of the University of Pennsylvania; Director, Center for Cognitive Therapy, Philadelphia, Pennsylvania.

Jeffrey R. Bedell, Ph.D. Associate Professor of Psychiatry, Albert Einstein College of Medicine of Yeshiva University; Psychologist, Sound View-Throgs Neck Community Mental Health Center, Bronx, New York.

Myron L. Belfer, M.D. Professor of Psychiatry, Harvard Medical School, Boston, Massachusetts; Chief, Department of Psychiatry, Cambridge Hospital, Cambridge, Massachusetts.

Arthur L. Benton, Ph.D. Professor Emeritus of Neurology and Psychology, University of Iowa College of Medicine, Iowa City, Iowa.

Karen Faith Berman, M.D. Director, Regional Cerebral Blood Flow Laboratory, National Institute of Mental Health, Clinical Brain Disorders Branch, National Institute of Mental Health Neurosciences Center at Saint Elizabeths, Washington, DC.

Wade H. Berrettini, M.D., Ph.D. Staff Psychiatrist, Clinical Neurogenetics Branch, National Institute of Mental Health, Bethesda, Maryland; Adjunct Assistant Professor of Psychiatry and Pharmacology, Jefferson Medical College of Thomas Jefferson University, Philadelphia, Pennsylvania.

Barry Blackwell, M.D., F.R.C.Psych. Professor and Chairman, Department of Psychiatry, University of Wisconsin Medical School, Milwaukee Clinical Campus; Chief of Psychiatry and Director, Behavioral Medicine, Sinai-Samaritan Medical Center, Milwaukee, Wisconsin.

Floyd E. Bloom, M.D. Adjunct Professor of Neurosciences, University of California at San Diego School of Medicine; Director, Division of Preclinical Neuroscience and Endocrinology, Research Institute, Scripps Clinic, La Jolla, California.

Mark J. Blotcky, M.D. Clinical Instructor in Psychiatry, University of Texas Southwestern Medical School at Dallas; Director of Residency Training in Child Psychiatry and Clinical Director, Timberlawn Psychiatric Hospital, Dallas, Texas.

William E. Boggiano, M.D. Clinical Assistant Professor of Psychiatry, Uniformed Services University of the Health Sciences F. Edward Hebert School of Medicine, Bethesda, Maryland; Staff Psychiatrist, Walter Reed Army Medical Center, Washington, DC.

Jonathan F. Borus, M.D. Associate Professor of Psychiatry, Harvard Medical School; Director, Residency and Fellowship Training in Psychiatry, Massachusetts General Hospital, Boston, Massachusetts.

Charles L. Bowden, M.D. Nancy U. Karren Professor of Psychiatry, University of Texas Medical School at San Antonio, San Antonio, Texas.

Michael D. Browning, Ph.D. Assistant Professor of Pharmacology, University of Colorado School of Medicine, Denver, Colorado.

Jack D. Burke, Jr., M.D., M.P.H. Acting Director, Division of Biometry and Applied Sciences, National Institute of Mental Health, Rockville, Maryland.

Robert N. Butler, M.D. Brookdale Professor of Geriatrics and Adult Development and Chairman of the Gerald and May Ellen Ritter Department of Geriatrics and Adult Development, Mount Sinai School of Medicine, New York, New York.

Robert W. Butler, Ph.D. Clinical Assistant Professor of Psychiatry, University of California at San Diego School of Medicine, La Jolla, California; Staff Psychologist, University of California, San Diego Medical Center, San Diego, California.

Magda Campbell, M.D. Professor of Psychiatry, New York University School of Medicine; Director, Division of Child and Adolescent Psychiatry, Department of Psychiatry, New York University School of Medicine; Attending Psychiatrist, University Hospital of the New York University Medical Center; Attending Psychiatrist, Bellevue Hospital, New York, New York.

Robert Cancro, M.D., Med.D.Sc. Professor and Chairman, Department of Psychiatry, New York University School of Medicine; Director, Department of Psychiatry, University Hospital of the New York University Medical Center, New York, New York; Director, Nathan S. Kline Institute of Psychiatric Research, Orangeburg, New York.

Dennis P. Cantwell, M.D. Joseph Campbell Professor of Child Psychiatry, University of California at Los Angeles School of Medicine; Director of Residency Training in Child Psychiatry, Division of Mental Retardation and Child Psychiatry, Neuropsychiatric Institute and Hospital, Los Angeles, California.

Ned H. Cassem, M.D. Associate Professor of Psychiatry, Harvard Medical School; Acting Chief of Psychiatry, Massachusetts General Hospital, Boston, Massachusetts.

David Charnow, M.A. Family and Community Education, Teachers College, Columbia University, New York, New York.

C. Robert Cloninger, M.D. Professor of Psychiatry and Genetics, Washington University Medical School; Director, Outpatient Services, Jewish Hospital of St. Louis, St. Louis, Missouri.

Ralph Colp, Jr., M.D. Assistant Professor of Clinical Psychiatry, Columbia University College of Physicians and Surgeons; Senior Consulting Psychiatrist, Mental Health Division, Columbia University Health Service; Senior Attending Psychiatrist, St. Luke's-Roosevelt Hospital Center, New York, New York.

Joseph T. Coyle, M.D. Distinguished Service Professor of Child Psychiatry and Professor of Psychiatry, Neuroscience, Pharmacology, and Pediatrics; Director, Division of Child Psychiatry, Johns Hopkins University School of Medicine, Baltimore, Maryland.

Allen C. Crocker, M.D. Associate Professor of Pediatrics, Harvard Medical School; Lecturer in Maternal and Child Health, Harvard School of Public Health; Director, Developmental Evaluation Clinic, Children's Hospital, Boston, Massachusetts.

John F. Curry, Ph.D. Associate Professor of Medical Psychology, Department of Psychiatry, Duke University School of Medicine, Durham, North Carolina.

Kenneth L. Davis, M.D. Professor and Chairman, Department of Psychiatry, Mount Sinai School of Medicine; Director, Alzheimer's Disease Research Center, Mount Sinai Medical Center, New York, New York; Director, Schizophrenia Biological Research Center, Veterans Administration Medical Center, Bronx, New York.

John M. Davis, M.D. Gilman Professor of Psychiatry, University of Illinois College of Medicine; Director of Research, Illinois State Psychiatric Institute, Chicago, Illinois.

Lynn E. DeLisi, M.D. Associate Professor of Psychiatry, State University of New York at Stony Brook School of Medicine, Stony Brook, New York; Director, SUNY Stony Brook Schizophrenia Evaluation Unit, Kings Park Psychiatric Center, Kings Park, New York.

James W. Dilley, M.D. Assistant Clinical Professor of Psychiatry, University of California at San Francisco School of Medicine; Project Administrator, UCSF-AIDS Health Project, San Francisco, California.

David F. Dinges, Ph.D. Clinical Associate Professor of Psychology, Department of Psychiatry, University of Pennsylvania School of Medicine; Co-Director, Unit for Experimental Psychiatry, The Institute of the Pennsylvania Hospital, Philadelphia, Pennsylvania.

John P. Docherty, M.D. Professor of Clinical Psychiatry, Tufts University School of Medicine, Boston, Massachusetts; Medical Director, Brookside Hospital, Nashua, New Hampshire.

Marian Droba, M.D. Clinical Assistant Professor of Psychiatry, University of Pennsylvania School of Medicine; Chief, Addiction Recovery Unit, Veterans Administration Medical Center, Philadelphia, Pennsylvania.

Marshall P. Duke, Ph.D. Professor of Psychology, Emory University, Atlanta, Georgia.

Maurice W. Dysken, M.D. Associate Professor of Psychiatry, University of Minnesota School of Medicine; Psychopharmacologist, Veterans Administration Medical Center, Minneapolis, Minnesota.

James Egan, M.D. Professor of Psychiatry and Behavioral Sciences, George Washington University School of Medicine and Health Sciences; Chairman, Department of Psychiatry, Children's Hospital National Medical Center, Washington, DC.

Carl Eisdorfer, M.D., Ph.D. Professor and Chairman, Department of Psychiatry, University of Miami School of Medicine; Professor of Psychology, University of Miami; Chief of Psychiatry, Jackson Memorial Medical Center, Miami, Florida; Director, Wien Center for Memory Disorders, Mount Sinai Medical Center, Miami Beach, Florida.

Alan M. Elkins, M.D. Professor of Psychiatry, University of Vermont College of Medicine, Burlington, Vermont; Chief of Psychiatry, Maine Medical Center, Portland, Maine.

Joseph T. English, M.D. Professor of Psychiatry and Associate Dean, New York Medical College, Valhalla, New York; Adjunct Professor of Psychiatry, Cornell University Medical College, New York, New York; Lecturer in Psychiatry, Harvard Medical School, Boston, Massachusetts; Director, Department of Psychiatry, St. Vincent's Hospital and Medical Center, New York, New York.

Spencer Eth, M.D. Assistant Professor of Psychiatry, University of California at Los Angeles School of Medicine; Clinical Associate Professor of Psychiatry, University of Southern California School of Medicine; Associate Chief of Psychiatry, West Los Angeles Veterans Administration Medical Center (Brentwood), Los Angeles, California.

Raymond A. Faber, M.D. Associate Professor of Clinical Psychiatry and Clinical Medicine, Division of Neurology, University of Texas Medical School at San Antonio; Director, Neuropsychiatry Program, Psychiatry Service, Audie L. Murphy Memorial Veterans Hospital, San Antonio, Texas.

Fawzy I. Fawzy, M.D. Associate Professor of Psychiatry, University of California at Los Angeles School of Medicine; Chief, Consultation-Liaison Service and Associate Director, Neuropsychiatric Institute and Hospital, Los Angeles, California.

Susan M. Fisher, M.D. Clinical Associate Professor of Psychiatry, University of Chicago Pritzker School of Medicine; Attending Physician, University of Chicago Hospitals and Clinics, Chicago, Illinois.

Jeannette E. Fleischner, Ed.D. Professor of Education and Chairman, Department of Special Education, Teachers College, Columbia University, New York, New York.

Jack M. Fletcher, Ph.D. Associate Professor of Psychology, University of Houston, Houston, Texas.

William J. Freed, Ph.D. Chief, Preclinical Neurosciences Section, National Institute of Mental Health at Saint Elizabeths Hospital, Washington, D C.

Frances Jackson Freeman, Ph.D. Adjunct Professor, Departments of Otolaryngology and Neurology, University of Texas Southwestern Medical School at Dallas; Research Scientist, University of Texas at Dallas, Callier Center for Communication Disorders; Director, Dallas Center for Vocal Motor Control, Dallas, Texas.

Warren J. Gadpaille, M.D. Associate Clinical Professor of Child Psychiatry, Department of Psychiatry, University of Colorado School of Medicine; Adjunct Professor, Department of Physical Education and Sports Sciences, University of Denver, Denver, Colorado.

Barry D. Garfinkel, M.D., F.R.C.P.(C) Associate Professor of Psychiatry, University of Minnesota Medical School; Director, Division of Child and Adolescent Psychiatry, University of Minnesota Hospital and Clinic, Minneapolis, Minnesota.

Katherine Garnett, Ed.D. Associate Professor of Special Education, Hunter College, City University of New York, New York, New York.

Robert H. Gerner, M.D. Associate Research Professor of Psychiatry, University of California at Los Angeles School of Medicine; Chief, Affective Disorders Research Unit, West Los Angeles Veterans Administration Center (Brentwood); Director, Center for Mood Disorders, Los Angeles, California.

Elliot S. Gershon, M.D. Chief, Clinical Neurogenetics Branch, National Institute of Mental Health, Bethesda, Maryland.

Alexander H. Glassman, M.D. Professor of Clinical Psychiatry, Columbia University College of Physicians and Surgeons; Chief, Clinical Psychopharmacology, New York State Psychiatric Institute, New York, New York.

Lynn R. Goldin, Ph.D. Research Geneticist, Clinical Neurogenetics Branch, National Institute of Mental Health, Bethesda, Maryland.

Thomas A. Gonda, M.D. Professor and Chairman, Department of Psychiatry and Behavioral Sciences, Stanford University School of Medicine, Stanford, California (deceased).

Donald W. Goodwin, M.D. Professor and Chairman, Department of Psychiatry, University of Kansas School of Medicine, Kansas City, Kansas; Consulting Psychiatrist, Veterans Administration Medical Center, Kansas City, Missouri.

Jack M. Gorman, M.D. Associate Professor of Clinical Psychiatry, Columbia University College of Physicians and Surgeons; Director, Biological Studies Unit, New York State Psychiatric Institute; Associate Attending Psychiatrist, Presbyterian Hospital, New York, New York.

James R. Gorman, M.S. Medical Scientist Training Program, Columbia University College of Physicians and Surgeons, New York, New York.

Roger L. Gould, M.D. Associate Clinical Professor of Psychiatry, University of California at Los Angeles School of Medicine, Los Angeles, California.

Igor Grant, M.D., F.R.C.P.(C) Professor and Acting Chairman, Department of Psychiatry, University of California at San Diego School of Medicine, La Jolla, California; Assistant Chief for Ambulatory Care, Psychiatry Service, Veterans Administration Medical Center, San Diego, California.

Jack A. Grebb, M.D. Assistant Professor of Psychiatry, New York University School of Medicine; Guest Investigator, Laboratory of Molecular and Cellular Neuroscience, The Rockefeller University; Assistant Attending Psychiatrist, Bellevue Hospital, New York, New York; Research Scientist, Nathan S. Kline Institute for Psychiatric Research, Orangeburg, New York.

Alan I. Green, M.D. Assistant Professor of Psychiatry, Harvard Medical School; Administrative Director, Commonwealth Research Center, Massachusetts Mental Health Center, Boston, Massachusetts.

Arthur H. Green, M.D. Associate Clinical Professor of Psychiatry, Columbia University College of Physicians and Surgeons; Attending Psychiatrist and Medical Director, Family Center and Therapeutic Nursery, Presbyterian Hospital, New York, New York.

Wayne H. Green, M.D. Associate Professor of Clinical Psychiatry, New York University School of Medicine; Unit Chief, Child and Adolescent Psychiatric Clinic, Bellevue Hospital; Assistant Attending Psychiatrist, University Hospital of the New York University Medical Center, New York, New York.

Stanley I. Greenspan, M.D. Clinical Professor of Psychiatry and Behavioral Science and Child Health and Development, George Washington University School of Medicine and Health Sciences; Supervising Child Psychoanalyst, Washington Psychoanalytic Institute, Washington, DC.

John H. Greist, M.D. Professor of Psychiatry, University of Wisconsin Medical School; Co-Director, Lithium Information Center and Anxiety Disorders Center, University Hospital, Madison, Wisconsin.

John G. Gunderson, M.D. Associate Professor of Psychiatry, Harvard Medical School, Boston, Massachusetts; Director, Psychotherapy and Psychosocial Research Program, McLean Hospital, Belmont, Massachusetts.

Andrew Guterman, M.D., Ph.D. Assistant Professor of Psychiatry and Neurology, University of Miami School of Medicine; Director, Memory Disorders Clinic, Jackson Memorial Medical Center, Miami, Florida; Chief, Psychiatric Services, Wien Center for Memory Disorders, Mount Sinai Medical Center, Miami Beach, Florida.

Thomas G. Gutheil, M.D. Associate Professor of Psychiatry, Harvard Medical School; Co-Director, Program in Psychiatry and the Law, Massachusetts Mental Health Center, Boston, Massachusetts.

Thomas P. Hackett, M.D. Eben S. Draper Professor of Psychiatry, Harvard Medical School; Chief of Psychiatry, Massachusetts General Hospital, Boston, Massachusetts (deceased).

John M. Hamilton, M.D. Deputy Medical Director and Director, Psychiatric Services, American Psychiatric Association, Washington, DC; Attending Psychiatrist, Howard County General Hospital, Columbia, Maryland.

Max Hamilton, M.D., F.R.C.P., F.R.C.Psych., F.B.P.S. Emeritus Professor of Psychiatry and Consultant Psychiatrist, General Infirmary and St. James's Hospital, Leeds, England (deceased).

Lennart Heimer, M.D. Professor of Otolaryngology and Neurosurgery, University of Virginia School of Medicine, Charlottesville, Virginia.

Fritz A. Henn, M.D., Ph.D. Professor and Chairman, Department of Psychiatry, State University of New York at Stony Brook School of Medicine; Director of Psychiatry, University Hospital, Stony Brook, New York.

Robert M. A. Hirschfeld, M.D. Chief, Mood, Anxiety, and Personality Disorders Research Branch, Division of Clinical Research, National Institute of Mental Health, Rockville, Maryland.

Jimmie C. Holland, M.D. Professor of Psychiatry, Cornell University Medical College; Chief, Psychiatry Service, Memorial Sloan-Kettering Cancer Center, New York, New York.

Thomas B. Horvath, M.D. Professor and Vice Chairman, Department of Psychiatry, Mount Sinai School of Medicine, New York, New York; Chief of Psychiatry, Veterans Administration Medical Center, Bronx, New York.

James I. Hudson, M.D. Assistant Professor of Psychiatry, Harvard Medical School, Boston, Massachusetts; Associate Chief, Biological Psychiatry Laboratory, Laboratories for Psychiatric Research, McLean Hospital, Belmont, Massachusetts.

David G. Inwood, M.D. Clinical Assistant Professor of Psychiatry and Director of Training in Child and Adolescent Psychiatry, State University of New York Health Science Center at Brooklyn; Assistant Attending Psychiatrist, Maimonides Medical Center, Brooklyn, New York.

Jerome H. Jaffe, M.D. Clinical Professor of Psychiatry, University of Maryland School of Medicine; Director, Addiction Research Center, National Institute of Mental Health, Baltimore, Maryland; Clinical Professor of Psychiatry, University of Connecticut School of Medicine, Farmington, Connecticut.

David B. Jarrett, M.D., Ph.D. Associate Professor of Psychiatry and Medicine, University of Pittsburgh School of Medicine; Director, Clinical Neuroendocrinology Program, Western Psychiatric Institute and Clinic, Pittsburgh, Pennsylvania.

Lissy F. Jarvik, M.D., Ph.D. Professor of Psychiatry, University of California at Los Angeles School of Medicine; Chief, Section on Neuropsychogeriatrics, Neuropsychiatric Institute and Hospital; Distinguished Physician, Veterans Administration Medical Center, Los Angeles, California.

James W. Jefferson, M.D. Professor of Psychiatry, University of Wisconsin Medical School; Director, Center for Affective Disorders and Co-Director, Lithium Information Center, University Hospital, Madison, Wisconsin.

John M. Kane, M.D. Professor of Psychiatry, Albert Einstein College of Medicine of Yeshiva University, New York, New York; Chairman, Department of Psychiatry, Long Island Jewish Medical Center, Glen Oaks, New York.

Harold I. Kaplan, M.D. Professor of Psychiatry, New York University School of Medicine; Attending Psychiatrist, University Hospital of the New York University Medical Center; Attending Psychiatrist, Bellevue Hospital, New York, New York.

Peter M. Kaplan, M.D. Fellow in Psychiatry and Psychopharmacology, Department of Psychiatry, New York University Medical Center, New York, New York.

Robert M. Kaplan, Ph.D. Professor of Community and Family Medicine, University of California at San Diego School of Medicine; Acting Chief, Division of Health Care Sciences, University of California, San Diego, La Jolla, California; Professor of Psychology, Adjunct Professor of Public Health, and Director, Center for Behavioral Medicine, San Diego State University, San Diego, California.

Ismet Karacan, M.D., Med.D.Sc. Professor of Psychiatry and Director, Sleep Disorders and Research Center, Baylor College of Medicine; Director, Research and Development, Veterans Administration Medical Center, Houston, Texas.

Toksoz Byram Karasu, M.D. Professor of Psychiatry, Albert Einstein College of Medicine of Yeshiva University, Bronx, New York.

Marvin Karno, M.D. Professor of Psychiatry, University of California at Los Angeles School of Medicine; Attending Psychiatrist, Neuropsychiatric Institute and Hospital, Los Angeles, California.

Steven E. Katz, M.D. Professor and Executive Vice Chairman, Department of Psychiatry, New York University School of Medicine; Director, Health Policy, New York University School of Medicine; Director of Psychiatry, Bellevue Hospital, New York, New York.

John S. Kennedy, M.D., F.R.C.P.(C) Assistant Professor of Psychiatry (Geriatric), Case Western Reserve University School of Medicine; Assistant Director, Alzheimer's Center, University Hospitals of Cleveland, Cleveland, Ohio.

Ronald C. Kessler, Ph.D. Professor of Sociology and Program Director, Institute for Social Research, University of Michigan, Ann Arbor, Michigan.

S. Peter Kim, M.D., Ph.D. Professor of Psychiatry and Pediatrics, Department of Psychiatry and Health Behavior, Medical College of Georgia; Attending Psychiatrist, Medical College of Georgia Hospital and Clinics, Augusta, Georgia.

J. David Kinzie, M.D. Professor of Psychiatry and Director, Psychiatric Clinical Service, Oregon Health Sciences University School of Medicine, Portland, Oregon.

Darrell G. Kirch, M.D. Medical Director, Neuropsychiatric Research Hospital, National Institute of Mental Health, Washington, DC; Clinical Assistant Professor of Psychiatry and Behavioral Sciences, George Washington University School of Medicine and Health Sciences, Washington, DC.

Melvin Konner, M.D., Ph.D. Samuel Candler Dobbs Professor of Anthropology, Emory University; Associate Professor of Psychiatry, Emory University School of Medicine; Affiliate Scientist, Yerkes Regional Primate Research Center, Atlanta, Georgia.

Melvin R. Lansky, M.D. Adjunct Professor of Psychiatry, University of California at Los Angeles School of Medicine; Staff Psychiatrist and Chief, Family Treatment Program, West Los Angeles Veterans Administration Medical Center (Brentwood); Faculty, Los Angeles Psychoanalytic Institute, Los Angeles, California.

Ruth L. LaVietes, M.D. Professor of Clinical Psychiatry and Pediatrics and Director, Pediatric Consultation-Liaison in Psychiatry, New York Medical College; Attending Psychiatrist and Director of Psychiatry, Mental Retardation Institute, Westchester County Medical Center, Valhalla, New York.

Lawrence W. Lazarus, M.D. Assistant Professor of Psychiatry, Rush Medical College; Associate Attending Psychiatrist, Rush-Presbyterian-St. Luke's Medical Center, Chicago, Illinois.

Marguerite S. Lederberg, M.D. Clinical Associate Professor of Psychiatry, Cornell University Medical College; Associate Attending Psychiatrist, Memorial Sloan-Kettering Cancer Center, New York, New York.

Robert L. Leon, M.D. Professor and Chairman, Department of Psychiatry, University of Texas Medical School at San Antonio; Chief, Psychiatry Service, Medical Center Hospital, Bexar County Hospital District; Consultant, Audie L. Murphy Memorial Veterans Hospital, San Antonio, Texas.

Leonard I. Leven, M.D. Research Assistant Professor of Psychiatry, New York University School of Medicine; Attending Psychiatrist, Bellevue Hospital, New York, New York.

Harvey S. Levin, Ph.D. Professor, Chela and Jimmy Storm Distinguished Professor in Surgical Research; Professor, Division of Neurosurgery, Departments of Surgery, Neurology, and Psychiatry, University of Texas Medical Branch at Galveston, Galveston, Texas.

Stephen B. Levine, M.D. Professor of Psychiatry, Case Western Reserve University School of Medicine; Medical Director, Center for Human Sexuality, University Hospitals of Cleveland, Cleveland, Ohio.

Dorothy Otnow Lewis, M.D. Professor of Psychiatry, New York University School of Medicine; Attending Psychiatrist, Bellevue Hospital, New York, New York; Clinical Professor and Attending Physician in Psychiatry, Child Study Center, Yale University School of Medicine; Attending Physician in Adult Psychiatry and Associate Attending Physician in Child Psychiatry, Yale-New Haven Hospital, New Haven, Connecticut.

Melvin Lewis, M.B., B.S.(London), F.R.C.Psych., D.C.H. Professor of Pediatrics and Psychiatry, Child Study Center, Yale University School of Medicine; Attending Physician in Pediatrics and Psychiatry, Yale-New Haven Hospital, New Haven, Connecticut.

Robert Paul Liberman, M.D. Professor of Psychiatry, University of California at Los Angeles School of Medicine; Chief, Rehabilitation Service, West Los Angeles Veterans Administration Medical Center (Brentwood); Director, Clinical Research Center for Schizophrenia and Psychiatric Rehabilitation; Director, Clinical Research Unit of Camarillo State Hospital, Los Angeles, California.

Mack Lipkin, Jr., M.D. Associate Professor of Clinical Medicine, New York University School of Medicine; Associate Attending Physician, University Hospital of the New York University Medical Center; Associate Attending Physician, Bellevue Hospital, New York, New York.

Don R. Lipsitt, M.D. Associate Professor of Psychiatry, Harvard Medical School, Boston, Massachusetts; Chairman, Department of Psychiatry, Mount Auburn Hospital, Cambridge, Massachusetts.

Steven E. Locke, M.D. Assistant Professor of Psychiatry, Harvard Medical School; Director, Computers in Psychiatry, Center for Clinical Computing and Department of Psychiatry, Beth Israel Hospital, Boston, Massachusetts.

Lars B. Lofgren, M.D. Clinical Professor of Psychiatry (Ret.), University of California at Los Angeles School of Medicine, Los Angeles, California.

James W. Lomax, II, M.D. Associate Professor of Clinical Psychiatry, Vice Chairman for Education, and Director, General Psychiatry Residency Program; Baylor College of Medicine, Houston, Texas.

John G. Looney, M.D. Professor of Psychiatry and Director, Child and Adolescent Psychiatry, Duke University School of Medicine; Director, Durham Community Guidance Clinic, Durham, North Carolina.

Alfred E. Mamelok, M.D., F.A.C.S. Clinical Associate Professor of Ophthalmology, Cornell University Medical College; Attending Surgeon and Chief, Uveitis Clinic, Manhattan Eye, Ear and Throat Hospital; Attending Ophthalmologist, New York Hospital; Section Chief of Ophthalmology, Doctors Hospital, New York, New York.

Theo C. Manschreck, M.D. Associate Professor of Psychiatry, Harvard Medical School and Massachusetts General Hospital; Director, Laboratory for Clinical and Experimental Psychopathology and Associate Psychiatrist, Massachusetts General Hospital, Boston, Massachusetts.

Richard C. Marohn, M.D. Professor of Clinical Psychiatry, Northwestern University Medical School; Faculty, Institute for Psychoanalysis; Attending Psychiatrist, Northwestern Memorial Hospital, Chicago, Illinois.

Joseph C. Masdeu, M.D. Chairman of Neurology, St. Vincent's Hospital and Medical Center, New York, New York; Professor of Neurology, New York Medical College, Valhalla, New York; Clinical Professor of Neurology, New York University School of Medicine; Attending Neurologist, Bellevue Hospital; Attending Neurologist, New York University Medical Center, New York, New York.

Miriam D. Mazor, M.D. Clinical Instructor in Psychiatry, Harvard Medical School; Senior Associate in Psychiatry, Beth Israel Hospital, Boston, Massachusetts.

Richard G. McCarrick, M.D. Clinical Associate Professor of Psychiatry, New York Medical College, Valhalla, New York; Adjunct Faculty in Health Administration, Graduate School of Management, The New School for Social Research; Assistant Director and Chief, Training and Education, Department of Psychiatry, St. Vincent's Hospital and Medical Center, New York, New York.

Thomas H. McGlashan, M.D. Director of Research, Chestnut Lodge Research Institute; Research Professor of Psychiatry, University of Maryland School of Medicine; Staff Psychiatrist, Chestnut Lodge Hospital, Rockville, Maryland.

Michael T. McGuire, M.D. Professor of Psychiatry, University of California at Los Angeles School of Medicine; Attending Psychiatrist, Neuropsychiatric Institute and Hospital, Los Angeles, California.

William T. McKinney, M.D. Professor of Psychiatry, University of Wisconsin Medical School; Attending Psychiatrist, University Hospital, Madison, Wisconsin.

W. Walter Menninger, M.D. Miles G. Seeley Professor of Psychiatric Education; Dean, Karl Menninger School of Psychiatry and Mental Health Sciences; Instructor, Topeka Institute for Psychoanalysis; Executive Vice President and Chief of Staff, The Menninger Foundation, Topeka, Kansas; Clinical Professor of Psychiatry, University of Kansas School of Medicine, Kansas City, Kansas.

Arthur T. Meyerson, M.D. Professor of Psychiatry and Chairman, Department of Mental Health Sciences, Hahnemann University School of Medicine; Chief of Psychiatry, Hahnemann University Hospital, Philadelphia, Pennsylvania.

Mark J. Mills, M.D., J.D. Clinical Professor of Psychiatry, University of California at Los Angeles School of Medicine; Director, Program in Psychiatry and Law, Neuropsychiatric Institute and Hospital, Los Angeles, California; President, Forensic Sciences Medical Group, Santa Monica, California.

Ronald T. Mitsuyasu, M.D. Assistant Professor of Medicine, Division of Hematology-Oncology, University of California at Los Angeles School of Medicine; Associate Director, UCLA-AIDS Clinical Research Center; Attending Physician, UCLA Medical Center Hospital, Los Angeles, California.

Richard C. Mohs, Ph.D. Associate Professor of Psychiatry and Director, Division of Psychology, Mount Sinai School of Medicine, New York, New York; Psychologist, Veterans Administration Medical Center, Bronx, New York.

Richard F. Mollica, M.D. Assistant Professor of Psychiatry, Harvard Medical School; Attending Psychiatrist, Massachusetts General Hospital, Boston, Massachusetts; Director, Indochinese Psychiatry Clinic, St. Elizabeths Hospital, Brighton, Massachusetts; Director, Harvard Program in Refugee Trauma, Harvard School of Public Health, Cambridge, Massachusetts.

John J. Mooney, M.D. Instructor in Psychiatry, Harvard Medical School; Staff Psychiatrist, Massachusetts Mental Health Center; Staff Psychiatrist, New England Deaconess Hospital, Boston, Massachusetts.

Constance A. Moore, M.D. Assistant Professor of Psychiatry and Medical Director, Sleep Disorders and Research Center and Director, Human Sexuality Program, Baylor College of Medicine; Attending Psychiatrist, The Methodist Hospital; Attending Psychiatrist, St. Luke's Episcopal Hospital, Houston, Texas.

John M. Morihisa, M.D. Professor and Associate Chairman for Research, Department of Psychiatry, Georgetown University School of Medicine, Washington, DC.

Kim T. Mueser, Ph.D. Assistant Professor of Psychiatry, Medical College of Pennsylvania; Staff, Eastern Pennsylvania Psychiatric Institute, Philadelphia, Pennsylvania.

Carol C. Nadelson, M.D. Professor and Vice-Chairman, Department of Psychiatry, Tufts University School of Medicine; Director, Training and Education, Department of Psychiatry, New England Medical Center Hospitals, Boston, Massachusetts.

John C. Nemiah, M.D. Professor of Psychiatry, Dartmouth Medical School; Attending Psychiatrist, Mary Hitchcock Memorial Hospital, Hanover, New Hampshire; Professor of Psychiatry Emeritus, Harvard Medical School, Boston, Massachusetts.

Vernon M. Neppe, M.D., Ph.D. Associate Professor of Psychiatry and Behavioral Sciences and Director, Division of Neuropsychiatry, University of Washington School of Medicine; Attending Physician, University Hospital; Attending Physician, Harborview Medical Center, Seattle, Washington.

Jeffrey H. Newcorn, M.D. Assistant Professor of Psychiatry, Mount Sinai School of Medicine; Coordinator of Residency Training in Child Psychiatry; Director, Child and Adolescent Inpatient Services, Mount Sinai Medical Center, New York, New York.

Grayson S. Norquist, M.D. Assistant Clinical Professor of Psychiatry and Assistant Dean for Student Affairs, University of California at Los Angeles School of Medicine; Attending Psychiatrist, Neuropsychiatric Institute and Hospital, Los Angeles, California.

Stephen Nowicki, Jr., Ph.D. Professor of Psychology, Emory University, Atlanta, Georgia.

Keith H. Nuechterlein, Ph.D. Associate Professor of Medical Psychology and Co-Chief, Cognition, Psychophysiology, and Neuropsychology Laboratory, Clinical Research Center for the Study of Schizophrenia, University of California at Los Angeles School of Medicine; Director, Aftercare Clinic, Neuropsychiatric Institute and Hospital, Los Angeles, California.

Charles P. O'Brien, M.D., Ph.D. Professor and Vice Chairman, Department of Psychiatry, University of Pennsylvania School of Medicine; Chief of Psychiatry, Veterans Administration Medical Center, Philadelphia, Pennsylvania.

Donald Oken, M.D. Clinical Professor of Psychiatry, University of Pennsylvania School of Medicine; Director, Consultation-Liaison Service, Department of Psychiatry, Pennsylvania Hospital, Philadelphia, Pennsylvania.

Robert L. Okin, M.D. Assistant Clinical Professor of Psychiatry, Harvard Medical School; Clinical Associate in Psychiatry, Massachusetts General Hospital, Boston, Massachusetts.

David G. Oldham, M.D. Professor of Psychiatry, University of Texas Southwestern Medical School at Dallas; Medical Director, Adolescent Psychiatry, Baylor University Medical Center, Dallas, Texas.

Martin T. Orne, M.D., Ph.D. Professor of Psychiatry, University of Pennsylvania School of Medicine; Director, Unit for Experimental Psychiatry and Senior Attending Psychiatrist, The Institute of the Pennsylvania Hospital; Adjunct Professor of Psychology, University of Pennsylvania, Philadelphia, Pennsylvania.

Herbert Pardes, M.D. Professor and Chairman, Department of Psychiatry, Columbia University College of Physicians and Surgeons; Director, New York State Psychiatric Institute; Director, Psychiatry Services, Presbyterian Hospital, New York, New York.

Robert O. Pasnau, M.D. Professor of Psychiatry, University of California at Los Angeles School of Medicine; Director, Adult Psychiatry Clinical Services, Neuropsychiatric Institute and Hospital, Los Angeles, California.

J. Christopher Perry, M.D., M.P.H. Assistant Professor of Psychiatry, Harvard Medical School, Boston, Massachusetts; Director of Research, Department of Psychiatry, Cambridge Hospital, Cambridge, Massachusetts.

Theodore A. Petti, M.D., M.P.H. Professor of Child Psychiatry, University of Pittsburgh School of Medicine; Attending Psychiatrist, Western Psychiatric Institute and Clinic, Pittsburgh, Pennsylvania.

Daniel A. Plotkin, M.D. Assistant Professor of Psychiatry, University of California at Los Angeles School of Medicine; Director, Geriatric Psychiatry Outpatient Clinic, Neuropsychiatric Institute and Hospital, Los Angeles, California.

Derek C. Polonsky, M.D. Assistant Clinical Professor of Psychiatry, Tufts University School of Medicine; Clinical Instructor in Psychiatry, Harvard Medical School; Attending Psychiatrist, Beth Israel Hospital, Boston, Massachusetts.

Harrison G. Pope, Jr., M.D. Associate Professor of Psychiatry, Harvard Medical School, Boston, Massachusetts; Chief, Biological Psychiatry Laboratory, Laboratories for Psychiatric Research, McLean Hospital, Belmont, Massachusetts.

Michael K. Popkin, M.D. Professor of Psychiatry and Medicine, University of Minnesota Medical School; Chief, Consultation-Liaison Psychiatry Service, University of Minnesota Hospital, Minneapolis, Minnesota.

Felix Post, M.D. Emeritus Physician, Maudsley Hospital and Bethlem Royal Hospital, London, England.

Robert M. Post, M.D. Chief, Biological Psychiatry Branch, National Institute of Mental Health, Bethesda, Maryland.

Warren R. Procci, M.D., Ph.D. Adjunct Associate Professor of Psychiatry, University of California at Los Angeles School of Medicine, Los Angeles, California; Director, Residency Education in Psychiatry, Harbor-University of California at Los Angeles Medical Center, Torrance, California.

Kurt Rasmussen, Ph.D. Post-Doctoral Associate in Psychiatry, Yale University School of Medicine, New Haven, Connecticut.

Darrel A. Regier, M.D., M.P.H. Director, Division of Clinical Research, National Institute of Mental Health, Rockville, Maryland.

Victor I. Reus, M.D. Associate Professor of Psychiatry, University of California at San Francisco School of Medicine; Medical Director, Langley Porter Hospital, San Francisco, California.

Sylvia O. Richardson, M.D. Clinical Professor of Pediatrics, University of South Florida College of Medicine; Distinguished Professor of Communication Sciences, College of Social and Behavioral Sciences, University of South Florida, Tampa, Florida.

Carolyn B. Robinowitz, M.D. Deputy Medical Director, American Psychiatric Association; Clinical Professor of Psychiatry and Behavioral Sciences, George Washington University School of Medicine and Health Sciences; Professorial Lecturer, Department of Psychiatry, Georgetown University School of Medicine, Washington, DC; Senior Lecturer, Uniformed Services University of the Health Sciences F. Edward Hebert School of Medicine, Bethesda, Maryland.

Carl R. Rogers, Ph.D. Resident Fellow, Center for Studies of the Person, La Jolla, California (deceased).

Jerrold F. Rosenbaum, M.D. Associate Professor of Psychiatry, Harvard Medical School; Chief, Clinical Psychopharmacology and Psychosomatic Medicine Units, Massachusetts General Hospital, Boston, Massachusetts.

Richard B. Rosse, M.D. Assistant Professor of Psychiatry, Georgetown University School of Medicine; Attending Psychiatrist, Veterans Administration Medical Center, Washington, DC.

Alec Roy, M.B. Staff Psychiatrist, National Institutes of Health, Bethesda, Maryland.

A. John Rush, M.D. Betty Jo Hay Chair in Mental Health, Department of Psychiatry, University of Texas Southwestern Medical School at Dallas; Attending Psychiatrist, Parkland Memorial Hospital, Dallas, Texas.

Benjamin J. Sadock, M.D. Professor and Vice Chairman, Department of Psychiatry, New York University School of

Medicine; Attending Psychiatrist, University Hospital of the New York University Medical Center; Attending Psychiatrist, Bellevue Hospital, New York, New York.

Virginia A. Sadock, M.D. Clinical Professor of Psychiatry and Director, Graduate Education in Human Sexuality, New York University School of Medicine; Attending Psychiatrist, University Hospital of the New York University Medical Center; Attending Psychiatrist, Bellevue Hospital, New York, New York.

Ruth C. Sanford, M.A. Adjunct Professor, C.W. Post Center, Long Island University, Greenvale, New York.

Paul Satz, Ph.D. Professor of Medical Psychology, University of California at Los Angeles School of Medicine; Chief of Neuropsychology, Neuropsychiatric Institute and Hospital; Director of Research, UCLA-Camarillo State Hospital, Los Angeles, California.

Thomas E. Schacht, Psy.D. Associate Professor of Psychiatry and Family Medicine, East Tennessee State University Quillen-Dishner College of Medicine, Johnson City, Tennessee; Research Associate, Vanderbilt Center for Psychotherapy Research, Nashville, Tennessee.

Malvin Schechter, M.S. Assistant Professor, Gerald and May Ellen Ritter Department of Geriatrics and Adult Development, Mount Sinai School of Medicine, New York, New York.

Marshall D. Schechter, M.D. Professor Emeritus of Child and Adolescent Psychiatry, University of Pennsylvania School of Medicine; Consultant in Psychiatry, Pennsylvania Hospital; Attending Psychiatrist, The Institute of the Pennsylvania Hospital; Attending Psychiatrist, Veterans Administration Medical Center, Philadelphia, Pennsylvania.

Stephen C. Scheiber, M.D. Executive Secretary, American Board of Psychiatry and Neurology, Deerfield, Illinois; Professor of Clinical Psychiatry, Northwestern University Medical School; Attending Physician, Northwestern Memorial Hospital, Chicago, Illinois; Attending Physician, Evanston Hospital, Evanston, Illinois.

Joseph J. Schildkraut, M.D. Professor of Psychiatry, Harvard Medical School; Director, Neuropsychopharmacology Laboratory, Massachusetts Mental Health Center; Director, Psychiatric Chemistry Laboratory, Department of Pathology, New England Deaconess Hospital, Boston, Massachusetts.

Daniel P. Schwartz, M.D. Medical Director, Austen Riggs Center, Stockbridge, Massachusetts; Lecturer in Psychiatry, Harvard Medical School, Boston, Massachusetts and Yale University School of Medicine, New Haven, Connecticut; Consultant in Psychiatry, Massachusetts General Hospital, Boston, Massachusetts.

Göran Sedvall, M.D. Professor and Chairman, Department of Psychiatry, Karolinska Hospital, Stockholm, Sweden.

Richard I. Shader, M.D. Professor and Chairman, Department of Psychiatry, Tufts University School of Medicine; Psychiatrist-in-Chief, New England Medical Center Hospital, Boston, Massachusetts.

David Shaffer, M.B., B.S., F.R.C.P., F.R.C.Psych. Irving Philips Professor of Child Psychiatry and Professor of Psychiatry and Pediatrics, Columbia University College of Physicians and Surgeons; Director, Child Psychiatric Services, Presbyterian Hospital, New York, New York.

Arthur K. Shapiro, M.D. Clinical Professor of Psychiatry, Mount Sinai School of Medicine; Attending Psychiatrist, Mount Sinai Medical Center, New York, New York.

Elaine Shapiro, Ph.D. Associate Clinical Professor of Psychiatry, Mount Sinai School of Medicine, New York, New York.

M. Tracie Shea, Ph.D. Head, Personality Disorders Program, Mood, Anxiety, and Personality Disorders Research Branch, Division of Clinical Research, National Institute of Mental Health, Rockville, Maryland.

Margaret Jo Shepherd, Ed.D. Professor of Education and Coordinator, Learning Disabilities Program, Teachers College, Columbia University, New York, New York.

James H. Shore, M.D. Professor and Chairman, Department of Psychiatry, University of Colorado School of Medicine; Superintendent, Colorado Psychiatric Hospital, Denver, Colorado.

Larry J. Siever, M.D. Associate Professor of Psychiatry, Mount Sinai School of Medicine, New York, New York; Director, Out-Patient Division, Veterans Administration Medical Center, Bronx, New York and Mount Sinai Hospital, New York, New York.

Peter E. Sifneos, M.D. Professor of Psychiatry, Harvard Medical School; Associate Director, Department of Psychiatry, Beth Israel Hospital; Consultant in Psychiatry, Massachusetts General Hospital, Boston, Massachusetts.

Austin Silber, M.D. Director, Psychoanalytic Institute; Clinical Professor of Psychiatry, New York University School of Medicine, New York, New York.

Larry B. Silver, M.D. Clinical Professor of Psychiatry, Georgetown University School of Medicine, Washington, DC.

Andrew Edmund Slaby, M.D., Ph.D., M.P.H. Clinical Professor of Psychiatry, New York University School of Medicine, New York, New York; Adjunct Clinical Professor of Psychiatry, Brown University Program in Medicine, Providence, Rhode Island; Adjunct Clinical Professor of Psychiatry, New York Medical College, Valhalla, New York; Psychiatrist-in-Chief, Regent Hospital, New York, New York; Medical Director, Fair Oaks Hospital, Summit, New Jersey.

Gary W. Small, M.D. Assistant Professor of Psychiatry, University of California at Los Angeles School of Medicine; Director, Geriatric Psychiatry Consultation-Liaison Service, Neuropsychiatric Institute and Hospital, Los Angeles, California.

Seymour Solomon, M.D. Professor of Neurology, Albert Einstein College of Medicine of Yeshiva University; Attending Neurologist and Director, Headache Unit, Montefiore Medical Center, Bronx, New York.

James J. Strain, M.D. Professor of Psychiatry and Director, Behavioral Medicine Consultation Psychiatry, Mount Sinai School of Medicine; Attending Psychiatrist, Mount Sinai Hospital, New York, New York.

Gordon D. Strauss, M.D. Associate Clinical Professor of Psychiatry, University of California at Los Angeles School of Medicine; Associate Director, Residency Education, Neuropsychiatric Institute and Hospital and West Los Angeles Veterans Administration Medical Center (Brentwood), Los Angeles, California.

Hans H. Strupp, Ph.D. Distinguished Professor of Psychology, Vanderbilt University, Nashville, Tennessee.

Norman Sussman, M.D. Clinical Associate Professor of Psychiatry, New York University School of Medicine; Director, Psychopharmacology Service, Bellevue Hospital; Assistant Attending Psychiatrist, University Hospital of the New York University Medical Center; Assistant Attending Psychiatrist, Bellevue Hospital, New York, New York.

Ludwik S. Szymanski, M.D. Assistant Professor of Psychiatry, Harvard Medical School; Director of Psychiatry, Developmental Evaluation Clinic, Children's Hospital, Boston, Massachusetts.

Zebulon C. Taintor, M.D. Professor and Vice Chairman, Department of Psychiatry, New York University School of Medicine; Chief of Staff, Manhattan Psychiatric Center; Attending Psychiatrist, Bellevue Hospital, New York, New York.

Alfonso Troisi, M.D. Visiting Research Scientist, University of California at Los Angeles School of Medicine, Neuropsychiatric Institute and Hospital, Los Angeles, California; Assistant Professor of Clinical Psychiatry, Catterdra di Clinica Psichiatrica, II Universita di Roma, Rome, Italy.

Gary J. Tucker, M.D. Professor and Chairman, Department of Psychiatry and Behavioral Sciences, University of Washington School of Medicine; Psychiatrist-in Chief, University of Washington Hospitals, Seattle, Washington.

Thomas W. Uhde, M.D. Chief, Unit on Anxiety and Affective Disorders, Biological Psychiatry Branch, National Institute of Mental Health; Clinical Associate Professor of Psychiatry, Uniformed Services University of the Health Sciences F. Edward Hebert School of Medicine, Bethesda, Maryland.

Louis Vachon, M.D. Professor and Chairman, Division of Psychiatry, Boston University School of Medicine; Psychiatrist-in-Chief, University Hospital, Boston, Massachusetts.

George E. Vaillant, M.D. Raymond Sobel Professor of Psychiatry and Director, Study of Adult Development, Dartmouth Medical School, Hanover, New Hampshire; Director, Study of Adult Development, Harvard University Health Services, Cambridge, Massachusetts.

Wilfred G. Van Gorp, Ph.D. Assistant Professor in Residence, University of California at Los Angeles School of Medicine; Chief, Neuropsychology Assessment Laboratory, West Los Angeles Veterans Administration Medical Center (Brentwood), Los Angeles, California.

Gary W. Van Hoesen, Ph.D. Professor of Anatomy and Neurology, Department of Anatomy, University of Iowa College of Medicine, Iowa City, Iowa.

Deborah L. Warden, M.D. Instructor in Psychiatry and Neurology, Georgetown University School of Medicine; Chief, Treatment and Evaluation Unit, Psychiatry Service, Veterans Administration Medical Center, Washington, DC.

Stanley J. Watson, M.D., Ph.D. Professor of Psychiatry, University of Michigan Medical School; Research Scientist and Associate Director, Mental Health Research Institute, Ann Arbor, Michigan.

Daniel R. Weinberger, M.D. Chief, Clinical Brain Disorders Branch, Intramural Research Program, National Institute of Mental Health; Associate Clinical Professor of Neurology and Psychiatry, George Washington University School of Medicine and Health Sciences, Washington, DC.

Myron F. Weiner, M.D. Professor and Vice Chairman, Department of Psychiatry, University of Texas Southwestern Medical School at Dallas; Director, Psychiatric Consultation-Liaison Service, Parkland Memorial Hospital, Dallas, Texas.

Richard D. Weiner, M.D., Ph.D. Associate Professor of Psychiatry, Duke University School of Medicine; Staff Psychiatrist, Veterans Administration Medical Center, Durham, North Carolina.

Elizabeth B. Weller, M.D. Professor of Psychiatry and Pediatrics and Director, Division of Child and Adolescent Psychiatry, Ohio State University College of Medicine; Medical Director, Pre-Adolescent Psychiatric Unit, Division of Child and Adolescent Psychiatry, Ohio State University Hospitals, Columbus, Ohio.

Paul H. Wender, M.D. Professor of Psychiatry and Director, Psychiatric Research, University of Utah School of Medicine; Attending Psychiatrist, University of Utah Hospital, Salt Lake City, Utah.

Peter C. Whybrow, M.D. Professor and Chairman, Department of Psychiatry, University of Pennsylvania School of Medicine; Psychiatrist-in-Chief, Hospital of the University of Pennsylvania, Philadelphia, Pennsylvania.

Robert L. Williams, M.D. D. C. and Irene Ellwood Professor and Chairman, Department of Psychiatry, Baylor College of Medicine; Co-Director, Sleep Disorders and Research Center; Chief, Psychiatry Service, The Methodist Hospital; Chief, Psychiatry Section, St. Luke's Episcopal Hospital, Houston, Texas.

William J. Winslade, Ph.D., J.D. Professor of Medical Jurisprudence and Psychiatry, University of Texas Medical Branch at Galveston; Director, Ethics Consultation Service, Institute for the Medical Humanities, Galveston, Texas.

Deane L. Wolcott, M.D. Associate Clinical Professor of Psychiatry, University of California at Los Angeles School of Medicine; Associate Director, Consultation-Liaison Psychiatry Service, Neuropsychiatric Institute and Hospital, Los Angeles, California.

Normund Wong, M.D. Clinical Professor of Psychiatry, University of California at San Francisco School of Medicine; Director, Affiliated Psychiatric Education, Letterman Army Medical Center; Member, San Francisco Psychoanalytic Institute, San Francisco, California; Member, Topeka Institute for Psychoanalysis, Topeka, Kansas.

Richard Jed Wyatt, M.D. Chief, Neuropsychiatry Branch, National Institute of Mental Health, Neuroscience Center, Intramural Research Program, Washington, DC.

George E. Woody, M.D. Clinical Professor of Psychiatry, University of Pennsylvania School of Medicine; Chief, Substance Abuse Treatment Unit, Veterans Administration Medical Center, Philadelphia, Pennsylvania.

Joel Yager, M.D. Professor of Psychiatry, University of California at Los Angeles School of Medicine; Director, Residency Education, Neuropsychiatric Institute and Hospital; Associate Chief of Staff for Residency Education, West Los Angeles Veterans Administration Medical Center (Brentwood), Los Angeles, California.

J. Gerald Young, M.D. Professor of Psychiatry, New York University School of Medicine; Attending Psychiatrist, University Hospital of the New York University Medical Center; Attending Psychiatrist, Bellevue Hospital, New York, New York.

CONTENTS

VOLUME ONE

VOLUME TWO

CHAPTER 1 NEURAL SCIENCE

1.1
INTRODUCTION AND OVERVIEW

JACK A. GREBB, M.D.

The neurosciences are fundamentally important to the clinical specialties of psychiatry, neurology, and neurosurgery because they explore the biology of neuronal tissues. Two subspecialty areas within psychiatry—neuropsychiatry and biological psychiatry—have particularly endeavored to integrate neuroscientific information with clinical psychiatry. It is unfortunate in some respects that these subspecialty concepts have evolved, since an appreciation for the basic neurosciences should infuse the clinical approaches of all professionals working with the mentally ill.

MISLEADING DICHOTOMIES There is a common tendency to divide and distinguish phenomena, even in the absence of adequate data. This tendency has had unfortunate consequences for the mentally ill. In recent history, people inflicted with diseases that were not understood (e.g., tuberculosis, cancer) have been ostracized from society. Once the conditions were understood as medical diseases, these outcasts entered the relative comfort of a medical model for their afflictions. Patients with mental illnesses are currently caught in a transitional phase in this process. The general acceptance of mental illness as a disease of the brain is currently hindered by at least five misleading dichotomies.

Neurology vs. psychiatry The clinical distinction between neurology and psychiatry is increasingly appreciated as awkward and artificial (Chapter 2). Neurology has traditionally focused on organic disorders with identifiable pathology, whereas psychiatry has focused on functional disorders without observable pathology. Regardless of intentions, the implication is that neurological disorders are real diseases, whereas psychiatric disorders are not. *Functional,* in this context, actually means that the organic pathophysiological basis has not been discovered yet—not that one does not exist. A better term for functional might be idiopathic.

The mind-brain dichotomy The mind and the brain share the same organ. *Mind* is what is called the personal experience of the brain or perhaps the experience of change in the brain. How can the complexity of the mind be explained by the brain? First, the brain is undoubtedly more complex than is currently known; second, perhaps minds are not as complex as is generally thought.

Nature vs. nurture There is no contest: nature is nurtured, and nurture has a nature. Nature and nurture are mutually interacting systems. It has been shown clearly that the environment (i.e., nurture) can affect biology at very basic molecular levels (e.g., branching of dendrites, activity of enzymes). Nurture itself can be seen as a reciprocal biological event. Human beings affect one another, and there exist biological changes parallel to the subjective experiences.

Structure vs. function All mental activities (behavior, thoughts, feelings) are paired with biological events in the brain. The techniques of basic neuroscience can potentially identify the structural correlates of mental activity at the level of genes and other molecules. The division between structure and function rests solely on which biological level is arbitrarily chosen as a cutoff point. A more accurate approach is to accept that each biological disorder, including mental illness, has a structural pathology at some level or assortment of levels, and that this structural abnormality is reflected as a disorder of function or regulation.

Biology vs. psychology This dichotomy is both a derivative of the mind-brain issue and an unfortunate offshoot of debates within the field of psychiatry. Biology, psychology, sociology, and other disciplines are explanatory systems for empirical observations. The level and descriptive lexicon used to describe behavioral phenomena can be varied. In a particular situation, one model might be more enlightening or clinically appropriate than another.

OVERVIEW OF NEURAL SCIENCES

The aim of this 15-section neural sciences chapter is to provide a brief introduction to the basic science principles that underlie the many biological theories, organic therapies, and research findings discussed in the chapters on specific clinical disorders. Therefore, the sections within this chapter do not systematically review the relationships between their topics and relevant clinical disorders. Rather, this chapter can either be read as an introduction to basic biological principles or used as a reference when reading about biological material in subsequent chapters.

NEUROANATOMY Classical neuroanatomy (Section 1.2) describes regions and connections in the brain based primarily on observations from gross neuroanatomy. Functional neuroanatomy (Section 1.3) is based more on data from studies defining the distribution of specific molecules (e.g., neurotransmitters) and from studies using advanced histochemical techniques that have defined more clearly the projection patterns of neuronal populations. Functional neuroanatomy is possibly more relevant to psychiatric disorders than is classical neuroanatomy; in fact, the insights of functional neuroanatomy are slowly eclipsing some of the previous tenets of classical neuroanatomy.

Neurons The *neuron,* or nerve cell, is the basic functional unit of the nervous system. Neurons vary widely in terms of size, shape, number of synapses, and chemical constituents. The cell body, also called the soma or perikaryon, typically gives rise to *axons* and *dendrites*. The axon arises from the cell body or the base of one of the main dendrites. The initial axon segment, the axon hillock, actually is the site of initiation for the action potential in many neurons. Enlargements at the ends of axons are called axon terminals, or *boutons,* and are the sites of presynaptic neurotransmitter release. Within the axon terminals are the *synaptic vesicles,* which contain neurotransmitter substances. There are different types of synaptic vesicles, varying in size, shape, and other visual characteristics. These different types often contain different neurotransmitters, and conceivably these vesicles respond differentially to stimulation of the axon terminal. There may be one or many dendrites (or none at all) emerging from the cell body. Dendrites are usually profusely branched, and most are studded with small spikes, the dendritic spines, which, along with somata and dendritic shafts, are the sites of synaptic connections.

Glia Glia, glial cells, or neuroglia are synonymous terms for a class of nonneuronal cells in the nervous system. There are four types of glial cells in the central nervous system (CNS)—astrocytes, oligodendrocytes, ependyma, and microglia—and two types in the peripheral nervous system—Schwann and satellite cells. The *astrocytes* provide structural support to neurons and are the major cell type in glial scar tissue in the CNS. The *oligodendrocytes* are the myelin-forming cells of the CNS and also may perform a nurturing role for neurons. Both astrocytes and oligodendrocytes are involved in phagocytosis. The *ependyma* line the brain ventricles and the central canal of the spinal cord. The surfaces of ependymal cells that border the ventricles are covered with cilia, whose beating facilitates the movement of cerebrospinal fluid (CSF). Although investigations of neurons have overshadowed interest in the glia, it is quite possible that glial cells have a more direct and critical role in neuronal activity than is currently believed.

Blood-brain barrier An important feature of the brain to which glial cells contribute is the *blood-brain barrier,* a semipermeable barrier between the blood vessels and brain that prevents many chemical compounds from passing between brain and blood. The ability of a molecule to cross the blood-brain barrier is based on its molecular size, electric charge, solubility, and the presence of specific transport systems for the compound. The endothelial cells of brain capillaries differ from other capillaries because they are virtually continuous with each other and lack the pinocytotic vesicles that have been implicated in transport of substances from one side of the membrane to the other. The biogenic amine neurotransmitters (e.g., dopamine) are metabolized within the CNS into acidic metabolites that are actively removed by a transport system in the choroid plexus. The drug probenecid (Benemid) is often used in psychiatric research because it blocks this transport system, causing a buildup in CSF of amine metabolites that then can be measured as part of a research protocol (e.g., clinical trials of a new drug).

Membranes All cells, including neurons and glia, are enclosed in cell membranes that function as a complex regulatory site. The membrane is a sea of phospholipids, organized as a bilayer with the hydrophobic ends of the lipid molecules pointing toward the middle of the membrane. Within this lipid bilayer are various types of protein molecules. Some proteins are embedded in the external or internal surfaces of the membrane. Neurotransmitter receptors (Section 1.4), for example, are proteins that are located partially on the outside surface of the membrane and transmit a message to another protein (e.g., an enzyme [Section 1.6]) that is located on the inside surface of the membrane. Other proteins, such as ion channels (Section 1.7), extend the entire width of the membrane.

Cerebrospinal fluid The CNS ventricular system is filled with CSF, produced by the choroid plexi in the cerebral ventricles. CSF leaves the ventricular system via the median aperture of Magendie and the two lateral apertures of Luschka and is then absorbed into the venous system through the arachnoid villi. Hydrocephalus results from a disorder of CSF drainage resulting in increased CSF pressure. This can often be seen in computed tomographic (CT) scans by the presence of dilated ventricles.

The CSF has a volume of approximately 125 ml in the normal adult, and approximately 500 ml are made each day. The total volume of CSF, therefore, is replaced approximately four times each day. The use of lumbar punctures to obtain CSF is routine in neurological practice. The CSF also is a source of research information in psychiatry because it reflects neurochemical activity in the brain. However, metabolites from the spinal cord may significantly contribute to the chemical content of CSF, and neurotransmitter metabolites from deep brain structures may not reach the CSF efficiently. Other considerations when evaluating research data based on CSF measurements are the possibilities of a vertical gradient in the concentration of the chemical within CSF and also of rhythmic variations of production of the chemical with time (e.g., diurnal variation).

NEUROTRANSMISSION Neurotransmission can occur either through chemical or electrical synapses. The role of electrical synapses, also called gap junctions, in the CNS is poorly understood. In contrast, a great deal is known about chemical synapses. Chemical neurotransmission classically involves a presynaptic neuron that releases a neurotransmitter that diffuses across a synaptic cleft, where it binds to a specific receptor that initiates a series of molecular events in the postsynaptic neuron. The three major classes of chemical neuromessengers are biogenic amines (also called monoamines) (Section 1.4), amino acids (Section 1.4), and neuropeptides (Section 1.5). The intraneuronal molecular events that occur preceding transmitter release and following receptor activation have recently been defined (Section 1.6).

Synapses The most conventional types of chemical synapses are the *axo-dendritic* and *axo-somatic* synapses, in which the axon of the presynaptic neuron synapses, with a dendrite or the cell body, respectively, of the postsynaptic neuron. Such synapses may be inhibitory, excitatory, or modulatory. In *axo-axonic* synapses, the presynaptic axon synapses with the axon hillock or axon terminal of the postsynaptic neuron. It is thought that these synapses are usually inhibitory. Two more recently discovered synapses are dendro-dendritic and dendro-axonic. Both of these synaptic types are probably involved in local modulation of synaptic function and do not elicit postsynaptic action potentials. One final complication of synapses is that nonsynaptic neurons probably exist as well. These are neurons with axon terminals that release neurotransmitters into the extracellular fluid or the CSF and therefore do not have synapses with specific neurons and may function in a paracrine fashion.

Receptors *Receptors* (Section 1.4) are proteins in the neuronal membrane that are, in part, exposed to the extracellular fluid and specifically recognize neuromessengers. To be classified as a receptor, the binding to this protein should be saturable, specific, and reversible. *Saturable* means that in experimental preparations it can be demonstrated that there is a finite number of the receptors present. *Specific* means that the receptor binds, relatively speaking, only the alleged neurotransmitter for that receptor. Binding to a functionally meaningful receptor is reversible, which means that the receptor must first bind, then release, the neurotransmitter so that the receptor subsequently can respond to another message. The term *putative receptor* is often used to describe a binding site that has not yet been definitively shown to have all the properties required of a receptor.

Receptors can be either postsynaptic or presynaptic. In an axo-dendritic synapse, for example, the receptors on the receiving dendrite are postsynaptic. Receptors on the axon itself are presynaptic. They are called either presynaptic autoreceptors if they bind the neurotransmitter released by their parent neuron or presynaptic heteroreceptors if they bind a neurotransmitter released by some other neuron.

The concepts of supersensitivity and subsensitivity are applied to receptors. When demonstrated appropriately, these properties signify that a specific postsynaptic neuron responds in either an augmented or attenuated fashion to a constant amount of neurotransmitter. Such regulation of synaptic response could come from three receptor-related changes. First, the number of receptors available for neurotransmitter binding could increase or decrease. Second, the binding affinity of the receptor for the neurotransmitter molecule could increase or decrease. Third, the molecular mechanism by which the receptor translates its message into the neuron could be more or less efficient.

Neuromessengers *Neuromessenger* is a generic term that includes neurotransmitters, neuromodulators, and neurohormones. The term *neurotransmitter,* however, is also commonly used to mean any type of chemical interneuronal message. More specifically, however, neurotransmitters are the classic neuromessengers that are rapidly released by the presynaptic neuron upon stimulation, diffuse across the synaptic cleft, and have either an excitatory or inhibitory effect on a postsynaptic neuron. *Neuromodulators* also bind to specific receptors, but are conceptualized as tuning or grading the response of the postsynaptic cell to the neurotransmitter. It obviously is somewhat arbitrary and artificial to decide how much tuning is merely modulation as opposed to actual transmission. *Neurohormones* are chemical messengers that are released by neurons into the bloodstream, rather than into the synaptic cleft or extraneuronal space. The differentiation of these three different neuromessenger types is usually less clear in actuality. Furthermore, any specific chemical may act in all three roles depending on the specific synaptic or neuronal system under consideration.

Other chemical messengers In addition to biogenic amines, amino acids, and neuropeptides, there are other chemical messengers that are the subject of active research investigations.

The *eicosanoids* include arachidonic acid and its metabolites—prostaglandins (PGs), thromboxanes, and leukotrienes. Although all of the eicosanoids are involved in neurochemical processes, the prostaglandins have been most studied in neuropsychiatric disorders. The eicosanoids differ from classical neurotransmitters in that they are not synthesized and then stored for future release; rather, they are synthesized de novo when needed. The PGs are subtyped into several series (D, E, F, etc.) and series subtypes (e.g., PGE_2). The PGEs have been hypothesized to have a role in the sedative, anticonvulsant, and analgesic effects of various medications. Lithium has been reported to decrease PGE_1 stimulation of adenylate cyclase, and tricyclic antidepressants and monoamine oxidase inhibitors (MAOIs) have been hypothesized to act through down-regulating the activity of PGE_2.

Adenosine is a nucleoside that functions as a neuromessenger. The adenosine receptors are linked to adenylate cyclase such that A_1 receptors inhibit cyclic adenosine monophosphate (cAMP) production and A_2 receptors stimulate cAMP production. Two other nucleosides, guanosine and inosine, may also function as neuromessengers.

ELECTROPHYSIOLOGY AND CLINICAL BRAIN IMAGING The electrophysiological properties of single neurons (Section 1.7) can largely be explained by the movements of four ions—sodium, potassium, chloride, and calcium—across the neuronal membranes. The effects of neuromessengers and psychoactive drugs are ultimately translated into changes in the fluxes of these ions. Several clinical tests—electroencephalograms, evoked potentials, and computerized mapping of brain electrical activity (Section 1.8)—measure the mass effects of these ionic changes.

Both gross anatomy and brain function can now be imaged in living human subjects (Section 1.10). CT and magnetic resonance imaging (MRI) can image gross anatomy. Positron emission tomography (PET), regional cerebral blood flow (rCBF), magnetic resonance spectroscopy, and single photon emission computed tomography (SPECT) measure various aspects of brain function.

PSYCHONEUROENDOCRINOLOGY AND PSYCHONEUROIMMUNOLOGY The nervous system, the endocrine system (Section 1.11), and the immune system (Section 1.12) are the three bodily systems that can communicate within themselves through complex chemical signals. It is now appreciated that each of these systems also can communicate with the other two, creating a triad of intercommunicating systems (Section 1.12). The neuroendocrine system may be the major mediator of environmental stress, and soon the neuroimmune system may help explain the pathophysiology of psychosomatic disorders. Someday, the seemingly straightforward division of disorders into neurological, immunological, or endocrinological may seem archaic.

CHRONOBIOLOGY AND PLASTICITY IN THE MATURE CNS Virtually every objective biological measure discussed in Sections 1.2 to 1.12 changes with time in a regular fashion. The study of these biological rhythms is called *chronobiology* (Section 1.13). The brain is a plastic, mutable organ that also evidences nonrhythmic changes (Section 1.14), such as changes in the neuronal shape, the number and quality of synaptic connections, and the intraneuronal molecular contents. Although, for all intents and purposes, mammalian neurons cannot divide in the adult, there remain remarkable mechanisms for moderating changes in the CNS.

GENETICS

Molecular genetics (Section 1.15) is the study of genes and gene expression at the basic chemical level. The techniques of molecular genetics have made it conceptually possible to diagnose, prevent, and treat mental disorders at this most basic molecular level. Although molecular genetics currently is one of the most exciting areas of neuroscience, *population genetics,* the study of the inheritance of phenotypes in groups of individuals, provides the historical and conceptual foundation for much of biologically oriented psychiatry.

RESEARCH STRATEGIES IN DESCRIPTIVE POPULATION GENETICS In addition to linkage studies (Section 1.15), there are five general types of studies in descriptive population genetics—pedigree analyses, family risk studies, twin studies, adoption studies, and high-risk studies. The validity of any of these types of investigations requires both an unbiased identification and an accurate diagnosis of all subjects studied.

Pedigree analysis Pedigree analysis involves the study of individual families that contain members who are affected by the disorder under investigation. Family trees can be constructed to diagram marriages, children, deaths, and affected members. Pedigree analysis can suggest hypotheses regarding whether disorders are inheritable and what the type of inheritance might be (e.g., dominant, recessive, X-linked). However, because of the small number of individuals who have been studied, as well as the biased ascertainment method and the possible role of nongenetic environmental influences, pedigree analysis is generally useful only for the generation of hypotheses that will subsequently be tested by other types of studies.

Family risk studies Family risk studies begin with the identification of an unbiased sample of patients with the disorder under investigation. These patients are referred to as the *probands* or *index cases.* The next step involves the identification of the various relatives (parents, sibs, children, grandparents, etc.) for each of the index cases. Psychiatric diagnoses can be made either through interviewing each relative (family study method) or reviewing records and interviewing other relatives (family history method). Although the family study method is more accurate and preferable, it involves much more time, money, and effort.

The goal of family risk studies is to compare the rates of diagnoses in various relatives (e.g., first-degree or second-degree relatives) with rates in the general population. Disorders with a genetic basis are usually expected to be more common in relatives of index cases than in the general population and more common in first-degree relatives than in second-degree relatives. The findings from family risk studies are reported as expectancy rates (the number of cases that exist or may arise during the lifetimes of the relatives). A variety of statistical methods (e.g., Weinberg method, Stromgren method) are used to calculate expectancy rates based on data from only one point in time. The data from family risk studies are useful in genetic counseling. Data from family risk studies do not generally help distinguish, however, between genetic and environmental influences on the development of psychiatric disorders.

Twin studies The study of twin pairs, of whom at least one is affected by the disorder of interest, is a method that does provide some information on the relative contribution of genetic and environmental (e.g., familial) influences on the development of psychiatric disorders. Valid twin studies require that the sample be unbiased, the disorder not be more common in twins than in single births, and that the determination of zygosity be accurate. The rates of psychiatric disorders can then be compared between the various groups studied according to decreasing degrees of genetic closeness: monozygotic twins, dizygotic twins, full siblings, half siblings, stepsiblings. The strongest support for a genetic basis of a disorder is present when monozygotic twins are significantly more concordant for the disorder than are dizygotic twins and when dizygotic twins are no more concordant than are nontwin siblings.

The interpretation of twin studies does require an understanding of the possible variations in the environmental influences on the twins. For example, the assumption that monozygotic twins raised in the same family will have identical environments is often incorrect. Environmental differences for monozygotic twins can begin in utero if the twins receive unequal placental circulation. Furthermore, whereas some parents will raise twins identically, other parents will make a special effort to differentiate their approach to each twin. It is perhaps these types of environmental differences that usually result in monozygotic concordance rates that are much less than 100 percent. In fact, very few genetic disorders of any body system demonstrate a 100 percent concordance rate in monozygotic twins.

Adoption studies Adoption studies assess the rates of disorders in children, including twins, who are raised apart from very early ages, preferably from infancy. The theory is that strong genetic influences should often evidence themselves regardless of the environment to which they are exposed. Two major designs have been employed. The first approach is to compare rates of illness in adopted children of affected biological parents with the rates of illness in adoptees who had healthy biological parents. For disorders with a genetic basis, adopted children of affected biological parents should have higher rates of illness than adopted children of normal biological parents, assuming that the two groups of adoptive parents are similar and mentally healthy. The second approach is to compare the biological and adoptive parents of affected adoptees with the parents of nonaffected control adoptees. For a genetic disorder, the biological parents should have the highest rate of illness, and the adoptive parents and the control parents should have equal rates of illness.

A variation of this design includes a group of affected adoptees whose biological parents are normal but whose adopted parents are affected. Potential problems with adoptive studies include a possible genetic basis for the decisions either to give up or take in a child, a nonrandom socioeconomic distribution of adoptions, and the effects of a difficult child on adoptive parents.

High-risk studies High-risk studies identify and prospectively follow children who have at least one biological parent who is affected by the disorder under study. Such studies can identify precursor signs of the disorder, important environmental variables affecting the expression of the disorder, and potential strategies for early intervention and prevention.

PARADIGMATIC SHIFTS

Despite efforts to maintain harmony between basic neuroscience disciplines and the psychological foundations of psychiatry, there remains a fundamental question regarding their integration. Will the tenets of psychology and descriptive psychiatry be used to test the discoveries of neuroscience, or will the discoveries of neuroscience be used to mold new ideas about human psychology and nosology? Although it is premature to take only one of these approaches, neuroscientific inquiry into the human brain must proceed with few preconceptions about how the brain works. The commonsense appeal of such concepts as conscious-unconscious, free will, and motivation may entrap or seduce the scientist from seeing more basic truths about brain function and mental illness.

HUMBLENESS IN NEUROSCIENCE

The brain is tremendously complex, and it is not yet understood how its molecular structure results in what is considered normal and abnormal mental functioning. The sections within this chapter present neuroscientific knowledge as it is currently understood. Neuroscientific knowledge, however, is growing and changing at a very fast rate. A reasonable approach to the field of neuroscience is to know as much as possible about what has already been demonstrated and to consider new information that may completely contradict what has previously been thought. Although the success and excitement of recent neuroscientific advances may invite intellectual arrogance, a humble attitude toward understanding the brain is still very much indicated.

REFERENCES

Arieti S, editor in chief: *American Handbook of Psychiatry*, ed 2, vol 8, *Biological Psychiatry*, P A Berger, K H Brodie, editors. Basic Books, New York, 1986.
Asbury A K, McKhann G M, McDonald W I, editors: *Diseases of the Nervous System*, vols I and II. Saunders, Philadelphia and Heinemann, London, 1986.
Cooper A M: Will neurobiology influence psychoanalysis? Amer J Psychiat *142:* 1395, 1985.
Cummings J L: *Clinical Neuropsychiatry*. Grune & Stratton, Orlando, FL, 1985.
Darnell J, Lodish H, Baltimore D: *Molecular Cell Biology*. Scientific American Books, New York, 1986.
Detre T: The future of psychiatry. Amer J Psychiat *144:* 621, 1987.
Emery A E H: *Methodology in Medical Genetics*. Churchill Livingstone, New York, 1976.
Goldstein G W, Betz A L: The blood-brain barrier. Sci Amer *255:* 74, 1986.
Hofer M: *The Roots of Human Behavior*. Freeman, San Francisco, 1981.
Kallmann F J: *Heredity in Health and Mental Disorder*. Norton, New York, 1953.
Kandel E R: From metapsychology to molecular biology: Explorations into the nature of anxiety. Amer J Psychiat *140:* 1277, 1983.
Kandel E R, Schwartz J H: Principles of Neural Science, ed 2. Elsevier, New York, 1985.
Kanof P D, Johns C, Davidson M, Siever L J, Coccaro E F, Davis K L: Prostaglandin receptor sensitivity in psychiatric disorders. Arch Gen Psychiat *43:* 987, 1986.
McIlwain H, Bachelard H S: *Biochemistry and the Central Nervous System*, ed 5. Churchill Livingstone, New York, 1985.
Mesulam M M, editor: *Principles of Behavioral Neurology*. Davis, Philadelphia, 1985.
Pardes H: Neuroscience and psychiatry: Marriage or coexistence? Amer J Psychiat *143:* 1205, 1986.
Pincus J H, Tucker G J: *Behavioral Neurology*, ed 3. Oxford University Press, New York, 1985.
Scientific American: The Brain. Sci Amer *241(3):* entire issue, 1979.
Scientific American: The Molecules of Life. Sci Amer *253(4):* entire issue, 1985.
Stiles G L: Adenosine receptors: Structure, function, and regulation. Trends Pharmacol Sci *7:* 486, December 1986.
Williams M: Purigenic receptors and central nervous system function. In *Psychopharmacology: The Third Generation of Progress*, H Y Meltzer, editor, p 289. Raven Press, New York, 1987.

1.2 MAJOR BRAIN STRUCTURES

GARY W. VAN HOESEN, Ph.D.
GEORGE F. ALHEID, Ph.D.
LENNART HEIMER, M.D.

SUBDIVISIONS OF THE BRAIN

The convention in adult neuroanatomy, as in nearly all aspects of anatomy, is to parcellate a complex or large structure into meaningful smaller parts. Embryologic development of the nervous system provides the initial impetus and has played a major role in shaping neuroanatomical thinking. For example, in the fourth week of embryonic development, the rostral part of the neural tube reaches the three-vesicle stage and consists of the *prosencephalon* in a fore position (forebrain), the *rhombencephalon* in an aft or hind position (hindbrain), with the *mesencephalon* (midbrain) between the two. Secondary changes lead to the formation of a five-vesicle structure with the prosencephalon forming two divisions (the *telencephalon* and *diencephalon*), the mesencephalon remaining static in terms of position, and the rhombencephalon dividing into a *myelencephalon* and a *metencephalon* (Fig. 1.2-1).

TELENCEPHALON The telencephalon gives rise to the largest adult derivative of the neural tube, namely, the cerebral cortex, whose genesis is one of the most phenomenal of all biological events. Massive subcortical structures, such as the *caudate nucleus*, the *lentiform nucleus*, and the *amygdaloid body*, are also of telencephalic origin.

DIENCEPHALON The diencephalon is composed of three subdivisions: the *epithalamus, thalamus*, and *hypothalamus*. The epithalamus, the smallest of the three, consists of the *habenular nuclei*, with an associated *habenular commissure*, and the *pineal gland*, or *epiphysis*. The hypothalamus and thalamus are, in part, divided by a shallow groove, the *hypothalamic sulcus*, which can be found as paired indentations along the lateral wall of the third ventricle. These are both complex structures composed of many different subdivisions.

MESENCEPHALON The mesencephalon, like the diencephalon, is composed of three distinct anatomical entities: a dorsally located *tectum*, the *tegmentum* in an intermediate location, and a *basal peduncular* region along its ventral surface. The tectum consists of two sets of paired elevations, the *superior* and *inferior colliculi*. Beneath these is the *cerebral aqueduct*, the small, narrow passage of communication between the third and fourth ventricles. It is surrounded by a distinct gray matter area known as the *central gray substance* or *periaqueductal gray*.

METENCEPHALON The anatomical components of the metencephalon are the *cerebellum* and the *pons*. The cerebellum is characterized by a highly enfolded and thin cortex that forms two distinct hemispheres and a midline *vermis*. The deep cerebellar nuclei—*fastigial, globose, emboliform*, and *dentate*—are gray-matter masses contained within the white matter of both the vermis and the cerebellar hemispheres. The cerebellum is connected to the brain stem by three pairs of

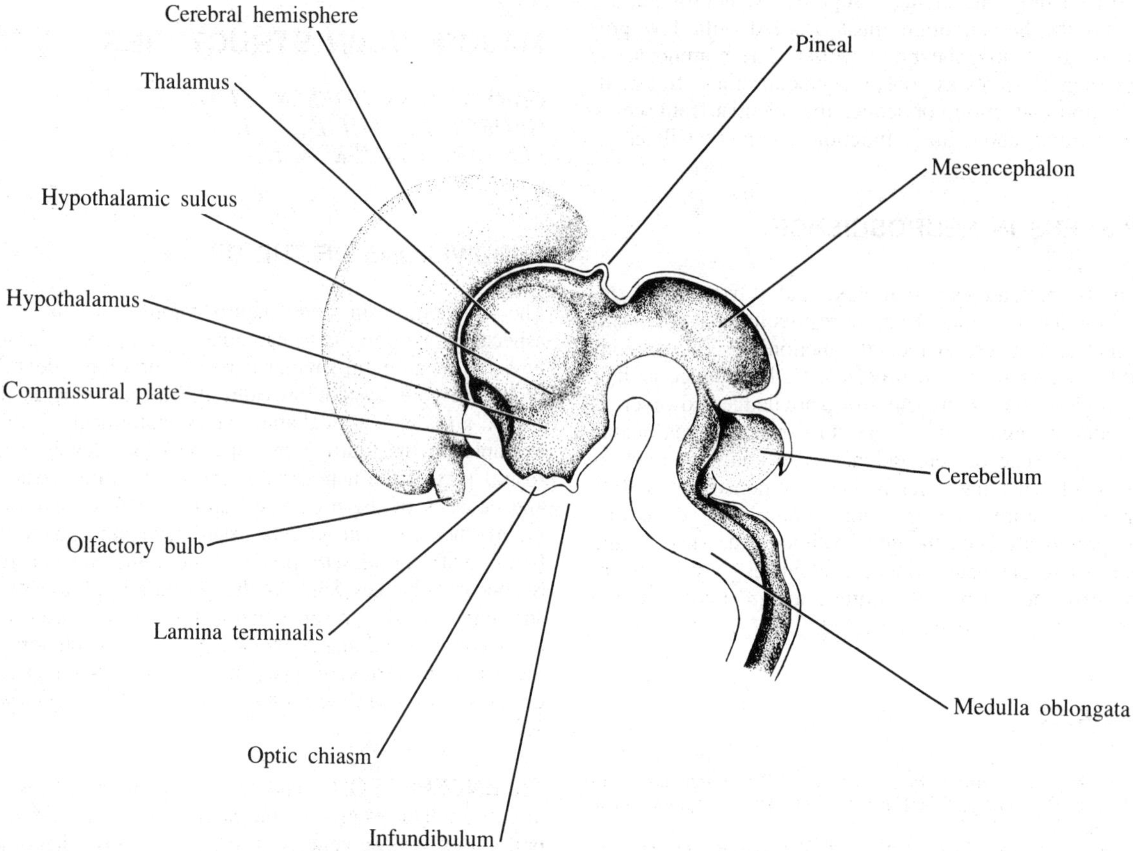

FIGURE 1.2-1. *Development of diencephalon. The medial surface of the brain in a 43-mm human embryo. The hypothalamic sulcus separates the thalamus from the hypothalamus. (Modified after Hines M: J Comp Neurol* 34: *73, 1922. From Heimer L:* The Human Brain and Spinal Cord. *Springer-Verlag, New York, 1983, with permission.)*

peduncles: the *superior, middle,* and *inferior cerebellar peduncles*.

The pons consists of the *pontine tegmentum* and the *basis pontis*. The pontine tegmentum is a caudal continuation of the mesencephalic tegmentum, whereas the more voluminous basal part of the pons owes its prominence to the massive pontocerebellar fiber system, which projects to the cerebellum and arises from the large nuclear complex, the pontine nuclei of the basis pontis.

MYELENCEPHALON The myelencephalon forms the *medulla oblongata* and is directly continuous with the cervical spinal cord. It contains distinct sensory and motor nuclei. The basal portion of the medulla oblongata is dominated by the pyramids, which contain the corticospinal tracts. Another prominent anatomical feature of the medulla oblongata is the *inferior olivary nucleus,* which forms a rounded prominence, the olive, next to the pyramid on the external surface of the upper medulla oblongata. Some of the relationships for the five-vesicle stage of neural development are illustrated in Figure 1.2-1.

EXTERNAL FEATURES OF THE BRAIN

For a review of human neuroanatomy, a logical starting point is to consider the gross structure of the cerebral hemisphere and, in particular, the major sulci and gyri that enable one to subdivide the cerebral cortex into lobes and smaller functional subdivisions, such as those related to language, sensation, and motor control.

LATERAL VIEW OF THE CEREBRAL CORTEX **Frontal lobe** As shown in Figure 1.2-2, the sulcal limits that define the frontal lobe are the *central sulcus* (or *fissure of Rolando*) posteriorly, and the *lateral* (or *Sylvian*) *fissure* ventrally. The precentral sulcus lies roughly parallel with the central sulcus, in a rostral position, and typically enables an unambiguous identification of the *precentral gyrus* (Brodmann's area 4) where motor representation for the contralateral body musculature is mapped. Other major sulci of the frontal lobe include the *superior frontal sulcus* and the *inferior frontal sulcus,* which divide the frontal cortex into *superior, middle,* and *inferior frontal lobules*. The inferior frontal lobule is parcellated further into two important branches of the lateral fissure. One branch, which ascends vertically, is known as the *anterior ascending* branch of the lateral fissure, and between it and the ventral part of the precentral sulcus is the so-called *pars opercularis* (area 44). Another branch, the *anterior horizontal* sulcus, extends in the direction of the frontal pole, and the cortical area between it and the anterior ascending sulcus forms the so-called *pars triangularis* (area 45). The pars opercularis and pars triangularis together form Broca's expressive speech area. Beneath the anterior horizontal branch of the lateral fissure is the orbital part of the frontal lobe, which overlies the orbit.

Parietal lobe In most human brain specimens, the parietal lobe, unlike the frontal lobe, is not defined precisely by primary sulci. Its anterior boundary is defined clearly by the central sulcus, and a prominent *postcentral sulcus* is seen typically running parallel to it. Between the central and the postcentral sulcus is the *postcentral gyrus,* where somatic sensation for the entire contralateral body surface, including the face, is mapped (areas 3, 1, and 2). The posterior border of the parietal lobe is typically clear-cut on the medial surface

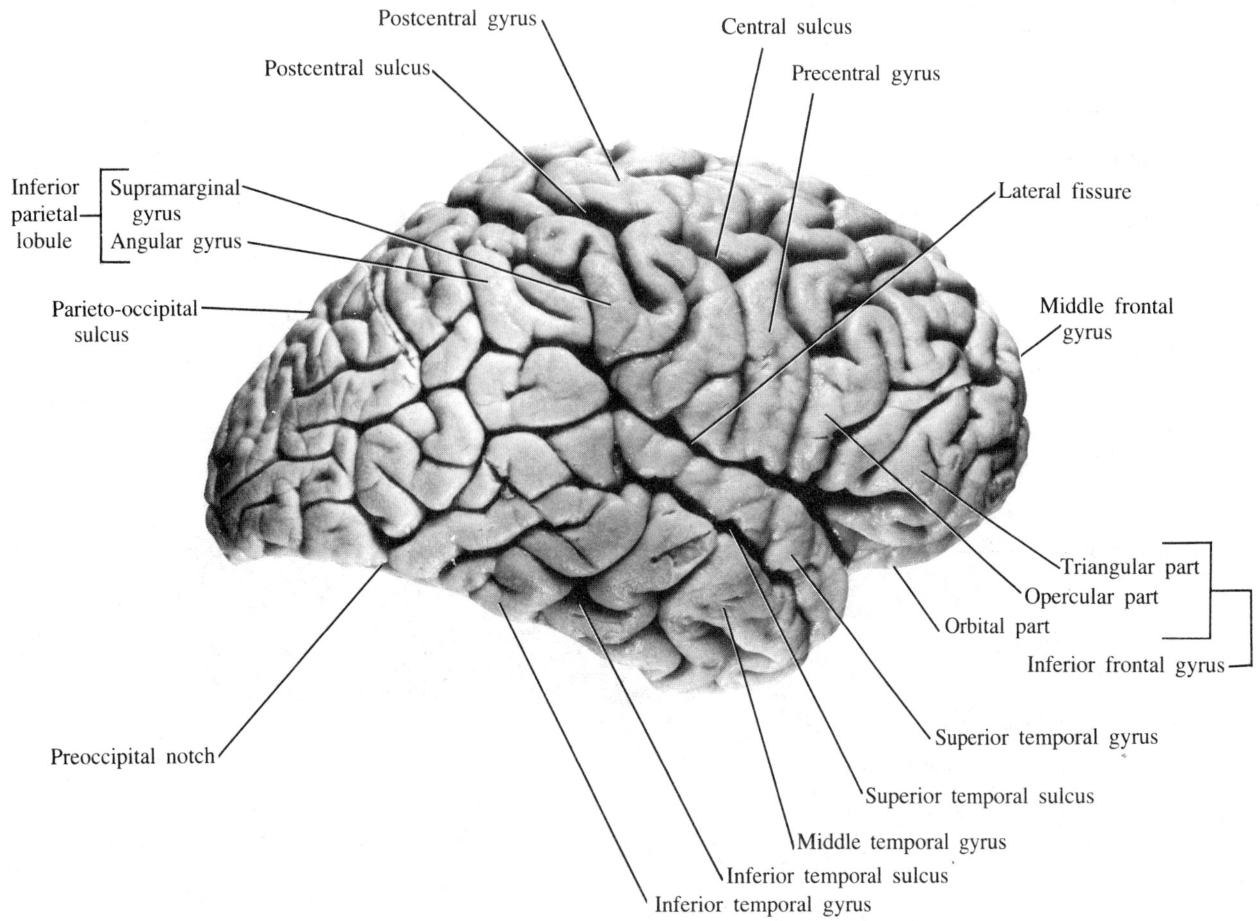

FIGURE 1.2-2. *Lateral surface of the brain.*

of the hemisphere where it is formed by the *parieto-occipital sulcus*. If this sulcus can be seen on the lateral surface of the hemisphere, a line connecting it to the *preoccipital notch* on the ventral extent of the hemisphere provides an arbitrary, but reasonable, approximation for the parietal boundary with the occipital lobe. The *intraparietal sulcus* is normally prominent in most specimens and courses more or less perpendicular to the postcentral sulcus. It divides the parietal lobe into a *superior parietal lobule* and an *inferior parietal lobule*. The inferior parietal lobule is important for sensory language functions and is formed by area 40, the *supramarginal gyrus*, and area 39, the *angular gyrus*. The former caps the posterior tip of the lateral fissure, whereas the latter either caps or lies in proximity to the posterior tip of the superior temporal sulcus.

Occipital lobe Only the polar portion of the lateral surface of the hemisphere forms the occipital lobe. Most of the occipital lobe and much of the primary visual cortex (area 17) lie on the medial surface of the hemisphere and will be described below.

Temporal lobe The temporal lobe is bounded dorsally by the lateral fissure and extends posteriorly to the arbitrary line between the parieto-occipital sulcus and the preoccipital notch. The superior temporal sulcus is a prominent feature and parallels the lateral fissure for much of its course. The superior temporal gyrus lies between this sulcus and the lateral fissure. The auditory cortex, areas 41 and 42, is located on the upper bank of the superior temporal gyrus, where it is mostly hidden from view in the depth of the lateral fissure. The *middle temporal gyrus* lies between the superior temporal gyrus and the *inferior temporal sulcus*. Beneath, or ventral to, the inferior temporal sulcus, a small rim of the *inferior temporal gyrus* can be observed, although much of it lies on the ventral surface of the hemisphere. The inferior temporal sulcus often consists of a series of discontinuous secondary sulci rather than a long, uninterrupted primary sulcus.

MEDIAL VIEW OF THE CEREBRAL CORTEX

Frontal lobe The superior frontal lobe on the medial surface of the hemisphere (Fig. 1.2-3) is demarcated ventrally by the *cingulate sulcus* and posteriorly by the medial continuation of the central sulcus. The latter can be subtle in many specimens, but usually can be found anterior to the *marginal* or *ascending ramus* of the cingulate sulcus, where it notches the medial surface. This landmark defines the location of the *paracentral lobule*. This important region represents the medial continuation of the pre- and postcentral gyri and contains the somatosensory representation for the contralateral lower extremity posterior to the central sulcus and the motor representation of the contralateral lower extremity anterior to it. Both areas receive their vascular supply from branches of the *anterior cerebral artery*. Both somatic representation and motor control for all of the other body parts lie within the vascular territory of the *middle cerebral artery*.

Parietal lobe The medial surface of the parietal lobe is defined by the central sulcus anteriorly and the parieto-occipital sulcus posteriorly. No clear boundary exists ventrally, and this cortex merges with the cortex of the limbic lobe and posterior cingulate gyrus. Topographically, the area is known as the *precuneus*.

Occipital lobe The medial surface of the occipital lobe is expansive, extending from the pole of the hemisphere to levels that approximate the splenium of the corpus callosum. The *calcarine fissure* divides the area into a dorsal area known as the *cuneus* and a ventral area known as the *lingual gyrus*. Area 17, the primary visual cortex, forms the upper and lower banks of the calcarine fissure. The visual field is mapped precisely onto this cortex.

Temporal lobe The temporal lobe is also expansive and is divisible into several regions by sulci that course in an anterior-posterior direction. The inferior temporal sulcus separates the cortex of the *inferior temporal gyrus* (lateral occipitotemporal gyrus) from the cor-

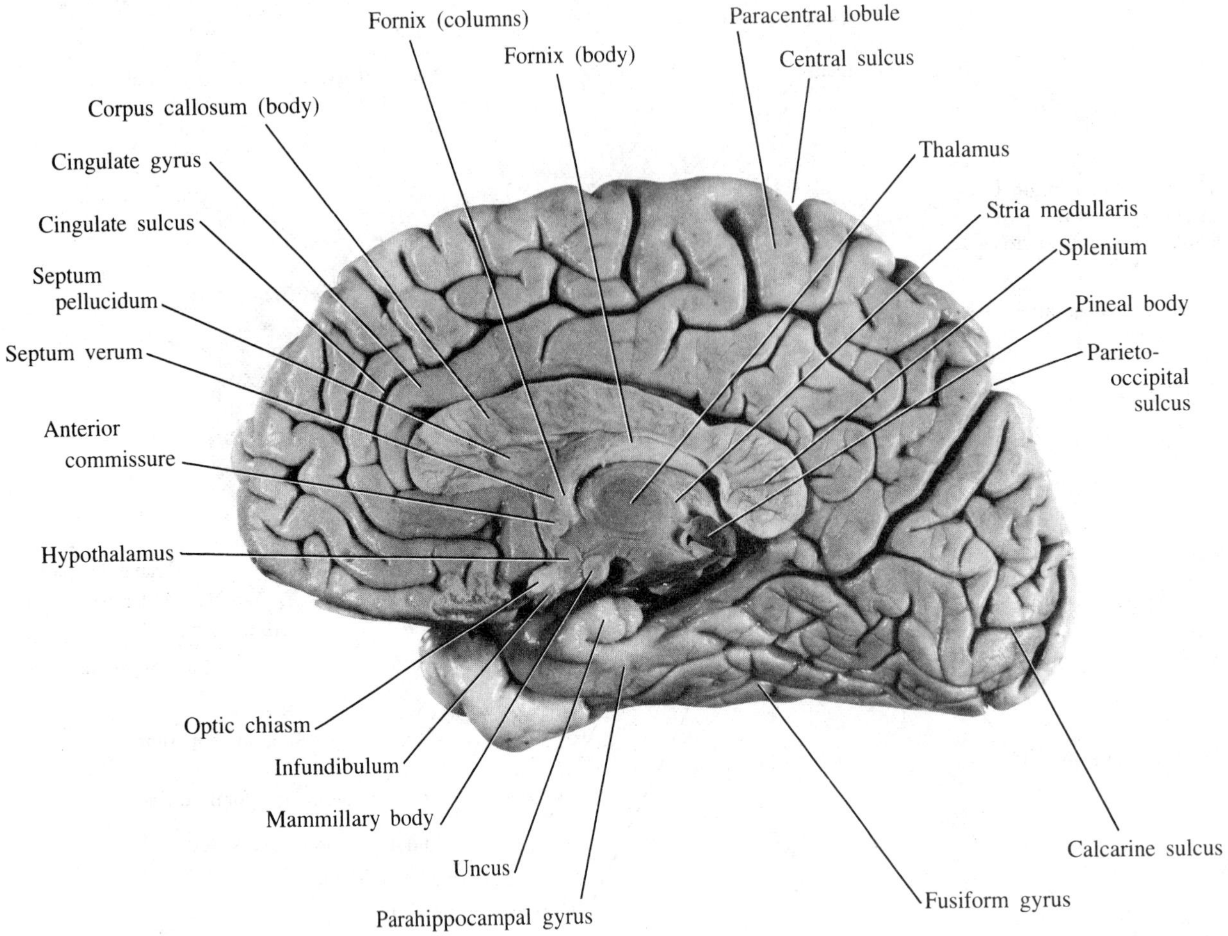

FIGURE 1.2-3. *Medial sagittal section of the brain.*

tex that forms the *fusiform gyrus* (medial occipitotemporal gyrus). The latter forms a large area in the human brain wedged between the lingual gyrus of the occipital lobe and the inferior temporal gyrus of the temporal lobe. Posteriorly, the *collateral sulcus* separates the occipitotemporal gyri from the parahippocampal gyrus, the fifth temporal gyrus and the most medial part of the temporal lobe. The *uncus* is a conspicuous part of the anterior parahippocampal gyrus. It receives the vast majority of olfactory bulb projections via the lateral olfactory tract. The uncus also contains the cortical amygdaloid nuclei and part of the hippocampal formation, which has become extruded from the temporal or inferior horn of the lateral ventricle. The remaining cortex of the anterior parahippocampal gyrus is the *entorhinal cortex,* area 28, which is connected intimately with the hippocampal formation.

Limbic lobe In the latter part of the nineteenth century, Paul Broca called attention to the fact that the limbus or edge of the cerebral hemisphere formed a continuous ring or band of cortex around the corpus callosum and upper brain stem that was uninterrupted by primary sulci. He coined the term *limbic lobe* to set this area apart from the other lobes. Paul MacLean expanded this concept and added subcortical gray masses and various interconnecting pathways with the cortex of the limbic lobe into what he termed a *limbic system.* The limbic lobe is purely cortical in terms of structure and contains nearly all of the nonisocortical areas of the cerebral hemisphere. These include cortical areas whose structure is less complex than the iso- or neocortex, which is characterized by six layers. Two major sulci aid in defining the limbic lobe. Anteriorly, and dorsally, the *cingulate sulcus* separates the *cingulate gyrus* from the medial and dorsal parts of the frontal lobe, thus paralleling the *corpus callosum* for much of its course. Anteriorly, the *subcallosal* portion of the cingulate gyrus lies immediately ventral to the *genu* of the corpus callosum. Posteriorly, the cingulate sulcus has a pronounced dorsal trajectory, referred to as the *marginal branch,* which forms the anterior boundary of the medial part of the parietal lobe, or precuneus. The lateral limit of the limbic lobe in the temporal area is formed by the *rhinal* and *collateral sulci*. Thus, the *cingulate* and *parahippocampal gyri* are the largest components of the limbic lobe, and both are delimited by long primary sulci. There are numerous bridging areas that link the cingulate and parahippocampal gyri together in a continuous ring of cortex. The *hippocampal formation,* which is a prominent part of the limbic lobe, is only barely visible from the external surface of the hemisphere. It is rolled up largely in the *inferior* or *temporal horn* of the *lateral ventricle*.

BRAIN STEM **Dorsal surface** The dorsal surface of the brain stem (Fig. 1.2-4) is obscured totally by the posterior part of the cerebral cortex and overlying cerebellum; it cannot be viewed adequately unless it is detached from the remainder of the hemisphere and the cerebellum is dissected away. Moreover, it is necessary to transect the *superior* and *inferior medullary veli* that cover and obscure the brain stem areas that form the floor of the fourth ventricle. The most anterior part of the brain stem is formed by the *thalamus* and, from a dorsal viewpoint, it has the appearance of paired football-shaped structures whose anterior ends are attached and whose posterior ends diverge laterally over the underlying mesencephalon. The dorsal portion of the third ventricle is present along the midline. Conspicuous fiber bundles course along the medial edge of the two thalami and along their lateral boundaries with the *striatum*. The medial fiber bundle is the *stria medullaris,* and the lateral fiber bundle is the *stria terminalis*. The *anterior thalamic nuclei* form a prominent protuberance at the anterior tip of the thalamus, and the *pulvinar nucleus* dominates its posterior part.

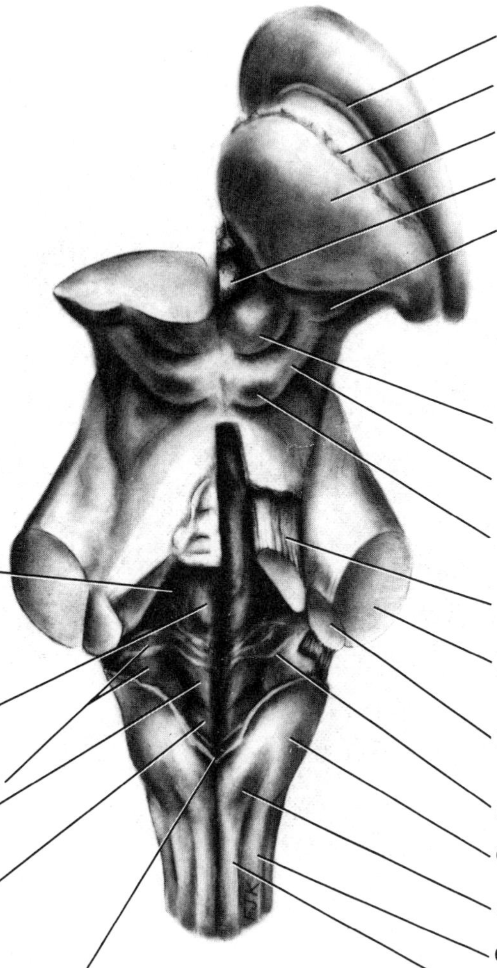

FIGURE 1.2-4. *Rhomboid fossa. The floor of the fourth ventricle, the rhomboid fossa, has been exposed by removing the cerebellum. (From Heimer L:* The Human Brain and Spinal Cord. *Springer-Verlag, New York, 1983, with permission. Drawing by F J Kabir.)*

The dorsal surface of the mesencephalon is characterized by the paired elevations that form the *superior* and *inferior colliculi*. Together these form the *tectum*. The *trochlear* or fourth cranial nerve exits the dorsal surface of the brain stem immediately posterior to the inferior colliculus. The dorsal surface of the pons forms the anterior part of the floor of the fourth ventricle and is characterized by the presence of the *facial colliculus*. This paired midline elevation is formed by the underlying nucleus of the *abducens* or sixth cranial nerve and the *facial* or seventh cranial nerve, which loops over the abducens nucleus.

Posterior to the facial colliculus, the *striae medullares* course at right angles to the midline across the floor of the fourth ventricle. They generally mark the point of transition between the pons and the medulla oblongata. The *hypoglossal nuclei* or the twelfth cranial nerve and the *dorsomotor nucleus of the vagus* or tenth cranial nerve form the remainder of the floor of the fourth ventricle. Their apex, or posterior limit, marks the position of the *obex* and the formation of the *central canal*. The remaining dorsal surface of the medulla resembles the dorsal surface of the cervical spinal cord. For example, the *posterior median sulcus* is conspicuous, as is the paired *fasciculus gracilis* and *cuneatus*. These large pathways, also called the *dorsal column system*, carry information related to discriminative touch and conscious proprioception for the body. They end in the *gracile* and *cuneate nuclei*, which appear as elevations on the surface of the medulla lateral to the obex.

Ventral surface Only a small component of the diencephalon can be seen from a ventral perspective (Fig. 1.2-5), and the area belongs entirely to the *hypothalamus*. Immediately posterior to the *optic chiasm*, the *tuberal* region of the hypothalamus can be seen with the associated pituitary gland. The *mammillary bodies* are immediately posterior to this location.

The *cerebral peduncles*, which encase the area on both sides, are the only portion of the mesencephalon that can be seen from the ventral surface. The *oculomotor* or third cranial nerve exits the mesencephalon in the region of the *interpeduncular fossa* between the cerebral peduncles.

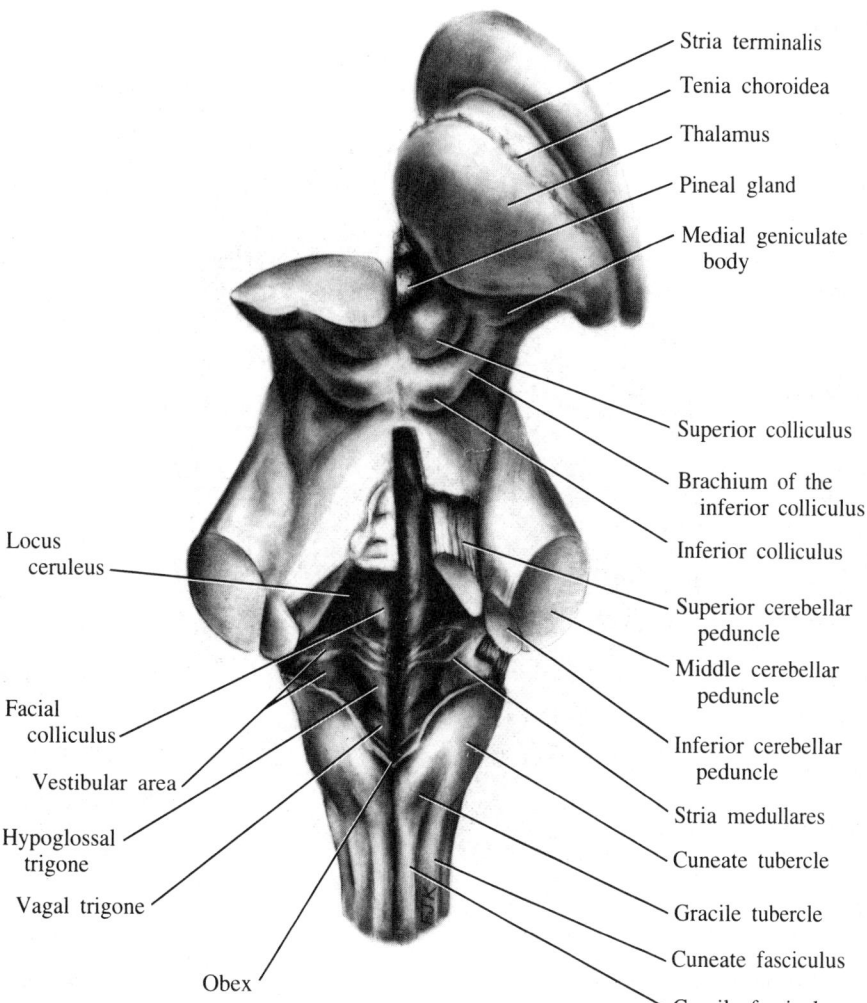

The base of the pons is a major feature of the ventral surface of the brain stem and contains along the midline a prominent *basilar groove*, which accommodates the *basilar artery*. The *trigeminal* or fifth cranial nerve is seen along the ventrolateral surface of the pons and is ventral to the middle cerebral peduncle. The pontomedullary junction is marked by many conspicuous features of the external anatomy of the brain stem. It is characterized by the presence of the abducens or sixth cranial nerve, which appears at the rostral border of

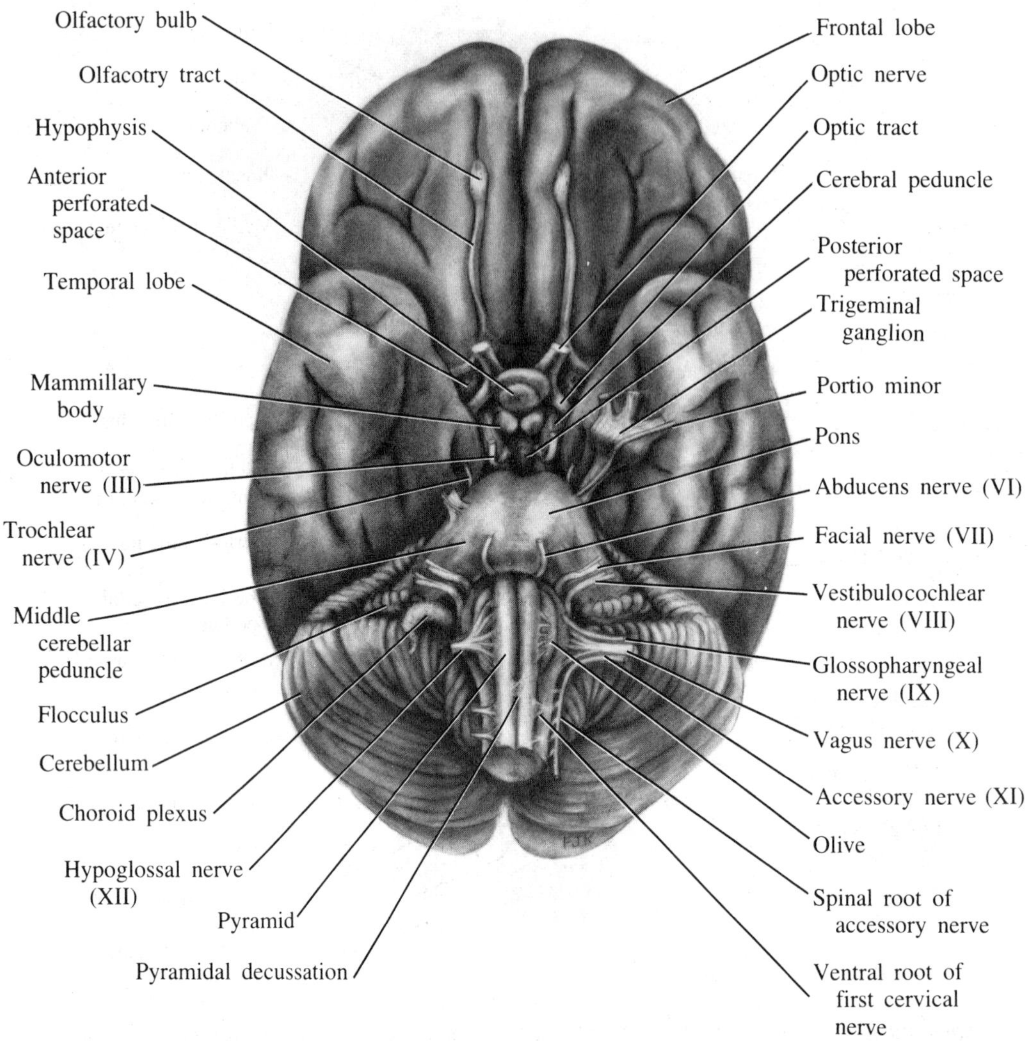

FIGURE 1.2-5. *Basal surface of the brain and the cranial nerves. (From Heimer L:* The Human Brain and Spinal Cord. *Springer-Verlag, New York, 1983, with permission. Drawing by F J Kabir.)*

the pyramid. The *facial* or seventh cranial nerve and the *vestibulocochlear* or eighth cranial nerve are seen in a position dorsal to the olive in the cerebellopontine angle. The ninth *(glossopharyngeal),* the tenth *(vagus),* and the eleventh *(spinal accessory)* cranial nerves are found along the lateral surface of the medulla in the *postolivary sulcus.* The twelfth *(hypoglossal)* cranial nerve exits the medulla between the pyramid and the olive along the *preolivary sulcus.*

CEREBELLUM The cerebellum (Figs. 1.2-6 and 1.2-7) is the largest structure of the *posterior cranial fossa* and is involved functionally in many aspects of motor control. In a general sense, its structure shares certain similarities with the cerebral cortex. For example, its surface is formed by a highly enfolded cortex connected to intrinsic subcortical nuclei that lie within a medullary core of white matter. Three paired cerebellar peduncles connect the cerebellum with the midbrain, pons, and medulla and convey the major input and output of the cerebellum. Three cerebellar sulci are essential features of cerebellar anatomy. The deep *primary fissure* on the superior surface of the cerebellum divides the cortex into a smaller *anterior lobe* and a larger *posterior lobe.* The *horizontal fissure* courses along the posterior edge of the cerebellum and divides its expansive surface area into superior and inferior regions. The inferior surface of the cerebellum also contains a major fissure called the *posterolateral fissure.* It courses behind the *flocculonodular lobe* and separates the paired flocculi and the midline nodulus from the inferior parts of the posterior lobe.

Another important feature of cerebellar anatomy concerns the fact that the more lateral parts of both the anterior and posterior lobes are adjoined along the midline by a contiguous region of cerebellar cortex known as the *vermis.* The nodulus of the flocculonodular lobe is also part of the vermis.

Three pairs of peduncles attach the cerebellum to the brain stem and link the structure to many parts of the *neuraxis,* either directly or indirectly. The inferior cerebellar peduncle provides both spinal and medullary input. The middle cerebellar peduncle is also largely an input system and carries fibers that arise almost exclusively from the *pontine nuclei* of the contralateral side. These nuclei receive a powerful input from the ipsilateral cerebral cortex and thus mediate a series of connections (corticopontocerebellar) that link the cortex of one cerebral hemisphere with the contralateral cerebellar hemisphere. The superior cerebellar peduncle is the major output pathway of the cerebellum and carries cerebellar efferents that arise largely from the deep cerebellar nuclei. This massive system decussates at the level of the inferior colliculus and terminates in the contralateral *red nucleus* and *ventrolateral thalamic nucleus.* The latter projects powerfully

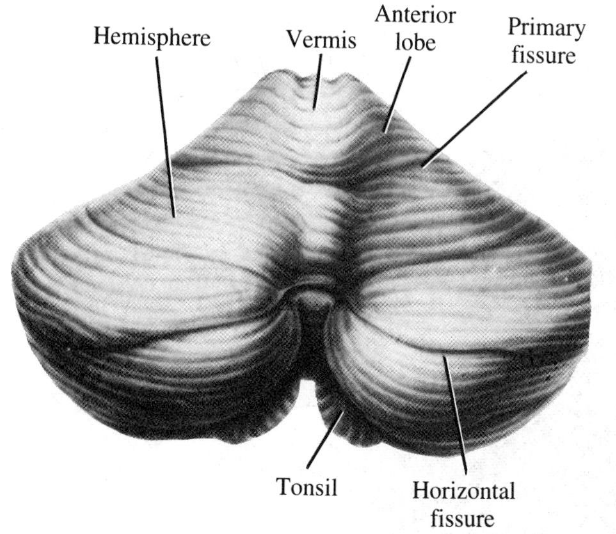

FIGURE 1.2-6. *Dorsal view of cerebellum. (From Nieuwenhuys R, Voogd J, van Huijzen C:* The Human Central Nervous System. *Springer-Verlag, New York, 1978, with permission of the authors and publisher.)*

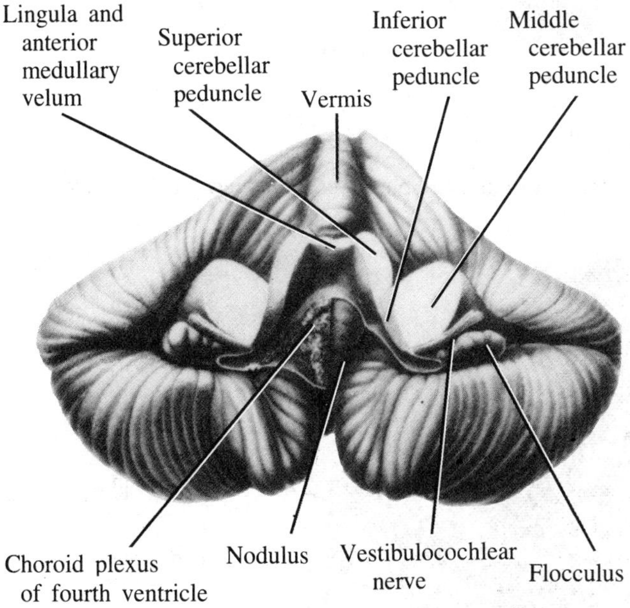

FIGURE 1.2-7. *Ventral view of cerebellum. (From Nieuwenhuys R, Voogd J, van Huijzen C:* The Human Central Nervous System. *Springer-Verlag, New York, 1978, with permission of the authors and publisher.)*

to the motor cortex; therefore, via these connections and those with the red nucleus, the output of the cerebellum can influence both the *rubrospinal* and *corticospinal* motor pathways.

INTERNAL STRUCTURES OF THE BRAIN

FOREBRAIN **Basal ganglia** Structures usually included in the basal ganglia are *caudate nucleus, putamen, globus pallidus, substantia nigra,* and *subthalamic nucleus*. The *lentiform nucleus* is sometimes used as a general term for the putamen and globus pallidus. These two structures, however, are characterized by great differences in histological structure and anatomical relationships, and a functionally more appropriate alignment is established between the caudate nucleus and putamen, which are referred to as the *striatum*.

STRIATUM Although the caudate nucleus and putamen are separated by the projection fibers forming the internal capsule, bridges of cells connect the two nuclei in many places, especially at more rostral levels (Fig. 1.2-8), where the caudate nucleus is especially voluminous. The large, rounded part of the caudate that forms the lateral wall in the anterior horn of the lateral ventricle is known as the head of the caudate. As if to emphasize the common origin of the caudate and putamen, there is a broad region of continuity between the two structures underneath the rostroventral part of the internal capsule. This area is often referred to as the *fundus striati* or *nucleus accumbens* and forms part of the ventral striatum (Figs. 1.2-9 and 1.2-10). Although the concept of the ventral striatum was introduced primarily on the basis of histological and connectional grounds, it is permissible, at least as a first approximation, to refer to the striatal parts below the level of the anterior commissure as the *ventral striatum*. Significant components of what is generally referred to as the *substantia innominata* in the human brain are in effect represented by striatal tissue that extends to the surface of the brain in the region of the anterior perforated space. In more caudal sections, putamen is still easily recognizable as the scoop of ice cream in the cone represented by globus pallidus (Figs. 1.2-10 and 1.2-11). The caudate nucleus, however, diminishes significantly in volume in a caudal direction and becomes the body of the caudate, which is located in the floor of the central part of the lateral ventricle. The body of the caudate tapers and sweeps downward in a semicircular fashion behind the internal capsule and then forward into the temporal lobe toward the region of the *amygdaloid body*, following closely the courses of the inferior or temporal horn of the lateral ventricle.

GLOBUS PALLIDUS AND VENTRAL PALLIDUM The *globus pallidus* is subdivided into an outer (lateral) and an inner (medial) segment by the *medullary lamina* (Figs. 1.2-10 and 1.2-11). It can easily be distinguished from the putamen in a freshly cut brain because of its pale color, which reflects the presence of many myelinated fibers. Whereas the medial and dorsal boundaries of the globus pallidus are well demarcated against the internal capsule, its ventral border is more difficult to define. Traditionally, only a small part of the globus pallidus was identified underneath the anterior commissure. However, recent studies with modern tracer techniques and immunohistochemical methods for the identification of pallidal markers (e.g., Substance P, enkephalin) have shown convincingly that the ventral striatum, as discussed above, is accompanied by a ventral extension of the globus pallidus—the *ventral pallidum*. The ventral pallidum occupies a rather extensive area underneath the temporal limb of the anterior commissure (see Fig. 1.3-5 in Section 1.3).

SUBSTANTIA NIGRA The *substantia nigra* is located primarily in the mesencephalon (Fig. 1.2-12). It is unique in the sense that it contains a large number of neuromelanin-containing neurons, which give the structure its characteristically dark color in unstained preparations, unless the individual suffered from Parkinson's disease, in which case the dark-colored band becomes pale as a result of substantial loss of neuromelanin-containing neurons. Melanin is a polymerized form of dopamine and norepinephrine metabolites, and the melanin-containing neurons in the substantia nigra do in fact represent the dopaminergic neurons in the pars compacta, which give rise to the ascending dopaminergic *nigrostriatal pathway*. This is only one of several pathways that tie the substantia nigra closely to the rest of the basal ganglia. But there seems to be an even more compelling reason to consider the substantia nigra as an integral part of the basal ganglia. Substantia nigra forms a tissue plate that extends throughout the mesencephalon and reaches rostrally to the neighborhood of the internal segment of the globus pallidus. Physiological and anatomical data suggest that the reticular part of the substantia nigra and the medial globus pallidus represent two parts of the same structure that is subdivided by the fiber bundles of the internal capsule in a fashion similar to the way internal capsule fibers have subdivided the striate body into caudate nucleus and putamen in the rostral forebrain.

SUBTHALAMIC NUCLEUS The subthalamic nucleus (Fig. 1.2-11) is a lens-shaped nucleus located on the medial side of the internal capsule beneath the thalamus. It is contiguous caudally with the substantia nigra and has close relations to the rest of the basal ganglia, especially to pallidal areas, including the pars reticulata substantia nigra.

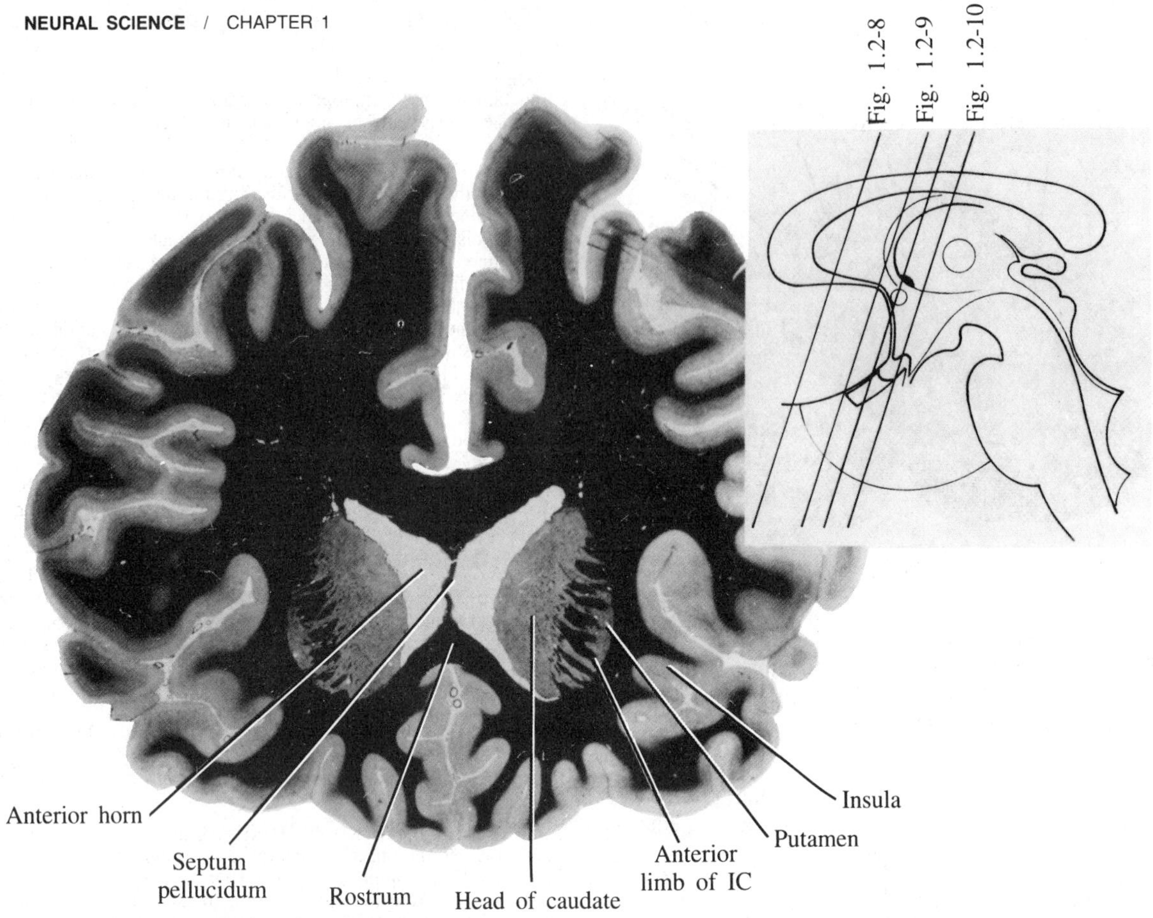

FIGURE 1.2-8. *Frontal section of the brain. (From Heimer L:* The Human Brain and Spinal Cord. *Springer-Verlag, New York, 1983, with permission. From the Yakovlev collection.)*

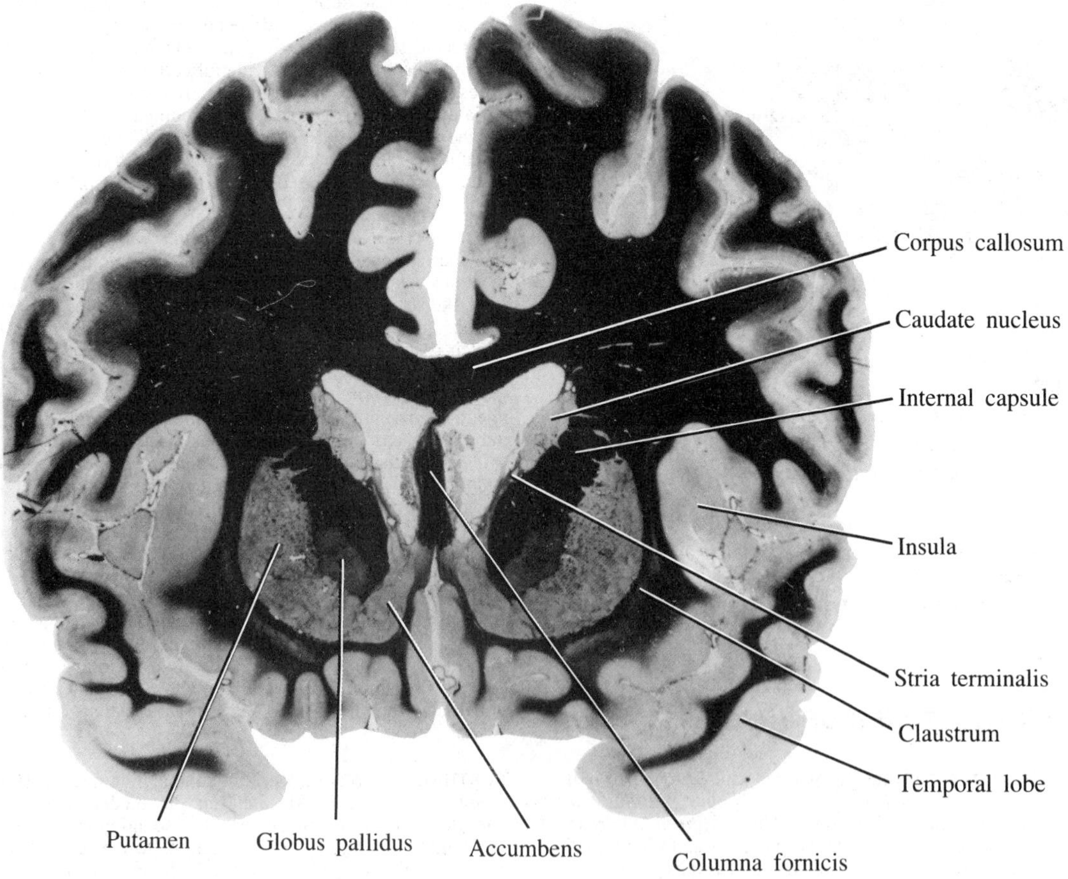

FIGURE 1.2-9. *Frontal section of the brain. (From Heimer L:* The Human Brain and Spinal Cord. *Springer-Verlag, New York, 1983, with permission. From the Yakovlev collection.)*

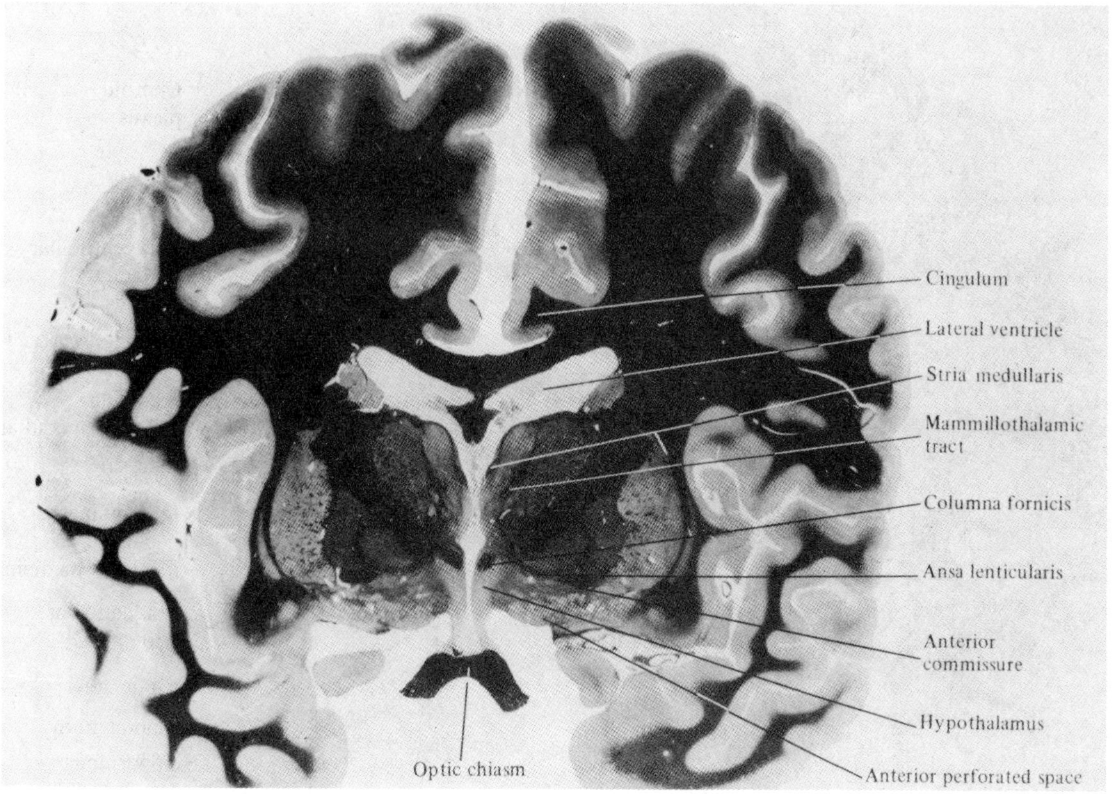

FIGURE 1.2-10. *Frontal section of the brain. (From Heimer L:* The Human Brain and Spinal Cord. *Springer-Verlag, New York, 1983, with permission. From the Yakovlev collection.)*

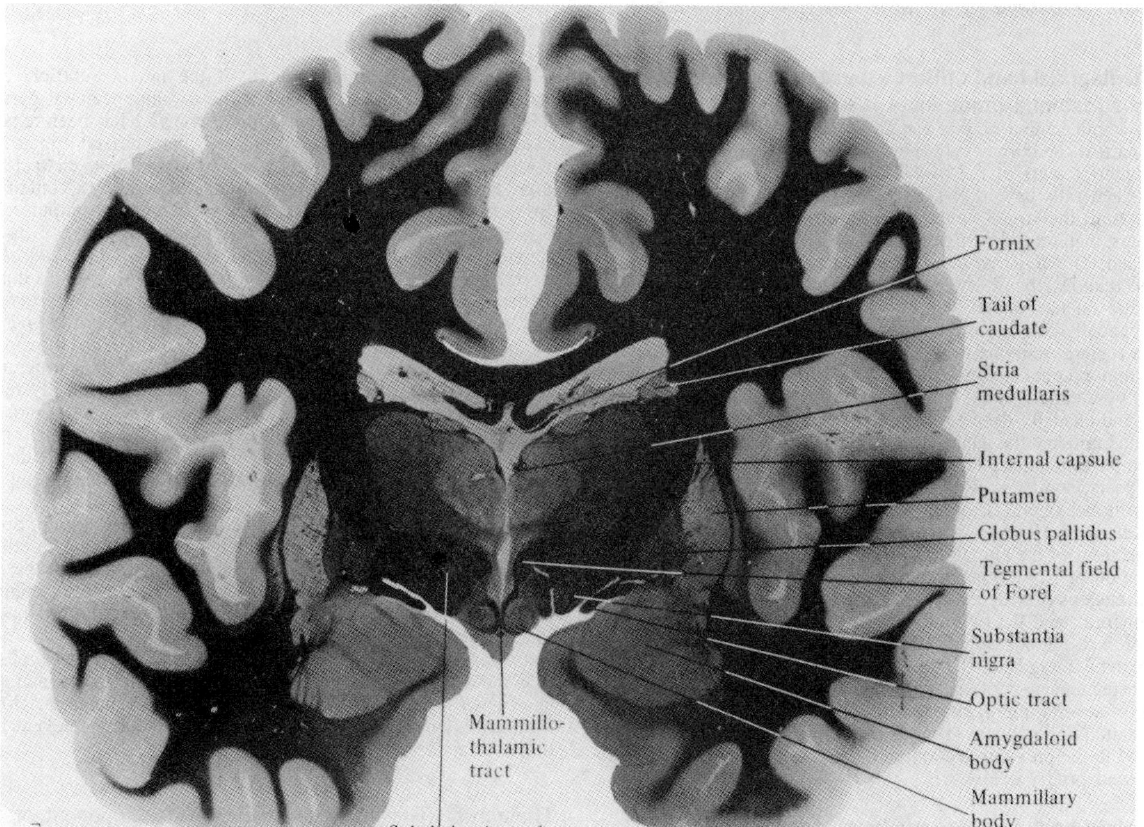

FIGURE 1.2-11. *Frontal section of the brain. (From Heimer L:* The Human Brain and Spinal Cord. *Springer-Verlag, New York, 1983, with permission. From the Yakovlev collection.)*

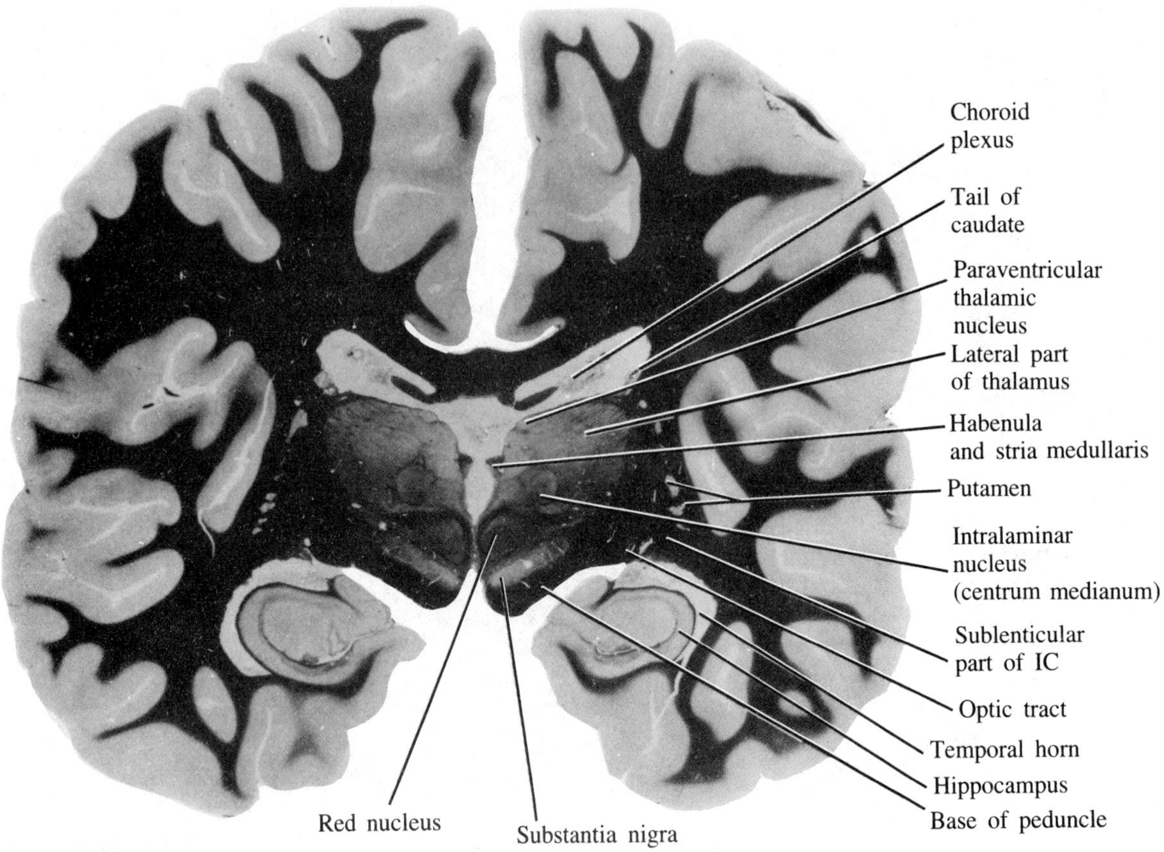

FIGURE 1.2-12. *Frontal section of the brain. (From Heimer L:* The Human Brain and Spinal Cord. *Springer-Verlag, New York, 1983, with permission. From the Yakovlev collection.)*

Septum, diagonal band of Broca, basal nucleus of Meynert, and the substantia innominata The *septum pellucidum* (Fig. 1.2-8) is a thin lamina of glia and fibers that stretches between the anterior part of the corpus callosum and the fornix, thereby separating the anterior parts of the two lateral ventricles. This part of the septum is generally devoid of nerve cells. However, the ventral parts of the septum, the "true" septum *(septum verum),* contain important cell groups that merge rostroventrally with the nucleus of the diagonal band. The *diagonal band nucleus,* and its accompanying fiber tract, the diagonal band, sweep downward in front of the anterior commissure on the medial side of the hemisphere and the nucleus extends caudally and laterally into an ill-defined but extensive basal forebrain region traditionally referred to as the *substantia innominata.* This region contains a heterogenous population of neurons and is traversed by a variety of axonal tracts. Substantia innominata extends laterally and caudally deep to the optic tract, between the basal surface of the brain and the lateral extension of the anterior commissure.

Substantia innominata has received considerable attention in the last few years, and the region is of considerable importance for those interested in behavioral disorders. One of its main components is the *basal nucleus of Meynert,* which can be easily identified in Nissl-stained sections of the human brain (Fig. 1.2-13) because of its dense accumulation of large hyperchromatic neurons. Many of the cells in the basal nucleus of Meynert and in the nucleus of the diagonal band are cholinergic, and the two nuclei together with cells in the medial septum project in topographic fashion to all of the cerebral cortex and the basolateral amygdala. The basal nucleus of Meynert, which is the most conspicuous part of the corticopetal system in the human, is only one of several important basal forebrain systems in the region of the substantia innominata. The *ventral striatopallidal system* was mentioned in the previous section, and the "extended amygdala" will be discussed briefly below.

Amygdaloid body and bed nucleus of stria terminalis The *amygdala* is a major telencephalic structure that dominates the ventromedial part of the temporal lobe and is located largely in front of the anterior tip of temporal horn of the lateral ventricle and immediately underneath the uncus of the parahippocampal gyrus (Fig. 1.2-11). Traditionally, the *amygdaloid complex* has been regarded as a key structure in the limbic system and characterized primarily by its close relationships to the hypothalamus. But this characterization alone is inadequate. In fact, the amygdaloid complex contains many different nuclei, each with its own specific input-output relations. However, it seems sufficient in this context to make a distinction among three basic territories or nuclear groups: a *basolateral group;* a *centromedial group,* which in the human is located as a dorsal cap on the large basolateral complex; and a smaller *cortical group,* which fuses with the olfactory cortex on the medial aspect of the parahippocampal gyrus. The basolateral amygdala, although subcortical by definition, is in many aspects reminiscent of a cortical structure. Like all cortical areas, the basolateral amygdala is reciprocally related to other cortical regions as well as to the thalamus, and its most extensive subcortical projection is directed toward the striatum, especially the ventral striatum, rather than to the hypothalamus. Like the cortex, the basolateral amygdala receives a powerful cholinergic input from the basal nucleus of Meynert.

The centromedial complex, unlike the basolateral group, does have significant relations with the hypothalamus as well as with other parts of the autonomic nervous system. It is continuous with the *bed nucleus of the stria terminalis,* which straddles the anterior commissure close to the midline. Centromedial amygdala and the bed nucleus of stria terminalis are interconnected via cell columns in the sublenticular substantia innominata and to a lesser extent via cells alongside the stria terminalis. The centromedial amygdala and the bed nucleus of stria terminalis together with these interconnecting cells form an extended amygdala, which is particularly relevant to emotional behavior.

Thalamus The thalamus, the largest component of the diencephalon, forms two large ovoid masses of gray matter, one on each side of the third ventricle, close to the center of the

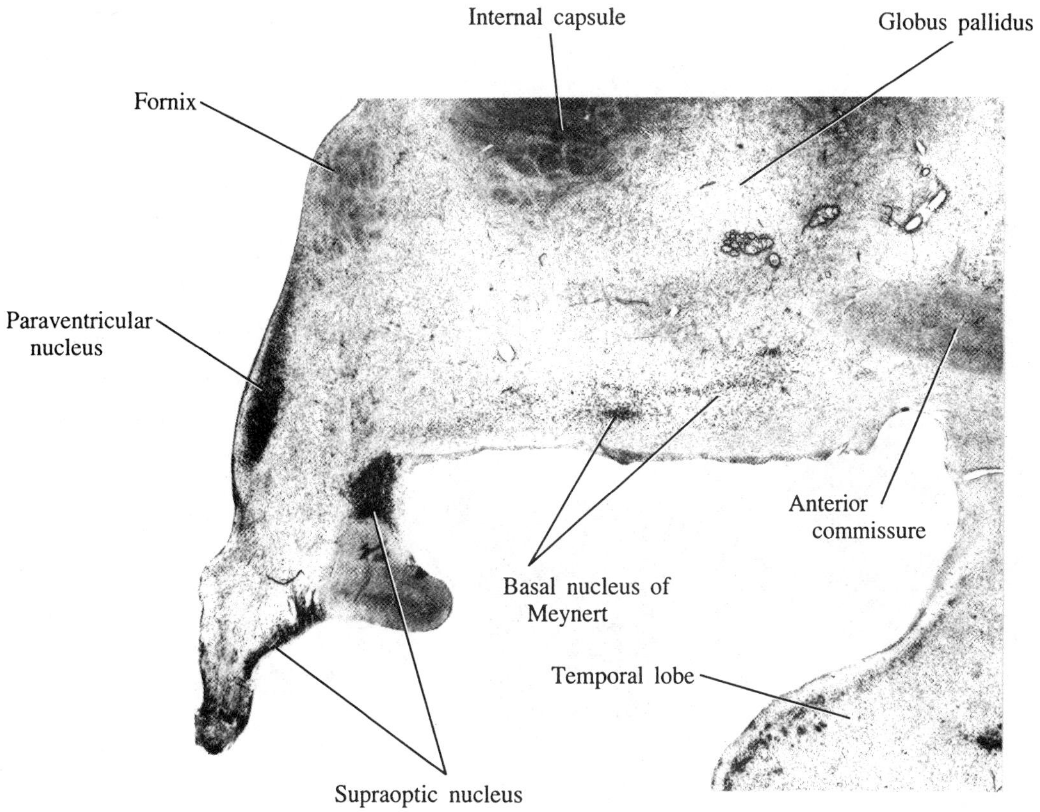

FIGURE 1.2-13. *Supraoptic and paraventricular nuclei. Nissl-stained cross section through the anterior hypothalamus of a human brain showing the circumscribed supraoptic and paraventricular nuclei, as well as the large dark-staining cells of the basal nucleus of Meynert. (From Heimer L:* The Human Brain and Spinal Cord. *Springer-Verlag, New York, 1983, with permission.)*

brain. It is always found along the medial side of the posterior limb of the *internal capsule* (Figs. 1.2-11, 1.2-12, 1.2-14, and 1.2-15). It is subdivided into anterior, medial, and lateral groups of nuclei by a vertically placed layer of white substance, the *internal medullary lamina,* which in its rostral part splits in a Y-shaped manner around the anterior nuclear group. A posterior bifurcation encases an *intralaminar group* of nuclei.

The functional diversity of the thalamus is reflected in its connections; there are a multitude of extrinsic thalamic pathways, and the different thalamic nuclei are characterized by specific afferent and efferent relations. In spite of this diversity among the thalamic nuclei, there is also a certain commonality, not only in the sense that all nuclei are confined to a single and easily identified nuclear mass, but also in regard to certain general principles of thalamic organization. One of the most widely known principles is depicted in Figure 1.2-16, which shows the reciprocal relations between the major thalamic relay nuclei and various parts of the cerebral cortex. In fact, all the nuclei of the dorsal thalamus project to the cerebral cortex, but not necessarily in such a well-delineated, specific topography as indicated for the major relay nuclei in the figure. On the contrary, the intralaminar nuclei—including the midline nuclei—do not project densely within the boundaries of one or even a few well-defined cortical fields; rather, they project diffusely to widespread areas of the cerebral cortex. Such nonspecific thalamic projections are thought to form an important link in the ascending activating system.

However, the thalamus is more than just a collection of relay stations where the impulses are passed along faithfully and without modification to the cerebral cortex. Although there is a general lack of associative connections between the different thalamic nuclei, the stimuli that reach the thalamus are being modulated not only by interneuronal circuits but also by *corticothalamic* input as well as by the *reticular thalamic nucleus,* which is represented by a sheath of γ-amino-butyric acid (GABA)-ergic neurons on the lateral and ventral aspects of the thalamus.

Hypothalamus The hypothalamus is a small, gray-matter region that forms the ventral part of the diencephalon. Its *tuberal region* and *mammillary nuclei,* immediately posterior to the optic chiasm, are the only parts of the diencephalon that can be seen from the external surface of the brain. The hypothalamus borders the third ventricle for much of its extent, and the hypothalamic sulcus, a small indentation along the lateral wall of the ventricle, demarcates its dorsal limit and borders with the thalamus (Figs. 1.2-3, 1.2-10, and 1.2-11). Dorsally, the lateral limit of the hypothalamus is formed partially by the internal capsule; rostrally and ventrally, it has a substantial spread laterally where it interdigitates with other basal forebrain systems, including the basal nucleus of Meynert. Convention places its anterior border at the level of lamina terminalis and the point where the anterior commissure crosses the midline. This is somewhat arbitrary since hypothalamic-preoptic areas merge anteriorly with the diagonal band and septal and substantia innominata areas. Like-

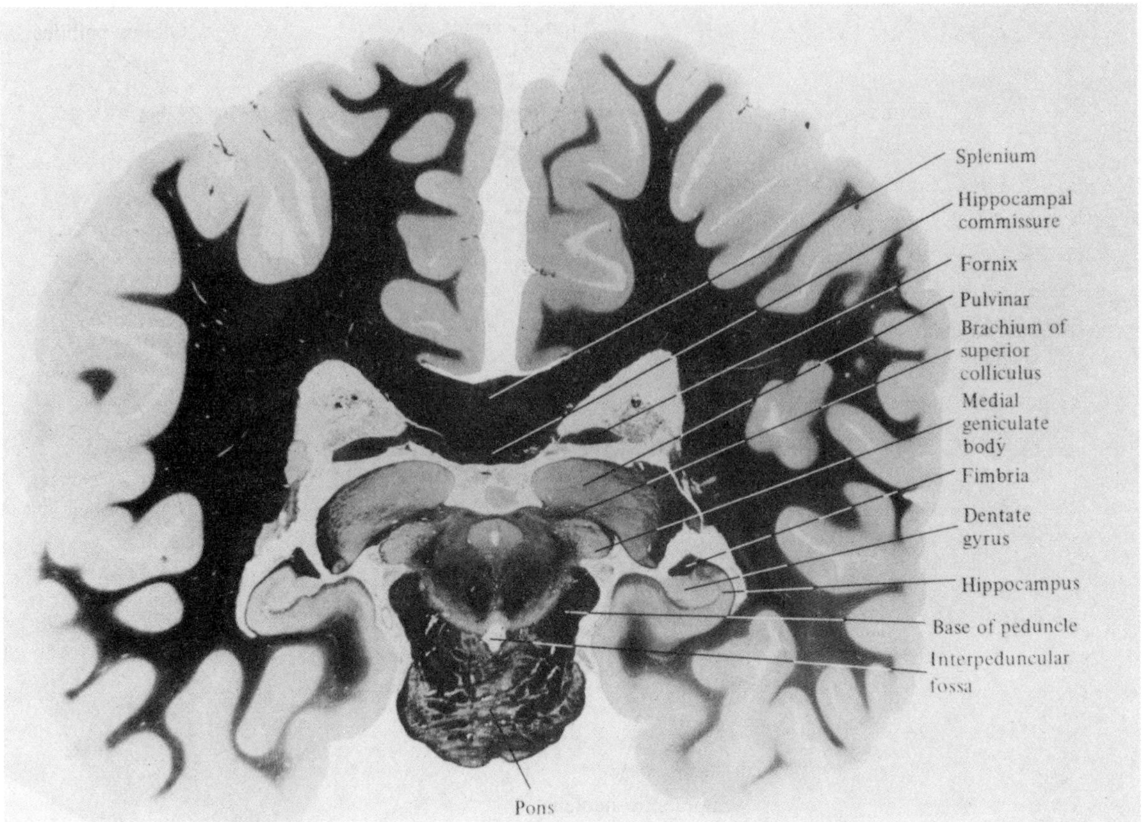

FIGURE 1.2-14. *Frontal section of the brain. (From Heimer L:* The Human Brain and Spinal Cord. *Springer-Verlag, New York, 1983, with permission. From the Yakovlev collection.)*

wise, the posterior limit of the hypothalamus is not well defined. It follows the third ventricle posteriorly to the midbrain at the level of the cerebral aqueduct and merges with the periaqueductal gray and midbrain reticular formation. The morphology of hypothalamic neurons has led some authors to suggest that this structure is best viewed as a diencephalic extension of the reticular formation.

Several hypothalamic nuclei are well known by virtue of their role in endocrine mechanisms or behavioral syndromes. However, the hypothalamus is not well understood in terms of cytoarchitecture, and much remains to be learned regarding its internal organization. Much research dealing with the hypothalamus-preoptic region has to do with areas rather than well-defined nuclei and even with scattered neurons that have a particular neurochemical or neurophysiological characteristic irrespective of their location.

HYPOTHALAMO-HYPOPHYSEAL RELATIONSHIPS The best-known hypothalamic nuclei are those that contain the neurosecretory neurons that give rise to the *hypothalamo-hypophyseal tract*. These arise from the *supraoptic* and *paraventricular nuclei* (Fig. 1.2-13) and terminate in the posterior lobe or neurohypophysis of the pituitary gland where they release oxytocin and vasopressin (Fig. 1.2-17). The latter is a well-known antidiuretic hormone and is released in response to changes in the osmotic pressure of circulating blood or extracellular space.

Hypothalamic control of the adenohypophysis or anterior lobe of the pituitary is more complex and involves the unique vascular loops of the median eminence, the interface between the neural portions of the diencephalon, and the glandular tissue of the anterior pituitary. Hypothalamic neurons transport a variety of releasing and inhibiting hormones to the portal vessels of the median eminence. These hormones are then transported to the capillary beds of the anterior pituitary, where they regulate the secretion of many essential hormones (Fig. 1.2-17).

HYPOTHALAMUS AND THE AUTONOMIC NERVOUS SYSTEM Although the hypothalamic control of endocrine mechanisms is well known and, in part, well understood, this diencephalic structure also plays a prominent role in the regulation of autonomic functions and diffuse behavioral mechanisms that protect the organism. For example, the *posterior, dorsomedial,* and *paraventricular hypothalamic nuclei* all project to *preganglionic parasympathetic centers* in the medulla and to *preganglionic sympathetic neurons* in the *intermediolateral cell column* of the thoracic spinal cord. These connections are thought to play critical roles in emotional reactions to integrated sensory events transmitted to the hypothalamus.

Behavioral mechanisms relating to thirst, hunger, sex, and aggression are thought to be localized in the hypothalamus, and there is little doubt that selective hypothalamic lesions can alter many aspects of behavior associated with these mechanisms. However, the hypothalamus has many connections with other brain areas that probably also play a role in such behaviors. Thus, a lesion in the hypothalamus that leads to behavioral changes may in fact compromise only one, albeit critical, component of an integrated neural system essential for the execution of a complicated behavior.

The hypothalamic control of autonomic and endocrine function is highly relevant in so-called psychosomatic disturbances, which are often a significant factor in the development of commonly known diseases (e.g., cardiovascular disorders, asthma, peptic ulcer, and eating disorders). Although the psychosomatic diseases are not generally referred to as hypothalamic disorders, it is by way of the hypothalamus that the psychosomatic disturbances are executed.

Internal capsule and forebrain commissures The white matter of the forebrain consists of myelinated fibers, which generally can be divided into three major groups: projection fibers, commissural fibers, and association fibers. Many of

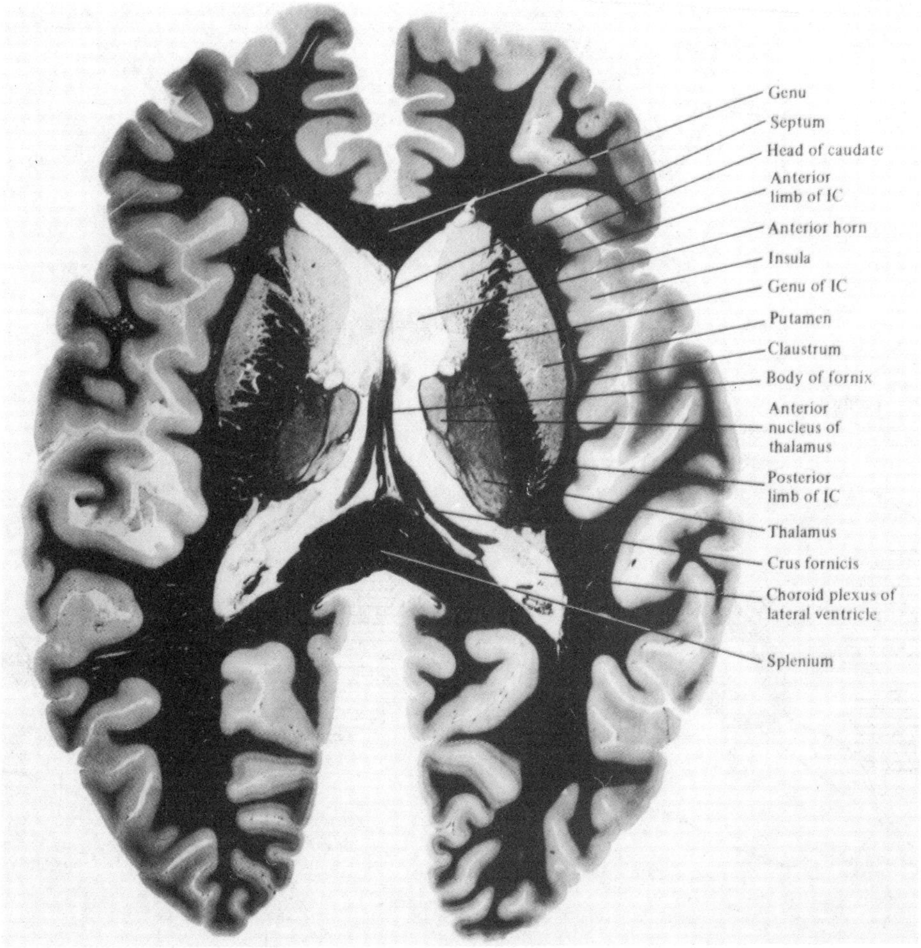

FIGURE 1.2-15. *Horizontal section. (From Heimer L:* The Human Brain and Spinal Cord. *Springer-Verlag, New York, 1983, with permission. From the Yakovlev collection.)*

the projection fibers connect the cerebral cortex with subcortical regions, and they are closely related to the internal capsule. The commissural fibers cross the midline and interconnect areas in the two hemispheres with each other. The largest of the commissures, the *corpus callosum,* interconnects neocortical areas in all lobes. The association fibers interconnect cortical regions within the same hemisphere; some are short fibers interconnecting adjacent gyri (i.e., arcuate fibers), whereas others form large bundles connecting the various lobes.

INTERNAL CAPSULE The extent and three-dimensional configuration of the *internal capsule* can be dramatically revealed in blunt dissections of the human brain (Fig. 1.2-18). Within the internal capsule, fiber bundles can be followed continuously from the upper part of the hemisphere to the base of the mesencephalon or even further down in the brain stem. The capsule is also prominently displayed in regular cross sections through the forebrain. It has a V-shaped form on horizontal sections (Fig. 1.2-15) with the apex pointing medially. The part of the capsule located between the head of the caudate medially and the lentiform nucleus laterally is called the *anterior limb.* It contains most of the fibers connecting the frontal cortex with subcortical regions. The angle of the internal capsule is known as the genu. The massive posterior limb separates the lentiform nucleus from the thalamus on the medial side and contains many important fiber tracts, including the corticospinal (pyramidal) tract and the sensory radiations carrying sensory impulses to the somatosensory cortex. The parts of the posterior limb that are located behind and underneath the lentiform nucleus are known as the *retrolenticular* and *sublenticular parts* of the internal capsule. They contain fibers of the optic and acoustic radiation. The internal capsule is supplied by striate and perforate arteries from the vessels that form the circle of Willis. They are often affected by cerebrovascular accidents and the small vessel disease of hypertension. Because the capsule contains a variety of important fiber tracts, a capsular lesion can exhibit a variety of different symptoms; however, the most common picture is that of a capsular hemiplegia.

CORPUS CALLOSUM AND OTHER FOREBRAIN COMMISSURES The corpus callosum, the largest fiber system in the brain, appears as a dorsally convex thick plate on midsagittal sections (Fig. 1.2-3). The different parts of the corpus callosum are referred to as the rostrum, genu, body, and splenium. The corpus callosum, which permits the transfer of information from one hemisphere to the other, is sometimes severed to prevent the spread or generalization of epileptic discharge from one hemisphere to the other.

Although the corpus callosum carries fibers from all lobes, many of the commissural connections between the temporal cortical areas cross in the *anterior commissure.* Another important forebrain com-

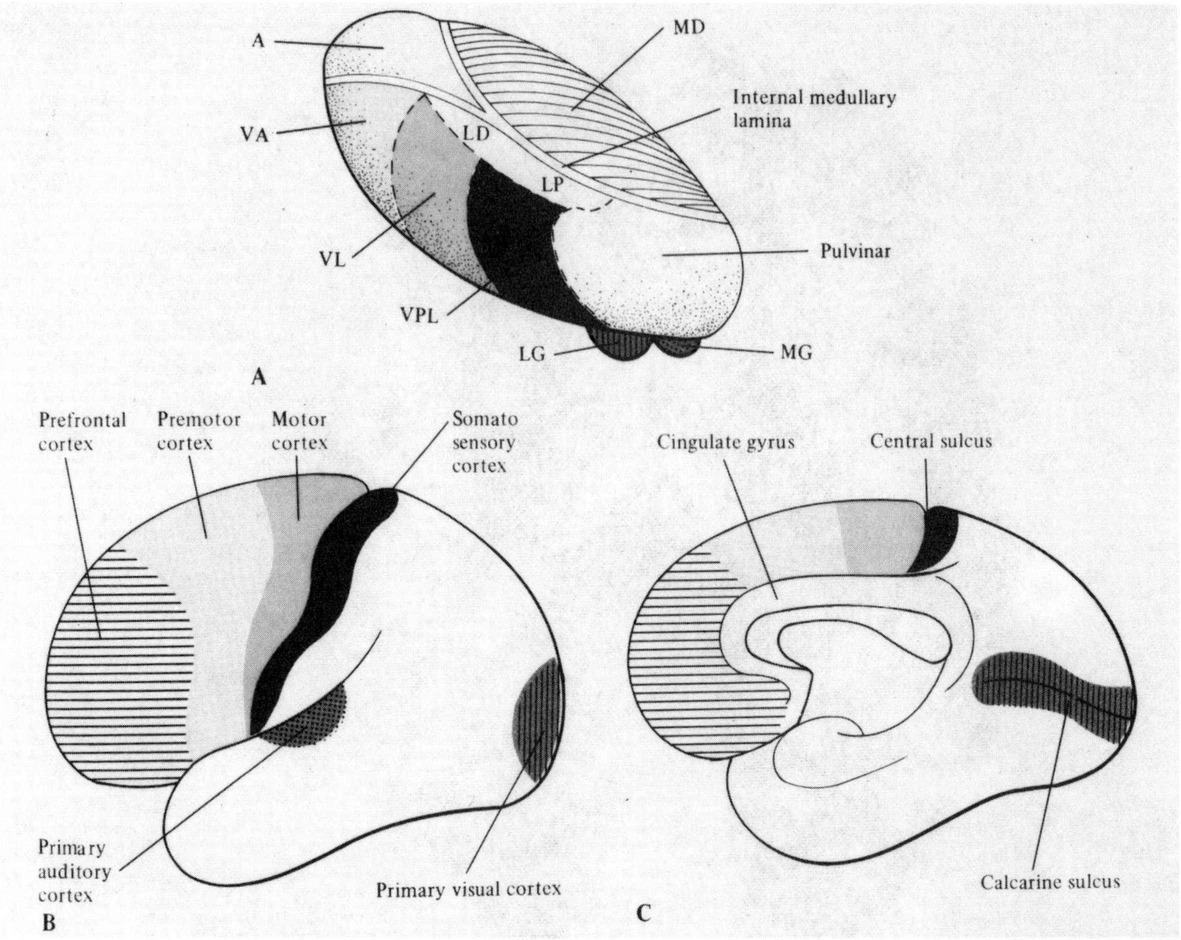

FIGURE 1.2-16. *Thalamocortical connections.* A. *Dorsolateral view of the thalamus showing the main subdivisions.* B. *Lateral surface of the cerebral hemisphere showing the main projection areas of the various thalamic nuclei.* C. *Medial surface of the cerebral hemisphere. (From Heimer L:* The Human Brain and Spinal Cord. *Springer-Verlag, New York, 1983, with permission.)*

missure is the *hippocampal commissure,* which carries information between the various parts of the parahippocampal gyrus in primates or hippocampus in nonprimates. The hippocampal commissure is located underneath the splenium of the corpus callosum. The hippocampal commissural fibers bridge the gap between the two fornices as each of them diverges laterally and sweeps downward behind the thalamus into the temporal lobe. Incidentally, the fornix constitutes another important landmark on a midsagittal section through the forebrain. It represents an important bundle of projection fibers between the hippocampus, septum, and hypothalamus. The prominent column of the fornix appears as a characteristic semicircular arch rostral to the *intraventricular foramen of Monro* before it disappears into the gray substance of the hypothalamus as it courses toward the mammillary body (Fig. 1.2-3).

BRAIN STEM **Mesencephalon** The midbrain, or mesencephalon (Fig. 1.2-19), is characterized by gray matter masses that have distinct motor and sensory functions. The nuclei that form the tectum and the superior and inferior colliculi illustrate such a statement. For example, the superior colliculus plays a role in visual-spatial behaviors relating to body position and eye movements. It receives input not only from the visual system but also from a variety of different sources, including other sensory systems. It gives rise to the tectospinal tract, which influences cervical motor neurons responsible for the innervation of neck and other axial musculature. This structure aids in coordinating the complex processes of integrating the eyes with neck movements in relationship to stimuli that require discrete, graded, and integrated responses, both in terms of the organism's position in space as well as the position of the stimulus in space.

The inferior colliculus is much less understood, but there is little doubt that it plays a key role in auditory processing. Most of the ascending auditory projection fibers are relayed in this structure en route to the *medial geniculate nucleus* (Figs. 1.2-14 and 1.2-15) and the primary auditory cortex. The *oculomotor nuclei,* which are located in the ventral part of the central gray substance underneath the superior colliculi, receive input from many levels of the neuraxis, including pontine, midbrain, and cortical areas. These nuclei are aggregations of lower motor neurons that control the extraocular musculature except the lateral rectus and the superior oblique muscles. A special parasympathetic nucleus within the oculomotor complex, the *Edinger-Westphal nucleus,* controls the pupillary aperture via the *ciliary ganglion.* The trochlear nuclei are located in the ventral part of the central gray substance underneath the inferior colliculis.

The tegmentum is dominated throughout its extent by the red nucleus, a major target of the motor cortex on the ipsi-

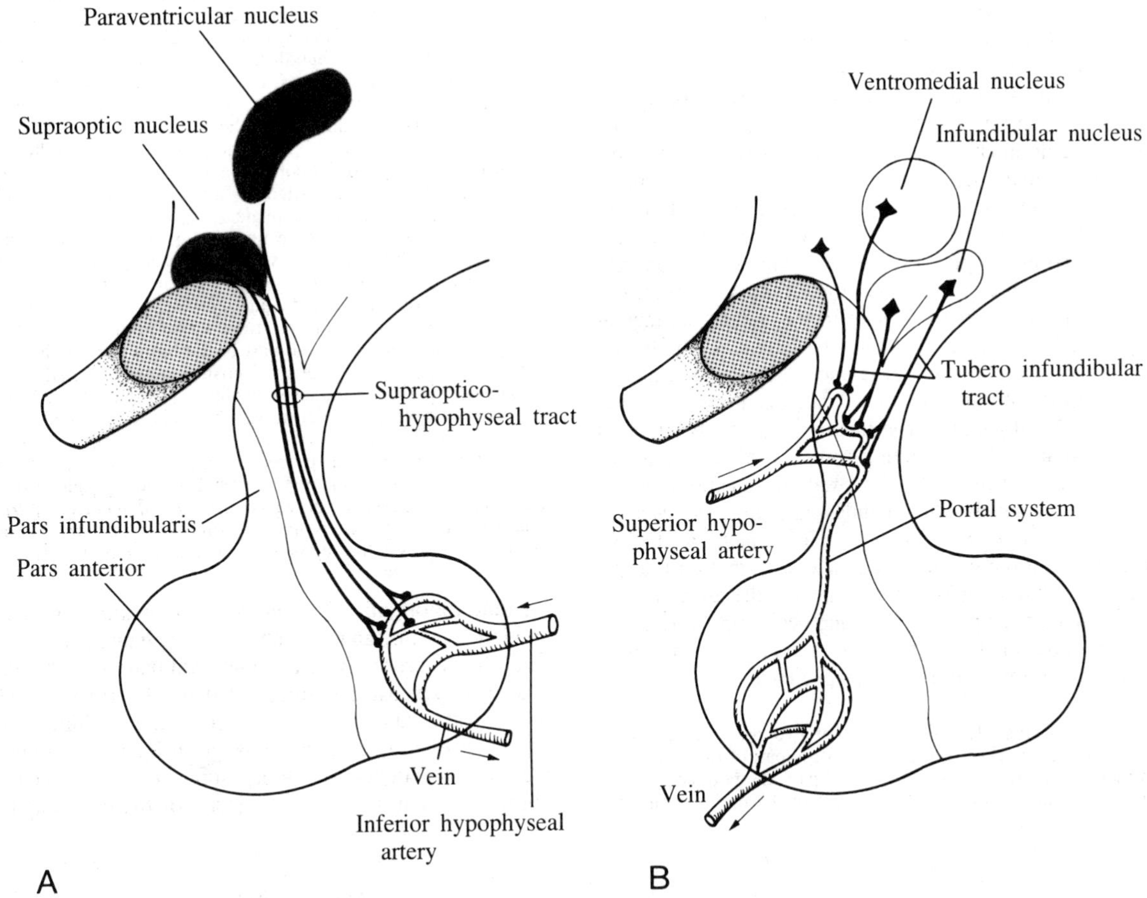

FIGURE 1.2-17. *Hypothalamohypophyseal pathways.* A. *Supraopticohypophyseal tract.* B. *Tuberoinfundibular tract and the hypophyseal portal system. (From Heimer L:* The Human Brain and Spinal Cord. *Springer-Verlag, New York, 1983, with permission.)*

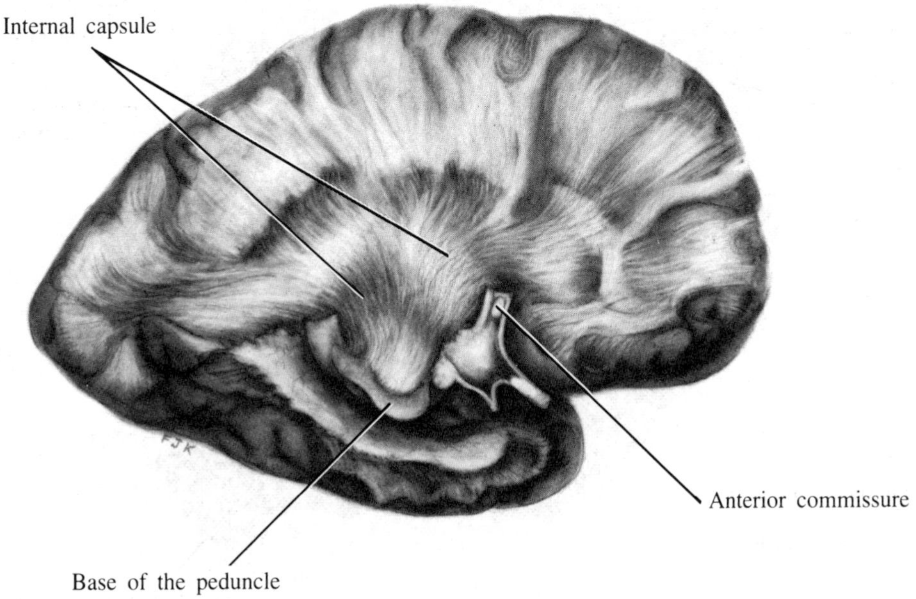

FIGURE 1.2-18. *Internal capsule and corona radiata. (From Heimer L:* The Human Brain and Spinal Cord, *Springer-Verlag, New York, 1983, with permission. Drawing by F J Kabir.)*

lateral side and the deep cerebellar nuclei, particularly the dentate nucleus, of the contralateral cerebellum. It gives rise to the *rubrospinal tract,* which crosses the midline in the *ventral tegmental decussation* and descends in the lateral funiculus of the spinal cord. Functionally, this pathway resembles the lateral corticospinal tract. The dorsal parts of the tegmentum are dominated by the ascending sensory pathways laterally and the main part of the reticular formation in a more medial location. Other important structures in the midline are the *raphe nuclei* and, further ventrally, the *ventral tegmental area*. The raphe nuclei give rise to the ascending serotonergic pathways, which are widely distributed in the forebrain, whereas the dopaminergic fibers from the ventral tegmental area project to the ventral striatum, the extended amygdala, and the frontal lobe. The ventral tegmental area is continuous laterally with the substantia nigra, which was discussed in the context of the basal ganglia. The massive base of the cerebral peduncles contains all descending motor corticofugal axons except those that terminate in the striatum and motor thalamus. At midbrain levels, this includes *corticospinal, corticobulbar,* and *corticopontine* axons. These have a distinct topography within the cerebral peduncle such that corticospinal and corticobulbar axons form the middle third of the peduncle, whereas tempo-, parieto- and occipitopontine fibers travel in its upper or dorsal third. Frontopontine axons travel in the ventral or lower third of the peduncle.

Pons The pons (Fig. 1.2-20) consists of two parts, a ventral or basilar part that is especially large in the rostral part of the pons close to the mesencephalon, and a smaller dorsal part, the pontine tegmentum, that is continuous with the tegmentum of the midbrain and the medulla oblongata. The basilar part contains large areas of gray matter, the pontine nuclei, which serve as relay stations for the massive *corticopontocerebellar fiber system,* as well as transversally and longitudinally running fiber bundles. The transverse bundles, the crossed pontocerebellar fibers, serve as the second link in the abovementioned corticopontocerebellar system and enter the contralateral cerebellar hemisphere through the large middle cerebellar peduncles, displayed along the lateral part of the pons. The longitudinal bundles represent primarily corticopontine axons and the corticospinal and corticobulbar tracts. The corticospinal axons form the pyramids along the base of the medulla oblongata.

Several of the cranial nerve nuclei (i.e., those of the fifth, sixth, seventh, and eighth cranial nerves) are located in the pontine tegmentum. Several of the nuclei are embedded in the reticular formation, but they are well delineated and their location is determined by a developmental plan according to which the motor nuclei are, in general, located in the medial part of the brain stem with the sensory nuclei in a lateral or dorsolateral position. An especially interesting arrangement is seen at the level displayed in Figure 1.2-20, where the fibers of the seventh cranial nerve, the facial nerve, make a dorsally directed detour over the abducens nucleus close to the floor of the fourth ventricle and then proceed in a ventrolateral direction where they exit the brain stem in the cerebellopontine angle (Fig. 1.2-5). The ascending sensory pathways, the *medial lemniscus, trigeminal lemniscus, auditory lemniscus,* and *spinothalamic tract* are located in the ventral part of the tegmentum in this part of the brain stem.

Medulla oblongata The *medulla oblongata* (Fig. 1.2-21) is continuous with, and resembles, the spinal cord macroscopically; however, the typical spinal cord pattern with a centrally placed gray substance surrounded by the fiber tracts of the white matter cannot be recognized in the medulla oblongata. Although there is a gradual change in internal morphology at the spinomedullary junction, some changes occur rather abruptly. For instance, the majority of the corticospinal tract

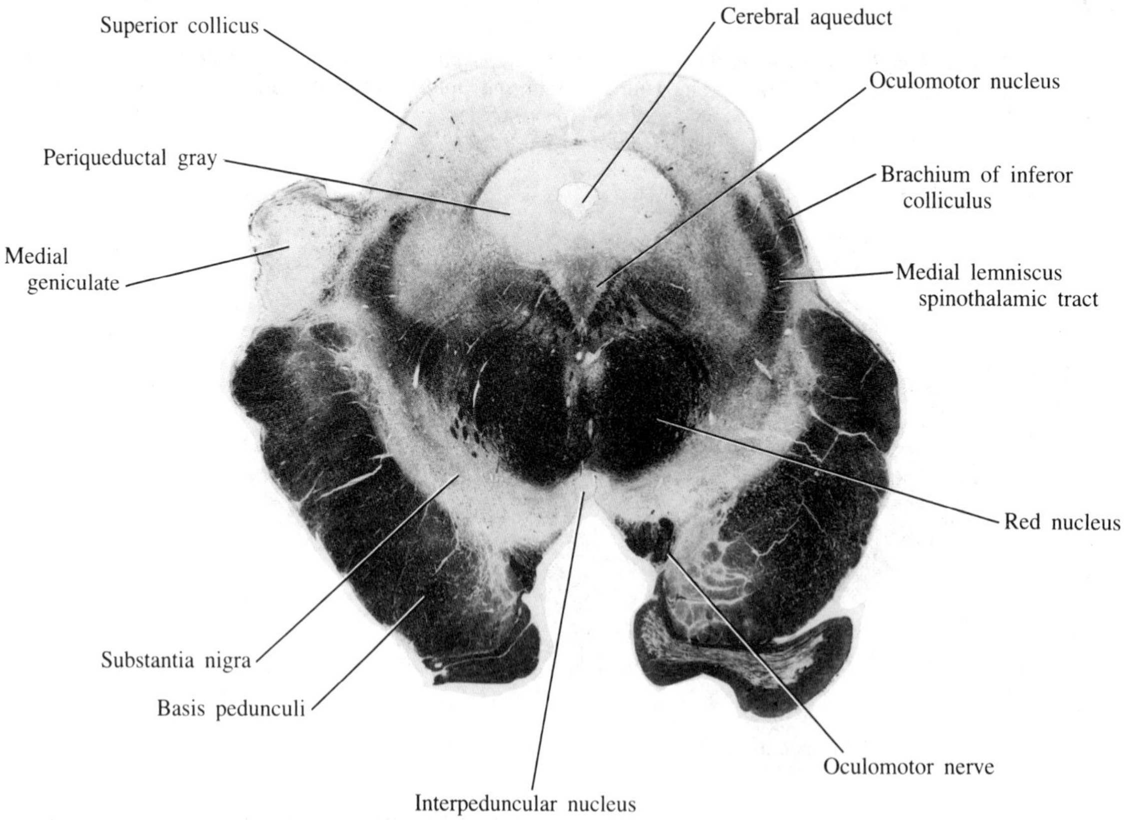

FIGURE 1.2-19. *Cross section of mesencephalon.*

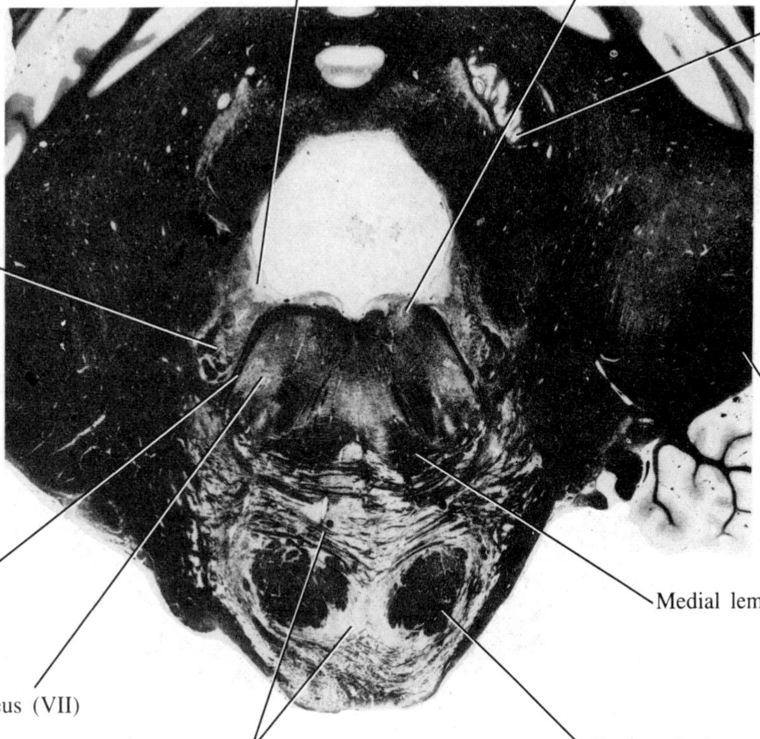

FIGURE 1.2-20. *Cross section through pons. (From Gluhbegovic N, Williams T H:* The Human Brain. *Harper & Row, New York, 1979, with permission.)*

fibers in the pyramids cross over the midline in the *pyramidal decussation* to form the *lateral corticospinal tract* that descends in the dorsolateral part of the spinal cord. Immediately above the pyramidal decussation, the sensory internal arcuate fibers from the dorsal column nuclei cross over the midline in the sensory decussation to form the medial lemniscus. The medial lemniscus ascends close to the midline in the medulla oblongata and gradually diverges laterally in the upper part of the brain stem in order to reach the *ventral posterior lateral* (VPL) *nucleus,* the sensory relay nucleus in the lateral part of the thalamus. On the lateral side of the medial lemniscus, the *inferior olivary nucleus* stands out as one of the most prominent structures in the ventral half of the medulla oblongata. This bag-shaped nucleus gives origin to a massive system of *olivocerebellar fibers,* which cross the midline and then enter the cerebellum through the inferior cerebellar peduncles, which can be identified dorsolaterally in the upper part of the medulla oblongata.

The *central canal* of the spinal cord is gradually displaced in a dorsal direction through the appearance of the large motor and sensory decussations until it finally opens up into the fourth ventricle in the upper half of the medulla oblongata, where part of its dorsal surface is represented by the floor of the ventricle. The gray matter underneath the floor of the fourth ventricle is represented by the reticular formation and a number of specific cranial nerve nuclei, including the hypoglossal nucleus, the dorsal motor nucleus of the vagus, and the *nucleus of the solitary tract* immediately below the ventricle, whereas the *nucleus ambiguous* is located more ventrally. Nuclei belonging to the *vestibular complex* border the inferior cerebellar peduncle in the most dorsal part of the medulla. The *dorsal* and *ventral cochlear nuclei* can be found on the lateral side of the inferior cerebellar peduncle a little higher up in the medulla oblongata, at the transition to pons.

VENTRICULAR SYSTEM

The ventricular system in the interior of the brain is formed by four communicating cavities: two lateral ventricles (one in each hemisphere), the third ventricle in the diencephalon, and the fourth ventricle beneath the cerebellum. Each of the ventricles contains a *choroid plexus* for the production of *cerebrospinal fluid* (CSF). The lateral ventricle is characterized by its horseshoe shape. It is divided into an anterior horn in front of the interventricular foramen, followed by a central part and a posterior horn that projects for a variable distance into the occipital lobe, and finally a temporal horn that curves downward behind the thalamus into the temporal lobe and ends blindly about 2.5 cm from the temporal pole and just behind the amygdaloid body. The CSF produced in the choroid plexus of the lateral ventricle escapes through the interventricular foramen of Monro into the third ventricle, which, in turn, is continuous with the fourth ventricle through the narrow cerebral aqueduct in the midbrain.

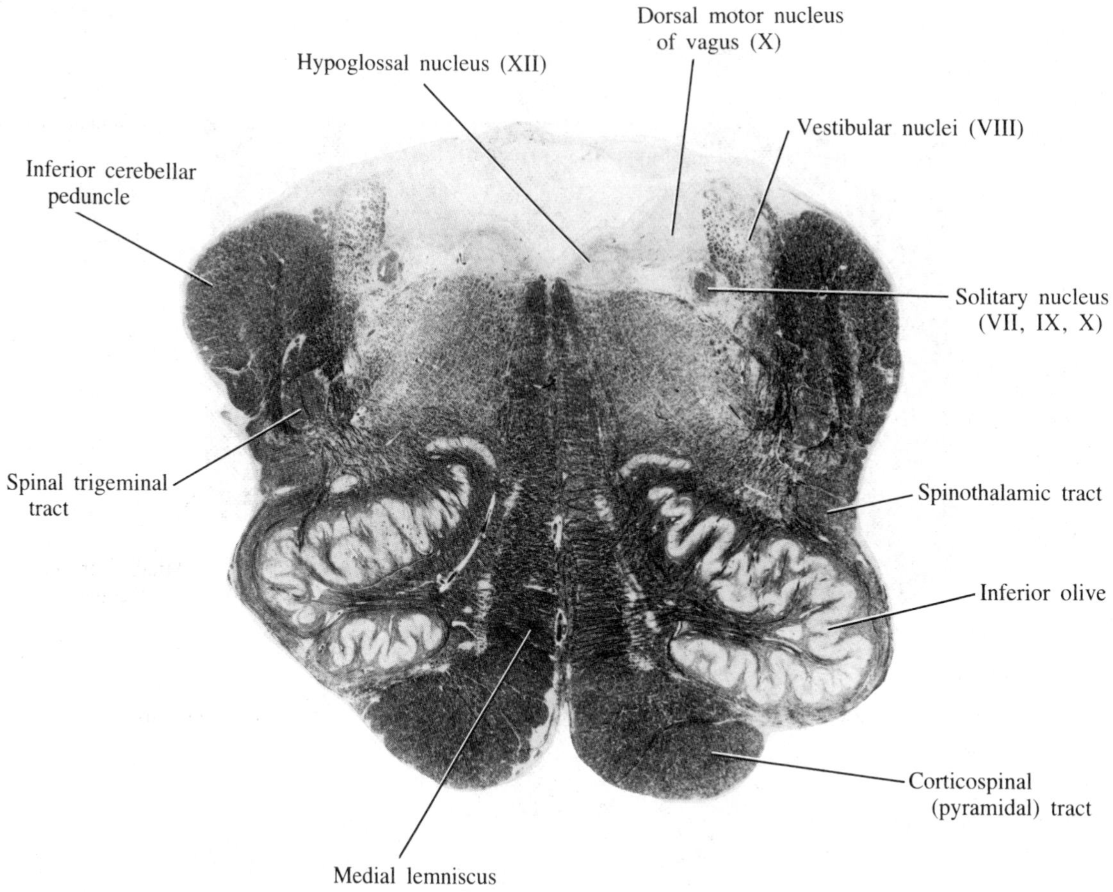

FIGURE 1.2-21. *Cross section through medulla oblongata. (From Gluhbegovic N, Williams T H:* The Human Brain. *Harper & Row, New York, 1979, with permission.)*

The third ventricle, which is located between the two thalami and the two halves of the hypothalamus, has three prominent recesses: the *optic, infundibular,* and *pineal recesses*. The fourth ventricle is shaped like a tent, with its top or apex *fastigium* projecting into the cerebellum. Although the fourth ventricle, like the third, contains a choroid plexus, most of the CSF is formed by the choroid plexus in the lateral ventricles. Having reached the fourth ventricle, the CSF enters the subarachnoid space through three apertures in the fourth ventricle; the *median aperture of Magendie* in the midline and the two *lateral apertures of Luschka* in the lateral recess. The median aperture is located in the angle between cerebellum and medulla oblongata and opens into the *cerebellomedullary cistern,* or *cisterna magna,* whereas the lateral aperture can be found in the cerebellopontine angle.

The flow of CSF is quite rapid; the total volume of CSF in the ventricle system and the subarachnoid space is about 125 ml, but it is estimated that more than four times that amount, or about 500 ml, is formed during a 24-hour period. An excessive amount of CSF in the ventricular system is referred to as *hydrocephalus,* which can occur with or without an increase of intracranial pressure. Hydrocephalus with increased intracranial pressure is most often caused by obstruction in the circulation of CSF. As indicated above, the ventricular system contains various passages—for example, the interventricular foramen and cerebral aqueduct—where a pathological process can easily block the flow of CSF.

VASCULAR SUPPLY OF THE BRAIN

Two major pairs of vessels supply the cranial contents—namely, the *vertebral* and *internal carotid arteries*. Although they are segregated in their peripheral course, anastomotic links, which form the *circle of Willis,* occur once they enter the cranium (Figs. 1.2-22 through 1.2-24).

INTERNAL CAROTID ARTERY SYSTEM

Middle cerebral artery The internal carotid artery has four major branches. The first and largest branch is the *middle cerebral artery,* which skirts across the *limen insulae* and courses in the *lateral fissure*. Secondary branches from this artery supply much of the lateral surface of the frontal lobe, including Broca's area and the motor representation for the face, arm, and upper body. The anterior and lateral parts of the temporal lobe are also supplied by this vessel, including *Wernicke's receptive speech area* and the primary auditory cortex in the *transverse temporal gyri of Heschl*. Parietal branches of the middle cerebral artery supply the areas of somatosensory representation for the face, arm, and upper body as well as the higher-order association cortices that form the *supramarginal* and *angular gyri*.

Anterior cerebral artery Another major branch of the internal carotid artery is the *anterior cerebral artery,* which supplies much of the medial surface of the hemisphere, including the motor and sensory representations for the leg.

Posterior communicating artery Two other major branches of the internal carotid artery need comment. One is the *posterior communicating artery,* which forms an anastomotic link

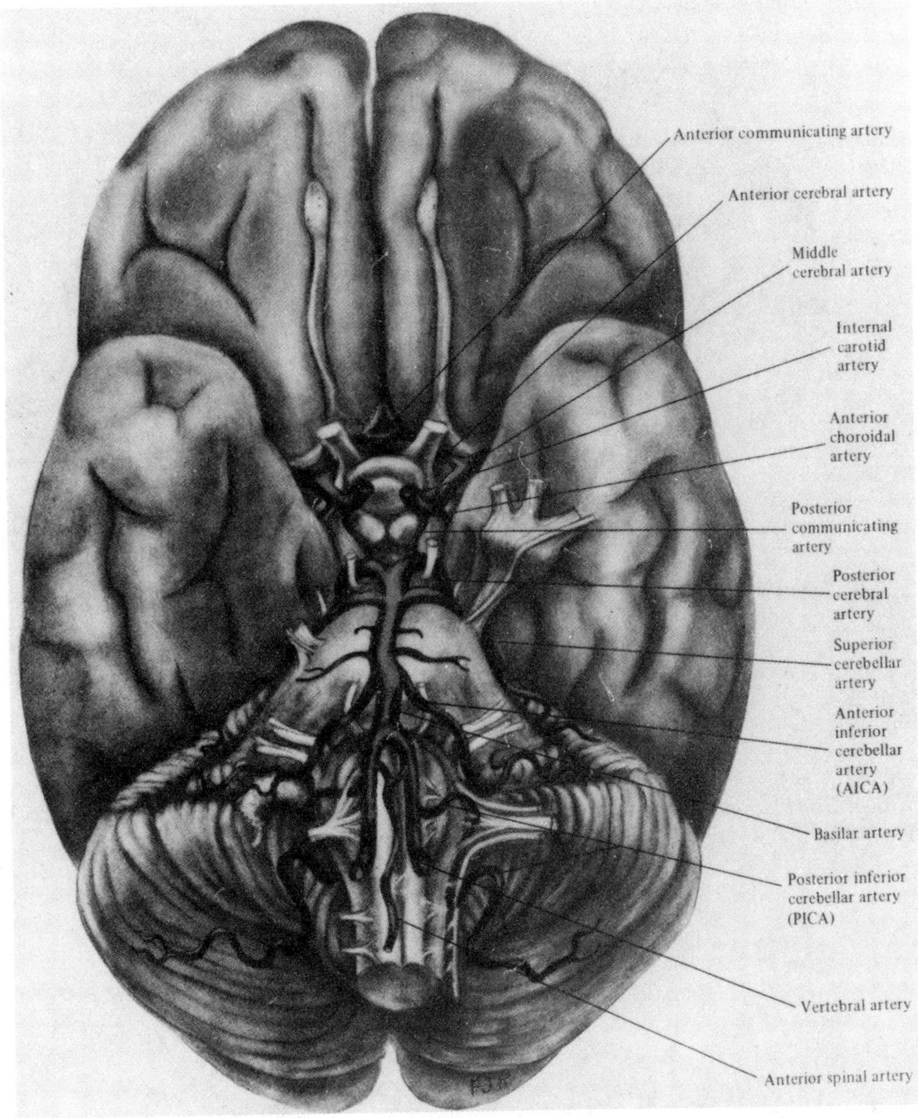

FIGURE 1.2-22. *Major arteries on the basal surface of the brain. (From Heimer L:* The Human Brain and Spinal Cord. *Springer-Verlag, New York, 1983, with permission. Drawing by F J Kabir.)*

with the *vertebral-basilar system* by linking with the *posterior cerebral artery*. Small penetrating vessels from the posterior communicating artery serve important diencephalic centers, such as the hypothalamus.

Anterior choroidal artery The *anterior choroidal artery* is another branch of the internal carotid artery of considerable importance. It supplies the anterior part of the parahippocampal gyrus, a large portion of the amygdala, the optic tract, the inner segment of the globus pallidus, the ventromedial part of the internal capsule and, in some cases, the lateral geniculate nucleus. This has been brought into sharp focus in recent years with such noninvasive scanning methods as computed tomography (CT), since many of the neurological signs of vascular disease in the anterior choroidal artery can mimic vascular disease in larger cerebral vessels.

VERTEBRAL-BASILAR ARTERY SYSTEM **Posterior cerebral artery** The vertebral-basilar blood supply to the brain is extensive and includes branches that supply that part of the cerebral cortex not supplied by the internal carotid system as well as much of the brain stem and cerebellum. The paired posterior cerebral arteries are a consequence of the bifurcation of the basilar artery and supply the ventral and posterior parts of the temporal lobe, nearly the entire occipital lobe, and a small portion of the posterior and superior parts of the parietal lobe. Many important penetrating branches of the posterior cerebral artery and posterior communicating artery supply the deeper structures of the brain, such as the thalamus and midbrain.

Cerebellar arteries Other branches of the vertebral-basilar system include the *superior cerebellar* and *anterior inferior cerebellar arteries*. These arteries, along with short and long circumferential vessels also originating directly from the basilar artery, supply much of the cerebellum and the midbrain and pontine portions of the brain stem. Vascular insufficiency of the basilar artery or one of its many branches may present a variety of different symptoms depending on the site of the lesion.

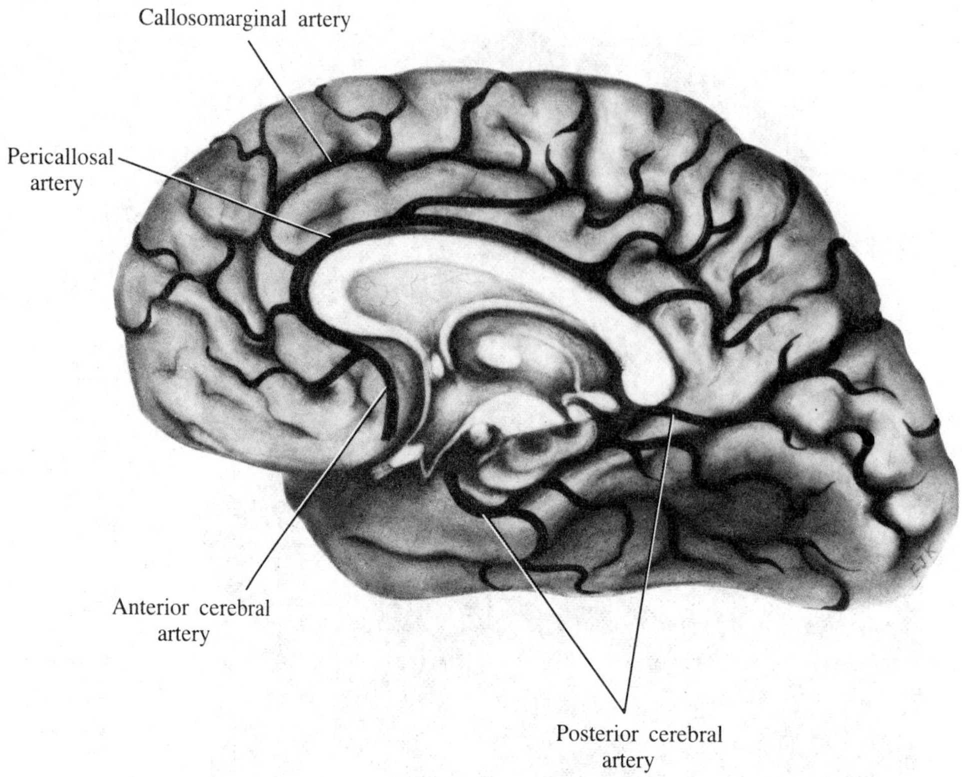

FIGURE 1.2-23. *Cortical distribution of anterior and posterior cerebral arteries. (From Heimer L:* The Human Brain and Spinal Cord. *Springer-Verlag, New York, 1983, with permission. Drawing by F J Kabir.)*

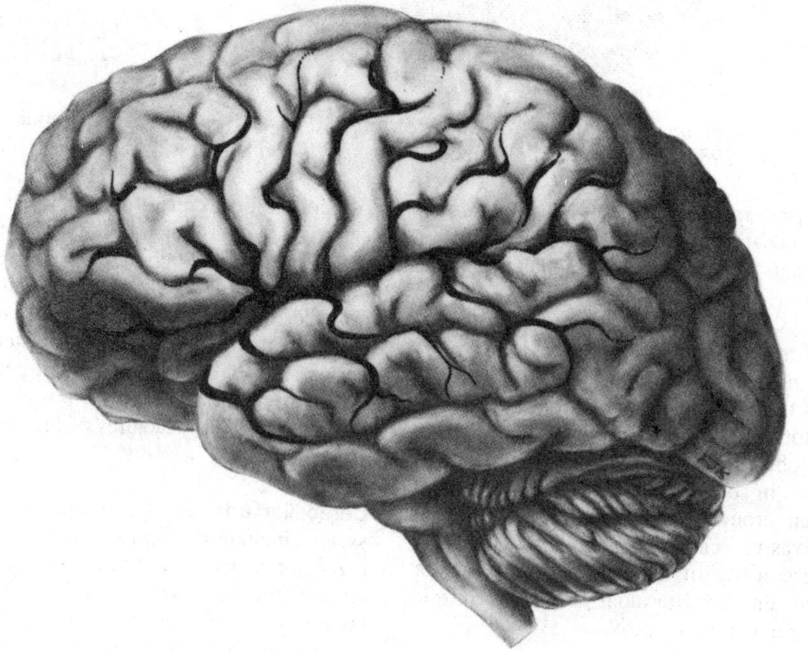

FIGURE 1.2-24. *Cortical distribution of the middle cerebral artery. (From Heimer L:* The Human Brain and Spinal Cord. *Springer-Verlag, New York, 1983, with permission. Drawing by F J Kabir.)*

A major vessel that is always a direct branch of the vertebral artery is the *posterior inferior cerebellar artery* (PICA). As the name implies, it supplies the inferior surface of the cerebellum but before doing so negotiates an S-shaped course on the lateral side of the medulla oblongata to which it gives off many penetrating vessels. Thus, it supplies such major medullary structures as the inferior and medial vestibular nuclei, the inferior cerebellar peduncle, the spinal trigeminal tract and nucleus, the nucleus ambiguous, the medullary reticular formation, and the spinothalamic tract. This latter crossed pathway carries pain and temperature sensation for the contralateral side of the body.

TABLE 1.2-1
Neurovascular Syndromes

Artery	*Typical Signs and Symptoms in Occlusion of Vessel*
Internal carotid artery	Varies according to compensatory capacity of circle of Willis. Often preceded by important warning signs, such as transient ischemic attacks (TIAs). Sensorimotor deficits usually most pronounced in face and arm, but also in leg if anterior cerebral artery is involved. Often speech disturbances if lesion on the left side. Large infarcts of one hemisphere are often fatal.
Middle cerebral artery	Commonly involved in cerebrovascular accidents. Contralateral hemiplegia and hemianesthesia, homonynous hemianopia, and global aphasia in most patients with left-sided lesion. Right-sided lesion may cause confusion and neglect for left side of body in visual and somatosensory spheres. Paralysis of conjugate gaze to opposite side.
Anterior cerebral artery	Occlusion distal to its connection with the anterior communicating artery results in contralateral hemiparesis and hemianesthesia in foot and leg. Large strokes affecting anterior cingulate cortex and supplementary motor area on either side may cause akinesia and mutism.
Posterior cerebral artery	Great variety of symptoms depending on site of lesion and collateral circulation. Occlusion of proximal part may cause hemianesthesia, transitory hemiparesis and agonizing pain (thalamic syndrome), as well as contralateral visual field defects and agnosias.
Basilar artery	Variety of different symptoms depending on site of lesion or branch occluded. Full-fledged basilar artery syndromes—with disturbances of consciousness, tetraplegia, impaired sensation and vision, disorders of eye movements, facial paralysis, and cerebellar ataxia—are usually fatal.
Vertebral artery and posterior inferior cerebellar artery (PICA)	Variable picture depending on the arrangement of nearby vessels. The classic lateral medullary syndrome of Wallenberg is characterized by loss of pain and temperature sensation for ipsilateral side of face and contralateral side of the rest of body ("crossed" syndrome), ipsilateral Horner's syndrome (miosis, ptosis, and decreased sweating), changes in phonation, disequilibrium, vertigo, and vomiting.

Anterior spinal artery The paramedian and medial parts of the medulla receive their vascular supply from the vertebral arteries. The midline core of much of the medulla is supplied by the *anterior spinal artery,* a single vessel that courses in the anterior median fissure of the medulla and spinal cord and forms from paired retrovertebral branches of the vertebral artery. It supplies the pyramids, the medial lemniscus, and the nucleus and rootlets of the twelfth or hypoglossal cranial nerve.

In summary, the brain's blood supply is derived from two major sets of vessels, the internal carotid and vertebral arteries. The systems are linked together via the posterior communicating artery. These vessels—along with the middle cerebral, anterior cerebral, and anterior communicating arteries—form the circle of Willis. This anastomatic circle of vessels on the base of the brain provides the opportunity for collateral circulation in the event of occlusion in one of the major arteries proximal to the circle. Penetrating vessels from these branches of the internal carotids and vertebral-basilar arteries supply deep structures of the cerebral hemisphere. A summary of the most common neurovascular syndromes is given in Table 1.2-1.

REFERENCES

Björklund A, Hökfelt T: *Handbook of Chemical Neuroanatomy,* vol 2. Elsevier, New York, 1984.

Björklund A, Hökfelt T, Kuhar M J: *Handbook of Chemical Neuroanatomy,* vol 3. Elsevier, New York, 1984.

Björklund A, Hökfelt T, Swanson L W: *Handbook of Chemical Neuroanatomy,* vol 5. Elsevier, New York, 1987.

Brodal A: *Neurological Anatomy.* Oxford University Press, New York, 1981.

Carpenter M B, Sutin J B: *Human Neuroanatomy.* Williams & Wilkins, Baltimore, 1983.

DeFrance J F: *The Septal Nuclei.* Plenum, New York, 1976.

Evered D, O'Conner M, editors: *Functions of the Basal Ganglia,* Ciba Foundation Symposium 107. Pitman, London, 1984.

Foote S L, Morrison J H: Extrahypothalamic modulation of cortical function. Ann Rev Neurosci *10:* 67, 1987.

Heimer L: *The Human Brain and Spinal Cord.* Springer-Verlag, New York, 1983.

Heimer L, Alheid G F, Zaborszky L: The basal ganglia. In *The Rat Nervous System,* vol 1, G Paxinos, editor, p 37. Academic Press, Orlando, FL, 1985.

Hobson, J A, Brazier A B: *The Reticular Formation Revisited: Specifying Function for a Nonspecific System.* Raven Press, New York, 1980.

Isaacson R L, Pribram K H, editors: *The Hippocampus,* vol 3. Plenum, New York, 1986.

Jones E G: *The Thalamus.* Plenum, New York, 1985.

Jones E G, Peters A, editors: *Cerebral Cortex,* vol 5. Plenum, New York, 1986.

McKenzie J S, Kemm R E, Wilcock L N, editors: *The Basal Ganglia.* Plenum, New York, 1984.

Morgane P J, Panksepp J: *Anatomy of the Hypothalamus,* vol 1. Marcel Dekker, New York, 1979.

Mountcastle V B, Plum F, Geiger S R, editors: *The Handbook of Physiology,* vol 4, *Intrinsic Regulatory Systems of the Brain.* American Physiological Society, Bethesda, MD, 1986.

Mountcastle V B, Plum F, Geiger, S R editors: *The Handbook of Physiology,* vol 5, *Higher Functions of the Brain.* American Physiological Society, Bethesda, MD, 1987.

Nauta W J H, Domesick V: Afferent and efferent relationships of the basal ganglia. In *Functions of the Basal Ganglia,* Ciba Foundation Symposium 107, D Evered, M O'Conner, editors, p 201. Pitman, London, 1984.

Nauta W J H, Feirtag, M: *Fundamental Neuroanatomy*. Freeman, New York, 1986.
Parent A: *Comparative Neurobiology of the Basal Ganglia*. Wiley, New York, 1986.
Paxinos G: *The Human Nervous System*. Academic Press, Orlando, FL, 1988.
Silverman A J, Pickard G E: The hypothalamus. In *Chemical Neuroanatomy*, P C Emson, editor, p 295. Raven Press, New York, 1983.
Sjölund B, Björklund A: *Brain Stem Control of Spinal Mechanisms*. Elsevier, New York, 1982.

1.3
FUNCTIONAL NEUROANATOMY

GEORGE F. ALHEID, Ph.D.
GARY W. VAN HOESEN, Ph.D.
LENNART HEIMER, M.D.

INTRODUCTION

In a brief discussion of functional neuroanatomy, it is not possible to cover every detail of brain organization from synapse to cell, to nuclear cluster, to system. The most salient features in the organization of the central nervous system (CNS) with respect to psychiatry have therefore been selected, and, as appropriate, more detailed references to more exhaustive reviews that focus on particular brain areas have been provided.

Knowledge about the structure of the brain and spinal cord has been derived largely from comparative studies of animals, with the vast majority of experiments having been performed on the laboratory rat. Although the general plan of the mammalian brain is well represented within this species, real and important differences among the species do exist. Confidence in the details of human CNS organization can be gained only by experiments with primates, and, when possible, by direct observations in human brains.

FOREBRAIN ANATOMICAL SYSTEMS Some of the more general features of brain architecture can be described by grouping several related areas into a single system whenever the criteria for inclusion or exclusion are more or less clearly stated. One result in taking this liberty is that some areas might be considered as belonging to more than one system, whereas other areas may not be rationally included in any broader system when their connections and functions are poorly understood. In general, brain systems are characterized by parallel input and output pathways, with varying degrees of internal processing. It must be true, of course, that individual subsystems of the brain are linked together. The external inputs and outputs of various subsystems that provide this linkage have been identified as much as possible.

Several forebrain systems are of special interest for the study of behavior. The dramatic expansion of the cortex in higher mammals culminating in the massive cortex of human brains has been taken as a priori evidence for its role in uniquely human endeavors, but there are few functions that the cortex serves entirely on its own. One of these functions is the increasingly elaborate differentiation of sensory information once it reaches primary cortical sensory areas. On the output side, the cortex is intimately connected with elaborate subcortical processing systems; some of these have access to motor areas in the brain stem to influence overt behavior. At the same time, they all provide feedback to cortex so that subcortically reprocessed information becomes intermingled with the total sensation of the internal and external environment.

In the basal forebrain, several functional anatomical systems are closely interconnected to the cortex and appear to be of vital importance to the more elaborate behavior attributed to the telencephalon. These are (1) the *striatopallidal system;* (2) an extended amygdala, which is a continuous band of neurons stretching from the *centromedial amygdala* into the *rostromedial forebrain;* (3) the *septum;* and (4) the *corticopetal basal forebrain* system of neurons, whose best-studied component is the magnocellular neurons that provide the massive cholinergic projection to cortex. Much more research needs to be done before the details of these systems can be described completely. Nonetheless, these systems have come into sharper focus as a result of intensive research during the past few years, and since they seem to be of particular importance in psychiatric disorders, they will receive special attention in this section of Chapter 1.

CEREBRAL CORTEX

CYTOARCHITECTURE The internal structure of the cerebral cortex was not studied effectively until the latter part of the nineteenth century, with the advent of suitable fixatives and stains. The *Golgi method,* in particular, was a major achievement in that it allowed an exquisite view of the cellular detail of the cortex. Many scientists capitalized on the pioneering studies of Nissl, who perfected a technique of staining neural cell bodies by the use of aniline dyes. By means of these procedures, all neural and glial cell bodies could be visualized, and the differing structure of the cortex could be compared and characterized by studying sequential sections. Several criteria were applied to parcellating the cortex. For example, attention was paid to the number of cell layers, the overall thickness of the cortex, the density of cells within a layer, the thickness of individual layers, and the predominant cell type within a layer. For Brodmann, this type of study led to the formulation of a cortical map with the cerebral cortex of the human brain parcellated in 51 different fields, each with a unique architecture (Fig. 1.3-1).

The differential cytoarchitecture of the cortex is the starting point for understanding its general principles of organization, both structural and functional. For example, each of the various sensory modalities is represented within the cortex, and each has a unique architecture (Fig. 1.3-2). The primary cortical sensory areas receive relayed input from specific thalamic nuclei, which convey direct or indirect lemniscal afferents that are linked to the periphery. In the case of the visual modality, retinal ganglion cells project to the *lateral geniculate nucleus,* which, in turn, gives rise to the optic radiation. This massive pathway terminates in Brodmann's area 17, the *primary visual cortex*. The medial geniculate nucleus receives auditory input from the inferior colliculus and gives rise to the acoustic radiation that terminates in Brodmann's areas 41 and 42, the *primary auditory cortex*. Lemniscal input carrying

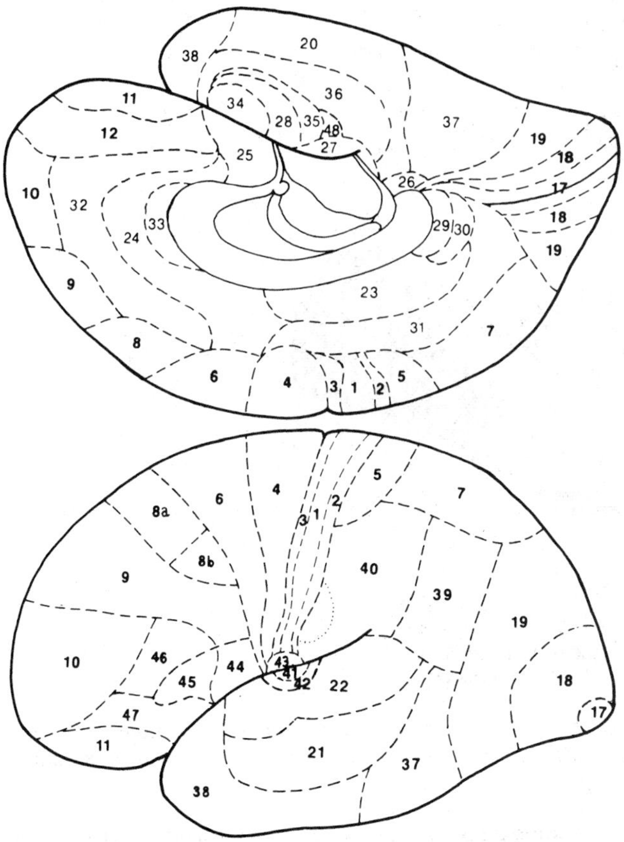

FIGURE 1.3-1. *Brodmann's areas. (From Romero-Sierra C:* Neuroanatomy, a Conceptual Approach. *Churchill Livingstone, New York, 1986, with permission.)*

somatic sensory information for the entire body terminates in the ventrobasal complex of the thalamus, which projects to Brodmann's areas 3, 1, and 2. All of the primary sensory areas are characterized by conspicuous cytoarchitectural features that set them apart from other cortical areas. Most notable is a highly dense and granular layer IV, populated by small stellate neurons. These neurons are the major recipients of the thalamic relay that terminates in the primary sensory cortex.

The major motor-related areas of the cerebral cortex comprise Brodmann's areas 4, 6, and 8 and, like the primary sensory areas, these brain areas have a distinct cytoarchitecture. These areas form the so-called agranular parts of the cerebral cortex, so named because they have poorly developed layer IVs and a paucity of small neurons. Pyramidal cells predominate in this cortex and they are especially well developed in layers III, V, and VI.

Although the primary sensory and agranular motor fields are important functional areas, and distinct anatomical parts of the cerebral cortex, they constitute a rather small percentage of the total cerebral cortex in the human brain. A vast amount of the human cerebral cortex, which generally has been termed *association cortex,* is best characterized as intermediate in structure—that is, having both a population of smaller granule or stellate neurons and a discernible population of larger pyramid-shaped neurons. Six well-differentiated layers are seen in Figure 1.3-3: (1) a largely cellular molecular or plexiform zone adjacent to the pia mater, forming layer I; (2) a narrow, but clear, external granular layer of smaller cells, forming layer II; (3) a wide outer pyramidal cell layer, forming layer III; (4) a compact internal granular layer, forming layer IV; (5) a conspicuous layer of larger pyramids, forming the internal pyramidal cell layer or layer V; and (6) an intermixed or multiform layer, forming layer VI. This laminar parcellation is valid for much of the nonagranular and nonprimary sensory parts of the cerebral cortex, although there are substantial regional variations. For example, two areas of cortex that conform to the general six-layered plan may have different densities of cells in layer III, or perhaps layer V is sharply defined in one area but less distinguishable from layer VI in another. These are the types of subtleties that are revealed by good Nissl stains and that became the basis for Brodmann's many subdivisions of the cortex.

It is useful to divide the association cortices into two categories. The primary association cortices that are located near the primary sensory cortices form one category. These receive short corticocortical connections from the primary sensory cortices. Such areas as Brodmann's areas 18 and 19 for the visual modality, area 22 for the auditory modality, and area 5 for somatic sensation are committed functionally to a single modality, and deficits due to their destruction are purely unimodal. The second category is the so-called nonprimary association areas, which, unlike the primary areas, appear to be functionally multimodal. Brodmann's areas 9, 10, and 46 in the frontal lobe and areas 39 and 40 in the parietal lobe are good examples. Deficits resulting from the destruction of these areas are usually more general in nature and subtend perceptual abilities that are not unique to information associated with a single modality.

The primary sensory cortices, the agranular motor cortices, and the association cortices can all be viewed as *neo-* or *isocortex,* and they conform in a general sense to the six-layered pattern. Other cortical areas do not. For example, much of the cortex of the limbic lobe is best termed "proisocortex." It has many characteristics of the isocortex, but its laminar arrangement is incomplete. For example, layer IV, the internal granular layer, may be missing entirely or be incipient, or layers V and VI may merge together into an undifferentiated layer of cells. Brodmann's areas 23 and 24 of the cingulate gyrus are good examples of proisocortex. The *periallocortex* is another atypical form of cortex. It is often characterized by an incomplete six-layered pattern, but it also has an unusual laminar distribution of neurons. Large, densely packed neurons may be present in layer II, for example; however, this is typically seen in only the deeper layers of the iso- and proisocortices. The presubicular and entorhinal cortices are good examples of periallocortex. The least typical of all cortical types is the allocortex. It has only two to three layers. The cortex of the hippocampus and olfactory cortical areas are the best examples of allocortex.

CONNECTIONS OF THE CEREBRAL CORTEX A tremendous amount is known about the connectivity of the cerebral cortex; however, only a survey is included here. In general, it is useful to parcellate these into three categories: *corticopetal projections,* which convey afferent input to the cortex from noncortical areas; *corticofugal projections,* which convey efferent output away from the cerebral cortex; and *association projections,* which link the cortex together within the hemisphere (intrahemispheric) or between the two hemispheres (interhemispheric).

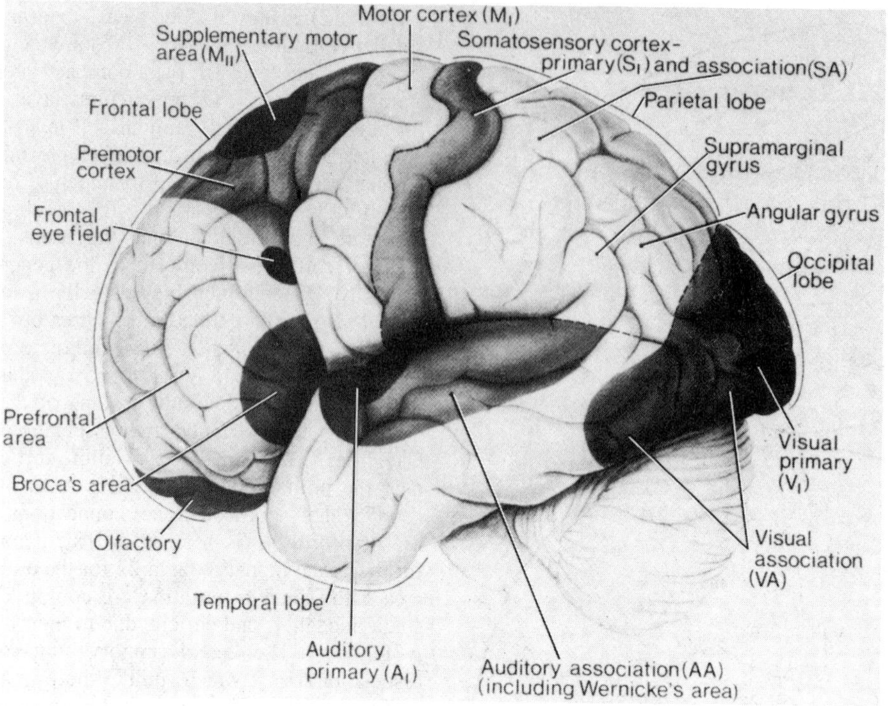

FIGURE 1.3-2. *Major functional areas of cortex. (From Pandya D N, Yeterian E H: Architecture and connections of cortical association areas. In* Cerebral Cortex, vol 4, *p 3, A Peters, E G Jones, editors. Plenum, New York, 1985, with permission.)*

Corticopetal connections THALAMOCORTICAL INPUT Projections from the various thalamic nuclei provide the single largest source of extrinsic input to the cerebral cortex (see Fig. 1.2-16), and there is a relatively rigid organization in functional terms. For example, sensory relay nuclei, such as the ventrobasal complex, medial geniculate nucleus, and lateral geniculate nucleus, project to the primary sensory cortices for somatic sensation, audition, and vision, respectively. Motor nuclei, such as the ventral anterior and ventral lateral nuclei project to the premotor and motor cortices. The anterior thalamic nuclei and the nucleus reuniens have extensive projections to the cortex of the limbic lobe, such as the cingulate, presubicular, entorhinal, and hippocampal cortices, and the pulvinar and mediodorsal nuclei project to association areas of the cerebral cortex. Pulvinar projections are especially extensive and terminate in association areas of all four lobes and in selective parts of the limbic lobe, such as the temporal polar and posterior parahippocampal cortices. The mediodorsal nucleus, on the other hand, projects to all parts of prefrontal association cortex, but not to other cortical areas.

TRANSMITTER-SPECIFIC INPUTS Several corticopetal projections are associated with well-known and well-studied neurotransmitters. For example, certain magnocellular neurons of the basal forebrain—such as those associated with the medial septum, diagonal band nuclei, and basal nucleus of Meynert—provide cholinergic input to the whole of the cortex. A relatively rigid topography has been delineated for these projections. Throughout the same area occupied by the cholinergic neurons are found corticopetal cells that use γ-aminobutyric acid (GABA) or somatostatin, although projections from these neurons may be less extensive in terms of the number of areas innervated. Noradrenergic and serotoninergic input to the whole cortex arise from the nucleus locus ceruleus and from the raphe complex, respectively. Dopaminergic input to the cerebral cortex has been identified, and at least some of it arises from neurons located in the ventral tegmental area of the midbrain. These have been thought to be directed primarily to frontal lobe areas. However, some recent evidence indicates that dopaminergic afferents can be found widely throughout the cortex.

AMYGDALOCORTICAL INPUTS In recent years, it has also been shown that the amygdala has extensive projections to several frontal lobe areas, the anterior cingulate cortex, the association cortices of the temporal lobe, and to some parts of the primary association cortex of the occipital lobe.

Corticofugal connections CORTICOTHALAMIC OUTPUT As discussed above, the thalamocortical projection system is sizable and is organized topographically and functionally. This is reciprocated by discrete projections that emanate from the cortex and project back to the thalamus. In large part, it appears that there is a faithful reciprocity and that the vast majority of corticothalamic projections arise from infragranular layers, particularly layer VI.

CORTICOSTRIATAL OUTPUT Projections from the cerebral cortex to the caudate nucleus and putamen form the corticostriate system; literally all of the cerebral cortex projects to the caudate nucleus and putamen. These projections arise principally from a subset of neurons located in layer V of the cortex, although other cortical layers (e.g., layer III) may contribute to this system. Some of the corticostriatal terminals also arrive as collaterals of descending cortical axons that pass through striatum en route to nonstriatal targets.

In general, the agranular cortices project primarily to the putamen, whereas sensory and association areas project predominantly to the caudate nucleus. Limbic cortical areas as well as prefrontal and temporal association areas project primarily to the ventral striatum, including the accumbens.

CORTICAL OUTPUT TO BASAL FOREBRAIN Several basal forebrain structures receive direct corticofugal projections from the cerebral cortex. For example, the septum and the nucleus of the vertical limb of the diagonal band of Broca receive hippocampal and subicular projections. The substantia innominata, presumably including the basal nucleus of Meynert, receives input from medial frontal, orbitofrontal, anterior insular, and temporal polar cortex.

The amygdala receives a massive cortical input that is derived from all types of cortex. These convey to the amygdala sensory association input from all modalities. For example, visual input reaches the amygdala via projections from the inferior and middle temporal gyri, auditory input is derived from the anterior half of the superior temporal gyrus, and somatosensory input arises from the insular cortex. A sizable olfactory input reaches the superficial amygdaloid nuclei via direct projections from the olfactory bulb itself and via relayed projections from the olfactory cortex. Finally, information related to taste arises from the cortex that forms the frontal operculum. In addition to sensory-related input, the amygdala also receives direct entorhinal and subicular cortex projections.

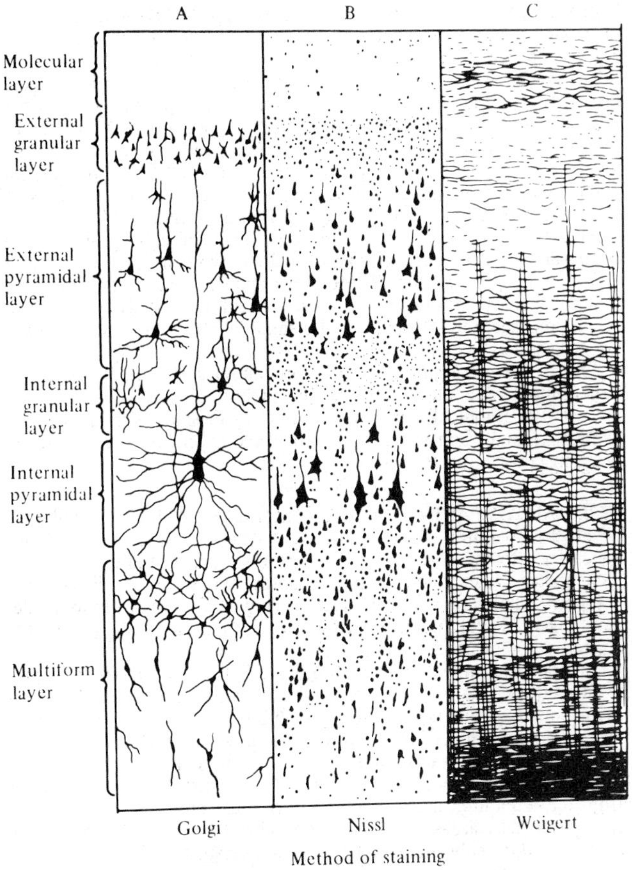

FIGURE 1.3-3. *Layers of the cerebral cortex.* A. *Golgi method.* B. *Nissl stain.* C. *Weigert myelin stain. (After Brodmann.)*

CORTICOPONTINE OUTPUT The corticopontine projection is the initial link in a bisynaptic neural system that links the cerebral cortex of one hemisphere with the cerebellar cortex of the contralateral hemisphere. These projections arise primarily from a subset of neurons in layer V of the cortex and terminate in the ipsilateral pontine gray matter. Unlike the corticostriate projection, which arises from all parts of the cerebral cortex, the corticopontine projection does not receive a strong contribution from certain association areas in the frontal and temporal lobes. Through this system the cortex has a major influence on the pontocerebellar pathway, which decussates in the pons, forms the middle cerebellar peduncle, and terminates in the contralateral cerebellar cortex.

CORTICOSPINAL OUTPUT The major motor, and to some extent sensory-related, pathway that leaves the cortex and terminates in the contralateral spinal intermediate and anterior horn zones is the corticospinal pathway. It takes its origin from pyramidal neurons in layers III and V, located in Brodmann's areas 4, 6, 3, 1, 2, 5, and 24. The function of this classical upper motor neuron system in humans is associated largely with fine coordinated movements of the extremities.

CORTICOBULBAR OUTPUT Corticobulbar projections are analogous in many ways to corticospinal projections; however, they arise from the face parts of the precentral gyrus and innervate the motor nuclei of cranial nerves and interneurons linked to them in the reticular formation. Unlike the corticospinal pathway, which crosses largely to the contralateral side in the pyramidal decussation of the lower medulla, corticobulbar projections innervate the motor nuclei of cranial nerves bilaterally either directly or indirectly. An interesting exception occurs in the case of those parts of the facial nucleus that innervate the muscles of facial expression for the lower face. These parts receive primarily contralateral innervation and, therefore, can be affected by diseases that alter upper contralateral motor neurons.

Association connections Although a significant part of the input to the cerebral cortex is derived from sources extrinsic to it, corticocortical pathways are very extensive and account for many of the connections formed with cortical neurons. Many varieties of such connections exist consisting of local circuit connections within a column of cortical neurons, short association connections that connect adjacent gyri or spatially separated areas within a cytoarchitectural field, and long association connections that link together different cytoarchitectural areas, often within different lobes.

The primary sensory cortices are the recipients of input from the lemniscal relay nuclei in the thalamus. These areas, in turn, give rise to short connections to primary sensory association cortical areas located nearby (Fig. 1.3-4*A*). In the case of visual projections this would entail projections from area 17 to areas 18 and 19; in the case of auditory projections it would entail projections from areas 41 and 42 to area 22; and in the case of somatic projections it would entail projections from areas 3, 1, and 2 to area 5. Each of the primary association areas then gives rise to projections to other parts of the association cortex, which have been referred to as secondary association areas. Typically, these projections are more widespread in their distribution. Beyond this point in the outflow of sensory information, cortical projections diverge substantially. For example, the secondary visual association areas of the temporal lobe (Brodmann's areas 20 and 21) project to frontal lobe areas (Fig. 1.3-4*B*) and to limbic cortical areas. The anterior parts of area 22 have a similar pattern of projections, as does the cortex of the inferior parietal lobule. Another

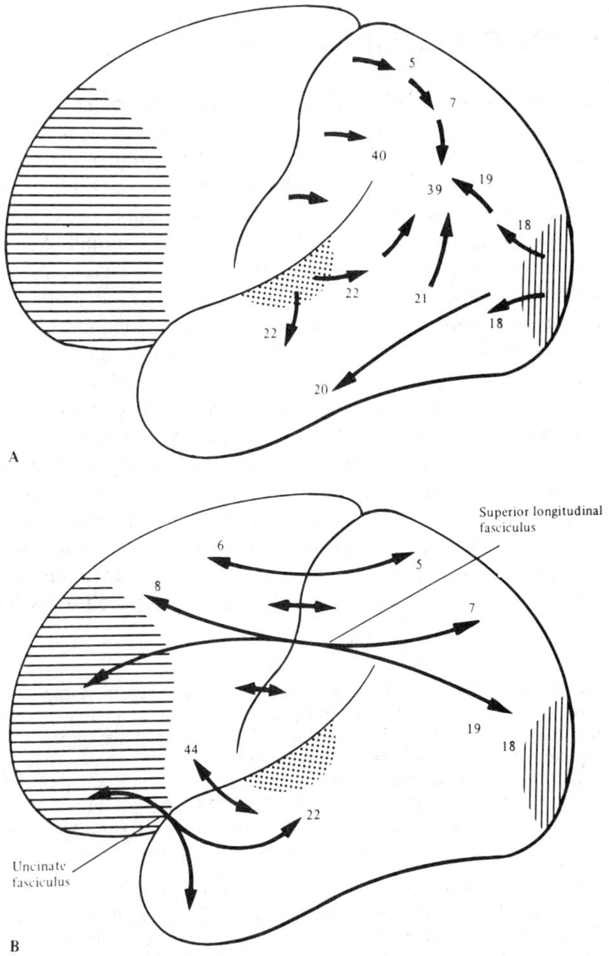

FIGURE 1.3-4. *Association pathways.* A. *Schematic diagram showing sequential processing of sensory information. Reciprocal connections to sensory areas are not shown.* B. *Examples of short and long association fibers providing the anatomical substrate for specific interactions between different cortical areas. (From Heimer L:* The Human Brain and Spinal Cord. *Springer-Verlag, New York, 1983, with permission.)*

feature of the divergence centers around the fact that each sensory association area may also send projections to a common cortical area where multimodal convergence occurs. Thus, it is fair to state that the major targets of sensory association area projections are the frontal cortex, the cortex of the limbic lobe, and multimodal areas located in the frontal, parietal, and temporal lobes. This entire sequence of projections has been referred to as the feed-forward system of cortical connections, and it is complemented by a feedback system of connections.

HIPPOCAMPAL CORTEX Connections of the hippocampus have been implicated as a pathological focus in global amnesias that are due to direct trauma or to the rather more occult processes that result in primary degenerative dementia of the Alzheimer type. Complex information from the limbic lobe, multimodal, and frontal lobe areas project to the entorhinal periallocortex, which projects in turn to the allocortex that forms the hippocampal formation. Numerous intrinsic connections link the various allocortical fields of the hippocampus together and to the subicular portion of the hippocampus. The hippocampus, including subiculum, projects to the septum, and the subiculum provides additional outputs to amygdala, nucleus accumbens, anterior thalamus, and mamillary bodies. Finally, the subiculum provides associative connections back to the limbic lobe and frontal cortical areas. The entorhinal cortex, in particular, relays this output to nearly the entire cortical mantle.

BASAL FOREBRAIN SYSTEMS

STRIATOPALLIDAL SYSTEM

It has only recently been appreciated that the striatopallidal system extends ventrally in mammals to include the *nucleus accumbens, olfactory tubercle,* and *rostral* portions of *substantia innominata* (Figs. 1.3-5 and 1.3-6). These areas process inputs from allocortical areas in much the same way that the dorsal striatopallidal system processes neocortical input. In the following discussion, the term "striatopallidal system" generally refers to both the *dorsal* and *ventral striatum,* as well as to the *dorsal* and *ventral pallidum*. In addition, the *subthalamic nucleus* and the *substantia nigra* are so closely related to the striatopallidal system that they are usually included as integral parts. The *pars reticulata* of substantia nigra, in particular, shares several features in common with the internal segment of the globus pallidus and in some respects may be treated as an extension of the internal segment; some significant differences, which are considered below, do occur, however. Altogether, the striatum, globus pallidus, subthalamic nucleus, and substantia nigra are alternatively referred to as the *basal ganglia*.

Structure The most common neuron in the striatum is medium-sized with four to seven primary dendrites and a relatively large number of secondary dendrites densely covered with spines in a typical "bottle brush" appearance; these account for more than 90 percent of the cells in the striatum, and they are the principal projection neurons of the striatum. Of the other cell types found within the striatum, the large cholinergic interneurons are most worthy of note; they are more or less evenly dispersed among the "medium spiny neurons."

Pallidal neurons are relatively large, fusiform cells with two to four long, thick, radiating dendrites containing few, if any, spines. These neurons have large, disk-shaped dendritic arborizations oriented perpendicular to striatal axons, so that each neuron may interact with large numbers of incoming axons. Despite the tremendous convergence of input on pallidal neurons, it has been shown that the topography of the various cortical areas appears to be roughly represented within the pallidum and its output. Since the striatum appears to have few, if any, long intrinsic horizontal association pathways, cortical output effectively terminates in vertical striatal columns, whose base may be approximated by the dendritic radius of individual pallidal neurons.

Input-output relations of the striatopallidal system The most significant afferents to the striatum are undoubtedly from the cortex. The entire cortex projects almost directly to underlying terminal zones in striatum. Somatomotor areas, for example, project primarily to putamen, whereas association areas primarily reach the caudate. Projections from allocortex (i.e., hippocampus and olfactory cortex) reach ventral striatal territories (i.e., the nucleus accumbens and olfactory tubercle, respectively). The cortex-like basolateral complex of the amygdala, discussed below, also sends afferents to striatum, projecting most densely to ventral striatum. Many of the *corticostriatal* projections may be collaterals of cells projecting to other subcortical targets. Association areas typically project to more than one area of striatum. These areas appear to be organized along functional lines, inasmuch as related cortical areas sharing reciprocal projections seem to terminate in the same locality within striatum but not necessarily on the same neuron.

The *thalamostriatal* projections are another important source of striatal input. The intralaminar nuclei (including some midline nuclei) project topographically in a continuous fashion to both dorsal and ventral striatum, and at least some of these axons may be collaterals of axons projecting to cortex.

STRIATAL COMPARTMENTS AND CHANNELS Although the ubiquity of the medium spiny neuron gives a somewhat homogenous appearance to the striatum in Nissl stains, recent studies using histochemistry, tract tracing, and receptor binding have disclosed a compartmentalization of the striatum (Fig. 1.3-7) that seems to depend on the discontinuous distribution of striatal afferents and on the clustering of projection neurons.

Several experiments with rats indicate that striatal input from prefrontal cortex and from the remainder of cortex appears to be channeled into two distinct striatofugal pathways. In the first instance, terminations from prefrontal cortex end on striatal cells projecting to *pars compacta* substantia nigra. These striatal cells are found within enkephalinergic receptor-rich "patches." In contrast, cortical afferents from the remaining areas of cortex terminate preferentially in "matrix" (nonpatch) areas of striatum on striatal neurons that project to *pars reticulata* substantia nigra. It is important to point out that the patches of enkephalin receptors do not coincide with striatal areas that are typically dense when immunostained for enkephalin; they may be complementary. The result of the channeling of output to pars compacta or pars reticulata seems to be that inputs from prefrontal cortex can affect the firing of large areas of striatum by means of their input on the origin of the nigrostriatal pathway. The second channel affects motor output more directly through striatal cells that project directly to globus pallidus and the pars reticulata substantia nigra. Although these channels have a degree of independence, there may also be some interchannel communication provided by somatostatinergic or cholinergic interneurons, or both. The channeling of striatal output is attractive in that it provides a functional rationale for the existence of striatal compartments, but it is based mainly on experiments in rats. It will be important to see whether such systematic channeling of impulses can be confirmed in primates.

PALLIDOFUGAL PATHWAYS The *external* pallidal segment projects rather massively to the subthalamic nucleus, to the *internal* pallidal segment, and to pars reticulata substantia nigra as well. The internal segment of the pallidum and pars reticulata substantia nigra appear to be the major output points for information processed by the basal ganglia. Both project to brain stem motor areas and to the thalamus, which provides feedback to premotor and supplementary motor cortex. The pars reticulata, in addition, sends collateral projections to the deeper layers of superior colliculus, providing an input to tectal cells that are important in the control of visual orientation. The output to the thalamus seems to be topographic; that is, rostrodorsal internal pallidum and rostromedial pars reticulata substantia nigra, which receive afferents from the caudate, project to the ventral anterior nucleus of the thalamus. The caudoventral pallidum and caudolateral pars reticulata, which receive afferents from putamen, project to the ventral lateral nucleus. The *pallidothalamic* projection also includes some axons that terminate in the centromedian and centrolateral nuclei. The internal pallidal segment additionally sends afferents to the habenular nuclei, particularly to the lateral parts; these projections arise from a population of neurons independent of those projecting to thalamus and brain stem. Although, most commonly, the output of pallidal areas has been analyzed in terms of its transthalamic feedback to motor cortex, it is important to realize that

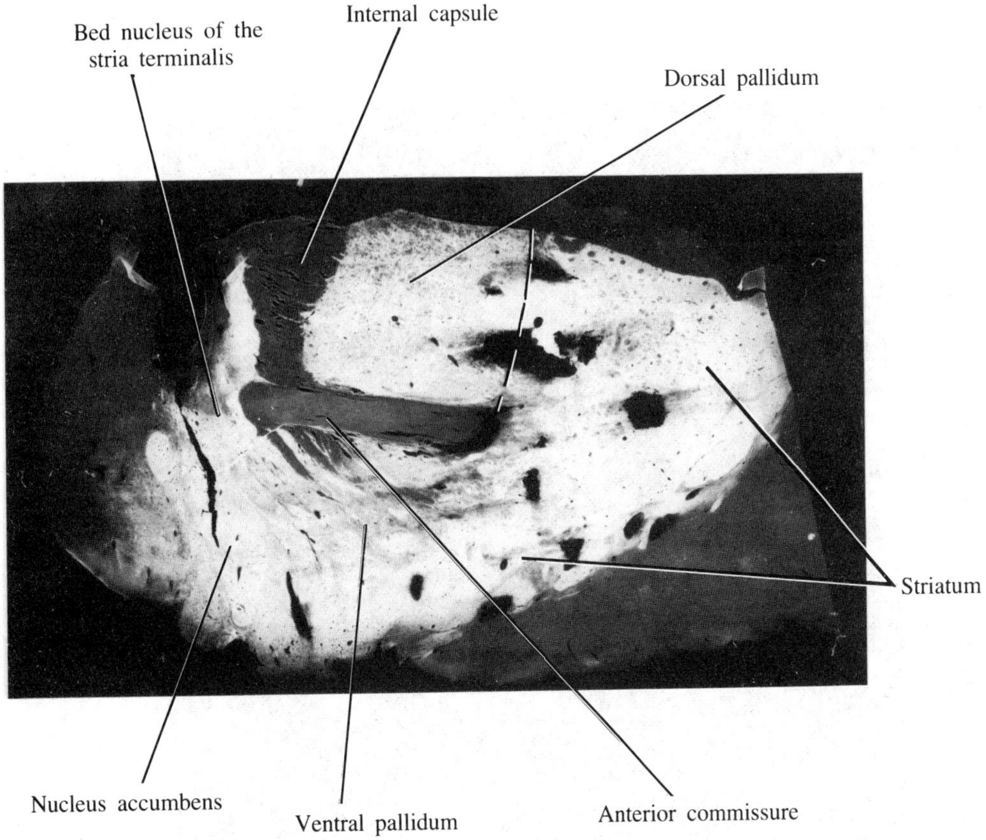

FIGURE 1.3-5. *Acetylcholinesterase-stained adult human brain showing ventral extension of striatum that reaches the base of the brain. Dark field from direct print of brain section. (Courtesy of H R Brashear, Departments of Neurology and Behavioral Medicine and Psychiatry, University of Virginia, Charlottesville.)*

double-labeling experiments have shown that a large percentage of neurons that project to thalamus also send a collateral axon to the brain stem. The implication is that the same information reaches both areas, and it is not necessary for striatopallidal information to go through cortex in order to affect movement.

VENTRAL STRIATUM Information seems to flow through ventral striatum in a fashion similar to that generally described for the dorsal striatum. The cortical input to the ventral striatum originates in allocortex (hippocampus and olfactory cortex) and also in association areas in the frontal and temporal lobes, as well as in the cortex-like basolateral complex of the amygdala. Ventral striatum, in turn, projects to the ventral pallidum. Significant differences, however, seem to exist between dorsal and ventral pallidofugal pathways. The majority of ventral pallidal projections reach the mediodorsal thalamus rather than the ventral thalamic complex. The mediodorsal thalamus, in turn, projects to prefrontal cortex, including the anterior cingulate area. In the rat, ventral pallidal projections have also been reported to reach the brain stem, although this pathway does not appear to be as substantial as that from dorsal portions of the pallidum. Moreover, this projection has not yet been demonstrated in the primate.

Ventral striatal projections from nucleus accumbens also reach the dopamine cells in the ventral tegmentum as well as cells in pars compacta of substantia nigra; however, few striatal projections, if any, seem to reach the substantia nigra from the medium-sized cells of the olfactory tubercle.

Striatal side loops and modifiers The striatopallidal system is characterized by a large number of feedback pathways or *side loops*. The subthalamic nucleus receives a massive projection from the lateral pallidal segment that it reciprocates while, in addition, it sends collaterals to both the medial pallidal segment and the pars reticulata substantia nigra. The reciprocal connections of the subthalamic nucleus with pallidal areas include at least some portions of the ventral pallidum. The subthalamic nucleus also receives direct excitatory afferents from motor and premotor cortex, in contrast to the inhibitory input it receives from the external pallidal segment.

The well-known dopaminergic *nigrostriatal* pathway is perhaps best characterized as a feedback to striatum from striatonigral axons synapsing on pars compacta cells. Pars compacta, however, does receive a variety of extrastriatal inputs, including those from the midbrain raphe and tegmentum, and possibly from hypothalamus. To a degree, the dopaminergic projection originating in the ventral tegmentum provides feedback to ventral striatum, reciprocating afferents from nucleus accumbens, which projects to pars compacta substantia nigra as well. However, the projections of the ventral tegmental dopamine cells are more widespread than just to ventral striatum and include prefrontal cortex as well as the extended amygdala and entorhinal cortex. The serotonergic neurons described below provide an important input to striatum that originates in the dorsal raphe. This might be considered a modifying striatal input because the elaborate branching pattern of the serotonin projections suggests that little in the way of a point-to-point transfer of information can occur. In contrast to the remainder of basal forebrain, the striatum is almost devoid of noradrenergic input. The exception to this is the medial portion of nucleus accumbens, which may represent a mixed zone of ventral striatum and extended amygdala, as will be discussed below.

AMYGDALA The amygdala is important in emotional behavior and learning. Few neurobiologists would disagree with this often-used statement, but few would have felt comfortable expanding on this premise until recently, because the amygdala has been rather reluctant to yield its secrets. At

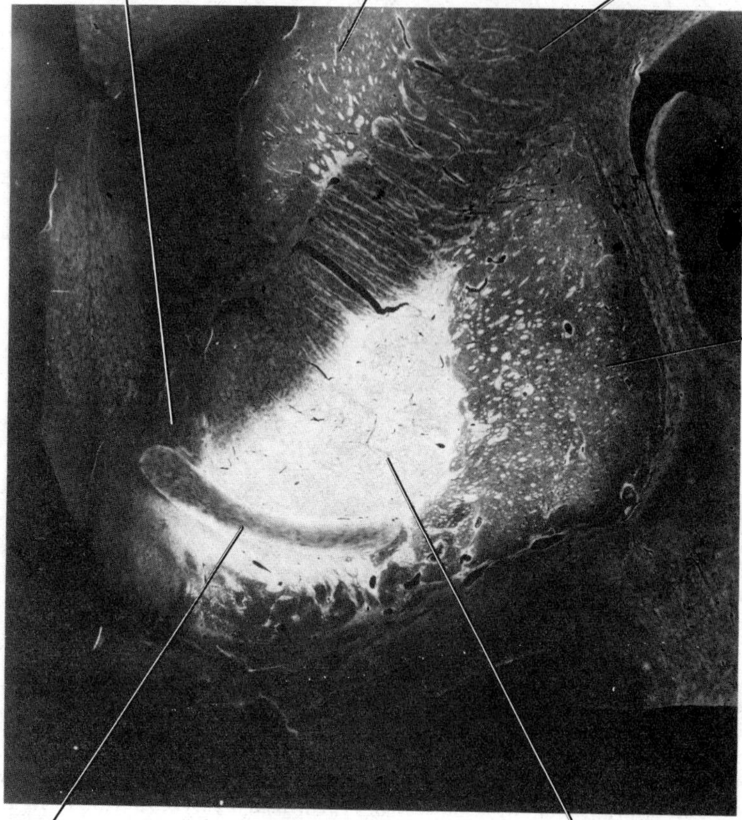

FIGURE 1.3-6. *Iron stain of adult human brain, showing the globus pallidus and its subcommissural extension (ventral pallidum). It should be noted that the ventral pallidum and ventral striatum (Figs. 1.3-5 and 1.3-11) occupy a large proportion of what has been termed the rostral part of substantia innominata; the caudal or sublenticular substantia innominata is, in general, occupied by the extended amygdala (see text and Figs. 1.3-9 and 1.3-11). Dark field from direct print of brain section. (Courtesy of R C Switzer III, Departments of Pathology and Medical Biology, University of Tennessee, Knoxville.)*

least one major impediment to research in this part of the basal forebrain is the complex array of subnuclei that constitute the amygdala. However, the situation has improved dramatically within the past decade; two lines of anatomical research have helped to regroup these nuclei in more manageable form.

Basolateral complex The basolateral complex of the amygdala, which in humans includes the *lateral, basolateral,* and *basal accessory* nuclei, functions in many respects as a cortical area. This was appreciated by earlier anatomists; for example, in 1941, Crosby and Humphrey termed the basolateral complex a *vicarious cortex* that is "comparable to the surface pallium except that it has a periventricular position and lacks the laminae characteristic of fully developed cortex." Although it is neither superficial nor laminated, it shares many features with cortical areas. For example, the principal output neurons of the basolateral complex appear to be pyramidal in form, and interneurons within the basolateral complex also resemble at least some of the stellate cells of cortex. Fusiform cholinergic interneurons that are indistinguishable from those in cortex have been observed in rats. The basolateral complex has reciprocal connections with other areas of cortex, most notably with temporal polar, insular, and prefrontal cortices. As with other areas of cortex, the basolateral complex sends direct projections to striatum, innervating zones similar to that of prefrontal cortex, and presumably using glutamate-aspartate as a neurotransmitter in this projection. The basolateral complex, like the cerebral cortex, receives a projection from both the cholinergic and noncholinergic corticopetal basal forebrain system of neurons. The basolateral complex does provide important input to the remainder of amygdala, but so do the other areas of cortex with which it is most closely related.

Extended amygdala A second line of research has resulted in a reevaluation of the *centromedial amygdala.* Biochemically, morphologically, and hodologically, the *bed nucleus of the stria terminalis* and centromedial amygdala are closely related. It has been observed recently that the centromedial amygdala forms one end of a larger structure, which is continuous through the caudal or *sublenticular substantia innominata* with the bed nucleus of the stria terminalis. For convenience, this larger structure may be termed the "extended amygdala." Within the extended amygdala two major subdivisions may be readily discriminated. A *central subdivision* consists of the central amygdaloid nucleus and its continuation through substantia

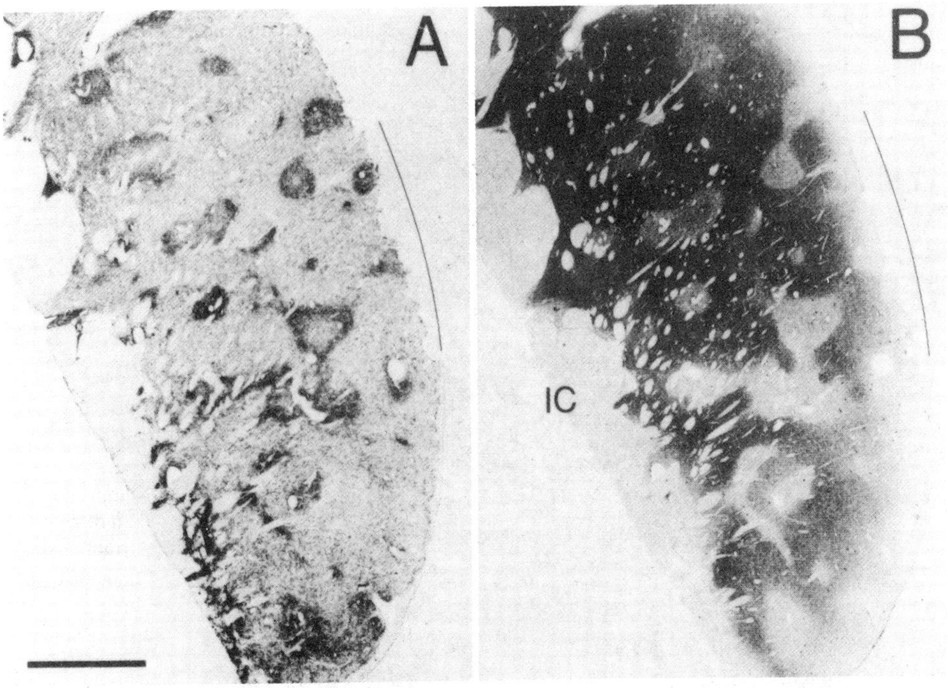

FIGURE 1.3-7. *Adult human striatum. Illustrating compartmental distribution of enkephalin immunoreactivity* (A) *which matches acetylcholinesterase poor striosomes (shown in* B*).* A *and* B *are from serially adjacent sections. (From Graybiel A M: Neurochemically specified subsystems in the basal ganglia. In* Functions of the Basal Ganglia. *Ciba Foundation Symposium 107, p 114. D Evered, M O'Conner, editors. Pitman, London, 1984, with permission.)*

innominata into the lateral part of the bed nucleus of the stria terminalis. A *medial subdivision* includes the medial amygdaloid nucleus and its continuation in substantia innominata into the medial part of the bed nucleus of stria terminalis. Both subdivisions also include path neurons along the dorsal course of the stria terminalis.

Afferents to both divisions of the extended amygdala arrive from the dopamine, norepinephrine, and serotonergic cells in the brain stem, but these terminations appear to be more dense within the central division. Both divisions of the extended amygdala also provide afferents to the corticopetal neuronal complex of the basal forebrain, with the most dense projection arising from the central amygdaloid group.

NUCLEUS ACCUMBENS AND EXTENDED AMYGDALA The nucleus accumbens, which is continuous with the rostral part of the bed nucleus of stria terminalis caudomedially (Fig. 1.3-8) and with the putamen and caudate nucleus dorsolaterally, may be related to the extended amygdala as well as to striatum. The medial portions of this nucleus, in particular, apparently include hypothalamic and brain stem projecting cells that are not typical of striatum in general but are quite characteristic of the extended amygdala. Biochemically, the nucleus accumbens also appears more similar to extended amygdala than to the rest of striatum. For example, norepinephrine concentrations are an order of magnitude greater in nucleus accumbens than in the remainder of striatum, and the same may be said for a variety of neuropeptides. On the other hand, both the medial and lateral portions of nucleus accumbens apparently project to ventral pallidum.

With the data presently available it is difficult to formulate a simple model of the relationships among striatum, amygdala, and accumbens, and it therefore may be reasonable to consider the nucleus accumbens as a mixed area of striatal and amygdaloid elements until more information becomes available about its detailed synaptology.

CONNECTIONS OF THE CENTRAL DIVISION OF EXTENDED AMYGDALA The central subdivision of the extended amygdala is best characterized by its reciprocal connections with brain stem viscerosensory and visceromotor areas, such as the nucleus of the solitary tract, the dorsal motor nucleus of the vagus, and the parabrachial nuclei. The descending projections include those to somatomotor areas, including the lateral reticular formation, as well as projections to the cervical spinal cord. The central amygdaloid division also sends efferents to the medial, and especially the lateral hypothalamus, perhaps via collaterals of descending projections. In general, the hypothalamus reciprocates these projections.

Cortical afferents arrive at the central division of the extended amygdala from the limbic lobe, including projections not only from olfactory cortex and posterior parahippocampal gyrus but also from orbitofrontal cortex and insular cortex. The basolateral amygdaloid complex, in addition, provides a massive input to the central division of the extended amygdala.

A variety of thalamic afferents reach the central division of extended amygdala particularly from the midline nuclei. Sensory information, however, may directly enter the central division. For example, the *medial geniculate* sends terminals directly to the central division, at least in rats, and this acoustic information is vital to the formation of classically conditioned emotional responses to auditory stimuli.

Intrinsic connections of the central division are quite striking; injections of anterograde or retrograde tracers within this complex label terminals or cells, respectively, throughout the remainder of the central division (Fig. 1.3-9), suggesting an unusual degree of internal association connections.

CONNECTIONS OF THE MEDIAL DIVISION OF EXTENDED AMYGDALA The medial subdivision is best characterized by its reciprocal connections with the medial "endocrine" hypothalamus, including medial preoptic area, paraventricular hypothalamic area, ventromedial hypothalamus, and premammillary nuclei. Direct cortical afferents also reach the medial division of extended amygdala, although these are less extensive than those arriving at the central division. These include projections from the limbic lobe (including olfactory cortex), hippocampus, and insular cortex.

SEPTUM The *septum verum* is an oblique pyramid of gray matter, with the base of the pyramid resting on the anterior commissure; the apex is formed by the columns of the fornix. The septum is reciprocally connected to the hippocampus and is continuous rostroventrally with the diagonal band. It receives input not only from the hippocampus but also from the hypothalamus and amygdala, as well as from monoamine cell

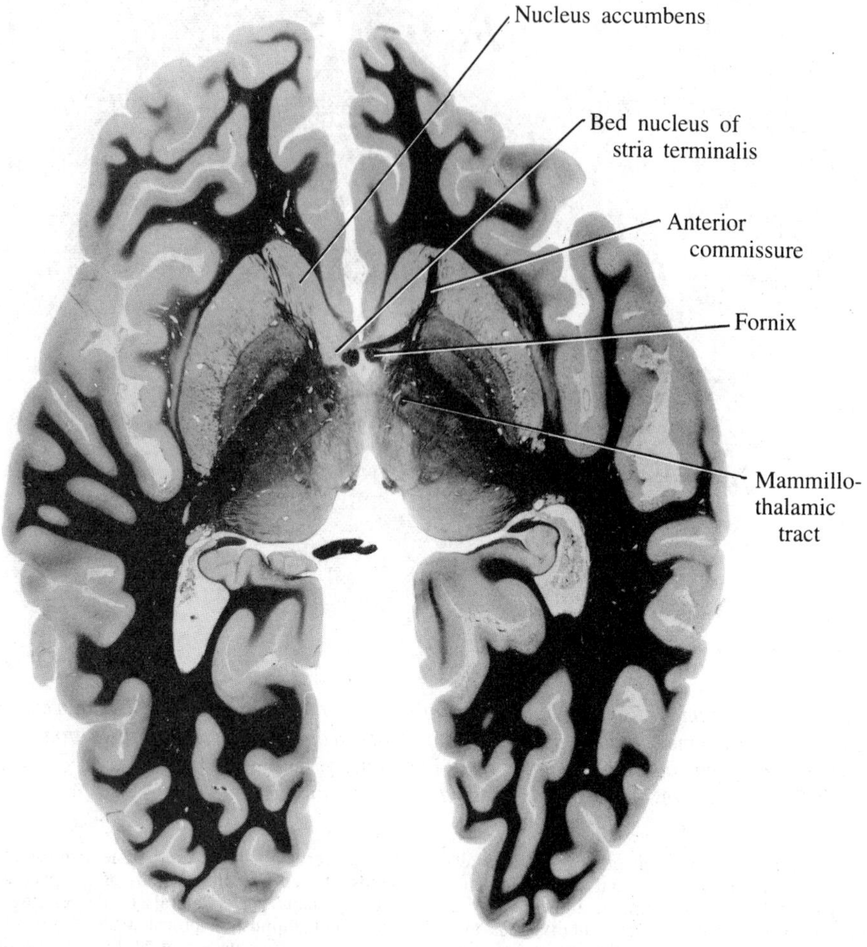

FIGURE 1.3-8. *Horizontal section of human brain through bed nucleus of the stria terminalis, nucleus accumbens, and putamen. Note that nucleus accumbens is contiguous with both the striatum and bed nucleus. (From the Yakovlev collection, with permission.)*

groups in the brain stem. The septal nuclei project to a variety of targets in hypothalamus and brain stem.

The *subfornical organ,* which is located underneath the ventrally coursing fornix fibers where it faces the ventricle, may also be included within the septal group in that it is interconnected with the septum verum and contains neurons that contribute to hypothalamic and subthalamic projections. It has a particularly rich set of efferent connections, including projections to the medial preoptic area, the paraventricular and supraoptic nuclei, the lateral hypothalamic area, and the zona incerta, as well as the extended amygdala and apparently the frontal cortex. The subfornical organ has been convincingly implicated in the initiation of drinking in response to circulating angiotensin II, and may be involved in other, nonbehavioral aspects of cardiovascular regulation.

BASAL FOREBRAIN CORTICOPETAL NEURONS

The *corticopetal basal forebrain system* was first identified by means of retrograde studies as a loose aggregation of neurons extending from the medial septum and diagonal-band nuclei caudally through the substantia innominata. This system also extends dorsally as scattered pockets of cells at the mediodorsal edge of the globus pallidus within and adjacent to the internal capsule, and in ventral parts of the internal and external medullary lamina of the globus pallidus. In the primate, this system includes, but is not limited to, the cells condensed into the prominent *basal nucleus of Meynert.* It was soon realized that the major portion of these cells use acetylcholine as a transmitter and that they account for a significant proportion of the cholinergic terminals in cortex. A loss of cholinergic activity, as measured by a decrease in the synthetic enzyme choline acetyltransferase, was one of the few metabolic abnormalities measurable in the postmortem brains of patients with primary degenerative dementia of the Alzheimer type, thus, there has been an intense research effort to understand the details of this corticopetal projection and its relations with the rest of the brain. As a result, the topography of the corticopetal projection is rather well known (Fig. 1.3-10), although the afferents to this system have proved more difficult to establish with certainty.

The fact that this neuronal group seems to cross several traditionally defined nuclear areas supports the view that afferents to the cholinergic cells are quite heterogeneous and dependent on the particular zone in which the cells are found. For example, the distribution of the cholinergic corticopetal cells overlaps both the dorsal and ventral pallidal areas and is intermingled or adjacent to the extended amygdala (Fig. 1.3-11). Hence, the cholinergic corticopetal cells may be closely related to either or both of these systems.

Although most authors have focused on the cholinergic portions of the corticopetal system, it is clear that not all the neurons in the extended aggregation of corticopetal cells use acetylcholine as a transmitter. The proportion of noncholinergic cells varies somewhat from area to area, with estimates as high as 90 percent of the cells projecting to neocortex using acetylcholine as a transmitter; a much lower proportion of cells projecting to allocortical targets are cholinergic. Not only has GABA been identified as an important noncholinergic transmitter in at least part of the corticopetal system, but it seems that somatostatin neurons are involved as well.

Given the fact that noncholinergic corticopetal cells are intermingled or adjacent to the cholinergic projection neurons of basal forebrain throughout much of their extent, it is perhaps somewhat premature to consider the cholinergic corticopetal cell group as an independent entity. The noncholinergic forebrain projection neurons seem to favor so-called limbic cortical areas in comparison with the cholinergic neurons, but their terminals overlap considerably, especially in areas, such as the hippocampus, olfactory cortex, and basolateral complex of the amygdala.

Finally, although the cortical projections from basal forebrain have received most of the attention, several recent reports have indicated that the cholinergic cells in this complex may also send projections to the mediodorsal and reticular nuclei of the thalamus, as well as to brain stem targets.

FUNCTIONAL CONSIDERATIONS Parallel processing in basal forebrain systems The striatopallidal system, extended amygdala, and septum appear to be quite different structures, especially in terms of their efferent pathways. However, it is interesting to note that there are superficial similarities in the synaptic processing of cortical information by the septum, striatopallidal system, and the central divisions of the extended amygdala (Fig. 1.3-12). In general, the cortical afferents to these structures appear to terminate on

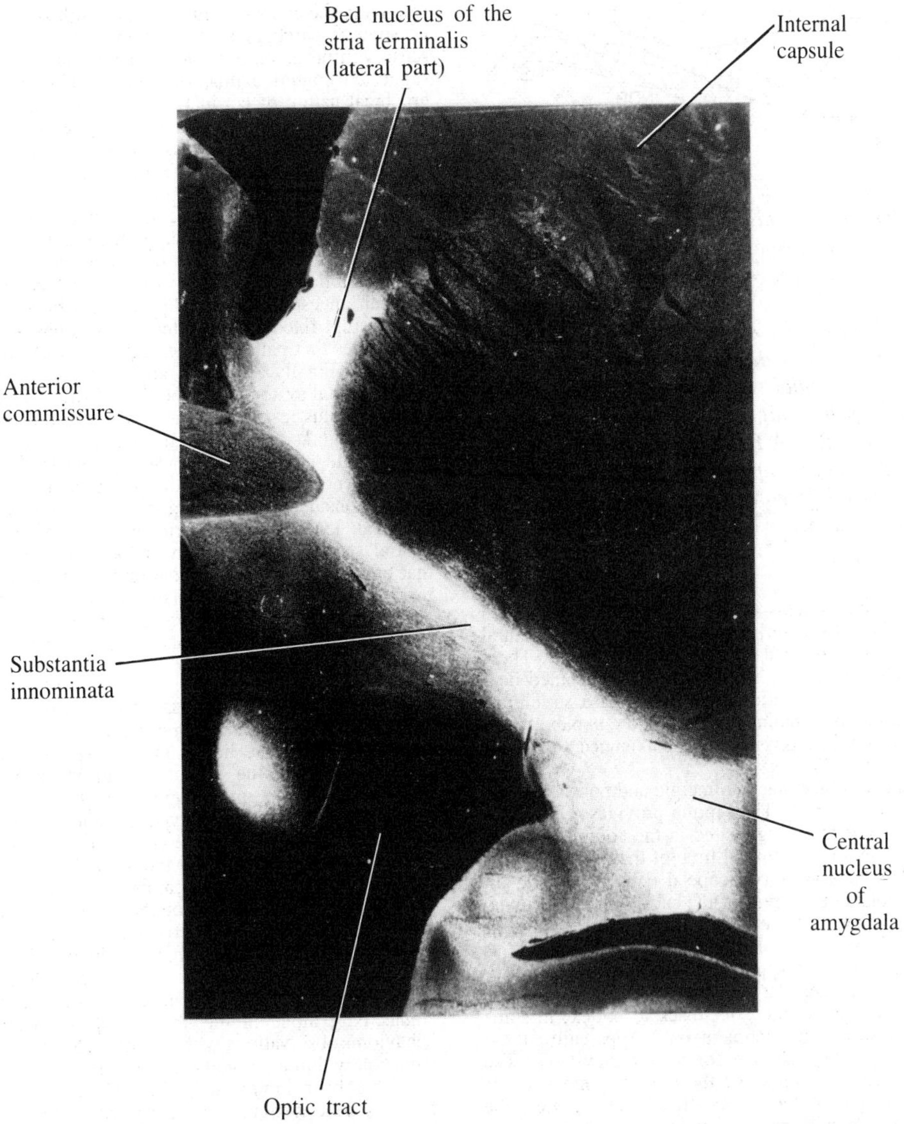

FIGURE 1.3-9. *Central division of extended amygdala. The entire extent of the central division of extended amygdala is labeled by an injection of ^{3}H-amino acids in the central amygdaloid nucleus. Dark-field autoradiograph. (Courtesy of G Van Hoesen.)*

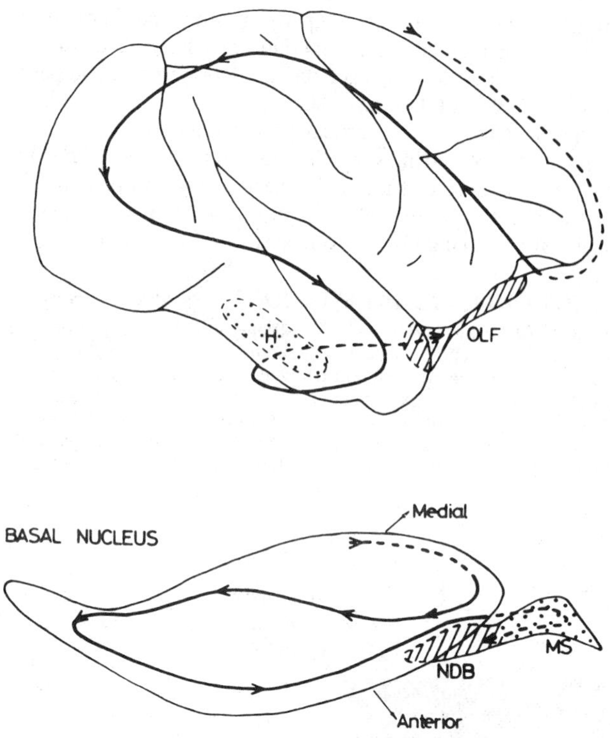

FIGURE 1.3-10. *Corticopetal basal forebrain projection system. Schematic diagram of projections from basal forebrain to cortex. The arrowheads are at corresponding points on each figure. In the cortex the allocortex of the hippocampus is shown by filled circles and the olfactory area by hatching. The same symbols are used in the diagram of the basal nucleus: hippocampus* (H); *medial septal nucleus* (MS); *nucleus of the horizontal limb of the diagonal band* (NDB); *olfactory allocortex* (OLF). *(From R C A Pearson, K C Gatter, T P S Powell: The cortical relationships of certain basal ganglia and the cholinergic basal forebrain nuclei. Brain Res* 261: *327, 1983, with permission.)*

medium-sized neurons that possess densely spiny dendrites. Such cells are located in the lateral septum, in lateral portions of the central subdivision of the extended amygdala, as well as in striatum. These cells, in turn, project to large cells with long sparsely spined dendrites that appear to be the main efferent cells for these structures. These are found in the medial septum-diagonal band complex, in the medial portions of the central subdivisions of the extended amygdala, and in the globus pallidus.

All of these areas seem to innervate cholinergic and noncholinergic cells providing feedback to cortex. The septum provides efferents to hippocampopetal neurons loosely aggregated in the complex formed by cells in the medial septum and vertical limb of the diagonal band. The extended amygdala innervates corticopetal cells within the diagonal band and the sublenticular areas of the substantia innominata. Whereas in primates the evidence for afferents to corticopetal cells from the striatopallidal system is slight, in nonprimates afferents from dorsal and ventral striatum appear to reach peripallidal corticopetal neurons. In subprimates, large cholinergic cells within the striatum itself appear to provide minor feedback to cortex, in some cases as collaterals of striatal projecting axons. Apparently, these ascending feedback loops are important for all three systems. The majority of the cholinergic feedback for the striatum, however, is targeted closer to the ouput of the corticostriatal system (i.e., the medium spiny neuron). Seen from this perspective, cognitive and motor functions of the forebrain may be modified by similar synaptic-neurotransmitter mechanisms. These are differentiated mainly by the level at which feedback affects behavioral plasticity.

Several other pathways seem to have parallels within these subcortical systems. The septum, extended amygdala, and striatum all appear to reciprocate connections with the dopamine cells of the tegmentum, although dorsal and ventral striatum receive the most dense dopamine terminations. In addition, the septum, striatopallidal system, and extended amygdala all receive serotonergic inputs from the brain stem; in contrast, significant noradrenergic inputs reach only the septum and extended amygdala. Both the septum and especially the extended amygdala also appear to have a greater variety of neuropeptide-containing cells and processes than does the striatum.

Striatopallidal functions The basal ganglia are best known for their motor functions; dysfunction of specific parts of the basal ganglia circuits may result in typical motor diseases, such as parkinsonism, Huntington's chorea, and hemiballismus. In parkinsonism, which is a consequence of dopamine depletion subsequent to dopamine cell loss in the substantia nigra, the major negative signs include akinesia and deficits in postural adjustments; however, in chorea, which involves direct damage to the striatum, or in hemiballismus, which results from damage to the subthalamic nucleus, movements are gated inappropriately.

Although clinical as well as physiological observations have led to the formulation of a role for the striatopallidal system in motor planning or in the initiation of movement, the exact role of the basal ganglia in the control of movement is still controversial. Most recently, some researchers have suggested that the basal ganglia act to gate sensory information relevant to movement. Alternatively, others have suggested cognitive functions for striatum. For example, the topographical nature of cortical inputs to striatum indicates that association and sensory areas of cortex may influence the striatum to the same degree as motor areas. The implication is that local areas of striatum should reflect the functions of overlying cortex; some experimental data do support this contention. On the other hand, in 1970, MacLean observed that the striatum is a well-conserved structure among vertebrates and suggested that it may function as part of a "reptilian brain" dedicated to functions, such as the rather more fixed and unemotional behavioral patterns that perhaps characterized our reptilian ancestors. Striatal lesions in submammalian species do, in fact, disrupt fixed action patterns, and it has been demonstrated even in primates that pallidal lesions interfere with species-specific display behavior. Finally, Mishkin and co-workers have argued that the striatopallidal system could be the substrate for learned motor habits. Such stimulus-response rather than stimulus-stimulus learning persists in patients with bilateral temporal lobectomies, who otherwise demonstrate global anterograde amnesia for cognitive tasks.

The ventral portion of the striatopallidal system may deserve special consideration with regard to the cognitive aspects of learning. Although some animal experiments support a role for portions of the ventral striatopallidal system in locomotor behavior, it is also true that one of the most prominent targets of the ventral pallidum is the mediodorsal thalamus. This latter nucleus has been implicated as the site of pathology in patients suffering from anterograde amnesia either as the result of Korsakoff's syndrome or from focal thalamic damage.

Limbic system and basal forebrain Both the septum and amygdala are included within current definitions of the *limbic system*. MacLean defines the limbic system (see Section 1.2) as the limbic lobe of cortex and the structures with which they have primary connections (e.g., septum, amygdala, and anterior thalamus), whereas others have identified the hypothalamus as the focus of the limbic system. Nauta and Domesick also have discussed a "limbic striatum" consisting, in particular, of the striatal areas receiving input from basolateral amygdala, hippocampus, and frontal cortex and from the ventral tegmental group of dopamine cells. The value in identifying a "limbic circuit" certainly derives from the goal of describing functional-anatomical systems that are involved in the phenomena of learning and emotion. However, it is not clear that this aim is furthered by a too generous inclusion of anatomical structures based on connectivity alone in the absence of behavioral data or based on behavioral observations without adequate anatomical justification for inclusion within a particular system. In this section, the term "limbic lobe" has been limited to the allocortical and periallocortical structures as described in the survey given in Section 1.2. The term "limbic system" is not used, in preference to anatomically defined structures that are characterized by similar afferent and efferent projections, as well as basically parallel steps for intrinsic synaptic processing of information.

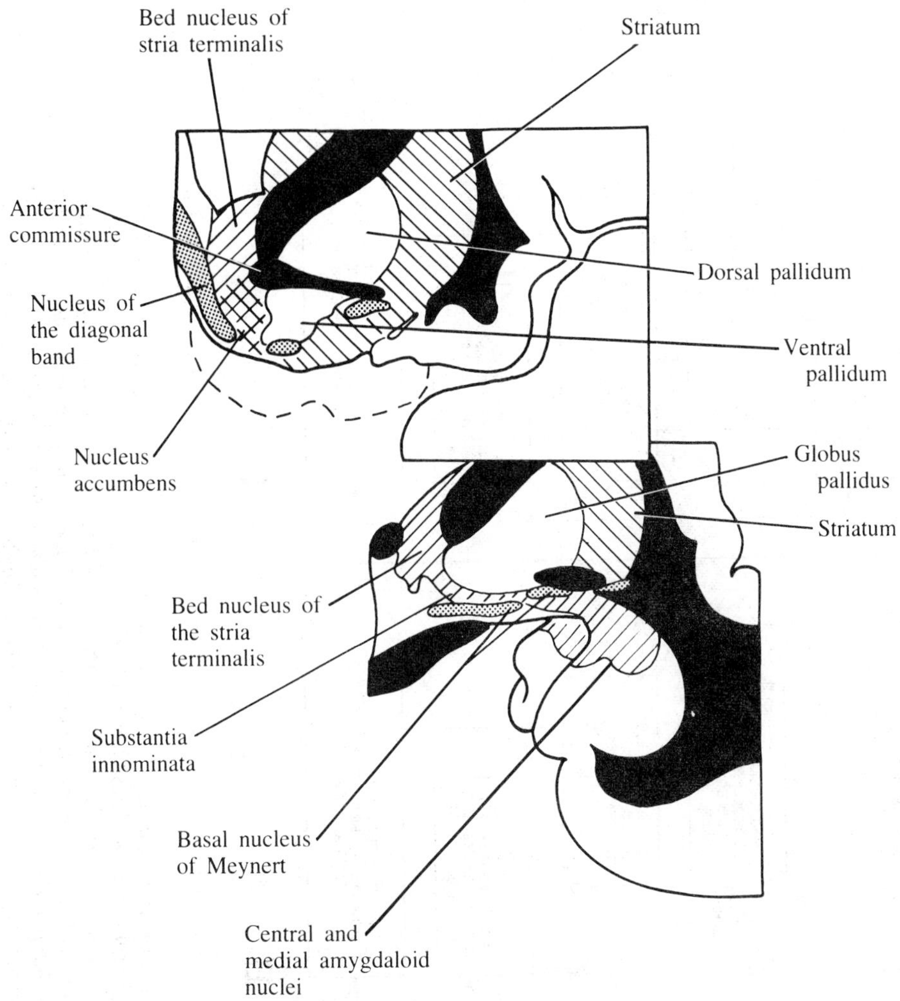

FIGURE 1.3-11. *Three basal forebrain systems. Schematic diagram of the relationship among the striatum \\\\\\, globus pallidus, "extended amygdala" /////, and cholinergic cells of the corticopetal basal forebrain system (stippled). Note that the area of the nucleus accumbens is a possible intermixed zone of ventral striatum and extended amygdala.*

Basal forebrain systems in memory The hippocampus has long been a focus of studies on human learning since the very dramatic demonstrations that bilateral hippocampal damage results in global anterograde amnesia. This result has been difficult to duplicate in animal experiments, in that global memory deficits have not been observed after bilateral hippocampectomy. In contrast, specific memory deficits in place or spatial learning have been found, as well as evidence for individual hippocampal neurons that fire phasically with respect to place cues. As a consequence, O'Keefe and Nadel, in 1978, proposed that the hippocampus may function as a cognitive map. Recently, however, Mishkin and co-workers have argued that global memory deficits, at least for cognitive tasks, could be obtained by combined hippocampal and amygdala lesions. Furthermore, lesions of the hippocampus alone produced more pronounced effects in spatial learning tasks while amygdalar lesions resulted in losses in cross-modal learning tasks.

In terms of basal forebrain anatomical structures, the basolateral complex of the amygdala is the recipient of connections from a wide variety of sensory association areas and therefore could provide a "cortical" substrate for cross-modal learning. In addition, both the hippocampus and basolateral complex provide important afferents to the extended amygdala. Thus not only would these important polysensory "cortical areas" be absent following combined hippocampal and amygdala lesions, but also an extensive deafferentation of the extended amygdala would result even when there is no direct damage by temporal lobe resections. This loss, in turn, would alter, if not silence, the output of the extended amygdala to the basal forebrain corticopetal neuronal system, thus disrupting the output of the corticopetal system even for areas of cortex not directly affected by the lesions.

Under normal circumstances the large number of intrinsic association fibers that seem to characterize the central division of extended amygdala and its output to the corticopetal cells of basal forebrain could provide at least one explanation for simultaneous activation of distal areas of cortex during the performance of learned tasks.

Extended amygdala and emotions The extended amygdala seems to be remarkably well equipped to function in integrating emotions with learning. The medial division of the extended amygdala incorporates sexually dimorphic subnuclei in temporal lobe, as well as in portions of the bed nucleus of stria terminalis that extend into anterior hypothalamus. The medial division also appears to be rich in receptors for circulating hormones and by means of its afferents to medial hypothalamus, seems to be particularly well suited to effect psychoendocrine responses to reproductive or stressful stimuli. Along with the central division of the extended amygdala it shares in the innervation of the corticopetal forebrain system; moreover, it sends projections into the central division, thus providing indirect feedback to wide areas of cortex.

The central division of extended amygdala seems more suited to the integration of visceral input with the external world. It also provides an important avenue for the transmission of such information to cortex and to effectors in hypothalamus and brain stem. For example, classically conditioned autonomic or behavioral responses are attenu-

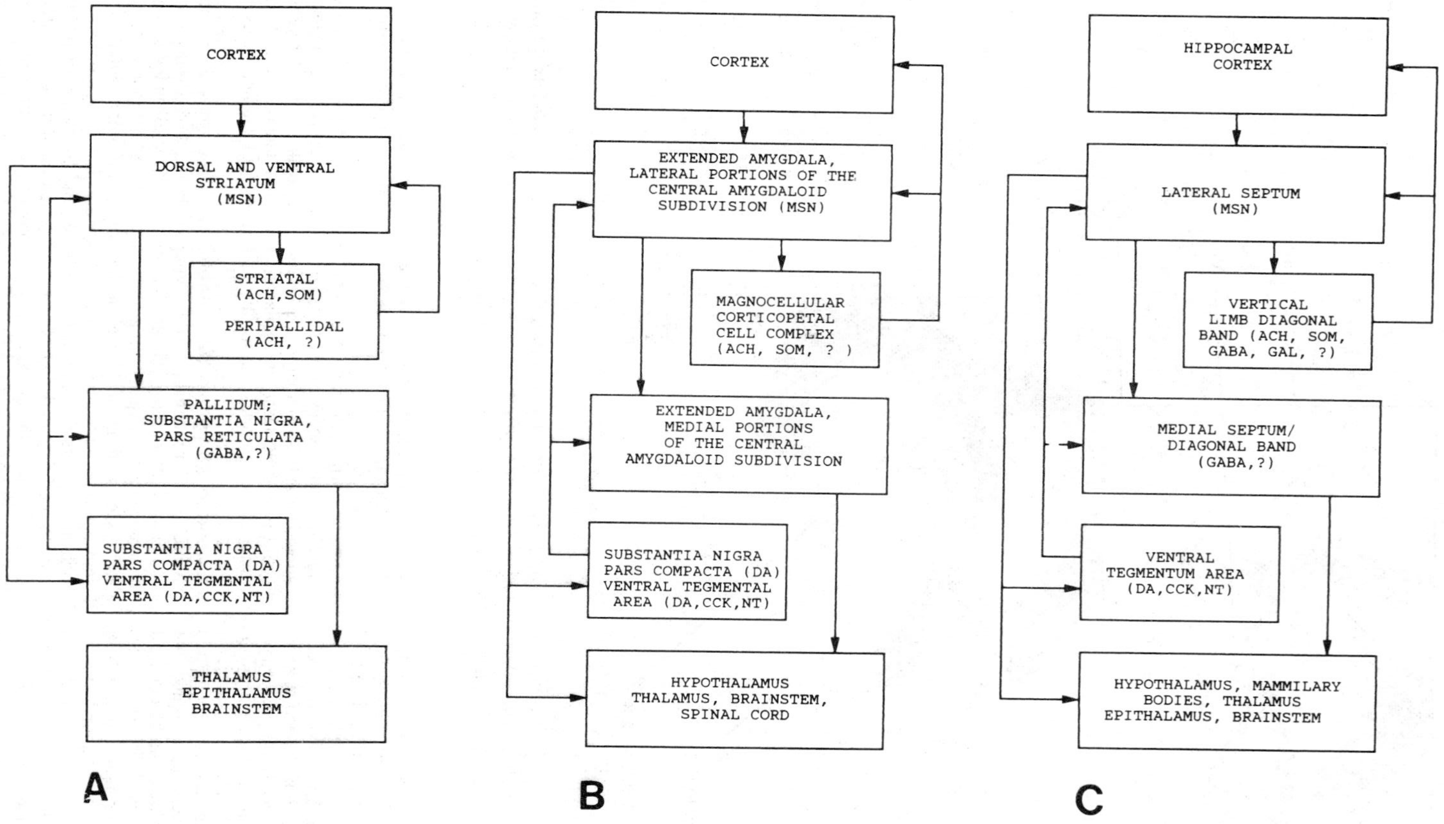

FIGURE 1.3-12. *Parallel processing in basal forebrain. Schematic diagram of parallel pathways in the striatopallidal system (A), the extended amygdala (B), and the septum (C).*

At each level depicted for all three systems, information is processed by cells with similar morphological characteristics. Cortical output is received by medium-sized densely spiny neurons (MSN) and relayed to large output neurons with long sparsely spiny dendrites (in pallidum, in extended amygdala, and in the medial septum-diagonal band complex). Feedback is provided by large neurons with long moderately spiny dendrites (within striatum itself, in the magnocellular corticopetal cell complex, and in the vertical limb of the diagonal band). For the striatopallidal system in primates, this feedback does not appear to reach cortex from the striatal interneurons, although such feedback may result from peripallidal corticopetal cells. Dopaminergic innervation to pallidal areas and to the medial septum-diagonal band complex is rather sparse and is therefore depicted by a broken line. For simplicity, several well-known projections including direct cortical and hippocampal efferents to diencephalon and brain stem are not depicted, nor are ascending afferents from these latter areas (other than the dopamine projections). Similarly, no attempt has been made to incorporate every class of interneuron that has been observed within these systems. Abbreviations: ACH = acetylcholine, CCK = cholecystokinin, DA = dopamine, GABA = γ-aminobutyric acid, GAL = galinin, NT = neurotensin, and SOM = somatostatin.

ated or eliminated after central amygdaloid lesions, although unconditioned autonomic responses are not affected. This appears to be caused by the loss of neurons intrinsic to the central division of the extended amygdala, since axon-sparing lesions with cytotoxins produce the same result.

In general, observations such as these, as well as observations based on the symptoms of patients with temporal lobe epilepsy or after electrical stimulation in the amygdala of such patients, suggest that the amygdala is crucial in evaluating the significance of external and internal events.

Basal forebrain and psychosis The observation that most antipsychotics block dopamine receptors has focused attention on the "mesolimbic" dopamine system described below as a possible site of dysfunction in schizophrenia. Along with ventral striatum, the extended amygdala, and particularly the central division, is a major recipient of dopamine terminals from the midbrain. These observations argue for the possibility that a primary dysfunction within the extended amygdala could contribute to the behavioral manifestations of schizophrenic patients. The direct auditory input to the central division, for example, could help explain the favored frequency of auditory hallucinations in schizophrenia. The likely involvement of the extended amygdala in limbic seizures would be consistent with the occurrence of psychotic symptoms in temporal lobe epilepsy. Finally, the course of the extended amygdala that follows from the medial dorsal part of the temporal lobe through the sublenticular substantia innominata and into the medial forebrain fits rather well with the most common locus of neuropathology in schizophrenics, as described in recent studies by Farley and co-workers and by Stevens. (See also Section 14.2a of this text.)

In principal, the septum could as well be the target of dopaminergic-blocking antipsychotics. The septum has close relations with the hippocampus, and the latter structure also appears to be structurally disorganized in schizophrenic brains. The hippocampus projects to both septum and nucleus accumbens, and this latter structure may represent, in part, the most rostral portion of the extended amygdala.

THALAMUS

The functions of the thalamus are diverse (Table 1.3-1). These functions include the relay of sensory information to cortex as typified by the ventrobasal complex and the medial and lateral geniculate bodies and the relay of motor information from the basal ganglia and cerebellum by way of the ventral anterior and ventrolateral nuclei. The major thalamic relay nuclei are reciprocally connected with cortex and project in a rather strict topographical manner to their cortical targets.

In addition to the specific relay nuclei, the remainder of the dorsal thalamic nuclei also project to cortex but carry information that is less clearly characterized. Of these, the anterior nuclei relay information from the mammillary nuclei of the hypothalamus and from the hippocampus to the limbic lobe, and particularly to the cingulate gyrus. The mediodorsal nucleus receives input from a variety of structures from the forebrain and brain stem and projects massively to the prefrontal association cortex. Descending afferents include those from olfactory cortex, entorhinal cortex, ventral pallidum, and amygdala, as well as projections from the reticular nucleus of the thalamus. In humans, lesions in the mediodorsal nucleus have been associated with profound anterograde memory loss.

The intralaminar nuclei project densely and topographically to striatum, and via collaterals of the same axons, project sparsely but diffusely to overlying cortex. Frontal cortex provides substantial afferents to the intralaminar nuclei, and this includes terminals from the prefrontal, motor, and premotor cortex; however, these cannot be considered reciprocals of the more widespread cortical projections of the intralaminar nuclei. Other afferents to the intralaminar nuclei arrive from the medial segment of the globus pallidus and from the pars reticulata substantia nigra, as well as from the spinal cord, the reticular formation, and the cerebellum.

TABLE 1.3-1
Major Thalamic Nuclei

SENSORY RELAY NUCLEI
Ventrobasal complex. *Ventral posterolateral* and *ventral posteromedial* nuclei relay somatosensory impulses from spinothalamic tract, medial lemniscus and trigeminal lemniscus, respectively, to somatosensory cortex (areas 3, 1, and 2) in postcentral gyrus with a high degree of place and stimulus specificity. *Basal ventromedial* nucleus relays impulses from the nucleus of the solitary tract.
Lateral geniculate body. This multilaminated nucleus receives impulses from the contralateral visual fields of both eyes via the optic tract and projects through the optic radiation to visual cortical areas 17, 18, and 19 in the occipital lobe.
Medial geniculate body. Consists of several nuclei that receive input from the inferior colliculus and other auditory centers in the brain stem, and project to the auditory cortex (areas 41 and 42) in the superior temporal gyrus, as well as to caudal striatum and to the central division of extended amygdala.
Lateral posterior-pulvinar complex. Receives significant input from the superior colliculus and pretectum and is reciprocally related to visual cortical areas, parieto-occipital frontal and temporal association areas. Provides for an extrageniculate visual pathway to the cerebral cortex, and is also involved in other, but little known, functions, including aspects of language functions.
MOTOR NUCLEI
Ventral anterior nucleus. Receives fibers from basal ganglia (globus pallidus and substantia nigra, pars reticulata) and projects to premotor cortex, especially the supplementary motor areas (area 6).
Ventral lateral nucleus. Receives fibers from basal ganglia and cerebellum and projects to motor cortex (area 4).
OTHER THALAMIC NUCLEI
Mediodorsal nucleus. Receives projections from a variety of structures in the forebrain (e.g., dorsal and ventral pallidum, diagonal-band nuclei, preoptic area, amygdala, and olfactory cortex) and the brain stem (e.g., superior colliculus) and is reciprocally related to the prefrontal association cortex. Although the mediodorsal nucleus is not a motor nucleus in strict sense, it may influence the planning of motor behavior. It is also related to important temporal-lobe structures including the hippocampus and has been implicated in olfactory function, learning, and memory.
Anterior nuclei. Receive significant input from the mammillary body via the mammillothalamic tract and are reciprocally connected with the cortex of the limbic lobe.
Intralaminar nuclei. In addition to their presumed role in arousal, motor and sensory functions have also been proposed for the intralaminar nuclei. These nuclei project topographically to the striatum as well as diffusely to widespread areas of the cerebral cortex, presumably forming one branch of the ascending activating system. The cortex partly reciprocates these projections, as does the basal ganglia via projections from the internal segment of globus pallidus and from pars reticulata substantia nigra. Afferents from the spinal cord, cerebellum, and reticular formation also reach the intralaminar nuclei.
Midline nuclei. Include the paratenial, paraventricular, rhomboidal, and medioventral (reuniens) nuclei. The first three project to striatum and are sometimes considered part of the intralaminar nuclei. The medioventral nucleus projects to virtually all areas of the limbic cortex.
Reticular nucleus. Receives collaterals from thalamocortical and corticothalamic fibers passing through the nucleus and feeds the information back to the thalamus. It also projects to the midbrain reticular formation and may be involved in sleep-arousal mechanisms.

HYPOTHALAMUS AND SUBTHALAMUS

The hypothalamus includes important nuclei related to neuroendocrine regulation, especially in its medial zone; in addition, it provides afferents to brain stem and spinal cord that are important in the discharge of integrated autonomic activity. In its cellular morphology and projections, the hypothalamus resembles the brain stem reticular formation, particularly in its lateral zone, where hypothalamic neurons commonly produce bifurcating axons. One axon branch descends to motor areas of the brain stem, and the second branch ascends to provide feedback to more rostral forebrain systems. Many of these axons appear to produce short collaterals along their ascending and descending course. The subthalamic area includes the zona incerta and the subthalamic nucleus. Whereas the subthalamic nucleus is an integral part of the striatopallidal system, the zona incerta seems to be more closely related to the hypothalamus, especially to its lateral corridor. As in the case of the hypothalamus, the zona incerta seems to possess a cellular morphology reminiscent of reticular neurons (i.e., cells possessing bifurcating axons with projections to the brain stem, spinal cord, and rostral forebrain).

MEDIAL HYPOTHALAMUS The medial hypothalamus contains most of the neurons concerned with regulation of the pituitary, as well as important efferent sources for projections to brain stem and spinal autonomic areas. In addition, the medial hypothalamus has extensive reciprocal connections with the medial division of extended amygdala. The hippocampus, either directly or via the septum, also sends afferents to medial hypothalamus.

Anterior medial hypothalamus The anterior portion of the medial hypothalamus contains the *medial preoptic-anterior hypothalamic continuum*, the *suprachiasmatic nucleus*, the *supraoptic nucleus*, and the *paraventricular nucleus* of the hypothalamus. The term "medial preoptic-anterior hypothalamic continuum," as it is used here, encompasses a collection of nuclei and areas including the *organum vasculosum of the lamina terminalis* (OVLT), the medial preoptic area, the anterior hypothalamic area, and the periventricular nucleus of the hypothalamus.

This complicated zone of the rostral hypothalamus has been implicated in a variety of functions including endocrine reflexes in reproduction, in male and female copulatory behaviors, as well as in maternal behavior and thirst. Central control of thermoregulation appears to be dependent on neurons in this general area that are both temperature-sensitive and the recipient of afferents conveying temperature information from the periphery.

The *lamina terminalis* is one of the circumventricular organs and structurally resembles the infundibulum (median eminence). Axons of hypothalamic neurons have been observed to terminate on capillaries in the OVLT, and this structure is thought to function additionally as a receptor area for hormonal feedback to the endocrine hypothalamus.

The *suprachiasmatic nucleus* has been identified as an endogenous timekeeper. This small nucleus receives afferents directly and indirectly from the retina in order to synchronize otherwise free-running circadian rhythms with the day-night cycle. At least some of its actions, particularly on hormonal rhythms, appear to be mediated by means of projections to the medial hypothalamus. Additional projections that have been observed to lateral septum, the habenula, interpeduncular nucleus, and superior colliculus may affect behavioral rather than endocrine rhythms.

The *supraoptic* and *paraventricular* hypothalamic nuclei (Fig. 1.2-14) are two of the best-studied structures of the hypothalamus. The magnocellular neurons found within the supraoptic and paraventricular hypothalamic nuclei, along with scattered clusters of large cells between these two nuclei, comprise the *hypothalamo-neurohypophysial* system. These cells send oxytocin- and vasopressin-containing fibers to the posterior neural lobe of the pituitary (Fig. 1.2-17). In addition to oxytocin and vasopressin, which are present in separate collections of neurons, several neuropeptides (e.g., glucagon, cholecystokinin, angiotensin II, corticotropin-releasing factor [CRF], leu- and met-enkephalin, dynorphin) are colocalized with either oxytocin or vasopressin in magnocellular neurosecretory neurons.

The paraventricular nucleus is a complex structure that includes several subgroups of small (parvicellular) neurons containing a variety of putative neurotransmitters, including not only vasopressin and oxytocin but also somatostatin (SOM), dopamine, leu- and met-enkephalin, neurotensin, substance P, angiotensin II, and CRF. Some of the parvicellular neurons project to the external layer of median eminence where they participate in the regulation of the anterior pituitary. Others are the source of extrahypothalamic projections from the paraventricular nucleus. Descending projections of the paraventricular nucleus reach several areas of the medulla and spinal cord, including especially such sympathetic and parasympathetic autonomic areas as the dorsal vagal complex, parabrachial nucleus, nucleus of the solitary tract, and intermediolateral cell columns of the spinal cord. Projections to the paraventricular nucleus come from both extrahypothalamic sources (e.g., the bed nucleus of the stria terminalis, subfornical organ, noradrenergic cell groups in the medulla, and parabrachial area) and from other hypothalamic nuclei, especially the dorsomedial nucleus.

The supraoptic and paraventricular nuclei play important roles in the integration of autonomic and endocrine responses regulating the cardiovascular system. The fact that both the paraventricular nucleus and supraoptic nucleus are receptor areas for circulating sex steroids suggests that these nuclei also participate in regulatory adjustments within the reproductive cycle. The paraventricular nucleus, in addition, has been implicated in a variety of other behaviors, including feeding and thirst, as well as in the organization of autonomic and endocrine responses to stress. The paraventricular nucleus, for example, is a sensitive target for local chemical stimulation of feeding by several different neurotransmitters, although some of these responses may be blocked by hypophysectomy.

The middle group of medial hypothalamic nuclei The middle zone of the medial hypothalamus includes the *ventromedial*, *arcuate* (infundibular), and *dorsomedial* nuclei.

The *ventromedial nucleus* and *arcuate nucleus*—together with the *periventricular nucleus* in anterior hypothalamus, the *paraventricular nucleus*, and neurons loosely scattered in the mediobasal hypothalamus—participate in the formation of the *tuberoinfundibular tract* that terminates on the hypophyseal-portal capillary system. This provides the neural link between the hypothalamus and the anterior pituitary. In terms of the various releasing and inhibiting factors that influence the secretion of anterior pituitary hormones, some neurosecretory cells appear to be somewhat localized, whereas others are scattered across various hypothalamic areas. Apparently, only a few cells containing neuropeptide-releasing factors occur within the ventromedial nucleus, but these releasing factors include growth hormone releasing factor (GRF) and inhibiting factor (SOM).

The paraventricular nucleus contains particularly high numbers of cells with CRF and thyrotropin-releasing hormone (TRH), but also cells containing GRF and SOM. Gonadotropin (lactating hormone-releasing hormone [LHRH]) cells appear throughout the medial hypothalamus but are most frequent in the medial preoptic complex of the rat. In primates, comparatively more LHRH cells are found posteriorly in hypothalamus, with increased numbers in the arcuate nucleus. It is well documented that hypothalamic dopamine neurons that project to the infundibulum inhibit prolactin release. In this respect it should be kept in mind that other putative transmitters such as GABA, acetylcholine, enkephalins, angiotensin II, and norepinephrine are also found within the infundibulum and may act to effect hormone release from anterior pituitary. In fact, at least six different transmitters are colocalized in various combinations with CRF within the paraventricular nucleus. Of these, neurotensin, angiotensin II, and cholecystokinin appear to increase corticotropin (adrenocorticotropic hormone [ACTH]) release.

The ventromedial hypothalamic nucleus, in addition to its output to the infundibulum, also projects to nearby hypothalamic areas, including the *dorsomedial nucleus*. One of the main output channels, however, is directed toward the mesencephalic periaqueductal gray substance, which probably serves as a relay station for projections to the medullary reticular formation, thereby giving rise to descending pathways to the sympathetic preganglionic neurons in the spinal cord. The ventromedial hypothalamic nucleus and other areas in the medial hypothalamus are also reciprocally connected with the extended amygdala.

In addition to its role in the neuroendocrine relay, the ventromedial nucleus is thought to function as an important relay in reproductive behavior and in ingestive behavior. However, this latter role for the ventromedial nucleus as a satiety center that tonically inhibits feeding remains controversial. Experimental lesions in the ventromedial area of the hypothalamus result in dramatic hyperphagia, but apparently not because of direct damage to the ventromedial nucleus inasmuch as lesions carefully confined to the nucleus are rather ineffective. It has been argued that the effective lesion may include the paraventricular hypothalamic nucleus; lesions at this latter site also result in overeating. The role of the medial hypothalmus in feeding may well be indirect. It depends in large part on the metabolic regulatory functions of this area, which are effected by both its neuroendocrine and autonomic projections. For example, medial hypothalamic lesions also result in increased fat deposition even when overeating is prevented. It has also been observed that lesions within the ventromedial hypothalamic area result in hyperinsulinemia, which appears to be the result of neural modulation of pancreatic function. Section of the vagus nerve appears to block both the hyperinsulinemia and overeating resulting from ventromedial lesions. Despite the shift away from a view of the ventromedial hypothalamic nucleus as a satiety center, it is clear that this general area, including the dorsomedial and ventromedial nuclei of the hypothalamus, is important in both the endocrine and autonomic physiology of energy metabolism.

Posterior medial hypothalamus The posterior part of the hypothalamus includes the *posterior nucleus* and the *mammillary complex*. The posterior nucleus apparently has some reciprocal connections with the extended amygdala and with the central gray of the midbrain. Efferents also include projections to the dorsal raphe and to spinal cord, with this latter projection arising at least in part from dopamine neurons within the posterior nucleus. The posterior nucleus is more developed in primates than in common laboratory animals, such as the rat. Perhaps, as a consequence, the functions of this area have been less thoroughly studied than have the other hypothalamic nuclei.

The mammillary complex is at the caudal border of the hypothalamus. Rostrally, the premammillary nuclei are reciprocally connected with the extended amygdala, whereas the lateral and medial mammillary nuclei are the recipients of a massive input from the hippocampus by way of the fornix. These nuclei project via the mammillo-thalamic tract to the anterior nuclei of the thalamus, and are reciprocally connected with the dorsal and ventral tegmental nuclei via the mammillo-tegmental tract.

The mammillary bodies have been thought to play some role in memory and emotions because of their input from the hippocampus and their output by way of the dorsal thalamic relay to the cingulate cortex. These nuclei are frequently damaged in patients with Korsakoff's syndrome along with damage that is more reliably found in mediodorsal thalamus. Their role in memory, however, is still controversial.

LATERAL HYPOTHALAMUS AND SUBTHALAMUS

The lateral preoptic-lateral hypothalamic (LPO-LH) continuum is only moderately populated by neurons, which are interspersed among the fibers of the medial forebrain bundle, the rostrocaudal extent of this area results, nonetheless, in a sizable population of neurons. The LPO-LH area shares a wide variety of reciprocal connections with the forebrain, caudal brain stem, and spinal cord. The physiology of this area is complicated by the fact that many axons traverse this area, which may or may not synapse locally. Descending fibers in lateral hypothalamus include axons from the central division of extended amygdala that synapse in hypothalamus but also descend to targets in the brain stem and spinal cord. Descending afferents to the LPO-LH area include axons from the septal area, including the subfornical organ. Ascending afferents to the lateral hypothalamic area include those from the monoamine cells in the brain stem—in particular from norepinephrine and serotonin cells, but presumably also from areas, such as the brain stem reticular formation, the parabrachial nuclei, and the nucleus of the solitary tract.

Neurons in the LPO-LH area resemble those within the brain stem reticular formation and are of moderately large size, with long dendrites generally oriented perpendicularly to the axons of the medial forebrain bundle, from which they receive collaterals and to which they contribute axons. Many of these cells give rise to axons that project rostrally to targets including cortex and, presumably, amygdala. These axons also send a caudal branch to brain stem and spinal cord. The neurons appear to contain a variety of neuropeptides, including α-melanocyte-stimulating hormone, met-enkephalin, and dynorphin, as well as somatostatin and angiotensin II. These neurons appear to be confluent with similar cells in the zona incerta and with cells extending into the perifornical area of the hypothalamus.

The LPO-LH continuum has been the subject of wide diversity of behavioral experiments. For example, stimulation within this continuum can result in feeding, drinking, or a variety of behaviors that depend on the environmental context. In addition, electrical stimulation administered to the lateral hypothalamus appears to be rewarding, and an animal will self-administer shocks to its own brain. Lesions in lateral hypothalamus result in aphagia, adipsia, and a variety of deficits in learned and unlearned behaviors. These observations have given rise to the notion of the lateral hypothalamic area as a feeding and drinking center or, alternatively, as a zone particularly involved in behavioral arousal. Despite the attraction in such formulations, many of the effects or deficits seen after lateral hypothalamic manipulations appear after similar manipulations of extra-hypothalamic areas that send axons through the hypothalamus. Examples include ascending monoamine pathways (particularly the dopaminergic tracts) and descending pathways from the basal ganglia.

Such observations suggest a rather extensive participation of forebrain systems in behavioral homeostasis and arousal. That the lateral hypothalamus and subthalamus may be parts of such systems is attested to by the observations that neurotoxin lesions of lateral hypothalamus or zona incerta, which presumably do not destroy axons of passage, also result in temporary aphagia, adipsia, and chronic disruption of responding to acute homeostatic challenges.

In summary, although some role for the LPO-LH continuum and the zona incerta in homeostasis can be supported, many of the observations can be the results of disruption of axons of passage. Before generalization to human behavioral systems can be safely made, much more research needs to be performed, especially on primates in which the trajectory of such axons may be different from those in the rat, which has been the subject of most experiments.

BRAIN STEM

The brain stem may be defined to include the mesencephalon, pons, and medulla oblongata. This is an area that is composed of many vital structures including: (1) important visual and auditory processing areas in the superior and inferior colliculi, respectively; (2) the midbrain relay nuclei of the basal ganglia— that is, the ventral tegmental area, the substantia nigra, and the area adjacent to the pedunculopontine tegmental nucleus; (3) the central, periaqueductal gray; (4) the reticular formation; (5) the neurons that provide the origin of the ascending and descending monoamine pathways; (6) the primary sensory and motor nuclei of the cranial nerves; and (7) the sensory and motor pathways of the spinal cord. Of these areas, the substantia nigra and the striatopallidal system have been discussed. The principal sensory and motor nuclei of the brain stem were described in Section 1.2, as were the superior and inferior colliculi. The central gray, which seems to be part of an endogenous "pain-inhibiting system," and the cerebellum are similarly excluded from further discussion.

RETICULAR FORMATION The reticular formation is composed mainly of neurons with long interlacing dendrites located in the central core of the brain stem. The axonal arborization of reticular neurons is particularly striking, with many cells sending bifurcating, long ascending and descending axon collaterals. The remainder of the cells send either long ascending or long descending axons. Along the course of reticular axons, perpendicular collaterals are issued in such a way that an intricate pattern of interconnections is created. This complex axonal arborization extends into the hypothalamic and thalamic targets of reticular cells as well.

Two main roles of the reticular formation have attracted special attention. The first is the descending control of motor mechanisms, and the second is the ascending influence on the level of consciousness and on attention.

Reticular formation and motor control Much progress has been made in recent years in the analysis of motor control functions within the brain stem. In general, descending afferents from the cortex, the striatopallidal system, the extended amygdala, the thalamus, and the hypothalamus all reach brain stem reticular areas and participate to varying degrees in the modulation of autonomic and somatic motor patterns. These afferents are supplemented by more or less direct sensory input from brain stem sensory nuclei, and include proprioceptive feedback from the spinal cord.

The afferents from the forebrain are targeted toward local units of the brain stem which have been identified with particular motor functions. However, the boundaries of these units often partially overlap with each other, and they are often composed of groups of neurons that are physically separate from one another. As a result, motor output units frequently do not correspond to identifiable cytoarchitectonic boundaries, nor are they confined to the reticular formation as strictly defined. Despite this limitation, it has been possible to describe, for example, brain stem-reticular areas related to locomotor control, vestibular and oculomotor functions, respiration, and cardiovascular reflexes.

Ascending influences of the reticular formation Decades of research have implicated the reticular formation in some of the most vital functions of arousal and consciousness. The reticular formation includes zones which actively induce sleep, as well as areas that are apparently essential for widespread cortical activation and behavioral arousal as a response to incoming stimuli. The ascending activating system was thought to act via connections to midline and intralaminar thalamic nuclei, together with the thalamic reticular nucleus. However, the reticular thalamic nucleus does not appear to have ascending cortical projections as was once thought, and is likely to act, rather, through its widespread descending connections with the remainder of thalamus. The intralaminar nuclei do indeed project diffusely to cortex, although their main target appears to be the striatum. Projections of the midline nuclei reach limbic cortical areas, but also the substantia innominata, where they could affect cortical firing via inputs to basal forebrain corticopetal cells or indirectly via terminations on cells of the extended amygdala.

Recently, it was suggested by Rye and co-workers that the *pedunculopontine tegmental nucleus,* which is mainly composed of cholinergic neurons, may provide the majority of the thalamic afferents from the reticular formation to rostral thalamus and could represent the most effective area of origin for the ascending activating system. It was noted, however, that both the *locus ceruleus* and *parabrachial* nuclei also contribute axons to the thalamus; these two areas also send massive projections ventrally through subthalamus and hypothalamus, which is known to be a second route for ascending activation. The locus ceruleus is an important source of noradrenergic fibers to much of the forebrain, whereas the medial and lateral parabrachial nuclei are apparently relays for gustatory and visceral information. Ascending fibers from the parabrachial nuclei terminate in thalamus, hypothalamus, and limbic areas of cortex, but most conspicuously in the extended amygdala.

Sleep is also actively induced from the territory of the reticular formation. Pharmacological studies have implicated the ascending serotonergic projections, as described below, especially from the rostral raphe nuclei, in actively inducing sleep. Cholinergic and noradrenergic systems together participate in waking and arousal and also in sleep phases when rapid eye movements (REM) and desynchronized electroencephalographies (EEGs) are present.

MONOAMINERGIC PATHWAYS Many psychotherapeutic agents affect the monoamine systems in one way or another, and much of what is known about the the pharmacology of psychoactive drugs depends on the understanding of the monoamine pathways in the brain. This knowledge is, in part, attributable to the early understanding of the role of the monoamines as neurotransmitters, as well as to the widespread projections of monoamine neurons. Although the monoamine pathways are often discussed as systems, it should be kept in mind that in almost every case, monoamine cell groups are widely dispersed in brain stem and more rostral areas of the brain. It is therefore unlikely that all the cells containing a given monoamine neurotransmitter serve a single function. Only the serotonin, dopamine, norepinephrine, and epinephrine pathways are discussed below.

Serotonin pathways The cells of origin of the serotonin terminals in the CNS are located principally in the raphe nuclei of the brain stem (Fig. 1.3-13). These form a more or less continuous collection of cell groups close to the midline, which begin at the most rostral end of the mesencephalon just dorsal to the interpeduncular nucleus and extend into caudal medulla. The cells in the rostral part of forebrain distribute widely to forebrain, often reaching widely dispersed areas via collaterals from a single axon. Most of the raphe nuclei contribute some fibers to cerebellum, whereas the serotonin cells in the medulla oblongata send projections to spinal cord. Serotonergic fibers are found in a dense plexus on most ventricular surfaces, and some serotonin fibers have been observed on blood vessels. Although the physiological significance of such vascular terminations is unknown, they appear to originate mainly from cells within the brain. In the rat, some serotonin neurons have also been observed on the ventricular surface, most frequently at the rostral part of the floor of the fourth ventricle. Finally, it should be mentioned that other transmitters are frequently colocalized with serotonin within raphe neurons. For example, GABA, substance P, and enkephalin- or thyrotropin-releasing hormone may be released at the same time with serotonin.

In addition to its potential role in the neural organization of sleep, serotonin has been implicated in a variety of functions, including reproductive behavior, aggression, and pain. Regarding pain, neurons within the raphe magnus send descending projections to substantia gelatinosa and electrical stimulation of raphe magnus results in analgesia.

Dopamine pathways The dopamine projections of the brain (Fig. 1.3-14) have been intensively studied, particularly the tegmental cell groups that make up the mesostriatal pathway originating from pars compacta substantia nigra and from cells in the ventral tegmental area. The ventral tegmental cells are distinguished from those of pars compacta in that they can contain a second putative neurotransmitter in addition to dopamine. For example, many dopamine cells of the ventral tegmental area were found to also contain cholecystokinin or neurotensin. The ventral tegmental dopamine cells may be thought of as an extension of the nigrostriatal projection system, in that the pars compacta substantia nigra projects to dorsal striatum, whereas the ventral tegmental area seems to provide most of the dopaminergic input to ventral striatum. It should be kept in mind, however, that the ventral tegmental area and related cells in the retrorubral field also send dopamine terminals to the extended amygdala, lateral septum, piriform cortex, entorhinal cortex, and prefrontal cortex. More recently, dopamine terminals have been reported in additional areas of cortex, but the origin and significance of such terminals is, at present, unclear.

The neurons of pars compacta project to striatum with a well-ordered medial-to-lateral topography. In contrast, individual neurons seem to arborize extensively within the rostrocaudal dimensions of the striatum. The result of this arborization is that rostrocaudal-oriented columns of dopamine cells within pars compacta appear to project to a given longitudinal segment of the striatum. Although the functional impact of this arrangement has not been well studied, the implication is that a given column of dopamine cells will affect striatal circuit activity across a broad range of corticostriatal inputs.

Other dopamine projection systems include the diencephalospinal system, the incertohypothalamic system, and the tuberohypophyseal system. The diencephalospinal system originates in dorsal and posterior hypothalamus and zona incerta, and projects to spinal cord, with

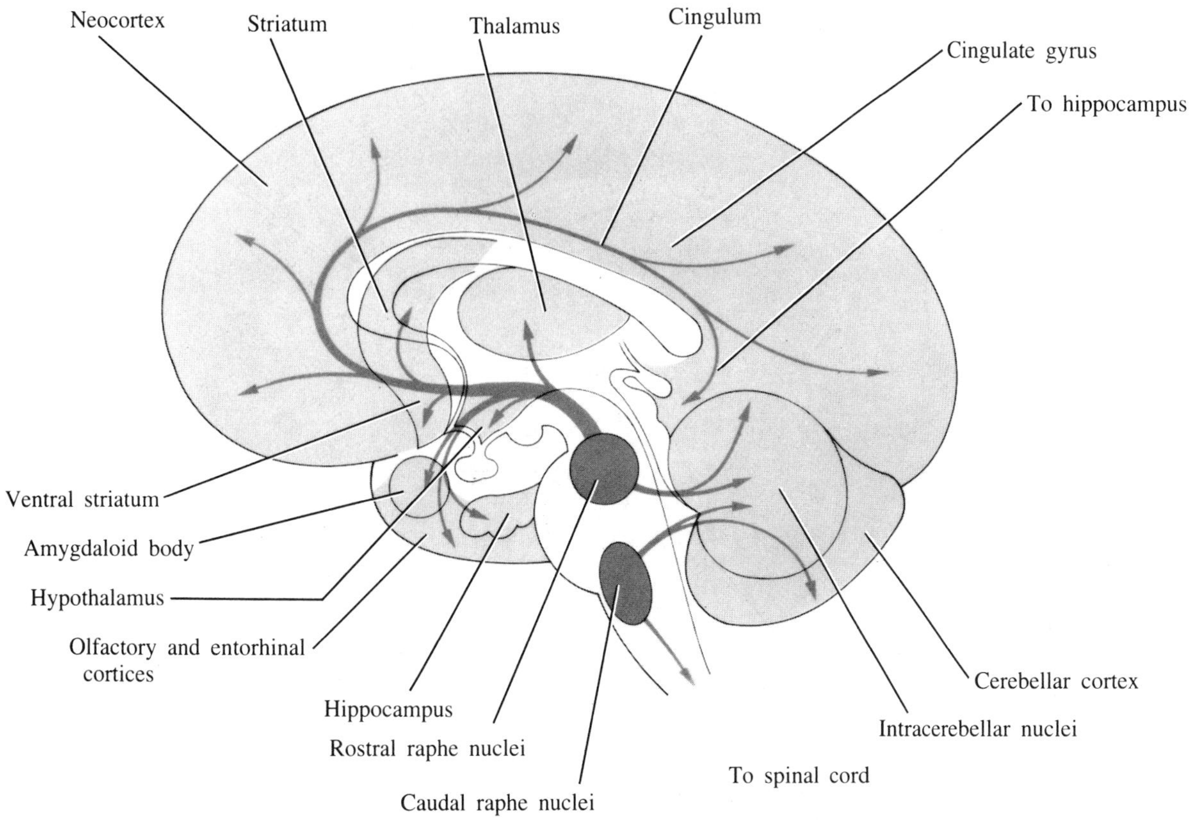

FIGURE 1.3-13. *Serotonergic pathways. The raphe nuclei form a more or less continuous collection of cell groups close to the midline throughout the brain stem, but for the sake of simplicity they have been subdivided into a rostral and a caudal group in the drawing. The rostral raphe nuclei project to a large number of forebrain structures. The fibers that project laterally through the internal and external capsules to widespread areas of the neocortex are not indicated in this highly schematic drawing. (From Heimer L:* The Human Brain and Spinal Cord. *Springer-Verlag, New York, 1983, with permission.)*

axons terminating in both the dorsal horn and in the intermediolateral cell columns. Rostral projections of this system may come from collaterals of descending axons and give rise to the periventricular dopamine system that reaches the periaqueductal gray, medial thalamus, and medial hypothalamus.

The incertohypothalamic system sends terminals into the zona incerta, rostral hypothalamus, and septum. The tuberohypophyseal system consists of cells in the arcuate and periventricular hypothalamic nuclei that project to the infundibulum and posterior and intermediate parts of the pituitary.

Dopamine cells that appear to be local interneurons have also been observed in the olfactory bulb and the retina, and it has been recently reported that dopamine cells may be observed in primates at the dorsal and lateral borders of the striatum.

Dopamine is clearly critical for the proper functioning of the striatum; however, the observation that the efficacy of antipsychotic drugs correlates with their ability to block dopamine receptors has also focused research on the role of dopamine in schizophrenia and possibly in mood disorders. Much of this research has presumed that the effective site for antidopamine antipsychotics is in the terminal areas targeted by the ventral tegmental dopamine cells.

Norepinephrine pathways Norepinephrine axons originate from cell groups in the pontine and medullary reticular formation (Fig. 1.3-15). These include cells in the locus ceruleus, the ventrolateral tegmentum, and the nucleus of the solitary tract, and near the area postrema. Highly collateralized axons characterize the norepinephrine cells of the brain stem, especially those in locus ceruleus and in lateral tegmentum. Both of these groups contribute to terminal fields in the brain stem and hypothalamus, although lateral tegmental cells seem particularly targeted to these areas, whereas the locus ceruleus seems more heavily targeted toward the thalamus and cortex. Descending noradrenergic axons reach both dorsal and ventral horns of the spinal cord, as well as the intermediolateral cell columns. Tracing experiments suggest that locus ceruleus neurons project to dorsal and ventral horn targets, whereas the lateral tegmental neurons send terminals to the intermediolateral cells. Finally, many noradrenergic terminals, apparently of central origin, terminate on small blood vessels, suggesting a possible role in cerebrovascular regulation.

Recent data suggest that afferents to the locus ceruleus are much more limited than previously supposed. In the rat, these arise from the region of the prepositus hypoglossal nucleus and the area of the nucleus paragigantocellularis, both of which are located in rostral medulla. The latter nucleus projects densely to the intermediolateral cell column and apparently responds to neutral polymodal stimuli, as well as to painful stimuli. The former nucleus has been implicated in the control of gaze.

The ascending noradrenergic projections have been suggested as a component in the ascending activating system, and many experiments can be interpreted to support this view. Descending projections of the locus ceruleus may participate in driving spinal oscillators that provide for locomotion.

Epinephrine pathways Although epinephrine concentrations are low in the CNS compared with the other monoamines, a system of epinephrine neurons has been demonstrated immunohistochemically. Two extended cell groups have been identified in the medulla oblongata, and these appear to provide the majority of epinephrine terminals observed in the forebrain, brain stem, and spinal cord. Both cell groups extend approximately (in the rat) from the level of the caudal tip of area postrema to the middle of the facial nucleus. The ventral group occupies the ventrolateral portion of the medulla, near or just ventromedial to the nucleus ambiguus. The dorsal group occupies a territory in or adjacent to the nucleus of the solitary tract and the dorsal motor nucleus of the vagus. Epinephrine terminals are found in low concentrations in the telencephalon, with terminals reaching the septum and medial portions of nucleus accumbens (particularly to the bed nucleus of the stria terminalis), as well

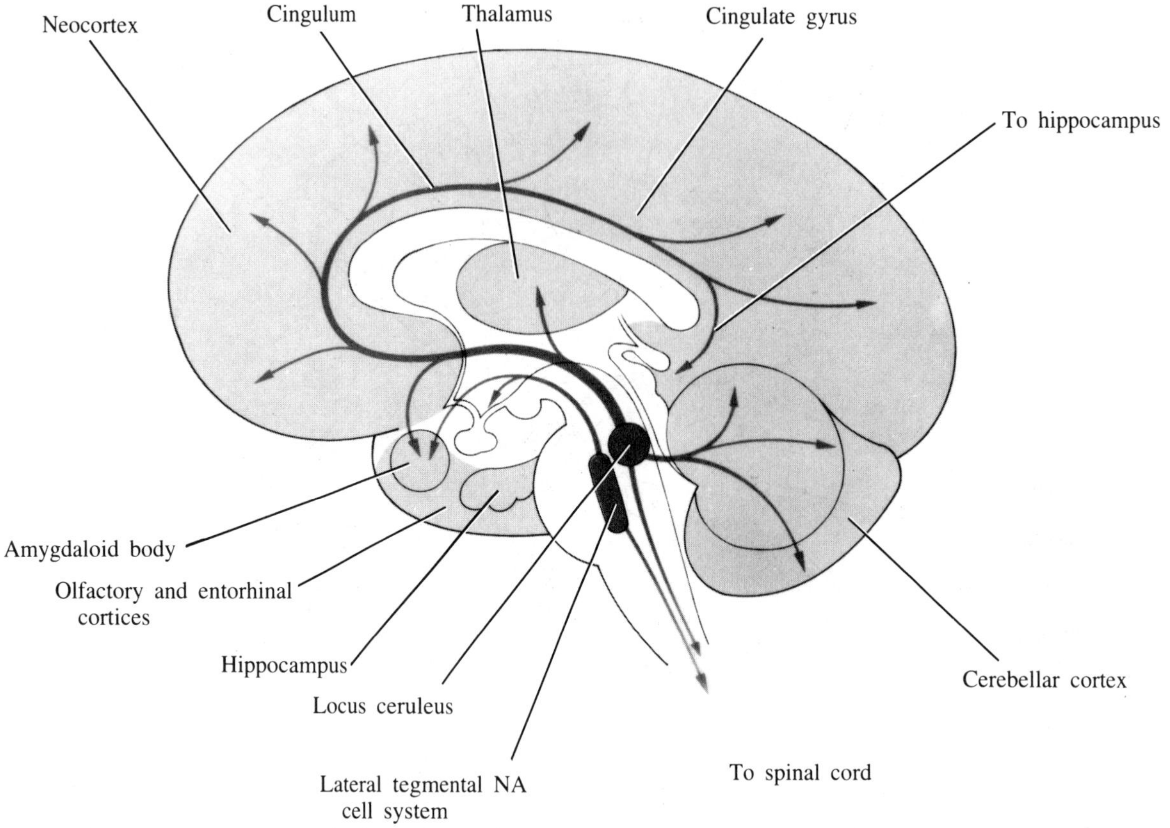

FIGURE 1.3-14. *Noradrenergic pathways. Locus ceruleus, which is located immediately underneath the floor of the fourth ventricle in the rostrolateral part of pons, is the most important noradrenergic nucleus in the brain. Its projections reach many areas in the forebrain, cerebellum, and spinal cord. Noradrenergic neurons in the lateral brain stem tegmentum innervate several structures in the basal forebrain including the hypothalamus and the amygdaloid body. (From Heimer L:* The Human Brain and Spinal Cord. *Springer-Verlag, New York, 1983, with permission.)*

as in substantia innominata and the central nucleus of the amygdala. In the diencephalon, moderately dense epinephrine terminals are found in medial and lateral hypothalamus, especially in the perifornical area. In the thalamus, moderate to dense terminals are found in the periventricular nucleus. Caudally in the brain stem, moderate numbers of epinephrine terminals are seen, particularly in the central gray, dorsal vagal complex, and locus ceruleus. Finally, epinephrine axons to the spinal cord appear to terminate most densely in the intermediolateral columns, with only few terminals outside this area.

REFERENCES

Alexander G E, DeLong M R, Strick P L: Parallel organization of functionally segregated circuits linking basal ganglia and cortex. Ann Rev Neurosci *9:* 357, 1986.

Alheid G F, Heimer L: New perspectives in basal forebrain organization of special relevance for neuropsychiatric disorders; the striatopallidal, amygdaloid, and corticopetal components of substantia innominata. Neuroscience: 1988.

Amaral D G: Memory: Anatomical organization of candidate brain regions. In *The Handbook of Physiology,* vol 5. V B Mountcastle, F Plum, S R Geiger, editors. American Physiological Society, Bethesda, MD, 1987.

deOlmos J, Alheid G F, Beltramino C A: The amygdala. In *The Rat Nervous System,* G Paxinos, editor, p 223. Academic Press, New York, 1985.

Fallon J H and Loughlin S E Monoamine innervation of cerebral cortex and a theory of the role of monoamines in cerebral cortex and basal ganglia. In *Cerebral Cortex,* vol 6. E G Jones and A Peters, editors, p 41. Plenum, New York, 1987.

Farley I J, Price K S, McCullough E, Deck J H N, Hornykiewicz O: Norepinephrine in chronic paranoid schizophrenia: Above normal levels in limbic forebrain. Science *200:* 456, 1978.

Gerfen C R, Herkenham M, Thibault J: The neostriatal mosaic: II. Patch- and matrix-directed mesostriatal dopaminergic and non-dopaminergic systems. J Neurosci *7:* 3915, 1987.

Geschwind N: Pathogenesis of behavior change in temporal lobe epilepsy. In *Epilepsy,* A A Ward, Jr, J K Penry, D Purpura, editors, p 355. Raven Press, New York, 1983.

Gray J A: *The Psychology of Fear and Stress,* ed 2. Cambridge University Press, Cambridge, 1987.

Graybiel A M, Ragsdale C W: Biochemical anatomy of the striatum. In *Chemical Neuroanatomy,* P C Emson, editor, p 427. Raven Press, New York, 1983.

Herkenham M: Mismatches between neurotransmitter and receptor localizations in brain: Observations and implications. Neuroscience *23: 1,* 1987.

Holstege G, Meiners L, Tan K: Projections of the bed nucleus of the stria terminalis to the mesencephalon, pons, and medulla oblongata in the cat. Exp Brain Res *58:* 379, 1985.

Holstege J C, Kuypers H G J M: Brainstem projections to spinal motoneurons: An update. Neuroscience *23:* 809, 1987.

Kapp B S, Pascoe J P, Bixler M A: The amygdala: A neuroanatomical systems approach to its contribution to aversive conditioning. In *Neuropsychology of Memory,* L R Squire, N Butters, editors, p 473. Guilford, New York, 1984.

Köhler C, Haglund L, Swanson, L W: A diffuse α-MSH immunoreactive projection to the hippocampus and spinal cord from individual neurons in the lateral hypothalamic area and zona incerta. J Comp Neurol *223:* 501, 1984.

LeDoux J E: Emotion. In *The Handbook of Physiology,* vol 5, *The Nervous System,* V B Mountcastle, F Plum, S R Geiger, editors, p 419. American Physiological Society, Bethesda, MD, 1987.

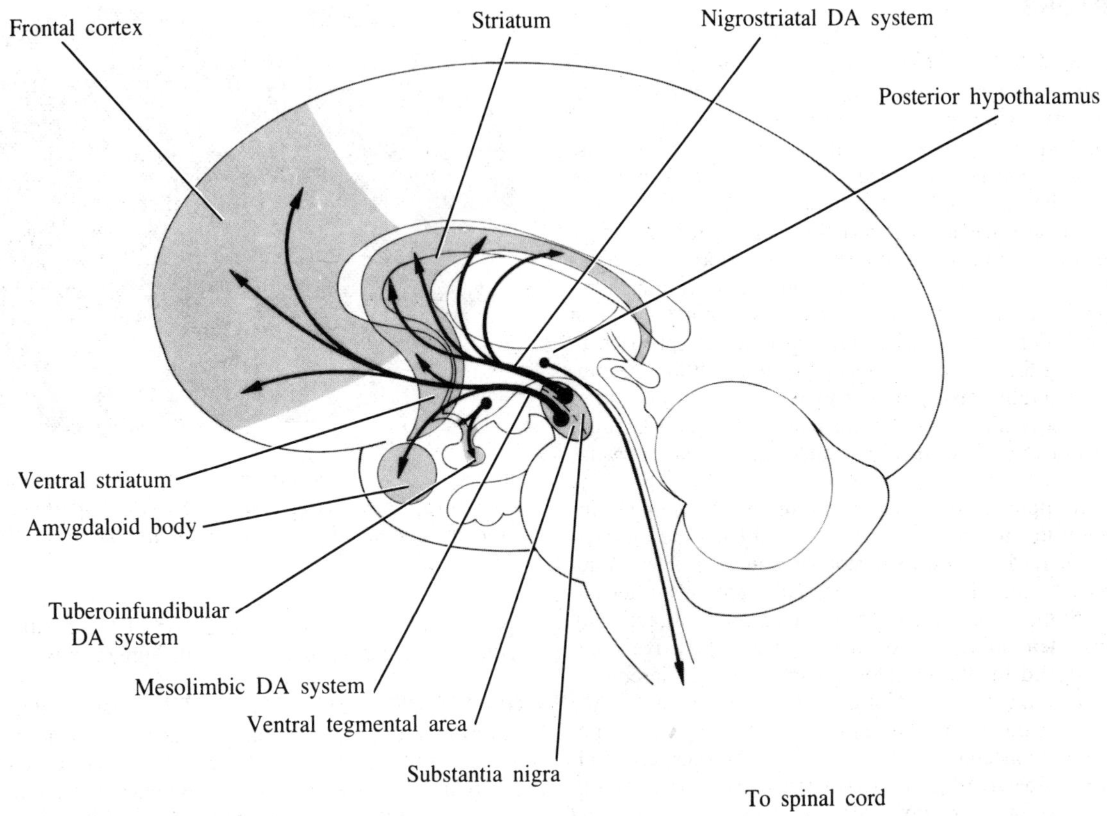

FIGURE 1.3-15. *Dopaminergic pathways. The nigrostriatal DA system originates in the substantia nigra and terminates in the main dorsal part of the striatum. The ventral tegmental area gives rise to the mesolimbic DA system, which terminates in the ventral striatum, amygdaloid body, frontal lobe, and some other basal forebrain areas. The tuberoinfundibular system innervates the median eminence as well as the posterior and intermediate lobes of the pituitary, and dopamine neurons in the posterior hypothalamus project to the spinal cord. (From Heimer L:* The Human Brain and Spinal Cord. *Springer-Verlag, New York, 1983, with permission.)*

Mesulam M-M, editor: *Principles of Behavioral Neurology*. Davis, Philadelphia, 1985.
Mishkin M, Malamut B, Bachevalier J: Memories and habits: Two neural systems. In *Neurobiology of Learning and Memory*, G Lynch, J L McGaugh, N M Weinberger, editors, p 65. Guilford, New York, 1984.
Price J L, Russchen F T, Amaral D G: The limbic region II: The amygdaloid complex. In *Handbook of Chemical Neuroanatomy*, vol 5, A Björklund, T Hokfelt, L W Swanson, editors, p 279. Elsevier, New York, 1988.
Rye D B, Saper C B, Lee H J, Wainer B H: Pedunculopontine tegmental nucleus of the rat: Cytoarchitecture, cytochemistry and some extrapyramidal connections of the mesopontine tegmentum. J Comp Neurol *259:* 483, 1987.
Saper C B: Diffuse cortical projection systems: Anatomical organization and role in cortical function. In *The Handbook of Physiology*, vol 5, V B Mountcastle, F Plum, S R Geiger, editors, p 169. American Physiological Society, Bethesda, MD, 1987.
Schneider, J S, Lidsky T I, editors: *Basal Ganglia and Behavior: Sensory Aspects of Motor Functioning*. Hans Huber, Toronto, 1987.
Stevens J R: Neuropathology of schizophrenia. Arch Gen Psychiat *39:* 1131, 1982.
Strick P L: Anatomical organization of multiple motor areas in the frontal lobe: Implications for recovery of function. In *Advances in Neurology*, vol 47, *Functional Recovery in Neurological Diseases*, S G Waxman, editor, p 293. Raven Press, New York, 1988.
Sverdlow N R, Koob G F: Dopamine, schizophrenia, mania and depression: Toward a unified hypothesis of cortico-striato-pallido-thalamic function. Behav Brain Sci *10:* 197, 1987.

1.4 RECEPTORS, MONOAMINES, AND AMINO ACIDS

JAY M. BARABAN, M.D., Ph.D.
JOSEPH T. COYLE, M.D.

INTRODUCTION

Rapid progress in recent years has greatly expanded the understanding of neurotransmitter and drug action in the brain. Ongoing research on the well-characterized monoamine and inhibitory amino acid neurotransmitter systems has generated new insights into the actions of many psychotropic drugs. Advances in the study of excitatory amino acid neurotransmitters have also brought these systems into the mainstream of psychopharmacology. Many of these recent developments stem from advances in neurotransmitter receptor research and underscore the importance of familiarity with fundamental concepts of receptor function for understanding key aspects of psychotropic drug action.

RECEPTORS

BASIC CONCEPTS *Neurotransmitter receptors* are proteins located on the external surface of the neuronal membrane that detect the neurotransmitter in the vicinity of the neuron and initiate a response to it. Detection of neurotransmitter is accomplished by a recognition site on the receptor that binds the neurotransmitter in a lock-and-key fashion. Binding of neurotransmitter to receptor then triggers a cascade of events affecting neuronal activity. Inasmuch as the recognition site of the receptor is the focal point of neurotransmitter action, this aspect of receptor function has received a great deal of attention. The classical pharmacological approach to characterizing these sites entails evaluating the ability of compounds structurally related to the endogenous neurotransmitter to elicit or block a response. In this manner, receptor agonists and antagonists can be identified and their potencies evaluated.

The development of radioligand-binding techniques for neurotransmitter receptors has greatly facilitated the pharmacological characterization of receptor recognition sites. With this approach, the binding of drugs and neurotransmitter analogues to the recognition site is monitored directly by measuring their ability to compete with a radioactive compound or ligand for the receptor-binding site and thereby reduce the amount of the radioligand bound. The higher the affinity that a compound possesses for the recognition site, the lower the concentration required to inhibit receptor binding of the radioactive ligand. Two parameters widely used to characterize drug interaction with receptors are the K_D and B_{max}. K_D is defined as the concentration of drug needed to occupy half of the receptors. For example, haloperidol (Haldol), a high-potency antipsychotic, has a lower K_D and therefore higher affinity for the D_2 dopamine receptor than chlorpromazine (Thorazine), a low-potency antipsychotic. Estimates of receptor density in a tissue sample, often abbreviated as B_{max}, can also be obtained with radioligand-binding techniques by extrapolating the maximal number of sites available with increasing concentrations of radioligand.

The basic concepts of receptor-ligand interactions have been developed by studying brain homogenates incubated in physiological buffers in the presence of the radioactive ligand. However, the binding of radioactive ligands to receptors can also be studied in tissue slices or brain sections. A thin brain section affixed to a microscopic slide can be incubated in a physiological buffer containing the radioactive ligand, which binds to the appropriate receptors. The excess radioligand is then washed away by incubation in fresh buffer, leaving the specifically bound ligand attached to the receptors. In this way, the distribution of radiolabeled receptors can be visualized at a microscopic level in the brain sections by exposing the sections to photographic film; at those precise cellular sites where radioactive ligand is attached to the receptor, silver grains appear on the photographic film, thereby revealing the cellular distribution of receptors in brain tissue sections (Fig. 1.4-1).

The successful exploitation of receptor autoradiography in brain tissue with radioligands set the stage for the exploitation of the same principles for the visualization of receptor distribution in the living human brain with *positron emission tomography* (PET). With this technique, positron radiolabeled ligands with very high affinity and specificity for brain receptors are injected into the patient. By exploiting computer-based techniques for resolving the radioactive emissions in space, relatively precise localization of the positron-emitting radioligands can be determined in human brain.

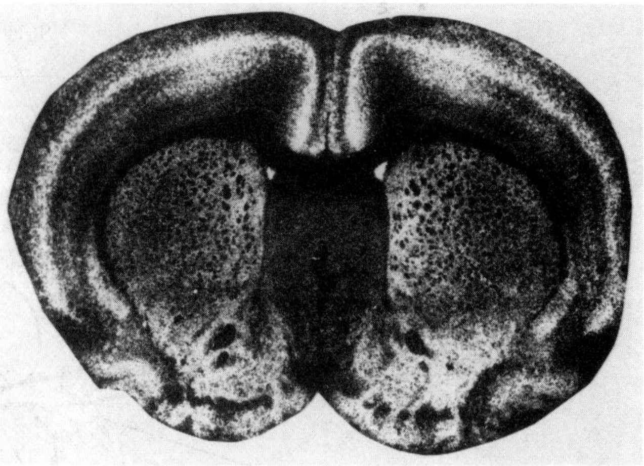

FIGURE 1.4-1. *Autoradiogram of 5-HT$_2$ receptor subtype demonstrating heterogeneous distribution of these receptors thought to be the site of action of hallucinogens. (Photograph courtesy of M Blue.)*

RECEPTOR HETEROGENEITY Pharmacological characterization of receptors has led to the identification of several distinct receptors capable of recognizing and responding to an individual neurotransmitter. Classic examples are norepinephrine, which stimulates both alpha (α) and beta (β) adrenergic receptors and acetylcholine, which acts at nicotinic and muscarinic receptors. Distinguishing receptor subtypes has been facilitated by the development of drugs that selectively antagonize one subtype and not the others. For example, propranolol (Inderal) blocks β-receptors but not α-receptors, whereas phentolamine (Regitine) blocks α-receptors but not β-receptors. Thus, the receptor subtype stimulated by a neurotransmitter determines its effect on the innervated neuron.

The ability to distinguish between receptor subtypes has refined our understanding of drug actions. For example, although it is well known that antipsychotic drugs block the actions of dopamine, it has become clear that of the two identified dopamine receptors, D_1 and D_2, the affinities of the antipsychotic drugs for the D_2 and not the D_1 subtype correlate closely with their clinical antipsychotic potency. Recent research on hallucinogens suggests that agonist activity at one of the receptors for serotonin, the 5-HT$_2$ receptor, accounts for the hallucinogenic activity of lysergic acid diethylamide (LSD) and mescaline-like drugs. Thus, with better definition of receptor subtypes, major advances are being made in the identification of the sites of psychotropic drug action. The availability of selective drugs also makes it possible to assess the involvement of particular receptor subtypes in the pathophysiology of psychiatric disorders.

RECEPTOR ACTIONS Two general classes of receptors have emerged based on the mechanism used to initiate neuronal response to neurotransmitters. One group of receptors conforms to the allosteric model of receptor action exemplified by the nicotinic acetylcholine receptor. For receptors of this type, agonist stimulation leads to a conformational or allosteric change in the receptor complex that opens a transmembrane ion channel formed by the receptor complex itself. For example, the nicotinic acetylcholine receptor consists of five proteins linked together by hydrogen bonds to form a macromolecular complex that spans the neuronal membrane. The core of this complex consists of a channel, which opens to allow the passage of ions when acetylcholine binds to the recognition sites. One of the γ-aminobutyric acid (GABA) receptors, designated as the $GABA_A$ receptor, functions in a similar fashion. Binding of GABA to the receptor opens a channel that allows chloride ions to pass through the neuronal membrane.

The second major class of neurotransmitter receptors responds to neurotransmitter stimulation in a different manner, by activating coupling proteins that are distinct from the receptor (Fig. 1.4-2). These coupling proteins link receptors of this class to other effector proteins within the cell, such as second-messenger-generating enzymes or ion channels. Since these coupling proteins use guanosine triphosphate (GTP) as a cofactor, they are known as GTP-binding proteins. For example, activation of adenylate cyclase by β-adrenergic receptors is mediated by one member of the GTP-binding protein family, G_s. Conversely, inhibition of adenylate cyclase by transmitter receptors is mediated by G_i, another GTP-binding protein. This decentralized form of receptor organization allows several neurotransmitters to activate a common pool of effector proteins; thus, adenylate cyclase can be activated by receptors stimulated by dopamine, norepinephrine, serotonin, and histamine. By contrast, the allosteric receptor configuration ensures that only one neurotransmitter can activate channels formed by the receptor complex.

These two classes of receptors are best suited for mediating different aspects of neurotransmission. In the allosteric class, the tight linkage between the neurotransmitter recognition sites and the ion channel are ideal for fast, precise signaling between neurons. Each neurotransmitter molecule bound activates one channel. By contrast, for the GTP-binding protein-linked receptors a slower sequence of events is triggered. For example, β-adrenergic receptor activation stimulates G_s, which, in turn enhances adenylate cyclase, setting into motion the cyclic adenosine monophosphate (AMP) second-messenger cascade. The involvement of many components in this response allows an incoming signal to be greatly amplified and distributed widely within the neuron. In this arrangement, speed and precision of the allosteric receptor have been exchanged for amplification and versatility.

RECEPTOR DYNAMICS Far from being static binding sites, receptors are constantly in flux, changing their sensitivity and number in response to developmental stage, innervation, functional activity, and exposure to drugs. The antecedent history of receptor stimulation plays an important role in the synthesis and turnover of receptors. A well-characterized example is the effect of denervation on the muscle nicotinic receptor; with the loss of cholinergic input, the number of nicotinic receptors increases on the muscle and they spread beyond the synaptic junction, resulting in supersensitivity. Persistent pharmacological blockade of receptors can produce a similar up-regulation in receptor number as is the case for D_2 dopamine receptors in striatum in response to chronic antipsychotic administration. Conversely, persistent activation of receptors causes a down-regulation, which is associated with a subsensitivity. Chronic administration of tricyclic antidepressants, which enhance central noradrenergic neurotransmission, results in a decrease in the number of β-adrenergic receptors in the cerebral cortex. The association of normal diurnal variations in neuronal activity with alterations in receptor number and sensitivity indicates the dynamic nature of receptor function.

An important means of regulating receptor sensitivity by drugs has been demonstrated for the $GABA_A$ receptor. In this instance, benzodiazepine action at a site near the GABA recognition site markedly increases the receptor affinity for GABA. However, not all changes in receptor activity are reflected in alterations of receptor K_D or B_{max}. The functional responses to neurotransmitter can be dramatically affected by changes beyond the neurotransmitter recognition site involving coupling of the receptor to second-messenger systems. For example, changes in the efficiency of the coupling by GTP-binding proteins may contribute to the dramatic changes observed in tolerance or supersensitivity to neurotransmitters and psychotropic drugs.

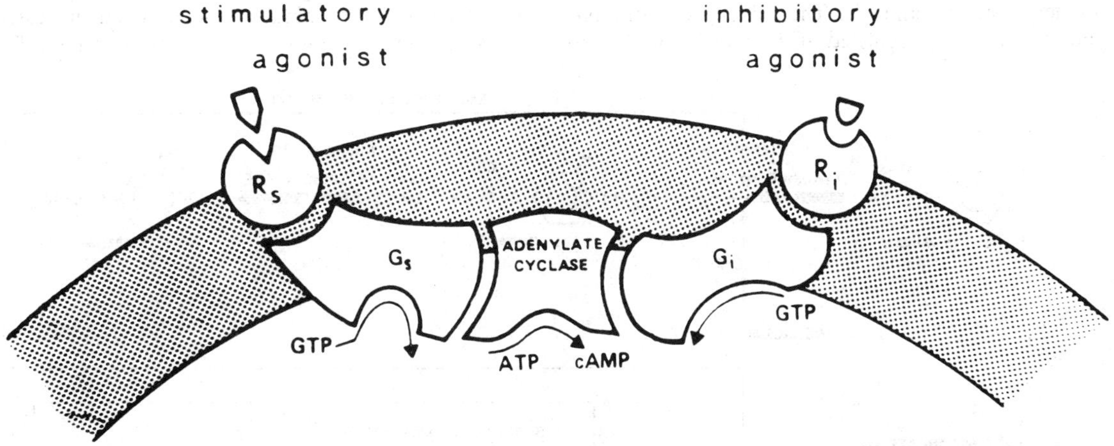

FIGURE 1.4-2. *Receptor regulation of adenylate cyclase. Stimulation of adenylate cyclase by transmitters is mediated by G_s, which couples stimulatory membrane receptors (R_s) to adenylate cyclase enhancing the formation of cyclic AMP from adenosine triphosphate (ATP). Activation of another set of membrane receptors (R_i), such as α_2-adrenergic receptors by clonidine (Catapres) or μ opiate receptors by morphine, inhibit adenylate cyclase activity via G_i. Both G_s and G_i are members of a larger group of GTP-binding proteins that link membrane receptors to enzymes or ion channels.*

MONOAMINES

NEUROTRANSMITTER LIFE CYCLE The identification of *monoamine* (also called *biogenic amine*) neurotransmitters in brain ushered in the modern era of psychopharmacology. Classic research in this field has elucidated the life cycle of these neurotransmitters and has demonstrated that many aspects, apart from the neurotransmitter-receptor interactions, are important sites of psychotropic drug action. For this class of neurotransmitters, synthesis proceeds by sequential enzymatic modification of simple, abundant precursor molecules, such as choline, tyrosine, or tryptophan. The completed neurotransmitters are stored within vesicles in the nerve terminal, released into the synaptic cleft, and act upon receptors located postsynaptically to transfer information across the synapse. In addition, in many cases they also may interact with receptors located presynaptically on the nerve terminal to regulate the release process. An intriguing aspect of the inactivation of this group of neurotransmitters is that it involves primarily a reuptake process that recycles the neurotransmitter or its immediate precursor in the case of acetylcholine.

CATECHOLAMINES The synthetic and degradative pathways for catecholamines are among the best understood of all neurotransmitters. The catecholamines include dopamine, norepinephrine, and epinephrine, the first two of which serve as precursors or as neurotransmitters in their own right, depending on the neuronal system. The catecholamine biosynthetic pathway is a tightly regulated sequence of enzymatic steps that ensures that a stable amount of neurotransmitter is available at the nerve terminal for release regardless of varying activity levels of the neurons. Catecholamine synthesis is entirely controlled within the nerve terminal where the requisite enzymes are concentrated.

The initial and rate-limiting step in the synthesis pathway is tyrosine hydroxylase (Fig. 1.4-3). Compared to subsequent steps, this enzyme exhibits a relatively low velocity and is virtually saturated by its precursor, the nonessential amino acid, L-tyrosine. Tyrosine hydroxylase converts tyrosine to the catechol dihydroxy-L-phenylalanine, or levodopa (Dopar, Larodopa). This product is rapidly converted to dopamine by aromatic amino acid decarboxylase in the cytoplasm of catecholaminergic nerve terminals. The velocity of catecholamine synthesis is rigidly regulated at the tyrosine hydroxylase step. This enzyme is subject to end product inhibition, and therefore when catecholamines exceed the storage capacity for the vesicles within the nerve terminal, the excess free catecholamines inhibit the activity of tyrosine hydroxylase and thus prevent further synthesis. When catecholamines are released on neuronal firing, this inhibition is removed. However, other factors come into play with increased demands for catecholamine release. Increases in the intracellular concentration of calcium resulting from repeated nerve terminal depolarization activates protein kinase C, which phosphorylates tyrosine hydroxylase and increases the velocity of the enzyme. During periods of sustained increase of catecholaminergic neuronal activity, additional enzymes in the synthetic pathway are synthesized in the neuronal cell body and transported down to the terminal.

In the dopaminergic neurons, the final step in the synthesis pathway is the decarboxylation of levodopa to dopamine. Noradrenergic neurons contain an additional enzyme located in the storage vesicle, dopamine-β-hydroxylase, which converts dopamine to norepinephrine. In the adrenal medulla and certain neuronal groups in the brain, an additional enzyme, phenylethanolamine-*N*-methyltransferase, catalyzes the conversion of norepinephrine to epinephrine. The amount of this enzyme in adrenal medullary cells is regulated by corticosteroids.

The primary mechanism for inactivation of synaptically released norepinephrine and dopamine is through reuptake by a transport process concentrated on the nerve terminals. Dopaminergic neurons possess a specific transport process for dopamine, and noradrenergic terminals possess a specific process for norepinephrine. The transport is driven by the gradient of sodium ions across the neuronal membrane (high outside, low inside). These two transfer processes have quite different pharmacological characteristics, so several drugs, such as desipramine (Norpramin), are selective inhibitors of norepinephrine uptake.

The catecholamines can also be enzymatically inactivated (Fig. 1.4-4). Monoamine oxidase (MAO), an enzyme localized to the external membrane of the mitochondria, the power packs of the cells, plays a major role in catabolizing catecholamines that are free in the nerve terminal cytosol and unprotected by the storage vesicles. Catecholamines synthesized within the nerve terminal are sequestered in vesicles by an energy-dependent pump, thereby protecting them from catab-

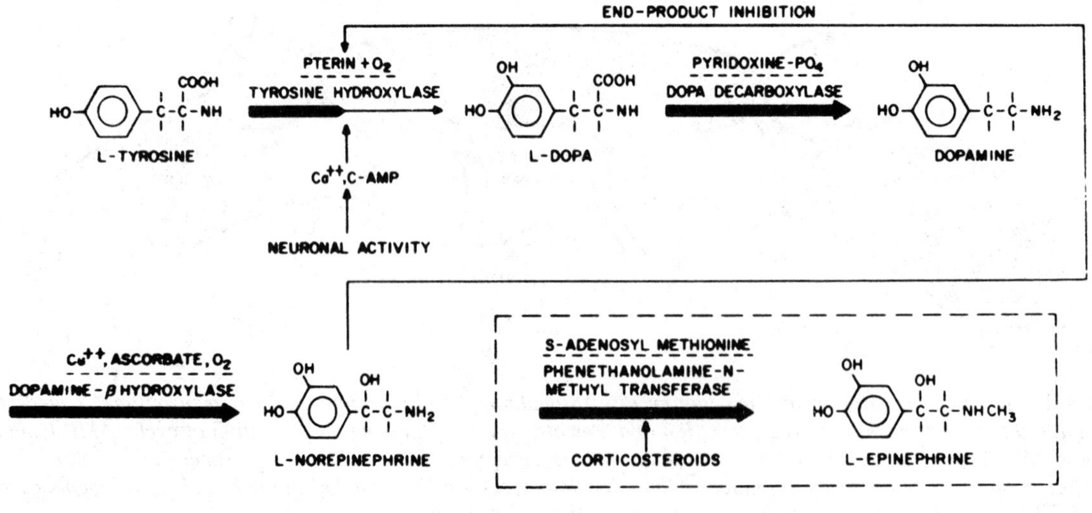

FIGURE 1.4-3. *Biosynthetic pathway for catecholamines.*

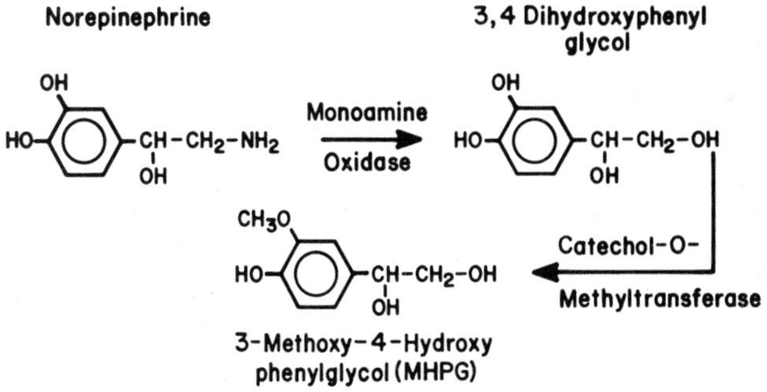

FIGURE 1.4-4. *Catabolism of norepinephrine.*

olism by MAO. Reserpine, an antihypertensive, inhibits the vesicular amine pump, causing the released catecholamines to be deaminated by MAO. Situated on the outer membranes of many different cell types is catechol-*O*-methyltransferase, which inactivates catecholamines that have diffused beyond the synaptic cleft by *O*-methylating one of the hydroxyl moieties. Unlike the catecholamine-synthesizing enzymes, which are restricted to catecholaminergic neurons, the catabolizing enzymes have a broad distribution in cells throughout the body. In fact, they serve a protective function due to their high activity in gut and liver by inactivating catecholamines and indirectly acting sympathomimetics, such as tyramine and phenethylamine, that are contained within the diet. For patients treated with MAO inhibitors, this enzymatic barrier is inactivated. As a consequence, ingestion of food containing large amounts of tyramine, such as aged cheeses and meats, by these patients results in direct access of the tyramine to the general circulation, which releases norepinephrine from sympathetic terminals, causing acute hypertension.

SEROTONIN *Serotonin* (also called 5-hydroxytryptamine [5-HT]) is synthesized from the essential amino acid, tryptophan, with tryptophan hydroxylase serving as the initial and rate-limiting step in the synthesis pathway (Fig.1.4-5). In contrast to L-tyrosine, the ambient levels of tryptophan are not saturating with regard to tryptophan hydroxylase. Thus fluctuations in tryptophan levels in blood and therefore in brain can affect the amount of serotonin synthesized by serotonergic neurons. Ingestion of foods rich in tryptophan will acutely increase brain serotonin synthesis, which accounts for their mild sedating effects. Following hydroxylation of tryptophan, it is rapidly converted to serotonin by decarboxylation by aromatic amino acid decarboxylase. As with the catecholaminergic neurons, the primary means of inactivation of serotonin released in the synaptic cleft is through a high-affinity uptake process on the serotonergic nerve terminals. This transport process is potently inhibited by tertiary tricyclic antidepressants, such as imipramine (Tofranil), and certain atypical antidepressants, such as fluoxetine (Prozac). In addition, intracellular serotonin not protected by vesicular storage is catabolized by MAO. Subtypes of MAO have been identified, with MAO_A acting primarily on serotonin and norepinephrine, and MAO_B catabolizing primarily phenethylamines, including dopamine.

HISTAMINE The recent visualization of histamine neurons in the brain has provided long-awaited confirmation of histamine's role as a neurotransmitter. The synthesis of histamine parallels that of other monoamines, inasmuch as it is produced from an amino acid precursor, histidine, by the enzyme histidine decarboxylase. As this enzyme is not saturated by circulating levels of histidine, administration of histidine increases brain histamine levels. In neurons, histamine metabolism proceeds by methylation to form methylhistamine, which, in turn, is further degraded by MAO.

ACETYLCHOLINE The life cycle of acetylcholine varies somewhat from the above-described theme. The synthesis of acetylcholine is catalyzed by the enzyme choline acetyltransferase, which transfers an acetyl group from acetyl CoA to choline. Acetylcholine released into the synaptic cleft is rapidly catabolized by acetylcholinesterase, which is found in high concentration on the external surface of cholinergic neurons, particularly in their synaptic cleft, as well as on the surface of many other cell types.

This broad distribution of acetylcholinesterase prevents acetylcholine from diffusing from the synaptic cleft and activating in an inappropriate fashion more distant cholinergic receptors. Cholinergic neurons, however, possess a sodium-dependent high-affinity uptake process for choline, so the choline liberated by the breakdown of acetylcholine in the synaptic cleft is efficiently reutilized for acetylcholine synthesis. In fact, this high-affinity transport process for choline appears to be the rate-limiting step controlling acetylcholine synthesis. Notably, the velocity of this transport process is dynamically regulated on the basis of antecedent activity of cholinergic neurons. Thus, when cholinergic neurons are

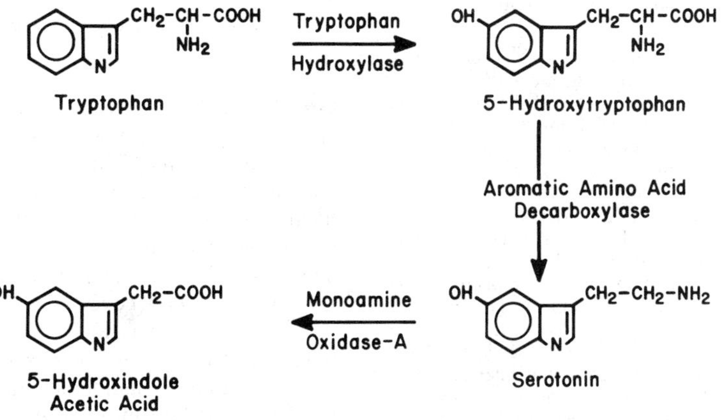

FIGURE 1.4-5. *Biosynthetic and catabolic pathway for serotonin.*

quite active in releasing acetylcholine, the velocity of the transport process increases to enhance the intracellular availability of choline.

MONOAMINE RECEPTORS Several distinct receptors have been identified for each of the monoamine neurotransmitters.

Adrenergic receptors Early classical studies on the peripheral sympathetic system established the existence of α- and β-receptors. More recent studies have revealed further important subtyping of these two major classes of adrenergic receptors. With regard to the β_1-receptor, the type concentrated in the heart, norepinephrine as well as epinephrine, serves as an agonist. The β_2-receptor exhibits greater sensitivity to epinephrine than norepinephrine and to *N*-alkyl-substituted catecholamines, such as isoproterenol. In the brain, β_1-receptors appear to have a high degree of localization to neurons, whereas β_2-receptors are more concentrated on glia and blood vessels. Specific agonists and antagonists for the β-receptor subtypes are presently available. As mentioned above, the β-adrenergic receptors are linked to G_s, which stimulates adenylate cyclase, producing a cascade of cell-specific responses due to the elevation of intracellular cyclic AMP.

The α-receptors have also been distinguished into two pharmacologically and physiologically distinct subtypes. The α_1-receptor, the receptor traditionally linked to smooth muscle contraction and glandular secretion in the periphery, exerts its intracellular effects through a second messenger system, the phosphoinositide system. The antihypertensive, prazosin (Minipress), is a potent and specific inhibitor of the α_1-receptor. When activated, α_2-receptors are associated with a decrease in peripheral and central noradrenergic activity. In part, this reflects the fact that α_2-receptors are coupled to a GTP-binding protein, G_i, which inhibits adenylate cyclase. In addition, presynaptic α_2-receptors on noradrenergic terminals inhibit the release of norepinephrine. The α_2-receptors have attracted considerable interest because clonidine, a potent antihypertensive, has also been found to reduce the physiological symptoms of the withdrawal syndrome in individuals addicted to opiates, nicotine, and alcohol.

Dopaminergic receptors Dopamine receptors have also been found to exist in two distinct subtypes. The D_1 receptor exerts its physiological effects through activation of adenylate cyclase by G_s. Although the transduction process mediating the effects of the dopamine D_2 receptor remains unclear, this receptor appears to be negatively coupled to adenylate cyclase through G_i. Although many antipsychotics have significant affinity for both dopamine receptor subtypes, several active drugs, such as haloperidol and molindone (Moban), are disproportionately weak antagonists of the D_1 receptor, suggesting that the D_2 subtype is the pertinent site for the therapeutic action of antipsychotics. Furthermore, the clinical potencies of a large number of antipsychotic drugs of diverse chemical structure parallel their affinities for the D_2 receptors as measured in vitro by radioligand-binding techniques. This correlation has prompted the widely accepted hypothesis that the D_2 dopamine receptor is the site of action of antipsychotics. The concomitant appearance of extrapyramidal neurological symptoms with antipsychotic treatment is also attributed to D_2 receptor blockade in the striatum.

Serotonergic receptors Serotonin receptors have been divided into 5-HT_1 and 5-HT_2 subtypes. The hallucinogenic actions of LSD have long been thought to involve interactions with brain serotonin systems, since both compounds share an indoleamine structure. Recent studies point to the 5-HT_2 receptor as the site of action of LSD, mescaline, and related hallucinogens. In animal model systems, selective 5-HT_2 receptor antagonists block behavioral responses to these compounds, and the affinities of a large series of hallucinogens for this receptor correlate closely with their human hallucinogenic potencies. The fact that 5-HT_2 receptors are selectively located in cortical regions suggests that activation of this branch of the serotonergic system can induce the hallucinogenic response, which has served as an intriguing model of clinical psychotic states. Research on 5-HT_1 receptors has led to the further subdivision of this class into three more receptor subtypes. Of particular interest to psychopharmacology have been studies relating the antianxiety action of buspirone (Buspar), a recently introduced nonbenzodiazepine anxiolytic, to its ability to stimulate 5-HT_{1a} receptors. Thus, more than one of the 5-HT receptors may be important sites of psychotropic drug action.

Histaminergic receptors Both histamine H_1 and H_2 receptor subtypes are present in brain. Classical antihistamines used for allergic symptoms are potent antagonists of H_1 receptors and exert marked sedative effects, presumably by blocking central H_1 receptors. Many phenothiazine antipsychotics are potent H_1 receptor blockers, and this property may underlie their prominent sedative effects. Cimetidine (Tagamet) and other H_2 receptor blockers are widely prescribed for their ability to suppress stomach acid secretion. Although cimetidine can produce an organic mental syndrome, especially in elderly patients, it remains to be determined whether this side effect stems from central H_2 receptor blockade. The H_1 and H_2 receptors provide an interesting example of how different receptor subtypes allow an individual transmitter to affect distinct intracellular second-messenger systems; H_1 receptors stimulate the phosphoinositide system, whereas H_2 receptors activate adenylate cyclase.

Cholinergic receptors With the discovery of pirenzepine, a muscarinic acetylcholine receptor antagonist that is effective in inhibiting gastric acid secretion without causing tachycardia, there was clear evidence of subtypes of muscarinic acetylcholine receptors. Stimulation of muscarinic acetylcholine receptors results in the activation of two distinct intracellular signaling systems, guanylate cyclase, which increases intracellular cyclic guanosine monophosphate (GMP), and phosphoinositide turnover. Whereas the muscarinic receptor subtype distinction between M_1 and M_2 are not readily translatable from the periphery to the brain, the brain M_1 site, which is quite sensitive to pirenzepine, appears to be linked to the phosphoinositide intracellular system, whereas the M_2 receptor appears to be negatively coupled to adenylate cyclase through a G_i protein. The development of more specific agonists and antagonists for the brain muscarinic receptors has been prompted by the evidence that cortical and hippocampal cholinergic systems play an important role in cognitive functions, especially recent memory. Consistent with this role of forebrain cholinergic neurons in cognitive functions, postmortem studies have revealed marked reductions in the presynaptic markers for cholinergic terminals in the hippocampus and cortex and loss of nucleus basalis cholinergic cell bodies in Alzheimer's disease.

AMINO ACID NEUROTRANSMITTERS

In contrast to the small number of monoamine neurons (less than 1 percent) in the central nervous system, the amino acid neurotransmitters account for the bulk of brain synapses (up to 70 to 80 percent). Both GABA and glycine are major inhibitory neurotransmitters, and the acidic amino acids, glutamate and aspartate, appear to be the major excitatory neurotransmitters. Together, these two classes represent the majority of synapses in most brain regions. Ironically, the universal excitatory effects of glutamate and its role in protein synthesis and ammonium metabolism hindered its acceptance as a neurotransmitter since it was not felt to have a selective neuronal localizaion or to possess specific excitatory properties.

GABA GABA is synthesized from glutamic acid by the enzyme glutamic acid decarboxylase, which requires pyridoxine as its cofactor. This enzyme is selectively localized to neurons that utilize GABA as their neurotransmitter, which include a host of systems, such as the stellate inhibitory interneurons in cortex, the striatal afferents to globus pallidus and substantia nigra, and the Purkinje cells in the cerebellum. GABA is catabolized by the enzyme GABA transaminase (GABA-T), which is located on the outer membrane of the mitochondria. The anticonvulsant, valproic acid (Depakene), is thought to exert its therapeutic effects in part by inhibiting GABA-T catabolism of GABA. The synaptic actions of GABA are primarily terminated by a sodium-dependent high-affinity reuptake process on the GABA-ergic nerve terminal. The inhibitory neurotransmitter, glycine, is restricted primarily to neurons in the brain stem and spinal cord, where it serves as the inhibitory neurotransmitter in the Renshaw cells.

The rapid onset of inhibition of neuronal activity through activation of glycine and GABA receptors reflects the fact that they are allosteric-type receptors whose recognition sites are coupled to chloride channels. Thus, the binding of these two inhibitory neurotransmitters to their receptors opens these channels, allowing chloride ions to flow into the neuron, thereby hyperpolarizing it and rendering it more resistant to excitation. Whereas the glycine receptor is specifically antagonized by strychnine, the GABA receptor is blocked by bicuculline, and both are potent convulsants.

The GABA receptor has been thrust to the center of psychopharmacological attention by the important discovery that benzodiazepines act at this receptor to exert their anxiolytic, sedating, and anticonvulsant effects. The benzodiazepines bind to a site on the GABA receptor that is closely linked to but distinct from the GABA recognition site. In so doing, they enhance the affinity of the recognition site for GABA, thereby potentiating its inhibitory action. Barbiturates, which have a more pervasive inhibitory effect in brain, appear to interact with sites directly related to the chloride channel, thereby prolonging the duration of its opening. These differences may account for the fact that benzodiazepines have a much lower propensity for depressing respiration than do the barbiturates. A second GABA receptor has recently been identified, the $GABA_B$ receptor, at which the antispastic agent, baclofen, appears to be a potent agonist.

Because the benzodiazepines modulate the $GABA_A$ receptor, there has been considerable interest in identifying potential endogenous agonists at the benzodiazepine receptors. Costa and his colleagues have isolated a protein from brain that interacts with these sites. Certain β-carbolines also exhibit benzodiazepine-like activity. Nevertheless, the existence of a physiologically active, endogenous benzodiazepine receptor agonist has not yet received compelling support.

Intensive research on the benzodiazepine-$GABA_A$ receptor interaction has led to several fascinating developments. A benzodiazepine antagonist has been discovered that reverses the actions of these drugs in a fashion analogous to naloxone's (Narcan's) blockade of opiate effects. Accordingly, it may be of clinical utility in treatment of toxic overdose with benzodiazepine. An unexpected offshoot of this work has been the introduction of benzodiazepine antagonists, which exert effects on the $GABA_A$ receptor that are diametrically opposed to the actions of standard benzodiazepine agonists. These inverse agonists reduce the inhibitory actions of GABA and, in limited clinical trials, induce severe anxiety, pointing to the possible role of GABA-ergic systems in the pathophysiology of anxiety disorders. Evidence has also accumulated that ethanol exerts its anxiolytic and sedative effects in part through enhancing $GABA_A$ receptor function. In animal studies, signs of severe ethanol intoxication can be reversed by a benzodiazepine analogue.

EXCITATORY AMINO ACIDS There is now reasonably compelling evidence that the acidic amino acids, glutamate and aspartate, serve as the major excitatory neurotransmitters in brain. This evidence is based on the demonstration of specific high-affinity sodium-dependent transport process for glutamate on excitatory terminals, the calcium-dependent evoked release of glutamate from these terminals, and the pharmacological similarities between the effects of the endogenous excitatory neurotransmitter and that of locally applied glutamate. Furthermore, recent studies using immunocytochemical techniques have demonstrated that several defined excitatory neuronal systems are markedly enriched in glutamate. Nevertheless, it is conceivable that in some of these excitatory pathways, neuropeptides containing glutamate or aspartate, rather than glutamate or aspartate themselves, may serve as the endogenous neurotransmitter.

The putative glutamatergic systems are widespread in the brain and include the pyramidal cells of cortex, the granule cells of the cerebellum, and primary sensory afferent systems. Although research on the psychopharmacological relevance of these excitatory systems is only at an early stage, there is reason to believe that drugs that reduce excitatory glutamatergic neurotransmission could exhibit anxiolytic, anticonvulsant, and sedating properties analogous to drugs that enhance inhibitory GABA-ergic neurotransmission.

Three major receptors mediating the effects of glutamate in brain have been identified and are named after their most potent and specific agonists. These include the *N*-methyl-*D*-aspartate (NMDA), the quisqualate, and the kainate receptors. Neurophysiological, autoradiographic, and pharmacological studies provide convincing evidence that these represent three distinct receptors with differing regional distributions in brain. All three appear to be linked to ion channels, through which sodium and other cations may flow to produce depolarization and excitation.

It is not unexpected that intracerebral injection of agonists for the excitatory receptors produces seizures. Activation of the kainate receptor is associated with a persistent syndrome of limbic seizures that reproduces the pathology of temporal lobe epilepsy. In contrast, agonists at NMDA and quisqualate receptors produce generalized tonic-clonic convulsions. Recently, a potent antagonist of NMDA receptors, aminophosphonoheptanoic acid (APH), has been shown to be among the most potent anticonvulsants known. This discovery has prompted increasing research into the development of other excitatory amino acid receptor antagonists as novel anticonvulsants. The psychopharmacological relevance of NMDA receptors has come to the fore with the discovery that phencyclidine (PCP) and related psychotomimetic anesthetics antagonize the excitatory effects of NMDA. Ligand-binding and neurophysiological studies suggest that the so-called PCP receptor may be part of the ion channel to which the NMDA receptor is coupled (Fig. 1.4-6).

Prolonged stimulation of the excitatory receptors by means of intracerebral injection of their stable, potent analogues results in a highly selective pattern of neuronal degeneration. Neurons with cell bodies in the area of the injection site degenerate, whereas axons passing through or terminating in this area from distant neurons and nonneuronal elements are spared. This response has been termed "excitotoxicity." Notably, the injection of kainic acid, and more recently, an endogenous metabolite of tryptophan, quinolinic acid, which acts at NMDA receptors, into the striatum of experimental animals reproduces the neuropathology of Huntington's disease, leading to the hypothesis that excitotoxic mechanisms may be involved in certain types of neurodegenerative disorders. This hypothesis has received very promising validation by the demonstration that NMDA antagonists can prevent the neurodegeneration that results from status epilepticus, profound hypoglycemia, and anoxia. Thus, these findings are suggesting neuropharmacological strategies that may prevent

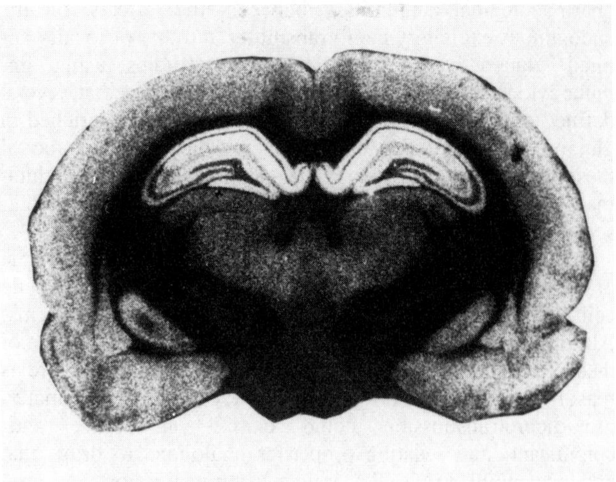

FIGURE 1.4-6. *Autoradiogram of PCP receptor demonstrating discrete anatomic localizations of receptors that can be visualized by applying receptor binding techniques to tissue sections. PCP binding sites are linked to excitatory amino acid receptors of the NMDA type. Regions of high receptor density are shown as white. (Photograph courtesy of B Largent and A Gundlach.)*

or markedly reduce the extent of brain damage following cardiac arrest and stroke.

TRENDS FOR THE FUTURE

Future characterization of neurotransmitter receptor heterogeneity by standard pharmacological techniques promises to lead to further insights into psychotropic drug action and the pathophysiology of psychiatric disorders. The application of newly developed molecular genetic techniques to neurotransmitter receptors has generated considerable excitement as genes for several receptors and GTP-binding proteins have already been cloned and sequenced. Intensive interest in this novel approach stems from the hope that defects in receptor structure and regulation related to psychiatric disorders may be uncovered in the foreseeable future.

REFERENCES

Charney D, Menkes D, Heninger G: Receptor sensitivity and the mechanism of action of antidepressant treatment. Arch Gen Psychiat *38:* 1160, 1981.
Collinridge G L: Long-term potentiation in the hippocampus: Mechanisms of initiation and modulation by neurotransmitters. Trends Pharmacol Sci *6:* 407, 1985.
Cooper J R, Bloom F E, Roth R H: *The Biochemical Basis of Neuropharmacology*. Oxford University Press, New York, 1986.
Cotman C W, Monaghan D T, Ganong A H: Excitatory amino acid neurotransmission: NMDA receptors and Hebb-type synaptic plasticity. In *Annual Review of Neuroscience,* vol 11, W M Cowan, E M Shooter, C F Stevens, and R F Thompson, editors, p 61. Annual Reviews, Palo Alto, CA, 1988.
Coyle J T, Price D L, DeLong M R: Alzheimer's disease: A disorder of cortical cholinergic innervation. Science *219:* 1184, 1983.
Coyle J T, Snyder, S H: Catecholamines. In *Basic Neurochemistry,* G J Siegel, R W Albers, B W Agranoff, R Katzman, editors, p 205. Little, Brown, Boston, 1981.
Gilman A G: Receptor-regulated G proteins. Trends Neurosci *9:* 460, 1986.
Lefkowitz R J, Caron M G, Stiles G L: Mechanisms of membrane-receptor regulation. New Eng J Med *310:* 1570, 1984.
Meldrum B: Excitatory amino acids and anoxic/ischaemic brain damage. Trends Neurosci *8:* 47, 1985.
Snyder S H: Dopamine receptors, neuroleptics and schizophrenia. Amer J Psychiat *138:* 460, 1981.
Snyder S H: Drug and neurotransmitter receptors in the brain. Science *224:* 22, 1985.
Suzdak P D, Glowa J R, Crawley J N, Schwartz R D, Skolnick P, Paul S M: A selective imidazobenzodiazepine antagonist of ethanol in the rat. Science *234:* 1243, 1986.
Tallman J F, Gallager D W: The GABAergic system: A locus of benzodiazepine action. Ann Rev Neurosci *8:* 21, 1985.

1.5
NEUROPEPTIDES: BIOLOGY AND REGULATION

STANLEY J. WATSON, M.D., Ph.D.
HUDA AKIL, Ph.D.

INTRODUCTION

The original concepts of neurotransmission in the central nervous system (CNS) involved "small molecules," substances such as acetylcholine and norepinephrine and, later, γ-aminobutyric acid (GABA) and several other amino acids. In the past 15 years, a whole new class of substances has been identified in nervous tissues as having neurotransmitter or neuromodulator roles. These substances, neuropeptides, are larger, more complex, and almost universally derived from protein precursor molecules. They encompass a substantial proportion of the transmitter activity in brain, involve every part of the central and peripheral nervous system, and are expressed in almost every known cell type. Their physiology is complex because they appear to modify a large proportion of normal behavior. The focus of this chapter is twofold: first, the presentation of general features of the biology of neuropeptide-producing cells; second, a more in-depth description of a single peptidergic system with special focus on anatomy, biochemistry, and regulation of adrenocorticotropic hormone (ACTH)/β-endorphin-producing cells.

PEPTIDES: GENERAL PROPERTIES

The chemistry of peptide structures is presented in Figure 1.5-1. The condensation of amino acids to form covalent peptide bonds is the structural basis of peptide synthesis. The biogenesis of peptides is carried out through a specialized cellular machinery, transcribing and then translating the genetic code and producing precursor proteins, which, in turn, are cleaved enzymatically to liberate biologically active peptides. Chains of amino acids in the form of peptides are capable of carrying enormous amounts of information. For example, each position in a peptide could be any one of 20 amino acids. Even a dipeptide could therefore be composed of 20 times 20 (i.e., 400) possible combinations. A short five-amino-acid peptide could have 20^5 (3,200,000) possible sequences. Many peptides are in the range of 15 to 45 amino acids in length, thus allowing for enormous coding potential. To date, a large set of peptides from nervous and endocrine sources have been described and sequenced (Table 1.5-1). This list of substances is by no means exhaustive, but it generally reflects those substances for which the authors had some means of searching (e.g., an accurate and sensitive bioassay). It may be of interest to the reader to realize that the naming of a peptide often derives from its first observed biological action rather than a summary of all of its actions. Although there are a large number of peptide systems in brain, brief mention will be made of six well-studied peptides.

Somotostatin was among the first neuropeptides described. The name came from its ability to inhibit release of growth hormone from pituitary. When its distribution was studied in brain, it was found to be extremely widespread, especially in cortical structures. Physiologically, somatostatin has been shown to exhibit powerful, broad spectrum inhibitory effects.

Neurotensin was first described as a material with vascular actions. Upon sequencing and after the development of specific antisera, it was seen to be widely distributed in brain. Physiological studies have emphasized its potent impact on dopamine systems in brain.

Substance P was first described early in this century. It also was one of the first peptides to be mapped and was found to be colocalized with serotonin. The assay for purification of this neuropeptide involved a peripheral response (saliva production).

Cholecystokinin was classically thought of as a gut hormone. It is closely related in the structure of its carboxyl end to gastrin (a true gut hormone). It has been described as a major CNS peptide with high cortical concentrations. There is, in contrast, no known gastrin in the CNS.

Arginine vasopressin (AVP) is the oldest, most classical neuropeptide. It is both a neuropeptide and a hormone. The same cell groups in brain (supraoptic nucleus and paraventricular nucleus of hypothalamus) project to hormonal targets (posterior pituitary) and to brain synaptic targets.

Corticotropin-releasing factor (CRF) was only recently sequenced. It was assayed and subsequently characterized using release of ACTH from anterior pituitary cells. It is an unusually long peptide (41 amino acids). The biology of CRF involves at least eight to 10 cell groups in brain, one of which is involved in the hormonal response to stress.

All of these six peptides, as well as most on the list (Table 1.5-1) have had the structure of their precursor proteins deduced using recombinant deoxyribonucleic acid (DNA) cloning methods (see Section 1.15). This list of peptides, and others in the list in Table 1.5-1, have often been investigated for their involvement in mental illnesses. In general, these studies are preliminary, yielding a few interesting hints, but difficult to confirm or expand.

When the various peptides and classical transmitters are anatomically mapped in brain a rather startling event is observed. A large number of these transmitters are found in the same cell types in combinations of twos and threes. Such *co-transmission* represents a radical departure from the traditional "one transmitter, one neuron" dogma of the early 1970s. Table 1.5-2 is a sample listing of examples of peptide co-transmission (e.g., peptide-peptide; peptide-acetylcholine). The implications of widespread co-transmission are far-reaching, the most obvious being that a cell with two (or more) transmitters can deliver a complex signal across the synapse. Instead of one substance turning a receptor on or off, there are several substances acting on their own receptors, and those receptors interacting with each other—all in the process of activation of the postsynaptic cell.

Although peptides and small-molecule transmitters may be colocalized in the same cell, they are actually synthesized by different routes. For example, the general route of

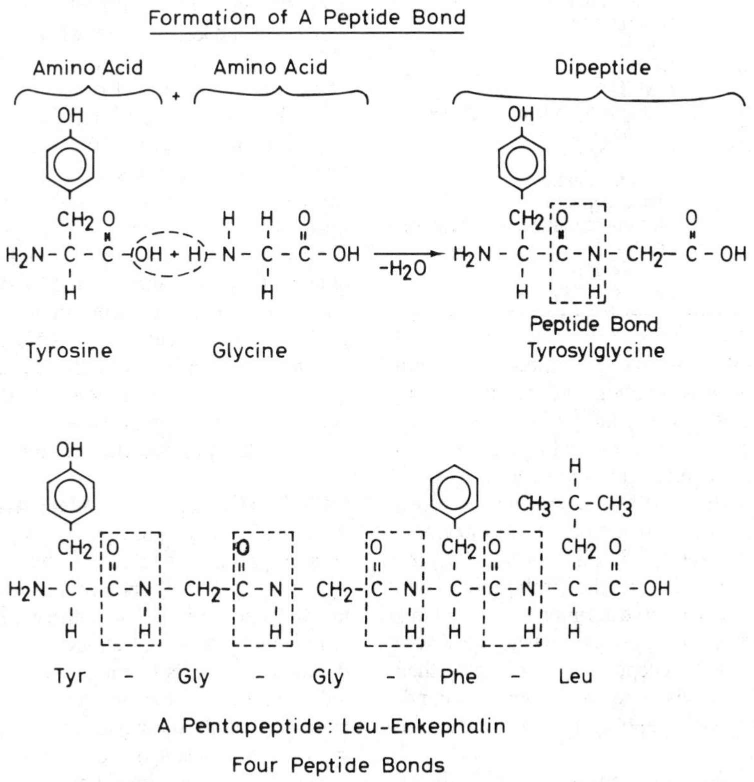

FIGURE 1.5-1 *Structural basis for peptide synthesis.*

TABLE 1.5-1
Peptides from Nervous and Endocrine Sources

Atrial-related peptides	Leumorphin
Atrial natriuretic polypeptide	α-neoendorphin
Atriopeptin I	β-neoendorphin
Atriopeptin II	Releasing factors and related peptides
Atriopeptin III	
Bombesin related peptides	Corticotropin-releasing factor
Alytesin	Growth hormone-releasing factor
Bombesin	
Neuromedin B	Leutinizing hormone-releasing factor
Neuromedin C	
Calcitonin-related peptides	Somatostatin
Calcitonin	Thyrotropin-releasing hormone
Calcitonin gene-related peptide	
	Tachykinins and related peptides
Katacalcin	
Gastrointestinal peptides	Eledoisin
Caeralin	Kassinin
Cholecystokinin	Neurokinin A (neuromedin L, substance K, neurokinin α)
Galanin	
Gastric inhibitory polypeptide	Neurokinin B
Gastrin	Phyllomedusin
Gastrin-releasing peptide	Physalaemia
Glucagon	Spantide
Insulin	Substance P
Insulin B	Uperolein
Insulin-like growth factor	Neurotensin-related peptides
Insulin-like growth factor	Neurotensin
Peptide YY	Neuromedin N
PHM-27	Pituitary peptides
Secretin	Oxytocin
Vasoactive intestinal peptide	Vasopressin
Kinin-related peptides	Growth hormone
Bradykinin	Leutinizing hormone
Liforin	Follicle-stimulating hormone
Ranatensin	Thyroid-stimulating hormone
T-kinin	Prolactin
Xenopsin	Pro-opiomelanocortin-related peptides
Miscellaneous neuropeptides	
Beta-casomorphin	ACTH
Dermorphin	β-endorphin
FMRF	β-lipotropin
GAWK	α-MSH
Head activator neuropeptide	β-MSH
Kytorphin	γ-MSH
Morphine tolerance peptide	Proenkephalin-related peptides
Neuropeptide Y	Amidorphin
Proctolin receptor peptide	BAM-12P
Urotensin II	Leu-enkephalin
Neoendorphin and dynorphin precursors	Met-enkephalin
	Metorphinamide (adrenorphin)
Dynorphin A	Peptide B
Dynorphin B (rimorphin)	Peptide E
Dynorphin 32	Peptide F

monoamine synthesis involves uptake of amino acids with their subsequent enzymatic modification and packaging. In contrast, peptide biosynthesis involves more direct activity by the nucleus and messenger ribonucleic acid (mRNA). In general, peptide mRNAs are copied from the gene, processed to mature mRNA. This mature mRNA is translated into a prohormone which is co-packaged with processing enzymes. As that packaged granule (or vesicle) is transported down the axon, the processing enzymes cleave the prohormone into smaller active fragments. At the nerve terminal, the contents of the granule are released into the synapse, where the active peptide fragments bind to their receptor. This receptor then activates the receptive cell via one of several second-messenger systems. Finally, the peptide itself is inactivated by a series of peptidases.

Peptide systems are therefore one step more closely linked to genomic regulation than are the monoamine systems. Yet, both require genomically regulated processing enzymes, and transport and release systems.

Thus, in the past decade, neurobiology has come to recognize the following:

That there is a very large number of bioactive peptides.
That peptidergic systems are widespread throughout the peripheral and central nervous systems, not just the hypothalamus.
That peptides are capable of acting as transmitters or modulators.
That peptide co-transmission is a common event.
That co-transmission suggests that complex information transmission across the synapse is the rule in brain.

The remainder of this section will focus on the endogenous opioid peptide systems in general, and on the ACTH/β-endorphin system in particular. The precursor for ACTH/β-endorphin is also known as pro-opiomelanocortin (POMC). The first subsection will deal with the basic information on the POMC-producing cells: their anatomy, molecular genetics, peptide processing, and receptors. However, the notions derived from the study of these systems appear to represent general principles applicable to almost all known neuropeptide systems. The final subsection will emphasize regulatory changes in peptidergic cells as a function of demand. The authors will emphasize the hypothalamo-pituitary-adrenal axis and its response to stress. Special focus will be placed on the regulatory cell biology of the anterior pituitary corticotroph because it controls the production and secretion of ACTH and β-endorphin in response to varying demands.

ENDORPHINS: BASIC PERSPECTIVES—ANATOMY AND BIOCHEMISTRY

Over the past decade, more than 15 peptides with opiate-like actions have been identified in nervous tissue. These peptides carry the generic name of *endorphins* (endogenous morphines) or endogenous opioids. These several peptides are now known to derive from three different protein precursors and related genes (Fig. 1.5-2). The proenkephalin, and prodynorphin/neoendorphin precursors each produce several copies of opioid peptides (the basic opioid-active peptide sequence is Tyr-Gly-Gly-Phe-Met [or Leu]). In contrast, the third opioid precursor, POMC, gives rise to ACTH, several copies of the melanocyte-stimulating hormone (MSH) sequence (α-, β-, and γ-MSH have a common amino acid core), and one copy of an opioid peptide (β-endorphin). Each of these three precursors, in different tissues and cell types, is capable of being cleaved into several active peptides. Figure 1.5-2 shows the main products that can be generated from each of the three precursors. Other patterns of peptide cleavage are also possible for all three precursors.

OPIOID RECEPTORS AND ANATOMY Generally, it is thought that the opiate-active peptides from these three precursors produce their effects by interacting with one of three opiate receptor subtypes found in nervous tissue, termed delta, mu, and kappa. These three receptors, when activated by either endogenous or exogenous ligands, appear to produce distinctly different physiological effects. For example, although μ-receptor activation at the proper brain sites is associated with analgesia, the activation of κ-receptors at the same sites may not be. Conversely, κ-receptor activation can result in hallucinations and dysphoria; these symptoms are rarely seen with μ agonists. The short sequences [Tyr-Gly-

TABLE 1.5-2
Examples of Peptide Co-Transmission

Coexistence of Classical Transmitters and Neuropeptides

Classical Transmitter	*Neuropeptide*	*Area (Species)*
Dopamine	Neurotensin	Ventral tegmental area (rat)
Dopamine	Cholecystokinin	Ventral tegmental area (human, rat)
Dopamine	Enkephalin	Carotid body (cat, dog, monkey)
Norepinephrine	Neuropeptide Y	Medulla oblongata (rat)
Norepinephrine	Enkephalin	Medulla oblongata (rat)
Norepinephrine	Enkephalin	Locus ceruleus (rat)
Norepinephrine	Enkephalin	Adrenal medulla (several species)
Norepinephrine	Somatostatin	Sympathetic ganglia (guinea pig)
Norepinephrine	Neurotensin	Adrenal medulla (cat)
Epinephrine	Enkephalin	Adrenal medulla (several species)
Epinephrine	Neurotensin	Medulla oblongata (rat)
Serotonin (5-HT)	Substance P	Medulla oblongata (rat)
Serotonin (5-HT)	TRH	Medulla oblongata (rat)
Serotonin (5-HT)	Enkephalin	Medulla oblongata (rat)
Acetylcholine	VIP	Cortex (cat)
Acetylcholine	Enkephalin	Cochlear nerves (guinea pig)
Acetylcholine	Somatostatin	Heart (toad)
Acetylcholine	Substance P + enkephalin	Ciliary ganglon (avian)
Acetylcholine	Neurotensin	Preganglionic nerves (cat)
Acetylcholine	Substance P	Pons (rat)
GABA	Somatostatin	Thalamus (cat)
GABA	Motilin	Cerebellum (rat)

Coexistence of Multiple Neuropeptides

Neuropeptides	*Area (Species)*
ACTH + β-endorphin	Anterior pituitary (several species)
Vasopressin + dynorphin	Hypothalamo-hypophyseal system (rat)
Oxytocin + cholecystokinin + enkephalin	Hypothalamo-hypophyseal system (cow)
Oxytocin + CRF	Supraoptic nucleus (rat)
LH/FSH + dynorphin	Anterior pituitary (rat)

Gly-Phe-Met (or -Leu)] found in the proenkephalin molecule interact most specifically with the δ-receptor subtype; whereas the prodynorphin or neoendorphin-produced peptides tend to prefer κ-receptors (or κ- and μ-receptors). β-endorphin is a mixed μ- and δ-preferring ligand. Figure 1.5-3 shows the differences in location of the three receptor subtypes in horizontal sections of rat brain. If one compares the above-mentioned receptor anatomy with the maps of the peptide-producing cells and fiber projections for all three peptide families (Fig. 1.5-4) one can readily see common areas of innervation between peptide families, and overlapping receptor locations. It is also possible to demonstrate two or three receptor subtypes in the same anatomical area. In fact, it is commonly hypothesized that one peptide precursor can produce peptides capable of interacting with several receptor subtypes. Thus, another type of complexity is added to our list.

PRO-OPIOMELANOCORTIN PROCESSING BIOCHEMISTRY If one focuses on the POMC system and the intricacies of its biochemistry, several key principles of neuropeptide biology can be uncovered. Figure 1.5-5 shows the structure of the pre-POMC molecule (a "pre-pro" structure includes the prohormone with a *signal* peptide at its amino terminal end; a signal peptide directs the cell to insert the protein into a granule for eventual secretion). The POMC molecule itself (without the signal peptide) is cleaved into several active peptide forms, depending on the tissue in which it is located.

For example, the corticotroph in the anterior lobe of the pituitary first cuts the lipotropin (LPH) molecule free from the rest of the precursor, followed by the cleavage of ACTH and then γ-3-MSH. All of these cleavages occur at dibasic sites (sites made up of two basic amino acids: lysine or arginine [e.g., Lys-Arg]). In the corticotroph there is very little further cleavage of LPH into β-endorphin, or ACTH into α-MSH. In contrast, POMC in the intermediate lobe of pituitary is further cleaved and further modified. These changes are called posttranslational modifications. The cleavage pattern in the intermediate lobe involves first the liberation of LPH, followed by a second dibasic proteolytic step, liberating β-endorphin and γ-LPH. ACTH is simultaneously separated from the amino terminal peptide and is further cut at dibasic sites liberating $ACTH_{1-13}$ and $ACTH_{18-39}$ (also known as corticotropin-like intermediate lobe peptide or CLIP). Finally, the amino terminus of POMC is processed into γ-3-MSH and a *joining peptide*. In most of these cases, the resulting peptides are then posttranslationally modified. The majority of β-endorphin molecules are acetylated on the amino-terminal tyrosine and shortened by four or five amino acids on its carboxyl terminal, resulting in six possible forms of β-endorphin (*N*-acetyl 1-31, 1-27, 1-26, and the nonacetylated versions of 1-31, 1-27, and 1-26). $ACTH_{1-13}$ can be mono- or diacetylated. It is also modified on its carboxyl end with the addition of an amide group. There are, therefore, six possible variants of this molecule as well (three possible amidation states). The majority of $ACTH_{1-13}$ in intermediate lobe is converted to *N*-acetyl-$ACTH_{1-13}$ amide; its alternate name is α-MSH. The CLIP molecule ($ACTH_{18-39}$) is known to be phosphorylated (the addition of a phosphate group), whereas γ-LPH is not thought to be further modified. Finally, both γ-1-MSH (the 11 amino acid piece) and the joining peptide are amidated.

Although adult human pituitary does not contain an intermediate lobe, similar processing patterns occur in human and rat brains. In addition, during development of primates, intermediate lobe-like processing patterns appear in the anterior lobe; simultaneously, the adrenal, at that developmental stage, has a higher sensitivity to α-MSH than to ACTH.

When one attempts to study this wide variety of peptide forms (cleaved and posttranslationally modified) from both lobes, a number of technical and conceptual problems are encountered. At a technical level, one has to separate the two sources (anterior from intermediate lobe) before beginning the

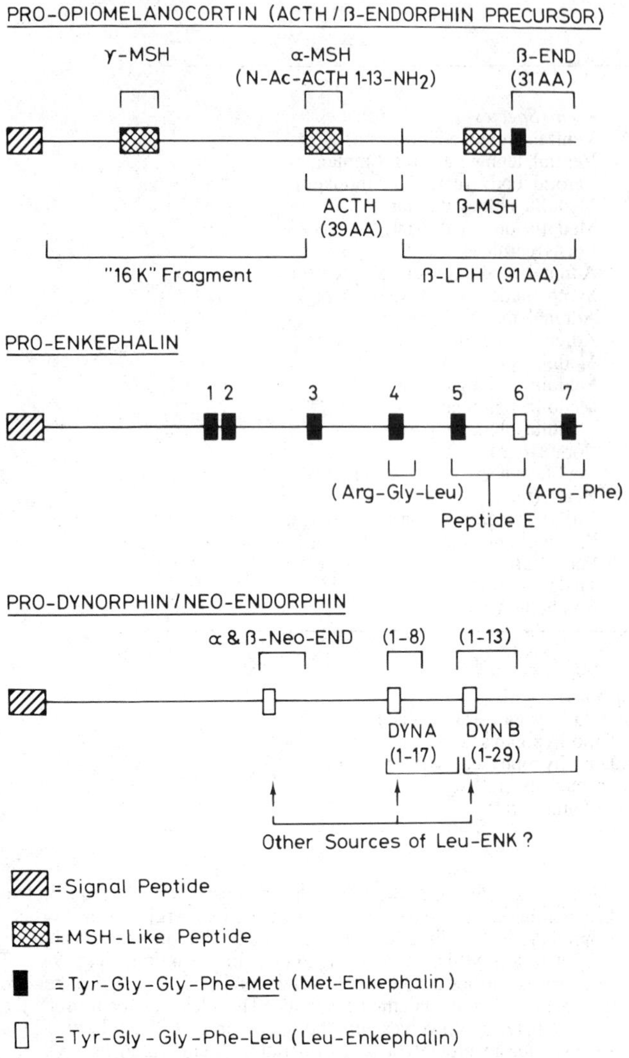

FIGURE 1.5-2 *Endogenous opioid peptide precursors.*

task of distinguishing and quantitating all the various forms of each type of peptide. More conceptually, however, one is faced with the question of determining why such complex cellular processing machinery was developed. What is the physiological purpose of all these peptides and their forms? What are their tissue targets? Although these peptide forms can now be separated and measured, an understanding of their physiology is far behind.

Thus, there are several points and principles demonstrated in this brief discussion of a prototypical set of peptide families:

Bioactive peptides with similar activities often occur.
They can be found in multiple copies in one precursor.
They can occur in totally separate precursors.
There are often multiple receptor subtypes for a defined physiological or pharmacological activity.
A single precursor can produce peptides capable of a broad spectrum of related and unrelated actions.
The anatomical locations of peptides and receptors are complex, often reflecting different anatomical projections to the same terminal area and different receptor preferences of the peptides in those terminals.
Peptide processing is quite tissue-specific and capable of a large degree of plasticity, resulting in a wide variation in the biological activity of the end product.

BIOLOGICAL REGULATION OF A PROTOTYPICAL PEPTIDE SYSTEM

This subsection is aimed at describing the mechanisms a particular neuropeptide-secreting cell uses to respond to demand for increased secretion, both acutely and chronically, and how it adapts to negative feedback. Before moving to the cell biology level, however, this subsection will briefly describe the major elements in a multipeptide, multihormone system located both within the CNS and in the periphery. The axis to be described is the limbic-hypothalamo-pituitary-adrenal (LHPA) axis as it responds to various types of stress.

OVERVIEW OF THE ENDOCRINE BIOCHEMISTRY OF THE LIMBIC HYPOTHALAMO-PITUITARY-ADRENAL AXIS Figure 1.5-6 shows the main structures associated with the LHPA axis. In general, the brain responds to various stressors by activating the hypothalamic neurons which secrete two major peptides—CRF and AVP. Both these peptides are released from several areas of brain in various physiological conditions. Of relevance to the present discussion, CRF and AVP are both produced in the neurons of the paraventricular nucleus of the hypothalamus. These cells project to the external layer of the median eminence, where they secrete their stress-responsive peptides into the portal capillary system, which also bathes the anterior lobe of the pituitary. In this small volume, AVP and CRF reach high enough concentrations to bind to their respective receptors on the POMC-producing corticotroph, thereby stimulating the release of ACTH, β-LPH, γ-3-MSH, and so on into the systemic circulation. The peripheral targets for β-LPH and γ-3-MSH are unclear, whereas ACTH causes the release of corticosteroids from the adrenal cortex. Corticosteroids modulate a wide variety of stress-responsive systems, and also play critical feedback roles in modulating all the components of the LHPA axis. In the brain, corticosteroids bind to a variety of sites, the main one appearing to be the pyramidal cells of the hippocampus. By a still undefined route, the hippocampus, along with direct corticosteroid actions, appears to inhibit the firing of AVP- and CRF-containing cells in the paraventricular nucleus. Corticosteroids can also act directly on the anterior pituitary corticotroph to dampen its POMC-secreting activities.

CELL BIOLOGY OF THE CORTICOTROPH The corticotroph system requires smooth functioning of several neuronal and endocrine cell types, involving a wide variety of transmitters, peptides, and hormones. Almost any element in this circuit is capable of yielding important information about the modulation of biologically secreted products. In the following paragraphs, the authors choose one cell, the POMC-secreting corticotroph in the anterior pituitary. Its receptors, its genes, its mRNA, and its peptides, as it responds to stress-related events, will be investigated.

A good start on such an exploration is the description of the main stress-responsive elements in the corticotroph (Fig. 1.5-7). The cell is located in loose groups in the anterior lobe and is bathed with portal capillary blood. Its surface is known to have at least three important receptors: AVP_r for AVP, CRF_r for CRF, and CS_r for corticosteroids. These blood-borne hormones can act on the cell to modulate a variety of its POMC synthesis and secretion controls. Following a single, acute stressful event, one specific type of cellular response follows. Since both AVP and CRF can stimulate POMC secretion and

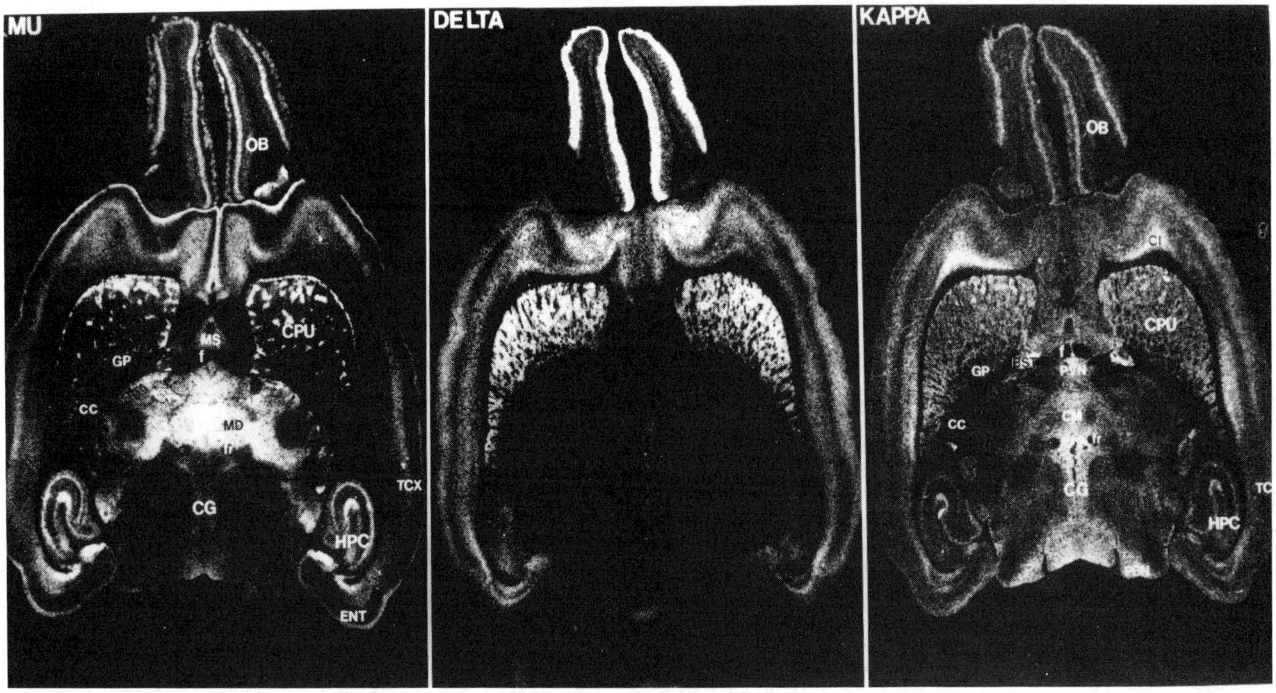

FIGURE 1.5-3 *Dark-field autoradiograms of horizontal rat brain sections labeling μ, δ, and κ opioid receptors. Note the three distinct receptor distributions.* Abbreviations: *incl. bed nucleus stria terminalis* (BST); *corpus callosum* (CC); *central gray* (CG); *claustrum* (Cl); *centromedial thalamus* (CM); *caudate-putamen* (CPU); *entorhinal cortex* (ENT); *fornix* (f); *fasciculus retroflexus* (fr); *globus pallidus* (GP); *hippocampus* (HPC); *mediodorsal thalamus* (MD); *medial septum* (MS); *olfactory bulb* (OB); *periventricular thalamus* (PVN); *temporal cortex* (TCX).

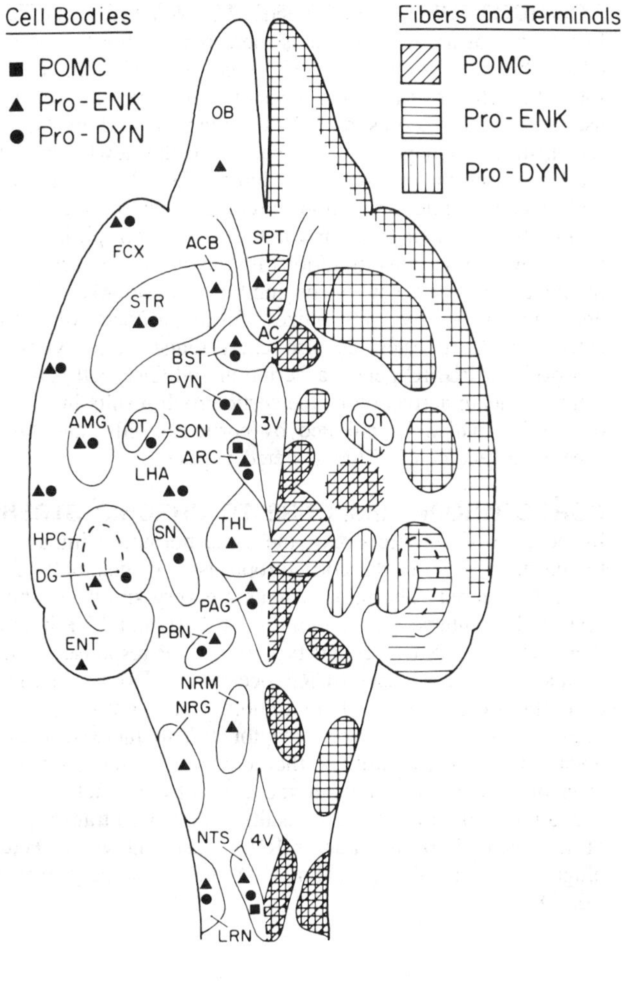

FIGURE 1.5-4 *This schematic horizontal view of the rat brain shows the distribution of opioid neuronal perikarya* (left) *and fibers and terminals* (right) *in selected structures. The distributions of the cell bodies or fibers are* not *meant to be quantitative.* Abbreviations: *pro-opiomelanocortin* (POMC); *pro-enkephalin* (Pro-ENK); *prodynorphin* (Pro-DYN); *third and fourth ventricles* (3V, 4V); *anterior commissure* (AC); *nucleus accumbens* (ACB); *amygdala* (AMG); *arcuate nucleus* (ARC); *bed nucleus of stria terminalis (BST); dentate gyrus* (DG); *entorhinal cortex* (ENT); *frontal cortex* (FCX); *hippocampus* (HPC); *lateral hypothalamic area* (LHA); *lateral reticular nucleus* (LRN); *nucleus reticularis gigantocellularis* (NRG); *nucleus raphe magnus* (NRM); *nucleus tractus solitarius* (TNS); *olfactory bulb* (OB); *optic tract* (OT); *periaqueductal gray* (PAG); *parabrachial nucleus* (PBN); *paraventricular nucleus* (PVN); *substantia nigra* (SN); *supraoptic nucleus* (SON); *septum* (SPT); *striatum* (STR).

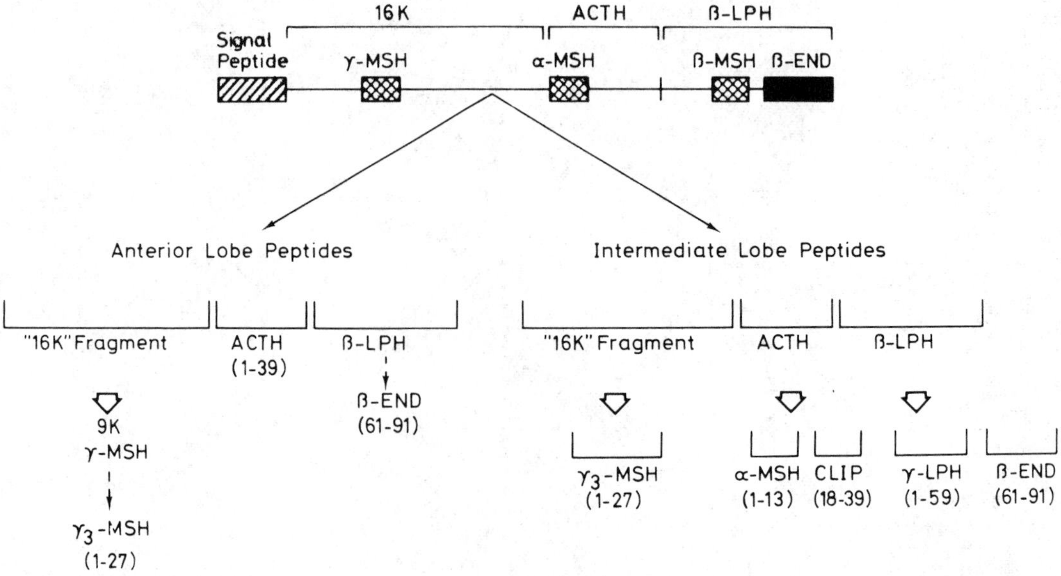

FIGURE 1.5-5 *Pro-opiomelanocortin: the ACTH/β-endorphin precursor.*

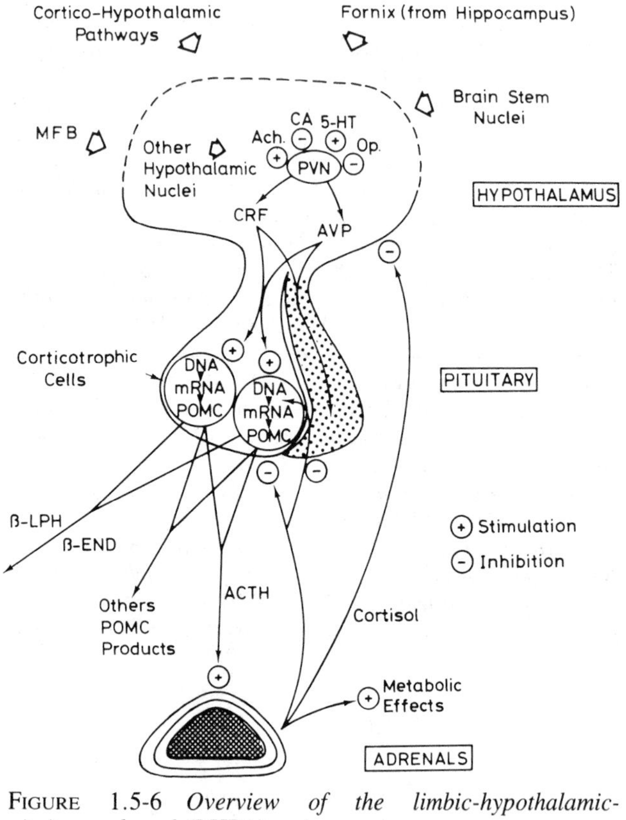

FIGURE 1.5-6 *Overview of the limbic-hypothalamic-pituitary-adrenal* (LHPA) *axis.*

both have their relatively specific receptors, it is reasonable to speculate that these receptors, though different in structural binding requirements, might interact with each other. It is known that AVP and CRF can potentiate each other in producing POMC release. There are currently no data on the biochemistry of the CRF_r-AVP_r interaction, but it is an area ripe for investigation. Following a brief stimulation of CRF_r, there is an increase in the content of cyclic adenosine monophosphate (cAMP) via adenylate cyclase in the corticotroph. Cyclic AMP can have a number of effects; one type of effect may be to stimulate the release of POMC peptides from their granules into the portal blood. A second, less immediate, effect of cAMP is on the POMC gene; it is discussed below under the chronic stress condition.

CORTICOTROPH RESPONSE TO ACUTE STRESS

In the case of an acute stimulus there is probably too brief a cAMP burst to stimulate POMC gene transcription. Therefore, the cell, after its short burst of POMC peptide release, uses its existing stores of POMC precursor and mRNA to replenish secreted peptide. Further, once the newly secreted ACTH causes the release of corticosteroids, these hormones will enter systemic circulation, circulate to the pituitary, and rapidly bind to their receptor within the corticotroph itself, as well as within neurons in various limbic areas. CS_r activation in the corticotroph causes the inhibition of POMC release, and physiologically antagonizes further effects of CRF_r activation. Corticosteroids also exert longer term types of feedback on POMC gene transcription and CRF cell activity. Thus, an acute activation of the corticotroph results in release of POMC, which is inhibited by corticosteroids, and fairly speedy replacement of the secreted peptide.

CORTICOTROPH RESPONSE TO CHRONIC STRESS

In the case of chronic stress, the same hormones impact on the corticotroph, but the corticotroph itself is eventually dramatically altered. The initial events are very similar to those seen in the acute stress situation in that CRF and AVP bind to their receptors, but a second type of cAMP response is now produced by the persistent CRF_r occupancy. Even in the face of corticosteroid feedback inhibition, CRF continues to be released and to activate its receptor and to increase cAMP levels. The indirect result is the activation of the regulatory sites on the POMC gene in the corticotroph nucleus. The activation of the POMC gene results in increased transcription of that gene into immature mRNA (also known as *h*eterologous *n*uclear RNA or hnRNA) and eventually mature mRNA.

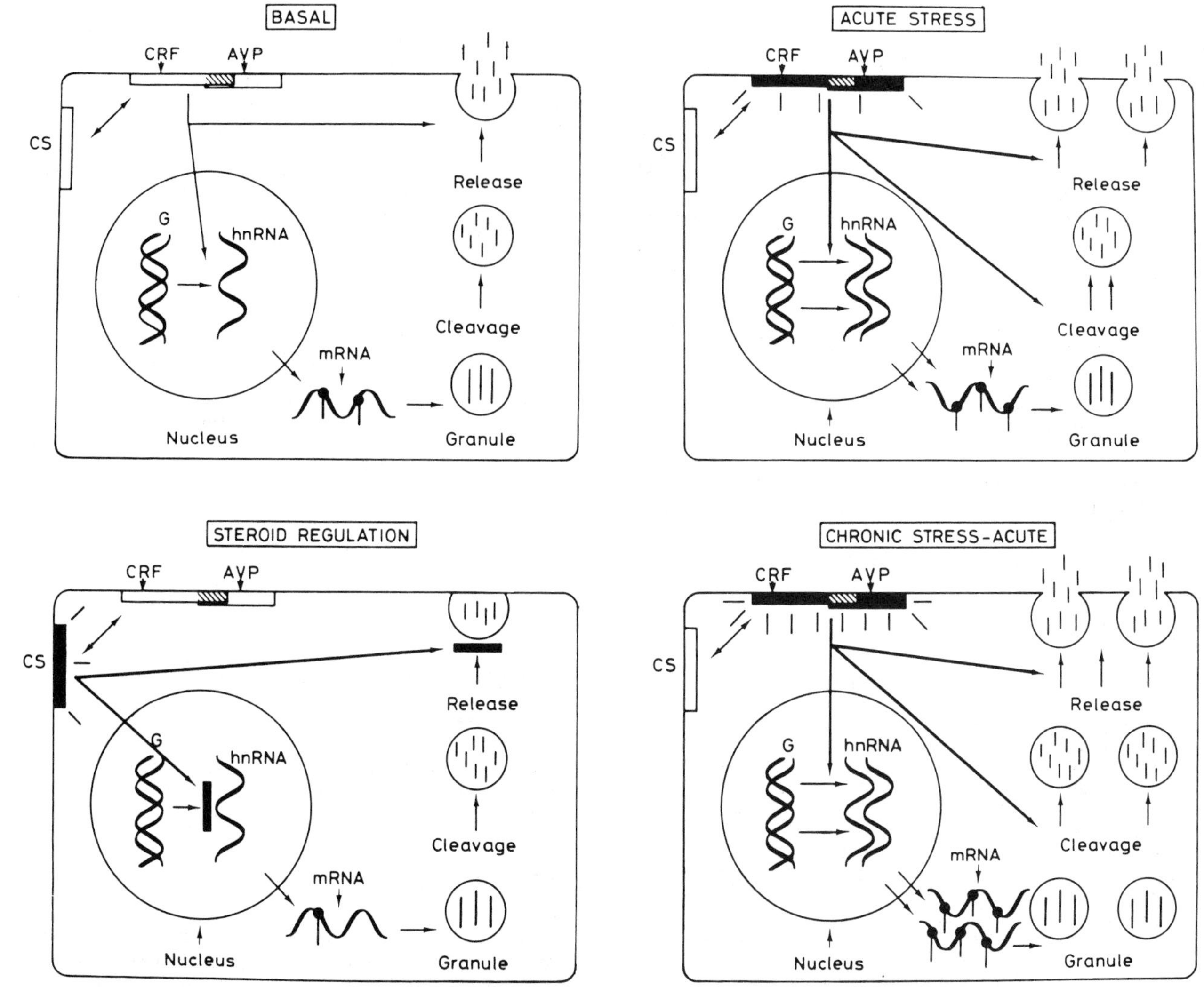

FIGURE 1.5-7 *Stress-responsive processes within corticotrophs.*

With continued stress and continued POMC gene transcription (over hours to days), the corticotroph gradually increases its supply of POMC mRNA in spite of continuing negative feedback from corticosteroids. Currently, it is thought that POMC gene expression is up-regulated by CRF, AVP, and so forth and down-regulated by corticosteroids. The cell is now capable of meeting increased synthesis demands to replace the continuously secreted peptide. Greater stores of POMC mRNA result in larger stores of the prohormone and the processed peptides. In addition, this chronic stress state leads to the alteration of several other aspects of the cell biology of the corticotroph. High levels of receptor occupancy may result in increased utilization of that receptor and its related second-messenger systems, thereby requiring increased gene transcription and mRNA levels for those proteins (CS_r, AVP_r, CRF_r, adenylate cyclase, etc.). Alternatively some systems (especially receptors) may be down-regulated by such heavy demand. Further, increased peptide production and release should also result in increased demand for ribosomes, processing enzymes, granule proteins, and the like. This net activity should also increase the requirement of the cell for energy and thereby increase its demand on mitochondrial energy sources. Thus, an enormous and varied set of demands are placed on a cell under these conditions.

One endocrinological observation that may be of interest is that when one compares the plasma levels of ACTH and cortisol in a naive animal under acute stress with those of a chronically stressed animal under acute stress, there are no differences found. In other words, both endocrine organs (the pituitary and the adrenal) deliver to the plasma the same amount of hormone under either condition. The glands themselves are often radically changed. They may be physically larger, and have more cells, more mRNA, and more hormone. The purpose of these complex changes appears to be to maintain the timing, concentration, and homeostatic balance of the secretory system.

The major points of this subsection on peptide system regulation are listed below. Many of these points are common to most endocrine and peptide systems. These principles are very much the same in the TRH/TSH/thyroid axis or the LHRH/FSH-LH/gonadal axis. The specific peptides and hormones may change, but the cellular regulatory responses are very similar.

Peptide cell regulation involves the interaction of several types of cellular elements.

Gene and mRNA expression and regulation are the critical set of initial events for peptides, enzymes, receptors, and coupling proteins.

Cell surface receptors can control both peptide secretion and gene transcription.
Interaction between release stimuli and feedback systems are central to total cellular activity.
Such cells can control their end products quite accurately, even with very different regulatory strategies and set points.

In sum, the cellular responses of a peptidergic system, even in this brief example, are truly multifacted, involve responses to both local and distantly produced stimuli, invoke rapid and brief responses as well as major long-term change, and can act at any level from the cytoplasm to deep within the nucleus.

If one rethinks the issues presented in this section, it should be possible to begin to understand the forces acting on peptidergic neurons and their means for responding to these demands. The principles outlined here are generally and broadly applicable to most peptide producing systems. One might well ask about the regulatory state of the POMC cell in an acutely ill melancholic patient versus the same patient after 3 months of illness, or even on recovery. Are these changes merely a reflection of chronic stress, or do they imply something about the nature of the disease?

REFERENCES

Akil H, Hughes J, Richardson D E, Barchas J D: Enkephalin-like material elevated in ventricular cerebrospinal fluid of pain patients after analgetic focal stimulation. Science *201:* 463, 1978.

Akil H, Watson S J, Young E, Lewis M E, Khachaturian H, Walker J M: Endogenous opioids: Biology and function. In *Annual Review of Neuroscience,* W Maxwell, E M Shooter, C F Stevens, R F Thompson, editors, vol 7, p 223. Annual Reviews, Palo Alto, CA, 1984.

Berger P A, Watson S J, Akil H, Elliott G R, Rubin R T, Pfefferbaum A, Davis K L, Barchas J D, Li C H: Beta-endorphin and schizophrenia. Arch Gen Psychiat *37:* 635, 1980.

Douglass J, Civelli O, Herbert E: Polyprotein gene expression: Generation of diversity of neuroendocrine peptides. In *Annual Review of Biochemistry,* C C Richardson, P D Boyer, A Meister, editors, vol 53, p 665. Annual Reviews, Palo Alto, CA, 1984.

Goodman R R, Snyder S H, Kuhar M J, Young W S III: Differentiation of delta and mu opiate receptor localizations by light microscopic autoradiography. Proc Nat Acad Sci USA *77:* 6239, 1980.

Hokfelt T, Johansson O, Goldstein M: Chemical neuroanatomy of the brain. Science *225:* 1326, 1984.

Hokfelt T, Johansson O, Ljungdahl A, Lundberg J M, Schultzberg M: Peptidergic neurons. Nature *284:* 515, 1980.

Holaday J W: Endogenous opioids and their receptors. In *Current Concepts,* p 4. Upjohn Company, Kalamazoo, MI, 1985.

Hughes J, Smith T W, Kosterlitz H W, Fothergill L A, Morgan B A, Morris H R: Identification of two related pentapeptides from the brain with potent opiate agonist activity. Nature *258:* 577, 1975.

Khachaturian H, Lewis M E, Tsou K, Watson S J: Beta-endorphin, alpha-MSH, ACTH and related peptides. In *Handbook of Chemical Neuroanatomy: GABA and Neuropeptides in the CNS,* Part I, A Bjorklund, T Hokfelt, editors, vol 4, p 216. Elsevier, New York, 1985.

Kowall N W, Beal M F: Cortical somatostatin, neuropeptide Y, and NADPH diaphorase neurons: Normal anatomy and alterations in Alzheimer's disease. Ann of Neurol *23*: 105, 1988

Loh Y P, Brownstein M J, Gainer H: Proteolysis in neuropeptide processing and other neural functions. In *Annual Review of Neuroscience,* W Maxwell, E M Shooter, C F Stevens, R F Thompson, editors, vol 7, p 189. Annual Reviews, Inc., Palo Alto, CA, 1984.

Lundberg J M, Hokfelt T: Coexistence of peptides and classical neurotransmitters. TINS *6*(8): 325, 1983.

Martin W R: Pharmacology of opioids. Pharmacol Rev *35:* 283, 1984.

Matthews J, Akil H, Greden J, Charney D, Weinberg V, Rosenbaum A, Watson S J: Beta-endorphin/beta-lipotropin-like immunoreactivity in endogenous depression: Effect of dexamethasone. Arch Gen Psychiat *43:* 374, 1986.

Millan M J, Herz A: The endocrinology of the opioids. Int Rev Neurobiol *26:* 1, 1985.

Palkovits M, Brownstein M J: Distribution of neuropeptides in the central nervous system using biochemical micro-methods. In *Handbook of Chemical Neuroanatomy: GABA and Neuropeptides in the CNS,* Part I, A Bjorklund, T. Hokfelt, editors, vol 4, p 1. Elsevier, New York, 1985.

Petrusz P, Merchenthaler I, Maderdrut J L: Distribution of enkephalin-containing neurons in the central nervous system. In *Handbook of Chemical Neuroanatomy: GABA and Neuropeptides in the CNS,* Part I, A Björklund, T Hokfelt, editors, vol 4, p 273. Elsevier, New York, 1985.

Roberts J L, Herbert E: Characterization of a common precursor to corticotropin and beta-lipotropin: Cell-free synthesis of the common precursor and identification of corticotropin peptides in the molecule. Proc Nat Acad Sci *74:* 4826, 1977.

Vale W, Speiss J, Rivier J, Rivier C: Characterization of a 41-residue ovine hypothalamic peptide that stimulates secretions of corticotropin and beta-endorphin. Science *213:* 1394, 1981.

Watson S J, Albala A, Berger P, Akil H: Peptides and psychiatry. In *Brain Peptides,* D T Kreiger, M Brownstein, J Martin, editors, p 349. Wiley, New York, 1983.

1.6
INTRANEURONAL BIOCHEMICAL SIGNALS

JACK A. GREBB, M.D.
MICHAEL D. BROWNING, Ph.D.

INTRODUCTION

This section describes some of the better-established intraneuronal biochemical processes that mediate the production by extracellular signals of specific responses within target neurons. More specifically, neurons contain many kinds of molecules that are involved in the transduction of extraneuronal signals (i.e., nerve impulses, neurotransmitters, hormones) into appropriate intraneuronal signals and the consequent cellular responses (e.g., increased synthesis of a neurotransmitter, potentiation of a synaptic connection).

Most of the molecules considered in this section are proteins—long chains of amino acids. Neurotransmitter receptors, cytoskeletal proteins, and ion channels are just a few examples of protein molecules that are involved in normal neuronal functioning. Proteins are the products of deoxyribonucleic acid (DNA) transcription and translation; genetic diseases are those in which certain proteins are abnormal or absent. Considerable attention should thus be devoted to discovering which proteins are abnormal in genetically based psychiatric disorders; however, it is estimated that there are more than 15,000 proteins that are unique to the human brain and not expressed elsewhere in the body. Thus, identification of the particular proteins involved in a particular disease could be an impossible task. Fortunately, research in the past decade has yielded much information about the types of molecules that play critical roles in neuronal functioning. This effort has been greatly aided by the discovery of a class of proteins known as phosphoproteins. The process of protein phosphorylation, which will be discussed in detail below, is the primary mechanism used by eukaryotic cells for regulation of protein activity. Phosphoproteins and related molecules, therefore, may well be pathophysiologically relevant to genetically based psychiatric disorders. The remainder of this section will focus on this class of proteins and the mechanisms by which the activity of phosphoproteins are regulated by extracellular signals.

THE SECOND-MESSENGER HYPOTHESIS

The understanding of the mechanism by which extracellular signals produce biological signals in target cells was greatly aided by the discovery by Earl Sutherland and colleagues in the late 1950s that epinephrine stimulates glycogenolysis in the liver by increasing the intracellular concentration of cyclic adenosine monophosphate (cAMP). When additional studies revealed that cAMP was the intracellular mediator for several hormonal responses, it was proposed that cAMP was an intraneuronal second messenger that mediated the biological responses to a variety of extracellular first messengers. Subsequently, Edward Krebs and colleagues discovered that the mechanism of action of cAMP in skeletal muscle was to activate a protein kinase, an enzyme that phosphorylates proteins. The addition of a charged phosphate group to a protein changes the three-dimensional structure of the protein molecule and thus changes its activity.

Subsequent studies have revealed that other second messengers besides cAMP are involved in mediating intraneuronal signals. There are three basic classes of second messengers: (1) *cyclic nucleotides* (cAMP, cyclic guanosine monophosphate [cGMP]); (2) *calcium ions;* and (3) *phospholipid metabolites* (inositol 1,4,5-trisphosphate [IP_3]; diacylglycerol [DAG], arachidonic acid). Although these second messengers are discussed separately, they actually are interrelated in the normally functioning neuron.

Except for neurotransmitters with receptors coupled directly to ion channels (Section 1.7), most monoamine, amino acid (Section 1.4), and neuropeptide (Section 1.5) neurotransmitters have their intraneuronal effects via a second messenger. In fact, many ion channels are also regulated by second-messenger systems (Section 1.7). In many cases, these second messengers produce the biological response in neurons by activating protein kinases and thus phosphorylating specific proteins. However, before protein phosphorylation is considered, some discussion of the way in which the first-messenger signal is transformed into an intracellular second-messenger signal is appropriate.

PRODUCTION OF SECOND MESSENGERS

CYCLIC ADENOSINE MONOPHOSPHATE The synthesis of the second messenger cAMP is regulated by first messengers that interact with specific receptors on the surface of the cell (see Fig. 1.4-2). The production of cAMP within a neuron can be either stimulated or inhibited when a neurotransmitter binds to a specific receptor subtype (Table 1.6-1). Cyclic AMP is produced from adenosine triphosphate (ATP) by the enzyme adenylate cyclase. The mechanism by which the receptor is able to activate adenylate cyclase involves a group of proteins known as G-proteins. Because G-proteins are involved in the production of several second messengers, these proteins will be discussed at the end of this section. Cyclic AMP activity is terminated by its conversion into 5'-AMP by phosphodiesterase.

TABLE 1.6-1
Neurotransmitter Receptor Subtypes That Utilize Phosphoinositide or cAMP Second-Messenger Systems

Receptor Subtype	*Phosphoinositide**	*cAMP**
Monoamines		
D_1		+
D_2		–
α_1	+	
α_2		–
β_1		+
β_2		+
5-HT_1		+
5-HT_2	+	
Muscarinic	+	–
H_1	+	
H_2		+
Purines		
A1		–
A2		+
Adenosine		
Amino acids		
GABA		+(B)
Glutamate	?	
Peptides		
Opioids		– (μ, δ)
Angiotensin II		–
LH/FSH		+
Glucagon		+
ACTH		+
Vasopressin	+ (V1)	+ (V2)
Substance K	+	
Neurotensin	+	
CCK	+	
Substance P	+	
Bradykinin	+	
TRH	+	
Nerve growth factor	+	
VIP	+	
Caerulein	+	

*Activation of second messengers is indicated by a "plus" sign (+) and inhibition by a "minus" sign (–).

CALCIUM Although most second messengers are molecules synthesized within the neuron, calcium is a second messenger that can be transported into the neuron from the extracellular space. Calcium can also be released into the cytoplasm from intraneuronal organelles (e.g., endoplasmic reticulum). The intraneuronal calcium ion concentration is very low (10^{-7} M) compared to extraneuronal concentrations (10^{-3} M), and very small increases in intraneuronal calcium concentrations can activate a large variety of proteins, including protein kinases. Thus, proteins involved in maintaining this calcium gradient (e.g., calcium pumps, calcium channels) play an important role in regulating neuronal signaling. In fact, a specific type of neuronal calcium channel (L channel) is a likely site of action for the calcium channel inhibitor drugs (e.g., verapamil [Isoptin, Calan]) that have been reported as clinically useful for some neuropsychiatric disorders.

Some proteins are activated directly by calcium, and others require that the calcium be associated with a calcium-binding protein. The calcium-activated potassium channel is an example of a protein that is activated directly by calcium. Calmodulin is the best-known example of a calcium-binding protein. Calmodulin has binding sites for four calcium ions; the calcium-calmodulin complex can activate a variety of proteins. Many antipsychotic drugs (e.g., trifluoperazine [Stelazine]) affect the activity of the calcium-calmodulin complex; however, the functional significance of this interaction for the clinical effects of antipsychotics is unknown.

PHOSPHOLIPID METABOLITES Just as adenylate cyclase converts ATP into an active second messenger, phospholipase C (a phosphodiesterase) converts phosphatidylinositol 4,5-bisphosphate (PIP_2), a phospholipid located in membranes, into two active second messengers: inositol 1,4,5-trisphosphate (IP_3) and diacylglycerol (DAG) (Fig. 1.6-1). Stimulation of phospholipase C occurs when neurotransmitters bind to specific receptor subtypes (Table 1.6-1). A receptor-mediated mechanism for inhibiting phospholipase C activity has not been identified. IP_3 binds to specific receptors on the endoplasmic reticulum and causes release of calcium into the neuronal cytoplasm. DAG is involved in the activation of protein kinase C and may also promote the activation of guanylate cyclase (see below). IP_3 is inactivated by a phosphatase to form IP_2 and IP; diacylglycerol is inactivated by DAG kinase. Lithium ions block inositol-1-phosphatase, an enzyme involved in the recycling of IP_3 back into PIP_2. There is some evidence that this effect of lithium is especially pronounced in neurons in which the phosphoinositide system is particularly active. Blockage of this enzyme could hypothetically reduce the responsiveness of such neurons to first messengers. This effect has been hypothesized to be the neurochemical basis for the therapeutic effects of lithium in bipolar disorder; however, the evidence for this remains controversial.

EICOSANOIDS Another enzyme, phospholipase A_2, can release arachidonic acid from membrane lipids. In turn, arachidonic acid can be metabolized into prostaglandins, thromboxanes, and leukotrienes. This entire class of compounds is called the eicosanoids, and comparatively little is understood about their functions in neurons. Arachidonic acid and its metabolites may function as second messengers. The prostaglandins are synthesized on demand, rapidly metabolized, and thought to have diverse effects on the modulation of both presynaptic and postsynaptic events. For example, prostaglandins mediate the hyperalgesia generated by postganglionic neurons. The observation that different subtypes of prostaglandins are distributed unevenly in various brain regions suggests that prostaglandins are physiologically important compounds with regionally specific functions. There is also substantial evidence that leukotrienes occur in the median eminence and other areas in the hypothalamus. It is also interesting that preformed stores of leukotriene C_4 have been identified in the hypothalamus. This contrasts with the prevailing notion that leukotrienes or related eicosonoids are synthesized on demand. In the brain, leukotriene C_4 can stimulate a rapid release of luteinizing hormone from rat anterior pituitary cells, which suggests a role for this eicosanoid as a neuromodulator.

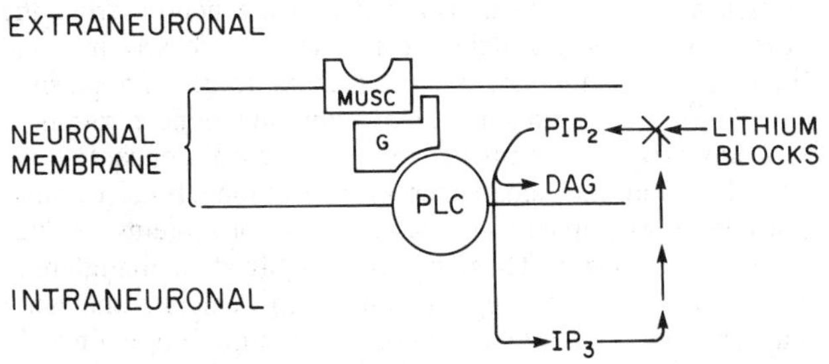

FIGURE 1.6-1 *Schematic representation of the phosphatidyl inositol second-messenger system. The muscarinic acetylcholine receptor provides one example of how a neurotransmitter can regulate the production of IP_3 and DAG. When the muscarinic receptor* (MUSC) *is stimulated by acetylcholine, phospholipase C* (PLC) *is activated via the activity of an as-yet-unidentified G-protein* (G). *Phospholipase C catalyzes the conversion of membrane-bound PIP_2 into IP_3 and DAG. IP_3 causes the release of calcium ions from endoplasmic reticulum. DAG is involved in the activation of protein kinase C. DAG is inactivated by DAG kinase. IP_3 is recycled back into PIP_2 via a series of enzymatic steps, the last of which is catalyzed by inositol-1-phosphatase. Lithium blocks the activity of inositol-1-phosphatase, and this effect may be the basis for the therapeutic effects of lithium in mood disorders.*

CYCLIC GUANOSINE MONOPHOSPHATE Cyclic GMP is synthesized by guanylate cyclase, and G-proteins of unknown types are thought to be involved in the regulation of this enzyme. In addition to its role in activating cGMP-dependent protein kinase, cGMP has been shown to play a pivotal role in the response of retinal photoreceptors to light.

G-PROTEINS Guanine-nucleotide-binding regulatory proteins (G-proteins, sometimes called N-proteins) are a family of membrane proteins that link receptor proteins to effector proteins. Receptor proteins specifically bind neurotransmitters (Section 1.4) and other first messengers; effector proteins can be either ion channels (Section 1.7) or enzymes (e.g., adenylate cyclase, phospholipase C). G-proteins are involved in the amplification and specificity of neuronal responses to first messengers. G-proteins are 10 to 100 times more abundant than receptor proteins. One receptor protein stimulated by its neurotransmitter can activate many G-protein molecules, thereby resulting in an amplified second-messenger signal. Because there is a family of G-proteins, each associated with one or more specific intraneuronal events, a single neurotransmitter could activate different second-messenger systems in different neurons according to which G-protein is associated with the receptors on each neuron. The fact that G-proteins are involved in the regulation of intraneuronal processes means that G-proteins could conceivably be involved in both drug actions and disease processes. For example, one study of postmortem brains from patients with schizophrenia reported data consistent with the notion that hyperdopaminergic activity in schizophrenia could be caused by an increased efficiency of the G-protein-mediated coupling between D_1 dopamine receptors and adenylate cyclase.

PROTEIN KINASES

All of the aforementioned second messengers (with the possible exception of the eicosanoids) are involved in the activation of protein kinases. As stated earlier, protein kinases are enzymes that transfer the terminal phosphoryl group from ATP to a target protein. Phosphate groups are removed from proteins by protein phosphatases. There are four recognized protein phosphatases in the brain: 1, 2A, 2B (also called calcineurin), and 2C. Some protein phosphatases are regulated by second messengers; other phosphatases are regulated by another class of molecules, phosphatase inhibitors, which, in turn, are regulated by second messengers.

Protein kinases are abundant in the brain, and protein phosphorylation is thought to be the major molecular mechanism for regulating the functions of proteins. Proteins are the "workhorses" of the neuron; the addition or deletion of phosphate groups is somewhat akin to an on-off switch for the

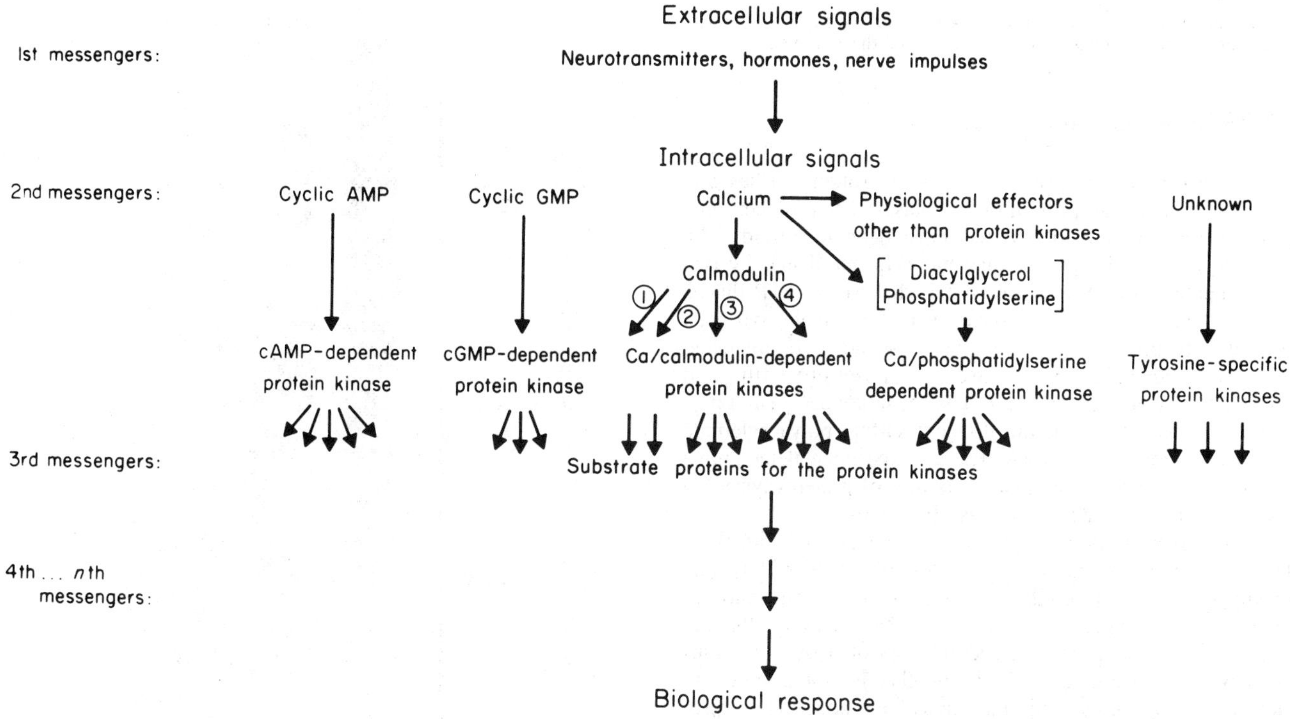

FIGURE 1.6-2 *Steps in the translation of extracellular signals into biological responses. Various first messengers stimulate the production within the neuron of three well-defined second messengers—cAMP, cGMP, and calcium. These second-messenger molecules, as well as some as-yet-unidentified signals, activate specific protein kinases that phosphorylate phosphoproteins. Phosphoproteins are the third messengers in what may be a succession of messengers that eventually result in a biological response (e.g., synapse formation). (Reproduced from Hemmings H C, Nairn A C, Greengard P: Protein kinases and phosphoproteins in the nervous system. In* Neuropeptides in Neurologic and Psychiatric Disease, *J B Martin, J D Barchas, editors, p 48. Raven Press, New York, 1986, with permission.)*

functioning of these proteins. There is abundant evidence that protein phosphorylation is involved in neuronal metabolism, excitability, neurotransmitter synthesis and release, growth, differentiation, and plasticity.

Proteins that are phosphorylated (i.e., phosphoproteins) can be conceptualized as third messengers (Fig. 1.6-2). Virtually all of the effects of cAMP are mediated through cAMP-dependent protein kinase (A-kinase). Many of the effects of cGMP are thought to be mediated through cGMP-dependent protein kinase (G-kinase). The effects of calcium as a second messenger can be mediated independent of protein phosphorylation; however, many effects are mediated through two types of protein kinases—calcium/calmodulin-dependent protein kinases (CaM-kinases) and calcium/phosphatidyl serine-dependent protein kinase (C-kinase). All of these kinases phosphorylate proteins on either threonine or serine residues. Tyrosine kinases phosphorylate proteins on tyrosine residues; however, the second messengers for tyrosine kinases are not known. There are several first messengers that appear to activate protein kinases directly without a second messenger intermediary, and there are also protein kinases that are independent of all known first- or second-messenger systems.

Many experiments have provided direct evidence in support of the hypothesis that first-messenger signals are mediated by the activation of protein kinases. These experiments have largely involved neurons from invertebrate organisms, such as the sea mollusks *Aplysia* and *Hermissenda* and the land snail *Helix*. The experiments have shown that the injection of purified protein kinases into individual neurons can mimic the effects of first messengers by duplicating the normal physiological responses. Additional experiments have shown that the effects of first messengers can be abolished by the injection of inhibitors of protein kinase activity.

SPECIFIC PROTEIN KINASES The various protein kinases provide an additional regulatory system for intraneuronal molecular events. Different protein kinases phosphorylate specific proteins, although one protein may also be phosphorylated by more than one kinase. A protein that is phosphorylated on more than one site may have varying levels of activity depending on how many phosphate groups have been added or removed.

A-kinase There are two types of A-kinase: I and II. The latter is more abundant in neurons. A-kinase is particularly concentrated at pre- and postsynaptic sites, and it is found in virtually all neurons.

G-kinase In contrast to A-kinase, G-kinase is unevenly distributed in brain. It has its highest concentrations in the cerebellum, where it is highly enriched in Purkinje cells.

CaM-kinases The CaM-kinases require the presence of a calcium/calmodulin complex for activity. There are five types of CaM-kinases in brain: CaM-kinase I, CaM-kinase II, CaM-kinase III, myosin light chain kinase, and phosphorylase kinase. CaM-kinase II is the most abundant of these in human brain and is found at both pre- and postsynaptic sites. CaM-kinase II may be identical with the so-called major postsynaptic density protein.

C-kinase C-kinase is maximally active in the presence of DAG, phosphatidylserine, and calcium. In the presence of DAG, however, the enzyme is not thought to need any more than basal intraneuronal concentrations of calcium to be maximally active. Phosphatidylserine is very abundant in membranes; therefore, the availability of DAG becomes a limiting factor for the activity of the C-kinase.

PHOSPHOPROTEINS

Phosphoproteins are phosphorylated by protein kinases and dephosphorylated by protein phosphatases. Over 70 neuronal proteins that are phosphorylated have been identified. The identification of phosphoproteins has been facilitated by two experimental procedures. The first is the use of ATP that is radiolabeled with ^{32}P, thus allowing proteins that have been treated with protein kinases in the presence of radiolabeled ATP to be identified by the use of radiosensitive film and quantitated by autoradiography. The second experimental procedure is the use of sodium dodecyl sulfate polyacrylamide gel electrophoresis (SDS-PAGE), an experimental technique that is able to separate complex mixtures of proteins based on their differing molecular weights (Fig. 1.6-3).

Neuron-specific phosphoproteins can be divided into three large classes. One class of phosphoproteins is widely and evenly distributed throughout the brain. These phosphoproteins are presumed to be involved in molecular events that are common to all neurons. The second class of phosphoproteins is unevenly distributed in the brain; that is, some areas are rich in these proteins, and other areas have none. These proteins are presumed to be involved in functions that are specific to a region or group of regions of the brain, such as the basal ganglia or limbic system. Finally, there are phosphoproteins that are found in only one brain area, and these are presumed to be involved in a function specific to a single type of neuron. By studying phosphoproteins and their distributions, it should be possible to develop a biochemical neuroanatomy of the brain based on the functional distribution of phosphoproteins.

Protein kinases are known to phosphorylate proteins for which a function is known, as well as proteins for which a function is not yet known. For proteins that have previously been identified, the study of their phosphorylation helps us understand how their functions are regulated within the neuron. Proteins for which functions are not known have been discovered using experiments in which stimulated in vitro brain slices were analyzed for proteins that had been phosphorylated by the stimulatory signal. Starting with this observation that a previously unknown protein is phosphorylatable, it is then possible to purify the protein and to study its structure and function. It is hypothesized that the study of such previously uncharacterized phosphoproteins could lead to the discovery of previously unknown regulatory processes in neurons.

PHOSPHOPROTEINS WITH KNOWN FUNCTIONS

Many proteins with previously known functions are phosphorylated by one or more of the protein kinases (Table 1.6-2). Two examples of such proteins are the β-adrenergic receptor and tyrosine hydroxylase. Phosphorylation of the β-adrenergic receptor may, in fact, be involved in the regulation of receptor sensitivity.

The phosphorylation of tyrosine hydroxylase is perhaps the best-understood example of regulation of a known protein by phosphorylation. Tyrosine hydroxylase is the rate-limiting enzyme in the synthesis of catecholamines (dopamine, norepinephrine, and epinephrine). Tyrosine hydroxylase is phosphorylated at different amino acid sites by A-, C-, and

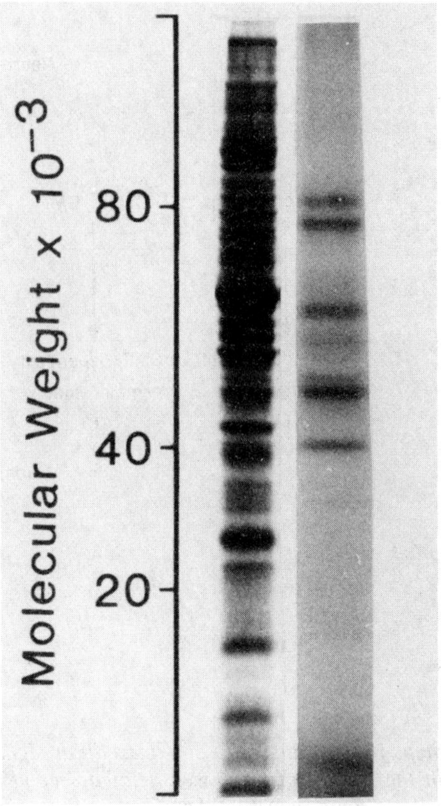

FIGURE 1.6-3. *Results obtained by using "back phosphorylation" and gel electrophoresis. The left lane is a photograph of a dried electrophoretic gel; the right lane is a photograph of a radiographic film that had been exposed to the gel on the left. The dark bands in the left lane represent proteins of different molecular weights as separated by gel electrophoresis and revealed by a protein-specific stain (Coomassie blue). The dark bands in the right lane represent only those proteins that had incorporated ^{32}P during the back phosphorylation assay. The number of different phosphoproteins in the back phosphorylated lane is much less than the total number of different proteins.*

TABLE 1.6-2
Examples of Proteins with Previously Known Functions That Are Phosphorylated by Protein Kinases

Enzymes involved in neurotransmitter synthesis	
	Tyrosine and tryptophan hydroxylase
Enzymes involved in cyclic nucleotide metabolism	
	Adenylate and guanylate cyclase, phosphodiesterase
Autophosphorylated protein kinases	
	A-, G-, C-, and CaM-kinases
Protein phosphatase inhibitors	
	Inhibitors 1 and 2
Proteins involved in regulation of transcription and translation	
	RNA polymerase
Cytoskeletal proteins	
	Microtubule-associated proteins, actin
Neurotransmitter and hormone receptors	
	Nicotinic, muscarinic, β-adrenergic, GABA, insulin, somatomedin C, immunoglobulin E
Ion channels	
	Sodium and potassium voltage-dependent channels

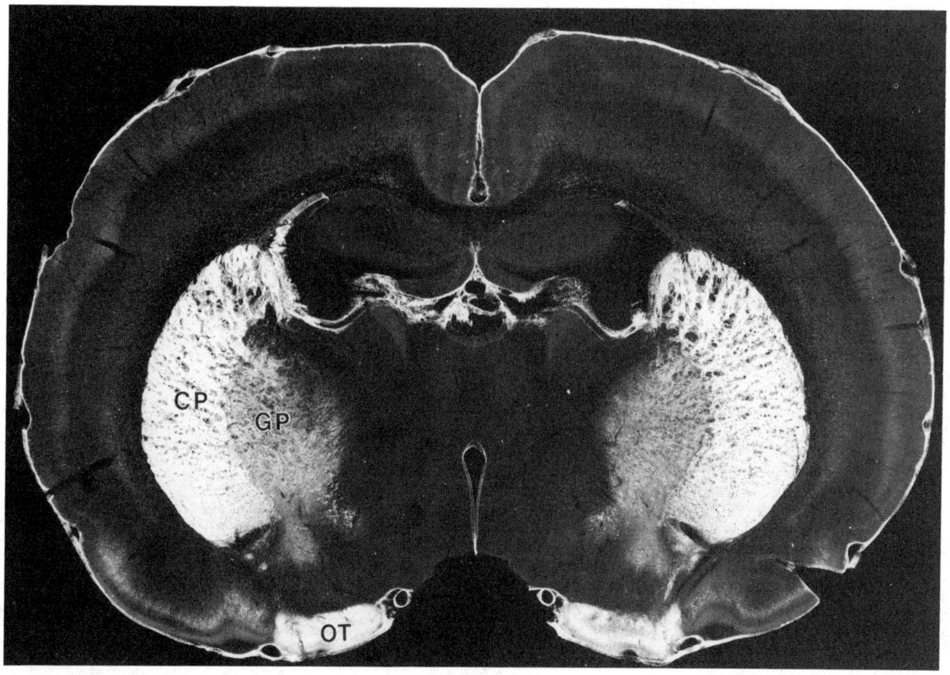

FIGURE 1.6-4. *Coronal section of a rat brain stained by immunocytochemical techniques for DARPP-32. The regions containing DARPP-32 are light areas. DARPP-32 is an example of a neuron-specific phosphoprotein that is localized to specific regions of the brain. Staining is most intense in the caudate-putamen* (CP), *globus pallidus* (GP), *and olfactory tubercle* (OT). *Much lighter staining is visible is other areas of the brain, including the cerebral cortex. The rim of bright staining surrounding the entire section is an artifact of the technique. (Figure courtesy of Charles Ouimet.)*

CaM-kinases. It appears, therefore, that activation of catecholaminergic cells leads not only to the release of catecholamines but also to the phosphorylation of tyrosine hydroxylase, thus resulting in increased synthesis of the catecholamines.

PHOSPHOPROTEINS WITH PREVIOUSLY UNKNOWN FUNCTIONS

DARPP-32 Dopamine- and cAMP-regulated phosphoprotein with a molecular weight of 32,000 daltons (DARPP-32) is especially enriched in the basal ganglia, particularly the medium-sized spiny neurons of the caudatoputamen (Fig. 1.6-4). DARPP-32 is found in neurons that receive dopaminergic input and is hypothesized to be associated specifically with the D_1 receptor. When phosphorylated by A-kinase, DARPP-32 functions as a protein phosphatase inhibitor, thereby prolonging the time other phosphoproteins are phosphorylated and resulting in a potentiation of their effects.

Synapsin I Synapsin I is thought to be involved in the process of neurotransmitter release. The dephosphorylated form of synapsin I binds to synaptic vesicles and may act to inhibit exocytosis (Fig. 1.6-5). When synapsin I is phosphorylated by A- and CaM-kinases, the synapsin I dissociates from the synaptic vesicles, and the synaptic vesicle is then free to fuse with the membrane and release its contents into the synaptic cleft. The validity of this model is supported by the recent demonstration that injection of unphosphorylated synapsin I into the giant synapse of the squid inhibited release of neurotransmitter from that synapse. Injection of CaM-kinase, which phosphorylates synapsin I, produced the opposite effect—namely, an increase in neurotransmitter release.

Protein III Protein III is a phosphoprotein that is also localized to synaptic vesicles. Less is known about the function of protein III than about synapsin I; however, it is clear that protein III and synapsin I are closely related in structure since most antibodies raised against protein III cross-react with synapsin I. One interesting fact about protein III is that an abnormal form of this protein has been found in a high precentage of brains of individuals who had alcoholism, a neuropsychiatric disorder that is known to have a strong genetic component. Although it is currently unknown what relationship the abnormal form of protein III has to alcoholism, this study does demonstrate how the study of molecules that play critical roles in normal neuronal functioning could lead to significant insights into the mechanisms of genetically based neuropsychiatric disorders.

REFERENCES

Augustine G J, Charlton M P, Smith S J: Calcium action in synaptic transmitter release. Ann Rev Neurosci *10:* 633, 1987.

Berridge M G, Irvine R F: Inositol triphosphate, a novel second messenger in cellular signal transduction. Nature *312:* 315, 1984.

Browning M D, Huang C-K, Greengard P: Similarities between protein IIIa and protein IIIb, two prominent synaptic vesicle-associated phosphoproteins. J Neurosci *7:* 847, 1987.

Browning M D, Huganir R, Greengard P: Protein phosphorylation and neuronal function. J Neurochem *45:* 11, 1985.

Dolphin A C: Nucleotide binding proteins in signal transduction and disease. Trends Neurosci *10:* 53, 1987.

Fisher E J, Agranoff B W: Receptor activation and inositol hydrolysis in neural tissues. J Neurochem *48:* 999, 1987.

Gispen W H, Routtenberg A, editors: *Progress in Brain Research,* vol 69, *Brain Phosphoproteins.* Elsevier, New York, 1986.

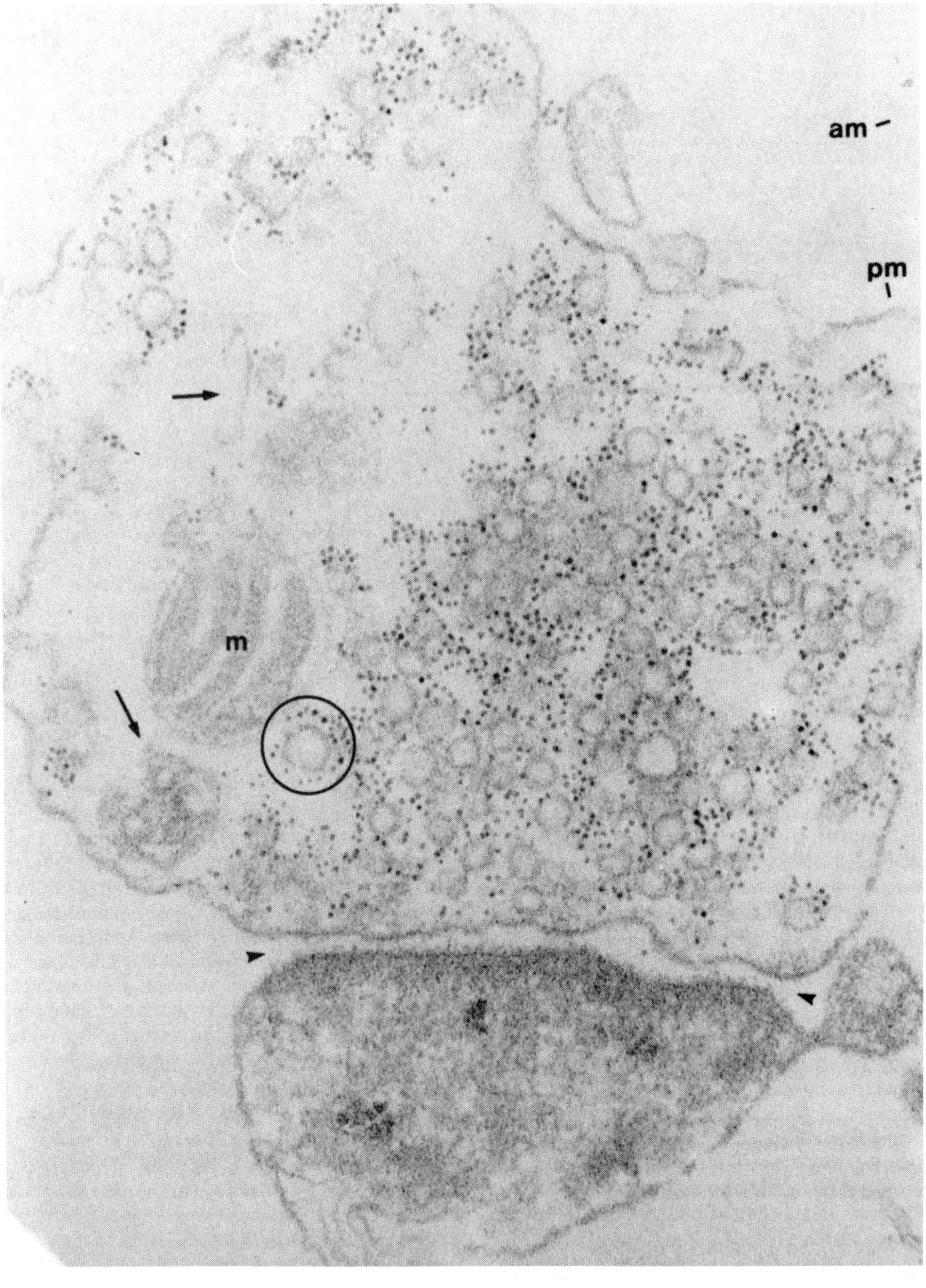

FIGURE 1.6-5. *Synapsin I. The electronmicrograph shows a nerve ending bounded by a plasma membrane* (pm), *facing a synaptic cleft* (arrowheads), *and containing mitochondria* (m), *synaptic vesicles* (circle), *and other vesicles* (arrows). *The tissue has been labeled for the presence of synapsin I by immunoferritin. It can be seen that most synapsin I is associated with synaptic vesicles, and some vesicles are actually surrounded by synapsin I* (circle). *(Reproduced from De Camilli P, Harris S M, Huttner W B, Greengard P: Synapsin I (protein I), a nerve terminal-specific phosphoprotein. II. Its specific association with synaptic vesicles demonstrated by immunocytochemistry in agarose-embedded synaptosomes. J Cell Biol* 96: *1360, 1983, with permission. Copyright © The Rockefeller University Press.)*

Greengard P, Browning M D, McGuinness T L, Llinas R: Synapsin I, a phosphoprotein associated with synaptic vesicles; possible role in regulation of neurotransmitter release. In *Molecular Mechanisms of Neuronal Responsiveness,* Y H Ehrlich, R H Lenox, E Kornecki, W O Berry, editors, p 135. Plenum, New York, 1987.
Hallacher L M, Sherman W R: The effect of lithium ion and other agents on the activity of myo-inositol-1-phosphatase from bovine brain. J Biol Chem *255:* 10896, 1980.
Hemmings H C, Nairn A C, Greengard P: Protein kinases and phosphoproteins in the nervous system. In *Neuropeptides in Neurologic and Psychiatric Disease,* J B Martin, J D Barchas, editors, p 49, Raven Press, New York, 1986.
Hirata F, Axelrod J: Phospholipid methylation and biological signal transmission. Science *209:* 1082, 1980.
McGuiness T L, Lai Y, Ouimet C, et al: Calcium/calmodulin-dependent protein phosphorylation in the nervous system. In *Calcium in Biological Systems,* R P Rubin, G B Weiss, J W J Putney, Jr, editors. Plenum, New York, 1985.
Nestler E J, Greengard P: *Protein Phosphorylation in the Nervous System.* Wiley, New York, 1984.
Nestler E J, Walaas S I, Greengard P: Neuronal phosphoproteins: Physiological and clinical implications. Science *225:* 1357, 1984.
Nishizuka Y: Studies and perspectives of protein kinase C. Science *233:* 305, 1986.
Ogorochi T, Naramiya S, Mizuno N, et al: Regional distribution of prostaglandins D_2, E_2, and F_{2alpha} and related enzymes in postmortem human brain. J Neurochem *43:* 71, 1984.
Rotrosen J, Wolkin A: Phospholipid and prostaglandin hypotheses of schizophrenia. In *Psychopharmacology, The Third Generation of Progress,* H Y Meltzer, editor. Raven Press, New York, 1987.
Wang J K Y, Walaas S I, Greengard P: Protein phosphorylation in nerve terminals: Comparison of calcium/calmodulin-dependent and calcium/diacylglycerol-dependent systems. J Neurosci *8:* 281, 1988.
Wolf M E, Roth R H: Dopamine autoreceptor stimulation increases protein carboxyl methylation in striatal slices. J Neurochem *44:* 291, 1985.
Worley P F, Baraban J M, DeSouza E B, et al: Mapping second messenger systems in the brain: Differential localization of adenylate cyclase and protein kinase C. Proc Nat Acad Sci USA *83:* 4053, 1986.
Worley P F, Baraban J M, Snyder S H: Beyond receptors: Multiple second-messenger systems in brain. Ann Neurol *21:* 217, 1987.

1.7 BASIC ELECTROPHYSIOLOGY

GEORGE K. AGHAJANIAN, M.D.
KURT RASMUSSEN, Ph.D.

INTRODUCTION

The basic electrophysiology of the central nervous system (CNS) is best approached at the level of the single neuron. From the vantage point of the single neuron, one can probe elementary processes occurring at the membrane level. Many neurotransmitters and related psychotropic drugs are known to control the opening or closing of specific types of ion channels located in neuronal membranes; the algebraic summation of these elementary ionic membrane events underlie and explain the firing patterns of single neurons. On another level, the firing of individual neurons can be viewed within the framework of neuronal systems and the behavioral processes subserved by these systems. The aim of this section is to give an overview of basic electrophysiology from a cellular standpoint, with a particular emphasis on relationships to neurotransmitters, psychoactive drugs, and behavior.

ELEMENTS OF ELECTROPHYSIOLOGY

On a qualitative level, the essentials of electrophysiology can be grasped relatively easily, at least to the extent of allowing the expert and nonexpert to share a common language as a basis for communication. In this regard, it is useful to have some familiarity with the methods commonly used by electrophysiologists—the tools of the trade. A brief treatment of these topics follows.

ION CHANNELS: THE BASIC FUNCTIONAL UNITS OF ELECTROPHYSIOLOGY All biological membranes, including those of neurons, possess specialized transmembrane proteins that form channels to allow the selective passage of one or another type of ion either into or out of the cell. The proteinaceous ion channels are embedded in a lipoidal matrix that confers the properties of electrical resistance and capacitance to the membrane. Because the neuronal membrane in its resting state offers considerable resistance to the passage of ions, a transmembrane potential can be established. This potential difference (or polarization) is maintained by ion pumps, such as the sodium pump, which establish a negativity of the inside of the cell with respect to the extracellular space. Thus, the polarized neuronal membrane is poised to respond electrically to any change in ionic permeability. The opening or closing of ion channels affects transmembrane potential E in accordance with Ohm's law, $E = IR$, by altering the product of current I, which in this case would be carried by ions, and membrane resistance R. In direct conformity with Ohm's law, an increased inward flow of positive ions (or outward flow of negative ions) would result in a decreased negativity of the transmembrane potential; this event is termed "depolarization," whereas the reverse (i.e., increased negativity of the membrane potential) is termed "hyperpolarization."

Neuronal membranes are especially well endowed with ion channels that can be controlled by either electrical or chemical means. Although no channel is perfectly selective, channels tend to be identified by the predominant type of ions for which they have some degree of selective permeability. In this regard, there are only four major ions to be concerned with: sodium (Na^+), potassium (K^+), chloride (Cl^-), and calcium (Ca^{2+}). *Electrically activated* (voltage-sensitive) ion channels are those whose opening or closing is controlled or gated by changes in the transmembrane potential of the cell. The ion channels responsible for the action potential are of this kind and they open when membrane potential depolarizes to a critical level termed *spike threshold.* The channels involved in generating the action potential are primarily those selective for Na^+. In addition, voltage-sensitive Ca^{2+} channels become activated during the action potential. A second major type of ion channel is *chemically gated;* that is, these channels are activated by neurotransmitter substances. However, it is now known that the distinction between electrically and chemically activated channels is not absolute and that the function of many voltage-dependent channels can be modulated by neurotransmitters.

What are the electrophysiological consequences of the opening or closing of ion channels? The answer to this question follows directly from the fact that pumping mechanisms establish an unequal distribution, inside to outside, of the four major ions that carry current in neurons. As a result, ions are in a position to flow down their concentration gradient; this situation creates a diffusional potential across a semipermeable membrane. The cell's transmembrane potential can either enhance or oppose the diffusional forces that drive the movement of ions. Na^+ and Ca^{2+} ions have a high outside-to-inside concentration ratio. Thus, at the *resting potential* of a typical neuron, which is normally negative inside with respect to outside by approximately –55 to –65 millivolts (mV), the opening of Na^+ or Ca^{2+} channels will result in an inward flow of these positive ions. At spike threshold (typically –55 mV), multiple voltage-sensitive Na^+ channels open in a kind of chain reaction to generate a massive but brief (0.1- to 2-msec) depolarization termed the "action potential" or "spike" (Fig. 1.7-1); Ca^{2+} ions also enter through their own voltage-sensitive channels during the action potential, contributing to the depolarization. The entry of Ca^{2+} ions along with Na^+ during the spike has several important implications: (1) Ca^{2+} functions as a second messenger in the cell (Section 1.6): (2) Ca^{2+} entry triggers the release of neurotransmitters at the nerve terminal (and in some instances in the region of the cell soma and dendrites); (3) Ca^{2+} activates a special kind of hyperpolarizing outward K^+ current, which produces a potential called an *afterhyperpolarization,* so named because it comes after the spike (Fig. 1.7-1). The afterhyperpolarization serves an intrinsic negative feedback function by transiently diminishing cell excitability.

The opening of Cl^- channels results in a hyperpolarizing effect due to the inflow of negative ions. Cl^- ions flow inward at resting potential, despite the inside negativity of the cell, because the high outside-to-inside ratio of Cl^- establishes a diffusional potential that exceeds the resting membrane potential. Moreover, the opening of K^+ channels has a hyperpolarizing effect because of the outward flow of these positive ions; the flow is outward because the diffusional potential of the high inside-to-outside ratio of K^+ ions exceeds the negativity of membrane potential at resting levels. Conversely, the closing of K^+ channels, some of which may be open at rest, results in depolarization.

In terms of overall cell function, the depolarizing effect of opening Na^+ and Ca^{2+} channels (or the closing of K^+ channels) causes an increase in cell excitability or spiking; the hyperpolarizing effect of opening Cl^- or K^+ channels leads to a decrease in cell excitability or spiking.

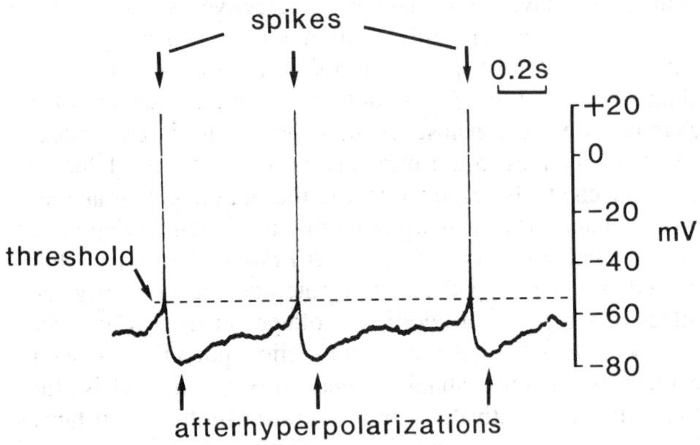

FIGURE 1.7-1. *An oscilloscope trace showing a repetitively firing neuron recorded intracellularly in vivo. This example was taken from a serotonergic neuron in the dorsal raphe nucleus of the rat midbrain. As can be seen from the trace, when membrane potential, in millivolts, reaches* threshold *(–55 mV), an all-or-none* spike *occurs. Following each spike there is an* afterhyperpolarization, *which moves the cell away from threshold into a more negative zone (near –80 mV). As the afterhyperpolarization decays, the cell again approaches spike threshold.*

THE BASIC TOOLS OF THE ELECTROPHYSIOLOGIST The common final output of fluctuations in channel openings are alterations in the rate of firing of neurons. Thus, firing rate represents an integration of multiple channel events at a membrane level. The firing rate of single neurons can be monitored with the use of microelectrodes, either etched metal electrodes or fine-tipped glass micropipettes. To measure firing rate, microelectrodes are positioned near the outside surface of a neuron; this technique is referred to as *extracellular recording*. Such recordings can be performed in the brain of the intact animal (in vivo) or in vitro in brain slices or cell culture. In vivo recordings may be done in anesthetized animals or in awake, behaving animals; the latter, called *chronic unit recording,* allows for observing correlations between neuronal activity and behavior.

A more direct approach to monitoring ion channels can be accomplished by means of *intracellular recording,* where the neuron is impaled by a very fine micropipette (usually filled with a K^+ salt because this is the major intracellular cation). By this means, transmembrane potentials or currents can be measured. Customarily, when membrane potential is recorded, current pulses of constant magnitude are periodically injected through the recording electrode to assess membrane *input resistance* (by Ohm's law the input resistance is the voltage deflection produced by the constant-current pulse divided by the value of the constant-current test pulse used). This is the so-called *current clamp* mode, which permits a direct assessment of membrane potential and membrane permeability (as indicated by changes in input resistance).

An even more direct method for monitoring permeability changes in ion channels is the *voltage clamp* technique. When intracellular recordings are made in the voltage clamp mode, membrane voltage can be set at a given constant value, which is termed the "command voltage" (feedback circuits inject sufficient hyperpolarizing or depolarizing current through the intracellular electrode to maintain command voltage). By this means, inward and outward transmembrane currents can be measured directly without the confounding variables of membrane resistance and capacitance. Finally, it is now possible to detect the opening or closing of a few ion channels, or even a single channel, by the *patch clamp* method, in which a small area of neuronal membrane is brought against the opening of a fire-polished micropipette to form an extremely high-resistance seal (gigaseal). Single-channel recording can be done only in neuronal preparations with naked membranes (i.e., those free of any glial covering), which occur in cell culture or in invertebrate ganglia. The validation of the existence of specific ion-selective channels and how they work rests on evidence obtained by this exciting new method.

ELECTROPHYSIOLOGY OF NEUROTRANSMISSION

SYNAPTIC POTENTIALS PRODUCED BY NEUROTRANSMITTERS Most agents that are suspected of acting as neurotransmitters have either an excitatory or inhibitory effect on firing rate if they are applied to neurons that have receptors for these substances. For several decades, the most popular technique for assessing the effects of putative neurotransmitters on the activity of CNS neurons has been that of *microiontophoresis*. In essence, this technique involves the use of multibarreled micropipettes in which all the tips are close together. Typically, one barrel is used to record neuronal spikes and the other barrels are used to apply, by the passage of current, minute amounts of transmitter or drug ions in the direct vicinity of the neuron being recorded. This procedure yields a useful characterization of the type of response (e.g., excitatory or inhibitory) produced by a substance when applied to a neuron.

However, the fact that a given neuron responds to a particular microiontophoretically applied exogenous substance does not itself prove that it receives an endogenous input utilizing that substance as a transmitter. It is an essential part of the physiological characterization of a transmitter, based on anatomical and histochemical data for the existence of a given neurochemical input (Sections 1.2 and 1.3), to stimulate electrically the pathway mediating this input. Of greatest value in this regard is the monitoring of postsynaptic responses by intracellular recording. By this means, either depolarizing or hyperpolarizing potentials can be elicited in the postsynaptic cell; the depolarizing responses are termed *excitatory postsynaptic potentials* (EPSPs) and the hyperpolarizing responses are termed *inhibitory postsynaptic potentials* (IPSPs). EPSPs and IPSPs are characteristically small, graded potentials that can either elicit or abort the occurrence of an all-or-none spike; in any given instance the outcome depends on whether the integrated action of multiple EPSPs and IPSPs produces a net shift of the cell membrane potential toward or away from spike threshold. Rate of onset and duration are other important characteristics of synaptic potentials. Some synaptic potentials are extremely rapid in onset and offset; others are slow in onset and of long duration. The physiological significance of a synaptic input can be viewed as a function of these rate characteristics. Fast synaptic events serve to transmit discrete messages, whereas slow synaptic potentials alter cell excitability with respect to other inputs over relatively long periods of time and are in this sense modulatory.

COUPLING OF RECEPTORS TO ION CHANNELS Neurotransmitter receptors do not necessarily interact directly with ion channels but can interact indirectly through a sequence of intervening biochemical steps mediated by second-messenger systems (Section 1.6). The electrophysiological implications of these various forms of coupling, depicted schematically in Figure 1.7-2, will now be considered.

Direct coupling The simplest and most direct form of coupling occurs when the transmitter recognition site (the "receptor" in the narrowest sense) is actually part of the protein complex that includes the ion channel itself (Fig. 1.7-2A). The classic example of this type of coupling is the nicotinic cholinergic Na^+ channel of the skeletal neuromuscular junction. Acetylcholine receptor sites are located on two of the five protein subunits that comprise this ion channel. When acetylcholine binds to these receptors there is an immediate conformational change in the channel protein complex, resulting in a rapid and marked increase in permeability to Na^+ as well as to other cations. The great advantage of direct coupling is rapidity of response, which is of obvious value in the transmission of excitatory impulses at the skeletal neuromuscular junction where speed is of the essence.

In the CNS, rapid, directly coupled excitatory neurotransmission is mainly subserved by a different class of substances, the excitatory amino acids (e.g., glutamate, aspartate) (Section 1.4). The prominent action of the excitatory amino acids is to produce a rapid onset and offset of depolarization. It is suspected that the amino acid receptor sites are closely associated with the protein complex that forms the ion channel—in all probability a type of chemically gated channel that is permeable to Na^+ and other monovalent cations. However, this has not been established directly (e.g., through purification and reconstitution of the protein subunits) as has been done in the case of the nicotinic cholinergic receptor. The excitatory amino acids have been proposed as the principal transmitters for many primary sensory neurons and pyramidal tract neurons (upper motor neurons), where it is advantageous to have rapid transmission with minimum delay. In addition to these fast excitatory effects, the excitatory amino acids, acting through a different receptor, produce a slow excitation by opening a special type of Ca^{2+} cation channel that is permeable to Ca^{2+} as well as to Na^+.

Receptors for the major inhibitory amino acids (i.e., γ-aminobutyric acid [GABA] and glycine) in the CNS also appear to be situated directly on the protein complex that forms the ion channel—in this case, Cl^- channels. Accordingly, inhibitory responses (i.e., IPSPs) believed to be mediated by GABA and glycine in the CNS are characterized by the rapidity of their onset and offset.

Transducer protein coupling and second-messenger systems Many receptors are not an intrinsic part of an ion channel but instead are coupled to macromolecules that belong to a family of membrane proteins characterized by their guanosine triphosphate (GTP)-binding properties—the so-called *G-proteins* or *N-proteins* (Figs. 1.7-2B and C). In a general way, G-proteins function as transducers, coupling receptors to various effector systems within the cell. Originally, it was assumed that the only function of G-proteins was to couple receptors to second-messenger systems. However, new evidence, primarily of an electrophysiological nature, has come to light indicating that G-proteins can couple receptors directly to ion channels without the intervention of any second messengers, such as cyclic adenosine monophosphate (cAMP) or the products of phosphotidylinositol turnover. The first evidence for G-protein coupling of neurotransmitter receptors to ion channels came from intracellular recordings in cultured heart cells where certain inhibitory effects of acetylcholine (acting through muscarinic receptors) were found to be mediated by a type of G-protein. One type of muscarinic inhibition is caused by an opening of a specific class of K^+ channels; the opening of K^+ channels is inhibitory because it produces a hyperpolarizing outward current.

A second muscarinic effect in heart cells is the inhibition of adenylate cyclase, resulting in a reduction of intracellular levels of cAMP. In heart cells, the opposite effect, an increase in the formation of cAMP, occurs through β-adrenergic receptors acting via the stimulatory G-protein (G_s); the resulting elevation of intracellular cAMP has an excitatory effect by opening Ca^{2+} channels. Acetylcholine, acting through the inhibitory G-protein (G_i) is able to interfere with the ability of β-adrenoceptors to stimulate adenylate cyclase. Thus, acetylcholine has a dual action on heart cells: direct inhibition through an opening of K^+ channels and a suppression of β-adrenergic excitation. Together, these effects can explain the powerful suppressant effect of acetylcholine on cardiac activity.

As is often the case, peripheral systems, such as the heart, serve as a good model for neurotransmitter actions in the CNS. Already, there is evidence in the case of several receptor systems in the brain (e.g., opiate, α_2, D_2 dopamine, $GABA_B$, and serotonin-1) for a G-protein coupling mechanism. These receptors evoke an opening of K^+ channels through the mediation of a G-protein and, in some cases, an inhibition of adenylate cyclase, probably through the same G-protein. The occurrence and clinical implications of G-protein abnormalities are just beginning to be recognized in general medicine (e.g., pseudohypoparathyroidism). The possibility that such abnormalities may occur in psychiatric disorders remains to be explored.

NEUROTRANSMITTERS: CLASSIFICATION ACCORDING TO ION CHANNEL Implicit in the discussion of how receptors are coupled to effector mechanisms is the notion that particular transmitters are linked, directly or indirectly, to specific types of ion channels. This suggests that a useful way of classifying neurotransmitters would be according to the types of ion channels that they regulate. Moreover, this allows for a degree of simplification given the fact that there are only four major types of ions to be concerned with: Na^+, K^+, Ca^{2+}, and Cl^-. A further simplification comes from the fact that openings of Na^+ and Cl^- channels are rapid, brief events since these channels are generally directly coupled to their neurotransmitter receptors. In contrast, the effects of transmitters on K^+ (and sometimes Ca^{2+} channels) are relatively slow and long-lasting events, inasmuch as they may involve mediation by transducer proteins and, in many instances, the further involvement of second-messenger systems. Such indirectly coupled, slow transmitter actions are often regarded as *neuromodulatory* since they do not fit the classical concept of neurotransmission as a rapid and direct opening or closing of ion channels.

There is much work in progress at this time aimed at determining the types of channels that are affected by various transmitter substances in the CNS. Table 1.7-1 summarizes data that have been accumulated up to this time on the predominant types of channels that are regulated by some of the major classes of transmitter substances known to exist in the mammalian nervous system. The table reflects the fact that the effect of a transmitter on ion channels may depend on which of its receptor subtypes mediates the response (e.g., nicotinic versus muscarinic). The more traditional classes of neurotransmitters (i.e., acetylcholine, monoamines, amino acids) are well represented on this list. In contrast, except for the opioids and somatostatin, there has not as yet been an extensive characterization of the actions of peptides on ion channels in the CNS. In the coming years, it can be anticipated that much new data on the physiological actions of neuropeptides will be forthcoming. It is also likely that the peptides, as well as the more traditional transmitters, have important trophic actions in addition to their relatively short-term effects on ion channels.

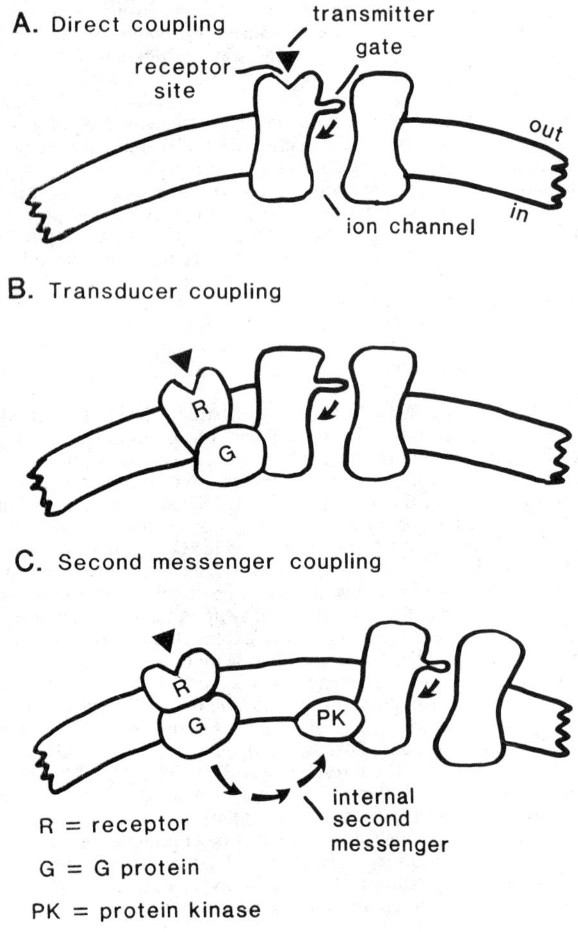

FIGURE 1.7-2. *Schematic representation of three forms of coupling that can occur between receptors and ion channels.* A. *Direct coupling, where the receptor site is located on the protein complex of the ion channel itself.* B. *Transducer coupling, where an intervening G-protein (the transducer) links the receptor to the ion channel.* C. *Second-messenger coupling, where a receptor is linked via a G-protein to a second messenger system (e.g., adenylate cyclase); the second messenger may then interact with the ion channel through a phosphorylation reaction catalyzed by a protein kinase.* B *and* C *are not mutually exclusive mechanisms and may occur simultaneously to give rise to a dual form of coupling that can link a receptor to more than one type of channel.*

ELECTROPHYSIOLOGY OF PSYCHOTROPIC DRUG ACTION

The actions of most psychotropic drugs can be ascribed to interactions with one or more neurotransmitter systems. This general finding is not very surprising in view of the fact that chemical neurotransmission represents the predominant mode of interneuronal communication in the mammalian nervous system. Any aspect of the process of neurotransmission is a potential site for the interaction of a drug with a neurotransmitter: synthesis, storage, release, receptor action, and inactivation (e.g., uptake, catabolism). A drug effect may manifest itself rapidly (e.g., the immediate blockade of a transmitter at its receptor) or only after a delay of several weeks (e.g., a long-term up- or down-regulation of a receptor). In either case, the ultimate effect of a drug will be to promote or impede the ability of a given transmitter to gate ionic conductances. The electrophysiology of some specific types of psychoactive drugs will be considered below.

ANXIOLYTICS The *benzodiazepines* (e.g., diazepam [Valium]) constitute the major type of antianxiety (anxiolytic) drug in clinical use today. The receptors that mediate the actions of benzodiazepines have a close association with

TABLE 1.7-1
Neurotransmitters and Ion Channels

Transmitter (Receptor)	*Ion*	*Channel Effect*	*Physiological Response*
Glutamate and asparate	Na^{+}*	Opening	Fast excitation
Acetylcholine (nicotinic)	Na^{+}*	Opening	Fast excitation
Acetycholine (muscarinic)	K^{+}	Closing	Slow excitation
Norepinephrine (α_1-adrenoceptors)	K^{+}	Closing	Slow excitation
Norepinephrine (α_2-adrenoceptors)	K^{+}	Opening	Slow inhibition
Serotonin (2 receptor)	K^{+}	Opening	Slow inhibition
Serotonin (1A receptor at motorneuron)	K^{+}	Closing	Slow excitation
Opioid peptides	K^{+}	Opening	Slow inhibition
Somatostatin	K^{+}	Opening	Slow inhibition
Glycine and $GABA_A$	Cl^{-}	Opening	Fast inhibition
$GABA_B$	K^{+}	Opening	Slow inhibition

*These channels are relatively nonspecific and are permeable to cations in addition to Na^{+}.

$GABA_A$ receptors, a subtype of receptors for the inhibitory amino acid GABA. In turn, $GABA_A$ receptors are closely associated with a particular subset of Cl^- channels that they activate (i.e., open). Together, these elements combine to form the benzodiazepine-receptor–GABA-receptor–Cl^--channel complex. Through this arrangement the benzodiazepines act indirectly (allosterically) to facilitate the ability of GABA to open Cl^- channels and, therefore, to produce inhibition on a cellular level. Thus, benzodiazepines, applied in small amounts by microiontophoresis to single neurons, have no effect by themselves, but they markedly enhance the inhibitory effects of GABA applied concurrently to the same neurons. Because GABA represents the most prevalent inhibitory transmitter system in the brain, it is to be expected that a facilitation of GABA's actions by benzodiazepines would affect many kinds of inhibitory functions. Thus, it is not surprising that the benzodiazepines have anticonvulsant as well as antianxiety properties. When used as anxiolytics, the anticonvulsant effects of benzodiazepines may be regarded as side effects. However, the abrupt cessation of long-term benzodiazepine treatment can result in withdrawal convulsions, indicating the development of tolerance and dependence. Therefore, a tapering of drug dosage is necessary when patients are being withdrawn from benzodiazepines. On a single-cell level, tolerance to benzodiazepines is manifested by a reduced responsivity of neurons to GABA or in a reduction in the ability of benzodiazepines to facilitate GABA inhibition.

ANTIDEPRESSANTS There are two major classes of antidepressants, the *tricyclics* (e.g., imipramine [Tofranil]) and the *monoamine oxidase inhibitors* (e.g., phenelzine [Nardil]). Members of both classes of drugs given acutely have immediate effects on the uptake or accumulation of monoamines. Most tricyclic drugs rapidly block the reuptake of serotonin or norepinephrine, or both. The monoamine oxidase inhibitors induce an accumulation of monoamines by blocking a major enzyme responsible for the degradation of these substances. The recognition of these actions represented important underpinnings of the *monoamine hypothesis* of depression. Stated in its most general form, this hypothesis proposes that depressive illnesses (particularly the major depressive disorders) arise from an impairment in either serotonergic or noradrenergic function.

However, any hypothesis based on the mechanism of action of antidepressants must take into account the well-known delay (typically 2 to 3 weeks) from the onset of drug administration to therapeutic response. This protracted time course is difficult to reconcile with the fact that the effects of drugs on amine uptake or metabolism are manifested within a matter of hours or days. Consequently, the attention of researchers has shifted away from the study of acute actions of these drugs to an examination of effects with a delayed onset, in parallel with the clinical time course. Single-cell recordings in certain postsynaptic regions of the rat brain have revealed that electrophysiological responses to serotonin, both inhibitory and excitatory, are progressively increased after 1 to 2 weeks of tricyclic drug administration. The inhibitory effects of serotonin are due to an opening of K^+ channels; conversely, the excitatory effects of serotonin result from a closing of K^+ channels. There is evidence that the receptors linked to an opening of K^+ channels belong to the serotonin-1 ($5\text{-}HT_1$) subtype. The enhancement of these electrophysiological actions cannot be explained by a blockade of serotonin uptake since it is also produced by certain atypical tricyclic drugs that do not block serotonin uptake. These studies suggest that serotonin receptor sensitivity itself is somehow enhanced in a time-dependent fashion after chronic antidepressant administration.

A new class of antidepressant drugs, distinct from the tricyclics, that are highly selective for blocking serotonin uptake (e.g., fluoxetine [Prozac]) do not appear to operate through sensitizing postsynaptic responses to serotonin. Instead, the selective serotonin uptake inhibitors, perhaps by maintaining high levels of serotonin extracellularly, induce a delayed desensitization of presynaptic serotonin receptors (serotonin autoreceptors); the monoamine oxidase inhibitors also appear to desensitize presynaptic serotonin receptors by this mechanism. Because presynaptic receptors have a negative feedback influence on serotonin release, their desensitization results in an overall enhancement of serotonergic transmission.

Single-cell studies with antidepressants have also revealed long-term changes in norepinephrine receptor sensitivity: α_1-adrenoceptor responses are enhanced and β-adrenoceptor responses are depressed. These findings are in accord with biochemical studies that show a down-regulation of β-adrenoceptors after chronic antidepressant drug treatment. The fact that the changes in β-adrenoceptors require an intact serotonergic neuronal network suggests an important interaction between these two transmitter systems. It remains to be determined whether these or other long-term alterations in receptor sensitivity contribute to the long-term therapeutic actions of the various classes of antidepressant drugs.

ANTIPSYCHOTICS Two major classes of antipsychotic drugs are the *phenothiazines* (e.g., chlorpromazine [Thorazine]) and the *butyrophenones* (e.g., haloperidol [Haldol]). Both types of antipsychotic drugs are potent dopamine receptor antagonists, and there is a good correlation between the affinity of these drugs for dopamine receptors and clinical efficacy. On this basis it has been proposed that dopamine receptor blockade is responsible for antipsychotic activity. Parkinsonian side effects of these drugs are clearly attributable to a rapid blockade of dopamine receptors in the extrapyramidal motor system. However, a true reduction in psychotic symptomatology may be delayed for several weeks or more. Thus, as in the case of the antidepressant drugs, it has been necessary to postulate long-term adaptive changes to account for the delayed clinical response. One long-term change known to be induced by antipsychotic drugs is dopamine receptor supersensitivity. This mechanism may be involved in the development of tardive dyskinesia, which is believed to be a manifestation of excessive dopaminergic transmission in the extrapyramidal motor system. However, as the emergence of tardive dyskinesia may be associated with an exacerbation of psychosis, dopamine receptor supersensitivity per se cannot account for antipsychotic activity.

An electrophysiological mechanism for delayed antipsychotic efficacy has been suggested on the basis of chronic studies in experimental animals. When antipsychotic drugs are administered acutely, there is an increase in the rate of firing of single neurons in nigrostriatal and other dopaminergic pathways. When antipsychotic drugs are given over a period of weeks, the numbers of dopaminergic neurons whose firing can be detected becomes progressively reduced. Paradoxically, the quiescent cells are unable to fire, not because they are hyperpolarized (i.e., below spike threshold) but because they are in a state of *depolarization inactivation* (hyperdepolarization), which results from excessive depolarization. The precise mechanisms underlying the slow development of depolarization inactivation are not known. However, it is known that the induction of depolarization inactivation depends on the intactness of neuronal feedback pathways that relay information from postsynaptic areas (e.g., the neostriatum) back to the dopaminergic cells of origin in the substantia nigra. The delayed reduction in the numbers of functional dopamine neurons correlates well with the delayed clinical response to antipsychotic drugs.

An alternative mechanism to account for delayed antipsychotic efficacy relates to actions of antipsychotic drugs at nondopamine receptors. For example, virtually all the typical antipsychotic drugs have some antagonist activity at a subset of serotonin receptors termed serotonin-2 (S-2 or 5-HT_2) receptors. There is electrophysiological evidence showing that the effects of psychedelic hallucinogenic drugs are mediated through an agonist action at serotonin-2 receptors. Moreover, clozapine (Clozaril)—a so-called atypical antipsychotic drug because it does not induce extrapyramidal side effects or tardive dyskinesia—has a higher affinity for serotonin-2 receptors than for dopamine receptors. Thus the action of antipsychotic drugs at serotonin-2 receptors may be important in either promoting therapeutic effects or suppressing the development of side effects. The chronic administration of antipsychotic drugs induces a long-term down-regulation of serotonin-2 receptors. A gradual reduction in the number of serotonin-2 receptors correlates with the delayed onset of therapeutic activity. However, it is not known as yet whether this down-regulation of serotonin-2 receptors plays a significant role in the therapeutic action of antipsychotic drugs.

HALLUCINOGENS The *psychedelic* ("mind-expanding") hallucinogens produce marked cognitive, affective, and perceptual disturbances while leaving orientation largely intact. There are two major structural classes of hallucinogens: the *indoleamines* (e.g., lysergic acid diethylamide [LSD]) and the *phenethylamines* (e.g., mescaline). Because of the striking similarities between the clinical states produced by these two types of hallucinogens, a unitary mechanism has long been sought to account for the actions of these drugs on the nervous system. There appears to be only one type of receptor for which indoleamine and phenethylamine hallucingens have shared affinity—that is, the serotonin-2 receptor. For both classes of hallucinogens, radioligand-binding studies have shown an extremely high correlation between hallucinogenic potency (in humans) and affinity for the serotonin-2 receptor. This receptor is highly concentrated in or near layer 5 of frontal and occipital (visual) cortex in the human brain. These regions of the brain are believed to subserve functions such as visual perception that are disordered by the hallucinogenic drugs.

Electrophysiological studies in experimental rats have identified several neuronal systems that are affected in a like manner by the indoleamine and phenethylamine hallucinogens. For example, noradrenergic neurons of the locus ceruleus, which are diffusely activated by sensory stimuli applied anywhere on the body, are affected in a unique way by these drugs; that is, the hallucinogens suppress their baseline firing while enhancing their responsivity to sensory stimuli. This pattern of effect is specific to psychedelic hallucinogens; no other types of drugs are able to mimic this effect. All of the shared physiological effects of the hallucinogens, including those in the locus ceruleus, can be blocked by drugs that are highly selective antagonists of the serotonin-2 receptor. As yet, the selective serotonin-2 antagonists have not been tested for their ability to block the effects of hallucinogens in humans.

DELIRIANTS Many chemical agents can induce a state of *delirium,* which is characterized by confusion, disorientation, hallucinations, and short-term memory deficits; this syndrome is typical of the so-called organic or toxic psychosis. In some cases, deliriants act by causing a generalized metabolic dysfunction of the brain. However, the belladonna alkaloids (e.g., atropine and scopolamine) and their synthetic congeners are particularly interesting because they can produce a delirium state through blocking one specific type of receptor in brain, the muscarinic cholinergic receptor. In addition, there are other classes of psychotropic drugs (e.g., tricyclic antidepressants and low-potency antipsychotics) that can produce clinically significant muscarinic receptor blockade to the extent that an overdose can present as a delirium.

Cholinergic neurons, arising from nuclei in the basal forebrain, have diffuse projections to regions of the brain (e.g., the hippocampus and neocortex) that are believed to subserve normal cognitive functions. Electrophysiologically, the tonic release of acetylcholine onto postsynaptic neurons in these regions can be viewed as maintaining an optimal state of excitability. On a cellular level, acetylcholine, acting at muscarinic receptors, enhances neuronal excitability by closing certain types of K^+ channels. The blockade of muscarinic receptors leads to a reduction in the excitability of vast numbers of neurons in the hippocampus and neocortex, resulting in a critical impairment in the ability of these neurons to process information arriving from other sources. If cholinergic transmission is restored by the administration of acetylcholinesterase inhibitors, the delirium produced by antimuscarinic drugs can be reversed completely. A degeneration of cholinergic neurons has been implicated in the pathogenesis of Alzheimer's disease, which shares some of the characteristics of the antimuscarinic delirium. However, other types of neuronal degeneration may also play a role in Alzheimer's disease, and the relative importance of degeneration in the cholinergic system in this condition has not been determined as yet.

SINGLE-CELL ACTIVITY AND BEHAVIOR

In the foregoing, much attention has been given to how various drugs or neurotransmitters can affect neuronal firing. Such studies are generally carried out in anesthetized animals or in vitro. The question now arises as to when, or under what conditions, neurons undergo a change in their firing rate in the awake, behaving animal. One way to examine this question is to record extracellularly from single cells in unanesthetized animals. This can be accomplished by implanting electrodes into the brain of an animal under surgical anesthesia, allowing the animal to recover from the surgery, and then monitoring neuronal activity during various spontaneous or induced behaviors. In this way, unit activity can be correlated with different behaviors without the confounding effects of anesthesia. Unit activity can be correlated with relatively simple spontaneous behaviors, such as sleeping or eating, or with more complex behaviors such as those occurring during operant or Pavlovian conditioning.

SINGLE-CELL CORRELATES OR COGNITIVE FUNCTIONS Some of the initial studies using chronic recording techniques examined the activity of movement-related neurons in the motor cortex of awake monkeys while the monkeys performed tasks involving various types of specific movements. Later, studies began to correlate the activity of neurons not just with specific types of movement but with various aspects of integrated behaviors. For example, studies performed in the behaving rat have shown that the firing pattern of certain cells in the hippocampus is directly related to the animal's position or location in the environment but is unrelated to the animal's movements in that location (i.e., "place" cells). One may have expected to find neurons of this type in the hippocampus, a structure that has been linked to memory and orientation, and whose malfunction, possibly through the disruption of cholinergic inputs, may result in the disorientation and short-term memory deficits seen both in Alzheimer's patients and after administration of deliriant drugs.

Other studies have examined the activity of neurons in relation to various complex cognitive capabilities used during the performance of operant tasks. For example, various types of neurons have been recorded in the prefrontal cortex of monkeys whose activity correlates with: (1) the animal's level of concentration during bar pressing for reward; (2) the behavioral significance and mnemonic representation of different stimuli; (3) the suppression or execution of a behavioral response; and (4) emotional processes, such as those occurring during the presentation of highly palatable (food) or aversive (a toy snake) stimuli. Again, it is interesting to note that one may have expected cells of these types to be found in the prefrontal cortex based on the deficits in cognitive function suffered by both humans and experimental monkeys following lesions in the prefrontal cortex.

CHRONIC UNIT RECORDINGS FROM CHEMICALLY IDENTIFIED NEURONS The interpretation of results obtained from chronic recording with randomly encountered cells (as in some of the above studies) is necessarily complex because of the heterogeneity of the cell types involved (i.e., different cell types with different responses are interspersed in the same region). Another approach to recording in behaving animals involves the study of homogeneous populations of neurochemically defined cells. Three types of neurochemically identified cells that have been studied in detail (mostly in the cat and monkey) are the serotonergic, dopaminergic, and noradrenergic cells. The cell bodies of these monoaminergic neurons are almost exclusively confined to nuclei in the brain stem, but they send projections to virtually all parts of the neuraxis and thus can affect many different parts of the brain simultaneously. By studying these monoaminergic cells with chronic recording techniques one can assess their functional relationships in a wide range of behavioral situations.

Serotonergic neurons In the dorsal raphe nucleus, serotonergic neurons discharge at a slow and extremely regular pace when the animal is in a quiet, resting state and increase their rate of firing when the animal exhibits motor activity. An early hypothesis for serotonergic function was in the active generation and maintenance of sleep. However, chronic unit recordings from serotonergic neurons in unanesthetized animals have failed to substantiate this idea. Serotonergic cells display a decrease rather than an increase in activity during the various stages of sleep. This decrease begins at the onset of slow-wave (non-rapid eye movement [REM]) sleep and progresses until serotonergic neurons become virtually silent during dream (REM) sleep. Another hypothesis has implicated serotonergic neurons in the response of the CNS to stress. However, when animals are exposed to both physiological and environmental stressors, serotonergic unit activity does not increase above a baseline rate. In general, serotonergic neurons observed in behaving animals discharge with a remarkable tonic regularity and are relatively unperturbed by a variety of manipulations, indicating that these neurons may serve to modulate a wide variety of homeostatic processes rather than directly mediate any of them. Such a modulatory role is consistent with data showing that drugs that act on serotonin receptors can affect broad functions ranging from mood to perception.

Dopaminergic neurons The activity of dopaminergic neurons, in contrast to that of serotonergic neurons, recorded in the substantia nigra is unrelated to the sleep-wake cycle. These cells discharge at a slow and somewhat regular pace with occasional bursts of activity when the animal is in a quiet, resting state, and their rate of firing remains remarkably constant through non-REM and REM sleep. During periods of increased motor activity dopaminergic neurons show slightly increased activity. In response to stress (e.g., physical restraint, loud white noise) substantia nigra dopaminergic neurons do not change their activity above a baseline rate. Based on biochemical studies, however, it may be expected that the activity of the other major dopaminergic systems, the mesolimbic and mesocortical (which have not as yet been examined by chronic unit recording), do become activated in response to stress.

One of the most dramatic changes in activity of dopaminergic neurons is a short-latency excitation followed by a long-lasting depression of activity that occurs during orientation to a novel or significant stimulus. The depression of activity appears to correspond to the period of fixation and suppression of movement. One of the best stimuli to evoke this orientation and concomitant change in unit activity is the entrance of the experimenter into the room where the animal is housed. In addition, changes in dopaminergic neuronal activity occur during rapidly executed large-body-mass movements (i.e., reaching movements), but not in relation to smaller movements. This type of response of dopaminergic cells supports the hypothesis that dopamine may play a permissive (rather than mediative) role in motor activity and would explain how a loss of dopaminergic cells could result in the loss of the ability to initiate motor function that occurs in parkinsonian patients.

Noradrenergic neurons The activity of noradrenergic neurons recorded in the locus ceruleus is positively correlated with the sleep-wake cycle. These cells discharge in a slow and somewhat regular manner when the animal is in a quiet waking state, increase their rate of firing when the animal becomes active (although this change is unrelated to any one particular movement), decrease their activity in non-REM sleep, and fall virtually silent in REM sleep. The activity of noradrenergic neurons seems to be most strongly related to stress and to stimuli that are perceived as stressful. In monkeys, noradrenergic neurons show a very dramatic and sustained increase in activity in response to human imitations of primate aggressive social signals, but only a transient increase in response to novel, but nonthreatening, stimuli. In cats, noradrenergic neuronal activity is dramatically increased in response to the physiological stress of hypotension or hypoglycemia as well as to the environmental stress of physical restraint or loud white noise. In contrast, the presentation of stimuli that are simply arousing but not stressful does not cause an increase in neuronal activity. This dissociation between stress and arousal is best shown using Pavlovian conditioning experiments. Noradrenergic neurons show dramatic increases in activity in response to the presentation of a tone that has been associated with the occurrence of a noxious event (i.e., a strong air puff to the face), but show no change in response to the presentation of a tone that has been associated with the occurrence of a rewarding event (i.e., delivery of a highly preferred food). Taken together, these studies suggest that central noradrenergic neurons play an important role in mediating adaptive responses to enteroceptive and external stimuli, particularly to those that are potentially threatening or stressful.

RELEVANCE TO PSYCHIATRY

It is inevitable that developments in neurobiology will have increasing relevance to psychiatry, both diagnostically and therapeutically. As presented elsewhere in this text, improved biochemical, electrophysiological, and imaging techniques are being introduced in the diagnostic evaluation of psychiatric patients. For example, positron emission tomography (PET) scanning can reveal alterations in brain metabolism or receptor density in specific brain regions or systems (Section 1.10). Such images reflect the state of activity or receptivity of clusters of individual neurons that operate within the labeled systems. Thus, a knowedge of electrophysiology at the single-neuron level is an essential component of the interpretation of information derived from brain imaging or other types of clinical biological assessment.

Similarly, it may be expected that an understanding of basic neurobiological mechanisms will play an increasingly important role in therapeutics. Not all depressions, psychoses, or anxiety disorders are likely to be identical in etiology or pathogenesis. As finer discriminations are made between pathophysiological subtypes, it will become possible to select more specific and efficacious treatments. For example, the drugs presently used in the treatment of schizophrenia have multiple neurochemical and physiological actions, no one of which may constitute the optimal therapy for a given type of patient. Moreover, extraneous actions of these drugs can induce serious and, occasionally, irreversible side effects, such as tardive dyskinesia. In the future, it can be anticipated that therapeutic drugs with greater selectivity of action will become available for clinical use. Increasingly, the discriminating use of such drugs will require a familiarity with differential mechanisms of action at a basic biochemical and electrophysiological level.

REFERENCES

Aghajanian G K, Sprouse J S, Rasmussen K: Physiology of the midbrain serotonin system. In *Psychopharmacology. The Third Generation of Progress*. H Meltzer, editor. Raven Press, New York, 1987.

Aghajanian G K, Wang Y-Y: Common α_2 and opiate effector mechanisms in the locus coeruleus: Intracellular studies in brain slices. Neuropharmacology *26:* 793, 1987.

Bunney B S: Antipsychotic drug effects on the electrical activity of dopamine neurons. Trends Neurosci *7:* 212, 1984.

Charney D S, Menkes D B, Heninger G R: Receptor sensitivity and the mechanism of action of antidepressant treatment. Arch Gen Psychiat *38:* 1160, 1981.

Cooper J R, Bloom F E, Roth R H: *The Biochemical Basis of Neuropharmacology*. Oxford University Press, New York, 1986.

Dolphin A C: Nucleotide binding proteins in signal transduction and disease. Trends Neurosci *10:* 53, 1987.

Einhorn L C, Johansen P A, White F J: Electrophysiological effects of cocaine in the mesoaccumbens dopamine system: Studies in the ventral tegmental area. J Neurosci *8:* 100, 1988.

Hille B: *Excitable Membranes*. Sinauer Associates, Inc, Sunderland, MA, 1984.

Jacobs B L: Central monoaminergic neurons: Single unit studies in behaving animals. In *Psychopharmacology. The Third Generation of Progress*, H Meltzer, editor. Raven Press, New York, 1987.

Kandel E R, Schwartz J H: *Principles of Neural Science*. Elsevier, New York, 1985.

McGeer P L, Eccles J C, McGeer E G: *Molecular Neurobiology of the Mammalian Brain*. Plenum, New York, 1986.

Meltzer H, editor: *Psychopharmacology, The Third Generation of Progress*. Raven Press, New York, 1987.

Nicoll R: The septo-hippocampal projection: A model cholinergic pathway. Trends Neurosci *8:* 533, 1985.

Noma A: GTP-binding proteins couple cardiac muscarinic receptors to potassium channels. Trends Neurosci *9:* 142, 1986.

Shepard G M: *Neurobiology*. Oxford University Press, New York, 1983.

Snyder S H: *Drugs and the Brain*. Scientific American Books, New York, 1986.

Spiegel A M, Gierschik P, Levine M A, Downs R W, Jr: Clinical implications of guanine nucleotide-binding proteins as receptor-effector couplers. New Eng J Med *312:* 26, 1985.

Tallman J F, Gallager D W: The GABAergic system: A locus of benzodiazepine action. Ann Rev Neurosci *8:* 21, 1985.

1.8
APPLIED ELECTROPHYSIOLOGY

RICHARD B. ROSSE, M.D.
DEBORAH L. WARDEN, M.D.
JOHN M. MORIHISA, M.D.

INTRODUCTION

The measurement of human brain electrical activity by the electroencephalogram (EEG) was first described in 1929 by the Austrian psychiatrist Hans Berger. His hope was that the EEG would help detect and characterize the disordered brain function of psychiatric patients. However, in the ensuing decades following Berger's discovery, no definitive EEG abnormalities have been identified for any functional psychiatric disorders. Additionally, many questions concerning the nature of the sources of the electrical activity detected from the human scalp by the EEG remain unanswered. Nevertheless, the EEG has become established as an important and valuable diagnostic tool in psychiatry and allied medical disciplines. It is useful in the workup of several organic brain conditions of relevance to psychiatrists, such as epilepsy, delirium, dementia, central nervous system (CNS) infections, metabolic abnormalities, intracranial masses, and head trauma. The EEG is also utilized in the assessment of brain death. Furthermore, the field of electroencephalography has been extended into sleep studies, EEG telemetry, evoked-potential (EP) testing, and computerized topographic mapping of electrophysiological data.

DETECTION AND MEASUREMENT OF BRAIN ELECTRICAL POTENTIALS

The electrical activity of the brain can be measured in a number of ways. These include recordings from scalp electrodes, from electrodes surgically placed on the surface of the brain (electrocorticography), and from electrodes surgically placed in the brain (depth electrodes). The latter two techniques may be used in patients who are being considered for epilepsy surgery. Basic science investigations also employ electrophysiological measurements from single neurons, generally utilizing animal systems that lend themselves more readily to these recording techniques. Information acquired from single nerve cell recordings has enhanced researchers' understanding of the exceedingly more complex system of the human brain.

Because of practical considerations, the brain's electrical activity is most often measured clinically by scalp electrodes placed outside the cranial cavity. Electrodes placed at some distance from the actual electrically active neurons themselves measure a summation of electrical potentials produced by many neurons. Brain electrical activity measured by scalp electrodes is generally felt to reflect the sum of excitatory and inhibitory postsynaptic potentials (EPSPs and IPSPs) from extensive groups of neurons. When using scalp electrodes, the activity of small groups of specific neurons can at best be only the subject of hypothetical speculation. The standard EEG amplifies the detected brain electrical activity so that the amplitudes of the electrical activity that are recorded from the scalp are usually in the range of 10 to 100 microvolts (μV).

PHYSICAL CONSIDERATIONS OF ELECTRICAL RESISTANCE Brain electrical activity is governed by certain basic laws of physics. For example, Ohm's law describes the relationship of voltage, current, and resistance. However, although brain electrical activity is governed by known principles, the brain and its coverings comprise a very complex case of these laws of physics. The brain is an organ of inhomogeneous components that is, at the cortical mantle, invaginated into numerous convolutions (gyri) and encased in cerebrospinal fluid, bone of varying thickness, and finally scalp. These substances exhibit disparate resistance properties. Clinicians and brain researchers alike must always appreciate the complexity of this system when trying to interpret surface electrical activity. Furthermore, in current conventional EEG recordings, the bone, skin, hair, and fluid that separate the brain from the scalp electrodes reduce the amount of electrical activity that reaches the electrodes. Increased wave amplitude might be noted in an area that has decreased resistance, as in the case of a skull defect resulting from prior surgery.

NEAR- AND FAR-FIELD RESPONSES The electrical activity detected from cortical sources directly under the scalp electrodes is sometimes referred to as the *near-field response*. Activity detected from sources more distant from the scalp electrodes (e.g., subcortical generators) is sometimes referred to as the *far-field response*. It is believed that the conventional clinical EEG primarily reflects near-field (cortical) activity, whereas certain electrophysiological measurements, such as the brain stem auditory evoked potential (BSAEP) as recorded from the scalp, are felt to reflect synchronous far-field electrical activity in auditory pathway neurons in the brain stem. The somatosensory-evoked potential (SEP) is believed to measure the near-field activity of the primary somatosensory cortex neurons underlying the recording electrodes. However, cortical activity as measured by EEG is believed to be affected often by certain subcortical (i.e., far-field) influences. For instance, the synchronization of brain α-activity of cortical origin has been hypothesized to be influenced by a subcortical pacemaker, perhaps located in the thalamus.

THE CONVENTIONAL EEG RECORDING

EEG TECHNIQUE The International 10-20 System The conventional EEG measures brain electrical activity from multiple electrodes placed in standardized positions on the patient's scalp. The electrodes are placed across the scalp in positions according to the International 10-20 System (Fig. 1.8-1). The International 10-20 System permits reproducible electrode placement across a variety of skull sizes. Additional reference electrodes are often placed on the ears (A_1 and A_2).

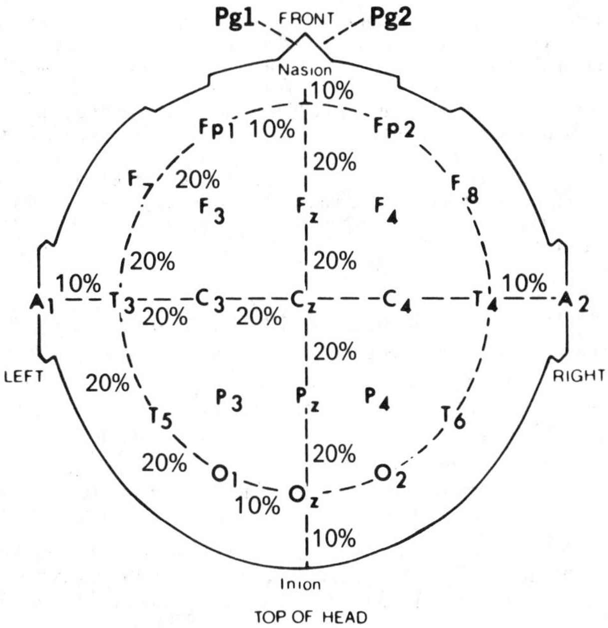

FIGURE 1.8-1. *The International 10-20 System for specifying EEG electrode placement. The system is based on measurements made from the nasion (depression at the bridge of the nose) to the inion (raised portion of the skull at the back of the head) and from the left to right auricular depressions (slight valleys just in front and above the earlobes). Electrodes are placed either 10 percent or 20 percent of these distances on the scalp as indicated in the figure. Frontal* (F); *central* (C); *parietal* (P); *occipital* (O); *midline* (Z); *nasopharyngeal lead* (Pg). *Odd-numbered subscripts are found on the left side of head; even-numbered subscripts are on the right side of head. (*Note: O_z *is a placement location not always associated with the conventional International 10-20 System, but it has been included here because this electrode location, which is based on the 10-20 system, is frequently utilized.)*

Monopolar vs. bipolar electrode arrangements The EEG measures patterns of brain electrical activity through the coupling of certain scalp electrodes into pairs, with the EEG displaying the electrical *potential difference* between the electrode sites. Each pair of electrodes relays a separate signal to an EEG "channel," with a conventional EEG tracing typically consisting of either 8 or 16 different channels. Generally, both *monopolar* and *bipolar* measurements are made during an EEG recording. A monopolar electrode arrangement usually involves the connection of a scalp lead to an indifferent, reference electrode (e.g., located on the ear lobes), with the subsequent measurement of the potential differences between the scalp and reference electrodes. The goal in selection of the reference electrode is to obtain as electrically neutral a recording location as possible. Some EEG investigators utilize an *average reference* system, which averages brain electrical activity obtained from many (or all) scalp electrodes. This average is then used as the reference to be compared with a single active scalp electrode. Bipolar recordings involve the interconnection of two scalp electrodes with the measurement of the potential differences between those two lead locations. Bipolar electrode arrangements can enhance visualization and characterization of spike and sharp wave discharges.

The EEG montage The particular combination of electrode pairs monitored at one point in time during an EEG recording is called the montage. Although the actual placement of the electrodes on the patient's head remains the same, the person operating the EEG machine may change the EEG settings so that the machine measures the voltage difference between different electrode pairs. Different montages provide specific information that focus on different aspects of brain electrical activity. The two main types of montages generally used are monopolar (or referential) and bipolar. A complete EEG recording can include different bipolar and monopolar montages. This allows for the most complete delineation of possible underlying pathology. The particular montage patterns employed during an EEG recording must be indicated on the EEG record in order to allow an accurate interpretation of the tracing. The montages utilized in the recordings of Figs. 1.8-2 through 1.8-5 are specified at the left of the figures.

CLINICAL INTERPRETATION

EEG frequencies The spectrum of EEG frequencies has been divided into various bands: *Beta* (β) activity occurs at frequencies equal to or greater than 13 Hz (cycles per second) ($f \geq 13$ Hz), *alpha* (α) activity at 8 Hz $\leq f <$ 13 Hz, *theta* (θ) activity at 4 Hz $\leq f$ $<$ 8 Hz, and *delta* (δ) activity at $f <$ 4 Hz.

In the normal eyes-closed resting adult EEG record, α-activity is present and usually most prominent over the occipital lobes (Fig. 1.8-4). Although α-activity is felt to be cortical in origin, a number of hypotheses have been proposed concerning the importance of subcortical influences. When the normal adult is stimulated or if the eyes are opened, α-activity essentially disappears and is replaced by higher-frequency β-activity. This disappearance of α-activity has been referred to variously as α-blocking, desynchronization, arousal response, or the alerting response. The EEG is normally performed with the subject's eyes closed.

Higher-frequency cortical activity (β-activity) seems to be largely asynchronous between adjacent cortical regions. As a result, the activity from surrounding brain areas tends to cancel itself out, interfering with detection and topographic localization. Abnormalities of β-rhythm can include the presence of focal or high-amplitude β-activity. Increases in β can represent a variety of pathological states, such as drug ingestion, or may reflect normal physiological processes.

The θ and δ EEG frequencies normally appear prominently during sleep. Drowsiness and hyperventilation can augment slowing of the EEG. Thus, the subject's level of alertness can alter the electrical activity reflected in the EEG. The EEG reader must also note the patient's age and level of arousal. For instance, the normal EEGs of infants might include much disorganized, slow-wave activity. EEG changes between infancy and young adulthood generally include decreasing

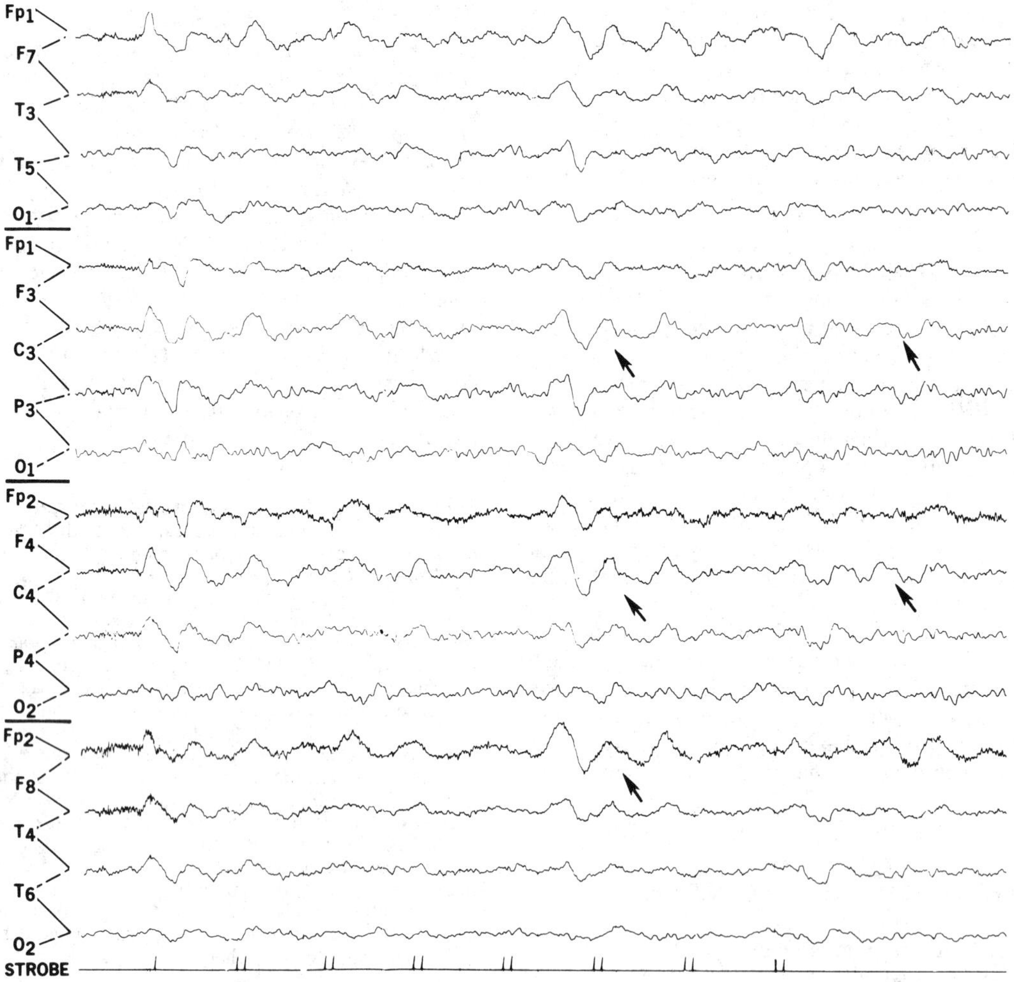

FIGURE 1.8-2. *Delta waves of 1–2 Hz evident in the frontal regions bilaterally, indicated by arrows. This rhythm is known as FIRDA (frontal intermittent rhythmic delta activity) and may be seen in patients with metabolic encephalopathies. The particular combinations of electrodes used while making the recording (called the montage) are indicated to the left of the figure. (Courtesy of Charlotte McCutchen, M.D., Veterans Administration Medical Center, Washington, DC.)*

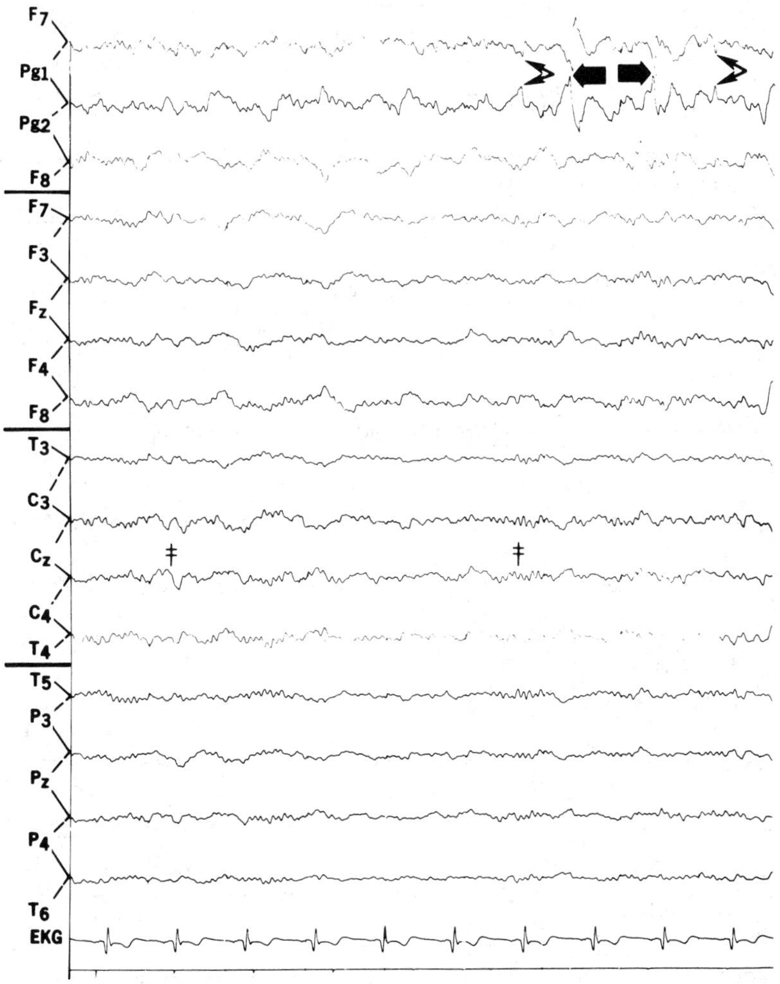

FIGURE 1.8-3. *An EEG recording performed after sleep deprivation using NP leads (top three lines). Sharp (wide arrow) and spike (thin arrow) wave discharges originating in the left mesial temporal area are evident on NP leads. Other leads show bilateral 14- to 15-Hz sleep spindles and vertex waves indicating stage II sleep (‡). Note the montage on the left of the figure. (Courtesy of Charlotte McCutchen, M.D., Veterans Administration Medical Center, Washington, DC.)*

amounts of δ activity, with increasing amounts of α-rhythm. Also, some physiologically normal EEG changes can be found in geriatric patients.

EEG abnormalities The clinical reading of the EEG involves the visual inspection of the many pages of EEG recording in order to characterize waveform amplitude, frequency, and EEG abnormalities. Waveforms can include regular rhythmical waves, spindles, irregular waves and wave complexes, as well as spikes and sharp waves. Abnormal EEG patterns can be divided into four main types: (1) δ-wave slowing, as manifested by prominent, low-frequency rhythms as seen in many patients with delirium (Fig. 1.8-2); (2) asymmetries of the EEG record (e.g., voltage and frequency asymmetry) when comparing homologous areas of the left and right sides of the head; (3) suppression of EEG amplitudes to low voltages (e.g., as might be seen in subdural hematoma); and (4) dysrhythmias, such as spikes and sharp waves (e.g., as might be seen in epilepsy). It is important to remember that many of these abnormalities may in certain situations represent normal physiological processes (e.g., slow waves during sleep).

Spikes and sharp waves A spike has been defined for clinical purposes as a pointed peak on the EEG record that is transient and clearly distinguishable from background activity. A spike should have a duration of less than 80 msec. Sharp waves are "spike-like" waves with durations greater than 80 msec (Figs. 1.8-3 and 1.8-5). The type of neuronal activity that is thought relevant to a discussion of spike wave activity is the paroxysmal depolarization shift (PDS). This category of neuronal activity has been suggested as responsible for the generation of epileptiform spikes on the EEG. During a PDS, neurons are thought to undergo depolarization of much greater magnitude than during the EPSPs of normally functioning cells. Furthermore, during a PDS, neurons are hypothesized to lose their ability to generate an action potential.

EEG artifacts Other tasks of the EEG reader include the search for EEG artifacts. Causes of EEG artifact can be divided into ex-

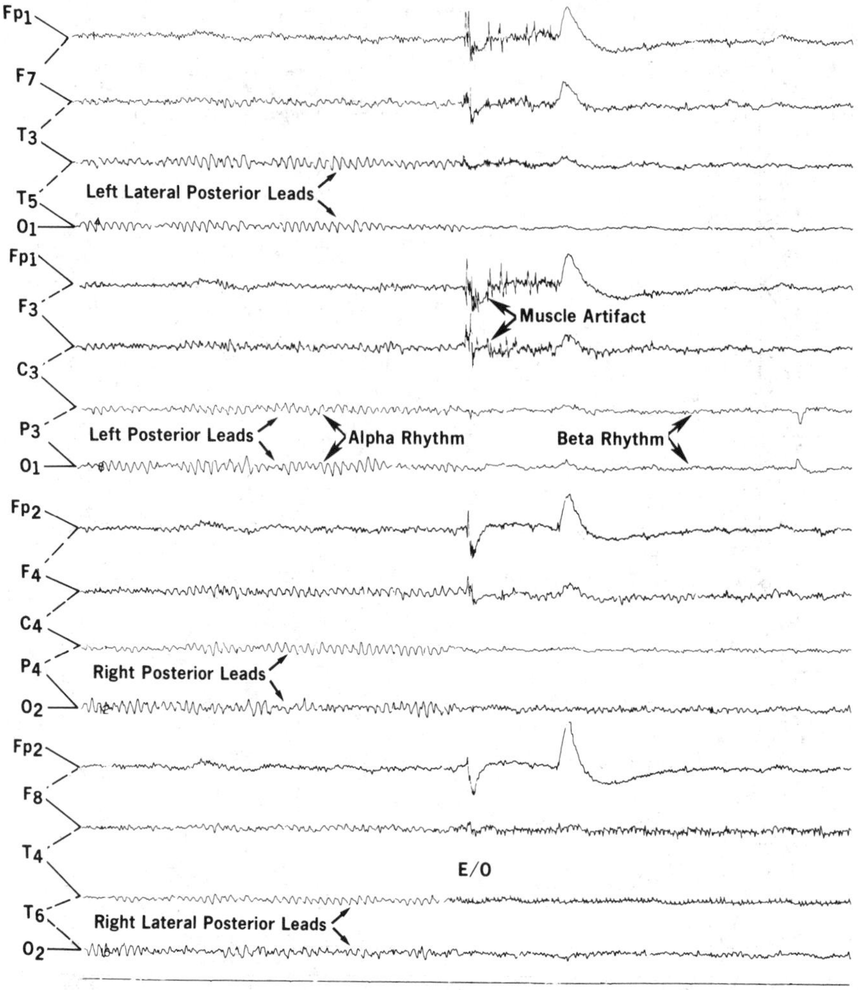

FIGURE 1.8-4. *A normal EEG tracing demonstrating well-formed posterior dominant alpha of 9–10 Hz. The α-rhythm attenuates with eye opening* (E/O) *and is replaced by lower amplitude, higher frequency (24- to 28-Hz) β-rhythm. Muscle artifact is identified during eye opening. The montage is indicated on the left of the figure. (Courtesy of Charlotte McCutchen, M.D., Veterans Administration Medical Center, Washington, DC.)*

ternal, instrumental, and physiological (Table 1.8-1). An example of an externally induced artifact is 60-Hz interference (e.g., from nearby electrical equipment). Instrumental artifacts include improper electrode placement, electrode loosenings, and defective electrodes. Sources of physiologically induced EEG artifact include the electrocardiogram (EKG), muscle activity (e.g., from the scalp), eye movement, swallowing, scalp electrodermal activity, and medication effects. Medication effects are particularly difficult to control in psychiatric patients, many of whom might be on psychotropic medications for prolonged periods of time. The EEG has been shown to be quite sensitive to some CNS–acting drugs, and even in some drug-free patients, the possible long-term effects of these psychoactive drugs cannot be completely excluded as a possible source of artifactual contamination.

SPECIAL EEG TECHNIQUES

Activation procedures An EEG activation procedure involves some manipulation, which may enhance or elicit abnormal EEG activity not present in the unactivated record. Activation procedures can involve: (1) sleep deprivation; (2) various provocative stimuli (such as photic stimulation with a flashing strobe light) or the presentation of specific stimuli suspected of precipitating a particular patient's seizure activity (e.g., reading, music, or startle stimuli), as well as certain chemical challenges (e.g., with such substances as pentylenetetrazol or procaine); and (3) hyperventilation. Experimental activation procedures include cognitive challenge tests and certain drug infusions.

Sleep deprivation is often requested on a second EEG if the initial routine EEG reveals no abnormalities. After sleep deprivation, the patient is more likely to fall asleep during the EEG procedure. During shifts in the level of consciousness while falling asleep, certain EEG abnormalities (e.g., spike and sharp-wave activity) can be more likely to appear on the EEG record.

TABLE 1.8-1
Major Types of EEG Artifacts

External
60-Hz interference
Instrumental
Electrode origin
EEG machine
Physiological
Sweating
Muscle movement, especially facial muscles
Eye movements and eyelid movements
EKG
Pulse
Iatrogenic
Medications

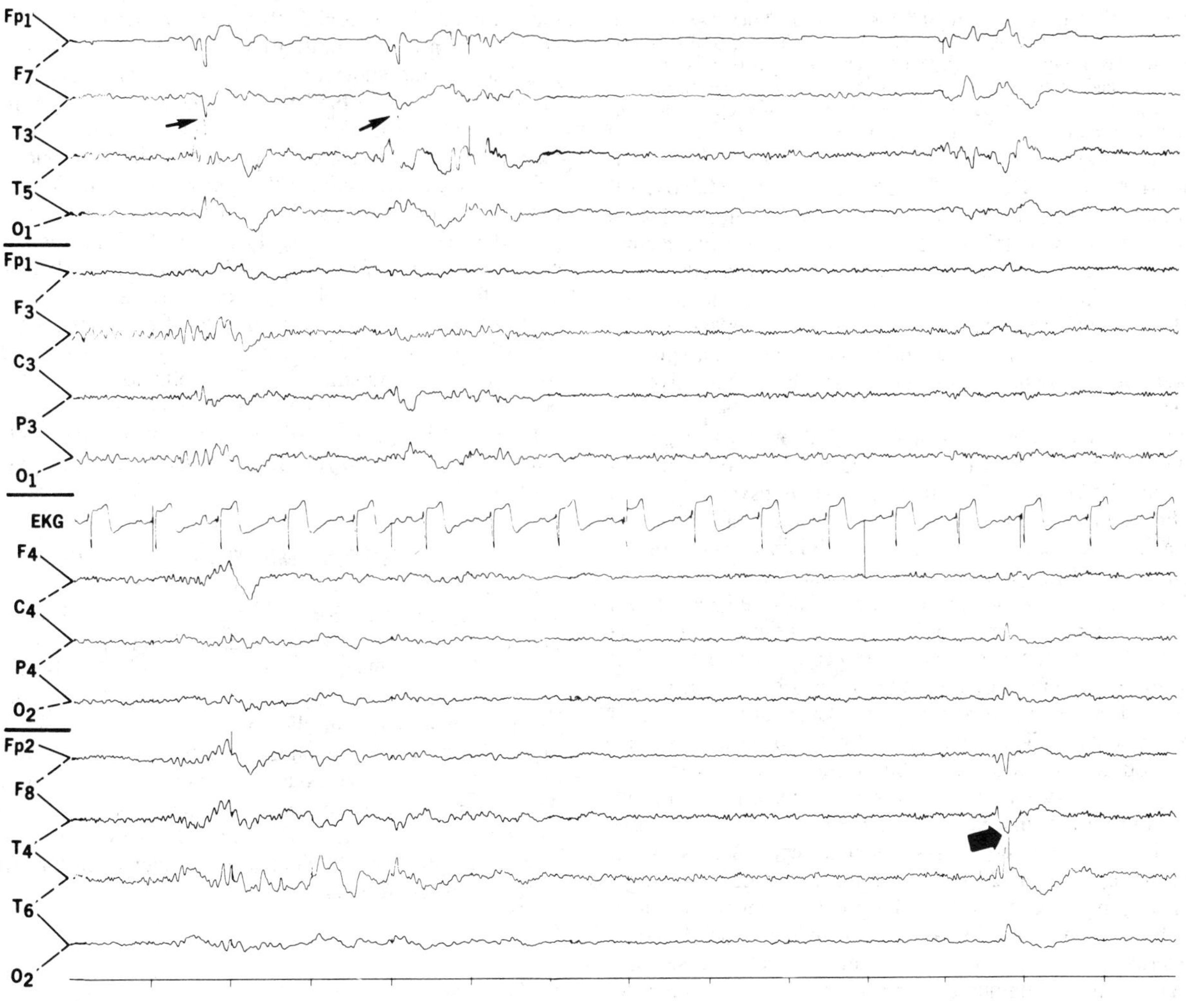

FIGURE 1.8-5. *This tracing demonstrates bilateral independent temporal lobe discharges. Left mid to posterior temporal lobe discharges with instrumental phase reversal are seen in the first part of the tracing (thin arrows); a right anterior to mid-temporal discharge with instrumental phase reversal is seen seconds later (wide arrow). An EKG tracing is recorded to ensure that the spike discharges are not EKG artifact. (Courtesy of Charlotte McCutchen, M.D., Veterans Administration Medical Center, Washington, DC.)*

Hyperventilation is usually performed for about 3 minutes. The forced hyperventilation of the subject generally results in a decrease of the EEG frequency with associated increases in wave amplitude, a response that is usually more prominent in children. Abnormal responses to hyperventilation include paroxysms of slow activity and the generation of spikes on the EEG.

Photic stimulation with a flashing strobe light might also demonstrate latent paroxysmal activity. Abnormal latent paroxysmal activity should not be confused with normal responses to a flashing light. Photoentrainment or photic driving is the physiological response in which brain activity, usually maximal over occipito-parietal areas, is noted at the same flash frequency as the strobe light. A photoconvulsive response is abnormal paroxysmal activity that is not synchronized with the stimulus and may persist after the cessation of photic stimulation. A photoconvulsive response may be accompanied by postural or facial changes (e.g., drooping eyelids). Some normal twitching of the facial and eye muscles in response to photic stimulation can result in muscle artifact on the EEG and should not be confused with epilepsy.

Special electrodes Other techniques of electrode placement, such as nasopharyngeal (NP) leads (inserted through the nares to rest touching the top of the nasopharynx), have been used to increase the diagnostic yield of the EEG, especially when temporal lobe pathology is suspected. NP leads were first used to record electrical activity from the basal forebrain structures, and they have continued to be used in the belief that they provide a more advantageous approach from which to record electrical activity from the inferior and mesial temporal lobes. Although there is no consensus concerning the absolute value of the EEG supplemented with NP leads in psychiatric patients, there clearly exist some occasions in which epileptiform activity will be observed only with NP leads (as with the patient in Fig. 1.8-3). Sphenoidal electrodes can also be positioned to obtain EEG data from the inferior aspects of the anterior temporal lobes. Sphenoidal electrodes are thought to be less prone to artifactual contamination than are NP leads, but they are more difficult to place and require specialized technical training of the practitioner.

Electrocorticograms and depth electrodes When needed, electrodes can be directly positioned over or implanted into brain tissue during a neurosurgical procedure for more direct measurements of brain electrical activity. The neurosurgical placement of electrodes is often done for the most accurate measurements possible in preparation for surgery to control a patient's epilepsy. The measurement of this electrical activity from deeper cortical or subcortical tissues requires the use of depth electrodes (i.e., intracerebral electrodes), as is done in depth EEG (DEEG). Abnormal brain electrical activity detected with the use of depth electrodes may not be detected when scalp electrodes alone are utilized. This can also be the case when an electrocorticogram (ECoG) is compared to a scalp EEG. In ECoG, the electrodes are placed directly on the underlying cortex as opposed to being placed on the scalp. The electrical activity as measured from the scalp is of decreased amplitude when compared to a concomitantly obtained ECoG or DEEG record.

APPLICATION OF THE EEG TO PSYCHIATRY

Indications As previously outlined, the conventional EEG is a useful tool for helping differentiate some organic mental disorders (e.g., dementia or delirium) from idiopathic psychiatric conditions. Investigators have also recommended that the EEG might be a part of a routine screening battery for psychiatric patients, if the patient's history reveals an episodic behavioral or mental disturbance possibly suggestive of epilepsy.

Indications for obtaining an EEG in a psychiatric patient might include: (1) a history of an episodic, paroxsymal behavioral disturbance; (2) a first episode of psychosis; (3) a youthful patient with a psychotic disorder (e.g., age less than 25); and (4) a history of possible brain injury or neurological disturbance (e.g., accidents, unconsciousness, infections, birth complications, seizure disorder). The clinician should note, however, that a normal EEG cannot be used to exclude completely a diagnosis of epilepsy in patients who have clinical histories of an episodic behavioral disturbance that is suggestive of a seizure disorder (e.g., secondary to a partial complex seizure). The EEG does not have absolute sensitivity in any clinical situation. Sampling error is also possible because the paroxysmal electrical activity may not have occurred during the time period of the EEG recording. In cases in which sampling error is suspected, repeat EEGs, sleep deprived EEGs, or 24-hour ambulatory recordings (e.g., telemetry) may be helpful. Prolonged EEG recordings may also be accompanied by a video camera, which records the patient's activities before, during, and after a seizure. Sometimes this technique has proved valuable in defining the seizure type (e.g., epileptic or psychogenic) and in objectifying abnormal behavior that may accompany epileptic activity.

EEG as biological marker There have also been attempts to utilize the EEG in the search for specific neurophysiological markers of idiopathic psychiatric disorders (e.g., schizophrenia, major mood disorders). Most of the studies converge on the finding of a greater prevalence of various EEG abnormalities (often called nonspecific abnormalities) in psychiatric patients than in normal individuals. Additionally, psychiatric patients appear more sensitive to activation procedures. However, no specific diagnostic patterns have been identified that would make the conventional EEG routinely useful in the definitive diagnosis of any specific idiopathic psychiatric condition. With advances in the application of computers to the analysis of EEG data, as employed in computerized topographic EEG techniques, it is hoped that the utility of the EEG will be increased for both the psychiatric clinician and the neuroscientist.

EVOKED POTENTIALS

There are specific EEG responses to certain types of sensory stimulation. These responses, however, are generally buried in background EEG activity in the conventional EEG recording. In evoked potential (EP) testing, a stimulus (of perhaps 20 to 200 msec in duration) from one sensory modality is presented to the subject repeatedly, and the EEG responses are recorded under standardized conditions. The brain electrical activity on EEG that follows each repeated stimulus is then averaged. It is therefore possible to average out most of the brain electrical activity thought not to be directly related to the evoking stimulus; hence, the nonstimulus-related background EEG activity is largely removed. What remains is a characteristic waveform, the *evoked potential*. EPs have also been referred to variously as averaged evoked potentials, cortical evoked potentials, or event-related potentials. The evoking stimulus can be visual, auditory, or somatosensory (although other modalities, such as olfactory, have been reported) leading to the elicitation of either visual evoked potentials (VEPs) (Fig. 1.8-6), auditory evoked potentials (AEPs) (Fig. 1.8-7), or somatosensory evoked potentials (SEPs).

EVOKED POTENTIAL MEASURES The EP waveform consists of negative and positive voltage peaks (or components) spread out along a time axis. EP studies typically investigate the presence, amplitude, latency, and shapes of various EP components, as well as other measures such as waveform variability. The *latency* of an EP component is generally measured from the onset of the stimulus to the point of maximum waveform amplitude (either positive or negative). Interpeak latencies are determined by measuring the time differential between peaks on the same EP. Waveshape variability is a measure of how much the waveform of the EP changes for the same subject without changes in the stimulus or recording conditions.

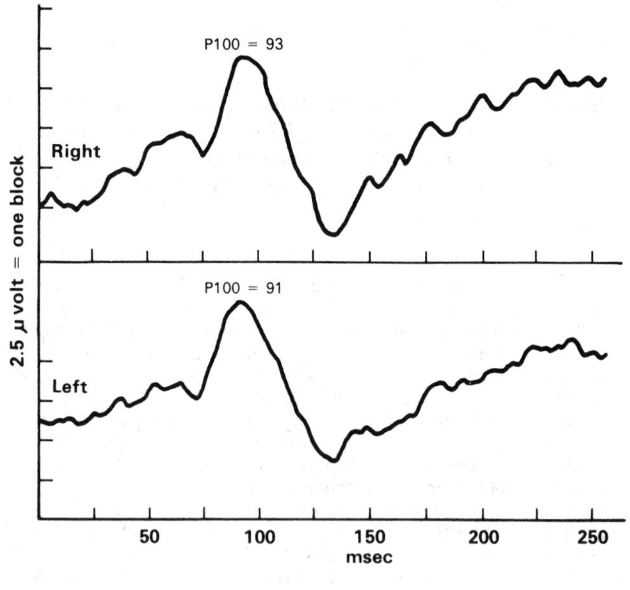

FIGURE 1.8-6. *Normal visual evoked potential bilaterally. The P100 is clearly identified. (Normal in this laboratory is a P100 of less than 112 msec latency and no more than a 6.5-msec difference between the right and left P100.) Each tracing is the computer-averaged representation of 400 individual pattern shift visual stimuli. (Courtesy of John Schwankhaus, M.D., Veterans Administration Medical Center, Washington, DC.)*

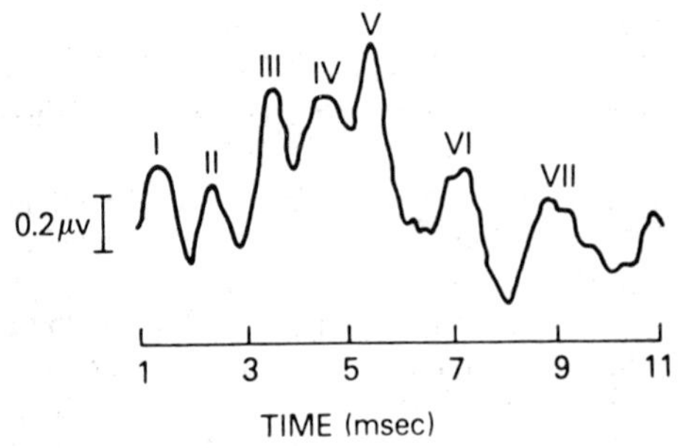

FIGURE 1.8-7. *Brain stem auditory evoked potential (BSAEP) recorded between the vertex and earlobe ipsilateral to the stimulated ear of a normal subject. The BSAEP was evoked by 60-dB SL condensation clicks, 50 μsec in duration, presented at a rate of 10 per second. Positivity of the vertex electrode is represented as an upward deflection. The seven waves of the BSAEP are labeled. (Courtesy of Connie C. Duncan, Ph.D., Unit on Psychophysiology, Laboratory of Psychology and Psychopathology, National Institute of Mental Health, Bethesda, MD.)*

SIGNIFICANCE OF EARLY, MIDDLE, AND LATE EVOKED POTENTIALS The early peaks (or components) have been generally defined as those peaks occurring within the first 50 to 80 msec poststimulus. It is thought that these early components probably represent electrical responses along afferent sensory pathways and primary sensory cortical areas.

Middle latency potentials have been defined as occurring between as early as 50 msec and as late as 250 msec after the stimulus, and the late potentials have been defined as occurring after 250 msec. In general, EP components occurring after 50 msec poststimulus are hypothesized to reflect certain cerebral events associated with cognitive or psychological processing. However, the specific anatomic generators of these EP components have not yet been well delineated. Although there remain certain unanswered questions concerning the accuracy of relating certain cognitive processes associated with specific EP components, there has been a growing body of research that supports some of these relationships. The hypothesized significance of the different EP components include attention, sensory filtering, categorization, and mismatch recognition. However, virtually every measure of these events seems subject to some artifactual contamination. Important variables that must be controlled include patient cooperation, motivation, task performance, level of alertness, fatigue, eye movement artifact, acuity for the sensory modality tested, and use of psychoactive substances.

EXAMPLES OF EARLY, MIDDLE, AND LATE EVOKED POTENTIALS **Brain stem auditory evoked potential** An example of commonly evaluated early EP components is the brain stem AEP, often abbreviated as BSAEP (Fig. 1.8-7) and also known as the brain stem auditory evoked response (BAER). These components comprise the earliest peaks of the AEP (i.e., within the first 10 msec poststimulus). These early components of the AEP are labeled with Roman numerals; a recording can be normal and not contain all the EP peaks (for example, the absence of II is a normal variant). Interpeak latency of I to III has been hypothesized to represent lower brain stem conduction and interpeak latency of III to V to represent upper brain stem conduction. For these AEPs, the interpeak latencies are thought to be more reliable and sensitive indicators of CNS disease than the absolute latencies (i.e., from time of stimulus to peak), which can be affected by the organs of sensation themselves.

N100-P200 complex An example of a middle latency EP that has been investigated in some psychiatric studies is the N100-P200 complex. The N100-P200 complex is reportedly augmented by increases in the intensity of the evoking stimulus.

P300 A commonly studied late positive potential is the *P300* (P is for positive voltage potential and 300 represents 300-msec poststimulus). The P300 has also been referred to as the *late positive wave* (LPW) or *late positive component* (LPC). To elicit a P300, the patient is typically presented with two different stimuli mixed in a sequence and is asked to respond to one (e.g., to the rarer of the two stimuli). The P300 occurs with a latency of approximately 300 msec (Fig. 1.8-8) after the rarer (or target) stimulus (only if the patient is paying attention). The amplitude of the P300 is inversely proportional to the probability of the evoking stimulus (Fig. 1.8-9). The P300 has also been observed after the unexpected omission of the target stimulus in a regular, predictable series or during the presentation of unexpected novel stimuli. The P300 distribution is widespread; its amplitude is usually maximal when measured at parietal locations, and some clinical neuroscience findings implicate a possible limbic origin. The specific generators underlying the P300 require further clarification, and the psychological and functional significance of the P300 is the subject of active investigation. The P300 has been hypothesized to be a manifestation of cognitive processes invoked by stimuli relevant to the organism. The amplitude of the P300 appears to vary directly with the attentional resources allocated to process a stimulus.

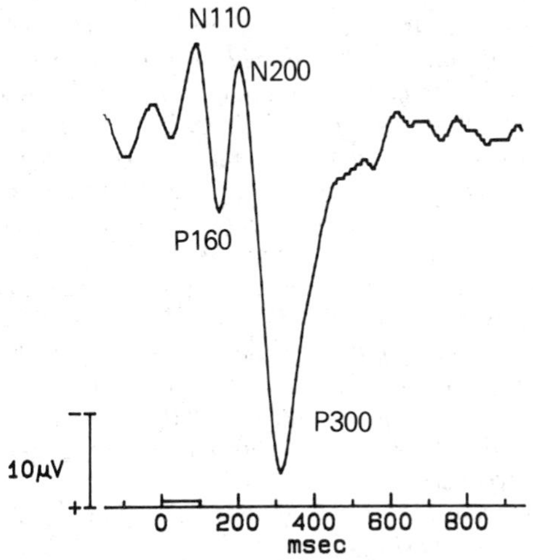

FIGURE 1.8-8. *An evoked potential (EP) elicited by a 50-dB SL tone pip presented with a probability of .10 in a choice reaction time task and recorded over the vertex in a normal subject. Onset of the 100-msec tone is represented by a 0 on the time scale. Positivity of the vertex electrode relative to the reference electrodes is plotted as a downward deflection. Major components of EP are labeled. Note the large P300 that was elicited by the low-probability task-relevant stimulus. (Courtesy of Connie C. Duncan, Ph.D., Unit on Psychophysiology, Laboratory of Psychology and Psychopathology, National Institute of Mental Health, Bethesda, MD.)*

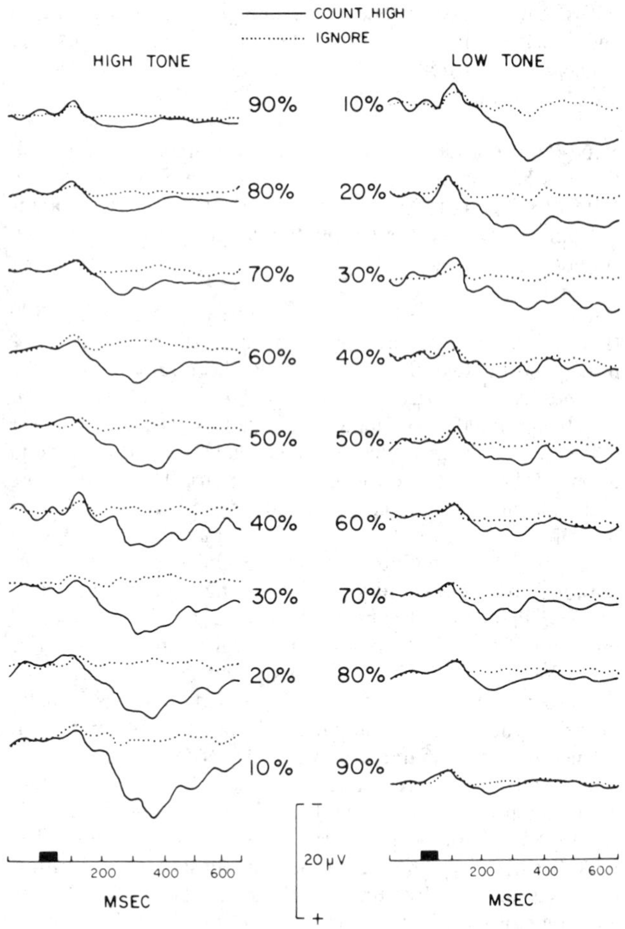

FIGURE 1.8-9. *Evoked potentials elicited by tone pips at nine different levels of probability, recorded from the midline parietal scalp area and averaged over 10 normal subjects. High- and low-frequency tones were presented in random order at complementary probabilities. Data in this figure are superimposed for two task conditions: Subjects either counted the high tones (solid lines) or ignored the tones while performing a word puzzle (dotted lines). Stimulus occurrence is indicated by a black rectangle on the time scale. Positivity of the parietal electrode with respect to the reference electrodes is plotted as a downward deflection. When the stimuli were task-relevant, the amplitude of the P300 was inversely related to probability. Note, however, that when the tones were irrelevant to the subjects-task, no P300 was elicited even by low-probability tones. (From Duncan-Johnson CC, Donchin E: Quantifying surprise: The variation of event-related potentials with subjective probability. Psychophysiol* 24: *456, 1977, with permission.)*

A number of variables have been found to affect the P300. For example, a reduced amplitude P300 has been found in several studies of schizophrenic patients, which has been interpreted by some investigators to represent abnormalities of attentional processes in these patients. Moreover, recent work suggests that this finding may be influenced significantly by stimulus modality and stimulus probability. Indeed, a recent study even raised the importance of state versus trait considerations in the evaluation of the P300 in schizophrenia. Such potentially confounding variables in the interpretation of electrophysiological data are characteristic of the evolving nature of this field and will hopefully be clarified by the eventual elaboration of relevant basic neuroscience principles.

CNV, PINV, and MRP Certain late or slower potentials, such as the *contingent negative variation* (CNV) and the *postimperative negative variation* (PINV), might be measured over a period as long as several seconds. The CNV is the negative shift in electrical potential that comes after a warning stimulus (S_1) and precedes an imperative stimulus (S_2). The subject must respond (imperative) in some fashion (e.g., by pressing a button) to the S_2. The PINV is the continuation of the negative potential after the S_2 has occurred. Prolonged PINVs have been reported to be associated with certain psychiatric disorders. Another EP, called the *movement-related potential* (MRP), also known as the *readiness potential* (RP) or the *Bereitschafts potential,* is the slowly increasing negative potential that occurs after the subject has been signaled to initiate a movement (e.g., lifting a finger). The negative potential begins 0.5 to 1 sec prior to the actual movement. The MRP is believed to reflect the preparation for movement, as it occurs only before active movement and is not seen prior to passive movements.

Selective attention effect Stimulus attention has been associated under certain experimental conditions with a negative shift (approximately 60 msec to as much as 500 msec after a stimulus) that is thought to be related to selective attention, and this phenomenon has been designated the *selective attention effect* (Nd). The integrity of the prefrontal cortex has been found to be important in such attentional processes, and abnormalities in attention have been noted in schizophrenia. In this context, it should be noted that recent clinical neuroscience investigations of schizophrenia using regional cerebral blood flow and positron emission tomography (PET) have provided evidence suggesting that the prefrontal cortex may play an important role in the pathophysiology of this disorder.

CLINICAL UTILITY OF EVOKED POTENTIAL STUDIES IN PSYCHIATRY As mentioned earlier, EP testing has some established indications in clinical neurology and neurosurgical practice, especially in the evaluation of demyelinating disorders, such as multiple sclerosis (Fig 1.8-10) and the intraoperative evaluation of nerve integrity during certain neurosurgical procedures. There is, however, no consensus as to the current clinical utility of EP testing in the evaluation of idiopathic psychiatric disorders. Table 1.8-2 lists some EP components that have been studied in psychiatric patients. EP studies are unique among electrophysiological and brain-imaging methodologies in the EP technique's ability to detect the cerebral processing of stimuli and information that takes place within milliseconds of the occurrence of the stimulus. Some cognitive processes of special interest to psychiatrists and neuroscientists occur on this chronological order of magnitude. Abnormalities of early, middle, and late EP components have been reported in psychiatric disorders, but none seem diagnostically definitive or of clear clinical usefulness as of this date. However, this is an area of active investigation. It is hoped that the value of EP testing to psychiatrists will be enhanced with additional careful clinical studies and by the application of advances in the computer analysis of EP data (e.g., computerized topographic EP mapping).

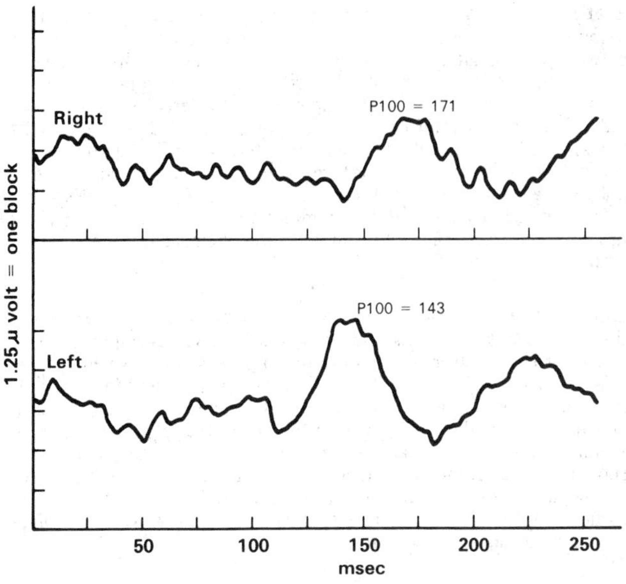

FIGURE 1.8-10. *Bilaterally abnormal pattern shift visual evoked potentials. Each eye reveals a prolonged latency of the P100, seen here in a patient with multiple sclerosis and a history of bilateral optic neuritis. (Courtesy of John Schwankhaus, M.D., Veterans Administration Medical Center, Washington, DC.)*

TABLE 1.8-2
Examples of EP Components of Possible Significance to Psychiatry

Early components (< 50 msec)
SEP N20-P30
Middle components (50–250 msec)
AEP N_1 (N100), P200 (N100-P200 complex)
VEP P200
Late components (> 250 msec)
P300
CINV
PINV

COMPUTERIZED TOPOGRAPHIC MAPPING OF ELECTROPHYSIOLOGICAL DATA

INTRODUCTION The amount of data generated by the conventional multielectrode EEG is enormous. This huge volume of data must generally be visually inspected page by page. Inasmuch as a routine EEG recording for an individual patient can involve more than 100 pages of EEG tracings (each containing data from multiple combinations of EEG electrodes), this sheer volume of EEG data has limited the clinical and research utility of the conventional EEG.

A number of attempts have been made to analyze this enormous amount of data. Indeed, topographic techniques to display EEG or EP data have been under development for more than three decades. With recent advances in solid-state electronics and computer software, the analysis of often unwieldly EEG data has evolved to the application of computer-assisted EEG systems that are capable of summarizing large amounts of EEG data, usually in the form of color-coded or gray-scaled topographic maps (Fig. 1.8-11). The technique by which this process is applied to both EEG and EP data has been called computerized topographic mapping of electrophysiological data. In addition, nonmapping EEG approaches utilizing computer analysis of the numerical indices generated by the computerized EEG have been developed.

The brain's electrical activity as portrayed in computerized topographic maps is detected and measured in a manner similar to conventional EEG recording. In these computerized EEG systems, the EEG data are generally recorded for subsequent computer analysis, from which various topographic maps are generated. The computer analysis of the EEG data generally employs a mathematical algorithm, specifically the fast Fourier transform, to quantitate the separate contribution of each of the various spectral frequency bands (i.e., δ, θ, α, β) for a particular EEG study. The contribution of each frequency band may be depicted numerically or in a map format that provides the topographic distribution of the brain's electrical activity.

Generation of topographic maps In topographic EEG mapping, the scalp electrode locations are generally the same as

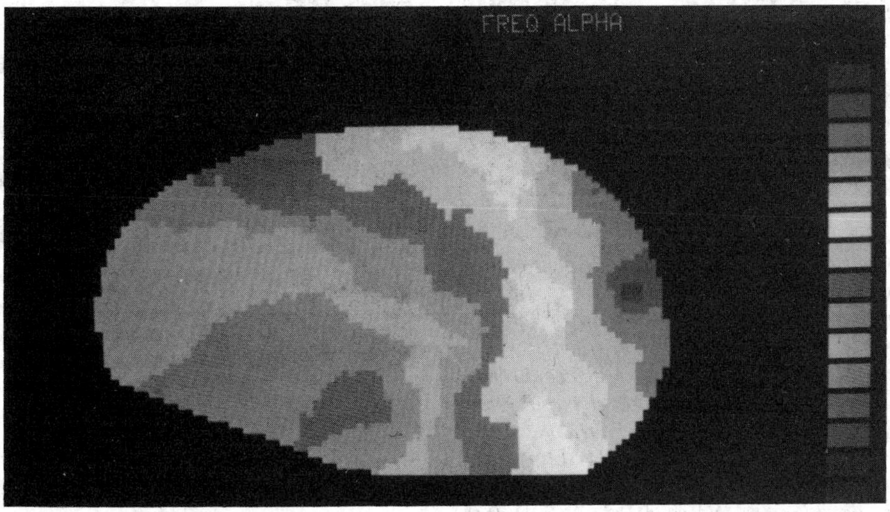

FIGURE 1.8-11. *Computerized EEG map depicting the topographic distribution of α-activity. The view in this figure is a profile view of one hemisphere of the head. This map delineates the occipital region as the area of greatest α-activity. (Courtesy of Richard Coppola, D.Sc., National Institute of Mental Health, Bethesda, MD.)*

described by the International 10-20 System (Fig. 1.8-1), although some computerized mapping systems employ extra scalp electrodes to augment the conventional 10-20 system. Current recommendations suggest the use of dedicated eye electrodes to effectively eliminate contamination by eye movement artifact.

Generally, in the development of a topographic map by a computerized EEG system, a multiarea grid matrix is laid over the data points provided by the scalp electrodes. The resultant grid matrix defines thousands of picture elements, or pixels, of the brain map. Each of these pixels is given a value by employing either a three- or four-nearest-neighbor interpolation algorithm. In this method, data from either three or four of the nearest electrodes are used to define the different colors (or shades of gray) to be assigned to the pixel, corresponding to a specific voltage range of brain electrical activity. The specific statistical algorithm or number of electrodes used in the interpolation varies among different computerized EEG systems. Additionally, some systems employ a mapping technique that is an approximate equal-areas projection, in which the projection of the area from the three-dimensional scalp is represented by an equal area of the two-dimensional computerized map. Such an equal-areas projection is felt to limit topographic gradient distortions and provide for more accurate anatomic comparisons of the data. Computerized EEG systems display data within graphic outlines of the head, either as if viewed from above or within a graphic outline of the head as if viewed in profile, thereby producing separate maps for the left or right hemispheres (Fig. 1.8-11).

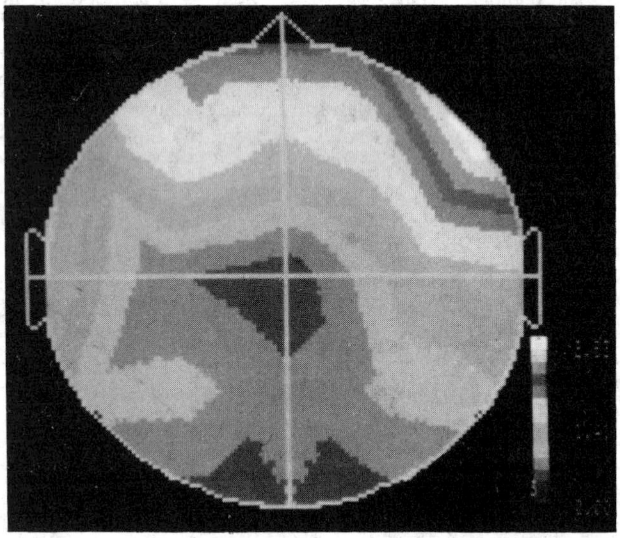

FIGURE 1.8-12. *Brain electrical activity map depicting statistical information comparing two groups of subjects. In this example, electrophysiological data from a group of schizophrenic patients with frontal atrophy (demonstrated by CT scan) are compared to data from a group of schizophrenic patients without frontal atrophy. In this map, electrophysiological differences between these two groups overlie the frontal regions of the brain. (Courtesy of John M. Morihisa, M.D., Department of Psychiatry, Georgetown University School of Medicine, Washington, DC, and Frank H. Duffy, M.D., Department of Neurology, Harvard Medical School, Boston, MA.)*

Statistical analysis In addition, topographic maps may be used to represent statistical relations between individuals and groups or between two populations of subjects (e.g., patients with schizophrenia as compared with control subjects). In this case, a *z*-transform or a *t*-transform is used to highlight regional differences between an individual and a group or between two groups (Fig. 1.8-12). This technique has been called significance probability mapping or *T*-statistic maps and represents a form of exploratory data analysis that does not address the overall significance of group differences. This issue may be investigated using multivariate discriminant analysis based on the electrophysiological measures delineated by these topographic approaches.

Computerized mapping of evoked potentials EPs for the entire cortical surface can also be topographically visualized using these computerized electrophysiological mapping systems. Generally, the EPs are averaged over epochs (time intervals) measured in milliseconds (e.g., 4 msec), and the EP data can be viewed for each epoch. As with the mapping of EEG data, the EPs are displayed within outlines of the head with different colors or gray tones corresponding to different EP voltage ranges (Fig. 1.8-13). Both positive and negative voltages can usually be visualized on the same map by assigning different color ranges to positive and negative (e.g., blue-purple as negative, orange-red as positive).

APPLICATION OF COMPUTERIZED TOPOGRAPHIC MAPPING TO PSYCHIATRY Work in this area of computerized mapping is still preliminary. In general, superior clinical utility has yet to be definitively demonstrated for computerized mapping systems over the standard EEG laboratory and this technique remains primarily a research tool at this time, although a number of commercially available computerized mapping systems are available.

Some advantages of computerized topographic mapping systems over other types of brain imaging research techniques (e.g., regional cerebral blood flow or PET) include: (1) the absence of radiation exposure; (2) greater chronologic resolution for the computerized electrophysiological mapping systems (specifically computerized EP mapping), which is of the order of milliseconds versus minutes with other brain-imaging techniques (e.g., PET); and (3) the generally lower cost of computerized EEG as compared with other brain-imaging procedures.

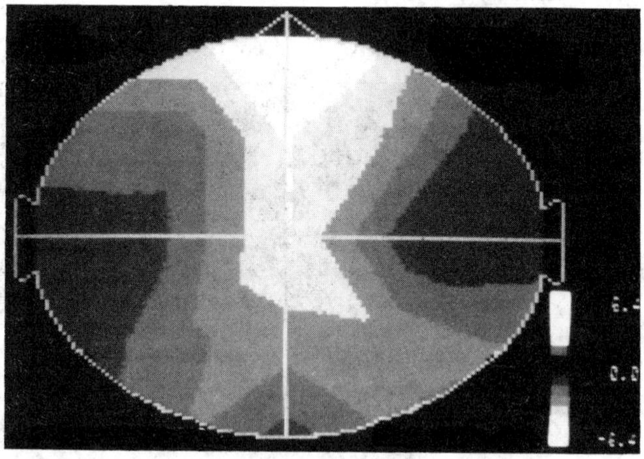

FIGURE 1.8-13. *Brain electrical activity map showing data from a visual evoked potential. This map summarizes brain electrical activity occurring 320 msec after a flash of light and represents an average of data collected from multiple presentations of this stimulus. (Courtesy of John Morihisa, M.D., and Frank H. Duffy, M.D.)*

As in conventional EEG and EP testing, computerized mapping procedures require vigilance for possible artifactual contamination of the data. Problems perhaps specific to computerized topographic systems include possible limitations or flaws in the software design (e.g., possible built-in erroneous assumptions, oversimplifications, or compromises), as well as possible mathematical or statistical inaccuracies. In addition, the compelling patterns delineated by color maps of electrophysiological data can invite overinterpretation beyond what can be justified by the available research data.

FUTURE DIRECTIONS

The potential for computerized topographic mapping techniques in both research and clinical settings is significant. More study and research in this area will be needed before computerized topographic mapping of electrophysiological data can be definitively added to the clinical armamentarium. However, the reader should understand that this field is rapidly evolving and changing, and some of the ideas and concepts that have been presented here will no doubt be subject to modification as individuals obtain more experience with these mapping techniques and new research in this field is reported.

Some directions for future research studies might include: (1) the application of computerized mapping systems in conjunction with other complementary brain-imaging methodologies; (2) application of new mathematical approaches to the statistical analysis of data; (3) use of specific cognitive activation procedures (e.g., drug infusions, specific cognitive challenges, such as the Wisconsin Card-Sorting Test); and (4) the development of new technologies, such as magnetoencephalography (MEG).

An example of this first strategy is demonstrated in Figure 1.8-12. Here the computerized evoked-potential data from patients with and without frontal cortical atrophy as demonstrated by computed tomography (CT) were compared. In the future, the utilization of computerized EEG systems in concert with other brain-imaging techniques, such as positron emission tomography (PET) or magnetic resonance imaging (MRI), might yield useful information about the brain.

Potential technical advances in the technique of magnetoencephalography (MEG) might provide an alternative, noninvasive method for directly recording both cortical and deeper subcortical electrical activity. MEG measures the very weak magnetic fields generated by the electrical activity of neurons and then converts the magnetic energy back to an electric signal. At this time, the detection of these very minute magnetic fields requires the utilization of a super quantum interference device (SQUID) that must be cooled to –260°C and is the subject of extensive research development. Refinement of MEG methodology is occurring at a number of medical centers worldwide, but the technology is still in its early stages.

Perhaps with the further elaboration and refinement of new methods, such as computerized electrophysiological techniques and MEG, Hans Berger's goal of measuring brain electrical activity to detect and characterize the underlying neuropathophysiology of psychiatric disorders may be more fully realized. However, the application of these new computerized imaging techniques must be shaped and guided by the growing body of neuroscientific research that has begun to elucidate the basic mechanisms of brain function.

REFERENCES

Baribeau-Braun J, Pincton T W, Gosselin J: Schizophrenia: A neurophysiological evaluation of abnormal information processing. Science *219:* 874, 1983.

Berger H: Uber das elektrenkephalogramm des menschen I. Arch Psychiat Nervenkr *87:* 527, 1929.

Buschbaum M S: Middle evoked potentials. Schizophr Bull *3:* 93, 1977.

Cooper R, Winter A L, Crow H J, et al: Comparison of subcortical, cortical, and scalp activity using chronically indwelling electrodes in man. Electroenceph Clin Neurophysiol *18:* 217, 1965.

Coppola R, Buchsbaum M S, Rigal F: Computer generation of surface distribution maps of measures of brain activity. Comput Biol Med *12:* 191, 1982.

Duffy F H, Burchfiel J L, Lombroso C T: Brain electrical activity mapping (BEAM): A method for extending the clinical utility of EEG and evoked potential data. Ann Neurol *5:* 309, 1979.

Duncan-Johnson C C, Donchin E: Quantifying surprise: The variation of event-related potentials with subjective probability. Psychophysiology *24:* 456, 1977.

Duncan C C, Morihisa J M, Fawcett R W, et al: P300 in Schizophrenia: State or trait marker. Psychopharmacol Bull *23:* 497, 1987.

Goldensohn E S: Neurophysiologic substrates of EEG activity. In *Current Practice of Clinical Electrocephalography,* D W Klass, D D Daly, editors, p 424. Raven Press, New York, 1979.

Grebb J A, Weinberger D R, Morihisa J M: Electroencephalogram and evoked potential studies of schizophrenia. In *Handbook of Schizophrenia,* vol 1, *The Neurology of Schizophrenia,* H A Nasrallah, D R Weinberger, editors. Elsevier, New York, 1986.

Hanson J C, Hillyard S A: Endogenous brain potentials associated with selective auditory attention. Electroenceph Clin Neurophysiol *49:* 277, 1980.

John E R, Karmel B Z, Corning W C, et al: Neurometrics. Science *196:* 1393, 1977.

Karson, C N, Coppola R, Morihisa J M, et al: Computed electroencephalographic activity mapping in schizophrenia. Arch Gen Psychiat *44:* 514, 1987.

Knight R T: Electrophysiology in behavioral neurology. In *Principles of Behavioral Neurology,* M M Mesulam, editor. Davis, Philadelphia, 1985.

Lopes da Silva F H, Van Rotterdam A: Biophysical aspects of EEG and MEG generation. In *Electroencephalography Basic Principles, Clinical Applications and Related Fields.* E Niedermeyer, F H Lopes da Silva, editors. Urban and Schwarzenberg, Baltimore, 1982.

Morihisa J M: Functional brain imaging techniques. In *American Psychiatric Association Annual Review,* no 6, R Hales, A Frances, editors. American Psychiatric Press, Washington, DC, 1987.

Morihisa J M, McAnulty G B: Structure and function: Brain electrical activity mapping (BEAM) and computed tomography (CT scan) in schizophrenia. Biol Psychiat *20:* 3, 1985.

Niedermeyer E, Lopes da Silva F: *Electroencephalography. Basic Principles, Clinical Applications and Related Fields.* Urban and Schwarzenberg, Baltimore, 1987.

Nunez P L: *Electric Fields of the Brain. The Neurophysics of EEG.* p 234. Oxford University Press, New York, 1981.

Roth W T, Horvath T B, Pfefferbaum A, et al: Late event-related potentials and schizophrenia. In *Evoked Brain Potentials and Behavior,* H Befleiter, editor, p 499. Plenum, New York, 1979.

Shagass C: Early evoked potentials. Schizophr Bull 3: *80,* 1977.

Shagass C: Evoked potentials in adult psychiatry. In *EEG and Evoked Potentials in Psychiatry and Behavioral Neurology,* J R Hughes, W P Wilson, editors. Butterworth, Boston, 1983.

1.9
BASIC SCIENCE OF SLEEP

CONSTANCE A. MOORE, M.D.
ISMET KARACAN, M.D., D.Sc.
ROBERT L. WILLIAMS, M.D.

INTRODUCTION

The scientific study of sleep has progressed more in the past 35 years—beginning with the discovery of rapid eye movement (REM) sleep and its association with dreaming—than in the previous two centuries. The greatest gains have ensued from the development of new technology, a multidisciplinary approach to evaluating sleep complaints, and a better understanding of the chemistry of the brain. Despite such significant accomplishments, the basic phenomenon of sleep remains enshrouded in mystery to sleeper and investigator alike. Researchers and clinicians are still perplexed by many unanswered questions. Why do organisms sleep? What biological need does this cyclical process fulfill? What is the purpose of dreaming? Why is disordered sleep often a forerunner or prominent symptom of mental or medical illness? The exploration of these enigmas has led current sleep research away from its former emphasis on the description of sleep and its stages, phenomenology, and ontology, to two main areas: (1) basic sleep mechanisms and sleep physiology and (2) sleep problems in clinical medicine. This section will discuss briefly these former emphases, but the focus will be on the exploration of mechanisms and physiology.

SLEEP PHYSIOLOGY

Sleep is a behavioral state composed of two relatively distinct parts, REM and non-REM (NREM), that are distinguished polygraphically by recording the electroencephalogram (EEG), electrooculogram (EOG), and chin electromyogram (EMG). In humans, NREM sleep consists of four stages. The relaxed, waking state with eyes closed is stage 0, characterized in most people by segments of *alpha* (α) (8 to 12.5-Hz [cycles per second])-brain wave activity, high muscle tone, and some eye movement (Fig. 1.9-1). Stage 1 comprises the transition into sleep, the "twilight" sensation, in which α-waves drop out and *theta* (θ) (4 to 7-Hz) waves begin (Fig. 1.9-2). Relatively low-voltage fast background activity is seen and vertex sharp waves may be present. Slow eye movements appear and EMG activity is not suppressed. In stage 2, EEG spindles (13 to 15 Hz) and high-voltage spikes called K-complexes appear (Fig. 1.9-3). The background consists of irregular θ waves. In stages 3 or 4, *delta* (δ)-waves, or slow waves (1.5 to 3 Hz) predominate. These two stages are differentiated mainly by the concentration of δ-activity; 20 to 50 percent identifies the sleep segment as stage 3 (Fig. 1.9-4), which becomes stage 4 when the proportion increases to at least 50 percent (Fig. 1.9-5). Growth hormone secretion is increased during stage 4 and the sleeper has a high threshold of arousal. After total sleep deprivation, there is a significant rebound effect of stage 4. Stages 3 and 4 are sometimes scored together as slow-wave sleep. Most dreaming occurs during REM sleep (Fig. 1.9-6). Although the EEG characteristics of this stage resemble stage 1, REM is unique in its extreme hypotonia as well as short bursts of phasic activity, such as REMs, blood pressure and heart rate variability, muscle twitches, and nocturnal penile tumescence (NPT). The sleeper is more likely to awaken after REM episodes than any other stage. After sleep deprivation, REM sleep significantly rebounds. In the healthy young adult, REM sleep represents about 25 percent, stage 1 about 5 percent, stage 2 about 50 percent, and stages 3 and 4 combined about 20 percent of total sleep time.

ONTOGENY Although some generalizations can be made about sleep EEG characteristics, the normalcy of sleep is relative to age. For example, the average 25-year-old adult has four to six sleep cycles during any given 8-hour sleep period in the following sequence: 1—2—3—4—3—2—REM. In this age group, the time from the beginning of one REM episode to the beginning of the next is about 90 minutes, and the duration of the first REM episode is about 15 minutes. Quantity of slowwave sleep decreases and duration of REM episodes lengthens in the third and fourth cycles of the night.

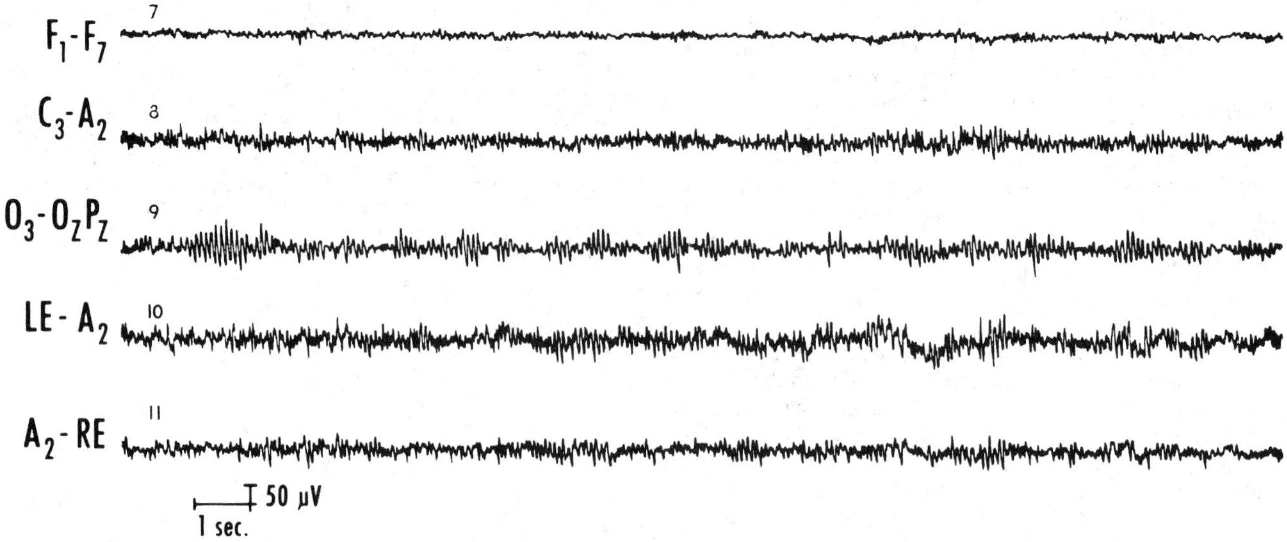

FIGURE 1.9-1. *Stage 0 EEG and EOG recording from a 29-year-old female.*

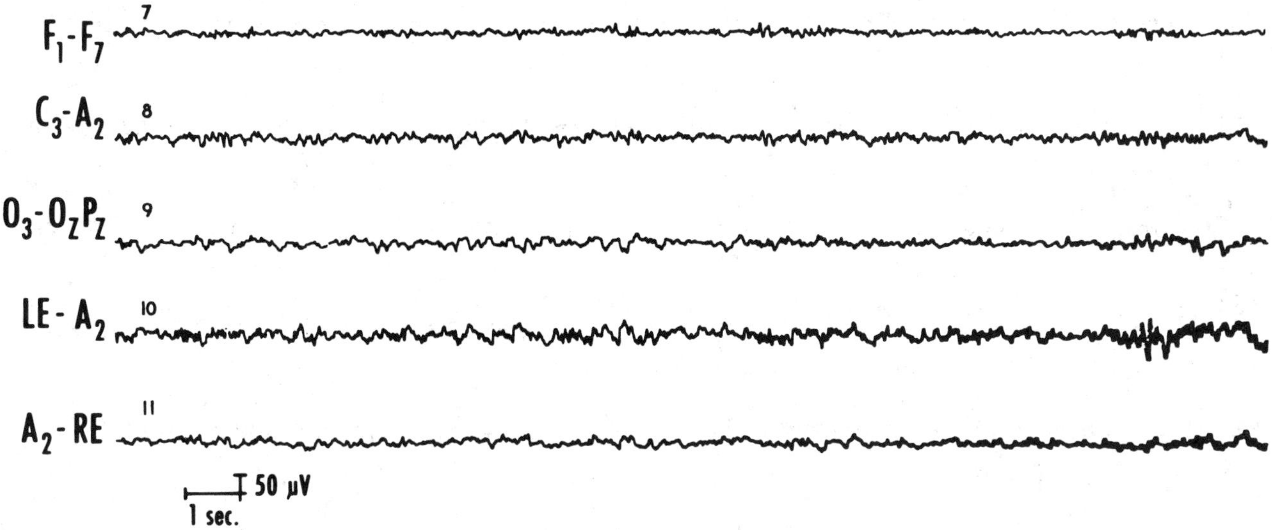

FIGURE 1.9-2. *Stage 1 EEG and EOG recording from a 29-year-old female.*

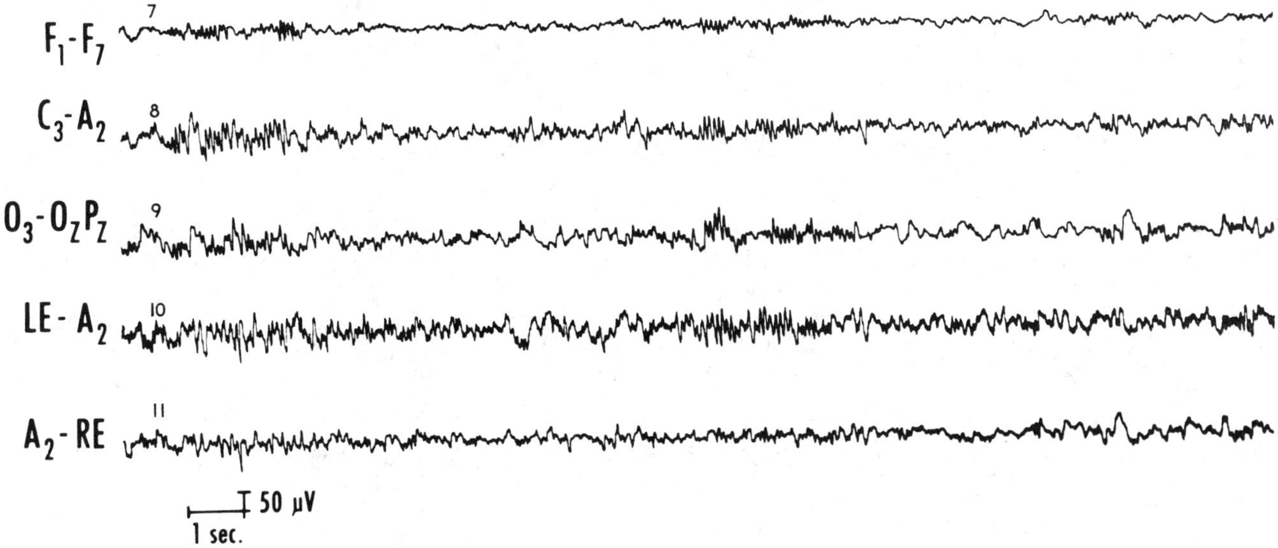

FIGURE 1.9-3. *Stage 2 EEG and EOG recording from a 29-year-old female.*

Sleep patterns, which can be recorded long before birth, gradually change throughout one's lifetime. The most distinct changes occur, however, after 3 years of age, after puberty, and after the fourth decade of life, particularly in men. Examining the sleep characteristics of males in 3 decades—young (20 to 29), middle-aged (40 to 49), and elderly (70 to 79)—will help demonstrate these age-related differences.

With advancing age, one may spend the same length of time in bed, but total sleep time decreases and the number of awakenings increases. Thus, the elderly person sleeps restlessly and lies in bed awake for longer periods. In addition, the proportion of the five sleep stages varies over a lifetime. Young men spend 15 percent of sleep in stage 4, and this amount dwindles to 3 percent in middle age and usually none in the elderly. Similarly, the amount of REM declines from a postadolescent high of 28 percent to 18 percent in old age. These trends seem to indicate that sleep becomes lighter and less refreshing with age (Fig. 1.9-7).

ACTIVITY IN ORGAN SYSTEMS Modern sleep research has refuted earlier beliefs that sleep constitutes a time of physiological deceleration. The entire body does not rest; instead, patterns of physiological activity merely redistribute according to sleep stage. Respiratory, esophageal, cardiovascular, erectile, and cerebral physiology exhibit marked changes during sleep.

Respiratory physiology Even in normal, healthy people, respiratory function declines during sleep. Mild alveolar hypoventilation accompanies sleep onset, an effect exacerbated in patients with chronic obstructive pulmonary disease (COPD). Respiratory rate and minute ventilation decrease during slow-wave sleep, whereas breathing is generally more rapid, shallow, and erratic during REM sleep. Further reducing respiratory function, especially during REM, is the partial collapse of the upper airway and decreased tone of the intercostal and genioglossal muscles. Lung secretions may be retained due to reduced coughing and mucociliary clearance during both sleep phases. While having little effect on healthy people, these changes may be life-threatening to patients with asthma, chronic obstructive

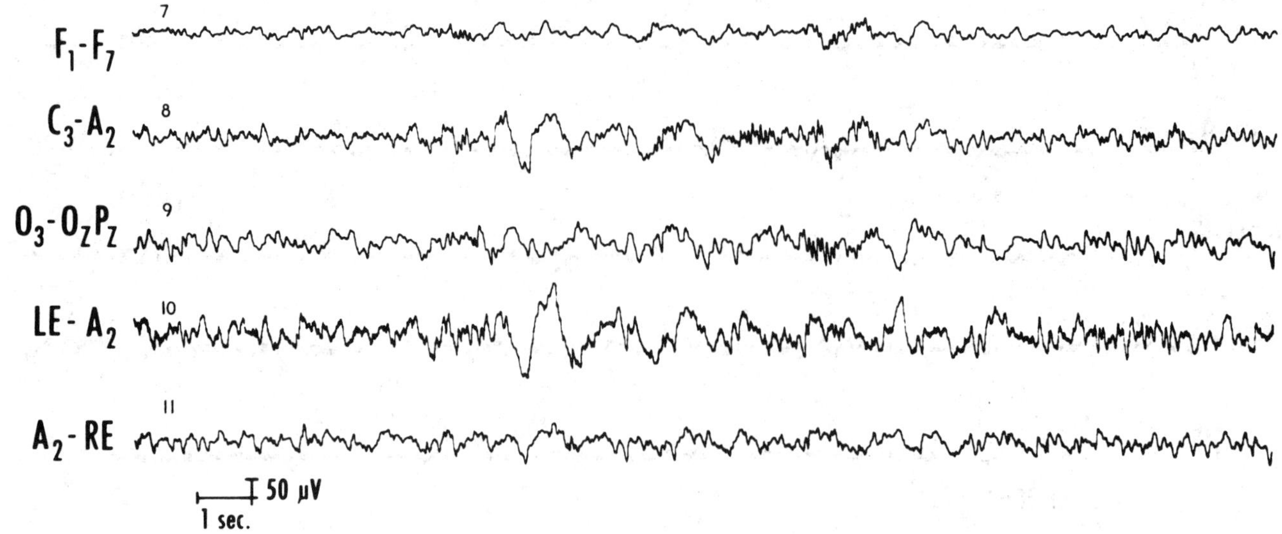

FIGURE 1.9.4. *Stage 3 EEG and EOG recording from a 29-year-old female.*

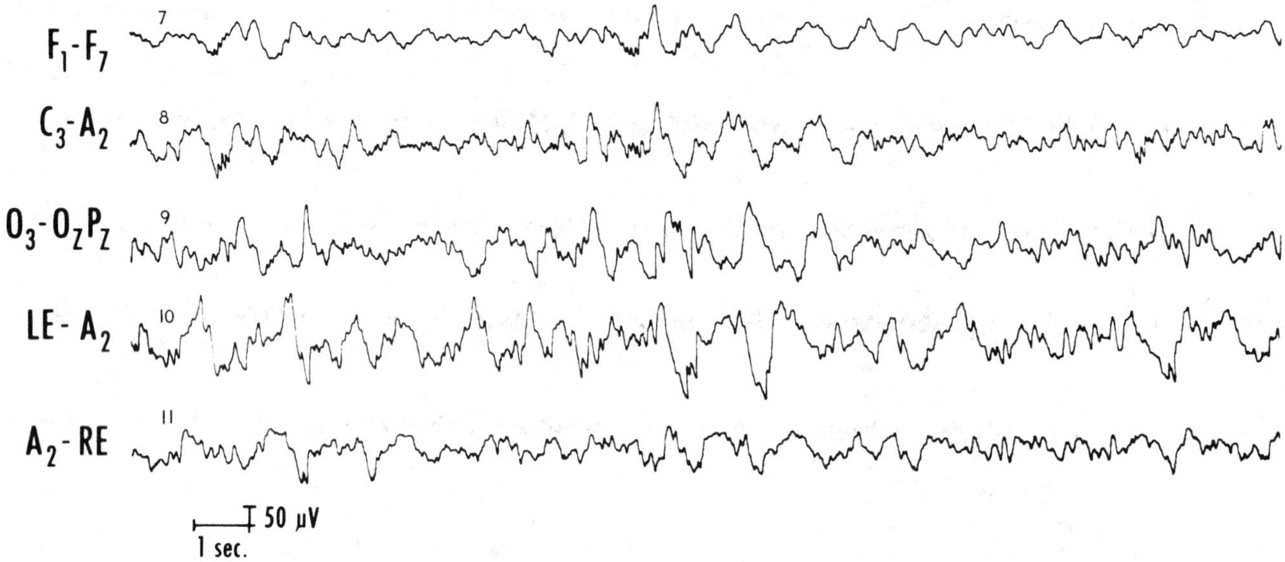

FIGURE 1.9-5. *Stage 4 EEG and EOG recording from a 29-year-old female.*

lung disease, sleep apnea, or other respiratory impairments. During REM, compensatory mechanisms that normally come into play when respiration is compromised during waking or NREM sleep are unresponsive. Thus, respiratory control during REM sleep is not subject to the vagal mediation that is so apparent during waking and NREM sleep. These REM-related defects have been ascribed to a suspension of homeostatic feedback regulation by the hypothalamus. Many studies of patients with sleep apnea indicate that sleep-related breathing disorders may involve a defective centrally regulated arousal mechanism.

Esophageal function Also associated with central arousal mechanisms is acid clearance from the esophagus during sleep. Because acid clearance during sleep is prolonged compared to during wakefulness, a person who does not awaken to swallow may suffer from esophagitis and pulmonary aspiration.

Thermoregulation The sleep stage having the most profound interaction with the physiological regulation of core body temperature is REM. When REM periods occur on the rising slope of the temperature cycle, they have a shorter latency and last longer. The regulation of body temperature is much different during REM sleep than during NREM sleep. At low ambient temperatures, body temperature tends to increase during NREM sleep and to decrease during REM sleep. Under conditions of high ambient temperatures, the opposite occurs. Thus, NREM sleep seems to be homeothermic, whereas REM sleep is poikilothermic. Studies of peripheral skin temperature measurements verify that vasomotor activity appropriately increases as the result of rising ambient temperature during NREM sleep, but it decreases during REM sleep. Likewise, lowering ambient temperature decreases vasomotor activity in NREM and increases it in REM. What could be responsible for this lack of appropriate homeothermic thermoregulatory response during REM sleep? Researchers hypothesize that the responsiveness of hypothalamic thermoreceptive structures is depressed during REM sleep. This explanation is consistent with the paradoxical findings during REM of other physiological processes, such as respiration.

Cardiovascular physiology Sleep-related cardiovascular function, though studied mainly in cats, is particularly relevant to humans

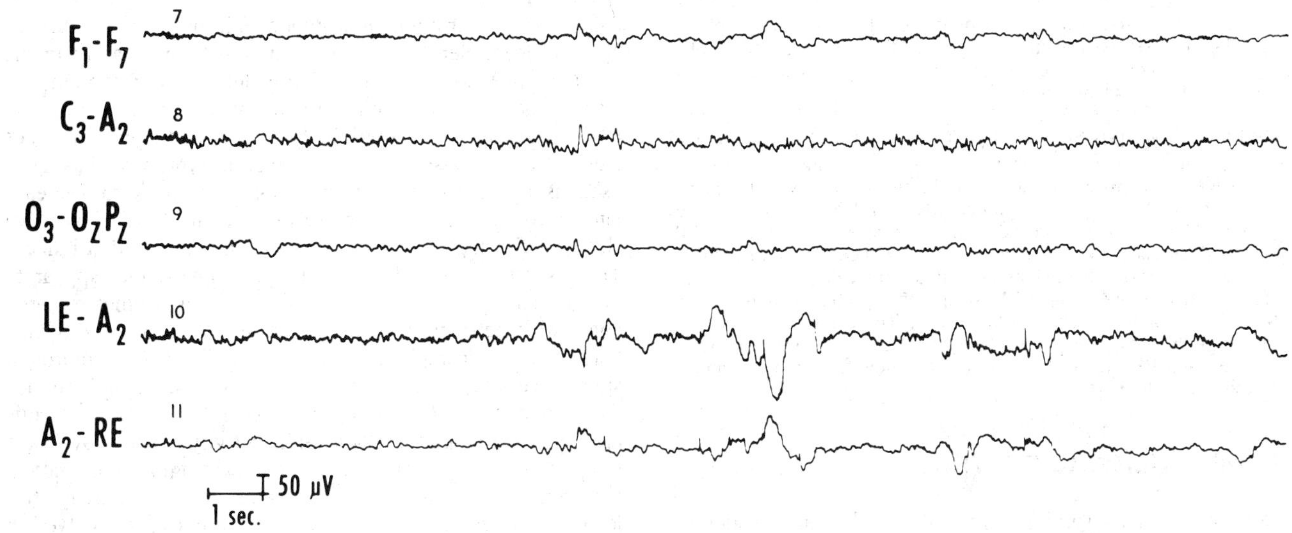

FIGURE 1.9-6. *REM EEG and EOG recording from a 29-year-old female.*

with cardiovascular disease. Although mean arterial blood pressure and heart rates decline about 10 percent and 6 percent, respectively, during both NREM and REM sleep, greater variability during REM has been hypothesized to precipitate stroke, myocardial infarction, angina, and dysrhythmias. Coinciding with the onset of rapid eye movements and muscle twitches, mean blood pressure increases briefly but sharply 30 to 40 mm Hg, whereas heart rate declines tonically. These changes during REM may be associated with marked vasodilation in mesenteric or renal vessels and vasoconstriction of blood flow to skeletal muscle. The danger of bradycardias and tachycardias is the least during slow-wave sleep, when heart rate and blood pressure reach their lowest and least variable levels. Despite these differences between REM and NREM sleep, most research of patients with coronary heart disease or arrhythmias indicates a decline in frequency of arrhythmias during sleep, with no significant difference between the two. Nevertheless, those cardiac patients who do display more severe electrocardiographic (EKG) findings during sleep should be identified and given higher doses of vasodilator and antiarrhythmic medications at night.

Sleep-induced erections Also part of the autonomic activity during REM sleep in healthy males of all ages are episodes of nocturnal penile tumescence (NPT). These episodes, averaging four 30-minute periods per night and declining with age, serve as a biological marker for erectile capacity. Abnormal frequency, duration, or rigid-

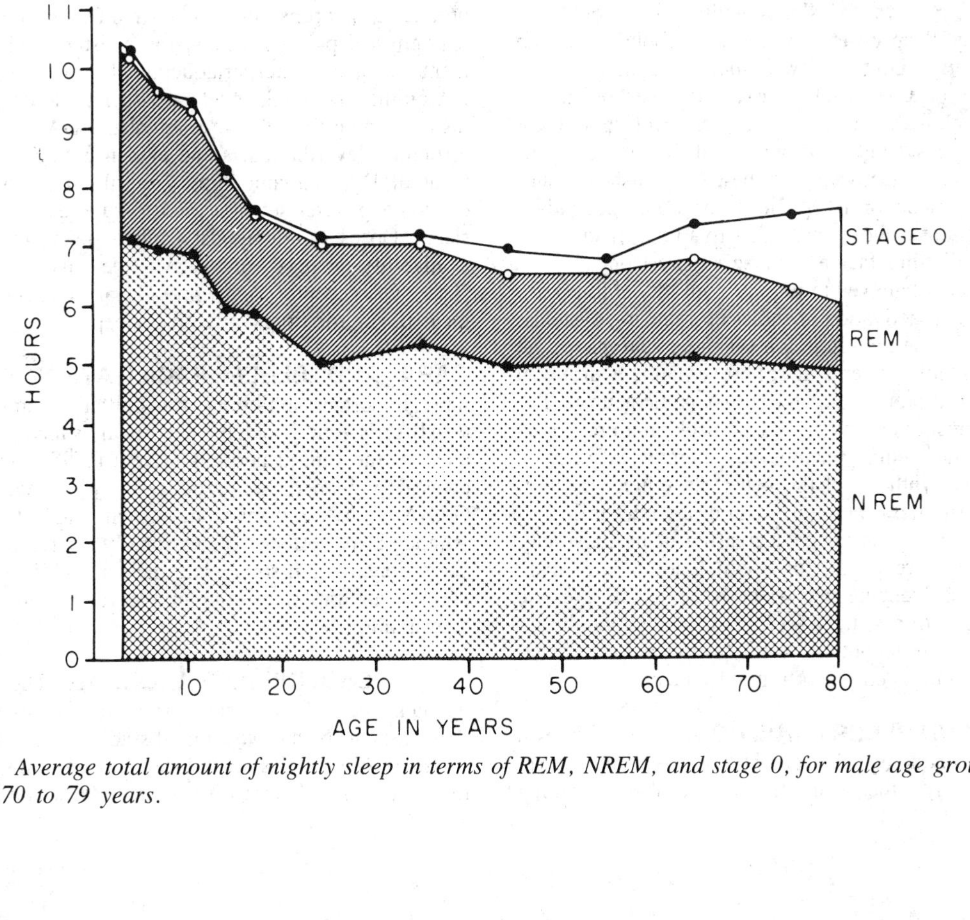

FIGURE 1.9-7. *Average total amount of nightly sleep in terms of REM, NREM, and stage 0, for male age groups from 3 to 5 years through 70 to 79 years.*

ity of NPT episodes during adequate REM sleep may implicate vascular disease, neuropathy, endocrinopathy, or drug and alcohol abuse as producing impotence, regardless of any psychological contributions to sexual dysfunction.

Cerebral circulation Increases in cerebral blood flow (CBF) indicate sites of highest metabolic activity in the brain during various stages of the sleep-wake cycle. Since the sleep-wake cycle is centrally regulated, this measure is particularly useful in helping sleep researchers better understand the function of sleep. Changes in CBF during sleep should imply corresponding changes in brain activity. Overall, studies of CBF in cats and humans indicate a global increase of cerebral activity during REM sleep and a global decrease during NREM compared with the waking state. These normative findings can help diagnose sleep disorders, such as narcolepsy, in which changes in CBF are in the opposite direction from those found in normal subjects.

NEUROCHEMICAL CONTROL MECHANISMS

Despite the many studies of animals and humans to identify the neurochemicals involved in the control of sleep, the neurotransmitters and peptides regulating the sleep-wake cycle can only be inferred. Complicating research is the lack of an animal species whose sleep EEG characteristics are equivalent to human sleep. Because sleep occurs spontaneously, it is difficult to prove that an experimental factor is actually the factor that induced sleep. Furthermore, the sleep induced may not be physiological sleep; that is, general anesthetics, sedatives, and neurotoxins may produce EEG changes reminiscent of slow-wave sleep and REM sleep that merely resemble true sleep. Certain chemicals facilitate but do not induce sleep.

A *sleep-facilitating factor* is not necessary, sufficient, or exclusive to produce sleep onset, but its presence may cause drowsiness, facilitate sleep onset, or increase sleep duration in the presence of sleep-inducing factors. Examples are sedative drugs, the postprandial state, and a comfortable sleep environment. Although removal of sleep-facilitating factors may temporarily delay sleep onset, a secondary rebound of sleep should occur. By contrast, *sleep-inducing factors* are endogenous and act directly on the executive mechanisms of sleep. Their administration at the receptor level should not only cause sleep onset but also increase slow-wave sleep or REM sleep, or both. Inactivation of these factors should suppress slow-wave sleep or REM sleep, or both. Secondary rebound should not follow these inactivation effects, nor should sleep-facilitating factors reverse suppression.

Sleep induction is believed to require both the inhibition of arousal systems and activation of the sleep-inducing systems. Neurotransmitters released from presynaptic neurons excite (depolarize) or inhibit (hyperpolarize) postsynaptic neurons by interacting with receptor sites on the postsynaptic neuron. The released neurotransmitter may also "feed back" onto receptors in the presynaptic neuron membrane, thereby influencing further release or synthesis of the neurotransmitter. In addition to neurotransmitters, hormones and drugs may influence neuronal activity by increasing or decreasing neurotransmitter synthesis, release, reuptake, or degradation. The main neurochemicals influencing the sleep-wake cycle are the monoamine neurotransmitters—serotonin, norepinephrine, and dopamine—γ-aminobutyric acid, acetylcholine, histamine, peptides, and sleep-promoting substances.

SEROTONIN AND SLEEP INDUCTION More is known about the sleep-inducing characteristics of serotonin than about those of any other neurotransmitter. The prevailing theory is that serotonin is a hypnogenic neurotransmitter for NREM sleep. Serotonergic neurons are found mainly in the median raphe extending from the medulla to the midbrain, but also in the medullary and mesencephalic reticular formation (RF). Applying serotonin directly to areas of the brain induces EEG sleep. The serotonin precursor L-tryptophan has been used as an effective hypnotic drug in humans to decrease latency to sleep onset, increase the percentage of slow-wave sleep, and in high doses, increase the amount of REM sleep. Thus, serotonin and the serotonergic raphe nuclei appear to play a major role in sleep induction, although other research concerning neuronal activity levels during sleep raises doubts that serotonergic raphe neurons are crucial for the control of slow-wave sleep and essential for readying other neurons for the production of REM sleep. One resolution proposed to this apparent contradiction of low-raphe activity during slow-wave sleep is that serotonergic systems dampen vigilance in waking and trigger slow-wave sleep by a short surge of activity, followed by a decrease in activity. Serotonin seems involved in the biosynthesis, storage, and liberation of other sleep-inducing factors when released during waking and sleep deprivation.

EFFECTS OF NOREPINEPHRINE ON AROUSAL AND RAPID EYE MOVEMENT SLEEP Noradrenergic neurons are located in the medulla and pons; the major source is the locus ceruleus. The reticular activating system also contains noradrenergic neurons. These neurons appear to be involved in tonic cortical arousal, which is reflected as low-voltage fast-EEG activity during both waking and REM sleep, but the extent of this influence remains unresolved. Researchers speculate that the occurrence of REM sleep probably does require norepinephrine (NE) neurotransmission.

DOPAMINE AND AROUSAL Central dopamine (DA)-producing neurons are found mainly in the hypothalamo-hypophyseal portal systems, the substantia nigra-ventral tegmental area, and the periaqueductal gray area. The effects of DA on the sleep-wake cycle are difficult to determine because distinguishing the relative roles of the DA and NE systems is difficult. Nevertheless, some evidence exists for the involvement of DA in maintaining arousal. DA agonists appear to delay sleep onset severely and to suppress stage 4 and REM sleep. Doses of antagonists and agonists that enhance DA availability decrease slow-wave sleep and, eventually, REM sleep. DA receptors may provide an important pharmacological target for drugs affecting sleep.

GABA AND SLEEP FACILITATION Considered the most important inhibitory transmitter, γ-aminobutyric acid (GABA) is found widely in cortical, subcortical, and spinal areas of the central nervous system (CNS). Sedation and decreased vigilance are produced by agents that facilitate GABA-ergic transmission, such as benzodiazepines. Although the effects of regionally increased GABA concentrations remain somewhat unclear, GABA is hypothesized to play an important role in the regulation of arousal and "dewaking."

ACETYLCHOLINE AND AROUSAL The production and maintenance of arousal probably involves cholinergic transmission. Numerous animal studies indicate that enhanced cholinergic transmission induces and prolongs REM sleep or its components. These effects are less definitive in humans.

HISTAMINE Although histamine (HA) is likely to be involved in the control of sleep and waking, it has received much less attention from researchers than other neurotransmitters. The highest levels of HA are found in the hypothalamus, basal ganglia, thalamus, and midbrain gray region. Its neuroregulatory role in sleep and waking has been inferred mainly from pharmacological studies in which the arousing effect of HA and the sleep-inducing actions of some H_1 receptor antagonists were described. Experiments in rats indicate that responses to decreased neuronal HA levels differ according to the phase of the light-dark cycle; this finding implies the involvement of HA with circadian rhythms, which will be discussed in the next subsection. HA also seems to inhibit the occurrence of REM sleep.

PEPTIDES AND SLEEP-PROMOTING SUBSTANCES

Also possibly involved in the regulation of sleep, especially slow-wave sleep induction, are certain brain peptides and sleep-promoting substances (SPSs) that accumulate in the brain during periods of prolonged wakefulness or sleep deprivation. These include delta sleep-inducing peptide (DSIP), arginine vasotocin (AVT), factor S, SPS, and vasoactive intestinal polypeptide (VIP). Protein synthesis may be necessary to trigger REM sleep.

CIRCADIAN RHYTHMS AND THE SLEEP-WAKE CYCLE

The sleep-wake cycle is a *circadian rhythm* in humans. It is genetically determined rather than learned and established some time after birth. Zeitgebers and endogenous rhythms are responsible for this periodicity. By entraining or synchronizing the pacemaker to a periodic cycle, a *zeitgeber,* or signal from the environment, helps establish the proper phasing of internal to external cycles. The light-dark cycle is the most important zeitgeber in animals. Knowledge of the time of day and other social cues are additional zeitgebers for humans. Zeitgebers are not essential, however, for circadian rhythms to continue operating. Even when zeitgebers are removed and biological rhythms are free-running, the human sleep-wake cycle generally develops about a 25-hour periodicity, which is close to the 24 hours of a normal circadian rhythm.

In humans entrained to a 24-hour circadian cycle, the sleep-wake, temperature, cortisol, growth hormone (GH), and prolactin (PRL) cycles are linked. Temperature falls with sleep onset and rises sharply at the end of the sleep period. GH is secreted mainly during slow-wave sleep. A large pulse of PRL secretion occurs shortly after sleep onset, and cortisol levels are at a nadir in early sleep and peak at the end of sleep.

Attempts to locate the circadian pacemaker have identified the suprachiasmatic nucleus (SCN) as one pacemaker. Lesions of the SCN bilaterally in rodents result in the loss of many circadian rhythms, including those of food intake, locomotor activity, pineal serotonin-*N*-acetyltransferase, adrenal corticosterone, and estrous cycle. Circadian sleep-wake cycles are abolished in SCN lesions in the rat, although the amount of time spent in waking, slow-wave sleep, and REM sleep remains the same. Lesions of the various afferent inputs do not produce arrhythmicity, but destruction of efferent fibers does. Furthermore, the SCN in rats shows a circadian rhythm in electrical activity that persists with little periodic change in continuous light or dark.

Evidence that circadian pacemakers are composed of multiple oscillators indicates that the SCN is not the sole circadian oscillator. One indication is that when zeitgebers are removed, different physiological rhythms may separate from one another and develop different periods of their own. In the free-running state, the temperature and cortisol levels separate from the sleep-wake cycle, whereas the GH and PRL linkage undergoes little alteration. Rhythms of rectal temperature and cortisol levels persist after SCN lesions in primates. The existence of more than one circadian oscillator is implied by these findings.

Also possibly involved in circadian cycling is the pineal gland. Mammalian pineal glands synthesize and release melatonin at various rates that are entrained by the 24-hour light-dark cycle. The enzyme that regulates melatonin synthesis, *N*-acetyltransferase, in rats shows a 50-fold increase in activity at night. This activity appears to be regulated by β-adrenergic receptors. Melatonin given to birds chronically exerts dose-dependent effects on the locomotor activity cycles. In birds, pinealectomy abolishes free-running locomotor activity rhythmicity in darkness but entrainment to light-dark cycles persists.

Abnormalities in circadian rhythms may reflect clinical depression. During major depression, rhythms of temperature, REM sleep, and cortisol may advance with respect to the sleep-wake or light-dark cycle. Imipramine (Tofranil), lithium, and clorgyline, which are used to treat mood disorders, all lengthen free-running rhythms in animals, thereby resynchronizing these biological phases.

The best-known example of asynchronous sleep-wake and other biological rhythms is jet lag. After flying east or west, many individuals have difficulty sleeping at a time that is now out of phase with some of their body cycles.

FUNCTIONS OF SLEEP

Examining neurochemical control mechanisms and circadian rhythms in relation to the sleep-wake cycle provides some insight into the nature of sleep but not the purpose or function of sleep. Studies of sleep deprivation and the differences between long sleepers (more than 9 hours required) and short sleepers (less than 6 hours required) demonstrate that sleep probably does serve some restorative functions.

One technique for determining the function of a system is to observe what deficits result from removing it. When people are deprived of sleep, physiologically they show central hypoarousal combined with autonomic hyperarousal. The waking EEG shifts away from α-frequencies toward lower frequencies. Pulse and respiratory rates often are more rapid. During recovery from sleep deprivation, the sleeper has much slow-wave sleep in the first hours and an increase in total REM time in succeeding hours or days. Social and environmental factors greatly influence the psychological effects of sleep deprivation. A task is more susceptible to the effects of sleep deprivation if it is long and dull, rather than difficult. As expected, confusion and fatigue increase, and alertness and vigor decrease. Such effects usually do not seriously impair productivity. After prolonged periods of sleep deprivation, however, hallucinations, delusions, and progressive confusion may occur. Attempts to deprive a person of REM sleep only by frequent awakenings are nearly futile, since REM will try to begin more and more often. Recovery sleep from these awakenings out of REM usually consists of a large rebound increase in REM. More irritability and social difficulties seem to ensue from REM deprivation, whereas greater physical lethargy follows slow-wave sleep deprivation.

The difference between long and short sleepers appears to be the amount of REM sleep required, since both groups exhibit equivalent amounts of slow-wave sleep. This suggests that although the need for a certain amount of slow-wave sleep is consistent among various groups of people, the need for REM sleep may vary widely. What distinguishes the high-need REM group from the low-need group may provide some clue to the purpose of this sleep state. Based on the results of quantitative psychological tests and psychiatric interviewers, researchers have concluded that in contrast to short sleepers, long sleepers exhibit minor psychopathology, such as mild depression or anxiety, and tend to be worriers and nonconformists. Short sleepers are nonworriers who are generally socially adept, ambitious, energetic, and satisfied with themselves and their lives. These findings suggest that more REM sleep may be needed to restore the brain after worrying, mild depression, or anxiety. The fact that a regular sleep requirement of less than 4 hours is seldom or never found suggests that normal humans require at least 4 or 5 hours of sleep daily.

Persons may require more or less sleep at certain periods of their lives. Occasionally, people require less sleep for months when they are involved in a very engrossing, satisfying pastime. Even more predictable is the increased sleep needed by people who are changing occupation, more mentally active than usual, depressed or upset, or undergoing a particularly stressful period. More sleep may also be needed after heavy physical labor and exercise or during pregnancy or illness.

A prevailing conclusion from such findings is that sleep has two closely related restorative functions: (1) NREM sleep involves the anabolism and synthesis of macromolecules of protein or ribonucleic acid (RNA), with some of these used during subsequent REM sleep; and (2) REM involves the formation of new connections in the cortex and NE systems ascending to the cortex, both of which are required for optimal attention, as well as repair, reorganization, and self-guidance during waking.

Due to these primary functions, sleep may secondarily serve as a physiological marker for disturbance in normal bodily functions. Disturbed sleep, especially frequent arousals from sleep, may provide early warnings of physical pathology (e.g., respiratory impairment, cardiovascular disease, gastrointestinal disease, erectile dysfunction) or psychopathology (e.g., schizophrenia, depression).

REFERENCES

Akerstedt T: Review article: Sleepiness as a consequence of shift work. Sleep *11:* 17, 1988.

Cespuglio R, Faradji H, Gomez M E, et al: Single unit recordings in the nuclei raphe dorsalis and magnus during the sleep waking cycle of semi-chronic prepared cats. Neurosci Lett *24:* 133, 1981.

Czeisler C A, Weitzman E D, Moore-Ede M C, Zimmerman J C, Knaner R S: Human sleep: Its duration and organization depend on its circadian phase. Science *210:* 1264, 1980.

Dement W, Kleitman N: Cyclic variations in EEG during sleep and their relation to eye movements, body motility, and dreaming. Electroenceph Clin Neurophysiol *9:* 673, 1975.

Drucker-Colin R, Sckurovich M, Sterman B M, editors: *The Functions of Sleep.* Academic Press, Orlando, FL, 1979.

Hartmann E: *The Functions of Sleep.* Yale University Press, New Haven, CT, 1973.

Inoue S T, Kawamura H: Persistence of circadian rhythmicity in a mammalian hypothalamic "island" containing the suprachiasmatic nucleus. Proc Nat Acad Sci USA *26:* 5962, 1971.

Karacan I, Goodenough D R, Shapiro A, Starker S: Erection cycle during sleep in relation to dream anxiety. Arch Gen Psychiat *15:* 183, 1966.

Koella W P, editor: *Sleep 1982: Sixth European Congress of Sleep Research.* Karger, Basel, 1983.

McGuinty D J, Drucker-Colin R: Sleep mechanisms: Biology and control of REM sleep. Int Rev Neurobiol *23:* 391, 1982.

Monnier M, Gaillard J M: Biochemical regulation of sleep. Experientia *36:* 21, 1980.

Orr W C, Robinson M G, Johnson L F: Acid clearing during sleep in the pathogenesis of reflux esophagitis. Dig Dis Sci *26:* 423, 1981.

Parmeggiani P: Integrative aspects of hypothalamic influences on respiratory brain stem mechanisms during wakefulness and sleep. In *Central Control Mechanisms in Breathing,* C von Euler, H Lagercrantz, editors, p 53. Pergamon, New York, 1979.

Passonneau J V, Hawkins R A, Lust W D, Welsh F A: *Cerebral Metabolism and Neurologic Function.* Williams & Wilkins, Baltimore, 1980.

Rechtschaffen A, Kales A: *The Manual of Standardized Terminology, Techniques, and Scoring System for Sleep Stages of Human Subjects,* NIH Publication no 204. National Institutes of Health, Bethesda, MD, 1968.

Suda M, Hayaishi O, Nakagawa H, editors: *Biological Rhythms and Their Central Control Mechanism.* Elsevier, New York, 1979.

Sullivan C, Lizar L, Murphy E, Phillipson E: Primary role of respiratory afferents in sustaining breathing rhythm. J Appl Physiol *45:* 11, 1978.

Townsend R E, Prinz P N, Obrist W D: Human cerebral blood flow during sleep and waking. J Appl Physiol *35:* 620, 1973.

Wauquier A, Monti J M, Gaillard J M, Radulovacki M R: *Sleep Neurotransmitters and Neuromodulators.* Raven Press, New York, 1985.

Webb W B, editor: *Biological Rhythms, Sleep, and Performance.* Wiley, New York, 1982.

Wheatley D, editor: *Psychopharmacology of Sleep.* Raven Press, New York, 1981.

Williams R L, Karacan I, Hursch C J: *Electroencephalography (EEG) of Human Sleep: Clinical Applications.* Wiley, New York, 1974.

Zales M R, editor: *Eating, Sleeping, & Sexuality: Treatment of Disorders in Basic Life Functions.* Brunner/Mazel, New York, 1982.

1.10
BRAIN IMAGING

GÖRAN SEDVALL, M.D.

INTRODUCTION

For the psychiatrist, observation has always been an important tool for obtaining indirect information concerning the feelings, emotions, and thoughts of patients. By the meticulous observation of a patient's behavior and careful listening to the verbal expression of a patient's inner life, the psychiatrist synthesizes a psychological model of the patient's mind. This is the current basis for the diagnostic and psychotherapeutic efforts of psychiatrists. For this synthetic work, the interpretation of the messages given by the patient and the psychiatrist's imagination are limiting factors for success in diagnosis and treatment. Needless to say, these procedures are highly subjective, and many psychiatrists have looked for objective methods to examine more directly what is going on in their patients' minds. For the medically oriented psychiatrist, the brain is the organ of the mind. Therefore, the objective analysis of anatomical and functional brain correlates to mental phenomena should be an indispensable tool for progress in the diagnostic and therapeutic work in psychiatry. However, not until the end of the 1970s did such techniques begin to have an impact on psychiatry.

Important methodological progress in this direction was made during the 1930s when pneumoencephalography and electroencephalography were developed. Both of these techniques allowed the objective recording of anatomical and functional features of the brain in relation to specific neuropsychiatric conditions. However, these methodologies soon turned out to be of limited value for understanding schizophrenia and mood disorders. In the past 50 years, knowledge concerning the chemical composition of the brain has developed dramatically. Many of the recently detected chemical neurotransmitter systems in the human brain have been implicated in the pathophysiologies of mental disorders. However, the lack of techniques for analyzing these mechanisms in the living human brain has been a major limitation for progress in clinical neuroscience.

In the early 1970s, advances in applied physics and computer science laid the background for the development of instruments that permitted, for the first time, the analysis of new aspects of brain anatomy and function in living patients. These technical achievments include: (1) computed tomography (CT); (2) emission tomography (ET); and (3) magnetic resonance imaging (MRI), also called nuclear magnetic resonance (NMR). These methods have been the subject of intensive technical development and have already had an impact on clinical psychiatric practice.

The present section will give a brief outline of the physical principles underlying the currently available imaging techniques. The scientific and practical value of these techniques for diagnosis and treatment of various psychiatric disorders will also be indicated.

IMAGING OF BRAIN STRUCTURE

COMPUTED TOMOGRAPHY The technique of CT is based on the physical principle that X-rays (i.e., photons) are absorbed in tissues as a function of the electron density, which is related to the chemical composition of the tissue. Some tissues with a high calcium content (e.g., bone) have a high X-ray-absorbing capacity (attenuation); soft tissues (e.g., brain) have little X-ray absorbance. Accordingly, the conventional skull X-ray (Fig. 1.10-1) gives a distinct image of the bone structure surrounding the brain but is virtually useless with regard to information concerning the structure of the brain. In conventional X-ray procedures, the tube and the detector (or the film) are fixed in position, and a single shot of X-rays is allowed to pass through the structure to be imaged. In CT, the information from a number of X-ray exposures of the tissue from different angles is used. This may be accomplished by moving the X-ray tube and the detector in a circular process around the head (Fig. 1.10-2). This procedure will markedly increase the sensitivity at low absorption or attenuation levels. The information from the detectors is subsequently fed into a computer. A mathematical algorithm is then used to reconstruct the tomographic distribution of the X-ray absorption in cross-sectional planes throughout the brain. The information from the detectors is broken down into a grid or matrix (80 × 80 units in early scanners, now as many as 540 × 540). Each position in this grid is given an attenuation number indicating the density of the small piece of tissue represented by that grid, called a *volume element* or *voxel*. The grid is ultimately projected onto an image screen on which the images can be studied and evaluated. The word "tomography" comes from *tomos,* the Greek word for cut. McCormack and Hounsfield, who developed the principle of computerized axial tomography (now called computed tomography), were awarded the Nobel prize in physiology or medicine in 1979. By means of this technique, the absorbance in many sections of the brain can be recorded (Fig. 1.10-3). In this way, soft tissues, such as the brain, can be imaged with a reasonably good contrast. In CT scan images, various shades of gray, black, or white can then be assigned to the density number corresponding to each voxel. Thus, cerebrospinal fluid with a density similar to water appears to be almost black, whereas bone appears to be white (Table 1.10-1).

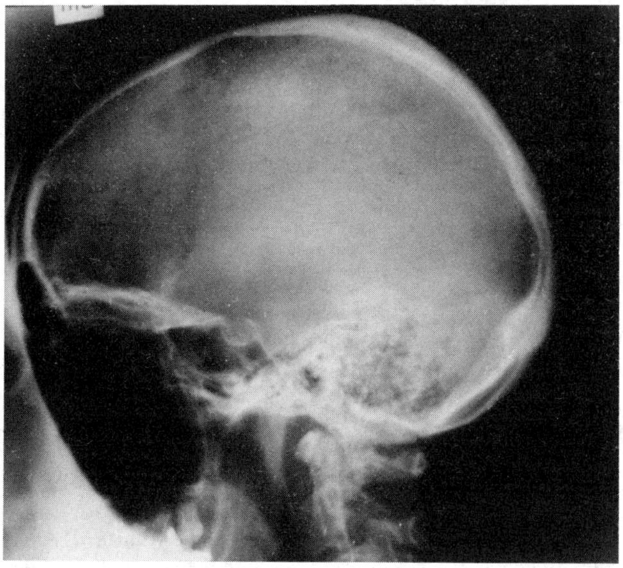

FIGURE 1.10-1. *Conventional skull X-ray of a 33-year-old man. Note that details of the brain structure cannot be distinguished.*

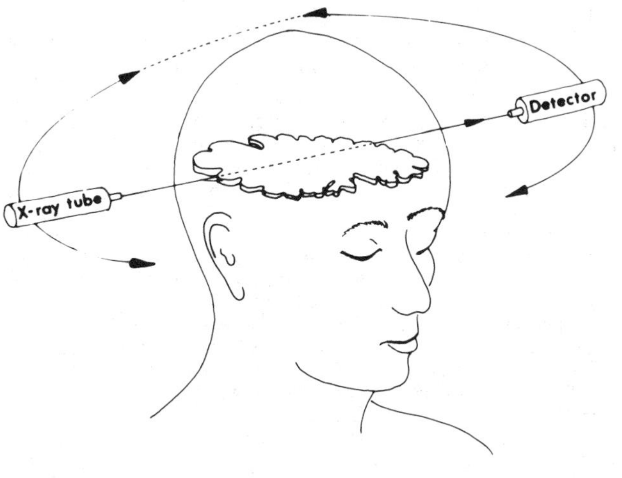

FIGURE 1.10-2. *Principles of computed tomography.*

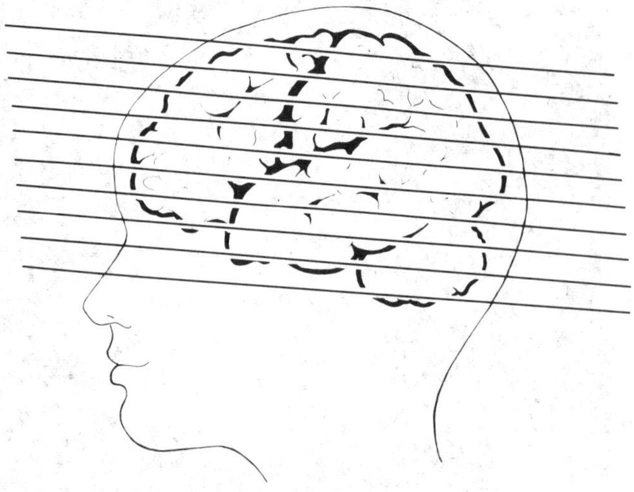

FIGURE 1.10-3. *Cross section through the head illustrating the planes of 10 CT scans parallel with the canto-meatal line.*

TABLE 1.10-1
Attenuation Values of Different Tissues in the Brain

Tissue	*Attenuation Value (Hounsfield units)*
Bone	+1,000
Gray matter	+ 46
White matter	+ 32
Cerebrospinal fluid	+ 8
Water	0
Fat	− 100
Air	−1,000

As shown in Figure 1.10-4*B*, the currently best available CT scanners can produce images of brain sections in which several details of the tissue structures can be visualized. Thus the outline of the ventricular system is easily distinguished from the brain tissue proper. The major sulci are clearly visualized as well. Although it is difficult to distinguish gray from white matter, several major brain nuclei in the basal ganglia and the thalamus can often be outlined because of their different X-ray-attenuating properties as compared with the surrounding tissues. To correct for brain size, several modifications of the *ventriculo-brain ratio* (VBR) have been used in measuring the size of the ventricular system in relation to the size of the brain. Currently available CT scanners have a resolution of approximately 2 mm. One current limitation of CT scanners is the fact that images can only be produced in parallel planes through the head (Fig. 1.10-3). The recent elaboration of computer techniques already allows the imaging of the brain of living patients through several geometrical planes. An ordinary CT scan examination of the brain takes about 10 minutes with the fastest machines available. It is expected that this time will be further reduced within a few years. The radiation exposure to the subject during an ordinary CT scan procedure is of the same order as that of an ordinary skull or chest X-ray. Conventional high-resolution CT scanners show morphological features of about 2- to 13-mm-thick sections through the brain.

Computed tomography in clinical psychiatry The importance of CT for the diagnosis of psychiatric disorders is most evident in relation to neurodegenerative disorders. Widened ventricles, widened sulci, and reduced size of the cortical gyri can be observed in presenile and senile dementia, many cases of schizophrenia, chronic alcoholism, and drug abuse. Since such alterations of brain morphology vary considerably with regard to the age of the patient, the duration of the disease, and other individual factors, it is doubtful whether CT scanning can be of diagnostic value as a single technique. There is also evidence from several studies that mentally normal subjects may have signs of marked cerebral degeneration on a CT scan. However, in the future, a more refined analysis of brain morphology with regard to normal values will likely supply information for morphological and biological dimensions in psychiatric diagnoses. For this to be accomplished, the development of standardized measures of various features of brain morphology are required.

Several studies have verified the occurrence of a higher VBR, reflecting increased size of the ventricular system in chronic alcoholism and many cases of schizophrenia. Alterations of the attenuation property of brain tissue in cases of schizophrenia have also been reported. Evidence for the occurrence of neocortical and cerebellar degeneration in schizophrenia has also been supplied by the CT technique. However, the effects of such factors as age and sex on these measures in healthy subjects have to be determined before their value can be ascertained for the diagnosis of neuropsychiatric disorders.

From a scientific point of view, knowledge of the relationships between the development of psychiatric symptoms and specific brain morphological measures will be of value for the further elucidation of etiological and pathophysiological mechanisms. The demonstration of increased frequencies of altered brain morphology in patients with alcoholism and schizophrenia by CT has illustrated the value of this technique for studying some biological aspects of these disorders. Before the development of CT scanning, the occurrence of morphological brain alterations in these disorders was generally not accepted by the scientific community (Fig. 1.10-5).

MAGNETIC RESONANCE IMAGING At first sight, a magnetic resonance image (MRI) is similar to the CT image, as shown in Figure 1.10-4 (see also Fig. 1.10-6). Both methods produce images of sections through the tissue; however, the two methods are based on completely different physical principles. The CT image reflects differences in absorption of X-rays. Anatomical MR images are produced as a function of the proton density in water, lipids, carbohydrates, and proteins of the tissue. The images also depend on the physical environment of the protons. It is possible to make pictures using other atomic nuclei than protons, but it is more difficult because signals from other nuclei are less intense than from protons.

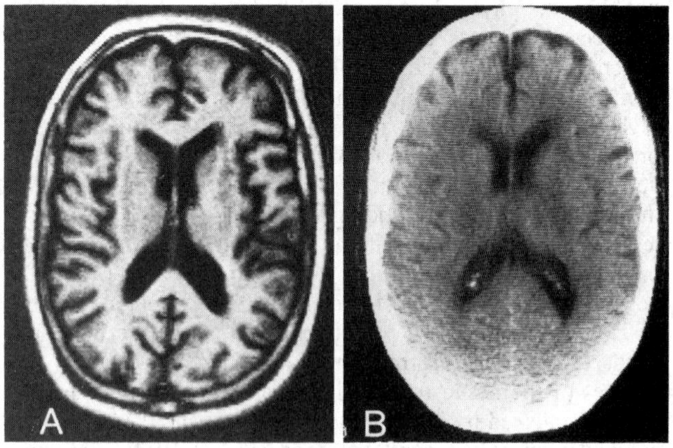

FIGURE 1.10-4. A. *MRI scan through the canto-meatal line of the same 33-year-old healthy man as in Figure 1.10-1.* B. *CT scan through the canto-meatal line of the same 33-year-old healthy man. Note that details of the brain structure cannot be distinguished as in the MRI scan shown in* A.

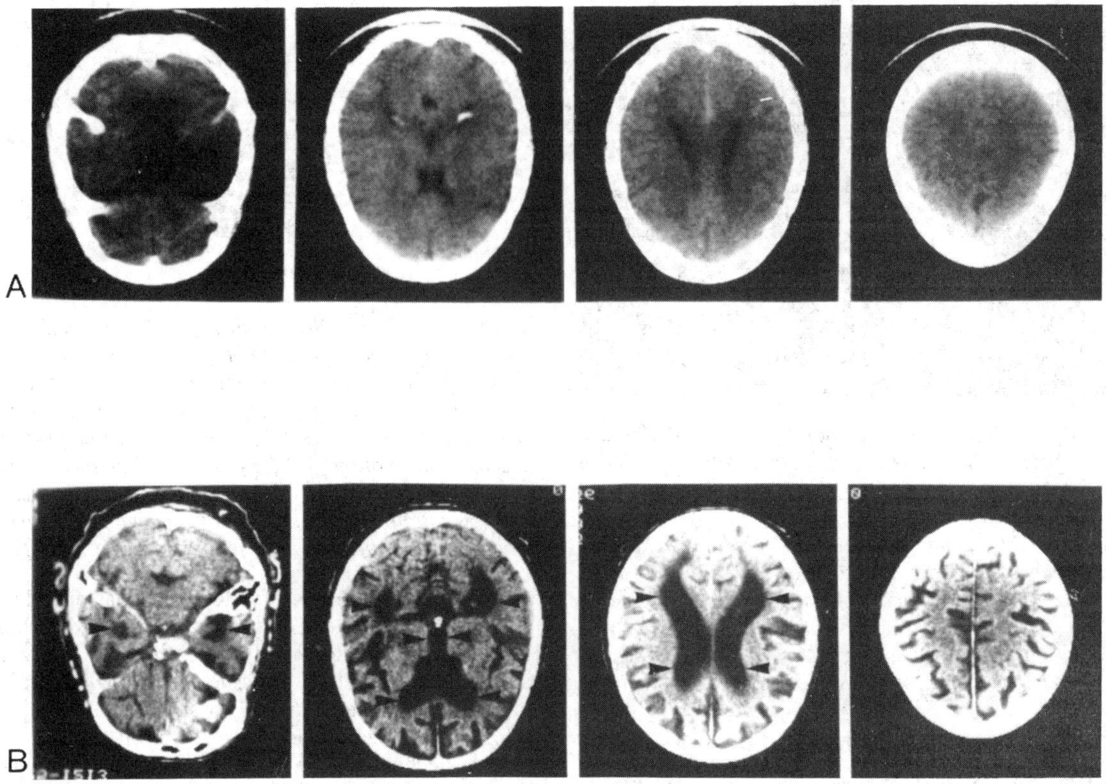

FIGURE 1.10-5. A. *CT scans of the brain from a 36-year-old healthy man.* B. *The corresponding investigation of the brain from a man of similar age who has abused alcohol for many years. From left to right the four images represent slices about 1 cm thick from the base to the vertex. The dark structures marked with arrows constitute the ventricular system, which has been widened as a result of the alcohol abuse. The other dark structures represent widened sulci between the gyri. These appear most distinct in the picture to the right. The widening of the sulci is a typical sign of age, but in this case, it has been markedly accelerated by the alcohol abuse. (The images were produced by Tomas Hindmarsh, Department of Neuroradiology, Karolinska Hospital.)*

Compared to the physical principles of other imaging techniques mentioned in this section, the principles of MRI are more complex. Some atomic nuclei have an impulse momentum such that the charges within the nucleus can be regarded as rotating around an axis; that is, the nucleus is said to have spin. When placed in a powerful magnetic field, nuclei show a *precessional* motion about the field direction. The precessional frequency will increase as the field strength increases. Precession is similar to the wobbling of a spinning top that has been displaced from the vertical. The axis of rotation describes a cone around the vertical axis, which is also the direction of the force of gravity (Fig. 1.10-7). The precessional frequency of the top is lower than the spin frequency. Accurate measurements of the angular momentum of various nuclei can be made by placing the nucleus in a magnetic field and increasing the field strength until the precession is in resonance with an additional oscillating magnetic field.

The magnetic moment of the proton is about 660 times as small as that of the electron. Bloch and Purcell and their colleagues were the first to recognize that under certain circumstances nuclei precessing in the radio-frequency range can give off a radio-frequency signal that could be detected by a radio-receiver. They also showed that certain atomic nuclei with an odd number of protons or neutrons, or both, tended to align themselves with a powerful magnetic field. If, for any reason, these atoms were displaced from the direction of the primary magnetic field, they tended to precess about the direction of the magnetic field at a specific and resonant frequency, known as the Larmor frequency. By having a magnetic field of the appropriate strength, the precession frequency is in the radio-frequency range for MR studies. Bloch and Purcell showed that a radio-frequency stimulus applied to the atoms at the right angle to the magnetic field caused the nuclei to precess at a wider and wider angle from the magnetic field. When the radio-frequency stimulus was discontinued, the precessing nuclei emitted a brief radio-frequency (i.e., MR) signal at the same frequency as the precession frequency (Fig. 1.10-8). This radio-frequency signal could be detected by using an appropriate antenna and radio receiver. Bloch and Purcell shared the Nobel prize in physics in 1952 for their discovery of the MR phenomenon.

Initial interest in the MR phenomenon centered on the discovery of *chemical shift,* a small but specific change of the resonant frequency of particular nuclei of different chemical compounds. In 1973, Lauterbur demonstrated that by using the principles from reconstruction of CT images, it was also possible to reconstruct images of MR signals measured in linear magnetic radiant fields in different directions. This is the basis for the reconstruction of two-dimensional MR images in different planes through the brain. The MRI method has subsequently developed very rapidly. The resolution has been improved and is now comparable or superior to that of CT. As in CT, the MR image is made of picture elements (pixels) generated by a computer. In CT, the numerical value of each pixel represents X-ray attenuation by a given volume element (voxel) of the tissue; in MRI, the numerical value of each pixel reflects the intensity of the MR signal coming from the voxel of tissue. The MR signal emitted by the tissue is the result of the resonance phenomenon rather than representing attenuation as with X-rays or reflection as with ultrasound of an external beam. Newer methods for reconstruction of images have also been developed. Currently, two-dimensional Fourier transformation reconstruction is used in which the Y-coordinate is phase-coded and the X-coordinate is frequency-coded.

An MR system consists of the following components: (1) a main magnet; (2) gradient coils; (3) a radio-frequency emitter and receiver; (4) a computer; and (5) a patient data retrieval system. The key to a good MR magnet is its homogeneity. Three types of magnets are used in medical MR systems—permanent magnets, resistive magnets, and superconducting magnets. There are different opinions

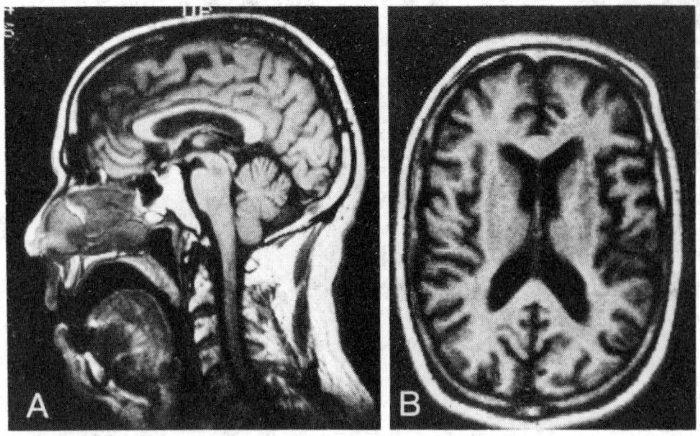

FIGURE 1.10-6. *Sagittal* (A) *and horizontal* (B) *MRI scans through the head of the same 33-year-old healthy man as in Figure 1.10-4. Both scans were obtained using inversion recovery* (IR), *which is* T_1*-dependent. Note the high contrast in the images. Sulci and gyri are well distinguished. The margin between gray and white cortical matter can also be determined. The sagittal section* (A) *also gives excellent images of the corpus callosum, the pituitary gland, and the cerebellum. (The images were produced by Tomas Hindmarch, Department of Neuroradiology, Karolinska Hospital.)*

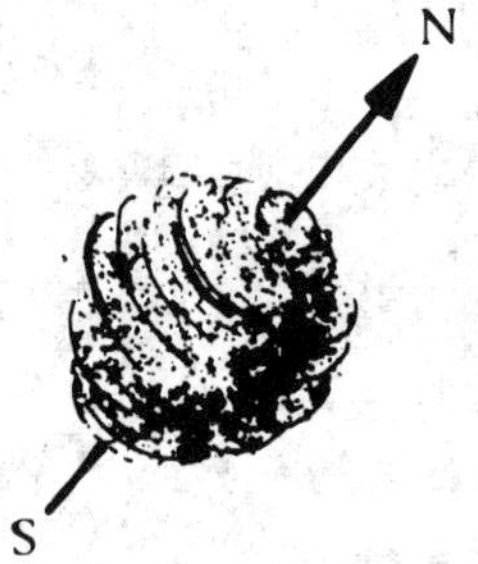

FIGURE 1.10-7. *Hydrogen nucleus. The nucleus of the most abundant isotope of hydrogen consists of a single, spinning proton. It possesses a magnetic moment and, therefore, behaves like a small bar magnet with north and south poles. When placed in a powerful magnetic field, the proton shows a precessional motion. Precession is similar to the wobbling of a spinning top that has been displaced from the vertical. The axis of rotation describes a cone around the vertical axis, which is also the direction of the force of gravity.*

regarding which field strength gives the best images from a diagnostic standpoint. It seems clear, however, that superconducting magnets up to 1.5 teslas give the sharpest images with the shortest time of measurement. The purpose of the gradient coils is to generate magnetic field gradients in three dimensions. The gradient coils are placed between the patient and the main magnet. There is great demand on the current generators for these coils as currents of the order of 20 amperes and potentials of 80 volts with very rapid (less than 1 msec) alternations of current direction are required. The coils are also subjected to mechanical strains—for example, it is the bumping of the gradient coils one can hear when an MR machine is used. The transmitter and the receiver coils can either be combined in one coil or divided so that the radio-frequency signal is emitted in a body coil and the signal is detected in a smaller head or surface coil. In order to handle the great amount of data, 32-byte minicomputers are commonly used. In order to perform the fast Fourier transformations for the image reconstruction, an array processor specially designed for rapid operations is used. The patient data retrieval system for an MR machine is similar to that of a CT scanner. There are one or more image screens on which the images can be studied and evaluated. There is also a multiformat camera for the transfer of the image to film and a magnetic tape station or disk memory for storage of images.

There are currently no specific rules as to how resolution, contrast, and noise should be measured in MRI. The development of MRI is currently at the same stage as when CT and γ-cameras were first used in the early 1970s. The major advantages of MRI as compared with CT are the avoidance of ionizing radiation and the fact that the imaging can be made just as well in transverse, sagittal, and coronal sections. In order to take an MRI image, a variety of different current frequencies (i.e., time and amplitude variation) are used to form the radio-frequency signal and the gradient magnetic fields. Currently, the most commonly used sequences are the following: (1) inversion recovery (IR), which is T_1-dependent (Fig. 1.10-8); (2) spin echo (SE), which is T_1- and T_2-dependent (Fig. 1.10-8); and (3) saturation recovery (SR), which is dependent on the proton density. An IR sequence gives information about contrast between tissues with different T_1 values. An SE sequence gives contrast between tissues with different T_1 and T_2 values. An SR sequence gives the density of protons in the tissue. T_1 and T_2 are *relaxation constants;* T_1 is spin-lattice relaxation and T_2 is spin-spin relaxation (Fig. 1.10-8).

This background information should indicate that MR imaging is a more dynamic procedure than CT scanning. Thus, the MR signal not only will give anatomical information but also will supply indications of local alterations in the chemical environment of protons in the brain. However, the chemical character of such alterations cannot ordinarily be determined by this technique.

The spatial resolution of MR images has already exceeded those from the best CT scanners. Thus, MRI has rapidly become an alternative to the conventional X-ray technique and to CT for the study of tissue morphology. If MRI medical imaging techniques continue to show no harmful biological effects, MRI may replace CT, the current flagship of modern medical technology. It is also likely that developments with regard to both modalities are likely to make CT and MRI useful as complementary methods for the determination of pathological tissue alterations. The attenuation coefficients given by CT when combined with measurements of proton density and relaxation numbers from MRI may add significantly to the information obtained with only one of the methods.

Magnetic resonance imaging in psychiatry The fact that the MRI signals are considerably affected by the chemical environment of the brain protons makes it possible to use the MRI technique for visualizing a number of cerebral disorders affecting the chemical composition of the brain. Because of the relatively low sensitivity of the method, only crude alterations of brain chemistry can be recorded by this technique so far. Therefore, the current use of MRI in psychiatry is related to its ability to give a detailed imaging of most anatomic aspects of the human central nervous system. Also, the diagnosis of tumors and degenerative conditions may turn out to be a useful application of this methodology in neuropsychiatry. As shown in Figures 1.10-4 and 1.10-6, a detailed imaging of the gyri and sulci of the cerebrum as well as an outline of the ventricular system, the brain stem, and the cerebellum can be obtained with modern MRI. It is also evident from Figure 1.10-4*A* that, as compared with the CT image of Figure 1.10-4*B*, the MR image gives more contrast, including the differentiation between gray and white brain matter. The skull X-ray of Figure 1.10-1 and the anatomical brain images of Figures 1.10-4 and 1.10-6 were all obtained from the same healthy human subject, and should give the reader a realistic view of the considerable progress that CT and MRI represent to the clinical neurosciences.

The MRI technique has been used to image brain morphology in patients with schizophrenia, primary degenerative dementia of the Alzheimer type, and chronic alcoholism. In principle, the alterations of brain morphology previously demonstrated by CT have been verified using MRI. Recently, this technique has also showed its uniqueness in demonstrating human immunodeficiency virus (HIV)-induced brain alterations in the early stages of this infection.

Since the MRI technique allows the imaging of structures down to the resolution level of about 1 mm from any angle, this method can be expected to generate considerable new information with regard to the detailed localization of many types of altered brain morphology occurring in neuropsychiatric disorders. It can be expected that the scientific establishment of such morphological alterations by MRI

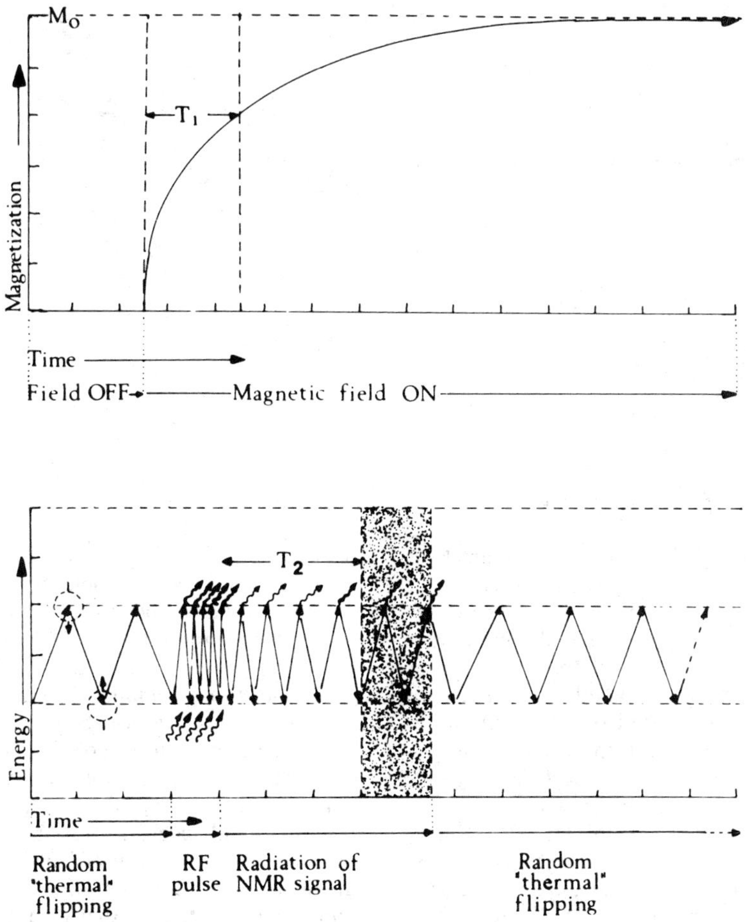

FIGURE 1.10-8. *Relationship between magnetization and proton energy in relation to radio-frequency pulse and the relaxation times* T_1 *and* T_2.

may also be useful as a new diagnostic dimension for the medical discipline of psychiatry. However, as with CT, standardization of routines for measurements, and studies in control populations have to be performed with MRI before the potential of this technique for diagnostic purposes in psychiatry can be fully evaluated.

IMAGING OF BRAIN FUNCTION

Embedded in the bone of the skull, the brain is one of the most encapsulated and protected organs of the body. In order to measure brain function in the living human subject, physical methods have to be used that can bring information about the inside of the head to the outside where external detecting devices can be localized. Electromagnetic waves (i.e., X-rays) and radio-frequency signals have the ability to penetrate bone tissue. Accordingly, these principles have been used in CT and MRI techniques in which a signal from the outside is transformed by the interior of the head into an outgoing signal that can be used for information retrieval by detector devices located outside the head.

Another possibility for obtaining information about events within the living brain is by introducing into the brain specific compounds labeled with radioactive isotopes emitting signals that can be recorded by detectors placed outside the head. By selecting such a compound that also participates in brain functions without fundamentally disturbing them, kinetic information about the fate of the compound may be used as an index of these functions in regions of the brain. For neuropsychiatrists, such a methodology may give more useful information than the previously mentioned anatomical imaging techniques since it will reflect biochemical and physiological events in the central nervous system. Several naturally occurring compounds have γ-ray-emitting isotopes. Gamma radiation easily penetrates the skull and brain tissue. If compounds participating in brain metabolism are labeled with γ-ray-emitting isotopes and introduced into the body, their localization within the tissues can be determined by an external detector system. When γ-rays hit certain crystals, they emit photons or light signals that can be recorded by a photomultiplier. By having a system of such scintillation detectors positioned around the head and by magnifying and feeding the information back into a computer system, images of the localization of the γ-ray-emitting isotope within sections of the brain can be recorded. This technique is called emission tomography (Fig. 1.10-9). Currently, two types of emission tomography are used for recording functional events in the central nervous system—single photon emission computed tomography (SPECT) and positron emission tomography (PET).

SINGLE PHOTON EMISSION COMPUTED TOMOGRAPHY In 1945, Kety and Schmidt opened up the field of functional studies of the human brain based on measurements

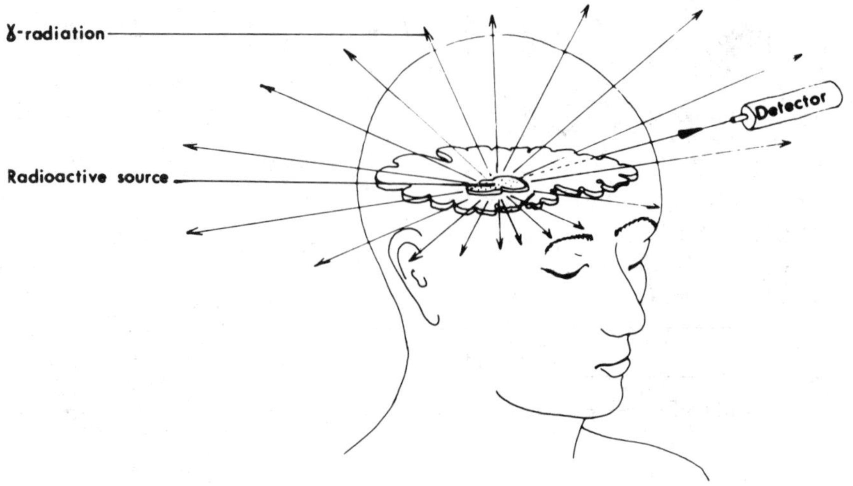

FIGURE 1.10-9. *Principles of emission tomography.*

of the cerebral blood flow (CBF). They recorded the uptake in brain tissue of an inert gas (nitrous oxide) and measured the arteriovenous differences of oxygen and glucose. These procedures allowed the first measurements of blood flow, oxygen consumption, and glucose metabolism in the living human brain. A few years later, Kety and Schmidt laid the general theoretical foundations for studies of blood flow with diffusible gases. They introduced what was then the only method—besides recording of the cerebral electrical activity—for measuring the cerebral functions more directly.

Normally, there is a tight coupling between CBF, glucose metabolism, and neuronal activity of the brain. Thus, CBF measurements could be used in normal and anoxic tissue as an indicator of cerebral metabolism and nerve cell function. In 1961, Lassen and Ingvar introduced regional cerebral blood flow (rCBF) measurements with intraarterial administration of isotopes of an inert radioactive gas, such as krypton (^{85}Kr) or xenon (^{133}Xe). They used the extracranial recording of γ-ray activity by scintillation detectors and measured the clearance of isotopes from regions of the brain. This marked another important step toward the study of regional brain function. Such measurements allowed Ingvar and his collaborators to describe a hypofrontal rCBF distribution pattern in chronic schizophrenic patients.

The introduction of SPECT in ^{133}Xe rCBF measurements by Stokeley and colleagues in 1980 enabled three-dimensional studies to be made of CBF. The SPECT technique has also been used to image dynamic functions of the cerebrospinal fluid (CSF) circulation. Using diethyltriaminepenta-acetic acid (DTPA) labeled with the γ-ray-emitting isotope of technetium (^{99}Tc), the kinetics of distribution of the compound after its intrathecal administration have been evaluated. This technique has also been used to study dynamic aspects of CSF circulation in patients with low-pressure hydrocephalus and schizophrenia. In one study, this technique was used to demonstrate that more than 30 percent of patients with chronic schizophrenia have evidence of altered CSF circulation.

POSITRON EMISSION TOMOGRAPHY The random occurrence of gamma radiation in nature creates a relatively high noise level for the detectors used in SPECT. The use of artificially produced positron emitting isotopes in PET gives an excellent opportunity to reduce random noise markedly. Positron-emitting isotopes can be produced by bombardment of natural elements with protons in a cyclotron. Positron-emitting isotopes are unstable. When disintegrating, they emit positrons—that is, positively charged electron-like particles (antimatter) (Fig. 1.10-10). The positron passes through the tissue until it encounters an electron. When these particles collide, they are annihilated, and simultaneously two γ-rays are emitted. The two γ-rays go in directions opposite to each other, and, thus, it is possible to detect them by placing coincidence-coupled scintillation detectors at 180° from each other in pairs in a ring. By this procedure, only signals arising from the simultaneous activation of the two opposite scintillation detectors can be used for image reconstruction of the distribution of radioactivity in the brain. A positron emission tomograph can be constructed following a design that is basically similar to that of the CT scanners. As in CT, image reconstruction is based on the use of grids in which each pixel element represents the radioactivity in a certain volume of tissue. An outline of the procedure is presented in Figure 1.10-10.

Positron-emitting isotopes of several of the so-called bioisotopes can be produced artificially in a cyclotron. Thus, positron-emitting isotopes of carbon, oxygen, nitrogen, and fluorine can be produced (Table 1.10-2). If the natural atoms of an organic compound are replaced by one or several corresponding positron-emitting isotopes, radioactive molecules are obtained, which can be used as tools for analysis of the participation of the molecule in a specific metabolic reaction. Thus, when such a compound is introduced intravenously, its fate in the living organism can be followed by PET. The PET technique was first applied in biochemical studies for the measurement of glucose consumption in the human brain by Reivich, Sokoloff, and their collaborators, who used glucose analogues labeled by positron-emitting isotopes of fluorine (^{18}F) or carbon (^{11}C). Thus, if, for example, ^{11}C-labeled glucose is introduced intravenously into a living human subject, the radioactive compound is taken up and distributed within the body, including the brain, in proportion to the flow of natural glucose molecules. Since the glucose molecule can be labeled to a very high specific activity (ratio of labeled molecules to unlabeled molecules), a large amount of signal-producing ^{11}C isotope may be present even though the total amount of glucose molecules in the tissue is not substantially altered; that is, tracer doses of the glucose marker can be used. By introducing the radioactivity measurements as they vary with time in regions of the brain and plasma into a

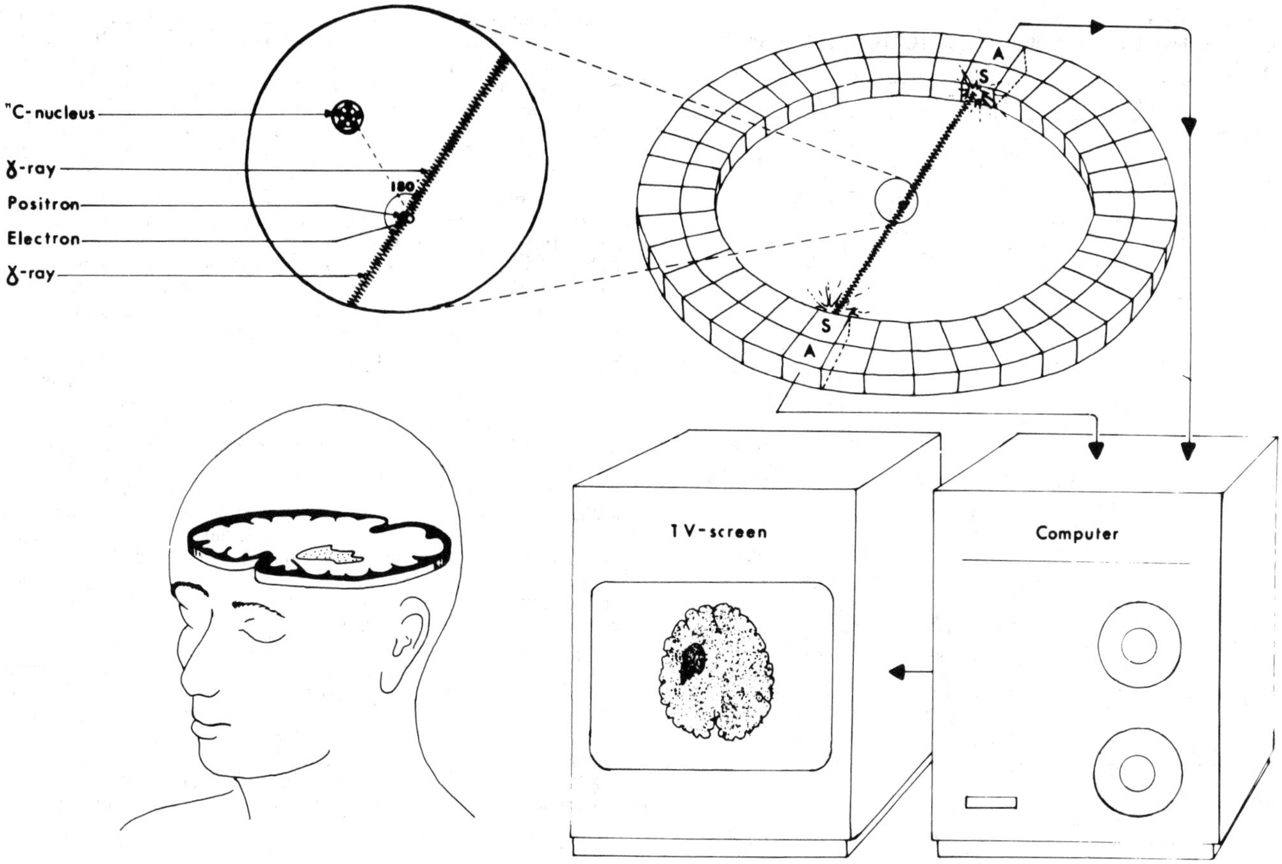

FIGURE 1.10-10. *Procedure for localization of a positron-emitting isotope (^{11}C nucleus) by the technique of PET. The γ-ray irradiation produced by the annihilation of the positron with an electron is recorded by a ring of coincidence-coupled scintillation detectors. The information from pairs of scintillation detectors is fed into a computer. Abbreviations: scintillation detector* (S); *amplifier* (A).

system of equations describing the fate of glucose molecules within plasma and brain compartments, quantitative data for glucose metabolism within small regions can be obtained after correction for the continuous formation of radioactive metabolites. A major advantage of the PET technique is that most of the positron-emitting isotopes are short-lived, with half-lives ranging from minutes to a few hours (Table 1.10-2). The short half-life will result in a relatively short-term exposure of patients to the ionizing radiation. Suitable tracer molecules for the determination of regional blood flow, blood volume, glucose metabolism, oxygen consumption, and protein metabolism have been developed. Some of these methodologies have been developed into quantitative procedures by Phelps and Mazziotta, among others.

Determination of neuroreceptor characteristics One of the more interesting possibilities of PET scanning is represented by the recent demonstration that neuroreceptor characteristics of the brain

TABLE 1.10-2
Positron-Emitting Isotopes Useful for Clinical PET Scan Studies

Element	*Isotope*	*Half-Life (minutes)*
Oxygen	^{15}O	2.1
Carbon	^{11}C	20.1
Nitrogen	^{13}N	10.0
Fluorine	^{18}F	110.0

can be studied in living human subjects by this technique. Brain function is currently believed to be based on the graded release of transmitter molecules interacting with specific receptor structures on nerve cells. Therefore, the possibility of recording transmitter events in the brain of living subjects should be of utmost interest to the clinical psychiatrist. This view is further emphasized by the well-known fact that most, if not all, of the currently clinically used psychoactive agents produce their effects by interacting with specific neurotransmitter receptors within the brain. Based on such evidence, a plethora of hypotheses have been proposed with regard to the possible role of disturbed neurotransmitter receptor functions of the brain in the pathophysiologies of various neuropsychiatric disorders. The neurotransmitters and some drugs interacting with their receptors have strong affinities for the receptors. This means that these compounds bind with weak, but significant, noncovalent binding forces to the receptors. The term *ligand* is often used for such compounds that bind to receptors. The availability of such ligands allows the possibility of using PET for analyzing the distribution and some characteristics of the neuroreceptors in living subjects by studying the biological fate of such ligands labeled with positron-emitting isotopes. This is the principle behind the first successful attempts by Wagner and his collaborators to demonstrate radioligand binding to neuroreceptors by the technique of PET in living human subjects. By the use of various mathematical models, it has been possible to obtain quantitative data for some neuroreceptor systems in the brain of living human subjects. This area is developing rapidly. Table 1.10-3 gives a list of ligands developed for imaging neuroreceptors in the human brain.

Figure 1.10-11 shows an outline of the principles for imaging neuroreceptors in the brain by PET. Briefly, the procedure involves the following steps. A precursor of the appropriate ligand is labeled with a positron-emitting isotope produced in an on-site cyclotron. A well-shielded radiochemistry laboratory is required for this purpose.

TABLE 1.10-3
Ligands Used for Visualization of Neuroreceptors by PET in Humans

Neurotransmitter	*Receptor*	*Ligand*
Dopamine	D_1	^{11}C-SCH 23390
	D_2	^{11}C-raclopride
		^{11}C-piquindone
		^{11}C-*N*-methylspiperone
		^{76}Br-spiperone
		^{77}Br-spiperone (SPECT)
		^{18}F-methylspiperone
		^{18}F-ethylspiperone
Serotonin	5-HT_2	^{11}C-*N*-methylspiperone
		^{76}Br-spiperone
		^{77}Br-spiperone (SPECT)
		^{18}F-methylspiperone
		^{18}F-ethylspiperone
GABA	$GABA_A$	
	$GABA_B$	
	BZ	^{11}C-Ro15-1788
		^{11}C-suriclone
Opiates	Opiate μ	^{11}C-carfentanil
		^{11}C-etorphine
Acetylcholine	Muscarinic	^{11}C-MQNB
		^{11}C-dexetimide
	Nicotinic	^{11}C-nicotine

After the chemical purification of the radioligand, a sterile injection solution is prepared and administered intravenously to a human subject placed in the positron camera. Most neuroreceptor ligands currently used are labeled by a rapid methylation of the desmethyl precursor using ^{11}C-methyliodide as an efficient reagent. The positron camera (Fig. 1.10-12) contains one or more rings of detectors. The information from these detectors allows the reconstruction of images of the radioactivity distribution within one or several sections through the brain of the subjects. With the four-ring camera depicted in Figure 1.10-12, images of four direct and three cross-planes can be reconstructed from the impulses generated in 384 scintillation detectors. These planes have a thickness of about 11 mm; the resolution within the planes is about 7 mm. Figure 1.10-13 shows images of the distribution of radioactivity in seven sections through the brain of a healthy subject after intravenous administration of the D_2 dopamine receptor ligand ^{11}C-raclopride. By this technique, it has been possible to study the distribution and binding characteristics of D_1 dopamine, D_2 dopamine, S_2 serotonin, and benzodiazepine receptors in the brain of living human subjects (Fig. 1.10-14). This technique has also been used in order to examine the possible alteration of D_2 dopamine receptor characteristics in the basal ganglia of schizophrenic patients. Using ^{11}C-labeled *N*-methylspiperone, Wong and colleagues reported a marked increase of D_2 dopamine receptors in the basal ganglia of drug-naive patients with schizophrenia. Although this finding could not be confirmed by Farde and co-workers, who used ^{11}C-raclopride as the ligand, this type of PET approach will, in all probability, soon answer several questions regarding the role of altered dopamine receptor functions in schizophrenia.

Several of the ligands binding to neuroreceptors in the brain are also useful for studying how psychoactive agents interfere with neuroreceptors in the brain of living patients. Figure 1.10-15 shows how clinical doses of chemically different types of antipsychotic drugs markedly interfere with the binding of the D_2 dopamine antagonist ^{11}C-raclopride in the basal ganglia of the brain. This technique can also be used to determine quantitatively the degree of dopamine receptor occupancy in relation to clinical antipsychotic

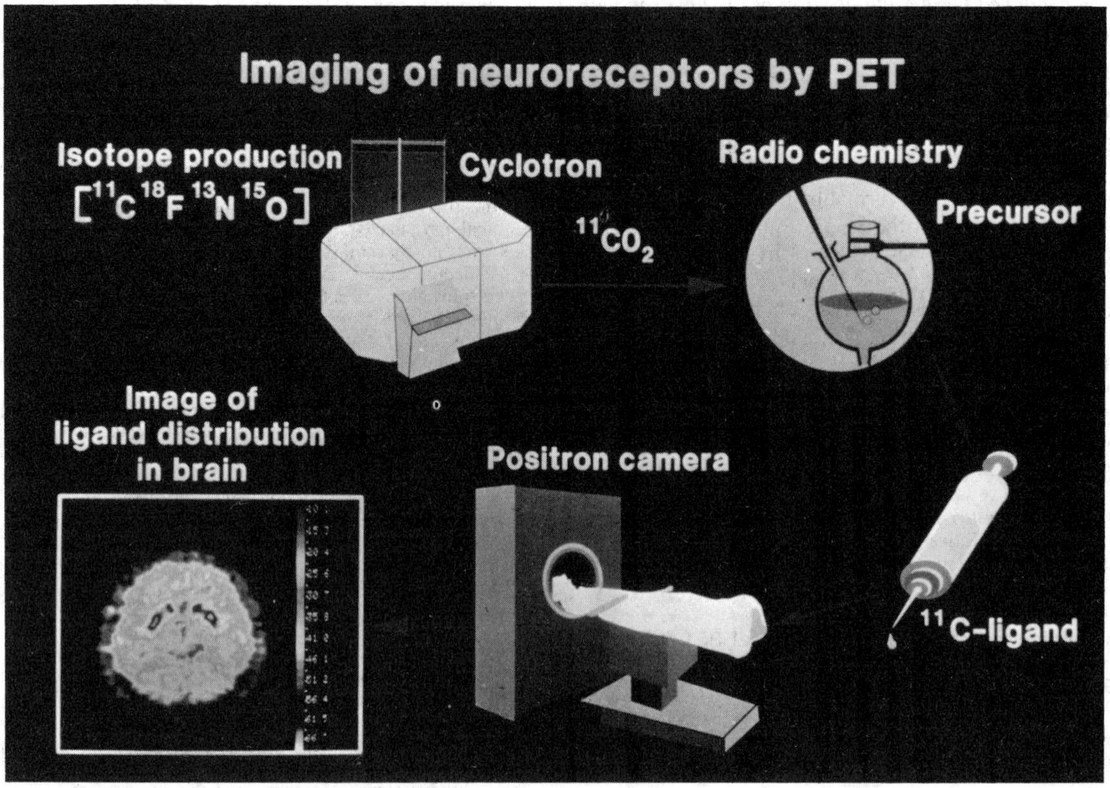

FIGURE 1.10-11. *Techniques for imaging of neuroreceptors in the brain by PET.*

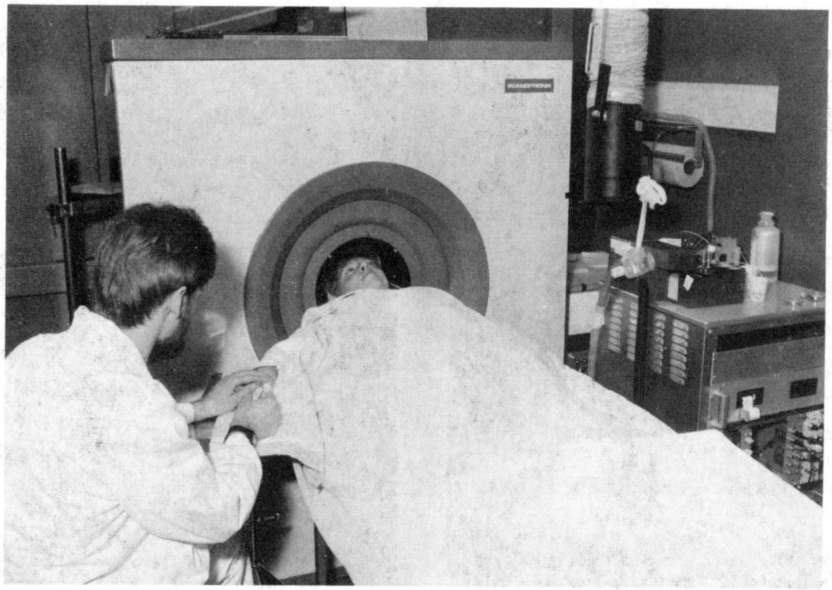

FIGURE 1.10-12. *Positron camera designed for brain studies (Scanditronix PC 384). This camera contains 384 scintillation detectors placed in four rings around the head. The data retrieval system consists of a VAX 750 computer.*

drug treatment. Farde and colleagues recently demonstrated that all the major classes of chemically different antipsychotic drugs produce 65 to 90 percent blockade of central D_2 dopamine receptors when given in clinical doses (Table 1.10-4). This effect was specific for the antipsychotic drugs since it was not induced by clinical treatment with the antidepressant drug nortriptyline (Pamelor). This technique accordingly gives a potential method for a further analysis of the relationships between D_2 dopamine receptor blockade antipsychotic effects and extrapyramidal side effects in antipsychotic-treated patients with schizophrenia.

Lately, it has also been possible to use the PET technique for demonstrating receptor occupancy during clinical benzodiazepine treatment (Fig. 1.10-16). It can be expected that this principle for studying neuroreceptors in living human subjects will be one of the major clinical applications of brain imaging in clinical psychiatry.

MAGNETIC RESONANCE SPECTROSCOPY As mentioned in the previous discussion of the principles of MR, several nuclei of natural atoms have resonance signals that are dependent on the chemical environment of the nucleus. Thus, chemical reactions affect the radio-frequency spectrum of the resonance signal. Accordingly, magnetic resonance spectroscopy (MRS) may prove to be valuable for the evaluation of some aspects of cerebral metabolism. MR spectra of phosphorus can already be obtained in vivo using a relatively high magnetic field strength. These spectra show distinct peaks for the phosphorus atoms of adenosine triphosphate (ATP), creatinine phosphate, sugar phosphate, and the inorganic phosphorus compounds. Animal studies have shown that increasing cerebral hypoxia results in a decrease in ATP, and a complete obstruction of blood flow leads to a loss of the ATP peaks. In addition, the shift in organic phosphate peaks can be used to indicate tissue pH. These facts make possible the quantification of some metabolic changes in the living brain by MRS. To achieve the goal of evaluating cerebral metabolism by measuring the relative amounts of ATP and creatinine phosphate, one may have to be satisfied with resolutions of relatively large volumes. There could also be health hazards from the powerful magnetic fields required for tissue energy state measurements. Further prospective studies of the health effects of these fields need to be performed.

TABLE 1.10-4
Dopamine D_2 Receptor Occupancy in Patients Treated with Psychoactive Drugs*

	Dose (mg)	*Receptor Occupancy (percent)*
Phenothiazines		
Chlorpromazine	100 b.i.d.	80
Thioridazine	100 t.i.d.	75
Trifluoperazine	5 b.i.d.	80
Perphenazine	4 b.i.d.	79
Thioxanthenes		
Flupenthixol	5 b.i.d.	74
Butyrophenones		
Haloperidol	4 b.i.d.	84
Melperone	100 t.i.d.	70
Diphenylbutyls		
Pimozide	4 b.i.d.	77
Dibenzodiazepines		
Clozapine	300 b.i.d.	65
Substituted benzamides		
Sulpiride	400 b.i.d.	82
Sulpiride	400 b.i.d.	73
Sulpiride	400 b.i.d.	68
Raclopride	4 b.i.d.	72
Raclopride	3 b.i.d.	65
Tricyclic antidepressants		
Nortriptyline	25 b.i.d.	-3

*Receptor occupancy is defined as the percent reduction of specific ^{11}C-raclopride binding in relation to the expected binding in the absence of drug treatment.

FUTURE DEVELOPMENTS IN BRAIN IMAGING

It seems likely that the further elaboration of CT and MRI techniques will supply anatomical images of brain structure in living human subjects with a resolution of about 1 mm with high contrast. Such a resolution level will be satisfactory for studying macroscopic alterations of the brain in neuropsychiatric disorders. Whether the analysis of brain anatomy will be significant for the improvement of diagnostic procedures or

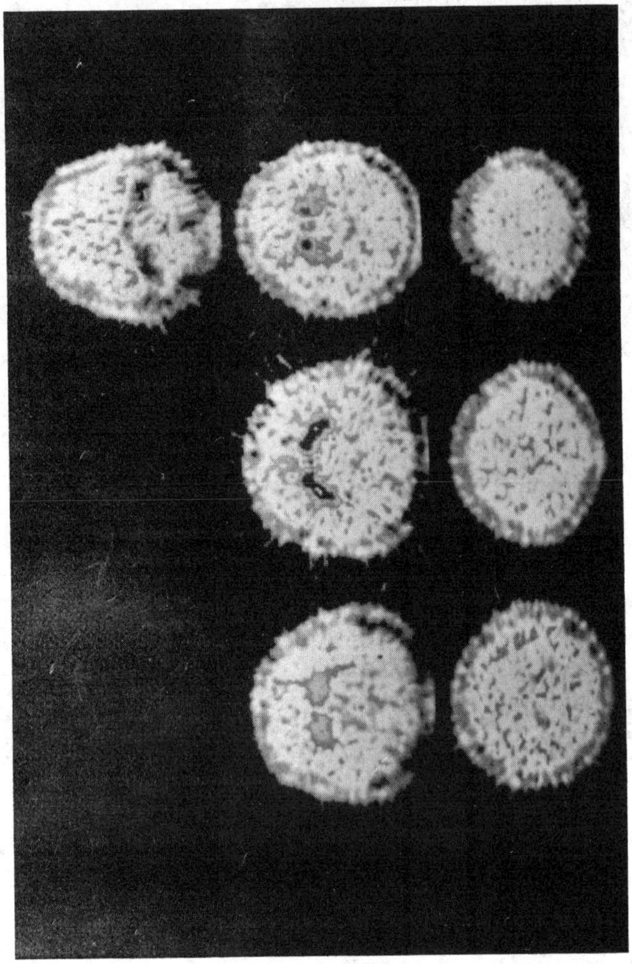

FIGURE 1.10-13. *PET scan images showing the distribution of radioactivity in seven sections through the brain after IV administration of the* D_2 *dopamine receptor ligand* ^{11}C*-raclopride. The images were obtained by accumulating radioactivity during the time period from 10 to 60 minutes after the injection of the tracer. Note the high accumulation of radioactivity in the* D_2 *dopamine receptor-rich basal ganglia, as indicated by black areas in center section of middle row. The section on the upper right is at the base of the skull; the section on the lower right is at the vertex.*

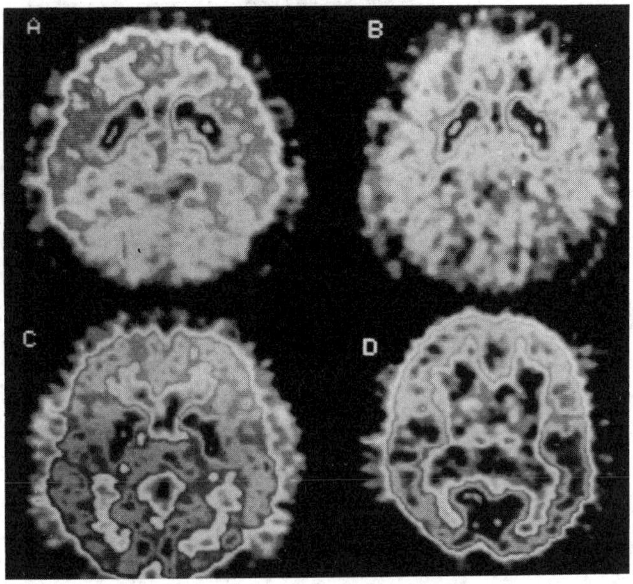

FIGURE 1.10-14. *PET scan images of midbrain sections of healthy volunteers after administration of four different neuroreceptor ligands.* A: ^{11}C *SCH 23390;* B: ^{11}C*-raclopride;* C: ^{11}C*-piquindone;* D: ^{11}C*-Ro 15-1788.* A: *Illustration of high density of* D_1 *dopamine receptors (as indicated by dark areas) in the major basal ganglia. The PET scan image also reflects the low but significant density of* D_1 *and 5-HT-2 receptors in the neocortex. (Gray areas around edge represent frontal and parietal cortex.)* B: *Illustration of the high density of* D_2 *dopamine receptors in the basal ganglia. The figure also illustrates the relative lack of* D_2 *dopamine receptors in all other areas of the brain.* C: *Distribution of* D_2 *dopamine receptors in the basal ganglia. The fairly high degree of accumulation of this ligand in nonstriatal tissues presumably reflects a fairly high nonspecific binding of this ligand.* D: *Illustration of the high density of benzodiazepine receptors in the occipital and parietal cortical areas of the brain. Because this is a black-and-white reproduction of a color image, the ventricular system also appears as black in this figure.*

treatment evaluation in psychiatry seems unlikely. However, anatomical studies of such disorders in large groups of patients may provide clues to the elucidation of the etiologies and pathophysiologies involved.

The development of functional brain images, however, may be more spectacular and of greater interest for clinical psychiatry. If MRI is able to supply us with a three-dimensional analysis of brain energy metabolism, it will intrude, to some extent, on the domain previously thought to be reserved for PET. It is possible that MRI will take over some of the functions of PET which has been used so effectively for the study of several aspects of brain physiology. However, the positron camera appears to have a far greater potential than MRI for the study of physiology because it covers a much wider range of metabolic processes. It permits the study of the kinetics of almost every substance of interest in brain physiology. Methods are already available for regional mapping of oxygen and glucose metabolism, cerebral blood flow, protein synthesis, neuroreceptor characteristics, and psychoactive drug disposition. These investigations can be carried out with extremely small amounts of the tracer, less than one picogram per cubic centimeter of tissue. Since these quantities are several orders of magnitude smaller than those needed for MR isotope studies, physiological or toxic actions of the tracers are unlikely.

The radiation dose given to the patient is the limiting factor in PET investigations. PET competes with the γ-camera and SPECT and has the added advantages of a greater potential for exact activity measurements and higher sensitivity. In recent years, SPECT has attracted considerable interest for three main reasons. It is less expensive to implement than PET; it can profit from the well-developed chemical agents available for the γ-camera; and it does not depend on an expensive cyclotron as does the PET technique. In the area of relative regional blood flow, the SPECT devices might become im-

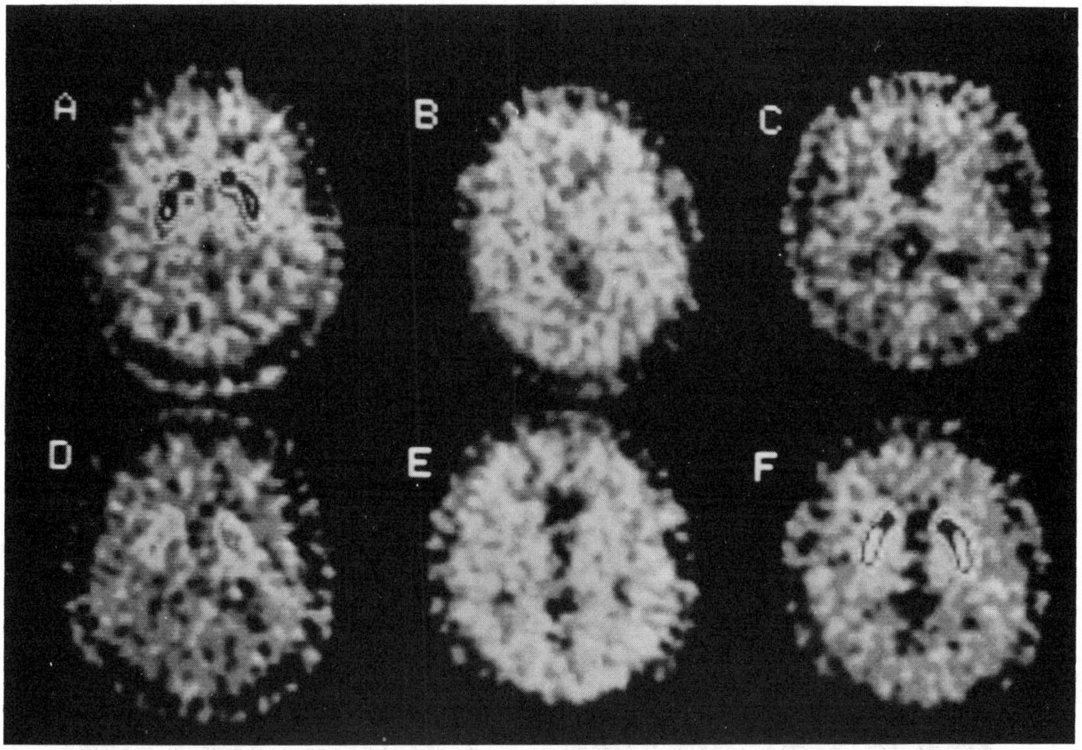

FIGURE 1.10-15 *^{11}C-labeled raclopride (100 mBq to each subject) binding in human brain.* A: *healthy volunteer;* B: *haloperidol (Haldol)-treated (8 mg per day) patient;* C: *fluphenthixol-treated (100 mg per week) patient;* D: *clozapine (Clozaril)-treated (600 mg per day) patient;* E: *sulpiride-treated (1600 mg per day) patient;* F: *same patient 2 weeks after complete withdrawal of drug. Note marked reduction of specific raclopride ^{11}C binding in basal ganglia (dark areas) during, but not after, withdrawal of drug treatment. White indicates the highest level of radioactivity, black the lowest.*

portant tools for routine clinical evaluation in the next few years. However, advances in technology and computer sciences are making positron cameras, as well as cyclotrons, less expensive and easier to handle. Moreover, an abundance of useful tracers labeled with positron-emitting isotopes will be available. PET will therefore also be a method to be considered seriously for routine nuclear medicine. The low resolution is the currently limiting factor in PET. Today, the best camera systems have a resolution of 2 to 4 mm. It can be expected that in a few years commercial instruments with down to 2 mm resolution will be available. With the elaboration of available tracers, it is very likely that within the coming decade several major breakthroughs with regard to imaging of metabolic alterations in neuropsychiatric disorders will show the clinically oriented psychiatrists that the PET technique will join the diagnostic armamentarium of psychiatrists. This methodology will very likely turn out to be highly useful for both diagnostic procedures and treatment evaluation in routine clinical psychiatry.

REFERENCES

Alavi A, Dann R, Chawluk J, Alava J, Kushner M, Reivich M: Positron emission tomography imaging of regional cerebral glucose metabolism. Semin Nucl Med *16:* 2, 1986.

Andreasen N C: Brain imaging: Applications in psychiatry. Science *239:* 1381, 1988.

Bergman H, Borg S, Hindmarsh T, Ideström C-M, Mutzell S: Computed tomography of the brain and neuropsychological assessment of male alcoholic patients. In *Proceedings of the Conference on Addiction Biochemical Aspects of Dependence and Brain Damage,* D Richter, editor, p 201. Oxford University Press, New York, 1979.

Bergstrand G, Larsson S, Bergström M, Eriksson L, Edner G: Cerebrospinal fluid circulation: Evaluation by single-photon and positron emission tomography. Amer J Neuroradiol *4:* 557, 1983.

Bergstrand G, Oxenstierna G, Flyckt L, Larsson S A: Radionuclear cisternography and computed tomography in 30 healthy volunteers. Neuroradiology *28:* 154, 1986.

Block F: Nuclear induction. Phys Rev *70:* 460, 1946.

Bradley W G, Newton T H, Crook L E: Physical principles of nuclear magnetic resonance. In *Modern Neuroradiology: Advanced Imaging Techniques,* T H Newton, D G Potts, editors, vol 2. Clavadel Press, San Anselmo, CA, 1983.

Greitz T: Brain imaging—The past, the present and the future. In *Modern Neurology. Advanced Imaging Techniques,* T H Newton, D G Potts, editors, vol 2, p 1. Clavadel Press, San Anselmo, CA, 1983.

Hounsfield G N: Computerized transverse axial scanning (tomography): Description of system. Brit J Radiol *46:* 1016, 1973.

Ingvar D H, Franzen G: Abnormalities of cerebral blood flow distribution in patients with chronic schizophrenia. Acta Psychiat Scand *50:* 425, 1974.

Johnstone E C, Crow T J, Frith C D, Husband J, Kreel L: Cerebral ventricular size and cognitive impairment of chronic schizophrenia. Lancet *2:* 924, 1976.

Kety S S, Schmidt C F: The determination of cerebral blood flow in man by the use of nitrous oxide in low concentrations. Amer J Physiol *143:* 53, 1945.

Kety S S, Schmidt C F: Effects of altered arterial tensions of carbon dioxide and oxygen on cerebral blood flow and cerebral

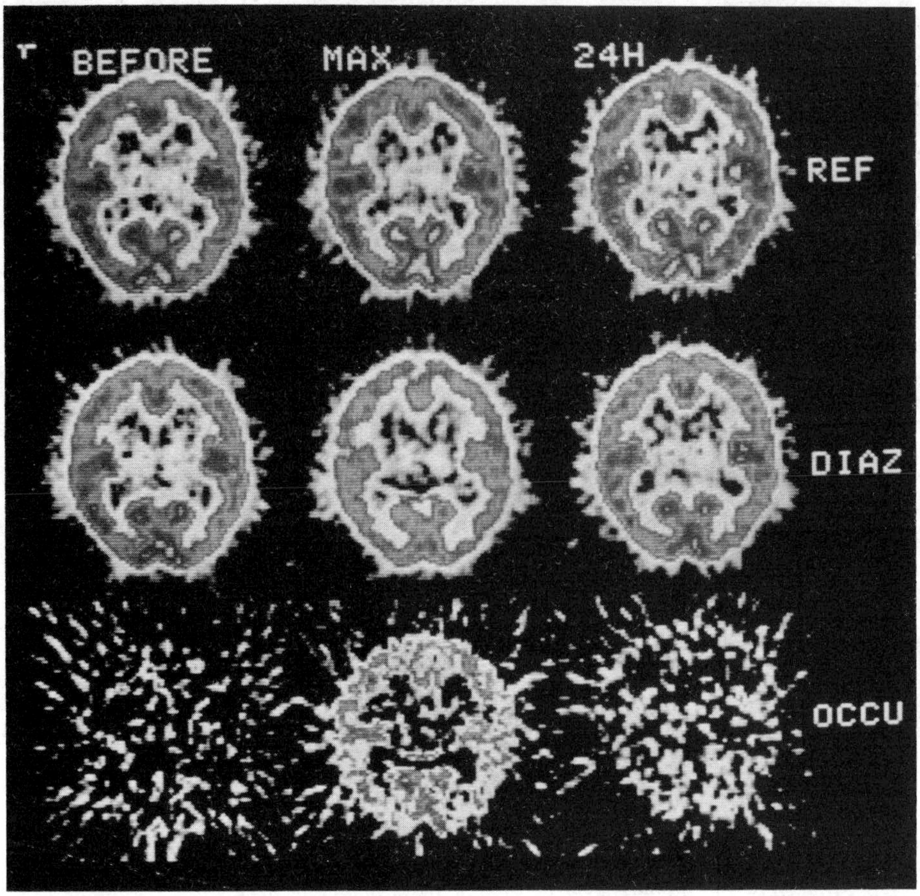

FIGURE 1.10-16. *PET scan images showing the distribution of radioactivity in a section through the brain of a healthy man after repeated IV injections of a tracer dose of the benzodiazepine antagonist ^{11}C-Ro 15-1788. Upper panel shows distribution of radioactivity before, 2 hours after, and 24 hours after administration of a placebo tablet. Middle panel shows distribution of radioactivity before, 2 hours after, and 24 hours after oral administration of 30 mg diazepam (Valium). Lower panel shows benzodiazepine receptor occupancy (radioactivity in middle panel subtracted from radioactivity in upper panel), before, 2 hours after, and 24 hours after oral administration of 30 mg diazepam. The results demonstrate that 2 hours after diazepam administration benzodiazepine, receptors are markedly occupied, and 24 hours after the benzodiazepine administration, only a faint tracer of receptor occupancy remains.*

oxygen consumption of normal young men. J Clin Invest *27:* 484, 1948.

Lassen N A, Ingvar D H: The blood flow of the cerebral cortex determined by radioactive krypton-85. Experientia *17:* 42, 1961.

Lauterbur P C: Image formation by induced local interactions: Examples employing nuclear magnetic resonance. Nature *242:* 190, 1973.

Lauterbur P C: Magnetic resonance zeugmatography. J Pure Appl Chem *40:* 149, 1974.

Leenders K L, Gibbs J M, Frackowiak R S J, Lammertssma A A, Jones T: Positron emission tomography of the brain: New possibilities for the investigation of human cerebral pathophysiology. Progr Neurobiol *23:* 1, 1984.

Oxenstierna G, Bergstrand G, Bjerkenstedt L, Sedvall G, Wik G: Evidence of disturbed CSF circulation and brain atrophy in cases of schizophrenic psychosis. Brit J Psychiat *144:* 654, 1984.

Phelps M E, Mazziotta J C: Positron emission tomography: Human brain function and biochemistry. Science *228:* 799, 1985.

Phelps M E, Mazziotta J C, Huang S-C: Study of cerebral function with positron computed tomography. J Cereb Blood Flow Metab *2:* 113, 1982.

Purcell E M, Torrey H C, Pound R V: Resonance absorption by nuclear magnetic moments in a solid. Phys Rev *69:* 37, 1946.

Raichle M E: Positron emission tomography. Ann Rev Neurosci *6:* 249, 1983.

Revely M A: CT scans in schizophrenia. Brit J Psychiat *146:* 367, 1985.

Sedvall G, Farde L, Persson A, Wiesel F-A: Imaging of neurotransmitter receptors in the living human brain. Arch Gen Psychiat *43:* 995, 1986.

Sokoloff L: Ann Neurol (suppl) *15:* S1, 1984.

Stokeley E M, Sveinsdottir E, Lassen N A, Ronner P: A single photon dynamic computer assisted tomography (DCAT) for imaging brain function in multiple cross sections. J Comput Assist Tomogr *4:* 230, 1980.

1.11 PSYCHONEUROENDOCRINOLOGY

VICTOR I. REUS, M.D.

INTRODUCTION

The term "psychoneuroendocrinology" reflects in its construction an appreciation of inextricable structural and functional relationships between the hormonal system and the central nervous system (CNS) and the behaviors that modulate and are derived from both. In the classical conception, hormones were defined as products of endocrine glands that were transported by blood to exert their action at sites distant from their release. A wealth of new data has dramatically altered this view, resulting in the recognition that the brain, in many ways, acts as an endocrine organ itself and that classical distinctions between the origin, structure, and function of nerve, as opposed to endocrine, cells are not valid. The term "paraneuron" has been utilized to refer to cells that possess neurosecretory or synaptic vesicle-like granules and that release substances traditionally identified as neurotransmitters or neurosecretions in response to relevant stimuli. Thus, substances usually considered hormones may have, in specific cases, modulatory effects on neurotransmission when released into a synapse, travel short distances in extracellular space to exert their actions on adjacent target cells, or be transported via blood to more distant sites.

Several hormonal compounds may interact in an overlapping manner to regulate secretory release. Structurally, hormones have been classified as proteins or polypeptides (e.g., adrenocorticotropic hormone [ACTH], β-endorphin, cholecystokinin [CCK]), as phenol derivatives (e.g., thyroxine, norepinephrine), and as steroids (e.g., cortisol, estrogen, testosterone) (Table 1.11-1). In general, most hormonal compounds appear to exert their effect in a tonic rather than phasic fashion, being diffused in a less precise manner than a neurotransmitter and over a longer time period. Theoretically, such a characterization would allow hormones to be more closely linked to integrated behavioral response. From a phylogenetic perspective, substances that act as hormones in mammals can be seen even in unicellular organisms. Accordingly, as organisms progressed in complexity, most hormones retained an incredible multiplicity and variability of functions, a quality that has been referred to as pleiotropy. A greater understanding of the scope of such effects may help link observations of specific endocrine dysregulation in major psychiatric syndromes to the more general physiological and metabolic alterations that characterize their presentation.

Hormones of widely differing chemical structure appear to exert their actions in a remarkably similar fashion. Contrary to earlier beliefs, primary receptor recognition sites for both peptide and steroid compounds can be found on the outer cell surface. Neurotropic effects may occur in milliseconds to seconds or involve intracellular receptors in a more delayed effector system. Lysosomal activation is integral to the propagation of the signal and to the internalization and migration to the nuclear compartment of the hormone-receptor complex. Within a matter of minutes to hours, genomic activation occurs and alterations in the rate of transcription and translation are evident. The end result is the induction of such gene products as enzymes or other cell proteins that actually effect the metabolic change.

TABLE 1.11-1
Classification of Hormones

Classification	*Examples*
Structures	
Proteins, polypeptides	ACTH, β-endorphin, TRH
Phenol derivatives	Thyroxine
Steroids	Cortisol, estrogen
Functions	
Autocrine	Self-regulatory effects
Paracrine	Local or adjacent cellular action
Endocrine	Distant target site

Interest in the relationship between behavior and neuroendocrine regulation stems from historical appreciation of behavioral changes occurring in the development of primary endocrine disorders and in association with exogenous hormonal treatment, from the development of technical methods sensitive to subtle alteration in endocrine function, and from a hope that such alterations in neuroendocrine function might serve as a window to the brain. The latter concept, that changes in hormonal level could serve as markers of parallel alteration in classical neurotransmitter regulation, has lost favor as the complexity of neuroendocrine systems has been unveiled and as the number of peptide hormones produced in specific anatomic sites in the brain itself has expanded.

Space limitations prohibit a definitive review of all the behavioral effects of hormonal compounds. Since there is heuristic merit to defining hormonal output as an independent rather than a dependent variable in relationship to behavioral pathology, this section is organized from that perspective. In each of the major systems discussed, critical effects on neuronal development and known roles in normal adult behavioral expression are considered initially, followed by a survey of behavioral effects of exogenous hormonal administration and psychiatric disorders associated with a known endocrine disease process. Documented dysregulation of these systems in psychiatric illness and any known effects of psychiatric drugs are also reviewed.

CORTICOTROPIN-RELEASING HORMONE, CORTICOTROPIN, AND CORTISOL

Since the earliest conceptions of the stress response by Selye, Mason, and others, investigation of hypothalamic-pituitary-adrenal cortex (HYPAC) function has occupied the central position in psychoendocrine research. Corticotropin-releasing hormone (CRH), corticotropin, and cortisol are all elevated in response to a variety of physical and psychic stresses and serve as prime factors in the maintenance of homeostasis and the development of adaptive response to a novel or challenging stimulus. Aside from generalized effects on arousal, distinct effects on sensory processing, stimulus habituation and sensitization, pain, sleep, and memory storage and retrieval have been documented. Autoradiographic evidence indicates that the principal neuroanatomical site of action for the central effects of pituitary-adrenal hormones lies within the limbic midbrain circuit and the ascending reticular activating system. The neurochemical mechanisms involved in the mediation of HYPAC effects on mood and mentation are complex, inasmuch as CRH release is regulated by inhibitory noradrenergic as well as stimulatory cholinergic and serotonergic systems, with additional influences by γ-aminobutyric acid (GABA)-ergic, opioid, and other peptide systems.

Observations of mood change in patients with Cushing's syndrome and Addison's disease engendered hypotheses that

HYPAC abnormalities might be involved in the genesis and character of primary mood disorders. These hypotheses were buttressed by the high incidence of induced depression and mania associated with exogenous glucocorticoid treatment. Disturbances of mood are found in more than 50 percent of patients with Cushing's syndrome, with psychosis or suicidal thought apparent in more than 10 percent of the cases studied. Cognitive impairments, principally in visual memory and in higher cortical functions, are common and have been related to the degree of hypercortisolemia present. In general, reductions in cortisol level dramatically result in a normalization of mood and mental status. In Addison's disease, apathy, social withdrawal, impaired sleep, and decreased concentration frequently accompany prominent fatigue. Again, glucocorticoid, but not electrolyte, replacement results in resolution of behavioral symptomatology.

Despite early attempts to utilize ACTH and corticosteroids therapeutically in schizophrenia, the most reproducible HYPAC abnormalities have been found in depression. In addition to a decreased sensitivity to suppression of cortisol by dexamethasone, many depressed patients show an augmented adrenocortical response to ACTH infusion, elevated basal ACTH secretion, and altered circadian rhythms of both ACTH and cortisol. Increased tissue levels of cortisol have been reported in postmortem examination of suicide victims, as have increased cerebrospinal fluid (CSF) levels of CRH, ACTH, and cortisol in hospitalized depressed patients. In some cases, cortisol release during hypoglycemia is attenuated. Parallel aberrant cortisol responses to infusions of clonidine (Catapres), physostigmine (Antilirium, Eserine), and 5-hydroxytryptophan have also been delineated. More recently, several groups have reported a blunted ACTH response to CRH infusion. Thus far, despite the array of reproducible abnormalities in this system in depression, no integrative underlying mechanism has been put forth.

Investigations employing concomitant assessments of neuroendocrine and monoamine neurotransmitter function have variably implicated enhanced central serotonergic, as well as diminished central noradrenergic, system responsiveness. The comparative absence of longitudinal, as opposed to cross-sectional, studies has contributed to a stasis in the understanding of such phenomena and the relative contributions of genetic, developmental, environmental, and psychological factors. The intriguing relationship between chronic stress and depressive disorders suggests that some psychiatric syndromes may not be disease states per se, but rather exist on a continuum with normal functioning. In support of such a conception are a variety of studies implying that although acute release of glucocorticoids may serve homeostatic needs, more prolonged activation can result in structural neuropathology and, speculatively, more lasting behavioral change. Some of the neuropathological sequelae of normal human aging parallel such stress-induced adaptations in the HYPAC system and may either produce or be secondary to changes in neuroendocrine function and stress responsivity.

ENDORPHINS, ENKEPHALINS, AND OTHER ENDOGENOUS OPIOIDS

Since the discovery of endogenous opiate receptors and their endogenous ligands in the early 1970s, research into the possible behavioral roles of such compounds has grown at a rapid pace. Thus far, effects on analgesia are the best documented, but effects on stress, regulation of appetite, learning and memory, motor activity, and immune function have significantly expanded scientific consideration of the functional principles that govern opioid localization and release. The recognition that there are at least three different receptor systems (μ, δ, and κ) may help to clarify which substances and systems are utilized under which physiological conditions.

In humans, several studies have found that levels of plasma β-endorphin can be correlated with measures of stress of surgery and pain. In addition, perceived stress associated with performance of mental arithmetic has been altered by opioid antagonists. Most commonly, opiate agonists have been found to increase—and antagonists to decrease—eating behavior, but attempts to translate such observed effects into clinical protocols investigating treatment in obesity and anorexia have produced mixed results. In one recent study, naloxone (Narcan) significantly reduced food consumption as well as self-ratings of hunger in normal obese individuals. Elevated levels of CSF opioid activity have also been reported in anorexia nervosa, with normalization following weight restoration. Despite some facilitatory effects of opiate antagonists on memory in animal studies, relatively little work has been done thus far in humans. Naloxone improved some measures of cognitive performance in patients with Alzheimer's disease, but was ineffective in depression.

In general, exercise increases release of endogenous opioids; this observation, together with the report that naloxone administered to runners resulted in an increase in pain and a decrease in enjoyment, have led to speculations of a linkage between exercise and mood change. Such conclusions, however, are premature in that additional specific and nonspecific effects on other neurochemical systems cannot be excluded. Initially, both a decrement and an excess in brain opiates were independently hypothesized to be etiologically related to mental illnesses, such as schizophrenia and depressive and anxiety disorders. However, enthusiasm for either of these positions has dwindled in the face of contradictory results. Increases in various endorphin compounds have been reported in plasma as well as in postmortem brain tissue of schizophrenic patients, but studies of acute and chronic opiate antagonist treatment show no consistent or reproducible effects on psychopathology. Similarly, initial reports of therapeutic effects of opiate analogue compounds have not been sustained in follow-up studies. The relationship between endogenous opiate systems and psychopathology is no clearer in studies of mood disorders.

Although some investigators document higher levels of plasma β-endorphin in mood-disorder patients, naloxone treatment has not been shown to result in improvement in mood; indeed, in one study utilizing extremely high doses, naloxone produced a consistent and significant worsening in objective and subjective measures of depression. Similar observations in manic patients suggest that nonspecific effects may be involved. Interpretation of these and other studies using similar methodology is confounded by a lack of understanding as to which opiate actions are due to circulating factors acting in the periphery and which to centrally released substances.

VASOPRESSIN, RENIN, AND ALDOSTERONE

Vasopressin or antidiuretic hormone (ADH) is a posterior pituitary hormone, which maintains plasma osmolarity through regulation of renal water excretion. ADH release is triggered by pain, emotional stress, dehydration, increased plasma osmolarity, or decreases in blood volume. ADH is secreted into the hypophyseal-portal circulation by neurons that originate in the paraventricular nucleus and terminate in the median eminence of the hypothalamus. Although the pathways by which pain, stress, and emotional activation result in ADH release are not well defined, there is evidence that ADH and other hypothalamic hormones, such as oxytocin, may in certain physiological situations act as secretogogues of ACTH and play a key role in the overall hormonal response to stress.

Animal studies using intracerebroventricular injections of extremely low doses of ADH have indicated that the hormone may enhance both consolidation and retrieval of memory, particularly that associated with aversive learning. Clinical studies employing longer-acting synthetic analogue compounds in assessments of attention, concentration, and memory in aged, depressed, or demented populations have resulted in more mixed results. Although positive results exist, the effect is small and has yet to be consistently reproduced.

Profound alterations in fluid ingestion and excretion have been observed in psychiatric patients throughout most of this century. Polydipsia occurs in 10 to 15 percent of hospitalized psychiatric patients and seems unrelated to diagnosis. In many cases, the syndrome is secondary to an inappropriate secretion of ADH. This may occur as a feature of the altered behavioral state itself and resolve with its treatment or, conversely, may be precipitated by a variety of antidepressant or antipsychotic agents.

CSF ADH levels in depressed patients are somewhat lower than in controls, and in bipolar patients are lower in the depressed than in the manic phase. The release of vasopressin in response to infusion of hypertonic saline has also been reported to be attenuated in depression.

The term *neurophysin* refers to a high-molecular-weight carrier protein that binds to vasopressin or oxytocin within neurosecretory granules in the posterior pituitary. In several recent studies, CSF levels of neurophysins related to both vasopressin and oxytocin have been noted as higher in bipolar depressed patients than in other psychiatric subjects; antidepressant treatment has also been associated with abolition of insulin-induced neurophysin release. There are relatively few direct studies of the aldosterone-renin-angiotensin system. In one protocol, manic-depressive patients manifested normal aldosterone levels in the face of high renin excretion.

THYROTROPIN-RELEASING HORMONE, THYROTROPIN, AND THYROID HORMONES

It is now well established that thyroid hormones are essential for the normal development of the CNS and that thyroid deficiency during critical stages of postnatal life will severely impair growth and development of the brain, resulting in behavioral disturbances that may be permanent if replacement therapy is not instituted. In adult life, thyroid hormones are involved in the regulation of nearly every organ system, particularly those integral to the metabolism of food and the regulation of temperature. Knowledge of the neurotransmitter modulation of thyrotropin-releasing hormone (TRH), thyroid-stimulating hormone (TSH), and thyroid release is still quite limited. There is general agreement that central noradrenergic systems are primarily stimulatory to TSH secretion and that central dopamine neurons inhibit TSH release. Thyroid hormones, in turn, are important regulators of central adrenoreceptor function, generally decreasing presynaptic noradrenaline release and increasing postsynaptic β-adrenoreceptor number. Hypothyroidism is associated with opposing effects. These changes parallel the alteration in α- and β-receptor sensitivity associated with pharmacological and electroconvulsive antidepressant treatments and may explain the therapeutic efficacy of supplemental thyroid hormone in treatment-resistant depression. In addition to its prime endocrine function, TRH has direct effects on neuronal excitability, behavior, and neurotransmitter regulation, particularly on central cholinergic systems located in the septo-hippocampal band and on mesolimbic and nigrostriatal dopamine systems. In lower animals, TRH possesses mild stimulant properties. Initial reports of its mood-elevating effects in normal human subjects led to a number of projects investigating its acute and chronic antidepressant effects in clinical populations. Despite some initial enthusiasm, the degree of mood alteration does not seem to be great nor is its occurrence reliable.

Given these observations, it is not surprising that alterations in behavioral function have been observed in patients with primary thyroid gland dysfunction, beginning with the earliest reports in the medical literature. Hyperthyroidism is commonly associated with fatigue, irritability, insomnia, anxiety, restlessness, weight loss, and emotional lability. Marked impairment in concentration and memory may also be evident. Such states can progress into delirium or mania or, alternatively, be episodic in nature. On occasion, a true psychosis develops, with paranoia a particularly common presenting feature. Despite these observations, it should be recognized that no predictable relationship between behavioral symptomatology and laboratory indices of thyroid function exists. In some cases, psychomotor retardation, apathy, and withdrawal rather than agitation and anxiety are the presenting features. Manic symptomatology has also been reported following rapid normalization of thyroid status in hypothyroid individuals and may covary with thyroid level in individuals with episodic endocrine dysfunction. In general, behavioral abnormalities resolve with a normalization of thyroid function and are responsive symptomatically to traditional psychopharmacological regimens. Caution should be exerted, however, regarding antidepressant treatment in hyperthyroid states because of possible synergistic cardiotoxicity. In several case reports, haloperidol (Haldol) has been linked to increasing thyrotoxicity and hyperthyroidism to an enhancement of the neurotoxic effects of antipsychotics.

The psychiatric symptoms of chronic hypothyroidism are generally well recognized. Most classically, fatigue, decreased libido, memory impairment, and irritability are noted, but a true organic psychosis or dementia-like state can also develop. Suicidal ideation is common and the lethality of actual attempts is profound. In milder, subclinical states of hypothyroidism, the absence of gross signs accompanying endocrine dysfunction may result in its being overlooked as a possible etiology of a mental disorder. Accordingly, the evaluation of basal TSH level or the TSH response to TRH infusion is necessary to arrive at the proper diagnosis. Several recent reports indicate an increased risk of rapid mood cycling in the course of treatment with tricyclic antidepressants or lithium in these individuals. In the majority of patients with primary hypothyroidism, an autoimmune etiology is implicated.

In parallel with psychiatric disorders resulting from primary thyroid dysfunction, a variety of disturbances in thyroid regulation have been noted in patient populations defined by classical psychiatric criteria. Most of the observations thus far have derived from investigations of individuals with mood disorders, although abnormalities have also been found in patients with anxiety or eating disorders, schizophrenia, and dementia. Several large-scale studies have shown that anywhere from 10 to 30 percent of patients presenting with acute psychiatric illness exhibit a transient state-dependent hyperthyroxinemia. Longitudinal studies are rare and more confusing. In one study, depressed patients showed increased T_4 levels in the acute phase compared with remission, and in another study, patients entering a depressive recurrence manifested lower free versus bound thyroxine quotients and higher TSH secretion than those who remained euthymic. Other investigators have reported decrements in free T_3 levels, elevation in TSH hormone, elevations in CSF reverse T_3, and a significantly increased prevalence of detectable titers of antithyroid antibodies in depressed patients compared with the normal population.

Perhaps the most widely replicated finding has been that of an alteration in thyrotropin response to TRH. A relative blunting of TSH release in response to TRH is observed in approximately 25 percent of hospitalized depressed patients. A significant augmentation of response can additionally be found in women who present with rapid cycling mood disorder. Initial enthusiasm for the utility of TSH response in the differential diagnosis of psychiatric disorders and as a trait marker for mood disorder have not been supported by recent studies. Blunted TRH test results occur in a significant percentage of patients with eating disorders, alcoholism, and schizophrenia. However, the test possesses some clinical utility in that an unchanged response following clinical recovery is associated with an increased risk of relapse. There is also initial evidence that the identification of an augumented TSH pattern serves as a useful predictor of antidepressant response to supplemental thyroid hormone in individuals with a history of treatment resistance. Although high levels of cortisol may serve to desensitize thyrotropic receptors, most studies that employ both assessments have found little relationship between TSH response to TRH and cortisol response to dexamethasone in individual depressed patients, indicating separate endocrine abnormalities.

The majority of psychoactive medications, with the exception of lithium and carbamazapine (Tegretol), have no clearly demonstrable effect on peripheral thyroid function. Lithium increases antithyroid antibodies, and inhibits iodine uptake into the thyroid, iodination of tyrosine, release of T_3 and T_4 from the thyroid, and peripheral breakdown of thyroid hormones. It also blocks the thyroid-stimulating effects of TSH through interference with adenylate cyclase and may, in certain circumstances, precipitate a rebound thyrotoxicosis. About 30 percent of patients receiving lithium will have an elevated TSH level during treatment, and approximately one-sixth of these will go on to develop frank hypothyroidism. Attention to subtle alteration in thyroid status induced by lithium treatment is important in the clinical evaluation of symptomatic complaints, such as fatigue, memory impairment, and anhedonia. Carbamazapine, an anticonvulsant shown to have antimanic properties akin to lithium, also decreases peripheral thyroid hormone levels while increasing TSH.

PARATHYROID HORMONE

The medical literature surveying behavioral manifestations of altered parathyroid gland function is quite rudimentary, somewhat surprisingly in view of the frequent and often profound neuropsychiatric changes that can result. In one large series, more than 60 percent of patients had mood disturbance, with 10 percent experiencing changes of psychotic proportion. In many cases, patients exhibited subtle personality changes that had developed over a course of years and were characterized by depression, reduced concentration, absence of initiative and spontaneity, fatigue, and, occasionally, irritability and suspiciousness. The majority of reports suggest that the behavioral pathology is more closely related to the degree of hypercalcemia than to the parathyroid hormone level, but patients with high levels of plasma calcium may have no observable behavioral pathology. Similarly, individuals with mild hypercalcemia may present with a profound disturbance. The mechanism by which calcium induces such changes is not understood. Primary hyperparathyroidism most commonly occurs secondary to a single parathyroid adenoma, the removal of which almost invariably results in a lysis of behavioral symptoms, regardless of severity or chronicity.

Lithium treatment can increase parathyroid hormone secretion and raise serum calcium, perhaps more frequently than generally recognized. In cases where such effects are associated with somatic or behavioral change, lithium discontinuation should result in rapid symptomatic improvement. On those occasions when this does not happen, a parathyroid adenoma is sometimes discovered fortuitously. Because there are no longitudinal studies, it is debatable whether this represents a coincidental finding or is secondary to the prolonged stimulatory effects of the drug.

PROLACTIN

Since its identification in 1970, the anterior pituitary hormone prolactin has been examined as a potential index of dopamine activity and receptor sensitivity in studies of CNS function in psychiatric patients, and as a correlate of stress responsivity or antipsychotic drug level. The secretion of prolactin is under direct inhibitory regulation by dopamine neurons located in the tuberoinfundibular section of the hypothalamus. The extent to which dopamine exerts its actions through direct effects on the pituitary as opposed to release of as yet unidentified inhibitory factors is controversial. Prolactin also inhibits its own secretion by means of a "short-loop" feedback circuit to the hypothalamus. In addition, prolactin-releasing factors have been identified. In humans, intravenous L-tryptophan infusion results in a robust increase in prolactin, suggesting an active involvement of serotonin in prolactin secretion. TRH stimulates prolactin secretion at doses comparable to those required to modulate TSH release, whereas endogenous opiates and somatostatin have stimulatory and inhibitory effects, respectively, on prolactin secretion in humans.

In both rats and humans, the lactotrophs of the anterior pituitary have been shown to be stress responsive, increasing release to such stimuli as immobilization, hypoglycemia, surgery, and cold exposure. There is also evidence that prolactin may mediate some of the effects of estrogen on the brain and potentiate such estrogen-dependent behaviors as sexual receptivity. Emotional stressors or psychological factors, such as novelty, result in a rapid twofold to threefold increase in prolactin level, but this habituates with repeated exposure. Studies in psychiatric populations have attempted to use prolactin response to infusions of dopaminergic agonists as an index of central neurotransmitter activity. Thus far, the conclusions to be drawn from this strategy are not clear since widely discrepant and contradictory results have been reported. Serum prolactin levels have also been positively correlated with severity of tardive dyskinesia, particularly in women who have been exposed to antipsychotic medication. In parallel with the findings reported in schizophrenic patients, assessments of prolactin level and rhythm in depression have produced contradictory results. Both diminished and enhanced prolactin responses to TRH have been documented, as well as both normal and elevated basal levels. A subgroup of depressed patients appears to have a blunted prolactin response to intramuscular methadone administration and an alteration in 24-hour rhythm of prolactin release. Although it is tempting to deduce from such reports that any relationship may be artifactual, support for a relationship between prolactin and psychopathology can be seen in studies of women with prolactin-secreting pituitary tumors. In addition to common symptoms of oligomenorrhea and galactorrhea, hyperprolactinemic patients commonly complain of depression, decreased libido, stress intolerance, anxiety, and increased irritability. These behavioral symptoms usually resolve in parallel with decrement in serum prolactin when either surgical or pharmacological treatments are employed.

GROWTH HORMONE

Most psychiatric studies of the regulation of growth hormone (GH) have utilized strategies similar to those described for prolactin. Accordingly, studies of GH response to various provocative stimuli, such as hypothalamic-releasing factors or psychotherapeutic drugs, have been seen as a means to evaluate central neurotransmitter function. Augmentation of GH secretion in response to luteinizing hormone-releasing hormone and TRH in adolescent schizophrenic (as opposed to normal) boys has, for example, been seen as reflecting an alteration in catecholamine and possibly prostaglandin regulation, which facilitate human GH secretion. In general, however, there is a large variation in GH response to dopamine agonists in schizophrenic patients. Many patients have a blunted response, a result that has been variably linked to length of illness, presence of negative symptoms, and platelet monoamine oxidase activity. Some prepubertal, as well as adult, patients with diagnoses of major depression show hyposecretion of GH during an insulin tolerance test, a deficit that has been interpreted as reflecting alterations in both cholinergic and serotonergic mechanisms. Attenuated GH responses to GH-releasing hormone and to clonidine have also been reported in depression. Secondary factors, such as weight loss, rather than a pituitary defect, may be responsible for such alterations in endocrine release. The stress responsivity of somatotrophs is well established but species dependent, with increases in circulating GH being noted in humans and inhibition of secretion in rodent studies. Case reports have documented reversible GH deficiencies and marked growth retardation and delay of puberty secondary to stressful experience. Administration of GH to individuals with GH deficiency appears to have a beneficial effect on cognitive function in addition to its more obvious somatic effects.

CHOLECYSTOKININ

Long known to be present in pancreas and the gastrointestinal tract, CCK has recently been identified in mammalian brain, with high concentrations found in the cerebral cortex, limbic system, and hypothalamus. In animal studies, CCK is involved in the regulation of such behavioral functions as inhibition of intake of both solid and liquid food, production of satiety, and pain relief. Of additional interest to psychiatry is the discovery that CCK coexists with dopamine in mesolimbic and mesocortical, but not nigrostriatal, dopamine systems. This finding suggests that CCK fragments involving the terminal octapeptide portion (CCK-8) might either be dysregulated in psychiatric syndromes thought to involve altered dopamine transmission or be used therapeutically in the treatment of these same syndromes. Additional support for a behavioral effect in humans can be seen in the finding that in rats, administration of CCK-8 results in a more rapid rate of habituation to the novelty of environmental stimuli. Unfortunately, although early reports found both reduced levels of CCK in the CSF of schizophrenic subjects and some antipsychotic-like activity of CCK analogue compounds, more recent double-blind controlled studies have failed to find any evidence of benefit when the peptide compounds have been administered parenterally. In humans, caerulein, an amphibian analogue of CCK, has been demonstrated to relieve both natural and experimentally induced pain, but studies of intravenous infusion of CCK-8 have thus far failed to show a significant decrease in binge-eating behavior of patients with bulimia nervosa.

SOMATOSTATIN

Somatostatin is a hypothalamic tetradecapeptide that is located principally in the nerve endings of the median eminence, but also in neurosecretory neurons located in the paraventricular nucleus. Somatostatin was named because of its action in inhibiting the release of immunoreactive GH, but it seems to have a specific anatomical localization with cholinergic neurons in mammalian brain. There is also evidence that somatostatin may be a primary agent in the negative feedback control of thyrotropin secretion.

In rats, somatostatin and an analogue compound have been found to delay the extinction of active avoidance behavior and to antagonize amnesia induced by electric shock, yet not affect spatial discrimination learning. In patients with primary degenerative dementia of the Alzheimer type, senile onset, CSF levels of somatostatin are decreased in parallel with acetylcholinesterase. Similar findings of lowered somatostatin in ventricular as well as lumbar CSF have been reported for patients with mood disorder and in some patients with schizophrenia. A significant negative relationship between CSF somatostatin and postdexamethasone plasma cortisol level in psychiatric patients, independent of diagnosis, has also been found by one group.

GONADOTROPINS AND SEX STEROIDS

Gonadotropin-releasing hormone (GnRH) is a decapeptide that was sequenced and synthesized by Schally and colleagues in 1971. GnRH administration results in the rapid release of luteinizing hormone (LH) and follicle-stimulating hormone (FSH) from the pituitary in healthy subjects and in some pathological states, such as acromegaly, an abnormal release of GH or prolactin. Behaviorally, GnRH has direct central stimulatory effects on sexual behavior and possibly enhances attention and alertness as well. The cell bodies of GnRH are located principally over the optic chiasm in the arcuate area, with projections to the median eminence, and in the lamina terminalis. GnRH release is stimulated by norepinephrine and inhibited through negative feedback of gonadal steroids.

Alterations of gonadotropin regulation have been linked to the behavioral expression of sexual dimorphism, with some investigators hypothesizing an alteration in gonadal endocrine function underlying male homosexuality and transsexualism. Studies of gonadotropin and sex steroid hormone regulation in depression indicate a slight decrease in circulating testosterone, as well as in LH and FSH levels in depressed male patients. These differences are state-dependent, with normalization paralleling clinical recovery. FSH responses to GnRH administration are reportedly reduced in schizophrenic patients, with abnormal increases in GH secretion occurring in a significant subset of patients. That conclusions of a primary defect may be somewhat premature can be seen in the finding that dopamine receptor blockers, such as antipsychotics, may also cause significant declines in FSH and LH concentrations.

There is increasing evidence that the mammalian brain is structurally sexually dimorphic and that gonadal steroid compounds contribute to such differentiation through effects on neuronal survival. Postnatally, circulating gonadal steroids appear to interact with psychological and social factors in the development and display of sexual behaviors. In various androgen deficiency states, aggressiveness and sexual libido are decreased, particularly if the hormonal decrement occurs prior to puberty. Conversely, there is some evidence, principally through studies of exogenous administration, that increases in androgen level result in increased sexual behavior and aggression. Mood-altering effects have not been widely studied, although double-blind trials indicating an antidepressant action and case reports documenting induction of hypomania exist. Estrogens can influence neural activity in the hypothalamus and limbic system directly through modulation of neuronal excitability and have complex multiphasic effects on nigrostriatal dopamine receptor sensitivity. Accordingly, there is clinical evidence that the antipsychotic effect of neuroleptics may change over the menstrual cycle and that the risk of tardive dyskinesia is, in part, dependent on estrogen level. Chronic estrogen treatment, in animal studies, results in a decrease in the number of type-1 5-hydroxytryptamine (5-HT_1) and β-adrenergic receptors and in an associated increase in 5-HT_2 receptors, changes that hypothetically are relevant to mood change in premenstrual and postpartum depressive syndromes. In uncontrolled studies, supplemental estrogen treatment has resulted in improved mentation in women with Alzheimer's disease, and in improved mood, rapid cycling, or akathisia in depressed females. Because of methodological problems and disagreement as to the exact nature and definition of the problem, little is still known about the relationship between menstruation and disorders of mood. The term "premenstrual syndrome" has been used indiscriminately, and biochemical hypotheses of proposed etiologies remain speculative and contradictory. Alterations in estrogen, progesterone, prolactin, adrenocortical, thyroid, cholinergic, serotonergic, and endorphin regulation have been individually proposed, with little evidence supporting one hypothesis over another.

OTHER HORMONES

In addition to the systems reviewed thus far, a variety of other hormones affect behavior. Their classification here should not be interpreted as their being of secondary importance, but rather, as a reflection of their more recent identification and the lesser amount of investigation accomplished to date.

Increasing interest in the behavioral effects of *melatonin* have derived from recognition that the pineal gland serves as a transducer though which environmental light affects neuronal activity and influences circadian rhythms. In animals, either artificial changes in day length or melatonin administration can result in the production of differential circadian rhythms and, functionally, in alterations of reproductive cycle. The finding that some patients experience depression only in fall or winter and respond beneficially to the administration of bright light has suggested that the mood symptoms may be due to an abnormal secretion of melatonin, since bright light is known to suppress plasma melatonin levels dramatically. Unfortunately, although some groups have found increased levels in such patients, other investigators record exactly opposite results, and light exposure that does not suppress melatonin secretion seems as effective as light that does. Administration of pharmacological doses of melatonin to normal subjects significantly decreases subjective alertness and briefly increases sleepiness. Since animal studies indicate that chronic treatment with several antidepressant drugs can decrease plasma melatonin, recent or current drug treatment may be partially responsible for the disparate results reported thus far. Melanocyte-stimulating hormone (MSH), an anterior pituitary peptide, controls the secretion of melatonin and, in some paradigms, exerts opposite effects on measures of behavior. Intraperitoneal administration of α-MSH delays extinction in a passive-avoidance response and increases emotional response. In a double-blind crossover trial in humans, an infusion of α-MSH resulted in a significant improvement in verbal memory, but little change in mood. Because phenothiazines increase pituitary MSH secretion and pigmentation in patients in proportion to their therapeutic potency in humans, it has been suggested that MSH peptides may possibly possess some therapeutic properties. A dose-related biphasic effect on mood has also been reported for MSH-release-inhibiting factor (MIF-I).

Neurotensin, a tridecapeptide found in the substantia nigra and limbic areas, as well as in the hypothalamus, appears to have a close neuroanatomical relationship with dopaminergic pathways. Although antipsychotic drugs alter neurotensin concentration in the caudate nucleus and nucleus accumbens, clinical studies of neurotensin concentrations in the CSF and postmortem brains of schizophrenic patients have produced contradictory findings.

Substance P, an 11 amino-acid peptide discovered originally in 1930, acts as an excitatory transmitter in primary afferent nerve terminals in mammalian spinal cord and may help regulate sympathetic noradrenergic function. In one study of psychiatric patients with mixed diagnoses, substance-P-related peptides were elevated in CSF in comparison to normal values. Depending on the pain paradigm utilized, administration of substance P can produce either hyperalgesia or analgesia.

REFERENCES

Akil H, Watson S J, Young E, Lewis M E, Khachaturian H, Walker J M: Endogenous opioids: Biology and function. Ann Rev Neurosci 7: 223, 1984.

Beumont P, Burrows G: *Handbook of Psychiatry and Endocrinology*. Elsevier, New York, 1982.

Brambillia F, Racagini G, DeWied D: *Progress in Psychoneuroendocrinology*. Elsevier, New York, 1980.

Cohen L M, Molitch M E: Psychiatric aspects of pituitary tumors. In *Psychiatric Medicine Update,* T C Manschreck, G B Murray, editors, p 87. Elsevier, New York, 1984.
Devaris D P, Mehlman I: Psychiatric presentations of endocrine and metabolic disorders. Prim Care *6:* 245, 1979.
Gold M S, Pottash A L C, Extein I: Hypothyroidism and depression: Evidence from complete thyroid function evaluation. JAMA *245:* 1919, 1981.
Halbreich U, Rose R: *Hormones and Behavior.* Raven Press, New York, 1987.
Hennessy J W, Levine S: Stress, arousal, and the pituitary-adrenal system: A psychoendocrine hypothesis. In *Progress in Psychobiology and Physiological Psychology,* J M Sprague, G N Epstein, editors, p 133. Academic Press, New York, 1979.
Majewska, M: Steroids and brain activity—essential dialogue between body and mind. Biochem Phamacol *36:* 3781, 1987.
Miles A, Philbrick D: Melatonin and psychiatry. Bio Psychiat *23:* 405, 1988.
Miller L, Sandman C, Kastin A: *Neuropeptide Influences on the Brain and Behavior.* Raven Press, New York, 1977.
Nemeroff C B, Calivas P W, Goden R N, Prange A J, Jr: Behavioral effects of hypothalamic hypophysiotropic hormones, neurotensin, substance P, and other neuropeptides. Pharmacol Ther *24:* 1, 1984.
Nemeroff C, Dunn A: *Peptides, Hormones and Behavior.* SP Medical & Scientific Books, New York, 1984.
Nemeroff C, Loosen P: *Handbook of Psychoneuroendocrinology.* Guilford, New York, 1987.
Pepper G M, Krieger D T: Hypothalamic-pituitary-adrenal abnormalities in depression: Their possible relation to central mechanisms regulating ACTH release. In *Neurobiology of Mood Disorders,* R Post, J Ballenger, editors, p 245. Williams & Wilkins, Baltimore, 1984.
Reus V I: Behavioral disturbances associated with endocrine disorders. Ann Rev Med *37:* 205, 1986.
Reus V I, Collu R: Endocrine effects of stress. In *Clinical Neuroendocrinology,* G Brown, R Collu, G R Van Loon, editors. Blackwell, London, 1988.
Rose R: Psychoendocrinology. In *Williams Textbook of Endocrinology,* J Wilson, D Foster, editors, p 653. Saunders, Philadelphia, 1985.
Sachar E J: *Hormones, Behavior, and Psychopathology,* Raven Press, New York, 1976.
Sapolsky R M, Krey L C, McEwen B S: The neuroendocrinology of stress and aging: The glucocorticoid cascade hypothesis. Endocrin Rev *7:* 284, 1986.
Wilson W H, Jefferson J W: Thyroid disease, behavior, and psychopharmacology. Psychosomatics *26:* 481, 1985.
Zandina J E, Banks W A, Kastin A J: Central nervous system effects of peptides, 1980–1985: A cross-listing of peptides and their central actions from the first six years of the journal Peptides. Peptides *7:* 497, 1986.

1.12
NEURAL, ENDOCRINE, AND IMMUNE INTERACTIONS

JAMES R. GORMAN, M.S.
STEVEN E. LOCKE, M.D.

INTRODUCTION

In the 1890s, I. G. Savchenko and then Y. E. London attempted to assess the role of the brain in modulating resistance to disease by examining whether removal of brain parts would modify infectious processes. In the first half of the twentieth century, a number of investigators attempted to determine whether immune responses could be modified by behavioral conditioning and neural influences. During the second half of this century, as modern immunology matured, evidence emerged that the immune system can regulate itself and can function autonomously. Most recently, pioneering research has again focused on interactions between the three major integrative systems of the body: the immune, nervous, and endocrine systems.

OVERVIEW OF THE IMMUNE SYSTEM

OVERVIEW OF IMMUNITY The immune system is the body's main line of defense against acquired diseases. The immune system can recognize and reject an enormous array of foreign environmental pathogens. In addition, immune cells can recognize and destroy self-cells (i.e., cells belonging to the same organism) that are virally infected or neoplastically transformed. All of these protective functions must be performed without damaging the host; therefore, exquisite mechanisms have evolved to distinguish between self and nonself. Structurally and functionally, the resulting system is comparable in complexity to the nervous system.

In humans, the immune system consists of about a trillion cells (most of which are lymphocytes) and about 10^{20} antibody molecules of tremendously diverse specificity. Antibody molecules are produced by a subset of lymphocytes. Antibodies act as cell-surface receptors on these lymphocytes and are also secreted and circulated systemically. The number of different antibody specificities is estimated to be about 10^8. Through this antibody diversity, lymphocytes and antibodies recognize structures of different molecular configurations, thereby allowing the immune system to distinguish between the molecular and cellular entities of self and nonself. Under certain conditions, the immune response can play a role in disease onset, through either an underactive immune response or an overactive immune response. Diseases associated with an underactive immune response include infectious diseases and some cancers, while an overactive immune response is associated with autoimmune diseases and allergies (Fig. 1.12-1).

HUMAN LEUKOCYTE ANTIGENS AND THE GENETIC CONTROL OF IMMUNITY Immunologists have clearly demonstrated that immune responsiveness to some *immunogens* (substances that the immune system recognizes and responds to as foreign) is genetically determined. The human genes most studied in this regard are the genes of the major histocompatibility complex, which encode a group of proteins called the human leukocyte antigens (HLA). The HLA proteins encoded by these highly variable genes serve as self-recognition elements for cells of the immune system; self-HLA proteins do not provoke an immune response, while nonself-HLA, or self-HLA in association with foreign immunogens, provokes vigorous immune responses. Certain HLA alleles probably confer susceptibility to a number of diseases associated with an underactive or overactive immune response to specific self- or foreign immunogens.

COMPONENTS OF IMMUNITY Collectively, the cells of the immune system are called *leukocytes,* commonly known as white blood cells. All leukocytes arise from precursor cells in the bone marrow called hematopoietic stem cells (Fig. 1.12-2). The human immune response includes two broad types: nonspecific immunity and specific immunity. *Nonspecific immunity* provides a first line of defense against

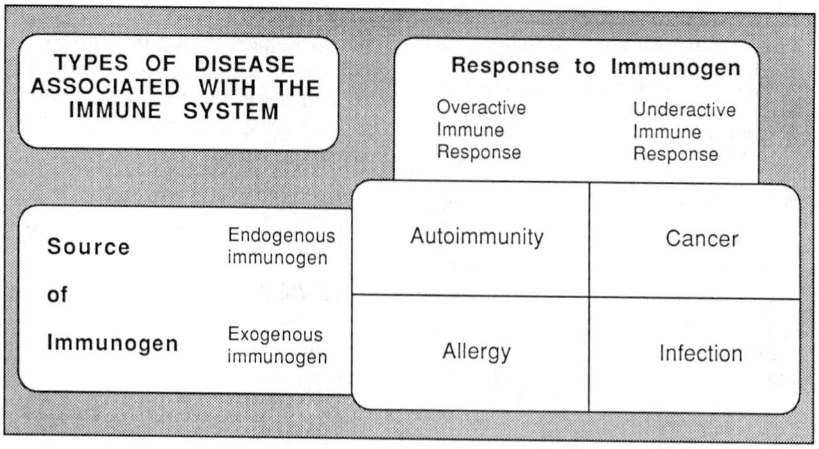

FIGURE 1.12-1. *Schematic diagram of four categories of disease that can be associated with underactive or overactive immune responses. An underactive immune response to an external immunogen may lead to infection, whereas an insufficient response to neoplastically transformed self-cells may allow certain tumors to progress. An overactive response to certain external immunogens produces allergies, whereas an excessive response to self-tissues can lead to autoimmunity. (From Locke S E, Colligan D:* The Healer Within, *p 26. E P Dutton, New York, 1986, with permission.)*

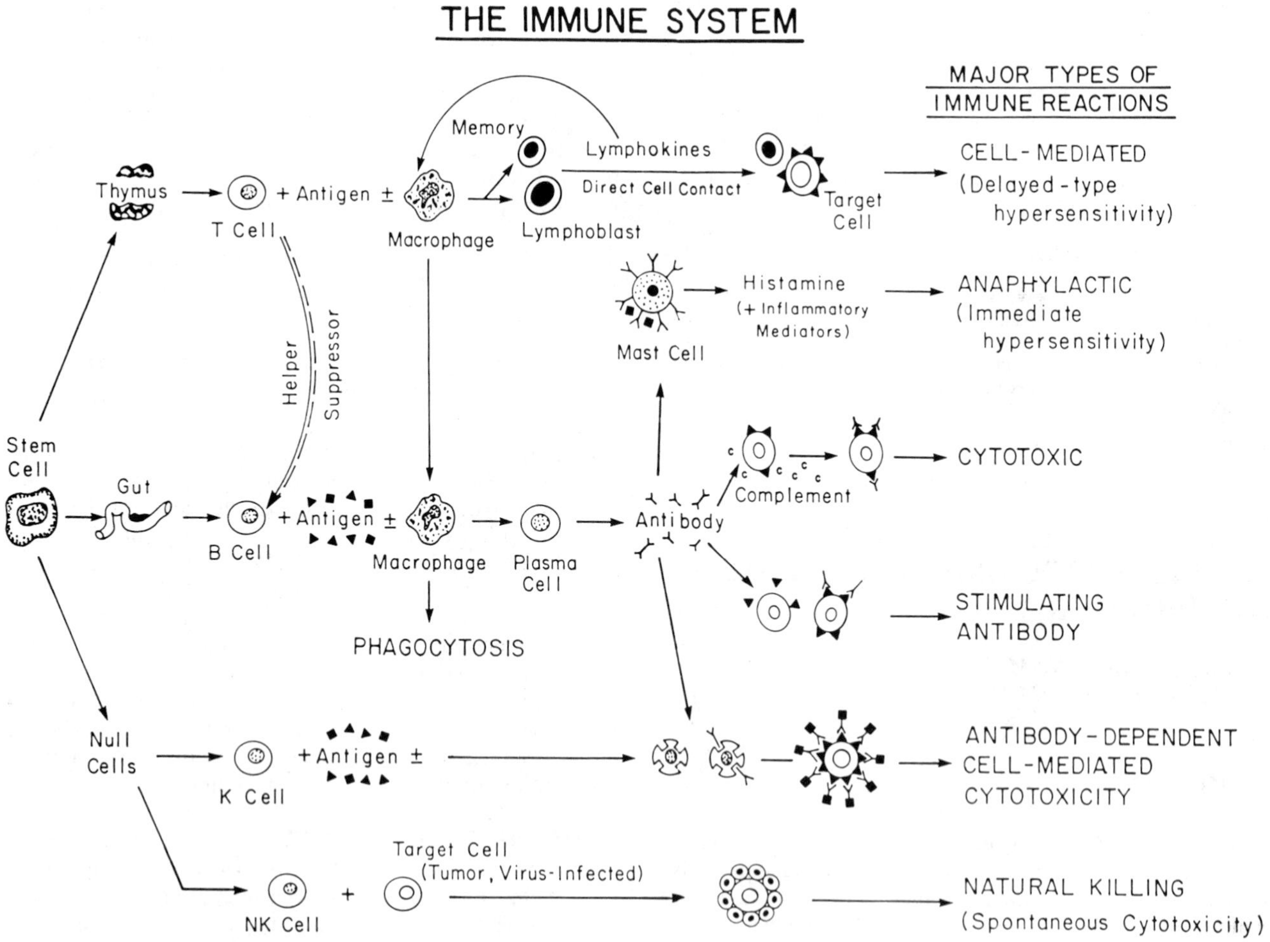

FIGURE 1.12-2. *Schematic diagram showing the development, interactions, and functions of the major classes of immune cells. (From Locke S E, Colligan D:* The Healer Within, *p 30. E P Dutton, New York, 1986, with permission; adapted from Ritts R E, Jr: Should we deem clinical immunology a new specialty? Med Opinion* 4: *11, 1975.)*

foreign particles and organisms, and is mediated by several cell types. For example, the *phagocytic cells,* such as blood *monocytes* and tissue *macrophages,* engulf and destroy many foreign particles and pathogens; likewise, the *polymorphonuclear granulocytes* aid in protection against a variety of microorganisms and, along with *mast cells,* play a major role in acute inflammation. In addition, a class of cells of undefined lineage, called *natural killer cells* (NK-cells), appears to provide a first line of defense against many virally infected or neoplastically transformed cells.

Specific immunity is distinguished from nonspecific immunity by the presence of specificity, learning, and memory. The term *specificity* denotes the fact that secreted antibodies and lymphocyte cell-surface receptors for immunogens are exquisitely sensitive to the three-dimensional configurations of different immunogens. Individual lymphocytes make and bear on the cell surface only one antibody or receptor type; each lymphocyte therefore responds to only one or a few closely related shapes. *Learning* and *memory* denote that once an individual is exposed to a specific immunogen, immune cells "learn" the shape of that immunogen and of that immunogen only; the next time the individual encounters the same immunogen, the immune system "remembers" the immunogen, and the response to that immunogen is stronger and more rapid. These phenomena of learning and memory act by a process called *clonal selection* (Fig. 1.12-3). The first time the immune system is exposed to a given immunogen, the immunogen stimulates only the tiny percentage of lymphocytes specific for the given immunogen. Each lymphocyte that recognizes the immunogen proliferates into a *clone* of identical cells, all making and bearing antibodies of the same specificity; some differentiate into antibody-secreting plasma cells, while others become long-lived memory cells. Like military reserves, these *memory cells* remain in readiness as inactive resting cells. They can be activated by a subsequent encounter with an identical immunogen, and because they greatly increase the number of lymphocytes that recognize the immunogen, they lead to more rapid and widespread lymphocyte proliferation and thus make the secondary response stronger and more rapid than the primary response. By this mechanism, the immunogen selects the proper lymphocytes and causes their proliferation into clones of effector and memory cells all specific for the immunogen.

The cells of specific immunity have been classically subdivided into B-lymphocytes, which mediate humoral immunity, and T-lymphocytes, which mediate cellular immunity

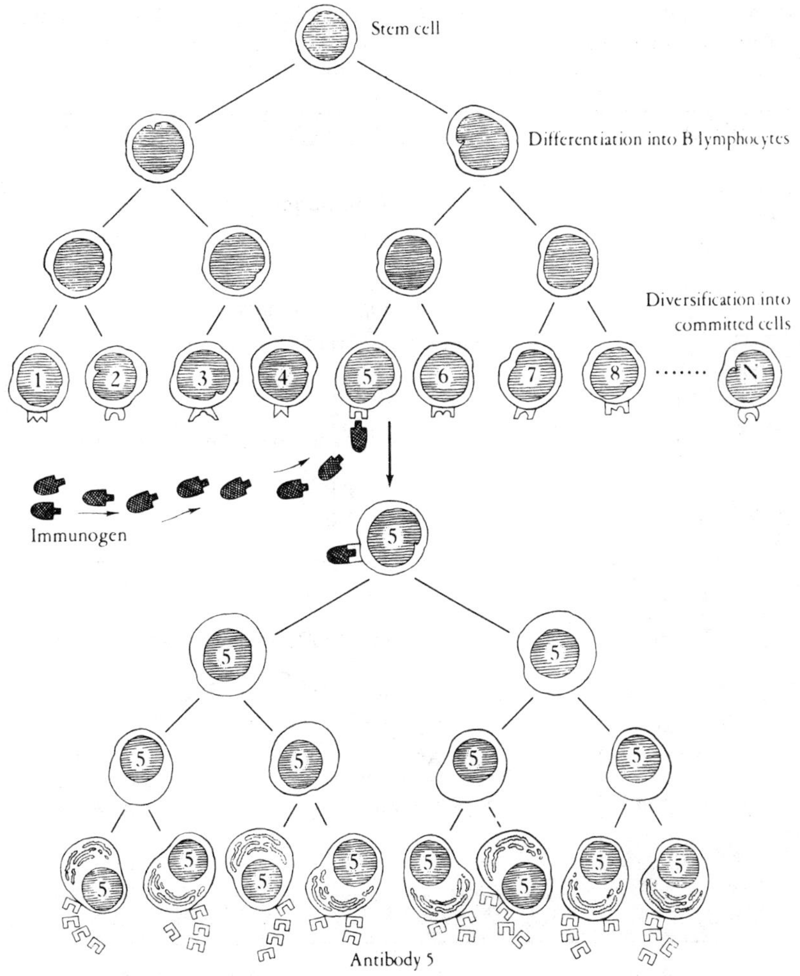

FIGURE 1.12-3. *Schematic diagram illustrating the clonal selection theory. A large repertoire of lymphocytes of diverse specificity, each present at low frequency, is randomly generated during cellular ontogeny. A given immunogen selects the lymphocytes that specifically recognize the immunogen and induces the proliferation of these specific lymphocytes, resulting in numerous identical copies (clones) of the lymphocyte specific for the given immunogen. (From Bellanti J A:* Immunology III, *p 137. Saunders, Philadelphia, 1985, with permission.)*

(Fig. 1.12-4). B-lymphocytes (called B-cells) arise from precursor cells in the bone marrow, and in humans, the site of their maturation is uncertain; T-lymphocytes (called T-cells) also arise from precursor cells in the bone marrow, then mature and differentiate in the thymus, and finally migrate to the periphery. Mature T- and B-cells continuously recirculate between the lymphatics, the lymph nodes, the blood vessels, and the spleen. Despite the classical distinction made between humoral immunity (classically considered to be mediated by B-cells and their soluble products) and cellular immunity (classically considered to be mediated by T-cells and their products), it is now clear that T-cells and B-cells interact and cooperate in most humoral immune responses and in some cellular immune responses. In addition, specific immunity is aided by macrophages and other nonlymphoid cells, which play a crucial role in the immune response; they ingest immunogenic proteins, process them, and reexpress protein fragments on their surface in association with self-HLA-molecules, allowing the immunogens to be recognized by T-cells. This function is known as antigen presentation, and the cells are referred to as *antigen-presenting cells*.

B-cells produce, bear on their surface, and secrete an enormously diverse repertoire of immunoglobulin (Ig) molecules, also referred to as antibodies. Each B-cell is genetically programmed during cellular ontogeny to make, bear, and secrete only one antibody specificity. B-cells and antibodies provide protection against bacteria, bacterial toxins, and viral reinfection. There are five classes of Ig—IgG, IgM, IgA, IgD, and IgE—that mediate different effector functions. (For example, IgE antibodies play a central role in immediate hypersensitivity reactions, such as asthma and anaphylaxis.)

T-cells are divided into several subsets, which perform different functions. The T-cell subsets produce many different soluble mediators, which are collectively referred to as cytokines. Examples include the interleukins, the interferons, B- and T-cell growth and differentiation factors, chemotactic factors, suppressor factors, and cytotoxic factors, such as lymphotoxin and tumor necrosis factor. Different subsets of T-cells mediate different effector functions. Cytolytic T-lymphocytes (CTLs) can destroy foreign tissue grafts and fungi or self-cells that are virally infected or infected with intracellular parasites; in addition, CTLs destroy some tumor cells and protect against the growth of some tumors. Regulatory functions mediated at least, in part, by T-cells include activation and amplification of the immune response (by T-helper cells) and suppression of the immune response (by T-suppressor cells). Human T-cells can be separated into two different subsets using anti-T_4 and anti-T_8 monoclonal antibodies. The subset that is recognized by the T_4 antibody expresses the T_4 molecule on its surface and is usually referred to as the helper-inducer subset. The other subset, which is recognized by the OKT_8 antibody, expresses the T_8 molecule on its cell surface and is usually referred to as the suppressor-cytotoxic subset.

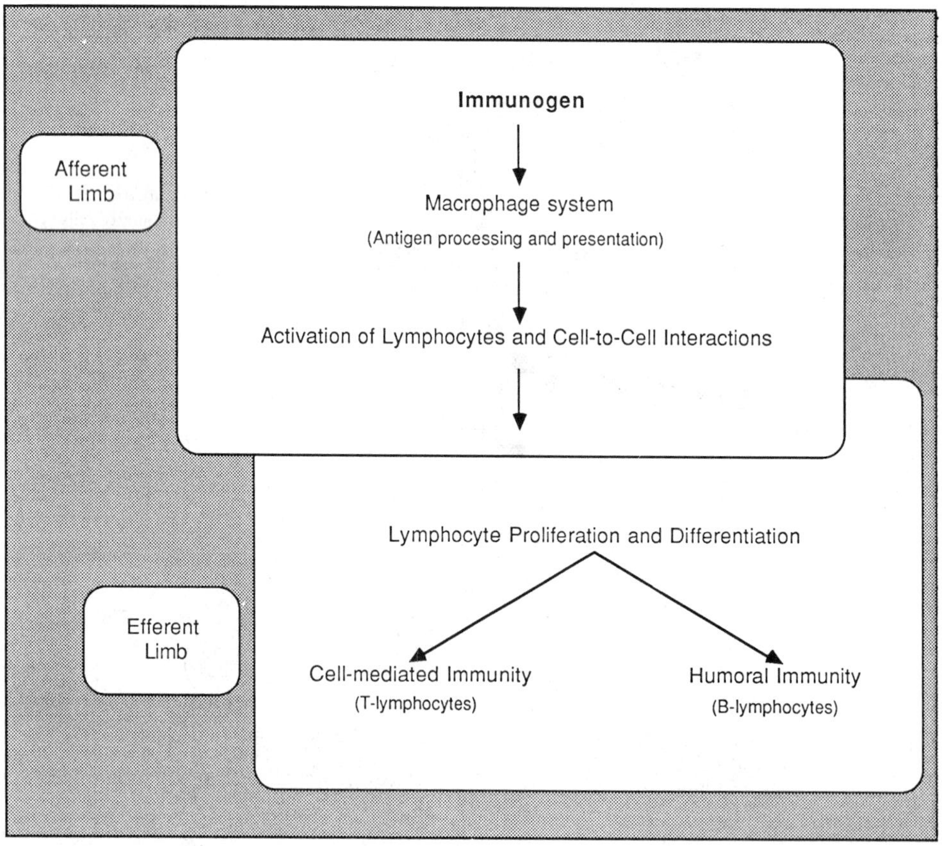

FIGURE 1.12-4. *Schematic diagram representing the major steps in the afferent and efferent limbs of the immune response. Immunogens are engulfed, processed, and presented on the surface of antigen-presenting cells. Lymphocytes and regulatory cells are activated, and lymphocytes proliferate and differentiate. B-lymphocytes mediate antibody responses (humoral immunity), and T-lymphocytes mediate cellular immune responses (cell-mediated immunity). (Adapted from Bellanti J A:* Immunology III, *p 13. Saunders, Philadelphia, 1985, with permission.)*

THE IMMUNE SURVEILLANCE HYPOTHESIS The *immune surveillance hypothesis* states that tumor cells carry "markers," which allow tumors to be recognized and rejected by the host's immune cells. It further hypothesizes that the evolutionary development of a cell-mediated immune response may have been driven by the need for a tumor surveillance system. Finally, it assumes that tumor cells arise frequently in a normal host and are rejected by immune cells; tumor cells that progress to clinical cancers are therefore hypothesized to result from the failure or circumvention of cell-mediated immunity. Although there is still substantial evidence both for and against it, the immune surveillance hypothesis has gained fairly wide acceptance among immunologists.

MEASURES OF IMMUNE FUNCTION A number of different assays measure the in vivo and in vitro functions of the immune system. In vivo assays are in some ways more straightforward to interpret in terms of their relevance to actual physiological processes. However, because in vivo systems contain many more variables, it is frequently more difficult to manipulate a single variable precisely in an in vivo assay; in addition, in vivo assays are often difficult and expensive to perform. Examples of in vivo assays of immunity in humans include skin tests that measure the delayed-type hypersensitivity (DTH) response mediated by T-cells and infectivity tests that measure the development of signs and symptoms of infection in subjects who have been deliberately exposed to a pathogen, such as a virus. In animal systems, additional in vivo assays are sometimes used, such as the growth of transplanted or virally induced tumors or the redistribution of immune cells to different organs upon challenge with immunogen.

In vitro measures are commonly employed by researchers in behavioral immunology in attempts to measure various parameters of immune function. Many researchers in behavioral immunology use these assays, although the relevance of these immune response parameters in predicting clinical susceptibility to disease remains uncertain. *Mitogens* are plant derivatives that nonspecifically stimulate proliferation of large numbers of B- or T-cells, or both. The most commonly used assay, and yet one of the least clear in its immunological and clinical implications, is the T- or B-cell proliferative response to mitogens. In vitro assay systems that are more obviously relevant to the in vivo interactions between immune cells, such as in vitro assays using cloned immunogen-specific lymphocytes, are starting to be used by some investigators. Several in vitro assays specifically measure the antibody response to a given immunogen; the most commonly employed are measures of antibody titer and measures of the number of antibody-producing plaque-forming cells. Other assays measure NK-cell activity or the cytotoxic activity of cytotoxic T-lymphocytes. Finally, some assays measure the absolute numbers or the percentages of different immune cells, including B-cells, T-cells, or T-cell subsets.

NORMAL VARIANCE IN BASELINE IMMUNE FUNCTION Disease-free individuals normally differ in their baseline responsiveness on a variety of parameters of immune function. Some sources of normal individual difference include genetic differences, nutritional and developmental factors, and age. Lunar, circadian, and ultradian rhythmicity of immune responsiveness also have been demonstrated.

BIOLOGICAL INTERACTIONS AMONG THE IMMUNE, NERVOUS, AND ENDOCRINE SYSTEMS

There is substantial experimental evidence that the nervous, endocrine, and immune systems are highly integrated with each other, routinely communicate with each other, mutually regulate various aspects of each other's responsiveness, and together contribute to the organism's homeostasis. The brain and the immune system are linked by at least two major pathways: (1) the autonomic nervous system and (2) the neuroendocrine system.

INTERACTIONS BETWEEN THE IMMUNE AND AUTONOMIC NERVOUS SYSTEMS **Neuroanatomy of immune tissues and cells** AUTONOMIC INNERVATION OF IMMUNE TISSUES Extensive anatomical studies, some as early as the mid-1800s, have identified autonomic fibers showing regional and specific innervation of both the vasculature and the parenchyma of the tissues (referred to as *lymphoid tissues*) that comprise immune organs. Lymphoid tissues innervated by noradrenergic sympathetic fibers include primary lymphoid tissues (bone marrow and thymus), encapsulated secondary lymphoid tissues (spleen and lymph nodes), and gut-associated lymphoid tissues (tonsils, appendix, and Peyer's patches of the small intestine). Recent immunohistochemical studies have also localized peptidergic fibers in lymphoid tissues. In recent neuroanatomical studies, some morphological patterns in this immune tissue innervation have been elucidated. Nerve fibers typically innervate both the blood vessels supplying immune organs and the parenchyma of immune organs (where fields of lymphocytes and other cells are localized within immune organs). The parenchymal fibers are usually found in areas of T-cells and plasma cells, rather than in nodular regions rich in B-cells. Noradrenergic fibers in the parenchyma are closely apposed to lymphocytes and macrophages, as well as to mast cells and eosinophils. Precisely how and to what extent this direct autonomic innervation of lymphoid tissues actually regulates immune function is not yet clear.

It has been known for some time that myelinated and nonmyelinated nerves innervate the marrow of long bones; in recent studies of mice, rats, rabbits, and monkeys, it has been shown in all cases that innervation extends to the regions of bone marrow where hematopoietic stem cells are found. This innervation includes fibers containing catecholamines and synapses containing acetylcholinesterase. There is one report of afferent connections from bone to brain. Two broad types of function have been postulated for this autonomic nervous system innervation of bone marrow. First, the autonomic nervous system may help regulate production of hematopoietic stem cells. The time course of development of neural inervation and hematopoiesis is consistent with this hypothesis. Second, these nerves may regulate the production of lymphocytes. Several types of evidence have been offered in support of this hypothesis. For example, catecholamine agonists stimulate, whereas acetylcholine agonists inhibit, bone marrow production of lymphocyte colony-forming units in irradiated mice. Localized central nervous system (CNS) stimulation can increase bone marrow production of reticulocytes, and brain lesions can affect bone marrow production of erythrocytes.

Autonomic innervation of both human and mouse thymuses by secretory, sensory, and vasomotor fibers, both catecholamine-positive and acetylcholinesterase-positive, has been recently reported (Fig. 1.12-5); the report of cholinergic innervation of thymus has not yet been replicated. Vasoactive intestinal peptide (VIP)-containing peptidergic fibers may innervate thymic cortex. Although the functions of this thymic innervation are not yet clear, several roles are possible. First, the time course of appearance of autonomic innervation in thymic development has led to speculation of a role for the autonomic nervous system in guiding the development and differentiation of lymphoid cells during ontogeny. This hypothesis is supported by experiments in which localized lesions of the CNS produce abnormal thymic development. Second, since thymocytes are specifically clustered in those thymus areas that are most densely innervated with autonomic fibers, the autonomic nervous system may help regulate both the migration of immature lymphocytes to the thymus and their distribution within the thymus. Third, thymic nerves may: (1) control the permeability of the blood-thymus barrier to the entry of prethymocytes and the exit

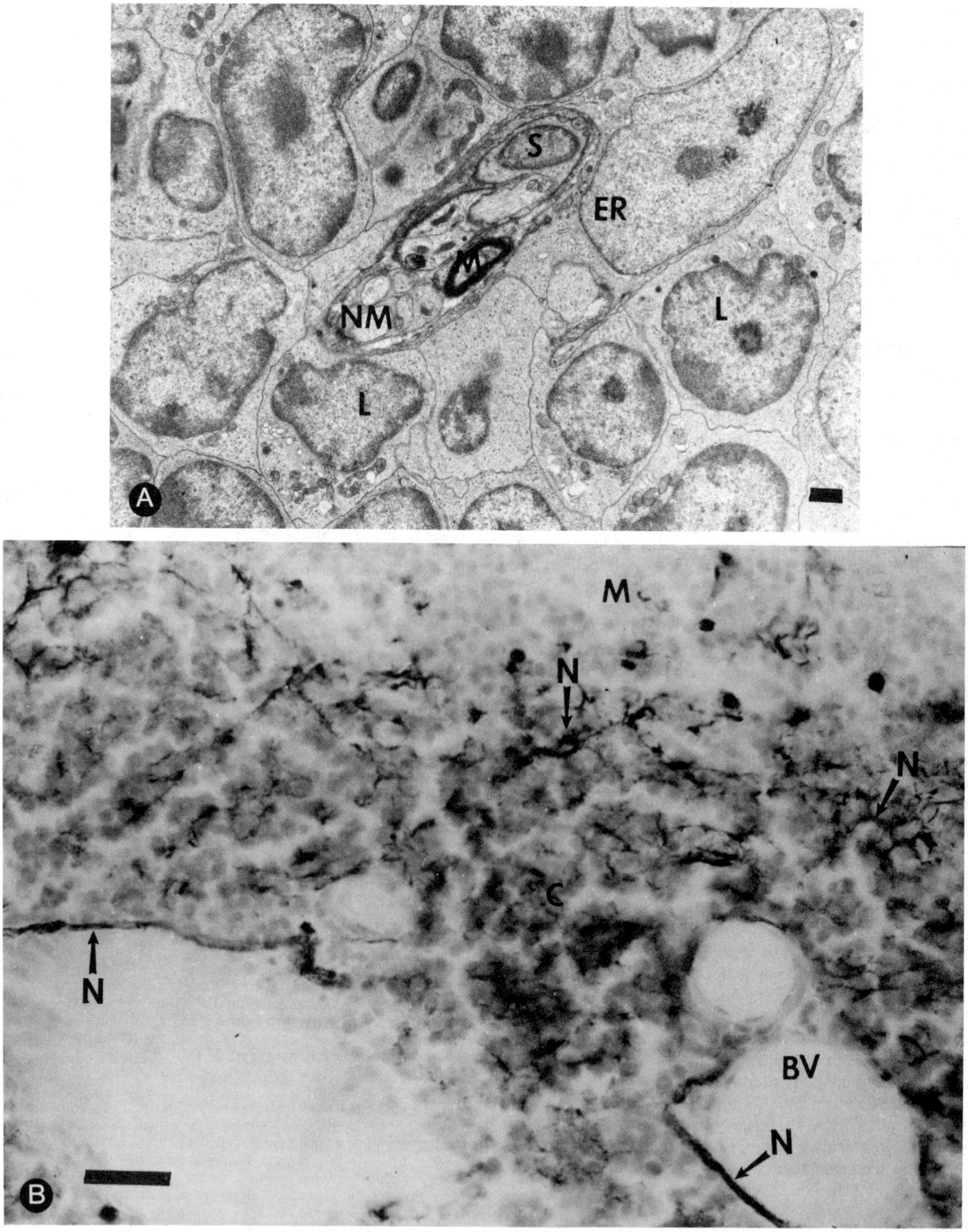

FIGURE 1.12-5. A: *Photomicrograph of acetylcholinesterase-positive nerve fibers derived from the vagus nerve located within the corticomedullary boundaries of the mouse thymus. Abbreviations: nerve* (N); *blood vessel* (BV); *cortex* (C); *medulla* (M). *Length of bar represents 100 microns (μm).* B: *Electron micrograph of a nerve bundle within the parenchyma of a thymus transplanted under the kidney capsule of a nude mouse. Abbreviations: Schwann cell* (S); *nonmyelinated nerve* (NM); *myelinated nerve* (M); *epithelial reticular cell* (ER); *lymphocyte* (L). *Length of bar represents 2 μm. (Courtesy K. Bulloch, Ph.D.)*

of T-cells; (2) influence T-cell differentiation via release of neurotransmitters or neuropeptides; and (3) modulate thymic hormone secretion, thereby affecting immune-neuroendocrine interactions.

In the mouse spleen, most sympathetic noradrenergic fibers terminate in the white pulp; both adrenergic and cholinergic fibers innervate the human spleen. Although most fibers are closely associated with blood vessels, some nerves clearly contact lymphocytes. Splenic white pulp appears to be innervated by peptidergic nerve fibers containing neuropeptide Y, methionine-enkephalin (met-enkephalin), cholecystokinin, and neurotensin. Although splenic nerves have been thought to function in contraction of the spleen, these nerve fibers may also help to regulate lymphocyte activity.

In the lymph nodes and lymphatic vessels, innervation by sympathetic and parasympathetic fibers is not as dense as in the thymus and the spleen. The existence, during embryogenesis, of distinct topographic relations between the lymph nodes, the lymphatic vessels, and the autonomic nervous system suggests that the autonomic nervous system may provide developmental signals for these lymphoid tissues. Lymph node innervation controls the flow of lymph and blood by regulation of vascular diameter. This innervation may also function in the neural modulation of lymphocyte behavior, and thus of immunity.

Autonomic fibers innervate the mucosa-associated lymphoid tissue of the gut, respiratory tract, and urinogenital tract, including the tonsils, appendix, and Peyer's patches. In the rabbit appendix, these autonomic fibers innervate areas containing both T-cells and plasma cells, and in rabbit Peyer's patches, nerve terminals make close contact with lymphocytes. An immunomodulatory function for the innervation of the tonsil has also been reported in several studies.

IMMUNE CELL RECEPTORS FOR NEUROCHEMICALS The cells and tissues of the immune system have surface or cytoplasmic receptors for a wide variety of neurohormones, neuropeptides, and neurotransmitters, as well as for other mediators affected by these neurochemicals (Table 1.12-1). Lymphocyte proliferation, differentiation, and effector function can be modulated, in part, by binding of these neurochemicals to lymphocyte receptors. Lymphocytes have receptors for acetylcholine (nicotinic and muscarinic subtypes), epinephrine, norepinephrine, histamine, and possibly dopamine. Human polymorphs have also been found to have β-adrenergic receptors. Immune cells have receptors for several central neurohormones, including adrenocorticotropic hormone (ACTH) and growth hormone, and probably for the endorphins and enkephalins. Immune-cell receptors have also been found for peripheral neuropeptides, including somatostatin, substance P, and vasoactive intestinal peptide. Finally, various cells of the immune system have receptors for a variety of hormones that, although not secreted directly by the nervous system, are nonetheless regulated by the nervous system. These include lymphocyte receptors for testosterone, insulin, glucagon, triiodothyronine, and corticosteroids (such as cortisol in humans). Monocytes have recently been found to have receptors for benzodiazepenes, and thymic epithelial cells have receptors for estrogen and dihydrotestosterone. The existence of autonomic innervation of lymphoid tissues and the presence of immune-cell receptors for numerous neurochemicals have sparked intensified interest in the pursuit of experiments to test directly whether the autonomic nervous system can modulate immune function in intact animals. In the hypothetical pathway, internal or external stimuli could stimulate autonomic nervous system activity either directly or via the CNS (Fig. 1.12-6).

TABLE 1.12-1
Effect of Hormones on the Immune System

	Direct Effect on			*Receptors on*		
Hormone	*RES*	*T-Cells*	*B-Cells*	*RES*	*T-Cells*	*B-Cells*
Steroids						
Glucocorticoids	+	+	+	+	+	±
Estrogens	+	+	+	±	+	0
Progestogens	0	±	±	0	±	±
Androgens	±	+	+	–	+	0
Catecholamines						
α-Adrenergic	+	±	0	+	–	0
β-Adrenergic	+	+	+	+	+	+
Neuropeptides and neurotransmitters						
Substance P	+	+	–	+	+	–
Vasointestinal peptide (VIP)	0	+	–	+	+	–
Neurotensin	0	+	–	0	+	–
Bombesin	+	0	0	+	0	0
α-Endorphin	0	+	+	0	+	+
β-Endorphin	+	+	+	+	+	+
Enkephalin	0	+	+	0	+	+
Peptide hormones						
ACTH	+	0	0	0	±	+
FSH/LH/hCG	–	±	–	0	0	0
PRL	0	+	±	±	±	±
hGH	+	+	±	±	±	±
TSH	–	–	–	0	0	0
Insulin	+	+	+	+	±	0
IGFs	0	±	±	0	+	+
PDGF, FGF, EGF	+	+	+	0	0	0
TGF α-, β-	+	+	+	0	0	0
Vasopressin	0	+	+	+	±	0
Oxytocin	0	+	+	+	±	0
Glucagon	+	0	0	0	0	0
Somatostatin	+	+	–	0	+	–
Angiotensin	+	+	0	+	0	0
Thyroid hormones						
T_3, T_4	0	±	±	0	0	0

Table from Keiss W, Hall N R: Psychoneuroimmunology and endocrine mediated evolution of the immune system. In *Handbook of Endocrinology*, D Hesch, editor. Klinik Der Gegenwart Series, Urban and Schwarzenberg, Munich, West Germany, 1989.
0 Insufficient data available
+ Established finding
– Clearly absent
± Controversial findings

Immunomodulation by the autonomic nervous system Several lines of evidence support the existence of a role for the sympathetic nervous system in neural modulation of immunity. It appears that intact noradrenergic innervation in lymphoid tissue is necessary for normal primary humoral and cell-mediated immune responses in vivo. Recent efforts to account for the different observed effects of sympathetic nervous system manipulations have produced evidence of strain and species differences, and differences due to developmental stage of sympathectomy. Likewise, addition of catecholamines to lymphocyte cultures has produced varied results, with reports of sympathetic agonists either inhibiting, enhancing, or not affecting various parameters of immune responsiveness. In vivo effects of catecholamine administration are also not clear. Therefore, although the cumulative evidence supports a potentially important role for immunomodulation by the sympathetic nervous system, substantial further work is required to clarify the precise nature and mechanisms of these putative in vivo sympathetic nervous system influences on immune responses.

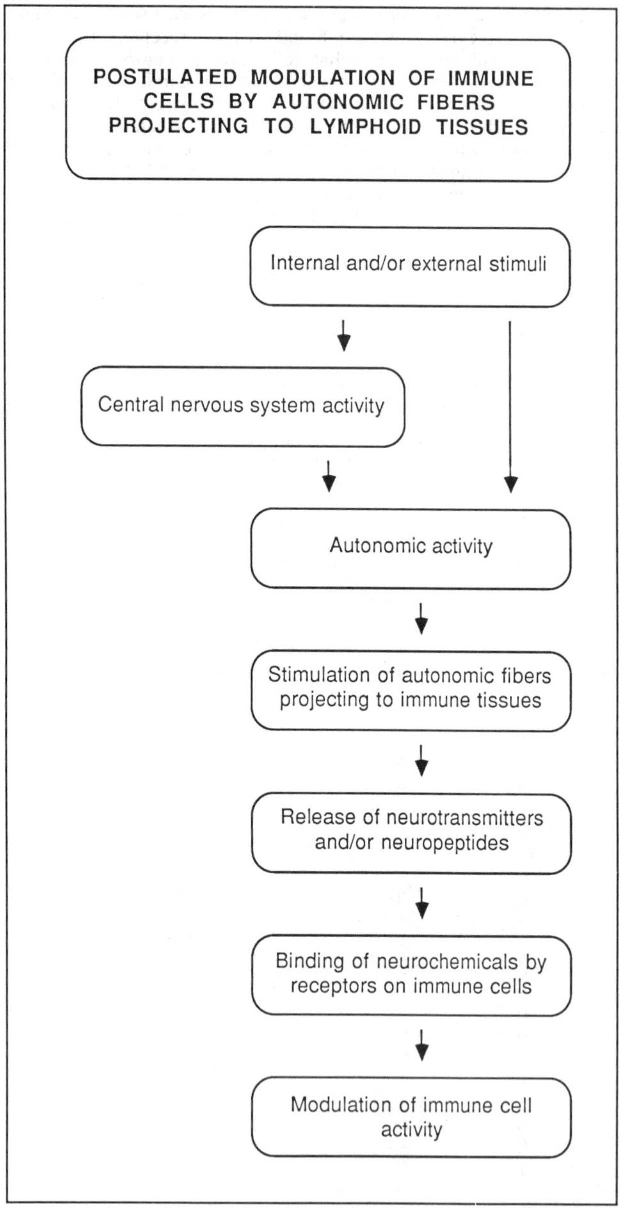

FIGURE 1.12-6. *Schematic diagram of steps in postulated pathway by which autonomic innervation of lymphoid tissue might play a role in directly modulating the function of immune cells.*

INTERACTIONS BETWEEN THE NEUROENDOCRINE AND IMMUNE SYSTEMS The endocrine system reacts to internal imbalances by secreting the hormones necessary to alter metabolic processes and restore homeostasis. It is known that the endocrine system is inextricably linked to the nervous system and to virtually every other physiological system. The endocrine system might therefore be expected to respond to the intrusion of nonself-molecules recognized by the immune system (immunogens). There is now considerable evidence that the immune and neuroendocrine systems are thoroughly integrated through the expression of a shared set of hormones and a shared set of receptors for these hormones.

A true regulatory circuit between the neuroendocrine and immune systems would require, at the very least: (1) an *afferent* pathway, by which the immune system could signal the neuroendocrine system when an immunogenic challenge occurs; (2) an *efferent* pathway, by which the neuroendocrine system could then regulate the developing immune response; and (3) a *feedback* mechanism, by which the immune system could signal to the nervous system that the efferent command had been received. Simple demonstrations of neurohormonal and neurotransmitter effects on immune cells do not constitute sufficient proof that the immune system is physiologically regulated by the neuroendocrine system. If such regulation exists, it should be possible to find phasic changes in neural and neuroendocrine activity that correspond with phasic changes in immune responses. These corresponding phasic changes in neural and neuroendocrine activity should be capable of influencing the activity of immune cells. Several pathways appear to exist for both the afferent (immune-neuroendocrine) and efferent (neuroendocrine-immune) arms of such a postulated circuit; in addition, the postulated phasic changes in neural and neuroendocrine activities capable of influencing immune cells actually appear to occur.

Afferent (immune-neuroendocrine) effects One afferent pathway by which the immune system appears to influence neuroendocrine activity is by immune-cell production of soluble factors, which can act on the hypothalamus to influence the hypothalamic-pituitary-adrenal (HPA) axis (Fig. 1.12-7). First, immunogenic challenge stimulates lymphocytes to release a factor that acts, via the HPA axis, to raise blood glucocorticoid levels. Then, the heightened glucocorticoid levels help to shut off the immune response by curtailing further clonal expansion of the immunogen-specific lymphocytes and by preventing the expansion of unrelated lymphocyte clones. Evidence for the existence of this circuit is as follows: The development of an immune response is accompanied by complex spatial and temporal changes in hypothalamic neuronal activity. Increased firing of individual neurons of the ventromedial hypothalamus occurs in a pattern that parallels the temporal development of the immune response. Norepinephrine synthesis in the whole hypothalamus is significantly decreased, corresponding with the peak of the immune response in the spleen. More specifically, the norepinephrine level in the paraventricular nucleus of the hypothalamus, but not in several other hypothalamic and brain stem nuclei, is decreased at the peak of the immune response.

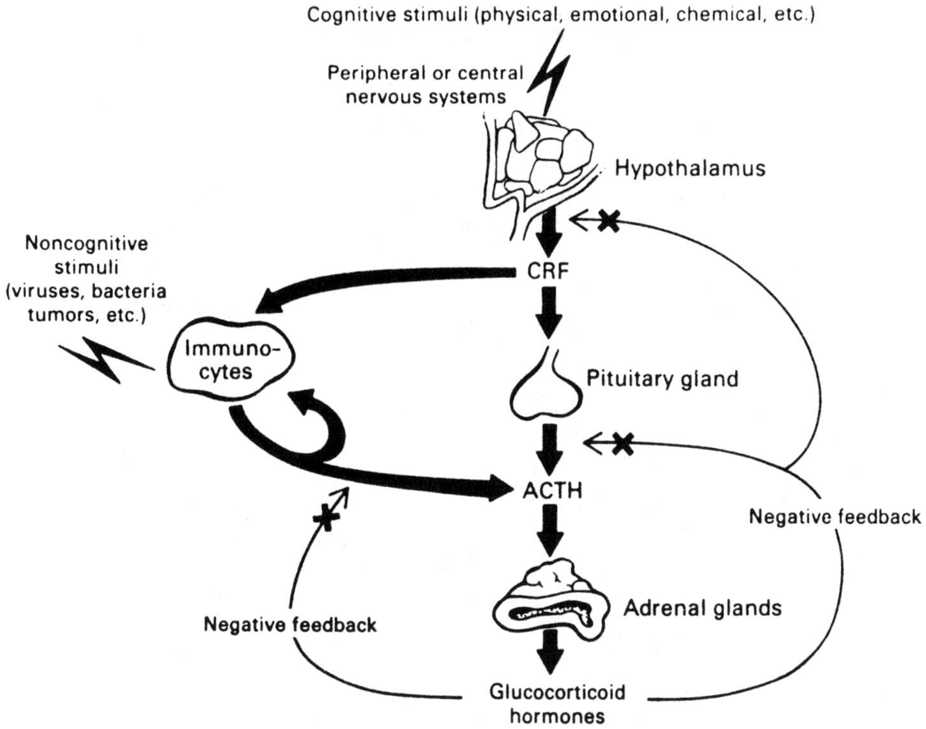

FIGURE 1.12-7. *Illustration of apparent connections between the hypothalamic-pituitary-adrenal axis and cells of the immune system. (From Blalock J E: Peptide hormones shared by the neuroendocrine and immunologic systems. J Immunol* 135: *859s, 1985.)*

Because this nucleus contains a large number of neurons that secrete corticotropin-releasing factor (CRF), the hypothalamic-releasing hormone for ACTH, it has been proposed that these paraventricular noradrenergic neurons may act as a key link in the immune-HPA-immune feedback circuit. At the peak of the immune response to an immunogenic challenge, the blood concentration of glucocorticoids reaches heightened levels, which can inhibit immune reactions. A nonpyrogenic factor found in the supernatants of lymphocytes stimulated in vitro can, when injected in vivo, double or triple blood glucocorticoid levels in the rat. Hypophysectomy completely eliminates this rise in blood glucocorticoid levels, suggesting that this factor may act to increase pituitary release of ACTH. Although several molecular candidates exist, the molecular species responsible for this activity has not yet been fully characterized. Thus, there is preliminary evidence for at least one complete brain-immune regulatory circuit.

A second afferent pathway by which the immune system may influence neuroendocrine activity is by immune-cell production of neuroactive peptides. For example, two immunoglobulin cleavage products, termed "tuftsin" and "rigin," can bind to opiate receptors, can cause analgesia when injected intracisternally, and can modify behavior when injected intraperitoneally. Likewise, ACTH and β-endorphin, which are derived from the precursor pro-opiomelanocortin (POMC), are now known to be produced by stimulated lymphocytes. The POMC gene is expressed in virus-infected spleen cells but not in uninfected spleen cells, as measured by the presence of POMC messenger ribonucleic acid (mRNA). The quantity of POMC mRNA produced by lymphocytes and its functional significance in lymphocytes remain to be determined. Currently, it appears that lymphocytes produce ACTH and β-endorphin in such small quantities that the peptides probably act primarily on nearby lymphocytes. Stimulation with mitogen or with CRF can reportedly induce immune-cell production of ACTH, while dexamethasone can suppress this production, suggesting the existence of induction signals and negative feedback similar to those that control the HPA axis. There are also reports that leukocytes can produce thyrotropin, vasoactive intestinal peptide, somatostatin, luteinizing hormone, and human chorionic gonadotropin. Finally, both macrophages and some tumor cells can produce the neuropeptide bombesin.

A third afferent pathway by which the immune system may influence neuroendocrine circuits is by the action of thymosin peptides. These thymic hormones, which are produced by thymic epithelial cells, function in the development and regulation of T-lymphocytes. Together, they help stimulate T-cell differentiation and function. They have also been reported to affect both the pituitary-adrenal and pituitary-gonadal axes, either directly or via the hypothalamus. Conversely, estrogen can bind to receptors in thymic epithelium and influence the release of immunomodulatory factors. Notably, some thymosins apparently act, probably via the HPA axis, to increase blood levels of ACTH and cortisol. Several of these peptides, which are found in thymus extract, have been purified, sequenced, and shown to have both immunomodulatory and endocrine activity (Fig. 1.12-8).

An intriguing view, consistent with the above evidence, is that the immune system may serve a sensory function, conveying to the nervous system general signals about the presence of such noncognitive stimuli as bacteria or viruses, which the nervous system cannot directly detect. These signals evoke neuroendocrine changes that may have physiological, immunological, and behavioral consequences. If this pathway is in fact active in vivo, then immune responses can

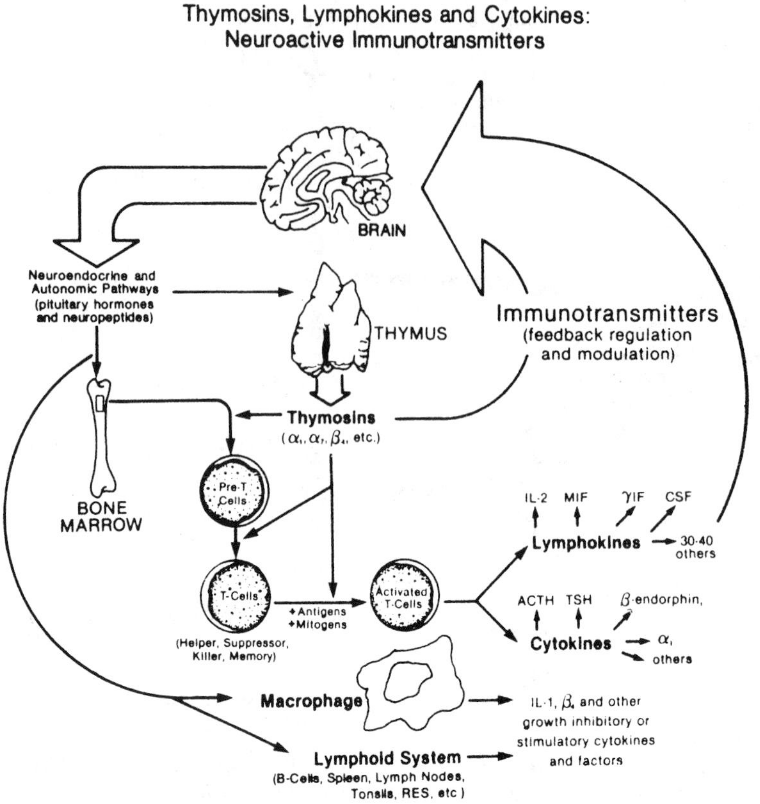

FIGURE 1.12-8. *Illustration of proposed role of thymosins in helping to mediate brain-immune interactions. (From Hall N R, et al: Evidence that thymosins and other biological response modifiers can function as neuroactive immunotransmitters. J Immunol* 135: *807s, 1985, with permission.)*

induce hormone release similar to that produced when stressful stimuli are perceived directly by the brain. In any case, the above evidence supports the existence of several afferent physiological pathways by which the immune system can influence nervous system and neuroendocrine activity.

Efferent (neuroendocrine-immune) effects Conversely, much evidence supports the view that the brain can influence immune responsiveness. Some of the early evidence for such efferent pathways came from extensive experiments in which specific brain regions of laboratory animals were lesioned or stimulated, and the animals' immune responses were then tested and compared to immune responses in control animals. These and subsequent studies by several different groups have shown that electrolytic lesions or electrical stimulation in discrete regions of the hypothalamus, the reticular formation, and the limbic system, and even the neocortex, can predictably enhance or inhibit leukocyte counts and function. Specifically, destruction of the posterior hypothalamic area impairs cellular immunity, primary antibody responses, and clearing of immunogen from the blood; conversely, stimulation of the same region enhances these functions. Discretely placed electrolytic lesions of the anterior and ventromedial hypothalamus decrease the numbers of nucleated spleen cells and thymocytes, and also decrease spleen-cell mitogen responsiveness, NK-cell activity, anaphylactic shock, and DTH. Similarly, discrete electrolytic lesions in many different regions of the limbic system, such as the amygdala, the hippocampus, and the mammillary bodies, suppress or enhance leukocyte numbers and function. Finally, lesioning the left cerebral cortex influences maturation of the T-cell lineage, production of T-cell-inducing factors, and NK-cell activity, but does not influence the activity of B-cells or macrophages. These lesions do not only affect immunity by altering the activity of the neurons that innervate lymphoid tissues. The lesions also appear to alter neuroendocrine activity, which apparently helps to modulate immunity in the intact normal organism.

The HPA axis has been the most frequently described neuroendocrine-immune pathway. In early investigations of "the stress response," prolonged stress profoundly affected immunological structure and function, resulting in enlargement of the adrenal gland, accompanied by involution of the thymus and lymph nodes. The mechanisms by which the hypothalamus influences immune functions include both the autonomic and neuroendocrine axes. The precise identification of those regulatory circuits that are physiologically significant remains a major challenge. Alteration of circulating glucocorticoid levels, induced by the HPA axis, is clearly the most established mechanism. Glucocorticoids can modulate the in vitro responsiveness of virtually every major immune-cell type, and every type of immune response. Rodent lymphocytes show more sensitivity to human steroids than do human lymphocytes; for this reason, early studies, in which human corticosteroids were applied to rodent lymphocytes, are difficult to interpret. However, since these species' differences in lymphocyte sensitivity to human corticosteroids have become understood, the effects of native endogenous rodent corticosteroids on rodent lymphocytes have been studied, and human corticosteroids have been studied for their effects on human lymphocytes. In vitro, low concentrations of native glucocorticoids stimulate, whereas high concentrations inhibit, lymphocyte proliferation and leukocyte phagocytic activity. In vivo, glucocorticoid effects are also well established and are probably attributable to both direct glucocorticoid effects on immune-cell responsiveness and to glucocorticoid-induced changes in lymphocyte migration patterns. In addition, the hypothalamic-pituitary system regulates homeostatic functions, such as temperature and electrolyte balance, which may affect immune function. Although the HPA axis is the most extensively studied efferent neuroendocrine-immune pathway, other such pathways are now thought to exist. Virtually all hormones, including many neurohormones and neurally modulated hormones known to be affected by stress, have been reported to enhance or inhibit various measures of immune function.

Increasingly, the pineal gland and its neurohormone melatonin have been implicated in immunomodulation. The pineal has been reported to exert an inhibitory effect on carcinogenesis and tumor growth. In humans, alterations in melatonin production have been associated with sleep and emotional disorders, with psychosomatic diseases, and with cancer. Early studies using surgical pinealectomy, which have now been confirmed and extended using chemical pinealectomy, have produced strong evidence that melatonin, which is known to influence sexual cycles as well as seasonal and circadian rhythms, also influences immune reactions. Chemical pinealectomy suppresses the cellular and humoral immune response to sheep red blood cells, and administration of melatonin eliminates the immune suppression in pinealectomized mice. Conversely, melatonin administered at the proper point in the circadian cycle enhances the antibody response to sheep red blood cells. This immunostimulatory effect of melatonin may operate by an opiatergic mechanism, because the effect can be completely blocked with the opioid antagonist, naltrexone (Trexan). Thus, the circadian release of melatonin by the pineal gland may buffer stress.

A wide variety of neuropeptides also affect immunity both systemically and locally in many complex ways. For example, physiological concentrations of both opioids and substance P have been shown to recruit independently the migration of macrophages in vitro. (This process of directional macrophage migration in response to a concentration gradient of soluble products is termed "chemotaxis." In vivo, the ability of immune cells to undergo chemotaxis in response to a wide variety of signals is believed to be the major mechanism by which immune cells accumulate at the site of an inflammatory reaction or immunogenic challenge.) A second example is that a variety of neuropeptides, many of them stress-related, can enhance or inhibit the measures of macrophage and lymphocyte function. ACTH can completely block the activation of macrophages to a tumoricidal state, and VIP and substance P can potentiate macrophage activation.

Within the past decade, a wide variety of assay systems have produced evidence that opioid peptides have multiple effects on the in vitro and in vivo function of immune cells. At physiological concentrations in vitro, both β-endorphin and met-enkephalin can each affect lymphocyte proliferation and monocyte chemotaxis. β-endorphin can also affect NK-cell activity, as well as the generation of primary antibody responses. The results from different experiments that have tested the in vitro effects of opioids on human lymphocyte proliferation have frequently conflicted; both enhancement and inhibition of lymphocyte proliferation have been reported. It now appears that either enhancement or inhibition of lymphocyte proliferation may be mediated by opioid peptides, depending on the individual lymphocyte donor. Based on a recent report that opioids can bind to some but not all HLA alleles, these interindividual differences in opioid effects may be based at least in part on immunogenetic (HLA) differences between individuals. Both β-endorphin and met-enkephalin have been shown in several different assay systems to be chemotactic for human monocytes.

Several different stress paradigms have been shown to elevate endogenous opioid levels in experimental animals. Stressors varying in seemingly minor detail can result in distinctly different forms of analgesia. For example, inescapable foot shock of constant intensity can elicit analgesia via opioid or nonopioid mechanisms depending on the temporal parameters of the foot shock. Prolonged, intermittent foot shock induces opioid analgesia (blockable by the opioid antagonist naloxone [Narcan]), whereas brief, continuous foot shock induces nonopioid analgesia (not blockable by naloxone). Rats exposed to the opioid form, but not rats exposed to the nonopioid form of foot shock stress, developed significant inhibition of NK-cell activity compared to unshocked rats, an effect that was reversible by the administration of an opioid antagonist. Similarly, rats exposed to the opioid-inducing form of foot shock before transplantation with a rat mammary tumor had reduced median survival time and percent survival, compared to unshocked rats and rats exposed to the nonopioid-inducing form of foot shock. Conversely, in a mouse neuroblastoma model, endogenous opioids appeared to inhibit tumorigenesis, based on several lines of evidence. These workers suggested that foot shock stress might result in a temporary increase in endogenous opioid levels, followed by a subsequent "overshoot" in which opioid levels might decrease below baseline, thereby allowing tumorigenesis to proceed at an increased rate; this overshoot effect has been seen following injection of β-endorphin into brain. In the same neuroblastoma system, it was shown that exogenous opiates and opiate antagonists could exert their effects by acting directly on opiate receptors borne by the tumor. Thus stress can result in the release of opioids, which have multiple and at times seemingly contradictory effects on both immune function and tumor growth.

Theoretically, opioids could exert their effects on immune responses and on tumor growth by several different possible routes (Fig. 1.12-9). Morphine and opioid peptides might

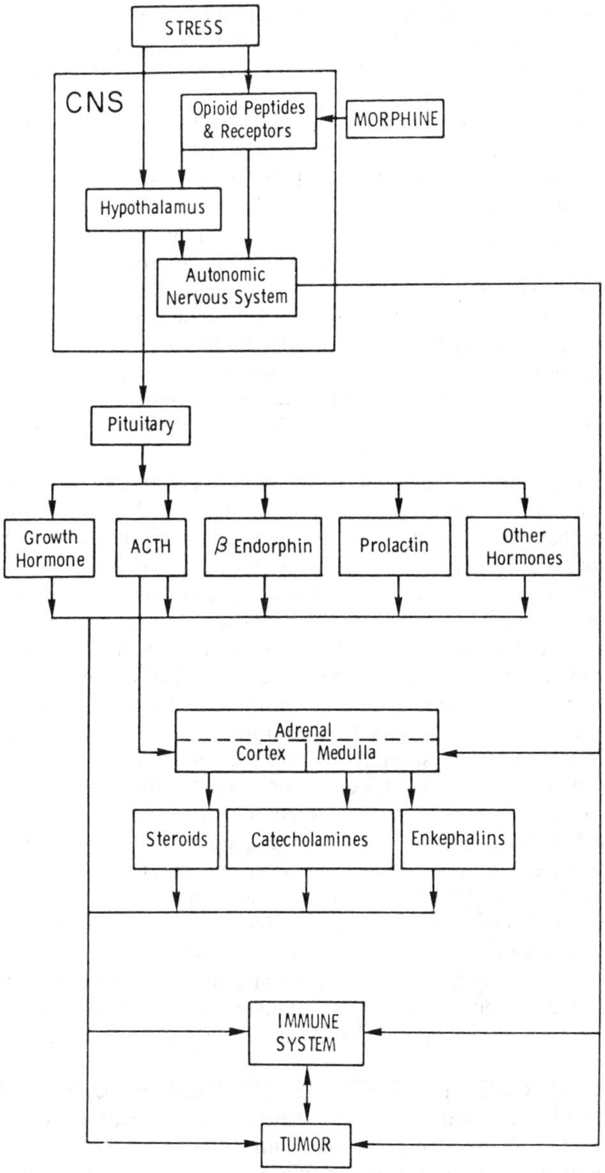

FIGURE 1.12-9. *Schematic diagram summarizing neural and neurohumoral mechanisms by which stress and morphine might affect the immune system and tumors. (From Shavit Y, et al: J Immunol 135: 836s, 1985.)*

directly alter immune function by binding to receptors on immune cells, which has been shown to occur in vitro. A second possibility is that opioids could alter immune function by altering the levels of other hormones, such as ACTH and corticosteroids. Finally, opioids are known to modulate the activity of the autonomic nervous system, which, in turn, could alter immune-cell activity via autonomic innervation of lymphoid tissue. Likewise, opioid peptides and exogenous opiates might alter tumor growth by directly binding to tumor-borne opioid receptors, as has been known to occur in some tumor systems. Alternately, opioid peptides could alter levels of tumor-promoting hormones, such as prolactin, which is secreted during stress and is known to promote the growth of many experimental mammary tumors. Finally, opioids could affect tumor growth by directly binding to immune cells and altering their responsiveness. Clarification of the actual in vivo pathways of opioid effects on immunity and on tumor growth will require further reductionist experimental approaches to establish the molecular mechanisms by which opioids can affect the responses of immune cells, the growth of tumor cells, the release of hormones, and the activity of the autonomic nervous system.

In preliminary clinical trials, met-enkephalin significantly elevated the number of lymphocytes, the number of active T-cells, and the number of cells in several T-cell subsets. In addition, there was a significant increase in T- and B-cell mitogen response in many, but not in all, individuals. Thus, endogenus opioid systems may play complex roles in the normal in vivo modulation of the immune system and also in the regulation of both in vitro and in vivo tumor growth in at least some tumor systems. The resolution of the enhancing and inhibiting effects of opioids on immune responses and a full understanding of the extent to which the immune effects of opioids are causally related to opioid effects on cancer growth will require further studies.

The development of the immune and neuroendocrine systems appears to be extensively intertwined. The molecular mechanisms for this developmental interdependency remain unknown. Of possible interest is the recent discovery of a lymphokine product of stimulated lymphocytes, which has been termed "neuroleukin." The gene for neuroleukin has now been cloned and sequenced; the protein product is neurotrophic for spinal and sensory neurons and also can support the growth in culture of sensory neurons and some embryonic spinal neurons. Conversely, the hormonal environment during development can strongly affect the development of both the immune and nervous systems. For example, clinical researchers have documented an association between left-handedness and autoimmune diseases, such as atopic diseases and autoimmune thyroiditis. It has been postulated that this association could result from the effects of abnormally high testosterone levels during fetal development. High testosterone levels may slow development of the right cortex, resulting in hemispheric dominance by the left cortex, and also may slow development of the thymus, resulting in immune abnormalities and, ultimately, in an increased incidence of autoimmune diseases.

OTHER NEURAL EFFECTS ON IMMUNE FUNCTION

Besides the autonomic and neuroendocrine pathways described above, there are other important neural effects on immune function that do not fit neatly into either of these two categories. They include conditioning effects on immune function and the effects of peripheral sensory neuropeptides on immune function.

Conditioning effects The suppression and enhancement of several measures of immune function by classical (Pavlovian) conditioning have been repeatedly demonstrated. Extensive experiments conducted in the Soviet Union, at least as early as the 1920s, produced considerable evidence that conditioning can alter nonspecific immunological defense reactions, such as leukocyte infiltration to the site of infection. In addition, several studies produced evidence, some conflicting, about the conditionability of antibody production. During the past decade, the study of conditioning effects has been significantly expanded. For example, in several experiments, animals were treated with an unconditioned stimulus (an immunosuppressive drug) paired with a conditioned stimulus (the taste of saccharin); when the same animals were subsequently reexposed to saccharin, a small but significant reduction in antibody titers of the conditioned animals was observed as compared with the appropriate control animals. Similar conditioning effects were subsequently demonstrated using several measures of cell-mediated immunity and were widely replicated under a variety of experimental conditions. To explore the possible biological and clinical significance of these effects in altering disease course, the effects of conditioned immunosuppression were investigated using a well-established mouse model of the autoimmune disease systemic lupus erythematosus. The substitution of conditioned stimuli for immunosuppressive therapy in conditioned mice significantly delayed the development of autoimmune disease and mortality. Similar results were obtained by two other groups of investigators who studied whether conditioning of immune responses could alter tumor growth rather than autoimmune disease. In one study, conditioned suppression of immune function enhanced tumor growth and increased the rate of mortality. In the other study, conditioned enhancement of NK-cell activity increased median survival time.

Sensory neuropeptide effects Neuropeptides released into tissues by sensory neurons in response to noxious chemical and physical insults rapidly elicit local and systemic responses similar to those of immediate hypersensitivity reactions (such as those seen in food allergies, hives, hay fever, asthma, and systemic anaphylaxis). Both substance P and somatostatin are present in different subsets of sensory nerves and can be released by these nerves following specific stimulation. Asthma is a disease involving hypersensitivity states of the lung. In guinea pigs with asthma, sensory nerves projecting to cells lining the lungs show abnormal secretion of substance P. This substance P secretion can be induced by noxious stimuli and by inflammatory reactions in pulmonary tissue, with the net result that the original hypersensitivity response is worsened. Conversely, the secretion of somatostatin generally inhibits the hypersensitivity response. Therefore, the hypersensitivity reaction may be increased or decreased depending on the mix of secreted sensory neuropeptides. In vivo, these sensory neuropeptides directly affect functions of leukocytes and macrophages via leukocyte cell-surface receptors for the neuropeptides. In vitro, these neuropeptides are selectively recognized by and can variously modify the activity of immune cells, including mast cells and basophils, which are involved in immediate hypersensitivity reactions. The immune complex disease arthritis is likewise accompanied by abnormal substance P release from sensory neurons projecting to cells lining the joints. Thus, sensory nerves may play an important role in modulating both some immediate hypersensitivity diseases, such as asthma, and some immune complex diseases, such as rheumatoid arthritis.

IMMUNE ABNORMALITIES AND MENTAL ILLNESS

If the nervous system and the immune system are physiologically integrated and help to regulate each other's activities, then some patients who show severe emotional and behavioral abnormalities should show immune abnormalities as well. Immune abnormalities have been reported in patients with major mental illness, especially schizophrenic patients, since the early 1900s. At least as early as 1912, one investigator suggested the possibility of an autoimmune component in schizophrenia. Immunological abnormalities in patients with schizophrenia or with major depression have been extensively studied. Often, the particular immune abnormalities appear to result from disordered immune regulation. Many questions remain about the issue of whether the observed immune abnormalities play any role in the onset of the accompanying mental illnesses. There have also been some studies of immunological abnormalities in other disorders, such as alcoholism, Alzheimer's disease, autism, cerebral atrophy, criminal behavior, dementia, mental retardation, Parkinson's disease, and senile dementia. Schizophrenia and major depression are the mental illnesses in which immunological abnormalities have been most thoroughly studied, and they will be the focus of this subsection.

IMMUNE ABNORMALITIES AND SCHIZOPHRENIA

Background and theoretical trends Conflicting reports have emerged in the past 25 years about immune abnormalities in schizophrenic patients. Both quantitative and qualitative changes in immunoglobulin levels, in humoral immunity to various immunogens, and in various parameters of cell-mediated immunity, such as lymphocyte morphology and mitogen-stimulated proliferation, have been reported in schizophrenic patients. Similarly, in each of these findings either conflicting or negative results, or both, have been reported. One of the fundamental questions that has stirred much controversy is whether such reported immune abnormalities are actually involved in producing the onset of schizophrenia. Instead, the abnormalities could simply accompany or follow the onset of the disease, as side effects or epiphenomena.

In the literature on schizophrenia, there are at least four hypotheses that relate the onset of schizophrenia to abnormalities of the immune system. These hypotheses propose that the onset of schizophrenia is mediated by one or several of the following factors: (1) autoimmunity, such as humoral or cell-mediated immune responses against brain or other self-tissues; (2) viral infection; (3) an immunogenetic defect in the HLA encoded by the major histocompatibility complex; and (4) an allergy or hypersensitivity to common food immunogens, such as cereal grains or wheat glutens. Published studies that have attempted to test these hypotheses now number in the hundreds. To date, the available evidence has neither convincingly proved nor convincingly disproved that any one of these four factors is important in the onset of the disease. Efforts to refine the experimental techniques and to integrate the available facts into a model of the disease process continue in many laboratories. Therefore, a brief overview will be presented of the types of ideas and evidence that have been offered to date.

Immunity and the onset of schizophrenia: Four hypotheses AUTOIMMUNITY AND SCHIZOPHRENIA Schizophrenia, like several well-established autoimmune diseases, is influenced by genetic, psychodynamic, and stress factors. Since the 1960s, there have been frequent reports that schizophrenic patients have a general increase in autoantibodies, including antibrain antibodies, antithymic antibodies, antinuclear factor (this finding is not limited to schizophrenic patients), and rheumatoid factor (also not limited to schizophrenic patients). In the early 1960s, animal models for the effects of antibrain antibodies were developed. Antibrain antibodies can affect the brain activity of rodents, lobsters, squid, and snails, resulting in a variety of functional abnormalities; these findings provided early support for the idea that antibrain antibodies might play a role in the onset and course of schizophrenia.

The possible presence of antibrain antibodies in schizophrenic patients has received substantial attention. During the late 1950s and the 1960s, one group reported a protein, eventually thought to be an antibody, in the sera of schizophrenic patients. Results from their own wide variety of experiments, along with the finding by other investigators that myasthenia gravis is of autoimmune origin, prompted these authors to propose that schizophrenia might result from the presence of antibrain antibodies.

Evidence has subsequently been produced both for and against the hypothesis that antibrain antibodies are the causative agent in schizophrenia. In at least two dozen studies conducted in different laboratories, antibrain antibodies have been found in the sera of some schizophrenic patients; several investigators testing the sera of both drug-free and medicated individuals have reported that the presence of the antibodies is not related to medication. The percentage of schizophrenic patients showing the presence of antibrain antibodies has varied from 20 to 70 percent, depending on the specific assay and the laboratory. Conversely, in at least six studies, no antibrain antibodies were found in the sera of schizophrenic patients. In a few studies, antibrain antibodies have even been reported in nonschizophrenic patients. Even if the finding of antibrain antibodies in the sera of some schizophrenic patients becomes consistently replicable, there remains the problem of why the antibodies are to date detectable in only a percentage of schizophrenic patients, as well as the related question of whether the antibodies actually play any role in causing the onset of the disease. One intriguing refinement of the original antibrain antibody hypothesis proposes that schizophrenia may be caused in whole or in part by antibodies to neurotransmitter receptors; for example, antidopamine receptor antibodies could act either as dopamine antagonists or dopamine agonists. Further work with increasingly sophisticated techniques will be necessary to determine the specific role, if any, played by antibrain antibodies in the onset of schizophrenia.

In addition to self-directed humoral immune responses mediated by antibrain autoantibodies, self-directed cell-mediated immune responses to brain immunogens have also been found in schizophrenic patients. For example, in one series of investigations, heightened cell-mediated immunity to human myelin basic protein was found in chronic, but not in acute, schizophrenic patients; this heightened response to myelin basic protein did not appear to be drug-induced. In the largest study of cell-mediated immunity to brain immunogens, a double-blind design was used to examine a group of more than 1,000 neuropsychiatric patients, including patients with dementia, mental retardation, cerebral atrophy, ethanol-induced brain deterioration, and schizophrenia. About 90 percent of every patient group, including drug-free dementia and mentally retarded patients, showed a delayed-type hypersensitivity (cell-mediated immunity) response to S-100 protein (found mostly in brain) and to neuron-specific enolase when these proteins were injected under the skin of the test patients. Thus, although it generally has been found that immune autoreactivity often accompanies schizophrenia, the role of autoimmunity in the onset and course of schizophrenia remains unclear.

VIRAL INFECTION AND SCHIZOPHRENIA The second hypothesis is that schizophrenia results from infection by a viral agent. To date, this hypothesis is based largely on many lines of controversial inferential evidence. Several different approaches have been used in attempts to find more direct evidence in support of the viral hypothesis. Some, but not all, investigators have reported heightened levels of antibodies to various viruses, such as herpes simplex virus (HSV) and cytomegalovirus (CMV), in the cerebrospinal fluid and in the serum of some schizophrenic patients. In perhaps the most direct approach, several groups have used sensitive assays to search for viral nucleic acid sequences or viral immunogens in postmortem brain tissue from schizophrenic patients. Most frequently, they have tested for the presence of the well-known neurotropic viruses, such as CMV and HSV. The results have been negative. Although many other viruses remain to be tested, no approach so far has produced compelling evidence that viral infection is important in the onset of schizophrenia.

IMMUNOGENETICS AND SCHIZOPHRENIA The third hypothesis is that specific, genetically determined immunological markers, such as HLA types, may be found for schizophrenia. A number of different investigators have reported different and at times conflicting associations. The most consistently reported finding has been an association between the HLA-A9 immunogen and paranoid schizophrenia; this association remains to be explained. Overall, numerous efforts have as yet produced no consistent, clear-cut genetic markers for schizophrenia.

FOOD ALLERGY, HYPERSENSITIVITY, AND SCHIZOPHRENIA The fourth hypothesis is that allergy or hypersensitivity to common food components, such as gluten, plays a causal role in the onset of schizophrenia in genetically predisposed individuals. The term "allergy" assumes immune-mediated mechanisms, whereas the term "hypersensitivity" implies that nonimmune mechanisms may be involved. The original evidence offered in favor of this proposal was indirect evidence from epidemiological analyses. Several approaches have been used to examine more directly whether a relationship exists between grain consumption and schizophrenia; so far, the findings have not been consistent.

IMMUNE ABNORMALITIES AND MAJOR DEPRESSION

Suppressed measures of immune function have been frequently observed in patients with major depression and have usually been considered a side effect of the disordered neuroendocrine regulation seen in these patients. In two initial studies, T- and B-cell mitogen responses were reduced in bereaved spouses during the weeks and months following bereavement. In a subsequent study, mitogen response was significantly reduced only in bereaved subjects with high scores on the depression subscale of the Hopkins Symptom Checklist.

At least a dozen controlled studies have attempted to examine directly the immune function of clinically depressed patients. Although some results have conflicted, the results of most studies, including a large recent study with expanded controls, have supported the hypothesis that a substantial percentage of depressed patients show suppressed responses on in vitro measures of cellular immunity (usually suppressed mitogen responses, the in vivo significance of which remains in question); the immunosuppression has been reported to subside as the depression is successfully treated. The observed changes in immunity may be mediated, in part, by increased blood levels of cortisol, or by autonomic influences on lymphoid tissue; however, other variables, such as smoking, alcohol consumption, diet, and sleep, are less easily measured or controlled. Further work is necessary to determine the mechanisms of the frequently observed correlation between major depression and suppressed measures of immune function in many depressed patients.

PSYCHOACTIVE DRUGS AND IMMUNE FUNCTION A number of commonly prescribed psychoactive drugs alter various parameters of immune-cell numbers and function in both humans and laboratory animals. Of these, only lithium consistently enhances immune function. Although in a few studies no immune effects from lithium treatment were reported, the vast majority of studies reported that lithium treatment enhances almost every measured parameter of immune activity. These parameters include lymphocyte response to mitogens, immunoglobulin synthesis, stem-cell proliferation, and leukocyte counts. In addition, there are several reports of decreases in HSV activity, upper respiratory infection, and other infections during lithium treatment. In fact, lithium has received much attention as a possible treatment for chemotherapy-induced leukopenia, which is usually reversed by lithium treatment. These immuno-enhancing effects may result from decreased suppressor T-cell activity. One adverse effect of this heightened immune activity is the occurrence of thyroid symptoms. It was found in one study that one-third of the tested outpatients under long-term lithium therapy showed the presence of antithyroid autoantibodies. Of these patients with antithyroid autoantibodies, one-quarter had goiter.

Many other psychoactive drugs have been found to inhibit different parameters of immune function to varying degrees. The drug that has received the most attention in this regard is chlorpromazime (Thorazine). In the most optimistic reports, it has been concluded that chlorpromazine induces only a transient decrease in leukocyte numbers, which rarely persists. In the majority of studies, adverse effects of chlorpromazine treatment have been reported. These have included decreased percentage and number of T-lymphocytes, decreased antibody production, decreased immunogen clearance from the blood, formation of antinuclear antibodies, inhibited lymphocyte responses to T- and B-cell mitogens, and a 20 to 30 percent decrease in DTH response. Another frequent finding is the presence of lupus-like circulating anticoagulant factors in chlorpromazine-treated patients. For example, in one study of 75 schizophrenic patients, among those treated with chlorpromazine for more than 2½ years, two-thirds had antinuclear antibodies and antinucleoprotein antibody; among all chlorpromazine-treated patients, one-third had significant depression in T-cell numbers. These authors concluded that extended chlorpromazine treatment produces one or more immune abnormalities in most patients. The clinical implications of these immune abnormalities are not yet well established. Many other antipsychotic drugs, including haloperidol (Haldol), trifluoperazine (Stelazine), and fluphenazine (Prolixin, Permitil), have been reported to suppress one or more parameters of immune function.

Treatment with tricyclic antidepressants at clinical dose levels has not been correlated with impaired in vivo immunity, although agranulocytosis and leukopenia have been reported occasionally as side effects. Leukopenia is also occasionally reported in patients treated with monoamine oxidase inhibitors. Interpretation of in vivo antidepressant effects is complicated by the evidence that drug-free depressed patients frequently show alterations in immune functions and in distribution of immune-cell subsets. In a recent in vitro study, desipramine (Norpramin), imipramine (Tofranil), and amitriptyline (Elavil) were examined for possible effects on NK-cell activity. Desipramine reversibly inhibited NK-cell activity at drug concentrations found in the serum of drug-treated patients, whereas the other two drugs were inhibitory at higher concentrations.

Some anxiolytics have also been tested for possible immune effects. The immune effects of benzodiazepine treatment have usually been tested in mice, and the results have varied. Future investigations may further clarify whether these apparent drug-induced alterations in immune function significantly affect disease resistance.

REFERENCES

Ader R, editor: *Psychoneuroimmunology*. Academic Press, Orlando, FL, 1981.

Ader R, Cohen N: CNS-immune system interactions: Conditioning phenomena. Behav Brain Sci *8:* 379, 1985.

Bennett C B, Bulloch K, Fox B H, Janković B D, Kerza-Kwiatecki A P, Monjan A A, Spector N H, Pierpaoli W, editors: *Neuroimmunomodulation: Proceedings of the First International Workshop on Neuroimmunomodulation,* International Working Group on Neuroimmunomodulation. National Institutes of Health, Bethesda, MD, 1985.

Cooper E L, editor: *Stress, Immunity, and Aging*. Marcel Dekker, New York, 1984.

DeLisi L E, Crow T J: Is schizophrenia a viral or immunologic disorder? Psychiat Clin N Amer *9(1):* 115, 1986.

Fabris N, Garaci E, Hadden J, Mitchison N A, editors: *Immunoregulation*. Plenum, New York, 1983.

Fox B H, Newberry B H, editors: *Impact of Psychoendocrine Systems in Cancer and Immunity*. C J Hogrefe, Lewiston, NY, 1984.

Frederickson R, Hendrie H C, Hingtgen J N, Aprison M H, editors: *Neuroregulation of Autonomic, Endocrine, and Immune Systems*. Martinus Nijhoff Publishing, Boston, 1986.

Goetzl E J, volume editor: Neuromodulation of immunity and hypersensitivity. J Immunol *135* (suppl): August 1985.

Guillemin R, Cohn M, Melnechuk T, editors: *Neural Modulation of Immunity*. Raven Press, New York, 1985.

Janković B D: From immunoneurology to immunopsychiatry: Neuromodulating activity of anti-brain antibodies. Int Rev Neurobiol *26:* 249, 1985.

Janković B D: Neuroimmune interactions: Experimental and clinical strategies. Immunol Letters *16:* 341, 1987.

Janković B D, Marković B M, Spector N H, editors: Neuroimmune interactions: Proceedings of the Second International Workshop on Neuroimmunomodulation. Ann NY Acad Sci. *496:* 1, 1987.

Korneva E A, Klimenko V M, Shkhinek E K: *Neurohumoral Maintenance of Immune Homeostasis*. University of Chicago Press, Chicago, 1985.
Lee S W, Tsou A-P, Chan H, Thomas J, Petrie K, Eugui E M, Allison A C: Glucocorticoids selectively inhibit the transcription of the interleukin 1-beta gene and decrease the stability of interleukin 1-beta mRNA. PNAS *85:* 1204, 1988.
Livnat S, Felten S Y, Carlson S L, Bellinger D L, Felten D L: Involvement of peripheral and central catecholamine systems in neural-immune interactions. J Neuroimmunol *10:* 5, 1985.
Lloyd R: *Explorations in Psychoneuroimmunology*. Grune & Stratton, New York, 1987.
Locke S E, Ader R, Besedovsky H, Hall N, Solomon G, Strom T, editors: *Foundations of Psychoneuroimmunology*. Aldine, Hawthorne, NY, 1985.
Locke S E, Hornig-Rohan M, editors: *Mind and Immunity: Behavioral Immunology*. Institute for the Advancement of Health, New York, 1983.
Neuroimmunomodulation. J Neurosci Res *18:* 1, 1987.
Pert C B: The wisdom of the receptors: Neuropeptides, the emotions, and bodymind. Advances *3:* 8, 1986.
Plotnikoff N P, Faith R E, Murgo A J, Good R A, editors: *Enkephalins and Endorphins: Stress and the Immune System*. Plenum, New York, 1986.
Smolensky M H, Reinberg A, editors: *Chronobiology in Allergy and Immunology*. Charles C Thomas, Springfield, IL, 1977.
Stein M, Schleifer S J, Keller S E: Psychoimmunology in clinical psychiatry. In *Psychiatry Update*, vol 6, R E Hales, A J Frances, editors, p 210. American Psychiatric Press, Washington, DC, 1987.

1.13 CHRONOBIOLOGY

DAVID B. JARRETT, M.D., Ph.D.

INTRODUCTION

The environment is predictably periodic, with day following night as reliably as spring follows winter. Inasmuch as living organisms have evolved in this rhythmic milieu, it should not be surprising that they have developed behavioral and physiological rhythms as part of their adaptation to the environment. These biological rhythms are pervasive in nature and were first formally described in 1729 by Jean Jacques d'Ortous de Marian, who observed that the heliotrope plant exhibited periodic leaf movements that persisted even in constant dark conditions. Over the past 250 years, it has become accepted that living organisms have an internal time-keeping mechanism, which serves two important physiological functions. The first, rather similar to the conductor of an orchestra, ensures that there is internal synchrony within the organism, and the second ensures that the organism remains synchronized with the environment in which it is living. Biological rhythms are ubiquitous and are recognized as patterns of behavior, such as the rest-activity cycle, reproductive cycle, and metabolic rhythms. *Chronobiology* has emerged as the scientific study of these biological rhythms and the mechanisms whereby they are regulated.

As already indicated, biological rhythms reflect the predictably rhythmic environment, and they have surprisingly stable periods, which may be shorter than (ultradian), the same as (circadian), or longer than (infradian) the 24-hour day. Although much attention has been focused on daily rhythms, there has been a growing interest in rhythms with annual cycles. The latter, which are typically associated with specific behaviors, such as migration or hibernation, also have physiological correlates that serve an important adaptive function. Since these rhythms track environmental time cues so accurately, it could easily be assumed that they are passive reflections of such periodic environmental changes as day length or seasons. However, it has been clearly shown that this is not the case because they persist in the absence of any external time cues. In addition, these rhythms are expressed in animals that have been bred under constant laboratory conditions in which there has been no exposure to their rhythmic natural environment. Perhaps even more striking is the fact that these rhythms breed true and persist as if the animals were living in the field. There can be little doubt that these endogenous rhythms are innate and allow the species to anticipate predictable changes in the environment, and, hence, they must have considerable survival value.

This internal temporal organization is a clear indication of how biological systems have adapted to and synchronized with the environment. The concept of internal constancy or homeostasis, as developed by Claude Bernard in 1878, should be revised to include both the programmed rhythmic changes in the internal milieu that anticipate the predictable events in the environment and the regulatory processes that modify the physiological responses to unpredictable events. In the latter case, strong negative feedback modulation ensures that random perturbations in the internal milieu are damped out and that biological rhythms are accurately preserved. The internal milieu of most organisms is obviously not constant, but varies in a highly ordered temporal fashion—a concept that has been termed "predictive homeostasis." Such homeostatic regulation in the healthy organism implies a high degree of order and synchronization both within and between each physiological regulatory system. The behavior observed in all living organisms is therefore a synthesis of the biological rhythms that are driven by the programmed endogenous time-keeping mechanisms and the adaptive behavior of the organism as dictated by the demands of the environment. In this context, it is important to point out that biological rhythms modulate the perception of external cues, as well as the behavioral and physiological responses to them. Thus, the responses elicited by a given stimulus will depend on the timing of the stimulus in relation to the endogenous biological rhythms.

The fact that biological rhythms are remarkably stable and appear to be independent of feedback control protects the biological clock from perturbations caused by adaptive homeostatic responses and ensures the predictive ability of the rhythm. In addition, the biological pacemaker is protected from unscheduled environmental perturbations and, in many species, is temperature-compensated. There is some evidence, however, that the hormonal milieu may modulate the circadian system, and, hence, the system may tend to become less stable with increasing age. It is reasonable to expect that disturbances in the regulation of these biological rhythms (as occurs in jet lag and shift work) will result in pathophysiological changes that may ultimately manifest themselves as clinical illness in the susceptible human.

PROPERTIES OF BIOLOGICAL RHYTHMS

All rhythms are part of a time series and have a characteristic period, amplitude, and waveform. The *period* is the time for one complete cycle of the rhythm (i.e., peak to peak); the

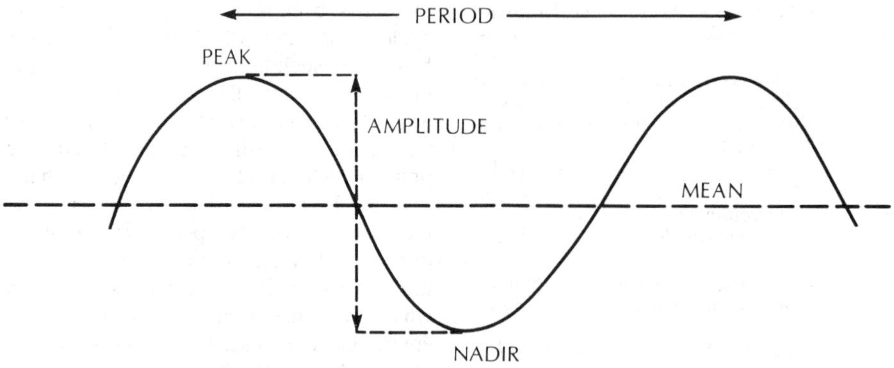

FIGURE 1.13-1. *Idealized biological rhythm showing the period (time from peak to peak), amplitude (peak to nadir deviation), and the mean value. In a cosinor analysis, the acrophase is the fitted peak value, the mesor is the mean of the fitted curve, and the amplitude is traditionally half of the deviation from the fitted peak to the fitted trough.*

amplitude is the measure of the rhythmic change (i.e., the deviation from the peak to the trough); and the *mean* is the average value across the rhythm (Fig. 1.13-1). The *phase* of the rhythm defines a point on the rhythm relative to an independent reference marker (e.g., the position of the peak relative to a predetermined time point). The period of the rhythm determines whether the rhythm is circadian (20 to 28 hours), ultradian (< 20 hours), or infradian (> 28 hours).

To characterize a biological rhythm fully, it is necessary to sample frequently across several cycles of the rhythm. This represents a major difficulty in clinical studies, although it is less of a problem in animal studies. Longitudinal sampling in the same animal is preferred, and the data gathered are then frequently analyzed using the cosinor technique.

The *cosinor technique* is an inferential statistical method in which it is assumed that the errors in the measurements are independent and identically distributed. The analysis provides a probability value that indicates the significance of the fit of the data by the method of least squares to a cosine curve. Three rhythm parameters can be derived from the cosinor analysis: The *acrophase,* which is the fitted peak value, can be referenced to an independent time point to characterize the phase of the rhythm; it frequently, but not always, corresponds to the maximum measured value. The *mesor* is the mean of the fitted cosinor curve, and the *amplitude* (as defined using the cosinor technique) is the distance between the mesor and the acrophase, which is actually half the peak-to-trough deviation. Biological rhythms invariably hold specific and reproducible phase relationships to each other, as judged by the relative positions of their acrophases.

CIRCADIAN RHYTHMS

The daily light-dark cycle is the most obvious environmental rhythm, and daily—or circadian—rhythms are present in most biological systems. In higher organisms, biological rhythms are most easily recognized as patterns of behavior; however, as the science of chronobiology has progressed, it has become apparent that these behavioral rhythms frequently have physiological substrates and correlates that can only be exposed experimentally. Some of the circadian rhythms that have been described include the sleep-wake cycle, body temperature regulation, patterns of activity, such as eating or drinking, and hormonal secretion. It is important to recognize that these rhythms, though synchronized with the environment, persist under constant conditions in the absence of any external time cues. This implies that the biological rhythms must be driven by an internal time-keeping mechanism. Bearing in mind the complexity of higher organisms, it is implicit that this time-keeping mechanism coordinate the internal milieu and, at the same time, synchronize the internal rhythms with the external environment.

The search for the circadian time-keeping mechanism or *pacemaker* started with the endocrine system, but when these rhythms persisted despite endocrine ablation, attention focused on the nervous system. By a long process of elimination, it was eventually established that destructive lesions in the ventromedial hypothalamus eliminated circadian patterns in activity, feeding, and drinking behavior in blinded rats maintained in a time-free environment (free-running condition). As will be discussed later, the neural substrate for the circadian system has been established, and then neurochemical and neurophysiological studies followed. Nevertheless, the mechanism whereby circadian signals are generated and propagated has not been established.

Although a biological clock permits the organism to anticipate predictable daily changes in the environment, this internal clock has an intrinsic period that does not accurately match the 24-hour rhythm of the environment. Indeed, it has been shown that it is advantageous for the intrinsic period of a pacemaker to differ from 24 hours, in order both to maintain a stable phase relationship with the environment and to adapt to alterations in the duration of the light cycle (photoperiod). The temporal organization of the internal milieu also depends on these pacemakers, which generate a rhythmic output. The critical component in the stability of circadian rhythms is the input to the pacemakers, which ensures that it and the internal milieu remain synchronized to each other and to the environment. As with all time-keeping mechanisms, there is a need for regular adjustment to keep the biological clock synchronized with the environment. In this regard, a variety of temporal environmental cues, such as the light-dark cycle and social contact, provide important circadian input to the clock.

THE SUPRACHIASMATIC NUCLEI

Following the identification of the central role of the hypothalamus in the regulation of circadian rhythms, it became apparent that there must be a neural pathway to provide temporal environmental cues to the hypothalamus. Eventually a *retinohypothalamic tract* (RHT) was identified. This is a unique monosynaptic projection from the retina to the *suprachiasmatic nucleus* (SCN) located in the ventromedial hypothalamus of the rat. It was subsequently found that bilateral destruction of the SCN resulted in the disappearance of the circadian pattern of corticosterone secretion in the rat. At the same time, it was found that bilateral lesions in the SCN also destroyed the classical circadian patterns of activity and drinking behavior in the rat. It is now clear that a large number of behavioral and physiological circadian rhythms are sustained by the SCN. The integrity of at least one SCN is essential for the coordination and the temporal organization of circadian rhythms. Bilateral destruction of the SCN in primates, rats, and hamsters, followed by exposure to constant conditions, results in disorganization of both behavioral and physiological circadian rhythms. Thus, the sleep-wake cycle, activity and drinking patterns, heart rate, and food intake are disrupted, as are the neuroendocrine rhythms in growth hormone secretion, glucocorticoid secretion, and *N*-acetyltransferase activity in the pineal gland. This disorganization of circadian rhythms is frequently associated with the appearance of ultradian rhythms. This association suggests that the SCN should be viewed as the coordinator and pacemaker of a potentially multioscillatory system.

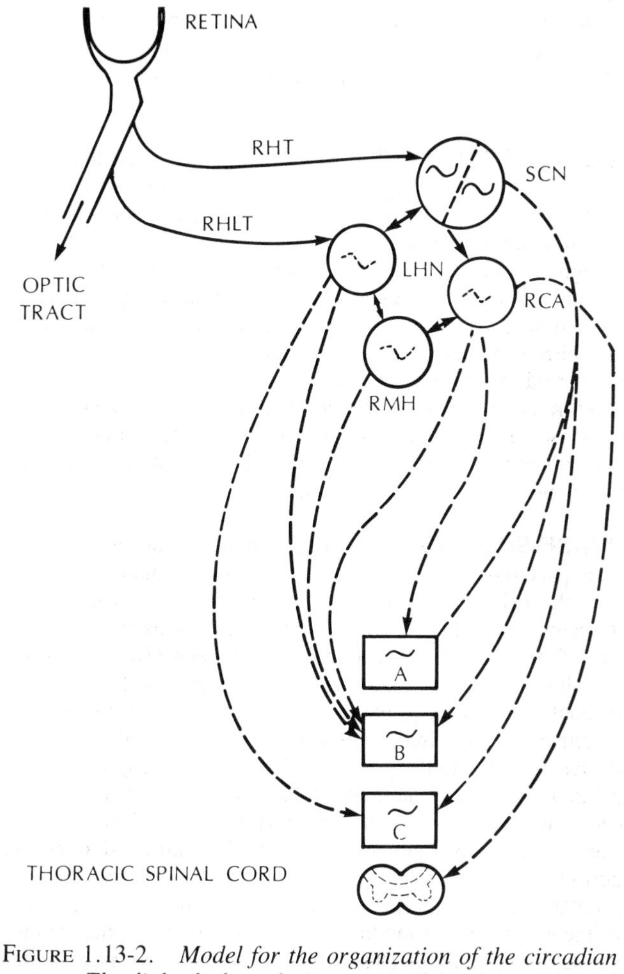

FIGURE 1.13-2. *Model for the organization of the circadian system. The light-dark cycle is perceived by the retina and information is relayed through the optic nerves and chiasm via the retinohypothalamic tract* (RHT) *and the retinolateral hypothalamic tract* (RHLT). *The RHT terminates in the ventrolateral region of the suprachiasmatic nucleus* (SCN). *Additional input to the SCN comes from lateral hypothalamic nuclei* (LHN) *which receive input from the RHLT, the ventromedial nucleus* (VMN), *and nuclei in the retrochiasmatic area* (RCA). *The efferent pathways pass to hypothalamic structures* (ABC), *which then function as secondary oscillators, being paced by the SCN. There is also a direct projection from the RCA to the interomediolateral cell column in the thoracic spinal cord. (Adapted from Moore R Y: The suprachiasmatic nucleus and the organization of a circadian system. Trends Neurosci* 5: *404, 1982.)*

NEUROANATOMY OF THE SUPRACHIASMATIC NUCLEI The SCN are small, bilaterally symmetrical nuclei that lie above the optic chiasm on either side of the third ventricle in the ventral hypothalamus. The nerve cell bodies comprising the nuclei are small (5 to 15 μm) and, in many species, are tightly packed, especially in the dorsomedial region. The nuclei receive fibers from the retina through the RHT, which is a bilateral projection from the optic chiasm. The RHT terminates in the ventrolateral aspect of the nucleus, with a preponderance of fibers coming from the contralateral retina. This is the most important afferent pathway for the regulation of circadian rhythms and is functionally distinct from the visual pathways. Lesions that destroy the RHT disrupt entrainment of the circadian system by the light-dark cycle. However, lesions in the optic pathways rostral to the optic chiasm are without effect on this entrainment, even though animals with these lesions are blind and have no visually guided behavior. The importance of this tract is underscored by the observation that it is an invariable feature of the mammalian visual system and is present in all mammals that have been studied.

Two other major afferent pathways have a functional role in the overall regulation of the circadian system. One of these originates in the raphe nuclei of the midbrain and the other is a bilateral projection from the ventral lateral geniculate nuclei; both of these projections also terminate in the ventral portion of the SCN. The nucleus receives additional inputs from other subcortical areas, and these inputs appear to play a modulating role. There are also projections between the nuclei, which probably serve to couple the circadian oscillators. The efferent pathways from the SCN are predominantly restricted to the hypothalamus, passing to the contralateral SCN and to the anterior, tuberal, retrochiasmatic, and periventricular regions of the hypothalamus, where they play a major role in determining the patterns of neuroendocrine and other physiological rhythms.

These data have been used to develop a neuroanatomical model for the organization of the circadian system, which involves pathways for signal transmission, processing, and output (Fig. 1.13-2). It has been suggested that the dorsomedial and ventrolateral components of the SCN function as coupled oscillators. The ventrolateral region receives the visual afferents and is the locus of entrainment. Apparently, efferent projections arise from both regions and permit separate control over different circadian rhythms.

DISTRIBUTION OF NEUROTRANSMITTERS IN THE SUPRACHIASMATIC NUCLEI The dorsomedial and ventrolateral regions of the SCN are distinguished by cell morphology, dendritic arborization, and immunohistochemically distinct cell populations. The dorsomedial region contains small bipolar neurons, which stain for vasopressin, somatostatin, and enkephalin-like material. In contrast, the ventrolateral region has larger multipolar neurons with extensive dendritic arborization and receives the retinal input. These cells stain for vasoactive intestinal peptide, bombesin, and neurotensin-like material, γ-aminobutyric acid (GABA) is distributed throughout the nucleus, and there are many local circuits. Studies of the afferent connections have shown that the projection from the raphe nuclei is predominantly serotinergic and that from the lateral geniculate nucleus contains neuropeptide Y. The neurotransmitter involved in the RHT is not known. Timed injections of neuropeptide Y into the area of the SCN in the hamster produce phase shifts consistent with a regulatory role for this peptide in the circadian system.

NEUROPHYSIOLOGY OF SUPRACHIASMATIC NUCLEI As would be expected of any intrinsic pacemaker, isolated SCN are capable of generating spontaneous rhythmic neural activity under constant conditions. Rhythmic multiunit activity has been recorded in isolated hypothalamic islands, an experimental procedure that effectively abolishes circadian rhythmicity in other parts of the brain. The activity within these islands can be entrained to the light-dark cycle, provided the neural connection between the SCN and the retina is intact. Spontaneous rhythmic activity within the SCN therefore can be modulated by the light-dark cycle, with activity being greatest during the day. Single-cell recordings from the SCN also show spontaneous rhythmic neural activity. This activity is entrained to the light-dark cycle in which the animals had been living. These studies have shown that this rhythmic activity is an intrinsic property of the SCN, and the rate of firing increases in response to light stimulation of the retina. Consistent with the neuroanatomical distribution of cells within the SCN, there appears to be a functional lateralization within the nucleus, with most of the spontaneous activity in the cells of the dorsomedial region. In addition, direct electrical and chemical stimulation of the SCN in the rodent is associated with a phase shift in the circadian system.

Further evidence for the primary role of the SCN in the regulation of the circadian system comes from the observation that not only is there spontaneous rhythmic neural activity within the SCN but also rhythmic metabolic activity. By the use of ^{14}C-2-deoxyglucose in either constant conditions or in a light-dark cycle, it has been shown that metabolic activity is highest during subjective day consistent with the increased neural activity recorded at that time.

ENTRAINMENT OF CIRCADIAN RHYTHMS

From a teleological perspective, biological rhythms serve an adaptive function, ensuring that the behavior and physiology of the organism are synchronized with the periodic environment. In the absence of any temporal or social cues from the environment, the circadian pacemaker will express its intrinsic period. This experimental condition is accomplished by placing an animal in temporal isolation with constant low-level lighting and allowing it to self-select meal and sleep times. Under these conditions, an animal is said to *free-run;* it is presumed that the monitored behavior and physiological parameters are being driven by the endogenous pacemaker. The expressed circadian period should be the intrinsic period of the pacemaker and is invariably longer than 24 hours. Indeed, in the largest reported study of humans, the mean free-running circadian period was found to be about 25 hours. This finding implies that there must be a coupling mechanism that links the pacemaker to the environment, and, therefore, time cues are perceived and registered, and the rhythms are synchronized with the environment. The process by which these biological rhythms are synchronized with the environment is termed *entrainment,* and the term *zeitgeber* (time giver) is used to describe the environmental time cues that synchronize these biological rhythms. The light-dark cycle is the most obvious circadian zeitgeber, although there are clearly multiple temporal cues in the environment.

To be classified as a zeitgeber, an environmental timing cue must reset and synchronize (i.e., entrain) a biological rhythm. This is usually demonstrated by exposing a free-running organism to the potential zeitgeber. The biological rhythm should synchronize with the zeitgeber so that their periods match and a stable phase relationship develops between the zeitgeber and the biological rhythm. Entrainment requires that the rhythm must be reset and synchronize with the zeitgeber. Following removal of the zeitgeber and exposure of the entrained organism to constant conditions, it should free-run from a phase position determined by the zeitgeber (i.e., the entrained rhythm) and not the rhythm prior to exposure to the zeitgeber.

If entrainment does not occur, then the biological rhythm has not been reset by the environmental cue, and under constant conditions, the organism will free-run from a position that would have been predicted from the rhythm prior to exposure to the new environmental time cue. The conclusion is that the intrinsic rhythm has been unaffected by the weak environmental cue, although the cue can still influence the expression of the rhythm.

There are two possible effects of an environmental cue on a biological rhythm. First, a weak environmental cue may interact with a biological rhythm and alter the phase without resetting the rhythm. This produces an apparent phase shift, so the rhythm appears to be synchronized with the environmental cue. However, on removal of the cue, the rhythm immediately reverts to its previous period and phase. This phenomenon has been termed *relative coordination.* Second, an environmental cue may have no effect on the phase of the rhythm and only distort the shape of the rhythm. On removal of the environmental cue, the biological rhythm immediately reverts to its previous period and phase, indicating that the environmental cue has simply distorted or *masked* the underlying rhythm.

RANGE OF ENTRAINMENT As might be expected, there are limits to the influence a zeitgeber can exert on a pacemaker. For every zeitgeber there is a range of periods over which it can entrain a biological rhythm. This means that even though a zeitgeber may be effective at certain times in the circadian period, as judged by the phase shift it produces; at other times, it is without effect. The maximum phase shift a zeitgeber can produce will determine the effective limits for the period to which a pacemaker can be entrained. This range of entrainment of a biological rhythm is determined by the response of the pacemaker to the zeitgeber; moreover, the strength of a zeitgeber is defined by the maximum phase shift it can produce within the circadian period.

PHASE SHIFTING If the endogenous period of the circadian pacemaker is 25 hours, the zeitgeber must be strong enough to shift the acrophase of the rhythm by 1 hour so that it occurs earlier than it would if the animal was free-running. This shift means that the acrophase has been *phase advanced* by 1 hour each day to maintain entrainment to a 24-hour day. In contrast, if the acrophase was shifted to a later time than would occur in a free-running condition, it would be *phase delayed* relative to the predicted time of its appearance. If the zeitgeber is actually able to produce a phase shift of 2 hours each day, then the limit of entrainment will be 23 to 27 hours. That is, the circadian system could be entrained over the period ranging from 23 to 27 hours and synchronized with such artificial environments. If the animal is exposed to a zeitgeber period outside this range, entrainment to that zeitgeber is not possible. The range of entrainment is also dependent on the intensity of the zeitgeber. It appears that the closer the zeitgeber is applied to the limit of entrainment, the stronger it needs to be to have any effect. In this regard, it has been shown that the range of entrainment to light can be extended in the human by increasing the intensity of the stimulus. Once outside the range of entrainment, a rhythm will continue to free-run, although it may be influenced or masked by external time cues.

ENTRAINING CUES As already indicated, in the absence of any time cues, biological rhythms express an intrinsic period; therefore, the pacemakers must be reset on a daily basis to maintain entrainment. Thus, for pacemakers with an intrinsic period shorter than that of the zeitgeber, the phase reference point would be reached earlier. Such a rhythm is phase advanced and must be delayed to maintain entrainment. The reverse is true for rhythms having intrinsic periods greater than that of the environmental time cue, and these rhythms must be phase advanced to maintain entrainment. The mechanism whereby this occurs is dependent on the phase relationship between the zeitgeber and the pacemaker, as well as on the strength of the zeitgeber and the sensitivity of the pacemakers to the zeitgeber.

It has become clear that there is a rhythm in the sensitivity of the pacemaker to the zeitgeber and, therefore, depending on when it is applied, it may produce a phase delay, phase advance, or be without effect. For light, subjective dawn and dusk have emerged as the critical times, with dawn being associated with a phase advance and dusk with a phase delay. The circadian system is relatively insensitive to light during daylight hours. The relationship between a zeitgeber and the phase shift it produces can be displayed graphically (Fig. 1.13-3), and such *phase response curves* have been established for a variety of species. These are difficult experiments because the animal should be in constant dark and free-running at the time of exposure to the zeitgeber pulse and again immediately afterward. This exposure will be followed by some transient disruption in the free-running rhythm before the new phase position will be clearly expressed. The zeitgeber pulse can be quite short and a phase shift can be produced by a single light pulse applied at a critical time in the circadian period.

In mammals, the light-dark cycle perceived by the retina appears to be the major circadian regulatory input or zeitgeber. In the presence of the zeitgeber, the SCN is entrained to the environmental input; however, in the absence of any zeitgebers, the SCN paces the endogenous biological rhythms at its own intrinsic rate. Using this model, any failure in entrainment would be due to either inadequate zeitgeber input, inadequate signal processing by the SCN, or failure in the output transmission from the SCN.

DEVELOPMENT OF CIRCADIAN RHYTHMS The SCN appears late in gestation, and metabolic studies using ^{14}C-labeled 2-deoxyglucose have demonstrated rhythmic metabolic activity in the SCN of fetal rats. This metabolic activity is in phase with that of the maternal SCN, with high activity during the day and reduced activity at night. This activity is paced by the maternal SCN, which is entrained by the environmental light-dark cycle, and ablation of the maternal SCN disrupts the timing of the developing fetal pacemaker. During the perinatal period, the maternal circadian system coordinates the circadian system of the neonate until it begins to react to the light-dark cycle. In the rat, the entrainment of the fetal SCN to the light-dark cycle occurs via the maternal circulation. The maternal circadian system entrains the SCN to the environment in both pre- and postnatal development. The subsequent development of biological rhythms and internal temporal organization is an ordered postnatal event. It appears that, in the human, there is a hierarchy in the development of rhythmic activity, starting with body temperature and followed by the sleep-wake cycle, which begins to appear earlier than it becomes entrained. The neuroendocrine rhythms appear later. It is apparent that animals do not need to experience 24-hour light-dark cycles during development to show circadian rhythms as adults. The implication is that the neuronal substrate of the SCN arises as genetically determined oscillators that become coupled during late development. In humans, the development of circadian rhythmicity depends more on maturity than on the time of exposure to environmental stimulation. Circadian rhythmicity is innate, as is the mechanism of entrainment. Free-running by neonates even in the presence of a light-dark cycle underscores the independence of rhythm generation from the environment.

MATHEMATICAL MODELS OF THE CIRCADIAN SYSTEM As the physiology of the circadian timing system has been unraveled, mathematical models inevitably would be developed in an attempt to describe biological rhythms, particularly those with a circadian period. Based on experimental data in the human, two different models have been proposed (Fig. 1.13-4).

The first model uses two coupled oscillators to explain the phenomenon of spontaneous internal desynchronization, which has been described in some human subjects maintained in temporal isolation for long periods of time. In this situation, there is a spontaneous

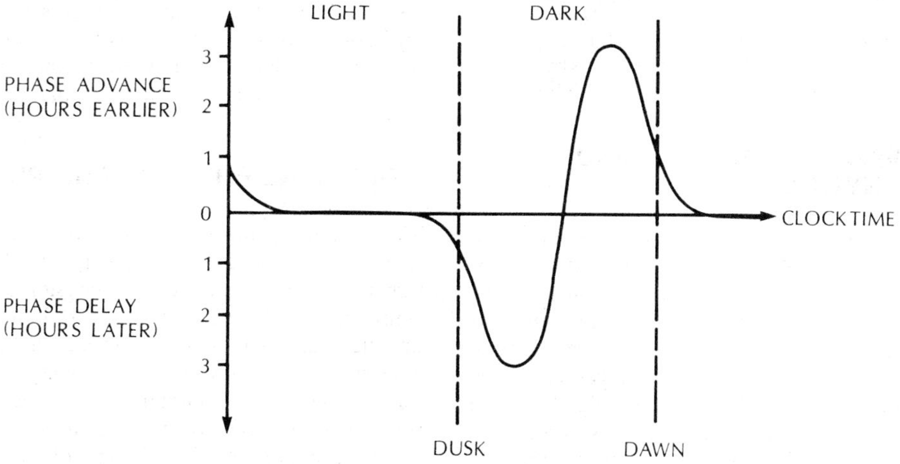

FIGURE 1.13-3. *Phase response curve for light as determined in most species. Free-running animals in constant dark are exposed to brief light pulses at discrete times during the circadian period and then allowed to free-run in constant dark. After the transients have been resolved, the new phase position of the rhythm is determined and plotted against the circadian period. In both diurnal and nocturnal animals, dusk is associated with a phase delay and dawn with a phase advance. The circadian system is insensitive to light pulses during the subjective day.*

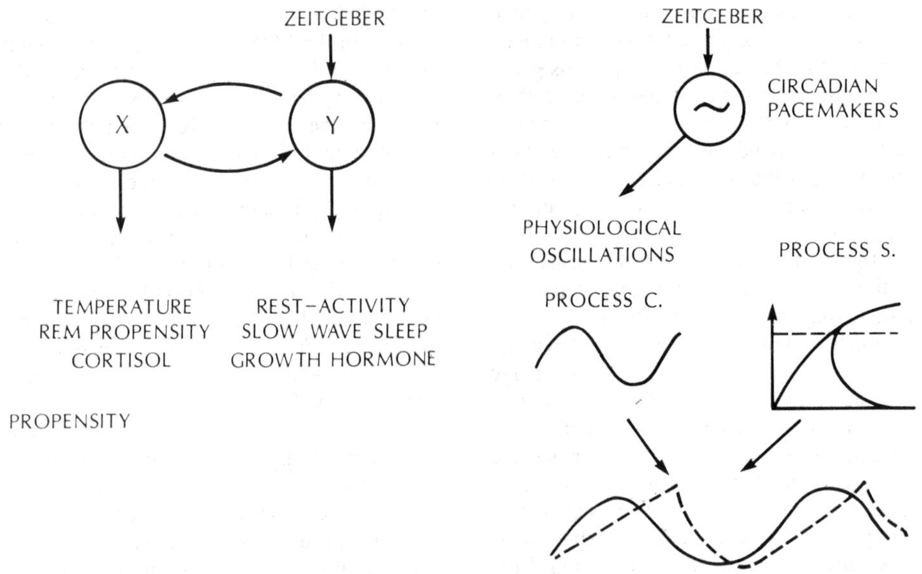

FIGURE 1.13-4. *Schematic representations of two mathematical models for the circadian system. On the left is the model showing two mutually coupled oscillators. The stronger X oscillator is coupled to the weaker Y oscillator, which, in turn, is coupled to the environmental zeitgebers. On the right, the alternate model envisages a circadian pacemaker that is coupled to environmental zeitgebers (process C). This pacemaker is entrained and the rhythms are represented by circadian physiological oscillators. In addition, there are a series of relaxation oscillators (process S) that generate tension over the circadian period. Once a threshold is reached, these oscillators decay, provided that process C is permissive.*

disassociation between the sleep-wake cycle and the rhythm in core body temperature, with the latter having a period of 24 to 25 hours and the former a period of approximately 33 hours. When desynchronized, the different circadian rhythms segregate into two clusters. The two-oscillator model suggests that there are two groups of circadian rhythms, each being driven by a separate, yet coupled, oscillator. Rapid eye movement (REM) sleep propensity, core body temperature, and cortisol secretion are driven by a strong oscillator. The other group of rhythms, typified by the rest-activity cycle, growth hormone secretion, and slow-wave sleep, are driven by a weaker oscillator, which is coupled to environmental zeitgebers.

The alternative model uses only one oscillator and a series of relaxation oscillators. This model invokes a multiple-oscillator concept, but utilizes only a single circadian pacemaker. In either case, it must be recognized that these models are mathematical and do not necessarily have any physiological substrate. It is clear that both models invoke at least one oscillator that is entrained directly by the environmental zeitgeber. As models, they permit the development of experimental protocols that can be used to test their validity.

PHOTOPERIODISM, SEASONALITY, AND CIRCANNUAL RHYTHMS

Although much attention has been focused on the circadian system, there are obviously other biological rhythms, many of which are infradian. Of these, the circannual rhythms may be the most prominent, and the presence of such rhythms was suggested by the expression of seasonal patterns of behavior in animals deprived of environmental photoperiodic time cues. The most obvious examples are the migratory and hibernating behaviors exhibited by some animals during predictable times of the year. There is little doubt that the seasonal changes in metabolism, reproduction, and behavior are determined by an endogenous circannual timing mechanism, which persists under constant conditions. As with the circadian system, the periods of these rhythms deviate from 12 months, and the need for an entrainment process is implied.

In addition to circannual cycles, most biological systems also display periodic changes that reflect alterations in the duration of light (photoperiod) to which the animal is exposed. These seasonal changes in photoperiod are best exemplified by the mammalian reproductive cycle. It is well known that gonadal regression is induced in hamsters by short photoperiods, and recrudescence takes place in long photoperiods. Initially, it was believed that it was the amount of light that determined the photoperiodic response, but it is now clear that the determinant is where the light falls in the circadian cycle. In addition to the circadian component, the pattern of the circadian secretion of melatonin by the pineal gland is instrumental in transducing photoperiodic information into physiological regulation. It is generally believed that the temporal pattern of melatonin secretion is important in determining photoperiodic responses, particularly in the hypothalamic-pituitary-gonadal axis. Thus, for the hamster, short photoperiod melatonin secretion is antigonadal.

BIOLOGICAL RHYTHMS AND PSYCHIATRY

There are many medical implications for chronobiology, and it is not unreasonable to expect that chronobiological disturbances are associated with physiological and behavioral consequences. In the human, most biological rhythms pass unnoticed unless they are perturbed, as happens in some disease states or shift work or following rapid transmeridianal travel. Under these circumstances, the intrinsic biological rhythms of the sleep-wake, performance, and cognitive ability cycles become exposed, and many of the psychological symptoms the human experiences, such as jet lag, can be presumed to occur because there is a mismatch between the internal biological rhythms and environmental time cues. Under these conditions, reentrainment will take place, but this does not happen rapidly, and it may be several days before the circadian system is once again synchronized with the environment. It must be remembered from the phase response curve that phase delaying a rhythm (as must happen following westward transmeridianal travel) is generally more rapid than a phase advance, because the endogenous period in the human is 25 hours and, thus, favors a phase delay.

PHASE ABNORMALITIES IN DEPRESSION Although some biological rhythms are easily exposed, others, such as core body temperature and hormone secretion, can be exposed only by sophisticated measurements. Notwithstanding, it is becoming clear that some, if not all, patients with a major depressive illness have a reversible disruption in the physiological regulation of the sleep-wake cycle and reductions in the amplitudes of the body temperature rhythm and circadian neuroendocrine secretory profiles. It can therefore be postulated that a depressive illness is frequently associated with a pathophysiological disturbance in the regulation of circadian biological rhythms. Much emphasis has been placed on dysregulation in the hypothalamic-pituitary-adrenal axis, but there are also disturbances in the regulation of the sleep-wake cycle and in the circadian secretion of growth hormone, prolactin, thyrotropin, and melatonin.

Two chronobiological hypotheses have been developed in an attempt to explain the biological disturbances described in depressed patients. Both hypotheses have focused mainly on disturbances in the sleep-wake cycle. The *phase advance hypothesis* suggests that the apparent phase shifts in the distribution of REM sleep, motor activity, cortisol secretion, and core body temperature result from a generalized phase advance of rhythms in depression. The phase advance hypothesis predicts an advance of the strong oscillator with respect to the weaker oscillator and the environment.

The other hypothesis focuses on the disturbance in slow-wave sleep seen in depressed patients. This hypothesis attributes the decrease in slow-wave sleep to a decline in process S (sleep propensity), which can best be modeled as a relaxation oscillator, whose tension increases during the waking period and decays during sleep. According to this model, depression is associated with a deficiency in process S that results in light, fragmented sleep, decreased slow-wave sleep, and a short REM latency. This hypothesis fails to explain why antidepressants prolong REM latency, but are not associated with an immediate increase in slow-wave sleep.

If the mood disorders are associated with disturbances in the regulation of the circadian system, it is reasonable to assume that treatment should be directed toward reentrainment. In the first instance, it can be argued that the nature of the chronobiological disturbance, if any, should be defined. Although a phase response curve for light has not been developed in the human, it is reasonable to assume that morning light will phase advance while evening light will phase delay. Indeed, when this principle is applied as light therapy to depressed patients with significant disturbances in the regulation of their sleep-wake cycle, many of them recover in 5 to 7 days. This recovery is sustained by continued exposure to bright light at dawn and at dusk.

Alternatively, sleep deprivation may also be invoked in much the same way, and this would be consistent with the hypothesis suggesting that there is a disturbance in the regulation of the sleep-wake cycle in depressed patients. It has been reported that phase delaying the sleep-wake cycle through sleep deprivation is associated with short-term remission from a depressive illness. Finally, antidepressant medications, including lithium ions, have been shown to slow the biological clock, again suggesting that this might be an important component in their therapeutic action.

REFERENCES

Aschoff J, editor: *Handbook of Behavioral Neurobiology*. Plenum, New York, 1981.

Bunning E: *The Physiological Clock*. Springer-Verlag, New York, 1973.

Daan S, Beersma D G M, Borbely A A: Timing of human sleep: Recovery process gated by a circadian pacemaker. Amer J Physiol *246:* 161, 1984.

Gillin J C: Sleep studies in affective illness: Diagnostic, therapeutic and pathophysiological implications. Psychiat Ann *13:* 367, 1983.

Karsch F J: Seasonal reproduction: A saga of reversible fertility. Physiologist *23:* 29, 1980.

Krieger D T, editor: *Endocrine Rhythms*. Raven Press, New York, 1979.

Moore R Y: The suprachiasmatic nucleus and the organization of a circadian system. Trends Neurosci *5:* 404, 1982.

Moore R Y, Card J P: Visual pathways and the entrainment of circadian rhythms. Ann NY Acad Sci *453:* 123, 1985.

Moore-Ede M C: Physiology of the circadian timing system: Predictive versus reactive homeostasis. Amer J Physiol *250:* R735, 1986.

Moore-Ede M C, Czeisler C A, editors: *Mathematical Models of the Circadian Sleep-Wake Cycle*. Raven Press, New York, 1984.

Moore-Ede M C, Czeisler C A, Richardson G S: Circadian timekeeping in health and disease. New Eng J Med *309:* 469, 1983.

Moore-Ede M C, Fuller C A, Sulzman F M: *The Clocks That Time Us*. Harvard University Press, Cambridge, MA, 1982.

Richter C P: *Biological Clocks in Medicine and Psychiatry*. Charles C Thomas, Springfield, IL, 1965.

Robertson L M, Takahashi J S: Circadian clock in cell culture: I. Oscillation of melatonin release from dissociated chick pineal cells in flow-through microcarrier culture. J Neurosci *8:* 12, 1988.

Rusak B, Zucker I: Neural regulation of circadian rhythms. Physiol Rev *59:* 449, 1979.

Stephan F K, Zucker I: Circadian rhythms in drinking behavior and locomotor activity of rats are eliminated by hypothalamic lesions. Proc Nat Acad Sci USA *69:* 1583, 1972.

Takahashi J S, Zatz, M: Regulation of circadian rhythmicity. Science *217:* 1104, 1982.

Turek F W: Circadian neural rhythms in mammals. Ann Rev Physiol *47:* 49, 1985.

Wehr T A, Goodwin F K, editors: *Circadian Rhythms in Psychiatry*. Boxwood Press, Pacific Grove, CA, 1983.

Wever R A: *The Circadian System of Man*. Springer-Verlag, New York, 1979.

Zucker I: Motivation, biological clocks, and temporal organization of behavior. In *Handbook of Behavioral Neurobiology*, E Satinoff, P Teitelbaum, editors, p 3. Plenum, New York, 1983.

1.14 NEURONAL DEVELOPMENT AND PLASTICITY

ANTHONY M. ADINOLFI, Ph.D.
WILLIAM J. FREED, Ph.D.

INTRODUCTION

This section will focus on the development of the central nervous system (CNS) and on the principles underlying neuronal plasticity during development and following brain injury. It is not intended as an exhaustive review of neuroembryology or of factors underlying structural and functional recovery. Instead, emphasis is placed throughout on defining, with appropriate examples from experimental literature, basic principles of neuronal development and on discussing current concepts of how the CNS responds to injury.

The cytoarchitecture of the mammalian brain is organized such that the more than 10 billion neurons occupy unique spatial distributions, and groups of cells constitute systems that subserve specific functions. Within these systems, neurons receive information along their dendritic and somatic surfaces, integrate and modify this information, and then transmit signals to target cells via their axons. This highly ordered morphology of neurons and their interconnections is called *neural specificity*. *Neural plasticity*, during development or recovery from injury, refers to events related to the establishment and maintenance of neural circuits that subserve specific functions. The questions as to how such specificity of structure and function arises during development and how stable these neuronal patterns are in the mature brain will be explored and emphasized in subsequent subsections.

DEVELOPMENT OF THE CENTRAL NERVOUS SYSTEM

The CNS is derived from a thickened area of embryonic ectoderm called the neural plate. In humans, formation of plate neuroectoderm is induced during the third embryonic week by, as yet poorly understood, factors from underlying notochordal and paraxial mesoderm. Immediately after formation, the neural plate is organized into discrete focal regions that are predestined to develop into the major parts of the brain.

Experiments with disaggregated mesodermal and ectodermal cells cultured at different ages suggest the involvement of one factor that primes the dorsal ectoderm to become the neural plate and another factor that, at different concentrations, determines the different brain regions. Thus, the neural plate becomes divided into subfields. Removal of an entire subfield from one embryo and transplantation into another will result in a permanent defect (e.g., forebrain missing) in the donor brain and in duplication of the transplanted part in the host brain. Once regional designation is assigned, it is permanent. By the middle of the fourth embryonic week, the neural plate has undergone an invagination midsagittally to form a neural groove, which subsequently fuses middorsally to form the neural tube.

Following the induction of the neural plate and the formation of the neural tube, regional specialization occurs, which begins near the end of the fourth week with the appearance of three primary brain vesicles called the prosencephalon or forebrain, mesencephalon or midbrain, and rhombencephalon or hindbrain. During the fifth week, the forebrain expands and divides into a telencephalon (which gives rise to the cerebral cortex and the basal ganglia) and a diencephalon (which gives rise to the thalamus and the hypothalamus). The midbrain remains unchanged, and the hindbrain divides into the metencephalon (pons and cerebellum) and the myelencephalon (medulla oblongata). These secondary swellings or vesicles result from rapid and disproportionate cell proliferation within the walls of the cephalic end of the neural tube. The caudal part of the neural tube gives rise to the spinal cord.

PROLIFERATION AND MIGRATION OF NEURONS

Theories about the origin of neuronal and glial cell lines have changed considerably during the past century. In the last decades of the nineteenth century, neurons and glial cells were thought either to arise from two separate cell lines or from a single line of precursor cells that separated after migrating away from the ventricular zone. Introduction of *thymidine autoradiography* in the 1960s led to the conclusion that neurons arise first, and, when neurogenesis is complete, dividing cells give rise to glial cells. Current techniques that employ cell-specific markers, such as *neuron-specific enolase* (NSE) and *glial fibrillary acidic protein* (GFAP), provide recent evidence that nerve and glial cell precursors coexist in the ventricular zone from the earliest developmental stages. Postmitotic cells migrate from proliferative zones in the ventricular and subventricular layers of the neural tube to form various brain regions, where they mature and establish synaptic connections. In a process similar to amoeboid movement, migrating cells are directed to their definitive locations in developing cerebellar and cerebral cortices along glial processes, which extend radially from the ventricular zone to the pial surface. Most radial glial cells are transitory, disappear after neuronal migration, and may become astrocytes. Support for the role of radial glial processes or fibers in migration stems from ultrastructural observations that neurons are intimately associated with glial fibers during migration and from studies of the Reeler mutant strain of mice in which the cerebellum and forebrain are malformed. Here, young neurons are arrested in their migration along radial glial fibers and later arriving neurons are unable to migrate into the cortical plate.

AGGREGATION AND MATURATION OF NEURONS

Once migrating neurons reach their proper location, they aggregate to form either laminar or nuclear masses. Cells of similar embryonic origin selectively adhere to one another, and when cell cultures from different brain regions are dissociated and mixed, they reaggregate only with cells from the same source. Often, these cells share a common birth date, which is defined as their last mitotic division and determined by thymidine autoradiography. Factors that promote aggregation of cells are believed to be large molecules on the cell surfaces that recognize and bind to similar cells. They are called cell surface ligands, and their specificity probably results from the presence of different ligands for different cell types. Two specific ligands, a retinal binding factor and a cerebral binding factor, have been identified for neurons of the retina and the cerebral cortex and have been shown to be associated with surface glycoproteins.

With few exceptions, most neurons generate their processes after migration to their final position in the CNS. Dendritic arborizations of neurons are genetically determined, and neurons grown in isolation have dendritic branching patterns that closely resemble those seen in the intact brain. Their final form is modified by local influences, such as the numbers and distribution of their axonal inputs. For example, Purkinje cell dendrites have a characteristic planar organization and are oriented perpendicular to their major axonal input, the parallel fibers of granule cells. If this input is disrupted, as seen in several mutant strains of mice (Weaver, Reeler, Staggerer) with granule cell depletion, Purkinje cell dendritic branching is much reduced and their planar organization is disordered.

AXONAL ELONGATION AND THE FORMATION OF SYNAPTIC CONNECTIONS The development of complex, yet highly specific, synaptic connections in the CNS is probably mediated by diffusible substances that guide growing axons to appropriate target neurons. The existence of such chemotrophic molecules was implied by early studies that showed that neuron survival depended on interaction with target tissues and that failure to establish appropriate synaptic connections led to cell death during development. With the discovery of nerve growth factor (NGF) nearly 40 years ago came evidence that growth and survival of neurons in sensory and sympathetic ganglia were mediated by diffusible molecules—in this case, a complex protein. Over the years, experiments have shown that natural and induced (by axon section) cell death was prevented by application of NGF; that exposing embryos to antiserum to NGF blocked the development of the sympathetic nervous system; and that NGF influences the direction of neurite outgrowth in tissue culture and, thus, may help shape synaptic interactions in the developing peripheral nervous system.

The trophic effects of NGF may not be limited to cells of neural crest origin, such as the catecholamine-containing neurons in sympathetic ganglia or the neurons in dorsal root ganglia. Although NGF has no effect on catecholaminergic neurons in the brain, it does act on cells that contain acetylcholine, such as those found in the basal forebrain and the septum. NGF increases the concentration of the enzyme choline acetyltransferase in these neurons, and antiserum to NGF recently has been shown to inhibit development of cholinergic neurons in fetal, but not in more mature, basal forebrain. Thus, NGF may be needed for the development of cholinergic neurons in the embryonic brain.

The search for other trophic factors has provided preliminary information on several substances that seem to promote survival of neurons and outgrowth of neurites in tissue culture. Factors that promote neurite outgrowth in culture may act directly on target cells or may stimulate extension of processes by modifying adhesion to the substrate. NGF is representative of the type of factor that acts directly on the growth cones at the ends of neurites. Neurite-promoting factors that enhance binding of cells to substrate have been found to be produced by chick cardiac muscle cells, bovine corneal endothelial cells, glial cells, and tumor cells (PC12 pheochromocytoma and schwannoma). These factors are normal constituents of the extracellular matrix, and analysis of their trophic properties suggests that most of the neurite-promoting activity is due to one of the components called laminin. When laminin is inactivated by antiserum, the neurite-outgrowth-promoting activity of these factors is lost.

Following the outgrowth of axons to the vicinity of their target sites, specificity of their synaptic connections is most likely achieved by recognition of surface molecules analogous to the trophic factors that allow axons to find appropriate pathways to target sites. Recognizing that the ability of axons to grow during development may be regulated by neurite-promoting glycoproteins located in the extracellular matrix, it has been postulated that the extracellular surfaces of synaptic membranes may contain a unique array of glycoproteins within the synaptic cleft that enhance synapse formation.

Axonal outgrowth during regeneration provides additional information about the behavior of growing axons. Peripheral axons regenerate after they are severed and often reinnervate their normal target tissue. However, severed central axons extend only short distances beyond a lesion and fail to reestablish appropriate synaptic connections. Nevertheless, central axons can grow long distances after injury, as has been shown by studies in which segments of sciatic nerves were transplanted to bridge central lesion sites in the brain or spinal cord. In these transplanted pieces of peripheral nerve, the axons degenerate and only the sheath (Schwann cell and basal lamina) remains. Apparently, this material forms an excellent substrate for the growth of brain axons, just as it does for axons of the peripheral nervous system. Therefore, the growth of neurites appears to be just as or more dependent on the substrate (i.e., the terrain to be traversed) as on the properties of the cells themselves.

Although the interaction of nerve cell surfaces with the surrounding environment plays a major role in determining whether nerve cells will grow and extend neurites, unquestionably there are internal events that also regulate the production of neurites by nerve cells. For example, when segments of peripheral nerve were implanted into the brain, the growth of some types of cells was stimulated, whereas other types of nerve cells that were equally close to the transplant were unaffected. Thus, various properties of nerve cells themselves—not only of their external environment—influence whether growth of neurites will occur.

Although relatively little is known about substances that influence nerve cells, it is becoming clear that they may have two kinds of effects. Some substances seem to increase the growth of neurites, whereas others specifically promote the survival of nerve cells. Although NGF has both kinds of effects, most other substances have only one. At least one substance that has nerve cell survival-promoting effects is produced following injury to the brain. The presence of this substance was initially detected in an experiment in which injury was induced in rats by removal of a part of the cerebral cortex. A piece of gelatin sponge was placed in the wound cavity and later removed. When pieces of this conditioned sponge were then placed into culture dishes with nerve cells, survival of the nerve cells was greatly enhanced. Secretion of this substance reaches a maximum at about 10 days after brain injury. Tissues transplanted into the site of an injury survive best when the transplantation also takes place 10 days after the injury. Similar substances are found in the cerebrospinal fluid of patients who had recently suffered brain injury. Perhaps secretion of such substances by the injured brain serves to protect nearby uninjured brain cells from secondary damage resulting from loss of their connections with the cells that have been directly injured or destroyed.

NEURONAL PLASTICITY DURING DEVELOPMENT

Accumulating evidence indicates that, under varying conditions, the CNS alters its structural and functional organization. This capacity for change, called neuronal plasticity, serves as a mechanism to shape neuronal circuitry during development, to change the way information is processed, and to compensate for injury. Morphological plasticity includes the adjustments to neuronal death and synapse elimination during development, as well as collateral sprouting of axons and reactive synaptogenesis following partial denervation of selective brain regions. Functional plasticity includes long-term postsynaptic potentiation and kindling. Both phenomena involve lasting changes in neuronal responses to stimulation and have served as models for learning at the synaptic level.

NEURONAL DEATH AND SYNAPSE ELIMINATION

During development, most regions of the CNS undergo a period of neuronal degeneration and death. Cell death occurs naturally and not only helps to determine the final size of a particular neuron pool and its projection field, but also helps to eliminate those neurons whose connections are inappropriate or temporary. In addition, selective elimination of axon collaterals and terminal branches without death of the parent cell helps to adjust the final wiring of synaptic pathways. These changes generally occur about the time when synapses are formed and are most likely the result of competition for limited target sites. Cell death reduces the population of neurons initially generated, and synapse elimination helps to determine the final number of axons that will contact each target cell. For example, a striking feature of the synaptic circuitry in the cerebellar cortex is that a single, climbing fiber contacts each Purkinje cell. In newborn rats, however, about half the Purkinje cells receive multiple climbing fibers and the one-to-one relationship becomes established by the second postnatal week. There is also ultrastructural evidence that about 50 percent of synapses degenerate spontaneously and are removed from spinal motor neurons during the second postnatal week.

Synaptic rearrangement hallmarks the development of the visual system. During embryonic and early postnatal periods, retinal projections redistribute from all parts to selective layers of the lateral geniculate nucleus. Likewise, neurons of the primary visual cortex are arranged in ocular dominance columns, such that discrete columns are dominated alternately by inputs from the right and left retinas in adults, whereas in fetal and newborn brains there is overlap of right and left retinal inputs to these columns.

COLLATERAL SPROUTING AND REACTIVE SYNAPTOGENESIS Neurons in many regions of the developing and mature CNS are capable of reorganizing or establishing new synaptic connections in response to injury. This process involves the formation of new preterminal axon branches (collateral sprouting), which form synaptic contacts at denuded sites (reactive synaptogenesis). These events are best illustrated where one of two convergent synaptic inputs has been interrupted. They were described, initially, following partial deafferentation of the septal nuclei and confirmed by similar studies of the optic tectum, red nucleus, and hippocampus. For example, retinal projections end, normally, in superficial layers, and visual cortical projections terminate in deeper layers of the superior colliculus. If one eye is removed at birth, the visual cortex sprouts to superficial layers; if the visual cortex is ablated at birth, retinal projections sprout to the deeper layers.

In the red nucleus, cerebellar inputs terminate on cell bodies and proximal dendrites, whereas projections from the sensorimotor cortex end on distal dendrites. Following destruction of the deep cerebellar nuclei, collateral sprouting of axons from cerebral cortex and formation of physiologically active synapses along somatic and proximal dendritic surfaces of rubral neurons occur. Finally, the dentate gyrus of the hippocampal formation receives ipsilateral input via the perforant pathway from the entorhinal cortex. These axons end on distal dendrites of granule cells, whereas association and commissural fibers from the contralateral hippocampus end on proximal dendrites of granule cells. Destruction of the ipsilateral entorhinal cortex results in sprouting of commissural and association fibers, which then reinnervate distal granule cell dendrites.

FUNCTIONAL PLASTICITY Functional plasticity of neuronal connections is evidenced by long-term postsynaptic potentiation and by kindling. *Long-term potentiation* consists of increased postsynaptic responses to a given stimulus, following a short train of high-frequency stimulation. *Kindling* is a process of repetitive stimulation, over long periods of time, which alters the pathway so that a stimulus that originally produced only a weak response then becomes able to trigger widespread seizure activity and convulsive behavior. Both long-term potentiation and kindling have served as models for learning at the synaptic level. Increased calcium ion concentration and increased neurotransmitter release from presynaptic axon terminals, coupled with increased sensitivity of postsynaptic receptors, may explain long-term potentiation. As yet, there is no clear explanation of the substrates underlying the kindling phenomenon. There is some evidence that activity in excitatory pathways is enhanced. For example, the entorhinal cortex sends a large excitatory projection to distal dendrites of granule cells in the ipsilateral dentate gyrus. Following daily stimulation for 21 days, the excitatory postsynaptic potentials are increased in strength. This change in activity of target cells is independent of input, and target cells retain their transformed properties after input has been excised. If kindling is established by perforant path stimulation and the entorhinal cortex is subsequently excised, the contralateral entorhinal cortex sprouts to fill some of the denuded distal dendritic sites. When the contralateral entorhinal cortex is stimulated, the kindled granule cells still produce convulsive discharges.

Finally, the environment in which an animal is reared influences neuronal morphology. It has been shown that the behavioral development in rats, which occurs postnatally and progresses from acquisition of simple reflexes to complex motor skills, corresponds with increases in the numbers of dendritic spines and increases in the size and thickness of their synaptic junctions. If newborn animals are subjected to enriched or complex environments, dendritic development and synaptic connectivity are stimulated. Conversely, rearing animals in deprived surroundings retards the development of axo-dendritic connectivity.

RECOVERY FROM CENTRAL NERVOUS SYSTEM INJURY

SIMPLER SYSTEMS Although the issue of recovery from injury to the mammalian brain is very complex, it is clear that substantial regrowth occurs following injury to the nervous system of lower animals and following injury to the peripheral nervous system of mammals. For example, the spinal cord of amphibia and the optic nerve of fish can regenerate successfully after being completely severed. Such complete regeneration of the spinal cord and optic nerve does not occur in mammals. The axon in mammals is completely dependent on the cell body for survival. But, in some lower animals, such as the leech, the axon can survive being completely severed from the neuronal cell body and eventually may become reunited with the parent cell.

In contrast, injured tracts in the mammalian CNS do not regenerate, except under unusual circumstances. In mammals, the simplest components of the nervous system, the peripheral nerves, show the most vigorous regeneration. The peripheral nerves have a relatively simple internal structure. These nerves consist of neurites, the Schwann cells, and the myelin produced by Schwann cells, as well as the basal lamina that covers each neurite. Within a peripheral nerve, there are no neurons or interconnections between adjacent cells, and each myelin-producing cell is dedicated to only one neurite.

When a mammalian peripheral nerve is crushed, but not completely severed, it will regenerate rapidly and effectively, resulting in an almost complete return of sensory and motor function. When the same nerve is severed completely, it will also regenerate rapidly but, in most cases, sensory and motor function will not recover or will recover only partially. This functional failure appears to be due to misrouting or scrambling of the regenerating axons; that is, even though the axons regenerate, individual axons do not reach their correct targets. When the nerve is crushed instead of severed, however, the basal lamina sheath of each fiber is preserved, and this basal lamina guides the regenerating fibers to their correct targets, resulting in functional recovery. Techniques that enable completely severed rat peripheral nerves to be reconnected with good functional recovery have been developed recently. These techniques involve minimizing the disturbance at the point of transection by supporting the nerve with a rubber cuff, by cooling the nerve and simultaneously altering the extracellular medium by bathing the nerves in a fluid that resembles intracellular medium, and by trimming the ends of the nerve with a vibrating razor blade while the nerve is frozen to obtain a sharp, clean-cut surface. This method results in consistent functional recovery following sciatic nerve transection in rats.

Thus, cutting and repairing a peripheral nerve usually leads to regeneration without functional recovery. If a peripheral nerve is simply crushed instead of severed or repaired under carefully controlled conditions, however, the regeneration will be successful because scrambling or misrouting is avoided. It is important to note that regeneration alone is not sufficient; correct organization is also necessary.

FUNCTIONAL RECOVERY FOLLOWING BRAIN INJURY It has long been recognized that behavioral deficits that result from brain injury have a tendency to diminish with the passage of time. This is what is meant by the term "functional recovery." The opposite outcome, lesion-induced behavioral deficits that gradually increase in severity with the passage of time, is unusual. In the early part of the twentieth century, the possibility that functional recovery was due to regeneration of damaged parts of the brain was seriously considered. It has become clear, however, that true regeneration is unusual in the CNS of mammals except for unusual circumstances, such as after transplantation of embryonic brain tissue or peripheral nerve into the brain. Nevertheless, more subtle forms of restructuring, such as collateral sprouting, are common in the CNS following injury. Current theories of functional recovery from brain injury thus fall into two general categories: (1) theories suggesting that there is no essential alteration in the microstructure of the CNS during functional recovery, and (2) theories postulating that a structural alteration of CNS circuitry underlies functional recovery.

Diaschisis The theory of *diaschisis,* or neural shock, suggests that lesioning of one brain area causes a temporary impairment of the functioning of associated, but undamaged, brain regions. Functional recovery is suggested to be due to the return of normal functioning in these associated brain areas. This concept was originated by Constantin von Monakow in 1914. Although von Monakow was unable to define diaschisis in physiological terms, he did state that diaschisis was not the result of edema or similar phenomena, but was propagated via neuronal pathways. The existence of diaschisis as a physiological phenomenon has not been established; moreover, direct evidence for diaschisis as a mechanism of functional recovery from brain lesions is lacking. There are, however, a number of experimental results that are at least consistent with a diaschisis explanation. For example, in some cases the deficits resulting from certain lesions can be reversed by a subsequent (or even a prior) lesion of a different brain area. A well-known example is that of a soldier who was unable to speak following a brain injury. Although he was retrained by a person with a Yankee accent, when he learned to speak again, it was with his original southern accent. Such observations are most parsimoniously explained in terms of diaschisis.

Compensation Behavioral compensation theories suggest that, following brain injury, animals learn to utilize new behavioral strategies, sensory modalities, or different muscle groups to achieve goals. Such theories hold that there are no changes in the functioning of specific brain areas, but that the animal is simply optimizing the capacity of its remaining resources.

Related to behavioral compensation theories are neuronal compensation theories. Such theories suggest that behavioral functions are redundantly represented in the brain by more than one brain area or system. Destruction of one brain area may cause an initial disruption, but it eventually leads to substitution of function by redundant circuits that were not "on line" prior to the lesion.

Denervation supersensitivity Unquestionably, a major form of neuronal plasticity is *denervation supersensitivity*. In the peripheral nervous system, denervation supersensitivity is a ubiquitous and easily produced phenomenon. When the innervation of peripheral excitable tissues, such as smooth muscle or glandular tissue, is removed either pharmacologically as with reserpine or surgically by denervation, sensitivity to the natural transmitter is increased 10- to 1,000-fold.

The primary cellular change that is responsible for denervation supersensitivity is a proliferation of synaptic receptors. This change is not specific for the denervated neurotransmitter, in that removal of one neurotransmitter innervation will result in changes in the sensitivity of most or all of the agents to which that cell is responsive, including both neurotransmitter agonists and nonspecific excitants, such as potassium ions.

Many examples of denervation supersensitivity have also been found for the CNS. For example, dopaminergic supersensitivity of striatal neurons can be induced by removing the dopaminergic input to the striatum by lesioning the substantia nigra or by chronic administration of antipsychotic drugs, such as haloperidol (Haldol), which block dopamine receptors. The magnitude of changes in sensitivity observed in the CNS is generally smaller than that observed in the peripheral nervous system. This result may be understood in terms of the greater multiplicity of inputs that are received by central neurons. In other words, neurons in the CNS may be less likely to be drastically altered through the loss of any single input.

The possible relevance of these phenomena to neuronal plasticity is quite obvious. The functioning of a partially destroyed pathway conceivably might be restored as denervation supersensitivity develops.

Regrowth theories of recovery of function It has long been recognized that some abortive growth of neuronal processes does take place following CNS injury. During the past 15 years, it has also become recognized that a form of neuronal growth termed "collateral sprouting" is a major form of structural reorganization of the CNS following injury.

Following an injury, CNS neurites may grow in two quite different ways. Regeneration consists essentially of elongation of neurites more or less along their original paths, whereas collateral sprouting involves extension of axon collaterals along new pathways to fill in terminal fields vacated by a lesion. Thus, collateral sprouting leads to formation of new circuits that are different from the original. It would be more conducive to functional recovery if vacated target areas were refilled with their original inputs through regeneration; however, collateral sprouting can be thought of as an alternative to regeneration—one that may succeed when regeneration fails.

Although lesions in many, if not all, areas of the brain induce collateral sprouting, it has been very difficult to demonstrate in any specific instance that behavioral recovery is caused by collateral sprouting. In some studies, a temporal association between sprouting and lesion recovery has been found. The hypothesis that collateral sprouting and lesion-induced synapse formation contribute to functional recovery from lesions is both reasonable and attractive. Although there is some support for this hypothesis, it is not conclusive at the present time. Moreover, sprouting under some circumstances is thought to cause maladaptive behaviors or spasticity. Thus, at the present time, a best guess would be that collateral sprouting contributes to functional recovery in some circumstances, but may not be a general mechanism for recovery of function.

Environmental enrichment and training effects One of the first studies of the effect of environmental enrichment reported that rats raised in enriched conditions (as pets) showed improved maze-learning performance as compared with rats raised under normal laboratory conditions. Later studies reported an increase in weights of the cerebral cortices of rats raised in enriched environments. Other studies have also reported increased rates of incorporation of amino acids into protein as well as a variety of other changes in animals raised in enriched environments. These changes are relatively general; that is, they are not specific for any single brain constituent, nor are these changes restricted to any single area of the brain.

Very few studies have investigated the effects of environmental enrichment on recovery from brain damage. One recent study employed the Morris water maze to assess recovery of function following cortical damage. Rats that were housed in an enriched environment (an outdoor enclosure) after cortical lesions showed substantially improved maze-learning performance compared to animals housed under deprived laboratory conditions. However, environmental enrichment did not alter the performance of neonatally lesioned rats.

There are very few controlled studies of effects of environmental enrichment or specific postlesion training on recovery from brain lesions in humans. This literature does suggest (1) that training following brain injury is most effective when instituted as soon as possible after the injury occurs, and (2) that the effects of training are relatively nonspecific; in other words, training does not selectively influence the skills that are retrained, but acts more as a general activation effect.

MANIPULATION OF NEURONAL PLASTICITY

A great deal of interest has been sparked recently by developments in the area of brain tissue transplantation, although, as early as 1917, there had been reports that brain tissue, as well as tissues from other parts of the body, could survive transplantation into the brain. In the early 1970s, several investigators began to explore the issue of brain tissue grafting and found that embryonic brain tissue, in particular, was amenable to transplantation.

INTRAOCULAR GRAFTING The anterior chamber of the eye is very similar to the brain as a site for tissue transplantation and has been a valuable model system. Transplantation of tissues to the anterior eye chamber permits studies of tissue development and trophic interactions. The presence of the iris as a target tissue also permits studies of neurite growth and reinnervation of the iris. For example, locus ceruleus grafts in the anterior eye chamber were found to innervate approximately one-third of the host iris. Sympathectomy did not alter this pattern. Severing the trigeminal nerve, however, caused the locus ceruleus grafts to reinnervate nearly the entire iris. Subsequent studies suggested that trigeminal nerve section caused a release of trophic substances in the iris that stimulate neurite growth from the locus ceruleus.

NIGROSTRIATAL SYSTEM The nigrostriatal dopamine system consists of dopamine-containing neurons located in the substantia nigra and the ipsilateral dopamine-containing projection to the corpus striatum. In animals, bilateral destruction of this system causes a syndrome of aphagia, adipsia, akinesia, and rigidity, leading to death within 1 to 2 weeks. Unilateral destruction of this system causes postural and sensory asymmetry, which can be accentuated by dopamine agonists, such as amphetamine and apomorphine. The resulting rotational behavior is frequently employed as a test for the severity of unilateral substantia nigra lesions. In humans, damage to this system causes Parkinson's disease.

The nigrostriatal system was chosen for many of the initial studies of brain tissue transplantation. It is possible to restore the dopaminergic innervation to the striatum by transplanting embryonic substantia nigra near the striatum, either to the lateral ventricle, to cavities in the cerebral cortex, or directly into the striatum as dissociated cells. These grafts have been shown, in a number of different experiments, to reverse or prevent many of the consequences of substantia nigra lesions in rats, including rotational behavior, sensorimotor neglect, adipsia, aphagia, and akinesia, depending on the transplantation technique employed. Recent preliminary reports also suggest that these techniques may be successful in primates.

ADRENAL MEDULLA GRAFTS A second means of producing recovery from substantia nigra lesions is through transplantation of adrenal medulla to the lateral ventricle. The chromaffin cells of the adrenal medulla produce dopamine as an intermediary in the synthesis of norepinephrine and epinephrine. After transplantation to the ventricle, the relative concentrations of dopamine in these cells is increased. Intraventricular adrenal medulla grafts also can decrease rotational behavior after substantia nigra lesions, but do not reinnervate the striatum. These grafts may function through secretion of catecholamines, which reach the striatum through diffusion or via the circulatory system.

Adrenal medulla grafts placed directly into the striatum survive poorly, both in rats and in primates. Such intrastriatal adrenal medulla grafts have been placed in patients with Parkinson's disease and transient clinical improvement has been observed. The fact that these improvements last no more than 1 month is consistent with the poor survival of adrenal medulla grafts in the striatum. However, there have been several recent reports of long-term improvement of patients with Parkinson's disease after adrenal medulla is transplanted into the striatum and exposed to the lateral ventricle.

SEPTOHIPPOCAMPAL CHOLINERGIC SYSTEM The cholinergic innervation of the hippocampus originates in the septum and reaches the hippocampus through the fimbria-fornix. This innervation can be removed by fimbria-fornix lesions. Analogous to nigro-striatal grafts, grafts of embryonic septum adjacent to the hippocampus can provide a new cholinergic innervation to the hippocampus and reverse some of the deficits in spatial maze performance caused by the lesions. These grafts also have been found to reverse spatial maze deficits in a subpopulation of aged rats with evidence of impaired hippocampal cholinergic function.

CORPUS STRIATUM GRAFTS Whereas Parkinson's disease is related to a loss of dopaminergic input to the striatum, Huntington's disease is characterized by a loss of neurons within the corpus striatum. A model of Huntington's disease in animals is produced by intrastriatal administration of the neurotoxins, kainic acid or ibotenic acid. Several investigators have reported that embryonic striatum transplanted into the damaged host striatum decreases the locomotor hyperactivity caused by these lesions. This finding has since been replicated by several other groups. This system is unusual in that these grafts were transplanted into the same location as the lesion. It is possible that these grafts in some way restored local circuits that were damaged by the lesions. It is also possible that grafts of this type act through secretion of a chemical substance that interacts with surrounding tissues or even through mechanical compression of the surrounding tissues. At present, the mechanism of action of brain tissue grafts in this system is unknown.

CORTICAL GRAFTS Embryonic neocortex is readily transplanted to the intact or lesioned cerebral cortex, and cortical grafts grow very large in comparison with other embryonic brain tissue grafts.

Lesions of the medial frontal cortex cause deficits in the performance of certain maze-learning tasks. Grafts of fetal cortex into the sites of these lesions have been found to improve behavioral performance on these tasks.

The fact that this effect was produced by late fetal grafts, but not by more immature tissue, suggested that something other than reinnervation was responsible for the behavioral effect. It recently has been found that grafts of glial cells into the site of cortical lesions produce behavioral recovery similar to that seen after brain grafts, which suggests that secretion of neurotrophic substances by these brain grafts is responsible for the behavioral effect.

REFERENCES

Ajmone-Marsan C, Matthies H, editors: *Neuronal Plasticity and Memory Formation*. Raven Press, New York, 1982.

Berg D K: New neuronal growth factors. Ann Rev Neurosci *7:* 149, 1984.

Bjorklund A, Stenevi U: Intracerebral neural implants: Neuronal replacement and reconstruction of damaged circuitries. Ann Rev Neurosci *7:* 279, 1984.

Cotman C W, editor: *Neuronal Plasticity*. Raven Press, New York, 1978.

Cotman C W, Nieto-Sampedro M: Cell biology of synaptic plasticity. Science *225:* 1287, 1984.

Cowan W M: Aspects of neural development. In *Neurophysiology III, International Review of Physiology,* R Porter, editor, vol 17, p 149. University Park Press, Baltimore, 1978.

Finger S, Almli C R: Brain damage and neuroplasticity: Mechanism of recovery or development? Brain Res Rev *10:* 177, 1985.

Fleming W W, McPhillips J J, Westfall D P: Post-junctional supersensitivity and subsensitivity of excitable tissues to drugs. Ergebn Physiol *68:* 55, 1973.

Freed W J, de Medinaceli L, Wyatt R J: Promoting functional plasticity in the damaged nervous system. Science *227:* 1544, 1985.

Greenough W T: Enduring brain effects of differential experience and training. In *Neural Mechanisms of Learning and Memory,* M R Rosenzweig, E L Bennet, editors, p 255. MIT Press, Cambridge, MA, 1976.

Haber B, editor: *Nervous System Regeneration*. Alan Liss, New York, 1983.

Hubel D H, Wiesel T N, LeVay S: Plasticity of ocular dominance columns in monkey striate cortex. Phil Trans Roy Soc London (B) *278:* 377, 1977.

Jessell T M: Adhesion molecules and the hierarchy of neural development. Neuron *1:* 3, 1988.

Levi-Montalcini R: The nerve growth factor: Its mode of action on sensory and sympathetic nerve cells. Harvey Lect *60:* 217, 1966.

Lund R D: *Development and Plasticity of the Brain. An Introduction*. Oxford University Press, New York, 1978.

Morell F, de Toledo-Morell L: Kindling as a model of neuronal plasticity. In *Kindling 3,* J A Wada, editor, p 17. Raven Press, New York, 1986.

Moscona A A: Surface specification of embryonic cells: Lectin receptors, cell recognition and specific cell ligands. In *The Cell Surface in Development,* A A Moscona, editor, p 67. Wiley, New York, 1974.

Rakic P: Organizing principles for development of primate cerebral cortex. In *Organizing Principles of Neural Development,* S C Sharma, editor, vol. 78, p 21. NATO ASI Series, Plenum, New York, 1982.

Teuber H-L: Recovery of function after lesions of the central nervous system: History and prospects. Neurosci Res Progr Bull *12:* 197, 1974.

Varon S, Manthorpe M, Williams L R: Neuronotrophic and neurite-promoting factors and their clinical potentials. Develop Neurosci *6:* 73, 1984.

Whishaw I Q, Zaborowski J-D, Kolb B: Postsurgical enrichment aids adult hemidecorticate rats on a spatial navigation task. Behav Neural Biol *42:* 183, 1984.

1.15 BASIC MOLECULAR GENETIC NEUROSCIENCE

FLOYD E. BLOOM, M.D.

INTRODUCTION

A genetic disease is one caused by variations in the chemical composition of genes, the basic units of heredity, that is sufficient to produce abnormal proteins (such as enzymes, intercellular signals, signal receptors, or structural proteins). Thanks to advances in molecular biology over the past decade, there has been rapid progress in the identification of many genetic abnormalities, not only at the functional level with detection of the specific abnormal gene products, but also at the level of abnormalities in the nucleic acid sequences of the gene itself and in the intermediary sequences of the messenger ribonucleic acid (mRNA). When applied to psychiatric diseases with a potential genetic basis, the ability to probe for fine features of genetic variation, therefore, can be applied at many molecular levels as well as at the more conventionally accessible levels of the gene products and the individual's phenotype (i.e., the expressed collection of genetic information, demonstrable as the physical makeup and behavior of the individual). Moreover, since all somatic cells more or less share the identical set of gene information, it is possible to probe for alterations in gene structure that affect the brain by examining the nucleic acid structure of peripheral cells, such as fibroblasts or white blood cells. This research capacity has greatly increased the sensitivity of detecting inheritable traits and also has widened the search for molecular explanations of these diseases.

In some cases, such as color blindness, hemophilia, or sickle-cell anemia, the genetic variation alone is sufficient to produce the disorder directly. In other cases, such as galactosemia or acute intermittent porphyria, certain exogenous dietary or environmental factors are required in addition to the abnormal gene to reveal the existence of the gene defect and defective gene product that results in disease.

Some genetic diseases can be successfully treated, whereas others are simply palliated; however, most remain untreatable. Nevertheless, even with no possibility of treatment, a rigorous genetic diagnosis can offer the patient or the patient's family insight into the cause of a disorder and provide a basis for genetic counseling of siblings and protection of future generations. Because of the complexity of the structural and chemical components of the brain, the function of this organ is highly susceptible to errors of genetic origin. However, many of these defects are so disruptive to the program of brain development that they are incompatible with survival. There is, at present, strong presumptive evidence of an inheritable basis for enhanced susceptibility to schizophrenia, mood disorders, psychosis, and alcoholism, even though the nature of the specific genes and gene products involved remains totally unknown. This section will consider the implications of genetically based psychiatric disorders in terms of the basic molecular analysis of the nervous system and complex behaviors.

GENETICS AND GENOMES

To appreciate the present state of genetic analysis of the nervous system with reference to psychiatric diseases, it is first necessary to review briefly some basic concepts of classical genetics as well as the modern molecular interpretation of those classical phenomena. The complete array of genetic information carried within every somatic cell of every organism is termed the *genome*. In humans, the genome consists of 22 pairs of chromosomes, called autosomes; these chromosomes show no sex-related differences. A twenty-third pair are the sex-determining chromosomes, X and Y, with females carrying XX and males carrying XY. Somatic cells, all of which carry the full complement of chromosomes, are termed *diploid;* that is, each chromosome exists as a pair, one of which was contributed by each parent's germ line. Dividing diploid cells maintain their diploidy through the process of mitosis, by which the genome is duplicated during the final stages of cell division. However, when spermatic or ovarian gametes undergo cell division in preparation for sexual reproduction, they execute a two-phase cell division process of meiosis, in which the pairs of chromosomes are separated into chromatids, and single sets of them (i.e., one of each of the 23 pairs) are included in each gamete (Fig. 1.15-1). The fusion of a haploid sperm and a haploid ovum into a fertilized zygote thus reunites the chromosomes into the full diploid number.

The laws of Mendelian genetics, first worked out more than 100 years ago on peas, established that there is a pair of *hereditary units,* later renamed *genes,* for each phenotypic trait (e.g., height, hair, eye and skin color, as well as many cognitive and emotional traits). Each member of a gene pair can exist in multiple alternative states, termed *alleles,* and each allele resides in an identical position on a particular

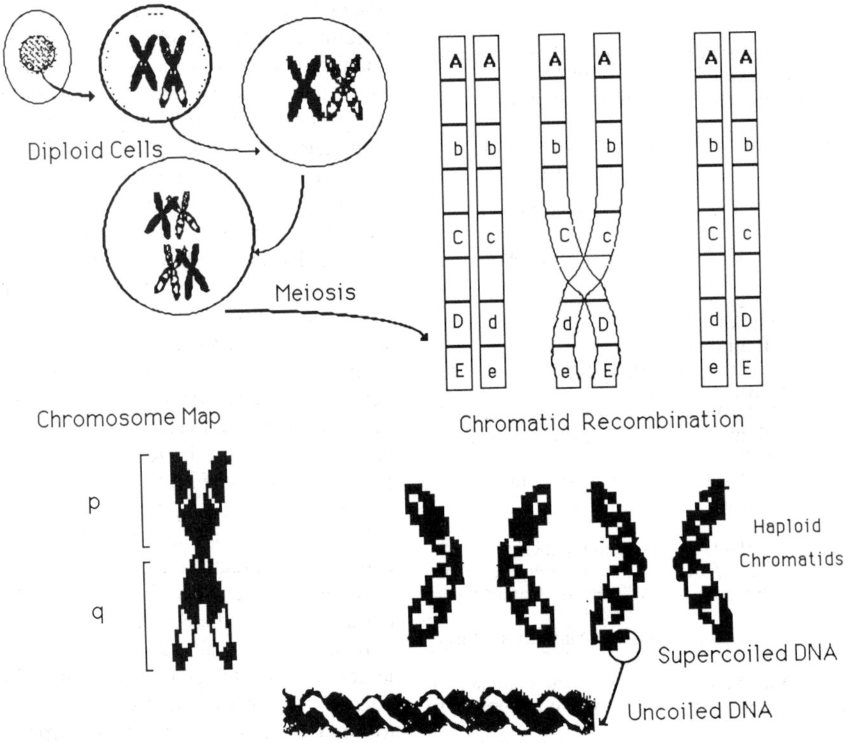

FIGURE 1.15-1. *A concordance among classical genetics, cell biology, and molecular analysis of the genome. Beginning at upper left, a typical active cell is shown with its chromatin dispersed. When cells can undergo cell division, which differentiated neurons cannot, the chromatin organizes into distinct chromosomes and replicates so that diploid cells maintain their full complement of 23 pairs of chromosomes. When germ cells undergo the two-phase process of meiosis, homologous chromosome pairs align, and homologous chromatids undergo contacts that can lead to recombination. At upper right is shown, in a more schematic fashion, adjacent zones of two chromatids bearing the genes for proteins* AA, bb, Cc, Dd, *and* Ee, *where* A–E *and* a–e *represent the dominant and recessive forms of the respective genes. Through crossover between the chromosome bands containing the genes for products* Dd *and* Ee, *the chromatids are reorganized such that the left chromatid carrying the alleles* A, b, *and* C *will now also contain* d *and* e, *rather than the* D *and* E *forms that originally existed. The complementary change has occurred through recombination on the right chromatid. When these chromatids now separate in meiosis, each chromatid in a haploid germ cell may pass on the new combination to the zygote if successful during fertilization. Below are shown more schematically a stained chromosome, with its paired short arms* (p) *and long arms* (q), *and the central centromere that connects the two illustrated chromatids. Individual haploid chromatids arising from this chromosome are shown at lower right. Should a sample of the supercoiled DNA within a chromatid be uncoiled from the chromatin threads, histones, and other nucleoproteins, the dual-helical chains of DNA can be recognized.*

member of a chromosome pair (Fig. 1.15–1). An individual is said to be homozygous for the trait when the two alleles are identical, and to be heterozygous when they are not. In heterozygous individuals, expression of one allele may dominate the other, accounting for dominant and recessive traits. A gene is termed *polymorphic* when two or more different alleles coexist in the population (e.g., the A, B, and D alleles of the human red blood cell groups). Polymorphisms are important exploitable attributes that are useful in gene-mapping studies.

In the early part of the twentieth century, microscopic observation of the giant chromosomes of drosophila, together with observation of the progeny, established that genes for physically detectable traits (e.g., eye color or wing shape) were linearly arranged on the chromosomes; during meiosis, genetic recombination could occur when adjacent members of duplicating chromosomes crossed over. The frequency with which the genes for specific traits remain linked through generations is inversely related to the distances that separate them on their chromosome; that is, closely spaced genes remain linked, but distantly spaced genes do not. The degree to which trait-controlling genes remain together through generations is exploited in the strategy of linkage analysis of genetic diseases, in which a trait (e.g., a particular human leucocyte antigen) or a functionally uncharacterized gene marker is correlated with the co-occurrence of the disorder. Since one member of each pair of alleles is contributed from each parent during fertilization, genetic recombinations that occur during meiosis can lead to extraordinary variation in the phenotypic expression of inherited traits (Fig. 1.15-1).

CHEMICAL STRUCTURE OF GENES

These general principles of Mendelian genetics and the ability of alleles to be segregated and sorted during meiosis independently of one another were well accepted by the 1920s. However, there was little progress in the genetic analysis of more complex biological problems and little understanding of the basis for the observable phenomena. Such remained the case until a resurgence of molecular research that began in the mid-1950s with the demonstration of the structure of the nucleic acid chains in deoxyribonucleic acid (DNA), which ultimately provided insight into how genetic information was encoded as well as decoded by the linear sequence of just four purine and pyrimidine bases. Molecular biological research further blossomed in the late 1970s with the recognition that genetic material from eukaryotes, higher animals, and bacteria could be combined experimentally to create new bits of genetic information and that these experimental engineering achievements could greatly facilitate analysis of gene expression and the identification of novel gene products, as well as markers of defective genes.

Based on those discoveries, it is possible to summarize current understanding of molecular genetic concepts as follows:

1. Genetic information is stored in the form of long, double-helical strands of DNA chains. Each individual neuron, or neuroglia, attains its specialized functional and structural status by expressing a subset of the genetic instructions contained in the genome that is identical to the genome in all other somatic cells. (Cells of the immune system offer a slight variation on this theme [Section 1.12].) In humans, it is estimated that each somatic cell carries about 6 feet of DNA, representing nearly 6 billion bases in length. To accommodate this much DNA within the nucleus of a cell that may measure less than 5 μm in diameter, the DNA chains are coiled and supercoiled around special protein elements of the nucleoplasm.

2. To express selective segments of the genome, the DNA-encoded information is converted, or transcribed, into a second similar molecular form as single strands of ribonucleic acid (RNA). Special proteins (RNA-synthesizing enzymes or polymerases) perform the transcription steps by opening the DNA double helix and reading the order of bases from the template strand (Fig. 1.15-2). It is hypothesized that specific sequences of DNA mark the initiation sites for transcription of the specific gene segments needed by specialized cell classes, such as those of the brain.

3. The primary RNA transcript of the selected genetic information is then edited. This process occurs in several rapid steps still under active investigation, during which the RNA is exported from the nucleus to the cytoplasm. The primary transcript—termed heterogeneous nuclear RNA (hnRNA) or, more descriptively, premessenger RNA—is longer than will be needed and contains segments of DNA transcription that have no known information.

4. The edited RNA transcript, or mRNA, is then translated by special cytoplasmic organelles, also made of RNA and proteins, called ribosomes (Fig. 1.15-3). Translation is a chemical language shift from the nucleic acid code of the RNA into the amino acid sequence of the protein that is to be expressed. Each set of three mRNA bases codes for an individual amino acid that is transported to the protein assembly site by another form of RNA, transfer RNA (tRNA). Since there are 64 possible combinations of triplet sets of the purine and pyrimidine bases and only 20 available amino acids, there is some redundancy in the amino acid codes for specific proteins. Other triplets code for the initiation of translation and for its termination.

5. In virtually all cells, the translated protein undergoes posttranslational processing. In neurons and other secretory cells, the structure of the protein may be modified to attain a folded, globular, or linear shape that allows it to become associated with the proper intracellular compartments (e.g., within the plasma membrane or within the cytoplasm) where it is intended to function.

NUCLEIC ACID INTERACTIONS

The cornerstone discovery of molecular biology was the formulation by James D. Watson and Francis H. C. Crick, in 1953, of the double-stranded helix model of DNA structure. The insightful model they developed provided a coherent integration of the X-ray crystallographic structure of partially purified DNA with the previously known quantitative chemical data that the purine-pyrimidine bases adenine (A)–thymidine (T) and guanine (G)–cytosine (C) were paired, such that the A:T and G:C ratios were unity, whereas the A–T:G–C were not. The Watson-Crick molecular model for DNA also accurately predicted the basic mechanism of DNA replication.

NUCLEIC ACID BASE PAIRING COMPLEMENTARITY In the Watson-Crick double helix, two right-handed helical polynucleotide chains coil around the same central axis, making a complete helical turn every 10 nucleotides (Fig. 1.15-2). In the interior of the helix, the purine and pyrimidine bases (A with T, G with C) are paired through hydrogen bonding of their complementary structures, placing the phosphate groups around the outside of the helix. The crucial structural feature for gene expression is the precise molecular complementarity between the primary sequences of nucleotide bases in one strand of the DNA helix with the antiparallel sequence of the second strand. The strand that encodes the genetic information is termed the *sense strand*. Wherever a particular base occurs in the sense strand, there will be a complementary base, and only that base in the antisense strand, such that A always pairs with T, and vice versa, and G always pairs with C, and vice versa.

The base pair complementarity allows for duplication of the genetic information in dividing cells. This is accomplished by enzymes known as DNA polymerases that open the helix and replicate each single strand back into double strands according

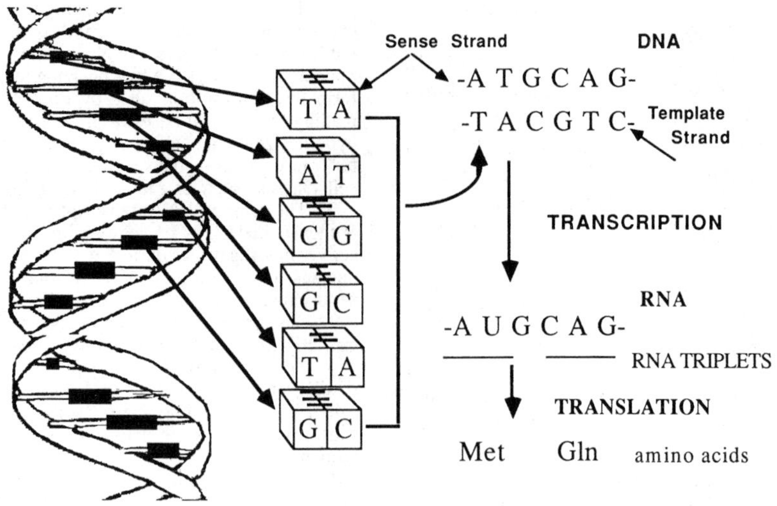

FIGURE 1.15-2. *The arrangement of bases within the DNA double helix, and the relationships among nucleic acid base pairs, RNA, and amino acids during the process of transcription and translation.*

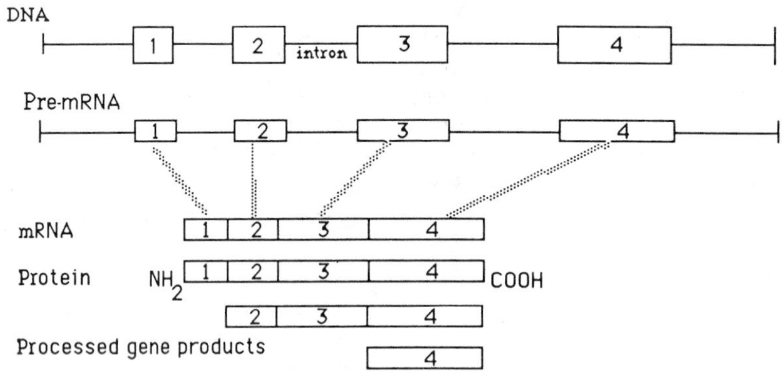

FIGURE 1.15-3. *The relationship between DNA base sequences in introns and exons (1–4), the resulting primary RNA transcript (pre-mRNA), the subsequently edited forms of mRNA, and the resulting proteins, which can then undergo posttranslational processing to yield small peptides (e.g., 4), or to add other chemical modifications to the final gene product molecule.*

to the single strand's template. The double-stranded complementarity also provides a means to repair the DNA, should it be damaged, since whichever single strand survives the damage can act as a template for the repair.

In a similar manner, the information-bearing or sense strand of the helical DNA chain is copied into a single-stranded complementary RNA during the process of transcription. This is done by making a single-stranded complementary copy of the DNA sense strand so that its sequence resembles closely that of the DNA antisense strand (Fig. 1.15-3). RNA differs chemically from DNA by the substitution of uridine for thymidine, and ribosephosphates for deoxyribosephosphates.

The affinity of the base pairs along sequences of a single DNA strand for their complementary base pair sequences in DNA or RNA is extraordinarily precise. In fact, it is so precise that small segments of natural or synthetic nucleotide chains can be used as probes for the detection of homologous sequences between large domains of DNA and RNA. (A nucleotide consists of one of the four bases, the deoxyribose or ribose-sugar, and the phosphate.) Because of the molecular complementarity that allows only the most exact sequence matches to hybridize, a probe will bind to a nucleic acid segment only when there is a long sequence of consistent match. The ability of a single-stranded nucleic acid to bind, or hybridize, to a complementary sequence is an essential component of many molecular biological techniques.

THE GENETIC CODE To translate genetic information from sequences of RNA into linear sequences of amino acids in proteins requires a strict code. The 20 or so amino acids commonly found in proteins are specified by various combinations of the four nucleotides. Through an ingenious series of experiments, it was demonstrated that sets of three RNA bases (triplets) provide the code words that specify the order of amino acids to be incorporated into protein (Fig. 1.15-2) and that other triplet sequences mark the point at which synthesis would begin or end or be modified in other ways.

INTERRUPTED DNA SEGMENTS FOR GENES Research conducted in the late 1970s, starting with the encoding of information in certain viruses and then supported by early analyses of the genes encoding the immunoglobulins and the hemoglobins, led to a major unexpected discovery: The genes of multicelled organisms (and some viruses, as it turns out) did not follow the principles that had been uncovered from the study of prokaryotes. Whereas the DNA coding regions of prokaryotes are found in the same linear sequences in which they are read during transcription, the higher organisms (and the viruses) have gene segments (exons) that are eventually expressed as proteins separated by intervening regions (introns) that are not found in mature mRNA.

This interrupted segmental DNA coding structure leads to two outcomes: (1) The primary gene transcript, formally termed the heterogeneous nuclear RNA (hnRNA), is a complete copy of the gene that contains intronic RNA sequences. These introns must be edited out before the mRNA can successfully direct protein synthesis by ribosomes (Fig. 1.15-3). The editing process consists of opening up the hnRNA, removing intronic segments, and resplicing the cut ends. (2) In some cells, including neurons, the composition of the transcribed mRNA can be further edited by splicing exon segments in or out of the mature mRNA. The editing-splicing process provides a means by which a single gene containing several exons can give rise to several different gene product proteins, in which certain protein domains may be shared and others will be unique (see Section 1.5).

When gene products share similar nucleotide and protein sequences, they are often referred to as a *structural family*. When structurally or functionally related gene sequences within functionally related protein families occur along adjacent segments of the chromosome, they are referred to as *gene clusters*. The genes for the hemoglobins, immunoglobulins, histocompatibility antigens, and certain pituitary hormones are organized in these linear clusters.

CLASSIFICATION OF GENETIC DISORDERS

Genetic variations that cause disease are conventionally classified as being Mendelian, chromosomal, or multifactorial. Classic Mendelian defects are based on small deletions, insertions, or inversions in a gene, which can then give rise to errors in transcription, translation, and processing as well as to abnormal functioning of the gene product. Although individuals with point mutation diseases are relatively rare, there are, in fact, many known genetically based diseases, although they do not include any psychiatric disorders. The chromosomal diseases are the congenital disorders, such as trisomy 21, which result from abnormalities of chromosome number or genetic expression during fertilization and early embryogenesis. Since these diseases are not necessarily caused by transmissible genetic defects, they will not be considered further in this section.

Much more relevant to psychiatric diseases, but less easily resolvable, are the multifactorial disorders, in which multiple genetic and environmental factors cooperate in the etiology and pathogenesis of the disease. The genetic roots of psychosis and alcoholism are represented in this large and important category, as are many other very serious disorders, such as non-insulin-dependent diabetes mellitus, essential hypertension, and most forms of atherosclerosis. The critical element here is that the presence of the gene defect per se is not adequate to induce the disease unless the individual is exposed to the necessary and complementary environmental conditions. Establishment of the genetic basis for a multifactorial condition requires detection and characterization of the possible gene defects and the number of these defects that may be required for disease expression, as well as the elucidation of the gene products and how they function under these conditions to result in long-latency disorders as complex as schizophrenia or alcoholism. To grasp the nature of such defects and the methods by which they can be detected, it is necessary to examine the basic strategies of molecular biology and the control of gene expression.

MOLECULAR BIOLOGICAL INVESTIGATION

The power of molecular biological methods is gained from several related, but independent, operational developments: (1) the ability to *clone* genetic information (i.e., to isolate a segment, purify it, and create large amounts of the purified selected sample); (2) the ability to obtain the molecular *sequence* of the nucleic acids that encode genetic information (i.e., to determine the complete molecular structure of genes); and (3) the ability to practice *genetic engineering* (i.e., to perturb and control gene expression and alter the structure of gene products by chemically modifying precise sites in the molecular structure of the genes).

GENE CLONING Molecular biologists have adopted many strategies in their quest to isolate gene sequences. A typical procedure begins with the isolation of mRNAs for all the genes that a particular brain or brain region is actively expressing. After obtaining partially purified cell fractions, enriched mRNAs are converted into DNA by the enzyme reverse transcriptase. The copied double-stranded DNA form (cDNA) can then be incorporated (inserted) into specific sites within an infectious vector, or plasmid, which is basically a circular segment of double-stranded DNA. In order to insert a cDNA into a plasmid, the circular structure of the plasmid is opened by bacterial enzymes (restriction endonucleases) that cleave DNA-specific nucleotide sequence sites. The typically chosen restriction sites for insertion are genes that code for some discernible functional property of the isolated plasmid, such as antibiotic resistance. Therefore, when insertion has been successful, loss of that functional property can be used to identify which plasmids have successful inserts. By cultivating the successfully infected bacteria so that each individual bacterium generates a colony of identical bacteria, each of which will bear identical replicates of the plasmid and its insert, the DNA is said to have been cloned. The cDNA then can be recovered from the plasmid through another exposure to the restriction enzyme that was used to open the plasmid for insertion. Thus, in relatively few steps, one can start with a mixture of mRNAs in widely differing proportions, purify them individually, and prepare virtually unlimited quantities of the complementary DNA.

DNA-RNA SEGMENT IDENTIFICATION The affinity of the base pairs for their complementary base pair sequences in DNA or RNA are so precise that small segments can be used as probes for the detection of homologous sequences of large stretches of DNA and RNA. This capacity arises because the molecular complementarity of the nucleic acid base sequences allows the probe to bind to its complementary structure only when there is a long sequence of consistent match. The ability of a single-stranded nucleic acid chain to bind, or hybridize, to its complementary chain sequence is an essential component of many molecular biological techniques. When DNA is fractionated by restriction enzymes and the resulting fragments are separated by gel electrophoresis, it is possible to transfer, or blot, the resulting fragments from the acrylamide gel to a nitrocellulose or nylon support, and then to analyze them for the ability to hybridize with cDNA or RNA probes. This method, referred to as a *Southern blot,* is named for the scientist who first described this method. When the starting material to be separated is RNA and the transfers onto nitrocellulose are probed with radioactive cDNA, this test is referred to as a *Northern blot.*

NUCLEIC ACID SEQUENCE DETERMINATIONS The final fundamental procedural development that has accelerated molecular biological methods is the ability to determine the sequence of nucleotide bases within DNA molecules. From these DNA sequences, it is possible to deduce the nucleotide sequences of RNA and thereby determine the amino acid sequence of the protein products. The structures of the DNA and proteins then can be analyzed, often via computer, to compare their sequences with previously characterized proteins or nucleic acids. Additional important clues to the functional features of the proteins may be inferred from the domains, hydrophobic and hydrophilic, and from other structural sites of possible posttranslational modification (e.g., protein phosphorylation).

GENETICS AND THE NERVOUS SYSTEM

The phenotype of an individual cell and the larger population of similar cells to which it is related almost certainly depends on the specific gene products that are expressed. These include the structural, metabolic, and regulatory proteins by which the cell establishes its own recognizable structural and functional properties. Neurons, the more complex neuronal ensembles, and the still more complex behaviors that these ensembles control, undoubtedly require many special-purpose proteins. These proteins may exist in limited amounts and may be expressed only at specific periods in neuronal development.

To purify such rare proteins by the methods that existed before molecular cloning, especially in the absence of a functional assay to guide the purification process, would require substantial patience and resources and a very large supply of the proper starting tissue. For example, for some of the very rare hypothalamic hypophysiotrophic-releasing factors (e.g., corticotropin releasing factor [CRF]), hundreds of thousands of hypothalami were required.

By converting the quest for the structure of specific proteins into a molecular biological quest for the mRNA or gene segment that encodes this protein, the experimental analysis becomes greatly facilitated. When functional assays can be used to purify a desired gene product enough to derive a partial amino acid sequence, that sequence can be used to synthesize all the possible nucleotide triplet sequences that could encode the protein. These synthetic oligonucleotides can then be used to probe a cDNA library to select a specific clone for a detailed sequence analysis.

Given the creativity with which molecular biological methods are being applied to cell biology, including the actions of psychoactive drugs on the nervous system, one senses that an exponential increase in the number of specific proteins that will be fully characterized is about to be experienced. The products of cDNA cloning can also be used to probe the regions around the exons to search for the molecular mechanisms for control of expression.

These specific gene probes can also be used to determine the position of the genes on the chromosomes. In a very simplified view, the gene probes obtained from cloning provide a means to examine the genome directly for the location of structural variations. This is in contrast to the previous methods that focused only on the gene products or on the individual phenotypes.

The new molecular methods have been able to exploit the DNA polymorphisms (i.e., variations) that exist within every species. In a typical approach, human DNA preparations are exposed to a single restriction enzyme, and the Southern blots that contain the gene fragments are compared for hybridization to specific oligonucleotide probes. When this test procedure is done with the DNA of several family members who have a specific illness, it is possible to make a correlation between the presence of the disorder and the so-called restriction fragment length polymorphisms. There can be considerable individual variation in nucleotide sequences, however, without disturbing the function of the encoded proteins. The ability to link specific fragments of DNA with the inheritance of genetic disorders helps to establish approximate locations of genetic mutations, such as the localization of a potential gene for Huntington's disease to human chromosome 4.

Similarly, gene marker probes can be used to locate the reactive chromosome in an in situ chromosome preparation. Many proteins have had their chromosomal location determined with this or related techniques. Since these cloning methods have been applied to the human chromosome, more than 800 locations for specific genes and genetic disorders that their variants represent have been mapped, most of them being on the relatively small X chromosome. However, there are vast expanses of the mammalian, and more critically the human, genome with no known markers of any kind. The pursuit of the molecular genetic bases for psychiatric diseases of the nervous system is particularly difficult since much less than 1 percent of the genome is associated with known nervous system markers (Table 1.15-1).

STRATEGIES FOR THE DETECTION OF BRAIN GENES

Much information remains to be learned about the genes for the organization, operation, and maintenance of the normal brain before one is able to begin to detect the genes whose expression and regulation may be abnormal in multifactorial genetic brain diseases. A major part of such future efforts will be the identification of yet unknown proteins used by the normal nervous system. The methods of molecular biological analysis may make these searches more heuristic by characterizing mRNA rather than by isolating the rare proteins of the nervous system.

For most tissue, including the brain, individual mRNA species are present in a wide range of concentrations, generally split into three classes: (1) high-abundance mRNAs present in thousands of copies per cell and assumed to encode the major secretory products (such as ovalbumin for cells of the oviduct, and immunoglobulin for immune system cells); (2) middle-abundance mRNAs (a few hundred copies per cell), such as for the vegetative and cell differentiation proteins that are required by all cells for their housekeeping operations; and (3) low-abundance mRNAs, of which there may well be a very large number of individual examples, occurring with a very few copies per cell, and varying considerably from cell type to cell type. Given these general categories, it is of interest to recognize the results of recent studies that indicate the heterogeneity of mRNAs expressed in the adult mammalian brain. Based on studies of the genetic complexity of brain

TABLE 1.15-1
Human Genome Assignments of Brain-Related Genes

Chromosome	*Position*	*Gene Marker*
1		Atrialnaturetic factor
1	p 36.12	Enolase 1
1	p 36	Microcephaly marker
1	q 31-32	Neuroblastoma marker
1	p32	Nerve growth factor
1	p 22	Retinitis pigmentosa marker
2		Pro-opiomelanocortin (POMC)
3	p23	Somatostatin
4	q 27-28	Huntington's disease marker G8
5		β-adrenergic receptor
6		Manic-depressive disease marker
6		Spinocerebellar ataxia
7		Neuropeptide Y
8	p (term)-q22	Gonadotropin-releasing hormone
9	p21-q11.2	Dopamine-β-hydroxylase
11		Calcitonin gene-related peptide (CGRP)
11	p 15.4-15.1	Insulin-like growth factor 2
11		Nerve cell adhesion molecule (NCAM)
11	q 23-term	Thy-1 marker
11		Tyrosine hydroxylase
12	p	Enolase 2
12	p 11-12	Phenylalanine hydroxylase (PKU marker)
12	q24.1	CD4 T-cell antigen
13		Retinoblastoma marker
14	q 14.1	Creatine kinase (brain type)
15	q 32	Coronavirus sensitivity
17	q 11	Pancreatic polypeptide
18	p 11.1-q.term	Gastrin-releasing peptide (neurotensin)
18		Myelin basic protein
19		Polio virus sensitivity
20	q	Vasopressin
22		Platelet-derived growth factor
X		HGPRT (Lesch-Nyhan enzyme)
X	q 26	Monoamine oxidase A
X	q13	Myelin proteolipid
X	q13-22	Retinitis pigmentosa, X-linked marker
X	p 11-13	Synapsin I

Table adapted from McCusick, V A: The morbid anatomy of the human genome. A review of gene mapping in clinical medicine. Medicine *65:* 1, 1986.

mRNAs, it was already considered that brain probably expresses severalfold more genes than other specialized tissues. However, exactly how much greater this expression was in the brain was not readily determinable by previous measurements. Using cloning methods to sample about 200 mRNAs in the brain randomly and to develop specific probes by which to compare the mRNA populations in the brain, liver, and kidney, it is now possible to deduce that well over half of the mammalian genome, some 30,000 genes, may be expressed either exclusively or in much higher frequency in the brain. Even scrupulous reading of encyclopedic texts on the chemistry of the brain can provide scarcely more than 500 proteins, either specific to or enriched in brain. Thus, it is clear from these figures that the ability to detect, diagnose, understand, and possibly treat or prevent genetic defects underlying genetically linked psychiatric disorders is just beginning.

REFERENCES

Cahill G F, Jr: Genetics and inborn errors of metabolism. In *Scientific American Medicine,* E F Rubenstein, editor, sec 9, chap VII, p 1. Scientific American Publishers, New York, 1983.

Cloninger C R, Reich T, Yokoyama S: Genetic diversity, genome organization, and investigation of the etiology of psychiatric diseases. Psychiat Develop *3:* 225, 1983.

Darnell J, Lodish H, Baltimore D: *Molecular Cell Biology.* Scientific American Books, New York, 1986.

de Duve C: *The Living Cell,* vol 2, p 284. Freeman, New York, 1984.

Gilbert W: Genes-in-pieces revisited. Science *228:* 823, 1985.

Gottesman I I, Shields J: *Schizophrenia—The Epigenetic Puzzle.* Cambridge University Press, New York, 1982.

Gurling H: Application of molecular biology to mental illness: Analysis of genomic DNA and brain mRNA. Psychiat Develop *3:* 257, 1985.

Gusella J F, Tanzi R E, Anderson M A, Hobbs W, Gibbons K, Raschtchian R, Gilliam T C, Wallace M R, Wexler N S, Conneally P M: DNA markers for nervous system diseases. Science *225:* 1320, 1984.

Maxam A M, Gilbert W: A new method of sequencing DNA. Proc Nat Acad Sci USA *74:* 5463, 1977.

McKusick V A: The morbid anatomy of the human genome. A review of gene mapping in clinical medicine. Medicine *65:* 1, 1986.

Milner R J, Sutcliffe J G: Gene expression in rat brain. Nucleic Acids Res *11:* 5497, 1983.

Rosenfeld M G, Amara S G, Evans R M: Alternative RNA processing: Determining neuronal phenotype. Science *225:* 1315, 1984.

Rosenfield M G, Crenshaw E B III, Lira S A, Swanson L, Borrelli E, Heyman R, Evans R M: Transgenic mice: Applications to the study of the nervous system. In *Annual Review of Neuroscience,* vol 11, W M Cowan, E M Shooter, C F Stevens, R F Thompson, editors, p 353. Annual Reviews, Palo Alto, CA, 1988.

Ruddle F H: A new era in mammalian gene mapping. Somatic cell genetics and recombinant DNA. Nature *294:* 115, 1981.

Sanger F, Coulson A R: A rapid method for determining sequences in DNA by primed synthesis with DNA polymerase. J Molec Biol *94:* 444, 1975.

Schmitt F O, Bird S J, Bloom F E: *Molecular Genetic Neuroscience.* Raven Press, New York, 1982.

Schuckit M A: Biological markers in alcoholism. Progr Neuropsychopharmacol Biol Psychiat *10:* 191, 1986.

Stryer L: *Biochemistry,* ed 2. Freeman, New York.

Sutcliffe J G, Milner R J, Gottesfeld J M, Reynolds W: Control of neuronal gene expression. Science *225:* 1308, 1984.

Watson J D, Crick F H C: Molecular structure of nucleic acids: A structure for deoxyribose nucleic acid. Nature *171:* 737, 1953.

Watson J D, Tooze J, Kurtz D T: *Recombinant DNA. A Short Course.* Freeman, New York, 1983.

CHAPTER 2 NEUROLOGY

2.1 NEUROLOGICAL EVALUATION

SEYMOUR SOLOMON, M.D.
JOSEPH C. MASDEU, M.D.

INTRODUCTION

This section of the chapter will concentrate on the clinical examination of the patient with neuropsychiatric signs or symptoms, followed by a description of different diagnostic procedures, such as electroencephalography (EEG) and imaging modalities. Sections 2.2 and 2.3 are reviews of the different disorders encountered in neurology, with particular emphasis on those entities more likely to be encountered by the psychiatrist: the organic mental disorders. In the revised third edition of the American Psychiatric Association's *Diagnostic and Statistical Manual of Mental Disorders* (DSM-III-R), a distinction is made between organic mental syndromes and organic mental disorders. Organic mental syndrome refers to a constellation of psychological or behavioral signs and symptoms without reference to etiology (e.g., delirium, dementia); organic mental disorder designates a particular organic mental syndrome in which the etiology is known or presumed (e.g., alcohol withdrawal delirium or primary degenerative dementia of the Alzheimer type). Although structured somewhat differently from DSM-III-R, Section 2.2 deals with neurological disorders, such as brain trauma and Alzheimer's disease. Section 2.3 deals with neurological syndromes, such as coma, epilepsy, and pain.

Diagnosis of neurological disease is reached through an adequate history and neurological examination. The neurological examination provides information on where to localize the lesion; the history indicates its most likely etiology. Often, use of neurophysiological or neuroimaging procedures confirms the diagnosis and provides valuable information for the management of the patient's problem. Neurophysiological diagnostic procedures include electromyography (EMG) and nerve conduction tests for the study of the peripheral nervous system, EEG for the study of brain activity, and evoked potentials (EPs), which provide information about both the central and peripheral nervous systems. Many neurological disorders are associated with long-term disability that can be psychologically devastating. In turn, psychological difficulties may manifest themselves in the form of motor or sensory impairments. Thus, an in-depth knowledge of the patient's psychological makeup and milieu are fundamental in the evaluation of neurological disease.

EVALUATION OF THE ADULT

HISTORY The historical account should include the source of the information and its reliability. The patient's age, sex, and handedness are best noted at the outset. A chronological résumé of the present illness is the essential feature of the history. Each complaint should be evaluated with regard to onset, duration, and frequency of occurrence; note should be made of both aggravating and alleviating factors. Specific qualities of the complaint should be evaluated. If pain is a chief complaint, the type of pain, its location, and its severity are to be recorded. The exact meaning of the symptom to the patient must also be elicited. *Dizziness,* for example, should mean a spinning sensation or a sensation of imbalance, but patients often use the term to denote such symptoms as nausea, malaise, or faintness. Other symptoms associated with the chief complaint must then be sought, and the course of the disease must be established.

The patient should be specifically questioned with regard to such neurological symptoms as headaches, dizziness, episodes of fainting or faintness, fits or convulsions, shaking or trembling, and unsteadiness or incoordination. Questions should be asked about past or present weakness, stiffness, paralysis, aches, pains, and numbness or tingling, either focal or generalized. Symptoms referable to the specific senses should be checked, such as a history of double vision, spots before the eyes, temporary blindness, or blurring of vision. Does the patient experience ringing in an ear or hearing impairment? Has the person noted any changes in the senses of taste or smell? Perversions in the sphere of these special senses may easily be neglected by the patient unless specifically questioned: "Do you ever smell or taste anything peculiar? Do you ever hear or see things out of the ordinary?" Visceral symptoms may reflect neurological disorders. Dysphagia or dysarthria are often the first manifestations of brain stem or muscle disease. Disturbances of bladder control or impotence in the male may herald spinal cord disease or an autonomic neuropathy. Change in sleep patterns may become symptomatic as narcolepsy or a sleep apnea syndrome. Symptoms of mental illness also should be sought. Incipient manifestations of a frontal lobe tumor, such as decreased drive, impoverished ability to plan ahead, and unusual moodiness may not become apparent during mental status testing but will be volunteered by the patient's relatives or professional acquaintances. Historical information from a witness is particularly useful when the disease is accompanied by transient impairment of the patient's alertness. Some persons with temporal lobe or other types of seizures are completely unaware of their occurrence.

Included in the past medical history should be queries as to trauma, surgery, and medical or psychiatric illness. Does the patient have a history of allergy, of exposure to toxins, or of weight gain or loss? Has there been use of medication or drugs, particularly in recent months? Defects in the patient's remembrance of previous illnesses may be sometimes overcome by inquiring about past hospitalizations.

Social history should include the person's occupation, sexual behavior, home environment, special interests, and drinking and smoking habits. Evaluation of present or potential support systems is critical in the case of disabling disorders. In the process of obtaining the family history, the question of consanguinity should be raised. In addition to the causes of death in near relatives, the history should note the presence of epilepsy, migraine, and other diseases, both mental and neurological.

PHYSICAL EXAMINATION The general physical examination often proves critical for the diagnosis of neurological disease. Findings of lung or breast cancer may provide the clue to explaining the patient's hemiparesis or recent onset of a seizure disorder, because both types of tumor often metastasize to brain. Similarly, neurological deficits associated with a changing heart murmur and splinter hemorrhages in the nail bed or conjunctiva suggest the diagnosis of subacute bacterial endocarditis with embolic brain infarction. Jaundice or spider angiomata point to liver failure as a likely cause of a patient's metabolic encephalopathy. Severe peripheral vascular disease, with absent peripheral pulses, is often associated with important atheromatous disease of the extracranial cervical arteries and thus with an enhanced risk of cerebral infarction. Differences in the pulse or blood pressure readings of the two arms suggest subclavian stenosis, which may give rise to vertebrobasilar insufficiency. Skin changes are characteristic in the so-called neurocutaneous syndromes. Café au lait spots and cutaneous neurofibromas bespeak neurofibromatosis, whereas sebaceous adenomas and depigmented spots accompany tuberous sclerosis. A brownish ring in the episcleral region is almost invariably present in neurologically symptomatic Wilson's disease, a disorder often attended by psychiatric manifestations.

NEUROLOGICAL EXAMINATION The degree of alertness should be recorded at the outset. If the patient is alert, the degree of attention, distractibility, and cooperativeness are pertinent. If consciousness appears depressed, is the patient drowsy, stuporous, or comatose?

Mental status Neurological disorders of the brain are likely to affect attention, memory, language, the ability to identify objects (loss of which is called *agnosia*), and the ability to perform different types of sequential movements (loss of which is called *apraxia*). Evaluation of these areas of cognition is particularly helpful in neurological diagnosis. Rather than use different tests in every new patient encounter, it is preferable to become well acquainted with a brief set of screening procedures. One such screening instrument for older patients is Folstein's mini-mental status questionnaire (Table 2.1-1), which should be supplemented with some of the tests for hemineglect described below. A standard for normal performance can be achieved that takes into account the patient's age and cultural background. Areas found abnormal should then be explored in greater detail.

Attention and neglect Attentional disturbances can be global or restricted to activities carried out in the right or left hemispace, called *hemineglect*. Global attentional disturbances blend as a continuum with disturbances of alertness. The extreme of inattention is stupor, when the patient has to be stimulated constantly to elicit any response. Milder degrees of inattention are often associated with a mental status that oscillates between listlessness and agitation (the latter often triggered by pain or by the perception of danger). Although they are apparently on opposite poles, both of these behavioral manifestations result from diminished cortical control. With less severe attentional disorders, tasks requiring a temporal or spatial program are likely to be interrupted or degraded in midstream. Inattention may become obvious as patients try to give an account of their complaints or as they perform a set of movements on command. Characteristically, when asked to touch the tip of their noses while keeping their eyes closed, patients with impaired attention are unable to maintain their eyes shut; they repeatedly open their eyes after having closed them at the insistence of the examiner.

Adequate attention is necessary for the performance of any cognitive or motor task; therefore, attention is best evaluated while carrying out the rest of the neurological examination. Milder attentional deficits will become obvious only as the examination progresses,

TABLE 2.1-1
Mini-Mental Status (MMS) Questionnaire

Orientation (Score 1 if correct)	
Name this hospital or building.	_____
What city are you in now?	_____
What year is it?	_____
What month is it?	_____
What is the date today?	_____
What state are you in?	_____
What county is this?	_____
What floor of the building are you on?	_____
What day of the week is it?	_____
What season of the year is it?	_____
Registration	
Name three objects and have the patient repeat them. Score number repeated by the patient. Name the three objects several more times if needed for the patient to repeat correctly (record trials ____).	_____
Attention and calculation	
Subtract 7 from 100 in serial fashion to 65. Max. score = 5	_____
Recall	
Do you recall the three objects named before?	_____
Language tests	
Confrontation naming: watch, pen = 2	_____
Repetition: "No ifs, ands, or buts" = 1	_____
Comprehension: Pick up the paper in your right hand, fold it in half and set it on the floor = 3	_____
Read and perform the command "close your eyes" = 1	_____
Write any sentence (subject, object, verb) = 1	_____
Construction	
Copy the design below = 1	_____

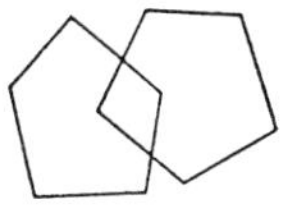

Total MMS Questionnaire score (Max. = 30)	_____

Table adapted from Folstein M F, Folstein S, McHugh P R: Mini-mental state: A practical method for grading the cognitive state of patients for the clinician. J Psychiat Res *12:* 189, 1975, with permission.

when the patient becomes a bit tired and accustomed to the examiner and to the examination procedure. Patients with attentional disorders, though able to repeat complex sentences, perform poorly in tests of verbal fluency. For instance, they are unable to state more than a few items when asked to name everything that can be found in a supermarket or as many words as they can think of beginning with the letter L. Impaired verbal fluency, despite intact sentence repetition, is also found with frontal lobe lesions. Most common causes of global attentional disturbances are toxic-metabolic encephalopathies, medication effects, and psychotic or mood disorders.

Hemineglect or, simply, neglect is the inability to report, to recognize, or to respond to stimuli on one side of space. Pointing to objects in either hemispace, performing commands that involve bringing the hand into the contralateral hemispace, or crossing off a particular letter embedded randomly in an array of letters are tasks that can be used to demonstrate hemineglect. Although more common with lesions of the right temporoparietal area or the thalamus, hemispatial neglect can be found with lesions of either hemisphere, particularly with those of an acute nature, such as an infarct or a seizure related to a tumor. Thus, hemispatial neglect strongly suggests a neurological disease, particularly when the patient is unaware of the deficit.

Emotional status The patient's emotional status, often closely related to the attentional status, should be noted. Important areas of observation include mood and its lability, degree of anxiety, distorted perception of reality (e.g., delusions, illusions, hallucinations), thought content, and appropriateness of social conduct. Behavior, neatness, mannerisms, and other forms of motor activity can be seen in a first interview; however, determination of the patient's insight, motivation, and special appetites may require more prolonged evaluation.

Orientation and memory Disorientation with respect to time generally is accompanied by poor recent memory. In addition to the questions exemplified in Table 2.1-1, the fund of information and recent memory can be tested by inquiring about recent national or international news. Memory for remote events should be tested when recent memory is impaired. Asking for the names of the presidents or for identification of popular figures or events in each of the past decades will prove helpful to identify the time frame of the patient's memory loss. In this regard, care should be taken not to mistake a language impairment (generally anomia) or attentional impairment for an impairment of memory. Memory loss or amnesia is generally caused by bilateral medial temporal disease (most often Alzheimer's disease, ischemia, herpes simplex encephalitis, or trauma) or by bilateral medial thalamic disease (most often ischemic or related to thiamine deficiency); Korsakoff's psychosis is the result. Anterograde amnesia can result from bilateral loss of a selective area of the hippocampus (cornu ammonis [CA]-1). Bilateral lesions anywhere in the limbic system can cause memory loss. Patients with amnesia, particularly those with thalamic lesions, may deny any difficulty with their memory and may make up stories to fill in their informational gaps (i.e., they confabulate).

Language disturbances THE APHASIAS Although language disturbances are often present in a mild to severe degree in psychotic patients, distorted grammar or marked comprehension difficulties are characteristic of dominant-hemisphere disease. Aphasia refers to the disturbance of spoken language, whereas the terms "alexia" and "agraphia" refer to impaired reading and writing, respectively.

Language is best tested by careful evaluation of conversational speech and of the ability to understand spoken language, followed by a test of the patient's ability to name objects presented to him or her (confrontation naming) and tasks that involve repetition of sentences (Table 2.1-1). Subsequently, reading and writing can be explored. If the patient is mute, the inability to articulate sounds, called *anarthria,* rather than aphasia, may underlie the mutism; large dominant-hemisphere or bilateral capsular lesions are most often responsible. Mute patients who write correctly are likely to have capsular lesions. Sparse but informative speech, which is agrammatical or telegraphic because of the meager use of function words, such as "the" or "with," generally results from an anterior perisylvian lesion; this is known as Broca's or nonfluent aphasia. Phonemic paraphasias, such as "shair" for "chair," may occur. The spontaneous speech of patients with posterior perisylvian lesions, known as Wernicke's or fluent aphasia or conduction aphasia, is fluent in the sense that sentences are produced without strain and contain small function words. Hyperabundant speech or logorrhea is occasionally present. Paraphasic errors are termed categorical ("table" for "chair"), associative ("throne" for "chair"), or asemantic ("wheelbase" for "chair"). An utterance, such as "wheelbase," is called a *neologism* (i.e., a new word).

Auditory comprehension is screened by having the patient perform on command a somewhat complicated task. A favorite from the times of the French School of Aphasiology is attributed to Pierre Marie. The patient, presented with three pieces of paper of different sizes, is asked to put on the floor the smallest one, to fold into two the largest one and to give to the examiner the middle-size piece of paper. Performance of such tasks may be impaired by cognitive deficits in spatial perception or praxis. If screening fails, other simpler tasks, even using pantomime to convey the message of the command, should be tried in order to isolate a verbal comprehension difficulty. Auditory comprehension is impaired in Wernicke's aphasia, but not in Broca's aphasia.

Testing the patient's ability to repeat sentences, such as "No ifs, ands, or buts about it," is important because with lesions in the perisylvian area of the dominant hemisphere, repetition is almost always impaired. Impairment of repetition with preserved spontaneous speech and comprehension is characteristic of *conduction aphasia.* Nonaphasic language disturbances present in some psychotic or attentional disturbances generally spare the ability to repeat. Repetition is also relatively spared with lesions in the mesial aspect of the frontal lobe or basal ganglia, which may give rise to a paucity of spontaneous speech, called *transcortical motor aphasia,* or in the pulvinar of the thalamus, which may give rise to an impaired comprehension and the production of neologisms, known as *transcortical sensory aphasia.* Confrontation naming, often impaired following damage of the inferior temporal or angular gyri of the dominant hemisphere, is unreliable as a localizing function. Impaired naming to confrontation is termed *anomia.* It may be the only language defect with a small lesion of the dominant hemisphere or with diffuse cerebral dysfunction, such as metabolic encephalopathy.

DISORDERS OF SPEECH Speech production may be abnormal even if the ability to construct meaningful sentences is intact, as in the case of the patient who is mute but can write correctly. The production of speech requires the timed execution of precise movements by the articulatory organs. Impairment of this mechanism results in a number of speech disturbances, known as *dysarthrias.* The speech may be imprecise (consonant sounds become blurred) and nasal, in which case the dysarthria is often due to bulbar palsy, resulting in weakness of the palate and tongue, or the speech may be slurred, as in the speech of someone who is intoxicated, in which case cerebellar disease is responsible. It may be monotone, as with Parkinson's disease. It may be somewhat explosive and poorly modulated, in which case a pseudobulbar palsy from bilateral corticobulbar involvement is most likely. Scanning dysarthria refers to production of each syllable individually, in a staccato fashion. This type of speech, common in multiple sclerosis, is related to damage of both the cerebellar and the cortical levels of speech control.

Stuttering is the interruption of speech flow by the tendency to repeat the initial syllable of a word. It is aggravated by emotional stress, but pathophysiological, as well as psychological, factors are thought to be operative. Stuttering may be due to defective lateralization of cerebral dominance for language. Occasionally, it is the sequela of organic bilateral cerebral disease.

Palilalia is the tendency to repeat the last word or words of a sentence. The repetition increases in frequency but fades in volume. This rare condition may occur with diseases of the basal ganglia, as in postencephalitic parkinsonism, and with bilateral cerebral lesions causing dementia. It also may be a manifestation of schizophrenia.

Cluttering is speech so rapid that words are run together and syllables may be omitted. The cause of this uncommon condition is unknown.

Dysphonia or *aphonia* is an impairment or loss of voice volume. Usually, the disturbance in phonation is due to local diseases affecting the respiratory system or vocal cords, or to neurological disease affecting the speech musculature or its innervation. Whispered speech is sometimes a neurotic manifestation. Hoarseness is usually due to structural changes of the vocal cords; it is rarely psychogenic. Quivering or wavering speech may be caused by palatal myoclonus.

Spastic dysphonia is caused by the contraction of speech musculature after normally speaking a few words or sentences; patients sound as if they are being strangled during attempts to continue conversational speech. Whispering is unaffected and shouting is easier than quiet speech. Spastic dysphonia begins in middle or late life and is probably due to extrapyramidal disease. Because organic disease is not evident, the condition is often falsely assumed to be psychogenic.

Mutism is the complete loss of vocal expression. If writing expression is normal, then mutism represents the extreme of anarthria when the patient, albeit not aphasic, cannot utter any sounds. However, a mute patient may not be able to write, as in the case of the *locked-in syndrome,* due to bilateral interruption of the corticobulbar and corticospinal tracts at the level of the basis pontis. Some vertical eye movements may remain and can be used to let the examiner know that the patient is indeed able to understand and follow commands. Another type of mutism is accompanied by a lack or paucity of any other spontaneous movements and by a failure to make any attempt at communication; this is known as *akinetic mutism.* Bilateral damage of the area where midbrain, hypothalamus, and thalamus converge, or of the medial aspect of the frontal lobes, is generally responsible for chronic akinetic mutism.

Alexia and agraphia *Alexia* denotes the inability to understand the meaning of written symbols; *dyslexia* is now reserved for particular difficulty in learning to read. The physician should ask the patient to read out loud and then follow up with questions to determine comprehension. *Agraphia* is a defect of expression in written language. When alexia and agraphia occur together, the responsible lesion is usually in the angular gyrus of the dominant hemisphere. This syndrome is regularly accompanied by difficulty in spelling words orally or in understanding words spelled out. Spelling is spared in the syndrome of alexia without agraphia, which results from pathology in the dominant medial occipital lobe and splenium of the corpus callosum.

In about 99 percent of right-handed persons and about 60 percent of left-handed persons, the left hemisphere is dominant for speech. Left-handed persons often present unusual language disturbances. For instance, patients with lesions of the left hemisphere may be totally alexic and agraphic, although they have completely normal oral language.

Agnosia *Agnosia* is a disorder of recognition. Partial damage of the primary sensory cortex or lesions in the secondary association areas cause agnosia. The type of agnosia depends on the type of primary area affected. *Visual agnosia* is an impairment in the ability to recognize objects visually in the absence of a loss in visual acuity or general intellectual functions that would account for it. With apperceptive visual agnosia, the patients behave as if blind, except that they avoid obstacles when walking. Such patients cannot name items presented to them, draw them, or match them to samples, and they cannot point to objects named by the examiner. They can distinguish small changes in the intensity or hue of a minute source of light. A milder deficit is associative visual agnosia. This term refers to the deficit of patients who cannot visually recognize objects, but can draw or point to them when they are presented in an array of different objects. The two disturbances are often associated with right-homonymous hemianopsia, alexia without agraphia, and color-naming deficits. They follow lesions of the mesial aspect of the dominant occipital lobe and splenium of the corpus callosum. Bilateral lesions of the inferomedial aspect of the occipital lobes with extension into the temporal lobe, in the region of the lingual gyri, cause inability to identify faces, termed *prosopagnosia,* and objects visually similar, such as a specific car in a parking lot. *Visual simultanagnosia* refers to the inability to appreciate the meaning of the whole picture or environment, although the elemental parts are well recognized. Patients with this deficit often have other components of the so-called Balint's syndrome, which follows bilateral parieto-occipital lesions in the convexity of the hemispheres and is characterized by (1) failure to shift gaze on command, called an apraxia of gaze; (2) optic ataxia, manifested by clumsiness of object-bound movements of the hand performed under visual guidance; (3) decreased visual attention, affecting mainly the peripheral visual fields and resulting in constriction of the fields to "tunnel vision"; and (4) visual simultanagnosia. Such patients may fail to see a match offered them a few inches away from the tip of the cigarette they are concentrating on.

Auditory agnosia denotes an impairment of sound discrimination with normal or near-normal pure-tone audiometry. It is caused by bilateral lesions of the superior temporal gyrus of Heschl. Different sounds, such as the ringing of a phone or the clapping of hands, cannot be distinguished or localized. Similarly, the spoken word cannot be identified (pure word deafness), although these patients may read and speak quite normally, but loudly on occasion. Some sounds of a normal intensity may be perceived as having an annoying quality. One such patient, unable to understand his wife's normal speech, disliked the sound of the television set and compelled her to turn the volume so low that she could not hear it.

Lesions of the postcentral gyrus cause contralateral impairment in the ability to identify an object by palpation; this is called *astereognosis*. Astereognosis is generally accompanied by impaired two-point discrimination and graphesthesia (the inability to recognize a letter or digit traced on the patient's skin).

More complex deficits of cortical integration are impairment of right-left discrimination and the inability to recognize body parts. *Gerstmann's syndrome,* indicative of dominant angular gyrus dysfunction, consists of finger agnosia, agraphia, right-left disorientation, and acalculia. *Anosognosia* (denial of illness), map disorientation, and confusion in space, but not time, are manifestations of nondominant parietal disease.

Apraxia *Apraxia* is a disorder of skilled movement that is not caused by weakness, sensory loss, abnormality of tone or posture, abnormal movements, intellectual deterioration, or poor comprehension. In the posterior parietotemporal areas, sensory information is integrated and projected to the premotor areas of the frontal lobe. Damage of this area may result in disturbances of sensorimotor integration. *Ideomotor apraxia* is the inability of patients to carry out motor activity on command, but they retain the ability to do so spontaneously. In testing a patient, commands are given referable to the extremities ("Pretend to comb your hair. Make a fist"), to the facial musculature ("Whistle. Show your teeth"), and to the axial muscles ("Stand up. Walk"). Apraxia of limb and face may occur independently of axial apraxia. Less common, *ideational apraxia* is the inability of patients to carry out a complex multistep command, although they are able to perform each step individually. These forms of apraxia are caused by lesions of the dominant hemisphere.

Impairment of visual spatial integration results in *constructional apraxia*. This defect may be uncovered by asking the patient to copy geometrical figures or to draw certain objects, such as a clock or a cube. *Hemispatial neglect* may also be evidenced by these tasks. Dressing apraxia often accompanies constructional apraxia. Nondominant parietal lesions are most often responsible for these disorders. *Motor impersistence* (the inability to maintain a static posture, such as a protruded tongue or a fixation of gaze) is also associated with disease of the nondominant hemisphere.

COGNITIVE AND EMOTIONAL SYNDROMES RELATED TO SITE OF ORGANIC DISEASE

The characteristics of cognitive and emotional symptoms depend, to a large degree, on the site of organic involvement. Having described the different symptoms and signs of cerebral disease, it is pertinent to list them by location.

FRONTAL LOBE SYNDROME The frontal lobe syndrome occurs mainly with lesions of the prefrontal and orbitofrontal cortex of the brain, and the clinical features are most striking when the disease is bilateral. The major defects are inattentiveness, defective ability to plan ahead, decreased social drive, and impaired appreciation of social nuances. Personality changes predominate. One form of this syndrome may simulate the personality of the sociopathic-antisocial person or the hypomaniac, but without the feeling of happiness. Loss of inhibition leads to inappropriate, silly, and child-like behavior; responses are boastful, jocular, or facetious (this is known as *witzelsuch*). A lack of concern and the loss of self-consciousness may result in aberrant erotic behavior, such as exhibitionism. Bursts of irritability and, sometimes, violence may occur. Another form of the frontal lobe syndrome simulates depression. Patients of this type are apathetic or abulic; they lack interest in their environment and no longer have the will to act. What may superficially appear as depression is not accompanied by sadness or morbid preoccupation. There may be emotional lability and alterations between these two forms of behavior, but both manifest impairment of affective responses and lack of concern and social awareness. Such patients cannot easily adjust to change.

Motor activity is diminished in patients with the frontal lobe syndrome, and there is loss of spontaneity and initiative. Activities having to do with personal habits of washing, dressing, and toilet are neglected; the patient may become incontinent; and motor impersistence and perservation often occur. Abulia may progress to akinetic mutism.

At first, the overall intelligence quotient (I.Q.) may be normal; some of the errors in the mental status examination may be due to inattention and unconcern. Later, cognitive functions become impaired, first affecting abstract thinking, judgment, and memory. Eventually, orientation for time and place are disturbed.

An important factor supporting the organic nature of the psychological disturbances described above is the history of change from the patient's previous status. Sometimes the change is an exaggeration of the former personality (e.g., a woman who is parsimonious and reserved may become miserly and paranoid). In other patients, the change is opposite to that of the lifelong personal traits (e.g., a quiet and introverted man may become garrulous and grandiose). The development of cognitive defects, dysphasia, or incontinence firmly establishes the organic nature of the disease.

PARIETAL LOBE DISEASE Parietal lobe lesions may cause agnosia, aphasia, or apraxia. Anosognosia and other agnosias occur with lesions of the nondominant cerebral hemisphere, especially the parietal lobe. Fluent aphasias and ideomotor apraxia are characteristic of dominant hemisphere lesions.

The clinical manifestations of parietal lobe lesions may be difficult to differentiate from mental and psychogenic phenomena. Fluent aphasias may be mistaken for dementia or schizophrenia. Bizarre symptoms, such as distortion of body image and other spatial disorders, may suggest psychosis. The inattention and unconcern of a patient with parietal lobe disease may be misinterpreted as the apathy and indifference of a conversion reaction. Variability of performance, especially with different examiners, further complicates diagnostic decisions.

OCCIPITAL LOBE DISEASE Occipital lobe lesions may cause simple or complex illusions and hallucinations that may be mistaken for psychosis. Illusions may consist of *metamorphopsia* (distortion in the shape or size of images) or alterations of color or movement. With a complex illusion, an object may take on strange affective qualities. Simple visual hallucinations consist of geometric figures or lights, which may be stationary or mobile. Complex hallucinations are of people or animals. Visual hallucinations may occur within one visual field, either in a hemianoptic field or in the normal field, or they may be generalized. Suggestion may influence the type of formed hallucination—such as the hallucination of seeing Santa Claus at Christmas. The intellectual and emotional backgrounds of the patient are also important factors in the type of hallucination. Visual hallucinations are not limited to lesions of the occipital lobe; they are as common with disease of the temporal lobe as with the occipital lobe. However, they rarely occur with lesions of the frontal lobe or retina. Although formed hallucinations are often of temporal lobe origin and unformed hallucinations are of occipital lobe origin, this differentiation is not invariable.

Cortical blindness occurs with disease of both right and left visual cortices. Denial of blindness, called *Anton's syndrome,* occurs when the disease extends to the visual association areas. The patients move about as if they can see, excusing and confabulating reasons for bumping into things. This condition may be misdiagnosed as hysteria, for the fundi and pupils are normal, and the patient either denies the blindness or is unconcerned. Concentrically reduced fields of vision of organic origin may also be misinterpreted as hysteria. Bilateral lesions may also cause *prosopagnosia* (inability to recognize faces), metamorphopsia, and Balint's syndrome. Unilateral lesions on the left side give rise to alexia without agraphia, generally accompanied by a right homonymous hemianopsia and visual agnosias, including color agnosia.

DISEASE OF THE TEMPORAL LOBE Irritative lesions of the temporal lobe evoke mental and emotional symptoms with or without associated psychomotor seizures. Disturbances of behavior, usually automatisms as part of seizure activity, are often difficult to differentiate from impulsive psychogenic behavioral disorders.

Disease of the temporal lobe may alter conscious, cognitive, and emotional states. Disorders of consciousness are manifested by dreamy states. Organic mental disorders are usually characterized by impairment of recent memory. Abnormalities of thought and behavior range from obsessions and compulsions to sensations of unreality or depersonalization to frank psychosis, especially paranoia. Affective symptoms are usually anxiety, depression, rage, or fear. Disturbances of time perception may occur; time may seem to stand still or rush by.

Temporal lobe lesions may cause illusions and hallucinations. Paracusia refers to perceptions of sounds as more or less loud than normal, which may be associated with altered timber or tone. Elementary hallucinations consist of blowing, whistling, or humming sounds, whereas complex hallucinations include voices or music. The patient may or may not recognize the unreality of these phenomena.

Auditory agnosias are usually associated with lesions of the secondary auditory cortex of the right temporal lobe, except for verbal agnosia (i.e., fluent aphasia). Amusia, the inability to recognize music, is usually part of auditory agnosia. Fluent aphasia, alexia, and agraphia due to lesions of the dominant hemisphere may be mistaken for psychogenic phenomena.

After bilateral temporal lobectomy, the Klüver-Bucy syndrome occurs in monkeys. These animals become unusually docile and tame. Apparent visual agnosia leads them to mouth and touch everything, perhaps for purposes of identification. These animals demonstrate severe memory loss and bizarre hypersexuality. Bilateral temporal lobe lesions in humans may cause symptoms similar to the monkeys, but in a considerably modified form, with aphasia, bulimia, or dementia. Lesions of the medial temporal lobes cause Korsakoff's syndrome, involving loss of ability to remember new data. Rarely, bilateral temporal lobe disease results in belligerence and aggressive behavior.

DISEASE AFFECTING OTHER CEREBRAL STRUCTURES **Disease of the brain stem reticular formation** Lesions within this complex system affect multiple functions, such as arousal, alertness, and awareness; neuroendocrine functions; sensory perception; and motor activity. Motor abnormalities range from akinetic mutism to generalized convulsive disorders.

Limbic system The limbic system consists of the following anatomic structures: amygdala, hippocampal region, fornix, mammillary bodies, anterior thalamic nucleus, and cingulate gyrus. In addition, the reticular formation of the midbrain, the hypothalamus, and the medial portion of the thalamus are intimately connected with the limbic structures. Lesions in one of the above structures affect the functions of others, and disease of one cannot always be differentiated from disease of another. Irritative lesions within the limbic system may initiate psychomotor seizures. Disagreeable olfactory or gustatory hallucinations and associated lip, tongue, and swallowing activities are initiated within cortical areas of the limbic system. Genital and sexual responses may also be caused by irritative lesions in this area. The autonomic aspects of emotion—especially those of rage, fear, and defense phenomena—may be similarly evoked. Lesions of the hippocampal gyri result in the inability to remember new data. Bilateral disease of the cingulate gyri causes apathy, akinesis, and mutism. Lesions of the septal area lead to reduction or absence of emotional expression. Diseases of the hypothalamic and medial thalamic regions, even more clearly than those of other structures, produce their effects by the release of facilitating or inhibiting mechanisms necessary for balanced human behavior. Bilateral disease of this area is often associated with emotional lability or spontaneous laughter or crying. In lower animals, lesions of the anterior diencephalon are associated with sham rage—sympathetic motor activity of rage, probably without appropriate change of affect. Extreme excitement, savageness, and increased feeding drive are also evoked. In humans, marked agitation or manic activity may occur with disease in this area. In contrast, lesions of the posterior diencephalon in animals are associated with unusual tameness and, sometimes, severe apathy. In humans, disease of this area causes apathy, hypersomnia, and akinetic mutism. Lesions of the medial thalamic region may cause cognitive defects of confusion, confabulation, amnesia, or dementia.

Disease of the lateroventral thalamus The thalamic syndrome is due to unilateral disease, usually infarction, of the thalamus. There is impairment of sensation over the opposite side of the body, but much more distressing is an extreme hypersensitivity to all forms of somatic stimuli. Spontaneous unpleasant sensations, often of an agonizingly painful nature, tend to be continuous. These sensations may be aggravated by such minor stimuli as the touch of clothing, as well as by visceral and affective stimuli. There may be a delay in perception of the stimulus, distortion in the quality of the sensation, and a spread of the sensation far beyond the point of stimulation. These peculiar features and the frequent paucity of objective signs sometimes lead to a mistaken psychogenic diagnosis. Deep cerebral lesions involving right and left corticobulbar pathways cause pseudobulbar palsy, attended by emotional lability or spontaneous laughing or crying without the associated emotional feeling.

Disease of the basal ganglia Lesions of the extrapyramidal system cause disturbances of motor function and involuntary movements that are aggravated by slight emotional stimuli. They are discussed in other parts of this section. Especially in their early stages, dyskinesias are sometimes mistaken for psychogenic tics. For example, the child with Sydenham's chorea is often initially criticized for restlessness. The tics, grunts, and coprolalia of Tourette's disorder were, until recently, considered psychogenic. Several features of Parkinson's disease may be mistaken for psychological disturbances. The early tremor of parkinsonism may be considered nervousness, particularly because it may occur only with slight emotional stress. The sudden freezing of activity may mistakenly be considered catatonia. Conversely, akathisia, the inability to maintain a resting posture, may be mistaken for neurotic restlessness. The bradykinesia of parkinsonism—decreased spontaneity of movement and speech, coupled with loss of facial expression—are frequently misinterpreted as withdrawal and depression. Patients with disease of the basal ganglia may become depressed and irritable; compulsive and obsessive features are common; and emotional lability and spontaneous laughing or crying may occur. Slowness of mentation may parallel slowness of movement, and intellectual deterioration occasionally progresses to severe dementia.

Disease of the corpus callosum Because the corpus callosum may be congenitally absent without obvious signs, the clinical manifestations seen with lesions of this area probably result from disease or dysfunction of neighboring structures. The left hand may be apractic; in rare instances, it may even perform activities independent of the patient's will (alien hand sign). The patient may be unable to imitate with the right hand the position in which the examiner has placed the fingers of the left hand.

Midbrain Ischemia or infarction of the midbrain may cause lethargy, inattentiveness, and apathy, and a mute state may occur. Peduncular hallucinosis refers to vivid hallucinations recognized by the patient as unreal. A bizarre disorientation may occur in which reality cannot be distinguished from dreams.

DISEASES OF THE RIGHT, NONDOMINANT HEMISPHERE The right hemisphere modulates affect, behavior, nonverbal communication, and complex spatial perceptual functions. The nondominant hemisphere is, in large part, responsible for integrating major central neural systems: the arousal and vigilant aspects of the reticular formation, the sensory and spatial data of the parietal lobe, the motor programs for activity of the frontal lobe, and the drive and motivational factors of the limbic system. Disease of the nondominant hemisphere may lead to severe disabilities. To the uninitiated, these defects may be mistaken for psychogenic phenomena. There are several disorders of mentation associated with right-hemisphere lesions, but note that these syndromes are often seen with bilateral cerebral disease.

Anosognosia is denial of illness or of body parts. Impaired perception or conception may apply to any affected body part, most commonly hemiplegia and blindness. The degree of anosognosia may be severe with explicit denial and confabulation. These patients claim that the paralyzed limbs are not theirs, or they acknowledge the limbs but deny the paralysis. The patients may ascribe their inability to move or get out of bed to some external interference. Anosognosia may be implicit and manifested by inattention or withdrawal; the patients will admit hemiplegia only if they are specifically queried, and they seem unconcerned. There is a sense of depersonalization, especially toward the affected part; patients may refer to themselves in the third person. There may be disorientation for body parts or defects in body schema, known as *autotopognosia*. The finger agnosia of Gerstmann's syndrome is a manifestation of autotopognosia. Reduplication of body parts or places or times may occur. Although typical of right-cerebral disease, denial of illness may also occur with lesions in the dominant cerebral hemisphere. The site of the brain damage determines the symptoms that are denied and the symbolic structure or language in which the denial is expressed. The mechanism of denial, however, is much more complex; it includes the integration of environmental factors, past experiences, premorbid personality, symbolic values, type of disability, and the degree of brain damage or dysfunction. When denial of illness is psychogenic, it is usually a reaction to some catastrophic event.

Motor impersistence refers to the inability to sustain motor activity. These patients cannot keep their eyes closed, maintain conjugate gaze, or sustain handgrip. Associated similar psychological phenomena are manifested by impulsivity in response to the speech or acts of others. Typically, a patient will begin to answer before the question is finished.

Abulia is the loss of will to act. There is a long latency between thought and action. In severe cases, the abulic patients lie or sit immobile, are virtually unresponsive, and may appear comatose. In its milder forms, patients lose their spontaneity and initiative.

Nonlinguistic elements of speech and communication are controlled by the right cerebrum. The meaning of speech is conveyed not only by words and syntax, but by prosody of speech (i.e., pitch, rhythm, accent, tone, emphasis, cadence, and timing of words). People know when other people are angry without attention to the words they speak. A right-cerebral lesion may impair the patient's ability to appreciate or express affective qualities of speech. There may be associated loss of the ability to recognize the attitude and emotional qualities of gestures, other body language, and facial expressions that color our communication. The ability to appreciate music and art may be lost or impaired. Doctors must use great care in evaluating the emotional state of these patients. Even when they attempt to express their emotions in words, the patients' speech and face appear bland, flat, and indifferent.

Impairment of spatial orientation is a major sign of nondominant cerebral disease. This defect may be manifested in different ways. Disorientation for place may occur; patients may not be able to find their room or house. Directional sense may be lost, whereby patients cannot read a map or follow a route. There may be a peculiar sense of reduplication; patients acknowledge that they are in a hospital yet insist that they are in the bedroom of their home. Inability to recognize familiar faces, or prosopagnosia, may be part of this syndrome. These phenomena are often misdiagnosed as dementia.

Constructional apraxia is manifested by the patients' inability to draw a clock, arrange sticks in a pattern, or copy a geometric figure, although they maintain the motor and sensory functions to do so. Dressing apraxia may be part of this syndrome. Patients may put on clothing inside out or attempt to put both feet into the same trouser leg. Patients with a left cerebral lesion will draw a house in proportion, but it will be very simple. Those patients with a right cerebral lesion will draw the house in detail, but the dimensions will be wrong and the lines will be skewed.

Spatial neglect is another manifestation of a nondominant cerebral lesion. There will be extinction of the left stimulus (e.g., touch, pain, visual, auditory) during bilateral simultaneous stimulation. The patient ignores the environment, including people, on the left side. (Physicians should always examine such patients on the attentive right side.) Despite normal visual fields, the patient may read only the left side of the headline.

Head and neck Inspection may reveal asymmetries of the head and unusual postures of the neck. On palpation of the scalp, exostosis may be noted, such as that overlying a meningioma. The superficial temporal and carotid pulses should be palpated and note be made of cervical lymph nodes. Auscultation over each eyeball—allowing the opposite eyelid to open greatly diminishes adventitious muscle sounds—may reveal bruits of a vascular malformation or of a carotid-cavernous fistula. Bruits over the carotid or subclavian arteries may also be indicative of stenosis of these vessels. The loudness of a bruit bears no direct relationship to the degree of stenosis, but the higher the pitch, the more severe the stenosis. Mobility of the neck to passive movement may be diminished after cervical injuries or with paraspinal infections. Restriction of neck flexion is a sign of meningeal irritation or of a posterior fossa mass.

Cranial nerves OLFACTORY NERVE (1) The patient is asked to identify familiar odors, such as coffee or tobacco. Each nostril is tested in turn. Loss of smell is most often due to chronic smoking or to other diseases of the mucous membrane. Neurological causes of impoverished smell include head trauma, which results in lesions of the olfactory bulbs, and olfactory groove meningioma.

OPTIC NERVE (2) Visual acuity is evaluated by having the patient read a Snellen chart or regular newsprint. Each eye should be tested individually, both with and without the patient's eyeglasses. If a deficit is encountered and corrective lenses are unavailable, have the patient read through a pinhole. Improved performance suggests a refraction defect. Ophthalmoscopy is then performed, and the appearence of the optic disk and retina should be noted. Pallor and sharpness of an optic disk are manifestations of optic atrophy. Hyperemia of the disk, blurring of its margins, disappearance of the physiological cup, venous engorgement, and absence of venous pulsations indicate the presence of papilledema.

The visual field of each eye can be tested by confrontation. The patient covers one eye, looks at one of the examiner's eyes, and counts the number of fingers presented by the examiner at the periphery of the field. Each quadrant and each half of the right and left visual fields are tested. Standard perimetry and the tangent screen examination are required to determine the exact peripheral and central visual fields.

An irregular central scotoma within one visual field is usually a residual of retrobulbar or optic neuritis, as seen in multiple sclerosis. Enlargement of the blind spot occurs in papilledema. Arcuate or ring defects in one eye indicate retinal or optic nerve involvement, often due to glaucoma. Bitemporal hemianopsia occurs with lesions of the optic chiasm. Homonymous hemianopsia is associated with a lesion of the opposite optic tract or optic radiations. Homonymous superior quadrantanopsia is associated with a lesion of the opposite temporal lobe, whereas involvement of the parietal lobe results in a homonymous inferior quadrantic defect. Homonymous hemianopsia with sparing of central vision (known as *macular sparing*) is due to a lesion of the opposite occipital lobe (Fig. 2.1-1).

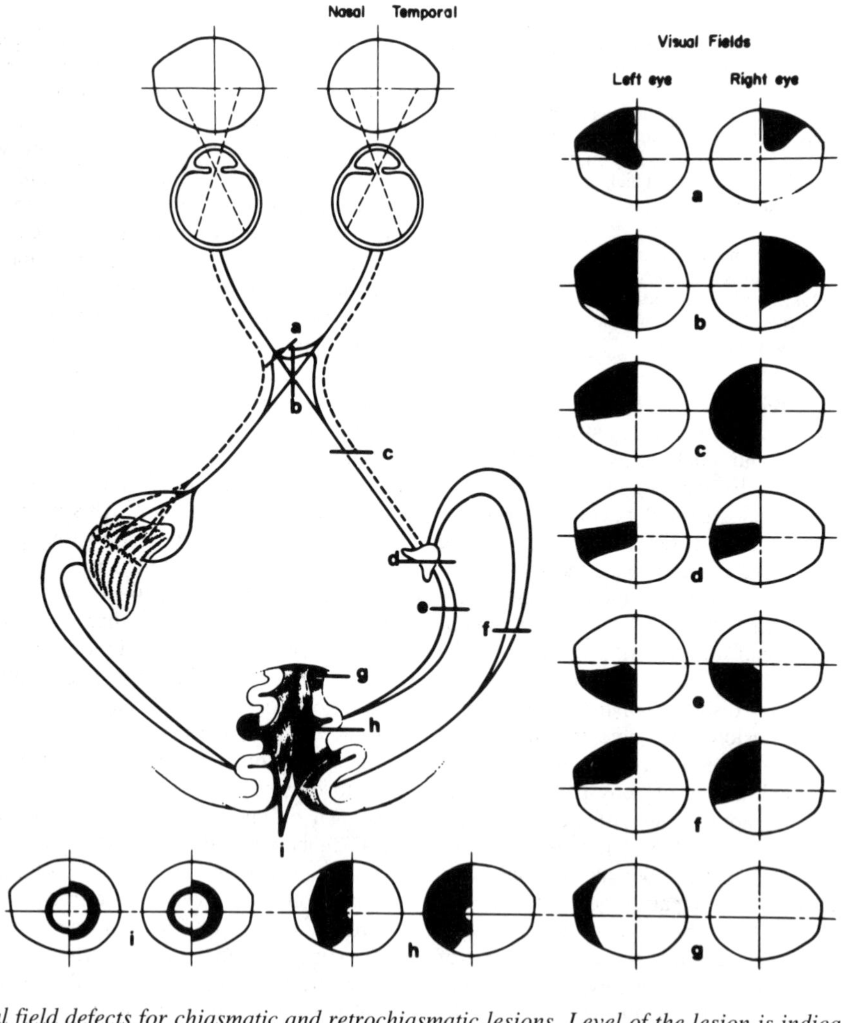

FIGURE 2.1-1. *Visual field defects for chiasmatic and retrochiasmatic lesions. Level of the lesion is indicated on the diagram to the left. Corresponding visual field defect is depicted to the right and at the bottom of the figure. (From Brazis P W, Masdeu J C, Biller J:* Localization in Clinical Neurology, *p 107. Little, Brown, Boston, 1985, with permission.)*

OCULOMOTOR, TROCHLEAR, AND ABDUCENS NERVES (3, 4, and 6) Because they supply the muscles of eye movement and, in the case of the oculomotor nerve, the constrictors of the pupil and the elevator of the eyelid, these nerves are tested together. The size, shape, and symmetry of the pupils are noted, and the response of the pupil to accommodation is tested by noting the pupillary constriction as the patient focuses from a distant object to one that is close. The reaction of the pupil to light can be seen by shining a light into each eye from the side. (Shining the light directly into each eye may cause the pupils to constrict because of accommodation.) Both direct and consensual pupillary reactions should be tested. A unilaterally dilated pupil may be the first sign of oculomotor nerve compression. Conversely, the pupil is usually spared when the oculomotor nerve is affected by diabetic neuropathy. Constriction of a pupil associated with ptosis and impairment of sweating over the ipsilateral forehead are manifestations of Horner's syndrome, indicative of a lesion in the ipsilateral sympathetic nerve pathway.

To determine the range of extraocular movements, the patient should be asked to look and then follow the movement of the examiner's finger in all directions of gaze. The examiner should pause briefly in every direction to look for nystagmus.

Except for congenital or long-standing cases, the patient complains of double vision (i.e., *diplopia*) when an extraocular muscle becomes paretic. At times, inspection cannot resolve which is the paretic muscle. The cover test should then be used. The patient is asked to fix on an object in the direction where the true and false images are farthest apart. The patient then alternatively covers each eye. The weak muscle belongs to the eye that suppresses the image that is the farthest out. For instance, if the images are farthest apart when gazing to the right with both eyes, either the left medial rectus or the right lateral rectus is weak. If covering the right eye suppresses the most distant image, the right lateral rectus is the weak muscle.

Ptosis of the lid is one sign of involvement of the oculomotor nerve, but the palpebral fissures may be asymmetrical from other causes. Disease of the facial nerve, for example, causing weakness of the orbicularis oculi muscle, results in a larger palpebral fissure on the side of the facial involvement. The patient's inability to move the eye up, down, or medially, with associated ptosis of the lid and dilation of the pupil, is a sign of complete loss of function of the oculomotor nerve. In lesions of the trochlear nerve affecting the superior oblique muscle, the patient has difficulty looking down and in; consequently, the head is tilted toward the shoulder of the opposite side. Disease of the abducens nerve, as the name implies, prevents abduction of the eye. In patients with conjugate gaze palsy, the eyes are generally deviated toward a destructive cerebral lesion and away from an irritative epileptogenic lesion, but only during the early ictal period. Low pontine lesions cause ipsilateral gaze palsy. High pontine lesions cause a medial longitudinal fasciculus syndrome (termed *internuclear opthalmoplegia syndrome*), wherein the eye on the side of the lesion has impaired adduction and the contralateral eye abducts and exhibits coarse nystagmus.

Nystagmus is due to disease of the oculovestibular system, spanning from the inner ear to the brain stem and cerebellum. Inner ear disease may evoke nystagmus that is horizontal or rotary. These types of nystagmus may also be noted with disease of the brain stem, but pure vertical nystagmus and monocular nystagmus are pathognomonic of brain stem disease. Nystagmus of vestibular origin increases when fixation is eliminated, as by use of strong lenses or when the eyes are closed; nystagmus of brain stem or cerebellar disease is most marked on fixation. Unidirectional nystagmus is a manifestation of labyrinthine disease; nystagmus elicited on gaze both to the left and to the right is indicative of brain stem or cerebellar disease.

TRIGEMINAL NERVE (5) Sensation of the face and cornea can be tested by observing the patient's blink response when a wisp of cotton lightly touches the edge of the cornea and by using the same wisp of cotton to test touch over the three divisions of the trigeminal nerve—forehead, cheek, and chin—and comparing the right side with the left side. Response to pinprick is tested in a similar distribution. When hypalgesia is mild, temperature impairment over the same distribution confirms the objective nature of the defect. Loss of corneal reflex may be the first sign of trigeminal nerve compression by an ipsilateral acoustic neuroma, and analgesia over one side of the face may be seen in brain stem infarction. The masses of the temporal and masseter muscles are palpated with the jaws tightly closed. An open jaw deviates toward a weakened external pterygoid muscle. The jaw jerk is elicited by tapping the middle of the chin with a reflex hammer while the patient's jaw is loosely open. Hyperactivity of this reflex may be indicative of bilateral damage of the corticobulbar tract above the level of the pons. The trigeminal nerve carries pain and touch sensations from the mucous membranes of the nose and mouth, but sensations of these areas need not be regularly tested.

FACIAL NERVE (7) The facial muscles are observed while the patients speak and by noting symmetry of blinking. The patients are then asked to show their teeth and wrinkle their foreheads. Sometimes, minimal asymmetries noted on movement of the face to command are exaggerated during the expression of emotion or other spontaneous activity. The strength of the orbicularis oculi muscle is tested by attempting to open the patients' eyelids against their resistance. Paralysis or weakness of all the facial muscles on one side, including those of the forehead, is indicative of damage of the ipsilateral lower motor neuron or facial nerve, as seen in Bell's palsy. If the forehead muscles are spared, the facial weakness is presumed to be caused by a contralateral lesion, such as a cerebral infarct, affecting corticobulbar pathways. The sensory portion of the facial nerve carries taste from the anterior two-thirds of the tongue. Sugar or salt in solution is placed on the left or right anterior portion of the protruded tongue, and the patients are asked to indicate the presence of taste by raising a hand. The rapidity of response on one side is then compared with the response on the other side. Taste is often unilaterally lost in patients with Bell's palsy, but not in patients with central nervous system (CNS) disease.

ACOUSTIC NERVE (8) The acoustic nerve is composed of the cochlear and the vestibular nerves. Auditory acuity may be tested by asking the patient to repeat words whispered into each ear. In Rinne's test, a vibrating tuning fork is placed on the mastoid portion of the skull behind the patient's ear. When the patient can no longer hear the sound, the fork is then placed next to the ear. Under normal circumstances, air conduction of sound is better than bone conduction. Both bone conduction and air conduction are impaired in the case of nerve deafness, but bone conduction is preserved in the presence of an air conduction defect. Weber's hearing test is performed by placing a vibrating tuning fork on the midline of the skull. If the sound is referred to one ear, the test is considered positive. When air conduction deafness is present because of middle ear disease, Weber's test lateralizes to the affected ear; if there is nerve deafness, the sound is heard in the normal ear. Audiometry is of value in precisely quantitating the hearing loss. When nerve deafness is suspected, the caloric test should be performed to evaluate the vestibular portion of the acoustic nerve. With the patient supine and the head raised 30°, injection of 4 to 15 ml of ice water into the external auditory canal normally evokes, within a few seconds, vertigo, nystagmus (with fast component to the opposite side), and past pointing to the stimulated side. When the acoustic nerve is compromised, loss of auditory acuity and of caloric response is evident on the involved side. Many refinements of audiometry, other tests of vestibular function, and brain stem auditory evoked responses may assist in differentiating lesions of the inner ear, the acoustic nerve, and the brain stem.

GLOSSOPHARYNGEAL AND VAGUS NERVUS (9 and 10) These two nerves are tested together. The gag reflex is tested by touching each side of the pharynx. Bilateral impairment of the gag reflex need not be abnormal, but loss of the gag reflex on one side and pulling up of the soft palate toward the normal opposite side are indicative of involvement of the ninth nerve. Hoarseness may be an indication of weakness or paralysis of a vocal cord. Difficulty in swallowing (i.e., *dysphagia*), when of neurological origin, is noted earliest with liquids and is indicative of bulbar (medullary) or pseudobulbar (upper motor neuron) disease. *Dysarthria* may also be bulbar (nasal speech), pseudobulbar (explosive speech), or cerebellar (speech of the drunkard). Staccato speech combines pseudobulbar and cerebellar elements. The glossopharyngeal nerve carries taste from the posterior third of the tongue, but this sensation is not usually tested. The autonomic functions of the vagus nerve, having to do with cardiopulmonary activity, are noted during the general physical examination.

SPINAL ACCESSORY NERVE (11) The *trapezius* muscle raises the shoulder. The *sternocleidomastoid* muscle turns the head to the opposite side. These muscles are tested by having the patient move them against the examiner's resistance. Lesions compressing the nerve at the jugular foramen or, less often, in the lower medulla cause weakness or paralysis. The trapezius and, less often, the sternocleidomastoid may also be affected by a contralateral cerebral lesion. The sternocleidomastoid muscle is often partially uncrossed in its supranuclear innervention; thus, a lesion in a cerebral hemisphere may affect the ipsilateral sternocleidomastoid muscle.

HYPOGLOSSAL NERVE (12) The protruded tongue is normally in the midline. It deviates to the weakened side—that is, ipsilateral to the lesion if the lower motor neuron is involved and contralateral to the lesion in upper motor neuron disease. If lower motor neuron disease is present, atrophy or fine fasciculations of the tongue may be seen on the side of involvement.

CRANIAL NERVE SIGNS OF CEREBRAL DISEASE Cranial nerve signs associated with infarct or tumor affecting one cerebral hemisphere are summarized in Table 2.1-2.

PSEUDOBULBAR PALSY This syndrome is characterized by symptoms mimicking disease of the medulla, but is attributable to bilateral disease of supranuclear corticobulbar fibers. Because most bulbar musculature has a bilateral cerebral representation, a unilateral supranuclear lesion does not cause lasting bulbar signs. Pseudobulbar palsy is most often caused by multiple small cerebrovascular lesions in or near the internal capsule or ventral pons. Dysarthria and dysphagia are most common. The patient's speech has a nasal, slurring, and often explosive quality, and voice volume is diminished. Chewing and swallowing are impaired, and food may accumulate in the mouth, with drooling of saliva and frequent choking. The patient's gait is often defective, particularly because of disequilibrium. All movements may be slow and poorly performed, the facial expressions may be flattened, and exaggerated emotional responses are prominent. Spontaneous laughing and crying frequently occur; they are involuntary and unassociated with appropriate emotions. Gag reflexes may be absent or preserved, and deep reflexes, including the jaw jerk, are often hyperactive.

Motor system A screening type of motor examination can be performed quickly when done in an orderly fashion. If motor abnormalities are noticed, a more detailed examination will disclose the nature of the disorder. Gait and station are examined first. Simultaneously, muscle bulk is inspected and any abnormal movements noted. The patient should then lie on an examining table to allow for accurate testing of muscle tone and reflexes. Testing of coordination of distal movements, evaluation of meningeal signs, and sensory testing will then conclude the neurological examination.

Gait and station Observe the patient rise from sitting on a low stool and walk in normal fashion as well as on heels, toes, and in tandem (touching the heel of one foot to the toe of the other). Muscle atrophy, deformities of the extremities or trunk, and abnormal movements should be recorded. Impairment of truncal equilibrium, due to midline cerebellar or thalamic disease, is manifested by increased lateral sway as the patient rises from a supine or sitting position. Rising from a low stool is hindered by proximal muscle weakness or by the impaired postural reflexes of parkinsonism. Walking on heels will be defective, with weakness of the anterior compartment of the lower leg, from either pyramidal or peripheral nerve disease. During heel and toe walking, mild pyramidal or cerebellar dysfunction becomes conspicuous. Unilateral pyramidal or hemiplegic gait is characterized by impaired dorsiflexion of the foot, which is externally rotated; and stiffness of the leg, held straight at the knee with resultant circumduction, a circling, scything-like movement of the leg. Cerebellar gait is broad-based and lurching. Tandem walking is impaired by posterior column, thalamocortical, or cerebellar disease. Vestibular disease or ipsilateral midline cerebellar disease, causing a tendency to drift to the affected side, may be revealed by having the patient take three steps forward and three backward while keeping the eyes closed. Star walking then results, as the tendency to veer to one side makes the patient progressively turn from the original path. Other causes of gait disturbance are outlined in Table 2.1-3. Arm swing may be lost with ipsilateral cerebellar or contralateral extrapyramidal or pyramidal disease.

The patient is then observed standing erect, with feet together, arms outstretched in front and supinated, first with eyes open, then with eyes closed. Inability to maintain an erect posture with the eyes closed, known as Romberg's sign, is usually indicative of posterior column disease or severe peripheral neuropathy, but the sign may be occasionally present with a cerebellar lesion. Impairment of postural reflexes in Parkinson's disease may be shown by the ease with which patients can be pushed from their standing base. Downward drift, flexion at the elbow and wrist, and pronation of the outstretched arm indicate disease anywhere along the corticospinal tract originating in the opposite cerebral hemisphere. The arm may drift laterally with cerebellar disease or proprioceptive loss.

TABLE 2.1-2
Cranial Nerve Signs of Unilateral Cerebral Disease*

Cranial Nerve	*Signs*
2	Contralateral homonymous hemianopsia
3,4,6	Conjugate deviation of eyes away from the side of the irritative lesion or toward the side of the destructive lesion
5	Contralateral impairment of pain and touch over the face and diminished corneal reflex
7	Contralateral paresis of the face, not including the forehead
11	Contralateral weakness of the trapezius muscle and ipsilateral weakness of the sternocleidomastoid muscle
12	Contralateral weakness of the tongue

*The numerals refer to the cranial nerves, but it is their supranuclear innervation that is affected.

Involuntary movements Involuntary movements are outlined in Table 2.1-4. Many of these conditions are discussed in Sections 2.2 and 2.3.

TREMOR Tremor may be associated with disease of the contralateral basal ganglia or ipsilateral cerebellar pathways. In contrast to the intention tremor of cerebellar disease, basal ganglia tremor occurs mainly at rest. Tremor is increased by emotional stress and disappears during sleep. Parkinsonian tremor has a rate of 4 to 7 Hz (cycles per second) and affects distal portion of the extremities. In the hands, the tremor produces a pill-rolling movement.

CEREBELLAR DISEASES In contrast with extrapyramidal disease, cerebellar disease does not usually cause tremor at rest, but rather during activity; it is an action or intention tremor.

Essential (familial) tremor affects the upper extremities and is both postural, with the arms outstretched, and present on precise action. It may be an exaggeration of normal physiological tremor.

Cerebellar outflow tremor, seen with lesions affecting the pathways of the dentate nucleus of the brachium conjunctivum, is a severe, coarse, rhythmic tremor enhanced by activity, but present even at rest.

HYPERKINESIAS Athetosis, chorea, dystonia, hemiballismus, and tics are generally grouped as basal ganglia disorders. Recent evidence indicates that dystonia may be due to brain stem disease.

Athetosis is manifested by slow, writhing, twisting movements affecting predominantly the distal portions of the extremities; associated similar movements of the face cause grimacing. Spasticity is present more often than hypotonicity. Athetosis is usually due to anoxia at birth.

Chorea is characterized by rapid, irregular, asymmetrical jerks of the extremities. The movements are purposeless, but may be turned into semipurposeful movements. Hypotonicity is usually present. In childhood, Syndenham's chorea is a manifestation of rheumatic fever; in adult life, the movements may be a sign of Huntington's chorea.

Dystonia musculorum deformans or torsion spasm is manifested by slow, writhing torsions of the trunk and the pelvic and shoulder girdles. Scoliosis and lordosis are common. Dystonic tremor, worse while lying down, is often pronounced. Dystonia or dyskinesia may occur as a complication of psychotropic medication.

Buccolingual dyskinesias are choreoathetoid movements of the mouth, jaw, and tongue; involuntary head and neck movements are often associated. Levodopa (Larodopa, Dopar) toxicity or psychotropic drug therapy are the most common causes. *Meige's syndrome* is the combination of blepharospasm and oromandibular dyskinesia. *Paroxysmal dystonic choreoathetosis* is a familial disease. Bursts of activity last from minutes to hours, recurring several times daily. *Paroxysmal kinesigenic choreoathetosis* is a rare condition but the movements occur very frequently because they are precipitated by voluntary activity.

Hemiballismus is characterized by unilateral violent, flailing movements of the extremities. The patients appear to be trying to throw their extremities away from their trunks. Usually a vascular lesion of the subthalamic nucleus causes this condition.

TABLE 2.1-3
Gait Disturbances

Neurogenic alterations of gait
  Upper motor neuron disease—spastic gait
    Hemiplegic gait—the lower extremity extended and circumducted
    Paraparetic gait of spinal cord disease—stiff legged and wide based
    Paraparetic gait of cerebral palsy (diplegia)—adductor spasm with scissoring (alternately crossing) extended lower extremities
  Lower motor neuron disease—steppage gait (The leg of the flaccid foot is raised higher than usual, and the foot slapped down to prevent stumbling over the toe.)
  Disease of the basal ganglia
    Parkinsonism—shuffling, small steps, festination (a tendency to accelerate)
    Choreoathetotic gait—intermittently irregular and jerking
    Dystonic gait—pelvic and truncal torsion
    Wilson's disease—both cerebellar ataxia and extrapyramidal features
  Cerebellar disease—staggering, with tendency to fall toward the side of the lesion
  Proprioceptive defect—ataxic, wide-based, worse at night or with the eyes closed
  Apraxia of gait—inability to walk, in spite of intact motor power and coordination (The patients do not know what to do with their feet; they seem to be glued to the floor.)
Nonneurological gait disturbances
  Limping gait—favors leg due to pain or orthopedic defect of lower extremity or back
  Mincing gait—restricted range of motion as in rheumatoid arthritis
  Waddling gait—proximal leg defects as with bilateral dislocations of the hips or muscular dystrophy
  Hysterical gait—bizarre and variable (The disability is often so great that, if the disturbance were organic, one would expect the patient to fall frequently, but the contrary is the case. Astasia-abasia is the inability to stand or walk in spite of adequate muscle strength and coordination.)

Tics are sudden, repetitive, irregular muscle contractions. They usually consist of grimacing, blinking, or other facial movements; twisting of the head and neck; or shrugging of the shoulders. *Tourette's disorder* is manifested by multiple tics and vocal outbursts, often coprolalia.

Torticollis, the involuntary turning of the head to one side, may be the first sign of, or a *forme fruste* of, dystonia musculorum deformans or of Tourette's disorder.

Myoclonus is a sudden, brief jerk or contraction of a muscle or muscle groups. The activity, faster than chorea, may be almost imperceptible, or it may be gross, affecting the entire body. Myoclonic activity may arise from disease or dysfunction of any part of the CNS. It may occur spontaneously or may be evoked by activity, known as action myoclonus. Cerebral anoxia is a common cause of myoclonus.

Asterixis is a repetitive flapping movement of the extended hands due to a sudden, brief loss of postural tone. This variety of myoclonus generally accompanies hepatic coma or other metabolic encephalopathies. Unilateral asterixis most often indicates involvement of the opposite thalamus or internal capsule.

Epileptic phenomena, such as focal motor seizures, are faster and more regular than chorea; unlike tremor, however, they are not rhythmic. *Epilepsia partialis continua* is manifested by continuous, mild clonic movements of a portion of one extremity, lasting for hours or days. Impairment of consciousness differentiates *status epilepticus,* often manifested by multifocal twitching, from most of the hyperkinetic disorders discussed above. Consciousness is also impaired when generalized myoclonus follows an episode of severe brain anoxia. Slow, clonic movements of the trunk and upper extremities may occur in petit mal status.

OTHER INVOLUNTARY MOVEMENTS *Hemifacial spasm* begins with blepharospasm and progresses to other muscles innervated by the facial nerve. It is usually due to vascular cross-compression of the facial nerve adjacent to the brain stem.

Restless legs syndrome is a nocturnal phenomenon wherein peculiar sensations—cramp-like, paresthetic, or vague pains—of the lower extremities evoke restlessness in the legs.

Fasciculations are fleeting twitches of a group of muscle fibers making up a motor unit. Unlike myoclonus, fasciculations are not powerful enough to move a joint, except the small ones in the hand. Fasciculations often indicate disease of the lower motor neuron, but they may normally occur with exposure to cold, fatigue, or anxiety.

Muscle tone With the patient lying on the examining table, consistency of the muscles is noted by palpation, tone is explored by passive motion of the elbows and knees, and reflexes are elicited. Palpation may elicit pain in a patient with myositis. Muscle consistency may be fibrous or rubbery in myopathies or after long-standing denervation. A prolonged contraction occurs when a myotonic muscle (thenar eminence or tongue) is briskly tapped. The handgrip of a myotonic patient is slow to relax.

Varieties of increased muscle tone include clasp-knife *spasticity* with an upper motor neuron lesion and *rigidity* (often of the cogwheel or lead-pipe type) with certain extrapyramidal diseases, such as parkinsonism. Spasticity is present only in flexion or in extension, whereas rigidity is present in both directions. The third type of increased muscle tone, characteristic of bilateral frontal lobe disease, is called *paratonia,* or *gegenhalten.* It feels as if the patient is actively opposing the action of the examiner. Paratonia is enhanced by brusquely moving the limb and disappears when the extremity is gently handled. One of the most effective ways of eliciting paratonia is by peremptorily asking the patient to relax. Muscle tone is decreased or flaccid with lower motor neuron lesions, hemispheric

TABLE 2.1-4
Involuntary Movements

Extrapyramidal diseases
  Parkinsonism
  Athetosis
  Chorea
  Dystonia
  Buccolingual dyskinesia
  Paroxysmal dystonic choreoathetosis
  Hemiballism
Cerebellar diseases
  Action, intention tremor
  Essential, familial tremor
  Cerebellar outflow tremor
Tics
  Common tics
  Tourette's disorder
  Torticollis
Hepatic and other metabolic diseases
  Wilson's disease
  Asterixis
Epilepsy
  Epilepsia partialis continua
  Status epilepticus
  Myoclonus (also see below)
Other involuntary movements
  Myoclonus
  Hemifacial spasm
  Restless legs syndrome

cerebellar disease, and, transiently, after a complete transection of the spinal cord or a massive cerebral infarct.

Reflexes Both muscle-stretch and superficial reflexes are influenced by disease of the segmental motor arc and of suprasegmental input playing on the segmental level; thus, they provide valuable information for the localization of disease of the central or peripheral nervous system. Muscle tone and reflexes often correspond closely. For instance, with upper motor neuron lesions, muscle tone is increased in the form of spasticity, and the muscle-stretch reflexes are hyperactive; with lower motor neuron lesions, both are depressed. Muscle-stretch reflexes are elicited by tapping the tendon of specific muscles. In the upper extremities, the muscles most commonly tested are the biceps (C5-6), brachioradialis (C6), triceps (C7), and flexors of the fingers (C7-8). In the lower extremities, the patellar (L2,3,4), medial (L4-5, S1) and lateral (L5, S1-2) hamstrings, and the Achilles (S1-2) tendons are tapped. In testing muscle-stretch reflexes, one must compare symmetrical muscles and apply the stimuli with equal intensity to relaxed extremities. Reflex reinforcement—by having patients clench their teeth tightly or pull against their hands hooked to each other by flexed fingers, called the *Jendrassik maneuver*—should be used when reflexes are not initially elicited by percussion. Reflexes are graded, taking into account the amplitude of the contraction, the multiplicity of response (single or clonic), and the degree of spread to other muscles, generally within neighboring segments. The scale is as follows: (0) absent even with reinforcement; (+) present with reinforcement only; (++) normoactive; (+++) marked spreading to neighboring muscles; and (++++) clonic responses. Hyperreflexia with clonus of the calf muscles can also be demonstrated by eliciting ankle clonus, when the foot is briskly dorsiflexed and kept in this position by gentle pressure. Hyperreflexia may be found in healthy individuals, particularly those who are thin and anxious. More important is the presence of asymmetric responses, but note that mild voluntary contraction of one side, as often seen in psychogenic weakness, can spuriously cause reflex hypoactivity on that side.

The *superficial reflexes* are tested by stroking the skin with a semisharp object. The four quadrants of the abdomen are tested (D7,8,9 upper; D11,12 lower). Stroking the medial aspect of the thigh elicits the cremasteric reflex (D12; L1). Stimulation of the perianal area evokes contraction of the anal sphincter, the anal reflex (S2,3,4,5).

Certain *pathological reflexes* are indicative of pyramidal tract disease. The Babinski sign is elicited by stroking the lateral aspect of the sole from the arch to and across the ball of the foot with a semisharp object. Flexion of the toes is the normal response; dorsiflexion of the big toe and spread of the other toes is the abnormal response. The Chaddock sign (stroking the lateral aspect of the dorsum of the foot), the Gordon sign (squeezing the calf muscle), and the Oppenheim sign (forcefully stroking the anterior surface of the shin) show toe responses like that of the Babinski sign. The Hoffmann sign is elicited by forcefully flicking downward the distal portion of the patient's middle finger. In a positive response, flexion and adduction of the thumb occur. The Hoffmann sign is another way of eliciting the finger-flexor reflex and has the same significance as muscle-stretch reflex hyperactivity.

Muscle strength Screening for muscle weakness is best performed by observing the patient arise to the standing position, walk, and perform activities of daily living, such as buttoning one's clothes. If atrophy, weakness, or clumsiness are noted or suspected, the affected region should be examined in greater detail by having the patient use the affected muscles against the examiner's strength. Voluntary muscle strength is impaired in certain patterns, corresponding to the site of the disease. Weakness of the distal portions of the extremities suggests neuropathy, whereas proximal weakness is characteristic of myopathy. If there is suspicion of nerve root or peripheral nerve involvement, the corresponding muscles are specifically examined. With spinal cord involvement, weakness of the lower extremities is common but may initially be masked by spasticity. In the presence of minimal unilateral upper motor neuron disease, such as a lesion in a cerebral hemisphere, slight weakness of the contralateral extremities may be manifested first in the extensor and supinator muscles of the upper extremity and in the flexor and internal rotator muscles of the lower extremity. Thus, with the patient's eyes closed and arms extended, a slight downward drift, flexion, and pronation of the affected upper extremity develops. In the prone position, upper motor neuron weakness is first manifested by a slight downward drift of the affected flexed lower leg, known as *Barré's sign*, and when supine, by a slight external rotation of the weakened leg and a slight foot drop. Documentation of the degree of weakness is important in establishing the course of the patient's illness. The muscle strength is graded as follows: normal—grade 5; able to resist the examiner—grade 4, good; able to resist gravity, but not the examiner—grade 3, fair; able to move only when gravity is eliminated—grade 2, poor; only a flicker of movement discernible—grade 1, trace; total paralysis—grade 0.

Coordination Coordination of axial movements is observed as patients walk or shift in bed. Coordination of distal movements is tested by having patients touch the heel of one foot to the knee of the other leg and then run the heel down the shin of the leg, first with eyes open and then with eyes closed. To test hand movements, patients' pointed index fingers alternately touch the tips of their noses and the examiner's pointed finger. The maneuver is repeated with eyes closed. Action or intention tremor and dysmetria may be observed by these maneuvers. In testing the ability to alternate movements rapidly, the patient taps the floor with each foot or pats the thigh alternately with palm and then dorsum of each hand. *Dysdiadochokinesis* is a defect in rapid alternating movements. Rebound phenomenon occurs with the inability to quickly check a movement. The phenomenon is tested by releasing, without warning, an extremity that has been forcefully restrained. Fine skills are observed when the patients write or button their clothes.

Defects in coordination and rebound of extremities suggest disease of the ipsilateral cerebellar pathways if the lesion is below the midbrain. Cerebellar involvement can be invoked only if weakness or sensory (position sense) loss in the affected limb is not responsible for the distal incoordination.

Summary of signs of cerebellar or cerebellar pathway disease

Defective equilibrium impairs stance and gait, with tendencies to deviate toward the side of the cerebellar lesion. Associated movements are also impaired on the affected side. Defective ipsilateral coordination is manifested by ataxia of the extremities, with intention tremor, dysmetria, past pointing, dysdiadochokinesis, and rebound phenomenon. There is associated ipsilateral decrease in muscle tone and pendular reflexes. Fatigability and slowness of movements are common. Dysarthria, especially of the scanning (staccato) type, and nystagmus may be present.

Sensory examination This portion of the examination is often the most difficult and frustrating. Both the patient and the examiner must be alert and cooperative. Because it is impractical to stimulate every square centimeter of the body, there must be some idea of the location of the neurological lesion for which the examiner is searching. In almost all instances, the patient is asked to differentiate a stimulus applied to a normal portion of the body from the same stimulus applied to a portion of the body that is presumably affected. Thus, in searches for a peripheral nerve defect, the patient compares a stimulus in the area of the presumed deficit with a similar stimulus over the opposite extremity. When the examiner is searching for polyneuropathy manifested by distal sensory impairment, the patient is asked to compare the sensation over the toes and feet or fingers and hands with a similar sensation over the more proximal portions of the extremities. In searches for a spinal level, the patient compares a stimulus below the presumptive sensory level with a stimulus above that level. When the examiner is investigating a possible intracranial lesion, the patient is asked to compare a sensation over the affected side of the body with a similar sensation over the presumably unaffected side.

During all sensory testing, the patient's eyes should be closed. *Superficial touch* sensation is examined by means of a wisp of cotton, *superficial pain* by a pin or a pinwheel. Sensitivity to *temperature* is tested by using test tubes containing hot and cold water; if test tubes are not readily available, the metal handle of a reflex hammer may be used. In an attempt to quantitate the degree of sensory impairment, the patient is asked to estimate the degree of defective sensation as a percentage of the 100 percent normal stimulus. Inconsistencies in the patient's responses and minor impairments—for example, 90 percent of normal—can usually be ignored. *Vibration sense* is evaluated by means of a tuning fork, with a frequency of 128 or 236 Hz, placed on bony prominences of the extremities. *Position sense* is examined by passively moving the distal phalanx of the patient's finger or toe and by asking the patient to indicate promptly the direction of movement. If the examiner grasps the sides of the digit, pressure on the finger or toe cannot be used by the patient in interpreting the direction of movement. The ability of the patient, while keeping the eyes closed, to maintain a stance or to reach the tip of the nose with the tip of the finger are also sensitive tests of proprioception.

Vibration and position sensations are carried by the posterior columns of the spinal cord, whereas superficial pain, touch, and temperature sensations are carried by the spinothalamic tracts. Any modality may be impaired by a lesion of its pathway from the peripheral nerve through the spinal cord and brain stem to the thalamus and parietal lobe.

Fine discriminatory sensations require the cerebral cortex for interpretation. The tests are performed with the patient's eyes closed. With a cerebral defect, especially a lesion of the parietal lobe, extinction of the stimulus on the opposite side of the body may occur when the right and left sides of the body are simultaneously stimulated by touches or pinpricks. Two-point discrimination is tested by simultaneously applying two stimuli close to each other and asking whether the patient can distinguish one or two points; this discrimination is best in the fingers. Stereognosis is tested by asking the patient to identify familiar objects placed in the hand. One tests graphesthesia by asking the patient to recognize letters or numbers written on the skin. Impairment of fine sensation prevents the differentiation of the textures of cotton, silk, and wool. It is clear that defects of these cortical sensory phenomena do not implicate the cortex if more peripheral sensory pathways are affected.

Autonomic nervous system Evaluation of vital signs is part of the general examination. Orthostatic changes in blood pressure often herald an autonomic neuropathy, such as caused by diabetes or amyloidosis, or a central disorder of autonomic regulation, such as the Shy-Drager syndrome. Particularly if there is a history of fainting spells, the blood pressure should be obtained with the patient supine, after rising to a standing position, and after 4 minutes of standing. The physiological pulse acceleration induced by rising to the standing position may be blunted in autonomic disorders. Regional autonomic disturbances, often caused by tumors or trauma that affect the sympathetic pathways, result in trophic changes that can be detected by inspection. The skin is erythematous, warm, sweatless, and mildly edematous. Hair may be lost. Affection of the cervical sympathetic chain, as by a Pancoast tumor of the lung, results in an ipsilateral Horner's syndrome. Determining the function of the bladder may require cystometric examination, but the tone of the rectal sphincter can be easily palpated. Cystometric examination is performed by recording intravesicular pressures after specific amounts of saline have been injected into the urinary bladder. The patient's sensations of fullness and desire to void are also noted. Special tests of autonomic function, including the Valsalva maneuver, tilt table studies, and determination of catecholamines in blood should be performed in cases of generalized autonomic dysfunction of unclear origin. Sleep disturbances that appear to have an organic basis should be evaluated by polygraphic recording during sleep and wakefulness.

NEUROLOGICAL SIGNS IN THE ELDERLY

The aging process affects neurological function. Certain signs that are usually considered evidence of disease may be of no clinical importance beyond the age of 50 or 60. When one or two of the responses to be noted occur in people over the age of 50, they are not considered evidence of disease, but three or more signs may be indications of a pathological process. As always, the findings on examination must be interpreted within the context of the entire clinical picture.

MEMORY The most common sign of aging is impairment of recent memory. This may be manifested by the inability to recall three unrelated words after several minutes of distraction or the inability to spell a simple word, such as "world," backward as well as forward. These findings are noted in about one-fourth of normal people between the ages of 50 and 80 and in one-half of those beyond that range. The other neurological signs occur in 5 to 10 percent of the population between the ages of 50 to 70 and rise to 25 to 50 percent in the older ages.

CRANIAL NERVE SIGNS Cranial nerve signs associated with senescence are referable to the eyes. The pupils tend to be small and sluggishly reactive. There is often some impairment of upward gaze, convergence, or Bell's phenomenon. Horizontal pursuit may be hesitant or jerking (cogwheel-like) rather than smooth. Impersistence of lateral gaze is sometimes noted.

MOTOR AND SENSORY SIGNS Examination of the motor system may reveal atrophy of intrinsic hand muscles and slight weakness of the muscles of the pelvic girdle. Resting muscle tone is often slightly increased with features of paratonia or gegenhalten. Slight dysmetria may be present on finger to nose or heel to knee tests and rapid alternating movements are slowed. The most common sensory sign on examination is decrease or loss of vibration sense at and below the ankles. Mild impairment of position sense, and pain and touch sensations are also occasionally noted.

REFLEXES Reflexes are often altered in the elderly. The abdominal reflexes are lost and the ankle jerks are diminished or absent. Dysinhibition of developmental reflexes, so-called release signs, are noted by the snout, grasp, or palmomental reflexes. The glabellar blink response and impairment of postural reflexes, characteristically seen in parkinsonism, often occur in the elderly.

EVALUATION OF THE CHILD

HISTORY A manner similar to that outlined for the adult is used for obtaining a child's history, but with different emphasis. In the child, a past history of trauma, encephalitis, meningitis, or neonatal seizures is particularly important because these conditions may more seriously affect the developing brain than the brain of an adult. The review of systems proves to be less helpful. The social history concentrates on environmental factors. The family history must be thorough.

The importance of the prenatal, perinatal, and postnatal history cannot be overemphasized. Was the mother's pregnancy normal, or was there a history of vaginal bleeding? Did the mother experience illness during the pregnancy, and what drugs, if any, did she take? Was the pregnancy full-term, or was the delivery premature? Was the labor unusually prolonged or in any other way abnormal? Was the delivery of the infant difficult or in any other way potentially traumatic? Did the infant cry immediately and have good color? What was the birth weight?

The assessment of the neurological status of the infant and child is primarily a measurement of the maturation of the nervous system. The child's developmental history is essential. The parents may not be aware of all the features in the infant's development, but they can often remember some of the following events.

Infants should begin to lift their heads while prone from the time of birth and begin to lift them well by 4 months of age. Babies should begin to smile at 2 months of age and laugh, as well as recognize their mothers by 4 months of age. Children should sit unsupported by 8 months of age and begin to crawl or creep between 10 and 12 months of age. They should wave "bye-bye" at 10 to 11 months of age. At 11 months of age, they should pull themselves up to the standing position and begin to walk with support at 12 months. The word "mama" becomes meaningful at 10 months of age, and by 1 year, an additional one- to three-word vocabulary should be evident. There is a wide range of normalcy; slow development of one or two features should not be taken as evidence of significant retardation. For example, although the average child walks without assistance soon after 1 year of age, retardation of gait is not considered to be present before 18 months of age.

Other history during the first year of life may also be pertinent. Was the baby colicky or were there other feeding problems? Did the infant sleep excessively; that is, was the baby an unusually good one? Or, alternately, was evidence of hyperactivity manifested during the baby's first year? The course of the patient's symptoms helps to differentiate a static encephalopathy, such as one due to birth injury, from a progressive disease, in which an initial period of normal development precedes the evidence of disease and deterioration.

EXAMINATION Even more important than the adult's is the child's general physical examination, for often it reveals the major clue to the diagnosis. The child, for instance, may exhibit the skin manifestations of a phacomatosis, the skeletal characteristics of mongolism, or the hepatosplenomegaly of lipidosis.

Observation of the young child may reveal asymmetries of the face or head, asymmetry of limb size or movement, or abnormal posture of the trunk or head and neck. In performing the neurological examination, one observes the child's social adaptability and language, motor activity, perception, postural reactions, and reflex activity. Other tests, as discussed for the adult, are integrated into this general pattern of examination.

EVALUATION OF THE PATIENT IN COMA

The first step in evaluating a patient in coma consists of insuring an open airway and of taking steps to stabilize the cardiovascular and respiratory states. The treatment of coma is discussed in Section 2.3. Important historical information includes exposure to sedatives or other toxic agents; past medical history, particularly cardiac disease, liver failure, and hypertension; possible head trauma; and the time course of the loss of consciousness. Coma of acute onset is often due to trauma, cardiovascular or cerebrovascular disease, intoxication, or heat stroke. Gradually developing coma is probably caused by meningoencephalitis, systemic infection, cerebral mass, or metabolic disease.

PHYSICAL EXAMINATION During attention to the vital functions, the heart, lungs, and abdomen are evaluated. The patient's breath odor and skin color may give important diagnostic clues. The breath may smell of alcohol, or its odor may be indicative of diabetic coma, uremia, or hepatic failure. The skin may be discolored (pale, cyanotic, jaundiced) or show signs of altered hydration (edema, dehydration) or of vascular changes (petechiae, bruises).

Respiratory rate and rhythm Cheyne-Stokes respiration is usually caused by metabolic disease or dysfunction deep within the cerebrum. Central, or neurogenic, hyperventilation is due to a lesion between the lower midbrain and the lower pons. Prolonged periods of apnea are associated with lesions of the mid- and lower pons. Ataxic, agonal respirations occur when respiratory centers in the medulla are affected.

NEUROLOGICAL EXAMINATION The neurological examination of the comatose patient helps to determine the site of disease affecting the brain, if not its cause.

Mental status The degree and type of responsiveness to stimuli (light, sound, superficial and deep pain) are documented. In a semicomatose state, the patient may make semipurposeful movements to ward off the stimulus. The comatose patient may reflexively withdraw from the stimulus; at a deeper state of coma, only decorticate or decerebrate activity can be evoked, as described below. Rather than labeling the degree of coma, it is better to describe the patient's response to a few reproducible stimuli, such as calling the patient's name or applying pressure to the fingernail bed. In this manner, the response over time can be evaluated successively by different examiners.

Psychogenic unresponsiveness The patient may hold the eyes forcibly closed and resist eye opening or may keep the eyes open in a fixed stare, interrupted by quick blinks. The pupils are of normal size and position and react to light unless a cycloplegic drug has been instilled in an attempt to visualize the fundi. The "doll's eye maneuver" elicits random or no eye movements. More helpful is caloric testing, performed by placing 10 ml of ice water into the external auditory canal. It normally gives rise to classic vestibular nystagmus with a quick component that indicates a state of alertness. In truly comatose patients, the quick component is absent, and the eyes deviate slowly to the side of the cooled tympanic membrane. Muscle tone and reflexes are normal in psychogenic unresponsiveness. The patient may hyperventilate or breathe normally. If the results are in doubt after the clinical evaluation, the EEG should prove helpful in differentiating psychogenic from organic or metabolic depression of consciousness.

Head and neck Nuchal rigidity may be evidence of meningitis or subarachnoid hemorrhage, but this sign often disappears in deep coma. Battle's sign and periorbital ecchymoses are indicative of basilar skull fractures.

Cranial nerves The optic fundi may reveal retinal hemorrhages or papilledema. A record of the size and reactivity to light of each pupil is essential. A unilaterally dilated and fixed pupil is often indicative of oculomotor nerve compression by herniation of the medial portion of the temporal lobe through the tentorium of the cerebellum. When all other signs of neurological function are absent, reactive pupils are characteristic of metabolic coma. (Important exceptions to this rule are caused by hypoxia; such drugs as the belladonna compounds, opiates, and glutethimide (Doriden); and eye disease or eye medication.) The pupils are unaffected by superficial cerebral disease; they become smaller, but remain reactive in diseases of the diencephalon. When a lesion affects the midbrain or medulla, the pupils are usually in midposition and are fixed, whereas a pontine lesion causes pinpoint pupils. The extraocular movements are tested by moving the patient's head and by noting changes in the position of the eyes relative to the orbits; these are known as doll's eye or oculocephalic maneuvers. Absence of such eye movement suggests brain stem disease, which can be confirmed by the absence of response after the instillation of 10 ml of ice cold water into the external auditory canal. If the brain stem is intact, cold caloric stimulation in a comatose patient evokes tonic conjugate deviation of the eyes to the side of the injection.

Motor and sensory systems Decerebrate posture is manifested by extensor spasticity of all extremities and occurs with extensive pontine-midbrain disease. Flexion contraction of the arms with extension of the legs is termed decorticate posture and is seen with bilateral deep cerebral lesions. These postures may occur spontaneously or may be evoked by stimuli. Asymmetry of movement of the face or extremities in reaction to painful stimuli, or asymmetry of muscle tone, may reveal the side affected by CNS disease. Similarly, asymmetry of corneal reflexes may be a clue to unilateral sensory impairment.

Reflexes Asymmetry of reflexes will help to lateralize the lesion. Bilateral pathological reflexes are common in comatose patients and of little diagnostic or prognostic significance.

ELECTROENCEPHALOGRAPHY

EEG is discussed in greater detail than are other diagnostic measures, not because it is a more useful test in the neurological evaluation of the patient, but because it is a test very commonly used by psychiatrists.

In obtaining the EEG, 21 electrodes are placed in standardized positions over the scalp and additional reference electrodes are placed on the ears. The tracing consists of 8 or 16 channels, each simultaneously printing out the difference in electrical potential transmitted by a pair of electrodes. This electrical activity reflects postsynaptic potentials of apically aligned neuronal dendrites in the cerebral cortex. Only the summation of inhibitory and excitatory potentials of large groups of neurons is recorded. Great amplification is required for purposes of recording; a 7-mm deflection of the recording pen is usually calibrated to correspond to 50 μV.

The waveforms recorded on EEG should be described in terms of frequency, amplitude, location, and duration of these transient events with distinct characteristics. Changes in morphology with sleep and with different stimuli, such as eye opening and hyperventilation, should be noted.

Depending on its frequency, EEG activity is classified as *delta* (δ) (slower than 4 Hz, or cycles per second), *theta* (θ) (4 to 7 Hz), *alpha* (α) (8 to 13 Hz), or *beta* (β) (faster than 13 Hz). EEG amplitudes, measured from peak to peak, range between 10 to 100 μV (generally, 10 to 50 μV in adults). Normally, the amplitude oscillates, giving a sinusoidal appearance to series of waves. With regard to location, it is important to note the distribution of the predominant frequencies, or background activity; their symmetry on both hemispheres; and the regions where transient events have the greatest amplitude. EEG waveforms that last for a brief period of time and stand out from the background are termed transient or paroxysmal events. The term "transient" generally denotes a wave or complex that is distinguished from the background pattern. The most common transients are spikes (duration from 20 to 70 msec) and sharp waves (pointed waves of 70 to 200 msec). "Paroxysmal" usually refers to epileptiform activity—the abrupt onset and termination of a series of transients.

NORMAL EEG IN THE ADULT In the awake adult, α-rhythms predominate in the posterior regions so long as the patient is relaxed, with eyes closed (Fig. 2.1-2*A*). Eye opening or intense mental activity, such as complex calculation, induce flattening of the α-rhythm (normal reactivity). In a subset of normal adults, particularly those with a tense nature, the α-rhythm is undetectable (Fig. 2.1-2*B*), but it may transiently appear upon eye closure. In right-handed individuals, the α-rhythms often have a slightly greater amplitude on the right side. Faster activities, within the β-range, predominate in the anterior regions and tend to be symmetric over both hemispheres.

Theta (θ) activity may be present in the temporal regions of normal people younger than 30 years or older than 70 years. The so-called rolandic- or MU-rhythm ranges between 7 and 11 Hz, is recorded over the central regions and has a spiky appearance, like a wicket or the letters "M" or "U." This rhythm, recorded in about 10 percent of individuals, is abolished by intended movement, particularly of the contralateral limbs. Lambda (λ) waves are sharp or sawtooth waves over the occipital areas and are evoked by visually scanning an object or a picture.

Delta (δ) activity and paroxysmal events are normally absent from the EEG of the resting awake adult. However, the wakeful pattern is altered by drowsiness or sleep and in response to stimuli, and varies from childhood to adult life.

During drowsiness, α-rhythm decreases in amplitude and slightly in frequency, becomes intermittent, and is finally replaced by low-voltage activity. This pattern is termed stage 1 sleep (Fig. 2.1-3*A*). With the advent of light sleep (stage 2), θ-activity appears within the low-voltage activity, and intermittent series of 14 Hz sleep spindles are seen (Fig. 2.1-3*B*). As stage 3 evolves, δ-activity occurs in 20 to 60 percent of the record, with decreasing amounts of θ-activity, and the frequency of sleep spindles diminishes from 14 to 12 to 10 Hz. In the deepest degree of sleep (stage 4), δ-activity grows slower and of higher amplitude and forms more than 60 percent of the tracing; sleep spindles no longer occur. Vertex transients are random sharp waves arising from the central areas of the cortex and are evoked by stimulation during sleep stages 1 and 2. K-complexes (Fig. 2.1-3*B*) are high-voltage waves followed by faster spindle activity, predominantly from the anterior cerebrum, and are evoked by stimulation in sleep stages 2 and 3.

During a normal night's sleep, periods of rapid eye movement (REM) sleep occur at approximately 90-minute intervals (Fig. 2.1-4). The EEG pattern of REM sleep is similar to that of stage 1 sleep, with low-voltage activity of mixed frequencies, but sawtooth waves representing eye movement activity are superimposed. Dreaming and inhibition of motor tone throughout the body, except for eye and sphincter muscles, are among the most dramatic events that occur during REM sleep.

During the EEG, hyperventilation is performed for 3 minutes. A build-up of slow activity—decrease in frequency and increase in voltage (Fig. 2.1-5, *left side*)—occurs during, and may persist for as long as 100 seconds, after the cessation of hyperventilation. This response is seen more commonly in children than in adults. A relatively low blood sugar and the erect posture increase the response to hyperventilation. The slow activity during hyperventilation is probably due to cerebral vasoconstriction evoked by hypocapnia.

Photic stimulation is attained by means of a bright flashing stroboscope held close to the patient's closed eyes. A driving response may normally be evoked over both occipital areas and consists of bilaterally symmetrical activity, synchronous with the flash frequencies, usually near or within the α-range (Fig. 2.1-6*A*). Sometimes, the evoked response is a subharmonic or a multiple of the flash stimuli. Photic stimulation may result in a photomyoclonic response characterized by twitches of the face and eyes, with associated muscle artifact in the EEG. This response should not be interpreted as a manifestation of epilepsy.

EEG CHARACTERISTICS OF CHILDREN The waking EEG after the first year of life reveals a gradual increase in frequencies of low-voltage slow activities, especially over the occipital

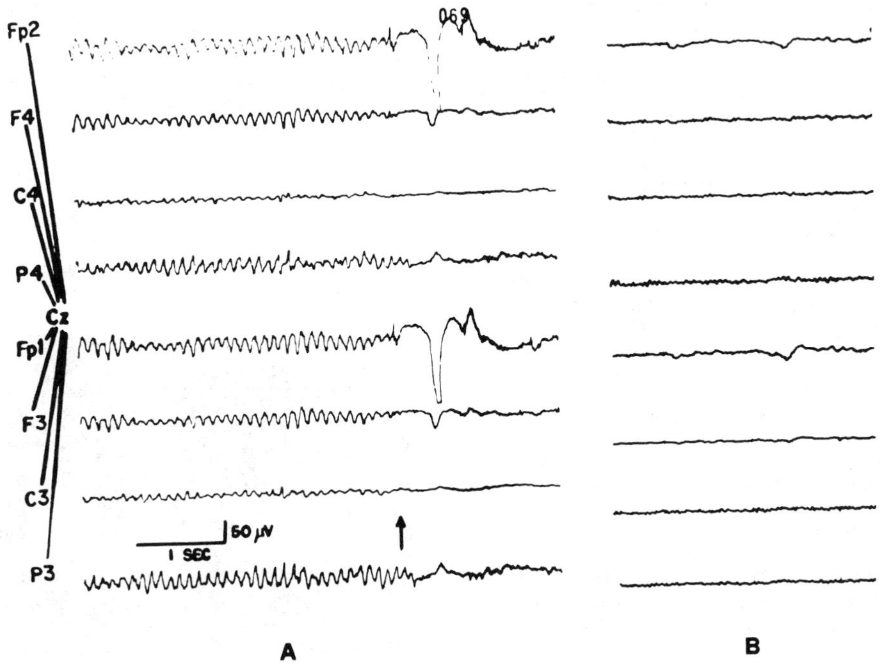

FIGURE 2.1-2. A. *The normal adult EEG. At the* arrow *the eyes of the patient were open: note the "blocking" of α-rhythm.* B. *The normal low-voltage fast adult EEG. The designation of electrode positions is that adopted by the International Federation of Societies for Electroencephalography and Clinical Neurology:* F_p *(frontal pole),* F *(frontal),* C *(central),* P *(parietal),* O *(occipital),* T *(temporal),* C_z *(vertex),* A *(ear). Even numbers as subscripts indicate the right hemisphere, odd numbers the left.*

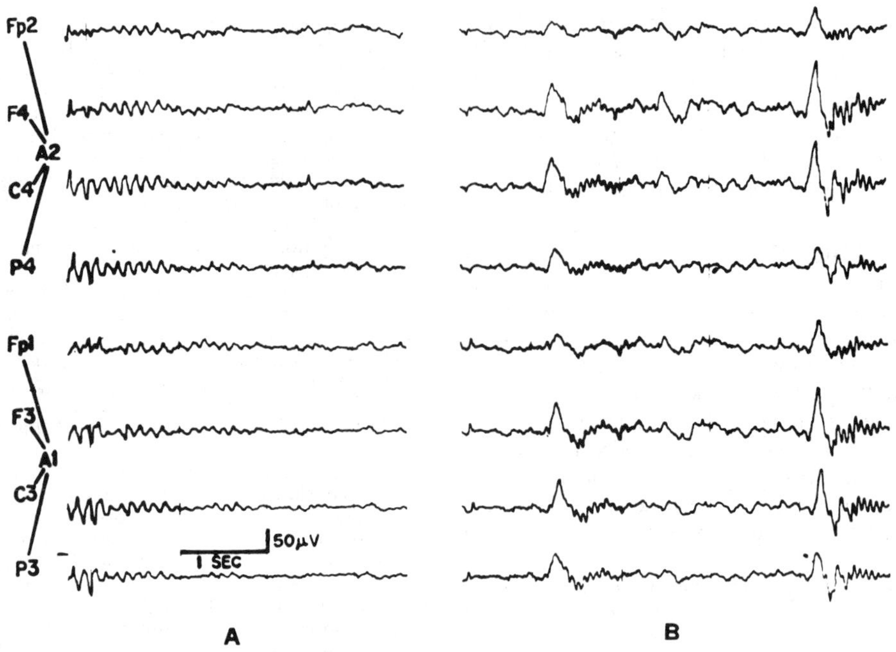

FIGURE 2.1-3. A. *The normal adult drowsy EEG. Note the dropping out of α-rhythm and its replacement by low-voltage activity.* B. *The normal sleeping EEG with θ-activity. 14-per-second sleep spindles, and bilaterally synchronous sharp waves of predominantly central origin (K-complexes).*

areas. Between 2 and 9 years of age, the background activity is polyrhythmic, with an increasing proportion of frequencies within the α-range as the child grows older (Fig. 2.1-7). Between 10 and 16 years of age, stable and dominant frequencies within the adult α-range predominate, and slow frequencies diminish as age advances.

Drowsiness after the first year of life is characterized by disorganization of the record with increases in voltage and in diffuse slow activity. The steady, slow activity of drowsiness usually disappears after 6 years of age. Paroxysmal bilaterally synchronous high-voltage slow activity during drowsiness rarely persists after 15 years of age.

During light sleep, the EEG reveals intermittent central sharp waves occurring in a bilaterally synchronous fashion. The second stage of sleep is manifested by 14-Hz sleep spindles. With moderately deep sleep, there is an increase in 4- to 6-Hz activity and then an increase in 2- to 3-Hz activity; 12-Hz sleep spindles are noted. In deep sleep, very high-voltage and very slow activity is seen without spindles or central sharp waves. Continuous or paroxysmal slow activity may follow the K-complex of arousal.

ARTIFACTS Unfortunately, because of the great amplification of electrical activity (50 million times), artifacts are frequently present and form a major pitfall in the interpretation of the EEG (Fig. 2.1-8). Muscle contraction and movement cause a great variety of artifacts (Fig. 2.1-8*A*), but are usually easily distinguished. Swallowing may cause a paroxysmal burst of muscle spikes (Fig. 2.1-8*B*). A defective electrode may cause artifacts resembling focal spikes or focal slow activity (Fig. 2.1-8*C*). The electrocardiogram, when superimposed on the EEG, may simulate spike-and-wave patterns. The almost imperceptible tremor of parkinsonism may cause paroxysmal spike-and-slow-wave artifact. Eye movement is a common source of artifacts that need not be limited to the bifrontal areas.

ABNORMAL CHARACTERISTICS OF THE EEG The following features are abnormal only when not accounted for on the basis of youth or a change in the conscious state of the patient, or in response to stimulation.

Frequency Activity slower than 8 Hz—that is θ- or δ-activity, particularly if occurring in series—is abnormal. Generalized slow activity is suggestive of diffuse organic disease or of a metabolic disorder. Focal slow activity (Fig. 2.1-9) is indicative of underlying organic disease, although small amounts of θ-activity over the bitemporal areas are of doubtful significance. Activity faster than α-rhythm (β-activity) is abnormal if focal, excessive, or of high amplitude. Generalized fast activity is seen in some drug intoxications. Unless a skull defect is responsible, focal fast activity usually results from epileptogenic organic disease.

Voltage Low-voltage, diffuse, slow activity may reflect severe cerebral disease from anoxia, encephalitis, or a toxic metabolic process. Low-voltage activity of a focal nature may result from pathology, generally a tumor or a subdural hematoma, interposed between the cerebral cortex and the recording electrodes. Activity progressively increasing in amplitude may precede a seizure.

Epileptiform activity Anterior temporal spike activity is most commonly associated with complex partial (psychomotor) seizures (Fig. 2.1-10). Small sharp spikes in the midtemporal region are considered a nonepileptiform variant. Other spike activity or spike-and-wave activity may be indicative of an underlying epileptogenic lesion. Multiple spike foci in children suggest seizure activity or mental or physical retardation. Spikes in children's EEGs may change

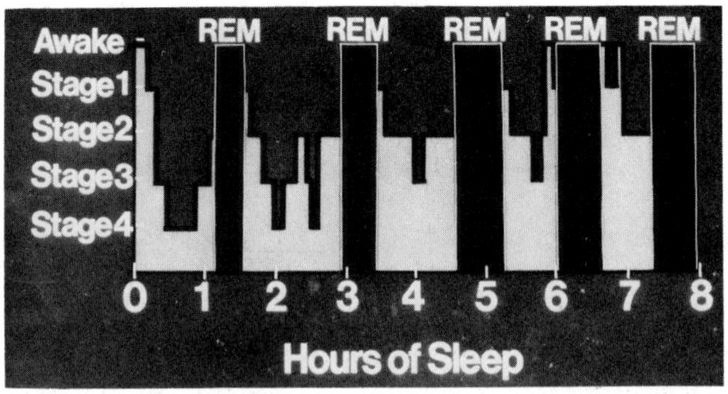

FIGURE 2.1-4. *Sleep stages of a typical night's sleep. REM, rapid eye movement. (Courtesy of M J Thorpy, MD, Montefiore Medical Center, New York.)*

location from one time to another. Positive 14- and 6-per-second spikes (Fig. 2.1-11*A*) may be associated with visceral phenomena or behavior symptoms, but are most often a normal variant.

Bilaterally synchronous paroxysmal slow activity is seen in patients with generalized convulsive disorders and in disease or dysfunction of deep midline structures. Generalized nonconvulsive, petit mal epilepsy is characterized by 3-per-second spike-and-slow-wave bilaterally synchronous paroxysmal bursts (Fig. 2.1-12). Spike-and-slow-wave bursts of faster frequencies often correlate with generalized convulsive, grand mal epilepsy (Fig. 2.1-13).

The determination of EEG abnormality depends on a large number of variables; however, only two examples are cited here. There may be many single slow waves in a normal record, but the same slow waves occurring in series are usually abnormal. Slightly slow activi-

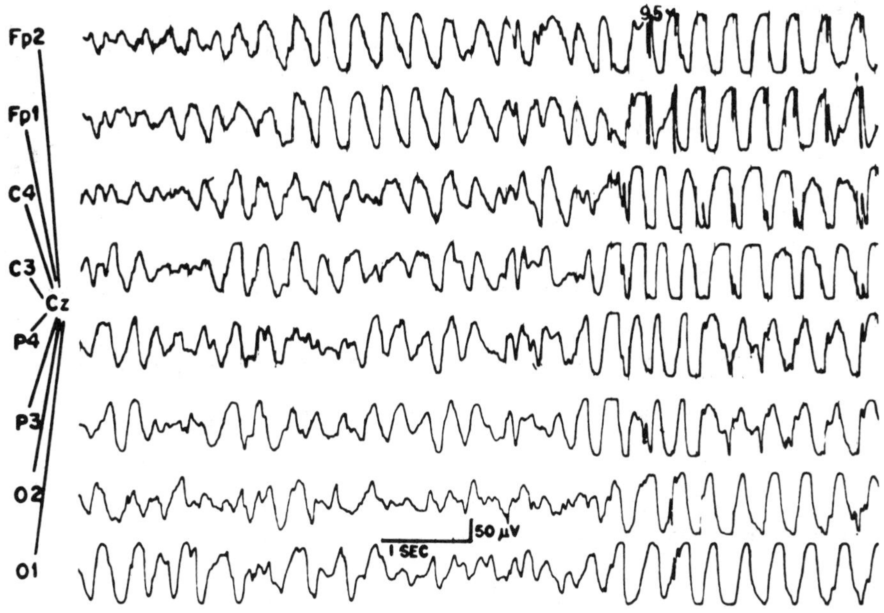

FIGURE 2.1-5. *Hyperventilation. On the* left, *the normal build-up of high-voltage slow activity in a 9-year-old child. On the* right, *the superimposed spike activity, alternating with the high-voltage slow waves, is an abnormal response.*

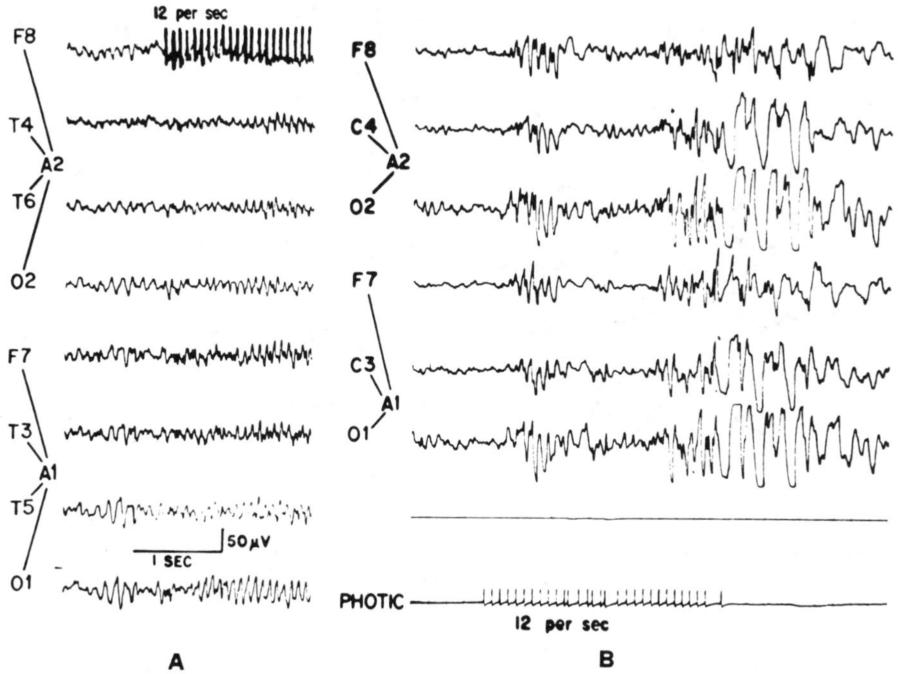

FIGURE 2.1-6. *Photic stimulation.* A. *The normal response. Photic stimulation has been superimposed on the F8 recording. Note the change from a slower background pattern to a 12-cycle-per-second rhythm synchronous with the photic flash.* B. *An abnormal response to photic stimulation. Polyspike-and-slow-wave activity is evoked and persists after cessation of the photic stimuli.*

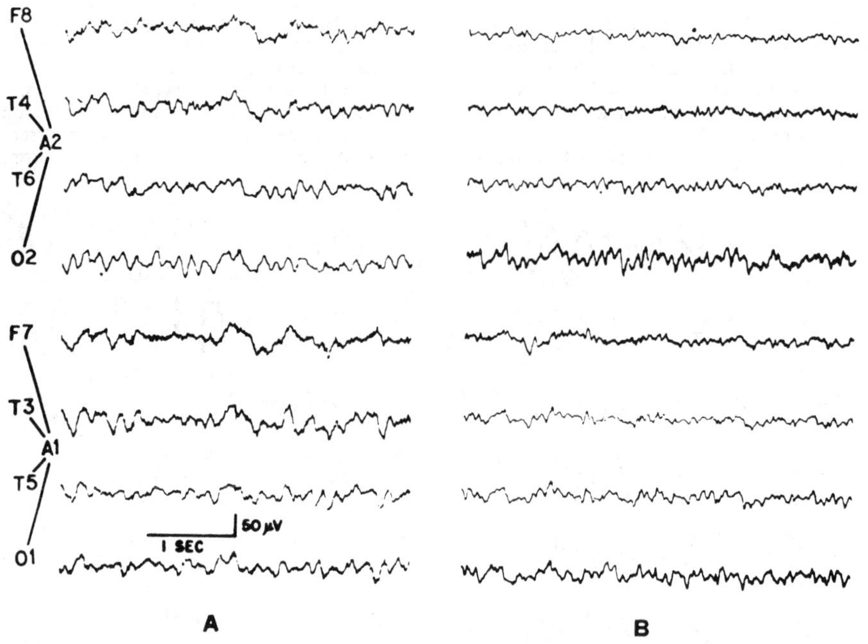

FIGURE 2.1-7. A. *The normal child's EEG, age 3 years.* B. *The normal child's EEG, age 9 years. Note the increase in frequency, but with persistence of scattered and underlying slow activity.*

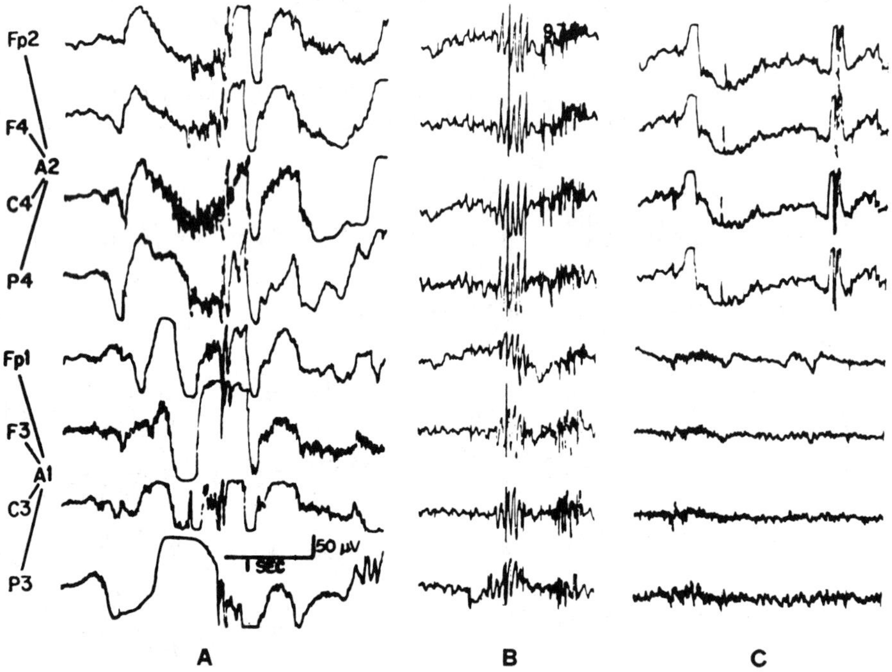

FIGURE 2.1-8. *Artifacts.* A. *A combination of movement and muscle artifact manifested by high-voltage irregular slow waves and very fast activity, respectively.* B. *Swallowing artifact, causing paroxysmal series of spikes followed by lower voltage very rapid activity.* C. *Right ear electrode artifact, producing a random irregular slow wave, a random spike, and an irregular spike-and-slow-wave complex.*

ties over the temporal areas may be normal, but the same activity over the occipital areas is often abnormal.

Abnormal EEG patterns in the first year of life Abnormal slow waves, fast activities, and spikes may occur in infants. In addition, an infant's record that is too well organized (i.e., the record appears more mature than expected for the age) is probably abnormal. Occipital spike activity in infants and children is often associated with seizures, prematurity, and visual defects. The following EEG abnormalities, peculiar to infants, carry poor prognoses for physical or mental development.

Hypsarrhythmia The pattern of hypsarrythmia, seen in patients with infantile spasms, is characterized by multifocal high-voltage, irregular spike-and-slow-wave activity occurring on a markedly disorganized background (Fig. 2.1-14). The EEG abnormality usually clears after 2 years of age and is rare after 4 years, but physical and mental retardation remain.

Extreme spindles Although they resemble sleep spindles, extreme spindles are of higher voltage, more continuous, and occur in a wider distribution. They are usually seen between 6 months and 5 years of age and are associated with brain damage.

DIAGNOSTIC VALUE OF EEG The EEG may be normal in the presence of organic brain disease, particularly if the lesion is deep, small, or old. For instance, the EEG is often normal early in the course of multiple sclerosis, when the lesions are small, scattered, and subcortical. In epilepsy, the duration of the record may not be long enough to detect intermittent paroxysmal abnormality. Attenuation of voltage when recording from the scalp may suppress EEG abnormality.

The response of cerebral electrical activity to injury or disease of

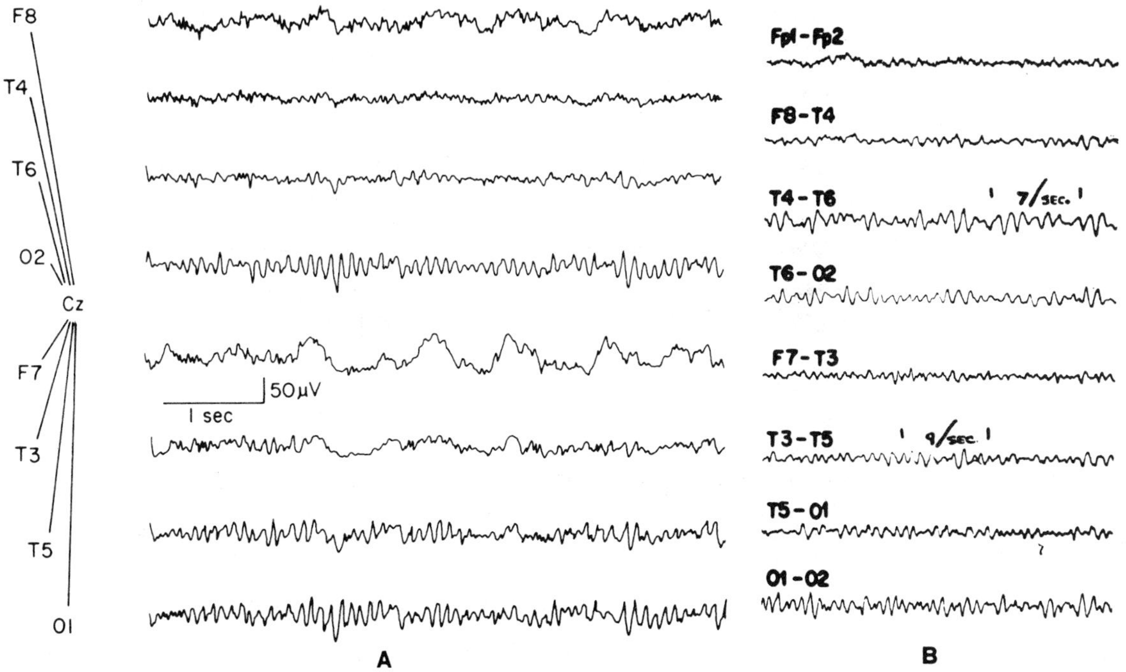

FIGURE 2.1-9. A. *Focal 2-Hz δ-activity from the F7 and T3 electrodes, indicative of a left anterior temporal lobe lesion, in this case a glioblastoma multiforme.* B. *Slightly slow activity of 7 Hz, predominantly from the T6 electrode, indicative of a right posterior temporal lobe lesion, in this case an infarct.*

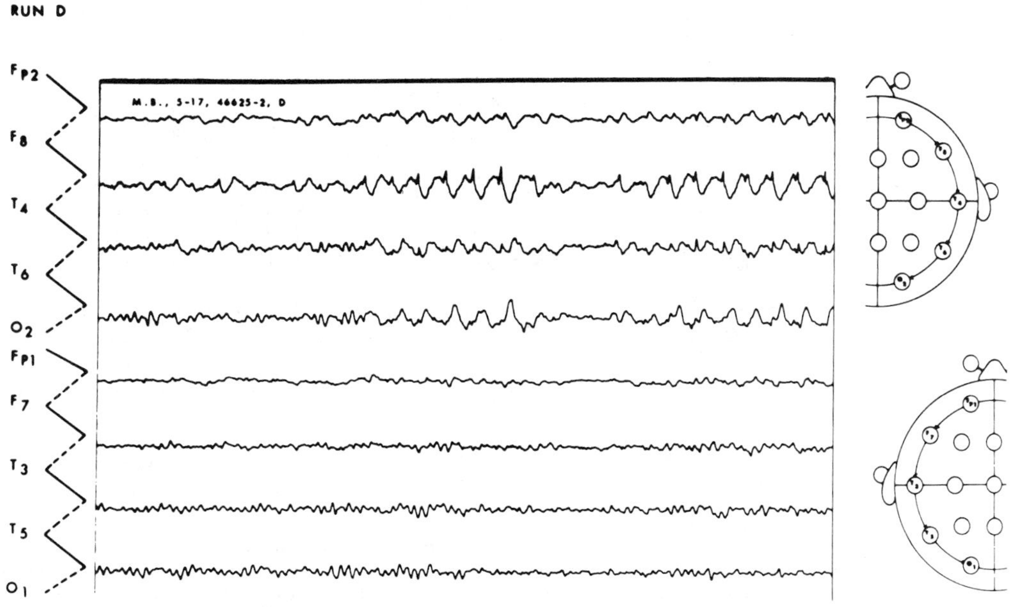

FIGURE 2.1-10. *Right temporal lobe spike-and-wave complexes, due to an underlying lesion. (From Goldensohn E S, Appel S H:* Scientific Approaches to Clinical Neurology. *Lea & Febiger, Philadelphia, 1977, with permission.)*

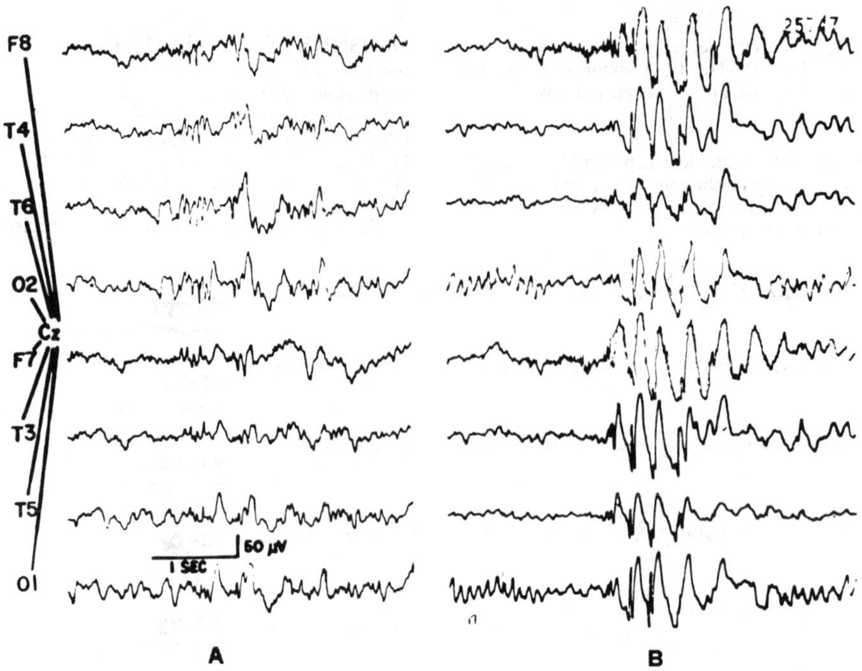

FIGURE 2.1-11. A. *14-per-second positive spikes seen in a 10-year-old child with behavior disorder and intermittent episodes of abdominal pain.* B. *Paroxysmal irregular spike-and-slow-wave bursts occurring in a bilaterally synchronous fashion at approximately 4 Hz, seen in another 10-year-old child with sudden paroxysms of abdominal pain (abdominal epilepsy).*

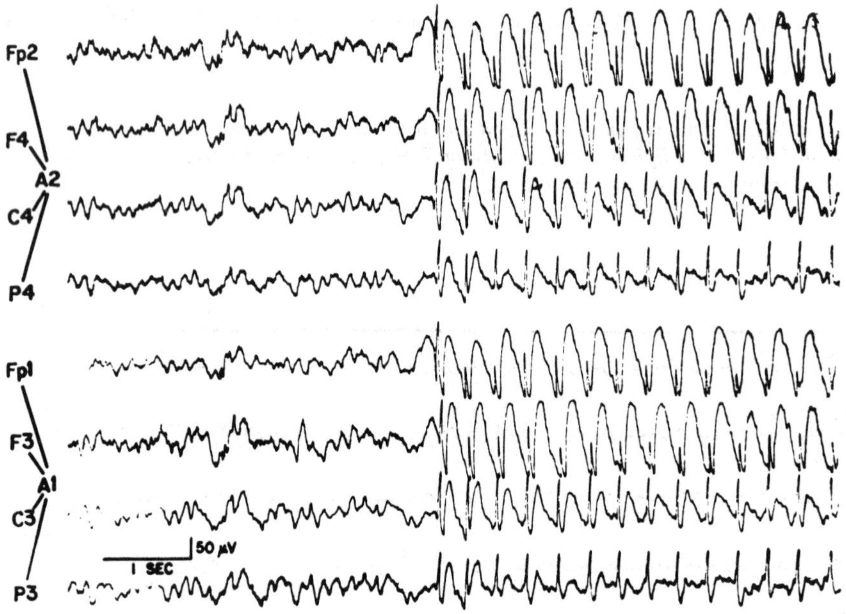

FIGURE 2.1-12. *Petit mal epilepsy characterized by bilaterally synchronous, 3-Hz spike-and-slow-wave activity.*

any type is relatively limited. EEG patterns are not pathognomonic of specific disease, with the possible exception of petit mal epilepsy. The initial response of the EEG to cerebral disease is slow activity or depression of voltage or both. As a rule of thumb, the lowest frequencies correspond to the most severe lesions. Spike or sharp activity is often a sequela of injury, and focal spike activity may indicate that an old lesion has become epileptogenic. Focal slow activity is indicative of an underlying anatomical lesion or, less often, a functional defect. The disease does not always exactly underlie the site of maximum EEG abnormality; for instance, a cerebral lesion may be associated with slow activity that is recorded predominantly over the occipital lobe in children or over the temporal lobe in adults.

Neoplastic cerebral disease A cerebral tumor is usually manifested by focal δ-activity (Fig. 2.1-9*A*). If the tumor is deep or causes increased intracranial pressure, diffuse activity, especially frontal intermittent rhythmic δ-activity (FIRDA), may occur. FIRDA may also be seen with other diseases affecting deep frontal or diencephalic structures. Infratentorial lesions in adults may similarly project FIRDA, whereas such tumors in children are often associ-

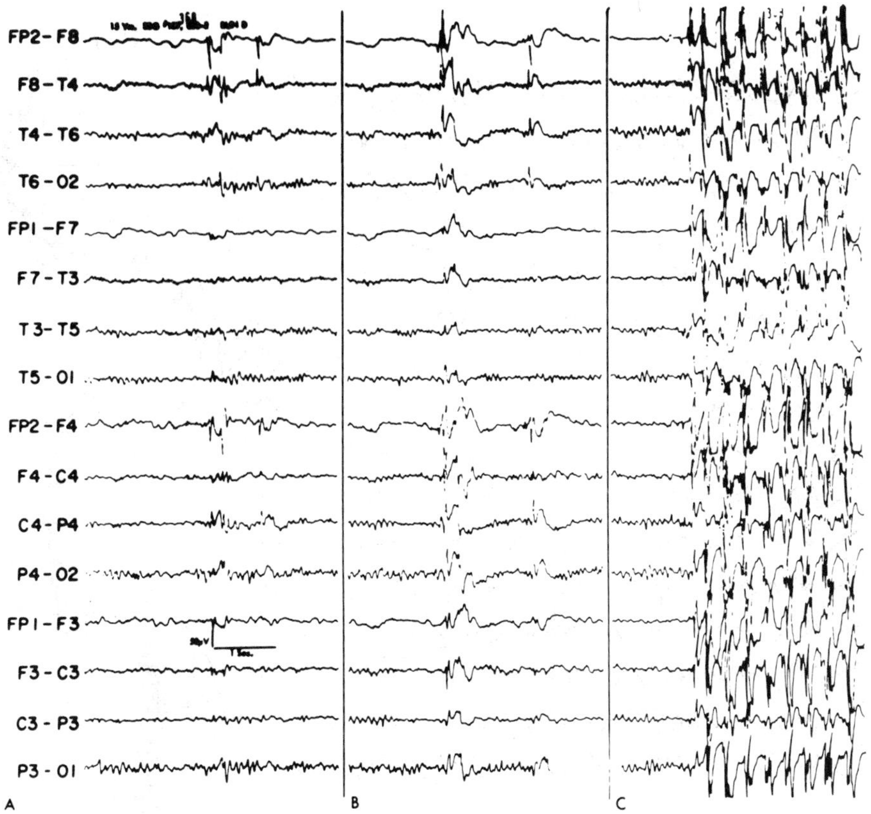

FIGURE 2.1-13. *Rapid spread from a focal discharge to generalized bilateral synchrony.* A: *Focal spiking at F8.* B: *Bilateral spiking.* C: *Generalized bilaterally synchronous spike-and-wave discharges. (From Goldensohn E S, Appel S H:* Scientific Approaches to Clinical Neurology. *Lea & Febiger, Philadelphia, 1977, with permission.)*

ated with bioccipital slow activity. The EEG is often normal in slowly growing extracerebral intracranial tumors, such as meningiomas.

Vascular lesions Cerebral infarction is usually associated with focal slow-wave activity (Fig. 2.1-9*B*). If the cerebral infarct is recent, large, or superficial, or if a hematoma is present, focal δ-activity may occur. Scattered small-vessel disease often results in diffuse or scattered θ-activity. A subarachnoid hemorrhage is often associated with diffuse slow activity, but focal slow waves sometimes may be the clue to the site of a ruptured aneurysm.

Inflammatory disease Inflammatory diseases affecting the cerebrum as a whole, such as meningitis and encephalitis, usually cause diffuse slow activity (Fig. 2.1-15*A*), with occasional focal qualities. An abscess, however, causes high voltage focal δ-activity. Serial studies may be helpful in evaluating meningitis in children; if improvement in the EEG does not occur after 2 weeks, one should suspect the development of sinus thrombosis, subdural empyema, or subdural effusion. Subacute sclerosing panencephalitis is often characterized by an unusual EEG pattern of sharp-and-slow-wave complexes occurring periodically every 2 to 8 seconds on a background of abnormally slow activity. In patients with Creutzfeldt-Jakob disease, the EEG rapidly evolves from diffuse slow activity to generalized spike or sharp activity, occurring characteristically in periodic fashion of about 1-second intervals (Fig. 2.1-16). In the early stages of herpes simplex encephalitis, pseudoperiodic lateralized epileptiform discharges (PLEDS) occur from one temporal or frontotemporal area with a background pattern of diffuse slow activity. Periodic discharges, whether generalized or PLEDS, may also occur in a variety of other diseases, particularly of vascular and traumatic origin.

Cerebral trauma Injury to the brain may produce focal or diffuse EEG abnormality (Fig. 2.1-15*B*) and sometimes paroxysmal slow activity. The paroxysmal slow activity may be attributable to the shearing effect of rotation of the cerebrum on its pedestal, the brain stem, with associated dysfunction of the diencephalon. A comatose patient manifesting α-rhythm or sleep spindles probably has severe brain stem injury. Diffuse slow activity soon after severe cerebral trauma may obscure focal slow activity overlying in an area of contusion. Focal depression of amplitude in a patient with head trauma raises the suspicion of an underlying subdural hematoma. Because a spike focus is usually the result of an old injury, an observation of such a focus on the day of the cerebral trauma or a few days later suggests that the abnormality is unrelated to the recent trauma.

Metabolic or degenerative diseases These illnesses usually cause diffuse slow activity in the EEG. Hepatic and other encephalopathies are manifested by bilaterally synchronous slow waves predominant over the anterior cerebrum, often accompanied by sharp and slow-wave forms called triphasic waves. The EEG is not a precise guide to the activity or severity of metabolic cerebral disease because clinical changes often precede changes in the EEG; however, the occurrence of triphasic activity and burst suppression patterns correlate well with depression of consciousness.

Drugs and toxic substances Toxins have a nonspecific effect on the EEG, causing either diffuse slow activity or diffuse fast activity or both. The drugs that may cause fast activity in the EEG are the sedatives (barbiturates, chloral hydrate [Notec], glutethimide), minor tranquilizers (meprobamate [Miltown], diazepam [Valium], chlordiazepoxide [Librium]), and stimulants (amphetamine). The anticonvulsants usually have little effect on the background pattern of the EEG. The phenothiazine derivatives and antidepressants cause fast activity at low dosages but, at high dosage, they may evoke slow activity; these drugs also potentiate EEG and clinical seizure activity in susceptible persons. Analgesics, narcotics, and hallucinogens have little effect on the EEG, unless consciousness is depressed or an organic mental disorder is evoked. Other drugs and noxious agents, if they affect the EEG, do so by causing slow activity. The patient in deep coma with diffuse fast activity in the EEG raises the strong suspicion of barbiturate narcosis (Fig. 2.1-15*C*). In a stuporous patient who has been taking anticonvulsant medication, the

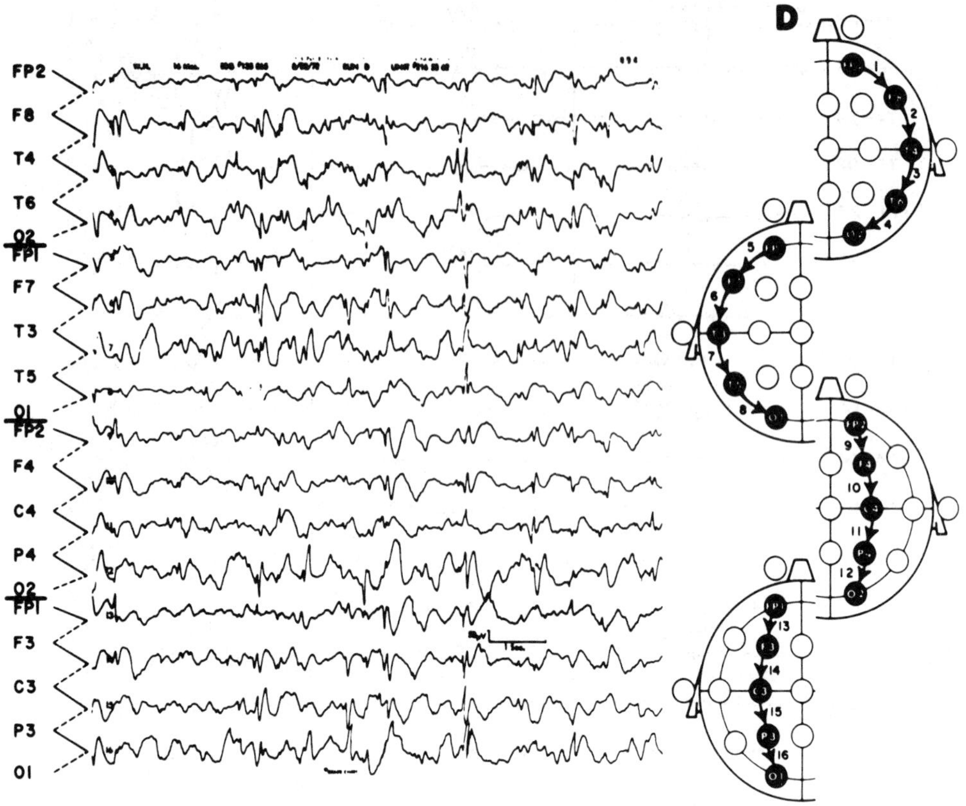

FIGURE 2.1-14. *Hypsarrhythmia in a 16-month-old child with tonic spasms. High voltage, spikes, spike-and-wave complexes, and slow waves occur both synchronously and asynchronously from all areas. (From Goldensohn E S, Appel S H:* Scientific Approaches to Clinical Neurology. *Lea & Febiger, Philadelphia, 1977, with permission.)*

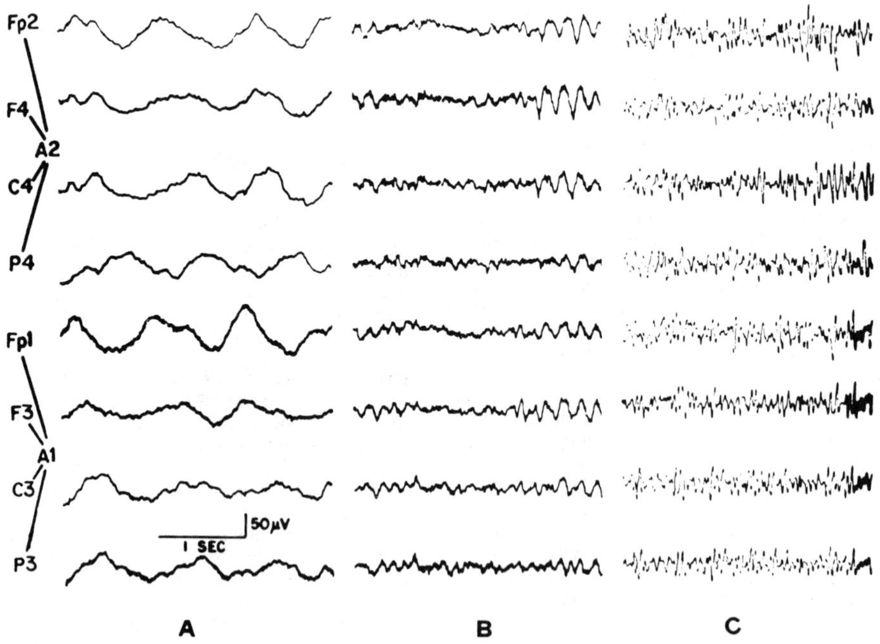

FIGURE 2.1-15. A. *Diffuse moderate- to high-voltage very slow (δ) activity seen in a patient with severe encephalitis.* B. *Diffuse θ-activity seen in a patient soon after cerebral trauma.* C. *Diffuse fast (β) activity seen in a patient with barbiturate intoxication.*

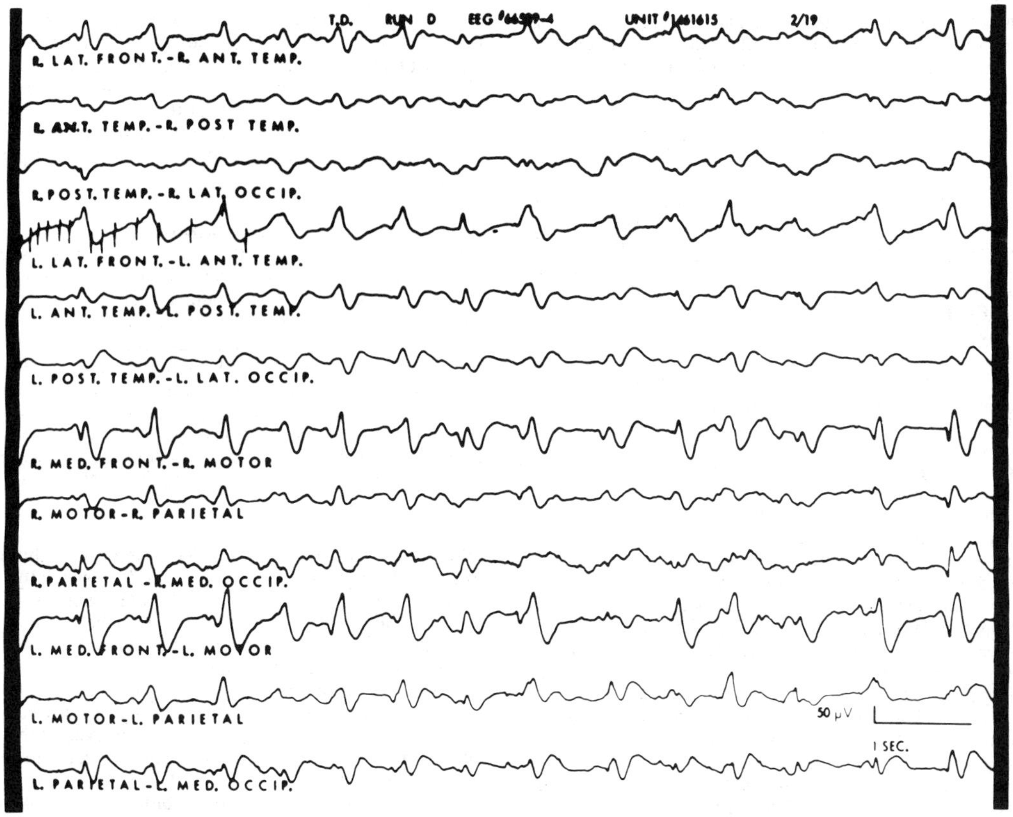

FIGURE 2.1-16. *Cruetzfeldt-Jakob disease. Periodic diphasic and triphasic waves recur at approximately 1-second intervals. (From Goldensohn E S, Appel S H:* Scientific Approaches to Clinical Neurology. *Lea & Febiger, Philadelphia, 1977, with permission.)*

EEG helps to differentiate subclinical (electrical) status epilepticus, which is manifested by almost continuous paroxysmal activity, from drug intoxication, which is evidenced by diffuse fast or slow activity.

Epilepsy The EEG is of greatest value in the diagnosis of epilepsy; after the history, the EEG is the most helpful factor. Paroxysmal abnormalities are characteristic. The EEG is most often abnormal in generalized nonconvulsive, petit mal epilepsy; almost all such cases reveal an abnormal EEG before treatment. The EEG may be normal in from 30 to 50 percent of other forms of epilepsy during the interictal period. Generalized, nonconvulsive, petit mal epileptic activity (Fig. 2.1-12) is characterized by generalized, bilaterally synchronous, symmetrical 3-per-second spike-and-wave bursts. A petit mal variant shows an EEG pattern of irregular spike-and-wave bursts slower than 3 per second, and it is associated with minor motor seizures that usually have an organic basis. Generalized convulsive, grand mal epilepsy (Fig. 2.1-13) is manifested by diffuse, bilaterally synchronous paroxysmal slow or spike activities or, most often, a combination of the two. Focal or partial convulsive disorders reveal focal spikes or sharp waves, often associated with slow activity; the most common example is a spike focus over an anterior temporal lobe in patients with partial complex, psychomotor epilepsy (Fig. 2.1-10). Partial seizures may become secondarily generalized when focal discharges lead to diffuse paroxysmal activity; the focal component may not be clinically evident (Fig. 2.1-13).

ABNORMAL EEGs IN NORMAL PEOPLE

Most electroencephalographers agree that 10 to 15 percent of the normal population have abnormal EEGs. The difference in statistics is attributable, in large part, to differences in the interpretation of those EEGs that lie on the borderline of normal—that is, diffuse slightly fast and diffuse slightly slow activity. At some time in their lives, those so-called normal people who have unequivocally abnormal EEGs probably experienced a subclinical disease or injury that caused persistent cerebral electrical changes (e.g., birth trauma without obvious signs or encephalitis manifested by no more than a headache and a common cold).

Except in epilepsy, the EEG is usually not a definitive test. The EEG should be used as any other laboratory tool, in association with all other factors, in an effort to establish as wide a base as possible for appropriate diagnosis and treatment.

ACTIVATION AND OTHER TECHNIQUES

Certain techniques may bring out abnormalities not previously evident or may exaggerate abnormalities noted in the resting EEG record.

Hyperventilation A response to hyperventilation is abnormal if spikes are associated with a paroxysmal series of slow activity (Fig. 2.1-5, *right side*) or if a focal spike or focal slow-wave pattern is evoked. Hyperventilation frequently brings out 3-per-second spike-and-wave paroxysms in patients with petit mal epilepsy.

Photic stimulation The response to photic stimulation is abnormal if focal paroxysmal spike-and-slow-wave activity is evoked or if the normal driving response occurs only over one hemisphere. Paroxysmal activity is abnormal if the response persists after the cessation of the photic stimuli; this is termed the *photoconvulsive response* (Fig. 2.1-6*B*).

Telemetry Patients with convulsive disorders can be monitored by telemetry. In this way, rarely occurring abnormal EEG discharges not revealed during standard recordings can be found. This technique also is valuable in differentiating psychomotor epilepsy from hysterical seizures.

Other techniques Differentiating hysterical seizures from true epilepsy is often difficult. Observations with split-screen television recordings of patient and EEG is the best way of differentiating the two. Sometimes, drugs are administered to evoke epileptogenic EEG activities.

Epileptogenic activity is often buried within the medial anterior temporal lobe, relatively far from scalp electrodes. Nasopharyngeal electrodes or, less often, sphenoidal electrodes may be placed much closer to the anterior temporal lobe and pick up electrical abnormality that otherwise may be too attenuated when standard electrodes are used. Nasopharyngeal recording will be abnormal in only 5 to 7 percent of patients with normal scalp recording. Temporal lobe foci are often detected on EEG in the transition between wakefulness and sleep. Thus, an EEG after sleep deprivation is often more helpful than nasopharyngeal recording in screening for temporal lobe epilepsy.

In patients being evaluated for surgical treatment of refractory seizures, electrodes may be implanted in the brain. Recordings may be carried out for hours or days in an attempt to define precisely the site and extent of the epileptogenic tissue.

Depth electrode recordings from nuclear structures within the brain are well-recognized techniques in the study of brain physiology in lower animals and have been used to a limited degree in humans during surgery for pain or movement disorders. The EEG is useful in monitoring depth of anesthesia and has been used to note changes in cerebral activity during cardiac and carotid surgery.

The EEG is an important research tool. It has been valuable in the study of the 24-hour sleep-wake cycle. Increasing knowledge of such sleep disorders as insomnia, narcolepsy, and sleep apnea has led to improved therapy. Because penile erection occurs almost invariably during REM sleep, its observation eliminates organic causes of sexual impotency. Polygraphic recordings, coupled with frequent blood sampling, have determined temporal episodic patterns for neuroendocrine secretions. Computerized frequency analysis of the EEG and computerized topography of the EEG are additional research modalities. More experience is needed to define their potential usefulness as diagnostic tools.

The determination of brain death has been necessary to permit the use of organs for transplantation and for other medicolegal purposes. With clinical neurological criteria of brain death, the complete absence of EEG activity over a defined period of time is part of this determination. EEG recording under these circumstances must follow specific guidelines in order to exclude technical causes of a seemingly flat tracing.

EEG IN PSYCHIATRY

The EEG is a relatively crude method of recording the sum effect of the electrical activity of millions of neurons. It is too much to ask this test to reflect psychological phenomena that represent the highest integrative function of the brain. Normal EEG patterns are best recorded when the cortex is least activated—that is, when the patient is resting comfortably with eyes closed and with an unstimulated mind. Activation of high cerebral function tends to disrupt the well-formed α-rhythm.

The EEG is abnormal in a larger percentage of patients with emotional illness than in the normal population, but a consistent type of abnormality is not present. Because specific EEG abnormalities do not correlate with specific emotional diseases, the EEG is of relatively little aid in the evaluation of psychological illness.

Intelligence There is no correlation between the EEG and normal or above-normal intelligence. In those people with intellectual deficits, EEG abnormalities are greater than in the normal population.

Personality Passive, dependent, submissive persons often show relatively high-amplitude α-rhythm in a large percent of the record. Aggressive, competitive persons, however, often have EEGs of low-amplitude, poorly formed α-rhythm. A tense and anxious person may have a low-voltage, fast EEG pattern or a relatively fast α-rhythm.

Behavior disorders of childhood The behavior disturbances most likely to be associated with EEG abnormalities are the disturbances of aggressive, impulsive types. Sometimes, children with episodic visceral complaints have accompanying psychological symptoms, and frequently their EEGs are abnormal. Similarly, personality disturbances are often seen in patients with convulsive disorders. Virtually every type of EEG abnormality has been reported with behavior disorders, with or without intermittent visceral symptoms. About 50 percent of children with behavior disorders reveal immature records, manifested by diffuse slow activity, maximal over the occipital and temporal lobes. Paroxysmal EEG abnormality may be associated with episodic visceral phenomena (e.g., abdominal epilepsy) (Fig. 2.1-11*B*). The significance of the 14- and 6-per-second positive spike pattern (Fig. 2.1-11*A*) is still controversial. This pattern is one of the most common EEG correlates of behavior disorders during childhood, but it is also found in about 10 to 30 percent of normal adolescents.

Personality disorders in adults Adults with personality disorders, particularly those with aggressive characteristics, often reveal prominent temporocentral or temporo-occipital slow activity over one or both hemispheres. These adults have a higher percentage of 14- and 6-per-second positive spikes than is seen in the normal population. Six-per-second spike-and-wave complexes are more common in adults and may be a variant of 14- and 6-per-second positive spikes in children. When spikes or other abnormal activities are seen from the anterior temporal lobe in adults with personality disorders, it is likely that many of these patients have psychomotor epilepsy or behavioral disturbances due to a mechanism operative in this type of epilepsy. In criminals, the highest incidence of EEG abnormalities is found in aggressive psychopaths.

Neuroses Anxiety causes a decrease in α-rhythm and an increase in low-voltage fast activity (Fig. 2.1-2*B*), especially over the central areas. Maturational defects in the EEG, such as increased percent time of bitemporal θ-activity, may also be present. Those persons who manifest obsessional phenomena and patients with psychosomatic complaints reveal EEG characteristics no different from those of the normal population.

Usually, the cerebral electrical activity of hysterical patients and of persons who have been hypnotized reacts exactly the same as that of normal people. Evoked potentials can be recorded in the EEG after pain stimulation of the hysterically analgesic extremity. Similarly, the α-rhythm of the EEG may be blocked by visual stimulation in a patient with hysterical blindness.

Mood disorders Patients with manic-depressive psychosis reveal a somewhat greater percentage of abnormal EEGs than does the general population: β-activities are especially prominent. Both probands and family members show a nearly 50 percent incidence of the small sharp-spike EEG variant. Depression seems to be more often associated with right-sided EEG abnormalities than would be expected on the basis of chance. Stage 4 sleep is reduced in depressed patients.

Schizophrenia It is not surprising that the reports of EEG characteristics in schizophrenia are as variable as its definition. Most schizophrenic patients have normal EEGs, but the percentage of abnormal EEGs, especially β-activity and paroxysmal abnormalities, is two or three times that found in the normal population. About 50 percent of autistic children have abnormal EEGs. Abnormality in the EEG is more likely to be present when there is a family history of psychosis or when the onset of the disease is early, the duration long, and the severity great. Paradoxically, the prognosis has been reported to be worse for schizophrenic patients with normal EEGs than for those patients having EEG abnormalities. The abnormal EEG in an apparently schizophrenic patient may have good prognostic implications if the correct diagnosis proves to be some other illness, generally a mood disorder. EEG abnormalities are most often seen in catatonia, least often in paranoia. Low-voltage slow activity is often seen in catatonic stupor, and paroxysmal patterns are seen more often in catatonic patients than in patients with other forms of schizophrenia. In schizophrenic patients, α-rhythm may not respond to visual or emotional stimuli; conversely, α-rhythm is absent during hallucinations.

Organic psychoses The EEG abnormality corresponds to the nature of the underlying lesion in the organic psychoses. Patients in the early stage of dementia due to cerebral degenerative diseases (e.g., Huntington's chorea and Alzheimer's disease) reveal a slowing of the frequency and decreased percent time of α-rhythm. As the disease advances, diffuse θ-activity or, less often, diffuse δ-activity may occur, sometimes with focal components. The severity of dementia does not necessarily correlate with the severity of the EEG abnormality, but the degree of EEG abnormality is most severe in those cases of dementia showing rapid progression.

The EEG is helpful in establishing the diagnosis of psychosis secondary to drug or metabolic encephalopathy, psychosis of brain tumor, psychosis with epilepsy, and dementia associated with Creutzfeldt-Jakob disease. A very abnormal EEG favors organic delirium versus paranoid agitated behavior, and severe dementia with associated psychomotor retardation versus the withdrawal and mute states of depression and schizophrenia.

Additional techniques of EEG study in psychiatry **Sedation threshold** The amount of amobarbital sodium (Amytal) required to produce a maximum degree of fast activity in the EEG is the sedation threshold. Unfortunately, there is not a sharp end point, and the degree of variation is too great for most diagnostic purposes. The sedation threshold is highest in patients with anxiety states, but it is also high in obsessive-compulsive patients and in chronic schizophrenic patients.

Depth electrode studies These studies have shed light on the anatomical and physiological substrate of emotion. Spike discharges and slow-wave activity in the septal region, the hippocampus, and the amygdala have been recorded in patients with schizophrenia and other psychoses. Bilateral bursts of high-voltage 2- to 5-Hz slow activity have been noted from deep ventromedial frontal areas in psychotic patients, but most of these patients had been tested after electroconvulsive therapy (ECT). High-voltage, fast spindles have been recorded from the hippocampus of patients during periods of strong emotion. The significance of these recordings with regard to psychological phenomena is uncertain.

Electroconvulsive therapy The EEG is useful in monitoring ECT, particularly when unilateral treatment is given, because generalized seizures are required for therapeutic benefit. The EEG confirms the generalized spike-and-wave afterdischarge of adequate duration (i.e., between 25 and 90 seconds). Longer seizures are associated with more amnesia and other untoward side effects. Slow activity after ECT is caused by secondary activation of inhibitory interneurons with hyperpolarization of neural membranes. More prolonged EEG abnormalities and rarely prolonged memory impairment are probably attributable to neuronal loss or dysfunction associated with failure of the vascular supply to meet the increased metabolic demands of the hyperactive electrically discharging brain. The severity of the EEG abnormality after ECT is a highly individual factor. With the first electric shock, there is usually quick return of the EEG to normal. After successive treatments, slow activity decreases in frequency, increases in voltage, and becomes more diffuse. The increasing slow-wave abnormality may be associated with organic mental signs. After several ECTs, the EEG usually returns to normal within days, weeks, or months; sometimes, however, it never returns to normal. Even when the EEG does not return to normal, clinical evidence of organic cerebral disease usually does not persist. Preexisting EEG abnormalities may predict a less favorable response to ECT.

Quantitative computer-based studies Quantitative EEG techniques include frequency analysis and topographic mapping using computer-based calculations and displays. These techniques are of research rather than clinical value.

EVOKED POTENTIALS

When a sensory impulse reaches the brain, a specific EEG response is evoked. This response, which is maximal in the cortical area appropriate to the modality and site of the stimulus, has a consistent latency, a specific waveform, and very low amplitude (0.1 to 20 μV). The deflections are labeled positive (P) or negative (N), and the latency is in milliseconds. By computer averaging techniques, the evoked responses of repetitive stimuli can be separated from the spontaneous EEG activity in which they are otherwise buried. These tests evaluate potentials evoked by stimulation of peripheral or cranial nerves: somatosensory evoked potentials (SSEP), visual evoked potentials (VEP), and brain stem auditory evoked responses (BAER). EPs are clinically useful in evaluating the functional integrity of the somatosensory or special sensory pathways. Different latencies and wave patterns help to localize lesions ranging from the end organ through the nervous system to the cerebral cortex. Often, defects in these pathways are not otherwise evident.

The most useful clinical application of VEPs is in the diagnosis of multiple sclerosis. The prolonged latency in the VEP may be the only residual evidence of demyelination within the visual system. In comatose patients, the BAERs are near normal with toxic or metabolic insults, but abnormal if structural lesions have occurred. By means of VEPs or BAERs, vision and hearing can be evaluated in infants, and psychogenic defects of these special senses can be differentiated from organic diseases. Lesions of sensory pathways from the peripheral nerve, nerve root, and spinal cord show different SSEP patterns. EPs are being used to monitor neural pathways when patients are anesthetized during surgery and to document brain death.

The EPs discussed thus far are recorded shortly (between a few and 100 msec) after the stimulus. These short-latency potentials lend themselves to diagnostic applications because they are readily obtained with simple stimuli and have little interindividual variability in their essential elements. Potentials obtained between 100 msec and 3 or 4 sec after the stimulus are more variable, and their relation to the stimulus is not as clear as the early components. The correlation between long-latency responses and behavior—or behavioral disturbances—is being studied. Neuronal activity has been recorded in the limbic system at the latency of P300. Two late potentials have attracted particular interest: The *novelty potential* (P300) is elicited when a novel stimulus is interspersed in a train of repetitive monotonous stimuli. The *readiness potential,* or contingent negative variation (CNV), is obtained by using random stimuli that call for a motor response. Both of these potentials contain a number of discrete subunits. Early components of CNV have maximal amplitude over the parietal cortex and may represent the last stage of the stimulus evaluation process, whereas later components have a frontal predominance and may correspond to resetting for a response. Substantially smaller amplitude of P300 has been reported in schizophrenic patients. An early negative potential (N120) has been found to be less well localized and less responsive to the intensity of the stimulus in schizophrenic patients as compared to normal controls. Preliminary studies of computerized topographic mapping of EEG and evoked responses have shown frontal lobe dysfunction in schizophrenia. The long-latency EPs and computerized topographic EEG mapping may have future clinical applications, but their significance is still being investigated.

ELECTRODIAGNOSIS OF PERIPHERAL NERVE AND MUSCLE DISEASE

Evoked responses can help in the evaluation of peripheral neuropathy, but nerve conduction studies are more specific. Electromyography is best suited for the study of motor neuron or myopathic disease.

NERVE CONDUCTION VELOCITY Nerve conduction velocity is determined with the use of two electrodes placed over the skin of the nerve and muscle to be tested. The time (as a measure of distance on the cathode ray oscilloscope) required for the impulse to travel between the stimulating proximal electrode and the distal recording electrode is tabulated. The speed of conduction between the known distance of the two electrodes is then calculated. Slow velocities are indicative of disease of the peripheral nerve. The conduction time through a simple, monosynaptic reflex arc can be measured and recorded in the lower extremities as the H-reflex. Motor diseases of the CNS influence reactivity of the lower motor neuron and may be evaluated by changes in the H-reflex. The H-reflex and the corresponding F-wave in the upper extremity are delayed or lost in disease of the proximal portion of the peripheral nervous system—namely, the nerve roots and plexi.

ELECTROMYOGRAM The electromyogram (EMG) is a record of electrical activity transmitted from a muscle by a needle electrode to a cathode ray oscilloscope and a loudspeaker. A normal muscle is electrically silent at rest. During contraction, normal action potentials are manifested by fast, moderate-voltage, well-modulated bursts of activity. Approximately 10 to 20 days after nerve injury, evidence of denervation can be found. A partially denervated and reinnervated muscle produces complex polyphasic, arrhythmic, high-voltage potentials during contraction. In addition, spikes of low-voltage, fast, random potentials, or fibrillations, are noted at rest. Disease of the anterior horn cells in the spinal cord or of nerve roots reveal fibrillation potentials with normal nerve conduction velocity. In muscular dystrophy, electrical activity during muscle contraction is faster and of lower voltage than normal potentials. Fibrillations and low-amplitude polyphasic potentials are recorded in polymyositis.

ELECTRO-OCULOGRAPHY (EOG) AND ELECTRONYSTAGMOGRAPHY (ENG) Evaluation of eye movement disorders, including nystagmus, is greatly facilitated by recording the speed and amplitude of eye movements. Ocular dysmetria of brain stem or cerebellar disease, elusive on clinical observation, becomes obvious when recorded. Nystagmus of labyrinthine end-organ disease is enhanced by eye closure and the loss of fixation; the opposite is true in brain stem or cerebellar disease.

NEUROIMAGING TECHNIQUES

Imaging of the human brain, enclosed in a protective, calcified structure, has been revolutionized by the advent of computer-assisted imaging modalities. First, X-ray *computed tomography* (CT) and, more recently, *magnetic resonance imaging* (MRI or MR) allow visualization of the brain parenchyma without the need of invasive procedures. From the 1930s until the 1970s, pathological distortion of brain anatomy had to be gleaned from shifts in the disposition of the blood vessels seen by angiography, or of the air-filled cavities seen by pneumoencephalography. Both of these procedures require the injection of contrast media.

Computer-aided imaging techniques are based on the determination of radiodensity (CT) or magnetic resonance (MR) properties of each of thousands of volume elements (voxels) of tissue making up the whole brain. In both modalities, the computer uses Fourier transformation to identify the individual components of a complex signal. In a simple, intuitive explanation of the basis of CT and MR, the computer is analogous to the brain in analyzing complex visual or auditory signals. As with CT, clinicians can construct three-dimensional images by looking at two perpendicular radiographs of an object. Similar to the way that the location and type of a musical instrument can be determined by analyzing the sound of an orchestra, the MR scanning technique can locate and provide tissue characteristics by using nuclear MR.

Other recent imaging procedures provide information about ongoing metabolic processes in the brain. *Positron emission tomography* (PET), of great interest in the domain of psychiatry, is being used as a research tool; however, it is too expensive for clinical work in most institutions. Information on regional changes of cerebral blood flow during various psychological tasks or with different disorders can be obtained with a more affordable technique, *single photon emission computed tomography* (SPECT). Conventional brain-imaging techniques that use radioisotopes, such as the static and dynamic brain scans, have limited use if CT and sophisticated angiographic techniques are available.

Imaging of the arteries supplying the brain is most accurately obtained with *angiography,* which requires arterial injection of a contrast medium. The major vessels also can be visualized by means of *digital intravenous angiography* (DIVA), which is easier to perform and less traumatic than arterial angiography. Noninvasively, the carotid arteries are studied with real-time ultrasound (Doppler) or with MR. Circulation of the cerebrospinal fluid (CSF) in the subarachnoid space is evaluated by radionuclide or iodinated contrast cisternography. Similar contrast material is used to visualize the subarachnoid space around the spinal cord during the performance of myelography. Myelography may soon be displaced by MR.

ROENTGENOGRAMS OF THE SKULL After the advent of CT, conventional skull roentgenography, known as skull X-ray, lost its position as a screening modality for head trauma and for the detection of abnormal calcifications in a variety of brain disorders. At the present time, it is mainly used to evaluate the region of the sella and the foramina at the base of the skull in cases where these structures may be eroded by neoplasms or infections; plain films may also reveal sinusitis.

COMPUTED TOMOGRAPHY Brain CT is indicated for the evaluation of any disorder that may cause a change in the anatomic appearance of the brain. Neoplasms, abscesses, and hemorrhagic lesions are particularly well visualized. Before performing CT, a contrast medium is often injected intravenously to allow better visualization of pathology. Increase in tissue density (contrast enhancement) occurs in areas where there is a breakdown of the blood-brain barrier (Fig. 2.1-17). The clearest indications for a contrast study include metastatic brain disease, early stages of brain abscesses, brain infarction and arteriovenous malformations. Kidney disease or allergic predisposition may preclude injection of the iodinated compound.

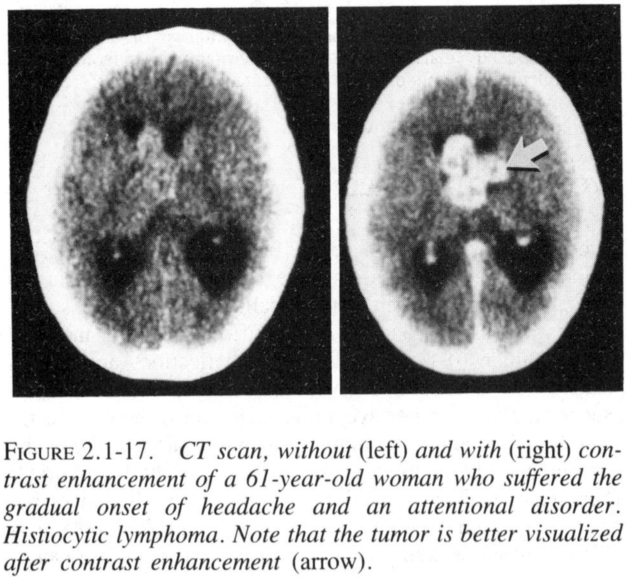

FIGURE 2.1-17. *CT scan, without* (left) *and with* (right) *contrast enhancement of a 61-year-old woman who suffered the gradual onset of headache and an attentional disorder. Histiocytic lymphoma. Note that the tumor is better visualized after contrast enhancement* (arrow).

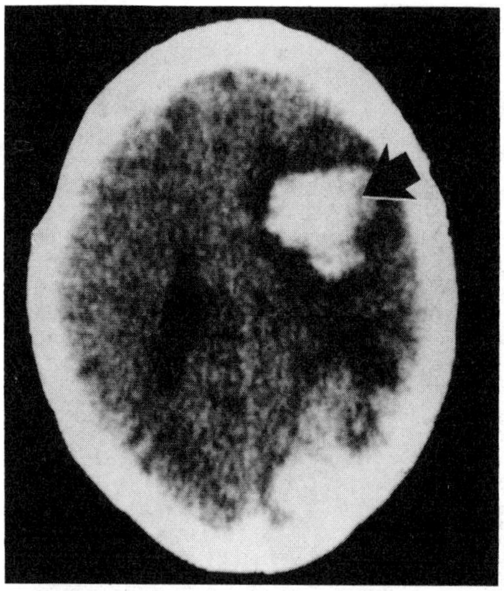

FIGURE 2.1-18. *CT scan showing an acute hemorrhage* (arrow) *in a metastatic lung carcinoma.*

An adequate knowledge of normal brain anatomy is needed to interpret abnormal CT images. On CT, lesions may appear with higher density (hyperdense), lower density, or the same density as the normal structures. In the last case, the lesion can be identified if it produces distortion of the normal anatomy. Fresh blood and calcium are hyperdense on CT (Fig. 2.1-18). Some very cellular tumors, such as lymphomas, have only slightly higher density than the surrounding tissue. Lesions containing increased water content, due to edema, appear hypodense on CT. Fat and air have very low densities (Fig. 2.1-19).

Regarding specific clinical problems in head trauma, CT will disclose not only skull fractures but also epidural or other hemorrhages that may have to be evacuated. The yield of CT is minimal for uncomplicated syncope, dizziness, or headache. New-onset generalized seizures in an adult are seldom associated with a positive CT; however, it will be abnormal in as many as 50 to 70 percent of patients with focal seizures or an abnormal neurological examination. Unless explained by a toxic-metabolic cause, the patient in coma warrants a CT to identify causes that range from a subdural empyema to a massive subarachnoid hemorrhage. Delirium occasionally results from a medial occipitotemporal infarct or other lesion identifiable on CT. Although it is generally performed as part of the evaluation of patients with progressive dementia, CT is seldom helpful in connection with this disorder. A tumor is found in 1 to 3 percent of patients with dementia. The ventricles are larger in groups of demented compared with nondemented elderly, but individual variability precludes good correlation of ventricular size and cognitive function. Among psychiatric patients with focal neurological findings or cognitive impairment, 20 to 50 percent have an abnormal CT. Nonspecific CT changes, particularly ventricular dilation, have been reported in a subgroup of patients with schizophrenia.

Psychiatric symptoms occasionally reflect treatable neurological disease, such as a neoplasm. On the basis of a cost-benefit analysis, the following indications for ordering CT in psychiatric patients have been proposed: confusion or dementia of unknown cause, movement disorder of unknown etiology, prolonged catatonia, anorexia nervosa, and first episode of personality change after age 50. Less clear-cut are two additional indications—namely, the first episode of a major mood disorder after age 50 and the first episode of a psychosis of unknown etiology.

Recent infarcts may be difficult to visualize on CT, particularly when they are small. Within the second week after the stroke, about 80 percent of infarcts may show increased density after the infusion of contrast media (contrast enhancement). After approximately 1 month, chronic infarcts usually appear as low-density areas, triangular with the base toward the skull when involving the cortex or rounded when in the deep nuclei (Fig. 2.1-20). White matter infarcts are ragged and tend to occur in the periventricular region and in the higher sections of the centrum semiovale.

Acute intracerebral hemorrhage is very well visualized on CT (Fig. 2.1-18). Its location and the presence of enhancement from an underlying vascular or neoplastic lesion aid greatly in the identification of the cause. In a few weeks, hemorrhages become isodense with the surrounding brain; they can then be detected by the mass effect they generate. Subarachnoid hemorrhages may pass undetected when the amount of blood that mixes with the CSF is small. In these cases, lumbar puncture is the next diagnostic procedure. An aneurysm or arteriovenous malformation occasionally may be visualized after contrast injection. Chronic subdural hematomas, sometimes causing dementia, may be isodense because of ongoing small hemorrhages into the mass of the organizing hematoma (Fig. 2.1-21).

In contrast to infarcts, the appearance of brain neoplasms on CT is more striking than expected from the clinical findings (Fig. 2.1-17). Estimation of the histological type is accomplished by taking into account the clinical history and the CT characteristics, including location, multiplicity, density, presence of blood or calcification, and the pattern of contrast enhancement. For instance, a tumor in the sella turcica with homogeneous enhancement and a small hypodense area representing a cyst is most likely a pituitary adenoma. A similar appearance accompanied by calcification suggests the diagnosis of craniopharyngioma.

Infections generally cause rounded hypodense areas, each surrounded by a ring-like area of contrast enhancement (Fig. 2.1-22). The ring portion of each lesion is thinner and more regular than the doughnut-like lesions due to neoplasms. Early in the course of a bacterial infection or throughout a viral infection, the affected area may be hypodense, with some degree of mass effect.

Congenital disorders often have a striking appearance on CT and should be carefully correlated with the clinical findings to avoid blaming the old static lesion for a new unrelated problem (Fig. 2.1-23).

MAGNETIC RESONANCE Some atomic nuclei (protons) within a strong magnetic field will align and rotate (precess) within the direction of the field. When these nuclei are then exposed to an alternating magnetic field of a radio frequency the same as that of the rotating nuclei, some of the nuclei will be forced to a state of higher energy level. The atomic nuclei absorb energy from the radio-frequency transmitter only at a resonance frequency that is specific for the element. When the radio frequency is stopped, the nuclei will re-emit energy and return to their former state. The T_1 and T_2 relaxation times are the energies emitted when atomic nuclei spin back to realign themselves after termination of their excitation by a radiofrequency pulse. T_1 refers to the interaction between the nuclei and the environment (lattice); T_2 refers to the interaction between the relaxing and unaffected nuclei. Computer analysis of the parameters of this emitted energy is used to portray a spatial image of the distribution of specific elements (e.g., hydrogen or phosphorus). In this way, not only detailed anatomy but also the biochemical state of the tissue can be evaluated. Imaging with CT provides information about one variable: tissue radiodensity. Four different tissue characteristics combine to form MR images: proton density, T_1 and T_2 relaxation times, and tissue flow (particularly CSF and blood). Only axial images can be directly obtained with CT, without repositioning the patient. MR yields images in any plane.

Although considerable experience has been accumulated over the past decade on the pathological patterns depicted by CT, the application of MR imaging is a nascent field. Swift technological improvements have occurred in image quality, blood flow imaging, use of paramagnetic labels, and the potential for spectrographic analysis of brain compounds. Many of these applications are at an experimental stage. At the time of this writing, MR imaging is mainly used to detect morphologic changes. In addition to providing greater anatomic definition (Fig. 2.1-24), MR has proved more sensitive than CT in a number of disorders, particularly multiple sclerosis and gliomas. MR studies avoid patient exposure to ionizing radiation, which renders MR more suitable than CT

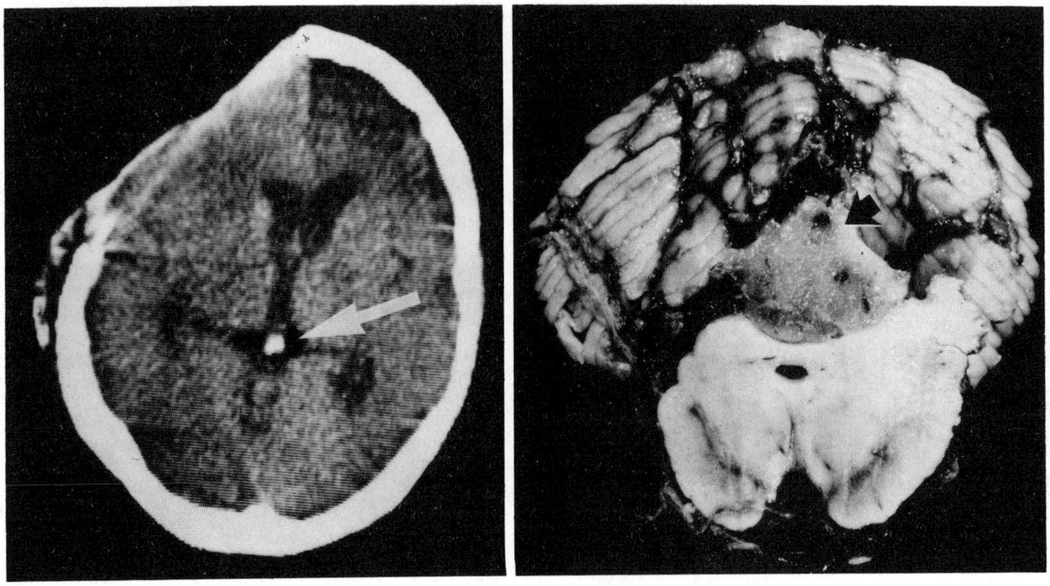

FIGURE 2.1-19. *CT scan* (left) *and pathology specimen* (right) *of a lipoma in the quadrigeminal plate cistern. Note that on CT the lesion* (arrow) *appears darker than the CSF.*

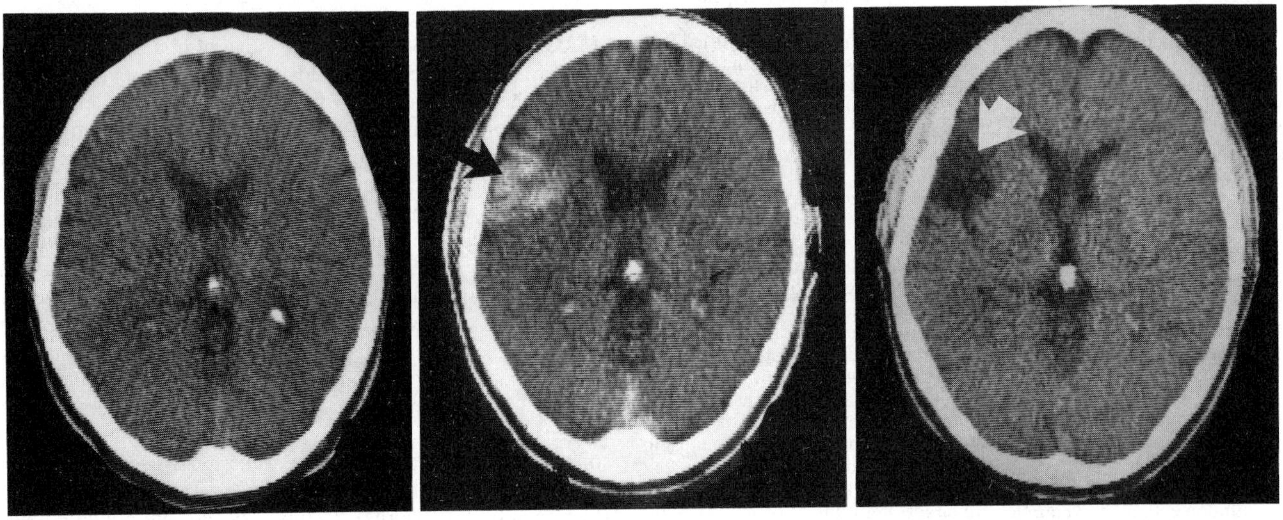

FIGURE 2.1-20. *CT scan of a 47-year-old man with an embolic infarction of Broca's area. Scan obtained 6 days after the stroke, without* (left) *and with contrast* (center). *The lesion is invisible without contrast and shows contrast enhancement* (black arrow). *Repeat scan 3 weeks after the stroke* (right) *shows the hypodense, area of chronic encephalomalacia* (white arrow).

as a screening procedure; however, MR is more costly than CT. Moreover, a strong magnetic field needed for MR prevents its use in studying patients who are monitored or maintained with equipment containing ferrous substances.

Since calcium gives no signal on MR, calcified areas appear dark on images obtained with this modality (Fig. 2.1-24). MR images may be obtained in order to maximize T_1 contrast (T_1-weighted images) or T_2 contrast (T_2-weighted images) among the different tissues. Section 2.2 contains examples of MR applied to the study of different disorders. Brain edema from ischemia, infections, tumors, or trauma appears hyperintense on T_2-weighted images. Brain infarcts appear hypointense on T_1-weighted images and hyperintense on T_2-weighted images. MR detects infarction earlier than CT, but CT may be more specific in revealing fresh blood within the infarct. The MR appearance of intracerebral hemorrhages depends on the stages of their evolution. In the first week, the center of the hemorrhage is hypointense on T_2-weighted images; hemorrhages older than 1 month are hyperintense on both types of images. Subdural hematomas are defined better with MR than with CT. MR is the undisputed modality of choice for the visualization of multiple sclerosis plaques, which appear hyperintense on T_2-weighted images. Areas of infection can be detected by MR as hyperintense lesions on T_2-weighted images, even before an abscess has resulted in the typical ring-enhancing pattern on CT. Neoplasms, particularly those in the temporal lobe that often result in behavioral abnormalities, are often visualized earlier with MR than with CT. Sagittal section capability and avoidance of bone-related artifacts render MR as the modality of

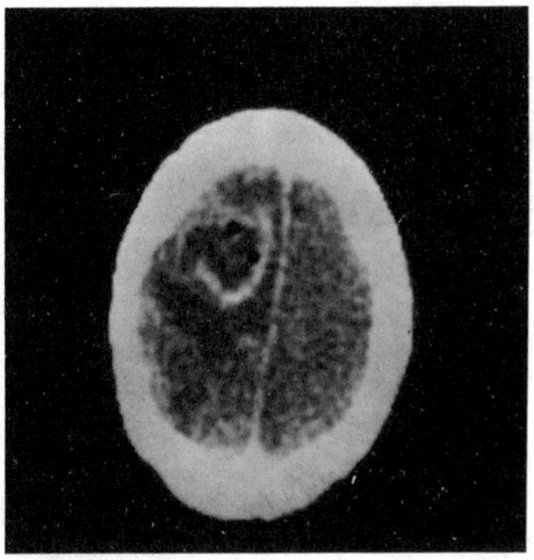

FIGURE 2.1-21. *Subdural hematoma. A chronic subdural hematoma over the right convexity has caused a ventricular shift from right to left. A small rim of increased density between the surface of the brain and the hematoma represents the membrane enclosing the hematoma. The hematoma has, for the most part, changed from dense blood clot to a less dense fluid.*

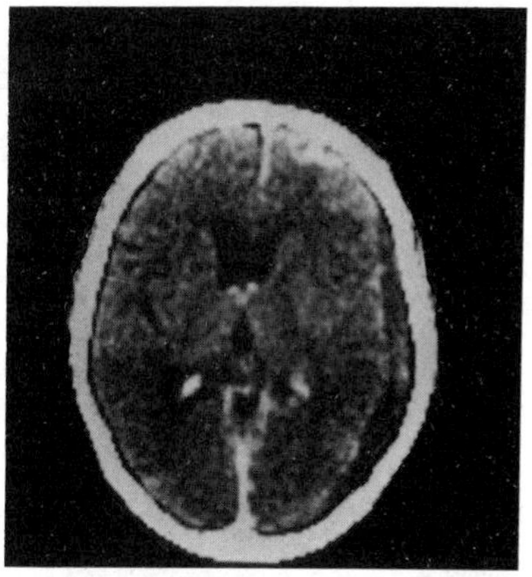

FIGURE 2.1-22. *Cerebral abscess. A large left frontal abscess is enclosed by a hypervascular capsule (density enhanced by intravenous contrast) and surrounded by a zone of edema (decreased density). The tiny markedly lucent zones within the lesion represent gas produced by bacteria and indicate that this mass is an abscess, rather than a neoplasm.*

choice for the study of disorders in the posterior fossa and at the cervico-medullary junction, such as the Arnold-Chiari malformation.

POSITRON EMISSION TOMOGRAPHY This technique is particularly well suited for the study of psychiatric disease. Although high cost limits its availability, PET may become more widespread when regional cyclotrons can provide short-lived tracers to community hospitals. For the performance of PET, a radiotracer is administered by inhalation or injection, which quickly participates in the metabolic processes of the brain. Positrons emitted by the radiotracer produce high-energy photons that can be detected by appropriately aligned scintillation detectors. As with CT and MR, algorithms are used to compute the site of origin of the detected photons and to reconstruct the tomographic planes. PET measures specific physiological processes, such as cerebral blood flow and metabolism, membrane transport, and, of particular interest in psychiatry, receptor-ligand interactions. The distribution of opiate receptors in the brain has been illustrated using [^{11}C] carfentanil (Fig. 2.1-25). PET studies of regional metabolism

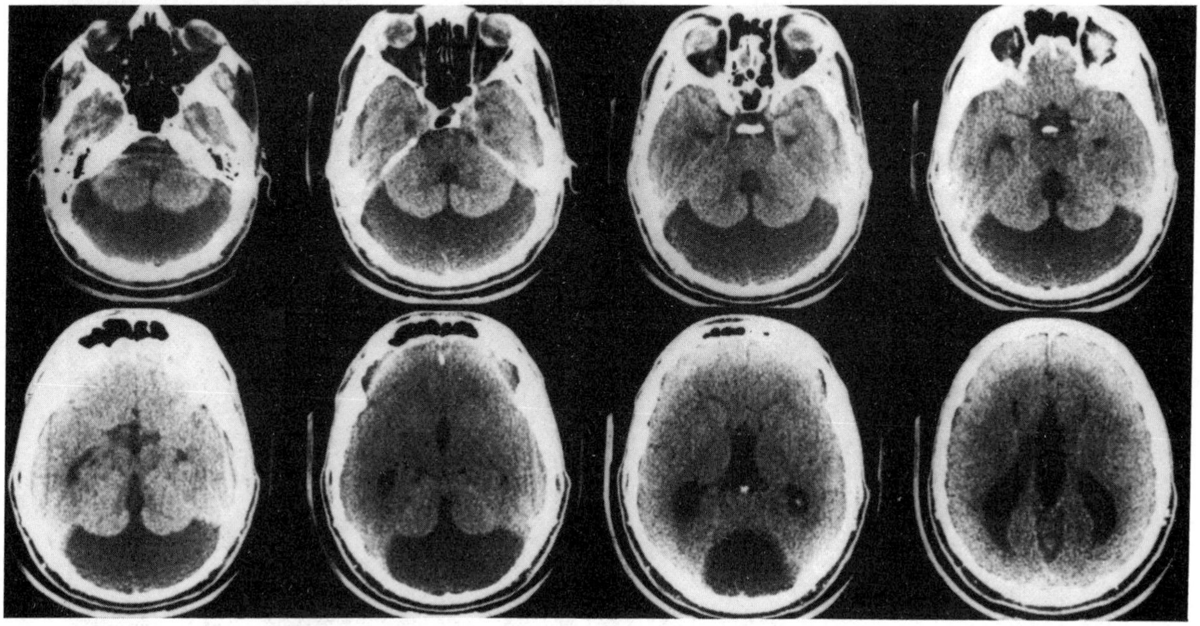

FIGURE 2.1-23. *CT scan of a 42-year-old man showing a Dandy-Walker malformation of the posterior fossa and agenesis of the corpus callosum. The scan was performed for headaches. Standard neurological examination was normal. Headaches were related to muscle contraction and improved with biofeedback therapy and psychotherapy. (From Masdeu J C, Dobben G, AzarKia B: Dandy-Walker syndrome studied by computed tomography and pneumoencephalography.* Radiology 147*:109, 1983. Copyright 1983 The Radiological Society of North America, with permission.)*

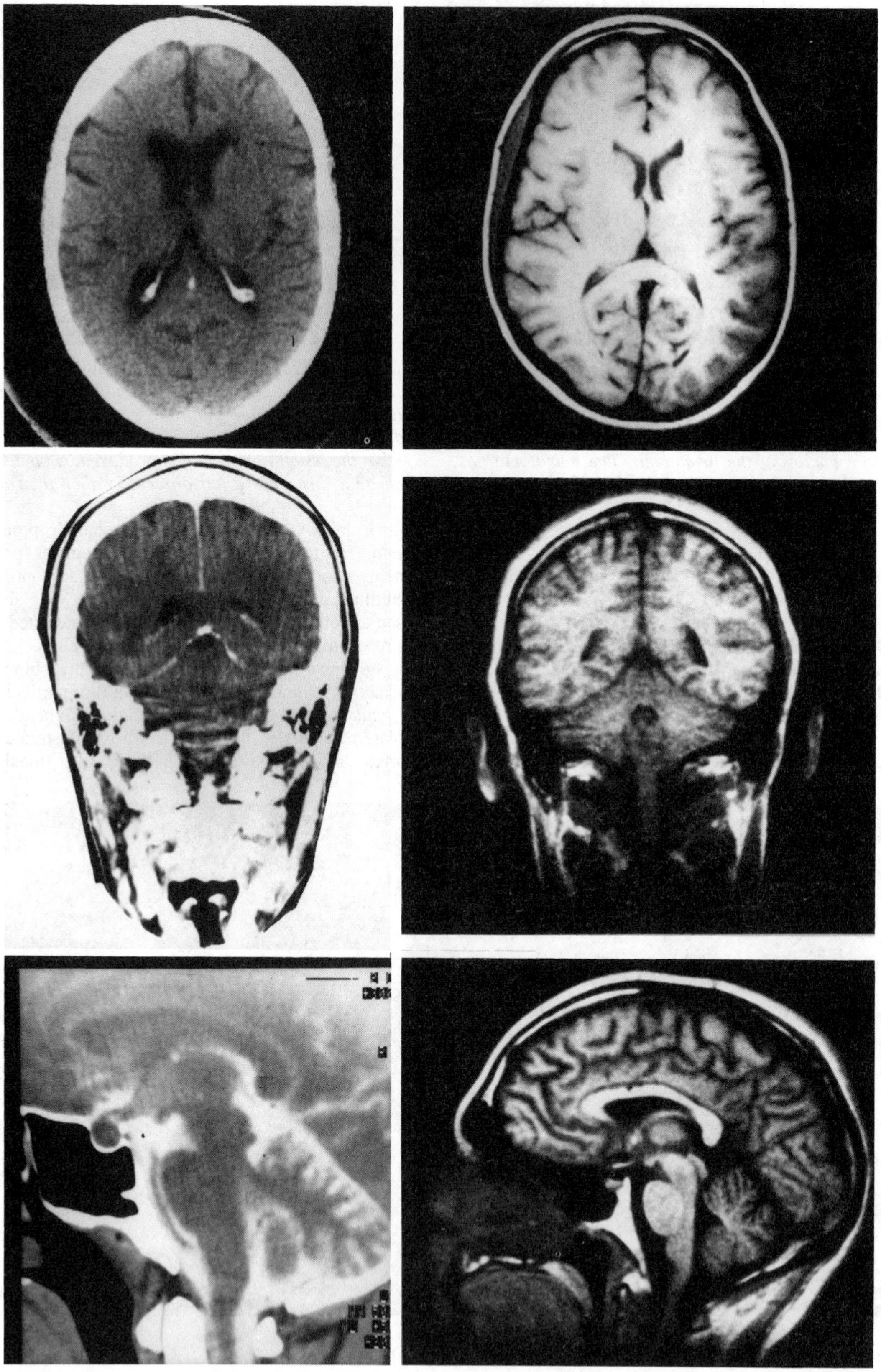

FIGURE 2.1-24. *X-ray computed tomography (CT) sections* (left) *compared with magnetic resonance (MR) imaging sections at similar levels* (right) *and at three different planes* (Top: *axial;* Center: *coronal;* Bottom: *sagittal*). *Sagittal CT performed with contrast media in the CSF. (From Gonzalez C F, Grosman C B, Masdeu J C:* Head and Spine Imaging. *Wiley, New York, 1985, with permission.)*

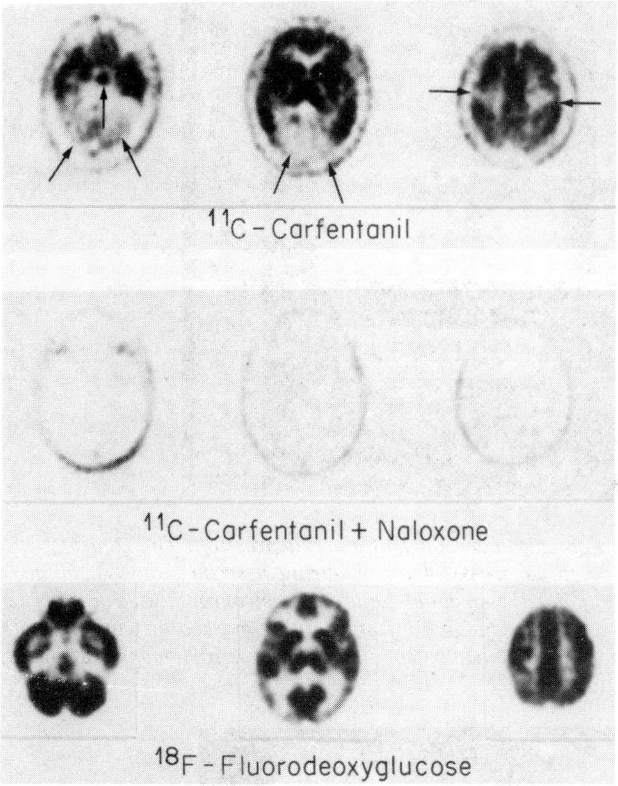

FIGURE 2.1-25. *Opiate receptors in human brain. The PET images in the* top *row were obtained 30 to 60 minutes after intravenous administration of 25 mCi of [^{11}C] carfentanil (80 ng/kg). The three images are 7.2, 4, and 0.8 cm above the canthomeatal line. Images in the* middle *row were acquired 30 to 60 minutes after intravenous administration of 1 mg per kg naloxone (Narcan) (+)-isomer, an opiate antagonist, and the same dose of [^{11}C] carfentanil used in first study. In the top row, a preferential accumulation of activity is seen in areas rich in opiate receptors, such as the thalamus, basal ganglia, and frontal cortex (*center *and* right *images) and pituitary gland (*left *image,* inner arrow*). Low activity is seen where opiate receptors exist in low concentration, such as the occipital cortex (*center *image,* arrows*), the postcentral gyrus (*right *image,* arrows*), and the cerebellum (*left *images,* arrow*). Images in the middle row demonstrate the low level of nonspecific binding when labeled carfentanil is blocked with (+)-naloxone. Approximately 90 percent of specific opiate receptor binding in the thalamus and basal ganglia is blocked. For comparison,* bottom *row of images are of local glucose utilization for approximately the same levels as the opiate receptor distribution study. (Carfentanil studies from J J Frost et al, Johns Hopkins University, and glucose utilization images from M E Phelps et al, UCLA School of Medicine. From Mazziota J C, Phelps M E: Positron emission tomography studies of the brain. In* Positron Emission Tomography and Autoradiography: Principles and Applications, *M E Phelps, J C Mazziota, H R Schelbert, editors, p 493. Raven Press, New York, 1986, with permission.)*

during specific mental activity yield a clearer understanding of the behavioral instrumentality of the different regions of the brain.

PET has proved to be of value for the study of a number of pathological conditions. In patients with temporal lobe epilepsy amenable to surgery, both temporal lobes often show seizure activity on EEG. PET helps to decide which one contains the primary focus and, therefore, should be surgically removed. On the affected side, metabolic rates are depressed in the interictal stage, but markedly enhanced during a focal seizure (Fig. 2.1-26). During electroconvulsive therapy, the seizure is attended by diffusely enhanced metabolic activity, followed by generalized depression (Fig. 2.1-27). PET has documented the effect of localized infarcts or tumors on the metabolic rates of related regions of the brain; hypometabolism extends well beyond the area of necrosis. In patients with primary degenerative dementia of the Alzheimer type, metabolic rates are abnormally low in the frontal, parietal, and temporal association cortex. Patchy areas of hypometabolism, larger than suggested by CT images, can be visualized in multi-infarct dementia. In Huntington's chorea, the caudate nucleus appears hypometabolic on PET well before it becomes atrophic on CT (Fig. 2.1-28). Frontal hypometabolism has been described in schizophrenic patients, particularly those patients exposed to antipsychotic drugs. In a small group of depressed obsessive-compulsive patients, reversal of frontal hypometabolism may occur as they improve with medication (Fig. 2.1-29).

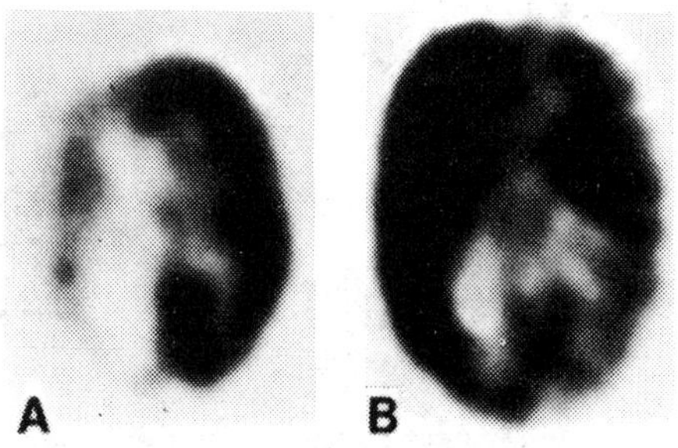

FIGURE 2.1-26. *Representative planes of section of interictal* (A) *and ictal* (B) *PET scans from a patient with partial seizures. Ictal activation of the entire left hemisphere occurred with nine seizures that originated electrically in the left parietal area and clinically spread to involve both sides of the body, the right side more than the left. (From Engel J, Kuhl D E, Phelps M E: Regional brain metabolism during seizures in humans.* Advances in Neurology *34:* 141. New York, Raven Press, 1983, with permission.)

CEREBRAL ANGIOGRAPHY Cerebral angiography is performed when the vessels of the brain have to be studied in detail. The most common indications include carotid artery disease, where the extent and disposition of atheromatous changes need to be known before carotid endarterectomy; aneurysms and arteriovenous malformations; definition of the blood supply of a tumor; and suspected vasculitis of the small arteries. By femoral catheterization, iodinated contrast material is injected in the carotid and vertebral vessels through their origins. Serial roentgenograms are obtained while the contrast successively opacifies arteries, capillary beds, and veins. Serious complications of arteriography, primarily brain ischemia or infarction, occur in fewer than 2 percent of studies. Complications often stem from displacement of atheromatous deposits by the catheter tip and from vascular irritation caused by the highly concentrated contrast media.

DIGITAL VENOUS ANGIOGRAPHY The large arteries—including the proximal portions of the intracranial territory, the large veins, and the venous sinuses—can be visualized by means of DIVA technique. Injection through an intravenous catheter is potentially less traumatic than arterial injection, but the contrast media reaching the cerebral bed is more diluted than with arteriography. The densities of roentgenograms obtained during DIVA are digitized by an optic scanner, both before and after contrast has filled the vessels. By means of a computer, densities corresponding to the skull and other

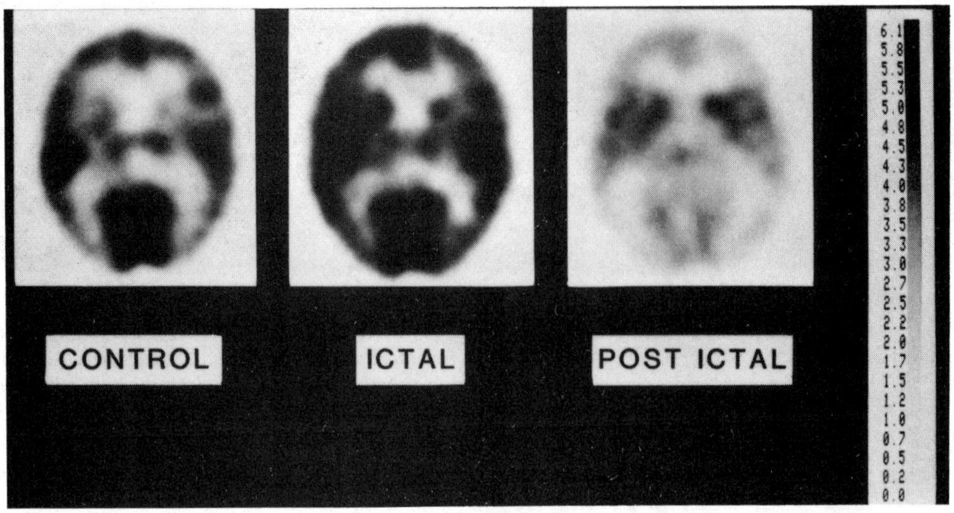

FIGURE 2.1-27. *Representative sections from three PET scans of a patient undergoing ECT for depression. The control scan* (A) *was obtained when the patient was not undergoing ECT. The ictal scan* (B) *obtained during a seizure shows a diffuse increase in local glucose utilization, whereas the postictal scan* (C) *obtained immediately after an electrographic seizure, at the beginning of the postictal EEG depression, shows a diffuse decrease in local glucose utilization, more marked for cortical than subcortical structures. (From Engel J, Kuhl D E, Phelps M E: Regional brain metabolism during seizures in humans.* Advances in Neurology, *34:* 141. New York, Raven Press, 1983, with permission.)

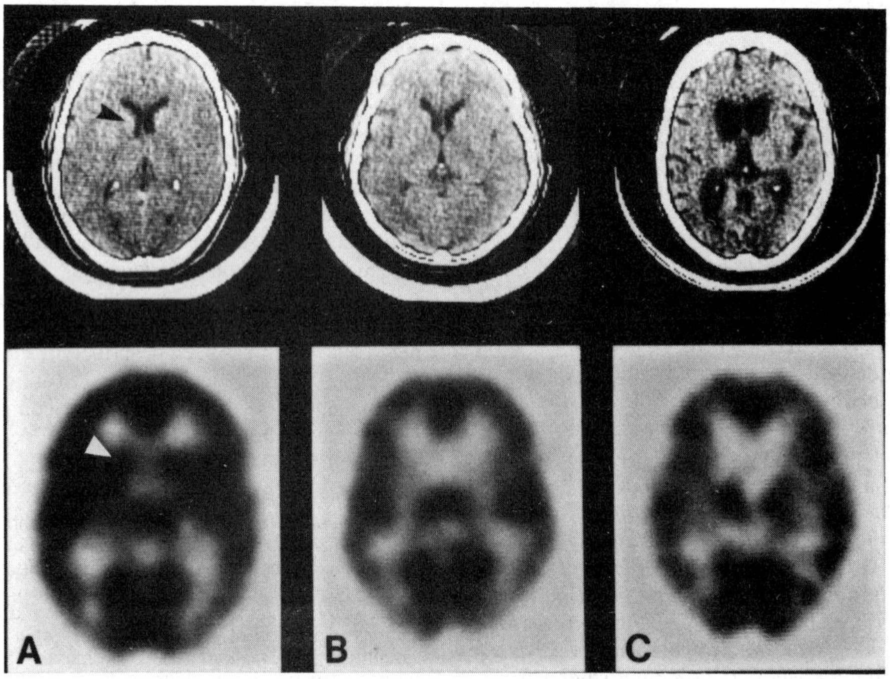

FIGURE 2.1-28. *Atrophy and local glucose utilization in Huntington's disease (HD) demonstrated by X-ray CT and PET images.* A. *Normal individual, showing the structural and metabolic appearance of the normal caudate nucleus and putamen* (arrow). B. *Patient with early clinical HD, depicting the normal structural appearance of the caudate nucleus on X-ray CT but profound hypometabolism of caudate and putamen bilaterally in the PET image.* C. *Patient with late HD, demonstrating both structural (cortical and subcortical atrophy) and functional abnormalities of the caudate and putamen bilaterally. Such studies show that the functional abnormalities (as measured by local glucose utilization) of the basal ganglia in patients with early HD precede structural cell loss sufficient to produce changes in the X-ray CT. (From Kuhl D, Phelps M, Markham C, Winter J, Metter J, Riege W: Local cerebral glucose metabolism in Huntington's disease determined by emission computed tomography of* ^{18}*F-fluorodeoxyglucose.* J Cereb Blood Flow Metab 1 *(suppl): 459, 1981, with permission.)*

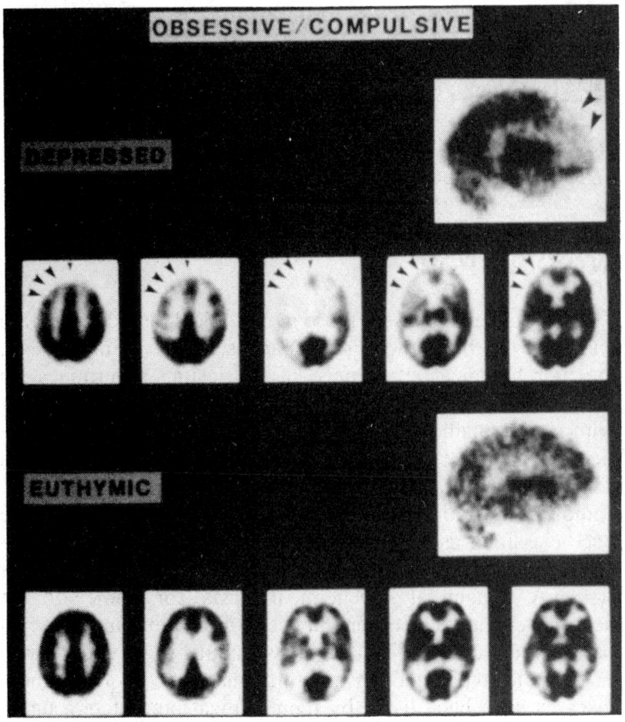

FIGURE 2.1-29. *PET scans showing fluorodeoxyglucose metabolism in a patient with obsessive-compulsive disorder and depression. Two larger images at the right are rectilinear scans demonstrating lateral view, whole brain glucose utilization. Decreased local glucose utilization was present in the left frontal and anterior cingulate cortices* (arrows). *Following drug therapy, which resulted in alleviation of the depressed mood, the patient became euthymic and the metabolic asymmetries resolved* (bottom row). *(Courtesy of L. R. Baxter et al, UCLA School of Medicine. From Mazziota, J C, Phelps M E: Positron emission tomography studies of the brain. In* Positron Emission Tomography and Autoradiography: Principles and Applications, *M E Phelps, J C Mazziota, H R Schelbert, editors, p 493. Raven Press, New York, 1986, with permission.)*

nonvascular structures present in the preinjection roentgenograms are subtracted from the postinjection images containing the contrast-filled vessels. Thus, despite the low concentration of contrast media, the vessels are greatly highlighted and visualized. This technique does not depict the small intracranial vessels well. The quality of images may be impaired by artifacts easily induced by motion, including swallowing, and in patients with impaired cardiac output.

ECHO-DOPPLER (DUPLEX) ULTRASOUND The intrathoracic and, particularly, the cervical portions of the carotid and vertebral arteries can be noninvasively studied by combining two ultrasonographic techniques: B-mode real-time bidimensional imaging and pulsed Doppler, also known as duplex imaging. Sonography may overestimate or underestimate the degree of stenosis in about 15 to 20 percent of patients examined. The fine characteristics of ulcerated plaques may not be well visualized. For this reason, either angiography or DIVA is preferred when carotid endarterectomy is strongly contemplated or in patients with a low risk for invasive procedures. Transcranial Doppler sonography has been introduced recently. It can provide important information concerning major arteries at the base of the brain.

CISTERNOGRAPHY Cerebrospinal fluid (CSF) circulation is abnormal in normopressure hydrocephalus, a potential cause of dementia. Normally, the CSF is secreted by the choroid plexus, exits the ventricular system, and bathes the spinal cord and the base and convexity of the brain. The CSF is reabsorbed into the superior sagittal sinus through the pachionian granulations. In normopressure hydrocephalus, impaired reabsorption into the venous sinuses causes a backing up of CSF and a reversal in its flow; it becomes reabsorbed through the ventricular wall. Evaluation of CSF circulation is most often performed by injecting a radionuclide of indium, ^{111}In, into the subarachnoid space through a lumbar puncture. Normally, the radionuclide appears over the brain convexity and parasagittal region within 24 hours and becomes undetectable within 48 to 72 hours. In instances of communicating or normopressure hydrocephalus, the radionuclide is not readily reabsorbed and diffuses into the lateral ventricles, where it can be detected after 48 hours. Cisternography can also be performed by following with serial CTs the transit of water-soluble radiodense media.

MYELOGRAPHY High-concentration, water-soluble radiodense solutions injected by lumbar puncture into the subarachnoid space allow visualization of the spinal cord and the spinal roots in roentgenograms. This study is often followed by CT to obtain a more detailed view of the affected areas on axial sections. Suspected disk disease was the most common indication for myelography; now, CT has become the procedure of choice for this condition. CT and myelography are being replaced by MR.

CEREBROSPINAL FLUID EXAMINATION

An invasive, uncomfortable procedure, the lumbar puncture (LP), should be performed only when clearly indicated. The indications include meningeal infection, encephalitis, neoplasms spreading to the meninges, pseudotumor of the brain, demyelinating disease, and subarachnoid hemorrhage with a negative CT. Dementia in the elderly is a dubious indication since it seldom results from syphilis or cryptococcal meningitis.

Serious complications of a lumbar puncture are rare. Papilledema or other evidence of increased intracranial pressure, particularly with a mass lesion in the temporal lobe or posterior fossa, is the major contraindication for this procedure. In the presence of increased intracranial pressure, LP may suddenly create a decreased pressure gradient across the tentorium cerebelli or foramen magnum, with consequent herniation of the medial temporal lobe or cerebellar tonsils. Resultant brain stem compression is often fatal. When in doubt, a CT is indicated to define intracranial pathology. Important determinations include pressure, color and clarity, cell count, protein and glucose values, serology, and in some instances culture and immunological studies.

The initial CSF pressure must always be measured with the patient horizontal and relaxed; pressures exceeding 180 to 200 mm of CSF are considered elevated.

In regard to color and clarity, CSF is normally indistinguishable from water, with which it should be compared. Bloody CSF may be due to a traumatic lumbar puncture. If this is so, the amount of blood in the CSF decreases in successive collecting test tubes, and the supernatant CSF after centrifugation is clear. Blood in CSF is usually due to subarachnoid hemorrhage or, less often, to an intracerebral hemorrhage that has ruptured into the ventricles or out to the subarachnoid space. Cerebral trauma and a subdural hematoma may be associated with blood in the CSF. Xanthochromia in CSF is the residual pigment of blood. Severe jaundice or unusually high protein causes a yellow discoloration of CSF. Turbid CSF may be due to meningitis, a slight amount of blood, or a highly elevated protein content.

An elevated white blood cell count—that is, more than three lymphocytes per mm^3—is indicative of inflammation or irritation of the meninges. If the cell count is elevated, the CSF should be smeared and stained, as well as cultured, for infecting organisms. A low-grade infection, such as CNS syphilis or aseptic meningeal irritation (e.g., a brain tumor near the meninges) may be manifested by 5 to 50 white blood cells, especially lymphocytes, per mm^3. Chronic meningitis, as caused by fungi, results in an elevation of white blood cells, predominantly lymphocytes, ranging from 50 to 500 per mm^3. Acute purulent meningitis is usually associated with pleocytosis of 1,000 to 15,000 white blood cells per mm^3, predominantly polymorphonuclear leukocytes. If a search for exfoliative tumor cells is to be made, the CSF must be immediately preserved in an equal volume of 50 percent ethyl alcohol.

Protein elevation of the CSF—more than 50 mg per 100 ml—may be seen in any organic neurological disease. As a rule of thumb, an elevation of protein of more than 100 mg per 100 ml is much more indicative of a cerebral neoplasm than of a cerebrovascular lesion. Fluid drawn below a spinal block usually contains protein elevated beyond 100 mg per 100 ml, and the CSF of meningitis may reveal similar findings. In multiple sclerosis, neurosyphilis, and subacute sclerosing panencephalitis, the CSF γ-globulin is usually elevated—that is, beyond 12 to 15 percent of the total protein. The finding of elevated myelin basic protein and the presence of oligoclonal bands of γ-globulin with agar gel electrophoresis, strongly support the diagnosis of multiple sclerosis.

The glucose content of CSF is normally 50 to 65 mg per 100 ml and corresponds to a value two-thirds that of the blood glucose at the time of the lumbar puncture. CSF glucose of less than 40 mg per 100 ml or less than half that of the simultaneously drawn blood glucose is abnormal and is found in meningitis of bacterial or fungal origin. Low CSF glucose may sometimes occur in noninfectious diseases that irritate the meninges, such as meningeal carcinomatosis, sarcoidosis, and subarachnoid hemorrhage.

A positive finding of CSF serological test is indicative of active CNS syphilis if the test is accompanied by an elevated white cell count and elevated protein in the CSF.

REFERENCES

Aminoff M J: *Electrodiagnosis in Clinical Neurology,* ed 2. Churchill Livingstone, New York, 1986.

Bickerstaff E R, editor: *Neurological Examination in Clinical Practice,* ed 4, Mosby, St. Louis, 1980.

Brant-Zawadzki M, Norman D, editors: *Magnetic Resonance Imaging of the Central Nervous System.* Raven Press, New York, 1987.

Brazis P W, Masdeu J C, Biller J: *Localization in Clinical Neurology,* Little, Brown, Boston, 1985.

Brodal A: *Neurological Anatomy in Relation to Clinical Medicine,* ed 3. Oxford University Press, New York, 1981.

Cadet J L, Rickler K C, Weinberger D R: The clinical neurologic examination in schizophrenia. In *Handbook of Schizophrenia,* vol I, *The Neurology of Schizophrenia,* H A Nasrallah, D R Weinberger, editors. Elsevier, New York, 1986.

Folstein M D, Folstein S E, McHugh P R: "Mini mental state." A practical method for grading the cognitive state of patients for the clinician. J Psychiat Res *12:* 189, 1975.

Freeman L M, editor: *Freeman and Johnson's Clinical Radionuclide Imaging,* ed 3. Grune & Stratton, Orlando, FL, 1984.

Gonzalez C F, Grossman C B, Masdeu J C: *Head and spine imaging.* Wiley, New York, 1985.

Health and Public Policy Committee, American College of Physicians: The diagnostic spinal tap. Ann Intern Med *104:* 880, 1986.

Illingworth R S: *The Development of the Infant and Young Child: Normal and Abnormal,* ed 8, Churchill Livingstone, New York, 1984.

Kandel E R, Schwartz J H, editors: *Principles of Neural Science.* Elsevier, New York, 1981.

Kaufman D M: *Clinical Neurology for Psychiatrists,* ed 2. Grune & Stratton, Orlando, FL, 1985.

Lawton-Smith J: *Neuro-ophthalmology Now!* Year Book, Chicago, 1986.

Lee S H, Rao K: *Cranial Computed Tomography and MRI,* ed 2. McGraw-Hill, New York, 1983.

Mayo Clinic: *Clinical Examinations in Neurology,* ed 5. Saunders, Philadelphia, 1981.

Mazziota J C, Phelps M E: Positron emission tomography studies of the brain. In *Positron Emission Tomography and Autoradiography: Principles and Applications,* M E Phelps, J C Mazziota, H R Schelbert, editors, chap 11, p 493. Raven Press, New York, 1986.

Mumenthaler M, Appenzeller O: *Neurologic Differential Diagnosis.* Grune & Stratton, Orlando, FL, 1985.

Niedermeyer E, da Silva F H L, editors: *Electroencephalography: Basic Principles, Clinical Applications and Related Fields.* ed 2. Urban & Schwarzenberg, Baltimore, 1987.

Rudge P: *Clinical Neuro-otology,* Churchill Livingstone, New York, 1983.

2.2 CLINICAL NEUROLOGY AND NEUROPATHOLOGY

JOSEPH C. MASDEU, M.D.
SEYMOUR SOLOMON, M.D.

INTRODUCTION

This section encompasses those neurological disorders that are characterized by pathological changes in the brain. Indeed, the morphological appearance of the lesions determines, in most instances, their etiological classification. Some disorders with varied pathological expressions, such as vitamin deficiencies, have been grouped together because they share a similar etiology. A large group of diseases with characteristic pathological findings but poorly understood etiology were once classified as neurodegenerative disorders. One such example is primary degenerative dementia of the Alzheimer type. A congenital biochemical basis for some of the neurodegenerative disorders has been discovered in the recent past, but the cause of the majority remains to be determined. In order to avoid making assumptions about etiology, these diseases have been listed by their clinical presentation under the heading of hereditary and idiopathic disorders. Specific pediatric disorders are discussed at the end of the section.

BRAIN HISTOLOGY AND COMMON PATHOLOGICAL CHANGES

Except for the vessels and microglial cells, the brain cells are derived from the primitive neuroectoderm. The most differentiated are the neurons, which do not reproduce after birth. Among the glial elements, astrocytes provide an interface between the neurons and the blood vessels. Oligodendrocytes elaborate myelin, critical in the fast conduction of axonal impulses. Ependymal cells line the ventricular surface. The extravascular space in the brain is separated by the blood-brain barrier from the systemic metabolic milieu. Anatomically, the blood-brain barrier is formed by the tight junctions of the endothelial cells in the brain capillaries.

Severe neuronal injury causes neuronal loss—that is, an absence of normally occurring neurons. Intermediate stages, with shrinkage of the cytoplasm and eosinophilia, may precede the complete disappearance of the neuron. In some disorders, microglia cluster on the injured neuron and remove it, a phenomenon known as neuronophagia. Less serious injuries, such as transection of the axon, may result in a glassy, swollen appearance of the neuronal cytoplasm. The nucleus is peripherally displaced, and the cytoplasmic reticulum (Nissl substance) appears indistinct (i.e., chromatolysis). Lipofuscin, an insoluble mixture of lipids and proteins, normally accumulates in the neuronal cytoplasm with advancing age, Abnormal accumulation of lipids occur in the lipid storage diseases, such as Tay-Sachs. Inclusion bodies are often viral and can occupy the neuronal nucleus (e.g., herpes simplex encephalitis) or the cytoplasm (e.g., rabies). Intracytoplasmic neurofibrillary tangles are characteristic of Alzheimer's disease and other neurodegenerative disorders.

The histological appearance of astrocytes is often helpful in making a diagnosis. Ischemia or other insults induce swelling of the astrocytes. These swollen astrocytes, referred to as gemistocytic astrocytes, may become multinucleated as well. Glial scars are often the last stage of brain repair after various injuries, ranging from ischemia to trauma. Microglial cells, similar to histiocytes or macrophages, also play an important role in the organization and repair of tissue damage in the brain. They participate in the inflammatory response to infections and act as scavenger cells (lipid-laden macrophages), removing lipoproteinaceous debris from a variety of lesions.

Gross and microscopic morphology is yielding to biochemical and immunological techniques as the main tools in unveiling the pathophysiology of various brain disorders. The correction of neurotransmitter abnormalities has changed the prognosis of several degenerative disorders, notably Parkinson's disease. Advanced techniques of molecular biology have recently allowed the identification of the genetic locus for Huntington's disease. Western blot and hybridization studies were instrumental in defining the acquired immune deficiency syndrome (AIDS) virus as the cause of dementia in patients afflicted with this disorder.

CEREBROVASCULAR DISEASE

Despite the recently documented drop in the incidence of stroke in the United States, cerebrovascular disease remains the leading cause of neurological mortality and the third most common cause of death in the United States, after heart disease and cancer. According to estimates from the American Heart Association for 1984, there will be approximately 500,000 new victims of stroke each year; the result will be a total of 1,830,000 stroke patients in the United States. About 15 percent of these patients will be institutionalized and half of the remaining patients will need considerable assistance at home. Death rates from stroke have fallen about 5 percent per year since 1969. Control of hypertension has been crucial in effecting this welcome trend. Small population studies indicate a decline in brain infarction and intracerebral hemorrhage, but not in the incidence of subarachnoid hemorrhage.

Stroke, the sudden onset of neurological dysfunction, is generally the pattern in which cerebrovascular disease presents. There are two broad categories of cerebrovascular disease: ischemic and hemorrhagic. Among the cerebrovascular syndromes presenting to a general hospital, about 11 percent are transient ischemic attacks (TIAs). Of the strokes, 63 percent are infarcts, and 37 percent are hemorrhages. Although large hemorrhages tend to produce a more cataclysmal clinical picture than infarcts, strokes due to small hemorrhages can be indistinguishable clinically from strokes due to infarcts; however, they can be easily separated by use of computed tomography (CT) or magnetic resonance imaging (MR or MRI). The clinical presentation, pathology, and treatment of ischemic and hemorrhagic cerebrovascular diseases will be reviewed. Several of the disorders producing ischemic diseases, such as subacute bacterial endocarditis, also cause hemorrhagic disease of the brain. Since many of these entities affect the brain by ischemia first, they will be discussed with the ischemic disorders.

Despite the great social impact of cerebrovascular disease, treatments of the majority of these disorders are still neither satisfactory nor standardized. Procedures touted for a while as stroke-preventing, such as anastomosis of the superficial-temporal to the middle-cerebral arteries, are being debunked by carefully controlled prospective studies. In the following discussion, conditions are emphasized that, albeit relatively uncommon, clearly benefit from therapy.

Stroke victims are prone to psychiatric disease. Adjustment disorders are to be expected in persons subjected to a sudden change in life-style because of their inability to use a limb or impaired communication abilities. In addition, depression appears to develop in left-hemispheric-damaged patients more than would be expected from the physical handicap alone. Delirium or dementia often occur after repeated strokes.

TRANSIENT ISCHEMIC ATTACKS A TIA is a brief episode of focal neurological dysfunction due to ischemia that tends to recur but leaves no evidence of cerebral infarction. Classically, a TIA is diagnosed if the deficit lasts for less than 24 hours; however, most TIAs last for a few minutes to an hour. When they last longer, there is a greater chance that the patient may have sustained an infarct. Retinal ischemia, causing amaurosis fugax, transient hand weakness or numbness, transient diplopia, and unilateral perioral numbness are common examples of focal symptoms. A sudden loss of muscle tone, causing a person to fall without loss of consciousness, called a drop attack, is thought to be a TIA within the vertebrobasilar arterial tree. Transient lightheadedness or syncope does not qualify as a TIA because they are not caused by focal cerebral ischemia. (These symptoms are often due to global cerebral ischemia, as in the case of critically diminished cerebral perfusion due to a bradyarrhythmia.) Before a transient neurological deficit is assumed to be a TIA, focal seizures need to be considered. Not infrequently, a tumor betrays its presence by transient weakness, often caused by a focal seizure in which the clonic component passed unnoticed. For this reason, a CT or MR should be performed in all patients with TIAs. These procedures may also disclose an infarct or a small hemorrhage, thereby ruling out a diagnosis of TIA.

TIAs are usually due to minute emboli that break away from atheromatous plaques within the internal carotid, vertebral, or basilar arteries. An atherosclerotic lesion is usually located just beyond the bifurcation of the common carotid artery. Less often, changes in the cardiovascular system, such as arrhythmia or hypotension, may induce a TIA in the territory of a stenotic artery.

Recurring TIAs in middle-aged patients may be related to a migrainous phenomenon. The diagnosis is most clear when the patient has had migraine in the past, cardiac examination is normal, and angiography is unrevealing. Some neurologists have postulated that even when there is no history of headaches, a mechanism akin to migraine is operational. On rare occasions, migraine leads to infarction; this is known as complicated migraine.

When carotid disease is present, examination may reveal bruits over the orbits or carotid arteries in the neck, diminished pulsation of the carotid artery or its temporal branch, or evidence of emboli in the retinal arteries. The clinical diagnosis of carotid artery disease may be supported by the findings of ophthalmodynamometry, ocular plethysmography, Doppler, and thermographic tests. However, arteriography is necessary before endarterectomy.

TIAs should not be taken lightly because they are followed by a stroke within the first few months in about 30 percent of the cases. In a final analysis, the management of a TIA depends on its mechanism. Many of the processes considered below as causes of cerebral infarction may be first manifested as a TIA. There is then time to disclose the damaging agent and do something about it before the patient becomes irreversibly paralyzed. Therefore, the mechanisms and management discussed under cerebral infarction apply to TIAs as well. Unfortunately, treatment is less than effective in many instances.

CEREBRAL INFARCTION Cerebral infarction is the necrosis of brain cells because of the lack of oxygen or, rarely, of glucose. Pure hypoxia is a rare cause of brain infarction; carbon monoxide poisoning and drowning are two examples. More often, there is impaired perfusion of the brain, as in the case of cardiac arrest. The most common causes of brain infarction are decreased perfusion due to stenosis or thrombosis of the cranial arteries and occlusion of cerebral arteries by embolism from the heart. Of all strokes presenting to a clinical service, about 63 percent are infarcts; 7 percent due to occlusion of a large artery; 14 percent lacunes; 10 percent embolic from the heart; 7 percent from other occlusive-embolic arterial disease; and 25 percent of unclear origin.

Cerebral blood flow (CBF) is regulated more by metabolic than by neural factors. The major metabolic factor regulating CBF is the blood carbon dioxide (CO_2) level. Increased cerebral metabolism generates more CO_2, and the subsequent increase in hydrogen ions evokes vasodilation and associated increase in CBF; decreased metabolism is associated with an opposite series of events. A less important factor is oxygen concentration; its effect on the arteries is the converse of the effect of CO_2. Autoregulation refers to the maintenance of stable CBF in the presence of blood pressure alterations. Cerebral vasodilation follows a drop in blood pressure, and vasoconstriction is associated with blood pressure rise. Regional CBF is altered in association with acute cerebrovascular disease and with other cerebral lesions. Autoregulation is lost in the areas of diseased brain and sometimes in other areas as well. Hypotension under these circumstances is not compensated by vasodilation; instead, decrease in CBF occurs. CO_2 accumulates in areas of acute infarction, and there is resultant local vasodilation, with loss of normal reactivity to further metabolic change.

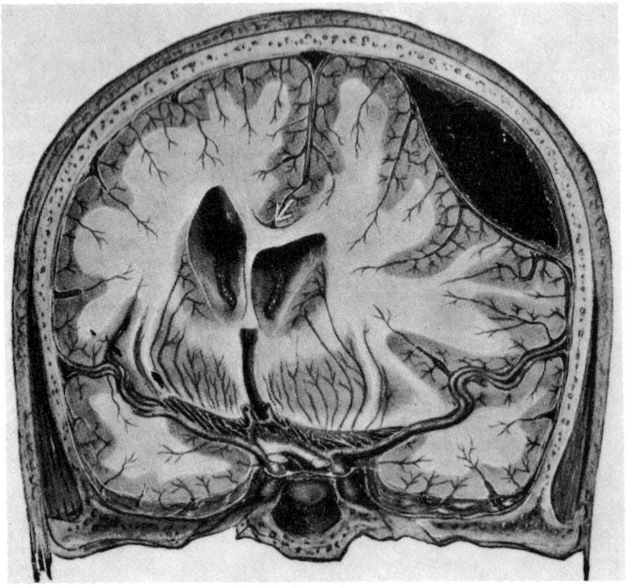

FIGURE 2.2-1. *Chronic subdural hematoma. The mass displaces the brain toward the opposite side. Note the arrangement of the peripheral arteries, piercing the brain from the convexity, and of the deep arteries, which arise from the proximal portion of the middle cerebral artery and supply the basal ganglia. (From Blackwood W, Dodds T C, Sommerville J C:* Atlas of Neuropathology, *ed 2, p 167. Williams & Wilkins, Baltimore, 1964, with permission.)*

Pathologically, the appearance of the infarcted area of the brain depends on the degree of damage, the nature of the insult, and the time elapsed between the acute insult and observation. Neurons are most susceptible to hypoxia. Glial cells and, finally, connective vascular tissue will be affected with progressively greater degrees of ischemic-hypoxic insult. Some areas in the brain are more susceptible to hypoxia than others. With diffuse hypoxia, ischemic changes are most prominent in Sommer's sector of the hippocampus, in layers 3 and 5 of the cortex, and in the Purkinje cells of the cerebellum. Hypercarbic hypoxia is often followed by bilateral damage of the globus pallidus.

An understanding of the arrangement of the intracranial vessels is essential for the diagnosis of focal ischemic disease. Two vascular systems can be distinguished: the peripheral or circumferential and the perforating (Fig. 2.2-1). Peripheral arteries, such as the distal branches of anterior and middle cerebral arteries, supply the cortex and subcortical white matter. The perforating vessels arise from major trunks: the lenticulostriate arteries from the middle cerebral artery, the thalamo-perforating arteries from the posterior cerebral artery, and the paramedian brain stem arteries from the basilar artery. They supply the basal ganglia, thalamus, periventricular white matter, and brain stem. The peripheral vessels run most of their course in the subarachnoid space, branching out into progressively thinner arteries. In contrast, the perforating vessels arise at right angles from a major trunk, where the perfusion pressure is high. Because of this disposition, peripheral vessels are more likely to be occluded by emboli, whereas perforating arteries suffer the ravages of arterial-wall arteriosclerosis, which is accelerated by chronic hypertension.

Cortico-subcortical infarcts generally have a triangular shape, with the base toward the cortex (Fig. 2.2-2). With severe ischemia, such as in the case of embolic infarction, damage of the capillary wall results in diapedesis of red and white blood cells into the surrounding tissue (Fig. 2.2-3). This phenomenon is most prominent in the gray matter and peaks toward the end of the first week (Fig. 2.2-4). The infarcted area becomes swollen within the first few hours. Cytotoxic edema, resulting from cellular damage, is maximum in about 2 to 3 days and may persist for longer than 3 weeks in the case of large lesions. If only the neurons have been affected, proliferation of astrocytes occurs in the area of damage; however, edema is likely to be more severe when all of the cellular elements are affected. The infarcted area then becomes more and more friable because of the action of proteolytic enzymes; new capillaries proliferate into it, scavenger cells clear away the necrosed tissue, and a fluid-filled cavity results. This process takes a few weeks for small, lacunar infarcts, but it may take many months for large infarcts.

The microscopic appearance of the infarct varies through the stages of organization. In the first few hours, the necrotic neurons have a shrunken body (which stains a vivid pink with eosin), microvacuoles, and a dark-staining nucleus. Within the first few days, the cytoplasm becomes uniformly eosinophilic and the nucleus appears triangular and shrunken. Depending on the local metabolic conditions and on the degree of tissue damage, neuronal vestiges may disappear or they may remain as incrustated darkly staining neurons. Glial nodules are the clusters of microglial cells, which perform the process of neuronophagia, or phagocytosis of neuronal debris. Among the glial cells, oligodendrocytes are more susceptible to hypoxia than are the astrocytes. With moderate anoxic insults, the astrocytes proliferate and become enlarged, with pink-staining cytoplasms and large, vesicular nuclei (plump or gemistocytic astrocytes). When the hypoxic insult is pronounced, all of the tissue elements die, including the capillaries. Lesser degrees of anoxia respect the capillary endothelial cells while destroying all of the other cellular elements. The endothelial cells themselves acquire vesicular nuclei, indicative of increased metabolic activity and protein synthesis; the tight junctions become loose and fluid, and cellular elements seep into the perivascular spaces (Figs. 2.2-2 and 2.2-3). Some of the cellular elements are red blood cells, which create a hemorrhagic appearance of recent infarcts. Others are macrophages, scavenger cells that soon become round, swollen with lipoprotein debris (lipid-laden or foamy macrophages). The endothe-

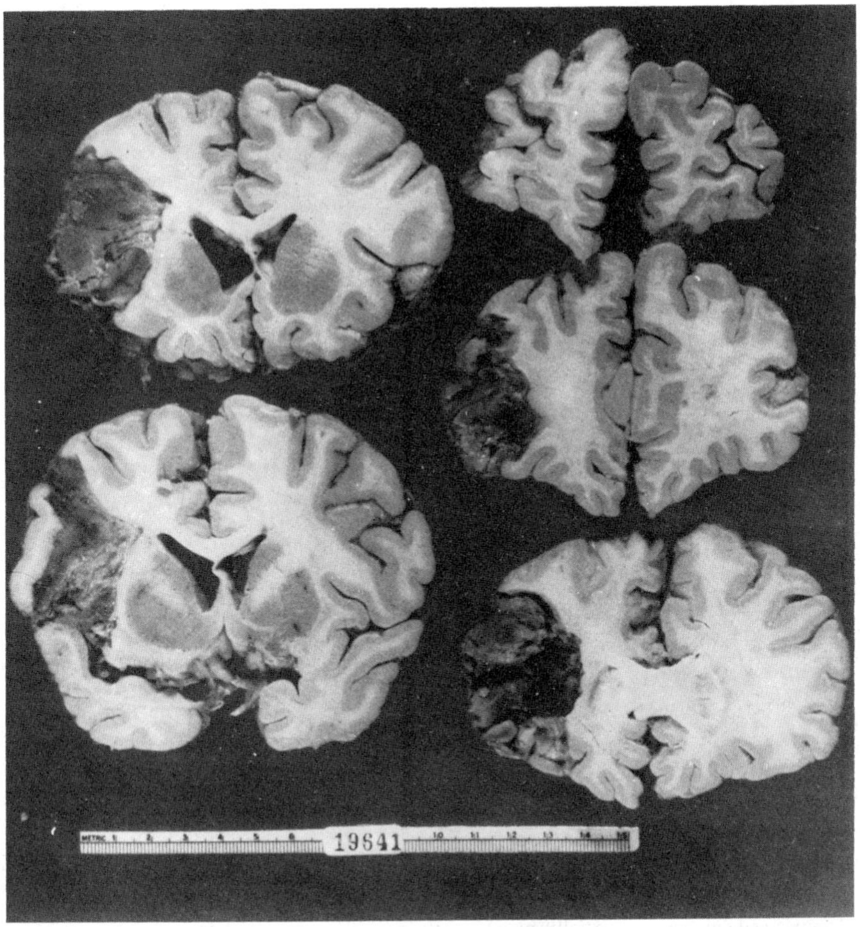

FIGURE 2.2-2. *Hemorrhagic infarct in the territory of the middle cerebral artery. (From Hirano A:* A Guide to Neuropathology, *p 52. Igaku-Shoin, New York, 1981, with permission.)*

lial cells proliferate, giving rise to new capillaries, which facilitate the penetration of scavenger cells into the necrotic tissue. After a week, most of the area metabolically active is constituted by neoformed capillaries and lipid-laden macrophages. Ultimately, this granulation tissue recedes, leaving a fluid-filled cavity.

The pathological characteristics, causes, and location of infarcts can be suspected clinically and confirmed by CT or MR. Infarcts may pass unnoticed on CT for a few days; contrast enhancement increases the yield, particularly after the first 5 days. Multiple infarcts with a cortical base, particularly in the territory of a branch of the middle cerebral or anterior cerebral arteries, strongly suggest embolic disease or arteritis.

Syndromes of major arteries The classical syndrome of internal carotid artery stenosis or occlusion is blindness of the ipsilateral eye, supplied by the ophthalmic branch of the internal carotid artery, contralateral hemiparesis, hemisensory impairment, homonymous hemianopsia, and—if the dominant hemisphere is affected—aphasia. Usually, only fragments of the complete syndrome are seen. Occlusion of the main trunk of the middle cerebral artery causes contralateral signs, as listed above. Occlusion of the anterior cerebral artery is associated with contralateral paresis of the lower extremity, and occlusion of the posterior cerebral artery results in contralateral homonymous hemianopsia. Sudden occlusion of the basilar artery is incompatible with life. More often, stenosis within the vertebral or basilar arteries causes ischemia or infarction of the brain stem, with a variety of ipsilateral cranial nerve signs and ipsilateral cerebellar signs, coupled with contralateral pyramidal tract signs or sensory signs or both. Of the many brain stem vascular syndromes, infarction within the distribution of the posterior inferior cerebellar artery is the most common; it is usually due to thrombosis of the adjoining vertebral artery. The resultant lateral medullary syndrome is characterized by ipsilateral ataxia and facial analgesia; contralateral analgesia of the trunk and extremities; nystagmus, ipsilateral Horner's syndrome, and paresis of the soft palate are often present. A fresh cerebellar infarct, manifested by ataxia with or without nystagmus, may act as a mass lesion; surgery is then necessary to prevent brain stem compression. CT is the chief diagnostic tool in verifying the clinical diagnosis of infarction.

Syndromes of small arteries Long slender infarcts, or lacunes, affecting the capsular and basal ganglia regions, are most often the result of lipohyalinosis of the wall of the perforating arteries. This process accompanies chronic hypertension. Pure motor weakness, dysarthria, or ataxia, with preservation of language and of visuospatial abilities, are characteristic of *lacunar disease*. Over time, lacunes tend to affect both cerebral hemispheres, resulting in gait apraxia, incontinence, or a pseudobulbar palsy. In *Binswanger's disease,* also known as subcortical arteriosclerotic encephalopathy, arteriosclerosis causes bilateral periventricular demyelination with multiple small infarcts. This disorder is attended by dementia and impairment of gait.

Incomplete infarcts in the distal distribution of the middle cerebral artery and in the periventricular white matter (watershed areas) are probably related to atheromatous disease of arteries in the neck or near the circle of Willis. Clinically, watershed infarcts may present with cortical findings (e.g., aphasias, agnosias) or give rise to weakness mimicking lacunar disease. CT is helpful in differentiating these lesions.

Management of ischemic disease Clinical differentiation of stroke is important because it will dictate the diagnostic workup and treatment. Unless precluded by a history of hypertension, dementia, or hemorrhagic disease, anticoagulation is indicated in a patient with embolic disease from a cardiac source (e.g., arrhythmia, valvular or other endocardial disease, cardiomyopathy with an akinetic segment). CT should be performed prior to anticoagulation to demonstrate the absence of intracranial hemorrhage. Lumbar puncture (LP) need not be done unless the clinical findings suggest meningitis or a subarachnoid hemorrhage as the cause of the stroke. Patients with a pure motor syndrome or other features of a lacunar stroke should not be anticoagulated. Treatment of hypertension is the best avenue for preventing lacunar strokes. Carotid endarterectomy may be considered

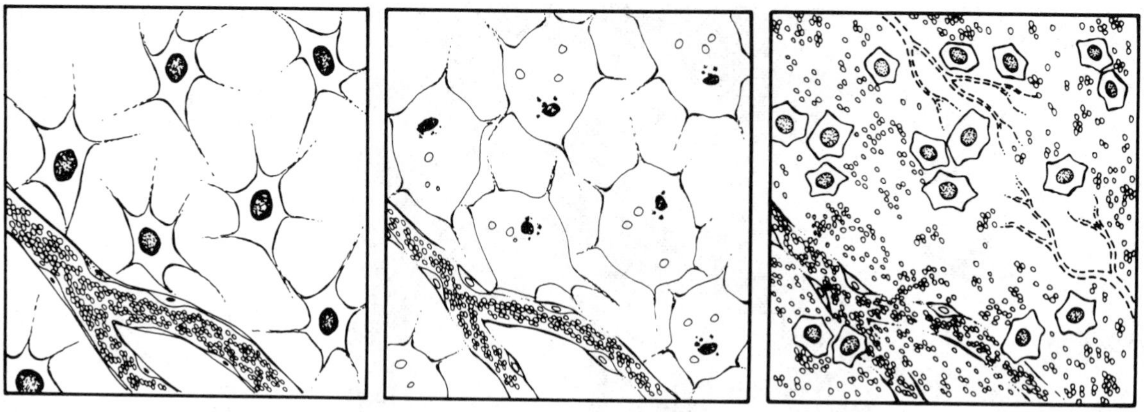

FIGURE 2.2-3. *Diagrammatic representation of the evolution of early changes after infarction.* Left: *Normal tissue.* Center: *Within the first 3 to 24 hours after infarction, intracellular edema and initial endothelial cell changes occur.* Right: *Around the second week after infarction there is marked extravasation of red blood cells and neovascularization. (From Gonzalez C F, Grosman C B, Masdeu J C:* Head and Spine Imaging, *p 300. Wiley, New York, 1985, with permission.)*

when carotid artery disease is suspected by the occurrence of TIAs or as the cause of a slight stroke. Digital subtraction angiography or conventional angiography will depict the surgical lesion. The usefulness of carotid endarterectomy for the prevention of stroke is unclear. A prospective clinical trial is under way to evaluate this widespread procedure. Most neurologists treat the first TIA with aspirin for its antiplatelet action. If TIAs persist, anticoagulant therapy may be substituted.

Unless anticoagulation is used, the acute treatment of stroke is mainly supportive. Aspiration is a major risk in patients with large infarcts, which decrease the level of alertness and impair the swallowing mechanism. Parenteral fluids should be used until the patient is clearly free from the risk of aspiration. Positional therapy (i.e., frequently turning the patient from side to side) is indicated to minimize the risk of pneumonia, with attendant hypoxia and enlargement of the area of infarction. Although patients should be mobilized, having a hemiplegic patient sit up unattended for long periods of time should be avoided because orthostatic hypotension may aggravate the infarct. For a similar reason, vigorous treatment of increased blood pressure is unwise. Mild hypertension, frequent after a stroke, is probably a protective mechanism to increase perfusion in areas marginally oxygenated. Hypervolemic hemodilution has been recently recommended to decrease blood viscosity and improve the microcirculation, but controlled trials have been inconclusive.

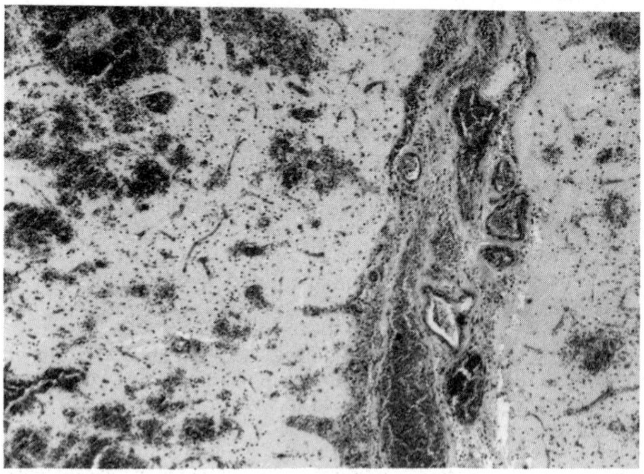

FIGURE 2.2-4. *Microscopic appearance of a 2-week-old infarct showing dilated, engorged vessels with pericapillary microhemorrhages. (From Gonzalez C F, Grosman C B, Masdeu J C:* Head and Spine Imaging, *p 299. Wiley, New York, 1985, with permission.)*

A referral for rehabilitation should be made at inception for any case in which a neurological deficit is expected to remain after the acute phase of the stroke. The psychological aspects of the care of the stroke patient cannot be overemphasized. Relatives may consider the behavior of stroke patients as "crazy" unless they are taught that it is consistent with the patients' misperception of reality or with their functional limitations. The problem is compounded because frequently the patients themselves are unaware of their deficits. For instance, a patient with bilateral occipital lesions may be blind and yet claim perfect vision (Anton's syndrome). Lack of understanding for this or other type of aberrant behavior confounds the relationship of the patient with others. Tact and knowledge about the nature of the neurological impairment is paramount for the design of an effective rehabilitation plan. Tricyclic drugs may alleviate the depression, especially noted in left-hemisphere-damaged patients.

HYPERTENSIVE ENCEPHALOPATHY This uncommon condition is caused by a sudden, severe rise in blood pressure, with associated cerebral vasoconstriction. Headache, seizures, and obtundation are common, but any variety of generalized, more than focal, signs may occur. Hypertensive retinopathy is invariably present. Petechial hemorrhages and edema affect the brain as well. Treatment with rapidly acting antihypertensive agents is mandatory.

INTRACRANIAL ARTERITIS Systemic noninfectious arteritis may affect the brain, causing multiple small-vessel occlusions and virtually any neurological sign or symptom. Aphasic and other behavioral syndromes, as well as seizures, are common. These diseases respond to corticosteroid therapy.

Temporal arteritis This disease, also known as giant-cell arteritis, occurs in elderly people and is manifested by headache in the area of a swollen, hard, and tender cranial artery of the scalp. It often involves other cranial arteries. Inflammation of the ophthalmic artery results in blindness in about 25 percent of untreated patients; involvement of other intracranial arteries causes stroke. Pain in the jaw muscles when chewing is almost pathognomonic of giant cell arteritis. *Polymyalgia rheumatica* is closely related to temporal arteritis and is manifested by muscle and joint aches and malaise. However, a paucity of objective signs often falsely raises the question of psychogenicity. An elevated sedimentation rate supports these diagnoses; temporal artery biopsy is required for proof.

Systemic lupus erythematosus In this condition, central nervous system (CNS) involvement may occur early, and 75 percent of patients develop neurological or psychological problems in the course of their illness. Seizures and psychosis are common.

Polyarteritis nodosa This disease typically manifests itself as an abrupt peripheral neuropathy in 30 to 50 percent of patients. Multifocal cerebral infarction is less common.

Takayasu's disease Arteritis of the aorta and its major branches (pulseless disease or Takayasu's disease) causes neurologial symptoms due to ischemia of the brain stem or cerebrum.

Granulomatous angiitis This disease of the brain is characterized by granulomatous inflammation with giant cells and fibrinoid necrosis of small leptomeningeal vessels, resulting in multifocal infarction. The diagnosis is made by meningeal biopsy, because the process may be restricted to brain vessels. A viral etiology (varicella-zoster) has been suspected, but there has been no proof. Prognosis is poor, and death often ensues in months; however, some patients have recovered after treatment with steroids or immunosuppressant drugs.

HEMATOLOGICAL DISORDERS Disease of the hematopoietic system may affect the brain in several ways. Sickle-cell anemia, thrombotic thrombocytopenic purpura, and disseminated intravascular coagulation may cause thrombosis or hemorrhage. Contraceptive medications may alter coagulation mechanisms and lead to infarction. Hemophilia is associated with hemorrhage, whereas polycythemia vera leads to infarction. Cerebellar hemangioblastoma is sometimes associated with polycythemia vera. Macroglobulinemia, multiple myeloma, and other dysglobulinemias cause neurological disease, not only by thrombosis or hemorrhage, but also by lymphocyte and plasma cell infiltration. Leukemia and the lymphomas similarly cause hemorrhage, thrombosis, or tumor cell infiltration.

VENOUS DISEASE Aseptic thrombosis of dural sinuses is sometimes seen in children who suffer from malnutrition or who have serious systemic illnesses. Thrombosis of a dural sinus is more often secondary to pyogenic infections. These lesions are manifested by increased intracranial pressure and congestion in the head or face area normally drained by the affected sinus and its contributory veins. Thrombosis of cortical veins may be a postpartum complication. Convulsive seizures and focal signs are due to passively congested cerebral tissue.

INTRACRANIAL HEMORRHAGE Nontraumatic brain hemorrhage constitutes about one-third of all strokes. In an older population, about three-fourths of the hemorrhages primarily occur in the brain parenchyma and secondarily may extend into the subarachnoid space. By contrast, in a younger population the majority of spontaneous intracranial hemorrhages are caused by aneurysms or arteriovenous malformations and have an important or even exclusive subarachnoid component.

PARENCHYMAL HEMORRHAGE The most common cause of spontaneous intracerebral hemorrhage is chronic hypertension. When exposed to chronic high blood pressure, the walls of the perforating arteries sustain hyalin degeneration of the media, lipohyalinosis, and in severe cases, fibrinoid necrosis. As discussed above, occlusion of the vessel and lacunar infarction may occur. In addition, microaneurysmal formation may lead to rupture of the vessel, with a resultant focal bleeding. Blood then dissects the brain tissues, following white matter and vascular tracts. Shearing of other small arteries results in further sources of bleeding. Hypertensive hemorrhages are located deep in the brain, involving, in order of frequency, the external capsule, putamen, thalamus, cerebellum, and pons (Fig. 2.2-5). A recently characterized cause of intracerebral hemorrhage in the elderly is amyloid angiopathy. Hemorrhages in this disorder tend to be multiple and involve the subcortical white matter (Fig. 2.2-6).

Intracerebral hemorrhages in nonhypertensives may arise from a small cryptic angioma or from a metastatic tumor—particularly lung carcinoma and malignant melanoma. Hemorrhage may also be the result of a bleeding diasthesis or of a toxic vasculitis, particularly in conjunction with amphetamine use. Unlike hypertensive hemorrhages, these lesions are lobar hemorrhages and tend to affect the cortical or subcortical regions. CT is the procedure of choice for the detec-

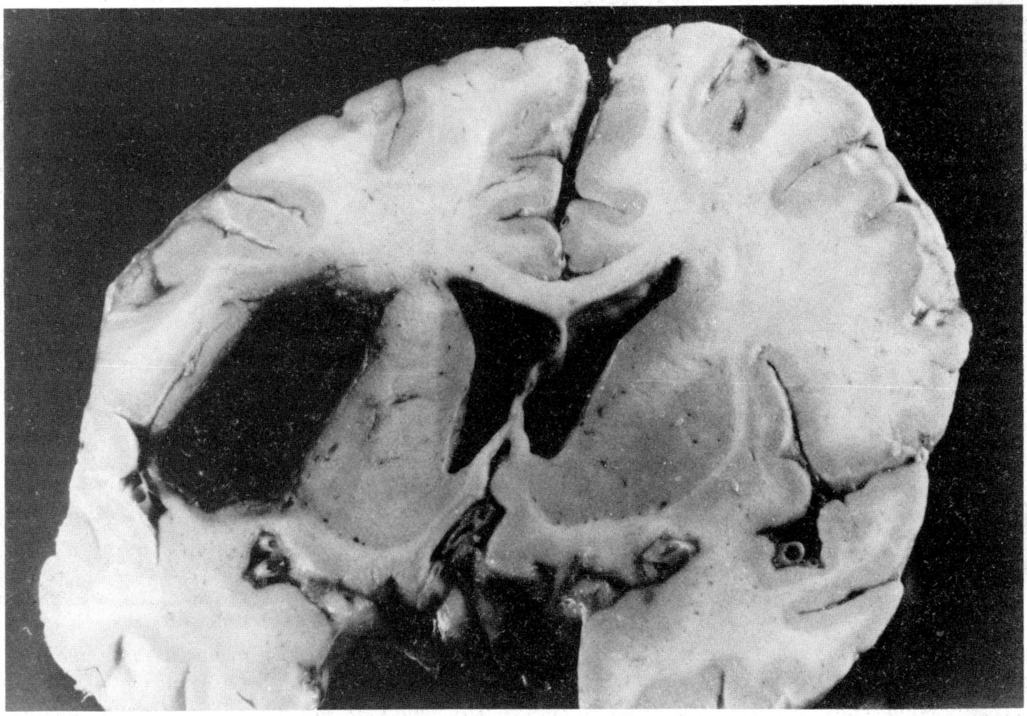

FIGURE 2.2-5. *Intracerebral hematoma. (From Hirano A:* A Guide to Neuropathology, *p 83. Igaku-Shoin, New York, 1981, with permission.)*

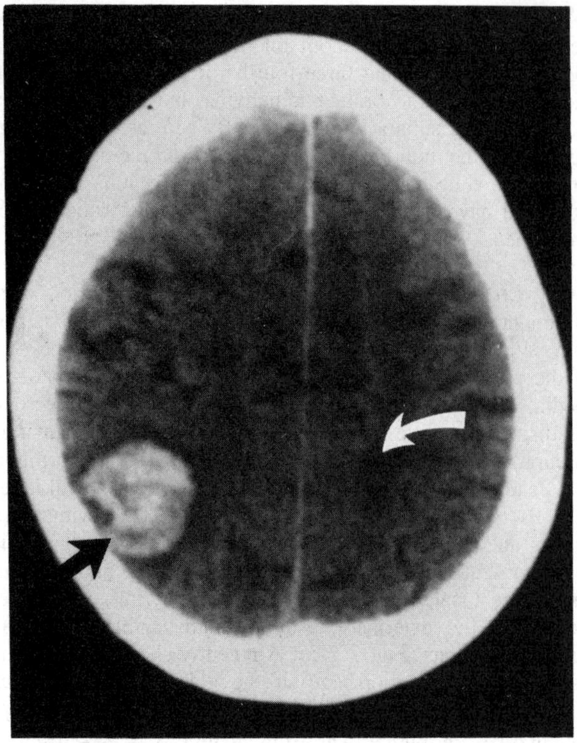

FIGURE 2.2-6. *Amyloid angiopathy. This 79-year-old woman, a hypertensive, had the sudden onset of inability to walk. Note the hemorrhage* (black arrow) *and the abnormally hypodense white matter* (white arrow). *(Courtesy of Charles Elkin, MD, Montefiore Medical Center, New York.)*

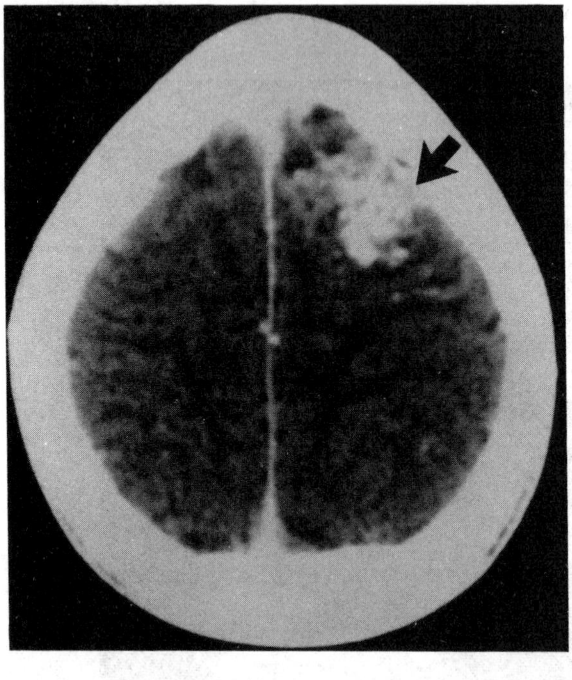

FIGURE 2.2-7. *Arteriovenous malformation* (arrow) *in a 16-year-old high school student brought to the emergency room after two episodes of twitching of the left arm followed by a generalized seizure. (Courtesy of Charles Elkin, MD, Montefiore Medical Center, New York.)*

tion of intracerebral hemorrhages. In addition, contrast enhancement may provide further diagnostic clues of an arteriovenous malformation (Fig. 2.2-7).

Small capsular or putaminal intracerebral hemorrhages tend to cause weakness without cortical signs of aphasia or agnosia. Large hemorrhages in the putamen cause hemiplegia and may impair the mental status as edema increases in the second or third day. Steroids are given to counter edema. Small thalamic hemorrhages cause transcortical sensory aphasia or neglect syndromes, in addition to a hemisensory loss. Large thalamic hemorrhages cause coma and often extend into the ventricular system (Fig. 2.2-8); their prognosis is poor. Cerebellar hemorrhages give rise to nystagmus, or other oculomotor signs, ataxia, and headache. Unless the hemorrhage is small, evacuation of the hematoma is mandatory to prevent compression of the brain stem. Temporal lobe hematomas should also be evacuated if their size is such that midbrain compression may result from hippocampal herniation. Surgical removal of other types of intracerebral hemorrhages is usually not indicated.

SUBARACHNOID HEMORRHAGE After trauma, ruptured aneurysms are the most common cause of subarachnoid hemorrhage; arteriovenous malformations are less likely. Most aneurysms develop from congenital defects in the media of the arterial wall, especially at the bifurcation of vessels in or near the circle of Willis (Fig. 2.2-9). Mycotic aneurysms are secondary to infection, usually from subacute bacterial endocarditis. Atherosclerosis or trauma may weaken an arterial wall and may lead to aneurysmal formation. The mortality rate of subarachnoid hemorrhage due to rupture of an aneurysm is close to 50 percent for each bleeding episode. The hemorrhage is manifested by the sudden onset of severe headache and, usually, loss or alteration of consciousness. Nuchal rigidity is found on examination. If blood from the ruptured aneurysm breaks into the parenchyma, focal neurological signs occur. Aneurysms may also cause signs by their

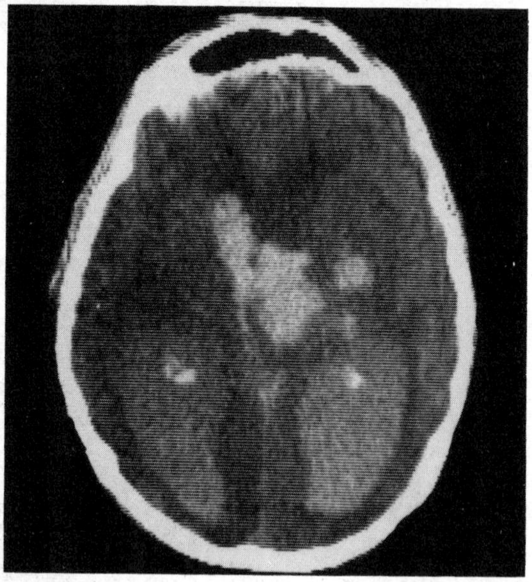

FIGURE 2.2-8. *CT showing a large thalamic hemorrhage that has ruptured into the ventricles. (From Gonzalez C F, Grosman C B, Masdeu J C:* Head and Spine Imaging, *p 334. Wiley, New York, 1985, with permission.)*

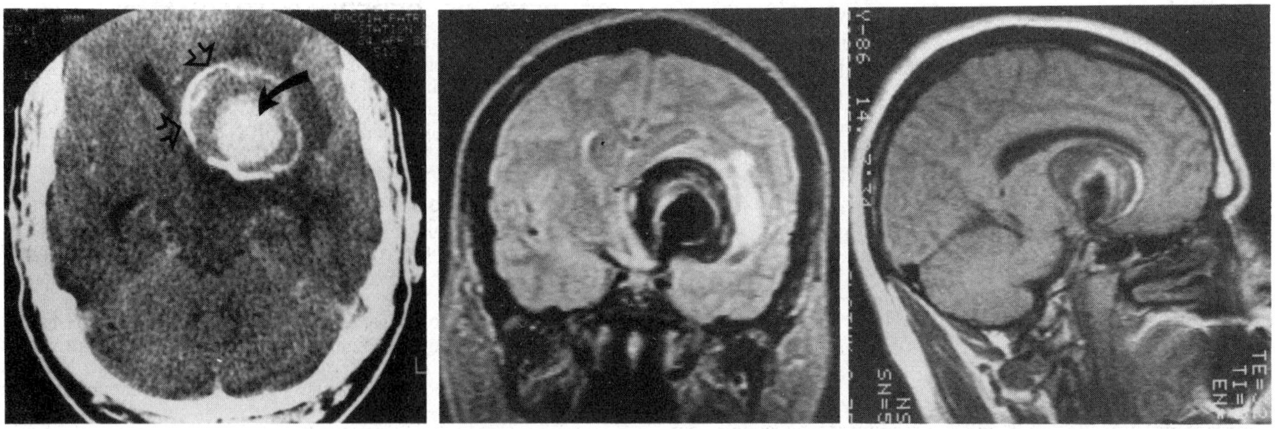

FIGURE 2.2-9. *Giant aneurysm in a 39-year-old man with headaches. Partially calcified wall appears white on CT* (left, open arrows). *Only the core contains circulating blood, which appears white on axial CT* (left, curved arrow) *and black on coronal* (center) *and sagittal* (right) *MR. (Courtesy of Charles Elkin, MD, Montefiore Medical Center, New York.)*

pressure on adjacent structures, such as the oculomotor nerve. CT often confirms the diagnosis without lumbar puncture (Fig. 2.2-10), but if the CT is negative, lumbar puncture will still reveal blood with xanthochromia of the supernatant cerebrospinal fluid (CSF). Angiography is necessary to define the vascular anatomy.

The treatment of choice for a cerebral aneurysm, if surgically accessible, is ligation of the neck of the aneurysm. Bed rest and control of blood pressure are the major features of initial conservative therapy. The ideal time for surgery after the onset of subarachnoid hemorrhage has not been established, but the present trend is to operate early if the patient is neurologically intact.

OTHER VASCULAR LESIONS

Arteriovenous malformation This congenital defect consists of a tangle of abnormal arteries and veins within the cerebrum (Fig. 2.2-7). Seizures may occur, and a bruit is frequently heard. If hemorrhage occurs, it is less acute than a hemorrhage following a ruptured aneurysm.

Sturge-Weber syndrome This syndrome is manifested by a facial wine-colored nevus, contralateral neurological signs, epilepsy, and glaucoma. Roentgenograms of the skull reveal curvilinear calcifications that have developed in an atrophic cortex underlying a meningeal angiomatous malformation (Fig. 2.2-11). Angioma of the choroid of the eye is often present.

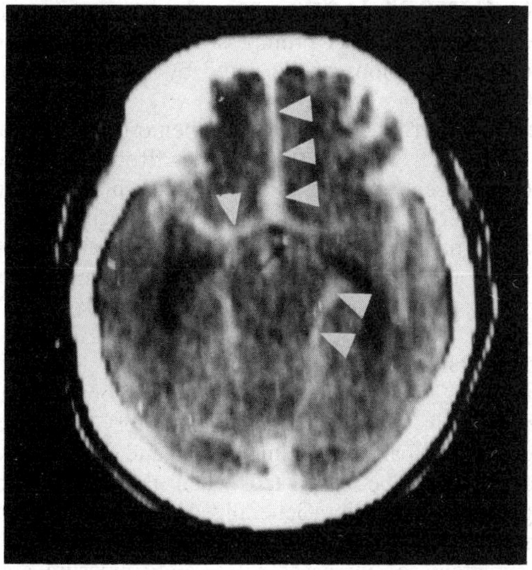

FIGURE 2.2-10. *Subarachnoid hemorrhage. On CT, the brain sulci and fissures, full of blood, are white* (arrowheads) *because blood has a high CT density as compared to brain.*

Carotid cavernous sinus fistula This lesion is due to rupture of the carotid artery within the cavernous sinus. It is manifested by pulsating exophthalmus, an ocular bruit, and ophthalmoplegia.

BRAIN TRAUMA

Acute head trauma may be minimal, causing a transient headache, or severe, rendering the patient comatose. Even if there are no residual focal signs, sequelae from trauma range

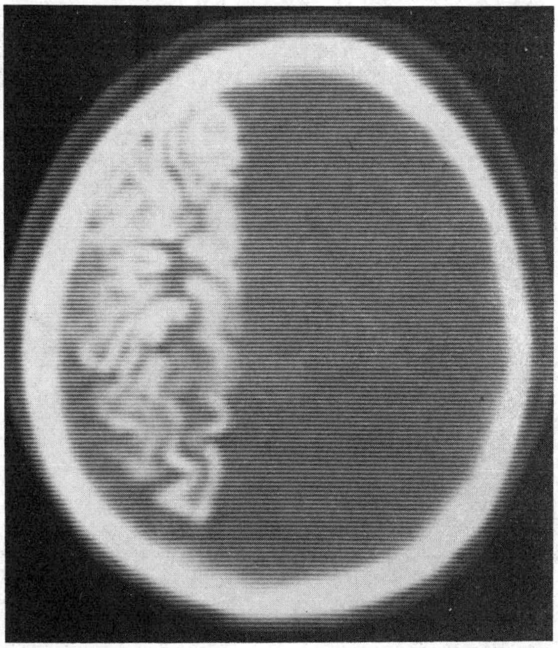

FIGURE 2.2-11. *Sturge-Weber malformation. CT without contrast media, showing the calcified cortex and arteriovenous malformation. The brain itself is not seen because the scan is displayed at bone-window level. (Courtesy of Charles Elkin, MD, Montefiore Medical Center, New York.)*

from the postconcussion syndrome to behavioral disturbances related to damage of the orbitofrontal and inferior temporal regions (Fig. 2.2-12). These areas are frequently traumatized because they overlie the rough bone of the floor of the anterior and middle fossas. Damage may also occur as the cerebral hemispheres rotate or are sheared at the midbrain junction. Delayed seizure disorders result in about half of the patients who have had severe head injuries. Head trauma in the past is a frequent cause of seizures in patients with chronic alcoholism.

In addition to life-threatening damage of the brain stem, other processes may contribute to poor responsiveness in a trauma patient. Such treatable causes as epidural and subdural hematomas should be immediately disclosed and treated. Steroids are particularly helpful in younger patients prone to brain edema. Ventilation should be maintained because hypercarbia causing vasodilation contributes to brain swelling.

Fractures of the base of the skull are notoriously difficult to detect in roentgenograms, but are often clinically evident by ecchymoses over the postauricular area (Battle's sign) or around the orbits (raccoon-eyes sign) or by blood behind the ear drum or in the outer ear canal. Fractures through the cribiform plate or the middle ear may cause rhinorrhea or otorrhea, respectively. Leakage of CSF through the skull is associated with risk of intracranial infection. Rhinorrhea of CSF can be distinguished from the secretion of nasal mucosa by the presence of glucose in the CSF.

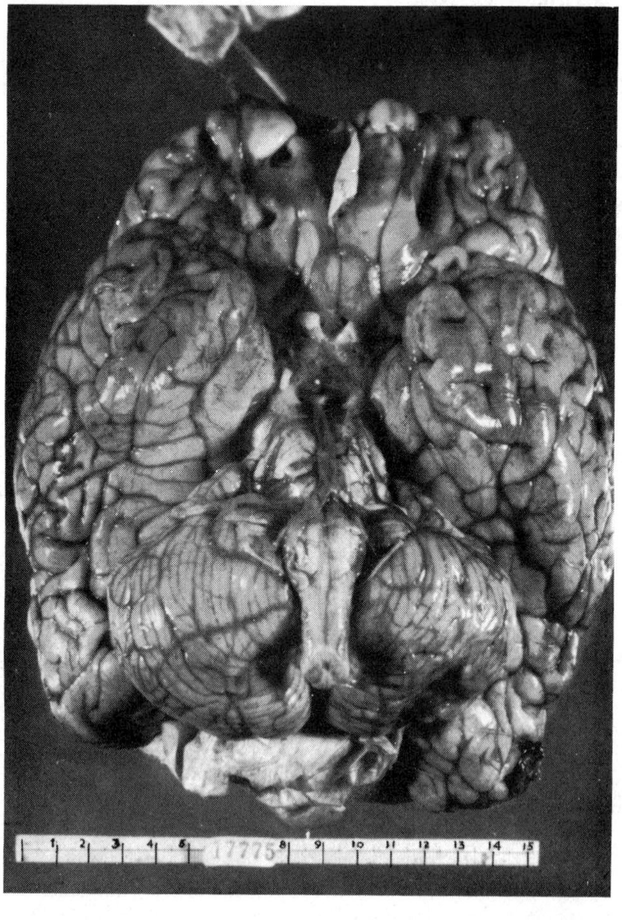

FIGURE 2.2-12. *Severe contusion of the frontal poles has resulted in their atrophy and distortion. (Courtesy of H M Zimmerman, MD.)*

DEGREES OF CEREBRAL TRAUMA **Cerebral concussion** This clinical term denotes unconsciousness with rapid recovery and lack of residual cerebral signs. Repeated cerebral concussion, however, may lead to irreversible brain damage, as seen in the punch-drunk boxer. Experimental studies and those few cases that have come to autopsy have revealed petechial hemorrhages and associated edema.

Cerebral contusion In a patient with cerebral contusion, residual signs of cerebral injury are noted after recovery of consciousness, but these signs usually show extensive improvement or complete clearing.

Cerebral laceration The patient with cerebral laceration has severe and often permanent signs of cerebral damage after prolonged unconsciousness. The lesion is often associated with a depressed skull fracture, and bony fragments may cause gross tears of the brain tissue.

Intracerebral hemorrhage, usually superficial, is frequently associated with severe head injury. The symptoms may simulate symptoms of a subdural hematoma, and surgical therapy may be warranted.

POSTCONCUSSION SYNDROME As the name implies, this condition may follow relatively minor, as well as major, head injuries. The syndrome is characterized by one or a variety of neurological symptoms, most often headache and dizziness. Other symptoms that are impossible to document are fatigue, impairment of concentration, and loss of work efficiency. Personality changes include irritability, emotional lability, and depression, often with associated insomnia and decreased libido. Anxiety and frustration are common. These patients complain of impairment of memory and attention; they have difficulty comprehending and formulating complex or abstract concepts. The postconcussion syndrome is difficult to evaluate because of the absence of accompanying objective neurological signs and normal laboratory studies. Most of the time, the symptoms have an occult neurophysiological mechanism rather than being solely an emotional phenomenon. Subtle abnormalities are often noted in studies of evoked potentials and in comprehensive neuropsychological tests. Evidence of axonal injury has been demonstrated with the electron microscope in experimental animals subjected to cerebral concussion.

DURAL HEMORRHAGES The clinical suspicion of a dural hemorrhage warrants prompt study by CT, MR, or angiography. The lesion can be cured by surgical evacuation.

Epidural hemorrhage An epidural hemorrhage is acute because of arterial bleeding, most often from rupture of the middle meningeal artery in its course through a fractured temporal bone. After an initial loss of consciousness caused by trauma, the patient awakens for a short time, and then lapses into stupor and coma as the growing hematoma compresses the brain.

Subdural hematoma A subdural hematoma is subacute or chronic (Fig. 2.2-1) and is due to bleeding from traumatically sheared veins in the subdural space. A history of trauma need not be present; particularly in infants and the elderly, this diagnosis should be suspected when there is progressive lethargy or hemiparesis. Generalized cerebral symptoms of depressed consciousness, impaired mentation, headache, and other symptoms of increased intracranial pressure are common. The most accurate lateralizing sign is ipsilateral pupillary dilation when the oculomotor nerve is compressed in the course of herniation of the medial temporal lobe through the tentorium of the cerebellum. Focal signs need not be present or may be falsely localizing. For example, a shift of the contralateral cerebral peduncle against the tentorium of the cerebellum may cause hemiparesis ipsilateral to the intracranial mass. Subdural hematomas are located predominantly over the frontal and parietal areas of the brain.

In the early stages, liquid blood or a black clot is present, but soon organization occurs. New capillaries and fibroblasts grow from the dura and enclose the hematoma with a false membrane. The new vessels within this membrane may exude serum or may rupture and cause additional bleeding, thus enlarging the total size of the mass. When fully encapsulated, the hematoma changes to brown and then to yellow fluid.

Subarachnoid hemorrhage and arteriovenous fistulas may result from trauma. Their manifestations are noted above.

OTHER FORMS OF TRAUMA When death occurs as a result of these injuries, the brain reveals petechial hemorrhages, edema, and zones of necrosis.

Electric shock Electric shock occurs by accidental contact with lines of moderate voltage and high amperage. Coma and almost any variety of central and peripheral nervous system signs may occur.

Electroconvulsive therapy (ECT) causes immediate and sometimes persistent symptoms. The seizure may cause alterations in blood pressure and heart rhythm; fractures are a thing of the past since the use of muscle-paralyzing agents. Although confusion and headache are common immediately after the patient awakens from ECT, these symptoms quickly clear. Memory impairment is the most common complaint following ECT. The memory difficulties often persist for weeks, but many patients complain that their memory is permanently defective. Amnesia averages 6 months retrograde and 2 months anterograde. Memory defects are least likely to occur if the ECT is administered unilaterally over the nondominant hemisphere, with pulsed rather than sine wave current and with the least number of treatments.

Radiation Progressive neurological symptoms and signs referable to an area of former radiotherapy are often correctly attributed to recurrent malignancy. Occasionally, however, the progressive deficit is the result of brain tissue necrosis caused by radiation. Radiation necrosis tends to involve the white matter, where the small arteries undergo fibrinoid necrosis. The symptoms usually begin from 6 to 18 months after radiotherapy.

INFLAMMATORY DISEASE OF THE BRAIN

Inflammatory disorders of the brain can be caused by microorganisms or by other immunological processes. In multiple sclerosis and other diseases, viral infections are thought to evoke an immunological response many years later.

INFECTIOUS DISORDERS Intracranial infection may spread from infected paranasal sinuses, ears, or mastoids through emissary veins or originate from organisms in the bloodstream. With the increasing use of immunosuppressive therapy, infection by opportunistic organisms has become more frequent. Cerebral infection is, nevertheless, relatively uncommon because of the blood-brain barrier. Focal breakdown in the blood-brain barrier may lead to the spread of infection from blood to brain, with abscess formation. Meningitis usually causes a generalized disturbance of the blood-brain barrier and allows infection to spread to superficial areas of the brain.

LOCALIZED INFECTIONS Brain abscess Sources of infection in the development of a brain abscess are the bloodstream, carrying organisms from a distant site, such as a chronic pulmonary infection or subacute bacterial endocarditis; infected paranasal sinuses, mastoids, or ears; and fractures of the skull. Patients with AIDS, patients receiving immunosuppressive drugs, and children with congenital cyanotic heart disease are particularly prone to develop brain abscesses. Toxoplasma gondii abscesses are common among AIDS patients. The symptoms and signs of a brain abscess are similar to those of a neoplasm of the brain. Headache is most common, but fever is often conspicuous by its absence. The brain abscess may expand as a tumor, may seal off and resolve, may rupture to the surface or into a ventricle, causing meningitis, or may lead to sinus thrombosis. The acute brain abscess appears as a pus-filled cavity surrounded by soft necrotic brain tissue and, beyond that, localized edema (Fig. 2.2-13). More chronic abscesses are walled off by thick, firm, fibrous tissue. CT or MR should be performed if a brain abscess is suspected. Lumbar puncture is nondiagnostic and may be dangerous. Abscesses require intensive antibiotic therapy and surgical evacuation if they are large and accessible.

Dural abscess Abscesses adjacent to the dura usually produce signs of a focal cerebral lesion and of increased intracranial pressure. The patient shows clinical evidence of an infection, and the CT shows the contrast-enhanced wall. A subdural empyema is most often secondary to middle-ear or paranasal sinus infection, but may follow a dural sinus thrombophlebitis. An extradural abscess is usually secondary to frontal sinusitis or mastoiditis. Because antibiotic therapy cannot adequately reach the lesion, immediate surgery is essential.

Sinus thrombosis This condition is most often caused by the extension of an infection, particularly from the ears or paranasal sinuses to the cranial venous sinuses. Cavernous sinus thrombosis usually arises from an infection of the face, nose, eye, or sphenoid or ethmoid paranasal sinuses. Transverse sinus thrombosis is secondary to middle-ear infection or mastoiditis. Superior longitudinal sinus thrombosis most often occurs from frontal sinusitis or is secondary to debilitating disease in the very young or the very old. Edema and congestion in the brain are accompanied by fever and by signs of increased intracranial pressure. Leg weakness and seizures are common. Antibiotics are the treatment of choice.

MENINGITIS Purulent or acute meningitis Purulent meningitis often begins as an upper respiratory infection, soon followed by the sudden onset of headache, usually with nausea and vomiting. Examination reveals an acutely distressed patient with high fever and nuchal rigidity; depression of consciousness soon occurs. The CSF is turbid; contains 1,000 to 15,000 white blood cells per mm^3, predominantly polymorphonuclear leukocytes; and has elevated protein and low glucose. The subarachnoid space becomes occupied first by a fibrinous exudate and later by a purulent exudate (Fig. 2.2–14). The exudate follows cerebral sulci or vessels, or both, along the base and over the convexity of the brain. There may be associated blockage of absorptive surfaces of the meninges or obstruction of the foramina of the fourth ventricle, with resultant hydrocephalus. If recovery is delayed, the purulent exudate may organize into a thick, gray membrane. On microscopic examination, one sees numerous polymorphonuclear leukocytes and large mononuclear cells within the exudate (Fig. 2.2–15). In the brain, perivascular infiltration of inflammatory cells is predominantly within the superficial perivascular (Virchow-Robin) spaces. The exudate following the blood vessels into the cortex may cause microabscesses.

Neisseria meningitides (meningococcus) and Diplococcus pneumoniae (pneumococcus) account for 85 percent of cases of meningitis in otherwise healthy adults. However, gram-negative bacilli, particularly *Escherichia coli* and *Listeria monocytogenes,* are the common offenders in the neonatal period, in the elderly, and in patients with serious medical disorders. *Hemophilus influenza* affects almost exclusively children and patients who have undergone recent surgery. Patients with head trauma or neurosurgical wounds are at risk for infection with nosocomial agents, such as Pseudomonas, Klebsiella, *E. coli,* Serratia, and Staphylococcus. Immunocompromised subjects are prone to meningitis by mycobacteria, *Cryptococcus neoformans, Toxoplasma gondii,* and cytomegalovirus.

When a bacterial meningitis is suspected, the diagnosis should be confirmed as soon as possible and treatment started, ideally within an hour of presentation. Failure to proceed swiftly results in bacterial proliferation and a marked increase in morbidity and mortality. The

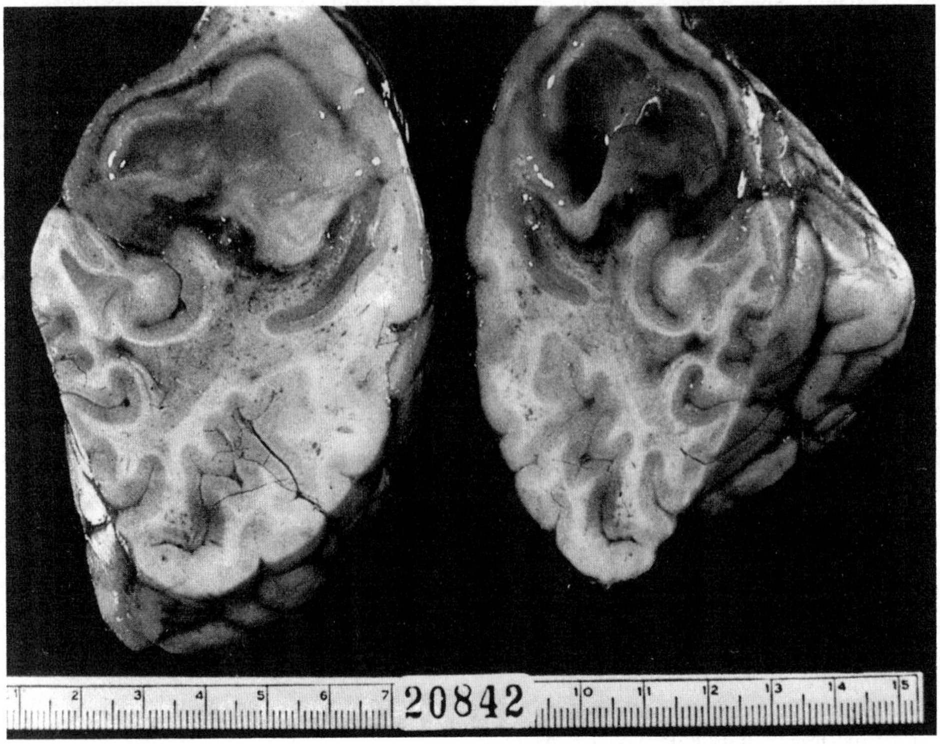

FIGURE 2.2-13. *Cerebral abscess. A demarcated cystic lesion is seen within the occipital lobe. The cavity contains purulent material. (From Hirano A, Iwata M, Llena J F, Matsui T:* Color Atlas of Pathology of the Nervous System, *p 39. Igaku-Shoin, New York, 1980, with permission.)*

CSF will show an increased white cell count and protein and a decreased glucose level. Identification of the organism is quickly accomplished by Gram-staining the centrifuged CSF and by identification of bacterial antigens with countercurrent immune electrophoresis (CIE). A stain for acid-fast mycobacteria should also be performed on the spun sediment of at least 10 ml of CSF if there is a history of tuberculosis or if the CSF cell count is mainly lymphocytic. Abnormal CSF samples should be sent for bacterial and fungal culture and for cryptococcal latex agglutination tests. Lumbar puncture should not be delayed while waiting for a CT unless the patient has focal findings or papilledema or there is a reasonable suspicion that a brain mass may be present, particularly a temporal lobe brain abscess. When any of these entities is suspected, empirical treatment with penicillin G, 3 to 4 million units intravenously (IV) every 4 hours should be started until the CT becomes available. Patients allergic to penicillin should be given IV chloramphenicol (Chloromycetin), 25 mg per kg every 6 hours. Ampicillin and chloramphenicol or cefotaxine (Claforan) is also the empirical therapy of choice in children younger than 5 years of age because of the risk of *H. influenza* meningitis. The elderly are treated with a combination of cefotaxime and ampicillin, both given IV at a rate of 2 g of each, every 4 hours.

Chronic meningitis The chronic meningitides are manifested by the gradual development of headache, stiff neck, malaise, and fever. Cranial nerve involvement is often present because of exudate at the base of the brain. Arteritis with thrombosis and infarction is another frequent complication, especially of tuberculous meningitis. The CSF usually contains 50 to 500 white blood cells per mm^3, predominantly mononuclear leukocytes; elevated protein; and low glucose.

Tuberculous meningitis The tubercle bacillus is the most common cause of chronic meningitis. At autopsy, a pale, glistening, web-like exudate is seen at the base of the brain. Sometimes, miliary tubercles (gray-white nodules) may be found in the cerebral sulci and fissures. Large granulomas, tuberculomas, may act as slowly growing brain tumors. Treatment of tuberculous meningitis consists of isoniazid (Nydrazid), rifampin (Rifadin), and ethambutol (Myambutol).

Cryptococcus meningitis *Cryptococcus neoformans* produces an exudate similar to that of tuberculosis at the base of the brain. Foreign-body giant cells contain the fungi and granulomatous nodules of cryptococci in the cerebrum may act as solid or cystic masses (Fig. 2.2-16). If the organism is not seen on India ink preparation, the diagnosis can be made by the more sensitive latex agglutination test for cryptococcus antigen in the CSF. Cryptococcus meningitis and other fungal meningitides, once invariably fatal, often respond to amphotericin B (Fungizone) and 5-fluorocytosine (Ancobon).

Other forms of chronic meningitis are caused by fungi or other nonbacterial organisms. Sarcoidosis and carcinoma may invade the meninges and present a picture similar to that of a chronic infectious meningitis.

Sarcoidosis This systemic disease is of uncertain origin. Sarcoidosis is characterized by granulomata composed of large epitheloid cells, unassociated with necrosis. Diverse neurological involvement may include paralysis of the facial nerve in association with uveitis and parotitis (uveoparotid fever); optic neuritis and peripheral neuritis; aseptic meningitis with low levels of CSF glucose; and granulomatous disease of the base of the brain, causing diabetes insipidus. Steroid therapy is beneficial.

Viral meningitides These diseases are usually benign. Lymphotic choriomeningitis and the meningitides of mumps, Coxsackie, and enteric cytopathogenic human orphan (ECHO) viruses are the most common.

ENCEPHALITIS Before the advent of AIDS, herpes simplex was the most common episodic encephalitis. Different arboviruses (e.g., eastern equine, St. Louis) accounted for most of the epidemic encephalitides. In institutions caring for AIDS patients, toxoplasmosis, the subacute encephalitis of AIDS, and cytomegalovirus encephalitis are now seen with increasing frequency.

The nonsuppurative encephalitides induce a slight to moderate meningeal congestion and the underlying edematous, hyperemic brain often has petechial hemorrhages. On microscopic examination, an inflammatory cellular infiltrate is seen within the tissue and perivascular spaces (Fig. 2.2-17). Inclusion bodies within neurons or glial cells suggest a viral origin. The diseased brain affected by slowly incubating viruses may show degenerative changes, rather than an inflammatory reaction.

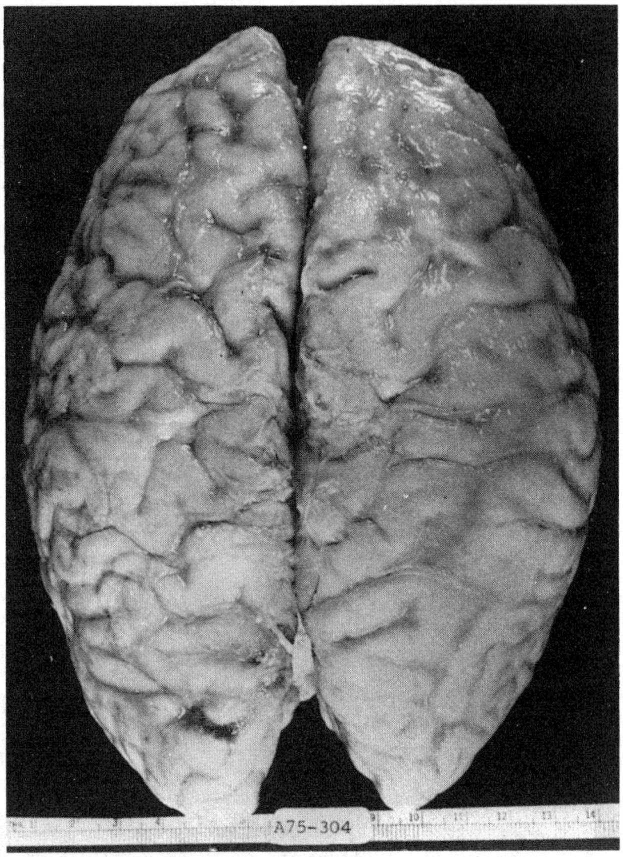

FIGURE 2.2-14. *Acute meningitis. The convexity of the brain is covered with a purulent exudate that fills the sulci. (From Hirano A, Iwata M, Llena J F, Matsui T:* Color Atlas of Pathology of the Nervous System, *p 10. Igaku-Shoin, New York, 1980, with permission.)*

Neurotropic viruses Neurotropic viruses cause encephalitis that may be manifested by no more than headache and fever. Seizures, somnolence, confusion, and sometimes, delirium, coma, and death can occur in the more severe cases. Papilledema, focal signs, and neck stiffness are common. Systemic involvement is manifested by malaise and upper respiratory tract or gastrointestinal symptoms. The CSF reveals 25 to 250 leukocytes per mm^3, mostly lymphocytes.

Infections caused by neurotropic viruses include those borne by arthropods: the equine encephalitides, St. Louis encephalitis, and Japanese B encephalitis. These diseases do not have distinguishing clinical or pathological characteristics. Some viruses are predisposed to affect one particular area of the CNS much more than other areas. Economo's encephalitis, in the 1920s, injured the basal ganglia, and postencephalitic parkinsonism resulted. Poliomyelitis attacks the anterior horn cells of the spinal cord. Herpes zoster affects the dorsal root ganglia or sensory cranial nerve ganglia.

Herpes simplex encephalitis After AIDS, this disease is the most common, severe sporadic encephalitis in the United States. It begins with fever and focal, especially temporal lobe, signs. Disorientation, paranoid ideation, and lethargy, with hemiparesis, develop and rapidly progress—seizures are common. The course often simulates that of a temporal lobe tumor. The electroencephalogram (EEG) reveals periodic sharp waves from a temporal area on a background of diffuse slow activity. The CSF has an increased white cell count and is often hemorrhagic. The diagnosis can be established by isolating the virulent type 1 virus from a brain biopsy. (The type 2 herpes simplex virus causes a more benign meningitis in adults and, in contrast to type 1, can be isolated from the CSF or from blood leukocytes.) Early treatment with acyclovir (Zovirax) is essential. At autopsy, hemorrhagic necrosis accompanies an inflammatory reaction that especially affects the cortex of the inferior frontal and temporal lobes (Fig. 2.2-18). Intranuclear inclusion bodies are seen under the microscope.

Rabies About 30 to 70 days after the bite of a rabid animal, rabies may occur. In addition to the usual features of encephalitis, rabies causes extreme agitation and severely painful spasms of the throat, with inability to swallow. Seizures, coma, and death are invariable in untreated cases. After rabies is found or strongly suspected in the attacking animal, treatment with an antirabies vaccine prevents the disease in most cases. In the brain infected by rabies, Negri bodies, which are oval acidophilic inclusion bodies, are seen in the cytoplasm of neurons (Fig. 2.2-19).

Slow viruses In recent years, some diseases formerly classified as degenerative have been found to be due to viruses having an extremely slow incubation period, often years. *Kuru*, which affects an isolated people in New Guinea, was the first disease in humans shown to be due to a slow virus.

CREUTZFELDT-JAKOB DISEASE This disease, also called *subacute spongiform encephalopathy*, has been transmitted from humans to chimpanzees after prolonged incubation and has been accidentally transmitted from human to human—most recently from infected batches of pituitary glands used to manufacture growth hormones. The illness begins in the fourth or fifth decade and is

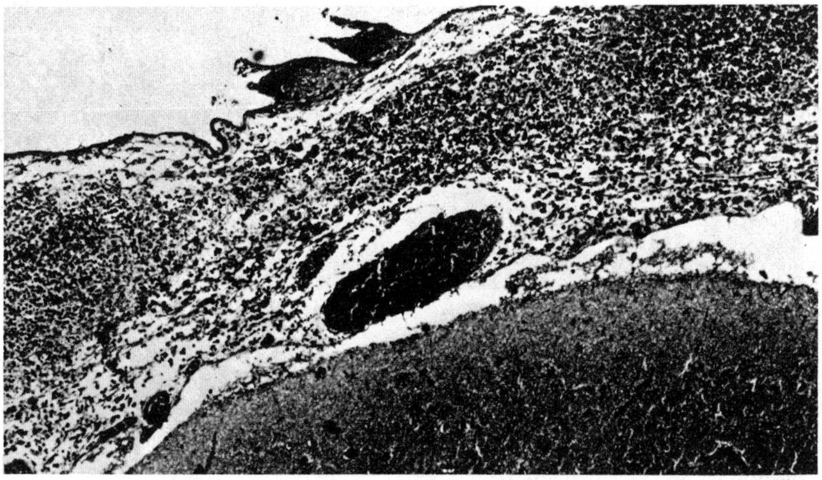

FIGURE 2.2-15. *Acute bacterial meningitis. The exudate in the leptomeningeal space, enclosed by the arachnoid membrane above and the pial surface below, is composed predominantly of neutrophils. (From Robertson D M, Dinsdale H B:* The Nervous System, *p 124. Williams & Wilkins, Baltimore, 1972, with permission.)*

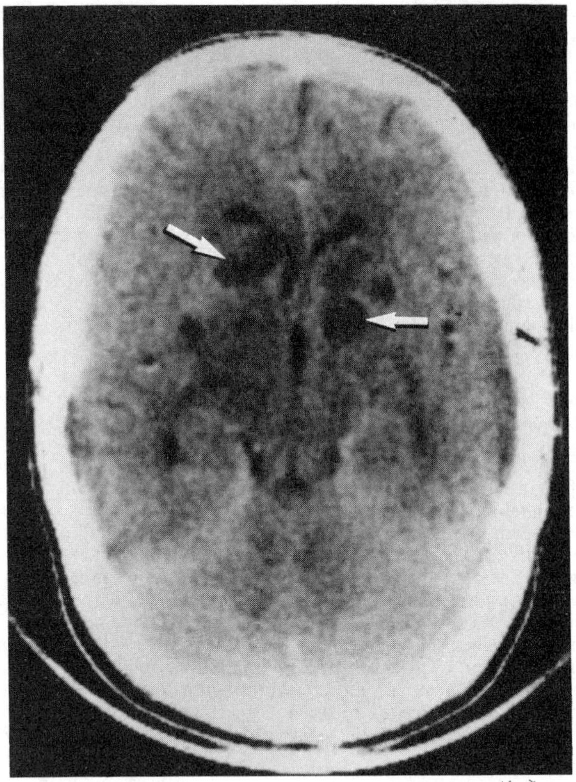

FIGURE 2.2-16. *Multiple cryptococcal abscesses* (arrows) *on CT. The patient had AIDS and a cryptococcal meningitis. (Courtesy of Charles Elkin, MD, Montefiore Medical Center, New York.)*

manifested by progressive dementia and motor signs of pyramidal, extrapyramidal, cerebellar, or lower motor neuron disease, with myoclonus, spasticity, tremors, atrophy, or fasciculations. The EEG shows periodic generalized spike activity. Death usually occurs within 3 to 12 months. The pathology is that of subacute spongiform encephalopathy. The disease predominantly affects neurons throughout the CNS, ranging from the cerebral cortex to the anterior horn cells of the spinal cord. Vacuolation affects the dendrites and axons, as well as astrocytes. A typical inflammatory response is not seen.

It is intriguing to consider how many other degenerative diseases may be due to a virus that has incubated for many years, and it is frustrating to consider how long it may take to prove or disprove this concept.

Conventional viruses causing slow infections Other viruses cause slow but progressive degeneration of the brain.

PROGRESSIVE MULTIFOCAL LEUKOENCEPHALOPATHY This disease occurs in late adult life and causes death in 2 to 6 months. It is due to papovavirus infiltration after immune mechanisms have been impaired, most often by a malignant lymphoma or by AIDS (Fig. 2.2-20). The disease is manifested by lethargy, progressive dementia, and multifocal cerebral signs. Under the microscope, zones of demyelination are scattered throughout the cerebrum. Monster-sized astrocytes and oligodendroglia are at the periphery of the demyelinated areas; nuclear inclusion bodies are characteristically found in oligodendrocytes.

SUBACUTE SCLEROSING PANENCEPHALITIS This illness, attributable to involvement of the CNS by the measles virus, begins insidiously in childhood or adolescence and causes progressive deterioration of the intellect and behavior. Within weeks or months, a variety of deficits occur, especially involving motor and visual modalities; seizures and myoclonic jerks are common. Decerebration, coma, and death supervene after a course of months to years. The clinical diagnosis is established by the findings of periodic sharp activities in the diffusely slow (EEG) and elevated γ-globulin, representing measles antibodies, in the CSF. On microscopic examination, intranuclear and intracytoplasmic eosinophilic inclusion bodies (Dawson bodies) are found in cortical neurons.

CYTOMEGALIC INCLUSION DISEASE The cytomegalovirus causes neonatal jaundice, thrombocytopenia, and pneumonia. Microcephaly and cerebral calcifications are seen. Survival is associated with cerebral palsy, hydrocephalus, and epilepsy. Cytomegalic inclusion disease, causing systemic illness, may also occur in older children, in adults who have AIDS, or in adults who have received immunosuppressive medications or who are otherwise debilitated. The viruses

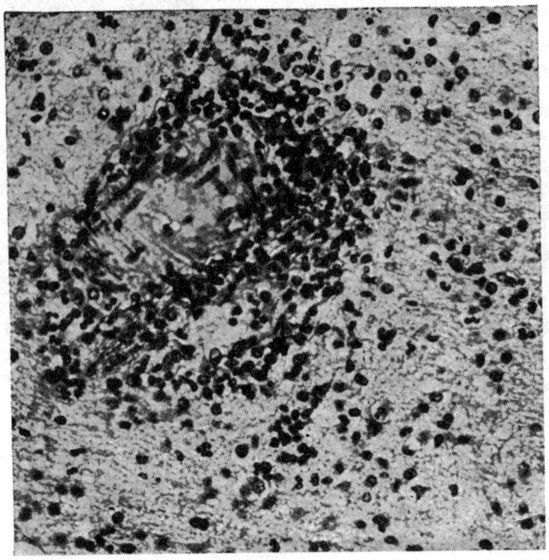

FIGURE 2.2-17. *Encephalitis. Polymorphonuclear and mononuclear leukocytes infiltrate and surround a blood vessel within an area of disintegrating white matter. Hematoxylin and eosin stain,* × *250. (From Blackwood W, Dodds T C, Sommerville J C:* Atlas of Neuropathology, *ed 2, p 77. Williams & Wilkins, Baltimore, 1964, with permission.)*

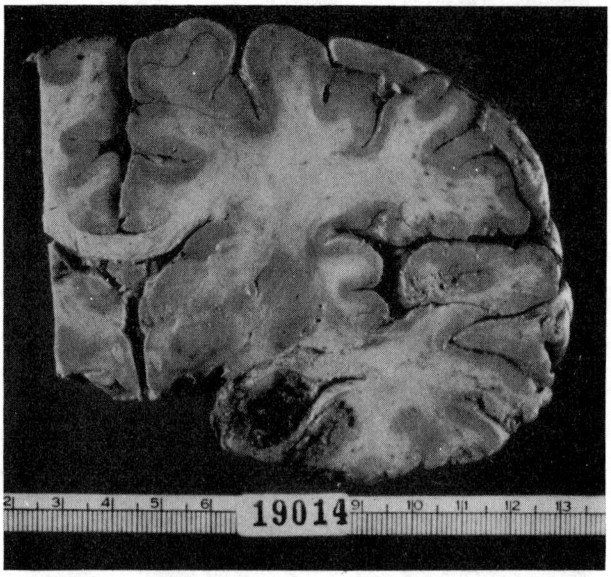

FIGURE 2.2-18. *Encephalitis, in this case, due to herpes simplex virus. Edematous brain tissue has compressed the ventricles. Hemorrhagic necrosis is seen in the inferior medial aspect of the temporal lobe. (Courtesy of H M Zimmerman, MD.)*

form intranuclear and intracytoplasmic inclusions in the viscera and in glial cells and neurons. Findings of such inclusions in large cells of urinary sediment or culture of the virus from CSF, urine, or biopsy material establish the diagnosis during life.

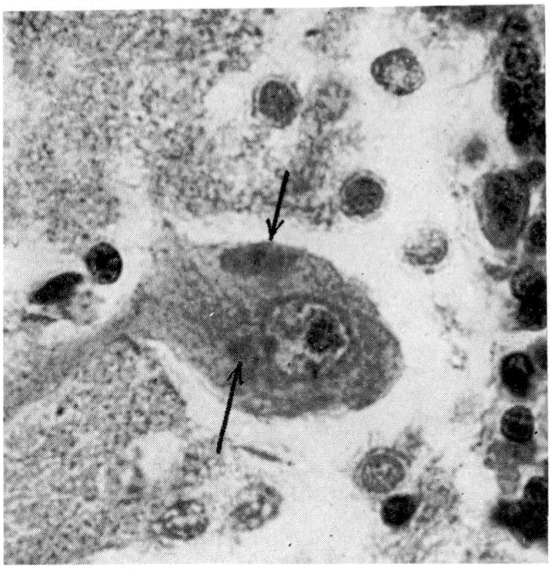

FIGURE 2.2-19. *Rabies. In a Purkinje cell of the cerebellum are rounded intracytoplasmic inclusions, Negri bodies* (arrows). *Hematoxylin and eosin stain, × 1,000. (Courtesy of T Poon, MD and A Hirano, MD.)*

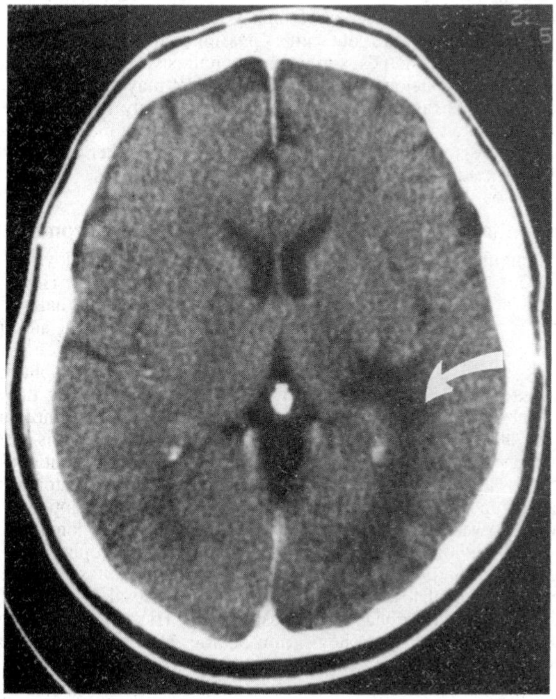

FIGURE 2.2-20. *Progressive multifocal leukoencephalopathy. CT scan of a 46-year-old man with AIDS who presented with progressive dementia. In addition to poor attention and memory, he had a left homonymous hemianopia. (Courtesy of Charles Elkin, MD, Montefiore Medical Center, New York.)*

Postinfectious or postvaccinal encephalitis Some encephalitides are a reaction of the brain to vaccination; exanthemata, such as measles and chicken pox, rheumatic fever, and other systemic inflammations.

ACUTE ENCEPHALOMYELITIS *Acute disseminated encephalomyelitis* suddenly occurs either during an infectious disease or a few days to 4 weeks after an infectious illness or vaccination; recovery may occur. *Acute hemorrhagic leukoencephalitis,* as the name implies, affects predominantly white matter, but it is probably a fulminating form of disseminated encephalomyelitis. This disease often follows a febrile illness and ends in death after a few days. These two illnesses are probably acute allergic demyelinating diseases with secondary reactive inflammation.

SYDENHAM'S CHOREA This form of chorea may occur in young adolescents or young primiparas (chorea gravidarum), but it most frequently occurs in children between 5 and 13 years of age. The onset may be manifested by no more than irritability or unusual restlessness. Choreiform movements of the extremities increase in prominence, and similar movements affect the face and the tongue. Emotional symptoms sometimes progress to delirium. The treatment of choice is bed rest in a quiet environment, with judicious use of sedatives. Prophylactic penicillin is warranted because this form of chorea is related to rheumatic fever.

ACUTE CEREBELLAR ATAXIA OF CHILDHOOD The abrupt onset of truncal ataxia, incoordination of limbs, and ocular dysmetria may occur in preschool children after a mild illness. Recovery takes place within an average of 2 months. The disease is either an autoimmune reaction or due to direct virus infection.

CENTRAL NERVOUS SYSTEM DISEASE CAUSED BY VISCEROTROPIC ORGANISMS Many organisms are viscerotropic and involve the nervous system as part of a generalized systemic infection. The following is an incomplete list of organisms that may infect the CNS.

Viruses Coxsackie, ECHO, mumps, and the Epstein-Barr (EB) virus of infectious mononucleosis cause generalized encephalitis.

Bacteria Most bacteria cause cerebritis associated with meningitis or preceding abscess formation. Generalized cerebral inflammatory changes may accompany typhoid, but associated arteritis sometimes results in focal infarctions. Tetanus, diphtheria, and botulism produce their effects by elaborating toxins. Mycoplasma pneumonia may cause encephalomyelitis and radiculitis.

Rickettsia Typhus and Rocky Mountain spotted fever produce generalized encephalitis; the associated arteritis may cause focal signs.

Protozoa Cerebral malaria due to occlusion of capillaries often causes delirium and other psychological manifestations, as well as other signs of general and focal cerebral disease. Toxoplasma infects infants *in utero* and causes hydrocephalus, convulsions, chorioretinitis and intracranial calcifications. It is often found in patients with AIDS.

Fungi Cryptococcosis is the most common fungus causing chronic basilar meningitis; however, coccidioidomycosis, histoplasmosis, nocardiosis, candidiasis, mucormycosis, aspergillosis, and other fungi also invade the brain on rare occasions.

Helminths In patients with trichinosis and schistosomiasis, granulomata occur; with cysticercosis and echinococcosis, cysts develop. All result in focal signs and seizures. Cysts frequently cause increased intracranial pressure.

Spirochetes The leptospira of Weil's disease may cause meningitis, usually mild. Syphilis was the most notorious disease in this category. Lyme disease is becoming increasingly prevalent and may account for otherwise unexplained psychiatric and neurological syndromes.

ACQUIRED IMMUNE DEFICIENCY SYNDROME The advent of AIDS has caused a remarkable increase in the frequency of brain infections. In some metropolitan general hospitals, the neurological complications of AIDS, often of an infectious nature, are only second to stroke as the most frequent lethal neurological disorder. From 40 to 60 percent of AIDS victims experience neurological complications, which are often the presenting complaint.

AIDS is caused by a new virus, human T-cell lymphotropic virus type III (HTLV-III), now termed *human immunodeficiency virus* (HIV). Transmission appears to be solely via body fluids, usually through sexual activity, through transfusions or inoculations of blood and blood products, and by transplacental transport. The antibodies of HIV can be detected by enzyme-linked immunosorbent assay (ELISA), and the presence of the virus is confirmed by the Western blot assay.

In the United States and in Central Africa, the problem is of epidemic proportions. Originally present in the male homosexual population and among users of IV drugs, the disorder has now been transmitted heterosexually in about 4 percent of the cases. Others at particular risk include hemophiliacs receiving Factor III concentrate and children or spouses of high-risk individuals.

The onset of AIDS is associated with lymphopenia and a reduction in the ratio of helper-suppressors to T-lymphocytes. The initial systemic symptoms may include fatigue, dyspnea, cough, diarrhea, anorexia, and weight loss. Depression may be associated with or antedate these symptoms. Lymphadenopathy and yeast infections are common. Multiple opportunistic infections develop, the most common of which are viruses (cytomegalovirus and herpes simplex), bacteria, (*Mycobacterium avium* and *intracellular*); fungi (*Cryptococcus neoformans* and *Candida albicans*), and protozoa (*Pneumocystis carinii* and *Toxoplasma gondii*). *Pneumocystis carinii* pneumonia is the most common illness in patients with AIDS.

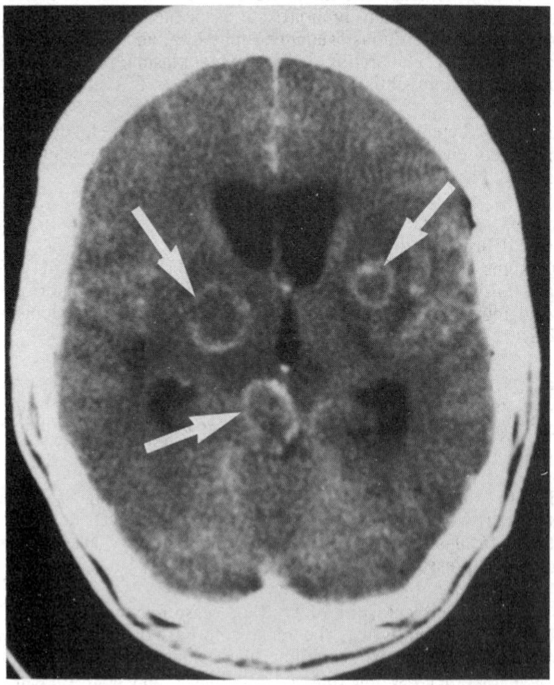

FIGURE 2.2-21. *Toxoplasmosis. Multiple ring-enhancing lesions on CT in an AIDS patient. (Courtesy of Charles Elkin, MD, Montefiore Medical Center, New York.)*

Kaposi sarcoma is particularly virulent in AIDS patients and rapidly spreads to viscera as well as to lymph nodes. Other lymphomas are common. Death usually occurs within 24 to 36 months; rarely, patients live as long as 5 years. Experimental therapy has been directed to drugs that inhibit reverse transcriptase, the enzyme necessary for replication of the retrovirus HIV.

Approximately half of AIDS patients suffer neurological complications during the course of their illness. In about one-third of these patients, neuropsychiatric manifestations herald the beginning of the disorder. Most common neurological complications of AIDS are infectious; commonest is toxoplasmosis, comprising about 30 percent of all the complications of AIDS. Probably just as common or perhaps even more frequent is the subacute encephalitis of AIDS, due to infection by the AIDS virus. Less frequent are cryptococcosis (13 percent), aseptic meningitis (6 percent), herpes simplex encephalitis (3 percent), progressive multifocal encephalopathy (1.5 percent), mycobacterial infections, and candidasis.

Toxoplasmosis *Toxoplasma gondii* is a frequent cause of encephalitis in immunosuppressed patients, particularly IV drug users with AIDS. Multiple brain foci are common, each containing a necrotic center with macrophage infiltrate. On light microscopy, the organisms are conspicuous in some of the macrophages. A common clinical presentation consists of headache, mild fever, and mental status changes, which vary according to the area of the brain that is affected. Prostration is less pronounced than with bacterial meningitis. Because of the risk of herniation with lumbar puncture, a CT or MR should be performed. The presence of one or several ring-enhancing lesions in a patient with AIDS is suggestive of toxoplasmosis (Fig. 2.2-21). Treatment with pyrimethamine and sulfadiazine should then be started. If the patient continues to deteriorate after 48 hours, a CT-guided stereotactic biopsy of one of the lesions should be undertaken to rule out other possible etiologies, most often cytomegalovirus, herpes simplex, tuberculosis, progressive multifocal leukoencephalopathy, or lymphoma; MR may reveal lesions not visible on CT (Fig. 2.2-22). Toxoplasma antibody titers should not be relied on to make the diagnosis, but an acute rise may signal acute toxoplasmosis and may warrant treatment even if other tests, including biopsy, are negative.

Dementia of acquired immune deficiency syndrome

Thought until 1985 to be related to infection by cytomegalovirus, this syndrome is now known to correlate with infection by the HIV. This virus causes an overt subacute encephalitis in about half of all patients with AIDS. Initial manifestations are apathy and psychomotor retardation, which may be mistaken for depression. Memory loss and attentional impairment in the absence of aphasia or apraxia has led to the classification of this disorder among the subcortical dementias. Preeminence of progressive cognitive impairment in the absence of impaired consciousness distinguishes this disease from encephalitis caused by toxoplasma or other conventional infectious agents. Paranoid delusions, delirium, or catatonia may occur; impaired gait and truncal movements may develop over the course of weeks or months. Global disorientation and coma precede death. Pathologically, there is diffuse cerebral atrophy with demyelination and spongiform changes in the centrum semiovale, as well as neuronal loss and glial nodules. The causal agent has been identified in macrophages and astrocytes. HIV antigen is found in CSF. CT imaging shows nonspecific atrophy. White matter hyperintensity on T_2 images may be visualized on MR. Treatable causes of encephalitis, such as toxoplasmosis, cryptococcosis, cytomegalovirus, and herpes, should be ruled out in these patients by MR and CSF examination.

Not all psychological symptoms in AIDS patients are due to disease of the brain. People in the high-risk group experience anxiety, obsessive-compulsive disorders, and hypochondriasis; fear of the disease is understandable. Once the diagnosis is made, even though asymptomatic, the patient may behave like a cancer patient. Denial and disbelief are followed by depression and anxiety. Hopelessness, feelings of guilt, fear of uncertainty, and anger are common.

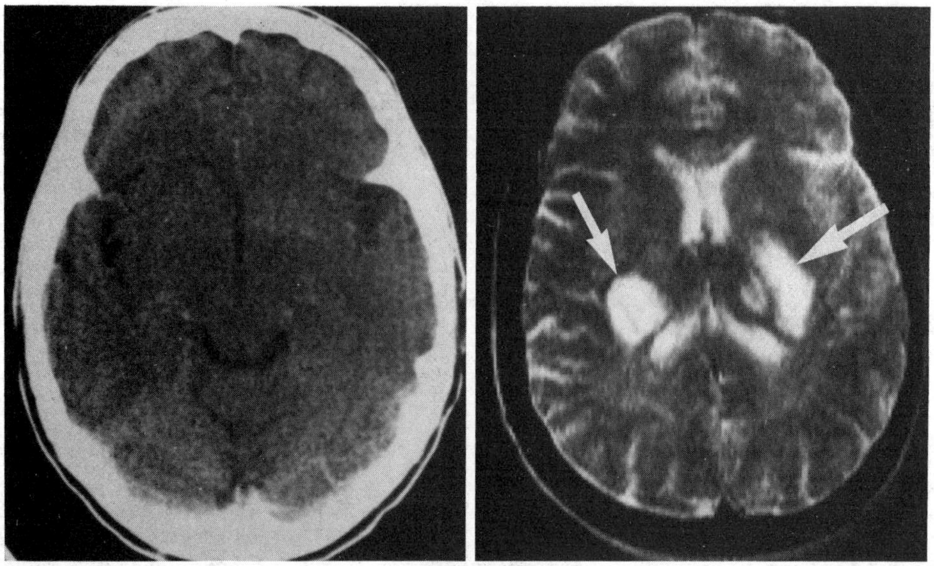

FIGURE 2.2-22. *CT with contrast* (left) *was normal in a 42-year-old woman with AIDS and bilateral weakness. MR showed bilateral lesions* (right, arrows). *(Courtesy of Charles Elkin, MD, Montefiore Medical Center, New York.)*

Other neurological complications There are several other complications of AIDS. Meningeal and cerebral lymphoma constitutes 9 percent of all complications—the most common, noninfectious neurological lesion. Cerebral infarction and hemorrhage occur infrequently. Myelopathy, peripheral neuropathies, or myopathic syndromes affect about one of every 10 AIDS patients. These changes may be due to viral infection or metabolic dysfunction secondary to nutritional deficiencies.

LYME DISEASE Lyme disease is caused by the spirochete *Borrelia burgdorferi* and is transmitted by ticks. The disease may occur in three stages. In the first stage, an oval erythematous skin lesion is noted with fever, malaise, headache, and other generalized systemic symptoms. In the second stage, weeks to months later, neurological or cardiological symptoms occur. The neurological symptoms are usually meningitis but may also include cranial neuropathies and radiculo-neuritides. The third and late stage occurs many months to years after the initial infection and is manifested by arthritis or a diffuse or multifocal encephalopathy. Lyme disease has replaced syphilis as the mimicker of other diseases. It must be considered when psychiatric or neurological symptoms develop and progress without obvious cause. In the second or third stages, antibody IgG titers are elevated. The disease is responsive to penicillin or tetracycline therapy.

NEUROSYPHILIS The *Treponema pallidum* may affect the blood vessels of the CNS, the interstitial tissue, or the neurons; these sites are not mutually exclusive. Within days or weeks after the secondary phase of lues, meningovascular manifestations may occur. In *luetic arteritis,* parenchymal involvement is secondary to thrombosis and infarction. *Luetic meningitis* presents the features of a chronic meningitis, with thickening of the meninges at the base of the brain. The luetic granuloma (gumma) acting as a brain tumor is virtually extinct. The therapy of choice for neurosyphilis is penicillin. A total dose of 6 to 9 million units is administered by intramuscular injection in divided doses over a period of 2 to 3 weeks.

Neurosyphilis is expressed as two chronic diseases: tabes dorsalis and general paresis. Both diseases occur 5 to 20 years after the primary infection. In both, miotic pupils unreactive to light (Argyll Robertson pupils) are found, although less often in paresis than in tabes. The CSF reveals elevated protein, increased lymphocytes, positive serological test and an abnormal colloidal gold curve; although in burnt-out tabes, the CSF is sometimes normal. Tests for specific treponemal antibodies, including fluorescent treponemal antibody absorption (FTA-ABS) or microhemagglutination assay (MHA), will eliminate false negatives.

General paresis is manifested by progressive dementia, with agitated, expansive, or depressive qualities. Slurred speech and minor tremors are common. The brain—predominantly the frontal lobes—is atrophic. The microscope reveals neuronal degeneration within the frontoparietal cortex. Hypertrophied microglia are seen as elongated rod cells, often filled with iron granules that stain brilliantly with Prussian blue.

Tabes dorsalis is characterized by demyelination of the posterior columns of the spinal cord and of the dorsal roots. The resultant position-sense loss causes ataxia, and the associated loss of deep pain sensation may lead to the development of painless traumatic arthropathies (Charcot joints). Optic atrophy and oculomotor nerve paresis sometimes occur. Pain is a prominent symptom. Lightning-like pains, usually in the extremities, and girdle pains, or paresthesias, are common; crises of severe pain may be referred to visceral areas.

PRESUMPTIVE IMMUNOLOGICAL DISORDERS

MULTIPLE SCLEROSIS The prevalence of this chronic demyelinating disease varies between 30 and 40 cases per 100,000 population. It usually begins between the ages of 20 and 40 years, and the disease is most prevalent in persons who have spent their childhood in the northern latitudes. It is postulated that a viral illness in childhood induces an autoimmune reaction many years later. The disease is multiple in space (i.e., in the CNS) and in time. Involvement of the optic nerve by retrobulbar neuritis causes unilateral blindness. Disease of the brain stem is often manifested by diplopia and nystagmus. Internuclear ophthalmoplegia, with nystagmus of the abducting eye and palsy of the adducting eye on lateral gaze, is usually due to multiple sclerosis affecting the medial

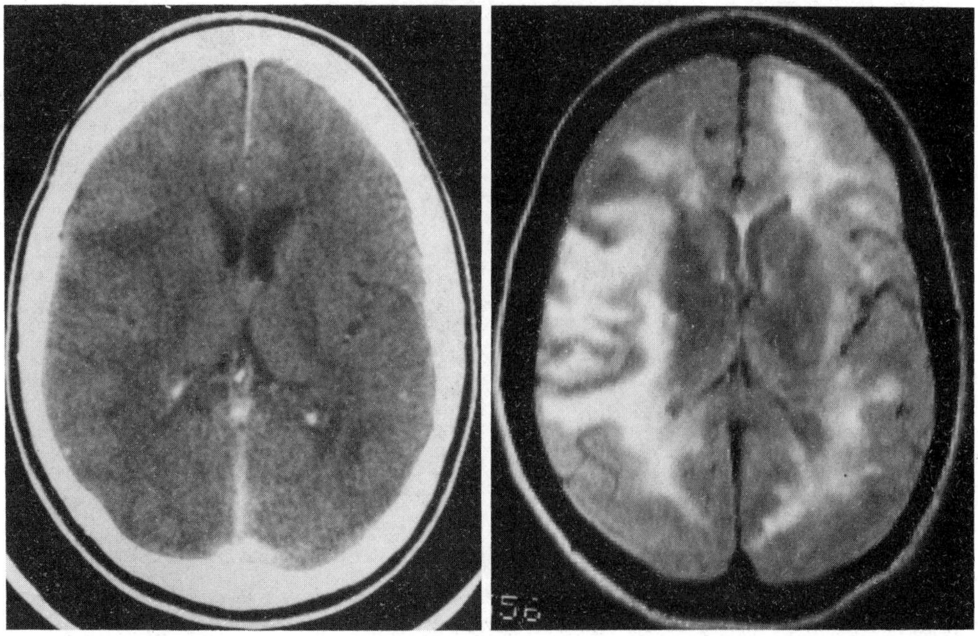

FIGURE 2.2-23. CT (left) *and* MR (right) *of a 32-year-old woman with remissions and exacerbations of a clinical picture consisting of bilateral weakness, inattention, and urinary incontinence. MR shows white matter lesions not visualized on CT. (Courtesy of Charles Elkin, MD, Montefiore Medical Center, New York.)*

longitudinal fasciculus. Cerebellar demyelination is manifested by ataxia, with intention tremor and scanning (staccato) speech. Spinal cord involvement results in paraparesis, with impaired sphincter control and impotence. A lesion of the motor or sensory pathways anywhere along their course between the cerebrum and the spinal cord may cause weakness or sensory defects. An organic mental disorder occurs infrequently; seizures, aphasia, and homonymous hemianopsia are rare. Because symptoms often outnumber the signs at the onset, the disease may be mistaken for neurosis. Conversely, signs may be found without associated symptoms. Relative euphoria, often present in these patients, may be misinterpreted as *la belle indifférence* of hysteria. The course is characterized by exacerbations and remissions of unpredictable severity, duration, and frequency.

Optic nerve disease, not otherwise evident, may be established by the finding of impaired color perception or a cecocentral scotoma in the visual fields. Abnormal evoked cortical potentials may verify disease of the visual or somatosensory pathways when signs are not present on neurological examination. MR imaging often reveals multiple white matter lesions in the presence of a negative CT (Fig. 2.2-23). Evaluation of CSF in patients with multiple sclerosis usually reveals elevation of the γ-globulin with an electrophoretic pattern of oligoclonal bands. The myelin basic protein is raised when the disease is active. Although adequate treatment is not available, steroids are considered of value in ameliorating the acute attack. Long-term immunosuppressive therapy may decrease the frequency of exacerbations.

Gross examination of the brain (Figure 2.2-24) reveals scattered gray, sharply demarcated plaques of demyelination, which are variable in size and shape and are most numerous in the areas adjacent to the ventricles. In recent areas of demyelination, microscopic examination shows destruction of myelin, swollen axis cylinders, and many fat-laden phagocytic cells. Old areas of demyelination (Figure 2.2-25) reveal complete myelin loss, with fragmentation of axis cylinders and the formation of a dense glial scar.

Neuromyelitis optica (Devic's disease) This disease is probably a variant of multiple sclerosis in which severe acute demyelination, often accompanied by ischemic changes, is limited to the spinal cord and the optic nerves. Steroids should be used to decrease the risk of cavitation in the spinal cord.

Reye's syndrome This condition occurs 2 or 3 days after a mild flu-like illness, mainly in children from 5 to 14 years of age. It has a high mortality rate. Vomiting is rapidly followed by delirium, seizures, and coma. Fatty disease of the liver and other viscera is associated with metabolic defects, especially hypoglycemia. Cerebral edema is prominent. Aspirin is implicated in the pathogenesis of Reye's syndrome.

OTHER PROBABLE IMMUNOLOGICAL DISORDERS

The causes of the following disorders are unclear.

Behçet's syndrome is manifested by recurrent uveitis and ulcers of mucous membranes. Meningoencephalitis occurs, and sometimes there is involvement of the brain stem or the spinal cord.

Vogt-Koyanagi-Harada syndrome is characterized by uveitis, deafness, and depigmentation of the skin and hair. Neurological manifestations are predominantly those of meningitis or encephalitis.

Reiter's syndrome is characterized by urethritis, conjunctivitis, and arthritis. Meningoencephalitis, cranial neuropathy, or peripheral nerve involvement occur on rare occasions.

DISEASES ASSOCIATED WITH SYSTEMIC MALIGNANCY

Subacute cortical cerebellar degeneration is manifested by progressive cerebellar signs and dementia. Death occurs within a few months. The disease is associated with carcinoma, most often of the bronchus or the ovary. Frequently, the neurological symptoms antedate evidence of the primary malignancy.

Progressive multifocal leukoencephalopathy occasionally occurs in patients with malignant lymphoma. The malignancy impairs immunological mechanisms and allows papovavirus infiltrations.

Encephalomyelitis rarely occurs as a remote effect of oat cell carcinoma of the lung. In a few cases, the disease has affected predominantly the limbic system, with associated recent memory loss.

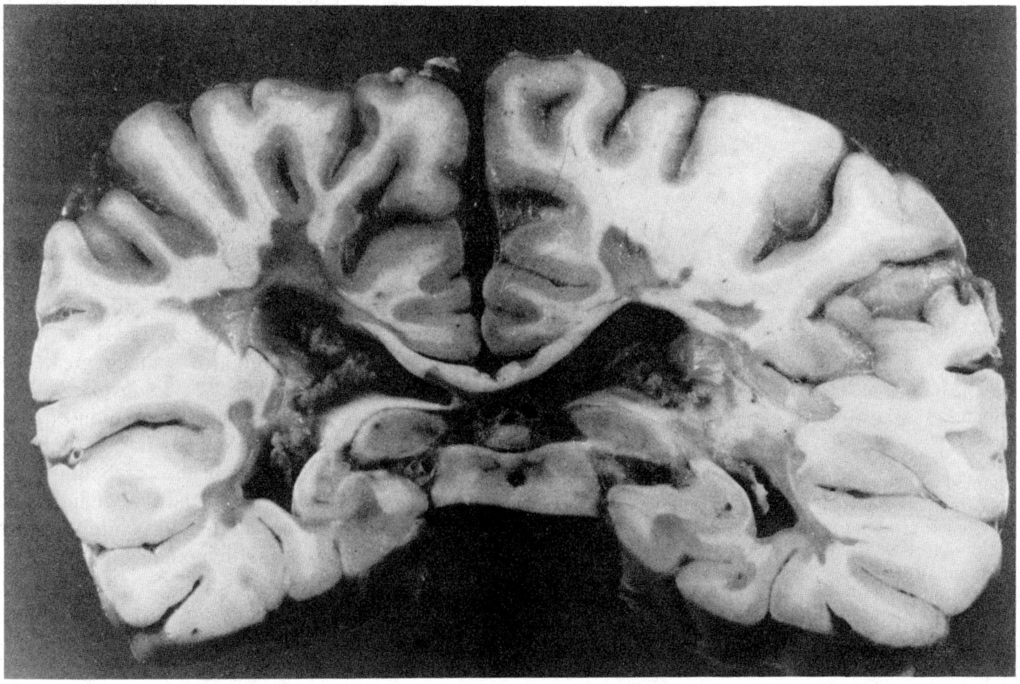

FIGURE 2.2-24. *Multiple sclerosis. Plaques of demyelination are predominant in the periventricular areas. (From Hirano A:* A Guide to Neuropathology, *p 61. Igaku-Shoin, New York, 1981, with permission.)*

A toxic *psychosis* sometimes occurs in patients with metastatic carcinoma of the lung, but without metastases to the brain. *Neuromyopathy* and degenerative changes within the spinal cord or medulla may also occur as remote effects of malignancy.

BRAIN NEOPLASMS

Primary brain tumors have a prevalence of about 20 cases per 100,000 population and are more frequent in males than in females. Metastatic brain disease is almost as common as primary brain neoplasms; about 10 percent of patients dying of systemic cancer harbor brain metastases. Brain lymphomas were a rarity before AIDS. Primary tumors of the CNS are the second most common malignancy in children and account for about 2 percent of all cancers. They are usually classified according to the cell of origin (Table 2.2-1). Among the primary intracranial tumors, medulloblastoma, astrocytoma, and ependymoma are predominant in young patients, whereas glioblastoma multiforme and meningioma occur mainly in the later decades of life. The relative frequency and peak age of incidence for different types of tumors affecting the brain are shown in Table 2.2-2.

Typically, brain tumors cause progressive symptoms and signs that reflect focal brain involvement, such as a hemiparesis or nonlocalized brain dysfunction, such as change in personality, impaired cognitive function, depression of consciousness, or generalized seizures. An organic mental disorder and personality changes are particularly prevalent in frontal brain tumors, but may occur with neoplasms in any area of the brain. With increased intracranial pressure, headache, vomiting, lethargy, and papilledema may occur, but these typical features are often absent. Visual acuity is impaired only late in the course of papilledema, due to intracranial hypertension, in contradistinction to optic neuritis, which may present an almost identical funduscopic picture, but with early blindness. Since the advent of CT, presentations lacking a progression of the neurological deficit are common because patients are scanned for relatively unimpressive deficits, such as transient diplopia or hand numbness. As a result, progressive focal findings related to tumor growth are not part of the presentation as often as in the past, when the major diagnostic tests were invasive (e.g., angiography or pneumoencephalography) and were used sparingly and later in the course.

Acute onset of symptoms is not uncommon. Seizures or, less likely, intratumoral hemorrhage are two mechanisms by which a tumor may suddenly betray its presence. A tumor must be a primary consideration when convulsions originate during adult life. Seizures are the presenting symptom of tumors in 15 to 20 percent of all cases. When seizures begin

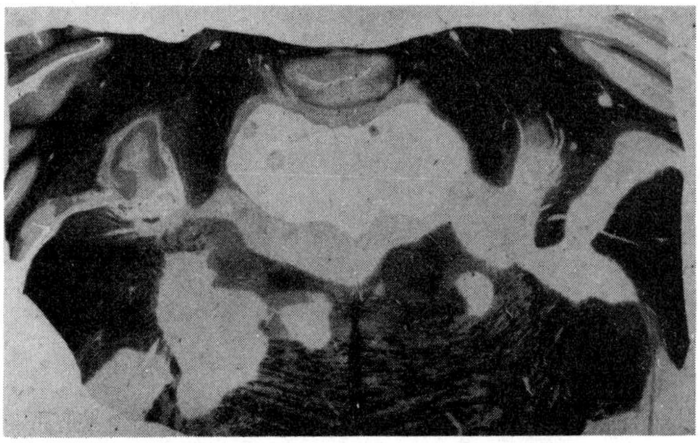

FIGURE 2.2-25. *Multiple sclerosis. Irregular, seemingly punched-out zones of demyelination are evident in this section through the level of the fourth ventricle. Myelin stain, × 2.6. (Courtesy of H M Zimmerman, MD.)*

TABLE 2.2-1
Histological Classification of Intracranial Tumors

A. *Congenital tumors of maldevelopmental origin*
  Teratoma; lipoma
  Epidermoid (cholesteatoma) and dermoid cysts
  Craniopharyngioma
  Neural hamartomas; Lindau's syndrome
  Tuberous sclerosis; neurofibromatosis
B. *Tumors of the meninges*
  Meningioma
  Primary sarcoma
C. *Tumors of the reticular tissue*
  Lymphoma
  Microglioma
  Reticulum cell sarcoma
D. *Tumors of the blood vessels*
  Hemangioblastoma
  Arteriovenous malformation
  Venous angioma
E. *Tumors of neuroectodermal origin*
  1. Gliomas
    a. Mixed glial components
      Glioblastoma multiforme
    b. Astrocytic group
      Astrocytoma; astroblastoma
      Polar spongioblastoma
    c. Oligodendroglia
      Oligodendroglioma
    d. Ependyma and its homologues
      Ependymoma; subependymoma
      Choroid-plexus papilloma
      Colloid cyst
  2. Neuronal and primitive neuroepithelium origin
    Medulloblastoma; medulloepithelioma
    Neuroblastoma
    Ganglioneuroma and ganglioglioma
    Retinoblastoma
F. *Pineal region tumors*
  Teratomas; lipoma; germinoma
  Pineocytoma; pineoblastoma
G. *Pituitary adenomas*
  Chromophobe
  Acidophil
  Basophil
H. *Tumors of the cranial nerves*
  Schwannoma
  Neurofibroma

in an adult, the incidence of brain tumor is 25 to 35 percent if the seizures or the EEG have focal qualities or if the patient is more than 50 years old. The incidence is as high as 50 percent if neurological signs also are found.

Intracranial tumors may originate in the brain parenchyma (intra-axial tumors) or in the structures surrounding the brain (extra-axial tumors). This distinction has practical implications because the histology, prognosis, and treatment of the two types differ.

INTRA-AXIAL TUMORS About 45 percent of all intracranial tumors are intra-axial tumors. In adults, they are almost always gliomas, particularly the malignant glioblastoma multiforme (Fig. 2.2-26). Since these tumors infiltrate the surrounding brain, complete surgical removal is impossible (Fig. 2.2-27). The pathogenesis of primary brain tumors is unclear. Chromosomal abnormalities, with an overrepresentation of chromosome 7 and an underrepresentation of chromosome 22 and the sex chromosome, have been identified in glial malignancies. These neoplasms contain an increased amount of receptors for growth factors and growth-factor-like substances. Growth factors are related to oncogene products, such as the transforming proteins of the retroviruses. Oncogenes are normally present in the nucleus; when activated, they free the cell from the normal constraints of cellular growth and differentiation, setting the stage for malignant changes. Oncogenes could be carried into the nucleus by a retrovirus.

The clinical manifestations of brain tumors vary according to the area of the brain involved. Frontal and temporal sites result in personality changes and dominant-hemisphere language disturbances. Tumors near the rolandic or central sulcus often give rise to jacksonian seizures in the contralateral limbs (Fig. 2.2-28). Occipital tumors cause hemianopic field defects. Cerebellar neoplasms manifest progressive ataxia on the same side as the lesion. Generally, the deficit is relatively minor, considering the size of brain displacement and involvement by the tumor depicted by CT or MR. An infarct of a similar size would produce a much greater deficit.

The common gliomas, *glioblastoma multiforme* and *astrocytoma,* as well as the less common *oligodendroglioma,* arise in the cerebral hemispheres in adults, but the astrocytomas are more likely to be in the cerebellum or brain stem of children. *Ependymomas* and the malignant *medulloblastomas* of the cerebellum are tumors of childhood, and their first signs may be intracranial hypertension caused by blockage of the ventricular system. A similar mechanism occurs with such rare tumors as *papilloma of the choroid plexus,* usually within the fourth ventricle, and *colloid cyst* of the third ventricle.

Metastatic tumors generally reach the brain through the bloodstream and most often from neoplastic deposits in the lung, either primary lung tumors or metastases (Fig. 2.2-29). Lung and breast cancer are the most common types of brain metastases (Fig. 2.2-28). Thyroid and kidney carcinomas, choriocarcinoma, and malignant melanoma (Fig. 2.2-30) are less frequent. Direct spread to the intracranial cavity occurs in the case of nasopharyngeal and other cancers of the head. Seldom, tumors of the pelvis or retroperitoneum, such as prostatic carcinoma, may reach the brain dura mater through the spinal epidural veins of Batson's plexus. Except in patients with AIDS, primary lymphoma of the brain is rare, but it seems to be growing in prevalence.

Hemangioblastomas are rare vascular neoplasms. They often arise in the cerebellum and evoke polycythemia. When associated with cystic disease of other organs and angiomatosis of the retina, the clinical picture is called *Hippel-Lindau's* disease.

EXTRA-AXIAL TUMORS Extracranial tumors tend to grow slower than primary brain tumors. These tumors have a clear plane of cleavage, which often facilitates complete surgical excision. Vasospasm, with attendant infarction and hemorrhagic complications, may occur, particularly when diagnosis has been delayed until the tumor is large. In the past decade, the use of the operative microscope has markedly improved the outcome of surgery for these lesions. Most common extra-axial tumors are the meningioma (Fig. 2.2-31), schwannoma (Fig. 2.2-32), and pituitary adenoma (Fig. 2.2-33). Metastatic tumors, particularly breast carcinoma, may also be extra-axial, affecting the meninges. Extra-axial tumors at the base of the brain cause cranial nerve deficits. Endocrinological disorders may reveal the presence of a pituitary adenoma (Fig. 2.2-33) or a craniopharyngioma (Figs. 2.2-34 and 2.2-35).

The most common sites for *meningiomas* are the sagittal sinus, sphenoid ridge, and over the convexity of the cerebrum. Symptoms are due to compression of underlying brain. A sphenoid ridge meningioma often causes exophthalmos, oculomotor palsy and optic atrophy; temporal lobe seizures may occur. Meningiomas often stimulate hyperostoses of the adjacent bone. The *schwannoma* most commonly arises from

TABLE 2.2-2
Characteristics, Treatment, and Prognosis of Intracranial Tumors

Tumor Type	*Per cent**	*M/F Ratio*	*Peak Age (yr)*	*Cell Type*	*Location*	*CT Findings*	*Treatment*	*Survival*
Intra-axial tumors								
Glioblastoma, anaplastic astrocytoma	28	2:1	50–70	Astrocyte	Temporal, frontal; 6% multicentric	Ring enhancement, hemorrhage	Subtotal resection; radiotherapy (RT); chemotherapy	Median: 1 year 25%: 18 months
Cerebral astrocytoma	7	2:1	30–50	Astrocyte	Hemisphere	Hypodense lesion	Surgery; RT if patient older than 40	Median: 5–7 years
Cerebellar astrocytoma	4	2:1	0–20	Astrocyte	Hemisphere	Cyst, mural nodule	Surgery	10 to > 40 years
Oligodendroglioma	5		30–40	Oligodendrocyte	Frontal, thalamus	Calcified (60%)	Surgery; RT	5 to > 10 years
Ependymoma	5		0–20	Ependymal cell	Ventricles	Mixed density, calcific. contrast enhancement	Surgery; RT	50%: 5 years
Medulloblastoma	5	2:1	0–10	Medulloblast	Midline cerebellum	Hyperdense lesion	Surgery; RT	40%: 5 years 30%: 10 years
Extra-axial tumors								
Meningioma	15	F>M	60–80	Meningocyte	Parasagittal; anterior fossa	Homogeneous enhancement; calcification	Surgery	5–20% surgical mortality
Schwannoma	7	1:2	20–60	Schwann cell	Cerebello-pontine angle	Homogeneous enhancement	Surgery	10–30% surgical mortality
Pituitary adenoma	10		30–50	Adenohypophyseal cell	Sella turcica	Homogeneous enhancement	Surgery; bromocryptine	5–20% surgical mortality
Craniopharyngioma	2	2:1	4–16	Epithelial cells	Suprasellar	Solid or cystic; irregular enhancement; calcification	Surgery	10–30% surgical mortality
Cholesteatoma	1.5		20–40	Epidermoid cyst	Cerebello-pontine; sella; subtemporal	Very low density (fat)	Surgery	20–40% surgical mortality

*Approximate frequency of specific tumor type among intracranial neoplasms (excluding metastases). These figures refer to clinically important lesions. Small extra-axial tumors (for instance, small pituitary adenomas) are more common than the figures quoted above.

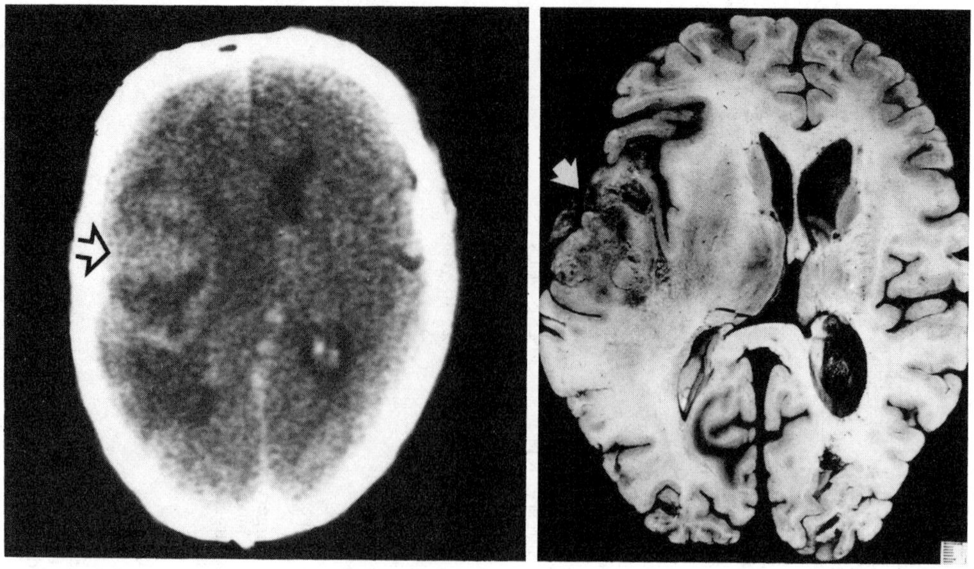

FIGURE 2.2-26. *Glioblastoma multiforme in the left temporal lobe of a 67-year-old man with an anomia. CT scan* (left) *showing a ring-enhancing lesion, which corresponds to the tumor in the pathological specimen* (right, arrow).

the sheath of the acoustic nerve. Symptoms result not only from involvement of the acoustic nerve and adjacent trigeminal and facial nerves, but also of the cerebellum.

Tumors of or near the pituitary may compress the endocrine-secreting cells of the pituitary and cause hypopituitarism. The *craniopharyngioma* and the *pituitary adenoma* that grow beyond the pituitary fossa compress the optic chiasm and result in bitemporal hemianopsia. Most pituitary adenomas secrete an excessive amount of prolactin and cause the syndrome of amenorrhea and galactorrhea. The rare *eosinophilic adenoma* produces excessive growth hormone, causing acromegaly in adults or gigantism in children. The adrenocortico-stimulating hormone of rare minute *basophilic adenomas* evokes Cushing's syndrome.

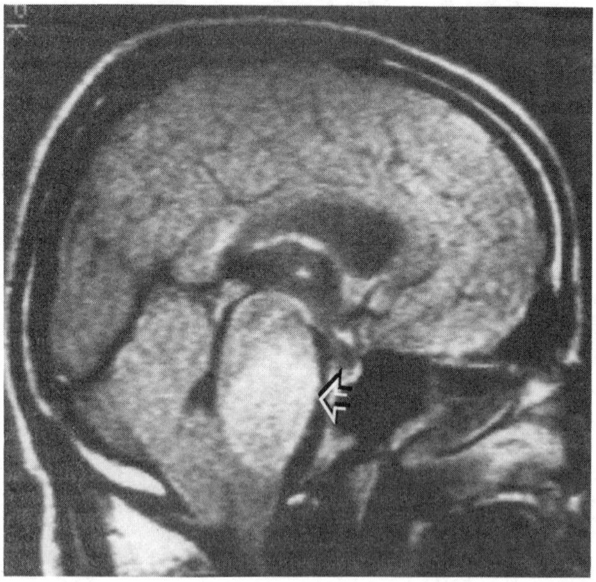

FIGURE 2.2-27. *MR of a pontine glioblastoma in a 33-year-old man with dysarthria, bilateral six-nerve palsy, and a right hemiparesis. The tumor is hyperintense on MR* (arrow). *(Courtesy of Charles Elkin, MD, Montefiore Medical Center, New York.)*

Chordomas are rare growths that arise from embyonic rests in the midline, usually along the clivus, and are manifested by signs of cranial nerve compression. *Cholesteatomas* develop from epidermoid tumors, but mastoid infections may cause a similar mass. These lesions are rare and most commonly arise in the cerebellopontine angles. The rare *pineal neoplasms,* usually teratomas and germinomas, occur most often in boys and cause paralysis of upward gaze (Parinaud's syndrome) by compressing the quadrigeminal plate; obstruction of the underlying aqueduct of Sylvius results in increased intracranial pressure and hydrocephalus.

DIAGNOSIS, TREATMENT, AND PROGNOSIS CT or MR are the procedures of choice to visualize brain tumors. MR is superior for intracerebral tumors, particularly gliomas. It also provides valuable information on the vascular supply and neighboring relationships of midline neoplasms and tumors at the cervicocranial junction. Temporal lobe and posterior fossa tumors, obscured on CT by bone-induced artifact, may become obvious on MR. Calcification is better seen with CT; calcified tumors tend to be benign and grow slowly. Diagnosis is based on tumor location, multiplicity, and density (CT) or intensity (MR) characteristics, coupled with demographic and other clinical information (Table 2.2-2).

The differential diagnosis between neoplasms and other lesions depends on careful evaluation of the clinical picture and imaging procedures. Cerebrovascular disease usually causes a more acute deficit, although carotid artery lesions can produce a stuttering course. Both strokes and tumors may have a sudden presentation. Subdural hematomas are diagnosed by CT or MR. Abscesses and granulomata often behave clinically as tumors do. They also may be difficult to differentiate on imaging procedures. Brain biopsy is then advisable, particularly considering the increasing frequency of infectious complications of AIDS.

Therapy for brain tumors depends on the tumor type and its location. Benign tumors at the base of the brain or convexity, such as meningiomas, pituitary adenomas, and acoustic schwannomas, should be resected surgically. Small asymp-

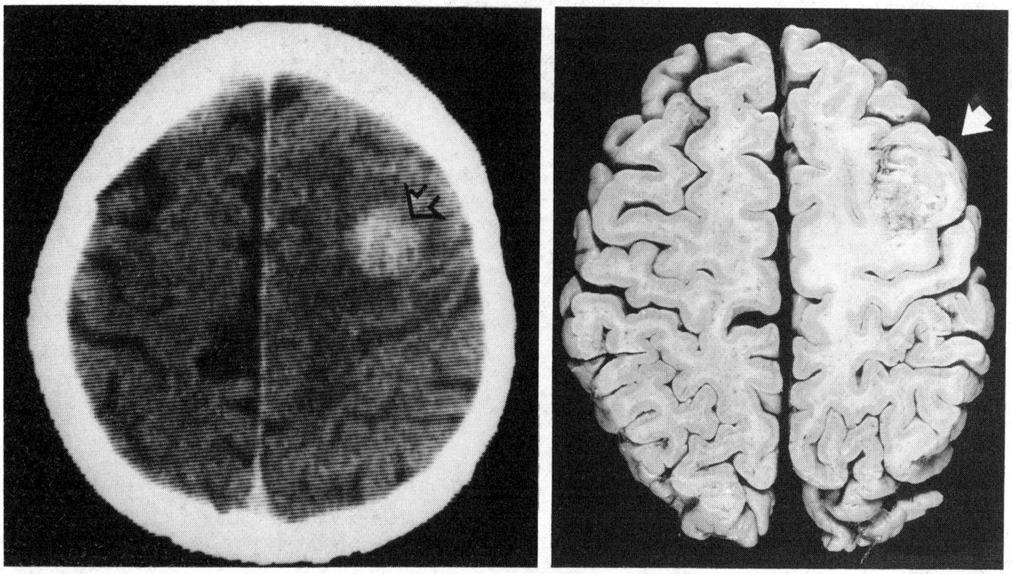

FIGURE 2.2-28. *CT* (left) *and corresponding pathologic specimen* (right) *showing a metastasis in the precentral gyrus from adenocarcinoma of the lung. (From Gonzalez C F, Grosman C B, Masdeu J C:* Head and Spine Imaging, *p 273. Wiley, New York, 1985, with permission.)*

tomatic meningiomas need not be removed. These lesions are often found incidentally at autopsy and on CT performed for other reasons. It is prudent to follow these small tumors by repeating the CT or MR within a year of discovery in order to assess the rate of growth. MR is the procedure of choice to visualize small intracanalicular auditory nerve schwannomas, which can be removed through the external auditory canal, obviating the need for a craniotomy. In the absence of MR, CT may be used, with air or iodinated contrast material injected into the subarachnoid space to better outline the internal auditory meatus. Prolactin-secreting pituitary adenomas can be treated with the dopamine agonist bromocriptine (Parlodel), useful in reducing the size of these lesions. When the endocrine effects of acidophilic adenomas or the continuous growth of prolactinomas prompt their removal, transsphenoidal microsurgery is preferred unless suprasellar extension of the tumor dictates an intracranial approach. If the large size of a pituitary adenoma precludes complete removal, radiation therapy should follow.

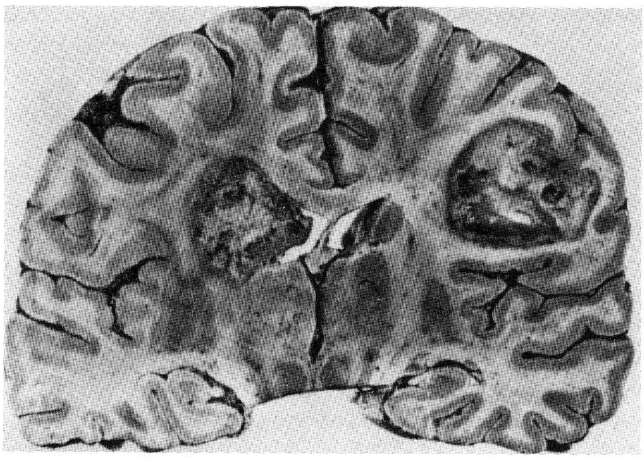

FIGURE 2.2-29. *Metastatic carcinoma (from the lung). The well-circumscribed masses contain necrotic cysts. (From Russell D S, Rubenstein L L:* Pathology of Tumors of the Nervous System, *ed 3, p 267. Williams & Wilkins, Baltimore, 1971, with permission.)*

For malignant gliomas, whole-brain radiation therapy plus a local boost to a total of 6000 rads (tumor dose) is given after subtotal resection of the tumor. Chemotherapy with a nitrosourea, (1,3-bis-(2-chloroethyl)-1-nitrosourea BCNU), is effective in extending survival for a few months. For diagnostic and therapeutic reasons, single metastases should be resected if they are accessible. Steroid and radiation therapies are useful in metastatic brain disease. Anticonvulsants should be given because seizures increase intracranial pressure.

Expected survival for the more common intracranial neoplasms is shown in Table 2.2-2. Prognosis for benign tumors depends on the extent of removal, location, and growth characteristics of the tumor. For malignant gliomas, good prognostic factors include age younger than 45 years, short duration of symptoms (less than 6 months), less malignant tumor histology (e.g., abscence of necrosis), and a normal level of consciousness after surgery. In 1970, the median survival time of patients with malignant gliomas was approximately 6 months. In current prospective clinical trials, the median survival time has been extended to 1 year and 25 percent of the patients survive longer than 18 months. Patients with metastatic brain disease generally succumb to the primary malignancy before the brain lesions recur. When such patients are treated with radiation therapy and steroids, their median survival time is 3 to 6 months.

FLUID, ELECTROLYTE, AND ENDOCRINE DISORDERS

Metabolic encephalopathies are manifested by one or more alterations in behavior, cognitive function, or consciousness; involuntary movements often occur. Disturbances of cognitive function range from mild absentmindedness to loss of all thought processes and disorientation. There may be slight drowsiness, stupor, or coma. Involuntary movements range from tremulousness to asterixis to seizures.

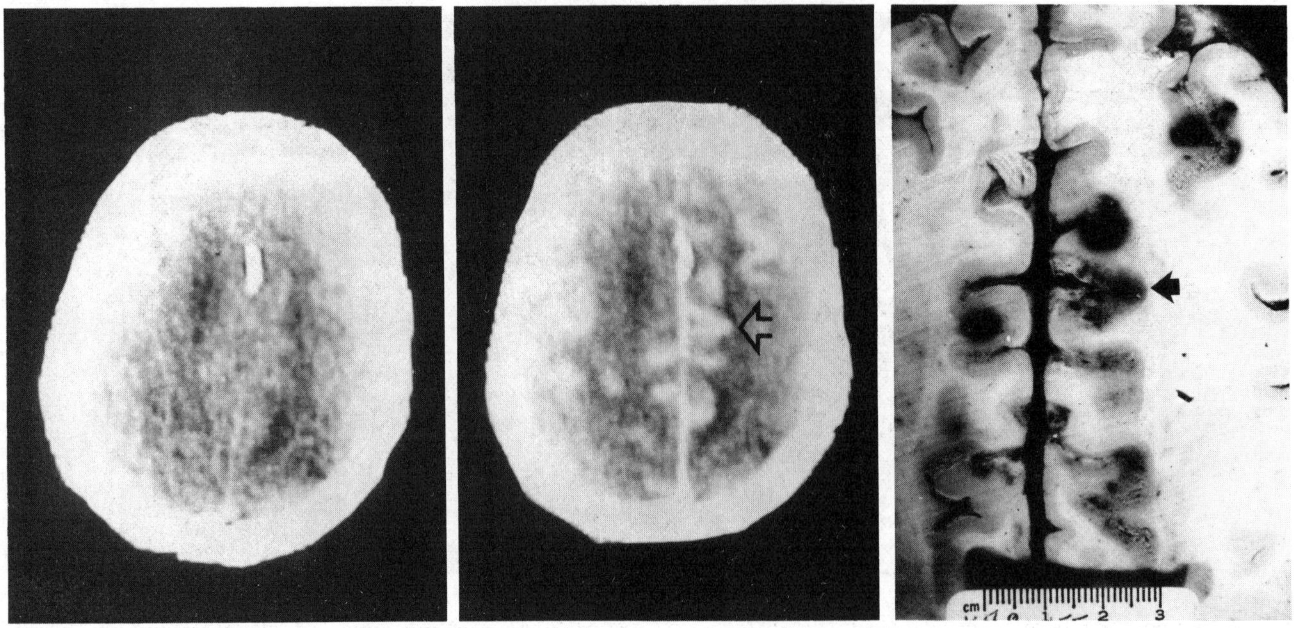

FIGURE 2.2-30. *Malignant melanoma metastatic to brain. CT scan, without* (left) *and with contrast media* (center), *and pathologic specimen* (right). *The tumor infiltrates the cortical ribbon* (arrows). *(From Gonzalez C F, Grosman C B, Masdeu J C:* Head and Spine Imaging, *p 268. Wiley, New York, 1985, with permission.)*

WATER AND ELECTROLYTE ALTERATIONS Both *dehydration* and *overhydration* may cause generalized weakness and encephalopathy. Overhydration may also result in cerebral edema with intracranial hypertension. *Hypernatremia* is usually associated with dehydration. It is often seen in stuporous patients or in others who have not been drinking normally. Diabetes insipidus may rapidly deplete water and is sometimes unrecognized in a comatose patient. Overhydration is often accompanied by *hyponatremia*. Renal disease, with defective excretion of water, or psychogenic polydypsia may cause this condition. *Inappropriate antidiuretic hormone secretion,* with disease or dysfunction of the hypothalamohypophyseal system, may occur in many neurological conditions and after the administration of psychotropic drugs. There is excessive renal excretion of sodium in spite of normal renal function. As a result, hyponatremia, water retention, and hypotonicity of body fluids occur. Fluid restriction, rather than sodium administration, usually corrects all but severe cases.

ACIDOSIS AND ALKALOSIS *Respiratory acidosis (CO_2 narcosis)* is due to respiratory depression, usually caused by drugs or diseases that depress brain respiratory centers or pulmonary disease. Drowsiness and weakness occur, and increased intracranial pressure may result from vasodilation. *Metabolic acidosis* is most often associated with diabetic ketoacidosis and uremic encephalopathy. The hyperpnea of Kussmaul's respiration accompanies lethargy, progressing to stupor and coma.

Respiratory alkalosis is caused by hyperventilation and occurs with hepatic encephalopathy or aspirin intoxication, but it is frequently psychogenic, associated with anxiety. The early symptoms are lightheadedness, feelings of unreality, and paresthesias. Palpitations, drowsiness, tremulousness, tremors, and, finally, tetany may occur. *Tetany* is manifested by carpopedal spasm or laryngospasm; neuromuscular irritability may be demonstrated by Trousseau's and Chvostek's signs. *Metabolic alkalosis,* usually due to excessive vomiting, also causes tetany. There may be associated generalized weakness, apathy, or delirium.

Potassium disorders Both *hyperkalemia* and *hypokalemia* cause flaccid paralysis and lethargy. Paralytic ileus also occurs with hypokalemia. Alterations in serum potassium affect the cardiac rhythm. Depletion of serum potassium may cause cardiac excitation and arrhythmias; excessive serum potassium more often causes heart block. Electrocardiogram (EKG) changes may be diagnostically helpful. Hypokalemia is associated with QT prolongation, a broad T wave, and a large U wave. Hyperkalemia may cause a tall T wave, flattened P wave and widened QRS complex. Hypokalemia is commonly caused by diuretics, renal disease, excessive adrenal steroids, or mineral loss due to gastrointestinal disease. Hyperkalemia is associated with renal disease or deficiency of adrenal steroids. Familial periodic paralysis (hypokalemic) and adynamia episodic hereditaria (hyperkalemia) are discussed later.

Magnesium alterations *Excessive serum magnesium* is usually due to renal insufficiency. It causes decreased neuromuscular responsiveness, respiratory depression, lethargy, and, finally, coma. *Magnesium depletion* often occurs with other deficiencies, especially potassium and vitamin. It is due to malabsorption and renal disease, as associated with alcoholism, diuretic therapy, and diabetic coma. Twitching, coarse irregular tremors, as well as weakness, paresthesias, tetany, and convulsions may occur. Other basal ganglion or cerebellar signs have been reported. Delirium and other features of encephalopathy may be noted.

Complications of hemodialysis A *dysequilibrium syndrome* occurs during dialysis when the osmotic gradiant between the brain and blood causes a shift of water into the brain and resultant cerebral edema. Most patients undergoing dialysis complain of headache. A small percentage of patients also experience nausea, muscle cramps, and changes in mentation, ranging from irritability to delirium or stupor, with or without convulsions.

Progressive encephalopathy may be associated with long-term (2 to 3 years) hemodialysis for chronic renal failure. The standard serum chemistries are not significantly changed, but a disorder of CNS metabolites is postulated. The condition is characterized by dementia, dyspraxia of speech, and abnormal motor activities—myoclonus, asterixis, grimacing, and seizures. The abnormalities are at first transient and occur during dialysis; then they become permanent and progress to death in 3 to 15 months. Aluminum toxicity from the dialysis fluid has been blamed for this condition.

Patients requiring chronic dialysis may also be subject to other neurological complications. Vitamin depletions may cause Wernicke's encephalopathy. Subdural hematomas may occur without obvious trauma.

Hyperalimentation This term refers to the maintenance of nutrition solely by parenteral means. *Hypophosphatemia* is its most common complication. Neurological side effects range from motor signs of weakness or paralysis to ataxia and seizures; in addition, numbness of hands and feet, as well as a diffuse sensory impairment, may occur. Coma with cerebral hemorrhage and death may supervene.

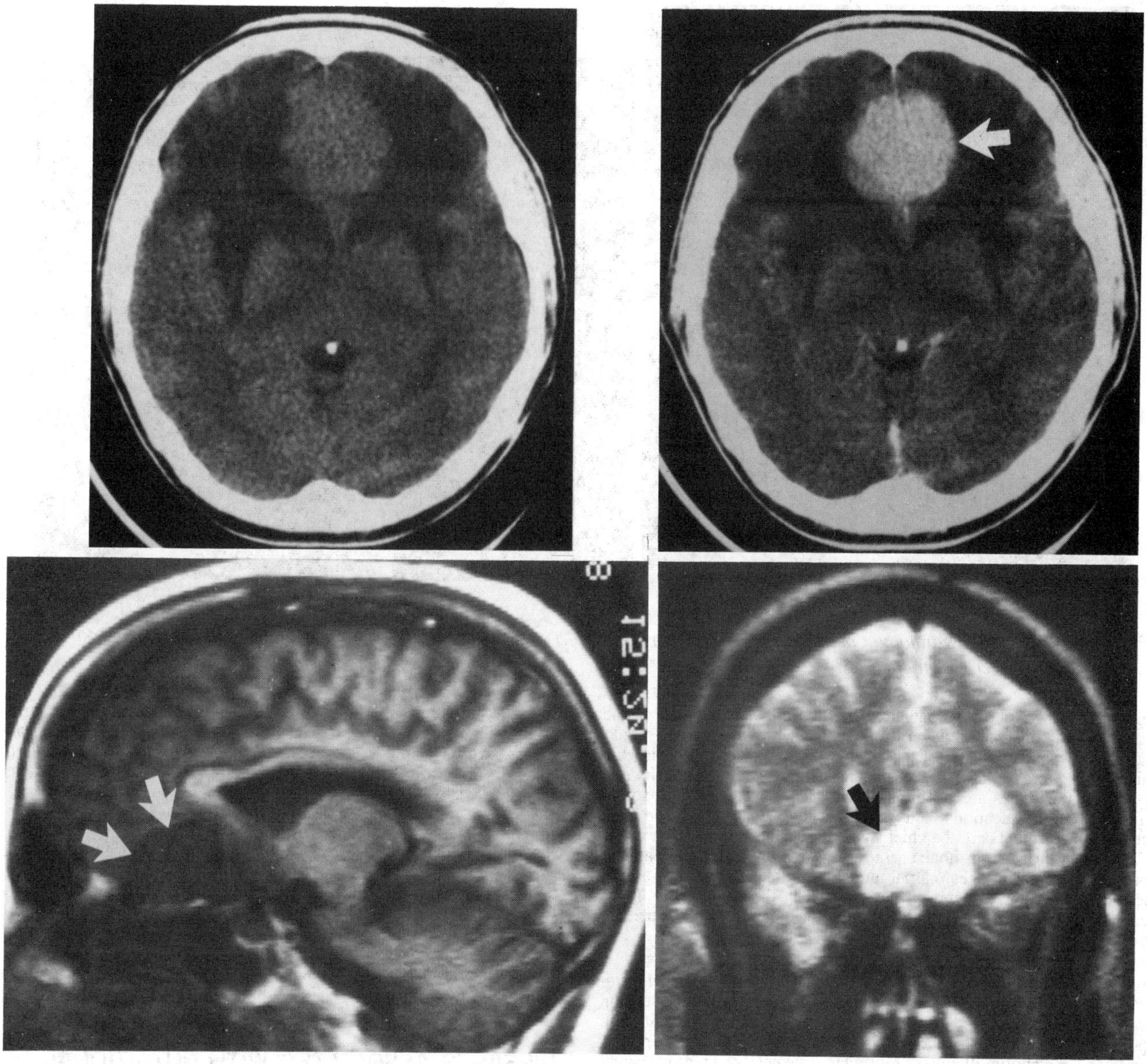

FIGURE 2.2-31. *CT* (top) *and MR* (bottom) *of two different subfrontal meningiomas. CT belongs to a 57-year-old man with a history of long-standing schizophrenia. Urinary incontinence was a recent development. The patient was oriented but had a flat affect. Meningiomata are better visualized with contrast on CT and on MR* T_2*-weighted images* (right-sided panels). *(Courtesy of Charles Elkin, MD, Montefiore Medical Center, New York.)*

ENDOCRINE DISORDERS **Parathyroid and calcium disorders** *Hyperparathyroidism* is associated with hypercalcemia. Excessive serum calcium is also seen in patients with vitamin D overdosage, renal and bone diseases, and malignancy. Hypotonic weakness and pain in the extremities are noted. In severe cases, personality changes, delirium, dementia, stupor, and coma may develop. Osteomalacia is seen in roentgenograms of bones. *Hypoparathyroidism* causes hypocalcemia with muscular cramps, hyperreflexia, tetany, and, finally, convulsions. Paresthesias are common. Increased intracranial pressure may occur, and mental changes range from nervousness to frank psychosis. Cataracts form when the disease is chronic; cerebellar or basal ganglion signs may also develop. Osteoblastic changes in bones and, sometimes, calcifications in the basal ganglia are evident in roentgenograms.

Pancreatic abnormalities *Hyperinsulinism,* causing hypoglycemia, is initially manifested by anxiety, perspiration, hunger, weakness, palpitation, and shortness of breath. Tremor, irritability, increasing confusion, delirium, or frank psychosis may follow. Muscular twitching, convulsive seizures, decerebrate rigidity, and coma are the final signs. The cerebral symptoms of *diabetes* are related to premature atherosclerosis. Diabetic coma (acidosis) has been noted above.

Pancreatic encephalopathy is manifested by agitation and confusion, progressing to delirium and coma. It is said to occur in association with acute pancreatitis, especially in alcoholics. However, there is doubt as to whether it represents a specific entity, rather than a combination of the effects of alcoholism, shock, and metabolic defects that accompany pancreatitis.

Thyroid dysfunctions *Hyperthyroidism* causes an increase in sweating, appetite, and fatigue, as well as tachycardia and dyspnea on exertion. Myopathy, especially quadriceps weakness and eye signs (e.g., exophthalmos, lid swelling, lid lag, and ophthalmopareses), are common. Fine tremor is noted; choreiform movements and, rarely, convulsions may develop. The disease is associated with emotional symptoms of anxiety, lability of affect, irritability, and agitation. Thyroid crisis may result in acute delirium and other symp-

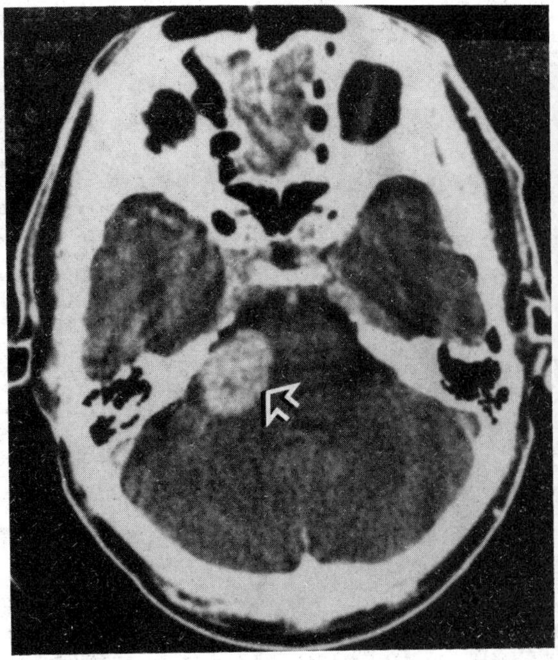
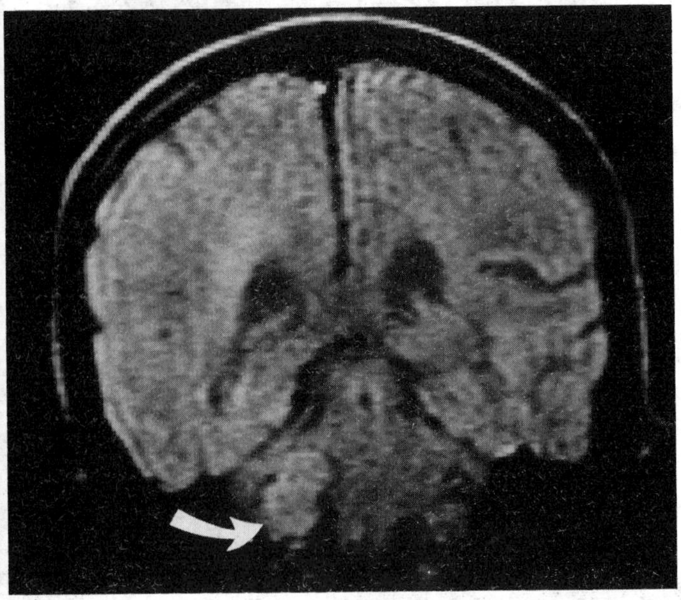

FIGURE 2.2-32. *Schwannoma, or acoustic neurinoma. Axial CT with contrast* (left) *and coronal MR* (right). *(Courtesy of Charles Elkin, MD, Montefiore Medical Center, New York.)*

toms of toxic psychosis. Apathetic hyperthyroidism rarely occurs and may lead to coma. *Myxedema* is associated with lethargy and weakness. The skin, especially of the face, is dry and puffy; the hair, thin and brittle (Fig. 2.2-36). There is decreased psychomotor activity and personality changes are common—most often depression, but sometimes paranoid ideations and frank psychosis. Memory and perceptual impairments are the chief signs of dementia. Headache, dizziness, dysarthria, and hoarseness are often present. Myopathies, pseudomyotonic reflexes, carpal tunnel entrapment neuropathy, and, less often, peripheral neuropathies may affect the extremities. Truncal ataxia sometimes occurs. Hypothermia and coma are terminal events.

Adrenal gland diseases *Primary aldosteronism (hyperaldosteronism),* a dysfunction of the adrenal cortex, causes hypertension with potential cardiac and cerebral complications. Polyuria and polydypsia may occur. There is associated hypokalemia, hypernatremia, and metabolic alkalosis. Muscular weakness or cramps, paresthesias, and headaches are common symptoms.

Cushing's syndrome (hyperadrenocorticism) causes obesity of the face, neck, and trunk, with purplish striae (Fig. 2.2-37). Amenorrhea, hirsutism, and loss of libido also occur. Patients with this disease frequently develop diabetes mellitus and hypertension. Weakness, fatigability, and personality changes are common.

Pheochromocytoma is a tumor of the adrenal medulla that causes paroxysms of severe hypertension. The encephalopathy evokes headache, dizziness, and paresthesias, as well as other encephalopathic features. Perspiration, palpitation, pallor, coldness of extremities, nausea, and vomiting may occur. Cerebral hemorrhage is a potential complication.

Addison's disease, decreased function of the adrenal cortex, is manifested by progressive asthenia, fatigue, weight loss, and weakness. Irritability, apprehension, and personality changes are common. Syncope and shock are associated with hypotension, and tremors or convulsions sometimes occur. Abdominal distress and pigmentation of the skin and mucosa are characteristic of this disease.

Adrenogenital syndrome, adrenal hyperplasia, is associated with virilization in children (congenital form), with masculinization in women and, sometimes, with feminization in men (acquired form, such as adenocarcinoma). There are no primary neurological symptoms.

Pituitary disorders *Hyperpituitarism,* due to an eosinophilic adenoma in an adult, causes acromegaly (Fig. 2.2-38). Arthralgias, muscular weakness, and personality changes frequently occur. The tumor in children is manifested by gigantism. Basophilic adenomas, even though minute, lead to Cushing's syndrome. *Hypopituitarism* causes apathy, asthenia, fatigue, and lethargy. The facies is often bland; the skin waxen, pale, and dry; and the body free of hair. There is associated hypofunction of other endocrine glands, especially the ovaries and testes; hypothermia and hypotension may occur. Minor emotional symptoms are common, but depression and frank psychosis sometimes occur. This condition in children results in dwarfism. *Pituitary apoplexy* is due to bland or hemorrhagic infarction of the pituitary and occurs in the postpartum period, with other systemic stresses, or in patients with a pituitary adenoma. There is acute hypopituitarism with headache, hypotension, and drowsiness; diabetes insipidus and hypoglycemia may supervene. Coma and death often occur unless prompt treatment with steroids or surgical transsphenoidal decompression is instituted.

DISEASES ASSOCIATED WITH NUTRITIONAL FACTORS

VITAMIN DEFICIENCY Vitamins, especially of the B complex group, are essential for neuronal metabolism.

Vitamin B complex *Thiamine (vitamin B_1) deficiency* may result in *beriberi,* with peripheral, predominantly sensory, neuropathy. In severe deficiency, mental symptoms and cerebral edema have been noted. Thiamine deficiency is a major factor in the cause of Wernicke's encephalopathy.

Niacin deficiency causes pellagra, although pellagra is truly a polyavitaminosis. The familiar triad is dementia, diarrhea, and dermatitis; delirium and convulsive seizures may also occur. Motor signs implicating the peripheral nerves, pyramidal tracts, cerebellum, or extrapyramidal system occur late, if at all. In the United States, pellagra is likely to be seen as a result of alcoholism.

Pyridoxine (vitamin B_6) deficiency may cause convulsions in infants. Vitamin B_6 deficiency does not occur in adults, except in those being treated with isoniazid, or hydralazine (Apresoline); the medications interfere with pyridoxine metabolism, and a sensory polyneuropathy may result.

Vitamin B_{12} deficiency causes pernicious anemia. The neurological syndrome of *subacute combined degeneration* is a disorder of middle or late adult life, which may develop within a few weeks or months. It may precede the anemia, especially when folate is used for treatment. Achlorhydria is present, the B_{12} level in the serum is de-

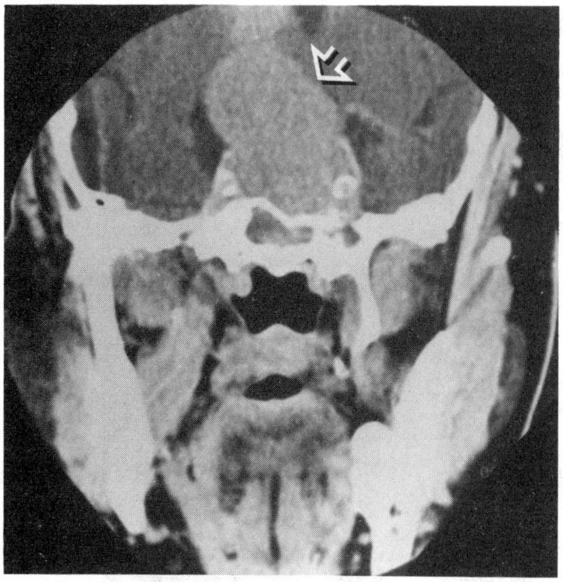

FIGURE 2.2-33. *Large pituitary adenoma, on contrast-enhanced coronal CT, in 68-year-old man with a 20-year history of headaches, impotence, and progressive visual loss. Most recent admission was due to delirium caused by hyponatremia. (Courtesy of Charles Elkin, MD, Montefiore Medical Center, New York.)*

pressed, and the Schilling test is diagnostic. The neurological signs implicating the spinal cord are spastic weakness and ataxia, due to demyelination of the lateral and posterior columns of the cord. Peripheral neuropathy is common. Cerebral manifestations are disturbances of personality or dementia.

Vitamin A deficiency This deficiency may cause mental retardation and hydrocephalus with papilledema. It occurs in infants and preschool children who do not drink milk.

Vitamin C deficiency *Scurvy,* when severe, is sometimes associated with intracranial bleeding.

Vitamin D deficiency This condition causes rickets in children and osteomalacia in adults. Anticonvulsant drugs may cause osteomalacia and rickets as well. Tetany or convulsions occur late in the course of rickets.

Vitamin E deficiency Hypolipoproteinemia in patients who have chronic fat malabsorption may result in a lack of vitamin E. The rare neurologic defects may include retinopathy, ophthalmoplegia, polyneuropathy, and spinocerebellar degeneration manifested by ataxia, dysarthria, and proprioceptive loss.

ALCOHOLISM The harmful effects of alcoholic beverages are twofold. Alcohol tends to be ingested to the exclusion of food, with resultant nutritional deficiencies, and alcohol has direct toxic effects on the nervous system. The syndromes related to alcohol toxicity are discussed later. The nutritional deficiencies, especially of the vitamin B complex group, may cause devastating encephalopathies.

Wernicke's encephalopathy This disease is characterized by eye signs (oculomotor or conjugate gaze palsies and nystagmus); ataxia, especially of gait; and mental aberrations (delirium, a confused apathetic state, or Korsakoff's syndrome). Consciousness may be depressed, and convulsions sometimes occur. Thiamine deficiency is the predominant cause, and prompt IV administration of this vitamin with glucose may be lifesaving. On examination of the brain (Fig. 2.2-39), petechial hemorrhages and necrosis are found in the upper brain stem and diencephalon, particularly in the mammillary bodies and periventricular nuclei.

Korsakoff's syndrome This condition is characterized mainly by recent, short-term memory loss. Long-term memory impairment, other manifestations of an organic mental disorder, and confabulation may occur. Delirium tremens frequently precedes the mental symptoms. Polyneuropathy and Wernicke's encephalopathy are usually superimposed. Korsakoff's syndrome may have causes other than nutritional deprivation. Ischemic lesions may permanently impair the memory centers in the dorsal medial thalamic nuclei, the medial

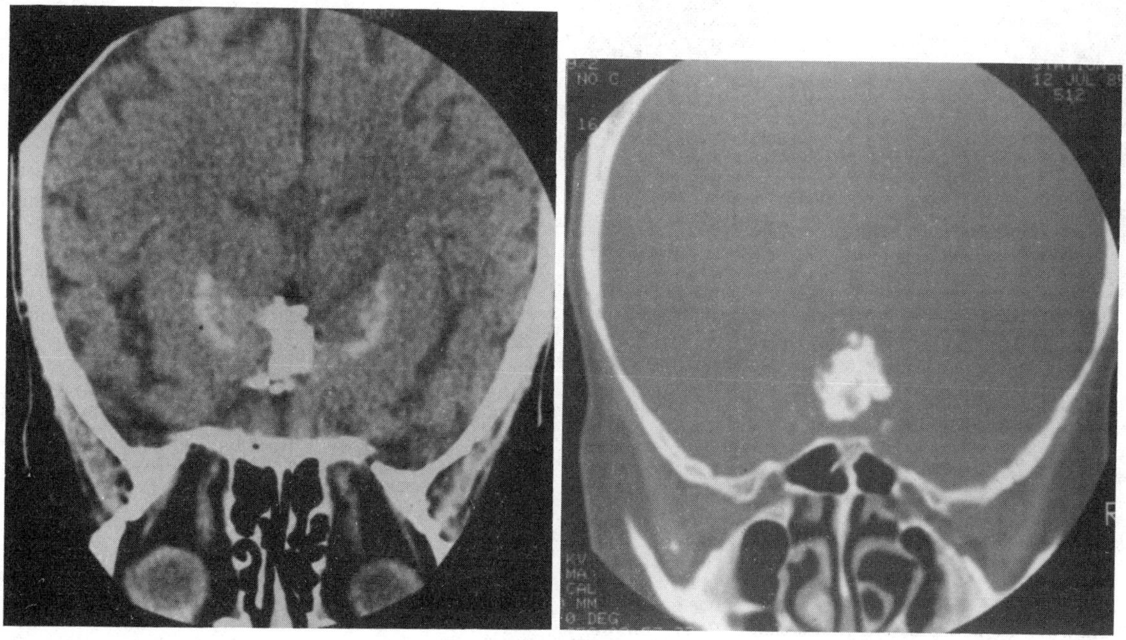

FIGURE 2.2-34. *Craniopharyngioma. CT scan (bone-window on the* right) *was obtained without contrast in a 47-year-old woman with panhypopituitarism. She had been treated with radiation therapy at age 6. Currently the tumor was calcified. (Courtesy of Charles Elkin, MD, Montefiore Medical Center, New York.)*

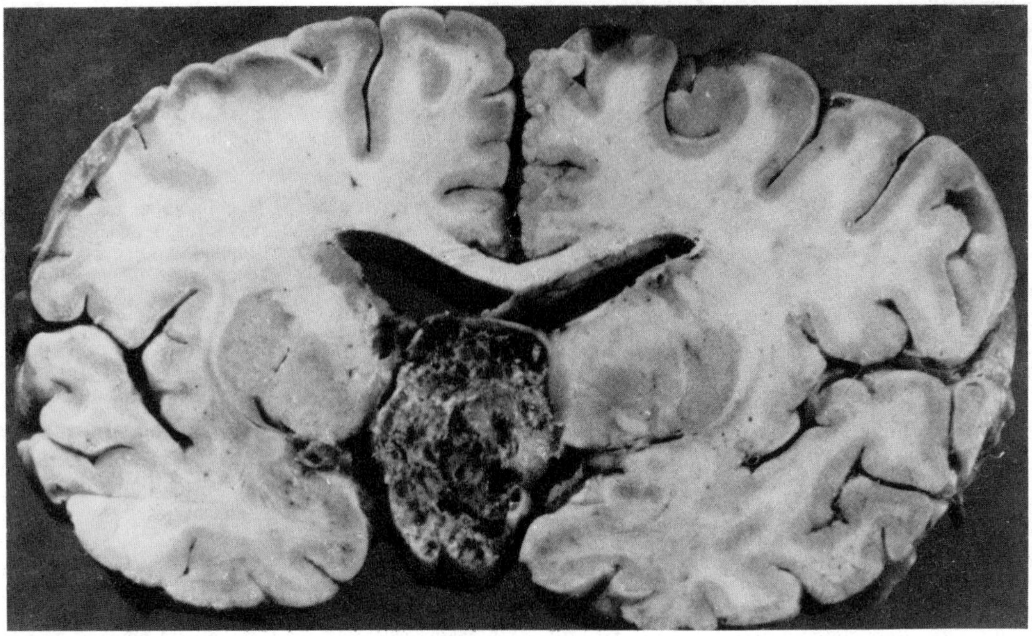

FIGURE 2.2-35. *Craniopharyngioma. The suprasellar tumor protrudes upward obstructing the third ventricle. (From Hirano A:* A Guide to Neuropathology, *p 84. Igaku-Shoin, New York, 1981, with permission.)*

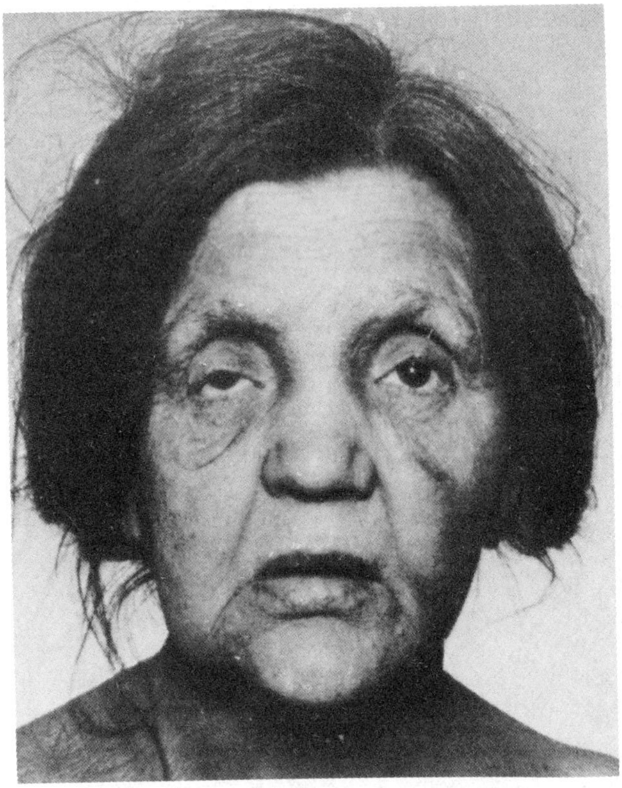

FIGURE 2.2-36. *Myxedema. The facial skin is puffy, the hair thin and brittle. The face has a dull, lifeless look. (From Spillane J D, Spillane J A:* An Atlas of Clinical Neurology, *ed 3, p 343. Oxford University Press, New York, 1982, with permission.)*

pulvinar, and the mammillary bodies. Even when Korsakoff's syndrome is associated with alcoholism, treatment with thiamine and glucose is less strikingly beneficial than in Wernicke's disease.

Alcoholic cerebellar degeneration Chronic alcohol abuse may lead to degeneration of the anterior cerebellar lobe and subsequent ataxia, predominantly affecting the trunk and legs. Examination may be normal until the patient is asked to stand and walk.

Central pontine myelinolysis This acute and fatal disease occurs mainly in adults. A history of chronic alcoholism is usually noted, but other causes of severe nutritional deprivation in gravely ill patients may lead to this disease. The chief manifestations are quadriplegia with brain stem signs; pseudocoma, the locked-in syndrome, may occur.

Marchiafava-Bignami disease This rare condition occurs in men of middle or late life who are chronic alcoholics. The clinical features are predominantly those of a frontal lobe syndrome, with psychomotor retardation; associated features may include delirium, seizures, and hallucinosis. Apraxia occurs more often than aphasia. Death occurs after 3 to 6 years, and autopsy reveals demyelination of the medial portion of the corpus callosum.

Other neurological illnesses Peripheral neuropathy is common in chronic alcoholics. Chronic neuropathy results in weakness and atrophy in the legs, much more than in the arms. Myelopathy, myopathy, and optic neuropathy may occur. Hepatic encephalopathy is discussed below.

TOXIC DISEASES AFFECTING THE BRAIN

Neuronal degeneration and demyelination are found in both acute and chronic toxic lesions. When metabolism is disturbed, death may occur without appreciable microscopic changes. The brain is affected in different ways by different

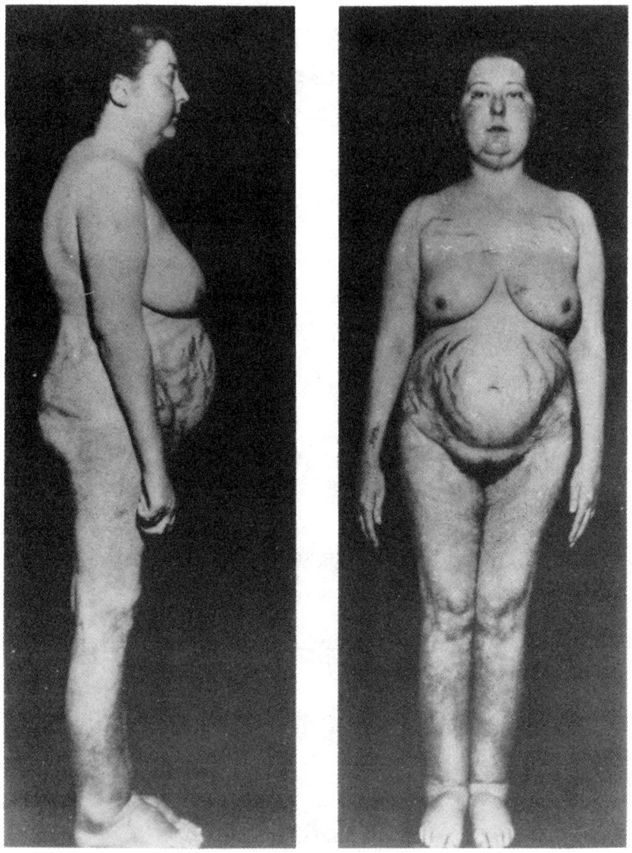

FIGURE 2.2-37. *Cushing's syndrome: Obesity and round face are evident. Hirsutism and abdominal striae are noted. (From Spillane J D, Spillane J A:* An Atlas of Clinical Neurology, *ed 3, p 365. Oxford University Press, New York, 198, with permission.)*

toxins. Heavy metals and organic toxins are protoplasmic poisons causing neuronal degeneration. Some heavy metals interfere with neuronal enzyme systems, whereas the toxin of botulism disturbs nerve impulse transmission. In addition to these direct effects on neuronal metabolism, nerve cells may be affected by systemic metabolic alterations caused by toxins. Toxins may evoke a direct inflammatory reaction or an arteritis. Anoxic poisons cause vasodilation and increased capillary permeability with petechial hemorrhages.

The toxic encephalitides present evidence of generalized cerebral dysfunction; focal signs are usually absent or minimal. In adults, early signs of intoxications are maladaptive behavior, impairment of judgment, and, often, belligerence. Later, symptoms of headache and dizziness are accompanied by lethargy, confusion, and delirium. Convulsive seizures may occur. Systemic signs depend on the offending agent; fever may or may not be present. Acute toxic encephalopathy in children is manifested by the sudden onset of fever, nausea, vomiting, stupor, delirium, or convulsions. The child may be flaccid, but more often manifests increased muscle tone, with stiff neck; papilledema may occur. In adults, and particularly in children, multiple factors may contribute to the acute toxic encephalopathy. The effect of the toxin itself, the high fever and its associated dehydration, the changes in serum electrolytes, other alterations in blood chemistry, and anoxia secondary to a convulsion or to respiratory deficits must all be considered.

ENDOGENOUS TOXINS The most common endogenous toxins are associated with uremia, diabetic acidosis, and hepatic failure. Porphyria is a rare disease in this category. Eclampsia was once thought to be due to toxins, but it is now recognized as a manifestation of uncontrolled hypertension.

Diabetic or uremic coma Lethargy and stupor precede coma. Delirium and seizures commonly occur in acute uremia; signs of meningeal irritation also may be noted. Kussmaul respirations are most often associated with diabetic coma. Distal polyneuropathy often occurs with uremia and, especially, diabetes.

Hepatic coma or hepatic encephalopathy In this disorder, insidious impairment of mental processes leads to stupor and coma. Sometimes, delirium and other evidence of toxic psychosis occur. Asterixis is characteristic of impending hepatic coma. The EEG often shows diffuse, slow activity, with bilaterally synchronous triphasic waves. Both asterixis and triphasic waves may occur with other metabolic encephalopathy.

Porphyria In this inherited disorder of porphyrin metabolism, an enzyme deficiency prevents the inhibition of porphyrin synthesis. The most common form affects young and middle-aged adults, more often women than men. The disease is characterized by episodic bouts of abdominal pain, other visceral symptoms, and peripheral neuropathy. Cognitive and emotional symptoms, as well as convulsive seizures, are common. Exacerbations may be precipitated by the ingestion of many agents, including alcohol and barbiturates. Porphobilinogen is found in the urine.

EXOGENOUS TOXINS These toxins may be grouped as alcohol, drugs, biological toxins, heavy metals, and industrial toxins. Only the most common poisons will be discussed.

Alcohol The most common of all toxins is ethyl alcohol. Methyl alcohol is much more toxic and causes blindness by particularly affecting the ganglion cells of the retina and optic nerve fibers. Acute ethyl alcoholic intoxication, simple drunkenness, is an all-too-well-recognized entity. There is deterioration of behavior and attention, change of mood and irritability, as well as signs of dysarthria, ataxia, and nystagmus. Rarely, assaultive behavior occurs, of which the patient may have no memory. Bouts of amnesia may occur during severe, acute alcoholic intoxication, termed *blackouts* by alcoholics. During these periods, consciousness is not impaired, but memory of events does not occur. This condition probably has a pathophysiological basis other than psychological repression. In its extreme form, acute intoxication may lead to coma. Encephalopathy may also occur as a result of alcoholic liver disease, rather than because of direct effects of alcohol.

Acute alcoholic hallucinosis Accusatory or threatening auditory hallucinations are accompanied by fear and apprehension. This condition may be a psychotic phenomenon liberated by alcohol, rather than a toxic reaction. In rare instances, this condition evolves into chronic alcoholic hallucinosis and may be mistaken for paranoid schizophrenia.

Alcoholic withdrawal syndromes Between 8 and 48 hours after relative or absolute withdrawal from alcohol, several phenomena may occur; the extreme form of these events is delirium tremens. Restlessness, tremulousness, or coarse tremors are often referred to as "the shakes" or "the jitters." They usually occur in the morning after a night's abstinence. Nausea, vomiting, and insomnia are commonly associated. Withdrawal seizures or "rum fits" are of the generalized tonic-clonic type, occur in chronic alcoholics, and are often a precursor of delirium tremens. Extreme psychomotor activity, with confusion, is associated with the shakes or seizures. Visual delusions, more often than auditory hallucinations, and associated anxiety are accompanied by autonomic dysfunctions (e.g., fever, perspiration, tachycardia, hypertension, hypotension). Intercurrent infection or in-

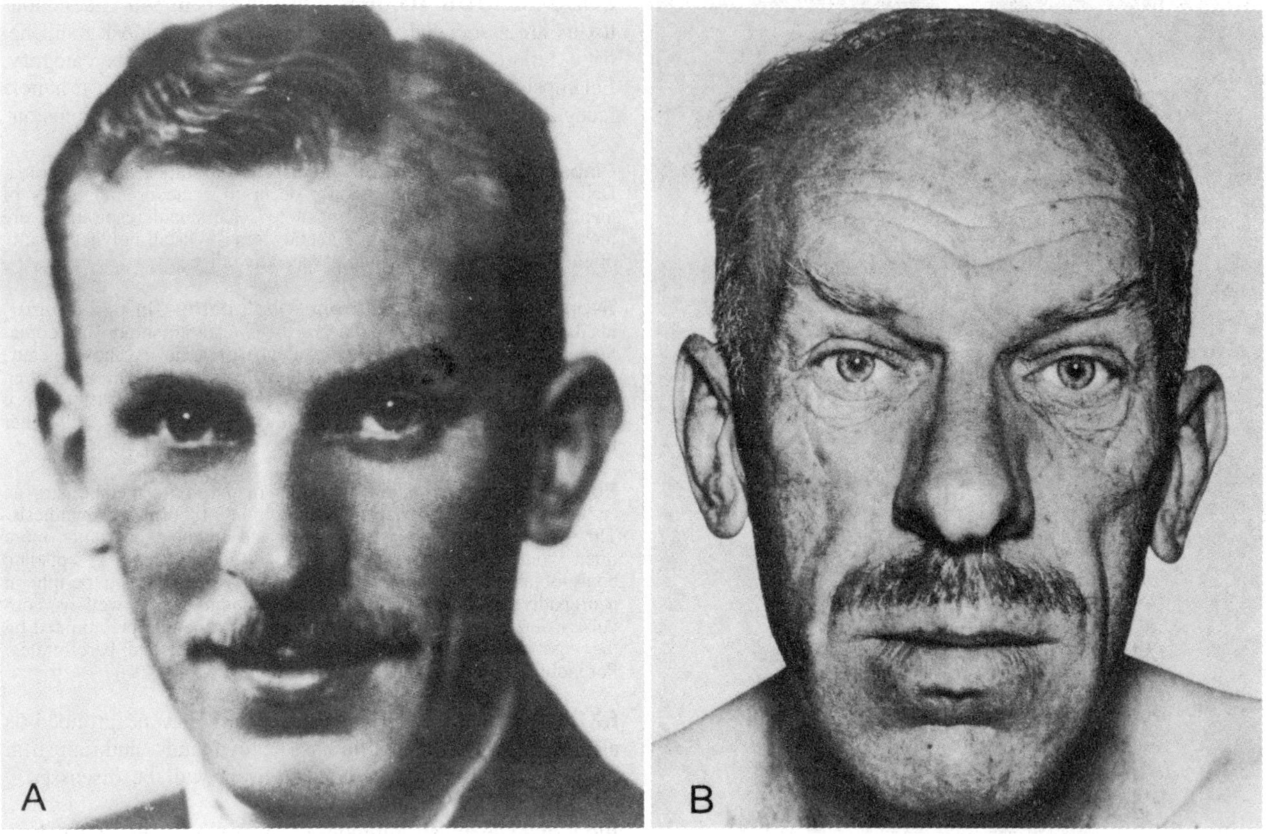

FIGURE 2.2-38. A. *Before onset of acromegaly.* B. *Acromegaly. Enlargement of the mandible, nose, and lips are obvious. (From Spillane J D, Spillane J A:* An Atlas of Clinical Neurology, *ed 3, p 356. Oxford University Press, New York, 1982, with permission.)*

jury, as well as alcoholic withdrawal, may precipitate delirium tremens 2 to 4 days later. Treatment consists of restoring fluid and electrolyte balances with vitamin supplementation while controlling hyperactivity with high doses of minor tranquilizers, such as chlordiazepoxide (Librium). If associated traumatic brain lesions are suspected, phenytoin (Dilantin) may be helpful for seizure control. The bout of delirium tremens usually subsides after 72 hours, but the mortality rate ranges from 5 to 15 percent.

Other disorders associated with chronic alcoholism Not all the disorders listed under alcoholic nutritional diseases have been proved to be attributable to specific nutritional factors. Other conditions of uncertain pathogenesis that are seen in chronic alcoholics are probably due to a combination of nutritional, toxic, and systemic factors. Alcoholic dementia with degeneration of personality and cognition may be attributed to the conjunction of repeated trauma, hepatic encephalopathy, and chronic Wernicke-Korsakoff syndrome.

Fetal alcohol syndrome Alcoholic abuse by a pregnant mother may adversely affect the fetus. At birth, such infants are shorter than normal and have a smaller head size. Congenital abnormalities of the face, palate, and hips and other joints may occur; moreover, cardiac and genital abnormalities are possible. The neonatal mortality is high, and mental retardation is common in the survivors.

Drugs There are hundreds of drugs that may affect the nervous system. The toxic effects of agents used to treat specific neurological disorders, such as parkinsonism and epilepsy, are discussed in the sections dealing with these diseases. Only the major drug categories most relevant to the psychiatrist are discussed here. This discussion of the features of drug toxicity is necessarily brief and includes mainly those factors that help to clinically distinguish one type of drug toxicity from another.

Habituating and addicting drugs Morphine, heroin, and other addicting opioids cause initial euphoria, then dysphoria and apathy with psychomotor retardation. With high dosage, depression of consciousness, respiration, and heart rate occur; impairment of attention and other cognitive features are associated. Miosis is an important clue. During the withdrawal period, either spontaneous or induced by naloxone (Narcan), there are autonomic signs of mydriasis, tearing, and rhinorrhea, with excessive perspiration, piloerection, and diarrhea. Tachycardia, fever, and slight hypertension are common. The patient yawns frequently but cannot sleep.

Cocaine is usually sold as the powder of the hydrochloride salt and is snorted intranasally. More recently, the alkaloid of cocaine (crack) has also become popular; it is almost pure cocaine. Crack is smoked (free-based) and produces an effect comparable to intravenous injection. There is an almost immediate, intense, euphoric effect; but within minutes, a dysphoric letdown occurs, leading to repeated doses and rapid addiction. During the euphoric state, the person is talkative and grandiose, with increased psychomotor activity, which may lead to agitation or maladaptive behavior. The CNS-stimulating effect of cocaine causes tachycardia and hypertension and may lead to fever, ventricular arrhythmias, intracranial hemorrhage, seizures, and death. Anxiety, tactile hallucinations, paranoid ideations, and depression have been noted.

The amphetamines induce excitement that may lead to delirium. On withdrawal, depression and sleep disturbances occur. Lysergic acid diethylamide (LSD), phencyclidine (angel dust), and mescaline evoke visual hallucinations, panic attacks, and schizophrenic-like behavior. Marijuana's effects, when mild, resemble alcoholic intoxication and, when severe, are similar to those of LSD.

Anoxic toxins Anoxic toxins prevent oxygen from reaching nerve cells by depressing respiration. In this group of anesthetics and hypnotics, the barbiturates are most commonly abused. Anoxic

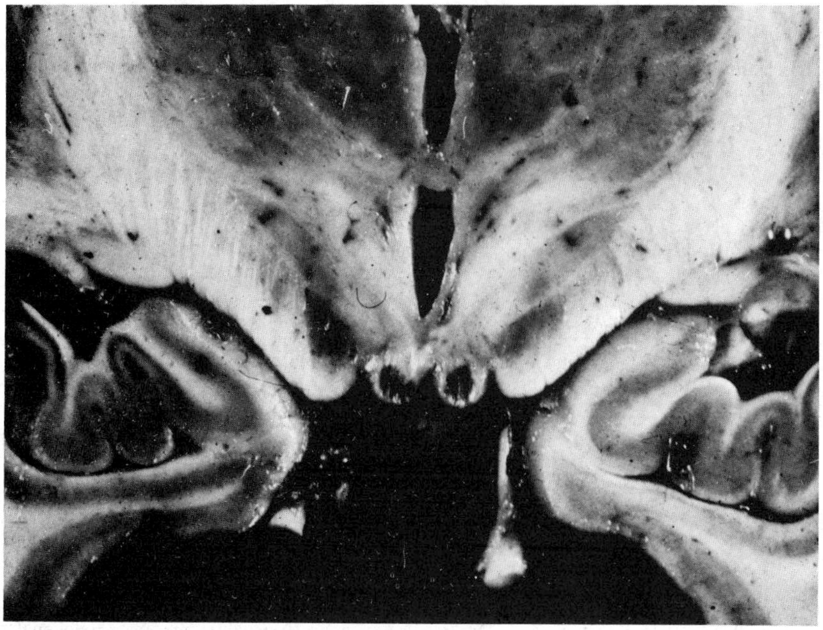

FIGURE 2.2-39. *Wernicke's encephalopathy. Bilateral hemorrhagic necrosis is seen in the mammillary bodies, and necrotic zones are scattered in the hypothalamus near the third ventricle. (From Robertson D M, Dinsdale H B:* The Nervous System, *p 71. Williams & Wilkins, Baltimore, 1972, with permission.)*

toxins may also prevent oxygen from being used by nerve cells. Carbon monoxide and cyanide are the best examples of this group.

Intoxication by barbiturates is manifested by the gradual depression of consciousness, leading to coma. In the early stages, impairment of cognitive functions, deterioration of behavior, and, occasionally, delirium occur. Depressed respiration is a prominent sign. During coma, preservation of pupillary reactivity may be the only sign of neural life. The duration of coma has greater prognostic significance than its depth. Diffuse, fast activity in the EEG may be an important clue in establishing the diagnosis; the determination of barbiturate levels in gastric contents, blood, or urine is definitive. Respiratory support is the most essential part of therapy. The signs of barbiturate withdrawal are similar to those of alcoholic withdrawal.

Psychotropic drugs Psychotropic drugs refer to the major tranquilizers: the antipsychotic agents and antidepressant compounds. The so-called minor tranquilizers are best labeled as antianxiety drugs and their toxic effects most closely resemble toxic effects of the barbiturates. Major psychotropic drug intoxication may cause neuronal damage, most pronounced in the basal ganglia, hypothalamus, and mesencephalon. Table 2.2-3 lists the clinical manifestations of the side effects and intoxications. This outline refers, for the most part, to major tranquilizers-antipsychotics, as exemplified by the phenothiazines; the butyrophenones have similar but usually fewer side effects. Most of these symptoms may also occur with antidepressant drugs, either tricyclic derivatives or monoamine oxidase inhibitors (MAOIs).

Sedation, postural hypotension, anticholinergic symptoms and extrapyramidal signs are the most common adverse effects of chlorpromazine (Thorazine). Sedation and hypotension are less likely with perphenazine (Trilafon), fluphenazine (Permitil), trifluoperazine (Stelazine), haloperidol (Haldol), thiothixene (Navane), or molindone (Lidone, Moban).

Extrapyramidal disorders are among the most common side effects of the major tranquilizers. Acute dystonia and akathisia usually appear at the onset of therapy. The dystonia usually affects the face, tongue, and neck, but oculogyric crisis and dyskinesia of the limbs may also occur. These reactions respond to parenteral diphenhydramine (Benadryl). Signs of parkinsonism appear after therapy is in progress. These phenomena are reversible and respond to lowering dosage or drug withdrawal and anticholinergic-antiparkinsonism medications.

Tardive dyskinesia is manifested by buccal-lingual-facial-masticatory involuntary movements, which may be accompanied by dystonic or choreoathetoid movements of the neck, trunk, and extremities. This phenomenon is common after long-term psychotropic therapy or after the discontinuation of such therapy; the disorder is often irreversible. Tardive dyskinesia is noted particularly in the elderly who have received high doses of antipsychotic agents, especially the phenothiazines or haloperidol. The disorder seems to be due to denervation hypersensitivity of dopamine receptors in the basal ganglia that had been chronically blocked by the tranquilizer. The dyskinesia can be inhibited by reinstitution of psychotropic medication. Reserpine, which inhibits dopaminergic transmission presynaptically, is preferred to phenothiazines or haloperidol. Acetylcholine precursors, such as deanol (Deaner) and choline, may be of some therapeutic benefit. Focal perioral tremor, known as *rabbit syndrome,* is another late side effect of antipsychotic drugs. It responds well to antiparkinsonian agents.

The *neuroleptic malignant syndrome* is an uncommon idiosyncratic reaction to antipsychotic medication, affecting men five times more often than women. It is manifested by extrapyramidal signs, including catatonic-like rigidity and tremulousness; hyperthermia, labile blood pressure, and other autonomic dysfunction; and obtundation. Death due to respiratory failure occurs in 20 percent of patients. Treatment with bromocriptine and dantrolene sodium (Dantrium) is more effective than anticholinergic-antiparkinson agents or the benzodiazepines.

The most frequent complications of the tricyclic antidepressant drugs are anticholinergic, cardiovascular, and neurological. Dryness of the mouth is more common than glaucoma, urinary retention, paralytic ileus, and impotence. Hypotension, especially the orthostatic type, occurs much more often than cardiac arrhythmias associated with heart block or tachycardia. Sedation is the major neurological symptom, but delirium may be evoked in the elderly. Weight gain is common. Muscle twitching, restlessness, and insomnia may progress to confusion, agitation, and toxic psychosis. The MAOIs may cause hypertensive crisis when taken in conjunction with tyramine-rich foods, sympathomimetic drugs (including over-the-counter cold remedies), tryptophan, levodopa (Larodopa, Dopar), and meperidine (Demerol). Hypotension, restlessness, insomnia, and afternoon sleepiness are common side effects; anticholinergic symptoms, tremors, and paresthesias are uncommon.

TABLE 2.2–3
Manifestations of Psychotropic Drug Side Effects or Intoxication

I. Toxic effects on the nervous system
  A. Mental and emotional reactions
    1. Impaired psychomotor function*
    2. Restlessness and excitement†
    3. Confusion and delirium
    4. Insomnia and bizarre dreams
    5. Increase in schizophrenic symptoms or in depression
  B. Autonomic and endocrine disturbances
    1. Alteration of vital signs
      a. Tachycardia,† bradycardia, or other cardiac arrhythmias
      b. Hypotension, especially orthostatic*†; hypertension† with sympathominetic drugs and tyramine-containing foods
      c. Depression of respiration
      d. Disturbed temperature regulation, both hypothermia and heat stroke
    2. Anticholinergic symptoms
      a. Dry mouth† and skin
      b. Paresis or paralysis of the bladder or bowel†
      c. Tachycardia and fever
      d. Dilated pupils
      e. Mental and motor signs (as above)
    3. Altered sexual factors
      a. Inhibition of ejaculation* and impotence† in men or, paradoxically, increase in libido in women
      b. Hyperprolactinemia with gynecomastia, lactation, and amenorrhea
      c. False-positive pregnancy test
    4. Other effects
      a. Weight gain,† peripheral edema†
      b. Hyperglycemia or hypoglycemia
      c. Nasal congestion, excessive perspiration
  C. Other neurological phenomena
    1. Lethargy, somnolence, fatigue*
    2. Involuntary movements*: dyskinesias, muscle spasms, parkinsonism, fine tremor,† akathisia, dystonia, tetanus-like syndromes
    3. Convulsive seizures
    4. Other neurological symptoms (headache, dizziness, weakness)
    5. EEG slow-wave or paroxysmal abnormality
    6. Peripheral neuropathy

II. Other systemic toxic reactions
  A. Primary reaction
    1. Cholestatic jaundice* and xanthomatous biliary cirrhosis, liver cell disease†
    2. Contact and other dermatitis,*† skin photosensitivity
    3. Blood dycrasias, eosinophilia, anemia, agranulocytosis, pancytopenia, thrombocytopenia
    4. Pigmentary retinopathy, melanin pigmentation of the cornea and lens
    5. Renal disease
    6. Gastrointestinal disturbances
    7. Questionable teratogenic effects
    8. Vagolytic quinidine-like effect in electrocardiogram
    9. Shock after electroconvulsive therapy
    10. Death due to overdosage
  B. Secondary effect on other modalities
    1. The potentiation of other drugs, such as sedatives, narcotics, anesthetics, amphetamines, hypotensive agents, digitalis, insulin; the potentiation of alcohol and its complications
    2. Sedation leading to hypostatic pneumonia and trophic ulcers

*Most common with antipsychotics.
†Most common with antidepressants.

The first side effects of lithium toxicity are nausea, fine tremor, fatigue, weight gain, polyuria, and thirst. Lithium predisposes to heat stroke. At toxic serum concentrations, vomiting, diarrhea, dizziness, ataxia, weakness, dysarthria, extrapyramidal effects, and blurred vision may be associated with changes in conscious and mental status. Lithium must be used with caution in patients with renal or cardiac disease. In the early stages of intoxication, drug withdrawal and sodium chloride with fluid replacement are indicated. In severe cases, hemodialysis is the treatment of choice. Damage to the cerebellar and basal ganglion pathways is rarely permanent.

Other drugs Neostigmine (Prostigmine) and other agents used for myasthenia gravis may cause excessive cholinergic activity because of their cholinesterase inhibition. The toxicity may be manifested by muscarinic effects of abdominal cramps, lacrimation, and incontinence; nicotinic effects of fasciculations, followed by generalized muscle weakness and paralysis; and CNS effects of headache, dizziness, personality changes, lethargy, and convulsions. Atropine and its related compounds produce a central anticholinergic effect with mental symptoms of amnesia, hallucinations, illusions of unreality, or delirium and with motor signs of weakness, ataxia, restlessness, excitement, or choreiform activity. The antineoplastic agents may affect any part of the nervous system. Vincristine (Oncovin) commonly causes peripheral neuropathy; 5-fluorouracil (Adrucil) may cause cerebellar dysfunction; high doses of methotrexate (Folex, Mexate) are associated with leucoencephalopathy. Penicillin may cause convulsions when administered in high dosage, and other antibiotics may injure cochlear or vestibular function. Salicylates are the most readily available antiinflammatory-analgesic agents and at toxic levels may cause respiratory alkalosis with global cerebral disturbance. Digitalis often causes visual symptoms. Halogenated anesthetics may trigger malignant hyperthermia, a life-threatening hypermetabolic myopathy rarely affecting familial susceptible individuals. Many other drugs used in medical practice have toxic effects on the brain, manifested by alterations in behavior and mentation.

Biological or bacterial toxins Tetanus, botulism, and diphtheria are the main diseases in this category.

TETANUS Tetanus is caused by the toxin of the *Clostridium tetani*. The toxin disinhibits impulses within the CNS. Symptoms usually occur 5 to 15 days after the patient has suffered a contaminated wound. Stiffness of jaw and neck muscles with tonic spasm (trismus), retraction of the corners of the mouth (risus sardonicus), and dysphagia are the first signs. Rigidity gradually develops with severe paroxysms of excruciatingly painful extensor spasms, especially of the trunk musculature (tetanic seizures). Consciousness is usually preserved.

BOTULISM The toxin of *Clostridium botulinum* blocks neuromuscular synaptic transmission, causing weakness, first affecting the intraocular and extraocular muscles, then bulbar structures, and soon the skeletal musculature. Death is due to respiratory paralysis. Symptoms begin 12 to 36 hours after eating contaminated food, most often foods preserved at home.

DIPHTHERIA *Corynebacterium diphtheriae* toxins cause weakness of the palate, paralysis of accommodation of the pupils, and laryngopharyngeal weakness. In 20 percent of cases, the neurological symptoms begin 5 to 12 days after the onset of diphtheritic pharyngitis. Weeks later, polyneuritis may occur.

Animal poisons The bites of snakes, spiders, and scorpions inject curare-like toxins that block neuromuscular transmission and cause respiratory failure. Lyme disease is caused by a spirochete transmitted by a tick bite. Days or weeks later, systemic symptoms of fever, malaise, and arthragias occur, followed by diverse neurological illnesses, including aseptic meningitis, encephalitis, mononeuritis, or polyneuritis.

Plant poisons Many hallucinogens are derived from plants; marijuana is the most common example. Certain wild mushrooms affect hepatic and renal metabolism with acute gastrointestinal symptoms or cause muscarine poisoning with acute parasympathetic stimulation. Convulsions, coma, and death often ensue. Lathyrism is common in India and North Africa where certain varieties of the chick pea are consumed to avoid starvation. Degeneration of the spinal cord results in spastic paraplegia. Ergot poisoning is rare, in spite of the common use of this alkaloid for postpartum uterine atony and for migraine.

Chronic overdosage may cause complications associated with vasoconstriction. Muscle spasm and fasciculations are common, but seizures or other serious neurological disorders are not.

Heavy metals Lead poisoning is one of the most frequent causes of acute toxic encephalopathy in young children. It usually occurs when infants chew paint off window sills and peeling walls in urban slum dwellings. Acute lead encephalopathy begins with vomiting, irritability, and clumsiness and progresses to irritability, seizures, stupor, and coma. The mortality rate is approximately 15 percent, and permanent morbidity occurs in 25 percent of patients. The diagnosis can be made by the finding of lead lines at the metaphyses of long bones or basophilic stippling of erythrocytes. Elevated lead levels in the blood and urine are noted, but fail to correlate with the severity of encephalopathy. Lead intoxication in adults is rare; it usually is manifested by abdominal pains and peripheral neuropathy, causing wrist drop. A black lead line may develop along gingival margins, and excessive lead is excreted in the urine after administration of EDTA (calcium disodium edetate).

Both acute and chronic arsenic poisoning results in an encephalopathy, peripheral neuropathy, or myopathy. Chronic mercury poisoning causes an encephalopathy with special predilection for the cerebellum; ataxia and involuntary movements are prominent. Chronic manganese poisoning, manifested as parkinsonism, mainly affects the extrapyramidal system. Other metals cause toxicity of the gastrointestinal or renal systems, with encephalopathy as a late or terminal event.

Industrial toxins There are hundreds of industrial poisons, but intoxications are most common on exposure to the organophosphates as in insecticides, such organic solvents as carbon tetrachloride, and inhalants such as toluene in glues and nitrous oxide. The organophosphates cause acute anticholinesterase symptoms and chronic motor neuropathy. Carbon tetrachloride and other organic solvents affect both the central and the peripheral nervous systems, but the primary changes in the CNS may be difficult to differentiate from the effects of severe liver and renal disease. Excessive inhalation of toluene or *n*-hexane occurs in adolescents who sniff glue. Cerebellar ataxia, disturbance of eye movements, neuritis of the optic and auditory nerves, as well as hallucinations, seizures, and coma may occur. Peripheral neuropathy follows chronic intoxication. Nitrous oxide, the gas most frequently abused for recreational purposes, causes sensory neuropathy.

HEREDITARY AND IDIOPATHIC DISORDERS OF THE BRAIN IN ADULTS

This subsection includes hereditary-metabolic defects manifesting in adulthood and a number of disorders for which the etiology remains to be elucidated. They all share a relatively slow progression over several years, tend to affect preferentially one or several of the neuronal systems (e.g., Parkinson's disease affects the nigral neurons, Huntington's chorea the striatal neurons) and used to be classified as degenerative disorders of the brain.

The biochemical basis of many of these disorders in adults (unlike similar disorders of children) remains unknown. Thus, a clinical rather than a biochemical classification has been chosen for this subsection. Although most of these disorders present a multitude of neurological manifestations, there is generally one that dominates the clinical picture, particularly early in the course. For instance, dementia is most prominent in Alzheimer's disease; however, late in the course the impairment of motor function may become pronounced. This tempo reflects the selective vulnerability of different types of neurons. Early involvement of cholinergic neurons in the nucleus basalis of Meynert and of hippocampal neurons accounts for the early loss of memory in Alzheimer's disease. Later in the disease, many other types of neurons are affected, and global impairment results. A classification by the most prominent symptom also indicates the region of the brain maximally affected, because the basic deficit, such as dementia or ataxia, reflects the localization of the pathology.

DEMENTIA

Alzheimer's disease This disorder accounts for most of the cases of primary degenerative dementia of the Alzheimer type, as defined in DSM-III-R:

> Dementia is of insidious onset and has a generally, progressive deteriorating course for which all other specific causes have been excluded by the history, physical examination, and laboratory tests. The dementia involves a multifaceted loss of intellectual abilities, such as memory, judgment, abstract thought, and other higher cortical functions, as well as changes in personality and behavior.

Alzheimer's disease is clearly age-dependent. Incidence is as high as 2.4 cases per 100 persons at risk per year in a population between 75 and 85 years, whereas it is less than 0.1 percent per year for subjects in their early 60s. Prevalence of severe dementia, enough to require full care, climbs from less than 1 percent in those younger than 65 to about 15 percent among the over-85 group. Alzheimer's disease accounts for more than half of the dementias. The proportion is even higher in older groups, where other causes of dementia, particularly multiple brain infarcts, are proportionally less common than in the fifth through seventh decades. Approximately 2 million persons in the United States have Alzheimer's disease; this figure will increase as the older segment of the population continues to expand.

Pathologically, Alzheimer's disease is characterized by neuronal degeneration and cortical atrophy. Neuronal loss particularly affects the hippocampal area, locus ceruleus, and notably the nucleus basalis of Meynert, which harbors cholinergic neurons with widespread cortical projections. Cholinergic (choline acetyltransferase) deficiency is linked to the memory loss characteristic of Alzheimer's disease. The putative peptide neurotransmitters somatostatin and vasopressin are reduced in large cortical neurons and in the hippocampus and basal ganglia, respectively. Remaining neurons may contain neurofibrillary tangles, particularly in the hippocampus and association cortex, where neuritic plaques are also prominent (Fig. 2.2-40). Granulovacuolar degeneration of pyramidal neurons and Hirano bodies may be present in the hippocampus.

The etiology of Alzheimer's disease is unknown. In a very small percent of cases, it is transmitted as an autosomal dominant trait. In rare families, Alzheimer's disease is caused by a defect of an autosomal dominant gene. By the use of genetic linkage to deoxyribonucleic acid (DNA) markers, the defective gene has been localized to chromosome 21. This is also the site of the gene that encodes the β-protein found in the amyloid plaques of Alzheimer's disease. In the great majority of cases, Alzheimer's disease seems to be sporadic. However, given the advanced age of presentation it is conceivable that a hereditary pattern may be missed in many cases. Other postulated causes include viral infection, disturbed immunity, abnormal protein synthesis, and neurotoxicity, particularly by aluminum and silica. Head trauma has been associated with an increased incidence of Alzheimer's disease; the brains of patients with dementia pugilistica also contain neurofibrillary tangles, albeit in a different distribution. Similar histological changes are also prematurely present in the brains of individuals with Down's syndrome.

The certain diagnosis of Alzheimer's disease can be reached only by histological examination. Clinical diagnosis is about 70 to 90 percent accurate. Diagnostic criteria include evidence of slowly progressive deficit in two or more areas of

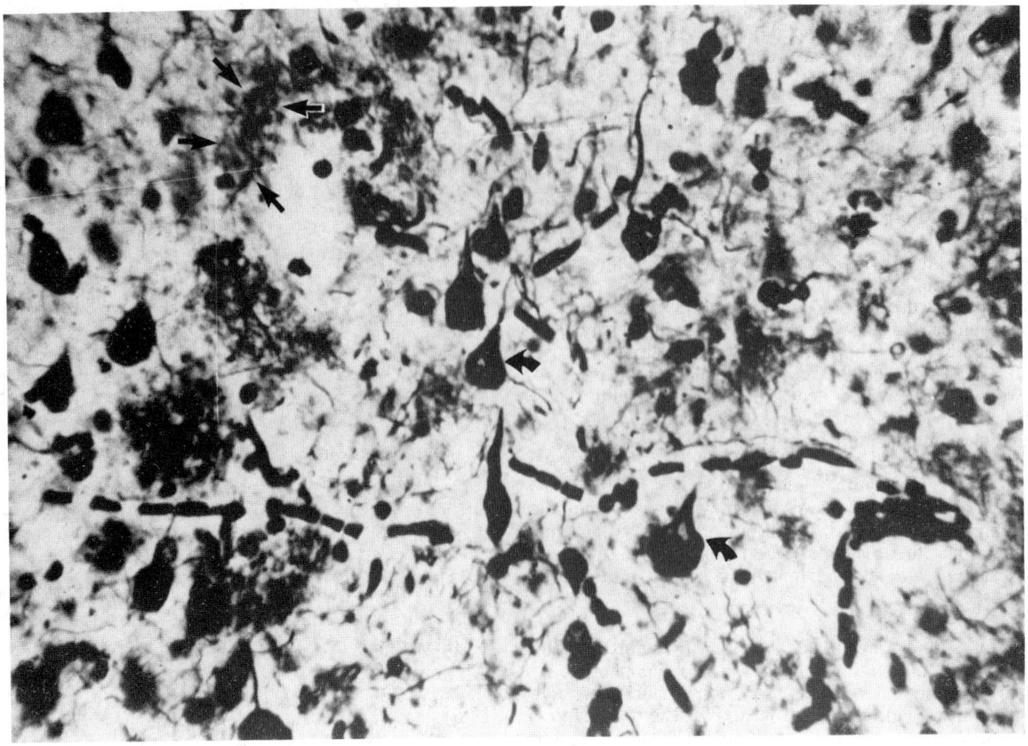

FIGURE 2.2-40. *Alzheimer's disease. Senile plaque (surrounded by* four arrows*) and neurofibrillary changes* (curved arrows) *are prominent. Silver stain. (From Hirano A:* A Guide to Neuropathology, *p 186. Igaku-Shoin, New York, 1981, with permission.)*

cognition, normal level of alertness, and absence of systemic disorders or other brain diseases that alone could account for the deficits. Aphasia, agnosia, or apraxia may be early signs. Seizures occur in 10 percent of cases. Documentation of the deficit and its progression can be made by using the Mini-Mental Status or similar tests, discussed in Section 2.1. If the patient is not fully awake and alert, delirium should be suspected. The differentiation is important because delirium often has a treatable etiology. Treatable causes of dementia should be ruled out by performing brain CT or MR, a serologic study for syphilis, thyroid function tests, and obtaining B_{12} and folate levels, as well as standard blood count and blood chemistries. Lumbar puncture should be performed after negative CT and biochemical studies if a chronic inflammatory meningoencephalitis is suspected or for cerebrospinal flow studies in cases of hydrocephalus. CSF proteins that may be markers of Alzheimer's disease are currently under scrutiny.

Differential diagnosis includes other causes of dementia. Ischemic brain disease is blamed for about 10 to 20 percent of the cases of dementia. Multi-infarct dementia differs from Alzheimer's disease by its abrupt onset, stepwise course, history, signs or CT or MR evidence of stroke, presence of hypertension, or other signs of atherosclerosis. A smaller proportion of cases of dementia may be due to midline or frontotemporal tumors, subdural hematoma, or hydrocephalus. CT or MR can help differentiate these processes from Alzheimer's disease. Toxins, including psychotropic drugs; infections, such as cryptococcosis, Whipple's disease, or Creutzfeldt-Jakob disease; chronic liver, lung, or renal failure; and vasculitis can occasionally mimic Alzheimer's disease. In younger patients, the subacute dementia of AIDS has become relatively common. Chronic dementia is often associated with other degenerative disorders discussed below. For instance, dementia develops in about one-third of patients with Parkinson's disease. However, parkinsonian features are common in the late stages of Alzheimer's disease and about 30 percent of brains of Alzheimer's disease victims contain histological changes of Parkinson's disease. The pseudodementia of depression in the elderly is discussed in Section 2.3.

Still in an experimental stage, oral tetrahydroaminoacridine (THA), a centrally active anticholinesterase, has been reported to improve memory and orientation in patients with mild to moderate Alzheimer's disease. Instructions on how to cope with the cognitive deficits and community support services should be available to the patients and their families. In the absence of adequate home support, institutional care should be provided.

Pick's disease This unusual disorder, characterized by progressive dementia, is often difficult to differentiate from Alzheimer's disease on clinical grounds. Pathological findings include marked atrophy of the frontal and temporal tips with preservation of the posterior third of the superior temporal gyrus (Fig. 2.2-41) or asymmetric atrophy of the parietotemporal association cortex. Neuronal loss, cytoplasmic neuronal swelling (Pick cells) and rounded argentophilic neuronal inclusion bodies (Pick's bodies) are seen under the microscope. Memory loss is less pronounced than in Alzheimer's disease, and the cognitive deficit is characterized by impaired social nuances and drive or an aphasic-apractic syndrome. CT or MR shows the characteristic polar distribution of brain atrophy.

DEMENTIA AND BASAL GANGLIA MANIFESTATIONS

Huntington's disease This disease is an autosomal dominant disorder of mid-life, characterized by early chorea and late dementia, although this sequence is not invariable. The disease has

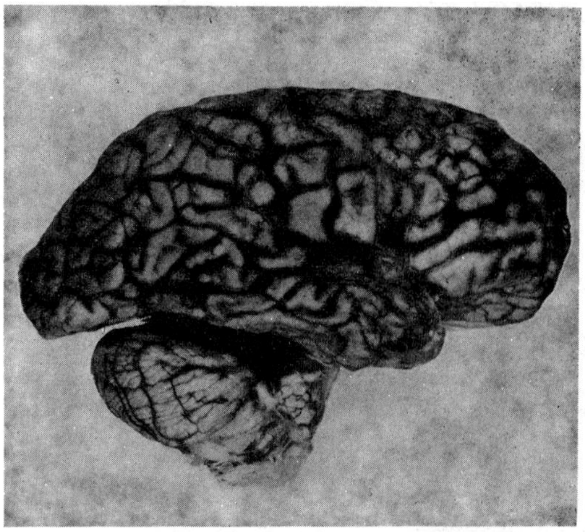

FIGURE 2.2-41. *Pick's lobar atrophy. There is prominent shrinkage of the temporal lobe with generalized atrophy of the middle and anterior aspects of the hemisphere. (From Blackwood W, Dodds T C, Sommerville J C:* Atlas of Neuropathology, *ed 2, p 113. Williams & Wilkins, Baltimore, 1964, with permission.)*

been traced to the G8 fragment of chromosome 4. In about 6 percent of the cases, clinical manifestations appear before the age of 15, but mean age of onset is approximately 40 years. Depression, impulsivity and emotional lability may herald the onset of the disease. Pathologically, the medium-size spiny cells of the striatum bear the brunt of the damage. These γ-aminobutyric acid (GABA)-ergic neurons send axons to the globus pallidus. Somatostatin is normal or increased and may play a role in the genesis of chorea. Clinical diagnosis requires the family history and is supported by the finding of atrophic caudate nuclei on CT or MR. The morphological changes are preceded by decreased metabolism in the caudate, visible with positron emission tomography (PET) (see Fig. 2.1-28). Chorea may be alleviated with the use of haloperidol; however, this medication may increase the patient's rigidity and tendency to fall.

Experimentally, predictive testing of relatives can be attained by determining the genotype at the G8 locus in DNA obtained from blood. This information, however, may have devastating effects. Positive test results may lead to disruption of family and personal life and an increased incidence of suicide, already high among patients with Huntington's chorea.

Progressive supranuclear palsy The rare disorder (about 150 patients reported) is characterized by supranuclear palsy of vertical gaze, parkinsonian features, and dementia. Onset is generally in the sixth or seventh decade, and death occurs in 2 to 12 years. Downgaze is more affected than upgaze, in contrast to the situation in Parkinson's disease. The eyes fail to move on volition, but can be deviated by the oculocephalic (doll's eye) reflex. Initial presentation is generally one of postural instability, with easy falling, and memory loss or depression. Axial rigidity and pseudobulbar findings are often prominent. The dementing syndrome consists of attentional impairment, emotional lability, and amnesia. Aphasia, apraxia, or agnosia are conspicuously absent ("subcortical dementia"). Histologically, neuronal loss and gliosis are particularly marked in the periaqueductal region of the midbrain, globus pallidus, subthalamic nucleus, substantia nigra, and dentate nucleus. Neurofibrillary tangles, different from those in Alzheimer's disease, are ubiquitous in the subcortical structures. CT shows generalized atrophy. Methysergide (Sansert) or bromocriptine has helped some patients.

Chronic hydrocephalus Hydrocephalus is characterized by ventricular enlargement, in excess of what is expected for the patient's age. Normally, CSF is secreted into the ventricles by the choroid plexus. From the lateral ventricles, CSF exits through the foramina of Monro, and travels through the third ventricle, Sylvian aqueduct, and fourth ventricle to egress through the foramina of Lushka and Magendi into the subarachnoid space at the base of the brain and around the spinal cord (Fig. 2.2-42). From the brain convexity, CSF ascends to the parasagittal region, where it reaches the superior sagittal venous sinus percolating through specialized rounded bodies known as pachionian granulations. Obstruction to the flow of CSF anywhere along this path results in ventricular enlargement. Lumbar CSF pressure is generally normal in chronic hydrocephalus caused by impaired resorption, a condition known as normopressure hydrocephalus. Ventricular enlargement can also occur when there is atrophy of the periventricular structures (i.e., hydrocephalus ex vacuo).

Hydrocephalus, a pathologic entity, may have different etiologies. In children, it is generally related to congenital malformations or tumors. Antecedent subarachnoid hemorrhage or a meningitis, with consequent fibrosis of the pachionian granulations, is most common in adults. In the elderly, hydrocephalus is often idiopathic. Possible etiologies include brain atrophy, possibly greater in chronic hypertensives, and decreased resorption through the pachionian granulations in the superior sagittal sinus. Atrophy of these granulations occurs with advancing age. In contrast to the case of acute hydrocephalus due to obstruction of the ventricular system by a tumor, headache is absent in patients with chronic hydrocephalus. The earliest and constant clinical manifestation is gait apraxia, a shuffling gait with a tendency for the feet to stick to the ground, sometimes referred to as magnetic gait; these patients can move their feet quite well when lying in bed. Bradykinesia, truncal akinesia, and rigidity are also

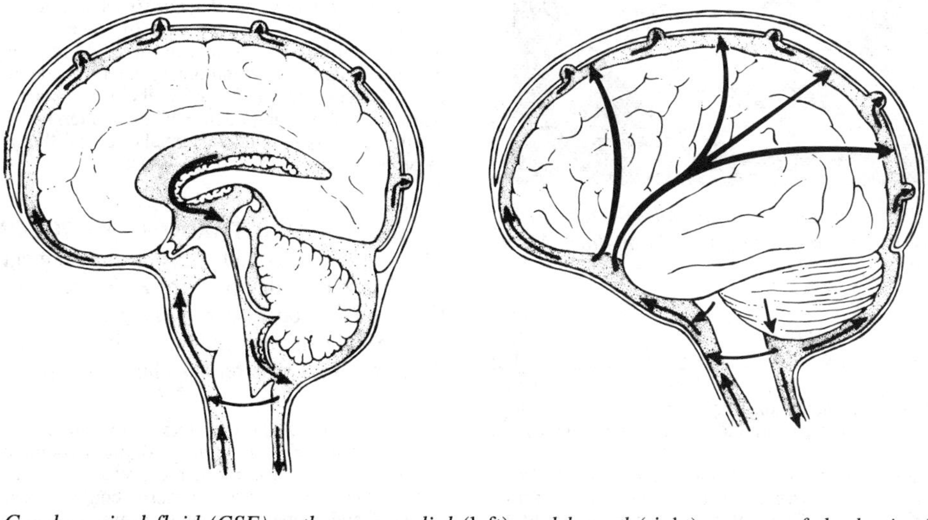

FIGURE 2.2-42. *Cerebrospinal fluid (CSF) pathways, medial* (left) *and lateral* (right) *aspects of the brain. From the choroid plexus in the ventricles CSF circulates over the brain base and convexity, reaching the venous sinuses through the Pachionian granulations. (Modified from Milhorat T H:* Pediatric Neurosurgery. *Davis, Philadelphia, 1978, with permission.)*

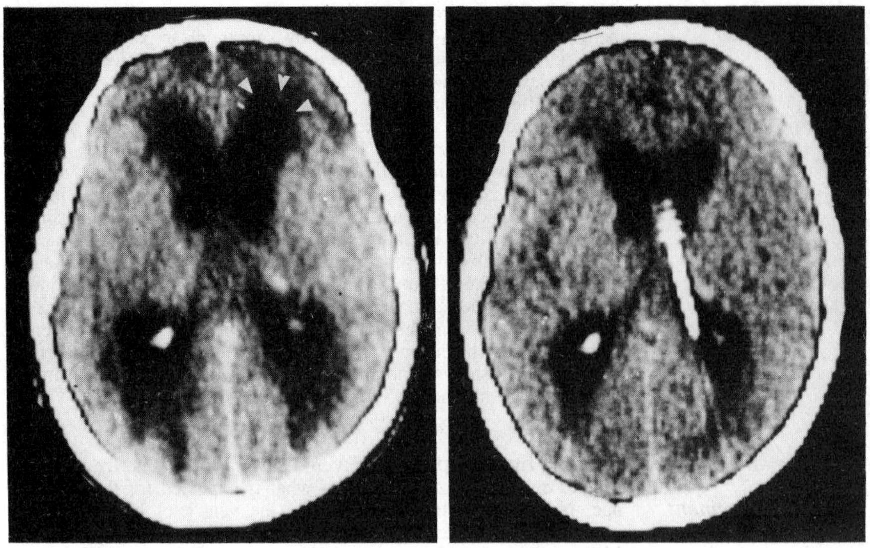

FIGURE 2.2-43. *Hydrocephalus from a cerebellar tumor obstructing the fourth ventricle. Note the dilatation of the ventricles before shunting* (left, arrowheads) *relieved after shunting* (right). *(From Masdeu J C, Chuman C M: Ventricular catheter in the cistern of the transverse fissure: A cause of shunt malfunction. Neurosurgery 5: 597, 1982, with permission.)*

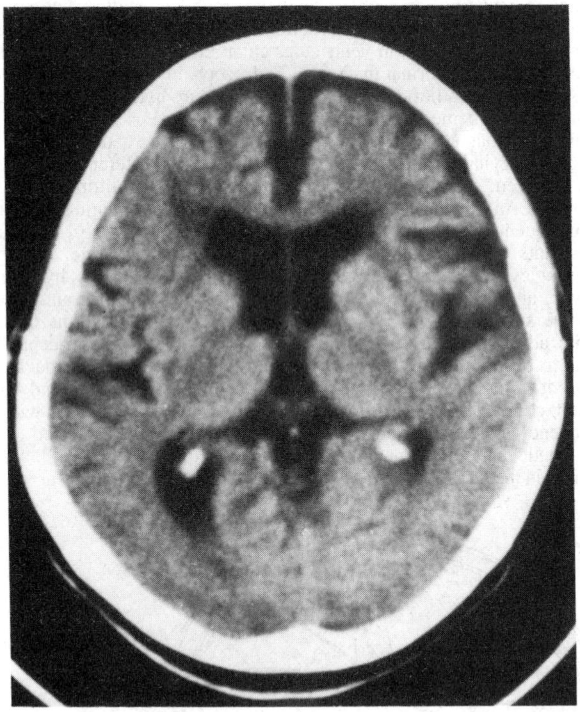

FIGURE 2.2-44. *Brain atrophy in a normal 79-year-old individual. (Courtesy of Charles Elkin, MD, Montefiore Medical Center, New York.)*

common. The clinical picture thus resembles parkinsonism, but patients with hydrocephalus often have, in addition, urinary urgency or incontinence. Changes in mentation may be minimal, but bradyphrenia, which involves impaired attention and verbal fluency, is common.

Diagnosis depends mainly on the clinical picture. CT or MR is used to document ventricular enlargement and to visualize possible tumors or other lesions in the CSF pathways. Caution should be exercised in interpreting ventricular enlargement in an elderly person with gait disturbances. In this situation, symptomatic hydrocephalus is rarely to blame, but both the clinical and radiological findings are due to age-related brain atrophy or to poorly understood disorders of the basal ganglia or white matter (particularly Binswanger's disease). In symptomatic hydrocephalus, the calloso-caudate angle tends to be rounded and the cortical sulci are obliterated by the cortical mantle being pushed toward the inner table of the skull (Fig. 2.2-43). By contrast, the cortical sulci are prominent in the aged brain or in atrophy with degenerative disorders such as Alzheimer's disease (Fig. 2.2-44). If symptomatic hydrocephalus is suspected, radionuclide cisternography (see Section 2.1) is performed to demonstrate abnormal CSF resorption. Although shunting of ventricular CSF to the abdominal or pleural cavities can relieve symptomatic hydrocephalus, it is helpful in only a small proportion of the elderly with gait abnormalities and urinary incontinence.

DEMENTIA + ATAXIA + PYRAMIDAL SIGNS *Adult-onset metachromatic leukodystrophy* is caused by a deficiency of arylsulfatase A. This very rare autosomal recessive disorder generally presents as a psychosis or progressive dementia. Spasticity and lively reflexes in the legs contrast with the absence of reflexes observed in the infantile form of the disease, where involvement of peripheral nerve is more severe. Urinary sulfatide excretion is increased. The diagnosis is confirmed by the finding of low leukocyte enzymatic activity of arylsulfatase A and of sulfatidase. No treatment is available.

Cerebrotendinous xanthomatosis is a rare, recessively inherited disorder caused by the deposition of cholestanol and the replacement of cholesterol by cholestanol in the CNS and peripheral myelin. The patients have tendon xanthomas, cataracts, dementia, and pyramidal paresis. Less consistent are cerebellar ataxia and peripheral neuropathy. CT shows hypodense white matter and low-density areas in the posterior fossa. Chenodeoxycholic acid therapy has been reported to arrest progression of the disease.

DEMENTIA + ATAXIA + MYOCLONIC SEIZURES

The rare disorders under this heading are autosomal recessively inherited, with onset in adolescence or early adult life. Creutzfeld-Jakob disease may present a similar clinical picture. Sialidosis also has a similar presentation, but without dementia and with retinal cherry-red spots.

Lafora-body disease differs from another form of myoclonic epilepsy, Unverricht-Lundborg (Baltic myoclonus), in its later age of onset (11 to 18 years) and the presence of dementia. Skin biopsy shows the characteristic Lafora bodies, acid-Schiff-positive inclusions constituted by polyglucosans.

Neuronal ceroid lipofuscinosis is a group of diseases characterized by the lysosomal accumulation of ceroid lipofuscin, demonstrable in neurons of the rectal mucosa and in eccrine skin cells. Psychiatric, cognitive, retinal, extrapyramidal, or cerebellar abnormalities may be more prominent than the myoclonic seizures. EEG shows marked photosensitivity.

Mitochondrial encephalomyopathy begins between the ages of 5 and 50 years. Dementia is frequent and may be associated with short stature, hearing loss, optic atrophy, and neuropathy. Ragged-red fibers are present on muscle biopsy.

BASAL GANGLIA MANIFESTATIONS

Parkinson's disease This condition is characterized by bradykinesia, rigidity, resting tremor, and impaired postural reflexes. Not all patients have the four clinical characteristics. Tremor may be subtle, particularly in the group with older-age onset. About one-third of patients in this subgroup tend to develop dementia. Prevalence is of 1.7 per 1,000. The disorder rarely begins before age 40 years, and incidence increases with advancing age. An environmental etiology is suggested by the finding of strong discordance between monozygotic twins. A syndrome identical to parkinsonism has been recently encountered among abusers of methylphenyl tetrahydropyridine (MPTP), a synthetic street drug sold as a heroin analogue. This finding has fueled intense research into possible environmental causes of Parkinson's disease. The increased incidence in farming areas has been blamed on the use of pesticides, but this claim has not been substantiated. Antipsychotic-induced parkinsonism is a well-known type of symptomatic parkinsonism. Rare causes include manganese or carbon monoxide poisoning. Pathologically, there is pallor of the substantia nigra (Fig. 2.2-45) caused by nigral neuronal loss. These neurons are dopaminergic and innervate the acetylcholine-rich striatum. In Parkinson's disease, dopamine is markedly decreased in the substantia nigra and striatum.

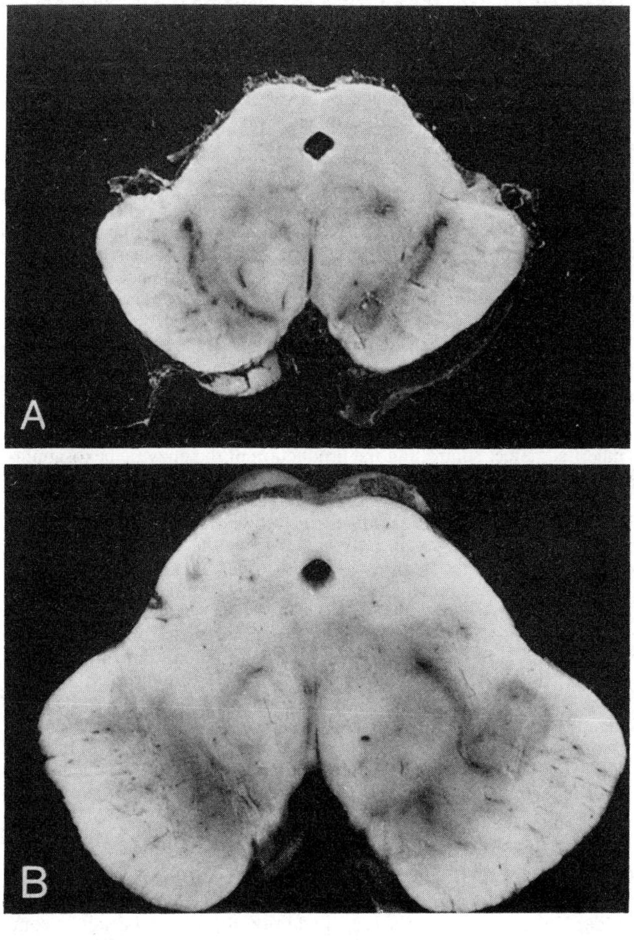

FIGURE 2.2-45. *Parkinson's disease.* A. *Normal midbrain with well pigmented substantia nigra.* B. *In Parkinson's disease, neuronal loss is associated with depigmentation in the substantia nigra. (From Hirano A, Iwata M, Llena J F, Matsui T:* Color Atlas of Pathology of the Nervous System, *p 58. Igaku-Shoin, New York, 1980, with permission.)*

Therapy should aim at the improvement of disabling or disturbing symptoms, most often bradykinesia or the tendency to fall. Although it can be aesthetically unpleasant, tremor is seldom a cause of dysfunction because parkinsonian tremor improves during movement. Therapy with anticholinergic medication such as trihexyphenidyl (Artane), useful in antipsychotic-induced parkinsonism, is not advisable in patients older than 70 because confusion related to memory loss is a common consequence. At a dosage of 100 mg b.i.d., amantadine (Symmetrel) often helps minor degrees of the disorder. Levodopa combined with a peripheral decarboxylase inhibitor, carbidopa (Sinemet), is the therapy of choice. Starting doses of 100 mg t.i.d. may be increased to the point at which the patient is functionally improved. Hyperkinesias, in the form of chorea or dystonia, are limiting dose-related side effects. Particularly after prolonged therapy, periods of profound bradykinesia may alternate with periods when the patient can move well or is hyperkinetic (on-off phenomenon or end-of-dose deterioration). Careful titration of levodopa, avoidance of protein intake during the day hours, or the addition of a direct dopamine receptor agonist, bromocriptine, may ameliorate this syndrome. Pump-regulated subcutaneous infusion of lisuride, another dopamine receptor agonist (not yet available in the United States), has been used to obviate the fluctuations of dopaminergic-agent blood levels that may contribute to the "on-off" effect. Parkinsonism resistant to levodopa may respond to small doses of bromocriptine (between 2.5 and 30 mg). Both levodopa and bromocriptine may induce orthostatic hypotension and a psychotic-hallucinatory syndrome. The most recent innovation in the treatment of this disorder is the experimental autotransplantation of portions of adrenal medulla into the caudate nucleus. The reported improvement is presumably due to dopamine release. Because only a small number of patients have undergone this experimental operation, its long-term usefulness is uncertain.

Striatonigral degeneration clinically resembles Parkinson's disease, but tremor is absent and there is no response to levodopa because the dopamine receptors in the striatum are lost as a result of striatal neuronal disease.

Dystonia musculorum deformans This disease begins during childhood but the patients live into adult age. Unlike later-onset dystonias, dystonia musculorum deformans is transmitted as an autosomal recessive trait. The brain lacks morphological changes, but the levels of norepinephrine are decreased in the posterior hypothalamus, subthalamic nucleus and locus ceruleus. High-dose anticholinergic medication or bromocriptine may help some patients.

Wilson's disease This condition is an autosomal recessive disorder of copper metabolism, manifested by hepatic dysfunction, dystonia, cerebellar ataxia, intention tremor, and psychiatric symptoms. Prevalence is about 25 per million. Age of onset is generally between 6 and 20 years, but onset into the fifth decade has been described. In about 20 percent presenting features are psychiatric, often with an abrupt onset. Deterioration of schoolwork, inappropriate social behavior, a severe neurosis or a syndrome similar to schizophrenia or manic-depressive psychosis may herald Wilson's disease.

Diagnosis is reached by finding low serum ceruloplasmin, 24-hour urinary excretion of copper greater than 100 μg, and high levels of copper in a liver biopsy, which shows findings of cirrhosis or "chronic active hepatitis." Slit-lamp examination should be performed if inspection of the corneoscleral junction fails to reveal the brownish Kayser-Fleischer ring that is present in most patients with neurological manifestations. CT or MR shows the symmetrical putaminal lesions (Fig. 2.2-46). Early treatment with dietary copper restrictions and D-penicillamine reverses the disorder.

Choreoacanthocytosis is a familial disorder characterized by chorea, tics, dystonic dysphagia, late dementia, muscle atrophy and absent reflexes. Blood smear shows acanthocytes.

BASAL GANGLIA, CEREBELLAR, AND AUTONOMIC MANIFESTATIONS

Shy-Drager syndrome This condition is manifested as orthostatic hypotension and other autonomic deficits, followed, after weeks or months, by cerebellar dysmetria and rigidity. Sleep apnea occurs late. Neuronal loss affects the intermediolateral column of the spinal cord, substantia nigra, and other nuclei in the brain stem and cerebellum. Hypotension is treated with

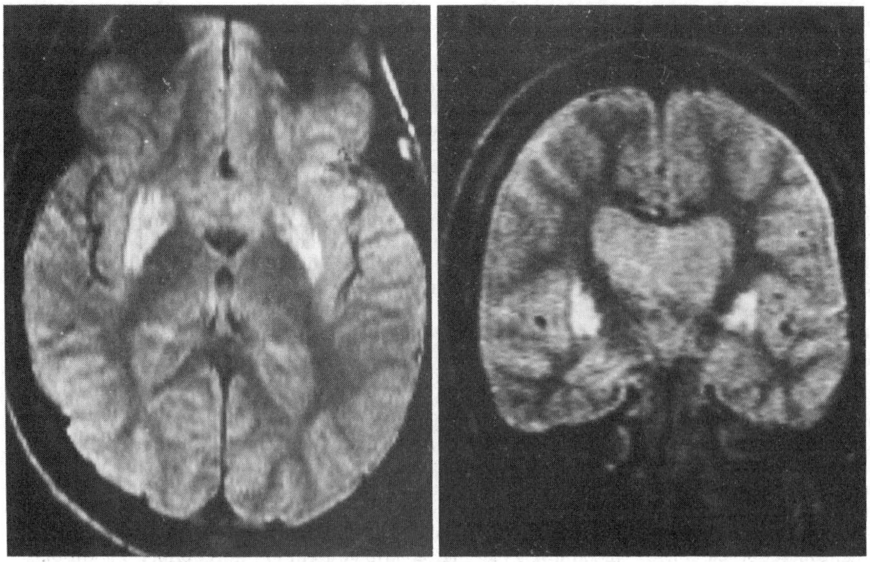

FIGURE 2.2-46. *Wilson's disease. Axial* (left) *and coronal* (right) *MR scans showing high-intensity lesions in the putamen of this 24-year-old man. (Courtesy of Charles Elkin, MD, Montefiore Medical Center, New York.)*

indomethacin (Indocin) or fludrocortisone (Florinef Acetate). Anticholinergic drugs or amantadine (Symmetrel) may improve the parkinsonian manifestations.

Olivopontocerebellar degeneration Like the Shy-Drager syndrome, the disease is characterized by widespread neuronal loss in many brain structures. Some authors classify the two disorders under the single label of multiple system atrophy. However, cerebellar ataxia precedes the onset of parkinsonian features in olivopontocerebellar degeneration, and orthostatic hypotension is mild. Onset is in the second through sixth decades. Supranuclear ophthalmoplegia is common. Pontocerebellar atrophy can be documented by CT (Fig. 2.2-47). The enzyme glutamate dehydrogenase is decreased in the fibroblasts of a subgroup of these patients.

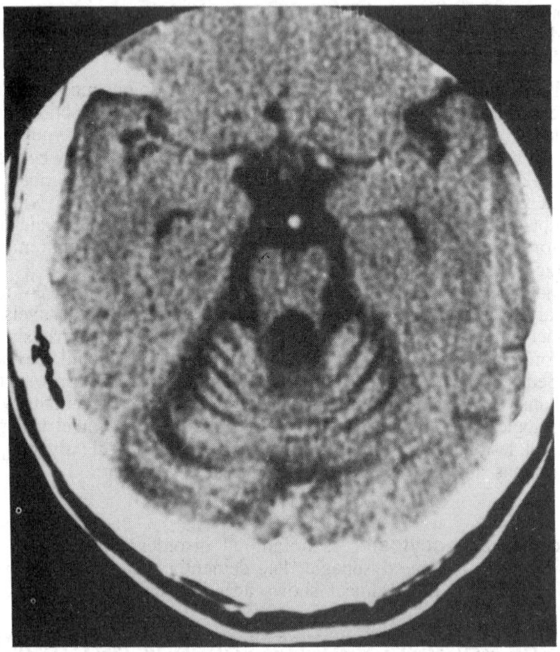

FIGURE 2.2-47. *Olivopontocerebellar atrophy. CT of a 49-year-old man. (Courtesy of Charles Elkin, MD, Montefiore Medical Center, New York.)*

CEREBELLAR MANIFESTATIONS Most of the ataxic syndromes with onset after the age of 20 correspond to the olivopontocerebellar atrophies or to ataxic-myoclonic syndromes described above. Rarely, autosomal dominant "pure" cerebellar ataxia has been reported, with onset after age 50. Another variety is episodic; the attacks of ataxia may be prevented with acetazolamide (Diamox) therapy.

CEREBELLAR AND SPINAL CORD OR PERIPHERAL NERVE MANIFESTATIONS The spinocerebellar degenerations comprise a heterogeneous group of disorders characterized by ataxia and sensory or motor manifestations of spinal cord disease. Some, like vitamin E deficiency, are discussed under the specific etiology. Others are the phenotype for a variety of biochemical disorders which manifest a more malignant course when surfacing during infancy or childhood. For instance, G_{M2} gangliosidosis can present as the infantile Tay-Sachs disease, deadly in the first year of life, or as a spinocerebellar syndrome with motor neuron disease findings. The different phenotype is explained by differences in the inherited defect controlling the production of the enzyme hexosaminidase, responsible for the metabolism of G_{M2} gangliosides. A multiple-locus, multiple-allele system explains the diverse clinical syndromes and is used to classify them. Adrenoleukomyeloneuropathy, with storage of long-chain fatty acids, is another genotype. In many other instances, the nature of the disorder underlying the spinocerebellar clinical picture remains to be determined.

Machado-Joseph's disease is a rare autosomal dominant disorder of young adults in which ataxia predominates. It is often associated with dementia, optic atrophy, supranuclear ophthalmoplegia, rigidity, chorea, dystonia, and pyramidal weakness or amyotrophy.

Refsum's disease, due to the accumulation of phytanic acid, is characterized by ataxia, retinitis pigmentosa, polyneuropathy, and an increased CSF protein. Hearing loss and skin changes similar to ichthyosis are common. Therapy consists of a restricted dietary intake of butter, animal fat, and vegetables, all rich in phytanic acid.

DISEASES WITH PREDOMINANT SPINAL CORD MANIFESTATIONS **Familial spastic paraparesis** This disease may be transmitted as an autosomal dominant or recessive disorder. Impaired position sense in addition to the paraparesis is common in the late-onset (after age 40) form of the disease. The progression is slow, over the course of years. Pathologically, the corticospinal tracts of the cord are affected, maximally at more caudal levels. Baclofen (Lioresal) is used to control spasticity.

Adrenoleukodystrophy Transmitted as an X-linked disorder, this disease is characterized by the accumulation of very-long-chain fatty acids in the adrenal cortex and cerebral white matter. In adults, the most common presentation is progressive spastic paraparesis; the female carriers may have a mild paraparesis. A peripheral neuropathy may also be present. Endocrine changes are consistent with Addison's disease. Severe demyelination occurs in the corticospinal tracts. The abnormal fatty acids can be measured in the serum or in skin fibroblasts. Treatment of the adrenal insufficiency does not prevent progression of the neurological disorder.

Friedreich's ataxia This familial disease occurs in late childhood. Its clinical manifestations are ataxia of the extremities associated with position-sense loss, areflexia, and bilateral Babinski's signs. Cerebellar cortical degeneration often occurs, and there are many other variations of this disease.

Amyotrophic lateral sclerosis This disease is the only one in this group not commonly hereditary (except among the natives of the Mariana islands). The illness begins in middle or late life and ends in death after 2 to 4 years. Spastic or flaccid progressive weakness, which is accompanied by atrophy and fasciculations, affects the extremities and bulbar musculature. More chronic variants of this disease are progressive spinal muscular atrophy, with major involvement of the anterior horn cells, and primary lateral sclerosis, with maximum involvement of the pyramidal tracts.

DISEASES PREDOMINANTLY OF THE PERIPHERAL NERVES

Charcot-Marie-Tooth disease or *peroneal muscular atrophy* is a hereditary, slowly progressive disease beginning in the first 3 decades of life. It is manifested by weakness and atrophy of the lower legs and lower third of the thighs, with distal sensory impairment. Similar, but less marked features affect the upper extremities. Charcot-Marie-Tooth disease is often associated with Friedreich's ataxia, just as Friedreich's ataxia may blend into the cerebellar degenerations.

DISEASES OF EARLY LIFE

One must marvel at the relative rarity of congenital disorders, in view of the complex process of embryonic maturation. Early developmental defects are due to abnormalities of the germ plasm; later, trauma, infection, and biochemical stimuli during embryonic life account for the majority of malformations. Defects vary with the embryonic stage of the maturation process, the site of neural involvement, and the severity and type of the underlying disturbance. The birth process is fraught with particularly traumatic and anoxic hazards. Infections and other illnesses in the neonatal period may cause irreparable damage.

Knowledge of neurochemistry and genetics has grown rapidly. Elevation of α-fetoprotein in maternal blood and in amniotic fluid obtained by amniocentesis leads to the prenatal diagnosis of neural tube defects, such as anencephaly and spina bifida. Fetal cells obtained by amniocentesis can be cultured and analyzed for chromosomal anomalies. Many inborn errors of metabolism responsible for physical and mental retardation or death are now detectable in the fetus and in carriers. Fetal blood sampled from the placenta may lead to the diagnosis of muscular dystrophy. The genetic counselor is able to make increasingly accurate predictions. In-utero therapeutic procedures can now be performed, such as shunting for hydrocephalus.

CEREBRAL PALSY

Cerebral palsy may be due to such prenatal factors as developmental anomalies and infections in utero to perinatal events, especially asphyxia and mechanical trauma at the time of birth, or to postnatal factors, such as kernicterus, infections, and injuries. Most often, the cause is indeterminate.

The manifestations of cerebral palsy depend on the site of maximum damage. Disease of the cerebral hemispheres and cortex causes bilateral spastic weakness. Lesions of the basal ganglia result in dyskinetic, athetoid, or choreiform movements. Defects of the cerebellum are associated with hypotonia and ataxia. The neurological signs may be minor or severe. Mental retardation occurs in a third of all children with cerebral palsy, and epilepsy is present in another third.

Kernicterus is caused by severe neonatal hyperbilirubinemia, usually due to maternal-fetal blood (especially Rh group) incompatibility and associated erythroblastosis fetalis. It is manifested during the first 2 weeks of life by jaundice, lethargy, opisthotonos, or seizures. Cerebral palsy with mental retardation, extrapyramidal signs, and deafness are the usual sequelae in those who survive.

DEVELOPMENTAL DEFORMITIES

Defects of the cerebrum Microcephaly—the reduction in the size of the cerebral hemispheres, with anomalies of face, limbs, and heart—may occur in the offspring of chronic alcoholic mothers. Porencephaly, a cavity within a cerebral hemisphere, need not manifest clinical signs. Patients with agenesis of the corpus callosum may have only subtle clinical findings.

Cervicocranial deformities These malformations include craniostenosis (premature closure of cranial sutures), basilar impression (elevation of the rim of the foramen magnum into the cranial cavity) and *Arnold-Chiari malformations.* The most common Arnold-Chiari defect is the extension of the medulla and the cerebellum through the foramen magnum, with the cerebellum overlapping the upper cervical spinal cord and associated meningomyelocele. Hydrocephalus is often associated with defects of the occipitocervical junction.

Dilation of the ventricles or the central canal **Hydrocephalus** Abnormal dilation of the ventricular system in the infant is associated with head enlargement and is usually due to congenital obstruction of the ventricular channels, such as stenosis of the Sylvian aqueduct. In patients with Dandy-Walker syndrome (see Fig. 2.1-23), atresia of the foramina of the fourth ventricle causes a cyst-like dilation of that ventricle and lesser enlargement of the other ventricles. Hydrocephalus is often seen in perinatal inflammatory diseases that prevent reabsorption of CSF and in neoplastic diseases that obstruct the outflow of CSF. Hydrocephalus is often associated with the cervicocranial deformities noted above or congenital defects of the meninges, such as meningocele (failure of the envelope of the meninges to close fully at the midline) or meningomyelocele (failure of the neural tube to close fully, with splitting of the spinal cord and the meninges).

Syringomyelia and syringobulbia The development of a cavity within the central portion of the spinal cord and the medulla may be congenital, although symptoms need not begin until the second or third decade of life. Benign cystic gliomas may present an identical clinical picture. Typically, loss of pain, but preservation of touch sensations, in the hands precedes other signs of neuraxial involvement.

CHROMOSOMAL ANOMALIES

Mongolism (Down's syndrome) This condition is due to trisomy of chromosome 21 and occurs most often when the mother is beyond the age of 35 or 40. In addition to severe mental retardation, alterations of the head and face include brachycephaly, flattened nose, large tongue, slanted and widely spaced eyes, and small ears. The bones, especially of the fingers, are shortened, and other deformities are common. Life is shortened by congenital anomalies of the heart or by intercurrent infections.

Sex Chromosomal Defects In *Klinefelter's syndrome,* which affects males, gynecomastia and aspermatogenesis occur, and mild mental retardation and psychosis are common. *Turner's syndrome* affects females and is characterized by retardation of growth and sexual development; these patients develop a webbed neck. An extra X chromosome is present in Klinefelter's syndrome, whereas an X chromosome is missing in Turner's syndrome.

PHAKOMATOSIS

Phakomatosis is a generic term for diseases affecting ectodermal tissue and neurocutaneous structures. These diseases are usually inherited as autosomal dominants with variable penetrance. The lesions become manifest in childhood and slowly progress.

Neurofibromatosis This condition, also known as *von Recklinghausen's disease,* is characterized by areas of skin hyperpigmentation (*café-au-lait* spots) and by cutaneous and subcutaneous tumors that become increasingly prominent in late childhood. Neuromas may also arise from the sheaths of spinal or cranial nerves, especially the acoustic nerves. Other neoplasms, such as meningiomas and gliomas, may affect the CNS. Glial hypertrophy may lead to hydrocephalus.

Tuberous sclerosis In infancy, this disease is characterized by convulsive seizures and mental retardation. During preschool years, sebaceous adenomas, depigmented spots, and other skin lesions occur. Numerous pale nodules project from the cortex or into the ventricles, like the gutterings of a candle (Fig. 2.2-48). The nodules may be noted in computed tomograms, and their calcifications may be seen in roentgenograms of the skull.

Vascular anomalies of the skin associated with neurological abnormalities *Sturge-Weber syndrome* is manifested by a congenital craniofacial vascular nevus and meningeal angioma. Double-contoured calcifications are present in the underlying atrophic cerebral cortex. The cerebral lesion often causes seizures and focal neurological signs.

Hippel-Lindau disease is characterized by hemangioblastomas of the cerebellum and retina; sometimes, the spinal cord or nerve roots are also affected. In addition to the associated neurological defects, polycythemia and cystic disease of other organs occur.

Ataxia telangiectasia, also called *Louis-Bar syndrome,* is a hereditary ataxia that becomes evident in the preschool years. Degeneration affects the cerebellar cortex, the peripheral nerves, and sympathetic ganglia; there is demyelination of the posterior and spinocerebellar tracts of the spinal cord. Telangiectatic lesions develop over the conjunctiva and the face. Impairment of immunoglobulin accounts for recurrent respiratory tract, paranasal sinus, and pulmonary infections.

Familial telangiectasia, also known as Rendu-Osler-Weber disease, affects the skin, mucous membranes, other organs, and occasionally the CNS. The telangiectasia appear in childhood and later in life. The lesion may bleed, but only rarely in the brain.

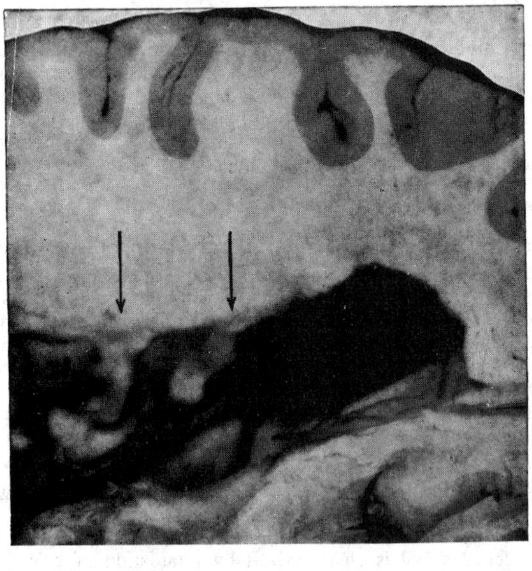

FIGURE 2.2-48. *Tuberous sclerosis. The* arrows *indicate nodules of glial tissue projecting into the lateral ventricle. (From Blackwood W. Dodds T C, Sommerville J C:* Atlas of Neuropathology, *ed 2, p 221. Williams & Wilkins, Baltimore, 1964, with permission.)*

ENDOCRINOPATHIES Hyperthyroidism during fetal life results in *cretinism,* with severe mental retardation. Abnormalities of parathyroid function in early life may cause tetany, choreiform activity, or seizures, and mild mental retardation.

INTRAUTERINE INFECTIONS Viruses, rather than bacteria, reach the fetus through the placental barrier at an early stage. Maternal rubella may cause cataracts, deafness, mental retardation, and congenital heart disease in the offspring. Syphilis, cytomegalic inclusion disease, and toxoplasmosis were discussed above.

Metabolic (Degenerative) Diseases Enzyme deficiencies, usually inherited as autosomal recessive diseases, have been found to be responsible for many of the disorders formerly considered degenerative diseases of childhood. Defects in the metabolic pathway disturb cell function, either by the accumulation of metabolites or the lack of a substrate. In lysosomal storage diseases, the accumulation of metabolites in the bodies of nerve cells may physically disturb the cell function, as in Tay-Sachs disease (Fig. 2.2-49), or the metabolites may be neurotoxic. The lack of substrate may block the metabolic pathway (e.g., phenylketonuria) or an alternate metabolic activity may be induced (e.g., hypoglycemia associated with galactosemia). The metabolic abnormalities may cause illness and death without appreciable change in the structure of the nervous system, but disease usually is evident in the white matter or the gray matter or both.

In Table 2.2-4, the metabolic and degenerative diseases are classified according to the type of tissue predominantly affected—that is, gray or white matter—and subdivided according to their main sites in the nervous system. Some diseases affect more than one tissue under which they are listed (e.g., Krabbe's disease affects neurons as well as white matter) or affects other areas of the nervous system in addition to their predominant site (e.g., subacute necrotizing encephalomyelopathy). On rare occasions, many of these diseases have their clinical onset in adult life.

Diseases of white matter In children, disease of white matter is often termed *leukodystrophy,* a term that implies a static condition caused by faulty myelin formation rather than progressive degeneration of demyelination, but this distinction is not always valid. In other diseases of white matter, there is the accumulation of abnormal lipids (lipidoses), as distinguished from degeneration of lipids (demyelination), but in certain diseases, such as metachromatic leukoencephalopathy, both processes occur. In many diseases of white matter, the pathogenesis is not known.

Diseases of gray matter The largest group of diseases in this category are the lysosomal storage diseases, in which the neurons' lysosomes become engorged with metabolites that they would normally degrade. Secondary demyelination often occurs. The lipid storage diseases, sphingolipidoses, are more common than mucopolysaccharidoses.

In establishing the clinical diagnosis, the most crucial aspect of the history is the determination of the course of the illness. Developmental regression signifies a dynamic disease, whereas lack of development often indicates a static embryonic lesion. There are many clinical manifestations of these diseases. Failure to thrive, mental retardation, and failure of neurological and physical development are common. Weakness progresses to paralysis and, terminally, to decerebrate rigidity. Myoclonic and other seizures occur. Blindness is more frequent than deafness. It has been customary to classify the diseases according to their respective defects of lipid, mucopolysaccharide, carbohydrate, or protein metabolism (Table 2.2-5). There are dozens of inborn errors of metabolism, and the list is expanding yearly.

These diseases are now diagnosed by quantitative analysis of specific metabolites or their enzymes. For want of the degradative enzyme, metabolites accumulate in excessive amounts in the cells' lysosomes and may be excreted in excessive amounts in the urine. Enzymes in skin fibroblasts can be assayed after cell culture and can be measured in blood serum, leukocytes, or amniotic fluid. Prenatal

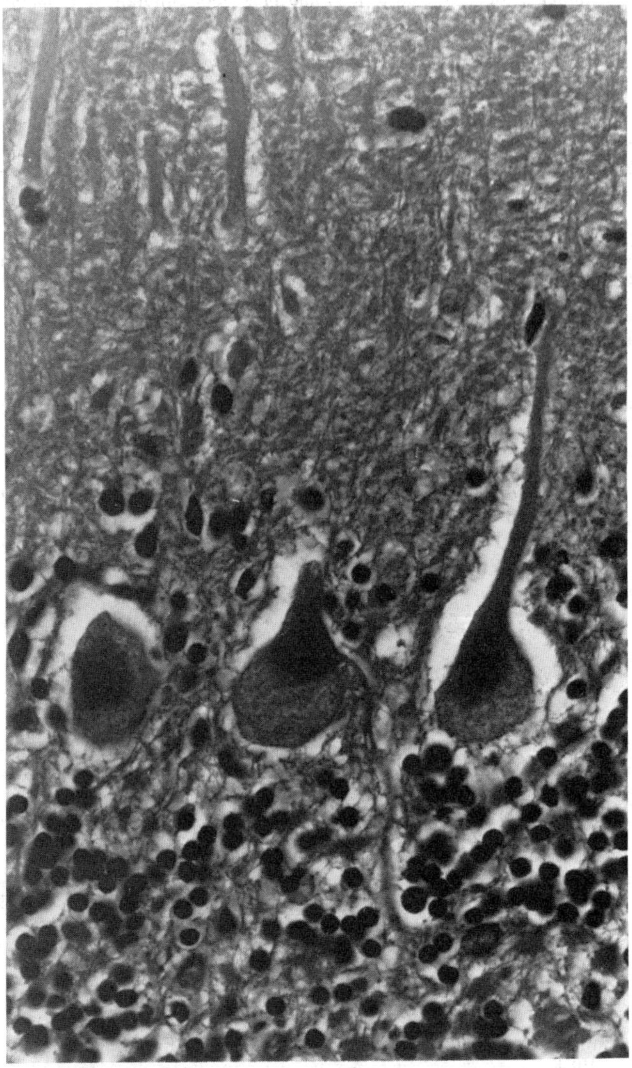

FIGURE 2.2-49. *Tay-Sachs disease. Lipid deposition swells the cytoplasm of the neurons. Hematoxylin and eosin stain. (From Hirano A, Iwata M, Llena J F, Matsui T:* Color Atlas of Pathology of the Nervous System, *p 93. Igaku-Shoin, New York, 1980.)*

TABLE 2.2-4
Metabolic and Degenerative Diseases of Early Life

I. Diseases affecting predominantly the white matter
  A. Central nervous system
    1. Metabolic diseases due to enzyme deficiencies
      a. Lipid diseases
        (1) Metachromatic leukodystrophy
        (2) Globoid cell leukodystrophy (Krabbe's disease)
      b. Amino acid diseases
        (1) Phenylketonuria
        (2) Other aminoacidurias
    2. Unknown pathogenesis
      a. Merzbacher-Pelizaeus disease
      b. Adrenoleukodystrophy (Schilder's disease)
      c. Other sudanophilic leukodystrophies
      d. Spongy leukodystrophy (Canavan's sclerosis)
    3. Immune or viral-induced demyelinations
      a. Postvaccinal and postinfectious diseases
      b. Multiple sclerosis
      c. Subacute sclerosing panencephalitis
  B. Peripheral and cranial nerves; spinal cord
    1. Metabolic diseases
      a. Refsum's disease
      b. Primary familial amyloidosis
      c. Fabry's disease
    2. Unknown pathogenesis
      a. Hereditary spastic paraplegia
      b. Peroneal muscular atrophy (Charcot-Marie-Tooth disease)
      c. Hypertrophic interstitial neuritis (Dejerine-Sottas disease)
      d. Hereditary sensory neuropathy
      e. Leber's optic atrophy
      f. Congenital deafness
II. Diseases of gray matter: neuronal disease
  A. Cerebrum
    1. Metabolic diseases due to enzyme deficiencies
      a. Lipid diseases
        (1) G_{M2} gangliosidosis (Tay-Sachs disease)
        (2) Niemann-Pick disease
        (3) Gaucher's disease
        (4) Other lipid storage diseases
      b. Mucopolysaccharidoses
        (1) Hunter's syndrome
        (2) Hurler's syndrome
        (3) Other mucopolysaccharidoses
      c. Carbohydrate diseases
        (1) Galactosemia
        (2) Gierke's disease
        (3) Other diseases of complex carbohydrates
    2. Other metabolic diseases
      a. Subacute necrotizing encephalomyelopathy (Leigh's disease)
      b. Alper's disease
      c. Copper malabsorption disease (Menkes' kinky-hair disease)
      d. Familial myoclonus
      e. Lipofuscinosis
  B. Basal ganglia
    1. Metabolic disease
      a. Wilson's disease
    2. Unknown pathogenesis
      a. Dystonia musculorum deformans
      b. Hallervorden-Spatz disease
  C. Spinal cord
    1. Unknown pathogenesis
      a. Progressive infantile spinal muscular atrophy (Werdnig-Hoffmann disease)
      b. Wohlfart-Kugelberg-Welander disease
III. Diseases of gray and white matter
  A. Spinocerebellar disorders
    1. Metabolic diseases
      a. Ataxia telangiectasis
      b. Bassen-Kornzweig syndrome
    2. Unknown pathogenesis
      a. Friedreich's ataxia
      b. Other spinocerebellar degenerative diseases

TABLE 2.2-5
Examples of Metabolic Diseases Due to Enzyme Deficiency

Disease	*Deficient Enzyme*
Lysosomal storage diseases	
Sphingolipidoses	
Gangliosidosis (e.g., Tay-Sachs disease)	Hexosaminidase A
Gaucher's disease	β-Glucosidase
Niemann-Pick disease	Sphingomyelinase
Krabbe's disease	Galactocerebrosidase
Metachromatic leukodystrophy	Arylsulfatase A
Mucopolysaccharidoses	
Hurler's syndrome	α-Iduronidase
Hunter's syndrome	Iduronate sulfatase
Deficiencies of metabolic substrate	
Carbohydrate diseases	
Galactosemia	Galactose 1-phosphate uridyl-transferase
Gierke's disease	Glucose 6-phosphatase
Amino acid diseases	
Phenylketonuria	Phenylalanine hydroxylase
Maple syrup urine disease	Decarboxylasing enzymes
Histidinemia	Histidase
Homocystinuria	Synthase, methyltransferase reductase

diagnosis is made by tissue culture of cells obtained by amniocentesis or by analysis of noncultured amniotic cells or fluid. Detection of carriers of disease has revolutionized genetic counseling. All regions routinely perform newborn screening tests for congenital metabolic disorders of hypothyroidism and phenylketonuria; in some states, tests are also performed for galactosemia, homocystinuria, and maple syrup urine disease. Treatment should be instituted as soon as possible after birth.

Riley-Day syndrome This rare dysfunction of the autonomic nervous system, also known as familial dysautonomia, is manifested during the first year of life, usually in Jewish children. The disease is characterized by defective lacrimation, excessive salivation and perspiration, blotchy skin, hypertension with postural hypotension, and defective temperature control. Motor retardation and emotional instability often occur. A decrease of serum dopamine β-hydroxylase has been noted in these patients.

DISEASES OF CHILDHOOD AND ADOLESCENCE DISCUSSED UNDER OTHER CATEGORIES

Neoplasms Brain tumors in children differ from those in adults in several aspects. About three-fourths of all childhood brain tumors affect midline structures, and more than half are in the posterior fossa—that is, the cerebellum, the brain stem, and the fourth ventricle. The most common sites above the tentorium are the third ventricle, the adjacent diencephalon, and the optic chiasm. Gliomas—particularly medulloblastomas, astrocytomas, craniopharyngiomas, and optic nerve gliomas—occur more often in children than in adults. Ependymomas, papillomas of the choroid plexus, and pinealomas develop predominantly in the young. The clinical manifestations are similar to those noted in adults but, because of their midline predominance, increased intracranial pressure is an early sign. In children less than 6 years of age, intracranial hypertension may cause separation of the sutures of the skull, resulting in cracked-pot resonance to percussion as well as head enlargement.

Vascular disease Cerebrovascular disease in childhood is likely to be congenital; the Sturge-Weber syndrome is described above. Congenital heart disease often causes embolic cerebral infarction and, less commonly, cerebral abscess. Subarachnoid hemorrhage in childhood is much more likely to be due to an arteriovenous malformation than to an aneurysm. Cerebral hemorrhage in a child is often associated with blood dyscrasia, especially leukemia. A debilitated child is more likely to develop sinus thrombosis than an adult. Acute hemiplegia, occurring in infants and preschool children, is probably of vascular origin; febrile illness is often the precipitating event, and convulsive seizures are common.

Toxic and inflammatory diseases Lead toxicity causes encephalopathy in children, but not in adults. Subacute sclerosing panencephalitis occurs almost exclusively in children. Acute cerebellar ataxia of childhood is probably of viral origin. Those diseases associated with childhood systemic infection include Sydenham's chorea and Reye's syndrome. The postvaccinal and postexanthemata encephalitides are usually childhood phenomena. Hemophilus meningitis, toxoplasmosis, and cytomegalic inclusion disease (also called inclusion body disease) were limited to children until the outbreak of AIDS.

Other syndromes beginning in childhood Of the epilepsy subtypes, infantile spasms, febrile convulsions, and petit mal are invariably diseases of children. Familial dysautonomia is congenital; Tourette's disorder and Kleine-Levin syndrome begin in childhood or adolescence. The most common muscular dystrophies begin in childhood, and the periodic palsies usually begin in childhood or adolescence. Werdnig-Hoffmann lower motor neuron degeneration and hereditary spastic paraparesis are the most common motor neuron diseases of childhood.

REFERENCES

Adams R D, Victor M: *Principles of Neurology*, ed 3. McGraw-Hill, New York, 1985.

Asbury A K, McKhann G M, McDonald W I, editors: *Diseases of the Nervous System*. Saunders, Philadelphia, 1986.

Baker A B, Joynt R J, editors: *Clinical Neurology*, Harper & Row, New York, 1986.

Barnett H J M, Mohr J P, Stein B M, Yatsu F M, editors: *Stroke: Pathophysiology, Diagnosis and Management*. Churchill Livingstone, New York, 1986.

Booss J, Thornton G F, editors: Infectious Diseases of the Central Nervous System. In *Neurologic Clinics*, vol 4. Saunders, Philadelphia, 1986.

Caplan L R: *Stroke: A Clinical Approach*. Butterworth, Stoneham, MA, 1986.

Haymaker W, Adams R D, editors: *Histology and Histopathology of the Nervous System*. Charles C Thomas, Springfield, IL, 1982.

Hirano A: *A Guide to Neuropathology*, Igaku-Shoin, New York, 1981.

Hollister L E: *Clinical Pharmacology of Psychotherapeutic Drugs*, ed 2. Churchill Livingstone, New York, 1983.

Martin J B, Reichlin S: *Clinical Neuroendocrinology*, ed 2. Davis, Philadelphia, 1987.

Menkes J H: *Textbook of Child Neurology*, ed 3. Lea & Febiger, Philadelphia, 1985.

Rosenberg R N, editor: *The Clinical Neurosciences*. Churchill Livingstone, New York, 1983.

Rowland L P, editor: *Merritt's Textbook of Neurology*, ed 7. Lea & Febiger, Philadelphia, 1984.

Sever J L, Gibbs C J: Retroviruses in the nervous system. Ann Neurol *23* (suppl): S1, 1988.

Swash M, Kennard C, editors: *Scientific Basis of Clinical Neurology*. Churchill Livingstone, New York, 1985.

Walton J N: *Brain's Diseases of the Nervous System*, ed 9. Oxford University Press, New York, 1985.

2.3 NEUROPSYCHIATRY AND BEHAVIORAL NEUROLOGY

SEYMOUR SOLOMON, M.D.
JOSEPH C. MASDEU, M.D.

INTRODUCTION

After a discussion in Section 2.1 of neuropsychiatric findings as they are elicited by the physician, Section 2.2 dealt with the different etiological factors operative in neurological disease. This section is a synthesis of findings and etiology; the clinical syndromes of neuropsychiatry are discussed and treatment is suggested.

Neurology and psychiatry were blended as one part of medical science, neuropsychiatry, in the 1800s; however, the two separated and grew increasingly distant after World War II, as neurology became the science of visible organic disease and psychiatry became the science of personality disorders. In recent decades, the two specialties are again coming together since the emergence of behavioral neurology and biological psychiatry. There is increasing recognition of the biochemical abnormalities responsible for many disorders of function of the central nervous system. These abnormalities may cause alterations of motor or sensory systems in the realm of neurology or changes in the integrative and psychological mechanisms in the realm of psychiatry. Behavioral abnormalities are often attributable to one or more of these factors. The understanding and treatment of patients with altered behavior often requires the skills of both neurologist and psychiatrist.

In this section, a discussion of disturbance of consciousness (coma and syncope) is followed by a review of epilepsy and sleep disorders. Impairment of cognition includes disorders of attention, memory, and language, as well as the more encompassing subjects of dementia and brain dysfunction in childhood. Review of motor function impairment emphasizes movement disorders, defects of motor tone, and weakness associated with peripheral nerve diseases and muscle diseases. Discussion of impairment of sensory function includes dizziness and headache as well as other pain syndromes. Finally, conditions common to psychiatry and neurology are reviewed, especially conversion reaction and those diseases causing symptoms without signs.

IMPAIRMENT OF CONSCIOUSNESS

The distinctions between different degrees of depressed consciousness are not always precise. Stuporous patients require vigorous and frequent stimuli to evoke a response that may be briefly mumbled or briefly purposeful. Semicomatose patients respond only by withdrawing appropriately from painful stimuli. Patients in coma respond with decorticate or decerebrate movements to deep pain or do not respond at all. The best way to record information about the degree of depression of consciousness is simply to describe the patient's responses to reproducible stimuli. See Section 2.1 for a discussion of the features differentiating organic from psychogenic impairment of responsiveness.

COMA Coma of acute onset is most likely due to trauma, cerebrovascular or cardiovascular disease, intoxication, heat stroke, or hypotensive shock. Gradually developing coma is probably due to meningoencephalitis or some other infectious process, a cerebral mass, a metabolic disease, or a disease causing gradual ischemia or hypoxia. The differential diagnosis is listed in Table 2.3-1. The examination of the comatose patient is discussed in Section 2.1.

Treatment In the unconscious patient, the immediate primary concern is maintenance of vital functions. Alterations in the rate and depth of respiration may be due to an obstructed air passage; tracheal intubation and artificial respiration may be necessary. Shock is the most common cardiovascular factor requiring treatment. The patient with tachycardia or bradycardia may need corrective medication or a cardiac pacemaker. High fever must be brought down by ice packs. Hypothermia may be secondary to hypoglycemia or hypothyroidism. The consideration of potential hypoglycemia and thiamine deficiency should be addressed by intravenous (IV) administration of 50 ml of 50 percent glucose and 100 mg of thiamine after blood has been drawn for analysis. If there is suspicion of narcotic overdosage, 0.5 mg of the narcotic antagonist naloxone (Narcan) should be given. Nutrition, hydration, and electrolyte balance must be maintained. Attention to the bladder and the bowels is necessary, and a retention catheter is usually required. The patient should be turned frequently to prevent pneumonia and decubiti. Sedatives are to be avoided; however, if extreme restlessness occurs, one of the phenothiazines may be used.

Laboratory evaluation Laboratory studies of the comatose patient should include evaluation of blood gases, blood count, urinalysis, standard blood chemistries, and serum thyroxine (T_4). Vomitus or gastric analysis and stool examination may be diagnostic. Toxicological studies, especially for barbiturates, may be helpful. A spinal tap is essential if there is suspicion of meningitis; otherwise, the tap is best deferred until after a computed tomography (CT) or magnetic resonance imaging (MR or MRI) has ruled out a mass lesion with a shift of midline structures. Roentgenograms of the chest and an electrocardiogram are essential. The treatments for some of these conditions are discussed in Section 2.2.

Atypical syndromes When the cause of coma is removed, the patient becomes alert. However, if residual damage of the alerting mechanisms has occurred, coma may evolve to a state called akinetic mutism. In the locked-in syndrome and with psychogenic unresponsiveness, the patient appears comatose but is not.

Akinetic mutism occurs with organic disease of the diencephalon, especially the caudal hypothalamus; bilateral mesial frontal lesions may cause a similar state. Most common causes of akinetic mutism are severe anoxic or hypoglycemic brain damage, infarction with an anterior communicating artery aneurysm, and brain trauma. Akinetic mutism often develops after the patient has been comatose for several days or weeks. The sleep-wake cycle returns, but the patient remains immobile, mute, and cannot voluntarily respond. The eyes may follow people about the room or may be diverted by sound. A painful stimulus sometimes evokes withdrawal or feeble movements. On rare occasions, the patient may repeat a sentence or a song (isolation of the speech area). In contrast to psychotic withdrawal, patients with akinetic mutism do not exhibit negativism or catatonic waxy flexibility. (Sometimes, however, the features of catatonia may occur with organic disease, such as encephalitis.) Usually a chronic condition, akinetic mutism may, in rare instances, improve and the patient may be left with an attention disorder. Treatment mainly consists in keeping the patients comfortable and free from infections. Since they cannot verbalize or point to express their needs, other indicators have to be used. Profuse perspiration or a sudden rise in blood pressure should alert the clinician to the possibility of pain, often from a full bladder, a decubitis ulcer, or pneumonia.

The *locked-in syndrome* is usually caused by an infarct or hemorrhage in the base of the pons. A de-efferented state results, with paralysis of the limbs and all of the cranial nerve musculature, except for the eye muscles. The conscious patient is locked into a helpless body but may be able to communicate with the eyes.

TABLE 2.3-1
Differential Diagnosis of Coma

- Toxic and metabolic diseases
  - Exogenous toxins
    - Alcohol
    - Narcotics
    - Medicinal drugs
    - Biological toxins
    - Heavy metals
    - Industrial toxins
  - Endogenous metabolites
    - Diabetes
      - Ketosis
      - Hyperosmolar, nonketotic
    - Uremia
    - Hepatic encephalopathy
    - Other endocrine and electrolyte disorders
- Infections
  - Systemic
    - Pneumonia
    - Septicemia
  - Intracranial
    - Meningitis
    - Encephalitis
- Vascular diseases
  - Systemic
    - Cardiovascular
    - Pulmonary
  - Intracranial
    - Hemorrhage
    - Ischemia or infarction
- Other etiological categories affecting the brain
  - Trauma
  - Tumor
  - Seizure disorders
  - Electric shock
  - Hyperthermia or hypothermia
- Psychogenic unresponsiveness
  - Hysteria
  - Catatonia
  - Depression withdrawal

SYNCOPE Syncope is brief loss of consciousness, usually no more than 15 seconds. The most frequent causes of syncope are vasovagal dysfunction, orthostatic hypotension, cardiac arrhythmia, and, much less often, vertebrobasilar artery insufficiency. The differential diagnosis is listed in Table 2.3-2.

TABLE 2.3-2
Differential Diagnosis of Syncope

- I. Primary brain mechanisms
  - A. Vascular causes
    - 1. Transient ischemic attack, within vertebrobasilar territories
    - 2. Subarachnoid hemorrhage
    - 3. Carotid sinus reflex (direct cerebral effect)
    - 4. Hyperventilation (causing vasoconstriction)
  - B. Other transient cerebral dysfunctions
    - 1. Epilepsy
    - 2. Concussion
    - 3. Severe vertigo (vasovagal response)
    - 4. Psychogenic factors
- II. Brain ischemia caused by cardiovascular factors (note that mechanisms under A and B are often associated with diseases under C and D)
  - A. Cardiac arrhythmia
    - 1. Bradycardia or heart block
    - 2. Vagal reflexes: vasovagal (carotid sinus), vagovagal (swallowing), oculovagal (eyeball pressure), viscerovagal (intrathoracic or intra-abdominal stimulus)
    - 3. Tachycardia: atrial or ventricular
  - B. Hypotension
    - 1. Orthostatic hypotension
      - a. Pathophysiological: after prolonged bed rest, pregnancy, exhaustion, prolonged standing, drugs
      - b. Pathological: idiopathic autonomic disease, diabetes mellitus, adrenal insufficiency, postsympathectomy, malnutrition
    - 2. Vagal reflexes—vasodepressor
      - a. Carotid sinus reflex
      - b. Severe pain
      - c. Emotional stimuli
  - C. Primary decrease in cardiac output
    - 1. Valvular disease, especially aortic stenosis (also hypertrophic subaortic stenosis, mitral insufficiency, and stenosis)
    - 2. Myocardial infarction
    - 3. Cardiomyopathy
    - 4. Other cardiac causes of heart failure
  - D. Secondary decrease in cardiac output
    - 1. Changes in intrathoracic pressure
      - a. Physiological: cough (tussive syncope), valsalva maneuver, positive pressure breathing
      - b. Pathological: pulmonary embolism, pneumonia
    - 2. Changes in peripheral resistance
      - a. Physiological: micturition, hyperventilation, vasodilator drugs
      - b. Pathological: sodium loss, hypovolemia, anemia
- III. Impairment of brain metabolism
  - A. Hypoxia: hypoventilation, lack of environmental oxygen, carbon monoxide, cyanide
  - B. Hypoglycemia
  - C. Other causes of metabolic encephalopathy

EPILEPSY

A seizure is a paroxysmal disturbance of cerebral function due to excessive neuronal discharge. Epilepsy is the recurrence of seizures and is manifested by transient somatic, visceral, or psychic phenomena or by all three and is usually associated with loss or alteration of consciousness. In the past, seizures were named for their clinical manifestations, hence the terms "grand mal," "petit mal," and "psychomotor." Later, epilepsy was classified by correlating electroencephalographic (EEG) features and clinical signs. With this classification, most forms of epilepsy are divided into two major groups: generalized seizures and partial or focal seizures.

GENERALIZED SEIZURES Seizures that are generalized at the onset affect the cerebrum as a whole, and the EEG paroxysms appear in a bilaterally symmetrical and synchronous fashion. Loss or alteration of consciousness almost always occurs. Many of these seizures have been termed "idiopathic" because an organic defect often cannot be found; a biochemical mechanism is postulated. Many cases are found to be due to specific toxic or metabolic disturbances or to diffuse or scattered organic cerebral disease. Most generalized seizures are subdivided into nonconvulsive and convulsive seizures.

GENERALIZED CONVULSIVE SEIZURES An aura is usually not part of a generalized convulsive seizure, also known as a tonic-clonic or grand mal seizure. Loss of consciousness is invariable, and tongue biting or incontinence is common. During the tonic phase, breathing is impossible and cyanosis ensues. Violent clonic jerks follow, which gradually decrease in frequency until all movements cease and the patient lies flaccid, still unconscious. After the seizure, the patient is drowsy and confused; there may be muscle aches. Generalized convulsive seizures show bilaterally synchronous polyspike and slow-wave bursts in the EEG.

GENERALIZED NONCONVULSIVE SEIZURES Petit mal seizures usually begin between the ages of 5 and 10 years and generally subside after puberty, but can persist into adult life. The most typical seizure is manifested by simple loss or impairment of consciousness, called petit mal *absence*. The seizures last only a few seconds, and begin and end abruptly without aura or sequelae. They typically occur many times a day. Slight rhythmic movements of lips, mouth, and head, as well as blinking, are often associated with altered consciousness, especially if the seizure persists for more than 10 seconds. Brief automatisms or decreased postural tone may occur. Hyperventilation often induces the absence. Petit mal status is characterized by a semistuporous state. Classical absences are not associated with organic disease. The EEG of petit mal seizures reveals rhythmic bilaterally synchronous and symmetrical 3-per-second spike-and-wave discharges.

Juvenile myoclonic epilepsy may also begin in young adults. Bilateral myoclonic jerks without alteration of consciousness occur most often soon after awakening. The myoclonic activity may be mistaken for nervousness or tics. These patients usually have grand mal or absence attacks as well. They are and remain neurologically intact.

Febrile convulsions Generalized convulsive seizures are often associated with fever before the age of 3 years. The high familial incidence (25 percent) and normal interictal EEG help to establish the benign nature of this condition. It should be distinguished from seizures precipitated by fever, but due to encephalitis or other cerebral disease.

Withdrawal seizures The so-called rum fit occurs in the chronic alcoholic from 6 to 48 hours after abstinence. About a third of these patients develop delirium tremens. Seizures may occur after withdrawal from many types of drugs. The onset of seizures after barbiturate withdrawal may be as early as the second day or as late as the second or third week.

Other generalized seizures Some generalized seizures are caused by serious cerebral disease and are relatively refractory to treatment. Myoclonic activity is often the sequela of cerebral anoxia or generalized ischemia. In young children, atonic or akinetic seizures are manifested by loss of postural tone and resultant drop attacks; later, tonic seizures may occur. In this atypical petit mal, known as *Lennox-Gastaut syndrome*, the EEG paroxysms are slightly slower and less rhythmic than in classical petit mal.

PARTIAL OR FOCAL SEIZURES With these seizures, the EEG shows spike discharges localized to cortical or subcortical regions of one cerebral hemisphere. Organic lesions would be expected in these disorders, but remediable diseases are found infrequently; constitutional factors are important. Seizures of this type may occur in children, but the incidence increases with age. Partial seizures are subdivided mainly into those with elementary, simple symptoms and those with complex symptoms.

Partial seizures with either simple or complex symptoms may spread from the initial discharging site to ever-widening adjacent areas and thus progress to generalized seizure activity; that is, the seizures become secondarily generalized. Jacksonian seizures begin as focal motor activity in one extremity, spread over the ipsilateral side, and finally, become secondarily generalized (grand mal). Sometimes, this progression is so rapid that the focal qualities may not be clinically apparent. The EEG, however, shows the evolution of a primary focus to secondary generalized paroxysmal activity.

Perinatal anoxic damage of the medial temporal lobe is often responsible for the onset of focal seizures in adolescents or young adults. Tumors or trauma predominate in adult life and cerebral infarction is the most common cause of new seizures in the elderly. Post-traumatic seizures erupt most often within 6 months after cerebral trauma, but they may occur many years later. The incidence of seizures after head trauma largely depends on the severity of the cerebral injury: usually 50 percent after cerebral laceration and 15 to 20 percent after contusion.

PARTIAL SIMPLE SEIZURES These seizures are usually focal motor in character and unassociated with impairment or loss of consciousness. They consist of clonic movements involving part or all of the musculature on the side contralateral to the discharging cerebral focus. In addition, adversive seizures are manifested by turning of the head, eyes, and body away from the side of the discharging lesion. Less common focal motor seizures include inhibitory seizures, characterized by loss of tone and strength, and seizures that cause arrest of speech. Other partial seizures of an elementary type are sensory and usually occur as an aura of a motor seizure, rather than as an isolated seizure state. There are rare somatosensory seizures with local pain over some part of the contralateral face, body, or extremities. Special sensory seizures include visual, auditory, olfactory, or gustatory phenomena. Vertiginous symptoms are sometimes of epileptic origin and may arise from the insula or medial temporal lobe. Autonomic symptoms occurring in a paroxysmal fashion are rare manifestations of partial seizures; the epileptogenic focus is usually in the insula or orbitofrontal cortex. Episodic abdominal pain (abdominal epilepsy) is the most common example.

COMPLEX PARTIAL SEIZURES Seizures that arise from the temporal lobe or associated limbic areas may evoke a complex clinical pattern. The aura of a seizure is its onset, not a warning of an impending event. The aura of complex partial seizures may be a visceral discomfort within the abdomen or the head; an emotional experience, such as anxiety; or illusions or hallucinations of the special senses: gustatory, olfactory, auditory, or visual. During the seizure, there is alteration of consciousness and thought processes; amnesia for the event is common; and aphasia may occur. Automatic stereotyped behavior is most characteristic and consists of smacking of the lips, chewing, or swallowing. These automatisms, coupled with psychological changes, warrant the term "psychomotor seizures." The behavior is often bizarre, partially or totally inappropriate, and may be semipurposeful. Simple automatisms may consist of fumbling with clothing, manipulation of the hands, or aimless stumbling about. More complex activities may be the pursuit of a previous line of habitual activity. During the seizure, patients may obey simple commands; less commonly, they may be antagonistic.

Ictal psychological and behavioral phenomena The psychic phenomena of partial complex seizures are often perceptual, characterized by illusions. Sensory illusions may be a distortion of any of the special senses, such as floors tilting or sounds echoing. There may be an alteration in self-awareness or déjà vu phenomena. Hallucinations, usually formed and complex, may be evoked by seizures. In contradistinction to schizophrenic hallucinations, the hallucinations of partial complex seizures are usually recognized as such by the patient. Seizures may cause alterations in mood or affect, especially fear and depression.

Sudden depression may occur as the aura of a seizure or as the major manifestation of a complex partial seizure. Particularly in young patients, complex partial seizures may be manifested by rapid alterations in mood; swings from depression to euphoria may occur within hours. If laughter occurs, it is not accompanied by appropriate affect. Bursts of anger or sexual sensations are rarely manifestations of epilepsy; sexual automatisms are sometimes associated with frontal lobe lesions. Disturbance of thought, especially forced thinking, may be a seizure manifestation. Automatisms are the most common type of psychomotor phenomena. Automatic behavior may follow the seizure or may constitute part or all of the seizure.

Complex partial seizures (psychomotor seizures) are difficult and sometimes impossible to differentiate clinically from similar behavioral disturbances of psychological origin, hysterical reactions (Table 2.3-3). Evaluation by simultaneous closed-circuit television and EEG recordings may resolve this diagnostic dilemma. An elevation of serum prolactin occurs after an epileptic seizure (except for some simple seizures), but not after a psychogenic seizure. The chief clinical differentiating features of complex partial seizures are the aura (especially olfactory hallucinations) and the postictal drowsiness and depression of mentation; there usually is amnesia concerning the episode. Seizures are usually of shorter duration than psychogenic events. Although the automatisms of the psychomotor seizure may be as bizarre as the psychogenic seizure, the epileptic seizures tend to be stereotyped for each patient. Aggressive activity and rage reactions are likely to be psychogenic. It is not unusual for hysterical seizures to occur in patients with complex partial epilepsy. Occasionally, a psychomotor seizure takes the form of schizophrenic-like behavior and may lead to the mistaken diagnosis of psychosis. The epileptic patient, however, has greater fluctuation of mental status, only spotty loss of associations, and attempts to maintain contact with reality; dysphasia or impaired perception may also be evident. The behavior during psychomotor seizures is stereotyped, occurs episodically, and usually lasts much less than 24 hours, all in contradistinction to schizophrenia. The gustatory or olfactory aura of temporal lobe seizures should not be mistaken for psychotic hallucinations or illusions, which are more likely to be auditory, to be of longer duration, and to have meaning for the patient. The autisms, withdrawals, bizarre thought content, and symbolic processes seen in schizophrenia are usually absent in epilepsy.

Postictal psychosis A confused and delirious state sometimes follows convulsions and may last for minutes, hours, or days. Overdosage of anticonvulsive medication may also cause a toxic psychosis.

VIOLENCE AND EPILEPSY Postictal agitation may evolve into violence if attempts are made to restrain the patient forcefully, but extreme violence is very rare as a manifestation of a complex partial seizure. Epileptics do not have a higher incidence of interictal violence than people with other diseases, and there is no greater prevalence of epilepsy in people convicted of violent crimes than in other convicts. The legal term "temporary insanity," if at all applicable to medicine, should be limited to acts during complex partial seizures. Epilepsy, as a defense in criminal cases, is being increasingly invoked. The proof should be neurological, not psychiatric. There must be evidence of aggressive behavior as a stereotyped automatism of temporal seizures documented by simultaneous television and EEG recordings.

TABLE 2.3-3
Epilepsy vs. Hysterical Fits

Feature	*Epilepsy*	*Hysteria*
Precipitating factors	None, or alcohol or drug withdrawal	Emotionally stressful event
Environment	Any place, any circumstance, occasionally nocturnal	Indoors, especially home, with people present
Onset	Sudden	Often gradual
Aura	Often unpleasant taste, lip smacking	Often hyperventilation or its symptoms
Seizure	Automatism or tonic-clonic	Struggling, thrashing, quivering, pelvic thrusting
Pattern	Stereotyped	Variable
Screaming	At onset	During attack
Talking	Rare	Often
Biting	Tongue	Lips, hands, other people
Micturition	Often	Rare
Sequelae	Drowsy, aches	Alert
Injury	Often	Rare
Memory of seizure	Amnesia is common	Recall of some events
Duration	Few minutes	Many minutes

INTERICTAL PERSONALITY Is there an epileptic personality? Most people with epilepsy are not psychologically disturbed, but there is a higher incidence of interictal psychological disturbances than in the general population. The mechanism of these changes in personality is controversial. In some cases, personality changes are caused by the disease or dysfunction that evokes seizures. This is especially true of seizures arising in the frontal or temporal lobe or other parts of the limbic system. Most changes can be explained by the interpersonal and environmental stresses of having to deal with chronic recurring seizures or the threat of seizures. The use of multiple anticonvulsant drugs may cause changes in personality as well as cognition. Behavioral abnormalities in some epileptic patients are believed to be due to a pathophysiological process rather than to life stresses. There are several factors in support of this concept. The behavioral traits of epileptics are stable, rather than episodic, and their severity correlates with the duration of epilepsy rather than with the frequency of seizures. Moreover, the personality defects are more common in patients with bitemporal lobe EEG abnormalities than in those who have a consistently unilateral temporal lobe focus. The limbic areas are particularly susceptible to kindling of new epileptogenic sites in lower animals. It is postulated that abnormally discharging temporal lobe neurons in epileptics over many years results in the formation of new neuronal bonds (hyperconnections) to the special sensory association areas of the cortex. As a result, enhanced emotional associations are made with what would ordinarily be emotionally neutral stimuli.

Impairment of cognitive function in epileptic patients is uncommon. When it occurs, it may be caused by an underlying organic cerebral lesion. Many years of anticonvulsant medication may depress mental faculties. Early age of onset, high frequency, and long duration of seizures are adverse factors.

The relationship between epilepsy and melancholia has been noted since the time of Hippocrates. Depression and epilepsy are common ailments, but their association is much greater than would be expected by chance. Depression is the most common clinical psychiatric diagnosis made in epileptic patients, and the depression scale of the Minnesota Multiphasic Personality Inventory (MMPI) is often elevated, especially if the seizures are of late onset. The rate of suicide is higher in epileptics than in the rest of the population, and patients with complex partial seizures are at highest risk. The relationship between depression and complex partial seizures has often been noted, but perhaps because these seizures are the most common type of epilepsy. Other common features in these patients are anxiety, fear, and irritability. Mania is rare. As noted above, swings of mood may be manifestations of complex partial seizures; This phenomenon is more often noted as an interictal manifestation of altered personality. Changes of mood may be more prevalent with decrease in seizure frequency.

Although tricyclic and monoamine oxidase inhibitor antidepressants lower the convulsive threshold, they are not contraindicated in epilepsy. When these drugs are used, however, the anticonvulsant as well as antidepressant drugs must be closely monitored. Nomifensine (Merital) has little effect on seizure threshold and has been advocated as the antidepressant of choice for epileptic patients. Electroconvulsive therapy (ECT) may be used for depressed patients with epilepsy if antidepressant medication and psychotherapy fail.

Certain behavioral traits have been seen in less than 10 percent of patients with chronic complex partial (temporal lobe and psychomotor) seizures. Abnormalities occur in the emotional overtones assigned to events and people. Activities with important emotional content, such as social interaction, religion, and sex, are distorted in these patients. The most common phenomena are viscosity of thought processes, deepening of emotions with stern moralism and idiosyncratic religious or cosmological beliefs, and diminished sexual drive. Viscosity refers to the tendency to adhere to each thought and action. There is preoccupation with excessive detail, and thought processes are circumstantial and perseverative. Hypergraphia is an obsessional phenomenon manifested by writing extensive notes and diaries. Verbosity is the verbal correlate. The intense emotions are often labile; thus, the patient sometimes may exhibit great warmth, whereas anger and irritability may evolve to rage and aggressive behavior on other occasions. A sense of grandiosity is less common than feelings of guilt, self-recrimination, and depression. Suspiciousness may extend to paranoia. A sense of helplessness may lead to passive dependency. These patients often have little insight. A stern moralism and associated humorless sobriety calls for strict attention to rules and associated desire to exact severe punishment for minor infractions. Religious beliefs tend to shift and are not only intense, but may be associated with idiosyncratic theological or cosmological theories. Libido is diminished, but sometimes sexual behavior is deviant.

A schizophrenic-like psychosis rarely occurs in patients with epilepsy. This psychosis is more common in complex partial seizures than in other forms of epilepsy, and there is some evidence implicating the left more than the right temporal lobe. The clinical features of this psychosis may be indistinguishable from schizophrenia, but in epileptics there is a greater tendency to preserve affect and to establish rapport, with less disorganization of thought. In schizophrenics without epilepsy, there is usually a past history of schizophrenic behavior or severe personality disturbance, and often there is a family history of psychosis.

A temporal lobectomy for intractable complex partial seizures usually diminishes traits of aggressiveness and impulsivity, and often ameliorates hyposexuality. There is usually little change in the hyperreligiosity, viscosity phenomena, or schizophrenic-like psychoses. The suppression of seizure activity with anticonvulsant medication sometimes increases the psychological abnormalities, and an increase in seizure frequency may ameliorate the psychosis.

DIFFERENTIAL DIAGNOSIS Most seizures are diagnosed by their distinguishing clinical characteristics. The diagnosis of a generalized convulsive (grand mal) seizure is supported by tongue biting or incontinence during the seizure, and subsequent drowsiness, confusion, or muscular aches. Generalized nonconvulsive (petit mal) epilepsy, however, is not associated with an aura or sequelae, and never begins in adult life. Complex partial seizures (psychomotor seizures) may be preceded by an aura of uncinate phenomena (olfactory or gustatory hallucinations) or by licking and smacking of the lips, and amnesia for the seizure is almost invariable. Although these seizures are extremely variable from one patient to another, they tend to be stereotyped for each individual. All of the above seizures are associated with loss or impairment of consciousness, which is most profound in grand mal, may be so brief as to be indiscernible in petit mal, and may be obscured by the complex automatism of a psychomotor seizure. Partial seizures with elementary symptoms are not associated with impairment of consciousness unless the seizure spreads to deep cerebral structures and becomes secondarily generalized.

Seizure activity may be mistaken for other conditions. The child during a petit mal seizure may be accused of inattention. What seems to be syncope may be a minor seizure. The fugue state of complex partial status epilepticus or the stuporous appearance of a patient in petit mal status may resemble amnesia of psychogenic origin. When hysterical seizures simulate grand mal epilepsy, the movements are more likely to affect the trunk than the extremities and usually mimic coitus.

Epilepsy in young children must be differentiated from other episodic phenomena: (1) *Breath-holding spells* occur from 6 months to 3 years of age and are provoked by crying. When crying begins, expiration is prolonged and the cry is held or breath is lost for about 15 seconds. Loss of consciousness then occurs for a few seconds, with flaccidity, rigidity, or, sometimes, brief clonic activity. (2) Very young girls may masturbate by squeezing their extended legs together in a tonic fashion. The child may be poorly responsive during this time and fall asleep afterward. (3) *Tics* are more complex and less stereotyped than myoclonic jerks and can be voluntarily controlled for a short period. (4) Similarly, psychomotor seizures are more stereotyped than paroxysmal behavioral disturbances and temper tantrums. (5) A child may be unresponsive during and briefly following somnambulism and night-terrors. These sleep disorders will be discussed below.

EVALUATION OF THE EPILEPTIC In the initial evaluation of patients with seizures, several laboratory studies are advisable in addition to the EEG. Severe anemia or leukemia, uremia, lues, and hypoglycemia may all present with seizures as the initial symptom.

CT or MR is indicated for every patient with onset of seizures after the age of 20 years. About 30 percent of all patients with severe epilepsy show changes, usually of atrophic nature, in CT or MR scans. Additional pathophysiological focal abnormalities are demonstrable with position emission tomography (PET) scanning. The probability of brain tumor is greatest when the onset of seizures is between the ages of 30 and 60; vascular disease is the most common cause of seizures after the age of 55.

TREATMENT **Medication** In most patients, epilepsy can be completely or adequately controlled by medication. One drug should be used and the dosage increased almost to the point of clinical toxicity before adding or substituting another drug. The drug must reach its serum plateau before its efficacy can be judged, and it takes about five elimination half-lives for the anticonvulsant to build up a stable serum concentration (Table 2.3-4). When a second anticonvulsant drug is added to a therapeutic regimen, it may inhibit or stimulate the metabolism of the first drug. Similarly, other medications may alter the pharmacokinetics of the drugs. In discontinuing an anticonvulsant, gradual withdrawal is mandatory.

The drug must be matched to the type of epilepsy. For partial seizures, both simple and complex (psychomotor), the drugs of choice are carbamazepine (Tegretol), phenytoin (Dilantin), or phenobarbital, which are also the primary drugs for generalized convulsive (grand mal) seizures; however, divalproex sodium (Depakote) is increasingly being used as the anticonvulsant of first choice. Ethosuximide (Zarontin) and divalproex sodium are most effective for generalized nonconvulsive seizures—that is, petit mal absences. When grand mal and petit mal occur in the same patient, and for juvenile myoclonic epilepsy, divalproex sodium is the drug of choice. Several other anticonvulsants may be used if the first-line drugs fail. Primidone (Mysoline) is effective for grand mal or psychomotor seizures, for seizures that are secondarily generalized, and for therapeutic failures of petit mal absence. Table 2.2-3 is a summary of the major anticonvulsants. Phenytoin may be started with a loading dose of 1,000 mg per day; the other anticonvulsants should be started at one or two tablets per day, with increases adjusted to the patient's responsiveness and serum concentrations.

TABLE 2.3-4
Anticonvulsant Medications

Drug	Size of Tablet or Capsule (mg)*	Dosage Range (mg per day)	Minimum Time Before Judging Efficacy (weeks)	Therapeutic Serum Concentration (mg per ml)
Phenobarbital (Luminal)	15, **30**, 60, 100	90–180	3–4	15–40
Phenytoin (Dilantin)	30, 50, **100**	200–500	2–4	10–20
Carbamazepine (Tegretol)	100, **200**	600–1,400	1–2	4–12
Ethosuximide (Zarontin)	**250**	750–1,500	1–3	40–100
Divalproex sodium (Depakote)	**250**, 500	750–3,000	4–6	40–150
Primidone (Mysoline)	50, **250**	500–1,500	3–4	5–12
Clonazepam (Klonopin)	**0.5**, 0.75	2–8	1–2	0.01–0.10

*Most common sizes are in boldface type.

When seizures persist for longer than 10 minutes (status epilepticus), maintenance of an open airway is the first objective. Blood chemistries are drawn, and IV glucose and vitamin B complex are administered, followed by an infusion of normal saline. An IV dosage of diazepam (Valium), 2 mg per minute, is given to a total of 10 or 20 mg, and phenytoin is infused at a rate of less than 50 mg per minute for a total dose of 1,000 to 1,500 mg. If the seizures persist for longer than 30 minutes, intubation will be necessary; phenobarbital is then administered IV, at 100 mg per minute, up to 1,500 mg. In addition to respiratory depression, the patient must be observed for cardiac arrhythmias and hypotension.

The anticonvulsant drugs are relatively safe, but side effects are common. Drowsiness, dermatitis, and gastrointestinal symptoms may occur with all medications. Depression of the bone marrow is rare. Certain toxic reactions are characteristic of specific drugs. Phenytoin causes nystagmus, ataxia, and drowsiness as blood levels increase; gum hypertrophy, megaloblastic anemia, and hirsutism may occur; rarely, syndromes simulate lupus erythematosus or lymphoma. Vertigo and nystagmus may occur with many anticonvulsants but are most prominent with primidone overdosage. Hematological toxicity with carbamazepine is rare, but it occurs more often than with phenytoin or phenobarbital; hepatic toxicity occurs more often with divalproex sodium than with phenytoin or carbamazepine. Both phenobarbital and clonazepam (Klonopin) may cause drowsiness and ataxia and, in children, hyperkinetic behavior. There is evidence of impairment of cognitive skills after years of phenytoin or barbiturate therapy.

Ancillary measures Several other medications may be appropriate in the treatment of epilepsy. Acetazolamide (Diamox) has anticonvulsant action, and other diuretics may be helpful, particularly for those women who experience an increase in seizure frequency associated with menstruation. Regulation of living habits is important. People with epilepsy should avoid overhydration, fatigue, and alcoholic beverages, although an occasional drink will do no harm. If a tranquilizer is needed, diazepam, which has anticonvulsant properties, or meprobamate (Miltown), or chlordiazepoxide (Librium), are preferred to phenothiazine compounds, which may lower the convulsive threshold. If a major tranquilizer is necessary, molindone (Moban) or haloperidol (Haldol) is recommended. Depression is not rare in epileptics, and antidepressant medication may be used with anticonvulsants.

Surgery Surgical resection of an epileptogenic scar or other cerebral lesion is considered when all conservative measures have failed. In patients with a single anterior temporal lobe focus, surgery is successful in significantly decreasing the frequency of seizures or completely halting them.

COGNITIVE IMPAIRMENT

ATTENTIONAL DISORDERS As discussed in the subsection on coma, the distinction between coma and impaired attention is often only a matter of degree. For instance, a patient with a mild hepatic encephalopathy will have an attentional impairment, which will gradually deepen and ultimately yield to coma as the liver failure worsens. In both coma and attentional disorders, the alerting mechanisms discussed in Section 2.2 are impaired. Patients who have recovered from coma following brain trauma or a subarachnoid hemorrhage are often left with an attentional syndrome. Disturbed attention results in poor performance in all aspects of cognition. Forward planning and the performance of spontaneous meaningful activity suffer most. Attentional abnormalities are best exemplified by the delirious state and by attentional disorders in children, both discussed below.

MEMORY AND AMNESIA Memory has several components that become explicit when there is amnesia. *Amnesia* is the loss of memory with preservation of other cognitive function. People with *anterograde amnesia* cannot learn new information, whereas people with *retrograde amnesia* cannot recall past events. Sometimes, memory loss is denied and the patient confabulates—that is, makes up stories. Amnesia is usually due to bilateral medial temporal lobe (medial hippocampus) disease as seen in early Alzheimer's disease, anoxia, ischemia (terminal basilar artery distribution), or herpes simplex encephalitis. Conditions that result in anterograde amnesia (with or without confabulation) appear to be due to the bilateral loss of a selective zone (cornu ammonis [CA]-1) of the hippocampus. Disease of the basal forebrain (orbitofrontal, septal, and hypothalamic areas) also causes amnesia, which may be associated with impaired consciousness.

Transient global amnesia In middle or late life, a sudden inability to remember present events (i.e., anterograde amnesia) lasts from 1 hour to several hours. The patient is bewildered and, not recalling answers, repeatedly asks the same questions. Retrograde amnesia for past hours or days also occurs, but old memories are preserved. As memory returns, the retrograde amnesia shrinks, but anterograde amnesia for the episode is permanent. Transient global amnesia is probably a transient ischemic attack of the medial temporal lobes.

Amnesia Amnesia is often psychogenic, a dissociative disorder, and its differentiation from memory loss due to organic disease may be difficult. Amnesia of organic origin is frequently abrupt (for example, post-traumatic or postictal) and often has both retrograde and anterograde components. These components gradually shrink as recovery occurs. When memory loss is psychological, it is often of vague onset and termination; if there is a retrograde component, it may be of inappropriately long duration. Recovery from organic amnesia is commonly incomplete and often is followed by confusion for hours or days; events during the illness are not recalled. After the patient with dissociative disorder has recovered memory, there is complete return to normal mentation; isolated events during the period of amnesia may be remembered. In organic disease, precipitating factors may be obvious (e.g., trauma) or occult (e.g., ischemia). A traumatic emotional experience may precipitate psychogenic amnesia, and the amnesia serves a psychological need. The behavior of a patient with organic loss of memory is often abnormal, and delirium is common. The patient with psychogenic amnesia usually behaves normally and has excellent contact with the surroundings. Amnesia of organic disease is often generalized, and all cognitive spheres, including language, may be affected. With hysteria, there often is selective loss of personal information, especially psychologically stressful topics; nevertheless, the forgotten painful events may influence actions. Amnesia of one's name and identity, while maintaining other orientation, language, and intellectual skills, is always a hysterical dissociation. Organic amnesia is frequently accompanied by objective neurological signs, whereas psychogenic memory loss may be accompanied by hysterical signs.

DISORDERS OF SPEECH AND LANGUAGE

Impairment of speech production The production of speech has to do with fluency, articulation, and voice volume. When other features of the neurological examination are abnormal, the organic basis is evident. Although several conditions have no known organic or pathophysiological mechanism, they are not necessarily caused by psychological disturbances. Dysarthria, stuttering, pallilalia, and dysphonia are discussed in Section 2.1.

Mutism, the loss of vocal expression, occurs in a variety of organic lesions. It is commonly the result of expressive aphasia or disease of the diencephalon. It may occur during petit mal or temporal lobe status epilepticus; on rare occasions, a catatonic-like stupor is caused by herpes encephalitis, tumors of the corpus callosum, or hyperparathyroidism. The absence of vocal output is a common manifestation of psychological illness. Mutism occurs during the acute phase of catatonic schizophrenia and in the end stage of chronic schizophrenia. It may also be evident in patients with paranoid distrust and with severe depression (rarely during a manic state). Hysterical aphonia sometimes occurs. Occasionally, a child will be selectively mute and speak only to his or her mother.

Disorders of language

Patients who have aphasia or dysphasia usually show other signs of organic cerebral disease. When aphasia occurs without other signs, it may be mistaken for psychological illness. For the examination and localization of aphasias, see Section 2.1.

Nonfluent dysphasia Slight word-finding difficulties are normal experiences and vary with such factors as education and speech habits. Word-finding difficulty may occur with such diverse psychological phenomena as anxiety, depression, and catatonic schizophrenia. In distinguishing schizophrenic from organic language impairment, careful evaluation reveals that thoughts, more than words, are blocked in schizophrenia. Schizophrenic patients are undisturbed and unconcerned by the change in language, but dysphasic patients are distraught by the inability to adequately express themselves. The circumstantiality of speech of the dysphasic patient's groping for expression may simulate circumlocution of the schizophrenic patient, but the latter is associated with inattention and lack of concern. The verbal output in schizophrenia is prolonged and the content bizarre, in contrast to dysphasic defects of language production. Unaccustomed errors in grammar and paucity of adjectives and adverbs are manifestations of expressive dysphasia, but syntax and vocabulary are intact in patients with psychological illness. The patient with expressive dysphasia usually shows a decrease in rate of speech and in length of phrase as well as impairments in rhythm and inflection; dysarthria may be present. All or some of these features may occur with depression, but the depressed patient appears sad, and the expressed thought content is morbid, self-deprecatory, and negative.

Fluent aphasia or dysphasia Fluent aphasia, whereby the patient is unable to understand speech, results in verbal output that has been called "word salad." Meaningless jumbles of words are spoken rapidly, and the speech often contains clichés, circumlocutions, neologisms, and other paraphasic errors. This "crazy" speech, if unassociated with other neurological signs, may be mistaken for schizophrenic behavior. This type of speech may evolve gradually in cases of chronic schizophrenia, in contrast to the acute onset of organic disease, such as cerebral infarction. As with expressive nonfluent aphasia, patients with fluent aphasia show some awareness of their difficulties and are often disturbed by them, in contradistinction to schizophrenic patients, who are unconcerned and often presume that the listener understands them. Accordingly, aphasic patients attempt nonverbal communication and may pause to allow the examiner to help them; not so with schizophrenic patients, who are less attentive to the examiner. Paraphasic words and neologisms are more common with fluent dysphasia than with schizophrenia. Severely disturbed schizophrenic patients may seem to have difficulty in the comprehension of spoken language, but they usually show some understanding of speech by carrying out some commands by incorporating some of the examiner's words into their own speech or by echoing the examiner.

Etiology of neurogenic language disturbances

Cerebral infarction is the leading cause of aphasia. Intracerebral hemorrhage less commonly results in aphasia, but complicated subarachnoid hemorrhage, accompanied by spasm of the intracranial vessels and cortical infarcts, often causes an aphasic syndrome. Trauma is another cause of sudden aphasia. These language impairments may be expected to improve over time. Progressive aphasia develops with dominant hemisphere tumors, with Alzheimer's disease, and with a number of unusual degenerative disorders, including Pick's disease, rare cases of motor neuron disease, and some cases of Creutzfeldt-Jakob disease. Dementia eventually develops in most of the progressive cases.

Prognosis and treatment of aphasia

Small infarcts in Broca's area or in the superior temporal gyrus may give rise to an acute, alarming language disturbance; as a rule, however, conversational speech becomes functional in a few days. Large perisylvian infarcts resulting in severe impairment of fluency and comprehension are generally attended by a persistent aphasia. In less serious cases, the greatest amount of improvement occurs in the first 2 or 3 months after onset; beyond 6 months, the rate of recovery drops; spontaneous improvement seldom occurs after a year. Patients with receptive or Wernicke's aphasia tend to reach a plateau more quickly than those with nonfluent, or Broca's aphasia. Speech therapy has been shown by several controlled studies to improve outcome, even many years after the stroke. The most frequently used forms of therapy are stimulation, programmed instruction, and melodic intonation. Well-structured home therapy is as effective as institutional therapy, particularly after the stage of accelerated improvement. Special social programs help to deal with the isolation of aphasic patients.

ORGANIC MENTAL SYNDROME

An organic mental syndrome is the impairment of cognitive function, wherein not only memory but any or all of the thought processes of perception and information processing are affected. Behavior is also affected in this condition. Sometimes, as in frontal lobe disease, behavioral changes precede intellectual deterioration. The terms "acute brain syndrome" and "chronic brain syndrome" had been used to connote reversible and irremediable cerebral diseases, respectively, but these relationships are not valid. For example, the acute syndrome of Wernicke's encephalopathy often causes permanent intellectual defects, and the chronic brain syndrome due to hypothyroidism is remediable. There are three major factors in the pathogenesis of an organic mental syndrome. First, and most important, are the location and the size of the lesion or the type and severity of the metabolic defect. The duration of the disease and its static or progressive course also have great bearing. The second factor pertains to the psychological and physical states of the patient. Both the previous personality and the emotional state at the time of the illness affect the symptoms. The age of the patient, the presence of systemic disease, and the preexistence of other cerebral disease are influential. Finally, environmental factors may be operative. Isolation and unfamiliar surroundings are destabilizing elements. Excessive environmental stimulation and sleep deprivation have similar untoward effects. The stresses of recent interpersonal relationships may modify the patient's reaction to organic disease.

DELIRIUM Delirium is an acute or subacute alteration in mental, motor, and autonomic function; it is usually reversible. Although the patient is alert, there is decreased awareness of or interest in the environment. The attentional impairment is reflected in poor performance in all areas of cognition, particularly orientation and memory. Behavior may be apathetic and withdrawn, but more often the patient is hyperactive, agitated, and incoherent. Fear or panic, illusions, and hallucinations often occur. Motor abnormalities may range from coarse tremor, asterixis, or multifocal myoclonus to convulsive seizures. Fever, tachycardia, and increased sweating are often present; hyperventilation or hypoventilation may occur. The autonomic changes depend on the underlying cause of delirium. The symptoms fluctuate markedly; they tend to be most severe at night since the sleep-wake cycle is disturbed. Delirium may last for hours or several days, even after the cause is corrected.

Etiology Virtually any organic brain disease may evoke delirium. The most common causes are intoxications by endogenous metabolites (hepatic or renal failure) or exogenous agents, especially alcohol and drugs. Febrile illnesses, vitamin deficiencies secondary to alcoholism, and severe exhaustion are frequent etiologies. Cerebral trauma, intracranial inflammation, and cerebral ischemia or hypoxia are less common. Older patients and patients with mild degenerative mental disorders are predisposed to the development of delirium.

Certain manifestations of delirium may be clues to the underlying cause. Delirium tremens, especially when associated with Korsakoff's syndrome, leaves little doubt about the diagnosis of chronic alcoholic intoxication. If depression of consciousness follows delirium, the toxic effects of sedatives or narcotics must be suspected. Delirium caused by alkaloids of the belladonna group is often associated with parasympathetic reactions and choreiform movements. The phenothiazine derivatives and other tranquilizers may cause dyskinesias with delirium. Amphetamine intoxication often produces euphoria preceding delirium. Cocaine intoxication evokes extreme excitement. Illusions and hallucinations are added to agitation with mescaline and lysergic acid diethylamide (LSD) toxicity.

Hallucinosis Organic hallucinosis refers to hallucinations without alteration of perception, consciousness, cognitive functions, or personality. In alcoholics, auditory hallucinations unrelated to delirium or other depression of consciousness and mentation may occur. These hallucinations may be unstructured sounds, such as clicking, ringing, or humming, but more commonly they manifest themselves as human voices that usually malign or threaten the patient. Although these phenomena are usually brief (minutes or days), they have been known, rarely, to occur for months. When the hallucinations become chronic, paranoid delusions become prominent, and the patient may be misdiagnosed as a paranoid schizophrenic, even though the past history is free of schizoid personality traits or a family history of schizophrenia. With lesions of the midbrain and subthalamus, visual hallucinations may occur *(peduncular hallucinosis)*, but they are recognized as unreal. Pontine lesions may cause auditory hallucinosis. These hallucinations are usually more complex than simple sounds but are less well formed than voices (e.g., the patient may hear an orchestra tuning up).

Differential diagnosis Delirium must be differentiated from nonorganic psychogenic states. Many symptoms are common to both. Changes in personality, with loss of interest in self and in the environment, and decreased attention and awareness, are often noted in organic and psychogenic disturbances. The patient's behavior may be aggressive, hostile, and accusatory; or restlessness, irritability, agitation, and excitement may occur. Disturbances of cognition are manifested by impairments of memory, judgment, orientation, and language.

Several clinical features help to differentiate acute organic cerebral disease from psychogenic illness. Patients with organic disease often give a history of failing memory, especially recent memory, but can provide adequate recall of events before the acute onset. Disorientation for time or date precedes that for place and person. If hallucinations occur with organic disease, they are likely to be visual. The change in personality is often abrupt, and there may be rapid fluctuations in mental state, behavior, or consciousness. The patient with a metabolic or toxic psychosis often manifests asterixis or myoclonus. The mental and personality changes of organic disease are likely to be worse at night and tend to improve with repeated reorientation. Within a few days, the patient with acute organic cerebral disease usually will either recover or show deterioration toward coma. Abnormal neurological signs and positive laboratory studies, such as abnormally slow EEG activity, usually establish the diagnosis.

Certain characteristics of an acute psychological disorder differ from features of organic disease. The onset of psychological illness is rarely abrupt and de novo. There often is a precipitating psychologically stressful event. The past history usually reveals a personality disturbance or prodromal phenomena, such as loss of interest, anorexia, and sleep disturbance. Sociability is lost early in the course of acute psychosis. Disorientation is more likely to be for place and person, rather than for time or date. The poor judgment of a neurotic is likely to be due to feelings of anger or fear. If present, tremors are usually fine. With the passage of time, additional evidence of a psychological disorder is likely to appear. The most common of these psychological illnesses are the mood disorders: the manic state and the agitated or stuporous state of a manic-depressive disorder. Mild depression frequently precedes a manic state. Schizophrenic hallucinations tend to be more auditory than visual; delusions are elaborate, thought processes bizarre, and mood inappropriate. The invariability of inconsistent responses of the patient with Ganser's syndrome is the differential clue.

Treatment Force must be avoided in caring for a delirious patient. Most patients can usually be moved by gentle means. (For example, several people gather together and gradually crowd the patient into a room.) A patient's room should be light, quiet, and bare of decoration. Personnel should repeatedly calm, reassure, and orient the patient. Restraints should be avoided, and sedation used sparingly. A solution of 10 ml of paraldehyde (Paral) in a glass of iced fruit juice is still favored by many physicians. Chlordiazepoxide, in doses ranging from 75 mg to 100 mg, may be given by mouth or injection. If more potent therapy is necessary, chlorpromazine may be used, but the phenothiazines should generally be avoided because they lower the convulsive threshold. The underlying cause must be determined and corrected. Prompt therapy of hypoxia, hypoglycemia, meningitis, or Wernicke's encephalopathy may be lifesaving. Fluid and electrolyte balance must be maintained, with special attention to glucose, potassium, and vitamin supplementation. Oral or IV administration is preferred to use of a nasogastric tube because the tube often evokes hyperactivity and frequently predisposes to aspiration pneumonia.

DEMENTIA Dementia is the impairment of memory, along with the deterioration of other intellectual functions. It is the most common disease of the elderly. One of every six people over the age of 65 is affected by this disorder, and the prevalence continues to increase with age. The first sign of dementia may be a reduction in adaptive ability accompanied by a change in personality. Interest in social activities gradually decreases, and work efficiency deteriorates. Emotional stability diminishes. Mental processes and physical activity slow down. With the patient's awareness of these changes, depression and anxiety may occur. The patient then becomes more self-absorbed and less sensitive to others. Memory for recent events, the ability to deal with abstract concepts, and judgment become defective. An early sign may be the abandonment of cognitive reaction (e.g., the patient stops playing bridge). Sedatives and alcoholic beverages may cause unusually marked lethargy. Vocabulary and past memories often remain adequate even when dementia becomes obvious. Thereby one may differentiate recent organic mental disorders from congenital or educational defects.

Further deterioration causes loss of inhibition, dress is less orderly, and speech is irrelevant, facetious, or circumstantial. Affect is flattened or emotional lability is prominent. All intellectual functions are further impaired, with particular difficulty in calculation and in orientation for time. Impulse control becomes impaired, and the patient may develop paranoid ideations, illusions, or hallucinations. Premorbid personality factors often come to the fore, and psychotic behavior may occur. Apathy, lethargy, and inappropriate sleep alternate with restlessness or agitation. Deficiencies are no longer recognized, and the previous anxiety is lost. Sedatives, tranquilizing medication, alcoholic beverages, intercurrent illnesses, or changes in the environment, such as hospitalization, often exacerbate the mental symptoms and may provoke delirium. Agitation after sundown is common.

The patient becomes unaware of friends and family. There may be confabulation or perseveration of speech and activity. Passivity or catatonic posturing may be noted; however, hyperactivity often occurs. The patient becomes relatively indifferent to noxious stimuli, but sometimes these evoke excessive infantile responses of crying or rage. The development of frontal release neurological signs includes grasp, snout, and suck reflexes; flexion of the trunk and extremities; and irregular stiffening of the limbs against passive movements, called *gegenhalten*.

Finally, the patient is totally incapacitated, incontinent of urine and feces, and unable to walk or talk. There is little or no response to auditory or noxious stimuli; if reaction occurs, it is generalized rather than specific. Terminally, overwhelmed by a systemic infection, most often pneumonia, the patient becomes stuporous and lapses into coma.

Cerebral site A subcortical location of dementia—as occurs with Huntington's chorea, Parkinson's disease, normal pressure hydrocephalus, multi-infarct dementia, and Wilson's disease—is associated with movement disorders and gait apraxia. Psychomotor retardation is prominent, with apathy slowly progressing toward an akinetic mute state. The cortical dementias, as exemplified by Alzheimer's disease and Creutzfeldt-Jakob disease, frequently manifest aphasia, agnosia, or apraxia.

Dementia vs. aphasia It may be difficult or impossible to differentiate dementia from global aphasia, and the two may coexist. Because dementia is more likely to be associated with diffuse rather than focal disease, the following signs are more often associated with dementia than with aphasia: inappropriate behavior, emotional lability or irritability, inability to deal with new concepts, depression of consciousness, urinary or fecal incontinence, and snout or grasp reflexes. The aphasic patient may show impaired comprehension by incorrectly carrying out a requested activity or by perseveration of speech; focal signs implicating the dominant cerebral hemisphere are most helpful.

Dementia and pseudodementia It is often difficult to differentiate dementia caused by organic or metabolic cerebral disease from pseudodementia resulting from depression of spirits. The term "pseudodementia" is based mainly on symptoms of impaired memory and disorientation, formerly thought to be diagnostic of organic disease. The two conditions have several features in common. Both impair psychological and cognitive functions. Affect is flat, or depression may be evident. In both dementia and pseudodementia, there is decreased concentration and poor attention; thought and action are slow. Apathy may alternate with irritability; disturbances of speech and sleep are common, and somatic complaints and delusions may occur. Evaluating the patient's thought content is often difficult because of the paucity of communication. The absence of verbal expression may be attributable to aphasia or the inaccessibility associated with agitation or hostility.

The differentiation of dementia from pseudodementia has important therapeutic implications. Patients with pseudodementia often respond well to treatment of depression. With restoration of normal mood, there is clearing of memory and orientation and of other seemingly organic signs. Features differentiating dementia and pseudodementia are listed in Table 2.3-5.

Depression in reaction to organic cerebral disease, such as a stroke or Parkinson's disease, is a frequent occurrence. This type of depression may be treated with mood-elevating drugs; however, ECT is often more beneficial and may have fewer side effects than drugs, particularly in treating the elderly.

Causes of dementia The differential diagnoses of dementia are listed in Table 2.3-6. Alzheimer's disease accounts for at least half of all cases of dementia (see Section 2.2). The next most frequent cause (20 percent) is cerebral vascular disease with small multiple infarctions. Brain tumors account for less than 5 percent of the dementias. From 30 to 60 percent of acquired immune deficiency syndrome (AIDS) patients have progressive dementia, related to direct invasion of the brain by human immunodeficiency virus (HIV). Dementia may be the sequela of many other acute and chronic diseases or injuries to the brain, but the incidence of these is only 1 or 2 percent of each. Most diseases causing dementia cannot be cured. The following conditions are amenable to successful treatment and should be sought: normal pressure hydrocephalus, most of the metabolic and some of the toxic diseases, cardiac emboli, arteritis, subdural hematoma, and some other mass lesions (neoplasm or abscess), chronic meningitides, and neurosyphilis.

Diagnostic evaluation About 10 percent of all patients with dementia have potentially treatable diseases, although half of this number have brain tumors, which are not always resectable. Establishing the cause of dementia is essential in an attempt to find a remediable disease. Systemic diseases may be discovered by the general physical examination, chest roentgenograms, electrocardiogram, blood count, urinalysis, and serum serological test for syphilis. The serum chemistries, serum thyroxine (T_4), and serum level of vitamin B_{12} determinations help to diagnose most of the metabolic and endocrine causes of dementia. The neurological examination may reveal evidence of an occult intracranial mass or chronic meningitis, but in most cases, these diseases are found by laboratory studies, CT, or MR. The cerebrospinal fluid (CSF) may be evaluated for evidence of chronic infection (e.g., cryptococcal meningitis or syphilis). EEG and isotope brain scanning are only occasionally useful.

Treatment In the treatment of the demented patient, one must preserve and enhance what functions remain. First, there is the task of correcting past neglect. Adequate nutrition, including vitamins and fluids, is essential. Rehabilitation may allow the ignored person to recover ambulation and other activities of daily living.

The correction and prevention of systemic disease is important because pain, fever, toxins, metabolic abnormalities, and dehydration have exaggerated effects on the impaired brain. Similarly, psychological stresses more readily disturb the demented personality than the normal personality. One must reduce demands on the patient who can no longer adequately perform former tasks at work or at home. Stressful environmental factors should be avoided. Instead, the familiar should be preserved, and the surroundings should be calm; routine activities should be maintained. Activity and social contact are to be encouraged. The services of a visiting nurse, a social worker, and an occupational and physical therapist may be integrated into family life.

Medications may be necessary for symptomatic relief, but the demented patient is often unusually sensitive to psychotropic and sedative drugs. Anxiety is best treated with diazepam or chlordiazepoxide. For agitation, such relatively nonsedating phenothiazines as perphenazine (Trilafon) or haloperidol may be necessary. Thioridazine (Mellaril) is also recommended; it is sedating, but is less likely to cause extrapyramidal symptoms. Amitriptyline (Elavil, Endep) or imipramine (Tofranil) are the drugs of choice for depression. Insomnia is difficult to overcome, but a small amount of promethazine (Phenergan) or diphenhydramine (Benadryl) or a short-acting hypnotic, such as temazepam (Restoril), may be useful.

BRAIN DAMAGE OR DYSFUNCTION OF CHILDHOOD The extent of neurological disability depends on the size, location, activity, focal or diffuse nature, and age of onset of the cerebral lesion. Age is a particularly important variable. Brain injury in the prenatal or neonatal period may cause severe and permanent damage, whereas a similar injury in an older child may be tolerated to a marked degree and with much greater recuperation. Difficulty in making the diagnosis of mental retardation is inversely proportional to the age of the patient. The diagnosis may be impossible in the newborn, unless there are obvious signs of cerebral disease.

TABLE 2.3-5
Comparison of Dementia Caused by Organic Disease and Pseudodementia Caused by Depression*

Dementia of Organic Disease	*Pseudodementia of Depression*
Age is nonspecific, usually adult	Elderly—60 years or older
Onset vague: months, years	Onset more precise: days, weeks
Course: slow; worse at night	Course: rapid and uneven; no nocturnal change
Past history of systemic illness or of drug or alcohol abuse	Past history of depression, mania, or somatic manifestations of depression
Often unaware of cognitive defect; unconcerned or denial of problem	Often complains of memory loss; distressed and emphasizes problem
Organic signs of neurological disease, such as dysphasia, apraxia, agnosia, incontinence	Psychological symptoms of sadness, self-accusation, preoccupation, anxiety, delusions; or somatic symptoms of depression
Greater impairment of cognitive features, such as recent memory and orientation for time and date	Greater impairment of personality features, such as confidence, drive, interests
Mental status examination shows spotty responses with some features much poorer than others; consistent on repeated exams	Mental status examination shows variability of impairment of different features on repeated exams
Behavior and affect consistent with degree of cognitive defect	Behavior and affect incongruent with degree of cognitive impairment
Cooperative but frustrated by struggle to perform well; relies on notes to remember	Poorly cooperative, with little effort to do well or remember
Responses to queries are approximate, confabulated, or perseverated	Responses to queries are often "I don't know"
Emphasizes trivial accomplishments	Emphasizes failures
Responses to funny or sad situations are normal or exaggerated; mood is shallow or labile	Little or no response to funny or sad circumstances; depression of mood
Neurological studies (CT and EEG) may be abnormal	Neurological studies usually normal

*The differences listed are not mutually exclusive, and there is considerable overlap between the two categories. Moreover, depression may be an early reaction to dementia.

Mental retardation This general term includes all forms of cognitive impairment with onset at birth or early age. All diseases of early life affecting the brain may cause mental retardation, but usually the cause is unknown. The term is used for a static encephalopathy, in contrast to deteriorating mental functions associated with hydrocephalus or brain neoplasm.

Emotional symptoms are common and are related to the type and extent of the cerebral lesion as well as to environmental stresses. Those patients with mild retardation are more capable of appreciating failure, experiencing frustration, feeling rejection, and feeling insecurity than are children with severe mental defects. However, severe organic disease may be associated with refractory behavioral abnormality.

Many neurological defects may be associated with early cognitive impairment. Speech retardation and subsequent speech disturbance are most common. Neuromuscular development is often retarded, and paresis, dyskinesia, or ataxia may be present. In patients with motor defects, cerebral palsy and mental retardation coexist, but the two disorders often occur independently. Sensory function is sometimes impaired, and defects of hearing and vision are common. Convulsive seizures often occur. Systemic defects may be manifested by unusual susceptibility to upper respiratory tract infections. Defective autonomic regulation may be manifested by excessive responses of temperature, pulse, or respiration to relatively minimal stress.

Attention-deficit hyperactivity disorder The terms "minimal brain dysfunction" or "slight brain damage" are no longer used, for they falsely connote a poor prognosis. Because disorders of attention and hyperactivity are the major manifestations, the term "attention-deficit hyperactivity disorder" (ADHD) is considered most appropriate. The condition is not caused by disease or injury but rather is a genetic disorder, predominant in boys beginning before the age of 7 and often familial. ADHD may include those children of normal or just below average intelligence with behavioral problems or learning disabilities, or both. Minor neurological abnormalities may be present.

ATTENTION DEFICITS Children with ADHD have difficulty in focusing and sustaining their attention; they are distracted by everything. Like younger children, they cannot discriminate unimportant from important stimuli in the environment. The degree of impairment of attention fluctuates, causing the uninformed observer to suspect psychological mechanisms. Defective attention impairs the ability to deal with abstract concepts and interferes with the learning process.

In a small percentage of children with ADHD, a phenomenon opposite to the above is present; these children are preoccupied with details. They show markedly decreased response to different stimuli, and their speech or actions may be perseverated.

BEHAVIORAL ALTERATIONS Deviations in motor activity are usually interrelated with defects in attention. Hyperkinetic impulsive behavior is the most common characteristic of ADHD, but it need not be present; therefore, caution should be exercised in making the diagnosis solely on this factor. Children with ADHD are constantly active and show lack of inhibition and impulse control. They touch everything and speak and act impulsively; behavior is disruptive, inappropriate, or antisocial. Emotional lability is often present. The child cries with minimal provocation; temper tantrums and panic are easily evoked. Because phenobarbital further depresses the attentional mechanisms, there may be an increase in hyperactivity after the administration of this drug. The drugs of choice in controlling hyperactivity are methylphenidate (Ritalin), pemoline (Cylert), and dextroamphetamine (Dexedrine). In a small percentage of cases, a decrease in physical activity may be a manifestation of ADHD.

LEARNING DIFFICULTIES Learning disabilities, either generalized or specific, are common in patients with ADHD, but are not necessarily part of the syndrome. Perceptual motor deficits often occur. The child may be poor in writing, drawing, and particularly in copying geometric figures. Concept formation is frequently disturbed. Learning deficits may be present in only one sphere, such as reading, spelling, or calculation. Scatter of performance on psychometric tests and differences from one time to another are often noted.

Dyslexia is the most common learning deficit. There are three major types of dyslexia. A specific language disorder is often present, of which anomia is the chief factor. In others, the problem is impairment of speech articulation and defective graphomotor coordination. The smallest group of patients has a disorder of visual-spatial perception. Differentiation of these types has therapeutic implications. The dyslexic who has a language disorder responds best to a phonics teaching program, while those children with defects of speech articulation and graphomotor coordination learn best by whole-word recognition.

NEUROLOGICAL SIGNS Children with ADHD often have equivocal or minimal ("soft") abnormal neurological signs. Defects in coordination are most common and are manifested by a generalized awkwardness (maladroitness), or poor finger coordination. Retarded speech or other speech defects may be noted. There is often right and left confusion. Mild somatic sensory defects or slight impairment of hearing or vision may be present. Occasionally, strabismus or other physical defects are evident. The EEG may show slight abnormalities.

Differential diagnosis of organic mental disorder of children

DEPRIVATION Potentially reversible symptoms and signs of organic mental disorder may be caused by malnutrition, avitaminosis, or anemia. Emotional deprivation, which occurs with the absence of the mother or mother figure or from lack of affection, may cause growth hormone deficiency and retardation. Retarded development may be caused by the deprivation of social stimuli. Early correction of these factors leads to a normal course of intellectual and personality development.

AUTISTIC DISORDER An infant with autistic disorder is unable to make contact with or respond to the environment; there is extreme aloofness. When picked up and cradled, the child does not cuddle or adapt. In contradistinction to this lack of relationship to people, there is an attachment to and fascination with inanimate objects. The child often shows an obsessive insistence on sameness and a corresponding aversion to new things. This marked inflexibility may be strongly defended by temper tantrums or rages. The child is often late in learning to walk and to speak.

SCHIZOPHRENIA Childhood schizophrenia may be first manifested as autism. Although the diagnosis of schizophrenia is sometimes made as early as the third or fourth year of life, diagnoses made before the age of 8 are questionable. In concert with the autistic child, the schizophrenic child does not respond to the environment, other children, or adults. Sometimes activity is diminished, but more often hyperactive behavior occurs. Repetitive movements, such as rocking and swinging, are common. Speech may be delayed in onset or develop in bursts. In contrast to retarded development, mental and physical features occasionally regress.

COMMUNICATION DEFECTS Speech retardation is sometimes the result of overindulgence. The child finds that verbal communication is not required because his or her needs are anticipated and immediately fulfilled. Deafness is a common cause of speech retardation and associated behavioral impairment. Unrecognized visual defects may retard mental development. Dyslexic children may be falsely considered brain damaged unless the reading and writing impairments are appreciated as specific and isolated phenomena.

OTHER PHYSIOLOGICAL DEFECTS The postictal state is associated with a dulling of mentation, and frequent seizures will prolong this condition. During petit mal or temporal lobe status epilepticus, the patient appears awake but with marked impairment of cognitive functions. Prolonged systemic illnesses in children are frequently associated with mental retardation. Hysteria and other psychogenic phenomena are occasionally misinterpreted as physical or mental retardation.

TABLE 2.3-6
Causes of Dementia

Degenerative diseases
- Alzheimer's disease
- Pick's disease
- Huntington's chorea
- Progressive supranuclear palsy
- Other basal ganglia and cerebellar degenerations
- Myoclonus epilepsy
- Communicating hydrocephalus
- Multiple sclerosis and other demyelinating disorders
- Parkinson's disease
- Myotonic dystrophy

Metabolic diseases
- Endocrinopathies
  - Myxedema
  - Hypoglycemia
  - Parathyroid disease
  - Hypopituitary disease
  - Adrenal disease
- Deficiency states
  - Vitamin B complex: Wernicke's syndrome, Korsakoff's syndrome
  - Niacin: pellagra
  - Vitamin B_{12} and folic acid: pernicious anemia
- Other metabolic diseases
  - Chronic liver disease
  - Chronic renal disease
  - Lipidoses
  - Wilson's disease
  - Porphyria
  - Remote effect of malignancy
  - Adult onset of leukodystrophies and neuronal storage diseases

Toxins
- Exogenous toxins
  - Alcohol
  - Drugs
  - Biological toxins
  - Heavy metals
  - Industrial toxins
- Endogenous metabolites

Anoxic-ischemic disorders
- Multiple small infarcts and lacunae
  - Atherosclerosis and hypertension
  - Emboli from the heart
  - Arteritis and collagen diseases
- Subarachnoid hemorrhage
- Repeated effects of hypoxia or ischemia of pulmonary, cardiovascular, or hematological disease
- Postanoxic encephalopathy

Trauma
- Subdural hematoma
- Repeated concussions and contusions (punch-drunk)

Tumors
- Neoplasm in a "silent" area of the brain, such as the frontal pole
- Neoplasm causing increased intracranial pressure without focal signs, such as in deep midline area

Infections
- Chronic (fungal) meningitis
- Neurosyphilis
- Creutzfeldt-Jakob disease
- Progressive multifocal leukoencephalopathy
- Occult brain abscess
- Encephalitis
- Acquired immune deficiency syndrome (AIDS)

IMPAIRMENT OF MOTOR FUNCTION

Motor function impairment may be expressed as a disorder of movement, muscle tone, or strength. Disorder of movement refers to the paucity of spontaneous movements, called *hypokinesia,* or an excess of movements, called *hyperkinesia.* Often a disturbance of muscle tone occurs in these syndromes, but occasionally the abnormal tone occupies center stage of the syndrome. Weakness is a frequent result of central nervous system (CNS) disease. Diseases causing these disorders were reviewed in Section 2.2. The present discussion centers on those features that may have psychological, as well as neurological, signs.

MOVEMENT DISORDERS Hyperkinetic activity and hypokinesis may be seen in both organic and psychological illnesses. There is controversy about the classification of some disorders. For example, tics may be a manifestation of neurological or psychological disease. Before the turn of the century, parkinsonism was considered a psychiatric illness. The tremor is precipitated or markedly aggravated by minimal stress and disappears when the patient is alone or asleep. Bradykinetic patients immobilized in a wheelchair may, nonetheless, quickly move their arms to protect themselves from a ball thrown at them and have been known to run out of their wheelchair when the house is on fire. Parkinsonism patients may find that their feet seem to be glued to the floor when they attempt to walk, but their gait may be close to normal once movement has begun. Some must perform a peculiar act, such as tapping the head with the hand, before walking begins. Other peculiar activities have been reported in patients with Parkinson's disease. The bizarre changes in activity, once attributed to the psyche, are now known to be associated with metabolic abnormality of dopamine metabolism in the nigrostriatal system of the brain.

Hypokinesis Bradykinesis and hypokinesis are common features of parkinsonism. On rare occasions, the immobility of parkinsonism is of such severity that it simulates coma or schizophrenic catatonia. With patience, the examiner is eventually able to evoke some slight response from the patient with parkinsonian akinesia. Akinesia is seen in the parkinsonian oculogyric crisis or the on-off phenomenon associated with levodopa therapy. Treatment of parkinsonism was discussed in Section 2.2. Inertia may be part of the apathy noted in patients with disease of the frontal lobes or the diencephalon. Paucity or slowness of movement, usually associated with slowness of thought, is seen with pseudobulbar palsy. Akinetic mutism and the locked-in syndrome, discussed in the section on coma, are also attended by hypokinesia. A paucity of truncal movements in the elderly may be related to disease of the periventricular white matter. Hydrocephalus may cause bradykinesia and is relieved by shunting ventricular cerebrospinal fluid (CSF) into the peritoneal or pleural cavities.

Catatonic schizophrenia is the prime example of hypokinesis resulting from psychological illness. In contrast to organic disease, the inert posture of catatonia is awkward and sometimes bizarre. Muscle tone has a variable wavy flexibility, rather than cogwheeling or rigidity. Abrupt changes in tone may occur with catatonia. Such changes are rare in organic disease except for parkinsonian oculogyric crisis or the on-off phenomenon.

Depression may simulate parkinsonism. In both conditions, there may be slowing and paucity of movement, small-stepped or shuffling gait, expressionless face, and weak voice. Constipation and sleep disturbance may occur in both. The mood and the thought content define the depressed patient, but, clearly, parkinsonism may evoke depression.

Stupor, coma, or akinetic mutism may be simulated by the withdrawal seen in schizophrenia or depression. The schizophrenic patient may resist eyelid opening or may withdraw from the examiner. In patients with psychotic pseudocoma, oculocephalic reflexes are not evoked, and the caloric response is that of the awake patient. At the onset, laboratory studies may be necessary to establish the presence of organic disease. In time, if the stuporous state is psychological, the patient will begin to speak. Then, the disordered thought of the schizophrenic patient and the sad mental content of the depressed patient will become evident.

Hyperkinesia Chorea, tremor, and other clinical findings encountered with movement disorders were discussed in Section 2.1. A normal physiological phenomenon is a slight tremor of the extremities that is not usually seen with the naked eye. Such physiological states as fatigue, anxiety, and fear and such pathophysiological states as thyrotoxicosis and alcoholic intoxication may make subclinical tremors more visible. These tremors are postural and noted when upper extremities are extended against gravity or when the head is supported by the neck in the erect position. *Familial essential tremor* is similar to an exaggerated postural physiological tremor, but activity (especially precise movement) increases tremor. This tremor becomes slower and coarser with age. Primidone or propranolol (Inderal) may alleviate familial essential tremor. The akathisia of parkinsonism is sometimes mistaken for psychogenic restlessness. The resting tremor of parkinsonism is of basal ganglion origin, whereas action tremor is associated with lesions affecting the superior cerebellar peduncle (cerebellar outflow tremor). Tremors of the midbrain origin may have resting, static, and intention qualities. Hepatic encephalopathy is associated with flapping tremors (asterixis).

The involuntary movements of chorea, athetosis, dystonia, and ballismus were once thought to be psychogenic because of their bizarre pattern—aggravation by emotional stress, amelioration during tranquility, and disappearance during sleep. Ballismus, almost always hemiballismus, occurs in adults and begins suddenly because of infarction of the corpus luysii. Ischemic hemiballismus tends to recede spontaneously within a few days or weeks. Sedation and support are the main therapeutic measures. Athetosis is the sequela of birth anoxia, kernicterus, and other congenital disorders. Therapy, largely limited to muscle relaxants, is of little use. At onset, chorea and dystonia are frequently mistaken for restlessness or nervousness. About 50 percent of patients with Huntington's chorea present with psychological symptoms. Treatment of chorea is aimed at the underlying cause. Sydenham's chorea and the chorea of vasculitides may benefit from steroids. Haloperidol usually provides symptomatic relief but, particularly in elderly patients, it may aggravate a proneness to falling. Torticollis is often a manifestation of dystonia—sometimes the only manifestation. The dystonia of Wilson's disease improves with copper-chelating agents. High-dose anticholinergic medication may improve childhood-onset dystonia.

Torticollis is the involuntary contraction of cervical muscles, predominantly the sternocleidomastoid, twisting the head to one side. This focal dystonia may be a manifestation of phenothiazine or similar drug toxicity, but most cases are of unknown pathophysiological origin. Psychogenic mechanisms are no longer thought to be the predominant cause. The results of psychiatric therapy are poor, but spontaneous remissions are common. Medications, such as trihexyphenidyl (Artane), baclofen (Lioresal), and carbamazepine, are of some benefit. Surgical therapy is warranted only in severe and intractable cases.

Buccolingual dyskinesia is a well-recognized complication of psychotropic therapy, but it may occur spontaneously in the elderly. Tardive dyskinesia often occurs after discontinuation of antipsychotics. Some patients respond to such dopamine-depleting agents as reserpine. The rare condition *familial paroxysmal choreathetosis* was thought to be hysterical until other families were reported with identical symptoms and signs. Phenytoin alleviates this disorder.

Essential blepharospasm occurs in late adult life, and this inability to keep eyes open may render the patient functionally blind. When associated with oromandibular dystonia manifested by bizarre grimacing, the term *Meige's syndrome* is applied. Spastic dysphonia (see Section 2.1) is often associated, and other dystonic phenomena sometimes occur. Although the cause is not known, these conditions are not psychogenic. Anticholinergic drugs or injection of botulinum toxin into affected muscles are useful therapies.

Myoclonic activity may range from the contraction of a single muscle to the synchronous contraction of the entire somatic musculature. Because consciousness is not lost, some of these activities may be incorrectly diagnosed as tics or psychogenic phenomena. Myoclonic activity is often evoked by movement, particularly when caused by hypoxic encephalopathy. Sometimes, it is only a specific movement or posture that precipitates the myoclonic activity. When this stereotyped sequence occurs, psychological interpretations may be falsely applied. The treatment of myoclonus depends on its etiology. Correction of an underlying metabolic encephalopathy or treatment of a tumor may improve the myoclonus. Clonazepam or divalproex sodium are helpful in the relief of postanoxic and epileptic myoclonus.

TICS Because of their uncertain pathogenesis, tics are still in the borderland between neurology and psychiatry. Tics are common in children and usually of little consequence; however, they are an integral part of Tourette's disorder and may be fragments of other diseases with hyperkinetic syndromes (e.g., the first sign of Sydenham's chorea). The patient may involuntarily suppress a tic, but for only a brief period, for it requires great effort and generates much tension. A consistent psychological profile or set of psychodynamics is not present in these patients.

TOURETTE'S DISORDER Tourette's disorder begins in childhood or early adolescence; hereditary factors are prominent. Multiple tics affect the head, neck, and extremities, along with involuntary vocalizations. The tics increase in complexity, and the vocalizations may progress from slight cough or grunt to barking or coprolalia. Tourette's disorder had been considered psychogenic because of the bizarre symptoms and absence of objective disease. It has a pathophysiological mechanism associated with dopamine-receptor hypersensitivity. The symptoms are ameliorated with administration of dopamine-blocking agents, such as haloperiodol or pimozide (Orap).

PSYCHOGENIC MOVEMENT DISORDERS Not all movement disorders are of neurological origin. Psychological disturbances may be manifested by activity ranging from slight, simple tics to complex behavioral disorders. Sometimes, the movements of such patients simulate orofacial dyskinesia, chorea, athetosis, or dystonia. When the schizophrenic patient has a movement disorder, it is usually stereotyped and frequently enacts a specific mannerism. Unusual movements of psychotic patients often include the handling of body parts or other objects.

Hyperactive behavior of organic origin is sometimes mistaken for the euphoria or mania of the manic-depressive. When neurological diseases cause hyperactivity, cognitive impairment is frequently present, as seen with delirium and the bizarre hyperkinetic behavior of a patient having a psychomotor seizure.

DISTURBANCES OF MUSCLE TONE

Hypotonia After any acute lesion of the corticospinal tract in the brain or spinal cord, the tone of the muscles may be flaccid until spasticity sets in. Transient absence of muscle tone and reflexes, known as *limp-man syndrome,* may result from a midbrain tumor. In this case, the pathophysiology is similar to cataplexy. Decreased muscle tone can be found in disorders of the cerebellar hemispheres, such as infarction, cerebellitis, and trauma. Severe muscle denervation or muscle atrophy associated with myositis can also cause flaccidity.

Hypertonia Increased muscle tone in the form of spasticity, rigidity, or paratonia can result from a variety of disorders and was discussed in Section 2.1. Increased tone is a prominent feature of the dystonias, discussed previously in this section. Hypertonia characterizes tetanus and the "stiff-man syndrome." Although not necessarily accompanied by ongoing muscle contraction, several muscle disorders accompanied by myotonia are also noted here.

STIFF-MAN SYNDROME In this condition, bouts of severe spasm of the somatic musculature last for hours or days. Trunk and abdominal wall muscles are particularly involved, and the syndrome may resemble tetanus. The spasms may or may not be painful. Stiff-man syndrome may be precipitated by minimal physical or emotional stimuli. The mechanism of this condition is unknown. Diazepam decreases the severity of the muscle contractions.

Myotonia Myotonia is characterized by prolonged muscle contraction, with delay of muscle relaxation, and is usually part of myotonic muscular dystrophy, also termed myotonia dystrophica. This is a hereditary disease, beginning in young adults, manifested by myotonic impairment of function and dystrophic muscle wasting of the face, neck, and extremities. Associated features include premature baldness, cataracts, testicular atrophy, other endocrinopathies, and mental deterioration. *Myotonia congenita* is also hereditary, but strength is normal and the associated features of myotonia dystrophica are lacking. *Paramyotonia* is slow muscle contraction and relaxation in association with cold; it also occurs with hyperkalemic periodic paralysis. Treatment with procainamide (Pronestyl), phenytoin, or quinine may ameliorate the myotonic phenomena.

WEAKNESS CAUSED BY PERIPHERAL NERVOUS SYSTEM DISEASE

Muscle weakness and atrophy can be due to disease of the anterior horn cell, peripheral nerve, motor endplate, or muscle. The diagnosis of motor neuron disease generally offers no problem. Weakness, atrophy, diffuse fasciculations, and relatively brisk reflexes all point to the diagnosis of amyotrophic lateral sclerosis. Fasciculations need not be an ominous finding. Benign fasciculations may be precipitated by anxiety, cold environment, or hyperthyroidism and are often present in the calves of elderly people.

Peripheral neuropathy Affection of the peripheral nerves often causes sensory deficits and pain, in addition to or with the exclusion of weakness. However, a brief discussion of peripheral neuropathies is included here because these entities may result in complaints easily mistaken as psychogenic. Neuropathies can affect one nerve (mononeuropathy), several single nerves (mononeuropathy multiplex), or all of the nerves symmetrically, usually with a distal predilection (polyneuropathy).

The most common mononeuropathies are due to compression or entrapment of a nerve in a region exposed to trauma, such as the ulnar groove at the elbow (ulnar neuropathy), the median nerve passing underneath the carpal ligament (carpal tunnel syndrome), or the point where the lateral cutaneous nerve of the thigh exits the abdominal cavity in close contact with the inguinal ligament (meralgia paresthetica). The type of deficit depends on the constitution of the nerve. Ulnar and median neuropathies have motor and sensory components: Hand grip is weakened, and there is tingling and numbness in the ulnar or median aspect of the hand. Meralgia paresthetica is a purely sensory syndrome: the patient complains of burning or boring pain on the dorsolateral aspect of the thigh. The disturbance can be improved by diminishing trauma to the nerve (weight reduction in the case of meralgia paresthetica) or by surgically decompressing or relocating the nerve. *Bell's palsy* is weakness or paralysis of sudden onset caused by idiopathic disease of the facial peripheral nerve. When the condition is severe, there is retroauricular pain. A short course of steroids is helpful.

Mononeuritis multiplex is most often due to diabetes or a vasculitis, such as polyarteritis nodosa. Infarction of the nerve as a result of disease of the vasa nervorum appears to mediate this type of neuropathy. Sudden onset of weakness in the distribution of a peripheral nerve is heralded by severe, usually transient, neuralgic pain. Sarcoidosis can also cause a mononeuropathy multiplex, but it often results in polyneuropathy. About one-third of patients with mononeuropathy multiplex have a chronic inflammatory demyelinating disease rather than an ischemic neuropathy. Treatment by blood sugar control or steroids depends on the etiology.

Polyneuropathy is manifested by complaints of weakness, pain, or numbness, generally most pronounced in the distal lower extremities. On examination, the reflexes are diminished and the sensory loss, if present, covers the foot or hand in a stocking or glove-like distribution. Pure motor neuropathies are generally caused by demyelination of the axon, and they can be acute or chronic. Acute weakness, occasionally mistaken for hysteria, is the hallmark of acute postinfectious polyneuropathy, or the Guillain-Barré syndrome. Diagnostic accuracy is important because these patients may quickly develop respiratory insufficiency, requiring intubation and intensive care. The Guillain-Barré syndrome tends to occur within 2 weeks of a viral or febrile illness. A few days into the course, the CSF shows a markedly elevated protein level but a normal cell count. Plasmapheresis early in the course of severe cases may shorten the convalescent period and result in a fuller recovery. Chronic or recurrent inflammatory polyneuropathy responds to steroid therapy. Another group of chronic motor neuropathies is transmitted as an autosomal dominant trait (e.g., peroneal muscular atrophy or Charcot-Marie-Tooth disease).

Polyneuropathy with motor and sensory findings is most often due to diabetes. Leprosy causes a sensorimotor neuropathy affecting the exposed areas of the skin. A pure sensory neuropathy may herald the presence of cancer. More frequent is the sensorimotor polyneuropathy of terminal cancer, which may have a nutritional or immune basis. Vitamin-deficiency neuropathies, as in chronic malnutrition and chronic alcoholism, can be painful. Since they are often accompanied by cerebellar dysfunction, the gait disturbance may be out of proportion to what would be expected from the degree of sensorimotor loss in the legs. A number of toxic substances, medications, and even vitamins when taken in large amounts, can cause polyneuropathy, which is often sensorimotor, but may be predominantly sensory [with piridoxine, metronidazole (Flagyl), cis platinum (Platinol)] or motor (dapsone, lead). Electromyography and nerve conduction studies are helpful in the diagnosis of the neuropathies and can be used to quantify progress. Treatment of these disorders includes removing the offending agent, correcting the metabolic disturbance (as in the case of diabetes or uremia), or furnishing the nutritional factors that are lacking. The burning sensation present in some of the painful neuropathies may be alleviated with a small amount of amitriptyline at bedtime.

MUSCLE DISORDERS

Myasthenia gravis Myasthenia gravis occurs most often between the ages of 20 and 40 years and affects women more often than men. Antibodies bind and inactivate the aceticholine receptor sites of the postsynaptic myoneural junctions. The thymus and thyroid glands are probably involved in the autoimmune mechanism, for there is an increased incidence of diseases of these organs in myasthenics. Excessive fatigability and weakness, predominantly of the muscles innervated by the cranial nerves, are the hallmark of myasthenia gravis. The upper extremities are involved to a lesser extent and the lower extremities are least affected. The most common initial symptoms are double vision, ptosis, dysphagia, and difficulty in chewing. The diagnosis is clinically established when brief disappearance or improvement of signs occurs within 30 seconds of an IV injection of edrophonium (Tensilon). There is a characteristic electromyographic pattern and acetylcholine receptor antibodies are elevated in the serum.

Maintenance therapy consists of pyridostigmine (Mestinon) or neostigmine (Prostigmin), but some of the toxic effects of these cholinesterase inhibitors may simulate an exacerbation of myasthenia. Thymectomy or steroid therapy usually permits reduction in the dosage of anticholinesterase drugs and may induce complete remission. Other immunosuppressive agents, such as cyclosporin (Sandimmune), have also been effective.

Myopathies Myopathies form a large group of disorders characterized by weakness, atrophy in the end stages, and relative preservation of the reflexes. Sensory function is intact. Acute muscle destruction, such as with alcoholic myopathy or some of the vasculitides, may be accompanied by muscle tenderness. In these cases, the level of creatine phosphokinase is greatly elevated. Increased levels of this enzyme are found in the myopathies, except in the most indolent ones. A number of myopathies are genetically determined; most of them are idiopathic. In myopathies with identified underlying metabolic defect, the process generally involves the pathways of muscle energy production. An exception is acid maltase deficiency. Among the acquired myopathies, the most common in adult life is polymyositis, an idiopathic condition. Other myopathies are due to infection by organisms, endocrine abnormalities, or injury by trauma or toxic substances.

Periodic paralysis The sudden onset of extreme weakness of the periodic paralyses can be mistaken for psychogenic weakness. They are associated with alterations of serum potassium. Spontaneous episodes of hyponatremia may also cause periodic paralysis without change in serum potassium levels.

Hypokalemic (familial) periodic paralysis Beginning in adolescence, this condition affects men more than women. Recurrent bouts of flaccid weakness or paralysis of somatic musculature occur, usually sparing the muscles innervated by the cranial nerves and the muscles of respiration. The symptoms persist for 2 to 24 hours. Potassium aborts the attack and is used prophylactically. Hypokalemic paralyses may also be associated with thyrotoxicosis, hyperaldosteronism, and potassium loss through the kidneys or gut.

Hyperkalemic periodic paralysis (adynamic episodica hereditaria) In contradistinction to familial (hypokalemic) paralysis, hyperkalemic bouts of paralysis usually begin in the first decade of life, equally affect both sexes, are of short duration, and are associated with paramyotonia. Calcium ameliorates the individual attacks. Acetazolamide and other diuretics are useful prophylactic agents.

DIZZINESS OR IMPAIRMENT OF EQUILIBRIUM

Patients must be asked to define the term "dizziness," for they often use the word synonymously with such feelings as faintness, malaise, and headache. Dizziness should indicate a disturbance of equilibrium (imbalance or unsteadiness) or vertigo (spinning sensation) or at least a sense of movement. The differential features of dizziness of labyrinthine or peripheral origin from dizziness due to CNS disease are listed in Table 2.3-7.

Diseases of the ear Dizziness is most often caused by diseases of the internal ear, although obstructions in the external or middle chambers of the ear sometimes provoke the symptom.

Labyrinthitis The most common cause of dizziness is disease or dysfunction of the labyrinth or the adjacent vestibular nerve. Many mechanisms have been implicated, including infection, allergy, vascular disease, trauma, tumor (especially cholesteatoma), drugs, and toxins. In most cases, the cause is indeterminate and the course is benign. Labyrinthitis is usually manifested by sudden imbalance or

TABLE 2.3-7
Comparison of Dizziness Caused by Labyrinthine Disease and CNS Disease

Labyrinthine Disease	*CNS Disease*
There may be a past history of bouts of dizziness or ear disease.	There may be a history of CNS disease, such as past symptoms of multiple sclerosis.
Episodes of dizziness are paroxysmal and of short duration.	Dizziness is less acute and more prolonged.
Dizziness is precipitated or aggravated by movements of the head, as when lying down or rolling over in bed.	Dizziness need not be aggravated by head movement. When due to vertebrobasilar artery insufficiency, dizziness may be precipitated by arising from bed or by neck movement.
There may be associated symptoms or signs of tinnitus, hearing impairment, difficulty in multiple-voice discrimination, or hyperacusis. Nausea and vomiting accompany dizziness.	There are often associated symptoms or signs of disease implicating the brain stem, such as diplopia, and sensory or motor signs. Nausea and vomiting are less common.
Nystagmus, when present during an attack, is horizontal more than rotatory and unidirectional; increases when fixation is eliminated, as by strong lenses; disappears when dizziness clears.	Nystagmus may be of any variety, but, when vertical, is pathognomonic of brain stem origin; not unidirectional; increases on fixation; may persist after dizziness has gone.
Ataxia, if present, occurs only during the attack.	Ataxia may be present without dizziness.
Tests:	*Tests:*
The caloric test may be normal or reveal decreased reactivity of the labyrinth. On repeated stimulation, there is increasing latency and exhaustion (decreasing duration and degree) of response.	The caloric response is usually normal, but may evoke nystagmus of perverted or incongruent type. Repeated stimulation evokes a consistent response.
Electronystagmography reveals increased nystagmus with eyes closed.	Electronystagmography reveals increased nystagmus with eyes open.
Audiometry often reveals defective acuity and, in Ménière's disease, recruitment of loudness of pure tones but impaired intelligibility of amplified speech.	Audiometry is usually normal.
Roentgenograms of the skull may reveal evidence of old mastoiditis or cholesteatoma.	Roentgenograms may reveal intracranial pathology.
Other laboratory features are usually normal.	The CT, MR, EEG, CSF, or angiogram may reveal abnormality.
Brain stem evoked potentials differentiate local ear or auditory nerve disease from CNS lesions.	Brain stem evoked potentials differentiate local ear or auditory nerve disease from CNS lesions.

vertigo, typically precipitated or aggravated by movement, lasting minutes or hours. Nausea and vomiting are the most common associated symptoms. The attacks usually recur with decreasing frequency and severity for days or weeks. Between the acute bouts, a sense of insecurity when moving or a poorly described feeling of ill-being is often present. These vague symptoms sometimes are mistaken for neurosis. Benign paroxysmal positional vertigo is precipitated by sudden movement of the head and lasts a few seconds. Repeated movements of the head are associated with increasing delay and exhaustion of the response. Vestibular neuronitis is of longer duration and not necessarily precipitated by sudden movement. Examination reveals unilaterally absent or decreased response to caloric stimulation.

Ménière's disease This condition is clinically distinguished from labyrinthitis by the addition of auditory symptoms, such as tinnitus or hearing difficulty. The auditory symptoms are present not only during acute bouts of dizziness, but also persist intermittently or continuously and grow progressively severe. On examination, there is impaired intelligibility of amplified speech and audiometric recruitment phenomena. Although the pathogenesis usually is unknown, all the causative factors listed for labyrinthitis are applicable to Ménière's disease.

Symptomatic treatment of labyrinthitis and Ménière's disease consists of rest, with as little movement of the head as possible. The antihistaminic agents dimenhydrinate (Dramamine), meclizine (Antivert), or cyclizine (Marezine) are of some benefit. If vertigo causes prolonged disability, surgery of the labyrinth or the vestibular nerve may be necessary.

Diseases of the eighth cranial nerve or brain stem The auditory nerve may be affected by meningitis, trauma, or tumor (especially acoustic neuroma). Hearing impairment is usually more prominent than dizziness. Acoustic neuroma is usually associated with an absent caloric response, nerve deafness, severe impairment of speech discrimination, and an enlarged internal acoustic meatus. Imaging techniques will reveal the mass. Disease of the vestibular nuclei and lesions in other areas of the brain stem cause dizziness. Other cranial nerve defects or long tract signs are usually present. Vascular and degenerative diseases, particularly multiple sclerosis, are more common than inflammatory and neoplastic diseases of the brain stem.

Diseases of the cerebellum and cerebrum The symptom of dizziness associated with lesions of the brain is likely to be faintness or lightheadedness, poorly described as dizziness. Disease of the temporal lobe sometimes causes vertigo, but less specific dizziness may occur with any anatomical or metabolic disease of the cerebrum or cerebellum, especially acute disease. Alcoholic toxicity is the most common example. Vascular diseases and the postconcussion syndrome are more common causes of dizziness than are cerebellar tumors, deficiency states, and inflammatory diseases.

Special audiometric measurements—such as loudness recruitment, speech discrimination, Békésy audiometry, short-increment sensitivity index, and auditory evoked responses—help to establish the site of disease: cochlear, retrocochlear (cranial nerve), brain stem, or temporal lobe.

Physiological dysfunctions Dizziness may be experienced just before syncope. Vertigo may occur with epilepsy; in rare instances, it may be the only manifestation of epilepsy. Dizziness and headache are the most common symptoms of the postconcussion post-traumatic syndrome.

Proprioceptive impairment Imbalance due to position sense defects may be misinterpreted by the patient as dizziness. This finding is common in the elderly and with diseases affecting the posterior columns of the spinal cord or peripheral nerves.

Diseases of the eye Extraocular muscle paresis may cause dizziness. Refractive error and glaucoma are rarely associated with this symptom.

Systemic diseases Any generalized illness may cause dizziness. Of the endocrine disturbances associated with dizziness, the most common are hypocalcemia, hypoglycemia, hypothyroidism, hypoadrenalism, and hyperadrenalism. Patients with systemic infections, hematological disease, deficiency states (especially pellagra), allergies, and toxic phenomena often complain of dizziness.

PAIN: DYSFUNCTION OF SOMATIC SENSORY SYSTEM

Pain is an unpleasant sensory and emotional experience associated with real or perceived tissue damage. The neural pathways of pain are complex. Pain impulses, carried by small-diameter myelinated and unmyelinated fibers in peripheral or cranial nerves, reach the perceptual centers in the brain after being relayed in the dorsal root entry zone of the spinal cord (and the corresponding zone of the brain stem), in the reticular nuclei of the brain stem, and in the thalamus. Substance P is the major biochemical transmitter of pain. The placebo response, once thought to be psychogenic, is now recognized as due to the elaboration in the brain of endorphins, endogenous opioid-like polypeptides. Impulses from mesencephalic periaqueductal gray matter and medullary raphe nuclei descend to inhibit pain at the root entry zone. Serotonin is an important neurotransmitter of this inhibitory system. Inhibition of pain impulses at the root entry zone may also occur by stimulation of afferent sensory peripheral neurons carrying touch and proprioception.

Because pain is a psychophysiological phenomenon, this subjective condition is difficult to evaluate, but there are several factors to be considered. The threshold of pain varies greatly from one person to another. At one end of the spectrum is the entity of congenital indifference to pain. At the opposite extreme are those with little tolerance for minor discomfort; in this group, psychogenic elements are often prominent. Attention and distraction are important factors influencing the appreciation of and reaction to pain. The difference between real and imagined pain is more semantic than physiological. It may be impossible to differentiate pain caused by organic disease or dysfunction from pain manifested as part of a psychological illness. Pain caused by a structural lesion (e.g., malignancy, ischemia, or neuritis) is usually accompanied by objective signs of the disease. Neuralgias, although usually not associated with signs of organic disease, clearly have a physiological basis, in that the pain follows the anatomical course of a nerve, nerve root, or nerve plexus. Pains resulting from disease or dysfunctions of the autonomic nervous system or the CNS do not follow a specific nerve distribution and may be confused with pain of psychological origin.

When pain is chronic, psychological factors inevitably complicate the clinical problem. The fact that pain may be ameliorated by suggestion or distraction does not mean that the pain is imagined. It is a common and disturbing fact that pain is often present without obvious cause and yet is due to organic, rather than psychogenic, dysfunction. The neurological examination is normal or may show only minimal defects in pains associated with migraine, cranial neuralgia, thalamic syndrome, phantom limb pain, whiplash injury, or reflex sympathetic dystrophy. The patient with chronic pain presents one of the most difficult therapeutic challenges. Elimination of the source of pain often cannot be accomplished. Analgesics sometimes fail to effect relief because the physician is too cautious to prescribe sufficiently high dosages. Psychotropic medications are often of more benefit than analgesics or narcotics. Tricyclic compounds and phenothiazines ameliorate chronic pain unrelated to their mood-lifting and tranquilizing actions. In some instances, it is necessary to interrupt pain pathways either by a chemical block or by surgical section of the nerve, nerve root, or spinothalamic tract. Depth electrode stimulation of the periaqueductal gray pain inhibitor center is rarely advisable. Psychotherapy is of great value in modifying pain perception and in helping patients cope with their illnesses. Other modalities—such as biofeedback, transcutaneous electrical stimulation, hypnosis, and acupuncture—are beneficial in selected cases.

HEADACHE

Headache is the single most common symptom, experienced by 75 percent of all Americans each year. Although headaches are rarely caused by serious organic disease, the symptom is often disabling. Chronic headaches interfere with interpersonal relationships at home, work, and play, and they take a high economic toll. About 90 percent of all headaches are either vascular (migraine or cluster) or tension (muscle contraction) headaches (Table 2.3-8). Psychological factors play a role in all patients with chronic pain, particularly in those with chronic headaches, but headaches are rarely the sole manifestation of depression, conversion, delusion, or hypochondriasis. Although a small percentage of headaches are due to organic disease or systemic dysfunction, there are dozens of causes of such headaches. They are best considered under categories of intracranial disease, disease of the head and neck, and systemic disease or dysfunction.

MIGRAINE Although migraine may begin at any age, the usual onset is adolescence or young adult life, and women with this ailment outnumber men by about four to one. Common migraine is characterized by one-sided throbbing pain of moderate to marked severity, lasting many hours to all day. The frequency may vary from a few per lifetime to several per week. Nausea and, when the attack is severe, vomiting are the most common associated features; sensitivity to light, noise, and odors usually accompany the attack. In the 10 to 15 percent of patients who experience classical migraine, symptoms of brain dysfunction precede the headache by 20 to 30 minutes. In contrast to a transient ischemic attack, the aura gradually evolves. The most common aura is visual, typically an expanding arc of zigzag, scintillating scotoma within a homonymous visual field; homonymous hemianopsia is often associated. Tingling of the extremities of one side may follow the visual symptoms or develop de novo; hemiparesis and aphasia are less common. Symptoms implicating the cerebellum and brain stem (basilar migraine) may also precede the headache, particularly in children. Rarely, the symptoms of brain dysfunction persist into and beyond the headache phase, very rarely resulting in cerebral infarction (complicated migraine). Ophthalmoplegic migraine with paresis of extraocular muscles is also rare. Many factors may precipitate or aggravate an attack; menstruation, relaxation after stress, and alcoholic beverages are the most common. Sometimes, migraine occurs only in association with the menstrual period (menstrual migraine). The poststress phenomenon is one factor explaining the higher occurrence of migraine during weekends and on vacations. Other aggravating factors are alteration in sleep pattern, missing a meal, and changes in barometric pressure. In approximately 10 percent of the patients, foods other than alcohol may provoke an attack. Migraineurs may be sensitive to almost any food, but the most frequently implicated are those containing tyramine (hard cheeses), phenylethylamine (chocolate), and nitrates (processed meats). During an attack, migraineurs prefer to lie down in a quiet, dark room, applying cold compresses or pressure to the area of the involved scalp. From 75 to 80 percent of patients with migraine have family members with this condition.

The acute attack of migraine is best treated with a prepara-

TABLE 2.3-8
Differentiating Features of Common Types of Headache

		Vascular Headaches	
	Muscle Contraction (Tension) Headache	*Migraine*	*Cluster Headache*
Sex	Male = female	Female > male	Male > female
Age of onset	Not specific	Puberty to menopause	20 to 50 years
Family history	Not specific	Often familial	Not familial
Quality of pain	Pressure, tightness, band-like, or not specific	Throbbing	Excruciating, boring, piercing, burning
Location of pain	Bilateral, occipital > frontal	Unilateral, often temporal	Unilateral orbital or adjacent head or face or both
Time of onset	Afternoon or evening more than morning	Early morning, often on weekends	Soon after onset of sleep, and daytime
Mode of onset	Gradual	Abrupt or gradual, often prodromata*	Abrupt
Duration	Hours, days, or weeks; often continuous	Hours, 1 to 2 days	20 minutes to 2 hours
Frequency	Not specific; chronic daily headache	Not specific	Cluster, such as one or more a day for 2 to 10 weeks
Precipitating aggravating factors	Emotional stress or not apparent	Emotional stress, menstruation, vasodilators; alcohol, certain foods; change in weather	Alcohol, lying down, REM sleep
Ameliorating factors	Nonspecific: relaxation, alcohol; Rx: analgesics, tricyclics	Rest, compression of scalp arteries; pregnancy; Rx: ergotamine, propranolol	Activity; Rx: oxygen, ergotamine, methysergide, lithium, steroids
Associated symptoms or signs	None or not specific symptoms—tenderness of scalp or neck muscles	Prodromata: scintillating scotomata, hemianopsia, other brain signs During attack: nausea, vomiting, photophobia, irritability; tender scalp	Ipsilateral redness and tearing of eye, stuffiness and discharge of nostril, ptosis and myosis
Personality traits	Competitive, sensitive, conscientious > perfectionistic	Perfectionistic, neat, efficient, restrained, ambitious > compulsive	Not specific > perfectionist

tion of ergotamine tartrate (1 mg), and caffeine (100 mg) (e.g., Cafergot) administered in a single dose. One or two doses at the onset of the attack and one or two every half hour until the attack has ceased is the standard therapy. No more than 6 mg of ergotamine tartrate per attack or 10 mg per week should be taken. The medication is usually taken by mouth, but it is even more effective by rectal suppository; it can also be administered by sublingual and inhalation compounds. Dihydroergotamine (DHE 45) may be administered parenterally for status migrainosus. An antinauseant is often prescribed with the ergot preparation. Isometheptine (as in Midrin) may be effective if the ergot preparation fails. A nonsteroidal anti-inflammatory agent, such as naproxen (Naproxyn), 750 mg, is also useful in aborting the acute attack. When migraine occurs two or more times a month, prophylactic agents are usually warranted. The treatment of choice is propranolol, beginning with 80 mg a day and increasing to 320 mg a day if necessary. Other β-adrenergic blocking agents have been useful. Small doses of an ergot preparation, such as ergonovine, 0.2 mg, or ergotamine tartrate, 0.3 mg (as in Bellergal), three times a day, are useful agents. Amitriptyline and other tricyclic compounds are beneficial alone as well as with other agents. Methysergide (Sansert), 2 mg tablets, three per day or more, is very effective, but it must not be taken for more than 5 to 6 months at a time because it may cause retroperitoneal or intrathoracic fibrosis. Calcium channel-blocking compounds are useful in migraine prevention. Cyproheptadine (Periactin) is of some value, as are the monoamine oxidase inhibitors.

The pathophysiology of migraine is not well understood. The pain appears to be associated with exudation of polypeptides through hyperpermeable dilated vessels in the scalp (and perhaps in the meninges) with the production of a sterile perivascular inflammatory reaction. Both pain and vasodilation may be initiated by substance P at the perivascular nerve endings of the trigeminal nerve. Decrease in cerebral blood flow accompanies the aura of classical migraine; however, this change is probably not due to vasospasm, as was thought in the past, but rather to the decreased metabolic demands of cortical neurons affected by a spreading depression of neuronal activity following a stimulus to the cortex. This phenomenon, of the spreading depression of Leao, was first described in lower animals. Increased aggregability of platelets has been noted in migraineurs, and the level of blood serotonin drops during an attack. These factors may be related to the cause of migraine or may be epiphenomena.

CLUSTER HEADACHE Cluster headache begins most often between the ages of 20 and 40—very rarely before puberty. Men are affected six to eight times more commonly than women. The headache is an excruciating, boring, burning—less commonly stabbing or throbbing—pain typically in the area of the orbit, but it may affect adjacent areas of the face or the head. Fortunately, the pain only lasts 20 minutes to 2 hours, but it recurs, invariably in the same area, one or more times every day for a series or cluster of weeks or months. The cluster of attacks then spontaneously stops, only to recur again months or a year or so later. Some unfortunate individuals do not experience a remission, but have chronic cluster headaches. Associated with the pain is ipsilateral redness and tearing of the eye, clogging of or secretion from the nostril, and, sometimes, a partial Horner's syndrome (ptosis and miosis); sweating of the face is often present. Cluster headaches typically awaken the patient during rapid eye movement (REM) sleep, but they may also occur at any other time during the night or day. Alcohol will precipitate an attack during the cluster period. In contrast to migraineurs, patients with cluster headache cannot lie quietly, but most often pace back and forth or sit up and rock to and fro. Chronic paroxysmal hemicrania is a variant of cluster headache that affects women. The attacks last only a few minutes, but recur a dozen or more times per day without remission.

The acute attack of cluster headache is treated with the same medications used to abort migraine. In addition, oxygen inhalation often aborts the headache within a few minutes. Prevention of cluster headache is usually attained by a combination of prednisone, 80 mg per day, and methysergide, 2 mg, three or more times per day. If this regime is ineffective, lithium, 300 mg, two or three times a day, will often prevent cluster headache; the lithium level must be maintained at 0.6 to 1.4 mEq per liter. If these regimes are ineffective, the second line of drugs are the others used for migraine prophylaxis. In addition, phenothiazine compounds may be beneficial. When all oral medications fail, a course of IV histamine diphosphate may be useful. As a last resort, a lesion may be placed in the ophthalmic division of the trigeminal nerve by radio-frequency coagulation or glycerol injection in an attempt to block the afferent pain pathway. Indomethacin (Indocin) is specific therapy for chronic paroxysmal hemicrania.

Although the mechanism of cluster headache is a mystery, virtually all of the symptoms of an attack can be explained by parasympathetic discharges through the nervus intermedius of the facial nerve. The circadian and circannular rhythm of these attacks, however, must be attributable to a disturbance of biological clocks within the CNS.

TENSION HEADACHE The terms "tension headache" and "muscle contraction headache" are used for the common headache experienced by almost everyone at one time or another. These headaches are brief and ameliorated with over-the-counter analgesics. Headaches sometimes increase in frequency and duration and become chronic daily headaches. Tension headaches usually begin in adolescence or young adult life and more often affect women. They do not have well-defined characteristics, and the diagnosis is often made by excluding organic diseases and vascular headaches. In its most typical form, a nonthrobbing, aching pain is experienced as a band-like sensation around the head. Similar pain over the back of the head, the vertex, and the bifrontal areas is also common, but this type of headache may occur in any area. Patients with these headaches may be sensitive to light and noise, but they usually do not have the gastrointestinal or other systemic symptoms that are associated with migraine. The term "tension headache" implies that emotional tension is a precipitating mechanism. However, many patients with this condition often seem to have the headache as a response to the normal stresses of everyday life rather than due to specific emotional events. In contrast to vascular headaches, alcohol may ameliorate these symptoms. There is a very high incidence of depression and analgesic abuse in patients with chronic daily headache.

The treatment of chronic daily headache begins with withdrawal from daily analgesics often being taken in large amounts. The medication of choice is amitriptyline or other tricyclic compounds used for their analgesic as well as antidepressant effects. Nonpharmacological therapy is stressed. Avoidance of those work habits that may cause muscle stress, the use of such relaxation techniques as biofeedback conditioning, and attention to underlying psychological factors are most helpful.

The terminology for this headache is unsatisfactory because the mechanism of pain in unknown. The term "muscle contraction headache" is used synonymously with tension headache, but there is a growing belief that muscle contraction of the scalp, face, or neck has little to do with this pain. Patients with tension headache often have migraine as well and the term "mixed headache" is then applied. Many chronic daily tension headaches seem to have evolved from increasingly frequent migraine. Because of these relationships, many believe that tension headache has a vascular mechanism akin to migraine. Others have postulated a dysfunction of central pain control in patients with chronic daily headache and have shown a decrease of β-endorphin in the CSF.

HEADACHES CAUSED BY INTRACRANIAL DISEASE Intracranial disease evokes pain either by traction or irritation of the meninges or the major blood vessels. The traction is usually due to generalized or localized increased intracranial pressure, although low pressure, as may occur following a lumbar puncture, also causes traction and headache.

The headache of a brain tumor does not have a specific quality, but is usually consistent in location, roughly corresponding to the site of the underlying mass. As expected with an expanding mass, the headache is of relatively recent onset and tends to increase in severity and duration until it becomes continuous. It is aggravated by change of position, coughing, or straining.

When the meninges are irritated by blood or infection (or, rarely, by malignancy), headache will usually be associated with nuchal rigidity. A subarachnoid hemorrhage resulting from a ruptured aneurysm is manifested by the sudden onset of the most severe headache ever experienced; there may or may not be associated loss or alteration of consciousness. The general and neurological examinations may be normal, but the typical history requires CT of the head and, if the latter is normal, a lumbar puncture. Except for subarachnoid hemorrhage, the diagnosis of intracranial disease is not made by the characteristics of the headache, but by the associated neurological or systemic symptoms and signs.

Vascular disease of the brain is frequently associated with throbbing headaches, which often precede the onset of cerebral infarction or hemorrhage. Headache occurs in 50 percent of patients with cerebral hemorrhage, in 30 percent with infarction or transient ischemic attacks and is not rare, even with lacunar infarcts.

THE POST-TRAUMATIC POSTCONCUSSION SYNDROME Relatively minor head injury, leaving the patient free of neurological signs, often results in a stereotyped group of symptoms, of which nonspecific headache is the most common. Associated dizziness is either a sense of lightheadedness or vertigo. Personality change is manifested by apathy or irritability or by depression or anxiety. The patient complains of easy fatigability, lack of motivation, difficulty in concentration, and associated memory impairment—all leading to poor work efficiency. Because the physical and neurological examinations are normal, these patients are often accused of malingering for secondary gains, especially related to litigation. Studies with experimental animals have shown that after even minor trauma, certain types of shearing forces may cause diffuse axonal injury, seen with the electron microscope. Trauma is a well-recognized cause of labyrinthine dysfunction. Evoked visual and brain stem auditory responses and psychometric studies have shown abnormalities in a high percentage of these patients, supporting the concept of an organic rather than a psychological mechanism.

DISEASES OF THE HEAD AND NECK Any disease of the head and neck may cause pain; trauma, infection, and neoplasm are usually obvious. The following discussion will emphasize those diseases that are not obvious because the routine general physical and neurological examinations are often normal.

Cranium and scalp Temporal (cranial) arteritis must always be considered when headache begins for the first time after the age of 55. The headache is usually over one or both temples in the area of a swollen, indurated, tender branch of the superficial temporal artery. Other branches of the external carotid artery are often affected, and the headache may be located over any area of the head. Ischemia of the muscles of mastication lead to pain on chewing. Eventually, intracranial arteries become involved. The ophthalmic artery is most commonly affected, causing blindness; infarction of the brain may occur. Polymyalgia rheumatica is the systemic manifestation of this disease. Scattered pains of muscles and joints may be associated with malaise. There may not be overt inflammation within the external carotid arterial tree and, as a result of a normal examination, these people may be labeled "old crocks," whose symptoms are psychogenic. The diagnosis of temporal arteritis is supported by an elevated erythrocyte sedimentation rate and confirmed on biopsy of a branch of the superficial temporal artery by the presence of an inflammatory infiltrate with giant cells. This condition responds promptly to steroids, and treatment will prevent blindness and stroke.

Diseases of the eye Pains associated with eye disease are not only in the eye, but often over the forehead. Retrobulbar neuritis, glaucoma, and orbital tumors cause pain in and about the eye. Eyestrain is usually associated with refractive error or paresis of extraocular muscles.

Diseases of the ear, nose, and throat Inflammatory diseases of these sites frequently cause local pain, but sometimes the pain is predominant in the head. *Sinus headache* is a common complaint and connotes chronic sinusitis. Most people who believe they have sinus headaches have tension headaches or migraine; chronic sinusitis is an uncommon cause of headache. Acute sinusitis, on the other hand, invariably causes pain overlying the affected paranasal sinus. Associated fever and malaise easily differentiate this condition from chronic sinusitis. Nasopharyngeal carcinoma may cause pain behind the nose, as well as congestion of the nasal passages. This radiosensitive tumor will extend to the base of the skull and cause cranial palsies. Biopsy is the only way of establishing an early diagnosis.

Dental diseases Diseases of the teeth are the most common causes of facial pain. Occasionally, pain in the temples and other areas of the head will be the first sign of dental disease. Temporomandibular joint (TMJ) dysfunction is discussed below.

Diseases of the neck Whiplash injuries of the neck may cause demonstrable lesions such as a fractured vertebra and a herniated intervertebral disk. More commonly, however, the injury tears muscles and ligaments. These lesions cannot be diagnosed by roentgenograms and, except for variable tenderness and restricted movement, show no abnormality on examination. Whiplash injuries cause pain over the neck, often radiating to the head. One must not assume that the complaint of prolonged pain without objective signs is an attempt to obtain secondary gains. Osteoarthritis of the cervical spine is a common disease, but there is no relationship between the severity of the arthritis and the production of pain. Many European headache specialists believe that cervical arthritis is a common cause of headache; their U.S. counterparts tend to downplay this relationship.

SYSTEMIC DISEASES Virtually any systemic disease may cause headache by evoking certain metabolic responses.

The headaches associated with systemic disease appear to have a vascular mechanism. Vasodilation may initiate a sequence of changes akin to migraine. Acute vasopressor responses also cause headache.

Vasodilating diseases Carbon dioxide (CO_2) is a potent vasodilator and may initiate a vascular headache. This complaint may occur with elevation of blood CO_2 or may be evoked in local tissues by hypoxia or ischemia, usually associated with respiratory or cardiac disorders. Intracranial hypertension due to increased blood volume may be caused by heart failure or obstruction of the superior vena cava. A headache initiated by vasodilation is often the consequence of endogenous metabolites and associated fever or exogenous toxins, including medications (e.g., nitroglycerine).

Vasopressor reaction Although headache occurs somewhat more often in patients with hypertension than in the general population, hypertension, per se, does not cause headache. Blood pressure must rise suddenly and to very high levels before headache occurs, as may be seen in patients with hypertensive encephalopathy resulting from pheochromocytoma or the malignant phase of essential hypertension. Vasopressor reactions also occur when patients taking monoamine oxidase inhibitors fail to heed warnings with regard to abstention from tyramine-containing foods, such as hard cheeses. Under these circumstances, cerebral hemorrhage, as well as hypertensive encephalopathy, can occur.

CRANIAL NEURALGIAS The cranial neuralgias are characterized by brief bouts of paroxysmal lancinating pain recurring within the anatomical distribution of a cranial nerve. The pain often is triggered by external stimuli and usually can be relieved by interrupting the affected nerve. No objective deficits can be elicited from the involved nerve on neurological examination. These illnesses occur most commonly in the elderly, perhaps because a tortuous artery cross compresses the nerve root adjacent to the brain stem. Gross pathology is usually not seen, but electron microscopy reveals subtle damage. A demyelinating plaque of multiple sclerosis at the entry zone of the nerve root may cause trigeminal neuralgia in youth.

Trigeminal neuralgia, also called *tic douloureux,* is manifested by stabs of severe pain within the distribution of the fifth cranial nerve, usually the second and third divisions. Pains are often precipitated by touching the affected side of the cheek and by hot, cold, or spicy foods stimulating the mouth. The pain is initially prevented by such medication as carbamazepine or phenytoin. Attacks of pain may later break through the medical barrier. Partial blocking of nerve roots at the gasserian ganglion by glycerol or radio-frequency coagulation usually produces lasting relief. Surgically decompressing the nerve root from the cross-compressing artery adjacent to the brain stem usually cures the disease.

Glossopharyngeal neuralgia is manifested by bouts of sharp pain in the areas of the tonsil, the base of the tongue, the throat, and deep in the ear. The pains may be precipitated by yawning or swallowing. Laryngeal neuralgia is probably a fragment of this syndrome.

Geniculate neuralgia causes lancinating pain deep in the ear and adjacent structures. It presumably is caused by dysfunction of the geniculate (sensory) ganglion of the facial nerve.

The pain of *occipital neuralgia* is mainly in the occipitonuchal area, and the greater occipital nerve is implicated. Nerve blocks and surgical section are usually beneficial.

OTHER CRANIOFACIAL PAINS Less well-defined pain syndromes are of uncertain cause. There may be a pathophysiological mechanism, but the pains often appear to be a neurotic manifestation.

Temporomandibular joint syndrome and myofascial pain dysfunction (MPD) These syndromes are often the same condition. About 75 percent of patients are women between the ages of 30 and 50. Pain in the area of the TMJ often extends to the head and face. In a minority of cases, disease may be demonstrated in the TMJ by roentgenograms or CT. In the majority of cases, the diagnosis is based on the history of pain aggravated by jaw movement, decreased range of jaw motion, and tenderness in the area of the TMJ or muscles of mastication; clicking or crepitus of the TMJ need not be pathological. The mechanism of occlusal dysfunction, initially believed to be the primary cause of TMJ syndrome, has given way to the concept of excessive contraction of the muscles of mastication, hence the term "myofascial pain dysfunction." As with other pain syndromes evoking the mechanism of increased muscle contraction, psychogenic factors are often present. Measures to rest the joint and muscles, prosthodontic devices to diminish jaw clenching and bruxism, and tricyclic analgesic-antidepressant compounds constitute the treatments of choice. In exceptional cases, surgery is required to correct obvious disease of the TMJ.

Atypical facial pain This term refers to a more or less constant facial pain, often with bizarre qualities and not confined to the anatomical distribution of the trigeminal nerve or of other specific structures. The syndrome is most common in women in their late thirties and forties with a long past history of facial discomfort. The pain often becomes the patient's only concern and may be completely disabling. These patients eagerly submit to unnecessary dental work and other types of surgery in an attempt to find relief. Although this condition is thought to be psychogenic, patients refuse to acknowledge underlying psychological mechanisms and respond poorly to medical, surgical, or psychiatric treatment.

PAIN ORIGINATING IN THE AUTONOMIC NERVOUS SYSTEM

Causalgia When dysfunction of sympathetic nerve fibers occurs during partial peripheral nerve injury, a peculiar burning hyperpathia affects a poorly demarcated zone of a hand or foot. There are associated trophic changes in the affected part with smoothened and reddened skin, excessive perspiration, swelling, and tapered digits. Sympathectomy is usually beneficial.

Reflex dystrophies Other reflex (sympathetic) dystrophies may follow minor trauma or may occur after disease of certain organs. These injuries cause not only pain, but also muscle contracture and atrophy, vasomotor changes (hypothermia, cyanosis, edema), and trophic changes of the bones, skin, hair, or nails. *Sudeck's atrophy,* post-traumatic osteoporosis, is one form of reflex dystrophy. The *shoulder-hand syndrome* is usually associated with coronary heart disease, although it may be seen with disease of other viscera. There is pain and restricted mobility of the affected upper extremity, with trophic and vasomotor changes in the skin, muscles, bones, and joints.

PAIN WITH CENTRAL NERVOUS SYSTEM MECHANISMS

THALAMIC SYNDROME The pain in this condition is over one part or one side of the body; it is spontaneous, continuous, and often indescribable. The threshold of superficial pain is slightly raised, but when the stimulus is felt, it is unusually painful or disagreeable, and the zone of pain may spread from the area of the stimulus over ever-widening adjacent zones. There may be delay in appreciation of the stimulus, but the resultant sensation may persist for an unusually long period of time. Because of the paucity of objective signs, psychogenic mechanisms may be falsely invoked. The thalamic syndrome is usually caused by an infarction of part of the contralateral thalamus after occlusion of the thalamogeniculate branch of the posterior cerebral artery. Many characteristics of the thalamic syndrome may occur in other lesions of sensory pathways within the CNS. Pain of CNS origin is extremely resistant to all forms of medical, surgical, and psychiatric treatment. Paroxysmal pain may respond to carbamazepine (Tegretol). For burning pains, combinations of antipsychotics and tricyclic antidepressants afford the best relief.

Phantom limb pain Transient awareness of a phantom limb is common after amputation, but in a small number of patients the sensation may not disappear or may become painful. The pain is initiated at the amputation stump and perpetuated in sensory CNS centers.

Postherpetic neuralgia Burning pain recurs 2 or 3 months after acute herpes zoster in 50 percent of patients over the age of 60 years. The pain persists for many months and is unresponsive to section of peripheral nerves or nerve roots. This neuralgia may be prevented by early treatment of the primary infection with corticosteroids or acyclovir (Zovirax). Amitriptyline (Elavil) is often useful.

Epilepsy Pain may rarely occur as an epileptic manifestation. It was discussed under focal or partial epilepsy.

PAINS OF POORLY UNDERSTOOD MECHANISM

Acroparesthesias Unpleasant, crawling, tingling, sometimes painful sensations may occur in the hands and arms mainly at rest during the night. The symptoms are diminished by rubbing or moving the extremities. The restless legs syndrome is probably related to this condition.

Post-traumatic pain Pain in the head, neck, and other injured body parts often persists for many months after an injury. Whiplash injury of the neck is the prime example. Lesions of the muscles, joints, or vertebrae may not be demonstrable. Although malingering for purposes of litigation is often suspected, it is usually untrue. The postconcussion syndrome has been discussed.

Referred pain Different areas of the body may be innervated by the same segments of the spinal cord. The interrelationship of neurons at these segments accounts for pain generated in one organ and experienced at ("referred" to) a distant site. Usually, nerve root pain will radiate from the proximal site of the root to a distal zone, but sometimes the peripheral pain will be the only clue of root disease.

SYNDROMES COMMON TO NEUROLOGY AND PSYCHIATRY

On many occasions, symptoms cannot be readily identified as organic or psychogenic. Physiological disturbances without objective pathologic lesions are often erroneously diagnosed as psychogenic. (When the metabolic mechanisms of the psychoses are discovered, will the psychoses fall into the province of biochemical neurology?) In diagnosing a clinical problem that could be either neurological or psychogenic, it is wise to err in favor of organic disease. For example, patients with headache suffer less from a search for a brain tumor that is not present than from the presumption and treatment of a psychiatric disorder that turns out to be caused by a brain tumor. On the other hand, pseudodementia caused by depression is often more remediable than is dementia of organic mental disease. As a rule of thumb, patients who insist that their multiple symptoms are organic often have a psychological basis for them. Paradoxically, patients who deny illness or search for a psychological cause often have organic disease. The features distinguishing organic from psychogenic impairment of responsiveness were noted in Section 2.1.

Conversion disorder Conversion disorder, commonly termed *hysteria,* is the presence of symptoms or signs that the patient erroneously believes to be of organic origin. Multiple and recurrent symptoms that do not conform to disease entities are also termed *somatization disorders*. The symptoms usually date back to youth, or a past history of psychosomatic phenomena is elicited. An emotionally disturbing event often is a precipitating factor. The symptoms allow the patient to avoid unpleasant situations or obtain outside support. Hysterical patients usually appear bland and indifferent to their defect *(la belle indifférence),* but some are anxious or their attitude is evocative of sympathy. The marked suggestibility of patients with conversion reaction leads to contradictory responses and changes in, or disproportion between, symptoms and signs.

Hysteria occurs most frequently in women; malingering most often in men. There is less tangible evidence of secondary gain in hysteria than in malingering. The symptoms may allow the hysterical patient to escape responsibility, whereas the malingerer may seek the settlement of a lawsuit. The only absolute proof of malingering, however, is the patient's confession. The signs of hysteria discussed below can usually be applied to malingering. These signs are not pathognomonic, in that they may sometimes be found in patients with organic disease.

Sensation Pain is the most difficult symptom to evaluate. Not only is it subjective, but pain from any cause has an affective component. Pain that is primarily psychogenic may be poorly described as to quality and site or elaborately depicted with unusually graphic qualities: "like someone pounding a nail in my head." Even though it may be the major focus of the patient's waking hours, psychogenic pain does not often disturb sleep.

Hysterical sensory phenomena are commonly manifested by analgesia—that is, total loss of sensation. Analgesia, in contrast to hypalgesia, is rare as an organic phenomenon. On the other hand, extreme hypersensitivity to examination may occur in patients with a conversion reaction, and responses may not vary with the intensity of the stimulus. Psychogenic sensory loss often has a glove or stocking distribution with a sharp border and affects all modalities. Hypalgesia and hypesthesia from peripheral neuropathy also have a glove-or-stocking pattern, but the borders are less distinct and there are gradations of increasing sensitivity in the distal-to-proximal direction. The sensory impairment of hysteria does not conform to the anatomical zone of a peripheral nerve or dermatome; in an extremity, the defect may be present only medially or laterally. Inconsistencies in sensory responses are frequently noted with conversion reactions. Patients may profess loss of superficial sensation and yet be able to identify objects placed in their hands. Complete loss of position sense may seem to be present on direct testing, and yet the patient uses the extremity well with eyes closed and does not show the pseudoathetosis of organic position sense loss.

Several tricks can be used to foil the malingerer and detect the hysteric. An unsophisticated patient may be asked to say "yes" when the pinprick is felt and "no" when it is not, but many patients will misunderstand the command and say "no" when they feel less. With the patient's hands crossed behind the back and fingers interlaced, quickly testing the sensation of right and left fingers may evoke inconsistent responses. Impairment of sensation that ends at the exact midline is characteristic but not pathognomonic of a nonorganic hemisensory defect. Normal sensation overlaps the midline when hemisensory impairment is due to organic origin. Vibratory sensation in a patient with conversion reaction may be experienced differently over the right and left halves of the same bone, such as the sternum or skull.

Motor function Psychogenic weakness usually varies with the effort of the examiner testing the strength of the affected part; the tested muscle may give way inappropriately. The patient may contract antagonistic muscles in an attempt to simulate weakness of protagonist muscles, and resistance of "paralyzed" muscles to passive movement is sometimes found. Covert observation of the patient, as when dressing, may reveal use of "paralytic" muscles. Inconsistencies may be found in the patient's responses when asked to move those fingers that are touched while hands are crossed behind the back with fingers interlaced. In hysterical hemiplegia, the face and tongue muscles are spared. With the patient supine and the examiner's hands under the patient's heels, downward movement of the hysterically paralyzed leg will be noted while the patient lifts the normal leg, which will fail to pull downward on attempts to raise the "paralyzed" leg (Hoover's sign). Psychogenic paralysis of wrist extension is noted to be false by the synergistic extension that occurs while making a fist. There may be lack of resistance on testing dorsiflexors of the feet, and yet the patient may be able to walk on the heels. In psychogenic paraplegia, the urinary and rectal sphincters are usually unaffected.

Coordination Defects of coordination seen in hysteria are often gross and bizarre. The hysterical ataxic gait often has a bouncing quality and, when falling, the patient may show normal dexterity in preventing the fall or may conveniently fall so as to prevent injury. In spite of marked ataxia on finger-to-nose and heel-to-knee tests, the patient may be able to write and normally perform fine movements. During the Romberg test, patients may sway only from the hips or fall en masse without attempting to catch themselves; distracting patients during the test may prevent falling. Associated movements, such as the normal swing of a "paralyzed" arm while walking, may be noted.

Reflexes Reflexes are usually normal in patients with conversion reaction. On the other hand, absent gag reflexes and decreased corneal reflexes may be normal. Symmetry of reflexes, whether diminished or hyperactive, lessens the likelihood of organic disease.

Special senses With the exception of vision, the special senses are usually not impaired as a conversion reaction. Occasionally, hearing loss is psychogenic, and then it is bilateral and complete. Such a patient makes no attempt to read lips. Rarely is the loss of sense of taste or smell hysterical; such defects are very difficult to differentiate from organic lesions. Psychogenic blindness is usually bilateral. When a patient is asked to look at a close object, convergence occurs in a patient with organic visual impairment, but not in the hysteric. Opticokinetic nystagmus can usually be evoked in patients with conversion reaction blindness. Hysterical amblyopia is often associated with tubular constriction of the visual fields, and the size of the retained visual field does not increase as the testing distance increases. In unilateral as well as bilateral hysterical blindness, the pupillary reaction is preserved.

Other modalities A large variety of other symptoms may be psychogenic. Dysphonia is the most common speech disorder of this nature; these patients may be able to cough loudly. Spastic dysphonia has been discussed and is not a conversion reaction. Psychogenic dysphagia, also called globus hystericus, may accompany dysphonia or occur independently. The symptom of a "lump in the throat" is usually not due to organic disease. Of the respiratory dysfunctions, hyperventilation is most often psychogenic. Urinary retention may have a psychological mechanism, but urinary incontinence rarely does. Tics and habit spasms, often classified as psychogenic, may be metabolic in origin or a manifestation of Tourette's disorder. Psychogenic fainting or bizarre behavior may be difficult to differentiate from vasomotor syncope or psychomotor epilepsy. Major hysterical convulsions are rare, but often simulate coitus. Table 2.3-3 lists the differences between hysterical fits and epilepsy. Amnesia of psychological origin has been discussed above.

Special tests Examination of the patient while asleep may reveal sensory or motor reactivity not evident while awake. The EEGs of patients with hysterical blindness usually reveal normal suppression of α-rhythm when the eyes are opened and driving response to photic stimulation. The EEG K-complex during sleep is a reaction to an auditory stimulus. The finding of normal evoked responses belies patients' claims of blindness, deafness, or somesthetic sensory loss. During an amobarbital (Amytal) test, psychogenic signs tend to disappear or diminish, whereas organic signs are exaggerated. The test is administered by infusing amobarbital IV at a rate of 100 mg every 30 seconds until nystagmus is evoked, usually at a dose of 250 mg to 300 mg. Psychometric tests are very useful in evaluating the patient for conversion reaction.

PSYCHOSOMATIC DISORDERS

Psychological factors often affect normal function. The term "psychosomatic" is applied when psychological factors, usually mediated through the autonomic nervous system, are a major element affecting physical conditions. These conditions may be associated with tissue damage, as in duodenal ulcers, asthma, or eczema; or, there may be physiological dysfunction, as exemplified by hyperventilation, psychogenic cough, cardiac neurosis, and pruritus. Psychosomatic disorders are distinguished from hysterical symptoms by mode of expression and degree of symbolism. Hysterical symptoms are mediated by the voluntary sensorimotor system, and they symbolically express an unconscious concept. Psychosomatic symptoms are autonomic responses to an unconscious process, and symbolism is not present. As with many classifications, this dichotomy is not always precise. Because hyperventilation may cause many neurological symptoms, it is discussed briefly here.

Hyperventilation Anxiety and other psychological phenomena may cause hyperventilation. This condition occurs most often between the ages of 15 and 30. Often, there is a past history of complex multiple symptoms, conversion disorder, or hypochondriasis. The symptoms evoked by hyperventilation are due to hypocarbia, which induces a decrease in cerebral blood flow and respiratory alkalosis. Tetany may occur, but more common neurological symptoms include faintness or impairment of concentration, headache or fullness in the head, vague dizziness or vertigo, visual disturbances, and paresthesiae of the hands, feet, or mouth. The swallowing of air, as well as hyperventilation, leads to such systemic symptoms as fullness in the chest or epigastrium, shortness of breath or palpitations, nausea and occasionally vomiting, sensations of heat, and cold sweat.

Sexual dysfunctions Most problems of a sexual nature are psychological rather than the result of organic disease.

Hyposexuality Most causes of impotence are psychological. When organic systemic or cerebral illness causes sexual dysfunction, it usually inhibits sexual drive and activity. Impairment of libido may be a sequela of temporal lobe diseases, including epilepsy. Decrease of sexual potency associated with hypothalamic lesions is probably due to hormonal dysfunction. Impotence is often caused by atherosclerosis of penile arteries, diabetic neuropathy, and spinal cord disease; endocrinopathy or local disease of the penis are rare causes. Organic causes should be sought when a man who had normal sexual function and has normal libido experiences impotence under all circumstances and stimuli. The vascular and neurological causes of impotence can be established by penile Doppler studies or arteriography and by neurological studies of the sacral segments of the nervous system. The difference between organic and psychological impotence can be established with certainty. Nocturnal penile tumescence is almost invariable during REM sleep. Documentation of this phenomenon in a man complaining of impotence is evidence of its nonorganic nature.

Hypersexuality Increase in sexual drive is rarely caused by organic disease. Hypersexuality may occasionally occur with temporal lobe epilepsy (either as a postictal event or after the seizures have been controlled) and as a sequela of encephalitis. Frontal lobe lesions may cause loss of inhibition, and the resultant increase in sexual activity is often inappropriate. On rare occasions, deviant sexual behavior, such as exhibitionism, may follow a temporal lobe resection. Also rare are diseases of the parietal lobe or thalamus that may heighten pleasurable genital sensations. Those rare young men with Kleine-Levin syndrome manifest uninhibited sexual activity during bouts of ravenous appetite. An increase in sexual desire is associated with some medications, such as amphetamines. Hypersexuality also has been imputed to such drugs as marijuana, and it may occur in women who require androgen hormone therapy. Other agents touted as aphrodisiacs probably achieve their effect either by removing inhibitions or by relieving anxiety or depression.

DRUG-INDUCED SYNDROMES

Psychiatric and neurological symptoms may be manifestations of drug toxicity. Psychotic reactions may be induced by drugs used to treat neurological and other systemic diseases. However, neurological as well as other medical reactions may be evoked by drugs used to treat psychosis.

Drug-induced psychological syndromes Drug intoxication may cause mild psychological syndromes manifested by slight changes in mood, including euphoria, depression, anxiety, or irritability. Impairment of sleep, alertness, and memory may occur. More severe reactions cause psychoses that resemble schizophrenia, with hallucinations, illusions or delusions (especially paranoid), and alterations of mood sufficiently severe to disturb the patient's functioning. Severe toxic reactions also include cognitive defects of memory, orientation, and language. There may be depression of consciousness or agitation. Symptoms of intoxication usually disappear after the drug is stopped. Some compounds cause symptoms when they are withdrawn. Withdrawal psychoses may occur days after discontinuing alcohol, barbiturates, or benzodiazepines.

Mild tranquilizers have replaced sedatives as the most frequently prescribed drugs in the United States. Abrupt withdrawal of barbiturates and—to a lesser extent—benzodiazepines may cause convulsions or delirium, as well as signs of acute psychosis. Severe depression may follow discontinuation of stimulants. Psychosis-simulating paranoid schizophrenia can be induced by an overdosage of amphetamines. Belladonna alkaloids and other anticholinergic agents are known to induce psychosis; symptoms of stimulation are more common than depression. Levodopa evokes a psychological reaction in 15 to 30 percent of patients; the most common features are confusion, delirium, depression, agitation, and delusions or hallucinations (usually visual, anthropomorphic, and menacing). Levodopa occasionally exacerbates or precipitates schizophrenia. Corticosteroids and adrenocorticotropic hormone (ACTH) often produce an elevation in mood and, occasionally, restlessness and agitation; high dosages may cause psychosis, especially manic behavior or paranoid thoughts. These reactions may be difficult to differentiate from the effects of the disease being treated—for example, lupus erythematosus. Nonnarcotic analgesics, even aspirin, may produce agitation and delirium.

Neurological syndromes induced by psychotropic drugs There are many neurological side effects of antipsychotic drugs. Extrapyramidal signs are the most common. Haloperidol and fluphenazine (Permitil, Prolixin) (Mellaril) are among the most troublesome in this respect; thioridazine is least likely to evoke an extrapyramidal reaction. Acute dystonia may occur at the onset of treatment with psychotropic drugs, especially in children after an initial dose of prochlorperazine (Compazine). Akathisia, another early toxic reaction, may be misinterpreted as psychotic agitation. Sometimes, the acute dyskinesias are mild; face, tongue, and neck movements may simulate the bizarre mannerisms of schizophrenia. The reactions may also be severe, with oculogyric crisis or opisthotonos, sometimes suggesting catatonia. Parkinsonian symptoms due to psychotropic medication are usually a late complication and may be indistinguishable from idiopathic Parkinson's disease. If tremor is asymmetrical, it is unlikely to be drug-related. The appearance of apathy, caused by bradykinesia and mask-like facies, may be mistaken for the withdrawal of depression or schizophrenia. These drug-induced extrapyramidal signs respond to anticholinergic drugs, such as benztropine (Cogentin) and trihexyphenidyl. Tardive dystonia occurs less often than tardive dyskinesia. The dyskinesias, manifested mainly by buccolingual movements, are noted late in the course of high-dosage psychotropic therapy, especially in the elderly or after drug withdrawal. These activities are less complex than psychotic mannerisms. Patients with early Huntington's chorea show more gait impairment and fewer abnormal oral movements than patients with drug-induced activity. The neuroleptic malignant syndrome (see Section 2.2) is manifested by extrapyramidal symptoms, depression of consciousness and hyperthermia, as well as by other autonomic dysfunctions.

The major antipsychotic medications lower the convulsive threshold, but seizures are a rare complication of such therapy, and the medication can usually be continued at the same or a slightly lowered dosage after adding an anticonvulsant drug. Drowsiness caused by psychotropic agents usually occurs early in the course of treatment and is soon tolerated by the patient. Psychomotor retardation caused by drug toxicity may be incorrectly attributed to bilateral or diffuse cerebral lesions. Alterations in sleep, such as insomnia, bizarre dreams, and somnambulism, sometimes occur with these medications; monoamine oxidase inhibitors cause insomnia and restlessness. Antipsychotic drugs may cause neurological symptoms because of their autonomic side effects. Orthostatic hypotension may cause syncope or other manifestations of cerebral ischemia. Urinary retention or paralytic ileus may be mistaken for primary urological, colonic, or neurological disease. Impotence, beginning with the impairment of ejaculation, may be an autonomic complication of psychotropic medication, particularly the piperidine phenothiazines. Ataxia may follow benzodiazepine therapy, and fine tremors are often noted in patients taking lithium. The toxic confusional states sometimes seen with these drugs may be related to their anticholinergic properties, which may also cause mydriasis, with blurring of vision. Other drugs have adrenergic properties causing miosis. Such compounds as thioridazine occasionally lead to impairment of visual acuity as a result of retinitis.

DISEASES CAUSING SYMPTOMS WITH FEW OR NO SIGNS

One of the most common errors in medicine is the assumption of psychological illness when the physician cannot find objective signs to explain the patient's symptoms. Further complicating the diagnosis are psychological reactions of the patient to the initial symptoms of organic disease. Depression, conversion disorder, or some other superimposed phenomenon may mislead the physician.

Symptoms of short duration Transient symptoms and the absence of localized signs may be mistakenly diagnosed as psychological. These features are often seen in pathophysiological diseases. The dysphagia of myasthenia gravis may be mistaken for globus hystericus; dysphonia and other fleeting and variable weaknesses of the cranial nerve musculature may be similarly misinterpreted. The generalized weakness of periodic potassium abnormalities, cataplexy, and sleep paralysis may also be misdiagnosed. Pitfalls in the diagnosis of epilepsy and syncope have been discussed.

Diseases that affect the structure of the nervous system may present symptoms of short duration. Transient ischemic attacks are the most common examples of such phenomena. Brief local or generalized symptoms may also be the first signs of a brain tumor. Transient sensory symptoms are most difficult to evaluate, but one is also hard put to interpret brief weakness described as "heaviness," momentary blurring of vision, and fleeting speech impairment. Subarachnoid hemorrhage is often manifested by headache without objective signs.

Multiple small cerebral lesions Pseudobulbar palsy is usually the result of small bilateral cerebral infarcts. The psychomotor retardation associated with this condition may be misinterpreted as depression of spirits. Spontaneous laughter or crying in patients with pseudobulbar palsy lacks the underlying emotion. Lesser gradations of this release phenomenon include emotional lability and crying or laughing with minimal provocation. All these symptoms are subject to misinterpretation with regard to psychogenic versus organic illness. Other diseases that cause multiple small infarcts, such as lupus erythematosus and minute emboli from endocarditis, may present as an acute psychotic disorder.

Multiple sclerosis is a common disease of youth, and symptoms often outnumber or precede signs. The relative euphoria often seen in patients with this disease may be mistaken for *la belle indifférence* of hysteria. The blindness of retrobulbar neuritis is not associated with abnormalities on ophthalmoscopic examination. Sensations of numbness and tingling, whether caused by a CNS lesion or an early peripheral neuropathy, may be particularly difficult to document because methods of measuring sensation during examination are much less sensitive than the fine perceptual discriminatory powers of the brain.

Occult focus of disease When the focal site of the organic disease is obscure, there may be a problem in differentiating organic neurological disease from psychiatric illness. This difficulty most commonly occurs with cerebrovascular diseases and mass lesions (neoplasm, abscess, hematoma). Focal diseases of the brain may be clinically silent in anterior aspects of the frontal or temporal lobe, in parts of the parietal lobe, over the surface of the brain, or affecting deep midline structures, including the ventricles. These lesions may cause generalized symptoms rather than specific focal signs. Headache, dizziness, lethargy, and personality changes associated with such diseases are often unaccompanied by objective signs. The most common intracranial mass that causes symptoms without signs is a chronic subdural hematoma, which is often present without a history of trauma. A meningioma over the convexity of the brain, an ependymoma growing into a ventricle, and an infiltrating diencephalic glioma are other examples of mass lesions affecting "silent" parts of the brain. An infarct or a neoplasm of the temporal lobe or other parts of the limbic system may be manifested solely by a disturbance of behavior. Hydrocephalus may cause slowing of thought and action before dementia or gait impairment. Cortical blindness due to infarction of the occipital lobes may simulate psychogenic blindness; in both conditions, the pupillary reactions and the optic fundi are normal, and the patient may be indifferent to the defect.

Encephalopathies Diseases that affect the brain as a whole often begin by disrupting the personality. Encephalitis and metabolic or toxic encephalopathies initially may be mistaken for psychosis or neurosis. As examples, psychotic reactions are associated with acute porphyria; schizophrenic behavior is seen in Wilson's disease; and autism occurs in children with neurolipidoses. There may be psychological manifestations of acute encephalitis and the postencephalitic state. Personality disorders and day-night sleep reversal may be postencephalitic sequelae. Oculogyric crises occurred years after von Economo's disease, a form of encephalitis.

Diseases causing dementia may start with changes in personality. Patients with Huntington's chorea often manifest psychological changes before the onset of dementia or chorea. Although Huntington's chorea may cause schizophrenic-like delusions and hallucinations or manic behavior, depression is much more common—first spontaneous, and later reactive to the other aspects of the illness.

The postconcussion syndrome Symptoms of headache, dizziness, easy fatigability, loss of libido, impairment of concentration, and poor work efficiency may occur without clinical evidence of disease. Impairment of memory and attention is accompanied by depression and anxiety. These symptoms often last for many months or years. This syndrome was considered to be a neurotic reaction to injury. The occurrence of these symptoms after minor trauma, the similarity of symptoms from one patient to another, and the frequent absence of appropriate psychodynamics have led to the belief that the postconcussion syndrome is a physiological disruption of brain function. That concept has been supported by subtle psychometric cognitive abnormalities and abnormal evoked potential tests. There is microscopic evidence of diffuse axonal injury in animal studies.

Diseases of the spinal cord, cauda equina, peripheral nerves, and muscles During their initial presentation, lesions at these sites may suggest a psychological illness. Loss of sexual potency may be the first sign of spinal cord disease in a man. Urinary retention is sometimes the only sign of cauda equina disease, especially in women. The glove-and-stocking sensory impairment of peripheral neuritis may be mistaken for a similar defect of hysteria. The pain of herpes zoster and the sense of weakness in the Guillain-Barré syndrome usually precede overt signs of these diseases. Muscle diseases may begin with pain as the chief or only symptom. Patients in pain resulting from whiplash injury of the neck or low back strain and patients with muscle cramps caused by metabolic diseases may be falsely accused of malingering or incorrectly diagnosed as neurotic. The stiff-man syndrome, with painful tetanic-like contractions of the trunk without obvious clinical or laboratory evidence of disease, may lead to the erroneous diagnosis of hysteria. Elderly people with polymyalgia rheumatica and cranial arteritis may be considered as cranks because their scattered vague aches, malaise, and headache are unassociated with objective signs. Their remarkable improvement following a course of steroid therapy rewards both patients and those doctors who tread carefully before discarding any of their patients' complaints.

REFERENCES

Bonica J J, editor: *Pain, Research Publications: Association for Research in Nervous and Mental Disease,* vol 58. Raven Press, New York, 1980.

Browne T R, Feldman R G: *Epilepsy: Diagnosis and Management.* Little, Brown, Boston, 1983.

Cooper J R, Bloom F E, Roth R H: *The Biochemical Basis of Neuropharmacology.* Oxford University Press, New York, 1986.

Cummings J L: *Clinical Neuropsychiatry.* Grune & Stratton, Orlando, FL, 1985.

Grant I, Adams K M: *Neuropsychological Assessment of Neuropsychiatric Disorders.* Oxford University Press, New York, 1986.

Green J B, editor: Borderland between neurology and psychiatry. In *Neurologic Clinics,* vol 2. Saunders, Philadelphia, 1984.

Katzman R, Terry R D: *The Neurology of Aging.* Davis, Philadelphia, 1983.

Kirshner H S: *Behavioral Neurology: A Practical Approach*. Churchill Livingstone, New York, 1986.
Lance J W: *Mechanism and Management of Headache*, ed 4. Butterworth, Stoneham, MA, 1982.
Marsden C D, Fahn S, editors: *Movement Disorders Two*. Butterworth, Stoneham, MA, 1986.
Martin J B, Reichlin S: *Clinical Neuro-endocrinology*, ed 2. Davis, Philadelphia, 1987.
Mesulam M-M, editor: *Principles of Behavioral Neurology*. Davis, Philadelphia, 1985.
Parkes J D: *Sleep and Its Disorders*. Saunders, Philadelphia, 1985.
Pincus J, Tucker G J: *Behavioral Neurology*, ed 3. Oxford University Press, New York, 1985.
Plum F, Posner J B: *The Diagnosis of Stupor and Coma*, ed 3. Davis, Philadelphia, 1980.
Reynolds E H, Trimble M R, editors: *Epilepsy and Psychiatry*. Churchill Livingstone, New York, 1981.
Roberts J K A: *Differential Diagnosis in Neuropsychiatry*. Wiley, New York, 1984.
Sternbach R A, editor: *The Psychology of Pain*. Raven Press, New York, 1986.

CHAPTER 3 CONTRIBUTIONS OF THE PSYCHOLOGICAL SCIENCES

3.1
PERCEPTION AND COGNITION

KEITH H. NUECHTERLEIN, Ph.D.
ROBERT F. ASARNOW, Ph.D.

INTRODUCTION

Many psychiatric symptoms involve disorders of such psychological functions as perception, attention, memory, planning, and self-regulation. For example, in the revised third edition of the American Psychiatric Association's *Diagnostic and Statistical Manual of Mental Disorders* (DSM-III-R), auditory hallucinations and marked loosening of associations are among the characteristic symptoms of schizophrenia; inattention and impulsivity are two characteristic symptoms of attention-deficit hyperactivity disorder (ADHD); and memory impairments are characteristic features of delirium, dementia, and anamnestic disorders. Perception, associative processes, attention, and memory are the subject matter of what is now called cognitive psychology. It is therefore not surprising that psychological studies of cognition have made important contributions to the description and understanding of psychopathology. This section is intended to provide a brief overview of these contributions. To familiarize clinicians with this discipline, the section has been organized around explicating the different types of contributions made by cognitive psychology to the understanding of two adult disorders (schizophrenia and mood disorder) and two childhood disorders (ADHD and autistic disorder) in which impairments in cognitive functioning are central features. After an introduction of the different topic areas, central concepts of cognitive psychology will be described.

HISTORY The influence of what is now called cognitive psychology on the description and understanding of psychiatric disorders can be traced back to the earliest attempts to produce a systematic psychiatric nosology. For example, Emil Kraepelin's seminal classification of psychiatric disorders was heavily influenced by his training with Wilhelm Wundt in what was then called experimental psychology. This influence is reflected in the distinctions Kraepelin made between different attentional functions: *Auffassung*, the passive registration of information, and *Aufmerksamkeit*, active, voluntary attention. Kraepelin noted that in dementia precox *Auffassung* appears to be disturbed only in the acute and terminal stages of the disorder. In contrast, disturbances in active, voluntary attention *(Aufmerksamkeit)* are a consistent feature of dementia precox.

As another example, Kraepelin's description of the loosening of associations in dementia precox reflects the influence of the experimental studies of thinking by Wundt, a leading proponent of the associationist theory of thinking. This influence of associational theories of thinking became even more prominent in Eugen Bleuler's descriptions of schizophrenic thinking, which explicitly describe schizophrenic thinking as a breaking of the associational processes. Carl Jung, who worked in Bleuler's clinic, modified the word association procedures developed in Kraepelin's laboratory for the objective measurement of associational processes.

Kraepelin and his colleagues employed a number of other techniques from experimental psychology to study psychiatrically ill patients, including: (1) studies of fatigue using ergograph work curves; (2) the psychopharmacology of alcohol and other drugs, in which the induction of miniepisodes of mental disorder by means of drugs anticipate the subsequent work in psychotomimetics; (3) psychomotor reflexes, voluntary movements, and handwriting movements; (4) plethysmographic plots of mental processes; (5) word association; (6) memory; and (7) reaction time.

Starting in the 1930s, a number of centers in the United States, particularly one developed by Joseph Zubin at the New York State Psychiatric Institute and one led by David Shakow at the Worcester State Hospital in Massachusetts, conducted programmatic investigations of patients with mental disorders using techniques from the field of experimental psychology.

CONTRIBUTIONS OF COGNITIVE PSYCHOLOGY TO PSYCHOPATHOLOGY There are a number of interrelated types of contributions that cognitive psychology and neuropsychology have made to our understanding of psychiatric disorders. The type of contribution, in part, varies depending on the nature of the disorder. For example, in disorders such as schizophrenia in which genetic predisposition plays an important role, psychological laboratory measures of attention have been used extensively as possible indices of genetic vulnerability to the disorder. In contrast, similar measures of attention have been used in neuropsychology to describe the nature of the cognitive impairments resulting from acquired central nervous system (CNS) insults like closed head injury. The applications of cognitive psychology capitalize on the sensitivity of higher cognitive functions to disruption by psychiatric disorders and neurological diseases that affect the CNS. In many instances, subtle impairments in cognitive functions antedate or are prodromata of full-blown psychiatric symptoms.

Perhaps the most fundamental contribution is the use of the constructs of cognitive psychology to describe more precisely the cognitive impairments that are central features of many psychiatric disorders. In this vein, the concepts of cognitive psychology complement phenomenological approaches to describing the symptoms of psychiatric disorders. For example, the descriptions contained in DSM-III-R of the nature of inattentiveness in children with ADHD were heavily influenced by theories of attention in contemporary cognitive psychology that emphasize the importance of filtering out extraneous stimuli.

A second, related contribution is the use of cognitive psychological measures to quantify cognitive impairments along a continuous dimension. This application weds the technology of cognitive psychology to the rigorous scaling methods that have been developed to quantify behavior. These scaling methods have emerged from psychology's long-standing interest in the measurement of individual differences. Pinnel and Binet's attempts to develop intelligence tests to provide continuous measures of general intellectual efficiency were forerunners of this enterprise. The "biometric" movement initiated by Zubin represents the most ambitious application of this approach to the field of psychopathology. This approach features the assessment of psychiatric patients across multiple dimensions, including personality; performance measures of sensation, perception, and learning; and psychophysiological indices. The application of tasks from the psychological laboratory to assessment of psychiatric patients has been facilitated greatly in recent years by the programming of such tasks for standardized presentation on microcomputers. An example of such a testing situation is shown in Figure 3.1-1.

Objective, quantitative measurements may be useful for symptoms whose description was originally influenced by concepts of cognitive psychology as well as for symptoms that were derived on a phenomenological basis but can be quantified through the use of methods devised in cognitive psychology. For example, a variety of tasks have been used to provide quantitative measures of the memory disorders found in patients with dementing disorders. The development of quantitative measures of cognitive functions associated with or isomorphic with particular psychiatric symptoms is of critical importance for attempts to detect relatively subtle, naturally occurring changes in clinical state and to measure the alteration of clinical state by a variety of somatic and behavioral treatments.

Subtle cognitive dysfunctions that can be detected by continuous measures may be useful as subclinical markers of a number of psychiatric disorders. For example, certain impairments in attentional functioning are observed in some of the first-degree relatives of schizophrenic patients (including the children and parents of schizophrenic probands). The ability to quantify functions that might represent subclinical markers of a disorder makes it possible to use some of the powerful methods of quantitative genetics to test specific models of transmission of psychiatric disorders with greater sensitivity than is possible when the dependent variable is a dichotomous classification of disease status.

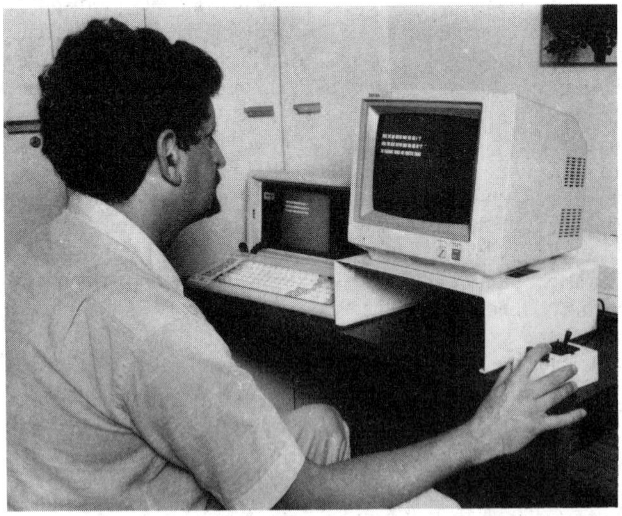

FIGURE 3.1-1. *Computerized assessment of perceptual and cognitive functioning with programs developed for Compaq Portable or IBM microcomputers with support from the MacArthur Foundation. (Courtesy of Keith H. Nuechterlein and Robert F. Asarnow.)*

The development of laboratory measures of the cognitive functions that are central features of a number of psychiatric disorders has also made it possible to exploit more fully the potential of some of the new brain-imaging procedures, such as positron emission tomography (PET) and topographic mapping of event-related potentials, to delimit the CNS substrate of the cognitive impairments associated with particular psychiatric disorders. Cognitive tasks can be used to stimulate or make demands on specific cognitive functions that are thought to be dysfunctional in particular disorders. Through use of brain-imaging techniques that record metabolic or electrical activity during the performance of these tasks, the brain regions associated with these impaired cognitive functions can be determined. Specific components of the event-related potential can also be examined to help isolate specific stages or levels of information processing that might be impaired in a particular psychiatric disorder.

Finally, parametric studies using cognitive psychological tasks can give a detailed, objective, functional characterization of the impairments of psychiatric patients that provides a bridge to the rapidly growing neurobehavioral literature on the CNS substrate of those functions in humans and animals with both focal and diffuse brain lesions. In this way, the methods and constructs of cognitive psychology provide an interface between phenomenological descriptions of the symptoms of psychiatric patients and the CNS systems that may mediate some of the cognitive impairments that are central features of a number of psychiatric disorders.

KEY CONCEPTS OF PERCEPTION, COGNITION, AND INFORMATION PROCESSING

Models of human information processing have been used increasingly to integrate and interpret the impairments of perception, cognition, and attention associated with a number of psychiatric disorders. *Information-processing models* emphasize the structures and processes by which individuals register, encode, select, maintain, transform, store, and retrieve information. Although information-processing models have deemphasized the boundaries among the traditional realms of sensation, perception, and cognition, some distinctions between these concepts can be made. *Sensation* typically includes the initial registration of stimuli at the peripheral sensory organs, the neural activity generated at these sites, and the conscious experience of very simple stimuli. Studies of sensory processing usually involve very simple, unpatterned stimuli without signal value (e.g., a neutral flash of light). Signal value denotes stimulus characteristics that carry informational content for the subject. *Perception* refers to the identification and initial interpretation of the stimulus based on its signal (or informational) value. Studies of perceptual processing usually use stimuli of intermediate complexity, such as visually presented lines, or single letters, or numerals, or auditorily presented patterns of tones, or single letters, or numerals.

The term "cognition" is sometimes used broadly to refer to

the whole range of processes addressed by information-processing models, which would encompass perception and higher levels of processing. However, in its usual narrower sense, *cognition* refers to the active translation, rehearsal, storage, or retrieval of information, or higher-order processing in which a broader context influences the processing of specific information. Thus, cognition involves the aspects of experience that require thinking and memory. Cognitive processing studies usually present very complex patterns of stimuli, such as words, sentences, or complex pictures.

In addition to the major realms of sensation, perception, and cognition, an important topic of information-processing models is *attention,* which can be best conceptualized as processes that control the flow of information processing. The concept of attention includes at least three functions: selection, capacity, and sustained concentration. Although information-processing models continue to evolve rapidly and many controversies over optimal conceptualization remain, some central concepts will be reviewed to provide a background for the summary of representative research on abnormal perceptual, cognitive, and attentional phenomena in psychiatric disorders.

SELECTIVE ATTENTION *Selective attention* refers to the mechanisms that lead to further processing of relatively few stimuli out of the multiple stimuli that impinge on the sensory apparatus at any one point in time. The assumption that incoming sensory information proceeds through a fixed sequence of information-processing stages was very important in early models of selective attention. Early models debated whether selection occurred early or late in the information-processing stage sequence. Complete rejection of unattended stimuli after early selection by a simple physical characteristic of a stimulus (e.g., masculine or feminine voice) could not account for the intrusion of some stimuli from unattended channels that have high adaptive or contextual significance (e.g., hearing one's name called while focusing on an opposite-sex voice). The efficiency of selection by a simple physical characteristic, in contrast, could not be easily accounted for if all stimuli were hypothesized to be processed until later information-processing stages. Thus, subsequent models of selective attention have suggested that stimulus selection can take place at several different stages or levels of information processing, depending on the characteristics of the target and nontarget stimuli.

Broadbent differentiates between three types of selection operations. *Filtering* involves selection of certain stimuli possessing a single distinctive physical feature (e.g., gender based on voice quality, spatial location). These stimuli are given preferential entry into a limited-capacity perceptual channel for further analysis. Selection of a voice from a person to the left of an individual's head as opposed to one from a person to the right is an example of filtering, because the single physical feature of spatial location can be used to differentiate the voices. *Categorizing* occurs within the limited-capacity channel and entails considering only those stimulus features that show it to be a member of a certain stimulus class. Thus, the visual stimuli "4," "four," and "IV" are grouped into the same information category despite the differences in their visual form. Finally, *pigeonholing* refers to applying a bias to the categories produced during the limited-capacity stage such that a certain category will be triggered by less perceptual evidence than would otherwise be demanded. Pigeonholing can influence processing of classes of stimuli based on more complex discriminations than those affected by filtering. For example, a person can be asked to search the content presented by simultaneous speakers to determine each time that words for digits 0 to 9 are presented, regardless of who says them. In this situation, mistaken identification of nondigit words as digit words would likely be increased due to having a bias toward selectively perceiving digit words. The clinical application of this version of Broadbent's model is evident in cross-sectional studies of deficits in schizophrenic adults that emphasize greater difficulty in pigeonholing than in filtering among actively symptomatic schizophrenic patients.

Another important model of selective attention has differentiated between two interactive ways of processing sensory inputs: preattentive processing and focal attention. *Preattentive processing* refers to a global, holistic pattern detection that occurs very rapidly (mostly in a parallel fashion) and early in information processing. A more detailed, slower analysis of segments of the stimulus field receiving *focal attention* follows preattentive processing. For example, in an array of letters C, I, O, and L, a person asked to find a single letter O would likely be able to locate very quickly, through preattentive processing, those letters that were either O or C because of the presence of rounded features. However, the more detailed analyses that are characteristic of focal attention would then be needed to discriminate between C and O. In this model, selective perception is the product of the degree to which stimuli are processed, rather than the result of rejection of some stimuli at a given stage of processing.

ATTENTION AS PROCESSING CAPACITY Another major conception views attention as a limited nonspecific *capacity* or pool of resources that can be allocated to specific processing tasks. Certain aspects of information processing that are completed through simultaneous or parallel processing require little or no processing capacity. Processes that demand processing capacity are identified by the limits they place on simultaneous performance of other cognitive operations.

In one influential processing capacity model, an individual can allocate the limited processing capacity to possible cognitive tasks fairly flexibly and can change allocation policy from moment to moment. Certain enduring rules of involuntary attention (e.g., allocate processing capacity to identify any novel stimulus) can influence allocation policy, as can momentary intentions such as those in most voluntary attention situations (e.g., select the message presented by a given speaker from among many simultaneous conversations at a cocktail party). The individual's evaluation of ongoing performance serves as a feedback mechanism to allow adjustment of the level of processing capacity allocated to a given task.

Allocation of processing capacity in this model varies with physiological arousal to influence task performance in an inverted-U fashion. At low levels of arousal, performance is impaired by allocation of too little processing capacity, which is in turn caused by failure to establish a task set or failure to evaluate performance quality. Moderate arousal levels are associated with optimal performance. At very high levels of arousal, performance is impaired by difficulty in making fine discriminations between relevant and irrelevant stimulus features, increased focus on dominant stimulus features, and increased lability of the allocation policy.

Models of information processing that posit a fixed sequence of processing stages lead to searches for a specific dysfunctional stage in the information-processing chain or a specific deficient elementary cognitive operation. Processing capacity models, in contrast, raise the possibility that decreased overall processing capacity, a deviant or unstable processing allocation policy, or abnormal regulation or level of arousal could cause many perceptual and cognitive anomalies in psychiatric disorders. A lowered allocation of nonspecific processing resources would be expected to impair performance in a wide variety of tasks that make extensive demands on processing capacity.

The difficulty level of a task is one of the factors that determine the processing capacity that a task requires. One scaling of the processing load of different tasks uses the amplitude of the task-evoked pupillary response as a physiological measure of mental effort or processing load. These momentary pupillary dilations serve as an index of overall processing load that is analogous to an electric meter that measures the total amperage required at a given moment by the various electrical devices in a house. A meaningful progression of processing load occurs both within and across cognitive task types (Fig. 3.1-2). Processing load increases from simple perceptual tasks to difficult perceptual discriminations to moderately complex memory, language, and reasoning tasks. The processing load of short-term memory tasks, which involve storing newly presented information in an active, working form for several seconds, varies greatly in direct relationship to the number of items stored for recall. Difficult quantitative reasoning tasks involve very high processing loads. Thus, within tasks that demand similar types of cognitive operations (e.g., short-term memory), processing load can vary substantially, depending on task difficulty level.

These different processing loads across and within perceptual and cognitive domains have important implications for the study of abnormal information processing. If perceptual and cognitive deficits in a psychiatric disorder involve restrictions on the overall level of available processing capacity, deficits will be expected across many types of effortful mental operations when the processing load exceeds the allocated processing capacity. Tasks that involve minimal processing loads will not be expected to show performance deficits.

Recent research indicates that cognitive operations may draw on several pools of processing resources, rather than a single one, because there is less interference between simultaneous performance on some combinations of effortful tasks than would be expected if all resources were from a single pool. If this multiple-resource model is adopted, an executive function that coordinates the allocation of resources to tasks assumes even greater importance.

SUSTAINED ATTENTION Sustained concentration and maintenance of alertness over time are the central concerns of the experimental psychology of *vigilance*. Vigilance or sustained attention tasks are characterized by a continuous demand for alertness and concentration to allow detection of relatively infrequent target stimuli at randomized intervals over a period of at least a few minutes, and often 30 to 60 minutes. In practice, most vigilance tasks involve discrimination of the occurrence of a target stimulus from the occurrence of other stimuli of a similar nature.

In clinical research, various versions of the continuous performance test (CPT) have been used as the principal measures of sustained attention. The group of vigilance tasks referred to as versions of the CPT involve monitoring a continuous series of stimuli (usually visually presented single digits or letters) in random order as they are presented briefly one at a time at about one per second for several minutes and pressing a response button each time that a predesignated stimulus occurs. The traditional sustained attention scores are (1) errors of omission or target misses and (2) errors of commission or responses to nontargets.

Some recent clinical studies of sustained attention have derived signal detection theory indices from the traditional raw error scores to delineate more clearly the processes that are malfunctioning in psychiatric populations. These concepts of signal detection theory will now be introduced to prepare the reader for subsequent discussions of vigilance findings within certain diagnostic groups. A distinction in *signal detection theory* between sensitivity and response criterion dimensions has proved useful for distinguishing two processes within normal vigilance performance. These two separate performance di-

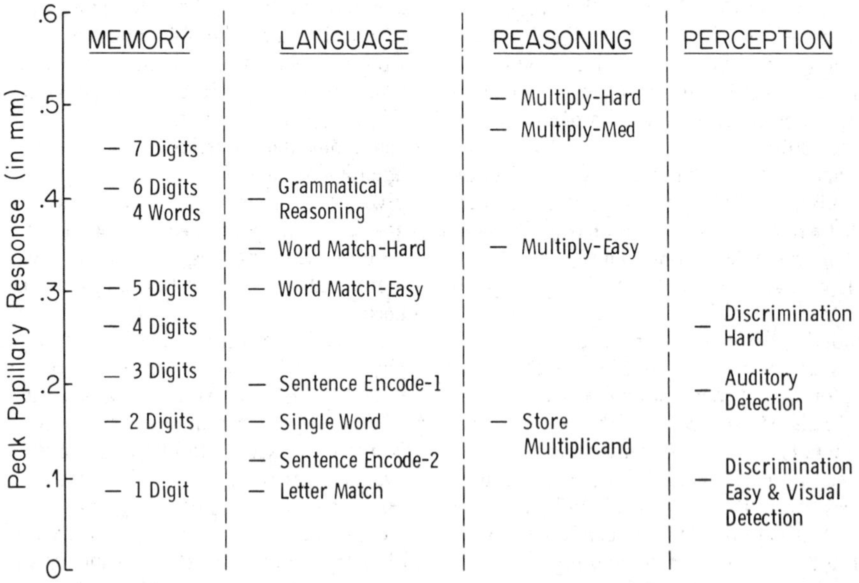

FIGURE 3.1-2. *Processing load of a range of cognitive tasks, as indexed by the peak amplitudes of the task-evoked pupillary responses. (Reprinted from Beatty J: Task-evoked pupillary responses, processing load, and the structure of processing resources. Psychol Bull 91: 276, 1982, with permission. Copyright 1982, American Psychological Association.)*

mensions are derived from joint consideration of the error tendencies represented by the two traditional scores of errors of omission and errors of commission. The first dimension, the subject's level of discrimination of the target (signal) stimuli from the nontarget (noise) stimuli, is called *sensitivity*. High sensitivity is usually characterized by a relatively high target hit rate (few errors of omission) and a relatively low false-alarm rate (few errors of commission). The second dimension, *response criterion*, indexes the amount of supportive perceptual evidence that the subject requires to decide that a stimulus is a target. A high, or "cautious," response criterion is typically characterized by a relatively low target hit rate but also a simultaneous low false-alarm rate. A low, "liberal" response criterion is indicated by a relatively higher hit rate but also a higher false-alarm rate.

A decrement in sensitivity over the course of a vigilance task is strong evidence of decreased sustained attention. Vigilance tasks produce sensitivity decrements over time in normal subjects only if the stimulus presentation rate is high and the targets involve either memory for successive stimuli or highly degraded (blurred) stimuli. A linkage can be made between the decrements in sustained attention within these types of vigilance tasks and the conception of attention as processing capacity that was discussed above. Target stimuli that require memory for successive stimuli or require difficult perceptual processing of multiple ambiguous features of individual, highly degraded stimuli involve relatively high levels of processing capacity. Thus, vigilance tasks that produce a decrement in sensitivity over time apparently entail a high demand on processing capacity. In contrast, vigilance tasks that are characterized either by slower stimulus presentation rates or by targets that are single, clearly focused, familiar stimuli do not produce decrements in sensitivity over time in normal individuals. Slower stimulus rates involve lower processing load. Similarly, detection of individual, clearly focused, very familiar target stimuli involves a process of encoding to a recognition level that occurs with very low demands on processing capacity. Thus, the decrement in sustained attention for normal subjects appears to be linked to vigilance tasks that impose a high level of momentary processing load.

The fact that task-evoked pupillary dilation, which indexes processing resource allocation, decreases as sensitivity decreases during vigilance also indicates a connection between processing resource allocation and sustained attention. This relationship implies that common neurophysiological systems may modulate the intensity of attention (the capacity dimension) and the maintenance of attention over time.

EPISODIC MEMORY: MULTISTORE MODELS In the domain of memory research, a distinction is often made between episodic and semantic memory. *Episodic memory* refers to storage and retrieval of information about specific events or episodes in one's life. It is autobiographical in nature and usually includes spatial-temporal information. One of the most influential theoretical frameworks for understanding episodic memory is the multistore model of Atkinson and Shiffrin, which includes the fundamental structural elements of the sensory register, the short-term store, and the long-term store. The *sensory register* stores sensory information in a preconscious, relatively complete form for a very short period (about 250 msec). This sensory information not only disappears rapidly, but can be erased by new information arriving from the senses.

Information from the sensory store and the long-term store are transferred to the *short-term store,* an active memory structure where conscious memory routines (e.g., rehearsal, chunking) are employed. *Chunking* refers to combining small physical units of sensory input (e.g., words) into meaningful larger units (e.g., meaningful phrases) to facilitate storage. The short-term store has very limited storage space. Thus, careful selection of information for processing by conscious memory routines is required. According to the multistore model, conscious manipulation of information occurs only in short-term memory. Information can be held in short-term memory as long as continuous attention is allocated to it, but without attention the information disappears after 15 to 30 seconds.

The third episodic memory structure, *long-term store,* is a repository for an unlimited quantity of information that is transferred from the short-term store and possibly also directly from the sensory register. Transfer of information into the long-term store is facilitated by control processes in the short-term store that relate the content to the existing contents of the long-term store.

SEMANTIC MEMORY AND SCHEMATA *Semantic memory* refers to storage and retrieval of knowledge regarding word meanings, language structure, procedures, attributes of objects, and structural relations between events. This knowledge is not connected to the unique context or episode in which it was acquired. For example, most adults understand that a red traffic light is a symbol for automobiles to stop and do not need to recall the specific episodes in which this information was acquired to make this interpretation. Similarly, well-known word meanings are retrieved without reference to the incidents in which they were learned. Organized encoding, perception, and interpretation of everyday experiences and events are heavily dependent on rapid access to semantic memory. Semantic memory provides a context within which events and experiences can be understood. The structure of semantic memory can be represented hierarchically at lower levels as a network of propositions and at higher levels as extended, complex units of knowledge called schemata.

Schemata have been the focus of substantial recent research within depression, as is reviewed later in this section. *Schemata* are prototypic abstractions of concepts and events based on prior experiences that allow current experience to be encoded in a coherent and unified summary fashion consistent with prior knowledge and expectation. Schemata help an individual infer missing information from the information gathered during an experience. Because schemata help to guide encoding of new information, they can also contribute to memory distortions through preferential selection, abstraction, interpretation, and integration of stimulus input. The probability that a given schema will be activated is dependent on motivational factors, the recency and frequency of prior activation, and the goodness of match between information input and the schema.

AUTOMATIC VS. ATTENTION-DEMANDING PROCESSING In addition to the focus on the memory *structures* in episodic and semantic memory that has just been described, recent research in cognitive psychology has emphasized a distinction between *processes* that draw on limited central processing capacity (attention) and those that occur automatically without capacity limitations. This processing distinction has been very influential in research on both memory and attention. Several theorists have made this differentiation, each using slightly different terms.

Posner characterizes *automatic processes* as mental operations that do not interfere with other mental processing and that occur without intention and without conscious awareness. Presentation of a familiar stimulus automatically activates a psychological pathway that results in temporary facilitation of processing of a subsequent identical or similar stimulus without inhibition of other stimuli. *Conscious attention* is a flexible, voluntarily directed, limited-capacity system that can be used to increase processing efficiency for certain stimuli at various stages of information processing. Conscious attention is allocated differentially to expected events and results in processing facilitation if the expected event occurs. However, unlike automatic processing, conscious attention will result in impaired performance if an unexpected event that requires processing occurs. This impairment is caused by the time needed to shift conscious attention away from the expected event and to the event that actually occurred.

Within the overall framework of a multistore memory model, a similar distinction between automatic and controlled processes has been proposed. *Controlled processes* are temporary sequences of mental operations in short-term memory that are under the individual's control and are activated by attention and involve processing capacity limitations. Controlled processes have the advantage of allowing flexible adaptation to situational demands, but they are relatively slow and are subject to interference by other simultaneous controlled processing. Intentional learning, rehearsal, and sustained concentration are examples of controlled processes. *Automatic processing* involves direct access to long-term memory, is not affected by limits on available processing capacity, and does not interfere with other simultaneous processing. Automatic processes activate a fixed sequence of mental operations in response to a specific input configuration without requiring attention. Although they are efficient because of the absence of interference with other processing, automatic processes are difficult to modify or suppress and are therefore not very useful in situations that require flexible responding. Automatic processes develop after extended practice with consistent stimulus-response combinations. The initial encoding of very familiar letter or number characters to the recognition level is an example of a process that is almost automatic for most adults. However, with sufficient practice, complex sequences of behaviors, such as initiating a braking response to a red traffic light, may also become automatic.

In memory research, others have made a similar distinction between automatic and effortful processes, which are viewed as a continuum rather than a dichotomy. *Effortful processing* refers to processing that involves demands on the central, limited-capacity system. Certain organismic conditions, such as old age and depression, are hypothesized to decrease processing capacity and thereby also influence effortful processes. *Automatic memory processes* are usually unaffected by variations in such states. Effortful operations, such as recall, rehearsal, and elaborative mnemonic activities, would be impaired by states that reduce processing capacity. Alternatively, relatively automatic processes such as simple stimulus recognition, coding of information about an event's frequency, and activation of a familiar word's meaning should not be disrupted by reductions in processing capacity.

SCHIZOPHRENIA

The number of systematic perceptual and cognitive studies of schizophrenia is so large that only a sampling of the methods and results can be presented here.

NATURE OF PERCEPTUAL AND COGNITIVE IMPAIRMENTS It is well documented that schizophrenic patients have impairments in certain aspects of perception, cognition, and attention, some of which have been tied to symptom clusters or subtypes of schizophrenic disorders. Numerous discrete cognitive processes have been examined in an attempt to find a specific impairment that underlies the cognitive symptoms of this disorder. As the reader will shortly see, the diversity of tasks that elicit impaired performance in schizophrenic individuals makes it difficult to isolate a specific underlying dysfunctional process.

Maintaining readiness to respond Schizophrenic individuals have consistently been shown to have difficulties in sustaining optimal readiness to respond to environmental stimuli. This deficit has been demonstrated on tasks in which the patient is asked to respond as rapidly as possible to a simple tone or light stimulus that appears several seconds after a warning stimulus. The time between the warning stimulus and the signal to respond is called a *preparatory interval*. When responses after regular fixed (predictable) and irregular (unpredictable) preparatory intervals are compared, process schizophrenic patients have been found to show a distinctive *crossover pattern* in which their responses to a stimulus after a predictable interval become slower than their responses to an unpredictable interval as the length of these intervals increases. Thus, when the mean reaction times to a stimulus are plotted as a function of the preparatory interval, the reaction times for brief preparatory intervals are shorter for the predictable than for unpredictable intervals, but the opposite occurs for long preparatory intervals, forming crossed functions. In contrast to normal subjects, process schizophrenic patients often cannot take advantage of the predictable timing of the onset of the stimulus to help maintain optimal readiness to respond. This crossover pattern is found frequently only in process schizophrenic patients, in temporal lobe lesion patients, and, to a lesser extent, in some aged persons.

Sustaining focused attention Versions of the CPT have been used to examine sustained, focused attention in schizophrenia. Chronic drug-free schizophrenic patients have been found to detect fewer target stimuli than chronic alcoholic or normal subjects. The CPT apparently taps a deficit with particular relevance to schizophrenia, because chronic alcoholic patients are more impaired than schizophrenic or normal subjects on certain other tasks, such as the Digit Symbol Substitution Test, a brief, self-paced, number-symbol transposition task. The relative specificity of CPT deficits to schizophrenic disorder is also indicated by evidence that hospitalized schizophrenic patients detect fewer targets than hospitalized patients with either schizoaffective disorder or major mood disorder. Recent research indicates that deficits in signal discrimination during a degraded-stimulus version of the CPT in schizophrenic patients are related to the presence of schizophrenic *negative symptoms*, such as blunted affect and anergia, as well as to certain schizophrenic forms of formal thought disorder.

Sustaining smooth pursuit eye tracking Abnormalities in smooth pursuit eye movements (SPEM) in schizophrenic patients have been viewed as reflecting disruption of an involuntary form of attention caused by failure of a modulating or inhibiting function. Although the relationship of these abnormalities to concepts of contemporary information-processing theory has not yet been fully worked out, these abnormalities are included here because of their prominence in current research on potential markers of vulnerability to schizophrenia. SPEMs are the movements that are used to follow a continuously moving object, as contrasted with the high-velocity saccadic shifts of the eyes that fixate the image of an object onto the fovea. Holzman and his colleagues have found that 50 to 85 percent of schizophrenic patients show abnormalities in such smooth pursuit movements as compared to about 8 percent of normal comparison subjects. The most common procedure involves having subjects track a small target moving horizontally in a sinusoidal pattern at a frequency of 0.4 Hz (cycles per second), but other target waveforms can also be used to detect these SPEM dysfunctions. Gross inattention or lack of cooperation do not explain the SPEM abnormalities. Multiple, discrete, small saccades have been found to intrude into the SPEMs of schizophrenic patients. Figures 3.1-3 and 3.1-4 show examples of deviant and normal SPEMs, respectively.

Selective attention In dichotic listening studies, different messages are presented to each ear and the subject is told to repeat aloud immediately *(shadow)* the message presented to one ear. Schizophrenic patients usually make more errors in shadowing of the attended message than comparison groups. Impaired shadowing performance when the nonshadowed ear contains a message with specific personal relevance suggests that altered stimulus selection based on conceptual categories affects schizophrenic selective attention. Some studies have also found that schizophrenic patients show greater intrusion of words from the message in the other ear. When analysis is at the phoneme level, this intrusion is present even in a dichotic listening task that should allow filtering by ear of presentation.

Initial sensory storage and readout Studies of these initial components of information processing have used a forced-choice span of apprehension task and backward masking procedures. The *forced-choice span of apprehension* involves asking a person to examine a visual array of letters that is presented very briefly to determine which one of two letters is included (e.g., a T or an F). Samples of letter arrays of four different sizes are presented in Figure 3.1-5. Symptomatic schizophrenic patients show a greater decrement

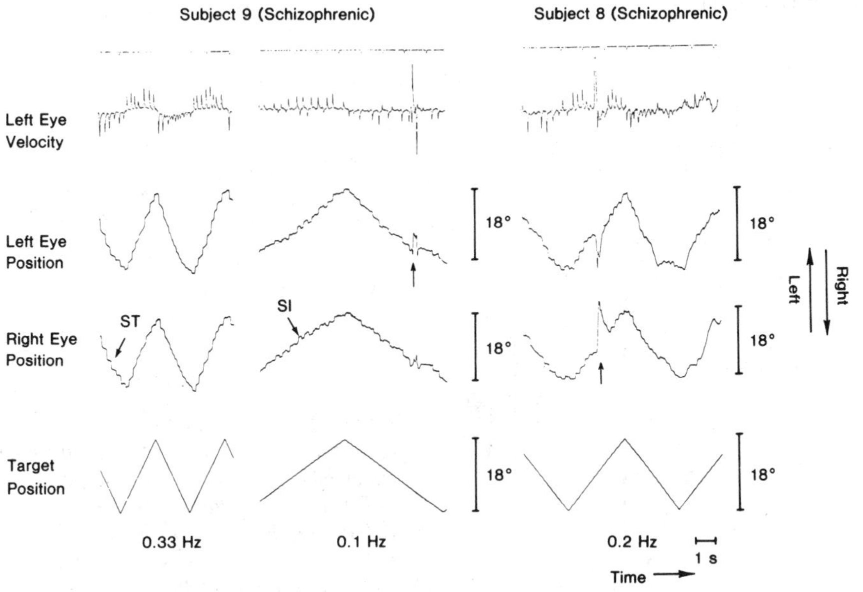

FIGURE 3.1-3 *Smooth pursuit eye movements of two schizophrenic patients tracking a target that moved in a triangular pattern. For subject 9, two tracking frequencies, 0.33 and 0.1 Hz, are shown. For subject 8, one tracking frequency is shown. Note the preponderance of saccadic intrusions (SI) in slow target condition and of saccadic smooth pursuit tracking (ST) in faster target condition.* Arrows *indicate eye blinks. (Reprinted from Levin S, Jones A, Stark L, Merrin E L, Holzman P S: Identification of abnormal patterns in eye movements of schizophrenic patients. Arch Gen Psychiat* 39: *1125, 1982, with permission. Copyright 1982, American Medical Association.)*

in the detection of the target letter when it appears within larger arrays (e.g., 10 to 12 letters) than when it appears within small arrays (e.g., 1 to 3 letters), compared to nonpsychotic psychiatric patients and normal subjects. Because changing the general similarity of target and distractor letters affects schizophrenic and normal subjects to a parallel extent, the schizophrenic deficit does not seem to involve primarily difficulty in discriminating target letters from similar distractor letters. Instead, an abnormally low limit on the number of letters processed before sensory storage fades, caused by slow letter processing or slowed initiation of letter processing, may be implicated. Like the CPT signal discrimination deficit, the span of apprehension deficit appears to be associated with negative symptoms of schizophrenia.

Backward masking studies involve presentation of a very brief visual stimulus (e.g., a letter) followed very shortly by presentation of another visual stimulus (the mask) in the same visual area, thereby limiting further processing of the initial stimulus. By varying the interval between the target and mask stimuli, it is possible to determine the interval needed to identify the target stimulus. Schizophrenic patients require an abnormally long interval between a target letter and a subsequent pattern mask to recognize the initial letter. The need for this longer interval suggests that schizophrenic patients take longer to process the target letter to a representational level with which the pattern mask cannot interfere. If schizophrenic patients are separated into those with a gradual symptom onset and poor premorbid social and occupational competence (poor prognosis) and those with rapid onset and good premorbid social and occupational competence (good prognosis), different patterns of backward masking performance are found. The stability of the backward masking impairment across repeated test sessions is greater in poor-prognosis schizophrenic patients with a family history of schizophrenia than in good-prognosis schizophrenic patients with a negative family history.

Poor-prognosis schizophrenic patients also need a longer stimulus duration to identify which of two letters is presented without a masking stimulus than do patients with good-prognosis schizophrenia, schizotypal personality disorder, depression, or manic disorder. The latter groups do not show this impairment in *critical stimulus duration*. It has been hypothesized that the increased stimulus duration without a mask involves deficits before or during sensory memory, while the need for longer target-mask intervals to allow target recognition with masking entails slowed processing after the sensory memory stage. Thus, poor-prognosis schizophrenic patients appear to show processing impairments that occur before or during sensory memory as well as after sensory memory.

Episodic memory Many schizophrenic patients have relatively normal ability to recognize which of a series of stimuli they have recently been presented *(recognition memory)*. The exception to this general rule occurs when the input to be remembered is not presented in a well-organized form, such as in the case of nonsense syllables. Abnormally poor recognition of nonsense syllables has been demonstrated, even in the absence of impaired word recognition. Nonsense syllables involve a higher processing load for short-term recognition memory because they require more information storage than the more familiar, redundant word items. This pattern of schizophrenic recognition deficit for stimuli with low association strength might indicate inefficient chunking of the elements for storage, which is a component of mnemonic organization.

In comparison to short-term recognition memory, the ability to *recall* recently presented stimuli is abnormally poor in schizophrenic patients. The deficit in recall is evident in auditory digit span and word span tasks, particularly under the distraction conditions. For example, it has been demonstrated that an opposite-sex voice reading irrelevant digits between the presentation of each relevant digit impairs recall of a series of digits in chronic schizophrenic patients. This distraction effect appears likely to extend beyond difficulties with high processing loads.

In contrast to the visual signal-discrimination deficit in the CPT and forced-choice span of apprehension, auditory distractibility in serial verbal recall has recently been found to be associated within schizophrenic samples with the degree of delusions, hallucinations, and positive formal thought disorder. Thus, the susceptibility of verbal memory impairment to distraction may be an underlying contributor to so-called *positive symptoms* of schizophrenia, a phrase that refers to the fact that hallucinations and delusions represent the presence of experiences that normally are absent.

Schizophrenic patients are particularly impaired by distractors relative to normal individuals, in the recall of the first items presented within a series of items within a trial. For example, when presented with a series of words to be remembered under distracting conditions, schizophrenic patients show impaired recall of the first presented words, but show normal recall of the last presented words. Active rehearsal serves to transfer the initially presented items to long-term storage. Recall of items in the initial positions requires this transfer to long-term storage. Thus, distraction in schizophrenic patients apparently interferes with active rehearsal. The more passive, relatively automatic processes used to recall items at the end of an item series are not disrupted by distraction to an abnormal degree.

Other evidence also shows that schizophrenic patients do not use

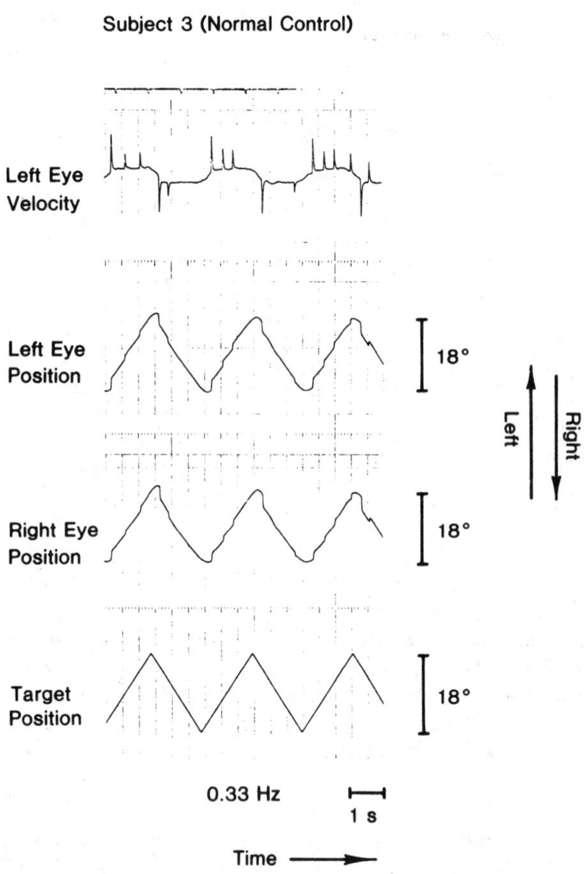

FIGURE 3.1-4. *Smooth pursuit eye movements of a normal control subject tracking a target that moved in a triangular pattern. Note only occasional saccadic smooth pursuit tracking and saccadic intrusions. (Reprinted from Levin S, Jones A, Stark L, Merrin E L, and Holzman P S: Identification of abnormal patterns in eye movements of schizophrenic patients. Arch Gen Psychiat 39: 1125, 1982, with permission. Copyright 1982, American Medical Association.)*

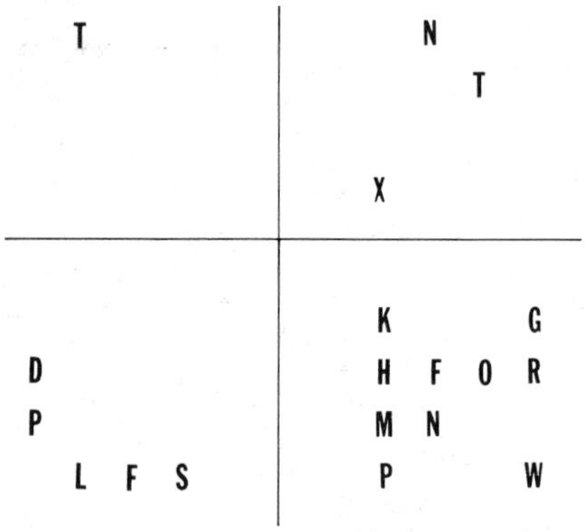

FIGURE 3.1-5. *Example of 1-, 3-, 5-, and 10-letter arrays for the forced-choice span of apprehension. The task is to detect whether a T or an F is present in the array during a very brief presentation. (Courtesy of Keith H. Nuechterlein and Robert F. Asarnow.)*

spontaneous, effortful, capacity-demanding processes, such as clustering by semantic categories in recall and other mnemonic organization strategies, to the extent that normal individuals do. However, appropriate mnemonic organization strategies can be elicited in schizophrenic patients with training. Thus, the limited use of active short-term memory strategies may be a result of insufficient allocation of processing capacity by executive functions rather than a result of defects in information-processing structures.

Relationships between cognition and language A subgroup of schizophrenic patients exhibits *formal thought disorder,* which refers to abnormalities in the form, rather than the content, of their thinking. Formal thought disorder includes marked loosening of associations, incoherence, and poverty of content of speech, among other symptoms. All of these symptoms are assessed through examination of the speech of the patient, which is inferred to reflect the form of thought. Formal thought disorder is not unique to schizophrenia, but is much more common in schizophrenia than in other psychiatric disorders, with the exception of manic states of bipolar mood disorder. Furthermore, the formal thought disorder in manic states has somewhat different characteristics than that occurring in schizophrenia. *Marked loosening of associations* refers to conceptual links between words or phrases that defy the culturally held norms to such an extent that the listener has difficulty seeing any connection. The type of loosening of associations that commonly occurs in schizophrenia is sometimes called *derailment* because the departures from a logical train of thought are so abrupt. *Incoherence* refers to the inability of the average listener to understand the meaning of the schizophrenic patient's discourse and subsumes a variety of more specific communication problems. Phrases of the patient's sentences may be meaningful, but because of vague referents, sudden shifts in frame of reference, illogical deductions, neologisms (idiosyncratic use of words or creation of new words), or other abnormalities, the overall understandability of the patient's message is very low. *Poverty of content of speech* involves speech that is relatively normal in amount but appears empty because of vagueness, overabstraction, or stereotyped repetitiveness; hence, it conveys essentially no meaning.

Several programs of research have suggested that abnormalities in basic cognitive functions may contribute to formal thought disorder. Some researchers have hypothesized that schizophrenic errors in language usage reflect such exaggerated influences of dominant word meanings that dominant meanings intrude into contexts in which subordinate meanings would be more appropriate. They have shown through multiple-choice tests that schizophrenic patients select dominant word meanings to an abnormal degree within passages in which a weaker meaning is the correct one. This failure to select weaker meanings of words when they are appropriate represents an inability to consider fully the context in which a word is being used. Thus, schizophrenic word usage may appear bizarre because, to a marked degree, words are used out of context.

Several studies have examined the schizophrenic tendency to use referents that the listener finds vague and unhelpful. The nature of this speech abnormality has been explored in referential communication tasks in which the speaker is asked to provide a verbal description of one colored disk that will allow a listener to discriminate it from other colored disks in a display. A first step was to examine the ability of schizophrenic patients to pick the appropriate colored disk based on a description that was generated by a normal individual, in an effort to determine whether schizophrenic patients shared a common word association structure with the normal population. Schizophrenic patients showed no impairment in their use of cues provided by normal speakers to pick the appropriate target disk, indicating that they have a word association structure that is similar to that of normal individuals.

However, when schizophrenic patients were asked to generate appropriate cues, neither normal nor schizophrenic listeners could pick the appropriate target disks. The impairment in generating appropriate cues was examined further to determine whether the deficit involved the initial sampling of possible descriptors or the editing of these descriptors for relevance to the situation and the listener. For example, if a navy blue disk was being described within a display of blue disks, the descriptor "blue" might be the association that was sampled first but would need to be edited out or elaborated in order to be helpful to the listener. As the discriminations among colored disks became more difficult, it was found that schizophrenic patients had particular difficulty editing the possible descriptors for relevance to the immediate needs of the listener. Thus, the cues were often strong associations to the target color, but lacked value in discriminating the target from nontarget colors. Thus, faulty self-editing of thinking may serve as one source of incoherence in schizophrenia. Furthermore, schizophrenic patients showed *perseverative chaining,* a speech pattern in which their immediately preceding descriptors, rather than the target disk, became the stimulus for their associations. Marked loosening of associations may be a clinical manifestation of such drifts in the effective stimulus for speech.

The difficulty in maintaining perspective on the informational needs of listeners that is found in schizophrenia has been examined within ongoing discourse. The conventional pauses before utterances have been found to be abnormally long in schizophrenic patients, suggesting that cognitive processes during these conventional pauses are disrupted. Many content switches and ambiguous referents in schizophrenic speech occur between phrases within sentences, points which require monitoring information in the prior phrase for continuity with information in the next phrase. Because schizophrenic patients have difficulties with the capacity-demanding, effortful processing in short-term memory that is required at these junctures, their problems in making transitions from one phrase to the next within speech may reflect these basic information-processing deficits. Thus, many abnormalities that are observed clinically in schizophrenic speech may be caused by fundamental deficits in more basic information-processing abilities.

PROGNOSTIC IMPLICATIONS Research to date suggests that information-processing performance has prognostic utility within the schizophrenic population. Overall performance levels across tasks with prominent perceptual-motor components, including reaction time tasks, have been found to be good predictors of patient status at the end of a 2-year period at a state hospital. The degree of rehabilitation and ability to leave the hospital was shown to be directly related to initial performance on the perceptual-motor tasks. Other studies that examined simple reaction time of unmedicated schizophrenic inpatients during the initial 2 to 3 weeks after hospital admission indicate that the overall speed of response is directly related to short-term improvement and to the number of days spent in psychiatric institutions over the subsequent 3 years. Simple reaction time was found to be independent of depressive mood, social class, and a prognostic rating scale based on social competence.

In one study, acute schizophrenic patients who later showed short-term clinical improvement had faster simple reaction times than those who did not improve, despite the fact that global symptom ratings and symptom profiles at the time of testing did not differentiate the two groups. These results may be interpreted as indicating that acute schizophrenic patients who show greater responsivity to task demands have a better short-term prognosis than other acute schizophrenic patients with the same level of acute symptomatology.

The prognostic utility of attentional difficulties for a 7-year follow-up period has also been demonstrated in one recent project that examined choice reaction times as well as inpatient ratings of attentional impairment, poverty of speech, incoherence, delusions, and hallucinations. The reaction time measures again showed predictive power. Among the inpatient ratings, the attentional impairment scale was found to be the most consistent predictor, with significant relationships to later hospitalization, social competence, employment steadiness, and a global outcome rating.

Some evidence indicates that antipsychotic medication may influence prognosis in schizophrenia partially through altering information-processing deficits. Studies using span of apprehension, CPT, and simple reaction time measures suggest that antipsychotic drugs may reduce positive symptoms in some schizophrenic patients by enhancing certain aspects of information processing. One recent study found that schizophrenic patients who made the greatest improvement on the forced-choice span of apprehension in the first weeks of antipsychotic medication treatment showed the greatest subsequent short-term reduction in conceptual disorganization.

INDICATORS OF VULNERABILITY TO SCHIZOPHRENIA Recent evidence suggests that certain deficits in the areas of attention, perception, and cognition occur in populations at risk for schizophrenia prior to the onset of psychotic symptoms and may serve, therefore, as indicators of vulnerability to schizophrenia. Children of schizophrenic parents have been the primary focus of these studies, but other first-degree relatives (parents and siblings of schizophrenic patients) and groups that show schizotypal traits have also been studied. Depending on the breadth of the diagnostic criteria that are used, first-degree relatives of schizophrenic patients have a 5 to 15 percent risk of developing schizophrenia compared with a general population risk of 0.5 to 1 percent. Some additional first-degree relatives who do not develop schizophrenia are also likely to have a genetic predisposition to the disorder. These considerations make first-degree relatives of schizophrenic patients a particularly informative group for detection of vulnerability indicators.

In some 7- to 16-year-old children of schizophrenic parents, anomalies in attentional functioning and information processing have been found on sensitive laboratory measures before the development of any psychotic symptoms. Deficient information processing has been found more frequently in children born to schizophrenic parents than in normal comparison groups. The observation that these information-processing deficits are present in a subgroup of children of schizophrenic parents is consistent with the genetic prediction that only some children of a schizophrenic parent are at truly high risk for schizophrenia.

Several measures have revealed abnormalities in children at high risk for schizophrenia. Versions of the continuous performance test that involve a high processing load have shown significant deficits in signal-noise discrimination (sensitivity) in three different samples of children of schizophrenic patients. Figure 3.1-6 shows the lower level of signal-noise discrimination (d') and lower target detection rate (hit probability) found among children of schizophrenic patients, as compared with representative normal children on a degraded-stimulus CPT. Individuals who report schizotypal personality characteristics, but no personal history of major psychiatric disorder, also show deficits in signal-noise discrimination on a high-processing-load CPT. Current evidence indicates that children of parents with nonschizophrenic psychiatric disorders do not show any significant abnormalities in discrimination of target and nontarget stimuli in these tasks, although some hyperactive children do show a signal-noise discrimination deficit combined with an abnormally low response criterion. Initial longitudinal evidence suggests that offspring of a schizophrenic parent who later show clinically significant deviance during late adolescence had signal-noise discrimination during a high-processing-load CPT at ages 7 to 12 that was lower than that of later nondeviant children of schizophrenic parents. Adding to the view that such deficits may be trait-like aspects of vulnerability to schizophrenia is evidence that a similar target detection deficit in the CPT is present in remitted schizophrenic outpatients.

In a series of studies, the forced-choice span of apprehension task that was described earlier has also yielded evidence of persistent deficits in early visual processing across children of schizophrenic parents, actively psychotic schizophrenic patients, relatively remitted schizophrenic patients, and individuals without a personal history of major psychiatric disorder who report schizotypal personality characteristics. Inasmuch as these target detection deficits occur with the larger perceptual array sizes, but not with the smaller arrays, it seems that processing load is an important factor. A recent study suggests that the span of apprehension performance of schizophrenic patients and of their biological mothers may be significantly correlated. Deviant performance on this task characterizes about 40 percent of schizophrenic patients in a nonpsychotic, relatively remitted state; therefore, this potential vulnerability factor may be particularly relevant to a subgroup of schizophrenic patients.

Susceptibility of effortful, verbal short-term memory processes to auditory distraction may also be related to vulnerability to schizophrenic disorder. Short-term recall has been found to be impaired among children of schizophrenic parents when a series of numbers is presented for memory under distraction conditions, as compared to conditions without distraction. This impairment seems to be specific to items in the early serial positions within item lists, which need

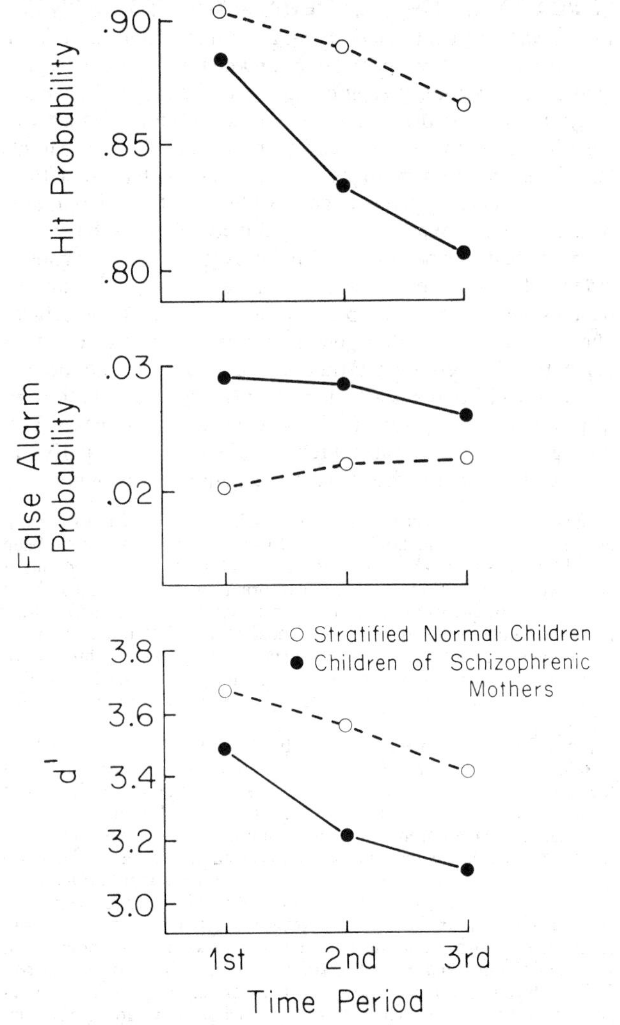

FIGURE 3.1-6. *Differences in hit probability, false-alarm probability, and signal-noise discrimination (d') at each of three time periods during the degraded-stimulus continuous performance test for 9- to 16-year-old children of schizophrenic mothers and stratified normal comparison children. Each time period equals 230 seconds. (Reprinted from Nuechterlein K H: Signal detection in vigilance tasks and behavioral attributes among offspring of schizophrenic mothers and among hyperactive children. J Abnorm Psychol 92: 4, 1983, with permission. Copyright 1983, American Psychological Association.)*

active rehearsal to be successfully recalled (Fig. 3.1-7). Children who have a parent with bipolar or unipolar mood disorder have not shown this specific pattern. A parallel deficit for recall of items in early serial positions has been found among actively psychotic as well as among partially recovered schizophrenic patients.

Evidence for the status of SPEM dysfunction as a vulnerability indicator and potential genetic marker for schizophrenia has come from studies of parents, siblings, and twins rather than children of schizophrenic patients. First-degree relatives of schizophrenic patients show an abnormally high frequency of poor smooth pursuit eye tracking. Research with twin pairs who were chosen because one twin had schizophrenia shows that concordance for poor smooth pursuit eye tracking is higher among monozygotic twins than among dizygotic twins. This finding supports genetic transmission of the eye-tracking dysfunction. Since SPEM dysfunctions have also been found in relatively remitted schizophrenic patients, these dysfunctions are not limited to the psychotic state. Furthermore, recent evidence supports the relative specificity of the SPEM dysfunction to families of schizophrenic patients as compared with families of mood-disorder patients.

Whether the deficits in information processing and attentional functioning detected by the promising vulnerability indicators just reviewed tap a common underlying process is not currently known. Furthermore, individuals at increased risk for schizophrenia need to be followed to determine their eventual diagnostic outcome in order to evaluate whether deviations in particular aspects of information processing, or a generalized deficit across perceptual and cognitive tasks that involve high momentary processing loads, are antecedents of schizophrenia. Studies that examine the mode of transmission of these deficits within families of schizophrenic patients are also of great current interest.

MOOD DISORDERS

Studies of perception, cognition, and memory in the major mood disorders can be divided into those examining the adequacy of processing information without affective content and those examining the processing of information with positive or negative content. The latter topic has been a very popular one in recent years, whereas the former one is more closely related to the research on information-processing deficits in schizophrenia that has just been reviewed. To facilitate comparison to the research on schizophrenia, research on processing of information with neutral content will be described first.

PROCESSING OF INFORMATION WITH NEUTRAL CONTENT Among the important themes of research in this area are (1) whether objective evidence can be found for the memory and learning deficits that are reported by depressed

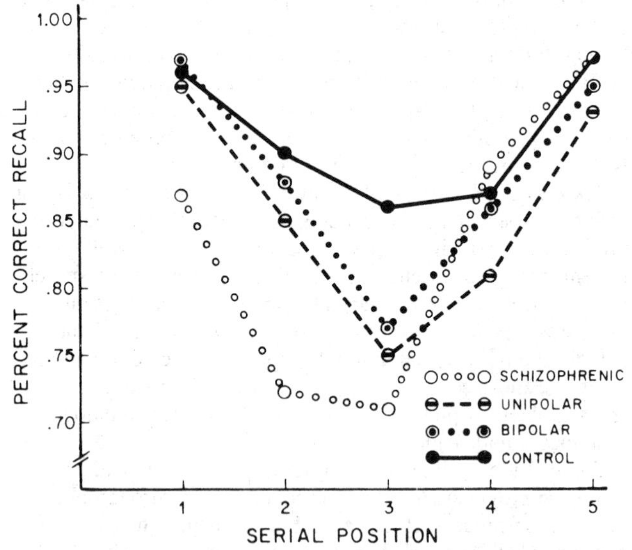

FIGURE 3.1-7. *Serial position curves by group for items presented during distraction. Groups are the 13- to 18-year-old offspring of schizophrenic, unipolar, bipolar, or normal control parents. (Reprinted from Harvey P, Winters K, Weintraub S, Neale J M: Distractibility in children vulnerable to psychopathology. J Abnorm Psychol 90: 298, 1981, with permission. Copyright 1981, American Psychological Association.)*

patients and (2) whether the flight of ideas and easy distractibility that characterize mania clinically are related to distinctive information-processing deficiencies on cognitive tasks.

Learning and memory deficits in depression The available data support the view that major depressive disorder is associated with some degree of learning and memory impairment. When compared to normal individuals, depressed patients show deficits in short-term memory. It has been shown that tasks demanding elaborate encoding of material to be remembered are particularly difficult for depressed patients. Similarly, although depressed patients show normal recall of easily organized information, they do not efficiently reorganize information to aid future recall when organization is not readily apparent. Although active organization of new material for later recall is deficient during major depressive periods, the retrieval from long-term memory of previously encoded information appears to be relatively intact. This pattern of cognitive processing during episodes of major depressive disorder may be linked to a reduction in the sustained cognitive effort necessary to complete active, elaborate transformations of stimulus input.

Another factor that is likely to influence the recall of information from short-term memory in depressed patients is an unusually cautious response style. In comparison to elderly normal individuals and elderly patients with dementia, elderly depressed patients have significantly higher response criterion scores for recognition memory, as determined by signal detection theory analyses. Thus, part of the memory deficit observed in depression is likely to be due to a style of not responding that something is remembered unless when one has a high level of confidence in the memory.

Johnson and Magaro have recently concluded, based on a review of available evidence, that memory impairment in depressive disorder is related to the current severity of the depressive state and is reversed when the depressive state resolves. They propose that the severity of the depressive state affects memory processes either by disrupting the creation of the memory trace or by lowering the level of effort used in encoding and storage.

Cognitive deficits in mania Patients with bipolar mood disorder who are in a manic state demonstrate flight of ideas, grandiose and overgeneralized thinking, and easy distractibility in clinical interviews. That manic patients show certain deficits in cognitive processing is suggested by their distinctive Rorschach inkblot responses. Recent research with the Thought Disorder Index has clarified the qualitative differences between manic and schizophrenic thought disorder. Manic patients are characterized by high scores in response categories representing combinatory thinking and irrelevant intrusions. Thus, manic patients show extravagant combinations and elaborations of ideas that are loosely held together, often interspersed with poorly integrated intrusions that appear playful or flippant. Schizophrenic patients, in contrast, are characterized by ideationally fluid thinking, interpenetration of ideas into each other, confusion, and use of peculiar words and phrases, without evidence of playfulness or extravagant elaboration.

Although the amount of research on manic performance of tasks drawn from cognitive psychology is rather limited at this point, some tentative observations can be made. Recent work with the forced-choice span of apprehension task has suggested that bipolar manic inpatients may not differ significantly from schizophrenic inpatients in accuracy of target detection within large letter arrays, although small sample sizes have limited the power of this comparison. Manic-depressive outpatients in relative remission in another study showed significantly better forced-choice span of apprehension performance than relatively remitted schizophrenic outpatients and generally did not differ significantly from normal subjects. This finding provides indirect evidence for possible state-related deficits in early visual information processing during mania. Similarly, recent visual backward masking studies, which also examine readout from initial sensory memory, have shown that pattern masks interfere with visual processing in psychotically disturbed manic inpatients to the same degree as in schizophrenic inpatients, but less disturbed manic patients do not display this susceptibility to pattern masking. Other findings indicate that poor-prognosis schizophrenic inpatients show interference from backward masking that persists across multiple testings. Although longitudinal study of psychotically disturbed manic patients is needed, the cross-sectional data suggest that their backward masking impairment may remit with the resolution of the manic state. Thus, early visual processing in bipolar patients appears to be disrupted in the acute manic state but may be less persistently disturbed than in schizophrenic patients.

Short-term recall during manic episodes seems to be disturbed by distraction in a fashion similar to that occurring in schizophrenia. Both manic and schizophrenic patients recall fewer words from word lists presented under auditory distraction conditions than from word lists presented without distraction. Bipolar manic inpatients have also been found to have more inefficient association networks and idiosyncratic learning patterns during manic phases than during nonmanic phases on serial learning tasks, random free recall tasks, and free association tasks. This pattern may lead to decreased efficiency of long-term memory during mania. The fact that performance on these tasks has been found to be related to severity of the manic state at the time of testing suggests that these memory deficits are reversible in bipolar patients with resolution of the manic phase, although much more longitudinal research is needed to examine this issue fully.

DIFFERENTIAL PROCESSING OF INFORMATION WITH POSITIVE VS. NEGATIVE CONTENT IN DEPRESSION In addition to identifying deficits in processing of nonaffective information, recent studies have examined whether differential memory encoding and retrieval occurs in depressive states as a function of positive versus negative content. The theoretical orientation of these studies derives from work on the role of schemata in semantic memory, as reviewed briefly earlier in this chapter. This research has been stimulated by one worker's cognitive theory of depression, which hypothesizes that negative (depressive) cognitive schemata serve to maintain depression by distorting the processing of information.

Consistent with the viewpoint that depressive cognitive schemata influence the processing of semantic information, several studies indicate that depressed individuals, compared to nondepressed comparison subjects, show enhanced encoding of negatively toned information relative to positively toned information. Many of these studies have employed a depth-of-processing paradigm, in which information with differing content is presented and recall accuracy is later examined in a free recall task. Information that is more deeply processed leaves a stronger memory trace and is more likely to be recalled. Instructions that emphasize the relationship of presented information to the self are viewed as particularly likely to yield encoding that is guided by the prevailing self-schema. Thus, for example, after rating each item on an adjective list for relevance to self, depressed patients have been shown to have better recall of adjectives with depressive content than adjectives with nondepressive content, whereas nondepressed patients and normal subjects recall more nondepressive than depressive self-referent adjectives.

Whether depressed individuals actually suppress encoding of positive semantic information is not clear based on current research, but studies of encoding of episodic information do indicate underestimation of frequency of positive events. Several studies have examined the accuracy with which depressed and nondepressed subjects recall reinforcement as compared to punishment within tasks in which rates of each type of feedback have been manipulated. Depressed individuals underestimate the frequency with which they are reinforced, whereas they either accurately estimate or overestimate the frequency of punishment.

Studies of retrieval of personal memories that were stored prior to the experimental situation also show the influence of current mood. Depressive inpatients with diurnal mood variations have been found to recall more unpleasant than pleasant memories during periods of high depression, but show the opposite pattern during periods of relatively low levels of depression. Similarly, induction of depressed or elated moods in college student subjects results in retrieval of more unpleasant memories during the depressed mood than during the elated mood, whereas more pleasant memories are recalled in the elated mood than in the depressed mood.

Thus, the bias to encode and retrieve information that is congruent with current mood state is generally consistent with the hypotheses of schema theory. The presence of a depressive self-schema results in differential encoding and retrieval of negative and unpleasant information as compared to positive and pleasant information, thereby making current experience more consistent with prior expectation than new input would dictate.

Less support is found for the hypothesis that the depressive self-schema is a stable cognitive structure that develops early in life and leads to depression when activated by life circumstances similar to those present at its development. Although this hypothesis has not been adequately tested in a prospective study, some evidence indicates that the enhanced processing of depressive information does not continue after the depressed mood lifts, as one might expect if the depressive self-schema was a stable cognitive structure. Furthermore, it has been argued that the fact that a transient mood state induced in college students yields content-biased encoding and retrieval that parallels that of clinically depressed patients suggests that the current mood state rather than a stable depressive self-schema might be the dominant factor. Thus, although the biased encoding and retrieval of information with negative content during depression seems to be increasingly well documented, the role that this phenomenon plays in the etiology of depressive disorder remains ambiguous. The success of cognitive therapy for depressive disorder, however, which attempts to reverse the content biases in information processing, might indicate that such biases do play a role in maintenance of at least some forms of depression.

ATTENTION-DEFICIT HYPERACTIVITY DISORDER

Studies of cognitive functions have made important contributions to our understanding of ADHD. Research conducted in the late 60s and early 70s on children with a diagnosis of hyperkinetic reaction by the second edition of the *Diagnostic and Statistical Manual of Mental Disorders* (DSM-II) revealed that, in addition to increased activity levels and impulsivity, these children consistently showed important cognitive deficits, particularly on tasks that measure attentional functioning. The third edition of DSM (DSM-III) recognized the importance of these attentional impairments by renaming the syndrome attention deficit disorder and by designating attentional problems as one of the three characteristic sets of symptoms of this disorder. DSM-III-R has continued the emphasis on attentional problems and reintegrated excessive activity into the name for this syndrome by calling it attention-deficit hyperactivity disorder. Easy distractibility and difficulty sustaining attention are among 14 characteristic behaviors of this disorder in DSM-III-R, and related cognitive attributes appear to contribute to several of the remaining characteristic behaviors.

Cognitive studies of ADHD children have had three interrelated purposes: (1) clarifying the nature of the cognitive deficit in ADHD children; (2) determining the extent to which cognitive deficits in ADHD children are caused by lack of mastery motivation and the failure to use appropriate problem-solving strategies; and (3) determining which cognitive deficits are remediated when ADHD children are given stimulant medications.

NATURE OF THE COGNITIVE IMPAIRMENTS Studies that demonstrated that hyperkinetic children have important problems in the regulation of attention show that they have, as Virginia Douglas wrote, "an inability to sustain attention and to inhibit impulsive responding on tasks or in social situations that require focused, reflective, organized, and self-directed effort."

These deficits in ADHD children are evident on a very wide range of cognitive tasks. Deficits on simple vigilance and reaction time tasks of a long and repetitive nature have been among the most thoroughly researched. Deficits are also found in perceptual tasks that require an organized, careful analysis of available cues. Other tasks that demand similar self-directed and self-sustained effort for rehearsal or evaluation of relevant information, such as intentional memory tasks and complex problem solving, also reveal deficits among ADHD children.

This line of investigation is exemplified by studies of vigilance in hyperactive children that have used modifications of the CPT. In one version, the child is required to respond to the letter "X" only when it is immediately preceded by the letter "A." Hyperactive children were found to make fewer correct detections and more incorrect responses (more "false alarms") than normal children; the robustness of these findings was confirmed by demonstrating them using both an auditory and visual CPT. In addition, hyperactive children showed a marked lowering of correct detections and increase in false alarms over time while normal children did not. Recently, using signal detection theory methodology, it was found that hyperactive children were particularly distinguished by a low, liberal response criterion factor measured across five CPT versions, which indicates that they responded to stimuli as relevant even when the perceptual evidence for their relevance was meager.

Parallel results have been obtained on other tasks that make demands on sustained attention, such as delayed reaction time (DRT). In DRT tasks, a warning signal is followed by a delay. A reaction signal is then presented. The child is instructed to respond as quickly as possible to the reaction signal by pressing a response button. ADHD children respond more slowly to the reaction stimulus. They also make more errors on DRT tasks, including responding before the reaction signal occurs, responding to the warning signal, and pushing more than once in response to the reaction signal. Thus, ADHD children not only have difficulty detecting the target stimuli, but also fail to inhibit inappropriate responses in tasks that demand sustained attention.

Although these studies have consistently found that ADHD children have impairments on tasks demanding sustained attention, they also highlight the complexity of these impairments. The tasks that elicit impaired performance from ADHD children are typically quite complex, making demands on a number of cognitive processes, including perceptual discrimination, inhibition of impulsive responding, and maintenance of a task set. They also involve noncognitive processes, such as modulation of arousal. To isolate the specific cognitive processes that might be deficient in ADHD, recent studies have attempted to determine which characteristics of tasks are responsible for eliciting impaired performance in ADHD children. Once the task manipulations that are critical in eliciting impaired performance are isolated, the nature of the cognitive processes that are impaired in ADHD can be inferred by drawing on our knowledge of the specific cognitive processes demanded by these task characteristics.

To this end, task parameters, such as the frequency of the target stimulus and the length of the interstimulus interval in a vigilance task or the saliency of the stimuli in a discrimination task, have been manipulated to determine which parameters enhance and which reduce performance differences between ADHD and normal children. For example, to contrast with the experimenter-paced CPT, a serial reaction time task was examined, in which the child's response to each stimulus causes the next stimulus for response to appear. When the sustained attention demands were reduced by having children control the presentation of trials in the serial reaction time task or when children were rewarded for sustaining attention through a partial reinforcement schedule during the serial reaction time task, the performance of ADHD children was comparable to that of normal controls. Conversely, the performance differences between ADHD and normal children can be increased by manipulating other task parameters. In many cognitive laboratory situations, ADHD children have been found to be no more distractible than normal children. However, when the irrelevant dimension was one that was highly salient within a speeded classification task, a greater distraction effect was found to occur for ADHD children than when the irrelevant dimension was not particularly salient. A similar finding is that engaging, appealing distractors elicited greater impairment in ADHD children than in normal controls on a task that required children to solve simple arithmetic problems presented for up to 3 seconds by a teaching machine.

The evidence to date indicates that a number of task manipulations can elicit performance deficits in ADHD children. The pattern of findings has led many investigators to conclude that there is not a single cognitive process impaired in ADHD. Rather, the deficient performance of ADHD children on certain cognitive tasks is thought to result from a constellation of interrelated primary impairments.

Douglas's list of the defective processes includes: "(1) the investment, organization, and maintenance of attention and effort; (2) the inhibition of impulsive responding; (3) the modulation of arousal levels to meet situational demands; and (4) an unusually strong inclination to seek immediate reinforcement."

ROLE OF PROBLEM-SOLVING OR MOTIVATIONAL DEFICIENCIES A second major question addressed by cognitive studies of ADHD children is the extent to which the cognitive impairment observed in ADHD children represents a failure to use efficiently general problem-solving strategies or task-specific strategies to help in performing a task or, alternatively, reflects an absence of intrinsic, effectance motivation to succeed on a task.

This line of inquiry was stimulated by widespread observation that ADHD children often fail to make use of knowledge and skills they possess that would help them perform on tasks; however, they often show surprising gains in performance when they work in the presence of authority figures and are given explicit encouragement. More systematic studies have revealed that the performance of ADHD children on cognitive tasks can be enhanced by: (1) teaching them both general problem-solving approaches and the specific operations required for doing a particular task, and (2) withholding rewards after errors while they are performing attention-demanding tasks. Deficiencies in the use of cognitive strategies and reduced mastery motivation may be secondary processes arising from the failure experienced by ADHD children in academic settings because of constitutionally determined primary deficits. These secondary processes, however, can impair future learning and lead ADHD children to fall increasingly behind their peers. Research to date suggests both the importance and feasibility of using cognitive training to teach ADHD children general problem-solving strategies.

EFFECT OF STIMULANT MEDICATION A third major thrust of cognitive studies of ADHD children has involved attempts to elucidate the mechanism of the therapeutic effect that stimulant medications have for many ADHD children. This research has focused on identifying the cognitive processes that are normalized when ADHD children are treated with stimulant medications such as methylphenidate (Ritalin). Early studies generally suggested that stimulants enhanced (for a brief period of time) the vigilance and reaction time performance of hyperactive children. The facilitative effect of stimulants on these tasks is not unique to hyperactive children; both normal adults and children also show enhanced vigilance performance when given stimulants. More recent studies have suggested that the cognitive effects of stimulants may be somewhat more dose- and task-specific than previously suspected. Stimulants enhance performance on many tasks, have little effect on other tasks, and even impair performance on certain tasks. For example, low doses of stimulants have been found to enhance the mean performance of ADHD children on a measure of cognitive impulsivity (the matching familiar figures test), on several CPT versions, on a paired associate learning task, and on a picture recognition task, but higher doses of stimulants have been found to have no effect on the matching familiar figure test and have even impaired the performance of ADHD children on a picture recognition task relative to their performance on placebo.

The research conducted to date does not isolate a unique cognitive process that is enhanced when ADHD children are given stimulant medication. Some evidence suggests that stimulants enhance performance by increasing the rate of cognitive processes that exist in the unmedicated condition. One group of researchers examined the free recall of word lists containing sets of either semantically or acoustically related words in hyperactive and normal children given low doses of stimulants or placebo. In the placebo condition, the groups did not differ significantly in the free recall of acoustically related words. The hyperactive children, however, recalled significantly fewer semantically related words than controls. Amphetamine treatment resulted in a marked increase of recall for both sets of words in both hyperactives and normals. The hyperactive children, however, showed their greatest increase in the recall of acoustically processed words, whereas the normal controls showed their greatest increase in the recall of semantically processed words. The researchers concluded that amphetamine seems to enhance the cognitive processes used by children in the unmedicated state rather than facilitating the utilization of other, sometimes more efficient, cognitive processes.

Other hypotheses that attempt to account for the apparent interaction between dose level and task demands in ADHD children have emphasized either the normal action of amphetamine drugs in inducing stereotyped behaviors, of which focusing of attention is an example, the modulating effect of amphetamines in increasing low rate behaviors and decreasing high rate behaviors, or an effect of amphetamines on self-regulatory processes.

Not only is the effect of stimulants on ADHD children somewhat task- and dose-specific, but as a group ADHD children are heterogeneous in their response to stimulants. Although the precise values vary depending on the definition of positive response, about 55 to 60 percent of ADHD children have a favorable response to stimulants in double-blind drug trials. This heterogeneity has led a number of investigators to assert that response to stimulant medication may be a useful basis for subgrouping ADHD children with different pathophysiology and etiology. It has been suggested that the most important clinical benefit that has emerged to date from the use of cognitive tasks in diagnostic drug trials is their utility in predicting which children will not benefit from stimulant medications rather than in predicting favorable response to stimulants. ADHD children who show little enhancement of cognitive performance during a drug trial tend not to have a favorable clinical response to stimulants.

AUTISTIC DISORDER

The earliest descriptions of autism emphasized the severe distortions of social functioning found in this disorder. Cognitive deficits were not regarded as important. Kanner described autistic children as having "innate inability to form the usual, biologically provided affective contact with people, just as other children come into the world with innate physical or intellectual handicaps."

Subsequent studies of autistic children suggested that there is a basic cognitive deficit in autistic children that is not secondary to social withdrawal. It has been argued that the cognitive deficit involves impaired language, sequencing, and abstraction abilities. The following five sets of evidence are cited by Rutter as suggesting that this cognitive deficit is the core of autism and that it may underlie many other autistic features:

1. The cognitive deficit is present in virtually all cases of autism.
2. There is a close association between the cognitive abnormalities and the social-behavioral features of autistic disorder. Discriminant function analyses showed that autistic disorder could be diagnosed almost as well by cognitive test performance as by behavioral or linguistic measures.
3. Follow-up studies have shown that intelligence quotient (I.Q.) and language functioning are the best predictors of psychosocial outcome in autistic individuals.
4. Behavioral treatment studies reveal that I.Q. and language competence are the autistic features least influenced by treatment, and thus suggest that the cognitive deficit is probably intrinsic to the autistic child's basic biological handicap.
5. Twin and family studies suggest that a predisposition to autistic disorder may be genetically transmitted. Rutter notes, "what is inherited is some form of cognitive abnormality, that includes but is not restricted to autism. The cognitive abnormalities linked with autism were rather varied in type, but most involved some form of language impairment."

The evidence of early, severe cognitive impairment in autistic disorder, in conjunction with studies of family history and prognosis that indicated little overlap with adult-onset psychosis, resulted in autistic disorder being removed from the rubric of psychosis (in DSM-II, it was included in the syndrome of childhood schizophrenia) and being designated as one of the pervasive developmental disorders in DSM-III and DSM-III-R. These disorders are characterized by severe disturbances in many basic areas of psychological development that occur at the same time.

Subsequent research has attempted to elucidate the nature of cognitive deficit in autistic disorder. A wide range of cognitive processes have been studied, including perception, discrimination learning, coding processes, attention, memory, and language functioning. A number of cognitive deficits that have been found cannot be accounted for by the general mental retardation found in most autistic children. The constellation of deficits includes hypo- and hyperresponsiveness to visual, auditory, and tactile stimuli, deficiencies in imitation learning, poor coding of auditory material, an inability to reduce information through the extraction of crucial features such as rules and redundancies, difficulties with symbolic material involving transformation and flexible recombination of incoming information, and a wide range of language problems. These deficits are juxtaposed with a number of intact cognitive processes including visual-spatial and musical abilities and rote memory. For example, a number of studies have found that nonretarded autistic children have superior performance on block design tasks. Figure 3.1-8 illustrates this pattern of deficient and intact abilities on the Wechsler Intelligence Scale for Children—Revised. Nonretarded autistic children show deficient performance on the comprehension subtest and superior performance on the block design subtest, a pattern that differentiates them from patients with childhood-onset schizophrenia.

Several investigators have interpreted this pattern of cognitive abilities and disabilities as reflecting left-hemisphere dysfunction in autistic children. Autistic children perform relatively well on tasks presumed to measure functions (visual-spatial and Gestalt) predominantly subserved by the right hemisphere of the brain while performing quite poorly on

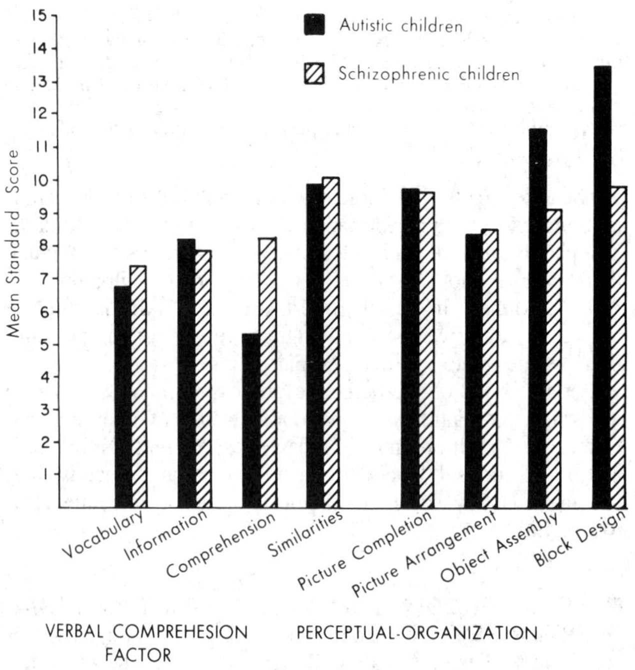

FIGURE 3.1-8. *Performance of nonretarded autistic and schizophrenic children on the subtests of the Wechsler Intelligence Scale for Children—Revised that load on the Verbal and Perceptual Organization factors. The standardization sample has a mean scaled score of 10 with a standard deviation of 2. (Adapted from Asarnow R F, Tanguay P E, Bott L, Freeman B J: Patterns of intellectual functioning in nonretarded autistic and schizophrenic children. J Child Psychol Psychiat* 28: *273, 1987, with permission.)*

tasks presumed to measure functions (language and symbolic representation) predominantly subserved by the left hemisphere of the brain.

Although the hypothesis of left-hemisphere dysfunction in autism has been heuristically useful for both stimulating and focusing research, Fein and associates conclude that

> The argument for a universal selective impairment of language in autism and for left-hemisphere involvement in this impairment is called into question by evidence that (a) language deficits and delays in autistic samples are very varied; (b) phonological and syntactic aspects of language may be more delayed than deviant; (c) abnormalities in prosodic and pragmatic aspects of language, as well as other behavioral features, suggest analogies to right-hemisphere-impaired patients; (d) aspects of perceptual functioning may also show delay and deviance; (e) only some autistic children show verbal deficits relative to perceptual performance; and (f) formal tests of verbal and visuospatial functions may be confounded by task demand and information-processing differences.

Many autistic children do not show the right-hemisphere advantages on measures of sensorimotor asymmetry and dichotic listening or the distribution of handedness predicted by the hypothesis that autistic children have a unilateral left-hemisphere dysfunction. Left-hemisphere dysfunction is found in a subgroup of autistic children and may be a useful marker for a subtype of autistic children.

A major focus of much current research concerns the nature of the cognitive-linguistic deficit found in autistic children. Is there a basic impairment in the processing of linguistic stimuli and/or deficit in mediational processes that cuts across the nature of stimuli to be processed? What is the CNS substrate of this deficit? Do insults or maldevelopment of the left hemisphere produce this deficit in a subgroup of autistic children?

Investigators have attempted to determine whether a particular set of cognitive-linguistic deficits index a vulnerability to develop autistic disorder. As noted above, family and twin studies reveal increased rates of cognitive and linguistic deficits among the relatives of autistic probands. A number of studies are attempting to determine whether the familial distribution of these impairments fits a particular model of genetic transmission.

Finally, there is a great deal of interest in the relation between the cognitive and social-affective disturbances found in autistic children. Are the cognitive deficits and disturbances in social-affective functions found in autistic children due to a common cause? Are the cognitive deficits primary to the social-affective disturbances? Do impairments in social cognition provide an interface between the cognitive and social-affective disturbances found in autistic children?

IMPLICATIONS FOR THE FUTURE

Advances in research on normal perception, cognition, and attention enhance our understanding of the deviant cognitive processes found in major psychiatric disorders. The conceptual distinctions that are currently receiving substantial research attention in experimental psychopathology include these contrasts: (1) automatic, parallel processes versus effortful, capacity-demanding processes; (2) initial sensory storage versus active, short-term memory; (3) semantic versus episodic types of long-term memory; and (4) sensitivity versus response bias components of performance within vigilance and memory.

Abnormalities in a number of basic attentional, perceptual, and cognitive processes have been identified in schizophrenic patients through the use of performance tasks. Research that has attempted to isolate the stage or level of information processing at which deficits occur has shown that schizophrenic patients have impaired stimulus detection in initial stages of visual processing and show decreased spontaneous use of active rehearsal and organizational strategies in short-term memory, particularly when distracting stimuli are present. However, appropriate mnemonic organization strategies can be adopted by schizophrenic patients with sufficient environmental inducement. This finding suggests that structural components of short-term memory are probably intact and that the impaired performance shown by schizophrenic patients on short-term memory tasks may be due to inadequate allocation of processing resources by executive functions. Behavioral and pharmacological treatment strategies aimed at enhancing and organizing allocation of processing resources may be a promising future direction.

Certain measures of attentional functioning have prognostic value within schizophrenia. For example, slowed simple reaction time has been shown in several studies to be a predictor of poor outcome. Several information-processing tasks have also been found to be useful measures of response to antipsychotic medication and may index processes that mediate medication effects. In addition, recent research indicates that measures of information processing and attentional functioning are among the most promising vulnerability indicators for schizophrenic disorders. Studies of first-degree relatives of schizophrenic patients and individuals with schizotypal personality characteristics suggest that potentially useful indicators of vulnerability include impaired smooth pursuit eye movement, poor discrimination of targets from nontargets in high-processing-load vigilance tasks, impaired early visual processing in forced-choice span of apprehension and backward masking tasks, and susceptibility of active, effortful processing in short-term auditory memory to distraction.

In the mood disorders, deficits in perception and cognition have been demonstrated during depressive episodes and in manic episodes. The evidence to date suggests that these abnormalities may be state-related and reversible.

Children who have ADHD show deficient performance on perceptual and cognitive tasks that involve inhibition of impulsive responses and maintenance of reflective, self-directed, effortful processing. ADHD might also involve poor modulation of arousal in response to situational requirements and abnormally strong needs for immediate rewards. The impulsive cognitive style may particularly distinguish ADHD children from other psychiatric groups that show deficits on tasks demanding high levels of effortful processing.

In autistic disorder, research has increasingly attempted to identify basic cognitive deficits that are not secondary to the social abnormalities that were initially thought to be the central features of this disorder. Among the cognitive deficits are difficulties in abstraction of rules, defective transformation and recombination of symbolic material, and impaired auditory coding. Many visual-spatial and musical abilities are intact in autistic children, however, which has suggested left-hemisphere dysfunction to some investigators. This hypothesis may apply mainly to a subtype of autistic children.

The specificity of various basic perceptual, cognitive, and attentional abnormalities to individual psychiatric disorders is receiving increasing research attention, but, in many cases, has only begun to be clarified. Some measures appear to tap relatively specific abnormalities, whereas others reveal deficiencies that seem to be relevant to a wide range of severe psychiatric conditions. The search for performance deficits that are relatively specific to given classes of psychiatric disorders is an evolving process that entails continuing theoretical and methodological developments within cognitive psychology and cognitive neuroscience and, at the same time, continuing redefinition of categories of psychiatric diagnosis.

Another critical area for the future is the development of more explicit models to link elementary perceptual and cognitive processes to development of specific symptoms. The emergence of attempts to demonstrate empirical links between specific performance deficits and symptom clusters within disorders, such as associations with positive versus negative symptoms in schizophrenia, is a step in this direction. A related encouraging development is the increasing emphasis on examining temporal relationships between elementary perceptual and cognitive processes and symptom development through repeated measurements within patients. These approaches have promise for increasing our understanding of fundamental cognitive processes underlying psychiatric symptomatology.

REFERENCES

Alba J W, Hasher L: Is memory schematic? Psychol Bull *93:* 203, 1983.

Asarnow R F: Schizophrenia. In *The Child at Psychiatric Risk,* R E Tarter, editor, p 150. Oxford University Press, New York, 1983.

Beatty J: Task-evoked pupillary responses, processing load, and the structure of processing resources. Psychol Bull *91:* 276, 1982.

Broadbent D E: *Decision and Stress.* Academic Press, Orlando, FL, 1971.

Douglas V: Attentional and cognitive problems. In *Developmental Neuropsychiatry,* M Rutter, editor, p 280. Guilford, New York, 1983.
Fein D, Humes M, Kaplan E, Lucci D, Waterhouse L: The question of left hemisphere dysfunction in infantile autism. Psychol Bull *95:* 258, 1984.
Holzman P S: Recent studies of psychophysiology in schizophrenia. Schizophr Bull *13:* 49, 1987.
Ingram R E, Reed M R: Information encoding and retrieval processes in depression: Findings, issues, and future directions. In *Information Processing Approaches to Clinical Psychology,* R E Ingram, editor, p 131. Academic Press, Orlando, FL, 1986.
Johnson M H, Magaro P A: Effects of mood and severity on memory processes in depression and mania. Psychol Bull *101:* 28, 1987.
Kahneman D: *Attention and Effort.* Prentice-Hall, Englewood Cliffs, NJ, 1973.
Kanner L: Autistic disturbances of affective contact. Nerv Child *2:* 217, 1943.
Knight R A: Converging models of cognitive deficit in schizophrenia. In *Nebraska Symposium on Motivation, 1983,* vol 31: *Theories of Schizophrenia and Psychosis,* W D Spaulding, J K Cole, editors, p 93. University of Nebraska Press, Lincoln, 1984.
Maher B A, Maher W B: Psychopathology. In *The First Century of Experimental Psychology,* E Hirst, editor, p 561. Erlbaum, Hillsdale, NJ, 1979.
Nuechterlein K H: Signal detection in vigilance tasks and behavioral attributes among offspring of schizophrenic mothers and among hyperactive children. J Abnorm Psychol *92:* 4, 1983.
Nuechterlein K H, Dawson M E: Information processing and attentional functioning in the developmental course of schizophrenic disorders. Schizophr Bull *10:* 160, 1984.
Posner M I: *Chronometric explorations of mind.* Erlbaum, Hillsdale, NJ, 1978.
Rapoport J L, Buchsbaum M S, Zahn T P, Weingartner H, Ludlow C, Mikkelsen E J: Dextroamphetamine: Cognitive and behavioral effects in normal prepubertal boys. Science *199:* 560, 1978.
Rutter M: Cognitive deficits in the pathogenesis of autism. J Child Psychol Psychiat *24:* 513, 1983.
Swanson J: What do psychopharmacological studies tell us about information processing in ADD(H)/Hyperactivity? In *Attention Deficit Disorder III,* L M Bloomingdale, editor. Spectrum Books, New York, 1985.
Sykes D H, Douglas V I, Morgenstern G: Sustained attention in hyperactive children. J Child Psychol Psychiat *14:* 213, 1973.
Tariot P N, Weingartner H: A psychobiologic analysis of cognitive failures: Structures and mechanisms. Arch Gen Psychiat *43:* 1183, 1986.
Weingartner H, Rapoport J L, Buchsbaum M S, Bunney W E, Ebert M H, Mikkelsen E J, Caine E D: Cognitive processes in normal and hyperactive children and their response to amphetamine treatment. J Abnorm Psychol *89:* 25, 1980.

3.2 PIAGET'S APPROACH TO INTELLECTUAL FUNCTIONING

STANLEY I. GREENSPAN, M.D.
JOHN F. CURRY, Ph.D.

INTRODUCTION

The following overview of Jean Piaget's developmental psychology will introduce his basic theoretical concepts and briefly summarize his model of stages of intelligence in childhood and adolescence. Recent cognitive theorists have emphasized the importance of the child's unique experiences and abilities as well as the importance of experimental context and task. In so doing, they have challenged and revised aspects of Piaget's model as well as a number of his specific conclusions. Yet, his essential theory and insights remain a basic foundation for inquiries into human intelligence.

Jean Piaget was born in 1896 in Neuchatel, Switzerland. After receiving a doctorate in biology at the age of 22, Piaget turned his attention to the study of human psychology. He worked at Bleuler's psychiatric clinic in Zurich and studied the works of Freud, Jung, and Adler. In spite of this early familiarity with the emotional side of human nature, Piaget decided that his predominant interest was in the acquisition of intelligence. What became Piaget's lifelong interest began with his work on the standardization of an intelligence quotient (I.Q.) test at the Binet Laboratory in Paris. Piaget found that he was less interested in whether children answered questions incorrectly than in how they arrived at their incorrect answers. His extensive observations of his own three children was the foundation for his theory on the development of intelligence. Piaget died in 1980, at the age of 84.

GENETIC EPISTEMOLOGY

Widely renowned as a child or developmental psychologist, Piaget considered himself primarily a genetic epistemologist. This self-designation reveals at once that Piaget's central project was not the articulation of a child psychology, as this term is generally understood, but rather an account of the progressive development of human knowledge.

On the classical question of the origins of knowledge, Piaget was neither a nativist nor an empiricist; however, his position should not be considered to be an amorphous form of interactionism. Piaget has spelled out in detail the nature of the interactionist position to which he ascribed. It is, in his words, a "constructivist structuralism," according to which the origin of mental structures is to be sought in the actions of the subject on objects as the subject strives to adapt to its environment. Structures, then, are constructed within the subject as a consequence of interactions between subject and object. What is innate is an intelligent functioning that makes possible the production of progressively more adequate structures of knowledge on the basis of abstraction from actions performed during the stages of development.

To take one example, the concept of space is a fundamental mental structure developed in the earliest period of children's lives. In earliest infancy, children are aware of not one homogeneous space, but of several heterogeneous spaces, each centered on a certain part of the child's body (e.g., visual space, tactile space). As children act on objects that may traverse these various spaces (e.g., a rattle occupying visual, tactile, and auditory space), they come to coordinate these individual spaces. Eventually, such actions representing displacements in space are organized into the general concept of space. This concept is a structure that can be described in logico-mathematical terms.

EQUILIBRATION For Piaget, the general criterion for intelligent functioning is *equilibration,* briefly defined as "a compensation for an external disturbance." Hans Furth described equilibration as "the factor that internally structures the developing intelligence. It provides the self-regulation by which intelligence develops in adapting to external and internal changes." At every level of development, the equilibration mechanism is operative in furthering adaptation, but as development proceeds toward the highest level of cognitive functioning, equilibration becomes progressively more adequate in enabling the organism to adapt to a wider range of internal and external disturbances. Piaget's notion of intelligence as adaptation is therefore essentially bound to an equilibration model of intelligent functioning.

ASSIMILATION AND ACCOMMODATION To explicate this equilibration model further, it is necessary to introduce the concepts of *assimilation* and *accommodation*.

The biological foundation of Piaget's developmental theory is nowhere more clearly evident than in his notions of assimilation and accommodation. These processes are taken to be *functional invariants* of all intelligent behavior. At every level of intellectual development, from infancy to adulthood, they are operative in the overall process of adaptation.

The assimilation-accommodation account of development stresses the interaction between organism and environment. A certain readiness is postulated as a condition within the organism necessary for change or development to take place. In Piaget's view, associationism (empiricism) in psychology has committed the fallacy of crediting one-half of the necessary conditions for learning with all explanatory power. A full account of human development must include not only the influence of stimuli on respondents (S → R), but also the influence of the responding organism on incoming stimuli (S ← R). Such an account is provided by Piaget's assimilation-accommodation viewpoint: "From a biological point of view, assimilation is the integration of external elements into evolving or completed structures of an organism. In its usual connotation, the assimilation of food consists of a chemical transformation that incorporates it into the substance of the organism."

Furth referred to assimilation as "an inward-directed tendency of a structure to draw environmental events towards itself." Assimilation is the conservative side of intellectual development. It assures continuity and coherence by incorporating new aliments into the mental structures. But it alone cannot account for growth or change within these structures. This is where the notion of accommodation comes into play.

Furth referred to accommodation as "an organism-outward tendency of the inner structure to adapt itself to a particular environmental event." Tuddenham pointed out the variations in accommodation relative to levels of intellectual development as follows: "At the lowest psychological level, accommodation refers to the gradual adaptation of the reflexes to new stimulus conditions—what others have called conditioning or stimulus generalization. At higher levels it refers to the coordination of thought patterns to one another and to external reality."

Accommodation occurs at points during the developmental periods when new data cannot be wholly assimilated to existing structures, and yet the data are not so entirely foreign to those structures that their existence can be ignored.

Following this line of thought it can be seen in what sense intelligence is defined by Piaget in terms of equilibration. The equilibration to which he refers is not a static, balanced system, but a dynamic or mobile equilibration between assimilation and accommodation.

STRUCTURALISM

Intelligence has been discussed in terms of an equilibration process involving assimilation of aliments to structures and accommodation of structures to new, somewhat different aliments. Before the stages of intellectual development through which this process passes can be analyzed, it is necessary to understand more fully the notion of intellectual structure as Piaget used it, and to take a more fundamental look at the origins and developmental forms of the cognitive structures.

The term Piaget used for cognitive structures is *scheme:* "A scheme is the structure or organization of actions as they are transferred or generalized by repetition in similar or analogous circumstances."

Schemes exist in the infant in the form of perceptual-motor behavior patterns (e.g., the grasping reflex). They also exist in mature intelligence, although, as Furth pointed out, the term "scheme" is more commonly used to refer to early structures. The general schemes of higher intelligence are referred to as *operations*.

The abstraction process that leads to the formation of cognitive structures is called *reflective* or *formal abstraction*. It is an abstraction from *actions,* according to which the similarities inherent in various behavioral acts are dissociated from their particularized contexts. According to Furth and colleagues, "More precisely, reflective abstractions are an enriching feedback into the structures of the organism from the most general coordinations of actions."

THE THEORY OF STAGES

The discussion to this point has been general, designed to provide a theoretical perspective on Piaget's work as a unique system of genetic epistemology. Forming an integral part of this system is a psychology of cognition, which seeks to answer descriptively the question of how knowledge develops and changes. To proceed further, a genetic framework must be adopted and the process of intellectual adaptation as it passes through the major periods of life must be examined. Therefore, Piaget's theory of stages in development will be reviewed, and the major characteristics of each stage will be outlined.

The stages of cognitive development that Piaget and his associates delineated on the basis of research are not defined merely by the dominance of some aspect that remains present in a less dominant manner throughout development. Rather, they constitute structured wholes and they can be defined by reference to a set of criteria.

Concerning his stages of cognitive development, Piaget was not entirely consistent in naming or enumerating them. His descriptions, however, are consistent, and the only possible source of confusion in relatively recent writings is whether the so-called preoperational period is to be considered apart from the period of concrete operations, in which it culminates. On the basis of Flavell's 1963 study and Piaget's 1983 summary, three major periods and one subperiod of intellectual development will be delineated (Table 3.2-1). Within these periods are found subdivisions referred to as stages. The major periods are:

1. The sensorimotor period, which extends from birth until approximately 1½ years of age. This period is divided into six stages, which will be described in general here with reference to the development of the concept of the permanent object.
2. A period of preparation for and acquisition of concrete operations. This period is initiated by the appearance of the symbolic or semiotic function and ends with the beginning of higher mental operations applied to concrete objects.
3. The period of formal operations, which begins at approximately 11 years of age. During this period, full adult intelligence develops as the operations are extended to apply to propositional or hypothetical thinking.

TABLE 3.2-1
Periods of Intellectual Development

Age (years)	*Period*	*Cognitive Developmental Characteristics*
0–1½	Sensorimotor	Divided into six stages, characterized by (1) inborn motor and sensory reflexes; (2) primary circular reaction and first habits; (3) secondary circular reaction; (4) use of familiar means to obtain ends; (5) tertiary circular reaction and discovery through active experimentation; and (6) insight and object permanence.
2–7	Preoperations subperiod*	Deferred imitation; symbolic play; graphic imagery (drawing); mental imagery; language
7–11	Concrete operations	Conservation of quantity, weight, volume, length, and time based on reversibility by inversion or reciprocity; operations: class inclusion and seriation
11 through end of adolescence	Formal operations	Combinatorial system, whereby variables are isolated and all possible combinations are examined; hypothetical-deductive thinking

*This subperiod is considered to be its own period by some authors.

THE SENSORIMOTOR PERIOD The sensorimotor period of intelligence is so named because the construction of mental structures or schemes is in no way aided by representations, symbols, or thoughts. Hence, the schemes are totally dependent on perceptions and bodily movements.

Stage 1 of sensorimotor development is marked by relatively few reflexes, which stand out against the background of the spontaneous general activity of the neonate. Among these early reflexes are the sucking reflex and the palmar reflex. These primitive reflexes take on the nature of the first scheme, through three types of assimilation: (1) reproductive (repeating the actions); (2) generalizing (repeating the actions on new objects); and (3) recognitory (performing different varieties of the actions on different objects).

Stage 2 is that of the first habits and the primary circular reaction. The first habits develop out of the original schemes as these are applied to objects in the environment or to parts of the infant's body, but without any differentiation between means and end. In a primitive state of consciousness, the infant is aware only of action sequences, and not even aware of self.

In stage 3 of the sensorimotor period, an initial distinction between means and ends becomes apparent, but in a very primitive sense. The infant repeats a particular action pattern that succeeded in achieving one end for the purpose of achieving many other (unrelated) ends. For example, a baby who succeeds in shaking a rattle by pulling a string may repeatedly pull the string in an attempt to effect other sounds or results.

In stages 4 and 5, infants use a variety of available means to obtain particular goals. The distinction between stages 4 and 5 lies in the relative creativity or newness of the means employed; the former is marked by use of already familiar means. Stage 5 is marked by a search for new means based on further differentiations of already known schemes and by the tertiary circular reaction. The latter differs from a secondary circular reaction in that the child no longer produces schemes that were effective in one situation to produce magically efficacious results in every situation. Instead, the child relies on real exploration and variation to test for effectiveness. Discovery is a hallmark of stage 5. For example, a child may use a stick to move an object that is not in reach.

Stage 6 is actually a transitional one leading into the preoperational subperiod. In this stage the child becomes capable of inventing new means, not by direct actions on objects, but by mental combination. Where discovery marked stage 5, insight is characteristic of stage 6. For example, a child, having seen the father bang on a drawer to loosen it up, may bang on a toy box to make it easier to open.

During the sensorimotor period, a number of extremely significant concepts are developed, including the child's concepts of space, time, and causality. These categorical concepts develop in a parallel process according to the sequence of the six stages outlined above. Above all, during the sensorimotor phase, the child develops the scheme of the permanent object, the first major victory of conservation and the foundation of all future knowledge.

The scheme of the permanent object The knowledge that objects in the external world have an existence independent of the child's actions on them or interactions with them is a major accomplishment of the sensorimotor period. Flavell has outlined Piaget's observations and interpretations of infants' reactions to the disappearance of interesting objects, the foundation for his theory of development of object permanence. In stages 1 and 2, for example, a child simply continues to look at the place where the object was last seen. In stage 3, if an object such as a spoon drops to the floor, the infant will look for it (e.g., by leaning over and looking at the floor). Stage 4 contains one of the most intriguing of Piaget's observations. If an object is repeatedly hidden at point A (in sight of the child) and then hidden at point B (also in sight of the child), the child searches for it at the original, rather than the current hiding place (A, not B). Stages 5 and 6 mark the child's increasing understanding of object permanence in that the infant is able to follow multiple displacements of the object through points in space, even if the object is hidden within another object.

THE PREOPERATIONAL SUBPERIOD AND THE SEMIOTIC FUNCTION The advent of the preoperational subperiod is marked by the appearance of what Piaget called the *semiotic function*. This is a new ability defined by Piaget and Inhelder as follows: "It consists in the ability to represent something (a signified something: object, event, conceptual scheme, etc.) by means of a signifier which is differentiated and which serves only a representative purpose: language, mental image, symbolic gesture, and so on."

In the sensorimotor period, a thing could be represented in a limited sense by a part of itself (e.g., the mother's voice might represent the presence of the mother in the room). However, such signifiers are indices undifferentiated from their significants. Symbols and signs are signifiers that are differentiated from their significants. They become available to the child only with the appearance of the semiotic function, with which representational thought becomes possible. As Furth pointed out, representation has first of all an active meaning in Piaget's theory. The child becomes capable of summoning up a symbol or sign to stand for a given significant. It is essential to point out that, for Piaget, representation is not of the essence of thought. It serves rather an auxiliary function.

Characteristic behavior patterns The semiotic function is heralded by five characteristic behavior patterns in evidence during the second year of life: (1) deferred imitation, or imitation that starts after the disappearance of the model; (2) symbolic play, or the game of pretending; (3) drawing, or graphic imagery; (4) mental image, which appears as an internalized imitation and not as a function of perception; and (5) verbal evocation of events not occurring at the time.

Each of these behavior patterns will be examined briefly to provide a better understanding of the origins of representational thought and the beginning of the preoperational subperiod of cognitive development.

IMITATION It is possible to follow the development of imitation through the same six sensorimotor stages that were delineated for the concept of object permanence. Piaget has done this in his volume *Play, Dreams and Imitation in Childhood*. For the purposes of this discussion, however, it is sufficient to point out that a radically new form of imitation occurs during the second year of life, *deferred imitation*. For example, children may put on their father's hat and walk as their father does, even hours after the father has gone off to work.

It should be recalled at this point that intelligence, for Piaget, is seen as an equilibration process in which assimilation and accommodation are in balance. Imitation, on the other hand, is behavior in which accommodation outweighs assimilation. According to Piaget, imitation is behavior in which "the subject's schemes of action are modified by the external world without his utilizing this external world." In imitation, the cognitive structures undergo temporary change without simultaneously incorporating new aliment.

SYMBOLIC PLAY A second new behavior pattern appearing at about this same time is *symbolic play*. In imitation, the imbalance between assimilation and accommodation is weighted in favor of accommodation; however, the opposite holds true in symbolic play, which is a lessening of the demand of the adaptive process.

Play, too, can be followed in its development through the six stages of sensorimotor intelligence, but the use of symbols in play is found only after the sensorimotor period. This is the type of play characterized by games of pretending. For example, a little girl will pretend that she is asleep, that a box is her pet cat, or that she herself is a church. In each of these cases symbols are generated "in order to express everything in the child's life experience that cannot be formulated and assimilated by means of language alone."

According to Piaget's theory, these symbols are created by the same process of imitation that gives rise to deferred imitation at this time. In fact, Piaget views imitation as the process underlying the development of the entire semiotic function. In symbolic play, then, symbols are generated by a process in which accommodation outweighs assimilation. But instead of being used accurately (i.e., to represent that from which they are derived), they are placed at the service of a process in which a liberating assimilation outweighs accommodation.

DRAWING A third behavior pattern associated with the rise of the semiotic function is *drawing*, or graphic imagery. Piaget sees in this activity elements of play and of imitation. In developmental terms, he considers drawing as "halfway between symbolic play and the mental image," appearing at about age 2 or 2½ years. It is playful activity in the sense that it is an end in itself, and is characterized by reproductive assimilation; in other words, the child enjoys producing drawings for their own sake. However, the graphic play also has accommodative elements especially as the child grows older and attempts to draw not just formless scribble, but some *thing*.

MENTAL IMAGE Very closely related to drawing is the *mental image* itself. Piaget sees the genesis of mental imagery as being tied to accommodative imitation. He explicitly denies that mental images can be the product of perception itself. They are a construction, something the child creates.

The mental image is not directly given by perceptual input; rather, it is constructed by the process of accommodation.

VERBAL EVOCATION OF EVENTS The fifth behavior pattern associated with the rise of the semiotic function has to do with language. It consists of the *verbal evocation of events* that are not present. Piaget gives the example of a little girl saying "Anpa, bye-bye" (Grandpa went away), while pointing to the path he had taken when he left. The parallel with deferred imitation is clear, but here the new representational ability is supported by the social system of language.

These five behavior patterns mark children's initiation into the preoperational subperiod. For Piaget, the semiotic function, which serves to enlarge the children's worlds to such a great extent—liberating them from the bonds of immediate space and time and enabling them to begin to manipulate symbols and to think rather than just to act on immediately present objects—finds its roots in imitation.

CONCRETE OPERATIONS A crucial difference between preoperational and concrete-operational thought is the presence within operative thinking of concepts of *conservation*. When concrete operations have been organized into a system, they enable the child to conserve—that is, "to discover what values do remain invariant . . . in the course of any given kind of change or transformation."

Conservation of quantity The clearest sign that a child remains in the preoperational subperiod is the absence of the concept of conservation. For example, if liquid is poured from a short, wide glass into a tall, narrow one, the preoperational child thinks its quantity has changed.

At the level of concrete operations, however, children are no longer overwhelmed by the perceptual discrepancy between the two configurations. They begin to reason about the transformation, and their correct judgments regarding the conservation of quantity of liquid are accompanied by explanations grounded in logical properties. It is assumed that children are not aware of the logic they utilize.

When problems of conservation begin to be solved, the child passes from the preoperational subperiod into the period of concrete operations, for which the former was a long time of transition and preparation. The progressive and continual structure building that takes place in the concrete operational period is evident in the increase, with development and age, in the scope of such concepts as conservation.

Conservation of substance At the age (on the average) of about 7 or 8, the child can solve the conservation-of-quantity problem mentioned above and can perform similar judgments in the conservation of substance of a lump of clay following a transformation in its shape. Between the ages of 9 and 10, the child discovers that the weight of a given object is also conserved even if its shape is transformed. However, it is not until approximately age 11 or 12 that children have a logical comprehension that the volume displaced by a given object is conserved even after transformation of the object's shape. Conservation entails logical certainty that one characteristic of an object remains invariant, while the object itself undergoes some type of perceived transformation.

Concept of cardinal numbers To take one more brief example, the concept of cardinal numbers develops from an initially nonconserving to a conserving stage. Preoperational children can be presented with two rows of dots in one-to-one correspondence; for instance, there is a row of six blue dots with a row of six red dots directly beneath them and in optical correspondence (i.e., imaginary vertical lines could be constructed between each red dot and its corresponding blue dot). If the experimenter destroys this optical correspondence by spreading out one of the rows of dots, the preoperational child will think the larger row now contains more dots. Only after conservation of cardinal number has been established as a logical necessity does the child maintain the numerical equivalence of the spread-out row. Clearly, preoperational concepts of number would provide inadequate bases for arithmetic skills. Thus, it is possible that a lag in the development of number conservation could underlie certain types of arithmetic-related learning disabilities.

OPERATIONS We have seen that notions of conservation are the mark of well-established concrete operational thinking. At this point, it is essential to discuss the meaning of *operation* in Piaget's thought. Operations, themselves, constitute essential thinking. For Piaget, an operation is an action that is: (1) interiorized, (2) reversible, and (3) part of an organized system of such actions.

The operations that form this system are, first of all, interiorized actions. In the sensorimotor period, external behavior patterns gave rise through a process of abstraction to the construction of sensorimotor schemes. In similar fashion, internal thinking patterns now give rise to operations. According to Furth, it is the generalizable aspects of actions, "those which can be found in any coordination of action," that enter into the construction of operations. To say that the crucial aspect of actions in this regard is their generalizability is to explain the importance of interiorization in the construction of operations. *Interiorization* refers to "the increasing dissociation of general form from particular content." In other words, the notions of generalizability and interiorization merely point out the process of abstraction which is at work. For example, a child adds two apples and three apples to obtain five apples. In another instance, a child adds seven blocks and one block to obtain eight blocks. In a third instance, a child combines the category of fathers with that of mothers to obtain the category of parents. The operation abstracted from these three mental actions is that of addition or combining, without reference to the particular content of numbers, objects, or categories.

Not only must an operation be interiorized action; it must also be reversible. The action of combining (addition) is not an operation until its relationship to the action of separating (subtraction) is comprehended. To understand reversibility is to understand the third criterion of an operation, its inclusion in a system.

The reversibility essential to operatory thought may be of either of two types: inversion or reciprocity. In reversibility by inversion, an action $+A$ is reversed by $-A$. For example, in the above conservation-of-quantity example, the pouring of liquid into container 2 ($+A$) may be mentally reversed—that is, mentally poured back into container 1 ($-A$).

In reversibility by reciprocity, a relation $A < B$ is reversed by a relation $B < A$. Referring again to the conservation-of-quantity example, let A stand for container 1, and B stand for container 2. Then, the rising height of liquid in container 2 ($A < B$) is offset by its narrower width ($B < A$).

Corresponding to these two types of reversibility are the two major categories of concrete operations: those pertaining to classes and those pertaining to relations. In the system of operations performed on classes, reversibility is by way of inversion; in those performed on relations, it is by way of reciprocity. For example, comparing sticks of different size relates to reciprocity; subtraction and addition relate to inversion.

Class inclusion The concrete operation demonstrating understanding of classes is the class inclusion task. In this task, a child is shown, for example, an array of pets (superordinate class) consisting of dogs and cats (subordinate classes). After counting the number of dogs, cats, and pets, the child is asked whether there are more dogs or more pets. Preoperational children cannot maintain in mind the superordinate class while perceiving only the subordinate classes. Thus, they fail the task frequently over a series of such arrays.

Relations The concrete operation that demonstrates an understanding of relations is seriation. Children are asked, for example, to arrange a set of rods in order, according to increasing size. Preoperational children may subgroup the rods, but will have difficulty completing an entire array along the dimension. They may understand smaller versus larger but have difficulty with comprehending the gradual nature of change.

We have dealt with the extensive period of a child's life that begins with the appearance of the semiotic function and continues until the establishment of concrete operations. What remains to be described is the third and final period in the intellectual development of the child. The logical structures of concrete operations are superseded by the structures of this last phase in cognitive development, formal operations.

FORMAL OPERATIONS The following discussion will describe the basic characteristics of the final period of intelligence, the period of *formal operations*.

The relationship between the real and the possible, which is characteristic of adolescent thinking, represents a reversal of that relationship in the thinking of the concrete operational child. Inhelder and Piaget note that the real has priority for the younger child, and that possibility is conceived of merely as a prolongation or extension of real operations "as, for example, when, after having ordered several objects in a series, the subject knows that he could do the same with others."

For the adolescent, however, the possible occupies a place of priority and the real is seen as a particular instance of it. "Henceforth, they conceive of the given facts as that sector of a set of possible transformations that has actually come about." This immediately presupposes that the adolescent can take a given empirical event (e.g., "the long, thin rod bends") and categorize it within a system of possible combinations of events (e.g., long rods or short rods, thin rods or thick rods, bending or not bending).

Three characteristics follow from this fundamental reorientation in thought: (1) Adolescent thought is hypothetical-deductive in nature; (2) it deals in propositions rather than in concrete events; and (3) it is capable of isolating variables and of examining all possible combinations of variables.

HYPOTHETICAL-DEDUCTIVE THOUGHT As a hypothetical-deductive form of thought, formal operational intelligence proceeds from the possible to the real. In this sense, it mirrors scientific reasoning. The implications of a propositional statement are drawn and then tested against reality. Rather than building up by induction from disparate concrete examples to a loose generalization, it operates systematically from general statement to particular instance via testable hypotheses. In Flavell's words, "To try to discover the real among the possible implies that one first entertains the possible as a set of hypotheses to be successively confirmed or infirmed. Hypotheses which the facts infirm can then be discarded; those which the data confirm then go to join the reality sector."

PROPOSITIONAL THOUGHT When it is said that formal operations deal in propositions rather than in concrete events, an increased freedom from immediate content is implied, with a correspondingly greater intellectual mobility. At one level, this freedom implies the ability to manipulate abstractions that have never been tied to concrete examples or events. The adolescent, for example, can perform a transitive inference ($A < B$, $B < C$; therefore, $A < C$) without any empirical demonstration of referents for the terms A and B. At another level this freedom implies that, having performed a concrete operation, the adolescent can abstract the results of that operation and perform further operations on them. For example, an adolescent can perform the concrete operation of combining two liquids to observe the color of the resultant mix and then take the result of this operation and systematically relate it to results of all other combinations of available liquids.

ISOLATING VARIABLES AND EXAMINING COMBINATIONS This example helps to explain the third characteristic of adolescent thought mentioned by Flavell: the isolation of variables and the examination of all possible combinations. Instead of dealing with disparate concrete experiments, hypothetical-deductive adolescents can organize their investigations into a coherent pattern a priori, then perform all relevant combinations of variables to test their hypotheses, in this way isolating causal factors. It should be quite clear from this brief description that Piaget's theory of formal operational cognition has focused on scientific thinking. For example, the weight, speed, shape, and size of an object may all be seen to have their relative contribution to the size of a hole the object will make when hitting the ground.

Preoperational children merely describe what they see, and causal thinking is expressed in an undifferentiated form ("It has to"). The concrete operational child can categorize and order the relevant variables independently, but has difficulty integrating the system of all relevant variables. The adolescent, however, can generate all possible combinations of relevant variables and can proceed to a systematic test of the importance of each variable.

A complete combinatorial system only makes its appearance during the period of formal operations. Instead of focusing on empirical givens, as the concrete operational child does, the formal operational adolescent constructs a hypothetical system, of which the empirical givens are members. Where the younger child was capable of classifying events according to the various categories of length, width, and weight, the adolescent counterpart uses this classification as a basis on which to abstract all possible combinations of variables. Having done this, the adolescent can then test hypotheses derived from the combinatorial system. In the problem at hand, the end result of this new ability is the capacity to test the causal significance of each individual factor in succession by holding all other factors constant.

Piaget interprets the rise of formal operational thought in the context of his equilibrium model of cognitive development. Thus, he considers neurological maturation and experience of the object and interpersonal world as necessary but not sufficient conditions to explain this qualitative improvement in thinking.

In essence, the equilibration explanation is as follows: During concrete operations, a number of qualitatively heterogeneous factors are constructed by the child, resulting in the achievement of conservation of the factor in question even in the face of perceptual transformations. Such factors include quantity, weight, volume, time, and length. Eventually, the child discovers that in many concrete instances the operation of these factors is interrelated. Thus, although they have been constructed mentally in relative isolation from one another, their presence in real objects is mixed. Thus, through experience with both impersonal and interpersonal objects, the child's concrete operational understanding of these factors is shown to be insufficient, and a more comprehensive, more intelligent understanding is stimulated.

EGOCENTRISM AND THE DEVELOPMENTAL PERIODS

Each of the major periods of cognitive development discussed above is characterized by a qualitative shift toward more comprehensive and more adaptive cognitive structures. In this sense, the adolescent is more intelligent than the infant. At the same time, however, each transition to a higher level of cognitive organization is initially accompanied by a lack of full differentiation between self and object. Each period has an early organizational phase, followed by the phase of accomplishment of cognitive developmental tasks. During the early organizational phase, the child's failure to differentiate fully the self from objects is manifest in behavior reflecting stage-specific forms of egocentrism. Elkind has summarized the process. Each developmental period has characteristic forms of egocentrism.

In the sensorimotor period, egocentrism refers literally to a lack of differentiation between self and object, as perceived in the lack of object permanence. The existence of objects independent of action patterns of the self is not acknowledged. In the preoperational subperiod, the capacity to engage in symbolic thinking is accompanied by initial failure to differentiate fully between symbols and their referents. This may be manifest, for example, in failure to differentiate such mental images as dreams from real objects. In the concrete operational period, the capacity to engage in logical operations is accompanied by an unrealistic certainty in which probability is not appreciated and mental constructions of the self are not differentiated from facts. Finally, at adolescence, the capacity to engage in hypothetical thinking and to understand other persons' points of view is accompanied by characteristic patterns of thought in which others are unrealistically presumed to be focusing on the self. As Elkind has pointed out, adolescent egocentrism is a "belief that others are preoccupied with (the adolescent's) appearance and behavior," when, in fact, it is the adolescent who is preoccupied with these topics.

PRESENT AND FUTURE RESEARCH

Piaget's approach to observing children has led to illuminating insights, and his theory of intellectual development is still the most comprehensive one available. Many followers of Piaget and more recent cognitive researchers, however, are now developing findings that bring into question many of the specifics of Piaget's theory. For example, several researchers propose that the type of instructions children are given will influence task performance. They further find that children prefer different tasks at different ages depending on areas of competence, and that Piaget's general postulates may not hold. They feel that each ability needs to be researched in its own right and that generalizations are difficult to make.

Nevertheless, Piaget's approach to discovering how the mind works is not just of historical importance. His model of adaptation is still quite compelling and his insights about the way in which mental abilities build on one another and progress with age, maturation, and experience will guide those who are refining the specifics of his area of inquiry for many generations to come.

The relationship of cognitive to emotional development is yet another challenging area. As developmental researchers refine and improve on Piaget's findings and formulations, the developmental model will be more frequently applied to social and emotional development and provide a basic foundation for clinical and educational intervention.

REFERENCES

Anthony E J: The system makers: Piaget and Freud. Brit J Med Psychol *30:* 255, 1957.

Elkind D: Egocentrism in adolescence. Child Develop *38:* 1025, 1967.

Elkind D: Piagetian psychology and the practice of child psychiatry. J Amer Acad Child Psychiat *21:* 435, 1982.

Flavell J: *The Developmental Psychology of Jean Piaget.* Van Nostrand, New York, 1963.

Flavell J: Concept development. In *Carmichael's Manual of Child Psychology,* P Mussen, editor, p 983. Wiley, New York, 1970.

Furth H G: *Piaget and Knowledge.* Prentice-Hall, Englewood Cliffs, NJ, 1969.

Furth H G, Youniss J, Ross B: Children's utilization of logical symbols: An interpretation of conceptual behavior based on Piagetian theory. Develop Psychol *3:* 36, 1970.

Greenspan S I: Intelligence and adaptation: An integration of psychoanalytic and Piagetian developmental psychology, Monograph 47/48. Psychol Issues: 1979.

Inhelder B, Piaget J: *The Growth of Logical Thinking from Childhood to Adolescence.* Basic Books, New York, 1958.

Piaget J: *Play, Dreams and Imitation in Childhood.* Norton, New York, 1951.

Piaget J: The stages of the intellectual development of the child. Bull Menninger Clin *26:* 120, 1962.

Piaget J: *The Early Growth of Logic in the Child.* Norton, New York, 1969.

Piaget J: *Structuralism.* Basic Books, New York, 1970.

Piaget J: Piaget's theory. *Manual of Child Psychology.* P Mussen, editor, p 103. Wiley, New York, 1983.

Piaget J, Inhelder B: *The Psychology of the Child.* Basic Books, New York, 1969.

Piaget J, Inhelder B: *The Origin of the Idea of Chance in Children.* Norton, New York, 1975.

Pinard A, Laurendeau M: "Stage" in Piaget's cognitive-developmental theory: Exegesis of a concept. In *Studies in Cognitive Development: Essays in Honor of Piaget.* D Elkind, J H Flavell, editors, p 121. Oxford University Press, New York, 1969.

Tuddenham R: Jean Piaget and the world of the child. Amer Psychol *21:* 207, 1966.

Wolff P H: The developmental psychologies of Jean Piaget and psychoanalysis, Monograph 5. Psychol Issues: 1960.

3.3
LEARNING THEORY

W. STEWART AGRAS, M.D., F.R.C.P.(C)

INTRODUCTION

Learning is central to an understanding of the genesis of psychiatric disorders and to their treatment. Much of the disordered behavior that characterizes the syndromes of interest to psychiatry is learned and maintained within a social context, particularly within the family. Psychotherapeutic treatment can be regarded as being educational in nature, enabling the individual to learn more adaptive coping behaviors and to extend personal control over problem behaviors. Thus, it is necessary for therapists to have a firm grasp of the principles of modern learning theory so that they can understand and modify problem behaviors in the most effective manner.

Psychological theories concerning learning have been developing since the turn of the century; experimental work, first with animals and then with humans, began to flourish. Among the building blocks of learning theory are respondent and operant conditioning. In *respondent* or *classical conditioning,* learning is thought to take place as a result of the contiguity of environmental events. When events occur closely together in time, it is likely that individuals will come to associate the two. In the case of *operant conditioning,* learning is thought to occur as a result of the consequences of one's actions, and the resultant effect upon the environment. As B. F. Skinner, the father of radical behaviorism, put it, "A person does not act upon the world, the world acts upon him." Skinner, in his definition of the sphere of interest of psychology, specifically eschewed the role of intervening variables such as thoughts. *Social learning theory* incorporates both the respondent and operant models of learning, but considers that there is a reciprocal interaction between the individual and the environment, in which not only does the environment determine aspects of behavior, but the individual can change the environment as well. Cognitive processes are viewed as important factors in modulating the individuals' responses to environmental events.

Psychoanalytic theory and practice developed concurrently with learning theory. A number of attempts have been made over the past half century to integrate these two theoretical approaches. For example, in 1950 Dollard and Miller reformulated many psychoanalytic concepts in terms of learning theory. But such attempts have not had a lasting influence on psychoanalytic thought or therapy. Instead, behavior therapies based on various aspects of learning theory have been developed over the past quarter century, and because of the experimental and hypothesis-testing emphasis deriving from learning theory, these therapies have become the mainstream of psychotherapy research. Nonetheless, psychoanalytic theory has raised many issues of consequence to learning theorists, and these issues will ultimately be addressed experimentally.

More recently, there has been much interest in the neurophysiological and biochemical components of learning. For example, research with simple organisms, such as Aplysia, a sea mollusk, has revealed that the learning of avoidance behavior alters the chemical structure of cells in the nervous system—and that when the avoidance is unlearned, these chemical changes are reversed. Thus, the foundation for understanding the neurochemistry of learning has been laid, and it is now clear that there is a *reciprocal* interaction between ongoing biological processes in the central nervous system and behavior changes resulting from environmental influences.

Since this section is aimed at laying the foundation for understanding the process of behavior change, particularly when directed toward the amelioration of disordered thought, feelings, and actions, the various behavior change procedures deriving from the different models of learning will be particularly emphasized. Since most therapies consist of an articulated package of procedures aimed at changing behavior and then maintaining that change, the singling out of particular procedures is somewhat artificial. Nonetheless, this approach is necessary to the understanding of the role of learning in the treatment of psychiatric disorders.

LEARNING DEFINED

Unfortunately, it is not easy to arrive at a satisfactory definition of learning because of the enormous variety in what can be learned—from simple descriptions of events, to complex motor skills, to information of various kinds. The basic concept is that the organism acquires new behaviors as a result of experience. To demonstrate learning it is necessary to test the organism's state of knowledge, present an experience of some kind, and then show that the state of knowledge has changed. Furthermore, it is necessary to conduct this experiment in such a way as to exclude other factors that might influence the state of the organism, such as drugs, fatigue, and the nature of the task. Innate behaviors, which are often species-specific, also need to be taken into account when evaluating acquisition, as do innate limitations in capacity to learn particular behaviors. Taking all these factors into account, here is a definition of *learning:* "the change in a subject's behavior to a given situation brought about by repeated experiences in that situation, provided that the behavior cannot be explained on the basis of native response tendencies, maturation, or temporary states of the subject."

To assess learning it is necessary to measure one or other aspect of performance: the accuracy of a motor skill, the ability to recognize or repeat words, and so on. It is, however, important not to confuse learning and performance. Performance may fail for a variety of reasons—for example, insufficient motivation to carry out the task. Thus, learning may have taken place but, given insufficient motivation, may not be demonstrable. By changing the motivating influences, the fact that the organism did learn something may be shown. State-dependent learning is another case in which performance may not betray learning. If a behavior is acquired under the influence of a pharmacological agent, and tests for learning are carried out in the absence of the drug, there may be little or no evidence of acquisition. On the other hand, if the learning test is carried out under the influence of the drug, performance may change and learning may now be demonstrated. Thus it is important to separate the concepts of learning and performance.

MODELS OF LEARNING

RESPONDENT LEARNING The idea that learning takes place when two events occur closely together in time has a long history, stemming from association theory developed by the British school of philosophical empiricism. Ivan Sechenov, a pioneer of Russian physiology, later developed the theory that voluntary behavior consisted of a chain of reflexes. But it was Ivan Pavlov and his co-workers, who over many years documented the parameters of this form of learning in carefully conceived experiments. *Respondent* or *classical conditioning* results from the repeated pairing of a neutral (conditional) stimulus with one that evokes a response (unconditional stimulus) such that the neutral stimulus eventually comes to evoke the response. The time relationship between the presentation of the conditional and unconditional stimuli was found to be important, varying for optimal learning from a fraction of a second to several seconds. In a well-established conditional reflex, stimuli similar to the original conditioned stimulus will also result in the response being emitted, albeit in weakened form. This is an example of *stimulus generalization. Extinction* occurs when the conditioned stimulus is presented repeatedly without the unconditioned stimulus until the response evoked by the conditioned stimulus gradually weakens and eventually disappears. Pavlov extended the notion of classical conditioning to the word, suggesting that similar laws governed thought and speech. One example is the generalization curve for imagined feared situations, in which galvanic skin response (an indicator of sympathetic nervous system arousal) increases with imagined approach to the phobic situation.

Later workers discovered that classical conditioning can be extended to a wide variety of organs and functions, including blood pressure, insulin secretion, secretion of urine, and the activity of various endocrine glands. This discovery is important because it forms a theoretical basis for the development of psychosomatic disorders and suggests that accidental learning may play a significant role in the development of such problems. An example of such learning is the conditioned nausea occurring with cancer chemotherapy, in which a variety of environmental cues are associated with the nausea produced by the drug and eventually come to elicit nausea. Such conditioning can be extinguished using *systematic desensitization,* a behavior therapy developed by Joseph Wolpe, one of the early translators of learning theory into therapy. In this therapy, the nausea-evoking scenes are repeatedly imagined in gradually increasing intensity while the patient is relaxed.

Pavlov's work was enthusiastically espoused by American psychologists such as John B. Watson, who demonstrated that classical conditioning could give rise to neurotic behavior in a now classic experiment. The subject of the experiment was Albert B., who was 11 months old. Watson demonstrated that a few pairings of a loud noise (*unconditional stimulus*), an event that caused the baby to cry, with the sight of a white rat (*conditional stimulus*), led Albert to avoid not only the rat, which had not caused fear before, but also related objects, such as cotton wool and sealskin, an example of stimulus generalization. This was the first experimental demonstration of the development of a phobia in the human, although, as discussed below, this account is much oversimplified.

Prepared learning Evidence that associations are learned more quickly to some stimuli than to others has led to the hypothesis that organisms are biologically prepared to acquire certain connections more rapidly than others. Fear learning would seem to be an example of this, since avoidance responses to pictorial stimuli, such as snakes, are easier to condition than avoidance to stimuli, such as flowers, and the fear response to snakes takes longer to extinguish than a response to flowers. Thus avoidance behavior characterizing fears and phobias may be based, in part, on biologically prepared tendencies toward rapid learning of avoidance to certain classes of potentially harmful environmental events, presumably an inborn protective mechanism. The range of human phobias is limited, which would not be the case were we equally able to form avoidances to any environmental event. Gastrointestinal conditioning demonstrates similar prepared features. A radiation dose sufficient to cause vomiting several hours after eating a particular food leads to a lasting aversion to that food. However, pairing electric shock with food causes only temporary avoidance. In the latter case, the aversive event is not in the same sensory modality as the unconditioned stimulus, and, hence, may not lead to prepared learning. The interesting feature associated with gastrointestinal conditioning is that learning takes place even after a long delay between the conditioned and unconditioned events, presumably as a protection against continued consumption of poisonous foods.

Although Pavlov became interested in how the theory and findings of classical conditioning could lead to psychopathology and developed such treatments as sleep therapy based on his theories, these developments have not had a major impact on the practice of psychiatry, mainly because of the lack of empirical studies verifying the utility of these treatments. Nonetheless, classical conditioning is viewed by most learning theorists as the foundation on which more complex forms of learning are built.

ENACTIVE LEARNING The notion that learning occurs as a consequence of action has a number of roots, for example, in the pioneering work of Edward L. Thorndike, whose learning theory dominated U.S. psychology for the first half of this century. A typical experiment devised by Thorndike would consist of placing a hungry cat in a cage with some form of latching device that, when correctly manipulated, would allow the cat to escape to a second cage for a bite of food. Thorndike noted that the cat gradually became more proficient at operating the latch as measured by the time taken to unlock the cage door. He also noted that the most efficient sequence of behavior gradually evolved, a process he called *trial-and-error* learning. In essence, Thorndike believed that the appropriate connections between stimulus and response were stamped in as a result of experience. These experiments raised such issues as motivation and reinforcement and led Thorndike to formulate the *law of effect,* which states that when a modifiable connection is made, the strength of the connection is increased if the connection is followed by a satisfying state of affairs.

B. F. Skinner and his co-workers, following up on Thorndike's work, made the effect of environmental events on behavior a central aspect of learning theory. The findings stemming from this area of inquiry have led to the discovery of many useful procedures to promote learning in a wide variety of species across a multitude of situations. In broad terms, Skinner considered that the environmenal consequences of actions determine which behaviors will be retained in an individual's repertoire, and also determine the level of probability that such behavior will be exhibited under certain circumstances. This is the sense in which he thought that the environment acts on humans to determine their behavior.

Consequences of behavior POSITIVE REINFORCEMENT refers to the process by which certain consequences of behavior raise the probability that the behavior will occur again. On the whole, positive reinforcers are viewed as pleasant (e.g., food, attention, praise, money). It should be noted, however, that events viewed as aversive by some might be reinforcing for others. For example, the behavior of some children will be reinforced by scolding, which, after all, is a form of attention. Many drugs appear to be positive reinforcers, including opioids, barbiturates, and stimulants, such as amphetamine and cocaine. Animals and humans self-administer these substances, reliably discriminating between the active drug and placebo. Complex patterns of behavior can be shaped in animals using drugs as reinforcers.

NEGATIVE REINFORCEMENT describes the process by which behavior that leads to removal of an unpleasant event strengthens that behavior. Negative reinforcers tend to be viewed as unpleasant. It is important to distinguish negative reinforcement from punishment. In the *punishment* paradigm, an event delivered consequent on the occurrence of a behavior reduces the probability that the behavior will occur again. Punishers are generally viewed as aversive events. It is also important to distinguish between the usual use of the term "punishment" and the technical use of the term given here. In the punishment paradigm, the punishing event is always delivered contingent on performance and demonstrably reduces the frequency of the behavior being punished. This is considerably different from the use of the term to denote imprisonment, for example, since the prison sentence follows long after the crime and may not affect future criminal behavior.

RECIPROCAL INFLUENCES Since much human behavior occurs within an interpersonal context, reciprocal influences will occur. An example of the way in which such reciprocal influences may give rise to complex behavior patterns is afforded by one study of predelinquent behavior. These observations of families suggest that predelinquent behavior patterns are set in motion by the excessive and inconsistent use of punishment on the part of parents. Thus, a mother may severely scold her small son, who in response may whine or have a temper tantrum. If the mother then responds by talking to the child to calm him down, the child in turn stops whining. Thus, the child's whining punishes mother's scolding and makes her less likely to scold in the future. Mother's attention to whining reinforces that unpleasant behavior on the part of the child. Such a behavior pattern, when well-established in the child, is viewed as unpleasant and aggressive by others and increases the likelihood that the child will be rejected by parents, peers, and teachers, thus initiating a complex series of events, such as poor school performance and joining a deviant peer group, which, in turn, highly predisposes to delinquent behavior.

SCHEDULES OF REINFORCEMENT Complex patterns of reinforcement lead to the development of both deviant and prosocial behaviors. Such behaviors may then be strengthened by the social environment or may be weakened over time as the individual matures and enters new social environments providing different reinforcement contingencies. Much is known about various *schedules of reinforcement,* defined as the pattern or frequency with which a reinforcer is delivered as a consequence of behavior. It is clear, for example, that *partial reinforcement,* in which reinforcement only occasionally results from a particular behavior, will maintain the behavior at full strength. Moreover, partially reinforced behavior may be particularly resistant to extinction. Since many deviant behaviors provoke attention from others, it is easy to see how they are maintained by the social environment. Much observational and experimental work, for example, has demonstrated that hospital staffs tend to reinforce their patients' abnormal behaviors by attending to them. When the staff learns to stop such attention, and to attend more frequently to adaptive behaviors, patient behavior improves. Similar findings have been made in the context of the school. Teacher attention has been shown to reinforce disruptive behavior in the classroom, and when such attention is withdrawn, the disruptive behavior decreases.

FIXED-INTERVAL SCHEDULE A *fixed-interval* (FI) reinforcement schedule refers to a situation in which a rewarding event is delivered contingent on the first required response after the elapse of a specified elapse of time—up to a 10-minute interval in most animal experiments. Such a schedule has two main effects on performance. First, the number of responses increases in inverse proportion to the interval of time; thus, responding will be twice as frequent on a 2-minute FI schedule as on a 4-minute FI schedule. Second, responding will tend to increase as the time for reinforcement draws near; thus, performance will tend to rise and fall in relation to the interval of reinforcement, a phenomenon known as *scalloping.* To eliminate this uneven performance, a *variable-interval* (VI) reinforcement schedule can be used. By varying the delivery of reinforcement randomly around a particular interval of time (e.g., 2 minutes), a steady rate of performance can be obtained. Thus variable interval schedules are useful in the clinical situation in attempts to increase the rate of performance of a particular behavior.

FIXED-RATIO SCHEDULE Reinforcement may also be delivered in relationship to the amount of behavior emitted by an organism. In the *fixed-ratio* (FR) schedule, reinforcement is delivered after so many responses have occurred, typically ranging from 5 to well over 100. On this schedule of reinforcement, organisms tend to show a low rate of behavior immediately following reinforcement followed by very high rates of responding. A smoother pattern of behavior is found with a *variable-ratio* (VR) schedule, in which reinforcement is delivered on a schedule randomly changing around a given ratio. The rate of responding on this schedule tends to be very rapid, since the fewer the pauses the faster will the organism contact the reinforcer. Although all of these schedules of reinforcement may have some use in the clinic, the most used is a *shaping* paradigm in which a particular behavior is changed in form by reinforcing components of the final behavior sequentially. For example, in teaching a mute schizophrenic to talk, the first behavior to be reinforced might be simply looking at the therapist, followed by any mouthing movement, followed by any vocalization (perhaps imitating the therapist), and, finally, simple words and sentences. A continuous reinforcement schedule might first be used, followed by a partial reinforcement schedule as each component behavior is first developed and then strengthened. Other schedules of reinforcement, such as a VR schedule, may be useful to generate and maintain a higher rate of speech once it is established. When speech is fully developed, artificial reinforcement can be phased out, since speaking should be more reinforcing than being mute. This is also an example of *chaining* of behaviors and reinforcement, since all the initial behavioral sequences are necessary for the final behavior of talking, and a more complex sequence of behaviors is gradually built up and reinforced. In the analysis of a problem behavior, it is often important to consider at which point in a behavioral chain to intervene.

Many problem behaviors seen in the human have been developed in animals using various schedules of reinforcement. Thus, head banging, a behavior seen frequently in retarded and autistic children, has been developed in monkeys with the use of reinforcement at a frequency and strength that the monkeys actually injure themselves. Although such experiments do not prove that similar behaviors seen in humans are learned, they do call attention to the powerful effect of reinforcement in developing deviant behavior and to the fact that many behaviors are developed and maintained in this way.

Reinforcement is a basic ingredient of most therapies, often given in the form of attention and praise contingent on certain behaviors. Skilled therapists of most persuasions use contingent verbal reinforcement, as has been demonstrated even in nondirective psychotherapy, so that certain therapeutic themes are strengthened. Other methods used in reinforcement paradigms include tokens exchangeable for goods or activities that cannot be bought or engaged in otherwise. What is reinforcing for one person may not be for another; thus, when reinforcement is used, it is important to observe and measure the behavior being reinforced to ensure that it is being strengthened. The data from a clinical example of the use of token reinforcement to increase social communication is shown in Figure 3.3-1.

The patient was a 21-year-old male who was extremely withdrawn. He spent most of his time in his hospital room, rarely approaching others or initiating conversation. Skilled psychiatric nursing care had not altered this behavior. As a first step in increasing conversational ability, reinforcement for approaching nurses was instituted. To accomplish this, the patient was first carefully observed, and it was noted that he enjoyed listening to radio and watching television. He was told that for every 2 minutes that he talked with the nursing staff during three daily sessions, he would earn a token that could be exchanged for 3 minutes of listening to the radio or watching television, and that this was the only way in which he would be able to engage in these activities. This is an example of the use of an FR schedule of reinforcement. The nurses, in turn, were instructed not to approach him during these three sessions, but to engage in conversation if he initiated and maintained it, thus reinforcing a chain of behaviors: approaching nurses, initiating conversation, and maintaining conversational behavior. They also timed the number of minutes of conversation using a stopwatch.

As can be seen in Figure 3.3-1, the patient engaged in little conversation with the nurses during baseline measurement. When the token system was introduced, he began to speak with the nurses for increasing lengths of time. In the third phase of this treatment program, he was given a free supply of tokens equivalent to what he had earned in the previous phase; thus, tokens were no longer contingent on his behavior. Under these conditions the amount of conversation gradually declined, an example of extinction. When the original reinforcement conditions were reintroduced during the final experimental phase, conversational ability steadily improved. Similar procedures were used to generalize this newfound conversational ability to other staff and patients, eventually allowing this patient to engage successfully in a rehabilitation program.

PREMACK'S PRINCIPLE *Premack's principle* states that a behavior engaged in at a higher frequency can be used to reinforce a lower-frequency behavior. In one experiment, Premack observed that children spent more time playing with a

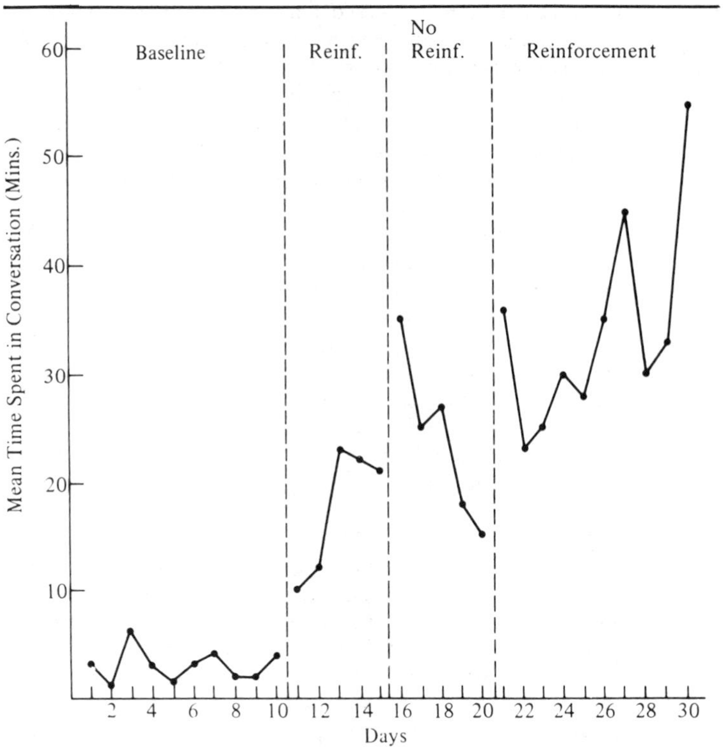

FIGURE 3.3-1 *The time spent by a withdrawn patient conversing with nurses during sequential experimental phases comprising baseline (measurement only); with reinforcement delivered in the form of tokens; after reinforcement was withdrawn; and, finally, when reinforcement was reinstated. The effect of positive reinforcement is demonstrated by an increase in conversation during the two phases in which tokens were delivered.*

pinball machine than eating candy when both were freely available. When he made playing with the pinball machine contingent on eating a certain amount of candy, the amount of candy eaten by these children increased. In a therapeutic application of this principle, schizophrenic patients were observed to spend more time sitting down doing nothing than working at a simple task in a rehabilitation center. When 5 minutes of sitting down was made contingent on a certain amount of work, then work output was considerably increased, as was skill acquisition.

As noted above, disordered behavior is often developed and maintained by reinforcement in the form of attention from others. In such cases, it is important to identify the reinforcer and to remove it from the patient's environment, thus leading to extinction of the undesirable behavior.

A clinical example of the use of extinction involved a girl of 13 with a phobia of sickness, who became anxious whenever anyone in her classroom sneezed, coughed, or claimed to feel ill. This preoccupation kept her from attending school regularly and prevented her from concentrating on her schoolwork; as a result, her grades began to fall. On careful history taking, her mother revealed that every night she would sit with her daughter, and for an hour or so reassure her, in response to her anxious questioning, that she would not become sick. Since this behavior on the mother's part appeared to be reinforcing the girl's fear and obsession with sickness, it was suggested that the mother discontinue this practice. She was also warned that her daughter would protest this and might become worse, in terms of being more demanding, before she improved. Removal of reinforcement often leads to a brief strengthening of the behavior being extinguished. For a few nights, her daughter hardly slept, complained for much of the night, and more frequently missed school. Eventually, her complaints diminished, she stopped talking about sickness, and her school attendance improved. Soon, her grades improved, and she began to enjoy school again, returning to her old friendships.

Punishment is less useful as a therapeutic procedure than either reinforcement or extinction, since it may produce unwanted side effects, such as aggressive behavior, and there is always the possibility of inflicting physical damage. For the most part, punishment is used only in situations in which the behavior to be changed threatens injury to the patient.

A clinical example of such a condition is infant rumination, in which babies regurgitate their feed mouthful by mouthful, which leads to malnutrition, dehydration, and not infrequently a threat to life. One approach to treatment is to use the principle of punishment, by making an unpleasant event contingent on each episode of regurgitation. In the case illustrated in Figure 3.3-2, lemon juice was used as the unpleasant event. As can be seen in the figure, during the baseline before treatment the infant ruminated between 40 and 70 percent of the time it was awake. Once the lemon juice was presented contingent on spitting up food, the frequency of rumination steadily declined. Punishment was then briefly removed, and rumination returned to baseline levels, demonstrating the efficacy of punishment. Reintroduction of punishment eventually led to virtual elimination of the behavior and a return to normal weight with no relapse at 1-year follow-up.

The use of punishment in a clinical situation should be carefully overseen and should follow certain rules. The behavior to be addressed should have been resistant to well-thought-out behavior change procedures involving the use of positive reinforcement. Behaviors incompatible with the problem behavior can often be reinforced, and, thus, the problem is eliminated. In addition, the behavior to be changed should be severely incapacitating and should threaten physical integrity (e.g., the self-injurious behavior of some autistic children). Punishment procedures that themselves cause tissue damage should not be used. The behavior to be changed should be observed, measured, and recorded (as shown in Fig. 3.3-2); in this way, the effects of punishment can be seen, as can the amount of punishment used. It is the usual experience that effectively used punishment will rapidly bring a behavior under control, and that incompatible behaviors can then more easily be built up with the use of positive reinforcement.

Antecedent events The notions of classical conditioning are incorporated into operant conditioning in the form of *stimulus control*. In this paradigm a particular environmental event

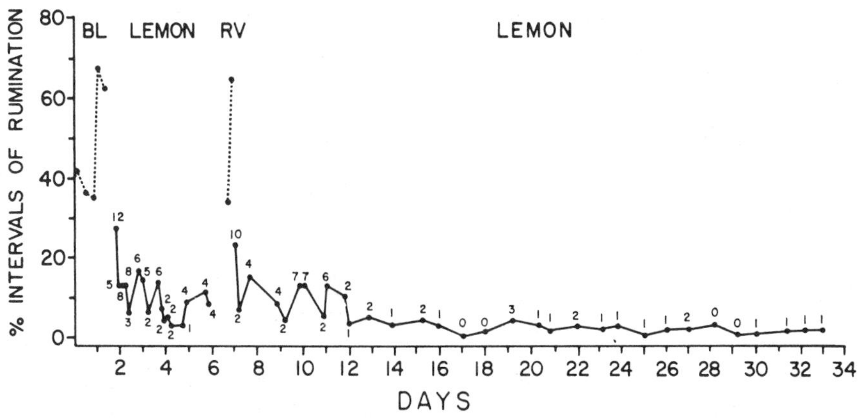

FIGURE 3.3-2 *The effect of punishment is shown in this experiment in which lemon juice was delivered contingent on rumination. The frequency of rumination was rapidly reduced and only increased when punishment was stopped during a brief reversal* (RV) *phase. The number of applications of lemon juice is shown by the numbers above each data point.*

regularly elicits a behavior that has been frequently reinforced in the presence of the particular event. In opiate addiction, for example, environmental cues regularly associated with drug taking can come to elicit conditioned cravings for the drug. Such cues are likely to evoke drug-taking behavior in addicts, even after prolonged abstinence in a hospital environment, thus leading to relapse. The stimuli eliciting a particular behavior can be changed through a process known as *stimulus fading*. In this procedure, behavior occurring under one stimulus, for example a red light, can be made to occur under a new stimulus condition (e.g., a yellow light), provided that the stimulus is slowly changed from red to yellow while the behavior is reinforced. Fading is a useful therapeutic procedure. In the introduction of a low-fat diet, for example, rather than going from whole milk to nonfat milk directly, it is easier to proceed by adding increasing amounts of low-fat milk and then nonfat milk to whole milk. In this way, the behavior of drinking milk is maintained as taste adapts to each mixture. Interestingly, once the stimulus fading has been completed, individuals find whole milk distasteful. In other words, the behavior of drinking milk is now controlled by the sight and taste of nonfat milk.

A MEDIATIONAL STIMULUS-RESPONSE MODEL OF BEHAVIOR Although the operant conditioning paradigm does not take into account the potential influence of variables that intervene between a behavior and its environmental antecedents or consequences, other learning theories do. In operant theory, there is little or no speculation about events that may intervene between an input into an organism and the behavior that then occurs. Clark L. Hull, one of the foremost theorists in the first half of the century, formulated a more complex theory of learning based on both respondent and operant conditioning, elaborating the explanation of the observed behavior with reference to habit and drive states. He viewed the learning occurring as a result of respondent conditioning as a special instance of reinforcement. In Hull's view, the food (unconditional stimulus) not only elicited salivation but also reinforced both the connection between the bell (conditional stimulus) and salivation, and salivation itself. In this sense, he abandoned the principle of contiguity thought to underlie classical conditioning. In turn, reinforcement was felt to produce its effects on behavior by reducing biologically based drive states (e.g., hunger or fear). In addition to biological drives, reinforcement could also work by reducing learned cravings, which are not dependent on reduction of a biological need. The concept of *reactive inhibition* was also important in Hullian theory; thus, any behavior repeatedly emitted would tend to build up inhibition, and, in turn, there would be a tendency to lower the rate of emission of the behavior. Thus, extinction was conceptualized as an active process in which inhibition was learned. The reason to formulate a set of intervening variables between an environmental event and observed behavior was that more complex behaviors could be explained with reference to reinforcement theory. Mediational theories of learning can more easily deal with the influence of cognitive events upon behavior. Thus, it would be expected that thoughts, symbolic representations of the feared events, should elicit physiological evidence of anxiety. As described earlier, galvanic skin response, an indicant of physiological arousal, does vary systematically when subjects are instructed to imagine their feared situations.

Many of the early behavior therapies, such as Wolpe's systematic desensitization developed to treat the anxiety disorders, based their procedures on Hull's learning theory or on later modifications of the theory. O. H. Mowrer, one of Hull's colleagues at Yale, proposed a two-step conditioning process that was hypothesized to underlie the development of fear and, by analogy, the phobic disorders. The first step involved the pairing of a stimulus situation with fear, while the second step involved reinforcing avoidance of the now feared situation by anxiety reduction. This view became known as *two-factor learning theory* and much influenced early models of neurotic behavior espoused by learning theorists and behavior therapists. Wolpe's desensitization procedure, for example, was assumed to reduce the conditioned fear response, thus leading to extinction of the phobic avoidance behavior. In this procedure, the relaxation response was assumed to be the mechanism for fear reduction using the principle of *reciprocal inhibition* (i.e., one cannot be anxious and relaxed at the same time). Physiological experiments suggest that such a mechanism may be operating in desensitization. However, the main effect of desensitization appears to be to motivate individuals to expose themselves to their feared situations, since such exposure has been demonstrated to be the central therapeutic feature of all psychotherapeutic treatments for phobia.

Whether exposure therapy should be regarded as an extinction paradigm (i.e., avoidance behavior and anxiety responses are being extinguished) or as a relearning of active approach behavior is not clear. However, modern theories regarding the origins of agoraphobia closely fit a two-factor model, since panic attacks (presumably of biological origin) occurring in various situations are hypothesized to lead to the avoidance behavior known clinically as agoraphobia through classical conditioning. Once the association has been learned, reentering the situation produces feelings of anxiety, which are relieved when the patient leaves the situation. Thus, phobic avoidance is reinforced.

SOCIAL-COGNITIVE LEARNING THEORY Despite the remarkable success of behavior therapies based on respondent and operant learning paradigms, it is clear that cognitive processes are extraordinarily important in the development and maintenance of human behavior and in the procedures used in the treatment of psychiatric disorders. *Social learning theory* incorporates the elements of respondent and operant conditioning, but views cognitive processes as important mediators in such learning. Thus, an interaction is postulated between environmental events, behavior, and personal and cognitive processes. Reinforcement is viewed not as automatically strengthening behavior, but as a source of information concerning future events that regulates behavior. Research has shown that classical conditioning is by no means automatic, but varies depending on the information provided in the experimental situation. Similarly, reinforcers that carry more information about future reinforcement contingencies produce stronger and more rapid effects on behavior than reinforcers that do not carry such information.

Expectancies Albert Bandura, one of the leading social learning theorists in the United States today, describes two main types of expectancies, *outcome expectancies,* defined as the degree of certainty that a particular behavior will result in a particular outcome, and *efficacy expectancies,* defined as the degree of confidence that individuals have in their ability to carry out a particular behavioral sequence. Such expectancies vary depending on the individuals' perception of the effectiveness of their behavior in producing the desired outcome. Thus, concepts central to social learning theory include goal setting, self-observation, observational learning, and self-regulation.

Instructional control of behavior Humans can learn by listening to or reading instructions. In addition, their past experience modulates their response to such instructions. Much research has been devoted to examining the effect of therapeutic instructions on the outcome of treatment. Such instructions modify both outcome and efficacy expectations of patients. It has been shown, both in traditional verbal psychotherapy and in behavior therapy, that therapeutic instructions exert a powerful impact upon the outcome of treatment. Different instructions give rise to different outcomes. In a study of systematic desensitization, for example, there was little improvement in a group of individuals who thought they were taking part in a physiological experiment, whereas another group of subjects who were told they were receiving therapy showed significant improvement. Apart from the therapeutic instructions, both groups received identical treatment procedures. The different instructional sets presumably produced differences in outcome expectancies. These differences altered what individuals attended to throughout the experiment, and, thus, efficacy expectancies and therapeutic outcome were affected.

Even more remarkable are the findings shown in Figure 3.3-3. In this experiment with hypertensive individuals, all participants were told that relaxation training would help them reduce their blood pressure. One-half of the group members were also told that their blood pressure would show reductions after three sessions of relaxation training given in one morning. The other half were told that they could expect reductions only after prolonged relaxation practice. As shown in Figure 3.3-3, there was no difference between the groups

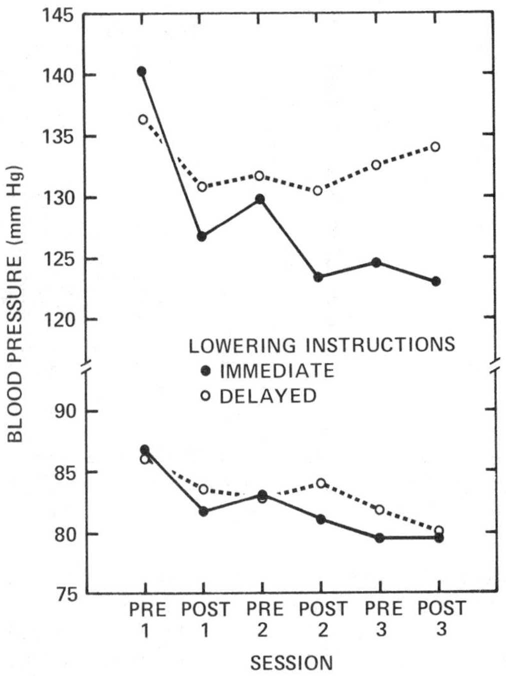

FIGURE 3.3-3 *The effect of two different expectancies on systolic and diastolic blood pressures of hypertensive individuals. Systolic blood pressure was markedly reduced in the group of patients told that relaxation training would lower blood pressure after only one or two training sessions, in contrast to those who were told to expect lowering only after prolonged training.*

in diastolic blood pressure. In systolic blood pressure, however, large and significant differences are shown; the group receiving immediate lowering instructions showed lower blood pressures, whereas the other group did not. The mechanism underlying this effect is unknown. It seems possible, however, that an expectancy of blood pressure lowering is needed to induce the biochemical changes necessary to lower blood pressure. This is an example of the complex interactions that occur between environmental events, in this case the instructions given to the patient, the patient's cognitive appraisal of the instructions, and neurochemical processes. Therapists tend to neglect the effect of therapeutic instructions, but experimental work suggests that the therapist should do everything to enhance the development of outcome and efficacy expectations.

Self-instruction In learning, children often repeat their teacher's instructions to themselves as they practice the task. Although it is not so apparent, adults often do the same thing. Self-defeating instructions and beliefs that may diminish self-efficacy are often encountered in clinical practice. Cognitive approaches to therapy focus on altering such self-instructions and other cognitive distortions, such as arbitrary self-imposed rules governing behavior. The first step in altering such cognitions is to explore and articulate the self-statement fully, and then by applying rules of logic to challenge the statement. It should be noted that cognitive change can also be brought about by altering performance, and it is extraordinarily difficult to separate the effects of cognitive and behavioral processes in therapeutic experiments. This difficulty is recognized by calling such therapies cognitive-behavioral. The bulk of the evidence suggests that a direct approach to behavior change leads to a superior outcome over the use of cognitive procedures alone. Nonetheless, self-instructions and beliefs influence the process of behavior change.

In the cognitive-behavioral approach to depression, for example, depressive cognitions about the uselessness of doing anything positive are challenged and corrected. In turn, this practice allows the patient to try out behaviors that result in positive reinforcement. The use of self-monitoring allows the patient and therapist to observe more accurately the positive effects of such new behaviors, thereby increasing self-efficacy and enhancing the probability of engaging in such behaviors again. Simultaneously, negative cognitions diminish, positive cognitions increase, and mood is enhanced.

Observational learning Humans also learn by observing others. Indeed, observational learning may be more important than other forms of learning during infancy and early childhood. Punishment, for example, not only reduces the probability that a particular behavior will occur, but also demonstrates a particular way of behaving toward others. Frequently, punished children will tend to use punishment in their interactions with others. The principle of observational learning has been used therapeutically, particularly with children, in a procedure known as *modeling*. Fearful children become less fearful when they watch other children behaving without fear in the same situation. Demonstrating a fearless approach to phobic situations may also be useful with adults to motivate approach to the feared object or situation. Similarly, parents can be taught more appropriate methods of interacting with their children by watching a skilled therapist use effective reinforcement procedures. In each case it should be noted that both a behavioral sequence and its consequences are being observed. Thus, observational learning involves the development of outcome expectancies dependent on the individual's interpretation of the consequences of the modeled behavior.

Goal setting and feedback Individuals set both long- and short-term goals for themselves. Research has shown that the setting of sequential short-term goals leads to better performance than setting a distant goal. Presumably, the reason is related to the reinforcing qualities of goal attainment, since it is known that reinforcing successive small steps is better than reinforcing the final behavior, at least until the behavior is well established. The definition of the goal is also important, since the attainment of well-specified goals is more easily recognized than the attainment of poorly defined goals. In general, it has been found that the higher the goal set, the better the performance. At the highest levels of goal setting, performance begins to decline, underlining the fact that unrealistic goals undermine performance. Goal attainment enhances self-efficacy and, in turn, affects future performance.

From a therapeutic viewpoint, research on goal setting suggests that the therapist should help the patient to define and set realistic, well-specified goals that signal small steps along the way to the overall goal. In this way, demoralization can be kept at bay by success. It is also important that patients set their own goals, since self-determined goals lead to better performance than goals imposed by others. Thus, teaching patients a problem-solving strategy that they may use in many situations is a useful aspect of most therapies.

Goal attainment is not the only indicator of improvement in performance. Behavior change itself, if observed by the individual, can provide information regarding progress toward a particular goal. This process, known as *informational feedback*, enhances performance in a wide variety of tasks, such as learning to shoot accurately at a target, driving an automobile, or the self-regulation of autonomic processes.

Experimental work has shown that removing informational feedback in a wide variety of therapeutic situations leads, at least temporarily, to setbacks. Information regarding therapeutic progress can be fed back to the patient in several ways. First, patients can observe their own progress when the desired behavior change is relatively linear. An example of such linear behavior change is approach to a phobic object or situation. Many behaviors, however, are more complex. In such cases, self-monitoring the behavior can enhance feedback. In addition, patients can plot the results of such feedback in graphical form, to examine progress over longer periods of time. Enhancement of information regarding progress is the central focus of biofeedback. In the typical *biofeedback* paradigm, processes that are not easily observed (e.g., blood pressure, small muscle contractions, and skin temperature) are made available for inspection by amplification. With sensitive and continuous feedback, the individual has the opportunity to learn to regulate invisible behaviors.

Information processing It is important to understand the way in which information about the environment is stored and activated in the central nervous system, since the microstructure of storage is likely to determine both normal learning mechanisms and disorders of learning. The advent of computers and robotics has led to the development of a number of new theories about such processes and to the building of models to explain, and even mimic, the way in which behavioral sequences are learned. Theoretical models of learning based on mathematical modeling and computer simulation have demonstrated that the processes underlying classical conditioning may occur in a single neuron. In one such model, it appears that neurons may learn to associate changes in the rate of firing of another neuron with changes in its own rate of firing. This theory suggests that it may be changes in the stimulus circumstances, rather than the stimuli themselves, that become associated in classical conditioning.

What is learned may be stored in memory as sequences of connected word concepts that, when retrieved, activate images, affect, and autonomic and motor behavior. In the case of phobia, for example, the sight of the phobic object will most strongly activate these action tendencies because it provides a full match with the most feared situation, whereas the sight of a picture, or a verbal description, of the object will only partially activate the sequences stored in memory. It has been shown that good visualizers will demonstrate more vigorous physiological responding to partial representations of a feared stimulus than will poor visualizers. In the case of simple phobia, it seems likely that a tight cluster of associated sequences is stored in memory; hence, only stimuli associated with the specific phobic situation will generate the full avoidance behavior. For agoraphobia, on the other hand, the memory sequences would seem to be more widely connected with other sequences, and, therefore, many situations will lead to activation of physiological arousal and avoidance behavior. Experimental methods to examine processing capacity and to test hypotheses concerning the likely structure of memory are available at both the human and animal levels, and it seems likely that such work will have important implications for the understanding of psychopathology.

THE ACQUISITION OF BEHAVIOR

One of the basic principles of learning theory is that behaviors are acquired and modified in a social context. Complex patterns of behavior are developed through the various processes that have been described in this section. Behaviors are acquired in the hurly-burly of family life, and reinforcement and punishment are often delivered in haphazard fashion. Some behavior patterns persist over years, whereas others are extinguished as a person's social environment changes. In addition, chance encounters may markedly influence one's life. While learning theory can account for the acquisition of many deviant behaviors, and symptom-like behavior has been developed in many learning experiments with animals, the delineation of the complex pattern of events that lead to the development of particular deviant behaviors poses difficult methodological problems. It is impossible to untangle learning histories by retrospective report, although such case histories can guide etiological hypotheses. Long-term prospective studies with multiple measures testing particular hypotheses are needed if progress is to be made in this difficult area.

From a clinical viewpoint, research during the past 25 years has set forth the major therapeutic components involved in the acquisition of more adaptive behaviors. Such components include therapeutic instructions; goal setting, including delineating small steps in the acquisition of desired behavior; modeling; providing practice opportunities; providing informational feedback regarding progress, reinforcement, and extinction; reframing of cognitive distortions; and the use of punishment. It is clear that different behavior problems respond to specific therapeutic packages containing many of the basic therapeutic procedures listed above. There is, however, no uniform therapy for all behavior problems. Research findings also suggest that different learning processes are involved in the acquisition and maintenance of behavior. This conclusion implies that once new and more adaptive behaviors are built up first in one situation, and then through carefully planned generalization training in a broad range of situations, the focus of therapy must shift to the maintenance of these new behaviors, using somewhat different strategies to prevent relapse.

THEORIES OF RELAPSE

One of the major problems facing therapists of all persuasions is that of patient relapse. Some instances of relapse can be easily understood; for example, the original environmental influences reinforcing symptomatic behavior may not have altered, and the patient's behavior is brought under their control once treatment has ended. This is an example of insufficient treatment; perhaps, for example, the family should have been brought into therapy. Sometimes, however, it denotes an impossible situation for the therapist, who is unable to alter a noxious psychological environment.

Less is known about the process of relapse than about the acquisition of behavior, and for the most part relapse has been studied in the addictive disorders, such as alcoholism and opiate addiction, and in related disorders, such as cigarette smoking and obesity. The basic theory concerning relapse involves situations that pose a high risk for engaging in the problem behavior, situations in which the behavior has occurred at a high frequency in the past. If such a situation is coped with successfully, then an individual will experience an increase in self-efficacy, and this increase will lead to a lower probability of relapse. The assumption here is that the individual has been taught or has developed usable coping skills. However, an individual who is deficient in coping with the high-risk situation will develop a positive expectancy regarding the beneficial effects of the substance and will then engage in initial use of the substance. This practice leads to an *abstinence violation* effect, which may be defined as the breaking of a self-imposed rule leading to a diminished sense of self-efficacy, negative cognitions and mood, and an increased probability of relapse. Several studies have found levels of self-efficacy to be predictive of outcome.

A fair amount is known about the characteristics of high-risk situations and the determinants of relapse, particularly for alcoholism, cigarette smoking, and the eating disorders. Physiological processes underlying the withdrawal syndrome are an important factor in relapse in many addictive disorders, since abstinence from the abused substance often leads to symptoms that are alleviated by the substance. As has been seen, cravings and urges may also be conditioned responses to environmental stimuli associated with use of the substance, whether it be alcohol, cigarettes, or food. These cravings may persist in specific circumstances for a very long time, thus increasing the probability of relapse. Such a scenario may also be true for bulimics, who crave their regular binge food particularly in specific stimulus circumstances (e.g., when alone at home). Research suggests, however, that symptoms of withdrawal and conditioned cravings are responsible for only a small proportion of the instances of relapse.

Such negative emotional states as depression, anxiety, and stress symptoms appear to be important determinants of lapses. More than half of the relapse episodes in alcoholism, cigarette smoking, and bulimia are associated with negative moods. Since the use of substances, such as alcohol, tends to relieve negative mood in the short term, the sequence of negative-mood onset and drinking alcohol will be learned. Future occurrences of negative mood triggered by stressors will then lead to drinking. It is not surprising, therefore, that factors militating against negative mood, such as adequate social support, tend to protect against relapse. Such support is most powerful when it stems from family or friends; however, therapeutic groups are also potential sources of support.

All treatments should contain relapse prevention procedures. The most important element of such a program is a careful analysis of the circumstances under which lapses occur during the treatment program, including events, cognitions, and moods. This will involve the use of self-monitoring combined with a problem-solving procedure to identify behaviors that are incompatible with relapse. Such behaviors are then practiced in high-risk situations, being refined through experience. Among promising techniques are extinction procedures aimed at breaking the connections between environmental cues and the cravings promoting relapse.

THE BIOLOGICAL BASIS OF LEARNING

The major experimental models for studying the biology of learning and memory are (1) identified neuronal pathways controlling specific behaviors in invertebrates (e.g., *Hermissenda* and *Aplysia californica*), (2) cerebellar neuronal pathways controlling the rabbit nicitating membrane and eyelid response, and (3) hippocampal neurons involved in long-term potentiation of behavioral sequences in vertebrates. Research conducted by Eric Kandel and his colleagues at Columbia University with *Aplysia californica* has been particularly well covered in the psychiatric literature. The details of this work are discussed below; however, the summary point is that it is now clear that there is a *reciprocal* interaction between central nervous system biological processes and environmental influences, resulting in the development and modification of behaviors.

The aplysia, a sea mollusk, is a useful animal to study because of the simplicity of its nervous system as compared to that of humans. The Aplysia contains approximately 20,000 neurons, and many of these are quite large and readily identifiable during repeated experiments. The specific behavior studied is a defensive reflex involving the withdrawal of the siphon of the snail when the animal is tactually stimulated. If the snail is touched repeatedly, it learns not to withdraw its siphon and gill, a process called habituation. If the snail receives a strong stimulus (e.g., an electric shock), it will become sensitized, such that even a previously subthreshold tactile stimulation will cause the animal to withdraw its gill and siphon. Furthermore, it is possible to condition the snail classically in such a way that it withdraws its siphon and gill to a conditioned stimulus. Habituation, sensitization, and classical conditioning of this reflex in the snail can be considered forms of learning and memory. Parallels have also been drawn between classical conditioning and phobias, as well as between a hypothetical lack of habituation and generalized anxiety.

The neuronal anatomical and chemical bases for these learning processes have been well worked out in this animal model. Sensory neurons receiving tactile information form excitatory synapses with the gill and siphon motor neurons that cause the withdrawal activity. Habituation, sensitization, and classical conditioning all involve neurochemical changes in the sensory neuron, resulting in alterations in the amount of excitatory neurotransmitter released. The neurochemical basis of habituation is that upon repeated stimulation of the sensory neuron (e.g., from repeated tactile stimulation), less calcium enters the presynaptic nerve terminal, resulting in less neurotransmitter being released and, thus, less activity of the motor neurons. Sensitization requires the presence of additional neurons, called facilitator interneurons, that synapse onto the sensory neurons. The sensitizing stimulus (e.g., an electric shock) causes the facilitator interneuron to release serotonin that binds to serotonin receptors on the sensory neuron. Activation of the serotonin receptors activate adenylate cyclase, producing cyclic adenosine monophosphate (AMP), thereby activating a cyclic AMP-dependent protein kinase, which, in turn, is believed to phosphorylate an S-type potassium channel. Phosphorylation of this potassium channel results in increased calcium influx during the action potential and increased neurotransmitter release. Although it is known that classical conditioning also results in an increased amount of neurotransmitter released by the sensory neuron, the neurochemical basis is less well understood at this time but may involve additional protein kinases.

Experimental work with young Aplysia has shown that the processes of habituation and sensitization develop at different times, with habituation preceding sensitization. This suggests that it may be possible to identify the separate biological processes which give rise to both of these important learning phenomena.

OVERVIEW

Enough is known about the processes of learning to account for the development of many behavior problems. Biological factors and learning processes interact in complex ways to produce psychiatric disorders. Such interactive processes are now becoming an important research area. As noted at the beginning of this section, all psychotherapies are based on the notion that a learning experience can beneficially affect problem behaviors. In this sense, learning theory is the basis for the practice of all psychotherapies.

REFERENCES

Agras W S: *Behavior Modification: Principles and Clinical Applications,* ed 2. Little, Brown, Boston, 1978.

Bandura A: *Principles of Behavior Modification.* Holt, Rinehart and Winston, New York, 1969.

Bandura A: *Social Foundations of Thought and Action: A Social Cognitive Theory.* Prentice-Hall, Englewood Cliffs, NJ, 1986.

Bandura A: Self-efficacy: Toward a unifying theory of behavioral change. Psychol Rev *84:* 191, 1977.

Brownell K D, Marlatt G A, Lichtenstein E, Wilson G T: Understanding and preventing relapse. Amer Psychol *41:* 765, 1986.

Clark G A, Hawkins R D, Kandel E R: Cell biological perspectives on learning, in *Diseases of the Nervous System,* A K Asbury, G M McKhann, W I MacDonald, editors. Saunders, Philadelphia, 1986.

Hilgard E R, Bower G H: *Theories of Learning,* ed 4. Prentice-Hall Inc, Englewood Cliffs, NJ, 1975.

Mischel W: Toward a cognitive social learning reconceptualization of personality. Psychol Rev *80:* 252, 1973.

Pavlov I P: *Conditioned Reflexes.* Clarendon, London, 1927.

Poling A: *A Primer of Human Behavioral Pharmacology.* Plenum, New York, 1986.

Rachlin H: *Introduction to Modern Behaviorism.* Freeman, New York, 1970.

Seligman M E P: Phobias and preparedness. Behav Ther *2:* 307, 1971.

Skinner B F: *Science and Human Behavior.* Macmillan, New York, 1953.

Watson J B, Rayner R: Conditioned emotional reactions. J Exper Psychol *3,* 1, 1920.

3.4 AGGRESSION

MICHAEL T. MCGUIRE, M.D.
ALFONSO TROISI, M.D.

INTRODUCTION

The neighborhood cinema features the latest movie on sex, greed, and revenge. A spy novel unfolds the story of a plot to assassinate a foreign agent. People are physically beaten and some die. . . . The gates to a nuclear power station open. Protesters throw stones. The police respond. Ten protesters and six policemen are injured. . . . A psychologically deranged killer stalks the streets at night. Eleven women are raped and murdered over a year. . . . Normally shy monkeys watch two men walk from the forest to their Land Rover. One man comes between an infant and its mother. He picks up the infant. The adult monkeys threaten. The man's companion fires his shotgun. Seven monkeys die.

Aggression, destruction, murder, rape, social protest, self-defense, assaultive behavior—it is called many things and is everywhere. Siblings hit each other; criminals shoot police; parents spank children; gangs fight in the streets; and husbands and wives slug it out. Aggression influences lives as much as love and friendship, thought and inspiration, or nutrition and sleep.

When investigating the causes of aggression among people with psychiatric disorders, mental health professionals ask: "Why does it occur?" "What causes it?" and "What can be done about it?" In trying to answer these questions, it is essential to attend to at least two facts: Aggression is common among persons *not* suffering from psychiatric disorders, and aggressive behavior can be biologically adaptive despite (often) social and ethical attitudes to the contrary.

DEFINITION AND CLASSIFICATION

Although many definitions of aggression have been put forth, the term is not easily defined; nor are any of the existing definitions satisfactory. The term subserves almost any behavior, and behavior that is aggressive in one context may be harmless in another. For the present, an inquiry into how aggression is classified will be more instructive than the pursuit of an acceptable definition. The classification systems shown in Table 3.4-1 illustrate this point. They not only hint at the difficulties inherent in trying to organize behavior not tied to a unitary concept (e.g., weaning) but also reveal how investigators have organized the multiple phenomena of aggression. One approach to classification is to categorize aggressive acts on the basis of observation (System 1 in Table 3.4-1); that is, behavior patterns similar in form are assigned to the same category. There are advantages to this approach. Descriptions and definitions are not dependent on inferences about the organization of behavior, the intentions of actors, or possible underlying physiological mechanisms. Definitions based on form of behavior are useful in studies of nonprimate species, in which behavioral repertoires are limited. With primates, however, aggressive acts vary enormously in both form and context. Thus, the utility of this approach for understanding human aggression is limited.

A second approach (System 2 in Table 3.4-1) emphasizes proximate or immediate events and mechanisms. A mechanism is a behavioral event (e.g., attack by another), psychological event (e.g., fear), or physiological event (e.g., rise in epinephrine) that, when it occurs, alters the probability of aggression. Many, if not most, investigators of aggression are interested in identifying mechanisms associated with aggression. Both single mechanisms and sequences of mechanisms have been postulated, such as: frustration → physiological-psychological change → increased responsiveness to aggression-eliciting stimuli → aggressive behavior. Classification by type of mechanism has clinical utility if mechanisms can be identified. In studies of humans, specific mechanisms have been difficult to identify, although considerable progress has been made over the past decade. Thus, this approach also lacks utility. The search for mechanisms remains a central focus in animal research, however.

Difficulties similar to those encountered in the search for mechanisms arise when aggression is classified in terms of either process concepts (e.g., developmental and genetic predispositions) or intuitively acceptable categories (e.g., dominance-related). System 3 in Table 3.4-1 is built partly on process concepts and partly on intuitively acceptable categories. Different process variables are postulated to interact in different ways, and different combinations affect different behaviors. The main limitation of this approach is that the number of possible permutations is so great that discussions of process often confuse as much as clarify. Moreover, categorization by intuition suffers from disagreements over the inclusion or exclusion of particular types of aggression in specific categories.

The study of aggression (tens of thousands of publications exist on the subject) has proved frustrating. In considerable part, frustration is due to the fact that investigators have defined aggression idiosyncratically, failed to clarify underlying concepts, or have interpreted the contributions of others in their own conceptual framework. In the clinical literature, in particular, the term "aggression" is so fraught with subjective assumptions (e.g., that it is a sure sign of psychopathology, that it is a negative attribute) that it runs the risk of becoming a useless term, not only clinically but as a referent in serious scientific discussion.

An obvious implication of the preceding discussion is that clinicians and investigators concerned with aggression must articulate definitions, underlying concepts, and their posited interrelationships. The term "aggression" is not specifically defined in the revised third edition of the American Psychiatric Association's *Diagnostic and Statistical Manual of Mental Disorders* (DSM-III-R). The definition used in this section is the following: Aggression is behavior intended to cause physical injury to others. Two concepts underlie this definition—one emphasizing function, and the other emphasizing mechanism. They will be discussed in detail below. The definition is descriptive, classifying disparate behaviors together by virtue of their short-term consequence: harm to others. There are limitations to the definition. For example, it excludes many behaviors that intuitively seem aggressive, such as verbal aggression, that do not result in physical injury; managerial styles that result in harmful psychological consequences to others; and premeditated social ostracism of others. The importance of these behaviors in day-to-day living should not be underestimated, nor should their effects on recipients' self-esteem, social status, and happiness. Because of space limitations, these forms of aggression will not be considered.

TABLE 3.4-1
Classification Systems for Aggression

System 1
Verbal
Physical against objects
Physical against self
Physical against others
System 2
Predatory attack
Intermale
Fear-induced
Irritable
Territorial defense
Maternal
Instrumental
Sex-related
System 3
Territorial
Dominance-related
Weaning-related
Parental (disciplinary)
Antipredatory
Moralistic

THEORETICAL FRAMEWORKS

Selecting a definition or identifying underlying concepts does not assure that clinical and research findings will be understood. A theoretical framework is necessary to facilitate data interpretation. A number of frameworks, each of which can muster supportive data, have been advanced to explain human aggression. Five are reviewed below.

FREUD'S VIEW In the Freudian view, aggression initially serves as a reaction to the blocking or thwarting of libidinal impulses. It occurs only in selected situations, and its incidence is expected to differ as a function of situational characteristics. Later, Freud introduced the concept of "Thanatos" or the "death force" instinct. If this instinct remains unrestrained, it results in self-destruction unless neutralized by libidinal energy or redirected either through sublimation or displacement. Because libidinal neutralization and sublimation are never complete, some aggressive energy is inevitably directed toward others. Variations on the Freudian view, especially those developed by Melanie Klein, have placed a greater emphasis on infantile aggression.

LORENZIAN VIEW In the view of *Konrad Lorenz,* sometimes referred to as the innate-tendency view, aggression that causes physical harm to others springs from a fighting instinct that humans share with other organisms. The energy associated with this instinct is spontaneously produced within organisms at a more or less continuous rate. The probability of aggression increases as a function of the amount of stored energy and the presence and strength of aggression-releasing stimuli. In this view, aggression is inevitable, and spontaneous eruptions sometimes occur.

ELICITED-DRIVE VIEW In the elicited-drive view, aggression stems mainly from external conditions that result in frustration, loss of face, and pain. These conditions arouse a strong motive to engage in harm-producing behaviors toward persons responsible for such conditions. Aggression is not inevitable in this view. However, given most imaginable living situations, it is likely.

AGGRESSION AS A LEARNED SOCIAL BEHAVIOR In this view, aggression occurs both because of aggressive responses acquired through experience and the rewards associated with aggressive behavior. Thus, aggression is not a consequence of built-in urges toward violence or because of aggressive drives; rather, it is more likely to occur in social situations in which aggression is rewarded or where a reward for aggression is anticipated. In this view, the causes of aggression are varied in scope, and different combinations of contributing variables (e.g., past experiences, specific social situations, degree to which needs are being met) are associated with different forms and intensities of aggression. This view is fundamentally different from the previous three or the evolutionary view described below. In effect, aggression is much like other complex behaviors in that it must be acquired.

EVOLUTIONARY BIOLOGY The fifth framework, evolutionary biology, is closely associated with the concepts of function and mechanism, and it is the framework that has guided the organization of this section. An evolutionary framework has been selected because, in the authors' view: (1) human aggression probably has evolutionary homologues (i.e., similar proximate mechanisms across closely related species); (2) it facilitates the integration of cross-species findings (the majority of research data on aggression comes from studies of nonhuman species); (3) other explanatory frameworks have had only partial success in improving the understanding of aggression; and (4) many of the elements of the four frameworks reviewed above can be included within the evolutionary framework.

An overview of the evolutionary framework is as follows: In order to survive, organisms must take in nourishment and eliminate waste products. They must distinguish between prey and predator and between potential mates and potential enemies, and they must evaluate situations for their potential danger. They must explore their environment and orient their sense organs appropriately as they take in information about the potentially beneficial and harmful aspects of their immediate world. At times, they will attempt to change their world or aggress against participants within it. The contexts within which, as well as the mechanisms by which, these functions are carried out will vary widely throughout the animal kingdom. However, the basic prototype functions are likely to remain invariant.

In the evolutionary framework, aggressive behavior is not viewed as the result of a specific process, such as a drive, an innate tendency, an eliciting stimulus, or something learned. Rather, like language acquisition, it is an evolved capacity that can be developed, and the development of aggressive behavior (or any other behavior system) generally subserves two ultimate evolutionary functions: survival and reproduction. Its short-term functions include: securing preferential or exclusive access to vital resources such as space, shelter, food, and mates; and defense of oneself, of those in whom one has direct genetic investment (e.g., offspring, parents), and of selected nonrelatives. Proximate mechanisms may be physiological, psychological, or contextual (e.g., threat by another).

Large amounts of data previously reported and interpreted in other conceptual frameworks can be subsumed within the evolutionary framework. For example, frustration associated with delays in acquiring preferred resources can result in aggressive behavior; direct physical or verbal provocation, when perceived as threats, also can result in aggressive behavior; physical pain or forced confinement, if perceived as compromising survival, likewise can result in aggression, and often among persons without a history of aggressive behavior; a variety of environmental influences, such as air pollution, excessive heat, excessive noise, and crowding are all likely to alter physiological states and increase the probability that frustration, provocation, pain, or confinement will be responded to with aggression.

Implications What are the implications of this framework for understanding aggression among humans? First, in many situations, aggression may be adaptive. As animals do, people often aggress in situations where essential functions are perceived to be compromised (e.g., competition for food or a mate, property encroachment, favors not repaid). Behavior that results in settling preferential or exclusive access to required or preferred resources often affects the probability that a person will be psychologically stable, physically healthy, and reproductively fit. Second, the form of aggression will differ in the situations described above. Defending against a predator may begin with throwing a rock, hand-to-hand combat, or waiting for a predator to behave in a certain way. Third, for any given instance of aggression, the contributions of physiological, psychological, and contextual variables will differ. It follows that in each instance of aggression the clinician and investigator must ask: "Is an aggressive patient acting as most normal people would or as a consequence of his or her psychiatric disorder?" "What are the proximate mechanisms?" "What contextual variables contribute to the behavior?" Answers to such questions determine whether an individual's aggression should be diagnosed as normal or abnormal.

DATA OF AGGRESSION

The data of aggression are plagued by a number of problems. Quality of reporting, often not the fault of investigators, is one type. Aggression is seldom seen because it usually occurs rapidly. People fume, hate, and plan revenge for months, but an aggressive act may last only a few seconds, and it often occurs in private. Post hoc discussions with persons who have aggressed or have been aggressed against often result in accounts of doubtful validity. Thus, there is some uncertainty as to the frequency, the form, and the importance of context in human aggression.

Physiological data raise another type of problem. Reports suggesting that persons who are frequently aggressive differ biochemically from nonaggressive controls demonstrate putative correlations but not causal relationships. Similar interpretive problems are encountered in trying to assess the degree to which psychological states are contributory. People in similar psychological states often act differently.

The limitations of our knowledge are brought into sharp focus when clinicians attempt to predict aggression among persons who are not chronic aggressors. Before-the-fact discussions suggest that approximately one in every ten adults wants to hurt a specific other. Approximately one adult in 50 will do so in any given year. Who the one might be and, more important, when and where such a person might act, cannot be accurately predicted by interview, biochemical analysis, psychiatric diagnosis, or the use of any other information now available.

The difficulties encountered in doing research on humans often attract investigators to animals, where experimental conditions and interventions can be controlled. Animal data clearly suggest that there are multiple functions to aggression as well as mutiple mediating mechanisms. Yet, animal research is not the only answer. As systematic as such research often is, there is good evidence that species differ in critical ways with respect to aggression.

RESEARCH IN AGGRESSION

This subsection begins with a review of reports of the prevalence of aggression among persons with and without psychiatric disorders. It is followed by a review and evaluation of data from different areas of research. The areas to be discussed include genetics, development, social context, psychological state, hormones and neurotransmitters, and neuroanatomy. These headings identify areas of current research interest. They differ with respect to the sources of available data (e.g., animal vs. human). The reader will note that the areas are independent of DSM-III-R categories. It is the authors' opinion that many psychiatric disorders currently listed in DSM-III-R will change over time. It follows that attempts to understand aggression in its own right should precede efforts to understand aggression in terms of specific psychiatric disorders. However, because of reporting conventions, some references to DSM-III-R categories are inevitable.

INCIDENCE OF AGGRESSION **In the population as a whole** A few statistics will help set a perspective. In 1983, in the United States, there were approximately 170,000 reported rapes or attempted rapes and 4,250,000 instances of reported assault. In 1975, the U.S. homicide rate was 10.2 per 100,000 persons; in 1960, it was 4.7 per 100,000 persons. These figures reflect a progressive increase in the frequency of reported homicide in the United States. Compared to the rate in other countries, the homicide rate in the United States is neither high nor low, with other countries ranging from 0.4 to 31.2 per 100,000 persons per year. These data suggest (despite reservations about reporting practices and changing legal defintions) that people are behaving more aggressively.

In persons with psychiatric disorders Few detailed studies of the prevalence of aggression among persons with psychiatric disorders are available, and definitions of aggression often differ among those studies. Generally, data are not sufficient to say for certain that the probability of aggression increases with specific psychiatric disorders. Available findings suggest that between 10 and 15 percent of persons admitted to psychiatric inpatient facilities have engaged in aggressive behavior (directed toward physically hurting others) in the year prior to their hospital admission. Persons suffering from psychiatric disorders but who are not admitted to inpatient psychiatric facilities also engage in aggressive acts. Thus, the percentages given above would likely be higher if all persons with psychiatric disorders could be sampled. Once persons become inpatients, the frequency of aggression appears to increase. Aggressive acts may occur in as many as 10 percent of inpatients in any 3-month period. It is not known whether this increase is attributable to more accurate reporting or to an interaction between hospitalization and aggression. Both factors seem likely, and the possible effects of commitment status and context variables (e.g., abuse of inpatients, restricted activities) remain to be determined.

PSYCHIATRIC INPATIENTS Psychiatric inpatients who are male, young, and diagnosed as suffering from schizophrenia, alcoholism, organic mental disorder, mental retardation, seizure disorder, and personality disorder are reported to be most aggressive. However, data supporting the higher incidence in such persons remains controversial, and sampling as well as interpretative errors are likely. In the authors' experience, once persons are labeled as aggressive (usually on the basis of historical information), it is nearly impossible to remove the label or to eliminate interpretative biases. Overall, persons with mood disorders are reported to engage in aggressive behavior less frequently than persons with the disorders listed above, although persons who are manic are more often aggressive than persons who are depressed. A summary of selected studies is presented in Table 3.4-2.

PSYCHIATRIC OUTPATIENTS Studies of outpatient populations report that 2 to 4 percent of newly evaluated outpatients have engaged in aggressive behavior during the year preceding evaluation. Among those patients who were aggressive, most appear to be suffering from a type of personality disorder or a nonpsychiatric disorder (e.g., epilepsy). These percentages also are likely to be lower than the actual rate of occurrence. Although data on this population are sparse, and characteristics of outpatient populations have significantly changed in recent years, the 2 to 4 percent figure for aggressive acts of outpatients is not significantly different from some reports of the incidence of aggressive acts for the population as a whole. Assuming that each person who aggresses does so only once, the earlier noted statistic of 4.25 million assaults in the United States during 1983 approximates the 2 percent figure for the entire population of the United States. Less severe forms of psychiatric disorders thus may not be associated with measurable increases in aggressive behavior. The low outpatient percentages, when compared with the relatively high inpatient percentages, would be expected if it is assumed that there is an interaction between psychological decompensation (generally, greater in inpatients than outpatients) and aggression.

SOME CHARACTERISTICS OF AGGRESSION The majority of adults with and without psychiatric disorders who commit aggressive acts are more likely to commit such acts against familiar persons, usually family members. This fact suggests that aggression is not indiscriminately directed. A possible exception to the familiar-person generalization is reported among adolescent males, who often aggress against casual acquaintances or persons who are unknown to them. The greater opportunities to aggress against unknown others as well as the greater likelihood that a casual acquaintance or unknown person will report aggression partially explain this finding.

TABLE 3.4-2
Summary of 13 Studies Examining Psychiatric Diagnoses of Patients Who Commit Violent Acts

Study	*Number of Subjects; Nonviolent Control Group; Diagnostic Criteria*	*Characteristics of Population Studied*	*Type of Study*	*Definition of Violence*	*Overrepresented Diagnoses*
1	100 violent patients; none; unspecified	Admissions over 15 months to a psychopathic hospital for homicidal threats	Retrospective review of admission records	"Homicidal threat": (1) verbal threat of assault (81%) or (2) physical assault (19%)	Personality disorder, schizophrenia, organic brain syndrome (OBS)
2	30 violent patients; none; unspecified	Admissions over a 3-month period to a community mental health center	Retrospective review of incident reports	Verbal threat of schizophrenia, affective disorder	Chronic alcoholism
3	1,004 (7% violent); yes; unspecified	Two-year survey of all incident reports of inpatients at a state hospital	Retrospective review of incident reports	In-hospital physical assaults of threats of	OBS, personality disorder
4	237 (33% violent); yes; DSM-II	Six-month survey of inpatients at a community mental health center, 34% schizophrenic	Retrospective review of admission records	In-hospital physical assaults	Schizophrenia
5*	9,365 (10% violent); yes; DSM-II	Admissions to several public hospitals over a 1-year period, 33% schizophrenic	Retrospective review of admission records	Physical assault listed as a problem at the time of admission on a checklist	Schizophrenia (paranoia), OBS, "other" (personality disorder mostly)
6	5,164 (7% violent); yes; DSM-II	Survey of inpatients hospitalized for over 1 month at two large state hospitals, 70% schizophrenic	Retrospective review of patients' records	In-hospital physical assault	Schizophrenia (nonparanoid), OBS, "other" (personality disorder mostly)
7	876 (11% violent); yes; DSM-II	Admissions over a 1-year period at two public hospitals, 30% schizophrenic	Retrospective review of admission records	Physical assault listed as a problem at time of admission on a checklist	Schizophrenia, OBS, "other" (personality disorder mostly)
8	222 (62.6% violent); none; unspecified	Consecutive admissions to a geriatric unit of a state hospital	Retrospective review of admission records	Physical assault or threats of assaults	Senile dementia, schizophrenia
9	68 assaults; none; unspecified	Survey of 115 psychiatrists connected to a medical school (about being assaulted by patients)	Retrospective review questionnaire sent to psychiatrists	Physical assault of therapists	Schizophrenia
10	103 violent patients; none; unspecified	Survey of 725 psychiatrists mostly in one U.S. city (about being assaulted by patients)	Same as above	Same as above	Schizophrenia, personality disorder
11	867 (10% violent); yes; unspecified	Consecutive admission to three wards of an acute-care municipal hospital (approximately 50% schizophrenic)	Two-year retrospective and 2-year prospective studies of arrest records	Arrest record for violent crimes involving direct bodily harm or potential for harm (i.e., burglary and robbery)	Drug dependency, alcoholism, schizophrenia
12	301 (24% violent); yes; unspecified	Admissions to a state hospital (73% schizophrenic)	Two-year retrospective study of arrest records	Arrest record for violent crimes involving direct bodily harm	Schizophrenia
13	2,152; yes; unspecified	All male admissions to a state hospital	Five-year retrospective; 5-year prospective study of FBI records	Arrest record for violent crimes including murder, manslaughter, rape, robbery, aggressive assault	Personality disorder

Table adapted from Krakowski M, Volavka J, Brizer D: Psychopathology and violence: A review of literature. Comp Psychiat *27*(2): 131, 1986, with permission.
*Approximately the same rates are observed in private hospitals.

Generally, the probability of aggressive behavior increases as persons become more psychologically decompensated, and perhaps also if the onset of a psychiatric disorder is rapid. Otherwise, very little is known about the relationship between the course of illness and aggression. Episodic decompensation may occur in persons who ingest large quantities of alcohol: greater than 50 percent of persons who commit criminal homicides and who engage in assaultive behavior are reported to have imbibed significant amounts of alcohol immediately prior to aggressing.

With the exception of antisocial personality disorder, efforts to identify specific personality disorders for aggressive patients have been unsuccessful. Aggressive patients comprise a heterogenous group of personality types. Persons with the primary diagnosis of personality disorder are sometimes reported to engage in aggressive behavior when not in emotional turmoil. Recent studies of the behavior of aggressive patients using cluster analytic techniques revealed four identifiable patient subgroups: two groups frequently engaged in violent acts but differed in severity of their violence; one group infrequently engaged in violent acts but, when individuals were violent, they engaged in severe violence; and one group had no history of violence. No specific within-subgroup etiologies were identified, and single subgroups often included persons with different psychiatric disorders.

The above findings, though tentative, suggest that psychological and physiological mechanisms mediating aggression remain largely intact during periods in which people suffer from psychiatric disorders. In turn, certain psychological-physiological states associated with disorders alter interactions between mechanisms, and these changes in interaction alter the probability of aggression. This view is in line with current evolutionary thinking, which holds that aggression is a phylogenetically old and highly selected behavioral system. The primary mechanisms of aggression (e.g., perception that one's survival is compromised, frustration in obtaining desired resources, elevated norepinephrine or reduced serotonin function) should be strongly buffered from intermittent physiological and psychological change. However, secondary mechanisms, such as suboptimal information processing, emotional states, and frustration tolerance (often altered in psychiatric disorders), are likely to be less well buffered, and changes in such mechanisms could significantly alter the probability of aggression. From this perspective, aggression is not an integral component of psychiatric disorders but a consequence of disorders.

Recently, there has been an increasing interest in sex differences in the predisposition for and frequency of aggression. For aggression classified as homicide, battery, assault with a weapon, or rape, the frequency among males clearly exceeds that of females. For domestic violence, in which one marital partner acts to hurt another, the frequency among males and females is about equal. Studies of persons who are hospitalized in psychiatric facilities over long periods of time indicate that the prevalence of male and female aggression is approximately equal. Recent reports of studies of African cultures show that, in many communities, not only is the prevalence of female aggression significantly higher than previously thought, but also the frequency of female aggression may exceed that of male aggression. The frequency of female aggression closely correlates with the scarcity of resources—in this instance, available males who are also good and predictable providers. When these findings are combined with those for male prevalence in homicide, battery, and rape in the United States, it seems clear that culture, sex, and context are important. Nonhuman primate studies are revealing on this point. Extrapolations to humans from field studies of nonhuman primates generally would lead to the prediction of greater frequencies of aggressive behavior among males than among females. However, there are important exceptions. For example, females are more aggressive toward unknown females of the same species than are males, females will engage in noticeably increased frequencies of aggression in establishing and maintaining female hierarchies and during periods in which adult males are contesting dominance status, and females are more likely to inflict serious injury on unknown females.

GENETIC DATA AND AGGRESSIVE BEHAVIOR

Genetic mechanisms in aggression are implicated by selected breeding in animals that can alter the severity of aggressive behavior. Among laboratory strains of rats, Sprague-Dawley rats are less aggressive than both the S3 strain (Tryon Maze dull) and wild rats. Similar differences apply to strains of dogs. It is not surprising, therefore, that questions dealing with possible genetic contributions to human aggression have been asked. Basically, three kinds of research approaches have been pursued: twin studies, pedigree studies, and what will be called chromosome-behavior studies.

STUDIES OF TWINS Research of monozygotic twins suggests that there is a hereditary component to aggressive behavior. Thus far, most studies have focused on nonpsychiatric populations. In these studies, concordance rates for monozygotic twins exceed those for dizygotic twins. A recent study by Rushton and colleagues measuring the frequency of altruistic and aggressive behavior in a large sample of monozygotic twins suggests that aggression is significantly influenced by genetic contributions. There are, however, many unresolved problems (e.g., statistical-interpretative, incidence reporting, assessment of severity of aggression) associated with data interpretation, and monozygotic twins often have different experiences (e.g., intrauterine, environmental, birth order, perinatal illnesses). Moreover, if twins are dizygotic, they often are raised differently (especially if they are of the opposite sex). When combined with animal data, the human evidence is suggestive enough to justify further investigation. However, a word of caution is in order: None of the studies reports data that would allow anyone to make strong predictions about the behavior of an unseen twin if one member of a monozygotic pair is known to be aggressive.

PEDIGREE STUDIES Perhaps the most compelling evidence that there is genetic loading for aggressive behavior has been provided by pedigree studies. On balance, these studies show that persons from families with histories of psychiatric disorders are more prone to develop psychiatric disorders and engage in aggressive behavior than are persons without such histories. A particularly interesting set of findings has been reported for isolated tribes in the Amazon Basin (Yamamomo) that suggest the inheritability of aggressive tendencies. Pedigree studies, however, are not without interpretive problems. Generally, studies report on instances in which subjects lived with their parents during childhood. Thus, the possible influences of parental, social, and educational experiences cannot be easily ruled out. Intelligence also may be a factor. Persons with low intelligence quotient (I.Q.) scores appear to have a higher frequency of deliquency and aggression than persons with normal I.Q. scores. However, I.Q.-related findings must be interpreted cautiously. Interpretations of genetic contributions thus remain tentative. Critical questions, similar to those suggested earlier, are raised by these studies. For example, what is it that is really being measured? Is it a specific predisposition to aggression, some type of metabolic imbalance, a learning disorder, or cumulative experience? Observed correlations between aggressive behavior and other atypical behaviors suggest that genetic predispositions for atypical behavior, including behaviors associated with psychiatric disorders, are associated with atypical physiological function, one consequence of which is an increase in the probability of aggression.

CHROMOSOME INFLUENCES Behavior research involving the influence of chromosomes has concentrated primarily in abnormalities in X and Y chromosomes, particularly the 47-XYY syndrome. Early studies suggested that persons with this syndrome could be characterized as tall, having below average intelligence, and more likely to be apprehended and in prison for engaging in criminal behavior. Subsequent studies suggest that, at most, the 47-XYY syndrome contributes to aggressive behavior in only a small percentage of the cases. Studies of the androgen and gonadotropin characteristics of 47-XYY persons also have been inconclusive and have not established that such persons are biochemically atypical.

Certain inborn metabolic disorders, genetic in origin, that diffusely involve the nervous system have been reported to be associated with aggressive personalities. Examples include Sanfilippo syndrome (increased mucopolysaccharide storage), Spielmeyer-Vogt syndrome (a diffuse neuronal storage disorder with increased ganglioside storage), and phenylketonuria.

The findings from genetic studies are suggestive but not conclusive. Moreover, many questions will not be easily resolved because of legal and ethical conditions governing studies of humans. Despite the fact that animals can be bred to be more or less aggressive, well-controlled studies demonstrating that genetic loading among humans is a significant contributing factor in aggression remain to be completed. At this point in history, human mating practices appear to be random enough (except in unusual situations) that repeated loading for aggressive tendencies is unlikely. What is more probable is that there are gene-environment interactions leading to particular types of physiological-psychological characteristics. Under specific circumstances, these characteristics are associated with an increased probability of aggression.

DEVELOPMENTAL DATA AND AGGRESSIVE BEHAVIOR

Age and sex interact with aggression in nonhuman primates. Submissive behavior is more prevalent than aggression in juvenile monkeys, and aggressive behavior increases with age, most dramatically among females. As animals get older, aggression generally becomes briefer in duration and more efficient. These profiles are at variance with what is observed among humans. Adolescent males, for example, often are more physically aggressive than adult males, although they may not be as aggressive verbally.

Nonhuman primate studies also show that randomly selected animals can be raised under conditions that predictably result in an increase in the frequency of aggressive behavior when such animals become adults. Reduction of social contact in early life results in an increased frequency of aggression being directed toward both the self and others. Once aggressive tendencies have developed, the frequency of aggressive behavior is not easily altered. From one perspective, growing up can be thought of as learning the rules of both social cooperation and selective aggression (i.e., aggression directed toward selected targets under specific conditions). Animals growing up in atypical environments appear to have insufficent opportunities to learn social rules as well as alternative ways of behaving.

It is possible to view neurotic and delinquent children as the two ends of a spectrum on which normal children are located somewhere near the middle. Delinquent children frequently are hyperaggressive; neurotic children frequently are hypoaggressive; and normal children generally are aggressive in specific contexts. Developmental contributions are implicated over this entire spectrum. Some studies report an increased frequency of aggressive behavior as well as criminality among persons who have grown up in families where they have witnessed parental discord, divorce, separation, death, multiple childhood placements, alcoholism, or child abuse, or combinations thereof. Other studies suggest, relative to national averages, that persons who engage in serious aggressive behavior (including killing) less often were adopted, foster, or runaway children, but more often were childhood thieves. Still other studies fail to support the idea that the developmental years of those adults who repeatedly aggress differ from those of adults who are not aggressive. In effect, within rather wide limits, different child-rearing practices or parental values are not predictive of aggressive behavior among offspring. Recent studies also question the relationship among the triad of enuresis, fire setting, and cruelty to animals as a significant predictor of aggressive behavior in adults. Thus, although evidence is suggestive, conclusive results are not available. An apparent exception to the preceding point is that of antisocial personality disorder. Adults diagnosed with this disorder are likely to have a history of serious conduct disturbance and aggression before age 15.

Two sets of findings emerge from developmental data. First, many of the upbringing conditions that mental health professionals have long suspected mold adult behavior (e.g., multiple childhood placement, parental discord) do not uniformly result in expected outcomes among adults. Again, the interpretation of findings cannot be easily divorced from methodological issues. For example, aggressive youngsters are likely to spend less time in any given foster setting. Second, in some instances, such as pre-antisocial personality disorder and extreme upbringing conditions (e.g., extreme and repeated physical punishment), signs of what is to come are present during the early years of development, or early experiences correlate with adult behavior. Such experiences do not correlate so well that alternative explanations need not be considered, however. These findings notwithstanding, it is still difficult to throw off the belief that upbringing conditions in some way contribute to specific adult behavior. There is no doubt that they do, but what needs to be specified is which conditions lead to which adult behavior. Thus, in considering etiology, one must keep in mind that two processes may work in parallel or they may not be relevant; that is, upbringing conditions may alter the probability of psychiatric disorders or aggressive behavior, or both, or not significantly influence such behavior.

SOCIAL CONTEXT AND AGGRESSIVE BEHAVIOR

Among nonhuman primates, alteration in social context often results in aggression. For example, overcrowding, the introduction of an unknown animal into an established social group, and the manipulation of social groups such that animals compete for dominance status all increase the frequency of aggression. The latter finding can be interpreted from a number of perspectives. A social learning approach is possible: Competition and associated aggressive behavior is learned; animals who reach adulthood have had the opportunity to see and engage in competition; thus, their aggressive behavior during periods of dominance competition is expected. An elicited-drive interpretation is also possible: The eliciting stimulus might be the opportunity for dominance. An evolutionary interpretation is possible as well: Animals will fight over who controls valued resources. Whatever the interpretation, extrapolation of such findings to humans is not uniformly straightforward. Most investigators who have looked at relationships between social context and aggression have failed to find correlations consistently. For instance, studies of crowding effects among humans often report contradictory findings. Epidemiological data suggest that aggressive behavior is more prevalent among persons who have experienced severe and prolonged poverty. Yet, low-status monkeys (a possible analogous state) are not necessarily more aggressive than high-status monkeys. Like many other variables with which mental health professionals must deal, social context variables sometimes seem to be critical; sometimes they do not. When they are, usually more than one variable appears to be relevant.

If one carefully examines social context findings, data often are surprising. For example, moderate aggression often appears to accompany the development of cooperation. In certain circumstances, aggression is an efficient means of resolving lingering disputes and changing the behavior of others. In such situations, aggression appears to stem from frustrations caused by others: Persons are aggressive toward others because the behavior of others is perceived to be essential to the well-being of the aggressor (e.g., competition over a mate or a job promotion). Although humans have devised good moral and ethical reasons for not being aggressive, it is difficult to overlook certain data: namely, that, in many instances, aggressive behavior is a far more effective means of altering others' behavior than is either verbal persuasion, the administration of drugs, or threats. Moreover, in many situations, it is difficult to judge whether aggressive behavior is a negative attribute, particularly if one considers increased cooperation or well-being of the person who is aggressed against as an outcome. In its cohesive form, aggression is generally expressed as reproachful and punishing behavior that has as its goals assisting a reunion and discouraging further behavior that endangers a relationship.

There is a body of evidence from animal studies showing that when two animals of the same species interact, certain deviations from normal behavior by one animal are associated with an increase in the probability of aggressive behavior by the other. This phenomenon can be readily demonstrated in rats, where one animal in a dyad is treated with a behavior-altering drug but the other is not. The untreated rat often responds aggressively. The same result has been observed with monkeys: Monkeys who have recovered from temporal lobe ablations and are returned to their groups often refuse to respond to threats and displays by other animals. After approximately a week, they are likely to be attacked by other group members. Recently, this model has been applied to humans taking into account variables that influence human behavior (e.g., history of relationships, knowledge of kinship). Findings suggest that people engage in certain types of trait identification (communicating to others who and what they are and how they are likely to act) and that this information (e.g., words, facial expressions, postures) is encoded by the receiver, who adjusts and responds accordingly. The process is bidirectional. This paradigm may be valuable in trying to understand contextual mechanisms of aggressive behavior among persons with psychiatric disorders; here, aggression can result either because of atypical trait communication (frequent among persons with psychiatric disorders) or because of atypical encoding (also frequent among persons with psychiatric disorders). For example, one of the consequences of psychological decompensation is that persons interpret events, generally interpreted as dissimilar, in a similar way. Thus, stimuli that do not ordinarily elicit aggressive responses may be perceived as dangerous, frightening, or the like. In such situations, the probability of aggression increases.

There are also situations in which the likelihood of aggression is increased because of the structure of social systems. This point can be demonstrated relatively easily in experiments with nonhuman primates. When animals unknown to each other are put together for the first time, they frequently aggress toward one another. Once hierarchial structures are established, both the frequency and severity of aggression declines. Analogous human situations may exist among families or organizations where structural variables either shift frequently or remain undefined. Clinicians who are responsible for the administration of residential homes and inpatient psychiatric facilities are sensitive to this point: Changes in patient work assignments, patient privileges, and staff responsibilities frequently result in outbursts of aggressive behavior among patients, particularly among long-term residents of such facilities. Psychiatric patients with severe chronic disorders not only have difficulty organizing new information but are also highly sensitive to cues related to space, resource access, and privileges. Changes in information, living rules, and personnel are likely to be perceived as threats and may heighten the probability of defensive aggressive responses.

PSYCHOLOGICAL STATE DATA AND AGGRESSIVE BEHAVIOR

Most mental health professionals have listened to patients who express inordinate amounts of anger toward others. What kinds of patients should one worry about? There are at least three answers to this question: Worry about patients who lack perspective on their anger (that is, patients who do not consider that their anger may reflect their tendency to misinterpret events in the world); worry about patients who continually want to hurt specific others, but in unspecified ways; and worry about those who have a history of episodic aggression. Patients with such characteristics show reduced attention to possible consequences of aggressive behavior and a failure to consider alternative ways of dealing with anger (Table 3.4-3). Another type of patient, one who fails to communicate anger to others, is worrisome for other reasons. Such persons often are highly dependent on the person toward whom they are angry, and unpredictable outbursts of anger occur frequently.

There have been numerous studies into the psychology of anger and aggression. These studies suggest that the principle causes of anger stem from how people interpret and value the behavior of others. Situations in which one is treated unfairly, in which others cause pain, in which others break rules that are normally followed, or in which one wishes to assert authority, are associated with anger. Although it is attractive to view anger as a psychological state linked with aggression, the frequency with which such feelings turn into aggression is still unknown. Other investigations have pointed to a correlation between the degree to which specific interpersonal expectations are not fulfilled and the probability of aggression. "The concept of prerogative or right as an important event the individual feels and, challenging a conspecific as an immediate eliciting stimulus constitute the linchpins of human angry aggression." Still other factors, including symmetry (aggressing toward an equal), asymmetry (aggressing toward an unequal), and motivation type (e.g., offensive, defensive, submissive), appear to influence both the form of aggression and its outcome.

PHYSIOLOGY AND AGGRESSIVE BEHAVIOR

Findings dealing with relationships between psychological states and physiological events reveal an increasingly complex picture. Angry thoughts result in significant increases in diastolic blood pressure and heart rate as well as slower recovery of systolic pressure following exercise. These effects are the opposite of relaxation and may result in physiological states that alter the probability of aggression. Studies of people who repeatedly aggress suggest that some persons use distraction to avoid aversive stimuli. The frequently stated hypothesis that aggression is more likely during increased arousal states is attractive, and although such states may be desirable because of the associated sense of feeling that one is in control of one's environment, arousal-related explanations can explain only part of the data. Studies suggest that persons who aggress may have higher, lower, or more volatile arousal states than controls.

Although most investigators suspect that there are important psychological contributions to aggression, one critical issue remains unresolved: Are the contributions similar both within persons and across persons? Alternate answers to this question have quite different clinical and research implications. The likely answer is that both types of similarity are present only occasionally. Research and clinical assessments of psychological contributions, therefore, should focus as much on dissimilarities as similarities.

HORMONES Aggression has been linked in animals with testosterone, progesterone, luteinizing hormone, renin, β-endorphin, prolactin, melatonin, pyro-glu-Asn-GlyOH, norepinephrine, dopamine, epinephrine, acetylcholine, serotonin, 5-hydroxyindoleacetic acid, and phenylacetic acid, among others. The list may reveal that very little is known; however, it may be that many of the hormones and neurotransmitters listed above are associated with aggression. The authors favor the latter interpretation because it is what is predicted with a multisystem interpretation of aggression. Given this view, a major issue to be resolved is that of identifying interactions between multiple physiological variables. Before discussing some of the more promising possibilities, the following point should be emphasized: None of the evidence for endocrine or neurotransmitter effects on human aggression is conclusive. Moreover, before a clear understanding of endocrine or neurotransmitter contributions is possible, studies that challenge these systems in a variety of contexts are essential.

Testosterone For nearly 3 decades reports have correlated elevated levels of testosterone with aggression. This relationship often is found among lower animals. Among nonhuman primates, correlations between elevated testosterone levels and an increased frequency of aggression sometimes, but not always, are present. Moreover, recent reports suggest that testosterone levels may rise only after aggression and sex (sometimes). Thus, studies over the past decade have been inconsistent in the sense that they have produced conflicting results with respect to a general testosterone-aggression correlation among humans. A possible exception concerns aggression associated with sexual assault: testosterone levels may be high in the vast majority of assaults. These cautious interpretations reflect a now well-supported view that primates differ from lower animals with respect to reliance on hormone elicitation of aggression as well as a better understanding of methodological difficulties associated with conducting well-controlled studies.

Other androgens A similar history applies to other testicular androgens and gonadotropins. Although details remain to be specified, available evidence suggests that the manipulation of intrauterine conditions, particularly those that increase masculinization, alters postbirth behavior. For example, the experimental administration of androgens to pregnant animals can result in offspring who are more aggressive than are nontreated control animals. Analogous situations may occur in humans in situations such as the adrenogenital syndrome. Although numerous studies have been conducted and have produced suggestive results, replication has been inconsistent. Much of the same may be said about the adrenogenital syndrome (mothers' adrenal cortex exposes the fetus to elevated adrenal androgens, resulting in masculinization) and the androgen insensitivity syndrome (in which there is defective binding of androgens to proteins, resulting in male offspring who have a female appearance). Despite early reports, neither group of individuals appears to be significantly more aggressive than normal controls, although increases in rough-and-tumble play in masculinized girls does seem to occur.

NEUROTRANSMITTERS The neurotransmitter data are still far from complete, and one view on the current state of knowledge may be summarized as follows: Generally, cholinergic and catecholaminergic mechanisms seem to be involved in the induction and enhancement of predatory aggression, whereas serotonergic systems and γ-aminobutyric acid (GABA) seem to inhibit this type of behavior. Affective aggression is evidently modulated by both the catecholaminergic and serotonergic systems. Dopamine seems to facilitate aggression, whereas norepinephrine and serotonin appear to inhibit it. Recently, serotonin has again gained attention as a potentially important mediating factor in aggression. It is well known that rapid declines in serotonin levels or function are associated with increased irritability and, in nonhuman primates, with increased aggression. Some human studies have suggested that cerebrospinal fluid of 5-hydroxyindoleacetic acid levels inversely correlate with the frequency of aggression, particularly among persons who commit suicide.

A number of other findings deserve mention because they are suggestive, although they are not yet adequately replicated. First, plasma concentrations of free and conjugated phenylacetic acid (the major metabolite of phenylethylamine) among prisoners serving sentences for violent crimes are reported to be significantly elevated over concentrations among nonviolent control prisoners. Second, a recent report has suggested that in mice there is a relationship between genotype, receptor binding, and behavioral sensitivity to androgen and estrogen. And third, among women, but not men, there may be a correlation between elevated prolactin function and hostility and aggression.

Considering drugs and chemicals, the following generalizations appear to hold: Small doses of alcohol inhibit aggression while large doses facilitate it; barbiturate effects are similar to alcohol effects; aerosols and commercial solvent effects (acute) also resemble alcohol effects; anxiolytics generally inhibit aggression, although paradoxical aggression is sometimes observed; opiate dependence (but not opiate intoxication) is associated with increased aggression, as is the use of stimulants, hallucinogens, and near toxic doses of marijuana. Among persons with psychiatric disorders who are aggressive, drug use or dependence should always be ruled out.

Despite the lack of conclusive data, there are good reasons to suspect direct neurotransmitter and hormone contributions to aggression. The fact that many types of aggression occur nearly instantaneously suggests that physiological systems capable of rapid action (e.g., neurotransmitter systems) are involved. The lack of conclusive findings may be the result of the diversity of forms and circumstances contributing to aggression and the methodological limitations of studies, especially human studies.

NEUROANATOMY AND AGGRESSIVE BEHAVIOR

Compared to surgically induced lesions, the subject of naturally occurring lesions is less emotional. Natural lesions will be discussed first. Anger, rage, and increased irritability are frequent during certain stages of Korsakoff's syndrome and

Huntington's chorea, both diseases that directly affect the brain. Encephalitis lethargica and rabies also are associated with increases in aggression. There is evidence suggesting that the following kinds of lesions are associated with increased aggression: irritable focus lesions; certain forms of epilepsy, particularly temporal lobe and psychomotor; temporal lobe tumors; anterior hypothalamic lesions; frontal lobe lesions; abnormal discharges in the medial amygdala and mesencephalic tegmentum; and dominant hemisphere lesions. Because subject samples often are small and the availability and the quality of lesion analysis differs across studies, the interpretation of findings is controversial. For example, although lesions establish that particular anatomical structures are important in mediating aggression, some structures may be more essential than others.

Animal studies point in several directions. Brain stimulation of the lateral and medial hypothalamus result in different types of aggression. Experimental studies of the amygdala suggests that it has a critical place in aggression. Surgical lesions of only a small part of the amygdala have resulted in members of normally aggressive species (e.g., wildcats) becoming quite tame.

The evidence on psychosurgery remains incomplete. There is some indication that there is an amelioration of aggressive behavior following radical ablation of the temporal lobes. Certainly this occurs in nonhuman primates. Other studies show that surgical lesions around the medial amygdala and the red nucleus tend to reduce recurrent aggressive behavior. Bilateral amygdalectomy is reported to reduce aggression and increase docility in 85 to 92 percent of extremely violent patients. Such percentages seem unusually high, however.

When the results of the preceding studies are considered from another perspective, it is clear that neural systems, not neural centers are involved in aggression. Thus, recent studies have focused on different areas of the brain and different circuitry that influence different types of aggression. These studies show that, among different species, lesions of the olfactory region, lateral septum, medial accumbems, medial hypothalamus, and dorsal and median raphe nuclei alter the form and probability of defensive and predatory aggression, but not social aggression.

TREATMENT

Determining whether a patient is likely to assault another person or commit homicide are critical clinical assessments. Important questions to be asked include: "Is the aggression likely to be situational (e.g., probable because of the presence of another or a particular situation)?" or "Is it seemingly independent of identifiable contextual variables?" Different answers to these questions imply quite different therapeutic interventions. For example, in situation-related aggression, altering situations as well as using drugs may be helpful. If aggression is assumed to be inevitable, hospitalization may be the only alternative. Table 3.4-3 summarizes the characteristics that one should look for and how they influence the probability of aggression, particularly homicide.

Given that one judges that a patient is likely to act aggressively, what are the treatment alternatives? It is probably clinically wise to assume, until there is more specific evidence, that the probability of aggression increases as a function of psychological decompensation. Generally, reduction of decompensation is most rapidly achieved through the use of drugs. Current reports suggest that different types of drugs as well as different types of clinical monitoring (e.g., blood pressure, electroencephalogram) are essential for optimal treatment in aggressive persons suffering from psychiatric disorders. These reports may be summarized as follows: Lithium is reported to be a drug of promise for some populations of violent patients (e.g., for the nonacute patient and for maintenance), especially adolescent, delinquent boys (controlled studies are lacking, however); anticonvulsants occasionally reduce seizure-induced forms of aggression and they may have the same effect among nonepileptics; antipsychotic medications appear to reduce aggression in both psychotic and nonpsychotic violent patients; antidepressants may be effective in reducing violence in some depressed patients; minor tranquilizers appear to have a limited role in reducing aggression; antiandrogen agents may be effective in the treatment of sex offenders; β-blockers and stimulants may be effective in aggressive children; and electroconvulsive therapy may be effective in selected patients.

At this writing, there is no specific antiaggressive drug available, although this statement may require retraction as a result of a number of new drugs currently under study. For example, current data from studies of "normal" nonhuman primates suggest that serotonin agonists significantly reduce aggressive behavior. What remains to be determined is whether such drugs reduce aggression among persons suffering from psychiatric disorders. The type of aggressive behavior reduced among nonhuman primates is normal aggression, part of the everyday existence of group-living animals. If aggression among persons with psychiatric disorders is an extension of this type of aggression (as the authors have suggested), such drugs are likely to be effective.

Dealing with aggression using psychotherapy techniques is a complex matter, and no standard formula is applicable. Therapists should first consider the possibility that a single episode of aggressive behavior, as contrasted with repeated violent aggressive behavior, may be normal. Aggression may be provoked in psychiatric patients by persons with whom they interact and social situations in which patients find themselves. A further consideration is the assessment of patients' tendencies to interpret events in ways that lead to anger or aggressive responses. With certain patients, tendencies to misinterpret can be altered through frequent interactions with a therapist.

Some additional points are worth considering because of their helpfulness in clarifying certain situations: Behavioral effects of drugs differ across social settings; catharsis (once thought to be tension-reducing) does not appear to decrease aggression; punishment occasionally works as a deterrent; and, generally, if there is an obvious biological component (e.g., brain lesion, seizure disorder), psychotherapy is unlikely to be effective.

ETHICAL ISSUES

Largely because of the enactment of recent laws, mental health professionals are no longer able to establish their ethical standards without reference to legal statutes governing certain types of professional conduct. The details or relevant laws and their means of enforcement differ from state to state. Nonetheless, certain ethical principles have general applicability in most states: If a patient is likely to harm others, there is a legal and ethical obligation to protect endangered others; if a patient is likely to harm himself or herself, there is an obligation to intervene in a medically appropriate way. Readers who wish details on these issues are

TABLE 3.4-3
Assessing the Risk of Committing a Homicide*

Clinical Characteristics	*Low*	*Medium*	*High*
Inimicality (past history):			
Family Life	Wanted child, good loving family	Some family disruption, loss of a parent or one-parent family	Early violence, battered child, poor parent model
Significant others	Several reliable family or friends available	Few or one available	None available
Daily functioning	Good in most activities	Moderately good in some activities	Not good in any activities
Life-style	Stable	Moderately stable	Unstable
Socioeconomic	Upper	Middle	Lower
Employment	Employed	Employment history fairly stable	Unemployed
Education	High school graduate or more (university or technical training)	High school dropout, can read and write	School dropout, semiliterate to illiterate
Housing	Lives in adequate housing, clean environment and space	Fair housing, some overcrowding	Poor housing, crowded, slums
Isolation or withdrawal	Able to relate well to others, outgoing	Mild, some withdrawal and feelings of hopelessness	Long history of being a loner, antisocial, withdrawn, hopeless, helpless feelings
Alcohol or drug use	Nondrinker, occasional social use	Social drinker or user to occasional abuse	Chronic abuse
Psychological help	No history of need for or use of psychiatric hospitalization	Some outpatient psychiatric help, moderately satisfied with self	History of psychiatric hospitalization, negative view of help
Personal history†	No history of violence or impulsive behavior	Occasional history of violence or impulsive behavior	Frequent history of violence or impulsive behavior
Perturbation (negative emotional states):			
Anxiety	Low, good emotional control	Occasional feelings of anxiety	Easily aroused to anxiety, high or panic state
Depression	Low	Occasional depression	Severe, chronically moody
Self-esteem	Good, has reinforcements from others	Usually good; has times of being put down and not able to handle	Chronically poor self-image
Hostility	Low	Some	Marked, aggressive
Impulse control	Controlled	Some impulsive acting out not physically violent	Feels need for violence
Constriction (narrowing of vision):			
Coping strategies and devices being utilized	Able to cope with stress and outside irritating influences; well-developed defense mechanisms	Usually can cope under most pressures; sometimes becomes constrictive in thinking and acts out	Becomes constrictive under most stress; acts out in destructive socially unacceptable ways
Disorientation and disorganization	None, is in good contact with what is happening	Little to moderate	Marked, losing contact with reality
Resources	Able to make good use of resources available	Some use, aware of most resources	Either unable to use resources available or recognize that there is help available
Cessation (stop the person causing the problem):			
Previous arrests	None	Has been arrested, has not served time	Multiple arrest history, served time in prison, would murder to avoid going back to prison
Previous homicide	None	Has exhibited aggressive behavior, been in fights but no attempt to kill another	Yes, looks at the killing of another as a feasible act
Homicide plan	None	Has held fleeting thoughts of killing another, no definite plan	Frequent or constant thoughts with a specific plan
Weapon available	None that person thinks of	Yes, person aware of weapons in immediate environment but not seriously considering use	Yes, and planning on use (a loaded gun should be considered as highly lethal)

*This table lists clinical characteristics of persons who are potential homicidal risks and relates characteristics to low-, medium-, and high-risk persons. No one clinical characteristic predicts homicide. However, the greater the number of clinical characteristics that are present in the medium and high categories, the greater the risk. Adapted from Allen N: *Homicide: Perspectives on Prevention*. Human Sciences Press, New York, 1979, with permission.

†Added by authors of this section.

advised to search out further expertise for areas in which they work. Criteria for seclusion and restraint are particularly pertinent with respect to this point.

REFERENCES

Allen N: *Homicide: Perspectives on Prevention*. Human Sciences Press, New York, 1979.

Averill J R: *Anger and Aggression. An Essay on Emotion*. Springer-Verlag, New York, 1982.

Baron R A: Aggression. In *Comprehensive Textbook of Psychiatry*, H I Kaplan, B J Sadock, editors, ed 4, p 213. Williams & Wilkins, Baltimore, 1985.

Blanchard D C, Blanchard R J: Affect and aggression: An animal model applied to human behavior. In *Advances in the Study of Aggression*, R J Blanchard, D C Blanchard, editors, vol 1, p 1. Academic Press, Orlando, FL, 1984.

Brain, P F: Biological explanations of human aggression and the resulting therapies offered by such approaches: A critical evaluation. In *Advances in the Study of Aggression*, R J Blanchard, D C Blanchard, editors, vol 1, p 63. Academic Press, Orlando, FL, 1984.

Brown, G L, Goodwin F K, Bunney W E Jr: Human aggression and suicide: Their relationship to neuropsychiatric diagnoses and serotonin metabolism. In *Serotonin in Biological Psychiatry*, B T Ho, J C Schoolar, E Usdin, editors. Raven Press, New York, 1982.

Kling, A S: The anatomy of aggression and affiliation. In *Emotion: Theory, Research, and Experience*, vol 3, p 237. Academic Press, Orlando, FL, 1986.

Krakowski M, Volavka J, Brizer D: Psychopathology and violence: A review of literature. Comp Psychiat *27*(2): 131, 1986.

Lion J R, Reid W H: *Assaults Within Psychiatric Facilities*. Grune & Stratton, Orlando, FL, 1983.

McGuire M T, Raleigh M J, Brammer G L: Sociopharmacology. Ann Rev Pharmacol Toxicol *22:* 643, 1982.

McKenna J J: Primate aggression and evolution: An overview of sociobiological and anthropological perspectives. Bull Amer Acad Psychiat Law, *11*(2): 105, 1983.

Plutchik, R: Universal problems of adaptation: Hierarchy, territoriality, identity, and temporality. In *Environmental and Population: Problems of Adaptation*, J B Calhoun, editor, p 223. Praeger, New York, 1983.

Raleigh M J, Brammer G L, McGuire M T, Yuwiler, A: Dominant social status facilitates the behavioral effects of serotonergic agonists. Brain Res *348:* 274, 1985.

Rushton J P, Fulker D W, Neale M C, Nias D K B, Eysenck H J: Altruism and aggression: The heritability of individual differences. J Personal Soc Psychol *50*(6): 1192, 1986.

Schiavi P C, Theilgaard A, Owen D R, White D: Sex chromosome anomalies, hormones, and aggressivity. Arch Gen Psychiat *41:* 93, 1984.

Singhal R L, Telner J I: A perspective: Psychopharmacological aspects of aggression in animals and man. Psychiat J Univ Ottawa, *8*(3): 145, 1983.

Tardiff, K: *The Psychiatric Uses of Seclusion and Restraint*. Washington, DC: American Psychiatric Press, 1984.

Tardiff K, Koenigsberg H W: Assaultive behavior among psychiatric outpatients. Amer J Psychiat *142*(8): 960, 1985.

Tardiff K, Sweillam A: Assaultive behavior among chronic inpatients. Amer J Psychiat *139:* 212, 1982.

CHAPTER 4 CONTRIBUTIONS OF THE SOCIOCULTURAL SCIENCES

4.1 ANTHROPOLOGY AND PSYCHIATRY

MELVIN KONNER, Ph.D., M.D.

INTRODUCTION

Traditional accounts of the relationship between anthropology and psychiatry have usually been limited to cultural psychiatry: the definition of culture, interactions between it and the individual, culture-specific syndromes, and cross-cultural differences in definitions of health, illness, and healing. These categories, important as they are, represent only a part of the interface between the two fields as it now potentially exists. When this interface was first extensively explored, during the 1930s and 1940s, psychoanalytic theory seemed the most promising domain in psychiatry, and it independently interested anthropologists as a powerful tool for the study of culture. The interaction between psychoanalysts or psychiatrists and anthropologists was both natural and fruitful.

It became clear that cultures differ in their definitions of health, illness, and healing, and also vary greatly in child-rearing patterns, social models and expectations, role opportunities, and other major variables that would be anticipated by psychodynamic theory to influence the etiology and course of psychiatric disorders. However, it is equally necessary to realize that both anthropology and psychiatry have been drastically transformed during the past 30 years, owing largely, though not exclusively, to the increasing importance of biology in each of those fields. The interface between them has become much more complex, and a new and more usable description of it is in order. The goal of this section is to reconceptualize in current terms the relationship between anthropology and psychiatry. (Parenthetical notes in the text refer by number to pertinent cases in the appendix.)

BIOLOGY, PSYCHOLOGY, AND CULTURE: HISTORICAL PERSPECTIVE

Psychiatry has been transformed from a primarily psychological to a truly biopsychological discipline. Inevitably, this change has been somewhat wrenching, and what is described as eclectic psychiatry is often a not very well-integrated amalgam of psychodynamics, psychopharmacology, and behavioral and clinical pragmatism. The transformation of anthropology during the same period has been parallel in important ways. As cultural anthropology pioneers Alfred L. Kroeber and Margaret Mead had recognized by the 1950s, the increasing delineation of cross-cultural variety must inevitably carry with it the potential for describing the invariant features of human behavior and mental life. This observation proved to be a prescient one, as the description of universals of language, culture, facial expression, parent-offspring interaction, and many other aspects of human life was soon possible. These universals constitute a part of what is meant by human nature, a term that must be considered again, after decades of disfavor, as having scientific legitimacy.

In the nineteenth century, it was not unusual for treatises on aspects of human psychology to refer to ethnographic data. Charles Darwin's 1872 book on facial expression cited the occurrence of certain expressions in primitive societies as evidence of their biological basis, and attempted to relate them to facial expressions in nonhuman animals in an evolutionary sequence. Edward Westermarck, whose theory of incest aversion is still read and tested today, appealed to ethnographic evidence to illuminate a deeper psychodynamic process he considered to be as universal as certain facial expressions. In the late nineteenth century, it was common for prominent anthropologists to attempt to array nonindustrial societies in an evolutionary sequence, whether of social complexity, religion, or language. And in the early years of the twentieth century, ethnological expeditions tested members of primitive societies for the presence of proposed perceptual universals.

These trends, which might be seen as early efforts to characterize human nature and its origins, were transformed by the development of modern social and cultural anthropology and by the parallel emergence of psychoanalysis. Anthropologists on both sides of the Atlantic, despite many differences of opinion, came to share a contempt for evolutionary sequencing of cultures, replacing this effort with accurate, if not exhaustive, descriptive characterizations of cultures as independent units. Proposed universals of human behavior or mental function were met with equal skepticism, and anthropologists still delight in the opportunity to say, "Not among my people they don't," a kind of statement that has been aptly called the anthropological veto.

Psychoanalytic theory Early generalizations by Jean Piaget and others were tested cross-culturally, but none elicited the same enthusiasm that was aroused by psychoanalysis. The British social anthropologist Bronislaw Malinowski attempted to demolish the universality of the Oedipus complex by describing a separation of male authority (vested in the mother's brother) from the object of male jealousy (the biological father) in his society in the Trobriand Islands (an argument still actively debated). With the skeptical encouragement of Franz Boas, the dean of American anthropology, disciples, such as Margaret Mead, attempted to test certain psychoanalytic convictions by means of cross-cultural comparison, and, at the same time, to use psychoanalytic and other psychodynamic theory to explain culture.

The fundamental theorem of this school was that cultures are distinctive because of distinctive patterns of child rearing, and that a unified approach combining psychoanalysis and cultural anthropology could explain culture and elucidate laws of psychological development simultaneously. During World War II, this approach reached its most exuberant florescence with dubious speculations about the national character of Russians, Japanese, Germans, and Americans, relating these speculations to nonquantitative, even anecdotal, observations of infant and child care. Sigmund Freud's method, difficult enough when applied to a single patient studied in a concentrated way for hundreds of hours over a period of years, was thus adopted for a completely distinct task, for which it was almost unquestionably inappropriate.

By the 1950s, the approach had generated research that to some extent delegitimized it through refinement and measurement. Both the assessment of adult psychological disposition and the objective description of child training were made quantitative, the first through projective testing and the second through direct behavior observation, with interviews supporting both approaches. Cora Dubois and Anthony F. C. Wallace demonstrated, through projective testing and interviewing, that even small-scale societies with relatively homogeneous cultures do not have something properly called basic personality (an entity corresponding to national character in large-scale societies). Individual variation in personality and character is great in every known culture, however primitive. At best, there is perhaps a modal personality (from the statistical concept of mode) shared by a substantial minority of a culture's members—as shown by Wallace for two distinctive native American groups. In any case, a culture must derive its distinctiveness from the particular mutual articulation of its various personality types, and the opportunities it provides for their expression, rather than from fundamental tendencies shared by a majority—a sort of symphony orchestra model of culture and personality.

Child training John Whiting and Beatrice Whiting, in the meanwhile, were trying to put the cross-cultural study of child training on a scientific foundation. A landmark 1953 study by John Whiting and Irvin Child demonstrated that themes in childhood experience of interest to psychoanalysts are correlated with similar themes in religion, folklore, and other cultural expressions (which they pointedly called projective systems) in a large cross-cultural sample. They focused on a culture's traditional explanations of illness and its treatment, reasoning that these particular beliefs might reflect chronic, shared anxieties. For example, cultures rated as causing high levels of anxiety to infants and children in relation to their oral needs (as through early weaning or the withholding of food as a form of punishment) tended to be the same cultures that used oral themes in the explanation of illness (for example, as a result of the ingestion of prohibited foods). Cultures in which child-training anxieties were high in the area of aggressive behavior tended to be those in which adults explained illness as an attack by a human sorcerer or an evil spirit.

The researchers recognized, however, that such correlations might arise from causes other than the ones most friendly to psychoanalysis, and also that childhood experience needed to be measured much more rigorously. The Whitings devoted the next 3 decades to such measurement in a number of societies around the world and developed a model of the influence of fundamental features of society—such as ecology, economy, and vulnerability to external attack—on child-training practices that might give rise to certain consistent adult predispositions. But it was rarely possible to establish causality in these relationships beyond the level of correlations, and many cultural anthropologists became disillusioned with such theories.

Cross-cultural diagnosis A parallel development relevant to cultural psychiatry was the attempt to study systematically the incidence of psychiatric disorders cross-culturally, an approach associated with the reputation of Jane Murphy and Alexander Leighton, among others. This attempt continues to be fruitful, but is beset by doubts about the cross-cultural validity of diagnostic categories. Recent attempts to rationalize nosology at the international and national levels reveal similar obstacles to cross-cultural diagnosis. Nevertheless, certain still-valid conclusions soon emerged from such work: First, both the general category of psychological deviance and at least several major syndromes appear to be characteristic of all cultures for which information is available; second, some psychiatric disorders appear to be relatively or largely culture-specific; and third, it is extremely difficult, if not impossible, usefully to compare incidence or prevalence of most disorders cross-culturally, much less to draw conclusions about the etiology of alleged cross-cultural differences in prevalence.

Medical anthropology Also by the late 1950s, the subdiscipline of medical anthropology had emerged and had established certain firm generalizations. The sick role, whether in relation to psychological or physical illness, occurs in all cultures but carries many different meanings and expectations. The same ailment, even what is apparently the same degree of physical pain, varies greatly in designation and interpretation, to the extent that some cultures recognize diseases unrecognized as abnormalities in others, and some encourage the expression of pain while others discourage it.

In early Christianity, which was a healing religion, the suffering of illness was to be borne, and could bring about a state of grace. Among the !Kung San, hunter-gatherers of the Kalahari, the sick person was under attack from the spirit world and an aggressive stance against the spirits might be appropriate. Among the Kaluli of New Guinea, a person's body is dark to the *sei,* an evil spirit that resides in another person, who is usually unaware of it. But if the person becomes upset or angry, or has a minor illness, the body may become bright to the *sei,* and the person may die as a result. A classic study of subcultural or ethnic group differences in American cities revealed that both Jewish and Italian patients feel free to express their pain whereas "Old Americans" do not. Italian-Americans are oriented to the pain itself and express confident gratitude toward the doctor when pain remits. Both Old Americans and Jews are more oriented to the prognosis, but the former are optimistic about it whereas the latter remain skeptical of the doctor.

Finally, the role and responsibility of the healer show a comparable degree of variation. The Christian physician—even the modern fundamentalist trained by Oral Roberts—joins healing to salvation. The !Kung healer enters a deep trance, risking life and limb as his soul leaves his body (and he runs off into the bush or dives into the fire) so he can berate the spirits on behalf of the sick person. The Kaluli heal by holding a violent dance in which dancers are given repeated second-degree torch burns by their hosts, in a spectacle that both celebrates and expresses the primary oppositions of human life. The *sei,* charmed by the life-enhancing ceremony, forgets his anger against the sick person. And as for American ethnic groups, every physician knows that their more traditional members may require different bedside manners. These sorts of findings have usually been presumed to have stronger implications in the realm of psychiatric illness and treatment than in other branches of medicine.

Current approaches The stage was now set for the transformation of anthropology that began in the 1960s. Although some cultural anthropologists drifted out of the stream of science altogether, finding their affinities with literary criticism and philosophy, the main body of the discipline became increasingly quantitative, scientific, and biological in orientation. The four subfields of traditional American anthropology—cultural anthropology, archaeology, linguistics, and biological anthropology—became, for many anthropologists, reunified in an enterprise that had been moribund since the late nineteenth century: the characterization of human nature and its evolutionary origins. Not every member of each subfield subscribed to this purpose, but it became once again a highly legitimate purpose, and the only one that could fairly be said to have the potential for unifying and invigorating anthropology as a whole.

This enterprise advanced on seven fronts simultaneously: (1) the adoption, extension, and testing of evolutionary theory, particularly as it applies to behavior; (2) the characterization of human origins as revealed in an ever-improving fossil record; (3) the systematic description and analysis of the behavior of nonhuman primates, both in order to test evolutionary theory and to make inferences about the behavior of humanity's protohuman ancestors; (4) the study of contemporary and recent hunting-gathering societies, with a view toward making inferences about behavior and social organization in the environment of human evolutionary adaptedness; (5) the rise of scientific archaeology, with its attempt to reconstruct the social worlds of past societies and relate them to the recent ones studied by cultural anthropologists; (6) the corresponding attempt by cultural anthropologists to understand ecological influences on stability and change in contemporary nonindustrial societies—for example, hunter-gatherer societies that become settled and gain access to cow's milk shorten their birth spacing, with many consequences for social structure and psychological development; and finally, (7) the characterization of cross-cultural universals of language, nonverbal behavior, and culture—including universals of abnormal behavior, of its classification, and of attempts at healing.

These approaches proceeded in parallel with the continued vigorous effort to document the extant, and unfortunately steadily disappearing, variety of human cultures. Some cultural anthropologists remain aloof from this unified enterprise, but they admit to being aloof from science as a whole. The majority of anthropologists who work within it are laying the foundations for a science of human nature—the results of which are of increasing significance to psychiatry.

BIOLOGICAL AND BEHAVIORAL EVOLUTION

The fossil evidence for human and protohuman evolution has accumulated steadily for more than 100 years. However, new discoveries are made each year that add details, and during the past 2 decades, biochemical taxonomy has further altered understanding. Many controversies remain. Thus, it is clear that the chimpanzee (although perhaps the pygmy chimpanzee *Pan paniscus* rather than the common chimpanzee *Pan troglodytes*) is the human being's closest relative, but estimates of the time of divergence of the human from the ape line range from as little as 5 to as much as 13 million years ago. It is clear that there were more than one contemporaneous species of hominids (protohuman-like forms) at around 2 million years ago, but there may have been as few as two or as many as four. It is clear that upright posture was established before most of human brain evolution took place, but the lag between the two and the role of tool using or tool making in brain evolution remains controversial.

There is therefore little to be gained for the purposes of psychiatry in closely following each argument in human paleontology. It will be decades before agreement is reached on many points that might be relevant to the understanding of the origins of human behavior. However, there is much to be gained from understanding (1) the general higher primate background of human evolution; (2) the environment of human evolutionary adaptedness, that of hunting and gathering; and (3) the principles of evolutionary adaptation as applied to behavior and reproduction. These three categories of knowledge can be defined in such a way as to be relatively resistant to future disruption by discoveries regarding the details of paleontology and evolutionary lineages.

HIGHER PRIMATE BACKGROUND All higher primates without exception are social animals with great learning capacity, and with the mother-offspring bond at the center of social life. This bond is always prolonged, as is the anatomical and behavioral course of individual development, including each phase of the life cycle as well as of the life span as a whole. Laboratory and field studies demonstrate the capacity for complex social cognition and learning, up to and including cultural transmission of social rank, tool-using techniques, and knowledge of location of food sources. Play, especially social play, is characteristic of all primate species, particularly during development, and there are various reasons to believe it to be an important opportunity for learning. As shown by Paul MacLean, the higher primate emphasis on both the mother-infant bond and play represents an intensification of the pattern established by the early mammals, and is essential to the understanding of the phylogeny of the limbic system and the emotions.

Primate groups generally include a core of genetically related individuals with associated nonrelatives. In most instances, the core is a matrilineage, stable over the life course of individuals; but in a few species, including the common chimpanzee, the core is a patrilineage, and the females are unrelated migrants. In any case, the distribution of acts of social support and generosity is preferentially toward genetic relatives, but not exclusively so. Monkeys and apes aid nonrelatives, and can usually expect reciprocal aid. Cooperation is ubiquitous, but so is competition, and one of the major purposes of cooperation is mutual defense against conspecifics. Conflict is frequent, with both sexes participating, but with males generally exhibiting more aggression than females.

Beyond these broad generalizations, great variation exists in social organization both between and within species. Monogamy is present in some South American monkeys and in gibbons, but in most species, larger group associations subsuming more temporary (although sometimes more than transient—see Case N1) associations between individual males and individual females are the rule. Among orangutans *(Pongo pygmaeus),* despite their relatively close relationship to humans, the usual social groupings are a female with her offspring, and (separate from those units) solitary males. The causes of this variation in higher primate social organization remain obscure, although some relevant evolutionary principles will be considered below.

Some generalizations may also be made about the nature and social context of individual development among monkeys and apes. Because the New World monkeys separated from the Old World monkeys and the apes approximately 40 million years ago, some of these generalizations do not apply to all New World monkeys. However, they do apply to all the *catarrhines,* a category that subsumes all Old World higher primates, including monkeys, apes, and humans. (The rationale for including humans in these generalizations will be clear in the next subsection.) The catarrhine mother-infant complex is characterized by (1) a hemochorial placenta, with exceptionally intimate maternal-fetal circulation; (2) single birth; (3) frequent nursing, at least four times an hour; (4) late weaning, at around 30 percent of the age at first estrus or menses; (5) direct mother-infant physical contact more than 90 percent of the time in the immediate postnatal months; (6) close mother-infant proximity at least until weaning; (7) gradual transition to a multiaged play group; and (8) variable but low direct involvement of adult males in most species.

One of the great advantages of interpreting primate field studies in relation to human behavior is the existence of an increasing body of laboratory data on the consequences of manipulation of early rearing conditions. These experiments provide an epistemological link between anthropological primatology and psychiatry. Although there are important species variations, it may be generally said that higher primates are sensitive to significant perturbations of the early social environment, such as isolation rearing or repeated involuntary mother-infant separation, and that these perturbations give rise to abnormalities of sexual, maternal, and aggressive behavior that in humans would be viewed as psychopathology.

In a number of species, isolation rearing gives rise to stereotyped behavior, such as rocking and self-directed aggression, and mother-infant separation gives rise to symptoms usually described as protest followed by depression. Even deprivation of contact with peers during development has produced abnormal behavior in many experiments. Apparent human analogues of these causal relationships, although difficult to interpret, have encouraged the use of primate models. Equally important, these experiments greatly enhance the interpretive value of field studies of higher primate behavior for psychiatry, and emphasize the extent to which the normal development of behavior in such animals has come to depend, in the course of evolution, on an intact social matrix.

Natural variation in stable individual behavior patterns (personality) occurs in free-ranging monkey and ape groups, and extends to variants that would be considered pathological if seen in humans, such as hyperaggressive, isolative, phobic, or depressed behavior. It is rarely possible to explore the etiology of such variants, but most cannot result from specific abnormalities of social rearing such as are deliberately instituted in typical laboratory experiments. Most variants are probably both genetic and environmental in etiology. Some abnormalities, such as severe depression—as in Case N2, an 8-year-old wild chimpanzee, after the death of its mother—may be incompatible with survival. Others, however, such as hyperaggressiveness—as in Case N3, a female chimpanzee that, together with her daughter, systematically and repeatedly killed the infants of other females—may actually enhance reproductive adaptation for the abnormal individual. This theoretical possibility is taken up in greater detail below.

HUNTING-AND-GATHERING ENVIRONMENT The above generalizations apply to the social and psychological world of protohuman higher primate species for a period of approximately 40 million years. Against this background hominids evolved during the past few million years, culminating in the emergence of our species within the past few hundred thousand years, and finally in the appearance of truly modern Homo sapiens about 30,000 to 40,000 years ago. The latest evidence from comparative studies of human mitochondrial deoxyribonucleic acid (DNA) indicates that all people living today originated from a small group of individuals who lived no more than 200,000 years ago—strongly arguing for the biological unity of humankind. Aside from the rise in intelligence, as indicated by increasing relative and absolute brain size as well as by increasing complexity of stone tools, one hallmark of the transition to hominids was a greater reliance on hunting. All monkeys and apes are largely vegetarian, and the instances of meat eating are instructive but relatively infrequent.

Among the most technologically primitive humans, whether in the fossil or ethnographic record, hunting is invariably of major importance. Most of the stone tools that have survived archaeologically were used in hunting or butchering, and the demands of hunting have long been held to be central to the emergence of human intelligence and social organization. Recent evidence has shown that the stone used for this purpose had to be traded over long distances, implying unexpectedly complex social networks earlier than 2 million years ago. Furthermore, even chimpanzees share meat after a kill (but not plant foods), and among human hunter-gatherers, adherence to elaborate regulations for such sharing of meat may be a life-and-death matter. Finally, with one noteworthy exception (the Agta of the Philippines, where women routinely hunt), all hunting-and-gathering societies in the ethnographic record have a division of labor by sex—men do almost all the hunting and provide the meat, and women supply most of the plant foods. For these reasons, among others, it may be that the advent of hunting accounted for some peculiarly human aspects of social life, but these features had to have been grafted to the already complex social life characteristic of nonhuman higher primates.

This traditional male-centered view, however, gives at most half of the story. In many hunting-and-gathering societies, plant foods gathered by women constitute much more than half of the diet. Plant foods are shared in these societies (although not beyond the immediate family) but are not shared by nonhuman primates. Postweaning mortality is much higher in nonhuman primate juveniles than in human children, and it has been speculated that the provision of children with plant foods by human mothers accounts for this difference. The early advent of upright posture may have had more to do with the need for females to carry plant foods as well as infants to a base camp than with any advantage that upright posture might confer in hunting. It may be that digging sticks and carrying devices for plants or infants were among the first tools invented, probably by women. These tools, however crucial to daily life, would not have been preserved in archaeological collections.

The psychodynamic theorist John Bowlby seems to have been responsible for the phrase "the environment of human evolutionary adaptedness," which aptly describes the hunting-and-gathering way of life. The phrase correctly implies that this environment is, or was, the context for which natural selection prepared human beings, and from which they departed only during the past 10,000 years, a short time in evolutionary terms. (The industrial revolution, in the same terms, happened only a moment ago.) From many studies of recent and current hunting-and-gathering peoples, combined with archaeological evidence of those of the distant past, it is possible to make certain generalizations about this context: (1) social groups are usually small, ranging in size from 15 to 40 people related through blood or marriage; (2) groups are nomadic, moving frequently to take advantage of changing subsistence opportunities, and are flexible in composition, size, and adaptive strategies; (3) daily life involves physical challenge, vigorous exercise, and occasional hunger, but with a usually dependable food base acquired by a moderate work effort, and with a marked division of labor by gender; (4) diseases, mainly infectious, produce high rates of mortality, especially in infancy and early childhood, with consequent frequent experience of loss; (5) virtually all of life's activities are carried out in a highly social context with people one knows well—often the same people for different activities; (6) privacy is limited, but creative expression in the arts is possible, and conflicts and problems are dealt with through extensive group discussions. (Case H1, a woman among the !Kung San of Botswana, illustrates some of these points.)

These generalizations describe the contexts in which almost all of human evolution and history have taken place, so it is often said that modern people are, in effect, hunter-gatherers wearing business clothes and pursuing their prey in skyscrapers. Simplistic observations about the consequences of this change are useless. Life in these societies was, and is, not simply more or less stressful; the stresses are quite different. Social density crudely measured is neither demonstrably higher nor lower, but strangers are rarely encountered and privacy or loneliness is unusual. A truly thoughtful set of observations and analyses of the differences between psychological conditions in modern and past societies—unaffected by the common biases either for or against such societies—could be imagined but has not yet been carried out.

Childhood experience Baby and child care can also be seen to be distinctive in such societies, and includes the following: (1) frequent breast feeding (up to four times an hour) and late weaning (up to 4 years of age); (2) close mother-infant contact, including extensive skin-to-skin carrying and adjacent sleeping until weaning (Fig. 4.1-1); (3) prompt response to infant crying and indulgent response to other infant and child demands; (4) a gradual transition from an intense mother-infant bond to a multiaged child-play group of mixed gender; (5) minimal assignment of responsibility in the sense of chores or schooling in middle childhood, with learning taking place through observation and play; (6) liberal premarital sexual mores with sex play throughout middle childhood gradually giving rise to adolescent sexuality, but with late menarche limiting opportunities for childbearing until the late teens.

These characteristics of hunter-gatherer childhood extend the patterns found among nonhuman higher primates. Some of these features, such as universal breast feeding and sleeping in the same room with the infant, usually in the same bed, can be generalized to all nonindustrialized societies. Other characteristics, such as a high degree of premarital sexual freedom, are significantly more applicable to hunting-and-gathering societies than they are to agricultural or herding societies. Either way, they are likely characteristics of the environment of human evolutionary adaptedness, and they accordingly suggest many hypotheses about the possible consequences of the departures from these patterns made by modern industrial societies. Few, if any, such hypotheses have been properly tested.

Largely because of morbidity and mortality, the hunter-gatherer pattern of childhood experience is not idyllic. But frustration and loss come mainly from inadvertent features of the environment rather than from parental attitudes. As for the outcome of these child care practices, both major and minor mental illnesses are present in such societies. All experience

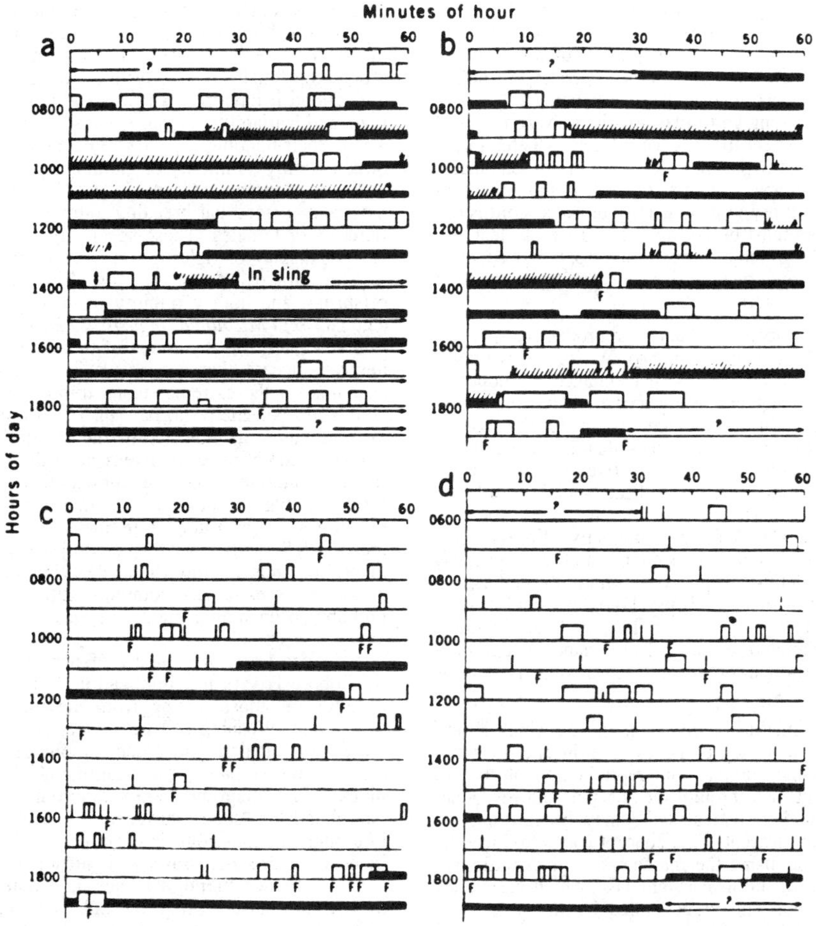

FIGURE 4.1-1. *Breast feeding in hunter-gatherers. A day in the life of each of four infants among !Kung San hunter-gatherers of northwestern Botswana in 1975.* (a) *A 4-day-old boy;* (b) *the same boy at 15 days;* (c) *a 12-month-old girl;* (d) *a 17-month-old boy. The long dark bars are sleep. The higher open bars and vertical lines are nursing bouts. (From Konner M, Worthman C: Nursing frequency, gonadal function and birth spacing among !Kung hunter-gatherers. Science 207*: 788, 1980, with permission.)

some level of violent conflict, including homicide. In one group, the !Kung San (Bushmen) of Botswana, homicide rates are higher than in American cities, belying the common description of this group as "the harmless people." Human behaviors often considered normal but undesirable, such as selfishness, deceit, adolescent rebellion, adultery, desertion, and child abuse, occur in such societies (Case H1), although it is impossible to compare the rates of such behaviors with those in other societies.

Such societies are fluid in their way, but life in them proceeds among a very small number of people, and the lack of privacy must constitute a stress just as crowding and high levels of contact with strangers may cause stress for today's society. Morbidity and mortality, as well as the stresses and uncertainties of the daily food quest, must also take their psychological toll.

NEO-DARWINIAN THEORY OF BEHAVIOR Since the late 1960s, an influential new field of evolutionary study known as *neo-Darwinian theory* or, more commonly, *sociobiology,* has emerged. This new set of principles has been quickly adopted by most investigators who study animal behavior under natural conditions, including ethologists and behavioral ecologists, and has also influenced many anthropologists and psychologists. Briefly summarized, the principles are as follows:

1. An organism is a gene's way of making another gene. Put more strictly, an organism is a way found by thousands of genes, through short- or long-term cooperation, to make copies of themselves. As long as it is admitted that there can be no forces operating in nature other than physicochemical ones, then it must be admitted that continued membership in an ongoing germ plasm is the only goal served by any given gene. To the extent that a gene influences behavior, it can only continue in the germ plasm if it maintains or enhances, through the behavior, the number of copies of itself in the gene pool of the next generation. (Contrary to a frequently repeated confusion, the fact that most behaviors must be multigenic and largely learned, and the cohesiveness of the genome through pleiotropy and epistatic and regulatory effects have only quantitative, not qualitative, bearing on the validity of this principle.)

2. Genes increase their number by enhancing reproductive success. Enhancing survival is only one way of doing so. Where the two goals are in conflict, as they often are, genes that enhance reproductive success will replace genes that enhance survival. The concept of fitness in evolutionary theory has no meaning except for the relative frequency of characteristics and of the genes that influence them. Fitness is a tautological dimension of reproductive success and has nothing necessarily in common with its medical, social, or athletic definitions, all of which can be achieved without an increase, or even with a decrease, in technically defined reproductive fitness. This principle has profound implications for medicine, and for psychiatry especially. We attempt to adjust people to a commonly understood professional standard of medical and psychological equilibrium, usually subscribed to by patients, their families, or both. In many particulars, this goal is unrelated to the goal of enhancing reproductive fitness, for which the human organism, like all organisms, was primarily designed.

3. Fitness is properly defined as *inclusive fitness,* by which evolutionary theorists mean the tendency of genes to influence their frequency not only through the survival and reproduction of the individual carrying them, but also through the survival and reproduction of other closely related individuals who may be carrying the same gene through common descent. This concept was introduced by W. D. Hamilton to account, using the mathematics of evolutionary genetics, for the existence of altruism in animals, which previously seemed to be something that should be culled by the process of natural selection. Thus, a newly defined subprocess of natural selection, called *kin selection,* was needed. If one twin dies to save an identical twin, then the frequency of any gene that helped predispose the first twin to that action will (all else being equal) be unaffected by the death. In general terms, such genes, or any genes predisposing an individual to self-sacrifice for a relative, should be favored under conditions where $b/c > 1/r$, where b is the benefit to the recipient, c is the cost to the altruist, and r is the degree of genetic relatedness, or the likelihood that any gene found in one individual is identical to the same gene found in another *by common descent.* This concept has been invoked to explain self-sacrifice of soldier ants for the colony, alarm calls of birds and ground squirrels, and nepotism in human beings, among many other phenomena of animal and human behavior. Other theories that have been brought to bear on the problem of altruism are reciprocal altruism and the prisoner's dilemma model of cooperation, neither of which requires that the altruist and the recipient be related. Reciprocal altruism assumes that the organism has some memory capacity and lives long enough to repay an act of generosity with a reciprocal one—directed preferentially toward the same individual. Unfortunately for this theory, it is difficult to make such a system resistant to the evolution of cheating. The prisoner's dilemma model makes the reciprocity simultaneous—in effect, it involves cooperation. The game consists of a situation in which two prisoners must either cooperate or not cooperate (defect). The game is arranged so that the reward is greatest if one person defects and the other person cooperates. However, if the game is repeated again and again, the second player will learn not to cooperate. When both defect, which they will soon do repeatedly, both gain much less than they would have if both had cooperated. It is not obvious what one should do in this situation, assuming that there will be many trials, but it has been shown empirically, through computer simulation, that the most successful strategy is tit for tat—doing what the other person did the last time—rather than consistent defection.

4. As argued by Robert Trivers from a suggestion of Darwin's, in species with two sexes in which there is a physiological or behavioral difference in the energy invested in individual offspring, the sex that invests more will become the scarce resource for which the other sex competes. In most mammals and in many birds, females exhibit greater investment, but direct male parental investment may be very high in some species. Species in which male parental investment is high tend to be those in which pair formation of a breeding male with a breeding female is long-lasting; sexual dimorphism, both morphological and behavioral, is low; male-male competition for females is low; and variability among males in reproductive success is low. These "pair-bonding" species, a category including 8,000 species of birds but only a minority of mammal species, may be contrasted with "lek" or "tournament" species, so called because they sometimes have annual seasonal breeding tournaments in which males compete fiercely for females. These species often have high sexual dimorphism for display or fighting (e.g., antlers or peacock feathers), a low tendency for pair formation, low direct male parental investment in offspring, and high variability in male reproductive success. In the elephant seal *Mirounga angustirostris,* for example, 4 percent of the males account for 85 percent of the copulations, a skewing of reproductive success that can result in a rapid rate of evolution and accounts for the extreme sexual dimorphism in this species. Human beings are considered to be near but not at the pair-bonding end of the continuum, as indicated by the amount of sexual dimorphism, the degree of direct male involvement in the care of offspring in a wide range of cultures, and the known distribution of human marriage forms. (Polygyny, in which one man marries more than one woman, is allowed or encouraged in most cultures in the anthropological record [708 of 849, or 83 percent] whereas the converse arrangement, polyandry, is rare [four of 849] and a double standard of sexual restriction is extremely common; still, most human marriages have probably been monogamous, at least in intent.)

5. A neo-Darwinian model of parent-offspring conflict advanced by Robert Trivers has implications for the nature of the family as profound as those arising from the theory of differential parental investment. Weaning conflict is very common among mammals, and there are equivalent phenomena among birds, even including tantrum behavior on the part of the weanling. If the evolutionary purposes of mother and offspring were isomorphic, then they should "agree" (shorthand for "should have been selected to act as if they agreed," implying no conscious intent) that a given level and duration of investment are necessary and sufficient, after which the mother should turn her attention to her next potential offspring. However, even if the current offspring and its unborn sibling have the same father, the offspring's reproductive success will be twice as great if it acts selfishly to maximize its own reproductive value, as compared with that of its sibling. Eventually, a point is reached at which the offspring's need for further maternal investment is outweighed by the inclusive fitness advantage gained through the birth of a subsequent sibling. But this point comes later for the offspring than for the mother, who is equally related to the weanling and the potential

unborn sibling. Although a naive model of the nature of the family assumes that it functions as a harmonious unit under ideal conditions, since supposedly that is how it was designed by evolution, it was not so designed. Like the breeding pair discussed above, the family is an association among individuals with overlapping but distinct evolutionary purposes. Its members naturally pursue individual goals that are sometimes at odds with each other's ultimate (not merely temporary) purposes, and their relationships are naturally conflictful rather than harmonious. This natural conflict is not the result of friction in what should or could be a smoothly functioning system, but is intrinsic.

6. Competition among unrelated individuals can be expected to be extreme at times. Virtually all animal species for which there is sufficient evidence have been seen to exhibit extremes of violent conflict, including homicide, in the wild. The belief that human beings are rare among animal species in that they kill their own kind is erroneous, and more evidence to the contrary accumulates every year. One particularly noteworthy phenomenon is *competitive infanticide,* already alluded to in relation to the wild chimpanzees (Case N3). The paradigmatic description is that of the Hanuman langur monkey of India, *Presbytis entellus.* Langur troops consist of a core of related females and their offspring, associated for periods of a few years or less with unrelated immigrant males. Occasionally, new males arrive and challenge the resident males. If the newcomers win and take over the troop, they drive their predecessors away, and proceed systematically to attack and kill resident infants under 6 months of age. The mothers of those infants then come into estrus again (much sooner than they would have if the infants had survived and continued to nurse) and are impregnated by the new males. Controversy has centered on whether this behavior is normal or is a response to crowding or other social stress. Such controversy misses the point that the behavior enhances the reproductive success of the new males at the expense of the old ones in either case, and can be expected to be favored by natural selection, whether or not it is called normal. Similar phenomena (for example, the killing of a number of infant chimpanzees by two unrelated females under natural conditions) have been observed in many species.

Value judgments Neo-Darwinian or sociobiological theory is sometimes presumed to include value judgments. This presumption merely repeats an ancient philosophical fallacy, according to which whatever is, is right. An extension of this fallacy would hold that sickle cell anemia or thalasemia must be accepted because natural selection has maintained them through balanced polymorphism, the heterozygotes being at an advantage in malaria resistance; or that myopia should not be corrected because natural selection in favor of sharp vision has relaxed in the human population since the end of the hunting-and-gathering era. Human judgments about what is desirable are separate from and take precedence over any observations or explanations of what exists in nature, although they may be enhanced by taking the facts of the natural world into account.

This caution applies equally to clinical and ethical judgments. Just as these two value judgments must be kept separate from each other, so each must be separated from Darwinian fitness, and one can imagine situations in which all three types of judgments would lead to different conclusions. Nevertheless, there is something satisfying about the fact that survival and reproduction—priorities reordered by the neo-Darwinians as reproduction and survival—show a certain symmetry with the goals of mental health as Freud defined them: *lieben und arbeiten,* or to love and to work.

CROSS-CULTURAL CONSTANCY AND VARIATION IN HUMAN BEHAVIOR

A MODEL OF CULTURE AND PERSONALITY Figure 4.1-2 shows how the elements of human social organization and culture may articulate with the universal characteristics of the human life cycle, especially its developmental phase, to produce the variation observed in the anthropological record. It is loosely based on a model developed by John and Beatrice Whiting to summarize their view of culture and personality after several decades of work in psychological anthropology.

This model carries on a tradition begun in the 1930s of assuming that (1) some aspects of society and culture are likely to determine the major features of childhood experience; (2) such childhood experience markedly influences the adult personality of the typical member of the society; and (3) some other aspects of society and culture are likely to be consequences of the typical adult personality and so of the childhood experiences. Phylogeny was not explicitly part of the Whiting model, but is added here as a result of considerations reviewed above, which will be extended and integrated with the rest of the model.

Even without the phylogenetic arrows, the model is explicitly Darwinian. The environment is considered primary, and the society and culture a response to the environment, much as in the longer course of evolution, individual morphology and innate behavioral capacities of different species are responses to the environment. (The addition of history to the model was a relatively late development; defined as it is in terms of borrowings and inventions, it does not change the basic conception of society and culture as responses to the environment.) *Maintenance systems* are the aspects of social organization most heavily influenced by the demands of adaptation, especially subsistence ecology and defense. These demands, according to the model, constrain the learning environment in childhood and adulthood, producing distinctive features of individual personality and behavior. Finally, *projective systems,* aspects of culture theoretically only indirectly dependent on the environment, are determined largely by the culture's particular collection of adult personalities.

Many studies in psychological anthropology have been inspired by this general type of model, which emerged initially from collaborations between anthropologists and psychoanalysts. Cross-cultural applications of psychoanalytic theory continue to be fruitful, as in the work of Robert LeVine *(Culture, Behavior, and Personality)* and Robert Paul *(The Tibetan Symbolic World),* both anthropologists who undertook psychoanalytic training, and in that of Robert Levy *(Tahitians),* who was a practicing psychiatrist before becoming an anthropologist. Melford Spiro's *Oedipus in the Trobriands* defends the concept of the putatively universal oedipal conflict against the old objection of Malinowski—that it could not occur in a society in which the traditional European father's role was split between the father and the mother's brother.

Most recent studies do not rely on psychoanalytic constructs, however, but on categories of behavior and child development that are easier to operationalize. Leaving phylogeny out for the moment, consider a cross-cultural study done by Whiting and Whiting in 1975, which exemplifies both the appeal and the limitations of the approach. The study was done using the *Human Relations Area Files,* one of the most important tools for quantitative research in anthropology. These files consist of nested samples of societies and cultures studied by anthropologists throughout the world, especially a core sample of 60 and a larger sample of nearly 200. Among criteria for inclusion are (1) quality of data, as indicated by training and language competence of the ethnographers, person-years of study at the field site, number of published pages, and other measures; (2) geographic and cultural representativeness of the entire known range of several thousand societies and cultures; and (3) mutual independence of influence, to maximize the likelihood that each society entered in the world sample will function as a statistically independent unit.

The Whitings analyzed a dimension they called "husband-wife intimacy," which they measured by three intercorrelated, independently rated dimensions: whether the husband and wife eat together; whether they sleep together; and how much the father is involved in the direct care of the children. All three dimensions vary markedly in the world cultural sample, but the covariance is high; that is, they vary

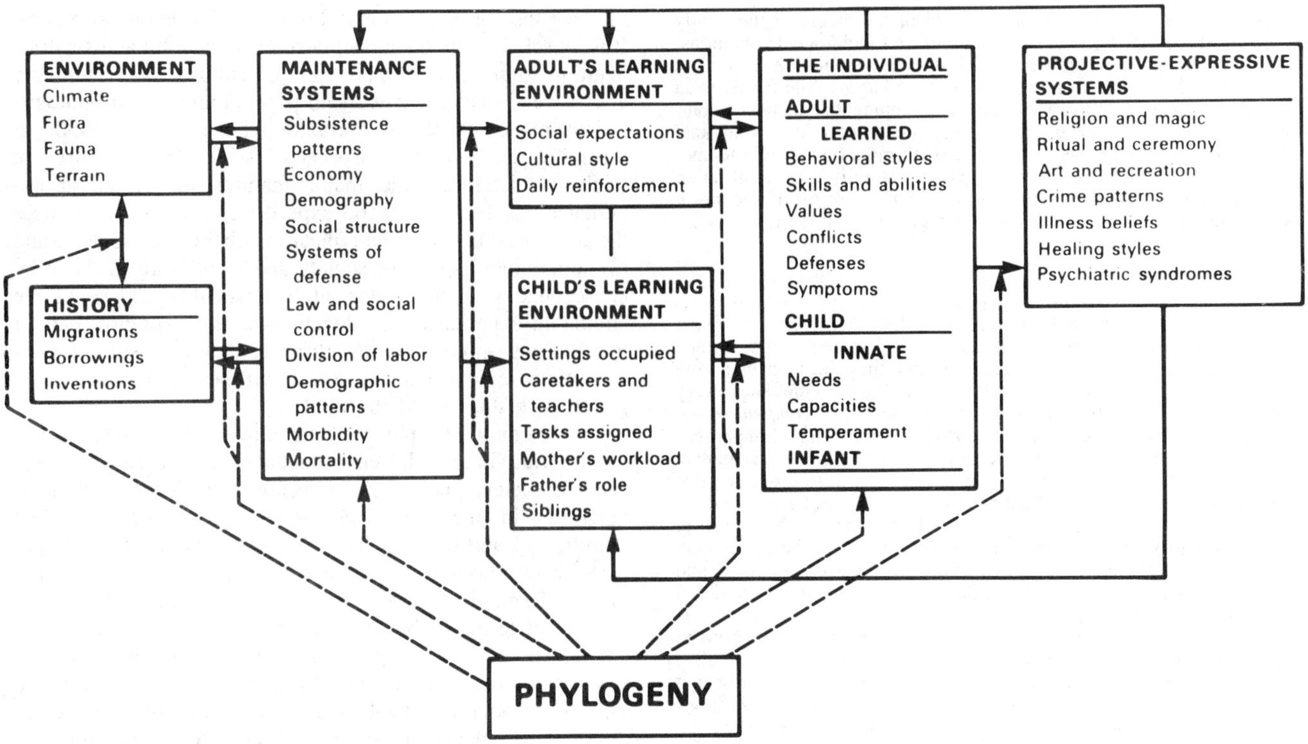

FIGURE 4.1-2. *A model of the interrelationships of child training, adult personality, and various aspects of society and culture, under the influence of phylogeny. Modified from a model of John and Beatrice Whiting.*

together. Furthermore, all three are related to a measure of how much the society is involved in war and preparations for war. At one extreme are the typical war-like cultures of the crowded highlands of New Guinea, for example, with collective houses in which men eat and sleep separated from women and young children, and to which teenage boys are sent to begin their training for belligerency. At the other extreme are non-war-like societies—such as the small, protected, island cultures of the south Pacific—which have high husband-wife intimacy and higher involvement of men with infants and young children.

The model is used to interpret these correlations as follows: Some societies are thrust into warfare because of demographic and geographic conditions; others are protected from attack by natural conditions. Distinct maintenance systems arise in the two types of society, with consequences for child care, such as bringing teenage boys into an all-male world that trains them for war and predisposes them to avoid contact with women and young children. In the realm of adult learning, being exclusively around other men reinforces a man's identification with war-like purposes. Projective systems, such as distinctive male dress and hair style, religious beliefs, and beliefs about male superiority (not directly incorporated in the study), would be seen as epiphenomena of the basic or typical male personality.

This study is appealing because fitting it to the model involves primarily commonsense assumptions about the relationships within and among the various systems. However, it remains an interpretation of correlations, and not an actual causal demonstration. It might be argued that in war-like societies, the first event was a historical accident—say, the advent of a very belligerent leader. This person may have invented men's houses and trained boys for war, which eventually led to a state of chronic belligerency toward neighboring societies. In this model, accepted by some historians and anthropologists, ideology and individual predisposition precede fundamental environmental adaptations. The model may seem plausible in the explanation of the structure and function of a given society at a given moment, but it is difficult to argue convincingly that regularities such as those observed in broad cross-cultural statistical analyses, involving scores or even hundreds of societies, could emerge from a collection of such ideological or historical accidents.

CHILDHOOD EXPERIENCE AND ADULT PREDISPOSITION The model has faced its most troubling difficulties not in the anthropological realm of the relationship between maintenance systems and ideology, but in the psychological realm of the relationship between childhood experience and adult predisposition. In the early 1970s, the developmental psychologist Jerome Kagan became involved in research in cross-cultural psychological development. This research led him to initiate a major challenge to one of the most fundamental assumptions not only of behavioral and social science but also of psychiatry and clinical psychology. The assumption was that childhood experiences, especially in early childhood, have different and more lasting effects on the formation of adult predispositions and abilities than do later experiences. Specifically, in studying cognition in infancy and childhood in a remote Guatemalan Indian village, he and his colleagues found that lack of stimulation and substantial deficits in infancy did not imply deficits in later childhood. In the United States, they found that being in day care for 8 hours a day throughout infancy did not affect available measures of cognition, attachment, or other dimensions of behavior. The research and judgment of many other experimental developmental psychologists also seem to challenge this assumption, which is fundamental to psychological anthropology and psychodynamic psychiatry, and to support the counterclaim that little if anything that happens in early life is irreversible in effect.

It is not possible to review the controversy here, but the essential features of it must be mentioned, as so much reasoning in psychological anthropology hinges on it. Psychodynamic clinicians routinely accept retrospectively collected interview data as evidence for the relationship between early environment and adult personality; rigorous experimentalists do not seriously entertain such data in relation to this particular question. Some investigators of child development do prospective studies using excellent measures that seem to show consequences of early experience on later development; skeptics argue that without random assignment of subjects, these studies produce mere correlations that can be readily explained without a particular causal effect of early experience. Research on the lasting effects of early deprivations or interventions, as long as they are not extreme, has generally failed to support such effects. This research includes follow-up studies of low Apgar scores, lack of stimulation in infancy, breast feeding as opposed to bottle feeding, day care in infancy, Head Start preschool interventions, and other variables. In general, the more rigorous the study and the longer the follow-up, the less is the detectable effect.

Counterarguments are also numerous. Specific measures used in childhood or adulthood may have been inappropriate, behavior under stress rather than baseline behavior may be the right outcome measure, random assignment of subjects is unethical, and so on. The fact remains that developmental psychologists, psychiatrists, and educators have failed to show to the satisfaction of reasonable skeptics that decisive lasting effects of early experience exist. They also have failed to show how such effects might operate or what they might specifically be, despite the strong beliefs of many clinicians about these relationships.

Animal models The only really decisive evidence concerning these processes comes from studies of animal models, which are given insufficient attention by some psychodynamic clinicians and cultural anthropologists. Animal studies using random assignment and rigorous control of other independent variables have repeatedly shown that early experience can make a lasting impression not only on behavior and psychological predisposition but also on neural and neuroendocrine structure and function.

In the jewel fish, early social experience changes the number and shape of the dendritic spines on the pyramidal neurons of the tectum. In the young of some bird species, imprinting (the formation of early attachments, normally to the mother) alters neuronal structure and glucose utilization in the hyperstriatum, and permanently determines not only the juvenile attachment the bird will form but also its adult sexual choice. Rats stimulated, stressed, or handled in infancy have faster rates of growth, larger bodies, and greater resistance to being killed by starvation, drowning, tumor injection, and other means. They are less fearful in strange situations, exploring more and defecating less, and they have improved learning ability compared with controls. All these effects are believed to be related to their altered pattern of corticosterone secretion from the adrenal cortex—a pattern in which secretion is low when stress is low but rises markedly when stress is high.

Male mice raised in isolation for 3 weeks after weaning are much more likely to fight when paired with another male than are controls raised in groups and then paired with strange males. Such isolation also results in altered levels, turnover, and related enzyme activities of monoamine neurotransmitters, although the precise relation of the neurochemical changes to the increased aggressiveness is not known. Rats of any age, including those near the end of the life span, can experience brain alterations in response to experiential enrichment: in the occipital region of the cerebral hemispheres, the thickness and weight of the cortex, the number and size of synapses, the complexity of dendritic branching and density of dendritic spines, and the activity of choline acetyltransferase are favorably affected.

In rhesus monkeys, closure of one eye for a few days during the first 6 months of life will result in permanent impairment of depth perception; incoming stimuli from the two eyes are at that time in competition for sites on binocularly responsive cells in the visual cortex, and removal of stimulation from one eye allows the other to take over all sites on the cells, which will then be unable to respond binocularly. In rhesus monkeys, as in several other species of monkeys and apes, isolation rearing results in a variety of permanent impairments of social and reproductive behavior, in the presence of pathological behavior such as stereotyped rocking and self-directed aggression at baseline, and in a lower threshold for the elicitation of such pathological behaviors by amphetamine, even in monkeys that have recovered from the isolation-induced syndrome. Even short separations of a week or so of rhesus monkeys have been shown to have lasting effects on the behavior in strange situations.

TRANSFERABILITY TO HUMANS The lessons to be drawn are complex. Most of these results cannot be transferred in a simple manner to humans, yet some principles may be transferable. For example, the fact that a variety of stimulating tactics in infancy in rats—some of which are simply stressors—have the same apparently positive effects must lead to caution in interpreting human early stress effects. The monocular closure experiment demonstrates that a particular distortion of input can, in a short time, produce permanent damage, even though closure of both eyes, a blanket deprivation, would have little permanent effect at the same age. If this could be extrapolated to human social and emotional development, it might vindicate psychodynamic thinking about early emotional trauma. The amphetamine challenge experiment shows that monkeys that have recovered behaviorally from early isolation still have neurochemical abnormalities that make them vulnerable to neuropharmacological challenge, suggesting that some psychodynamic theorists may be right in thinking that the behavioral measurements of developmental psychologists do not necessarily get at the underlying structure of the psyche.

Given the number and variety of these and related findings, and the fact that they range over the whole of the vertebrate phylogenetic tree, only an assumption of the most unlikely discontinuity between the nature of human brain and behavioral development and that of animals can support the expectation that similar effects in human development will not be shown. Such effects, when properly delineated, will form the core of a new body of theory in both clinical psychodynamics and psychological anthropology. To believe that such effects exist is reasonable, but to hold strong specific beliefs about how early experience and cultural variations in child care influence adult personality, in the absence of clear evidence, can only impede the growth of knowledge about these processes.

CROSS-CULTURAL UNIVERSALS OF HUMAN BEHAVIOR, MIND, AND CULTURE Although the main enterprise of cultural anthropology in general, and of psychological anthropology in particular, has been the description and analysis of cross-cultural variation, that enterprise has always had an inevitable, even if tacit, complement: the characterization of features of human behavior that do not vary or that vary relatively little. The concept of universals has at least five different meanings: (1) behaviors, such as coordinated bipedal walking or smiling in social greeting, that are exhibited by all normal members of every known society; (2) behaviors that are universal within an age or sex class, such as the Moro reflex in all normal neonates, or the ejaculatory motor action pattern in all postpubertal males; (3) population characteristics that apply to all populations but not all individuals, such as the sex difference in physical aggressiveness; (4) universal features of culture rather than of behavior, such as the taboos against incest and homicide, or the institution of marriage, or the social construction of illness and attempts at healing; and, finally, (5) characteristics that, although unusual or even rare, are found at some level in every population, such as homicidal violence, thought disorder, depression, suicide, or incest.

The list of characteristics that describe these five categories is a long one, much longer than the prominent anthropologists of the early heyday of cross-cultural study would have predicted. (The ethologist Irenaus Eibl-Eibesfeldt has been responsible for the description of many further remarkable constancies in nonverbal communication and social relationships.) The search for societies without violence, or without gender differences that go beyond reproduction, or without mental illness, or even without the ability to make and use fire, has been a vain one. Although there is convincing documentation of variation in the incidence or context of expression of most human behaviors, the existence of a large core of always-present, if variable, features constitutes a demonstration of the reality of human nature and its validity as a scientific construct. It should be emphasized that these universals are fundamental to the nature of the human species in a deeper way than are the previously considered features found in human hunter-gatherers but departed from by later types of society: Universals are features found in all societies regardless of environment or subsistence ecology, and, thus, are likely to be related to human nature in an even more intrinsic way.

Traditional cultural anthropologists have shown little or no interest in such universals, viewing them as trivial or outside their subject matter. This attitude is like being interested in population variations in blood pressure, but not in the Starling curve, or like being interested in the height difference between the Watusi and the Pygmies, but not in the common mechanism of action of growth hormone. The elucidation of universal features of human behavior and culture is increasingly being recognized as one of the central tasks of the discipline, and one likely to enhance, not hinder, the analysis of cultural variation. Even many cultural anthropologists have attempted to delineate such universals as symbol systems and mental structures whose common underlying characteristics link widely disparate kinds of art, language, and ritual—an intellectual strategy owing much to that of psycholinguists, who have found common functional features of all languages that transcend specific manifestations.

With regard to the model in Fig. 4.1-2, the delineation of universal features of human behavior is central to the elucidation of the effects of phylogeny, shown in dotted lines in the diagram. Phylogeny is shown as directly affecting the box representing the individual, especially the "innate needs, drives, and capacities." But most of its effects on the system are modeled as occurring through its influence on other arrows. That is, natural selection operating on ancestral organisms created not only individuals with certain needs, drives, and capacities, but also equations ("if-then" statements) relating the environment to the social system, the social system to the individual, and so on. To refer again to the study of husband-wife intimacy, phylogeny appears to have provided a system in which separating men from women and small children enhances their effectiveness as warriors. It does not mean that they must be warriors or that they must be aloof from their wives, but that choosing aloofness may increase effective belligerency, and perhaps the converse. The universal characteristic here is not only a phenotypic characteristic (males are more aggressive than females), but also an underlying mechanism relating two sets of characteristics to each other (the difference is exaggerated by gender separation).

Recent applications In the past decade, the application of neo-Darwinian or sociobiological theory to ethnological materials has produced many findings that seem to bypass the complex questions of the relationships among society, culture, and individual development. For example, societies in which young men inherit land from their mothers' brother are more lax about the prevention of female adultery than are societies in which young men inherit from their fathers; in societies in which polygyny is allowed, wealthier men tend to have more wives; in small-scale societies in which adoption of children is common, it tends to follow patterns predicted by genetic relatedness. Investigators making these findings usually declare that they do not claim any direct genetic basis for these variations in human behavior, and some of the most egregious confusion about sociobiology stems from a failure to appreciate this distinction between the propositions of neo-Darwinian theory and those of traditional behavioral genetics or molecular genetics.

Even in a nonhuman species such as the redwing blackbird *Agelaius phoeneceus,* males who sing in richer territories mate with several females instead of one. The mechanism of this flexible adaptive system, known as a *facultative adaptation,* must be quite different in blackbirds, however, than that in human beings (although it would probably underestimate blackbirds to assume that in them the system is under tight genetic control). The wings of insects come from thoracic tissue, the wings of birds from forearm structures, the wings of bats from fingers, and the wings of humans from technology. These four adaptations to the problem of flight arrive at similar functions through extremely different developmental processes. The same will prove to be true of adaptations in social behavior.

INCEST For example, sociobiologists (and classical evolutionists and geneticists before them) predicted that incest would be avoided in most sexually reproducing species to avoid the appearance of maladaptive homozygous recessive individuals. But adults on the verge of mating must recognize close kin. In insects and in some vertebrates, such recognition depends on pheromones. In humans, the unlikelihood of that mechanism has led to a search for other ontogenetic explanations. The anthropologist Arthur Wolf, motivated by considerations apart from sociobiology, has shown conclusively that in traditional China, where young girls sometimes lived with the families of their intended spouses (also children), the resulting marriages had a much higher rate of failure and infertility than did other arranged marriages. He has further identified a sensitive period of contact for the effect to occur. Similar findings emerge from studies of the marriage rate among Israeli kibbutz cohort members.

The conclusion is that the familiarity breeds contempt hypothesis of incest, introduced by Westermarck in the last century, receives support. The implication is that human beings achieve inbreeding avoidance through a psychological mechanism influenced by cultural choice, even though the evolutionary effects may ultimately be the same as in species that rely on pheromones for their own incest avoidance. In such analyses, the purposes and methods of psychological anthropology and sociobiology are joined, and the study of human behavior is much better served than it is by sterile debates about nature and nurture.

UNIVERSALS AND VARIATIONS IN PSYCHOSOCIAL GROWTH Freud postulated, and present-day child psychiatry continues to accept in altered and disputed forms, a universal sequence of emotional development on which the social environment of the family could be claimed to operate to produce enduring traits of emotional disposition. Beyond some very general elements, such as the existence of infantile sexuality, the formation of an attachment to a primary caretaker who is usually the mother, and the ubiquity of conflicts and jealousies within the family, this allegedly universal sequence has never found empirical support; hence, unresolvable disputes have arisen among different schools of child psychoanalysis, along with the enduring skepticism of outsiders. Extensive cross-cultural studies of human behavioral and psychological development have not produced evidence relevant to these particular models, but they have produced extensive evidence supporting some more empirically grounded putative universals of psychosocial growth. In the absence of knowledge of neuropsychological development, psychoanalytic theory postulated a libidinal theory of neural development that many question. However, the growing body of actual knowledge about neural and neuroendocrine development can now begin providing an anatomical foundation for a parallel function, the newer, more empirically sophisticated, studies of psychosocial growth.

These studies have been reviewed elsewhere and can only be briefly summarized here. Among the well-established cross-cultural universals of psychosocial development, the following are the best supported, and in most cases can be plausibly related to putative underlying neural or neuroendocrine maturational events: (1) the emergence of sociality, as heralded by social smiling and sustained mutual gaze, during the first 4 months of life, in parallel with the maturation of the basal ganglia and cortical motor circuits; (2) the emergence of strong attachments, as well as of fears of separation and of strangers, in the second half of the first year of life, in parallel with the maturation of the major fiber tracts of the limbic system; (3) the emergence of language during the second year and after, in parallel with the maturation of the thalamic projection to the auditory cortex among other circuits; (4) the emergence of a sex difference in physical aggressiveness in early and middle childhood, with males on the average exceeding females, a consequence in part of prenatal androgenization of the hypothalamus; and (5) the emergence of adult sexual motivation and functioning in adolescence, in parallel with and following the maturation of the hypothalamic-pituitary-gonadal axis at puberty, against the background of the previously mentioned prenatal androgenization of the hypothalamus.

Other cross-cultural developmental universals, such as increased babbling in the second half of the first year and progress through the first three or perhaps four of the six stages in Lawrence Kohlberg's scheme of moral development in childhood, are neither as well established nor as plausibly related to underlying maturational events as are the five advanced above. Although the neuropsychology underlying even these five is at an early stage of elucidation, their cross-cultural universality has been well established, and, in each case, extensive experimental evidence supports the maturational nature of the process in behavioral development. They thus constitute a first approximation of the true structural basis of psychosocial development, which Freud was groping for with his theory of libidinal development in the nervous system.

The universals also constitute a firm basis for the future understanding of how variations in social experience, whether clinical or cross-cultural, act on the maturing psychosocial competence to produce potentially lasting variations. In each of the five processes mentioned, cross-cultural differentiation of the maturing competence begins almost as soon as the maturation occurs. In some cases, there is sufficient evidence to state provisional rules relating environment to differentiation, for example, "Infants whose smiles are favorably responded to will smile more," or "All children will acquire languages with similar cognitive and social functions, but with whatever particular semantic content is presented." In others, such as the differentiation of the strength of attachment in different cultures, it has been difficult thus far to discern any plausible relationship to the characteristics of the social and emotional world that preceded the attachment, despite the expectation of such relationships.

Unfortunately, the more interesting developmental events are more refractory to explanation. However, the increasingly detailed and reliable description of the maturational constants underlying psychosocial growth will provide a steadily firmer place on which to stand while attempting to appreciate the true, and undoubtedly large, role of cultural and individual experience.

CROSS-CULTURAL PSYCHIATRY

Cross-cultural psychiatry as practiced by both anthropologists and psychiatrists has consisted of three closely related enterprises: (1) *psychological anthropology,* using psychodynamic and other psychological theory to interpret the relationships among elements of society and culture; (2) *comparative psychiatry,* using formal epidemiological or less formal observational and clinical methods to describe and analyze cross-cultural variation in incidence or prevalence of syndromes and symptoms; and (3) *medical anthropology,* using traditional anthropological methods to elucidate cross-cultural variation in the social and cultural construction of illness from disease, and in the elaboration of healing or care-taking roles and relationships. The first has already been described; the remainder of this subsection will be devoted to the other two.

COMPARATIVE PSYCHIATRY Comparative psychiatry has been a difficult enterprise under the best of circumstances. The revised third edition of the *Diagnostic and Statistical Manual of Mental Disorders* (DSM-III-R) was developed in an attempt to rationalize and reduce the wide variations in diagnostic styles found even among major medical centers in the United States. Ongoing debates, which will lead eventually to the fourth edition of the *Diagnostic and Statistical Manual of Mental Disorders* (DSM-IV), show that much disagreement still exists. The international equivalent of this manual, under the supervision of the World Health Organization, is quite different, and is subject to similar controversy. Yet, one often reads statements about the prevalence of psychiatric disorders in different countries and cultures that seem to presume the nonexistence or unimportance of such nosological controversy.

For example, it is often said that the incidence of schizophrenia is roughly similar in all countries, with ½ to 1 percent incidence the figure usually cited. England and the United States alone—two English-speaking countries with excellent medical cooperation and communication—have had major differences in the definition of schizophrenia that would preclude any meaningful statement about whether the incidence of this syndrome or disorder is roughly similar or very different in the two countries. And this comparison takes place under ideal conditions of communication, relatively free of doubt about differences in the age and mortality of the populations, the likelihood of case location, the quality and integrity of hospital records, and other factors that plague the cross-cultural epidemiological study of even the best-defined diagnoses in medicine and surgery.

The implication often drawn from this roughly constant cross-cultural incidence of schizophrenia—namely, that it supports a genetic basis for the disorder—is incorrect. Most known genetic diseases have marked population variation in their incidence that is well known to physicians and anthropologists. Various categories of evidence support some genetic hypothesis of schizophrenia defined in almost any way, but the alleged cross-cultural constancy in incidence, even if true, is not one of them. (Perhaps it merely reflects a cross-cultural constancy in the threshold for labeling a thought disorder as serious or chronic.)

Cross-cultural incidence and prevalence When the discussion turns to questions of incidence in small-scale societies, such as those most often studied by anthropologists, the size of the cohort is simply too small to support meaningful comparative study. Still, two generalizations about the cross-cultural incidence and prevalence of psychiatric disorders can be made, regardless of the scale of the societies under comparison.

SYMPTOM CLUSTERS First, the major psychiatric symptoms and symptom clusters, including those at the core of the major disorders and syndromes variously defined, appear to exist in all societies. These symptoms include anxiety, mania, depression, suicidal ideation, major thought disorder, paranoia, somatization, and many other diagnoses or components of diagnoses on Axis I of DSM-III-R. In addition, it includes a range of normal and abnormal personality types that is comparable to the range exhibited by the diagnoses on Axis II.

These disorders frequently manifest themselves as folk illnesses, with labels that subdivide the range of symptom patterns differently than psychiatrists do. Some cultures fail to label at all, but recognize the abnormality, and even its treatability. And many give labels surprisingly close to cross-national comparisons of Western psychiatric diagnoses. Jane Murphy's research among the Eskimo of northwest Alaska and the Yoruba of rural Nigeria provides several illustrations. People in both of these cultures clearly recognize a syndrome resembling schizophrenia—an idiosyncratic severe thought disorder, chronic or chronically recurring, that markedly impairs social functioning. The Eskimo call it *nuthkavihak* and the Yoruba *were* (in English, "crazy" or "insane"). Its victims are responded to with a mixture of compassion and fear, and treated with persistent attempts at decent maintenance as well as restraint. The syndrome is carefully distinguished from shamanistic thought disorder, which is believed to be voluntary, despite temporary hallucinations and delusions.

In the realm of nonpsychotic symptomatology, both cultures recognize and have labeled such complaints as insomnia, night terrors, agoraphobia, anxiety, and claustrophobia, and considered them treatable by folk healers, but neither has a general label corresponding to "neurosis." Each culture has a word (*kulangeta* in Eskimo, *arankan* in Yoruba) for the rare individual who would be called a sociopath by psychiatrists (DSM-III-R antisocial personality disorder), and each considers the condition untreatable.

Folk views of human character make quite subtle distinctions even in very simple societies. Case H2 is that of a man who, in a culture in which all men had extensive homosexual experience, was recognized by the culture as deviant in his devotion to such experience, and (although not labeled there) would perhaps merit the diagnosis of ego-dystonic homosexuality in DSM-III. Case H3 is that of a Guatemalan Indian woman who experienced an isolated episode of what would perhaps be called a brief reactive psychosis and which received the folk label *colera*. Yet, years later, when she was mature, she was recognized as having special powers in a positive sense, an excellent long-term adaptation given her history.

CULTURE-BOUND SYNDROMES Second, the cross-cultural distribution of some disorders is so skewed that the differences can probably be accepted even without strictly reliable epidemiological methods. These so-called culture-bound or culture-specific syndromes should be referred to as syndromes usually found in one or more particular cultural settings. Thus, the disorder not only may have a label, social construction, explanation, or mental content that is culturally unique (which is true of virtually every diagnosis defined by any society), but it is so bound up with its cultural meaning that it essentially would not exist (would be something else) in the absence of the particular cultural framework.

Psychiatric tradition in Western culture includes at least two diagnoses that are probably in this category. Conversion disorder remains in the DSM-III-R classification but appears to have been a much more common condition in the bourgeois society of the late nineteenth century than in any other cultural context, and it is possible that it was, to some extent, a specific interaction of individual predisposition with the cultural expectations of that subculture. Anorexia nervosa, in the past few decades an increasingly common disorder among middle-class adolescent and postadolescent females, appears likely to be evoked by particular cultural conditions that affect body image and self-expectation. Both disorders were or are strongly culturally constructed and subject to spread through psychocultural communication. In addition, several DSM-III-R substance use disorders have been, if not culture-bound, certainly highly skewed in their patterns of subcultural distribution within our society.

The following are among the frequently cited syndromes believed to be characteristic of one or a few specific non-Western cultural settings: (1) *amok,* a condition among traditional Malay men in which a period of brooding is followed by an outburst of frenzied, often homicidal, violence ending in exhaustion and amnesia; (2) *pibloktoq,* an "Arctic hysteria" described among the Eskimo of northern Greenland, characterized by irritability followed by up to half an hour of wild excitement and dangerous and inappropriate behavior ending in seizures, and finally some hours of stuporous sleep ending in amnesia; (3) *latah,* an extreme "startle reaction" to a novel stimulus that especially affects middle-aged women in Southeast Asia, consisting of disorganized speech and action, echolalia, and echopraxia, among other symptoms; (4) *koro,* another Southeast Asian malady consisting of extreme anxiety with the mental content of fear of involution of the genitalia and fear of death; and (5) *windigo,* a psychosis among the Algonkian Indians in which the fear of becoming a cannibal through possession by the windigo, a mythic creature, is a prominent feature of the thought disorder.

Still other culturally defined syndromes seem insufficiently distinctive to merit inclusion among culture-bound syndromes, yet have a folk definition and cultural content that make it seem inadequate simply to translate them into a DSM-III-R diagnosis. *Nervios,* a syndrome first described for Costa Rica but common elsewhere in Latin America (loosely translated as "nerves," and perhaps related to North American symptom patterns that go by that folk label), consists of complaints of headache, insomnia, loss of appetite, fears, anger, trembling, falling, disorientation, fatigue, and despair. It is common, is considered hereditary, and legitimizes psychological complaints (allowing secondary gains) in a culture that otherwise resists them. *Susto,* a condition of general malaise and anhedonia resulting from a severe fright, is another example of a widespread Latin American folk diagnosis. In modernizing sub-Saharan Africa, many male students experience what they call *brain fag*—headache, visual difficulties, agnosia, and chronic fatigue—which, despite its seemingly humorous name, causes much anguish.

In all these "diagnoses"—certainly the folk illnesses, but also the more distinctive culture-bound syndromes—the uniqueness can be questioned by any experienced psychiatrist, and in some (such as the *windigo* psychosis) the very existence of the disorder is in dispute. In none has the disorder been sufficiently well studied either to permit the firm assignment of a DSM-III-R or other standard diagnosis, or to establish firmly the need for a new diagnosis. However, given the protean nature of human mental life in health and disease, it is not unlikely that the complex biopsychosocial dynamics of mental illness would produce some entities in some cultures that fall outside the range of DSM-III-R. Premature assignment of DSM-III-R diagnoses to these syndromes may prevent important discoveries about the mechanisms of psychiatric disorder. Such mechanisms may not be culturally determined. *Pibloqtoq,* for example, has been variously hypothesized to be the result of hypothermia, hypocalcemia, and hypervitaminosis A, among other proposed (including cultural) causes. Its elucidation might be precluded by a smug assurance that it is not unique. (Similar attitudes delayed the recognition of the causes of the New Guinea neurological disorder *kuru* and of pellagra.) Labeling theory provides a set of cultural mechanisms that explain some symptoms and syndromes as the result of learning. It is known that people admitted to psychiatric hospitals in the United States take on characteristics that the staff expect them to have, an experience that should be even more possible in a traditional society. The existence of voodoo death alone indicates the power of culturally defined symbols to produce illness, and some culture-bound syndromes and folk illnesses may be in a similar category. But it must also be noted that the great range of variation in human cultural and social life would have been expected to produce more and different exotic syndromes than these few disputed entities—unless there were fundamental biological constraints on the way the human mind and behavior break down.

MEDICAL ANTHROPOLOGY Dispute about the question of completely distinctive culture-bound syndromes misses an important point about this material. Whether or not such syndromes are homologous with DSM-III-R diagnoses already established, they have a distinctive psychiatric reality by virtue of the cultural definitions, expectations, and responses that surround them. In this sense, the most prosaic symptom or disorder in DSM-III-R may become exotic when it appears in any other culture. Even medical and surgical illnesses undergo a similar transformation in non-Western cultural or subcultural settings.

The presence of an actual underlying biological disease is not at issue here, but it is clear that culture changes the meaning of the biological reality in ways that directly affect the physician's behavior. The differential diagnosis and treatment of a diffuse abdominal or lower back pain, for instance, will be altered in cultures that have elaborate beliefs about discomfort in those areas, whether the physician likes it or not. The differential diagnosis of ideas of reference or paranoid delusions will be even more subject to such cultural differences; moreover, the psychiatrist's role in consultation and liaison may make the circumstances of cultural expectation more critical for psychiatry than for most other fields of medicine.

Medical anthropology is a subfield of anthropology devoted to culture-bound syndromes as well as to non-Western concepts and systems of healing. Although it has not often been done, it is not difficult to reconcile this kind of cross-cultural variation with the evolutionary perspective. Nonhuman primates have many response patterns that in a human being would be labeled abnormal by a psychiatrist (Cases N1–N3), and it is likely that if the primates could speak, the range of such phenomena would seem even wider than it does now. Still, their abnormal behaviors, such as prolonged grief after a loss, or isolative behavior, or excessive violence, produce social effects and responses. Even medical illnesses and wounds are responded to by other group members with caretaking attempts.

Thus, it is hardly surprising that all human cultures have made some attempt to define abnormal conditions of body and mind and to respond to them with healing. Disease in general was probably the most important selective force operating on the ancestors of human beings during evolution, and it is inconceivable that cultural creatures with increasing intelligence should fail to try to do something about it. Although it can be argued that some of the most primitive attempts at healing may have had some biological effectiveness, one does not have to go to that length to conclude that the placebo effect of the mere attempt, for the patient, and the calming effect for others who might be frightened or saddened by the patient's condition, would constitute an adaptive response that could enhance survival and reproduction.

Explanatory model of illness Medical anthropologists draw a distinction between *disease* and *illness,* disease being the underlying biological reality (to the extent that one exists) and illness the result of the social construction of the disease. Although it has proved difficult to introduce the specific terminology for this distinction into typical medical environments where the two terms are used interchangeably, every health care professional will recognize the validity of the distinction. The social construction, or illness, involves a series of intersecting or nested *explanatory models* for the disease, held or promulgated variously by the patient, the family, the physician, other health care personnel, and the larger culture as represented, for example, by religious authority or the law. Medical anthropologists have argued for the addition of an Axis VI to what will become DSM-IV. On this axis, the cultural or subcultural explanatory model offered by the patient or the patient's family would be recorded. This modification would strike most physicians who have worked in different cultures, or even with patients from different subcultures, as potentially valuable.

Among traditionally oriented people in modern Taiwanese culture, for example, patients with syndromes that psychiatrists would call anxiety neuroses routinely attempt to define their symptoms as primarily somatic, and hold a somatopsychic rather than psychosomatic explanatory model of the syndrome (Case H4). This explanation is not psychobiological, but is a cruder reasoning from vaguely defined aches, pains, and pressures in particular body parts to the symptoms of psychological distress. The patient's relationships with the family, not in the sense of remote, early, formative effects, but in the sense of currently acting ones, are held to be strongly operative. Patients and families often refer to the balance or loss of yin and yang to explain their symptoms, and may also visit either a Taoist priest or a shaman, who provides a spiritual formulation of the disorder and undertakes to help placate the gods alleged to have caused the problem or to drive away ghosts or evil spirits. In addition, herbalists with various theories of particular illnesses sell their wares openly to patients. All these explanatory models may influence a single patient attempting to get help.

In a much less complex culture, that of the !Kung San (Bushmen), hunter-gatherers of Botswana, a person who is ill either medically or psychiatrically will usually be viewed as being the target of some motivation (anger, capriciousness, grief) of either a god or the spirit of a dead relative. The community, consisting of a small band of relatives, responds by convening a trance dance, which is both the central religious experience of the culture and the main approach to healing. Women sit around the fire clapping and singing while men dance in a circle around them and gradually enter trances, during which their souls theoretically may separate from their bodies and which make them capable of healing. In one case of malaria (which the !Kung recognize as a separate diagnosis) in a young woman, a healer in trance traveled to the world of the spirits, where he found her father, recently dead, holding her in his arms. Through vigorous argument, he convinced the father that he was being selfish in taking such a young woman away from the living, and this effort was believed to have healing efficacy.

Such psychological insight is not unusual in the traditional healing systems of non-Western cultures, and as long as the patient is made aware of the explanatory model, some genuine effect, corresponding to what might be called a placebo effect, bedside manner, counseling, or even psychotherapy, is not implausible. In some cases, the anticipation of Western psychological theories and techniques is remarkable, as in a form of group discussion for the purpose of dream analysis found among the seventeenth century Iroquois. Explanatory models in other cultures are not so benign. Many cultures have theories of witchcraft or voodoo in which some individuals are believed to put curses or hexes on others. These theories not only serve as explanatory models of conventional illness, but they have been found to be capable of causing distress, illness, and death in people who believe that they are the targets of such curses. Some of these cases may be coincidences, and the others remain a challenge to medical science, perhaps especially to psychiatry.

Psychiatric disorders may be even more subject to spiritualistic explanation than medical or surgical disorders. In many cases, not only the behavior and situation of the patient but also those of other individuals involved, such as the healer or the witch, are of psychiatric interest. Healers are often respected but marginal individuals in traditional societies (the !Kung are exceptional in that many can heal) and may have attained healing power through trances, hallucinations, self-starvation, substance use, or other processes that psychiatrists would consider to be in their province, and which are often of great psychological interest. Theories that relate shamanism to mental illness (specifically acute schizophrenia, but the arguments would apply as well to manic-depressive illness or borderline personality disorder), either individually or familially, have been advanced; if true, they would help to explain the maintenance of these conditions in the human population during the course of evolution. (Among the !Kung San, a young woman with a recurring thought disorder that may have been either bipolar illness or remitting schizophrenia was the daughter of a woman whose trance and healing powers were legendary.)

Conversely, in some societies, psychiatric disorders evoke an explanatory model that labels their victims witches who are held responsible for other people's illnesses and misfortunes. (Some recent Soviet psychiatric practices, recognized as abuses by the World Psychiatric Association, appear to have reversed this phenomenon, giving psychiatric diagnoses to individuals who are healthy by all criteria except political cooperativeness.)

These and many other examples demonstrate that explanations of illness, including culture-specific symbol systems, as well as behaviors and relationships involved in healing, vary greatly across cultures in ways that are of direct concern to psychiatry. Closer attention to these variations can aid psychiatrists and other physicians in a myriad of daily tasks, involving consultation, liaison, compliance, hypochondria, factitious disorders, placebo effects, abuse of the health care system, and other problems. As for the core of disorders for which psychiatrists are directly responsible—psychoses, neuroses, substance use, personality disorders, and more acute reactive symptomatology—only a purely psychopharmacological explanation, such as is not really tenable for any disorder, could lead to the conclusion that non-Western approaches must be devoid of value. Any other currently accepted psychiatric explanatory model—psychodynamic, existential, cognitive, behaviorist, family-dynamic, or community based—must lead to serious consideration of the possible effectiveness of non-Western explanatory models and their resulting treatments.

CASES FROM THE ANTHROPOLOGICAL LITERATURE

Each of the following cases illustrates several different, usually disparate, arguments. The first three cases are from the nonhuman primate literature, and the remainder from the cross-cultural literature. They depart from the conventions of case history writing in several ways, the most noteworthy being that each case is both a context (a different species or culture) and an individual; thus, the context is introduced before the individual is described. Although the individuals selected are unusual in some way against the species or cultural background, their inclusion does not necessarily imply a presumption of diagnosable psychiatric abnormality.

CASES FROM THE NONHUMAN PRIMATE LITERATURE

Case N1 Barbara Smuts's book *Sex and Friendship in Baboons* exemplifies the complex interactionist outlook advocated at the level of nonhuman primates. Resting firmly on a groundwork of evolutionary theory, it nevertheless recognizes the extreme complexity of social behavior and its determination in the individual life cycle. Characteristically, in this species (olive baboons, *Papio cynocephalus anubis,* a large, ground-living, Old World monkey considered highly relevant to human behavior), sexual relationships are frequently inseparable from male-female friendships, and are properly thought of as nonexclusive sexual friendships. Foreign males immigrate to troops and must form friendships with females that may eventually become sexual, a process that takes months to a year or more.

One male, whom she called Ian, was a mature (10-year-old) immigrant to her main study troop who never made this transition. He "had great difficulty establishing relationships with females." He almost always provoked alarm in them, and unlike most males his age, did not seem to know how to calm them by sitting at a distance and making friendly sounds and gestures. Instead, he pursued them, frightening them further, and even eliciting screams that brought a group response, which drove him from the troop. Eventually, he failed to integrate and disappeared. (Another male his age who had arrived at the same time, and who had the appropriate behavior toward females, was by then fully absorbed into the troop.) It is not known what individual life history led to his behavioral inadequacy, which may have been genetic or environmental, or both. The negative impact on his reproductive success seems clear.

Case N2 Jane Goodall's studies of *Pan troglodytes,* the chimpanzee species that is at least the second closest animal relative of humans, culminated in her masterwork, *The Chimpanzees of Gombe: Patterns of Behavior*. This book summarizes 25 years of study of known groups of wild chimpanzees, whose relationships are subtler and more complex than those of baboons, and details not only life histories but family histories up to three generations long. Among many other observations were the responses of 11 young individuals up to 9 years of age (the approximate age of female sexual maturity) to the deaths of their mothers. Classic behavioral depression and other abnormalities were characteristic of the younger individuals, most of whom did not survive, but the severity of the grief reaction was inversely proportional to age, and three of the four that were between the ages of 7 and 9 showed few effects.

The fourth, called Flint, has become famous for his extreme grief reaction. When he was 5 years old, his infant sibling died, and he had resumed dependence on his mother that was extreme for his age, including riding on her back and sleeping in her nest. This dependence, which eventually became mutual, continued until her death 3½ years later, at a stage of development roughly equivalent to that of a human 12-year-old. He lingered near her body for many hours, and became increasingly lethargic over the next 6 days. He was out of sight for 4 days, and when seen again, was in a markedly deteriorated physical condition that worsened until his death, 2 weeks later, of autopsy-proved gastroenteritis and peritonitis. It has been speculated that psychoimmunological vulnerability induced by an abnormal grief reaction may have played a role in his death, but in any case, his dependency was definitely abnormal.

Case N3 Another chimpanzee in Goodall's study, a female known as Passion, also became well known for abnormal behavior. She was first identified in 1961 before coming into estrus, and was in the study until her death of "an unknown wasting disease" in 1982. In 1965, she gave birth to an infant, Pom, and exhibited "inefficient and indifferent maternal behavior." Despite this indifference, Pom survived and a close and lasting bond formed between the two. Beginning in 1970, Passion became increasingly isolative, spending most of her time with her own offspring, eventually three in number. In 1971, she suffered an eye injury that resulted in 2 weeks of monocular closure and evident pain, with a runny nose and eyes and a whitish patch on the iris. Eye healing was apparently complete but her nose continued to run for more than 10 years. Although most chimpanzee hunting is done by males, four of seven bushbuck fawns seen to be captured were killed by females, two of these by Passion in 1977.

Her truly divergent behavior, however, was cannibalistic infanticide. Of six chimpanzee infants killed by adult chimpanzees, three were killed by males in the course of attacks on the mothers, and later eaten, and three were killed systematically, with attacks on the infant only, by Passion, with the cooperation of her adolescent daughter Pom. They also made unsuccessful attempts on two other infants. Without their close cooperation, it would have been impossible for them to overpower the infants' mothers, but Passion was clearly the leading force. The pair may have taken seven other infants in addition, unobserved. These events took place between 1974 and 1977, and it is not known why they began or why they stopped. Pom gave birth herself in 1978, but the infant died about 2 years later, at which point the mutual dependency of Passion and Pom intensified. Infanticide with and without cannibalism has been observed in many species, and in several other studies of chimpanzees, but it is very unusual, and Passion's devoted pursuit of it so far is unique in the literature.

CASES FROM THE CROSS-CULTURAL HUMAN LITERATURE

Case H1 Marjorie Shostak's *Nisa: The Life and Words of a !Kung Woman* describes in intimate and psychologically rich detail, in autobiographical narrative and commentary, the life history of an essentially normal woman among hunter-gatherers in northwestern Botswana. The outlines of the culture and child-rearing pattern fit the model described for hunter-gatherers in general. Nisa was the third child (a second died in infancy) of a then stably married couple living traditionally. She describes her life as idyllic until weaning at around age 3, shortly before the birth of her younger brother, which she attended and whom she claims to have saved from infanticide by her mother. She describes intense sibling rivalry with her brother (e.g., continuing attempts to nurse) and attributes her small stature and other problems to allegedly early weaning. Her father fought violently with her mother but they remained together until Nisa was in adolescence. She was married several times premenarcheally and (despite a culturally typical pattern of sex play throughout childhood) had a stormy introduction to adult sexuality, but her parents tolerated her flight from her husbands.

She remained with her fourth husband, Tashay, and eventually had four children, two of whom died in infancy and early childhood, and another of illness in his youth; the fourth, a girl, was killed by her own husband shortly after they were married. These losses, along with Tashay's death soon after the birth of their third child when Nisa was in her late 20s, shaped her adulthood. She had occasional contacts with lovers both before and after Tashay's death, a habit she had not given up by the time she was interviewed at ages 50 and 55, despite two further marriages, of which her current one was quite stable. Her menopause near age 50 caused a period of sadness and self-assessment, but at 55 she had accepted her childlessness and was bringing up her younger brother's two children. She was vibrant, mildly eccentric with an at times bawdy sense of humor, eloquent on both her own life and the culture, open to new relationships, including the interview relationship with its probing self-exploration, and proud of having surmounted difficulty and tragedy with a willingness to go forward and a continuing joy in life.

Case H2 Gilbert Herdt's book *Guardians of the Flutes* is the best known of a series of ethnographies on cultures in a region of New Guinea ("the semen belt") where male homosexuality is a virtually universal aspect of adolescent development, and the symbolic framework involves centrally the belief that semen must be absorbed—usually through fellation, although also, in some cultures, through anal intercourse—in order for a boy to become a man. Among the Sambia studied by Herdt, boys engage in homosexual activity exclusively beginning at age 7 to 10 and continuing until they are married in their late teens or early 20s. They must suck the penises of postpubertal boys as often as possible until they go through puberty, after which they are fellated very frequently by younger boys. This ritual proceeds in an atmosphere of extreme misogyny and of hypermasculine preparations for warriorhood and hunting. At the end of this period, they marry and become exclusively heterosexual husbands and fathers in almost every case—a challenge to several theories of homosexuality, and an answer to the obvious Darwinian objections to such an apparently maladaptive pattern.

The psychoanalyst Robert Stoller and Herdt published an aberrant case, Kalutwo, who had married four times by his mid-30s; the marriages were infertile, and perhaps unconsummated. He was the illegitimate son of an older widow and a man married to someone else who did not take the widow as his second wife. Stigmatized, Kalutwo was raised by his mother, who was bitter against men, and he had no contact with his father. He showed unusually keen enjoyment of fellatio, had unusually strong homoerotic feelings and attachments, and committed the serious indiscretion of continuing to fellate even younger boys after he had reached puberty. Although he acted tough, he never displayed true masculine achievements such as war injuries or acts of courage. Stoller and Herdt argue for a classic psychoanalytic provenance of homosexuality in this case, but that, regardless of etiology, Kalutwo "would be a homosexual anywhere, independent of the culture's erotic customs," which in themselves do not produce characterological or even stable homosexuality.

Case H3 Benjamin Paul—and until her death, Lois Paul—studied the community of San Pedro la Laguna, a small Zutuhil (Mayan Indian) village in highland Guatemala, for more than 45 years, with periodic field trips beginning in 1941. In this traditional community, with relatively little contact with the Hispanic culture of the country, many ancient beliefs and rituals remained functional, including strong, well-defined roles for shamans (male) and midwives (female), the latter being spiritual as well as obstetric adepts.

Maria, who was 18 when the Pauls met her in 1941, was an attractive woman who had had two failed marriages and had a 9-month-old daughter. Her father, one of six shamans in a village of 2,000 people, and who was considered an expert on insanity, was also lazy, opportunistic, and given to drinking. Her mother, stable and dutiful, had lost three infants before Maria was born. Maria was somewhat sickly and was cared for attentively until the birth of two siblings in succession (at 15 months and between 2 and 3 years) displaced her. She became her father's companion for some years, but he eventually changed toward her, becoming punitive and scolding. She had intense rivalry with her next younger sister, eventually over the same boyfriend. Although she was considered masculine in her competitiveness, disobedience, and general willfulness, she was seductive, charming, and a popular dancer. She was vivacious with occasional morose lapses, witty with a flair for the gruesome, gossipy, and irresponsible. She fell in love and eloped, leaving her baby with her parents (cause for a lawsuit in this culture), but soon was fighting with her new husband.

One night, he struck her, and she suffered an attack of *colera,* essentially an adult temper tantrum believed to result from swelling of the heart as a result of bad blood, with symptoms of gasping and suffocation. Later that night, she lapsed into a state of unconsciousness ("cold and stiff as though dead for good," according to her husband and his father) so seemingly hopeless that the case was rejected by a shaman. She awoke spontaneously after 2 hours and began to wail that spirits of the dead were surrounding her and trying to take her. She was unresponsive to people and events, and talked only to the spirits. She was labeled *loca* (crazy), and her father was called because of his expertise in insanity. He took her (and most of her and her husband's families) to a more powerful shaman in a neighboring village. His advice (although spiritual) subdued many intense family conflicts and reoriented the kinship network to a common effort against the spirits trying to take Maria. She continued to have auditory hallucinations and delusions of persecution for about a week (with content seemingly related to her life situation, such as an insistence that she nurse the babies in the spirit world). She had one further dramatic episode, in which she beat and attempted to castrate her husband, but then remitted, and remained free of these symptoms thereafter. Her symptoms were defined in spiritual terms and treated as such.

Maria continued to have marital difficulties and eventually left the village with a fifth husband. In 1962, when she was in her late 30s, she complained of various physical symptoms, which she attributed to bewitchment and to her powers. A shaman treating her divined that she was being called to be a midwife. This profession, which she adopted with enthusiasm, made a great virtue of her eccentricities, and even her ideas of reference and persecution. Her younger sister, who had always been much more conventional and stable and had stayed in their hometown, became a midwife at about the same time through a more conventional route, but one that also involved illness (a protracted grief reaction, with anorexia, in the wake of their mother's death) and ideas of reference, though in a milder form than Maria's. The latter, in accordance with recommended practice, avoided sex after becoming a midwife and encouraged her husband to find lovers, but in a conflict with him and one of his mistresses, she became ill again. She was bedridden with abulia and anorexia for weeks, until cured by miraculous intervention in a dream.

Case H4 Arthur Kleinman's study of traditional healing in Taipei, a large urban community in Taiwan, is one of the few such efforts conducted by someone trained in both psychiatry and anthropology. Intensive observations of patients with medical as well as psychiatric symptoms and syndromes were made with a focus on the various traditional attempts at healing. Mr. Chen was a 44-year-old, lower-middle-class master woodworker who was a member of the ethnic subgroup Hakka within the Chinese majority. He complained of a feeling of pressure in his chest, general anxiety, weakness, malaise, and neck tension, intermittent for 16 years. He traced the problem to a time when he was in financial difficulties, lonely, and unhappy, but he was not helped by Western-style physicians, who could not identify his illness, or by Chinese-style physicians, who provided a diagnosis and an explanation and prescribed various remedies. He believed that his illness was physical, not psychological, but he also believed a fortune teller who told him that he had "bad fate" because he was being bothered by an ancestor, and that he had to find out who this was. This advice made a great impression on him, and he reasoned that it was his biological mother, who had been divorced from his father when Mr. Chen was 4 years old, and whom his father had forbidden him to visit on her deathbed. He propitiated her ghost, and his symptoms disappeared. He was free of them for 10 years.

Six years prior to Kleinman's interview, however, they had reappeared and had waxed and waned since. They then returned strongly, at a time when his business was at a crucial juncture, and a series of negative tests by Western-style physicians resulted in a diagnosis of neurasthenia. Finally, he visited a shaman with whom Kleinman was working. A full mental status examination revealed marked anxiety and somatic preoccupation but no other abnormalities, with limited insight into the nature of the illness, and resulted in a diagnosis of chronic anxiety neurosis. The shaman performed several rituals, but the milieu of the shrine seemed as important to the patient as the rituals, and the main thrust of the visit was that he should devote himself to the service of the god and return to the shrine frequently. After five nightly visits and much effort, he entered a subjectively described trance state, threw himself around violently, and eventually collapsed—a pattern that would become habitual, though more controlled. Two days after his first trance, he was evaluated at home by Kleinman, who found him greatly improved both objectively and subjectively. "My overall impression was . . . that his former anxiety had been largely, and perhaps entirely, relieved." This improved state continued on periodic follow-up for 2 years, during which the patient became increasingly involved with the life of the shrine and eventually became a leader who entered trances nightly.

Case H5 In *Saints, Scholars, and Schizophrenics,* her superb study of the cultural context of mental illness in a remote rural area of western Ireland, Nancy Scheper-Hughes explored the unusually high prevalence of serious mental illness in this region. She documented the relentless generations-long series of social stresses in the population, impoverished and condemned to farm very poor land. Dwindling and losing its traditions as its young people, especially women, emigrated, the populations experienced a breakdown of respect for the elders of the community, and lost its time-honored tolerance of people with strange visions. These stresses occurred against the background of a culture and child-rearing pattern characterized by severe sexual repression; canings, ridicule, and scapegoating of children; and both longing for and fear of intimacy. Thematic Apperception Test (TAT) and Draw-a-Person test results with psychiatric patients were consistent with her emphasis of these themes. Without denying the basic biological nature of vulnerability to schizophrenia, Scheper-Hughes argues persuasively that these sociocultural stresses account in part for the unusually high prevalence of schizophrenia and other serious mental illnesses. Two cases illustrate certain characteristic female and male themes.

Kitty was a 20-year-old hospitalized for the first time with a diagnosis of schizophrenia, which began during a brief period of emigration to work in a low-grade London pub. She was the second youngest in a large family, with an alcoholic, occasionally brutal, father and a compulsively religious and sexually repressed mother. Kitty became hysterical over her task of recycling leftover beer slops into fresh glasses, which she equated with the whoring behavior of her "Black Protestant" English clients, who recycled their defiled sexuality into their wives in a similar way. During her illness, she was obsessed with themes of polarity, such as order–disorder, female–male, pure–impure, Catholic–Protestant, and Celt–Anglo.

Patrick was a 34-year-old farmer, fourth in a family of seven and the youngest son, carrying the diagnosis of chronic schizophrenia. His parents had imposed on him a guilty sense that he must stay and care for them in their old age, and he had remained unmarried and celibate in a dying village from which most young women had fled. In the hospital, he rarely spoke, and usually remained still. His spotty responses on the TAT described the figures as statues or as "pictures of a picture." In talking of his relationship with his parents, he said, "I am their dead son."

These cases and others cited by Scheper-Hughes demonstrate the power of cultural context to invest a severe thought disorder with specific content, but also may be relevant to explaining the high prevalence of severe mental illness in traditional rural western Ireland during the 1970s.

REFERENCES

Bowlby J: *Attachment and Loss* (3 vols). Hogarth Press, London, 1969–77.

Cheney D, Seyfarth R, Smuts B: Social relationships and social cognition in nonhuman primates. Science *234*: 1361, 1986.

Eibl-Eibesfeldt I: *Human Ethology*. Aldine Press, New York, 1988 (translation of *Die Biologie des Menschlichen Verhaltens: Grundriss der Humanethologie*. Piper, Munich, 1984).

Goodall J: *The Chimpanzees of Gombe: Patterns of Behavior*. Harvard University Press, Cambridge, MA, 1986.

Kagan J: *The Nature of the Child*. Basic Books, New York, 1984.

Kenny M G, editor: New approaches to culture-bound mental disorders. Soc Sci Med *21*(2): 162, 1987.

Kleinman A: *Patients and Healers in the Context of Culture*. University of California Press, Berkeley, 1980.

Kleinman A, Good B, editors: *Culture and Depression: Studies in the Anthropology and Cross-Cultural Psychiatry of Affective Disorder*. University of California Press, Berkeley, 1985.

Konner M: *The Tangled Wing: Biological Constraints on the Human Spirit*. Harper & Row, New York, 1983.

Konner M: Universals of psychosocial growth in relation to brain myelination. M.D. Thesis, Harvard Medical School, Harvard-MIT Joint Program in Health Sciences and Technology, 1985.

Lee R, DeVore I: *Man the Hunter*. Aldine, Chicago, 1968.

LeVine R: *Culture, Behavior, and Personality*. Aldine, Chicago, 1973.

Levy R: *Tahitians: Mind and Experience in the Society Islands*. University of Chicago Press, Chicago, 1973.

MacLean P D: Brain evolution relating to family, play, and the separation call. Arch Gen Psychiat *42*: 405, 1985.

Munroe R H, Munroe R L, Whiting B B, editors: *Handbook of Cross-Cultural Human Development*. Garland STPM Press, Chicago, 1981.

Murphy J M: Psychiatric labeling in cross-cultural perspective. Science *191*: 1019, 1976.

Pastner C M: The Westermarck hypothesis and first cousin marriage: The cultural modification of negative sexual imprinting. J Anthropol Res *42*: 573, 1986.

Paul B: Mental disorder and self-regulating processes in culture: A Guatemalan illustration. In *Personalities and Cultures: Readings in Psychological Anthropology,* R Hunt, editor, p 150. Natural History Press, New York, 1967 (orig. 1953).

Paul L: Careers of midwives in a Mayan community. In *Women in Ritual and Symbolic Roles,* J Hoch-Smith, A Spring, editors, p 129. Plenum, New York, 1978.

Scheper-Hughes N: *Saints, Scholars, and Schizophrenics: Mental Illness in Rural Ireland*. University of California Press, Berkeley, 1979.

Schieffelin E L: *The Sorrow of the Lonely and the Burning of the Dancers*. St. Martin's Press, New York. 1976.

Shostak M: *Nisa: The Life and Words of a !Kung Woman*. Harvard University Press, Cambridge, MA, 1981.

Simons R C, Hughes C C, editors: *The Culture-Bound Syndromes: Folk Illnesses of Psychiatric and Anthropological Interest*. Reidel, Boston, 1985.

Smuts B: *Sex and Friendship in Baboons*. Aldine, New York, 1985.

Spindler G D, editor: *The Making of Psychological Anthropology*. University of California Press, Berkeley, 1978.

Stoller R J, Herdt G H: Theories of origins of male homosexuality. Arch Gen Psychiat *42*: 399, 1985.
Trivers R L: *Social Evolution*. Benjamin Cummings, Menlo Park, CA, 1985.
Whiting B B, Edwards C P: *Children of Different Worlds: The Formation of Social Behavior*. Harvard University Press, Cambridge, MA, 1988.
Whiting B B, Whiting J W M: *Children of Six Cultures: A Psychocultural Analysis*. Harvard University Press, Cambridge, MA, 1975.
Whiting J W M, Whiting B B: Aloofness and intimacy between husbands and wives. Ethos *3*: 183, 1975.
Wolf A; Childhood association and sexual attraction: A further test of the Westermarck hypothesis. Amer Anthropol *72*: 503, 1970.

4.2 SOCIOLOGY AND PSYCHIATRY

RONALD C. KESSLER, Ph.D.

INTRODUCTION

Sociology is the behavioral science that studies the organizing principles of social life, the broad societal and world-historic forces that shape these principles, and the effects of these principles on individual and organizational action. A basic premise of sociological inquiry is that there are fundamental constraints on individual action that must be understood if one wants to know why people do the things they do. An understanding of motivation is not enough because motives are shaped by social forces. Social influences intervene in even a more fundamental way, by determining the range of behavior options considered to be possibilities.

One of the earliest sociological investigations to study societal influences on individual action was Emile Durkheim's work on suicide. Durkheim, working in the late nineteenth century, was one of the first to document consistencies in suicide rates. He noted that married people had lower suicide rates than the unmarried; that men committed suicide more often than women; that there were consistent cross-cultural differences in suicide rates—all patterns that exist today. Durkheim argued that such patterns could not be explained on the basis of personality differences, and so broader social determinants must be at work. His analysis of these differences was highly speculative because he had only gross statistical data with which to work. Nonetheless, his provisional explanation, emphasizing the importance of stress, social support, and integration into networks that provide meaning and purpose to life, has a remarkably current ring of truth.

Contemporary sociology continues to be relevant for psychiatrists in a number of ways. Over the past decade, sociologists have studied the sociocultural determinants of mental health and illness, social factors in psychiatric help-seeking, attitudes toward the mentally ill, and mental health care organization. In each of these areas, an interdisciplinary body of theory and research exists, with contributions made not only by sociologists but also by psychiatrists, psychologists, and epidemiologists. The research findings and methodological issues of each area will be reviewed in turn. Although not exclusively the purview of sociologists, a distinctive sociological perspective is apparent and will be emphasized throughout.

SOCIAL AND CULTURAL DETERMINANTS OF MENTAL ILLNESS

Research on social and cultural factors in psychopathology has been dominated during the past decade by an interest in the health-damaging effects of stressful life experience. The first part of this section examines attempts to conceptualize, measure, and estimate the effect of stress on mental health. The analysis then turns to recent research on vulnerability factors that modify the impact of stress.

RESEARCH ON LIFE EVENTS Although the hypothesis that stress can cause mental disorder is an old one, serious population-based research on this topic has only been conducted during the past 2 decades. Most of this research has utilized a life event inventory to measure stress and estimate its effects. Early work of this type was limited to case-control studies in which retrospective reports about life events were obtained from psychiatric patients and controls. More recent work has been based on general population samples and longitudinal designs.

Documenting causality It has proved much more difficult than initially anticipated to document a causal association between life events and mental illness. The main problem is methodological—that an events–illness association could reflect an influence of the illness on the events rather than the converse. Job loss, divorce, and many of the other major events that make up life event inventories might occur as a result of a preexisting neurotic personality, and there is no certain way of discounting this possibility in the nonexperimental studies that are the mainstay of stress research. Recent studies have tried to deal with this problem by focusing on those events that are unlikely to be caused by prior disorder (e.g., death of a loved one), but such events form a comparatively small subset of all events that may contribute to mental health problems.

Despite this difficulty, some clear findings have emerged about the effects of life events. Early work on schizophrenia demonstrated a "triggering" effect of undesirable events, that negative events can precipitate a psychotic breakdown for schizophrenic patients. However, no evidence was obtained to suggest that stressful events play a more fundamental role in determining who becomes schizophrenic.

Researchers next turned to general population studies of nonspecific psychological distress. The relationships documented in these studies were extremely small, accounting for no more than a few percentage points of the variation in the outcome variables. Subsequent studies found at least two reasons for this result. First, much of the distress measured in these screening scales is chronic, and, therefore, unrelated to events that occur at a particular time. Second, the life event inventories used to assess stress are too coarse to capture the important dimensions of stress that are associated with emotional disorder.

These two problems can be avoided by focusing on recent-onset cases of depression or anxiety disorders and obtaining detailed information about the context of events experienced over a standard retrospective recall period. Such research shows clearly that severe life events substantially increase the risk of major depressive disorder and generalized anxiety disorder.

To detect substantial effects of life events, it is critical to obtain detailed information about the contexts of all events that preceded the disorder. The emotional effects of an event vary enormously depending on its context. Job loss, for example, differs in its meaning depending on whether the family has financial resources, whether chances for equivalent reemployment are high, and whether the unemployed person was committed to a particular line of work. With this detailed information on hand, it is fairly easy to predict who will become depressed by a job loss.

The difficulty is that it is hard to obtain the kind of detailed information one needs to reconstruct the context of every event experienced by a large sample of respondents. Studies using the most sophisticated methods of life event assessment thus have been small, and the results consequently have been variable. One method of circumventing this problem has been to conduct more intensive investigations of adjustment to particular events in special samples of people who have undergone the same stressful experiences.

EFFECTS OF CRISES Most early work in this area was conducted by clinicians who were primarily interested in developing an understanding of some crisis—job loss, rape, widowhood, life-threatening illness—that could guide them in their intervention efforts. For this reason, studies of specific life crises have consisted mainly of relatively small, descriptive studies focused on how people react to the crisis and how these reactions change over time.

Most of this research has centered on emotional reactions. The findings show that these reactions are characterized by extreme variability. Although it is widely believed that emotional distress must be expressed in order to resolve a crisis, particularly a serious emotional loss, people who show little distress soon after the crisis continue to score low in distress. Evidence also does not support the widely held view that people undergo predictable states of emotional reaction as they attempt to deal with a crisis, or that those people who progress through stages in a particular order achieve better adjustment than other people who are grappling with the same life problem.

Careful comparative studies have demonstrated that people who experience bereavement, rape, or a life-threatening illness have higher rates of psychopathology than people who have not been subjected to such an event. Furthermore, there is evidence that between 20 and 40 percent of the people who experience a major life crisis do not recover emotionally with the passage of time. Among the bereaved, for example, one study found 30 percent to have a bad outcome on a combined assessment of psychological distress, social functioning, and physical health measured 2 to 4 years after the loss.

Little basis exists for making predictions about the conditions of an event that account for why a particular person will or will not recover. The early clinical studies did not systematically discriminate among the contexts that differentiate people who experience the same event. However, during the past few years, as social scientists have begun to focus on adjustment to particular life crises, efforts have begun to specify the dimensions of crises that make them stressful. Preliminary studies have documented that the differential impact of particular events can be explained in part by individual differences in the way these dimensions coalesce in particular instances. For example, job loss seems to promote anxiety and depression on several dimensions, including increased financial strain and heightened reactivity to unrelated stresses. As a result, the most serious emotional effects of job loss are found among people who lack financial reserves and who experience some other major stress—such as one of their children developing a life-threatening illness—during the period of unemployment. It is likely that the next decade will see a major expansion of related research that delineates much more clearly the contextual features of particular stressful experiences that predict healthy adjustment and recovery.

RESEARCH ON CHRONIC STRESS Research on the relationship between chronic stress and emotional disorder is much less well developed than work on life events. It is easier to determine whether or not an event has occurred than to measure objectively the existence of an ongoing stressful situation. It is also easier to make a causal interpretation about the effect of a discrete event than of a chronic stress. Because of these difficulties, many researchers have favored life event measures over chronic stress measures.

This favoritism does not imply that life events are more important than chronic stresses. Recent research suggests that chronic stresses are more predictive of psychological disorders in community surveys. More reliable procedures for measuring this kind of stress and for studying its effects remain for future research.

The most finely developed work of this sort to date concentrates on job stress. Naturalistic studies have documented that time pressure, closeness of supervision, job insecurity, and a variety of other job dimensions are associated with depression, anxiety, and substance abuse. Based on these results, more focused studies of such high-risk occupations as assembly line work and air traffic control have been undertaken.

These studies have described particular constellations of job conditions associated with emotional disability. For example, several large studies have linked the combination of high job demands (e.g., a job in which workers must rush to meet important deadlines) with low decision latitude (i.e., low control over either the pace or organization of work) to both emotional disability and cardiovascular disease.

Many major corporations have now agreed to carry out job redesign experiments aimed at modifying some of these health-damaging job conditions. These efforts, motivated partly by a desire to increase worker productivity, are providing an unparalleled opportunity to study the effects of chronic stress. These experiments should yield important new knowledge about the determinants of chronic job stress and about effective strategies for changing work environments to reduce the most pernicious kinds of stress.

RESEARCH ON VULNERABILITY FACTORS The evidence clearly demonstrates that only a small minority of people who are exposed to stressful life experience develop clinically significant emotional disorders. In fact, emerging evidence indicates that stressful encounters can sometimes promote coping. For these reasons, the major thrust of current research on life stress is to identify variables that may help explain differences in stress responsiveness. Some investigators have emphasized enduring physiological or psychological characteristics, whereas others are interested in such psychosocial resources as cognitive flexibility, effective problem-solving behaviors, interpersonal skills, financial assets, and social support.

Research on vulnerability factors represents an important

new direction in work on the relationship between social factors and psychopathology. Full consideration of this research cannot be undertaken here, and so the following discussion centers on one factor that has generated particular interest among sociologists—social support.

The term *social support* has been widely used to refer to the mechanisms by which interpersonal relationships protect people from the deleterious effects of stress. The popularity of the term was triggered by a series of influential review papers in the mid-1970s that demonstrated a consistent relationship of psychiatric disorders with such factors as marital status, geographic mobility, and social isolation. Although highly inferential in their arguments, and not always clear about their definition of the concept, these authors generated a great deal of scientific interest in the possibility that support can have health-promoting effects.

Over the intervening years, the initial enthusiasm has been replaced by a more critical examination of the issues and evidence. Various types of support have been identified and distinctions have been made empirically among the effects of these various dimensions. Several different functions of support have been identified, such as the expression of positive regard, expression of agreement with the person's beliefs or feelings, encouragement of ventilation, and provision of advice or information. The question of whether each of these aspects of support is associated with vulnerability to psychiatric disorders has been addressed in a number of ways, the most important of which are considered next.

Clinical studies Research comparing the social networks of psychiatric patients and normals shows that psychotics have very tight kin-based networks, and neurotics have loose and sparse networks, as compared with controls. These network structures might be causally implicated but it is equally likely that they are results of the disorders.

This causal ambiguity has been resolved to some degree by research in which the supportiveness of social networks at the time of illness onset was assessed to predict subsequent relapse. The most important work in this tradition was that of sociologist George Brown and his colleagues in London, who isolated a pattern of "expressed emotion" characterized by hostile feelings and intrusiveness on the part of the families of schizophrenic patients, which is strongly associated with poor prognosis after discharge. More recent work based on Brown's model has resulted in the design of family interventions that have been effective in altering this expressive style. This work has been experimentally evaluated and shown to reduce relapse among first-episode schizophrenics. Parallel research on relapse for major depression has begun, but lags far behind the research on schizophrenia.

Normal population and case-control studies Whereas research on the relationship between support and the course of illness has focused on the direct effects of support, most recent research has concentrated on the ability of support to ameliorate the impact of stress on health. For example, it has been shown that the impact of life events in provoking episodes of major depression is reduced among individuals who have an intimate, confiding relationship with a friend or relative. In one of the studies documenting this association, nearly 40 percent of the stressed women without a confidant became depressed compared with only 4 percent of those women with access to a confidant. This result has been replicated in several community surveys and case-control studies.

Although these studies provide suggestive evidence, serious methodological problems make the results difficult to interpret. The most serious problem is that there is virtually no way to rule out the possibility that some predisposition to become depressed accounts for the presumed buffering effect—that individuals who are predisposed to becoming depressed under conditions of stress are also, for reasons related to this predisposition or its personality correlates, less likely than other people to form close, confiding personal relationships.

As investigators have come to recognize this problem, they have instituted studies that include measures of presumed confounding variables. It is too early to draw any definitive conclusions from this new series of investigations, but preliminary evidence shows that personality does have some effect on support. A group of investigators from Australia has shown that trait neuroticism disrupts close, supportive relationships, and is also associated with the exacerbation of stress effects. When neuroticism was statistically controlled in their analyses, the buffering effect of social support was explained away.

Although methodological problems prevent one from concluding too much from this single study, it clearly calls into question a simple interpretation of support buffering effects. Other personality factors may also be implicated. New studies under design to investigate this possibility might lead to a revision of the currently optimistic view about the importance of support.

Experimental interventions As researchers have come to recognize the methodological shortcomings of naturalistic social support studies, experimental support interventions have become popular. Most of these interventions, which have been implemented in hospital settings, have examined the effect of support on such outcomes as preoperative anxiety, recovery from surgery, and compliance with medical regimens. Support interventions have also been instituted to facilitate coping with such life crises as widowhood, rape, and job loss.

These interventions have operationalized support in many different ways, although all of them have involved both emotional and informational interactions with support providers. Most have been provided by health care professionals and have been modest in scope, generally with limited resources and involving a small number of sessions. Nonetheless, in the vast majority of cases, these manipulations have been effective in fostering adjustment to life crises.

This result strongly suggests that social support may protect against emotional disorders that have been linked to life crises. However, the intervention experiments carried out to date have not been designed to illuminate the mechanisms through which this influence occurs. Furthermore, as most of these interventions were multifaceted, it is impossible to determine from them which aspects of support are most effective.

Future directions in research on social support The evidence suggests that social support may play an important part in protecting against both the onset and the continuation of psychopathology. A clearer understanding of these influences will require research advances in several directions. One advance would involve further specification of components and characteristics of support, including its differential effects according to who provides it. A related issue pertains to the effects of negative social interactions. The literature clearly suggests that interactions between psychiatrically impaired individuals and their social networks are not merely unsupportive but are openly conflictual. It would be useful to assess negative social exchanges as risk factors for onset and prolongation of psychiatric disorders. In the few studies that have compared positive and negative elements of social interaction, the negative elements have uniformly been more strongly related to mental health outcomes. There is a need to know more about the relative importance of positive and negative components as stress buffers and risk factors.

A more balanced perspective will also require researchers to concentrate on the provider of support as much as on the recipient. Some beginning efforts along this line have been made in studies of the psychiatrically impaired. Attention has focused on the part played by family environments in maintaining the disorder. However, little is known about precisely what behaviors of the disordered person tend to provoke nonsupportive responses from family members.

GROUP DIFFERENCES IN PSYCHIATRIC DISORDER A large part of sociological research on psychopathology has traditionally been concerned with structural correlates of psychiatric illness such as social class, sex, race, and urbanicity. Recent research has centered on these same associations in a way that reflects the contemporary issues reviewed above.

The most obvious hypothesis to test in examining such associations is that differential exposure to stress explains group differences in mental illness. After over a decade of research, however, it is now clear that this hypothesis can be rejected. Although it is true that people in comparatively disadvantaged positions in society (e.g., women, lower-class persons, nonwhites) are exposed to more stress than their advantaged counterparts, this differential exposure cannot explain their higher rates of anxiety, depression, and nonspecific distress in general population samples.

Vulnerability factors have taken center stage in research on group differences. This research has shown consistently that there are group differences in vulnerability to stress and that this factor plays an important role in explaining differences in rates of psychiatric disorder.

Vulnerability to stress might come about in any of numerous ways, and current research on group differences is centrally concerned with these processes. Although this is a new area, some initial results are worth reporting with regard to research on social class, gender, and race.

Social class One of the oldest and most firmly established associations in psychiatric epidemiology is the one between social class and mental illness. People in socially disadvantaged positions have been shown to have higher rates of psychiatric disorder than their more advantaged counterparts. This difference has been reflected both in treatment statistics and in higher rates of nonspecific distress in community surveys.

Early work on social class and psychopathology was based on the influential work of Hollingshead and Redlich, which defined social class in terms of a "two-factor index" that combined information on educational attainment and occupational prestige. Their research studied patterns of social class variation in psychiatric hospitalization. They documented clearly that lower-class people have both a significantly higher probability of hospitalization and remain hospitalized longer than their middle-class counterparts. Subsequent work has used the term *social class* to describe measures as diverse as family income, occupational prestige, education, and even the Marxian concept of "class" that distinguishes workers from owners. The most recent descriptive work on this issue shows that it is important to discriminate these various measures rather than combine them as Hollingshead and Redlich did. The evidence now suggests that income (among men) and education (among women), rather than class, are the primary correlates of psychopathology. Furthermore, the effect of income is actually due to personal earnings rather than to total family income, which implies that financial adversity is not the central operating factor.

Until the early 1970s, the dominant line of thinking in the literature on class and mental illness was that lower-class people were exposed to more stressful life experiences than those of more advantaged social status, and that this differential exposure accounted for the negative relationship between class and mental illness. This view was challenged for the first time in the Midtown Manhattan Study, in which an attempt was made to demonstrate empirically that the lower-class excess of mental health problems could be accounted for by greater exposure to stressful life experiences. Although this attempt was unsuccessful, a more complex association was documented: that stressful life experiences have a greater capacity to provoke mental health problems in the lower classes than in the middle class. Subsequent work has shown that this class-linked vulnerability to stress accounts for the major part of the association between social class and major depression as well as between social class and nonspecific distress.

There are several ways in which this vulnerability might come about. One of the most plausible explanations is that some type of selection or drift of incompetent copers to the lower classes might lead to the relationship between class and vulnerability. Another explanation is that one's experience as a member of a particular class leads to the development of individual differences in coping capacity as well as to differences in access to interpersonal coping resources.

Evidence is available consistent with both of these hypotheses. Most of the evidence for the drift hypothesis comes from studies of major mental illnesses, primarily schizophrenia. These studies show that the early onset of a disorder can reduce one's chances of socioeconomic achievement—a fact that seems to be true primarily for people who become ill before becoming established in a career. At the same time, less severe disorders do not seem to interfere with socioeconomic achievement.

Evidence for the linkage of vulnerability factors and class is widespread. Lower-class people are disadvantaged in their access to supportive social relationships. Evidence also indicates that personality characteristics associated with vulnerability to stress, such as low self-esteem, fatalism, and intellectual inflexibility, are more common among lower-class people. To date, the major efforts in this area have been confined to the study of social support. The most influential work here has been that of the English sociologist George Brown, who documented that lower-class people have fewer confidants than those in the middle class, and that this contributes to their vulnerability to undesirable life events. This finding has been replicated in several investigations, but more work needs to be done to investigate in parallel fashion the importance of coping strategies and personality characteristics. At the same time, as most investigations of class and stress have focused on life events, a more serious investigation of ongoing stressful situations may help us to develop a more complete understanding of the relationship between class and psychopathology.

Gender Community surveys show that adult women are twice as likely as men to report extreme levels of psychiatric distress. In community surveys of psychiatric cases, women are between two and three times as likely as men to report a history of mood (affective) disorder. Although other types of psychopathology are as common among men as among women and still others are more prevalent among men, most research has emphasized mood disorders and nonspecific distress in community samples.

Much research on sex differences in nonspecific distress has been done during the past 10 years or so. Two lines of research can be discriminated, with the first based on indirect assessments of role-related stress. For the past decade, the dominant perspective has held that women are disadvantaged relative to men because their roles expose them to more chronic stress. Because of the difficulties in measuring chronic stress objectively, empirical analysis has used indirect assessments based on measures of objectively defined role characteristics or constellations of multiple roles to document this relationship.

The second line of research on sex differences has examined stressful events. This work has shown that there is a significant interaction between sex and undesirable events in predicting distress, with women appearing more vulnerable than men to the effects of stressful events. Several different hypotheses have been advanced to account for female vulnerability to stress, including the arguments that females are disadvantaged in access to social support, in the use of effective coping strategies, and in personality characteristics.

Although aggregate analyses of life event inventories show that women are, on average, more vulnerable than men, there are some events for which this is not true. Research on widows, for example, shows that women adjust to spousal death better than men. Women also adjust as well as or better than men to divorce, and financial difficulties do not affect women as much as men.

A challenge for future research will be to reconcile the discrepancy between these studies of particular life events and aggregate life event surveys. The only attempt that has been made to do this was a meta-analysis of several large-scale community surveys in which the effects of different types of events were assessed separately. This analysis also found no evidence that women are more distressed than men by such major life crises as job loss, divorce, or widowhood. Their greater vulnerability is primarily associated with events that happen to people close to them—death of a loved one other than a spouse being the most commonly reported event in this regard.

The greater impact of network events on women can be interpreted in several ways. One component of this difference is probably linked to the fact that women provide more support to others than men and that this creates stresses and demands that can lead to psychological impairment. Another interpretation is that women might be more empathic than men, or might extend their concern to a wider range of people. These and other possibilities need to be investigated in the future, since the role played by network events appears to account for a very substantial part of the overall sex-distress relationship.

Race Much of the research on race differences in psychopathology has focused on black–white differences. Research is also increasing on the comparison of Americans of Mexican and of Anglo-Saxon heritage. These two bodies of research are reviewed briefly below.

Some authors who have examined treatment statistics argue that blacks have higher rates of treatment for psychosis than whites, but studies that focus on a broader array of disorders are more ambiguous. Most careful reviews state that no black–white difference exists in overall treatment rates. Although community surveys paint a much more consistent picture, with blacks clearly evidencing higher average levels of distress than whites, statistical control for the fact that blacks generally have lower socioeconomic levels than whites accounts entirely for this race difference regarding nonspecific distress.

This demonstration implies that minority status and the life experiences associated with it are not in themselves instrumental in creating mental health problems once socioeconomic factors are controlled. This observation can be understood from several different aspects. The viewpoint most actively pursued in the literature is that minority status, although related to experiences of prejudice and discrimination, is also related to structural resources that can help protect against the adverse mental health effect of these stresses.

There is a long tradition that emphasizes the stress-buffering effect of group solidarity among members of deprived groups. Theoretically, this effect may stem from at least two sources: (1) the group provides cognitions that identify responsibility for their deprivation with structural conditions, thus removing any self-blame for their lack of financial achievement; and (2) the group provides emotional support that can buffer the effects of life stress in a variety of ways.

Some beginning attempts have been made to investigate this counterbalancing effect of group solidarity on the mental health of blacks. However, this work has been hampered by the fact that the stresses of minority status have not been measured explicitly. In particular, only one study of race differences in exposure and response to life events has been reported in the literature, and this study found both greater exposure and vulnerability to undesirable events among nonwhites. Other researchers have inferred from available data that blacks are exposed to more stresses than whites, by virtue of their disadvantaged social status, but there have been no attempts to measure stress explicitly.

Evidence has been presented that indirectly supports the view that blacks develop cognitions that shield them from the self-esteem assaults that can come with some types of stress. Specifically, the relationship between personal efficacy and self-esteem is much weaker among blacks than among whites. Perhaps a group ideology that explains low personal efficacy as a result of discrimination negates the damaging effects that feelings of low efficacy would otherwise have. More work is needed on this possibility, and on extensions that would take into consideration vulnerabilities to particular types of stress situations.

Consistent evidence exists that Americans of Mexican heritage are underrepresented in treatment statistics relative to their proportions in the population. Furthermore, community surveys of Anglo-Hispanic differences in nonspecific psychological distress report mixed results, with no consistent evidence for a difference in the levels of distress experienced by members of the two groups.

The underrepresentation of persons of Mexican origin in treatment groups and the inconclusiveness of normal population surveys have been the source of much speculation. Minority scholars share the general view that Mexican Americans have much greater mental health needs than these statistics show, and that further research should attempt to measure that need accurately and to study the determinants of underutilization. Considerable research also has been conducted on the possibility that minority communities and family structures provide protective resources that bolster the mental health of Hispanics. Most of this work focuses on the relationship between group identification and mental health. The general view is that acculturation leads to heightened psychological distress by exposing individuals to conflicting values and pulling them away from the traditionally supportive environment that buffered them from the effects of life stress. Consistent with this hypothesis, Mexican-American mental patients are more often seen to be in a conflicted position between traditional Mexican values and the more mainstream values of American society as compared with nonpatients.

Systematic evidence is lacking about how minority families foster identities and provide nurturant environments. Personal identity is created in the context of an early childhood environment where a child's most significant interactions take place with people of the same race or ethnicity. Group identity, in comparison, takes place later as a result of contacts with the larger society. There is currently a great deal of interest in the parallel developments of these two identities and the conditions under which they are tied to each other. The ability to develop a deeper understanding of minority mental health hinges on unraveling these developmental processes and their implications for self-attributions, supports, and coping efforts.

PSYCHIATRIC HELP-SEEKING

Needs-assessment surveys show that most people with serious emotional problems do not seek professional help, although this attitude is changing, as people increasingly accept the view that emotional problems should be treated by a mental health professional. Nonetheless, informal helpers are still appealed to most often in times of emotional turmoil. Furthermore, a person seeking professional help is more likely to turn to a primary care physician than a mental health specialist. This choice is partly a result of the lack of mental health specialists in some areas of the country, but other variables are also involved.

Most of our direct knowledge about these other determinants comes from general population surveys that ask respondents about emotional problems they might have had and whether they sought professional help for these problems. These surveys have documented several consistent attitudinal, demographic, and system-dependent determinants of help-seeking.

Sociologists have been particularly interested in structural determinants, the strongest and most consistent of which is social class. A positive correlation between social class and help-seeking has persisted even though community mental health centers and other inexpensive treatment facilities have reduced the financial barriers to care. In the most recent surveys, education has emerged as a stronger predictor of help-seeking than income, which suggests that some cultural facilitating factors are more important than financial resources in accounting for the influence of social class.

Women are much more likely than men to seek mental health care, even given the higher prevalence of disorder among women. Sociological research over the past few years has made considerable progress in understanding this sex difference by showing that women are more likely to recognize their problems than men, and that this recognition of a problem is the main point in the decision-making process that discriminates men and women. Once either men or women recognize that they have a problem, they do not differ in their likelihood of obtaining professional help. The subject of why women are more likely to recognize their problems is currently under study.

The most recent studies of help-seeking suggest that the determinants of utilization differ markedly from one community to another, a fact that suggests indirectly that alternatives play a major part in determining who will seek treatment. It is likely that this result will lead to greater emphasis on comparative case studies of particular communities.

It is interesting to note that most careful case studies of help-seeking document that the critical point in the process is deciding that help is needed. The difficulty is that most people do not have any conception of when a personal problem is big enough to warrant professional care. As social scientists come to appreciate the great importance of problem definition, more sophisticated theories are being developed about how people make sense of symptoms. Recent research has suggested that people operate on the basis of schemas for explaining particular kinds of illnesses. These schemas contain lay accounts of the cause, course, symptoms, and prophylaxis for various illnesses. Research has already shown that a number of different schemas exist for particular medical conditions, and that characteristics of the schema held by a particular person provide important insights into the person's help-seeking and compliance habits. Although systematic research into schemas for psychiatric disorder is in its infancy, it is likely to become a major area of investigation over the next decade.

COMMUNITY RESPONSES TO THE MENTALLY ILL

ATTITUDES Attitudes about the mentally ill have been charted in public opinion surveys since the 1950s. Dislike and fear have remained high among the attitudes surveyed. Negative attitudes are particularly pronounced among people who are poorly educated and among the elderly. Men consistently report more negative attitudes than women.

The core concerns about persons who are mentally ill revolve around their presumed unpredictability and dangerousness. These concerns have some basis in reality, as patients released from state psychiatric hospitals have evidenced comparatively high arrest rates. However, most crimes committed by released patients are property crimes that do not involve violence.

Intensely negative attitudes about the mentally ill may be part of a larger cluster of beliefs, attitudes, and values characterized by an absence of sympathy for people who need help, a deep-seated distrust of people and institutions who are different, and a rigid outlook on what is right and wrong. People with this orientation cannot easily be swayed by rational arguments to change their views.

Fortunately, most people have much less intense negative feelings that can be modified on the basis of experience, and as they become more knowledgeable, learn to make finer distinctions about kinds of mental illness and treatment. Visits to a psychotherapist, for example, have much less stigma attached than hospitalization for a mental illness. Private hospitalization seems to be less stigmatizing than public hospitalization. Drug therapies are perceived as evidence of greater disorder and so provoke more fear and distrust of the patient than of a person who has undergone insight therapy. For a similar reason, treatment by a psychiatrist invokes more negative attitudes than consultation with a psychologist, social worker, or member of the clergy.

Survey data suggest that attitudes of community members can be influenced by contact with the mentally ill. Survey respondents who report knowing someone who has a history of mental illness are, in general, less negative than people who report no personal contact. It is difficult to sort out cause and effect here, because negative attitudes might be associated with failure to report to an interviewer the mental illness of a close relative.

Family studies and studies of the reintegration of former patients into their old work roles show that contact with their former co-workers and associates promotes positive attitudes about the mentally ill. Seeing a former patient perform adequately in a normal role is particularly important in this regard. Self-disclosure by the former patient about what it was like to have a mental illness and to be hospitalized also helps promote normalization and acceptance by reducing the aura of mystery that otherwise surrounds the illness.

Much less is known about how to change negative attitudes in the general population. Studies of the mass media show that the stereotyped depictions of former patients that commonly appear on television and in movies reinforce negative public perceptions about the mentally ill. Whether sympathetic treatments of mentally ill people in the mass media might change these negative attitudes, or whether informational campaigns making use of the mass media could increase public knowledge about mental illness, is less understood.

This last issue is attracting considerable interest, however, with several large mass media campaigns under development to increase public awareness, recognition, and treatment of mental illness. The largest of the campaigns is the D/ART (Depression Awareness, Recognition, and Treatment) Program being designed by the National Institute of Mental Health to inspire increased voluntary help-seeking for major depression. This program will be evaluated to learn more about the kinds of message strategies and information channels that most effectively lead to attitude and behavior changes. One can anticipate that this evaluation will yield important new information about the influence of the mass media on attitudes about mental illness.

COMMUNITY REACTIONS TO SHELTERED CARE HOMES Negative attitudes about the mentally ill are important for a number of reasons, including the fact that they inhibit help-seeking for personal problems. In this subsection, one consequence is considered that has been the subject of recent sociological attention—the organizational effect of negative attitudes on attempts to establish group homes for the mentally ill.

Sociologists have done a great deal of research on collective action, and community opposition to group homes has become one of the mobilization activities studied by those working in this tradition. This research clearly indicates that middle-class neighborhoods are much more resistant to having group homes in their midst than are working-class neighborhoods. This greater resistance can be traced to effective mobilization efforts. In particular, efforts to meet and organize local opposition are effected more quickly in middle-class neighborhoods. A person or a committee is more likely to be selected to act on the neighborhood's behalf and multipronged political actions are more likely to occur here.

Community attitudes also play an important part in the success of group homes in fostering readjustment among deinstitutionalized patients. Ethnographic research shows clearly that patients are aware of the accepting or rejecting attitude climates in their neighborhoods, which influence their social functioning. Most sheltered care homes eventually succeed in establishing themselves, and the ease with which the residents of these homes adjust to life in the community depends to a large degree on community acceptance—and the conflict that can attend the creation of the home does not make a good foundation on which to build such acceptance. In general, public opinion surveys show that contact with former patients who are strangers exacerbates whatever fears and uncertainties community residents already have, particularly in cases where conflict arose about the establishment of the group home.

These issues have been neglected in most sociological studies of community opposition to group homes. Such studies generally concentrate on structural determinants of neighborhood mobilization and on strategies available to agencies for diffusing this opposition. Research is urgently needed on what happens next, after the home is opened and the residents have to live in the neighborhood. As noted earlier, the evidence demonstrates that contact with a former mental patient who was known prior to hospitalization can foster positive attitude changes, especially when the former patient can be seen performing adequately in normal roles. A challenge for the future is to create structured situations that will facilitate contact between residents of sheltered care homes and their neighbors in such a way that these kinds of positive attitude changes can occur.

THE ORGANIZATION OF MENTAL HEALTH SERVICES

RESEARCH ON INTERORGANIZATIONAL COORDINATION Research on complex organizations is one of the liveliest areas in sociology today as a result of the enormous organizational changes in American society and the innovative work of social theorists in developing new frameworks within which to understand these changes. The mental health care delivery system has been a favorite example used by these theorists to test new ideas about interorganizational linkage, as it provides unique opportunities to study a decentralized system consisting of many overlapping organizations that have complex coordinating links.

This work is too new to have developed any broad theoretical perspectives or clear understanding of the complex relationships among the organizational networks that make up the community mental health system. It has contributed a number of informative case studies, however, which collectively document that the failures of the system can be traced to inconsistencies in the rationalities of the different organizational actors it comprises. Each decision-making unit in the system functions in a way that promotes the success of a particular organization, but no mechanisms are in place to guarantee the success of the entire system.

Among the various lines of research that demonstrate these inconsistencies is the use of intensive case studies that map out the relations that develop among different community agencies in particular areas. These studies show that many of the interorganizational arrangements involving community mental health agencies are poorly coordinated. Historical analyses indicate that this lack of coordination results from the cumulation of many different specific decisions that seemed rational from a narrow perspective at the time they were made but lack any overall plan or purpose. The challenge for researchers is to combine these case studies into a comparative analysis that pinpoints the fundamental coordinating mechanisms that facilitate rationality in the relations among community organizations. This kind of work is currently the subject of intense interest among organizational sociologists.

A related series of studies has attempted to trace the influences of state and national policy initiatives on community-based organizations and systems. Studies have been done, for example, on how strategic decision-making in local organizations is affected by considerations concerning the future actions of state and national funding agencies. These studies show that state or national initiatives to develop community-based programs often set in motion local processes of adaptation with consequences that were not intended by the policy makers who developed the programs. Current research is moving in the direction of comparative studies aimed at isolating characteristics of particular community systems that determine the directions local responses take.

ORGANIZATIONAL FACTORS IN SERVICE DELIVERY Another kind of organizational research extends the work on job stress reviewed earlier by studying the influence of organizational structure on the health, well-being, and productivity of its members. Some of this work has studied the structural components of mental health care organizations that affect staff satisfaction with their work. A few studies have also examined the impact of organizational structure on patient outcomes. All of this work has been naturalistic rather than experimental, and comparative rather than based on case studies of individual treatment settings.

Some of the more interesting findings include the fact that staff satisfaction and productivity are positively associated with decision latitude. Patient functioning in long-term mental hospitals is also positively associated with the decision latitude of lower-level staff. Other correlates of good patient functioning include high staff job satisfaction and high staff participation in treatment decisions. Patient functioning in acute-care inpatient settings is positively associated with an active management style; functioning of patients in community-based shelter care homes is likely to be better when the homes are small, have flexible rules, and require patients to take some responsibility for the activities of daily living.

As this litany of results suggests, there is as yet no overarching theoretical framework that integrates the specific findings into a coherent model of organizational influence on staff and patient functioning. This is an important goal for the next decade. Integrative work of this type will be facilitated by the insights sociologists are obtaining from job redesign experiments in industrial settings. Similar experiments in treatment settings are much less common, although innovative experiments are now under way to change the structures of community-based shelter care homes in an effort to reduce the problems of staff burnout and turnover. It is likely that the success of these organizational redesign efforts will determine whether similar experiments are carried out in a wider range of treatment settings.

EVALUATION OF COMMUNITY MENTAL HEALTH SERVICES Another level of organizational research is the evaluation of local mental health services. The development and maintenance of an effective community-based system require a cyclical process of service planning, implementation, evaluation, and feedback. The first step in this process is usually some kind of needs assessment, identifying the mental health problems in the community and establishing priorities for the creation of services to address these problems. Such an assessment is vitally important to organizational success by monitoring demand for services and pinpointing needs not recognized by community residents.

The most direct way to conduct such an assessment is by means of large-scale community surveys. Unfortunately, such surveys are very expensive and most local service organizations are unable to afford them. As a result, a number of innovative approaches have been devised to obtain more indirect information about need at a lower cost. These techniques include systematic interviews with key informants, the establishment of citizen advisory councils, the use of national statistics on need profiles in conjunction with small-area social indicators on community demographics, and extrapolation from data on demand for services to estimates about need for services.

Once programs are developed, research can also be important in evaluating effectiveness and targeting areas that must be changed to increase effectiveness. Program effectiveness relies on at least two levels of research. The first level focuses on success in attracting participants to the program; the second level's focus is on success in helping people with their problems. Behavioral scientists have been more active in the first research area than in the second area.

Research on success in attracting program participants emphasizes acceptability, accessibility, and awareness. Acceptability refers to how willing community residents are to use the new service. Accessibility involves the ease with which the program can be reached. Time, distance, transportation, and financial barriers are all important to consider here. Awareness relates to community knowledge that the service exists and that it is appropriate for particular needs. An understanding of local culture is required to develop programs that are sensitive to these issues and sociological research can be critically important in obtaining such knowledge. This is usually accomplished through ethnographic research or by other strategies that increase the sensitivity of program staff to local norms and customs.

Research that evaluates the effectiveness of programs is much less common. Several factors account for this inadequacy of research, including the substantial costs of implementing a carefully controlled study of treatment effectiveness, the high level of methodological sophistication required to carry out such an investigation, and the potential threat to clinicians and program administrators of openly studying whether their services are actually therapeutic. Sociologists and other behavioral scientists have the expertise to do this work. It is of great importance to obtain accurate evaluations of treatment effectiveness. Sadly, this remains an underdeveloped area of investigation.

THE SOCIAL CONTEXT OF PROFESSIONAL ACTIVITY It is apparent that the medical profession is undergoing enormous change, engendered by such things as diagnostic related groups and other new payment arrangements, shifting of care from inpatient to ambulatory settings, diversification of the medical care industry, increasingly overt competition among providers, and the growing importance of third-party payers.

These changes are part of broader societal forces that include the aging of our population, and cohort shifts that have led to massive expansion in the plant facilities of the medical care industry, as well as to a marked increase in the number of physicians in the marketplace.

Sociologists have been keenly interested in the implications of these trends for the future of medicine. Several perspectives can be distinguished among the views of the social theorists who have turned their minds to this issue.

One perspective holds that physician domination of the health care system is too firmly established to be shaken by the changes in social context that are taking place. The legal subordination of nurses, pharmacists, and other medical care professionals to the physician is cited as critical in this regard, as are the exclusive licensing powers granted to physicians as gatekeepers of the medical care system.

An opposing view is that the medical profession is in a period of declining power as a result of the resurgence of consumerism in medicine. The greater number of medical patients who suffer from chronic conditions rather than acute ones, created by medical successes in the period since World War II in prolonging the lives of patients with life-threatening chronic illnesses, creates an interest group of lay people who acquire considerable technical knowledge about their own afflictions, band together to form self-help groups, and sometimes challenge the professionals who care for them. The technical diversification of medical procedures and the increasingly important contributions to health care by technician-specialists who are not physicians are also thought to play a part. With changes in the organization of professional care, new systems of ownership and management have promoted competition among physicians, which inevitably brings with it increased consumer control. Finally, the more dominant position of large insurers consolidates the bargaining position of consumers in a way that has never before been witnessed. These views are particularly relevant to psychiatrists, because the existence of auxiliary mental health specialists, such as clinical psychologists and psychiatric social workers, has no counterpart among other medical specialties.

Another perspective on the changing nature of medical practice involves the proletarianization of medical work. More and more physicians are working as salaried employees in large, bureaucratically managed organizations, and this is especially true of psychiatrists. Furthermore, these organizations are instituting managerial styles orchestrated by the graduates of business schools rather than of medical schools. Along with these changes have come changes in procedures for professional control. Formal review procedures are being applied to a wider range of professional behaviors. Within particular institutions, mechanisms are being developed to monitor and control the technical decisions of clinicians. All of these trends will result in increasing external control of the domain of professional practice.

The shape that psychiatric practice will take in the future is difficult to forecast, and the conflicting views of social scientists who specialize in this kind of prognostication demonstrate considerable uncertainty. It is likely that, over time, a more complete set of findings will develop to increase understanding of the changes that are taking place today, and perhaps even to extrapolate these understandings into a perspective that can be used to help prepare or modify the place of psychiatrists in the future medical care system.

REFERENCES

Aiken L H, Mechanic D: *Applications of Social Science to Clinical Medicine and Health Policy*. Rutgers University Press, New Brunswick, NJ, 1986.

Brown G W, Harris T: *Social Origins of Depression*. Free Press, New York, 1978.

Cohen S, Syme L, editors: *Social Support and Health*. Academic Press, New York, 1985.

Falloon I R H, Boyd J L, McGill C W: *Family Care of Schizophrenia*. Guilford, New York, 1984.

Greenley J R: Social factors, mental illness, and psychiatric care: Recent advances from a sociological perspective. Hosp Comm Psychiat *35:* 813, 1984.

Henderson S, Burne D G, Duncan-Jones P: *Neurosis and the Social Environment*. Academic Press, New York, 1981.

Kahn R L: *Work and Health*. Wiley-Interscience, New York, 1981.

Kessler R C, Price R H, Wortman C B: Social factors in psychopathology: Stress, social support, and coping processes. Ann Rev Psychol *36:* 531, 1985.

McHugh S, editor: *Illness Behavior: A Multidisciplinary Model*. Plenum, New York, 1986.

Scott W R, Black B L, editors: *The Organization of Mental Health Services*. Sage, Beverly Hills, CA, 1986.

Silver R L, Wortman C B: Coping with undesirable life events. In *Human Helplessness,* J Garber, M E P Seligman, editors, p 279. Academic Press, New York, 1980.

CHAPTER 5 QUANTITATIVE AND EXPERIMENTAL METHODS IN PSYCHIATRY

5.1
EPIDEMIOLOGY

DARREL A. REGIER, M.D., M.P.H.
JACK D. BURKE, JR., M.D., M.P.H.

INTRODUCTION

This section is intended to assist clinicians, administrators, and other mental health research investigators in understanding the contributions of epidemiology to their respective fields.

DEFINITION Mental disorder epidemiology is the quantitative study of the distribution and causes of mental disorder in human populations. This definition has several important components.

Population focus Population groups, rather than individuals, constitute the basic unit of analysis. Although individuals within population groups must be accurately diagnosed, the unique scientific questions addressed by epidemiology begin with descriptions of how mental disorders are distributed across different population subgroups.

Quantitative methods Because of its focus on the health status of population groups, epidemiology has often been referred to as the basic science of public health. Higher than average disease rates in population groups are referred to as epidemics from the Greek *epi* (upon) and *deme* (the people). Although there are many clinical, journalistic, or political ways of describing the impact of an illness on the population, it is the province of epidemiology to provide a quantitative assessment of the frequency with which illnesses affect different segments of the population at different times. Quantitative statistical methods are the means by which differences in the frequency of disorders in population groups are assessed.

Correlates It is a basic tenet of scientific faith that pathological states are not randomly distributed in the population, but rather are differentially associated with physical, biological, social, and temporal characteristics of human beings and their environment. Epidemiologists seek to discover characteristic factors that may define populations with excessively high rates of a mental disorder. This approach is used initially to narrow the range of characteristics associated with a disorder and ultimately to identify characteristic risk factors, which, if altered, will interrupt a causal network producing a disorder.

SPECIAL FEATURES Despite great efforts in the past 30 years, both in the United States and elsewhere, progress in psychiatric epidemiology has been slow because of several methodological problems that are just now being overcome.

Nosology The relative quiescence of epidemiological mental health research over the past generation may be attributed in part to limits on the state-of-the-art in the clinical research field of nosology. The grouping of morbidity states for quantitative analysis requires that classification of disorders be explicit and reliably applied across large populations. If mixed conditions are included under one diagnostic category, risk factors associated with one of the component disorders will have their statistical association diluted and, thus, fail to be recognized by the epidemiological method.

A limiting factor in psychiatric nosology has been the heavy reliance on manifestational criteria (e.g., signs, symptoms, clinical course, and treatment response manifestations) as opposed to causal criteria (e.g., toxins, trauma, and metabolic defect). Dependence on manifestational criteria in the absence of convincing causal factors increases the likelihood that heterogeneous groups may be combined in one diagnosis. This problem is shared by the rest of clinical medicine, which attempts to move beyond a diagnosis based on such symptoms as fever, to a specific etiological agent or anatomical defect. The new descriptive approach to psychiatric nosology has been an important intermediate stage that will facilitate more rigorous investigations of causal factors in clinical and epidemiological studies.

Case identification methods One special difficulty has been in developing a technique to obtain standardized psychiatric assessments of a large sample of individuals, so that the presence of clinically meaningful mental disorder can be determined. Without clearly defined nosological categories, it has been difficult both to define a case and to develop case identification (diagnostic) techniques that are appropriate for large-scale population studies. Such techniques require explicit criteria if clear communication to other researchers and reliable administration are to be feasible. In the absence of reliably administered assessment methods, epidemiologists have often used self-report questionnaires that assess the dimensions of psychological and psychophysiological symptoms. Cut-off scores on various symptom scales have been calibrated with symptom profiles of patients under treatment. Thus, subjects in the general population could be assessed in terms of their probability of having disorders similar to those seen in clinical settings. The absence of face validity of many such questionnaires, the lack of diagnostic specificity, and the tautological assumption that mental disorders under treatment should define the full spectrum of all types of mental disorder led to clinician apathy about epidemiological survey results. In recent years, however, standardized clinical interview methods have been adapted for use in epidemiological surveys—a development that offers major new opportunities for mental disorder epidemiology.

Risk factors At a more advanced level of investigation, another difficulty has been to determine what psychosocial and biological factors are likely candidates for identifying high-risk groups for particular psychiatric disorders; once identified, these factors must also be measured in objective ways as part of an epidemiological study.

The relative paucity of clearly defined and modifiable risk factors available for study has led to an overdependence on associations with descriptive and relatively unmodifiable factors such as age, sex, and ethnic status. Although presumably modifiable factors, such as stressful life events, have recently emerged, the mechanism of multifactorial interaction between individual susceptibility and stress has not yet been fully explicated.

Chronic disease epidemiology paradigm Other difficulties in psychiatric epidemiology are shared with the epidemiology of chronic medical diseases. These characteristics include a dependence on manifest criteria and incomplete information on the subsequent temporal aspects of clinical course; uncertainty about the time at which causative factors may have affected the individual; an undefined lag time between the onset of a pathogenic influence and the occurrence of the disorder; and the absence of any generally accepted concept as to a time when the disorder may be considered to be eradicated in a patient with a history of the illness. Although these characteristics do not apply to all mental disorders, they are shared by many in the fields of cancer, cardiovascular disease, and rheumatological disease epidemiology.

Future directions Recent advances in the classification and standardized diagnosis of mental disorders have made it possible to initiate a new series of population studies that can serve as a baseline for future investigations. In the next decade, as understanding of biological, psychosocial, and other cultural factors increases, risk factor studies of new power and scope will become possible. The careful attention to basic methodological issues in past research has brought psychiatric epidemiology to an exciting frontier, with a promise of future advance.

USES OF EPIDEMIOLOGY

There are essentially three sequential levels of investigation on which the various applications of epidemiology depend. These levels can be grouped according to their basic intent as follows:

1. Descriptive: studies that produce basic estimates of the rates of disorder in a general population and its subgroups.
2. Analytic: studies that explore the basis of variations in illness rates among different groups in order to identify risk factors that may contribute to the development of a disorder.
3. Experimental: studies that test the presumed association between a risk factor and a disorder and that seek to reduce the occurrence of illness by controlling the risk factor.

At each level of investigation, information is obtained that can be used to improve clinical practice and to plan public health policies. If the past difficulties with nosology, case-identification techniques, risk factor specification, and chronic disease paradigms can be addressed in the future, it may be possible to realize more fully the potential applications of epidemiology that were identified by J. N. Morris. These seven basic uses can be discussed in relation to the three stages of epidemiological inquiry in order to demonstrate the important applications of epidemiological knowledge, even in the earliest studies at the descriptive level of investigation.

DESCRIPTIVE LEVEL **1. Community diagnosis** The starting point for epidemiological research is to estimate rates of illness in a defined population. This task of community diagnosis provides a baseline for understanding the burden of illness in the population, the mix of disorders present, and the extent to which untreated cases exist. These basic rates are needed before more elaborate studies of risk factors can be undertaken, and they are important for health planners who want to know what kind of treatment services may be needed in the community, especially if untreated cases are to be brought into the health care system in the future.

When the President's Commission on Mental Health examined U.S. mental health issues in the late 1970s, two fundamental questions that were addressed were the extent of mental illness in the population and the role of health services in providing treatment to those individuals with mental disorders. In view of the previous difficulties in obtaining valid estimates for these figures, the best answer that could be given was based on a synthesis of information from a variety of studies. The composite picture of the situation is shown in Figure 5.1-1, which demonstrates where the 32 million Americans who were estimated to have a mental disorder at some point during 1975 were seen within the health care or other human services sectors.

2. Completing the clinical picture More precise answers to such questions about community diagnosis and basic rates of illness can be obtained only if a standardized assessment procedure is available that can be used to ascertain the diagnostic status of the large number of individuals who are sampled in a study. If this case ascertainment can be done well, then epidemiological studies will benefit clinical understanding, as well as the field of public health. The full clinical picture of the disorder can be studied by characterizing subclinical or mild cases, by studying relatives to determine the familial occurrence of the condition, and by following the progression of the illness to determine its course and prognosis in a comprehensive sample. The value of this effort rests on the fundamental rule of epidemiology, which is to sample individuals from a geographically defined population without the bias that may arise if a sample is drawn only from patients seen in particular treatment settings. For example, with the new classification of schizophrenia and related disorders in the revised third edition of the *Diagnostic and Statistical Manual of Mental Disorders* (DSM-III-R), it will be important to determine the associated features for each condition, the prognosis, and the course of the illness in longitudinal studies.

3. Identification of syndromes Similarly, it may be that some conditions occur in a population sample that have not previously been recognized in studies whose samples are drawn only from clinical populations. The opportunity to identify new syndromes in the population is provided by both representative sampling from the population and the application of thorough, standardized assessment procedures for all individuals in a sample. Whether epidemiological investigations can also be used to demonstrate that old syndromes are invalid is an intriguing notion, but still controversial. One example of such a debate has been the decision to omit a category for involutional melancholia from the third edition of the *Diagnostic and Statistical Manual of Mental Disorders* (DSM-III) and DSM-III-R because of findings based on epidemiological data.

ANALYTIC LEVEL **4. Assessing individual risks** Once the basic rates of illness are established, it is possible to identify groups in the population with unusually high rates of illness. This comparative analysis provides a variety of hypotheses for testing to see if some characteristics of the more commonly affected group can be linked to a causal chain for the illness. For example, an early finding of psychiatric epidemiology in the 1930s was that rates of schizophrenia appeared to be higher among low-income, inner-city residents. The first problem in assessing such a finding is to determine whether it reflects a potentially higher risk of developing schizophrenia among those who live in such conditions, or whether those who have schizophrenia move into such areas through downward social mobility. This question still awaits a definitive resolution.

Even if the place of residence seems to be an antecedent characteristic rather than a consequence of the disorder, it is still necessary for investigators to pursue the study of possible risk factors that may underlie the apparent association between this group characteristic and the disorder. It may be that particular features of poverty, poor housing, or population density may be risk factors; that genetic, nutritional, or other familial risks are higher in people who live in such areas; or that toxic or infectious agents are the true contributors and occur more commonly in such areas.

Moving from the demonstration of higher rates in a particular group to more targeted studies of putative risk factors for individuals is an essential but difficult step in the progression of epidemiological investigations.

5. Historical study Identification of risk factors may be made easier if some historical variation can be shown. This type of evidence may help strengthen the arguments for studying one or another putative risk factor. For example, to judge from a 25-year study of one community in Sweden, depression may be increasing and dementia may be decreasing in an industrialized Western society. For depression, other findings indicate that psychosocial and other environmental factors may be important risk factors.

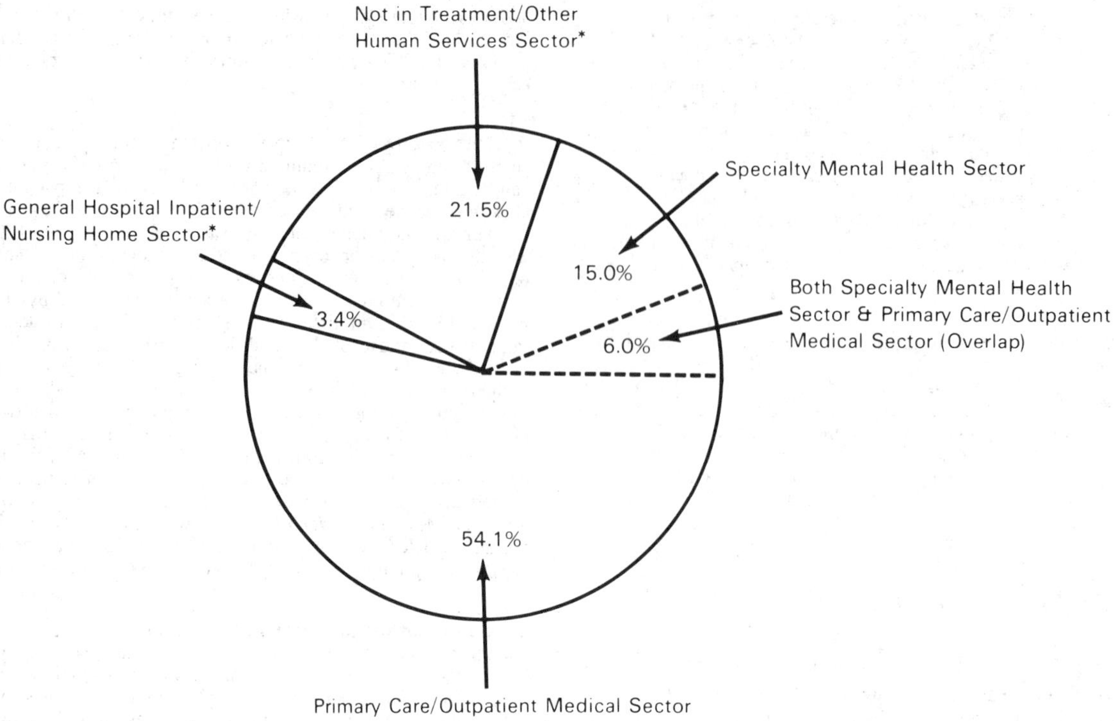

Note: Data relating to sectors other than the specialty mental health sector reflect the number of patients with mental disorder seen in those sectors without regard to the amount or adequacy of treatment provided.

*Excludes overlap of an unknown percent of persons also seen in other sectors.

FIGURE 5.1-1. *Estimated percent distribution of persons with mental disorder, by treatment setting, in the United States in 1975.*

EXPERIMENTAL LEVEL **6. Identifying causes** As risk factors are demonstrated, epidemiologists can help to reduce the contributing causes of the disorder by intervening in the causal chain that links a risk factor to the occurrence of disorder. Undertaking studies to modify a risk factor and to assess the effect of this intervention in reducing onset of illness is a long-term goal of epidemiologists. This type of investigation promises to elucidate opportunities for primary prevention of mental disorders by intervening to reduce the chances that high-risk individuals will develop an illness. One important benefit of the quantitative, population-based method of epidemiological investigation is that it can be used to measure the impact of preventive interventions being tested. Such an assessment is important both to determine the benefits of the intervention for high-risk individuals and to assess the magnitude of any unintended negative effects of the program.

7. Working of health services Although the epidemiological method is usually taken as a guide to primary prevention of disorders, it can also be used for secondary prevention—early diagnosis, and the prompt, effective treatment of persons who have already developed signs of the illness. The contribution of epidemiology to understanding the working of health services is often thought to refer to the descriptive level of study (with estimates of treatments provided and unmet need for service), but a wider perspective demonstrates that the three-stage epidemiological method can be applied to patient populations in clinical settings as well as to general populations in the community.

With a parallel to primary prevention based on assessment and reduction of risk factors, a scheme for secondary prevention can also be devised. Once the prevalence of clinical disorders is determined, as has been done with depression among primary care patients, it is possible to assess the extent of early diagnosis and prompt, effective treatment. Despite the common occurrence of depressive disorders in primary care patients, recent studies in the United States and elsewhere have suggested that these disorders often are not diagnosed or treated.

Interventions to improve clinical practice through secondary prevention can be tested, just as primary prevention intervention efforts would be tested in the traditional epidemiological model. Research of this type, with application of the three stages of epidemiological research to clinical populations, is known as clinical services research.

EPIDEMIOLOGICAL METHODS

It is believed that the greatest potential benefits to the mental health field lie not in past examples, but in providing a conceptual framework for future applications of epidemiological methods. An intelligent reading of many clinical and basic neurobiological research studies, as well as epidemiological studies, should be facilitated by this quantitative conceptual framework.

As noted earlier, epidemiology has several important characteristics, including a population-centered research strategy that requires an adequate sampling plan. Especially in psychiatry, epidemiological research also depends on advances in the nosology of mental disorders, which were necessary before acceptable case-identification instruments could be developed. With these prerequisites met, quantitative research in psychiatric epidemiology has become possible.

SAMPLING One of the most powerful features of the epidemiological method is that two desirable conditions about the sample of people under study can be met: A suitable reference population or universe can be defined, and individuals in the study can be related to this defined universe in a specified way. If these conditions are satisfied, the results of the study can be generalized to the universe.

In this discussion, the universe will be taken as the hypothetical population to which the investigator wishes to generalize results; the study population will be taken as the operational equivalent of the universe that will actually be studied by the investigator. A universe may be all residents of a delimited area whereas a study population may consist of those listed as customers of a local electric utility. The study population should be as equivalent to the specific universe as possible.

Once the study population has been defined, and is judged equivalent to the universe, its members can be assessed to determine their risk or illness status. All members of the study population can be assessed in a total count, if money, time, and other resources are adequate. Usually, though, it is necessary to select a few representative members of the study population to form the study sample.

Sampling design The fundamental principle of sampling is to select subjects in such a way that the sample results will be representative of the entire study population, assuming equivalence to the intended universe. To assure that the sample does represent the entire study population, the members of the study sample must be selected without bias and with a known probability of selection. The basic case is the simple random sample. All members of the study population are rostered, and a sample is selected randomly.

Sample selection Consider, for example, a study population of 3,000 individuals that can be listed in this way: The investigator has planned to examine about 300 subjects, which is a 10 percent sample of the study population. Using a random selection procedure, such as choosing subjects by a table of random numbers, the investigator can select, on the average, one in every 10 individuals to be in the study. In simple random samples, every member of the population has an equal and known probability of being selected for the sample, in this case a one in 10 chance. With large numbers chosen, random selection tends to produce a sample that in the aggregate reflects the composition of the study population. In the above example, if the distribution of females in the 3,000 population members is 60 percent, it will be roughly the same in the sample; the larger the total number of people chosen for the sample, the more likely it is that all the characteristics in the study population will be reflected accurately in the study sample.

Sample size The drive to reproduce overall population characteristics in the sample by random selection is one reason that large sample sizes are desirable; another reason is that estimates of rates or other statistics are more precise when a large number of individuals is used as the basis for estimation.

Point estimate Study sample A, drawn by the investigator as described above, is clearly not the only one that could be drawn from the study population. With a different starting point in the table of random numbers, a different series of 300 individuals would be selected for the study sample. This second sample can be called B. Its composition will also reflect, roughly, the characteristics of the overall population of 3,000; the proportion of females in sample B will also be about 60 percent, but it probably will not be exactly the same proportion as was calculated for sample A. If the investigator drew repeated samples, and continued to calculate the proportion of females in each sample, these various sample estimates of the proportion of females in the overall population would form a range of values tending to center around the true population value of 60 percent. The estimate produced from a sample is called a *point estimate* of the proportion of females in the study population.

Standard error Although this repeated sampling of 300 individuals from the total population of 3,000 can be easily described, it is almost never feasible in a world of limited time, money, and researchers. If the first sample has been drawn at random, it is possible to calculate a statistic—the standard error of the proportion—that describes how much variation exists in a large series of repeated samples, composed of 300 subjects, that could theoretically be selected from a given population. With this standard error, which is easily calculated using data from one sample, it is possible to calculate a range of values that allows investigators to say that 95 times out of 100 the true proportion of females lies within this range. This range is known as the "95 percent confidence interval," and it has become customary for authors to report this range along with the point estimates of characteristics they have assessed in their samples. Larger numbers of individuals permit more stable point estimates, which means that the confidence interval is smaller than it is with only a few subjects in the study.

Confidence interval uses Confidence intervals are quite helpful in comparing rates of illness. Suppose that in this sample of 300 subjects, the investigator assessed the presence of major depression and wanted to compare rates for all high school graduates with those who have less education. The point estimates may look different (e.g., 3.0 percent for graduates and 9.5 percent for nongraduates). A valid comparison requires a consideration of how rough these point estimates may be in terms of the true population-based rates of illness.

Calculating 95 percent confidence intervals helps the investigator to determine if the apparent difference in rates is due to the roughness of the point estimates or to a true difference. With such a small sample, the confidence intervals may be large, say 0.3 to 5.7 percent for graduates and 4.8 to 14.2 percent for nongraduates; there is an overlap, so the differences may be due to variability of point estimates associated with sampling from the population. Because the 95 percent confidence intervals are large enough to overlap, it may not be possible to say that the difference in point estimates of 3.0 percent and 9.5 percent is a real one. When confidence intervals overlap, a definitive comparison of point estimates can be made by a statistical test, such as the chi-square test. Larger numbers of subjects in the sample lead to smaller confidence intervals around point estimates, so there is a premium on having enough subjects. Statistical power analysis allows investigators to plan their studies so that they can be sure of a reasonable chance of having enough subjects to support confidence intervals that are smaller than the anticipated differences in the most important rates that will be compared.

Stratified sampling In many cases, unfortunately, simple random sampling is not useful. In the example being considered, suppose that the investigator wanted to look at subgroups—for example, college graduates—that occurred in the population much less commonly than high school graduates and nongraduates. Rather than collapsing the college graduates into a category with all who finished high school, the investigator may want to be sure that the study sample includes enough subjects who are college graduates. With the equal probability of selection entailed in the simple random sampling, college graduates would only be as common in the sample as they were in the study population.

A more complicated approach to sampling would be to roster the 3,000 individuals in three separate groups or strata, rather than in a single listing, and then to sample each stratum separately. The investigator could decide to have 100 subjects from each educational stratum. If the study population contained 1,500 persons who were nongraduates, the probability of selecting any one of them for the study would be 100 out of 1,500, or about 0.07. If the college graduates numbered only 500, the probability of selection would be 100 out of 500, or 0.20.

This type of sampling is called stratified random sampling, and it requires slightly more complex statistical techniques than simple random sampling does to calculate point estimates and confidence intervals for proportions. In stratified random sampling, each subject is weighted according to the selection probability; estimates can be obtained for specific strata as well as for the total study population.

Cluster sampling One problem with these sampling strategies is that individual members of the study population must be listed in order to be sampled. Such a listing may be possible for small populations whose members can be identified, such as patients seen in a clinical setting, but is usually not possible for large populations, especially of community residents. An alternative is to use lists of groups, or clusters, of individuals. The only roster of units that can be sampled in a community may be a list of census tracts or a map of city blocks. Once a sample is chosen, all the households within the selected block can be listed, and a sample of households can be selected. After the households are chosen, the people who live in them can be entered into the study. Cluster sampling is often the only feasible method, because lists of individuals in a population cannot always be obtained, and it is more efficient than simple or stratified random sampling of individuals in enrolling a large sample. However, it produces less precise estimates (i.e., larger confidence intervals).

In studies of the total population, cluster sampling can become quite complicated. Selection of clusters can be done within several different types of strata—households and institutions, urban and rural—and some individuals can be sampled at higher rates, for example, the elderly or children. In these cases, calculation of selection probabilities and the associated efforts to produce confidence intervals and more sophisticated statistical comparisons become highly complex, and they require special computer packages that are available in only a few research centers.

NOSOLOGY Before acceptable case-identification instruments can be developed in epidemiology, it is necessary to write diagnostic criteria that can be unambiguously interpreted. Once these clear explicit statements of the requirements for each disorder are available, it is possible to create examination protocols based on such statements.

Proposed sets of explicit criteria for psychiatric diagnoses were first published in the 1970s, with the St. Louis research criteria and Research Diagnostic Criteria (RDC). In 1980, DSM-III adopted the approach of writing explicit criteria to use as the basis for clinical practice and for epidemiological and other research; it proved very useful and has been extended in DSM-III-R.

CASE ASSESSMENT Information about a subject can be collected in several ways. Medical records often are used for patients seen in clinical settings; they provide essential documentation about prior course of the illness, other disorders or preexisting risks, and the type and course of the treatment provided. For some studies, the diagnoses shown in these records are used to identify patients with rare disorders.

Records in central data banks can be important both for very rare disorders and for studying patterns of treatment in a defined area. Case registers are now maintained on a national basis for specific types of cancer. They provide a roster of patients with the disorder, and also information that can be used to test hypotheses about risk factors or other features of the illness in the future. For more common disorders, geographically based case registers furnish a record of all those in the population who received treatment for the disorder on a longitudinal basis. For 2 decades, a register of all patients seen in mental health treatment facilities in Monroe County in New York has been used to describe population treatment patterns in an urban community. A similar register was also maintained through the late 1970s for the state of Maryland.

The most important source of information about a subject in the study is often a direct interview, an examination, or both. Until the late 1970s, the major obstacle in psychiatric epidemiology was the lack of an acceptable case-assessment instrument to identify subjects with mental disorders that could be used in studies of the total area population.

CRITERIA FOR ASSESSMENT INSTRUMENT Several criteria must be satisfied by an assessment instrument before it can be used successfully in studies of human subjects.

Safety The assessment of subjects should not cause them harm; if risks do exist, the benefits of the study must outweigh the potential harm. Anyone participating in such a study must do so voluntarily after being informed of the nature and extent of potential risks, and must be able to withdraw at any time. These requirements are enforced by institutional review boards for the protection of human subjects at an investigator's institution. At present, there is no reason to believe that participation in epidemiological studies that include a diagnostic psychiatric interview harms either adults or children.

Feasibility With research funds becoming more limited, it has been increasingly important to develop assessment procedures that yield adequate information about large numbers of subjects without being unduly time consuming, burdensome for subjects, or dependent on a highly skilled examiner whose services are expensive. For total population surveys that include large enough samples, it has become prohibitively expensive to use highly trained mental health clinicians to perform psychiatric interviews. Alternatives are needed before such major studies can begin.

Reliability One of the most important psychometric properties of assessment instruments is reliability. Although it has several aspects, *reliability* usually refers to the assessment instrument's capacity to give consistent results when used by different examiners or at different times.

Validity An instrument that has acceptable levels of interrater (defined below) and test-retest reliability can be assessed to determine if it is measuring what it intends to measure. This property is called *validity*.

These two properties, reliability and validity, are so important that a more extensive discussion of their role in evaluating case-identification instruments is provided.

RELIABILITY The property of yielding equivalent results when used by different examiners with the same subject is known as *interrater reliability*. The property of producing equivalent results when used for the same subject on different occasions is called *test-retest reliability*. Although these two properties are necessary, they are not sufficient for an instrument; for example, a diagnostic interview, at least hypothetically, could show high interrater and test-retest reliability but give consistently wrong results. Accuracy would be attenuated without consistency, however, so demonstration of acceptable levels of reliability is usually required of any assessment instrument proposed for use in an epidemiological study before the study begins. Several measures of reliability are available; to a large extent, choice of the proper measure depends on the type of information the assessment instrument uses. In the simplest case, consider an interrater reliability pretest of a diagnostic interview that used two examiners to assess the presence or absence of a disorder in a series of 100 individuals. A two-way table can be used to summarize the results from the two interviewers.

PROPORTION OF SUBJECTS CLASSIFIED BY TWO RATERS

	Examiner A		
Examiner B	*Present*	*Absent*	*Total*
Present	$a = 0.07$	$b = 0.08$	$B_1 = 0.15$
Absent	$c = 0.11$	$d = 0.74$	$B_2 = 0.85$
	$A_1 = 0.18$	$A_2 = 0.82$	1.00

Po = proportion of agreement observed = $a + d = 0.81$
Pc = proportion of agreement by chance = $A_1 \times B_1 + A_2 \times B_2 = 0.724$
$\kappa = (Po - Pc)/(1 - Pc) = (0.81 - 0.724)/(1 - 0.724) = 0.31$

A simple measure of agreement for these dichotomous data is the proportion of observed agreement, or the percent of patients the two examiners agreed had or did not have the disorder. In this instance, the results indicate 81 percent agreement; however, this measure is not recommended.

In comparing two judgments, some agreements can be expected to occur by chance alone, without regard to how consistent the interview may be. To adjust for the potential contribution of these chance agreements, a better measure of agreement is kappa (κ). Calculation of kappa, as shown in the table, yields a value of 0.31. Another advantage of kappa is that its confidence interval can be calculated for a determination of how stable the point estimate is of kappa's true value.

The kappa statistic can be used to measure agreement between the raters at different levels of information. Judgments about any disorder considered in the interviews; about just one of the specific disorders, as in the example; or about an individual item for a specific disorder can be described using kappa. As the levels become broader, the reliability is likely to improve, because there are more ways to qualify as having any disorder than there are as having an individual symptom. Another reliability feature as measured by kappa is that its value depends on how common the particular condition is in the study sample. For less common disorders with a frequency below 5 percent, kappa's value will be so low in most cases that some investigators suggest not calculating it for these conditions.

For data that are expressed as ratings on an ordinal scale, other statistical measures are appropriate, including an intraclass correlation coefficient using analysis of variance techniques. Kappa also can be calculated for complex situations, like shifting numbers of multiple examiners and when some items are weighted in importance.

Acceptable reliability has become an expected feature of psychiatric assessment instruments, especially diagnostic interviews, because substantial research has demonstrated that routine clinical diagnoses are not reliable. The classic demonstration of this inconsistency was the U.S.-U.K. Diagnostic Project, which showed that psychiatrists in New York and London used the same diagnostic terms in widely varying ways, both for their own patients and for patients interviewed on videotape and shown to both groups. One result of this study was to produce standardized interview schedules that were designed to reduce the most important sources of inconsistency in diagnostic assessments. These included the following:

1. *Information variance:* Examiners collect different types of information about patients.
2. *Observation variance:* Examiners interpret the subject's answers and nonverbal behavior in different ways.
3. *Criterion variance:* Examiners evaluate information about the subject according to different diagnostic rules.

Development of standardized interviews has resulted in a major advance by reducing, but not eliminating, these sources of inconsistency. Two other sources of variance remain: (1) *subject variance,* when the subject has different conditions at different times, and (2) *occasion variance,* when the subject is in a different stage of the same condition, or at least reports different information about it.

VALIDITY Reliability is assessed by comparing agreement between examiners or between examinations. Validity testing requires a demonstration that the test results are accurate, ideally by comparison with a well-known standard of truth. Naturally, in a new field that has just begun developing standardized instruments because clinical examinations have been shown to be unreliable, there is no gold standard to use as an absolute measure of truth in diagnostic assessment. In practice, the choice of any acceptable criterion instrument to use as a standard of comparison in any validity testing of a new diagnostic instrument is one of the most difficult aspects of the study.

A simple validity study would involve administration of the test instrument and, independently, of the criterion instrument to each subject, with the order of administration changed randomly to be sure that one instrument does not influence the results of the other. Different statistical measures are calculated to measure validity than are used for reliability. In reliability tests, no assumptions are made that one examiner is more likely than another to obtain the true answer, so a simple comparison of their agreement is made. In validity testing, however, the criterion instrument is assumed to produce the truth, and the measures calculated are designed to indicate how well results from the new instrument being tested match the results from the criterion instrument. A two-way table is constructed, as shown:

Truth (Criterion Instrument Results)

New Instrument	*Disorder Present*	*Disorder Absent*	*Total*
Disorder present	$a = 35$	$b = 8$	$a + b = 43$
Disorder absent	$c = 5$	$d = 52$	$c + d = 57$
	$a + c = 40$	$b + d = 60$	100

$$\text{Sensitivity} = \frac{a}{a + c} = \frac{35}{40} = 0.875$$

$$\text{False negative} = \frac{c}{a + c} = \frac{5}{40} = 0.125$$

$$\text{Specificity} = \frac{d}{b + d} = \frac{52}{60} = 0.87$$

$$\text{False positive} = \frac{b}{b + d} = \frac{8}{60} = 0.13$$

Sensitivity is a measure of the new instrument's ability to detect the true cases of disorder identified by the criterion instrument. The false-negative rate is the proportion of true cases missed by the new instrument.

Specificity is a measure of the new instrument's ability to identify the true noncases identified by the criterion instrument. The false-positive rate is most commonly measured as the proportion of true noncases that are mistakenly called cases by the new instrument.

These measures allow basic judgments to be made about the new instrument's ability to identify cases that it is designed to identify. Higher values of sensitivity and specificity are always desirable. For a given instrument, there are tradeoffs between these two values. The only way to improve both sensitivity and specificity without a trade-off is to improve the instrument itself.

Another useful measure related to validity is the proportion of apparent cases, as detected by the new instrument, that are true cases, as determined by the criterion measure. This proportion is the *positive predictive value* (PPV). Of the 43 individuals who appeared to be cases in the example, only 35 were true cases, so the PPV = 35/43 = 0.814. This measure is affected by the base rate, so it is especially difficult for diagnostic tests to achieve a high PPV with rare disorders.

Criterion validity These measures are all based on a type of validity known as criterion validity, because results of the test instrument are compared with results of another similar, but presumably more accurate, instrument. If the new instrument had been compared with a criterion that would be administered at some point in the future, the method would have been predictive criterion validity.

Face validity Types of validity other than use of a criterion have been described. The simplest type is face validity, which refers to a judgment that the new instrument makes sense to an investigator. Standards for this type of validity are usually not clear; however, it does have some usefulness in increasing the acceptability by clinicians and subjects of a new and unusual instrument.

Content validity This term refers to a systematic examination of the new instrument, by an expert in the area, to ensure that its items cover the types of information that would be needed for later interpretation and scoring of the examination; it is especially important for such instruments as standardized diagnostic interviews that are intended to collect information to be used with a set of explicit diagnostic criteria.

Procedural validity This term was recently introduced to refer to tests of whether a particular type of examiner (e.g., a nonclinician) can use the new instrument and produce the same results as a skilled examiner (e.g., a research psychiatrist). Because this concept involves both a comparison between examiners, as in reliability testing, and a comparison with a criterion, as in criterion validity testing, investigators have reported both kappa and sensitivity-specificity measures for these studies.

Construct validity The most important concept of validity is construct validity, which refers to the demonstration that the thing being measured exists in the way that the instrument designed to measure it assumes that it does. Establishing construct validity for a mental disorder is a difficult problem for research, and this concept will be described later.

Ideally, safety, feasibility, reliability, and validity will be examined before an instrument is used to assess subjects in an epidemiological study. In practice, the difficulty in picking a criterion instrument with its own validity already established means that only the first three factors—safety, feasibility, and reliability—can be well studied for psychiatric assessment instruments. In an effort to establish at least minimum standards for new instruments, they can be assessed for content and procedural validity, and comparison with other, similar instruments can be made. Although these other instruments cannot be used as legitimate criterion instruments, they can provide useful comparisons if they have met the same standards, including reliability and content validity, as the new instrument being studied.

DESCRIPTIVE STUDIES

Once an appropriate sampling plan and acceptable assessment instruments are available, epidemiological investigations can begin to explore the distribution of disorders in the population. For rare disorders, a total area population survey may be unrewarding, but for most psychiatric illnesses, the starting point is an area survey to determine basic measures of frequency of the illness.

In epidemiological studies, with an emphasis on careful sampling to produce results that can be extended to the universe of interest, the results based on the number of cases with a disorder are expressed not in raw numbers but in terms of population rates. In general, these rates are proportions that require both a numerator, the number of cases, and a denominator, the total number in the population, including cases and noncases.

$$\text{Rate} = \frac{\text{Cases in the population}}{\text{Total population (includes cases and noncases)}}$$

This rate is actually a proportion, a fraction that includes cases in both the numerator and the denominator. Some writers reserve the term "rate" to refer to an instantaneous change, and express it using methods of calculus. To simplify that concept, the term "average rate" can be used for measures that involve rates over specified time periods.

Point prevalence Most surveys in psychiatric epidemiology have examined the prevalence of disease in the population. The term "prevalence" encompasses several types of rates, but always refers to patients who have the disorder at a specified time, regardless of how long ago the disorder started. The basic measure is point prevalence rate, which refers to the proportion of individuals in the population who have the disorder at a specified point in time; this point can be a day on the calendar, such as April 1, 1990, as in the national census, or it can be a point defined in relation to the study assessment, such as day of interview, regardless of the calendar date.

$$\text{Point prevalence rate} = \frac{\text{Cases at } t_o}{\text{Population at } t_o}$$

Although a day is often taken as the definition of a point in time, the use of diagnostic criteria that require multiple symptoms to cluster, with a minimum duration of symptoms, has led in some instances to extension of the point measure backward in time to refer to the previous week or month. Moving the concept of a point to include a period beyond 1 month prior to the interview is not advisable, because it can lead to confusion and raises methodological problems, which will be discussed in relation to lifetime prevalence.

To establish a point prevalence rate for depression, an investigator would sample the residents of a circumscribed area, administer an assessment instrument that detects a depressive illness current at that time, and calculate the rate as the proportion of the sample with current depression. Because such a study of a large sample would take several weeks or months to conduct, the rate in that case would probably be based on a point at the time of the interview, rather than asking subjects to report their symptoms retrospectively to the starting date of the field survey. (Unless a simple random sample were chosen, the investigator would also need to weight the sample results to reflect the overall population figures according to an individual's probability of selection.)

Incidence In epidemiological research, incidence also has a specific meaning; it refers to a rate that includes only new cases whose illness started within a clearly defined time period. The most common time period is 1 year; thus, the annual incidence rate is the usual rate reported. A study of incident cases is more difficult than a study of prevalent cases. To be done most carefully, a study of incidence requires at least two examinations of each subject in the sample, one at the start and one at the end of the designated time period.

The initial assessment is needed to determine which members of the sample already have the disease; they are not eligible to become new cases because they already have the illness, so they will be omitted from the numerator of new cases counted at the end of the study. They are also excluded from the denominator, because they are not part of the population considered at risk of developing a new case of the disorder. At the start of the study, the numerator is set to zero; at the end of the study, those individuals who have developed the illness will be counted as cases. If, at the second examination, the assessment instrument is unable to provide retrospective coverage of the entire time period being used, such as 1 year, it is necessary to resurvey the population at risk more often than just at the end of the period. In some cases, it is useful to consider the possible recurrence of illnesses that individuals have once had, for example, a second episode of major depression. A broader concept of total incidence includes those with a new episode of illness, regardless of whether there have been previous episodes.

An alternative way to study incidence is to conduct a single examination of subjects, as if it were the end of the time period chosen for study, and to ask them to recall their disease status at the beginning of the time period. Besides problems of recall, this simpler design has the problem of systematically omitting some categories of new cases, including those who died during the time period and cannot be sampled and those who left the circumscribed geographic area for other reasons.

This description of incidence rates is the traditional one, but more precise concepts of incidence have been developed. These take into account change over time and the possible loss to follow-up of individuals in the at-risk population. The term "incidence density" (ID) refers to an average incidence rate over the time period of interest:

$$ID = \frac{\text{Number of incident cases in one year}}{\text{Population-time (person-years of observation)}}$$

Because some members of the at-risk population sample will develop the disease and some will drop out of the study (e.g., by moving without a forwarding address or by dying from an unrelated illness), the denominator is calculated in terms of a person-time figure, such as person-years of observation, until the individual leaves the at-risk population. This calculation depends on knowing when during the year an individual develops an illness or otherwise leaves the at-risk population. If, for 1,000 people being followed, 20 are lost at the end of 6 months and another 100 develop disease at the end of 6 months, the person-time figure for observation of at-risk, disease-free individuals is (880 × 1 year) + (20 × 1/2 year) + (100 × 1/2 year) = 940 person-years and

$$ID = \frac{100 \text{ persons (cases)}}{940 \text{ person-years}} = 0.1064 \text{ per year (or 0.1064 cases per person-year)}$$

One advantage of this more precise approach is that in stable populations, the point prevalence rate can be related in a simple way to the incidence density: $P = ID \times D$, where D is the average duration of illness before its termination through death or recovery. A stable population is one that is stable in size and age distribution and has constant incidence and prevalence rates.

Incidence rates are clearly more difficult to calculate, and they require more extensive data collection than point prevalence rates. Point prevalence rates reflect the accumulated burden of chronic cases of very long duration, however, so incidence figures based on new cases in a specified time period are more useful in analytic studies of risk factors. Point prevalence surveys are most useful for descriptive purposes, as in portraying the frequency of illness in a community population and relating disease frequency to potential need for services.

OTHER PREVALENCE RATES

Although point prevalence and annual incidence rates are the fundamental measures used for descriptive and analytic studies in epidemiology, other types of prevalence figures have also been described and have some usefulness.

Period prevalence Period prevalence rate is a term used to summarize the number of people who have a disorder at any time during a specified time period. The numerator of the proportion includes any existing cases at the start of the period, plus any new cases that develop the illness during the time period. For a 1-year period, the annual period prevalence rate is approximately equal to the point prevalence rate (existing cases/population at the start) plus the annual incidence rate (new cases in a year/population at risk). This measure has less value than the separate expression of its two components of point prevalence and annual incidence rates. It may be useful, however, for services research studies where annual treated prevalence rates are contrasted with annual true prevalence rates.

Lifetime prevalence Lifetime prevalence rate is a measure of individuals considered at a particular point in time who have ever had the illness under study. It may be useful to describe conditions that remit but that can often recur, such as major depression, but the use of this rate entails at least three potential problems:

1. It is almost always based on subject recall, which can be inaccurate.
2. It covers subjects over the full age range represented in the study population, including many who have not yet completed the age period of highest risk for onset of the disorder. It is possible to report lifetime rates separately for specific age groups, but this figure may be misleading for some purposes if no provision is made for the fact that death rates may be different for people with the disease at earlier ages than for those without the disease.
3. Used in a summary way, it does not allow for the fact that incidence rates may have changed over the years. Therefore, different age groups may have true differences in rates that are obscured both by using an overall rate and by the possible differences in mortality between cases and noncases.

Several alternatives to the lifetime prevalence rate, as determined from a point prevalence survey, have been described. One method uses a life table approach to estimate age-specific lifetime rates based on age-specific incidence and mortality figures. For psychiatric disorders, this detailed age-specific information is rarely available. Another method calculates lifetime risk by including persons in a birth cohort with and without the disorder who died, or otherwise dropped out, before the age designated as cutoff. This latter method also can be used to impute probable risk for those without illness who have not yet reached the cutoff age. This approach is most useful as an expression of risk, rather than actual development, of illness, and is especially important for genetic studies, which must include children and deceased relatives.

Treated prevalence This term usually refers either to a point prevalence or an annual period prevalence rate that is determined by counting all residents in a defined geographic population who receive treatment for a given disorder.

Administrative prevalence A more restricted form of treated prevalence has been used for studies that include, as their population denominator, registered patients at a clinical facility, rather than all area residents. This form of treated prevalence, with registered patients as the denominator population, has been called administrative prevalence. It does present difficulties, because the denominator depends on registration status, rather than being based on those who perceive the study facility as their usual source of care. Also, the numerator is assumed to be all treated cases in the population, although some may seek care elsewhere.

ANALYTIC STUDIES

Measures of disease frequency allow comparisons to be made among groups within the study sample. If one group has high rates of a disorder compared with other groups, then a search for factors that lead to the higher rate of disorder can be undertaken. Many studies of disease frequency have shown that women have higher rates of unipolar major depression than men. From this consistent finding, based on group comparisons, it is possible for investigators to formulate hypotheses about what factors place women at higher risk. Whether these putative risk factors are biological or psychosocial, they can next be studied in targeted investigations to see if women with the presumed risk factor have higher rates of major depression than women without them. To make comparisons among groups, and later among those groups with and without suspected risk factors, investigators have several options for study design.

Cross-sectional prevalence survey One approach to examining the apparent higher frequency of major depression among women is to conduct a sample survey of the total population in an area and calculate the point prevalence rates for men and women. These rates can be compared, and, as an example, it may be found that women have twice the point prevalence rate of men. If the investigator had examined characteristics that were suspected to be risk factors, such as use of oral contraceptives, it would also be possible to compare the rates among women who used this medication and those who did not.

Such a design has been used for this purpose, but has several drawbacks. As shown in the discussion on incidence rates, point prevalence is affected both by the rate of developing an illness, as reflected in the incidence rates, and by the duration of the illness after it develops. If men and women with major depression had different average durations, they would have different point prevalence rates, even with identical incidence rates; it is conceivable that the point prevalence rate for women could be twice the rate for men simply because those women who developed major depression had more chronic forms and tended to accumulate in the population. A second problem with this cross-sectional design is that it may be difficult to know whether women with the suspected risk factor (e.g., use of oral contraceptives) had been using the medication before they became ill, as would be required if there were a causal chain leading to major depression.

Incidence study and relative risk To isolate the frequency of onset from the duration once developed, and to assess possible risk factors accurately, studies of incidence rates are much more useful.

The fundamental measure to compare two groups is the relative risk (RR), a form of risk ratio:

$$RR = \frac{\text{Incidence rate in group with risk factor}}{\text{Incidence rate in group without risk factor}}$$

In terms of the usual two-way table, this RR can be expressed as follows:

Incident Series of Cases

	New Cases	*Noncases*
With risk factor	*a*	*b*
Without risk factor	*c*	*d*

$$RR = \frac{a}{a+b} \div \frac{c}{c+d}$$

If the RR is greater than 1.0, the group with the suspected risk factor does have a higher incidence rate of the disorder. In this study design, risk factor status (e.g., use of oral contraceptives) could be examined at the start of the time period for all those without the disorder; these subjects could be reexamined during or at the end of the period, or both, to assess the development of the illness, as well as continued use of the medication.

Prospective cohort study This design assesses incidence rates and RRs. A cohort is a group formed by sampling from a single, well-specified population, such as residents of a circumscribed area. It allows extension of study findings to the universe of interest, and as a prospective study, it allows determination of risk factor status in noncases that are followed to identify newly developed cases.

Case-control study For very rare disorders, or sometimes for exploratory studies of possible risk factors, a study using identified cases, rather than potential cases, may be used. This design is called a case-control study. It recruits cases already diagnosed, usually by monitoring records at clinical facilities, such as hospitals; this method of sampling cases assumes that everyone with the disorder is likely to present for medical attention and to be accurately diagnosed. It also assumes that all relevant facilities are monitored, or else that no differences exist in persons who stay at home or use different facilities.

One problem is that the universe from which these cases are drawn cannot be specified, at least in customary terms, such as geographic area of residence. Another problem is that a comparison group of noncases is not easy to specify. To compensate, often a comparison group is drawn from other patients in the same facility, and a second one is drawn from community residents in the area presumably served by the hospital. It is conceivable that either one of these comparison groups could be drawn from a universe different from the hypothesized one that is reflected in the sample of cases.

In these case-control studies, ascertainment of possible risk factors is usually possible only by retrospective report of the subjects, unless prior documentation exists, as in medical records.

Odds ratio Because incidence rates cannot be calculated in such a case-control design, the typical calculation of risk ratio must be altered. Instead of a relative risk, the odds ratio is calculated for case-control studies:

	Cases	*Noncases*
Possible risk factor present	*a*	*b*
Possible risk factor absent	*c*	*d*

$$\text{Odds ratio} = \frac{a}{b} \div \frac{c}{d} = \frac{ad}{bc}$$

Bias Analytic studies to assess risk factors can be flawed by three types of bias:

1. *Selection bias*. If a study sample is not drawn properly, it may not accurately reflect the study population; also, the study population may not be equivalent to the universe of interest. In case-control studies, a special problem is that the selection of cases may be distorted if the clinical diagnoses used to determine eligibility are not accurate.
2. *Observation bias*. If the assessment instruments are invalid, information about subjects will be wrong. In case-control studies, examiners who know the case or noncase status of subjects can be influenced in assessing the risk factors being studied.
3. *Confounding bias*. In a particular study sample, some other causal factors of the disorder may be related to the risk factor being studied. This effect can be examined and some adjustments can be made during data analysis.

These potential flaws can affect the validity of a study's findings, in terms of whether the findings are representative of the intended universe. A second question is whether the findings considered applicable to this particular universe also apply to other possible universes; for example, does a risk factor studied in one local community have the same association to disease in other types of communities? The answer to this second question is a matter of judgment until equally valid replications are performed.

Risk factors and causality Epidemiological data demonstrate an association between risk factors and a disorder. Because an association does not indicate causality in a particular direction, the desire to study human illness has led epidemiologists to consider standards of evidence that may support an interpretation of a causal connection between a risk factor and a disorder.

1. *Temporality*. Unless the risk factor precedes the disorder, it cannot cause the disorder. Clear demonstration of the prior occurrence of a risk factor strengthens the possibility of causality.
2. *Consistency*. Repeated demonstration of a risk factor's relationship to a disorder in multiple studies strengthens the possibility that a risk factor may be causative.
3. *Magnitude of association*. A large risk ratio tends to support an interpretation of a causality, as does demonstration of a dose-response effect.
4. *Plausibility*. If a possible causal mechanism can be postulated within the framework of existing knowledge, it may lend credibility to the interpretation of a causal relationship; however, in new fields where knowledge is growing, this criterion may not be so relevant.
5. *Specificity*. If a proposed risk factor can be associated with a single disorder and no others, that association may strengthen belief in a possible causal relationship. Some factors, such as adverse life events, may lead to a variety of disorders, however, so that the failure of specificity does not discredit a potential risk factor.
6. *Experimental intervention*. Experiments to control a risk factor may support a causal role for the factor if the occurrence of disease is reduced; however, with such an experiment, it is possible that unintended or unknown factors may have been the true responsible agents and may have been affected by the intervention.

EXPERIMENTAL STUDIES

An important goal of psychiatric epidemiology is to reduce the burden of illness. With a population-based approach, epidemiological investigations are especially well suited to assessing the impact of broad efforts to reduce the occurrence of illness, or its duration and associated disability.

Population attributable risk For primary prevention—the effort to reduce the onset of a disorder in those persons at risk for developing it—a measure of the potential impact of controlling an established risk factor is derived from the attributable risk (AR), the risk difference measure based on incidence rates (IR) for those persons with and without the risk factor.

$$AR = (IR \text{ with risk factor}) - (IR \text{ without risk factor})$$

The proportion of cases in the population that may be caused by a risk factor is the population AR:

$$\text{Population } AR = \frac{IR_{\text{total population}} - IR_{\text{without}}}{IR_{\text{total population}}}$$

If the incidence rate in a population is twice as high as the incidence rate for those population members without the risk factor, then the population AR will be 50 percent; this figure means that half the cases can be assumed to have the disorder because the risk factor has led to development of the illness.

When the more precise figures of incidence density are used, this measure has been called the "etiological fraction." In some instances, it may be possible to demonstrate that a "protective factor" has caused a lower rate of illness among those persons exposed to it; then the formula is reversed to show the "preventive fraction." Studies of low dental caries rates in areas with fluoridated water provide an example. Calculation of the etiological fraction from observational studies indicates the maximum benefit likely to occur with an intervention that is designed to reduce the pathogenic effect of the risk factor. Demonstration that an intervention has been effective rests on a controlled design, with calculation of a preventive fraction based on those persons with a risk factor receiving the intervention, and those with the risk factor who did not experience the intervention.

Preventive applications In addition to studies that test interventions to prevent a disorder from occurring, this method can be used for secondary and tertiary prevention as well. Secondary prevention is aimed at reducing the prevalence of illness by reducing its duration in those who have just developed it. Factors that tend to prolong an episode of illness can be targeted in primary prevention efforts.

Reduction of disability produced by a disorder, or tertiary prevention, can also be assessed, even if full recovery does not occur. Such studies would need to use instruments assessing severity of illness, and not simply a dichotomous present-absent rating for a disorder. Studies with this design are commonly used in controlled clinical trials to assess the effectiveness of new therapies to reduce duration until recovery, or reduce severity in those persons without full recovery.

Primary prevention efforts are especially difficult to study, because it is not clear how to choose large groups to study, how to demonstrate that they have received the intervention, and how to ensure that no other unplanned intervention actually produced any improvement that took place. Even if these conditions are met, it may be difficult to demonstrate that the intervention was effective for the reasons postulated, and that its costs, including any unintended negative consequences, did not overwhelm any benefits realized.

EPIDEMIOLOGICAL METHOD IN PSYCHIATRY

Special problems have delayed progress in psychiatric epidemiology. Although the general field of epidemiology has advanced to the point of being most concerned about such issues as controlling confounding bias in risk factor studies and developing ways to measure the impact of preventive interventions, methodological concerns for studies of mental disorders are more basic. They have centered on difficulties in applying complex sampling techniques, in developing acceptable case-assessment instruments, and in identifying potential risk factors that merit study in large-scale investigations. The most important of these problems has been the development and application of case-assessment instruments for large-scale studies.

Case assessment The major obstacle to valid identification of cases in large samples of nonclinical populations has been the lack of an explicit set of criteria for diagnostic classification systems. In using systems, such as the first edition of the *Diagnostic and Statistical Manual of Mental Disorders* (DSM-I), investigators were forced to rely on their own detailed descriptions of symptom patterns in order to achieve a meaningful classification of cases. During the 1960s and 1970s, this effort to use detailed specifications for disorders became more widespread and led psychiatry to produce more explicit statements of empirically based criteria for specific mental disorders. Until explicit diagnostic criteria were widely accepted in the publication of DSM-III and DSM-III-R, investigators had limited alternatives that were rarely used in clinical practice when selecting criteria and related instruments to identify cases.

The most common approach was to employ a self-report questionnaire, usually with a concentration on psychophysiological symptoms, that could yield a score based on positive answers by the subject. These scores were intended to reflect the probability that a subject had a diagnosable mental disorder, with higher scores indicating a greater likelihood. In most cases, a cutoff score was calculated to separate the sample into two groups—the cases and the noncases. (In some studies, these scales and other information were also reviewed by clinicians, who attempted to give an overall judgment about the subject's psychiatric status.)

The second major effort to develop standardized assessment instruments was to produce diagnostic interview protocols with acceptable interrater reliability. The first such protocol was the Present State Examination (PSE), an interview form that concentrates mainly on psychotic conditions and that has been used in major international studies, such as the U.S.-U.K. Diagnostic Project, the International Pilot Study of Schizophrenia, and other studies of schizophrenia supported by the World Health Organization and the National Institute of Mental Health (NIMH). The PSE is intended for use by skilled clinicians, usually psychiatrists, who have been trained in its administration; after training, the interviewers are commonly expected to participate in a pretest of any investigation to demonstrate adequate levels of interrater reliability.

The PSE does have drawbacks. As it is limited to coverage of the 1-month period prior to interview, historical information is not obtained. The very features that generate its capacity to be used reliably—an explicit glossary of psychopathological concepts to guide examiners, and a careful computer program (CATEGO) to score the interview—also may not reflect the diagnostic practices of any particular school of psychiatry; the authors of PSE-CATEGO are careful to present it as a nondiagnostic classification system that is not directly tied to any existing classification scheme. Although general outlines of the complex CATEGO algorithms have been published, detailed study by others has been undertaken only recently.

The PSE was not designed to yield diagnostic labels according to an established classification system, because the lack of explicit criteria in the early 1970s made it difficult to determine unambiguous standards for a given category. Only with the advent of formally stated, sufficiently detailed criteria for a range of psychiatric diagnoses was it possible to construct interviews that attempted to perform a diagnostic assessment and to assign subjects to specific categories of disorder. The notable success of the PSE encouraged the development of new diagnostic interviews.

When the St. Louis research criteria and the Research Diagnostic Criteria (RDC) were formulated in the 1970s, they were accompanied by interview schedules that investigators would use to assess subjects in a study. These instruments were the Renard Diagnostic Interview (RDI) for the St. Louis criteria and the Schedule for Affective Disorders and Schizophrenia (SADS) for the RDC. Because these schedules required skilled clinicians to spend up to 3 months learning them, and because epidemiological studies would need a large number of such high-level interviewers, they were not used much in community surveys. An important exception was use of the Schedule for Affective Disorders and Schizophrenia, Lifetime version (SADS-L) in a follow-up study of 511 community residents in New Haven, Connecticut. That study demonstrated that the SADS-L could be used successfully in such epidemiological studies of community subjects.

Stimulated by that demonstration of feasibility and usefulness, and aware that DSM-III would adopt the approach of using "operationalized criteria," as in the St. Louis and RDC systems, NIMH epidemiologists sponsored development of a fully structured interview that could be used by nonclinicians to assess a large number of subjects according to DSM-III criteria. This new instrument, the NIMH Diagnostic Interview Schedule (DIS), was based on the RDI and SADS interviews and was written by the authors of those two earlier interviews.

Structure of the DIS To allow nonclinicians to administer the DIS reliably, the interview contains the exact wording to be used for each question; examiners need only read the question aloud for each item being assessed. Once a question is answered positively, several types of probes are used to determine whether the item can plausibly be counted toward a psychiatric diagnosis. A severity criterion, based on having told a physician or other professional about the symptom, or on having experienced life interference as a result of the symptom, is used to separate common and insignificant problems from clinically meaningful phenomena. If the symptom has always occurred as a result of physical illness or injury, or in relation to medication, alcohol, or drugs of abuse, it is coded as being explained by those conditions, and not by a psychiatric illness.

These two features are intended to assure consistency, accuracy, and selectivity in the assessment of positive reports of symptoms. Interviewer observations are used only for behavior-related psychotic conditions, and extensive use of marginal notes and examples is encouraged to allow editors and reviewing clinicians to judge any uncertain items.

Another effort to achieve reliability and accuracy is the use of a computer program to score the information and make diagnostic assignments; this program is written in a familiar language and in a straightforward style; so that clinicians can easily interpret the scoring algorithms. Questions on the interview are formulated to allow criteria to be assessed for categories specified in the RDC and St. Louis systems, as well as DSM-III; however, only selected DSM-III categories are covered.

Unlike the PSE, which concentrates on the 1-month period prior to the interview, the DIS assesses the occurrence of symptoms at any time in the patient's lifetime. This lifetime approach allows a diagnosis of some disorders where symptoms accumulate to a threshold (e.g., somatization disorder, antisocial personality disorder), of disorders where history is important in the diagnosis (e.g., schizophrenia, bipolar disorder), and of prior episodes of recurring disorders (e.g., major depression). This approach also permits estimation of age of onset for subjects in a study as well as identification of subjects with a history of multiple disorders. Once a diagnosis is established on the lifetime basis, its most recent occurrence is dated. A modification of the DIS also permits dating of the most recent experience with any positive symptoms.

Several aspects of the DIS have been noted as potential weaknesses. Because it minimizes examiner observation and judgment, it is limited to a great extent to subject self-report; self-reports may not be adequate for assessment of disorders such as schizophrenia and mania. Eliciting these self-reports of symptoms on a lifetime basis means that poor recall may also affect the validity of symptom reporting; this possibility has been raised particularly for subjects with previous psychotic conditions. Although many aspects of the history of an illness can be obtained, such as age at onset and symptoms during worst episode (for recurrent illnesses), some aspects of the course cannot be determined; this limitation is especially clear for questions about onset and progression of symptoms for a particular episode. It is also possible that inevitable variations in training and editing procedures may show that there is an effective ceiling on the degree of standardization that can be achieved in multisite studies.

Characteristics of the DIS In the large epidemiological study that it was designed to support, the DIS has proved to be a feasible and safe instrument. It has been administered to about 20,000 subjects in five parts of the country, and the refusal and dropout rates for those subjects who agreed to start the DIS have been less than 1 percent.

Because the RDI and SADS interviews have been demonstrated as reliable for current and lifetime reports in a range of subjects, and because the DIS is similar to them, but with more structure and with a computer program to score information, it was decided to perform interrater reliability studies at a higher level, called "procedural validity." In this first test, agreement was measured between two examiners, a nonclinician and a psychiatrist. Acceptable levels of agreement were reached, and further field testing was undertaken in the context of the epidemiological studies.

Criterion validity for a diagnostic interview, especially one based on a new classification system, is hard to test, because there are no other validated interviews to use. The desire to apply a routine clinical judgment by psychiatrists using the clinical method suffers from the possible effects of information, observer, and criterion variance that led to the development of standardized interview schedules 20 years ago. One alternative is to use similar instruments that apply the same standards of evidence and to use scoring procedures based on the same system of diagnostic criteria. The purpose of these studies is not to validate the DIS, but to understand better any discrepancies with the comparison instrument. That approach has been taken in the NIMH multisite epidemiological studies, with repeat interviews of some subjects to allow comparisons to be made with three alternative instruments: a semistructured interview loosely based on the PSE, a SADS-L modified to meet DSM-III criteria, and a DSM-III criteria checklist used by psychiatrists who readminister the DIS.

Construct validity This concept—which, at least theoretically, is the most important form of validity for an assessment instrument—refers to a demonstration that an instrument does measure what it intends to measure, that the entity exists and can be quantified by the instrument. Various proposals have been made in the psychological literature for ways to accomplish this task for a range of purposes. In psychiatric epidemiology, the question involves more than whether an instrument detects a given disorder as specified by a classification system's rules. In practice, application of these rules cannot be performed independently of a specified, reliable assessment instrument; therefore, the question of construct validity of the diagnostic entities constructed by a system of classification arises.

As psychiatric nosology has advanced, ways to establish validity for a diagnostic entity have been considered. The first requirement suggested has been to demonstrate that a clinical picture with characteristic features can be described for the disorder, and then that these features can be used to separate the disorder from others that may resemble it. The second type of evidence, which can be derived from external criteria, includes biological variables, such as those obtained from biochemical and neuroanatomical studies; psychosocial and personality styles, including methods for coping with adverse life events; familial and genetic variables, such as patterns of transmission of the disorder in relatives; clinical course and outcome variables, such as stability of the diagnosis over time, response to treatment; epidemiological variables, such as systematic occurrence in certain groups or places; and multivariate statistical analysis to demonstrate separation from and relationship with other disorders in terms of these variables.

Ideally, such studies would be based on assessments by several different commonly used instruments to determine which technique most capably identified homogeneous groups of subjects with little overlap with groups of other disorders. Besides the DIS, these studies await both the development of other DSM-III-R assessment instruments and the capacity for supporting such an expensive set of research tasks.

STUDIES OF HISTORICAL IMPORTANCE

Given the conceptual framework and methodological tools already described, it is appropriate to discuss how major psychiatric epidemiological studies illustrate these principles. Although such a presentation could be organized by the study design, use of findings, case-identification method, and other variables, the population group from which the samples were drawn will be the basic organizational framework. The reason for this approach is to emphasize the primacy of the population group as the basic unit of analysis in epidemiology, as well as to illustrate that a variety of descriptive, analytic, and experimental studies may be appropriate with any population group, provided that the selection characteristics of the group are clearly defined and considered in the design. The population groups to be considered include (1) the treated populations in specialty mental health settings, (2) patients registered in general medical practice settings, (3) noninstitutionalized community populations, and (4) specific mental disorders within defined populations.

Definition of the study population group frequently affects decisions on the type of mental disorder criteria used, interviewer selection, interview method, and the descriptive or analytic variables used. Although within the public health framework, epidemiological surveys would proceed from a community population to general medical practices and then to specialty mental health treated populations, the reverse order more frequently has been the rule. This pattern is found in the rest of medicine, where the most frequent progression is from clinical observation to the laboratory for more intensive study, with the laboratory, in this case, being large population groups. The choice of treated populations arises from the relative ease of defining this population group, the availability of highly trained personnel to conduct assessments, and the existence of extensive diagnostic and other related information in the medical records.

The impetus for proceeding from specialty mental health surveys to general practice surveys has been to broaden the population base, so that it is more representative of the total community. In so doing, it is still possible to retain highly trained physicians for case identification and longitudinal medical-record data in order to increase the pool of information about subjects beyond the amount that could be obtained in cross-sectional studies. Although general practice surveys have a broad population base, some selection bias may affect the dependent variables of syndromes and diagnoses, as well as the associated descriptive and independent risk factor variables. Because a major goal of epidemiological studies is to generalize about the frequency, characteristics, and course of a given mental disorder in the entire population, limitations on such generalization result whenever the population base from which the disorders are drawn is narrowed. The association of causal or descriptive variables with disorders also may be confounded by the tendency of some variables to be strongly associated with persons' going to general practitioners or psychiatrists regardless of the presence of a mental disorder.

SPECIALTY MENTAL HEALTH SECTOR TREATED POPULATIONS

Social class and mental illness One of the most prominent specialty mental health treated prevalence surveys was that of A. B. Hollingshead and F. C. Redlich in the early 1950s. By exhaustively surveying every mental health facility and private office practice psychiatrist who treated any patient in the New Haven area, the researchers were able to define an overall mental disorder, 6-month treated prevalence rate of 8 per 1,000 population in the community. The rates vary, however, from between 5 and 7 per 1,000, in social classes I through IV, to a treated prevalence rate of 17 per 1,000, in the lowest social class V. These patients were assessed by clinicians employing a protocol report form that depended on their using unspecified clinical judgment methods and unspecified criteria for specific diagnoses. Social class was a principal descriptive variable used to stratify frequency of diagnoses and the frequency of treatment setting use (Table 5.1-1). Although careful attention was given to controlling for potential confounding variables of age, sex, or mental disorder type, a strong association was found between higher social class, less severe disorders, and private office treatment settings. This was contrasted with the concentration of severe disorders in both the lower social classes and the long-stay public mental hospital institutions. New cases coming into treatment settings (treated incidence) made up only one-eighth of the total 6-month prevalence, with a much narrower range of about 1.0 per 1,000, for classes I through IV, to 1.4 per 1,000, for social class V. Incidence rates were less discrepant across the social class groups than prevalence rates, which indicates that there was a longer duration of disorders in the lower social classes, that is, prevalence/incidence equals duration. This finding could be partially explained by the diagnostic distribution across social classes that showed a gradient increase in the proportion of psychotic to neurotic disorders from classes I through V.

This study may be seen as a combined descriptive and analytic epidemiological study of treated prevalence and incidence of mental disorders, in which the community population was examined only for social class and other demographic variables. As such, it provided treatment rates and showed strong associations between social class and the frequency, severity, and treatment setting of patients with mental disorders. The absence of standardized assessment procedures in the total population made it impossible to determine if diagnoses were reliably assessed across treatment settings; if social class was associated with mental disorders or only with treatment frequency; or if social class was related in any etiological way with the presence of mental disorders, or if it merely concentrated more direct risk factors within this population group.

Despite its methodological limitations, this study had a major impact on the collective social conscience of the day and may be seen as a classic example of the power of simple frequency and descriptive variable associations to have important administrative and health policy effects while generating, but not testing, hypotheses about etiology. Implications of social class determined treatment, and the possibility that community characteristics might have a role in the etiology of mental disorders supported major public policy decisions in the United States to expand specialty mental health services and the community mental health center legislation.

TABLE 5.1-1
Classification of Social Class by Hollingshead and Redlich

Class	*Characteristics of the Sample in New Haven, Conn.*
I	Class I, the highest social class, was composed of the community's business and professional leaders. Members of this group were well educated; they frequently had a history of attending private schools and both men and women had at least some college education. They earned the highest incomes, or lived on inherited wealth, and resided in the "best" areas of New Haven.
II	This class was composed of adults who had been upwardly mobile in their lives, and had jobs as managers or lower-ranking professionals. Their incomes were comfortable, but they had little accumulated wealth. Almost all of the adults had attended college, and they attributed their success to educational attainment.
III	The men in this class held administrative or semiprofessional positions or were skilled manual workers; many of the women worked in clerical or sales positions. They had economic security with some savings; most were high school graduates.
IV	In class IV, the men were skilled and semiskilled workers, and almost all women were employed in factory, clerical, or sales positions. Adults had usually left high school before graduating. Their incomes went for living expenses, and despite efforts to save, they had little, if any, savings accumulated.
V	In the lowest social class, employable adults were unskilled and semiskilled workers with low salaries. They had no savings and faced a constant struggle to cope with financial or social crises. Few of the adults had completed the ninth grade.

National reporting program An additional source of treated prevalence data is available from the NIMH National Reporting Program (NRP). This program complements the U.S. Public Health Service National Health Survey, which consists of periodic health examinations and facility surveys conducted by the National Center for Health Statistics (NCHS) and other Public Health Service agencies. Components of the NIMH NRP include the state and county hospital annual census, the inventory of specialty mental health facilities, and the sample patient surveys drawn from the universe of facilities. Routine data on office-based psychiatrists are drawn from the NCHS National Ambulatory Medical Care Survey.

The annual Census of State and County Mental Hospitals describes age, sex, and diagnostic composition of resident patients present in these hospitals at the end of each calendar year, and admissions during the year. A comprehensive inventory of all mental health facilities records information on the staffing and organizational characteristics of these facilities as well as on the caseload and capacity, including number of episodes of care. *Episodes* are defined as residents at the beginning of the year, plus all admissions in the year. As some patients may have more than one admission in a year, this indicator is slightly inflated over annual treated prevalence rates. Finally, the sample patient surveys provide more detailed information on patient characteristics, including diagnoses, length of stay, and type of treatment received.

Besides being the major source of national service use data, NRP has provided an invaluable source of longitudinal trend data on patients under treatment in the specialty mental health sector. For example, the decreased number of residents in state hospitals during the period of deinstitutionalization, from a 1955 high of 559,000 to a 1984 level of 116,000, can be documented (Fig. 5.1-2). Also, the shift in care from one type of facility to another can be analyzed. In 1955, 1.7 million episodes of care were delivered and 49 percent of these were inpatient episodes in state and county mental hospitals; by 1983 (the last year for which data are available), 6.9 million episodes were delivered and only 7 percent of these were inpatient episodes in state and county mental hospitals, with 12 percent in general hospital psychiatric units, 3 percent in private psychiatric hospitals, 2 percent in Veterans Administration medical centers, 3 percent in other inpatient settings, and 73 percent in all outpatient psychiatric services (Fig. 5.1-3).

Such data illustrate the value of treated prevalence data in describing the workings of the health care system. They also demonstrate how treated prevalence rates reflect administrative and policy decisions that affect patterns of treatment.

PRIMARY CARE SETTINGS

Because primary medical care settings reflect a much broader population base than do specialty settings and yet retain the potential for engaging patients in treatment, many epidemiological investigations have examined mental disorders in general medical populations. Various studies in the United States have indicated that at least 70 percent of the noninstitutionalized population uses general medical services over the course of a year, so general physicians are in a position to screen for mental disorders for a much larger proportion of the population than the

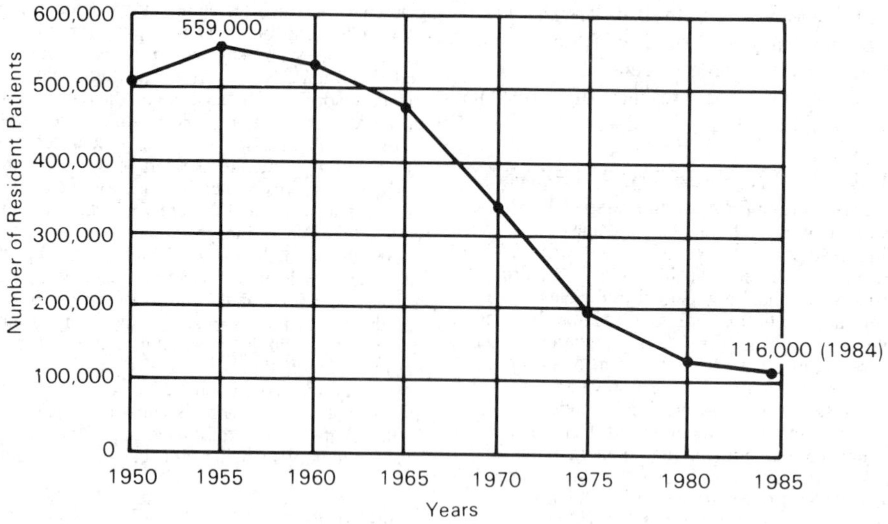

FIGURE 5.1-2. *Number of resident patients at year end in state and county hospitals.*

1 to 5 percent who may be seen in specialty mental health services during that time.

Recent studies of mental disorder in primary care patients have used contemporary diagnostic interviews to demonstrate that from 20 to 30 percent of patients visiting primary care offices have a current mental disorder. However, some of these same studies suggest that few of these disorders are recognized, diagnosed, or treated by the primary care clinician. A major public health campaign has been developed by NIMH to increase the awareness, recognition, and treatment of the most common of these conditions, depression. This effort, known as the Depression/Awareness, Recognition, Treatment Program (D/ART), will provide educational materials to the general public, primary care clinicians, and mental health specialists.

COMMUNITY POPULATION STUDIES To overcome the problems of selection bias and unreliability of routine clinical diagnosis in treatment settings, epidemiologists rely most heavily on direct surveys of community residents. Prior to World War I, epidemiological studies used institutional records or key informants to generate prevalence estimates of mental disorders. More recent studies have utilized direct interviews of community residents, with the information recorded on structured protocols by nonclinicians. Three studies conducted in the 1950s were classic investigations that attempted to generate prevalence estimates of mental disorders in accordance with one or more of the major diagnostic practices in use at the time. Two of them, the Stirling County, Canada, and the Midtown Manhattan studies, also examined specific etiological hypotheses about the causal relationship of socioenvironmental factors to the occurrence of mental disorders.

Stirling County The study of Stirling County, directed by A. Leighton and continued by J. Murphy, was begun over 30 years ago. From the 20,000 residents of a rural county in Canada, 1,010 adults were sampled. Independent variables, hypothesized to be causally related to mental disorders, were cultural and community characteristics. The dependent variables were mental disorders defined in accordance with the newly developed DSM-I, and were rated in terms of the presence or absence of 32 detailed symptom patterns, as well as of impairment levels and the need for psychiatric attention. Trained field workers surveyed this population sample with a structured psychiatric interview, which was clinically evaluated later by two psychiatrists. Additional information was gathered from all county general practitioners, who served as key informants for obtaining more detailed medical, psychological, and social data about each sample member.

Estimates of the lifetime prevalence of these dependent variables included rates of 57 per 100 population for all DSM-I conditions, 24 per 100 for these conditions associated with significant impairment, and 20 per 100 for these conditions in need of psychiatric attention; this last rate is regarded as the most clinically meaningful estimate. Higher rates of disorders were found in communities characterized by social disintegration, although the exact causal factors within these gross environmental descriptive categories could not be specified.

Midtown Manhattan The Midtown Manhattan Study of T. A. C. Rennie, L. Srole, and their colleagues also began in the early 1950s. From an area of midtown Manhattan that had a population of 110,000 adults, a sample of 1,660 adult residents was selected. The independent variables included various measures of stress, immigration status, social class, occupation, and marital status, with the dependent variables being a measure of impairment in adult life function, rated on a six-point gradient scale from "none" to "incapacitated."

Psychologists and social workers utilized a structured psychiatric interview to obtain information from respondents, which was subsequently rated by two psychiatrists. The most celebrated findings were that 81.5 percent of the population was shown to have at least mild impairment from psychological symptoms and 23.4 percent had significant impairment. Although correlations were found between sociodemographic and social stress variables with levels of impairment, one of the most significant results of this study was a debate about the dependent variable measure of mental health status. If less than 20 percent of the population could be identified as mentally healthy, the clinical usefulness of mental disorder definitions was open to question. The importance of using more rigorous criteria for diagnoses was immediately apparent to more medically oriented epidemiologists.

Baltimore A third major study was undertaken in Baltimore, Maryland, where the entire noninstitutionalized population was sampled, including children. This study was a two-stage morbidity survey in which the first stage consisted of household interviews by census interviewers and was followed by a second-stage clinical examination for 809 subjects, who were stratified by level of disability. General medical internists and pediatricians conducted a medical history and examination, followed by a psychiatrist's rating of all protocols with psychological symptoms or impairment related to mental disorders.

Because this was a morbidity survey to identify the prevalence of individuals with chronic medical or mental disorders for purposes of improving services, no attempt was made to test etiological hypotheses. Diagnostic categories provided in the International Statistical

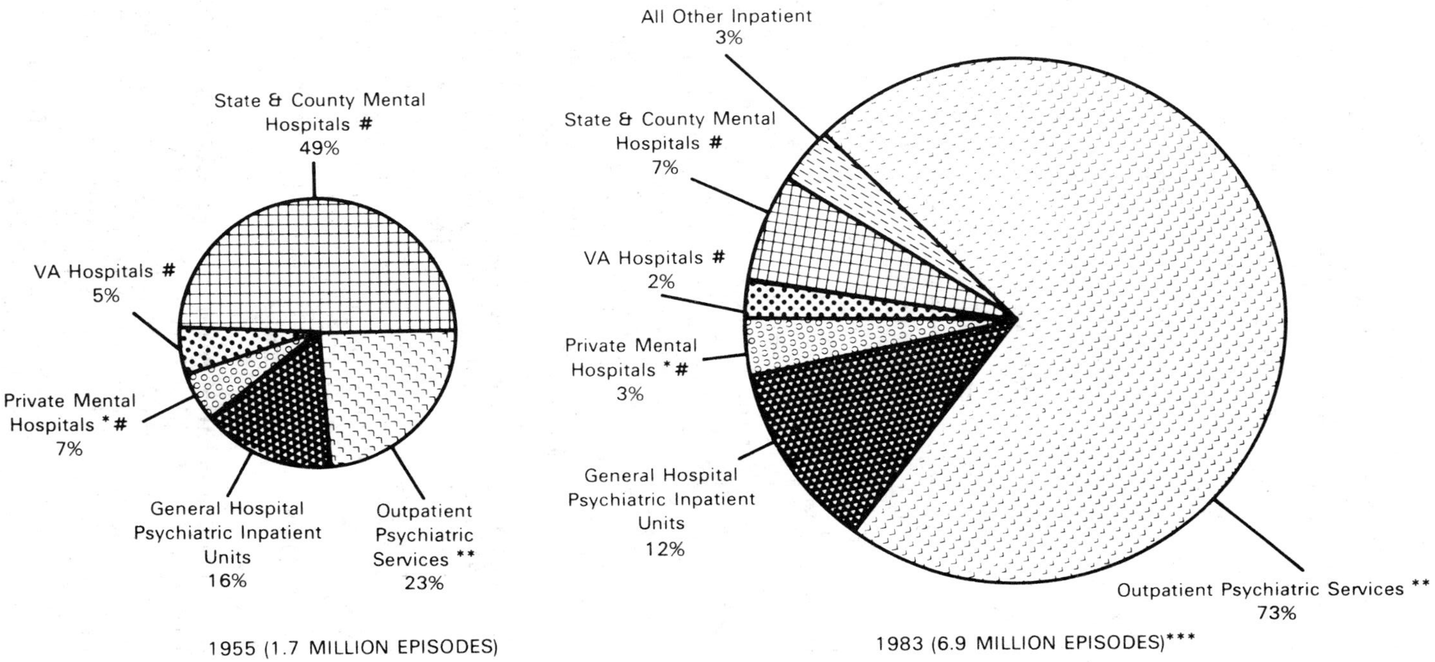

* Includes residental treatment centers for emotionally disturbed children

\# Inpatient services only

** Includes free-standing outpatient services as well as those affiliated with psychiatric and general hospitals

FIGURE 5.1-3. *Percent distribution of inpatient and outpatient care episodes in mental health facilities, by type of facility, in the United States in 1955 and 1983. (From Mandenscheid R W and Barrett S A: Mental Health United States 1987, DHS Pub No (ADM) 87-1518, US Government Printing Office, Washington, DC, 1987.)*

Classification of Diseases (ISCD) were used for all physical and mental disorders, although no effort was made to assess the reliability or validity of assessments. A point prevalence rate of 10.9 percent was found for all ISCD mental disorders, with 1.4 percent of the population exhibiting moderate or severe impairment.

CASE-CONTROL AND CASE-REGISTER STUDIES

Population samples are especially important for avoiding selection bias, but they are difficult to use for rare disorders or to generate hypotheses about possible risk factors. Case registers have been maintained for rare disorders that are serious and likely to come to medical attention, such as rare forms of cancer. Over the past 2 decades, case registers of psychiatric cases have been maintained at great effort in Maryland; in Monroe County (Rochester), New York; in Oxford, England; and in Mannheim, West Germany. These have been especially useful in providing information about schizophrenia, one of the most difficult disorders to study in population surveys because of its relatively rare occurrence and the difficulty in assuring an accurate diagnosis.

Danish adoption study One of the most prominent case-control studies in psychiatric epidemiology is that of S. S. Kety and colleagues begun in 1964. They studied a defined population of 5,483 adoptees, registered from 1924 through 1947, in the city and county of Copenhagen, Denmark. At that time, the adoptees ranged from 17 to 40 years of age. Of the total population, 507 were known to have been admitted at some time to a psychiatric hospital, and 33 of this group were assessed as having a diagnosis within a spectrum of schizophrenic disorders. An equal number of matched adoptees who had no history of mental hospitalization were identified for comparison.

For these cases and comparison adoptees, a systematic search of available records was conducted to assess the rate of schizophrenia-like conditions in their biological relatives. Of the 150 biological relatives of the schizophrenic adoptees, 8.7 percent had a diagnosis of schizophrenia, compared with 1.9 percent of the 156 biological relatives of the comparison group of adoptees. The highly significant difference in these rates indicated a genetic contribution to the presence of schizophrenia in the index cases, since environmental influences had been removed through adoption. As of this time, the genetic mechanism that increases passive susceptibility or causes active expression of particular genes has not been identified.

Experimental epidemiology Prospective trials have been used to test the effect of treatments among identified cases, with cases randomly assigned to experimental or control groups to control for possible selection bias. Longitudinal designs allow comparisons of rates of expected outcome between the control and experimental subjects. Similar clinical trial designs are being used to test preventive interventions in high-risk populations.

CONTEMPORARY EPIDEMIOLOGICAL STUDIES

STUDIES USING THE SCHEDULE FOR AFFECTIVE DISORDERS AND SCHIZOPHRENIA As the SADS interview was being developed for clinical studies in the mid-1970s, and was shown to be appropriate for both patients and normal controls in those studies, investigators began testing the feasibility of employing it in large, population-based studies of community residents and primary care patients. In a follow-up of 1,095 adults first studied in New Haven in 1967, J. K. Myers and M. W. Weissman conducted interviews with 511 who were still available for study in 1975 to 1976. They found that 15.1 percent of the sample had a definite RDC mental disorder at the time of the interview; these results attracted special interest in the research community by demonstrating that it was possible to conduct community-based studies using assessment instruments that produced clinically meaningful diagnoses.

After this successful study was carried out, NIMH investigators designed a study for primary care settings that also employed the SADS-L (Lifetime); this study demonstrated that nearly 28 percent of patients had a current RDC disorder, and that fewer than one in 10 of these disorders had been recognized by primary care clinicians.

STUDIES USING THE PRESENT STATE EXAMINATION Following successful use of the PSE in nine centers of the World Health Organization's International Pilot Study of Schizophrenia, in both developing and developed countries, European investigators began conducting studies of the general population using the PSE as the core assessment instrument. Although the PSE by itself does not generate diagnoses, it provides information that can be related to disease categories in the International Classification of Diseases (ICD) for the month preceding the examination. Among the multiple studies conducted with the PSE, five have been conducted in reasonably comparable ways and permit comparison of results for depressive and anxiety disorders (Table 5.1-2). Since these disorders typically show female predominance, whereas such disorders as alcohol abuse and dependence that are more common among males are not assessed in detail by the PSE, it is common for these studies to show that the total rate of disorder among females is higher than among males; such conclusions need to be qualified according to the range of disorders covered in the study, however. In general, Athens, Greece, and Camberwell, England showed generally equivalent rates of depressive conditions, and higher than those found in Canberra, Australia, and Edinburgh, Scotland; the highest rates by far are those from two Ugandan villages, and they are still unexplained. Rates of anxiety conditions among females are reported to be quite high in Athens.

An especially interesting finding was reported by the investigators in Edinburgh, who incorporated ratings of RDC criteria into their interview protocol that was built around the core items of the PSE. As noted in Table 5.1-2, they showed that PSE-derived categories of depression and anxiety in their sample of women were roughly comparable in frequency to the studies done in Canberra and Camberwell. However, their rates of depression and anxiety by RDC criteria in the sample, using information from the same interviews, were much higher, compared with those found in the New Haven cohort follow-up study that had used the SADS interview. This finding highlights the need to achieve greater diagnostic comparability in epidemiological investigations, particularly for international comparisons.

THE NIMH EPIDEMIOLOGIC CATCHMENT AREA PROGRAM The Epidemiologic Catchment Area Program (ECA) of the NIMH grew out of a combination of scientific developments and historical events within the mental health field. Of the scientific developments, none was more critical than the emergence of operational criteria for diagnoses that recently culminated in DSM-III and DSM-III-R. A logical extension of such criteria has been the construction of standardized clinical instruments to elicit reliably information on the presence of requisite symptom patterns from research subjects. Modification of one such instrument for epidemiological research produced a lifetime version of the SADS, which is based on the RDC. This modified instrument was shown to be feasible in a relatively small third wave of the New Haven epidemiological survey in 1975.

TABLE 5.1-2
Rates of ICD-equivalent disorders from the PSE in general population surveys

	Depression		*Anxiety*		*All Disorders*		
Location	*Males*	*Females*	*Males*	*Females*	*Males*	*Females*	*Total*
Athens	4.3%	10.1%	3.9%	12.1%	8.6%	22.6%	16.0%
Canberra	2.6	6.7	4.1	3.0	7.0	11.0	9.0
Camberwell	4.8	9.0	1.0	4.5	6.1	14.9	10.9
Edinburgh	-	5.9	-	2.8	-	8.7	-
Uganda	17.0	21.0	2.8	4.0	23.6*	27.0*	25.3*

*Rates calculated from tabular data published by authors.

In addition to the development of operationalized diagnostic criteria and standardized instruments, the 1978 President's Commission on Mental Health demonstrated major gaps in the knowledge of specific mental disorder population rates and how such disorders are treated. By synthesizing information from the NIMH NRP, mentioned above, psychiatric case registers, general practice epidemiological surveys, the Baltimore morbidity survey, and various other data sources, it was possible to provide conservative estimates of overall annual prevalence rates and the health care sector where individuals with such disorders received care. This analysis of secondary epidemiological and services research data resulted in mental disorder point prevalence rate estimates of 10 per 100 U.S. population, an annual incidence rate of five per 100 population, and an annual period prevalence rate of 15 per 100 population. On the basis of treated prevalence data, it was estimated that only 3.1 per 100 population were seen by any mental health specialist in the course of 1 year and that the majority (54 percent of the 15 per 100 population) were seen exclusively in the general medical outpatient sector. The total estimated distribution of the 15 per 100 population with mental disorder is shown in Table 5.1-3.

Fundamental deficits in knowledge of specific mental disorder frequency rates, the proportion of those treated and untreated, and the locus of treatment became readily apparent. The recommendation to proceed with a new wave of epidemiological and services research studies received favorable response from the NIMH leadership when the need was buttressed with evidence that the new diagnostic criteria and prototype standardized instruments could be applied for epidemiological purposes.

METHODOLOGY The NIMH ECA program is a multisite epidemiological and health services research study that assesses mental disorder prevalence, incidence, and service use rates in about 20,000 community and institutional residents. The survey uses the new DIS, previously mentioned.

The essential features of the research design include geographically defined community populations of at least 200,000 residents, from which stratified random probability samples are drawn to obtain completed interviews from approximately 3,000 adult (age 18 and over) community residents and 500 institutional residents. Participants include Yale University, Johns Hopkins University, Washington University, St. Louis University, Duke University, and the University of California at Los Angeles. Several of these sites have oversampled special populations, including the elderly and minority groups.

Following the sample selection, each subject is interviewed by a trained lay interviewer with the DIS and service utilization questions. A longitudinal design feature includes at least two face-to-face interviews (1 year apart) and one intervening telephone or face-to-face interview to assess service use as well as change in symptom or diagnostic status. Data collection has now been completed from all five sites and results have been presented from 18,571 persons interviewed in the first-wave community samples. U.S. estimates have been made by first weighting each person in proportion to the person's probability of selection in the individual catchment area site, and subsequently weighting each person in proportion to the person's representation in 36 age by sex by race-ethnicity groups in the 1980 U.S. census of noninstitutionalized adults age 18 and over.

The 1-month rates for all ages are provided to document the current state-of-the-art point prevalence rates using the DIS case-identification instrument. Standard errors are provided to illustrate the relative stability of these estimates of DIS-defined DSM-III disorder prevalence rates.

It is important to emphasize that these specific disorder rates allow multiple disorders for each individual and do not include any exclusionary diagnoses that were allowed by DSM-III. Although DSM-III would exclude a diagnosis of panic disorder if schizophrenia were present, the current diagnostic algorithms of the DIS do not unduplicate diagnoses based on exclusions.

RESULTS Current 1-month point prevalence rates (with standard errors in parentheses) are presented in Table 5.1-3 for the U.S. estimates derived from the combined data collected in all five sites. These data, which are weighted to the 1980 U.S. census noninstitutionalized population, provide a major advance in our ability to estimate U.S. rates over what was available at the time of the President's Commission on Mental Health. In addition to providing overall prevalence rates of DIS/DSM-III disorders, it has also been possible to identify sociodemographic correlates of these disorders that identify groups having relatively high or low rates of these disorders.

Table 5.1-3 shows that 15.4 percent of the U.S. population can be estimated to have had one or more DIS/DSM-III disorder in the 1 month before the interview. There is a small but significant difference between overall rates for males (14.0 percent) and females (16.6 percent), although these differences cease to be significant when age, marital status, race-ethnicity, and socioeconomic status variables are controlled. A summary rate of 11.5 percent, which excludes persons with only substance use disorders or severe cognitive impairment, is included to facilitate comparison with the PSE-based studies, which also exclude these disorders. When these disorders are excluded, the rates for males (8.2 percent) and females (14.6 percent) are close to the median rate (Camberwell) of the PSE-based studies of males (6.1 percent) and females (14.9 percent). These data show the importance of including alcohol and drug abuse disorders in epidemiological studies,

TABLE 5.1-3
One-Month Point Prevalence Rate Estimates per 100 U.S. Community Residents for Selected DIS/DSM-III Disorders, NIMH Epidemiologic Catchment Area Program (ECA).* Data Combined from Five Sites and Weighted to 1980 Census of U.S. Population.

	Rate per 100 Community Population		
Disorder	*Total* (*N* = 18,571)	Male (*N* = 7,618)	Female (*N* = 10,953)
Any DIS/DSM-III disorder covered	15.4 (0.4)[†]	14.0 (0.5)	16.6 (0.5)
Any disorder except severe cognitive impairment or substance use	11.5 (0.3)	8.2 (0.4)	14.6 (0.4)
Schizophrenic/schizophreniform disorders	0.7 (0.1)	0.7 (0.1)	0.7 (0.1)
Schizophrenia	0.6 (0.1)	0.6 (0.1)	0.6 (0.1)
Schizophreniform disorder	0.1 (0.1)	0.1 (0.0)	0.1 (0.0)
Affective disorders [mood disorders]	5.1 (0.2)	3.5 (0.3)	6.6 (0.3)
Manic episode	0.4 (0.1)	0.3 (0.1)	0.4 (0.1)
Major depressive episode	2.2 (0.2)	1.6 (0.2)	2.9 (0.2)
Dysthymia	3.3 (0.2)	2.2 (0.3)	4.2 (0.3)
Anxiety disorders	7.3 (0.3)	4.7 (0.3)	9.7 (0.4)
Phobia	6.2 (0.2)	3.8 (0.3)	8.4 (0.3)
Panic	0.5 (0.1)	0.3 (0.1)	0.7 (0.1)
Obsessive-compulsive disorder	1.3 (0.1)	1.1 (0.1)	1.5 (0.2)
Substance use disorders	3.8 (0.2)	6.3 (0.4)	1.6 (0.2)
Alcohol abuse/dependence	2.8 (0.2)	5.0 (0.4)	0.9 (0.1)
Drug abuse/dependence	1.3 (0.1)	1.8 (0.2)	0.7 (0.1)
Somatization disorder	0.1 (0.0)	0.0 (0.0)	0.2 (0.1)
Antisocial personality disorder	0.5 (0.1)	0.8 (0.1)	0.2 (0.1)
Cognitive impairment—severe	1.3 (0.1)	1.4 (0.1)	1.3 (0.1)

*The Epidemiologic Catchment Area Program (ECA) is a series of five epidemiological research studies performed by independent research teams in collaboration with staff of the Division of Biometry and Epidemiology (DBE) and the Division of Clinical Research (DCR) of the National Institute of Mental Health (NIMH). The NIMH principal collaborators are Darrel A. Regier, Ben Z. Locke, and Jack D. Burke, Jr.; the NIMH project officers are Carl A. Taube (1978–1985) and William Huber (1985–). The principal investigators and coinvestigators from the five sites are: Yale University, UO1 MOH 34223—Jerome K. Myers, Myrna M. Weissman, and Gary L. Tischler; Johns Hopkins University, UO1 MH 33870—Morton Kramer, Ernest Gruenberg, and Sam Shapiro; Washington University, St. Louis, UO1 MH 33883—Lee N. Robins and John Helzer; Duke University, UO1 MH 35386—Dan Blazer and Linda George; University of California, Los Angeles, UO1 MH 35865—Marvin Karno, Richard L. Hough, Javier I. Escobar, M. Audrey Burnam, and Dianne M. Timbers.
[†]Numbers in parentheses represent standard errors.

particularly when accurate rates for males are desired. Because diagnostic exclusions were not used, it is possible for subjects to have more than one diagnosis—hence, the sum of the rates for individual disorders will equal more than the overall rate.

Schizophrenia Schizophrenia was found in 0.7 percent of the population, with equal rates for men and women. The highest rates were found in the age group 25 to 44 (1.1 percent), followed by a rate of 0.8 percent in the age group 18 to 24. Significantly higher rates were found among those who were separated and divorced (1.5 percent) and in lower socioeconomic groups—an odds ratio of eight was identified for the lowest socioeconomic class as compared with the highest class.

Affective disorders Affective (mood) disorders were found at an overall rate of 5.1 percent, and were significantly higher in females (6.6 percent) than males (3.5 percent). Although these rates are consistent with previous studies, such as the median (Camberwell) for those using the PSE, specific biological or social factors that may account for this sex ratio discrepancy have not yet been identified. The age group of 25 to 44 years had the highest rates (6.4 percent) of any age group, with significantly lower rates in the 65+ age group (2.5 percent). Of all the sociodemographically defined groups, the separated or divorced marital status group was associated with the highest overall level of mood disorders at 11.1 percent compared with a rate of 4.1 percent for the married group. Rates for major depressive episode were also found in 2.2 percent of the population and manic episode, necessary for bipolar-I diagnostic criteria, was found in 0.4 percent of the population. Dysthymia, which requires a 2-year duration of symptoms for DSM-III criteria, was only identified on a lifetime basis at 3.3 percent, but is included in the current 1-month prevalence rates because of the higher probability of recalling more recent episodes and to avoid a serious underestimate of mood disorders. For example, the Camberwell study found a higher rate of total mood disorders (7.0 percent), and the same ratio of males (4.8 percent) to females (9.0 percent).

Anxiety disorders As a group, the anxiety disorders contain the highest overall prevalence (7.3 percent), with women (9.7 percent) having significantly higher rates than men (4.7 percent). Phobic disorders, which include simple phobias, social phobias, and agoraphobia, constitute the largest single diagnosis. Within the five sites, this disorder had the highest prevalence rates and the greatest variation between sites, ranging from a 4 to 5 percent level in three sites (New Haven, St. Louis, Los Angeles) to a level of 11 percent for two sites (Baltimore and Durham). The marked discrepancy in this one diagnosis has led the investigators to examine whether any of the following types of bias exist: observational bias (differences in interviewer training or questionnaire construction); selection bias (differences in characteristics of subjects); or confounding bias (whereby another factor, such as socioeconomic status, may be related to both a causal factor of phobia and the population of subjects with high rates of this disorder). Once these analyses of bias have been completed, it would be appropriate to consider environmental or other variables associated with the geographically defined population in Baltimore and Durham that are not found in the other three sites. Of the remaining anxiety disorders, it is of interest to note that panic disorder (0.5 percent) and obsessive-compulsive disorder (1.3 percent) are also found somewhat more frequently in women.

Substance use disorders Overall substance use disorders are found in 3.8 percent of the population, with markedly higher rates in men (6.3 percent) than in women (1.6 percent). Alcohol abuse or dependence rates (2.8 percent) show a significant difference between men and women, with males having over five times the rate for women. Sex ratios of this magnitude are found in only one other disorder, antisocial personality disorder, which has a low prevalence rate and a male to female ratio of 4 to 1. In contrast, drug abuse or dependence (1.3 percent) had male rates that were slightly more than two times higher than those for women. Although further analyses will proceed on the alcohol abuse or dependence category, the finding of a higher male to female ratio for alcoholism in comparison with the higher female to male ratio for depression and anxiety disorders has led other investigators to question whether a similar underlying biological disorder results in a differential phenotypical manifestation of depression or anxiety disorders in females and alcoholism in males because of social-role expectations. Population, genetic, and neurobiological research may eventually find measurable risk factors to test this hypothesis by case-control methods.

Somatization disorder The only somatoform disorder covered in the DIS is somatization disorder, which is closely related to Briquet's syndrome in the Feighner (St. Louis) criteria for mental disorders. It is found almost exclusively in females (0.2 percent), which, in the absence of any in males, results in an overall population rate of 0.1 percent.

Antisocial personality disorder This disorder is found predominately in men (0.8 percent), with a female rate of 0.2 percent and an overall population rate of 0.5 percent. It is also a disorder found predominately in the age group under 45 years (0.8 to 0.9 percent) and is associated with a separated or divorced marital status (1.1 percent) compared with married (0.5 percent). Lower socioeconomic status (SES) levels III and IV (0.7 to 0.9 percent) have higher rates compared with higher SES levels I and II (0.2 to 0.3 percent).

Severe cognitive impairment Cognitive impairment is not a DSM-III diagnosis, but is determined by a score of 0 to 17 on the Mini-Mental Status Examination. A major objective of this component of the DIS is to identify subpopulations with a high probability of having organic mental disorders, including such dementias as Alzheimer's disease, delirium, or other organic syndromes that affect cognition. Low scores of 0 to 17 on the Mini-Mental Status Examination indicate severe cognitive impairment, scores of 18 to 23 refer to mild impairment, and scores of 24 to 30 represent little or no impairment. In order to assess the range of disorders included and the sensitivity and specificity of the screening instrument for a detailed criterion assessment, detailed psychiatric and neurological examinations have been conducted on the sample of subjects with these disorders at the Baltimore site.

Summary rates As mentioned, the diagnostic algorithms for computing these rates allow for multiple diagnoses and do not apply DSM-III's exclusion rules. Summary rates are used to present the total number of individuals in the population with any one of these disorders, and they are included for comparative purposes. It should be emphasized that these summary rates do not identify the total rate of mental disorder in the population, but only identify that proportion having one of the DSM-III disorders and cognitive impairment identified by the DIS.

DISCUSSION A major benefit of data obtained from the ECA program will be to advance the understanding of nosological categories by examining how the combination of different symptom patterns correlates with external measures of validity-stability of disorder over time, longitudinal course, use of treatment services, and analytic variables that may be obtained by more in-depth case-control studies. The next major advance will be an opportunity to examine the DIS instrument in comparison with other clinical reevaluation instruments, such as the modified PSE, the SADS-L, and DSM-III-R checklists administered by psychiatrists. An improved screening instrument, as well as the identification of unique strengths and deficits of standardized clinical interviews, should be an important outcome of these analyses. Finally, where the same general methodology has been used across populations, the opportunity to compare results has provided for immediate replication of results—something that has never been feasible in the past. Greater confidence in the epidemiological findings should then allow for more creative applications of the instruments to identify risk factors and potential preventive and treatment intervention studies.

FUTURE OF MENTAL DISORDER EPIDEMIOLOGY

The previous material has identified recent advances in the fundamental scientific and technical underpinnings of mental disorder epidemiological research. These advances include the development of operational criteria that facilitate reliable application in large population groups. Although questions remain about the validity of DSM-III-R diagnoses based largely on manifestational rather than causal criteria, the explicit nature of the criteria renders them susceptible to empirical hypothesis testing. Removal of presumed etiological criteria from mental disorder diagnoses will actually facilitate research on the scientific veracity of etiological hypotheses. Epidemiological studies using DSM-III-R criteria will produce external validating criteria to assess the degree to which groups identified with specific disorders are homogeneous with regard to biological, demographic, social, and clinical course characteristics. Stability of mental disorder rates in populations with similar characteristics will support the validity of the diagnoses, whereas variations in rates may lead to additional subtyping, or even etiological clues.

The emergence of standardized interview instruments, such as the DIS, has also facilitated development of such standardized international epidemiological instruments as the Composite International Diagnostic Interview (CIDI), sponsored by the World Health Organization and the U.S. Alcohol, Drug Abuse, and Mental Health Administration—an instrument that combines elements of the DIS and PSE. In addition, the emergence of more clinical standardized interviews will improve clinical research and provide better criterion standards for assessing the DIS performance in large-scale populations.

With the above improvements in nosological and case-identification tools for epidemiological research, it will be necessary to extend the full range of epidemiological methods to new population groups, including those in other cultures. Further refinements in the basic tools for childhood disorders and culture-specific disorders should expand research opportunities in these understudied groups.

Once the intrinsic research base of epidemiology is more secure, it will be possible to extend the interface with other research fields, including service systems, clinical services, and clinical and neurobiological research areas. Many potential etiological or clinical service improvement risk factors emerging from these other research areas will require validation in large population studies using experimental epidemiological research designs.

The full potential of mental disorder epidemiology for health policy applications has yet to be realized. Improvements in the data base should facilitate future mental health service resource allocations, refine prevention efforts, and improve the safety and effectiveness of specific treatments for those persons who have a mental disorder and now reside in the often undifferentiated mass within institutions and communities.

REFERENCES

Bebbington P, Hurry J, Tennant C, Sturt E, Wing J K: Epidemiology of mental disorders in Camberwell. Psychol Med *11:* 561, 1981.

Burke J D: Diagnostic categorization by the diagnostic interview schedule (DIS): A comparison with other methods of assessment. In *Mental Disorders in the Community: Findings from Psychiatric Epidemiology*, J. E Barrett, R M Rose, editors, p 255. Guilford, New York, 1986.

Commission on Chronic Illness: *Chronic Illness in the United States*, IV: *Chronic Illness in a Large City: The Baltimore Study*. Harvard University Press, Cambridge, MA, 1957.

Dean C, Surtees P G, Sashidharian S P: Comparison of research diagnostic systems in an Edinburgh community sample. Brit J Psychiat *142:* 247, 1983.

Fleiss J L: *Statistical Methods for Rates and Proportions*, ed 2. Wiley, New York, 1981.
Henderson S, Duncan-Jones P, Byrne D G, Scott R, Adcock S: Psychiatric disorder in Canberra: A standardized study of prevalence. Acta Psychiat Scand *60:* 355, 1979.
Hollingshead A B, Redlich F C: *Social Class and Mental Illness*. Wiley, New York, 1958.
Kety S S, Rosenthal D, Wender P H, Schulsinger F: The types and prevalence of mental illness in the biological and adoptive families of adopted schizophrenics. In *Transmission of Schizophrenia*, D Rosenthal, S S Kety, editors. Pergamon Press, London, 1968.
Kleinbaum D G, Kupper L L, Morgenstern H: *Epidemiologic Research: Principles and Quantitative Methods*. Lifetime Learning Publications, Belmont, CA, 1982.
Leighton D C, MacMillan A M, Harding H S, Macklin D B, Leighton A H: *The Character of Danger*. Basic Books, New York, 1963.
Lilienfeld A M, Lilienfeld D E: *Foundations of Epidemiology*, ed 2. Oxford University Press, New York, 1980.
Mavreas V G, Beis A, Mouyias A, Rigoni F, Lyketsos G C: Prevalence of psychiatric disorders in Athens: A community study. Soc Psychiat *21:* 172, 1986.
Morris J N: *Uses of Epidemiology*, ed 2. Williams & Wilkins, Baltimore, 1964.
Orley J, Wing J K: Psychiatric disorders in two African villages. Arch Gen Psychiat *36:* 513, 1979.
Regier D A, Goldberg I D, Taube C A: The de facto U.S. mental health services system: A public health perspective. Arch Gen Psychiat *35:* 685, 1978.
Regier D A, Myers J K, Kramer M, Robins L N, Blazer D G, Hough R L, Eaton W W, Locke B Z: The NIMH Epidemiologic Catchment Area Program: Historical context, major objectives, and study population characteristics. Arch Gen Psychiat *41:* 934, 1984.
Regier D A, Boyd J H, Burke J D, Rae D S, Myers J K, Kramer M, Robins L N, George L K, Karno M, Locke B Z: One-month prevalence of mental disorders in the U.S.: Based on five epidemiologic catchment area (ECA) sites. Arch Gen Psychiat *45:* 977, 1988.
Srole L, Langner T S, Michael S T, Opler M K, Rennie T A C: *Mental Health in the Metropolis: The Midtown Manhattan Study*. McGraw-Hill, New York, 1962.
Thompson E A: Genetic Epidemiology: A review of the statistical basis. Stat Med *5:* 291, 1986.
Weissman M M, Klerman G L: Epidemiology of mental disorders: Emerging trends in the United States. Arch Gen Psychiat *35:* 705, 1978.
Weissman M M, Myers J K, Harding P S: Psychiatric disorders in a U.S. urban community: 1975–1976. Amer J Psychiat *135:* 459, 1978.

5.2 INTERDISCIPLINARY ANIMAL RESEARCH AND ITS RELEVANCE TO PSYCHIATRY

WILLIAM T. McKINNEY, M.D.

INTRODUCTION

Previous editions of this textbook included several sections that were highly relevant to what will be covered in the present section. Among the topics covered by these sections were sensory deprivation, sociobiology, ethology, animal models, the ethology of communicative behavior, aggression, and experimental disorders. In the present edition, it was decided to have one integrated section dealing with the various actual and potential linkages between animal behavioral research and clinical psychiatry.

The objective of the first part of this section is to discuss the basic rationale for using animals in psychiatric research and to outline a conceptual or philosophical framework for evaluating such research. These general principles will be illustrated by providing an overview of research being conducted utilizing animals to study specific aspects of several psychiatric illnesses. The disorders that will be used for this purpose are mood disorders, schizophrenia, and anxiety disorders. Other disorders could have been chosen, but the main goal is not to provide a comprehensive discussion of animal models of each of the psychiatric syndromes but rather to highlight certain trends that affect the interface between the various disciplines that are involved with the study of animal behavior and clinical psychiatry. The field of animal modeling is an active one despite controversies surrounding its continued development. The special contributions of animal models, in relation both to clinical research and to basic research, will be discussed. These are increasingly important interfaces for psychiatrists to be aware of over the next several years.

The next two parts of this section will focus on the interface between clinical psychiatry and ethology and on psychiatry and sociobiology. These extremely important interfaces are rarely discussed in any detail in psychiatry training programs. As these fields are large, somewhat arbitrary decisions have been made regarding the choice of topics to be covered. The attempt here will be to present those topics that seem most relevant to clinical psychiatrists.

ANIMAL MODELS IN PSYCHIATRY

HISTORY Ivan Pavlov is often said to have been the originator of research relevant to animal modeling of human psychopathology in general. His use of clinical terms, as well as the experimental techniques used in his studies, may seem foreign to most psychiatric clinicians. However, of central importance is the fact that his work represented one of the first moves away from the correlational method of behavioral analysis to the experimental study of psychopathology.

As H. D. Kimmel has said:

> The significance of this change in direction may best be comprehended in relation to its two most important implications. First, the completely correlational method of behavioral analysis, which was the empirical foundation of all earlier systematic efforts to understand psychological abnormality, including everything from Hippocrates' humors and Gall's prominences to the ingenious psychoanalytic theorizing of Freud, could now be supplemented, if not altogether supplanted, by a direct experimental approach which was much less fraught with the dual dangers of loose conjecture and empirical untestability. Second, and historically of possibly greater significance, the continuity of animal morphology, physiology, and behavior, already beginning to assume a position on center stage in man's philosophical thinking, received a new extensive thrust from the early Pavlovian findings since for the first time even such "uniquely human" phenomena as emotional breakdowns were seen to occur in subhuman animals.

Pavlov was followed by a number of other workers and it is difficult to know what conclusions to draw about this early history of the field of experimental psychopathology research. Some who have reviewed it have not seen it as a particularly noteworthy beginning. However, the early pioneers may have been more successful than it appears in developing certain principles that seem to be being rediscovered today. These include the following:

1. The demonstration that psychopathology could be experimentally studied in animals in addition to the strictly correlational studies done previously in humans.

2. The demonstration of the importance of both careful behavioral observations and serendipity. Although it is true that most of the early workers did not use the more sophisticated and quantifiable behavioral scoring techniques now available, they were keen observers and literate in their descriptions.

3. The repeated proposal of an interactive model of psychopathology. The role of the temperament of the animals, along with a variety of social and neurobiological variables, was repeatedly stressed in the early literature. The concept of individual variability was part of the early work, and investigation of the sources of such variability continues to be an important area of research.

4. The development of the principle that there could be a persistent internal response, even after the inducing stimulus is no longer present. This development remains a major contribution to the understanding of a number of forms of psychopathology.

5. The recognition of the importance of unpredictability and uncontrollability. Systematic investigations of these phenomena continue today.

6. Experimental paradigms led to the development of another basic principle that is still important today, namely, that adaptive behavioral processes provide the foundation on which maladaptive behavior patterns are built in the presence of altered environmental demands. Adaptive mechanisms of animals and humans are fragile and share a tenuous relationship with the environment. Either internal changes in the organism (e.g., with drugs or other altered neurochemistry) or changes in the external environment (e.g., separation, the imposition of uncontrollability) can lead to serious behavioral changes. These behavioral changes can, in turn, lead to neurobiological changes and the development of a vicious circle. The study of these interactions is becoming a cornerstone of animal modeling research in depression and other forms of psychopathology.

One of the problems with the early history of experimental psychopathology was that clinical terms were applied far too loosely and prematurely to a set of behavioral changes induced by methods that seemed to bear only a faint resemblance to inducing conditions for human syndromes. The result was a certain amount of skepticism and cynicism about the whole field by clinicians.

The work of Harry Harlow, in particular, helped to stimulate interest by clinicians in the field of primate behavioral research. Harlow died on December 6, 1981, at the age of 76. With his passing, the field of primatology lost one of its most prominent scientists.

Harlow's research with primates began in about 1930 with observations of primates at the local zoo. He soon discovered that monkeys and apes were much smarter than rats, and that tests designed to study rodent learning did not begin to tap their intellectual capabilities. It became apparent that more challenging or complex learning tasks and a better physical environment in which to test his primates were needed. Harlow attacked these two basic problems with what was to become characteristic vigor, and the two results were the Wisconsin General Test Apparatus (WGTA) and a primate laboratory.

The WGTA brought to the study of primate learning capabilities a means by which a large number of discrete learning tests could be rapidly presented in highly standardized fashion to subject after subject. Studies of primate learning proliferated in the years that followed, and a battery of discrimination learning and memory tasks was developed that provided a standardized "intelligence test" for monkeys. Harlow then proceeded to study cortical localization of learning capabilities by lesioning different primate brain areas and noting subsequent differential patterns of deficits in their performance on the test battery.

In the late 1940s, Harlow achieved a major conceptual and methodological breakthrough with his discovery of learning sets. He showed that rhesus monkeys presented with long series of six-trial, two-choice discrimination problems soon learned to achieve near-perfect performance on the second and subsequent trials of each problem. He was able to demonstrate unequivocally that the monkeys had acquired a strategy for problem solving. What the monkeys had learned was an abstract concept ("learning to learn," in his words), rather than the product of simple associative learning.

Harlow's interest in the processes underlying primate learning extended to two different lines of research. The first line involved motivation. In an effort to understand the factors that influenced learning performance, he discovered major inconsistencies with classic notions of drive reduction. It was not readily apparent why monkeys should solve puzzles more effectively when motivated by mere curiosity than when driven by hunger or thirst, but they did. Convinced that drive reduction and other motivational theories in vogue in psychology and psychiatry at that time could not possibly account for most of a monkey's behaviors, he began to look for alternative formulations.

At about the same time, Harlow began studies of the ontogenic development of learning capabilities in rhesus monkey subjects. This task required both devising a new battery of age-sensitive learning tests and acquiring suitable subjects. The latter requirement led to the establishment of a captive breeding colony and a nursery capable of hand-rearing large numbers of baby monkeys.

Next came the cloth- and wire-covered surrogate mothers and the entrance of primatology into clinical psychiatry. Infant rhesus monkeys reared with a choice between a wire surrogate that fed them and a cloth surrogate that did not overwhelmingly preferred the cloth "mother." Contrary to prevailing wisdom, "contact comfort," as Harlow termed it, was much more instrumental than feeding in bonding these infants to their surrogates. Harlow's discoveries with the surrogates sounded the end for drive reduction theory and revolutionized thinking concerning the socialization process in children. They also opened up the field of primate social development to serious scientific inquiry. Eventually, Harlow shifted the major focus of his research to the study of social behavior and its development, both normal and abnormal. He developed the concept of affectional systems, the idea that social ontogeny involves the establishment of qualitatively different types of social relationships with a variety of others in the social network—parents, siblings, peers—as one grows up. At the same time, he studied the consequences of blocking the formation of different affectional systems via social isolation rearing or disrupting the attachment bonds once formed by experimental separations. These studies clearly established the overwhelming importance of early social experiences for the development of species-normative adult social activities, including reproduction and maternal behavior.

Harlow spent his last years at Wisconsin expanding on the twin themes of normal and abnormal social behavior. He, along with Margaret Harlow, was instrumental in establishing the "nuclear family" living unit in which adult male-female pairs and various offspring could live together in a laboratory but in a situation rich in stimulation compared with the more typical laboratory environment.

Harlow made a career of using rhesus monkey subjects to study human capabilities and problems not easily researched in humans themselves, and many of the fundamental concepts he developed, which were the source of considerable controversy at the time, are now fully incorporated into developmental theories.

RATIONALE FOR USING ANIMALS IN PSYCHIATRIC RESEARCH

The following reasons for including animal modeling research as part of a comprehensive psychopathology research program are illustrative rather than comprehensive. Issues concerning the development, practical use, and potential benefits of animal models are also summarized in Table 5.2-1.

1. Many of the critical questions about the origins of human psychopathology cannot be studied directly in humans. By using animal preparations, it is possible to control inducing conditions rather precisely and to study the behavioral and neurobiological effects on both a short-term and long-term basis. For example, in relation to depression, prospective studies examining the effects of developmental events on behavior and on neurobiology can be done much more easily in animals. The timing and exact nature of certain alterations in development can be specified and the short- and long-term consequences studied. This aspect of modeling research is relevant to the question of developmental vulnerability based on early experiences and the mediating mechanisms of this vulnerability.

A particular line of research where animal preparations have a special contribution to make is in the conduct of prospective studies examining the effects of developmental events on behavior and neurochemistry. The interactions between these variables can be studied in a controlled and prospective manner. Animal preparations have been developing in the past decade that make such investigations feasible and will facilitate the movement beyond correlation and retrospective analysis to cause-and-effect studies.

2. The underlying mechanisms associated with specific behaviors and patterns of behaviors can be studied more directly in certain animal species. Animal models potentially make possible the dissec-

TABLE 5.2-1
The Development, Practical Use, and Potential Benefits of Various Types of Animal Models

Criteria for Development	*Use in Research*	*Benefits*
Similarity of inducing conditions	Treatment screens	New treatments
Similarity of behavioral syndromes	Study of developmental determinants	Help to define the syndrome in humans
Similarity of neurobiological mechanisms	Study of underlying mechanisms	Identification of at-risk individuals
Similarity in response to clinically effective treatments	Study of interactions between social and biological components	Development of improved diagnostic tests
Other criteria appropriate for the specific model		

tion of underlying mechanisms in a more direct way than is possible in human clinical research and complement ongoing efforts in this regard in human protocols. More direct, and potentially more invasive, studies of neurobiological mechanisms can be done, although such procedures will need to be suited to both the species and the overall purpose of having the experimental paradigm in the first place.

Not all procedures are justified on ethical or economic grounds in all species. The questions have to be clear and specific, especially in proposing such studies in higher-order primates. Nevertheless, the time is ripe for a vigorous effort in this area. It will need to involve multiple laboratories, much as collaborative human studies of psychopathology often involve many centers. The area of experimental psychopathology in animals has become complex enough that this type of collaborative approach needs to be undertaken. For example, different strategies and approaches need to be employed with several species, and techniques now generally available in only one laboratory need to be applied to many of these preparations. Attention needs to be given to how to do what kinds of mechanism studies in a given species. Molecular or submolecular studies may be indicated in some preparations, but this may not be the only reasonable way to approach mechanism studies, for example, in a socially behaving species. This frontier area is very controversial, in that basic neuroscientists sometimes want certain types of mechanistic studies to be done, but to do them in the way requested would vitiate the social behavioral studies. Continued dialogue is necessary, and it is hoped that it will be less acrimonious than it is at present. The issues are complex but probably solvable with enough discussion and the development of some collaborative protocols across laboratories that take advantage of complementing expertise.

Single variables can be evaluated in terms of their main effects and in terms of the nature of their interaction with each other. For example, the nature of the interactions among genetic, developmental, social, and biological variables can be studied in various combinations in different species. In human clinical research, multiple variables interact simultaneously, and it has been impossible to sort them out in any quantifiable way.

3. The ability to isolate specific behavior patterns in animals and to study their origins, pathophysiology, and responsiveness to treatment techniques is important. Typically, in clinical work one is dealing with a broad range of behaviors that occur together, and it is impossible to study one or two in isolation and to understand them more completely. The many examples include anhedonia, stereotypic rituals, social withdrawal, and altered learning and cognitive abilities. If one can begin to understand these and other particular aspects of psychopathological syndromes better, it might be possible to expand the understanding of situations where they typically occur together.

4. Animal models have played an important role in the preclinical evaluation of drugs. This topic, which relates to the empirical or predictive validity of animal models, will be discussed further with regard to the general kinds of animal models.

A related aspect of the use of animal models is their contribution in helping to foster a better understanding of the mechanism of the action of drugs in altering specific behavior patterns. This assistance goes beyond a mere global prediction of whether drugs work or do not work and relates to studying the behavioral effects of agents with relatively specific mechanisms of action.

5. Animal models can also be used to help understand the mechanisms of established treatment techniques. They potentially make possible the investigation of the mechanisms in terms not only of pathogenesis but also of treatment responsiveness. That is, why do some drugs work whereas others do not? What are the mechanisms of action of electroconvulsive therapy in depression? Why are certain behavioral interventions effective and others are not?

6. Animal models also permit the understanding of a specific behavior or set of behaviors in terms of the developmental and social context as well as pathophysiology. Rather than just focusing on global syndromes, one can investigate certain behaviors as to their origin, context, and responsiveness to certain interventions.

7. Animal modeling research, especially with primates, has led to the development of improved behavioral, ethologically based rating methods that can now be used in clinical research settings to evaluate social interactions, as between mother and infant or among peers.

ILLUSTRATIVE ANIMAL MODELS

Mood disorders

Pharmacological models In this approach, drugs are administered to animal models in order to reproduce some of the phenomenology of human depressive syndromes. A related approach is to use certain drugs to produce a set of changes in animals that do not necessarily bear much phenomenological similarity to human depression but have high empirical validity in terms of predicting clinical drug responses. In reviewing this area, R. D. Porsolt speaks of yet a third class of animal models. This class is heterogeneous and, although not based on drug-induced changes, has been found useful in predicting and characterizing antidepressant activity. This third type of model may have empirical validity in terms of drug screening, but in terms of induction techniques or behaviors, it seemingly bears little relationship to human depression (e.g., muricidal behavior, the bulbectomized rat syndrome, and kindled amygdaloid convulsions).

Among pharmacologically induced models, the syndrome induced by reserpine and related compounds has been the most widely used. Reserpine, when given to animals of various species, produces a characteristic set of behaviors, including ptosis, hypothermia, inactivity, social withdrawal, and sedation. The other historical context for the interest in this animal model came from the clinical observation that drugs containing reserpine were reported to induce depression in humans who took them for the treatment of hypertension. This clinical observation, at least in its initial form, has been called into question on the basis of recent evidence. It appears that humans who become depressed while taking reserpine-containing drugs have a history of depression, and presumably have a vulnerability in this area.

The reserpine syndrome as an animal model of depression has been reviewed extensively. In addition, a number of related compounds have been used to induce symptoms qualitatively similar to those produced by reserpine, though a number of factors are different, such as the speed of onset, duration, and central and peripheral effects. Initially, it was thought that most clinically active antidepressant drugs antagonized some or all of the symptoms induced by reserpine. In general, this is true, but there are a number of inconsistencies. The reserpine syndrome is not a unitary entity, but involves many different effects. For example, ptosis antagonism, although probably a peripheral effect, seems to identify the greatest number of clinically effective antidepressants, including several of the newer antidepressants, some of which are regarded as false negatives in other reserpine procedures. In evaluating the empirical validity of this model, one must be specific about which behavior is involved. Some behaviors could have high empirical validity in terms of predicting clinical drug response, although the mediating mechanism might not even be central in origin. Reserpine has so many different neurochemical effects that one cannot reason directly from such studies to possible mechanisms associated with the behaviors produced, let alone human depression.

Several other pharmacologically induced models have been developed. One is the amphetamine withdrawal model. Animals subjected to repeated amphetamine treatments, which are then stopped, evince a number of effects, including decreases in motor activity and self-stimulation behavior. These effects have been reported to be reversed to a certain extent by amitriptyline (Elavil), imipramine (Tofranil), mianserin, and pargyline (Eutonyl), when given on an acute basis, but especially when given on a chronic basis. Another proposed pharmacological model is clonidine (Catapres)-induced behavioral depression. Clonidine, an α-adrenergic receptor stimulant, is thought to act at presynaptic receptor sites to reduce the release of norepinephrine, resulting in hypothermia, analgesia, and marked sedation. Clonidine-induced hypoactivity has been proposed as a test for antidepressant drugs. Although it is not clear as to which drugs will work in this model, it may play a role in screening for antidepressants that might be inactive in other models.

Another class of procedures widely used in pharmacology involves the potentiation by antidepressants of the behavioral and other effects of amines or their precursors. These procedures do not attempt to mimic the clinical condition, but are based on theories about the role of the amines in depression. Thus, they are designed to show how these amines interact with each other and are influenced by antidepressant drugs. By such routes, important information can be obtained that may ultimately have a bearing on mechanism questions, and can be tested in more highly developed behavioral models. Examples of such procedures include the potentiation by antidepressants of the various central effects of amphetamine and yohimbine.

Pharmacologically induced models have been, and continue to be, important for screening clinically effective drugs. Thus, in evaluating them, attention should be paid primarily to their empirical or predictive validity. Each has false negatives and false positives, but by using several such tests in a battery, it may be possible to achieve an even higher degree of empirical validity.

In the case of all empirically based tests, it should be kept in mind that the mechanism by which the drug presumably acts in the animal preparation is not necessarily the same as its mechanism of action in human depression. Too many variables can intervene, and additional types of animal preparations may be necessary to assist with mechanism questions.

Separation models Disruption of attachment bonds, whether in humans or nonhumans, has been established as a very stressful event. Humans and many animal species are in their most stable condition when they have developed secure social attachment systems. Disruption of such systems almost invariably leads to the development of grief reactions and can precipitate clinical depression in some vulnerable individuals. Many developmental, social, and neurobiological variables are known to influence the reaction to separation. However, determining the influence of these different variables in humans, and how they interact with one another, has been extremely difficult. For these and other reasons, investigators have turned to animal models for a more systematic study of the effects of separation.

BEHAVIORAL RESPONSES TO MATERNAL SEPARATION The earliest work on separation in animals began in the 1960s with the short-term separation of pigtail macaque infants from their mothers at the ages of 5 and 7 months, and then reuniting them with their own or another mother. A number of laboratories conducted significant investigations of separation beginning in the 1960s and continuing to the present. The behaviors seen following separation have been divided into two categories, labeled "agitation" or "protest" and "depression" or "despair." Figure 5.2-1 shows a rhesus monkey recently separated from its mother and in the "depression" or "despair" stage.

The protest and despair response seen in many primate species following maternal separation has, arguably, been likened to the responses in human children diagnosed as having anaclitic depression or observed in institutions (usually hospitals or nurseries) where they were unavoidably separated from their mothers and families. The stages of response of human infants to maternal separation have been described as protest, despair, and denial (later changed to detachment). These stages have played a key role in the development of the theory of primary separation anxiety.

As animal researchers extended this original work on the response to maternal separation, it became apparent that the response of the infants was influenced by a number of parameters, including the species, age, and social conditions.

The reaction to maternal separation in primates represents a true biobehavioral syndrome. Not only are there significant behavioral effects as described above, but there are also major neurobiological changes.

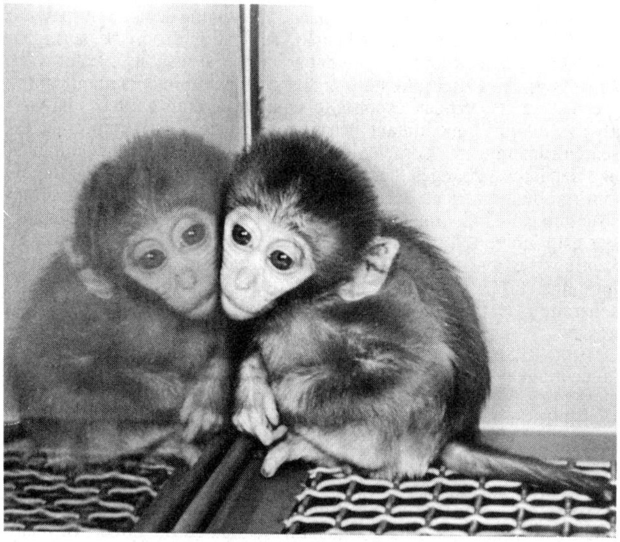

FIGURE 5.2-1 *A rhesus monkey recently separated from its mother in the depression or despair stage.*

PHYSIOLOGICAL RESPONSES TO MATERNAL SEPARATION Pigtail macaque infants undergoing maternal separation have been studied using totally implanted multichannel biotelemetry systems to monitor heart rate, body temperature, and sleep physiology before, during, and after the separation. In these studies, the biological mother was usually removed from a group living situation and the infant was left in the group. Attachment bonds have been found to be as central to the development of monkeys as they are to people, with disruption of these bonds leading to serious changes. In one study, for example, the infant's heart rate and body temperature increased significantly immediately after maternal separation. These changes were most pronounced early in separation and diminished as the separation continued. Beginning with the first night, both the heart rate and body temperature showed marked decreases from baseline levels and the behavioral patterns became more depressive-like. During reunion, both the heart rate and body temperature returned to normal, although some infants exhibited a lower heart rate well into the reunion. An increased incidence of cardiac arrythmias as a result of maternal separation has also been reported. Significant sleep changes have included increased sleep latency, more frequent arousals, less total sleep, and a disruption of rapid eye movement (REM) sleep.

In other research, neurochemical effects were examined in rhesus monkey infants that were in the protest stage following maternal separation. Positive findings included elevated serotonin levels in the hypothalamus, and significantly higher levels in the adrenal gland of all of the major enzymes involved in catecholamine syntheses. Resting levels of norepinephrine (NE) and dopamine (DA) were unchanged in any of the brain regions examined. This study measured resting levels of these substances at one point in time, and thus gives no information about possible dynamic changes occurring over time. However, it provides additional confirmation of the powerful effects of disrupting the maternal attachment bond. The syndrome is neither transient nor mild.

Squirrel monkeys, when separated from their mother or from a surrogate, show a marked increase in the pituitary-adrenal response. Initially, it was reported that there was an identical physiological response whether the infant was separated from a mother or from a surrogate. The monkey mother also showed an elevated corticoid response to separation. This latter finding is interesting in that the mother's responses to infant removal have been very minimally described in most studies because investigators have been preoccupied with assessment of the infant. The mother has been typically described as upset acutely but as getting over it very quickly. The infant's corticoid response was felt to be due to the separation itself rather than to the new cage in which it was housed during the separation phase, and this finding has been supported by data from a number of studies. The presence of a familiar animal during the separation phase did not alter the corticoid response, suggesting that the disruption of the specific attachment bond between mother and infant was the main cause of the increased corticoid levels.

Physiological and behavioral changes following separation may not occur simultaneously. For example, separation from the surrogate results in a behavioral response but no corticoid response. Later work appears to show that infants of highly dominant mothers manifest the greatest adrenocortical response to separation, and that they may not always exhibit concomitant behavioral changes. This important research illustrates the complexity of understanding the neurobiological and behavioral changes that might accompany separation. It is important to obtain adequate baseline behavioral profiles of both the group structure and individual behavioral assessments.

Desipramine (Norpramin) has been reported to be effective in preventing the response to maternal separation in primates, and imipramine has a similar therapeutic effect on the responses to peer separation.

OTHER RESPONSES TO MATERNAL SEPARATION When infant lagur monkeys were separated from their mothers at 6 to 8 months of age, all infants showed changes in social behavior. The reactions varied from minimal to severe, including two deaths. All infants sought substitute caretaking during the separation and adopted a major substitute caretaker. Most infants remained with the substitute even when the mother returned.

Some researchers have used distress vocalizations in various animals as an index of separation and have studied the effects of many pharmacological agents on these vocalizations. In general, the distress vocalizations are reported to be relieved by morphine and made worse by the narcotic antagonist naloxone (Narcan) when these drugs are given as single injections. A variety of opiate-like peptides have been tested and all have been reported to be effective in decreasing distress vocalizations in separated animals when injected into the vicinity of the fourth ventricle in quite low doses. Additional maternal separation studies have been done using canine puppies, guinea pigs, and chicks. From these studies, researchers have developed the theory that brain endorphins may play a critical role in the mediation of social bonds, and that when these bonds are disrupted by separation, a syndrome much like that following narcotic withdrawal is produced.

PEER SEPARATION Rhesus monkeys and most other primate species develop strong, complex social bonds, and paradigms have been developed that involve experimental disruption of these bonds in peers of various ages, including adults. In general, the behavioral reaction to peer separation is quite similar to that following maternal separation in terms of the classic protest-despair response. Furthermore, when peer groups are formed and separations are repeated, the response is seen with each separation. Not surprisingly, a number of variables can influence the nature of the response, including age, rearing conditions, housing conditions before, during, and after each separation, and treatment with pharmacological agents. Significant individual variability can be related to a number of developmental and neurobiological variables. For example, cerebrospinal fluid (CSF) NE appears to be a trait-related marker predicting a more severe response to separations. Animals with lower CSF NE respond to separation with more huddling and self-directed behaviors than animals with higher levels. By contrast, CSF homovanillic acid (HVA) and 5-hydroxyindoleacetic acid (5-HIAA) are state-related markers that reflect the behavioral response to separation no matter how this response is obtained.

Pharmacological agents can affect the response to peer separation. Imipramine will reverse the reaction to peer separation and prevent the reaction to future separations as long as the monkeys are kept on it. They return to more typical separation behavior when the drug is withdrawn. Amphetamine modifies the behavioral response to separation in a very similar manner to imipramine, but the overall effects of the two drugs on group social behavior can be distinguished. α-Methylparatyrosine, which blocks tyrosine hydroxylase and thereby lowers NE and DA levels, can exacerbate the response to peer separation at very low doses—doses so low that they have no effect when the monkeys are living as a stable social group. It is only when one combines the stress of separation with low-dose α-methylparatyrosine that one sees other effects of the drug in this paradigm. Parachlorphenylalanine, which blocks serotonin synthesis, has no effect. Low doses of alcohol alleviate the peer separation response whereas high doses make it worse.

RESEARCH APPLICATIONS With regard to proposed depression models, the rationale for separation studies in animals is that the bulk of evidence strongly suggests social separations as risk factors that cut across types of depressions. Animal studies represent one way of studying these risk factors. Although many factors are involved in depression, separations appear to be important events for vulnerable individuals and so are worthy of additional investigation. An even more important context in which to view separation studies is that they may be prototypes for the study of stressful events in general. With the recent advances in knowledge of both developmental and neurobiological influences on behavior, it becomes increasingly important to have some experimental paradigms in which the interactions between neurobiological factors and social risk factors can be examined. This type of animal preparation provides the opportunity to control social and developmental variables and to do prospective studies of both behavioral and neurobiological parameters. The long-term effects of early alterations can be examined in a much shorter period of time. One can obtain repeated measurements of neurobiological variables, as in the CSF, in a way that cannot be carried out in humans and in relationship to specific units of behavior. One can also evaluate the effects of drugs on parameters similar to those being studied in humans, and determine what these changes mean with regard to specific social behaviors. The role that specific neurotransmitter systems play in influencing specific units of social behavior, including responses to separation, can also be clarified. Humans are fundamentally social creatures, and an understanding of the social origins of psychopathology and how they are related to neurotransmitter systems becomes possible in this kind of preparation.

Learned helplessness This animal model has been extensively studied for more than 15 years. It relates closely to some important aspects of clinical depression, particularly cognitive aspects, such as a negative conception of the self, negative interpretations of one's experiences, and a negative view of the future. These cognitive aspects are reflected in feelings of helplessness and hopelessness. Whether these phenomena are primary or secondary is a moot point for the present discussion—the point is that they occur as core aspects of depression frequently enough to be worthy of further study. Both etiological theories and therapeutic approaches have developed from this cognitive view of depression.

In the original experimental study with animals, dogs were placed in one of three situations. In the first situation, they were put in harnesses and subjected to electric shock that they could terminate by touching a panel. Not surprisingly, they learned to escape the shock rather quickly. In the second situation, the dogs were prepared as in the preceding situation, but when the shock was given, they were unable to terminate it. Finally, to control for the effect of the shock itself, dogs were put in harnesses but were not shocked at all. In phase 2 of the study, dogs were given electric shock while unharnessed in a shuttle box. Normally, dogs have no difficulty learning to avoid the shock by going to the other side of the box, which proved to be true for the dogs that had been exposed to escapable shock while in the harness. However, the dogs that had been exposed to inescapable shock failed to learn that they could escape from the electric shock in phase 2 by jumping over a barrier that separated the two sides of the shuttle box. They were described as being initially agitated in reaction to the shock but, rather than run around frantically until they discovered that they could escape the shock by crossing the barrier, they would sit or lie down, quietly whining—that is, they acted as if they were "helpless" and incapable of escaping. The interpretation was that something had happened during the earlier experience to make them unable to cope with the present situation, and that this something was the inescapable shock. One explanation was that they had learned during their initial experience that outcomes were not contingent on their behavior. No matter what they did, it did no good; they "learned to be helpless."

In an attempt to reverse this state, attempts were made to retrain the dogs by trying to coax them across the barrier. This strategy was very difficult, and ultimately it was found that the only effective way was to drag the dogs across the barrier forcibly and thus terminate the shock. It took many such efforts before most of the dogs could learn this response and be able to do it by themselves when placed in the shuttle box.

RESEARCH APPLICATIONS The literature on learned helplessness is enormous and, as in the case of separation models, controversial. However, one set of recent findings merits closer scrutiny and illustrates clearly how experimental paradigms in animals can be used to investigate the interrelationships between behavioral events and neurobiology, an interface critical to understanding human psychopathology. Again, as in the separation models, one does not have to agree with the validity of the model itself to appreciate the value of this kind of work in a spectrum of research approaches aimed at understanding specific aspects of human depression.

Severe, inescapable trauma, for example, has been found to produce a deficiency in central noradrenergic activity, namely, depletion of locus ceruleus NE levels. However, studies have shown that if the subjects were able to control the noxious experiences, they did not develop the noradrenergic deficiency and were able to respond quite efficiently. When the drop in noradrenergic activity was prevented by treatment with drugs, the learned helplessness phenomenon did not occur. Unfortunately, these kinds of data have sometimes been cited as evidence that the concept of learned helplessness is not valid. Another view is as follows.

One is talking about a phenomenon on several different levels simultaneously, and it is an experimental paradigm that permits this, which may prove to be its greatest contribution. A major finding has shown that a state that is clearly induced behaviorally is associated with major changes in certain neurobiological systems, and that if these changes can be prevented, one can prevent the behavioral state, which results from certain well-described behavioral manipulations, or reverse it once developed. It would be interesting to learn if behavioral reversal of the syndrome leads to reversal of the biological changes, or if reversal of the biological changes alone (once the syndrome is set in motion) will reverse the behavioral aspects. Investigators know that in human depression not all of the significant behavioral and cognitive changes are necessarily reversed with drugs, which presumably alleviate whatever underlying biological alterations might be present. One sometimes has to deal directly with the altered cognitions and behaviors, as well as the underlying neurochemistry. The evidence of a complex interplay between a cognitive-behavioral state and neurobiology is exciting and clearly warrants further investigation.

Other exciting work going on in the learned helplessness area mainly relates to this interface between the behavioral state and underlying neurochemical substrates. Several such substrates may prove to be important as more are studied, and it will be critical to ascertain their interaction with behavioral variables.

Chronic stress models In these paradigms, rats are subjected to a chronic stress regimen that is designed to be unpredictable with regard to the stimulus properties of the stress, as well as the time of stress delivery. Stressors are administered over a period of 21 days but separated from each other by 1 or 2 days, and at various points in the circadian cycle. Stressors include switching of cage mates, removal from double housing to single housing for 24 hours, 30 minutes of scrambled unpredictable foot shock, 46 hours of food deprivation, 46 hours of water deprivation, a cold water swim, shaker stress, and tail pinch. After these 21 days, the rats are tested in an open field test situation, where they do not exhibit normal open field activity or the usual response to an acute stress. The decreased exploratory behaviors can be reversed by a variety of drugs, including monoamine oxidase inhibitors (MAOIs) and tricyclic antidepressants, as well as by electroconvulsive therapy (ECT). Amphetamine and scopolamine are ineffective. Thus, the model appears to have good pharmacological specificity and is one in which studies of the neurobiological substrates could readily be done. This approach emphasizes the combined influence of chronicity and unpredictability in producing the behavioral alterations.

Changes in dominance in hierarchy Another proposed model reflects the importance of dominance in the relationships of many nonhuman primates. It has been postulated that changes in the stability of this dominance arrangement cause behavioral alterations. It is hypothesized that the behavior that occurs in association with gaining higher dominance ranking may be elation, and with falls in one's position in the hierarchy, depression. Depression, in this theory, is postulated to be adaptive as it prevents the descending animal from fighting back. It has been reasoned that, if this is so, one could try to induce depression by altering the dominance hierarchy in some nonhuman primates. This theory rests on limited data as the evidence for particular behavior patterns occurring in association with specific changes in the hierarchy is fragmentary. Dominance hierarchies are not easy to manipulate. However, recent work concerning dominance and serotonin metabolism will be interesting to follow in this regard. This work is not concerned primarily with animal models of depression, but it does involve manipulation of the dominance hierarchy, careful behavioral observations, and study of the serotonin system. Evidence that would be helpful in determining whether there is any merit in this theory could come from field studies, but data about this theory from such studies are sparse. It must be concluded that this model is largely untested at this point.

Intracranial self-stimulation models Another proposed animal model of depression is the reward-reduction model using self-stimulating animals. The involvement of catecholamines in the mediation of intracranial self-stimulation (ICSS) has been well established, though there is controversy regarding their relative importance. In general, agents that enhance the effects of catecholamines tend to increase ICSS responding, whereas those that impair catecholamine actions tend to depress ICSS response rates. However, the actions of tricyclics in this model appear anomalous as they do not enhance ICSS responding despite their well-documented antidepressant action and their effects on catecholamine systems. These drugs tend to decrease the rate of responding and to raise the reward threshold. In view of this fact, attempts have been made to find an animal model in which tricyclics potentiate ICSS responding. One such model has been suggested in which reinforcement requires more and more effort. In these progressive fixed ratio schedules, responding typically drops gradually to zero. Antidepressants have been reported actually to enhance responding. However, efforts to replicate this work have been unsuccessful. Rats that had electrodes chronically implanted in the medial forebrain bundle were trained in progressively increasing fixed ratio schedules. Two tricyclic antidepressants (imipramine and protriptyline [Vivactil]) were given but neither resulted in response enhancement. Thus, additional work is indicated to evaluate more fully the reward-reduction model involving ICSS as an animal model of depression. It is worth pursuing, however, in view of the important finding that anhedonia is a key feature in many cases of severe depression. It would be valuable to have an animal model in which the mechanism and pharmacology of this sign could be studied.

Conditioned motionlessness This proposed model involves pairing a buzzer (conditioned stimulus) with a tetrabenazine injection (unconditioned stimulus) for at least 11 trials. Following conditioning, some rats exhibited motionlessness after the presentation of the buzzer alone. Imipramine attenuated the conditioned motionlessness. Subsequent neurochemical studies of these rat preparations supported the conclusion that the motionlessness observed was associated with an excess of functional serotonin at the synaptic cleft. This motionlessness after tetrabenazine is not blocked by imipramine. When the conditioned response is reversed by imipramine, however, the biochemical data resemble those for control subjects.

Behavioral despair This model involves the use of a test based on the observation that when rats or mice are forced to swim in a restricted space from which they cannot escape, they eventually cease their attempts to escape and become immobile. It has been suggested that this characteristic behavioral immobility reflects a state of despair in the rats or mice. The immobility is reduced by most clinically active antidepressants, as well as by nonpharmacological treatments such as ECT, REM sleep deprivation, or exposure to an enriched environment. The effects can be seen after acute administration, but more marked effects are seen after repeated treatments with lower doses. The drug effects do not appear to be caused by increased motor activity as the doses used generally decrease motor activity. Antidepressants seem to prolong the escape-directed behavior observed at the beginning of a test session, whereas psychostimulants or anticholinergics cause a generalized behavioral stimulation. These potential false positives can be distinguished from the effects of true antidepressants. However, as with all models, there are both false positives and false negatives. False-positive results have been reported with antihistamines, subconvulsant doses of convulsants, and some neuropeptides. False negatives have been found with clomipramine (Anafranil) in rats and salbutamol in rats and mice.

This model was developed mainly for drug screening and thus must be evaluated in terms of its empirical validity, which seems at least as good as that of most drug-screening models. At a theoretical level, its relationship with learned helplessness or uncontrollability models needs to be clarified. Mechanism studies remain to be done.

Schizophrenia

Is it possible to produce an animal model for schizophrenia? Several authors have suggested standards that should be satisfied if a particular preparation is to qualify as an adequate animal model. These criteria have been mostly drug related; for instance, clinically effective antipsychotic drugs should reverse the abnormal behaviors, and clinically ineffective drugs should not.

There should be no argument about the need for animal models of psychiatric diseases, in general, and for schizophrenia, in particular. Although significant progress is being made in clinical research on schizophrenia, the development and utilization of suitable animal preparations could enable many kinds of studies that, for ethical and practical reasons, are impossible to do in humans.

It should be noted that there are no animal analogues for many of the core signs and symptoms of schizophrenia. Clinicians, as well as animal researchers, need to pay careful attention to ways of making schizophrenic signs and symptoms operational, possibly through a more ethological analysis of human schizophrenia than has so far been done. If different types of human schizophrenia could be analyzed ethologically, the same, or a similar, system could then be applied to the development of animal models, and analogues for specific behaviors might then become more feasible. There also needs to be a major conceptual shift away from the idea that one can develop an animal model of schizophrenia. It is more likely that one is talking about developing animal preparations for studying specific but limited aspects of schizophrenia and to better understand some fundamental issues. Figure 5.2-2 summarizes some of the existing animal models of schizophrenia along with some future approaches.

Drug-related animal models AMPHETAMINE MODEL The amphetamine model has attracted a considerable amount of attention in relation to schizophrenia and hyperactivity because amphetamine psychosis in humans can closely mimic paranoid schizophrenia.

Do the data indicate, as some investigators have suggested, that animals become schizophrenic when they are given amphetamine? Clearly, the paranoid delusions have no direct measurable analogue in the animal model, although inferences have been made from certain behaviors. Some investigators have reported that animals are hypervigilant when given amphetamine, as shown by their increased alertness and visual attention to other animals in their environment. Subordinate rats actively withdraw from social interactions, retreat to strategically defensible positions in their environment, and remain hypervigilant. Some have theorized that this behavior may be a manifestation of paranoia.

When given to rats, cats, and monkeys, amphetamine produces stereotypical behaviors, and many researchers believe that this aspect is particularly intriguing. It should be remembered that stereotypical behavior is not included in any list of major human schizophrenic symptoms, and, thus, a model is being proposed that is mainly based on a behavior that is nonspecific and nondiscriminating for schizophrenia. However, from the standpoint of empirical validity, drugs that have antipsychotic properties in humans block the amphetamine-induced stereotypical behavior in both animals and people. This finding has been related to the possible dopaminergic mechanisms in schizophrenia on the basis of the idea that amphetamine-induced stereotypical behavior in animals is mediated by increased dopamine turnover.

Some investigators have tried to separate the stereotypical behavior from the increased locomotor activity produced by amphetamine by relating the behavior to the release of striatal DA that is significantly increased with repeated amphetamine administration. By contrast, the increased locomotor activity is thought to be mediated by NE. Tolerance develops in locomotor activity with repeated doses of amphetamine, but not to the effects on stereotypical behaviors. This kind of approach attempts to distinguish the different types of amphetamine-induced behavioral alterations in animals and to elucidate the neurochemical mechanisms that may be involved.

Other researchers have examined the effects of amphetamine on a variety of behaviors in rats and have focused on locomotor activity and stereotypy. A progressive augmentation of both behaviors with repeated drug administration has been reported. The duration of stereotypy was not necessarily increased, but the onset of stereotypy was. These data were interpreted to mean that long-term amphetamine administration tended to produce increased preservation of progressively more focused and restricted behaviors. A similar phenomenon has been reported in rhesus monkeys.

PHENYLETHYLAMINE MODEL Another proposed drug-induced model of schizophrenia involves phenylethylamine (PEA), a neuroamine that is an endogenous component of mammalian brain and is most highly concentrated in the limbic system of the human

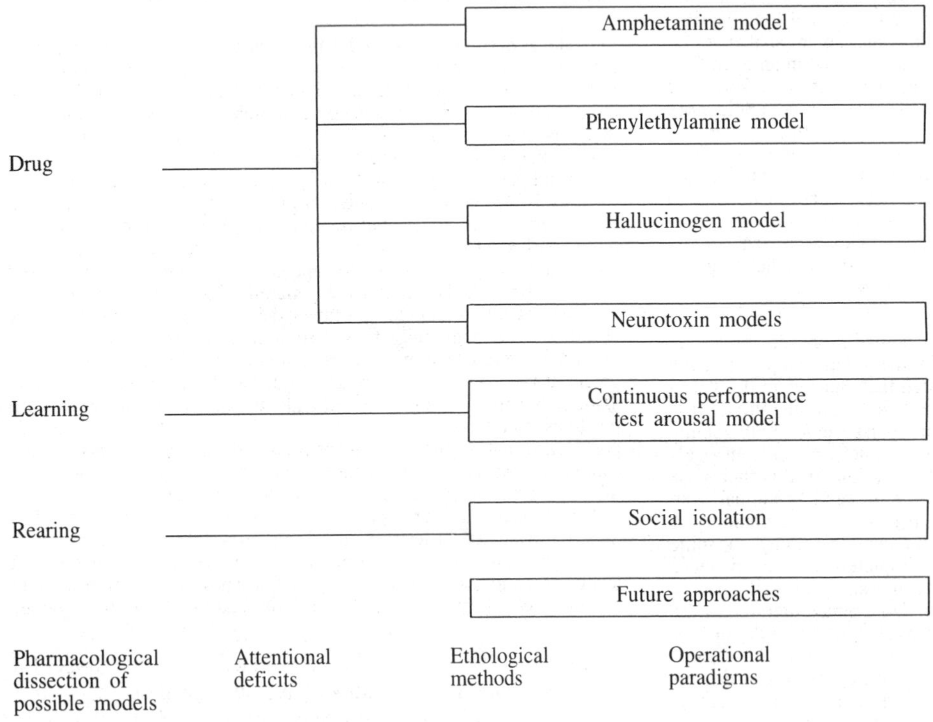

FIGURE 5.2-2 *Existing animal models of schizophrenia and future approaches.*

brain. This drug, too, produces stereotypies that closely resemble those produced by amphetamine.

HALLUCINOGEN MODEL Many animal experiments using hallucinogenic agents have been very productive in promoting the understanding of the behavioral pharmacology of these compounds, but they have not provided convincing animal models of schizophrenia. As the phenomenology of hallucinogenic-induced states in people was more carefully compared with the symptomatology of schizophrenia, the suggested behavioral isomorphism became less persuasive.

NEUROTOXIN MODELS One hypothesis concerning the etiology of schizophrenia is that it results from impairment of structural integrity of the noradrenergic reward mechanism, and that this impairment is chronic and at least partially irreversible. 6-Hydroxydopamine (6-OHDA) is said to be the aberrant metabolite that causes schizophrenia on the basis of the following evidence obtained from animal studies:

1. When injected into certain brain sites in animals, 6-OHDA decreases stimulation and other rewarded behaviors, and this effect is long lasting.
2. Prior treatment with chlorpromazine (Thorazine) blocks the behavioral deficits as well as the depletion of NE induced by 6-OHDA.

Nondrug animal models AROUSAL It has been postulated that patients with schizophrenia operate at excessive arousal levels and that impaired attention resulting from this hyperarousal constitutes a major deficit. By training rats on an operant task thought to be analogous to a test of attention used to study schizophrenic patients, attempts have been made to produce an animal model for this attentional deficit—that is, the continuous performance test. Low levels of electrical stimulation to the reticular formation in rats cause the animals to make errors similar to those made by schizophrenic patients. In general, those drugs with antipsychotic properties are most effective in reversing the deficit.

PRIMATE SOCIAL ISOLATION Isolation seems to share some components with schizophrenia, as illustrated in Figure 5.2-3, but one should be extremely cautious about such linkages until additional studies have been done.

There is, as yet, no single compelling animal model of schizophrenia. The most studied model is the amphetamine model, which is effective mainly in mimicking stereotypy. Because stereotypies are not a prominent diagnostic feature of most schizophrenic patients, it is difficult to estimate where this pharmacological behavioral analogy may lead.

The phenylethylamine model relies heavily on the stereotypical analogy and on comparisons with the amphetamine model. Simply because an antipsychotic drug blocks the stereotypical effects of phenylethylamine does not validate that syndrome as a model of schizophrenia, because it may reverse the stereotypical behavior for reasons unrelated to its antipsychotic activity in humans. Although this characteristic does not eliminate such animal models for drug screening, it also does not establish their validity.

The connection between lack of responsiveness to brain self-stimulation after 6-OHDA damage of noradrenergic pathways and the impaired reward responsiveness in human schizophrenic patients may prove to be an important variable. The relevance of the social isolation syndrome as an animal model of schizophrenia has yet to be established; nevertheless, it is such a dramatic and severe syndrome that further investigation may reveal additional similarities or clarify the relationship of this syndrome with other forms of psychosis. Perhaps one of the most fruitful areas to pursue in animal research is the attentional deficit that seems to characterize many aspects of schizophrenia. Although difficult to produce in animals, this deficit is potentially testable.

There are two potentially productive approaches toward creating animal models of schizophrenia. The ethological approach would focus on a specific behavioral analysis of schizophrenia. These data could, in turn, provide the foundation for comparisons with other species. The second approach would involve creative operational paradigms for animals based on the present level of analysis of human schizophrenia and move away from attempts to develop global models of the disorder.

Anxiety disorders It is well known to clinicians that anxiety can be either a symptom or a specific syndrome. The literature on animal models is often very confusing in this regard. In some work, anxiety seems to be used synonymously with neuroses; in other paradigms, what is being studied seems more akin to fear or to certain kinds of learning behavior. In any case, it is important to keep in mind the core features of the human syndrome.

In the case of anxiety, one must evaluate proposed models according to how they behaviorally resemble human anxiety and to treatment responsiveness criteria. Neither in itself is completely satisfactory, but investigators do not know enough about the etiology, pathogenesis, or mechanisms of human anxiety to use them as validating criteria for animal models. Some of the proposed animal models of anxiety may help clarify these issues.

Most approaches to animal modeling of anxiety utilize variations of operant conditioning paradigms, and validity is evaluated on an empirical basis—that is, how well do clinically effective antianxiety agents work in the paradigms and how specific is the response? In general, a number of the approaches have high empirical validity. Although they may not bear any relationship to the etiology or pathogenesis of human anxiety, they may still have merit in the context of this aspect of animal modeling.

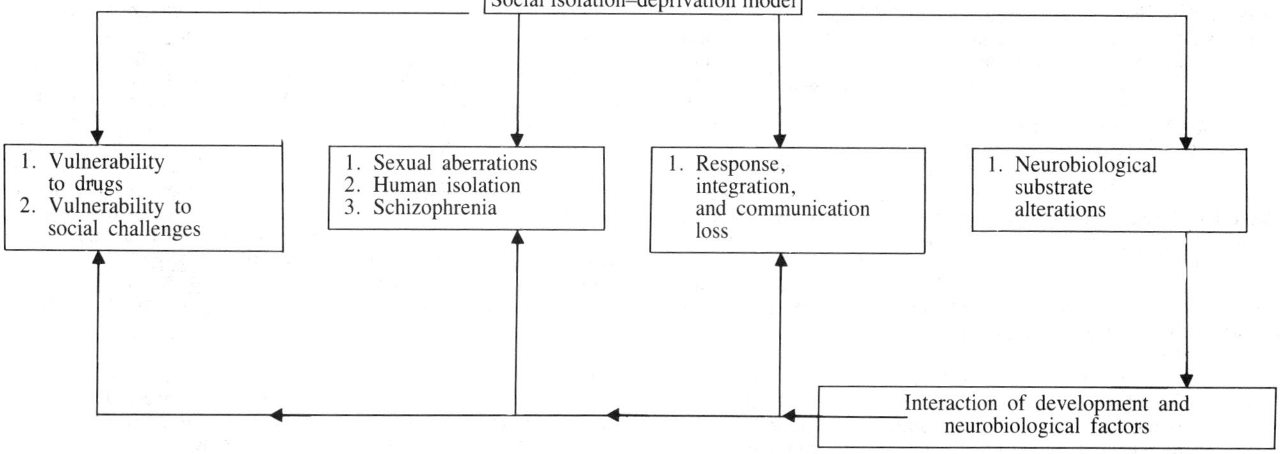

FIGURE 5.2-3 *Applications of the social isolation–deprivation model of human psychopathology.*

The assessment of behavior is of vital importance in the development of any animal model—and anxiety is no exception. One cannot talk to animals; thus, what defining characteristics of human anxiety (symptom or syndrome) should researchers attempt to measure in animals? The inducing conditions for many forms of human anxiety are unknown, and so it is impossible to use these conditions as a criteria. Also, not enough is known about its mechanisms to use anxiety as a criterion. Therefore, only behavioral similarities and treatment responsiveness criteria remain.

OPERANT CONDITIONING PARADIGMS The basic strategy with these models is to use operant techniques to elicit a behavior with a high frequency of occurrence. After the response is well established, the behavior is suppressed by punishing it when it occurs. The analogy to fear is the conditioned association between the behavior and the punishment. Potential antianxiety drugs are evaluated according to their ability to restore responding to what it was at their presuppression levels.

The Geller Conflict Test, one of the best known of such tests, is widely used in screening for potential antianxiety drugs. In the original Geller paradigm, rats were trained on a multiple variable interval (VI) 2-minute continuous reinforcement (CR) schedule for milk reinforcement; that is, there was a two-component operant behavior schedule. In VI portion, signaled by one stimulus, bar pressing is reinforced at variable intervals, with the mean interval being 2 minutes. In the CR portion, signaled by a different stimulus, every bar pressing is reinforced. When foot shock is given concurrently with the positive reinforcement, response rates are suppressed. Drug-induced increases in the rate of punished responding are interpreted as an index of antianxiety activity whereas decreases in unpunished responding are interpreted as indicating depressant activity. In other words, the type of behavior that originally has a high frequency of occurrence but is subsequently suppressed by certain manipulations is highly sensitive to the benzodiazepines and meprobamate (Miltown), but not to chlorpromazine. In general, this test, along with many modifications of it, identifies clinically active anxiolytic agents, predicts their clinical potency, and is generally insensitive to stimulant, antipsychotic, antidepressant, or analgesic drugs. It seems to work in different species, and to be relatively independent of the schedules of positive reinforcement or punishment. Thus, this operant conflict approach has high empirical validity in terms of predicting clinical drug responsiveness.

This model, involving conflict behavior, has been used to evaluate several biochemical hypotheses concerning the mechanism of action for the antianxiety, or what is termed the "emotional analgesic," properties of benzodiazepines. With the increasing interest in the possible neurobiological substrates of anxiety, the availability of a paradigm in which the mechanism of drug action can be explored simultaneously with measures of operant behavior is necessary for future research in this area. Over the past few years, with the identification of benzodiazepine receptor sites, evidence has begun to accumulate that these receptors may mediate the therapeutic effects of such drugs. The relationship of these receptor sites for benzodiazepines to the understanding of the neurobiological mechanisms of anxiety states is complex and remains an active and exciting area of investigation. The involvement of various neurotransmitter systems with these receptor sites is important to understand, and the continuing development of experimental systems in which these complex interrelationships can be studied would be helpful. A number of theories, especially with regard to the γ-amino-butyric acid (GABA) and the serotonin systems, purport to account for the effects of the anxiolytic drugs. However, anxiety has many different components, and different neurotransmitters may be involved with each. For example, the muscle relaxant or anticonvulsant properties may be neurochemically mediated in one way but the anxiolytic effects as revealed in conflict paradigms may be mediated by other neurotransmitters. It is important to have careful behavioral descriptions available along with the specific neurochemical technology.

ALTERATION OF LOCUS CERULEUS FUNCTION The locus ceruleus is a brain structure with a very high density of NE-containing neurons plus numerous projections to other brain regions. Various techniques to alter its function provide one way to learn more about the function of one noradrenergic system in the brain. The system has been studied in the cat, macaque monkey, and squirrel monkey with such techniques as electrical stimulation, ablation, and pharmacological probes. Significant species differences are found in the catecholamine-containing cells in the brain stem, in addition to significant variations in behaviors. Cross-species reasoning from such studies is difficult, but a recent set of studies in nonhuman primates may be particularly relevant to animal models of anxiety.

Increasing locus ceruleus function, whether by electrical stimulation or with drugs, led to an increase in threat-associated behaviors, whereas decreasing locus ceruleus function decreased threat-associated behaviors. These behavioral effects are said to be consistent with the critical role of the locus ceruleus in mediating anxiety and fear.

It has been argued that the behavioral measures associated with locus ceruleus function in primates are the same ones that change with environmental stimuli associated with fear in humans, and that they are lessened by diazepam (Valium). However, this approach does not permit a distinction between fear as a response to an externally threatening situation and anxiety, which typically is less related to a specific environmental precipitant. This problem arises with much of the animal modeling of anxiety literature, where anxiety, fear, and learning are often used interchangeably.

The general conclusion is that the locus ceruleus is essential, though not sufficient, for the behavioral and physiological expression of anxiety. Other areas are required. The locus is likened to an alarm system.

STUDIES OF APLYSIA It has been proposed that not only anxiety as a general state, but several specific subcategories of anxiety, can be modeled in the sea snail, Aplysia. It is contended that the molecular basis of anxiety can be studied in this type of animal preparation with its relatively simple nervous system. This approach has attracted interest because it offers the possibility of more direct approaches to studying the cellular mechanisms of behavior. Behavior in such a preparation has a very different meaning from that in some of the previous models. It is not social behavior and is closest to a variant of conditioning paradigms that has been utilized for some time in the animal modeling field.

In Aplysia, classically conditioned fear has been said to model anticipatory anxiety, and what is termed "long-term sensitization" to model chronic anxiety.

Many workers have speculated about the relationship of aversive conditioning paradigms in animals to human anxiety. The situation in which the conditioned stimulus serves as a cue predicting the occurrence of the unconditioned stimulus and various behavioral changes take place, presumably in anticipation of the unconditioned stimulus, has been likened by investigators to anticipatory or signaled anxiety. In the sea snail, for example, exposure to the extract of shrimp elicits the withdrawal and reflex responses. The term "chronic anxiety of long-term sensitization" has been widely used to describe the state when there is repeated exposure to the unconditioned stimulus alone without any cueing or prior exposure to the conditioned stimulus. Researchers have speculated about the role of the unpredictability of uncontrollability as a factor in mediating this response.

SOCIAL MANIPULATIONS It is in the area of social manipulations that one encounters such terms as fear, anxiety, agitation, stress, and neurosis being used interchangeably, with resultant confusion. For example, the initial stage of reaction to separation has historically been labeled the "agitation or protest" stage. More recently, it has been conceptualized in an anxiety context. The first phase is characterized by the infant's being very active behaviorally. It has also been found that infants have marked activation of the pituitary adrenal system and an increase in the enzymes involved in catecholamine synthesis. These findings and others support the view of separation as a very powerful event from both behavioral and neurobiological standpoints and are consistent with a large body of literature regarding the behavioral and biological effects of a variety of stressors. To what extent this initial stage of reaction responds to anxiolytic pharmacological agents and how specific this response may be are not known.

PHOBIAS AND OTHER ANXIETY DISORDERS In a recent review of this area, one is reminded of the distinction between fear, which comes from an old English term for sudden calamity or danger, and anxious, which is from the Greek root meaning press tight or strangle. Fear is described as an emotion produced by present or impending danger. The cause is apparent. Anxiety, on the other hand, is an emotion of which the cause is vague or less understandable. Fear can lead to one's either "freezing up" or becoming mute. Much stress literature reports the same thing—for example, rats freezing up in an open field—as being caused by stress.

The relationship between conditioning models and theories and anxiety and phobia models in animals has a number of shortcomings when extended to human phobias. Many animal experiments that assume conditioned fear, as well as avoidance conditioned by trauma, are models of human phobic (or anxiety) reactions. Although it is true that such induction techniques do produce fear of relatively specific stimuli and enable one to study the variables that are important for the learning of fear in humans, rarely can the initiation of a human phobia (or anxiety) be ascribed to a definable event (i.e., a definable unconditioned stimulus).

It is contended that research on animals has little to impart about human anxiety, which exists internally and symbolically, often without observable motor or autonomic concomitants. Anxiety is difficult to define. Some investigators feel that Pavlovian or Skinnerian conditioning paradigms are useless for modeling human phobias (anxieties). Human phobias and anxiety just do not fit into conditioning language or paradigms. It has been argued that conditioning language makes assumptions about etiology and treatment that are not borne out in practice, and that the terminology is difficult to apply to clinical events.

One other approach to the study of phobias involved the development of two lines of pointer dogs. One line was bred for fearfulness and lack of friendliness toward people and the other for the opposite characteristics. The basic hypothesis of this work was that inheritance would determine, in large part, many behavioral characteristics of the dog, including susceptibility to breakdown under acute and chronic stress. Through this process of selection and inbreeding, it was possible to establish the two lines of dogs and to study their behavior on a number of parameters. Throughout 10 generations, about 80 percent of each litter were similar in temperament to the parents. The phobic line of dogs was extremely timid, avoided humans, and showed decreased exploratory activity. They showed an excessive startle response, and had a slower heart rate and an increased incidence of atrioventricular heart block. Interestingly, even the dogs with the most severe disturbance could learn operant conditioning bar pressing, but it was necessary to facilitate this process with benzodiazepines—the most efficacious drugs. Both amphetamine and cocaine disrupted the behavioral responses of genetically nervous dogs to a far greater extent than the stable dogs.

PSYCHIATRY AND ETHOLOGY

Several authors over the years have suggested that work in the biological science of ethology might be useful in psychiatry and, of course, three ethologists shared a Nobel prize in medicine. John Bowlby has been taking an ethological approach to psychiatry for many years, and as early as 1957, suggested that such an approach might be useful in psychiatric research. Other authors who have written about this interface between ethology and psychiatry generally approached the topic by defining ethology, presenting its vocabulary, describing its methodology, and suggesting conceptual and specific applications of ethological findings to psychiatry.

Despite these writings and others about this interface, ethological methods and research findings have had little impact on psychiatry, although it would seem that ethology does have much to contribute to psychiatry, and psychiatry to ethology. The failure of this collaboration to materialize appears to be the result mostly of artifactual factors, rather than of an intrinsic incompatibility between ethological and psychiatric approaches.

The roots of ethology lie in the natural science of biology, in particular, zoology. The principal philosophical tenet is a naturalistic one, that is, that studies of behavior should emphasize the study of behavior in natural settings.

Its historical origin in biology and the emphasis on the study of behavior in context have led to ethology's being largely an observational, nonexperimental science. Several authors have contrasted this characteristic with the field of comparative psychology, which has different historical origins and emphases. Research in ethology has at times seemed indistinguishable from that in comparative psychology, as ethologists have utilized various techniques, from studying naturally occurring phenomena, to introducing experimental factors into a natural setting, to actually working in a laboratory. Researchers usually consider these occasional excursions into the laboratory as attempts to refine mechanisms of behavior, always cognizant of the fact that the behavior evolves in a natural setting.

A glossary of some of the key ethological terms is provided in Table 5.2-2.

It has been suggested that psychiatric research and practice might benefit from the careful observational techniques ethologists employ in describing both specific behavioral patterns and the context in which the behaviors occur. These techniques would be applicable to both nonverbal and verbal behavior, as well as to the communicative aspects of each. A more general methodological issue relates to the utilization of the scientific method in research. In particular, it has been stressed that the ambiguity in the interpretation of findings in psychiatric research could be reduced by a greater usage of operational definitions of behavior. One example is the definition of attachment behavior as any behavior that results in an increased proximity between two (or more) members of a species, rather than its being defined in more global terms that make inferences about the internal states of the individuals involved.

Another aspect of ethology that has been stressed in previous approaches to the interface between psychiatry and ethology has been that of the phylogenetic origins of behavior. Ethologists are involved in the comparative study of behavior and in carrying out such studies derive hypotheses based on phylogenetic assumptions. In the same way in which hypotheses are derived in the comparative study of anatomy, behavior can also be studied using the comparative method. The underlying assumption is that the behavioral patterns being studied have evolved as a result of mutation and natural selection in the same way as anatomical systems.

The more recent use of cybernetics, both control theory and information theory, in the understanding of behavioral systems in ethology has been paralleled to some extent in psychiatry. Therefore, the cybernetic approach is an aspect of ethology that may be useful to psychiatry and also a potential theoretical bridge between the two fields.

One area frequently cited with regard to the application of ethological methodology and theory to psychiatry has been that of the attachment system. The research on separation and on the relationship between separation and depression is a corollary of the work on attachment systems.

Another area commonly suggested where ethological research might be useful in psychiatry is that of aggression, particularly in the study of hierarchical and territorial behavior.

A certain natural relationship between psychiatry and ethology results from their parallel positions within their respective broader disciplines. The medical sciences are based principally on the biological sciences. Psychiatry is the area within medicine most concerned with the study of behavior, and ethology is in an analogous position in biology. However, ethology is still not commonly taught or utilized in training programs in psychiatry or child psychiatry in the United

TABLE 5.2-2
Selected Glossary of Ethological Terms

Action-specific energy	Energy associated with the innate releasing mechanism, and specific to a particular behavior pattern, which builds up if the releasing stimulus is not present to activate the behavior pattern, and conversely is depleted by repetition.
Aggression	Intraspecific conflict manifested by physical attack or social signaling.
Appetitive behavior	Phase of behavior involving the active seeking of sign stimuli, and thought to be driven by "action-specific energy" accumulating through inactivity of the specific behavior pattern.
Consummatory response	Phase of behavior whereby the energy driving the appetitive phase is released. Involves the perception of sign stimuli, the activation of the innate releasing mechanism (IRM), and the performance of the fixed action pattern (FAP).
Critical period	The time during which imprinting must occur, usually shortly after birth or early in life. Also, "sensitive period."
Displacement activity	A set of behavior patterns occurring alongside an unrelated set of behavior patterns. Originally, "irrelevant" movements from one behavioral system occurring in the presence of powerful but thwarted drive from another behavioral system.
Ethology	The biological study of behavior. From the Greek *ethos,* meaning custom, usage, manner, habit. The modern usage is attributed to Oskar Heinroth, Lorenz' teacher.
Fixed action pattern (FAP)	A genetically determined behavior pattern, which is initiated by stimuli particular to the pattern and which consists of species-specific stereotyped movements.
Imprinting	A specialized form of learning occurring early in life and often influencing behavior later in life. The exposure to the stimulus situation must occur during a particular period, the "critical period," and the exposure can be of short duration and without obvious reward. The learning is particularly resistant to change.
Innate	Genetically determined behavior patterns, in theory not influenced by experience.
Innate releasing mechanism (IRM)	Sensory mechanism selectively responsive to specific external stimuli and responsible for triggering the stereotyped motor response.
Instinct	A developmental process resulting in species-typical behavior.
Redirection activity	The venting of one drive from two or more incompatible, but simultaneously activated, drives on some third animal or object.
Ritualization	Process of a behavior pattern being incorporated through evolution into a primary signaling function, frequently with exaggeration and embellishment of some of the movements.

States. Why is this so? Nikko Tinbergen, one of the three ethologists to share the Nobel prize for physiology or medicine in 1973, has delineated three conditions that, in his view, have contributed to the relative lack of communication between psychiatrists and ethologists.

The first condition refers to communication difficulties that arise because of differences in scientific language. Second, there are obvious differences in the education of students in the two disciplines. The third point mentioned by Tinbergen is the likelihood that different types of people enter ethology as graduate students than enter medical school and subsequently train in psychiatry. But even if the people themselves are not particularly different, the caricatures and the personal expectations of them by others can contribute to the gap that inhibits communication between psychiatrists and ethologists.

In 1973, the Nobel prize in medicine was awarded to three ethologists: Karl von Frisch, Konrad Lorenz, and Nikko Tinbergen. This occasion highlighted the importance of ethology for medicine and its special relevance for psychiatry in a manner not dissimilar to the relationship between molecular biology and medicine. The contributions of these three ethologists that are particularly relevant to psychiatry are summarized below. Special acknowledgment is given to Borje Cronholm, whose monograph describes their important basic research.

KARL VON FRISCH Von Frisch, who was born in 1886, conducted studies on changes of color in fish and demonstrated that fish were capable of learning to distinguish among several colors and that their sense of color was fairly congruent with that of human beings. He later went on to study the color vision of bees.

Von Frisch's subsequent research was almost entirely concerned with the behavior of bees, and he is most widely known for his analyses of how they communicate with each other—that is, their language, or what is known as their dances. His description of this exceedingly complex behavior of bees has prompted an investigation of information systems of other animal species.

KONRAD LORENZ Born in 1903, Lorenz is known for his studies of animals, mainly birds, which he allowed to remain free but trained them so that they would not be disturbed by his presence. Lorenz was a systematic observer who brilliantly described behavioral traits exhibited by animals. Many of his conclusions have been verified in experimental studies by himself and by other researchers. His interest focused from the beginning on instinctive actions, meaning certain movements performed in a proscribed manner and provoked by certain key stimuli. These forms of behavior are now termed "fixed motor patterns." Lorenz showed that, in several animal species, when a fixed motor pattern has been provoked, it proceeds automatically. It seems to be genetically programmed and, once started, is not affected by the environment. Fixed motor patterns presumably develop as a result of evolution, through the pressure of selection. Lorenz studied these patterns in several species, including jackdaws, ducks, and geese.

According to Lorenz, fixed motor patterns are provoked by stimuli specific to each pattern, which are termed "key stimuli." These stimuli can be assumed to correspond to a particular organization of the central nervous system, originally termed "das angeborene auslosende Schema," and later, at Tinbergen's suggestion, as "the innate releasing mechanism" (IRM). This mechanism is assumed to react to key stimuli by prompting or releasing corresponding fixed motor patterns. Lorenz has emphasized that not only instinctive actions but all kinds of learning have their basis in the genetically programmed equipment of the individual.

Lorenz is perhaps best known by psychiatrists for his studies of *imprinting*. Briefly, imprinting implies that, during a certain short period of development, a young animal is highly sensitive to a certain type of stimulus that then, but not at other times, provokes a specific behavior pattern. Lorenz described how newly hatched goslings are programmed to follow a moving object, whereupon they rapidly become imprinted to follow this and possibly similar objects. Typically, the mother is the first moving object the young sees, but should it see something else first, the gosling will follow it. For instance, a gosling imprinted by Lorenz followed him and refused to follow a goose. Imprinting is an extremely important concept for psychiatrists to understand in their effort to link early developmental experiences with later behaviors.

Lorenz also studied the forms of behavior that function as sign stimuli—that is, as social releasers—in communications between individuals of the same species. Many of the signals have the character of fixed motor patterns in that they appear automatically and the reaction of other members of the species is equally automatic.

Lorenz is also well known for his interest in problems of aggression. He has written about the practical function of aggression, such as the defense of their territory by fish and birds. Aggression among members of the same species is common, but Lorenz has pointed out that, in normal conditions, it seldom leads to killing, or even to serious injury. Although the animals attack one another, a certain balance appears between tendencies to fight and flight, with the tendency to fight being strongest in the center of the territory and the tendency to flight strongest at a distance from the center.

In many of his works, Lorenz has tried to draw conclusions from his ethological studies of animals that can also be applied to human problems. Many of his suggestions are by now well known and provocative. The postulation of a primary need for aggression in humans, cultivated by the pressure of selection, is a primary example. This need might have served a practical purpose at an earlier time when human beings lived in small groups that had to defend themselves from other groups. Competition with neighboring groups became the most important factor of selection. However, Lorenz has pointed out how this need has survived the advent of weapons that can be used not merely to kill individuals but to wipe out all human beings.

NIKKO TINBERGEN Tinbergen, who was born in 1907, conducted a series of experiments to analyze various aspects of animal behavior. He also was successful in quantifying behavior and in obtaining measures of the power or strength of different stimuli in eliciting specific behavior. Tinbergen's first studies were of the digger wasp, *Philantus*. He determined that these insects dig individual nests, where they deposit captured bees to nourish their larvae. He was also able to show that they find their way back to their nests with the aid of various landmarks. Above all, they rely on their visual sense and learn the landmarks by means of an endogenously programmed aerial circuit.

Tinbergen's well-known studies of the various key stimuli that can provoke fixed motor patterns and of how they work together have been very valuable. Different stimuli can provoke the same motor pattern with different degrees of intensity. Particularly elegant is his analysis of the properties of the beak of the herring gull, which encourages its young to solicit food. For example, underneath, where the beak is narrow and yellow, there is a contrasting red patch against which the young peck. By using dummies of different shapes and colors, and with different degrees of contrast, he was able to measure the different degrees of force with which the stimuli prompted the young to peck.

Tinbergen's discovery of what are termed "displacement activities" represents another key contribution. These activities have been studied mainly in birds. For example, in a conflict situation, when the need for fight and the need for flight are of roughly equal strength, birds sometimes do neither. Rather, they display behavior that appears to be irrelevant to the situation. For example, a herring gull defending its territory can start to pick grass. Displacement activities of this kind will vary according to the situation and the species concerned. It is well known that human beings can engage in displacement activities when under stress.

In one of his later works, Tinbergen, together with his wife, studied early childhood autism. They began by observing the behavior of autistic and normal children when they meet strangers, which is analogous to the techniques used in observing animal behavior. In particular, they observed in animals the conflict that arises between fear and the need for contact, and noted that it can lead to behavior that is similar to that of autistic children. They hypothesized that in certain specially predisposed children, fear can greatly predominate and can also be provoked by stimuli that normally have a positive social value for most children. This innovative approach to studying infantile autism has opened up new avenues of inquiry. Although their conclusions regarding preventive measures and treatment must be considered tentative, the methodology illustrates another way in which ethology and clinical psychiatry can relate to each other.

CONSIDERATIONS FOR FUTURE STUDY The remainder of this section looks at aspects of the interaction that will continue to be difficult, but through which both psychiatry and ethology can be broadened.

This first aspect is methodology. Recent years have seen a beginning in the study of child behavior by ethological techniques. These techniques are similar to techniques used during the past quarter of a century in the study of primate behavior, and they involve operational definitions of specific behaviors and the careful observation and recording of their occurrence.

The second aspect of the interaction between psychiatry and ethology that can lead to a broadening in perspective is the relative differences in interest in normal and abnormal behavior. The focus in medicine and psychiatry tends to be on the abnormal, whereas ethologists generally study the parameters of normal behavior for a given species. In a general sense, ethologists and psychiatrists are both interested in differences in adaptation—the ethologist in species differences as related to varying ecological niches, and the psychiatrist in intraspecies differences in response to varying life situations. There has been a growing awareness in recent years of deficiencies in the objective understanding of normal human development, and more interaction with ethology could be useful in improving this situation.

The third issue that an interaction with ethology will force psychiatry to confront is that of the uniqueness of the human species. In psychiatry, it is often assumed that humans are so different from other species that the study of these species is of little use in understanding human behavior. Although a phylogenetic point of view is acknowledged in human anatomy and physiology, it is certainly not emphasized in psychiatry. Psychiatrists are interested in studying ontogeny, but in only one species, and this is where an interaction with ethology would be difficult, but broadening, in terms of considering phylogeny as well.

The fourth rough edge to be considered is the size of the behavioral units of interest to each area. Historically, ethologists have been interested in thoroughly studying the specifics of behavior to the point of a microscopic dissection, and recently, at the other extreme, through a more global approach. Psychiatry has been more interested in the behavior that takes place between these two extremes; that is, psychiatrists are not concerned about specific measurements of facial expression or difficulties in adaptation facing human beings today, but with the general behavior of individuals, families, and groups. Exceptions to this generalization include behavior modification at the more specific end of the spectrum and general systems theory at the more global end.

Inasmuch as ethology is a biological science, one might expect that of the 30 or more schools of thought within psychiatry, it would be in the area of biological psychiatry where the integration with ethology would be most likely to occur. However, it is perhaps the irony of ironies that, with the exception of the utilization of certain animal models for the understanding of the mechanism of action of a few psychopharmacological agents, biological psychiatrists have been among the least interested in utilizing the rich findings of this particular area of biology. Rather, biological psychiatry has tended to be quite reductionistic with its use of animal models. There is a growing body of literature on the effect of psychopharmacological agents in various species, but without much consideration of such factors as the phylogenetic status of the animal, its prior experience, and the effect of these agents on the animal in a natural setting.

The school of thought within psychiatry that comes closest to an ethological perspective is that of psychoanalysis. The libidinous and aggressive drives about which Sigmund Freud and others have written are quite analogous to the behavioral states studied in ethology. Much of the ethological literature has dealt with courtship and mating behavior, as well as aggression, whether expressed in hierarchical behavior or in territoriality. Much of Tinbergen's work dealt with the problem of achieving reproductive success when tendencies for courtship and tendencies of aggression occur simultaneously between prospective mates. Bowlby has articulated the natural relationship between psychoanalytic and ethological thought, and his work demonstrates the usefulness of doing so. It both has increased knowledge of the specific components of attachment behavior and broadened the understanding of their existence.

It is felt that the difficulties at the interface between psychiatry and ethology are, for the most part, surmountable. These include vocabulary, education, and caricatures of people in their respective fields, as well as some occasional territoriality. It is felt that the real differences in approach and methodology, the relative difference in interest between normal and abnormal behavior, the degree of willingness to accept a phylogenetic approach, and the breadth of behavior being studied, can all contribute to a widened perspective for psychiatry, and ethology as well, if the interaction between the two is increased.

PSYCHIATRY AND SOCIOBIOLOGY

As E. O. Wilson said in his classic book, *Sociobiology: The New Synthesis:*

Sociobiology is defined as the systematic study of the biological basis of all social behavior. For the present, it focuses on animal societies, their population structure, castes, and communication, together with all of the physiology underlying the social adaptations. But the discipline is also concerned with the social behavior of early humans and the adaptive features of organization in the more primitive contemporary societies. Sociology *sensu stricto,* the study of human societies at all levels of complexity, still stands apart from sociobiology because of its largely structuralist and nongenetic approach. It attempts to explain human behavior primarily by empirical description of the outermost phenotypes and by unaided intuition, without reference to evolutionary explanations in the true genetic sense. It is most successful, in the way descriptive taxonomy and ecology have been most successful, when it provides a detailed description of particular phenomena and demonstrates first-order correlations with features of the environment. Taxonomy and ecology, however, have been reshaped entirely during the past 40 years by integration into neo-Darwinist evolutionary theory—the "Modern Synthesis," as it is often called—in which each phenomenon is weighed for its adaptive significance and then related to the basic principles of population genetics. It may not be too much to say that sociology and the other social sciences, as well as the humanities, are the last branches of biology waiting to be included in the Modern Synthesis. One of the functions of sociobiology, then, is to reformulate the foundations of the social sciences in a way that draws these subjects into the Modern Synthesis. Whether the social sciences can be truly biologized in this fashion remains to be seen.

Sociobiology is at the same time a new and an old discipline. Perhaps formally ushered in with Wilson's 1975 book, its component parts are much older and include, among others, evolutionary biology, ethology, behavioral genetics, and ecology. It is basically a field that attempts to use the principles of some of these and other fields to better understand animal, including human, behavior. A subset of the field, called human sociobiology, is specifically devoted to understanding human behavior from the standpoint of these other disciplines.

Said in its simplest form, the field of sociobiology emphasizes the evolutionary or phylogenetic basis for understanding behavior of all animals, including humans. The more familiar ontogenetic framework within which psychiatrists generally work is viewed as not sufficient for understanding human behavior patterns. Evolution is seen as involving changes in the genetic makeup of a population over time, with natural selection being the mechanism by which this occurs.

The concept of natural selection is thus central to an understanding of sociobiology for psychiatrists. It is a large and complicated topic but the fundamentals of the concept can be traced back to Darwin. One way to understand this concept is that living things tend to behave in ways that maximize the number of offspring that they bear, the idea being that this increases the total number of genes in the future gene pool. Thus, natural selection operates by differential reproductive success, and certain behaviors survive across generations at the expense of others based on this success. Another way to conceptualize this point is in terms of ultimate and proximate mechanisms of behavior. As Barlow has said, ultimate explanations are those that treat the *why* aspect of behavior and result in a relative increase in genetic representation in the next generation. Ultimate explanations deal with the adaptiveness of behavior. They can be distinguished from proximate explanations, which center on mechanisms and are sometimes called *how* explanations. In psychiatry, such explanations often relate to neurobiological or ontogenetic developmental mechanisms. The concept of ultimate mechanisms relates to the evolutionary basis for certain behavior patterns and has been a central concern for sociobiology. Failure to distinguish between these two different explanations for behavior can inspire acrimonious debate. In other words, behaviors that survive are those that have evolutionary success. As Barash and Lipton have said, "Survival of the fittest refers only to the survival of genes that confer adaptive advantages on their possessors, not to a genetic prescription for bloody conflicts among individuals or societies."

A sociobiological perspective on behavior does not imply that individuals consciously choose certain behavior patterns because they are more likely to result in greater evolutionary success. Rather, natural selection results in their behaving in certain ways without being aware of the motivation for doing so. In a very crude sense, people are driven by evolutionary pressures to behave in certain ways (ultimate causes of behavior). Such pressures do not determine the exact content or specifics of the behavior, which may be more developmentally, neurobiologically, or socially determined. However, evolutionary factors may set constraints on flexibility, although they are certainly not deterministic in a rigid sense. Sociobiologists would typically talk about the interactive nature of behaviors and how they result from a combination of evolutionary (i.e., genetic) influences and other experiences (i.e., developmental, etc.).

The concepts of a psychobiological approach as they relate to an integrative framework for understanding human psychopathology mesh well with modern-day sociobiological thinking. The latter brings into focus for clinical psychiatry the role of evolutionary perspectives in understanding human behavior and attempts to expand the framework from a strictly ontogenetic one or one within a generation. With the increasing emphasis on the genetic basis of major forms of psychiatric disorders, it becomes important to have this kind of framework to begin to understand emerging data sets.

The sociobiological literature has included discussions of several specific topics that may be of special interest to clinicians—including altruism, mate selection and reproduction, parenting strategies, social competition (i.e., aggression and dominance), and strategies of spatial competition (i.e., territorial issues).

Barash commented in his 1977 book that sociobiology was a "whole new way of looking at behavior. It is the application of evolutionary biology to social behavior, an approach that has proven successful in animal studies and that may hold promise for a greater understanding of human behavior as well." He highlighted the basic organizing principle of sociobiology as being evolution by natural selection.

Barash also summarized the complex relationship between sociobiology and other related fields as follows: Ethology is viewed as the biological study of animal behavior. Its orientation has been evolutionary from the start, with emphasis on evaluating and understanding the diversity of behaviors in free living animals and on species-specific and genetically mediated behaviors. Ethology has had a tendency to emphasize a historical approach, especially the identification of behavioral homologies and phylogenies based on the proposition that behavior has evolved just like structure.

In his view, psychology has operated largely independently of the ideas of evolution, whereas sociology and anthropology have had an ambivalent relationship with Darwinism; at times, these fields seem to have embraced a conception of human behavior that is strongly environmentally determined and everything can be attributed to early experience, socialization, cultural norms, and the like.

Sociobiology not only has brought a perspective to the behavior of nonhuman animals, but, in the case of human behavior, the increasing recognition that behavior, even complex social behavior, has evolved and is adaptive.

Sociobiology has been extremely controversial. As A. L. Caplan has said, if all it amounts to is the utilization of population, genetic, and evolutionary models to explain the history of some behavioral phenomena in a few species of organisms, why all the fuss? However, sociobiology makes broader claims that have been hotly disputed:

1. Sociobiological models must be utilized in any attempt to explain the presence of universal types of behavioral tendencies, trends, and patterns throughout the animal kingdom.
2. Humans are social animals subject to the mechanisms of evolutionary change, and, therefore, the biology of sociobiology has much to impart about the origin and nature of human behavior. Human social behavior and organization can only be understood in the light of their evolutionary history and utility.
3. Some researchers have argued that those disciplines that are explicitly concerned with human social behavior, anthropology, economics, political science, sociology, and so on cannot achieve a scientific understanding without incorporating the biological models of sociobiological science.

In other words, what is controversial are questions regarding the scope, validity, accuracy, and implications of sociobiological thinking for human behavior.

The stakes are high with regard to the future of animal research in psychiatry, and, consequently, of the ability to conduct some of the highly important studies relevant to human psychopathology.

REFERENCES

Barash D P: *Sociobiology and Behavior*. Elsevier, New York, 1977.

Barash D P, Lipton J: Sociobiology. In *Comprehensive Textbook of Psychiatry,* H I Kaplan, B J Sadock, editors, ed 4, vol 2, p 70. Williams & Wilkins, Baltimore, 1985.

Caplan A L: *The Sociobiology Debate*. Harper, New York, 1978.

Cronholm B: *Ethology, Psychiatry, and Psychosomatic Medicine*. Laboratory for Clinical Stress Research, Karolinska Sjukhuset, Stockholm, Sweden, 1974.

Kandel E: *Cellular Basis of Behavior*. Freeman, San Francisco, 1976.

Kanner M: *The Tangled Wing*. Harper & Row, New York, 1982.

Kimmel H D: *Experimental Psychopathology: Recent Research and Theory*. Academic Press, New York, 1971.

Kornetsky C, Markowitz R: Animal models and schizophrenia. In *Model Systems in Biological Psychiatry,* D Ingle, H Shein, editors. MIT Press, Cambridge, MA, 1975.

Kraemer G W: Causes and changes in brain norepinephrine systems and later effects in response to social stressors in rhesus monkeys: The cascade hypothesis. In CIBA Foundation Symposium, nos. 126 and 127, *Antidepressants and Receptor Function*. Wiley, New York, 1986.

Kraemer G W, McKinney W T: The overlapping territories of psychiatry and ethology. J Nerv Ment Dis *167:* 3, 1979.

Marks I: Phobias and obsessions: Clinical phenomena in search of a laboratory model. In *Psychopathology: Experimental Models,* J Maser, M Seligman, editors. Freeman, San Francisco, 1977.

Matthyse S, Haber S: Animal models of schizophrenia. In *Model Systems in Biological Psychiatry,* D J Ingle, H Shein, editors. MIT Press, Cambridge, MA, 1975.

McGuire M T, Fairbanks L: Ethology: Psychiatry's bridge to behavior. In *Ethological Psychiatry,* M T McGuire, L Fairbanks, editors. Grune & Stratton, New York, 1977.

McKinney W T, Moran E: Animal models. In *Handbook of Affective Disorders,* E S Paykel, editor, p 202. Churchill Livingstone, Edinburgh, 1982.

McKinney W T, Moran E: Animal models of schizophrenia. Amer J Psychiat *138:* 478, 1981.

Pavlov I P: *Lectures on Conditioned Reflexes*. International Publishers, New York, 1928.

Porsolt R D: Pharmacological models of depression. In *The Origins of Depression: Current Concepts and Approaches,* J Angst, editor. Springer-Verlag, Berlin, 1983.

Porsolt J D: Psychoanalytical analysis of some behavior models of depression. Psychiat Psychol *2:* 150, 1986.

Redmond E A: Alterations in the function of the nucleus locus coerulus: A possible model for studies of anxiety. In *Animal Models in Psychiatry and Neurology,* I Hanin, E Usdin, editors. Pergamon, New York, 1977.

Snyder S: Amphetamine psychosis: A model schizophrenia mediated by catecholamines. Amer J Psychiat *130:* 161, 1973.

Suomi S J, Levy H: In memoriam: Harry F. Harlow. Amer J Primatol *2:* 319, 1982.

Weiss J M, Goodman P: Neurochemical mechanisms underlying stress-induced depression. In *Stress and Coping,* P McCabe, N Schneiderman, editors, vol 1. Erlbaum, Hillsdale, NJ, 1984.

Wilner P: The validity of animal models of depression. Psychopharmacology *83:* 1, 1984.

Wilson E O: *Sociobiology: The New Synthesis*. Belknap Press, Cambridge, MA, 1975.

Zegans L: An appraisal of ethological contributions to psychiatric theory and practice. Amer J Psychiat *124:* 729, 1967.

5.3
STATISTICS AND EXPERIMENTAL DESIGN

IGOR GRANT, M.D.
ROBERT M. KAPLAN, Ph.D.

INTRODUCTION

Descriptive statistics are used to organize, summarize, and describe observations. They might include summaries of symptom checklist scores for a selected group of neurotic patients, a summary of neuroendocrine data for a group of schizophrenic patients, or a descriptive summary of the correlation between watching television violence and behaving aggressively. *Inferential statistics* are required for drawing general conclusions about probabilities on the basis of a sample. There are many uses of inferential statistics. Statistical inference might be used, for example, to make statements about the eating habits of U.S. citizens on the basis of study of a small fraction of the American people or to decide whether to attribute differences between two groups to chance or to nonchance factors.

The purpose here is to address the informed consumer rather than the expert biomathematician. Thus, an effort has been made to explain a broad range of topics and to avoid the sorts of mathematical treatment that would put this work beyond the interest or expertise of most readers.

DESCRIPTIVE STATISTICS

Descriptive statistics are used to summarize observations and to place these observations within context. The most common descriptive statistics include measures of central tendency and measures of variability.

The three commonly used measures of central tendency are the mean, the median, and the mode. The *mean* is the arithmetic average, the *median* is the point representing the 50th percentile in the distribution, and the *mode* is the most common score. Sometimes the measures are the same but, on other occasions, they can be different.

The mean, median, and mode will be the same when the distribution of scores is normal. The *normal distribution,* shown in Figure 5.3-1, is a theoretical distribution of scores that is symmetrical. Under most circumstances, the mean, median, and mode will not be exactly the same. The mode is most likely to misrepresent the underlying distribution and is rarely used in statistical analysis. Typically, investigators choose between the mean and the median as a measure of central tendency. The major consideration is how much weight should be given to extreme scores. The mean takes into account each score in the distribution; the median finds only the halfway point.

Table 5.3-1 shows how the mean and median might have very different values. The table lists weights of two groups of college women. There are five women in each group, but four of them are in both groups (Sally, Sue, Leslie, and Dana). The fifth member is Allison in group 1 and Bertha in group 2. These two women have very different weights. As the example shows, the median is exactly the same in the two groups. However, the estimation of the mean is affected by

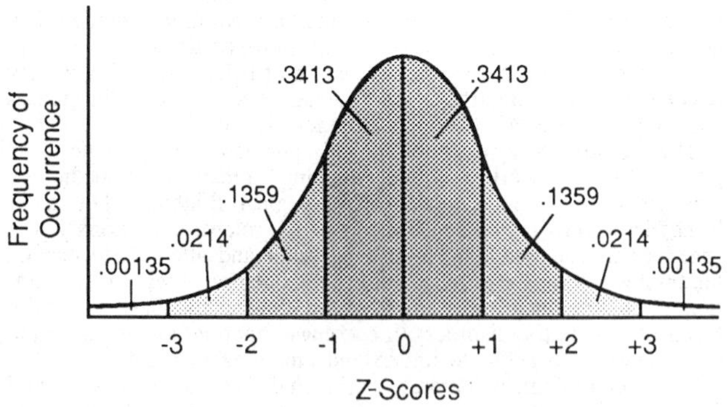

FIGURE 5.3-1. *The normal distribution and areas under the normal curve for Z-scores from –3 to +3.*

the addition of the extreme case. Because the mean best represents all subjects and because of desirable mathematical properties, the mean is typically favored in statistical analysis.

Despite the advantages of the mean, there are also some advantages to the median. In particular, the median disregards outlier cases. The mean moves further in the direction of the outliers. Thus, the median is often used when the investigator does not want scores in the extreme of the distribution to have a strong impact. The median is also valuable for summarizing data for a measure that might be insensitive toward the higher ranges of the scale. For instance, a very easy test may have a ceiling effect but does not show the true ability of some test takers. A ceiling effect occurs when the test is too easy to measure the true ability of the best students. Thus, if some scores stack up at the extreme, the median may be more accurate than the mean. If the high scores had not been bounded by the highest obtainable score, the mean might actually have been higher.

As noted above, the mean, median, and mode are exactly the same in a normal distribution. However, not all distributions of scores have a normal or bell-shaped appearance. The highest point in a distribution of scores is called the modal peak. A distribution with the modal peak off to one side or the other is described as skewed. The word skew literally means "slanted."

The direction of skew is determined by the location of the tail or flat area of the distribution. Positive skew occurs when the tail goes off to the right of the distribution. Negative skew occurs when the tail or low point is on the left side of the distribution. Figure 5.3-2 illustrates the normal distribution, or distribution that has positive skewness, and one that has negative skewness.

TABLE 5.3-1
Mean and Median for Weights (in Pounds) of Two Groups of College Women

Group 1		*Group 2*	
Woman	*Weight*	*Woman*	*Weight*
Sally	95	Sally	95
Sue	100	Sue	100
Leslie	105	Leslie	105
Dana	110	Dana	110
Allison	115	Bertha	275
	Mean $\bar{X}$ = 105		Mean $\bar{X}$ = 137
	Median Md = 105		Median Md = 105

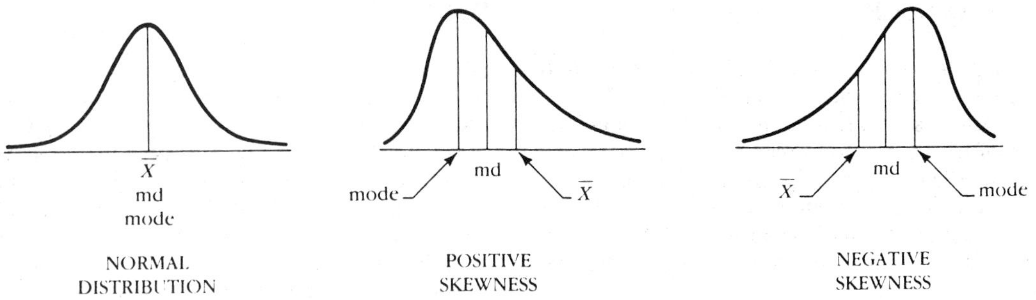

FIGURE 5.3-2. *Examples of normal distribution, positive skewness, and negative skewness.*

The mode is the most frequent score in the distribution. In a skewed distribution, the mode remains at the peak. The mean and the median shift away from the mode in the direction of the skewness. The mean moves furthest in the direction of the skewness, and the median typically falls between the mean and the mode. The relative positions of the mean, median, and mode in normal and skewed distributions are shown in the figure.

VARIABILITY

Measures of central tendency, such as the mean and median, are used to summarize information. They are important because they provide information about the average score in the distribution. Knowing the average score, however, does not provide all of the information required to describe a group of scores. In addition, measures of variability are required. The simplest method of describing variability is the range. The range is simply the difference between the highest score and lowest score. Another statistic, known as the interquartile range, describes the interval of scores bounded by the 25th and 75th percentiles. In other words, the interquartile range is bounded by the range of scores that represent the middle 50 percent of the distribution.

In contrast to ranges, which are used infrequently in statistical analysis, the variance and standard deviation are used commonly. Since the mean is the average score in a distribution, the sum of the deviations around the mean will always equal zero. Yet, in order to understand the characteristics of a distribution of scores, some estimation of deviation around the mean is important. Summing deviations will always yield zero. However, the squared deviations around the mean can yield a meaningful index. The *variance* is the sum of the squared deviations around the mean divided by the number of cases. It is described by the formula:

$$\sigma^2 = \frac{\sum (X_i - \bar{X})^2}{N}$$

where σ^2 is the variance, Σ is the sum, X_i is the score of the ith case, $\bar{X}$ is the mean for the population, and N is the population size.

The variance is a very useful statistic and is commonly employed in data analysis. However, its calculation requires finding the squared deviations around the mean rather than the simple deviations around the mean. Thus, when the variance is calculated, the result will always be in squared units. Taking the square root of the variance puts the units back into their original metric. The square root of the variance is known as the *standard deviation*. The standard deviation is an approximation of the average deviation around the mean. Although the standard deviation is not technically equal to the average deviation, it gives an approximation of how much scores deviate from the mean on the average.

SAMPLES AND POPULATIONS

The methods discussed so far describe populations. The *population* is defined as the entire collection of a set of objects, people, events, and so on, in a particular context. In other words, population refers to the collection of all items on which statements will be based. This might include all schizophrenic patients in a particular hospital, or all depressed individuals in a community.

In statistics, means and standard deviations for populations are typically estimated from observations taken from samples. A *sample* is a subset of observations selected from the population. It might be unusual for an investigator to describe only schizophrenic patients in a particular hospital, and it is unlikely that an investigator will measure every depressed person in a community. More frequently, statements are made about populations on the basis of samples. On the basis of a random and unbiased sample of individuals from a community, the mean of the population can be estimated. The formulas for estimating the standard deviations for samples differ slightly from those used for populations. The denominator in the radical, $N - 1$, is used for sample statistics instead of N, which is used for population statistics. Thus, the definitional formula for the standard deviation of a sample is

$$S = \sqrt{\frac{\sum (X_i - \bar{X})^2}{N - 1}}$$

The computational formula for a sample standard deviation is

$$S = \sqrt{\frac{\sum X^2 - \frac{(\sum X)^2}{N}}{N - 1}}$$

The computational formula does not require the calculation of each deviation from the mean. Instead, it uses the sum of the squared scores and the square of the summed scores. These scores can be easily obtained using spreadsheet programs for microcomputers.

STANDARDIZED SCORES

One of the problems with means and standard deviations is that their meanings are not independent of context. For example, if the mean of some set of scores is 57.6, it still does not convey all of the information necessary for an interpretation. Other metrics are designed for more direct interpretation. The *Z*-score is a transformation into standardized units that are easier to interpret. The *Z*-score is the difference between the score and the mean, divided by the standard deviation

$$Z = \frac{X - \bar{X}}{S}$$

In other words, a *Z*-score is the deviation of a score, *X*, from the mean, $\bar{X}$, expressed in standard deviation units. If a score is equal to the mean, its *Z*-score is zero. Consider the example of a score of 4 taken from a sample with a mean of 5.75 and a standard deviation of 2.11. The *Z*-score would be

$$Z = \frac{4 - 5.75}{2.11}$$

$$= \frac{-1.75}{2.11}$$

$$= -0.83$$

This means that the observed score (4) is 0.83 standard deviation below the average score or that the score is below the mean, but its difference from the mean is slightly less than one standard deviation. In other words, the deviation is less than the average deviation around the mean.

The standard normal distribution is of central importance in statistics and psychological testing. The normal distribution is derived from binomial probability. A binomial event has one of two outcomes—like the results of a coin flip. Using an infinite number of binomial events, a probability distribution can be generated, as shown in Figure 5.3-1. This distribution might be the theoretical frequency distribution of "heads" in an infinite series of coin flips.

On most occasions, the units on the *x*-axis of the normal distribution are in *Z* units. Any variable transformed into *Z* units will have a mean of 0 and a standard deviation of 1. Figure 5.3-1 shows the areas under the normal curve associated with these *Z* units. For example, 34.13 percent, or 0.3413, of the cases fall between the mean and one standard deviation above the mean. Since 50 percent of the cases fall below the mean, it can be concluded that if a score is one standard deviation above the mean, it will be in the 84th percentile rank (50 + 34.13 = 84.13). A score that is one standard deviation below the mean would be in the 16th percentile (50 − 34.14 = 15.87).

Translation of *Z*-scores into percentile ranks is accomplished using a table for the standard normal distribution. Certain Z-scores are of particular interest in statistics and psychological testing. The Z-score 1.96 represents the 97.5th percentile in a distribution and −1.96 represents the 2.5th percentile. A *Z*-score less than −1.96 or greater than +1.96 falls outside of a 95 percent interval bounding the mean of the *Z*-distribution. Some statistical definitions of abnormality view these defined deviations as cutoff points. Thus, an individual who, on some attribute, is more than 1.96 *Z*-scores from the mean might be regarded as abnormal.

McCALL'S T

There are a variety of other systems by which raw scores can be transformed to give them more intuitive meaning. One system was established in 1939 by W. A. McCall, who originally intended to develop a system to derive equal units of mental quantities. McCall suggested that a random sample of 12-year-olds be tested and that the distribution of their scores be obtained. Percentile equivalents then were to be assigned to each raw score, showing the percentile rank in the group for the persons obtaining that raw score. After this assignment had been accomplished, the mean of the distribution would be set at 50, to correspond to the 50th percentile. In McCall's system, the standard deviation was set at 10.

In effect, what McCall generated was a system that is exactly the same as standard scores (*Z*-scores) except that the mean in McCall's system is 50 rather than 0 and the standard deviation is 10 rather than 1. A *Z*-score can be transformed to a *T*-score by applying a linear transformation.

$$T = 10Z + 50$$

The *T*-score system is commonly used in psychological tests. For example, the Minnesota Multiphasic Personality Inventory uses McCall's system. Thus, a score of 60 on any subscale is one standard deviation above the mean. A score of 60 places an individual in approximately the 84th percentile relative to the standardization sample. The score of 70 or above is more than two standard deviations above the mean, and, thus, might be considered unusual in relation to the normative population.

CONFIDENCE INTERVALS

In most statistical inference problems, the sample mean is used to estimate the population mean. Each sample mean is considered to be an unbiased estimate of the population mean. Although the sample mean is unlikely to be exactly the same as the population mean, repeated random samples will form a sampling distribution of sample means. The mean of the sampling distribution is an unbiased estimate of the population mean. However, taking repeated random samples from the population is also difficult and expensive. Instead, it may be necessary to estimate the population mean on the basis of a single sample, by creating an interval around the sample mean.

The first step in creating this interval is finding the standard error of the mean. The *standard error of the mean* is the standard deviation divided by the square root of the sample size. Statistical inference is used to estimate the probability that the population mean falls within some defined interval. Sample means are distributed normally around the population mean, and so the sample mean is probably near the population value. However, it is possible that the sample mean is an overestimate or an underestimate of the population mean. Using information about the standard error of the mean, it is possible to put a single observation of a mean into context.

The ranges that are likely to capture the population mean are called *confidence intervals*. Confidence intervals are bounded by *confidence limits*. The confidence interval is defined as a range of values with a specified probability of including the population mean. A confidence interval is typically associated with a certain probability level. For example, the 95 percent confidence interval has a 95 percent chance of including the population mean. A 99 percent confidence interval is expected to capture the true mean in 99 of each 100 cases. The confidence limits are defined as the values for points that bound the confidence interval.

Creating a confidence interval requires a mean, a standard error of the mean, and the Z value associated with the interval. It is accomplished using the formula

$$CI = \bar{X} \pm Z_{\alpha} S_X$$

Consider the 95 percent confidence interval, which is obtained by taking the mean plus or minus the standard error of the mean multiplied by the Z-score for the 95 percent interval, or 1.96.

If smaller sample sizes are involved, it may be advisable to use another sampling distribution instead of the standard normal distribution. For example, it is common to use the t-distribution for creation of confidence intervals for smaller samples.

T-TESTS

In experimental sciences, comparisons between groups are very common. Usually, one group is the treatment, or experimental, group and the other group is the untreated, or control, group. If patients are randomly assigned to these two groups, it is assumed that they differ only by chance prior to treatment. Then measurements are taken after the treatment to determine whether the groups differ. The task of the statistician is to determine whether any observed differences between the groups following treatment should be attributed to chance or to the treatment. The t-test is commonly used for this purpose. The several different types of t-tests are summarized in Table 5.3-2. The table also shows the formulas used to calculate the t-values.

TABLE 5.3-2
Different Types of *t*-Tests

1. Comparison of a sample mean with a hypothetical population mean
2. Comparison between two scores in the same group of individuals
3. Comparison between observations made on two independent groups

Formulas:

1. $$t = \frac{\bar{X}_1 - \mu}{S_{\bar{X}}}$$

where $\bar{X}_1$ is the sample mean, μ is the hypothetical population mean, and $S_{\bar{X}}$ is the standard error of the sample mean.

2. $$t = \frac{\bar{D}}{\frac{S_D}{\sqrt{N_1}}}$$

where $\bar{D}$ is the mean of the differences between pairs of observations and $\frac{S_D}{\sqrt{N_1}}$ is the standard error of differences, as defined as

$$\sqrt{\frac{N \sum D^2 - \left(\sum D\right)^2}{N - 1}}$$

3. $$t = \frac{\bar{X}_1 - \bar{X}_2}{S_{\bar{X}1-\bar{X}2}}$$

where $\bar{X}_1$ is the mean of sample 1, $\bar{X}_2$ is the mean of sample 2, and $S_{\bar{X}1-\bar{X}2}$ is the standard error of the difference between means.

Most statistical tests have a common logic. All of these procedures are based on a ratio of observed to expected differences. The top half of the ratio is the observation. For the t-test, the numerator is usually the observed difference between means. The bottom half of the ratio is the standard error for that same observation—an estimate of the extent to which the means would be expected to differ by chance alone. The standard error of the mean is the standard deviation of the sampling distribution; that is, an approximation of the average deviation that would be expected in estimating the population mean from a sample. Consider the t-test for differences between independent means. For this test, the numerator is the observed difference between these independent means. The bottom half of the equation is the standard error of the differences between means. In other words, the observed differences between means are divided by an approximation of the average deviation that would be expected as a result of sampling error. If the ratios are large, then the numerator—the observed deviation—is greater than would be expected by chance. If the ratio is small, then the numerator or difference between groups is equal to or less than what might be expected by chance. The rationale is quite similar for other types of t-tests. For example, the t-test on paired observations compares the deviations between pairs (numerator) with the standard error for these deviations (denominator).

ANALYSIS OF VARIANCE

In psychiatric and psychological studies, researchers are often interested in comparing the means of more than two groups. For example, they may wish to compare the depression scores of persons in three groups: major mood disorders, schizophrenia, and nonpatient controls. The t-tests described above are suitable only for two-sample problems. When there are three or more samples, and the data from each sample are thought to be distributed normally, analysis of variance (ANOVA) may be a technique of choice.

Mathematically, it can be shown that if two or more samples are drawn from the same population, then the variances (S^2) of the several samples will all be estimates of the population variance (σ^2). Furthermore, the ratio of the variances derived from two samples of the same population will form a distribution that has been termed the F-distribution. The shape of this distribution depends on the size of each sample (or, more accurately, on $N - 1$ for each sample, which represents the degrees of freedom (df) associated with each sample; df $= N - 1$ because once the mean is known and all but the very last observation is specified, then the very last observation must be invariant).

When two or more samples are being compared, two sources of variance must be considered. For simplicity, consider the three-sample problem. For example, depression scores of patients with mood disorders (X_a) are to be compared with those of schizophrenic patients (X_s) and with controls (X_c). The task is to evaluate the hypothesis (null hypothesis) that the patients with mood disorders, schizophrenic patients, and the controls have been sampled from the same population with respect to depression scores. This population will have a mean depression score $\bar{X}$. The mean scores for the three groups will probably not be exactly the same (even if they come from the same population), but they will vary around X. This variance, termed *between samples variance,* is calculated in the ANOVA procedure.

The between groups variance provides an estimate of the difference between group means. How is it determined whether this variability is meaningful or random? To index between groups variance, an independent estimate of variability is used. Within each of the groups, the variability of individual scores around their own group mean provides an estimate of how depression scores are expected to vary by chance. When aggregated across groups, the variance of individual scores around their group means becomes an estimate of error, or *within samples variance*. The *F* ratio then becomes a fraction in which the numerator is the between samples variance estimate and the denominator is the within samples variance estimate. The larger the *F* ratio, the more likely it is that the null hypothesis can be rejected, namely, that the mood-disordered, schizophrenic, and control subjects came from the same population with respect to depression scores. Critical values of *F*, for various degrees of freedom at desired levels of significance, can be obtained from standard *F* tables.

So far, the discussion of ANOVA has considered only a one-way classification, that is, only one grouping factor (in the example above, diagnostic classification) has been considered. In a good deal of psychiatric research, subjects will actually be classified in several different ways, giving rise to a two-factor model, a three-factor model, and so on. For example, in the analysis of depression scores, one might wish to divide subjects not only by diagnostic classification (mood disorders, schizophrenic patients, control normals), but also by sex. The result would then be a 3 × 2 factorial design (three diagnoses by two sexes). *F* ratios can then be computed for each of the two *main effects* (i.e., diagnosis and sex). A main effect is a statistical difference that is independent of the influence of other variables. In this way, it is possible to determine whether there are significant differences in depression between diagnostic groups and also between men and women. The factorial design permits each of these assessments to be used independently. Typically, studies are designed so that these independant variables are orthogonal or uncorrelated.

If a situation involves two or more factors or classifications, then an *interaction* may occur. Interactions describe joint effects of two or more variables. For example, female patients with mood disorders may have higher depression scores than female patients with schizophrenia or controls, but the differences among diagnostic groups may be smaller for males. This effect might be even greater than would be expected by taking into account the independent contributions of diagnosis and sex. Such a systematic variation in depression scores as a function of both sex and diagnosis is termed an interaction. An interaction is literally a difference of differences. In this example, the difference in depression score attributable to diagnostic groupings is larger for female than for male patients. Once again, an *F* ratio can be computed for the interaction effect.

Table 5.3-3 illustrates the results of a two-way ANOVA. In this study, Beck depression scores were obtained for 10 patients with mood disorder, 10 with schizophrenia, and 10 controls. Half of the patients in each group were women. The raw scores indicate that there were differences between patients and controls and between men and women. The question is, are these differences greater than would be expected by chance (defined as occurring less than 5 percent of the time as a result of chance)? The ANOVA computation indicates that the *F* ratio for the diagnosis effect ($F_{2/24} = 100.79$, $p < 0.001$) is greater than the tabled value of *F* (5.61) at the 0.01 significance level for 2 and 24 df. Thus, there is a diagnosis main effect. Similarly, for gender, the *F* ratio exceeds the tabled value for 1 and 24 df at the 0.01 level (tabled value = 7.82). Finally, the *F* associated with the interaction is also larger than the tabled 0.05 level (3.40) for 2 and 24 df, demonstrating systematic influence of the combination of sex and diagnosis on Beck scores (i.e., women with mood disorders had significantly higher Beck scores than would be predicted from considering diagnosis and sex alone).

TABLE 5.3-3
Summary of 2 × 3 ANOVA for Sex by Diagnostic Group

Data:

	Controls (*N* = 10)	Schizophrenic Patients (*N* = 10)	Mood-Disorder Patients (*N* = 10)
Men (*N* = 15)	2	8	11
	4	9	9
	3	8	16
	1	7	12
	2	6	10
Women (*N* = 15)	4	12	20
	4	11	16
	2	9	18
	3	11	16
	6	13	22

ANOVA Summary Table*

Somse	*MS*	*df*	*F*	*p*
Diagnosis main effect	354.433	2	100.787	<.001
Sex main effect	116.033	1	32.995	<.001
Interaction	18.433	2	5.242	<.02
Error	3.52	24		

*MS = mean square, df = degrees of freedom, *F* is the *F* ratio, and *p* is the probability level.

CHI-SQUARE (NONPARAMETRIC STATISTICS)

The methods covered thus far are *parametric* because they are used to estimate population parameters, such as the mean and the standard deviation. Use of these methods requires assumptions about population characteristics. For example, one of these assumptions is that the variable under study is normally distributed within the population from which the sample is drawn. Although for most applications in basic statistics, violations of this assumption have relatively little impact on a statistical test, there are circumstances in which substantial bias will be introduced. To address this problem, there is another family of statistical procedures that does not make assumptions about population distributions. These procedures are called *nonparametic*, or distribution-free techniques. Many research workers prefer nonparametric methods because they rest on fewer assumptions. These techniques are also appropriate to the analysis of data that do not have continuous numerical properties, for example, data that exist as categories, ordinal data (e.g., clinical ratings of severity on a six-point scale), or ranked data.

The most commonly used nonparametric test for categorical data is the chi-square. The chi-square statistic is used to evaluate the relative frequency or proportion of events in a population that fall into well-defined categories. For each category, there is an expected frequency that is obtained from knowledge of the population or from some other theoretical perspective. There is also an observed frequency for each category. The observed frequency is obtained from observations made by the investigator. The chi-square statistic expresses the discrepancy between the observed and the expected frequency. The formula for chi-square is

$$\chi^2 = \frac{\sum (O - E)^2}{E}$$

where O is the observed frequency and E is the expected frequency.

An example of a situation in which chi-square is used might be to evaluate the association between sex and diagnosis of major depression. The investigator would consider whether each male and each female in a sample did or did not carry the diagnosis. Under the null hypothesis, the expected frequency for major depression would be assumed to be equal for men and women. The chi-square test would be used to evaluate the 2 × 2 table.

There are also nonparametric alternatives to problems that suggest the possibility of using a *t*-test or ANOVA, but where the properties of the data render application of parametric statistics inappropriate. For a two-sample experiment, the Mann-Whitney U Test may be preferable to the *t*-test, whereas for problems involving three or more samples, the Kruskal-Wallis procedure can replace the ANOVA. Both of these nonparametric methods involve transformation of the data into ranks.

TYPES OF ERRORS

When the null hypothesis is rejected, the observed differences between groups are deemed improbable by chance alone. For example, if drug A is compared with a placebo for its effects on depression and the null hypothesis is rejected, the investigator concludes that the observed differences most likely are not explainable simply by sampling error. The key word in these statements is *probable*. The odds are on the side of the investigator making the statement. However, what are the chances that the statement is incorrect?

In statistical inference, there is no way to say with certainty that rejection or retention of the null hypothesis was correct. There are two types of potential errors. A *type I error* occurs when the null hypothesis is rejected when it should have been retained. A *type II error* occurs when the null hypothesis is retained and it should have been rejected.

TYPE I ERROR Type I errors arise when the null hypothesis is rejected when it should have been retained. This error might be seen when a researcher decides that two means are different, that the treatment works or that groups are not sampled from the same population. Yet, in reality, the observed differences are due only to sampling error. In a conservative scientific setting, type I errors rarely should be made. There is great disadvantage to advocating treatments that really do not work. The probability of a type I error is denoted with the Greek alpha (α). Because of this desire to avoid type I errors, statistical models have been created so that the investigator has control over the probability of a type I error. At the 0.05 significance or alpha level, a type I error is expected to occur in 5 percent of all cases. At the 0.01 level, it may occur in 1 percent of all cases. Thus, at the 0.05 alpha level, one type I error is expected to be made in each of 20 independent tests. At the 0.01 alpha level, one type I error is expected to be made in each 100 independent tests.

TYPE II ERROR The motivation to avoid a type I error might increase the probability of making a second type of error. In this case, the null hypothesis is retained when it actually was wrong. For example, an investigator may reach the conclusion that a treatment does not work when actually it does. The probability of a type II error is symbolized by the Greek beta (β). Table 5.3-4 shows four possible outcomes broken down in a 2 × 2 table. In the left column are the decisions the researcher made about the null hypothesis. The hypothesis can be rejected or retained. Across the top of the table is the real world or actual situation. The researcher does not know this, but hypothetically it can be said that this is the decision that should have been made. Teachers often refer to it as "God's model," implying that there is a correct decision that could have been made but it is beyond one's capability of knowing.

Consider the entries in the table. The upper left box shows that the null hypothesis is rejected even though it is true. This is a type I error. It will occur with a probability of alpha, or the significance level for the test. For example, at the 0.05 alpha level, the probability of this type of error is five in 100. The other type of error is given in the bottom right box in the table. Here the decision is not to reject the null hypothesis although in the real world the hypothesis was false. This error is a type II error with the probability of beta.

Not all decisions are incorrect. The table also shows two boxes where the researcher made the correct decision. In the lower left box, the decision was to retain the null hypothesis, and the null hypothesis was true. This is a correct decision, and it occurs with a probability of $1 - \alpha$. Finally, in the situation portrayed in the upper right box, the investigator decided to reject the null hypothesis, and indeed it was false. This decision is a correct decision with a probability of $1 - \beta$. The upper right cell is of particular interest; it is often called the power of the test.

Statistical power There are several maneuvers that will help gain control over the probability of different types of errors and correct decisions. One type of correct decision is the probability of rejecting the null hypothesis and being correct in that decision. *Power* is defined as the probability of rejecting the null hypothesis when, in the real world, it should have been rejected. Ultimately, the statistical evaluation will be more meaningful if it has high power. It is particularly important to have high statistical power when the null hypothesis is retained. In other words, retaining the null hypothesis with

TABLE 5.3-4
Four Possible Outcomes of Decisions Concerning the Null Hypothesis

		"God's Model" What Actually Is True	
		H_0 is true *It should have been retained*	H_0 is false *It should have been rejected*
Researcher's decision	Reject H_0	Type I error $p = \alpha$	Correct decision $p = 1 - \beta$ (also called the power of the test)
	Retain H_0	Correct decision $p = 1 - \alpha$	Type II error $p = \beta$

high power gives the investigator more confidence in stating that differences between groups were nonsignificant. One factor that affects the power is the sample size. As the sample size increases, power increases. In other words, the larger the sample, the greater is the probability that a correct decision will be made in rejecting or retaining the null hypothesis. Tables are available that show the relation between sample size and power. These tables are very helpful in the planning of experiments.

Another factor that influences power is the significance level. As alpha or significance increases, the power increases. For instance, if the 0.05 level is selected rather than the 0.01 level, there will be a greater chance of rejecting the null hypothesis. However, there will also be a higher probability of a type I error. Reducing the chances of a type I error also reduces the chances of correctly identifying the real difference (power). Thus, the safest manipulation to affect power without affecting the probability of a type I error is to increase the sample size. The only problem with very large sample sizes is that statistical tests can sometimes detect very small differences that, although statistically significant, may be clinically trivial.

It is worth noting that not all statistical tests have equal power. Some statistical methods are more powerful than others, which means that the probability of correctly rejecting the null hypothesis is higher with some statistical methods than with others. Nonparametric statistics are typically less powerful than parametric statistics, for example.

CORRELATION

Quite commonly, clinicians or researchers are interested not so much in how samples might differ, but in how variables that represent characteristics of some particular sample or population are related to each other. For example, one might wish to know the relationship between an oral dose of haloperidol (Haldol) and plasma level, between rapid eye movement (REM) sleep latency and Beck depression scores, or between volume of the third ventricle and degree of amnesia. Figure 5.3-3 provides results from a clinical study in which plasma haloperidol was determined 1 hour after each of 10 single oral doses of the drug. The distribution of points in the scatter plot suggest that these data could be modeled in terms of a straight line, termed a *regression line*. The question becomes, how well can plasma levels be predicted from oral dose? In statistical terms, then, how much of the total variation in plasma haloperidol is attributable to the oral dose, and how much can be explained by other factors (e.g., age, diet, body mass)?

The regression line that expresses the relationship between plasma haloperidol (y) and oral dose (x) can be expressed by the equation $y' = a + bx$, where y' is the predicted value of plasma haloperidol taken from the regression line, a is the intercept of the line on the y-axis, and b is the slope of the regression line.

Once the regression line has been fitted to the data, the next question becomes, what is the strength of the linear relationship between plasma haloperidol and oral dose? The strength of the association is expressed as the ratio of the variance in y that is attributable to its relationship to x divided by the total variance in the model. This ratio has been designated r^2. In Figure 5.3-3, the r^2 was computed as 0.86—which means that 86 percent of the total variation in plasma haloperidol can be attributed to its relationship to the oral dose, and 14 per-

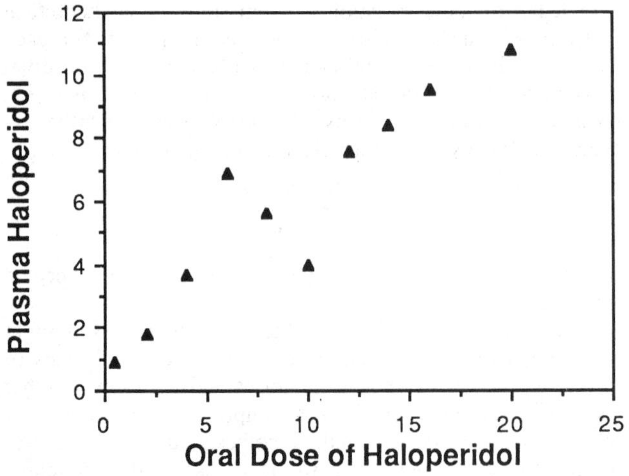

FIGURE 5.3-3. *Hypothetical relationship between oral dose of haloperidol and plasma concentration of haloperidol. The linear relationship accounts for 86 percent of the variance.*

cent of the variation is due to unexplained factors, including measurement error and characteristics of subjects.

Customarily, the strength of the linear relationship between two variables is actually reported as the correlation coefficient (product moment correlation, Pearson's r, or simply r). The correlation coefficient is the regression coefficient when both x and y variables are expressed in standardized or Z units. The regression coefficient allows a translation between X and Y in natural units. It is the amount of expected change in Y for each unit change in X. For example, the equation $Y = 3.25 + 0.5X$ suggests that each unit change in X is expected to correspond with a 0.5 change in Y. The value 3.25 is the intercept, or the value of Y when X is 0. The correlation coefficient is also the square root of r^2. In the example above, $r = 0.93$. To determine whether a product moment correlation falls outside the bounds of chance, one can compute a t statistic using a standard formula that takes into account the number of degrees of freedom. In the case of a correlation between two variables, the df $= n - 2$, where n is the number of pairs. In the above example, t was computed as 7.03, which exceeds $t = 2.90$, the critical value of $\alpha = 0.05$ for 8 df. Thus, it can be concluded that the r is significantly larger than would be expected by chance. The formulas for the correlation coefficient and the translation of r to t are

$$r = \frac{N \sum XY - (\sum X)(\sum Y)}{\sqrt{[N \sum X^2 - (\sum X)^2][N \sum Y^2 - (\sum Y)^2]}}$$

$$t = r\sqrt{\frac{N - 2}{1 - r^2}}$$

where N is the number of cases and X and Y are scores on measured variables.

CAUTIONS IN INTERPRETING THE CORRELATION COEFFICIENT Several issues need to be borne in mind in interpreting the correlation coefficient. First, it is important to inspect the data that are being modeled. For example, the linear correlation between plasma concentration of an anti-

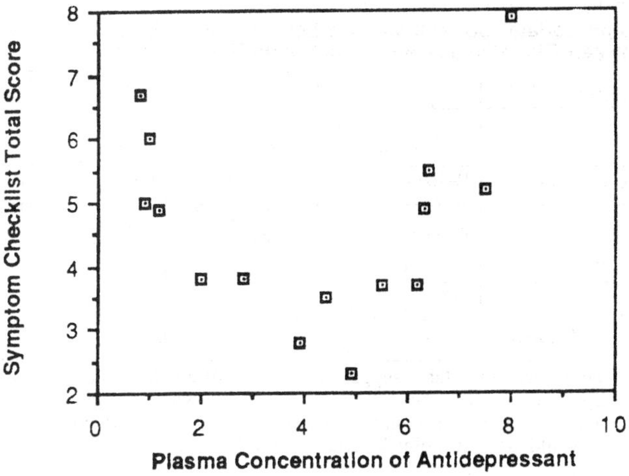

FIGURE 5.3-4. *The systematic U-shaped relationship between plasma concentration of antidepressant and scores on a symptom checklist is not detected by Pearson Product Moment Correlation Methods, which are designed to describe linear relationships.*

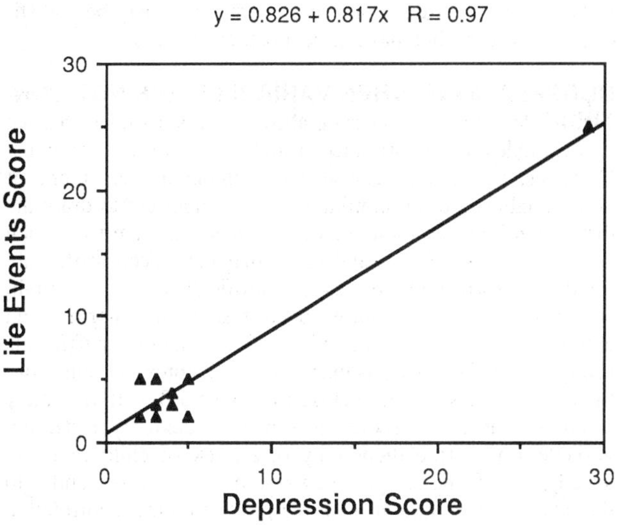

FIGURE 5.3-6. *The same data as Figure 5.3-5 with the addition of one outlier. A single outlier can have a significant effect on estimates of linear correlation.*

depressant and score on a symptom checklist is low in Figure 5.3-4. This correlation does not result because the variables are unrelated, however. The data are best modeled as a U-shaped function rather than as a straight line. Correlation coefficients can be biased by a single extreme value, as illustrated in Figures 5.3-5 and 5.3-6. Figure 5.3-5 shows the correlation between scores on an inventory of life events and a self-rated depression checklist. As the figure shows, there is only a very weak correlation between the scores ($r = 0.11$). Figure 5.3-6 displays the same relationship with the addition of a single "outlier." This one case had many life events and a high depression score. With the addition of this one extreme point, the correlation bounces to 0.97. The example illustrates the sensitivity of correlational methods to extreme scores. Investigators should inspect their data to avoid spurious high correlations caused by outliers.

Figure 5.3-7 illustrates another problem of interpreting the meaning of the correlation. Here, data collected from two samples were pooled and a product moment correlation was computed. Although it apparently was significant, an inspection of the scatter plot shows that this apparent linear relationship is explained by the fact that the two samples differed in their mean scores for memory errors and third ventricle width (i.e., the samples came from different populations), but that within each sample, there was no relationship between the two variables.

The range of variability in data also will determine the size of the correlation coefficient. For example, if the range of variability is very restricted (i.e., there is not much "play" in the scores), then the observed value of Pearson's r will be constrained near 0. The level of r at which a significant value is attained also depends on the size of the sample. In extremely large samples (e.g., hundreds or thousands of sub-

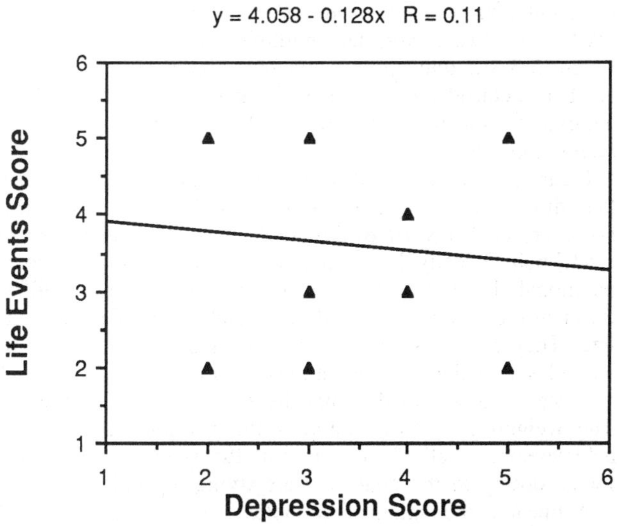

FIGURE 5.3-5. *Scatter plot of depression and life events scores.*

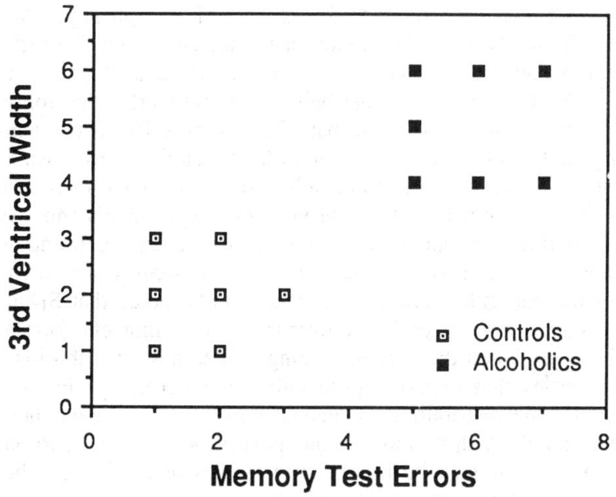

FIGURE 5.3-7. *Example of ecological correlation, a correlation that must be interpreted with caution. The correlation between memory and third ventricle width is low in both alcoholic and control groups. However, after merging both groups, a significant correlation appears. The fact that the correlation from the pooled samples is significant does not demonstrate a true association between ventricle width and memory.*

jects), even tiny values of r (e.g., $r = 0.07$) may be statistically significant but have little practical meaning.

CORRELATIONS WHEN VARIABLES ARE NOT CONTINUOUS In the discussion above, it was assumed that the two variables being correlated, x and y, both were continuous. However, correlations can also be computed even if one or both variables are not continuous. It is important to draw the distinction between dichotomous variables that are true, such as male versus female, and those that have been artificially divided to form dichotomies. An artificial dichotomy might be the division of a continuous test score into normal and abnormal categories. The types of correlation coefficients used to find the relationship between dichotomous and continuous variables are summarized in Table 5.3-5. If variable y is continuous (e.g., score on a manual dexterity test), but variable x is a true dichotomy (e.g., sex of children being tested), and if one assigns the value of 0 to one sex and 1 to the other, then computation of the product moment correlation will yield a special statistic called the *point biserial correlation*. The point biserial r can be interpreted in the same way as the standard product moment correlation. The relationship between a continuous variable and an artificial dichotomy is evaluated using the *biserial coefficient*.

If one is correlating variables both of which are dichotomous, then entering these scores into the formula for computing the correlation coefficient yields another statistic called the *phi coefficient* (ϕ). The phi coefficient is related to the more commonly known chi-square described earlier. In fact, it can be shown that $\chi^2 = N\phi^2$, where N is the number of cases.

The significance of phi thus can be determined by computing $N\phi^2$ and referring to a chi-square table with 1 df. When both variables are artificial dichotomies, another coefficient known as the tetrachoric r is used.

RANK ORDER CORRELATION Sometimes it is difficult to assign precise values to observations. For example, a clinician might wish to relate the amount of belligerence exhibited by drug-abusing patients to the strength of their phencyclidine (PCP) abuse habit. The notion of belligerence might be difficult to quantify, though it might be possible to rank the patients from most to least belligerent. Similarly, the notion of "strength of drug abuse habit" might be difficult to quantify, but it might be possible to order the subjects from heaviest to lightest user. A rank order correlation coefficient can then be computed that has been termed Spearman's rho. By computing a Z value, using formulas that can be found in standard texts, it is possible to evaluate the significance of rho for the particular sample size. It should be noted that Spearman's rho may be preferred over the product moment correlation even when the variables being related have distributional properties that depart significantly from normality. For example, the distribution of alcohol consumption among those who regularly drink has a strong positive skew. Rank correlation methods may be preferred in studies of alcohol use because of this nonnormal distribution.

MULTIVARIATE ANALYSIS

Multivariate analysis considers the relationship between combinations of three or more variables. For example, the prediction of number of psychiatric readmissions of schizophrenic patients from the linear combination of age, premorbid adjustment, presenting symptoms, and treatment history would be a problem for multivariate analysis. The field of multivariate analysis is a technical one, and it requires an understanding of linear and matrix algebra. However, a schematic representation of the techniques may help place them into context, and show the basic similarity of approaches that might, at first glance, appear quite different.

Fundamentally, multivariate techniques involve manipulation of matrix data, that is, data organized in columns and rows. The data in columns are called variables and the data in rows, observations. More specifically, multivariate analyses operate on matrix columns.

Figures 5.3-8*A* through 5.3-8*E* illustrate how this family of techniques is related. Figure 5.3-8*A* represents multiple regression. Here, variable y is being predicted from a linear combination (L_x) of variables x_1, x_2, and x_3. In Figure 5.3-8*B*, there are two predictors (x_1, x_2) and also two outcome (dependent) variables (y_1, y_2). This figure illustrates the basis of *canonical correlation*, that is, finding the relationship of the linear combinations of two or more predictors (L_x) and two or more outcomes (L_y) simultaneously. In Figure 5.3-8*C*, there is one outcome (y), but rather than being continuous, it has discrete levels. This figure illustrates *linear discriminant analysis*. In Figure 5.3-8*D*, the predictors x_1 and x_2 are dichotomous, but the outcomes y_1, y_2, and y_3 are continuous—a representation of *multivariate analysis of variance* (MANOVA) with two factors and multiple outcome variables. In Figure 5.3-8*E*, only the relationships among the x variables are being considered, and new linear combinations of these are expressed as the factors L_{x_1} and L_{x_2}. This figure illustrates *factor analysis*.

Clearly, there is a great deal more to multivariate analysis than this set of schematics has considered. The central point, however, is that what distinguishes these techniques is the model being specified more than the statistical theory or computational detail that underlies them. The various methods differ in the number and kind of predictor variables they utilize. They are the same in that they all transform groups of variables into linear combinations. A linear combination of variables is a weighted composite of the original variables. The weighting system combines the variables in order to achieve some goal. The different multivariate techniques differ according to the goal they are trying to achieve.

A linear combination of variables is expressed as:

$$Y' = a + b_1X_1 + b_2X_2 + b_3X_3 + \cdots + b_kX_k$$

TABLE 5.3-5
Appropriate Correlation Coefficients for Relationships Between Dichotomous and Continuous Variables*

Variable Y	Variable X		
	Continuous	*Artificial dichotomous*	*True dichotomous*
Continuous	Pearson r	Biserial r	Point biserial r
Artificial dichotomous	Biserial r	Tetrachoric r	Phi
True dichotomous	Point biserial r	Phi	Phi

*The entries in the table suggest which type of correlation coefficient is appropriate given the characteristics of the two variables. For example, if variable Y is continuous and variable X is true dichotomous, one would use the point biserial correlation.

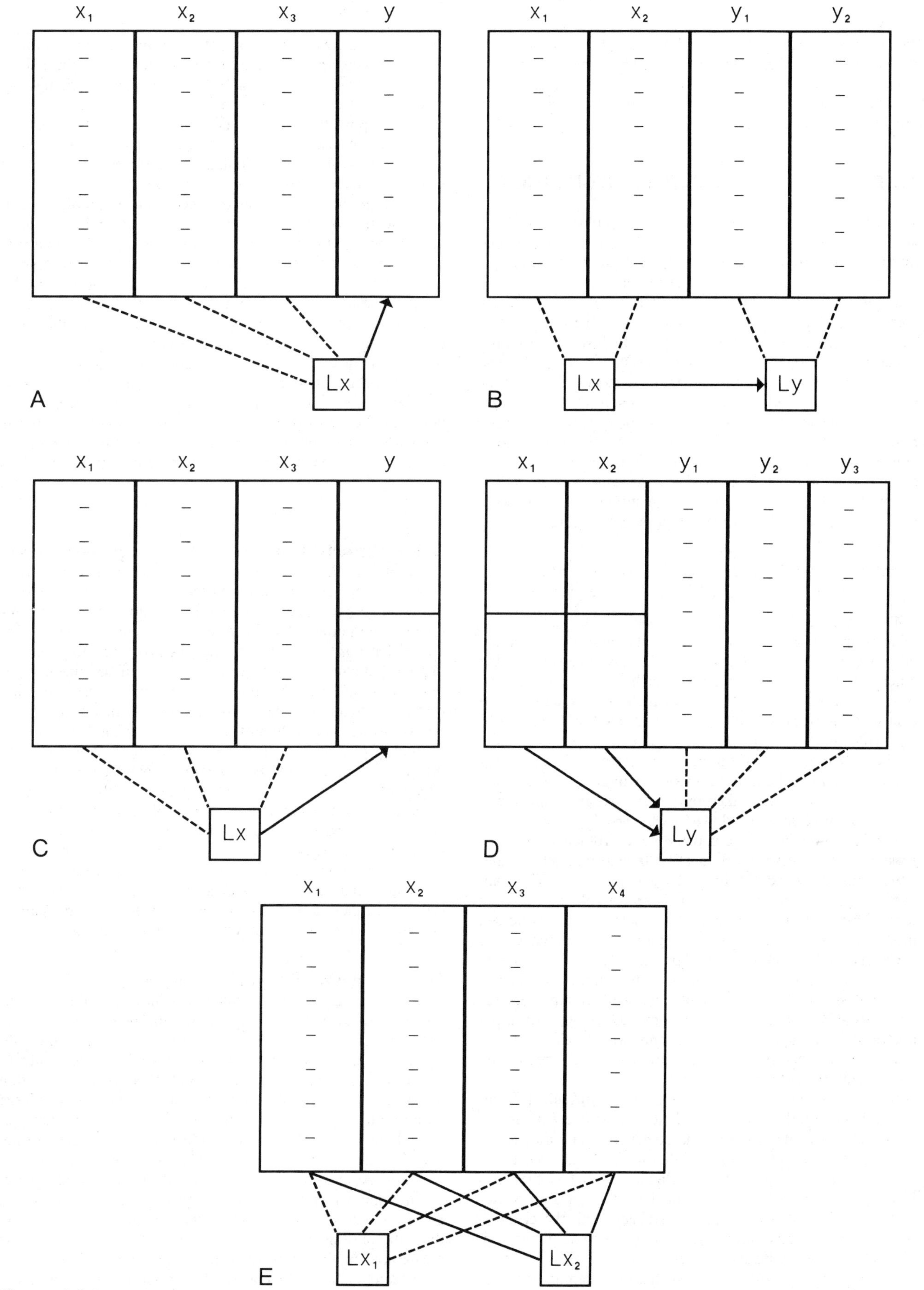

FIGURE 5.3-8. *Schematic representations of multivariate models. (Adapted from Van de Geer:* Introduction to Multivariate Analysis for the Social Sciences. *Freeman, San Francisco, 1971.)*

where Y' is the predicted value of Y, a is a constant, X_1 to X_k are variables and there are k such variables, and the b's are regression coefficients. The entire right side of the equation creates a new composite variable by transforming a set of predictor variables.

AN EXAMPLE USING MULTIPLE REGRESSION

Variables that are important in this combination will be associated with larger regression coefficients. An example using multiple regression might help to illustrate this concept. Suppose the objective is to predict the number of psychiatric hospitalizations from three variables: income, rating by psychiatrists, and age. This type of multivariate analysis is called *multiple regression,* and the goal of the analysis is to find the linear combination of the three variables that provides the best prediction of number of hospitalization episodes. The correlation is found between the criterion (hospital admissions) and some composite of the predictors (income plus psychiatrist rating plus age). The combination of the three predictors, however, is not just the sum of the three scores. Instead, a computer algorithm is used to find a specific way of adding the predictors that will make the correlation between the composite and the criterion as high as possible. A weighted composite might be:

Admissions = 0.3 (Z-scores for income) + 0.6 (Z-scores of psychiatrist ratings) + 0.03 (Z-scores for age)

This example suggests that psychiatrist ratings are given more weight in the prediction of hospital admissions than the other variables. The rating is multiplied by 0.6, whereas the other variables are multiplied by much smaller coefficients. Age is multiplied by only 0.03, which is very close to no contribution. Because any number multiplied by 0 will be 0, age will almost drop out of the equation.

The reason for using Z-scores for the three predictors is that the coefficients in the linear composite will be greatly affected by the range of values taken on by the variables. Income is measured on a scale of dollars, whereas the range in age might be 15 to 70. To compare the coefficients with one another, all of the variables must be transformed into similar units. This task is accomplished by using Z-scores. The standardized coefficients attached to these variable Z-scores are termed β or β weights. When the variables are not expressed in Z units, the coefficients or weights for the variables are expressed in their natural units. For example, if one wanted to find an equation that could be used to estimate someone's predicted level of success on the basis of certain personal characteristics, there would be some advantages to using coefficients that applied to the untransformed values. In this case, the weights in the model are called raw regression coefficients (sometimes called b's).

Interpreting regression coefficients can be difficult. In addition to being a reflection of the relationship between a particular variable and the criterion, the coefficients are affected by the relationships among the predictor variables. When the predictor variables are highly correlated with one another, it is difficult to evaluate their individual coefficients. Two predictor variables that are highly correlated with the criterion will not both receive large regression coefficients if they are highly correlated with each other.

Suppose that income and a psychiatrist's ratings are both highly correlated with readmission. However, these two predictors also are highly correlated with each other. In effect, the two measures seem to be of the same construct (which would not be surprising because the psychiatrist might include income in the overall appraisal). The psychiatrist's rating may receive a lower regression coefficient because some of its predictive power is already taken into consideration through its association with income. This problem is known as multicolinearity. Regression coefficients are most easily interpreted when the predictor variables do not overlap.

The strength of the association between the predictors and the outcome is expressed, as in simple correlation, as a correlation coefficient, usually termed multiple R. Note that the uppercase R is conventionally used in multiple regression rather than the lowercase r typically used in bivariate correlation. Squaring R provides an estimate of the amount of variance in Y explained by predictors X. There are methods for determining the significance of R. It is also possible to compute an "adjusted R" that takes numbers of subjects and variables into account—which is desirable because the replicability of the regression model becomes less likely if there are too many predictor variables in relation to number of subjects from which such observations derive. Generally speaking, as the ratio of subjects to variables begins dropping below 10 to 1, confidence in the replicability of the regression should dwindle.

DISCRIMINANT ANALYSIS Multiple regression is appropriate when the criterion outcome variable is continuous. However, in many cases, the criterion is a set of categories. For example, the question might arise as to what linear combination of demographic, historic, and symptom variables differentiates positive symptom and negative symptom schizophrenic patients. The task would be to find the linear combination of variables that provides a maximum discrimination between categories. One appropriate way to model this problem is through application of linear discriminant analysis. The technique attempts to find that linear combination of predictors that achieves the best separation between positive and negative symptom cases. A chi-square model can be computed to assess the significance of the solution. If an apparently successful classification is achieved, it is important to determine the generalizability of the model through one of several techniques and *cross-validation*. Cross validation is a procedure that requires two separate samples. The discriminant function equation is developed for the first sample and then tested for accuracy in the second sample.

FACTOR ANALYSIS Discriminant analysis and multiple regression analysis are techniques that find linear combinations of variables that maximize the prediction of some criterion. Factor analysis is used to study the interrelationships among a set of variables without reference to a criterion. It might best be thought of as a data-reduction technique. It is often desirable to reduce responses to a large number of items or a large number of tests to more manageable chunks. The task in correlation is to find the best fitting line through the points created by a two-dimensional scatter diagram. As more variables are added in multivariate analysis, the number of dimensions increases. A three-dimensional plot is shown in Figure 5.3-9. Scatter diagrams for more than three dimensions can only be imagined. Consider that points are plotted in the space created in these many dimensions.

In factor analysis, a matrix of correlations between every variable and every other variable is created. Then the linear combinations of the variables that describe as much of the

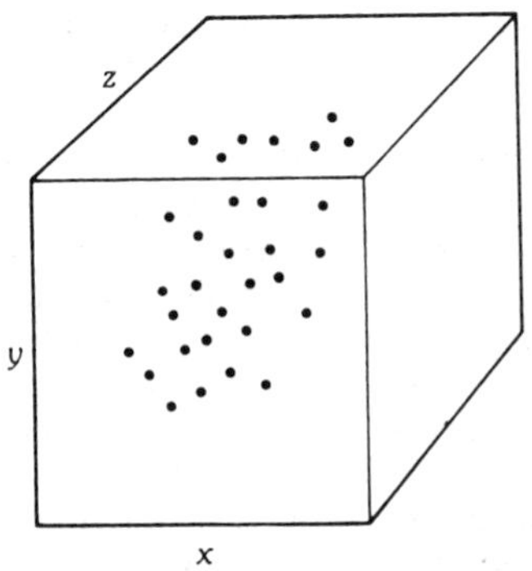

FIGURE 5.3-9. *A three-dimensional scatter plot might be represented by this box. In addition to plotting points on the X- and Y-axes, they must also be located with respect to a third axis, the Z-axis. Although it is difficult to show more than two dimensions on a flat page, a three-dimensional figure can be thought of as a box.*

interrelationships between the variables as possible are obtained. These linear combinations of the variables are called *principal components,* and the goal in creating them is to describe as much of the association between the variables as possible. As many principal components as there are variables can be obtained. However, each principal component is extracted according to mathematical rules that make it independent of or uncorrelated with all of the other principal components. The first component will be the most successful in describing the variation among the variables, and each succeeding component will be somewhat less successful. Typically, only a few components that account for larger proportions of the variation are extracted for further study.

Once the linear combinations or principal components have been found, the correlation between the original items and the factors are obtained. These correlations are called *factor loadings*. The expression "item 7 loaded highly on factor I" means there was a high correlation between item 7 and the first principal component. By examining which variables load highly on each factor, the factors come to be interpreted and named.

Factor analysis is a complex and technical method, and there are many options the user must consider. For example, investigators frequently use methods that help them get a clearer picture of the meaning of the components by transforming the variables in a way that pushes the factor loadings toward the high or low extreme. These transformation methods involve rotating the axes in the space created by the factors, and so have been labeled methods of *rotation*. These rotation methods can improve the scientific utility of the factor solution. There are several options for methods of rotation, and there are other options concerning the characteristics of the matrix that originally is entered into the analysis.

EPIDEMIOLOGICAL MEASURES

A variety of epidemiological measures is commonly used in psychiatric research. Epidemiological studies typically focus on outcomes expressed as morbidity and mortality. Morbidity rates are divided into two major types: incidence and prevalence. Incidence refers to the rate at which new cases are occurring. Incidence is defined as the number of new cases that occur within a specific population within a defined time interval. Typically, the incidence rate is expressed per 1,000 in the population. Conceptually it is

$$\text{Incidence rate per 1,000} = \frac{\text{New cases per unit of time}}{\text{Persons exposed or at risk per unit time}} \times 1{,}000$$

Prevalence rates describe the number of diagnosed cases at a particular point in time.

$$\text{Prevalence rate per 1,000} = \frac{\text{Cases at specific time point}}{\text{Persons in population at specific time point}} \times 1{,}000$$

Prevalence rate is equal to the incidence rate times the duration of the disease. For example, if the average duration of dementia were 5 years and its incidence were three per 1,000 per year, the prevalence would be 15 per 1,000. Epidemiologists often make a distinction between point prevalence and period prevalence. Point prevalence refers to the number of cases at a defined time period, such as the year 1987. Period prevalence is relevant to a time interval. Period prevalence begins with an estimate of prevalence at the beginning of some time period and includes all new cases accumulated until the end of that defined period.

OBSERVATIONAL STUDIES Virtually all research designs common to clinical and experimental research are used in psychiatry and behavioral sciences. Observational studies do not attempt to manipulate variables in a systematic fashion. Instead, inferences are made on the basis of an ongoing series of observations. Some of the most common observational studies include the cohort study, the panel study, and the case-control study.

Cohort study In a cohort study, groups of people who share some common characteristics are followed over the course of time. These studies, which are often prospective, resample the same population of individuals on repeated occasions. However, the participants in the study may not be the same on repeated observations.

Panel study A panel study is similar to a cohort study. However, the panel study has the stricter requirement that the same individuals who were in the original sample are followed at each repeated assessment. An example of a panel study is that conducted by R. and L. J. Jessor. These investigators were interested in alcohol, drug abuse, and deviant behavior among college students. A group of students was evaluated during their first year of college in 1969. The same group was restudied in 1970, 1971, 1972, and 1973. The investigators were able to report, for example, that marijuana use increased between the first and junior years in college. However, it leveled off during the senior year.

Cohort and panel studies are considered to be *longitudinal* designs. Longitudinal studies make inferences about changes over the course of time.

Cross-sectional studies differ from longitudinal studies in that they examine different groups of individuals at the same point in time. To make inferences about drug use in college, for example, the cross-sectional method would require sampling of each current class. Then entering students could be compared with sophomores, juniors, and seniors. These individuals would not be members of the same class or birth cohort.

Case-control study This methodology compares a group of people with a diagnosed disease (cases) with one or more groups that have not been given the same diagnosis. Case-control studies are typically *retrospective* because they make inferences about events that have caused currently diagnosed cases. Longitudinal studies are often *prospective* and have the advantage of documenting antecedents of new cases.

Observational studies often use correlational and multivariate statistical techniques. Variables that are uncontrolled through the experimental design are often adjusted for using statistical methods. In contrast to observational studies in which important variables are not controlled, experimental studies typically involve the systematic manipulation of variables.

EXPERIMENTAL STUDIES Mental illnesses have a natural history, and in most instances their course fluctuates considerably without treatment. One of the difficulties in determining the effects of an intervention is that the intervention may take place at a crisis time. Patients with mood disorder, for example, might seek psychiatric care on days when they are most depressed. If the exacerbation of the illness is self-limiting (as in the case of mood disorders), the patient's condition will improve spontaneously. A control group can help sort out the effects of treatment from other factors. Here, a group receiving the intervention under study is compared with the control group to determine whether there are differences attributable to the intervention.

It is widely accepted among medical and biobehavioral scientists that a control or comparison group is required to establish causal inference. In some cases, investigators are willing to accept quasi-experimental data in which an ad hoc control group is used, or where there is a stable baseline of observations prior to an intervention. However, several authors have argued that an experiment characterized by a single observation, an intervention, and a second observation is virtually impossible to interpret from a causal perspective.

For experiments using control groups, random assignment to treatment and control conditions is desirable. Simply stated, randomized clinical trials remove several sources of bias. The value of randomized clinical trials has been emphasized in a series of review articles. In 1982, H. Sacks, D. C. Chalmers, and H. Smith reviewed six therapies for which approximately equal numbers of randomized clinical trials and nonrandomized trials had been reported in the literature. They found that 79 percent of the studies in which patients were not randomly assigned to groups reported that the therapy was better than the control regimen. In contrast, the same therapies were found to be effective in only 20 percent of the studies in which patients had been randomly assigned to the treatment or control condition. In a related review, Chalmers and his colleagues analyzed 145 papers that were divided into three categories: those in which the randomization process was blinded, those in which the randomization was unblinded, and those in which assignment to treatment or control was by a nonrandom process. Review of these studies suggested a systematic relationship between the rigor of the experimental design and the probability of finding a treatment benefit. There was a significant treatment benefit in 58 percent of the studies in which the subjects were not randomly assigned. The same benefit was observed in 24 percent of the unblinded randomized studies and in approximately 9 percent of the blinded randomized studies.

There are many sources of bias in studies that do not use control groups and the end result is frequently an overestimate of the effects of the therapy under study. These biases are reduced in experimental studies, but the rigor of the experimental design is systematically related to the chances of finding a treatment benefit. Valid scientific inferences must be built on a solid experimental foundation.

ISSUES IN RESEARCH STUDIES

UNRELIABILITY ATTENUATES RELATIONSHIPS

Reliability is the extent to which the test or measure is free of measurement error. Measurement error is the discrepancy between an observed score and the true value for a particular attribute. Under most circumstances, it is assumed that the error is random and independent of the true score. Reliability is estimated in various ways. If the measure is supposed to be stable over the course of time, such as a personality trait, reliability can be assessed by examining the correlation between scores on the same test for the same individuals when the test is administered at two different points in time. Other forms of reliability consider the internal consistency of a test. For example, a measure designed to tap depression may be composed of many items, each of which is an independent assessment of the general depressive attribute. A test is more reliable if responses to these independent items are correlated with one another. Measures of internal consistency, including the Kuder-Richardson 20 and coefficient alpha, are typically correlation-like indexes with ranges from 0 to 1.0. The nearer the reliability coefficient is to 1.0, the higher is the reliability of the test.

The definition of an acceptable level of reliability depends on the purpose of the test. It has been suggested that reliability estimates in the range of 0.70 to 0.80 are high enough for most purposes in basic research. In many research studies, the investigator only needs an approximate estimate of whether two variables are correlated. If the result looks promising, it may be worth the extra time and effort to make the research instruments more reliable. Increasing the reliability beyond 0.90 may increase expense and respondent burden.

In clinical settings, high reliability is extremely important. When tests are used to make important decisions about individual patients, it is essential that classification error be minimized. Thus, a test with a reliability of 0.9 might not be good enough.

A number of procedures are available to increase the reliability of a test. For example, increasing the number of items tends to increase the reliability of a measure. A prophecy formula is available that permits the estimation of the specific number of items that need to be added in order to achieve a defined level of reliability. A second strategy is to factor analyze the items. In this way, homogeneous subsets of items can be obtained. Selection of items from these homogeneous subsets increases the reliability of the test.

The effect of low reliability on correlations has been well documented in the psychometric literature. Observed correlations between two variables are attenuated when either or both variables are measured with error. The expected observed correlation between two variables measured with error is defined as the true correlation times the square root of the product of their reliabilities or

$$r = tr\sqrt{r_{11}r_{22}}$$

where r is the expected observed correlation, tr is the expected true correlation, r_{11} is the reliability of the first measure, and r_{22} is the reliability of the second measure.

Consider the example of the association between a measure of life stress and a measure of social support. The Schedule of Recent Experiences (SRE) has an observed reliability of 0.55. The Arizona Social Support Interview Schedule has an observed reliability of 0.52. Suppose that the true correlation between these measures were a substantial 0.50. However, because each measure contains measurement error, the observed correlation between the two measures would be 0.27. In a study with 50 participants, the investigator would fail to find a significant correlation between these two variables, even though there is a substantial association.

MULTIPLE COMPARISONS It is common in psychiatric research to use multiple outcome measures. Investigators believe that this approach is beneficial because psychiatric outcomes are complex and a multitude of measures are required to capture them. However, the use of multiple measures creates other statistical biases. When multiple comparisons are made, the probability of finding at least one difference by chance increases. At the 0.05 significance level, one significant difference is expected for each 20 independent tests (or 5 percent of all comparisons). Thus, a certain number of significant differences between groups are expected by chance alone. Multiple comparisons problems occur under two circumstances. First, they may be common when the investigator is comparing multiple groups on the same outcome measure. The number of possible comparisons is equal to

$$j\ (j - 1)/2$$

where j is the number of groups.

For example, with six groups, the number of comparisons would be 15. This difficulty is avoided by using such methods as ANOVA with appropriate follow-up tests, such as the Neuman-Keuls Test.

The problem of multiple outcome measures is more difficult to deal with. The probability of finding at least one significant difference among uncorrelated outcome variables by chance is defined as:

$$\text{Probability of 1 or more type I errors} = 1 - (1 - \alpha)^c$$

where c is the number of tests.

As the number of tests increases, the investigator can expect to find more spurious results. For example, the probability of finding at least one spurious statistical difference in five contrasts is 0.23. For 10 contrasts, the probability is 0.40, and for 20 tests, the probability is 0.64. In other words, the chances of drawing the wrong conclusion about the null hypothesis can become quite high when multiple comparisons are performed.

There are several remedies for this situation. One should always be aware of difficulties associated with multiple comparisons tests. To avoid false conclusions, some investigators adjust the significance level to be more conservative. This adjustment is the basis for the Bonferroni inequality, a common procedure to correct for multiple comparisons. Under this procedure, if α were originally set at 0.05, but 10 comparisons were performed, then the adjusted α would be α/N = 0.005, where N was the number of comparisons. However, such adjustments may be problematic because some of the adjustments are so conservative that the null hypothesis is rarely rejected (i.e., a type II error may be introduced). Another approach is to use multivariate techniques that take multiple comparisons into consideration, or to reduce the data set to a smaller number of manageable dimensions. For example, if 20 neuropsychological tests were administered to 200 subjects, factor analysis might be used to reduce the neuropsychological domain to three or four factors.

SAMPLE SIZE ISSUES Generally speaking, there are fewer biases in studies with large sample sizes as compared with studies with small sample sizes, although a large sample size does not ensure that conclusions will be meaningful. Further, many studies with small sample sizes have appropriate internal validity. For studies attempting to estimate prevalence or incidence rates, representativeness is more important than sample size. In a famous case, the *Literary Digest* attempted to forecast the outcome of the 1936 presidential election race between Roosevelt and Landon. The magazine drew its sample from its readers, from automobile registrations, and from telephone directories. In 1936, all of these sources overrepresented the wealthy, most of whom were Republicans. The poll showed that Landon (the Republican) would win by a landslide. The results of the election were just the opposite. Roosevelt won by one of the greatest margins in U.S. history. Thus, survey results are of little value if the sample is not random. There was no problem with the size of the sample in the *Literary Digest* poll, which was very large. In contrast, election day polls using as few as 2,000 respondents to represent all of the voters in the United States have been repeatedly shown to be very accurate. Relatively small samples can be of great value if they are drawn in a random and representative fashion.

Most statistical tests take sample size into consideration. Thus, the probability of rejecting the null hypothesis by chance when the sample size is 10 is 0.05 if the 0.05 alpha level is used. The probability of rejecting the null hypothesis by chance in a sample size of 10,000 is also 0.05 at the 0.05 level. In other words, there is an inherent correction for sample size. It is commonly asserted that studies that reject the null hypothesis but have a small sample size are of little value. However, obtaining a significant difference with a small sample size often requires that the experimental effect is significantly stronger than obtaining the effect at the same alpha level with a larger sample. Thus, demonstrating treatment efficacy with a sample size of 10 per group might require that the treatment effect account for 30 percent or more of the variance in the outcome variable. Obtaining the same significance level with a large sample size, say 300, might only require that 1 or 2 percent of the variance be accounted for.

SELECTIVE BIASES Among the various biases found in psychiatric research, the following are identified as common flaws.

Selective attrition One of the major problems is that many studies involve follow-up of patients, who may be available only on a selective basis. For example, it has been demonstrated that, in treatment studies, those who are available for follow-up are not a representative sample from the original population. It is common for those available for follow-up to be among those who succeeded in the treatment program. This problem can be particularly severe in studies where the loss to follow-up is different for treatment and for control subjects.

Detection bias A common problem in studies of the etiology of disease is that those with the diagnosis may be examined differently than those who have not already been given this label. If at all possible, it is valuable to blind the observers.

EX-POST FACTO DESIGN PROBLEMS One of the most common designs in biomedical research is the case-control study known in the research methodology literature as the ex-post facto design. In these analyses, the investigator already knows that the groups being compared differ in some respect. Typically, individuals who have a diagnosed disorder are compared with a matched group of individuals who have not been placed in the same diagnostic category. The matching occurs for a limited number of variables, and the investigator attempts to determine whether the two groups differ on various prior or current exposures to causal factors. The case-control study is also known as the case-referent study or the case-comparison study design. An example of this design might be a comparison between patients with a diagnosis of paranoid schizophrenia (cases) with people without schizophrenia (controls). Prior history for the two groups might be compared.

In contrast to true experiments, the case-control or ex-post facto method has many deficiencies. In effect, the investigator clearly knows that the two groups differ on at least one variable. The observation that the groups differ on other variables implies relatively little about causation. In effect, these designs represent parallel correlational studies.

Often, in case-control studies, an investigator will match patients on a particular variable or use the variable as a covariate or covariable. If the matching variable or covariate fails to change the difference between the cases and controls, it is assumed that this variable does not explain the underlying basis of the condition. However, there are many rival explanations for the failure of covariables not to explain an observed relationship. One important explanation is that the covariates are measured with error or that the match has been imperfect. To the extent that these problems occur, the effect of adjustment will be greatly attenuated. Thus, the fact that a covariable does not have an effect does not necessarily mean that the covariable is unimportant in the observed relationship.

COMPUTER APPLICATIONS

The availability of computer software has greatly facilitated the execution of most statistical techniques. Statistical software, such as the Statistical Package for the Social Sciences (SPSS) and the UCLA Biomedical Research Package (BMD), have been extensively tested and are highly recommended. In addition, a growing number of well-tested software packages for microcomputers is becoming available. One program, known as SYSTAT, allows many technical operations to be performed on a microcomputer. Such developments, which create easy access to highly sophisticated statistical methodologies, represent both opportunities and dangers. On the positive side, no serious researcher need be concerned about an inability to utilize precisely that statistical technique that best suits the researcher's purpose, and to do so with the kind of speed and economy that was inconceivable just 2 decades ago. The danger is that some investigators may be tempted to employ after-the-fact statistical manipulations to salvage a study that was flawed to start with, or to extract significant findings through the use of progressively more sophisticated multivariate techniques. Such ex-post facto ransacking of data bases does not advance knowledge. Rather, progress in psychiatry will depend increasingly on careful crafting of hypotheses, experimental design, and appropriate statistical modeling.

A brief definition of commonly used statistical terms is listed in Table 5.3-6.

TABLE 5.3-6
Statistical Terms

Analysis of variance (ANOVA): A set of statistical procedures designed to compare two or more groups of observations.

Canonical correlation: A multivariate technique for simultaneously finding the relationship of linear combinations of two or more predictors and two or more outcomes.

Chi-square: A set of statistical procedures used to evaluate the relative frequency or proportion of events in a population that fall into well-defined categories.

Confidence interval: An interval that is likely to capture the population mean with a specified level of confidence. For the 95 percent confidence interval, the chances are estimated to be 95 in 100 that the true mean falls within that interval.

Correlation: A statistical index of the relationship between variables. The most common correlation coefficient is the Pearson Product Moment Correlation. This index of bivariate association varies between −1.0 and 1.0.

Dependent variable: The phenomenon of interest in a research study, often called the outcome variable.

Descriptive statistics: Methods used to summarize, organize, and describe observations. Examples include the mean, standard deviation, and variance.

Discriminant analysis: A multivariate method for finding the relationship between a single discrete outcome and a linear combination of two or more predictors.

Factor analysis: A data reduction technique used to reduce a large number of variables to a smaller number of linear combinations of variables.

Incidence rate: The rate at which new cases of a disease or a condition are occurring. The incidence rate per 1,000 persons in the population is the number of new cases that occur within a defined unit of time, divided by the persons exposed or at risk during the same time unit, multiplied by 1,000.

Independent variable: A variable studied in relation to an outcome or dependent variable. In experiments, the independent variable is controlled by the experimenter.

Inferential statistics: Methods used for drawing general conclusions about probabilities on the basis of a sample.

McCall's T: A specialized standard score with a mean of 50 and a standard deviation of 10.

Multiple regression: A form of multivariate analysis in which a scaled variable is correlated with a linear combination of independent or predictor variables.

Multivariate analysis: Methods for considering the relationship of three or more variables. Multivariate methods include multiple regression, discriminant analysis, canonical correlation, and factor analysis.

Multivariate analysis of variance (MANOVA): A multivariate technique that uses an ANOVA design but includes multiple dependent variables.

Nonparametric: Statistical methods that do not require restrictive assumptions about population distributions.

Null hypothesis: The hypothesis that observed differences or variation in scores can be attributed to random sources. When the null hypothesis is rejected, observed differences between groups are deemed to be improbable by chance alone.

Population: The entire collection of a set of objects, etc., having the same definition.

Power: The probability of rejecting the null hypothesis when, in the real world, it should have been rejected. Power is the probability of identifying a true difference.

Prevalence rate: The number of diagnosed cases of a disease or a condition at a particular point in time. The prevalence rate per 1,000 is defined as the cases at a specific point in time, divided by the number of persons in the population at a specific point in time, multiplied by 1,000.

Probability: A quantitative statement of the likelihood that an event will occur. A probability of 0 means that the event is certain not to occur; a probability of 1.0 means the event will occur with certainty.

Random variable: A variable for which the variation is determined by chance.

Sample: A subset of observations selected from a population.

Standard deviation: The square root of the variance. The standard deviation gives an estimate of the average deviation around the mean.

Standardized or Z-score: The deviation of a score from its group mean expressed in standard deviation units.

t-test: A statistical procedure designed to compare two sets of observations.

Type I error: The error that occurs when the null hypothesis is rejected when it should have been retained.

Type II error: The error that occurs when the null hypothesis is retained when it should have been rejected.

Variance: An estimate of variability. The sum of the squared deviations around the mean, divided by the number of cases.

REFERENCES

Chalmers T C, Celano P, Sacks H, Smith H: Bias in treatment assignment in controlled clinical trials. New Eng J Med *309:* 1358, 1983.

Cook T D, Campbell D G: *Quasi-experimentation: Design and Analysis Issues for Field Studies*. Rand-McNally, Chicago, 1979.

Darlington R B, Carlson P M: *Behavioral Statistics: Logic and Methods*. Free Press, New York, 1987.

Draper N R, Smith H S: *Applied Regression Analysis*. Wiley, New York, 1981.

Jessor R, Jessor L J: *Problem Behavior in Psychosocial Development*. Academic Press, New York, 1977.

Kaplan R M: *Basic Statistics for the Behavioral Sciences*. Allyn & Bacon, Newton, MA, 1987.

Kaplan R M, Sacuzzo D P: *Psychological Testing: Principles, Applications, and Issues*, ed 2. Brooks/Cole, Monterey, CA, 1989.

Kirk R E: *Experimental Design*. Brooks/Cole, Monterey, CA, 1982.

McCall R: *Fundamental Statistics for Psychology*, ed 3. Harcourt, Brace, Jovanovich, New York, 1980.

Marasculio L A, McSweeney M: *Nonparametric and Distribution-free Methods for the Social Sciences*. Brooks/Cole, Monterey, CA, 1977.

Sacks H, Chalmers D C, Smith H: Randomized versus historical controls for clinical trials. Amer J Med *72:* 233, 1982.

Smith M B, Glass G D: *Research and Evaluation in Education and the Social Sciences*. Prentice Hall, Englewood Cliffs, NJ, 1987.

Tabachnick B G, Fidell L F: *Using Multivariate Statistics*. Harper & Row, New York, 1983.

Van de Geer J P: *Introduction to Multivariate Analysis for the Social Sciences*. Freeman, San Francisco, 1971.

CHAPTER 6 THEORIES OF PERSONALITY AND PSYCHOPATHOLOGY

6.1 CLASSICAL PSYCHOANALYSIS

NORMUND WONG, M.D.

INTRODUCTION

Formidable advances have been made in biological and social psychiatry, but psychodynamic psychiatry remains a cornerstone of modern psychiatry. Psychoanalytic theory serves as the bedrock of psychodynamic thinking, offering the most comprehensive and profound understanding of human behavior and experience. Although the theory has expanded and changed considerably since Freud's time, most of his germinal contributions have remained, attesting to their validity and importance.

It must be pointed out here that any synthesis of the innumerable psychoanalytic concepts invariably runs the risk of oversimplification, as well as the possible loss of the nuance and sensitivity characteristic of psychoanalytic thinking. Furthermore, an adequate understanding of these concepts may be impeded by a lack of familiarity with free association, the principal tool of classical psychoanalysis. Whereas most fields of medicine acquire data in a systematic and organized manner, in the study of psychoanalysis, the analysis relies on the patient's spontaneous and uncensored verbal productions. Therefore, in order to become proficient in psychoanalysis, analysts are required to undergo their own analysis, to participate in formal coursework, and to engage in supervised clinical work.

Originally, classical psychoanalysis referred primarily to Freud's libido and instinct theories; today, it has evolved to include concepts from ego psychology, object-relations theory, development psychology, and, most recently, self-psychology. Nevertheless, it continues to be based on the free association method of investigation to yield clinical data and to afford the material from which its key concepts are derived.

BASIC HYPOTHESES OF PSYCHOANALYSIS

As with many theories of personality functioning, psychoanalytic theory seeks to understand the basis of all behavior. It differs from other theoretical schools in that it considers the motivational forces as deriving from unconscious mental processes. The founder of psychoanalysis, Sigmund Freud, elucidated two fundamental hypotheses of psychoanalytic theory—the existence of an unconscious mind and the concept of psychic determinism, or causality. Unconscious mental processes occur with great frequency and are present in normal as well as abnormal mental functioning. Examples of unconscious phenomena may be found in dreams, selective forgetting, errors in everyday life, and posthypnotic events. According to the concept of psychic determinism, nothing happens by chance. Essentially every psychic event is determined by previous ones. Discontinuity does not exist in mental life. These two hypotheses are intimately related, and it is not possible to consider one without the other.

Freud then evolved a third concept that was central to psychoanalytic theory—the mechanism of repression, or the unconscious selective forgetting of events or things that are too painful or objectionable for the conscious mind to acknowledge. Freud developed the concept of repression in connection with his studies of psychopathology, believing that the repression of sexuality was connected with the development of neuroses. But greater and more complex theoretical considerations were to build on this conclusion. Freud observed the development of infantile sexuality and, calling on his knowledge of perversions, he hypothesized that the sexual instinct must follow a complicated developmental sequence that can be subject to fixations and distortions.

A profound thinker, Freud conceptualized a model of mental structure and the economics of mental functioning, as well as its dynamics. Initially, he divided the mind into three regional or topographic areas: the unconscious, the preconscious, and the conscious. Later, dissatisfied with this model, he evolved the structural, or tripartite, model of the ego, id, and superego. In typical fashion, Freud continued to modify and elaborate his concept of the psychic apparatus, mental functioning, and the origins and nature of psychopathology.

HISTORY

SIGMUND FREUD Sigmund Freud was born on May 6, 1856, in Freiburg, a town in Moravia that is now part of Czechoslovakia. When he was 4 years old, his father, a Jewish wool merchant, moved the family to Vienna. Freud lived most of his life there, where he was educated and practiced until fleeing to England in 1938 in the face of Nazi persecution. He died a year later, in 1939.

Medical training During Freud's rather erratic career as a medical student from 1873 to 1881, he was exposed to the teachings of Charles Darwin and his associates and to the investigations of Helmholtz. Thus, emphasis was placed on natural law, the unity of science, and scientific rigor as opposed to the romanticism and the mysticism that prevailed in Europe following the Napoleonic wars. While in medical school, Freud studied in the laboratory of Ernst Brücke, one of the founders of the Helmholtz school of physiology. This scientific movement advocated that the only forces active in biological organisms were the physiochemical forces inherent in matter, which were reducible to the forces of attraction and repulsion. Furthermore, according to the Helmholtz school, all biological organisms were phenomena of the physical world, being systems of atoms, and were governed by physical forces that responded to the principle

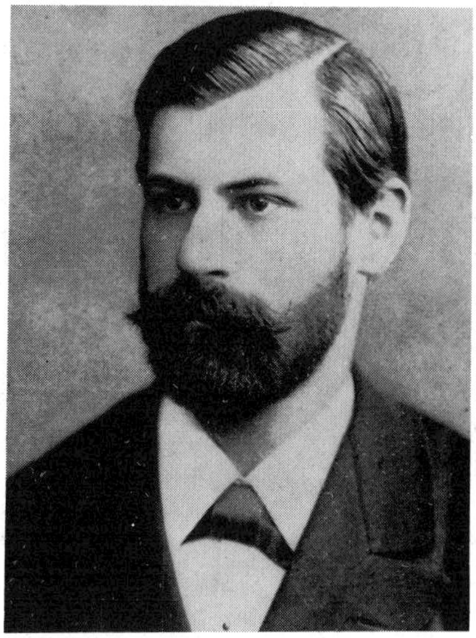

FIGURE 6.1-1. *Sigmund Freud as a young man. (Austrian Information Service, New York.)*

of conservation of energy, which had been postulated in 1842 by Robert Mayer.

Two other of Brücke's assumptions influenced Freud's research. Brücke believed that the mind and body were organized according to the principles of psychophysiological parallelism. He was also convinced that the nervous system had no spontaneous central activity and that the model of neural functioning was the reflex arc. The nervous system functioned mostly as a passive device that remained in a state of rest until it was stimulated by outside energies and reacted in such a way as to keep incoming stimuli to a minimum.

Medical career For a year after his graduation from medical school, Freud continued to work in Brücke's laboratory, developing the physiological framework into which he attempted to place his psychological theories. Throughout his lifetime, Freud tried to apply Brücke's principles to the study of the nervous system and later to the mind. He came to the threshold of a unitary theory of the neuron, a fundamental doctrine that was studied only a few years later by Santiago Ramon y Cajal and Wilhelm Waldeyer.

Despite doing creditable work in histology and neuroanatomy and displaying a liking for research, Freud was forced by financial considerations to leave the laboratory setting in 1892. He joined the staff of the General Hospital in Vienna as a general physician, initially on the surgical service and then in Theodor Meynert's psychiatric clinic. Although Freud shared the general opinion that Meynert was a gifted brain anatomist, he was not impressed with Meynert's skills as a psychiatrist. However, his study of Meynert's amentia (acute hallucinatory psychosis) provided Freud with insight into the mechanism

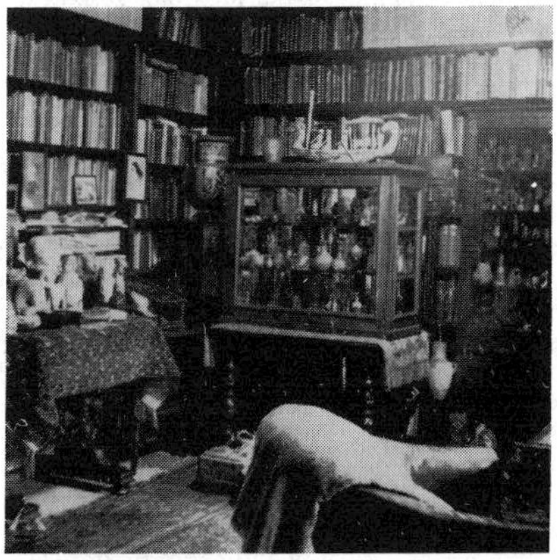

FIGURE 6.1-2. *Sigmund Freud's office in Vienna. (Austrian Information Service, New York.)*

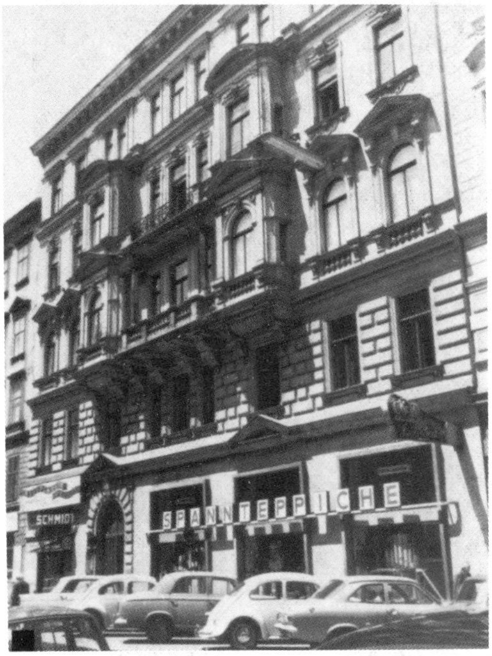

FIGURE 6.1-3. *Berggasse 19, the build in which Freud had his offices and which now houses the Freud Museum. (Austrian Information Service, New York.)*

of wish fulfillment that would become part of his own theory of the unconscious.

Neurological career Freud furthered his knowledge of brain disorders while on Meynert's service, and he received permission to use the laboratory to study the brain of the neonate. As a result of his work there, he decided to specialize in neurology rather than engage in private practice. In 1885, he received a traveling grant and went to Paris to study at the Salpêtrière under Jean-Martin Charcot, the great French neurologist. During his 5 months in Charcot's clinic, Freud observed a wide variety of neurological syndromes. However, at this crucial phase in his career, he was most impressed by Charcot's very

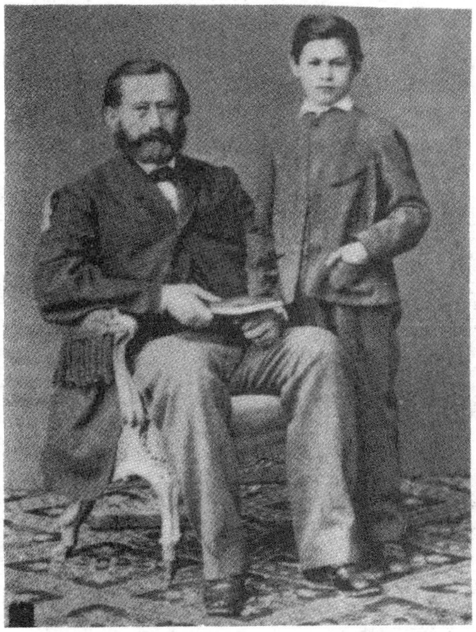

FIGURE 6.1-4. *Sigmund Freud and his father. (Austrian Information Service, New York.)*

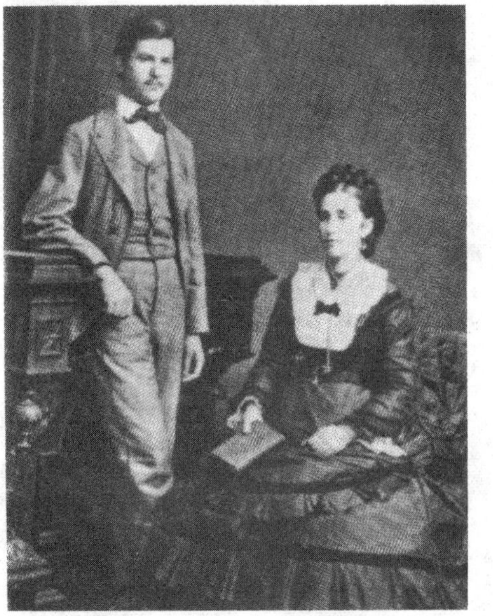

FIGURE 6.1-5. *Sigmund Freud and his mother in 1872. (Austrian Information Service, New York.)*

different and radical approach to hysteria. In contrast with the prevailing thought that hysteria was a conscious pretense, a product of a vivid imagination, or a display of malingering, Charcot regarded hysterical phenomena as reflecting disease of the nervous system and worthy of scientific study.

Charcot offered no psychological explanation for hysterical phenomena other than that the symptoms were of psychogenic origin, although he believed that a congenital degeneration of the brain accounted for the entity. The symptoms, he postulated, were caused by ideas held by the patient and so could be cured by ideas. Freud, however, believed that such phenomena might be psychogenic because hysterical paralyses, seizures, and other symptoms could be induced artificially by hypnotic suggestion.

In 1886, Freud returned to Vienna, determined to devote his time to the clinical practice of neurology. Retaining a deep interest in hypnosis, Freud spent several weeks studying in A. A. Liébault's clinic in Nancy, France. Liébault, a country doctor, was using hypnotic sleep to relieve patients of their neurotic symptoms via suggestion.

Because of his exposure to Charcot's methods, Freud was particularly interested in the work of Hippolyte Bernheim, an associate of

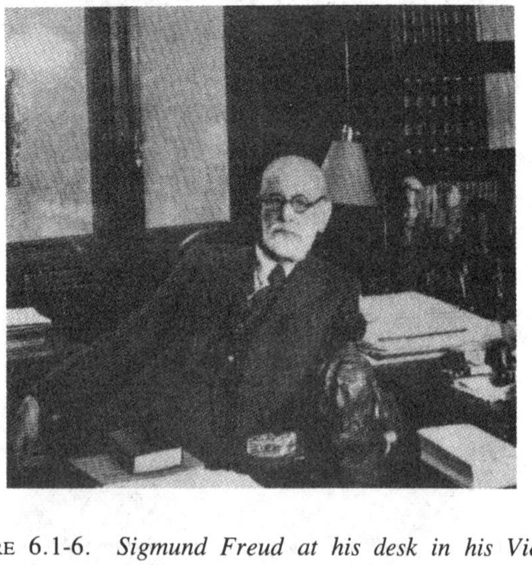

FIGURE 6.1-6. *Sigmund Freud at his desk in his Vienna office. (Austrian Information Service, New York.)*

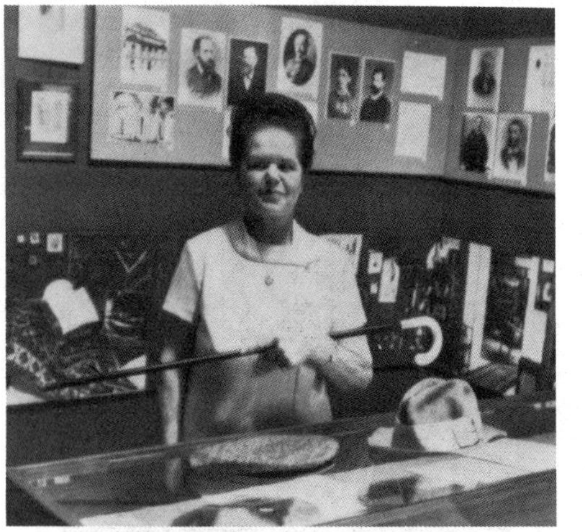

FIGURE 6.1-7. *Mrs. Paula Fichtl, Freud's last maid, with some personal items: hat, cane. (Austrian Information Service, New York.)*

Liébault. Bernheim, using hypnosis as a therapeutic modality, found hysterical phenomena in a wide variety of patients with neurotic disorders and in normal individuals as well. As Freud observed the relationships Liébault established with his patients and the dramatic results Bernheim was able to achieve through the use of hypnotic suggestion, he was struck by the possibility that powerful unconscious processes were operative in human motivation and behavior.

Despite his avowed intentions to give up his laboratory studies, Freud, in 1891, wrote a book titled *Aphasia,* which challenged Wernicke and Lichtheim's localization schemes of this disorder, offering instead a functional hypothesis that explained the subvarieties of aphasic disorders in terms of the radiating associational pathways. In 1891 and 1893, he published two exhaustive clinical reports on the paralyses of children. The first study, which dealt with unilateral paralysis, was written in collaboration with Dr. Oscar Rie, a pediatrician; it is considered a classic and remains widely accepted by neurologists. The second work was a comprehensive study of the central diplegias in children.

The Project During the period 1895 to 1897, Freud embarked on an ambitious plan to try to explain the physical roots of mental phenomena. Greatly influenced by the Brücke-Helmholtz School, he attempted to apply the laws governing physics and chemistry to psychology, also using the theory of neurons that derived from his neurohistological studies. Freud tried to describe the mind in terms of neurons and their synapses.

In his *Project,* Freud explained that the functioning of the nervous system could be described by two closely related principles. First, invoking his principle of inertia, he stated that neurons tend to discharge nervous excitation. According to this principle, pain is related to excessive nervous excitation, and pleasure is a result of its discharge. The primary function of the neuronic system is to discharge excitation that impinges on the nervous system to maintain psychic equilibrium from either internal or external sources. Specific pathways are selected for such discharge.

Freud also felt that the functioning of the nervous system was regulated by the principle of *constancy,* a concept traceable to the principle of the conservation of energy postulated by Mayer and Helmholtz in which the sum of forces remains constant in an isolated system. It was linked to Herbart's hypothesis that mental processes tend to strive for equilibrium, a concept later described by Cannon as homeostasis. In 1892, together with Breuer, Freud derived the following definition of constancy: "The nervous system endeavors to keep constant something in the functional condition that may be described as 'the sum of excitation.' " The principle of constancy was later to serve as the economic foundation for Freud's instinct theory.

Many of Freud's speculations in his *Project* were confirmed by neuropsychological studies, but it proved premature in its attempt to relate mental and psychological phenomena. Freud was too advanced for his time and lacked the instruments and preliminary data necessary to prove his contentions. However, two objectives were achieved through the work on his *Project:* His psychological principle of inertia was later transposed to the psychologically defined pleasure–unpleasure principle, and it demonstrated Freud's deep belief that ultimately his psychological theories would have a biological basis. The impact of his *Project* can also be seen in his work with Breuer in a *Preliminary Communication* (1893), which influenced some of their ideas about hysteria, as well as in *Studies on Hysteria* (1895), which entertained the notions of cerebral excitation and discharge of affect. Finally, in one of Freud's most widely recognized works, the seventh chapter of *The Interpretation of Dreams* (1900), he proposed a model of the mind that had direct connections to the earlier concepts of mental functioning formulated in the *Project*.

EVOLUTION OF PSYCHOANALYSIS

During the decade from 1887 to 1897, psychoanalysis evolved as a method of investigation, a therapeutic technique, and a scientific discipline. The body of knowledge and basic propositions first evolved through Freud's collaborative work with Breuer and then expanded through his own theoretical efforts and investigations.

COLLABORATION WITH BREUER: THE CASE OF ANNA O. During his career as a practicing neurologist, many of Freud's patients presented with psychoneurotic problems rather than neurological difficulties; as a result, he became deeply interested in clinical psychopathology. Joseph Breuer, a distinguished older colleague in the Viennese community with whom he had formed a friendship while working at Brücke's Institute of Physiology, became a decisive influence on Freud. Breuer related the details of his famous case of "Anna O." (Bertha Pappenheim) which he developed during the period spanning from December 1880 to June 1882. This case was one of the bases of the development of psychoanalysis. Freud became convinced of the power of unconscious memories and suppressed affects in the production of hysterical symptoms.

Anna O. was an attractive, highly intelligent woman of 21 years of age who developed a variety of symptoms in connection with the fatal illness of her father, to whom she had been greatly attached. Among these were paralysis of three extremities with contractures and anesthesias, severe disturbances of sight and speech, inability to take in food, and a distressing nervous cough for which Breuer had been consulted. Furthermore, she possessed two distinct states of consciousness: one was fairly normal and the other was that of a naughty and troublesome child. Anna O. effected the transition between these personalities by autohypnosis, which Breuer subsequently supplemented with hypnosis. Anna had shared with her mother the duties of nursing her father until his death. She was able to share with Breuer the intense emotions she had experienced while caring for her father. On one occasion, relating the details of the first appearance of a particular symptom resulted in its complete disappearance, much to Breuer's surprise. Seizing on the value of this experience, Anna O. continued discussing one symptom after another, terming the procedure "the talking cure."

For over a year, Breuer spent hours with this unusual patient. His wife became increasingly resentful and jealous of the time he was devoting to Anna O., which provoked such a strong reaction in Breuer that he abruptly terminated the treatment. Shortly afterward, he was called back to discover that Anna had become as ill as in the beginning. Furthermore, she was now in the throes of an hysterical childbirth (pseudocyesis), the termination of the phantom pregnancy that she had developed in response to Breuer's ministrations. Unnerved by this event, Breuer managed to calm her by hypnotizing her but fled her home in a cold sweat, withdrawing from any further participation in Freud's investigations into the unknown regions of the mind.

FREUD'S TECHNICAL EVOLUTION: USE OF HYPNOSIS When Freud opened his practice in 1887, he began to employ hypnosis extensively with his patients. In the beginning, he used hypnosis to help patients become free of their symptoms by means of hypnotic suggestion. He was frequently disappointed, however, to learn that the symptoms reappeared during the wakening state. Increasingly dissatisfied by the contradiction, superficiality, and ineffectiveness of the hypnotic approach, Freud was eager to learn what lay behind his patients' symptoms.

Intrigued by Breuer's recital of the case of Anna O., he employed the *cathartic method* in conjunction with hypnosis in order to retrace the origin of the symptom. The first time he applied this approach was in 1889 in the case of Frau Emmy von N., a woman about 40 years old who suffered from a variety of hysterical complaints that included mild deliria, hallucinations, anesthesia and pain in her leg, and an ovarian neuralgia. She also manifested alterations of moods, phobias, and abulias. Because he felt that her hysterical phenomena were of traumatic origin, his treatment goal was limited to the removal of symptoms through recovery and verbalization of the suppressed feelings with which they were associated—a method now known as *abreaction*. Also, Freud revealed in his clinical account that inhibited sexuality may have played a role in the origin of the patient's symptoms.

Because the transitory beneficial effects of this approach lasted only as long as the patient had contact with the physician, Freud was dissatisfied. He realized that therapeutic gains depended on the personal relationship between the physician and the patient and that improvement often reversed itself when the relationship was dissolved. His suspicions were confirmed when one of his patients awoke from a hypnotic trance and suddenly flung her arms around his neck. From that point on, he realized that the special relationship that proved so effective therapeutically had an erotic basis; 20 years later, he stated that transference phenomena had always seemed to him to be impregnable proof of the sexual origin of the neuroses. For these and other reasons, Freud became dissatisfied with the use of hypnosis. He believed that hypnosis concealed and prevented the investigation of the transference and resistance phenomena, permitted and even encouraged acting out to please the hypnotist instead of seeking understanding of the origins and significance of symptoms, and worked temporarily at best. In addition, Freud found that many of his patients were refractory to hypnosis. He later attributed this to a reluctance to remember and identified the concept of resistance. Also, he was determined to develop a treatment method that did not rely on whether or not the patient was hypnotizable. When in 1896 he had refined the technique of free association, he was never to employ hypnosis again.

CONCENTRATION METHOD AND DEVELOPMENT OF FREE ASSOCIATION While treating Elisabeth von R., a patient who appeared refractory to hypnosis, Freud recalled a remark by Bernheim that things experienced in hypnosis were apparently forgotten and that at any time they could be recalled if the treater insisted forcibly that the patient knew them. Thus, Freud attempted a concentration technique with the patient requiring her to be on a couch with her eyes closed, concentrate her attention on a particular symptom, and try to recall memories that might reveal the symptom's origin. He exerted pressure on her forehead with his hand and reassured her that some thoughts and memories would come to her when he questioned her. After repeated attempts using this method, the patient brought out what had occurred in her mind but commented, "I could have told you that the first time, but I didn't think it was what you wanted." After this experience, Freud informed patients to ignore all censorship, an early step toward the technique of free association. On yet another occasion, Elisabeth von R. reproached him for interrupting her flow of thoughts with his questions, causing Freud to take yet another step toward the method of free association.

By the late 1890s, Freud had come to realize that the urging, pressing, and questioning that were part of the concentration method disrupted rather than aided the free flowing thought. These procedures were abandoned and eventually patients no longer were requested to close their eyes. However, the use of the couch remains a part of the classical analytic technique.

RESISTANCE Early in his practice, Freud discovered that his patients seemed reluctant or were unable to recall memories that later proved to be etiologically significant. He termed such reluctance, which took place in the treatment setting, "resistance." These initial observations were further supplemented by data derived from his clinical investigations. He found that, in most of his patients, resistance could not be explained by a reluctance to cooperate or by a refusal to follow the rule of free association. In fact, many patients among those most distressed by their illness were the ones most bothered by this phenomenon. Freud concluded that resistance was the result of the pressure of active forces in the mind, of which the patients themselves were often unaware, that excluded from consciousness painful or embarrassing material. He described this active force as repression, one of the fundamental ideas of psychoanalytic theory.

REPRESSION To Freud, repression was at the core of symptom formation. He described its mechanism in the following manner:

> A traumatic experience or a series of experiences, usually of a sexual nature, that had occurred in childhood had been "forgotten" or "repressed" because of its painful or unacceptable nature, but the excitement associated with the incident was not extinguished and traces persist in the unconscious in the form of repressed memories. The memories remain quiescent until revived by a contemporary event, such as a disturbing love affair. At this point, the successful repression fails and the patient experiences what Freud termed "the return of the repressed." The original sexual excitement is reversed and surfaces via a new path in the form of a neurotic symptom. The symptom is a result of a compromise between the repressed desire and the "dominant mass of ideas constituting the ego."

Freud's concepts of resistance and repression grew out of his work during the 1890s with conversion hysteria. He proposed that symptoms arose as a compromise between a repressed impulse and the repressing forces. In cases of hysteria, impulses that were not allowed access to consciousness would be channeled into paths of somatic innervation, producing such symptoms as paralysis, blindness, and disturbances of sensation. Such symptoms as obsessive-compulsive phenomena and even paranoid ideation were seen as compromise formations. Therefore, psychoanalytic treatment during this time focused on helping patients recall repressed sexual experiences so that the excitations attached to them could become conscious and be discharged through verbalization.

THEORY OF INFANTILE SEXUALITY During the 1890s, Freud placed great emphasis on the role of sexual seduction in the etiology of the psychoneuroses, especially when such seduction took place in early childhood and before puberty. He believed that in hysteria, the subject was passive during the sexual trauma, whereas in obsessive neurosis, the subject actively pursued the sexual experience. Up to this point, Freud literally believed the "tales of outrage" committed by fathers, caretakers, and nursemaids, and paid little attention to the child's own psychological life in the elaboration of these tales. Later, he radically shifted his view for reasons not clearly known. However, three reasons have been postulated: (1) He gained additional insight as a result of further investigation into the role of fantasy in childhood. (2) Through his own self-analysis, he came to realize how children can distort reality to conform to their wishes. (3) He may simply have begun to question whether there could be so many seductive and wicked parents in sophisticated Vienna. In a letter to his friend Wilhelm Fliess, in September 1897, he shared his doubts about the reports of seduction by his patients and suggested how sexual fantasies regularly involved the theme of parents.

This new insight proved depressing to Freud, who had struggled intensively to prove the seduction hypothesis on which his theories were based. He was able to see the new possibilities for the study of psychological factors. A dynamic theory of infantile sexuality in which the child's psychosexual life occupied a dominant role was to replace the static concept, which portrayed the child as an innocent victim whose eroticism was prematurely disrupted by seductive adults. Psychoanalysis had taken a new direction, coming into its own as a depth psychology. In the course of its early evolution, Freud, its founder, had turned to the study of dreams, struggled with his self-analysis, proposed a theory of the mind, originated studies of infantile sexuality, and examined the origins and nature of the neuroses. The period of initial exploration was brought to an end, and psychoanalysis as it is known today was beginning.

THERAPEUTIC AND THEORETICAL CONTRIBUTIONS Within the span of a decade, the fundamental concepts of psychic determinism and the operation of a dynamic unconscious were laid out. A theory of psychoneurosis based on psychic conflict and on the repression of memories of traumatic childhood experiences was established, and the important role of childhood sexuality in the production of psychological symptoms was revealed. Of paramount importance, the technique of free association was developed, a technique applicable to a wide range of mental phenomena that were poorly understood before Freud's discovery. Freud realized that the applications of psychoanalysis need not be restricted to the study of psychopathological conditions, and that it provided an approach to the study of dreams, creativity, wit, and other phenomena encountered in normal life.

FRAMEWORK OF PSYCHOANALYTIC THEORY

In essence, psychoanalytic theory is divided into the theory of the instincts, or drives, and the psychic apparatus that deals with the instincts. The *source* of the instinct refers to the part of the body from which it arises, to the somatic process that gives rise to stimuli that are represented in mental life as affects, or drive representations. The *impetus*, or pressure, refers to the amount of force or energy created by the instinctual stimulus. The *aim* refers to the action-directed tension release or to the achievement of satisfaction. Finally, the *object* is the recipient, either person or thing, of the satisfaction-seeking action that enables the instinct to discharge the tension and gain instinctual pleasure.

THEORY OF INSTINCTS

In the beginning, Freud unceasingly attempted to maintain psychoanalytic theory on a firm biological foundation, but the lack of scientific data and the inadequacy of scientific investigative tools induced him to abandon his efforts. His theory of the instincts, however, represents one of his most important attempts to link psychological and biological phenomena; for Freud, instincts bridged the mental and organic spheres. His use of the term "instinct" is not always consistent. For example, Freud used the term "libido" both to refer to the somatic process underlying the sexual instinct and to denote its psychological representation. Some of the confusion may stem from the fact that the German *Triebe* cannot be accurately translated into English. *Triebe* are defined as powerful, imperative strivings, such as sexuality and self-preservation, within living organisms that are rooted in their physical nature. On the other hand, instinct, in the Darwinian sense, implies innate inherited, unlearned, biologically useful behavior. Thus, Freud's *Triebe,* which has been variously translated as instinct, drive, or instinctual drive, should not be confused with the word "instinct" as it applies to zoology.

The clearest definition of *Triebe* appeared in Freud's 1915 paper "Instincts and Their Vicissitudes," in which he stated, "An 'instinct' appears to us as a concept on the frontier between the mental and the somatic, as the psychical representative of the stimuli originating within the organism and reaching the mind, as a measure of the demand made upon the mind for work in consequence of its connection with the body." Although instinct plays a distinctive role in psychoanalytic theory, the relationship between psychological and somatic processes is still unclear and difficult to elucidate. Psychoanalysis must restrict its theoretical constructs to the psychological parameters of human behavior. Thus, attention has been shown to the work of ethologists, such as Lorenz and other researchers in animal behavior, in efforts to learn more about instincts.

CLASSIFICATION OF INSTINCTS

During the early years of psychoanalysis, the development of instinct theory was closely related to the clinical phenomena that Freud was investigating. His dualistic classification of the instincts was postulated from the beginning. Although he proposed an instinct of self-preservation in the 1890s, Freud was primarily concerned with the sexual drive, reflecting his preoccupation with the role of sexual factors in the origins of hysteria and the psychoneuroses. As psychoanalytic theory continued to evolve, the relationship between the instincts and his clinical findings became further separated. In his classification of the life and death instincts, for instance, Freud was preoccupied with abstract forces in nature but he did not support his concepts with clinical evidence.

Ego instincts Until 1910, Freud's predominant interest was in the sexual basis of the neuroses, and he paid little attention to the self-preservative or ego instincts. However, his growing interest in the phenomena of self-love or narcissism resulted in a greater emphasis on the ego instincts. He saw narcissism as an essentially libidinal instinct and called the remaining aspects ego instincts, which were regarded as nonsexual and devoted to self-preservation. The ego instincts were also considered to be associated with repression. In addition, Freud believed that mental conflict could produce symptom formation and neurosis and resulted from the clash between libido, or the sexual instinct, and the ego, or the nonsexual instincts. This conception was not abandoned until he had developed a comprehensive theory of the mental structures, particularly the ego and the mechanisms of defense.

Libido Freud regarded the sexual instinct as a psychophysiological process that had both mental and physiological manifestations. He used the term *libido* to refer to "that force by which the sexual instinct is represented in the mind." The sexual instinct did not originate in finished form, as is seen in the stage of genital primacy; it undergoes a complex process of development during which it manifests itself in a number of ways other than through sexual union. The libido theory refers to the investigation of all of these manifestations and the paths they follow during the course of development. Infantile sexuality exemplifies the many facets of libidinal expression.

Aggression Initially, Freud thought of aggression in terms of sadism, which he defined as one of the sexual components or instincts that are evident during each phase of psychosexual development. Because there are nonsexual aspects of sadism as well, he originally included sadism among the ego instincts to explain the impulse to attack in order to defend oneself. It was only further along in his thinking that Freud realized that sadism has both sexual and nonsexual aspects. To resolve this difficulty, he differentiated between aggression and hate, and he assigned these to the ego instincts, and he placed the libidinal aspects of sadism with the sexual instinct. Sadism could also be regarded as a fusion of the sexual and aggressive instincts, as in the case of thwarted desire with its admixture of love and hate.

Freud had problems with the explanation of the self-destructive elements in depressed patients, the self-inflicted injuries in his masochistic patients, and the aimless, destructive behavior normally exhibited by small children. Because these aggressive impulses did not satisfy the criteria for ego instincts, he was forced to conceive of aggression as a separate instinct in *The Ego and the Id* in 1923. The source of the instinct, he said, is largely in the skeletal muscles and the aim of aggression is destruction. The aggression that appears in response to frustration of libido is secondarily provoked.

This new formulation of aggression reflected Freud's disappointment about the inherent goodness of humans, and also stimulated his thinking about the role of aggression in mental disorders and how aggression became neutralized or detoxified. These processes were left to Heinz Hartmann and Robert Waelder to explain 40 years later.

Life and death instincts In 1920, Freud introduced his theory of the dual life and death instincts, eros and thanatos in *Beyond the Pleasure Principle*. This classification of instincts is decidedly more abstract and has broader applications than his concepts of libido and aggression. The life and death instincts were regarded as the forces underlying the sexual and aggressive instincts. Although the death instinct was, in itself, not clinically verifiable, Freud felt that it could be demonstrated by clinical phenomena through the *repetition compulsion* or the tendency of individuals to repeat past behavior despite the suffering associated with such behavior.

He defined the term *death instinct* as the tendency of organisms to return to an inanimate state. *Eros*, or the *life instinct,* referred to the tendency of particles to reunite, or for parts to bind to one another, to form greater unities. Freud offered sexual reproduction as an example. The death and life instincts were analogous to catabolism and anabolism. And because the ultimate destiny of all biological matter, except for the germ cells, is to return to an inanimate state, Freud considered the death instinct to be the dominant force. Even today, Freud's death instinct has been most severely criticized. One of the major criticisms is that although all cells eventually deteriorate and die, it is a large step to draw from that the conclusion that the total organism prossesses a drive or instinct toward death.

PLEASURE AND REALITY Early in his career, Freud believed that the instincts were governed by regulatory principles that pertained to all internal and external stimuli affecting the organism. In 1895, in his *Project,* he called attention to the constancy principle, that is, the tendency of the organism to maintain a particular level, or state, of equilibrium. This concept, along with the death instinct, was related to the *Nirvana principle,* which proposed that the organism strives to discharge internal tension and to seek a state of rest. In 1911, he described two basic principles of mental functioning that grew out of the need to maintain a state of equilibrium, and which he termed the pleasure and the reality principles. These principles may be readily observed in clinical phenomena.

The *pleasure principle* is considered to be inborn and refers to the tendency of the organism to avoid pain and to seek pleasure through the discharge of tension. It persists throughout life, is modified by the reality principle, and requires the delay or postponement of immediate pleasure or gratification, with the aim of achieving even greater pleasure in the end. The *reality principle* is a learned function that is closely related to the maturation of the ego functions. As such, it may be impaired during ego development, resulting in the production of various mental disorders.

INFANTILE SEXUALITY

In 1905, Freud's *Three Essays on the Theory of Sexuality* appeared, in which he introduced his ideas about the development of sexuality. Contrary to common belief, Freud's notions did not cause an uproar, as Vienna at the time was exposed to a great deal of popular literature that dealt with a wide range of sexual problems. However, it was Freud's exposition concerning the development of sexuality in children that even today is unacceptable to many people.

Basically, Freud used the term "sexuality" to refer not only to the erotic life of the individual, but also to cover those activities and sensations that are pleasurable and afford sensual gratification. He formulated a developmental theory of childhood sexuality from his investigations into the actual neuroses (hypochondriasis, neurasthenia, and anxiety), which highlighted the importance of sexual factors in their etiology, and from his self-analysis, which he began in 1897. He concluded that these phenomena were not restricted to neuroses, but that individuals in the normal course of development underwent the same sequence.

Freud observed that infants exhibit erotic activity from birth and, in brilliant fashion, he described for the first time the different stages of development during the first 4 years of life. The fifth year marks the beginning of the latency period, when sexual development seemingly comes to a stop until the child reaches puberty at approximately 11 years of age. Then there is rapid growth of the genital organs, with an accompanying resurgence of the sexual drive, and the child begins final preparations for the adult sexual role.

PSYCHOSEXUAL DEVELOPMENT As described by Freud in *Three Essays on the Theory of Sexuality,* the earliest manifestations of infantile sexuality are basically nonsexual, arising in relation to such bodily functions as feeding and bowel and bladder control. Each of these stages of development were thought to build on and subsume the accomplishment of the preceding phases—the oral, the anal, and the phallic. The oral phase occupies the first 12 to 18 months of the infant's life, followed by the anal phase to about 36 months; the phallic phase takes place from ages 3 to 5.

Erotic activity in the phallic phase is initially linked with urination. The urethral phase was only briefly touched on by Freud but was elaborated on by later writers. Infantile urethral eroticism is closely interwoven with pregenital eroticism. Because the differences between sexes often become apparent during urination, urethral eroticism may appear in combination with the castration complex. During the urethral phase, the primary eroticism is pleasure in urination, as well as a secondary urethral-retention pleasure with resulting conflicts revolving around it. Although the original aims of urethral eroticism are autoerotic ones, they may be turned toward objects with sexually exciting fantasies about urinating on objects or being urinated on by objects. Shame is frequently the specific counterforce directed against urethral-erotic temptations, whereas ambition, described as an outcome of these conflicts, represents the fight against such shame.

In boys, Freud postulated that phallic erotic activity is a preliminary stage for adult genital activity. In males, the penis remains the principal sexual organ throughout the course of psychosexual development, but the female has two principal erotogenic zones—the vagina and the clitoris. Freud felt that during the infantile genital period, the clitoris was the chief erotogenic focus but that after puberty, erotic primacy was transferred to the vagina. Recent sexual studies have questioned the validity of the primacy of the vagina although classic analysts still retain this view.

Karl Abraham, one of Freud's followers, made valuable contributions to the basic psychosexual stages. The oral period was divided into a sucking and biting phase; the anal phase into an anal-sadistic and an anal-erotic phase; and the phallic period into an earlier phase of partial genital love, the true phallic phase, in contrast with the later mature genital phase.

Throughout each of the psychosexual stages, there were said to be specific erotogenic zones, which, on stimulation, gave rise to erotic pleasure. From his clinical investigations, Freud postulated the existence of three additional phases of genital masturbatory activity—during early infancy, during the phallic phase, and again during puberty.

VICISSITUDES During the child's earliest years, the mucous membranes of the mouth, anus, and external genitalia become the appropriate primary focus of the child's erotic life. This focus varies depending on the phase of psychosexual development, but in normal adults, sexual activity ultimately is dominated by the sexual zone. Nevertheless, the pregenital erotogenic functioning of the oral and anal zones continues to play a role in sexual activity, specifically during foreplay. Stimulation of these zones elicits pleasure that precedes coitus. In normal adults who have attained mature genital potency, the sexual act culminates in the pleasure of orgasm.

The erotic impulses arising from the pregenital zone were described by Freud as component or part instincts. Examples of activities associated with these part instincts are kissing, stimulating the area surrounding the anus, or even biting the love object during lovemaking. There may be displacement of genital excitement to the eyes, and looking and being looked at (scoptophilia) may become the prime focus of pleasure. Normally, in the course of development, the component instincts are repressed or serve a restricted role in sexual foreplay.

Ordinarily, the total sexuality of the young child is undifferentiated and encompasses all of the part instincts (polymorphous perverse sexual instincts). But in the normal adult, these part instincts usually become subordinate to the primacy of the genital region. If this process does not take place, psychopathology may result. And if the libido becomes too attached to one of the pregenital erotogenic zones or a part instinct becomes predominant, the result may be a perversion—such as fellatio or voyeurism—which would replace the normal act of intercourse. The persistent attachment of the sexual instinct to a particular phase of pregenital development is known as *fixation*.

NEUROSIS AND PERVERSION Freud discovered that in the psychoneuroses, only a limited number of normal sexual impulses are repressed, and the repression is responsible for neurotic symptoms. Usually, the repressed impulses are the same impulses as in the perversion except that they are expressed overtly. Thus, he regarded the neuroses as the negative of perversions. However, the situation proved more complex. Freud could not explain why a part instinct might become repressed and provoke a neurotic symptom response in one individual whereas in another it would become overt and produce a perversion. Although the theory of sexuality described the various zones of libidinal stimulation and excitement, it could not explain the outcome of a fixation for a given person. The answer to this problem had to await the further development of analytic theory, such as the elucidation of defense mechanisms, the functions of the ego and superego, and the nature and role of anxiety in mental functioning.

DEVELOPMENT OF OBJECT RELATIONS

Psychoanalysis has focused increasing attention on the importance of early disturbances of object relationships in later psychopathology. Disturbances in the relationship between the child's affect and the significant objects in the environment, especially the mothering object, have long-lasting and profound effects. Freud proposed the basic notion of an object relationship being intimately connected with the functioning of the sexual instinct. Drive discharge and object attachment are closely interwoven aspects of instinctual phenomena. He made constant reference to the significance of the relationships children had with crucial figures in the environment. Furthermore, he firmly believed that the choice of a love object in adult life, the nature of the love relationship, and object relationships in other areas would depend largely on the nature and quality of the child's object relationships during the early formative years of life.

DURING PREGENITAL PHASES Current research on neonates has demonstrated that they respond selectively to stimuli and prefer complex instead of simple patterns of stimulation. Infants seek sensory stimulation, have distinct biases or preferences with regard to sensations, and appear to be constantly evaluating their world. However, at the beginning of life, infants do not respond specifically to objects. Before they can distinguish between their own impressions and those derived from external objects, their perceptual and cognitive apparatuses must attain a certain level of development and a greater degree of differentiation of sensory impressions and integration of cognitive patterns.

The helplessness in human infants continues longer than in any other species. Unless they are cared for by external caretaking objects, they cannot survive or obtain relief from the painful disequilibrium of inner physiological states. Only when infants can begin to grasp the fact of their separate existence can object relationships of the most primitive kind begin to be established. In the beginning, infants cannot distinguish between their own lips and their mothers' breasts, nor can they associate the satiation of hunger pangs with the presentation of the extrinsic breast. The infant's responses to noxious and pleasurable stimuli are relatively undifferentiated early in life. Current research shows that by the age of 8 weeks, the infant experiences many affects, such as joy, interest, distress, and perhaps surprise and anger. By 2 to 3 months of age, the infant can recognize and expect a characteristic constellation of events.

In classical psychoanalytic theory, infants are believed to be aware only of their inner tension and relaxation, are unaware of the external object, and long for the object only to the extent that the disturbing stimuli persist and the yearning for satiation is unsatisfied in the absence of the object.

ORAL PHASE The infant first becomes aware of external objects through the experience of unsatisfied need along with the experience of frustration in the absence of the breast and the need-satisfying discharge of tension from the presence of the breast. The first psychological awareness of an object arises from the longing for a familiar experience that provides gratification of most needs but happens not to be immediately available. Tension and hunger force the recognition and acceptance of an outside world and the first awareness of reality. The infant judges reality in terms of something that provides satisfaction by being swallowed, or, if it produces tension, by being spit out.

The mother becomes recognized as the source of nourishment and the provider of the erotogenic pleasure that the infant obtains from sucking. She becomes the first love object. The child's focus, during the oral phase, on successive erotogenic zones with the emergence of associated partial instincts will influence the attachment to crucial figures in the environment and the feelings of love and hate toward them. A basically nurturing and warm bond between mother and child during the oral stage sets the stage for trusting and affectionate relationships with others in later life.

Mishaps that may occur during the oral phase may cause later impairment of object relations. Such mishaps include rejection by the mother, undue frustration experienced by the infant, and distortions in the early mother–child relationship.

Sucking and biting The oral stage has been further subdivided into a sucking and a biting phase. Fixation on biting at this point may manifest itself as excessive dependency and cannibalistic impulses toward objects. Early in the infant's life, there is both a biological bond to the mother and a psychological relationship. First to develop is the biological tie between mother and child that satisfies the child's physiological needs. Most analysts feel that the psychological component of the mother–child dependence may take many months to develop and requires some differentiation between self and object in the child's experience. The primitive affective responses of pleasure and unpleasure appear to many to be states of physiological homeostasis rather than an affective response to an object as a separate entity. The oral phase is generally regarded as occupying the first year and a half of life.

From an object-relations perspective, Margaret Mahler has named the first phase of psychobiological development the autistic phase, in which the infant basks in a state of absolute primary narcissism and is unaware of the mother. The predominant feeling of the infant is one of self-contained pleasure, which lasts only as long as there is a lack of differentiation between self and object. The task of the autistic phase, according to Mahler, is to achieve homeostatic equilibrium of the infant within the new extramural environment using predominantly somatopsychic mechanisms.

A stage of dim awareness that need satisfaction cannot be provided by the self but must come from outside the self signals the beginning of Mahler's symbiotic phase, which occurs between 2 and 6 months of age. During this period, the infant behaves and functions as though the infant and mother are an omnipotent system and essentially a dual unity within a common boundary. These boundaries are temporarily differentiated in the state of affect hunger but disappear again with need gratification. Gradually, the child forms more stable part images of the mother, such as breasts, face, and hands. Only when the specific or whole object becomes important to the child as a need-satisfying function can one regard the child as developing beyond the level of need-satisfying relationships and toward the attainment of object constancy. It should be emphasized that from the perspective of infantile sexuality or psychosexual stages of development, the oral phase is primarily focused on libidinal drive and stresses the predominance of the oral zone as the main erotogenic zones, whereas Mahler's object-relations perspective, or concept of need-satisfying relationships, is not so concerned with drive development but rather with the characteristics of object involvement and object relationships.

ANAL PHASE Whereas the infant is relatively passive during the oral phase of development, with the onus on the mother to satisfy demands, the child is expected to accede to the demands of toilet training during the anal period. The task is both complicated and pleasurable; initially, there is the pleasurable sensation of excretion, and later, there is the erotic stimulation of the anal mucosa through retention of the fecal mass.

A connection between anal and sadistic drives is evident during this period. The object of the anal-sadistic activity is the feces, whereas the "pinching off" is regarded as the sadistic act. In psychopathology, people may treat others as they previously treated feces. The sense of power over the environment that evolves from sphincter control represents another sadistic element. Often, in the struggle for cleanliness, the child exercises power over the parents by either giving up or refusing to give up feces.

Because elimination and pleasurable retention do not require assistance from an outside object, the initial anal strivings are autoerotic. Thus, during this state of development, the act of defecation is invested with a sense of omnipotence; the feces, which represent the producer of pleasure, become libidinized. Although external, they represent part of what was once the child's body. The feces become an ambivalently viewed object with the child tending to reintroject what was once eliminated. On the one hand, the feces are loved and retained or reintrojected; on the other, they are hated and pinched off.

The object strivings during the anal phase may be altered when pleasurable anal sensations are influenced by objects in the external environment. The stimulation associated with diaper changes and cleansing of the anal area and conflicts over toilet training exert a significant influence. The ambivalence associated with the feces in conjunction with early external influences may instill compulsive neatness in patients who regress to this pregenital phase. Obsessive-compulsive individuals who are fixed at this stage characteristically have the need to dominate and are rigid and pedantic. Their feelings are characterized by ambivalence, with simultaneous wishes to control and retain the object and to expel and destroy it. The anal phase traditionally takes place between the ages of 18 and 36 months.

During approximately the same time, Mahler's third developmental period, that of the separation and individuation phase, is still evolving. During the first or differentiation subphase, the child gradually differentiates from the symbiotic matrix, with the first signs apparent at 4 or 5 months of age, and is described as "hatching" from the symbiotic matrix. With further differentiation and separation from the mother, the second, or practicing, subphase of the separation and individuation phase begins. The early practicing period appears at about the age of 7 months, when the infant develops the ability to move physically away from the mother by crawling, creeping, or climbing. However, leaving the protective orbit of the mother creates risks and uncertainties, and frequently the infant adopts the pattern of visually "checking back to mother" and returning for physical contact in the form of "emotional refueling."

In the practicing period proper, at approximately 10 to 18 months of age, the toddler has attained free upright locomotion. Three other interrelated developments are also noticeable—rapid body differentiation from the mother, the establishment of a specific bond between mother and child, and the growth and functioning of autonomous ego apparatuses and dependence on the mother. By the middle of the second year (from about the ages of 15 to 22 months), the child has entered the third, or rapprochement, subphase. The danger or crisis in the rapprochement subphase is that of separation anxiety. Although seeking to be separate, autonomous, and omnipotent, the child becomes aware of the need for and dependence on the mother. Thus, ambivalence is characteristic of the middle part of the rapprochement subphase. The mother's availability and reassurance of her continuing love and support are crucial as the child seeks to become more independent. When the aims of the rapprochement subphase have been attained, the child enters the fourth and final phase of the separation and individuation process.

The fourth, or consolidation, phase (from 18 to 36 months of age) is characterized by emotional object constancy with significant development in the structuralization and integration of the ego and internalization of parental demands reflecting the development of superego precursors.

PHALLIC PHASE The phallic phase ushers in the beginnings of the oedipal level of development, the completion of the work of separation-individuation, and the attainment of object constancy. Object constancy is characterized by the capacity to differentiate between objects and to maintain a meaningful relationship with a specific object whether or not one's needs are satisfied. It implies the stability of object cathexis and the capacity to maintain positive emotional attachments to an object in the face of frustration of needs and wishes. Ambivalent feelings toward the particular object can be tolerated and the object is valued for qualities it possesses beyond its need-gratifying functions. When object constancy has been attained, complex and significant internal developments have taken place concerning the consolidation of relatively autonomous ego functions and their harmonious integration with drive derivatives.

Furthermore, in contrast to the pregenital phases of development where the child's libidinal activity is mostly autoerotic, or where sexual impulses are directed toward the child's own body, the fundamental task of finding a love object occurs in the phallic or genital period, at which time the pattern for later object choices is established.

OEDIPUS COMPLEX

The Oedipus complex occurs during the third to fifth years, as the sense of gender identity becomes consolidated and the child realizes the significance of anatomical sexual differences. Events at this time set the stage for the predisposition of the adult psychoneuroses. The Oedipus complex represents the climax of the development of infantile sexuality. Early in his studies of the unconscious mind, Freud discovered in his patients and in his own self-analysis regularly recurring fantasies of incest with the parent of the opposite sex and jealousy and murderous rage directed against the parent of the same sex. Drawing an analogy between such fantasies and the Greek legend of Oedipus, who unknowingly killed his father and married his mother, Freud called the constellation the Oedipus complex.

CASTRATION COMPLEX In normal circumstances, the Oedipus complex in boys is resolved by the castration complex; oedipal strivings are relinquished because of castration anxiety. However, a girl already lacks a penis, and as a result, she turns to her father because of his possession of one. Instead of fearing castration, the little girl is more distressed by the fear of the loss of love.

Resolution for boys Boys evince a strong erotic interest in the mother, with a concomitant wish to possess her exclusively. Such feelings become manifest around the age of 3 and reach a climax in the fourth or fifth year of life. Not surprisingly, the boy becomes greatly enamored with his mother; he wants to sleep with her, proposes marriage, and takes advantage of any opportunity to see her naked. He cannot tolerate any competition for his mother's affection, and particularly wants to eliminate his chief rival, her husband and his father. However, fearful of anticipated retaliation for aggressive wishes toward his father, he develops anxiety. Specifically, he begins to feel that if he continues to show interest in his mother, his penis may be removed. In *The Passing of the Oedipus Complex,* Freud identified the thought of losing the penis in this situation as the castration complex. He suggested that the narcissistic concern over losing the penis superseded the erotic attachment to the mother. To gratify his wishes to possess his mother would endanger his penis. The anxiety evoked by his aggressive desires toward his father finally causes the boy to renounce his oedipal love for his mother. In turn, the boy comes to identify with his father, and he incorporates his father's prohibitions. In the process, the boy internalizes the castration complex, until it is reactivated at puberty.

A boy's feelings toward his parents are far from simple; at times, he may love his father and hate his mother, especially when frustrated by her. He may also love or hate both parents. Because of the bisexual nature of the libido, the situation may become very complex. Whereas the boy may wish to kill his father, his archrival, and possess his mother, he may resent his mother's demands on his father and her interference with the father–son relationship. A negative Oedipus complex may arise when the boy's love for his father prevails and hatred for his mother occurs for disturbing the father-son relationship. Both the negative Oedipus complex, to some degree, and the more familiar positive orientation are normally present.

Resolution for girls For a girl, the resolution of the Oedipus complex is more complicated. Like the boy, the girl forms an initial attachment to her mother, who fulfills her vital needs. But unlike the boy who retains the mother as his predominant love object throughout life, the girl must shift the primary attachment from her mother to her father in order to prepare herself for her future sexual role. The girl's renunciation of the preoedipal attachment to the mother cannot be explained simply as a consequence of ambivalence or aggression found in the mother–child relationship during particular phases of development, as boys engage in a similar relationship. The crucial difference is to be found in the anatomical differences between the sexes. During the phallic period, the girl discovers that her clitoris is inferior to its male counterpart, the penis. The little girl reacts to this finding with an intense sense of loss and narcissistic injury, and with envy of the male. The mother engenders hostility for bringing the girl into the world less well equipped than a boy. And with her discovery that her mother also lacks this vital organ, the girl's devaluation of the mother becomes even more pronounced. To compensate for the missing penis, the girl turns to her father in the hope that he will give her a penis, or a baby in place of the penis. However, the Oedipus complex is resolved when the girl realizes that her mother disapproves of her wishes toward her father, along with her father's failure to comply.

The classical Freudian model of feminine psychosexual development is undergoing significant revision. Culturally, apart from constitutional differences, societal and parental attitudes toward the sexes have changed. Freud saw women as basically masochistic, weak, dependent, and lacking in moral conviction and character. He explained these defects as the failure in oedipal identification with the phallic father because of female castration. Today, most analysts regard Freud's formulations of a passive female libido, arrest in ego and superego development, and incapacity for sublimation as outdated and inaccurate. Male and female ego and superego development are different, but one is not superior to the other. Because women are different, their psychology is also different, and a new view of feminine development is gradually emerging.

SIGNIFICANCE OF OEDIPUS COMPLEX Freud regarded the Oedipus complex and its resolution—or, more accurately, its lack thereof—as the nucleus for the formation of later neurosis. Furthermore, the development of character and personality is profoundly affected by the various admixture of libidinal fixations, object orientations, and identifications with which the child emerges from the oedipal situation.

It should be emphasized that at puberty there is a resurgence of incestuous oedipal feelings in both sexes and the important task is the withdrawing of the libido from the parents and attaching it to other, more suitable love objects. Finally, with parenthood, fathers and mothers once again experience early relationships with their parents through identification with their own children.

LINES OF DEVELOPMENT

This discussion would be incomplete without some mention of Anna Freud's lines of development, first described in 1965. According to her, development lines can be traced for a stated area of the personality and its functioning. The developmental level achieved by the child in any given area reflects the outcome of interactions between drive and ego-superego development and the influences within the environment. A developmental line traces the course of interactions among the elements of maturation, adaptation, and structuralization. Anna Freud acknowledges the importance of Hoffer's work on the internal milieu, Mahler's developmental concepts, and some aspects of Melanie Klein's object-relations theory in her understanding of development.

One line that details the series of relationships with objects extending from primary infantile dependence to early adult independence and self-reliance includes the following elements:

1. A biological unity existing in the mother–infant couple where the mother's narcissism extends to the child and the child includes the mother in an internal narcissistic milieu. The whole is further subdivided into the autistic, symbiotic, and separation-individuation phases. Potential points of danger for developmental disturbances are present during each individual phase.
2. The part-object, or need-fulfilling, anaclitic relationship, which is founded in the urgency of the child's physical needs and drive derivations and is intermittent and fluctuating. Objects are cathected, or invested with psychic energy, under the impact of imperative desires but withdrawn once satisfaction has been achieved.
3. The stage of object constancy enabling a positive inner image of the object to be maintained regardless of satisfaction or dissatisfaction.
4. The ambivalent relationship of the preoedipal, anal-sadistic stage, characterized by ego attitudes of clinging to, torturing, dominating, and controlling the love objects.
5. The object-centered phallic-oedipal phase, manifested by possessiveness of the parent of the opposite sex or of the same sex, rivalry with and jealousy of the parent of the same sex, protectiveness, curiosity, the offering of admiration, and the appearance of exhibitionistic attitudes. Anna Freud called attention to a masculine, phallic-oedipal relationship to the mother in girls that preceded the oedipal relationship to the father.

6. The latency period, with transfer of libido from parental figures to contemporaries, community groups, and outside authority figures, as well as to impersonal ideals and aim-inhibited, sublimated interests. Not uncommonly, fantasies during this stage manifest disillusionment with and denigration of the parents, with the familiar family romance and twin fantasies.
7. A preadolescent prelude to the adolescent revolt, with a regression to early attitudes and behavior—which tend to be of a part-object, need-fulfilling, and ambivalent type.
8. The adolescent struggle revolving around denying, reversing, loosening, and shedding ties to infantile objects. There is a defense against pregenitality and the establishment of genital supremacy and the transfer of libidinal cathexis outside the family to persons of the opposite sex.

The perspective afforded by this line of development proves extremely useful in assessing object relations in the various forms of adult psychopathology.

CONCEPT OF NARCISSISM

The concept of narcissism has developed broad theoretical and treatment implications since Freud. And even today, narcissism is an extremely complex and confusing area. As Freud once wrote to Karl Abraham, "The narcissism was a difficult labor and bears all the marks of a corresponding deformation." He concluded: "I have a very strong feeling of vexation at its inadequacy." Throughout his career, Freud made contributions to this topic. In 1905, he described the first of more than 19 clinical phenomena in which narcissism played a vital role, showing a connection between narcissism and autoeroticism and between hypochondriasis and organ inferiority via the concept of an ego libido that arose from sexual and other body organs. *On Narcissism,* which appeared in 1914, contained the first systematic discussion of narcissism.

THEORETICAL BASIS The term "narcissism" comes from the classic myth of Narcissus, who fell so in love with his own reflection in a pool of water that he drowned in his attempt to embrace his image. Freud used the concept of narcissism to explain the first attachment of the libido to the ego. It played a major role in his thinking about libido, about instinct, and about the origins and functions of the ego. For example, he concluded that in cases of dementia precox (schizophrenia), the libido was withdrawn from persons and objects in the external environment and turned inward. This detachment of libido from outside objects accounted for the loss of reality in these patients. In his 1914 paper, he stated that the detached libido had been reinvested in the patient's own ego and resulted in the production of megalomaniacal delusions; the libidinal investment appeared to be reflected in the patient's grandiosity and omnipotence.

Freud was aware that narcissism not only characterized psychotic patients but could be found in neurotics and in normal persons under certain conditions. In states of physical illness and in hypochondriasis, for instance, the libido is frequently withdrawn from outside objects, interests, and activities. The most common example of the withdrawal of libido from the external environment can be found in sleep. Here, the detached libido during dreams, with their emotional vividness, was seen as the libidinal cathexis (concentration of libidinal energy) of the fantasy representations of the dreamer. Perversions, especially homosexuality, were regarded by Freud as representing narcissistic object choices. He also found manifestations of narcissism in the myths and beliefs of primitive people, explaining these as the projection of the magical omnipotence of their own thought processes onto external events. Children exhibit obvious narcissism through their renounced self-interest and intense beliefs about the magical omnipotence of their thoughts.

NARCISSISM AND OBJECT RELATIONS Freud believed that a state of primary narcissism exists at birth. In such a condition, the total amount of libido is stored in the ego. This state continues until the ego begins to invest the presentation of objects with libido, thus changing narcissistic libido into object libido. Narcissism that was once attached to external objects but now withdrawn from those objects and placed into the service of the ego is termed "secondary" narcissism and object libido is transformed into ego libido.

This postulate has been questioned by recent research that has shown that neonates soon after birth can respond to stimuli in their surroundings in complex and organized ways. Thus, it becomes questionable as to whether an absolute state of primary narcissism actually exists. It was Freud's belief that the neonate was entirely narcissistic, with all the libidinal energies devoted to the demands of physiological needs and the preservation of well-being. This self-investment was termed *ego libido.* As the infant comes to realize that the source of pleasure or relief from tension comes from the principal caretaker, narcissistic libido is withdrawn from the self or ego and redirected toward the external object. This transformed libido was called *object libido.* The development of object relations parallels the shift from primary narcissism to object attachment.

Some narcissistic libido is present normally throughout adult life; a healthy and well-integrated narcissism is, in fact, essential for the maintenance of a sense of well-being or self-esteem. It is also subject to fixations and developmental vicissitudes, which may result in pathology. Under the threat of actual or perceived injury or trauma, object libido may be withdrawn from objects and reinvested in the ego. Freud called this regressive libidinal ego reinvestment *secondary narcissism.* This formulation has caused considerable confusion in the understanding of narcissistic libido. Heinz Hartmann considered it more accurate to regard narcissistic libido as attached to the self rather than to the ego. Theoretical controversy, however, continues to rage over the psychoanalytic notion of the self.

Analysts also do not agree as to what constitutes normal and pathological narcissism. Some analysts view narcissism as always pathological and clinically detrimental, whereas others believe that it is not pathological and is extremely important to psychological growth. Perhaps the individual most responsible for this perspective is Heinz Kohut, who was the principal contributor to *self-psychology* and a major force in proposing a newer perspective in the understanding of narcissism.

Kohut's developmental lines Essentially, Kohut and his followers agree with Freud that the infant begins life in a state of self-contained, undifferentiated primary narcissism. Unlike classic Freudians, however, Kohut feels that there are three developmental lines for narcissism. One line starts from the original experience of perfection or absolute bliss, to which the grandiose self is assigned. In the second line of development, the infant strives to maintain the original state of perfection by assigning it to an idealized parent image, an admired omnipotent, transitional selfobject. In the third line of development, as in the classical formulation, part of the basic pool of primary narcissism is transformed into object love. The differentiation of the two basic archaic narcissistic configurations, the grandiose self and the idealized parent image, takes place simultaneously with the emerging differentiation between self and objects from the original state of primary narcissism. It is the dependence of the infant on an external object with the consequent setting of limits on the infant's sense of self-sufficiency and omnipotence that propels this forward movement. Furthermore, the child's need to preserve a sense of security maintains the residue of infantile grandiosity as manifested by the grandiose self, as well as maintaining a situation of dependence and a protective symbiosis with a powerful and idealized object, the idealized parent image.

Creation of selfobjects As development proceeds, these two basic narcissistic configurations undergo progressive modification and gradual integration into the psychic structure. According to Kohut, this narcissistic development progresses through the continual creation and re-creation of a sequence of selfobjects. The child relates to objects not as independent entities but as modified objects to represent specific components from the child's own emerging self-organization. These external objects are invested with significant degrees of narcissistic cathexis influenced by self-derived elements and become selfobjects.

Such selfobjects serve to maintain the child's internal narcissistic equilibrium, which is continually readjusted in response to narcissistic vulnerabilities during various phases of the developmental process. During the course of development, the child's dependence on the mother and the quality of the selfobject relationship undergoes a shift, so that the child becomes less vulnerable to the loss of the mother and more susceptible to the loss of the mother's love. However, the child's state of narcissistic equilibrium and coherence in the self continues to depend on the relationship with the mother. As growth continues, the evolving psychic structures reach a state that maintains a sense of inner continuity and cohesiveness of the self-organization where the potential loss of the object, or even of the loss of love of the object, may occur. Other narcissistic disappointments, although felt, do not disrupt this sense of cohesiveness of the self-organization.

At each stage in the developmental progression, the grandiose self and the idealized parent image undergo alterations and the degree of narcissistic investment is modified in more modulated and realistic directions. At each state, there is a proportional transformation of these narcissistic structures into stable and autonomous structures. Gradually, the grandiose self is modified to allow the child to maintain a sense of self-esteem and pride in accomplishment, even when confronted with unavoidable disappointments and limitations. A mature sense of stable and secure self-esteem, pride in accomplishments, ambition, and resiliency arises, and the individual is able to tolerate severe losses and narcissistic disappointments. Similarly, the idealized parental image is progressively modified in the direction of a realistic and attainable ego-ideal that is gradually internalized and is reflected in the acquisition of meaningful values and personal ideals.

At any stage of the developmental process, however, the elements of archaic narcissism can be disrupted and undergo a variety of pathological vicissitudes. Consequently, various narcissistic disorders may arise, ranging from severe narcissistic vulnerability with the threat of disillusion and fragmentation of the self to more stable forms of narcissistic vulnerability where the loss of self-cohesion is minimal. In its most mature and realistic expression, narcissism is transformed into the capacity for creativity, empathy, humor, and wisdom, and ultimately for the acceptance of the inevitability of death.

APPLICATION TO INFANTILE SEXUALITY How is narcissism different from and related to autoeroticism? In primary narcissism, the self and object are undifferentiated; in autoeroticism, eroticism is attached to the person's own body or body parts. Autoeroticism implies the absence of any specific object involvement. A child who is frustrated in attempts to acquire the love object (mother) or the part object (breast), seeks gratification by using personal body parts (thumbsucking) as if they were the desired objects. Autoeroticism and narcissism are similar in that the libidinal energies are directed to the individual and little heed is paid to the external environment. Both conditions are also associated with the earliest and most primitive stages of the infant's development.

Autoeroticism and primary narcissism overlap, even though they emphasize different aspects of the primitive libidinal condition. However, autoeroticism is quite distinct and different from secondary narcissism in that the former refers specifically to the self and not to the subject's body or its parts.

The vicissitudes of narcissism intermingle and operate throughout all the phases of psychosexual development. In Robert Waelder's scheme, levels of self-love or narcissism may be phase-appropriate to erotogenic zones. For example, during the oral period, narcissism may manifest itself as a wish for affection or to be given to. During the phallic phase, narcissism expresses itself as the wish to be admired. Furthermore, phase-specific narcissistic injuries may take place at each stage of psychosexual development. Characteristically, these injuries are determined both by the vicissitudes of object libido and by the developmental state of the psychic apparatus. For instance, oral deprivation during the oral phase can be viewed as a narcissistic insult that helps undermine the infant's sense of inner worth. Another narcissistic insult, the disappointment of oedipal wishes during the oedipal period, may leave the individual with a sense of inadequacy or inferiority or a lack of values.

CHOICE OF LOVE OBJECT Early object relationships play a crucial role in the later choice of a love object. Freud discovered that the concept of narcissism helped his understanding of the basis for the choice of a love object in adult love. A love object might be chosen "according to the narcissistic type," in which case the person resembles the subject's idealized or fantasied self-image. Or the object chosen might be an "anaclitic type," that is, the person would resemble someone who cared for the subject during the early years of life. People who have an enormous degree of self-love, such as especially attractive men or women, have, according to Freud, an appeal beyond their esthetic attraction. They supply for their admirers the narcissism that was painfully renounced in the process of turning toward object love. A homosexual object relationship represents yet another example of a narcissistic object choice that is based on sexual resemblance.

The concept of narcissism occupies a prominent position in psychoanalytic theory. As the notion gradually evolved, it became obvious that concepts of the individual and the individual's body and ego could no longer be used interchangeably. Further understanding and advances in psychoanalytic theory required a clearer definition of the concept of self and ego. Ambiguities in the concept of the ego were exposed and underscored the need for a systematic study of its development, structure, and functions. Attention to narcissistic phenomena has enlarged the understanding of a variety of mental disorders, and assisted in the exploration of normal psychological phenomena.

THE THEORY OF DREAMS

SIGNIFICANCE OF DREAMS Dreams continue to occupy a major position in psychoanalytic practice and theory, and have been extensively studied along physiological and psychodynamic lines. Although much has been learned about the various stages of the sleep cycle and sleep disorders, the psychoanalytic understanding of the dream process and the dream experience continues to draw heavily from Freud's discoveries as presented in *The Interpretation of Dreams* in 1905.

Through the development of the technique of free association and the refocus on the significance of fantasy experiences after he abandoned the seduction hypothesis, Freud began to appreciate the significance and value of investigating dreams. His self-analysis was also heavily dependent on a study of his own dream experiences. *The Interpretation of Dreams* was perhaps Freud's greatest work, and continues to serve as the basic text for the student interested in dreams. In this work, Freud concluded that the dream, like a psychoneurotic symptom, is a conscious expression of an unconscious fantasy or wish that is otherwise not readily accessible to the individual in waking life. The dream images represent unconscious wishes or thoughts disguised by symbolization, displacement, and repression.

Although dreams were considered to be a normal manifestation of sleep or the unconscious state, they were later shown to resemble the pathological thoughts of psychotic patients in the waking state. Freud believed that in order to disguise or exclude unconscious wishes from consciousness and to transform unconscious wishes into disguised conscious forms in the dream, a censor had to exist in the mind. The censor acted in the service of the ego, providing a self-preservative function in accordance with his logic that reason and volition ruled these functions. As ego psychology developed, the activities of the censor and the defense mechanisms normally seen in dreams (repression, displacement, condensation, and symbolism) were included among the many functions of the ego and superego that are beyond a person's conscious awareness.

ANALYSIS OF DREAM CONTENT The analysis of dreams requires the elicitation of material that has been repressed or excluded from consciousness by the defensive activities of the ego. The dream, as it is recalled by the dreamer, is the result of the unconscious mental activity that occurs during sleep, and that may, because of its intensity, threaten to interfere with sleep. One of the functions of the censor is to act as the guardian of sleep so that, instead of being awakened, the sleeper dreams. Freud considered the conscious experiencing of thoughts during sleep as dreaming.

Sleep research since Freud's time has shown that a wide variety of cognitive activity occurs during sleep. Some of the cognitive activity is in agreement with Freud's descriptions of dream activity (stage 1 rapid eye movement [REM] periods of the sleep–dream cycle), but much of it is more realistic, brief (non-REM sleep periods), and consistently organized along logical lines. The experienced content of the dream is the so-called *manifest* dream. The unconscious thought and wishes that threaten to awaken the sleeper are known as the *latent* dream content. The unconscious mental operations through which the latent dream content is transformed into the manifest dream is known as the *dream work*. Freud showed that the approach to dream interpretation was to move from the manifest content of the dream by way of free association to arrive at the latent dream content in order to provide the core meaning.

Freud believed that a variety of stimuli initiated dreaming. Today, however, it has been demonstrated that dreaming occurs in conjunction with the psychic patterns of central nervous activities during certain phases of the sleep cycle. Thus, what Freud considered initiating stimuli are more likely to be incorporated into the dream content and may influence the dream thoughts instead of initiating the dream.

Nocturnal sensory stimuli Sensory impressions, such as pain, hunger, thirst, or urinary urgency, may help to initiate a dream during sleep. To illustrate, a tired student, who must get up early for school, may, instead of disturbing his sleep (and leaving his warm bed), dream that he has bathed and dressed and is in the classroom. Freud's explanation that the activity of dreaming preserves and safeguards sleep, although one of the functions of the dream, no longer fully accounts for the considerably more complex functioning of dreams in contemporary psychiatry.

Day residues The residue of thoughts, ideas, and feelings left over from the preceding day, or even several days, before the dream remains active in the unconscious, and, like sensory stimuli, can be incorporated into the manifest dream. Not infrequently, the day residue is amalgamated with unconscious infantile drive and wishes, which disguise the infantile impulse and allow it to remain as the driving force behind the dream.

Repressed infantile drives The essential elements of the latent dream content are felt to arise from one or several impulses emanating from the repressed part of the unconscious. According to Freud, the driving forces behind the dream activity and process of dream formation are the infantile wishes, usually stemming from the preoedipal and oedipal levels. Although nocturnal stimuli and the day residue may form part of the dream content, they are significant insofar as they are associated with and are connected with one or more repressed wishes from the unconscious emerging in the form of a dream. Freud believed that a link had to exist between the day residue and the repressed content in order to incorporate events from the waking state into the dream content. His belief has been challenged with newer discoveries from sleep research, but much of what he initially observed continues to have clinical validity.

Dreams of early childhood are unique because the distinction between infantile, or early, and current conflicts are not much different. Dreams of young children appear to be less disguised and there is less distinction between latent and manifest content of dreams because of the child's immature ego and defenses.

DREAM WORK Freud maintained that every dream represents a wish fulfillment. Although readily observable in early childhood, the infantile wish or impulse becomes concealed and disguised in the manifest dream in later childhood and adult life. The dream work comprises several processes that transform the latent content into the manifest dream.

Dream formation During the state of sleep, the process of repression lets up and latent wishes and impulses press for discharge and gratification. Because mobility is blocked, the repressed wishes and impulses are discharged via the mechanisms of thought and fantasy. Latent material may be represented in two ways. First, these latent wishes or impulses can be shown through thoughts, impressions, or memories that are expressed in visual terms. Generally, thoughts and other experiences occurring during the day, or even several days earlier, may serve this function. Sound or other nocturnal stimuli during sleep may be linked with repressed wishes and impulses and manifest themselves as auditory, tactile, olfactory, or gustatory hallucinations.

Why are these unconscious wishes and impulses repressed? The answer is that they prove unacceptable to the ego. Nevertheless, such wishes or impulses continually press for discharge, and in order to bypass the dream censor, they often tag along with innocent or neutral images. Such images may appear trivial or unimportant but are dynamically associated with highly meaningful latent wishes. To enable these neutral images to surface in the dream, the dream work consists of several mental mechanisms that elaborately disguise the latent wishes.

Symbolism The dreamer substitutes innocent images that resemble the original part of the body or other highly cathected objects in one or more essential features. Symbols tend to be concrete and sensory, to represent a condensed expression of the idea or concept, and to be more primitive and repressed in terms of mental development. Symbols have unconscious meanings, and some seem to have a common, almost universal, meaning; for example, money can symbolize feces or a house may symbolize the female genitalia or womb.

Displacement In displacement, energy (cathexis) is transferred from an original object to a substitute or symbolic representation of the object. The substitute object is relatively neutral, or less invested with affective energy, and is more acceptable to the dream censor. Whereas in symbolization one object is substituted for another, in displacement, the distortion of unconscious wishes is facilitated by the transfer of affective energy from one object to another. The aim of the unconscious impulse, however, is unchanged. An example of displacement would be where the father may be represented visually by an unknown male figure to whom less emotional significance is attached. Yet, the dreamer continues to harbor the same affective responses toward the father.

Condensation In the mechanism of condensation, several unconscious wishes, impulses, or attitudes can be combined and attached to a single image in the manifest dream. A frightening animal may represent not only the dreamer's father but also some aspects of the mother, and the dreamer's own primitive impulses as well. Conversely, in the manifest dream content, a single latent wish or impulse may be expressed through multiple images or representations. Condensation provides the dreamer with a flexible and economic means of facilitating, compressing, or expanding the manifest dream that draws on latent or unconscious wishes and impulses.

Projection The process of projection enables the patient's unacceptable impulses or wishes in the dream to appear to emanate from another person. The person to whom the unacceptable impulses are ascribed in the dream is frequently the person toward whom the dreamer's own unconscious impulses are directed. For instance, a man who has strong, hostile feelings toward a male friend may dream that his friend is angry with him. He has projected his own unacceptable wishes onto another person and allowed their expression in the manifest dream.

Secondary revision Developmentally early modes of thinking utilizing symbolism, displacement, and condensation are characteristic of *primary process* thinking present in dreams. However, the absurd, bizarre, and illogical characteristics of dreams are subject to secondary revision, or the intellectual process employed by the mature ego to lend coherence and rationality to the manifest dream. Logical mental operations characteristic of the *secondary process* are introduced into the dream. Through these processes, the ego attempts to mold the manifest dream into a semblance of logic and coherence. It tries to make the manifest dream sensible, much as it tries to make sense of all impressions that enter its domain.

TYPICAL DREAMS **Anxiety dreams** Freud's basic theory of dreams preceded his development of a comprehensive theory of the ego. Thus, his early studies of dreams placed importance on their functions in the discharge or gratification of instinctual drives or wishes through the dreams' hallucinatory contents. But dreams also attempt to spare the subject psychic pain or tension. Initially, Freud thought that the mechanisms of symbolism, displacement, condensation, projection, and secondary revision facilitated the discharge of the latent impulses. Later, he realized that these devices are primitive defense mechanisms of the ego that also attempt to prevent the direct discharge of instinctual drives in order to protect the dreamer from the excessive anxiety and pain that would result from such discharge. These mechanisms may also be overwhelmed or fail in their protective function. Anxiety may be so severe that the sleeper is partially awakened or made uncomfortable. Thus, elements of the latent dream content may succeed in making its way into the manifest content and, despite the dream work, present themselves in a recognizable manner that is too threatening for the ego to tolerate. The ego reacts to the direct expression of repressed impulses with severe anxiety and the person experiences psychic discomfort.

Punishment dreams In punishment dreams, the ego anticipates condemnation from the superego should elements of the latent content of the dream break through the disguise of the manifest dream. In anticipation of the consequences engendered by the loss of the ego's control of the instincts during sleep, a compromise is frequently achieved between the repressed wish and the superego that results in the production of the punishment dream. However, other functions are subsumed by the punishment dream. Some analysts feel that these dreams represent a desire to relive earlier periods, when satisfactions were to be found, despite the psychic discomfort. In addition, the punishment dream may represent a repetitive attempt on the part of the dreamer to master traumatic events that have overwhelmed the ego in the past.

EARLY THEORY OF THE MIND

As discussed in the *Project,* published after Freud's death, his earliest theory of the mind was based on neuropsychological concepts derived from the Helmholtz school, which, in turn, was influenced by Newtonian physics. Freud tried to utilize the scientific and philosophic thinking of the period. Early in his career, he attempted to formulate a theory of the mind in terms of shifts of energy or quantities of excitation between neuronal systems. Lacking the scientific tools to confirm his postulates, Freud was forced to abandon his biological premises but he continued to believe that psychical processes depended on physiological interaction.

One can also trace in Freud's thinking antecedents of nineteenth century psychology and philosophy. His conceptualization of the unconscious corresponds to that put forward 70 years earlier by the German philosopher Johann Herbart, to whose theories Freud was exposed at the gymnasium. Herbart contended that unconscious mental processes were dominated by a constant conflict of ideas that varied in intensity. Furthermore, although opposing ideas could drive others from the conscious mind, they continued to assert themselves as disturbances.

Freud was also influenced by a number of his teachers, including Gustav Fechner, who based his philosophy on Herbart's theories. Fechner believed in the notion of unconscious processes that attained consciousness once they reached a certain intensity. Similarly, Brücke, with whom Freud worked, maintained that movements in the nervous system would cause ideas to arise. Another prominent German psychiatrist was Wilhelm Griesinger, who proposed that ideas could be kept out of the conscious and that bodily organs influenced the unconscious mind, one of the hypotheses that Freud used to explain dreams. Another influential figure in Freud's training was Theodor Lipps, who believed in the existence of unconscious mental processes. Similarly, Theodore Meynert, Freud's professor of psychiatry, thought that the mind and brain were interchangeable and suggested the presence of a controlling agency that inhibited or held back intrusive and undesirable activity of the brain. Although influenced by these writers, Freud was unique in basing his theory of the mind on clinical observations indicating the existence of a dynamic unconscious, and then, as a clinician, applying his theory to clinical practice.

TOPOGRAPHIC MODEL

The topographic model of the mind first emerged in 1900 in the seventh chapter of *The Interpretation of Dreams,* and although it has largely been supplanted by the structural model, it still is useful in understanding dreams and in classifying mental events according to their degree of awareness. This model divides the mind into three regions: the unconscious system (UCS), the preconscious system (PCS), and the conscious system (CS), each of which has unique characteristics.

THE UNCONSCIOUS The unconscious system can be viewed as the total of all those mental contents and processes at a given moment outside the sphere of consciousness and includes aspects of the preconscious. It can be thought of in dynamic terms as describing the mental contents and processes placed out of consciousness by a censoring or repressing counterforce called a *countercathexis*. The unconscious refers to a component subsystem within the topographic model that includes the dynamic unconscious, within which thinking and memory traces are governed by primary process. The following features are characteristic of the unconscious:

1. Unconscious content only becomes conscious through the preconscious, which censors or represses unacceptable or threatening drive representations or wishes. These elements become conscious when the censor is overpowered.
2. Primary process thinking and primary process are the predominant forms of mental activity. The primary process is characterized by a striving for immediate discharge of drive energy and an extreme mobility of drive cathexis. Primary process thinking contains the absence of negatives, the presence of conditionals, the coexistence of contradictions, and a lack of time sense, and employs the mental mechanisms of displacement, condensation, and symbolization. It freely uses allusion and analogy. Primary process thinking is characteristically found in very young children and in persons with severe mental illness. However, ready access to primary traces also may be associated with creativity.
3. Generally, the unconscious contains wishes or drive derivatives pressing for fulfillment that are the dynamic force behind neurotic symptoms and dreams.
4. Memories and fantasies in the unconscious can be retrieved when the energy pressing them is removed and then recathected during the analytic treatment process.
5. The unconscious is closely associated with the instincts. At this stage of the development of the topographic model, the instincts were thought to consist of sexual and self-preservative drives. The mental representatives and derivatives of the instinctual drive, particularly those of the sexual instincts, were placed in the unconscious. Accordingly, the dynamic unconscious is regulated by the demands of the pleasure principle.

THE PRECONSCIOUS This term was originally used by Freud to describe those mental contents capable of easily becoming conscious with the focusing of attention. The preconscious system is not present at birth but develops in childhood and parallels the course of ego development, later described in Freud's structural theory. The preconscious region of the mind interfaces with the unconscious proper and the conscious, with access to both. However, contents of the unconscious can reach consciousness only by becoming linked with words and thus becoming preconscious. The preconscious maintains the repressive barrier and censorship function of wishes and desires. Secondary process thinking exists in the preconscious and is characterized by a delay of instinctual discharge, the binding of mental energy in accordance with external reality, and an avoidance of unpleasure.

THE CONSCIOUS Freud regarded the conscious as a type of sense organ of attention registering stimuli from the outside world and from within the organism via the preconscious. Through attention, or the employment of neutralized psychic energy, a person becomes aware of external stimuli and internal perceptions. Before 1923, Freud thought that the conscious controlled motor activity and was instrumental in determining the distribution of psychic energy. The conscious commanded little attention from Freud and remains of lesser concern to contemporary psychoanalysts.

DYNAMICS OF MENTAL FUNCTIONING

In the last chapter of *The Interpretation of Dreams,* Freud compared the psychic apparatus to a compound optical instrument, such as a telescope or microscope, made up of many optical elements arranged consecutively. The psychic apparatus was thought to be composed of various psychic components arranged consecutively, with the perceptual or sensory system at one end and the motor system at the other, flanking the memory and association systems. In early childhood, particularly, perceptions are modified and stored in the form of memories. As in the model of the reflex arc, the mental energy associated with unconscious ideas seeks discharge through thought or motor activity, moving from the perceptual to the motor end during the waking state. However, under particular conditions, such as sleep or external frustration, the flow of psychic energy may be reversed, moving from the motor to the perceptual end. This reversal of the normal direction of energy was called *topographic regression*. Manifestations of this phenomenon included the appearance in dreams of early childhood impressions as originally perceived and the presence of hallucinations in severe mental disorders.

The model of the mind as a reflex arc was later abandoned by Freud, but he retained the principal concept of regression, which was modified in his theory of neurosis. In neurosis, libidinal frustration results in a reversion to earlier modes or objects of instinctual discharge or to earlier levels of fixation. This kind of reversion was called libidinal or instinctual regression.

DEFICIENCIES OF TOPOGRAPHIC THEORY

In contemporary psychoanalysis, several concepts from Freud's topographic theory are still accepted despite Freud's gradual recognition that his early theory of the mind was inadequate to explain some striking clinical conditions. These retained concepts include Freud's hypotheses of primary and secondary thought processes, the importance of wish fulfillment, the recognition of the process of regression during periods of stress and frustration, and the existence of the dynamic unconscious. However, the topographic model proved to be deficient in two important areas. First, Freud came to realize through his psychoanalytic work with patients that many of the defense mechanisms they employed were not readily accessible to consciousness and had to be considered unconscious resistances. The mechanisms also did not fit easily or logically into the preconscious or unconscious regions. For example, one of the principal defenses, repression, could not be considered preconscious, as that region of the mind was, by definition, easily accessible to consciousness. Second, he realized that some of his patients manifested an unconscious need for punishment or guilt. Again, according to the topographic model, the moral agency should have resided in the preconscious region, which was easily available to consciousness, but which proved not to be the case. From a clinical perspective, the topographic theory proved to be mechanically cumbersome, overly simplistic, and inadequate to account for the complex phenomena of unconscious moral guilt and the striving for punishment.

TRANSITION TO STRUCTURAL THEORY

Even during the early stages in the development of psychoanalysis, Freud had associated certain mental activities with the functioning of the ego and superego, entities he was to elaborate on in his structural theory. Because he was primarily concerned with establishing the existence and operation of unconscious mental processes, Freud paid little attention to conscious activities until he recognized that not all unconscious processes could be relegated to the instinct, and that some aspects, later attributed to the mental functioning of the ego and superego, were unconscious as well. He then devoted his efforts to a study of these structural components. Freud's contributions to ego psychology do not match the significance of his earlier psychoanalytic discoveries; however, he developed a basic framework of ego psychology that would later be expanded, refined, and applied clinically.

HISTORY OF EGO PSYCHOLOGY

The concept of the ego is best understood within the context of the historical development of psychoanalysis. The evolution of ego psychology can be divided into four phases. The first phase ended in 1897 and coincided with the development of early psychoanalytic formulations. The second phase is usually recognized to be the period from 1897 to 1923, and has been considered as the development of psychoanalysis proper. The third phase lasted from 1923 to 1937, during which time Freud developed both his theory of ego psychology and his later theory of anxiety. The fourth phase of ego psychology began with Freud's death and represents the contributions of Hartmann, Kris, Rapaport, Erikson, and other contemporary psychoanalysts who shifted the focus from ego function to the broader social and cultural perspectives of ego functioning and development.

EARLY CONCEPTS OF THE EGO During the initial phase of the development of psychoanalysis, the concept of the ego was ill defined and imprecise. The ego referred to the dominant place of the individual's conscious thoughts and values versus repressed impulses and wishes. It was thought to be mainly concerned with defense, a term synonymous with repression at that time. In the language of the *Project,* Freud saw the ego as an organization that existed to control the passage of quantities of excitation. In psychological terms, he conceived of the ego as a defense against impulses and wishes that were unacceptable to consciousness. These impulses or ideas were thought to be primarily of a sexual nature, and, Freud believed, originated from premature sexual trauma and actual seduction. It was the memories of the trauma that aroused unpleasant affect and evoked a defensive response, causing a repression of the original thoughts. In turn, the repression of ideas caused a damming up of energy and produced anxiety. A contradiction of the function of the ego became apparent with this early conceptualization. The ego functioned to reduce tension and avoid unpleasant affects aroused by sexual thoughts; yet, according to this hypothesis, the process would also produce anxiety, an equally unpleasant affect. When Freud relinquished his seduction theory in 1897, he also suspended his thinking about the function of the ego.

HISTORICAL ROOTS During this second phase, Freud devoted much energy to the study of the instinctual drives and their transformations, paying little attention to the ego. References to defense or defensive functioning were infrequent. But because of the confusion in Freud's early theory of the instincts and contradictions in his theory of the mind, he had to reexamine the nature and functioning of the ego.

In 1915, in his *Instincts and Their Vicissitudes,* Freud explored the vicissitudes to which the sexual instinct was subjected as it sought expression—including reversal into its opposite (a sadistic impulse might become masochistic), turning on one's own self, repression, and sublimation. From the perspective of ego psychology, each of these vicissitudes could be viewed as a defense mechanism. Thus, the instinct was invoked in defense, but this was a task properly belonging to the ego. The same contradiction arose with regard to the ego or self-preservative instincts that were responsible for repression.

In accordance with topographic theory, since neither the preconscious nor the ego instincts were solely responsible for regression or censorship, how was repression achieved? Freud attempted to answer this question by explaining that ideas are maintained in the unconscious through the withdrawal of libido. Furthermore, as unconscious ideas constantly push to become attached to libido in order to reach consciousness, the withdrawal of libido is a repetitive process. Freud described this continual withdrawal of libido as an anticathexis or countercathexis. Logically, it followed that to be consistently effective against ideas in the unconscious, the countercathexis had to be permanent and operate on an unconscious basis. This function was assigned to the ego, resulting in an increased understanding of the ego's role and development at this stage.

FREUD'S EGO PSYCHOLOGY Freud's contributions to the theory of the ego can be seen in *The Ego and the Id* in 1923. The ego was viewed as the coherent organization of mental processes and functions. Primarily organized around the perceptual conscious system, it also included the structures responsible for resistance and unconscious defenses. The ego was also depicted as a weak, passive agency and a resultant of pressures from the id, superego, and reality. Furthermore, the ego was felt to be genetically derived from the id, and later was depicted as a helpless rider on the id's horse, going wherever the id wished.

In *Inhibitions, Symptoms and Anxiety* in 1926, Freud introduced the concept of signal anxiety that was an autonomous function of the ego for the initiation of defense. The ego was no longer regarded as subservient to the id but could turn passively experienced anxiety into active anticipation. In addition, the ego now had a variety of defenses at its disposal to deal with the id impulses.

Freud's further elaboration of the reality principle included the ego function of adaptation, which enabled it to control instinctual drives when real danger prompted these drives into action. As the ego matured, the reality principle gradually became substituted for the pleasure principle. Although the reality principle aimed at the reduction of tension as much as did the id, it also considered the requirements, possibilities, and limitations of the environment, addressing the prospect of attaining greater pleasure in the future. During this third phase of development, the concept of the ego was radically changed. Now the ego was seen as a powerful regulatory force responsible for the integration and control of behavioral responses; the adaptive functioning of the ego in relation to reality was brought into prominence; and in his 1937 publication, *Analysis Terminable and Interminable,* Freud made explicit the assumption that from the start the ego evolved independently of the id. The notion of primary ego autonomy was further elaborated on by Hartmann and his followers, leading to the development of the fourth phase.

SYSTEMATIZATION OF EGO PSYCHOLOGY The third phase can be thought of as culminating in Anna Freud's work on the defense mechanisms of the ego whereas the beginning of the fourth phase is marked by the contributions of Heinz Hartmann on the ego and adaptation. Hartmann's work focused primarily on the autonomy of the ego and the problem of adaptation. He emphasized the independent genetic roots of the ego and laid the foundation for the notion of epigenetic maturation. According to the epigenetic principle, all growing organisms possess a ground plan out of which the parts arise. Each part has its time of social ascendancy until all the parts have arisen to form a functioning whole.

Hartmann brought the perspective of adaptive functioning into prominence as one of the basic metapsychological assumptions in psychoanalytic theory. This paved the way for the development of the concept of egotization, which afforded a broader perspective for psychoanalysis as a general psychology. Egotization encompassed the experimental and clinical aspects of psychology but could also interact with scientific disciplines involved in the study of human behavior.

As the process of egotization occurred, some psychoanalysts felt that a split had been created, leaving the id as the dynamic source of psychic energies and the ego as the container for the noninstinctual, nondynamic structural apparatus. Personality functioning and its dysfunction seemed inhuman and overly mechanized. The id came to be seen as a seething cauldron in which the instinctual energies no longer possessed the representational or directional qualities previously ascribed to them by Freud.

Also during the fourth phase of ego development, the role of reality reemerged as a significant factor in psychoanalytic thinking because of the emphasis placed on a person's adaptive functioning and interaction with the personal and social environment. The concern with reality has been reinforced by the direction provided by the work of Erik Erikson, who examined the adaptation of the individual throughout the life cycle, and by object-relations theory, which focuses on the interaction between the child and important figures early in the child's environment. The object-relations approach emphasizes the deficiencies of the environment rather than the internal vicissitudes of the instincts or constitutional defects in explaining the genesis of psychopathology. Also of significance in an object-relations approach is the fact that many of the theories are drawn from studies of character disorders and persons with personality organizations that are more primitive and show deeper levels of ego defects than the type of patients traditionally studied by psychoanalysts.

STRUCTURE OF THE PSYCHIC APPARATUS

The contemporary psychoanalytic model of the mind is the structural or tripartite theory, which divides the psychic apparatus into the id, ego, and superego. Each has different and distinct functions. The main distinction made is between the ego and the id. The id operates according to primary process and is the focus of the instinctual drives. It follows the dictates of the pleasure principle and pays no heed to the reality principle. In contrast, the ego is a coherent organization of functions, and one of its main tasks is to avoid unpleasure or pain by regulating or appraising the discharge of instinctual drives such that they conform to the demands of the external world. The superego, the third component of the psychic apparatus, also assists in the regulation of id discharges. It contains the internalized moral values, prohibitions, and standards of the parental imagos (image).

THE ID Freud was not the first person who used the term "id." It was used originally by Georg Groddeck, an internist who believed in psychoanalysis. Originally, the id stood for all that was ego-alien. It was conceived of as a completely unorganized primordial reservoir of energy, derived from the instincts and under the domination of the primary process. The issue of the organization of the id remains unresolved among psychoanalytic theorists. Freud clearly felt that the instinctual drives of the id had a vectorial and representational component and that the drives were organized according to the primary process. Thus, the id may have a form of organization as the instinctual drives do not operate at random.

The id is not synonymous with the unconscious, as certain defenses or functions of the ego acting against unconscious instinctual pressures are also unconscious; to a great extent, the superego itself also operates on an unconscious level.

Origins of the id Freud proposed that at birth the neonate is endowed with an id with instinctual drives seeking gratification. The infant lacks the capacity to delay, control, or modify these drives. At the beginning of life, the infant is completely dependent on caretaking persons in the environment.

THE EGO The conscious and preconscious functions, such as the use of words, ideas, or logic, are associated with the ego. However, early in the psychoanalytic setting, certain ego phenomena, specifically repression and resistance, were found to be unconscious. The need became apparent for an expanded concept of the ego as an agency that could retain a close relationship to consciousness and yet perform a variety of unconscious operations in relation to the drives. Thus, with this broadened scope of the ego, consciousness was acknowledged to be an exclusive quality of the ego, but it is only one of the characteristics of the ego. Perhaps the most complete definition of the ego is the one given by Freud in his 1938 *An Outline of Psychoanalysis:*

> Here are the principal characteristics of the ego. In consequence of the pre-established connection between sense and perception and muscular action, the ego has voluntary movement at its command. It has the task of self-preservation. As regards external events, it performs that task by becoming aware of stimuli, by storing up experiences about them (in the memory), by avoiding excessive strong stimuli (through flight), by dealing with moderate stimuli (through adaptation), and finally by learning to bring about expedient changes in the external world to its own advantage (through activity). As regards internal events, in relation to the id, it performs that task by gaining control over the demands of the instincts, by deciding whether they are to be allowed satisfaction. By postponing that satisfaction to times and circumstances favorable to the external world or by suppressing their excitations entirely. It is guided in its activity by consideration of the tension produced by stimuli, whether these tensions are present in it or introduced into it.

In essence, the ego controls motility, perception, and contact with reality, and through the mechanisms of defense available to it, the inhibition of primary instinctual drives.

Origins of the ego The newly born infant has no ego, or the most rudimentary of egos, if one defines the ego as a coherent system of functions for mediating between the instincts and the outside world. The neonate demonstrates a complex array of capacities and sensory and motor functions, but there is little coherent organization.

It was Freud's belief that the id undergoes modification as a result of the effect of the external world on the drives. But the pressures of external reality also enable the ego to appropriate the energies of the id to do its work. As the ego forms, it brings the influences of the external world to bear on the id, replaces the pleasure principle with the reality principle, and so contributes to its own further development. In essence, Freud placed great emphasis on the role of the instincts in ego development, and especially on the role of conflict. Initially, the conflict is between the id and the outside world; later, it is between the id and the ego.

Later contributors, such as Hartmann, Kris, and Loewenstein, modified the theory of the development of the ego. Hartmann postulated the existence of primary autonomous ego functions that developed independently of the drives and conflict. He and his collaborators suggested that the ego does not develop and differentiate from the id as such, but that both the ego and id rise from a common undifferentiated matrix. The rudimentary apparatuses underlying the primary autonomous ego functions, such as perception, motility, memory, and intelligence, are present from birth. It follows, therefore, that there may be genetically determined differences in ego functions. In 1937, Freud advanced such a hypothesis but the work of Hartmann and his colleagues expanded on the concept. Furthermore, Hartmann elaborated on the role of the rudimentary ego apparatus in the infant's interactions with the object and the environment to satisfy instinctual needs and drives. The coordination between these elements formed the basis for Hartmann's postulates about the adaptive functions of the ego, that is, the role of the ego in mediating between external reality and the needs and demands of the id and the superego. To function at an optimal level, the organism requires a balance of these forces.

Functions of the ego The ego is best viewed as a substratum of the personality; it is not synonymous with the self, personality, or character. It is an agency, or an organization of functions that have in common the task of mediating between the instincts and the outside world.

The list of basic ego functions suggested by various authors differs to some degree and a comprehensive description of all the ego functions must be arbitrary. The following descriptions focus on those activities generally conceded to be basic and fundamental to the operation of the ego.

1. *Control and regulation of instinctual drives*. As the ego develops, it has greater capacity to delay immediate discharge of wishes and impulses to assure its integrity and to function as the mediator between the id and the outside world. The development of the capacity to delay or to postpone instinctual discharge, similar to the capacity to test reality, parallels the progression in early childhood from the pleasure principle to the reality principle.

Correspondingly, the shift from the pleasure to the reality principle is closely related to the development of secondary process thinking, which aids in the control of drive discharge. The change from prelogical primary process thinking to the logical and more deliberate secondary process thinking is one of the means by which the ego is able to postpone or delay the discharge of instinctual drives. For instance, the fulfillment of representation in fantasy of instinctual wishes obviates the need for urgent action that might not be in the best interests of the individual. Another example would be the use of thought or verbalization to anticipate consequences and to understand the meaning of an impulse to best serve one's realistic functioning. The ego's capacity to control instinctual life and to regulate thinking is closely associated with its defensive functioning.

As part of its adaptive function, the ego is highly instrumental in the use of *signal affects*. The ego uses anxiety, guilt, shame, depression, and other states as signals of instinctual or other dangers adaptively to mobilize defenses to prevent the disruptive and overwhelming breakthrough of threatening instinctual contents. Not only does the signal function of such affective states act in the service of mobilizing defense, but it becomes an essential part of the ego's emerging capacity to tolerate the pain and frustration that contribute to the building up and maintaining of ego structural apparatuses—which, in turn, contribute to the regulation of instinctual drives. Furthermore, the ego's increasing capacity to tolerate moderate amounts of anxiety and other dysphoric affects within manageable limits minimizes the defensive interference of introjective configurations to allow for nonconflictual and independent operation of ego-consolidating identification or other synthetic processes.

2. *Relation to reality*. Among the ego's principal functions is its capacity to maintain a relationship with the external world. This relationship can be divided into three aspects: the sense of reality, reality testing, and adaptation to reality. The sense of reality occurs simultaneously with the development of the ego. The infant becomes aware of the reality of body sensations and then develops the capacity to distinguish reality outside the body. Reality testing refers to the ego's capacity for objective evaluation and judgment of the external world. The primary autonomous functions of the ego, such as memory and perception, are especially significant.

Reality testing is extremely important in the ego's ability to interface with the outside world, and impairment of this function is generally seen in severe mental disorders. The capacity to test reality develops slowly and is closely related to the progression from the pleasure to the reality principle. This capacity, the ability to distinguish fantasy from actuality, is subject to regression and temporary deterioration in children of grade-school age when they are faced with sexual conflict or intense instinctual wishes. Such regression, however, should not be confused with the breakdown of reality testing that accrues in adult psychopathology. The adaptation to reality refers to the capacity of the ego to utilize a person's resources to develop satisfactory resolutions to changing circumstances on the basis of previously tested judgments of reality.

The ego may retain good reality testing with regard to perception and grasp, but the individual's full resources may not be adequately utilized in the situation as it is perceived. Adaptation should be distinguished from adjustment, in which there is an accommodation to reality at the expense of particular resources or potentialities of the individual. Adaptation is more closely allied to the concept of mastery, both with respect to external tasks and in the control of the instincts.

Finally, adaptation to reality is an activity closely related to the defensive functions of the ego. Thus, in the obsessive-compulsive person, isolation of affect may serve important inner needs to curb instinctual drives. However, from another perspective, such affective isolation may be highly adaptive in enabling an individual to deal successfully with the complexities of external reality, as in the case of a surgeon in the operating room.

3. *Object relationships*. The capacity to form mutually satisfying relationships is one of the fundamental functions of the ego. The significance of object relationships in normal psychological development and in psychopathological conditions was not fully appreciated until relatively late in the evaluation of classic psychoanalysis. The development of the child's capacity for relationships with others, progressing from a state of narcissism to social relationships, first within the family and then within the larger community, has been addressed. Much emphasis has been placed on the early stages in the relationship with the need-satisfying object and on object constancy, which begins when the infant is approximately 6 months of age. The development of object relationships may be disturbed by a number of factors, such as retarded development, regression, or inherent genetic defects or limitations in the capacity to develop object relationships. Finally, the development of object relationships is closely related to the concomitant evolution of drive components and the phase-appropriate defenses that accompany them.

4. *Synthetic function of the ego*. Described by Herman Nunberg in 1931, the synthetic function of the ego refers to the ego's integrative capacities. It concerns the overall organization and functioning of the ego and involves other ego functions throughout the course of its operations. More specifically, the ego synthetic function refers to the ego's tendency to bind, unite, coordinate, and create. It also includes its capacity to simplify or to generalize.

5. *Primary autonomous ego functions*. As early as 1937, Freud referred to primal, congenital ego variations, but this concept was expanded and clarified by Hartmann. Primary autonomous ego functions are ascribable to rudimentary apparatuses present at birth that develop independently of conflict with the id in what Hartmann has termed the *average expectable environment*. On his list of primary autonomous ego functions, Hartmann included perception, intuition, comprehension, thinking, language, particular phases of motor development, learning, and intelligence. Initially evolved as conflict-free, these functions can become involved in conflict in the course of development. If, for example, overly aggressive and competitive impulses intrude on the impetus to learn, the ego may react with inhibitory responses and symptoms.

6. *Secondary autonomous ego functions*. According to Hartmann's concept of secondary autonomy, the conflict-free sphere of ego functioning derived from the primary autonomous structure can be enlarged when functions are withdrawn from the dominance of the drives. A mechanism that arose originally in the service of defense against instinctual drives may become an independent structure. Thus, the apparatus may come to serve functions other than the original defensive function. For example, an early obsessive-compulsive defense against the wish to soil may become pleasurable in its own right and be employed conflict-free in the individual's

chosen vocation as an accountant. This change of function, described by Hartmann, may occur as a result of neutralization, a generalization of Freud's concept of sublimation or desexualization. In neutralization, there is desexualization of libidinal drives or the deaggressivization of aggressive drives, providing the ego with independent energies and functions that arise without drive interference.

7. *Defensive functions of the ego*. In his initial psychoanalytic formulations, and even later, Freud equated the mechanism of expression with defense. Repression was directed primarily against impulse drives or drive representations, and especially against direct expressions of the sexual instinct. Upon the development of the structural theory, the function of defense was shifted to the ego. But only after Freud had formulated his second theory of anxiety was it possible to study the operations of the various defense mechanisms, or their mobilization in response to danger signals. And not until Anna Freud published *The Ego and the Mechanisms of Defense* was there presented a systematic and comprehensive study of the defenses. She took the strong position that everyone employs a characteristic repertoire of defense mechanisms, although of varying degrees. From her studies of children, she was not only able to explain their inability to tolerate excessive instinctual stimulation but to examine the processes whereby the intensity of drives at various developmental stages evoked defense-producing anxiety in the ego. In her clinical work with adults, she was able to derive a useful source of information about the ego's defensive operations.

Genesis of defense mechanisms During one's early developmental stages, the defenses emerge as a precipitate of the ego's struggles to mediate between the pressures of the id and the confines and requirements of outside reality. And at each phase of libidinal development, the associated drive components arouse characteristic ego defenses. For example, the mechanisms of introjection, denial, and projection are seen with oral incorporative or oral sadistic impulses, whereas reaction formations, such as shame and disgust, develop in relation to anal impulses and pleasures. Furthermore, the defense mechanisms from earlier phases of development may persist into later phases. Consequently, if the defense associated with pregenital periods of development predominate in adult life over more mature mechanisms, such as repression or intellectualization, the personality retains an infantile cast.

The kinds of defenses characteristically employed by a person to deal with stressful situations contribute to the person's character. Character traits, such as excessive orderliness or tidiness, although closely related to defenses, are distinguished from them by their total functioning in the general behavior of the individual and in situations that are not associated with conflict. Defenses, in themselves, are not pathological. They serve an important function in maintaining normal psychological well-being.

Psychopathology may arise as a consequence of one or several possible alterations of normal defensive functioning. In the case of hysteria, the defense of hysteria is overwhelmed by excessive sexual stimulation. In response to the upsurge in previously repressed impulses, more desperate efforts at renewed repression take place, resulting in phobic symptoms or conversion phenomena. The hysterical individual shows exaggerated development of and excessive resort to certain defenses, reacting in adulthood as though the dangers from infantile impulses were of the same dangerous magnitude. Such hypertrophy of certain defense mechanisms is characteristic of obsessional personalities and obsessive-compulsive neurotics. Then, too, the ego and its defenses may exhibit faulty development with an overreliance on the mechanisms of denial, projection, and distortion that are more characteristic of the early oral phases of development. In such cases, the defensive patterns interfere with the individual's ability to form meaningful object attachments, to engage in satisfactory heterosexual relationships, and to deal successfully or comfortably with competition at work. Finally, when the defenses fail, a breakthrough of direct instinctual expressions may occur with noticeable regression in the ego's capacity to control mobility, thinking, or affect as is exemplified in the schizophrenias.

Classification of defenses The ego defenses can be classified in a number of ways, none of which has taken into consideration all of the relevant factors. A developmental classification can be used where defenses are classified according to the libidinal phase in which they arise. Denial, projection, and distortion would be assigned to the oral stage of development and to the corresponding state of narcissistic object relationships. But some defense mechanisms, such as regression, cannot be categorized in this manner. In addition, some basic developmental processes, such as introjection and projection, may also serve defensive functions under certain conditions.

The defenses may be classified on the basis of the kind of psychopathology with which they are commonly seen. Thus, the hysterical defenses would include dissociation, repression, conversion, somatization, and isolation; however, defensive operations are not limited to pathological conditions. The defenses also may be divided into simple or complex mechanisms, into immature or mature defenses, or into psychotic or neurotic defenses.

Psychoanalysts disagree as to the actual number of defense mechanisms. According to Freud, defense mechanisms should possess the following properties: (1) they are a major means of managing instinct and affect; (2) they are unconscious; (3) they are discrete; (4) they are dynamic and reversible; and (5) they can be adaptive as well as pathological. A brief classification and descriptions of some basic defense mechanisms commonly recognized are given in Table 6.1-1.

THE SUPEREGO Last of the structural components to develop, the superego owes many of its origins to the ego. The superego has been called the heir to the Oedipus complex, and is greatly influenced by the resolution of the oedipal conflict. It is primarily concerned with moral behavior and also is involved in neurotic conflict. Structurally, neurotic conflict is understood as the struggle between the ego and the id. The superego may ally itself with the ego by imposing guilt feelings, or it may side with the id against the ego, especially when the individual shows marked regression.

Historically, the notion of the superego first appeared in 1896 with Freud's *Further Remarks on the Defense Neuro-Psychoses*, in which he described obsessional ideas as "self-reproaches which have reemerged in transmuted form and . . . relate to some sexual act that was performed with pleasure in childhood." In his early discussions of dreams, Freud mentions the activities of a self-criticizing agency that acts as a censor to deny unacceptable ideas entry into consciousness on moral grounds. The concept of a special self-critical agency can be traced to his 1914 paper "On Narcissism," in which he spoke of a hypothetical state of narcissistic perfection existing in early childhood where the child was the child's own ideal. But as the child grew up, this perfect image was destroyed because of the admonitions of others and the child's own self-criticism. To compensate for this lost narcissism, or to recover it, the child "projects before him" a new ideal or "ego-ideal." Having arrived at this point, Freud proposed the existence of another structural component, a special agency whose function it was to watch over the ego to make sure that

TABLE 6.1-1
Classification of Defense Mechanisms

	Narcissistic Defenses
Projection	A person attributes his or her own feelings and wishes to another individual because of intolerable inner feelings or painful affects. Characteristically present in psychotic states, especially paranoid syndromes, projection is also widely used under normal conditions. In psychoses, projection takes the form of frank delusions about external reality, usually persecutory in nature, and includes the perception of one's own feelings toward another and subsequent acting on the perception.
Projective identification	Unwanted aspects of the self are deposited into another person such that the individual projecting feels at one with the object of the projection. The extruded aspects are modified by and recovered from the recipient. This defense allows one to distance and make oneself understood by exerting pressure on another individual to experience feelings similar to one's own.
Primitive idealization	Through this mechanism, external objects that are viewed as either "all good" or "all bad" are unrealistically endowed with great power. Most commonly, the "all good" object is seen as omnipotent, or ideal, while the badness in the "all bad" object is greatly inflated.
Splitting	External objects are divided into "all good" and "all bad" accompanied by the abrupt shifting of an object from one extreme category to the other. Sudden and complete reversal of feelings and conceptualizations about a person may occur. The extreme repetitive oscillation between contradictory self-concepts is another manifestation of this mechanism.
Denial	This defense is used to avoid becoming aware of some painful aspect of reality. There may be a massive denial of the event itself, its memory, or only the affect associated with a particular idea or experience. Refusing to acknowledge what one sees or hears and negating the experience is an example of denial. Denial may be used in normal or pathological states. The excessive use of denial may precipitate a psychosis and the denied reality may be replaced by a fantasy or delusion.
Distortion	External reality is grossly reshaped to satisfy inner needs. Examples of distortion include hallucinations, wish-fulfilling delusions, megalomaniacal beliefs, and sustained feelings of delusional superiority or entitlement. There may be a merging or fusion with another person. Distortion can be highly adaptive, as manifested in religious beliefs.
	Immature Defenses
Acting out	The individual expresses an unconscious wish or impulse through action to avoid being conscious of the accompanying affect. The unconscious fantasy is lived out impulsively in behavior, thereby gratifying the impulse rather than the prohibition against it. Acting out involves chronically giving in to an impulse to avoid the tension that would result from the postponement of expression.
Blocking	A temporary or transient inhibition of thinking occurs in blocking. Affects and impulses may also be involved. Blocking closely resembles repression but differs in that tension arises when the impulse, affect, or thought is inhibited.
Hypochondriasis	Reproach arising from bereavement, loneliness, or unacceptable aggressive impulses toward others is transformed into self-reproach and complaints of pain, somatic illness, and neurasthenia. An illness may also be exaggerated or overemphasized for the purpose of evasion and regression. In hypochondriasis, responsibility can be avoided, guilt may be circumvented, and instinctual impulses are warded off. Because hypochondriacal introjects are ego-alien, the afflicted individuals experience dysphoria and a sense of affliction.
Introjection	Although vital to the developmental stages of the individual, introjection also serves specific defensive functions. The process of introjection involves the internalization of the qualities of an object, and when used as a defense, it can obliterate the distinction between the subject and the object. Through introjection of a loved object, the painful awareness of separateness or the threat of loss may be avoided. Introjection of a feared object serves to avoid anxiety when the aggressive characteristics of the object are internalized, thus placing the aggression under one's own control. A classic example is identification with the aggressor. An identification with the victim may also take place, where the self-punitive qualities of the object are taken over and established within one's self as a symptom or character trait.
Passive-aggressive behavior	Aggression toward others is expressed indirectly through passivity, masochism, and turning against the self. Manifestations of passive-aggressive behavior include failures, procrastination, or illnesses that affect others more than oneself.
Projection	At higher levels of functioning, projection may take the form of misattributing or misunderstanding motives, attitudes, feelings, or intentions of others. It includes severe prejudice, rejection of intimacy through suspicious hypervigilance to external danger, and a keen awareness of injustices.
Regression	Through this device, the person attempts to return to an earlier libidinal phase of functioning to avoid the tension and conflict evoked at the present level of development. It reflects the basic tendency to gain instinctual gratification at a less-developed period. Regression is a normal phenomenon as well, as a certain amount of regression is essential for relaxation, sleep, and orgasm in sexual intercourse. Regression is also considered an essential concomitant of the creative process.
Schizoid fantasy	Through fantasy, a person indulges in autistic retreat in order to resolve conflict and to obtain gratification. Interpersonal intimacy is avoided and eccentricity serves to repel others. The individual does not fully believe in or insists on acting out the fantasies.
Somatization	Psychic derivatives are converted into bodily symptoms and there is the tendency to react with somatic rather than psychic manifestations. In desomatization, infantile somatic responses are replaced by thought and affect; in resomatization, there is regression to earlier somatic forms in the face of unresolved conflicts.

TABLE 6.1.1 (*Continued*)

	Neurotic Defenses
Controlling	An excessive attempt exists to manage or regulate events or objects in the environment to minimize anxiety and to resolve inner conflicts.
Displacement	An emotion or drive cathexis from one idea or object is shifted to another that resembles the original in some aspect or quality. Displacement permits the symbolic representation of the original idea or object to be assumed by another idea or object that is less highly cathected or evokes less distress.
Dissociation	A temporary but drastic modification of a person's character or of one's sense of personal identity takes place to avoid emotional distress. Fugue states or hysterical conversion reactions are common manifestations of dissociation. Dissociation may also be found with counterphobic behavior, overactivity, and the use of pharmacological highs or religious joy.
Externalization	A more general term than projection, externalization refers to the tendency to perceive in the external world and in external objects elements of one's own personality, including instinctual impulses, conflicts, moods, attitudes, and styles of thinking.
Inhibition	In inhibition, limitations or renunciation of ego functions occur consciously, alone or in combination, to evade anxiety arising out of conflict with instinctual impulses, the superego, or environmental forces or figures.
Intellectualization	Closely allied to rationalization, intellectualization is the excessive use of intellectual processes to avoid affective expression or experience. Undue emphasis is focused on the inanimate in order to avoid intimacy with people, attention is paid to external reality to avoid expression of inner feelings, and stress is excessively placed on irrelevant details to avoid perceiving the whole.
Isolation	Isolation refers to the splitting or separation of an idea from the affect that accompanies it but is repressed. Social isolation refers to the absence of object relationships.
Rationalization	Rational explanations are offered by an individual in an attempt to justify attitudes, beliefs, or behavior that might otherwise be unacceptable. Such underlying motives are usually instinctually determined.
Reaction formation	Through this mechanism, an unacceptable impulse is transformed into its opposite. Reaction formation is characteristic of obsessional neurosis, but it may occur in other forms of neuroses as well. If this mechanism is frequently used at any early stage of ego development, it can become a character trait on a permanent basis, as in an obsessional character.
Repression	An idea or feeling may be expelled or withheld from consciousness in repression. Primary repression refers to the curbing of ideas and feelings before they have attained consciousness; secondary repression excludes from awareness what was once experienced at a conscious level. The repressed is not really forgotten in that symbolic behavior may be present. This defense differs from suggestion by effecting conscious inhibition of impulses to the point of losing and not just postponing cherished goals. Conscious perception of instincts and feelings is blocked.
Sexualization	An object or function is endowed with sexual significance that it did not previously have, or possessed to a lesser degree, in order to ward off anxieties associated with prohibited impulses or their derivatives.
	Mature Defenses
Altruism	Through this mechanism, the individual undergoes a vicarious experience by means of constructive and instinctually gratifying service to others. It includes benign and constructive reaction formation. Altruism is distinguished from altruistic surrender, where a surrender of direct gratification or of instinctual needs takes place in favor of fulfilling the needs of others to the detriment of the self, and the satisfaction can only be enjoyed vicariously through introjection.
Anticipation	Realistic anticipation of, or planning for, future inner discomfort that is goal-directed implies careful planning or worrying, and premature but realistic affective anticipation of dire and potentially dreadful outcomes.
Asceticism	In this defense, pleasurable effects of experiences are eliminated. There is a moral element in assigning values to specific pleasures. Gratification is derived from renunciation and asceticism is directed against all base pleasure perceived consciously.
Humor	This defense permits the overt expression of feelings and thoughts without personal discomfort or immobilization and does not produce an unpleasant effect on others. It allows the individual to tolerate and yet focus on what is too terrible to be borne; it is different from wit, a form of displacement that involves distraction from the affective issue.
Sublimation	Impulse gratification and the retention of goals are achieved, but the aim or object is altered from one that may have been socially objectionable to a socially acceptable one. Sublimation allows instincts to be channeled rather than blocked or diverted. Feelings are acknowledged, modified, and directed toward a significant object or goal and modest instinctual satisfaction occurs.
Suppression	In suppression, a conscious or semiconscious decision to postpone attention to a conscious impulse or conflict takes place. Issues may be deliberately cut off but they are not avoided. Discomfort is acknowledged but minimized.

Table adapted from Vaillant G E: *Adaptation to Life*. Little, Brown, Boston, 1977; Semrad E: The operation of ego defenses in object loss. In *The Loss of Loved Ones*, D M Moriarty, editor. Charles C Thomas, Springfield, IL, 1967; and Bibring G L, Dwyer T F, Huntington D S, Valenstein A: A study of the psychological process in pregnancy and of the earliest mother-child relationship: II. Methodological considerations. Psychoanal Stud Child *16:* 25, 1961, with permission.

it was measuring up to the ego-ideal. Thus, the superego evolved from the formulation of the existence of an ego-ideal and a special monitoring agency to ensure its preservation.

The ego-ideal The existence of the superego is once again brought up in 1915 in Freud's *Mourning and Melancholia,* where he speaks of "one part of the ego" which "judges it critically and, as it were, takes it as the object." Freud believed that this agency, which is split off from the rest of the ego, is what is commonly called the conscience. Freud stated that this self-evaluating agency acts independently, can become diseased, and is to be regarded as a major institution of the ego. In 1921, he termed this self-critical agency the ego-ideal and considered it responsible for the sense of guilt and the self-reproaches that are typical in melancholia and depression. By then, he no longer distinguished between an ego-ideal, or ideal self, and a self-critical agency, or the conscience.

In 1923, in *The Ego and the Id,* Freud assigned both the ego-ideal and the conscience to the superego. He believed that the operations of the superego were mostly unconscious because patients suffering from a severe sense of guilt punished themselves more harshly on an unconscious level than they did consciously, and that neurotics felt better when they were punished and had been suffering from guilt. These findings supported Freud's contention that such patients suffered from an unconscious need for punishment. In later works, Freud elaborated further on the relationship between the ego and the superego. He concluded that guilt feelings arose from tension between these two agencies and that the need for punishment was a manifestation of this tension.

In *Civilization and Its Discontents,* in 1930, Freud elaborated on the relationship of the superego to the aggressive instinct. Specifically, he believed that when an instinct undergoes repression, its libidinal aspects may be transformed into symptoms and its aggressive components are transformed into a sense of guilt.

Finally, Freud correlated the development of the superego with the evolution of culture and interpersonal relationships in society. In such moral precepts as "Love thy neighbor," aimed at controlling aggression, the cultural superego exerts external pressure on the individual much as the personal superego dictates internally. Freud believed that the cultural superego that represents the ideals of civilization evolved from the impact of the personalities of great leaders, "men of overwhelming force of mind or men in which one of the human compulsions has found its strongest and surest, and therefore often its most one-sided, expression." Freud recognized that certain limits on individual satisfaction were necessary in keeping with the demands of civilization, but he lamented deeply the degree of which individual instinctual gratification had to be renounced in order to conform to the social requirements of the larger group. Recognizing that his application of individual psychology to society as a whole was by analogy, Freud posed his ideas rather tentatively, but unfortunately they have often been expanded on a rather superficial level in discussions of the neurotic culture of the time.

Origins of the superego The superego appears on the resolution of the Oedipus complex, although primitive forerunners are evident pregenitally. As described earlier, during the oedipal period, the little boy wishes to possess his mother and the little girl her father. The parent of the same sex is seen as a substantial obstacle. The frustration of the child's positive oedipal wishes by this parent evokes intense hostility that is expressed in overly antagonistic behavior and through thoughts of killing the parent who stands in the way. Similar feelings are extended to brothers and sisters who compete for the love of the desired parent.

The child's hostility is unacceptable to the parents, and eventually it becomes intolerable to the child as well. Also during this phase, the boy's sexual explorations and masturbation may engender parental disapproval that may be underscored by a real or implied threat of castration. The little boy's observation that women and girls lack a penis convinces him of the reality of castration. As a result, he turns away from the oedipal situation to enter into the latency stage of psychosexual development. At this time, he renounces the sexual expressions of the infantile phase.

When girls become conscious of the fact that they lack a penis, they seek to redeem the loss by obtaining a penis (or a baby) from the father. Girls soon renounce their oedipal strivings because they fear the loss of their mother's love and are disappointed over their father's failure to gratify their wish. The latency phase is less defined in girls, and they continue to express their interest in family relations through play. Frequently, in their games, they act out the roles of wife and mother.

Evolution of the superego With the dissolution of the Oedipus complex, there is the concomitant abandonment of object ties and a rapid acceleration of the identification process. To a certain extent, the child identifies with the parent of the opposite sex after renouncing oedipal object ties, but for the most part, the strivings toward masculinity in boys and toward femininity in girls leads to a stronger identification with the parent of the same sex. However, the bisexual potential of boys and girls complicates the issue. A child may emerge from the Oedipus complex with varying degrees of masculine and feminine identifications. Such identifications play a significant role in the individual's character formation and later object choices.

In terms of superego formation, the identifications with both parents become integrated to form a precipitate within the ego that interacts with other contents of the ego as a superego. The identification with parents is further reinforced in the child's struggles to repress instinctual aims that were directed toward them, and the act of renunciation provides the superego with a prohibitive character. Then, too, the child's superego is shaped by an identification with the parents' superego.

Because the superego evolves to a large extent as a result of repression of the instincts, it is more closely related to the id than to the ego. Whereas the ego originates to a greater extent through interactions with the external world, the superego's origins are more internal. Throughout the latency period and beyond, one continues to build on early identifications via contacts with authority figures and admired persons who become incorporated into one's moral standards and values, aspirations, and ideals.

As the child moves into the latency period, conflicts with the parents continue but are generally less intense. They are more internal and occur between the ego and the superego. Standards, restrictions, and punishments previously imposed by the parents are now internalized in the superego, which, even in the absence of parents or external authorities, judges and guides behavior from within.

The young superego is initially rigid and overly punitive, but with further growth, it is usually modified to permit an adult sexual object choice. The adolescent period becomes a unique developmental challenge with the heightening of sexual and aggressive drives. Abandoned incestuous ties to the parents and the undermining of the superego are once again revived. The upheaval and rebellious acting-out behavior of teenagers can be understood in terms of the instinctual release that the superego has previously curbed. From another perspective, this behavior also can be seen as a deflection from the more threatening attachment to the parents to representatives in the external environment. In the case of the ascetic, oversubmissive, or intellectual adolescent, one sees a superego that has responded to the threat posed by these heightened drives with increased vigilance and intensified instinctual renunciation. One of the major tasks of adolescence, therefore, is to modify the development of the superego. The pregenital precursors of the superego are believed to provide the very rigid, strict, and aggessive qualities of the superego. These characteristics stem from the projection of the child's sadistic drives and primitive concept of justice based on retaliation that was formerly attributed to the parent. The strict emphasis on absolute cleanliness and propriety frequently found in obsessive-compulsives and very rigid individuals is based to some extent on the sphincter morality of the anal period. It should be noted that Melanie Klein's postulate that the Oedipus complex, including the superego, is established by the first year of life, derives from another theoretical framework and should not be confused with the classical psychoanalytic concept of pregenital precursors of the superego.

NATURE OF ANXIETY

One of Freud's most important contributions to psychoanalytic thinking was his conceptualization of anxiety, on which many analytic concepts rest. Initially, Freud's theory of anxiety emphasized the biological origins of the sexual instinct. From his clinical studies in the 1890s, he attributed pathological anxiety to a disturbance in sexual function. But Freud believed that different etiological factors were responsible for anxiety in specific oedipal identifications with the parents. With successful modification, the individual should be able to make a love-object choice that is not entirely dictated by the need for a parent substitute or to rebel against internalized images.

Of continuing interest has been the role of the drives and object attachments formed in the preoedipal period in clinical entities. Syndromes Freud called the actual neuroses (neurasthenia, hypochondriasis, and anxiety neuroses) had a physical basis, whereas the psychoneuroses (hysteria, phobias, and obsessional neuroses) were attributable primarily to psychological factors.

It was Freud's early contention that an increase in sexual tension, thought to be a physiological event, leads to an increase in its mental representation, libido, which is linked to various ideas and emotions. In the completed act of sexual intercourse, sexual tension is discharged somatically with a decrease in libido. But in the actual neuroses, abnormal sexual practices, such as coitus interruptus, prevent the adequate discharge of sexual tensions and the concomitant psychic elaborations. Freud maintained that this interference gave rise to anxiety. In contrast, anxiety in the psychoneurotic states was attributed to psychic conflict that interfered with normal sexual functioning. It was not until 1926 that Freud modified his original theory of anxiety.

MODIFICATIONS Many analysts have objected to Freud's first hypothesis regarding the somatic or toxic aspects of sexual functioning as being naive. Today, however, neurobiological findings lend some credence to Freud's somatic basis for anxiety. Biological dysregulation in some individuals with hyperactive alerting systems related to a failure of γ-aminobutyric acid (GABA) activity may be a significant factor in the production of anxiety. However, much remains to be learned.

Nevertheless, a somatic etiology to explain anxiety has certain inherent limitations. It contradicts a basic tenet in the psychoanalytic conceptualization of the psychoneuroses. If, in the psychoneuroses, anxiety is the result of sexual repression, the repression must have preceded anxiety. The question of what caused the repression also arises. Freud had contradicted himself. He had stated earlier that repression occurred in response to unbearable affects, which would, of course, include the affect of anxiety.

Freud's original theory did not account for the anxiety that appears in response to real danger, or objective anxiety. This anxiety may seem indistinguishable from that found in neurotic states and it is not related to the accumulation of sexual tensions. Freud soon acknowledged that a comprehensive theory of anxiety had to take into account its relationship to goals of self-preservation. The function of anxiety had to be considered. In his later theory of anxiety, Freud attempted to resolve the limitations in his first theory but he did not discard the essential relationship between thwarted sexuality and anxiety in certain neuroses.

NEW THEORY OF ANXIETY

Freud's second theory of anxiety appeared in 1926 in *Inhibitions, Symptoms and Anxiety,* when he had replaced the topographic model with the structural model. The ego assumed greater importance, with less emphasis on the role of drives in anxiety and the biological approach was set aside. The new theory focused on the function of anxiety in relation to internal and external threats to the organism. Real or external anxiety and neurotic or internal anxiety were now viewed as occurring in response to a danger to the organism. In real anxiety, the threat comes from a known danger outside of the person, whereas in neurotic anxiety, the danger is precipitated by an unknown and not necessarily external source.

A SIGNAL OF DANGER In his new theory, Freud identified two types of anxiety-provoking situations. The first kind took as its prototype the phenomenon of birth, where anxiety was a result of excessive instinctual stimulation that overwhelmed the organism's binding capacity. In this situation, the individual is in a state of helplessness and the excessive accumulation of instinctual energy penetrates the protective barriers of the ego, producing a state of trauma. Although such traumatic states most frequently are seen in infancy or childhood, when the ego is relatively undeveloped, they may also arise in adults who experience psychotic turmoil or in panic states when the ego organization is dangerously overwhelmed.

The second, and more common, situation occurs typically after the defensive organization has matured and when anxiety develops in anticipation of dangers and not as their result. This anxiety is subjectively experienced as similar to the anxiety over a past danger. The affect of anxiety serves a protective function by warning the subject of the approach of danger. Signal anxiety, which may be produced at a subconscious or unconscious level, signals the ego to mobilize protective measures to avert the danger and prevent a traumatic situation. The dangers may arise from either external or internal sources, such as the potential overwhelming of the defenses by instinctual drives. Defense mechanisms can be brought to bear against real or imagined dangers from without or within to guard against or reduce the degree of instinctual excitation.

According to this revised theory of anxiety, the appearance of neurotic symptoms indicates a partial failure of the psychic apparatus to cope with excitation or stimuli. The defensive activity of the ego has not succeeded in adequately containing the threatening drive manifestations or danger. In the case of phobias, the danger that arises from within becomes externalized and is perceived as though it had originated in the external world. The appearance of a neurotic symptom is seen as a failure in the defensive function of the ego, resulting in a partial distortion of the relationship of the ego to the external environment. In psychotic states, there is a drastic breakdown in ego defensive functioning where greater distortions of the ego take place to accommodate the distortions of the outside world as perceived by the patient.

CHARACTERISTIC DANGER SITUATION During each stage of the child's development, characteristic danger situations may arise that are specific or appropriate to issues pertinent to that particular phase. The earliest danger situation is the loss of the primary object, the person on whom the child is entirely dependent, which occurs when the child is the most immature and helpless psychologically and physiologically. Later in development, the fear of losing the object's love exceeds the fear of losing the object itself.

Most prominent during the phallic phase is the fear of bodily injury or castration. There is great anxiety over the potential loss of a narcissistical and highly invested part of the body. The common fear during the latency period is that the parental representations, expressed via the superego, will cease to love, will be angry with, or will punish the child. Anxiety is seen during each of these phases. Although each of these determinants of anxiety is appropriate to a particular phase, they can exist side by side. Moreover, anxiety with regard to a particular danger situation might not be felt until the developmental phase with which that situation was associated has passed. The persistence of earlier forms of anxiety has important implications for the understanding of psychopathology, reflecting neurotic fixations at earlier stages of development. Frequently, one finds in patients a persistence of these characteristic conflicts from earlier stages.

THE THEORY'S IMPLICATIONS Freud's new theory of anxiety was a very meaningful concept that allowed a much broader application and had greater explanatory power. It represented a decisive shift in Freud's thinking about the ego. When he introduced his structural theory in 1923, he saw the ego as a relatively weak and fragile agency that responded passively to the powerful drives of the id and the severe demands of the superego. However, with the introduction of the signal theory of anxiety, the perception of the ego changed. In his new theory, Freud emphasized that the appearance of anxiety before repression was operative, pointing out that the ego exerted some control over the forces of the id. The ego was also endowed with a degree of autonomy in the exercise of certain functions.

A variety of psychological phenomena can now be more easily understood, but several fundamental questions remain unanswered. Little is known about the conditions or circumstances by which the ego becomes overwhelmed. More knowledge is needed about the quantitative and qualitative factors that determine whether a certain amount of anxiety will stimulate ego development through mobilization and arousal of the individual's ego potential, or whether the same amount of anxiety will impede ego development by engaging the existing ego defense in excessive conflict.

Many analysts agree that anxiety is an important stimulus to structural development. Therefore, one of the important indices of intrapsychic development and ego integration is the individual's capacity to tolerate anxiety. During the process of growth, the ego must develop the capacity to use increasing degrees of anxiety to draw on inner resources to gain mastery and control. This aspect of the new theory of signal anxiety has significant treatment implications regarding how inner growth and change come about in patients.

Operating under his new theory of anxiety, Freud refocused his attention on the concept of defenses. Having gained insight into the nature of anxiety, he was able to formulate the operation of the defense mechanisms. He now regarded repression as only one of the possible defenses employed by the ego, although it remained a cardinal defense. The ego was no longer seen as a passive agency, feeble by comparison with the demands of the id and the outside world. The ego served as a scout, capable of signaling danger situations in advance and having at its disposal a variety of responses to danger, whether from within and from without. In its new role, the ego actively interfaced with the demands of the drives and the outside world.

PSYCHOANALYTIC CONCEPT OF CHARACTER

The concept of character varies widely, having moralistic, literary, sociological, and general meanings. In psychoanalysis, character refers to the unique combination of elements within a person's psychic organization that reflects the basic features of personality structure and style. Many theoretical propositions have been advanced concerning the meaning of character. When Freud was developing his instinctual theory, he pointed to the relationship between certain character traits and their psychosexual components. Obstinancy, orderliness, and parsimoniousness were linked to anality; ambition was related to urethral eroticism; and generosity was associated with orality. In his paper on "Character and Anal Eroticism," Freud concluded that permanent character traits represented "unchanged prolongation of the original instincts, or sublimation of those instincts, or reaction formation against them."

He made an important distinction in 1913 between neurotic symptoms and character traits. According to Freud, neurotic symptoms arise as a result of the failure of repression with the return of the repressed. Character traits, on the other hand, are attributable to the successful employment of repression or of the defense system, particularly through the persistent use of reaction formation and sublimation. In 1923, Freud, with increased understanding of the mechanism of identification and his formulation of the ego as a coherent system of function, clarified the relationship of character to ego development. He observed that the replacement of object attachment by identification, which established the lost object inside the ego, also contributed significantly to character formation. Late in 1932, Freud stressed the importance of identification with the parents in the construction of character, making particular reference to superego formation.

Freud's disciples also made important contributions to the concept of character. Karl Abraham investigated the relationships among oral, anal, and genital eroticism and various character traits. Wilhelm Reich added to the psychoanalytic understanding of character in the 1920s when he described the close relationship between resistance to treatment and the patient's character traits. In fact, Reich's observation that resistance characteristically appeared in the form of these specific traits anticipated Anna Freud's formulations describing the relationship between resistance and typical ego defenses.

CURRENT CONCEPTS OF CHARACTER Character and character traits are included among the properties of the ego, superego, and ego-ideal, although they are not synonymous with any of them. The focus has been extended from an interest in specific character traits to a consideration of character and its formation in general. Contemporary analysts regard character as a pattern of adaptation to instinctual and environmental forces that is typical or habitual for a given person. The character of a person refers largely to directly observable behavior and style of defense, and of acting, thinking, and feeling. The concept of character is employed by most psychiatrists and psychoanalysts.

EVOLUTION OF CHARACTER The interplay of multiple factors helps to form character and character traits. Innate biological predisposition also plays a role in character formation in the form of instinctual and ego anlage. Perhaps the major determinant in the development of character is the early interaction of id forces with ego defenses and environmental influences, especially the parents. In addition, early identifications and imitations of other human beings play a significant role in character formation. Important, too, is the developing capacity of the ego to tolerate delay in drive discharge and to neutralize instinctual energy stemming from early identifications and defense formations, which determine the later emergence of character traits such as impulsiveness. A particularly close association has been observed between character traits and the development of the ego-ideal. Over the past decade, attention has been focused on the developmental vicissitudes of narcissism and their impact on the formation of the ego-ideal. The exaggeration of certain character traits at the expense of others may lead to character disorders in later life. Such distortions in the development of character traits may produce a vulnerability or predisposition to psychotic decompensation.

IDENTITY The concept of identity is discussed at this point because of the close association with the terms identity and the self. Erik Erikson's formulations of the notions of identity and identity formation still have not attained a clear or definite position in psychoanalytic theory. The specific relationships among ego, self, character, and personality have yet to be defined to the satisfaction of most psychoanalysts. Even Erikson's own use of the term "identity" varies; at one time it specifically refers to the ego and at another to the total personality organization. More important are the questions raised about its connection to the current concept of the self. Some workers feel that the notion of identity can help bridge the psychology of character and the psychology of the self.

In essence, Erikson's notion of identity refers to a complex set of implications, including a conscious sense of individual identity or subjective self-experience, an unconscious striving for continuity of personal character, the result of ego synthesis, and a sense of inner solidarity consistent with the ideals and identity of a social group. According to Erikson, the achievement of identity is assigned to the adolescent period:

> Identity formation, finally, begins where the usefulness of identification ends. It arises from the selective repudiation and mutual assimilation of childhood identifications, and their absorption in configuration, which in turn is dependent on the process by which a new society (often subsocieties) identifies the young individual, recognizing him as somebody who had to become the way he is, and who, being the way he is, is taken for granted.

Taken in this light, identity refers to a specific aspect of self-organization and functioning, and denotes the phase of the subjectively experienced sense of self. Simultaneously, it is an attempt to articulate the role of the self vis-à-vis the object world.

CONCEPTS OF THE SELF In general, the notion of the self has come to be roughly equivalent to the concept of the person. It was Hartmann who attempted to clarify the ambiguity latent in Freud's use of the term "Ich." Hartmann distinguished the ego from the self by assigning the respective terms to different frames of reference. The ego referred to the specific intrapsychic agency with a frame of reference and action occurring within the intrapsychic agency and in relationship to the superego and the id. In contrast, the self had its proper frame of references in relationship to the notion of an object.

In a further effort to elaborate on and clarify the theoretical implications of the self, other thinkers have defined the self in representational terms, referring specifically to the self-representation, a subordinate function of the ego. But another point of view places the self as a structural organization that is seen as a fourth agency in addition to the ego, id, and the superego. As a further extension, some theorists define the self to include the tripartite structures as well as additional structural aspects.

The self can be viewed from a number of perspectives. It can be regarded as agent or as object, or described in locational terms, such as what is inside or outside of the mind or the psychic structure, and whether parts of the self are internalized or externalized. The view of self as an object of inner experience fits with the representational vision of the self, whereas the structural perspective is most congruent with the self as agent, as a source of psychic integration and activity, and as synonymous with the initiating source of personal action and awareness.

Certainly, the self as agent comes closest to the concept of a personal ego in structural theory.

Most psychoanalysts believe that the psychology of the self will occupy a permanent place in theory and practice, but the theory remains in a state of flux. Although an attractive concept, the organization of the self and of the tripartite entities cannot be simply identified. The self-organization operates at a different level of psychic organization than do the structural entities, which are defined as organizations of specific functions. These structures are less personalized, or anthropomorphized.

One of the often-voiced criticisms of the structural theory is that it has difficulty in integrating and explaining complex experiential states. There is no room for the experience of one's own self as an integrated and relatively autonomous self-originating focus of action. The concept of the self can fulfill the role of providing a subjective experience of self as an active and organizing principle with the intrapsychic apparatus.

OBJECT-RELATIONS THEORY

The increasing emphasis in contemporary psychoanalytic understanding on object-relations theory stems from the elaboration of a systematic ego psychology, with its focus on a better understanding of the adoptive functions of the ego and the intimate involvement of the ego with reality. The following are a few of the significant contributors to this theory.

MELANIE KLEIN Melanie Klein is generally acknowledged as a pioneer in presenting an object-relations viewpoint. Originally trained by Abraham in Berlin, she began extensive investigations of childhood pathologies in the 1920s in an attempt to document and refine his views on mental development and its pathological deviations. Much of Klein's focus was on the death instinct, generally regarded as a stepchild in psychoanalytic theory. She is best known for her studies on the developmental vicissitudes of the superego, elaborating on the fantasies and behaviors of severely disturbed children with an analysis of the child's internal psychic world and its development.

In Klein's view, the superego developed independently of biological influences and was heavily influenced by the nature of the child's relationship with the parents and the problems of the primary instincts. She paid great heed to the processes of introjection and projection, which are derived from the drives and their interactions with the primary objects of the child's early experience. For Klein, drives were defined as containing many of the properties of the ego as customarily understood in ego psychology. Drives are primarily relationships. This emphasis on the relationship with objects and a detailed delineation of the child's inner fantasy world in terms of the vicissitudes of the introjects provided Klein's basis for an object-relations perspective of development.

To Klein, internal objects were either good or bad, and the intrapsychic struggles between them and the individual were as meaningful as the conflicts involving objects outside of the person. External and internal objects are not clearly distinguished, according to Klein, because external object relations are influenced by the projective content derived from the internal object relations.

Many important theoretical and clinical innovations can be attributed to Klein. She called attention to the early relationships between the infant and the mother preceding the full development of the Oedipus complex in later childhood, and she introduced the concept of early introjects and identification. Klein contributed to the study of dynamic processes in psychotic, neurotic, and normal mental functioning with her formulations of primitive persecutory anxieties, early defenses dominated by splitting and its elaborations, and depressive anxiety and separation. She developed play techniques and described the insidious workings of greed and envy and their centrality in creating intransigent resistances in the psychonalytic situation.

Klein has been criticized for her vigorous interpretation of all forms of aggressive or destructive intent as manifestations of the death instinct; for her indiscriminate grouping together of all intrapsychic content; for her lack of scientific rigor in equating theoretical inferences with observations; and for predating the emergence of intrapsychic structures or agencies generally believed by other theorists to arise only in later developmental stages, such as the origin of the superego in the first year of life.

Although Klein emphasized the world of internal objects rather than the ego, and especially the role of instincts in the intrapsychic dynamics, rather than the agents themselves, subsequent object-relations theorists have shifted the emphasis from the instincts to a focus on the objects and the external environment.

W. R. D. FAIRBAIRN Another object-relations theorist deserving of mention is W. R. D. Fairbairn, who, in 1931, began to introduce personal object relations into classic psychoanalytic theory. Fairbairn considered the ego to be the core phenomenon of the psyche, as the real self and the dynamic center of the personality. He made a radical shift from emphasis on the instinctual drives to almost sole attention to the ego, where everything in human psychology became an effect of ego functioning. Libido and the instincts in general were regarded as object-seeking. Erotogenic zones became channels that mediated the primary relationships with objects, particularly influencing the relationships with early objects that had been internalized. Klein exerted considerable influence on Fairbairn's work.

Although he retained much of her language, Fairbairn shifted the meanings of Klein's terms. He emphasized the primary world of real others and the compensatory nature of internal objects, and he pointed out the destructiveness of parental deprivation. His most notable contributions to psychoanalysis were his descriptions of the conflicts accompanying the child's earliest relationships with significant others, the internalization of disturbing effects of such relationships, and the importance of the resulting internal object relations in all forms of psychopathology.

Fairbairn also differed from Klein in a number of other significant aspects. Fantasy for Klein was the earliest and most basic activity of the mind and constituted the direct manifestation of the instincts themselves. For Fairbairn, it was substitutive and not primary. From the start, the child is oriented toward reality and relations with others; fantasy represents a compensation for a failure of these actual relations. For Klein, the internal object world occurred naturally and as a continuing accompaniment of all experiences. But for Fairbairn, internal objects were compensatory substitutes for unsatisfactory relationships with real, external objects. According to Klein, internal objects develop around images that are part of the instincts a priori. For Fairbairn, the content of internal objects derived from real, external objects. To Klein, the root of psychopathology lay in the instincts, especially the death instinct, and aggression. But to Fairbairn, psychiatric disorder occurred because of maternal deprivation. Anxiety arises from the need to maintain the tie to the object despite the deprivation and psychopathology that emerged from ego's self-fragmentation in the service of preserving the tie and controlling its ungratifying aspects.

Much of Fairbairn's theorizing was based on his experience with schizoid patients. He believed that, unlike the more neurotic patient, the schizoid individual had to deal not with control of threatening impulses toward objects, but with the problem of forming any object relations. Confounded by the inconsistency in primary objects, the schizoid suffers a loss of internal unity and helplessness. Internalized objects are split into good and bad objects that cannot be amalgamated. Within the ego itself, a radical split occurs.

In essence, Fairbairn's object-relations theory differs from classical theory in the following basic ways: First, the ego is whole or total at birth and then becomes split or loses inner unity if it encounters early bad experiences in object relationships. In classical theory, the ego initially is seen as undifferentiated and unintegrated, and only achieves unity during the course of development. Second, according to Fairbairn, the libido is the primary life drive and the ego's source of energy in the search for relatedness with objects. Third, instead of viewing aggression as an independent instinct, he regarded aggression as a natural defensive reaction to the frustration of the libidinal drive. Fourth, the resulting structural ego pattern emerging from the lost pristine ego unity involves ego splitting and the formation of internal ego-object relations.

MICHAEL BALINT Michael Balint, an analysand and disciple of Ferenczi, offered another relational-structure model. From Balint's perspective, object relations are present from the beginning of life. In fact, the search for the primary love object underlies virtually all psychological phenomena. Balint did not believe in the concept of primary narcissism. From the very beginning, the infant wishes to be loved totally and unconditionally. Balint suggested that when the mother–infant tie is severed too early, the remainder of one's life is devoted to a search for restitution with the "final aim of erotic striving" to obtain passive object love. All psychological motivations are drives representing secondary, compensatory derivatives of the failure to receive sufficient primary love.

Balint differed from Fairbairn in not abandoning drive-structure theory, maintaining that libido is both pleasure-seeking and object-seeking. Like Fairbairn, he studied personality disorders that are more primitive and difficult to treat than the usual neurotic disorders. Thus, both theorists examined levels of early or preoedipal developmental failure.

Balint also had a different understanding of the analytic process. According to him, the first level of material centers around intrapsychic conflicts regarding the genital stage and can be approached with adult language. At the second, deeper level, interpretations using the conventional meaning of words are no longer perceived as meaningful to the patient. Balint believed that at this level of preverbal experience, attempts to describe the child's experience in adult language are bound to fail.

Phases of aggression Balint also described two phases of regression: benign and malignant. Benign regression, or a regression to a level of primitive relationship with the primary objects, is gradual and modulated in keeping with the patient's capacity to tolerate and integrate the resulting anxiety. Empathic responses from the analyst and recognition of this regression enable the patient to undergo the experience and to keep the anxiety within manageable limits. At the level of the basic fault, or early disturbance of object relations, the relationships with infantile objects can be reworked in the hope of changing the patient's basic assumptions that govern the interaction with the object world. The analyst, in order to be effective, provides empathic acceptance and recognition of the regression. The concept of primary love is applied at the deep level to describe the withdrawal of libido from the frustrating object in an attempt to recover the inner harmony in which it is possible to reestablish the conditions of early care and tranquility. The patient seeks basic recognition from the analyst similar to that denied by significant objects early in life.

Malignant regression tends to be precipitous and extreme and represents a need for gratification of instinctual craving. In such an event, traumatic anxiety may overwhelm the ego and prevent the reworking of fundamental disturbances in object relationships. The basic fault is recreated, blocking the development of conditions necessary for therapeutic revision.

D. W. WINNICOTT D. W. Winnicott provided a blend of Freudian and Kleinian thought in the form of a radically different developmental theory. An innovative and influential contributor to object-relations theory, he focused mostly on the conditions that make it possible for a child to develop awareness as a separate person. Winnicott believed that the infant begins life in a state of unintegration with unconnected and diffuse experiences, and that the mother provides the relationships that enable the incipient self of the infant to emerge. A holding environment is supplied by the mother within which the infant is contained and experienced. During the last trimester of pregnancy and for the first few months of the baby's life, the mother is in the state of primary maternal preoccupation, absorbed in fantasies of and experiences with her baby. According to Winnicott, the mother plays a vital role in bringing the world to the child and in offering empathic anticipations of the infant's needs. In this intimate relationship, the infant hallucinates the mother's presence and the content of the conjured material comes closer and closer to the real world.

Winnicott theorized that healthy development requires a perfect environment, albeit a brief one. The maternal preoccupation provides a close and accurate sensitivity to the baby's needs and gestures with the mother functioning as a mirror. Only if the mother is able to resonate with the infant's needs can the baby become attuned to its own bodily functions and drives that afford the basis for the gradually evolving sense of self.

As closely intertwined as mother and infant are, the latter must also be provided the proper conditions for the development of the capacity to be alone. The ability of the mother to offer a nondemanding presence when the infant is not making demands or experiencing needs makes it possible for the infant to experience a state of "going-on being" out of which needs and spontaneous gestures emerge. In Winnicott's words, "It is only when alone that the infant can discover his own personal life."

When the infant's hallucinatory omnipotence is well established, it becomes necessary for the infant to learn the reality of the outside world as well as to experience the limits of personal powers. The mother's failures and decreasing maternal preoccupation force the child to come to terms with reality reinforced by the push toward separateness. As the infant continues to develop, the mother correspondingly responds to any gestures but there is increasingly greater differentiation and interaction.

Winnicott describes two kinds of maternal failures that result in a fragmentation within the infant and a split between a true self and a false self on a compliant basis. The mother may fail to actualize the hallucinatory creations and needs of the infant in excited states, or she may interfere with the child's formlessness and unintegration in quiescent states. The true self, the source of spontaneous needs, images, and gestures, becomes hidden to avoid psychic annihilation, and the false self develops to protect the true self by complying with environmental demands and offering an illusion of personal existence. The result is an overactivity of the mind and a separation of cognitive processes from any affective grounding. A variety of severe character psychopathologies may result.

Transitional objects The notion of transitional objects was introduced by Winnicott to describe transitional phenomena as an aspect of the developmental process. The transitional object represents a way station between hallucinatory omnipotence and the acceptance of objective reality. Transitional objects, usually a favorite toy or a blanket, help the child negotiate the gradual shift from the experience of subjectivity to the sense of objectivity. They represent the child's first object possessions that are regarded as separate from the emerging self or the first "not me" possessions. Winnicott saw the object as a substitute for the maternal breast, which is the first and most significant external object to which the infant relates. Finally, the transitional object exists in an intermediate realm contributed to by both the external reality of the object and the child's own subjectivity. Transitional experiencing, in addition to being a developmental interlude, remains an important realm in healthy adult life. It is within this sphere of experience that art, religious experience, and creativity may roam.

Good-enough mothering For Winnicott, the emergence of a healthy, true self is contingent largely on the specific environmental conditions subsumed under the term "good-enough mothering." If nurtured in a nonimpinging environment, the true self should exhibit "the inherited potential which is experiencing a continuity of being, and acquiring in its own way and at its own speed a personal psychic reality and a personal body scheme." Yet, Winnicott admitted that despite all attempts to allow the emergence of the true self, "at the center of each person is an incommunicado element, and this is sacred and most worthy of preservation."

From a theoretical stance, Winnicott insisted that infants can only be described or understood in relation to the functioning of the mother, and that the earliest object relation consists of interactions between developmental needs within the child and maternal offerings supplied by the mother, which are entirely separate from drive gratification. Instincts exist but they occupy a secondary and peripheral status in development. Mental health is gauged by the relative integrity and spontaneity of the self. Psychopathology takes place where there are corruption and constriction in the movement and expression of the self. Psychosis, therefore, is seen as an environmentally caused disorder with a deficiency from the outside. Regression is not defined as a return to points of libidinal fixation or to specific erotogenic zones of gratification, but as a retreat to a point where the environment has failed the child. Furthermore, regression is not seen as dangerous, but rather as a search for missing relational experiences.

A nonclassical approach Winnicott's perspective of psychoanalytic treatment deviated markedly from the classical approach; he believed that psychoanalysis should supply the missing parental provisions and fulfill early developmental needs. Only if the appropriate facilitating environment is provided can the true self be attained and allowed to continue its growth.

Although aligned with Klein in some respects, Winnicott disagreed with her belief that object relations are derived from inherent, constitutional sources. From his perspective, they are rooted in and are constituted from the mother's interactions as a caretaker and from her character. He also reformulated some of Klein's hypotheses, viewing anxiety and guilt in the depressive position as being more directly related to the real person of the mother than did Klein. Although he acknowledged the existence of an inner world, internal objects, primitive greed, and the importance of fantasy, Winnicott disagreed with Klein's assumption that the infant has a priori knowledge of the father's penis, that birth is experienced in terms of the progression of aggression, and that the death instinct is a vital and necessary concept.

Winnicott redefined aggression as a life force almost synonymous with activity and devoid of anger or hate. He saw the Oedipus complex not as a conflict between drive and social reality, but as a conflict between love and hate. A sharp difference in focus between Freud and Winnicott is seen in the former's emphasis on the division between drives and regulatory functions and the latter's focus on the different forms of relation between self and others. Winnicott also believed that psychopathology is rooted in relational difficulties in contrast to the classical view that illness is based on the conflict arising between drive and defense. According to Winnicott, neurosis is understood as an inherent illness in life and in living as a whole person, who must deal with universal instinctual conflicts and constitutional excesses and deficiencies, as well as balances and imbalances.

EDITH JACOBSON The contributions of Jacobson warrant mention because they contain a mixture of object-relations and metapsychological concepts. Her complex descriptions of developmental psychology and severe psychopathology, revisions of classicial metapsychology, and descriptive clinical work with severely disturbed patients have had a significant effect on the work of contemporary psychoanalysts.

Developmentally, Jacobson views the infant's experience of pleasure or unpleasure as the core of the relationship with the mother. She suggests that this experience leads to specific developmental crucial relationships to the object. Satisfactory experiences lead to the formation of good or gratifying images whereas unsatisfactory experiences create bad or frustrating images. These images of the mother, along with their emotional attitudes, form the beginning of internal object relations. But the object-related attitudes acquire a motivational power of their own, independent of the search for drive gratification.

According to Jacobson, inadequate responses from the mother to the infant's needs frustrate and disappoint the infant. Frustration refers to drive demand in contrast to disappointment, which refers to the quality of the nascent object relationship. Disappointment results in devaluation of the object, which results in the discharge of aggressive drive energies in frustrating situations. Disappointment and subsequent devaluation create the desire to expel, to get away from, and to separate from the noxious object.

Similarly, pleasurable experiences give rise to specific attitudes toward the object. Experiencing pleasure, the infant values the object, and desiring to possess the source of the pleasure, attempts to merge with it. A sequence of attitudes toward the object arises that have a dynamic life of their own relatively independent of the drive demands on which they are generically based, and are understood as transactions between the self and the object world.

Jacobson attributes a causative, functional significance to relations with others. She regards the pathology of mood disorders, borderline states, and overt psychoses as derivatives of disturbances of self and object representations. The vicissitudes of the self and the object and their mutual relations depend on the actions of the ego and influence ego development. The ego and the self and object images exert a reciprocal influence on one another's development as well.

In Jacobson's view, the concept of fixation refers to modes of object relatedness and not to modes of gratification. Normal and pathological development are based on the evolution of images of the self and others. Early and austere disappointments that arise before the consolidation, differentiation, and instinctual investment of the self and object representation will result in an aggressive devaluation of the object to include a corresponding devaluation of the as-yet-undifferentiated self. Idealized self and object images will merge into a wished-for but unattainable goal, and a corresponding devaluation of other merged, hated self and object representations. The idealized images are believed to give rise to a precocious ego-ideal, whereas the superego itself will comprise archaic self and object representations that are unduly harsh, eventuating in depressive or psychotic psychopathology. Thus, development is conceptualized by Jacobson in terms of instinctual states and according to stages of ego maturation and object relations.

View of disappointment In contrast to other object-relations theorists, Jacobson's view of disappointment in the object is not synonymous with maternal failure. For her, disappointment is always relative to a specific, drive-determined demand rather than a global striving for contact or engagement. Jacobson differs from drive-theory proponents with regard to the concept of *primary narcissism* with her definition that it refers to "the earliest infantile period, preceding the development of the self and object images, the stage during which the infant is as yet unaware of anything but his own experiences of tension and relief, of frustration and gratification." Primary narcissism is no longer an instinctual vicissitude, but is defined in terms of object relatedness. Traditional drive concepts are viewed in experiential and relational terms. With regard to the energetic hypothesis, she postulates an initial state of undifferentiated energy that only later acquires libidinal or aggressive qualities, "under the influence of external stimulation of psychic growth and the opening up and increasing maturation of pathways for outside discharge." Furthermore, the two drives are "psychobiologically predetermined and are promoted by internal maturational factors as well as by external stimuli."

The traditional drive concept of orality is expanded by Jacobson to include the stimulation, gratification, and frustration occurring during the first few months of life; the understanding that the child's oral needs create a bond with the mother; and the fact that the oral drive serves as an organizing principle through which the infant orders the entire range of earliest experiences with caretakers. To Jacobson, orality becomes a mode of experience through which self-representations and representation of the mother emerge, accompanied by object-directed aims. During this period, merger fantasies and wishes to expel or to separate serve as the foundation for all subsequent object relations. The early fantasized transactions between infant and mother take place through the processes of introjection and projection.

Concept of the ego In Jacobson's complex conceptualization of the ego, as it matures, it integrates early pleasure–unpleasure experiences into partial primitive images of the self and the object. Subsequent events continue to be experienced as gratifying or frustrating. Such experiences influence the transactions within the representational world, and are also influenced by the level of ego development. A mature ego can resist the merger fantasies following realistic gratification, but, conversely, periods of refusion can weaken the ego functions of perception and reality testing and lead to an earlier, less-differentiated ego state.

By the second year of life, with further maturation of the ego, the child is able to distinguish specific features of the love object and develops an awareness of time and the future. The child is able to entertain the notion of being like the admired object rather than of becoming the object. During this phase, ambivalence and competitive strivings emerge. Aggression promotes the process of intrapsychic separation. But an excess of gratification or frustration can promote regressive merger fantasies. Under favorable conditions, selective identification, or the tendency to be like the object, gradually replaces the tendency toward refusion.

With further development, the child learns to differentiate between realistic and wishful self-images, aided by competition among peers and with the father. Competition fosters the desire for likeness to rivals, and the concomitant discovery of anatomical differences between the sexes contributes to identity formation. Stable ego identification and the establishment of an ego-ideal also take place at this stage. Jacobson differs from Freud by viewing the ego-ideal as the arena in which fusion between ideal self and ideal object images can partly compensate for the lost fantasies of merger. Along with the formation of the ego-ideal, the sense of identity develops, spurred by a desire for likeness to others and one's own internal standards. The development of the superego follows, and takes place in three phases. The early superego consists of archaic, sadistic images formed on the basis of introjective and projective processes; then the ego-ideal comes into being with the fusion of the ideal self and ideal object images; and finally, the mature superego contains the realistic, internalized parental demands, prohibitions, values, and standards.

Affects Jacobson is at variance with Freud's concepts regarding affects. Whereas Freud located affect within the system ego, Jacobson sees some affects as arising from intrasystemic tensions and others as resulting from intrasystemic tensions. Therefore, sexual excitement and rage emerge from the id, object love and hate from the ego, and shame and disgust from tensions between the ego and id. Guilt is the result of tensions between the ego and superego.

Most important, she stresses that affects are experiences to be understood in experiential terms and they cannot be derived from underlying quasibiological processes. The pleasure principle, as redefined by Jacobson, does not aim at the mere lowering of drive quantity, but it directs the course of biological swings around a middle axis or medium level of tension. The pleasure–unpleasure principle cannot be considered an economical principle, but it is not independent of psychoeconomic laws. Jacobson also revises the constancy principle and accords it the function "to establish and maintain a constant axis of tension and a certain margin for the biological vacillations around it." It does not, therefore, operate to keep the level of tension as low as possible as in the classical stance. Jacobson thus offers the explanation that the pleasure principle and the constancy principle actually oppose each other, as the pleasure principle acts to control the swings around the axis of tension and the constancy principle attempts to return the level of tension to that axis. Conflicts between the two principles are resolved by the reality principle.

Jacobson was especially skillful in treating severely disturbed patients by employing modifications of psychoanalytic technique. She feels it is interpretation that produces change in treatment, and does not attribute her technical modifications to the improvement in her patients. A deeply empathic and highly sensitive clinician, she recorded many observations about the idealizing and self-object transferences that were highlighted by later writers to form the basis for the departure from classical technique and to be considered curative in their own right.

OTTO KERNBERG Although he retains the language of drive theory, Kernberg considers his work to be an object-relations theory. He departs from the traditional classical theory in several ways. For Kernberg, the object should mean the human object. He sees human beings as social by nature, emphasizing that "the condensation of aggression and libido into internalized object relations constitute the intrapsychic nurturing of instinctual needs in terms of man's social nature." His statement that in the earliest state of undifferentiation, there is an external object present, although its representation is fused with that of the self, it rejects the concept of primary narcissism. Kernberg does not distinguish between psychic structures and mental representations. The id is created by the ego's regressive capacities, and the id's contents, rather than being biological givens, are configurations of self and object representations. Above all, the self is supraordinate to the ego, thus denying the inclusive nature of the tripartite model of the psychic apparatus. Kernberg qualifies the nature and aims of the drives to a considerable extent. In his theory, drives are psychological systems that organize early experience and then channel it into future motivational aims. Affects become the early and primary motivational forces and the dual instincts of libido and aggression arise from the already object-directed affective states of love and hate.

Kernberg derived much of his theory from his clinical experiences with severely disturbed patients. Most of his inferences were obtained from a study of the transference characteristically shown by these patients. In contradistinction to neurotic patients where intense transferences evolve slowly over the course of treatment, very disturbed patients become intensely involved over short periods, and reveal chaotic reactions and strikingly contradictory attitudes with corresponding, rapidly fluctuating self and object images.

Defense mechanisms A predominance of primitive defense mechanisms, especially splitting, is responsible for the rapid alternation of transference paradigms. The primitive mechanisms of defense that are well described by Kernberg include primitive idealization, devaluation, projection, and projective identification. That the transference paradigms can emerge with such great ease is explained by their nonmetabolized state. Metabolized object relations, in contrast, are allied to such phenomena as transmuting internalization, depersonalization, and internalizations. In psychic metabolism, unlike physical metabolism, the process is reversible and in a repressed state. But with the disturbed patients described by Kernberg, early unmodulated relationships in the transference occur more quickly because adequate metabolization has never taken place. Kernberg explains that because adequate psychic structures have not been developed, the information cannot be sufficiently processed. Analytic treatment should strive to address the splitting and contradictory state of mind to allow the patient to integrate split-off images to form a more unified version of the self and others. The early ego is very weak and organizes experience according to "good" or "bad," the affective coloring that accompanies it. The good and bad experiences remain separated because of ego weakness.

The early experiences, initially unintegrated and split and later employed for defensive responses, are relational configurations. In Kernberg's theory, these configurations are composed of three parts—the image of the object, an image of the self, and the affective coloring determined by the drive derivative present at the time of the interaction. These three components form an internalization system from which experience and the psychic structures are constructed.

Internalization systems are of three kinds, and each reflects the situation at a particular phase of development. Kernberg builds on Jacobson's basic framework with some modifications, changing some terms, and placing greater emphasis on the interaction of relationships with others. He also has a different understanding of the nature of the drives. The most primitive and early form of internalization is termed introjection. At this stage, there is internalization of the least organized and differentiated self and object images accompanied by the least modulated affective coloration. The intermediate level of internalization is called identification, where the child recognizes a personal role and the action of the object in interactions. The image of the object plays a specific role; there is an image of the self perceived in a complementary role; and affect is determined by a modulated drive derivative. The mature level of introjection is ego identity, a concept borrowed from Erikson to denote the overall organization of identifications and introjections that operates under the principle of the synthetic function of the ego. The components of this system are a consistent conception of the object world, a consolidated self as an ongoing organization, and mutual recognition of this constancy by the child and the objects.

Interpersonal exchanges As the child develops, the ego normally experiences greater difficulty in maintaining splitting operations. Opposite-valence self and object images are combined into good and bad object representations, leading to the presence of ambivalence and object-directed affects of guilt, concern, and mourning. Concomitant ideal-self and ideal-object representations develop. Four components are involved in interpersonal exchanges: a real and an ideal self and a real and an ideal object. Eventually, the ego-ideal is established. An integrated ego comes into being with the appearance of higher-level defense mechanisms. Rejected selfobject–affect units that are found unacceptable by the ego are repressed.

Superego, ego, and id Kernberg follows Jacobson closely in describing the establishment and consolidation of the superego. He sees the superego as consisting of three layers. The first layer contains early, hostile object images that reflect the child's projective processes; the second is composed of the ego-ideal formed by fixed ideal self and ideal object representations; and the third is made up of the integrated realistic parental images to include their values, prohibitions, and demands.

Some of Kernberg's positions warrant further comment. For one, he implies that experience precedes the structuralization of the ego. The ego as a structure comes into being with the use of introjection for defensive purposes. His stance is at variance with classical drive theory, which maintains that maturation and development of the structure ego precedes the crucial experiences of object relations. For another, he believes that the dynamic unconscious is composed of rejected introjection and identification systems, and that it is formed on the consolidation of the ego's repressive capabilities. The id is therefore composed of self-images, object images, and their associated affects, but he does not elaborate on the nonrepressed portion of the id. Following Kernberg's logic, the appearance of the structure ego precedes that of the structure id. For him, the formation of psychic structure is akin to Fairbairn's representating and integrating aspects of interpersonal relationships that lead to structure.

The drives Originally, Kernberg adhered to the classical concept of drives. In his later conceptualizations, however, drives only appear to manifest themselves in the context of internalization of interpersonal experience. Good and bad self and object relationships become associated, respectively, with libido and aggression. The inference is that goodness and badness in relational experiences precede drive cathexis. Not only do object relations constitute the building blocks of structure, but they are also the building blocks of the drives. In turn, the drives become higher-level systems that organize object relations into integrated motivational systems or into libidinal and aggressive aims. Good and bad affective experiences eventually become the basis for the motivational forces of libido and aggression. In contrast to Freud, who considered such blocks innate biological givens, Kernberg sees the blocks as originating from the vicissitudes of the development of internalized object relations. In his formulation of love and hate, Kernberg is at odds with drive theorists who contend that the two affects evolve out of the drives as a consequence of object cathexis; to Kernberg, however, these object-directed attitudes precede and give rise to the drives.

PSYCHOANALYTIC PSYCHOPATHOLOGY

THEORY OF NEUROSIS By 1906, Freud had attained an understanding of the psychological processes underlying the mental disorders and could classify them. His theory contained most of the major elements of the current psychoanalytic concepts of psychopathology. Freud's further contributions and those of his followers yielded only minor revisions and additions to his early theories. These theories continue to emphasize the investigation of causative factors rather than the description of symptoms that is prevalent in general psychiatry.

HISTORICAL EVOLUTION **Early concepts** On the basis of his treatment of cases of hysteria, Freud concluded that hysterical symptoms were caused by unconscious memories of past events. Furthermore, those memories were accompanied by strong emotions that had not been adequately expressed or discharged. Thus, Freud concluded that hysterical symptoms were caused by psychic traumata in persons congenitally or genetically predisposed to the development of such phenomena.

Freud believed that the symptoms of neurasthenia, an actual neurosis, were caused by excessive masturbation or nocturnal emissions. In contrast, anxiety neurosis was produced by sexual stimulation that was not allowed adequate discharge, such as the practice of coitus interruptus and lovemaking without sexual gratification. Even up to 1906, Freud was convinced that the symptoms of neurasthenia and anxiety neurosis were the result of somatic disturbances in sexual metabolism.

Later concepts When Freud came to realize that psychic conflict was a major element in the production of psychoneurotic disorders, he had to revise and expand his earlier ideas about phobic, hysterical, and obsessional neuroses. Previously, Freud had hypothesized that neurosis was a psychic consequence of a sexual seduction that had occurred at a young age. Although he later corrected this assumption, he maintained the position that the roots of psychoneurosis lie in a disturbance in early sexual development. But he also acknowledged that the patient's sexual makeup and heredity were etiological factors in the neurosis.

Freud's realization that infantile sexuality is a normal phenomenon enabled him to elucidate the origins of the sexual perversions and their relationship to both normal and psychoneurotic functioning. He concluded that, in the normal course of events, some components of infantile sexuality are repressed and others are integrated into the adult pattern of sexuality at puberty with resultant genital primacy. He found that excessive repression earlier in life would cause a failure of repression in later life and the appearance of neurotic symptoms when unconscious infantile sexual impulses break through.

Freud's study of dreams also influenced his thinking about the psychoneurotic process. To Freud, the manifest dream represented a compromise between one or more repressed impulses and the psychic forces opposing their admission into conscious awareness. He concluded that previous symptoms represented a similar compromise, with one exception. Whereas the latent or instinctual wish underlying the manifest dream may or may not have a sexual origin, the repressed impulses producing the neurotic symptoms are always sexual. However, the meaning of neurotic symptoms, like the elements of the manifest dream, are found in their latent or unconscious content.

CURRENT CONCEPTS Neuroses arise under the following conditions: (1) Inner conflict is produced by fears or guilt in response to the danger of emerging drives. (2) Sexual drives are involved in this conflict. (3) The conflict has not been worked through or realistically resolved; the drives seeking discharge have been expelled from consciousness through repression or other defense mechanisms. (4) The drives have been rendered unconscious but have not been deprived of their power and have surfaced as compromise formations or neurotic symptoms. (5) Only an inner conflict will lead to neurosis in adolescence or adulthood.

Traditionally, the term "neurosis" has been applied to hysteria, obsessional neuroses, and phobias. Modern psychoanalytic nosology now includes the depressive, traumatic, and impulse neuroses, and other symptomatic states.

ETIOLOGY During its development, the psychic apparatus is subject to a multitude of vicissitudes that affect its eventual state of functioning in adult life, such as maternal deprivation, failure to form necessary identifications, excessive frustration or overindulgence, or lack of capacity to express drives. Maternal deprivation during the critical early months may greatly impair a person's development. Overindulgence or excessive frustration may obstruct the formation of the necessary identifications and the ego may be hampered in its ability to mediate between the instincts and the environment. If drive discharge is limited, one is faced with an inability to obtain pleasure and to assert oneself. The lack of capacity for the reasonable expression of drives, especially the aggressive ones, may lead to overly self-destructive behavior when the drives are turned on the self. Disordered functioning of the superego may occur with parental inconsistency, excessive harshness, or undue permissiveness. The ego's capacity for sublimation may be thwarted by unresolved instinctual conflicts, resulting in excessive inhibition of its autonomous functions.

If the ego has been weakened in early childhood, a traumatic event in later life may strain its resiliency and overwhelm its defenses. A large amount of libido is then required to master the excitation. But if the libido thus mobilized has been withdrawn from the supply normally applied to external objects and is taken from the ego itself, ego strength is further diminished, producing a sense of depletion.

Thus, neuroses may be precipitated by experiences that disturb the balance between the warded-off impulses and the defending forces. An increase in the warded-off drives may be absolute, as at puberty or the climateric, because of the physiological intensification of sexual drives at these times. There may be a relative increase in a particular warded-off drive at the expense of other instinctual forces, as in the case of conscious or unconscious arousal, or the temptation of a particular wish.

Infantile longings can be revived with the formation of a neurosis, or regression may take place as a result of excessive disappointments or frustrations of adult strivings. Finally, previously effective defenses may be overwhelmed and a neurotic, or even psychotic, illness may be precipitated by a decrease in the warding-off forces because of fatigue, intoxication, or physical illness. When the warded-off instincts cannot be tolerated in consciousness, the ego must form symptoms and modify its objectives so that the unfulfilled strivings become less urgent.

SECONDARY GAINS The primary gain or purpose achieved by the formation of a neurotic illness is to reduce conflict and tension. Secondary gains or advantages from the illness may also be observed, such as evoking sympathy and attention from others, manipulating the external environment, or being materially compensated. The secondary gains can become so valuable that the patient may prefer to retain the neurosis rather than to lose it.

Each type of neurosis has its distinct form of secondary gain. In phobias, there is a regression to childhood where one was protected; in conversion hysteria, the patient derives much attention, and even material advantages; and in compulsive neuroses, there is narcissistic pride in the illness. In the psychosomatic diseases (organ neuroses), there is denial of psychic conflicts by displacing them onto the physical sphere and the elicitation of attention and sympathy. Even in psychosis, where the warding-off of painful drives or ideas leads to severe regression, the patient may satisfy extreme dependency needs by requiring care from others.

SYMPTOMATIC NEUROTIC STATES **Hysteria** Hysterical states may show predominantly conversion symptoms or conversion reactions. Conversion hysteria occurs more frequently in women and is characterized by somatic symptoms resembling those of physical disease, such as headaches, convulsions, paralysis, anesthesia, and other types of bodily disturbances in the absence of actual physical illness. If present in a very mild form in an otherwise well-adjusted personality, these symptoms are positive indications for analytic treatment. In addition to permanent symptomatic relief, analysis of the underlying conflicts ordinarily leads to permanent changes in the personality. In individuals with extremely infantile personalities, or in chronic cases of hysteria where the secondary gain from the symptoms is too great to renounce, analytic treatment is difficult or not effective.

The dissociative types of hysteria are characterized by the fact that a constellation of recent mental events, such as memories, feelings, or fantasies, are beyond the patient's conscious recall, but remain psychically active. Common forms of dissociative hysteria are somnambulism, localized or general amnesias, fugue states, and multiple personality. Other varieties of dissociative phenomena include automatic writing, Ganser's syndrome, trance states, and some kinds of mystical experiences.

SYMPTOMATOLOGY Hysterical phenomena are more frequently seen in hospital emergency rooms and medical wards than in office clinical practice, and are considered to be pantomimic expressions of complicated fantasies related to the child's notions of parental sexual relations. The hysterical seizure is thought to express pregenital actions that are regressive substitutes for the original oedipal fantasies. However, some attacks are not specifically sexual and may manifest themselves as convulsions, mood outbursts, explosive laughing, or crying spells. Bizarre symptoms may accompany the seizures, including the abrupt appearance or disappearance of such physical needs as hunger or thirst, the need to urinate or to defecate, or respiratory disturbances.

PATHOGENESIS Classically, conversion hysteria develops as a defense against threatening libidinal stimulation and transforms psychic excitation into physical channels. This intervention represents a genitalization of a particular part of the body associated with repressed unconscious wishes directed toward the love object. Etiological factors include a fixation at the phallic stage of psychosexual development, a tendency to libidinize thoughts and images, and extreme frustration relative to intense, unconscious fantasies.

The physical symptoms are distorted expressions of instinctual impulses that previously had been repressed. The symptoms are more than somatic expressions of affect; they are specific representations of thoughts that can be translated through the process of free association from their somatic language into words. The syndromes of conversion are unique to each individual.

The specific type of distortion is determined by the historical events that created the repression. The choice of the afflicted region is influenced by unconscious sexual fantasies and by the corresponding erotogenicity of the involved part, by physical injury, or by a change in the body part that renders it vulnerable by the nature of the situation in which repression occurs. Certain organs are known to express symbolically the unconscious drive in question. Hysteria imitates a wide variety of diseases, thus considerably complicating the clinical picture.

Phobic states Often considered forms of anxiety hysteria, phobias are abnormal fears caused by conflict arising from an increase in sexual excitation attached to an unconscious object. Fear is avoided by displacing the conflicts onto an object or situation outside of the individual. Once displacement has been accomplished, the readiness to develop anxiety becomes bound to the specific situation that precipitated the initial anxiety attack. Situations duplicating or symbolically representing the original event will create anxiety. To ward off the anxiety, the ego resorts to states of inhibition, such as impotence or frigidity, or avoids the objects that have become connected with conscious conflict through historical association or their symbolic significance.

Phobic anxieties may be manifested in various ways. Frequently, the connections between the feared situation and the original instinctual conflict become increasingly disguised as the degree of displacement from the original context increases. Typically, the feared situation or object has a specific unconscious symbolic significance, a forbidden gratification, a punishment for an unconscious impulse, or a combination of these. Young children commonly complain of phobic anxieties with the stirring up of instinctual impulses. Phobic reactions usually are seen in adults during sexual or aggressive crises that may be contributed to by fixations at the phallic stage, sexual frustrations, or external factors that weaken the ego's ability to handle anxiety or increases in libidinal excitement.

SYMPTOMATOLOGY The clinical symptoms of a phobic state are determined by the patient's history, the nature of the drives warded off, and the mechanisms of defense. Phobias about germs and touching are often a defense against anal-erotic temptation. Fear of open places and stage fright may be defenses against exhibitionistic wishes, whereas fears of high or closed spaces, falling, or riding in cars or airplanes may defend against pleasurable sensations connected with stimulation involving equilibrium.

PATHOGENESIS The list of phobias is long. The original instinctual conflict becomes more concealed as the degree of displacement increases and as the original offensive idea is further removed from consciousness. In "Little Hans," Freud's famous case, the boy's fear of a horse instead of his father helped him avoid hatred for his father, whom he loved, but by whom he also felt threatened. In Freud's "Wolf Man," projection from an internal onto an external danger that existed in the patient's imagination provided an additional advantage. Wolves appear in picture books, which need not be opened, or at a zoo, where one does not have to go. The object or the situation from which the phobic patient flees primarily represents the threatening parents, but there is also flight from the patient's own impulses. The fear of castration, perceived as an external threat, arises primarily as a result of the child's own phallic impulses.

Usually, phobic patients have attained a fairly coherent self-organization and their internal psychic agencies are well established. The conflicts are mainly of a phallic nature, although individuals with phobias about dirt and contamination may be defending against anal impulses. Persons who harbor a single phobia manifest a greater capacity to tolerate and master anxiety, whereas those with mutiple phobias, or those who are polysymptomatic, may suffer from a defect in ego development stemming from pregenital levels of development. Among people who are especially susceptible to phobic generalization are agoraphobics, or persons who fear open or public places.

Obsessional neurosis The obsessional neuroses are frequently found in men. In the obsessional patient, internal structure predominates and provides powerful control over drive impulses and their associated affects. The psychic structure is excessively rigid and fragile, having been established prematurely on an insecure base. The basic conflicts remain prephallic because of fixations at the anal-sadistic level and in retreat from castration anxieties. Treatment of obsessional neurosis is generally more difficult and protracted compared with the other neuroses as it represents serious disturbances in total life adjustment. The extent to which the fixations and conflicts have interfered with ego development determines how much regression these patients can tolerate without severe consequences. The undoing of obsessional defenses in some individuals may precipitate rapid regression to near-psychotic levels, with the appearance of delusional obsessional thoughts and incapacitating compulsive behaviors.

Obsessional ideas were described by Freud as self-reproaches that have reemerged from repression in transmuted form. He believed that they relate to some sexual act that was performed with pleasure in childhood. Usually, a period of apparent health or successful defensive functioning precedes the onset of the illness. The illness is distinguished by the return of repressed memories in the form of obsessive-compulsive symptoms, or the failure of the character defenses. The emerging obsessional ideas are derivatives of the warded-off drive or present as impulses. The patient may be aware of the ideas but not the original drives because the energy associated with the original impulse has been diverted, usually to a neutral idea.

SYMPTOMATOLOGY The obsessional or obsessive-compulsive neurosis is characterized by persistent recurring thoughts (obsessions) and repetitively performed behavior (compulsions) that bear little relation to the patient's realistic needs and are experienced as foreign or intrusive. The syndrome is characterized by rumination, doubting, and irrational fears. When the intruding thoughts or the repetitive acts are interfered with, morbid anxiety arises. Additional features of this disorder are a strong tendency toward ambivalence; regression to magical thinking, especially in relation to the obsessional thoughts; and rigid and punitive superego functioning. Ordinarily, the conflicts involved lie closer to the prephallic phase of psychosocial development than to the phallic-oedipal phase.

PATHOGENESIS Obsessional neuroses arise from the separation of affects from ideas or behavior through the defense mechanisms of undoing and isolation, by regression to the anal-sadistic level, or by turning the impulses against the self. In general, obsessional states can be regarded as states of affective insufficiency. The affect attached to a painful idea is displaced onto some other indirectly associated idea that is more acceptable. This idea then becomes invested with an inordinate quantity of affect.

The obsessional syndrome can also be understood as a regression to anal-sadistic levels as a defense against intolerable oedipal impulses and conflicts. The regression is motivated by castration anxiety, and object relations tend to have a sadomasochistic quality. From a developmental perspective, these patients have not resolved their conflicts during the anal stage of development and they struggle with problems of controlling parental figures, autonomy, and issues connected with toilet training. Control and ambivalence and the need to establish and maintain a sense of autonomy are dominant elements in the obsessional syndrome.

Depressive states In 1917, in *Mourning and Melancholia,* Freud conceptualized the basic psychoanalytic approach to depressive states. He described the mechanism of introjection of the lost object and the redirection of the ambivalence, originally directed to the object, against the now internalized object that had become part of the self. Essentially, the aggressive impulses originally directed toward the ambivalently viewed object were turned on the self.

In 1953, Edward Bibring provided a further understanding of depression, pointing out the common theme in depressive states of the undermining or diminution of self-esteem. Depressed patients view themselves as helpless and powerless and as victims of loneliness. They feel isolated and lack love and affection. Moreover, they see themselves as weak, inferior, or failures in life, incapable of controlling or directing their inescapable fate. Neurotic depressions generally involve a reactive component and are to be distinguished from the more severe depressive disorders, such as psychotic depressive states or the manic-depressive illnesses. In the latter conditions, the degree of repression is more severe and reality testing and interpersonal function are seriously impaired.

SYMPTOMATOLOGY Mood disturbances with resulting sadness, unhappiness, and hopelessness are prominent in depressed patients. There is a loss of interest in usual activities or difficulties in concentration. The patient feels lonely, empty, guilty, worthless, or inadequate, as well as extremely self-derogatory and self-critical. Because the patient frequently craves emotional support or reassurance, the depressive symptoms serve the purpose of eliciting sympathy and support from the environment. However, the complaints may be so hostile and demanding that they become self-defeating by alienating potential sources of affection. Suicide is a frequent component of depressive conditions, and suicidal ideas must be assessed as to their intensity or severity. Usually, the seriousness of the suicidal intent is related to the degree of hopelessness that the patient feels.

PATHOGENESIS A depressive neurosis usually sets in as a reaction to loss or failure, such as the death of a loved one or a disappointment with the love object. Failure to live up to one's own standards or to gain specific vocational or personal goals may also trigger a depression, causing a loss of self-esteem.

A number of factors affect self-esteem. First, an individual may have a poor self-image stemming from early pathological development of the self-concept, if reared in an unfavorable family environment. Second, excessive superego aggression can cause guilt, with the lowering of self-esteem. Fixation of the superego at an archaic or infantile mode, or a regression to this level of functioning, predisposes the person to depression, with a corresponding decrease in self-esteem. Third, self-esteem depends on the nature and level of integration of the ego-ideal. If the ego-ideal is unrealistic, excessive demands are placed on the ego, resulting in feelings of inadequacy. Fourth, the maintenance of self-esteem also depends on the integration of the individual's actual abilities and the functioning of the ego to meet the demands of the ego-ideal.

Depressed patients may have a significant number of oral instinctual and narcissistic elements, particularly when the demands of the ego-ideal are determined by primitive narcissistic wishes that are grandiose and excessive. Failure in self-esteem may also be traced to pregenital levels of development.

The psychoanalytic treatment of depression is most successful in cases where the depression is reactive and does not result from excessive fixations at pregenital levels. When the depressive symptoms are removed by treatment, other characterological problems may have to be confronted, such as a narcissistic disorder. A strictly psychoanalytic approach is contraindicated for excessively depressed individuals or for persons with long-standing depressions.

Impulse neuroses In these neuroses, impulses are ego syntonic and irresistible. These patients are intolerant of tensions and the pathological impulses bring about a distorted instinctual satisfaction of a sexual or aggressive nature. Tension is perceived as traumatic and the impulsive actions are aimed at discharging the tension. Impulse neurotics are fixated at pregenital levels with undifferentiated strivings for sexual satisfaction and security. They are dependent on being loved and react to frustration with violence. They wrestle with tendencies toward violence and to repress all aggressiveness through the fear of loss of love. To impulse neurotics, objects are not persons but deliverers of supplies. Impulse neurotics fall into the symptomatic categories of kleptomania, pyromania, addiction to gambling, drug addiction, alcoholism, and running away.

Psychosomatic disorders These disorders are characterized by functional and sometimes anatomical alterations. Originally known as organ neuroses, they are generally considered psychosomatic or psychophysiological disorders, although the revised third edition of the *Diagnostic and Statistical Manual of Mental Disorders* (DSM-III-R) now lists them vaguely as psychological factors affecting physical condition. They include peptic ulcer, ulcerative colitis, and asthma.

Classically, psychosomatic disorders have been kept separate from hysterical conversion syndromes. Conversion phenomena characteristically affect the peripheral sensory or motor nervous system, or the special sense organs, and represent the transformation of psychic or symbolic conflicts into physical forms of expression. In the psychosomatic disorders, the vegetative nervous system is involved and an imbalance of sympathetic and parasympathetic regulation of organ systems occurs. There can be acute and chronic involvement of the organ systems, producing transient symptomatic episodes (migraine, asthmatic attacks) or chronic disease (ulcers, colitis).

PATHOGENESIS Many psychiatric theories have been advanced to explain the origin of psychosomatic disorders. An extension of Freud's original ideas about the genesis of hysterical disorders postulates that psychosomatic symptoms are affect equivalents that represent dammed-up emotions or their symbolic representations. They lack adequate discharge through speech or behavior and instead find expression along somatic pathways, resulting in a structural or functional alteration in an organ or organ system. Thus, anger, sexual excitement, or anxiety may be expressed via the intestinal, respiratory, or circulatory system.

Attractive as it may appear, the theory of affect equivalents is considered an oversimplification of the complex interrelationships between somatic and psychological processes in these disorders. Although all affects are carried out by motor or secretory means, physical manifestations of any given disease may be seen without a clearly established etiological relationship to specific psychological experiences. Because the psychosomatic disorders themselves may produce psychological adaptive responses, it is difficult to determine whether the emotional disorder preceded the physical, or vice versa.

CURRENT ISSUES Much remains to be learned about the intricate interrelations between hormonal physiology and instinctual phenomena. Present-day workers in the field of psychosomatic medicine recognize the complex interplay between a genetic predisposition to these disorders, stress, and the influence of inhibited specific affects that lead to certain hormonal secretions and changes in physical functions, and eventually to alterations in organ tissue. Recent evidence indicates that the brain interacts with and modulates the immunological systems such that the somatic symptoms may be greatly influenced by the social milieu.

The psychosomatic disorders encompass a considerable variety as to type of illness, severity of anatomical alteration, and degree of psychogenic involvement. Certain organic illnesses with psychosomatic symptoms may accompany a psychoneurosis, and may be cured incidentally to the major problems of the mental illness. With the resolution of emotional conflicts in analysis, one frequently sees the disappearance of various menstrual disorders, sterility, and circulatory and gastrointestinal symptoms.

Some psychosomatic disorders function as substitute symptoms for an underlying psychotic process. Thus, psychoanalysis is definitely contraindicated when the psychogenic components and the personality organization are at very primitive levels, as the induced regression and the undoing of defenses can have a harmful effect and uncover or precipitate the underlying psychotic process.

CHARACTER DISORDERS In the psychoanalytic sense, character refers to the individual's habitual mode of bringing into harmony the tasks presented by the internal demands and the external world. A precise description of pathological character types is difficult to provide as discrete personality types are rarely found in pure form. Yet, contemporary psychoanalysis now deals more extensively with the diagnosis and treatment of character types than with any other aspect of psychopathology. Today, patients' symptomatic complaints may be relieved early in the analysis and then the problems of the underlying character structure become the focus of treatment.

A particular character pattern or type becomes pathological when its manifestations are exaggerated to the point that behavior becomes destructive to the individual or to others, or when the functioning of the person becomes so disturbed that it is a source of distress. Deeply imbedded in the organization of the person's personality, characterological traits tend to be lifelong. The character types are commonly classified according to their symptomatic expression. Among the more typically encountered disorders are the following.

Hysterical character Hysterical characters tend to sexualize all relationships, are highly suggestible, and are inclined to irrational emotional outbursts, chaotic behavior, dramatization, and histrionic activity. Hysterical characters need not be associated with hysterical symptoms, such as conversion or dissociative phenomena. However, hysterical symptoms may be found in a variety of character types, in addition to hysterical personalities.

Phobic character These persons avoid situations they yearned for originally. Thus, certain external situations are avoided, as is true of neurotic phobic behavior. Internal reactions, such as rage or love, or all intense feelings, may also be subject to phobic avoidance.

Compulsive character Reaction formations are characteristic of these individuals. Typically, they attempt to overcome sadism with kindness and politeness and to conceal pleasure in dirt by rigorous cleanliness. Significant degrees of obsessional and compulsive ritualization may be present. Because they employ the defense of isolation, there is lack of adequate affective response and their modes of feeling are restricted. Object relations are of an anal-sadistic nature.

Depressive character The manifestations of the depressive neurosis are present but exist in a more enduring and chronic, low-keyed basis. Long-standing feelings of low self-esteem and worthlessness are characteristic of this syndrome. Frequently, there is a history of early object loss or severe deprivation. Most often, the depressive neuroses are concerned with object loss or narcissistic injury whereas the depressive character relates particularly to ego deficiencies and inadequacies.

Cyclical character These individuals experience periodic mood swings from depression to varying degrees of elation. Cyclical characters are especially concerned with unresolved oral needs and conflicts. Basically depressive characters, they are able to mobilize manic defenses analogous to the cyclic alternation between depressive and manic phases in manic-depressive psychosis.

Passive-aggressive character Hostile or destructive feelings and intentions are expressed through passive or submissive behavior. Passive-aggressive characters usually direct such behaviors toward others on whom they feel dependent or to whom they feel subordinate. Manifestations include disinterest, withdrawal, negativism, obstructionism, insufficiency, procrastination, sabotage, perfunctory behavior, errors of omission, indifference, foot dragging, lack of initiative, literalness in compliant behavior that frustrates the outcome, and a variety of other passive behaviors. The individual denies any hostile or negative intent, although there may be periodic angry outbursts.

Narcissistic character Narcissistic characters present an excessive degree of self-reference in their interactions with others, an intense need to be loved and admired, and apparently contradictory attitudes of an inflated self-concept and an inordinate need for tribute and admiration. Experiencing little empathy for others, narcissistic characters have a shallow emotional life. They lack new sources of reward to feed their self-regard, and easily become restless, bored, and disinterested. Their relationships with others are often exploitative and manipulative. They feel justified in controlling and possessing others and do so without guilt. Idealizing individuals from whom they expect narcissistic rewards, they depreciate, devalue, and treat with contempt those from whom they cannot expect such rewards. Often charming and engaging, they possess a ruthlessness and coldness. Although they appear to be dependent, they characteristically harbor a deep distrust of others. Feelings of inferiority and insecurity frequently alternate with feelings of importance, specialness, and omnipotence.

Narcissistic characters suffer from disturbances in the organization of the self. Archaic objects are highly cathected with narcissistic libido and have not been integrated with the rest of the personality organization. Because of the intense investment in the self, these individuals lack the capacity for mature object relatedness and functioning. In addition, their realistic adaptation is interfered with by the predominance of primitive narcissistic demands. Narcissistic characters have achieved a cohesive and organized self and are not threatened by the possibility of irreversible decompensation of the self organization or of narcissistically cathected objects, but they are affected primarily by a fear of loss of the object or the object's love, and secondarily by castration anxiety.

If the objects threaten punishment, abandonment, or withdrawal of love, the result is a narcissistic imbalance or defect in the patient. The maintenance of self-cohesiveness and self-esteem depends on the presence of a rewarding and approving object that provides narcissistic supplies.

Schizoid character Schizoid characters often present with symptoms of a depression. Feelings of being isolated and cut off are common. They complain of feeling apart or estranged from people and things, and of events and things being unreal, and they experience diminished interest in events and people. Life is seen as futile and meaningless. Unlike true depressives, schizoid characters lack an inner sense of anger and guilt. The depressives are still object related, but schizoid individuals have renounced their object ties. External relationships have been rendered empty by a massive withdrawal of libidinal attachment. Depleted of vital feeling and the capacity for action, the patient's ego seems to become unreal. To the outside world, schizoid characters appear uninvolved and without feeling. However, the schizoid state may alternate with depression. Their main defense against anxiety is to remain emotionally out of reach, inaccessible, and isolated. Schizoid characters attempt to cancel external object relations and to live in a detached and withdrawn manner. They face the dilemma of destructive love and the anxiety of destroying and losing the love object by being so devouring, greedy, and needy. A schizoid individual can exist neither in a relationship with another nor alone without risking the loss of both the object and the self. Thus, love relationships are seen as mutually devouring and destructive.

The schizoid character often overlaps with the narcissistic character in terms of the clinical description and dynamics. The cold and isolated self-sufficiency of the schizoid frequently masks an inner grandiosity indicative of severe pathological roots in the grandiose self.

Masochistic character For some people, pain is a necessary prerequisite to enjoying pleasure. In the masochistic character, pain becomes a means of assuaging the superego and expiating guilt. At times, the punishment is received in advance to compensate for a misdeed that has not yet been committed. These individuals avoid pleasure or even seek painful experiences, or only permit pleasure if it is associated with pain. There appears to be an inability to avoid misfortune, and in more severe conditions, self-destructive behavior is present. Masochism is frequently found in depressive individuals.

Additional underlying dynamics of masochistic behavior include the infantile desire to maintain omnipotent control of the universe. Masochistic characters may harbor the fantasy that pain and frustration are not the inevitable consequence of things over which they lack control but the result of their own behavior. They will abruptly break off relationships to ward off the threat that others might leave first, resign from a job lest they be fired, and volunteer for unpleasant jobs rather than risk being drafted for them.

Another common dynamic of the masochistic character relates to the safety and comfort provided by the familiar. Future masochists may have experienced love only if they had been subjected to frequent punishment and abuse and may feel insecure if they lack punishment for any length of time. Such individuals seek out situations that re-create early experiences and become uncomfortable if they cannot reestablish the role of the victim.

Masochistic behavior can provide immense secondary gain. Patients may get satisfaction from the sympathy of others who feel sorry for their misfortune and misery. Therefore, there may be a sense of moral superiority associated with the suffering for a good cause and they may feel the exaltation associated with sainthood. Frequently, suffering can impose a heavy burden on those involved with the sufferer, and the aggression directed against the self can be a most effective means of attacking others.

Finally, masochism can serve as a defense against depression. Masochists may actually take pride in their plight, often denying their own role in their difficulties, which they project onto the outside world.

Borderline personality disorder These patients possess a stable form of personality organization that is intermediate between neurotic levels of integration and the more primitive psychotic forms of personality structure. Many borderline patients, especially those manifesting affective lability and dysphoric trends, have a higher genetic affinity with mood disorders. They possess a typical constellation of symptoms and defenses and a characteristic pattern of defects in their object relations.

In the more primitive forms, borderline patients manifest a variety of neurotic symptoms and character defects. Chronic and diffuse anxieties are common. Neurotic symptoms include numerous phobias, obsessive thoughts and behaviors, conversion symptoms, dissociative reactions, hypochondriacal complaints, and paranoid traits. Promiscuous and perverse sexuality may be present. The personality organization may be infantile, and there are episodic outbreaks of impulsive behavior. Use of alcohol or drugs for the relief of tension and for gratification is a common feature.

Narcissism is often a predominant element in their character structure, and these patients appear very much like narcissistic characters. Paranoia based on projection of rather primitive rage is frequently seen. There may be severe underlying depressive-masochistic pathology. Paranoid and depressive-masochistic traits may be closely related and can alternate in these patients.

The inner core of the borderline personality reveals a weakness in the structure of the ego, which is indicated by a marked lack of tolerance for low degrees of anxiety, poor impulse control, lack of suitable channels for sublimation, poor capacity for neutralization of aggression, and a generalized shift toward primary process thinking.

A characteristic defense of borderline patients is splitting, which involves the separation between the good introjects derived from satisfying object experiences and the bad introjects stemming from frustrating or rejecting object relationships. Splitting originates at a preambivalent level of development and prevents the child from integrating the objects into ambivalent objects. The persistence of splitting prevents the neutralization of aggressive drive components and maintains a persistent ego weakness.

Developmentally, the borderline patient has not achieved a level of triadic oedipal conflicts characteristic of psychoneurotic individuals or higher-order character disorders. Preoedipal issues and concerns persist and the developmental vicissitudes of affective one-to-one relationships with parents remain unresolved. Parental introjects are not regarded as separate and whole objects, thus impeding the development of oedipal involvement. Mahler suggested that the most likely phase in which the borderline fixations and defects take place is the rapprochement subphase of the separation-individuation stage of infant development. Some developmental theorists regard the maintenance of separate and contradictory self-configurations as the later cause of faulty integration and syntheses rather than attributing these failures to the continued process of defensive splitting as advocated by Kernberg.

Different levels of borderline functioning exist. Some patients maintain good levels of ego functioning and only experience emotional difficulties in relatively restricted contexts in which they regress to borderline functioning. Such patients appear neurotic, or even normal, on the surface, and only show borderline characteristics as a result of severe stress or analytic regression. They are regarded as higher-order forms of character pathology within the borderline spectrum. Borderline patients at the lower end of the spectrum have diffusely organized ego functioning, readily show splitting, tolerate anxiety and frustration poorly, regress easily, and act out frequently in destructive and self-defeating ways.

Perversions The perversions include homosexuality, fetishism, transvestism, exhibitionism, voyeurism, and sadomasochism. The general mechanism of the perversions is thought to be a defensive flight from castration anxiety connected with fears of oedipal retaliation. In homosexuality, there is a flight from the positive oedipal configuration, in which the parent of the opposite sex is loved and the parent of the same sex is feared, to the negative oedipal constellation, in which the opposite sex is feared and the same sex is loved. In fetishism, anxiety is evaded by displacing the instinctual libidinal impulses to an inanimate object that symbolizes parts of the body of the loved person. Neurotic interest is invested in an object or body part that is inappropriate for normal sexual gratification. The fetish symbolizes the female phallus, and its use is related to a fantasy denying the danger of castration caused by the anatomical differences between the sexes. The fetishist employs splitting, in which one part of the mind is realistically aware of the lack of a penis in the female, but another part of the mind unconsciously asserts that the female does, in fact, possess a phallus. The transvestite experiences sexual excitement by dressing in garments of the opposite sex. The male transvestite seeks an identification with the phallic mother and the female transvestite attempts, through her behavior, to deny the lack of a penis. Other forms of perversions are seen as avoidances of the threat of castration anxiety.

The perversions are manifestly sexual in character, and on the release of the pathological impulses, orgasm is achieved. Anxiety at pregenital and phallic levels, bisexuality, identifications, structural considerations, and environmental circumstances all contribute to the genesis of perversions. In 1974, C. W. Socarides found that the defense against castration anxiety in the perversions results in a regression to pregenital levels, with a failure in the normal developmental process, thus preventing the integration of early instinctual expressions into the normal heterosexual phallic adjustment. Anxiety from early developmental failures can contribute to the formation of perversions. For example, homosexuality not only may be a reflection of genital-level phallic conflicts, but also the result of early symbiotically based difficulties in separating from the mother, producing an intense feminine identification. Another cause may be the overwhelming anxiety resulting from fears of engulfment and the loss of the sense of self in attempts to form intimate relations with a woman. Socarides cautions that the diagnostic assessment of the perversions requires a careful evaluation of underlying ego strengths and earlier developmental achievements.

Kernberg and character pathology A contemporary and inclusive division of character pathology was provided in 1970 by Kernberg, who grouped these disorders according to their structural development. At the higher level, patients possess a relatively well-integrated but severe and punitive superego. There is an integrated ego, an established ego identity, a stable self-concept, and a stable representational world. However, the defensive operations are excessive and repressed, and center around unconscious conflicts. The character defenses are mostly of an inhibitory or phobic nature, or they are reactions against repressed instinctual needs. Because of the excessive use of neurotic defense mechanisms, the ego is constricted and limited. Overall social adaptation is not grossly impaired. These higher-order character disorders have deep, fairly stable object relationships and are capable of expressing guilt, mourning, and a variety of affective responses. Although their sexual or aggressive drive derivatives, or both, are partially inhibited, the instinctual conflicts are at a level where the infantile genital phase and oedipal conflicts clearly predominate. There is no pathological condensation of genital sexual strivings with pregenital, aggressively determined strivings. Higher-level character disorders include the hysterical, obsessive-compulsive, and depressive-masochistic characters.

The intermediate level of character pathology includes people with a defective integration of the superego, which tolerates contradictory demands between sadistic, prohibitive superego nuclei and primitive, magical, and idealizing nuclei. These patients have a decreased capacity for experiencing guilt and may exhibit paranoid trends, contradictions in their value systems, and severe mood swings. Poor integration of the superego is reflected in contradictory unconscious demands on the ego and the appearance of pathological character defenses to include reaction formations against instincts, with partial expression of instinctual impulses. The ego employs the major defense of repression along with such defenses as intellectualization, rationalization, and undoing. According to Kernberg, these patients show dissociative trends, defensive splitting of the ego in limited areas, projection, and denial. Oral conflicts are prominent, although the genital level of libidinal development has been reached.

In this group, Kernberg includes the oral types of character pathology, such as the passive-aggressive, sadomasochistic, and some infantile and narcissistic personalities.

Kernberg's lower level of character pathology encompasses individuals with more severe structural deficits and their developmental consequences. Superego integration is minimal and there is a marked propensity to project primitive, sadistic superego nuclei. The capacity for experiencing guilt and concern is grossly impaired, and there is constant fluctuation in self-criticism. According to Kernberg, lower-level character disorders commonly include paranoid traits and employ projective identification. The synthetic function of the ego is seriously impaired and primitive dissociation or splitting defenses are prominent. The character defenses are chiefly of an impulsive, instinctively infiltrative kind with contradictory, repetitive behavior patterns. These patients have little need for secondary rationalization of pathological character traits, and lack an integrated ego and the capacity to tolerate guilt. They are unable to integrate libidinal and aggressively determined self- and object images and their relationships are of either a need-gratifying or a threatening nature. Relationships are also of a part-object type and object constancy has not been reached. Identity diffusion is present because of the absence of an integrated world of total internalized objects and a stable self-concept. The lack of an integrated libidinal and aggressive striving results in decreased neutralization of instinctual energy and creates a severely restricted conflict-free ego.

Character disorders in this category include the infantile, antisocial, and many narcissistic personalities. Also included are the more chaotic impulse-ridden and "as-if" characters, patients with multiple sexual deviations combined with drug addiction or alcoholism and pathological object relationships, and other forms of schizoid and paranoid personalities.

Prognosis In general psychiatry and in psychoanalytic practice, neurotic character disorders are seen in treatment more commonly than the symptomatic neuroses. The character disorders constitute a large portion of the population suitable for analysis. Psychoanalytic treatment produces a far more complete and fundamental reorganization of the neurotic personality than any other current psychotherapeutic technique. Aside from the character neuroses, the usefulness of psychoanalysis as a treatment modality is limited.

The more allied their character disorders are to hysterical or obsessive-compulsive neuroses, the more treatable they become. Persons with character disorders should be considered for psychoanalytic treatment to the extent that the disorders are a conspicuous and persistent source of concern for the patient and for family, friends, and co-workers. Such complaints include temper outbursts, nagging and constant complaints against others, feelings of inferiority, repeated job changes, recurrent unresolved work problems, a series of unhappy love affairs, an inability to derive pleasure from work or recreation, failures in forming friendships, marital discord, and general feelings of dissatisfaction.

Some character disorders have a better prognostic outcome with treatment than others. Narcissistic characters, in general, can receive significant help and be transformed to some extent by analysis, but their prognosis is extremely variable, and in many cases, guarded. The prognosis is better if psychoneurotic problems exist along with the narcissistic traits. The prognosis is especially poor for very dependent personalities who are extremely unassertive and are fixed in passive relationships. Mild schizoid characters may also benefit from psychoanalysis, but as is the case with some severe forms of character pathology, such patients require special parameters or modifications. Patients falling into the special categories include moderately paranoid individuals, alcoholics, drug addicts, and antisocial personalities. Contraindications for classical psychoanalytic treatment include patients with excessive infantile demands, an inability to tolerate frustration or to delay gratification, previously impaired ego functions, or a defective sense of reality.

Much interest has been focused on borderline patients. Although some are candidates for unmodified psychoanalysis, the majority require the use of treatment parameters. Particular issues of concern are their high narcissistic expectations and sense of entitlement. Resort to manipulations to gain needed gratification is commonplace and suicidal gestures are to be expected. Also characteristic of the borderline patient is the intense and chaotic transference that alternates between an excessive idealization and dependence and the devaluation of the therapist and impulsive withdrawal from therapy.

PSYCHOANALYTIC THEORY OF PSYCHOSIS Freud originally studied paranoid symptomatology as a manifestation of the psychotic process. His understanding of the symptoms of paranoia was facilitated by the discovery of unconscious homosexuality and the mechanisms of projection. Considerable insight into these mechanisms was acquired through his careful analysis of the Schreber *Memoirs,* an autobiographical account of Schreber's paranoid psychosis and his intricate delusional system. Freud had no contact with Schreber, who never recovered from his psychotic decompensation and finally died in a mental institution.

Freud's analysis of the Schreber case was an attempt to improve the basic theory of repression and the notion of the return of the repressed into the paranoid material. In paranoia, he postulated, the need to project coincided with an unconscious impulse to homosexual love, which was denied by the patient. Paranoid delusions stood for sexual conflicts concerning individuals of the same sex that had been projected onto some other object or force, which was then perceived as persecuting or threatening.

Other analysts emphasized the intimate relationship of paranoid symptoms to infantile fantasies in which the feces are personalized and considered dangerous entities that are powerful and highly threatening to the patient. Karl Abraham demonstrated the relationship between paranoia and the stage of development where the emotions are focused on a particular part of the object's body, rather than on the total person. He also observed that paranoid psychosis resembled certain phases of melancholia where the patient's fantasies indicate a desire to incorporate the object. Paranoid psychosis differs from melancholia in that hostility is directed against only a part, and not the entire object. The paranoid patient has fantasies that this incorporated part-object can be destroyed and eliminated by defecation.

Further understanding of paranoid psychosis has emerged through the concurrent demonstration of the relationships among primitive fantasies of aggression, overwhelming anxiety, and the need to project. Why homosexuality becomes so intense, threatening, and intolerable to paranoid patients remains unanswered. More recent studies of paranoid psychosis have tended to shift the emphasis away from homosexual dynamics and onto broader and more complex issues. Such issues include defects in ego development and primitive narcissistic trauma with resulting narcissistic rage as factors in the origin of paranoid states.

Narcissism in the psychoses In *On Narcissism,* published in 1914, Freud stated that psychosis was characterized by the patient's incapacity for emotional interest in people and things. But the psychotic process did not represent a total depletion of libido; rather, it involved a redistribution of libido that was normally directed to object love and self-love. According to Freud, energy was withdrawn from object relationships, producing an abnormally excessive interest in the self and increasing the cathexis of both bodily functions and the psychic attributes of the self. Also, the psychotic patient's use of language indicated a higher cathectic interest in verbal symbols than in the object that the words represent. Many symptoms of psychosis can be considered phenomena secondary to the primary loss of capacity for object attachment, and represent rudimentary and primitive efforts to reestablish and reconstitute a relationship with external objects.

The psychotic regression to earlier levels of functioning and development is shown in prelogical thought patterns and the pleasurable experiences that do not require reciprocal relationships between the patient and another person. Psychotic states are conditions of extreme and archaic narcissistic disorganization. The narcissism is of an extremely primitive and oral variety, and frustration of the psychotic patient's narcissistic demands may result in primitive and highly destructive rage. Conspicuous in the clinical picture of most psychotic patients are fragments of the intact personality and incomplete phases of psychotic regressions, along with efforts at restitution.

Current concepts Following Freud's suggestions, subsequent investigations of the psychoses have examined the conflicts between the individual and the environment. Recent work has focused on the disturbances and disorganizations in ego functioning that impair the patient's relationship with reality. The psychoses are thought to arise from defects in the ego's integrative or synthetic capacities, or capacity for fusion, and, consequently, from limitations on the ego's capacity to neutralize instinctual energies. Additional considerations include the ineffectiveness of ego functions for establishing real object relations and the impairment of functions essential for controlling intense infantile wishes.

The psychotic adjustment employs defenses that normally predominate at early levels of development of personality organization. Psychotic defenses tend to be of a primitive and narcissistic type, such as denial, distortion, and projection. These defenses are reflected in flight, social withdrawal, and simple inhibition of impulses or blocking. The primitive mechanisms are much less organized than the higher-order mechanisms of repression or reaction formation. In contrast to the neurotic, the psychotic individual fears detection by others, rather than suffering from guilt that normally occurs in later childhood and maturity. In psychotics, there exist limited patterns of imitation and introjection. Such patterns normally derive from emotional relations and early reactions to people who played a conspicuous role in the development of the psychotic's ego capacities.

Greater understanding and more effective therapeutic techniques must await the accumulation of further knowledge regarding the primitive ego of the child and the phases and processes that influence development. Current approaches have focused on the defects of object relations at these earliest phases and their debilitating effect on ego development. Studies of the ego's capacity to sublimate and neutralize primitive drives, and of the factors that interfere with the development of this crucial ego capacity, have enhanced the understanding of the pathogenesis of psychosis.

Modifications in the free association method have made possible approaches to a variety of psychotic states, and to the problem of vulnerability and the predisposition to psychosis. However, such concepts and approaches are in their initial stages. In addition to psychodynamic considerations, there are probable constitutional, biochemical, and genetic factors that influence the basic predisposition to the development of psychosis.

Hypochondriasis The actual neuroses (hypochondriasis, neurasthenia, and anxiety neuroses) have ceased to be a significant part of psychoanalytic nosology. These clinical syndromes are recognized as phases of ego regression or phases in a return to optimal ego functioning. Hypochondriasis rarely appears as an isolated neurosis. Frequently, it accompanies some other psychopathological condition, such as a compulsive neurosis or depression, or it appears as a state in the development of or recovery from a psychotic condition. Sadistic and hostile impulses, which are withdrawn from objects and represented as organic complaints, may play a pronounced role in hypochondriacal syndromes. The typical hypochondriac is a conspicuously narcissistic, seclusive, monomaniacal person, who is often in a transitional stage between reactions of a more hysterical character and those that are delusional and clearly psychotic. Hypochondriasis, with its excessive cathexis of bodily function and concern over organic states, has been regarded as one of the classic narcissistic neuroses. Further psychoanalytic study of infantile development may contribute to the understanding of this common clinical picture.

Psychotic depression (melancholia) Initial insights into the various forms of affective repressive states were formulated by Freud as early as 1915. In *Mourning and Melancholia,* Freud emphasized the topographic regions of the psychic apparatus involved in melancholic states, the regression of libido, and the abandonment of the unconscious cathexis of objects. His views differed from those of Abraham, who stressed the importance of anal sadism and maintained that its role in severe depressions was comparable to that of anal eroticism in obsessional neuroses. Abraham pointed out that anal-sadistic impulses contribute to many other clinical syndromes as well. Freud, however, emphasized the fact that the pain in mourning was limited to the loss of an external object, but in melancholia, it is the ego itself that is impoverished because it has experienced an internal loss. Thus, melancholic depressions may or may not be precipitated by an actual loss. As a concomitant of loss, the melancholic suffers a shattering fall in self-esteem. Because the ego seems poor and empty, it is deserving of reproach and attack from the superego.

The early formulations of both Freud and Abraham concerning melancholia and depression emphasized the frustration in object love, accompanied by narcissistic traumata that reinforced early oedipal disappointments and the introjection of an ambivalently loved parental image. These concepts still have clinical validity.

Abraham's continued investigations within the framework of infantile libidinal development, particularly focusing on the oral phase, led to further understanding of the mechanisms involved in depressive states. He suggested that the conflicts of depressed patients centered around oral and anal-sadistic impulses, and pointed out that persons who were prone to depressions often had a severe underlying character structure.

SYMPTOMATOLOGY The symptoms of depression are ubiquitous because it is a natural reaction to life events. Consequently, it is the excessive duration of depressive affects and their domination of the person that establish a depressive state as pathological. Psychotic depressions are characterized by their greater intensity and by the degree of fragmentation and helpless vulnerability of the ego response to the depressive affect. In psychotic states, the intensity of the aggression released is of a more punitive quality and, consequently, the depressions are almost always accompanied by profound suicidal ideas or serious suicide attempts. Psychotic depression has been described as a basic affective state in which the ego feels incapable of fulfilling its aims or aspirations, although these aims persist as desired goals. The ego is thus thrown into a state of continuing and total helplessness. Persons prone to depression often display a pseudoindependence and self-assurance that is, in reality, a reaction to early severe deprivation and a defense against the loss of further deprivation or rejection.

PATHOGENESIS Karl Abraham formulated the concept of primary depression to designate severe narcissistic injury that had occurred in early childhood as a result of disappointments in object relations. Later, Sandor Rado's studies of the effect of various vicissitudes of the nursing situation on the infantile ego showed the relationships between the etiology of depression and oral frustration and aggression, particularly at the oral level. John Bowlby's studies of the relationship between early maternal deprivation and the susceptibility to severe depression documented some of these early trends. Jacobson has discussed the impact on the young child's ego formation when there is early disillusionment about parental omnipotence, and the subsequent devaluation of parental images. Disillusionment and devaluation of the parents lead to a destruction of infantile self-esteem as a result of the early introjection of the idealized, good parental objects, and give rise to a primary depression, which is repeated whenever the adult is similarly disappointed or disillusioned. Thus, early ambivalent relationships with parental figures play a decisive role in the etiology of depressive states.

This basic concept has been expanded by other authors. Otto Fenichel ascribed the general predisposition to depression to an oral fixation that would determine the later response to narcissistic trauma, and he also discussed the possibility that shocks to the self-esteem in early childhood may secondarily create a decisive oral fixation. According to Melanie Klein, the achievement of a whole-object relationship is regularly accompanied by anxiety, together with a definite and specific vulnerability to depression in the event of object loss. Her view, however, implies a greater incidence of infantile psychosis than can actually be shown to exist.

MECHANISM OF DEPRESSION Depression normally occurs in the face of real or fantasied disappointments or disillusionments. However, the oral dependent person who requires constant narcissistic supplies from external sources is most likely to manifest depression in its most severe form. The prototype of depression is deprivation of vital narcissistic supplies. The availability of such supplies in the form of love, affection, or care is most significant for healthy development at the oral stage.

Later in development, with the internalization of parental images, which are derived from the resolution of the oedipal situation, the struggle to secure love from the need-gratifying object takes place at the intrapsychic level. The ego now seeks the approval of the superego and attempts to live up to the ideal standards of the ego-ideal. The earlier struggle for gratification from external sources now takes place intrapsychically. The child experiences this internalized need-satisfying object as initially frustrating and prohibitive, and displays a correspondingly hostile attitude toward the object. The later superego develops a critical and aggressive dimension from the quality of this early and crucial relationship. The failure to abandon or modify early narcissistic expectations of the immature ego may lead to unrealistic ego-ideal expectations that result in depression. The severe self-reproaches of depressed persons represent the ego's efforts to gain the favor of the superego through devaluation of the self when early object relationships were defective. Infantile intrapsychic conflicts may be revived in the face of object loss. Once the mechanisms described are set into operation by frustration and loss in adult life, depression arises.

Manic-depressive psychosis Persons with manic-depressive illness show an infantile, narcissistic dependency on the love object. To fend off feelings of worthlessness, the person requires a constant supply of love and moral support from a highly valued and idealized love object. The object may be a person, an organization, or a cause with whom or with which the patient can identify or feel a sense of belonging. As long as this object exists, the patient is able to function effectively and enthusiastically. However, because of strong, self-punitive tendencies, the manic-depressive's object choice is masochistically determined and bound to cause disappointment. Thus, the patient actually sets the stage for the illness. The ambivalence of the manic-depressive individual evolves from representations of the overvalued, idealized parental love objects, which extend to the whole world. As a result, disappointment in the love object causes impairment of the patient's ego functioning at every level.

DEPRESSIVE PHASE Frequently, the depressive phase of the manic-depressive psychosis resembles paranoia as the patient's fantasies contain a similar desire to incorporate the object. Paranoia, however, differs from depression in that hostility in the former condition is directed toward a part of the object, such as the breasts, penis, or buttocks, rather than the whole. Also, the fantasies in paranoia harbor the belief that the incorporated part object can be symbolically destroyed and eliminated by defecation. The paranoid defense can be seen as compensation for the inner sense of vulnerability and worthlessness that characterizes the basic depressive state. By means of the paranoid delusional system, the underlying depressed condition may be countered by bolstering the self-esteem or by restoring the fundamental object that was lost. Thus, the paranoid posture can serve as an alternative to the manic defense.

Mania occurs when the depressive phase subsides and gives way to a state of temporary elation. This transition takes place under a variety of conditions: first, when the narcissistically important goals and objects seem to be attainable once again; second, when they have become sufficiently modified or reduced to be within reach; third, when they are renounced completely; and fourth, when the ego recovers from its narcissistic shock and regains its self-esteem, with or without a change in objects and goals.

MANIC PHASE Initially, mania was approached from the libidinal standpoint, but later studies have stressed the role of structural components of the psychic apparatus and the importance of object relationships and their intrapsychic representations. Mania represents a means of avoiding awareness of inner depression and includes a denial of painful internal reality and a flight into the external world. Because mania is a denial of the underlying depressive affects, manic patients cannot permit themselves to empathize with others and they are frequently emotionally isolated.

A brief mention of B. Lewin's work is of help in a further understanding of the dynamics of elation. He focused on the oral-libidinal and oral-aggressive elements in mania and described, in structural terms, the fusion of ego and superego (ego-ideal) in elation and the prominent use of projection, denial, and introjection as major defenses. Lewin compared mania to a waking dream. In economic terms, the abundance of energy characteristic of elation represents a concomitant depletion in the energy available for reality testing or for coping with superego demands.

Schizophrenia Originally, Freud postulated that the onset of schizophrenia signified a withdrawal of libido from the outside world. He postulated that this libidinal energy was subsequently absorbed into the ego, thus producing a state of megalomanic grandiosity, or it was returned to the outside world in the form of delusions.

Recent interest in schizophrenia has focused on the intense ambivalence typical of these patients, their persecutory anxiety, and the infantile ego mechanisms that they characteristically use in their relationships with objects. The failure of these mechanisms results in the patient's decompensation or regressed state. Both Freud and Fenichel emphasized two stages that are especially conspicuous in the clinical picture of schizophrenic regression: the break with reality and the attempt to reestablish contact with reality.

CLINICAL CONCEPTS Object relationships in schizophrenia are based on the wish to possess the parental object or its substitutes through merger or fusion. Primitive introjective mechanisms, fixation at the early oral stage of libidinal development, and multiple impairments of ego functions are seen in this syndrome. Frustration of basic libidinal needs or factors that weaken ego resiliency, such as physical illness or increased emotional or performance demands on the patient, may precipitate the acute psychotic episode.

Schizophrenic regression may also be caused by poorly warded-off homosexual and pregenital impulses, particularly those of a sadistic and destructive nature. Controversy exists as to whether such states of libidinal upheaval precede the schizophrenic regression or are secondary to such regression. Upon the onset of the psychosis, early sources of libidinal excitation cannot be mastered, and they flood the ego and overwhelm it. If the libido returns to the ego, a megalomanic picture will result. If the sadistic impulses are projected onto the external world, as in paranoid schizophrenia, the once ambivalently loved person or representative will be perceived as the persecutor.

CLASSICAL PSYCHOANALYTIC TREATMENT

DIAGNOSIS Psychoanalytic treatment attempts to integrate the theory of psychic functioning with therapeutic usage. Two key considerations must be recognized before attempting treatment, namely, making a correct diagnosis and determining the analyzability of the individual. Diagnosis holds a central place because the decisions regarding the appropriate application of psychoanalytic treatment depend on the accuracy and precision of the diagnostic process. Psychoanalytic diagnosis is concerned with the evaluation of potential analyzability, selection of appropriate patients for analytic treatment, predictive value for assessing the nature of the patient's conflicts and predictable levels and areas of pathological impairment, and prognosis. The diagnostic issues relate in a very intimate and immediate way to the difficulties of the analytic process.

Psychoanalysts focus their attention to a great extent on the underlying motivation and dynamic considerations that enable the therapist to understand the nature of the patient's difficulties and to begin assisting the patient in dealing with them. The labeling of patients has received little emphasis. Over the years, analysts have concerned themselves increasingly with sophisticated refinements in assessing the levels of libidinal fixation and development in the evaluation and determination of patterns and heterogeneity of ego development. Sophisticated diagnostic means of assessing patients' strengths and weaknesses and the levels of developmental impairment, retardation, deficits, and regression have emerged. Diagnostic concern has shifted from symptomatic levels to complex personality evaluations that rely on structural and genetic data about symptomatic or dynamic issues.

Because the analytic approach emphasizes the patient's inner experience, particularly conflicts and related fantasies, the degree of ego autonomy and the susceptibility of ego functions to regression and the quality of the patient's object relationships are very important. One of the most significant places for further evaluation is within the context of the therapeutic relationship, specifically in the evaluation of the transference. Adequate time to assess the relationship to the patient is required before the analyst can gain a sufficient sense of the patient's capacity for object relatedness.

ANALYZABILITY The question of analyzability remains of central importance. In psychotherapy, patients frequently develop a treatment relationship that provides symptom relief by maintaining contact with the therapist. In this manner, they can avoid serious regression and maintain a reasonable level of adjustment and functioning. But the continuing availability of the therapist may be necessary and treatment may be interminable. A crucial question is the extent to which patients are capable of internalizing and identifying with the therapist. The potential for internalization requires a capacity for tolerating depressive affects and regressive forms of anxiety that might be experienced in the face of threatened loss. Patients who lack this capacity do not meet the criteria for analyzability.

Potentially analyzable patients have been able to reach a developmental level at which a genuine triangular conflict has been experienced. They have been able to sustain significant object relations with both parents through the latency years following the resolution of the oedipal conflict. Classical psychoanalysis is the treatment of choice for potentially mature adults whose difficulties revolve around the mastery of internal conflicts.

Other factors enter into the criteria for analyzability. At least normal, and perhaps superior, intelligence is preferred, if not required. Commonly associated with intelligence is the ability to verbalize one's thoughts. Verbalization implies the capacity of the individual to attach mental images to words to describe inner experiences. Secondary trust, the capacity of the patient to transfer or yield control to others, is necessary. The capacity to develop a transference neurosis and motivation for change, despite both pain and secondary gain, should exist. The potential for analyzability is enhanced when patients, although seeking relief from specific pain, are also aware that their thoughts, feelings, and behavior interfere with object relationships. Patients should desire self-understanding and an appreciation of the meaning of the present and past in order to prevent recurrences of their conflicts. There must be the capacity to regress in the service of therapy involving the reopening of intrapsychic conflicts previously sealed off by maladaptive defenses; the capacity to experience affect and feelings during treatment; the ability to deal with silence; the potential to minimize resistance; and the capacity for "psychological mindedness."

S. Applebaum, in 1973, defined *psychological-mindedness* as a state of mind characterized by four components: (1) the capacity to perceive the relationships among thoughts, feelings, and actions; (2) the potential and desire to learn the meanings and causes of experience and behavior; (3) the ability to direct psychological thinking to one's own psychic life rather than other objects; and (4) the capacity to integrate with the psychoanalytic process (basic trust and the therapeutic alliance).

Additional factors Among other elements that must be taken into account if an analysis is to be successful are the capacity to transform insight into adaptive behavior, the ability to free associate, the necessary control to avoid acting out, and certain extrinsic considerations such as the patient's physical health, age, financial resources, and physical availability. Concurrent somatic illness may limit a patient's energies for intensive analytic therapy, and personality and behavioral changes may no longer be possible to effect in some older patients. Moreover, a commitment of money over a significant period of time is required and the patient must intend to remain in the geographic area for the number of years necessary to see treatment to completion.

Diagnostically, patients who meet the criteria for analyzability fall into typical patterns of neurotic difficulty. The most common difficulty in analyzable women is in the area of heterosexual object relations, usually reflected in a hysterical form of personality organization. A common difficulty for analyzable men is likely to be in the area of work inhibitions. Men tend to present with symptoms of an obsessive, rather than a hysterical, nature. Patients with an obsessional neurosis or obsessional character usually have little difficulty in engaging in the analytic situation, but few of them are able to develop the overt and analyzable transference early in the analysis. Hysterical patients are either very good or very difficult patients. For them, the development of a transference neurosis is relatively easy and quick, but it is more difficult to engage them in the analytic situation.

The presence of hysterical symptoms alone is not a sufficient indicator of analyzability. Hysterical symptoms are frequently seen in borderline or more primitive patients. Analyzable hysterics have experienced a genuine triangular conflict developmentally and have been able to maintain significant object relations. They possess the capacity to recognize and tolerate internal reality and conflicts, and they are able to distinguish accurately between internal and external reality. They have been able to develop a mastery of ambivalence, particularly in the early relationship with the mother. This mastery provides a defensive organization that can buffer the significant ego regressions during the stressful analytic situation. Many analyzable hysterical patients reveal a combination of hysterical and obsessive characteristics, or a mixed neurosis.

Less analyzable hysterics fail to demonstrate the development of relatively stable and ego-syntonic obsessional defenses, and show inconsistent achievement in their work and in the maintenance of friendships. They tend to be passive and fearful of dependent wishes. These patients have greater difficulty in establishing a stable analytic relationship.

HYSTERICAL PATIENTS Hysterics with underlying depressive character structure are generally unable to mobilize their inner resources during developmental crises. Some may be analyzable, but long and difficult analyses are to be expected. Suffering from low self-esteem, these hysterical women patients tend to devaluate their own femininity. Although they may have experienced some triangular conflict, there may be excessive idealization of the father. They may also recognize and tolerate considerable depression, but they have failed in the area of routine mastery. Thus, they also tend to be passive and to feel helpless and vulnerable. All of these patients present serious problems in the terminal phases of analysis and may drift into an interminable analytic situation. The intensity, depth, and chronicity of the depression in these patients are critical. If excessive, the prognosis is less optimistic.

Primitive hysterics usually present a florid clinical picture and are incapable of tolerating a genuine triangular conflict. Their transference fantasies are intensely sexualized and they entertain the possibility of real gratification. They cannot distinguish between internal and external reality, and consequently have difficulty in establishing a therapeutic alliance and in differentiating it from the transference neurosis. These patients do not meet the criteria for analyzability.

Occasionally, male patients present with a predominately hysterical personality organization. Like the women described above, these men may be placed along a continuum from essentially neurotic to the more primitive character constellations. The assessment of analyzability is consistent with that described for women, although there is, because they are male, a difference in the underlying dynamics.

OBSESSIONAL PATIENTS These patients present different problems. Failure to form oedipal attachments is more likely to result in obsessional symptoms or an obsessional character structure in the male than in the female. The analyzability of obsessional patients does not depend on the content or severity of the presenting symptoms, but on the degree to which they can tolerate the instinctual regression necessary for the development of a transference neurosis. Obsessional patients tend to develop conflicts in such areas as love versus hate, activity versus passivity, and omnipotence versus helplessness. The resolution and mastery of these conflicts are crucial developmental tasks.

The resolution, particularly, of the conflict of love and hate and the tolerance of ambivalence are among the important developmental tasks in the achievement of healthy self-object differentiation and early identifications. The successful resolution of this conflict renders the patient more accessible to analysis. Analyzable obsessional patients must have sufficient tolerance for conflicting emotions to endure the alternation between love and hate that emerges in the transference neurosis. Furthermore, the patient must be able to separate transference feelings from the analytic relationship and to tolerate their ambivalence in order to allow themselves to maintain the therapeutic relationship. An important distinction exists between the developmental failure to integrate emotions and perceptions and the regressive impairment of previously established integration during neurotic symptom formation. Obsessional intolerance of conflict and ambivalence may reflect either developmental cause.

The major unresolved conflict in analyzable obsessional men derives from the triangular oedipal conflict. However, reaction formations can be established before the onset of the genital oedipal situation. Premature consolidation of obsessional defenses and the early crystallization of personality may form an impediment to the emergence of the triangular conflict. Thus, the presence of hysterical or obsessional symptoms is less important in evaluating the potential for psychoanalysis than the degree to which certain major developmental steps have been accomplished and the quality of object relations.

TOLERANCE OF ANXIETY AND DEPRESSION The capacity to tolerate anxiety and depression is another major concern in evaluating analyzability. Tolerance of depression involves a dual developmental task: (1) toleration of painful reality that cannot be immediately modified and (2) the subsequent mobilization of resources in available areas of achievement and mastery. The masculine ideal of competitive striving and mastery reinforces the second phase of this developmental task, so that analyzable obsessional men should have a relative intolerance for passivity and depression. For women, however, passivity rather than activity is central to the image of femininity. Women may have more difficulty in dealing with the second phase of the developmental task, whereas men are more likely to have difficulty with the first phase.

The evaluation of depression and the patient's capacity to bear and master it are crucial items. Depression is a frequent presenting symptom in patients suffering from hysterical and obsessional neuroses. Depressed patients often turn out to be analyzable neurotics, but a preliminary course of psychotherapy is often necessary to reestablish a sufficient level of self-esteem and the mobilization of coping resources to facilitate development of a positive therapeutic alliance. The therapeutic response allows the therapist to evaluate carefully the patient's capacity to tolerate depressive affects without significant regression, as well as the capacity to mobilize resources for active coping.

ANALYTIC PROCESS

In his initial psychoanalytic approach, Freud believed that recognition by the analyst of the patient's unconscious motivations, the communication of this knowledge to the patient, and comprehension of this by the patient would of itself effect a cure. This belief was his basic doctrine of therapeutic insight. Further experience, however, showed Freud the fallacy of these expectations.

Freud found that his discovery of the patient's unconscious wishes and his ability to impart these findings to the patient so that they were accepted and understood were insufficient. Although insight permitted clarification of the patient's intellectual appraisal of problems, the tensions for which the patient sought treatment were not alleviated. Freud began to realize that the success of treatment depended on the patient's ability to understand the experience on an emotional level and to retain and use that insight. Thus, if the experience recurred, it would elicit another reaction that would no longer be repressed, and the patient would have undergone a psychic economic change.

Freud continually refined his technique on the basis of his clinical experience and theoretical understanding. Psychoanalysis became recognized as a specific method for reaching and modifying phenomena that give rise to conflict. As one of its goals, psychoanalysis attempts to bring repressed material into consciousness to enable the patient to gain greater self-understanding and to find more realistic solutions to conflicts. Freud's formula for this process was, "Where id was, ego shall be."

Psychoanalysis attaches minimal importance to the immediate relief of symptoms or to guidance and moral support from the therapist. The goal of treatment is to pull the neurosis out by its roots, rather than to prune off the top. To accomplish this objective, it is necessary to break down the deep pregenital crystallization of id, ego, and superego, and to bring the unconscious material near enough to the surface of consciousness to enable it to be modified and reevaluated in the light of reality. This method distinguishes classical psychoanalytic treatment from the other psychodynamic forms of psychotherapy.

The patient is unaware of the psychic mechanisms the mind uses to deal with conflict. By isolating the basic problem, the patient is protected against what seems to be unbearable suffering. No matter how it may impair functioning, the neurosis is preferable to the emergence of unacceptable wishes and ideas. In the analysis, all the forces that permitted the original repression are mobilized again and emerge as a resistance to this threatened encroachment. Despite vigorous efforts to cooperate consciously in the analysis, and no matter how painful the neurotic symptoms may be, the patient automatically defends against the reopening of old wounds with every resource of defense and resistance available.

The regression induced by the analytic situation allows for a resurgence of infantile conflicts and the formation of a transference neurosis. The revived conflicts are manifested through the repetition compulsion. The regression is an attempt to return to an earlier state of real or fantasied gratification, but it can also be viewed as an effort to master previous traumatic experiences. Regression and the development of transference are preliminary conditions for the mastery of unresolved conflicts, but they also represent unconscious wishes to return to an earlier state of narcissistic gratification. The analytic situation must contend with this duality and its associated tensions.

As in any developmental crisis, the risk of deterioration in the analysis must be balanced against the promise of growth and mastery. Patients who are unable to achieve analytic regression cannot attain a good therapeutic result. It is the therapeutic alliance that serves as the balancing element between potentially constructive and destructive regression. A stable therapeutic alliance is the buffer against excessive ego regression and also provides the basis for potential growth.

Phases of the analytic process

The analytic process can be divided into three phases, each of which requires different capacities and developmental aptitudes in the patient to negotiate it successfully. The first phase relates to the patient's capacity to enter into, establish, and sustain a therapeutic alliance. To attain this phase, the patient must develop a special object relationship that will flavor the nature and quality of the therapeutic alliance. The second phase involves the patient's ability to develop a transference neurosis, to work it through, and to analyze it. The evolution of the transference neurosis involves a reopening and reworking of the oedipal conflicts. The third phase entails the patient's capacity to tolerate separation and loss and to integrate the resolution of these issues effectively into the pattern of positive identification with the analyst. This terminal phase deals more directly with the areas of autonomy and independence.

TREATMENT TECHNIQUES The analytic technique is adapted to the idiosyncrasies of each patient's developmental capacities, needs, and defenses. It also varies according to the stage of the analysis. The technical goal of the first phase is to establish the analytic situation; it differs from the aim of the second phase, which is to promote regression to allow for the development of the transference neurosis and to resolve it. In turn, the treatment technique of the third phase differs from the first two in dealing with the problems of termination.

Free association The cornerstone of psychoanalytic technique is the process of free association. The patient is instructed in this method and encouraged to apply it throughout the analysis. In addition to providing content for the treatment, free association promotes the regression and passive dependence connected with establishing and working through the transference neurosis. Free association is enhanced by techniques that also induce regression, such as lying on the couch, not being able to see the analyst, and having the analysis conducted in an atmosphere of quiet tranquility.

Frequently, the process of free association must be modified according to the patient's defensive needs or the developmental progression occurring within the analysis. The analytic process is complex, difficult to conceptualize, and must be understood in the context of the relationship between the analyst and the patient. More is required of the patient than simply the act of freely associating; the patient cannot just lie back passively and expect the analyst to do most of the work. The patient is called on to mobilize basic ego resources in the service of mastery, to gain insight, and to utilize executive and synthetic capacities. Ultimately, the patient must be able to function more actively in the analytic relationship. The degree to which the patient mobilizes these capacities varies from phase to phase of the analytic process.

Resistance Efforts on the part of the patient to say everything that comes to mind are never completely successful. No matter how willing and cooperative the patient may be in trying to freely associate, resistance exists throughout every analysis. Patients correct themselves, make slips of the tongue, stammer, remain silent, and fidgit. They may raise irrelevant questions, intellectualize, be late for appointments, and find excuses for not keeping them. They may be critical of the underlying premises of analysis, their minds may become blank, or they may resort to censoring their thoughts as irrelevant and uninteresting.

The development of resistance in analysis is automatic and independent of the patient's will. The powers of resistance are unconscious, and the emotional forces that give rise to resistance oppose those that produce the transference neurosis. Resistance during the second phase of treatment becomes of paramount importance because of the the emergence of the transference neurosis. The quality and significance of the resistance during the other phases of the analysis are quite different.

The resistance of the patient enables the analyst to evaluate and become familiar with the defensive organization of the patient's ego and its functions. Not only do these patterns provide valuable data to the analyst, but they become the channels through which the patient can be approached therapeutically. In helping the patient gradually to discover and work through the defenses, both parties come to understand what it is that the patient must defend against.

Transference may itself be a form of resistance as the wish for immediate gratification in the analysis can circumvent and postpone the desired goals of treatment. The wish for immediate gratification runs counter to the demands of the analysis for tolerance of anxiety, delay of gratification, and emotional growth. Consequently, the analysis of resistance, and particularly transference resistance, becomes a primary objective of the analysis.

As noted above, the nature of the resistance changes from phase to phase of the analysis. In the initial phase, the patient's resistance tends to be directed against the establishment of the treatment situation and entering into a meaningful relationship with the analyst. In the second phase, resistance is concerned with keeping the underlying conflicts unconscious and working against the induced regression of the analytic process. In the terminal phase, resistance works in the interest of clinging to the passive and dependent regressed relationship with the analyst.

Interpretation Interpretation is the chief tool available to the analyst to reduce resistance. In the early stages of the development of psychoanalytic treatment, the sole purpose of interpretation was to inform the patient of unconscious wishes. Later, it was to assist the patient in understanding the resistance to self-awareness. Today, the analyst's function as an interpreter is not limited simply to paraphrasing the patient's verbal reports, but can include indicating at appropriate moments what is not being reported. Analytic interpretation does not afford immediate symptomatic relief; on the contrary, it may produce a heightening of anxiety and the emergence of further resistance.

If a correct interpretation is given at the proper time, the patient may react immediately, or after a period of emotional struggle during which new associations are offered. These associations often confirm the validity of previous interpretations and add significant data that disclose motivations and experiences previously not revealed. Progress is made in the analysis by employing appropriate interpretations to help the patient gain insight independently by reducing the unconscious resistance to such self-awareness. The most effective interpretations are those that are timed in such a way as to meet the emerging and half-formed insights offered by the patient. The analyst must gauge the capacity of the patient at any one moment to hear, assimilate, and integrate the content of a given interpretation.

Interpretations cannot be considered in isolation from the total gestalt of the analytic situation and process. Ideally, an interpretation should take place within the context of the therapeutic relationship. It is well recognized that benefits produced by virtue of the analyst's exhortations or unilaterally provided insights are only temporary. To be most effective and to be of lasting therapeutic value, interpretations should be arrived at by a delicate dialectic arising from the mutually facilitated and growing awareness of both the patient and the analyst.

ROLE OF THE ANALYST In the initial phase of the analysis, the analyst's task is to facilitate the establishment of the analytic situation and the therapeutic alliance. At this stage, the quality of the patient's interactions with the analyst are heavily influenced by the patient's personality and its interaction with the analyst's personality. Although transference phenomena are present from the beginning, more realistic aspects of the patient's personality and the interaction with the analyst must be considered. Some patients develop a transference readiness before the beginning of the analysis and move quickly into transference issues, in which case the analyst must help the patient build the foundation for a firm therapeutic alliance. The more severe the patient's psychopathology, the more significant is the work of the first phase. When the therapeutic alliance is firmly and securely established, the more regressive aspects of the treatment situation can be addressed with greater confidence and less risk of harmful regression.

In the middle phase, which deals with the transference neurosis, the analyst uses techniques and approaches calculated to induce greater regression in the patient. Whereas in the beginning of the analytic process the analyst is like a mother adapting to the innate disposition of the child, during the second phase, the analyst becomes more like the parent who can recognize the child's incestuous fantasies without gratifying them. The transference regression invokes a recapitulation of the mother–child relationship.

The relative passivity of the analyst conveys to the patient an avoidance of permissive as well as authoritative expressions and allows for interpretations of the patient's dynamics as they emerge through free association. By maintaining such a posture, the analyst can clarify the way in which the patient's ego defenses operate to inhibit or preclude free association.

Finally, the analyst needs to respond to the patient in terms of the therapeutic alliance and of the transference material. While reacting intuitively to the patient's affect, particularly the basic need to feel accepted and to be understood as a real person, the analyst must recognize and interpret, at the appropriate moment, those wishes and fantasies that are derived from the transference neurosis.

Transference The patient's free associations reveal the hidden patterns of mental organization and fixations at immature levels. When the patient's fantasies and events are shared in the analytic setting, the analyst becomes invested with some of the accompanying emotions. Feelings originally directed toward early objects are displaced onto the analyst, who becomes loved or hated much as the original object was loved or hated. The patient's feelings toward the analyst to an increasing extent replicate the feelings toward significant persons in the patient's life. This special type of object displacement is known as transference.

As unresolved childhood attitudes emerge and function as fantasied projections toward the analyst, the analyst becomes for the patient a phantom composite figure who represents various important persons in the patient's early environment. Those earlier relationships that remain unresolved are reactivated with some of their original vigor. Gradually, patients see themselves as they really are, with unfulfilled and contradictory needs. The use of transference as a dynamic therapeutic force and the analysis of its unconscious sources are unique to classical analysis.

Transference neurosis As stated earlier, the transference neurosis usually develops in the second phase of analysis. The patient is engaged in a continuing battle with the analyst, and it becomes apparent that the most compelling reason for continuing the analysis is the desire to attain some kind of emotional satisfaction from the analyst. At this point in the treatment, the transference emotions are more important to the patient than the permanent health sought initially. Major unresolved and unconscious problems of childhood begin to dominate the patient's behavior. They are now reproduced in the transference with all their original emotion. The patient strives unconsciously to recapture what was taken away in childhood.

The transference neurosis is driven by three outstanding characteristics of instinctual life in early childhood: the pleasure principle, ambivalence, and repetition compulsion. The emergence of the transference neurosis in treatment is a gradual process, except in those patients with a propensity for transference regression. The life of the patient is analyzed until the original infantile conflict is fully revealed. Only then does the transference neurosis begin to subside. At that point, entry into the third phase of analysis is noted.

Termination of the analysis occupies the third period of the analysis. Again, it is a gradual process, and is not even complete with the last session. If the analysis was fairly thorough, thereafter, at times of emotional crisis, the patient may resolve, without assistance, those areas of conflict that were not entirely worked through with the analyst. Part of the patient's ability to accomplish this resolution depends on the patient's capacity for internalization and effective identification with the strengths and objectivity of the analyst. The patient experiences less need for introspection and self-analysis and is gradually able to deal with life on a more mature and satisfactory basis than was possible previously.

Therapeutic alliance The therapeutic alliance is based on the collaborative relationship that the patient establishes in the interaction with the analyst. Real personality characteristics of both the patient and the analyst contribute to this interaction. The distortions or misperceptions the patient brings to the relationship may not all be due to the transference, but may be determined by the patient's personality structure, which relates to the capacity to achieve and maintain a stable object relationship.

For this reason, the analyst's attempts in the beginning to clarify the patient's anxiety, expectations, and feelings about the analyst should not be regarded as transference interpretations. The purpose of such interventions is to support and to reinforce the patient's capacity to establish a meaningful therapeutic alliance. The alliance provides the stable and positive relationship between analyst and patient that enables them both to engage productively in the work of the analysis. It permits a split to take place in the patient's ego; the observing part of the patient's ego can ally itself with the analyst in a working relationship, which allows it gradually to identify positively with the analyst in analyzing and modifying the pathological defenses put up by the ego against internal danger situations.

The analyst's own personality has an important influence in establishing the therapeutic alliance. The analyst enters the analytic process as a real person and not merely as a transference object. These real characteristics can interfere with the achievement of a basic working relationship and with the satisfactory working through in the analytic process. The maintenance of the therapeutic alliance requires that the patient be able to differentiate between the mature and infantile aspects of the experience in the relationship to the analyst. The therapeutic alliance serves a dual function—as a significant barrier to regression of the ego in the analytic process and as a fundamental aspect of the analytic situation against which the wishes, feelings, and fantasies evoked by the transference neurosis can be evaluated and measured.

The therapeutic alliance derives from the modifications of specific ego resources related to the capacity for object relations and reality testing. The analyst must elicit the patient's capacity to establish such a relationship that will be able to withstand the inevitable distortions and regressive aspects of the transference neurosis.

MODIFICATIONS IN TECHNIQUES Psychoanalytic treatment typically extends over a period of years and requires patience on the part of both the analyst and the patient. The classical analytic method constitutes the best experimental situation yet devised for studying the complex features of human nature.

Rigid adherence to the fundamental mechanistic principles of psychoanalytic technique is an impossibility. At times, the immediate environmental situation may be so serious for the patient that the analyst must pay attention to its practical implications. Those patients whose early childhood was extraordinarily deficient in love and affection, so that they suffer from a basic developmental defect in their capacity for a one-to-one relationship, and, consequently, in their ability to sustain a therapeutic alliance, must be given more support and encouragement than is strictly advocated in the use of psychoanalytic techniques.

The nature and degree of the analyst's active interventions in the opening hours of analysis are still matters of discussion and controversy. The transference neurosis usually develops slowly and gradually. Attempts at premature interpretation may not be productive, and may even be counterproductive. Such attempts may create a tendency to prolonged silences, lack of responsiveness, rigidity, and, later, the relative lack of participation in the treatment situation by the analyst. Sometimes, problems with the transference in the subsequent stages of analysis can be attributed to a failure to establish a meaningful alliance in the initial stages of treatment. Thus, suitable interventions of the analyst in the early stages of treatment can be a help to the patient in establishing a constructive therapeutic alliance.

Very narcissistic or more borderline patients must establish a strong personal tie and significant feelings of attachment to the analyst before they can develop sufficient interest and motivation for analytic treatment. Moreover, such an object alliance for these patients is an absolute necessity if the destructive effects of excessive regression are to be avoided. However, experience suggests that every deviation from strict analytic technique that such special conditions compel tends to prolong the treatment and considerably increases its problems.

Modifications in psychoanalytic technique are called parameters, and they remain a source of discussion and controversy among analytic therapists. A significant contemporary trend is the increasing tendency of analysts to treat more difficult and complex cases; thus, the necessity for introducing modifications in various aspects of the treatment process increases correspondingly.

RESULTS OF TREATMENT

The impartial and objective evaluation of the therapeutic effectiveness of psychoanalysis is a complex and difficult issue. Some patients claim to have been analyzed when, in fact, no such procedure was undertaken, or the analysis was conducted by someone assuming the role of analyst who lacked a proper understanding of analytic science and technique or the rigorous training and supervision required. Other patients, after being in analysis for a very short time, have discontinued treatment on their own initiative or when advised by the analyst that they were not suitable candidates for analytic treatment. To date, no controlled studies are available that have objectively and scientifically evaluated the results of psychoanalytic therapy.

No analyst can ever eliminate all of a patient's personality defects and neurotic features, no matter how thorough or successful the treatment. An essential criterion of the effectiveness of treatment is the mitigation of the rigors of a punitive superego. In evaluating therapeutic change, psychoanalysts do not regard the alleviation of symptoms as the most significant aspect of the therapy, although it is important. Perhaps an even more meaningful index of the value of psychoanalysis is the absence of the illness and the lack of need for further treatment. However, the chief basis for evaluation remains the patient's general adjustment to life; that is, the capacity for attaining reasonable happiness, contributing to the happiness of others, dealing adequately with the normal vicissitudes and stresses of life, and entering into and maintaining mutually gratifying and rewarding relationships with others.

Specific criteria for judging the effectiveness of treatment include a reduction in the neurotic need for suffering, a lessening of neurotic inhibitions, a decrease in infantile dependency needs, and an increased capacity for responsibility. Other criteria are successful relationships in marriage, work, and social settings, and the capacity for sublimation and for creative and adaptive application of the patient's own potentialities. But the most important indication of the success of treatment is the release of the patient's normal potential, which has been blocked by neurotic conflicts, for further internal growth and the development of a mature, functioning personality.

A synthesis of the various developmental theorists, among whom are Margaret Mahler, John Bowlby, Sigmund Freud, Erik Erikson, and Jean Piaget, is provided in Table 6.1-2.

Some of the material in this section was derived from the chapter by William W. Meissner, S. J., M.D. on *Classical Psychoanalysis* that appeared in the fourth edition of the *Comprehensive Textbook of Psychiatry*.

REFERENCES

Abraham K: *Selected Papers for Psychoanalysis*. Basic Books. New York, 1953.

Bibring G L, Dwyer T F, Huntington D S, Valenstein A: A study of the psychological process in pregnancy and of the earliest mother-child relationship: II. Methodological considerations. Psychoanal Stud Child *16:* 25, 1961.

Brenner C: *Psychoanalytic Technique and Psychic Conflict*. International Universities Press, New York, 1976.

Brenner C: Working through: 1914–1984. Psychoanal Q *56:* 88, 1987.

Eagle M N: *Recent Developments in Psychoanalysis*. McGraw-Hill, New York, 1984.

Ellenberger H: *The Discovery of the Unconscious*. Basic Books, New York, 1970.

Federn P: *Ego Psychology and the Psychoses*. Basic Books, New York, 1952.

Fenichel O: *The Psychoanalytic Theory of Neurosis*. Norton, New York, 1945.

Freud A: *The Ego and the Mechanisms of Defense*. International Universities Press, New York, 1966.

Freud A: *Normality and Pathology in Childhood: Assessments of Development*. International Universities Press, New York, 1965.

Freud S: *Standard Editon of the Complete Psychological Works of Sigmund Freud*. Hogarth Press, London, 1953–1966.

Gill M M: *The Collected Papers of David Rapaport*. Basic Books, New York, 1967.

Greenberg J R, Mitchell S A: *Object Relations in Psychoanalytic Theory*. Harvard University Press, Cambridge, MA, 1983.

Hartmann H: *Essays on Ego Psychology*. International Universities Press, New York, 1964.

TABLE 6.1-2
A Synthesis of Developmental Theorists

Age (Years)	*Margaret Mahler*	*John Bowlby*	*Sigmund Freud*	*Erik Erikson*	*Jean Piaget*
0–1	Normal autistic phase (birth to 4 weeks) · State of half-sleep, half-wake · Major task of phase is to achieve homeostatic equilibrium with the environment Normal symbiotic phase (3–4 weeks to 4–5 months) · Dim awareness of caretaker, but infant still functions as if he and caretaker are in state of undifferentiation or fusion · Social smile characteristic (2–4 months) The subphases of separation-individuation proper First subphase: differentiation (5–10 months) · Process of hatching from autistic shell, i.e., developing more alert sensorium that reflects cognitive and neurological maturation · Beginning of comparative scanning, i.e., comparing what is and what is not mother · Characteristic anxiety: stranger anxiety, which involves curiosity and fear (most prevalent around 8 months)	Phase I (birth to 8–12 weeks) · Infant's ability to discriminate one person from another is limited to olfactory and auditory stimuli · To any person in infant's vicinity, infant will: - orient to that person - have tracking movements of the eyes - grasp and reach - smile - babble - stop crying on hearing voice or seeing face · These behaviors, by influencing the adult's behavior, are likely to increase time the baby is in proximity to mother (adult) Phase II (8–12 weeks to 6 months or much later, according to circumstances) · Continuation of phase I activities but more marked in relation to mother more specifically	Oral phase (birth to 1 year) · Major site of tension and gratification is the mouth, lips, tongue - includes biting and sucking activities	Basic trust vs basic mistrust (oral sensory) (birth to 1 year) · Social mistrust demonstrated via ease of feeding, depth of sleep, bowel relaxation · Depends on consistency and sameness of experience provided by caretaker · Second 6-months teething and biting moves infant "from getting to taking" · Weaning leads to "nostalgia for lost paradise" · If basic trust is strong, child maintains hopeful attitude	Sensorimotor phase (birth to 2 years) · Intelligence rests mainly on actions and movements coordinated under "*schemata*," (Schema is a pattern of behavior in response to a particular environmental stimulus.) · Environment is mastered through *assimilation* and *accommodation*. (Assimilation is the incorporation of new environmental stimuli. Accommodation is the modification of behavior to adapt to new stimuli.) · *Object permanence* is achieved by age 2 yrs. Object still exists in mind if disappears from view: search for hidden object · Reversibility in action begins

TABLE 6.1-2
continued

Age (Years)	*Margaret Mahler*	*John Bowlby*	*Sigmund Freud*	*Erik Erikson*	*Jean Piaget*
1–2	Second subphase, practicing (10–16 months) · Beginning of this phase marked by upright locomotion—child has new perspective and also mood of elation · Mother used as home base · Characteristic anxiety: separation anxiety Third subphase: rapprochement (16–24 months) · Infant now a toddler—more aware of physical separateness, which dampens mood of elation · Child tries to bridge gap between himself and mother—concretely seen as bringing objects to mother · Mother's efforts to help toddler often not perceived as helpful, temper tantrums typical · Characteristic event: rapprochement crisis: wanting to be soothed by mother and yet not be able to accept her help · Symbol of rapprochement: child standing on threshold of door not knowing which way to turn in helpless frustration · Resolution of crisis occurs as child's skills improve and child able to get gratification from doing things himself	Phase III (6–7 months and continues throughout second and into third year) · Attachment to mother figure evident · Following departing mother · Greeting her on her return · Using her as base from which to explore · Waning of friendly, undifferentiated responses to others · Treating of strangers with caution, alarm, withdrawal Phase IV (from 24 months and beyond) · Mother figure seen as independent · Object, persistent in time and space · More complex relationship with mother develops—"partnership" between mother and child develops where child acquires insight into mother's feelings and motives · child observes mother's behavior and what influences it	Anal phase (1 year to 3 years) · Anus and surrounding area is major source of interest · Acquisition of voluntary sphincter control (toilet training)	Autonomy vs. shame and doubt (muscular-anal) (1–3 years) · Biologically includes learning to walk, feed self, talk · Muscular maturation sets stage for "holding on and letting go" · Need for outer control, firmness of caretaker prior to development of autonomy · *Shame* occurs when child is overtly self-conscious via negative exposure · *Self-doubt* can evolve if parents overly shame child (e.g., about elimination)	Preoperational phase (2–7 years) · Appearance of *symbolic* functions, associated with language acquisition · *Egocentrism:* child understands everything exclusively from own perspective · Thinking is illogical and magical · Nonreversible thinking with absence of conservation - *Animism:* belief that inanimate objects are alive (i.e. have feelings and intentions) - "*Immanent justice*": belief that punishment for bad deeds is inevitable
2–3	Fourth subphase: consolidation and object constancy (24–36 months) · Child better able to cope with mother's absence and engage substitutes				

TABLE 6.1-2
continued

Age (Years)	*Margaret Mahler*	*John Bowlby*	*Sigmund Freud*	*Erik Erikson*	*Jean Piaget*
	· Child can begin to feel comfortable with mother's absences by knowing she will return · Gradual internalization of image of mother as reliable and stable · Through increasing verbal skills and better sense of time, child can tolerate delay and endure separations				
3–4			Phallic-oedipal phase (3–5 years) · Genital focus of interest, stimulation, and excitement · Penis is organ of interest for both sexes · Genital masturbation common · Intense preoccupation with *castration anxiety* (fear of genital loss or injury) · *Penis envy* (discontent with one's own genitals and wish to possess genitals of male) seen in girls in this phase · *Oedipus complex* universal: child wishes to have sex and marry parent of opposite sex and simultaneously be rid of parent of same sex	Initiative vs. guilt (locomotor genital) (3–5 years) · *Initiative* arises in relation to tasks for the sake of activity, both motor and intellectual · *Guilt* may arise over goals contemplated (especially aggressive) · Desire to mimic adult world; involvement in oedipal struggle leads to resolution via social role identification · Sibling rivalry frequent	
4–5					
5–6			Latency phase (from 5–6 years to 11–12 years) · State of relative quiescence of sexual drive with resolution of Oedipal complex		

TABLE 6.1-2
continued

Age (Years)	*Margaret Mahler*	*John Bowlby*	*Sigmund Freud*	*Erik Erikson*	*Jean Piaget*
			· Sexual drives channeled into more socially appropriate aims (i.e., schoolwork and sports) · Formation of *superego*: one of three psychic structures in mind which is responsible for moral and ethical development, including conscience · (Other two psychic structures are *ego,* which is a group of functions mediating between the drives and the external environment, and · the *id,* repository of sexual and aggressive drives · The id is there at birth and the ego develops gradually from rudimentary structure present at birth)		
6–11				Industry vs. inferiority (latency) (6–11 years) · Child is busy building, creating, accomplishing · Receives systematic instruction as well as fundamentals of technology · Danger of sense of inadequacy and inferiority if child despairs of his tools/skills and status among peers · Socially decisive age	Concrete (operational) phase (7–11 years) · Emergence of logical (cause-effect) thinking, including reversibility and ability to sequence and serialize · Understanding of part/whole relationships and classifications · Child able to take other's point of view · Conservation of number, length, weight, and volume
11+			Genital phase (from 11–12 years and beyond) · Final stage of psychosexual development—begins with puberty and the biological capacity for orgasm but involves the capacity for true intimacy	Identity vs. role diffusion (11 years through end of adolescence) · Struggle to develop *ego identity* (sense of inner sameness and continuity) · Preoccupation with appearance, hero worship, ideology · *Group identity* (peers) develops · Danger of *role confusion,* doubts about sexual and vocational identity · *Psychosocial moratorium,* stage between morality learned by the child and the ethics to be developed by the adult	Formal (abstract) phase (11 years through end of adolescence) · Hypothetical-deductive reasoning, not only on basis of objects but also on basis of hypotheses or of propositions · Capable of thinking about one's thoughts · Combinative structures emerge, permitting flexible grouping of elements in a system · Ability to use two systems of reference simultaneously · Ability to grasp concept of probabilities

Table by Sylvia Karasu, M.D. and Richard Oberfield, M.D.

Jacobson E: *The Self and the Object World*. International Universities Press, New York, 1964.
Jones E: *The Life and Work of Sigmund Freud,* 3 vol. Basic Books, New York, 1953–1957.
Kernberg O F: *Borderline Conditions and Pathological Narcissism*. Jason Aronson, New York, 1975.
Kohut H: *The Analysis of the Self*. International Universities Press, New York, 1971.
Mahler M S, Pine F, Bergman A: *The Psychological Birth of The Human Infant*. Basic Books, New York, 1975.
Menninger K, Holzman P S: *Theory of Psychoanalytic Technique*. Basic Books, New York, 1973.
Rangell L: *A core process in psychoanalytic treatment*. Psychoanal Q *56:* 222, 1987.
Rothstein A, editor: *The Interpretation of Dreams in Clinical Work*. International Universities Press, Madison, 1987.
Semrad E: The operation of ego defenses in object loss. In *The Loss of Loved Ones,* D M Moriarty, editor. Charles C Thomas, Springfield, IL, 1967.
Storrow R D, Brandchaft B, Atwood G E: *Psychoanalytic Treatment An Intersubjective Approach*. Analytic, Hillsdale, NJ, 1987.
Vaillant G E: *Adaptation to Life*. Little, Brown, Boston, 1977.
Weiss J, Sampson H: *The Psychoanalytic Process. Theory, Clinical Observation and Empirical Research*. Guilford, New York, 1986.

6.2 ERIK H. ERIKSON

LARS B. LOFGREN, M.D.

INTRODUCTION

During the more than 5 decades he has spent in the United States, Erik H. Erikson deeply influenced not only psychiatry, psychoanalysis, and other professions that use psychological interaction and therapy methods, but also the general understanding of the human situation and how it develops. He can be regarded as one of the most influential psychoanalysts in the world. That his influence extends across the boundaries of psychoanalysis and psychiatry is demonstrated by the fact that *Newsweek* magazine devoted a cover and feature story to Erikson on December 21, 1970. Although the crises of youth and adolescence may take a central place in his thinking, he has also contributed to a deeper understanding of the problems of women and minorities, and of authority conflicts in general.

If Erikson did not actually found the school of psychohistory, he has provided important tools for such endeavors and given them a new respectability. His study of Gandhi provides a new understanding of nonviolence. His emphasis on the importance of the actual historical situation has counteracted the tendency of psychoanalysts and psychologists to isolate themselves in laboratory-like conditions. Although many psychoanalysts still regard his views as controversial, their power and effect are indisputable.

HIS LIFE

Erik (Homburger) Erikson was born on June 15, 1902, in Frankfurt-am-Main, which is now in West Germany (Fig. 6.2-1). Both parents were Danish. His biological father was absent during his childhood and he grew up in the home of his mother's second husband, Theodor Homburger, a German-Jewish pediatrician. The Homburgers seem to have kept the fact of his actual parentage from him for a long time—a "loving deceit," as he later called it. Thus, the man who was to introduce the concept of identity crisis grew up as a blond, blue-eyed Dane among the Germans, a gentile among the Jews, and a Jew among the gentiles. His performance at school, the Humanistische Gymnasium in Karlsruhe, was not remarkable, except for his artistic gifts. After a year of peregrination, he began to study art in earnest in Karlsruhe, Munich, and Florence.

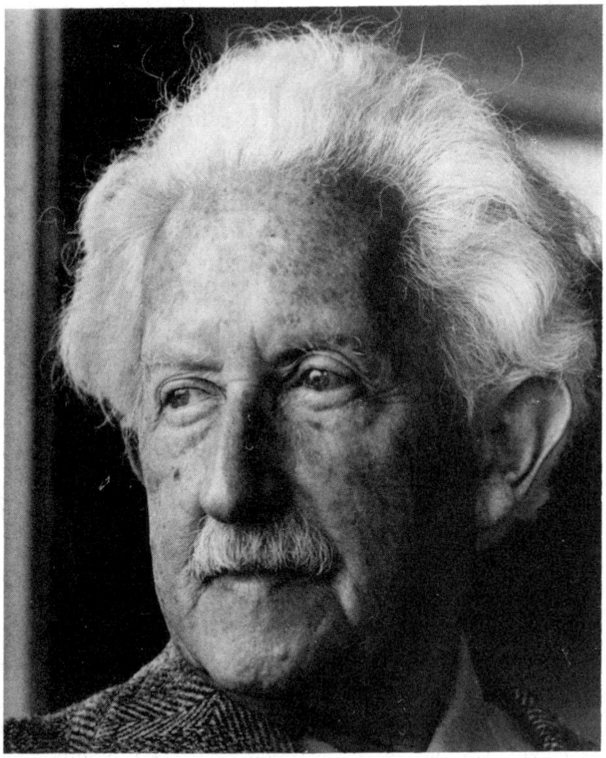

FIGURE 6.2-1 *Erik Erikson.*

Erikson's life reached a turning point in 1927, when Peter Blos, later to become a world-famous child psychologist, invited him to participate in setting up an informal school for the four children of Dorothy Burlingham, a New York professional then in analysis with Freud. The approach used by Erikson and Blos was strongly influenced by the radical pedagogical theories in Europe at this time; it offered the children freedom and responsibility in a very different way from the classical German school. Through this work, Erikson met Anna Freud, with whom he later entered into analysis. His training in analysis ended with graduation from the Vienna Institute in 1933, and shortly afterward he left Europe to escape the increasing threat of fascism in Italy and the Nazis in Germany.

It should be noted that Erikson did not receive any formal university education on the graduate or postgraduate level, a fact that seems to create some anxiety in persons with many academic merits. The change of his name from Homburger to Erikson took place after his arrival in the United States. His children did not like the somewhat unfortunate associations with the word "Homburger," and suggested that as they were Erik's children, the name "Erikson" would be appropriate. The assumption that the name has some direct connection with his Danish roots is thus incorrect.

In 1929, Erikson married Joan Mowast Serson, a Canadian woman with a strong interest in the arts. His friendship with Hanns Sachs, an important member of Freud's inner circle, helped him to become established at Harvard University, where he soon gained a reputation as a brilliant clinician and thinker. One of the features of Erikson's life is a tendency never to stay very long in one place ("Travel light" is one of his mottos), and in 1936, he joined the Institute of Human Relations at Yale University. At this time, he began his important research on the Sioux culture in South Dakota, with its emphasis on the cultural influences on child development. Similar work with the anthropologist A. L. Kroeber took him to the Yurok Indians in California.

In 1942, Erikson joined the faculty of the University of California at Berkeley. Here, he wrote the papers that later became *Childhood and Society*. He also began a major research project, a longitudinal study of a group of children. This work was interrupted in the later years of the troubled 1940s, when Erikson refused to sign the loyalty oath then required by the University of California.

Work at Riggs In 1950, Erikson joined the Austen Riggs Center in Stockbridge, Massachusetts, then directed by Robert P. Knight, one of the great psychiatric-psychoanalytic clinicians of the twentieth century. The presence of such prominent thinkers as Margaret Brenman, Merton Gill, David Rapaport, and Roy Schafer, and the close ties to the Yale psychoanalytic group, created an atmosphere highly conducive to creative work. Joan Erikson participated actively in the therapeutic work of the institute, creating a movement-dance class and an arts and crafts program decisively different from art and occupational therapy. The years at Riggs saw many important contributions from Erikson, especially *Young Man Luther*. In 1960, he was invited to join Harvard as a lecturer in psychiatry and professor of human development. Here, Erikson's creativity reached full fruition. Before he retired from Harvard in 1970, many of his most prominent works had been published or conceived.

One cannot understand Erikson's work without taking into account his marriage to Joan. Not only has she served as his editor, but their relationship is one of the rare unions between a man and a woman in which both have the ability to stimulate and enhance creativity in the other. Joan has flourished as a jeweler and has published an important book about Saint Francis. It is in recognition of the importance of their relationship that Erik Erikson very often uses the terms "we" and "our" about his work.

The Eriksons are currently living in Cambridge, Massachusetts.

THEORY OF PERSONALITY

THE HEALTHY PERSONALITY Freud posits three parts of the mental apparatus: id, ego, and superego. The id can only wish, and the wishes are the psychological representatives of the drives that operate on the boundary between the somatic and the psychological. The superego contains injunctions, rules, and prohibitions stemming from the parents, and thus also indirectly from the prevailing culture. The ego has the task of mediating between the id, the superego, and reality, essentially an executive and observing stance.

Erikson's model is also tripartite. He recognizes much of Freudian psychology, but his point of view represents an expansion of the older model. For Erikson, the understanding of the person must involve three different aspects: somatic, ego, and cultural-historical.

Freud stated that the ego is formed by precipitates of abandoned object relations. These relations rest firmly on the basis of constitutional drives. Erikson assumes that relationships of various kinds have a profound influence on the development of the ego. For Erikson, the person's (parent's, object's) actual specific qualities—both personal and cultural—are of greater importance than Freud, at least overtly, ascribed to them. Simply put, one can say that Freud created a dynamic psychology in a static milieu, whereas Erikson's milieu is fervently dynamic.

Erikson follows Freud in recognizing that some bodily zones dominate during different phases of development—in the earliest phase, the mouth, later the anus, and finally, the genital area. Erikson adds that these zones also give rise to certain specific patterns of behavior, which he calls *modes*. Thus, the dominating mode during the dominance of the oral zone is *incorporation*. The dominating mode during the anal phase is *elimination-retention*, and during the phallic aspect of the genital phase, it is *intrusion*.

The development of these modes is *epigenetic*, a term borrowed from embryology. It means that if a particular anlage does not manifest itself during the appropriate phase, it cannot reach full development; the moment has passed. In addition, later development is disturbed. If the anlage for the eye does not become manifest at the proper time, facial development will suffer. In the same way, a disturbance of the incorporative mode will lead to difficulties in the development of the eliminative-retentive mode, and so on.

What has been said so far is an oversimplification. The incorporative mode is paralleled by an ejective one—spitting out. Pyloric stenosis might make such an ejective mode dominant. The development of the teeth changes the nature of incorporation by adding an element of biting off, or biting into, representing a beginning of an intrusive mode. The mouth can also be clamped shut and prevent any incorporation at all. When the first coordinated movements are possible, grasping and moving actively to the mouth become important components of this mode.

The modes do not disappear as development proceeds, but an echo of earlier phases remains in later ones. The mode dominating the anal phase is eliminative-retentive, but the incorporative aspect can color the processes, and in male homosexuality it becomes quite apparent. The intrusive aspect of the genital-phallic period exists in both sexes, but in the female it must be combined with incorporation via the vagina. If such an incorporative aspect is absent in a girl, the full development of female sexuality becomes difficult or impossible. But the intrusive mode has to remain in a woman in a nondominating way to be used for constructive penetration into time and space. In the man, the inclusive aspect has to remain in some form to make it possible for him to take in and to hold. Because people also have to get rid of certain things, the ejective mode has to remain functional but not dominant in both sexes, and so on. In order for modal vestiges to remain in a functional and productive way, each stage requires a rather exquisite balancing of various modal possibilities to ensure good functioning. Each stage can be seen as a life crisis that has to find a good solution in order for development to proceed favorably.

In the solution of this series of crises, the environment is of crucial importance. The family of the growing child has to be finely attuned to the needs of a particular phase and its functional mode. If such an understanding is lacking, the incorporative mode may be disturbed, for instance, by an attempt to force food past firmly closed lips. And not only does the family need a fine sense for the particular modal needs of a certain stage, but its response must also make sense in terms of the culture in which the interaction takes place in order to avoid later alienation.

THE LIFE-CYCLE STAGES If a person suffers from gastric cancer, the pathology, pathophysiology, and clinical picture will not be very different whether that person is Chinese, black African, or Caucasian. The same thing is true of a small baby suffering from a blood disorder. The medical-technological action built on pathophysiology ideally will be the same in any case. However, the reaction of the patient and family, to a large extent will be determined by the cultural situation. To a certain degree, it will be necessary for the physician to deal with this aspect in order to initiate or maintain the treatment. Still, to many clinicians, the cultural situation will appear to be a side issue.

For Erikson, the person in the historical-cultural situation is the all-encompassing concern; only in this context is real understanding possible. Attempts to look at the person atomistically lead to viewing fragments instead of functioning parts.

In order to understand Erikson's view of the life cycle, it is necessary to define certain terms. (Zones and modes have already been defined, as has epigenesis.)

Crisis This term is used in the old sense of a turning point, where further development can go in different directions. Thus, the crisis in lobar pneumonia—to most physicians a purely historical concept—represented the point at which, rather suddenly, the patient would enter on the road either to recovery or to a fatal outcome. In the same way, every life stage has its specific crisis, where a good outcome means possibilities for further undisturbed development and a bad outcome always means a certain measure of arrest and disturbance.

Reality In Erikson's usage, this philosophically knotty term becomes "the world of phenomenal experience, perceived with a minimum of distortion of customary validation agreed upon in a given state of technology and culture." This definition seems to be close to the aspect of perception and memory that is referred to in describing a patient's quality of reality testing.

Actuality In Erikson's thinking, actuality is a very important concept. It seems to be related to, or included in, the wider concept of reality. Many important aspects of actuality are, however, probably unconscious, or at least preconscious. A first definition is "the world of participation, shared with a minimum of defensive maneuvering and a maximum of mutual activation." A crucial term is "mutual activation," because the ego gains its strength from a vast network of mutual influences. Sometimes this network weakens the ego, as, for instance, when the situation allows little or no mutuality. Actuality is a convergence point for outer conditions and inner states. Whereas reality testing concerns undistorted perception of reality, actuality is related to action unhampered by acting out. (Acting out is used here in a conventional psychodynamic way: an attempt to solve an internal conflict by alloplastic actions, effecting a change in the environment. The action, though not entirely reality oriented, is not bizarre enough to appear psychotic. Examples are driving a car at breakneck speed after an altercation with one's boss or skiing down dangerous trails to prove to oneself that one is not a coward.) Actualities are codetermined by an individual's stage of development, by personal circumstances, and by historical and political processes. Actuality is thus a central concept for understanding human beings' place and fate in the world. In a certain period, actuality encompasses a myriad of vital mutualities. All, of course, are also part of reality, but, as can be seen, a very dynamic and special aspect of it.

For the ego, actuality is of prime importance. An optimal network of mutuality activates the ego to a state of active ego tension in actuality. The absence of this beneficial interaction may lead to a state of *ego inactivation,* which is a state in which solution of the relevant life crisis cannot take place. Thus, in a certain way, actuality becomes a question of an ego quality. However, the concept contributes to the understanding of stages where the ego is not yet fully developed.

Virtue For Erikson, virtue is tied to its old English usage as representing inherent strength or active quality. The word was often used to indicate the good quality in a medicine or liquor, and for Erikson, virtue indicates certain human qualities of strength, at best "developed from stage to stage and imparted from generation to generation."

As depicted in Table 6.2-1, the understanding of a particular life stage involves the following factors: (1) psychosexual stage, (2) organ mode (rudimentary in adult life), (3) psychosocial stage, and (4) virtue. To these factors should be added (5) related psychopathology and (6) related elements of social order.

AGES OF MAN The melancholy Jaques in Shakespeare's *As You Like It* delineated seven ages of man, beginning with the infant "mawling and puking in his mother's arms."

Jaques: All the world's a stage,
And all the men and women merely players;
They have their exits and their entrances;
And one man in his time plays many parts,
His acts being seven ages.
As You Like It (William Shakespeare)

Erikson differs from the melancholy Jaques in that he describes eight stages, from trust versus mistrust to integrity versus despair. These stages are shown in Figure 6.2-2.

Stage 1: Trust vs. mistrust Within the limits of the infant's psychological abilities, the infant must experience that he or she has arrived in a world he or she can trust, in which help, care, and love are available. The mother thus must understand the incorporative mode and its ramifications, and how to deal with the firmly closed mouth, and later, with the dawning interest in biting. But the problem is not confined to the mutuality of mother and child. The mother's dealings with the child have to make sense, not only in terms of the wider family, but also in terms of the culture in which the family is living. In other words, the child is involved in an actuality in which this seemingly feeble creature shows an amazing ability to engage the environment. The child not only changes the family, but the surrounding society to ensure a continued existence. In addition, a social rejuvenation emanates from the child, indicating even a change of the future. This expansion of the field is very characteristic for Erikson. If all goes well, the infant will attain *hope,* which is the earliest virtue. Hope here might be easiest to define by its opposite; anyone who has seen a hopeless child will understand. The hopelessness can be seen as a state of (ego?) inactivation resulting from a faulty actuality. "Hope is the enduring belief in the attainability of fervent wishes, in spite of the dark urges and rages which mark the beginning of existence." Although basic mistrust as a dominating force means absence of hope, it also has a dynamic aspect. The child must learn not to trust everything in this world; that is, not everything can be put in the mouth and enjoyed or grasped with impunity.

The related psychopathology comprises the psychotic depressions, schizophrenia, and addictions. The related elements of social order are faith and organized religion. The first beginnings of an identity are "I am what I hope I have and give."

Stage 2: Autonomy vs. shame and doubt In this second stage of childhood, the anus is the leading body zone. The associated organ mode is holding on and letting go. Toilet

TABLE 6.2-1
An Overview of the First Three Psychosexual Stages with Their Organ Modes and Psychosocial Stages. Rudiment of Ego-Strength Corresponds to Virtue as Used Elsewhere in This Text. The Psychopathology Relates to Severe Disturbances of the Relevant Life Crisis. Table from Erikson E: *Insight and Responsibility,* p 186, Norton, New York, 1964, with permission.

Psychosexual Stage	*Organ Mode*	*Psychosocial Stage*	*Rudiment of Ego-Strength*	*Related Psychopathological Mechanisms*	*Related Elements of Social Order*
Oral–sensory–cutaneous	Incorporative	Basic trust vs. mistrust	Hope	Psychotic Addictive	Cosmic order
Muscular–anal–urethral	Retentive–eliminative	Autonomy vs. shame and doubt	Will	Compulsive Impulsive	Law and order
Phallic–locomotor	Intrusive	Initiative vs. guilt	Purpose	Inhibitive Hysterical Phobic	Ideal prototype

training must never be just a contest of will between mother and child. The mother must understand the need of the child both to oppose and to submit, and relate this need to the wider field in which she lives; in other words, a functioning actuality must be created. If it is not, a state of (ego) inactivation might take over, creating a sense of defeat with deep feelings of shame and doubt. The shame, an emotion not well understood, may result from being observed when one is not ready, or in incontinence. The doubt has much to do with *will*. Will is the virtue of this stage, "the unbroken determination to exercise free choice as well as self-restraint, in spite of the unavoidable experience of shame and doubt in infancy." The development of the muscular system and the increased motility is of much help in the growth of *will*. The intensity of a compulsive doubt can lead to doubt "whether one ever really willed what one did, or really did what one willed." This leads to a related pathology, which is situated in the compulsive and impulsive area, as a student of Freud might have guessed. The social elements here are law and order. The developing identity can be expressed by the phrase, "I am what I can will freely."

Stage 3: Initiative vs. guilt At this age, the genital zone takes the lead, creating phallic-intrusive—and, to some extent, inclusive—concerns. In both sexes, the intrusive mode is a dominating one, an exploration of time, space, and fantasy with new vigor. In other words, this age is the oedipal age. The awakening sexual interests must be met by the parents' ability to regulate the situation in a way that retains ego tension, an actuality that avoids ego inactivation with its accompanying paralysis and guilt. Various mechanisms provide the superego with new force, and conscience starts to govern initiative. The restraining force of conscience is balanced by the development of a new virtue, *purpose*. Play is an important stage for the exercise of purpose, and one of the prerequisites for a fortunate development of play is the existence of a family in an exemplary form—which presupposes a healthy relationship with the prevalent culture. "Purpose, then, is the courage to envisage and pursue valued goals uninhibited by the defeat of infantile fantasies, by guilt, and by the fear of punishment." The related pathology comprises inhibition, hysteria, and phobic states, or, in other words, the classical transference neuroses. The social elements connected to this age have to do with *ideal prototypes:* the heroes, kings, and queens of reality and fairy tale. "I am what I can imagine I will be."

Stage 4: Industry vs. inferiority Every child in every culture now enters a period of instruction that is more or less institutionalized. The emotional intensity of the previous periods is followed by a period of relative quiescence. No body zone takes the lead and the oedipal rivalry is supplanted by attempts at cooperation. The danger is that this new feeling of industrious learning will be destroyed by a feeling of inferiority, which may have little to do with actual ability. The reason instead may be that the learning situation does not recognize the historical actuality that can make learning a creative endeavor. Once again, what is learned must make sense in the context of the family and the wider culture.

Competence is the leading virtue in this period, a conglomeration of traits that make industry worthwhile in the civilization in which the child lives and acts. An unfortunate path leads from industry to what might be called "craft idiocy," when the activity itself dominates, crowding out playfulness, artistry, and goal seeking. From this point on, there no longer is a directly related psychopathology; regressive processes determine the malfunctioning. "Competence, then, is the free exercise of dexterity and intelligence in the completion of tasks, unimpaired by infantile inferiority." And it must be related to a prevailing technological ethos, "I am what I can learn to make work."

Stage 5: Identity vs. role confusion The richest and most extensive parts of Erikson's writings deal with adolescence, youth, and identity formation. Some of his salient points are as follows.

All through childhood, the ego is formed by successive identifications building on the introjection mechanism. Children continually lose their love objects; the child and mother of today are not the same as the child and mother of yesterday. The lost objects are taken into the ego and become its building blocks (as Freud pointed out).

When adolescence begins, the childhood way of living must be given up, and the task becomes one of reconciling the changes in the body and in one's social position with one's previous history and the identifications that are precipitated in the ego. What is formed is an identity, which is something definitely more than the sum of identifications. Thus, it contains the beginning elements of what later becomes a social role in its various aspects. There must be a reasonable congruence between how young people see themselves and how society perceives them. At this point in life, various initiation ceremonies take place to confirm that the former child

VIII							INTEGRITY vs. DESPAIR
VII						GENERATIV-ITY vs. STAGNATION	
VI					INTIMACY vs. ISOLATION		
V Temporal Perspective vs. Time Confusion	Self-Certainty vs. Self-Consciousness	Role Experi-mentation vs. Role Fixation	Apprenticeship vs. Work Paralysis	IDENTITY vs. IDENTITY CONFUSION	Sexual Polarization vs. Bisexual Confusion	Leader- and Followership vs. Authority Confusion	Ideological Commitment vs. Confusion of Values
IV			INDUSTRY vs. INFER-IORITY	Task Identi-fication vs. Sense of Futility			
III		INITIATIVE vs. GUILT		Anticipation of Roles vs. Role Inhibition			
II	AUTONOMY vs. SHAME, DOUBT			Will to Be Oneself vs. Self-Doubt			
I TRUST vs. MISTRUST				Mutual Recognition vs. Autistic Isolation			
1	2	3	4	5	6	7	8

FIGURE 6.2-2 *A rather complete formulation of Erikson's view of the components and antecedents of identity. Note how identity takes a central place in the diagram. Row V illustrates both what remains of earlier stages in a successful identity formation and the possible disturbances. Column 5 shows both the successful and the negative forerunners of identity in earlier stages. (From Erikson E:* Identity: Youth and Crisis, *p 94, Norton, New York, 1968, with permission.)*

now has a place among the adults. The sexual identity must be firmed up; it must be made clear that the young person is indeed fully a man or a woman. The endless discussions in this era between boys and girls serve to answer the questions: What does it mean to be a woman? A man? How does a man view a woman and a woman a man? How can men and women be different and still love each other without fear? Fortunate, indeed, is the youngster who can keep the sexual experimentation of the age within bounds, because, at this stage, the genitals may be functioning adequately, but the emotions are not ready for full mutuality. This period is also the time when the young person has to examine a negative identity, the developmental possibilities to avoid: being called the coward, schlemiel, sissy, dyke, bully, criminal, and so on. The job facing the young person is undoubtedly simpler in a homogeneous culture than in most of the world of today.

ROLE CONFUSION The task can become overwhelming and miscarry, leading to role or identity confusion. A role confusion always engenders some degree of alienation and can be carried so far that the young person actually assumes what should have been a negative identity—instead of a young worker and learner, a delinquent in a street gang, where time perspective is partially lost and where a firm sexual identity is replaced by promiscuity, barely hiding weak potency and low strength.

The virtue to guide the young person through adolescence is *fidelity,* "the ability to sustain loyalties freely pledged in spite of the inevitable contradictions of value systems. It is the cornerstone of identity and receives inspiration from confirming ideologies and affirming companions." The workable fidelity is one that makes it possible for the youngster to take his or her place in society, and not the kind of alienated and rudimentary loyalty found in a street gang. Identity and fidelity are necessary for ethical strength—morals instead of morality—but are not enough in themselves; the final shape has to be helped by the presence of ideal figures.

Adolescence is also a time when the past and future history of the community take on a new significance. In order for the young person to do the deeds that will place him or her in an acceptable social context, the historical actuality must make this possible. This *psychohistorical actuality* is "the sum of historical facts and forces which are of immediate relevance to the adaptive anticipations and to the maladaptive apprehensions in the individuals involved." The difficulties attendant in this actuality cannot be dealt with by an attempt to diagnose irrationalities via sterile reality testing, but must involve a creative understanding of the unconscious factors always involved in societal or group processes. Still, as a result of many factors, alienation rather than fidelity and psychohistorical adaptation becomes a real possibility. Such factors include fears aroused by discoveries and inventions that may seem to be more in service of death than life and anxieties aggravated by the decay of existing institutions that seem increasingly meaningless before the real threat of an existential vacuum.

Psychiatrically, it is important to recognize that the psychopathology that can be rather rampant during this struggle does not in itself constitute a mental illness but a tumultuous developmental stage. Erikson's point that diagnosis of, for instance, a psychosis should be avoided until the person is well into his or her 20s seems to be well taken. What looks like a psychiatric disorder may be a chaotic moratorium, a phase where development is held in abeyance until the next step can be taken. Many adolescents need a moratorium before they can progress, and the concept is of prime importance in understanding the psychology of youthful development.

Stage 6: Intimacy vs. isolation Real intimacy with a person of the opposite sex requires a firmly developed sexual and personal identity, with the kind of control of boundaries that makes it possible to soften and abolish boundaries in certain areas and hold them firm in others. Only then are sexual mutuality and orgasmic potency possible. For anyone whose identity is brittle or incomplete, intimacy creates a fear of fragmentation or submersion. Isolation is then the alternative. The virtue of this period is *love,* a concept very different from infatuation. This is the kind of love Freud had in mind when he talked about "Lieben und arbeiten" (to love and to work) as a signifier of normality.

Stage 7: Generativity vs. stagnation Love and intimacy reach their fulfillment in generativity, which basically means the ability to create a new generation. The actuality that the person encountered in childhood must now be revived in the service of the next generation. Many forms of creativity must be subsumed here, but all of them have their opposite in *stagnation,* the barren state of inhibited creativity and empty pursuits. The virtue that is prominent in this stage is *care,* the ability to nurture and promote development, whether of children or some other creation.

Stage 8: Integrity vs. despair Finally, everyone at some point must face the eventuality of not being and accept the fact that death is inescapably a part of life. This stage is the period of life when, ideally, interest leaves egotistical concerns and expands to encompass life itself in its various manifestations. At the end of life, some individual aspects lose their prominence so that an aging Chinese fisherman and an aging Western physicist become more alike in their final concerns. The virtue that combines the two is *wisdom,* which can avert despair over a wasted life. It seems to follow that wisdom should not be achieved too early; a youth in the midst of an identity crisis would probably be hampered by it. Lately, Erik and Joan Erikson, together with Helen Kivnick, have formulated views on old age, life stage 8, which are not only important for understanding this stage, but also help in understanding more fully the problems encountered in earlier stages.

The main problem in old age remains how to face not being, to be by having been, and still be able to reach integrity and avoid despair. The key word in this connection is *vital involvement*. The Eriksons also point out that old age actually can be divided into roughly two stages: one comprising the time from retirement up to age 85 and the other from the age of 85 to death. The problems are different in these two periods.

Retirement poses considerable problems for most people. Much of one's creativity, or generativity, is vested in one's work situation, as are one's identity, industry, and, for many persons, the intimacy with fellow workers. To retain autonomy while being employed and salaried requires constant dynamic problem solving, and the issue of trust versus mistrust certainly is partly played out around the boss or organization. Every life stage requires a reformulation and solution of the crises from earlier life, but old age perhaps more than any other.

The new contribution deals mainly with aging people who remain in their accustomed location. Eventually, one has to know more about people, who, in a way almost exclusively American, leave home, friends, and accustomed environment behind in order to relocate in some sunny spot filled with old-timers or who take off in a recreational vehicle (RV) to fulfill a new American dream of dying on wheels, as Erikson once put it.

What was once generativity now tends to become grandgenerativity as concern is shifted from immediate family to grandchildren. This also helps to fill out the identity of a retired person as an ancestor to laudable descendants, even if sometimes denial must occur when the reality is painful. In this age, flexibility is sometimes surprisingly good, and many aging persons find satisfying objects for their industry. Lifelong intimacy with a beloved spouse certainly helps keep despair at bay, but it must also be recognized that loss of such a spouse may lead to constant grief and essential loneliness. Some problems of old age are simply not solvable, and every aging person probably relies to some extent on denial. To retain autonomy and at the same time receive help for waning abilities—physical, spiritual, and economical—requires considerable mental strength. For many old people, trust and hope are tied to religious beliefs, which may be revived after having been set aside during a more active life stage; however, secular solutions are also possible, including faith in nature, life itself, and the eternal chain of generations, and a belief that the good in human nature somehow will triumph.

As aging continues with increasing feebleness, perhaps especially after age 85, solutions tend to become simpler, but may be no less difficult. The identity of being alive, or not yet dead, may come to dominate, and the main problems for generativity, industry, and autonomy may become just how to perform minimal daily chores in order to stay alive.

The Eriksons point out how society is essentially unprepared to meet the demands of a rapidly increasing cohort of the old and very old. However, a great responsibility remains with the individual. Everyone must recognize that growing old requires active preparation that maybe cannot start early enough.

ATTEMPT AT A TIMETABLE It must be clear that the crisis trust–mistrust takes place in infancy and probably either is solved or becomes manifest during the first year. In the same way, autonomy–shame and doubt have much to do with the development of the motor system and the ability to control the sphincters, perhaps from the end of the first year at the very earliest up to the age of 2 to 3 years. Initiative–guilt has to do with the oedipal period from 3 to 4 or 5 years of age. After that period, the child enters the latency period, and this period, with the accompanying crises of industry–inferiority, lasts to the onset of puberty. The time boundaries have already become much more indistinct; the onset of psychological puberty is too individually different to allow any firm time limit. The same thing is true of the remaining crises; intimacy–isolation belongs to early adulthood and generativity–stagnation to psychological middle age, but any attempt to establish time boundaries here is very difficult.

Taking these factors into consideration, the following very approximate timetable can be set up:

1. Basic trust versus mistrust—from birth to 1½ to 2 years of age.
2. Autonomy versus shame and doubt—from 1½ to 2½–3 years of age.
3. Initiative versus guilt—roughly corresponding to the classical oedipal age, 3 to 5 years of age.
4. Industry versus inferiority—latency and grammar school age, 5 or 6 to 11–13 years, the onset of psychological puberty.
5. Identity versus identity confusion—from the onset of puberty to young adulthood, age 13 to 18–21 years.
6. Intimacy versus isolation—from 16 to 18 years to the middle 20s.
7. Generativity versus stagnation—from the middle 20s to the later 40s or beginning 50s; cessation of fertility in woman helps form the boundary here.
8. Integrity versus despair—from the 50s to the end of life. But if a man in his late 50s fathers a new child, one must assume at least a partial revival of the generativity versus stagnation situation.

In reading this timetable it should be kept in mind that not only is development continuous, but it does not have any real nodal points. Thus, although a particular life crisis may dominate at a certain age, there are other times when one must assume that one life crisis is waning at the same time that the next life crisis is waxing.

ABNORMAL DEVELOPMENT

Erikson's schemata and classical psychiatric nosology come together at some nodal points. If basic mistrust is too strong or untempered by basic trust, no well-functioning internal objects can be established and some form of schizophrenic psychosis will become manifest. If the objects are there but are severely malfunctioning and split, some form of depressive psychosis may be the result. Addiction also belongs here. One can think of an addict as a person with a very prominent incorporative need. This person is, however, so lacking in trust that he or she turns from dangerous human beings to chemical substances. At the same time, the protective function of basic mistrust is missing and toxic substances are incorporated. Analogously, if shame and doubt dominate over autonomy, obsessive-compulsive symptomatology can be expected. Excessive guilt in the next stage may well lead to what in later diagnostics were called anxiety hysteria and phobic states. Beyond this stage, the connection with classical nosology becomes obscure and regressive processes dominate.

This problem, however, has different aspects. Consider a child who develops excessive doubt in the autonomy stage. According to the epigenetic principle, this doubt will lead to disturbances in later stages. In the industry stage, for one, the child may be too doubting to be able to muster the convictions that are necessary for learning. If one doubts that two and two make four, arithmetic is going to be very difficult. The child may, without being clinically sick, overemphasize the industry itself. The result is an extremely industrious child who is not achieving (Fig 6.2-2, row IV, column 5). In the same way, a youth with a defective identity may be unable to reach real intimacy and so will fail in the generative role of parent. And all these processes most often take place on a subclinical level. It is in understanding these states that Erikson's thinking is especially valuable.

TREATMENT

A child therapist or family therapist sometimes encounters a situation where it is clear that one of the early life crises can be brought to a more favorable solution by direct intervention. Such cases are probably rare. Usually, therapists have to deal with situations that are far removed from the real time of the therapy. It is difficult to imagine an actual ongoing difficulty that would lead to the development of despair in senescence; the causes can probably be found in earlier stages.

The treatment of psychotic states is dealt with elsewhere in this textbook. With regard to milder disturbances, Erikson has not formulated any new techniques. All kinds of psychotherapy operate essentially in two phases:

1. The understanding phase. The therapist understands the patient's situation and conveys this fact to the patient. During this phase, positive transference will develop.
2. The explanatory phase. During this phase, the therapist uses interpretations congruent with the system applied to the therapeutic situation (Freudian, Jungian, etc.). If this procedure leads to a change in the situation, one will have to go back to phase 1, and so on.

The more disturbed the patient, the longer phase 1 should last. If a therapist has to deal with a disturbed youth, understanding that the youth essentially is experiencing an identity crisis will certainly help to establish phase 1. The patient will feel understood. When the time comes for the therapist and the patient to explain what is going on, utilization of phase 2 will be more successful in effectuating a beneficial change, because concepts adumbrating the central identity conflict will make sense to the youth. At the same time, the therapist will feel less anxious, and it will be easier to maintain a professional stance.

The paradoxical conclusion to draw from the above is that many essentially subclinical conflicts constitute strong indications for psychotherapy, and persons with such states make the best use of psychological treatment methods.

Erikson's historical writings show the relevance of his theories for understanding greatness in its psychohistorical actuality. Such works as *Young Man Luther* and *Gandhi's Truth* (which cannot be covered here) illustrate the power of his theory as an aid in understanding personal crises. Further study of Erikson's theories will certainly lead to a better understanding of human beings, both as leaders and as patients.

REFERENCES

Coles, R: *Erik H. Erikson. The Growth of His Work.* Little, Brown, Boston, 1970.

Erikson E H: *Childhood and Society,* ed 2. Norton, New York, 1963.

Erikson E H: *Young Man Luther.* Norton, New York, 1958.

Erikson E H: The roots of virtue. In *The Humanist Frame,* J Huxley, editor. Harper, New York, 1961.

Erikson E H: *Insight and Responsibility.* Norton, New York, 1964.

Erikson E H: *Identity: Youth and Crisis.* Norton, New York, 1968.

Erikson E H: *Gandhi's Truth.* Norton, New York, 1969.

Erikson E H: *Life History and the Historical Moment.* Norton, New York, 1975.

Erikson E H: *Toys and Reasons: Stages in the Realization of Experience.* Norton, New York, 1977.

Erikson E H, editor: *Adulthood.* Norton, New York, 1978.

Erikson E H, Erikson K T: The confirmation of the delinquent. Chicago Rev *10:* 15, 1957.

Erikson E H, Newton H: *In Search of Common Ground.* Norton, New York 1973.

Erikson E H, Erikson J M, Kivnick H G: *Vital Involvement in Old Age.* Norton, New York, 1986.

Erikson J: *Saint Francis and His Four Ladies.* Norton, New York, 1970.

Evans R I: *Dialogue with Erik Erikson*. Harper & Row, New York, 1967.

Maier H W: *Three Theories of Child Development*. Harper & Row, New York, 1965.

Pulver S E: The manifest dream in psychoanalysis: A clarification. J Amer Psychoanal Assoc *35:* 99, 1987.

Stern D A, Fromm M G, Sacksteder J L: From coercion to collaboration: Two weeks in the life of a therapeutic community. Psychiatry *49:* 18, 1986.

Stewart C T: The developmental psychology of Sandplace. In *Sandplace Studies—Origin, Theory and Practice,* K Bradway et al, editors. C. G. Jung Institute, San Francisco, 1981.

Tähkä V: On the early formation of the mind. I: Differentiation. Int J Psychoanal *68:* 229, 1987.

CHAPTER 7 THEORIES OF PERSONALITY AND PSYCHOPATHOLOGY: OTHER PSYCHODYNAMIC SCHOOLS

MYRON F. WEINER, M.D.

INTRODUCTION

The practitioners–theorists discussed in this section all lived most of their adult life in the twentieth century, and were imbued with a psychological optimism that contrasted with the biological reductionism of the nineteenth century. All emphasized a positive view of patients' ability to become more effective in dealing with life's problems. Each person to be discussed has influenced the view of normal personality development, psychopathology, and therapy. They are listed in Table 7-1 by their order of birth, their country of origin, and the nation in which they eventually settled.

Except for Adolf Meyer, all were trained in psychoanalysis. All were physicians, except Melanie Klein and Otto Rank. Adler, Jung, Rank, Reich, and Rado had strong personal involvements with Sigmund Freud. There are many interesting paradoxes in this widely disparate group of personalities and approaches to life's problems. Adolf Meyer, who was trained as a neuropathologist, encouraged the psychoanalytic exploration of schizophrenia. Jules Masserman, a psychoanalyst, performed experimental studies of animals to probe the biological underpinnings of mental disorders. Both Meyer and Masserman (who had also been a student of Meyer) emphasized a broad approach to the treatment of mental disorders that encompassed a variety of biological and psychological treatments. Wilhelm Reich, having made a valuable psychoanalytic contribution to the understanding of character defenses, eventually espoused a bizarre biological theory of mental disorders. Melanie Klein, while emphasizing innate aggression as the biological root of emotional disorders, recommended the treatment of adults and children with all types of emotional disorders by an unmodified psychoanalytic technique.

Alfred Adler was the first to deal with the social and interpersonal contributions to psychopathology, involving parents in the treatment program for their children. Adler was followed by Karen Horney, who emphasized the culturally determined nature of psychopathology. She described much of ordinary human emotional misery as the product of miscarried attempts to meet needs for survival and security, and considered Freud's libido theory of neurosis too narrow.

TABLE 7-1
Influential Psychodynamic Practitioner-Theorists of the Twentieth Century

Adolf Meyer	1866–1950	Switzerland; United States
Alfred Adler	1870–1937	Austria; United States
Carl G. Jung	1875–1981	Switzerland
Sandor Rado	1880–1972	Hungary; United States
Melanie Klein	1882–1960	Austria; England
Otto Rank	1884–1939	Austria; United States
Karen Horney	1885–1952	Austria; United States
Harry Stack Sullivan	1892–1947	United States
Wilhelm Reich	1897–1957	Germany; United States
Jules H. Masserman	1905–	United States
Eric Berne	1910–1970	Canada; United States

Harry Stack Sullivan, a contemporary of Horney who worked with more disturbed patients, also concluded that psychopathology had its roots in interpersonal relationships. In contrast to Melanie Klein, who compressed the formative experiences and emotional reactions of life into the first year, Horney and Sullivan suggested a more prolonged period of development, extending into adult life. More recently, the interpersonal view of emotional disorder was popularized by Eric Berne as "games" characterized by ulterior transactions and payoffs.

Carl Jung held that Freud's libido theory and Adler's will to power are not mutually exclusive, but are polarities that require integration into the personality through a process that emphasizes transcendence and integration over analysis and rational understanding. Otto Rank emphasized each individual's ability to create his or her own destiny, describing the creation of one's own psychological being as the ultimate form of art. Rado, who is the least well known of the group, reformulated Freud's theory into an adaptational schema.

There is much overlap between the theories and therapeutic techniques to be presented. Indeed, much of what is presented as a unique theory is but a restatement of other theories in terms more acceptable to its author. The attraction of these theories is their internal consistency and the ease with which they explain many clinically observable phenomena. Melanie Klein's descriptions of primitive mental processes fit very well with clinical observations of schizophrenia, severe mood disorders, and borderline personality disorder. Karen Horney's description of neurotic processes fits everybody. The therapies, for the most part, fit the theories. Unfortunately, none of the therapies described has been evaluated for effectiveness other than by anecdotal positive reports from its practitioners.

From this plethora of theories and treatment approaches it becomes obvious that no single theory can encompass all human thinking or behavior in all settings and that no psychological treatment is universally applicable. Instead, each individual and setting must be considered as having many communalities with others and as having its own uniqueness.

ADOLF MEYER

Adolf Meyer (1866–1950), a Swiss immigrant to the United States, was the most influential American psychiatrist in the first half of the twentieth century (Fig. 7-1). His contributions to psychiatry include his emphasis on the interrelationship of symptoms and the individual person's psychological and biological functioning, his biographical–

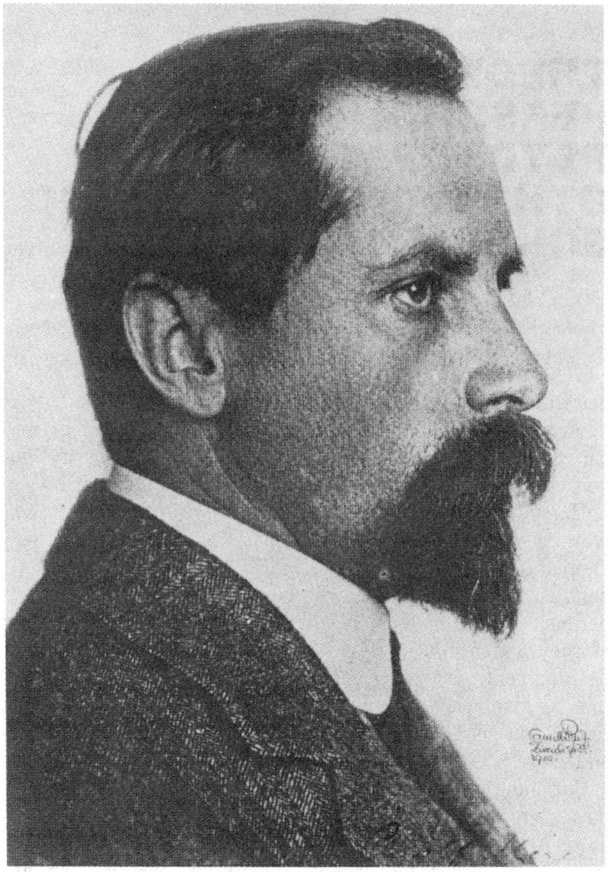

FIGURE 7-1. *Adolf Meyer. (Courtesy of National Library of Medicine, Bethesda, MD.)*

historical approach to the study of personality, his support of the psychotherapeutic treatment of schizophrenia, his advocacy of social action for mental health, and his attempts to bring psychiatric patients and their treatment out of isolated state hospitals into the community. During his tenure there as professor of psychiatry from 1909 to 1941, Johns Hopkins became the world's most important psychiatric training center.

PSYCHOBIOLOGY Meyer's psychobiological approach used biographical study to understand the whole person in a life situation. Meyer observed behavior, formulated predictable conditions under which those behaviors may occur, and tested and validated methods for their modification. Instead of using psychological or metapsychological constructs to account for his observations, he emphasized the soundness of common sense, and thus justified involving many professions, including teachers and the clergy, in working for community mental health.

Meyer believed that multiple biological, social, and psychological forces contribute to the growth and development of the personality, and emphasized a basic tendency toward integration. He held that a biographical (as opposed to phenomenological) approach to personality study provides a practical guide for eliciting individual data, a means of organizing those data, and a method for checking and reevaluating data elicited under varying conditions. In his clinical psychiatric examination, Meyer focused on pertinent details in the patient's life history; the patient's physical, neurological, genetic, and social status; and the correlation between those variables and personality factors. He made a differential diagnosis and formulated an individualized therapeutic plan. The study of all the factors in a person's life that played a positive or negative role in the patient's adjustment was called distributive analysis. The formulation of better coping methods, based on the patient's understanding of past maladaptation, was termed distributive synthesis.

Treatment Psychobiological therapy aims to help a person, hampered by abnormal internal and external conditions, to make the best adaptation possible to life and to change. Psychobiological treatment begins with distributive analysis and concludes with distributive synthesis. Meyer believed that treatment begins at the initial doctor–patient contact, with the patient's exposition of the problem. The first step in distributive analysis is the evaluation of the patient's assets and liabilities by studying the patient's life history, utilizing current data provided by the patient and supplemented by later reconstructions of past experiences.

Meyer recognized the need to obtain the cooperation of the healthy part of the patient's ego and believed that the healthier aspects of the patient's personality should be the starting point for treatment. Therapy is a service performed on the patient's behalf; the therapist uses every available means to assist the patient, including psychological, biological, and environmental measures. At first, the therapist focuses on the patient's sleep habits, nutrition, and regulation of daily routines, and also helps the patient describe any difficulties in specific detail, with the therapist using the patient's concepts and language to communicate suggestions and advice.

Problems are dealt with as conscious issues through face-to-face conversation. The psychiatrist focuses on the patient's present situation and reactions to everyday difficulties, as well as the patient's long-term life adjustment. At the beginning of each session, the patient is encouraged to discuss any experiences that took place since the last interview, beginning with obvious and immediate problems. When deeper relevant material is brought out later in therapy, those problems are explored in greater detail.

Guided by their psychiatrists, patients investigate their personality problems and their relative importance, reconstruct the origin of their conflicts, and devise healthier behavioral patterns. They may be asked to formulate their life stories by means of a life chart to demonstrate their understanding of their difficulties' origin and the means that might be used to resolve them and to prevent their recurrence.

Meyer believed that psychotherapy helps patients modify unhealthy adaptations. Those modifications, in turn, lead to personal satisfaction and proper adjustment. In the process of this "habit training," the psychiatrist advises, suggests, and reeducates, always focusing on the patient's current life situation.

ALFRED ADLER

Vienna-born physician Alfred Adler (1870–1937) was one of the original four members of Freud's group (Fig. 7-2). He was forced by Freud to resign from the Vienna Psychoanalytic Society after 9 years, in 1911, after Freud had made him its president a year earlier. Adler disagreed with Freud over the libido theory, the sexual origin of neurosis, and the importance of infantile wishes. Adler's personality theory includes the concepts of striving for self-esteem and for a feeling of superiority instead of inferiority in social situations. It includes social embeddedness, and an aptitude for social interest that must be consciously developed. His major social contribution was the establishment of numerous child guidance centers in Vienna public schools.

Replacing drive psychology with value psychology, Adler termed his system *individual psychology* and founded a society and journal by that name. Today, Adlerian societies exist in many countries as part of the International Association of Individual Psychology.

PERSONALITY THEORY Adler saw the human being as a unified biological entity whose psychological processes, including drives, perception, memory, and dreaming, all fit the person's life-style—the person's unique, self-consistent way of meeting the world.

Foreshadowing Rank, Adler saw human destiny as a product of choice and will. A person creates ideals and goals that enable him or her to make choices. Every person moves toward a chosen goal, even if unaware of the goal. Goal

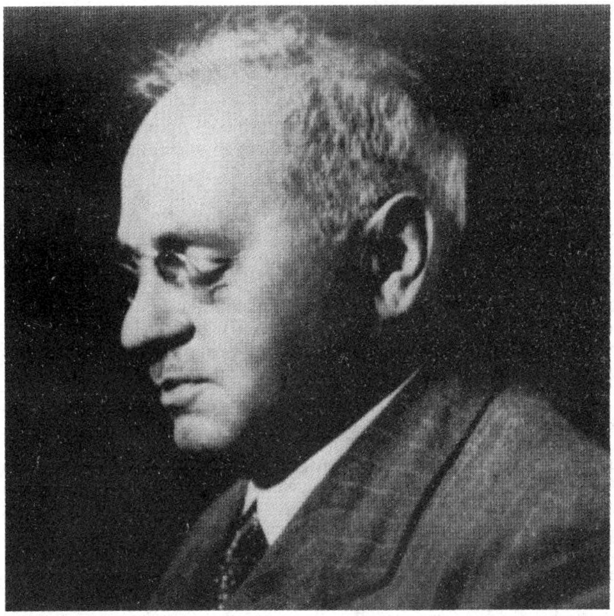

FIGURE 7-2. *Alfred Adler. (Courtesy of Wide World Photos.)*

striving is moving from a feeling of relative inferiority to a feeling of superiority, and always includes wanting to be a worthy human being. The striving to move from a sense of inferiority to a feeling of superiority is part of the general human tendency to sharply dichotomize and categorize as a means of simplifying reality. Normal persons are aware that their categories are not literal, but neurotic and psychotic persons attempt to force their rigid categories onto the world and operate on an all-or-nothing basis. Neurotic persons try to raise their self-esteem by depreciating others. That tendency is at the root of sadism, hatred, quarrelsomeness, intolerance, and envy. Another important device of the neurotic is avoiding action or decisions that may lead to defeat.

Human beings live within larger relational systems from which arise the life problems of vocation, general social relations, and love and marriage. Social interest is the main factor in a person's success or failure to solve life problems; it is expressed in cooperation and in feeling positive about and comfortable in the world. Social interest, of course, requires action.

Normal personality and adaptation Normal inferiority feelings are the cause of all improvements in human life. The abnormal person has low social interest and low activity, becomes discouraged, and continues to feel inferior. The ideal normal person has high social interest and activity and strives for superiority.

The child's development of self-esteem and social interest is hindered by imperfect organs (organ inferiority) and childhood diseases, pampering, and neglect. Children with imperfect organs and childhood diseases easily become self-centered. A child's life-style is greatly affected by the child's position in the family, including birth order. Adler suggested that the firstborn, having lost the position of only child, is often conservative, feeling that those in power should remain in power. The second child, wanting to equal the first, often wants power to change hands. The youngest can never be displaced, but is always the youngest. The birth order can be played out in many different ways, but early responses to one's birth order position become part of one's life-style.

THEORY OF PSYCHOPATHOLOGY For Adler, functional disorders result from erroneous or mistaken ways of living (life-styles) that can be changed through self-understanding. The mistaken life-style includes mistaken opinions about oneself and the world and mistaken goals, all strongly connected with underdeveloped social interest. Adler described it as the pampered life-style, the style of a person who expects from others, presses them into service, evades responsibility, and blames circumstances for personal shortcomings, but actually feels incompetent and insecure. Persons with mistaken life-styles may go through life without a crisis if their social interest is unchallenged. Confrontation with such a task triggers the development of symptoms, which are self-esteem-protecting excuses for avoiding life problems. Neurotic persons, having more social interest than psychotic persons, acknowledge their social obligations, but allow their symptoms to block them from their goals. Psychotic persons, in contrast, cut themselves off completely from the world of others.

PSYCHOTHERAPY Adler did not look for hidden meaning in patients' communications. He took them as metaphors for patients' subjective reality. Symptoms are ways to cope with life problems in accordance with patients' mistaken opinion of themselves and the world—an opinion of which they often are not aware. Conscious and unconscious processes do not conflict, in Adler's view. Both serve the life plan; they are different means to the same ends.

Therapeutic process The Adlerian therapist establishes and maintains a good relationship with patients; gathers data to understand patients' life-styles; helps patients become aware of their life-styles; and reorients and reeducates patients.

Patients are encouraged to stop working for symbolic successes and to strive for socially useful goals. They are shown by means of their life histories and recollections how they became discouraged from useful enterprises, and are encouraged to develop social interest. Social interest leads to solidarity with others, and that solidarity stimulates more courage in facing life. Self-esteem and courage are also increased by recognizing a person's special skills and helping the person learn new skills. Thus, dance, music, art, and work may be part of the treatment.

When specific obstacles that discouraged the development of a useful life-style are uncovered, the patient is encouraged to remove those obstacles. For example, if a person is troubled by a lack of physical prowess, an exercise or physical improvement program may be helpful. The therapist attempts to understand the patient's life-style, including erroneous ideas and goals and methods of attaining them. The therapist helps the patient see the falseness of the ideas and goals so that they can be changed. For that purpose, early recollections, position in the birth order, day and night dreams, and the precipitating environmental factors are explored.

Adler was less concerned with life events or memories than with how the person responds to them. Because memories are active choices, not merely the result of imprinting, it is unimportant whether a memory is objectively true. Adler also suggested that the therapist's interpretations need not be factually correct. They need only help the patient build a constructive perception of the self and the world. For Adler, the dream has no latent content; it is a metaphorical expression of the dreamer's concerns.

Adler's special techniques were related to his general holistic and dialectical approaches. In particular, he used the technique of reframing symptoms in the context of the patient's life-style, in reference to the patient's situation and its larger social context. For example, Adler interpreted indecision and ambivalence by changing from the subjective to an objective frame. When a person fails to decide, nothing happens. Therefore, indecision is a way to maintain the status quo—the hidden goal of the discouraged patient.

Adlerian therapists listen and observe dialectically. They ask themselves what opposites can be inferred from patients' statements and actions. Considering oneself too good for any occupation may mean not good enough. Wearing shabby clothes may be an expression of conceit. Harm inflicted on oneself may be linked to attempts to hurt others. When patients complain about what others do to them, the therapist may ask, "And what did you do to them?"

Adler also used paradoxical communication—overtly giving one suggestion while hoping to provoke an opposite response. In dealing with an indecisive person, Adler might warn against doing anything rash. Thus, he prescribed the patient's symptom and helped the patient bring it under voluntary control.

Adler used an educational approach that appealed to the rational aspect of his patients' personalities, employing other techniques as needed to move his patients toward more productive ways of thinking and living.

CARL JUNG

Carl Jung (1875–1961) was the only member of Freud's inner circle trained formally as a psychiatrist (Fig. 7-3). He initially pursued empirical research in schizophrenia through his word association test. Later in his career, he explored religious and mystical experiences as paths to understanding the human mind. Jung founded a school of psychotherapy that he named *analytic psychology*. He nevertheless acknowledged his indebtedness to Freud for his libido theory and his discovery of the unconscious and to Adler for his theory of the will to power. He saw these theories as complementary instead of antagonistic, and united them in his own theory of complexes.

PERSONALITY THEORY

Complexes Mental activity consists of behavior, emotion, cognition (thinking and ideas), and imagery, such as dreams, fantasies, and hallucinations. Mental activity is built around *complexes*—groups of ideas associated with particular emotionally toned events or experiences. The core of a complex is an archetype (see below for definition), for example, the archetype of the mother or father figure. The energy of a complex is derived from its affective tone. The more intense the affective tone, the more a complex impels to action.

Jung's theory of complexes derived from word association studies. He noted that complexes could be demonstrated in word association experiments by observing subjects' responses, such as perseveration, prolonged reaction time, absence of overt reaction, and mistakes or amnesia in the reproduction of the responses to the stimulus words. He called these reactions *complex indicators*. In elucidating the complex, Jung confirmed Freud's theory of the unconscious. One evokes complexes in others as part of ordinary social communication. Complexes can be positive or negative, intense or mild. An intense complex usually evokes strong emotion, imagery, and a tendency to action.

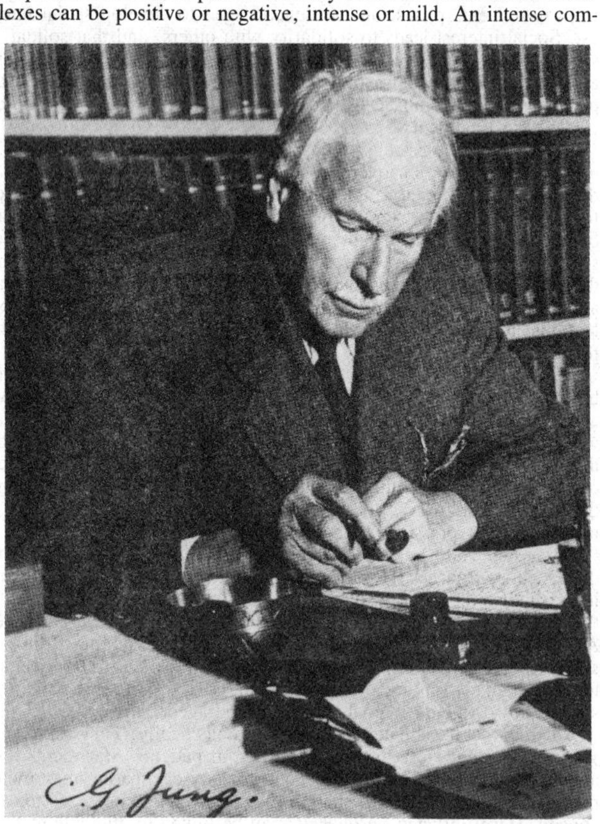

FIGURE 7-3. *Carl Gustav Jung. (Courtesy of National Library of Medicine, Bethesda, MD.)*

The ego is the master complex controlling conscious life and connecting external reality with the intrapsychic world. It is based on the archetype of the self. Other complexes that make up the psyche tend to align with or oppose the ego. The more conscious complexes may "sink into unconsciousness" and dissociate as other complexes rise to consciousness and dominate awareness.

For example, a father complex can be stimulated by someone who represents a father figure or by a stimulus that evokes such memories. This complex, formerly dormant in a person's unconscious or preconscious life, comes to the fore and tends to dominate consciousness. The emotions or affective tone, the imagery related to the meaning of "father" for this person, and the multiple memories and ideas relating to the person's experiences with an actual father are expressed. At a later time, when the ego is in ascendency, much of what was thought, felt, and experienced, or even acted on, may be forgotten or only dimly remembered.

Complexes are thought to exist in complementary pairs. A complementary relationship between complexes evolves from the beginning of psychic life. In addition, complexes are self-perpetuating. They select from life situations that which confirms their own version of reality. In their integrated state, bipolar complexes are experienced as within the individual, even when there is a great tension of opposites. The immature psyche of children tends to project complexes, especially the more primitive ones, onto other objects or persons. Hence, bipolar complexes play a part in the interactional field between human beings, as well as between the conscious and the unconscious within the individual.

Some complexes are more conscious, more developed, and more identified and aligned with the ego, whereas others are more alien, distant, and primitive. These latter complexes are projected onto suitable objects in the environment when those objects have characteristics and complexes themselves that are similar to the projected complex, from which projective and introjective processes evolve. A person may introject and identify with a complex that is being stimulated and projected by another person. Individuals also may project complexes that are fully developed but unintegrated within themselves to other persons and may thus enter into relationships with their own complexes. Individuals may introject complexes that are being stimulated or projected by others in the environment, identify with them, and bring their own unconscious, similar complexes into action. Thoughts, feelings, actions, and imagery are expressed by individuals as they demonstrate these complexes; however, these persons may be unaware of what has been taken in from other persons. Projective identification can be enacted in the same way. The undeveloped or charged pole of a bipolar complex is transferred to another person, who identifies with it and acts on it in the relationship.

More powerful and primitive complexes are more emotionally charged, and have a greater tendency to become autonomous. At times, complexes behave like partial personalities in opposing or actually controlling the ego. An extreme example is a seance, in which a medium brings forth spirits and other entities as "other personalities from the dead." These entities are considered to be splinter psyches or projected complexes. Personification of figures in dreams and highly excited mental states gives a striking demonstration of the dramatis personae of the complexes. A complex can be so strong that it invades and takes possession of the ego—which, from Jung's point of view, explains animism and states of possession in primitive cultures.

Archetypes Complexes have two components. The outer shell is related to the immediate personal experiences and associations, and affects experiences in an individual's life. The deeper aspect—the nuclear element—has nonpersonal or transpersonal features. For this nuclear element, Jung coined the term "archetype"—(*arche,* meaning the beginning or primary cause, and *type,* the imprint). He saw this component as an inherited predisposition to perceive and experience typical or nearly universal situations or patterns of behavior, analogous in physiological terms to the effect of the organization of the cerebral cortex, which enables and organizes perception.

The *archetype* is defined as a system of readiness to respond to environmental cues from a dynamic nucleus whose concentrated psychic energies seem to be autonomous and powerful. For example, in studying Freud's oedipus complex, Jung noted personal twists and manifestations of the complex and also universal forms and themes. He saw the archetype as having a psychosomatic dimension with two aspects—one linked to physical drive and instincts, and the other, a psychic one, related to primary fantasy images. Jung defined the archetypal image as "the instinct's image of itself." He suggested that there are as many archetypes as there are typical situations in life. The inherited brain structure causes a tendency to respond in certain universal, typical ways. However, these behavioral forms or patterns are without content until personal experience through relationship with significant objects brings them into expression and comprehension in a manner analogous to the development of visual perception. Jung emphasized that archetypes are not inherited ideas, but the inherited possibility of form and expression that find a particular mode in an individual's life that fits with the person's particular experience.

The unconscious Jung divided the unconscious world of the psyche into the personal unconscious and the collective unconscious. The *personal unconscious* is related to the complex, and its aspects are related to personal acquisitions and experiences. The *collective unconscious* is related to the archetypal core of the complex—the inherited possibilities of form and functioning universal for all humankind given specific expression in each individual's life. Mythological associations and motifs were the common comparisons Jung elucidated in studying these forms. Later, he also used the term "the objective psyche" instead of the collective unconscious. The newborn infant psyche is not a tabula rasa, but is a repository for all of humankind's evolutionary and ancestral past. He concluded, in agreement with modern neurophysiology, that the psyche is equipped from birth with latent structures and adaptational modes that exist prior to the emergence of consciousness. These influence ego structure and function. He felt that this psyche was the source of all instincts and creative impulses, along with the spiritual heritage of humankind.

Jung also emphasized that the personal unconscious is made up of material that at one time had been conscious but was either forgotten or repressed, much as Freud described. He noted that this area of the psyche is essentially made up of complexes, which may never have been conscious. These archetypal images can only be perceived and experienced as they clothe themselves in the garments of outer experiences through personal associations.

If, for example, one were to describe the mother complex with the archetypal image of the great mother at its center, one might find the names, experiences, and attitudes of personal mothering figures—a person's real mother, foster mother, or caretakers who affected the person in a variety of ways. Further, the person, through fantasy or dreams, or in extreme mental states, might produce an image of a huge woman, or even an animal, with many breasts. This image would represent an archetypal image of the universal all-giving nourishing mother, a motif that can be found in many cultures. This image of a mother with many breasts is universal in nature, suggesting an unlimited capacity for nurturance. The image speaks to a basic element of mothering that is circumscribed and comprehended only in specific individual experiences, with personal associations added to it.

A basic principle of analytical psychology is that the psyche, like all other living systems, attempts to stay in balance. This principle, the *law of compensation*, is particularly true in the relationship of conscious to unconscious life. For example, when the development of attitudes or experiences in conscious life is extreme or overintense, a counterbalancing reaction occurs in the unconscious in the form of juxtaposing bipolar complexes that are in opposition to or in great tension with each other. For example, a neglected child deprived of mothering might produce fantasy or archetypal images of the great mother with many breasts to compensate for what is missing in conscious life. The unconscious product of the great mother image would signal that the archetypal core of the bipolar complex of child–mother had been activated; there would be suggested a need for mothering and nourishment to restore a psychic balance. If the mothering image were one of an animal creating a nest for its young, this image might suggest a different kind of mothering necessary for the child, rather than the one suggested by the image of many breasts.

The symbol Jung made a unique contribution to the understanding of psychological symbols. Instead of defining a symbol as something representing something else that was known, he saw the symbol as the best possible expression of an unknown truth. Further, he found that symbols often have the quality of images that unite conscious and unconscious life where disparate sets of opposites within the world of complexes exist. The symbol reveals a potential for unification and integration. Symbols often express primordial images of the collective unconscious attempting to unite with the personal unconscious to bring about a needed integration and balance.

Personality structure The basic personality has at its center the ego, a complex that occupies the center of the field of consciousness and has a high degree of continuity and identity. With the ego, he described several universal complexes. The *persona* is a complex that mediates between the external objective world and the ego. The persona, a name derived from the masks worn by ancient Greek actors, is the public personality presented by individuals in their everyday lives.

The *shadow* complex is an alter ego image. This complex contains repressed or primitive emotions, thoughts, feelings, and images. It is often negative, but also has many potential positive elements.

The *anima* and *animus* are two other complexes or part personalities that do not ordinarily have personal connections or identity with the ego. They are contrasexual images within a person's own inner world. For a man, this contrasexual complex is the anima, or the totality of expressions of his relationships with women. For a woman, it is the animus, or her contrasexual experience of men. In primitive societies, these structures are often called the "soul image." The function of the anima or animus is to connect the ego to the inner world, or, if in the projected form, to persons or objects in the outer world.

The self Finally, Jung described the self as the central archetype that stands in greatest contrast to the ego. If the ego were considered as a complex, its nuclear element would be the self. The ego is small, personal, and immediately related to consciousness. The self is more all-encompassing and impersonal. Jung distinguished between the ego and the self, and believed that the self embraces the ego. This archetypal image suggests the innate potential for wholeness, as well as an ordering principle operating outside the bounds of consciousness directing the overall activity of psychic life. This concept of the self may be Jung's greatest difference from Freudian and other psychologies, in that out of the unconscious arise not only chaos and disorganization, but also integration, order, and individuation. In dreams, fantasies, and altered states of consciousness, the self appears as images of the super or ideal personality that give direction. Self-images, or images of totality and wholeness, can be observed in childhood play and fantasy life. The child may have a unitary self or basic psychosomatic entity out of which the ego evolves, and not the converse.

The model for ego and self can best be seen in early infancy with an infant and mother—the mother carrying the image of the self and the child that of ego. This ego–self axis or dynamic relationship, or both, may evolve through the developmental stages from infancy, childhood, and adolescence to adult life with different significant others in juxtaposition to the ego. Through the first half of life, there is a constant tendency for the ego to attempt to identify with the self and to appropriate its power in its own attempt at differentiation and growth. In the process, it does become one sided and at times inflated with an unrealistic sense of its power that in fact reflects borrowed images of the self. At other times, it can be cut off from the self, and states of alienation and depression ensue.

Individuation The developmental task of the second half of life is for the ego to relinquish its dominance in the field of consciousness and to give way to new integrated patterns dictated more by the self, in preparation for eventual death. For this developmental process, Jung coined the term "individuation," the need for individuals to evolve uniquely and to fulfill the spiritual propensities common to all humanity. In many cases, individuation may require withdrawing from one's early identities related to conventional successful standards and seeking new paths, even though the pursuit may be in opposition to one's previous position in life. Paradoxically, the change often leads to broader and more mature collective relationships, as well as to inner creativity.

Psychological types Jung's type theory has three axes and represents the principal ways of adapting and understanding behavioral, affective, cognitive, and imagery productions of the psyche. The extroversion–introversion polarity suggests a mode of object relationship. *Extroverts* orient themselves to the outer object primarily, and then return to include and adapt themselves to understanding the interaction. Extroverts are oriented to people, objects, and outer situations; they are likely to see subjective activity only in the light of external reality and object relationships. *Introverts,* however, orient themselves to the inner world, especially to the internal world of objects or complexes and imagery. Their energy flows inwardly first, and then to outer reality. For this reason, introverts are often seen as unadaptable and selfish. They attend to their inner world first and then examine how the outer objects can fit in and adapt to it.

The perceptive axis of *sensation and intuition* addresses how psychic reality is perceived and taken in. Jung postulated the perceptive axis of sensation as the psychic function that takes in the specifics in the here and now. Intuition, however, suggests a mode of apprehending psychic reality in which wholes, rather than parts, are taken in. The intuitive person tends to blur details but catch the overall picture. The old saying "He can't see the forest for the trees" suggests the perceptual mode of sensation. The sensation function would examine each tree in detail and build up a composite of perceived reality, whereas the intuition would tend to see the overall configuration of the forest before moving on to the specifics of individual trees.

Jung utilized the polarity of *thinking and feeling* to deal with information processing and judgment. In thinking, data are judged according to principle and logic. Feeling refers to making judgments through nonlogical processes oriented to value and appreciation, especially as they pertain to individual relationships. For example, a thinking-type host at a social gathering may judge how to greet guests by referring to the basic principles of good etiquette according to tradition or a set or code of values. A feeling-type host would consider the type of guests present and how they interact, or look for the affective quality most comfortable at the time.

These three axes come together to type each individual. For example, an extroverted-sensation-thinking type is oriented to outer objects in the real world, with a tendency to perceive details and to organize them into a logical structure based on past value systems made up of principles of behavior. Sensation acknowledges that something exists. Thinking tells what it is; through feeling its value is noted and through intuition its possibilities for ultimate meaning can be ascertained.

Everybody has all of the various combinations within their psyches. Each person has, however, one set of functions that is better developed than others. This superior function is the strongly developed type that one evolves outwardly in the growth to adulthood and develops from early life, with constitutional factors playing a contributing part. Inferior or less-developed functions are also present and clamor for attention through growing-up years. In the second half of life, adults attempt to integrate or broaden and deepen an understanding of their inferior functions. These less-developed functions appear in ego-alien complexes and are often projected onto other persons or situations. By attempting to reclaim these projections and to understand their inferior functions, mature adults gain a greater degree of completeness or personality wholeness. Thus, Jung's psychological-type theory suggests a specific tool related to ego functions that is a guide for the individuation process and realization of each person's potential.

PSYCHOPATHOLOGY Jung defined *neurosis* as a dissociation of the personality as the result of complexes. He meant that when one complex in bipolar relationship to another—particularly the ego—becomes extreme, the emotional suffering generated by this conflict becomes intolerable, and anxiety cannot be contained. This splitting makes it impossible to affirm the totality of one's nature; hence, neurotic dissociation, and possibly illness, evolves, especially if the condition becomes fixed. Individuals thus maintain their psychic equilibrium by living out two incompatible complexes, one more ego identified and the other more ego alien, usually experienced in projection, as noted earlier in the dynamic interplay of complexes.

Jung specifically pointed out the dissociability in hysteria with its tendency for splitting, even to the evolution of part personalities. In his theory of the complexes, he observed that consciousness is not a unified phenomenon. He felt that when a negative pathological complex becomes incompatible with consciousness, it becomes powerful and highly autonomous, and moves in opposition to the ego or ego-identified complexes. In this phenomenon of hysterical dissociation, and especially in multiple personalities, complex theory is very clear. Clinically, ego or part personalities or complexes are functioning along with shadow personalities that are destructive and antithetical to conscious ego attitudes, standards, desires, and goals. Also, contrasexual ego-alien complexes (anima or animus) are functioning. Finally, there are figures that function as archetypal images of the self that have an overriding healing and integrative function, and attempt to control the resulting chaos. Each personality engendered in this hysterical dissociation becomes a living manifestation of a complex that operates autonomously. Neurosis in its varying forms is similar to hysterical dissociation. Symptom expression is different, but the same mechanisms of complexes and their incompatibility are emphasized.

Psychological typing also helped Jung to identify certain psychopathological conditions. Extroverts tend to develop hysterical or psychopathic symptomatology, whereas introverts tend to develop dysthymia, anxiety, and obsessional neuroses. Often, the pathogenic complex will appear in the form of one's inferior functions, where primitivity and affectivity are strikingly and compensatorily overwhelming. These observations led Jung to a further conception about psychopathology that is fundamental to his point of view—that pathology may also represent the germ of wholeness or health. In other words, the real need may be to integrate the alienated complex in the unconscious. By accepting the suffering necessary to make that integration with consciousness, the bipolar split can be healed. This integration often requires the painful rearrangement of conscious attitudes, habits, and modes of living. Therefore, psychopathological symptoms per se were not viewed by Jung as something necessarily to be eliminated, but to be integrated into conscious life.

Some expressions of the inferior functions are not equated with psychopathology at all. These inferior developmental expressions must be looked on as just that—as inferiorities that need to be integrated and allowed a place in conscious life. For example, persons who are highly developed intellectually may find that their thinking functions are overburdened and overdeveloped. The law of unity and homeostasis in their own psyches may induce within them involuntary expressions of their feeling functions, which might be experienced, for example, through extramarital liaisons, in which these persons, usually controlled, become very emotionally labile, infantile, and sad. On exploration, these excesses and extremes may reveal unresolved losses during early years with a mothering person and an inability to find intimacy with a woman. Here, a neurotic dissociation may cause multiple incompatibilities in these individuals' psychic lives that need reconciliation. The inferior function of feeling has to be integrated into their own lives to enrich and enhance the process.

THERAPY Most practitioners of Jungian analysis work with their analysands face to face, primarily on a once-a-week basis. With the emphasis on reintegration, symbolism, and dreams, Jungian analysis seems well suited to helping educated persons deal with the problems of midlife. Having achieved a professional identity and established a firm family role, they often begin to ask: "Who am I and what is my connection to the rest of human history?"

Such persons, often strongly given to self-criticism, may be relieved to hear themselves described, not in terms of psychopathology, but in terms of a normal attempt to become fully united with themselves and the rest of humankind.

SANDOR RADO

Sandor Rado (1890–1972) was born and trained in Hungary (Fig. 7-4). He helped Sandor Ferenczi organize the Hungarian Psychoanalytic Society, and later became an analysand of Karl Abraham and a faculty member of the Berlin Psychoanalytic Institute. Rado emigrated to the United States in 1931, and in 1945, at Columbia University, he became the director of the first psychoanalytic institute to be established in a university medical school.

ADAPTATIONAL PSYCHODYNAMICS Rado developed a unified, systematized theory of human behavior. His theory of adaptational psychodynamics viewed the organism as a biological system operating under hedonic control. A psychologically healthy person's psychic apparatus performs its adaptive functions effectively. Psychological illness or disordered behavior is a failure of the organism's psychological equipment to perform its adaptive function.

Although Rado strongly emphasized the predominance of learning, disciplinary, and cultural factors over instinctual factors as causes of disordered behavior, he was also aware of the significance of biological factors, and suggested an underlying genetic-biochemical aberration in schizophrenia.

Levels of integration Rado postulated four hierarchical levels of human mental integration: hedonic, emotional, emotional thought, and unemotional thought. Those levels follow the phylogenetic evolution of the brain toward increased cortical influence over its more primitive portions. At the *hedonic* level, pain signals that the organism is being damaged and motivates it to move away. Pleasure indicates that the organism is being benefited and elicits a moving toward or clinging. Pain and pleasure also have secondary effects. The disorganizing effect of persistent pain indicates to the organism that it is failing, and thereby reduces self-esteem. Pleasure, in contrast, indicates success, and thereby raises self-esteem.

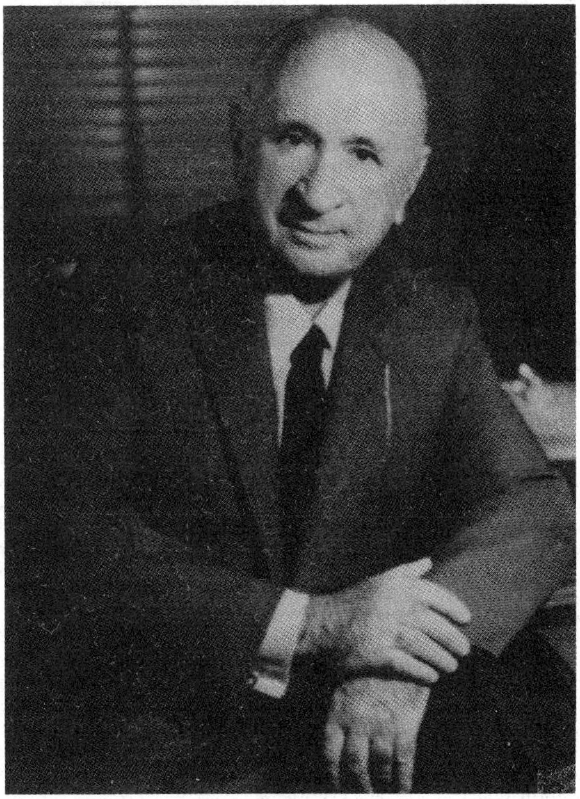

FIGURE 7-4. *Sandor Rado. (Courtesy of New York Academy of Medicine.)*

The *emotional* level of mental integration consists of the emergency emotions and the welfare or tender emotions. The emergency emotions, fear and rage, are responses to actual or anticipated pain or damage; they prepare the organism for flight or fight. Welfare emotions, such as love and pride, are responses to actual or anticipated pleasure or benefit; they prepare the organism to cling to or to possess the pleasurable stimulus.

Daily living is carried on primarily at the hedonic and emotional levels, and much effort is required to counteract emotional thinking. The emergency emotions of fear and rage that equip humans for adaptation or survival are far stronger than the welfare emotions that stimulate trust, cooperation, and affectionate exchange.

Fantasies, dreams, prejudices, and much of everyday thinking are based on *emotional thought,* which is essentially an intellectual expression of underlying feelings and so has little to do with objective reality. Illusions, delusions, and hallucinations are also examples of emotional thought. Its principal characteristic is its justification and reinforcement of the emotion from which it springs. *Unemotional* or *rational thought,* the equivalent of Freud's reality principle, makes it possible for a person to delay action and gratification, tolerate pain, forego present pleasure for future gain, and control emotional responses.

Conscience The conscience facilitates cooperation and curbs destructive competition. It stimulates healthy psychological development, but also produces pathological behavior. The development of conscience is based on the dependent child's need and wish to remain in the parents' good graces. The process begins with the child's delegation of the child's own omnipotence to the parents. The child's belief that the parents see and know all causes the child to fearfully anticipate inescapable punishment. That aspect of guilt makes conscience a powerful behavior regulator. The mature conscience, operating unconsciously and automatically, rewards good behavior and thus raises self-esteem. It punishes bad behavior by guilt, which lowers self-esteem. Conscience has other negative aspects. A child who misbehaves experiences painful guilty fear, a sense of being bad and a fear of inescapable punishment. Guilty fear has the reparative function of stimulating expiatory behavior. The child admits the wrongdoing and accepts punishment to restore the parents' positive feelings, which, in turn, relieves the painful guilty fear and raises self-esteem.

Pain-dependent or masochistic behavior is a form of expiatory behavior resulting from strong guilty fears. Those fears motivate the person to seek punishment in advance, which permits satisfaction of the formerly prohibited desire.

Discipline and the development of conscience are complicated by the buildup of rage that occurs when a child obeys or submits to his or her parents. That repressed rage, constantly seeking discharge, presents a serious problem to both the individual and society.

Concept of self Rado substituted the term "action-self" for ego. A child's first or primordial concept of self is that of an omnipotent, magical being. When children discover that their actual powers are limited, they repress their magical notions. On the way to developing a more realistic concept of self, children delegate their omnipotence and magical powers to their parents, whom they suppose will use those powers for the children's benefit. Rado conceived of the organism appreciating itself as a "proven provider of pleasure." That emotional appreciation of self is the basis of self-esteem or pride.

Treatment Rado defined psychological health as the relative predominance of the welfare emotions in a person who is reasonably independent and self-reliant. The emotionally healthy person stimulates pleasurable feelings in others that set up a chain of positive feelings by reinforcing the person's own pleasurable feelings. The emergency responses are still active but find nondestructive outlets in some form of activity or through dreaming.

Psychotherapy aims to alter the patient's emotional organization and increase self-reliance. Emotional reeducation increases the influence of the welfare emotions on behavior and reduces the influence of the emergency responses. The patient is also encouraged to relinquish dependency that causes and results from neurotic behavior and is helped to become reasonably self-reliant. The adaptational approach stresses exploration of the past to increase understanding of the present, not to reconstruct the past as such. Rado deemphasized the recovery and analysis of unconscious memories, placed less emphasis on the value of insight, and emphasized the patient's present, actual behavior. Rado also thought that the man agement of transference in classical technique infantilized the patient. He tried to avoid developing a transference neurosis and encouraged greater educational activity by the therapist.

MELANIE KLEIN

Melanie Klein (1882–1960) was a lay analyst who strongly influenced psychoanalysis in England. One of the first object relations theorists, she developed an elaborate theory of psychosexual development and psychopathology based on intrapsychic and interpersonal events presumed to occur in the first year of life. Her theory of psychopathology, based on the idea of excessive innate aggression, is used to explain every type of psychopathology from neurosis to psychosis.

There are many readily apparent flaws in Kleinian theory, including her attribution of complex thought processes to infants, her telescoping of intrapsychic development into the first year of life, and her inattentiveness to the role of environmental and interpersonal events in personality development. A pioneer in the treatment of child analysis, Klein excluded parents from the treatment because she believed that the fundamental problem was intrapsychic.

Kleinian therapists are criticized for using unmodified psychoanalytic technique with the entire spectrum of psychiatric illness despite the repeated clinical observation that psychotic and borderline patients worsen with such treatment. Their penchant for early, deep interpretations has been viewed by some critics as a form of indoctrination instead of self-exploration.

Nevertheless, Melanie Klein has shown the importance of early object relations, demonstrated superego functioning early in life, and described the primitive defenses characteristic of borderline personality disorder and psychosis.

PERSONALITY THEORY Klein agreed with Freud's life instinct–death instinct theory, viewing inborn aggression as an extension of the death instinct. The death instinct manifests as oral sadism, which, projected outward from birth as a fear of devouring objects, gives rise to fantasies of a bad, destructive, devouring breast. Oral sadism is reinforced by the trauma of birth, and later by fantasized or real frustrations. Both death and life instincts are expressed from birth on by unconscious fantasy; the contents of the fantasies represent the self and objects under the influence of crude, primitive emotions, the prototypes of love and hate.

Envy, greed, and jealousy derive from oral aggression. Envy is expressed by the fantasy that the frustrating object, originally the breast, willfully withholds. Oral envy expresses the hatred of that withholding object and the wish to spoil it, to make it less desirable. Envy gives rise to greed, and later to penis envy. Eventually, envy evolves into the envy of others' creativity and into guilt over one's own creativity because of the fear of envy attributed to others. Jealousy develops later, from triangular situations typical of oedipal conflicts. A third person is hated because that person preempts the love and libidinal supplies from the desired object.

Klein postulated that from the time of birth the ego expels all experiences of tension and displeasure in an effort to preserve a purified pleasure principle within the ego. These experiences are then projected onto persecutory objects.

The life instinct or libido is expressed from birth in pleasurable contacts with gratifying objects, primarily the good breast. Those objects are invested with libido and are introjected as internal objects infused with emotions representing libido. The breast activates the life instinct and is its first object; fantasies about the good, gratifying breast are introjected as the core ego identification or good inner objects. Projection of the good inner object on newly experienced objects is the basis of trust, learning, and knowledge. Gratifying experiences reinforce basic trust, shape the expression of libido, and influence the balance of life and death instincts.

Gratitude is the predominant emotion linked with the expression of libido. It expresses libido directed to external good objects that are also secured inside as good internal objects. Gratitude is connected with the emotion of trust, which, in turn, is based on the secure enjoyment of the good breast. Gratitude decreases greed because it leads to satisfaction with what has been received, rather than to the attempts to spoil that occur with envy. Gratitude is the origin of authentic generosity, which contrasts with reactive generosity, a defense against envy that eventually ends in feelings of being robbed.

For Klein, both life and death instincts were linked with object relations. Although the death instinct is largely projected as paranoid fears, part of it fuses with libido, giving rise to masochistic tendencies.

Theory of the ego The ego experiences and defends against anxiety, uses the mechanisms of introjection and projection, develops and maintains object relations, and has integrative and synthetic functions. The ego's response to expression of the death instinct is *anxiety*. Anxiety is also reinforced by the separation caused by birth and by the frustration of bodily needs. Anxiety becomes fear of persecutory objects, and later, through reintrojection of aggression in the form of internalized bad objects, the fear of inner persecutors. Inner persecutors are the origin of primitive superego anxiety. The content of persecutory fears relates to the level of psychosexual development. Oral fears of being devoured give way to anal fears of being controlled and poisoned, and then to oedipal fears of castration.

Introjection and *projection* are the primary processes of growth and of ego defense. They integrate the ego and neutralize the death instinct. Both good and bad experiences are projected. The projection of inner tension states and of painful external stimuli gives rise to paranoid fears. The projection of pleasurable states gives rise to basic trust. The introjection of good experiences is the origin of good internal objects, the basic stimulus for ego growth.

External stimuli invested with libido or aggression become primitive objects. Objects are, at first, part objects, but become whole objects. The Kleinian term "part object" refers to partial aspects of real persons (such as the breast) that are perceived by infants as if they were the entire person to whom the infants are relating.

Splitting is the active separation of good from bad experiences, perceptions, and emotions linked to objects. The good breast is separated from the bad breast, and the good internal object is separated from bad internal objects. For Klein, the predominance of part object relationships in earliest life was a consequence of the maximal operation of splitting mechanisms. Only later, when splitting mechanisms decrease, does synthesis of good and bad aspects of objects and ambivalence toward whole objects occur. The good breast and the bad breast are the first objects involved in the earliest unconscious fantasies. Introjection and projection create both good and bad internal and external objects; splitting mechanisms keep both internal and external objects separate in terms of libido and aggression. Part object relations characterize the earliest stage of development, the paranoid-schizoid position; whole object relationships characterize the depressive position.

Internalization of the good object is the basis for the growth of an integrated ego; the total projection of bad objects preserves a purified pleasure ego. Later, the synthesis of good and bad part objects into total or whole objects further contributes to ego growth and to the integration of the experience of reality. The predominance of aggression over libido interferes with ego integration. Under those circumstances, there is excessive *idealization,* a primitive defensive operation that preserves all-good internal and external objects. Excessive aggression also leads to overdevelopment of splitting mechanisms to protect the good internal and external objects from contamination. To the extent that splitting interferes with the accurate perception of reality, it fosters denial of reality. Although Klein accepted the influence of environmental factors in stimulating excessive aggression, she emphasized the constitutionally determined strength of the death instinct reinforced by the ego's excessive anxiety formation and low anxiety tolerance.

Paranoid-schizoid and depressive positions The paranoid-schizoid position and the depressive position, characteristic of the first and second halves of the first year of life, become stimulated at various times in life as defensive constellations, and are involved in conflicts related to all psychosexual levels.

The paranoid-schizoid position is characterized by splitting, idealization, denial, projective identification, part object relationships, and a basic fear (persecutory anxiety) about self-preservation. Persecutory fears stem from oral-sadistic and anal-sadistic impulses. If persecutory fears are not excessive, the paranoid-schizoid position evolves into the next developmental phase, the depressive position, in the second half of the first year.

When aggression is particularly strong and there is a predominance of bad objects, a secondary splitting of bad objects into fragments may take place, and those fragments may be projected into multiple external objects, giving rise to multiple persecutors. Splitting mechanisms may persist and determine a general fragmentation of affective experience, leading to depersonalization or to a general affective shallowness.

Idealization exaggerates the all-good quality of internal and external objects and satisfies fantasies of unlimited gratification (the inexhaustible breast) to protect against frustration and aggression. Idealized external objects also protect against persecutory objects. The flight toward an idealized inner good object may protect the person from an unbearable reality at the cost of impaired reality testing and may give rise to exalted or messianic psychotic states. The mechanism of idealization persists and evolves during the depressive position into idealization of the good object, based on a defense against guilt related to the object. In that case, the internal aggression toward the good external object is acknowledged, rather than split off, and the object is idealized so it will not be destroyed by the aggression. This depressive kind of idealization leads to overdependence on others. The existence of inner aggression and of the bad aspects of needed objects is denied, leading to a general impoverishment of reality experience and reality testing.

Projective identification is the prototype of all projective mechanisms and involves projecting split-off parts of an internal object into another person. One aim of projective identification is the forceful entry into the external object. Projective identification deals mainly with the projection of bad inner objects and bad parts of the self. The object onto which the projection has occurred is perceived as persecutory and must be controlled. Once the infant's own sadistic impulses are perceived as coming from the persecutory object, the need to control the object expresses the defense against persecutors and the acting out of primitive sadism toward the object.

SUPEREGO THEORY Klein argued for an early origin of the superego, and also stated the oedipal issues active in first year of life were the basis of the oedipal constellation.

Klein thought that superego development begins as part of the depressive position, that excessive superego pressures impair working through the depressive position and cause regression to the paranoid-schizoid position. The superego derives from split-off and projected bad objects that are later introjected. Guilt derives from the reintrojection of projected sadism. The superego is the synthesis of bad inner objects with the demand aspects of introjected whole objects. Beginning with the depressive position, there is a simultaneous introjection of objects into the ego and the superego; the prohibitive and demanding aspects of those objects determine the internalization into the superego. The normal predominance of love over hate and the subsequent internalization of predominantly good and demanding whole objects into the superego neutralize the bad inner objects; nevertheless, even under ideal circumstances, there is a contamination of the predominantly good superego objects by the bad objects.

Thus, the superego has a persecuting, demanding quality. The more idealized the good objects are internalized in the superego, the more perfectionistic are superego demands. Without excessive idealization of internalized good objects, superego pressures may protect the good inner objects of the ego. Under pathological circumstances, those pressures are expressed as the unremitting harshness of infantile and childhood morality.

Normally, the superego idealizes good inner objects and makes realistic demands for improvement and reinforcement of the reparative and sublimatory trends of the ego. It determines the crucial nature of the need to preserve the good inner objects and regulates ego functions by depressive anxieties reflecting the guilt or despair over dangers to the good internal objects.

Early stages of the Oedipus complex The longing for oral dependency on the mother is displaced onto the father; the longing for the good breast becomes a longing for the father's penis. In both sexes, this normal process is exaggerated when there is excessive oral frustration, thus prematurely initiating the negative Oedipus complex or feminine position in boys and setting the stage for the early development of positive oedipal striving in girls. The bad breast is also displaced to the bad penis. Oral-sadistic fantasies may be reinforced by envy of the parents' enjoyment of sex, determining the projection of sadistic fantasies onto the primal scene and distorting the sexual relations with primitive aggressive oral fantasies. The consequences of that development are the elaboration of fantastic, primitive images such as the devouring phallic mother, representing regressive castration fears in boys, a dangerous vagina, or a dangerous penis.

In boys, the predominance of the reparative, good image of the father's penis fosters the development of the positive Oedipus complex—a predominance of trust in a good oedipal father, and a reparative, sublimatory conception of sex, giving the mother a good penis. In contrast, when sadism predominates, there is excessive development of castration anxiety, and boys perceive the oedipal father as dangerous. Under those circumstances, it is more difficult for boys to achieve a positive oedipal identification with their fathers, and they are predisposed toward sexual inhibition and fear of women.

In girls, the predominance of good oral experiences reinforces normal oedipal development and genital desires—the expectation of a good penis resulting from the experience of the good breast. Excessive oral aggression in girls may bring about unconscious fantasies of robbing the mother of the father's love, penis, and babies, and may bring on unconscious fears that the primitive oral-sadistic mother will retaliate, thus determining a renunciation of the positive oedipal relationship.

Castration fears in boys derive from oral-sadistic desires to destroy the father's penis, and the castration fear is a projection of those impulses. Guilt over aggression toward the father reinforces repression of genital oedipal impulses. In girls, the Oedipus complex derives from the mother's having taken possession of the father's penis. The oral and genital desires for the father's penis combine, and penis envy constitutes a derivative of early envy of the mother's breast. Penis envy thus derives from oral sadism and is not a primary envy of male genitals, or, for that matter, a primary feature of female sexuality. Envy of the opposite sex occurs in both sexes. In her later years, Klein assumed an inborn knowledge of the genitals of both sexes, with the primitive oral and genital fantasies influencing experiences and conflicts from the first year of life on.

At about 6 months of age, splitting processes decrease, and the child becomes aware that the good and the bad external objects are one. At that point, infants recognize their own aggression toward the good object and recognize the good aspects of the object they attack, which they had perceived as bad. Projection is then only partially successful. Infants' attacks on the whole (good and bad) object also bring to awareness their own bad internal parts. In contrast to the persecutory fears of the paranoid-schizoid position, the predominant fear in the depressive position is of harming the good internal and external objects.

The basic fear about the survival of good inner and external objects is depressive anxiety or guilt, the primary emotional reaction of the depressive position. The preservation of good objects becomes more important than the preservation of the ego. Internal bad objects that are no longer projected constitute the primary superego, which attacks the ego with guilt feelings. Within the superego, bad internal objects may contaminate good internal objects that, because of their demanding or standard-setting nature, have also been internalized into the superego, bringing about demands for perfection.

Working-through mechanisms Under normal conditions, the mechanisms of reparation, increased reality testing, ambivalence, gratitude, and mourning permit working through the depressive position.

Reparation, the origin of sublimation, is the normal effort to reduce guilt over having attacked the good object by trying to repair the damage, expressing love and gratitude to the object, and preserving it.

Increased reality testing stems from the decrease of splitting mechanisms and from the growing capacity to evaluate whole objects and the total self, in contrast to the split self. The infant fears that the good mother has been lost or destroyed because of the infant's greed and destructive fantasies. The sorrow and concern over the mother and other objects with whom the infant repeats those processes bring about an increasing focus on the integration of reality and a reintrojection of objects then perceived as whole and alive, reassuring the survival and stability of good internal objects. The mother's and the infant's reality testing reinforce each other. Children, through being loved, are helped to preserve both their faith in their inner goodness and their good inner objects.

The infant's awareness of love and hate toward the same object brings about the capacity to experience ambivalence and, optimally, a predominance of love over hate in reaction to whole objects.

Klein believed that normal mourning reactivates the guilt of the depressive position. The difference between the depressive position of infancy and normal adult mourning is that during the period of weaning, the real, good mother is still present and helps the infant to reconstitute and consolidate good internal objects.

PSYCHOPATHOLOGY Fixation at the paranoid-schizoid level determines various types of psychopathology. The psychoses combine denial of reality, excessive projective identification, and pathological splitting that leads to fragmentation. Escape into an idealized inner object leads to autistic exalted states; generalized splitting and reintrojection of multiple, fragmented objects lead to confusional states. The predominance of fear of external persecutors, derived from objective identification, is characteristic of paranoia; the projection of persecutors onto the patient's own bodily zones, organs, and functions determines hypochondriacal syndromes. Schizoid personalities have shallow emotions, an incapacity to tolerate guilt feelings in depth, a tendency to experience objects as hostile, and a combination of internal withdrawal from object relations and artificiality in surface social adaptation.

The major pathological developments of the depressive position are pathological mourning or excessive development of manic defenses. *Pathological mourning* results from the loss of the good external and internal objects caused by their fantasized destruction. In pathological mourning, both the external and the internal good objects appear to die because of sadistic attacks. The bad internal objects produce a primitive, sadistic superego, evoke excessive guilt, and give rise to the feeling that all good objects are dead and the world is empty of love. The sadistic superego is characterized by cruelty, demands for perfection, and hatred of instincts. Efforts at compensation fail; the idealization of the object only increases further guilt and despair; and the self-reproaches of the depressed person are directed not against the object, but against the self (ego) and the internal impulses. Suicide may embody the fantasy of protecting the good object by destroying the bad self. In depressive psychosis, unconscious fantasies of a total destruction of inner world objects are manifested by hypochondriacal delusions, or fantasies of destruction of the whole world by means of projection. In defending against pathological, intolerable mourning, paranoid fears may avert pathological guilt and depression. Psychotic depression results from the pathological development of all these defensive operations and the inability to work through the depressive position.

Hypomanic and manic syndromes indicate the pathological predominance of manic defenses. Manic defenses include omnipotence, identification with the superego, introjection, triumph, and manic idealization. Omnipotence is based on identification with an idealized and powerful good object and the denial of other aspects of internal and external reality.

Identification with the superego is an identification with the sadistic superego. Depressive guilt and aggression are denied and projected outward; external objects are considered and treated as the hated, depreciated, bad self. Pathological development of introjection may be expressed as an object hunger linked with the denial of the danger to and from objects. The implicit fantasy is that, because there are so many objects, a few less do not matter. Manic triumph is expressed clinically as conscious triumph over the world, an exalted state of power. The exaggeration of idealization of the self may be represented by exalted states reflecting fantasies of merging with good, fantastically idealized objects.

TREATMENT Kleinians deal with patients' material by interpretation. Interpretations are primarily transference interpretations, and the same unmodified psychoanalytic technique is used with all patients. The analysis focuses on interpreting unconscious paranoid-schizoid and depressive unconscious fantasies representing both the content and the defensive operations at primitive levels of the mind. Kleinian analysts interpret at the level of the patient's maximum unconscious anxiety, which means interpreting material at deep levels from the earliest stages of treatment. Klein believed that all anxiety-producing situations reactivate persecutory and depressive anxieties, so that primitive defenses and fears influence all interpretive work with the transference.

Klein thought that children develop a full-fledged transference to the analyst, projecting onto the analyst split-off aspects of their parental images and of internal objects from the past. She observed and interpreted children's play in her office (50 minutes, 5 days a week) as a symbolic expression of their conflicts and anxieties, avoiding reassuring the children in any way except by analyzing the transference. The Kleinian analyst participates in a child's play only to the extent required by a full expression of a certain fantasy; and the analyst interprets the meaning of the child's anger or frustration when repetitive games, which serve the repetition compulsion, sadistic control, or acting out, are interrupted by the analyst's shift into an exclusively interpretive stance. Hannah Segal, a Kleinian analyst, recommends avoiding the temptation to "reeducate" patients directly and stresses the child's capacity to understand interpretations of unconscious meanings if they are couched in simple terms.

Kleinian therapists have been particularly interested in treating patients in whom primitive levels of conflicts and defenses predominate. Given their focus on the need to explore the splitting of love and aggression and the vicissitudes of integrative efforts to deal with them, Kleinians interpret both negative and positive aspects of the transference, emphasizing the early interpretation of negative transference features.

OTTO RANK

Otto Rank (1884–1939) was the only nonmedical person in Freud's inner circle (Fig. 7-5). He added a broad world view to the psychoanalytic movement during its early years. Later, he developed his own theory of personality and broke from psychoanalysis.

THE RANKIAN DIALECTIC To Rank, birth is the prototypical traumatic event in life. It causes primal anxiety that is dealt with by primal repression. All developmental crises are based on the terror of leaving the womb and the wish to return to a state of primal bliss.

The polarities of union–separation and likeness–difference are the core of the Rankian growth process. In uniting with

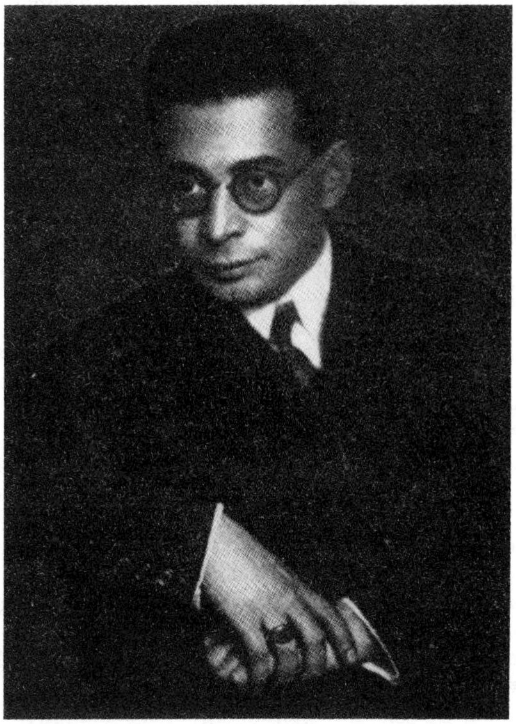

FIGURE 7-5. *Otto Rank.*

another person or persons, one discovers and affirms likeness to others. Through union and seeing one's reflection in a relationship with another person, one's likeness to others and self-worth are established. Separation leads to the discovery of self-identity. That discovery often comes as a shock when one person is suddenly cut off from another because of an error or an impulsive act. But in standing alone, one can see oneself in clear relief and has a chance to discover and affirm one's uniqueness.

Likeness and difference, and union and separation are in a dialectic relationship—a blending of opposites held in tension. A person's ability to move in any direction depends entirely on how certain the person is of the opposite direction. Movement toward another human being is only possible if one is certain of one's identity, which is discovered in separation; movement away from people is only possible if one is internally certain of one's belonging.

Rank believed that moving from union to separation is an act of will. In willing to engage with another person, each person experiences the depth of his or her need for belonging; in choosing to move out into the unknown (negative will assertion), each person affirms and claims his or her own uniqueness. In order to attain personal maturity, the will must overcome the forces that inhibit movement toward and away from people—guilt, death fear, and life fear. Every willed act produces guilt. Moving toward union causes guilt over needing someone else or needing to use someone for one's own growth. Moving away stimulates guilt for abandoning someone whom one has used and may need again.

A person can become lost in uniting with another person. Rank called that smothering, engulfing encounter the death fear. The more a person is unsure of his or her own identity, the greater is the fear of dying by such smothering. To move away from other people carries an opposite danger and fear. Separation has the danger of overshooting the pull of the union, which Rank called the life fear. With each union, one abandons one's own will to another's will to enjoy brief happiness, unaware of one's difference from the other person. The experience is then abandoned in a new rebirth experience. Fear of the unknown outcome of each movement is the price paid for growth.

This process of personality growth through movement into and out of relationships has familial, societal, artistic, and spiritual phases. Each phase contains one or more major movements toward union with significant others or with the world at large, and major rebirth experiences through separation by will affirmation. Each person needs to yield to a love relationship, setting aside personal differences to experience the unity of the self with others and to experience self-worth and a release from difference. That yielding to another's will terminates when the will asserts its separateness and renewed perception of difference. Another rebirth of the will and a new affirmation of individuality occur.

The prime mover in the Rankian dialetic is will. The will is a creative force that cannot be reduced to more basic elements. It is a first cause, not a means for discharge or inhibition of aggressive or sexual impulses in the Freudian sense or a will to power in the Adlerian sense. Will begins in childhood as negativeness or counterwill—the child indicating through words or behavior what he or she will not do. This basic expression of the personality can be abetted or warped. Neurotic persons fail to recognize their own will because of guilt over what they will or because they rationalize or deny what they will. Neurotics are described as persons of strong will who cannot acknowledge what they will or even that they will. The essential problem of therapy is to remove the blocks to recognizing and assuming responsibility for one's own will. The neurotic is regarded as an artist manque—a person who is potentially superior because of a strong will but who fails to use that will in the service of the ultimate artistic creation, the person's own personality.

Treatment The Rankian therapeutic process is a time-limited rebirth experience in which the patient makes dramatic leaps, and not a slow process of acquiring insight that is followed by adjustment or behavior change. In treatment, patients reenact in the relationship with the therapist all the past struggles with relationships, especially the problem of intimacy. In the encounter with the therapist, they experience and work through those feelings, especially the death fear. Resistance is viewed positively as patients' assertion of will against the therapist. Rebirth occurs after the patient–therapist relationship has affirmed a patient's innate self-worth. Using their inner strength for self-affirmation, patients relinquish their dependency on the therapist and claim their uniqueness as individuals. In that process, they overcome the life fear by acknowledging and expressing their fullest potential.

In therapy, patients move through phases analogous to the process of personality growth, first moving into a relationship with the therapist as a prototype of a particular person in each patient's life and of universal humanity, with whom they must unite. The first rebirth occurs as patients claim their own individuality personally and as a unique part of universal humankind. The second phase begins as they discover the physical universe and their likeness to it. After that phase, they claim their distinctiveness as creators within the cosmic reality as the creative artist is born. In the emergence of the self, they move to the final phase of growth as they unite with the ideological, philosophical, and spiritual reality. That phase is followed by the final birth of the ethical ideal—self-fulfilled human beings who no longer need to create in order to prove their right to exist.

The process of therapy is not aimed at understanding the historical self, but at an experience of the self in the present as expressed in the struggle with the therapist who helps the patient free his or her will. The struggle of the patient against the therapist is recognized as a legitimate expression of the positive life force of will and not as a resistance to be overcome. Thus, each therapeutic endeavor is an ad hoc process that takes place in whatever area the patient's will is stifled, denied, or rationalized and not fully owned.

KAREN HORNEY

Karen Horney (1885–1952) developed a psychoanalytic theory of human behavior and character structure that was based on a view of humans as continually striving to evolve and to realize themselves within their culture, family climate, and environment—the same major factors that produce neurotic behavior (Fig. 7-6).

PERSONALITY THEORY Each person is a unique combination of biological endowments living in a specific, highly personal environment of family and culture, and striving to develop his or her own particular potentialities.

Everyone has a *real self,* a source of energy, aliveness, and spontaneity; a sense of who one is; a dynamic psychological core that gives a sense of identity. It enables individuals to make choices and to accept responsibility for their consequences. It endures despite change and growth. *Self-realization,* the natural unfolding and development of human potential into activities and relationships, leads to healthy activities in which individuals move toward others to express love and trust, against others to express healthy opposition and to master their environment, and away from others to become self-sufficient.

Conditions during childhood are often unfavorable to healthy growth, but there is always the potential for healthy growth if blockages are removed. Parents may not provide the warmth and acceptance needed for a child to gain a sense of trust, causing anxiety over survival and deflecting the child's energies toward psychological survival. Under those conditions, children often do not develop in a healthy, spontaneous way, and a deformation of character or a character neurosis develops.

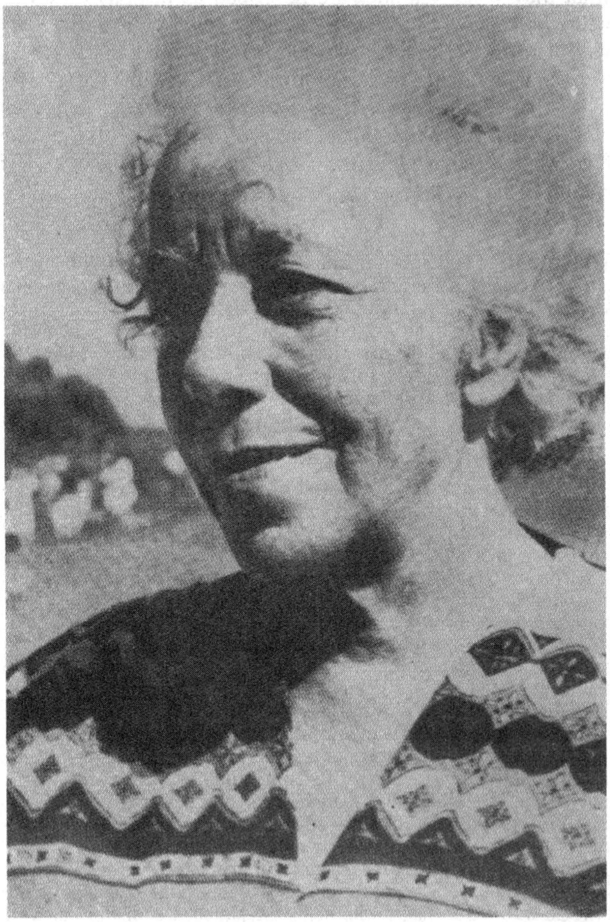

FIGURE 7-6. *Karen Horney. (From the National Library of Medicine, Bethesda, MD.)*

Horney doubted the prevailing Freudian notion that women are biologically predestined to be submissive and to suffer. She recognized that much of what was considered normal female behavior, such as fearfulness, dependence, submissiveness, and self-effacement, was culturally determined. Typical male and female character structures are the product of cultural forces and are not genetically determined.

HORNEY'S THEORY OF NEUROSIS Horney defined neurosis as a disturbance in relation to the self and others. Although some persons experience specific symptoms, such as phobias, compulsions, and anxiety states, most seek help because they are unhappy, feel blocked and unfulfilled in their work, or feel unable to form or maintain satisfactory relationships. Many persons are driven by feelings of hopelessness and despair to pursue superficial accomplishments that leave them dissatisfied and unfulfilled. These feelings and symptoms express a complex, self-perpetuating system of defensive patterns against basic anxiety that starts early in childhood. This system that persons develop in their efforts to survive forms the neurotic character structure.

Search for safety Children attempt to alleviate their anxiety, to make life safer and more predictable, and to achieve satisfaction. They search for affection and approval, become angry and hostile, or withdraw. A child in moving toward others identifies with his or her feelings of helplessness; in moving against others, accepts and takes for granted a hostile environment; and in moving away from others, accepts the impossibility of communicating or becoming involved with others. After trying all three strategies, the child eventually employs the way that is rewarded or accepted by the environment, but at the expense of meeting other needs. If clinging and helplessness succeed in appeasing important adults, the child avoids expressing hostility or needs for separateness. If anger and rebelliousness gain respect or a sense of power, needs for closeness are not acknowledged. If emotional withdrawal produces a sense of safety and is permitted by the adults, the child stops attempting to gain closeness or to express aggression.

As a result, only one aspect of the child's being is acknowledged and cultivated. The child no longer explores or expresses a full range of feelings and impulses, but limits them to what is acceptable to others. Despite a sense of safety, a new sense of precariousness develops. Instead of the security the child hopes to gain, there is danger from within that requires constant vigilance and leads to greater restriction of genuine feelings and impulses. As long as those unfavorable external conditions persist, feelings or impulses that give rise to conflicting behavior are repressed. Conflicting feelings are driven deeper until the child is no longer conscious of them, and is left instead with a diffuse sense of discomfort, anxiety, apprehension, and a shaky sense of self. The child can no longer trust his or her own feelings, but has shifted the point of reference outside the self and is torn by conflicting needs and desires. Patterns of behavior rigidity, and cause ever-increasing restrictions and blockages to growth. They crystallize into the complex, relatively fixed attitudes toward self and others that are called neurotic trends.

CHARACTER TYPES Horney proposed three main neurotic trends based on three predominant modes of relating to others.

Compliant, self-effacing type When the predominant defense against anxiety is moving toward others, their approval is needed to relieve anxiety. Compliant, self-effacing persons shape their personality so as to not provoke disapproval or rejection. They depend on others and turn to them for advice. Thus, such persons become sensitive to others' needs, are agreeable, and try to be unselfish. They subordinate themselves to others, take second place, and avoid the limelight. They avoid assertiveness. They value goodness, sympathy, and unselfishness, and feel that everyone can be won over by love. These kind, helpful, sensitive persons live in constant inner turmoil. Because they do not speak up for themselves, others often take advantage of them. They may work unceasingly for others, but fear reaching out for themselves. Ordinary disagreement is almost unbearable, as they panic at the slightest possibility of rejection.

Aggressive, expansive type In moving against others, this type of person seeks security through power and mastery. Such persons strive for control over others and for mastery over themselves and the environment. They come to feel superior to others by achieving success and by exploiting others' vulnerabilities. By seeing the world as fiercely competitive, they rationalize their aggressive behavior. They develop toughness and endurance, but equate tenderness with weakness and repress tender feelings. Their partner's love is less important than admiration and submission. Persons of this type often achieve outward success because of their prodigious efforts at mastery and self-control.

Detached, resigned type In moving away from others, these persons attempt to remove themselves from conflict and avoid their dependent and aggressive feelings. They develop a strong need for privacy and become hypersensitive to any feelings or involvements; they become onlookers. They avoid competition and deny any need for others. These persons consider their uniqueness a measure of superiority. Stressing their self-sufficiency, their greatest value is their so-called freedom.

AUXILIARY METHODS TO RELIEVE INNER TENSION Rigidly developing one of the three basic interpersonal styles suppresses the other two basic directions of interpersonal behavior. The submerged and contradictory impulses are still active, thus producing *basic conflict*. The person attempts to reduce conflict by using auxiliary approaches to artificial harmony. These approaches consist of mental mechanisms, such as blind spots, compartmentalization, and rationalization, and the use of complex adjustment techniques; and excessive use of self-control, arbitrariness, elusiveness, cynicism, and externalization.

Idealized image In adolescence, neurotic persons use imagination and fantasy to create an idealized image that promises to end their painful feelings and to provide self-fulfillment. The idealized image is formed by harmonizing through rationalization, enhancement, distortion, and exaggeration traits that they aspire to and admire. Those personal qualities, traits, attitudes, and values, originally developed as survival techniques, force neurotics to override their genuine feelings, wishes, and thoughts, and leave them increasingly alienated from their core selves, with only a vague sense of identity. Creating the idealized image, however, smooths over all the contradictions, conceals the defensive nature of their behavior, and magically restores a sense of wholeness. Energy formerly used for healthy self-realization is used in the pursuit of actualizing an idealized self.

For example, love-oriented, excessively dependent persons experience their fear of healthy self-assertion as saint-like humility, consideration of others, and the wish not to hurt others' feelings. Power-oriented persons rationalize exploiting others as proof of their superior intelligence and capabilities. They create the image of a conquering hero, a natural-born leader. Freedom-oriented persons create an image in which fear of emotional involvement and the deadening of their feelings become serenity and self-sufficiency.

Because the idealized self exists only in the imagination, neurotic persons are vulnerable to interpersonal confrontation or contact with reality. To protect themselves, they are driven to prove that the image is really themselves. They drive themselves to actualize and demonstrate that idealized self through compulsive perfectionism in which nothing short of flawless excellence is satisfactory. Neurotic perfectionism is reinforced by stringent "shoulds." Neurotic persons are also obsessed and driven by neurotic ambition. They must be first, and they take revenge on others whom they feel have thwarted, humiliated, or prevented them from actualizing their idealized self.

Claims As additional support for their idealized self, neurotics expect others to treat them with the respect their position commands. Horney called those expectations and demands on others "claims." Neurotic persons believe they are that glorified idealized self and feel that they deserve, and are entitled to, special benefits and considerations. Frustration of neurotic claims produces disproportionate anger, righteous indignation, resentment, and vindictiveness.

Shoulds Neurotic persons also demand from themselves that they live up to their idealized self. These "shoulds" require perfection, regardless of realistic conditions. To reduce the unbearable inner pressure of shoulds, these individuals externalize them and experience them as arising from others. At the same time, they try to dilute the pressure of shoulds by insisting that others live up to the same unrealistic demands that they make on themselves. They become critical of others and sensitive to criticism.

Self-hatred Intensifying the shoulds is the self-hatred generated when the person experiences the terror of failing to fulfill relentless inner demands. Self-hatred, shoulds, and claims operate only because there is an idealized self. They reinforce and support neurotics' beliefs in the self they have created.

Neurotic pride and the pride system *Neurotic pride*, a substitute for healthy self-confidence, results when one glorifies aspects of one's idealized image. When their pride is hurt by others, as when their idealized image is questioned, neurotic people respond with rage and seek to avenge that injury by achieving vindictive triumph over the offender.

Neurotic pride and self-hatred, with their supporting forces of claims and shoulds, form an armor or *pride system* that protects the idealized self. Just as cults defend their special beliefs by keeping their followers from engaging in free discussions with others, the pride system prevents exploration of the idealized self. Any attempt to reduce the elements of the pride system is perceived as an attack on the person. But despite the armor of this system, neurotics are not at peace. They are still vulnerable and in inner conflict with the very forces that protect them. The conflict between the forces of healthy self-realization and the pride system is the *central inner conflict*.

Another major conflict is within the pride system itself. Neurotic pride and claims identify themselves with the glorified idealized image; self-hatred and shoulds are involved with the weaknesses and unacceptable traits of the despised image. Conflict arises when neurotics try to satisfy both forces at the same time. To relieve that inner tension and anxiety, they move away from the center of the conflict and thus become further alienated from their real selves.

Alienation One of the most serious consequences of neurotic development is alienation. Alienation from self results from repeated, active denial and the repression of genuine feelings and impulses. As this process continues, such persons lose touch with the very core of their being, as well as the ability to determine and act on what is right for them. They feel lost, uncertain, and confused. If alienation is extreme, they may feel deadened and empty inside.

ANALYTIC TREATMENT Horney focused on the ongoing neurotic process. She did not consider adults to be repeating childhood experiences, and she did not focus on recovering childhood memories. Horney stressed that neurosis is a dynamic, complex, self-perpetuating structure. Ongoing neurotic patterns require careful analytic work to free patients from their blockages to healthy growth. Horney stressed the importance of dreams and, in her later works, the patient–analyst relationship as part of the analytic process. She was one of the earliest analysts to understand that analysts have feelings about patients, and that those feelings must be identified and worked with constructively.

Horney saw psychoanalysis as a cooperative venture that enables patients to liberate themselves from their neurotic character structure and to mobilize their forces for creative living and self-realization. She felt that it was the analyst's responsibility to assist patients in becoming liberated from the forces that retard healthy growth and movement toward self-emancipation, which she called *blockages*.

Blockages are neurotic patients' persistent attempts to resist change. In the initial phase of analytic therapy, blockages are identified and examined so that patients can become aware of them and make efforts to free themselves. This is the *disillusioning process*. The first phase of the disillusioning process emphasizes uncovering, identifying, and clarifying two major groups of blockages.

Horney called the first group of safety-oriented defenses *protective blockages,* defenses activated to prevent the anxiety caused by self-awareness. They resist the therapist's exploring and clarifying the compulsive nature of the patient's present behavior patterns. Protective blockages include silence, lateness, cancellation of sessions, self-narcotization with drugs or alcohol, expressed disappointment or deprecation of the analyst's values, pseudocompliance, and the use of self-accusation to prevent further insights and exploration by the therapist.

The second major group of defenses is *positive-value blockages*. They are used to prevent self-awareness and to allow patients to feel satisfied with themselves. These blockages reinforce patients' personal philosophies, which sustain and support their idealized self.

In the first phase of the disillusioning process, the analyst actively identifies and clarifies these two types of obstructive force. Protective blockages can be explored safely early in the analysis. Blockages that defend the idealized image require more careful handling. Neurotic patients have built up their entire sense of well-being on idealized images, and they respond to premature examination of their values with great fear.

Qualities of the analyst To help free patients from their neurotic conflicts and to mobilize their constructive forces toward self-realization, therapists need maturity, a belief in the constructive resolution of conflict, and an ability to communicate their hope to patients overwhelmed by self-hatred and hopelessness. Therapists also need to communicate their respect for patients' struggles. By listening, clarifying, and providing directions, they help patients to develop alternative solutions to conflicts. Alienation is reduced so that patients can own their feelings and are helped to regain their spontaneity and to find their own core selves.

Horney recognized that each human being is a unique combination of hereditary endowments and environmental influences. Thus, she stressed flexibility in technique in response to the therapist's sensitive perception of where the patient is at any moment. Because the emphasis was always on reducing forces that obstruct healthy growth, rigid adherence to the frequency of sessions and the use of the couch were deemed less important than in classical analysis.

Change in analysis and mobilizing constructive forces

Horney believed that simple behavioral change is not sufficient. Behavioral change can occur coercively, through imitation or coercion, or because of fear of the therapist's disapproval. To be lasting, the change must be based on true attitude change, which takes place only through a reorientation of values in an open atmosphere that permits patients' self-assessment as free individuals with the choice to discover and select personal values consonant with their real self. That reorientation begins after the disillusioning phase of treatment. When patients begin to question their present set of values and goals and the idealizing process begins to fade, they are ready to revise their values and to develop other sets of values that are less rigid and more appropriate to their real lives. Dreams, which always play a prominent part in the early part of the treatment, are very useful in the latter phase. Horney viewed dreams as bringing patients closer to the reality of themselves. They are attempts to solve conflicts in either a neurotic or a healthy way, and can show constructive forces at work even when they are hardly visible otherwise.

In the phase of mobilizing constructive forces, patients experience central inner conflict—the struggle between the pride system and the real self. That inner conflict produces psychic turbulence, pain, and hate. When there is successful resolution of central inner conflict, patients can move toward the final phase, the discovery and creative use of their spontaneous real inner self.

HARRY STACK SULLIVAN

Harry Stack Sullivan (1892–1949) synthesized Freud's appreciation of the unconscious with Adolf Meyer's view of mental disorders as dynamic patterns and types of reaction to life stresses (Fig. 7-7). Like Jung, he spent his first professional years working with mentally ill persons.

His contributions to theory include his formulations concerning the mother–child interaction, the child's modes (prototaxic, parataxic, and syntaxic) of experiencing, and the concept of dynamisms. He saw anxiety as the chief disruptive force in interpersonal relationships and as the root of serious problems in living. Sullivan's contributions to therapy are based on his thesis that psychiatry is the study of interpersonal relations, that mental disorders result from and are perpetuated by inadequate communication, and that, in a bipersonal field, each person contributes to the overall quality of the relationship. Thus, Sullivan saw individuals as the product of their real or fantasied interactions with others and not as the product of their drives and conflicts.

PERSONALITY THEORY In defining psychiatry as the study of interpersonal relationships, Sullivan established the base unit of observation as the field of interaction between self and real or fantasied others. He eschewed the Freudian model of an individual operating on inborn drives who is secondarily affected by the environment. Just as persons depend on and interact with the surrounding environment for physical nurturance and protection, they need others to help them grow and develop psychologically and socially.

Sullivan postulated that human life requires interchange with an environment that includes interpersonal relationships and culture. Human personality, in Sullivan's terms, is the

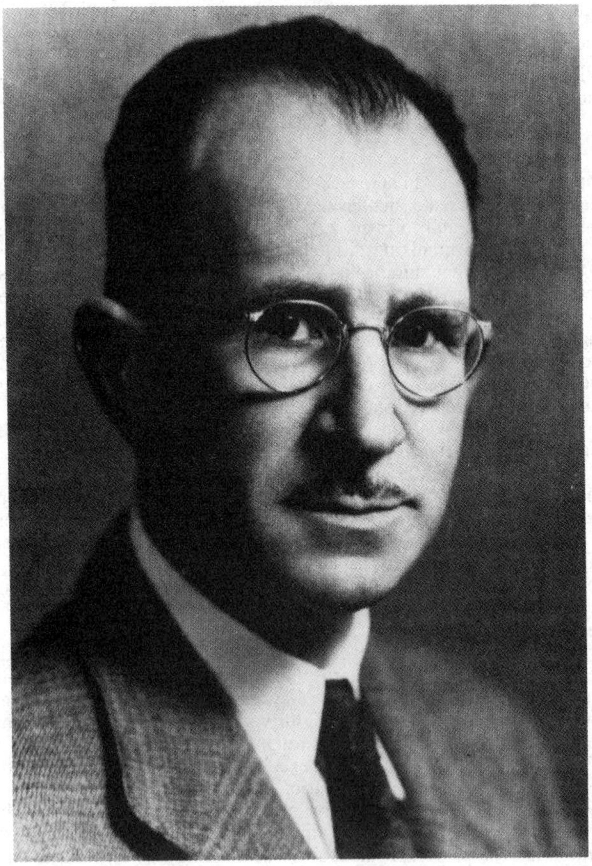

FIGURE 7-7. *Harry Stack Sullivan. (Courtesy of John Wiley, New York.)*

relatively enduring pattern of recurrent interpersonal operations that characterize a human life. Human personality is not static. It reflects the organization of experience at successive stages of development, and is also subject to modification throughout life.

Sullivan's theory of personality development is based on the vicissitudes of fulfilling biological and security needs. *Biological needs* refer to food, sleep, shelter, the physical presence of another human being, and sexual expression. *Security needs* are connected with uniquely human pursuits, such as financial security or personal recognition, reflecting the indoctrination into and adoption of cultural values that operate by preserving or enhancing self-esteem. Self-esteem or self-respect, in turn, can be defined as a sense of power in dealing with others.

Needs arising in the infant's internal physicochemical milieu are experienced as tensions that give rise to signals from the infant to the mother, such as crying and movement. The mother responds with a tension of her own (experienced as tenderness), thus relieving the infant's tension. If this process takes place relatively smoothly, the infant experiences a pleasant emotional state and the ground is prepared for an eventual sense of security based on the ability to involve a significant person in the fulfillment of one's needs. The experiencing of such possibilities and accomplishing them in successive stages of development enhance the sense of interpersonal competence.

If, instead, the mothering one becomes anxious because the infant's tension reduces her self-esteem ("If I were an adequate person, my baby wouldn't cry"), a sense of discomfort or dysphoria, later to be known as "anxiety," is transmitted to the infant, regardless of whether the infant's biological needs are fulfilled. This transmitted anxiety results in a diminished sense of security. To explain how anxiety is transmitted, Sullivan postulated an *empathic linkage* between the infant and the mothering one. The amount of anxiety transmitted does not coincide with the intensity of the biological need for food or drink. It has to do with the anxiety evoked in the mothering one. The infant's anxiety represents the miscarriage of an "integrative tendency" in an interpersonal situation. It becomes registered as a feeling that was unpleasant and one that the infant is not equipped to handle effectively or to eliminate. It can be revived on subsequent occasions of a similar nature, and is the main conditioning factor for the development of what Sullivan first called self-dynamism and later the self-system.

A *dynamism* is a relatively enduring pattern of energy transformation. Every person develops varied interwoven and overlapping patterns in relation to the important zones of interaction with the environment, such as oral and anal zones, and in relation to important needs, such as hunger and sexual need. The interpersonal field is made up of the interacting dynamism of two or more persons. Some dynamisms in this context are *conjunctive* (such as the need for intimacy) and lead to the integration of a situation and the reduction of tensions. Dynamisms involving anxiety can be *disjunctive* and lead to the disintegration of an interpersonal situation. At other times, dynamisms are not operative because there is no corresponding dynamism with which they can mesh.

Self-dynamism or *self-system* is the configuration of energy in interpersonal processes aimed at avoiding anxiety. This dynamism is essential for maintaining or enhancing the sense of security and gratifying needs for satisfaction. Originating in the wish to avoid discomfort induced in the infant by the mothering one's anxiety, self-dynamism assumes its function when anxiety results from disapproval by a significant person. As the self-dynamism grows, it functions in accordance with its state of development from the start. Self-dynamism accounts for a sort of tunnel vision that allows into awareness only the processes compatible with the approval of significant persons, thus minimizing the occurrence of anxiety. Within the personality, as earlier defined, self-dynamism favors the development of a sense of *self* that reflects the positive appraisals of others, and is, therefore, a comfortable way of thinking of or personifying oneself. The rest of the personality, which comprises all other kinds of impulses and performances, remains outside awareness.

The self-system employs *security operations*. Security operations vary in their efficiency and their means of dealing with anxiety. *Apathy* is an early security operation that reduces need awareness if strong discomfort was experienced in their fulfillment. A kindred process is *somnolent detachment*, a reduced susceptibility to the interpersonally induced tension of anxiety. Both of these processes presuppose a temperamental endowment that allows them to occur without undue damage to the infant. Another early security operation is *sublimation*, the unconscious substitution for a behavior pattern that encounters anxiety or collides with the self-system of a socially more acceptable activity pattern that satisfies the part of the motivational system that caused the trouble.

Selective inattention, the most frequently used security operation, arises in children after parental appraisals, approvals, and disapprovals become articulated in understandable speech. It concentrates on whatever has proved conducive to security by minimizing anxiety and enhancing approval, and keeps anything else not likely to achieve these aims outside of awareness. Selective inattention operates outside of awareness, but can be brought into awareness easily if presented by a well-disposed observer participating in the interaction. Selective inattention may be useful and healthy. Its potentially pathogenic aspect is its excluding from awareness the most relevant aspects of successful integration of an interpersonal situation, instead of the least relevant ones.

Unlike selective inattention, which maintains or enhances security rather than frustrating needs, *dissociation* or *dissociating processes* exclude from awareness motivational systems or needs for satisfaction, so that a large and important part of actual or potential living becomes isolated from the self-system. *Dynamisms of difficulty*, arising from these dissociating tendencies, are emergency measures pertaining to strongly felt or anticipated anxiety at various developmental stages. They include obsessionalism, with its substitutive and avoidant tendencies; various raw emotions—anger, pride, envy, jealousy—and the way in which they become integrated within the personality; the paranoid dynamism, essentially based on the transfer of blame and the use of projection; and the schizophrenic dynamism, reflecting the failure of the self-system and of dissociation itself to maintain an integrated personality organization.

Modes of experiencing Sullivan outlined three overlapping sequential modes of experiencing during the process of maturation: prototaxic, parataxic, and syntaxic. Prototaxic refers to experiences that occur before language symbols are used, parataxic refers to the use of private or autistic symbols, and syntaxic refers to experiences that can be shared with others through mutually acceptable symbols. Arrest or persistence in the two immature modes may account for certain peculiarities of personality or for specific forms of pathology. The modes of experiencing are important in acquiring learning skills and parallel the achievement of interpersonal competence.

The simplest mode is *prototaxic experience*, a series of momentary states of the sensitive organism, each making its own impact without any sense of sequence or connection, or of causation or prediction. Sullivan spoke of "prehensions" by the infant in the first months of life while it remains undifferentiated from its environment. He considered such experience as involving a zone of interaction of the infant (oral, anal, or other) with the environment. The *zone of interaction* refers to areas or channels through which the tension of needs and its way of relief are sensed in conjunction with the outside, although no specific knowledge of the latter is yet present. The prototaxic mode of experience can be inferred in later life when something has been perceived that affects one in a highly impressive way, but the experience cannot be adequately communicated to another. It can also be found in the cosmic, fusing experiences of schizophrenic persons.

The maturing infant begins to distinguish between the self and the world and to discriminate between zones of interaction and their involvement in meeting various needs. In the *parataxic mode of experience*, events and situations are recorded as momentary states of the organism, but their occurrence is given a serial or parallel meaning or symbolization. Visual and auditory channels begin to predominate and to contribute to connections, including recall and foresight, without logical or demonstrable consistency. These connections serve the budding self-system and the wish to avoid anxiety. Similarities, actual or apparent, are viewed as samenesses. Causality is established through happenstance and coincidence rather than rational examination or validation. Parataxic experience may give a sense of predictive power. Sullivan used the term "parataxic distortion" to refer to remnants of the parataxic experience as observed in later life situations, when one deals with others as if they were like significant persons in one's early life situations and in ways that formerly seemed to garner approval and freedom from anxiety. Stripped of its hierarchically regressive elements and those of libidinally gratifying preoccupations, this concept is similar to transference—less suggestive of actual regression, but more indicative of stunted progression in the integration of interpersonal relations.

The desirable outcome of healthy development is the *syntaxic mode of experience*. It reduces the elements of prototaxic and parataxic experience in interpersonal exchanges, relies on logical, sequential, internally consistent, and recurrent modifiable thinking regarding people and events, and allows for consensual validation. *Consensual validation* underlies the syntaxic mode of experiencing. Consensus means that a symbol has the same meaning to at least two persons involved in significant interaction. It becomes further validated in subsequent and repeated interactions with significant persons.

DEVELOPMENTAL ERAS

Infancy In infancy, which comprises the period from birth to the acquisition of language, the important zones of interaction are primarily the oral and then the anal and urethral zones. Specific differences obtain in what is seen or heard or otherwise "prehended" and vary according to the stage of maturation of the organism.

In later infancy, with the infant's differentiation from the mothering one and the addition of new symbols, whether words or gestures, "personifications" begin to develop. Achieving fulfillment of needs with relative freedom from anxiety results in the personifications of "good mother" and "good me." A moderate degree of anxiety accounts for the personifications of "bad mother" and "bad me" and a tendency toward security operations that put outside awareness anything pertaining to these personifications. Extremely disruptive instances of anxiety may result in the "not me" personification, with attendant dissociation instead of selective inattention, resulting in whole sets of impulses and feelings becoming an isolated, foreign, and unknown entity within the personality.

Childhood The years from about 2 to 5 are a time of learning through the acquisition of understandable speech. Autistic language yields to the adults' demands for more understandable language. Children learn to accept compromises that impoverish the highly individualistic elements of their experience but enrich their abilities to communicate with others effectively, and thus gain a sense of increasing interpersonal competence.

Learning through language also tends to fuse earlier personifications, such as "good mother" and "bad mother," into one mothering person. Although this fusion is made for convenience and communication in interpersonal situations, children may continue to experience the separate personifications within their own personalities. This usage may result in piecemeal dealings with and expectations of the other person. The perpetuation of such separate personifications in later life may usually be found in the histrionic personality.

Childhood is also the period when undue expectations for acceptable performances and prohibition of unacceptable ones, both actual and in fantasy, make adults appear to children as enemies who interfere with gratification. This development, parallel to the continued dependency on the significant person, may lead to conflicting feelings and contradictory reactions. To the extent that angry and hateful elements accrue and prevail in the interaction, children come to expect anxiety or pain when the need for tenderness is felt, even if they use the time-honored means to achieve the right or desirable responses. This reaction accounts for a subsequent development in which children stop using what they have learned to use to elicit the needed tenderness and proceed with self-defeating behaviors, as if they feel that whatever they do will not really matter in the interpersonal exchange. This "malevolent transformation" can be observed in certain character traits and in various psychopathological states, including obsessionalism, paranoia, and some depressions.

The juvenile era This era begins with the fifth year of life and is characterized by the need for peer relations and the spreading of authority to, or the sharing of it by, new figures other than family members. Earlier lonely or solitary preoccupations become shared with peers. One learns to compete with others and to cooperate with them while avoiding disapproval and seeking approval. Compromise (without compromising self-esteem) becomes the order of the day. This may prove difficult if there is considerable persistence of malevolent transformation in the juvenile or if there is anxiously experienced parental malevolence toward the juvenile's dealings with peers or new authorities.

Preadolescence The period of preadolescence, from roughly 8 to 12 years of age, is marked by the need for interpersonal intimacy. Such intimacy presupposes collaboration between two persons based on a common bond and concern with the recognition and enhancement of each other's worth and self-esteem, so that the other's welfare matters as much as one's own. Collaboration differs from the cooperation of the juvenile era, when children follow rules to preserve their own prestige and feeling of worth in the eyes of parents or valued peers. In preadolescence, a new type of interest develops in one particular other person of the same gender, the "chum," with whom mutual validation of personal worth is possible, with whom experiences can be shared, and misconceptions about the self can be corrected.

Adolescence This period is ushered in by the advent of true genital interest, felt as lust. Now, the prevalent zones of interaction and areas of stimulation and satisfaction are the genitals and the so-called erogenous zones. Sullivan saw significant differences between male and female in terms of physiological maturation and attendant needs for satisfaction. He viewed those differences pragmatically, and remarked that they should not be the basis of invidious comparisons that lead to conclusions about inferiority or inadequacy. He was aware of the effect of culturally conditioned stereotypes and discriminations, as already evidenced in the experiences of the juvenile era. As a possible common denominator, Sullivan postulated three needs associated with early adolescence, partly contradictory but also intricately connected, and likely to extend into later development. These needs are the continuing need for personal security, meaning freedom from anxiety; the need for intimacy, meaning collaboration with at least one other person; and the need for satisfaction of lust, involving genital activity for the achievement of orgasm.

Late adolescence, if reached with relatively successful resolution of the above conflicts, will be a period of refining the consensually dependable aspects of interpersonal situations, thus enhancing the syntaxic mode of experience. Assuming personal responsibility in adopting social concerns and standards rather than perpetuating opportunistic mimicking or paying of lip service both indicates and enhances self-esteem. Continued growth is promoted and foresight expands, allowing the late adolescent to foresee a career line.

PSYCHOPATHOLOGY

Sullivan described a series of syndromes based on character traits that reflect persistence in or arrest of ways to protect self-esteem through successive stages of development. The degree to which one relies on such ways, and the extent to which they prove interpersonally effective or successful, accounts for the maintenance of mental health or the development of mental illness. The outcome depends on internal and external emotional pressures that persons experience at certain points in their lives. When a clinical disorder is manifested, its characteristic symptoms often parallel basic character traits that have become pathogenic; however, this is not always the case. Depending on the ability of certain character traits to meet the stress of unexpected or untoward events, the clinical manifestations of a particular disorder can differ from the traits of the character matrix. Thus, a basic histrionic personality may be found to underlie obsessive-compulsive manifestations, and an obsessive character may show histrionic symptoms. Persons who function in obsessive ways may develop a full-blown paranoid disorder when their basic modes of coping fail to maintain their self-esteem. Paranoid or schizoid individuals can display histrionic behavior.

Sullivan viewed clinical diagnosis as having a purely pragmatic function, serving as a starting point for the psychiatrist. He deplored diagnostic labeling. Instead, he believed in the application of two frames of reference. The first frame is Meyerian, in which each case is viewed in terms of liabilities and assets and one sees how the main difficulties in living compare with the degree of ability shown in dealing with complex situations. The second frame of reference consists of determining from data directly or indirectly offered by the patient the likely "grounds for therapeutic operations" and the possibilities for change conducive to a better life. Formal diagnosis and presumed fixed prognosis can obscure the collection of meaningful data about patients because what one looks for and expects to find may differ from anything else that can be found there.

TREATMENT The patient–therapist relationship involves a contractual arrangement and implicit and explicit roles. It requires that one person reveal data to another person, who uses them skillfully. The patient's characteristic patterns of living are identified and elucidated, the contribution to problems is ascertained, and potential favorable changes are explored in the patient–therapist interaction. *Participant observation* is an important requisite in psychiatric interviewing and psychotherapeutic intervention. The psychiatrist is inextricably involved in each interview, as observer and as participant, constantly influencing the developments in the field of inquiry and continuously aware of his or her influences on them.

Sullivan delineated stages of psychotherapeutic interviewing. At the *inception,* the preliminary contractual elements are established and the respective roles stipulated. During the *reconnaissance,* the patient's recurring patterns and their successful and problematic aspects are identified. This stage is followed by the *detailed inquiry,* aimed at uncovering the mostly parataxic processes contributing to the patient's difficulties and suggesting areas where subsequent inquiry can shed light. This lengthy stage of therapy entails constant reexamination of earlier elicited information and the way the data fit into or reflect each patient's development history. The detailed inquiry includes continued elements of validation, some of which are the reciprocal emotions of patient and therapist with regard to states of agreement and disagreement; delays between apparent understanding and evident inability to use it for desirable change; persistence of conflict or attempts at its resolution; and an overall assessment of progress, obstacles to it, and the potential for further gains. The last stage is *termination* or *interruption,* indicating the reaching of optimal or limited goals, depending on the evolution of the contract between the patient and therapist and their mutual views as to its fulfillment. Patients are helped to leave the therapeutic situation with as many advances toward a syntaxic mode of experience as are possible for them. Their continued growth is based on such achievement and the concomitant further broadening of their self-system.

Throughout, Sullivan pointed to the resourceful use of the therapist's skill and knowledge about interpersonal events and their impact, including intuition and inquiry, that minimize disruptive anxiety. He cautioned against inferences being taken for facts and insisted on verifying the products of the uncovering process.

He thought that only interpersonal activities are subject to real and participant observation and amenable to change. He saw optimal human development, natural or remedial, not as opportunistic, but as allowing choice for the best use of one's abilities in the face of recurring opportunities for further growth. In this sense, he even dreamed of conjunctive developments that could spread to groups and to the world at large, seeing culture and society not as an enemy of individuals, but as a reality of existence and an area of mutually contributory interaction.

Psychoanalyst Leston Havens has extended Sullivan's emphasis on the bipersonal field in psychotherapy. As did Sullivan, Havens decries the passive analytic stance, especially in dealing with character pathology. He deemphasizes interpretation as the mutative element in psychotherapy and indicates that the transference must, in many situations, be managed in a way that does not threaten the integrity of the patient or demean the patient as a person. In Haven's interpersonal approach, the language of the therapist is of utmost importance, placing the therapist with patient when necessary, distancing the therapist from the patient's projections when necessary, and also opposing the patient when clinically indicated. The therapist's empathy and attentive following of the quality of the patient–therapist interaction guide the therapy more than the formal diagnosis of the patient's psychiatric disorder.

WILHELM REICH

Wilhelm Reich (1897–1957), a brilliant man who became mentally ill in his later years, was one of Freud's most controversial followers (Fig. 7–8). Reich maintained and extended Freud's early (and later discarded) view that neurosis results from the damming up of sexual energy, and suggested that neurotic symptoms and deviant character traits result from the blockage of normal orgasm. Because neurotic symptoms do not fully discharge sexual energy, they are difficult to eradicate, and the residual energy appears as bodily tension.

Reich believed that sexual energy can also be converted into anxiety, and that undischarged energy can be released as sadism or aggression. He held that ejaculation is not a measure of true orgastic potency. A truly orgastically potent person is totally involved with the other person and achieves total release of tension and pressure in the course of the orgasm. For Reich, such orgastic potency is rare in societies that have strong barriers against sexual expression. He believed that the orgastically potent person is truly attached to the partner and that such relationships involve self-regulation of sexual desires.

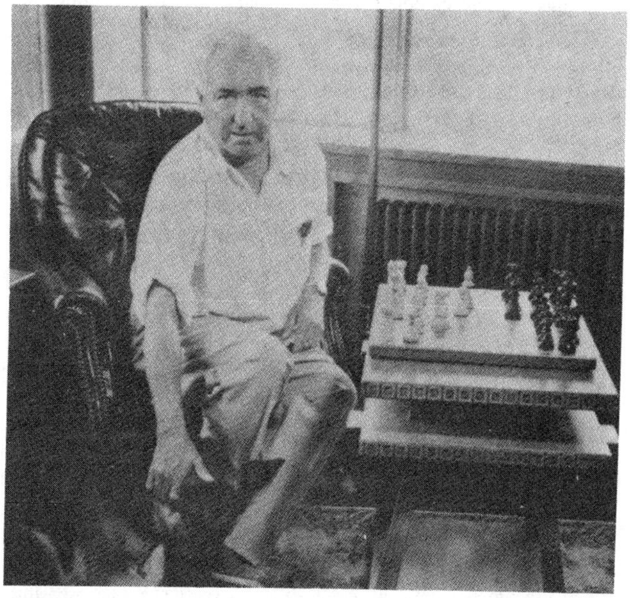

FIGURE 7-8. *Wilhelm Reich at home. (Courtesy of Farrar, Straus & Giroux, New York.)*

PERSONALITY THEORY Reich generally accepted Freud's view of personality formation, but added descriptions of interpersonal and physical behavior peculiar to each personality character type. Reich regarded those aspects of characterological behavior as part of one's character armor, with which one defends oneself against internal and external dangers. Those behaviors are important because they must be dealt with in treatment before the analysis of infantile experiences can proceed meaningfully.

In many people, habitual interpersonal behaviors or character traits defend against id impulses. Such defensive character traits are involuntary, repetitive, ego-syntonic reactions to certain situations that prevent the emergence of repressed impulses. The ingratiating person, for example, may be defending against hostile, self-assertive impulses, just as the hostile, self-asserting person may be defending against passivity and dependence. Character traits also manifest in the voluntary musculature as characteristic postures, such as excessive stiffness or fluidity of movement.

Hysterical character To Reich, the hysterical character has the least character armoring and the most lability of function. Most typical of the hysterical character is sexual or seductive behavior. The body movements of the hysterical person tend to be soft and rolling. The overall impression is one of superficiality, excitability, and flightiness. There is, however, a characteristic fearfulness and skittishness, together with high suggestibility and a tendency to easy disappointment.

According to Reich, the character armor of the hysterical person helps defend against his or her genital impulses, which are too easily aroused. The hysterical person's seductive behavior is an attempt to flush out dangerous stimuli so that they can be avoided. Thus, when a man responds positively to a female hysteric's seductive postures and remarks, she retreats and becomes hostile, unaware of her provocation and vehemently denying it when it is brought to her attention.

Persons with a hysterical character structure sublimate poorly and are not motivated toward intellectual achievement or sustained endeavors because they spend most of their time and energy avoiding dangerous situations and people.

Compulsive character Persons of this character type show inordinate concern for orderliness; are given to circumstantial, ruminative thinking; and exhibit indecision, doubt, distrust, restraint, and overcontrol. In the emotional domain, a substantial block exists between thoughts and feelings. Indeed, many of the compulsive character's behaviors, such as ruminative thinking and indecision, derive from that affect block. Affective cues allow one to assign priorities to one's actions, to make decisions, and to sense when one is becoming a bore. The compulsive character is insensitive to those cues.

In contrast to the physical lability and movement of the hysterical character, the compulsive person is tense and restrained. Facial and bodly muscles are tense. The compulsive person often sits, walks, and stands almost ramrod straight.

The compulsive character defends against loss of control over aggressive, sadistic impulses by attempting to eliminate uncertainty. Even a minor break in routine or pattern can cause great concern; the compulsive character fears the punishment and guilt that expression of instinctual impulses would stimulate if they were accidentally aroused.

Phallic-narcissistic character Outwardly, phallic-narcissistic persons appear cold, reserved, and bristly. They are outspoken and provocative, and often hold positions of power and authority in society. Reich held that phallic-narcissistic men have a partial or complete identification with the phallus (in women, with the fantasy of having a penis). Phallic-narcissistic men think of the phallus as a symbol of power and aggression. Reich argued that such men have strong erectile potency but are unable to experience true orgasmic potency. To Reich, they are frustrated at the genital exhibitionistic level of development and have a basically hostile attitude toward women.

Masochistic character Persons of a masochistic bent have a sense of lifelong suffering and tend to complain and to engage in self-damaging and self-deprecating words and actions that also provoke and torture others.

Reich argued against the traditional analytic interpretation that the masochistic person experiences displeasure (pain) as pleasure. He believed that the reverse is true and that the masochistic person finds pleasure painful. Masochists would rather have someone beat them than love them because beatings are less painful than love. Reich argued that the masochistic character has an inordinate craving for love but a low tolerance for accepting it. In proving themselves unlovable, masochists avoid the pain of being loved but are frustrated in their need for love. Masochists are in the impossible position of being hurt the most by that which they want and need the most.

TREATMENT Reich's major contribution to therapeutic practice was his indication of the need to analyze character resistances as a precondition for psychoanalysis proper. Reich thought that interpersonal issues between the patient and the therapist must be resolved before a patient can follow the basic rule of free association. He held that the character armor of the patient appears less in what the patient says than in how the words are said and the actions done. The words "I hate you" can be said aggressively and intrusively or quietly and passively. What the person says has to be interpreted in relation to the way it is said. In Reich's view, character armor is an interpersonal defense of the ego that can be used against the analyst and against treatment. Such defenses are more amenable to interpretation than those defending against id impulses and are therefore the starting point of treatment. Reich used face-to-face therapy and also attempted to deal directly with the muscular tension he called character armor. He sought to relax patients by interpreting their muscular patterns and by physical manipulation. That type of therapy, called *vegetotherapy* by Reich, is still practiced by Reich's followers under the name of *bioenergetics*.

JULES H. MASSERMAN

Jules H. Masserman, M.D. (1905–), the originator of the biodynamic approach, studied psychobiology with Adolf Meyer and psychoanalysis with Franz Alexander at the Chicago Institute for Psychoanalysis (Fig. 7-9). Biodynamics integrates the biological and dynamic aspects of all behavior. Based on his experimental studies with animals, Masserman believes, as did Horney, that all behavior originates in efforts toward individual and species survival; that each organism's patterns of adaptation result from its genetic potentialities, their various paths and speed of maturation, and its unique experiences. He finds that most frustrations are met by flexibly readjusting coping techniques or substituting goals, and that when an organism's coping capacities are overloaded by environmental uncertainties and adaptational conflicts, severe and persistent behavior changes result.

PSYCHOLOGICAL THEORY Humans defend against psychological disorganization and traumatization by three basic Ur-defenses: belief in their physical invulnerability, the fantasy that other humans are potential friends and helpers, and faith in a celestial order. They strive for physical survival, social belongingness, and cosmic identity. Environmental frustrations, cultural conflicts, or unpredictabilities in any of these physical, interpersonal, and philosophical modes of adaptation cause physiological dysfunction, social maladaptation, and existential suffering.

LABORATORY INVESTIGATIONS OF THERAPEUTIC MODES In the laboratory, Masserman has shown that pathological behavior can be induced by feeding-related

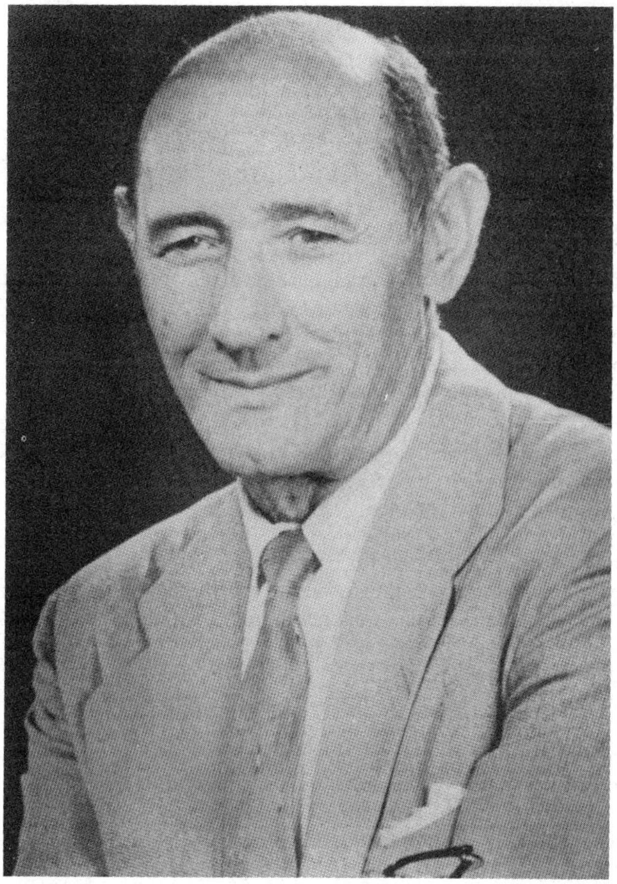

FIGURE 7-9. *Jules H. Masserman.*

stresses in monkeys, cats, and dogs—a process he calls *neurotigenesis*. The animals' means of recovery parallel the ways in which humans recover from emotional disturbances. Some laboratory animals retest formerly frustrating feeding mechanisms and work through related neurotic inhibitions and behavior in a manner similar to humans' reexploration and mastery of traumatic physical or social experiences. Other animals respond to certain therapeutic measures. For example, a hungry animal can be slowly pushed toward highly attractive food in an open reward box until its feeding and related inhibitions are overcome by its hunger. A fearful, inhibited animal placed with normal responders to the feeding situation often becomes less inhibited, as do humans in response to positive group influences. In some animals, however, the increased conflicts between attraction and aversion cause agitation and panic.

An experimenter can also retrain a neurotic animal by gentle steps: first, to take food from the experimenter's hand; next, to accept food in the experimental apparatus; then, to open the feeding box while the experimenter stays nearby; and finally, to work the formerly traumatizing switch and feed itself without further help. In terms of psychotherapy, the patient directs his or her needs for help to a therapist, who uses this transference patiently and wisely to reassure, guide, and support the patient in reexamining conflicting desires and fears, recognizing previous misinterpretations of reality, and exploring new ways of living until the patient is sufficiently successful and confident to proceed without such assistance.

TREATMENT Biodynamic therapy aims to relieve patients' immediate somatic, social, or psychological distress; to help patients realize that their former concerns or behavior patterns are no longer necessary; to guide patients into more satisfactory and profitable modes of behavior; and to help them evolve a comfortable and creative philosophy of life. To accomplish those ends, Masserman suggests a flexible schedule of therapeutic sessions that fit patients' needs and resources; judicious combinations of all forms of therapy, including specific guidance and use of drugs and physical treatment; and concentration on patient's physical, social, and attitudinal problems in the here and now with a probing of history only sufficient to clarify outmoded continued childhood patterns of behavior in and out of the therapeutic situation. He suggests joint sessions with family, friends, employers, and others to help clarify and improve a patient's interactions, and emphasizes salutary and realistic behavioral changes as the only valid indication of progress.

Masserman describes the essential parameters of psychiatric therapy as rapport, relief, review, reorientation, rehabilitation, resocialization, and recycling.

Masserman has also made a contribution to the general welfare of humanity that transcends his interest in the treatment of mental disorders. He has been an important physician spokesperson against nuclear weaponry and for the responsible use of human intelligence for the optimum benefit of all humankind.

ERIC BERNE

Eric Berne (1910–1970), who had a keen sense of humor and of history, received training in classical psychoanalysis and was particularly influenced by psychoanalyst Paul Federn (Fig. 7-10). Berne's personality did not lend itself well to the practice of psychoanalysis. As a result, he terminated his training before its completion and formulated an approach to psychopathology and psychotherapy whose basic premise was that psychopathology is developed and

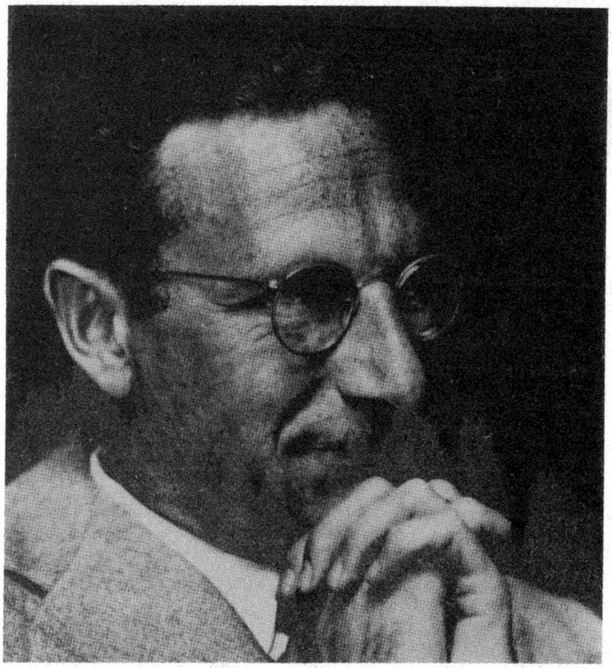

FIGURE 7-10. *Eric Berne. (Courtesy of Wide World Photos.)*

maintained in the context of relationships, and that through changing those relationships, more rewarding and satisfying ways of living can be established. He called his theory and treatment technique transactional analysis—now a worldwide movement with its own organization and publication *(The Transactional Analysis Journal).* Transactional Analysis is best understood in terms of ego states, transactions, games, strokes, scripts, and contracts.

EGO STATES Berne defined an *ego state* as a conscious cohesive system of feelings and thoughts, with a related set of behavior patterns. Each person's ego states consist of a *Child* ego state, which represents archaic elements that become fixed in early childhood but remain active through life; an *Adult,* which objectively appraises reality; and a *Parent,* an introject of the person's actual parents' values.

Berne emphasized that an archaic intuitive faculty lodged in the Child can be cultivated by the psychotherapist. A potent therapist resurrects the dormant aspect of the imaginative child. Thinking that is too adult and rational decreases the efficiency of the Child. The same holds true for prejudicial Parental thinking. Creativity based on intuition works best when the Child predominates and when the Adult and the Parent are reduced in influence.

Certain types of psychopathology are related to the structure of ego states. Delusional thinking is a breakdown of the functional barriers between the Adult and the Child, in which fantasy and archaic imagery in the Child become mixed with the Adult. For example, "People are following me," is a Child statement of fantasy and archaic ideas of importance, contaminating the actual Adult observation of people in the environment. Another major type of ego-state pathology is exclusion, the inability to cathect the different ego states freely. Thus, one remains in a Parent or Child ego state.

TRANSACTIONS AND GAMES Berne defined a *transaction* as a stimulus from an ego state of one person and the corresponding response from an ego state of another person. *Games* are stereotyped repetitive ulterior transactions with well-defined psychological payoffs. Berne devised a formula to which all games conform, in which a con and a gimmick lead to a response that is followed by a switch and a payoff. The con, or invitation to engage, is effective only if there is a gimmick that stimulates the respondent's greed, fear, or other emotional vulnerability. The response indicates that the respondent is engaged, after which the initiator makes a switch and obtains a payoff. Berne used an example from a therapy group to illustrate the differences between an aboveboard transaction and a game. In an aboveboard transaction, a group member asks, "Will I get well, doctor?" The therapist replies that there probably will be significant improvement. The patient, feeling reassured and more comfortable, says, "Thank you." The same transaction in the form of a game goes as follows:

Patient: Will I get well, doctor? (The con is the apparently straightforward question; the gimmick is the appeal to the therapist's narcissism.)
Therapist: I think you will. (The response indicates that the therapist is hooked into the game.)
Patient: What makes you think you know so much? (The switch.) Therapist says nothing, but squirms uncomfortably. (The payoff; making a fool of the therapist.)

STROKES The term "strokes" is equivalent to reinforcement. Words, glances, and other human recognitions are symbolic strokes, and the developing child learns ways to maximize the number of strokes received from the mother, father, and siblings. Ideally, strokes are obtained in a loving and positive way, but in certain families negative strokes are exchanged. Even negative strokes can be important for survival, at least temporarily, because they are better than none at all. Berne observed that stroke deficit leads to increased game playing.

SCRIPTS Success or failure in life is determined by a person's conformity to important early decisions. One becomes a winner or a loser, or develops a banal script. The life decisions that determine scripts are lodged in the Child ego state as a result of repetitive or especially strong parental injunctions, but they can be altered by redecision.

TREATMENT Berne's simple model of the mind was well received by a lay public that was pleased to learn how people create their interpersonal reality. His theory stimulated the publication of many self-help books. At a professional level, he emphasized the need for patients and therapists to agree on explicit goals for treatment, and urged therapists to examine their own role in the treatment process. He provocatively stated on many occasions that if the patient was not cured during the first session, the therapist should try to determine what went wrong. In that way, he emphasized resolving issues and getting treatment done instead of the patients continuing to make progress in a protracted treatment in which neither patient nor therapist knows where either is heading.

Berne's preferred therapeutic medium was group therapy. The active interaction that occurs in groups quickly brings out the typical interpersonal games of group members. As the ulterior transactions in games are ascertained, group members are helped through direct teaching and modeling to find better ways to meet the needs that have been met through the ulterior transactions. They are also helped to give up childish satisfactions, such as delight in frustrating others, in favor of adult satisfactions, such as loving and being loved by others.

Some of the material in this section was derived from the chapters by Otto F. Kernberg, M.D., on *Melanie Klein,* C. Jess Groesbeck, M.D., on *Carl Jung,* Miltiades L. Zaphiropolous, M.D., on *Harry Stack Sullivan,* and Alexandra Symonds, M.D. and Martin Symonds, M.D., on *Karen Horney* that appeared in the fourth edition of the *Comprehensive Textbook of Psychiatry.*

REFERENCES

Adler A: In *The Individual Psychology of Alfred Adler: A Systematic Presentation in Selections from His Writings,* H L Ansbacher, R R Ansbacher, editors. Basic Books, New York, 1956.
Adler A: In *Problems of Neurosis: A Book of Case Histories,* P. Mairet, editor. Harper & Row, New York, 1964.
Berne E: *Transactional Analysis in Psychotherapy.* Grove Press, New York, 1961.
Berne E: *Games People Play.* Grove Press, New York, 1964.
Havens L L: *Making Contact: Uses of Language in Psychotherapy.* Harvard University Press, Cambridge, MA, 1986.
Horney K: *The Neurotic Personality of Our Time.* Norton, New York, 1937.
Horney K: *Neurosis and Human Growth.* Norton, New York, 1950.
Jung C G: *Memories, Dreams, Reflections.* Random House, New York, 1961.
Jung C G: *Two Essays on Analytical Psychology.* Princeton University Press, Princeton, NJ, 1966.
Jung C G: *Symbols of Transformation,* ed 2. Princeton University Press, Princeton, NJ, 1967.

Karpf F B: *The Psychology and Psychotherapy of Otto Rank*. Philosophical Library, New York, 1953.
Klein M: Mourning and its relation to manic-depressive states. In *Contributions to Psycho-Analysis, 1921–1945*, M Klein, editor. Hogarth Press, London, 1948.
Klein M: Notes on some schizoid mechanisms. In *Developments in Psycho-Analysis,* M Klein, P Heimann, S Isaacs, J Riviere, editors, p 292. Hogarth Press, London, 1952.
Masserman J H: *Behavior and Neurosis*. Hafner Press, New York, 1963.
Masserman J H: *Theories and Therapies of Dynamic Psychiatry*. Science House, New York, 1973.
Meyer A: *Collected Papers of Adolf Meyer,* 4 vols. Johns Hopkins University Press, Baltimore, 1948–1952.
Meyer A: *Psychobiology: A Science of Man*. Charles C Thomas, Springfield, IL, 1957.
Mullahy P, editor: *The Contributions of Harry Stack Sullivan*. Hermitage House, New York, 1952.
Rado S: *Psychoanalysis of Behavior,* vols 1 and 2. Grune & Stratton, New York, 1956, 1962.
Rank O: *The Trauma of Birth*. Harper & Row, New York, 1973.
Reich W: *Character Analysis*. Farrar, Straus & Young, New York, 1949.
Segal H: *Melanie Klein*. Viking Press, New York, 1980.

CHAPTER 8 THEORIES OF PERSONALITY AND PSYCHOPATHOLOGY: SCHOOLS DERIVED FROM PSYCHOLOGY AND PHILOSOPHY

MARSHALL P. DUKE, Ph.D.
STEPHEN NOWICKI, JR., Ph.D.

INTRODUCTION

In his writings on the history and philosophy of science, Thomas Kuhn described two basic paradigms, which, he believed, characterized all true scientific disciplines. The first of these, *paradigm as a set of shared methods,* refers to the accepted experimental and scientific procedures by which a science goes about gathering data about the phenomena within its purview. The second type of paradigm, *paradigm as a set of shared beliefs,* refers to the global perspectives adopted by significant numbers of investigators within a science. These global perspectives provide guidance for the development of hypotheses, theories, and applications emerging from the specific paradigm. For example, some ancient peoples believed that abnormal behavior was caused by spirit possession; given this view, a reasonable treatment involved efforts to drive out the evil spirits. Among these efforts might be forcing the afflicted person to drink a potion composed of lamb's blood, cattle dung, and wine, or drilling a hole (or trephine) in the person's skull so that the spirits could escape. When viewed out of context, these activities certainly would not be considered therapeutic; however, when seen as derivations from a global belief about the way normal and abnormal behaviors arise, the procedures seem to follow logically. The concept of global belief and its relationship to therapeutics is embodied in the interconnection between theory and practice in the history of psychotherapy. Theories are derived not only because they help to achieve greater understanding of people's behavior, but because they guide professionals toward the development of effective treatment strategies. Similarly, methods of intervention (be they as commonsensical as Hippocrates' prescription of some quiet time in the country in the treatment of depression or as seemingly incongruous as the induction of a seizure through electric shock for the same symptom) do not emerge from thin air; they are among the natural consequences of a theory of behavior, a global belief.

Throughout the history of psychology and philosophy, numerous perspectives to explain behavior have emerged. Some of these perspectives have grown to the magnitude of theories; others have risen and then diminished in importance. All, however, have the potential to produce theoretically consistent therapeutic procedures, and the worth of these therapeutic procedures is in many ways tied intimately to the worth of the theories from which they grew.

PHILOSOPHICAL FOUNDATIONS OF MODERN PERSONALITY THEORIES

Modern accepted theories of personality and psychopathology are characterized by sophisticated conceptualizations and supported by research, but many of their roots may be traced back to nonscientific ancient philosophers. Plato has been credited with proposing one of the earliest conceptualizations of mental disorder. In the fifth century B.C., he proposed that there were only two kinds of mental disorders—madness and ignorance—and that both were attributable to physical factors:

> The disorders of the soul, which depend upon the body, originate as follows. We must acknowledge disease of the mind to be a want of intelligence; and of this there are two kinds; to wit, madness and ignorance. In whatever state a man experiences either of them, that state may be called disease; and excessive pains and pleasures are justly to be regarded as the greatest disease to which the soul is liable. For a man who is in great joy or in great pain, in his unreasonable eagerness to attain the one and to avoid the other, is not able to see or to hear anything rightly; but he is mad, and is at the time utterly incapable of any participation in reason. He who has the seed about the spinal marrow too plentiful and overflowing, like a tree overladen with fruit, has many throes, and also obtains many pleasures in his desires and their offspring, and is for the most part of his life deranged, because his pleasures and pains are so very great; his soul is rendered foolish and disordered by his body; yet he is regarded not as one diseased, but as one who is voluntarily bad, which is a mistake. The truth is that the intemperance of love is a disease of the soul due chiefly to the moisture and fluidity which is produced in one of the elements by the loose consistency of the bones. And, in general, all that which is termed the incontinence of pleasure is deemed a reproach under the idea that the wicked voluntarily do wrong. For no man is voluntarily bad; but the bad become bad by reason of an ill disposition of the body and bad education, things which are hateful to every man and happen to him against his will. And in the case of pain too in like manner the soul suffers much evil from the body.

In the true spirit of the Kuhnian description discussed above, Plato also derived a method of treatment from his global belief about personality and psychopathology:

> I dare say that you have heard eminent physicians say to a patient who comes to them with bad eyes, that they cannot cure his eyes by themselves but that if his eyes are to be cured, his head must be treated; and then again they say that to think of curing the head alone, and not the rest of the body also, is the height of folly. And arguing in this way they apply their methods to the whole body, and try to treat and heal the whole and the part together. Did you ever observe that this is what they say. . . .

> For all good and evil, whether in the body or in human nature, originates . . . in the soul, and overflows from thence, as if from the head into the eyes. And therefore if the head and body are to be well, you must begin by curing the soul; that is the first thing. And the cure, my dear youth, has to be effected by the use of certain charms, and these charms are fair works; and by them temperance is implanted in the soul, and where temperance is, there health is speedily imparted, not only to the head, but to the whole body.

A contemporary of Plato, Hippocrates, the Father of Medicine, also theorized about mental disorders, some of which he termed the "sacred diseases." Hippocrates' global belief was that all behavior was biologically based, that in the imbalance among the four bodily humours—blood, black bile, yellow bile, and phlegm—could be found the sources of individual personality variation as well as abnormal behavior patterns. Hippocrates suggested methods whereby these humours could be returned to balance, thereby restoring the person to normal. Because of the restrictions placed on dissection of the human body at the time, Hippocrates could not acquire a proper understanding of the brain and nervous system; nevertheless, his beliefs rested clearly on a biological foundation:

> Thus is this disease formed and prevails from those things which enter into and go out of the body, and it is not more difficult to understand or to cure than the others, neither is it more divine than other diseases. And men ought to know that from nothing else but thence [from the brain] come joys, delights, laughter and sports, and sorrows, griefs, despondency and lamentations. And by this, in an especial manner, we acquire wisdom and knowledge, and see and hear, and know what are foul and what are fair, what are bad and what are good, what are sweet, and what unsavory; some we discriminate by habit, and some we perceive by their utility. By this we distinguish objects of relish and disrelish, according to the seasons; and the same things do not always please us. And by the same organ we become mad and delirious, and fears and terrors assail us, some by night and some by day, and dreams and untimely wandering, and cares that are not suitable, and ignorance of present circumstances, desuetude, and unskillfulness. All these things we endure from the brain, when it is not healthy, but is more hot, more cold, more moist, or more dry than natural, or when it suffers any other preternatural and unusual affliction.

In addition to Plato and Hippocrates, both Epicurus (341–270 B.C.) and Cicero (106–43 B.C.) were noted early personality theorists. Rather than being believers in a biological paradigm, however, they clearly favored a psychological (cognitive) basis for personality and psychopathology. Epicurus, for example, wrote:

> How comes it, that Father whose Son is killed, is not a whit less cheerful or merry, if he know not of death of his son, than if he were yet alive in health? . . . Certainly, if Nature itself were the Author of that sadness, the Father's mind would be struck with a sense of loss of his Son in the same moment wherein he was slain. . . .
>
> Hence it is a perspicuous Truth, that those things for which the mind becomes malcontent and contristate, are not Real Evils to us; forasmuch as they are without the orb of our Nature, and can never touch us immediately or of themselves, but by the mediation of our own Opinion . . . It is Reason alone which makes life happy and pleasant, by expelling all such false Conceptions or Opinions, as may any way occasion perturbation of mind.

Similarly, Cicero believed that neglect of reason was the cause of mental disturbances:

> The cure of grief, and of other disorders, is one and the same, in that they are all voluntary, and founded on opinion; we take them on ourselves because it seems right so to do. Philosophy undertakes to eradicate this error as the root of all our evils: Let us therefore surrender ourselves to be instructed by it, and suffer ourselves to be cured; for whilst these evils have possession of us, we not only cannot be happy, but cannot be right in our minds.

ANGELICUS AND MAIMONIDES Following these early philosophers, there was little major change in views of mental disorder until the eleventh century, A.D. It was at, and after, this time that such people as the Christian theologian Bartholomaeus Angelicus and the Jewish philosopher Moses Maimonides proposed their views of madness and its cure.

In 1275, Angelicus proposed a completely naturalistic explanation and treatment:

> Madness cometh sometimes of passions of the soul, as of business and of great thoughts, of sorrow and of too great study, and of dread: sometime of the biting of a wood hound, or some other venomous beast: sometime of melancholy meats, and sometime of drink of strong wine. And as the causes be diverse, the tokens and signs be diverse. For some cry and leap and hurt and wound themselves and other men, and darken and hide themselves in privy and secret places. The medicine of them is, that they be bound, that they hurt not themselves and other men. And namely, such shall be refreshed, and comforted, and withdrawn from cause and matter of dread and bury thoughts. And they must be gladded with instruments of music, and somedeal be occupied.

Angelicus' approach represents a good example of the intimate relationship between theory and practice of psychotherapy. Without the theoretical belief in naturalistic causes of madness, Angelicus' treatments might sound preposterous, even bizarre; given his theory, one can understand why he treated people as he did, even though today his treatments seem unusual.

Rather than a naturalistic perspective, Maimonides (1135–1204) assumed a more spiritual and moral basis for personality and psychopathology. He scorned the use of physical treatments, and prescribed cures that were much more psychological:

> Let us take, for example, the case of a man in whose soul there has developed a disposition [of great avarice] on account of which he deprives himself [of every comfort in life], and which, by the way, is one of the most detestable of defects, and an immoral act, as we have shown in this chapter. If we wish to cure this sick man, we must not command him merely [to practice] deeds of generosity, for that would be as ineffective as a physician trying to cure a patient consumed by a burning fever by administering mild medicines, which treatment would be inefficacious. We must, however, induce him to squander so often, and to repeat his acts of profusion so continuously until that propensity which was the cause of his avarice has totally disappeared. Then, when he reaches that point where he is about to become a squanderer, we must teach him to moderate his profusion, and tell him to continue with deeds of generosity, and to watch out with due care lest he relapse either into lavishness or niggardliness.

THE CONTRIBUTIONS OF MESMER Although the thoughts and methods of Maimonides were somewhat controversial in their time, they eventually came to be recognized as important contributions to the awareness of behavior and its underpinnings. The same could be said of Anton Mesmer, who lived during the eighteenth and nineteenth centuries. In many ways, Mesmer was a forerunner of the modern era of psychotherapy. His theoretical notions regarding animal magnetism and the power of the moon were clearly in error, but his therapeutic efforts based on suggestion, trust, and belief in a healer were certainly akin to many modern therapeutic practices. As such, his ideas may be seen as being among the major philosophical foundations for modern theories of personality and psychotherapy. A historian of psychotherapy, Jan Ehrenwald, described Mesmer's importance quite well:

> Anton Mesmer (1734–1815), the Austrian-born physician, discoverer of "animal magnetism" as a new principle of psychotherapy, was a contemporary of Philippe Pinel, the great French reformer of psychiatry and advocate of more humanitarian care for the mentally ill. But the gulf between the two men seems unbridgeable. Mesmer was little concerned with mental disease. He regarded all illnesses as the manifestations of disturbances in a mysterious ethereal fluid

which linked together animate and inanimate things alike, and which made man equally subject to the influences of the stars and to those influences emanating from Dr. Mesmer himself. This is what Mesmer described as animal, in contrast to "ordinary," magnetism. His theories thus reach back to ancient astrological concepts. But it was in his practical approach to the patient that Mesmer hit upon a discovery of prodigious consequences. It was the discovery that by applying what he believed to be magnetic passes or other manipulations, he was capable of inducing peculiar trance-like conditions—or else convulsive crises—in his patients. Sometimes these magnetic influences resulted in spectacular cures of such apparently organic disorders as blindness, convulsions, paralyses or "congestions" of the liver or spleen.

One of the by-products of Mesmer's labors was his discovery of a peculiar "rapport" between the therapist and his patient. This too he ascribed to the operation of his all-pervading animal magnetism. He was not aware of the essentially psychological nature of the bond. One of his patients, a Miss Paradis, aged eighteen, whose blindness he claimed he had cured with his magnetic method, apparently fell in love with him. Mesmer himself, caught in the trap of her devotion—her "positive transference"—incurred the wrath of her outraged family and the censure of the medical profession. As a result of the ensuing scandal he had to leave his beautiful mansion in Vienna with its famous fishpond and magnetized trees. He fled to Paris in 1778. There he rose once more to fame-and-notoriety until in 1784 the French Academy of Science passed a devastating verdict on the claims made by him and his pupil Dr. d'Eslon.

The committee included such famous names as Jean Sylvain Bailly, Benjamin Franklin and Dr. Guillotin. They found that his results were essentially based on his patients' imagination or due to mechanical friction, imitation and the like. But there is one important fact which the learned committee (and subsequent equally learned committees) failed to realize: Mesmerism, although it was founded on thoroughly unscientific premises, was, in effect, a new method of psychotherapy. It was the first step toward the development of scientific hypnotism, hypnoanalysis and our current psychoanalytic methods of treatment.

History has been more generous in acknowledging Mesmer's share in this development than the various committees appointed to investigate his claims. There are few authors in the annals of mental healing whose contributions to the field have been quoted by so many as those of the discoverer of animal magnetism. But few have been read so little.

Following the work of Mesmer, the more recent and sophisticated ideas of Bleuler, Freud, and the other psychoanalysts came on the therapeutic scene. Somewhere between the late eighteenth century and the mid-nineteenth century, philosophy gave birth to its scientific offspring, psychology, and the theories of personality and psychopathology that continued to emerge smacked much more of the science of psychology than of the discipline of philosophy.

EARLY THEORISTS OF PERSONALITY AND PSYCHOTHERAPY

Many of the historically influential perspectives on personality and psychotherapy continue to be important as parts of current theories. This continuity serves as evidence that the nature of psychological inquiry is a process existing over time rather than at any given point in time.

GORDON ALLPORT **History** Born in Indiana, Gordon Allport (1897–1967) received his B.A. and Ph.D. degrees at Harvard University. He studied in Germany and England before he returned to the United States to pursue a teaching and research career. Allport was probably the first person to teach a personality course at a U.S. college or university. A very active figure in the development of American psychology, he served as president of the American Psychological Association (APA) in 1939. For his services to the discipline of psychology, he was given the APA's Distinguished Scientific Award in 1964. In 1967, Allport was rated as having the greatest impact on the field of psychology (except for Freud).

Concepts One of the first clearly recognizable personality theorists, Allport is often credited with defining the field in his 1937 book, *Personality*. He believed in the integrity of the individual and saw the study of the individual as being at the very heart of the study of personality. Presaging many modern personality theorists, Allport emphasized the need for the eclectic study of people's behavior. He felt that personality was not purely within the purview of psychology or psychiatry, but that religion, the liberal arts, and many other areas of inquiry also had much to offer.

At the core of Allport's theory of personality was the self, which was considered to be the primary focus of growth and development and the source of psychopathology. Allport believed that the self developed through a number of stages, beginning with the early self in infancy and progressing through awareness of body, self-identity, ego enhancement, self-extension, and self-image (in adolescence), to a sense of rational self and a goal-directed self (in adulthood). The sense of self as a "becoming" entity was termed the *proprium* by Allport; it was considered to be the basic source of personality unification and integrity maintenance.

Besides the "self," Allport also considered *traits* to be major units of personality structure as well as important forces in human motivation. He described these characteristic ways of behaving as existing at both the population level (common traits) and the individual level (personal dispositions). Further, these traits could fit within one of three levels of potency in determining behavior—cardinal, central, or secondary. *Cardinal traits* are broad qualities of people that characterize the majority of their behaviors; an example would be morality. A *central trait* is less general, but still covers a broad set of qualities; an example would be reliability. Finally, the most specific characteristics are seen as *secondary traits*, being tied most clearly to situations; an example might be athletic aggressiveness. Taken together, these types of traits result in a personal disposition that Allport considered the essence of personality.

Although traits per se were considered crucial elements of personality by Allport, specific or normal traits were not his primary concern. Many kinds of traits could be associated with a well-functioning individual; for Allport, the key term was not "normality versus abnormality" but "maturity versus immaturity." Mature persons were considered able to relate warmly and effectively to others, and were emotionally secure, accepting, and aware of themselves and the outside world. Such people typically manifested verve, enthusiasm, insight, and humor, and appeared to have a unified philosophy of life. The absence of these characteristics was typically associated with immaturity and the immature personality experienced more frustrations and difficulties in functioning.

Treatment applications Given his personality theory, Allport saw abnormal behavior as being a reflection of maladaptive traits, or of a poorly developed sense of self, or both. Under this view, treatment efforts would be directed at helping individuals to assess and rectify their self-development and to direct them toward the development of more effective personality styles.

HENRY MURRAY **History** Born in New York, Henry Murray (1893–1988) trained as a physician at Columbia University. He spent his early postgraduate years studying embryology and biochemistry in the United States and England and received a Ph.D. degree in biochemistry from Cambridge University. However, his studies and personal experiences led him to focus on psychology. He returned to the United States and became actively involved in the newly developing Harvard Psychological Clinic, the social relations department at Harvard, and the Boston Psychoanalytic Society (which he helped to found). Murray received both the Distinguished Scientist Award and the Gold Medal Award of the APA.

Concepts Joining Allport as a major contributor to early personality theory, Murray coined the term "personology" for the study of personality. As an advocate of interdisciplinary approaches to the study of human behavior, Murray believed that the study of personology should involve physical and social, as well as psychological, emphases. For him, personology represented an opportunity for the broad and creative study of people's behavior patterns; he was open to bold theorizing and innovative methodologies throughout his career.

Murray conceptualized personality as a hypothetical structure composed of internal and external *proceedings* (units of time during which attention is focused on particular events or circumstances). Ongoing behavior was seen as a reflection of these proceedings, some of which represented planned, goal-oriented activities, and others of which indicated reactions to spontaneously occurring events. Murray believed that people were continuously faced with conflicts between internal and external demands and that, in many ways, personality represented a systematic, integrated, and holistic compromise among the many forces affecting each individual.

In Murray's system, internal forces are called *needs* and external forces (pressures) are called *press*. Behavioral units are called *actones* and are seen as being expressed in various patterns termed *vectors*. Both inherent or primary needs, such as food, water, sex, and elimination, as well as learned or secondary needs, like achievement, dominance, nurturance, and affection, interact to produce specific behaviors. In addition to interacting with each other, primary and secondary needs also interact with the pressures of the outside world in the form of *alpha press* (the reality of the outside world) or *beta press* (the subjective interpretation of that reality). For example, to a person with a high need for achievement, a steep cliff may represent a real danger (alpha press), but also may be seen as a challenge (beta press). Over the course of development, Murray theorized, needs and press combine to become *themas*, or powerful motivational components that tend to characterize people over long periods of time. Murray believed that the thema was the proper molar unit for study by personologists. To uncover these themas, he developed the widely used Thematic Apperception Test (TAT), which, through a projective modality, allowed for analysis of dominant themas in people's functioning.

Although Murray's conceptualization of motivation and his belief in personology were quite new in their time, he was also quite strongly tied to the earlier psychoanalytic view of behavior and personality development. Like Freud, Murray believed in a tripartite psychic structure of id, ego, and superego. Each of these components was seen in essentially the same way as Freud saw them, except for the superego, which Murray appears to have seen as more changeable throughout life. Murray also believed in a stage theory of development paralleling Freud's. However, in addition to the oral, anal, and phallic stages, Murray added the *claustral stage*, a tranquil period of prenatal existence, and the *urethral stage*, which occurs between the oral and anal phases and is characterized by urethral eroticism. Again following Freud, Murray proposed that various patterns of adult personality could be traced to lack of resolution of a particular psychosexual developmental stage. Reflecting his added concepts, he hypothesized that the claustral complex was characterized by passive dependency with a tendency to withdraw while the urethral complex was marked by extreme ambition, narcissism, and a prominent concern for achieving immortality. It should be noted that the urethral complex is also sometimes known as the Icarus complex because of the pattern of behavior associated with it.

Treatment applications Murray's conceptualization of psychopathology derives from his view of normal behavior. That is, either there has been some form of maldevelopment of the id-ego-superego structure, a fixation at or lack of resolution of one of the psychosexual stages, or a maladaptive needs–press conflict or thema. His Freudian-based ideas do not yield a new conception of abnormality, and so they will not be expanded on here. Rather, the focus will be on need–press conflicts. When needs are in conflict with one another or do not mesh properly with the demands of the outside world, people experience tension. For example, people who have a strong need for dominance and an equally intense need for affiliation may experience internal conflicts when the realities of the outside world allow for satisfaction of one need, but not both. According to Murray's thinking, therapeutic interventions focus on identifying the conflicting or inordinately intense needs and on changing beta press (people's own interpretations of the world). Anticipating the present-day cognitive theory approaches, Murray suggested that helping people to interpret the world correctly can often significantly alter their troublesome reactions to it.

KURT LEWIN

History Born in Prussia, Kurt Lewin (1890–1947) received his Ph.D. degree at the University of Berlin in 1914. He subsequently rose to professorial rank at the university, where he was closely associated with the founders of Gestalt psychology. Because his fame had become international, when Hitler came to power, Lewin moved permanently to the United States and taught at both Cornell University and the University of Iowa. The last 12 years of Lewin's life were spent at the Massachusetts Institute of Technology as professor and director of the Research Center for Group Dynamics.

Concepts Murray was not alone in his belief that personality resulted from an interaction of environmental and intrapersonal factors. Lewin, the founder of *field theory*, agreed, theorizing that people function within *fields*, defined as "the totality of coexisting facts which are conceived of as mutually interdependent." Lewin offered a formula to reflect his belief that behavior was determined by an interaction between personality and environment.

In Lewin's formula, $B = f(P, E)$, where B refers to behavior, P refers to the person, and E describes the environment. Person–environment interactions take place in what Lewin called the *life space*, a dynamic area in which are placed all factors affecting an individual at a given point in time. The life space is separate from the rest of the internal and external world. Further, the environment component does not necessarily reflect the real world, but rather represents a psychological environment as the person experiences it. Within the life space, people are motivated by *needs* that result in tension, which may be reduced through action or thought. Depending on need states, the life space takes on *valences*, which may be either positive, neutral, or negative. Without conflicts, people will approach positively valenced goals, avoid negatively valenced goals, and ignore neutral goals. However, sometimes goals are in conflict; for example, there may be two positively valenced objects in different parts of the life space—the person cannot approach one without distancing himself or herself from the other. The result is a *dynamic conflict*, which produces increased tension, and this tension, in turn, leads to efforts to restore system equilibrium. Lewin described a number of common types of conflict, several of which are depicted in Table 8-1. In the methods available or used to deal with such conflicts may be found the sources of the rich variety of normal and abnormal behavior variation.

From the Lewinian perspective, an individual's behavior results from an interaction of many factors. In anticipation of modern systems theory, he believed that to understand a person (or group—Lewin introduced the term "group dynamics"), one must understand how internal perceptions and external system membership affect that person. Adjustment represents the ability to satisfy basic needs within the confines and context of one's life space. In contrast, maladjustment involves the inability to resolve the significant conflicts. Conflicts can be internally generated, externally generated, or both, and are necessary, but not sufficient, determinants of

TABLE 8-1
Common Conflicts Within Lewin's Field Theory

Approach-approach conflict: There are two positively valenced goals; however, only one can be attained at the given moment. A choice must be made, for example, between chocolate ice cream and strawberry ice cream.

Avoidance-avoidance conflict: There are two negatively valenced goals; neither is desirable and the individual desires to avoid both. Typically, there is an intense desire to "flee the field," as in the situation where a person must go through a painful procedure in order to reduce the pain of a decayed tooth.

Approach-avoidance conflict: There are both positive and negative valences associated with one goal and the individual both is drawn to it and repulsed by it. The individual must either lose the good, if the choice is to avoid, or face the bad, if the choice is to approach, as in an adolescent standing up to a bully.

Double (multiple) approach-avoidance conflict: There are two (or more) goals, each of which has both positive and negative valences. The individual must choose which to move toward, knowing that to move toward the good of one also results in the loss of the positive aspects of the other. An example would be choosing which of several potential dates to ask to a major social event.

maladjustment. For maladjustment, people must be unable to resolve conflicts that result in inordinately high or chronic states of tension (anxiety).

Treatment applications Psychotherapy based on Lewin's thinking follows logically from his basic notions. Psychotherapists must help people to identify their needs, to increase or clarify the resources in their life space for meeting those needs, and to learn better ways of resolving conflict.

Although its implications for the understanding of individual behavior are great, Lewin's field theory has had its most significant impact on the study of group behavior. Coining the now widely used term "group dynamics," Lewin theorized that groups needed to be studied through the interrelationships among their parts. In addition to being affected by their members, groups are affected by cultural, political, and economic factors; to fully understand any group's process, all of these factors must be considered. Lewin also noted that the relationship between a group and its members is bidirectional; not only do its members affect the group, but the group affects its members. Through controlled, systematic application of the group's effects on its members, Lewin was able to bring about a number of changes in members' levels of sensitivity and abilities to work with others. Under the auspices of the National Training Laboratory, these specialized training, or T, groups evolved as a major outgrowth of Lewin's global view of human behavior.

RAYMOND CATTELL

History Although Raymond Cattell (1905–) has had a tremendous effect on U.S. psychology, he did not come to the United States until he had completed his formal education in England, where he received his Ph.D. and doctor of science degrees from the University of London. During the first 3 decades of his academic career, most of which was spent at the University of Illinois, he was responsible for 22 books and monographs, 12 tests, and 250 articles. His productivity continued after his retirement in 1973. Cattell was a founder and first president of the Society for Multivariate Experimental Psychology. In 1953, he was awarded the Wenner-Gran Prize of the New York Academy of Sciences.

Concepts Lewin's emphasis on the environment as a source of behavioral variation suggested that people respond differently depending on situations, and thus consistency in behavior may stem from consistency in environments. An alternative view is that behavioral consistency derives from some set of consistent traits to be found within individuals. Although Allport described such qualities, Cattell was one of the first persons to study them systematically. More than anyone else, Cattell was responsible for the "scientizing" of personality research and theory. He distinguished among three methods in personality research: bivariate, clinical, and multivariate. Of these three methods, he proposed that the multivariate was the most desirable. The bivariate method, in which two variables were isolated for study, was rejected because of its piecemeal nature and limited reflection of the real world. Clinical research methods, although more naturalistic, were decried because they lacked rigor and objectivity. It was the multivariate approach that Cattell fancied most as he believed it combined the holism of the clinical method with the objectivity of the controlled bivariate designs, and from it he developed his trait theory of personality and his scientific methods of measuring individual differences.

Cattell proposed two types of personality traits—surface traits and source traits. *Surface traits* are an infinite number of simple sets of behaviors that tend to occur together. An example would be the characteristic way in which a person acts when with a close friend. By contrast, *source traits* are more limited in number and represent the underlying building blocks of personality. It is out of source traits that the specific components of surface traits are derived. Cattell developed the 16-PF Inventory to measure 16 source traits (Table 8-2) in normal populations and the Clinical Analysis Questionnaire to measure source traits that are more often found in abnormal populations. True to his empirical beliefs, Cattell proposed that psychopathology can be indicated by extreme scores or specific patterns of scores on his objective measures. It should be clear that his approach laid the foundation for the later development and wide usage of other objective tests, such as the Minnesota Multiphasic Personality Inventory (MMPI). For example, Cattell identified eight primary factors involved in neuroses—ego weakness, submissiveness, desurgency, threctia, premsia, guilt proneness, inadequate self-sentiment development, and ergic tension.

Cattell also proposed that there are forces motivating the appearance of trait-based behaviors. Specifically, he proposed 10 biologically based drives called *ergs,* and a number of culturally based motives called *sentiments.* The ergs include hunger, thirst, sex, gregariousness, parental protectiveness, curiosity, fear, acquisitiveness, self-assertion, and narcissistic sex. Representative sentiment sources are career, religion, parents, and the self.

Like Lewin, Cattell believes that conflict is a major source of psychopathology. However, for Cattell, conflict takes place when differing ergs or sentiments act on an individual. The degree of conflict is determined by the relative strengths of these competing drives. Cattell even quantified conflict into a dynamic specification equation, which represents the overall conflict present in an individual personality.

Treatment Treatment of conflict depends not so much on the observed symptom picture as on the various source traits that combine to produce maladaptive behaviors. It is Cattell's contention, for example, that although the surface traits of neurosis may be similar among individuals, the source traits may vary. As treatment involves changing source traits, psychotherapy may differ for different people who have the same symptom pattern. Specific treatment focuses on the correction of primary neurotic factors, such as ergic tension, inadequate self-sentiment development, guilt proneness, and submissiveness.

WILLIAM SHELDON

History From his rural background in Rhode Island, William H. Sheldon (1899–1977) rose to prominence in American psychology. His undergraduate education was at Brown University, and he went on to obtain both a Ph.D. and an M.D. degree from the University of Chicago. He taught at a number of prominent universities, including Wisconsin and Harvard. He trained

TABLE 8-2
Brief Descriptions of Some Primary Source Traits Found by Factor Analysis

	Technical Labels			
Low-Score Description	*Low Pole*	*High Pole*	*Standard Symbol*	*High-Score Description*
Reserved/detached/critical/cool	Schizothymia	Affectothymia	A	Outgoing/warmhearted/easy-going/participating
Less intelligent/concrete thinking	Low general mental capacity	Intelligence	B	More intelligent/abstract thinking/bright
Affected by feelings/emotionally less stable/easily upset	Lower ego	Higher ego	C	Emotionally stable/faces reality/calm
Phlegmatic/relaxed	Low excitability	High excitability	D	Excitable/strident/attention seeking
Humble/mild/obedient/conforming	Submissiveness	Dominance	E	Assertive/independent/aggressive/stubborn
Sober/prudent/serious/taciturn	Desurgency	Surgency	F	Happy-go-lucky/heedless/gay/enthusiastic
Expedient/a law to one's self/bypasses obligations	Low superego strength	Superego strength	G	Conscientious/persevering/staid/rule-bound
Shy/restrained/diffident/timid	Threctia	Parmia	H	Venturesome/socially bold/uninhibited/spontaneous
Tough-minded/self-reliant/realistic/no-nonsense	Harria	Premsia	I	Tender minded/dependent/overprotected/sensitive
Trusting/adaptable/free of jealousy/easy to get on with	Alazia	Protension	L	Suspicious/self-opinionated/hard to fool
Practical/careful/conventional/regulated by external realities/proper	Praxernia	Autia	M	Imaginative/preoccupied with inner urgencies/careless of practical matters, Bohemian
Forthright/natural/artless/sentimental	Artlessness	Shrewdness	N	Shrewd/calculating/worldly/penetrating
Placid/self-assured/confident/serene	Untroubled adequacy	Guilt prone	O	Apprehensive/worried/depressive/troubled
Conservative/respecting established ideas/tolerant of traditional difficulties	Conservatism	Radicalism	Q-1	Experimental/critical/liberal/analytical/free thinking
Group dependent/a joiner and sound follower	Group adherence	Self-sufficiency	Q-2	Self-sufficient/prefers to make decisions/resourceful
Casual/careless of protocol/untidy/follows own urges	Weak self-sentiment	Strong self-sentiment	Q-3	Controlled/socially precise/self-disciplined/compulsive
Relaxed/tranquil/torpid/unfrustrated	Low ergic tension	High ergic tension	Q-4	Tense/driven/overwrought/fretful

Table from Cattell R B: Personality theory derived from quantitative experiment. In *Comprehensive Textbook of Psychiatry,* ed 3, vol 1, H I Kaplan, A M Freedman, B J Sadock, editors, p 852. Williams & Wilkins, Baltimore, 1980, with permission.

with both Jung and Kretschmer, both of whom had a significant effect on his constitutional personality theories.

Concepts Although personality was considered a basically psychological and experiential phenomenon by many of the early theorists, a few thinkers believed that it was determined by biological–physical factors. These constitutional theorists, exemplified by such writers as Sheldon and Ernst Kretschmer, believed that a significant relationship exists between physical condition and behavior. Constitutional theories have their roots in biological approaches, such as Hippocrates' theory of bodily humours, eighteenth and nineteenth century physiognomy (the relationship between character and outward appearance), and late nineteenth century phrenology.

Sheldon believed that there were three basic *somatotypes,* or courses of bodily development, through which individuals pass in a dynamic fashion throughout their lives. These three processes are *endomorphy, mesomorphy,* and *ectomorphy*. Endomorphic people are thought to develop predominantly from the inner or endodermal embryonic layer. They are round bodied and tend to be heavier than the other types. Mesomorphy is believed to arise out of the middle or mesodermal embryonic layer and is marked by overdevelopment of muscular tissue and athletic physique. Finally, the ectomorph, related to emergence from the external or ectodermal layer, is characterized by increased development of skin surface and nervous system; such persons are fragile, thin, and linear. Sheldon believed that few pure forms of these somatotypes existed, but that each person represented each of the three types to some degree. He developed a somatotype scoring system in which a number from 1 to 7 was assigned to each somatotype component, in the order of endomorphy, mesomorphy, and ectomorphy. For example, 117 would describe an almost pure ectomorph, and 333 would apply to a person who had some characteristics of all three body types.

In addition to describing body form, Sheldon believed that his typology could also explain personality patterns. Each somatotype was seen as being associated with a particular set of behaviors. Endomorphic persons were described as possessing a viscerotonic temperament; they were seen as relaxed, friendly, tolerant, positive, food and comfort loving, and extraverted. Mesomorphs possessed a different set of qualities, termed a somatotonic temperament. These persons were described as bold, risk seeking, assertive, dominant, callous, action oriented, and macho. Finally, the ectomorphic person possessed a cerebrotonic temperament, marked by restraint, apprehensiveness, tension, secretiveness, and introversion. To the degree that each somatotype was represented physically, each of these sets of characteristics was represented in the personality; in this manner, the rich variety of normal personality patterns could be understood within Sheldon's framework.

Treatment applications From the point of view of constitutional theory, maladjustment arises from two sources. First, there may be a genetic predisposition to a particular extreme and maladaptive somatotype and its accompanying personality characteristics. Second, there may be a failure to accept the personality pattern required by one's bodily structure. This problem can result in poor self-image, self-hate, conflict, anxiety, or depression. Therapeutic intervention based on constitutional theory involves such rather global efforts as social programs to improve heredity, thereby avoiding the development of maladaptive somatotypes, and individual help in adjusting to one's body structure.

KURT GOLDSTEIN **History** Born and educated in Germany, Kurt Goldstein (1878–1965), after receiving his M.D. degree from the University of Breslau, studied neurological disorders in both Frankfort and Berlin. He directed a series of long-term studies of soldiers who suffered brain injuries during World War I. In 1935, Goldstein left Germany to come to the United States and Tufts Medical School. Although he retired from Tufts in 1945, he remained active as a clinician and teacher in New York City until his death.

Goldstein received numerous honors during his lifetime. He gave the William James lectures at Harvard University in 1939 and was awarded an honorary doctorate by the University of Frankfurt in 1958. He also was one of the founders of the Association for Humanistic Psychology.

Concepts Whereas Sheldon and the other constitutional theorists seemed to focus most heavily on specific constitutional characteristics, it was clear to other thinkers that one could not really separate physical components from mental or psychological aspects of behavior. Such a global belief, termed the *holistic* or *organismic* approach, found one of its earliest proponents in the theoretical work of Goldstein. After studying thousands of people who had suffered some form of organic brain damage, Goldstein put forth the proposal that people are complex, self-regulatory systems capable of healthy development toward maturity so long as they are presented with an environment filled with minimally threatening opportunities that stimulate growth. Anticipating some of the later humanistic points of view, Goldstein also believed that people were motivated by a drive toward *self-actualization* and needed to be free to express themselves in their own preferred ways. However, rather than seeing the thwarting of free expression as the source of pathology, it was Goldstein's belief that behavioral disturbances were efforts on the part of individuals to restore their total being to a state of natural and rightful integrity.

Goldstein's views of personality and psychopathology stemmed from his basic belief about the nature of human beings. He assumed that each individual possesses a genuine creative power, which is manifested in the need that he believed underlies all human behavior—the need for self-actualization. Although the need to self-actualize is universal, Goldstein contended, everyone is different because of each person's unique set of expressions of this drive. According to one's likes and skills, one develops a special set of behaviors and characteristics that represent movement toward a state of self-actualization. The degree to which a person succeeds or fails to achieve this desired state depends on three major concepts—coming to terms, figure and ground, and abstract versus concrete behavior.

To function effectively and to grow, Goldstein believed, people needed continuously to come to terms with, or adjust to, environmental challenges (mildly threatening events). As their ability to deal with the variety of these challenges increases, so also do their chances for self-actualization. A major source of challenges may be found in the constant shift between figure and ground in the environment. Individuals must develop the capacity to shift smoothly between what is important at a given moment (figure) and what is contextual (ground), and to integrate an appropriate response to ongoing situations. Inability to shift between figure and ground (that is, to perceive the world accurately) is associated with maladaptive patterns of behavior.

Coming to terms with the environment and shifting figure and ground certainly are important concepts, but many believe that Goldstein's most significant contribution lies in his focus on abstract versus concrete reactions to situational demands. He proposed that the ability to react with appropriate abstraction or concreteness as situations demand is a cardinal requirement for self-actualization. Thought, consideration, evaluation, and the like were considered abstract reactions, whereas overt behavior was considered concrete. Psychological maturity was characterized by the ability to adopt what Goldstein termed an *abstract attitude,* a pattern of coming to terms with situations that involved taking several points of view into account when making decisions, shifting easily from one point of view to another when necessary, being able to derive common properties of seemingly disparate situations, and planning ahead effectively. Failure to adopt this abstract attitude was considered by Goldstein to be the most prominent indicator of disruption in the process of self-actualization.

Treatment applications Goldstein proposed that psychopathology represented a disruption in the process of self-actualization, a failure to come to terms with environmental situations (for example, denying that one's capacities have been limited by brain damage), a breakdown in figure–ground shifting (as in the inability to identify the salient characteristics of situations), and the ascendence of a concrete approach to problem solving instead of an abstract stance (as in using drugs or alcohol or acting out in some other way rather than dealing with problems through higher mental processes). Traditional psychiatric symptoms often appear as a result of what Goldstein called *catastrophic reactions,* designed to maintain the integrity of the organism; examples of such reactions would be the total withdrawal sometimes seen in psychotic individuals or the rigidly ordered and deviation-free patterns sometimes adopted by those with milder disturbances. In general, Goldstein believed that the same processes motivate and underlie health and illness. The difference between the normal and the abnormal individual is that the abnormal person comes to terms with the world in ways that block self-actualization, whereas the healthy person comes to terms in ways that promote self-actualization or prevent its disruption.

Goldstein's organismic approach to personality derived from his belief that all aspects of living, whether normal and adjustive or abnormal and maladaptive, could be understood only from the perspective of a total organism. No subsystem of human functioning exists in isolation; each subsystem (including physical, familial, social, cultural, and psychological) affects and is affected by each of the others. Goldstein called this interrelationship *holocenosis* and proposed that it provided a way of understanding the psychological aspects of the behavior patterns found in the brain-damaged persons with whom he worked. From this holistic point of view, symptoms have functional significance for the entire organism, not just one malfunctioning part. It would follow, therefore, that treatments focused only on circumscribed problem areas would be inadequate.

GARDNER MURPHY **History** Although Gardner Murphy (1895–1979) was born in the Midwest, he received his graduate training and spent his professional life in the Northeast, obtaining his Ph.D. degree from Columbia University and continuing his postdoctoral training at Harvard University. His many professional activities included being a consultant to the United Nations at the invitation of the Indian government. He was president of the APA (1972), director of research at the Menninger Foundation, and a professor of psychology at George Washington University. His broad range of activities and persistent efforts to help others gained him the Gold Medal Award of the American Psychological Foundation in 1972.

Concepts Sharing with Goldstein the belief that a full understanding of personality is only possible through the integration of psychological and biological factors, Murphy proposed the *biosocial theory* of behavior. He was an intentional eclectic, believing that theorists should draw from all areas of psychology and experience in the effort to understand personality development and psychopathology; in his early years, this philosophy led him to an involvement with social psychology, learning theory, and Gestalt psychology, and, in his later years, to parapsychology and transpersonal theory. Beginning with his classic text (with Friedrich Jensen) *Approaches to Personality,* published in 1923, Murphy carried his eclectic approach to the highest level of development.

Murphy's biosocial theory of personality, published most completely in 1947, is based on his belief that people are biological organisms that maintain a reciprocal relationship with their material and social environments. Personality is considered to be a result of the dynamic interaction between internal and external forces:

> Man is a nodal region, an organized field within a larger field, a region of perpetual interaction, a reciprocity of outgoing and incoming energies. [A person is] a structured organism-environment field, each aspect of which stands in dynamic relation to other aspects. . . .

Other theorists (notably Lewin) had proposed similar concepts regarding the person-environment interaction, but Murphy was singular in his heavy commitment to the biological aspects of behavior. As C. Hall and G. Lindzey so tersely put it: "The facts and principles of genetics, embryology and biochemistry are as central for Murphy as are the facts and principles of experimental psychology, sociology and cultural anthropology."

Murphy proposed that personality is first of all a function of inherited physiological dispositions, which, in the form of organic traits, result in the development of certain tissue needs or tensions; these needs, he proposed, were "the ultimate elements in personality structure." Through the process of learning (conditioning), these organic traits are reworked into symbolic traits so that, for example, the tissue-based need for food evolves into a drive to obtain the means to acquire food. Social factors also come into play at this point because society and culture also determine the manner in which the physiological needs are satisfied. Through the process Murphy called *canalization* (after Janet), only certain forms of goal-attainment behavior are acceptable. Thus, for example, only certain foods will be considered acceptable and only specific modes of attaining those foods will be included in the behavioral repertoire. Murphy proposed that all personality traits are organic traits that have been conditioned and canalized into specific forms of behavior—which is the essence of his biosocial theory.

Other important concepts in Murphy's theory are roles, the self, and ego. By a *role,* Murphy meant a fixed way of satisfying tissue needs that is forced on a person by the culture. The *self* was defined as a person's perceptions and conceptions of his or her whole being, "the individual as known to the individual." In fact, Murphy conceived of a multiple of selves dealing interactively with one another, sometimes in concert, other times in conflict. Finally, the *ego* in Murphy's system defined a system of habitual activities that enhanced or defended the self; among these were classic defense mechanisms such as identification, rationalization, and compensation.

The development of personality was seen by Murphy as a three-stage process. In the first stage, that of undifferentiated wholeness *(the global stage),* the individual reacts to situations and stimulation as a whole, such as the infant who becomes generally disrupted in response to hunger in the same manner as in response to other discomfort. In the second stage *(the differentiated stage),* separate responses and need satisfaction modes become differentiated and are clearly distinguishable. In the third and final stage *(the integrated stage),* the differentiated functions are blended together in an organized and coordinated unity. Murphy believed that the achievement of the third stage of development was certainly desirable, but he also noted that under varying circumstances of situation or adjustment, people could regress to earlier stages. In part, this regression was associated with maladaptive behavior patterns, but it could also be part of normal responses to tissue needs, learning, or canalization.

Treatment applications According to his views of personality structure and development, it appears that Murphy would consider faulty learning and canalization to be involved in the development of psychopathology. The limits placed on behavior by society would play a part in many forms of maladaptive functioning, as would the learning of inappropriate ways to resolve organic tissue demands. Similarly, absence of integrated development also would appear to be involved in an incomplete or inappropriate set of behaviors.

In his later years, Murphy attempted to expand his eclecticism to incorporate the parapsychological approach in his theory. He believed, for example, that telepathy and clairvoyance might be more normal than typically thought. He proposed that they were so rarely observed because people tend to avoid these experiences through personal insulation from one another. He suggested that openness to mystical and transpersonal experiences could increase the potential biologically possible in people. These later views, although not as widely accepted as his earlier formulations, were quite consistent with Murphy's approach to personality. He believed throughout his life that all areas of human experience could be and should be applied in the effort to understand personality.

B. F. SKINNER **History** Born in a small town in Pennsylvania, B. F. Skinner (1904–) attended a small college in upstate New York. After graduation, he spent 2 years traveling before he entered Harvard University to pursue a Ph.D. degree in psychology. Skinner took a number of teaching positions after receiving his doctoral degree in 1931, and eventually ended up at Harvard in 1948. During his long and active career, Skinner has been a productive writer and lecturer. A professor emeritus at Harvard, Skinner has received numerous honors, including the Distinguished Scientific Award of the APA and the President's Science Award.

Concepts As has been the case with the majority of the foundation theorists discussed thus far, Skinner also may be seen as the source of a major modern approach to personality and psychopathology. It was Skinner's seminal work in *operant learning* that laid much of the groundwork for many of the current methods of behavior modification, programmed instruction, and general education. His global beliefs about the nature of behavior have been applied more widely, it might be argued, than those of any other theorist, except, perhaps, Freud. His impact has been impressive in scope and magnitude.

Skinner's approach to personality is more a derivation of his basic beliefs about behavior than it is a specific theory of personality per se. To Skinner, personality is not different from other behaviors or sets of behaviors; it is acquired, maintained, and strengthened or weakened according to the same rules of reward and punishment that alter any other forms of behavior. *Behaviorism,* as Skinner's basic theory is most commonly known, is concerned only with observable, measurable, and operationalizable behavior. Many of the abstract and mentalistic hallmarks of other dominant personality theories have little place in Skinner's framework; concepts, such as self, ideas, and ego, are considered unnecessary for the understanding of behavior and are shunned. There is no mind as such, but only a learning brain affected by stimuli in the internal and external environment. Through the process of operant conditioning and the application of basic principles of learning, such as variable and ratio intermittent reinforcement schedules, discrimination, stimulus generalization, aversive conditioning, extinction, spontaneous recovery, shaping, and other laboratory researched phenomena (Table 8-3), people are believed to develop sets of behavior that characterize their responses to the world of stimuli with which they are faced in their lives. This set of responses is called personality.

Adaptive personality patterns represent behaviors that effectively yield positive reinforcement in the environment. Thus, a set of social skill behaviors that result in frequent dates with the opposite sex might be considered a reflection of effective personality. Nonreinforced, weak behaviors or inappropriately reinforced behaviors may be observed in persons who experience problems in functioning. For example, the low energy level of the depressed person may be seen as a result of nonreinforcement of active involvement with others; similarly, the self-stimulation of the severely disturbed child may be seen as a result of the absence of environmental reinforcement for more appropriate behavior. Regardless of the specifics of the behavior, the operant view would be that the pattern can be understood without invoking any abstract, nonobservable concepts, and can be altered through manipulation of the same sorts of stimuli and reinforcers that led to the development of the behavior in the first place.

Treatment applications In conceptualizing psychopathology, a major difference between the behavioral view and most others extant today is captured in the comparison between the so-called psychological model of mental disorder and the medical model. In brief, the medical model asserts that abnormal behavior patterns are signs or symptoms of some underlying (psychological) disease process in much the same way that a fever, chills, and painful swallowing are signs of an underlying streptococcal infection. In this view, in order to reduce the symptoms, one must cure the underlying cause. Among the underlying causes for psychological problems, for example, are lack of existential awareness and blocking of self-actualization. By contrast, in the psychological model, symptoms are viewed as patterns of behavior that do not necessarily reflect an underlying disorder, but that have developed and are maintained according to the definable rules of learning and reinforcement. In this perspective, the symptoms can be treated directly without concern for identifying and curing an underlying disease process. Herein lies the basis for the wide variety of behavior modification techniques that are part of the modern psychiatric armamentarium.

LATER THEORISTS—THE HUMANISTIC, EXISTENTIAL, COGNITIVE, AND PERCEPTUAL PERSPECTIVES

As the history of psychology and psychiatry progressed, newer theoretical orientations emerged that, in most instances, rested on the foundations represented by the earlier theories. However, in addition to the theories associated with particular individuals, there arose in the middle part of the twentieth century some rather well-defined schools of thought that were

TABLE 8-3
Important Concepts and Principles in the Behavioral Approaches to Personality, Psychopathology, and Psychotherapy

Aversive conditioning: A procedure in which punishment or aversive stimulation is used to reduce the frequency of a target behavior.
Avoidance learning: A form of operant learning in which an organism learns to avoid certain responses or situations.
Classical conditioning: The association of a neutral stimulus with an unconditioned stimulus such that the neutral stimulus comes to bring about a response similar to that originally elicited by the unconditioned stimulus.
Conditioned response (CR): In classical conditioning, the response elicited by the conditioned stimulus.
Conditioned stimulus (CS): In classical conditioning, the originally neutral stimulus that comes to be associated with the unconditioned stimulus and eventually elicits a conditioned response.
Continuous reinforcement: A schedule of reinforcement in which every time a response is emitted, a reward is administered.
Covert reinforcement: A method of increasing behavioral frequency by using the imagination of pleasant events as a reinforcement.
Covert sensitization: A method of reducing the frequency of behavior by associating it with the imagination of unpleasant consequences.
Discrimination learning: A process whereby the tendency toward stimulus generalization is counteracted and responses are made only to specific stimuli.
Experimental neurosis: An abnormal behavior pattern produced in animals through application of classical or operant conditioning techniques.
Extinction: Reduction of frequency of a learned response as a result of cessation of reinforcement.
Fixed interval schedule: A reinforcement schedule in which a reward is given after a specific amount of time has passed.
Fixed ratio schedule: A reinforcement schedule in which a reward is given after a specific number of responses have been emitted.
Habituation: A simple form of learning in which the response to a repeated stimulus lessens over time.
Higher-order conditioning: In classical conditioning, the establishment of a new conditioned stimulus through association with an established conditioned stimulus.
Instrumental learning: Operant conditioning.
Law of effect: The principle that behaviors followed by pleasant consequences are strengthened, and those followed by negative consequences are weakened.
Modeling: Observational learning.
Negative practice: A method for reducing the frequency of behavior by intense repetition of the response.
Observational learning: Learning new behaviors by observing others responding and receiving some form of consequence; vicarious learning.
Operant conditioning: A form of learning in which behavioral frequency is altered through the application of positive and negative consequences.
Partial reinforcement: A schedule of reinforcement in which rewards are not given each time a response is made, rendering a learned response highly resistant to extinction.
Primary reinforcer: A stimulus that increases the probability of behaviors it follows.
Reinforcer: A stimulus that increases the frequency of responses it follows.
Respondent learning: Classical conditioning.
Secondary reinforcers: Stimuli that gain the power to reinforce behavior through association with primary reinforcers.
Shaping: An operant procedure in which a desirable behavior pattern is learned via successive reinforcement of approximations to that behavior.
Spontaneous recovery: The increase in strength of an extinguished behavior after the passage of a period of time.
Successive approximation: See Shaping.
Unconditioned response (UCR): In classical conditioning, a response that occurs spontaneously to the unconditioned stimulus.
Unconditioned stimulus (UCS): A stimulus that, without any training, produces specific response.
Variable interval schedule: A reinforcement schedule in which a reward is given after varying periods of time have passed.
Variable ratio schedule: A reinforcement schedule in which a reward is given after a varying number of responses have been emitted.

ascribed to by significant numbers of professionals. Thus, although there were major individual theorists such as the humanistic existentialists Rogers, Perls, Fromm, and Maslow, and the cognitive theorists Ellis and Lacan, there were also movements, such as the general humanistic–existential perspective and the perceptual approach.

THE HUMANISTIC–EXISTENTIAL MOVEMENT As exemplified by the ideas of Carl Rogers, Rollo May, Ludwig Binswanger, Frederick (Fritz) Perls, Abraham Maslow, Erich Fromm, and Irwin Yalom, humanistic–existential conceptualizations of personality are built on the general belief that people have inherent capacities to become healthy, fully functioning individuals. Psychopathology is typically seen as a result of the interruption of people's growth toward goodness and health. Psychotherapy, it then follows, would need to involve efforts to free individuals so that they might once again grow and function in an unimpeded manner. Although differing in some specifics, humanistic–existential theorists tend to see people as biological, social, and psychological beings whose primary task is to search for, and establish, meaning in their lives. As reviewed by S. Kobasa and S. Maddi, the ideal or fully functioning individual within the existential perspective is the authentic person.

> [This person] exercises vigorously the psychological needs or functions of symbolization, imagination, and judgment and allows these to influence his biological and social experiences. He is well integrated and demonstrates originality and change. Having accepted the givens of his past and present, his basic orientation is toward the future and its associated uncertainty. Uncertainty leads him to experience anxiety, but he accepts this anxiety as a necessary concomitant of vigorous living. He is aided in this acceptance by courage.
>
> The *unauthentic person,* in contrast, inhibits the expression of distinctively human psychological needs; he sees himself as a player of predetermined social roles and the embodiment of biological needs. His behavior is fragmentary and stereotyped and often includes exploitation of others, a rigidly materialistic attitude, and feelings of worthlessness and insecurity. He fears the uncertainty of the future; shrinking from it, he defines himself solely in terms of his past or present, in spite of resultant feelings of guilt and regret.

In general, existentialists perceive psychopathology as a result of continuing experiences of failure in unauthentic individuals (authentic persons can grow from failure). Therapeutic intervention within the existential perspective is directed at bringing people from a state of inauthenticity to authenticity. Kobasa and Maddi state:

> To move toward authentic being, the client must learn to begin and exercise symbolization, imagination, and judgment and thereby to achieve consciousness of his or her life as being partially under his or her control. He must begin to express these cognitive capabilities in his biological and social experiencing, moving thereby toward subtlety, taste, intimacy, love, and constructive social action. He must accept responsibility for the decisions he makes and attempt to tolerate anxiety so that he can choose to change and grow and thereby avoid accumulations of the guilt of missed opportunities. To learn to tolerate anxiety, he must begin to trust himself and to develop a generic set of goals which can lend direction to personal change. But he must also grow in ability to accept givens and inevitabilities, so that he is clear about what practical possibilities should be pursued.

Using various techniques such as focusing deeply on past memories, independence training, and paradoxical intention (in which patients are encouraged to exaggerate rather than try to suppress troublesome symptoms), existential therapists attempt to help people to make full use of their cognitive affective capacities.

Although Kobasa and Maddi's description of existential theory is applicable to the broad range of such approaches, there are specific differences among the many perspectives. Four representative theorists are Carl Rogers, Frederick Perls, Erich Fromm, and Abraham Maslow.

CARL ROGERS **History** Raised in a midwestern farm environment, Carl Rogers (1902–1987) spent his undergraduate years pursuing a career in agriculture. However, after graduation, he attended the Union Theological Seminary in New York to study for the ministry, but again changed career directions after taking psychology courses at Columbia University. Rogers received his Ph.D. degree in psychology from Columbia Teachers College in 1931. Work with abused children in Rochester for the next 12 years helped Rogers accumulate a variety of clinical experiences. These experiences would help him to develop his theory of psychological development. For the rest of his professional career, Rogers spent his time vacillating between academic and clinical involvements. He left his tenured position at the University of Wisconsin in 1964 to take a more clinically oriented position with the Western Behavioral Sciences Institute in California. Rogers was active in the training of clinical and counseling psychologists. For his research and training work he was awarded the Distinguished Scientific Contribution Award of the APA in 1966.

Concepts Carl Rogers's name is most clearly associated with the *person-centered theory* of personality and psychotherapy. In this view, major emphasis rests on the concepts of self-actualization and self-direction. Specifically, people are born with a capacity to direct themselves in the healthiest way, toward a level of completeness called *self-actualization.* From his person-centered approach, Rogers viewed personality not as a static entity composed of traits and patterns, but as a dynamic phenomenon involving ever-changing communications, relationships, and self-concepts. Utilizing this definition of personality and much research, Rogers proposed a number of principles regarding normal and abnormal human behavior (Table 8-4).

Treatment An examination of these principles suggests that Rogers believed that people can and must develop freely, and that hindrance to this development in the form of conditional acceptance

TABLE 8-4
Basic Principles of Rogers's Person-Centered Approach

With regard to the basic nature of individuals:

1. Each person has an inherent tendency to actualize unique potential.
2. Each person is born with an inherent bodily wisdom that enables differentiation between experiences that actualize and those that do not actualize potential.
3. It is crucially important to be fully open to all experiences.
4. Significant others are important in helping people to experience fully.
5. Experiencing becomes more than bodily sensing as the child grows older.
6. Through complex interactions with one's own body and with other persons, each individual develops a concept of self.
7. One can sacrifice the wisdom of one's own experiencing to gain another's love.

With regard to the continuing growth and maintenance of personality:

8. A rift can develop between what is actually experienced and the concept of self.
9. When the rift between experiencing and self is too great, anxiety or disorganized behavior results.
10. Validating experiencing in terms of others can never be completed.
11. All maladjustment, of whatever degree, comes about through denial of experiences discrepant with the self-concept.
12. Perhaps the most persistent denial of oneself is by finding one's value by adopting a role, rather than accepting oneself as one is.
13. To be accepted by others in terms of one's own reality rather than the realities of others facilitates the acceptance of one's realities.

Table based on Holdstock T, Rogers C: Person-centered theory. In *Current Personality Theories,* R Corsini, editor. Peacock, Itasca, IL, 1977, with permission.

from the outside world can lead to psychopathology. Given that he saw discrepancies between actual and perceived experience of the self as being basic to the development of maladjustment (principles 8, 9, and 10), it would follow that Rogers's treatment approach would be designed to reduce these discrepancies. With regard to his approach, Rogers has stated: "It began to occur to me that unless I had a need to demonstrate my own cleverness and learning, I would do better to rely upon the client for the direction of movement in the process."

Rather than direct the therapeutic process, the client-centered therapist's responsibility is to produce an atmosphere in which clients can recontact their strivings for self-actualization, renew their sense of self-acceptance, and begin once more to grow. The therapist uses three processes to accomplish this task: accurate empathic understanding, unconditional positive regard, and genuineness or congruence. *Accurate empathy* describes the therapist's temporarily "living in the person's life," sensing the client's feelings, and communicating what is sensed back to the client. To do this effectively, therapists must be able to lay aside their worldly concerns and enter the client's world totally without prejudice. By *unconditional positive regard,* the second therapeutic process, Rogers meant the total nonjudgmental acceptance of clients as they are. Such acceptance helps clients to regain a sense of their own worth. Finally, *genuineness* describes the attitude in which therapists are totally open about, as well as to, their own experiences with clients. Therapists are responsible for communicating their own feeling state about the client regardless of whether it is positive or negative. Through these three fundamental conditions of therapy, the person-centered therapist can apply the humanistic theory of Carl Rogers in an effective and productive manner.

For a further discussion of Carl Rogers's theories, see Section 30.3, Client-Centered Psychotherapy.

FREDERICK PERLS **History** Frederick (Fritz) Perls (1893–1970) was born, raised, and educated in Berlin. He was trained in neurology by Kurt Goldstein and in psychoanalysis by Ernest Jones. Perls left Germany during the 1940s and went to South Africa, where he founded the South African Institute for Psychoanalysis, and wrote the beginning framework for what was later to become Gestalt therapy. Perls came to the United States in 1946 and established a private practice and the New York Institute for Gestalt Therapy. In the 1960s, he also created the Gestalt Institute in Vancouver, Canada.

Concepts Although ostensibly derived from the early Gestalt psychology of Wertheimer, Kohler, and others, the Gestalt theory of Fritz Perls is much more akin to existential and Freudian theory than to the classical psychology of perception. The use of the term "Gestalt" in Perls's thinking reflected his belief in the wholeness of experience and the transcendence of a sum over its parts. In addition to this conceptual position, a second major similarity to the classical Gestaltists was seen in Perls's focus on figure and ground in psychological (social, interpersonal, cultural) as well as perceptual arenas. His belief that awareness of relevant and salient "here and now" phenomena is crucial to effective functioning became a basic tenet of his theory of personality and psychopathology and the therapeutic techniques deriving from them. W. Thetford and R. Walsh describe the importance to Perls of figure and ground quite clearly:

> In healthy persons, the shifting of figure and ground is a smooth, continuous process. In neurotic persons, the process suffers from considerable impairment. Lacking the ability to make sharp distinctions between figure and ground, neurotics have cluttered fields, and their differentiations are uncertain. They become confused and do not know what they really want. They cannot distinguish between the important and the unimportant, between the relevant and the irrelevant . . . their reactions become stereotypical and repetitive, rather than spontaneous and problem centered.

Perls's theory of pathology and his Gestalt therapy method derived from his holistic view of personality. Generally, he believed that personality is multilayered. The outer layer, or clique, includes superficial and polite interactions, such as perfunctory greetings. The next deeper level is the role-playing layer, which is composed of automatized behavior patterns that accompany such roles as mother, student, and salesperson. Next is the impasse layer, where individuals experience a sense of nothingness and fear as they face the world without the buffers of their comfortable (and comforting) clique and role layers. Beyond the impasse layer lies the implosive-explosive layer where people become aware of strong emotions that are either expressed outwardly (exploded) or intensely sensed inwardly (imploded). Finally, past these outer ("phony") layers is the layer of genuine personality. It is at this level that people are in contact with whom they really are and can allow their inborn self-regulating mechanisms to guide them toward positive growth.

For Perls, a key to getting into contact with the genuine layer of personality is awareness. In the disturbed person, the spontaneous personality of a positively actualized individual is replaced by a deliberate, externally molded and rigid pattern. The task of the therapist is to help patients to free themselves from the shackles of deliberate behavior by achieving an integrative awareness and acceptance of their own thoughts, actions, and feelings. In this way, Perls was very similar to Rogers. However, Perls suggested more directly a number of techniques that can be used to accomplish awareness.

Treatment applications In Gestalt psychotherapy, patients are guided through the experience of encountering themselves via a number of therapeutic interpersonal and intrapersonal communication techniques developed by Perls and his followers. The techniques are designed to increase people's awareness of the entire set of factors (total Gestalt) affecting them at any time. To achieve this level of awareness (intellectual as well as physical), a very active therapist uses specifically designed games or exercises, which may include reifying and talking with abstract concepts and feelings (such as depression, anxiety, guilt, addiction, a deceased parent, or a lover), role reversals, group experiences, and marathons. Perls's view was that any number of techniques could be effective, so long as the goals of total awareness and contact with the genuine personality layer were achieved.

ERICH FROMM **History** Erich Fromm (1900–1980) received his Ph.D. degree from the University of Heidelberg in 1922. He continued his training at the Berlin Psychoanalytic Institute and later founded the Frankfurt Psychoanalytic Institute. After coming to the United States in 1933, Fromm joined with others to form the William Alanson White Institute. Consistent with his educationally varied background, the institute allowed Fromm to combine his knowledge of sociology, psychology, philosophy, and psychoanalysis. After many years of private practice, Fromm moved to New Mexico and developed psychoanalytic training programs there and in Mexico before retiring to Switzerland.

Concepts Although formally trained as a psychoanalyst, Fromm evolved during his long career as a social philosopher and personality theorist into what he termed a *dialectical humanist*. In his early years, his writings had a distinct Marxist air, but later he focused increasingly on Eastern and Western religious philosophies as the bases for his theorizing about human behavior.

Fromm believed that the basic problem for all human beings is to overcome isolation and separateness from others. The powerful sense of one's total isolation from the rest of the world was seen to be at the core of a basic need to reunite with one's self and others. According to Fromm, each person (and society or culture, for that matter) begins in a state of peace with primary ties to, and complete dependence on, a mother (or nature). As time goes on, however, and growth occurs, primary ties are inevitably disrupted or broken and a key process called *individuation* is initiated. Once individuation begins, there can be no return to primary ties and the safety of total dependency, although there continues to exist a wish and drive toward this end. However, even though people would like to regain their dependency and avoid facing their true isolation, they must accept the fact of their inherent separateness and continue on toward a state of responsible independence. The process of movement toward an acceptance of this independence, or freedom, is at the center of Fromm's theory of personality, psychopathology, and psychotherapy.

Fromm noted that people are partly animal and partly human, but their human side leads them to an awareness of, and a need to deal with, impending disease, unavoidable losses, and their own deaths. In people's reactions to their awareness of these paradoxes of life, Fromm contended, may be found some important sources of individual differences. For example, some individuals may try to halt the process of individuation by avoiding (escaping from) freedom through establishing unhealthy dependency or pseudoprimary relationships with others. Other people may develop a false sense of individuated identity characterized by pseudothoughts, pseudointerests, and a pseudo-self. Fromm believed that only by accepting one's true separateness and facing its attendant anxiety can people ever be fully born and grow.

In addition to remaining involved in the process of individuation, certain needs must also be met as the individual develops. Major among these needs are (1) the need for relatedness, or a deep sense of unity with others; (2) the need for transcendence, or a rising above the animal in oneself; (3) the need for rootedness and identity, or the sense of belonging and acceptance of one's own uniqueness; and (4) the need for a frame of orientation or a frame of reference through which one can meaningfully and stably perceive one's self and the outside world.

Although individuation is necessary for the satisfaction of basic needs, not all people achieve this desired level of development. Rather, because of the intense anxiety associated with accepting total freedom, they may adopt one or more mechanisms of escape, which can result in what Fromm terms *unproductive orientations* to life. In the most extreme form of unproductive orientation, one escapes from freedom through a psychotic pattern of total withdrawal and fantasy. However, most examples of the processes of escape fall into three more common and less drastic categories—the authoritarian solution, the destructive solution, and the automation conformity solution. In the first of these solutions, people escape from freedom by establishing a symbiotic relationship with another, who is seen as responsible for what the individual does and feels. In the second solution, attempts are made to destroy indiscriminately any source of stress or judgment that might result in an individual being held accountable. Finally, in automation conformity, people escape from their own freedom by trying to be as much like others as possible, thereby denying their own individuality and isolation. Fromm considered this third form of escape mechanism the most common in modern society.

Once they have turned away from individuation and its associated freedom, people move toward one of four types of unproductive adjustments to life, each of which reflects their dominant escape mode. *Receptive characters* are passive people who are friendly, optimistic, and approval seeking. They are actually seeking powerful others who will take care of them and make decisions for them. *Exploitative characters* try to take things from others rather than assuming responsibility for getting the things on their own; they may be aggressive and demanding and may resort to crime and cunning to get what they want. The *hoarding character* is typically thrifty, distant, and aloof. Such a person minimizes the number of situations in which freedom must be exercised by keeping things just as they are. Finally, Fromm described the *marketing character,* who may be seen as a manipulative, utilitarian conformist who equates material success with individuation. Such people buy and sell their personalities much like commodities and, like chameleons, alter themselves to fit ongoing situations.

Fromm considered unproductive orientations and adjustments to be maladaptive, claiming that the only way really to overcome the basic challenge of separateness is through what he termed the *productive orientation*. The productive orientation is mature, courageous, and fulfilling, and is marked by the presence of *productive love*. In its ultimate form, productive love represents an integration of brotherly love, mother's love, self-love, love of others, and love of God (both a theistic and nontheistic concept for Fromm). At the highest level of development, all these forms of love become indistinguishable and the ultimate solution to isolation is achieved. If people can love others as themselves, they can overcome their aloneness through total acceptance of their own freedom and individuality.

Treatment applications As much a philosophy as a school of personality theory, Fromm's perspective has given rise to a specific view of psychopathology and psychotherapy. For Fromm, the disturbed individual is one who has moved too deeply into an unproductive orientation, one who cannot deal effectively with the need for individuation, one who sacrifices basic needs in an effort to escape from freedom, and one who cannot love either self or others. To the disturbed individual, other people become utilitarian objects that are used to fend off the threat of freedom rather than love objects that can help people to reach once again their original state of inner peace. To overcome their difficulties, people require a therapeutic experience in which they accept the fact of their separateness and refuse to let anxiety force them to halt their individuation or drive them into unproductive orientations to life.

ABRAHAM MASLOW

History Born in Brooklyn, New York, and educated at the University of Wisconsin, Abraham Maslow (1908–1970) combined training in Watsonian behaviorism and animal learning into a foundation for his later theorizing on human behavior and experience. Always a prodigious writer and lecturer, Maslow was on the faculty of Brooklyn College until 1951 and at Brandeis University until 1969. During these years, Maslow accumulated many honors, among them the presidency of the APA in 1967.

Concepts Very much in the holistic tradition of early theorists such as Goldstein and Murphy, Maslow believed that the scientific narrowing of psychology that occurred in the middle of the twentieth century was resulting in the study of only partial aspects of human behavior and personality. In response, he proposed a humanistic psychology in which soft concepts, such as individuality, morality, ethics, goodness, beauty, identity, authenticity, and human potential, stood equal and complementary to traditional hard variables, such as reaction time, stimulus, response, and traits. In addition, Maslow also believed that psychology focused too strongly on the needs and development of disturbed personalities and not enough on the development of healthy, well-functioning people. He proposed that the sick personality was different in many ways from the healthy personality and did not merely represent the absence of healthy functions. Similarly, the healthy personality was seen as more than simply one marked by the absence of disturbance; Maslow thus set out to describe more fully than his predecessors and contemporaries the process of development and maintenance of the healthy personality.

HIERARCHICAL ORGANIZATION OF NEEDS Arguably, his greatest contribution to the history of psychology was his proposal of a hierarchical organization of needs (Fig. 8-1). In this hierarchy, basic or instinctual needs are believed to be universal and intrinsic; among

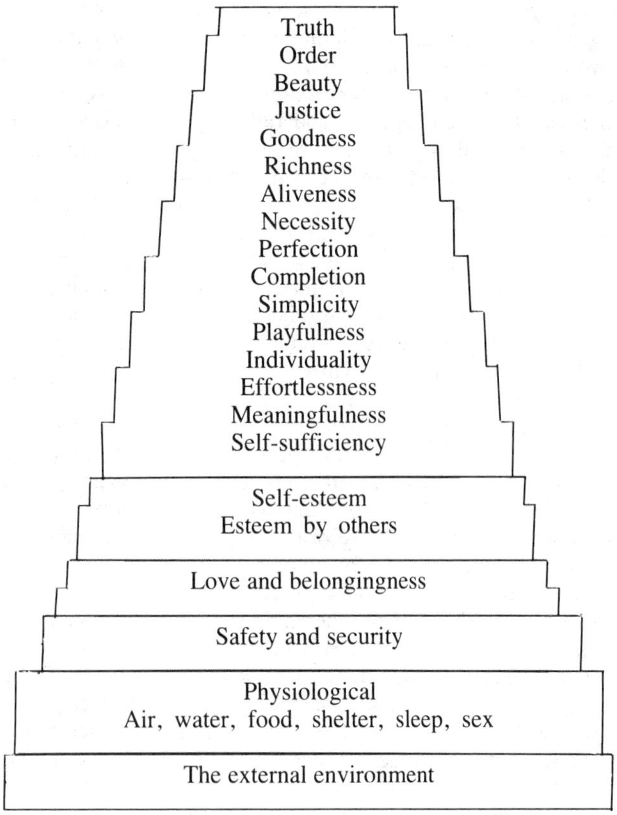

FIGURE 8-1 *Maslow's hierarchy of human needs.*

these needs are the survival-oriented needs with clear physical bases, such as hunger and thirst. Only when these basic needs are fulfilled do higher-level, less powerful needs become motivators for behavior; the first set of these higher-level needs to emerge includes the needs for shelter, for affection and belonging, and for self-esteem. The needs described to this point fall into a category Maslow labeled *D-needs* or *deficiency needs* because they involve the maintenance of a stable, secure, and protected individual and are invoked whenever a deficit or loss is experienced or threatened. However, given the satisfaction of these D-needs, Maslow proposed that a second set of higher-level needs, *B-needs* or *growth-oriented needs,* came to play a primary motivational role. B-needs include the need for freedom, beauty, justice, goodness, and altruism, and are considered abundancy motives; that is, they are not sought after because they reduce a deficit, but because they represent something that is valuable and worthwhile to achieve.

In Maslow's early thinking, the highest need level in his hierarchy was the *need for self-actualization,* or the achievement of one's complete potential. Later, he placed above self-actualization the desire for *self-transcendence,* a state in which B-needs become so important that people are willing to forego their basic needs (e.g., to go without food or water or security) in order to achieve higher goals such as justice and freedom.

In Maslow's view, human behavior may be seen as a reflection of fundamental and inherent conflicts between B-needs and D-needs. As the satisfaction of the deficiencies associated with the D-needs often requires dependence on others, these needs can render people more dependent and insecure, forcing them to behave very conservatively in order to "keep their supply lines open." Such behavior is clearly contrary to the growth orientation associated with the B-needs, which draw people toward independence, self-sufficiency, and self-direction. The continuous process of reconciling D- and B-need conflicts results in a form of bipolarity of life—regression versus advancement, maturity versus immaturity, and safety versus growth. Though such conflicts are sometimes stressful, they are seen as a necessary part of a healthy life. However, when these conflicts are resolved via distortion of basic needs by transforming them into unattainable neurotic needs, people can become bogged down and cannot grow toward self-actualization.

For Maslow, all forms of human behavior may be conceptualized in terms of the dynamic interaction between D- and B-needs. Any specific behavior will reflect the differential degree to which a D- or B-need is the predominant motivational force. In Maslow's example of behaviors associated with the "need to know," this interaction between context and level of need is clarified. At the D-need level, knowledge-seeking behaviors may reflect a desire to reduce the sense of insecurity associated with the fear of the unknown. At the B-need level, the same behaviors may reflect a desire to seek greater awareness of art or other forms of beauty for their own sakes. To Maslow, in fact, the entire purpose of education, of psychotherapy, even of life, is to shift the balance from D-needs to B-needs. Psychopathology or maladaptive functioning is the result when this process is thwarted or derailed.

SELF-ACTUALIZATION According to Maslow, the culmination of a balanced approach to life is self-actualization. Self-actualized people are described as realistically oriented, spontaneous, problem centered, creative, independent, and generally accepting of themselves and others. At times, they are also able to transcend even this high state of functioning and to reach levels of clarity, understanding, euphoria, holism, and integration with the universe called *peak experiences.* These rare, mystical events were believed to be a hallmark of healthy individuals. Maslow believed that peak experiences were possible for all people, but that most individuals were too fearful of their power and potential life-changing consequences to allow them to happen. It became a goal of the therapeutic approaches deriving from Maslow's theory to free people to move toward self-actualization and to make it possible for them to feel the peak experiences that could result in their turning away from aggressiveness and destructiveness and coming closer to their true selves and a sense of their own being.

ALBERT ELLIS

History Albert Ellis (1917–) did not become interested in psychology as a career until after he had graduated from City College of New York (1934) and tried to be a writer. He graduated from Columbia University with a Ph.D. degree in 1947 and developed his rational-emotive approach to psychotherapy during his tenure as the chief psychologist at Menlo Park State Hospital in New Jersey. By 1959, Ellis's theoretical system was developed to the point where he could start the Institute for Rational Emotive Therapy in New York City, of which he is still the director.

Concepts The basic notions of the cognitive theorists are that thought, perception, and language play major roles in human functioning, and that, prior to responding to them, internal and external situations are "filtered" through cognitive structures composed of beliefs, attitudes, and expectations. These cognitive structures may vary in meaning, adaptability, and flexibility. Generally, from the cognitive point of view, psychopathology involves some problem in language, perception, and thought, and treatment must focus on these factors rather than on the more ethereal emphases of the humanistic theorists.

Albert Ellis developed and is the driving force behind the theory (and philosophy) of rational-emotive therapy. It is his position that "men are not disturbed by things, but by the view they take of them" (Epictetus) and that "there is nothing either good or bad, but thinking makes it so" (Shakespeare).

Ellis's perspective involves situations (A), beliefs (B), and reactions (C). He believes that it is not what really happens (or does not happen) (A) that causes people to respond as they do (positively or negatively); rather, their reactions to events in the world (C) actually result from B, their beliefs about what has happened. Thus, the same event can result in different reactions, depending on one's beliefs. For example, a student may receive a grade of 80 on an important exam. If the student believes that it is necessary to get 90 in order to be approved of by parents or teachers, the student is likely to be very upset. In contrast, a student who believes that just passing (60) is a fine goal is likely to be very happy about receiving an 80. The reaction stems from the belief, not from the actual event.

Treatment In developing rational-emotive psychotherapy, Ellis proposed that there are a number of common irrational beliefs that cause people trouble (Table 8-5). Therapeutic efforts are focused on altering these beliefs through which events are translated and which result in negative emotional reactions. Thus, the rational-emotive therapist will question concepts, ideas, and other sources of rules that people live by. Ellis's philosophy is clear: Change people's beliefs and such symptoms as depression and anxiety will simply disappear.

THE PERCEPTUAL THEORISTS Related to the ways in which people think about the world are the ways in which their perceptions of the world determine their adjustment. Perceptual theorists believe that it is not the specifics of the real world that determine one's reactions to it or behaviors in it, but rather one's perceptions of that world. In that each person perceives some things as others do, there will be commonalities in human behavior. In that each person also perceives some things in unique ways, there will be individual differences among people. Gardner Murphy, an early proponent of the perceptual view, wrote:

> If we understand the differences in perceiving we shall go far in understanding the differences in the resulting behavior. The relation between the outer world and the individual is gravely misconstrued by the assumption that this world registers upon us all in about the same way, that the real differences between people are differences in what is done about this world. The contemporary point of view . . . has involved emphasis upon the basic notion that every individual lives in a more or less "private world" . . .; there is no standard objective world except through our slow yielding to a rather painful compromise process . . . that is less coercive, less "final," than the private world.

In a further refinement of the perceptual view, R. Blake and colleagues note:

> Each individual begins with certain physical structures, including the receptor, central, and effector nervous systems as well as the skeletal, respiratory, digestive, and other systems. These several part-systems in unitary organization constitute the more important structures involved in perception. The selective manner in which these part-systems are utilized in perception, however, is largely determined by the unique interaction between the individual and the cultural media which he has passed through and of which he is a part at present. Thus, the way one sees reality is contingent not only on the capacity of his given physical structure for detecting stimulus configurations and integrating information about stimuli but also on modifications in the use of the structure which derive from the impact of experience. The summed effects result in the individual's having more or less appropriate response patterns ready in order to cope with each of a myriad of specific stimulus configurations.

TABLE 8-5
Ellis's Listing of 11 Basic Irrational Thoughts

1. It is essential that one be loved by virtually everyone in the community.
2. One must be perfectly competent, adequate, and achieving to consider oneself worthwhile.
3. Some people are bad, wicked, or villainous, and therefore should be blamed and punished.
4. It is a terrible catastrophe when things are not as one wants them to be.
5. Unhappiness is caused by outside circumstances and the individual has no control over it.
6. Dangerous or fearsome things are causes for great concern and their possibility must be continually dwelt on.
7. It is easier to avoid certain difficulties and self-responsibilities than to face them.
8. One should be dependent on others and must have someone stronger on whom to rely.
9. Past experiences and events are the determiners of present behavior and cannot be eradicated.
10. One should be quite upset about other people's problems.
11. There is always a right and perfect solution to every problem, and it must be found or the result will be catastrophic.

Table from Ellis A: *Reason and Emotion in Psychotherapy*. Copyright 1962 by Lyle Stuart, Inc., with permission.

From the viewpoint of the perceptual theorists, therefore, to understand personality, one must understand perception at physical, developmental, psychological, linguistic, sociological, and cultural levels. Thus, a blind person perceives the world differently from a sighted person; a child, differently from an adult; an upper-class person, differently from a lower-class individual; a South Sea Islander, differently from an urban dweller; a person who speaks English, differently from one who uses an Eskimo dialect. These variables all contribute to the rich variety of personality patterns, but they are also implicated in the development of psychopathology and, in turn, psychotherapeutic approaches.

Perceptual theorists view psychopathology as stemming from false interpretations of the world, from tendencies to understand situations in ways that are not veridical. Thus, a normal person might perceive a friend's inquiry regarding one's health to be a sign of warmth and concern, whereas a paranoid person might perceive the question as part of a plan to expose the individual to some dreaded disease. Similarly, a normal individual might see the dawn of a new day as exhilarating, whereas a depressed person might see it as the beginning of another opportunity for failure.

The relationship between perception and behavior is a complex, circular one; it is not usually possible to determine which comes first, but that determination is not always necessary for psychotherapy. From the perceptual theorist's perspective, psychotherapy is a process whereby the interactions between individuals and their environments are reorganized. Although identified most clearly with the humanistic school of thought, Carl Rogers has noted the importance of perceptual changes in psychotherapy:

> If we think of perception as a complex phenomenon involving the raw data of immediate experience and the learnings we bring to it from the past, then therapy is a process whereby a safe exploration permits the person to separate and differentiate the elements of this phenomenon. He can feel the immediate experience of himself in this relationship. He can also experience the meaning which past learnings would tend to cause him to see in himself in this relationship. Where there is discrepancy, the perception becomes reorganized in terms of the immediate experience. He can be what he is and can recognize that past learnings would frequently cause him to see himself as something he is not. He acquires a new confidence as he rests his perceptions more securely upon the data of his senses. Perception of self thus becomes what it should be, an adequate hypothesis for living, soundly based on the available evidence, and alterable in the light of new evidence.
>
> But . . . when the individual has reorganized his perception of self, he has reconstructed the most significant learned element that he brings to any experience. Thus we find that, when the self is perceived in reorganized terms, it affects not only the future perception of self but the way the individual perceives his wife, his friends, other persons, the campus buildings, the counselor's face, and even that holy of psychological holies, the unstructured and ambiguous ink blot. It is thus, the writer believes, that psychotherapy reorganizes perception by providing a relationship in which the individual's most basic perception, his perception of himself, can change.

JACQUES LACAN History Born in Paris and trained as a psychiatrist, Jacques Lacan (1901–1982) also studied philosophy and structuralism while becoming a psychoanalyst. Although a member of the Psychoanalytic Society of Paris, he resigned during the 1950s and founded his own institute, the Freudian School of Paris. The institute became a major training facility.

Concepts Although an adherent to the psychoanalytic tradition, Lacan may be included among the cognitive theorists because he occupies a unique and controversial position between the intrapsychic concepts of Freud and the linguistic structuralism and semiotic perspectives of Levi-Strauss, Roman Jakobson, and de Saussure. Whereas Freud, for example, saw the unconscious as a seething cauldron of needs, wishes, and instincts, Lacan saw it as a sort of language that helps to structure the world. To Lacan, the "world of words creates the world of things." To understand personality, according to Lacan, one must be able to understand it from a structural linguistic perspective, from the view that all internal and external behaviors have sign value or meaning. Because of his controversial position and often difficult-to-follow writing, *Psychology Today* magazine described Lacan as the "most controversial Freudian since Freud." His ideas have galvanized professional opinion about him. In a history of psychoanalysis, for example, R. Fine states:

> Lacan is the most colorful postwar figure on the French psychoanalytic scene. . . . He is another of the many charismatic figures in the history of psychoanalysis, worshipped by his followers, ignored by the rest of the world. . . . He centers his theory of psychoanalysis around language. Two of his main pronouncements are: the unconscious is structured like a language; and the unconscious is the discourse of the Other. Lacan also . . . inveighs against behaviorism, dynamic psychiatry, ego psychology, and culturalism. He sees himself . . . as a structuralist. Some of his ideas may turn out to have value, but on the whole he seems too confused and disorganized to be able to make any real contribution to the mainstream of psychoanalytic thought.

Regardless of his detractors, Lacan appears to have attempted to place psychoanalytic thinking into the mainstream of modern linguistics and semiotics. To Lacan, basic Freudian concepts could be reconceptualized as parts of a linguistic structure. Instinctual energies, for example, are merely linguistic signs. Primary process thoughts are actually uncontrolled free-flowing sequences of meaning. Secondary process thought is the organization of free-flowing meaning into structured and intentional meaning. Symptoms are signs or symbols of underlying processes and the role of the therapist is to interpret the semiotic text of the personality structure.

As did Freud, Lacan conceived of development as a series of stages that need to be traversed successfully if a person is to be able to function normally. Lacan's most basic phase is the *mirror stage;* it is here that infants learn to recognize themselves by taking the perspective of others. Once this recognition is possible, an ego develops that incorporates the person's objective view of himself or herself via the role perspective of others. In this sense, the ego is not a part of the self, but something outside of and viewed by the self. Lacan proposed that this phenomenon is the basis for the self-alienation and rejection that play roles in later psychopathology. In view of his conceptualization of the self and ego as symbols, Lacan believed that, in intrapsychic discourse, the ego comes to represent parents and society, for example, more than it represents the actual self of the individual. In such a circumstance, there is not a "full discourse" between the ego and the "set of relationships" Lacan called the "real subject." A classic semiotic query may help in understanding Lacan's position—When you "talk to yourself," who is speaking and who is listening? From Lacan's perspective, it seems that there can be great conflict and turmoil within people if these multiple entities are in conflict.

Treatment Given his theory of development and personality, Lacan's therapeutic approach involved the transcendence of incorrect or fantasied relationships with significant others and the cessation of self-alienation. Among his most controversial beliefs was that the resistance to this transcendence can be reduced by cutting short the traditional 50-minute therapy hour. Although his methods and beliefs are difficult for many to understand and accept, it is also the case that Lacan is considered to have been the most influential of modern European psychoanalytic theorists.

EMERGING THEORIES OF PERSONALITY AND PSYCHOPATHOLOGY

The theories discussed to this point reflect an effort to highlight those conceptualizations that have stood the test of time and have made significant contributions to the history of personality theory. Often the decision to include or exclude a particular perspective was most difficult, but the selection of more recent theories was even more harrowing. Here, it was necessary to select, without the test of time, emerging perspectives that seem promising or seem noteworthy within the perspective of continuity from earlier models of behavior. It is here that bias will inevitably occur and where the authors must simply describe what they consider to be important steps in the development of personality theory.

A PSYCHOEVOLUTIONARY APPROACH TO PERSONALITY AND PSYCHOTHERAPY Most theories of personality that have developed out of the disciplines of psychology and philosophy have been based on an effort to answer the question, "What is personality?" However, recently there has been a move toward a psychoevolutionary perspective on behavior in which, in addition to "what" questions, "why" questions are also asked. Thus, in answer to the question, "Why do we have emotions?" R. Plutchik has proposed a psychoevolutionary theory of emotions. Similarly, some theorists have begun to ask, "Why is there a pattern of behavior called personality?" And: "What purpose does such a pattern serve in the survival of the human species?" One answer to the question may be found in Duke's situational stream theory.

The situational stream hypothesis builds on the notion that the defining and shared characteristic of living and behaving organisms is the existence of a continuous, unstoppable stream of behaviors. Further, it is proposed that the source of this continuous stream of behaviors is a parallel stream of situations to which the organism reacts in a continuous manner. All behavior is seen as representing a reaction to some situation. The unstopping stream of behavior, therefore, may be thought of as an unstopping series of reactions to a continuous stream of situations.

If the whole of the human behavioral system is seen as continuous in nature, it follows that its subsystems would either be continuous as well or be involved in some way in the maintenance of continuity in the general system. Thus, it should be possible to conceptualize such behavioral subsystems as memory, cognition, sensation, perception, motor activity, communication, and personality and social behavior as continuous in their own right. For example, one cannot stop the sensory system, one cannot not think, one cannot not communicate, one cannot will the cessation of autobiographical memory, one cannot not develop an association between two contiguous stimuli, a living organism cannot not be involved in some motor activity (even if totally still), and so on. Each of the continuous subsystems may be seen as playing some role in the assessment of, reaction to, or production of the situational (and, hence, behavioral) stream.

In that there cannot not be a behavior in a living thing, there cannot not be a situation in existence at a given time. Situations may be complex and composed variously of one or more of four different types of specific components. These are depicted in Fig. 8-2.

From the perspective of the personality theorist, the most important situation is type EI, the pattern in which situations that are experienced as externally produced are in fact internally caused. In this frame of reference, personality is defined as a set of behaviors that produces in other people situations that they then respond to in a familiar way. The personality pattern serves the purpose of defining the individual's interpersonal world and of stabilizing that world from situation to situation. The person who smiles at people finds that they smile in return, leaving the impression that the world is a friendly place. Similarly, the person who approaches all situations in a helpless way finds that others tend to run things, making the individual in question feel inferior and resentful and unable to muster up courage to take charge of the next situation. (It must be noted that given their stimulus value, people are considered situations in much the same way as other environmental stimulus configurations.)

In order to maintain the continuity of behavior (of the situational stream), several mechanisms of stream maintenance have been proposed. Among these are *stream-altering activities,* in which, through patterns such as the classic defense mechanisms, people modify or distort situations so that they may be responded to (even though, at times, maladaptively), and *stream-escape mechanisms,* in which people utilize strong emotions, such as anger or anxiety, to redefine a situation that otherwise cannot be dealt with effectively.

Given that personality represents a set of behaviors that produces situations in others, it follows that psychopathology may be seen as a reflection of such things as (1) an inability to produce effective and affiliative reactions in others; (2) feelings associated with the production of maladaptive situations in others (for example, depression associated with self-produced avoidance by others); or (3) ineffective methods of maintaining the ongoing situational stream (fantasy or self-stimulation behavior occurring when the individual is in a basically unstructured situation). From this perspective, much of what is traditionally considered to be the focus of psychotherapeutic efforts may be changed. Rather than conceptualizing anger, for example, as something that must be expressed and worked through, it is seen as an instrumental pattern that serves the purpose of removing people from situations with which they cannot deal. The therapeutic task, then, is to aid the person to develop situation-producing activities that can resolve the troublesome situations; the anger, theoretically, should simply disappear. In similar fashion, other common psychopathological patterns may also be reinterpreted within the situational stream theory framework.

While relatively new, the psychoevolutionary perspective on personality represents a theoretical development that has emerged more recently in the ongoing process of psychological and psychiatric science. However, basically novel approaches are not the only perspectives appearing on the scene. Integrations of well-established, seemingly irreconcilable (or, at least, markedly different) views have also evolved.

INTEGRATED VIEWS OF PERSONALITY AND PSYCHOTHERAPY Discussions of varying perspectives on personality and psychotherapy typically involve separation of opposing views and an emphasis on differences rather than similarities. To be sure, this approach serves a reasonable heuristic purpose and, as long as it reflects the existent state of theory and practice, it is a legitimate enterprise. However, since personality theory, like any scientific endeavor, is a dynamic process existing over time, as well as in time, it is not uncommon for once-separate theories to blend or move in various ways toward one another. Two examples of this phenomenon are (1) the rapprochement of the humanistic view of Carl Rogers and the psychoanalytic view of Heinz Kohut; and (2) the growing confluence of attitudes between behavioral and psychoanalytic perspectives on personality, psychopathology, and psychotherapy.

Source of Situation	Experience of situation: Internal	Experience of situation: External
Internal	Type II (headache, an idea, daydream)	Type IE (alarm clock, a reaction *of* others)
External	Type EI (a math problem, an injury, a reaction *to* others)	Type EE (time, place, weather)

FIGURE 8-2 *Components of the situational stream matrix. (From Duke M: The situational stream hypothesis. J Res Personal,* 21: *239, 1987, with permission.)*

Rogers and Kohut In a comparison of the work of Rogers and Kohut, E. Kahn stated that Heinz Kohut "has been able to provide a bridge between psychoanalysis and humanistic psychology." Kahn notes that, although a psychoanalyst, Kohut integrated a number of Rogers's concepts into his psychotherapeutic approach. For example, whereas Rogers described an atmosphere of unconditional positive regard, Kohut talked of a "therapeutic ambience" of acceptance and focus on the here and now. Further, both theorists emphasized the subjective experiential life of people; both considered the "self" as a primary entity in both adjustment and maladjustment in people; both stressed the importance of significant others (Kohut's selfobjects) in the development and maintenance of normal and abnormal personality; both considered empathy from others as a primary source of psychological health and healing.

Rogers's theory is more widely known and was discussed earlier, and so a brief discussion of Kohut's position seems in order. As a person grows, Kohut believed, the self acquires a psychological structure through a process called transmuting internalization, in which the inevitable frustrations of life lead to the development in an individual of qualities once found only in important selfobjects. Through this process, for example, in an empathic relationship with parents or other selfobjects, people develop three "sectors" of self—exhibitionistic needs, idealizing needs, and alter ego or twinship needs.

Exhibitionistic needs revolve around people's views of themselves and the development of self-acceptance. They lead, in the healthy individual, to feelings of self-esteem, ambition, and assertiveness. Idealizing needs stem from a desire to have heroes and all-powerful selfobjects; when these needs are frustrated, people develop their own healthy ideals, values, and principles to guide them through life. Finally, the need to be like others, to twin, to be a "person among other persons," leads to the development of skills and talents that allow for acceptance and integration into groups.

Kohut's view of the development of psychopathology focused on the empathy, or lack thereof, of selfobjects of childhood. According to Kohut, if normal structuralization is impeded, the self begins to lose its inherent cohesion and becomes fragmented. If this process occurs, individuals are not fully able to soothe themselves or to properly regulate self-esteem or interpersonal relationships; further, individuals become especially vulnerable to psychological injury and experience feelings of inner emptiness or depression. In an effort to deal with these situations, people may seek external sources of support, such as other people or drugs, or may develop maladaptive attempts at self-stimulation or soothing, such as abnormal sexual behavior, aggressive behavior, or fantasy.

Given his theory of psychopathology and personality, Kohut's view of psychotherapy focused on the strengthening of the structure of the self. In his perspective, the essential therapeutic force is the "reconstructive-interpretive approach" where pathological childhood experiences are revived and worked through. The therapist becomes the selfobject for the individual, and through dealing with this new selfobject, the transmuting internalization that did not occur in childhood takes place in the psychotherapeutic arena.

Although Kohut's ideas derived from a psychoanalytic foundation and Rogers's ideas from a humanistic perspective, both are similar in that they focus on the importance of the relationship between the therapist and the client as a primary source of psychological healing. Rogers spoke of a drive toward self-actualization and Kohut of the need for transmuting structuralization. Rogers spoke of unconditional positive regard and Kohut of psychotherapeutic ambience. Further, both focused heavily on the interpersonal aspects of the therapeutic endeavor, each emphasizing the importance of interpersonal, as opposed to intrapsychic, factors in the development of psychopathology.

Behaviorism and psychoanalysis Rogers was not the only theorist whose ideas have recently become intertwined with psychoanalytic thinking. Although John Dollard and Neal

Miller made an early attempt to reconcile behavioral and psychoanalytic approaches, only recently does there seem to be a growing and significant number of clinicians and theorists who perceive this set of "strange bedfellows" as a viable combination. S. Messer has provided an intriguing description of a psychotherapeutic intervention viewed from both behavioral and psychoanalytic perspectives. He concludes that many of the concepts of psychoanalysis are now frequently integrated into behavioral approaches under different names. For example, what a psychoanalyst might consider an unconscious fantasy, a cognitive behavior therapist might view as a schema, a traditional behavior therapist might view as a reciprocally inhibitory reaction to an unpleasant situation, and a social learning theorist might consider to be a learned reaction to some parental attitude. Regardless of the terminology, Messer believes that the actions of the therapist are in many cases remarkably similar. Even the hallmark of psychoanalysis, unconscious thought, has been referred to among some experimental cognitive psychologists as "unconscious processing."

Although he has found differences as well as similarities, Messer's efforts result in his suggesting that behavior therapists take into account some of the important principles of psychoanalytic therapy, and vice versa. For example, his advice to behavior therapists includes suggestions that (1) clients cannot be the sole determinant of therapeutic goals; (2) behavior therapists spend more time exploring clients' mental content; (3) behavior therapists should not always require or expect rationality among their clients; (4) behavior therapists should be more attuned to the possible unconscious character and childhood origins of behavior; and (5) behavior therapists should be on the alert for ambivalent and negative reactions that clients may have toward them per se.

Messer suggests that psychoanalytic therapists understand that (1) goals can and should be delineated in psychoanalytic therapy; (2) behavioral change often precedes insight as opposed to following it; and (3) unconscious fantasies may be seen as sources of self-perception. Moreover, they should (4) acknowledge the role of external realities, both past and present, for the client; (5) give more credence to the clients' own abilities to control their affect; and (6) allow their own human qualities to shine through and realize that, in addition to the content of their interactions, the relationship they have with their clients is part of their therapeutic effectiveness.

In both instances described here, there appears to have been a blending of theory that has emerged over time. According to the Kuhnian notion, one could expect that, rather than being anomalous, such theoretical blends may become more common as the process of personality theory moves ahead. And rather than being seen as signs of failure, these emerging integrated views of behavior are testimony to the vitality of the sciences of psychology and psychiatry.

REFERENCES

Alexander F, Selesnick S: *The History of Psychiatry*. New American Library, New York, 1966.

Allport G: *Personality: A Psychological Interpretation*. Holt, New York, 1937.

Blake R, Ramsey G, Moran B: *Perception: An Approach to Personality*. Ronald Press, New York, 1951.

Cattell R: *Personality and Motivation Structure and Measurement*. New World Book, New York, 1957.

Corsini R: *Current Personality Theories*. Peacock, Itasca, IL, 1977.

Duke M: The situational stream hypothesis. J Res Personal *21:* 239, 1987.

Ellis A: *Reason and Emotion in Psychotherapy*. Lyle Stuart, Northvale, NJ, 1962.

Ehrenwald S: *The History of Psychotherapy*. Jason Aronson, New York, 1976.

Fine R: *A History of Psychoanalysis*. Columbia University Press, New York, 1979.

Fromm E: *The Anatomy of Human Destructiveness*. Holt, Rinehart and Winston, New York, 1973.

Goldstein K: *The Organism: A Holistic Approach to Biology Derived from Pathological Data in Man*. American Book, New York, 1939.

Hall C, Lindzey G: *Theories of Personality*. Wiley, New York, 1957.

Holdstock T, Rogers C: Person-centered theory. In *Current Personality Theories,* R Corsini, editor, p 125. Peacock, Itasca, IL, 1977.

Kahn E: Heinz Kohut and Carl Rogers. Amer Psychol *40:* 893, 1985.

Kobasa S, Maddi S: Existential personality theory. In *Current Personality Theories,* R. Corsini, editor, p 243. Peacock, Itasca, Il, 1977.

Kuhn T: *The Structure of Scientific Revolution*. University of Chicago Press, Chicago, 1970.

Lewin R: *Field Theory in the Social Sciences*. Tavistock Publications, London, 1963.

Maslow A: *The Farther Reaches of Human Nature*. Viking Press, New York, 1971.

Messer S: Behavioral and psychoanalytic perspectives at therapeutic choice points. Amer Psychol *41:* 1261, 1986.

Murray A: *Exploration in Personality*. Oxford University Press, New York, 1938.

Perls F: *Gestalt Therapy Verbatim*. Real People Press, Lafayette, CA, 1969.

Rogers C: Perceptual reorganization in client centered therapy. In *Perception: An Approach to Personality,* R Blake, G Ramsey, editors. Ronald Press, New York, 1951.

Sheldon W, Stevens S, Tucker W: *The Varieties of Human Physique: An Introduction to Constitutional Psychology*. Harper & Row, New York, 1940.

Skinner B: *Science and Human Behavior*. Macmillan, New York, 1953.

Thetford W, Walsh R: Theories of personality and psychopathology: Schools derived from psychology and philosophy. In *Comprehensive Textbook of Psychiatry*, ed 4, H Kaplan, B Sadock, editors, p 459. Williams & Wilkins, Baltimore, 1985.

CHAPTER 9 DIAGNOSIS AND PSYCHIATRY: EXAMINATION OF THE PSYCHIATRIC PATIENT

9.1 THE PSYCHIATRIC INTERVIEW, HISTORY, AND MENTAL STATUS EXAMINATION

ROBERT L. LEON, M.D.
CHARLES L. BOWDEN, M.D.
RAYMOND A. FABER, M.D.

THE PSYCHIATRIC INTERVIEW

INTRODUCTION A psychiatric interview is a purposeful encounter between physician and patient. The purposes are many, but they can be subsumed under two major headings: gathering necessary information to assess the patient's condition and establishing a therapeutic doctor-patient relationship.

In modern medicine, treatment proceeds from accurate diagnosis. As more precise treatments are developed, the diagnosis must be more accurate. Before an accurate assessment can be made, a productive doctor-patient relationship must be established. It is becoming more difficult to do so as technological advances in medicine lead physicians away from the human factors in their patients. Body fluid analysis, electroencephalogram (EEG), electrocardiogram (EKG), and various imaging techniques give physicians previously undreamed-of information, about which patients may be unaware. It is often tempting to treat the disease found by this objective laboratory data rather than the person with the illness. Even the language of physicians urges them in this direction. "The patient presents with . . ." is not a statement that helps to understand a sick, troubled person. Patients actually present themselves to physicians for help.

A therapeutic relationship between physician and patient will dramatically improve compliance with whatever regimen is prescribed and will aid in gathering data. It will help patients to feel better and will aid in the curative process. Even one meeting between doctor and patient can be therapeutic. Doctor-patient encounters cannot be rigidly divided into diagnosis and therapy. This must occur to some degree, but the division is not clear-cut. There are a few instances of strictly evaluative interviews.

THE DOCTOR-PATIENT RELATIONSHIP Psychiatrists need to approach each patient with an understanding of the dynamics and complexities of the human experience and how it contributes to the doctor-patient interaction from the first moment of the encounter. A knowledge of personality development is essential for this understanding, because what the patient brings to the psychiatrist's office is influenced by his or her previous experiences. Doctor-patient interactions, whether they be psychotherapeutic or related to medication, will be influenced by these experiences.

Patient factors Patients, unless coerced to come, perceive a need for help, whether because of a specific problem or a vaguely defined uneasiness.

Beyond the immediate problem, patients come with a variety of feelings and concepts stemming from their society, culture, and past idiosyncratic personal experience. They have certain ideas about how to relate to physicians. Though present in everyone, these ideas are most easily seen in patients from a different culture. For example, many new immigrants from less developed Asian or Latin American countries may not come to a psychiatrist expecting to discuss emotions. Instead, they may expect help for perceived physical complaints. They may not discuss their depression in terms of feeling sad and unhappy, but rather as the physical correlates of depression. Well-educated Americans, in contrast, may expect to discuss feelings with their psychiatrist or may have unrealistic expectations for personality change.

Social and cultural expectations are inextricably intertwined with early life and family experience, since culture is expressed to the child through the family. Nevertheless, in order to understand patient reactions, it is helpful to separate these forces and to understand both as much as possible. The reactions to psychiatrists that have been shaped by early experience with family and significant others are called transference reactions. Each patient brings a whole set of feelings, reactions, and behavioral patterns into initial and subsequent encounters with his or her doctor. Since doctors are seen by society as authority figures, the reactions of patients will be determined, in part, by past experiences with authority figures. All imaginable reactions are possible, from a feeling of confidence in approaching the psychiatrist as an equal in an egalitarian relationship—a more mature and preferred approach—to a passive, completely dependent role assumed by individuals who take little responsibility for themselves.

All reactions and approaches to the psychiatrist will have both conscious and unconscious elements, and in both spheres there are motivations for and against working with the psychiatrist. Resistance to working with the psychiatrist has both conscious and unconscious elements. There may be conscious distrust based on past experience or a conscious reluctance to reveal oneself. There is also a deeper layer of resistance in the unconscious that is fueled by repressed conflicts.

While recognizing that all patients show varying amounts of resistance, the psychiatrist also should be alert to the aspects of the patient's conscious and unconscious motivations that are asking for help. This request for help is present along with resistance to the psychiatrist and is the basis for developing a therapeutic alliance. A therapeutic alliance is based on the help-seeking, and often more mature, aspects of the patient's personality, and allows patient and therapist to explore what are often difficult subjects.

Whatever a patient's approach to psychiatrists may be, it should be evaluated and taken into account in developing a therapeutic relationship.

Doctor factors Physicians are also a product of their culture and past experience and bring predetermined feelings and behavior patterns to encounters with patients. A number of factors can affect the doctor-patient relationship adversely. Culturally determined prejudice is one, either outright prejudice against individuals as representative of a particular group or, more likely, subtle prejudice of which doctors are unaware. It may take the form of expecting individuals of a particular group to react in a certain way—for example, the idea that young, single welfare mothers do not care how many more children they have.

Just as patients have transference reactions, psychiatrists have countertransference reactions, which emanate from past experience and can be detrimental to a productive doctor-patient relationship; therefore, it is important for psychiatrists to be constantly alert to their feelings and preconceived ideas. If psychiatrists are aware of their feelings and attitudes, they can usually compensate for them, but the ones that are outside of awareness may be destructive. For this reason, psychotherapy or psychoanalysis is helpful for the professional work of psychiatrists and is considered to be a training, as well as a therapeutic, experience. Learning about one's own attitudes and feelings as they relate to patients is a lifelong task that should be part of the continuing education of all psychiatrists.

Approach to the patient With wayward feelings and prejudices acknowledged, the psychiatrist is free to approach the patient in a nonjudgmental manner and with an open mind. When this approach is used, patients are more likely to take the initiative in expressing their troubles. The object is to allow the patient to express thoughts and feelings in the manner the patient deems important. Support and empathy on the part of the psychiatrist are required if the patient is to be comfortable in expressing feelings.

In the first interview, patients are usually anxious but still are willing to tell their story. They need some encouragement and need to feel that they will not be judged adversely. Psychiatrists need not agree with everything they are told or condone actions described, but they should listen, encourage patients to speak candidly and without censoring, and express support for what their patients are trying to do in the interview—that is, express their problem the way they see that problem. Much valuable material can be lost if psychiatrists are too controlling early in the interview.

Listening, being nonjudgmental, being aware of one's own feelings, and being supportive and empathetic with the patient's own efforts is a difficult task. With the exception of a few "natural psychiatrists," it does not come easily. It must be learned and then practiced with a constantly self-critical eye. Experienced and accomplished psychiatrists make the process look easy, but beginners find that there are many pitfalls. Most physicians only listen for the things they want to hear and discourage patients from saying anything else. Platt and McMath reviewed more than 300 clinical interviews performed by physicians with patients on a medical service. They found the physicians were not listening when the patients were expressing a feeling or discussing a problem that did not interest the doctor at that moment. Psychiatrists, especially those beginning to learn to interview, also have this problem. For example, they want the interview to proceed in an orderly manner, starting with the chief complaint and continuing with present illness, past history, and mental status examination. Patients may not have this order in mind at all. When the order deviates, many psychiatrists attempt to force patients into the predetermined pattern. This is a common way that patients' communications are stopped or discouraged.

When a 31-year-old woman was asked what brought her into the hospital, she said she had had a religious experience and then began talking about troubles with one boyfriend and how another was jealous. She then talked about how her father had molested her, but the psychiatrist still did not know the events that brought her to the hospital. Insistence on an orderly sequence of chief complaint and present illness so early in the interview would have discouraged the discussion of the rich material in the past history that was in the forefront of the patient's mind. As a matter of fact, this insistence might have stimulated a hostile reaction to the therapist, in part based on the early disturbed relationship with the patient's father.

The setting in which the interview takes place is an important factor in helping patients to feel relaxed and in encouraging them to express themselves in their own way. It is best that there be a quiet room where confidence is assured. The psychiatrist and the patient should both have a relaxed seating arrangement. The authors recommend that the barrier of a desk not be interposed between the psychiatrist and the patient. A desk serves to reinforce the image of authority on the part of the psychiatrist and may even obstruct his or her full observation of the patient's body language. If the ideal setting cannot be achieved, a satisfactory interview can still occur if the psychiatrist can convey a relaxed, confident, and open manner to the patient.

Healing powers of the doctor-patient relationship The healing powers of the doctor-patient relationship have been recognized since ancient times. Unfortunately, many nonmedical charlatans make use of interpersonal relationships as a way to dupe the unsuspecting who are seeking help. The doctor-patient relationship does not take the place of specific treatments for specific diseases, but it does accomplish many things for physicians. First, it simply helps the patient to feel better and thereby relieves some of the suffering. It helps the patient to develop a sense of trust and hope. It allows the patient to explore problems, and it makes it easier to comply with any medical regime.

There is evidence that the doctor-patient relationship actually improves the results of many medical treatments. Studies of schizophrenic patients demonstrate that improvement from psychotherapy plus medication was superior to either treatment alone. Other studies have demonstrated that disorders, such as ulcerative colitis, asthma, and peptic ulcer, respond better to a combination of medication and psychotherapy than to medication alone. Surgeons are acutely aware that the patient's psychological state influences the outcome of surgery and the healing process. There is ample evidence from many fronts that mental state can have a profound influence on neurochemical and other bodily processes. The influence of the physician on the patient's mental state comes about through the doctor-patient relationship. It is the responsibility of the psychiatrist to initiate and nurture that relationship so that it quickly may become therapeutic.

THE INTERVIEW Because of preconceived notions stemming from the transference and social and cultural factors already noted, psychiatrists may not know how their actions will be interpreted by their patients. Therefore, psychiatrists should be aware of all aspects of their behavior. This does not mean that psychiatrists should be stiff and formal, but they should tailor their behavior to the needs of the particular patient.

The patient coming to the initial interview is usually anxious and fearful. There may be hidden fears, as well as resentment and hostility if the patient was unhappy about coming. Some patients may have a feeling of great relief from having come to someone who will help them and are ready to relinquish all autonomy to the "all-knowing and all-powerful" physician.

Whatever the patient's motivation, both apparent and under the surface, the psychiatrist should attempt to infer as much as possible from the patient's behavior and respond accordingly. There are many possible responses, which will develop through knowledge and experience. For example, with an overly anxious patient, one may want to acknowledge the anxiety early in the interview, give the patient a chance to discuss it, and then give a more detailed explanation of what will happen. For the more defensive, perhaps somewhat paranoid, patient a more formal and less intrusive approach is indicated.

The psychiatrist should start the interview in a professional manner by introducing himself or herself and addressing the patient by that person's surname. There are exceptions to this, of course—for example, if the patient is known beforehand or if the patient is a teenager. Older people should be addressed by surname in the beginning as a sign of respect. This practice starts the interview with the proper tone. As the interview progresses, the psychiatrist might ask how the patient prefers to be addressed. The psychiatrist should attempt to put the patient at ease in the beginning with a friendly remark and some comments on the purpose of the interview if appropriate.

At the beginning of the interview, the patient will wait for the psychiatrist to indicate how to proceed. What the psychiatrist says, does, and the nonverbal cues given are crucial to the progress of the interview and may have a profound effect on the entire doctor-patient relationship. A collaborative relationship between doctor and patient holds the most diagnostic and therapeutic promise. To achieve this end, the patient must be given some autonomy. Autonomy is given in the beginning through a nondirective approach to the interview. Patients are asked to start in their own way and tell their story the way they want. A more directive approach, in which one begins by asking specific questions, getting an answer, and then going to another question, has a place in psychiatry and in general medicine, but it is not the best way to start an interview that will gather the most data and at the same time initiate a therapeutic doctor-patient relationship.

With the nondirective approach, an interview is started with a general question and the patient is allowed to proceed as the psychiatrist makes encouraging comments and asks general nonspecific questions. Some situations in which this approach is not indicated will be discussed later. The initial approach is to ask what brings the patient to the clinic or hospital. This question is usually sufficient for the patient to begin and continue with the chief complaint. Some patients need more encouragement and a little more structure to begin, so one might briefly review any previous information (if known) about the patient or explain more about what will happen in the evaluation. If the patient is reluctant to begin, one must not immediately take over the responsibility for developing that patient's story. It is important for the psychiatrist to make it clear that the patient's story as that patient feels it and wants to tell it is important.

As the patient proceeds, listening and intervening at the proper time and in the proper way becomes an active process. It is in this way that the psychiatrist exerts control of the interview and guides the process according to which areas are important. The psychiatrist, in effect, has a road map that guides active participation with the patient in the interview.

Once the patient begins to talk, the psychiatrist must make decisions at every point along the way as to how to participate in the process. Simply listening is one form of participation. A nod of the head or "uh-huh" is another kind. A clarifying question is another. Occasionally, when it is desirable to move to another topic, a question on another subject will be asked. Each of these forms of participation by the psychiatrist evokes a response from the patient, and the response will be different depending on what the psychiatrist does. This is why it is important that the psychiatrist be aware of these responses and what motivates them.

A general dilemma faced in the interview is whether or not to ask a clarifying question or for more information when the patient is talking about something important. For example, a man says, "I'm living with this woman now. She's very attached to me, but I don't have the intellectual stimulation I had with my first wife." The questions raised by this statement are numerous. To mention a few: How long was he married? How many wives has he had? Why does he stay with the woman he is living with now? How does he feel about her? How old is she? To ask any one of these questions early in the interview might detract from the story as it is unfolding in the patient's mind. And how it unfolds may be important information. The other information may well come out later in the interview. If not, questions can be asked then that will be less disruptive to a therapeutic doctor-patient relationship.

Ideally, as the interview progresses, a working relationship usually will be established with the patient. In such an ideal situation, the patient discusses feelings and important relationships, the psychiatrist occasionally asks a question or asks for clarification, and the patient is prompted toward more exploration.

Problems with a directive interview Directive questions are necessary at certain points in psychiatric interviews, and structured interviews now have an important place in psychiatric evaluation. Too much structure and direction too early in the interview may cause important psychodynamic information to be lost. Interviews that are entirely directive usually produce answers to specific questions, but they do not easily lead to an understanding of the patient's feelings about interpersonal relationships. The psychiatrist asks a question, the patient answers and may talk longer, but when the psychiatrist asks another question and another, the patient answers each question in turn and then waits for the next question. Spontaneity is lost. Things that may come into the patient's mind in a more free-floating interview are also lost because they are never permitted to come up. Furthermore, the patient has been permitted to assume less responsibility in the therapeutic doctor-patient relationship. The interview that is entirely directive makes the patient a passive partner. This situation is difficult to correct if a later long-term psychotherapeutic relationship is indicated. The interview that is predominantly directive may produce facts, even a large number of facts, but it tends to obscure feelings, which require a more open atmosphere for expression. And it is the expression of feelings that gives the psychiatrist an understanding of the depth and quality of a patient's psychological life. It is this psychological life that the psychiatrist deals with, even though it is often dealt with at an organic level.

Developing a history using a nondirective approach The patient's opening statement after being encouraged to talk usually contains much information and should be listened to carefully. The opening statement is not just a declaration of the patient's problem but is also a presentation of how the patient wants to be viewed by the psychiatrist; it is a complex set that presents a composite of request for help, the patient's relationship to the world, and his or her transference image of the psychiatrist. It provides a preliminary view of defense mechanisms. A great deal of material is packed into the patient's early remarks. The psychiatrist need not respond to everything but should make mental notes of as much material as possible.

As the patient talks, the chief complaint, present illness, and past history begin to unfold, and the psychiatrist enters into a kind of exploratory journey with the patient. In part of this journey, the psychiatrist will help the patient explore areas not explored before and perhaps make connections and associations not previously made or thought of. Other parts of the exploration will consist of the patient's presentation of material deemed important—some for the benefit of the psychiatrist and some because the patient needs to tell someone.

The role of the psychiatrist is to encourage the process for the benefit of the patient and to obtain an adequate psychiatric evaluation, which can often be accomplished by allowing the story to be told with as little interruption as possible. A general rule is to allow the patient to talk freely as long as important and pertinent information is being presented. This may be material the patient "just has to get out," and the patient may not feel free to go on to anything else until this happens. Usually, however, the patient is trying to give the psychiatrist an understanding of the problem and will bring in much important information if allowed to do so.

As the patient talks, the psychiatrist can show interest in certain areas by both verbal and nonverbal behavior. A nod or a question suggests to the patient that this is an area worth exploring. Some initial interviews will proceed in an orderly manner through chief complaint, present illness, and past history; others will not. The way the patient unfolds the material is important in allowing the psychiatrist a glimpse of the patient's associations—what the patient believes is connected and related and what may be connected but without the patient's awareness. An insistence by the psychiatrist on an order of procedure may disrupt these associations, and important material may be lost.

Outline for history While the patient is talking, the psychiatrist through his or her own knowledge and experience can put the material in proper perspective. The psychiatrist should have an outline of what is important to learn about the present illness, medical history, and past history. One such outline is shown in Table 9.1-1. In this outline, childhood history is organized from a developmental point of view. It allows the view of childhood experiences at crucial developmental phases. There are other ways that this material may be organized. A complete psychiatric report is described in Section 9.2.

Many psychiatrists who treat only adult patients minimize the importance of childhood experience and many may not include this in their review of history. This omission is unfortunate, because one cannot be a complete psychiatrist without understanding how the personality of the patient one is seeing at the moment has been shaped, and this shaping occurs through past experience with important people in that patient's earlier life.

Emotions in the interview Although feelings are important, they can be overlooked in the evaluation. In many psychiatric illnesses, the primary problem lies in the disturbance of emotion; in others, it may be cognition; and, in still others, it is a combination of both. With some patients, feelings are evident and present on the surface; with many patients, however, they are not, and it is up to psychiatrists to explore their presence. Outlines for the initial interview and history taking often do not provide for this exploration, so psychiatrists must always be prepared to ask patients how they feel about what is being discussed at the moment.

It is also important to determine how the individual patient handles feelings and whether or not the patient can understand the connection between feelings and thought content and other behavior. Many patients cannot understand this, and it is an important bit of data to be aware of early in the evaluation and treatment process. For example, many obsessive-compulsive patients cannot make the association between feeling states and thought content. Their major defense mechanism is the isolation of feelings from thought, but this may not be readily apparent unless psychiatrists specifically inquire what patients' feelings are about certain topics that they discuss. Sometimes the opposite is true, and the material presented by patients is primarily that of feelings and emotions; in this case, it is necessary to discover to what these feelings are connected.

Some patients have emotions that not only are easily expressed in the interview but actually interfere with the interview process and the doctor-patient relationship. These patients are often extremely anxious or hostile. In such cases, it is important to acknowledge the situation early in the interview and attempt to deal with it. Some statements reflecting the feelings that patients are having—such as "It appears that you are angry or upset about this interview. Can you tell me more about it?"—often serve to calm patients and allow them to proceed in a more productive manner. Simply allowing the emotions to obscure the interview situation is helpful neither to patients nor psychiatrists. In addition to acknowledging the anxiety and allowing the patient to discuss it, it may be helpful to go into more detail about the purpose of the interview and what happens when people see psychiatrists. Sometimes this information must be repeated because in the patients' anxiety they may not have been able to comprehend what was first said. The demeanor of psychiatrists with both anxious and hostile patients is very important. Psychiatrists certainly do not respond with like feelings—that is, show anxiety or hostility. A calm and reassuring manner on the part of psychiatrists may be the most important factor in allowing the interview to proceed in a more orderly fashion.

The open-ended interview discussed here will not be adequate for all patients. Some patients cannot respond to it and will require more structure. The open-ended approach can be modified to include the structured interview described in the next section. There are a few patients who cannot relate at all to this nondirective approach. For example, mildly retarded patients will not be able to think abstractly and, therefore, will not grasp the nuances of the interview as it has been described. With these patients, psychiatrists must take a more direct approach, often asking specific questions.

TABLE 9.1-1
An Outline for Psychiatric History

I. Identification and demographic information
   A. Name, address, phone number
   B. Age
   C. Sex
   D. Place of birth
   E. Marital status
   F. Ethnic group
   G. Occupation
   H. Education
II. Present illness
   A. Presenting complaint, problem, or problems (i.e., what the patient claims is the distress or symptom that prompted the visit to the psychiatrist)
   B. Onset, course, and duration
   C. Events temporally associated with onset, exacerbation, and remissions
      1. Other medical problems
      2. Socioeconomic problems
      3. Problems with interpersonal relationships
      4. School or work situation
   D. Developmental period associated with onset
   E. Personality changes prior to or at onset of illness
   F. Change in feelings about important people
   G. Special things to look for: changes in eating habits, interests, routines, sleep patterns, feelings about work
   H. Why does the patient come now?
   I. Past and present treatments and treatment results
III. Medical history
   A. Other current medical problems
   B. Past medical history
   C. Drug history
   D. Systems review
   E. Family medical history and history of mental illness, alcoholism, deviant behavior, and so on
IV. Psychosocial history: significant interpersonal relationships, feelings, and significant events from birth to present
   A. Infancy
      1. Circumstances surrounding birth
      2. Relationship of father and mother
      3. Socioeconomic situation of the family
      4. Health of the mother and father
      5. Principal caretaker or mothering figure
   B. Toddler and preschool phase
      1. Developmental milestones—walking, talking
      2. Significant family events
      3. New siblings
      4. First memories
   C. Middle childhood
      1. School
         a. Intelligence and successes and failures in schoolwork
         b. Problems with teachers
         c. Other school-related activities
   D. Adolescence
      1. Peer relationships
      2. Relationships with opposite sex
      3. School
         a. Academic
         b. Other activities
      4. Relationships with parents
      5. Aspirations
      6. Successes and failures
      7. First use of alcohol and drugs
   E. Adulthood
      1. Work
      2. Social relations
      3. Sexuality and marriage
      4. Family relationships
      5. Economic circumstances
      6. Changes with increasing age
      7. Alcohol and drug use
   F. Outlook and plans for the future in family, work, and social relationships

Note taking Although obtaining a good and complete psychiatric record is important, it may be somewhat in conflict with the ability of psychiatrists to concentrate on the behavior of patients during interviews. It is often necessary for psychiatrists to take some notes, but it should not interfere with their concentration on the patient and their ability not only to listen attentively but also to observe all of a patient's nonverbal behavior. Psychiatrists should not attempt to complete the write-up during a session, but rather jot down enough information to permit adequate recall of the material. The important thing to remember in note taking is that the doctor-patient relationship needs to be established, and this result requires a fully attentive psychiatrist who can respond appropriately.

Other factors affecting the interview There must be ample time for the patient to develop his or her story, ample time for the psychiatrist to obtain information necessary for an evaluation, and ample time for a therapeutic relationship to begin. The time necessary for this depends on the patient, the problem, and the amount of previous information. Usually, a complete evaluation takes more than one interview. The 45- to 50-minute psychotherapeutic hour is a good rule of thumb when considering the time necessary for the initial interview. Some patients need more time. For other patients, less time may be needed if there will be follow-up interviews soon to complete the evaluation.

Whatever time is given, it should be free of interruptions from phone calls or other matters that take the psychiatrist's attention away from the patients. It is generally agreed that only emergency calls should be accepted during an interview. Any interruption will disrupt the patient's flow of thought and associations, the doctor's attention and associations, and impair the developing doctor-patient relationship.

Frequently, justifiably concerned relatives accompany the patient to the interview. They may often request to talk with the psychiatrist, or the patient may make such a request. Relatives or significant others often have information that can be helpful to the evaluation. How relatives are handled may have an important effect on the doctor-patient relationship and on subsequent therapy. Usually, it is best to see the patient first, complete the interview, and then, after assuring the patient that no confidential information will be divulged, ask permission to see the relative. Almost always permission is given; but if not, one must abide by the patient's wishes unless the patient is clearly psychotic and has severely impaired judgment. It is often helpful to see the relative or relatives separately from the patient and then see patient and relatives together. Some patients may be so disturbed or so anxious that it is necessary first to see patient and relatives together. This approach may relieve some anxiety, and then the patient can be seen alone.

STRUCTURED PSYCHIATRIC INTERVIEW APPROACHES

OVERVIEW OF STRUCTURED PSYCHIATRIC INTERVIEWING

Structured psychiatric interviewing entails two features that distinguish it from open-ended approaches. The first is the elicitation of the key information based on systematic inquiry into specific historical and symptomatic information. This process may entail preformatted questions or may involve only a general description of the topic area, with the exact line of inquiry left to the clinician. The second feature is that structured methods provide for scoring the information obtained. In research, this practice allows for the quantification of scores and the development of statistical norms. Before specific structured interviewing techniques and examples are discussed, it is useful to review the rationale out of which these approaches developed.

RATIONALE FOR STRUCTURED INTERVIEWS

Criterion differences Historically, diagnostic precision in psychiatry has been poor. An example of this was the overdiagnosis of schizophrenia by U.S. psychiatrists when compared with European psychiatrists, prior to the implementation of the third edition of the American Psychiatric Association's *Diagnostic and Statistical Manual of Mental Disorders* (DSM-III). Studies have suggested that a major reason for this poor level of agreement lay in individualized, even idiosyncratic, differences in the criteria that two otherwise similarly competent psychiatrists might have used to establish a particular diagnosis. Thus, if one psychiatrist is satisfied with hallucinations alone as a sufficient criterion for schizophrenia, the rate of his or her diagnosis of schizophrenia will be substantially higher than that of a psychiatrist who requires the full criteria found in DSM-III. Recognition of the principal role of criterion-based differences in the poor interrater reliability of psychiatric diagnosis was a major motivating force to the development of the Research Diagnostic Criteria (RDC), from which DSM-III was developed. By defining explicitly what criteria, in number, severity, and duration of symptoms, meet the threshold requirements for a particular diagnosis, criterion variance has been substantially reduced.

Treatment specificity The past quarter century has seen the development of many specific and quite effective psychiatric treatments. Thus, in contrast to an earlier time when most treatment was nonspecific, or involved a generally invoked psychotherapy, diagnosis now matters keenly. In other words, if one lacks any specifically effective treatment for a disorder, and treatment is likely to be more similar than different regardless of the diagnosis, there is little incentive to distinguish among diagnostic possibilities. As an example, panic disorder was not a considered entity 25 years ago; therefore, few psychiatrists inquired in a sufficiently specific way to identify that disorder. It is now recognized that there are differences between panic disorder and generalized anxiety disorder in the development of symptoms, severity of episodes, illness course, and responsiveness to drugs. As a consequence, physicians who previously never considered panic disorder began to recognize it frequently. In little more than 5 years, major changes in everyday clinical thinking resulted.

Similarly, recognition that psychotic symptoms may accompany bipolar depression and manic disorders, new clinical epidemiological data about studies of schizophrenia, and the dramatic effectiveness of lithium in bipolar disorders resulted in a heightened interest in classification of psychotic disorders. As a result, many patients once diagnosed as schizophrenic have been more accurately rediagnosed as having bipolar disorders. Accordingly, treatment has been changed to lithium, which is generally more effective in such disorders than antipsychotic drugs.

Differences in patient response Open-ended interview strategies often do not work well with certain patients. Unsophisticated patients in particular are less likely, even when clearly encouraged, to give a full account of their illness. They are more likely to respond briefly to open-ended questions and wait for the physician to ask more questions. In addition to socioeconomic considerations, differences in personality and the fear of the implications of a set of symptoms may cause a patient to be verbally underproductive.

Studies of patient expectation and response Studies of patients in both diagnostic and therapeutic interviews further support an important role for structured ways of obtaining and providing information. Cox and his co-workers observed that the quality of information obtained in diagnostic psychiatric interviews was positively correlated with the use of more probe questions per topic and more requests for detailed information. Open-ended questions, coupled with frequent use of repetitions immediately after a patient's statement, resulted in more feedback from informants.

Studies in the area of adherence to treatment provide strong support for providing information about the illness and its treatment to the patient in a more systematic manner. Physicians had underestimated patients' desires for information and discussion about their illnesses and their treatment. Compliance was improved when the patients' expectations of what they wanted to know about their illness were met. Furthermore, compliance was improved when doctors provided proportionately more of the information in a therapeutic visit than did the patients.

Detailed instruction about a treatment regimen also improves compliance. About half of patients told to take a medication "with meals" misinterpreted the instruction to mean before meals, sometimes as long as an hour before the meal.

Differences linked to diagnosis Structured interviews are sometimes indicated principally because of the patient's particular disorder. As a rule, psychotic patients and patients with organic mental disorders are not effectively interviewed by open-ended techniques. These patients tend to be made anxious or become more disorganized in their thought processes in the absence of structure and well-defined boundaries in the interview situation. For both groups of patients, questions that ask explicitly for small bits of information are indicated. Their effectiveness is often aided by providing substantial feedback to patients and helping them establish structure in other ways, such as indicating the length of time of the interview.

Depressed patients often fail to provide spontaneously an adequate account of their illness, either because of psychomotor retardation and hopelessness or a wish to present an artificially cheerful, less-impaired face to the world. For either reason, specific inquiry about all historical, functional, and symptomatic aspects of depressive disorders is important. An additional reason for structured questions is that the patient may not have associated problems in certain areas with the basic disorder. For example, the patient may not spontaneously tell of waking during the night, or increased somatic complaints, simply because he has not linked them to his conception of depression. Inquiry about suicidal ideas nearly always requires a somewhat structured approach and should be made in all patients with depression, even if there is no apparent suicidal risk. A family history of suicide or previous suicidal behavior by the patient increases risk. Evidence of impulsivity, or of rigidly set, unrealistically high goals for oneself are additional warning signs. Patients with interview evidence of hopelessness or resignation are at greater suicidal risk. Patients who have made major changes in their life, who have recently put their life affairs in order for their demise, or otherwise planned for their suicide are also at increased risk.

Potentially violent patients should be approached with some of the same attitudes and strategies used with suicidal patients. Indicating that one is interested in and capable of dealing with the patient's capacity for violence is important. It conveys that one is accustomed to the unpleasant, as well as the pleasant, in life. Specific inquiry about previous violent acts committed and violence experienced as a child is important. One should determine under what conditions the person feels he or she would resort to violence. With violent patients, corroboration of their history of or propensity for violence through interview of relatives and friends is important. For violent patients, structure of the interview and treatment setting is also necessary. Although most interviews should first be one to one, the interviewer should have another person present. Other structured precautions include leaving the room's door open and sitting between the patient and the door. The interviewer needs to explicate that the patient is free to hold any feelings but is not free to act in a violent manner. Furthermore, the structure of the treatment unit and the actions of the staff will be used to lend the person support in efforts to maintain control.

Patients with somatoform disorders also require a type of structured interviewing. A major reason for this is that patients are often so identified with their physical complaints that the needed information about reactions of others to their problems, effect on work, or other responsibilities and symptoms indicative of associated depression or anxiety is not obtained without specific inquiry.

Although nondirective approaches are important in interviewing family members, there are several circumstances in which more structured approaches are valuable. A spouse may so closely identify with the plight of the patient that anxiety overwhelms the ability to provide coherent, useful information. Relatives may try to insinuate themselves into the treatment in a way that will be counterproductive. Relatives may not realize that certain kinds of information are best provided by an observer. For example, a spouse may be better able to describe the social interaction or the level of activity of the patient, but not the patient's thoughts or feelings. In each of these circumstances, relatively specific questions may accomplish more and be more time-efficient.

Differences linked to interview purpose The nondirective approach taken in a psychiatric interview often must be modified, depending on the aim and circumstances of the interview. An emergent crisis situation requires more focused questions and less inquiry into areas ancillary to the crisis at hand. The principal objective in an emergent situation is to establish sufficient information to begin treatment or otherwise make a disposition. A comprehensive initial evaluation has different objectives and methods. Usually the urgency is lower, facilitating the thorough exploration of the patient's illness, plus all of the background information that aids in understanding the context of the illness and, finally, a formulation for the patient. Even for an initial evaluation the amount and type of information varies, depending on the chronic or acute nature of the illness and the existence of previous records. Consultative evaluations are usually structured around the questions or objectives for which the consultation was requested.

The consultative evaluation, whether office-based or on the hospital ward, has other structured characteristics that are necessary for its success. Not only must the questions and needs of the requesting physician be understood, but the findings and treatment experience to that point should serve as an essential background to evaluation of the patient. In the hospital setting, additional information from nurses and others involved in the patient's care is often a prerequisite to an effective recommendation. Furthermore, the consultative evaluation needs to be prefaced by a discussion with the patient to determine what he or she expects of the consultation and thereby establish a reasonably mutual understanding. Finally, the degree to which the interview objective is problem identification rather than the conduct of treatment will substantially affect the role of structured psychiatric interview approaches.

GENERAL STRATEGIES FOR STRUCTURED INTERVIEWING

The majority of structured interviewing strategies are ones that can easily and flexibly be included in a wide variety of interview situations. An overriding principle is that in the conduct of the interview, psychiatrists will explicitly inquire about every symptomatic or historical area pertinent to the objectives of the interview. Such inquiry will usually be intended to establish relatively detailed information in each area. This approach is substantially different from one in which it is asserted that if information is important, patients will mention it—and if not mentioned, it is either normal or unimportant. This structured approach also requires that physicians do not assume anything from the patient's looks or behavior. For example, based on information already obtained, the psychiatrist in question may have concluded that this particular patient cannot have suicidal ideas, or hallucinations, and thus omit direct questioning in the area. Experience with structured interviews shows that a direct question in the area may result in a positive answer even though clinical judgment would have deemed it highly improbable—even in patients with whom close doctor-patient relationships have been established. At times, the approach may require psychiatrists' overcoming a sense of apology for asking patients about a seemingly irrelevant area.

The form and sequence of structured questions is straightforward. A general probe question of the area is asked. If the definition of a term is unclear, examples are provided. If patients respond affirmatively, subsequent questions establish the severity, frequency, context, and associated features of the behavior or feeling. To illustrate with the topic of depressed mood, an opening question is, "Do you ever feel downhearted, sad, or blue?" If patients respond affirmatively, subsequent questions would include: "How often do you feel (substitute patient's phrase for depressed mood here)? Is the feeling the same throughout the day, or are there times in the day in which you feel better, worse? Are there any things happening in your life to cause you to feel this way? Is this the same way that I would feel after a close relative died? How long have you been feeling this way? Is the feeling at its worst right now?"

Usual principles of patient interviewing apply to structured approaches. In particular, the first probe in an area should be relatively open ended, so as not to shut off the patients' responses. Thus, psychiatrists would avoid a question, such as, "You haven't thought about suicide, have you?" A more satisfactory question would be, "In the past week, have you thought about, considered, or attempted to take your own life?" Questions that help patients establish a temporal relationship are often useful (e.g., "Did you first become depressed before or after you lost your job?"). Other types of multiple-choice questions can be effective when used judiciously with poorly communicative patients ("Did the nervousness come on suddenly, or gradually build up?"). The descriptive statement followed by a question is useful for symptom areas that may be misunderstood, or which are likely to be emotion-laden ("Some people hear noises or voices when there is no one present. Does that ever happen to you?").

Certain types of directive questions should be avoided. So-called double-barreled questions ("Have you had any crying spells or felt faint?") tend to produce ambiguous answers. Accusatory or leading questions almost never help ("He doesn't wet the bed, does he?").

Although there have been relatively few objective studies of what does and does not work in interviewing, the evidence available is helpful, especially in addressing common concerns that physicians have about structured approaches. The concern that obtaining more factual data will impede the expression of feelings by patients is not borne out by studies. Indeed, emotional expression is generally greater when more factual information is obtained if physicians are receptive to emotional expression.

This lack of impedance of emotional expression is important to recall in follow-up treatment that combines pharmacotherapy and psychotherapy. It is easy to fall into a trap of essentially listening to patients describe the events of the immediate past interval period, or their associations in psychotherapy, without any systematic inquiry about target symptoms and side-effect areas. A similar problem results when the last 5 minutes of a session are left for a hurried inquiry about drug effects. Although it is true that psychiatrists gain valuable and essential information from observing patients' styles, level of animation, clarity of speech, and manner of relating, this information is not adequate in itself. Specific inquiry about the key symptomatic features of a patient's illness, the exact pattern of taking medications, and function in areas in which side effects frequently result is important. Patients will often acknowledge, on direct questioning, information that was omitted out of embarrassment, anxiety, or oversight. The practice of inquiring systematically conveys to patients the thoroughness of one's assessment. It also may aid educationally, causing patients to be more self-observant in the areas inquired about in subsequent intervals between appointments.

LIMITATIONS OF STRUCTURED TECHNIQUES Structured interviews are rarely best conducted in a particular fixed sequence of topics. Whereas this may be important for certain research purposes, clinically it is often preferable to allow patients to commence telling their stories, using the open-ended techniques described earlier in this section. One should prioritize the information obtained, with emphasis on those areas of principal importance. Phrased differently, it is less important that an interview schedule be pursued unbendingly than that all subject areas eventually be addressed. This approach allows one to take advantage of chance associations and may result in the emergence of otherwise unavailable material.

Structured interviews do not ensure that all information will be forthcoming. Patients may still deny, fail to remember, or not adequately comprehend the question asked. However, it is surprising how often patients who do not volunteer information, especially in such areas as suicide and drug dosage, will acknowledge the truth when queried.

Structured and open-ended interviews should not be viewed as incompatible; both have important roles in psychiatric practice. Many psychiatric interviews can and will contain elements of both types of interviews, with psychiatrists selecting the strategy best for the situation at hand.

OVERVIEW OF SPECIFIC STRUCTURED INTERVIEWS A number of formal structured psychiatric interviews have gained increasing use. Although these interviews are principally used in research settings, several are valuable for certain clinical conditions. The impetus for the development of some of these rating instruments is briefly reviewed here, and the principal features of some of the more widely used schedules are discussed.

One major impetus to the development of standardized diagnostic interview schedules was to ensure that the criteria used by one psychiatrist to establish a diagnosis would be identical to those used by another. In that way, when patients were referred to as having, say, obsessive-compulsive disorder, other investigators and clinicians would know with some confidence what symptoms those patients exhibited. This system, now embodied in the revised third edition of the *Diagnostic and Statistical Manual of Mental Disorders* (DSM-III-R), has its roots at least as early as the works of Emil Kraepelin and Karl Jaspers. In the 1960s, a group of investigators, many at Washington University, addressed these questions. The Feighner criteria developed there led to the RDC, which were the basis for DSM-III. In an effort to standardize diagnostic procedures further, an interview schedule was developed with the assistance of the National Institute of Mental Health (NIMH) Clinical Research Branch Collaborative Program on the Psychology of Depression to define the symptom areas and to provide a rating schedule of symptom severity and specific questions to elicit the information needed to make a diagnosis by the RDC. This instrument, the Schedule for Affective Disorders and Schizophrenia (SADS), is still extensively used in a wide range of psychiatric studies. An example of the symptom definition, severity ranking, and probe questions is shown in Table 9.1-2. The probe questions developed for instruments such as the SADS can often be used to advantage by the practicing psychiatrist in a clinical setting. The reason is that in developing the probe questions, attention was given to phrases that would not be ambiguous, that were effectively asked in a wide range of settings and patients, and that resulted in responses pertinent to the item being rated. A shorter version, utilizing those items sensitive to change with treatment, is also used (SADS-C). Another example of a principally diagnostic instrument is the Diagnostic Interview Schedule (DIS). The DIS also yields a DSM-III diagnosis, but utilizes a rigidly structured series of questions to which the answers are "yes" or "no". Administered by trained nonclinicians, it has been utilized principally in large-scale epidemiological studies.

The Structured Clinical Interview for DSM-III-R (SCID) is designed to approximate an experienced clinician's diagnostic interview. Although specific probe questions are utilized, many are intended to elicit open-ended responses rather than simple agreement that a symptom is present or absent, as in the DIS. The scoring is coded to indicate what meets or exceeds the diagnostic threshold or what is present but at a diagnostic subthreshold level. Both the DIS and the SCID are essentially diagnostic, not severity-determining, instruments.

The largest group of structured interviews are those designed principally to assess symptom severity in a particular area. The Hamilton Depression Rating Scale (HAM-D) and the similarly constructed Hamilton Anxiety Rating Scale for Anxiety (HAM-A) are among the scales longest in use. A similar scale used to assess psychotic disorders is the Brief Psychiatric Rating Scale (BPRS). These scales divide symptomatology reflective of disorders in the respective areas into 17 to 24 areas. Each area is defined in a brief accompanying description. The 4- or 5-point ratings for each item are linked relatively closely to the descriptions. There are no required

TABLE 9.1-2
Depression Item from Schedule for Affective Disorders and Schizophrenia

Subjective feelings of depression based on verbal complaints of feeling depressed, sad, blue, gloomy, down in the dumps, empty, "don't care." Do not include such ideational aspects as discouragement, pessimism, or worthlessness; suicide attempts or depressed appearance (all of which are to be rated separately).	0	No information
	1	Not at all
	2	Slight (e.g., only occasionally feels "sad" or "down")
How have you been feeling? Describe your mood.	3	Mild (e.g., often feels somewhat "depressed," "blue," or "downhearted")
Have you felt depressed (sad, blue, moody, down, empty, as if you didn't care)? (Have you cried or been tearful?) (How often? Does it come and go?) (How long does it last?)	4	Moderate (e.g., most of the time feels "depressed")
	5	Severe (e.g., most of the time feels "wretched")
How bad is the feeling? (Can you stand it?)	6	Extreme (e.g., most of the time feels extreme depression, which "I can't stand")
	7	Very extreme (e.g., constant, unrelieved, extremely painful feelings of depression)

Table from the Schedule for Affective Disorders and Schizophrenia, Robert L. Spitzer and Jean Endicott, Biometrics Research, New York State Psychiatric Institute, 722 W. 168th Street, New York, NY 10032.

probe questions, although guidelines for scoring and suggested interview strategies have developed over the years.

These ratings have the particular advantage that the overall score of a patient is closely linked to severity of illness. Thus, a group of depressed patients, all of whom had HAM-D scores of 20 or greater before entering treatment, would be considered at least moderately ill. Similarly, improvement to a score of 6 or less would be considered to reflect a generally recovered, largely symptom-free status. Use of such severity ratings greatly facilitates large-scale clinical studies and facilitates the interpretation of a study by readers, or comparing one study with another. Each of these rating scales can also be used to derive a score in a single area, such as sleep disturbance. Clinicians or investigators who are interested in the effect of a treatment on a particular symptom complex may use such rating forms to obtain that information.

A different, though complementary, approach to assessment of overall severity or change is use of a global measure. Of the several global scales, the Global Assessment of Functioning Scale has particularly wide use, in part because of the detailed structured criteria given for scoring in each decile range between 1 and 100. A global scale may in certain circumstances provide greater sensitivity than a scale composed of a large number of individual items. As an example, a schizophrenic patient may retain fixed delusions of grandeur and influence, even though, in terms of overall social interaction and ability to function in routine daily life, the patient is substantially improved. A global scale will often reflect this improvement better than a scale weighted toward psychotic items, such as the SADS-C or the BPRS.

Self-rating scales are intended to provide the patients with a comprehensive view of their symptoms. The Self-Report Symptom Inventory—Revised (SCL-90), the Zung Self-Rating Depression Scale, and the Beck Depression Inventory are examples of such scales. An advantage of such scales is that they can be obtained conveniently and without substantial professional expense. They can be useful in screening whether patients meet criteria for severity in a particular area. They should be particularly sensitive to the rating of subjective feeling states, such as sadness or guilt, which cannot be observed directly by clinicians. A limitation of self-rating scales is that patients, unlike professional staff, cannot be trained to a common standard of interpretation. Therefore, patients who tend to minimize all symptoms may respond substantially differently from otherwise equally ill persons who on self-report amplify their symptomatology.

Nurse-rated scales are available for many psychiatric disorders. The Affective Disorders Rating Scale (ADRS) and the Nurse Observation Scale for Inpatient Evaluation (NOSIE), which is relatively detailed in psychotic symptomatology but limited in the areas of depression and anxiety, are examples of nurse-rated scales. The strength and principal rationale for such scales is that certain symptoms, such as socialization and expressed anger, are better rated based on observed behavior rather than during a psychiatric interview or by self-report.

This brief review of some commonly used rating scales indicates that the critical question regarding their use is not whether they are of value, but what advantages and limitations they have for a particular objective in a particular setting.

As clinical and epidemiological advances in understanding about psychiatric disorders proceed, psychiatrists can envision an increasingly important role for structured psychiatric questions and comprehensive rating instruments. In part, this will be because patients will be unlikely, unless prompted, to make some of the associations that link events to symptoms and thus facilitate definitive diagnosis.

Two examples from the area of mood disorders are illustrative. Recent evidence indicates that seasonal factors influence the development of depression, generally in patients with features analogous to bipolar disorder. Unless specifically inquired for, patients may not have made this association. Similarly, reduced time spent asleep, independent of cause, may precipitate and serve as the harbinger of a manic state. Specific, focused questions about such symptoms may be critical to establishing the information needed for accurate diagnosis.

MENTAL STATUS EXAMINATION

The mental status examination is a formal procedure that describes patient behaviors that are evident at the time of the interview. It provides an objective record important both for diagnosis and for assessing the course of a disorder and its subsequent response to treatment. Careful and precise descriptions of phenomena, without speculations and inferences, are necessary in recording the mental status examination. The mental status examination is to be interpreted in conjunction with historical information, a physical examination, and laboratory studies. If considered without regard to other relevant data, erroneous conclusions may result, as in the following example:

A patient who has exhibited hyperactivity, rapid speech, persecutory delusions, and irritable mood meets inclusion criteria for a manic episode. After being administered antipsychotic medication, the patient may be misdiagnosed as having schizophrenia, paranoid type, because the clinical presentation has evolved to include paucity of speech, psychomotor slowing, constricted affect, and persecutory delusions. Antipsychotic drug effects are misconstrued as blunted affect. An additional error results from failure to perform an adequate physical examination on initial presentation to note dilated pupils, tachycardia, and hypertension, suggesting autonomic hyperactivity, a workup of which would include urinary drug testing, which would have revealed the presence of amphetamine metabolites. Consequently, the final diagnosis would be organic mood disorder secondary to amphetamine intoxication.

The following are components of the mental status examination:

1. Appearance
2. Activity
3. Mood and affect
4. Speech and language
5. Thought content
6. Perceptual disturbances
7. Insight
8. Judgment
9. Neuropsychiatric functions

Each of these parameters must be described for a mental status examination to be complete.

APPEARANCE The appearance of patients, including apparent age, obvious physical stigmata, general state of physical health, overt emotional displays, manner of relating, and level of cooperation, should be recorded. Facial expressions may convey happy, sad, anxious, or perplexed states of mind. Melancholic patients exhibit both an omega sign (a furrowed brow caused by sustained contraction of the corrugator muscle) and Veraguth's folds (an upward, inward peaking of the upper eyelids). Schizophrenic and organic patients may be dirty and disheveled, being both unaware of and unconcerned about their appearance. Schizophrenic patients may appear to be gangly, dysplastic, and poorly coordinated. Manic patients are the most colorful and bizarre in appearance. Head decoration with scraps of debris, excessive jewelry, and layers of mismatched clothing are all common among manic patients. Slick, au courant garb is common among antisocial personalities and drug abusers. Current social trends must be respected when assessing appearance, however, inasmuch as multicolored dyed hair, pins through the earlobe, and bones through the nasal septum may all be acceptable in some subcultures.

ACTIVITY Disturbances of motor activity may be classified as increased, decreased, and catatonic patterns. Increased motor activity is divided into hyperactivity and agitation. Hyperactivity, for example, is a supranormal degree of purposeful, goal-directed activity. It typically includes increased hand gestures used to punctuate ideas being conveyed. Agitated behavior includes increased purposeless, goalless behaviors, such as foot tapping, scalp rubbing, handwringing, pacing, alternately sitting and standing, and carphologic movements (picking at clothing and bed linens). Agitation can occur as a manifestation of confusion in delirium or dementia, an intense mood in anxiety states, psychoses, or mood disorders, or it may represent antipsychotic-induced akathisia.

Decreased activity or psychomotor retardation is manifested by a diminution of movement, speech, and thinking. It includes excessive speech latency before answering a question. Such slowing and paucity of activity is seen in dementias (especially subcortical dementias), lateral-convexity frontal lobe damage, depression, and schizophrenia. Extreme psychomotor retardation is designated as stupor. Patients appropriately designated stuporous are mute, immobile, and unresponsive to vigorous, even painful, stimuli.

Observable symptoms of catatonia may be gross or subtle and require skillful elucidation. Odd, repetitive movements may be called mannerisms if they seem to be part of a goal-directed activity, or they may be designated stereotypes if they are without discernible goals. Automatic obedience is a category of catatonic behavior, wherein verbal instructions are overriden by tactile or visual stimuli (e.g., the patient shakes hands with the examiner contrary to firm verbal instructions whenever the examiner's right hand is extended). Other examples of catatonia include *Mitmachen,* in which, despite instructions to the contrary, the patient will allow a body part to be put into any position without resistance to light pressure, then returns the body part to the original resting position when the examiner releases it.

In ambitendency, a lesser form of negativism, the patient makes a series of tentative back-and-forth movements that approach but never reach a goal, such as shaking hands or walking to a particular location. *Echopraxia* is the automatic copying of the examiner's movements or posture, whereas *echolalia* is the automatic repetition of the examiner's utterances. *Catalepsy* is the prolonged sustaining of an awkward posture or position. If the examiner encounters plastic resistance like the bending of a wax rod when moving the patient's arm, which will then be maintained in an odd position, the entire phenomenon is termed waxy flexibility or *flexibilitas cerea*.

MOOD AND AFFECT *Mood* is a sustained subjective feeling state, which can be described by qualities including (but not limited to) happiness, sadness, worry, anxiety, irritability, anger, detachment, and indifference. The patient's appearance may or may not be congruent with the mood described. *Affect* refers to more transitory and immediate emotional expressions with described mood content as one component. Other aspects of affect include: (1) range, which is constricted if a spectrum of moods is not elicitable, or expanded if excesses of joyfulness or sadness are seen; (2) intensity, which can be increased as in vituperative, invective speech with dogmatic insistence regarding self-convictions, or diminished when patients appear shallow and vacuous with little conviction in their statements; (3) stability versus nonunderstandable, rapid changeability or lability; (4) appropriateness of affective display to the content of speech and thought; and (5) relatedness, which is the ability to establish rapport and interpersonal connectedness.

To assess mood and affect fully, the clinical interview must cover a variety of topics in sufficient depth and breadth. If the interview is limited to an enumeration of symptoms, a comprehensive analysis of affect is impossible. Questions pertaining to patients' individually experienced joys and disappointments must be asked. Asking about personal losses and reactions to such losses is invaluable, as are questions concerning loved ones and career successes. By inquiring about hobbies and interests, different aspects of affect should be elicited, as well as information about drive and motivation and whether anhedonia is currently present. It is important to distinguish apathy without sadness from the sad and lowered mood present in depressions and grief states.

The expression *emotional* (or *affective*) *blunting* can be best applied to apathetic, indifferent patients whose affects are diminished in intensity and constricted to a narrow neutral range. Such patients do not display sadness or happiness, have no depth to their convictions, lack relatedness to the examiner, and lack concern for other people. If manifested to an extreme degree, the condition may be designated flattened affect. Although this symptom typifies many chronic schizophrenic patients and comprises the core of the so-called negative or Type II subtype of schizophrenia, it is also characteristic of a number of neurological conditions. Sometimes confused with affective blunting is motor dysprosody, which typically follows lesions caused by anterior right cerebral hemisphere strokes. It is marked by monotonous, sparse speech without affective or inflectional coloring; however, patients so afflicted can experience strong and painful emotions. With such patients, examiners can be misled into minimizing the dysphoria that is present and neglect to treat depressions, with their attendant morbidity and mortality risks.

Inappropriate affect with lability is characteristic of pseudobulbar palsy, in which patients laugh while describing depression or cry while claiming to be happy. Increased mood intensity is most often seen in manics, antisocial and borderline personalities, paranoid states, and some epileptics with limbic system foci. Frontal lobe disturbances can show a plethora of affective problems, including a silly, shallow inappropriate jocularity, irritability, emotional lability and impulsity, and apathy and indifference.

SPEECH AND LANGUAGE The speech and language productions of patients frequently provide examiners with an indirect view of their thoughts, since thoughts as such cannot be directly observed. Formal speech or language abnormalities can reflect brain pathology or a psychiatric disorder, or both. Neglecting to assess fully the form of communications by patients can be a critical error because the form of speech and language can be of diagnostic significance and must be examined separately from content.

Speech fluency should also be noted. Mutism, excessive latency of response, paucity of speech, dysarthria, anomia, agrammatism, and paraphasic errors are all pathological. Loud, insistent speech (pressured speech) is characteristic of mania.

Describing the form of a patient's language productions can be difficult, especially if the accompanying content is colorful, bizarre, or otherwise distracting. The following are generally referred to as types of formal thought disorders, although they are technically language disorders. *Circumstantiality* is overly detailed, circuitous speech that arrives at its intended goal. *Tangential* speech initially seems to address the intended point but veers away from it and never reaches that point as it progresses. *Blocking* is the patient's cessation of speech before the goal is reached, with the usual explanation that the mind went blank. If speech resumes on a completely different topic, *derailment* is present. In *loosening of associations,* there is a continued shifting of topics, which, if it progresses to near incoherence, is termed *word salad.* Impaired understandability due to idiosyncratic word usage, irrelevancies, abrupt change of subject, or lack of logical connection between words, phrases, or sentences occurs principally in psychotic disorders. When the disconnectedness from reality is emphasized, the terms *dereistic* and *autistic thinking* are often applied. These disturbances should not be rated if they are due to a nonpsychopathological cause, such as lack of education or dialect. Differentiating manic flight of ideas from schizophrenic loosening of associations can be exceedingly difficult. Manic speech will include *clanging,* or association by sound, be diverted by external stimuli, or occur in rapid and pressured fashion. In both conditions, incoherence may be reached and they cannot be differentiated. Answers that are totally unrelated to a question are *non sequiturs. Verbal preservation* can be either themes, phrases, or words that are inappropriately and repeatedly present in the flow of speech.

THOUGHT CONTENT Disorders of thought content range from transient preoccupations to intractable delusions. *Ruminations* commonly accompany states of depression and anxiety. They represent mood-congruent concerns, which abate when the underlying condition diminishes. *Obsessions* are unwanted and unwarranted ideas, images, or impulses that repeatedly and incessantly intrude into conscious awareness. They induce an intense dysphoria and are often accompanied by *compulsions*—stereotyped actions, which typically include counting, checking, washing, or rearranging rituals and are themselves the source of anxiety if not performed in a specific manner.

Phobias are unrealistic fears of specific objects, locations, or situations, which are avoided with great effort. If confronted with the object of their avoidance, phobic patients develop anxiety in a degree proportionate to the fears they harbor.

Delusional ideas represent a particular form of cognitive intransigence. These unshakable beliefs are not in keeping with a particular patient's social, cultural, or religious background. They may by chance be true, as is occasionally the case with delusions of infidelity, but almost always delusions are false and often outlandish. A primary delusional idea is one which cannot be understood as arising from preexisting psychopathology, such as hallucinations or an aberrant mood. If a primary delusional idea develops fully and suddenly, as an immediate enlightenment, it is termed an autochthonous delusion. It is therefore important to ask how patients became aware of any delusional ideas. The examiner should not challenge a patient's delusional ideas. Sometimes, on hearing a delusional idea, it may be useful to react with mild surprise or disbelief at the ideas expressed in order to assess the fixity of these beliefs. If examiners are nonplussed by a blatantly bizarre statement, patients with partial insight regarding their delusions may conclude that that examiner is patronizing and insincere. Patients may also be asked as to how they think the average person would regard such ideas in an attempt to assess the patients' insight regarding their delusions.

An *overvalued idea* is a useful term for a delusion-like idea that inappropriately preoccupies a patient but is not bizarre and about which the patient maintains insight. For example, a so-called survivalist adheres obsessively to the belief in total self-sufficiency. Overvalued ideas have been associated with a broad spectrum of psychiatric disorders.

Delusions of persecution, loosely known as paranoid delusions, include delusions of self-reference *(ideas of reference),* in which people take undue notice of or talk about the patient, and delusions of being influenced by outside forces or of being poisoned. Persecutory delusions may be elicited from guarded patients by asking whether they feel they are singled out from the populace at large for some type of maltreatment. Patients who are delusional will emphasize their uniqueness in being harassed. Grandiose delusions typify manic states. Somatic or hypochondriacal delusions include the conviction of having fatal diseases, infestations, or degeneration of internal organs. The *Capgras' syndrome* is the delusion that a significant person (often the spouse) has been replaced by an identical-appearing impostor. A related though rarer condition is the *Fregoli syndrome,* wherein patients believe a persecutor has taken on the appearance of familiar persons. *Erotomania,* or *Clérambault's syndrome,* is the delusion that a stranger, usually a celebrity, is in love with the patient. Delusions of guilt, poverty, and even nihilism *(Cotard's syndrome),* wherein patients feel they no longer exist or have a body, are usually found in psychotic depressions and understood as extreme manifestations of lowered self-esteem.

There are two additional contexts for using the term "delusion" besides delusional ideas. In a delusional mood, patients are convinced that something in their environment has changed, so they are preoccupied with fears of impending, though unspecified, adverse occurrences. This state occurs in many psychiatric conditions and can culminate in the formation of an explanatory delusional idea. A delusional perception is a Schneiderian (see below) first rank symptom of schizophrenia. This phenomenon has two components: a normal perception, which is then immediately followed by a delusional conclusion. An example would be concluding to be the descendant of a celebrity after seeing a Rolls-Royce automobile.

Schneiderian symptoms are those that the late German psychiatrist, Kurt Schneider, believed were diagnostic of schizophrenia in the absence of organic mental disease. It is now known that these symptoms can sometimes occur in manic, depressive, and neurological psychoses. In *experiences of influence,* patients believe that their thoughts, speech, or actions are being controlled by some outside agency that cannot be resisted or overcome by the patient.

In *experiences of alienation,* patients perceive thoughts, feelings, speech, and body parts as not belonging to them. They will describe, for instance, that some thoughts that come into their minds are qualitatively distinct from their own usual thoughts. This phenomenon is called thought insertion. In *thought broadcasting,* patients are convinced that their thoughts are audible to anyone in their vicinity. This is typically accompanied by secondary delusional explanations involving radar or mental telepathy. Finally, *complete auditory hallucinations* are loud, clear, lengthy voices perceived as coming from an external source. Subtypes include hearing two or more voices converse about the patient in the third person, voices continually commenting on the patient's actions, and thought echo, in which a patient's thoughts are repeated audibly.

PERCEPTUAL DISTURBANCES Any sensory modality may be affected with minor or severe perceptual aberrations. *Illusions* are perceptions that are misinterpreted (e.g., shadows are mistaken for threatening figures). Distortions of the intensity or quality of stimuli may occur as in hyperacousis, micropsia, and macropsia, the latter two of which are examples of dysmegalopsia, or distorted visual perceptions.

Such occurrences on falling asleep *(hypnagogic)* or arising *(hypnopompic)* are not pathological.

Hallucinations are sensory experiences occurring without external stimulation. Pseudohallucinations have been variously defined and consist of hallucinations accompanied by the insight that they are unreal. Elementary hallucinations consist of flashes of light, noises, or sounds that are not formed into a coherent organization. Functional hallucinations occur only when there is a concurrent real perception in the same sensory modality (e.g., hearing voices only when the water in a shower is running). Autoscopic hallucinations occur when patients have a visual hallucination of themselves. Extracampine hallucinations occur outside of a known sensory field (e.g., seeing objects through a solid wall).

The apperception of oneself can be disturbed in many psychiatric and neuropsychiatric conditions. Body image is distorted in patients with anorexic and bulimic eating disorders, schizophrenia, and borderline personalities. In *depersonalization,* patients feel that they have lost their personal identities and therefore feel strange and unreal regarding their persons. In *derealization,* they feel that the environment has changed and it is unreal. This condition is sometimes characterized by the description of feeling as though one were an actor on a stage—one step removed from reality. Although visual hallucinations may predominate in organic mental disorders, no hallucinations, in and of themselves, are pathognomonic for any specific psychiatric or neurological condition. It is important to inquire about perceptual disturbances of touch, taste, and smell, as well as hearing and vision, inasmuch as multiple types of hallucinations are more the rule than the exception in psychiatric disorders. Tactile hallucinations of insects crawling under the skin, termed *formication,* often accompanies drug-induced psychotic states.

In initial inquiries about major forms of psychopathology, such as hallucinations or delusions, it is best to start asking rather general questions, such as "Have you noticed anything unusual happening around you?" or "Are you concerned about matters that other people are probably unaware of?" This allows the patient to elaborate on concerns without suggestions as to what the examiner is looking for. Negative responses by the patient will require more focused inquiries, however.

INSIGHT AND JUDGMENT *Insight* refers to subjective awareness of the pathological nature of psychiatric symptoms and behavioral disturbances. Lack of insight is characteristic of psychotic states. Assessing the development of insight is a particularly useful way of determining recovery in psychotic disorders. Lack of insight or denial of illness is termed *anosognosia* in the neurological literature, where it is classically associated with right parietal lobe lesions. This phenomenon spans a spectrum that includes denial of hemiparesis or blindness to minimization of problems, indifference to the disability *(anosodiaphoria),* and a calm mental attitude toward any disability *(la belle indifférence).* The extent of insight present is a strong predictor of compliance with treatment plans, whether pharmacological or psychosocial.

Insight correlates strongly but not absolutely with judgment, in that lack of insight predicts poor judgment, but the presence of insight does not assure sound judgment. The assessment of patients' judgment is fraught with difficulties. Questions about mailing letters, reacting to fires in theaters, or walking in Central Park are used; however, inquiries about occupational, financial, and other life situations may be more germane. (What are the patient's specific long- and short-term career plans? How does the patient intend to manage financially on leaving the hospital?) Consideration of the patient's social and financial background is always necessary when evaluating such responses and determining mental competence, which often needs to be assessed in patients with significant psychopathology.

Suicide potential is assessed by asking a graded hierarchy of questions beginning with feelings of hopelessness, feeling life is not worth living, thoughts about death, wishing to die in one's sleep, thoughts of taking one's life, and having a means and plan to commit suicide. If the latter is the case, the next inquiry should be to establish how long that patient is willing to live before acting on his or her plan.

Determining a particular patient's potential to harm others is even more problematic. Patients should be asked whether they have any intention of deliberately hurting another person. If a specific victim is identified, psychiatrists have a legal duty to warn that third party. Command hallucinations to inflict harm must be taken seriously, although in most instances they do not lead to overt violence.

NEUROPSYCHIATRIC EVALUATION Central nervous system abnormalities may first be manifested as behavioral disturbances; therefore, a comprehensive mental status examination should include an evaluation of higher cognitive functioning.

Cognitive functioning is best considered as a hierarchy. Basic qualities are levels of consciousness, followed by ability to sustain attention and concentration, followed by language functions, then memory, then abstraction, calculation, praxis, and other higher functions. If a lower level of dysfunction is found, it may not be possible to judge the integrity of higher functions in the hierarchy. Thus, delirious patients may have difficulty in correctly naming common objects but cannot be said to have aphasia.

A number of screening batteries are available to evaluate cognitive functioning. The most widely used in psychiatric settings is the mini-mental status (MMS) questionnaire, which contains 30 items and takes about 10 minutes to complete. These items screen for orientation, immediate recall, attention and concentration, naming, reading, writing, verbal repetition, and copying ability. A score of 23 or below will generally indicate the presence of dementia or delirium. False positive scores can be found in the elderly, persons lacking formal education, and depressed, usually elderly, individuals with pseudodementia secondary to amotivation and decreased concentration. False negative scores can be found in highly educated professionals with early dementias and in patients with right-hemisphere lesions. It is therefore important to realize that the MMS is only a screening tool, with limitations in its sensitivity and specificity. When patients err on any item on the MMS, it is important to evaluate the type of error thoroughly and determine more precisely the extent of any dysfunction.

For example, if the pencil or watch is misnamed, examiners should elicit the naming of other common objects (e.g., shirt, sleeve, tie, jacket). Conversely, if a patient has some dysfluency of spontaneous speech, yet names the pencil and watch correctly, it is worthwhile to further test naming ability. Since naming the parts of an object is more difficult than naming the whole object, patients may be asked to name the band, buckle, crystal, and stem of a watch to determine naming difficulty more precisely, although such errors will not be reflected in the MMS score itself. (See Table 2.1-1 in Section 2.1 Neurological Evaluation, for a copy of the MMS.)

The Aphasia Screening Test (AST) is a component of the Halsted-Reitan neuropsychological test battery. The AST can be used alone as a brief cognitive screening tool. Contrary to its name, it does not examine exclusively for aphasia and, in fact, draws heavily on visuospatial and copying abilities.

The Set Test has been found useful in separating demented

from nondemented elderly. Subjects are asked to name 10 fruits, 10 animals, 10 colors, and 10 cities. Each category should be completed in 1 minute. A cumulative response of 15 or less is highly suggestive of dementia or delirium, whereas a score of 25 or more makes significant cognitive dysfunction unlikely. Persons scoring in the broad gray area between 16 and 24 require further investigation.

The Neurobehavioral Cognitive Status Examination is a very useful screening instrument that assesses language, constructions, memory, calculations, and reasoning as well as level of consciousness, orientation, and attention.

Sensorium Sensorium refers primarily to the *level of consciousness,* as well as to integrative and perceptual functions, such as orientation, memory, attention, and general awareness. Lower levels of consciousness can be accurately assessed using the Glasgow Coma Scale. This instrument examines impaired consciousness based on the patient's capability of eye opening and verbal and motor responses to graded stimuli. Level of consciousness is identified as comatose, stuporous, drowsiness, alertness, or hyperalertness.

If a patient is not fully alert, the examiner should specify the amount of stimulation needed for arousal, as well as the duration of time the patient can maintain attention.

Attention and concentration After determining that a patient is awake and alert, utilizing the Glasgow Coma Scale if a precise determination is required, attention and concentration are the basis of further testing of cognitive functioning. The latter functions are most easily assessed by digit span, serial sevens, spelling backward, and the "A" test. Patients should be able to repeat immediately at least five digits forward and four digits in reverse order. Numbers should be presented at a rate of one per second in a nonpatterned manner. Serial sevens requires rudimentary subtraction ability but it mainly tests the ability to sustain the task in mind and keep track of sequential answers after beginning at 100 and repetitively subtracting 7 from each new remainder. After first spelling a simple five-letter word, patients are asked to spell that same word backwards. In the "A" test, patients are asked to tap with one hand whenever the examiner says the letter A. Letters are then stated in random order, sometimes bunching the letter A and sometimes not saying "A" for a period of time. No errors of omission or commission are expected. In motivated patients, attentional errors may be indicative of delirium, dementia, depression, any psychosis, or mental retardation.

Language This complex, critical, uniquely human function follows next in the cognitive hierarchy. Language components include fluency, comprehension, naming, repetition, reading, writing, and prosody.

Fluency is assessed from spontaneous conversation with the patient. Prolonged latency of response or excessive pauses should be noted. These typify depressions, dementing states, and nonfluent aphasias. Fluency can be evaluated by asking patients to name as many animals as they can in 1 minute. Scores of 12 or more are expected. Patients can also be asked to name as many words as they can beginning with the letter F, then A, then S, allowing 1 minute per letter. Again, scores of 12 or more per letter are expected.

Language comprehension is tested by asking a graded series of questions requiring elementary responses (e.g., "point to the floor, door, and window"). Further testing can be accomplished using common objects but using more complex phrasing (e.g., "after touching the pen, then touch the keys with a coin"). Correct performance is obviously predicated on intact concentration and appropriate motivation, as well as language comprehension.

Repetition failure on a nondysarthric, linguistic basis usually is secondary to left perisylvian fissure lesions. Standard phrases and sentences that can be used include "Methodist Episcopal," "The president lives in Washington," and the more complex "No ifs, ands, or buts."

Naming errors may be noted in patients' spontaneous speech. These can include descriptive *circumlocutions* (avoidance of specific low-frequency nouns with circuitous phrasing of descriptive features of target word), *neologisms* (words of the patient's invention [e.g., "verbitrage" in reference to ordinary conversation]), *literal paraphasias* ("gub" for "gun"), *verbal paraphasias* ("spoon" for "fork"), and *stock words* (repetitively using the same real word inappropriately).

Reading ability is highly dependent on educational attainment. Patients may be given sentences to read both silently and aloud and then tested for their comprehension of the material. Writing is conventionally assessed by having patients write a sentence of their own composition. Grammar and elementary meaning are considered.

Prosody refers to the affective intonations that accompany language. Aprosodic speech is monotonic and without inflections. It typically follows right frontal cortical lesions. Right temporoparietal lesions are associated with comprehension dysprosody. To evaluate this function, examiners speak the same words but with different intonations, which patients are asked to identify (i.e., happy, sad, surprised, angry, and questioning tones). Any stock phrase can be used, such as "Richard and Linda Thompson performed well." Quite different meanings can be conveyed by emphasizing a given word in the sentence in a particular way. Patients with comprehension dysprosody cannot distinguish such differences in meaning. Patients with motor dysprosody cannot convey different meanings when asked to articulate the same sentence in the manner described.

Memory and higher cognitive functions *Memory* can be divided into immediate, recent, and remote functions. Immediate memory is more appropriately considered an attentional function, which has previously been discussed. Recent memory refers to the ability to learn and recall new information. *Orientation* to time and place assesses recent memory, as does having the patient learn three unrelated words and recalling them after 5 minutes. Orientation to person refers to the patient's ability to state his or her name correctly, as well as the names of known persons in the patient's immediate environment (e.g., spouse or doctor). If patients cannot spontaneously recall the words, clues as to category or first letter for each word should be given. Thus, if patients can then identify the correct answer, it establishes that learning took place but that forgetfulness supervened. Remote memory is tested by asking about past historical events that are verifiable, such as meaningful personal material including place and date of birth, grammar school attended, and social security number. Amnesias related to a specific event, such as traumatic brain injury or electroconvulsive therapy, are separated into retrograde and anterograde components. *Retrograde amnesia* refers to the forgetting of material learned before, whereas *anterograde amnesia* refers to the inability to learn new information after a traumatic event. In patients with amnesia, examiners should establish whether there is a temporal gradient of notable preservation of more remote memories with disproportionate loss of more recent material.

Constructional or copying difficulty is often referred to as *constructional apraxia.* Increasingly complex two- and three-dimensional figures are presented for patients to copy. Mild to moderate impairment is associated with diffuse brain dysfunction, whereas more severe impairment tends to be associated with right parietal lobe damage. For more detailed assessment, the complex Rey-Osterreith figure with its detailed scoring system can be utilized.

Calculating ability is tested by having patients perform simple arithmetic, such as figuring the change they would receive from a dollar bill after spending 27 cents or figuring the number of nickels there would be in $1.35 worth of nickels. *Abstracting ability* is determined by asking the meaning of idioms, proverbs, and similarities between objects in the same class. Examples include "cold shoulder," "Rome wasn't built in a day" (anything worth doing is worth doing well), and "car-airplane" (means of transportation). Both calculating and abstracting abilities are highly dependent on educational attainment, employment field, and social milieu. To assess these abilities more properly, an estimation of general intelligence is helpful.

General intelligence can be gauged by patients' vocabularies, complexity of concepts they use, and progressively more difficult questions about current events. Although they are heavily culture-bound, questions pertaining to popular TV shows or sports events, as well as names of the governor or vice president, can provide an adequate estimation of intelligence. Intellectual functioning may be overestimated if a patient's vocabulary or educational background is particularly strong. Therefore, a formal examination of the several areas of intellectual competence is often needed. The reliability of the clinical assessment will be lower than that obtained with formal psychological testing, where standardization of questions and of scoring can be accomplished. With this background, examiners can usually determine whether their patients' abstracting abilities are impaired. However, one cannot reliably conclude that patients are psychotic or evidencing cognitive decline solely on the basis of this evaluation. *Abstracting ability* does not develop fully until early adolescence, is closely linked to educational accomplishment, and may appear impaired if the person is not fluent in the language used. Testing abstracting ability is further made difficult by the two sometimes overlapping types of information provided: concreteness and personalization. *Concreteness* indicates thinking that is determined by, and not proceeded beyond, some immediate experience or attribute. Concrete responses principally indicate limited intellectual ability (e.g., apples and bananas both have peels). In contrast, personalized responses, especially of an idiosyncratic or bizarre quality, principally reflect a psychotic thought process. Simpler questions about proverbs and similarities should be asked first, in part, to reduce performance anxiety stemming from difficulties answering the questions.

Apraxia is the inability to perform a skilled act without basic disturbances of strength, coordination, or sensation. In ideomotor apraxia, patients cannot perform on command acts that can be performed spontaneously. Commands should include those for buccofacial ("drink through a straw"), limb ("hammer a nail"), and whole-body movements ("stand like a boxer"). Ideational apraxia is the inability to perform an organized motor sequence, although the individual components can be performed separately. It can be tested by asking patients to show how they would fold a letter, place it in an envelope, and then seal and stamp the envelope. Apraxias are indicative of significant brain dysfunction, often of the left hemisphere.

Localizing brain dysfunction using mental status examination is sometimes possible, but one cannot be absolute even with classic syndromes, such as Broca's or Wernicke's aphasia. Classic, severe neuropsychological dysfunction can occur without any identifiable abnormality of brain structure or function; however, abnormal functions related to damage in specialized brain areas may be demonstrated.

Patients with damage to the orbitofrontal regions of the frontal lobe are irritable, labile, tactless, and seem hypomanic except for the shallowness of their feelings. Typically they do not exhibit primary cognitive dysfunction. Apathy and indifference associated with damage to the frontal convexity are considered to be the classic frontal lobe disturbances. Such patients perseverate when copying figures and have difficulty programming alternating or progressive patterns, such as copying the examiner's tapping a surface with the fist, palm, then side of hand. Copying the letters m and n alternating in script can be difficult for such patients. They also tend to generate inadequate word lists when asked to name as many animals as possible within 1 minute. Abstraction and proverb interpretation are impaired.

Damage to Broca's area results in a nonfluent aphasia, with anomia, sparse agrammatism, deficits in reading, writing, and repetition, but with comprehension relatively spared. A classic depressive syndrome has been reported to occur frequently following left frontal cerebral infarction.

Damage to the right frontal lobe analogous to Broca's area is associated with the previously discussed motor dysprosody. Finally, catatonia is associated more with frontal lobe damage than with any other regional brain pathology. The same loose correlation holds for many neurological soft signs, including grasp, palmomental, snout, and glabellar reflexes.

Language comprehension impairments are characteristic of Wernicke's aphasia, which is associated with damage to the posterior third of the left superior temporal gyrus. Associated findings include impaired naming, repetition, reading, writing, and fluent paraphasic speech. Behaviorally, patients tend to develop excessive anxiety and suspiciousness. Unilateral damage to the right (nondominant) temporal lobe can be associated with impaired repetition and recollection of musical rhythms.

Any diffuse brain damage, but parietal lobe damage in particular, is associated with visuospatial dysfunctions, such as copying difficulty (constructional apraxia) and geographic disorientation. When such dysfunction is particularly severe, the right (nondominant) parietal lobe is most likely to be affected. Other nondominant parietal dysfunctions include dressing apraxia, anosognosia (denial or minimization of illness), prosopapnosia (impaired facial recognition), and left-sided spatial neglect.

The foregoing material will rarely be covered in entirety in the mental status examination of any individual patient. However, at least screening each area described is mandatory. The mark of skilled clinical psychiatrists is their ability to screen these areas efficiently and then pursue in depth any deviancies or deficiencies that are discovered.

It is incumbent on the examining psychiatrist to assess the veracity of information provided by the patient. Collateral histories by relatives or friends frequently illuminate unclear issues that pertain to better patient understanding. Inexact information can stem from deliberate untruths, biased recollections, faulty memory, or underlying psychopathology (e.g., manic grandiosity, depressive pessimism, or schizophrenic delusions). It serves no useful purpose to accept less than a complete and accurate data base when examining patient needs.

REFERENCES

Alexander M P: Clinical determination of mental competence. Arch Neurol *45:* 23, 1988.

Cox A, Hopkinson K, Rutter M: Psychiatric interviewing techniques. II. Naturalistic study: Eliciting factual information. Brit J Psychiat *138:* 283, 1981.

Cummings J L: *Clinical Neuropsychiatry*. Grune & Stratton, Orlando, FL, 1985.

Folstein M F, Folstein S E, McHugh P R: Mini-mental state: A practical method for grading the cognitive state of patients for the clinician. J Psychiat Res *12:* 189, 1975.

Hamilton M, editor: *Fish's Clinical Psychopathology,* ed 2. John Wright & Sons, Bristol, England, 1985.

Hopkinson K, Cox A, Rutter M: Psychiatric interviewing techniques. III. Naturalistic study: Eliciting feelings. Brit J Psychiat *138:* 406, 1981.

Kiernan R J, Mueller J, Langston J W, VanDyke C: The neurobehavioral cognitive screening examination: A brief but quantitative approach to cognitive assessment. Ann Intern Med *107:* 481, 1987.
Leon R L: *Psychiatric Interviewing: A Primer.*, ed 2. Elsevier, New York, 1989.
Lishman W A: *Organic Psychiatry*, ed 2. Blackwell Scientific Publications, Oxford, England, 1987.
Luborsky L, Singer B, Luborsky L: Comparative studies of psychotherapies. Arch Gen Psychiat *32:* 995, 1975.
MacKinnon R A, Yudofsky S C: *The Psychiatric Evaluation in Clinical Practice*. Lippincott, Philadelphia, 1986.
Malan D H, Heath E S, Bacal H A, Balfour F H G: Psychodynamic changes in untreated neurotic patients. II. Apparently genuine improvements. Arch Gen Psychiat *32:* 110, 1975.
May P R A: When, what, and why: Psychopharmacotherapy and other treatments in schizophrenia. Comp Psychiat *17:* 183, 1976.
Miller L: "Narrow localization" in psychiatric neuropsychology. Psychol Med *16:* 729, 1986.
Platt F W, McMath J C: Clinical hypocompetence: The interview. Ann Intern Med *91:* 898, 1979.
Roca R P: Bedside cognitive examination. Psychosomatics *28:* 71, 1987.
Sims A: *Symptoms in the Mind: An Introduction to Descriptive Psychopathology*. Baillieré Tindall, London, 1988.
Strub R L, Black F W: *The Mental Status Examination in Neurology*, ed 2. Davis, Philadelphia, 1985.
Strull W M, Lo B, Charles G: Do patients want to participate in medical decision making? JAMA *252*(21): 2990, 1984.
Taylor M A: *The Neuropsychiatric Mental Status Examination*. S.P. Medical and Scientific Books, New York, 1981.
Taylor M A, Abrams R, Faber R, et al: Cognitive tasks in the mental status examination. J Nerv Ment Dis *168:* 167, 1980.
Waitzkin H, Stoeckle J D: The communication of information about illness. Advances Psychosom Med *8:* 180, 1972.

9.2 PSYCHIATRIC REPORT

HAROLD I. KAPLAN, M.D.
BENJAMIN J. SADOCK, M.D.

The following summary represents an outline the clinician or student may use in writing a psychiatric report.

I. Psychiatric history

A. Preliminary identification: name, age, marital status, sex, occupation, language if other than English, race, nationality, and religion insofar as they are pertinent; previous admissions to a hospital for the same or different conditions; person or people with whom the patient lives

B. Chief complaint: exactly why the patient came to the psychiatrist, preferably in the patient's own words; if this information does not come from the patient, note who supplied it

C. Personal identification: brief, nontechnical description of the patient's appearance and behavior as a novelist might write it

D. History of present illness: chronological background and development of the symptoms or behavioral changes culminating in the patient's seeking assistance; describe precipitating stress, if present, at the time of onset; personality when well; how illness has affected patient's life activities and personal relations—changes in personality, memory, speech; psychophysiological symptoms—nature and details of dysfunction; location, intensity, fluctuation; relationship between physical and psychic symptoms; extent to which illness serves some additional purpose for the patient when dealing with stress—secondary gain; whether anxieties are generalized and nonspecific (free-floating) or specifically related to particular situations, activities, or objects; how anxieties are handled—avoidance of feared situation, use of drugs or other activities for distraction

E. Previous illnesses

1. Emotional or mental disturbances: extent of symptoms and incapacity, type of treatment, names of hospitals, length of illness, effect of treatment, compliance
2. Psychosomatic disorders: hay fever, rheumatoid arthritis, ulcerative colitis, asthma, hyperthyroidism, gastrointestinal upsets, recurrent colds, skin conditions
3. Medical conditions: following the customary medical review of systems, if necessary; syphilis, use of alcohol or drugs; at risk for acquired immune deficiency syndrome (AIDS)
4. Neurological disorders: history of craniocerebral trauma, convulsions, or tumors

F. Past personal history: history (anamnesis) of the patient's life from infancy to the present to the extent that it can be recalled; gaps in history as spontaneously related by the patient; emotions associated with these life periods—painful, stressful, conflictual

1. Prenatal history: nature of mother's pregnancy and delivery: length of pregnancy, spontaneity and normality of delivery, birth trauma, whether patient was planned for and wanted, birth defects
2. Early childhood (through age 3)
   a. Feeding habits: breast-fed or bottle-fed, eating problems
   b. Early development: walking, talking, and teething; language development, motor development, signs of unmet needs, sleep pattern, object constancy, stranger anxiety, maternal deprivation, separation anxiety, other caretakers in home
   c. Toilet training: age, attitude of parents, feelings about it
   d. Symptoms of behavior problems: thumb-sucking, temper tantrums, tics, head-bumping, rocking, night-terrors, fears, bed-wetting or bed-soiling, nail-biting, masturbation
   e. Personality as a child: shy, restless, overactive, withdrawn, persistent, outgoing, timid, athletic, friendly, patterns of play
   f. Early or recurrent dreams or fantasies
3. Middle childhood (3 to 11): early school history—feelings about going to school, early adjustment, gender identification, conscience development, punishment, peer relations, nightmares, phobias, bed-wetting, fire-setting, cruelty to animals
4. Later childhood (puberty through adolescence)
   a. Social relationships: attitudes toward siblings and playmates, number and closeness of friends, leader or follower, social popularity, participation in group or gang ac-

tivities, idealized figures; patterns of aggression, passivity, anxiety, antisocial behavior

b. School history: how far the patient progressed, adjustment to school relationships with teachers (teacher's pet versus rebellious), favorite studies or interests, particular abilities or assets, extracurricular activities, sports, hobbies, relationships of problems or symptoms to any school period

c. Cognitive and motor development: learning to read and other intellectual and motor skills, minimal cerebral dysfunctions, learning disabilities—their management and effects on the child

d. Adolescent emotional or physical problems: nightmares, phobias, masturbation, bedwetting, running away, delinquency, smoking, drug or alcohol use, anorexia, bulimia, weight problems, feelings of inferiority

5. Psychosexual history (childhood through adolescence)
   a. Early curiosity, infantile masturbation, sex play
   b. Acquisition of sexual knowledge, attitude of parents toward sex, sexual abuse
   c. Onset of puberty, feelings about it, kind of preparation, feelings about menstruation, development of secondary sexual characteristics
   d. Adolescent sexual activity: crushes, parties, dating, petting, masturbation, nocturnal emissions, and attitudes toward them
   e. Attitudes toward opposite sex: timid, shy, aggressive, need to impress, seductive, sexual conquests, anxiety
   f. Sexual practices: sexual problems, homosexual experiences, paraphilias, promiscuity
6. Religious background: strict, liberal, mixed (possible conflicts), relationship of background to current religious practices
7. Adulthood
   a. Occupational history: choice of occupation, training, ambitions, conflicts; relations with authority, peers, and subordinates; number of jobs and duration; changes in job status; current job and feelings about it
   b. Social activity: does patient have friends, is patient withdrawn or socializing well; kind of social, intellectual, and physical interests; relationship with same-sex and opposite-sex persons; depth, duration, and quality of human relationships
   c. Adult sexuality
      i. Premarital and extramarital sexual relationships
      ii. Marital history: common-law marriages, legal marriages, description of courtship and role played by each partner, age at marriage, family planning and contraception, names and ages of children, attitudes toward raising children, problems of any family members, housing difficulties if important to the marriage, sexual adjustment, areas of agreement and disagreement, management of money, role of in-laws
      iii. Sexual symptoms: anorgasmia, impotence, premature ejaculation, lack of desire
      iv. Attitudes toward pregnancy and having children; contraceptive practices and feelings about them
      v. Sexual practices: paraphilias, such as sadism, fetishes, voyeurism; attitudes about fellatio, cunnilingus, and coital techniques; frequency
   d. Military history: general adjustment, combat, injuries, referral to psychiatrists, veteran status, disciplinary action

G. *Family history:* elicited from patient and from someone else because quite different descriptions may be given of the same people and events; ethnic, national, and religious traditions; other people in the home: descriptions of them—personality and intelligence—and what has become of them since the patient's childhood; descriptions of different households lived in; present relationships between patient and other people who are in the family; role of illness in the family; history of mental illness and treatment

H. *Current social situation:* where does patient live—neighborhood and particular residence of the patient; is home crowded; privacy of family members from each other and from other families; sources of family income and difficulties in obtaining it; public assistance, if any, and attitudes about it; will patient lose job or apartment by remaining in the hospital; who is caring for children

I. *Dreams, fantasies, and value systems*
   1. Dreams: prominent ones, if patient will tell them; nightmares
   2. Fantasies: recurrent, favorite, or unshakable day-dreams; hypnagogic phenomena
   3. Value systems: whether children are seen as a burden or a joy; whether work is seen as a necessary evil, an avoidable chore, or an opportunity; concept of right and wrong

II. Mental status: sum total of the examiner's observations and impressions derived from the initial interviews

A. *General description*
   1. Appearance: body type, posture, bearing, clothes, grooming, hair, nails; healthy, sickly, angry, frightened, apathetic, perplexed, contemptuous, ill at ease, poised, old looking, young looking, effeminate, masculine; signs of anxiety—moist hands, perspiring forehead, restlessness, tense posture, strained voice, wide eyes; shift in level of anxiety during interview or abrupt changes of topic
   2. Behavior and psychomotor activity: gait, mannerisms, tics, gestures, twitches, stereotypes, picking, touching examiner, echopraxia, clumsy, agile, limp, rigid, retarded, hyperactive, agitated, combative, waxy
   3. Speech: rapid, slow, pressured, hesitant, emotional, monotonous, loud, whispered, slurred,

mumbled, stuttering, echolalia, intensity, pitch, ease, spontaneity, productivity, manner, reaction time, vocabulary

4. Attitude toward examiner: cooperative, attentive, interested, frank, seductive, defensive, hostile, playful, ingratiating, evasive, guarded, level of rapport

B. Mood, feelings, and affect

1. Mood (a pervasive and sustained emotion that colors the person's perception of the world): how does patient say he or she feels; depth, intensity, duration, and fluctuations of mood—depressed, despairing, irritable, anxious, terrified, angry, expansive, euphoric, empty, guilty, awed, futile, self-contemptuous
2. Affective expression: how examiner evaluates patient's affects—broad, restricted, depressed, blunted or flat, shallow, anhedonic, labile, constricted, fearful, anxious, guilty; amount and range of expression; difficulty in initiating, sustaining, or terminating an emotional response
3. Appropriateness: is the emotional expression appropriate to the thought content, the culture, and the setting of the examination; note examples of inappropriate emotional expression

C. Perceptual disturbances

1. Hallucinations and illusions: does patient hear voices or see visions; content, sensory system involved, circumstances of the occurrence; hypnagogic or hypnopompic hallucinations
2. Depersonalization and derealization: extreme feelings of detachment from oneself or from the environment

D. Thought process

1. Stream of thought: quotations from patient
   a. Productivity: overabundance of ideas, paucity of ideas, flight of ideas, rapid thinking, slow thinking, hesitant thinking; does patient speak spontaneously or only when questions are asked
   b. Continuity of thought: do patient's replies really answer questions; are they goal directed and relevant or irrelevant; is there a lack of cause-and-effect relationships in patient's explanations, are statements illogical, tangential, rambling, evasive, perseverative; is there blocking or distractibility
   c. Language impairments: impairments that reflect disordered mentation, such as incoherent or incomprehensible speech (word salad), clang associations, neologisms
2. Content of thought
   a. Preoccupations: about the illness, environmental problems; obsessions, compulsions, phobias; plans, intentions, recurrent ideas about suicide, homicide; hypochondriacal symptoms, specific antisocial urges; specific questions should always be asked about suicidal ideation
   b. Thought disturbances
      i. Delusions: content of any delusional system, its organization, the patient's convictions as to its validity, how it affects patient's life; somatic delusions—isolated or associated with pervasive suspiciousness; mood-congruent delusions—in keeping with a depressed or elated mood; mood-incongruent delusions—not in keeping with the patient's mood; bizarre delusions, such as thoughts of being controlled by external forces or thoughts being broadcast out loud
      ii. Ideas of reference and ideas of influence: how ideas began, their content, and the meaning the patient attributes to them
      iii. Abstract thinking: disturbances in concept formation; manner in which the patient conceptualizes or handles ideas; similarities, differences, absurdities, meanings of simple proverbs, such as, "A rolling stone gathers no moss"; answers may be concrete (giving specific examples to illustrate the meaning) or overly abstract (giving generalized explanations); appropriateness of answers should be noted

E. Sensorium and cognition

1. Consciousness: clouding, somnolence, stupor, coma, lethargy, alertness, fugue state
2. Orientation
   a. Time: does patient identify the day correctly; can patient approximate date, time of day; if in a hospital, does the patient know how long he or she has been there; does patient behave as though he or she is oriented to the present
   b. Place: does patient know where he or she is
   c. Person: does patient know who the examiner is and the roles or names of the persons with whom he or she is in contact
3. Concentration: subtract 7 from 100 and keep subtracting sevens; if patient cannot subtract sevens, can easier tasks be accomplished—4 times 9, 5 times 4; whether anxiety or some disturbance of mood or consciousness seems to be responsible for difficulty
4. Memory: impairment, efforts made to cope with impairment—denial, confabulation, catastrophic reaction, circumstantiality used to conceal deficit; whether the process of registration, retention, or recollection of material is involved
   a. Remote memory: childhood data, important events known to have occurred when the patient was younger or free of illness, personal matters, neutral material
   b. Recent past memory: the past few months
   c. Recent memory: the past few days, recall of what was done yesterday, the day before; what was eaten for breakfast, lunch, dinner
   d. Immediate retention and recall: ability to repeat six figures after examiner dictates them—first forward, then backward, then after a few minutes' interruption; other test questions; did same questions, if repeated, call forth different answers at different times; digit span measures; other mental

functions, such as anxiety level and concentration

e. Effect of defect on patient: mechanisms patient has developed to cope with defect

5. Information and intelligence: patient's level of formal education and self-education: estimate of the patient's intellectual capability and whether patient is capable of functioning at the level of basic endowment; counting, calculation; general knowledge; questions that have some relevance to the patient's educational and cultural background

F. Judgment

1. Social judgment: subtle manifestations of behavior that are harmful to the patient and contrary to acceptable behavior in the culture; does the patient understand the likely outcome of his or her behavior and is the patient influenced by this understanding; examples of impairment
2. Test judgment: patient's prediction of what he or she would do in imaginary situations; for instance, what patient would do if he or she found a stamped, addressed letter in the street

G. Insight: degree of awareness and understanding the patient has that he or she is ill

1. Complete denial of illness
2. Slight awareness of being sick and needing help but denying it at the same time
3. Awareness of being sick but blaming it on others, on external factors, or on organic factors
4. Awareness that illness is due to something unknown in patient
5. Intellectual insight: admission that patient is ill and that symptoms or failures in social adjustment are due to patient's own particular irrational feelings or disturbances without applying that knowledge to future experiences
6. True emotional insight: emotional awareness of the motives and feelings within patient and the important people in his or her life

H. Reliability: estimate of examiner's impression of patient's veracity or ability to report the situation accurately

III. Further diagnostic studies

A. Physical examination

B. Additional psychiatric diagnostic interviews

C. Interviews with family members, friends, or neighbors by social worker

D. Other tests as indicated: electroencephalogram, computed tomography scan, positron emission tomography, laboratory tests, tests of other medical conditions, reading comprehension and handwriting tests, tests for aphasia

IV. Summary of positive findings: mental symptoms, laboratory findings, psychological test results, if available; drugs patient has been taking, including dosage and duration of intake

V. Diagnosis: diagnostic classification according to the revised third edition of the American Psychiatric Association's *Diagnostic and Statistical Manual of Mental Disorders* (DSM-III-R)—nomenclature, classification number, diagnoses to be ruled out; DSM-III-R uses a multiaxial classification scheme consisting of five axes, each of which should be covered in the diagnosis; for a further discussion of Axes I, II, and III, see Chapter 11, Classification of Mental Disorders.

A. *Axis I:* consists of all clinical syndromes (e.g., mood disorders, schizophrenia, generalized anxiety disorder)

B. *Axis II:* consists of personality disorders and specific developmental disorders

C. *Axis III:* consists of any existing medical or physical illness (e.g., epilepsy, cardiovascular disease, gastrointestinal disease)

D. *Axis IV:* refers to psychosocial stressors (e.g., divorce, injury, death of a loved one) relevant to the illness (Table 9.2-1); a rating scale with a continuum of 1 (no stressors) to 6 (catastrophic stressors) is used (Tables 9.2-2 and 9.2-3)

E. *Axis V:* relates to the highest level of functioning exhibited by the patient during the previous year (e.g., social, occupational, and psychological functioning); a rating scale with a continuum of 9 (superior functioning) to 1 (grossly impaired functioning) is used (Table 9.2-4); Table 9.2-5 summarizes Axes IV and V of DSM-III-R.

TABLE 9.2-1
Types of Psychosocial Stressors

To ascertain etiologically significant psychosocial stressors, the following areas may be considered:

Conjugal (marital and nonmarital): e.g., engagement, marriage, discord, separation, death of spouse.

Parenting: e.g., becoming a parent, friction with child, illness of child.

Other interpersonal: problems with one's friends, neighbors, associates, or nonconjugal family members, e.g., illness of best friend, discordant relationship with boss.

Occupational: includes work, school, homemaking, e.g., unemployment, retirement, school problems.

Living circumstances: e.g., change in residence, threat to personal safety, immigration.

Financial: e.g., inadequate finances, change in financial status.

Legal: e.g., arrest, imprisonment, lawsuit, or trial.

Developmental: phases of the life cycle, e.g., puberty, transition to adult status, menopause, "becoming 50."

Physical illness or injury: e.g., illness, accident, surgery, abortion. (Note: A physical disorder is listed on Axis III whenever it is related to the development or management of an Axis I or II disorder. A physical disorder can also be a psychosocial stressor if its impact is due to its meaning to the individual, in which case it would be listed on both Axis III and Axis IV.)

Other psychosocial stressors: e.g., natural or man-made disaster, persecution, unwanted pregnancy, out-of-wedlock birth, rape.

Family factors (children and adolescents): In addition to the above, for children and adolescents the following stressors may be considered: cold, hostile, intrusive, abusive, conflictual, or confusingly inconsistent relationship between parents or toward child; physical or mental illness in a family member; lack of parental guidance or excessively harsh or inconsistent parental control; insufficient, excessive, or confusing social or cognitive stimulation; anomalous family situation, e.g., complex or inconsistent parental custody and visitation arrangements; foster family; institutional rearing; loss of nuclear family members.

Table from DSM-III-R *Diagnostic and Statistical Manual of Mental Disorders,* ed 3, revised. Copyright American Psychiatric Association, Washington, DC, 1987. Used with permission.

VI. **Prognosis:** opinion as to the probable future course, extent, and outcome of the illness; specific goals of therapy

VII. **Psychodynamic formulation:** causes of the patient's psychodynamic breakdown—influences in the patient's life that contributed to present illness; environmental, genetic, and personality factors relevant in determining patient's symptoms; primary and **secondary gains; outline the major defense mechanisms used by the patient**

VIII. **Treatment plan:** modalities of treatment recommended, role of medication, inpatient or outpatient treatment, frequency of sessions, probable duration of therapy; type of psychotherapy: individual, group, or family therapy; symptoms or problems to be treated

TABLE 9.2-2
Axis IV: Severity of Psychosocial Stressors Scale: Adults

		Examples of Stressors	
Code	*Term*	*Acute Events*	*Enduring Circumstances*
1	None	No acute events that may be relevant to the disorder	No enduring circumstances that may be relevant to the disorder
2	Mild	Broke up with boyfriend or girlfriend; started or graduated from school; child left home	Family arguments; job dissatisfaction; residence in high-crime neighborhood
3	Moderate	Marriage; marital separation; loss of job; retirement; miscarriage	Marital discord; serious financial problems; trouble with boss; being a single parent
4	Severe	Divorce; birth of first child	Unemployment; poverty
5	Extreme	Death of spouse; serious physical illness diagnosed; victim of rape	Serious chronic illness in self or child; ongoing physical or sexual abuse
6	Catastrophic	Death of child; suicide of spouse; devastating natural disaster	Captivity as hostage; concentration camp experience
0	Inadequate information, or no change in condition		

Table from DSM-III-R *Diagnostic and Statistical Manual of Mental Disorders,* ed 3, revised. Copyright American Psychiatric Association, Washington, DC, 1987. Used with permission.

TABLE 9.2-3
Axis IV: Severity of Psychosocial Stressors Scale: Children and Adolescents

		Examples of Stressors	
Code	*Term*	*Acute Events*	*Enduring Circumstances*
1	None	No acute events that may be relevant to the disorder	No enduring circumstances that may be relevant to the disorder
2	Mild	Broke up with boyfriend or girlfriend; change of school	Overcrowded living quarters; family arguments
3	Moderate	Expelled from school; birth of sibling	Chronic disabling illness in parent; chronic parental discord
4	Severe	Divorce of parents; unwanted pregnancy; arrest	Harsh or rejecting parents; chronic life-threatening illness in parent; multiple foster home placements
5	Extreme	Sexual or physical abuse; death of a parent	Recurrent sexual or physical abuse
6	Catastrophic	Death of both parents	Chronic life-threatening illness
0	Inadequate information, or no change in condition		

Table from DSM-III-R *Diagnostic and Statistical Manual of Mental Disorders,* ed 3, revised. Copyright American Psychiatric Association, Washington, DC, 1987. Used with permission.

TABLE 9.2-4
Axis V: Global Assessment of Functioning Scale (GAF Scale)

Consider psychological, social, and occupational functioning on a hypothetical continuum of mental health-illness. Do not include impairment in functioning due to physical (or environmental) limitations.

Note: Use intermediate codes when appropriate—e.g., 45, 68, 72.

Code	
90–81	**Absent or minimal symptoms** (e.g., mild anxiety before an exam), **good functioning in all areas, interested and involved in a wide range of activities, socially effective, generally satisfied with life, no more than everyday problems or concerns** (e.g., an occasional argument with family members).
80–71	**If symptoms are present, they are transient and expectable reactions to psychosocial stressors** (e.g., difficulty concentrating after family argument); **no more than slight impairment in social, occupational, or school functioning** (e.g., temporarily falling behind in schoolwork).
70–61	**Some mild symptoms** (e.g., depressed mood and mild insomnia) **OR some difficulty in social, occupational, or school functioning** (e.g., occasional truancy, or theft within the household), **but generally functioning pretty well, has some meaningful interpersonal relationships.**
60–51	**Moderate symptoms** (e.g., flat affect and circumstantial speech, occasional panic attacks) **OR moderate difficulty in social, occupational, or school functioning** (e.g., few friends, conflicts with co-workers).

TABLE 9.2-4
Continued

50–41	**Serious symptoms** (e.g., suicidal ideation, severe obsessional rituals, frequent shoplifting) **OR any serious impairment in social, occupational, or school functioning** (e.g., no friends, unable to keep a job).
40–31	**Some impairment in reality testing or communication** (e.g., speech is at times illogical, obscure, or irrelevant) **OR major impairment in several areas, such as work or school, family relations, judgment, thinking, or mood** (e.g., depressed man avoids friends, neglects family, and is unable to work; child frequently beats up younger children, is defiant at home, and is failing at school).
30–21	**Behavior is considerably influenced by delusions or hallucinations OR serious impairment in communication or judgment** (e.g., sometimes incoherent, acts grossly inappropriately, suicidal preoccupation) **OR inability to function in almost all areas** (e.g., stays in bed all day; no job, home, or friends).
20–11	**Some danger of hurting self or others** (e.g., suicide attempts without clear expectation of death, frequently violent, manic excitement) **OR occasionally fails to maintain minimal personal hygiene** (e.g., smears feces) **OR gross impairment in communication** (e.g., largely incoherent or mute).
10–	**Persistent danger of severely hurting self or others** (e.g., recurrent violence) **OR persistent inability to maintain minimal personal hygiene OR serious suicidal act with clear expectation of death.**

Table from DSM-III-R *Diagnostic and Statistical Manual of Mental Disorders,* ed 3, revised. Copyright American Psychiatric Association, Washington, DC, 1987. Used with permission.

TABLE 9.2-5
Summary of DSM-III-R Axis IV and Axis V Characteristics

Axis IV. Severity of Psychosocial Stressors

Axis IV provides a scale, the Severity of Psychosocial Stressors Scale (Table 9.2-3), for coding the overall severity of a psychosocial stressor or multiple psychosocial stressors that have occurred in the year preceding the current evaluation and that may have contributed to any of the following:

(1) development of a new mental disorder
(2) recurrence of a prior mental disorder
(3) exacerbation of an already existing mental disorder (e.g., divorce occurring during a major depressive episode, or during the course of chronic schizophrenia)

(Note: Post-traumatic stress disorder is an exception to the requirement that the stressor has occurred within a year before the evaluation.) The current disorder that is related to the psychosocial stressor may be either a clinical syndrome, coded on Axis I, or an exacerbation of a personality or developmental disorder, coded on Axis II. In some instances the stressor is anticipation of a future event, e.g., imminent retirement.

Although a stressor frequently plays a precipitating role in a disorder, it may also be a consequence of the person's psychopathology—e.g., alcohol dependence may lead to marital problems and divorce, which can then become stressors contributing to the development of a major depressive episode.

Rating the severity of the stressor. The rating of the severity of the stressor should be based on the clinician's assessment of the stress an "average" person in similar circumstances and with similar sociocultural values would experience from the particular psychosocial stressor(s). This judgment involves consideration of the following: the amount of change in the person's life caused by the stressor, the degree to which the event is desired and under the person's control, and the number of stressors. For example, a planned pregnancy is usually less stressful than an unwanted pregnancy. Even though a specific stressor may have greater impact on a person who is especially vulnerable or has certain internal conflicts, the rating should be based on the severity of the stressor itself, not on the person's vulnerability to the particular stressor. If a vulnerability to stress exists, it will frequently be due to a mental disorder that is coded on Axis I or II.

The specific psychosocial stressor(s) should be noted and further specified as either:

predominantly acute events (duration less than 6 months)

predominantly enduring circumstances (duration greater than 6 months)

Examples of predominantly acute events are entering a new school or beginning a new job, having an accident, and death of a loved one. Examples of predominantly enduring circumstances are chronic marital or parental discord, and persistent and harsh parental discipline. The distinction between these two types of stressors may be important in formulating a treatment plan that includes attempts to remove the psychosocial stressor(s) or to help the person cope with it (them). Furthermore, there is evidence that predominantly enduring psychosocial stressors are more likely to predispose children to develop mental disorders than predominantly acute events.

In evaluating the stressors that may have contributed to the development of the current episode of illness, more than one may be judged to be relevant, but rarely should more than the four most severe be recorded. When more than one stressor is present, the severity rating will generally be that of the most severe stressor. However, in the case of multiple severe or extreme stressors, a higher rating should be considered. Each of the stressors should be noted and listed in the order of their importance.

Separate examples are given in Table 9.2-1 for adults and for children and adolescents. These may be used as general guides for making the severity rating, the context in which the stressor(s) occurs being taken into account.

The code "0" should be used either when there is inadequate information about the presence or absence of psychosocial stressors to make a more definitive rating, or when the use of this axis is not appropriate because there has been no change in the person's condition (e.g., the person is being reevaluated after several months in the hospital because of a change of therapists).

Axis V. Global Assessment of Functioning

Axis V permits the clinician to indicate his or her overall judgment of a person's psychological, social, and occupational functioning on a scale, the Global Assessment of Functioning Scale (GAF Scale), that assesses mental health-illness (Table 9.2-4).

Ratings on the GAF Scale should be made for two time periods:

(1) Current—the level of functioning at the time of the evaluation.
(2) Past year—the highest level of functioning for at least a few months during the past year. For children and adolescents, this should include at least a month during the school year.

Ratings of current functioning will generally reflect the current need for treatment or care. Ratings of highest level of functioning during the past year frequently will have prognostic significance, because usually a person returns to his or her previous level of functioning after an episode of illness.

Table from DSM-III-R *Diagnostic and Statistical Manual of Mental Disorders,* ed 3, revised. Copyright American Psychiatric Association, Washington, DC, 1987. Used with permission.

9.3 TYPICAL SIGNS AND SYMPTOMS OF PSYCHIATRIC ILLNESS

HAROLD I. KAPLAN, M.D.
BENJAMIN J. SADOCK, M.D.

INTRODUCTION

The terms "signs" and "symptoms" refer to specific events: *Signs* are objective findings observed by the clinician (e.g., tachycardia or motor hyperactivity); *symptoms* are subjective complaints listed by the patient (e.g., palpitations or anxiety). Psychological symptoms can be ego-syntonic or ego-dystonic; that is, they can be experienced either as acceptable and compatible or as unacceptable and alien. In general usage, the terms "signs" and "symptoms" tend to be used interchangeably. It is especially difficult to maintain the distinction in psychiatry. Patients may not complain of any symptoms (e.g., the symptoms are ego-syntonic), but those around them believe their behavior to be strange, and it is that strange behavior that constitutes the signs of illness. Conversely, patients experiencing hallucinations may vigorously complain about what they believes they hear (the symptoms are ego-dystonic), but there are no observable signs of hallucinatory activity. Unlike certain medical conditions, there are few, if any, signs or symptoms that are pathognomonic of specific psychiatric disorders. Moreover, physical disease may first present with psychiatric symptomatology, thereby compounding the difficult task of making an accurate diagnosis. A *syndrome* is a group of symptoms that occur together and constitute a recognizable condition, and the term "syndrome" is less specific than "disorder" or "disease." Most psychiatric disorders are, in reality, syndromes.

In the outline that follows, a comprehensive list of various signs and symptoms are given, each with a precise definition or description. The student of human behavior needs to be familiar with each sign and symptom, some of which are traced from their roots in essentially normal behavior. Psychiatric diagnosis is more than just signs and symptoms. It involves recognizing prodromal and residual phases of illness: the phases before acute illness presents and after remission of florid symptoms occurs. It involves how patients think, feel, and act; the degree to which they are alert and oriented; how well they observe and remember; their personal eccentricities; and the ways in which they relate to other persons in the family—at work, at play, and in the community. Table 9.3-1 is an alphabetical listing of signs and symptoms discussed in this section.

I. Consciousness: state of awareness

Apperception: perception modified by one's own emotions and thoughts

Sensorium: state of functioning of the special senses (sometimes used as a synonym for consciousness)

A. Disturbances of consciousness

1. Disorientation: disturbance of orientation to time, place, or person
2. Clouding of consciousness: incomplete clear-mindedness, with disturbance in perception and attitudes
3. Stupor: lack of reaction to and unawareness of surroundings
4. Delirium: bewildered, restless, confused, disoriented reaction associated with fear and hallucinations
5. Coma: profound degree of unconsciousness
6. Coma vigil: coma in which the patient appears to be asleep but ready to be aroused (also known as akinetic mutism)
7. Twilight state: disturbed consciousness with hallucinations
8. Dream-like state: often used as synonym for complex-partial or psychomotor epilepsy
9. Somnolence: abnormal drowsiness seen most often in organic processes

B. Disturbances of attention: attention is the amount of effort exerted in focusing on certain portions of an experience; ability to sustain a focus on one activity

1. Distractibility: inability to concentrate attention; attention drawn to unimportant or irrelevant external stimuli
2. Selective inattention: blocking out only those things that generate anxiety

C. Disturbances in suggestibility: compliant and uncritical response to an idea or influence

1. *Folie à deux* (or *folie à trois*): communicated emotional illness between two (or three) persons
2. Hypnosis: artificially induced modification of consciousness, characterized by a heightened suggestibility

II. Emotion: a complex feeling state—with psychic, somatic, and behavioral components—that is related to affect and mood

A. Affect: the experience of emotion expressed by the patient and observed by others. Affect has outward manifestations that can be observed. Affect is variable over time, in response to changing emotional states

1. Appropriate affect: the normal condition in which emotional tone is in harmony with the accompanying idea, thought, or speech; also further described as broad or full affect, in which a full range of emotions is appropriately expressed
2. Inappropriate affect: disharmony between the emotional feeling tone and the idea, thought, or speech accompanying it
3. Blunted affect: a disturbance in affect manifested by a severe reduction in the intensity of externalized feeling tone
4. Restricted or constricted affect: a reduction in intensity of feeling tone, less severe than blunted affect but clearly reduced
5. Flat affect: absence or near absence of any signs of affective expression; voice monotonous, face immobile
6. Labile affect: rapid and abrupt changes in emotional feeling tone, unrelated to external stimuli

B. Mood: a pervasive and sustained emotion, subjectively experienced and reported by the patient; examples include depression, elation, and anger

1. Dysphoric mood: an unpleasant mood
2. Euthymic mood: normal range of mood, implying absence of depressed or elevated mood

TABLE 9.3-1
Index to Signs and Symptoms of Psychiatric Illness*

Abstract thinking	IV, A, 11
Acrophobia	IV, E, 10c
Affect	II, A
Aggression	III, A, 14
Agitation	II, C, 4
Agnosia	V, A
Agoraphobia	IV, E, 10d
Alexithymia	II, B, 12
Algophobia	IV, E, 10e
Ambivalence	II, C, 8
Amnesia	VI, A, 1
Anhedonia	II, B, 10
Anorexia	II, D, 1
Anosognosia	V, A, 1
Anxiety	II, C, 1
Apathy	II, C, 7
Aphasic disturbances	IV, D
Apperception	I
Appropriate affect	II, A, 1
Astereognosia	V, A, 4
Attention	I, B
Auditory hallucination	V, C, 3
Autistic thinking	IV, A, 8
Automatism	III, A, 8
Automatic judgment	IX, B
Autotopagnosia	V, A, 2
Bizarre delusion	IV, E, 3a
Blocking	IV, B, 13
Blunted affect	II, A, 3
Catalepsy	III, A, 4a
Cataplexy	III, A, 5
Catatonia	III, A, 4
Catatonic excitement	III, A, 4b
Catatonic posturing	III, A, 4e
Catatonic rigidity	III, A, 4d
Catatonic stupor	III, A, 4c
Cerea flexibilitas (waxy flexibility)	III, A, 4f
Circumstantiality	IV, B, 3
Clang associations	IV, B, 12
Claustrophobia	IV, E, 10f
Clouding of consciousness	I, A, 2
Coma	I, A, 5
Coma vigil	I, A, 6
Command automatism	III, A, 9
Compulsion	III, A, 11e; IV, E, 9
Concrete thinking	IV, A, 10
Condensation	IV, B, 7
Confabulation	VI, A, 2c
Consciousness	I
Constipation	II, D, 5
Constricted affect	II, A, 4
Conversion symptom	V, B
Critical judgment	IX, A
Déjà entendu	VI, A, 2e
Déjà pensé	VI, A, 2f
Déjà vu	VI, A, 2d
Delirium	I, A, 4
Delusion	IV, E, 3
Delusional jealousy	IV, E, 3n
Delusion of control	IV, E, 3m
Delusion of grandeur	IV, E, 3j
Delusion of infidelity	IV, E, 3n
Delusion of persecution	IV, E, 3i
Delusion of poverty	IV, E, 3f
Delusion of reference	IV, E, 3k
Delusion of self-accusation	IV, E, 3l
Dementia	VII, B
Depersonalization	V, B, 4
Depression	II, B, 9
Derailment	IV, B, 10
Derealization	V, B, 5
Dereism	IV, A, 7
Diminished libido	II, D, 4
Dipsomania	III, A, 11e(i)
Disorientation	I, A, 1
Distractibility	I, B, 1
Disturbances associated with conversion and dissociative phenomenon	V, B
Disturbances associated with organic brain disease	V, A
Disturbances in content of thought	IV, E
Disturbances in form of thinking	IV, A
Disturbances in speech	IV, C
Disturbances in suggestibility	I, C
Disturbances of attention	I, B
Disturbances of communication	III, A
Disturbances of consciousness	I, A
Disturbances of memory	VI, A
Dream-like state	I, A, 8
Dysarthria	IV, C, 6
Dysphoric mood	II, B, 1
Dysprosody	IV, C, 5
Echolalia	III, A, 1
Echopraxia	III, A, 2
Ecstasy	II, B, 8
Egomania	IV, E, 5
Eidetic images	VI, A, 4
Elevated mood	II, B, 6
Emotion	II
Erotomania	IV, E, 3o
Euphoria	II, B, 7
Euthymic mood	II, B, 2
Excited	III, A, 4b
Expansive mood	II, B, 3
Fausse reconnaissance	VI, A, 2a
Fear	II, C, 3
Flat affect	II, A, 5
Flight of ideas	IV, B, 11
Fluent aphasia	IV, D, 7
Folie à deux (folie à trois)	I, C, 1
Formal thought disorder	IV, A, 5
Free-floating anxiety	II, C, 2
Fugue	V, B, 6
Global aphasia	IV, D, 6
Glossolalia	IV, B, 14
Grief	II, B, 11
Gustatory hallucination	V, C, 6
Hallucinations	V, C
Hallucinosis	V, C, 12
Hyperactivity (hyperkinesis)	III, A, 11b
Hypermnesia	VI, A, 3
Hypersomnia	II, D, 3
Hypnagogic hallucination	V, C, 1
Hypnosis	I, C, 2
Hypoactivity (hypokinesis)	III, A, 12
Hypochondria	IV, E, 7
Hypnopompic hallucination	V, C, 2
Hysterical anesthesia	V, B, 1
Illogical thinking	IV, A, 6
Illusions	V, D
Impaired insight	VIII, C
Impaired judgment	IX, C
Inappropriate affect	II, A, 2
Incoherence	IV, B, 5
Initial insomnia	II, D, 2a
Insight	VIII
Insomnia	II, D, 2
Intellectual insight	VIII, A
Intelligence	VII
Irrelevant answer	IV, B, 8
Irritable mood	II, B, 4
Jamais vu	VI, A, 2g
Jargon aphasia	IV, D, 5
Judgment	IX
Kleptomania	III, A, 11e(ii)
Labile affect	II, A, 6
Lilliputian hallucination	V, C, 9

TABLE 9.3-1
Continued

Logorrhea	IV, C, 2
Loosening of associations	IV, B, 9
Macropsia	V, B, 2
Magical thinking	IV, A, 9
Mannerisms	III, A, 7
Memory	VI
Mental disorder	IV, A, 1
Mental retardation	VII, A
Micropsia	V, B, 3
Middle insomnia	II, D, 2b
Mimicry	III, A, 13
Monomania	IV, E, 6
Mood	II, B
Mood-congruent delusion	IV, E, 3c
Mood-congruent hallucination	V, C, 10
Mood-incongruent delusion	IV, E, 3d
Mood-incongruent hallucination	V, C, 11
Mood swings	II, B, 5
Motor aphasia	IV, D, 1
Motor behavior (conation)	III
Mourning	II, B, 11
Multiple personality	V, B, 7
Mutism	III, A, 10
Negativism	III, A, 4g
Neologism	IV, B, 1
Neurosis	IV, A, 2
Nihilistic delusion	IV, E, 3e
Noesis	IV, E, 11
Nominal aphasia	IV, D, 3
Nymphomania	III, A, 11e(iii)
Obsession	IV, E, 8
Olfactory hallucination	V, C, 5
Overactivity	III, A, 11
Overvalued idea	IV, E, 2
Panic	II, C, 6
Paramnesia	VI, A, 2
Paranoid delusions	IV, E, 3h
Paranoid ideation	IV, E, 4
Perception	V
Persecutory delusion	IV, E, 3h
Perseveration	IV, B, 6
Phobia	IV, E, 10
Physiological disturbances associated with mood	II, D
Posturing	III, A, 4e
Poverty of content of speech	IV, C, 4; IV, E, 1
Poverty of speech	IV, C, 3
Preoccupation of thought	IV, E, 4
Pressure of speech	IV, C, 1
Prosopagnosia	V, A, 5
Pseudodementia	VII, C
Pseudologia fantastica	IV, E, 3p
Psychomotor agitation	III, A, 11a
Psychosis	IV, A, 3
Reality testing	III, A, 4
Restricted affect	II, A, 4
Rigidity	III, A, 4d
Retrospective falsification	VI, A, 2b
Ritual	III, A, 11e(vi)
Satyriasis	III, A, 11e(iv)
Selective inattention	I, B, 2
Sensorium	I
Sensory aphasia	IV, D, 2
Simple phobia	IV, E, 10a
Sleepwalking	III, A, 11d
Social phobia	IV, E, 10b
Somatic delusion	IV, E, 3g
Somatic hallucination	V, C, 8
Somnambulism	III, A, 11d
Somnolence	I, A, 9
Specific disturbances in form of thought	IV, B
Stereotypy	III, A, 6
Stupor	I, A, 3; III, A, 4c
Synesthesia	V, C, 13
Syntactical aphasia	IV, D, 4
Systemized delusion	IV, E, 3b
Tactile (haptic) hallucination	V, C, 7
Tangentiality	IV, B, 4
Tension	II, C, 5
Terminal insomnia	II, D, 2c
Thinking	IV
Thought broadcasting	IV, E, 3m(iii)
Thought insertion	IV, E, 3m(ii)
Thought withdrawal	IV, E, 3m(i)
Tic	III, A, 11c
Trailing phenomenon	V, C, 14
Trend of thought	IV, E, 4
Trichotillomania	III, A, 11e(v)
True insight	VIII, B
Twilight state	I, A, 7
Unio mystica	IV, E, 12
Verbigeration	III, A, 3
Visual agnosia	V, A, 3
Visual hallucination	V, C, 4
Volubility	IV, C, 2
Waxy flexibility	III, A, 4f
Word salad	IV, B, 2
Xenophobia	IV, E, 10g
Zoophobia	IV, E, 10h

*This table lists in alphabetical order the signs and symptoms of psychiatric illness discussed in this section. The numbers and letters in the right-hand column refer to the place in the outline where each term is defined.

3. Expansive mood: expression of one's feelings without restraint, frequently with an overestimation of one's significance or importance
4. Irritable mood: easily annoyed and provoked to anger
5. Mood swings: oscillations between periods of euphoria and depression or anxiety
6. Elevated mood: air of confidence and enjoyment; a mood more cheerful than normal but not necessarily pathological
7. Euphoria: intense elation with feelings of grandeur
8. Ecstasy: feeling of intense rapture
9. Depression: psychopathological feeling of sadness
10. Anhedonia: loss of interest in and withdrawal from all regular and pleasurable activities, often associated with depression
11. Grief or mourning: sadness appropriate to a real loss
12. Alexithymia: inability or difficulty in describing or being aware of one's emotions or moods

C. Other emotions

1. Anxiety: feeling of apprehension from the anticipation of danger, which may be internal or external
2. Free-floating anxiety: pervasive, unfocused fear not attached to any idea
3. Fear: anxiety resulting from consciously recognized and realistic danger
4. Agitation: anxiety associated with severe motor restlessness, also known as psychomotor agitation
5. Tension: increased motor and psychological activity that is unpleasant

6. Panic: acute, episodic, intense attack of anxiety associated with overwhelming feelings of dread and autonomic discharge
7. Apathy: dulled emotional tone associated with detachment or indifference
8. Ambivalence: coexistence of two opposing impulses toward the same thing in the same person at the same time

D. Physiological disturbances associated with mood: signs that refer to somatic (usually autonomic) dysfunction of the individual, most often associated with depression (also called vegetative signs)

1. Anorexia: loss of or decrease in appetite
2. Insomnia: diminished or lack of ability to sleep
   a. Initial: difficulty falling asleep
   b. Middle: difficulty sleeping through night without waking up and difficulty falling back to sleep
   c. Terminal: early morning awakening
3. Hypersomnia: excessive sleeping
4. Diminished libido: decreased sexual interest, drive, and performance
5. Constipation: inabilities or difficulties involved with defecating

III. Motor behavior (conation): the aspect of the psyche that includes impulses, motivations, wishes, drives, instincts, and cravings, as expressed by a person's behavior or motor activity

A. Disturbances of communication

1. Echolalia: psychopathological repeating of words or phrases of one person by another; tends to be repetitive and persistent; may be spoken with a mocking or staccato intonation
2. Echopraxia: pathological imitation of movements of one person by another
3. Verbigeration: meaningless repetitions of specific words or phrases
4. Catatonia: motor anomalies in nonorganic disorders
   a. Catalepsy: general term for an immobile position that is constantly maintained
   b. Excited: agitated, purposeless motor activity, uninfluenced by external stimuli
   c. Stupor: markedly slowed motor activity, often to a point of immobility and seeming unawareness of surroundings
   d. Rigidity: assumption of a rigid posture, against all efforts to be moved
   e. Posturing: voluntary assumption of an inappropriate or bizarre posture, generally maintained for long periods of time
   f. Cerea flexibilitas (waxy flexibility): the person can be "molded" into a position, which is then maintained; when the examiner moves the person's limb, the limb feels as if it were made of wax
   g. Negativism: motiveless resistance to all attempts to be moved or to all instructions
5. Cataplexy: temporary loss of muscle tone and weakness precipitated by a variety of emotional states
6. Stereotypy: repetitive fixed pattern of physical action or speech
7. Mannerisms: stereotyped involuntary movements
8. Automatism: automatic performance of acts representative of unconscious symbolic activity
9. Command automatism: automatic following of suggestions (also called automatic obedience)
10. Mutism: voicelessness without structural abnormalities
11. Overactivity
    a. Psychomotor agitation: excessive overactivity, usually nonproductive and in response to inner tension
    b. Hyperactivity (hyperkinesis): restless, aggressive, destructive activity
    c. Tic: involuntary, spasmodic motor movements
    d. Sleepwalking (somnambulism): motor activity during sleep
    e. Compulsion: uncontrollable impulse to perform an act repetitively
       i. Dipsomania: compulsion to drink alcohol
       ii. Kleptomania: compulsion to steal
       iii. Nymphomania: excessive and compulsive need for coitus in female
       iv. Satyriasis: excessive and compulsive need for coitus in male
       v. Trichotillomania: compulsion to pull out one's hair
       vi. Ritual: automatic activity compulsive in nature, anxiety-reducing in origin
12. Hypoactivity (hypokinesis): decreased activity or retardation, as in psychomotor retardation; visible slowing of thought, speech, movements
13. Mimicry: simple, imitative motor activity of childhood
14. Aggression: forceful goal-directed action that may be verbal or physical; the motor counterpart of the affect of rage, anger, or hostility

IV. Thinking: goal-directed flow of ideas, symbols, and associations initiated by a problem of tasks and leading toward a reality-oriented conclusion; when a logical sequence occurs, thinking is normal. Parapraxes (lapses from logic, also called "Freudian slips") are considered part of normal thinking

A. Disturbances in form of thinking

1. Mental disorder: clinically significant behavioral or psychological syndrome, associated with distress or disability, not just an expected response to a particular event
2. Neurosis: mental disorder in which reality testing is intact and symptoms are experienced as ego-dystonic (distressing and unacceptable); behavior does not violate gross social norms; relatively enduring or recurrent without treatment; see authors' note below for current usage of this term
3. Psychosis: inability to distinguish reality from fantasy; impaired reality testing, with creation of a new reality
4. Reality testing: the objective evaluation and judgment of the world outside the self

5. Formal thought disorder: disturbance in the form of thought instead of the content of thought; thinking characterized by loosened associations, neologisms, and illogical constructs; thought process is disordered, and the person is defined as psychotic
6. Illogical thinking: thinking containing erroneous conclusions or internal contradictions; is psychopathological only when it is marked, and when not attributable to cultural values or to intellectual deficit
7. Dereism: mental activity not concordant with logic or experience
8. Autistic thinking: thinking that gratifies unfulfilled desires but has no regard for reality; preoccupation with inner, private world; term used somewhat synonymously with dereism
9. Magical thinking: a form of dereistic thought; thinking that is similar to that of the preoperational phase in children (Piaget), in which thoughts, words, or actions assume power (e.g., they can cause or prevent events)
10. Concrete thinking: literal thinking; limited use of metaphor without understanding of nuances of meaning; one-dimensional thought
11. Abstract thinking: ability to appreciate nuances of meaning; multidimensional thinking with ability to use metaphors and hypotheses appropriately

B. *Specific disturbances in form of thought*

1. Neologism: new words created by the patient, often from combining syllables of other words, for idiosyncratic psychological reasons
2. Word salad: incoherent mixture of words and phrases
3. Circumstantiality: indirect speech that is delayed in reaching the point, but eventually gets from original point to desired goal; characterized by an overinclusion of detail and parenthetical remarks
4. Tangentiality: inability to have goal-directed associations of thought; patient never gets from desired point to desired goal
5. Incoherence: speech that, generally, is not understandable; running together of thoughts or words with no logical or grammatical connection, resulting in disorganization
6. Perseveration: persisting response to a prior stimulus after a new stimulus has been presented, often associated with organic brain disease
7. Condensation: fusion of various concepts into one
8. Irrelevant answer: answer that is not in harmony with question asked
9. Loosening of associations: flow of thought in which ideas shift from one subject to another in a completely unrelated way; when severe, speech may be incoherent
10. Derailment: gradual or sudden deviation in train of thought without blocking; sometimes used synonymously with loosening of associations
11. Flight of ideas: rapid, continuous verbalizations or plays on words producing constant shifting from one idea to another; the ideas tend to be connected and, in the less severe form, may be intelligible to a listener
12. Clang associations: association of words similar in sound but not in meaning; words have no logical connection, may include rhyming and punning
13. Blocking: abrupt interruption in train of thinking before a thought or idea is finished; after brief pause, person indicates no recall of what was being said or was going to be said (also known as thought deprivation)
14. Glossolalia: the expression of a revelatory message through unintelligible words (also known as "speaking in tongues")

C. *Disturbances in speech*

1. Pressure of speech: rapid speech that is increased in amount and difficult to interrupt
2. Volubility (logorrhea): copious, coherent, logical speech
3. Poverty of speech: restriction in the amount of speech used; replies may be monosyllabic
4. Poverty of content of speech: speech that is adequate in amount but conveys little information because of vagueness, emptiness, or stereotyped phrases
5. Dysprosody: loss of prosody, or normal speech melody
6. Dysarthria: difficulty in articulation, not in word finding or in grammar

D. *Aphasic disturbances (disturbances in language output)*

1. Motor aphasia: disturbance of speech due to organic brain disorder in which understanding remains but ability to speak is lost (also known as Broca's nonfluent aphasia or expressive aphasia)
2. Sensory aphasia: loss of ability to comprehend the meaning of words or the use of objects (also known as Wernicke's fluent or Wernicke's receptive aphasia)
3. Nominal aphasia: difficulty in finding correct name for an object
4. Syntactical aphasia: inability to arrange words in proper sequence
5. Jargon aphasia: words produced are totally neologistic; nonsense words repeated with various intonations and inflections
6. Global aphasia: combination of a grossly nonfluent aphasia plus severe fluent aphasia
7. Fluent aphasia: inability to understand the spoken word; fluent, but incoherent, speech is present

E. *Disturbances in content of thought*

1. Poverty of content of speech: speech that gives little information due to vagueness, empty repetitions, or obscure phrases
2. Overvalued idea: unreasonable, sustained false belief maintained less firmly than delusional thinking
3. Delusion: false belief, based on incorrect inference about external reality, that is not consistent with patient's intelligence and cultural background and cannot be corrected by reasoning

a. Bizarre delusion: an absurd, totally implausible, very strange false belief (e.g., invaders from space have implanted electrodes in the patient's brain)
b. Systematized delusion: false belief or beliefs united by a single event or theme (e.g., patient is being persecuted by the CIA, FBI, Mafia, or his or her boss)
c. Mood-congruent delusion: delusions whose content is mood-appropriate (e.g., a depressed patient who believes he or she is responsible for the destruction of the world)
d. Mood-incongruent delusion: delusion whose content has no association to mood or is mood-inappropriate (e.g., a depressed patient who believes he or she is the new Messiah)
e. Nihilistic delusion: false feeling that self, others, or the world is nonexistent or ending
f. Delusion of poverty: false belief that one is bereft, or will be, of all material possessions
g. Somatic delusion: false belief involving functioning of one's body (e.g., belief that one's brain is rotting or melting)
h. Paranoid delusions: includes persecutory delusions, as well as delusions of reference, control, and grandeur (this is to be distinguished from paranoid ideation, which is suspiciousness of less than delusional proportions)
i. Delusion of persecution: false belief that one is being harassed, cheated, or persecuted; often found in litigious patients who have a pathological tendency to take legal action because of imagined mistreatment
j. Delusion of grandeur: exaggerated conception of one's importance, power, or identity
k. Delusion of reference: false belief that the behavior of others refers to oneself; that events, objects, or other people have a particular and unusual significance, usually of a negative nature; derived from ideas or reference in which one falsely feels one is being talked about by others; differs from an idea of reference, in which the false belief is not as firmly held as in a delusion
l. Delusion of self-accusation: false feeling of remorse and guilt
m. Delusion of control: false feeling that one's will, thoughts, or feelings are being controlled by external forces
   i. Thought withdrawal: delusion that one's thoughts are being removed from one's mind by other people or forces
   ii. Thought insertion: delusion that thoughts are being implanted in one's mind by other people or forces
   iii. Thought broadcasting: delusion that one's thoughts can be heard by others, as though they are being broadcast into the air
n. Delusion of infidelity (delusional jealousy): false belief derived from pathological jealousy that one's lover is unfaithful
o. Erotomania: delusional belief, almost exclusively in women, that a man is deeply in love with them (also known as Clérambault's syndrome)
p. Pseudologia fantastica: a type of lying, in which the person appears to believe in the reality of his or her fantasies and acts on them

4. Trend or preoccupation of thought: centering of thought content around a particular idea, associated with a strong affective tone, such as a paranoid trend or suicidal preoccupation
5. Egomania: pathological self-preoccupation
6. Monomania: preoccupation with a single object
7. Hypochondria: exaggerated concern over one's health that is not based on real organic pathology, but rather on unrealistic interpretation of physical signs or sensations as abnormal
8. Obsession: pathological persistence of an irresistible thought or feeling that cannot be eliminated from consciousness by logical effort, which is associated with anxiety
9. Compulsion: pathological need to act on an impulse, which, if resisted, produces anxiety; repetitive behavior in response to an obsession or performed according to certain rules, with no true end in itself other than to prevent something from occurring in the future
10. Phobia: persistent, irrational, exaggerated, and invariably pathological fear of some specific type of stimulus or situation; results in a compelling desire to avoid dreaded stimulus
    a. Simple phobia: circumscribed fear of a discrete object or situation (e.g., fear of heights or flying)
    b. Social phobia: fear of public humiliation, as in fear of public speaking, performing, or eating in public
    c. Acrophobia: fear of high places
    d. Agoraphobia: fear of open places
    e. Algophobia: fear of pain
    f. Claustrophobia: fear of closed places
    g. Xenophobia: fear of strangers
    h. Zoophobia: fear of animals
11. Noesis: a revelation in which immense illumination occurs in association with a sense that one has been chosen to lead and command
12. Unio mystica: an oceanic feeling, one of mystic unity with an infinite power

V. Perception: process of transferring physical stimulation into psychological information; mental process by which sensory stimuli are brought to awareness

A. *Disturbances associated with organic brain disease:* agnosia—an inability to recognize and interpret the significance of sensory impressions
   1. Anosognosia: denial of illness
   2. Autotopagnosia: denial of a body part
   3. Visual agnosia: inability to recognize objects or persons
   4. Astereognosia: inability to recognize objects by touch
   5. Prosopagnosia: inability to recognize faces

B. *Disturbances associated with conversion and dissociative phenomenon:* somatization of repressed material or the development of physical symptoms and distortions involving the voluntary muscles or special sense organs; not under voluntary control, and not explained by any physical disorder

1. Hysterical anesthesia: loss of sensory modalities resulting from emotional conflicts
2. Macropsia: state in which objects seem larger than they are
3. Micropsia: state in which objects seem smaller than they are (both macropsia and micropsia can also be associated with organic conditions, such as complex partial seizures)
4. Depersonalization: a subjective sense of being unreal, strange, or unfamiliar to oneself
5. Derealization: a subjective sense that the environment is strange or unreal; a feeling of changed reality
6. Fugue: taking on of a new identity with amnesia for the old; often involves travel or wanderings to new environments
7. Multiple personality: one person who appears at different times to be in possession of an entirely different personality and character

C. *Hallucinations:* false sensory perceptions not associated with real external stimuli; there may or may not be a delusional interpretation of the hallucinatory experience; hallucinations indicate a psychotic disturbance only when associated with impairment in reality testing

1. Hypnagogic hallucination: false sensory perception occurring while falling asleep
2. Hypnopompic hallucination: false sensory perception occurring while awakening from sleep
3. Auditory hallucination: false perception of sound, usually voices, but also various noises, such as music or rustling leaves
4. Visual hallucination: false perception involving sight, consisting of both formed images (e.g., people) and unformed images (e.g., flashes of light)
5. Olfactory hallucination: false perception in smell
6. Gustatory hallucination: false perception of taste, such as unpleasant taste due to an uncinate seizure
7. Tactile (haptic) hallucination: false perception of touch or surface sensation, as from an amputated limb (phantom limb) or crawling sensation on or under the skin (formication)
8. Somatic hallucination: false sensation of things occurring in or to the body, most often visceral in origin (also known as cenesthetic hallucination)
9. Lilliputian hallucination: false perception in which objects are seen as reduced in size
10. Mood-congruent hallucination: hallucination whose content is consistent with either a depressed or manic mood (e.g., a depressed patient hears voices saying he or she is a bad person; a manic patient hears voices saying he or she is of inflated worth, power, knowledge)
11. Mood-incongruent hallucination: hallucination whose content is not consistent with either depressed or manic mood (e.g., in depression, hallucinations not involving such themes as guilt, deserved punishment, or inadequacy; in mania, not involving such themes as inflated worth or power)
12. Hallucinosis: hallucinations, most often auditory, that are associated with chronic alcohol abuse and occur within a clear sensorium (as opposed to delirium tremens [DTs])
13. Synesthesia: sensations or hallucinations caused by other sensations (e.g., an auditory sensation is accompanied by or triggers a visual sensation; a sound is experienced as being seen or a visual experience is heard)
14. Trailing phenomenon: perceptual abnormality associated with hallucinogenic drugs in which moving objects are seen as a series of discrete and discontinuous images

D. *Illusions:* misperceptions or misinterpretations of real external sensory stimuli

VI. Memory: function by which information stored in the brain is later recalled to consciousness

A. *Disturbances of memory*

1. Amnesia: partial or total inability to recall past experiences, may be organic or emotional in origin
2. Paramnesia: falsification of memory by distortion of recall
   a. *Fausse reconnaissance:* false recognition
   b. Retrospective falsification: recollection of a true memory to which the patient adds false details
   c. Confabulation: unconscious filling of gaps in memory by imagined or untrue experiences that patient believes but that have no basis in fact
   d. *Déjà vu:* illusion of visual recognition in which a new situation is incorrectly regarded as a repetition of a previous event
   e. *Déjà entendu:* illusion of auditory recognition
   f. *Déjà pensé:* illusion that a new thought is recognized as a thought previously felt or expressed
   g. *Jamais vu:* false feeling of unfamiliarity with a real situation one has experienced
3. Hypermnesia: exaggerated degree of retention and recall
4. Eidetic images: visual memories of almost hallucinatory vividness

VII. Intelligence: the ability to understand, recall, mobilize, and constructively integrate previous learning in meeting new situations

A. *Mental retardation:* lack of intelligence to a degree in which there is interference with social and vocational performance: mild (intelligence quotient [I.Q.] of about 50 to 70), moderate (I.Q. of about 35 to 50), severe (I.Q. of about 20 to 35), or profound (I.Q. below 20); obsolescent terms are idiot (mental age less than 3 years), imbecile (mental age of 3 to 7 years), and moron (mental age of about 8)

B. *Dementia:* organic and global deterioration of intellectual functioning without clouding of consciousness

C. *Pseudodementia:* clinical features resembling a dementia not due to organic brain dysfunction, most often caused by depression

VIII. Insight: ability of the patient to understand the true cause and meaning of a situation (such as a set of symptoms)

A. *Intellectual insight:* understanding of the objective reality of a set of circumstances, without the ability to apply the understanding in any useful way to master the situation

B. *True insight:* understanding of the objective reality of a situation coupled with the motivation and emotional impetus to master the situation

C. *Impaired insight:* diminished ability to understand the objective reality of a situation

IX. Judgment: ability to assess a situation correctly and act appropriately within that situation

A. *Critical judgment:* ability to assess, discern, and choose among different options in a situation

B. *Automatic judgment:* reflex performance of an action

C. *Impaired judgment:* diminished ability to understand a situation correctly and to act appropriately

AUTHORS' NOTE ON NEUROSIS

A neurosis is a chronic or recurrent nonpsychotic disorder that is characterized mainly by anxiety, which is experienced or expressed directly or altered through defense mechanisms; it appears as a symptom, such as obsession, compulsion, phobia, or sexual dysfunction, among others. According to the third edition of the *Diagnostic and Statistical Manual of Mental Disorders* (DSM-III), a neurotic disorder is defined as:

> A mental disorder in which the predominant disturbance is a symptom or group of symptoms that is distressing to the individual and is recognized by him or her as unacceptable and alien (ego-dystonic); reality testing is grossly intact. Behavior does not actively violate gross social norms (though it may be quite disabling). The disturbance is relatively enduring or recurrent without treatment, and is not limited to a transitory reaction to stressors. There is no demonstrable organic etiology or factor.

In the revised edition of DSM-III (DSM-III-R), there is no overall diagnostic class of neuroses; however, the following DSM-III-R diagnostic categories are considered neuroses by many clinicians, and the reader will note that DSM-III-R uses the term "neurosis" in parentheses for some of these conditions.

Anxiety disorders (or anxiety and phobic neuroses) These include agoraphobia without history of panic disorder, social phobia, and simple phobia; panic disorder (with or without agoraphobia), generalized anxiety disorder, and obsessive-compulsive disorder (or obsessive-compulsive neurosis); and post-traumatic stress disorder.

Somatoform disorders These disorders include somatization disorder, conversion disorder (hysterical neurosis, conversion type), somatoform pain disorder, hypochondriasis (or hypochondriacal neurosis), body dysmorphic disorder, and undifferentiated somatoform disorder.

Dissociative disorders (hysterical neuroses, dissociative type) These disorders include psychogenic amnesia, psychogenic fugue, multiple personality, depersonalization disorder (or depersonalization neurosis), and dissociative disorder not otherwise specified.

Sexual disorders This broad category includes paraphilias and sexual dysfunctions. In common use, these categories have been considered neurotic disorders.

Dysthymia This disorder, also known as depressive neurosis, is now classified in DSM-III-R as a type of mood disorder.

In summary, the term "neurosis" encompasses a broad range of disorders of different signs and symptoms. As such, it has lost any degree of precision except to signify that the person's gross reality testing and personality organization are intact. A neurosis, however, can be and usually is sufficient to impair the person's functioning in a variety of areas.

REFERENCES

Andreasen N C: The clinical assessment of thought, language, and communication disorders. I. The definition of terms and evaluation of their reliability. Arch Gen Psychiat *36:* 1315, 1979.

Bender M D: *Disorders of Perception.* Charles C Thomas, Springfield, IL, 1952.

Bensen D F, Blumer D, editors: *Psychiatric Aspects of Neurological Disease,* vol 2. Grune & Stratton, Orlando, FL, 1982.

Bleuler E: *Dementia Praecox: The Group of Schizophrenias.* International Universities Press, New York, 1950.

Campbell R J: *Psychiatric Dictionary,* ed 5. Oxford University Press, New York, 1981.

Cavenar J O, Brodie, H K M: *Signs and Symptoms in Psychiatry.* Lippincott, Philadelphia, 1983.

Fenichel O: *Psychoanalytic Theory of Neuroses,* Norton, New York, 1945.

Frances A J, Hales R E: *Annual Review,* vol 5. American Psychiatric Press, Washington, DC, 1986.

Geschwind N: Aphasia. New Eng J Med *284:* 654, 1971.

Hellerstein D, Frosch W, Koenigsberg H W: The clinical significance of command hallucinations. Amer J Psychiat *144*(1): 219, 1987.

Solomon C M, Holzman J P S, Levin S, Gale H J: The association between eye-tracking dysfunctions and thought disorder in psychosis. Arch Gen Psychiat *44*(1): 31, 1987.

Spitzer R L, Skodol A E, Williams J B W: *Case Book Diagnostic and Statistical Manual of Mental Disorders.* American Psychiatric Association, Washington, DC, 1988.

9.4 PSYCHOLOGICAL ASSESSMENT OF PERSONALITY OF ADULTS AND CHILDREN

ROBERT W. BUTLER, Ph.D.
PAUL SATZ, Ph.D.

INTRODUCTION

A basic assumption underlying practice and research in the mental health professions is that people behave in a relatively organized, recognizable manner. It is possible to subcategorize organized behavior into at least two levels: trait and personality. A *trait* may be considered a disposition or tendency to act in a certain manner, be it hostile, kindly, passive, or whatever. *Personality* can be defined as a complex patterning of traits. In general, traits can be assumed as varying in strength both across individuals and within the individual, depending on situational parameters. Following this, Sundberg defined the assessment of personality as "the set of processes used by a person or persons for developing impressions and images, making decisions, and checking hypotheses about another person's pattern of characteristics which determine his or her behavior in interaction with the environment."

Although the activity of personality assessment has undoubtedly gone on throughout the ages, the introduction of the scientific method to personality assessment can be traced to Francis Galton and his studies of individual differences, reported in 1869. Since that time, eminent psychiatrists and psychologists, including Emil Kraepelin, Carl Jung, Hermann Rorschach, Raymond Cattell, and Henry Murray, as well as many present-day researchers, have worked toward advancing the ability to measure components of personality accurately and reliably, especially as they relate to the causative aspects of behaviors.

Though not without its critics, formal personality assessment continues to play an integral role in clinical practice. The essential question in clinical psychiatry is "How can the patient be helped?" Personality assessment provides information on the individuals' strengths and weaknesses, on how and why they are in their current situation, and on their prognosis. Valuable information regarding diagnosis is a frequent result of a thorough personality evaluation. Formalized assessment over the course of psychotherapy can be useful in documenting changes, both positive and negative.

In research methodology, the necessity for reliable and valid dependent and independent variables is readily apparent. Well-constructed personality assessment devices are required for any research question that deals with traits, behaviors, and personality—and with human characteristics in general. Research in the area of psychotherapy outcome is receiving increased attention. Personality assessment plays a primary role during the selection of outcome variables for this type of research.

Most therapists and researchers do not deny the need for measurement of personality. Formal psychological testing has been shown useful in the areas of treatment, diagnosis, prognosis, and research. There is disagreement, however, about the appropriate manner in which personality should be measured. Methodologies available for measurement are varied and tend to reflect the theoretical orientation of their developer and user.

THEORETICAL FOUNDATIONS

The manner in which one measures personality will be dictated, in large part, by how one conceptualizes personality and its development. In any discussion of personality assessment, it is essential that certain issues in the study of personality theory be considered.

STATE VS. TRAIT In the earlier definitions of personality and personality assessment, the concept of a trait was included. Anxiety as a trait implies that it will be a relatively enduring behavior pattern across time, perhaps waxing or waning, dependent on environmental conditions at the time of assessment. Another approach to personality assessment involves the direct sampling of occurring behavior without inferring the presence of a construct, such as a psychological trait. This state, or interactive behavioral, approach to personality assessment tends to decry the existence of chronic characterological anxiety and to be more involved in identifying the situational demand characteristics that are eliciting anxious behavior on the part of an individual. Enduring characteristics are de-emphasized unless behavioral triggers are present.

NOMOTHETIC VS. IDIOGRAPHIC A nomothetic approach to personality emphasizes the need to have a reference point to which an individual will be compared. Psychological normality is viewed from a lens that considers the person in relation to the human species in general. If the majority of the population reports some anxiety during public speaking, this level of anxiety becomes the reference criterion for whether speech anxiety is a potentially problematic, or abnormal, behavior. An idiographic approach to personality, in contrast, would place much less emphasis on normative groups. Whereas the nomothetic approach holds that prior to making a statement on whether anxiety in an individual is disabling, one needs to know how anxious the average person is, the idiographic approach is largely concerned with the fact that anxiety has been reported or observed on an individual basis. The anxiety is then examined in relation to how it affects the individual's functioning—psychologically, symptomatically, interpersonally, and otherwise.

DYNAMIC VS. EMPIRICAL The dynamic approach to personality emphasizes the importance of underlying causative agents that determine the nature of observable behaviors. Analytic theories of personality embody this approach and typically place less significance on specific symptomatic behavior per se, but rather consider symptoms in relationship to the nature of an individual's personality structure. Constructs that are relatively unobservable become necessary in the explanation of behavior determinants.

At the opposite pole of this continuum, the empirical approach to personality de-emphasizes underlying constructs, such as ego functions and object relations, that mediate behavior; instead, this approach views current behavior as a function of past learning. The properties of reward and punishment take on explanatory roles, and directly observable behavior is given primary importance in understanding the structure of personality.

METHODOLOGICAL ISSUES IN PERSONALITY ASSESSMENT

Traditionally, psychological personality assessment has been conducted by self-report, but this technique is not the only way in which to sample human behavior. One may obtain information from other informants, directly observe behavior, or observe behavior in contrived situations. In an ideal situation, one would assess personality by all of the above modalities; however, such comprehensive assessment is rarely possible because of time and financial constraints. If it were possible, an assumption probably would be made regarding intermethod agreement; that is, the person's behavior would be consistent across assessment modalities. Although this type of agreement is desirable in most assessment situations, its absence does not per se necessarily represent a problem in personality assessment. Any measurement of personality will be colored by the patient's reactions to the assessment method and also the assessor. Often, this type of information can provide valuable information. In general, it is best to assess a facet of personality by at least two different methods in order to maximize valid information.

Personality is rarely viewed as a unitary concept; rather, it is generally considered as having dimensions. It is necessary to determine what dimensions and how many are to be assessed. There is no simplistic answer or heuristic approach to this issue. Typically, the dimensions assessed are dictated by the specific question being asked or the need of the clinician to reduce the amount of data to be accumulated and digested. Also entering into the decision on what amount of information is required for an adequate and accurate assessment of personality are incremental validity studies. Research has suggested that, beyond a certain point, additional psychological testing can impair the accuracy of the assessment. It also may be the case that parsimony in rating personality along various factors and dimensions is preferable.

RESPONSE SETS Response sets refer to attitudes or styles in responding to personality questionnaires. For the most part, these sets appear to be problematic with objective inventories; however, they are also potential error sources with projective and behavioral assessment. A socially desirable response set is indicative of patients who attempt to present themselves in a favorable light. Conversely, "faking bad" refers to an opposite response set; that is, patients attempt to present a more dismal outlook than is the case. Some of the more well-constructed objective personality measures, such as the Minnesota Multiphasic Personality Inventory (MMPI) and the California Personality Inventory (CPI), have built-in scales designed to detect the presence of these types of response sets. Other response sets that may prove problematic involve a tendency to "yea say" or acquiesce to questions, or a tendency to "nay say" or exercise denial. Again, a well-constructed assessment device will control for these potential problems by careful wording of questions and balancing scoring properties.

One way to deal with response sets and to obtain as realistic and accurate a description of the patient as possible is by concealment of the true nature of the assessment. This approach, however, raises ethical issues that cannot be ignored. As a general rule, human dignity and the basic rights of the patient cannot be compromised. Although the specific nature of concealment might be appropriately defended, the patient needs to be informed regarding the process of deception, if it is involved. Patients always have the right to refuse to respond to questions or stimuli that they find objectionable. However, it is important that the evaluator be aware that this is occurring.

INDIVIDUAL VS. GROUP SETTING Psychological methods of personality assessment are most frequently administered in an individual as opposed to group setting. Some methods of assessment, particularly the objective "paper-and-pencil" questionnaires, lend themselves well to group administration, and this technique is permissible. Other methods, such as the projective Rorschach technique, would never be administered in a group setting by a competent psychologist. In general, the decision to administer personality assessment techniques in a group or individual setting rests with the assessor. Any thorough assessment of personality functioning will include a clinical interview with the patient on an individual basis. Thus, if a group format is utilized for the administration of various assessment techniques, it needs to be supplemented with individual patient contact. In this sense, no complete personality evaluation occurs in a group setting.

The next subsections describe various measurement tools designed to quantify personality. In recent years, personality assessment has experienced a period of regrowth. This renewed interest in assessment has resulted in the development of new and innovative measurement instruments and methodologies. The areas of objective and behavioral assessment have been at the forefront of this renaissance. Advances in projective assessment have generally involved increased attention toward psychometric soundness in measurement. In reviewing psychological methods of personality assessment, the authors have attempted to highlight these advances for the purpose of providing the physician with the most current information possible. The emphasis is on new developments that show promise in providing quality information. Coverage of more traditional assessment modalities has not been sacrificed, however, inasmuch as the goal is a comprehensive review of personality assessment.

As indicated previously, one's theory of personality will play a substantial role in the assessment devices selected and utilized. If a clinician or researcher believes that human behavior is a function of prior learning that interacts with the present environment, then behavioral personality assessment using checklists, rating scales, self-reports, and other such techniques are likely to be used to the exclusion of projective or objective methods. If one feels that personality is comprised of traits that interact with the environment, and thus a nomothetic orientation is preferred, then objective personality assessment is more appropriate. Finally, if a dynamic, idiographic orientation to personality theory is held, then projective assessment becomes the method of choice. Table 9.4-1 provides a summary of the relationship between theory and methodology in psychological personality assessment.

ADULT PERSONALITY ASSESSMENT

OBJECTIVE PERSONALITY ASSESSMENT The objective orientation to personality assessment is characterized by reliance on structured, standardized measurement devices, which are typically of a self-report nature. *Structured* refers to the tendency toward straightforward test stimuli, such as direct questions regarding the persons' opinions of themselves, and unambiguous instructions regarding completion of the test. *Standardization* refers to the tendency for test administration and scoring to be invariant across time and examiners.

TABLE 9.4-1
Relationship Between Theory and Method in Personality Assessment

Theoretical Orientation	*Theoretical Approach*	*Preferred Method*
Psychodynamic	Idiographic Trait Dynamic	Projective
Cognitive-behavioral	Idiographic State Empirical	Behavioral
Psychometric-interpersonal (interactional)	Nomothetic State or trait Empirical	Objective

The objective approach to personality assessment is strongly nomothetic, and most tests of this nature are norm referenced. In a norm-referenced test, the patient's responses to various questions are typically quantified, summed, and compared to a reference group of normal (e.g., nonpsychiatric) persons. The degree to which the patient deviates from the mean of this criterion reference group is noted and interpreted.

Objective personality tests can be used to measure state or trait behaviors. The tests have a clear empirical bias and are not typically used to formulate dynamic interpretations of personality structure. Proponents of objective personality assessment generally place considerable emphasis on the psychometric qualities of their assessment tools. Effort is expended to ensure that the tests possess adequate reliability (consistency of scores across time) and validity (actual measurement of the proposed construct)—characteristics deemed essential of all psychological tests.

Test development The development of objective personality tests most frequently follows one of three general approaches. *Rational development* involves the utilization of confirmatory test items or questions based on personality theory. Specifically, the test developer will construct items or questions that are designed to assess directly aspects of personality that have been predicted to exist by theoretical constructs. The Millon Clinical Multiaxial Inventory (MCMI), Edwards Personal Preference Schedule (EPPS), and Eysenck Personality Questionnaire (EPQ) are examples of tests that have utilized this approach. *Empirical development* involves contrasting groups of individuals in order to find those items that successfully identify the construct in question. This approach is largely atheoretical. The MMPI and CPI are examples of empirically derived personality tests. The *factor analytic* approach utilizes advanced statistical methods, which are applied to large groups of test items to reduce them into homogeneous, internally consistent scales or subgroups. The approach is largely a mixture of empirical and theoretical thinking. The initial item pool is typically selected on the basis of some theoretical notion of personality; however, the statistical procedures define the resultant measurement scales. The scales themselves are typically labeled only after inspection of the test items that have been shown to be highly intercorrelated. Comrey Personality Scales (CPS) and the 16 Personality Factor Questionnaire (16 PF) exemplify the factor analytic approach to test construction.

These differences in test construction become important to the professional who requests personality evaluation of a patient, particularly in regard to the referral question. For example, if knowledge regarding degree of depression is requested without concern for qualitative theoretical issues, then an empirically derived test, such as the MMPI, would be satisfactory. However, if the physician desired not only information on severity of depression but additionally, perhaps, the extent to which the patient's cognitive status was characterized by depression, then a rationally developed test, such as the Beck Depression Inventory (BDI), would be more appropriate. A note of caution needs to be raised regarding factor analytically developed objective personality tests. As mentioned above, the construct that these types of tests purport to measure is generally defined and named by inspection of the test items that comprise them. These definitions and labels are provided by the test developer. The test consumer may or may not agree with the test constructor on this issue. Although this problem may occur with any personality test, it is more frequently an issue with the factor analytically derived instruments. In any event, it behooves the consumer of psychological personality evaluations to have at least a basic familiarity with the specific measurement tools that form the basis of the assessment. In this way, one will be more comfortable with the information provided and also more assured of receiving the type of information requested.

Minnesota Multiphasic Personality Inventory The MMPI is a 566-item, group form, paper-and-pencil personality test. It was developed in the early 1940s, and items were selected using an empirical approach to test construction. Subsets of the test items are used in the scoring of 3 validity scales, 10 clinical scales, and 4 special scales. These scales are described in greater detail in Table 9.4-2.

The original intent of the MMPI was as an aid to clinical diagnosis—hence the diagnostic labels on the clinical scales. Items for these scales were selected by comparing relatively discrete groups of diagnosed patients to nonpsychiatric subjects (most frequently relatives of patients and visitors to the hospital). Those items that successfully differentiated the normals from the clinical groups were selected for the various scales. As a product of this empirical construction, scale items can be grouped into obvious (those items with high face validity) and subtle (those items with rather low face validity). The presence of both high and low face validity items in a personality test results in a potentially useful method of assessing the possibility of malingering, embellishment of symptomatology, and denial. *Face validity* refers to the degree to which the test taker believes that the question is measuring what the test developer intended. Thus, obvious items on the depression scale of the MMPI quite clearly assess aspects of depression to the responder, whereas subtle items generally appear to have little relationship to what people believe depression entails. Comparison of subtle versus obvious item endorsement on MMPI protocols often provides important clinical information.

Numerous additional scales have been developed from the MMPI items—some utilizing the empirical approach, others utilizing rational and factor analytic approaches. Many of these special scales are considered experimental in nature because there is too little research-based evidence to document their reliability and validity. A sample of MMPI results is reproduced in Table 9.4-3.

Although the MMPI was initially viewed as a diagnostic aid (i.e., a patient with a major depressive disorder would show an elevation on the depression scale), the advantages of a configural approach to interpretation quickly became apparent. The configural approach, which involves interpretations based on the patterning of the entire profile, has become the preferred method and has increased the effectiveness of the MMPI as a personality measurement device. Various researchers have identified numerous personality correlates of different MMPI scale configurations, frequently using the two highest scales as the basis for core interpretive statements. Actuarial research of this nature has also served as the basis for computerized interpretative services. These services, though not a substitute for a comprehensive personality evaluation, can assist the clinician in hypothesis formulation. Computerized services are especially useful when the MMPI is to be interpreted by a person knowledgeable in all aspects of the MMPI and the nature of the development of the computerized program. "Blind" use of these services by professionals not trained in the use of the MMPI is clearly inappropriate and, perhaps, even unethical.

The fact that the MMPI is the most widely used and researched psychological personality measurement device is undoubtedly one of its major strengths. Several hundred research papers on the MMPI appear in the literature each year, and it has been utilized extensively in cross-cultural clinical and research applications. The huge body of literature generated has resulted in a catalog of MMPI correlates on a wide variety of clinical cases, providing descriptive, predictive, diagnostic, and prognostic information. Another strength of the MMPI is its atheoretical nature, a characteristic that probably increases its usefulness over a broad spectrum. The presence of validity scales designed to assess test-taking attitude, in addition to clinical and personality information, is a distinct advantage that the MMPI maintains over many personality assessment tools.

Critics of the MMPI point to the outdated normative data on which interpretive statements are still being made. The MMPI is certainly in need of revision with current normative data, and this process is

TABLE 9.4-2
MMPI Validity and Clinical Scales

Validity

L: Lie Scale A nonempirically derived "social desirability" scale. Items tend to reflect behaviors that are considered socially desirable, but rarely practiced. The score can suggest defensiveness, illiteracy, psychosis, or personality processes, depending on various factors.

F: Infrequency Scale Measures a tendency to endorse selected items that are statistically rare responses (less than 10 percent of the original normal sample). Useful in identifying illiteracy, malingering, panic, confusion, psychosis, and personality processes.

K: Suppressor Scale It is used to adjust mathematically certain clinical scales in order to decrease false positives and negatives. The scale is also useful in determining overall test-taking attitude and is an indication of personality variables.

Clinical

1: Hypochondriasis This scale reflects somatic concerns and preoccupation with bodily functioning. Interpretation needs to take into account factors such as age and actual health status. As with all MMPI scales, interpretation is furthered by looking at its relationship with other scales.

2: Depression Scores on this scale tend to be reflective of depression as a mood disorder, or "neurotic" depression. The fact that the scale is quite sensitive to situational variables suggests that it may be a good index of state personality status.

3: Hysteria Items on this scale involve the identification of classical histrionic symptoms including the presence of physical symptoms coupled with indifference, denial, repression, and inhibition. The scale does not necessarily measure other more popularly conceived traits, such as lability and melodramatic attitude.

4: Psychopathic Deviance This scale was developed to assess the amorality and asociality aspects of psychopathy rather than the criminal or antisocial. Its meaning is very dependent on other scale configurations. The scale provides good information on the quality of interpersonal relationships.

5: Masculinity-Femininity Although it was originally developed to identify homosexuality, the scale is rarely used for this purpose, although it does provide information on gender identity. The scale reflects a variety of personality and interest areas, such as dependency, sensitivity, intellectuality, and tendencies toward introspection.

6: Paranoia Developed by the empirical identification of "classic" paranoids, the scale thus assesses vigilance, sensitivity, delusional thought, distrust, and suspicion. Except for the paranoid areas, the members of the original criterion group were considered functional in other areas of their lives.

7: Psychasthenia A very diverse scale designed to measure anxiety and obsessive-compulsive traits. Endorsed items can reflect fear, obsessive-compulsive symptomatology, interpersonal hostility, tension, specific phobias, and impaired concentration.

8: Schizophrenia Reflects the more acute "positive" symptoms of psychotic breaks with reality rather than the more chronic "negative" symptoms. The scale also assesses alienation, impaired self-identity, and isolation.

9: Hypomania Measures the rather "classic" symptomatology of mania, including elated and unstable mood, psychomotor excitement, and flight of ideas. It also appears to reflect narcissistic personality traits. In general, the scale will provide information on the degree of drivenness of the person's personality characteristics. It has a strong age component.

0: Social Introversion Provides information on social withdrawal, shyness, leadership, talkativeness, levels of gregariousness, and, to a lesser degree, self-concept and neurotic tendencies. It is, perhaps, more two-dimensional and bipolar (introversion versus extroversion) than the other scales.

Special

A: Anxiety The first general factor extracted from factor analytic studies on the MMPI. It is thought to reflect generalized endorsement of psychopathology.

R: Repression The second factor that is found on factor analytic studies of the MMPI. It can be conceptualized as measuring the tendency to engage in denial.

ES: Ego Strength Provides an index of how functional the patient may be in terms of work and other social areas, regardless of level of psychopathology.

MAC: McAndrews Alcholism Scale Estimates degree of addiction proneness, especially with alcohol and opiates. Especially sensitive to daily substance abuse rather than episodic abuse.

Table produced with the assistance of Alex Caldwell, Ph.D.

TABLE 9.4-3
MMPI Results of a Male Patient with an Antisocial Personality Disorder

	Validity Scales	*T*-Score (Mean = 50, Standard Deviation = 10)
	L	40
	F	66
	K	68
	Clinical Scales	***T*-Score (*K*-corrected as appropriate)**
1	(Hypochondriasis)	44
2	(Depression)	51
3	(Hysteria)	62
4	(Psychopathic Deviance)	87
5	(Masculinity-Femininity)	43
6	(Paranoia)	53
7	(Psychasthenia)	48
8	(Schizophrenia)	63
9	(Hypomania)	78
0	(Social Introversion)	40
A	(Anxiety)	40
R	(Repression)	63
ES	(Ego Strength)	65
MAC	(Alcoholism)	82

reportedly under way. Nevertheless, continued research with the present inventory helps to maintain its timeliness. The MMPI is rather long, and it is not uncommon for patients to complain about the length of the test and some of the personal questions. Several abbreviated versions of the MMPI have been developed to decrease administration time. These versions are generally considered unsatisfactory because of the resultant compromises in reliability and validity. In general, careful and sensitive administration techniques will offset patient compliance problems.

Millon Clinical Multiaxial Inventory (MCMI) The MCMI is a 175-item, true-false, paper-and-pencil personality inventory developed by Theodore Millon and co-workers in the late 1970s. The test allows for scoring and interpretation on 11 scales, which represent personality disorders from the third edition of the American Psychiatric Association's *Diagnostic and Statistical Manual of Mental Disorders* (DSM-III). The test also contains a brief validity scale and nine scales designed to assess reactive symptom disorders, which the test authors claim are of a less enduring nature than the personality scales. The scales are described in detail in Table 9.4-4.

Unlike the MMPI, which was empirically derived and is relatively atheoretical, the MCMI is based on Millon's theory of personality and psychopathology. Test items were developed by Millon's co-workers for the purpose of ensuring that the MCMI measured theory-derived variables. The inventory was also constructed so as to assist in arriving at DSM-III diagnoses. Since the MCMI represents a relatively new method for assessing personality traits, there is currently very little published research available beyond the initial validation studies. The inventory embodies a number of potential advantages, such as its brevity, theoretical underpinnings, and concordance with

TABLE 9.4-4
MCMI Clinical Scales

Personality Disorders (Axis II)

Scale 1: Schizoid Assesses the probability (as do the other scales of the MCMI) that an individual meets DSM-III diagnostic criteria for schizoid personality disorders. Symptoms include indifference, insensitivity, affect deficit, and apathy.

Scale 2: Avoidant Includes the measurement of characteristics of dysphoria, alienation, aversion to interpersonal behavior, and hypersensitivity.

Scale 3: Dependent Assesses trait characteristics of docility, submissiveness, initiation difficulties, poor self-image, and naivete.

Scale 4: Histrionic Assesses lability of affect, sociability, seductiveness, immaturity, inability to delay immediate need gratification, and a dissociative cognitive style.

Scale 5: Narcissistic Measures the presence of inflated self-image, exploitiveness, expansive thinking, imperturbability, and deficits in social conscience.

Scale 6: Antisocial (Aggressive) High scores suggest hostile affect, vindictiveness, power-oriented life style, malevolence, poor impulse control, and an inability to benefit from punishment.

Scale 7: Compulsive Key trait characteristics of a high score include restrained affect, conscientiousness, adherence to social conventions, conforming, cognitive constriction, and behavioral rigidity.

Scale 8: Passive-Aggressive Prominent personality traits include labile affect, contrariness, disillusionment, interpersonal ambivalence, and a discontented self-image.

Scale S: Schizotypal Assesses for the presence of social detachment, eccentricity, nondelusional autistic thinking, depersonalization, emptiness, emotional flatness, and anxious wariness.

Scale C: Borderline The salient characteristics of those scoring high on this scale are intense moodiness, dysregulated activation, self-destructive behavior, dependency anxiety, and ambivalence between thought-affect and action.

Scale P: Paranoid This scale measures the enduring traits of vigilant mistrust, distorted thought, criticalness, and provocative interpersonal behavior.

Clinical Syndromes (Axis I)

Scale A: Anxiety A high score suggests apprehension, phobias, tension, indecision, and psychophysiological symptoms.

Scale H: Somatoform Assesses the degree to which psychological conflict is likely to be channeled physically, and overall preoccupation with health.

Scale N: Hypomanic Measures the presence of unstable mood, restlessness, overactivity, pressured speech, impulsiveness, irritability, and other manic-type behavior.

Scale D: Dysthymia An elevation on this scale is likely to suggest despondency, guilt, discouragement, futility, and other symptoms of depression. The scale does not necessarily reflect extreme severity and, instead, implies preserved ego strength.

Scale B: Alcohol Abuse This scale provides a probability index for the presence or history of alcoholism.

Scale T: Drug Abuse This scale extends Scale B to include substance abuse, in general, and also implies poor impulse control and unconventionality.

Scale SS: Psychotic Thinking A high score on this scale suggests disorganized-regressed behavior, hallucinatory experiences, delusions, and inappropriate affect.

Scale CC: Psychotic Depression A high score suggests the presence of severe depression that is usually of incapacitating proportions.

Scale PP: Psychotic Delusions Elevations indicate that the individual is suffering from delusions, usually persecutory or grandiose in nature. Accompanying belligerency is common.

Table produced with the assistance and permission of Theodore Millon, Ph.D.

DSM-III terminology. Unfortunately, some of its potential advantages may turn out to be disadvantages. The test is likely to be useful only if Millon's theories continue to receive support. Additionally, an important consideration involves the current revision of DSM-III (DSM-III-R) as well as the likelihood of further revisions of psychiatric nomenclature. Although minimal changes in personality diagnosis are reflected in DSM-III-R, two new personality disorders were presented for research purposes, and they are not currently assessed by the MCMI. The MCMI will require continual updating and revision so as to not become outdated. For a standardized personality test, this is an expensive and time-consuming process. In any event, the method's primary usefulness at this time seems to involve the identification and description of personality disorders and related symptom constellations. The MCMI is undergoing constant revision, with attention directed to increased usefulness at clinical levels. The authors and publishers of the MCMI regularly sponsor seminars and symposia on the inventory and should be credited for attempts at stimulating research effort. Until recently, only computerized interpretative reports were available. Now, however, hand scoring keys are available for individual use. Certainly, this is an instrument that deserves close scrutiny, inasmuch as its future as a personality measurement device appears bright. For now, interpretation needs to be tempered by its recent development and therefore lack of extensive supportive research. A sample MCMI profile is reproduced in Table 9.4-5.

Other methods Of all the techniques used in the psychological assessment of personality, objective questionnaires are probably the most prolific. What follows is a brief description of some of the more popular self-report measures of personality. It should be reiterated that the body of research supporting the validity of these questionnaires is considerably less than that found with the MMPI. However, it does not necessarily follow that the MMPI will be a more appropriate measure in all cases. Many objective personality inventories have a limited, but sound, foundation, on which reliable and valid estimates of personality processes can be formulated.

The *16 Personality Factor Questionaire* (16 PF) is a factor analytically developed inventory that rates personality on 16 dimensions, examples of which are Dominant, Impulsive, Warm, Insecure, and Self-Disciplined. These factors were derived from data analyses using numerous self-reports, ratings, and performance tests. In a sense, the developmental procedure for this test involved proposing a theory of personality (16 pervasive dimensions) that originated from factor analytic studies, as opposed to the more common procedure of conceptualizing a theory of personality and then developing a test to validate the theory. The 16 PF comes in numerous forms and has had a wide range of research conducted on its usefulness with different populations. On the surface, this thoroughness appears to be an advantage; in reality, however, the data generated are extremely extensive—hence, somewhat confusing—and a high degree of sophistication is required for accurate application and interpretation. The dimensions assessed by the 16 PF are thought to represent basic psychological processes and not necessarily elements of psychopathology. For this reason, it is most commonly used in describing personality attributes of normal individuals in nonclinical settings, such as counseling centers, and for research projects with students. Outside of those individuals who have an active interest in the theory behind it, the 16 PF inventory does not have a high degree of support or widespread usage.

The *California Personality Inventory* (CPI) is an MMPI-type personality inventory designed for use in counseling situations as opposed to use with clinical, more pathological, populations. The test was developed by empirical means, much the same way as the MMPI, and rates personality on 16 principal dimensions such as Sociability, Tolerance, and Intellectual Efficiency. The CPI has generated a strong body of research and is quite widely used in counseling settings, such as university clinics. Its usefulness also may extend to less severe psychopathology, such as patients with adjustment disorders or life crises.

The *Jackson Personality Inventory* (JPI) is an example of psychometric sophistication in objective personality inventory construction. The test was developed to minimize overlap among the 15 dimensions of personality that it measures (Anxiety, Conformity, Risk Taking, Social Avoidness, etc.). Test construction also minimizes possible contamination from social desirability and other response sets. Although the JPI embodies features that reflect some of the more recent advances in objective test development, its clinical usefulness remains to be seen. Because test construction and normative data are based on college students, the JPI's applicability outside this population can be seriously questioned.

TABLE 9.4-5
Sample MCMI Profile of a Patient with a Narcissistic Personality Disorder

MCMI

MILLON CLINICAL MULTIAXIAL INVENTORY
By Theodore Millon

MCMI Hand-Scoring Profile

NAME ____________

AGE ______ RACE ________ DATE TESTED ___/___/___

REASON FOR REFERRAL ____________

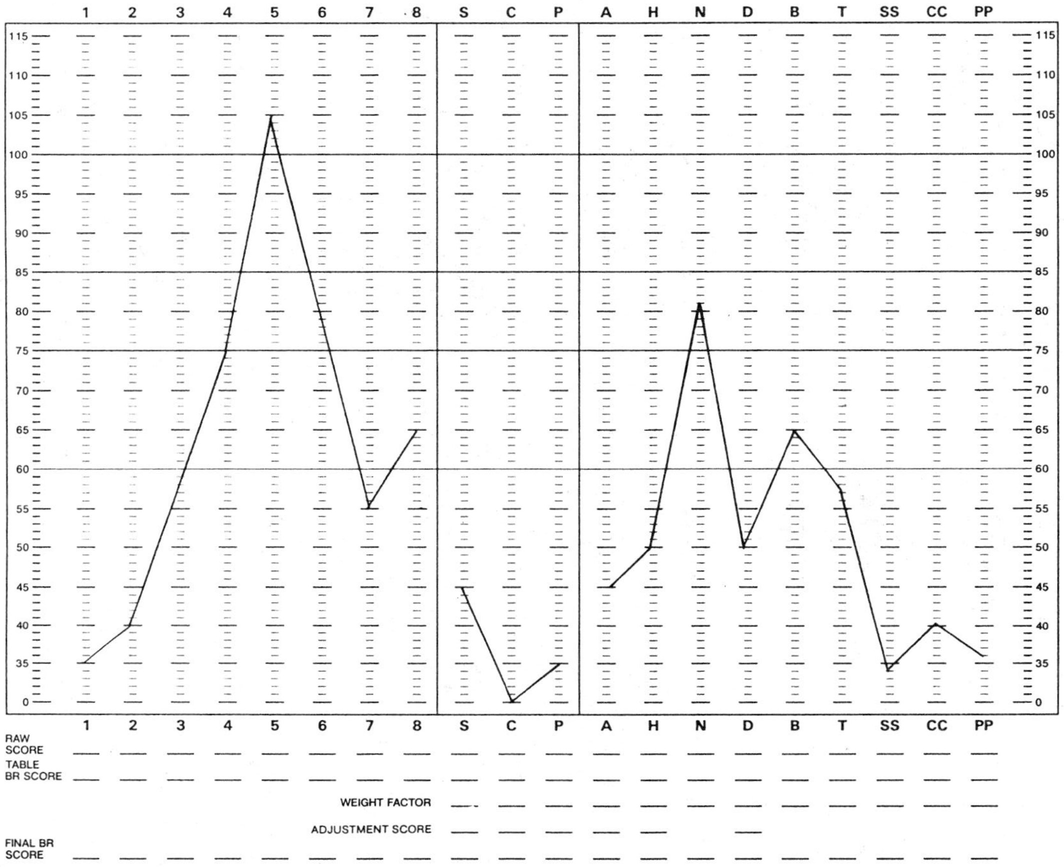

SUM 1-8 ________

TOTAL RAW SCORE SCALES 1-8	WEIGHT FACTOR
< 94	Invalid
94	+16
95	+15
96	+14
97	13
98	12
99	11
100	10
101	9
102	8
103	7
104	6
105	5
106	4
107	+3
108	+2
109	+1
110-131	0
132	-1
133	-1
134	-1
135	-2
136	-2
137	-2
138	-3
139	-3
140	-3
141	-4
142	-4
143	-4
144	-5
145	-5
146	-5
147	-6
148	-6
149	-6
150	-7
151	-7
152	-7
153	-8
154	-8
155	-8
156	-9
157	-9
158	-9
159	-10
160	-10
161	-10
162	-11
163	-11
164	-11
165	-12
> 165	Invalid

45117

Current status Objective personality assessment is particularly useful if one is interested in the nomothetic basis of personality attributes, that is, "How does my patient compare to others on these dimensions?" The psychometric characteristics of these measures make them well suited for empirical research; hence, in contrast to projective tests, they are more suited to answer such questions as "Which form of medication or psychotherapy is most likely to benefit this patient?" or "What is the most appropriate diagnosis for this patient?" The most widely used objective measure of personality, the MMPI, has long been in need of revision, especially in regard to normative data. Revising a test this widely utilized is truly a herculean task and runs the risk of invalidating the diverse interpretative literature that has been accumulated. It should be mentioned that a broad-scale revision of the MMPI recently has been undertaken; however, the results of these efforts are unlikely to become available for another few years. Objective assessment has been criticized by some for its reliance on normative samples. The key issue seems to be in determining an appropriate normative group. A frequently voiced recommendation is for test users to collect normative data representative of their local population. Although this suggestion offers a partial solution to the problem, it is usually logistically and practically unfeasible. Some of the more popular objective techniques are summarized in Table 9.4-6.

PROJECTIVE PERSONALITY ASSESSMENT The projective approach to personality assessment is defined by the use of unstructured, often ambiguous, test stimuli. A basic assumption is that when confronted with a vague stimulus and required to respond to it in some manner, individuals cannot help but reveal information about themselves—not only in the

TABLE 9.4-6
Objective Measures of Personality

Name	*Description*	*Strengths*	*Weaknesses*
Minnesota Multiphasic Personality Inventory (MMPI)	566 items, true-false; self-report format; 17 scales (numerous special scales)	Provides wide range of data on numerous personality variables; strong research base	Tends to emphasize major psychopathology. In need of revision with current normative data
Millon Clinical Multiaxial Inventory (MCMI)	175 items, true-false; self-report format; 20 scales	Brief administration time; corresponds well with DSM-III-R diagnostic classifications	In need of more validation research. No information on disorder severity
16 Personality Factor Questionnaire (16 PF)	True-false; self-report format; 16 personality dimensions	Sophisticated psychometric instrument with considerable research conducted on nonclinical population	Limited usefulness with clinical populations
California Personality Inventory (CPI)	True-false; self-report format; 17 scales	Well-accepted method of assessing patients who do not present with major psychopathology	Limited usefulness with clinical populations
Jackson Personality Inventory (JPI)	True-false; self-report format; 15 personality scales	Constructed in accord with sophisticated psychometric techniques; controls for response sets	Unproven usefulness in clinical settings
Edwards Personal Preference Schedule (EPPS)	Forced choice; self-report format	Follows Murray's theory of personology; accounts for social desirability	Not widely used clinically because of restricted nature of information obtained
Beck Depression Inventory (BDI)	Self-report on Likert-type format; measures depression	Follows Beck's theory of depression quite well; widely used	Assesses mood and thought well but inadequate on neurovegetative symptoms
State-Trait Anxiety Inventory (STAI)	Self-report on Likert-type format; measures anxiety	Allows for differentiation of state and trait anxiety; well researched	STAI items are quite transparent
Psychological Screening Inventory (PSI)	130 items, true-false; self-report format	Produces 4 scores, which can be used as screening measures on the possibility of a need for psychological help	The scales are short and have correspondingly low reliability
Eysenck Personality Questionnaire (EPQ)	True-false; self-report format	Useful as a screening device; test has a theoretical basis with research support	Scales are short and items are quite transparent as to purpose; not recommended for other than a screening device
Adjective Checklist (ACL)	True-false; self-report or informant report	Can be used for self or other rating	Scores rarely correlate highly with more conventional personality inventories
Comrey Personality Scales (CPS)	True-false; self-report format; 8 scales	Factor analytic techniques used with a high degree of sophistication in test construction	Not widely used; factor analytic interpretation problems
Tennessee Self-Concept Scale (TSCS)	100 items, true-false; self-report format; 14 scales	Brief administration time yields considerable information	Brevity is also a disadvantage, lowering reliability and validity; useful as a screening device only

way in which, or process by which, the ambiguity is confronted, but also in the content of their response.

Test stimuli for projective assessment devices, but not necessarily scoring and interpretation, are typically standardized. The Rorschach inkblot technique, for example, probably the most widely used projective method, currently has six different systems by which the test can be scored and interpreted. Although the different approaches overlap to some degree, there are considerable differences ranging from a strong psychoanalytic orientation to a more empirical, perceptual-cognitive approach. The net result of these different approaches is that one can never be sure what type of interpretation is being used when one requests an evaluation that includes projective tests. This problem is further manifested because many scoring and interpretative approaches to projective personality assessment have weak empirical research foundations.

The projective approach is essentially idiographic in nature, and most commonly the tests are not interpreted by comparing a person's responses to a set of criterion-referenced normative data. More typically, interpretation is based on a theory of human behavior and personality, and it is assumed that individuals bring with themselves certain needs, characteristics, defenses, and other qualities that will become apparent through the testing process.

Projective assessment also tends toward a dynamic bias, and a frequent assumption is that patients will project information about their need status onto the stimuli and that these projections will be symbolic of internal dynamics. Most commonly, these dynamics are interpreted on the basis of analytic or interpersonal-environment theories. This emphasis on personality theory and dynamics tends to focus projective assessment more onto the trait aspects of human behavior; however, state variables can be elucidated.

With some exceptions, the classic projective approach to personality assessment has tended to eschew firm adherence to measurement psychometrics. The unstructured nature of the test stimuli has been postulated to render empirical reliability and validity research more difficult. Fortunately, this situation has changed somewhat over time in view of the current emphasis on scientific methods in personality assessment. Nevertheless, the idiographic nature of projective methods tends to make them less psychometrically sophisticated than the objective measures of personality.

A number of semistructured situations and projective-type stimuli have been developed, including perceiving inkblots, drawing pictures, and telling stories on the basis of presented pictures. Brief descriptions of some of the more popular projective techniques follow.

Rorschach test The Rorschach technique of projective assessment consists of 10 plates with inkblots printed on them, one of which is shown in Figure 9.4-1. It was introduced by Hermann Rorschach in 1921 and had been extensively studied by a number of psychologists by the 1950s. Interest in the technique has waxed and waned over the years, never reaching the zenith it achieved during this initial period of development.

There are essentially six major schools of administration, scoring, and interpretation of the Rorschach technique. Despite differences among the various approaches, there are commonalities. Typically, administration is characterized by a brief orientation to the task, which is purposely nondirective. The plates are presented to the patient one at a time, and the individual's percepts are recorded verbatim. Interaction with the assessor is kept to a minimum. On completion of this phase, the cards are then re-examined, one at a time, with more directive questioning by the examiner in order to allow for accurate coding of the responses. Table 9.4-7 contains examples of responses to Rorschach stimuli.

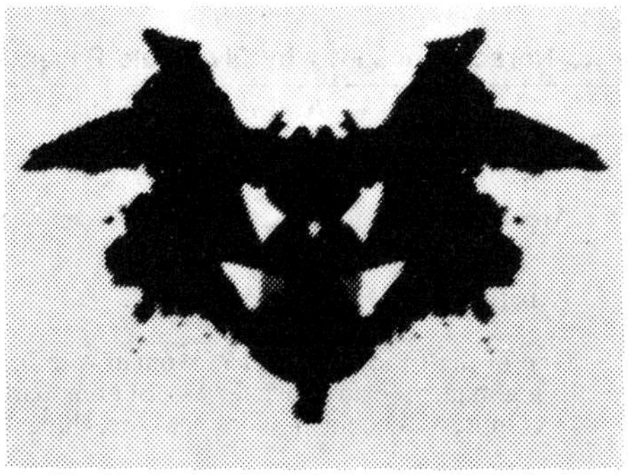

FIGURE 9.4-1. *Plate I of the Rorschach Test. (From Hans Huber Medical Publisher, Berne, with permission.)*

Although scoring systems vary, the patient's responses are typically coded under three general categories: location, determinants, and content. Location refers to what portion of the blot was utilized. Determinants are those aspects of the blot that are salient to the patient's percepts. These determinants include the use of form, color, and shading. Aspects of the percept that are not necessarily present in the actual blot, such as perceived movement or three-dimensionality, are also coded. Finally, content refers to the specific character of the percept, such as human, animal, or nature.

As is true of coding a Rorschach protocol, interpretation is a complex and time-consuming process. Rorschach method proponents maintain that the technique provides information on the patient's level of functioning, maturity, reality testing, interpersonal relationship style, ability to organize the environment and marshal resources, balance of activity and passivity, and emotional responsiveness. The Rorschach technique is also frequently used in the assessment of psychosis, suicidality, depression, anxiety, and other clinical syndromes and disorders. Table 9.4-8 provides an example of interpretative hypotheses based on Rorschach responses, and Table 9.4-9 illustrates diagnostic considerations.

The Rorschach method has generated a wide body of research literature; however, the complexity of the technique has hindered the development of a comprehensive, cohesive data base. This problem has been addressed in recent years through increased efforts toward uniformity in scoring and interpretation, and scientific validation. In general, however, research evidence supporting the validity of the Rorschach is mixed; and, although the test remains widely used, its psychometric properties are less sophisticated than nonprojective personality assessment approaches.

The fact that most individuals enjoy having the Rorschach administered to them can be seen as a strength of the method. The ambiguity of the stimuli and the unstructured means of administration can provide invaluable information on how a patient copes with these types of situations. Additionally, interpretative validity may be improved by more frequent use of the technique and increased clinical experience.

Thematic Apperception Test (TAT) The TAT, developed by Henry Murray, consists of 20 cards with pictures on them. The pictures vary in content, most containing one or more characters, with different degrees of ambiguity. The patient is requested to construct a story that has a beginning, middle, and ending on the basis of the stimulus card. Rarely are all 20 cards administered; typically, a number are selected in order to "pull" for certain material. The basic assumption is that the person will project his or her personality into the story. Information is obtained regarding the patient's beliefs, needs, traits, attitudes, and motives—in general, a broad spectrum of behavior and cognition.

Administration of the TAT is quite straightforward and, as with the Rorschach method, most patients find the task relatively nonthreatening and even enjoyable. Scoring of the TAT is by no means standardized, and numerous methods exist. Most scoring systems involve rating "need" states or levels, following from Murray's theory of personality. Murray believed that personality is effectively described by analyzing an individual's most powerful needs, such as achievement, affiliation, dominance, and play in relation to environmental "press"—that is, attributes of environmental stimuli that either facilitate or impede the efforts of a person to reach a specified goal.

Although scoring systems exist, the most typical process of interpretation is quite impressionistic and informal. In general, the

TABLE 9.4-7
Response to Rorschach Card I by Five Male Patients*

	Free Association	*Inquiry*
Patient A:	A bug with two witches attached to it.	This whole thing in the middle, just the way it looks. [Points] Just the wings here. Looks like a witch.
	Also a halloween mask. About all I can see.	That—the whole thing. The eyes, the mouth [White space] [?] Nothing else about it.
Patient B:	A bat, a bug.	Bat. [Whole] The blackness and the wings. Bug—that was just a pure reference to the color. I just see it as unpleasant.
	One of the furies. A headless woman with black wings, grasping hands, claws, whatever. Bottom part of her torso is compressed, held in, like she's reaching forward.	Furies. [Whole] The central portion could represent legs pressed together. She represents a figure of death launching forward, and the head gets lost. Sort of snake-like, and the outer parts are reaching forth at the shadow of the earth.
Patient C:	It looks like a monster bat. It has pincers. And an ass over here.	The whole thing. It has wings. It's kind of ragged, that's all. [Top center] Arches. Just shaped that way. Feel uptight, knowing I'm taking a test [?] Shape, two mounds.
	And a butterfly.	Whole object. The wings, the shape. I just feel I want to get out of here.
Patient D:	Two dancers and two children in between them like they're dancing around them.	[Whole] Head, cape, clothing, legs. Matching heads. A pair of children or a pair of dancers since it's symmetrical, one on one side and one on the other.
Patient E:	Looks like a bat? That's all I can make of it.	Whole blot. The middle makes it look like a body. And it looks like he has a tail and two short feet.

*This table gives the Rorschach responses, both free associations and inquiries, given to Card I by five male patients. These extracted test responses are reported primarily to illustrate the range given by different patients to the same stimulus. As such, these responses may not themselves always delineate the varying DSM-III-R diagnoses represented.

Patient A: 26 years old, multiple psychiatric hospitalizations within past 4 years. Unable to care for himself, believing himself controlled by a force that makes him act inappropriately. Suffers from chronic delusions, obsessional thinking, and social withdrawal. Schizophrenia.

Patient B: 23 years old, long history of social isolation, repetitive self-destructive behavior, depression, and inability to function academically. Has shown depersonalization and derealization phenomena but no admitted delusions or hallucinations. Schizotypal personality disorder.

Patient C: 28 years old, complaints of chronic and overwhelming anxiety, feelings of loneliness, and ambivalence about homosexual identification. History of excessive use of psychotropic medication. Borderline personality disorder.

Patient D: 20 years old, presently hospitalized for manic episode, with history of two clear-cut manic and depressive episodes, followed by remissions. Bipolar mood disorder.

Patient E: 33 years old, hospitalized on neurology service for organic mental disorder assumed to be related to occupational hazard: mercury poisoning. Prior history of behavior difficulties.

Table from Carr A C: Psychological testing of personality. In *Comprehensive Textbook of Psychiatry,* ed 4, H I Kaplan, B J Sadock, editors, vol 1, p 523. Williams & Wilkins, Baltimore, 1985.

TABLE 9.4-8
Psychologist's Interpretation of Patient's Responses to Rorschach Card I

1. It looks sort of like a cat's face. (Inquiry: The way the ears came up like this. The way the jaws puffed out. Looks like he's smiling. It's a real sinister smile. It looks sort of like a Chelsea grin. The eyes look devilish. He's sticking his tongue out and he's cross-eyed.) 2. First I thought it was two people here in the middle with their hands up, but I had no idea what these things on the side were. They're standing side by side like they're Siamese twins. You know what it looks like these two people are doing? They are trying to keep these walls open by pressing against it. (Inquiry: The whole blot. There are two heads and two hands. Or it could be one person with no head doing the same thing. The way they have their arms up they're facing out against the wall trying to keep them open. It's as if the walls were closing in on them trying to smash them.)	To be noted is that the patient does not give the usual, conventional response ("bat" or "butterfly") to what typifies a new situation. Closest to a common response is the center detail initially perceived as Siamese twins, rather than as a person (more usual). Strong affective attributes are projected onto a blot that is generally perceived as innocuous, suggesting that she experiences such reactions herself or that she perceives these qualities as coming from others. While the form accuracy of these responses is satisfactory (implying that the capacity to test reality is maintained), difficulties with her relationship with reality and feelings of reality are suggested ("walls were closing in on them"). Identity and symbiotic issues are highlighted by her reference to Siamese twins. Because the center area is assumed sometimes to elicit association to the mother-figure, it may be offered as a highly speculative inference that a Chelsea [Cheshire?] grin (a grin for which the face and body disappeared) may reflect the role of the mother's disappearance during the patient's difficulties. (In reality, the mother had died when the patient was 5 years old. The patient—now 20—makes a great deal of this loss, viewing it as related in some unknown way to her own suicide attempts and other difficulties. On one occasion during the onset of her decompensation, she was certain she saw her mother at a distance in a department store.) The history of interpersonal difficulties is marked, with distrust and jealousy of women and vulnerability to disillusionment and oversensitivity to rejection by men. By DSM-III-R criteria, the patient had been diagnosed as borderline personality disorder.

Table from Carr A C: Psychological testing of personality. In *Comprehensive Textbook of Psychiatry,* ed 4, H I Kaplan, B J Sadock, editors, vol 1, p 524. Williams & Wilkins, Baltimore, 1985.

TABLE 9.4-9
Schizotypal Versus Affective Rorschach Content

Schizotypal	*Affective*
Bizarre and idiosyncratic themes (boundaries blurred, fused body parts, crude primary process thinking: "An explosion with blood all over," "a worm coming out of a rabbit's eye," "a butterfly merged with a rabbit").	Themes of barrenness, depression, death ("desert," "setting sun," "dead animal"), or of elation, gaiety, excitement ("circus," "dance," "party").
Quasihuman percepts often unconventional, distorted, unreal, unworldly ("weird animal," "man from another planet").	Quasihuman percepts more conventional, often playful ("fairy," "Santa Claus," "puppets").
Themes of transformation and paranoid suspicion or concealment ("caterpillar changing into a moth," "eyes looking out," "mask").	Themes of oral supply and deprivation ("food," "mouth," "kissing"). Polarities reign (up-down, flying-falling, young-old).
Sexual content often reflects perverse sexuality; confused sexual identification ("she also has a penis, as well as breasts").	Sexual content often ultrafeminine or ultramasculine, hypersexual ("erection," "she looks pregnant").
Logic disturbed by formal thought disorder—associations are private ("I can't tell if it's a man or two women").	Logic disturbed by flight of ideas—associations are public ("two women with a butterfly between them—call them Madame Butterfly").

Table from Carr A C: Psychological testing of personality. In *Comprehensive Textbook of Psychiatry,* ed 4, H I Kaplan, B J Sadock, editors, vol 1, p 524. Williams & Wilkins, Baltimore, 1985.

TABLE 9.4-10
Sentence Completion Test Stimuli

I often wish ______________________________

____

When I was young ______________________________

____

It makes me angry when ______________________________

____

My mother ______________________________

____

Most people ______________________________

____

stories are examined with particular attention directed toward recurrent themes that might provide evidence of mood, conflict, interpersonal relations, and so forth.

The TAT was initially developed as an assessment device designed to measure trait behavior. Research, however, has tended to indicate the opposite. The TAT appears to be more sensitive to state-dependent variables. TAT usage has tended to decline over the years, most probably because of the relatively lengthy time required for administration and interpretation. Nevertheless, there are a significant number of clinicians who adhere to thematic test analysis. For these individuals, the TAT seems to be the method of choice.

Sentence completion test The sentence completion method is perhaps the least vague and most structured projective personality assessment technique. Patients are presented with the first few words or stem of a sentence and requested to complete it as they feel it best describes themselves. It is essentially an open-ended self-report inventory, and most items have a fairly obvious "pull" in terms of the type of information that is being sought. For this reason, patients who choose to be less than open may produce rather uninformative protocols, above and beyond the fact that they are resistant to the task. In a similar fashion, sentence completion tasks are quite susceptible to malingering and response sets. With one exception, *Rotter's Incomplete Sentence Blank,* scoring for the various tests is poorly standardized, and interpretation is solely on the basis of clinical intuition. With a cooperative patient, however, considerable information can be gleaned on both state and trait personality variables.

In addition to information on personality variables, a patient's sentence completion protocol often provides valuable additional information because, most typically, patients write out their responses. A brief review of the protocol can assist in formulating hypotheses regarding written language development, presence or absence of academic difficulties, and evidence of possible early learning disabilities. As is the case with most projective measures, the relatively ambiguous stimuli are also particularly well suited toward eliciting symptoms of a psychotic thought process. Examples of sentence completion test stimuli are presented in Table 9.4-10.

Other methods Similar in technique to the Rorschach method is the *Holtzman Inkblot Technique* (HIT), developed in order to rectify some of the psychometric difficulties found with the former. The HIT consists of 45 inkblot plates (there are two sets for alternate-form assessment, if desired) and the subject provides only one response per card. Though certainly an interesting concept, the HIT is not widely used, and research documenting its validity with clinical populations has been surprisingly limited. Additionally, Rorschach and HIT scoring and interpretation methods do not appear to be directly comparable, a shortcoming that has probably hindered research progress.

Figure drawings have long been used as projective personality assessment devices. A basic assumption is that in drawing figures, such as a person or a house, the patient will introject interpersonal, psychic, and familial conflicts onto the drawing. Perhaps the most widely used figure drawing technique is the *Draw-a-Person* procedure. Patients are presented with a blank sheet of paper and instructed to draw a picture of a person. The projective hypothesis implies that patients will symbolically introject their own personality characteristics onto the drawing. Scoring procedures are available for estimating intelligence; however, they are generally used only with mentally retarded persons or children. Manuals are also available that present guidelines for dynamic and analytically oriented interpretations of personality style and functioning. This technique has some degree of intuitive attractiveness, and on a case study basis one can find some remarkably valid profile interpretations. On the whole, however, the technique enjoys very little research to support most interpretative claims.

A variant of figure drawing that has also been used as a projective method is figure copying, most commonly done with *Bender-Gestalt* cards as stimuli. Some researchers have developed rather elaborate rules and interpretative strategies for inferring the personality characteristics of a patient on the basis of their Bender-Gestalt reproductions. This technique never developed a broad support base, and currently its practice is quite limited. A lack of empirical support for many interpretative claims is certainly a contributory factor in the infrequent use of figure reproduction as a projective assessment technique.

Current status Psychological measurement of personality via projective techniques has a long and rich history. Until recently, much of the interpretive schemata that have been developed have relied on clinical lore rather than sound empirical investigation. This situation is changing, especially in reference to work on the Rorschach technique. However, researchers and clinicians who advocate a more scientific approach to personality assessment have tended to eschew projective techniques in favor of behavioral and objective methods, which are more quantifiable, face and content valid, and conducive to sound psychometric principles. Although this trend may have created a decrease in projective usage in many circles, the techniques are by no means obsolete. Projective assessment is firmly adhered to by many practitioners, and this situation is unlikely to change in the near future. A summary of the more widely used projective techniques is presented in Table 9.4-11.

BEHAVIORAL ASSESSMENT OF PERSONALITY

Behavioral assessment of personality is a relatively recent outgrowth of a neobehavioral movement in clinical psychology. This movement has emphasized the use of scientific methodology in addressing clinical problems. Growing dissatisfaction with traditional personality assessment methodologies is also characteristic of the neobehavioral movement. Traditional testing of personality involves the measurement of theoretical constructs, which are then utilized in the prediction of overt behavior. In objective personality assessment, for example, such constructs as anxiety, sociability, and narcissism are frequently measured. The projective approach to assessment also purports to quantify such concepts as ego strength and neurotic dysfunction. Behavioral assessment, however, favors direct measurement of criterion behaviors within specified situations. The behavioral assessment of ego strength would involve measuring behaviors, such as amount of time spent in productive work, rather than ego strength per se. Adherents to this approach point out that behavioral procedures are more parsimonious, consistent with empirical research evidence, and conducive to direct empirical testing. The basic rationale appears to rest on findings that indicate that the best predictor of future behavior in a given situation is past behavior in the same type of situation. Behavioral assessment techniques are varied and include methods, such as direct observation, self-monitoring, psychophysiological measurement, interviews and questionnaires, and critical-event sampling.

The behavioral assessment of personality tends to be a highly structured process in which the assessor informs the patient of the purpose of the testing, what information is requested, and how it will be sought. Ambiguity is avoided unless the criterion behaviors to be measured involve the manner in which the patient copes with an unstructured situation. For example, a behavioral approach to this type of assessment situation would be quite similar to comments on behavior that a Rorschach assessor might make regarding a patient's responses when confronted with the ambiguous Rorschach stimuli (e.g., Did the patient request much information regarding "rules," become very anxious, or refuse to cooperate?). The approach is also very idiographic in nature.

Frequently, behavioral assessment is highly goal directed. Rather than attempting to describe a patient in terms of dynamics, defense mechanisms, traits, or diagnosis, the assessor is more interested in problematic behaviors, on an individual level, that require treatment (e.g., reduction in frequency or strength). For example, if a patient presents with an anxiety disorder, the behavioral assessor is not necessarily concerned with dynamics, diagnosis, or degree of anxiety in comparison with the rest of a population. Behavioral assessment will focus on measurable target behaviors that represent the discomfort that the patient is experiencing, be it increased perspiration, escape-avoidance behaviors, self-report of subjective distress, or increases in heart rate and blood pressure. The assessor determines which stimuli appear to elicit these responses, places the patient in an actual or analogous situation, and measures the responses. In selecting target or criterion behaviors to measure, the assessor considers such issues as frequency, intensity, duration, centrality to the patient's functional life, subjective distress, values, and potential risk and destructiveness of the behaviors.

The behavioral assessment process is particularly geared toward effective empirical intervention, perhaps more so than any other method of personality assessment. This process appears to be a function of the emphasis on determining which stimuli or variables elicit the target behaviors and the close relationship between behavioral assessment and behavioral therapy. The identification of variables and stimuli that serve to elicit the target behaviors has been labeled the most important purpose of any psychological assessment, particularly when assessment is to have a direct impact on treat-

TABLE 9.4-11
Projective Measures of Personality

Name	*Description*	*Strengths*	*Weaknesses*
Rorschach Test	10 stimulus cards of inkblots; some colored, others achromatic	Most widely used projective device and certainly the best researched; considerable interpretative data available	In terms of validity, the Rorschach remains an enigmatic device; as often as it proves useful, it fails
Thematic Apperception Test (TAT)	20 stimulus cards depicting a number of scenes of varying ambiguity	A widely used method that, in the hands of a well-trained person, provides valuable information	No generally accepted scoring system results in poor consistency in interpretation; time-consuming administration
Sentence Completion Test	A number of different devices available, all sharing the same format with more similarities than differences	Brief administration time; can be a very useful adjunct to clinical interviews, if supplied beforehand	Stimuli are quite obvious as to intent and subject to easy falsification
Holtzman Inkblot Technique (HIT)	Two parallel forms of inkblot cards with 45 cards per form	Only one response is allowed per card, making research easier	Not widely accepted and rarely used; not directly comparable to Rorschach interpretative strategies
Figure Drawing	Typically human forms but can involve houses or other forms	Quick administration	Interpretative strategies have typically been unsupported by research
Make-a-Picture Story (MAPS)	Similar to TAT; however, stimuli can be manipulated by the patient	Provides idiographic personality information via thematic analysis	Minimal research support; not widely utilized

ment. Behavioral assessment is frequently serial in nature and is conducted periodically throughout a treatment program in order to objectively document its effectiveness. This type of assessment tends to be a reciprocal feedback process, wherein modifications of assessment or treatment, or both, depend on the results of measurement.

As should be apparent, behavioral assessment has a rather strict empirical orientation and emphasizes state-dependent behaviors. Although it is not entirely atheoretical in nature (the recognition of inferential concepts, such as cognition, has become the rule with behavioral therapists rather than the exception), the method does avoid measuring personality constructs that require an additional level of inference that may not necessarily increase treatment effectiveness from a behavioral viewpoint.

Before some of the more commonly employed behavioral assessment methods are described, it should be noted that the aforementioned comments will tend to portray the behavioral assessor and therapist as cold, unfeeling scientists who rarely interact with their patients on a level other than aloof observer. This misconception is a common one because of the historical aspects of the technique and the reliance on scientific methodology. Behaviorists typically bring the same degree of warmth, empathy, and concern into assessment and treatment settings as any other mental health professionals, regardless of orientation.

Interviews The interview is perhaps the most common and frequently utilized assessment technique. Almost any assessment of personality begins with a clinical interview of some sort. The behavioral approach to interviews involves structured and semistructured formats designed to maximize information regarding overt behavior, behavior-environment interactions, quantifiable information, and potential causative factors. Many clinicians, researchers, and diagnosticians have adopted these techniques, at times without realizing the background and orientation that form the foundation for structured and semistructured interviews.

The *Brief Psychiatric Rating Scale* (BPRS) is an 18-dimension rating scale that is filled out on a patient on the basis of a semistructured interview. Each dimension represents a domain of psychiatric symptomatology, such as Anxiety, Hostility, Affect, Guilt, and Orientation, and is rated on a seven-point Likert scale from "not present" to "extremely severe." Although several of the domains tend not to be directly observable behaviors, the manner in which they are assessed is sufficiently structured to qualify as a behavioral assessment. The BPRS is a brief, rather easily learned technique and provides a quantitative score that reflects global pathology. It has been found useful in providing a somewhat crude barometer of a patient's overall benefit from treatment and as a dependent variable in many research protocols, particularly medication outcome studies. On the negative side, the BPRS does not provide much information on specific behavior because so many divergent symptom complexes are summated. A copy of the BPRS is reproduced in Table 9.4-12.

The widely used *Hamilton Depression Rating Scale* is scored on the basis of a semistructured interview. The patient is rated on depression-related symptoms, including psychomotor retardation, insomnia, mood, and insight. Several forms with different numbers of symptom ratings exist, leading to some confusion at times as to what exactly has been assessed. The summated score obtained correlates

TABLE 9.4-12
Brief Psychiatric Rating Scale

DIRECTIONS: Place an X in the appropriate box to represent level of severity of each symptom.

PATIENT ______________________
RATER ______________________
NO. ______________________
DATE ______________________

	Not Present = 0	Very Mild = 1	Mild = 2	Moderate = 3	Mod. Severe = 4	Severe = 5	Extremely Severe = 6
	0	1	2	3	4	5	6
1. Somatic concern—preoccupation with physical health, fear of physical illness, hypochondriases.	☐	☐	☐	☐	☐	☐	☐
2. Anxiety—worry, fear, overconcern for present or future.	☐	☐	☐	☐	☐	☐	☐
3. Emotional withdrawal—lack of spontaneous interaction, isolation, deficiency in relating to others.	☐	☐	☐	☐	☐	☐	☐
4. Conceptual disorganization—thought processes confused, disconnected, disorganized, disrupted.	☐	☐	☐	☐	☐	☐	☐
5. Guilt feelings—self-blame, shame, remorse for past behavior.	☐	☐	☐	☐	☐	☐	☐
6. Tension—physical and motor manifestations or nervousness, overactivation, tension.	☐	☐	☐	☐	☐	☐	☐
7. Mannerisms and posturing—peculiar, bizarre unnatural motor behavior (not including tic).	☐	☐	☐	☐	☐	☐	☐
8. Grandiosity—exaggerated self-opinion, arrogance, conviction of unusual power or abilities.	☐	☐	☐	☐	☐	☐	☐
9. Depressive mood—sorrow, sadness, despondency, pessimism.	☐	☐	☐	☐	☐	☐	☐
10. Hostility—animosity, contempt, belligerence, disdain for others.	☐	☐	☐	☐	☐	☐	☐
11. Suspiciousness—mistrust, belief that others harbor malicious or discriminatory intent.	☐	☐	☐	☐	☐	☐	☐
12. Hallucinatory behavior—perceptions without normal external stimulus correspondence.	☐	☐	☐	☐	☐	☐	☐
13. Motor retardation—slowed weakened movements or speech, reduced body tone.	☐	☐	☐	☐	☐	☐	☐
14. Uncooperativeness—resistance, guardedness, rejection of authority.	☐	☐	☐	☐	☐	☐	☐
15. Unusual thought content—unusual, odd, strange, bizarre thought content.	☐	☐	☐	☐	☐	☐	☐
16. Blunted affect—reduced emotional tone, reduction in normal intensity of feelings, flatness.	☐	☐	☐	☐	☐	☐	☐
17. Excitement—heightened emotional tone, agitation, increased reactivity.	☐	☐	☐	☐	☐	☐	☐
18. Disorientation—confusion or lack of proper association for person, place, or time.	☐	☐	☐	☐	☐	☐	☐

Table reproduced with permission of John E. Overall, Ph.D.

highly with degree of depression severity. The rating scale is highly effective in monitoring depressed state over time and is useful as an index of treatment effectiveness. A weakness of the Hamilton scale is its overemphasis on biological and neurovegetative depressive symptoms. If used, it probably should be paired with an additional assessment device more focused on the mood, affective, and cognitive changes that are known to accompany major depression. (See Table 9.8-4 in Section 9.8, Psychiatric Rating Scales, for a copy of the Hamilton Depression Rating Scale.)

The *Schedule for Affective Disorders and Schizophrenia* (SADS) is a structured interview that has been well received by diagnosticians and researchers. Its primary purpose appears to be as a diagnostic tool, although scores on nondiagnostic symptom complexes can be obtained. An excerpt from the SADS is reprinted in Table 9.4-13. The SADS interview process is highly structured for both the assessor and assessee, and it has proved itself to be a valuable diagnostic adjunct for a wide variety of purposes. Its use significantly improves diagnostic reliabilities, and it also serves as a useful index of behavioral change. Although the full SADS interview is somewhat time-consuming, there is a subform, the SADS-C, which only measures current psychopathology. Use of the SADS-C after initial evaluation reduces time considerations significantly if repeat assessment is desirable. The SADS, as do many structured and semistructured interview techniques, tends to focus more on the presence of pathology and not necessarily on individual strengths that the patient may be showing. This emphasis does not mean that the SADS embodies an inherent weakness. Rather, for a balanced assessment, pathology as well as strength needs to be measured. An example of a method that balances patient attributes is the *Global Assessment Scale* (GAS), developed by the authors of the SADS scales. The GAS provides a quantified index of overall current health and illness that allows for evaluations reflecting positive attributes. It is typically scored after a semistructured interview. The global nature of the rating does not allow for the assessment of relatively discrete behaviors. (See Table 9.2-4 in Section 9.2, Psychiatric Report, for an updated version of the GAS, called the Global Assessment of Functioning Scale [GAF]).

Questionnaires The questionnaire is not the exclusive domain of behavioral assessment; in fact, it is quite well represented by objective personality assessment. However, when the goal of a questionnaire becomes oriented toward the measurement of overt, observable behaviors, then the questionnaire becomes an instrument of the behavioral assessor.

A large number of focused questionnaires have been developed for behavioral assessment purposes. These questionnaires address many diverse target behaviors, such as social skills deficits, anger, marital functioning, obsessive-compulsive behaviors, sexual functioning, ingestive disorders, fears and phobias, and menstrual dysfunction. With few exceptions, questionnaires developed for behavioral assessment lack psychometric sophistication. Despite these shortcomings, questionnaires are quickly administered and can be useful as long as one is aware of the particular instrument's psychometric limitations.

One widely used self-report questionnaire that meets the criteria of a behavioral assessment device is the *SCL-90-R*. The SCL-90-R is a 90-item checklist on which the respondent indicates degree of distress being experienced on a wide range of symptoms. The checklist can be scored so as to provide a unitary index of global pathology or to provide quantitative measures on nine factors, which include Somatization, Interpersonal Sensitivity, Hostility, Paranoid Ideation, and Psychotocism. The effectiveness of the SCL-90-R in documenting change accurately has been demonstrated in a number of clinical and research settings, and it is generally considered one of the better standardized behavioral assessment questionnaires.

Observation Observation is perhaps the assessment methodology that is most in keeping with the purpose and orientation of behavioral assessment. Observation as an assessment can be naturalistic or analogue in nature. Naturalistic observation involves observing the patient's behavior in real-life settings and recording data on target behaviors. If possible, more than one observer is utilized, and behavior is recorded independently in order to verify interrater reliability. Because this process can be time-consuming and costly, time sampling is often employed. Time sampling typically involves setting out 15- or 30-minute segments of time throughout the day and observing during those periods, rather than continuously throughout the day.

Analogue observation techniques follow the same general model as naturalistic observation; however, the environment is contrived rather

TABLE 9.4-13
Excerpt from the Schedule for Affective Disorders and Schizophrenia.

HALLUCINATIONS

Hallucinations are perceptions in the absence of identifiable external stimulation. For the purpose of this assessment, hallucinations are recorded here only if they occurred when the subject was fully awake, and neither febrile nor under the influence of alcohol or some drug. Hallucinations should not be confused with illusions, in which an external stimulus is misperceived, or normal thought processes which are exceptionally vivid. Always get the subject to describe the perception in detail. A rating of "suspected" indicates that the rater suspects, but is not certain, that the subject has experienced the particular kind of hallucination noted, as for example, when it is not clear if the subject is describing an illusion rather than a true hallucination. If the hallucination occurred in the setting of a "religious experience," inquire to determine if this is an expected perception that is idiosyncratic to the subject.

If there is no evidence from the case record, informants, or from your interview to suggest hallucinations, ask the following questions and any others from the section on hallucinations which you think are appropriate.

Has there been anything unusual about the way things looked, or sounded, or smelled?

Have you heard voices or other things that weren't there or that other people couldn't hear, or seen things that were not there?

☐ If there is still no evidence to suggest hallucinations, check here and skip to Bizarre Behavior, page 32.

Experienced auditory hallucinations of voices, noises, music, etc. (Do not include if limited to hearing name being called.) *The (sounds, voices) that you said you heard, did you hear them outside your head, through your ears, or did they come from inside your head?* *Could you hear what the voice was saying?* *(Did it talk about you or repeat your thoughts?)* *Did you hear anything else? What about noises?*	0 1 2 3	No information Absent Suspected or likely Definite
Auditory hallucinations in which a voice keeps up a running commentary on the subject's behaviors or thoughts as they occur. *Did the voice describe or comment on what you were doing or thinking?*	0 1 2 3	No information Absent Suspected or likely Definite
Auditory hallucinations in which 2 or more voices converse with each other. *Did you hear 2 or more voices talking with each other?*	0 1 2 3	No information Absent Suspected or likely Definite
Nonaffective verbal hallucinations spoken to the subject. A voice or voices are heard by the subject speaking directly to him, the content of which is unrelated to depressed or elated mood (although he may be depressed or elated at the time). Rate absent if limited to voices saying only 1 or 2 words. Examples: A woman heard voices telling her that she was having a baby and should go to the hospital. A man heard a voice telling him he was being watched by his neighbors for signs of perversion.	0 1 2 3	No information Absent Suspected or likely Definite

Table reproduced with the permission of Robert Spitzer, M.D., and Jean Endicott, Ph.D.

than real. Whenever observation occurs with the patient's awareness, behavior will be altered. Any subsequent alteration in behavior that is reactive to the observation decreases the probability that a true sample of naturally occurring behavior has been obtained. With analogue observation, this becomes even more problematic because the observation technique itself is directly apparent to the patient. Despite these problems, analogue observation techniques are probably used more frequently than naturalistic techniques because of time and cost factors. Additionally, naturalistic observation is quite difficult to carry out logistically with target behaviors that need to be observed in outpatient settings.

A commonly utilized form of analogue observation is role playing. Role playing has been used extensively in the area of social skills training, and research suggests that its effectiveness as both an assessment and treatment methodology is promising. Typically, with the aid of assistants, an analogue situation will be acted out with the patient playing a central role. The situation will be constructed so as to elicit certain target behaviors. Role playing as a form of assessment is likely to be expanded into other areas if results continue to support its reliability and validity.

Self-monitoring Self-monitoring engages patients in recording data regarding their own target behaviors. If a patient is cooperative and a reliable informant, this deceptively simple technique can provide much valuable information. It can be particularly useful when the target behavior is one that occurs with a low frequency, making observation techniques difficult. It is less expensive and time-consuming than observational methods. However, just as individuals' behavior will be altered simply by knowing they are being observed, a change can be expected by asking patients to observe themselves.

Psychophysiological measurement In addition to assessing overt and covert behavioral characteristics and responses to stimuli, physiological responding can provide important information. It is now well recognized that physiological responding may be quite different from behavioral observations, and often this information is needed for a thorough assessment, particularly with stress-related disorders. Some of the more frequently used modalities of assessment include heart rate, blood pressure, galvanic skin resistance, muscle tension, and peripheral body temperature.

In general, the psychophysiological modality used will be dependent on the target behavior in question (e.g., anxiety and pulse rate, headache and muscle tension). Psychophysiological recording can be quite useful with some patients who complain subjectively of disorders, such as anxiety, but show little outward behavioral symptomatology and are unable to accurately identify discrete precipitating stimuli. In addition to initial assessment, psychophysiological recording has treatment applications, especially as an index of therapy effectiveness.

Psychophysiological assessment is not without its drawbacks, most prominently cost. This is mitigated somewhat by the newer, less expensive, compact recording devices. Nevertheless, equipment does tend to be expensive, bulky, and in need of frequent calibration.

Current status Behavioral personality assessment is gaining rapid acceptance, particularly among adherents to behavioral, empirical, state-oriented interventions. It is readily applicable to treatment monitoring, a decided advantage given the current emphasis on psychotherapy treatment effectiveness.

Weaknesses of behavioral assessment include its relative youthfulness as a method in assessing personality and, in some instances, a lack of adequate attention to the psychometric principles of establishing reliability and validity. Perhaps more importantly, the fact that the behavioral approach to personality measurement is somewhat atheoretical may disinterest many clinicians and researchers, particularly those of a more dynamic orientation. Indeed, there are those who maintain that behavioral formulations and personality theory are contradictory terms. Although an atheoretical approach is contrary to the scientific method, the techniques of behavioral assessment appear useful, regardless of orientation. For example, a psychiatrist with a dynamic orientation may wish to conduct a research project on therapy outcome. The psychiatrist will probably be interested in projective techniques as dependent variables. The psychiatrist would also likely want to use dependent variables that directly measure observable symptomatology and that have readily established reliability and validity. Behavioral assessment offers a clear advantage over traditional projective methods for these purposes. The point is that although orientation and theory do dictate one's approach to a large degree, one should not become blinded by theory. A summary of various behavioral methods in personality assessment is found in Table 9.4-14.

CHILD PERSONALITY ASSESSMENT

The assessment of personality with children and adolescents raises a number of issues and methodological problems unique to this particular population. Although the general approach to personality measurement (i.e., objective, projective, behavioral) does not necessarily change, one needs to exercise considerable caution in drawing inferences from the resultant information obtained. For example, the dynamics behind a child's production of a percept on the Rorschach may well be, and most probably are in many instances, quite different from the dynamics involved with adult perception.

In the same way that theory dictates the orientation of personality assessment with adults, it does so in children's assessment. Depending on one's theoretical position, interpretation of test results in child personality assessment needs to take the developmental process into consideration. This requirement is especially important in the dynamic and analytic theories of personality, and hence in projective methods of personality assessment. Although, in classical Freudian theory, the first few years of life are generally considered the most important for the formation of the personality, it is acknowledged that developmental stages continue to be in operation up through adolescence. A prolonged developmental process suggests that the significance of a child's projective assessment protocol may change quite drastically, depending on theoretical personality development constructs. Additionally, cognitive development plays a major role in accounting for changes in children's perceptions, quite independently of personality. A considerable body of research indicates that children's Rorschach perceptions will change as a function of cognitive maturity throughout the developmental span. A knowledge of these changes is essential for valid and reliable interpretations. For example, although it is quite normal for a child's Rorschach protocol to contain an abundance of animal content, its meaning takes on new significance if this same percentage is seen in an older adolescent or adult.

Also of importance is language and academic development. This aspect becomes particularly important with self-report and interview techniques. Although it is necessary at any age to ensure that the patient is able to read adequately when personality questionnaires are utilized, children's reading abilities vary dramatically as a function of grade level and age. Hence, one needs to exercise care in the administration of children's inventories. In general, children are less likely or less able than adults to use language as a means of coping or expression regarding inner conflicts. Methods for eliciting valid information from a child are frequently different from those used with adults. Specific training in these areas is essential prior to conducting comprehensive personality assessments with children.

In assessing aspects of personality development and status with children, it is generally prudent to use the parents or caregivers as a primary source of information. With children, a thorough assessment of familial dynamics is essential. The impact of parenting and familial issues is clearly pertinent while the child is in the home. Any assessment of child personality, regardless of orientation, must directly address structural and interactive aspects of children with their parents and their families in general. School relationships also pro-

TABLE 9.4-14
Behavioral Measures of Personality

Name	*Description*	*Strengths*	*Weaknesses*
Brief Psychiatric Rating Scale (BPRS)	Semistructured interview	Quick administration and established reliability and validity	Provides only a global pathology index
Hamilton Depression Rating Scale	Semistructured interview	Quick administration and established reliability and validity	Over-emphasis on biological and neurovegetative symptoms of depression
Schedule for Affective Disorders and Schizophrenia (SADS)	Structured interview	Two versions are available, thereby allowing for relatively brief repeated assessments; increased diagnostic efficacy	The lifetime form is rather lengthy; some training is required for administration
Global Assessment Scale (GAS)	Rating from observation and report	Quick and easily administered index of overall functioning, which takes into account strengths as well as weaknesses	The index is somewhat oversimplified
Present Status Exam (PSE)	Structured interview	Assesses a wide variety of symptoms	Somewhat lengthy and training required for accurate administration
SCL-90-R	Questionnaire	Brief yet reliable and valid; provides a global index of dysfunction in addition to subscores	Strict focus on pathology without adequate assessment of strengths
Direct observation	In vivo, naturalistic observation	Actually samples behaviors in question in the most direct manner possible	Expensive and time-consuming process; observation itself may alter behavior
Analogue observation	Role playing with observation	Decreases cost and time restraints of direct observation	Observation process may alter behavior
Self-monitoring	Patient records data on behaviors in question	Inexpensive methodology, which has been shown to be beneficial	Patient compliance is essential; also, self-monitoring in and of itself may alter the behavior
Psychophysiological recording	EEG, heart rate, GSR, and muscular electrical activity are most common modalities	Objective measures that provide additional information and require minimal patient compliance	Expensive technology, requiring considerable upkeep

vide valuable information on the child's personality, much in the same way that the work environment is an important source of behavioral information regarding personality with adults.

Prior to discussing some of the more widely used techniques in child personality assessment, the need for special training with children should be emphasized. Not only is a strong background in general clinical assessment needed, but additional training in developmental psychology and child psychiatry is essential as well. In addition to the issues raised above regarding critical differences in approach, children present unique problems on clinical assessment. As a general rule, they are less able to inhibit impulses and have less ability to maintain attention and concentration in the absence of new and interesting stimuli.

As many clinicians will attest, it is not uncommon for parents to bring in children without fully explaining to them the purpose of the visit. This lack of communication often creates unnecessary confusion, anxiety, and lack of trust in the child, which renders the assessment process more difficult. Furthermore, if the examiner does not adequately explain the purpose of the evaluation in such a way that the child is able to comprehend it, the child's orientation toward the personality assessment may be compromised. Related to this issue are parental interpretations of the child's behavior. By the time the parents decide to seek professional help, they may no longer be objective in their observations of the child. Thus, there is an inherent problem in objective personality assessment approaches—namely, that these questionnaires are typically completed by adults.

Language skills, insight, judgment, and moral reasoning are all less developed in the child. For these reasons, children are more likely either to deny or to maximize their problems. The child is frequently lacking in the more advanced abilities of introspection and abstract thought. Hence, it is extremely difficult for children to evaluate their own behavior objectively—a herculean task for most adults—and to compare and contrast their own situation with what might be considered normative.

This brief review of some of the major issues regarding personality measurement with children should alert the reader to the complexities of this area of assessment. It is apparent that a high level of specialized skill is necessary to obtain a valid personality assessment with children.

As mentioned earlier, the basic approaches to personality assessment with children can be grouped into three major orientations—objective, projective, and behavioral—in much the same way as with adults. A major difference is in the areas of objective assessment and, to a lesser degree, behavioral assessment. In these two assessment modalities, significant others are used as informants more frequently than patient self-report. This use of reporting by others has necessitated the development of innovative psychometric methods. In objective assessment, for example, new instruments are incorporating validity indexes specifically designed to account for the use of informants rather than the patients themselves (e.g., Personality Inventory for Children). Additionally, multivariate psychometric techniques have been applied in order to present a representative but parsimonious taxonomy of childhood psychopathology that accounts for informant reporting (e.g., Child Behavior Checklist). Advances in behavioral assessment with children have generally mirrored those used in adult assessment. The area of projective assessment with children, however, has tended to remain somewhat static, as will be seen.

OBJECTIVE PERSONALITY ASSESSMENT The *Child Behavior Checklist* (CBC) is a formalized rating scale that, though similar to behavioral assessment techniques, embodies a number of sophisticated psychometric qualities that enable it to be considered an objective method. The CBC was constructed following a multivariate taxonomic paradigm, yielding a typology of child psychopathology that avoids both diagnostic overlap and forced choices between multiple categories. Specifically, children receive scores that indicate the degree to which they are similar to criterion groups and different from normative groups in all symptom clusters. Additionally, the taxonomy itself is highly efficient.

The CBC is filled out by a knowledgeable informant who rates the child's behavior on each of a wide variety of areas (118 items) using a three-point scale: "never" a problem, "sometimes" a problem, and "frequently" a problem. The items are summed into nine scales, including Schizoid, Depressed, Hyperactive, and Delinquent. The various scales load onto two general factors, Internalizing and Externalizing. A sample protocol is presented in Table 9.4-15. These scales and factors comprise the taxonomy of the CBC. Test norms are available for both boys and girls between the ages of 4 and 16 years. The CBC contains a number of additional questions and items that are designed to measure social adjustment and interpersonal skills. The CBC has a number of strengths. It is quickly filled out and the wording is easily understood; thus, it is useful for a wide variety of parents, teachers, and significant others. Research indicates that it possesses satisfactory reliability and, although only several validity studies have been reported, overall results are quite positive. The rating scale can be scored according to three separate sets of norms within each sex (ages 4 to 5, 6 to 11, 12 to 16). Since the CBC is a relatively new instrument, less information on profile interpretation is available than with other tests. Largely for this reason, the CBC has been considered as a screening instrument until more specific, detailed interpretative strategies can be developed. Because the CBC is filled out by a knowledgeable significant other, there is a potential for error attributable to the respondent's relationship with the child. In order to obtain as true a picture of the child's behavior and personality as possible, the CBC should be completed by as many different raters as possible (e.g., mother, father, teacher, sibling). In such cases, one is able to determine the degree of convergence or divergence among the significant caregivers in the child's life. Convergence in this sense also provides evidence of reliability, whereas divergence may provide estimates of error in reliability or misperceptions in how the parents or caregivers see the child. This latter information can be particularly useful in treatment planning.

The *Personality Inventory for Children* (PIC) is another example of a behavioral rating scale that was closely modeled after adult objective personality inventories. The full PIC contains 600 behavioral and personality descriptors that sum onto a number of dimensions, including Adjustment, Ego Strength, Depression, Social Skills, and Delinquency. There are published short forms of the PIC which, though sacrificing some information, tend to make the assessment process more manageable. The PIC was constructed using a variety of psychometric techniques, such as empirical keying and rational development, in much the same way as the MMPI clinical, validity, and experimental scales were constructed. The PIC is appropriately used with children and adolescents between the ages of 6 and 16.

A prominent strength of this instrument is the inclusion of control scales, which are designed to provide information on the possible presence of a response bias on the part of the informant. Although this feature is certainly an advantage, one needs to keep in mind that even with validity scales, the PIC information is based on a rating by another individual. Specifically, one is not looking at a child's self-perceptions but rather at another person's perceptions of the child. These perceptions will be colored to an unknown extent by the relationship between the child and the rater. In this sense, the control scales do not eliminate this problem but put some limits on the degree of acceptability of the error variance. The PIC has been criticized for having an imbalance between extensive test construction literature and a relative dearth of validity and interpretative research. As one prominent psychologist has commented, the PIC is probably best thought of as an experimental personality inventory at this time. It holds considerable promise as a relatively objective assessment device; however, interpretative statements need to be tempered because of these research problems. A sample profile of the PIC is reproduced in Table 9.4-16.

Adolescent norms have been published for the MMPI. Also available are case history data on a number of adolescent MMPI profiles. This information is helpful; however, use of the MMPI with adolescents remains rather restricted because of the limited amount of research on the MMPI with adolescents. Thus, interpretative comments rest on much less firm ground than those involving adult patients.

PROJECTIVE PERSONALITY ASSESSMENT The Rorschach technique can be used with adolescents, but it is rarely used with younger children. As mentioned earlier, it is extremely important that the clinician interpreting a Rorschach protocol from a child or adolescent be knowledgeable about developmental norms for the various Rorschach responses. What is considered a pathological response in an adult may represent a typical or nondeviant response in a child or adolescent.

The *Children's Apperception Test* (CAT) consists of 10 cards that depict animal figures in a number of settings. The cards present various scenarios that are designed to elicit or "pull for" rather specific information. For example, one of the cards is a scene at a dinner table and another shows a young child sleeping in a room that somewhat ambiguously shows another bed, which presumably represents the parent's bed. The CAT has a definite analytic orientation and is most appropriately used for personality assessment in which a more dynamic interpretation of the child's personality is desired. The method is used in much the same way as the TAT. Although the CAT is somewhat dynamic in its orientation, it also can elicit considerable information concerning familial relationships, which are extremely important in child personality assessment. Published research on validity and interpretation is available, but the test has not been extensively researched or widely utilized on a clinical basis.

Play therapy techniques can be used with children in order to observe behavior and make inferences regarding personal-

TABLE 9.4-15
Revised Child Behavior Profile of a 9-Year-Old Male with a Diagnosis of Attention-Deficit Hyperactivity Disorder

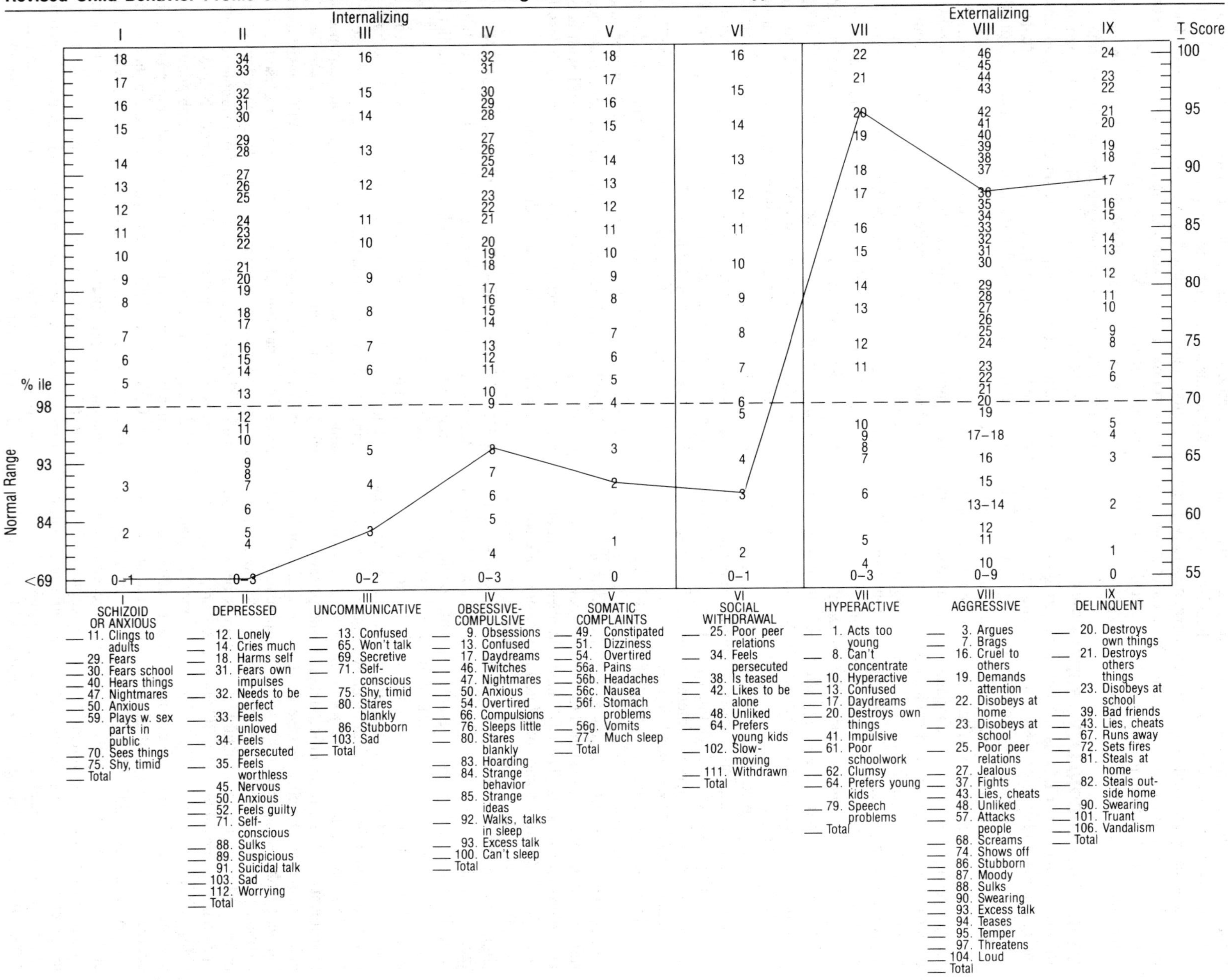

TABLE 9.4-16
Sample Profile of a 13-Year-Old Male with a Diagnosis of Dysthymia

MALE
Ages 6-16

Personality Inventory for Children

PROFILE FORM

R.D. Wirt, Ph.D.; D. Lachar, Ph.D.; J.K. Klinedinst, Ph.D. and P.D. Seat, Ph.D.

Published by:

WPS WESTERN PSYCHOLOGICAL SERVICES PUBLISHERS AND DISTRIBUTORS 12031 WILSHIRE BOULEVARD LOS ANGELES, CALIFORNIA 90025
A DIVISION OF MANSON WESTERN CORPORATION

Child's Name: ____________ Informant: ____________

Birthdate: ____________ Age: ______ Relation to Child: ____________

School Grade: ____________ ID: ____________ Date Tested: ____________

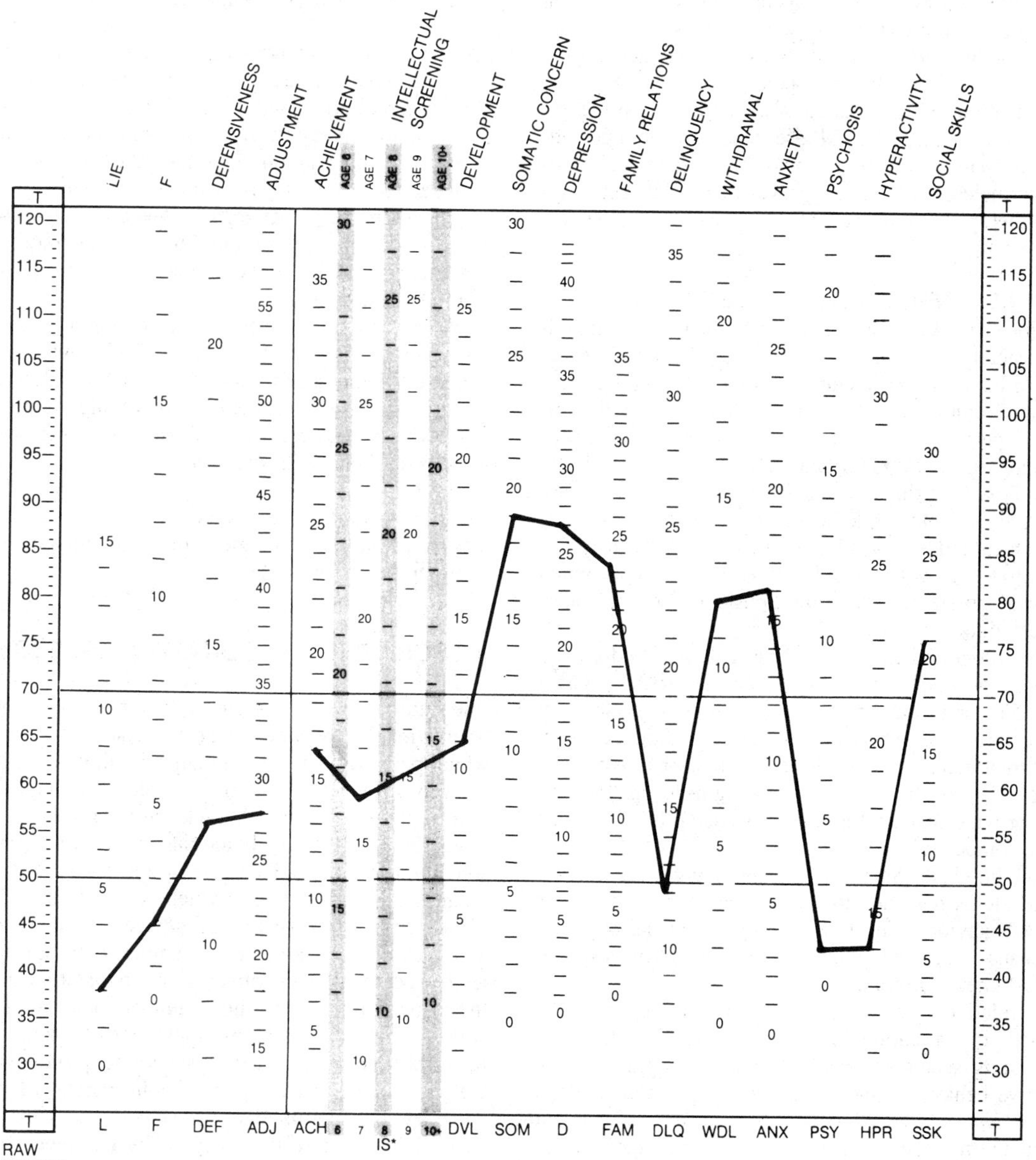

RAW SCORES ___ ___ ___ ___ ___ ___ ___ ___ ___ ___ ___ ___ ___ ___ ___ ___

*This scale is not a substitute for an individual intellectual assessment administered to the child.

W-152C

2 3 4 5 6 7 8 9 Printed in U.S.A.

ity structure. Although this process is very similar to the behavior assessment procedure of analogue observation, its use is closely connected with clinicians and researchers who have a more dynamic background and are more prone to view the child's interaction with various play therapy stimuli as projective in nature. Most typically, the child is presented with various dolls designed to represent both the child and also parental and sibling figures. The child's behavior is observed in play with the dolls and oftentimes the child is asked to make up a story using the dolls as characters. The story is recorded on the assumption that the child will project his or her own internal and family dynamics into the story. Empirical research on play therapy assessment techniques is somewhat sparse; however, the procedure is rather widely used by dynamically oriented clinicians.

The Blacky Pictures (BP) consist of a set of cards that depict dog figures in various settings and scenarios. They are specifically intended to cull intrapsychic conflict information from the child and provide data congruent with Freudian theory. The pictures represent such psychoanalytic conflict arenas as castration anxiety and oedipal conflicts. A rather structured set of questions is asked of the child after presentation of the stimulus card. The BP are rarely used and considered not more than a curiosity by many researchers and clinicians. Nevertheless, it might prove beneficial for psychoanalytic therapists to investigate the potential usefulness of the BP.

BEHAVIORAL PERSONALITY ASSESSMENT The theory, rationale, and technique of child behavioral assessment are basically identical to the methods described earlier for adults. In addition to the emphasis that behavioral assessment places on empirical validation, methods used with children must be particularly sensitive to the developmental process. At young ages, self-report and self-monitoring are rarely utilized, and other ratings and behavioral observations are more appropriate. As the child becomes more mature, a greater range of techniques is available. As with adults, a multimethod approach is advocated in order to obtain as much information as possible, given time considerations and other practical restraints.

A relatively popular behavioral rating scale for children and adolescents is the *Behavior Problem Checklist* (BPC), which consists of 55 items that are rated on a three-point severity scale. Scores are obtained on four dimensions: Conduct, Personality, Immaturity, and Socialized Delinquency. Although the BPC does a respectable job of assessing psychopathology, it does not provide much information on the child's strengths or areas of competence.

The *Louisville Fear Survey* (LFS) is a rating scale comprised of 81 items designed to assess a wide variety of fear and anxiety behaviors. The LFS is useful with many young children because fear syndromes and disorders, such as school phobia, are rather common.

Another relatively common syndrome in children is hyperactivity or attention-deficit hyperactivity disorder. Numerous rating scales are available for quantifying aspects of hyperactive behavior. One of the most popular methods is the *Conners Hyperactivity Rating Scale*. The scale is designed to be completed by teachers and provides a brief, but reliable and valid, estimate of hyperactive behavior.

A number of self-report assessment scales have been developed for children and adolescents. There are scales available for measuring anxiety, depression, fear, and anger. If used with caution, these techniques can be quite helpful, especially when combined with either observation or other ratings, or preferably both. Within behavioral assessment, self-report measures have tended to be underutilized. There has been a long-standing bias against self-reports largely because they do not assess directly the behavior in question. This bias is changing and there is growing recognition that self-reports represent behaviors worthy of attention.

CURRENT STATUS The assessment of personality with children and adolescents is an area that has broadened in recent years. Advances are evident in the behavioral assessment areas and also in work that has increased the psychometric sophistication of inventories using an informant or other report format. This psychometric sophistication has resulted in test instruments that provide data that closely approximate data found with adult objective assessment techniques.

An exciting outlook on multiaxial assessment of personality with children has been recently proposed. This proposal suggests that childhood assessment needs to cover five axes: parental perceptions, teacher perceptions, cognitive measures, physical conditions, and the clinician's assessment. This multiaxial approach results in a more complete assessment, which maximizes information regarding the child's strengths and weaknesses, as well as aspects of convergence and divergence, in the perceptions of the caregivers. Additionally, it allows for the use of multimodal assessment devices and can incorporate objective, behavioral, and even projective methods if desired.

While personality assessment of children is similar in many respects to that of adults, there are important differences. The major differences and cautions have been described earlier. What is necessary to reiterate is that a high degree of specialized skill is required to administer and interpret child personality assessment instruments.

Child psychiatry, in general, is a growing subdiscipline. As attention toward children increases in the mental health professions, continued advances in personality assessment with children can be expected.

INTEGRATIVE PERSONALITY ASSESSMENT

The authors have emphasized the importance of theoretical orientation in the assessment of personality. The manner in which personality is conceptualized will dictate, in large part, the way in which it will be assessed. Although this assertion is true, it needs to be acknowledged that many clinicians and researchers take a very functional, pragmatic approach to personality assessment. This type of approach is often referred to as integrative assessment, which is simply the administration of a variety of assessment devices from more than one approach or orientation. For example, both objective and projective personality instruments are frequently administered to the same patient, with the examiner then integrating the results of these two different approaches to personality assessment. The examiner will inspect the protocols for similar themes and discrepancies in the interpretative process. The value of this multimodal approach to assessment lies in the rich clinical picture that is typically obtained. If interpretive conclusions are verified across modalities, then their validity is strengthened. If discrepant results are obtained, an explanation is sought. Is the patient confused or malingering? Is one of the tests providing invalid information and, if so, why? Or, perhaps most commonly in situations where divergent results are obtained, is there some degree of truth to both sets of results? In any event, one generates hypotheses regarding the cause of discrepant results and seeks out data to support or refute these hypotheses.

Incremental validity is a very important issue in integrative personality assessment. Incremental validity involves the degree to which additional measures of personality functioning either increase or decrease the validity of the psychologist's interpretative statements. Research has indicated that, in terms of clinical judgment, increasing information beyond a certain critical point not only fails to increase assessment validity but may even begin to have detrimental effects on the evaluation. This effect appears to be a more serious problem with clinical judgment than with actuarial systems of interpretation. Actuarial systems use mathematical formulas in which one is able to state with some degree of certainty how much margin of error may be present on an interpretative statement. In constructing the formula, one knows exactly when to stop including information because the error margin will begin to increase in size. This mathematical accuracy in many instances appears superior to judgments and impressions made on the basis of clinical experience. For these reasons, the interpreter of psychological personality tests needs to exercise considerable caution in drawing summary conclusions on the basis of integrative assessment.

Integrative assessment can, and frequently does, provide a broad range of information useful for clinicians of varied orientation. Hence, it maximizes the report's usefulness, particularly in clinics where the patient may be seen by more than one team member. Integrative assessment also allows for the conceptualization of the patient on more than a unitary level.

FUTURE DIRECTIONS

A number of general trends in personality assessment can be identified, and it is likely that the field will continue to move in these directions. There is a continued emphasis on psychometric purity, meaning well-established reliability and validity—not only for objective devices, but also for projective and behavioral assessment methods. Greater attention to environmental and situational determinants of behavior is also reflective of the current movement in personality assessment. Although this approach has resulted in somewhat of a decrease in intrapsychic, analytic-type assessment, by no means are these methods obsolete. Regardless of the approach, continued emphasis on lower-level, more meaningful, and directly observable interpretations is likely.

The field of personality assessment has continued to emphasize the importance of the individual and the individual's view of his or her own psychological status. At times, this position reaches a level at which diagnostic categorization is ignored. There will probably always be those who hold that diagnosis in the mental health fields is inappropriate, reductionistic, and even, perhaps, harmful to the patient. It is unlikely that this position will become mainstream; actually, it is more reflective of those who advocate a more idiographic approach to personality assessment. Diagnosis remains an integral part of a thorough assessment and does not preclude greater attention to individual needs, wants, and desires. As Zubin, a psychologist, has remarked, "Diagnosis should be a design for action." Within such a model, a diagnosis is much more than a label and provides the impetus for broad-spectrum treatment planning.

Behavioral assessment has continued to grow in popularity, and its usage is increasing. Because behavioral assessment incorporates cognitive factors and pays greater attention to dynamic social interactions, its usefulness is likely to expand. Personality assessment that is directed toward providing a barometer of a patient's symptom changes is becoming more and more important, particularly in view of the greater focus on treatment accountability over the past few years. The fact that behavioral assessment techniques are particularly well suited for these purposes may also contribute to their increased use and development.

The traditional psychological battery for personality assessment remains the mainstay in clinical psychology. This situation is most probably not going to change in the near future, and psychological methods likely will be supplemented with behavioral methods rather than replaced by them. However, many of the traditional assessment devices, such as the MMPI and Rorschach technique, have remained unchanged for many years. Continued efforts to update normative data, make contemporary changes, and reestablish reliability and validity on these traditional measures can be expected.

Finally, personality assessment with children is a specialty area that is growing by leaps and bounds. As test developers continue to take into account the problems unique to child assessment, methods are likely to improve and become more innovative. An example is the multiaxial system of assessment, which systematizes an integrative assessment paradigm for children. Such innovations in child assessment will undoubtedly have a beneficial effect on personality assessment methodology with adults.

REFERENCES

Achenbach T M: *Assessment and Taxonomy of Child and Adolescent Psychopathology*. Sage, Beverly Hills, 1985.

Anastasi A: *Psychological Testing*, ed 5. Macmillan, New York, 1982.

Barlow D, editor: *Behavioral Assessment of Adult Disorders*. Guilford, New York, 1981.

Buros O K, editor: *The Eighth Mental Measurements Yearbooks*. University of Nebraska Press, Buros Institute of Mental Measurements, Lincoln, NE, 1978.

Butcher J N, Keller L S: Objective personality assessment. In *Handbook of Psychological Assessment*, G Goldstein, M Hersen, editors, p 307. Pergamon, New York, 1984.

Carr A C: Psychological testing of personality. In *Comprehensive Textbook of Psychiatry*, ed 4, H I Kaplan, B J Sadock, editors, p 514. Williams & Wilkins, Baltimore, 1985.

Cronbach, L J: *Essentials of Psychological Testing*, ed 4. Harper & Row, New York, 1984.

Dahlstrom W G, Welsh G, Dahlstrom L: *An MMPI Handbook: Volume 1, Clinical Interpretation*. University of Minnesota Press, Minneapolis, 1972.

Erdberg P, Exner J E: Rorschach assessment. In *Handbook of Psychological Assessment*, G Goldstein, M Hersen, editors, p 332. Pergamon, New York, 1984.

Goldfried M R, Kent R N: Personality assessment: A comparison of methodological and theoretical assumptions. Psychol Bull *77*: 409, 1972.

Goldfried M R, Stricker G, Weiner I: *Rorschach Handbook of Clinical and Research Applications*. Prentice-Hall, Englewood Cliffs, NJ, 1971.

Haynes S N: Behavioral assessment of adults. In *Handbook of Psychological Assessment*, G Goldstein, M Hersen, editors, p 369. Pergamon, New York, 1984.

Holt R R: *Assessing Personality*. Harcourt Brace Jovanovich, Orlando, FL, 1971.

Kleinmuntz B: *Personality and Psychological Assessment*. St. Martin's Press, New York, 1982.

Korchin S J, Schuldberg D: The future of clinical assessment. Amer Psychol *36:* 1147, 1981.

Lambert M J, Christensen E R, DeJulio S S, editors: *The Assessment of Psychotherapy Outcome*. Wiley, New York, 1983.
Meehl P E: *Psychodiagnosis: Selected Papers*. Norton, New York, 1977.
Millon T: *Millon Clinical Multiaxial Inventory Manuals*, ed 3. Interpretive Scoring Systems, Minneapolis, 1983.
Ollendick T H, Meador A E: Behavioral assessment of children. In *Handbook of Psychological Assessment*, G Goldstein, M Hersen, editors, p 351. Pergamon, New York, 1984.
Overall J E, Gorham D R: The Brief Psychiatric Rating Scale (BPRS): Recent developments in ascertainment and scaling. Psychopharmacol Bull *24:* 97, 1988.
Shneidman E S, Joel W, Little K B, editors: *Thematic Test Analysis*. Grune & Stratton, Orlando, FL, 1951.
Sundberg N D: *Assessment of Persons*. Prentice-Hall, Englewood Cliffs, NJ, 1977.
Wolman B, editor: *Handbook of Clinical Diagnosis of Mental Disorders*. Plenum, New York, 1978.
Zubin J, Eron L, Schumer, editors: *An Experimental Approach to Projective Techniques*. Wiley, New York, 1965.

9.5 NEUROPSYCHOLOGICAL AND INTELLECTUAL ASSESSMENT OF ADULTS

HARVEY S. LEVIN, Ph.D.
ARTHUR L. BENTON, Ph.D.
JACK M. FLETCHER, Ph.D.
PAUL SATZ, Ph.D.

INTRODUCTION

Neuropsychological assessment applies the methods of experimental and clinical psychology to the analysis of the cognitive and behavioral disturbances produced by injury, disease, or abnormal development of the brain. These procedures, which are employed both in clinical evaluation and in research, may be viewed as constituting a refinement and extension of certain aspects of the neurological examination. The same behavioral and mental capacities (e.g., orientation, memory, language functions) that are evaluated in the neurological examination are also evaluated in a more precise and objective manner by neuropsychological assessment. Neuropsychological tests are standardized techniques that yield quantifiable and reproducible results that are referable to the scores of normal persons of an age and demographic background similar to those of the individual tested.

The scientific origins of clinical neuropsychology include the investigation of brain-behavior relationships (particularly with respect to cerebral localization of higher functions), the establishment of experimental psychology laboratories, and pioneering studies of individual differences in ability that anticipated the emergence of intellectual assessment techniques. Contributions by Paul Broca and Carl Wernicke to the clinicopathological correlation between aphasia and lesions situated in the left hemisphere were followed by studies of apraxia, visuospatial deficit, memory disorder, and cognitive impairment related to frontal lobe injury. Controversies surrounding the issue of cerebral localization of higher function kindled interest in developing techniques to evaluate specific neurobehavioral deficits. A second influence on the development of neuropsychology was the establishment of experimental psychology laboratories in universities toward the end of the nineteenth century. Sir Francis Galton's measurement of individual differences in cognitive, motor, and sensory capacities during the late nineteenth century and development of standardized tests for evaluating intelligence by Alfred Binet and Theodore Simon at the turn of the century also anticipated the emergence of clinical neuropsychology. The demand for evaluating sequelae of brain injuries sustained by large numbers of servicemen in each World War provided further impetus for neuropsychological testing.

Until recently, extrapolation of neuropsychological methods developed in studies of patients with localized lesions to psychiatric disorders was constrained by difficulty in demonstrating morphological, neurophysiological, or neurochemical features of these conditions that could be related to the behavioral findings. Advances in neuroimaging, neuropharmacology, and neurophysiology have expanded the opportunities to characterize cerebral abnormalities in psychiatric disorders and to investigate their relationship to neuropsychological impairment. In recognition of the recent increase in neurobehavioral research and clinical applications in neurology and psychiatry, this section focuses on testing of adults. Section 9.6, by Fletcher and his colleagues, is devoted to neuropsychological and intellectual testing of children. These two sections on neuropsychology encompass a broad range of procedures in addition to intellectual assessment. Personality assessment was discussed separately in Section 9.4.

PURPOSES OF THE NEUROPSYCHOLOGICAL EXAMINATION

The major role of neuropsychological test procedures is that of providing an accurate and unbiased estimate of various aspects of a patient's behavioral capacity. The results can contribute to differential diagnosis and serve as a guide to clinical management and as a baseline for monitoring changes in clinical status. The indications for neuropsychological assessment are as follows:

1. To identify the presence and nature of early or mild disturbances of cognitive function in patients when other neurodiagnostic studies and mental status examinations have yielded equivocal findings.
2. To aid in the differentiation of depression or other causes of behavioral impairment from brain disease. Presented with complaints of memory impairment or slowness in thinking in a patient who is depressed or paranoid, the psychiatrist may be unsure of the possible contribution of neurological changes to the clinical picture. Indications for neuropsychological testing may be particularly evident when the findings of the neurological examination and ancillary procedures are either negative or equivocal. The differential diagnosis of incipient dementia from depression is a case in point, particularly when computed tomography (CT) fails to yield definitive results.
3. To evaluate the deficits and preserved functions in patients with neurological disease or injury in order to assist in planning for rehabilitation, including recommendations for speech therapy, training to ameliorate visual neglect, and cognitive retraining. Serial assessment in nonprogressive conditions, such as head injury, documents the patient's rate of recovery and potential for returning to work.
4. To assess the neurotoxic effects of alcohol and drug abuse, including improvement and residual deficits after detoxification. Chronic alcohol abuse can result in cognitive and memory defects, which resolve to a varying degree depending on the duration of abstinence.
5. To evaluate the effects of surgical intervention for epilepsy, cerebrovascular disease, and hydrocephalus. Drug therapy for neurological and psychiatric disorders can also be monitored by neuropsychological procedures. Serial administration of parallel forms of memory tests has been employed to investigate the effects of

cholinergic agents and other drugs on primary degenerative dementia of the Alzheimer type.

6. To evaluate school problems and developmental delay in order to differentiate between mental subnormality, emotional disturbance, and specific learning disability (Section 9.6).

7. To provide objective data for research; neuropsychological tests are particularly useful in psychiatric investigations involving behavioral variables.

TEST BATTERIES VS. FLEXIBLE STRATEGY

Strategies of neuropsychological assessment may be categorized as (1) "fixed battery" (i.e., administration of a comprehensive, invariant series of tests) or as (2) flexible or "adjustive," involving the selection of tests according to the reason for referral, pertinent clinical data, indications of deficits observed during an interview (e.g., hesitancy in speech), the patient's ability to cooperate, and the results of preliminary tests that may suggest the presence of specific deficits. Either strategy can provide a profile of abilities (i.e., intellectual, linguistic, mnemonic, perceptuomotor) and, in practice, many neuropsychologists integrate complete test batteries or selected components with other procedures.

While acknowledging the potential usefulness of both fixed battery and flexible strategies in neuropsychological consultation in psychiatry and neurology, the authors maintain that the examiner should be trained to conceptualize the neuroanatomical and neurobehavioral implications of the diagnostic entities under consideration. The neuropsychologist should be capable of interpreting patterns of test scores in view of principles of lateralization and localization of cerebral function and to take account of factors that adversely affect performance (e.g., fatigue, adverse drug effects, cultural deprivation, anxiety, rumination, and depression) and possibly mimic the neuropsychological impairment found in patients with demonstrable cerebral lesions. Clinical exigencies related to unusual neurobehavioral syndromes or extenuating circumstances might require an experimental approach to the individual patient that deviates from a standard battery. Although the Wechsler Adult Intelligence Scale (WAIS) is the most widely employed test battery, it is used primarily to evaluate intellectual level and is supplemented by tests that measure specific abilities. Consequently, this review of neuropsychological tests is organized according to function; components of batteries are included with their respective functions.

TESTS OF SPECIFIC ABILITIES

INTELLECTUAL FUNCTIONS

Development of intellectual assessment techniques To assess individual differences in mental ability in schoolchildren and more accurately identify students who could benefit from assignment to a training school because of mental retardation, the French psychologist Alfred Binet and physician Theodore Simon developed a scale in 1905, which they standardized on 100 schoolchildren and a sample from an institution for the retarded. The 30 items comprising the 1905 scale of intelligence were arranged in ascending order of difficulty. In a 1908 revision, Binet and Simon introduced the concept of mental age (M.A.), which they estimated from performance on test items that could be passed by a majority of children at each age level. The intelligence quotient (I.Q.) was proposed by William Stern in 1912 as a quantitative index of a child's mental age (M.A.) relative to chronological age (C.A.). This ratio I.Q. was computed by the formula

$$\text{I.Q.} = \frac{\text{M.A.}}{\text{C.A.}} \times 100$$

For example, a 10-year-old child with an I.Q. of 100 answered as many items correctly as the average 10-year-old child, whereas an I.Q. greater than 100 implied that the child correctly responded to items that were typically answered at a higher age level. In contrast, a child whose ceiling score corresponded to items that were usually answered by younger children obtained an I.Q. below 100.

The ratio I.Q. was incorporated in the 1916 revision of the Binet-Simon scale by Lewis Terman of Stanford University. Terman expanded the scale and standardized it on a sample of approximately 1,000 children and 400 adults who were selected in an attempt to obtain a cross section of the American population. The Stanford-Binet was widely adopted for applications in education and psychiatry. Although the I.Q. ratio was retained by Terman in his 1937 revision of the Stanford-Binet, developmental studies revealed that standard deviations of obtained I.Q.s varied with age and were inconsistent with the representative value of 16 I.Q. points. This finding was inconsistent with the underlying assumption of ratio I.Q. that mental age is directly proportional to chronological age across the age span. By implication, the ratio I.Q. could no longer be regarded as equivalent from one age to another.

David Wechsler, an American psychologist, employed statistical criteria rather than mental age in his Wechsler-Bellevue I, which he introduced in 1939. If the same I.Q. score of 100 was assigned to the different mean raw scores obtained on the same I.Q. test by various age groups and a standard deviation (σ) of 15 I.Q. points was used, it was possible to compare I.Q. scores directly across various ages and evaluate intraindividual changes over time. The Wechsler-Bellevue I was revised in 1946 and was replaced by the WAIS in 1955, which retained the deviation I.Q. Moreover, Wechsler's influence was reflected in the 1960 revision of the Stanford-Binet Intelligence Scale, which substituted the deviation I.Q. (mean = 100, σ = 16) for the ratio I.Q. based on mental age.

In contrast to the primary concern of Binet (and later Terman) with assessment of general intelligence by incorporating heterogeneous items into a single scale, the Wechsler-Bellevue included a separate Verbal Scale and a relatively nonverbal Performance Scale, each of which consisted of five subtests. As chief clinical psychologist at Bellevue Hospital in New York City, Wechsler had extensive experience with non-English speaking patients for whom the heavily verbal Stanford-Binet was highly unsuitable. The Wechsler-Bellevue yielded a Verbal I.Q., a Performance I.Q., and a Full-Scale I.Q. for individuals in the age range of 10 through 60 that could be compared to the distribution of scores obtained in persons of similar age.

The WAIS, which was revised in 1981 as the WAIS-R, and the Wechsler Intelligence Scale for Children-Revised (WISC-R) are the most widely used tests for assessment of cognitive functioning. Although the Wechsler scales were not originally designed to assess cognitive impairment associated with cerebral disease (and they have shortcomings in this respect), they have the advantage of standardization on large normative populations and yield highly reliable results when the findings of different examiners are compared. These test batteries have been translated for use with Spanish-speaking patients.

Distribution and correlates of I.Q. scores Standardization of the Wechsler scales over a wide age range of normal subjects permits conversion of raw scores to standardized scores that yield a mean I.Q. of 100, with a standard deviation of 15 (Fig. 9.5-1). Accordingly, 68 percent of the population have I.Q.s (85 to 115) within one standard deviation of the mean, and 95 percent of the population have I.Q.s (70 to 130) within two standard deviations of the mean. As depicted in Figure 9.5-1, the average (or normal) range is defined by an I.Q. of 90 to 110, whereas I.Q. scores of at least 120 are considered to be superior. In preparing reports, psychologists frequently utilize percentiles to clarify the interpretation of I.Q. scores (note in Fig. 9.5-1). Thus, a WAIS I.Q. of 100 corresponds to the 50th percentile, an I.Q. of 110 is at the 75th percentile, and a 90 I.Q. falls at the 25th percentile. Accordingly, an individual with a measured I.Q. of 80 has performed on a level that is exceeded by 91 of every 100 adults of comparable age (i.e., the 9th percentile). In contrast, a measured I.Q. score of 119 implies that fewer than 10 out of 100 persons would perform at a higher level on the WAIS.

According to the American Association of Mental Deficiency (AAMD), a range of mental retardation is defined by

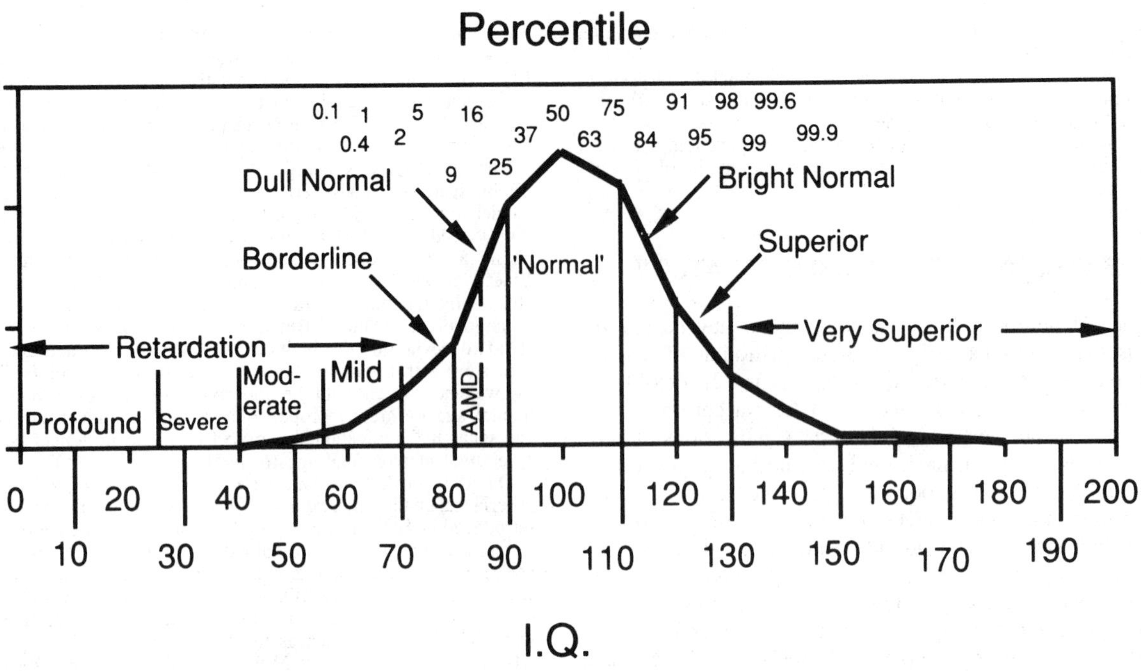

FIGURE 9.5-1. *The distribution of Wechsler Adult Intelligence Scale I.Q. categories. (Adapted from Matarazzo J D:* Wechsler's Measurement and Appraisal of Adult Intelligence, *ed. 5, p 124. New York, Oxford University Press, 1972, with permission.)*

an I.Q. less than 70, which corresponds to the lowest 2.2 percent of the population (Fig. 9.5-1). Consequently, about two out of every 100 persons have an I.Q. score consistent with mental deficiency, which can range from mild to severe.

Clinical interpretation of measured intelligence necessitates concurrent assessment of the individual's adaptive behaviors as reflected by performance of everyday and social activities. Psychologists often obtain information from the individual (parent or guardian in the case of a child or institutionalized person) concerning performance of roles in the home, at school, and in the workplace to interpret how intellectual capacities are utilized. For example, the Vineland Scale of Social Maturity, which is based on information obtained from a relative (usually a parent), is a standardized scale that provides an age-equivalent level of performance in areas such as communication and social relationships. Thus, the psychologist can ascertain whether performance of various roles is commensurate with the estimate of intellectual capacity as reflected by the I.Q. score.

The importance of integrating information obtained from the clinical history and evaluation of adaptive behavior with the results of intellectual assessment is reflected by the correlation coefficients of I.Q. with various criteria of educational and occupational attainment (Table 9.5-1). Although the validity coefficient for mental retardation is high, intellectual assessment demonstrating an extreme deviation in I.Q. is required for this diagnosis. Similarly, the impressive correlation between I.Q. and the ratings assigned by a panel of judges for prestige of various occupations encompass extreme endpoints (e.g., from ditchdigger to physician). In contrast, Table 9.5-1 shows relatively modest correlations between I.Q. score and job success (4 percent of the variance accounted for) or socioeconomic status (16 percent of the variance). Given the narrower range of intellectual functioning within occupations, it is clear that noncognitive variables, such as motivation, personality, and employment opportunity, are contributory.

Reliability of I.Q. scores Test-retest reliability (stability) in adults tends to be high for the Stanford-Binet and the Wechsler I.Q. scales. Reliability coefficients typically reach the 0.80 to 0.90 range. Retesting individuals 18 years and older rarely reveals marked changes in I.Q. that exceed the measurement error of the test. On the average, the reliability coefficient for the WAIS is approximately 0.89 for Verbal I.Q., 0.85 for Performance I.Q. and 0.90 for Full-Scale I.Q. In 1981 Wechsler reported that the reliability coefficients for the WAIS-R were 0.95, 0.94, and 0.89 for the Full-Scale, Verbal, and Performance I.Q.s, respectively, in one sample; and 0.96, 0.97, and 0.90 in a second sample over a 2- to 7-week retest interval. An implication of these findings for clinical applications is that a substantial change in I.Q. scores is atypical in adults. However, the test-retest reliability is somewhat lower over periods of several years. Caution about extrapolating from an I.Q. score obtained several years ago is especially warranted when the initial assessment was completed during early childhood, because marked changes in I.Q. are more common in the pediatric age range.

Clinical Interpretation of Verbal, Performance, and Full-Scale I.Q.s The WAIS and WAIS-R are comprised of two major scales: Verbal and Performance. Subtests of the Verbal Scale include Information (range of general information), Comprehension (practical reasoning and interpretation of proverbs), Similarities (abstraction and verbalization of the properties common to objects), Arithmetic (calculation of problems presented orally), Digit Span (repetition and reversal of numbers given orally by the examiner), and Vocabulary (definition of words). The Performance Scale includes Digit Symbol (a timed visuomotor coding test), Picture Completion (identification of details missing in line drawings of familiar objects and living things), Picture Arrangement (sequential arrangement of cartoon drawings to depict a theme), Block Design (timed construction using mosaic blocks of designs conforming to pictures presented on cards), and Object Assembly (timed construction of puzzles).

In contrast to the Verbal Scale, which largely reflects retention of previously acquired (and frequently overlearned) factual information, the Performance Scale emphasizes visuospatial capacity and visuomotor speed on relatively novel problems. Neurologically normal—

TABLE 9.5-1
Exemplars or Validity Coefficients of I.Q.

Exemplars	*Correlation*
IQ with adaptive behavior measure	
IQ × mental retardation	0.90
IQ × educational attainment (in years)	0.70
IQ × academic success (grade point)	0.50
IQ × occupational attainment	0.50
IQ × socioeconomic status	0.40
IQ × success on the job	0.20
Related variables	
IQ × independently judged prestige of one's occupation	0.95
IQ × parents' educational attainment	0.50

Table from Matarazzo J D: *Wechsler's Measurement and Appraisal of Adult Intelligence,* ed 5. Williams & Wilkins, Baltimore, 1972, with permission.

but culturally disadvantaged—persons may obtain a relatively low Verbal I.Q. (e.g., because of a limited range of information and vocabulary), whereas it is not unusual for highly educated and widely read persons to have a particularly high Verbal I.Q. The Performance Scale is less dependent on formal education but appears to be more sensitive to normal aging. The discrepancy between Verbal I.Q. and Performance I.Q. is generally less than 15 points.

A correction for age is introduced in the calculation of both the Verbal Scale and Performance Scale I.Q.s on the basis of the score distributions of normal subjects at different ages. Age-corrected standard scores are also available for each subtest, thereby facilitating intraindividual comparison of abilities. Thus, the cognitive efficiency of a 70-year-old patient is evaluated in terms of Verbal, Performance, and Full-Scale I.Q. scores that are corrected for age and by a profile of age-corrected standard scores on the subtests. Consequently, senile dementia is suspected when the Verbal or Performance I.Q. is significantly below expectation in view of the patient's estimated premorbid ability.

From a clinical standpoint, the Full-Scale IQ derived from the WAIS (or its predecessor, the Wechsler-Bellevue) is a moderately useful index of general intellectual impairment associated with cerebral disease provided that other explanations (e.g., depression, deficient motivation) for defective scores can be excluded. The Performance Scale I.Q. is about equal in efficiency to the Full-Scale I.Q. as a predictor of the presence of cerebral damage.

Disproportionate impairment on the Verbal Scale is primarily associated with left-hemisphere damage (assuming the patient is right-handed) when aphasic disorder is present, but this disparity is unimpressive in nonaphasic cases. Specific impairment on the Performance Scale occurs in patients with right-hemisphere (particularly posterior) lesions whose relatively intact language and normal Verbal I.Q. often contrast with marked impairment of visuoconstructive ability (e.g., block construction), neglect of the left visual field, or difficulty in visual guidance of movement. However, exceptions to the correspondence between the direction of the Verbal-Performance discrepancy and lateralization of brain injury are not rare, and additional testing is necessary in many cases.

Parietal lobe lesions in either hemisphere can compromise visuospatial ability (especially on constructional tasks), and subtle right-sided hemiparesis can slow coding speed and thus lower the Performance I.Q. in a patient with left-hemisphere disease. For reasons that are not entirely clear, conditions that produce diffuse cerebral disturbance or multifocal lesions (e.g., closed head injury, dementia of the Alzheimer type) frequently result in lower Performance I.Q. than Verbal I.Q.

A striking Verbal-Performance disparity is illustrated by the following case example:

The WAIS results were recorded about 18 months following the onset of primary degenerative dementia of the Alzheimer type in a 58-year-old physician. He obtained a Verbal I.Q. of 100 (corresponding to the population mean but considerably below estimated premorbid level) as compared to a Performance I.Q. of 66 (more than two standard deviations below the population mean). This wide Verbal-Performance discrepancy, which reflected the patient's complete failure to assemble even the simplest block design, was essentially unchanged when he was retested 12 and 16 months later. Manifestations of the patient's visuospatial impairment included topographic disorientation (e.g., he would become lost while driving) and a subjective report of visual disturbance.

However, striking exceptions, such as receptive language deficit during the early stage of primary degenerative dementia of the Alzheimer type, have been documented. Positron emission tomography (PET) in patients with presumptive Alzheimer's disease and normal subjects has disclosed that asymmetry in hemispheric metabolism corresponds differentially to specific cognitive functions; that is, left-hemisphere metabolism was related to verbal skills, whereas right-hemisphere metabolism was related to visuospatial ability.

A physical handicap, neurological deficit, abnormal behavior, or cultural differences may necessitate modification of standard testing procedures or substitution of other cognitive tests. Tests, such as the Leiter Scale and Raven's Progressive Matrices (for deaf patients or patients with auditory agnosia), or the Peabody Picture Vocabulary Test (for patients unable or unwilling to speak or cooperate with the WAIS), circumvent these limitations. Failure to recognize factors other than cognitive impairment that limit performance on specific standardized tests of intelligence may result in a spurious inference of subnormality or dementia.

BRIEF COGNITIVE TESTS AND RATING SCALES In response to pressure for rapid cognitive evaluation or screening and increased awareness of the age-related prevalence of dementia, there has been a proliferation of brief tests (10 to 30 minutes) that purportedly provide an estimate of intellectual level. Many of these procedures are designed to assess cognition in elderly normal subjects or to provide a measure of the severity of dementia in the presenium or senile periods. The Mini-Mental State of Folstein, Folstein, and McHugh and the Mattis Dementia Rating Scale include assessment of verbal, visuospatial, and mnemonic functions. These measures are useful for monitoring the course of moderate to severe dementia in patients who might not be otherwise testable. However, these brief cognitive tests lack the age-based standardization across their various subtests and range of difficulty necessary for the initial evaluation of older persons suspected of an incipient dementia. The claims of a strong correlation between scores on brief cognitive tests and the WAIS (or WAIS-R) are based primarily on patients exhibiting obvious deterioration or on studies with insufficient sample size. Moreover, excessive false-positive errors have been reported for elderly persons with low levels of education, while false-negative errors may occur in detection of right-hemisphere pathology. Detailed reviews of brief cognitive tests have been published. Provided that the clinician is aware of the limitations of these procedures, they can serve as useful screening tests.

Qualitative features of patients' behavior during neuropsychological testing and an interview can provide clinically useful information with respect to differential diagnosis and serial assessment of treatment efficacy. Behavioral manifestations, such as distractibility, inaccurate self-appraisal, and unrealistic planning, that reflect cerebral disease or injury can be difficult to evaluate with conventional neuropsychological tests. The structure provided by many neuropsychological techniques might enable patients to compensate for behavioral changes secondary to focal lesions in the frontal lobes or limbic system, whereas findings might be equivocal in patients with mild diffuse or multifocal cerebral insult. In contrast, such patients might exhibit maladaptive functioning in their occupational and psychosocial roles. To facilitate the documentation of clinical observations obtained during neuropsychological testing, interviewing, and other situations,

TABLE 9.5-2
Neurobehavioral Rating Scale

DIRECTIONS: Place an X in the appropriate box to represent level of severity of each symptom.

	Not Present	*Very Mild*	*Mild*	*Moderate*	*Mod. Severe*	*Severe*	*Extremely Severe*
1. Inattention/reduced alertness—fails to sustain attention, easily distracted; fails to notice aspects of environment, difficulty directing attention, decreased alertness.	☐	☐	☐	☐	☐	☐	☐
2. Somatic concern—volunteers complaints or elaborates about somatic symptoms (e.g., headache, dizziness, blurred vision), and about physical health in general.	☐	☐	☐	☐	☐	☐	☐
3. Disorientation—confusion or lack of proper association for person, place, or time.	☐	☐	☐	☐	☐	☐	☐
4. Anxiety—worry, fear, overconcern for present or future.	☐	☐	☐	☐	☐	☐	☐
5. Expressive deficit—word-finding disturbance, anomia, pauses in speech, effortful and agrammatic speech, circumlocution.	☐	☐	☐	☐	☐	☐	☐
6. Emotional withdrawal—lack of spontaneous interaction, isolation, deficiency in relating to others.	☐	☐	☐	☐	☐	☐	☐
7. Conceptual disorganization—thought processes confused, disconnected, disorganized, disrupted; tangential social communication; perseverative.	☐	☐	☐	☐	☐	☐	☐
8. Disinhibition—socially inappropriate comments and/or actions, including aggressive/sexual content, or inappropriate to the situation, outbursts of temper.	☐	☐	☐	☐	☐	☐	☐
9. Guilt feelings—self-blame, shame, remorse for past behavior.	☐	☐	☐	☐	☐	☐	☐
10. Memory deficit—difficulty learning new information, rapidly forgets recent events, although immediate recall (forward digit span) may be intact.	☐	☐	☐	☐	☐	☐	☐
11. Agitation—motor manifestations of overactivation (e.g., kicking, arm flailing, picking, roaming, restlessness, talkativeness).	☐	☐	☐	☐	☐	☐	☐
12. Inaccurate insight and self-appraisal—poor insight, exaggerated self-opinion, overrates level of ability and underrates personality change in comparison with evaluation by clinicians and family.	☐	☐	☐	☐	☐	☐	☐
13. Depressive mood—sorrow, sadness, despondency, pessimism.	☐	☐	☐	☐	☐	☐	☐
14. Hostility or uncooperativeness—animosity, irritability, belligerence, disdain for others, defiance of authority.	☐	☐	☐	☐	☐	☐	☐
15. Decreased initiative or motivation—lacks normal initiative in work or leisure, fails to persist in tasks, is reluctant to accept new challenges.	☐	☐	☐	☐	☐	☐	☐
16. Suspiciousness—mistrust, belief that others harbor malicious or discriminatory intent.	☐	☐	☐	☐	☐	☐	☐
17. Fatigability—rapidly fatigues on challenging cognitive tasks or complex activities, lethargic.	☐	☐	☐	☐	☐	☐	☐
18. Hallucinatory behavior—perceptions without normal external stimulus correspondence.	☐	☐	☐	☐	☐	☐	☐
19. Motor retardation—slowed movements or speech (excluding primary weakness).	☐	☐	☐	☐	☐	☐	☐
20. Unusual thought content—unusual, odd, strange, bizarre thought content.	☐	☐	☐	☐	☐	☐	☐
21. Blunted affect—reduced emotional tone, reduction in normal intensity of feelings, flatness.	☐	☐	☐	☐	☐	☐	☐
22. Excitement—heightened emotional tone, increased reactivity.	☐	☐	☐	☐	☐	☐	☐

TABLE 9.5-2
(continued)

23. Poor planning—unrealistic goals, poorly formulated plans for the future, disregards prerequisites (e.g., training), fails to take disability into account.	☐	☐	☐	☐	☐	☐	☐
24. Lability of mood—sudden change in mood which is disproportionate to the situation.	☐	☐	☐	☐	☐	☐	☐
25. Tension—postural and facial expression of heightened tension, without the necessity of excessive activity involving the limbs or trunk.	☐	☐	☐	☐	☐	☐	☐
26. Comprehension deficit—difficulty in understanding oral instructions on single or multistage commands.	☐	☐	☐	☐	☐	☐	☐
27. Speech articulation defect—misarticulation, slurring or substitution of sounds which affect intelligibility (rating is independent of linguistic content).	☐	☐	☐	☐	☐	☐	☐

Table developed by H S Levin, J E Overall, K E Goethe, W High, and R A Sisson, with permission.

Levin and colleagues developed the Neurobehavioral Rating Scale (Table 9.5-2), which is a revision of Overall and Gorham's Brief Psychiatric Rating Scale.

In a study of 101 patients with closed head injuries of varying severity and chronicity who were given a structured interview and mental status examination, Levin and his colleagues used a principal components analysis to derive four factors from the 27 scales shown in Table 9.5-2. The investigators found that three factors—metacognition (i.e., the capacity for self-evaluation of abilities, monitoring, regulating impulses, formulating realistic plans), cognition-energy (i.e., conceptual organization, memory), and language (expressive, receptive, articulation)—were sensitive to the severity of brain injury. Somatic complaints and anxiety, the fourth factor, tended to be equally or even more impressive in patients who had sustained relatively mild injuries. Follow-up neurobehavioral data based on ratings obtained at least 6 months postinjury confirmed that the most severely injured patients exhibited greater conceptual disorganization, inaccurate self-insight, diminished initiative and motivation, and poor planning. These neurobehavioral sequelae, which reflected difficulty in interpretation of proverbs, perseveration, difficulty in filtering tangential material, and failure to appreciate the cognitive defects resulting from injury, have been shown in numerous studies to impose an immense burden on family members and result in chronic disability. Whether the profile of qualitative behavioral manifestations of traumatic brain injury is distinctive as compared with other etiologies of brain damage awaits further research.

REASONING, CONCEPT FORMATION, AND PROBLEM SOLVING Decades ago, Kurt Goldstein emphasized that, apart from any specific intellectual defects that might be present, the patient with cerebral disease is likely to show cognitive impairment of a general nature, which he designated as "loss of the abstract attitude." He characterized the deficit as a loss of the capacity to reason abstractly and lack of flexibility in problem solving or in adapting to changed situations. Goldstein particularly implicated frontal lobe disease in producing these deficits. Although later research failed to support this localization of lesion associated with impaired abstract reasoning, the role of frontal lobe pathology in compromising the use of feedback to guide behavior and to solve problems has gained wide acceptance.

Investigators have operationalized the capacity for concept formation primarily in respect to sorting tests. The first clinical application was the color form sorting test, in which the patient is presented with a random array of forms (square, circle, triangle) of different colors (blue, yellow, green, red) and asked to "put those together that belong together." The crucial feature of performance that is evaluated is whether or not the patient is able to sort the forms according to a clear principle—that is, by shape or color. If the patient does separate the stimuli in accordance with one principle or another, the stimuli are once again presented in a random array and the patient is asked to "sort them in another way," interest being focused on whether or not the patient's approach is sufficiently flexible to shift the sorting strategy. This particular color form sorting test has proved in practice to be a relatively simple task that identifies only patients with gross impairment in reasoning and problem solving.

The Wisconsin Card-Sorting Test has proved to be a more informative procedure than earlier tests for assessing abstract reasoning and flexibility in problem solving. Stimulus cards differing in color, form, and number are presented to the patient for sorting into groups according to a principle preestablished by the examiner. While sorting the cards, the patient is told whether each response is correct or incorrect. The number of trials required to achieve 10 consecutive correct responses is recorded. When (or if) the patient has mastered the task, the examiner once again changes the principle of sorting, and the number of trials required to achieve correct sorting is recorded. The procedure is repeated a number of times, and measures of the capacity for abstract thinking (i.e., the number of trials required to achieve a solution) and of flexibility in problem solving (i.e., perseverative errors on successive sorting) are derived from the patient's performance. Nelson reduced the length and ambiguity of the Wisconsin Test while preserving its sensitivity and relative specificity to frontal lobe disease.

To illustrate the sensitivity of the Wisconsin Card-Sorting Test, Figure 9.5-2 depicts the short-form protocol of a 28-year-old mechanic (R. H.) who had sustained a midline frontal depressed fracture and left frontal subdural hematoma after the explosion of a tire that he was repairing. When R. H. was tested 16 months after injury, he had an excessive number of both perseverative and nonperseverative errors. Note his tendency to persist in a response strategy after the examiner has requested him to shift to a new principle of card sorting.

It has been shown that patients who have undergone frontal lobe excisions for amelioration of epilepsy exhibit a more impressive deficit on the Wisconsin Card-Sorting Test as compared with patients with posterior surgical lesions. The basis for their failure appeared to be an excessively strong perseverative tendency (i.e., rigidity in approach) rather than defective abstract reasoning per se. Other workers have recently shown that chronic schizophrenic patients ex-

SCORING SHEET FOR CARD-SORTING TEST – SHORT FORM

Card Number	Sorting Category	Errors	Card Number	Sorting Category	Errors
1	F		25	N	
2	N	X NP	26	N	
3	F		27	F	X NP
4	N	X NP	28	F	X P
5	N	X P	29	F	X P
6	F		30	F	X P
7	N	X NP	31	N	
8	N	X P	32	N	
9	N	X P	33	N	
10	N	X P	34	N	
11	N	X P	35	N	
12	F		36	N	
13	N	X NP	37	F	X NP
14	N	X P	38	N	X NP
15	N	X P	39	F	X NP
16	N	X P	40	F	X P
17	F		41	N	X NP
18	N	X NP	42	N	X P
19	F		43	N	X P
20	F		44	N	X P
21	F		45	N	X P
22	F		46	N	X P
23	F		47	F	X NP
24	F		48	F	X P

SORTING CATEGORY

C = Color
F = Form
N = Number

ERROR TYPE

NP = Nonperseverative
P = Perseverative
U = Unique

ERRORS

Cards used 36-48	48
Number of categories 0-6	2
Perseverative errors 0-48	18
Nonperseverative errors 0-48	11
Unique errors 0-48	00
Total number errors 0-48	29

FIGURE 9.5-2. *Modified card-sorting protocol of a 28-year-old man who had sustained a left frontal subdural hematoma associated with a severe closed head injury 18 months previously (Glasgow Coma Scale score = 5). Numerous perseverative errors (i.e., continuing to sort according to the previous principle after the examiner has requested the patient to shift to a new strategy) are present. The patient's task was to sort the cards correctly according to the initial principle (e.g., form) for six consecutive cards and then to shift to a new sorting principle at the request of the examiner. Although the patient sorted according to form initially, he failed to follow through with consecutive responses until trials 19 to 24. Correct sorting was limited to the categories of form and number, whereas color was omitted.*

hibited on the Wisconsin Card-Sorting Test impaired performance related to reduced cerebral blood flow in their frontal lobes, whereas differences in other cortical regions were less impressive. The hypofrontal pattern in the schizophrenic patients was specific to the Wisconsin Card-Sorting Test, whereas their cerebral blood flow was comparable to the control group values during performance of other tasks.

The Categories Test of the Halstead-Reitan Battery requires the patient to solve novel problems by selecting a relevant dimension, such as color or shape, in response to stimuli that are presented in a visual display. A booklet version of the test also has been developed. Although the Categories Test is sensitive to brain damage, deficient performance on this test is not as specific to frontal lobe involvement as impaired Wisconsin Card-Sorting Test performance.

A self-administered paper-and-pencil measure of conceptual thinking is provided by the Shipley Abstractions Test, which requires the patient to complete logical sequences. Correct responses to the Abstraction portion of the test demands a grasp of the underlying principles. Because performance on a test of this type is related to educational background, an accompanying vocabulary test is also given to the patient, and a comparison is made between performances on the two tests. A low abstraction score in relation to vocabulary level is interpreted as reflecting impairment in conceptual thinking. Interpretation of proverbs is often included in the mental status examination. Gorham developed a proverbs test that has been used to study patients with cerebral disease.

What may be termed the organizational aspects of problem solving are assessed by maze tests, such as those of Porteus and Benton and co-workers. These tasks demand both temporal and spatial integration of behavior while bringing into play such personal characteristics as playfulness and impulsivity. They have been found to be fairly effective in identifying patients with cerebral disease. However, the idea that a deficit on this type of task is specific to frontal lobe damage has not proved to be accurate. Patients with postrolandic lesions in the right hemisphere are likely to perform as poorly as those with frontal lesions.

MEMORY AND ORIENTATION **Memory** It is customary to distinguish between two types of memory: (1) immediate or short-term memory (STM), which persists for up to 30 seconds (e.g., forward digit span) and has a capacity limited to about seven plus or minus two chunks (or alternatives) of information; (2) long-term memory (LTM), which involves the consolidation of the supraspan information into a relatively permanent store that is subsequently retrievable. Remote memory refers to retention of information about events in the distant past (i.e., months or years ago). Recent memory (i.e., retention of experience over hours or days) is usually evaluated by informal procedures concerning orientation of the patient's environment—for example, a breakfast menu. Whether remote memory and recent memory are parts of a temporal continuum of LTM or are distinct types of memory is still debated. However, there is considerable evidence that both LTM and remote memory are biologically distinguishable and clinically dissociable from STM. Memory theorists have recently distinguished between episodic memory (e.g., for a telephone message in a specific spatiotemporal context) and semantic memory—that is, overlearned information that becomes part of a knowledge base (e.g., the first president of the United States).

SHORT-TERM MEMORY Immediate memory is often preserved in amnesic patients who are unable to learn and retain information beyond the limits of their forward digit span. Consequently, the finding of a normal digit span does not exclude the possibility of a memory deficit. Conversely, investigation of depressed patients has disclosed that they tend to exhibit disproportionate impairment of STM relative to LTM. This dissociation presumably reflects the disruptive effects of rumination on attention as opposed to amnesic disorder. In one study, patients hospitalized for depression also exhibited difficulty in encoding material as reflected by their underutilization of clustering related words and failure to impart organization to a word list as compared with normal controls. When information was presented in an organized or structured form, recall performance by depressed patients was normal. It was postulated that hypoarousal or disrupted activation mitigated the use of these active encoding strategies by depressed patients.

To explain the relatively preserved retention of motor skills in amnesic patients, investigators have proposed that procedural memory (knowing how) can be dissociated from declarative (knowing what) memory, both in performance and in neural substrate. Investigators have shown that procedural memory is relatively preserved after electroconvulsive therapy (ECT) and in patients with primary degenerative dementia of the Alzheimer type. The usefulness of these concepts for routine clinical memory testing remains an open question.

Visual STM is evaluated by having the patient draw designs after they have been removed from view (Fig. 9.5-3). In contrast to immediate recall of digits, memory for designs tests are among the more sensitive behavioral measures of the presence of brain damage. The probable reason is that the task of copying complex designs from memory is one that makes demands on the perception of spatial relations and on visuographic skill as well as on attention and immediate retention. Consequently, a patient's reproductions may be defective for one or more reasons. Reproduction of designs from STM was one of three neuropsychological tests selected and cross-validated by a discriminant analysis of patients with primary degenerative dementia of the Alzheimer type versus normal elderly. Recent research has also shown that short-term visual memory on the Benton Visual Retention Test is impaired in schizophrenic patients with negative symptoms (i.e., flat affect, asocial, inattentive) as compared with cases with only positive symptoms (e.g., delusions, hallucinations). By comparing the accuracy of the patient's reproductions from memory to the results of copying a parallel form held in view, the examiner can determine whether or not non-mnemonic factors contribute to the patient's apparent memory failure.

LONG-TERM MEMORY The Wechsler Memory Scale is the most widely used memory test battery for adults. It is a composite of verbal paired associate and paragraph retention, visual memory for designs, orientation, digit span, rote recall of the alphabet, and counting backward (which combined form the Mental Control subtest). This scale yields a Memory Quotient (M.Q.), which is corrected for age and generally approximates the WAIS I.Q.; amnesic conditions, such as the alcoholic Korsakoff's syndrome, are characterized by a disproportionately low M.Q. but a relatively preserved I.Q. The practice of combining the scores of these heterogeneous subtests to obtain a composite M.Q. has been criticized, but the availability of subtest norms and the addition of delayed recall tests of the paragraphs and paired associates to the Wechsler Memory Scale have enhanced its popularity among clinicians. The Memory for Paragraphs and Mental Control subtests were recently found to be among the most efficient neuropsychological measures in differentiating patients with mild degenerative dementia of the Alzheimer type, senile onset from normal subjects. However, many examiners and investigators prefer to employ specific tests of LTM that elucidate the component processes and strategies rather than the Wechsler Memory Scale.

A procedure that has been used occasionally in clinical and investigative work is assessment of a patient's capacity to learn a series of digits that is longer (supraspan) than his or her immediate span. This procedure provides a direct measure of learning and of long-term retention in contrast to digit span, which reflects immediate recall. One investigator reported instances of a marked disparity in performance in learning a series of digits just longer than the span. Many brain-diseased patients had an unremarkable digit span (e.g., six or seven digits) but were unable to learn an eight- or nine-digit span in 10 trials. Comparing forward digit span and the learning of a lengthy series of digits in patients with either known or presumed hippocampal dysfunction and in normal subjects, it was found that there was no significant difference in digit span performance, but that there was a large and significant difference in serial digit learning. This digit-learning procedure was used to investigate performance differences between older normal subjects and amnesic patients; it was noted that the normal subjects performed unremarkably, whereas the amnesic patients showed gross impairments. Finally, it was found that administration of the anticholinergic drug scopolamine produced a transient impairment of supraspan performance (LTM) in young subjects but had a negligible effect on their digit span. Normative data have been published on a digit-learning task that has been standardized for clinical use.

Other verbal techniques to evaluate LTM include recall of word lists and recognition of words that are presented repeatedly. One investigator modified the usual recall procedure (presenting the complete list on each trial) by selectively presenting only those words that the patient had failed to recall on the preceding trial (i.e., selective reminding).

A number of investigators have employed parallel forms of this selective reminding test to assess the effects of cholinergic (and other) medications on the memory deficit of patients with primary degenerative dementia of the Alzheimer type. Figure 9.5-4 compares the retrieval from long-term memory in three Alzheimer patients tested under conditions of baseline, lecithin alone, and the combination of physostigmine (Antilirium, Eserine) and lecithin. Long-term memory retrieval improved to within the range of age-matched controls under the combined physostigmine-lecithin condition.

Recent research has shown that schizophrenic patients with positive symptoms exhibited a more severe verbal memory deficit on the selective reminding test as compared with schizophrenic patients with primarily negative symptoms. In contrast, the direction of the group difference was opposite on a test of visual retention. Parallel forms of the selective reminding test are available for repeated assessment of memory.

The recently developed California Verbal Learning Test provides an opportunity to compare LTM under conditions of high versus low

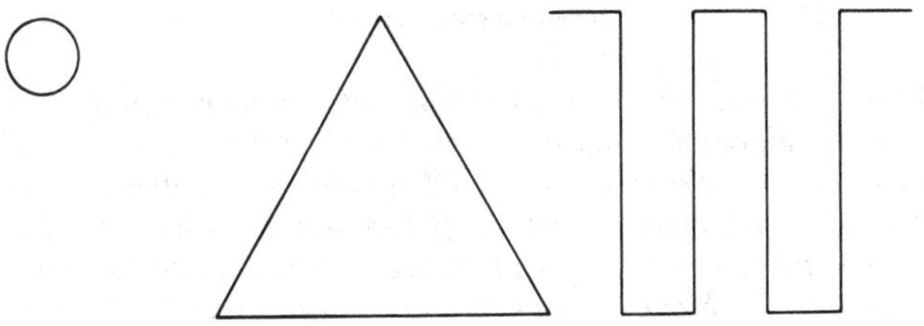

FIGURE 9.5-3. *Test item from the Benton Visual Retention Test. The most frequently employed testing condition involves presentation of each geometric figure for 10 seconds, after which the patient attempts to draw them from memory. (From Benton A L:* The Revised Visual Retention Test: Clinical and Experimental Applications, *ed 4. Psychological Corporation, New York 1974, with permission.)*

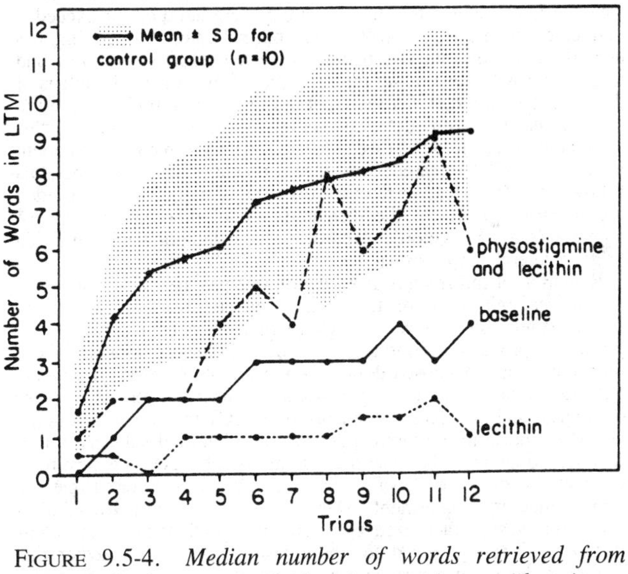

FIGURE 9.5-4. *Median number of words retrieved from long-term memory storage for three patients with primary degenerative dementia of the Alzheimer type tested under conditions of baseline (no medication), subcutaneous injection of physostigmine combined with lecithin and subcutaneous injection of a noncentrally active anticholinergic (placebo) drug combined with lecithin (indicated as lecithin in lower portion of graph). Parallel forms of the selective reminding test were employed in titration of the physostigmine dosage which preceded this randomized crossover trial. (From Peters B H, Levin H S: Effects of physostigmine and lecithin on memory in Alzheimer disease. Ann Neurol* 6: *219, 1979, with permission.)*

interference. Effects of interference on verbal LTM have also been studied using the Rey Auditory Verbal Learning Test, whereas the relative involvement of STM versus LTM in the Brown-Peterson distractor (i.e., counting backward before recall) technique has been debated. In comparison with nonverbal techniques, verbal LTM procedures facilitate the investigation of aiding recall by providing phonemic or semantic cues. Normative tables of word frequency and concreteness are available to develop parallel forms, but their equivalence must be tested directly. Specific or disproportionate impairment of verbal LTM accompanied by relatively preserved visuospatial LTM is characteristic of unilateral left-hemisphere lesions.

Apart from detecting deficits indicative of cerebral disease and evaluating the efficacy of treatment, interpretation of memory test findings based on normative data can be reassuring to patients complaining of forgetfulness, which may stem from diminished concentration, rumination, and mild depression. The diagnostic utility of normal findings is illustrated by the selective reminding protocol of the following patient.

V. R., a 41-year-old programmer, was referred for neuropsychological assessment by a neurologist because of her year-long history of memory problems and diminished work efficiency. The patient retrieved all 12 of the words by the seventh trial (total consistent retrieval from long-term storage summed across 12 trials was 119 vs. a mean of 113.4, σ = 23.3, for normal adults of similar age). She correctly recalled all 12 of the words after a 30-minute delay. A detailed social history and personality assessment revealed that the patient frequently ruminated about marital problems and was mildly depressed, but she had been reluctant to seek psychiatric treatment. The memory test findings were not only reassuring to patient V. R. but convinced her of the necessity for therapeutic intervention.

Visuospatial material has generally been employed to test nonverbal memory using both recall and recognition procedures. The stimuli of these predominantly research tests have included faces, random designs, and sequences of tapping an array of blocks and pictures of objects. Specific impairment of visuospatial memory with relative sparing of verbal LTM is consistent with right-hemisphere pathology.

Evaluation of LTM over long retention intervals (e.g., days) is usually impractical in clinical testing. It was found that patients with alcoholic Korsakoff's syndrome could recognize pictures presented a week earlier provided that the initial exposure duration far exceeded that given to normal subjects. This normal rate of forgetting has recently been confirmed in patients with Korsakoff's syndrome and in a patient with penetrating injury of the left dorsomedial nucleus of the thalamus provided that the input duration was sufficiently long to compensate for their deficient initial learning. In contrast, this recognition procedure has disclosed rapid decay of memory in patient H. M. with bilateral hippocampal lesions and in depressed patients following ECT. These distinctive forgetting functions have provided preliminary support for the differentiation of diencephalic type of amnesia (e.g., Korsakoff's syndrome) from temporal lobe amnesia (e.g., bilateral hippocampal lesions).

Retention of information from the remote past has been studied by testing recognition or recall of news events, titles of previously broadcast television shows, and photographs of persons who became prominent primarily during a specific period (year or decade). These procedures have disclosed deficits in the remote memory of patients with Korsakoff's syndrome, patients with amnesic disorders of other etiologies, and in depressed patients given ECT (a reversible deficit). However, these tests require pilot testing of normal subjects before widespread adoption because the assumption of previous exposure to the material may not be valid. Some investigators reported that the remote memory impairment exhibited by patients with Korsakoff's syndrome was characterized by a temporal gradient in which retention was relatively spared for the oldest information. Whether this finding reflects a progressive impairment of acquiring new information or retrograde memory loss is uncertain. In contrast, demented patients typically exhibit defective remote memory without a temporal gradient.

To investigate further the clinical observation of "shrinking retrograde amnesia" in patients with closed head injuries recovering from post-traumatic amnesia, the authors administered the remote memory test (based on recognition of titles of previous television programs) to patients undergoing rehabilitation after acute hospitalization for closed head injury. Although the results provided evidence for impaired remote memory both during and after resolution of post-traumatic amnesia, the authors found no evidence of a temporal gradient (Fig. 9.5-5*A*). However, relative preservation of older memories was demonstrated on a recall test for personally salient information covering various periods of the patients' lives before their injuries (Fig. 9.5-5*B*). Although remote memory tests can be useful in clinical neuropsychological assessment, the assumption of prior exposure to the material (e.g., televison programs) over the presumed time periods must be verified.

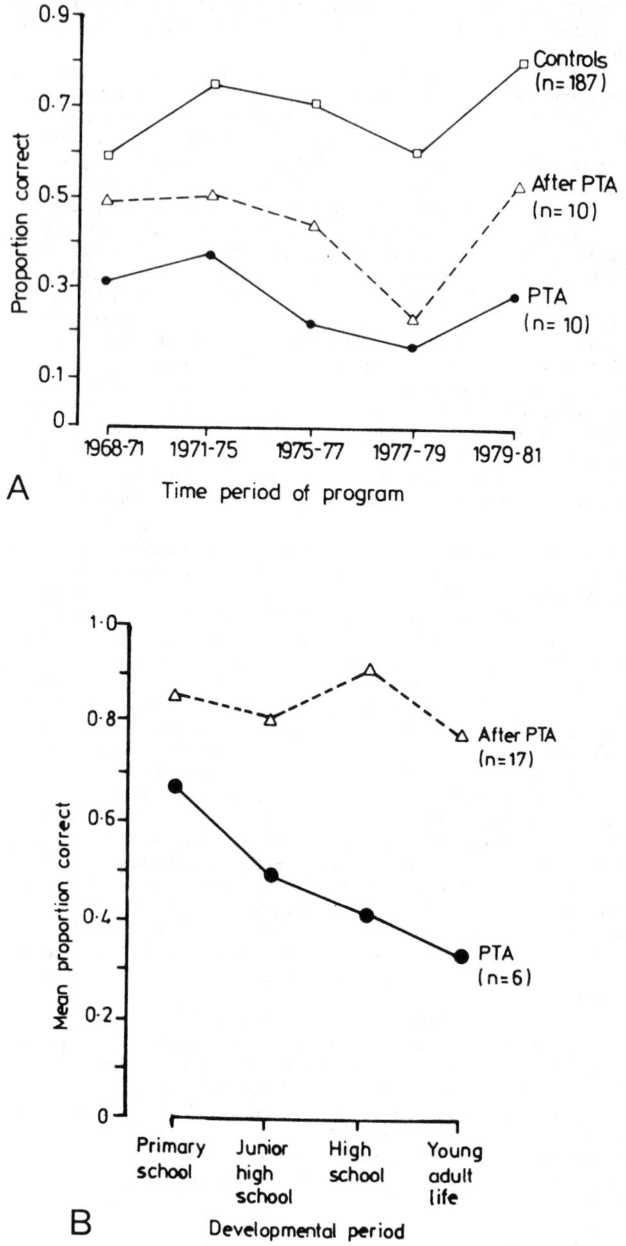

FIGURE 9.5-5. A. *Mean proportion of correct recognition of titles of television programs plotted against the time period of broadcast for closed head-injured patients tested after resolution of post-traumatic amnesia (PTA) and in patients studied during PTA. Normal control subjects were studied for comparison.* B. *Mean proportion of correct recall of autobiographical information plotted against developmental periods for head-injured patients in PTA and after PTA. The information was verified through interviews with a relative. (From Levin H S, High W M, Meyers, C A, Von Laufen A, Hayden M E, Eisenberg, H M: Impairment of remote memory after closed head injury. J Neurol Neurosurg Psychiat 48: 556, 1985, with permission.)*

Orientation Quantitative assessment of orientation is useful both in the detection of cerebral disease and in monitoring the rate of recovery (e.g., resolving post-traumatic amnesia after closed head injury; restoration of memory after ECT and during the transition from coma to normal consciousness in patients with metabolic, toxic, or vascular disorders). Using the schedule of questions shown in Table 9.5-3, for which data on control patients were obtained, defective performance in nearly one-fourth of a group of patients with cerebral disease has been found. Temporal disorientation was more common in patients with bilateral lesions (39 percent) as compared with groups with left-hemisphere lesions (20 percent, excluding aphasics) or right-hemisphere lesions (7 percent). In comparison with quantitative assessment, errors in the clinical judgment of orientation are generally of the false-negative type—that is, depicting a mildly disoriented patient as "oriented times three." Temporal orientation is rather vulnerable to the influence of cerebral disease, and an objective assessment procedure can disclose a degree of disorientation that is usually not detected by the impressionistic methods typical of the routine clinical examination.

ATTENTION AND VIGILANCE Attention deficit can contribute to impaired performance on various neuropsychological tests, particularly learning and memory tasks. Attention is generally viewed as multidimensional, including selectivity, coherence (limiting the number of stimuli attended to), sustained monitoring of the environment (vigilance), and the capacity to shift attention. Impaired attention may be disproportionately affected in conditions, such as closed head injury, metabolic and toxic disorders, epilepsy, and schizophrenia. Subcortical lesions may also lower the level of activation and diminish sustained attention. It has been suggested that the right parietal region integrates the various modalities of input and coordinates attention. Consistent with this view, Norman Geschwind has reported that infarctions in the distribution of the right middle cerebral artery frequently cause a confusional state.

In view of the vulnerability of attention and concentration in cases of cerebral disease or of injury, it is remarkable that no battery of tests is generally available to test various types of attention. At the present time, psychologists primarily use tests that were designed for other purposes. Integration of clinical observations with test data is essential to appreciate the salient features of attention deficit (e.g., distractibility). Attention and information processing can be evaluated by a number of widely employed clinical procedures, for example, the Arithmetic, Digit Symbol (coding), and Digit Span subtests of the WAIS, WISC, the Mental Control section of the Wechsler Memory Scale, the Reitan Trail Making Test, and cancellation tests in which the patient marks only designated letters (targets) interspersed with other letters (nontarget or distractor items) in lengthy sequences.

The Continuous Performance Test (CPT), an experimental task that involves rapid identification of a target and withholding response to distractor stimuli, permits analysis of both the accuracy and latency of response. The CPT, which is one of the few tests designed to assess attention, has been widely employed in psychopharmacological research and in studies of attentional deficit in schizophrenics. In an adjustive version of the CPT, a microcomputer changes the rate of presentation according to the patient's performance. The shortest interstimulus interval at which responding is still accurate is the primary performance measure.

TABLE 9.5-3
Temporal Orientation Test

Questions
1. What is today's date? (patient is required to give day, month, and year)
2. What day of the week is it?
3. What time is it now? (examiner makes sure that patient cannot look at watch or clock)

Scoring
- A. Day of week: 1 point off for each day removed from correct day
- B. Day of month: 1 point off for each day removed from correct day
- C. Month: 5 points off for each month removed from correct month
- D. Year: 10 points off for each year removed from correct year
- E. Time of day: 1 point off for each 30 minutes removed from correct time

Table from Benton A L, Van Allen M W, Fogel M L: Temporal orientation in cerebral disease. J Nerv Ment Dis *139:* 110, 1964, with permission.

Information-processing tasks Measures of information-processing rate, which include the Paced Auditory Serial Addition Task of Gronwall and Wrightson and the serial subtraction of sevens, are derived from cognitive models of limited-capacity, effortful processes. Slowing of information processing may contrast with relatively preserved performance on untimed tests (e.g., memory recall) or tasks that require relatively low effort, such as attending to frequency of presentation. Impaired serial addition with progressively more rapid representation of numbers is a frequent consequence of closed head injury and may be present for several weeks, even after apparently mild injury. Although normal persons often make one or two errors on serial sevens, the inability to complete serial subtraction or making more than five errors is generally confined to patients with cerebral disease. Experimental investigations have employed vigilance tasks in which a subject responds to the presence of an unpredictable recurring stimulus while ignoring other stimuli. Choice reaction time—that is, response to a button or key corresponding to a specific imperative stimulus that varies across trials—provides a measure of selective attention comparable with simple reaction time—that is, responding to the same button or key in each trial when an invariant stimulus comes on. The microcomputer permits convenient administration of these experimental tests, which were previously rather tedious to administer. Attention and vigilance tests are particularly useful in assessing patients who wish to return to an occupation in which reduced efficiency or impaired alertness would pose a safety hazard.

Language functions Clinical assessment of language and ideomotor praxis based on current understanding of their neuroanatomical organization may yield findings suggestive of the locus of a lesion without the aid of detailed testing. Demonstration of subtle language deficit, comparison of performance in different modalities (e.g., visual versus tactile naming), and serial evaluation of recovery from aphasia are facilitated, however, by standardized, quantitative procedures. Standardized aphasia test batteries provide profiles of percentile scores of functions, such as verbal fluency (retrieval of words beginning with a designated letter), repetition, naming, and receptive ability (Table 9.5-4). Writing and reading are usually also assessed. Language batteries, which permit intraindividual comparison and identify problems to be remediated in speech therapy, include the Boston Diagnostic Aphasia Battery, the Multilingual Aphasia Examination, the Neurosensory Center Comprehensive Examination for Aphasia, and the Western Aphasia Battery.

These language tests frequently disclose defects in word finding, naming, and the comprehension of complex commands that are not appreciated in patients without obvious aphasia. For example, it was reported that verbal fluency was among the triad of neuropsychological tests that efficiently discriminated patients with senile dementia from normal controls. Several of these batteries provide correction for age, sex, and educational level, factors that are difficult to weigh in a brief clinical examination. The Boston Naming

TABLE 9.5-4
Percentile Rank Scores of Four Aphasic Patients on Selected Tests of the Multilingual Aphasia Examination*

	Type of Aphasia Disorder			
Test	*Broca†*	*Wernicke‡*	*Amnesic§*	*Conduction§*
Visual naming	20	4	50	89
Sentence repetition	24	3	98	45
Word association	6	2	76	64
Oral comprehension	70	0	90	90
Reading comprehension	64	64	83	83

*Percentile rank scores based on the distribution of scores of a reference group of aphasic patients.
†Note dissociation between levels of expression and comprehension in this patient.
‡Note relative sparing of reading ability in these patients.
§Note contrasting patterns of levels of naming and repetition in these patients.

Test of Kaplan, Goodglass, and Weintraub is a standardized procedure for naming pictures of objects, which is graded in difficulty and available in parallel forms. Administration of the Boston Naming Test has disclosed that anomic disturbance is frequently present in patients with primary degenerative dementia of the Alzheimer type.

Administration of language tests can also be useful in differential diagnosis of psychiatric disorder in patients with neurological complaints, as illustrated by the following case example:

A 49-year-old executive was referred for neuropsychological assessment because of a history of "stammering speech" and dysnomia, which were episodic and associated with headaches. History of hypertension and a reported family history of Alzheimer's disease raised concern, as did the possibility of an epileptic basis for the patient's complaints. Although he initially had difficulty in naming line drawings on the Multilingual Aphasia Examination and his speech was occasionally halting, this problem appeared to be a manifestation of anxiety rather than aphasic disorder. Consistent with this interpretation, the patient achieved nearly a perfect performance on the Boston Naming Test administered later in the examination. This highly variable naming ability cast doubt on the likelihood of a left-hemisphere abnormality to account for the patient's speech problems. Monitoring the patient's electroencephalogram by telemetry revealed no evidence of abnormal cerebral activity during an episode of halting speech.

The Boston Diagnostic Aphasia Examination includes a speech rating scale that is useful for comparing to test scores and a brief schedule of items for assessing ideomotor praxis—that is, symbolic buccofacial and limb movements to exhibit gestures and to demonstrate the use of imagined or real objects. Spelling to dictation is tested by oral response, writing, and using block letters as part of the Multilingual Aphasia Examination.

The Token Test of De Renzi and Vignolo has proved to be a sensitive technique for detecting impairment in language comprehension, even in patients without clinically evident aphasic disorder. This test consists of oral commands on different levels of complexity, involving the manipulation of tokens that vary in shape, color, and size. The commands employ familiar words only, and the difficulty level is determined by the semantic content of the command (e.g., "Put the small red circle on the large black square"). The Token Test can demonstrate impairment in verbal understanding not only in patients with clinically evident receptive aphasia but also in patients with lesions of the left hemisphere who are not apparently aphasic on a mental status examination. In contrast, patients with lesions confined to the right hemisphere perform on a normal level (provided that the tokens are placed in the right visual field to mitigate neglect of the left visual field). Thus, the test brings to light a latent or minimal aphasia in at least some ostensibly nonaphasic patients with disease of the hemisphere dominant for language.

Intrepretation of receptive language performance on the Token Test is facilitated by concurrently examining verbal memory, the presence of visual (object and color) agnosia or neglect, and auditory screening to differentiate a receptive language deficit from failure secondary to memory, perceptual, or sensory impairment. Axial commands not involving visual search and manipulation of objects (e.g., "look up," "do birds fly?") are also useful to avoid misinterpretation of the Token Test and to determine the aspects of language comprehension that are preserved.

In practice, the examiner may select those subtests of an aphasia battery that are most relevant to the referral question. Modification of standard test administration and use of neurolinguistic tasks are also frequently necessary to examine the presence of a hemispheric disconnection syndrome (e.g., writing and tactile letter identification with the nonpreferred hand) and to distinguish modality-specific anomia (e.g., visual-verbal disconnection) from agnosia. Impairment of verbal learning and memory, which is a frequent residual of aphasia, should be investigated in follow-up examinations. Qualitative features (e.g. clang associations) of nonaphasic, disturbed language in chronic schizophrenia can be useful in differentiating these patients from cases with left hemisphere structural lesions.

AFFECTIVE EXPRESSION AND LATERALIZATION

Review of the clinical literature on emotional manifestations of cerebral disease has revealed that pathological laughing, inappropriate euphoria, and mania are closely related to right-hemisphere lesions, particularly involving the posterior region. In contrast, pathological crying is more strongly associated with left-hemisphere disease. However, the relationship of lateralization and localization of brain infarct to poststroke depression has been inconsistent in recent studies. Bilateral lesions have been implicated in labile transitions from one emotional state to another.

Experimental studies concerning the evocation and identification of emotion in speech have disclosed that patients with right-hemisphere lesions who exhibit visual neglect are frequently impaired in the expression and processing of affect. A double dissociation emerged whereby these patients performed above the level of left-hemisphere-damaged patients on tasks involving the semantic content of the same sentences.

A woman sustained extensive right-hemisphere injury in a motor vehicle accident 10 years earlier at the age of 26. In contrast to well-preserved linguistic abilities, tape recordings of her speech showed minimal variation in affect and prosody when she was asked to inject specific affective tones while reciting sentences that were emotionally neutral. Moreover, she had a corresponding deficit in identification of the affect expressed in tape-recorded sentences. Impoverished affect was also evident in the patient's facial expression, whereas she exhibited appropriate social behavior. Similar differences between left- versus right-hemisphere-damaged patients have been reported for processing affective material presented visually. An implication of these studies for clinical practice is the possibility that right-hemisphere disease should be considered in a differential diagnosis of patients exhibiting inappropriate or improverished affect.

VISUOPERCEPTIVE CAPACITY Many tests designed to disclose behavioral deficits associated with cerebral disease involve the processing and interpretation of visual information by the patient. For the most part, this emphasis on vision has been merely a matter of convenience in that the primary interest of the examiner has been in the assessment of cognitive processes that are presumed to be essentially independent of sensory modality. At times, however, the focus of interest may be on the status of higher level (essentially nonverbal) visual function, as contrasted to audition or somesthesis. These visual tasks are of a diverse nature: Some assess complex visual discrimination; others assess the capacity to integrate visual information into meaningful percepts; others assess the ability to differentiate between figure and background; and still others require a search process necessary to select the design that matches a model or sample.

Visual form discrimination These tests are useful to establish that a rudimentary form of visual discrimination is preserved in patients who exhibit gross deficits on more complex tests. Benton and colleagues have developed a multiple-choice visual form discrimination test that is useful in the evaluation of patients.

Complex visual discrimination Although the inability to recognize familiar faces (prosopagnosia) is an uncommon disorder, defective discrimination of unfamiliar faces is a common finding in patients with right-hemisphere or bilateral lesions. The Facial Recognition Test, in which the patient is required to identify a photograph of a face presented in a front view when it is included in various displays (e.g., side view or front view with shadows) produces a high frequency of failure in patients with posterior right-hemisphere lesions. Performance is generally intact in patients with left-hemisphere lesions (provided that receptive language is not seriously limited) and patients with relatively acute schizophrenia. The percentage of cases with impaired performance in patients with focal lesions is shown in Table 9.5-5. Similar testing procedures (using complex stimuli other than faces) have also disclosed deficits in patients with unilateral right-hemisphere damage.

Color discrimination Determination of a patient's capacity for color perception is useful for both clinical and research purposes. The Ishihara and Dvorine plates involve identification of embedded numbers or lines that differ in hue from the background. An achromatic condition obtained by presenting black-and-white photocopies is a useful control for isolating the defect in color perception. The Farnsworth-Munsell Test involves sorting hues according to saturation. This lengthy test is not feasible for use with patients exhibiting severe cognitive deficit. Finally, color object matching requires the patient to select the characteristic color of a familiar object, such as a banana. These tests permit a distinction to be drawn between color agnosia and visual-verbal disconnection (e.g., secondary to infarction of the left posterior cerebral artery involving the splenium).

Visuospatial tests Impairment in spatial thinking, as reflected in defective localization of objects in space, judgment of distance and direction, and geographical orientation, has long been regarded as a specific sign of disease of the right hemisphere. Numerous tests have been devised to probe for this type of deficit. One such test, which has been found to demonstrate failing performance in an impressive proportion of patients with right-hemisphere disease, requires matching the slopes of visually presented lines or pairs of lines. As depicted in Figure 9.5-6, the patient points to or verbally identifies the lines of the display that correspond to the angular orientation of each pair of lines. In agreement with the results on facial recognition, it has been found that the scores of patients with right-hemisphere lesions are frequently defective, whereas patients with left-hemisphere disease perform within the normal range.

Hidden-figure and figure-ground tests The capacity to discriminate figure from background under conditions of stimulus competition is typically assessed by hidden-figure, embedded-figure, or mixed-figure tests. Examples of the stimuli employed in hidden-figure tests are shown in Figure 9.5-7. It has been found that performance on this type of task is determined by factors that transcend the visual modality, since defective figure-background discrimination is shown by patients with and without visual field defects and with lesions in any region of either cerebral hemisphere. However, impairment in performance is particularly closely associated with aphasic disorder.

TABLE 9.5-5
Facial Recognition: Relative Frequency of Defective Performance

Group	*Number of Subjects*	*Defect (percent)*
Normal subjects	286	3.5
Right anterior	23	26
Right posterior	36	53
Left anterior nonaphasic	15	0
Left posterior nonaphasic	14	0
Left anterior, aphasic without comprehension defect	5	0
Left posterior, aphasic without comprehension defect	8	0
Left anterior, aphasic with comprehension defect	17	29
Left posterior, aphasic with comprehension defect	27	44

Table from Benton A L, Hamsher K deS, Varney N R, and Spreen O: *Contributions to Neuropsychological Assessment: A Clinical Manual*. Oxford University Press, New York, 1983, with permission.

Visual matrices Raven's Progressive Matrices require the patient to select from a multiple-choice pictorial display the stimulus that would complete a design in which a part is omitted. The difficulty of the discrimination increases over trials in this lengthy test. A briefer, less difficult version (Colour Matrices) is especially useful for patients who are unable to complete the standard test, which can require 30 to 45 minutes. Impaired performance is associated with poor visuoconstructive ability and with posterior lesions of either hemisphere, but receptive language deficit may be contributory in patients with dominant hemisphere damage. Raven's Progressive Matrices have also been employed to estimate intellectual level. In view of the modest correlation of performance with the WAIS I.Q., this practice is justified only in patients unable to take the WAIS, as in cases of bilateral motor weakness or non–English speakers.

Constructional praxis Constructional praxis refers to the assembly or articulation of parts to make a single entity or object. Thus, it implies combinatory or organizing activity in which the relationships among the component parts of the spatial entity must be appreciated if their synthesis is to be achieved correctly. Impairment in constructional praxis is usually regarded by neurologists as a more or less specific disability rather than as simply an expression of generalized mental defect. However, visuospatial and visuoconstructive deficits are frequently prominent during the early stages of primary degenerative dementia of the Alzheimer type. Assessment of verbal skills and concept formation is necessary to exclude global mental deficit. In any case, defective constructional performance is quite commonly encountered in patients with cerebral disease, and tests assessing this type of activity merit a place in diagnostic batteries.

Tasks that have been developed to assess constructional ability include construction of mosaic patterns of blocks, arranging sticks, block designs using three-dimensional models, and copying designs by drawing. Whether all these tasks actually measure the same ability is uncertain. Some patients show considerable intraindividual varia-

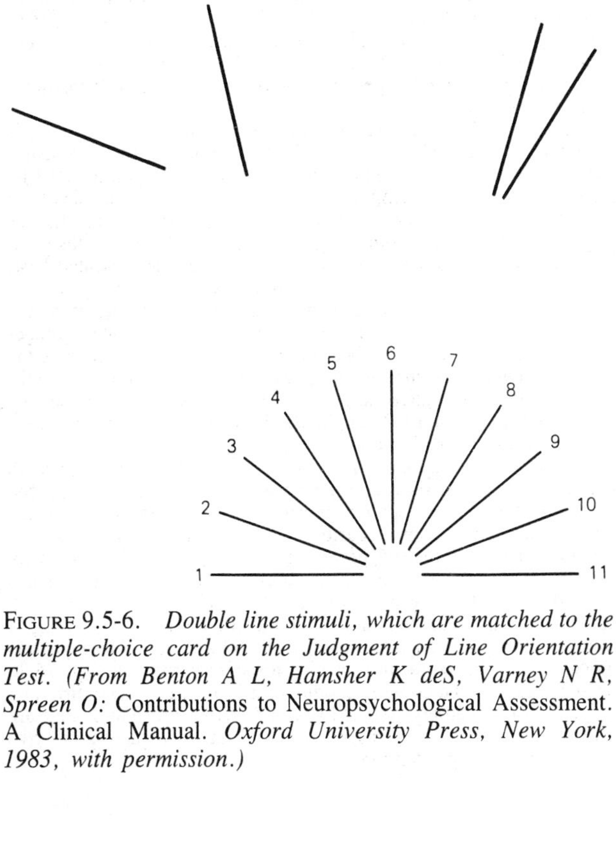

FIGURE 9.5-6. *Double line stimuli, which are matched to the multiple-choice card on the Judgment of Line Orientation Test. (From Benton A L, Hamsher K deS, Varney N R, Spreen O:* Contributions to Neuropsychological Assessment. A Clinical Manual. *Oxford University Press, New York, 1983, with permission.)*

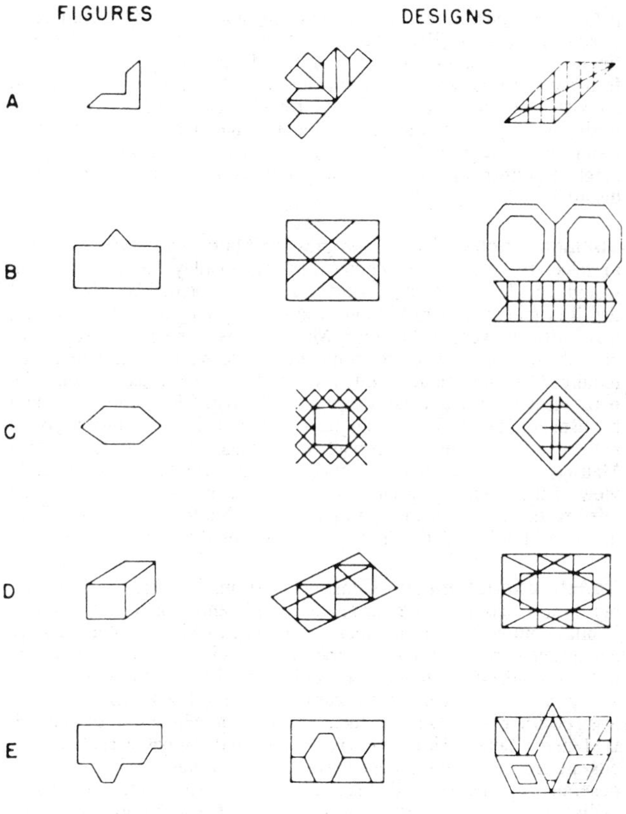

FIGURE 9.5-7. *Sample items from a hidden-figures test. (From Lezak M D:* Neuropsychological Assessment. *Oxford University Press, New York, 1983, with permission.)*

tion in performance, failing in one task but succeeding in another. Studies of the interrelations among various constructional performances in patients with cerebral disease have yielded positive correlations of modest degree, with evidence for at least two types of constructional praxis. Assembling tasks, such as block design construction and three-dimensional block building, appear to form one type, whereas the graphic performance of copying designs constitutes another type.

The most widely employed graphic test of constructional praxis is the Bender (Visual Motor) Gestalt Test. Appropriate for administration to both children and adults, this test was developed in 1938 by Lauretta Bender, who employed it to assess maturational levels in children. The test material for the Bender consists of nine figures (Figure 9.5-8) adapted from designs used by Wertheimer in his studies of Gestalt psychology. Item A in Figure 9.5-8 is presented first, followed by items 1 through 8 in numerical order. The patient is given a sheet of unlined paper and asked to copy each design as the card is left in view. To evaluate the ability to plan the spatial arrangement of the designs on the sheet of paper, the examiner informs the patient that nine designs will be presented. There is no time limit. Availability of normative data, including the manual developed by Elisabeth Koppitz in 1963, facilitates the interpretation of this measure of visuoconstructive ability.

Maturational changes in visuoconstructive ability are reflected in Figure 9.5-9, which shows the percentage of children who produced the level of response depicted or better. Instances in which correct production of the design occurred are denoted by a blank box. For example, it is seen that 95 percent of 11-year-old children correctly copy items A, 1, and 4. Note that adults typically copy all designs correctly, with the exception of item 1.

Clinicians also test the patient's reproduction of the Bender designs from memory after an interval of 45 to 60 seconds. Although this procedure can be useful in revealing a memory problem that would be undetected by the copying condition, it is advisable to confirm any suspicion of a memory deficit by administering procedures that are specifically designed for this purpose and have adequate normative data for evaluating retention.

Impairment in constructional performance is frequently one of the most prominent deficits in patients with a right-hemisphere lesion. Visuoconstructive deficit is most commonly present in patients with posterior lesions, but right frontal lesion sites have also been reported in affected cases. As noted for visuoperceptive deficit, impaired constructional performance by left-hemisphere-damaged patients is usually associated with aphasia. Consequently, a relatively specific visuoconstructive deficit in a nonaphasic patient is consistent with a nondominant hemisphere lesion. Qualitatively distinct errors in constructional performance have also been implicated in right- versus left-hemisphere-damaged patients. Two types of errors in constructing block designs from three-dimensional models are primarily (if not exclusively) found in patients with documented cerebral disease. These errors include the "closing-in" phenomenon, which refers to the patient utilizing part of the model to be copied in making his or her construction (Fig. 9.5-10*A*). Partial or total failure to build the left half of the construction is indicative of unilateral spatial inattention or neglect associated with right-hemisphere disease (Fig. 9.5-10*B*). A detailed description of visual neglect is given below. In contrast, global impairment of both visuospatial and verbal abilities is associated with bilateral or diffuse cerebral disease.

Visual neglect Inattention or neglect of the left visual field is a frequent consequence of right posterior lesions, particularly in cases of parietal involvement. Failure to search for and manipulate stimuli in the left visual field may produce a defective level of performance. The presence of neglect may be apparent by observing the patient perform daily activities (e.g., failure to attend to persons or objects on the left side), but the degree of inattention can be assessed by line bisection, drawing a clock, block construction, finding geographical locations on a map, or a test of crossing lines scattered throughout a page. As patients recover from right-hemisphere vascular or traumatic lesions, manifestations of their visual neglect in spontaneous behavior may resolve despite persistent signs on visuoperceptive and constructional tests (Fig. 9.5-10*B*).

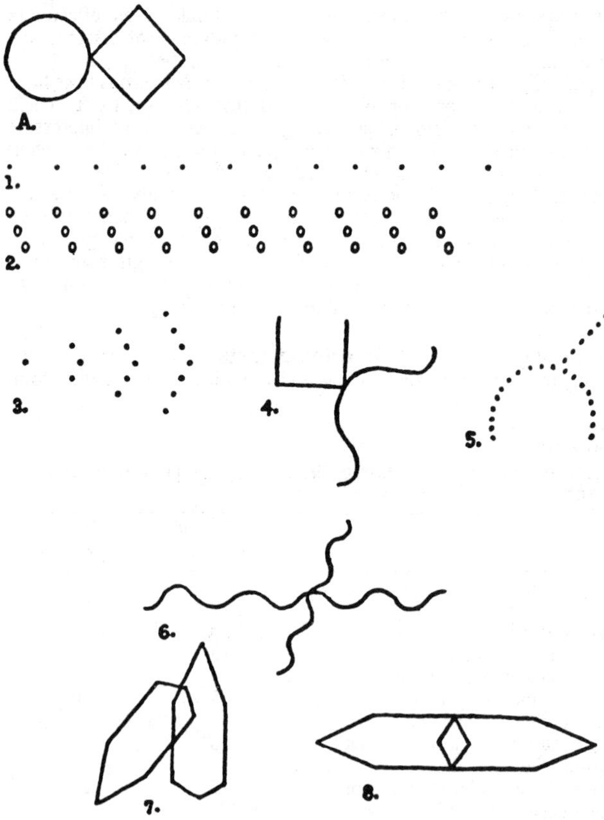

FIGURE 9.5-8. *Designs comprising the Bender (Visual Motor) Gestalt Test. (From Bender L:* A Visual Motor Gestalt Test and Its Clinical Use. *American Orthopsychiatric Association, New York, 1938, with permission.)*

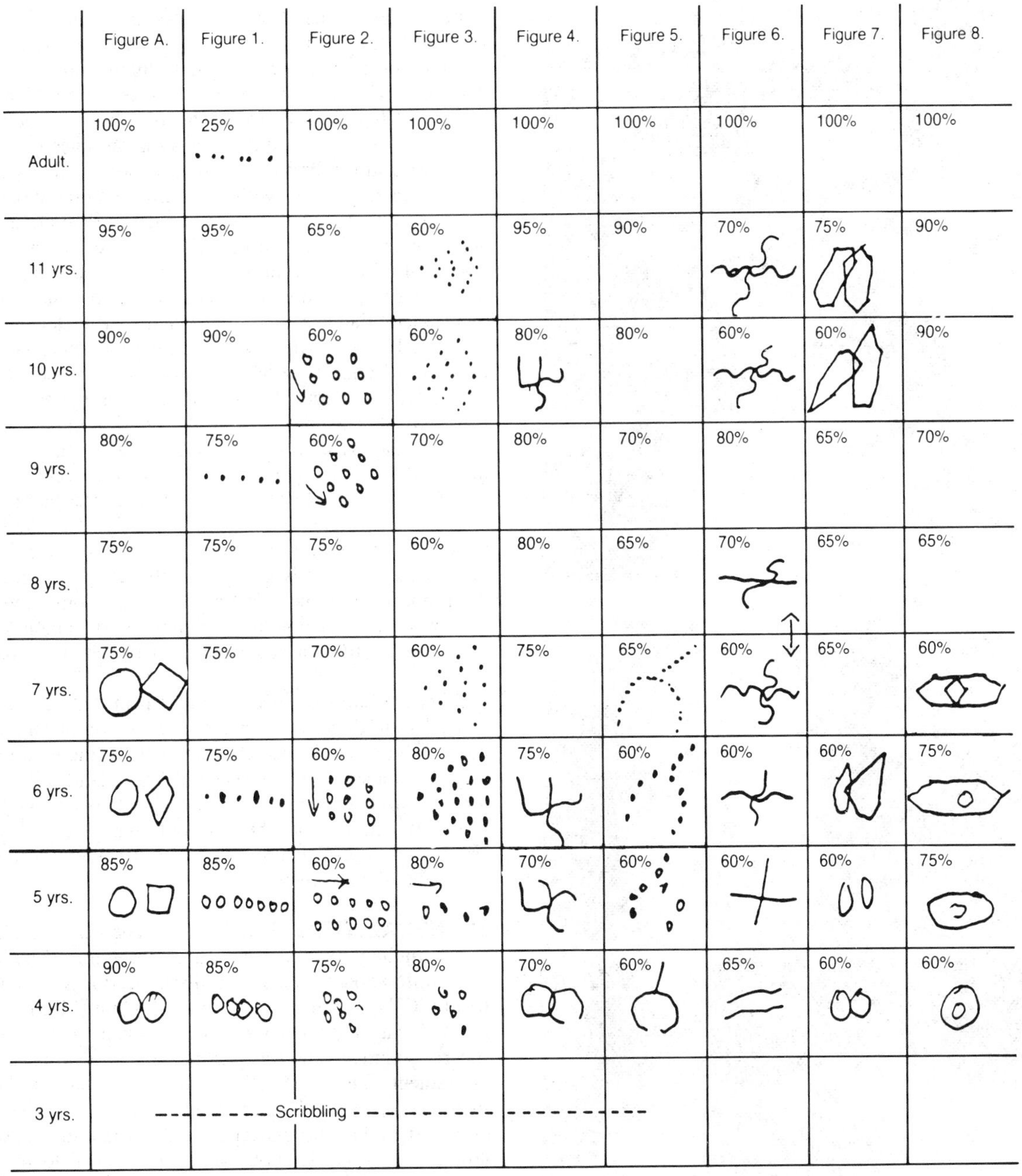
Figure A. Figure 1. Figure 2. Figure 3. Figure 4. Figure 5. Figure 6. Figure 7. Figure 8.
Adult. 100% 25% 100% 100% 100% 100% 100% 100% 100%
11 yrs. 95% 95% 65% 60% 95% 90% 70% 75% 90%
10 yrs. 90% 90% 60% 60% 80% 80% 60% 60% 90%
9 yrs. 80% 75% 60% 70% 80% 70% 80% 65% 70%
8 yrs. 75% 75% 75% 60% 80% 65% 70% 65% 65%
7 yrs. 75% 75% 70% 60% 75% 65% 60% 65% 60%
6 yrs. 75% 75% 60% 80% 75% 60% 60% 60% 75%
5 yrs. 85% 85% 60% 80% 70% 60% 60% 60% 75%
4 yrs. 90% 85% 75% 80% 70% 60% 65% 60% 60%
3 yrs.
Scribbling

FIGURE 9.5-9. *Percentage of children who could produce the type of response shown or better in copying the figures on the Bender (Visual Motor) Gestalt Test. Note the progressive maturational changes as reflected by increased ability to accurately reproduce the designs. (From Bender L:* A Visual Motor Gestalt Test and Its Clinical Use. *American Orthopsychiatric Association, New York, 1938, with permission.)*

AUDITORY PERCEPTION Auditory tasks include discrimination of words for the evaluation of learning disability in children, recognition of familiar nonverbal sounds to assess auditory agnosia, and appreciation of rhythm and tonal memory on Seashore's Test. Specific impairment of judgment of rhythm and tonal memory has been associated with right temporal lobe lesions. Auditory tasks used to assess processing of affective information were described previously.

SOMATOSENSORY PERCEPTION Somatosensory perception can be assessed by the Tactual Performance Test (TPT), which involves assembly of a form board in the absence of vision. The TPT is one of the most sensitive tests comprising the Halstead-Reitan Battery. A series of filaments of graded thickness are used to assess tactile thresholds in patients with lesions involving parietal cortex. Tactile form perception can be evaluated by presenting a series of textured geometric designs to each hand in the absence of visual cues and asking the patient to identify the corresponding design presented in a multiple-choice visual format. Protocols for localization of single and double simultaneous tactual stimulation of the fingers and right-left discrimination have been developed to detect cerebral disease, particularly of the parietal lobes. Inability to name objects as they are palpated may result from a corpus callosum lesion, particularly in the case of unilateral left tactile anomia.

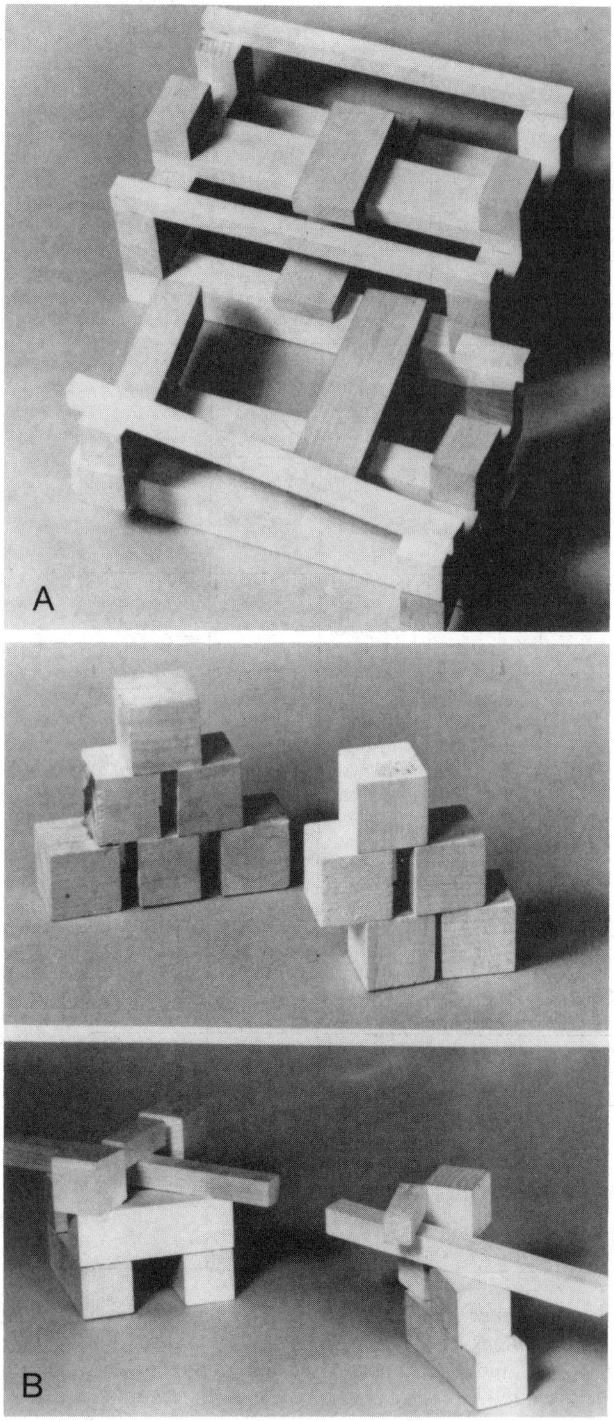

FIGURE 9.5-10. *Examples of "closing-in" error (A) and neglect of left side (B) on the three-dimensional constructional praxis test. (From Benton A L, Hamsher K deS, Varney N R, Spreen O:* Contributions to Neuropsychological Assessment. *Oxford University Press, New York, 1983, with permission).*

PSYCHOMOTOR FUNCTIONS A salient neurobehavioral effect of cerebral disease is slowness both in initiating behavior and in responding to external stimuli. For example, researchers found that in tests of reaction time, 40 percent of a group of brain-damaged patients were retarded on either simple tasks (e.g., pushing same button or key to onset of the same stimulus each trial) or tasks involving choice (e.g., pushing button or key corresponding to the onset of one of several randomly selected lights). Significant retardation is defined here as a response speed exceeded by 95 percent of control patients. Moreover, retardation in reaction time appears to be a deficit that reflects the presence (and possibly the size) of a cerebral lesion, independent of its locus. Thus, for example, patients with unilateral cerebral disease show reaction time retardation on the side ipsilateral, as well as contralateral, to the side of lesion. Studies of the effects of unilateral cerebral lesions on reaction time have disclosed more severe psychomotor retardation in patients with right-hemisphere damage than in patients with left-hemisphere damage. However, the results bearing on hemispheric asymmetry in reaction time have been inconsistent across studies. Similarly, the effects of task complexity on reaction time have been variable across studies of patients with unilateral lesions.

Investigations of diffuse or multifocal brain damage have indicated a positive relationship between task complexity and degree of deficit. Residual psychomotor retardation is a persistent effect of closed head injury in young adults and is related to the duration of coma and to task complexity. Slowing of reaction time is also positively related to age, but it is disproportionately increased by dementia. Some investigators employed the reaction time paradigm to demonstrate psychomotor retardation and attentional deficit in schizophrenic patients.

Other measures of speed of movement that have been used clinically are finger tapping and quickness in placing pegs in a board. There is evidence that the value of these simple speed tasks as indices of the presence of brain damage (particularly for comparing the performance of the two hands) compares favorably with that of other types of clinical tests. These tests can also be useful in assessing the efficacy of drugs in the treatment of movement disorder.

TRANSCALLOSAL FUNCTION The dissemination of research findings obtained in commissurotomized patients and the proliferation of reports on disconnection syndromes verified by CT or magnetic resonance imaging (MRI) of the corpus callosum have encouraged assessment of the interhemispheric communication as part of clinical neuropsychological assessment. These procedures are particularly indicated in suspected cases of alexia without agraphia and other features of visual verbal disconnection and in anterior callosal syndromes, such as ideomotor apraxia confined to the left upper extremity. Corpus callosum dysfunction also has been suggested in schizophrenia, but evidence for this view is equivocal.

Figure 9.5-11 illustrates the modalities and tasks employed by Sperry and Gazzaniga to study the effects of commissurotomy. Similar procedures have also been used to evaluate patients with alexia without agraphia arising from occlusion of the left posterior cerebral artery or surgical division of the splenium. As depicted in Figure 9.5-11, naming objects explored haptically by the left hand without the aid of vision and duplication of hand gestures (shown to the ipsilateral visual field or passively formed by the examiner) by the contralateral hand depend on the integrity of the anterior callosal pathways.

Tachistoscopic presentation of visual information to each visual field is employed to evaluate the capacities of the contralateral hemisphere for processing linguistic and emotive information in commissurotomized patients. Dichotic listening (i.e., simultaneous presentation of competing auditory in-

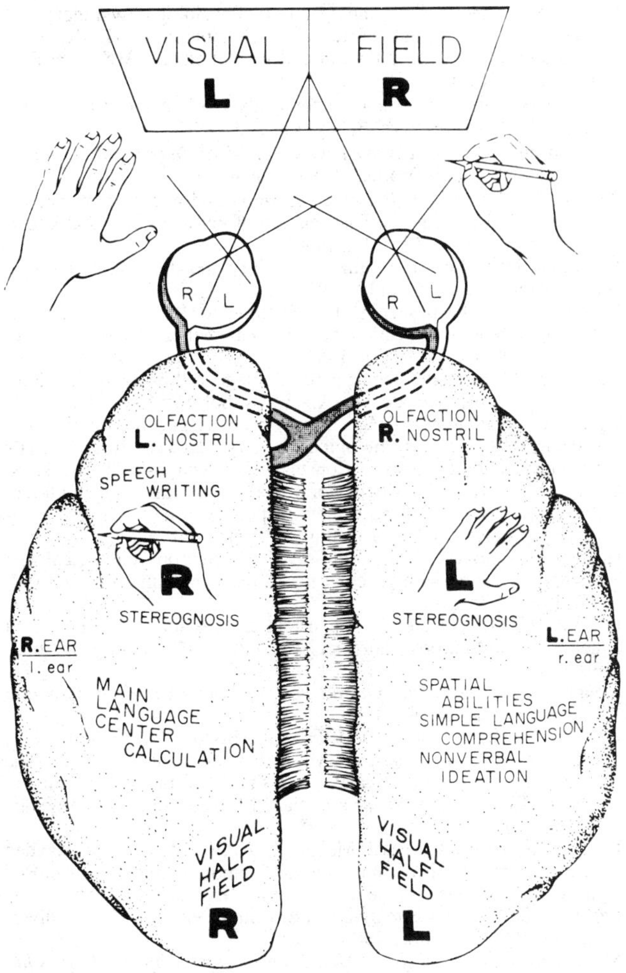

FIGURE 9.5-11. *Effects of commissurotomy on separation of neurological functions. This illustration is based on cortical lesion data and the results of studies of split-brain patients. (From Sperry R W: Lateral specialization in the surgically separated hemispheres. In* Hemispheric Specialization and Interaction, *B Milner, editor. MIT Press, Cambridge, MA, 1975, with permission).*

put to the two ears) may disclose markedly reduced monitoring of verbal information presented to the left ear when the corpus callosum is interrupted. This technique has been employed to investigate the efficiency of right-hemisphere functioning before and after treatment for depression, an illness that has been linked to nondominant hemisphere dysfunction. These procedures for assessment of callosal functioning have been extended to diverse problems, including traumatic injury to the corpus callosum, interhemispheric communication in psychiatric disorder, and agenesis of the callosum.

NEUROPSYCHOLOGICAL TEST BATTERIES

HALSTEAD-REITAN BATTERY (HRB) The basic battery in its present form consists of the following five tests:

1. *Category test.* This is a test of abstract reasoning and hypothesis testing in which the subject has to discover through trial and error the correct principle (e.g., number, spatial position) embodied in successive presentations of pictorial stimuli. The correct principle is changed across seven subtests.

2. *Tactual Performance Test (TPT).* The subject is required to place the variously shaped blocks of the Seguin-Goddard Form Board without the aid of vision. Time taken to place the blocks is the critical response measure. An incidental test of retention follows in which the subject is required to draw the board from memory. The number of blocks correctly drawn is the memory response measure. A spatial localization measure is derived from the accuracy of drawing the relative positions of the blocks from memory. The TPT is presumed to assess several abilities, including motor speed, use of tactile and kinesthetic cues, learning, and incidental memory (no forewarning is given that the drawing test follows).

3. *Rhythm Test.* This test, which is adapted from Seashore's Test of Musical Talent, requires the subject to judge whether two auditory rhythmic patterns (30 pairs) are the same or different. The Rhythm Test is interpreted as a measure of nonverbal auditory perception, attention, and sustained concentration.

4. *Speech Sounds Perception Test.* The subject is required to identify spoken nonsense syllables from four visually presented alternatives. This test assesses auditory-verbal perception, attention, and concentration.

5. *Finger Oscillation.* The subject taps a mechanical counter at maximum speed for 10 seconds per trial with the index finger of each hand. Absolute motor speed and right-left asymmetries are measured.

The HRB yields seven scores from which an Impairment Index is derived by dividing the number of defective scores (based on normative data) and dividing by seven. Additions to this core examination include the Trail Making Test, which measures the time required to draw a line between scattered circles in alphabetic (Trail A) or alphanumeric (Trail B) sequence, various modifications of the Aphasia Screening Test of Halstead and Wepman, a somatosensory examination including finger gnosis, graphesthesia, stereognosis, and double simultaneous stimulation, and a measure of grip strength using a dynamometer. The Wechsler Memory Scale, or other memory tests (see subsection on memory), are also commonly administered because the HRB is limited in this respect to an incidental recall trial on the TPT.

The HRB has the advantage of providing a uniform profile of scores that must be weighed against the considerable time required for administration. Although the results adequately differentiate brain-damaged from neurologically intact persons, the differential diagnosis of psychiatric versus neurologic disorder is unimpressive. Specifically, schizophrenic patients tend to perform above the level of subacutely brain-damaged patients, but not differently from chronic brain-damaged groups. Moreover, the pattern of deficits on the HRB is similar in brain-damaged and schizophrenic patients. It should be noted that similar conclusions have emerged when other tests have been subjected to studies attempting to discriminate patients with schizophrenia from patients with confirmed brain damage. In point of fact, neuropsychological tests are more useful for neurobehavioral investigations of schizophrenia than in routine differential diagnosis. The brief tests of sensory and motor function on the HRB appear to contribute to the assessment of lateralization of lesion, but the degree to which other components contribute information beyond the WAIS results is uncertain.

Luria's neuropsychological investigation Christensen has developed a set of materials comprising a text, manual of instructions, and test cards that represent the techniques employed by Luria and his conceptualization of cortical functions. These procedures have been reorganized into 10 sections according to specific functions (e.g., motor, sensory, visual, language skill). Items are also derived from standardized tests, such as Kohs blocks and hidden figures that Luria used, and from the mental status examination (e.g., digit span, serial sevens).

The complex motor tasks developed by Luria are particularly innovative and least redundant with other neuropsychological tests. The motor tests include commands requiring the patient to make a hand response that is the alternate of the examiner's hand movement (e.g.,

"Tap once when the examiner taps twice") and a "go–no-go" discrimination (e.g., "Squeeze the examiner's hand at the word 'red'; do nothing at the word 'green' "); alternating commands (e.g., "Raise the right hand in response to one signal, the left hand to two signals"). This test battery has other unique features, including detailed assessment of arithmetic and short-term memory for hand postures.

Christensen's adaptation of Luria's methods is a potentially useful adjunct to the clinical neuropsychological examination, particularly in respect to motor integration. Although many of the tests are not sufficiently difficult to detect subtle deficit, they can be used with severely impaired patients. Insufficient normative data and omission of tests of functions, such as verbal memory, discourages total reliance on this battery.

LURIA-NEBRASKA NEUROPSYCHOLOGICAL BATTERY In contrast to Luria's strategy of modifying his methods of study according to the research question and the capabilities of his patients, Golden and co-workers developed a battery that incorporates items and the categories in Christensen's manual. These scales include: Motor, Rhythm, Tactile (cutaneous and kinesthetic), Visual (spatial), Receptive and Expressive Speech, Writing, Reading, Arithmetic, Amnestic, and Intellectual. Golden and colleagues added a pathognomonic scale consisting of the items drawn from the other scales that they found to be maximally sensitive to brain dysfunction. The authors also added right- and left-hemisphere scales, reflecting items that measure unilateral sensorimotor function. In practice, a profile of transformed standard scores (after correction for age and education) is used in interpretation of the patient's performance.

Golden's adaptation and modification of a portion of the techniques employed by Luria (as compiled by Christensen) and standardization for clinical use have raised methodological questions. Lezak concluded from her review of the Luria-Nebraska that "the examiner must be extremely cautious about drawing conclusions based on the scores and indices of this battery as presently constituted."

Clinical tests and experimental tasks developed by neuropsychologists have contributed immensely to recent neurobehavioral studies of neurological and psychiatric disorders. In clinical practice, the usefulness of neuropsychological testing depends, to a great extent, on the examiner's knowledge of the disorder in question and both the sensitivity and the specificity of the individual measures and test batteries. Although different strategies of neuropsychological testing can often provide the psychiatrist with information pertinent to diagnosis and clinical management, the amount of information gained generally reflects the training and experience of the neuropsychologist. Positive neuropsychological findings in psychiatric patients can be frequently explained on a basis other than acquired cerebral lesions, whereas negative results hardly rule out a structural brain abnormality. Further research is needed to elucidate diagnostic implications of neuropsychological findings in psychiatric patients.

REFERENCES

Bender L: *A Visual Motor Gestalt Test and Its Clinical Use*. American Orthopsychiatric Association, New York, 1938.

Benton A L: *The Revised Visual Retention Test: Clinical and Experimental Applications*, ed 4. Psychological Corporation, New York, 1974.

Benton A L: Reaction time in brain disease: Some reflections. Cortex *22:* 129, 1986.

Benton A L, Hamsher K deS, Varney N R, Spreen O: *Contributions to Neuropsychological Assessment: A Clinical Manual*. Oxford University Press, New York, 1983.

Berman K F, Zec R F, Weinberger D R: Physiologic dysfunction of dorsolateral prefrontal cortex in schizophrenia. II. Role of neuroleptic treatment, attention and mental effort. Arch Gen Psychiat *43:* 126, 1986.

Buschke H: Selective reminding for analysis of memory and learning. J Verb Learn Verb Behav *12:* 543, 1973.

Christensen A-L: *Luria's Neuropsychological Investigation*, ed 2. Ejnar Munksgaards Vorlag, Copenhagen, 1979.

Cohen N J, Squire L R: Preserved learning and retention of pattern-analysis skill in amnesia: Dissociation of knowing how and knowing that. Science *210:* 207, 1980.

Drachman D A, Leavitt J: Human memory and the cholinergic system. Arch Neurol *30:* 113, 1974.

Eslinger P J, Damasio A R, Benton A L, Van Allen M: Neuropsychologic detection of abnormal mental decline in older persons. JAMA *253:* 670, 1985.

Gazzaniga M S: Right hemisphere language following brain bisection: A 20-year perspective. Amer Psychol *38:* 525, 1983.

Golden C J, Hammeke T A, Purisch A D: Diagnostic validity of a standardized neuropsychological battery derived from Luria's neuropsychological tests. J Consult Clin Psychol *46:* 1258, 1978.

Grant D A, Berg E A: A behavioral analysis of degree of reinforcement and ease of shifting to new responses in a Weigl-type card-sorting problem. J Exp Psychol *38:* 404, 1948.

Heaton R K, Baade L E, Johnson K L: Neuropsychological test results associated with psychiatric disorders in adults. Psychol Bull *85:* 141, 1978.

Heilman K M, Bowers D, Valenstein E, Watson R T: The right hemisphere: Neuropsychological functions. J Neurosurg *64:* 693, 1986.

Koppitz E M: *The Bender Gestalt Test for Young Children*. Grune & Stratton, Orlando, FL, 1983.

Levin H S, High W M Jr, Goethe K E, Sisson R A, Overall J E, Rhoades H M, Eisenberg H M, Kalisky Z, Gary H E Jr.: The neurobehavioral rating scale: Assessment of the behavioral sequelae of head injury by the clinician. J Neurol Neurosurg Psychiat *50:* 183, 1987.

Levin H S, High W M Jr., Meyers C A, Von Laufen A, Hayden M E, Eisenberg, H M: Impairment of remote memory after closed head injury. J Neurol Neurosurg Psychiat *48:* 556, 1985.

Lezak M D: *Neuropsychological Assessment*, ed 2. Oxford University Press, New York, 1983.

Matarazzo J D: *Wechsler's Measurement and Appraisal of Adult Intelligence*, ed 5. Williams & Wilkins, Baltimore, 1972.

Mesulam M M: A cortical network for directed attention and unilateral neglect. Ann Neurol *10:* 309, 1981.

Milner B: Effects of different brain lesions on card sorting. Arch Neurol *9:* 90, 1963.

Nelson A, Fogel B S, Faust D: Bedside cognitive screening instruments. A critical assessment. J Nerv Ment Dis *174:* 73, 1986.

Peters B H, Levin H S: Effects of physostigmine and lecithin on memory in Alzheimer disease. Ann Neurol *6:* 219, 1979.

Reitan R M: Theoretical and methodological bases of the Halstead-Reitan Neuropsychological Test Battery. In *Neuropsychological Assessment of Neuropsychiatric Disorders*, I Grant, K M Adams, editors, p 3. Oxford University Press, New York, 1986.

Sackeim H A, Greenberg M S, Weiman A L, Gur R C, Hungerbuhler J P, Geschwind N: Hemispheric asymmetry in the expression of positive and negative emotions. Neurologic evidence. Arch Neurol *39:* 210, 1982.

Sperry R W: Lateral specialization in the surgical separated hemispheres. In *Hemispheric Specialization and Interaction*, B Milner, editor. MIT Press, Cambridge, MA, 1975.

Sternberg D E, Jarvik M E: Memory functions in depression. Improvement with antidepressant medication. Arch Gen Psychiat *33:* 219, 1976.

Storandt M, Botwinick J, Danziger W L, Berg L, Hughes C P: Psychometric differentiation of mild senile dementia of the Alzheimer type. Arch Neurol *41:* 497, 1984.

Terman L M, Merrill M A: *Stanford-Binet. Manual for the Third Revision*. Houghton Mifflin, Boston, 1960.

Wechsler D: *WAIS-R Manual*. Psychological Corporation, New York, 1981.

Weingartner H, Cohen R M, Murphy D L, Martello J, Gerdt C: Cognitive processes in depression. Arch Gen Psychiat *38:* 42, 1981.

Wexler B E: Cerebral laterality and psychiatry: A review of the literature. Amer J Psychiat *137:* 3, 1980.

9.6 NEUROPSYCHOLOGICAL AND INTELLECTUAL ASSESSMENT OF CHILDREN

JACK M. FLETCHER, Ph.D.
HARVEY S. LEVIN, Ph.D.
PAUL SATZ, Ph.D.

INTRODUCTION

Neuropsychological approaches to the assessment of children are currently of great interest to practitioners in psychology, psychiatry, neurology, and education. Recent years have seen the publication of a variety of chapters and major texts on child neuropsychology, many of which have assessment as their major focus. Unfortunately, as is true in any area of rapid development, confusion can prevail as to the nature and purpose of neuropsychological assessment. Some practitioners, for example, emphasize the value of assessment for differential diagnosis of disorders that are functional or organic in nature. This emphasis in especially apparent in applications to psychiatry and the evaluation of emotionally disturbed children. Other approaches emphasize the value of neuropsychological assessments for determining cognitive impairments and strengths in an individual child, with remedial plans often emerging from these evaluations. These approaches include treatment as a major goal of the assessment.

Regardless of the approach, perhaps the most general view focuses on a process of evaluating individual children. In this view, neuropsychological assessment is seen as the administration and interpretation of a set of psychometric tests measuring a broad range of specific cognitive abilities necessary for success at school and in the community. These procedures are interpreted statistically according to psychometric properties of the tests as well as the context of the child's performance (e.g., school expectations, motivation, and emotional factors). Performance on these tests may have relationships with brain functions and, as such, may permit organismic inferences based on the emerging body of brain-behavior relationships in children. Regardless of these levels of inference, the assessment should lead to a remedial plan addressing the habilitation of the child from cognitive and behavioral (emotional) perspectives.

PURPOSES OF NEUROPSYCHOLOGICAL ASSESSMENT

Neuropsychological procedures have been applied to a broad range of childhood problems, including various neurological disorders (e.g., head injury, hydrocephalus, epilepsy), learning and attentional disorders, and emotional disorders. Regardless of the nature of the presenting disorder, key questions often revolve around possible cognitive impairments and their influence on school performance and behavior. Although neuropsychologists may attempt assessment to assist with decisions concerning the extent to which brain status or a particular neurological disorder contributes to the presenting problem, the focus is on identifying and measuring cognitive strengths and weaknesses as the basis for developing a remedial plan. As such, the purposes of neuropsychological assessment often overlap with other assessment-oriented disciplines (e.g., education). What distinguishes child neuropsychology from other assessment disciplines is the emphasis on a broad range of cognitive functions and an interest in brain-related bases of behavior.

REFERRAL QUESTIONS There are a variety of questions that lead to referral of a child for neuropsychological evaluation. The most general questions concern school performance, with issues revolving around the degree to which the child's academic performance is related to a learning disability or brain injury as opposed to other factors operant in the child's environment (e.g., family problems, curriculum). Other frequent questions concern children with problems in conduct and behavior at home and school. The question is often the degree to which cognitive dysfunctions contribute to the behavior problem. In addition to traditional psychological treatments, it may be necessary to remediate the cognitive problem and even to adjust the psychological intervention according to the child's capacity for processing information.

Referrals come from many sources, including parents, school personnel, psychiatrists, neurologists, and other health care providers. Upon referral, contact is made with the parents with an explanation of the nature and purpose of the evaluation. For children, early involvement of the family is critical. If the family is not centrally included in the evaluation, it will be difficult to identify relevant variables (e.g., parenting skills, marital dissatisfaction, finances) that contribute to the child's difficulties. In addition, any interventions must reflect the family's ability to respond. There is little point in recommending services that the family cannot afford or is categorically opposed to because of poor previous experiences.

If a referral is made in which there are questions concerning the etiology of a child's disability that are beyond a neuropsychologist's expertise, the referral questions should be discussed and clarified. For example, children sometimes are referred by educators who are concerned that a distractible child has a seizure disorder. This question cannot be determined by a neuropsychological evaluation. In this example, the evaluation should be completed only if there is a question about attention, learning, or behavior. Neuropsychological evaluations may provide data that assist with diagnosis, but are not in and of themselves diagnostic of medical disorders. This question of seizure disorders should be referred to a pediatric neurologist for a neurological evaluation. For more general questions, such as whether a child with a severe behavioral disorder who shows no evidence for overt neurological disease has an organic problem, the concerns and observations that led to the referral should be carefully discussed. However, the question should be posed as the extent to which constitutional and environmental factors contribute to the presenting disorder. Neuropsychologists rarely make specific statements concerning either etiology or pathology, or both, solely on the basis of psychometric procedures. In addition, the question is often trivial, inasmuch as the answer rarely has known treatment consequences in the behavioral domain.

The primary responsibility of the child neuropsychologist is the identification of the cognitive and behavioral correlates (and consequences) of emotional, learning, and neurological disorders. The results should be translated into a remedial plan for allied professionals (e.g., physicians) and for potential sources of intervention (e.g., educators). One advantage of an emphasis on cognitive processes is the focus on behavior and the de-emphasis of "neurologizing" about children. Terms, such as "organic brain syndrome" or "minimal brain injury," are generally empty and meaningless, with little implication for intervention. Nonetheless, such concepts are frequently proposed as the basis for referral, particularly when the etiology of the present problems is not known. In accepting such referrals, the neuropsychologist must establish that the assessment is an ability-oriented evaluation designed to help formulate the problem and determine specific approaches for intervention. Information may be derived that will contribute to an understanding of etiology, but this information must be evaluated in conjunction with other sources of diagnostic information. Neuropsychology offers a careful analysis of ability structure and the many factors influencing the child's behavior and does not establish (in isolation) physical diagnosis or etiology.

CLASSIFICATION ISSUES AND NEUROPSYCHOLOGICAL INFERENCE To explicate the critical issue concerning this view of the purpose of neuropsychological evaluation, consider referrals that simply ask for an assessment of the presence or absence of a brain-related disorder. With adults, the primary manifestations of many neurological diseases are behavioral in nature (e.g., memory loss in dementia). This is less true in children, in whom relationships of behavior and neurological disease are less well known and possibly more indirect. Unfortunately, despite this problem, determining whether a child has a brain-related disorder is often made on the basis of behavioral signs. The tendency to infer brain dysfunction in children based solely on behavioral signs has a long history in psychology, child psychiatry, and neurology. In recent years, the conceptual framework underlying this way of thinking about childhood disorders, particularly those disorders characterized by an absence of evidence for neurological disease, has been widely criticized across disciplines. These concerns apply specifically to common learning, attentional, and behavior disorders in which brain injury is excluded by history and current presentation (e.g., attention-deficit hyperactivity disorder, developmental reading disorder).

The notion that certain childhood learning and behavioral disorders are brain related is a viable hypothesis. For example, various forms of brain injury have been observed to produce changes in a child's ability to learn as well as patterns of behavior. Where problems have arisen is the tendency to view behavioral signs as ipso facto evidence of underlying brain dysfunction.

History The history of such thinking can be represented as the "concept of cerebral dysfunction." In the early 1900s, Sir George F. Still attributed certain cases of impulsive behavior to an unobservable brain disorder. The notion was that when environmental causes could be ruled out as contributory, these children must have a brain dysfunction that is simply not measurable. Similarly, the organic psychiatrists Kahn and Cohen argued in the 1930s that certain cases of impulsive, acting-out behavior represented brain-related disorders. The cases they observed had histories of head injury, measles encephalitis, or other neurological disorders from which physical recovery was sufficient to eliminate classic neurological signs of brain damage (e.g., hemiparesis). It was argued that this history supported the presence of what Kahn and Cohen felt was a distinct brain damage syndrome that could not be explained by then current psychoanalytic explanations focusing on the environment.

The "Straussian movement," popular in the 1940s and 1950s, is the most contemporary influence on the concept of cerebral dysfunction. On the basis of observations of mentally retarded children, Robert Strauss and associates argued that children who displayed impulsive, hyperactive behavior had minimal brain injury. This term was subsequently expanded to include children with achievement deficiencies. Strauss emphasized that the pattern of behavior in and of itself was sufficient evidence for the diagnosis of minimal brain injury, even in the absence of evidence or history of brain injury. In the 1960s, various federal task forces adopted Strauss's concept and modified the notion of minimal brain injury into definitions of minimal brain dysfunction and a corresponding achievement-oriented definition of specific learning disability.

Cerebral dysfunction and differential diagnosis The concept of cerebral dysfunction and the accompanying definitions have been widely criticized. The assumptions underlying this concept suggest that: (1) brain injury produces unitary forms of behavioral disorder; (2) there is a continuum of brain injury and, thus, if serious forms of injury result in death or intellectual retardation, mild forms result in learning and behavioral problems; and (3) there is an isomorphic relationship between behavior and the brain, so that certain behavioral signs are direct indicants of brain dysfunction. Each of these assumptions is false and misleading, with numerous logical fallacies (e.g., the isomorphism hypothesis) as well as a general absence of empirical evidence supporting either the hypothesis of unitary forms of behavioral disorder or a continuum of brain injury. The concept of minimal brain dysfunction is now frequently disregarded and does not appear in major neurological and psychiatric classifications, such as the revised third edition of the American Psychiatric Association's *Diagnostic and Statistical Manual of Mental Disorders* (DSM-III-R). Similarly, although the concept of specific learning disorders remains popular (and is inherent in DSM-III-R), this concept has also been widely criticized because available definitions have not yielded empirically validated criteria for diagnosing learning disability.

The concepts of cerebral dysfunction and differential diagnosis pervade both observational and test-based assessments of children. Since there is no evidence for unitary patterns of behavior attributable to brain injury, observing that a child is overactive and inattentive does not provide direct evidence that there is a brain-related etiology. Similarly, the presence of paraclassical or soft neurological signs on physical examination has not been established as a reliable indicator of a biological basis for the disorder. Indeed, studies comparing learning-impaired and attentionally impaired children with conduct-disordered children on soft signs and electroencephalogram (EEG) findings have yielded null results.

In a sense, the goal of these types of studies is to infer the status of the child's central nervous system (CNS). Such inferences require a set of empirically validated behavior-brain relationships, which have been well developed for many adult disorders. These relationships, however, can only be established when independent assessments of the child's behavior and CNS have been made. When such correlations are established, they pertain only to that patient population and cannot be extrapolated ipso facto to other populations. For example, brain-injured children may generate certain patterns of test responses. Observing a similar pattern in a child with no demonstrable injury does not validate an inference to the same type of injury. The pattern only indicates that the hypothesis is viable. Behavior in children is too variable and complex, and current understanding of the CNS and relationships with children's behavior is not sufficient, to permit this type of loose and careless reasoning.

Treatment implications Given these problems, it is not surprising that many contemporary approaches to child neuropsychological assessment have moved away from differential diagnosis toward more rounded approaches emphasizing treatment. The emphasis is not so much on deciding whether the problem is brain related, which is a relatively straightforward decision. Rather, the emphasis is on a detailed assessment of the ability structure of the child. From this assessment, decisions are made concerning prognosis and remediation plans. With this approach, a broad range of childhood disorders can be valuably served, ranging from children with various forms of brain injury to non–brain-injured children with learning and behavioral problems.

Many neuropsychologists are now engaged in systematic studies of children, particularly learning and attentional disorders, head injuries, and various emotional disorders. It is entirely possible that specific neuropsychological patterns can be defined within these large groups that have treatment and prognostic implications. Through such studies it is becoming increasingly possible to identify characteristic forms of cognitive disability that often overlap across groups. By studying the relationship of these profiles with variables describing the etiology and pathology of the disorders, clinicians may be able to derive a greater understanding of brain-behavior relationships in children. However, a major focus of clinical neuropsychological assessment of children will continue to center on the nature of ability strengths and weaknesses with an emphasis on treatment.

From this point of view, child neuropsychological assessment is a methodology for defining and remediating cognitive adaptational problems in children. This emphasis departs from traditional uses of psychometric tests for differential diagnosis. For example, the Bender-Gestalt, a perceptual-motor copying test for children, is frequently scored according to whether errors are emotional or neurological indicators. Using neuropsychological tests for this type of differential diagnosis assumes that (1) disorders of childhood can be easily categorized as organic or functional and that (2) specific treatment recommendations stem from these independent diagnoses. Neither assumption is correct. Classification issues in child psychiatry have not been adequately resolved to permit these types of etiological distinctions based on psychometric tests, behavioral observation, or even some features of the physical examination. Regardless of organic or functional categories, all children benefit from a careful assessment of abilities, with treatment planning following this assessment independently of diagnosis. For example, some emotionally disturbed children have difficulty learning in school. Even if the child's problems stem primarily from the emotional area, an assessment of school-related abilities may be useful in improving the child's response to instruction. A child who is stronger in visual-spatial skills may benefit from an approach to reading instruction that de-emphasizes phonetic decoding of words in favor of a sight-based approach. Such an approach may help reduce response to frustration and improve motivation. Similarly, most brain-injured children require careful instruction-oriented evaluations for school planning. However, if the child also presents a conduct problem, a behavioral program addressing these problem behaviors may be useful. Treatment plans can be developed from assessment results for both brain-damaged and emotionally disturbed children. The problem is not differential diagnosis, but the need for a careful assessment of adaptive strengths and weaknesses.

APPROACHES TO NEUROPSYCHOLOGICAL ASSESSMENT Specific methods for the neuropsychological assessment of children vary across settings and practitioners. Some neuropsychologists prefer the use of modified versions of standard neuropsychological batteries, such as the Halstead-Reitan Neuropsychological Battery. These neuropsychologists have systematically applied these procedures to thousands of children with learning disabilities, brain injuries, and emotional problems. Specific interpretative relationships across these disorders, along with remedial plans, have emerged from these applications. Other neuropsychologists focus on traditional intellectual, language, and perceptual tests and use them as the basis for assessment. The goal is to identify syndromes and develop intervention plans for children.

Another approach provides an explicit focus on measuring specific cognitive skills. Traditional instruments are employed, but these child neuropsychologists also use measures of cognitive skills drawn directly from the experimental literature on normal child development. Measures of phonological awareness for assessing reading difficulties in children are used because of the extensive evidence that these processes are highly related to reading proficiency. With head-injured children, various memory tests sensitive to the effects of head injury are employed. Others outlined several language tests for assessing learning-disabled and brain-injured children derived from contemporary psycholinguistic theories of the organization and development of language.

All approaches have contributed to the expanding knowledge base on the neurobehavioral correlates of various childhood disorders. Although the specific tests may vary across practitioners, the principles, goals, and methods of interpretation are quite similar. First, in each approach, psychometric tests are administered to help define the nature of the problem (e.g., intellectual, learning, attentional, language, or motor disability). Second, each approach administers other measures of cognitive skills that are correlated with the disorder. For example, children with reading problems often have difficulty with language skills. An attempt then is made to define the exact nature of any language deficiencies in the context of other cognitive skills. Third, an assessment is made of environmental variables that might impinge on the child's performance on the tests and on habilitation potential. A child who is inattentive, unmotivated, or easily frustrated may not display true potential on psychometric tests. Cultural variables are well known for their influence on intelligence tests and have similar effects on other cognitive tasks. For remediation, family resources may limit options in terms of various available services. Fourth, these three levels of analysis are compared with historical and current medical data to establish relationships of the child's ability structure and CNS integrity. Fifth, a remedial plan is developed on the basis of the results of the assessment. This plan will typically highlight areas for intervention, provide methods for remediation, and, if necessary, identify potential agents of intervention (e.g., special education).

ASSESSMENT MODEL. Figure 9.6-1 provides a schematic overview of the various levels of analysis that are common to neuropsychological assessment of children. This model divides the assessment process into four components:

1. The *manifest disabilities* represent the problems leading to the assessment, learning (e.g., school-based problems), language difficulties, and problems with conduct. Assessing the manifest disability requires interview of the child, parent, and teacher; developmental and medical histories; behavioral observation; and psychometric assessment.
2. *Basic competencies* are core skills (memory, attention, language) that correlate with the manifest disability. These skills are assessed with neuropsychological tests.
3. *Moderator variables* are social, environmental, and motivational factors that influence the covariation of the manifest disability and basic competencies. These variables determine the child's ability to cope and adjust to the presenting disorder.
4. *Biological indices* represent neurological influences on the relationship of manifest disabilities and basic competencies. The lesion of an aphasic child, severity of a closed head injury, and family history of learning disability are examples of biological variables that would influence ability development.

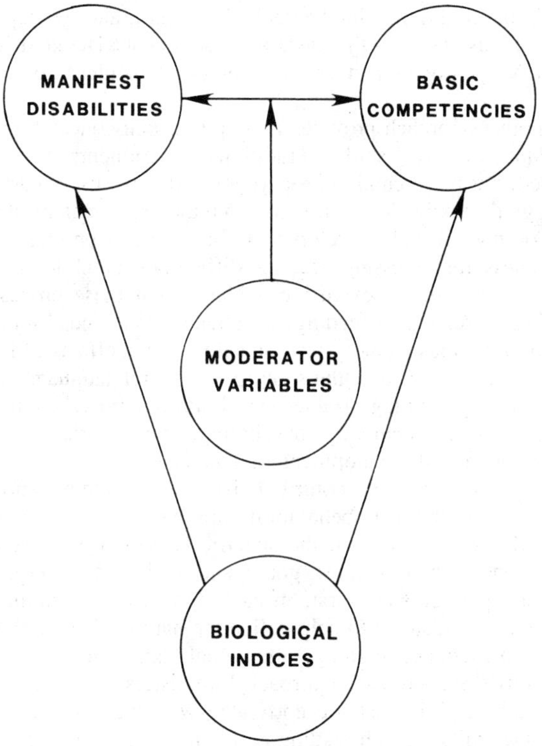

FIGURE 9.6-1. *Model for neuropsychological assessment of children.*

The four components in Figure 9.6-1 can be represented as three levels of analysis. At the first level, the neuropsychologist attempts to understand the relationship of the presenting problems (manifest disabilities) and a set of core skills (basic competencies). At the second level of analysis, the influence of external factors on the interaction of the manifest disabilities and basic competencies is considered. Children do not develop problems in isolation of the environment and internal variables, such as attitude and motivation. At the third level, attempts are made to understand how various CNS variables influence the relationship of the manifest disabilities, basic competencies, and moderator variables. The biological indices are assumed to influence behavior, but the question is the degree to which the influence is apparent in the child's ability structure. The analysis of the nature of the presenting problems begins at the level of behavior and proceeds to a more biological level. The purpose is to understand the relationship of these four components at behavioral and biological levels of analysis, not to make simplistic inferences concerning CNS status.

DEVELOPING A REMEDIAL PLAN Byron Rourke and colleagues have conveniently outlined the various steps in developing and implementing a remedial plan (Fig. 9.6-2). This model outlines seven steps underlying the development and implementation of an intervention plan.

The first step is a consideration of the interaction of the child's ability structure and variables related to brain status, representing the product of the evaluation process outlined in Figure 9.6-1. At this step, results of the neuropsychological assessment are formulated and decisions on the impact of brain status on adaptive function are made. This relationship is hardly direct and must be made on a case-by-case basis.

In step 2, immediate and long-term demands of the environment are considered. These demands—which represent such problems as the nature of the school environment, academic expectations, and how demands change as the child ages—represent major considerations for the implementation of an intervention plan. They vary with age and stage of treatment, and, therefore, the treatment plan must be individualized and flexible.

Steps 3 and 4 represent attempts to develop hypotheses about prognosis (step 3) and the ideal short- and long-term treatment plan (step 4). This part of the plan should be written so that the results of any intervention can be evaluated against hypothesized outcomes and goals. Step 5 concerns the availability of treatment resources, including not only the presence of certain types of intervention, but also family variables (e.g., finances, child rearing) that influence the family's capacity to participate in the developing habilitation plan. Along with the variables reviewed in step 2, step 5 represents what was described in Figure 9.6-1 as *moderator variables*: factors that influence the covariance of ability structure, biological variables, and the child's disability. In step 6, the most realistic remedial plan is formulated and implemented based on what is ideal (step 4) and possible (steps 2 and 5). Step 7 concerns the need to continue to follow the child with repeat assessments and modifications of the treatment plan.

This model highlights the major considerations involved in clinical neuropsychological practice with children. Assessment instruments and interpretations may vary, but these are relatively minor considerations so long as basic reliability and validity criteria are met. The model in Figure 9.6-2 allows the clinician to move beyond the assessment and to develop a specific plan for treating the child. This plan may involve other disciplines and resources, but it stems from the assessment.

TESTING PROCEDURES The specific instruments used by child neuropsychologists vary across setting. What is common is the use of measures of (1) intelligence; (2) academic achievement; (3) behavioral adjustment; and (4) various cognitive and motor skills.

Intelligence tests Table 9.6-1 summarizes some of the major tests used to assess intelligence in children. Each of these tests includes different scales that typically yield composite scores addressing verbal and nonverbal performance skills. The scales, in turn, are composed of various subtests that vary according to the nature and demand of the actual tasks. All of these tasks yield an overall composite intelligence quotient (I.Q.), with separate scores for verbal, performance, and other subtest combinations making up the scales. These tests have national standardizations across age cohorts and yield statistically derived scores that permit an estimate of the child's rank in the population. In general, scores of 100 are considered average, with scores below 70 representing the lowest 2 percent of the population. Children scoring below 70 are often candidates for the diagnosis of mental retardation, provided that they also show comparable decrements in adaptive and social functioning. Table 9.6-2 presents a classification of I.Q. scores commonly used to designate intellectual levels in children.

The specific tests vary in terms of constituent subtests, type of national standardization, and the underlying concept of intelligence. For example, the Stanford-Binet was one of the earliest measures of intelligence. Previous versions of the Stanford-Binet yielded only a single composite I.Q. score and were frequently criticized for inadequate standardizations. More recently, the Stanford-Binet was redesigned into a new format yielding a composite I.Q. score as well as scores for four separate scales (Verbal Reasoning, Abstract-Visual Reasoning, Quantitative Reasoning, Short-Term Memory). This version was only recently released, and data concerning its utility as an intelligence test have been sparse. However, the format and

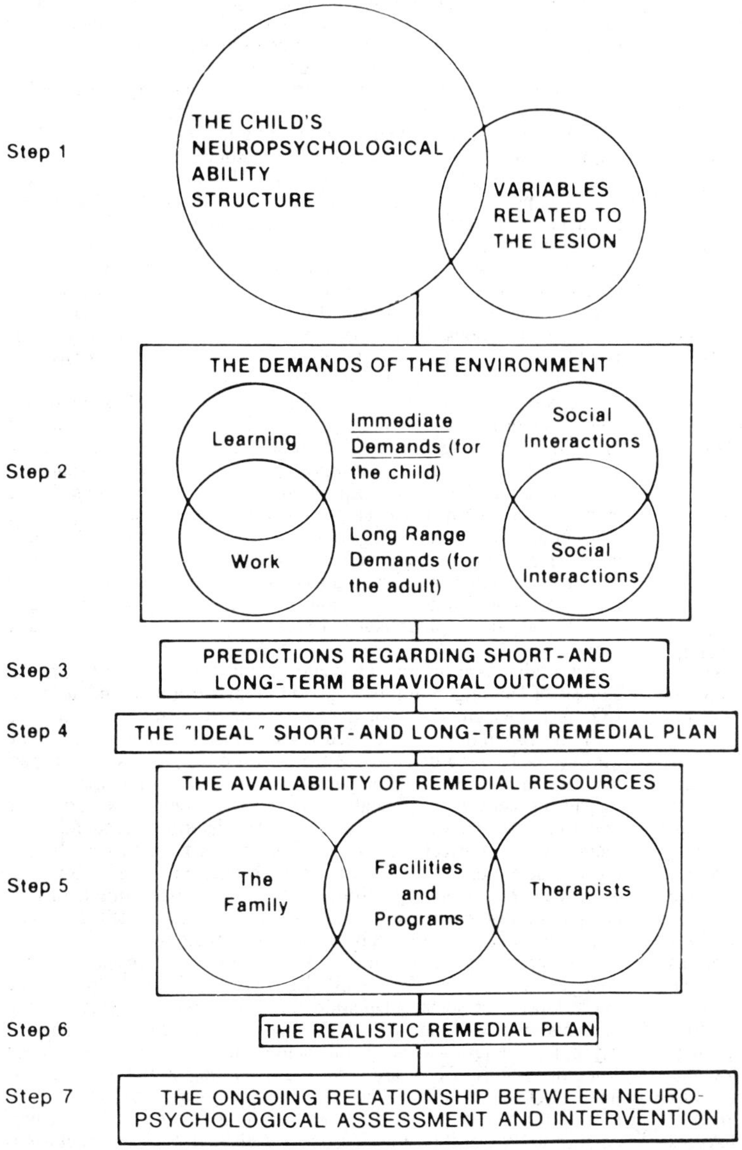

FIGURE 9.6-2. *Model for development of habilitation plans for children.*

standardization are clearly superior to earlier versions of the Stanford-Binet.

The recently developed Kaufman Assessment Battery for Children (K-ABC) conceptualizes intelligence according to a model of cognitive processing distinguishing simultaneous and sequential processing skills. Hence, subtests are designed according to whether the task requires the child to process information along one of these two dimensions. In addition to an overall score, composites for simultaneous and sequential processing subtests are provided.

The McCarthy Scales of Children's Abilities is a more traditional test that is unique because (along with the Bayley Scales of Infant Development) it yields a separate composite for fine and gross motor skills. The McCarthy also yields an overall composite (General Cognitive Index) and separate scores for Verbal, Perceptual-Performance, Quantitative, and Memory scales. The McCarthy is often used instead of the Wechsler Preschool and Primary Scales of Intelligence (WPPSI) because of its broader age range, ability coverage, and psychometric characteristics.

For children over 6, the most widely used intelligence measure is the Wechsler Intelligence Scales for Children-Revised (WISC-R). This test contains 12 subtests. Six of the subtests comprise the Verbal scale, and six comprise the Performance scale. The Verbal subtests consist of measures of general information, oral arithmetic, abstract reasoning, and vocabulary. Performance subtests consist of measures of constructional skills (block building, puzzle assembly), motor learning, and other tests. In addition to a composite Full-Scale I.Q. (FSIQ), separate Verbal (VIQ) and Performance (PIQ) intelligence quotients are obtained. The Verbal I.Q. is composed of the Information, Comprehension, Arithmetic, Similarities, and Vocabulary Subtests. The Performance I.Q. is represented by the Picture Completion, Picture Arrangement, Block Design, Object Assembly, and Coding subtests. Digit Span and Mazes are supplemental subtests that are not used to compute I.Q. scores. The different subtests and their measurement characteristics are contained in Table 9.6-3, which also provides the Kaufman interpretation of the subtest. This interpretation is based on factor analytic studies of the WISC-R.

Tests of I.Q. have many advantages. Comparisons between the child's performance on subtests requiring primarily verbal and performance skills may indicate processing deficits in these areas. Because I.Q. tests measure several abilities and are well standardized, these procedures can be used to estimate a child's general range of mental functions. Finally, in conjunction with assessments of adaptive behavior, standardized I.Q. test results are of value in supporting placement recommendations and in surveying areas in which the child's skill may be relatively intact. However, these tests also have limitations, particularly when used by insufficiently trained practitioners or for purposes for which they were not designed.

Mental retardation The definition and classification of mental retardation used in DSM-III-R correspond closely to criteria developed by the American Association for Mental Deficiency. Establishing the presence of mental retardation requires scores below the 3rd percentile of the population scores (i.e., scores less than 70)

TABLE 9.6-1
Intelligence Tests for Children

Infancy to 2.5 years
  Bayley Scales of Infant Development
  Cattell Infant Intelligence Scales

2.5 to 6 years
  Stanford-Binet Intelligence Test (2.5 years to adult)
  Wechsler Preschool and Primary Scales of Intelligence (WPPSI) (4 to 6.5 years)
  McCarthy Scales of Children's Abilities (2.5 to 8.5 years)
  Kaufman Assessment Battery for Children (KABC) (2.5 to 12.5 years)

6 to 16 years
  Wechsler Intelligence Scales for Children-Revised (WISC-R)

TABLE 9.6-2
Classification of Intelligence Test Scores

I.Q.	*Classification*	*Percentile Rank*
Above 129	Very superior	98–99
120–129	Superior	91–97
110–119	High average[1]	75–90
90–109	Average[1]	25–74
80–89	Low average[1]	9–24
70–79	Borderline	3–8
Below 70	Mentally deficient[1]	1–2

[1]Editor's note: High average is also known as bright normal; average is also known as normal; low average is also known as dull normal; and mentally deficient is also known as retardation. These are equivalent terms used in other classifications, which many workers, including the authors, believe to be pejorative.

on measures of intelligence and adaptive behavior. Criteria for the diagnosis are usually legally mandated. Because of the influence of cultural factors on I.Q. scores, the need for a systematic assessment of the child's socialization, communication skills, and overall capacity for everyday functioning cannot be overemphasized. To illustrate, consider a recently developed, well-standardized measure of adaptive behavior, the Vineland Adaptive Behavior Scales. The Vineland can be used from birth through adulthood. It has a national standardization and yields composite scores that are scaled in the same way as WISC-R I.Q. scores (i.e., average of 100, with units of 15 for the standard deviation). The Vineland is administered through a nondirective interview of parents or primary caretakers and covers activities of the child in four domains: Communication, Daily Living, Socialization, and Motor. Each of these domains includes a variety of age-appropriate items that represent behaviors or skills the child may or may not habitually demonstrate. Through the interview, the examiner can complete these items and then obtain standardized scores for each domain and for the child's overall level of adaptive behavior. Research is just beginning on the validity of the Vineland, but standardization and reliability are far superior to other current measures of adaptive behavior. The need to assess both intelligence and adaptive behavior for the diagnosis of mental retardation cannot be overemphasized.

Learning disabilities DSM-III-R provides definitions for two types of learning disabilities involving reading and arithmetic. These definitions parallel current legislation requiring discrepancies in measured I.Q. and academic achievement (usually one standard deviation) in order to establish the presence of a learning disability and the child's eligibility for special education.

Table 9.6-4 lists three of the many measures of academic achievement. These well-known tests are commonly used in evaluating learning-disabled children. Each of the tests measures basic skills in reading, spelling, and arithmetic, but vary in how these skills are assessed. The Wide Range Achievement Test-Revised (WRAT-R) consists of three subtests involving word identification, written spelling of single words, and computational arithmetic. The Peabody Individual Achievement Test (PIAT) and Woodcock-Johnson have similar tests of word identification. However, the PIAT measures arithmetic and spelling skills through a multiple-choice format that does not require writing. The Woodcock-Johnson has measures of computational and mental arithmetic and of written spelling. It also measures grammar and punctuation skills and content areas in science, social studies, and humanities. Both the PIAT and Woodcock-Johnson measure comprehension in reading. The PIAT uses a multiple-choice format in which the child silently reads a sentence and then selects one from four pictures representing the meaning of the sentence. For the Woodcock-Johnson, the child silently reads a sentence or passage with a missing word. Comprehension is measured in terms of the child's ability to supply the missing word.

It should be apparent that there are a variety of methods by which academic skills can be evaluated. Oftentimes, the detection of a learning disability depends on the type of measure used to assess academic proficiency. For example, reading disorders in children are frequently manifested by problems in decoding words. Comprehension problems can accompany decoding difficulties. However, children can perform poorly on comprehension tasks for a variety of reasons that may not reflect a reading disorder (e.g., lack of motivation, poor memory). Arithmetic disabilities often involve paper-and-pencil computations. If arithmetic proficiency is assessed only by the PIAT (which does not require paper-and-pencil computations), an important disability may be overlooked.

The validity of definitions of learning disability based on discrepancies in I.Q. and achievement mandated by law and embedded in DSM-III-R is questionable. The problems generally stem from the absence of well-accepted definitions of these disorders. Many researchers argue that the criteria are arbitrary and do not stand up to empirical validation. For example, there is little evidence suggesting that children with academic problems who meet DSM-III-R criteria are different from non–mentally retarded children with similar levels of academic achievement who do not show discrepancies relative to I.Q. (i.e., slow learners). The notion of specific disabilities is also widely questioned, since isolated areas of proficiency are generally rare.

The problems in using I.Q.-achievement discrepancies for the diagnosis of learning disability may stem in part from the limitations of I.Q. tests, which were not designed with the idea of diagnosing learning disabilities. Intelligence tests cannot be viewed as a pure measure of learning potential. Performance on I.Q. tests reflects past learning history as well as genetic endowment. In terms of discrepancies between I.Q. and academic achievement, it should be noted that the same basic deficiencies that determine academic problems may also affect I.Q. scores. This problem challenges the frequent practice of defining learning disabilities in terms of an I.Q.-achievement discrepancy. Similarly, the statistical limitations of computing discrepancies between moderately correlated I.Q. and achievement tests have received too little attention.

Another shortcoming is that I.Q. tests do not survey all possible areas of competency. The WISC-R, for example, fails to measure many aspects of social adaptation, nonverbal problem solving, and information-processing skills. Correlations between many neuropsychological test and academic achievement remain robust, even when the effects of I.Q. are extracted from the correlations. Furthermore, I.Q. tests were designed to predict learning or achievement outside of the test situation, rather than as measures of distinct processing skills. For this latter reason, it is difficult to draw conclusions regarding basic skills from performance on these tests. Individual I.Q. subtests often measure combinations of skills that provide few clues as to the nature of an individual's component mental abilities. Finally, I.Q. test results have not always been found useful for determining the treatment or remedial approach that is most likely to be successful for a given child. There is no reason to believe that educational strategies beneficial to children with lower I.Q. scores are any different from strategies that would be recommended for children with average or above-average I.Q. scores. Although the results of I.Q. tests can be useful in the assessment of children, these results may be of relatively limited value and must be interpreted with caution. The use of I.Q.-achievement discrepancies as the sole criteria for diagnosing learning disabilities is especially suspect.

Brain-injured children Unlike mentally retarded and brain-injured children, intelligence tests should not be used alone to diagnose brain damage in children. These tests are sensitive to the effects of brain injury, but there are no uniform patterns of performance that provide adequate criteria for the presence or absence of brain damage. Indeed, the limitations of intelligence tests for learning-disabled children also apply to children with brain injury. Unfortunately, the presence of brain injury and disruption of cognitive and motor abilities is sometimes not sufficient for placement of children in special education. Eligibility guidelines often follow those designed for non–brain-injured children with learning disabilities. Consequently, I.Q. tests may be required if placement recommenda-

TABLE 9.6-3
Subtests of the WISC-R

Subtest	*Scale*	*Operation*	*Kaufman Factor**
Information	Verbal	Retrieval of basic facts	VC
Comprehension	Verbal	Answer questions about social situations	VC
Arithmetic	Verbal	Oral arithmetic	FD
Similarities	Verbal	Abstract reasoning	VC
Vocabulary	Verbal	Oral vocabulary	VC
Digit Span	—	Forward and backward digit repetition	FD
Picture Completion	Performance	Recognition of missing elements of picture	PO
Picture Arrangement	Performance	Rearrange pictures depicting social situations	PO
Block Design	Performance	Block construction	PO
Object Assembly	Performance	Puzzle construction	PO
Coding	Performance	Incidental motor learning	FD
Mazes	—	Completion of mazes	PO

*VC = verbal comprehension; PO = perceptual organization; FD = freedom from distractibility.

tions are to be accepted by an educational institution. Unfortunately, tests, such as the WISC-R, are frequently overemphasized with brain-injured children and may lead to inappropriate decisions concerning placement in special education as well as the effects of brain injury on the child's capacity for adaptive functioning. The reason is that the I.Q. scores may be reduced and thereby prevent qualification for special education. Despite the reduction, I.Q. tests are not sensitive to all manifestations of the brain injury, providing an incomplete assessment of the child.

Intelligence tests are often sensitive to the behavioral effects of brain injury. However, these procedures are not sensitive to all aspects of a child's cognitive functioning. For example, the WISC-R provides a limited and largely indirect assessment of memory and attentional skills, which are frequently impaired in head-injured children. Consequently, it is not surprising that the use of I.Q. tests with brain-injured children is often unfair and prevents their entry into necessary special education classes. Indeed, some workers have found that children with head injury often show a decrement in I.Q. scores after injury, with subsequent recovery. However, recovery of memory skills often lags. If the child is evaluated shortly after injury, the I.Q. scores will be reduced and the needed discrepancy will not be established. Basic academic skills in reading and spelling are often not immediately affected by head injury. Reading problems often emerge several years after injury, reflecting the cumulative influences of the child's subtle learning deficiencies. As this example illustrates, results of I.Q. tests may be useful with brain-injured children but may provide a limited view of the child, and, hence, there may be direct consequences for placement and intervention.

There are numerous studies of intellectual development and recovery in brain-injured children. For example, children with head injury often show good recovery of WISC-R Verbal I.Q. scores, but slower recovery of Performance I.Q. scores. Congenitally hydrocephalic children often show better development of Verbal I.Q. than Performance I.Q. There is relatively little decrement in I.Q. scores in many cases of infectious diseases. However, studies of abrupt unilateral lesions in children (e.g., vascular anomaly) tend to show more disruptions of Verbal I.Q. In general, these findings seem to reflect the predominance of diffuse, subcortical brain disease in children, which seems more related to Performance I.Q. scores.

NEUROPSYCHOLOGICAL TESTS The specific tests used by neuropsychologists varies considerably across settings. The common element is the attempt to measure a variety of skills in several key areas. To illustrate, Tables 9.6-5 and 9.6-6 outline the tests used, respectively, by Rourke and associates and by Fletcher. A brief description of measurement characteristics are provided, but more specific descriptions should be obtained from the primary sources.

What is common in these tables is the division of the tests into major areas. Rourke considers tests of tactile-perceptual, visual-perceptual, language, problem solving, motor, and other skills. Like Rourke, Fletcher provides tests of language, visual-perceptual, somatosensory (tactile), and motoric skills. Rourke also includes measures of problem solving and concept formation, whereas Fletcher emphasizes memory and learning, as well as attentional skills. In fact, Rourke has tasks in the "other" category with memory components (Tactual Performance Test) and attentional skills (Underlining Test), so there is additional overlap. Some tests are identical, but the commonality is the attempt to measure a broad range of abilities and the nature of the constructs identified as important in assessment. Some of the tests also overlap with those described in the chapter on adult neuropsychology in this textbook. The tests in Tables 9.6-5 and 9.6-6 have normative information so that they can be administered to patients of different ages. However, the actual tests used with children and adults may differ in their level of difficulty. It is not assumed that the measurement characteristics and usefulness of the tests are the same for children and adults. It is often misleading to simply take tests developed for adults and apply them to children (or the elderly) without considering task difficulty and differences in measurement characteristics.

TABLE 9.6-4
Tests of Academic Achievement

1. Wide Range Achievement Test-Revised (WRAT-R)
2. Peabody Individual Achievement Test (PIAT)
3. Woodcock-Johnson Psycho-Educational Test Battery

The interpretations of these tests vary, depending on the nature of the assessment question and the child's presenting disorder. Furthermore, specific tests may be added or deleted depending on the presenting question and the results of the assessment. Tests are generally selected to measure abilities identified as an important correlate of school functioning, adaptive behavior, or known lesion. The process by which the results are interpreted and used on behalf of the child are outlined in Figures 9.6-1 and 9.6-2.

Arithmetic disabilities Arithmetic disabilities in children are poorly understood. Although there have been many studies of children with reading problems, there has been relatively little research on children who experience difficulty mastering arithmetic skills. This state of affairs is surprising because a fairly large number of school-age children manifest difficulties with arithmetic (about 6 percent). In fact, there may be more arithmetic-disabled children than reading-disabled children (about 4 percent). This difference probably reflects the fact that most children with reading problems also have problems with arithmetic. Moreover, although the incidence of children impaired only in arithmetic (but not reading) is high, very few children are impaired only in reading (but not arithmetic).

There are many types of arithmetic disabilities in children. For example, children who have motivational deficiencies can display poor grades in arithmetic. However, these children often do well on standardized tests of arithmetic achievement and present with little

TABLE 9.6-5
Modified Version of the Halstead-Reitan Neuropsychological Test Battery for Children Used by Rourke

I. Tactile-perceptual
- A. Reitan-Klove Tactile-Perceptual and Tactile-Forms Recognition Test
  1. Tactile Imperception and Suppression
  2. Finger Agnosia
  3. Fingertip Number-Writing Perception (9–15 years) Fingertip Symbol-Writing Recognition (5–8 years)
  4. Coin Recognition (9–15 years) Tactile-Forms Recognition (5–8 years)

II. Visual-perceptual
- A. Reitan-Klove Visual-Perceptual Tests
- B. Target Test
- C. Constructional Dyspraxia Items, Halstead-Wepman Aphasia Screening Test
- D. WISC Picture Completion, Picture Arrangement, Block Design, Object Assembly subtests
- E. Trail Making Test for Children, Part A (9–15 years)
- F. Color Form Test (5–8 years)
- G. Progressive Figures
- H. Individual Performance Test (5–8 yr)
  1. Matching Figures
  2. Star Drawing
  3. Matching V's
  4. Concentric Squares Drawing

III. Auditory-perceptual and language-related
- A. Reitan-Klove Auditory-Perceptual Test
- B. Seashore Rhythm Test (9–15 years)
- C. Auditory Closure Test
- D. Auditory Analysis Test
- E. Peabody Picture Vocabulary Test
- F. Speech-Sounds Perception Test
- G. Sentence Memory Test
- H. Verbal Fluency Test
- I. WISC Information, Comprehension, Similarities, Vocabulary, Digit Span subtests
- J. Aphasoid Items, Aphasia Screening Test

IV. Problem solving, concept formation, reasoning
- A. Halstead Category Test
- B. Children's Word-Finding Test
- C. WISC Arithmetic subtest
- D. Matching Pictures Test (5–8 years)

V. Motor and psychomotor
- A. Reitan-Klove Lateral Dominance Examination
- B. Dynamometer
- C. Finger Tapping Test
- D. Foot Tapping Test
- E. Klove-Matthews Motor Steadiness Battery
  1. Maze Coordination Test
  2. Static Steadiness Test
  3. Grooved Pegboard Test

VI. Other
- A. Underlining Test
- B. WISC Coding subtest
- C. Tactual Performance Test
- D. Trail Making Test for Children, Part B (9–15 years)

TABLE 9.6-6
Neuropsychological Assessment Procedures for Evaluation of Basic Competencies Used by Fletcher

Construct	*Test*	*Operation*
I. Language		
	A. Word Fluency	Retrieval of words to letters
	B. Rapid Naming	Naming of common pictured items
	C. Auditory Analysis	Breaking words into phonological segments
	D. Token Test	Comprehension of sentences
	E. Peabody Picture Vocabulary Test	Comprehension of single words
II. Visual-spatial and constructional		
	A. Beery Visual-Motor Integration	Copying of geometric figures
	B. Recognition-Discrimination	Matching of geometric figures
	C. 3-D Block Construction	Construction of three-dimensional block arrays
III. Somatosensory		
	A. Stereognosis Test	Lateralized haptic processing of sandpaper figures
IV. Motor-sequential		
	A. Finger Tapping	Lateralized fine motor speed: tapping key
	B. Grooved Pegboard	Lateralized fine motor speed and dexterity: peg insertion
	C. Trail Making Test	Sequential motor speed: number and number-letter connection
V. Memory and learning		
	A. Paragraph Recall	Memory for passages
	B. Continuous Recognition Memory Test	Recogniton of previously presented pictures
	C. Verbal Selective Reminding	Word list learning
	D. Nonverbal Selective Reminding	Memory for dot locations
VI. Attention		
	A. Continuous Performance Test	Selection of target stimuli from sequentially presented stream of stimuli

impairment in neuropsychological or information-processing skills. Children with reading problems often have difficulty with arithmetic. These children, whose reading problems may be related to language-processing difficulties, have special difficulty with word problems. They also forget number facts and procedures necessary for the successful execution of mechanical or computational arithmetic. These errors may reflect problems with verbal memory and the child's more general language-based learning disability.

The purpose of the neuropsychological evaluation is to determine (1) whether arithmetic disability is a central feature of the manifest disability and (2) the nature of basic competency deficits underlying any arithmetic disability. This process should lead to an explanation of the nature and type of problem, along with a remedial plan.

Of special interest are children whose primary learning impairment occurs in computational arithmetic as assessed by the WRAT-R or Woodcock-Johnson. These children are characterized, in part, by severe impairment of basic computational arithmetic skills. However, in contrast to reading-disabled children who also show arithmetic deficits, these children have excellent decoding skills with good abilities in word recognition and spelling. They generally have a nonverbal learning disability.

Nonverbal learning disabilities are characterized by problems in (1) computational arithmetic and writing, (2) social competence, and (3) nonverbal cognitive skills. In computational arithmetic, errors reflect poor spatial organization, procedural errors, inattention to visual detail, and graphomotor problems. Writing is often poor, although thematic maturity may be at grade-appropriate levels. This part of the assessment is typically completed with achievement tests, such as the WRAT-R, and represents an assessment of the manifest disabilities (i.e., problems with school achievement).

Social competency problems are often apparent in the development of social skills, particularly in unfamiliar or unstructured interpersonal situations. Anecdotal clinical descriptions include a poor understanding of other people's feelings and difficulty inferring emotions from behavior. These problems may not reflect any particular problem with their capacity for empathy, but may stem from difficulties interpreting facial expressions and gestures secondary to poor visual-spatial skills. Children with nonverbal learning disabilities also display body posture and facial expressions incongruent with their affect, and sometimes they show a poor understanding of appropriate interpersonal boundaries. They often talk excessively, a characteristic that reflects their well-developed automatic language skills. Although their vocabulary may be highly developed, language content sometimes seems empty, irrelevant, and tangential. These children rely heavily on their verbal skills in interpersonal (and learning) situations and may tend to underattend to nonverbal cues.

More generally, children with nonverbal learning disabilities seem poorly organized and unfocused. They are sometimes described as inattentive and distractible, but this behavior may reflect their poor organizational skills and reduced capacity for self-directed behavior. These children often have problems initiating activities, particularly if the task is perceived as difficult, and they elicit considerable structure and direction from external figures (e.g., teachers, parents) with their verbal skills. The social component of this disability is not well understood, but is important because it represents a direct consequence of the child's information-processing disability. In other words, the nature of the cognitive problem leads to predictable problems with social competence and interpersonal behavior. This type of social problem contrasts with the reduced self-esteem, frustration, and low achievement motivation often associated with reading disabilities as secondary or indirect consequences of the effects of repeated failure. The assessment of this component involves the manifest disability (in some children) as well as the moderator variables that influence adaptation to school and home. Interviews, personality tests, and behavior ratings are frequently employed and help distinguish the arithmetic-impaired child from those with primary problems in attention or psychological adjustment.

PERFORMANCE ON NEUROPSYCHOLOGICAL TASKS In addition to the problems with computational arithmetic and social competency, arithmetic-impaired children also display characteristic difficulties on neuropsychological tasks (i.e., basic competencies). This pattern helps differentiate arithmetic-disabled children from reading-disabled children, as illustrated in Figure 9.6-3. This figure shows the performance of groups of 9- to 14-year-old reading-disabled (group 2) and arithmetic-disabled (group 3) children on selected measures used by Rourke (Table 9.6-5). The children's scores have been converted into standard scores with a mean of 50 and a standard deviation of 10. A comparison of the group averages in the six areas measured by the tests shows that group 2 (reading-disabled) children have significant difficulty on measures of verbal and auditory-perceptual skills, but approximate average levels in other ability domains. In contrast, group 3 (arithmetic-disabled) children perform at age level on verbal and auditory-perceptual tasks, but display significantly impaired performance on measures of visual-perceptual, psychomotor, tactile-perceptual, and conceptual abilities. In general, arithmetic-disabled children have difficulty on nonverbal processing tasks, including bilateral psychomotor and somatosensory deficits that tend to be more apparent on the nondominant hand. They can also have difficulties on tasks using novel or unfamiliar material or that require the development and application of problem-solving strategies in an unfamiliar task, even when the material to be processed can be verbally coded.

If the same groups of children had been examined using the procedures outlined in Table 9.6-6, similar patterns would have emerged. The reading-disabled children would display problems on language-related tasks, including verbal memory skills. The arithmetic-disabled children would have primary difficulties on tasks involving visual-spatial and constructional skills, somatosensory, motor, and nonverbal memory. Figure 9.6-4 displays results from a comparison of selective reminding tasks for verbal and nonverbal material in reading- and arithmetic-disabled groups. The verbal task, shown in Figure 9.6-5, involves learning a list of animal names, whereas the nonverbal tasks involve memory for dot locations. Two scores are provided for each task, representing long-term storage (LTS) and consistent long-term retrieval (CLTR). Figure 9.6-4 shows that reading-disabled children have difficulty on the verbal task (particularly CLTR), whereas arithmetic-disabled children have difficulty on both the LTS and CLTR on the nonverbal task.

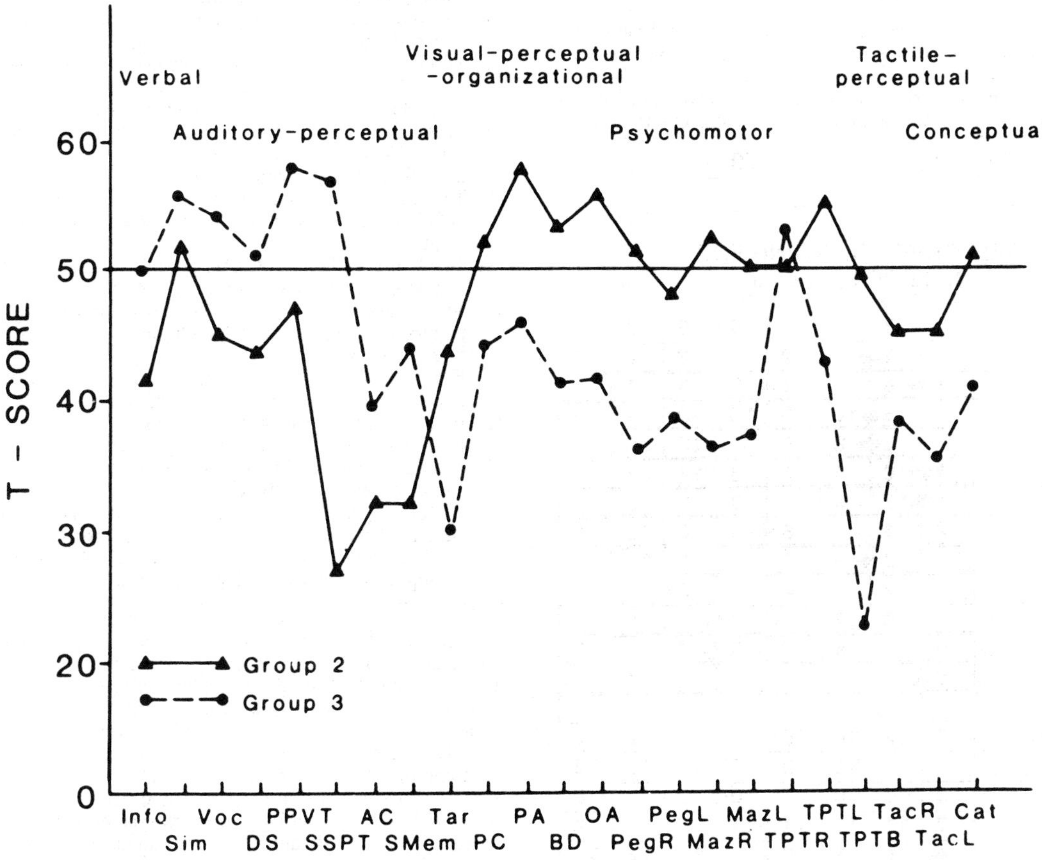

FIGURE 9.6-3. *Performance on Modified Halstead-Reitan Neuropsychological Battery by group 2 (reading-disabled) and group 3 (arithmetic-disabled) children.*

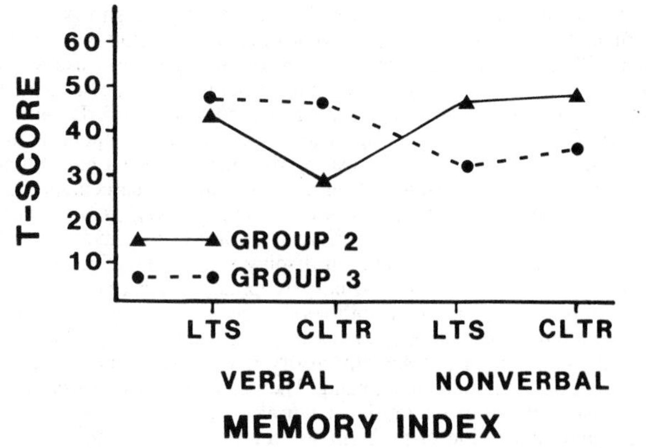

FIGURE 9.6-4. *Performance on verbal and nonverbal selective reminding tests by group 2 (reading-disabled) and group 3 (arithmetic-disabled) children.*

TREATMENT For each individual child, the neuropsychologist would carefully assess the variables depicted in Figure 9.6-1 and develop a plan as outlined in Figure 9.6-2. For arithmetic-disabled children, this plan would address the three components of the disability: educational, cognitive, and social. Tables 9.6-7 and 9.6-8 outline some of the educational and behavioral recommendations that might be used in developing the plan. Didactic, compensatory approaches are generally emphasized. Intervention should not attempt directly to remediate the child's processing deficits. Such attempts may improve the deficient skill, but they may not generalize to the academic or behavioral deficit. Instead, remediation should address the specific academic and behavioral problems manifested in the classroom or adaptive functioning area (e.g., peer relations) with an approach that emphasizes the child's strengths and helps develop compensatory mechanisms.

Table 9.6-7 discusses ways of dealing with the arithmetic and graphomotor components of the disability, whereas Table 9.6-8 focuses on the social competence problem that is characteristic of many children with nonverbal learning disabilities. There are three guiding principles underlying remediation efforts with these children. First,

NAME Control ♀ DATE 2-79

AGE 9 EDUC 3

SELECTIVE REMINDING FOR CHILDREN ≤ 12 y.o.

	1	2	3	4	5	6	7	8
Dog		1	2	2	3	2	2	2
Fox	1	6	1	1	2	1	1	1
Horse		5	10	9	10	3	3	3
Lion		2	8	10	1	12	8	12
Elephant	3	10	6	3	8	11	7	7
Bear	4	12	9	6	7	9	9	4
Rat	2	11		5	9	10	10	9
Raccoon		3	3	8	11	8	12	6
Goat		4		4		6	11	8
Squirrel	7	8	7		4	5	5	10
Beaver	5	9	4		5	4	6	5
Turtle	6	7	5	7	6	7	4	11
Total Recall	7	12	10	10	11	12	12	12
LTR	7	11	10	9	11	12	12	12
STR	0	1	0	1	0	0	0	0
LTS	7	11	11	11	11	12	12	12
CLTR	4	8	8	9	11	12	12	12
Random LTR	3	3	2	0	0	0	0	0
Presentations	12	5	0	2	2	1	0	0

FIGURE 9.6-5 *Verbal selective reminding test for children.*

TABLE 9.6-7
Educational Interventions for Children with Specific Arithmetic Disabilities

1. Emphasize reading comprehension skills to reduce excessive reliance on decoding skills.
2. Emphasize drill and repetition for short periods of time (with rewards), particularly in the graphomotor area.
3. Prior to any copying task, teach the child to read the material and verbally rehearse while copying.
4. Teach the use of appropriate aids (e.g., calculator) to older children.
5. Teach mechanical arithmetic in a systematic, verbal, step-by-step fashion. Typical problems include difficulties with (a) spatial organization; (b) misreading visual details; (c) procedural errors; (d) failure to shift set across different problems; (e) graphomotor difficulties with number formation; (f) forgetting or misuse of number facts; (g) poor logical grasp of number concepts.
6. Don't frustrate. Allow "dependency." Provide external structure. Be aware of the intervenor's role in preparing the child for adult life.
7. Provide adjuncts (e.g., calculators) as a compensatory device and as a teaching device.
8. Ensure appropriate attentional skills. Focus on methods of preventing careless errors.

TABLE 9.6-8
Interventions for Children with Social Competency Deficiencies

1. Observe the child's behavior, especially in novel or complex situations that are new and unfamiliar.
2. Didactic presentations of social behaviors can be useful, especially in adolescents.
3. Work with the child in a systematic, step-by-step fashion: Use a parts-to-whole verbal teaching method.
4. Ask the child to provide verbal feedback in a systematic, repetitive fashion when teaching any task.
5. Teach the child appropriate strategies for dealing with particularly troublesome situations that occur frequently.
6. Promote the generalization of learned strategies and concepts.
7. Teach the child to refine and use appropriate verbal expressive skills. Content may be irrelevant, but verbal mediation and rehearsal facilitate generalization.
8. Teach the child to make better use of organizational skills. When deficient, these skills must be exercised to promote development.
9. Teach the child to interpret visual information when there is competing auditory information, particularly in novel situations.
10. Teach appropriate nonverbal behavior, particularly in interpersonal situations, so that children can use and interpret gesture, body posture, etc.
11. Facilitate structured peer interactions. Teach the rules of interactional behavior in real-life situations.
12. Promote, encourage, and monitor systematic explorative activities, since the child will often resist new activities.
13. Facilitate older children's understanding of the nature of their adaptive behavior deficiencies.
14. Facilitate parental understanding of the nature of the child's adaptive behavior deficiencies. Provide explicit direction regarding the child's developmental needs. Avoid excessive psychologizing or nondirective interventions. Don't frustrate.

interventions should be as verbal as possible, including those for computational arithmetic. In completing arithmetic problems, verbal rules and routines should be emphasized. Children should rehearse steps verbally as they work arithmetic problems. Similarly, social competence skills can be improved if these behaviors are taught verbally, emphasizing repetition and rehearsal. These children will learn appropriate social behavior less effectively if time-based contingent maneuvers are used (e.g., time-out) or if training is done through a sequential contingent reward system. However, if appropriate social behavior is taught through language as a set of rules, the children have a better chance of developing appropriate social behavior. Since they often talk excessively, it may be helpful to encourage silent rehearsal and subvocalization.

Second, highly concrete and systematic teaching methods should be used. A parts-to-whole method, in which different activities (educational or behavioral) are broken into a set of component steps leading up to a sequence of activities, should be maximally effective with these children. The children should not be expected to break down new activities into these components. Rather, the components and necessary strategies and techniques should be presented to them and taught verbally with rehearsal and repetition. These children should not be expected to work independently, without structure and without external guidance. Otherwise, the experience will only be frustrating to them.

Third, arithmetically disabled children have significant organizational problems. They often do not understand how to approach a problem, particularly if it is unfamiliar, and may seem confused, unattentive, or unmotivated. These difficulties do not always stem from attentional deficits; rather, they reflect intentional deficits secondary to the more general problems with organization, which may lead to difficulties in initiating new behavior. In more extreme cases, such behavior can be misinterpreted as conduct problems and lead to excessive punishment that merely frustrates the child and exacerbates confusion and task avoidance. It is often tempting in these instances to remove structure from the child in an attempt to reduce dependency and increase responsibility. Such an approach is the opposite of what arithmetically disabled children need. Instead of being reduced, structure should be enhanced. These children may seem dependent when in fact they are attempting to elicit structure, which is a highly adaptive behavior. Hence, always be aware of the difficulties these children have in organizing themselves and initiating new behavior, and be prepared to provide organization and structure when needed.

These principles are derived primarily from anecdotal clinical experience with one type of arithmetically disabled children (i.e., nonverbal learning disability). Other children with arithmetic problems that are language based will require alternative approaches. In addition, the value of these principles awaits empirical validation that is often lacking in applying educational methods to the remediation of learning disabled children. Additional research is sorely needed, particularly given the poor adult prognosis for some children with primary arithmetic disabilities.

TABLE 9.6-9
Interventions for Attentionally Impaired Children

1. Help the child structure the task so that it is possible to proceed in a step-by-step manner.
2. Reduce distractions. Seat the child in front side row, thus reducing the number of close contacts. In a reading group, place the child at the end of the group.
3. Use some physical contact with the child, which may be a hand on the shoulder, or directing of arm and hand movements.
4. Redirect the child: "Go back and do this." Redirecting will usually elicit a more favorable reaction from the child than will simply stopping an activity.
5. Avoid teaching at a frustration level. Teach at a tolerance level at which it is easy for the child to work and at a level that is challenging for the child.
6. Be sure the child completely understands what is being taught.
7. Relate new situations to those the child already knows well.
8. Teach when the child is well motivated and ready to work.
9. Present the lesson in a vivid manner so that it stands out from background activities.
10. Keep the work area neat. Provide only the task on which the child is working.
11. Be calm. Try to avoid anger, irritation, or rejection toward the child. Speak softly so that the child must listen carefully.
12. Be firm. Do not allow the child to escape a task that you know he or she is capable of performing.
13. Be consistent. Do not alternate between giving in to the child and being firm about completing a goal.
14. Use simple commands and directions. Do not talk too much.
15. Never ask, "Do you want to do this?" Say, "Do this." You must structure the situation.
16. Reward "on-task" behavior with operant methods in small units of time (e.g., 5 minutes initially with an increase to 10 minutes later on). Avoid giving the child lengthy assignments (e.g., a worksheet with 20 problems). Give 5 to 10 problems at a time.
17. Keep in mind that with all children it is best to discontinue an activity at the highest point of their interest and then come back to the activity at a later time.
18. With children who have these difficult behaviors, there are frequently *many* behaviors that should be changed. Establish priorities.

Head injuries Neuropsychologists are commonly asked to evaluate children who have sustained traumatic injuries to the brain. Manifest disabilities typically involve difficulties in learning at school, accompanied by conduct problems at home or school, or both. Basic competency deficits vary across individual children. The most frequent deficits occur on (1) performance-based intelligence tests; (2) speeded motor tasks (e.g., rate of finger tapping); (3) subtle aspects of language (e.g., naming); and (4) memory and attention (e.g., selective reminding tasks). Moderator variables involve the availability of rehabilitation resources in the school and community, the child's response to the injury (e.g., depression), and the family's finances and capacity for dealing with an injured child.

Memory and attentional skills are the most frequent long-term sequelae of head injury in children. Tables 9.6-9 and 9.6-10 summarize recommendations derived from Yvilsaker that might form the basis for a treatment plan addressing these components of a head-injured child's difficulties. The management and habilitation of a head-injured child typically requires an interdisciplinary team. In addition, the plan must be frequently revised as the child recovers and the pattern of neuropsychological strengths and weaknesses changes. Behavioral changes are varied and common after head injury and must be dealt with on a case-by-case basis.

Head injury provides an example of how to evaluate biological indices in neuropsychological assessment. An evaluation of injury data should include an analysis of the nature and impact of the injury (i.e., etiology). Primary pathophysiological effects of head trauma include both multifocal, generalized injury caused by stretching of axonal fibers and the more specific mass effects of contusional injury. A host of potential secondary pathophysiological effects require careful evaluation. Head injury is associated with multiple complications, including hypoxia, increased intracranial pressure, and shock, all of which must be managed by the neurosurgeon during the acute phase of recovery. An evaluation of the child's condition should include review of clinical neurological status, duration of post-traumatic amnesia (PTA), and coma duration. Serial review of recovery in the intensive care unit, along with cerebral imaging procedures, will help elucidate the influence of secondary effects as well as late changes in the CNS (e.g., atrophy, degeneration of white matter) that occur with head injury and potentially influence behavior.

TABLE 9.6-10
Interventions for Memory-Impaired Children

1. Use self-question (e.g., "Do I understand? Do I need to ask a question? How is this meaningful to me? How does this fit with what I know?"). Periodically look for GMCs (gaps, misconceptions, or confusion) by summarizing or explaining and checking back with speaker, a written source, or reference material.
2. Build "frames" or background for new information that is of particular significance or interest. Read summaries, general textbooks, and ask knowledgeable person about topics of special interest.
3. Use a study guide for extended discourse material (e.g., SQ-3R procedure-survey, question, read, recite, review).
4. Make charts and graphs of important relationships in textual material.
5. Use external memory aids (e.g., tape recorder, logbook, notes, memos, written or pictured time lines).
6. Rehearse: Covert or overt; auditory-vocal or motor (pantomine).
7. Organize: Scan for or impose some order on incoming information.
8. Mnemonics: Method of loci, rhymes, imagery (meaningful and novel associations).
9. Use diagrams or forms that facilitate deeper encoding of information and its subsequent retrieval.
10. Relate the information to personal life experiences and current knowledge. Use semantic knowledge of basic scripts (e.g., going to a restaurant, buying groceries) to help reconstruct previous events.
11. Project and describe situation in which target information will be needed or used.
12. At retrieval, reconstruct environment in which information was received.
13. Verbalize visual-spatial information (e.g., "X is to the left of Y"). Visualize verbal information in graphs, pictures, cartoons, or action-based imagery.
14. Keep items in designated places.

The value of reviewing injury data has been demonstrated in several studies correlating indices of head injury with specific measures of cognitive development obtained after injury. These studies show that injury severity is the overriding correlate of recovery. Variables related to severity of injury—including coma duration, indices of depth of coma, and length of PTA—are most consistently associated with recovery. Longer periods of coma are clearly associated with poorer outcomes. The presence of brain stem abnormalities, including oculomotor and oculocephalic signs, is associated with poorer outcome on global ratings of recovery focusing on mortality and general quality of life. Higher levels of intracranial pressure are associated with poorer mortality rates and lower scores on global ratings of outcome in some studies. The locus of injury documented through cerebral tomography has not been consistently related to recovery. However, focal injury may have specific effects on the child's recovery.

This example illustrates the need to consider neurologic sources of variation in completing neuropsychological assessments of children, particularly if actual CNS injury is involved. Note that the presence of brain injury is generally known prior to referral. The task of the neuropsychologist is to establish behavioral and cognitive consequences and the relationship of the injury and environment to recovery. Treatment recommendations depend on the nature of basic competency deficits, but would be similar to those outlined in Tables 9.6-9 and 9.6-10.

Emotionally disturbed children Children who have primary problems with emotional functioning often have difficulty with cognitive and motor skills. These difficulties may contribute to problems implementing a treatment plan. Neuropsychological tests can be useful for establishing the extent to which a particular behavioral

TABLE 9.6-11
Clinical Management Tool for Language-Processing Deficits

I. Behavioral manifestations
  A. Receptive (listening) problem
    1. Does not seem to understand what is being said.
    2. Does not respond appropriately to verbal commands. Behavior doesn't match command.
    3. Child looks distractible when being given verbal commands.
    4. Child seems to forget what has been said to him or her (does not understand).
    5. Asks many questions in order to understand what is going on.
  B. Expressive (talking) problem
    1. Poor language usage. Speaks in one-word or short sentences.
    2. Does not use language to describe affects or experiences. Has trouble telling about feelings and needs.
    3. Has difficulty communicating needs.
    4. Stammers because of word retrieval problems. Uses gestures or jargon instead.
    5. Uses incomplete sentences so that listener has to fill in material.
    6. Disorganized speech, talks in circles.
    7. Speech is hard to understand because of articulation problems.

II. Management techniques and approaches
  A. Receptive problem
    1. Get child's attention (i.e., use eye contact, call name).
    2. Speak clearly and slowly.
    3. Speak in short statements.
    4. Repeat if necessary, leaving one word blank for child to fill in.
    5. Have child repeat what was said to ensure understanding.
    6. Provide list of things to be done, which child checks off upon completion.
    7. If child cannot read, use pictures.
    8. Provide running commentary of what child or you are doing.
  B. Expressive problem
    1. Listen to what child is saying rather than how child is saying it, then check out what you thought child said.
    2. Include the child in group activities but do not force participation.
    3. If child's communication is unclear, ask for different word or gestures.
    4. Provide child with verbal response, leaving a word to fill in.
  C. Handling Time-outs (receptive and expressive)
    1. Use visual cues to warn child that a time-out is imminent.
    2. Avoid "why" questions. Instead verbalize briefly what you think the child is feeling. Focus on the child's emotions and feelings. Use facial expressions and gestures.
    3. Before time-out is over, and when child is calm, briefly review what caused time-out.
    4. When time-out is over, let child communicate perception or feelings nonverbally by drawing pictures, by using play equipment, by modeling with clay, or through drama.

TABLE 9.6-12
Clinical Management Tool for Visual-Spatial Processing Deficits

Behavioral manifestations

1. Difficulty understanding cause-and-effect relationships. (These children have poor ability to develop insight and to learn from past experiences.)
2. Difficulty organizing and modulating behavioral responses to a broad range of environmental events and expectations.
3. Difficulty initiating activity, planning an approach to tasks, and carrying out intentions. (These youngsters are frequently seen as having problems attending—as lazy, disorganized, and poorly motivated.)
4. Difficulty interpreting social situations.
   a. Interpeting impact of their behavior on other people.
   b. Understanding gestures, social cues, spatial boundaries. (These youngsters often appear undersocialized and unempathic.)
5. Difficulty conceptualizing passage of time. (These children are frequently seen as oppositional.)
6. Difficulty responding well to lengthy time-out procedures.
7. Difficulty orienting themselves in space. (These children have a poor sense of direction and get lost easily.)
8. They tend to be concrete, but have the potential to develop more abstract abilities using language.
9. Difficulty recalling visually perceived information. (These children do not learn well by watching others.)
10. Some of these children are tactually defensive and become disorganized or fearful when touched.
11. These children process information best verbally.

Management Techniques and Approaches

1. Encourage these children to talk about experiences to others and, even more important, to themselves.
2. Engage them in a verbal dialogue, in which you relate an experience, then leave out parts and have them fill in or ask questions about the event.
3. Structure the environment to assist them in organizing time and procedures.
4. Post a written daily schedule with provisions for checking off activities as completed.
5. Use procedure charts for more complicated activities.
6. Label drawers and shelves to assist the child in organizing living spaces.
7. Establish clear-cut behavior expectations and consequences for misbehavior. Verbally explain cause-effect sequence after consequences have been administered.
8. Facilitate adaptation to changes in the environment by preparing the patient beforehand.
9. When possible, rehearse new situations prior to actual participation.
10. Facilitate an awareness of time concepts by making references to familiar events or by using a timer or clock.
11. Consider alternative disciplinary procedures. For example, having the child write 50 times: "I will not ___." Or if writing skills are poor, record on a tape: "I will not ___."
12. When going to new places, accompany the child and talk about landmarks that will aid them in finding their way. These children will need multiple tours.
13. These children frequently need to be told what is happening in social situations and need more specific directions concerning how to respond.
14. Consider structured social skills training.
15. If the child appears uncomfortable when touched, de-emphasize touching and hugging. Express feelings verbally.

problem reflects emotional or cognitive factors, or both. The evaluations are conducted in much the same way as with any other child, but with more emphasis on the assessment of emotional problems. School-related difficulties with learning would be dealt with in a manner similar to that developed for children with primary learning disabilities with accommodations according to the emotional factors operant in the case (i.e., moderator variables).

It is not always recognized that cognitive problems can contribute to the implementation of a psychotherapeutic program. In other words, children with language or visual-spatial processing deficits may have difficulty adapting to certain components of the treatment plan. Tables 9.6-11 and 9.6-12 outline a series of clinical management tools that were developed at a residential treatment center for children with significant emotional disturbances (Southwest Neurobehavioral Institute in San Antonio, Texas). These recommendations stemmed from an interdisciplinary assessment of the child that included a neuropsychological evaluation. As these tables indicate, the child's participation in milieu as well as procedures for setting limits on behavior and specific aspects of therapy were modified depending on the presence of basic competency deficits in language or visual-spatial skills. Other recommendations were made for academic problems (Table 9.6-7) and for other deficits (e.g., attention-deficit hyperactivity disorder).

The clinical management tools in Tables 9.6-11 and 9.6-12 each begin with a set of behavioral manifestations. The purpose of this portion of the tool is simply to translate the consequences of cognitive deficits into everyday behavioral terminology. Since a number of staff members work with the child, jargon is avoided in favor of descriptions of potential problems. These descriptions will not fit every child, but represent ideal cases. The staff is trained to observe the child using the results of the assessment and to develop specific descriptions for each case.

The second part of the description provides examples of program modifications that may prove useful to the child. These modifications apply to the milieu and influence setting of limits and discipline for various behavioral problems. Psychotherapeutic procedures may also be modified, depending on the nature of the problem. Classroom management (as well as instructional techniques) could also be modified after the results of the neuropsychological assessment are obtained.

This example demonstrates the major point of this section. The goal of an assessment is to develop habilitative plans for children regardless of diagnosis or presenting problem. In the case of head injury and emotional disturbance, the presence of CNS injury or severe emotional disorders is known prior to the evaluation. For all three examples, the neuropsychological evaluation helps establish the nature of the problem and the contribution of central processing deficiencies, behavioral and environmental factors, and CNS status. Simplistic causal statements are avoided in favor of a broader formulation of the nature of the child's problem. Through this formulation, a habilitative plan is developed and coordinated with other disciplines. Questions concerning brain status can be addressed, but only in the context of other evaluative technologies, the child's history, and current presentation. Neuropsychological testing is a component of the assessment, but a thorough evaluation of the child requires a broader focus by skilled practitioners, with a major emphasis on using the assessment to treat the child's disorder. Such an approach will make the best use of testing data and will benefit the child most fully.

REFERENCES

Dennis M: Neuropsychological assessment: New facts and new concepts. In *Behavioral Assessment of Childhood Disorders,* J Call, R Cohen, S. Harrison, L Stone, editors, vol 5, p 146. Basic Books, New York, 1985.

Fletcher J M: Neuropsychological assessment of brain-injured children. In *Behavioral Assessment of Childhood Disorders,* L Terdal, E Mash, editors, ed 2. Guilford, New York, 1988.

Fletcher J M, Levin H S: Neurobehavioral effects of brain injury in children. In *Handbook of Pediatric Psychology,* D Routh, editor. Guilford, New York, 1988.

Fletcher J M, Taylor H G: Neuropsychological approaches to children: Towards a developmental neuropsychology. J Clin Exp Neuropsychol *7:* 24, 1984.

Kaufman A: *Intelligent Testing with the WISC-R.* Academic Press, New York, 1979.

Matarazzo, J D: Psychological assessment of intelligence. In *Comprehensive Textbook of Psychiatry,* H I Kaplan, B J Sadock, editors, ed 4, vol 2, p 502. Williams & Wilkins, Baltimore, 1985.

Rourke B P, Bakker D J, Fisk J L, Strang, J D: *Child Neuropsychology: An Introduction to Theory, Research, and Clinical Practice.* Guilford, New York, 1983.

Rourke B P, Fisk J, Strang J D: *Neuropsychological Assessment of Children: A Treatment-Oriented Approach.* Guilford, New York, 1986.

Rutter M: Psychological sequelae of brain damage in children. Amer J Psychiat *138:* 1533, 1981.

Rutter M: Syndromes attributed to "minimal brain dysfunction" in childhood. Amer J Psychiat *139:* 21, 1982.

Sattler J M: *Assessment of Children's Intelligence and Special Abilities,* ed 2. Allyn & Bacon, Boston, 1982.

Satz P, Fletcher J M: Minimal brain dysfunctions: An appraisal of research concepts and methods. In *Handbook of Minimal Brain Dysfunctions: A Critical Review,* H E Rie, E D Rie, editors, p 669. Wiley, New York, 1980.

Sparrow S S, Fletcher J M, Cicchetti D V: Psychological assessment of children. In *Psychiatry,* J O Cavenar, editor, vol 2, chap 21. Lippincott, Philadelphia, 1985.

Taylor H G, Fletcher J M, Satz P: Neuropsychological assessment of children. In *Handbook of Psychological Assessment,* G Goldstein, M Hersen, editors. Wiley, New York, 1984.

Wilson B: Neuropsychological assessment of pre-school children. In *Handbook of Clinical Neuropsychology,* S Filskov, T J Boll, editors, vol 2. Wiley, New York, 1986.

Yvilsaker M, editor: *Head Injury Rehabilitation: Children and Adults.* College Hill Press, San Diego, 1985.

9.7 MEDICAL ASSESSMENT AND LABORATORY TESTING IN PSYCHIATRY

DARRELL G. KIRCH, M.D.

INTRODUCTION

Recent advances in the basic neurosciences and in clinical psychiatric research not only have been accompanied by increased interest in the biological substrate of mental disorders, but also have given rise to a renewed emphasis on the role of laboratory tests in psychiatric practice. This role extends beyond the traditional one of using the clinical laboratory to rule out various physical disorders, and now involves tests that are proposed to have utility in psychiatric diagnosis, choice of treatment, and clinical monitoring of response. Unfortunately, however, laboratory testing has not had a widespread effect on clinical psychiatric practice as yet. The following will provide an overview of general aspects of laboratory testing, a discussion of medical assessment of the psychiatric patient, and a summary of specific laboratory tests that have been applied to psychiatric disorders by researchers and clinicians.

HISTORY Many would attribute the recent emphasis on laboratory tests in psychiatry to the biological revolution that has taken place over the past 3 decades. It is incorrect, however, to view the current surge of interest in psychiatric laboratory tests as a new phenomenon. In fact, it may be more accurate to describe the relative inattention to the use of the laboratory on the part of many psychiatrists in the earlier part of this century as an unfortunate detour. Historically, many of the pioneers in the study of mental disorders were intensely interested in the potential of correlating psychopathological phenomena with quantifiable biological measures.

About 200 years ago, Franz Joseph Gall, a German anatomist, postulated a link between various mental functions and protuberances on the skull, the system known as phrenology. During roughly the same period, Vincenzo Chiarugi, as described in his multivolume *Medical Treatise on Insanity*, studied the brain at autopsy in cases of psychosis.

In the late nineteenth and early twentieth centuries, there were dramatic advances in delineating both the normal histology and the neuropathology of the brain, including pioneering studies by Alois Alzheimer, Theodor H. Meynert, Camillo Golgi, Ramón y Cajal, and Franz Nissl. This work included observations on changes in the brain in cases of psychosis as well as in more traditional neurological disorders. In 1871, Ewald Hecker described postmortem abnormalities in a case of hebephrenia. At the turn of the century, Emil Kraepelin emphasized the importance of direct neuropathological studies of brain tissue in cases of psychosis.

In 1913, Joseph W. Moore and Hideyo Noguchi discovered the spirochete, *Treponema pallidum,* in brain tissue from patients with general paresis. Various laboratory tests, in turn, made it possible to diagnose neurosyphilis reliably, thereby facilitating a specific medical subtyping of one group of psychotic patients.

The discovery of X-rays made it possible to obtain images of the skull and, in 1919, Walter E. Dandy described the technique of pneumoencephalography. Studies conducted in the first half of this century using this approach reported the presence of cerebral ventricular enlargement in some patients with schizophrenia. This work predated by several decades the technological advance of computed tomographic (CT) brain scanning, which has been used more recently in research replicating this structural finding.

As scientific discoveries led to the development of new clinical laboratory techniques, investigators have applied these tests to patients with mental illnesses. As a result of the introduction of laboratory tests, some disorders have moved from the realm of the psychiatrist into that of the internist, neurologist, and other specialists. The selected historical precedents cited above should not be ignored. The intellectual tradition in psychiatry in the past has been, and in the future should continue to be, one of seeking out and creatively using newly developed techniques to measure biological parameters that may be relevant to mental function.

FEAR OF BIOLOGICAL REDUCTIONISM On the part of clinicians not accustomed to the use of the laboratory, there may be a measure of apprehension regarding the increased emphasis on laboratory tests in psychiatric research and practice. The expressed concern often is that such an emphasis opens the door to a form of biological reductionism, which, in turn, diverts attention from the cultivation and maintenance of skills in observing and interviewing, resulting in a lack of rapport with the patient and an erosion of clinical proficiency. It is probably quite true that laboratory tests will never be found that objectively measure the complex psychodynamic issues so crucial to understanding many patients. It certainly must be acknowledged that the laboratory cannot replace the development of clinical acumen, whether in psychiatry or any other medical specialty. Nevertheless, laboratory tests may eventually provide the clinician with important information about the brain in any given patient.

SEARCH FOR BIOLOGICAL MARKERS Much of the current discussion involving laboratory tests in psychiatric research and practice is couched in terms of discovering biological markers for mental disorders. The term "marker" must be used with some caution. Unfortunately, it may cause some to view laboratory tests as ends in themselves, creating the impression that tests may be found that will mark with absolute certainty the correct diagnosis or the appropriate treatment in any subject. In fact, even the best laboratory tests have clear limitations involving sensitivity and specificity, as discussed below.

Laboratory tests are markers only in the sense of indicating an association (that may be present to a greater or lesser degree) between a biological measure and a given clinical disorder. Moreover, that association between the marker and the disorder may or may not be etiologically or pathophysiologically relevant. Biological markers in the form of clinical laboratory tests simply serve as tools to aid, rather than eliminate, the decision-making process.

SENSITIVITY, SPECIFICITY, AND PREDICTIVE VALUE

Test results are simply data, and the interpretation of data requires caution. The appropriate interpretation of medical laboratory tests, particularly those that are proposed as diagnostic devices, demands that certain definitions be clearly understood. Table 9.7-1 summarizes some key concepts.

Sensitivity refers to the ability of the test, by an abnormal result, to identify correctly individuals who actually have a given disorder (i.e., the ratio of true positives to the sum of true positives plus false negatives). *Specificity* refers to the ability of the test, by a negative result, to exclude correctly individuals who do not actually have the disorder (i.e., the ratio of true negatives to the sum of true negatives plus false positives). The *predictive value* of an abnormal test refers to the percentage of individuals with an abnormal test result who actually have the disorder in question (i.e., the ratio of true positives to the sum of true positives plus false positives).

In practice, laboratory tests never have perfect sensitivity or specificity. In fact, the sensitivity and specificity will vary with the cutoff value used by different laboratories to distinguish a normal from an abnormal test result. The choice of a particular cutoff value involves a trade-off between sensitivity

TABLE 9.7-1
Sensitivity, Specificity, and Predictive Value

Sensitivity
= probability of a positive test in one who has the disorder

$$= \frac{\text{true positives}}{\text{true positives} + \text{false negatives}} \times 100\%$$

Specificity
= probability of a negative test in one who does not have the disorder

$$= \frac{\text{true negatives}}{\text{true negatives} + \text{false positives}} \times 100\%$$

Predictive value of a positive test
= percentage of all positive tests that are true positives

$$= \frac{\text{true positives}}{\text{true positives} + \text{false positives}} \times 100\%$$

Predictive value of a negative test
= percentage of all negative tests that are true negatives

$$= \frac{\text{true negatives}}{\text{true negatives} + \text{false negatives}} \times 100\%$$

and specificity, with the former increasing as the latter decreases. Moreover, the predictive value of any diagnostic test will vary significantly with the actual prevalence of the given disorder in the population being tested. The higher the prevalence of the disorder, the greater the predictive value of a positive test. Thus, even though a test may have a relatively high sensitivity, it could fail as a screening test if the prevalence of the disorder is low in the population being examined. It can be seen that the results of each test not only must be integrated with the results of the history and examination for that individual, but also must be interpreted in terms of the actual sensitivity, specificity, and predictive value of the test in the specific patient population to which it is applied.

GENERAL FUNCTIONS OF LABORATORY TESTING

The emphasis on biological markers has created a tendency to focus on tests as diagnostic instruments. In fact, as outlined in Table 9.7-2, tests may serve a number of functions other than that of facilitating diagnosis.

DIAGNOSIS Diagnosis itself may be either etiological or descriptive. For example, a chest X-ray in a patient with a productive cough and fever may reveal pulmonary infiltrates consistent with the descriptive diagnosis of pneumonia. A sputum specimen submitted to microbiological laboratory analysis, however, would be required to yield an etiological diagnosis identifying a specific pathogen. Moreover, tests may serve not only to point toward a specific diagnosis, but also to quantify the severity of the disorder and indicate the prognosis in a given case, as in the use of cytology to determine the specific cell type in a cancer.

The state of knowledge regarding diagnosis in psychiatric disorders unfortunately remains almost exclusively on the descriptive level. Diagnoses are based on clusters of signs and symptoms and in most cases the etiology and pathophysiology of the syndromes described in the revised third edition of the American Psychiatric Association's *Diagnostic and Statistical Manual of Mental Disorders* (DSM-III-R) remain unknown. Nevertheless, even though they may say nothing regarding the actual cause of the disorder, biological tests for which abnormal values are consistently associated with a particular psychiatric diagnosis would be extremely valuable. They could aid in establishing the diagnosis in questionable cases, facilitate screening of at-risk populations, and help in guiding treatment as discussed below. Most important, biological tests are used to facilitate research that eventually may refine psychiatric diagnoses and reveal pathophysiology, moving the understanding of these disorders out of the realm of mere description and into that of etiology.

TABLE 9.7-2
Functions of Laboratory Testing

Diagnostic assessment
Descriptive diagnosis
Etiological diagnosis
Assessment of severity
Prediction of course
Treatment decisions
Assessment of need for treatment
Choice of treatment modality
Prediction of treatment response
Treatment monitoring
Assessment of treatment compliance
Evaluation of treatment efficacy
Identification of side effects
Determination of treatment endpoint
Population screening
Research

TREATMENT DECISIONS The process of establishing the diagnosis itself is clearly crucial in making initial treatment decisions. For example, in addition to facilitating the diagnosis of pneumonia, the presence of pulmonary infiltrates on a chest X-ray may help the physician decide to treat a febrile patient with an antibiotic. In addition, laboratory tests may be of value in terms of facilitating the choice among different treatment modalities, or may yield information that permits predictions of the efficacy or side effects of a given treatment.

In the case of psychiatric disorders, treatment decisions are often made that entail significant risks and financial costs for the patient, including choices regarding hospitalization, the prescription of psychopharmacological agents, and the use of electroconvulsive therapy (ECT). The value of tests that will facilitate these decisions is apparent.

TREATMENT MONITORING Even when the decision to treat is made and the modality has been selected, the need to monitor the patient remains. This is the function of laboratory testing most widely employed in psychiatry at this time. Treatment monitoring is a complex process that includes, but also extends beyond, the task of assessing the efficacy of the treatment in resolving the illness. When treatment is pharmacological, monitoring the effective level of the drug in the blood may be important. In some cases, monitoring can be accomplished directly by measurement of drug concentrations. In other cases, it is done indirectly—for example, by quantifying an effect of the drug, such as enzyme inhibition. The measurement of drug concentrations in the blood may also provide objective confirmation of patient compliance. Finally, insofar as no treatment is without risk to the patient, tests that monitor side effects (e.g., thyroid function tests in a patient on lithium) may be crucial to the ability of the physician to make ongoing decisions regarding the risk versus benefit of any given treatment.

In addition to the specific patient-oriented functions described above, laboratory tests also may be of value in screening populations for epidemiological purposes. Moreover, the role of the laboratory in clinical research is fundamental. Routine clinical tests typically are the ultimate product of extensive research studies by basic and applied medical investigators.

MEDICAL ASSESSMENT OF THE PSYCHIATRIC PATIENT

ROLE OF THE PSYCHIATRIST Many psychiatrists see some of the key elements of the medical assessment, in particular the physical examination, as lying outside their realm of responsibility. This notion has become institutionalized in various forms, including the manner in which some patients are referred for "medical clearance" to "rule out organic disorders" prior to entering psychiatric treatment. It certainly may be appropriate in some cases for psychiatrists to rely on family practitioners, internists, and other physicians to perform the detailed medical examination that many patients require as part of the initial diagnostic process. What is inappropriate, however, is the attitude that once this task has been performed by another physician, ongoing attention to organic issues is not required of the psychiatrist. Even if they do not personally perform the medical examination, psychiatrists must bear in mind that diagnosis, assessment, and treatment are ongoing processes that necessitate continuing awareness of all aspects of the patient's medical status. Medical problems may have been missed on an initial examination, diagnoses may be incorrect, psychiatric treatment may result in unexpected medical complications, or new unrelated medical problems may arise while a psychiatric disorder is being treated.

A number of studies have indicated that a significant proportion of psychiatric patients have unrecognized medical problems. One study of 2,090 psychiatric outpatients found that 43 percent had one or more physical illnesses, almost half of which were undiagnosed at the time of referral. In another survey of 100 patients admitted to a state hospital, 46 percent were found to have a previously unrecognized medical problem that either caused or worsened their psychiatric symptoms. Unrecognized medical problems may be particularly common in patients who are older, who are poor, or who have a severe psychiatric disorder.

Even after a thorough medical evaluation has been performed, with negative findings, the psychiatrist must bear in mind that the patient in no way becomes immune to the subsequent development of active medical problems. In this sense, the patient is never absolutely medically clear and the need for ongoing medical observation is never completely ruled out.

INTEGRATION OF THE HISTORY, EXAMINATION, AND LABORATORY TESTS The basic principles of medical practice apply to psychiatry no less than to other specialties. Proper evaluation of the patient requires the following: (1) acquisition of a thorough *history* from the patient and, when indicated, other individuals and records; (2) *examination* of the patient by means of casual observation, formal interviewing (including the mental status examination), psychological testing (when indicated), and the physical examination; and (3) *laboratory testing*. This sequence of the history, followed by the examination and then laboratory testing, is important in most cases. The history should determine the specific extent and content of the formal examination, with both, in turn, indicating which laboratory tests are appropriate.

Psychiatric and medical history The history taken from a psychiatric patient must include past hospitalizations and medical-surgical problems, current medications, a review of systems, and a family medical history. The history in cases of substance abuse must include illicit substances and both over-the-counter and prescription medications. In cases of suspected exposure to environmental toxins, thorough geographical and occupational data are crucial. If the history includes a report of a recent physical examination, the actual extent of that assessment must be determined even for patients medically cleared in an emergency room. Patients may not distinguish a rigorous examination from a cursory assessment of a localized complaint, such as a pharyngitis or abdominal pain.

Examination The formal and informal aspects of the mental status examination are discussed elsewhere in this text. With regard to performing a physical examination on a psychiatric patient, the physician must be sensitive to the anxiety, sexual concern, or even paranoia that may be aroused. Patients with psychosis or organic mental syndromes may be especially vulnerable. A reassuring approach and clear explanations during the examination are likely to have direct therapeutic benefit. When a physical examination of a psychiatric patient is indicated by the history, it should rarely be deferred, and then for only as brief a time as possible. Clearly, an acutely psychotic patient may not allow a thorough assessment. Nevertheless, even in such a case, an attempt must be made to assess vital signs and gross neurological function. In addition, an effort should be made to obtain data from family members or clinical records regarding recent medical problems. Finally, in cases where the history and physical examination raise questions of a significant organic mental syndrome, neuropsychological testing should be considered.

Laboratory tests The blind application of laboratory screening tests is usually of limited clinical utility and may actually represent a waste of scarce resources. In contrast, the choice of specific laboratory tests should follow only from a thoughtful assessment of the history and examination. Moreover, the results obtained from the laboratory are meaningful only insofar as they are integrated with these other data. By maintaining rigor in evaluating the patient, the physician maximizes the information available and increases the likelihood of correct decisions regarding diagnosis and treatment.

Many psychiatric units have all admissions, regardless of their history and physical examination, undergo a routine screening. In many cases, this includes a chest X-ray, electrocardiogram (EKG), urinalysis, complete blood count, glucose, blood urea nitrogen, creatinine, bilirubin, hepatic enzymes, and thyroid function tests. Depending on the setting, a tuberculosis skin test and syphilis serology may be included. In contrast, psychiatric patients entering outpatient treatment often have no laboratory evaluation of any kind. This creates the potential for overusing screening tests with a resulting low yield in inpatients and for missing important medical problems in outpatients.

As an alternative, it is recommended that for each patient all tests be ordered on an individual basis, taking into account the current history and physical examination, the results of any tests recently performed, and which treatments are being considered. By this approach, the initial evaluation of a 50-year-old inpatient or outpatient with depression and multiple somatic complaints who had not been seen by a physician recently should include a thorough physical examination and all the routine screening tests listed in the preceding paragraph. In contrast, in the evaluation of an otherwise healthy 21-year-old patient with marked anxiety following the breakup of a relationship, all laboratory tests might be deferred initially pending the results of crisis intervention. Specific features of the presenting illness should alert the psychiatrist to the need for further medical evaluation. These features include a known history of a significant medical disorder that may be chronic or recurring, prominent somatic symptoms, atypical symptoms that do not fit the profile usually seen in psychiatric disorders, and evidence of delirium or dementia on the formal mental status examination. In some cases, consideration of a specific treatment will dictate the tests to be ordered, such as the need to evaluate a complete blood count, electrolytes, glucose, thyroid function, blood urea nitrogen, creatinine, urinalysis, and an EKG in any patient prior to starting lithium.

NONPSYCHIATRIC DISORDERS PRESENTING WITH PSYCHIATRIC SYMPTOMS A key feature in the descriptive criteria listed for many of the individual diagnoses in DSM-III-R is a phrase specifying that the patient's condition not be attributable to another known organic factor. As described in detail elsewhere in this text, there is a well-defined differential diagnosis for each clinical psychiatric syndrome. Specific laboratory tests should be ordered only insofar as they facilitate narrowing of this differential diagnosis. It is imperative that the psychiatrist be versed thoroughly in the broad range of medical disorders that may mimic the psychiatric disorders in DSM-III-R by presenting with disturbances in behavior, mood, or cognition. Table 9.7-3 provides a list of illnesses that commonly manifest psychiatric symptoms.

Some of these disorders, in particular endocrine dysfunctions, may present with affective features, such as the anxiety seen in hyperthyroidism, the depression that may accompany hypothyroidism, or the appearance of panic attacks in a patient with pheochromocytoma. In other cases, a prominent feature may be a gradual personality change, such as the lability that sometimes accompanies multiple sclerosis or the indifference that might be seen with a slowly growing frontal lobe tumor. In some disorders, the symptoms may create the appearance of an acute or chronic psychosis, such as phencyclidine (PCP) intoxication that mimics an acute exacerbation of schizophrenia. It must also be borne in mind that a patient already in treatment for a known psychiatric disorder may be experiencing a new superimposed medical illness. For example, the acute onset of confusion in a patient with chronic schizophrenia could be associated with self-induced water intoxication, neuroleptic malignant syndrome, anticholinergic toxicity, or any one of a number of other organic factors.

TABLE 9.7-3
Medical Disorders That May Present with Psychiatric Symptoms

Neurological
Cerebrovascular accidents (hemorrhage, infarction)
Head trauma (concussion, post-traumatic hematoma)
Epilepsy (especially complex partial seizures)
Narcolepsy
Normal pressure hydrocephalus
Parkinson's disease
Multiple sclerosis
Huntington's disease
Endocrine*
Hypo- or hyperthyroidism
Hypo- or hyperadrenalism
Hypo- or hyperparathyroidism
Hypoglycemia
Diabetes mellitus
Panhypopituitarism
Pheochromocytoma
Gonadotrophic hormonal disturbances
Metabolic or systemic
Fluid and electrolyte disturbances
Hepatic encephalopathy
Uremia
Porphyria
Hepatolenticular degeneration (Wilson's disease)
Hypoxemia (chronic pulmonary disease)
Hypotension or hypertensive encephalopathy
Toxic
Intoxication or withdrawal associated with drug or alcohol abuse
Side effects of prescribed or over-the-counter medications
Environmental toxins (volatile hydrocarbons, heavy metals, carbon monoxide, organophosphates)
Nutritional
Vitamin B_{12} deficiency (pernicious anemia)
Nicotinic acid deficiency (pellagra)
Folate deficiency (megaloblastic anemia)
Thiamine deficiency (Wernicke-Korsakoff syndrome)
Trace metal deficiency (zinc, magnesium)
Nonspecific malnutrition or dehydration
Infectious
Acquired immune deficiency syndrome (AIDS)
Neurosyphilis
Viral encephalitides (especially herpes simplex)
Brain abscess
Viral hepatitis
Infectious mononucleosis
Tuberculosis
Systemic bacterial infections (especially pneumonia) or viremia
Autoimmune
Systemic lupus erythematosus
Neoplastic
Central nervous system primary or metastatic tumors
Endocrine tumors
Pancreatic carcinoma

*Most endocrine disorders may be either endogenous or caused iatrogenically by the administration of hormones or other drugs.

LABORATORY TESTS USED IN PSYCHIATRIC DISORDERS

In recent years, as advances in the basic sciences have been quickly translated into routine clinical laboratory techniques, psychiatric researchers have studied a number of laboratory tests for utility in making diagnostic or treatment decisions. Some of these tests have attained an accepted, albeit limited, role in selected clinical situations. Many have not proved to be useful. Most, however, require extensive further study prior to any firm conclusions regarding their actual utility and limitations in patient care. It often is extremely difficult to know whether a biological abnormality identified by research in psychiatric patients is pathogenically linked to the trait of the disorder, a transient event related to the state of the patients, an artifact of drug treatment, or simply an epiphenomenon of no relevance whatsoever.

Those tests that are most commonly cited as revealing biological correlates of psychiatric disorders are discussed below and listed in Table 9.7-4, grouped according to the type of laboratory technique utilized. Particular emphasis is placed on those tests that currently have some role in the diagnosis or treatment of the disorders in DSM-III-R.

BRAIN IMAGING **Computed tomography (CT)** Because the standard skull X-ray is so unrevealing regarding the structure of the brain itself, the advent of computer-enhanced brain-imaging techniques was of particular importance to psychiatry. The CT scan, by virtue of its greater structural resolution and lower risk, has virtually replaced older, more invasive techniques, such as pneumoencephalography and cerebral angiography. With regard to psychiatric disorders, a number of CT research studies have reported the finding of ventricular enlargement or cortical atrophy, or both, in some patients with schizophrenia. However, it must be emphasized that the CT scan of the brain does not represent a routine diagnostic test for schizophrenia. Increased ventricular size in schizophrenia is a statistical finding and is neither sufficiently sensitive nor specific to be a test for that disorder.

Nevertheless, the psychiatrist may often utilize CT scanning to rule out structural pathology resulting from tumors, infections, vascular events, and degenerative disorders. It has been proposed that reasonable indications for CT scanning in psychiatric patients are: (1) a first episode of psychosis; (2) a first episode of personality disturbance or mood disorder in a patient over 50; (3) delirium or dementia of unknown origin; (4) anorexia nervosa; (5) the emergence of abnormal involuntary movements; and (6) an extended catatonic episode. In most cases, the physician can obtain the desired information via a CT scan performed without the injection of a contrast medium, thereby minimizing the risk and cost of the procedure for the patient. Contrast scans should be used only in cases in which the patient has focal signs or symptoms or when a possible lesion is noted on the noncontrast scan.

Magnetic resonance imaging (MRI) It is likely that MRI of the brain will soon supplant the CT scan. The lack of radiation exposure, the higher resolution of tissue structure, and the potential for measuring physiological variables make MRI an extremely powerful technique. Although its applicability to psychiatric disorders is being studied, MRI is already of clinical utility in the diagnosis of certain neurological disorders, such as the early identification of plaques in multiple sclerosis.

Primary degenerative dementia (Alzheimer's and Pick's diseases) and multi-infarct dementia are included as mental disorders in DSM-III-R, and CT or MRI may show signs of these disorders in the form of cortical atrophy. In such cases, these techniques already have established clinical utility in psychiatric practice.

Other imaging techniques Newly developed imaging methods include *positron emission tomography* (PET), *regional cerebral*

TABLE 9.7-4
Laboratory Tests Used in Psychiatric Research and Practice

Imaging
- Computed tomography (CT)*†
- Magnetic resonance imaging (MRI)*†
- Positron emission tomography (PET)
- Regional cerebral blood flow (rCBF)
- Single photon emission tomography (SPECT)

Electrophysiology
- Electroencephalography (EEG)*†
- Polysomnography (PSG)*†
- Computed tomographic mapping of the EEG (CTM/EEG)
- Stimulus-evoked responses†
- Electroretinogram (ERG)
- Smooth pursuit eye tracking

Endocrinology
- Cortisol function and the dexamethasone suppression test*†
- Thyroid function and the thyrotropin-releasing hormone stimulation test*†
- Other peptides (prolactin, growth hormone, melatonin, cholecystokinin, somatostatin)†

Biochemistry
- Catecholamines (dopamine, homovanillic acid, dihydroxyphenylacetic acid, norepinephrine, 3-methoxy-4-hydroxyphenylglycol)
- Indoleamines (serotonin, 5-hydroxyindoleacetic acid)
- Other neurotransmitters and neuroregulators (acetylcholine, histamine, amino acids, prostaglandins, opioid peptides)
- Enzymes (dopamine-β-hydroxylase, monoamine oxidase, tyrosine hydroxylase, catechol-*O*-methyltransferase, adenyl cyclase)
- Receptor density and affinity

Determination of drug concentrations
- Lithium*
- Anticonvulsants*
- Tricyclic antidepressants*
- Antipsychotics*

Toxicology
- Drugs of abuse*†
- Alcohol*†
- Environmental toxins*†

Hematology, serology, immunology, and microbiology
- Complete blood count†
- Cellular immune function†
- Cerebrospinal fluid protein and immunoglobulin profiles†
- Microbiological cultures and sensitivity†
- Antibody titers (viral and autoimmune)†
- Allergic skin testing
- Interferon and interleukin activity

Genetics
- Chromosomal karyotypes*†
- Genetic linkage studies
- Genetic markers (HLA histocompatibility antigens)

Neuropathology
- Postmortem histopathology

*Tests with clinical utility in disorders listed in DSM-III-R.
†Tests useful in identifying nonpsychiatric medical disorders that may present with psychiatric symptoms (Table 9.7-3).

blood flow (rCBF), and *single photon emission tomography* (SPECT). These have the potential not only for visualizing brain structure, but also for revealing some aspects of brain function in vivo. The use of these techniques in research studies has revealed intriguing findings. For example, a number of studies have indicated relative functional hypoactivity of the frontal lobes in schizophrenia. Nevertheless, these techniques remain far from attaining general clinical applicability in routine psychiatric diagnosis or treatment.

ELECTROPHYSIOLOGY

Electroencephalography (EEG) The electroencephalogram has been available as a clinical tool for more than 50 years. Distinct advantages in the ongoing development of electrophysiological laboratory tests include their relatively low cost and low risk compared with brain-imaging techniques, which involve complex and expensive equipment and, in some cases, significant exposure to radiation. EEG has proved invaluable in terms of identifying certain neurological problems—in particular, epilepsy and focal structural lesions. Specialized EEG techniques, such as the use of sleep deprivation, hyperventilation, photic stimulation, nasopharyngeal leads, and even implantation of depth electrodes, may aid in identifying otherwise silent epileptiform discharges.

The specific utility of the EEG in psychiatric disorders, however, remains limited. The major clinical application has been to patients with schizophrenia. EEG abnormalities in psychosis were first reported more than 40 years ago, but numerous studies utilizing both the traditional EEG and stimulus-evoked responses in schizophrenia and bipolar disorder have not yielded a finding with sufficient sensitivity or specificity to have routine clinical utility. Nevertheless, a sleep-deprived EEG with nasopharyngeal leads may aid in ruling out an epileptiform process contributing to the psychosis in a patient presumptively diagnosed as having schizophrenia. An EEG is indicated in schizophrenic patients who are younger, are presenting with their first psychotic episode, or have a history of a cerebral injury. Finally, relatively nonspecific EEG findings may be observed late in the course of Alzheimer's disease, in some cases of mental retardation, or in drug intoxication.

Polysomnography (PSG) PSG involves monitoring of the EEG, electromyogram (EMG), eye movements, and vital signs during sleep. It has the potential for aiding in the diagnosis of sleep apnea, periodic nighttime movements, and other sleep disorders that may be associated with behavioral symptoms. The psychiatrist should consider obtaining a PSG study in any patient with either insomnia or hypersomnia that cannot be explained on the basis of an identified medical or psychiatric disorder. Sleep research in depressed patients has indicated a strong association between some variables, especially shortened rapid eye movement (REM) sleep latency and major depression. However, a significant number of depressed patients have normal or increased REM latency, and shortened REM latency is found in other psychiatric disorders, drug and alcohol withdrawal, sleep deprivation, and other conditions. At this point, measurement of REM latency does not have a role as a routine diagnostic test for depression or as a device for monitoring antidepressant treatment.

Computed tomographic mapping of the EEG (CTM/EEG) With regard to newer electrophysiological research techniques, there is much current interest in CTM/EEG, in which a computer is utilized to make summary surface maps of cortical electrical activity in specified frequencies. This technique has been used to examine various diagnostic groups and to study the EEG response after sensory stimuli or pharmacological challenges. Again, although some associations between particular CTM/EEG patterns and certain psychiatric disorders have been reported, these findings have not been sufficiently replicated to make CTM/EEG a routine diagnostic test.

Other electrophysiological techniques The *electroretinogram* (ERG), is a means of measuring retinal electrical activity that is hypothesized to reflect central nervous system (CNS) dopaminergic function. Research remains in the early stages. Numerous studies of *smooth pursuit eye-tracking movements* have noted abnormalities in a significant number of patients with schizophrenia and bipolar disorder (and in their relatives in some cases), leading some investigators to postulate that eye-tracking abnormalities represent a vulnerability marker for psychosis. Smooth pursuit abnormalities, however, are not of clinical diagnostic utility at this time. Electrophysiological recording of stimulus-evoked potentials may be of value in some neurological disorders, as in the case of visual evoked response (VER) abnormalities in multiple sclerosis. Likewise, EMG and nerve conduction studies may assist in the identification of myopathy and peripheral neuropathy.

ENDOCRINOLOGY

Another area of intense investigation has been that of neuroendocrine systems. Given that essential mechanisms involved in hormonal modulation reside in the limbic-hypothalamic-pituitary axis of the CNS, it has been reasonable to assume that alterations in endocrine systems, either in terms of basal hormone concentrations or response to pharmacological challenges, may serve as correlates of major psychiatric disorders. Most extensively studied (and also debated) in this regard have been the cortisol and thyroid hormone systems. With regard to both, it is important to note, as shown in Table 9.7-3, that endocrine disorders involving either increased or decreased hormonal function may initially present with psychiatric symptoms.

Dexamethasone suppression test (DST) There are a significant number of patients with depression (40 to 60 percent, depending on the diagnostic classification utilized) who have abnormally high levels of plasma cortisol in response to a modified DST. This abnormality is referred to as nonsuppression. Proponents of the clinical utility of this test assert that an abnormal DST lends support to the diagnosis of major depression. Moreover, some studies have indicated that failure of the DST to normalize after somatic treatment for depression may indicate a higher likelihood of relapse. However, the area of neuroendocrine testing in psychiatry has been marked by controversy, and early enthusiasm regarding the utility of the DST has now been tempered by a more realistic assessment of the key issues of sensitivity, specificity, and predictive value. Caution is warranted if the DST is used to assist in making diagnostic or treatment decisions in clinical settings. In particular, it is essential to bear in mind the ability of a number of other medical conditions and many commonly prescribed drugs, as listed in Table 9.7-5, to yield false-positive or even false-negative results when using the DST. Moreover, a number of studies have shown that approximately 7 percent of normal control subjects are nonsuppressors in response to the DST. When confronted with an unclear case, the clinician may use an abnormal DST to provide additional weight in support of the diagnosis of major depression and the initiation or maintenance of antidepressant treatment. The DST does not supplant a carefully gathered history and thorough examination in the diagnosis of depression, however, nor can it be used as a screening device for depression in an unselected population.

The generally accepted procedure for the DST in psychiatric patients involves an oral dose of 1.0 mg of dexamethasone, a synthetic glucocorticoid, taken at 11 P.M. For inpatients, blood samples are typically drawn the next day at 4 P.M. and 11 P.M., while for outpatients a single 4 P.M. sample is usually collected. These blood samples are analyzed for plasma cortisol concentrations. Normally, the single 1.0-mg dose of dexamethasone at 11 P.M. will suppress plasma cortisol concentrations, causing them to remain below 5 μg per dl for the next 24 hours. Plasma concentrations elevated above this level indicate nonsuppression, a positive test result. There may be variation in the assays available (with competitive protein binding and radioimmunoassay the preferred methods), and any DST plasma cortisol concentrations in the range of 4 to 7 μg per dl must be interpreted with caution.

Thyrotropin-releasing hormone stimulation test It also has been shown that in some cases of depression, even in the presence of normal routine thyroid function indices, there may be a decreased response of plasma thyroid-stimulating hormone (TSH) after the administration of thyroid-releasing hormone (TRH). In some cases

TABLE 9.7-5
Causes of Falsely Positive or Negative Results on the Dexamethasone Suppression Test

False Positives	*False Negatives*
Cushing's syndrome	Addison's disease
Weight loss or malnutrition	Hypopituitarism
Obesity	Slow dexamethasone metabolism
Pregnancy	
Alcohol abuse and withdrawal	Drugs
Anorexia nervosa	Synthetic corticosteroids
Temporal lobe epilepsy	Indomethacin
Dementia	High doses of benzodiazepines
Diabetes mellitus	
Infection	High doses of cyproheptadine
Trauma	
Carcinoma	
Renal or cardiac failure	
Renovascular hypertension	
Cerebrovascular accident	
Antipsychotic withdrawal	
Drugs	
High doses of estrogens	
Narcotics	
Sedative-hypnotics	
Anticonvulsants	

of primary hypothyroidism, the baseline level of TSH is increased. The clinical implications of a blunted TSH response, as with an abnormal DST, must be interpreted carefully in terms of sensitivity and specificity. The primary indication for using a TRH stimulation test in psychiatry is in cases of treatment-resistant depression. A blunted TSH response (especially in conjunction with an abnormal DST) may aid in confirming the diagnosis of major depression and supportcontinued antidepressant treatment. An increased baseline TSH (in conjunction with other thyroid indices) might, in turn, identify some cases of hypothyroidism mimicking a depressive disorder, cases that should respond to thyroid replacement therapy.

The TRH stimulation test is conducted in patients who have fasted overnight. In the usual procedure, the patient remains at bedrest and an intravenous line is started at approximately 8:30 A.M. and kept open by a saline drip. At 8:59 A.M., blood samples are collected for baseline thyroid indices, including TSH. At 9:00 A.M., synthetic TRH (protirelin) is administered intravenously, a dose of 500 μg being given over 30 seconds. Transient side effects, including gastrointestinal or genitourinary symptoms, a warm sensation, mouth dryness, a metallic taste, or chest tightness, may be observed after the infusion. Plasma samples for determination of TSH concentrations are then collected 15, 30, 60, and 90 minutes after infusion. A normal response to TRH will consist of an increase in plasma TSH of 5 to 15 μU per ml above baseline. A response of less than 5 μU per ml above baseline after TRH infusion is generally considered to be blunted and may be consistent with a major depression. Using this definition of blunting, an abnormal test is found in approximately 25 percent of patients with depression. Some laboratories consider a response below 7 μU per ml to be blunted, and correspondingly find a higher frequency of abnormal tests in patients with depression. It should be readily apparent that the TRH stimulation test involves potential discomfort to the patient and significant time and expense to administer, factors to be weighed carefully prior to seeking this additional laboratory information.

Other hormones and peptides Baseline levels of growth hormone, prolactin, melatonin, the gonadotrophic hormones, opioid peptides, somatostatin, and cholecystokinin have all been studied in psychiatric disorders. In the case of growth hormone and prolactin, response of the hormone to administration of apomorphine and other agents has also been examined. In spite of many interesting research findings, tests to measure these other endocrine functions currently remain outside the realm of general clinical applicability to psychiatric disorders, although they obviously have utility in identifying certain endocrine dysfunctions.

BIOCHEMISTRY Since early in this century, when theories were first advanced regarding chemical transmission in the nervous system, there has been ongoing interest in establishing correlations between various biochemical parameters and psychiatric disorders. As assays became available for specific biochemical constituents of blood, urine, and cerebrospinal fluid, they were typically applied to studies of psychiatric disorders. With the advent of effective psychopharmacological treatments and an accompanying increase in the understanding of neurotransmitter and receptor mechanisms, the focus turned more specifically to the catecholamines, indoleamines, and other neurotransmitters and neuromodulators. This, in turn, led to the elaboration of aminergic hypotheses for both schizophrenia and mood disorders and stimulated a plethora of research studies examining the concentrations of amines and their metabolites in the body fluids of groups of patients.

In spite of decades of intense research, however, these biochemical assays of neurotransmitters have not yet reached the level of general clinical applicability in psychiatry. For example, in spite of the tenacity of the dopamine hypothesis of schizophrenia, there currently is no established clinical role for measuring concentrations of dopamine or its metabolites, including homovanillic acid (HVA), in schizophrenic patients. Some investigators have noted an association between suicidal or aggressive behavior and decreased levels of the serotonin metabolite 5-hydroxyindoleacetic acid (5-HIAA) in the cerebrospinal fluid. This test, however, is not appropriate for clinical use at this time. Other researchers have reported that urinary excretion of 3-methoxy-4-hydroxyphenylglycol (MHPG), a metabolite of norepinephrine, is decreased in some cases of depression, especially in bipolar patients. Some investigators have asserted that patients with lower total urinary MHPG in a 24-hour collection are more likely to respond to tricyclic antidepressants, such as desipramine (Norpramin), that have primarily noradrenergic effects. This hypothesis remains controversial, however, having not been supported in some research studies.

Numerous other proven and putative neurotransmitters and neuroregulators, including acetylcholine, histamine, amino acids, peptides, and prostaglandins, have been intensively investigated. Moreover, in addition to measuring neurotransmitters and their metabolites, the enzymes involved in their metabolic pathways have been studied, including tyrosine hydroxylase, monoamine oxidase, and dopamine-β-hydroxylase. Receptors, which represent another link in the chain of neurotransmission, have also been the subject of extensive research. Studies of this type have generally made use of peripheral measures (e.g., platelet enzyme activity or receptor binding).

Although research studies of these neurochemical variables have reported numerous abnormalities, no reliable routine laboratory test of neurotransmitters or metabolites has been found to enhance decisions regarding diagnosis or treatment in patients with psychiatric disorders. Nevertheless, in spite of the failure of the measures described above to reach daily clinical practice, the crucial role of neurotransmitters in CNS function ensures that active investigation in this area will continue.

MEASUREMENT OF THERAPEUTIC DRUG CONCENTRATIONS For most psychiatrists, measurement of drug concentrations is the area of laboratory testing with which they are most familiar. This is particularly true with regard to lithium, an ion that is easily measured, for which there is a well-defined narrow therapeutic range of serum concentrations, and that may be associated with significant adverse effects. In addition to routine monitoring of steady-state serum lithium concentrations, models exist for the prediction of ultimate steady-state concentrations by a determination of the lithium concentration after a single acute dose. Similarly, it is advisable to monitor routinely blood concentrations of anticonvulsants, such as carbamazepine (Tegretol), that may be given to psychiatric patients.

Measurements of concentrations of the tricyclic antidepressants and, more recently, antipsychotics have also become available. Inasmuch as these drugs generally have a larger therapeutic index than lithium, determinations of concentrations are typically not required in routine treatment. The primary indication for determination of antidepressant or antipsychotic concentrations is in cases where poor treatment response or adverse reactions raise questions regarding toxicity, compliance, or unusual pharmacokinetics, such as slow or fast metabolism leading to excessively high or low concentrations. For some drugs—in particular, the tricyclic antidepressant, nortriptyline (Pamelor)—a *therapeutic window* may exist, meaning that above or below a certain range of drug concentrations a less than optimal clinical response can be expected. Because of their large therapeutic index, sedative-hypnotic agents do not usually require routine monitoring of blood concentrations. Nevertheless, given their abuse potential, they may be the subject of qualitative toxicological screening.

TOXICOLOGY The role of toxic substances in producing CNS effects and behavioral symptoms may be profound, whether through voluntary consumption in the case of drugs and alcohol or inadvertent exposure to substances, such as heavy metals. Because of the prevalence of substance abuse, drug screening has become a routine part of the psychiatric admission process in some settings. Especially in cases of unexplained delirium, dementia, or personality change, intentional or environmental exposure to toxic agents must be part of the differential diagnosis. As indicated in DSM-III-R, a number of specific organic mental syndromes are directly attributable to the toxicity of substances. Not only must toxicity be a consideration, but in many cases the absence of the drug (i.e., a withdrawal state) may explain the observed signs and symptoms. In addition, drug abuse commonly involves more than one substance, and often only a sound alliance with the patient and a diligently gathered history will reveal the extent of substance abuse.

Certain methodological considerations must be borne in mind when laboratory toxicological tests are performed to identify a specific drug or to screen for a range of substances. Relevant factors include the substance (or substances) involved, the time elapsed since the last use or exposure, the body fluid (i.e., blood or urine) chosen for testing, and the extraction process and analytical method used by the laboratory. Attention must be paid to each of these factors to minimize the likelihood of obtaining false-positive or false-negative results. For example, most drugs are much more concentrated in urine than in serum, but cleaner extractions are in general more easily obtained from serum than urine. Thin-layer chromatography is relatively inexpensive and provides rapid qualitative screening for a number of substances, whereas gas chromatography and other methods are much more sensitive, but also are more time-consuming and expensive. It is readily apparent that it often is prudent to consult with the laboratory specifically prior to collecting a sample from a patient and choosing an analytical method for toxicological testing.

HEMATOLOGY, SEROLOGY, IMMUNOLOGY, AND MICROBIOLOGY As is the case in every other area of laboratory investigation, there have been numerous studies utilizing tests of this type in psychiatric disorders, and many abnormal findings have been reported. Examples in schizophrenia research range from decreased wheal response after histamine injection to increased cerebrospinal fluid immunoglobulin concentrations. Investigators have hypothesized a viral or autoimmune pathophysiological basis for some of the major psychiatric disorders, especially schizophrenia. Recently, some researchers have postulated an association between persistent Epstein-Barr virus infection and some cases of chronic depression with prominent fatigue. Moreover, there is a growing body of basic research indicating complex interactions between the CNS and the cellular and humoral components of the immune system. However, none of these reported abnormalities in psychiatric disorders has been sufficiently replicated to yield a routine laboratory test for clinical psychiatric diagnosis or treatment.

GENETICS Laboratory tests of genetic factors may be of several types: gross chromosomal assessments (e.g., to identify XO, XXY, or trisomy 21 karyotypes); genetic linkage studies; or identification of genetic markers (e.g., human lymphocyte antigens or ABO blood group markers). One group of mental disorders in which chromosomal assessments have established utility is mental retardation. Chromosomal abnormalities may be associated with profound cognitive and behavioral disorders, as in the case of Down's syndrome or the fragile-X syndrome. In terms of genetic linkage studies directed at establishing the chromosomal locus of certain disorders, recent research involving large family groups in which many members are affected by Huntington's disease has localized the defect to chromosome 4. This finding, in turn, paves the way for a genetic test for carriers of the gene in this devastating neurological disorder. Likewise, recent studies indicate that, in some early-onset cases of Alzheimer's disease, the disorder appears to involve a genetic abnormality located on chromosome 21. In some cases of bipolar disorder, the locus of the genetic abnormality may be on chromosome 11 or the X chromosome.

Genetic linkage studies and genetic markers have been the topic of much recent psychiatric research, but have not yet demonstrated clinical utility in psychotic or mood disorders. Nevertheless, given the patterns of some degree of apparent familial transmission in a number of psychiatric and neurological disorders and the emergence of powerful new techniques in genetic research, the vast potential of studies in this area is readily apparent.

NEUROPATHOLOGY The principle of correlating gross and microscopic pathological findings with clinical signs and symptoms (using either biopsy material or postmortem specimens) is a crucial element in medical research and practice. It is perhaps unfortunate that the autopsy has been largely abandoned in clinical psychiatric practice in the United States. Postmortem neuropathology has been part of the tradition of psychiatry insofar as the pioneers in this field examined the brain searching for histopathological correlates of psychosis. The fact that they did not find pathognomonic lesions associated with specific disorders probably diverted attention from this area.

In recent psychiatric research, postmortem material has been more commonly used in neurochemical studies of schizophrenia, mood disorders, and suicide. The goal has been to identify abnormalities in tissue concentrations of amines and metabolites, in enzyme activity, or in neurotransmitter receptor density and binding affinity. In spite of intense study, the findings regarding biochemical alterations in postmortem tissue studies of various psychiatric disorders have been ambiguous.

Currently, there is a reawakening of interest in postmortem morphological examination of the brain in psychiatric disorders. This trend is especially noticeable with regard to schizophrenia, largely as a result of the structural and functional abnormalities observed by research studies using CT and other forms of brain imaging in this disorder. This new wave of neuropathological studies has been facilitated by the establishment of research "brain banks" to provide specimens for investigators and by the use of computer-based quantitative microscopy that allows automated assessment of large numbers of microscopic fields in the search for subtle structural abnormalities. The use of neuropathological studies in schizophrenia or mood disorders is not currently directly relevant to clinical practice. However, the definitive diagnosis of some forms of dementia, including Alzheimer's disease, is dependent on neuropathological verification.

THE LABORATORY'S ROLE

The laboratory has a role in clinical psychiatry no less than in any other medical specialty. Above all, the psychiatrist is obligated to understand the judicious use of the history, the examination, and laboratory tests to identify patients who have medical disorders presenting with cognitive, affective, or behavioral changes, so that these patients are not mistakenly diagnosed and treated as having a primary mental disorder.

The role of the laboratory in psychiatry may expand even more rapidly during the next few years as researchers continue to apply state-of-the-art basic scientific techniques to psychiatric disorders. As this occurs, the need will become greater than ever for practicing psychiatrists to understand the nuances of rigorously interpreting laboratory data in terms of test sensitivity, specificity, and predictive value. Only then will they be able to integrate these data with the results of interviews and examinations to form a coherent picture of diagnosis and treatment needs.

REFERENCES

Arana G W, Baldessarini R J, Ornsteen M: The dexamethasone suppression test for diagnosis and prognosis in psychiatry. Arch Gen Psychiat *42:* 1193, 1985.

Burrows G D, Norman T R, editors: *Psychotropic Drugs: Plasma Concentration and Clinical Response*. Marcel Dekker, New York, 1981.

Carroll B J: Dexamethasone suppression test: A review of contemporary confusion. J Clin Psychiat *46*(2,2): 13, 1985.

Galen R S, Gambino S R: *Beyond Normality: The Predictive Value and Efficiency of Medical Diagnoses*. Wiley, New York, 1975.

Garattini S, Tognoni G, editors: Biological markers in mental disorders (symposium). J Psychiat Res *18:* 327, 1984.

Gold M S, Pottash A L C: *Diagnostic and Laboratory Testing in Psychiatry*. Plenum, New York, 1986.

Greden, J F: Laboratory testing in psychiatry. In *Comprehensive Textbook of Psychiatry*, ed 4, p 2028. Williams & Wilkins, Baltimore, 1985.

Griner P F, Glaser R J: Misuse of laboratory tests and diagnostic procedures. New Eng J Med *307:* 1336, 1982.

Hall R C W, editor: *Psychiatric Presentations of Medical Illness: Somatopsychic Disorders*. SP Medical and Scientific Books, New York, 1980.

Hall R C W, Beresford T P, editors: *Handbook of Psychiatric Diagnostic Procedures*, vols 1, 2. SP Medical and Scientific Books, New York, 1984, 1985.

Koranyi E K: Morbidity and rate of undiagnosed physical illnesses in a psychiatric clinic population. Arch Gen Psychiat *36:* 414, 1979.

Lake C R, Ziegler M G, editors: *The Catecholamines in Psychiatric and Neurologic Disorders*. Butterworth, Boston, 1985.

Loosen P T, Prange A J: Serum thyrotropin response to thyrotropin-releasing hormone in psychiatric patients: A review. Amer J Psychiat *139:* 405, 1982.

MacKinnon R A, Yudofsky S C: *The Psychiatric Evaluation in Clinical Practice*. Lippincott, Philadelphia, 1986.

Martin R L, Preskorn S H: Use of the laboratory in psychiatry. In *The Medical Basis of Psychiatry*, G Winokur, P Clayton, editors, p 522. Saunders, Philadelphia, 1986.

McIntyre J S, Romano J: Is there a stethoscope in the house (and is it used)? Arch Gen Psychiat *34:* 1147, 1977.

Stahl S M, Kravitz K D: A critical review of the use of laboratory tests in psychiatric disorders. In *Biological Psychiatry*, P A Berger, H K H Brodie, editors, vol 8, p 1048, *American Handbook of Psychiatry*, S Arieti, editor-in-chief, ed 2. Basic Books, New York, 1986.

Usdin E, Hanin I, editors: *Biological Markers in Psychiatry and Neurology*. Pergamon, New York, 1982.

Weinberger D R: Brain disease and psychiatric illness: When should a psychiatrist order a CAT scan? Amer J Psychiat *141:* 1521, 1984.

Wells C, Duncan G: *Neurology for Psychiatrists*. Davis, Philadelphia, 1980.

9.8
PSYCHIATRIC RATING SCALES

JACK A. GREBB, M.D.

INTRODUCTION

Psychiatric rating scales, also called rating instruments, provide a method of quantifying aspects of a patient's psyche, behavior, and relationships with individuals and society. The measurement of pathology in these areas of an individual's life may initially seem much less straightforward than the measurement of pathology—hypertension, for example—seen by other medical specialists. Nevertheless, many psychiatric rating scales have been developed that are able to measure carefully chosen features of well-formulated concepts. Moreover, without utilizing these rating scales, psychiatrists are left with only their clinical impressions, which are difficult to record in a manner that allows for reliable comparison and communication in the future. Without psychiatric rating scales, quantitative data in psychiatry are quite crude (e.g., length of hospitalization or other treatment, discharge and readmission to hospital, length of relationships of employment, the presence of legal troubles).

There are several confusing aspects of nomenclature and connotation involving psychiatric rating scales. First, psychiatric rating scales are often referred to as objective measures. Traditionally, information from professionals is considered to be objective, whereas information from patients or other nonprofessional informants is considered subjective. However, since there are self-rated (i.e., patient-rated) psychiatric rating scales, it is not accurate to consider all psychiatric rating scales as objective information. Rather, psychiatric rating scales provide quantitative measures of both objective and subjective information. Second, although the term "psychiatric rating scales" would seem to be quite broad, it is not usually meant to include either diagnostic rating scales or traditional neuropsychological tests; however, the distinction between these terms is variable and confused. Psychological tests for the assessment of intelligence are covered in Sections 9.5, Neuropsychological and Intellectual Assessment of Adults, and 9.6, Neuropsychological and Intellectual Assessment of Children, and tests for the assessment of personality are covered in Section 9.4, Psychological Assessment of Personality of Adults and Children.

Psychiatric rating scales are useful in research, clinical care, and teaching. Their major use is in research studies designed to assess the effects of treatments or to describe patient populations. All clinicians need to know enough about these scales to be able to assess the merit of published clinical research that utilizes psychiatric rating scales as the dependent measures. Rating scales can also be used to document change in the psychiatric state of patients in the clinical setting. Such documentation can potentially be used for therapeutic effect with the patient, and use of psychiatric rating scales may become more common as third-party insurance companies require more evidence of treatment efficacy for individual patients. Finally, rating scales can be of pedagogical value, since they can serve as a mechanism of teaching students to look carefully and rationally at subsets of complex behavioral syndromes.

TYPES OF RATING SCALES

It is possible to discuss different types of rating scales based on who is doing the rating (e.g., patient, nurse, doctor) and the source of rated material (e.g., observations of the patient on the ward, information from an interview). Each of these types has advantages and disadvantages. Although some clinicians believe otherwise, it is usually advantageous to have information from several sources covering a range of relevant areas; therefore, several different types of rating scales may be employed in an individual situation. Most of these different types of scales can now be completed utilizing a computer program. Many such programs are interactional with the user and can improve the cataloging and analysis of data from the scales.

SELF-REPORT (PATIENT-RATED) SCALES Self-report scales are appealing because they report the opinion of the consumer of psychiatric treatment. Self-report scales are also the most direct way of assessing subjective internal states (e.g., guilt) that would require a high level of inference on the part of an outside rater. Another type of patient-rated scale is the self-monitoring inventory, in which a patient records the frequency and severity of a particular thought, feeling, or behavior. Although self-monitoring in a naturalistic setting provides relevant information, the act of self-monitoring may affect the targeted symptom. Self-report scales are also more sensitive than other-rated scales in detecting more subtle pathology, such as mild depression. Other advantages of self-report scales include the limited professional time and expense required and the ability to have patients mail self-report scales to the doctor to facilitate follow-up.

There are several disadvantages to self-report scales. Many patients may not be willing to complete such scales; therefore, research studies based on self-report scales are biased in that they report on a subset of patients who are willing to complete the scales. Patients who are too ill, have severe memory and attention problems, or cannot read would not be able to complete these scales. Self-report scales are subject to variability based on educational level, social level, and cultural background of the patient. Some patients might answer self-report scales falsely because of their psychopathology, desire for secondary gain, or legal problems. It is difficult, therefore, to report on the reliability and validity of self-report scales, inasmuch as such measures vary with the particular test group and the purpose of administering the scale.

INFORMANT-RATED SCALES Informant-rated scales can be completed by relatives, friends, or significant associates of a patient. Informant-rated scales have many of the same advantages and disadvantages as patient-rated scales. Informant-rated scales can, however, add valuable information about the patient's behavior in a naturalistic setting, including information regarding a patient's interpersonal and functional abilities. Moreover, many informants will be able to compare the patient's present behavior with earlier premorbid behavior, thereby potentially increasing the sensitivity of informant-rated scales to detect pathology. The limitations of informant-rated scales include the requirement that there be an informant who is willing to cooperate, as well as the potential biases and motivations of the informant.

PROFESSIONAL-RATED NATURALISTIC OBSERVATIONS These scales are completed by professionals based on observations of the patient on the ward, in a therapy activity (e.g., occupational therapy), or some other therapeutically related setting. Although the setting observed is usually not as naturalistic as the one for informant-rated scales, increased objectivity is offered by the professional rater. These scales can be quite useful in assessing the behavior of severely ill children and adults who are unable to complete self-reports and who often give very little information during an interview. These scales usually require a significant amount of professional time since they involve the professional's observing the patient for a specified period of time. The behaviors rated, therefore, need to be frequent and obvious enough to be measured accurately. Also, as with self-monitoring inventories, the process of observing a behavior may affect its characteristics.

PROFESSIONAL-RATED INTERVIEWS Professional-rated scales can be based on unstructured, semistructured, or structured interview formats of either patients or other informants. During the interview, the professional can encourage cooperation, clarify questions, and otherwise use his or her clinical judgment to aid in completing the scale. However, the use of clinical judgment and an excessive amount of inference can decrease the reliability and validity of a scale. The use of completely structured interviews in which the specific order and wording of questions is standardized can reduce this variability. A disadvantage of structured interviews is that they can be more awkward than standard clinical interviews, especially when the therapist knows the patient and is required by the structured format to ask questions to which the answer is already known. This problem can usually be overridden, however, by explaining the specific purpose of the interview to the patient. Major causes of low reliability in scales based on unstructured interviews are the differing theoretical approaches, interviewing styles, and experience of the interviewers. Paradoxically, it is often the less experienced clinicians, such as medical students and residents, who are better able to complete these scales reliably since they are more inclined to follow the directions and not to exercise their clinical judgment.

CHOOSING AND USING A RATING SCALE

A rating scale should be chosen on the basis of its ability to measure the specific clinical variable, the abilities and availabilities of the patient and rater, and the clinical setting. The appropriate choice of a rating scale requires a clear conceptualization by the therapist regarding the target symptoms to be assessed. The final choice of a scale should usually be made after several similar scales are considered. There is no one best scale to rate each specific disorder. The rater should complete the rating scale only after reading relevant introductory material and having any questions answered. It is ideal to have new raters rate 5 to 10 patients who are also rated by experienced raters. This technique can provide an informal measure of interrater agreement, though not interrater reliability. The use of practice ratings also controls for variances in the recent clinical experiences of the raters. For example, a psychiatrist who has just transferred from an emergency room to an outpatient clinic is likely to underrate the severity of illness in outpatients if he or she compares them directly to emergency room patients.

CHARACTERISTICS OF RATING SCALES

Rating scales can be specific or comprehensive, and they can measure both internally experienced (e.g., mood) and externally observable (e.g., behavior) variables. Specific scales measure discrete thoughts, moods, or behaviors, such as obsessive thoughts or temper tantrums; comprehensive scales measure broader abstractions, such as depression or anxiety. The broadest type of rating scale measures the overall severity of illness, such as the Global Assessment of Functioning Scale (GAF Scale; see Table 9.2-4 in Section 9.2, Psychiatric Report). This scale comprises Axis V in the revised third edition of the American Psychiatric Association's *Diagnostic and Statistical Manual of Mental Disorders* (DSM-III-R).

Classic items from the mental status examination are the most frequently assessed items on rating scales. These items include thought disorder, mood disturbances, and gross behaviors. Another type of information covered by rating scales is the assessment of adverse effects from psychotherapeutic drugs. Social adjustment (e.g., occupational success, quality of relationships) and psychoanalytic concepts (e.g., ego strength, defense mechanisms) are also measured by some rating scales, although the reliability and validity of such scales are lowered by the absence of agreed-on norms, the high level of inference required on some items, and the lack of independence between measures. A final area of material covered by rating scales is positive mental health. Although it was formerly thought that positive mental health was merely the mirror image of mental illness, several studies have shown that positive mental health and mental illness may be somewhat independent. Furthermore, the inclusion of items regarding positive mental health may increase the predictive validity of the rating scales.

Other characteristics of rating scales include the time period covered, the level of judgment required, and the method of recording the answers. It is absolutely critical that the time period covered by a rating scale be specified and that the rater adhere to this time period. For example, a particular rating scale may rate a 5-minute observation period, a week-long period of time, or the entire life of the patient. The most reliable rating scales require a limited amount of judgment or inference on the part of the rater. Whatever the level of judgment required, clear definitions of the answer scale, preferably with clinical examples, should be provided by the developer of the scale and be read by the rater. The actual answer might be recorded as either a dichotomous (e.g., true or false, present or absent) or continuous variable. Continuous items may ask the rater to choose a term to describe severity (absent, slight, mild, moderate, severe, extreme) or frequency (never, rarely, occasionally, often, very often, always). Although many psychiatric symptoms are thought of as existing in dichotomous states, for example, the presence or absence of delusions, most experienced clinicians know that the world is not so simple.

In the development of rating scales, a particular method is chosen to summarize the data gathered from each item in the questionnaire. Although the user of the scale usually just adds up the numbers, the developer of the scale had to have completed either a factor analysis or to have developed a method of converting the data into T-scores. When developing a scoring system, it is not possible simply to collapse all items into one score since the different items may not be correlated. A factor analysis involves the completion of a matrix (i.e., chart) of correlations between each item and all other items. This matrix is then reduced to a smaller number of variables, called factors, that have a correlation, called a loading, with each other factor. T-scores are a method of comparing the results from a rating scale for an individual with a reference group and often involves the conversion of the raw score into a percentile.

RELIABILITY AND VALIDITY

RELIABILITY The reliability of a rating scale is a measure of the consistency with which subjects are discriminated from one another. The reliability of a scale is not proved merely by demonstrating that several different raters assign the same patients the same scores; that would be a demonstration of interrater agreement. Reliability is best reported as a correlation coefficient, r, which is a number from 0 to 1. Zero represents a chance correlation, whereas 1 represents perfect agreement. It is inadvisable to use rating scales with a correlation coefficient less than 0.7 as reported in the literature.

Different types of reliability are interrater reliability, test-retest reliability, and internal consistency. Interrater reliability is a measure of the agreement between clinicians who evaluate the same series of patients. Test-retest reliability assesses the stability of the scale in producing the same results with time; test-retest reliability is based on the assumption that the factor being measured is stable within the time period. The internal consistency of a rating scale is a measure of the degree to which items in the scale covary. Ideally, different items and factors of a rating scale measure different aspects of the same phenomenon.

VALIDITY Validity refers to the concept of whether the test measures what it purports to measure. There are four types of validity to consider regarding rating scales—content, concurrent, predictive, and construct. Content validity is a measure of the extent to which the scale assesses appropriate aspects of the target concept. This level of validity is more relevant for the developers of scales than for the users, who should be more interested in concurrent validity. Concurrent validity is a measure of the correlation between the rating scale and some external measure, such as diagnosis. Concurrent validity is reported as a correlation statistic, epsilon (ϵ), with 0 representing complete overlap of distribution and 1 representing complete separation. The ability of a scale to assess change is a type of concurrent validity, and it is important not to assume that every scale can validly be used sequentially to record clinical change. Few scales have been designed to have predictive validity, and even fewer have actually been demonstrated to have prognostic significance. Finally, construct validity requires the demonstration that the explanatory concepts account for the variability of the scale.

SPECIFIC CLINICAL SITUATIONS

This subsection includes selected rating scales. Since rating scales should be individually chosen for each research or clinical situation, this selection does not represent a compilation of the best scales, but rather, typical examples of rating scales. In addition, these scales are designed primarily to assess severity and change of symptoms in patients who are already diagnosed as having a mental disorder. These scales are not designed for diagnostic use or for application on groups of normal subjects.

SCHIZOPHRENIA AND PSYCHOSIS The major aspects of the schizophrenic syndrome that can be measured by rating scales are positive symptoms, negative symptoms, thought disorder, and impact on functioning. The positive symptoms and, to a lesser extent, other symptoms of schizophrenia can be measured by comprehensive scales, such as the Brief Psychiatric Rating Scale (BPRS; see Table 9.4-12 in Section 9.4) or the Nurses' Observation Scale for Inpatient Evaluation (NOSIE, Table 9.8-1). The BPRS is a clinician-rated scale that is completed based on information from unstructured interviews and observations of the patient's present condition. The NOSIE was developed to be based on behavior of hospitalized psychiatric patients observed over a 3-day period. The total score is the sum of the scores for each item; however, some items are scored 0 = 4, 1 = 3, 2 = 2, 3 = 1, and 4 = 0. Another comprehensive rating scale is the Schedule for Affective Disorders and Schizophrenia (SADS). Negative symptoms can be measured using the Negative Symptom Rating Scale (NSRS, Table 9.8-2) or other available negative symptom scales, such as the Scale for the Assessment of Negative Symptoms (SANS). Thought disorder can be rated separately using such scales as the Scale for the Assessment of Thought Language and Communication (TLC) or the Thought Disorder Index (TDI). The Quality of Life Scale (QLS) provides a measure of the impact of deficit symptoms on the patient's daily life. Finally, the Chestnut Lodge Prognostic Scale for Chronic Schizophrenia may have a predictive validity. See Table 9.8-3 for the sources of the rating scales used for schizophrenia and psychosis mentioned above.

MOOD DISORDERS There are many more scales for assessing depression than for assessing mania. Different scales for depression emphasize the cognitive, physiological, behavioral, or affective components of this syndrome. The two most commonly used comprehensive scales are the Beck Depression Inventory (BDI), which emphasizes cognitive aspects, and the Hamilton Depression Rating Scale (HAM-D, Table 9.8-4), which emphasizes the more physiological aspects. The BDI is a patient-rated scale in which patients are asked to answer each item based on the past week. The HAM-D is a clinician-rated scale that is based on an unstructured interview and any other information available to the clinician. It was designed for use with patients who are already diagnosed as having a depressive disorder. The total score is a sum of the scores on all items; a score of zero indicates the absence of the symptoms measured in the scale, and a score of 74 indicates the maximum presence of the symptoms. The HAM-D score is sometimes reported as double the total score, producing a range from 0 to 148.

Other rating scales used for depression are the SADS, Standard Assessment of Depressive Disorders (SADD), Zung Self-Rating Scale for Depression, Caroll Rating Scale for Depression, Montgomery-Asberg Scale, Raskin Depression Rating Scale, and Inventory to Diagnose Depression. Many of the symptoms of gross mania will be measured by the BPRS, NOSIE, or SADS. Two specific scales for mania are the Mania Rating Scale and the Manic-State Rating Scale. See

TABLE 9.8-1
Nurses' Observation Scale for Inpatient Evaluation

Directions: On the following pages you are asked to rate the behavior of this patient. There are 80 items, which cover a wide range of activities. You are to base your ratings on the patient's behavior during the last 3 days only. For each item you are to estimate whether in the last 3 days the description of the patient's behavior was true:

0 Never
1 Sometimes
2 Often
3 Usually
4 Always

Indicate your choice by placing a circle around the correct number before each item.

0	1	2	3	4	*1. Is sloppy. (NEA)
0	1	2	3	4	2. Is impatient. (IRR)
0	1	2	3	4	3. Accuses others of wanting to hurt him. (DEP)
0	1	2	3	4	*4. Ignores the activities around him. (INT)
0	1	2	3	4	5. Cries. (DEP)
0	1	2	3	4	6. Demands the attention of the doctors. (DEP)
0	1	2	3	4	7. Has temper tantrums. (IRR)
0	1	2	3	4	8. Resists suggestions and requests. (IRR)
0	1	2	3	4	9. Shouts and yells. (IRR)
0	1	2	3	4	10. Is excited, noisy, and hilarious. (IRR)
0	1	2	3	4	11. Gets along with other patients.
0	1	2	3	4	12. Talks freely with volunteer workers or other visitors. (INT)
0	1	2	3	4	13. Shows curiosity and interest in activities around him. (INT)
0	1	2	3	4	14. Keeps busy during the day.
0	1	2	3	4	15. Conforms to hospital routine. (COO)
0	1	2	3	4	16. Is cheerful and optimistic. (INT)
0	1	2	3	4	17. Hoards things (carries things hidden in paper bags, hides things under bed, etc.).
0	1	2	3	4	18. Hits others.
0	1	2	3	4	19. Shaves himself. (COM)
0	1	2	3	4	20. Speaks in short phrases only (3 or 4 words at a time).
0	1	2	3	4	21. Looks sad.
0	1	2	3	4	*22. Needs help in dressing. (COM)
0	1	2	3	4	*23. Needs help in using the toilet. (COM)
0	1	2	3	4	24. Helps out when asked. (COO)
0	1	2	3	4	25. Plays cards with others.
0	1	2	3	4	26. Sits unless directed into activity.
0	1	2	3	4	27. Knows where he is. (COM)
0	1	2	3	4	28. Cooperates with other people. (COO)
0	1	2	3	4	29. Talks about himself.
0	1	2	3	4	*30. Stays by himself. (INT)
0	1	2	3	4	*31. Is hesitant and uncertain in making up his mind. (COM)
0	1	2	3	4	32. Jokes with others. (INT)
0	1	2	3	4	33. Gets angry or annoyed easily. (IRR)
0	1	2	3	4	*34. Wets or soils his clothes or bedding. (COM)
0	1	2	3	4	35. Asks for a pass to leave the hospital.
0	1	2	3	4	36. Talks about happenings on the ward. (INT)
0	1	2	3	4	37. Answers when spoken to.
0	1	2	3	4	38. Hears things that are not there. (PSY)
0	1	2	3	4	*39. Seems content and satisfied. (DEP)
0	1	2	3	4	40. Keeps his clothes neat and clean. (NEA)
0	1	2	3	4	41. Takes part in back and forth conversation. (INT)
0	1	2	3	4	42. Complains about the food and care. (IRR)
0	1	2	3	4	43. Tries to be friendly with others. (INT)
0	1	2	3	4	44. Becomes easily upset if something doesn't suit him. (IRR)
0	1	2	3	4	45. Assumes strange expressions, postures, or movements. (PSY)
0	1	2	3	4	46. Refuses to do the ordinary things expected of him.
0	1	2	3	4	47. Is irritable and grouchy. (IRR)
0	1	2	3	4	*48. Has trouble remembering. (COM)
0	1	2	3	4	49. Makes his own bed. (COM)
0	1	2	3	4	50. Refuses to speak.
0	1	2	3	4	51. Can be drawn into conversation. (INT)
0	1	2	3	4	52. Laughs or smiles at funny comments or events. (INT)
0	1	2	3	4	53. Volunteers to help out around the ward. (COO)
0	1	2	3	4	54. Claims that he is being controlled by people or unusual forces. (DEP)
0	1	2	3	4	*55. Is messy in his eating habits. (NEA)
0	1	2	3	4	56. Starts up a conversation with others. (INT)
0	1	2	3	4	57. Says he feels blue or depressed. (DEP)
0	1	2	3	4	58. Combs his hair. (COM)
0	1	2	3	4	59. Talks about his interests. (INT)
0	1	2	3	4	60. Takes part in recreation.
0	1	2	3	4	61. Sees things that are not there. (PSY)
0	1	2	3	4	62. Is friendly with someone on the ward. (INT)
0	1	2	3	4	63. Has unusual speech (mixes up words, makes up new words, repeats sounds, words, or phrases in a meaningless or mechanical manner). (PSY)
0	1	2	3	4	64. Shows inappropriate feeling or lack of feeling.

TABLE 9.8-1 *(continued)*

0	1	2	3	4	65. Reads newspapers and magazines.
0	1	2	3	4	*66. Has to be reminded what to do. (COM)
0	1	2	3	4	67. Sleeps, unless directed into activity.
0	1	2	3	4	68. Says that he is no good. (DEP)
0	1	2	3	4	*69. Has to be told to follow hospital routine. (COM)
0	1	2	3	4	70. Seems to enjoy life. (INT)
0	1	2	3	4	71. Pays attention when spoken to.
0	1	2	3	4	72. Washes himself. (COM)
0	1	2	3	4	*73. Has difficulty completing even simple tasks on his own. (COM)
0	1	2	3	4	74. Is alert and attentive.
0	1	2	3	4	75. Talks, mutters, or mumbles to himself. (PSY)
0	1	2	3	4	*76. Appears confused or puzzled. (COM)
0	1	2	3	4	*77. Is slow moving and sluggish. (COM)
0	1	2	3	4	78. Giggles or smiles to himself without any apparent reason. (PSY)
0	1	2	3	4	79. Quick to fly off the handle. (IRR)
0	1	2	3	4	80. Keeps himself neat and clean. (NEA)

Table from Honigfeld G, Klett C J: The Nurses' Observation Scale for Inpatient Evaluation. Psychol Rep *21:* 65, 1965, with permission.
*Item receives reflected score (0 = 4, 1 = 3, 2 = 2, 3 = 1, 4 = 0).

TABLE 9.8-2
Negative Symptom Rating Scale

Rater:______________________ Patient:______________________ Date:______________________

Not Rated (NR)	*Normal 0*	*Mildly Impaired (–) 1–2*	*Moderately Impaired (–) 3–4*	*Severely Impaired (–) 5–6*
I. Speech content	More than 5 ideas, elaborated	4–5 ideas	2–3 statements	1 statement or mute or nonsense
II. Judgment and decisions	Good grasp of reality, independent decisions	Slow, incomplete judgment	Vague judgment	Uncertainty, ambivalence
III. Memory—Correct recall after 10 minutes	5 words	4 words, or 5 with prompting	2–3 words	No words or 1 word with prompting
IV. Attention—Correct subtraction in 30 seconds serial 3's	> 10	5–10	2–4	0–1
V. Orientation	3	2	1	0
VI. Grooming—Clothing, face, hands	Clean, appropriate	Clean, untidy	Stained, disheveled	Soiled, uncared for
VII. Motivation—Plans, constructive activity	Without need for supervision	Needs reminders	Needs ongoing supervision	Needs active assistance
VIII. Motion—Amount, speed (task, make 5 steps back and forth)	Completes task without hesitation	Lag; mild slowing	Sluggish; needs encouragement	May only stand up or remains motionless
IX. Emotional response	Full affect range	Mildly constricted range of affect	Blunted affect	Flat affect
X. Expressive relatedness	Freely initiates	Does not initiate but readily engages	Avoids interaction, no warmth	Withdrawn, seclusive, mechanical requests
TOTAL				

The scoring principles are as follows: (1) The range of the scale lies between "0" and "–6" for each item. A score of "0" represents the average individual's healthy, adaptive exercise of occupational functioning, social relations, self-care, constructive use of time, and efficient mental performance. The normal behavior range declines to a score of "–2" and may overlap with soft signs of pathology, which means that even normal controls may score as mildly impaired on negative symptoms. A score of "–6" in most cases represents the complete lack of the assessed function and is a strong indication of severe and pervasive pathology. A rating of NR (not ratable) is used when the rater cannot get enough information to rate that item confidently. This is different from a rating of "0," which means that the rater possesses enough information to describe the behavior defined under that point on the scale. (2) Although there might not be a perfectly linear gradient in the way the points of the scale are being defined from "0" to "–6," should the rater hesitate between two neighboring scores, the one that stands closer to "0" is to be marked. (3) As a rule, the ratings represent the *best* of the patient's functioning during a rating period. (4) A *rating period* is the time span within which the raters collect the data necessary for completing one assessment. (5) Most of the data will be derived directly, during the rater's interview with the patient. On those items for which the patient does not provide sufficient information, the staff will be asked to provide a patient's cross-sectional behavioral profile at the time the assessment is being completed. Each rating should *not* be influenced by the rater's knowledge of the patient's performance during the previous ratings.

The rater's assessment guidelines provide a raw evaluation of four clusters of the patient's mental functions: (A) thought processes; (B) cognition; (C) volition; (D) affect/relatedness. They will be scored on scoring sheets, an example of which is provided below. The definition of each function and the guideline for each score are as follows:

TABLE 9.8-2 (*continued*)

(A) Thought Processes:

I. Speech content: Evaluates the *amount* of coherent, verbally expressed thoughts or personal ideas, regardless of their basis in fact. An absence of expressed thoughts may call for prompting on the rater's part.
0 The patient's speech contains *many ideas* (e.g., > 5) which sound clear, have meaning, and are readily volunteered.
(–) 1–2 The patient can coherently voice *several* personal, distinct *ideas (4–5)* but keeps quiet most of the time and seldom initiates discussion of them.
(–) 3–4 The patient expresses only *2 to 3 personal statements* and is usually speechless, even when urged to talk.
(–) 5–6 The patient is either *mute* or the speech is so disorganized that one cannot clearly recognize *a single thought.*

II. Judgment and decisions: Assesses the patient's capacity to use personal judgment and to make decisions within the ordinary requirements of daily living. It is assumed that the rater engages in a conversation with the patient, although when that is not possible the patient's attitudes/actions are to be rated. For expedited rating, judgment questions may be offered to the patient (i.e., should you receive cash as a gift, what would you do with this money? What are your current needs?).
0 The patient's judgment sounds logical, clear, and sensible. Decisions are made *independently, efficiently,* and in keeping with the patient's needs.
(–) 1–2 The patient's judgment is *marginal,* leaves a lot of loose ends, and may require *mild supervision* with more complex issues. Decision making may stall to a halt in difficult circumstances.
(–) 3–4 The patient needs a *lot of assistance* in making any reasonable decision for himself. Presents all issues in a *vague* manner.
(–) 5–6 The patient is incapable of judging or making own decisions, even with help. *Constant uncertainty* and *ambivalence* may be primary symptoms.

(B) Cognition:

III. Memory: Evaluates the patient's ability to register information and retrieve it after 10 minutes. After explaining the procedure to the patient, the rater presents to the patient, only once, 5 words representing objects, at 1-second intervals, and immediately asks the patient to repeat them. The rater then asks the patient to remember those words for 10 minutes, at which time the patient is again asked to recall the words. Only if the patient fails to recall should the rater use some clue and/or encouragement to elicit more. During the 10-minute interval, the patient is assessed on the following 7 items of the scale.
0 The patient recalls all *5 words* without difficulty.
(–) 1–2 The patient recalls *4 words,* or may recall the fifth word after prompting.
(–) 3–4 The patient recalls *2–3 words,* in spite of prompting.
(–) 5–6 The patient does *not* recall *any* of the words, or may recall 1 after prompting.

IV. Attention: Measures the patient's ability to focus his concentration on simple mental tasks such as serial 3's. The rater asks the patient to subtract "3" outloud serially, starting from 100 for 30 seconds. In order to exclude practice effect, the rater may change the starting point to another 2- or 3-digit number. The task is administered by the rater and the patient is instructed that only the number of correct subtractions counts and there will be no penalty for wrong answers. The rater will tell the patient that the procedure is to be timed and will notify the patient when the timing starts.
0 The patient correctly does *over 10* serial subtractions.
(–) 1–2 The patient correctly does *only 5–10* serial subtractions with some hesitation.
(–) 3–4 The patient stalls, performs in a halting manner, and can do only *2–4* serial subtractions.
(–) 5–6 The patient is unable to subtract more than once.

V. Orientation: Measures the patient's capacity to register occurrences within the surrounding environment, to react to them, and to know of the effect the events may have on him. It evaluates the patient's orientation, reality testing, and adaptive skills in a social environment.
0 The patient is oriented to time, place, and person (× *3*). Appears to follow conversation or action, participates actively and appropriately in activities, and can easily elaborate on what is going on in the community in which the patient lives.
(–) 1–2 The patient is oriented (× *2*). May have the day of the week or month wrong, but is oriented to the month of the year and the year, person, and place. Has trouble following conversation and may fall behind others when participating in activities. May seem mildly confused.
(–) 3–4 The patient is oriented to person, but is confused about time and place. May lose track of scheduled activities including personal needs and requires reminding. May have difficulty recognizing some people, but responds somewhat to reality testing and orientation by another.
(–) 5–6 The patient is totally disoriented and *confused.* May recognize only a few key people.

(C) Volition/Motivation:

VI. Grooming: Evaluates the care taken by the patient to maintain personal appearance, including clothing, hair, face, hands, and fingernails.
0 The patient is appropriately dressed with *clean* clothing, combed hair, a clean face and hands, and clipped fingernails.
(–) 1–2 The patient's clothing is clean, but *untidy,* and some neglect of shaving, makeup, or nail care may be visible.
(–) 3–4 Clothing may be stained and *disheveled,* hair is poorly combed, and facial and hand cleanliness have been neglected.
(–) 5–6 The patient and the patient's clothing are grossly *soiled,* with *no attempt* at self-care.

VII. Motivation: Evaluates the patient's ability to plan and carry out tasks of daily living and other constructive activities.
0 The patient's living space, possessions, and clothing are clean and well organized. Plans and carries out work or school tasks *without supervision.*
(–) 1–2 Encouragement and *reminders* are needed for the patient to maintain living space and clothing. Without supervision, the patient becomes unfocused and inefficient at work, school, or other activities.
(–) 3–4 *Ongoing supervision* is required even for the performance of tasks of daily living. The patient is unable to make plans or carry out work or school assignments, even with supervision.
(–) 5–6 *Active physical assistance* is required even for simple tasks such as bathing, dressing, and eating. The patient is apathetic.

VIII. Motion: Evaluates the amount and speed of large, voluntary body movement. The patient is asked to stand up and take 5 steps, turn around, and return to the chair.
0 The patient *completes* the entire task briskly with *no hesitation.*
(–) 1–2 The patient shows a *lag* in starting the task and/or *mild slowing* of gait.

TABLE 9.8-2 (*continued*)

(–) 3–4 The patient is *very sluggish,* but able to complete the task. The patient may require encouragement.
(–) 5–6 The patient may slowly stand up, but cannot complete the task or remains immobile.

(D) Affect/Relatedness:

IX. Emotional response: Evaluates the *range* of emotional expression and the promptness with which the patient is able to react to emotional stimuli such as humor (e.g., jokes), frustration (e.g., limit setting), aggravation, danger, etc.

0 The patient reacts *swiftly* to emotional stimuli. Can be easily seen readily laughing, crying, expressing anger or fear, with voluntary movements and gestures, showing a full emotional range in both intensity and quality.
(–) 1–2 The patient is seen reacting *slowly* to emotions. Can often be seen smiling, weeping, looking upset or anxious, but there is a distinct gap between stimulus and reaction. *Little* movement or gesture accompanies the emotional reaction.
(–) 3–4 The patient *rarely* appears moved by the emotion (e.g., eyes at times may look teary without weeping; voice may be raised for an *instant* or a smile may last for a second) and then one would wonder what led to the change in affect. No other manifestations of emotion are present. The affect is *blunted*.
(–) 5–6 The patient's affect is *flat* regardless of circumstances. Cannot be seen expressing emotion at all. Speech sounds monotonous.

X. Expressive relatedness: Evaluates the spontaneity, amount, and sincerity of interactions between the patient and others in the environment. Both verbal and nonverbal communication (including eye contact, facial expression, and gestures) are to be assessed.

0 The patient *freely initiates* contacts and relates in a genuine and animated fashion.
(–) 1–2 The patient *does not initiate* conversation, but when engaged relates in an appropriate manner. He interacts with more than one "friend."
(–) 3–4 The patient may *actively avoid* or cut short interactions. He can be engaged in a conversation but evokes no clear feeling of warmth.
(–) 5–6 The patient shows *no meaningful interactions* verbally, with no expression of thoughts or feelings and no eye contact. At best, his interactions consist of simple, mechanical requests for material items. He is withdrawn and seclusive.

Table from Iager A-C, Kirch D G, Wyatt R J: A negative symptom rating scale. Psychiat Res *16:* 27, 1985, with permission.

TABLE 9.8-3
Rating Scales Used for Schizophrenia and Psychosis

Scale	*Source*
Brief Psychiatric Rating Scale	Psychological Reports *10:* 799, 1962
Schedule for Affective Disorders and Schizophrenia (SADS)	Archives of General Psychiatry *35:* 837, 1978
Scale for the Assessment of Negative Symptoms (SANS)	The University of Iowa Press, 1983
Scale for the Assessment of Thought Language and Communication (TLC)	The University of Iowa Press, 1978
Thought Disorder Index (TDI)	Archives of General Psychiatry *40:* 1281, 1983
Quality of Life Scale (QLS)	Schizophrenia Bulletin *10:* 383, 1984
Chestnut Lodge Prognostic Scale for Chronic Schizophrenia	Schizophrenia Bulletin *13:* 277, 1987

Table 9.8-5 for the sources of the rating scales used for the mood disorders mentioned above. In addition, see Section 17.3, Mood Disorders: Clinical Features, for more discussion of rating scales for mood disorders.

ANXIETY DISORDERS The history of anxiety scales starts with scales that rated normal anxiety, then moves to scales that rated overall pathological anxiety, and most recently has moved toward scales that measure aspects of anxiety disorders specifically defined in DMS-III-R. An example of a more comprehensive general anxiety scale is the Hamilton Anxiety Rating Scale (Table 9.8-6). Other such scales are the Sheehan Anxiety Scale (Fig. 9.8-1), Brief Outpatient Psychopathology Scale, Physicians Questionnaire, Covi Anxiety Scale, and Anxiety States Inventory. Examples of more DSM-III-R-specific scales for phobias are the Sheehan Phobia Scale (Fig. 9.8-2), Fear Questionnaire, Mobility Inventory for Agoraphobia, and Social Avoidance and Distress Scale. A scale for panic disorder is the Sheehan Panic and Anticipatory Anxiety Scale (Fig. 9.8-3). The Leyton Obsessional Inventory and Maudsley Obsessional-Compulsive Inventory can be used for obsessive-compulsive disorder. The Fear Thermometer and the Impact of Events Scale can be useful in assessing post-traumatic stress disorder. Other than the generalized comprehensive anxiety scales, there are no scales developed yet specifically for generalized anxiety disorder. See Table 9.8-7 for the source of the rating scales used for anxiety disorders mentioned above.

DEMENTIA AND GERIATRIC PATIENTS A widely used scale that assesses dementia is the Brief Cognitive Rating Scale (BCRS, Table 9.8-8), and a comprehensive scale for the assessment of primary degenerative dementia of the Alzheimer type is the Global Deterioration Scale (GDS, Table 9.8-9). The BCRS is a clinician-rated scale based on information from a semistructured interview format. Patients are given a score of 1 to 7 in each of five cognitive areas. The GDS is a seven-point clinician-rated scale that is based on all available clinical data including information from an unstructured interview. The GDS is used to stage the clinical course of Alzheimer's disease rather than to diagnose the condition. Both the BCRS and GDS are useful for charting the clinical course of the disease. In the completion of rating scales on patients with dementing disorders, it is particularly important to have additional sources of information, such as relatives or employers, whenever possible. Two scales that address the functional and more remediable pathology of Alzheimer's disease are the Behavioral Pathology in Alzheimer's Disease Rating Scale (BEHAVE-AD) and the Functional Assessment (FAST) instrument for primary degenerative dementia of the Alzheimer type. Other scales for dementia are the Geriatric Mental State Inventory and Alzheimer's Disease Assessment Scale. The Plutchik Geriatric Rating Scale and the Parkside Behavior Rating Scale are useful in assessing institutional adjustment. See Table 9.8-10 for the sources of the rating scales used for dementia and geriatric patients mentioned above.

TABLE 9.8-4
Hamilton Depression Rating Scale

Clinic No.________ Date________ Rating No.________ Code Number________
Sex________ Age____ Patient's Name ________________________________
Patient's Address ____Tel __________

Item	*Range*	*Score*
1. Depressed mood	0–4	
2. Guilt	0–4	
3. Suicide	0–4	
4. Insomnia initial	0–2	
5. Insomnia middle	0–2	
6. Insomnia delayed	0–2	
7. Work and interest	0–4	
8. Retardation		
9. Agitation	0–4	
10. Anxiety (psychic)	0–4	
11. Anxiety (somatic)	0–4	
12. Somatic gastrointestinal	0–2	
13. Somatic general	0–2	
14. Genital	0–2	
15. Hypochondriasis	0–2	
16. Insight	0–4	
17. Loss of weight	0–2	
	Total Score	
Diurnal variation (M.A.E.)	0–2	
Depersonalization	0–4	
Paranoid symptoms	0–4	
Obsessional symptoms	0–4	

Table from Hamilton M: *Personal communication to the editors,* Feb. 1988.

The scale is designed to measure the severity of illness of patients already diagnosed as suffering from depressive illness. It is obviously not a diagnostic instrument because that requires much more information (e.g., previous history, family history, precipitating factors).

As far as possible, the scale should be used in the manner of a clinical interview. The first time the interview should be conducted in a relaxed, free, and easy manner, giving the patients time to unburden themselves and giving them the opportunity to speak of their problems and ask whatever questions they wish. It may then be necessary to obtain further information by asking them questions. At subsequent assessments, the interview can be briefer and more to the point.

An observer rating scale is not a checklist in which each item is strictly defined. The raters must have sufficient clinical experience and judgment to be able to interpret the patients' statements and reticences about some symptoms, and to compare them with other patients. They should use all sources of information (e.g., from relatives and nurses).

The scale consists of 17 items, the scores on which are summed to give a total score. There are four other items, one of which (diurnal variation) is excluded on the grounds that it is not an additional burden on the patient. The last three are excluded from the total score because they occur infrequently, although information on them may be useful for other purposes.

The method of assessment is simple. For some symptoms it is difficult to elicit such information as will permit of full quantification. If present, score 2; if absent, score 0; and if doubtful or trivial, score 1. For those symptoms where more detailed information can be obtained, the score of 2 is expanded into 2 for mild, 3 for moderate, and 4 for severe. In case of difficulty, the raters should use their judgment as clinicians.

TABLE 9.8-5
Rating Scales Used for Mood Disorders

Scale	*Source*
Beck Depression Inventory	Archives of General Psychiatry *4:* 561, 1961
Standard Assessment of Depressive Disorders (SADD)	Psychological Medicine *10:* 743, 1979
Zung Self-Rating Scale for Depression	Archives of General Psychiatry *12:* 63, 1965
Caroll Rating Scale for Depression	British Journal of Psychiatry *138:* 194, 1981
Montgomery-Asberg Scale	British Journal of Psychiatry *134:* 382, 1979
Raskin Depression Rating Scale	Journal of Nervous and Mental Disease *148:* 87, 1969
Inventory to Diagnose Depression	Archives of General Psychiatry *43:* 1976, 1986
Mania Rating Scale	Journal of Clinical Psychiatry *44:* 98, 1983
Manic State Rating Scale	Archives of General Psychiatry *25:* 256, 1971

CHILD AND ADOLESCENT PATIENTS Many adult psychiatric rating scales have been modified for children and adolescents. For example, the Global Assessment Scale (GAS) has been modified for children as the Children's GAS (CGAS, Table 9.8-11). The CGAS is designed for children aged 4 to 16, and scores above 70 indicate normal functioning. The CGAS is a clinician-rated scale that is based on a 1-month period of functioning.

ADVERSE EFFECTS OF DRUGS An example of this type of scale is the Systematic Assessment for Treatment Emergent Events (SAFTEE), which comes in two forms—

TABLE 9.8-6
Hamilton Anxiety Rating Scale

Instructions: This checklist is to assist the physician or psychiatrist in evaluating each patient as to his degree of anxiety and pathological condition. Please fill in the appropriate rating:

NONE = 0 MILD = 1 MODERATE = 2 SEVERE = 3 SEVERE, GROSSLY DISABLING = 4

Item		*Rating*	*Item*		*Rating*
Anxious mood	Worries, anticipation of the worst, fearful anticipation, irritability	______	Somatic (sensory)	Tinnitus, blurring of vision, hot and cold flushes, feelings of weakness, picking sensation	______
Tension	Feelings of tension, fatigability, startle response, moved to tears easily, trembling, feelings of restlessness, inability to relax	______	Cardiovascular symptoms	Tachycardia, palpitations, pain in chest, throbbing of vessels, fainting feelings, missing beat	______
Fears	Of dark, of strangers, of being left alone, of animals, of traffic, of crowds	______	Respiratory symptoms	Pressure or constriction in chest, choking feelings, sighing, dyspnea	______
Insomnia	Difficulty in falling asleep, broken sleep, unsatisfying sleep and fatigue on waking, dreams, nightmares, night-terrors	______	Gastrointestinal symptoms	Difficulty in swallowing, wind, abdominal pain, burning sensations, abdominal fullness, nausea, vomiting, borborygmi, looseness of bowels, loss of weight, constipation	______
Intellectual (cognitive)	Difficulty in concentration, poor memory	______	Genitourinary symptoms	Frequency of micturition, urgency of micturition, amenorrhea, menorrhagia, development of frigidity, premature ejaculation, loss of libido, impotence	______
Depressed mood	Loss of interest, lack of pleasure in hobbies, depression, early waking, diurnal swing	______	Autonomic symptoms	Dry mouth, flushing, pallor, tendency to sweat, giddiness, tension headache, raising of hair	______
Somatic (muscular)	Pains and aches, twitching, stiffness, myoclonic jerks, grinding of teeth, unsteady voice, increased muscular tone	______	Behavior at interview	Fidgeting, restlessness or pacing, tremor of hands, furrowed brow, strained face, sighing or rapid respiration, facial pallor, swallowing, belching, brisk tendon jerks, dilated pupils, exophthalmos	______

ADDITIONAL COMMENTS: ______

Investigator's signature:

Table from Hamilton M: The assessment of anxiety states by rating. Brit J Med Psych *32:* 50, 1959, with permission.

TABLE 9.8-7
Rating Scales Used for Anxiety Disorders

Scale	*Source*
Brief Outpatient Psychopathology Scale	Journal of Clinical Pharmacology *9:* 187, 1969
Physicians Questionnaire	Psychopharmacologia *17:* 338, 1970
Covi Anxiety Scale	Psychopharmacology Bulletin *18:* 69, 1982
Anxiety States Inventory	Psychosomatics *12,* 371, 1971
Fear Questionnaire	Behavioral Research and Therapeutics *17:* 263, 1979
Mobility Inventory for Agoraphobia	Behavioral Research and Therapeutics *23:* 35, 1985
Social Avoidance and Distress Scale	Journal of Consultative and Clinical Psychology *33:* 448, 1969
Acute Panic Inventory	Archives of General Psychiatry *41:* 764, 1984
Leyton Obsessional Inventory	Psychological Medicine *1:* 48, 1970
Maudsley Obsessional-Compulsive Inventory	Behavioral Research and Therapeutics *15:* 389, 1977
Fear Thermometer	Journal of Consultative and Clinical Psychiatry *15:* 488, 1983
Impact of Events Scale	Psychosomatic Medicine *41:* 209, 1979

TABLE 9.8-8
Brief Cognitive Rating Scale (BCRS)

Name of Patient or Code Number ______________________ Medication: ______________

Age: ______________________ Sex: Male______ Female______

Diagnosis: ______________________ Date:______________

Axis	*Rating (circle highest score)*	*Description*
Axis I: Concentration	1	No objective or subjective evidence of deficit concentration.
	2	Subjective decrement in concentration ability.
	3	Objective signs of poor concentration (e.g., on subtraction of serial 7's from 100).
	4	Definite concentration deficit for persons of their background (e.g., on subtraction of serial 4's).
	5	Marked concentration deficit (e.g., giving months backward or serial 2's from 20).
	6	Forgets the concentration task; frequently begins to count forward when asked to count backward.
	7	Marked difficulty counting forward to 10 by 1's.
Axis II: Recent memory	1	No objective or subjective evidence of deficit in recent memory.
	2	Subjective impairment only (e.g., forgetting names more than formerly).
	3	Evident deficit in recall of specific recent events. No deficit for major events.
	4	Can't recall major events of previous weekend or week.
	5	Unsure of weather: may not know current president or current address.
	6	Occasional knowledge of some recent events.
	7	No knowledge of any recent events.
Axis III: Past memory	1	No subjective or objective impairment in past memory.
	2	Subjective impairment only; can recall primary school teachers.
	3	Some gaps in past memory on detailed questioning.
	4	Clean-cut deficit. The spouse recalls more of the patient's past than the patient.
	5	Major past events sometimes not recalled (e.g., names of schools attended).
	6	Some residual memory of past (e.g., may recall country of birth or former occupation).
	7	No memory of the past.
Axis IV: Orientation	1	No deficit in memory for time, place, identity of self or others.
	2	Subjective impairment only. Knows time to nearest hour, location.
	3	Any mistake in time > 2 hours; day of week > 1 day; date > 3 days.
	4	Mistakes in month > 10 days or year > 1 month.
	5	Unsure of month, year, or season; unsure of locale.
	6	No idea of date. Identifies spouse but may not recall name. Knows own name.
	7	Can't identify spouse; may be unsure of personal identity.
Axis V: Functioning and self-care	1	No difficulty, either subjectively or objectively.
	2	Complaints of forgetting location of objects. Subjective work difficulties.
	3	Decreased job functioning evident to co-workers. Difficulty in traveling to new locations.
	4	Decreased ability to perform complex tasks (e.g., planning dinner for guests, handling finances).
	5	Requires assistance in choosing proper clothing or in shopping.
	6	Requires assistance feeding, toileting, bathing, or ambulating.
	7	Requires constant assistance in all activities of daily life.

Table from Reisberg B, Schneck M K, Ferris S H, Schwartz G E, DeLeon M J: The brief cognitive rating scale (BCRS): Findings in primary degenerative dementia (PDD). Psychopharmacol Bull *19:* 47, 1983, with permission.

NCS Trans-Optic® MP08-72504-321 A2203

Project ID	Investigator ID	Today's Date: Month	Day	Year	Visit	Patient ID	Birth Date: Month	Day	Year
0 0 0 0	0 0 0 0	Jan					Jan		
1 1 1 1	1 1 1 1	Feb					Feb		
2 2 2 2	2 2 2 2	Mar	0 0	0 0	s 0 0	0 0 0 0 0 0	Mar	0 0	0 0
3 3 3 3	3 3 3 3	Apr	1 1	1 1	b 1 1	1 1 1 1 1 1	Apr	1 1	1 1
4 4 4 4	4 4 4 4	May	2 2	2 2	w 2 2	2 2 2 2 2 2	May	2 2	2 2
5 5 5 5	5 5 5 5	Jun	3 3	3 3	f 3 3	3 3 3 3 3 3	Jun	3 3	3 3
6 6 6 6	6 6 6 6	Jul	4 4	4 4	4 4	4 4 4 4 4 4	Jul	4 4	4 4
7 7 7 7	7 7 7 7	Aug	5 5	5 5	5 5	5 5 5 5 5 5	Aug	5 5	5 5
8 8 8 8	8 8 8 8	Sep	6 6	6 6	6 6	6 6 6 6 6 6	Sep	6 6	6 6
9 9 9 9	9 9 9 9	Oct	7 7	7 7	7 7	7 7 7 7 7 7	Oct	7 7	7 7
		Nov	8 8	8 8	8 8	8 8 8 8 8 8	Nov	8 8	8 8
		Dec	9 9	9 9	9 9	9 9 9 9 9 9	Dec	9 9	9 9

Form # 8

Page # 1 of 2

Investigator's Initials X ______

Patient's Initials X ______

SHEEHAN CLINICIAN RATED ANXIETY SCALE

INSTRUCTIONS: Blacken the appropriate circle. IN RATING, CONSIDER:

1. Frequency
2. Severity of average symptoms
3. Description of last significant occurrence

HOW SEVERE HAS THE PATIENT'S SYMPTOM BEEN OVER THE PAST WEEK?	Absent	Mild	Moderate	Severe	Very Severe
1. Spells of dyspnea/hyperventilation/smothering.	○	○	○	○	○
2. Spells of choking sensation/lump in throat.	○	○	○	○	○
3. Spells of PVCs/tachycardia.	○	○	○	○	○
4. Chest pain/pressure.	○	○	○	○	○
5. Sweating.	○	○	○	○	○
6. Spells of dizziness/faintness, lightheadedness.	○	○	○	○	○
7. Spells of rubbery legs.	○	○	○	○	○
8. Spells of imbalance.	○	○	○	○	○
9. Nausea.	○	○	○	○	○
10. Derealization.	○	○	○	○	○
11. Depersonalization.	○	○	○	○	○
12. Spells of paresthesias/numbness.	○	○	○	○	○
13. Hot flashes or cold chills.	○	○	○	○	○
14. Spells of tremor/shaking.	○	○	○	○	○
15. Spells of fear of dying or impending danger.	○	○	○	○	○
16. Feeling of mental decompensation (self-control/sanity).	○	○	○	○	○

← Changes: date & initial in box at left in line with the change.

CONTINUED ON BACK

Form # 8 Page # 2 of 2

SHEEHAN CLINICIAN RATED ANXIETY SCALE (cont'd.)

HOW SEVERE HAS THE PATIENT'S SYMPTOM BEEN OVER THE PAST WEEK?	Absent	Mild	Moderate	Severe	Very Severe
17. Situational panic/anxiety attacks (3+ symptoms from those listed above).	O	O	O	O	O
18. Unexpected panic/anxiety attacks (3+ symptoms above).	O	O	O	O	O
19. Unexpected limited symptom attacks (1 or 2 symptoms above).	O	O	O	O	O
20. Anticipatory anxiety episodes.	O	O	O	O	O
21. Phobias.	O	O	O	O	O
22. Dependent on others.	O	O	O	O	O
23. Tension/nervousness/anxiety.	O	O	O	O	O
24. Signs of anxiety at interview (tremor, facial pallor, dilated pupils, respiration or sighing, restlessness, fidgeting, swallowing, burping, increased pitch and speed of speech).	O	O	O	O	O
25. Spells of increased sensitivity to sound, light, or touch (startle).	O	O	O	O	O
26. Diarrhea.	O	O	O	O	O
27. Hypochondriasis.	O	O	O	O	O
28. Tires easily.	O	O	O	O	O
29. Pains in head/neck/back.	O	O	O	O	O
30. Initial insomnia.	O	O	O	O	O
31. Middle insomnia.	O	O	O	O	O
32. Waves of depression with little or no provocation.	O	O	O	O	O
33. Emotional lability.	O	O	O	O	O
34. Obsessive thoughts.	O	O	O	O	O
35. Compulsive rituals.	O	O	O	O	O

Changes: date & initial in box at right in line with the change.

FIGURE 9.8-1. *Sheehan Clinician Rated Anxiety Scale. (From Sheehan D V, with permission.)*

NCS Trans-Optic® MP08-72503-321 A2203

Project ID	Investigator ID	Today's Date: Month	Day	Year	Visit	Patient ID	Birth Date: Month	Day	Year
		Jan					Jan		
		Feb					Feb		
0 0 0 0	0 0 0 0	Mar	0 0	0 0	s 0 0	0 0 0 0 0 0	Mar	0 0	0 0
1 1 1 1	1 1 1 1	Apr	1 1	1 1	b 1 1	1 1 1 1 1 1	Apr	1 1	1 1
2 2 2 2	2 2 2 2	May	2 2	2 2	w 2 2	2 2 2 2 2 2	May	2 2	2 2
3 3 3 3	3 3 3 3	Jun	3 3	3 3	f 3 3	3 3 3 3 3 3	Jun	3 3	3 3
4 4 4 4	4 4 4 4	Jul	4 4	4 4	4 4	4 4 4 4 4 4	Jul	4 4	4 4
5 5 5 5	5 5 5 5	Aug	5 5	5 5	5 5	5 5 5 5 5 5	Aug	5 5	5 5
6 6 6 6	6 6 6 6	Sep	6 6	6 6	6 6	6 6 6 6 6 6	Sep	6 6	6 6
7 7 7 7	7 7 7 7	Oct	7 7	7 7	7 7	7 7 7 7 7 7	Oct	7 7	7 7
8 8 8 8	8 8 8 8	Nov	8 8	8 8	8 8	8 8 8 8 8 8	Nov	8 8	8 8
9 9 9 9	9 9 9 9	Dec	9 9	9 9	9 9	9 9 9 9 9 9	Dec	9 9	9 9

Form # 15

Page # 1 of 2

Investigator's Initials X

Patient's Initials X

PHOBIA SCALE
(Sheehan after Marks & Mathews)

Phobias are situations or things that people fear and avoid. In completing Item 1, list the 4 feared situations or things (phobias) that you most want treated. List only phobias, not physical symptoms.

In the FEAR score rows, fill in the circle describing how much fear you would experience if you had to face each thing/situation now.

In the AVOIDANCE score rows, fill in the circle describing how often you would try to avoid each situation/thing if you had to face it now.

HOW MUCH DO YOU FEAR AND AVOID	FEAR: Not at all		Mildly		Moderately			Markedly			Extremely	AVOIDANCE: Never	Sometimes	Often	Very Often	Always
1. Main phobias you want treated																
A (specify)	0	1	2	3	4	5	6	7	8	9	10	0	1	2	3	4
B (specify)	0	1	2	3	4	5	6	7	8	9	10	0	1	2	3	4
C (specify)	0	1	2	3	4	5	6	7	8	9	10	0	1	2	3	4
D (specify)	0	1	2	3	4	5	6	7	8	9	10	0	1	2	3	4
2. Going far from home alone	0	1	2	3	4	5	6	7	8	9	10	0	1	2	3	4
3. Sudden unexpected attacks of panic/anxiety that occur with little or no cause	0	1	2	3	4	5	6	7	8	9	10	0	1	2	3	4
4. Traveling on buses, subways, trains, or in cars	0	1	2	3	4	5	6	7	8	9	10	0	1	2	3	4
5. Crowded places, e.g., shopping, sports events, theaters	0	1	2	3	4	5	6	7	8	9	10	0	1	2	3	4
6. Large open spaces	0	1	2	3	4	5	6	7	8	9	10	0	1	2	3	4
7. Feeling trapped or caught in closed spaces	0	1	2	3	4	5	6	7	8	9	10	0	1	2	3	4
8. Being left alone	0	1	2	3	4	5	6	7	8	9	10	0	1	2	3	4
9. The thought of physical injury or illness	0	1	2	3	4	5	6	7	8	9	10	0	1	2	3	4
10. Hearing or reading about health topics or disease	0	1	2	3	4	5	6	7	8	9	10	0	1	2	3	4
11. Eating, drinking, or writing in public	0	1	2	3	4	5	6	7	8	9	10	0	1	2	3	4
12. Being watched or being the focus of attention	0	1	2	3	4	5	6	7	8	9	10	0	1	2	3	4
13. Being with others because you are self-conscious	0	1	2	3	4	5	6	7	8	9	10	0	1	2	3	4
14. Specific situations other than those listed above that frighten you	0	1	2	3	4	5	6	7	8	9	10	0	1	2	3	4

Changes: date & initial in box at left in line with the change.

CONTINUED ON BACK

Form #
15

Page #
2 of 2

DO NOT WRITE IN THIS AREA

15. Specify furthest distance you can go alone.

0	0	0	0	○ Yards
1	1	1	1	○ Miles
2	2	2	2	
3	3	3	3	
4	4	4	4	
5	5	5	5	
6	6	6	6	
7	7	7	7	
8	8	8	8	
9	9	9	9	

Can you rate the present OVERALL state of your phobias, using the scale below?

No phobias present — 0
Mildly distressing or restricting — 1, 2, 3
Moderately distressing or restricting — 4, 5, 6
Markedly distressing or restricting — 7, 8, 9
Extremely distressing or restricting — 10

DO NOT WRITE IN THIS AREA

Changes: date & initial in box at right in line with the change.

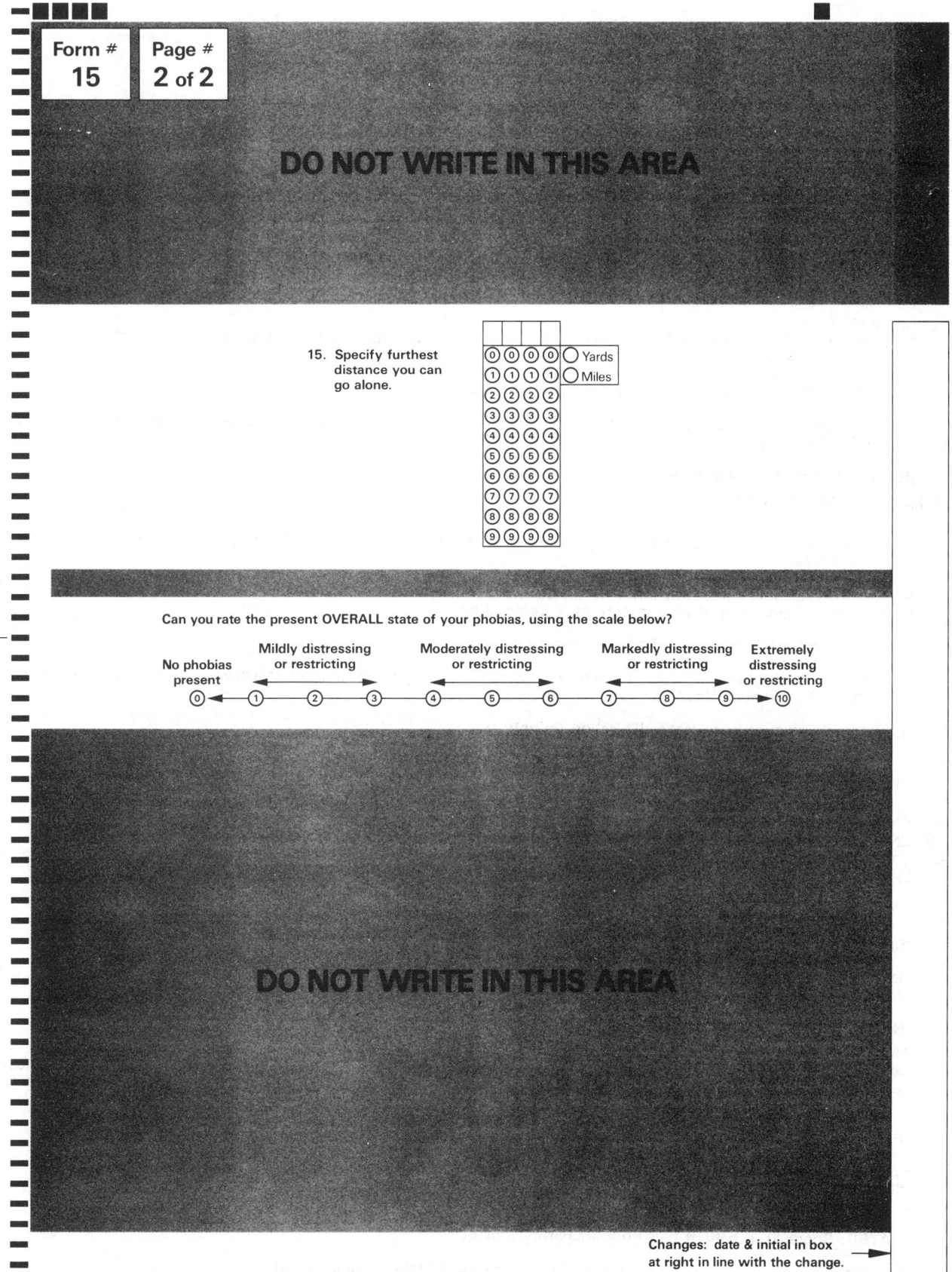

FIGURE 9.8-2. *Sheehan Phobia Scale. (From Sheehan D V, with permission. This scale was adapted from the work of I M Marks and A Mathews and modified for use in the United States by D V Sheehan. Those interested in the original work can consult the book* Living with Fear *by I M Marks, McGraw-Hill, 1978.)*

Now I will be asking you several questions about how you have been feeling in the past week. First of all, let me ask you about panic attacks, that is, when you suddenly feel frightened or extremely uncomfortable and have at least 4 of the symptoms on this list.

[RATER: Hand patient Symptom List.]

During the past week, how many panic attacks have you had?

A. PANIC ATTACKS

1. SITUATIONAL
   How many of these attacks occurred when you were in or just about to go into a place or situation that in your experience is likely to bring on an attack? **[Number/Week]**

   How long did most of these attacks last? **[Duration (mins)]**

   How bad were most of these on a scale of 1 to 10 with 1 being the least and 10 being the most anxious or uncomfortable you can imagine? **[Intensity]**

   [RATER: Score '0' if patient had no attacks]

2. UNEXPECTED
   So all the others were unexpected: that is they occurred when you were not in a place or situation that is likely to bring on an attack? **[Number/Week]**

   How long did most of these attacks last? **[Duration (mins)]**

   How bad were most of these attacks on the 1 to 10 scale, 1 being the least and 10 being the most uncomfortable you can imagine? **[Intensity]**

   [RATER: Score '0' if patient had no attacks]

B. LIMITED SYMPTOM ATTACKS

1. SITUATIONAL
   In the past week did you suddenly have **only** 1 2 or 3 of the symptoms on that list, without having a full panic attack with 4 or more symptoms?

   [RATER: If yes, have patient describe worst attack and go over list to make sure that there were no more than 2 symptoms. If there were, it may qualify as a panic attack.]

   During the past week, how many times has that happened?

   How often did this happen when you were in or just about to go into a place or situation that in your experience is likely to bring on an attack? **[Number/Week]**

   How long did most of these last? **[Duration (mins)]**

   How bad were most of these on the 1 to 10 scale, 1 being the least and 10 being the most uncomfortable you can imagine. **[Intensity]**

   [RATER: Score '0' if patient had no attacks]

2. UNEXPECTED
   So all the other times these limited attacks were unexpected, that is, they occurred when you were not in a place or situation that from your experience was likely to bring on an attack?

   During the past week, how many times have these unexpected attacks happened? **[Number/Week]**

   How long did most of these last? **[Duration (mins)]**

   How bad were most of these on the 1 to 10 scale, 1 being the least and 10 being the most uncomfortable you can imagine? **[Intensity]**

   [RATER: Score '0' if patient had no attacks]

3. ANTICIPATORY ANXIETY
   Now I would like to ask you about something different. In the past week what percent (%) of the time have you worried about having a panic attack or of going into a situation that in your experience is likely to bring on an attack, when you were not actually having one? **[% time]**

   [RATER: That is when patient is not having a panic attack or a limited symptom attack]

   When you were worrying about having a panic attack or of going into a situation that in your experience is likely to bring on an attack, how anxious or nervous were you on a scale of 1 to 10, with 1 being the least anxious you can imagine and 10 being the most anxious you can imagine? **[Intensity]**

   [RATER: Score '0' if patient had no anticipatory attack]

   How many episodes did you have of these in the past week? **[No. in past week]**

FIGURE 9.8-3. *Structured interview for rating the Sheehan Panic and Anticipatory Anxiety Scale. (From Sheehan D V, with permission.)*

TABLE 9.8-9
Global Deterioration Scale (GDS) for Age-Associated Cognitive Decline and Alzheimer's Disease

GDS Stage	*Clinical Phase*	*Clinical Characteristics*	*Psychometric Concomitants*
1 No cognitive decline	Normal	No subjective complaints of memory deficit. No memory deficit evident on clinical interview.	Average or above average performance for age and WAIS vocabulary score on 3 of 5 Guild memory subtests.
2 Very mild cognitive decline	Forgetfulness	Subjective complaints of memory deficit, most frequently in following areas: (a) forgetting where one has placed familiar objects; (b) forgetting names one formerly knew well. No objective evidence of memory deficit on clinical interview. No objective deficits in employment or social situations. Appropriate concern with respect to symptomatology.	Below average performance for age and WAIS vocabulary score on 3 of 5 Guild subtests.
3 Mild cognitive decline	Early confusional	Earliest clear-cut deficits. Manifestations in more than one of the following areas: (a) patient may have gotten lost when traveling to an unfamiliar location; (b) co-workers become aware of patient's relatively poor performance; (c) word and name finding deficit become evident to intimates; (d) patient may read a passage or a book and retain relatively little material; (e) patient may demonstrate decreased facility in remembering names on introduction to new people; (f) patient may have lost or misplaced an object of value; (g) concentration deficit may be evident on clinical testing. Objective evidence of memory deficit obtained only with an intensive interview conducted by a trained geriatric psychiatrist. Decreased performance in demanding employment and social settings. Denial begins to become manifest in patient. Mild to moderate anxiety accompanies symptoms.	One standard deviation or greater below average performance for age and WAIS vocabulary score on 3 of 5 Guild memory subtests. Often no errors on the Mental Status Questionnaire (MSQ). Frequent mistakes on 3 or more items on MSQ.
4 Moderate cognitive decline	Late confusional	Clear-cut deficit on careful clinical interview. Deficit manifest in following areas: (a) decreased knowledge of current and recent events; (b) may exhibit some deficit in memory of one's personal history; (c) concentration deficit elicited on serial subtractions; (d) decreased ability to travel, handle finances, etc. Frequently no deficit in following areas: (a) orientation to time and person; (b) recognition of familiar persons and faces; (c) ability to travel to familiar locations. Inability to perform complex tasks. Denial is dominant defense mechanism. Flattening of affect and withdrawal from challenging situations occur.	Deficits evident on brief MSQ assessment.
5 Moderately severe decline	Early dementia	Patient can no longer survive without some assistance. Patient is unable during interview to recall a major relevant aspect of their current lives; e.g., their address or telephone number of many years, the names of close members of their family (such as grandchildren), the name of the high school or college from which they graduated. Frequently some disorientation to time (date, day of week, season, etc.) or to place. An educated person may have difficulty counting back from 40 by 4's or from 20 by 2's. Persons at this stage retain knowledge of many major facts regarding themselves and others. They invariably know their own names and generally know their spouses and children's names. They require no assistance with toileting or eating, but may have some difficulty choosing the proper clothing to wear.	
6 Severe cognitive decline	Middle dementia	May occasionally forget the name of the spouse on whom they are entirely dependent for survival. Will be largely unaware of all recent events and experiences in their lives. Retain some knowledge of their past lives but this is very sketchy. Generally unaware of their surroundings, the year, the season, etc. May have difficulty count-	5–10 errors on MSQ.

TABLE 9.8-9 (*continued*)

		ing from 10, both backward and sometimes, forward. Will require some assistance with activities of daily living, e.g., may become incontinent, will require travel assistance but occasionally will display ability to travel to familiar locations. Diurnal rhythm frequently disturbed. Almost always recall their own name. Frequently continue to be able to distinguish familiar from unfamiliar persons in their environment. Personality and emotional changes occur. These are quite variable and include: (a) delusional behavior, e.g., patients may accuse their spouse of being an impostor; may talk to imaginary figures in the environment, or to their own reflection in the mirror; (b) obsessive symptoms, e.g., person may continually repeat simple cleaning activities; (c) anxiety symptoms, agitation, and even previously nonexistent violent behavior may occur; (d) cognitive abulia, i.e., loss of willpower because an individual cannot carry a thought long enough to determine a purposeful course of action.
7 Very severe cognitive decline	Late dementia	All verbal abilities are lost. Frequently there is no speech at all—only grunting. Incontinent of urine; requires assistance toileting and feeding. Lose basic psychomotor skills, e.g., ability to walk. The brain appears to no longer be able to tell the body what to do. Generalized and cortical neurological signs and symptoms are frequently present.

Table from Reisberg B, Ferris S H, de Leon M J, Crook T: Amer J Psychiat *139:* 1136, 1982, with permission.

TABLE 9.8-10
Rating Scales Used for Dementia and Geriatric Patients

Scale	*Source*
Behavioral Pathology in Alzheimer Disease Rating Scale (BEHAVE-AD)	Journal of Clinical Psychiatry *48* (5, supp): 9, 1987
Functional Assessment (FAST) instrument for primary degenerative dementia of the Alzheimer type	Hospital and Community Psychiatry *36:* 593, 1985
Geriatric Mental State Inventory	International Journal of Aging and Human Development *7:* 13, 1976
Alzheimer's Disease Assessment Scale	American Journal of Psychiatry *141:* 1356, 1984
Plutchik Geriatric Rating Scale	Journal of the American Geriatric Society *18:* 491, 1970
Parkside Behavior Rating Scale	British Journal of Psychiatry *117:* 157, 1970

TABLE 9.8-11
Children's Global Assessment Scale (for Children 4–16 Years of Age)*

Rate the subject's most impaired level of general functioning for the specified time period by selecting the *lowest* level which describes his/her functioning on a hypothetical continuum of health–illness. Use intermediary levels (e.g., 35, 58, 62).

Rate actual functioning regardless of treatment or prognosis. The examples of behavior provided are only illustrative and are not required for a particular rating.

Specified time period: 1 month

100–91 **Superior functioning** in all areas (at home, at school, and with peers), involved in a range of activities and has many interests (e.g., has hobbies or participates in extracurricular activities or belongs to an organized group such as Scouts, etc.). Likeable, confident, "everyday" worries never get out of hand. Doing well in school. No symptoms.

90–81 **Good functioning in all areas.** Secure in family, school, and with peers. There may be transient difficulties and "everyday" worries that occasionally get out of hand (e.g., mild anxiety associated with an important exam, occasionally "blow-ups" with siblings, parents, or peers).

80–71 **No more than slight impairment in functioning** at home, at school, or with peers. Some disturbance of behavior or emotional distress may be present in response to life stresses (e.g., parental separations, deaths, birth of a sib), but these are brief and interference with functioning is transient. Such children are only minimally disturbing to others and are not considered deviant by those who know them.

70–61 **Some difficulty in a single area, but generally functioning pretty well** (e.g., sporadic or isolated antisocial acts, such as occasionally playing hooky or petty theft; consistent minor difficulties with school work; mood changes of brief duration; fears and anxieties which do not lead to gross avoidance behavior; self-doubts). Has some meaningful interpersonal relationships. Most people who do not know the child well would not consider him/her deviant but those who do know him/her well might express concern.

60–51 **Variable functioning with sporadic difficulties or symptoms in several but not all social areas.** Disturbance would be apparent to those who encounter the child in a dysfunctional setting or time but not to those who see the child in other settings.

50–41 **Moderate degree of interference in functioning in most social areas or severe impairment of functioning in one area,** such as might result from, for example, suicidal pre-

TABLE 9.8-11 *(continued)*

occupations and ruminations, school refusal and other forms of anxiety, obsessive rituals, major conversion symptoms, frequent anxiety attacks, frequent episodes of aggressive or other antisocial behavior with some preservation of meaningful social relationships.

40–31 **Major impairment in functioning in several areas and unable to function in one of these areas,** i.e., disturbed at home, at school, with peers, or in the society at large (e.g., persistent aggression without clear instigation; markedly withdrawn and isolated behavior due to either mood or thought disturbance; suicidal attempts with clear lethal intent). Such children are likely to require special schooling and/or hospitalization or withdrawal from school (but this is not a sufficient criterion for inclusion in this category).

30–21 **Unable to function in almost all areas,** e.g., stays at home, in ward, or in bed all day without taking part in social activities OR severe impairment in reality testing OR serious impairment in communication (e.g., sometimes incoherent or inappropriate).

20–11 **Needs considerable supervision** to prevent hurting others or self, e.g., frequently violent, repeated suicide attempts OR to maintain personal hygiene OR gross impairment in all forms of communication, e.g., severe abnormalities in verbal and gestural communication, marked social aloofness, stupor, etc.

10–1 **Needs constant supervision** (24-hour care) due to severely aggressive or self-destructive behavior or gross impairment in reality testing, communication, cognition, affect, or personal hygiene.

Table from Shaffer D, Gould M S, Brasic J, Ambrosini P, Fisher P, Bird H, Aluwahlia S: A children's global assessment scale (CGAS). Arch Gen Psychiat *40:* 1228, 1983, with permission.
*An adaptation of the Adult Global Assessment Scale of R L Spitzer, M Gibbon, J Endicott.

TABLE 9.8-12
Abnormal Involuntary Movement Scale (AIMS) Examination Procedure

Patient identification: ______________________ Date ________
Rated by: ______________________

Either before or after completing the examination procedure, observe the patient unobtrusively at rest (e.g., in waiting room).

The chair to be used in this examination should be a hard, firm one without arms.

After observing the patient, he or she may be rated on a scale of 0 (none), 1 (minimal), 2 (mild), 3 (moderate), and 4 (severe) according to the severity of symptoms.

Ask the patient whether there is anything in his/her mouth (i.e., gum, candy, etc.) and if there is to remove it.

Ask patient about the *current* condition of his/her teeth. Ask patient if he/she wears dentures. Do teeth or dentures bother patient *now?*

Ask patient whether he/she notices any movement in mouth, face, hands, or feet. If yes, ask to describe and to what extent they *currently* bother patient or interfere with his/her activities.

0 1 2 3 4	Have patient sit in chair with hands on knees, legs slightly apart, and feet flat on floor. (Look at entire body for movements while in this position.)
0 1 2 3 4	Ask patient to sit with hands hanging unsupported. If male, between legs, if female and wearing a dress, hanging over knees. (Observe hands and other body areas.)
0 1 2 3 4	Ask patient to open mouth. (Observe tongue at rest within mouth.) Do this twice.
0 1 2 3 4	Ask patient to protrude tongue. (Observe abnormalities of tongue movement.) Do this twice.
0 1 2 3 4	Ask the patient to tap thumb, with each finger, as rapidly as possible for 10–15 seconds; separately with right hand, then with left hand. (Observe facial and leg movements.)
0 1 2 3 4	Flex and extend patient's left and right arms. (One at a time.)
0 1 2 3 4	Ask patient to stand up. (Observe in profile. Observe all body areas again, hips included.)
0 1 2 3 4	*Ask patient to extend both arms outstretched in front with palms down. (Observe trunk, legs, and mouth.)
0 1 2 3 4	*Have patient walk a few paces, turn and walk back to chair. (Observe hands and gait.) Do this twice.

*Activated movements

TABLE 9.8-13
Other Rating Scales

Scale	*Source*
Child and adolescent patients	
General reference for adult scales that have been modified for children	Psychopharmacology Bulletin *21:* entire issue, 1985
Adverse effects of drugs	
Systematic Assessment for Treatment Emergent Events (SAFTEE): General Inquiry (GI) Systematic Inquiry (SI)	Psychopharmacology Bulletin *22:* 343, 1986
Quality of life	
Patterns of Individual Change Scale (PICS)	Archives of General Psychiatry *42:* 703, 1985

General Inquiry (GI) and Systematic Inquiry (SI). The SI records all problems, not just those that may have been presupposed to be related to the specific drug treatment. Not surprisingly, the SI is more likely to identify adverse effects than the GI. Another example of a scale for drug adverse effects is the Abnormal Involuntary Movement Scale (AIMS, Table 9.8-12).

QUALITY-OF-LIFE SCALES There are also many scales for assessing the quality of the environment, the degree of social stressors, and the nature of the living situation. Although it is often difficult to demonstrate reliability and validity for these scales because of the wide variation in what is considered optimal or normal in these areas, the scales can be applied when confined to relatively restricted sociocultural groups. Other recently developed scales have attempted to assess characteristics that might be relevant to demonstrating the effectiveness of psychotherapy. One example of such a scale is the Patterns of Individual Change Scale (PICS). Table 9.8-13 lists the sources of the scales presented in these final three subsections.

REFERENCES

Bartko J J, Carpenter W T: On the methods and theory of reliability. J Nerv Ment Dis *163:* 307, 1976.

Bird H R, Canino G, Rubio-Stipec M, Ribera J C: Further measures of the psychometric properties of the Children's Global Assessment Scale. Arch Gen Psychiat *44:* 821, 1987.

Buros O K, editor: *Personality Tests and Reviews*. Gryphon Press, Highland Park, NJ, 1970.

Comrey A L, Backer T E, Glaser E M: *Sourcebook for Mental Health Measures*. Human Interaction Research Institute, Los Angeles, 1973.

Endicott J, Spitzer R L: Psychiatric rating scales. In *Comprehensive Textbook of Psychiatry*, ed 3, H I Kaplan, B J Sadock, editors, Williams & Wilkins, Baltimore, 1980.

Fyer A J, Mannuzza S, Endicott J: Differential diagnosis and assessment of anxiety: Recent developments. In *Psychopharmacology: The Third Generation of Progress,* H Y Meltzer, editor. Raven Press, New York, 1987.

Goldberg L R: Objective diagnostic tests and measures. Ann Rev Psychol *25:* 102, 1974.

Guy W: *ECDEU Assessment Manual for Psychopharmacology*. U.S. Department of Health, Education, and Welfare, Washington, DC, 1976.

Hargreaves W A: Systematic nursing observation on psychopathology. Arch Gen Psychiat *18:* 518, 1968.

Hargreaves W A, Attkisson C C, McIntyre M H, Siegel L M, Sorensen J E, editors: *Resource Materials for Community Mental Health Program Evaluation, Part I. Elements of Program Evaluation.* National Institute of Mental Health, Bethesda, MD, 1974.

Hughes J R, O'Hara M W, Rehm L P: Measurement of depression in clinical trials: An overview. J Clin Psychiat *43:* 85, 1982.

Kearns N P, Cruikshank C A, McGuigan K J, Riley S A, Shaw S P, Snaith R P: A comparison of depression rating scales. Brit J Psychiat *141:* 45, 1982.

Levine J, Ban T A: Assessment methods in clinical trials. In *Psychopharmacology: The Third Generation of Progress,* H Y Meltzer, editor. Raven Press, New York, 1987.

Lyerly S B: *Handbook of Psychiatric Rating Scales,* ed 2. National Institute of Mental Health, Bethesda, MD, 1973.

Raskin A, Jarvik L S: *Psychiatric Symptoms and Cognitive Loss in the Elderly*. Wiley, New York, 1979.

Riskind J H, Beck A T, Brown G, Steer R A: Taking measure of anxiety and depression. J Nerv Ment Dis *175:* 474, 1987.

Sartorius N, Ban T A, editors: *Assessment of Depression*. Springer-Verlag, New York, 1986.

Spitzer R L, Cohen J: Common errors in quantitative psychiatric research. Int J Psychiat *6:* 109, 1968.

Waskow I G, Parloff M B: *Psychotherapy Change Measures: Report on the Clinical Research Branch—NIMH Outcome Measures Project*. National Institute of Mental Health, Bethesda, MD, 1975.

Wittenborn J R: Reliability, validity, and objectivity of symptom-rating scales. J Nerv Ment Dis *154:* 79, 1972.

10 CLINICAL MANIFESTATIONS OF PSYCHIATRIC DISORDERS

JOEL YAGER, M.D.

INTRODUCTION

Psychiatric disorders express themselves in every dimension of human physiology, perception, emotion, thought, and behavior, and it is rare, if not unheard of, for only one dimension to be affected during times of faulty adaptation and breakdown. Because of the large number of signs, symptoms, and symptom complexes, it is important to consider several perspectives from which the clinician can organize this wide array of phenomena. Contemporary psychiatry has had some success at organizing patterns of signs and symptoms discussed in this chapter into recognizable syndromes and disorders that have predictable courses, treatment responses, and prognoses; nevertheless, such classification is still preliminary, and a great deal of psychiatric data, clinical thinking, and empirical work remain at the level of signs and symptoms, many of which are poorly understood at present.

This chapter discusses normal processes that affect human coping and adaptation, current framework for understanding maladaptive phenomena, and the abnormal phenomena that occur in psychiatric disorders.

COPING AND ADAPTATION

Coping has been defined as the physiological, emotional, cognitive, and behavioral efforts used to manage the constantly changing external and internal demands that tax or overwhelm the ordinary resources of a person. Coping behaviors are necessary to satisfy basic physiological needs, such as those for air, water, food, sleep, and sex. At a higher level, coping is necessary to satisfy interpersonal needs for affiliation related to attachment, affection, love, dependency, power, and submission. Other human needs satisfied by adequate interpersonal coping include acquiring a sense of reality, provided by belief systems that help to organize and add meaning and coherence to the world; social validation, as in being useful to other people; self-esteem; and personal safety.

The developmental tasks that confront people and that require new adaptations vary throughout the life cycle. Familiar examples involving adults in American culture include the demands of the teenage years and early adulthood to establish personal identity, life-style, and values and the need to separate from parents while developing new relationships with peers and sex partners. The tasks of the early 20s and 30s typically concern the choice of career, the development of a nuclear family or an equivalent relationship, child bearing and child rearing, and the general tasks of productivity and self-sustenance. People in their 30s and 40s frequently re-evaluate their adult life situations and rededicate themselves to existing patterns or commit to changing career, relationships, or values. Challenges of later adulthood relate to consolidating career, raising older children who will soon separate from their parents, and grandparenting. Also to be dealt with are the parents' illnesses and deaths, personal physical decline and aging, new familial and social roles that accompany retirement, the loss through death of family and friends, and the inevitability of one's own death.

The person who has a physical or psychiatric illness must master additional problems: dealing with pain, incapacity, and disfigurement; dealing with treatment environments, treatment procedures, health caregivers, and the overall system of medical care; dealing with the new external realities attendant upon illness and disability, such as changes in income, career, family relationships, social roles, and friendships; inevitable changes in aspirations and expectations from life and in self-concept.

Each of these coping tasks, in health and in illness, requires a person to appraise, evaluate, and make judgments about the situations, plan courses of action, carry them out and evaluate their effectiveness, and determine the costs and benefits of various actions. Successful coping requires the relative integrity of the biophysiological substrate; of the perceptual and cognitive apparatus necessary for perception, classification, discrimination, planning, and judgment; of the emotional apparatus that assures well-modulated and adequate levels of arousal without disruptive hyperarousal; and of the motor system needed to perform activities. Overwhelming stressors or weaknesses in any part of this system can preclude successful adaptation.

Under ordinary circumstances, while coping one's way through life, each person constructs a series of cognitive schemes, expectations, and plans that organize and impel behavior. These schemes are influenced by physiological drives, motivational states, and attendant emotions. Activities, such as searching for a mate—or, more mundanely, yearning for a girlfriend or boyfriend—fall into this category. More elaborate and far-reaching cognitive schemes may have equally powerful effects. Conceiving an elaborate social or industrial program, scientific theory, symphony, or novel—concepts whose activities fulfill needs for personal expression and mastery—may organize and define a person's behavior for years or for an entire lifetime. Disruptions of these ongoing, meaningful, major organizing themes in life that stem from unanticipated stressors may demand more accommodation and change than a person can muster and may provoke maladaptive breakdown and psychiatric disturbance.

Successful coping includes a variety of behaviors directed toward the problems at hand. These have been divided into problem-focused and emotion-focused coping behaviors. *Problem-focused* coping refers to activities through which problems are confronted directly. For example, a patient or family confronted with the diagnosis of schizophrenia may choose to become fully informed about the problem, consult the best experts in the field, and determine other activities that are likely to help the family deal with expected problems. *Emotion-focused* coping refers to activities that reduce the degree of emotional arousal and subjective distress that occur during periods of upset. In order to carry out effective problem-focused coping, one's emotional tone must be aroused and vigilant but not so hyperaroused or hypervigilant as to be disorganizing or so hypoaroused or hypovigilant as to be inadequate to motivate action. Emotion-focused coping includes use of the classical unconscious mechanisms of defense that modulate anxiety and of cognitive self-statements that either increase or reduce arousal. For example, a medical student facing a critical examination may attempt to calm down by repeating such self-statements as, "Don't worry, you've been through worse exams. Only 10 percent of the class flunks out of medical school, and you know 20 other students in the room who aren't as smart as you are." Task-irrelevant behaviors are somatically mediated tension-reducing activities that serve as another form of emotion-focused coping. For instance, a pitcher in a World Series baseball game, in order to settle down to pitch effectively, may execute a large number of fidgety mannerisms, most of which are not signals to other players. Another type of emotion-focused coping is the attempt to imbue with meaning otherwise chaotic, perplexing, and incomprehensible phenomena. For example, a young adult faced with a diagnosis of metastatic cancer might strive to find underlying philosophical or spiritual meaning: "I must have developed this because I was bad" or, "I guess God wanted me to appreciate what really matters in life and not think about so many hedonistic issues." The same mechanism—imbuing a system with meaning in order to bind overwhelming anxiety—has been postulated to be at work in the formation of some delusions.

The coping apparatus may be overwhelmed, and psychiatric disturbances may appear because of vulnerabilities in biological, psychological, or social systems, or the imposition of excessively burdensome physiological, psychological, or environment stressors.

PREDISPOSING VULNERABILITIES **Genetic and intrauterine factors** Familiar genetic vulnerabilities attend Down's syndrome, bipolar mood disorder, schizophrenia, and alcoholism. The fetal alcohol syndrome illustrates how alcohol in the intrauterine environment may impair subsequent development. Other constitutionally facilitated early developmental problems likely to increase subsequent psychiatric morbidity include speech and language difficulties and attention deficit disorders. These problems may presage later development of various adult psychiatric disorders and personality problems. Deafness, affecting as it does a major portion of the perceptual apparatus, also is associated with a high prevalence of psychiatric disturbances.

Temperament Considerable research demonstrates that by birth infants differ widely in temperament—in spontaneous activity levels and in threshold, intensity, and duration of reactions to external stimuli; in regularity or irregularity of certain biological rhythms, such as sleep; in tendencies to approach or withdraw from new stimuli and in speed and degree of adaptation to them; in attention span and distractability; in persistence of behavior; and in qualities of mood. On the basis of such early behaviors, children have been described as having easy or difficult temperaments and as being quick or slow to "warm up." Temperament is not immutable. There are discontinuities over time, and the development of temperament is at least, in part, a function of the goodness of fit with the parents. Nevertheless, early temperamental differences do correlate with behavioral problems, at least through early childhood. The extent to which they may persist and influence subsequent adaptation is not entirely known.

Constitutional factors Other persistent variations in normal personality development have been described that seem to be constitutionally related and that may influence subsequent resilience or vulnerability. Introversion, extroversion, and neuroticism appear to be relatively enduring and stable personality dimensions. Different aspects of intelligence, such as those related to conceptual, mathematical, musical, kinesthetic, and interpersonal abilities, have been postulated as having separate genetic determinants and patterns of development. The type A and B personality patterns as well as hardy, sensitive, fussy, irritable, phlegmatic, optimistic, and pessimistic characters have all been described as generally lifelong qualities that originate in early childhood.

COGNITIVE STYLES *Cognitive style* refers to how persons tend to approach and handle information—how information is appraised, sorted, broken down into components, reassembled, and used. Cognitive style has been related to the extent to which the individual deals with percepts as independent elements rather than as parts of a larger context or gestalt and to the degree of differentiatedness, rigidity, or flexibility with which thoughts, percepts, or cognitions are appraised (i.e., how complex, analytic, simplistic, or vague the pattern of thinking is). Individuals approach problems with different strategies. Some are open in their thinking, whereas others are restricted; some are intuitive, whereas others are logical; some rapidly scan an overall picture and rapidly find complete patterns based on few cues, whereas others tend to consider information systematically, element by element, and do not easily come to closure. A person with an obsessional cognitive style usually thinks analytically and in great detail, whereas a histrionic person usually thinks in global, impressionistic terms.

COPING STYLES As there is a variety of cognitive styles, so are there several *coping styles*. Coping style also reflects tendencies in information processing, particularly those involving appraisal of threats and psychological and behavioral tendencies and styles of engaging or avoiding problems. Some individuals tend to be generally vigilant and approach problems head-on; others tend to deny or avoid problems. Some tend to change the environment (alloplastic), whereas others try to change themselves to fit into a situation (autoplastic). Some act quickly and decisively—or impulsively; others act slowly and deliberately—or are habitually indecisive. These patterns may reflect differences in basic tendencies toward fight, flight, and withdrawal responses in the face of conflict. None of these styles is inherently good or bad, and each may be adaptive in certain situations. The manner in which a given individual copes with problems differs from situation to situation and is often multidimensional. Individuals do not employ the same coping style identically in response to every major stressor, but one may have characteristic action tendencies when faced with certain types of problems: an individual may typically try to repair the most complicated and unfamiliar machinery but assiduously avoid any unpleasant contacts with authority figures.

The implication of these style differences is that individual capacities to tolerate frustration, postpone gratification, and side-step or rush into difficulties vary with temperament and development. Certain styles may be more vulnerable to breakdown in certain circumstances. The avoider may do much better than the attacker in one situation, and vice versa. The more flexible the repertoire of coping behaviors, the more likely is successful adaptation and the less likely is the development of psychiatric disturbance.

PHYSIOLOGICAL STRESSORS Physiological vulnerability may result from longstanding problems or from newly acquired ones. All metabolic, toxic, infectious, and other causes of physical illness produce increased vulnerability to psychiatric disturbance. Studies have shown higher utilization of psychiatric services by those who are physically ill and higher than expected prevalence of physical disease among the psychiatrically impaired. In one study of 658 patients seen consecutively in a community mental health center, almost 9.1 percent had medical problems that were thought to have induced the psychiatric disturbance, and 28 percent of them were patients initially diagnosed as suffering from a functional psychosis. The tragic circumstances brought about by human immunodeficiency virus (HIV) infections leading to seropositivity, acquired immune deficiency syndrome (AIDS), and AIDS related complex (ARC) illustrate vividly how physical stressors can lead to psychiatric disturbances. Many patients with these conditions have psychiatric disturbances, and their complex symptoms challenge the best clinicians. These patients' psychiatric symptoms may represent organic changes that are a direct effect of the virus on the central nervous system (CNS), expectable psychological adjustment responses to an overwhelming, life-threatening disorder, or the emergence of latent or quiescent primary psychiatric disorders provoked by the stressors.

ENVIRONMENTAL STRESSORS There is a complex relationship between the development of psychiatric symptoms and the occurrence of various life events, particularly threatening, unpredictable, and uncontrollable negative events. In general, such undesirable life events predispose a person to develop psychiatric symptoms. This is especially likely if the person already has a psychiatric disturbance. Catastrophic events, such as incarceration in a concentration camp, cause enduring psychiatric disturbances in a high percentage of survivors, though individual responses vary widely. The stress-related consequences of combat also vary widely, so that some heavily exposed combat veterans develop long-lasting post-traumatic stress disorder (PTSD) and others develop very few persistent symptoms. Bereavement, divorce, and major physical injuries affect some people profoundly and others hardly at all, in the long run. During development, there may be critical periods when certain stressors are most traumatic. For example, the loss of a parent at a very young age is likely to be more traumatic and to have more profound and lasting effects than the loss of a parent by an adult child.

The combined impact of negative life events and poor social supports is important in the pathogenesis of at least some psychiatric disturbances. One British study found that women who were depressed were much more likely to have lost a mother at an early age, to be relatively housebound with three or more young children, and to lack a good confiding relationship with a spouse or boyfriend. In that study at least, biological vulnerability to depression seemed less important than the accumulation of negative life circumstances in the development of the disease. People who are ordinarily very competent in all role functions may fall apart completely when a supportive spouse who has bolstered them and taken care of many of their needs suddenly dies. As a group, psychiatric patients who are having acute episodes of depression have experienced more major uncontrollable losses, such as the death of a spouse, in the year prior to onset. Nevertheless, not all psychiatric disturbance is attributable to easily identified provocative negative life events; indeed, some negative life events that at first glance appear to precede a serious psychiatric disturbance may, in fact, occur only after the onset of the disturbance. For example, someone who attributes an episode of depression to having been fired from a job several months previously may already have been functioning suboptimally at that time and have been fired as a consequence of a depression-induced decline in role function.

Certain environmental features can counter the effects of environmental stressors and protect against breakdowns. Stable families and other social supports, good financial circumstances, and the like offer some protection. Research has shown that individuals with psychiatric disturbances have fewer social supports than normal controls. This may be due to friends' and relatives' withdrawal from deviant behaviors or to the disturbed individual's withdrawal from deleterious family and social relationships. In contrast, physically ill persons have more social support persons than others, perhaps reflecting their ability to recruit help in times of need. Of course, the quality as well as the quantity of social supports is important. As has been demonstrated in schizophrenia and mood disorders, for example, negative relationships even in close families may have harmful effects both in initiating and in sustaining psychiatric disturbance.

The negative impact of a physiological or environmental stressor is closely related to its personal meaning. For example, the amputation of a cancerous breast is likely to be much more distressing to a woman whose self-esteem is threatened by her physical disfigurement than to one whose self-confidence is more secure.

CHARACTERISTICS OF PSYCHIATRIC SIGNS AND SYMPTOMS

Signs and symptoms signal the presence of disorders. *Signs* are abnormalities directly observable by an examiner—spontaneously appearing disturbances and those elicited through physical, mental status, and laboratory examinations. *Symptoms* are past or present disturbances noted by the patient that are not necessarily directly observable by an examiner. Signs and symptoms are said to be present when the limits of normal variability of a given parameter (e.g., body temperature) are surpassed. Exactly what constitutes "normal" varies from culture to culture, from context to context, and from observer to observer. A behavior that may be defined as symptomatic in one context may be perfectly acceptable and within bounds in another.

Signs and symptoms are defined by abnormalities in amplitude (e.g., excesses or deficits), duration, intensity, timing, and modifiability of physiological events, perceptions, emotions, thoughts, and motor activities. Ordinarily, most behaviors are carefully regulated by tight sets of physiological controls and social rules. When observable behaviors deviate even slightly from the acceptable limits, this is quickly sensed by laypersons as well as professionals, and because deviance ordinarily implies threat, observers usually notice the deviance readily.

Deviations in amplitude, duration, and intensity can occur in facial expressions, gestures, postures, vocalizations, language, and other expressions of emotion and thought. A small increase in the rate of speech, an intrusion into one person's conversation by another who does not allow proper pauses, a gesture that comes just a bit too close to a face, an excessively rigid or distant stance, or a gaze that is too staring or too avoidant—each signals social insensitivity and alerts the observer to deviance.

OBSERVER SUBJECTIVITY In the absence of standardized criteria, observer subjectivity strongly influences the perception of signs and symptoms, and clinicians inevitably use their personal emotional and visceral responses—their intuitions—as part of psychiatric information gathering. Such intuition deserves respectful study and understanding. The information that stimulates these intuitive responses requires precise identification, verifiable description, and proper evaluation for clinical significance; simple trust based on faith is not sufficient. Thus, a clinician's sense that a patient is angry and potentially violent may result from the patient's subtle (but verifiable) body language and tone of voice, or it may be a countertransference distortion by the clinician that is not prompted by signs from the patient.

Clinician subjectivity is often seen in the use of the word "inappropriate," one of the more commonly misused and abused (often as a pejorative) terms in psychiatry. Appropriateness depends heavily on context, and what is proper in a given context is often highly subjective. Appropriate behavior in California may be inappropriate in Boston. What one clinician views as inappropriate laughter, for example, may be anxious defensive laughter or a subculturally acceptable expression of tension or anxiety, as is peculiar to some Asian groups.

Most psychiatric discourse occurs at the level of signs and symptoms. Patients and their families complain about signs and symptoms. Clinicians are most aware of signs and symptoms. Current treatments usually ameliorate signs and symptoms rather than disorders. Although contemporary psychiatry strives to organize groups of signs and symptoms into coherent syndromes and disorders for which predictions regarding pathogenesis, treatment, and prognosis can be made, current science has been, at best, partially successful in this regard. Consequently, many of the signs and symptoms seen clinically remain unexplained and have been classified poorly at best, lumped into syndromic wastebaskets.

NONSPECIFIC SIGNS AND SYMPTOMS Psychiatry has cardinal but nonspecific signs and symptoms that are analogous to such phenomena in general medicine as rubor, calor, and dolor. These signs and symptoms, including disturbances such as sweating and palpitations with autonomic arousal, perceptual disturbances such as hallucinations, cognitive disturbances such as delusions and thinking disorders, and mood disturbances such as persistent depressed mood, indicate the relatively limited number of final common pathways through which higher CNS function and psychological disturbances can be expressed. For example, hallucinations may result from structural brain injuries such as those in the temporal lobe, from the ingestion of chemicals such as lysergic acid diethylamide (LSD) or amphetamines, or from prolonged sensory deprivation, as well as from functional psychoses. Similarly, persistent depressed mood may result from some antihypertensive medications or from multiple unrelenting aversive life events, among other causes.

In general medicine, fevers are delineated as precisely as possible to provide clues to the underlying cause: the fevers of abscesses, malaria, tuberculosis, and other entities vary from one another in distinctive ways. Until the underlying cause is identified, a fever is currently classified as fever of unknown origin. Signs and symptoms in psychiatry deserve the same conceptual respect. As the imperfect understanding of pathogenesis requires that syndromes and disorders be classified imprecisely, and as interventions are often directed toward target symptoms rather than overall disorders, it would seem wise to define the picture of psychiatric signs and symptoms as carefully as possible but to use labels, such as hallucinations of unknown origin, delusions of unknown origin, or depression of unknown origin, when the pathogenesis is unclear. Given the fact that so many psychiatric signs and symptoms are not pathognomic, a somewhat algorithmic approach to their workup may be justified. For example, a person with vivid hallucinations may well require a drug screen and other physiological tests, even though the overall picture suggests a diagnosis of schizophrenia.

In spite of the fact that individual signs and symptoms may be organized into syndromes and disorders, they often have courses of their own. Thus, in the appearance or the resolution of a disorder, certain associated signs and symptoms may appear very early and may persist after all the others have waned. In some cases, certain signs and symptoms that are commonly associated with a given disorder may fail to appear. Each sign and symptom may have its own pattern and variability of response to treatment. In the treatment of schizophrenia, for example, some patients experience a rapid resolution of hallucinations but have persistent delusions without any other thinking disorder, whereas others may have no residual hallucinations or delusions but still have a prominent thinking disorder.

SYMPTOM CATEGORIES Symptoms have been categorized in various ways. According to how enduring they are and what evoked them, symptoms may be defined as trait or state phenomena. *Trait* symptoms are enduring characteristics of the person: A person who is temperamentally jittery and excitable, anxious in a variety of settings over long periods of time, is said to have trait anxiety. *State* symptoms occur only in relation to specific physiological or situational stimuli, (e.g., an episode of anxiety that is expected to resolve once a life crisis is past). Symptoms have also been divided into primary and secondary phenomena on the basis of current understanding of their centrality to a given disorder. Thus, Bleuler viewed thought disorder as a primary symptom in schizophrenia and hallucinations and delusions as secondary symptoms, that is, attempts by the patient to cope with the primary thinking disorder. Hughlings Jackson, an eminent neurologist of the nineteenth century, divided symptoms into those which represent true deficits and those which represent pathological release phenomena. In this view, the destruction of an inhibitory system or one that modulates and controls behavior might release pathological behavior. For example, a disturbance in the capacity to delay action by exerting judgment might result in impulsive behavior; a disturbance in the capacity to inhibit emotional expression might result in an outburst of rage.

Many signs and symptoms can be conceptualized as attempts at restitution, ineffective attempts to cope with some underlying problem. Illusions or delusions are often experienced in states of intense physiological arousal, attenuated consciousness, and ambiguous external stimulation, in which cases these phenomena may represent attempts of the frightened person to make sense of ambiguous, threatening stimuli.

CONTEXT The context in which psychiatric signs and symptoms are evoked is important to understanding them. Some signs and symptoms persist regardless of the surroundings, for example, guilty ruminations in major depression with melancholia. Some are remarkably state-dependent, that is, they are manifested only in specific settings or are dependent, for example, on the person's level of sexual frustration, hunger, sleep deprivation, or intoxication. For example, certain hallucinations or memories may be present only during states of drug or alcohol intoxication; in some patients, urticaria (hives) may erupt only during states of anger as a psychophysiological response. Interpersonal context is also important. Some persons become violent only when involved in sadomasochistic relationships or in certain group settings, such as adolescent gangs. Human behavior is extremely malleable under the influence of group and social pressures. In gangs, social pressures for conformity and expectations for aggressive behavior may provoke or release pathological behaviors that might otherwise never be expressed by gang

TABLE 10-1
Biopsychosocial Features In an Illustrative Syndrome of Depression

Biological	*Psychological*	*Behavioral*	*Interpersonal and Social*
Current Vegetative Symptoms	*Current*	Paucity of movement	Stops working
Anorexia	Depressed mood	Occasional agitation	Avoids family
Weight loss	Apathy	Drinks more alcohol than usual	Has burdensome financial problems
Constipation	Guilt	Buys a pistol	Recent death of friend
Impotence	Low self-esteem	Irritable and withdrawn	Disengages from major role functions as spouse, parent, member of community
Sleep disturbance	Hopelessness	Elicits sympathy from children	Shuns caregivers and interested members of community
Diurnal variation in mood	Helplessness	Elicits criticism and hostility from spouse	Faces pending litigation
Diminished libido	Suicidal thoughts	Refuses medication	Has responsibility for aging mother
	Delusions of having sinned		
Laboratory	Slow thinking		
Positive dexamethasone suppression test			
Abnormal TRH stimulation test	*History*		
Decreased REM latency	Early death of father		
	Repeated defeats in business, school		
History	Lifelong "crotchety" temperament		
Seasonal variation in syndrome			
Similar syndrome in identical twin			
Treatment with antihypertensives			

members individually. Acts of torture and other atrocities, like those sometimes carried out by terrorists and totalitarian states, occur much more rarely outside of social surroundings and microcultures that condone such behavior or when the tormentors must act entirely as individuals.

For many reasons—the intermittent nature of many psychiatric signs and symptoms, the potential unreliability of patients, the subjective biases that influence the clinician's perception of signs and symptoms—complete assessment of a psychiatric patient requires consultation with family, friends, co-workers, and other professional observers, to supplement the history, as well as observation of the patient over time, when possible.

THE NEED FOR A COMPREHENSIVE PERSPECTIVE The biopsychosocial model of disease reminds clinicians that a disorder may be characterized by psychiatric disturbances in any or all of these spheres. Figure 10-1 illustrates some of the issues that have been associated with each of these dimensions. In practice, common psychiatric syndromes often manifest in each of these dimensions (Table 10-1). Table 10-2 lists some of the clinical hypotheses currently used by clinicians, as they attempt to link collections of signs and symptoms into various syndromes and consider them with regard to treatment options.

Because the amount of information gathered in a thorough assessment of a psychiatric disorder is potentially overwhelming, the clinician often tends to limit the fields of vision and appreciate only part of the available information; the clinician's theoretical orientation and other personal and cultural factors also limit what is perceived. Research has demonstrated that clinicians tend to perceive primarily the signs and symptoms that are most in accord with their theoretical points of view and with the tools they have available to treat psychiatric disorders, a phenomenon known as *concept-driven perception.* The theoretical biases of clinicians seem to be related both to the microcultures of their training programs and to their own personality traits. Such differences may lead one clinician to see a major mood disorder, to be treated with medication, where another sees a pervasive personality problem with dysthymia, to be treated with psychotherapy, and to use different technical terms to label roughly the same phenomena. A psychodynamic psychiatrist might see psychomotor retardation where a neuropsychiatrist sees bradykinesia; a psychodynamicist might see depressed affect and muted speech where a neuropsychiatrist sees mask-like facies

TABLE 10-2
Common Current Clinical Hypotheses Used to Assess Signs and Symptoms: Ways of Understanding the Patient's Problems

Biologically derived hypotheses
1. As an organic mental disorder
2. As an affective (mood) disorder
3. As a nonaffective functional psychosis
4. In relation to the abuse of drugs or alcohol
5. As a disorder other than those listed in 1 through 4, above

Psychodynamically derived hypotheses
1. As being related to personality style
2. As being related to a precipitating event and its dynamic meaning
3. As a manifestation of unresolved grief
4. As a developmental crisis
5. As being related to ego functioning and related psychodynamic issues

Socioculturally derived hypotheses
1. As resulting from the nature and social impact of stressful life events
2. As being related to the extent, nature, and accessibility of social support
3. As being related to definitions of and responses to breakdown in the sociocultural grouping
4. As being related to the patient's motivation, treatment goals, and the dynamics of the entry process to help seeking
5. As social communication

Behaviorally derived hypotheses
1. As disordered thinking, feeling, or acting that is the result of specific antecedent events
2. As disordered thinking, feeling, or acting resulting from reinforcing consequences of the behaviors
3. As disordered thinking, feeling, or acting in response to sociocultural and biological events
4. As a deficit of behaviors (rather than as disordered behaviors) in the areas of thinking, feeling, or acting
5. By an analysis of areas of effective functioning

Table adapted from Lazare A: Hypothesis testing in the clinical interview. In *Outpatient Psychiatry, Diagnosis and Treatment,* A. Lazare, editor, p 131. Williams & Wilkins, Baltimore, 1979, with permission.

and aprosodic speech; the psychodynamicist might see ruminative thought where a neuropsychiatrist sees forced thinking; a psychodynamicist might see a grimace where a neuropsychiatrist sees a tic. Given the extent to which words themselves shape our concepts of reality, the consequences of using these different labels for very similar phenomena may be significant. Figure 10-2 illustrates concept-driven perception in which each clinician who adheres to a prominent contemporary point of view perceives only some of the potentially available phenomena related to a psychiatric disorder. Although there is overlap, each observer also perceives information not appreciated by the others. At the same time, some information that may be highly relevant to diagnosing or treating the disorder may be missed by all the observers; so, clinicians 100 years from now will be able to detect signs and symptoms not appreciated by anyone today.

In what follows, complex behaviors and higher mental functions are considered first as normal phenomena and then as they manifest abnormally. Although convention and simplicity require that the individual signs and symptoms be linked, for purposes of discussion, to specific categories of mental processes, such as perception, cognition, or emotion, in actuality many involve several categories simultaneously.

PHYSICAL MANIFESTATIONS OF PSYCHIATRIC DISORDER

Not only are physical diseases and psychiatric disorders closely associated, but many primary psychiatric disturbances produce signs and symptoms that manifest physiologically. The physiological apparatus of all drive states, including energy level, sleep, appetite, and sexual behavior, can be affected in psychiatric disturbance.

There is a wide range of normal energy levels. Some people fatigue easily throughout life and have "weak constitutions," whereas others appear to be blessed with almost boundless energy and little need for sleep. Deviations beyond such ordinary limits generate concern.

Fatigue is a common nonspecific symptom that occurs with both somatic and psychiatric disorders. Many patients with fatigue find themselves referred to psychiatrists by their physicians as depressed or neurotic after routine workup rules out anemia, hypothyroidism, and other frequent somatic causes. Among adolescents, in particular, fatigue can be a troubling and sometimes solitary symptom. For reasons that are as yet poorly understood, fatigue lasting months and even years may follow certain viral infections, such as mononucleosis and Epstein-Barr virus. Recently a new postviral syndrome of prolonged fatigue has been described that affects previously healthy young women, often vigorous runners, many of whom live in the western United States. Neurological evaluations generally have been negative, but some cerebrospinal fluid viral antibody titers have been elevated.

Fatigue may also reflect sleep disturbances, such as that caused by sleep apnea. In this condition, typically middle-aged patients complain of fatigue without obvious physical cause. A spouse may report severe snoring and periods when breathing stops. The condition results from soft palate abnormalities that cause intermittent airway obstruction throughout the night; patients awake repeatedly to find themselves gasping for air. Surgical intervention may be necessary to correct the condition.

The pathophysiology of fatigue states is still poorly understood, and although some primary care physicians may dismiss patients' mysterious complaints and refer them to psychiatrists, it would be foolish for psychiatrists to accept such complaints as psychogenic without adequate documentation of positive psychiatric findings.

SLEEP DISTURBANCES Sleep disturbances include insomnia and hypersomnia (excessive sleep). Insomnia is a common and sometimes chronic symptom. Frequently it is induced iatrogenically through sedative-hypnotics or other medications that, when discontinued, result in disturbed sleep. Insomnia is common in states of depression, anxiety, and pain and also as an independent symptom.

The hypersomnia seen in certain states of depression must be differentiated from fatigue states mentioned above and from hypersomnolence seen in some toxic and metabolic states. In *narcolepsy,* the patient has sudden attacks of irresistible sleepiness, which may be one symptom of a clinical tetrad that includes *cataplexy* (sudden attacks of profound generalized muscle weakness leading to physical collapse in the presence of alert consciousness), *sleep paralysis* (waking from sleep with a sensation of being totally paralyzed that may persist for minutes), and *hypnagogic hallucinations* (vivid visual hallucinations that occur at the point of falling asleep). Narcoleptic attacks are often precipitated by unusual states of arousal (e.g., cataplexy may immediately follow unrestrained laughter or orgasm). Daytime sleepiness may reflect sleep apnea. Periodic hypersomnia also occurs in the Klein-Levin syndrome, a condition typically affecting young men, in which periods of sleepiness alternate with confusional states, ravenous hunger, and protracted sexual activity. Intervals of days, weeks, or months may pass between these episodes.

APPETITE AND WEIGHT DISTURBANCES Increased appetite and weight may occur in some neurological disorders involving the hypothalamus and temporal lobes and also in mania, atypical depressive disorders, and bulimic syndromes. Loss of appetite, true anorexia nervosa, is often accompanied by changes in taste (e.g., foods begin to taste different or bitter and to have a fainter or unpleasant aroma). In addition to somatic and neurological conditions, anorexia nervosa may occur in primary and secondary mood disorders, in syndromes of drug and alcohol dependence, and in the late stages of anorexia nervosa, when confusion about proprioceptive sensations may occur.

DISTURBANCES IN SEXUAL DRIVE The normal range of sexual drives is very great. Some individuals are naturally lusty, whereas others have limited sexual desire. Diminished sexual drive with impotence may be seen in a variety of neurological, metabolic, and other somatic syndromes. Psychiatric disorders noted for diminished sexual drive include primary mood disorders, schizophrenia, substance abuse disorders, and marital conflicts.

Increased sexual activity may be seen in some neurological, drug-induced, and psychiatric disorders. Patients with mania and some with schizophrenia exhibit hypersexual behavior that is extraordinary for them. Some patients with satyrism and nymphomania may have heightened sexual drive, but such sexual activity is usually compulsive and unsatisfying.

Altered sexuality, including perversions such as fetishes, sadomasochism, and pedophilia, may be seen as isolated psychiatric syndromes. In individuals whose previous sexual behavior was within the bounds of social propriety for their

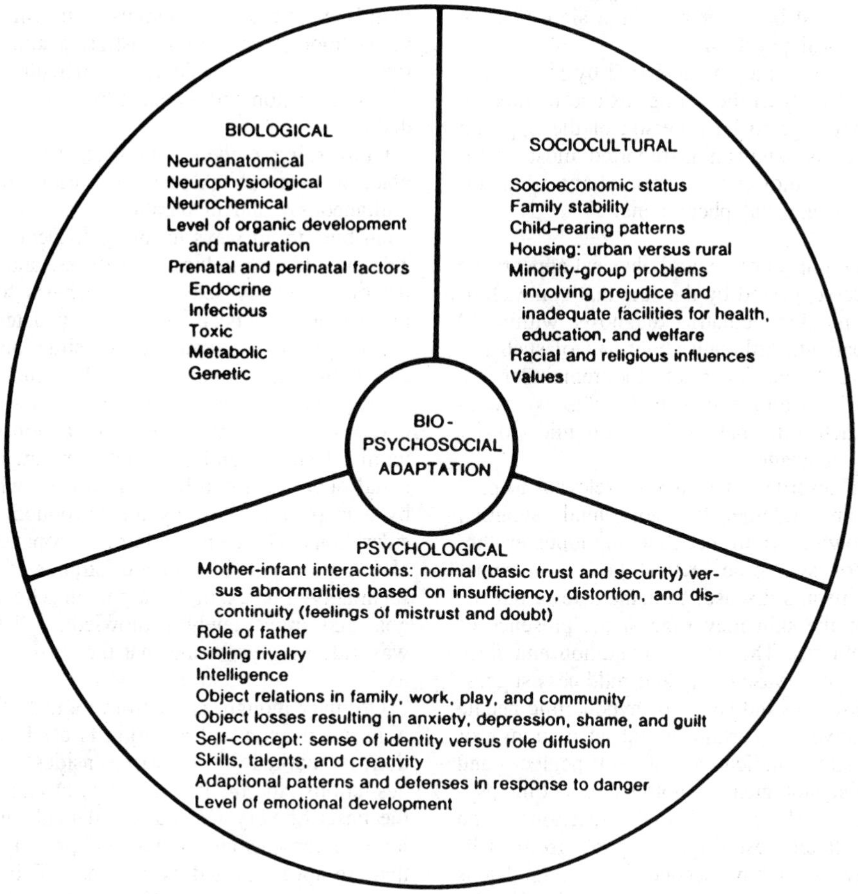

FIGURE 10-1 *Biological, psychological, and social forces interact and affect the psychiatric health of an individual. (Modified after Richmond JB, Lustman SL: Total health: A conceptual visual aid. J Med Educ* 29: *23, 1954; with permission.)*

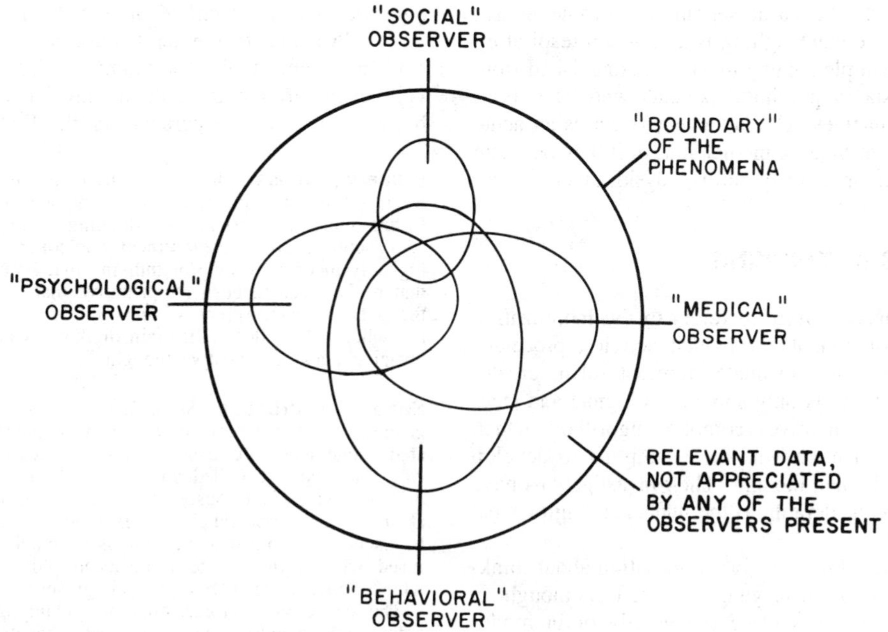

FIGURE 10-2 *Clinical data processed by four observers with different theoretical orientations. (From Yager J: Amer J Psychiat* 134: *736, 1977. Copyright 1977, The American Psychiatric Association, with permission.)*

group, inappropriate sexual behavior may be a sign of early brain disease or functional psychosis.

Transsexualism is a syndrome characterized by the feeling that one was born into a body of the wrong sex and marked by the desire from an early age to be a person of the opposite sex. Male-to-female transsexualism is reported most often. Both psychodynamic and biological theories have been advanced to explain these unusual phenomena.

APPEARANCE The impact of general physical appearance and body language are suggested by the fact that some clinicians formulate an initial psychiatric diagnosis within 30 seconds of seeing a patient. Although about half of such initial impressions prove to be incorrect, the remainder are validated by psychiatric history and mental status exam, revealing just how much information is communicated by appearance and body language.

Among the physical disorders that may be relevant to psychiatric conditions are acromegaly, congenital syphilis, Cushing's disease, Down's syndrome, systemic lupus erythematosus, fetal alcohol syndrome, Klinefelter's syndrome, phacomatoses, and Wilson's disease, to name a few, but the general appearance of the skin may suggest the presence of occult psychiatric problems. The general condition and flush of the skin may reveal hypervascularity and ruddiness suggestive of alcoholism, abscesses indicative of hypodermic needle abuse, tattoos indicative of certain group affiliations, or weathering and wasting indicative of self-neglect and malnutrition. Psychophysiological symptoms reflecting psychiatric disturbance include urticarial reactions and neurodermatitis, the latter resulting, in part, from self-excoriation, destructive scratching secondary to compulsions and unrelenting sensations of discomfort. The patient's odor may reveal lack of self-care, alcoholism, diabetic ketosis, or another condition that can have mental manifestations.

Examination of the head and neck may reveal exophthalmos or puffy eyelids suggesting thyroid disease, marked pupillary dilation with anxiety or stimulant abuse, miosis with narcotic abuse, abnormal pupillary pigments in Wilson's disease, salivary gland enlargement in bulimia nervosa, and necrosis of the nasal septum in cocaine abuse, among other signs. Frequent sighing is a common respiratory sign in depression. Simple sighing must be distinguished from respiratory dyskinesia in psychotic patients who have been treated with phenothiazines. The latter may occur as an acute dyskinesia due to antipsychotic medication, or it may be a late manifestation and component of tardive dyskinesia.

DISTURBANCES IN THINKING

NORMAL THINKING *Thinking* refers to the mobilization of the ideational components of mental activity, processes used to imagine, appraise, evaluate, forecast, plan, create, and will. Human thought is only sometimes logical and categorical. Most thought involves complex algorithms which have so far eluded scientists who are attempting to develop computer models of human thought. Their investigations have nevertheless added considerably to the understanding of what ordinary thinking is.

Although most available objective information about thinking comes from the study of language as it reflects thought, a great deal of thinking takes place preverbally or in modes other than those of ordinary language. Thinking occurs in images, music, kinesthetic sensations, and in symbols other than linguistic ones. Attempts to transmit preverbal and nonverbal thought are often frustrating and unsatisfactory. Creative artists have considerable difficulty describing the inner states of tension and inchoate awareness from which ideas are distilled.

Converging evidence suggests that human thought takes place in a multitrack fashion, various processes working simultaneously and in parallel to assess, solve problems, and contribute in all ways to thought. Deductive analyses operate side by side with inductive analyses, and the solutions that the person ultimately selects as the basis for action are usually those that have been most rapidly determined or those that seem to be most adaptive to the situation. Competing tendencies within individuals may reflect such competing analyses of a given problem, especially when solutions are not clear cut. When a potential course of action is judged to be both highly desirable and potentially threatening, in more or less equal degrees, a conflict state arises, which is resolved only by a leap of faith or by the introduction of still other considerations. The common human propensity for self-deception also reveals that simultaneous strands of thought are analyzed separately. For example, a person who fails to accomplish a goal may immediately acknowledge, "I knew all along that I was kidding myself and that the goal was beyond my capacity."

Ordinary thought is far from logical. The stream of thought is intruded upon and attention is easily distracted. Conversation is marked by recurring asides, interruptions, delays, hesitations, and the loss of ideas. Decisions are often made on the basis of very few cues and inadequate evidence: people jump to conclusions. Beliefs and prejudices are zealously held that are not supported by evidence. Thinking in stereotypes is more common than thinking in logical categories. From an evolutionary perspective, thinking in stereotypes and by approximation has probably been very adaptive, more so than thinking in strictly defined categories. The human tendency to think in stereotypes rather than categories also accounts for the fact that clinicians tend to make diagnoses by approximation and intuition and feel less comfortable using formal lists of criteria, such as those in the revised third edition of *Diagnostic and Statistical Manual of Mental Disorders* (DSM-III-R). Provided that other features are present, many clinicians are comfortable, for example, diagnosing anorexia nervosa even through the patient may have lost 13 percent of body weight, not 15 percent per the DSM-III-R criterion.

Primary process Historically, psychiatrists have tended to follow Freud's concept of primary process and secondary process thinking. In this model, *primary process* thinking uses symbol, metaphor, imagery, condensation, displacement, and concretism—the jumbled and logically incoherent style of thinking that Freud saw in dreams and that he believed to be more primitive than logical, language-based thought. Primary process thinking represents what has been metaphorically called right brain thinking, which is associated with visual images and creative thought.

Secondary process *Secondary process* thinking refers to language-associated thought in which the sequence of time is appreciated, statements are causally linked, clearly delineated abstract categories exist, and deductive rules of logic may be applied. Individuals vary enormously in the extent to which they can think abstractly and appreciate complex thought. Many students develop headaches and find that their minds go blank or that they feel confused when trying to read advanced philosophy or mathematics whose concepts seem beyond their grasp.

The capacity for forecasting and planning also varies greatly among among individuals, so much so that it has been viewed as a separate measure of intelligence. Studies of chief executive officers of multinational corporations have demonstrated that they often possess abilities to think in elaborate detail about complicated plans that extend decades into the future; most normal persons have difficulty in being able to imagine a detailed future beyond several years, or even several months. Such differences may have clinical significance. In a prospective study of adolescent girls attending a birth control clinic, it was found that girls with more elaborate future orientations were more likely to comply with birth control advice and not become pregnant than were those with poorer abilities to elaborate future schemas.

Normal secondary process thinking is characterized by predictability, coherence, and redundancy. In interpersonal communication, words are backed up by nonlexical vocalizations (inflections) and gestures that provide important contextual cues and a sense of overall coherence to the communication. Ideas follow one another in a sequence that is understandable to the listener. In the state of so-called normal psychological regression, as in the free associative method of psychoanalysis, the individual can willfully surrender the controls that maintain secondary process thinking and switch to the less controlled mode of primary process thinking, in which the associations of thought are dictated by emotional associations based on incidental parts of a thought or on relatively trivial similarities. Thoughts from several different streams can be intermingled, and associated melodic aspects of speech, such as fluency, rate, pitch, volume, and intensity, may be altered from usual patterns of communication.

Formal thought disorders are said to exist when the degree of disruption of thought exceeds that normally tolerated and the individual lacks the capacity to reinstate control over primary process thinking. The fact that almost every type of thought disorder can be temporarily induced in normal people under experimental conditions or with fatigue suggests that clinical thought disorders may be release phenomena; that is, such disorders may indicate the absence of those overriding control systems that ordinarily sift, evaluate, and regulate the form and flow of thought before it reaches consciousness.

Current systems for classifying thought disorders are primarily descriptive and are not informed by knowledge of pathogenetic mechanisms, because the underlying processes that govern thought are not understood. Furthermore, conventional classification separates form and flow from the content of thought, but many thought disorders typically include both form and content abnormalities. Thus, while delusions contain disturbances of thought content, they also have elements of rigidity and imperviousness of thought.

FLOW AND FORM DISTURBANCES Normal variations in the flow and form of thought are considerable. Some persons' thoughts flow rapidly, easily, productively, and with great precision; others' are expressed slowly and methodically and take form with difficulty. Pathological thinking and speech can be unusually slow or accelerated. Slowing of thought (and of movement) occurs in *psychomotor retardation,* a feature of major depressive disorders and hypothyroidism. *Thought blocking,* the sudden loss of an idea as if it dropped out of consciousness, can be a normal occurrence. In pathological conditions, such as schizophrenia, thought blocking may be accompanied by the perception that the thought is actually being stolen from the mind by some alien force.

Fast talking that is within normal limits is seen in some extremely talkative persons, sometimes referred to as "motor mouths," who exhibit mild logorrhea. Type A personalities and other energetic people speak rapidly and explosively. *Pressure of speech,* in which thoughts pour out at a very rapid rate, may attend excited states such as hypomania, thyrotoxicosis, and intoxication with caffeine, amphetamine, or cocaine. More rapid racing of thoughts may lead to *flight of ideas,* in which the flow of thought and the rate of speech are extremely rapid and thoughts are so jumbled as to lose some coherence. In flight of ideas, typical of manic states, the patient in a state of high emotional arousal leaps rapidly from topic to topic, but the point of association is usually comprehensible to the examiner (i.e., the story more or less makes sense, although it is told with rapid-fire delivery). At its extreme, such thinking may be incoherent. Flight of ideas must be differentiated from the rapid-fire, loosely associated thoughts that accompany states of catatonic excitement, in which an observer may fail to perceive any connection between thoughts and the patient may seem far less responsive to the environment.

Disturbances in the continuity of thought may take several forms. *Circumstantial speech* reveals thinking marked by multiple digressions. The speaker ultimately comes to the point, but in a very roundabout way. The stream of thought is interrupted; the associations are understandable but seem beside the point to the observer; and the speaker ultimately and without prompting is able to return to the main point of the statement. It has been suggested that digressive circumstantial speech may sometimes be a defensive maneuver by a speaker who is "playing for time": the speaker may start out to make a specific point, forget the intended point, stall for time by talking about other things, recollect the original idea, and finally get back on track.

Tangential speech wanders away from the intended point, moving to areas that are less and less relevant and never returning to the original idea. The speaker becomes derailed, possibly owing to anxiety, forgetting the initial purpose of the statement. The person who *talks past the point* (*vorbeireden,* a form of tangentiality) never quite gets to the central idea. *Perseveration* refers to the repetition of a sentence or phrase, sometimes several times over, after it is no longer relevant; it is as if the person has become stuck on a saying or word. Perseveration is usually due to organic mental disorder. *Stereotypy* refers to the repetition of a phrase or a behavior in many different settings, irrespective of context.

Loose association describes speech in which thoughts seem to the observer to have no logical relation to one another, although in the patient's mind they may be connected by a private logic. According to Bleuler, this classical thought disorder is a central feature of schizophrenia. In extreme cases, the associations of sentences and even phrases are incomprehensible, and syntax—the rules of grammar by which phrases are organized into sentences and words into phrases—may be disrupted. *Word salad* is the stringing together of words that seem to have no logical association, and *verbigeration* describes the complete disappearance of understandable speech, which is replaced by strings of incoherent utterances.

Clang association refers to a sequence of thoughts stimulated by the sound of a preceding word. For example, a manic patient said, "I'll kill with a drill or a pill—God, I'm ill—what swill." In *echolalia* the patient repeats a sentence just uttered by the examiner. Repetition of only the last word or phrase uttered is called *palilalia,* a symptom found most often in chronic schizophrenia.

Disturbances in the complexity of thought Abstract thinking is the ability to assume a mental set, to keep simultaneously in mind all of the aspects of a complex situation, to move from feature to feature as indicated by the situation, and to extract common properties. Normal persons show great individual variation in the ability to engage in abstract thinking. Many highly intelligent professionals, for example, feel totally surpassed by the virtuoso displays of abstraction achieved by intellectual giants, such as Einstein. *Concrete thinking,* typically seen in organic mental disorders, is a disturbance in the ability to form abstract concepts, generally illustrated by literal mindedness and the inability to abstract the commonality of members of a group, for example, the fact that a flea and a tree are similar in that they are both living things. Schizophrenic patients exhibit more highly selective disturbances of abstraction. It has been suggested that literal-minded thinking in schizophrenia may be a defensive maneuver to avoid responsibility or blame for "bad thoughts."

THOUGHT CONTENT The normal content of thought, the buzzing, booming stream of consciousness that constitutes the stuff of everyday life, is composed of awareness, concerns, beliefs, preoccupations, wishes, and fantasies occurring with various degrees of clarity, vividness, differentiation, imagination, and strength. Normal thought is often illogical, containing many beliefs and prejudices that, though they clearly contradict one another, are nevertheless held with passion and conviction.

Belief systems are the scaffolding of thought, chains of impressions and expectations around which plans and behaviors are organized. Belief systems may be attitudinal, setting general expectations and biases about the world that inform how incoming information is processed; examples are optimism, pessimism, and paranoia. Even some unsubstantiated beliefs are embraced passionately, such as religious convictions. Some beliefs are evanescent and fleeting; others are pervasive, tenacious, and influential. Some beliefs are unique and private, whereas others are shared by another person, a family, or a society.

Contents in the stream of thought that are perceived as being consistent with a sense of self, compatible with the individual's self-image, are called *ego-syntonic*. Other thoughts that appear just as naturally may be at variance with an individual's central values and may seem *ego-alien* or *ego-dystonic*. An ego-dystonic impulse to kill someone, being inconsistent with one's predominant value systems, may generate a counteractive ego-syntonic thought such as, "You really don't mean it."

Imaginative fantasy is an important component of normal thought, starting in earliest childhood. The vivid, eidetic imagination of a young child can produce vivid fantasies in which children become fully immersed, almost as if in hypnotic states. During latency many children develop imaginary companions as playmates. In later years, such imaginative thinking may be the essence of the creative reverie. Artists, writers, and creative scientists may retain access to these forms of thinking more readily than others. Meditative states of mind may facilitate the emergence of imaginative insights. Such thinking may also occur in dreams.

Intrusive reveries are common in the usual adult stream of consciousness. For example, a 90-minute daytime cycle has been demonstrated that involves oral fantasies of eating and smoking; it is probably reflective of basic rest and activity cycles (BRACs) related to rapid-eye-movement (REM) cycles of sleep. Some men experience intrusive sexual thoughts throughout the day (in one study, as often as once a minute). Elaborate wish-fulfilling daydreams are quite common during periods of specific deprivation, such as starvation.

Repeated and intrusive thoughts attain pathological status when they interfere with the normal events of life. Obsessional styles of thought are marked by attention to detail and great concern for the possible resonances and implications of a particular thought. Such styles of thinking may take the form of preoccupation with strict adherence to established rules, values, or beliefs in a way that strongly controls personality and behavior. An obsessional style may be highly adaptive for a surgeon or an astronaut; however, obsessionality can be maladaptive. In *scrupulosity,* the person rigidly adheres to rules even when such adherence is self-destructive and shortsighted for all concerned. *Religiosity,* a preoccupation with religious beliefs and rituals, is seen in some patients with complex partial seizures, in some religious cultists, and in other orthodox and fundamentalist faithful. Theoretically, such preoccupations may serve as psychological defense mechanisms that bind anxiety and prevent the emergence of other unwelcome ideas. *Obsessional thoughts* are rigid and repetitive and may concern any aspect of mental life. They may be devoted to any motivation—power, love, lust, altruism, or destructiveness. Some self-enhancing obsessional thoughts initially may be welcome and well tolerated, but even these, when excessive, become bothersome and ego alien. Objects of obsession may be erotic objects, competitive striving, or religious thoughts. Destructive obsessions may involve self-mutilation, suicide, homicide, jealousy, revenge, and similar issues. Unrelenting morbid obsessions, called *ruminations,* typically are seen in melancholia, where a morbid set of thoughts may be experienced repeatedly, like a tape endlessly replayed.

A 62-year-old melancholic man was constantly plagued by the thought that he was a terrible man and that the FBI would shortly be coming to arrest him. He paced agitatedly for hours, expecting every knock at the door or ring of the telephone to be the one announcing the FBI.

Sufficiently powerful obsessional thoughts often generate compulsive behaviors. Ego-alien obsessional thoughts and ruminations, those concerning forbidden impulses for example, frequently stimulate reaction formation, the assumption of thoughts and behaviors intended to undo the damage generated by such anxiety-producing impulses. So, for example, it has been speculated that a hand washing compulsion represents reaction formation against impulses to soil or perform other unacceptable behaviors. Some persons perform compulsive behaviors with little or no conscious awareness of the accompanying obsessional thoughts.

DISTURBANCES IN THOUGHT CONTENTS *Ideas of reference* are false, personalized interpretations of events, beliefs that occurrences or remarks refer specifically to oneself when, in fact, they do not.

A psychotic young man enlisted in the army immediately after seeing a billboard poster of Uncle Sam pointing his finger and saying, "Uncle Sam wants you." The man was convinced that Uncle Sam was directing his recruiting plea directly and solely toward him, and he felt compelled to oblige.

Phobic thoughts involve irrational fears; phobias may be simple or complex. Although some phobic thoughts are obsessional, others emerge only in the presence of specific phobic stimuli, such as snakes. In *simple phobias,* persistent, irrational fears are provoked by specific stimuli. Phobic persons almost always avoid phobic stimuli, in order to suppress anxiety. Some common simple phobias are fear of dirt, excrement, snakes, spiders, and heights. Behavioral, psychodynamic, and biological theories have all been advanced as causes of phobias. Some well-known phobias, such as fears of animals or of injections, have been thought either to result from early traumatic events and to develop along the paradigm of classical Pavlovian conditioning, or to represent displacements of early psychodynamic conflicts. Certain phobias may be closely related to biological factors. Some monkeys that have never been exposed to snakes panic when placed in the presence of a snake, a response that obviously has adaptive value, so it has been suggested that some human phobic responses represent exaggerations of adaptive behaviors shaped by evolution.

Complex phobias are more elaborate; they involve fears related to broader situations. Agoraphobia, the best known, is fear of being in open spaces. One current formulation suggests that agoraphobia can be understood as a defensive response to panic attacks: Persons who are terrified of having panic attacks in social settings and public places refuse to leave their own homes, hoping to reduce the likelihood of panic attacks by avoiding places where they were once triggered and where they might feel exposed and embarrassed. *Neophobia* is a general fear of novelty—in situations or people. It may be related to temperament and to the need of some individuals to keep stimulation and arousal to a minimum.

DELUSIONS *Delusions* are fixed false beliefs, strongly held and immutable in the face of refuting evidence. Delusional thoughts must be understood in the context of other strongly held beliefs and convictions, many of which are not fully supported by evidence, for example, some religious and political beliefs. One of the mind's primary functions is to generate beliefs, including myths and meaning systems. These beliefs provide the individual with a sense of personal and group identity and with ways of understanding reality. They are most noticeable when shared untestable beliefs often form the basis for group cohesion as in religions and cults. Some groups adhere to cherished beliefs despite an abundance of plausible contrary evidence, for example, fundamentalist sects that take literally the biblical creation story. In the face of contrary evidence or grave personal threat, individuals often cling to their primary beliefs as matters of faith (i.e., alternative, irrefutable bases for understanding). The strong faith with which religious, political, and nationalistic convictions are held, even at the cost of death, shows the power that untestable beliefs can have over behavior.

Delusions lie at the extreme of the following continuum of distorted beliefs: First there is the strongly held belief, not necessarily implausible, that a person is unwilling to disregard, in spite of contrary evidence: "I don't care what you show me, I know that he's a crook!" Next are unrealistic, firmly held private beliefs that the individual sometimes considers to be implausible: "Well, most of the time I *know* that I have cancer in spite of what the physicians tell me, but sometimes I wonder if it's all in my head." Finally, the definitive delusion, a privately held, immutable thought, usually idiosyncratic and bizarre, that remains a firm conviction in spite of evidence to the contrary: "My intestines are rotting and causing people to die all around."

Delusions are not seen only in isolated individuals. Shared delusions may occur in couples (*folie à deux*) and in families (*folie à famille*). Many psychiatrists would consider group delusions to be present in some cults as well, but exactly where the cut-off points occur with such beliefs held by larger, more traditional and well-organized religious, political, and other groups is arguable. The content of delusions is highly influenced by culture. Whereas centuries ago delusions of persecution often concerned persecution by the devil and had religious connotations, persecutory delusions today more often take on political and social perspectives.

An 18-year-old man presented with the belief that he was controlled by a computer aboard an Enterprise-like starship, an elaboration from the television series, *Star Trek*. He was convinced that all of his thoughts, actions, and feelings were being programmed aboard the starship which was located light years away and, therefore, could never be detected by anyone.

An electrical engineer believed that his brain was actually that of a robot, a fancy piece of equipment. He drew up blueprints illustrating just how the mechanism worked through detailed circuitry. The fact that no such equipment was visible on radiographs of his head in no way dissuaded him, because he knew that the wiring was much too fine to be detected by mere x-rays. The patient's delusion appeared, disappeared, and reappeared, depending on how much he complied with treatment. The psychosis responded very well to phenothiazines, and during remissions he totally denied the existence of the delusional beliefs, saying that the whole thing was "a bad dream" and functioned very well, except for a somewhat isolated life-style. When he stopped taking medications, the full-blown delusional system would return, identical from one episode to the next. The sequence resembled that of a repetitive dream, or what would be expected if the delusion were a state-dependent belief.

Patients with bipolar disorder exhibit the same phenomena: The same delusions reappear with each manic or depressive episode. During intermittent eurthymic periods, these delusions are usually inaccessible or only faintly remembered and are usually minimized or denied by the patient.

Table 10-3 lists some characteristics by which delusions have been classified, and Table 10-4 lists some classic types of delusions. *Simple delusions* contain relatively few elements, whereas *complex delusions* may contain extensive elaborations of people, spirits, motives, situations, and arrangements.

A chronic schizophrenic man with a simple delusion believed that a little angel named Hilo (i.e., "High-Low") sat on his shoulder and looked after him. He could not see Hilo and Hilo never spoke, but he nevertheless knew that Hilo was forever with him, knowledge that the patient found comforting. The patient's behavior in no way revealed the presence of this delusion.

Systematized delusions are usually restricted to well-delineated areas and are ordinarily associated with a clear sensorium and absence of hallucinations. They are often isolated from other aspects of behavior. In contrast, *nonsystematized delusions* usually extend into many areas of life, and new data—new people and situations—are constantly incorporated to further support the presence of the delusion. The patient usually has concurrent mental confusion, hallucinations, and some affective lability. Whereas the patient with a closed systematized delusion system may go about life relatively unperturbed, the patient with a nonsystematized delusion frequently has poor social functioning and behaves in response to the delusional beliefs.

An agitated inpatient was convinced that the FBI was following and attacking him. Although he gradually accepted the good intentions of the ward staff, at one point when he became upset and the ward staff had to restrain him, he suddenly turned and with a frightened start said, "Ah, now I realize that you're all part of the FBI."

Complete delusions are those held utterly without doubt. In contrast, *partial delusions* are those about which the patient entertains doubts. Such doubts may be seen during the slow development of a delusion, as the delusion is gradually given up, or intermittently throughout its course.

A 30-year-old woman believed that she was to bear the next Messiah. She was convinced that a stranger was going to impregnate her through the ether and that she would give birth to Christ and thereby help save the world from nuclear destruction. At times she wavered in her conviction, but she said that giving up the belief left her feeling empty and sad. She said that without the delusional belief her life was meaningless, that she was worthless and a failure. The contribution that the delusional belief made to supporting and maintaining her fragile self-esteem was evident. Giving up the delusion was too much for her to bear, so she repeatedly retreated to the safety and positive esteem afforded by the delusion. She had enough insight to occasionally joke about her need to hold on to the delusion, saying that she was simply following advice she'd seen printed on a tee shirt: "I've tried reality and now I'm looking for a good fantasy."

TABLE 10-3
Characteristics of Delusions

Simple vs. complex
Complete vs. partial
Systematized vs. nonsystematized
Primary (autochthonous) vs. secondary
How they affect behavior

TABLE 10-4
Some Classic Types of Delusions

Delusions of persecution
Delusions of grandeur
Delusions of influence
Delusion of having sinned
Nihilistic delusions
Somatic delusions
Delusion of doubles (*doppelgänger*)
Delusional jealousy (Othello syndrome)
Delusional mood
Delusional perception
Delusional memory
Delusions of erotic attachment (Clérambault's syndrome)
Delusions of replacement of significant others (Capgras' syndrome)
Delusions of disguise (Fregoli's syndrome)
Shared delusions (folie à deux, folie à trois, folie à famille)

Primary or *autochthonous delusions* take form in an instant, without identifiable precipitating events, as if full awareness suddenly bursts forth in an unexpected flash of insight, like a bolt from the blue. Such delusions may be quite elaborate.

A 17-year-old boy, characteristically a loner, came to the dinner table one evening and announced that he had to leave home and climb Mount Everest in order to save the world. This knowledge had come to him instantaneously, in a moment of sudden illumination. He denied that anything in particular had been troubling him beforehand, and his family had observed no recent changes in his behavior. He had never before had any interests in mountain climbing or altruistic pursuits.

In contrast, *secondary delusions* emerge slowly, usually following a period of emotional turmoil. Secondary delusions may play a restitutive, anxiety reducing function by imposing meaning on terrifying chaos. Neuroendocrine studies of patients with psychotic anxiety that show a correlation between a fall in corticosteroid secretion—a sign of diminishing physiological distress—and the development of delusional beliefs support this theory.

A 42-year-old woman became progressively tense and restless over a period of 3 to 4 weeks and impulsively flew from New York City to California "to find myself." She arrived in a state of bewilderment and gradually developed an awareness that she was the illegitimate sister of a well-known movie star; she also sensed that telepathic messages had been influencing her all along in her frantic move. With this realization she camped in front of the movie star's house, trying to get him to accept her as a sister. As her conviction in this belief grew, her confusion diminished considerably.

Patients vary considerably in the extent to which they act on delusional thoughts. *Delusions of influence,* those in which the patient perceives himself or herself as a passive victim forced to carry out the orders of an irresistible force, may result in dramatic self-destructive or aggressive behavior, as illustrated by the murderer who called himself Son of Sam. This psychotic killer murdered a series of people in New York and claimed that he was the powerless agent of a force that required him to commit the acts. Some patients may take bold or destructive action on their own initiative in efforts to protect themselves or others from delusionally anticipated events.

DISTURBANCES IN JUDGMENT

Judgment is a complex and diverse group of mental functions that includes analytic thinking, social and ethical action tendencies, and depth of understanding or insight. Analytic thinking includes the capacity to discriminate and to weigh the pros and cons of potential alternative actions. Social and ethical action tendencies are closely related to culture and upbringing, and possibly to constitutional factors as well. Insight may reflect intelligence, learning, and cognitive style.

Impairments in judgment occur in many psychiatric disturbances. Anxiety states, intoxications, fatigue, and even group pressure can cause temporary impairments in judgment in otherwise normal persons. Organic brain damage and functional psychoses may chronically impair any aspect of judgment in any person, regardless of premorbid character. Poor role models and deviant social backgrounds may lead to social and necessarily ethical action tendencies that are quite different from those of the examiner but that do not necessarily represent impaired judgment. Thus, someone raised in a criminal environment may have superb analytic judgment and self-awareness, which are, however, put to illegal use.

Judgment may be impaired in one dimension and spared in others. Individuals may retain sound ethical judgment when their analytic capacities fail or may retain excellent analytic abilities for nonpersonal matters while lacking insight into personal situations or behaviors. Thus, some people who could provide socially appropriate responses to traditional mental status examination questions about what one would do in a movie theater if fire broke out or what one would do with a stamped and sealed addressed envelope found in the street might, at the same time, be incapable of assessing the pros and cons of receiving a medication or electroconvulsive therapy, or of crucial clinical issues related to capacity to provide informed consent, or of having insight into their own states of health or illness. Judgments related to personal situations relevant to adaptation are clearly the most important to evaluate.

The term *insight,* usually in the context of self-awareness, has been used in a variety of ways. Basic insight refers to a superficial awareness of one's situation (e.g., that one is ill). A deeper level of insight is operating when there is the intellectual appreciation of what is going on (e.g., "I have hallucinations and delusions, and my doctors have told me that I am schizophrenic and must take medication"). Still deeper levels of insight reflect more complete cognitive and emotional appreciation of a situation (e.g., "I realize that I have schizophrenia, that it impairs my judgment and social function at times, and that I will have to take medications if I am to minimize my symptoms and try to make the most of my life. I feel profoundly disappointed about this affliction, because it prevents me from achieving some of the goals I've always wished for. Nevertheless, I have to do my best to get over my disappointment and hurt feelings so that I can get whatever I can out of life").

DISORDERS OF CONSCIOUSNESS

Consciousness can be defined as awareness of the self and environment. For many scientists and philosophers consciousness is the most interesting and perplexing phenomenon in all of human existence. If it were not for consciousness, biological organisms could probably be understood, more or less, as self-regulating automata, perhaps ultimately as elegant computers or robots; however, consciousness—as an emergent property of complex biological nervous systems, as a poorly understood property of an even more mysterious and complex universe, or as a property understandable only in religious and spiritual terms—remains unexplained and, at least from a scientific point of view, unexplainable. Consciousness does not seem to be simply an all-or-none phenomenon.

LEVELS OF CONSCIOUSNESS *Levels of consciousness,* defined as alertness and awareness of the environment, vary widely under normal conditions, and in pathological states even more remarkable properties are seen, for example, co-consciousness and multiple consciousness.

The experiments of Sperry and colleagues involving patients with commissurotomies of the corpus callosum have demonstrated the existence of two virtually separate systems of consciousness, which seem to operate side by side. For example, when in the course of a dull experiment the picture of a nude woman was flashed only to the right brain (the left visual field) of a commissurotomized patient, the subject verbally denied being aware of anything unusual, but at the same time, started to squirm and blush, remarking, "Oh, you have some machine!" Similarly, when a cup was presented to the right brain only, the patient denied seeing anything but was able with the left hand to pick out the cup from an assortment of objects. This literal splitting of verbal awareness from visual-spatial awareness in the brain produces behavior that is at least superficially similar to that of patients who deny being consciously upset by an event but who demonstrate visceral responses. While the formulation is too simplistic, the separate consciousness for logical-verbal and for spatial-visual awareness demonstrated in split-brain experiments may be crude analogues for more highly differentiated and discrete types of awarenesses and modes of information processing. Furthermore, the very fact that there are separate, and to some extent competing, modes of consciousness may increase the likelihood of psychological distress, because they are capable of yielding internally conflicting views of reality.

PSYCHOLOGICAL AND PHYSIOLOGICAL FACTORS In ordinary states of alert consciousness, individuals are able to deploy adequate amounts of attention to their surroundings and to reflective thought. Anxiety and other states of excessive emotional stimulation can produce distractibility and reduce attention span. Normal persons vary enormously in their ability to pay attention in different settings without being distracted; individual variations may reflect differences of temperamental and cognitive style, as was discussed earlier.

A sense of increased consciousness with heightened alertness, awareness, and sharper thinking may be experienced in states of high arousal or threat. In pathological levels of arousal seen in mania, catatonic excitement, and intoxications with amphetamines or cocaine, attention may fragment. On the other hand, illness or fatigue diminishes the sense of alertness and attentiveness, and thereby diminishes consciousness. As normal fatigue passes into dozing, attention and alertness fade so that intrusive visual images with primary process thinking may appear, as in the *Silberer phenomenon,* which occurs in hypnagogic states. In this phenomenon, a visual image suddenly appears that may represent a verbal thought in a condensed symbolic form. The thought, "Too many cooks spoil the broth," for example, may be represented by a picture of many people in chef's hats standing around and stirring a huge stew pot. This diminished state of alertness fades into light sleep and then into the other stages of sleep.

Consciousness involves, among other things, the experience of a continuous environment in time and space and of a sense of self. The experience of time and its passage may be altered by shifts in the level of awareness and by emotional states, such as boredom, concentration, pain, and discomfort. The experience of time and space may also be altered by hypnosis, marijuana, or psychedelic drugs.

The sense of self, a complex group of processes, is a fundamental aspect of consciousness. Components of the sense of self include the reality and integrity of self, the constancy and durability of self, body image, and various self-evaluations including self-esteem, self-love, ideal self, and self-purpose. Any or all of these qualities may be disturbed in psychiatric disorders, and the regulation of these self systems is of considerable interest to contemporary psychoanalysts.

Disturbances in the level of consciousness can occur in various states of intoxication and disease. *Clouding of consciousness* is marked by diminished awareness of sensory cues and diminished attentiveness to the environment and to the self. Secondary process thinking is most notably compromised, and more primary process thinking emerges into consciousness. The level of consciousness may fluctuate rapidly, in relation to the internal physiological state or to the degree of external stimulation. In alterations of consciousness, confusion may occur with disorientation to time, place, or person. The patient is usually highly distractible and unable to pay attention to a single stimulus. Such distractibility is typical of children with attention-deficit hyperactivity disorder and hyperactive behavior. Psychostimulants, such as methylphenidate (Ritalin), that increase the alertness of these children have the seemingly paradoxical effect of calming them down; it is as if patients with attention-deficit hyperactivity disorder are initially set or tuned at suboptimal levels of consciousness and are then elevated into the normal range by the stimulants.

Drugs with strong central anticholinergic properties, such as scopolamine, and some seizures and other delirious conditions can induce *twilight states,* dream-like states of wakeful consciousness in which attention is poor, there is an admixture of primary and secondary process thinking, and patients fade in and out of alertness. Dream-like experiences intrude into the stream of conversation. In a schizophrenic person, such thinking appears as loose associations and autistic thought.

Stupor is a state of diminished consciousness in which the patient remains mute and still although the eyes remain open and may follow external objects. Stupor is sometimes seen in catatonia. Catatonic states can be produced by a large number of neurological disorders involving the basal ganglia, limbic system, diencephalon, and frontal lobes; by systemic metabolic disorders and toxic and drug reactions; and, finally, by the schizophrenias, periodic catatonia, and, rarely, mood disorders. *Torpor* is a condition in which the patient is drowsy, falls asleep easily, and shows a narrowed range of perception and slow thinking. In the most extreme impairment of consciousness, *coma,* there is no evidence of mental activity at all. The patient appears essentially to be functioning on a decorticate or decerebrate level. In *akinetic mutism,* or *coma vigil,* patients with profound brain stem lesions appear to be awake with their eyes open, but there is no evidence of consciousness.

Mystical states of consciousness may occur in normal and pathological conditions. Intense meditation and peak or epiphanic experiences, reported by more than 10 percent of normal subjects in community surveys, may produce a sense that the self dissolves or expands, that the self fuses mystically with the cosmos, that time stops, and that universal meaning becomes clear. These perceptions may be accompanied by a sense of rejuvenation and renewed personal identity, ineffability, intense emotionality, and concurrent perceptual changes. Such experiences do not ordinarily last more than a few minutes. Many people have sought and some claim to have achieved these states through the use of psychedelic agents such as mescaline and LSD.

Hypnosis Hypnosis offers interesting insights into alterations of consciousness in normal persons. Studies suggest that up to 80 percent of people are hypnotizable and that the achievable depth of hypnosis varies from person to person. Some people are capable of achieving only light trance, whereas others easily slip into deep trance and exhibit remarkable hypnotic phenomena. Hypnotism occurs when the subject is in a state of heightened, not diminished, attention. Electroencephalographic (EEG) studies have shown hypnotized subjects to be fully awake and alert. The heightened concentration probably accounts for unusual levels of sensory and motor performance seen under hypnosis and self-hypnosis.

Hypnotic phenomena include hypnotic anesthesia, sustained motor behaviors and acts of strength ordinarily beyond the individual's capacity, and distortions of memory (both hypermnesia and amnesia). Several phenomena that reveal the multiple nature of consciousness, for example co-consciousness, are also demonstrable. Experiments have shown that even when a subject in deep trance has achieved profound hypnotic anesthesia and can, for example, keep a hand submerged in ice water for longer periods of time than usual, part of the hypnotized subject's consciousness continues to register exactly how painful the experience actually is and can signal the research about the pain by finger movements, without the subject having any conscious awareness or disturbance. This phenomenon, called the hidden observer, has also been seen in postsurgical patients who, under hypnotic trance after surgery, have been able to accurately recall conversations in the operating room that occurred while the subjects were under deep general anesthesia. Dissociative and psychosomatic phenomena have also been induced with hypnosis. Posthypnotic suggestion, for example, can prompt subjects to carry out complex actions without any hint that they are doing so because of previous hypnotic instructions. It has been suggested, not entirely facetiously, that many normal daily activities are conducted in a trance-like posthypnotic state, and although these activities are attributed to conscious intention, they may in fact be carried out in response to a previous suggestion. Urticaria (hives) can be hypnotically induced and made to disappear. When plantar warts have been successfully eradicated with hypnosis, researchers have documented a hypnotically induced reduction of the blood supply to their bases. It has recently been appreciated that yoga masters can exert remarkable control over basic bodily functions through self-hypnosis. As yet, little is known of the full extent to which heightened concentration may influence physiological regulation.

Suggestibility Pathological suggestibility may be seen in several clinical conditions. Automatic obedience has been described in *echolalia* (the automatic repetition of a sentence or phrase just uttered by another person), *echopraxia* (the automatic mimicking of a movement performed by another person), and *waxy flexibility* (maintaining for a prolonged period of time a posture in which one is placed), symptoms common in catatonic forms of schizophrenia. In situations of group delusions and sometimes in cults, passive individuals adopt the delusional beliefs of stronger ones. In epidemic hysteria, which was described so beautifully among young women at the Salem witch trials in Arthur Miller's *The Crucible*, distorted and even delusional perceptions and beliefs may sweep over a group that has been aroused by a charismatic leader.

Conative functions Closely tied to the sense of self are the *conative* functions, those relating to intentionality or will, including such functions as will power and self-directedness. Although strong senses of self, will power, resolve, and self-assurance are ordinarily indicative of psychological health and mature autonomy, single-minded willfulness may be adaptive or maladaptive, depending on a person's goals and circumstances. An act of extraordinary will may lead to remarkable accomplishment or take a self-destructive turn; furthermore, there is often a fine line between extraordinary willpower and obsessively controlled behavior. For example, patients with anorexia nervosa initially have the conscious experience of willing and controlling their intake of food. In the course of the disorder, however, the sense of willfulness is replaced by one of passivity, of being subjugated by obsessional thoughts and compulsive behaviors that assume control of the eating behavior.

Passivity phenomena are common in obsessional and compulsive disorders, in which patients experience intrusive, ego-alien thoughts and engage in irresistible ego-alien behaviors. In the presence of disrupted ego boundaries and the fragmented sense of self that occurs in some psychotic states, extreme examples of passivity phenomena can be observed, including *thought insertion*, the feeling that thoughts are being placed into the mind by an alien force, and *delusions of control* and *delusions of influence*, in which patients experience their own activities as being completely controlled by outside forces.

A woman with anorexia nervosa felt as if she were under the watchful eye of harsh, critical beings. Whenever she transgressed by eating more than she felt they would allow her on a given day, ordinarily 200 or 300 calories, she had the irresistible urge to harm herself by taking handfuls of laxatives. She felt that if she refused to take the laxatives to eliminate excess calories and to punish her transgression with severe abdominal cramps and diarrhea, she would go crazy.

An 18-year-old man with a 4-year history of obsessive-compulsive disorder described that whenever he walked past an electrical outlet he felt his hand irresistibly drawn to touch the openings. He constantly fought this tendency, which he found exhausting, and he avoided places where outlets were prominent.

A 43-year-old schizophrenic man described a delusion in which all of his thoughts and movements were under the control of a homunculus who resided in his abdomen. The central homunculus consisted of two beings, one encapsulated within the other; the man was the zombie-like third shell of this nested set of creatures. He felt that he was simply the receptacle of thoughts coming from the core homunculus and that all of his behavior was controlled as is that of a robot.

DISSOCIATIVE PHENOMENA *Dissociation* refers to the splitting off from one another of ordinarily closely connected behaviors, thoughts, or feelings. Thoughts can be dissociated from feelings or from behaviors. *Dissociative states* are those in which complex behaviors take place outside the awareness of one's predominant consciousness and include trances, fugues, blackouts, multiple personalities, and dissociative frenzies. Although dissociative states are ordinarily thought to be functional in nature, they may be more common among patients with subtle brain function disturbances, particularly those with partial complex seizures. In one series, one-third of patients with complex partial seizures had dissociative phenomena including multiple personality. In these patients the dissociative phenomena were not related to the seizure activity but to interictal alterations.

As occurs in posthypnotic amnesia, elaborate activity can occur in dissociative states and the subject will have no memory for what transpired during the trance state. This amnesia is functional in nature and can be reversed by hypnosis or drug-facilitated disinhibition (for example, sodium amytal infusion). *Blackouts* are periods of amnesia in alcoholism or other intoxications or following head trauma. An alcoholic blackout period may last for hours to days, after which the person has no recollection of what transpired, although observers attest to the fact that, during this period, multiple complicated behaviors were carried out. Although memory of the blackout is lost to the predominant consciousness, reintoxication may reawaken memories of what actually happened during the previous blackout, indicating that memories registered during these blackouts may be state dependent. *Fugue states* are prolonged dissociative periods, which in some cases go on for years. Dissociative amnesia may follow catastrophic events, such as traumatic, gruesome combat, or less momentous events that a given person prefers to forget—in order to preserve self-esteem by denying some shameful, immoral, or illegal act.

A 22-year-old soldier returning from Vietnam claimed to have no memory for his last month in combat. He had been assigned to a squad conducting a long-range patrol; only three of eight men returned alive. Through repeated amytal interviews conducted in a supportive setting, gradually, and with great emotion, he recalled that his squad had been ambushed; that early in the fire fight he had killed two or three 12- or 13-year-old Vietnamese boys who were in the attacking group; and that at a certain point he turned and ran away, leaving behind one or two of his wounded buddies, pleading for help.

Automatic behaviors *Automatic behaviors* are complicated activities, such as writing or speaking, out of supposed trance states without awareness of what one is doing. Case records have described many long, creative works presumably produced by persons in states of automatic behavior. For example, the *Course in Miracles,* a complicated, esoteric, widely read quasi-psychological Christian spiritual tract, is said to have been written by a Jewish psychology professor from New York City who perceived that she was ordered in a trance state one day to take down the book in dictation. The series of Seth books by Jane Roberts are also said to have been written down while the author was in trance states. On occasion, automatic behaviors have resulted in intellectual or artistic achievments of a quality far above the previously demonstrated capacities of the individual. In one famous case, an undistinguished piano teacher in the Midwest started falling into trances and wrote out entire symphonies in the manner of major eighteenth- and nineteenth-century composers, works of artistic invention that were far beyond her usual talents and what anyone imagined she could produce. Edgar Cayce, a well-known figure purported by some to have been a prophet and healer, had all of his visionary diagnostic and prophetic insights during trances from which he would awaken without recollection. While suspicion of fraud surrounds some of these reports, enough cases have been sufficiently well documented to substantiate the existence of automatic phenomena.

Multiple personality *Multiple personality* is a dramatic and extreme instance of a dissociative state that usually occurs in persons who as young children were severely and repeatedly brutalized by cruel parents. A number of different and somewhat independent personalities are elaborated within the victim. The development of such dissociated alternative personalities is thought to be a last-ditch psychological defense against an inescapable and unbearable traumatic situation. Famous cases, such as *The Three Faces of Eve* and *Sybil*, demonstrate that relatively few or large numbers of distinct personalities may reside within a single person. The personalities may be of different ages and even of different sexes. Some are aware of the others; some are not. Typically, the presenting personality is a drab character who may suffer headaches and periods of blackout or amnesia and who is unaware of the other personalities. A second personality is usually vivacious and uninhibited. Most multiple personality patients also have a component personality that has a transcendent view of all the others and that serves in successful treatment as the facilitator for the reintegration of all parts of the personality. This transcendent aspect of personality, reminiscent of the hidden observer described in hypnotic states, provides further support for the notion that ordinary human consciousness may be composed of different strands of consciousness that are woven together and usually regulated by an overriding integrative mechanism. In a sense, everyone experiences different states of mind, in which they may seem to themselves and others to be virtually different persons, the proverbial Dr. Jekyll and Mr. Hyde. A person awakened suddenly from sleep or when hungry may have a predictably irritable, snappy, critical, and humorless personality; but, with rest and food, consciousness may rapidly shift to that of a content and jovial personality. The latter personality may have relatively little awareness of the former, perhaps because that unpleasant state of mind is being repressed.

Depersonalization and derealization *Depersonalization* refers to the experience of being estranged from oneself, one's body, and the environment. The person observes occurrences involving the self from the perspective of a detached outsider. In *derealization,* although the sense of self is preserved, one has the feeling that everything going on is unreal. Momentary experiences of depersonalization and derealization occur frequently in normal persons, particularly under conditions of fatigue or acute situational distress, such as bereavement, or upon receiving a terminal diagnosis or surviving a serious accident.

Some people saved from imminent death by wild animals or firing squads have subsequently reported feelings of derealization or depersonalization that occurred in the moments just prior to the anticipated death accompanied by feelings of calm. Such reactions may serve as last-ditch defense mechanisms or they may parallel those of animals under attack by predators, which, once a fatal outcome is inevitable, have been observed to calm down, stop struggling, freeze, and apparently allow themselves to be killed.

Somnambulism *Somnambulism,* sleepwalking, is one of several disorders of nocturnal arousal occurring during stage 4, slow-wave sleep, representing automatic behaviors with incomplete wakefulness. Patients who walk or talk in their sleep (*somniloquy*) or suffer from night terrors (*pavor nocturnus*) execute automatic behavior in a confused state. Contrary to popular belief, these phenomena are not related to dreams in REM sleep.

An obese 35-year-old woman, who was attempting to diet, in the middle of the night experienced sleepwalking episodes, observed by her roommate, during which she went to the refrigerator and ate whatever was available, including raw flour and uncooked grains. She was sound asleep during these episodes. Her mother reported a history of sleepwalking since early childhood.

Disturbances in sense of self Disturbances in one's relationship to the self may take several forms. Inconsistencies in the sense of identity may be severe, like those in schizophrenia or multiple personality, or less severe, like those in many personality disorders. One's relation to other persons and even to oneself may be disruptively erratic, as in borderline personality disorders. The *as-if personality* type typically adapts characteristics of persons who are particularly important to the individual or characteristics the individual believes would at the moment please those persons. In adopting these characteristics, the as-if personality does not appear to be acting, but experiences and manifests the assumed traits in a genuine and enduring manner, at least for a while. A change in relationships and situations usually prompts the as-if personality summarily to discard previously held traits and to assume new ones that better fit the new circumstances. Woody Allen's character Zelig is a caricature of this phenomenon.

Patients with pseudologia fantastica and the impostor syndrome demonstrate extreme examples of inconsistency in the sense of self. In *pseudologia fantastica* the patient compulsively spins out webs of lies, ordinarily self-aggrandizing ones. In the *impostor syndrome,* such fantasies are acted out by liars and impostors who seem to wish fervently that the fantasies they portray are their reality, as if they cannot accept themselves and would be overwhelmingly ashamed to be known for who they actually are. The impostor compulsively adopts the identities of others and may, for example, show up properly attired at diplomatic functions and society galas and interact with the other guests under the assumed identity. Some famous impostors have in this way insinuated themselves repeatedly into inner circles of society and government.

A 22-year-old soldier was found in a military stockade after he tried to hang himself. He claimed that as a Green Beret he had been captured and held prisoner by the Viet Cong, had managed to escape, and had since been severely depressed and suicidal. He provided an elaborate and detailed account of his military experiences, naming dates, places, units, and personnel. Members of the staff who had been to Vietnam became suspicious because of irregularities in his story and confronted the soldier, who stuck steadfastly to his story. Even with repeated amytal interviews, conducted to the point of his falling asleep, he maintained his account with great consistency. When his family was contacted they revealed that not only had the soldier never been to Vietnam but that his history of acting as an impostor went back to early high school, when he repeatedly wore varsity sweaters and tee shirts in efforts to impress his peers, even though he was not on the varsity teams. During basic training at another army post, he acquired Green Beret uniforms with appropriate medals and stripes and often paraded around in that manner, in spite of the fact that he had been arrested on several occasions by the military police for posing as a Green Beret. When confronted by the staff with this obvious fabrication, he blandly acknowledged, "Well, I guess you're right." He had little remorse and could provide little further explanation as to why he felt the compulsion to behave in this strange way. His mental status was otherwise unremarkable. Psychological testing, including a full battery of projective tests and the Minnesota Multiphasic Personality Inventory (MMPI), revealed no evidence on these measures of psychotic thinking.

Other disorders *Munchausen's syndrome* is a syndrome of factitious illness. Patients repeatedly and compulsively present themselves for medical care with feigned or self-induced illness. The self-induced conditions may be so serious as ultimately to cause death: Some patients inject themselves with feces to produce systemic infections that will warrant hospitalization and intensive care. When the self-induced nature of the illnesses is found out, medical staffs often become enraged at these patients. The patients rarely accept or cooperate in psychiatric care, so few have been adequately studied. Most do not appear to be psychotic, but there seems to be a disturbance of personality structure.

Self-esteem is thought to reflect how one measures up to the desired self-image. To the extent that what one sees in oneself approximates what one would like to be, self-esteem is positive. Negative self-esteem is characteristic of chronic dysphorias, primary and secondary depressions, and situational failures. Superficially inflated self-esteem may be seen with narcissistic traits and personality disorders. *Ego ideals* represent fantasies of the optimal person one could ever wish to be. Although some simply regard the ego ideal as unattainable and are content to live as imperfect human beings, others strive to approximate the ideal, often in a driven manner, sometimes successfully but sometimes clearly and unhappily pursuing the impossible. *Body image* is an individual's mental representation of his or her own body; it may be realistic or quite distorted. Some formerly obese persons who lose a great deal of weight continue to think of themselves as fat for months or years. Emaciated patients with anorexia nervosa may perceive themselves to be fat. Since a great deal of self-esteem is tied up in body image, many people spend considerable effort attempting to perfect their bodies and adorning them. *Phantom limb* phenomena are hallucinations of lost body parts. It has been suggested that these phenomena result from the brain's persistent sensory expectations for stimulatory input from the missing parts, something like neural supersensitivity states that follow drug withdrawal and denervation.

Delirium, the acute confusional state, is usually characterized by relatively abrupt onset and short duration of clouded, reduced, and fragmented attention; impaired memory and learning; perceptual and cognitive abnormalities, such as hallucinations and delusions; disrupted sleep; and other autonomic dysfunctions. The EEG usually shows diffuse slowing. Typical motor abnormalities include an increase in general restlessness, fine and course tremors, and myoclonic jerks. Autonomic disturbances commonly include tachycardia, fever, elevated blood pressure, diaphoresis, and pupillary dilation.

DISORDERS OF ORIENTATION

Orientation refers to the person's awareness of time, place, and person. Accurate orientation requires the integrity of attention, perception, memory, and ideation. Impairments occur primarily in the organic mental disorders (i.e., structural and toxic metabolic brain abnormalities).

Normal individuals vary tremendously in their attention to the details of time and in the extent to which their bodies automatically keep time. Some people have extremely reliable built-in clocks, by which they can awaken themselves at precise times or accurately gauge the passage of time with uncanny accuracy, even in the absence of external cues, in a psychotherapy session, for example. Others have great difficulty making judgments about time and may develop pathological lateness or habitually schedule more activities than could ever be accomplished in the time available. Benign disorientation to time is common. After a few days in a hospital bed, most people do not know exactly what the day or date is, because they are not attending to or receiving the usual cues.

Pathological time disorientation can be mild or severe, with inaccuracies of estimation ranging from days to years. The dates reported by disoriented individuals may have personal significance, such as those of births, marriages, or deaths.

Because spatial cues are generally more available and obvious than temporal cues, disorientation to place often signifies a greater degree of cognitive impairment than disorientation to time. Disoriented persons may know, more or less, the type of place they are in without knowing the specific place—patients may recognize that they are in *a* hospital without being able to name *the* hospital.

A 42-year-old alcoholic man in delirium tremens, examined in a California hospital in the 1980s, was asked the date and where he was. He replied, "I'm standing on a street corner in Kansas City in 1966 minding my own business. Why don't you mind yours!"

Disorientation to person, a lack of awareness of one's own identity, usually is seen only in advanced dementias, such as primary degenerative dementia of the Alzheimer type, in some severe psychotic conditions, or in dissociative states. In organically induced postconcussion amnesia, global transient amnesia, and, presumably, functional fugue states, knowledge of one's own identity may disappear, and a person may remain unidentified for an indefinite period, until the memory for self returns.

DISTURBANCES OF MEMORY

Memories for different senses and perceptions vary. One person may have prodigious musical memory but less powerful verbal, conceptual, mathematical, visual, or kinesthetic memory. Careers have been established on the basis of unusual capacities to remember in one or another of these dimensions. In early life, many children are capable of powerful eidetic imagery and are able to remember certain things virtually in photographic detail. The so-called photographic memory of some adults is a highly adaptive aptitude.

The physicist Nicolas Tesla was reportedly able to visualize complete schematic diagrams and engineering plans, obviating the need to draw blueprints. He could see things in three dimensions, spin them around and view them from any angle, and essentially work out in his mind complicated design problems of the sort that are now possible only with computers.

Exceptionally detailed verbal memories have been associated with obsessional cognitive styles. When individuals with extraordinary memories complain of memory loss, ordinary memory tests may be inadequate to detect their deficits, as their relative memory loss may have reduced their capacities to a point within the range of most normal people.

A 62-year-old scientific executive with an extraordinary verbal memory enjoyed intimidating his therapist by reminding her, virtually verbatim, of dialogues of psychotherapy sessions 2 to 4 years in the past. He would recount these events in great detail, always announcing the exact time and date of the session. "As you recall, Doctor, on Monday, October 20, 1974, at 4:00 P.M., we discussed my marriage. At that point I mentioned that my wife was unhappy with my behavior, and you asked if I had any thoughts about it. Well I've been thinking about that since." Session notes verified the accuracy of his recall. This capacity remained intact even following a course of electroconvulsive therapy (ECT) for severe depression, after which the patient complained that his memory was much poorer than it had been.

Memory function has been divided into three stages, registration, retention, and recall. *Registration* refers to the capacity to add new material to memory. This material may be sensory, perceptual, or conceptual and may come from the environment or from within the person. Newly registered material is transferred incrementally from immediate to short-term memory to long-term memory. *Immediate* memory lasts for a few minutes; *short-term* or *recent* memory, for several minutes to up to a few days (the time involved in new learning and its early consolidation); *recent past* memory, for several months; and *long-term* or *remote* memory, for longer periods of time. Different physiological processes mediate each of these stages of memory. Processes that affect immediate or short-term memory often spare long-term memory. Disturbances in memory occur through interruption of registration, retention, or recall.

DISTURBANCES IN REGISTRATION Registration and short-term memory retention are usually impaired in disorders that affect vigilance and attention, such as head trauma, delirium, intoxication, psychosis, spontaneous or induced seizures, anxiety, depression, and fatigue. A variety of other metabolic and structural brain disturbances can affect memory as well, particularly lesions affecting the mammillary bodies, hippocampus, fornix, and closely associated areas. Patients with impaired attention and concentration who are able to demonstrate immediate recall may not be able to retain or retrieve items from short-term memory.

DISTURBANCES IN RETENTION *Retention* refers to the ability to hold memories in storage. The processes by which memories are transferred from short-term to long-term stores are unknown. It is thought that large numbers of neurons are involved in any specific memory and that reverberating circuits are formed in which memory traces are held by means of changes in proteins, synaptic connectivity, or both. The retention of memories is impaired in a number of organic brain diseases, such as dementias of the Alzheimer type and the Wernicke-Korsakoff syndrome. The latter, which ordinarily results from chronic thiamine deficiency seen with alcoholism, is associated with pathological alterations in the mammillary bodies and thalamus.

DISTURBANCES IN RECALL Disturbances in recall can occur even when memories have been registered and are in storage. At times, failure to recall may signify that the memory traces themselves have disappeared and are no longer retrievable. However, difficulties in recall can occur separately as in the everyday event of forgetting the name of a person or object, only to remember it spontaneously hours or days later. In normal forgetting, more remote events are less well remembered than recent ones, and important events are most vividly retained in memory. Under usual conditions, forgotten events can be recalled with prompting, associative memories, or other forms of stimulation, such as hypnosis.

Amnesias are either organic or functional disturbances in recall. Organic amnesias may be anterograde or retrograde. *Anterograde amnesia* is memory loss for events that occur after consciousness is regained and for some time thereafter; it follows head trauma or states of cerebral physiological imbalance. Patients who receive ECT frequently have anterograde amnesia lasting for an hour or more following treatments. *Retrograde amnesia* refers to the loss of memories that were registered prior to the traumatic event. This amnesia extends backward in time for variable periods. As memory is regained, the more remote memories usually return first: A patient originally amnesic for a 3-month period prior to an accident may ultimately be left with only a day or an hour of amnesia for events just prior to the accident. In organically caused retrograde amnesias, remote memories are usually intact while amnesia may exist for more recent events. This contrasts with functional amnesia, in which the time periods of forgotten events may be more spotty or selective.

Hypermnesia, unusually detailed and vivid memory, may occur in gifted persons, in association with obsessive-compulsive or paranoid personality traits, and in hypnotic trance. Although many forgotten memories can be recalled in hypnotic trance, research has shown that retrospective falsification and distortion may also occur under hypnosis. (Memories recalled under hypnosis usually are not accepted as evidence in court.) Retrospective falsification of memory is called *paramnesia* or *fausse reconnaissance*.

Confabulation is another common form of paramnesia in which the patient fills gaps in memory with fantasy. These fantasies may be experienced by the patient and communicated to observers as being so real that it may be necessary to consult outside informants to assess their validity. Confabulation is most prominent in certain alcohol amnesic syndromes, such as Wernicke-Korsakoff syndrome.

A 40-year-old chronically alcoholic man whose memory on mental status exam was found to be markedly impaired frantically demanded to be released from the hospital, saying that his wife had just been in an auto accident and he had to rush to another hospital to see her. He stated this with sincere conviction and appropriate fearful concern, and it was clear that for the patient, at least, the story was very real. In fact, his wife had been dead for 15 years. The patient told the same story over and over, always with evident conviction, in spite of the fact that the staff confronted him with the reality that his wife had been dead for years. The patient was never influenced by their assertions, as he could not register new memories. But, although his past memory was patchy at best, the story of his wife's emergency could be recalled repeatedly.

Déjà vu is the sense that one has seen or experienced before what is transpiring for the first time; it is a false impression that the current stream of consciousness has previously been recorded in memory. Related phenomena are *déjà entendu,* a sense that one has previously heard what is actually being heard for the first time, and *déjà pensé* a feeling that one has at an earlier time known or understood what is being thought for the first time. Experiences of *jamais vu, jamais entendu,* and *jamais pensé* involve feelings that one has never before seen, heard, or thought (respectively) things that, in fact, one has. These phenomena are all common in everyday life but may be more frequent in states of fatigue or intoxication and in other psychopathological states.

The *rule of Pitres* applies to people who have spoken several languages prior to incurring a brain injury from which aphasia results. Ordinarily, but not always, the first language to return is the mother tongue, the language learned as a very young child.

Patients with depressive disorders may complain of poor memory. In the face of such subjective complaints, actual deficits are sometimes difficult to document, but the complaints may reflect changes in memory that are still within the normal range. That is, patients who previously enjoyed remarkable memories, particularly those with obsessional traits, experience diminished but still quite serviceable memory when depressed. Similarly, a small percentage of patients who have had ECT for depression complain of prolonged retrograde and anterograde memory problems, some of which can be documented with objective tests. However, recent evidence suggests that, for some patients with depressive disorders, faulty memory may be an ongoing element regardless of treatment and that some of the memory difficulties attributed to ECT may be components of the depressive syndrome itself.

DISTURBANCES IN PERCEPTION

Normal perception requires that the individual organize sensations coming from the outside world into coherent, comprehensible events. The sense organs all contribute to organized perceptions, and although in states of sensory deficit such as blindness, deafness, and anesthesia, perception is impaired, perception is still possible because humans generally perceive information about an object through several sensory modalities. The intensity of sensation and perception is affected by vigilance and attention. Highly focused attention, such as intense concentration or hypnosis, may result in unusually acute sensation and perception—hypesthesia, hyperacusis, or extraordinary visual acuity. Focused attention may also result in failure to sense or perceive: Deep anesthesia and negative hallucinations induced by hypnosis are simply induced failures to perceive what exists in the world.

Humans usually operate in what has been called an "average expectable environment," an environment in which a certain type and level of sensory input is expected and for which the nervous system is primed. Excessive or inadequate stimulation in any sensory modality, or levels at input that are extraordinary, can provoke distorted perceptions in most normal people. For example, total sensory deprivation produced in carefully controlled artificial environments may elicit visual and auditory illusions and hallucinations.

Individuals vary in the levels of arousal and sensory input they require for comfort. Some seek a great deal of intense and novel stimulation and even thrive on risk taking; others are inclined to reduce stimulation and avoid novel experiences. Such variation may reflect basic differences in temperament and changes that occur with age.

ILLUSIONS Perceptual distortions in the estimation of size, shape, and spatial relations are common even in the absence of psychiatric disorders, especially when the subject is fatigued or excessively aroused. *Illusions* are misinterpretations of sensory cues, as when a child in a dark bedroom at night sees monsters emanating from shadows on the walls or hears ghosts in the sounds of the wind. *Pareidolia* are voluntary playful and whimsical illusions that can be seen when one looks at ambiguously defined or evanescent images, such as clouds, flames in a fireplace, or patterns of sand or water. Both the onset and termination of these perceptions are entirely voluntary. *Trailing* is another visual illusion, the perception that an object moving steadily in space is followed by temporally distinct after-images of itself. The effect is that of a series of stroboscopic photos. This phenomenon may occur with fatigue and is typically seen with marijuana or mescaline intoxication.

HALLUCINATIONS A further degree of perceptual disturbance, *hallucinations* are perceptions experienced in the absence of corresponding sensory stimulus. They are experienced as immediate, vivid, and independent of will, and are often, at least momentarily, felt to be real. Hallucinations can affect any sensory system and sometimes occur in several concurrently. In conditions where perception is altered, combinations of illusions and hallucinations, and often delusions as well, are frequently experienced together. In some studies, 90 percent of patients with hallucinations have also been shown to have delusions, and, alternatively, about 35 percent of patients with delusions also have hallucinations. About 20 percent of patients have mixed sensory hallucinations (mostly auditory and visual), which may accompany functional as well as organic conditions. A given external stimulus or set of stimuli may evoke very different perceptual distortions in different persons.

Three scientists floated in sensory deprivation tanks for long periods of time. One experienced a few illusions and no hallucinations; the second had many illusions and a few faint auditory and visual hallucinations; and the third had vivid, dramatic, and complex visual and auditory hallucinations.

Some young teenage boys routinely sniffed airplane glue as a group. One saw spots in front of his eyes that ceased with blinking or with pressure on his eyeballs. A second hallucinated a large globe that remained in front of his eyes for several hours. A third hallucinated a huge evil eye, which he came to view as the eye of an angry god he identified as the glue god. He described this in vivid detail to the other gang members, who, after further glue sniffing, began to see the same hallucination and confirmed this vision. As a group, these teenagers began to worship and follow the "glue god," which was subsequently conjured up on repeated occasions through glue-mediated hallucinations.

Hallucinations are experienced by many normal people under unusual conditions. *Hypnagogic* and *hypnopompic* hallucinations are common, predominantly visual hallucinations that occur during moments of falling into and emerging from sleep, respectively. In acute bereavement, up to 50 percent of grieving spouses have reported hallucinating the voice or presence of the deceased, and following amputations, phantom limb hallucinations are common. These observations suggest a "supersensitivity deprivation" hypothesis that might explain such hallucinations and associated ones: When deprived of important and anticipated perceptual stimuli, the mental apparatus may overinterpret any sensory stimulation as evidence of the presence of the needed objects.

A perceptual release theory suggests that hallucinations emerge from the combined presence of intense states of internal arousal and diminished sensory input (including poor attention and poor capacity to sort out relevant from irrelevant input). Thus, diminished input from the environment (as in sensory deprivation) or reduced capacity to attend to and take in the input (as in delirious states) heighten the likelihood that internal sensations, images, and thoughts will be interpreted as originating in the environment.

Hallucinations vary according to sensory modality, degree of complexity of the hallucinated experience, perceived location of the hallucination (e.g., inside or outside the body), the degree to which the person believes that the hallucination is actually real, and the degree to which the hallucination influences the person's behavior.

Visual hallucinations range from simple and elemental—flashes of light or geometric figures—to elaborate visions, such as a host of angels.

A terrified 37-year-old man in acute delirium tremens glanced agitatedly about the room. He pointed out the window and said, "My God, the Spanish Armada is on the lawn! They're about to attack!" He experienced these hallucinations as real, and they persisted intermittently for 3 days before abating. Subsequently, the patient had no memory of this experience.

Stimulation of one sensory modality sometimes evokes perceptual distortions in another. Marijuana and mescaline intoxication, for example, have been associated with *synesthesia,* an experience in which sensory modalities seem fused. This is also a normal experience for many people. Music may be experienced visually, the sound fusing with visual illusions; a tactile sensation may be experienced as a color (i.e., a hot surface may feel red).

In certain religious subcultures visual hallucinations may be experienced as normal. In one fundamentalist Pentecostal church, worshipers danced themselves into a frenzy, and without using any drugs several participants shared visions of the Virgin Mary at the altar.

Autoscopic hallucinations are hallucinations of the self being located elsewhere in the room, usually somewhere in front of the actual self. Such hallucinations may stimulate the belief that one has a double (*dopplegänger*). Reports of near-death, out-of-body experiences, in which persons see themselves rising to the ceiling and looking down at themselves in a hospital bed may be autoscopic hallucinations. *Extracampine* hallucinations are visual hallucinations experienced as located outside the field of vision, ordinarily behind the head. In *Lilliputian* hallucinations, the individual sees figures in very reduced size. They may be related to the perceptual distortions of *macropsia* and *micropsia,* respectively the perception of objects as much bigger or smaller than they actually are.

Several types of auditory hallucinations have been described. *Second-person hallucinations* involve the speaker and the subject. In severe mood disorders, two-person auditory hallucinations are common and are usually derogatory.

A 63-year-old woman with melancholia, pacing back and forth, held her hands over her ears. She was plagued by a voice that kept screaming at her, "You're a whore! You're no good! You should drop dead!" The voice disappeared after a course of ECT.

The person with *complete auditory hallucinations,* or *third-person hallucinations,* hears conversations between two or more parties about the person who is hallucinating, almost in the fashion of a Greek chorus discussing the individual. These are a feature of some schizophrenic persons.

A 17-year-old schizophrenic woman described hearing between three and seven voices talking about her all the time. The major voices belonged to Moses, Jesus, and Buddha discussing whether she was a good person. The other voices were those of minor prophets and the devil, who argued about her virtues and faults.

Command hallucinations are those in which the patient is ordered by voices to do things. They are often frightening as they involve acts of violence toward self or others, such as, "Jump off the roof," or "Pick up the knife and kill your mother." These voices vary in insistence and persistence, and patients differ in their capacities to ignore the commands. Patients with marked passivity may be helpless in the face of command hallucinations and may feel impelled to carry out the orders. The presence of command hallucinations is ordinarily a very troubling clinical sign; this symptom and the patient's ability to resist must be assessed very carefully. Occasionally, command hallucinations are harmless or even beneficial.

A young schizophrenic girl constantly hallucinated the voice of Joan of Arc. The voice encouraged her to go to school, to ignore taunts and insults of family members, and to try to deal constructively with her irritable mother.

Audible thoughts refer to hallucinated voices that speak aloud what the patient is thinking (from the German *gedankenlautwerden,* "to think loud words"). These voices may anticipate the patient's thoughts by a few moments, speak them concurrently, or repeat them after the patient has already spoken them.

Haptic hallucinations are hallucinations involving touch. Simple haptic hallucinations, such as the feeling that bugs are crawling over one's skin (*formication*) are common in alcohol withdrawal syndromes and in cocaine intoxication. When unkempt and physically self-neglectful patients complain of these sensations, it is important to rule out the presence of real stimuli, such as lice. Some tactile hallucinations, having intercourse with God, for example, are highly suggestive of schizophrenia, but may also occur in tertiary syphilis and other conditions, or may be stimulated by local genital irritation. *Olfactory* and *gustatory* hallucinations, involving smell and taste, respectively, have most often been associated with organic brain disease, particularly with the uncinate fits of complex partial seizures.

The term "pseudohallucination" has been used in several ways. Jaspers defined *pseudohallucination* as a perception experienced as coming from within the mind (i.e., not at the boundary or outside the mind). Thus, according to Jasper, loud voices, which are alien and ascribed to other beings but which the patient knows are actually within the mind rather than out in space, are pseudohallucinations. Hare used the term "pseudohallucination" to describe hallucinatory experiences whose validity the patient doubts, phenomena analogous to partial delusions. For consistency it is probably best to use the term "pseudohallucination" in Jaspers' sense, referring to experiences perceived as arising within the mind, and to reserve the term *partial hallucination* for those hallucinatory experiences about whose validity the patient has some doubt. *Functional hallucinations* are rare hallucinations that occur only in connection with a specific external perception, for example, in the presence of a sound such as running water, or of a color or in a particular place. However, unlike illusions, the hallucinated sights and sounds are not elaborations of the perceptions, but are simply triggered only in that specific context.

A patient with schizophrenia described returning repeatedly to a running brook near his parents' country home. When in the presence of the brook, he heard the voice of God calling out to him. He determined that this was his "holy place." He denied hearing hallucinations in any other setting.

Ictal hallucinations, occurring in the presence of seizure activity, ordinarily last only seconds to minutes. They are usually relatively elemental experiences, but they may contain elaborate images including fully remembered visions. The patient ordinarily experiences some dimming of consciousness or a twilight sleep while the hallucinations are being experienced.

Migrainous hallucinations are reported by about 50 percent of patients who suffer migraine headaches. Most are simple visual hallucinations of geometric patterns, but fully formed visual hallucinations, sometimes with micropsia and macropsia, may also occur. This complex has been called the Alice in Wonderland syndrome after Lewis Carroll's descriptions of the world in *Through the Looking Glass,* which mirrored some of his own migrainous experiences. In turn, these phenomena closely resemble visual hallucinations induced by psychedelic drugs, such as mescaline.

A *flashback* is the vivid re-experience of highly charged past events, usually replays of hallucinations that were induced initially by psychedelic drugs. Of several types, similar to those of migrainous hallucinations, they may be simple or complex geometric patterns, or they may consist of previously experienced elaborate drug-induced hallucinations. Flashback phenomena may be state dependent. For example, visual hallucinations initially experienced with mescaline or LSD are more likely to be subsequently experienced as flashbacks when the subject is smoking marijuana. In post-traumatic stress disorder, some complex, intrusive flashback-like images may attain hallucinatory vividness. Images often include horrifying memories of traumatic events, which may force themselves repeatedly into consciousness until they are acknowledged and worked through.

Hallucinosis is a state of active hallucination occurring in a patient who is alert and well oriented. This condition is seen most often in alcoholic withdrawal, but it may also occur in acute intoxication and other drug-mediated states.

A 30-year-old woman being treated for depression with a monoamine oxidase inhibitor snorted cocaine at a party. For the next 3 days, she described having vivid hallucinatory experiences while being all the while in an alert state. She managed to drive her car throughout this time, though with some difficulty. In her psychiatrist's office she alternated between relating coherently to the psychiatrist and responding to her complex, dream-like visual and auditory hallucinations.

The specificity of hallucinations While some clues about diagnosis may be obtained from the type and pattern of hallucinations present, the relationship of hallucinations to specific psychopathological conditions overlaps sufficiently so that exact diagnoses cannot be made solely on the basis of the type or pattern of hallucinations alone. Hallucinations in schizophrenia can occur in every sensory system, including smell and taste. Olfactory hallucinations usually raise suspicions about the presence of brain disease, but they are also reported in depressive psychosis, when the smell of rotting flesh may be experienced. Complete auditory hallucinations, once suggested as being peculiar to schizophrenia, have also been reported in mania and in several neurological disorders, including complex partial seizure conditions.

BODY IMAGE DISTORTION Body image, a function of self-awareness and consciousness, has perceptual and ideational components. Distortions of the body image may reflect primarily perceptual distortions or combinations of disturbed perception and appraisal. Body image disturbances can occur as normal responses to abrupt changes in the body (e.g., following amputation), in brain disease, and in functional psychiatric disorders. Phantom limb phenomena are classic body image problems in which an amputated limb is felt to be still present; the limb may even itch or be painful. This sensation may diminish gradually over time: the phantom feels as if it is receding into the stump. Many normal American women (as well as eating disorder patients) perceive themselves to be much fatter than they actually are.

Agnosias, lack of awareness of body parts, may accompany brain damage, most often of the nondominant parietal lobe. Patients with obvious deficits may deny that any deficit exists at all (*anosognosia*), or the denial may be limited to half of the body (*hemiagnosia*), usually the left side. The hemidepersonalization syndrome is a much less common disorder (*hemisomatognosia*) in which patients feel that one limb is missing, again usually on the left side. In duplication phenomena, patients feel as if part or all of them has doubled (e.g., that they have two heads or two bodies). These phenomena are rarely seen in schizophrenia, complex partial seizures, and migraine.

Dysmorphophobia refers to conditions in which patients distort and are very unhappy with the shape of a particular body part. There are fine lines between perceptual distortions and realistic but unhappy appraisals of the body, and given the high social values placed on physical appearance, in some social circles, cosmetic rhinoplasties, face lifts and other cosmetic surgeries are extremely common. Patients with borderline personality disorders may develop dysmorphophobias in relation to hair, breasts, the shape of the nose, or the shape of the entire body, as in some anorexia nervosa patients.

A 27-year-old woman with a history of borderline personality disorder, anorexia nervosa, and bulimia nervosa often became acutely suicidal following visits to her hairdresser. Whenever the hairdresser cut off a fraction of an inch more hair than she believed was proper, the patient suddenly felt that her hair was so short that she became very ugly, and she believed that everyone else could see it as well. She felt ashamed to be seen in public and would hide out in her bedroom for days or weeks until she felt presentable again.

Hypochondriacal complaints also combine perceptual and ideational distortions. Selective hypervigilance to bodily sensations may result in a higher likelihood of perceptions of unpleasant and potentially pathological body experiences among the so-called worried well, hypochondriacal populations, and patients with somatization disorder (Briquet's syndrome).

DISTURBANCES OF MOOD

Definitions of the terms mood, affect, and emotion vary from author to author. The most common convention, recommended here, defines *mood* as a sustained feeling tone or range of tones, pleasurable or unpleasurable, experienced by a person for periods of time lasting for hours to years. *Affect* is the moment-to-moment feeling state, sometimes rapidly shifting, that can be observed by the clinician. Mood has been compared to the range of a musical instrument and affect to the specific notes played within a song. *Emotions* have been defined as moods and affects that are connected to specific ideas. In common parlance, and often professionally as well, these words are sometimes used interchangeably. The term "mood disorders" in DSM-III-R has replaced "affective disorders" to describe the same group of psychiatric syndromes.

Moods, affects, and emotions can be described by a number of important qualities: intensity (shallow to deep); range (broad to narrow); stability (rigid to labile); reactivity to external events (none to much); periodicity (periodic to aperiodic); congruence with thought content (congruent to incongruent); speed of resolution (rapid to slow); and viscosity (evanescent to persistent). The lifelong predominant mood is one component of temperament. Thus, a person may be described as having a calm, buoyant, irritable, depressive, anxious, or hypersensitive temperament.

Moods, affects, and emotions serve as internal and external signal systems. With respect to the external world, they signal the state of the individual and often elicit necessary help and support from the environment. A baby's face communicates its state of need, tension, or contentment, thereby recruiting appropriate maternal interventions. Internally, moods, affects, and emotions let individuals know how well or how poorly they are doing, indicating how far and in what direction they are on the continuum from how they currently see themselves to how they would like to see themselves (i.e., the discrepancy between self-appraisal and self-expectations). For example, if individuals desire to master an important goal and feel that they have a reasonably good chance of doing so, their emotional state in relation to this goal will be pleasant. If something seriously threatens the likelihood that they will achieve the goal, they may become fearful and anxious. If something intervenes to assure that they will never achieve the goal, so that there is an insurmountable gap between their desires and the likelihood of success, they may feel hopeless. If they see themselves doing better than expected with regard to achieving the goal, they may feel elated. In addition to serving as signal systems, emotional states of nonspecific tension, arousal, or anger usually imply that some activity will be necessary to secure their discharge or release.

In addition to having intrapsychic determinants, emotional states and their expression are regulated by biological and cultural influences. Biologically, in addition to constitutional contributions to emotional temperament, emotions are affected by periodic shifts and by drive-related processes. For example, emotional lability occurs premenstrually in some women, with varying periodicity in cyclothymic individuals, and in relation to need states such as hunger, sleepiness, and sexual frustration. Physiological disinhibition in the expression of emotions may result from intoxications or from brain injury, as in frontal lobe disturbances which result in emotional lability or emotional incontinence. Mood shifts have also been related to environment-related physiological influences, such as seasonal changes in light and the prevalence of negative ions in the air.

Cultural regulation is significant in the expression of emotion. Although facial expressions for basic emotions are similar in all cultures studied, the range and style of emotional expression in relation to specific events varies greatly from culture to culture and from family to family. Some cultures and families are stiff-lipped and inhibit the open expression of emotion, whereas others encourage emotional display. Marked differences exist among cultures in the emotional expression of acute grief, fear, pain, and affection.

Ten types of basic emotion have been defined: interest-excitement, enjoyment-joy, surprise-startle, distress-anguish, anger-rage, disgust-revulsion, contempt-scorn, fear-terror, shame-humiliation, and guilt. In describing perplexity, most people signify highly complex emotions—jealousy, loneliness, embarrassment, vengefulness, pettiness, self-righteousness, smugness, and so forth. Poets are often more capable than clinicians of describing and discriminating among these emotional nuances. A dictionary contains many more negatively than positively tinged words to describe human emotions, perhaps owing to the fact that negative emotions pose greater threats than positive ones and therefore merit more vigilance and attention.

Emotional states motivate a variety of coping behaviors, leading to drive reduction, satisfaction, and achievement. Unpleasant states of arousal and emotion are also dealt with through the emotion-focused coping mechanisms mentioned above—the classical psychological defense mechanisms, cognitive self-regulation, and mood modification through use of chemical substances. Individuals sometimes deliberately display false emotions in social situations, attempting to hide their true feelings. Similarly, people try to hide certain unacceptable feelings from their own awareness through self-reception, mediated by denial, repression, or dissociation. Ambivalent persons often alter their emotional state between feeling positive and negative about a given object or idea. *Alexithymia* is a term used to describe persons who ordinarily express very little emotion or fantasy, even in relation to situations likely to generate strong emotions in most people.

ANXIETY The term *anxiety* has been used in reference to an emotional state, a response syndrome, and to specific psychiatric disorders. As a disagreeable emotional state, it often signals anticipated or impending threat. Anxiety has affective features and autonomic, visceral, perceptual, cognitive, and motor manifestations as well. The emotion of anxiety is usually associated with autonomic hyperarousal and attentive hypervigilance, in which the internal and external environments are monitored intensively for information relevant to the sense of threat. Anxious patients are more prone than others to startle in response to unanticipated stimuli, such as loud sounds. The *startle response* consists of rapid orienting in the direction of the stimulus, a sudden surge in pulse and blood pressure, a readiness for movement, usually flight, and an affective state of fright. In contrast to *fear,* the emotional state that exists when a source of threat is precise and well known, anxiety is said to occur when the threat is not well defined. *Free-floating anxiety* is a condition of persistently anxious mood in which the cause of the emotion is unknown and large numbers of diverse thoughts and events all seem to trigger and compound the anxiety. Many common psychiatric symptoms are thought to develop as efforts to control and reduce anxiety.

Individuals differ considerably in their proneness to anxiety. *Trait anxiety* refers to a lifelong pattern of anxiety as a temperament feature. Such persons are generally jittery, skittish, hypersensitive to stimuli, and psychophysiologically more reactive than others. Biological differences in susceptibility to anxiety are suggested by the fact that lactate infusion can differentiate patients with anxiety disorders from others, perhaps through lactate's effects on ionized calcium and the production of alkalosis. β-adrenergic autonomic nervous system reactivity may be greater in anxiety-prone patients than in others. In contrast to trait anxiety, *state anxiety* refers to acute, situationally bound episodes of anxiety that do not persist beyond the provoking situation.

Anxiety states are characterized by feelings of apprehension, restlessness, tension, and dread and may include perceptual distortions, experiences of depersonalization and derealization, poor attention span with distractibility, disruption in the flow of thought, tremor, pacing, and autonomic symptoms, including palpitations, tachycardia, hypertension, hyperventilation with lightheadedness, perspiration, pupillary dilation, and diarrhea.

Attempts have been made to separate the subjective mental experience of anxiety from the peripheral physiological responses that accompany it. The James-Lange theory of anxiety suggested that the anxiety reaction results, in part, from the person's subjective response to the concurrent peripheral manifestations of anxiety; that is, anxiety may be heightened through a positive feedback loop in which anxious persons perceive their own physical symptoms of anxiety, such as tachycardia and diaphoresis, and in response become even more anxious. The use of β-blocking agents to reduce and control autonomic symptoms, such as tachycardia, has been partially successful in the treatment of some anxiety states. Nevertheless, subjective feelings of dread are not eliminated by blocking peripheral anxiety symptoms.

Anxiety states, perhaps the most common nonspecific responses to distress, can result from numerous physical and psychological conditions. A sizeable percentage of patients who present with "anxiety neurosis" are found to have concurrent medical conditions that can account for at least some of the anxiety symptoms. Many endocrine, autoimmune, metabolic, and toxic disorders are known to generate anxiety. It is important to differentiate the response of the patient to an underlying condition (i.e., secondary anxiety or anxiety reaction) from symptoms of anxiety that may be generated by the condition itself. In psychiatric populations, anxiety syndromes are prevalent among patients with organic mental disorders and psychoses. In patients with schizophrenia, anxiety must be differentiated from *central akithesia,* a common and often overlooked syndrome of subjective restlessness and agitation resulting from antipsychotic medication. The coexistence of anxiety symptoms and depression in major depressive disorders is substantial; one-half to two-thirds of patients with agoraphobia-panic disorders have ordinarily merited a diagnosis of major depressive disorder at some point in their lives. Many patients with severe anxiety turn to drugs including benzodiazepine and other sedatives and alcohol for symptom relief. Dependence on these substances is common, and attempts to discontinue their use are frequently thwarted by a return of anxiety resulting both from medication withdrawal and a return of the original symptoms.

From a psychological point of view, anxiety frequently signals conflict between opposing desires, wishes, or beliefs, and major disequilibria generated by negative life events. *Role strains,* conflicts between the major social roles that form a person's identity—spouse, parent, child, wage earner, professional, community member—are common causes of anxiety states. The more important the conflict is, the less obvious is the resolution, and the greater is the associated anxiety. For example, anxiety symptoms may emerge for the first time when a person is confronted with an unavoidable unhappy choice, such as between sustaining a marriage or accepting career advancement that requires a major move unacceptable to the spouse. At times, these conflicts may escape conscious awareness: The person may feel anxious and not know why. Anxiety syndromes frequently result from a combination of several factors. A person in a job conflict facing an important deadline may try to alleviate initial anxiety symptoms by overwork, then ingest caffeine or amphetamines as stimulants to keep going, then become physically exhausted and fatigued and ultimately use alcohol excessively. Each of these elements contributes separately to an anxiety state.

Certain life situations are commonly associated with anxiety: *Stranger anxiety* or *separation anxiety* develops when an infant 6 to 8 months old begins to recognize the difference between mother and others. Development of anxiety symptoms and school phobias when a child starts school may indicate separation fears both in the child and the mother. *Performance anxiety* or *stage fright* includes symptoms of anxiety which may escalate to episodes of panic when public performance is required. Many successful professional performers routinely experience panic attacks before performances.

Panic attack is a circumscribed episode of severe state anxiety lasting minutes to hours, characterized subjectively by feelings of utter terror and fear that one will die or go crazy and physiologically by the many somatic symptoms of anxiety mentioned above, which are sometimes accompanied by severe chest pain, marked shortness of breath, exhausting fatigue, and fainting. These attacks may occur in isolated fashion without apparent cause, or during particularly stressful life situations, or they may cluster in specific anxiety disorders.

A promiscuous 31-year-old homosexual male developed panic attacks when he discovered a blue discoloration on his skin which he assumed to be Kaposi's sarcoma secondary to AIDS. For several days, he was tense, preoccupied, apprehensive, and unable to sleep. When he finally saw a physician and learned that the skin lesion was something trivial, he was greatly relieved and his panic attacks and pervasive anxiety abated. However, he remained extremely vigilant for other signs of ill health, anticipating that he might still develop AIDS.

Efforts to reduce anxiety take many forms. Psychological defense mechanisms, such as repression, projection, denial, intellectualization, reaction formation, and somatization, constitute attempts to bind, divert, and reduce anxiety. Hallucination and delusion formation, compulsive behavior, addictions, and perversions all may reduce anxiety. The idea that many different symptoms develop as means of anxiety reduction is consistent with both psychodynamic and behavioral theorists, but these theories are still inadequate to account for the specificity of symptom formation. For example, it is unclear why some individuals rapidly develop a host of neurotic defenses to ward off anxiety, whereas others suffer prolonged intense anxiety that is not quickly transformed into other types of symptoms.

DEPRESSION Like anxiety, the term *depression* has been used variously to describe an emotional state, a syndrome, and a group of specific disorders. In these contexts, depression has autonomic, visceral, emotional, perceptual, cognitive, and behavior manifestations, as illustrated in Table 10-1. Nonpathologically, most people experience brief episodes (hours to days) of depressed mood, demoralization, pessimism, and low energy following a disappointment or loss. For the majority, personal resilience, alternative coping options, and supportive social networks help alleviate these brief depressive states and prevent them from becoming chronic. Some individuals have a chronically depressed mood, tend to view the world as a difficult, inimical place and themselves as victims, and lack hope for the future. The extent to which constitutional, developmental, and ongoing aversive life events each contribute to this stance is unknown. Persons who in early life were deprived and traumatized may be less resilient and more prone to depression than others. Repeated failure and the impact of unrelenting, uncontrollable, and unpredictable negative life events may set the stage for learned helplessness in humans just as it does in animals. As with anxiety, *state depression,* an acute depressive response pattern, is a common reaction to major unwelcome and undesirable disruptions of life.

Normal *bereavement* must be distinguished from depression. In bereavement, dealing with a major loss such as the death of a spouse or child, persons experience sadness, pining, and yearning but do not ordinarily have feelings of guilt, unworthiness, and self-reproach that characterize depression. Convulsive crying does not always accompany depression; in fact, many depressive syndromes are marked by tearless apathy. Feelings of helplessness and hopelessness may be temporarily present in bereavement, but they ordinarily pass with time. In uncomplicated cases, the process of bereavement takes 3 to 6 months in the acute phase, and up to a year for complete resolution. Bereaved persons are more likely to feel physically ill and seek general health care than in better times, and older widowers are more liable to die than are age-matched nonbereaved controls. Altered immune responses have been demonstrated in the acutely bereaved, but their clinical significance is unknown. *Pathological grief reactions,* bereavements that last more than a year, may be seen when the surviving spouse was excessively dependent on the deceased and is unable to obtain support—emotional, financial, etc.—elsewhere or when the survivor is unable to grieve fully because of markedly ambivalent feelings toward the deceased. *Impacted grief* is said to be present when the initial grief response is inadequate owing to the overwhelming nature of the loss or to the presumed inability of the bereaved to assimilate the loss because of developmental immaturity. The inadequate expression of grief in incomplete bereavement is thought to be pathogenetic in many subsequent psychiatric disorders. For example, impulsive acting out by an adolescent who in childhood lost a parent is often assumed to be due to unresolved grief.

Many biological events contribute to the emergence of depression. Depressive syndromes are often seen in cerebrovascular disease. They are more common with frontal than posterior lobe lesions and more severe with left- than with right-sided lesions. Loss of the prosodic components of speech (i.e., inflections, emphasis) occurs with certain types of brain lesions and may contribute further to the appearance of depression as the voice assumes a flat, monotonous quality. Depression may appear in a variety of endocrine, metabolic, and other systemic disorders and is frequently provoked in patients taking reserpine or α-methyldopa for hypertension, especially if there is a history or family history of depression. Depressive disorders, particularly bipolar disorder, may be more prevalent among artistic and creative people than among others, perhaps reflecting cyclothymic constitution. Strong genetic contributions have been demonstrated for bipolar disorder and for some unipolar disorders.

Cognitive features of depression include feelings of worthlessness, helplessness, and hopelessness—the expectations that no one and nothing can help now or is likely to help in the future. The individual may also be irritable, angry, blaming, remorseful, or apathetic and may have suicidal ideation or ruminations. In severe depressive disorders with melancholia, psychotic features include hallucinations and delusions along with unrelenting psychomotor retardation or restless, ruminative agitation and pacing. *Vegetative symptoms* are those involving somatic systems. In depression these include appetite disturbances—self-indulgent, unrestrained overeating, or anorexia—and hypersomnia or insomia, the latter characterized by a decrease in REM latency, restless interrupted sleep, and early morning awakening. Difficulty falling asleep can also occur in mixed states of anxiety and depression. Loss of libido and constipation are also common.

Suicidal phenomena are of particular concern, and suicide is not uncommon in untreated severe depressive disorders. However, many persons who have no clearly diagnosable depressive disorder commit suicide as well, mostly patients with schizophrenia or organic mental, personality, or substance abuse disorders who are in severe adverse life situations from which they see no escape. Suicide is perceived as the only way out of hopelessness.

Suicidal persons differ in seriousness of intent, precision of planning, and likelihood of success. In the assessment of suicide potential, the patient should be examined in detail regarding suicidal fantasies, perturbation (the degree of emotional upset), strength of impulse to act suicidally, and lethality of plan. Vague fantasies or wishes to be dead ("I'd be better off dead") are less lethal than a plan to drive a car off a cliff or access to a loaded pistol when there is a need to quickly resolve a feeling of profound distress. Since the decision to suicide provides the demoralized victim with a way to regain some measure of control over events, the very act of making the decision and formulating a suicide plan may relieve anxiety and depression. For this reason a sudden, seemingly inexplicable improvement in mood in a severely depressed person should be regarded with suspicion and investigated. Suicidal persons are also known to give away belongings and to make final estate plans before carrying out a suicide. Such activities in a depressed person should arouse concern.

Suicidal gestures are also common among impulsive depressed and self-hating persons, for whom they serve as cries for help that may enlist desired social support. A history of suicide gestures is one of the better predictors of successful suicide in the future, and such gestures should not be taken lightly. Nonsuicidal self-destructive behavior, such as self-mutilation and repeated unnecessary risk taking, are also common in depressive syndromes. Subintentional suicide may result when suicidal gestures go awry or when reckless behavior, such as taking unnecessary risks in combat or driving while drunk, proves fatal.

Other depressive phenomena In geriatric populations, the effect of depression on cognition may be so profound as to produce *pseudodementia,* a syndrome in which the profound but reversible loss of attention and memory disturbances mimic dementia. Depressions in children are often associated with learning disabilities, hyperactive behavior, and impulsivity. However, typical depressive syndromes with psychomotor retardation and vegetative symptoms also appear. *Masked depressions* or *depressive equivalents* refer to a variety of psychological and psychosomatic symptoms thought to result from hidden depression or unresolved grief.

Anaclitic depression refers to a helpless and withdrawn response like that of an infant to the loss of a caretaker which follows initial responses of protest and intense crying. With continued deprivation, the infant enters the phase of despair, becomes morose, ceases crying, and appears to feel hopeless. Some waste away and die. Anaclitic depression in later life is a helpless and withdrawn state in a highly dependent person who seems to fall apart after losing a major source of support. *Existential depressions* result when individuals no longer find meaning in their activities and lose their sense of purpose. The loss of a sense of meaning may occur in primary depressions or in response to major disappointments and unfortunate life situations.

PLEASURABLE MOODS Pleasurable moods include euphoria, elation, exultation, and ecstasy. They are marked by feelings of well-being and expansiveness, optimism, capability, pleasure, and grace. Such moods are normally experienced when life is going very well, when long-sought goals are achieved, and in states of love, religious fervor, and spiritual transcendence. Peak experiences and experiences of mystic fusion are often accompanied by feelings of exultation and ecstasy. Sexual pleasure and some chemically mediated states of altered consciousness may also induce these feelings.

Hypomania exists when pleasurable feelings are excessive, prolonged, and accompanied by unusually high energy. *Mania* is a more extreme state in which judgment and sleep are impaired. In manic states, the mood is usually markedly elevated, expansive, and jocular, but it may easily become irritable or angry. Hyperactivity, pressured speech, flight of ideas, and cognitive disturbances occur. Manic states occur in primary mood disorders, such as bipolar mood disorder, or as a secondary response to a variety of physical and toxic conditions. Secondary manias may follow specific cerebral insults, accompany systemic disorders, or occur following ingestion of some drugs, including amphetamines, antidepressants, bromocriptine (Darlodel), isoniazid, hydralazine, and cimetidine (Tagamet), to name but a few. Up to 12 percent of patients treated with levodopa (Larodopa) and bromocriptine for parkinsonism develop mania. Approximately 10 percent of patients who have syphilitic general paresis develop mania. Mania is the second most common neuropsychiatric disturbance induced by steroids, occurring in 30 percent to 35 percent of patients who develop steroid-induced behavioral disorders. A majority of the brain lesions that produce manic behavior are located in the right cerebral hemisphere.

IRRITABILITY, HOSTILITY, ANGER, AND RAGE This spectrum of aggressive emotions is characterized by heightened vigilance in response to a sense of threat and by a tendency to act, usually to aggressively engage the threatening stimulus. To varying degrees, physiological tone is heightened in preparation for fight. Assertiveness, the adaptive aspect of these emotions, includes a sense that something needs to be done and feeling willing and competent to do something about it, often resulting in constructive action. The manner and extent to which aggressive emotions can be expressed varies from society to society and situation to situation, and they are among the most carefully regulated emotions because of their potential destructiveness.

Individual differences in the tendency toward experiencing and expressing irritability, anger, and rage are temperamental, developmental, and cultural in origin. Some infants are more irritable from birth. It has been postulated that subtle birth injuries and early brain anoxia may increase violence-proneness in later life.

The pathological childhood triad of bedwetting past the age of 6, setting fires, and torturing animals has been associated with subsequent violent behavior in adults. The irritable, hostile, violence-prone person communicates this attitude in body language. Studies of *body buffer zones,* the amount of physical space individuals require around themselves in order to feel comfortable, show that violence-prone individuals require more personal space than others. Violent persons feel threatened when approached too closely, particularly from the rear. Suggesting some biological contributions to the genesis of violence, one review of EEG patterns of criminals and persons with antisocial personality disorders revealed that, in 25 out of the 30 studies reviewed, 30 percent or more of the subjects had EEG abnormalities, and, in more than a third of the studies, 50 percent or more of the subjects had abnormal EEGs.

Psychological and social contributions are strong as well. Violence in families breeds violence, and it has been clearly demonstrated that battered children grow up to be battering adults. Cultural norms for the expression of violence differ considerably. In some socioeconomic and ethnic groups, violent gangs organize the energies of large numbers of adolescent youth. For some, violent behavior is an adolescent socialization pattern necessary to prove one's manhood. Differences among gang members occur in the degree of impulsivity, lack of inhibition, destructiveness, and socialization of violent behavior. Like other social organizations, violent gangs have detailed rules that inhibit the expression of violence. Some extremely unpredictable and unsocialized violent persons, loners, are too violent to be contained even in gangs.

Impulsive violence may be provoked by a number of external stimuli and situations. Alcohol is perhaps the most common disinhibitor of violence. Situations of intrafamilial violence, the most common setting for homicide, are frequently related to alcohol intoxication. In the syndrome of *episodic dyscontrol,* explosively violent behavioral episodes typically erupt after a person has had some alcohol, a phenomenon known as *pathological intoxication.* In these often ferocious and destructive outbursts, the individual may confront or provoke any potential target for violence, even a total stranger, but girlfriends, wives, and parents are frequent victims. Patients with episodic dyscontrol commonly have histories of violent sexual behavior including rape and, often while intoxicated, of speeding and reckless driving, sometimes chasing down, stopping, and attacking other motorists who they feel "got in their way."

A 35-year-old man who had been jailed repeatedly for assaultive behavior appeared in the Emergency Room, intoxicated. He was edgy and threatening, trying to provoke staff members into a fight and asserting that he had previously injured several policemen and security guards in similar situations. His wife confirmed the history. Ushered into a seclusion room and sedated, he pounded on the walls, bruising his hands, until he fell asleep. The next morning he was sheepish and apologetic, saying that he could hardly remember the events of the previous night. He had a childhood history of attention-deficit hyperactivity disorder.

A 35-year-old schizoid man, who had been battered as a child, avoided intimacy with people, fearing that he would be unable to relate well. He bought two dogs, hoping to teach himself to be socialized. To his horror, he found that he became jealous when one dog paid attention to the other rather than to him, and he sadistically beat the dog, realizing all the time that he was repeating the pattern of his father's abuse of him. While beating the dog, he would imagine feeling the same sadistic rage that his father must have felt toward him.

Temper tantrums Immature individuals with persistent personality problems may fail to develop mechanisms to inhibit temper tantrums they displayed as children. Particularly if childhood tantrums produced the desired results, learned tantrum behaviors may persist into adult life. Although such individuals may be extremely pleasant and sociable when things are going well, they often lack the capacity to tolerate frustration and are easily provoked by threats to self-esteem and self-image and by not having their own way. In these situations, they may act like bullies and lose their tempers easily, exhibiting aggressive behavior—glaring, snarling, yelling, shouting, intimidating, pouting, sulking, and sometimes being physically violent.

Displaced rage When circumstances prevent the expression of rage directly against the persons or institutions provoking frustration, other outlets for aggression are often found. Such displacement behavior is frequently seen in nonhuman species. Acts of violence that are either calculated or wanton may result. Cruelty to animals and fire setting may persist as adult forms of destructive behavior. Rape, an act of control, intimidation, terror, and humiliation, may also serve to displace frustrations that cannot be expressed more adaptively.

Sadism may occur with or without explicit sexual gratification. Calculated cruelty conducted seemingly without anger or emotional arousal may reflect inadequate development of social morality of individual conscience, as in the conduct of torture and some cold-blooded murders. In some societies and under specific circumstances at certain times in history, such activity has been socially sanctioned, indicating that, at least in many people, there are few inborn inhibitions against cruelty or violence.

The *Medea syndrome* refers to infanticidal impulses in psychotic (usually schizophrenic) mothers.

Self-mutilation The self may be the target of aggression, as when certain aspects of the self, such as inescapable destructive, impulsive, or compulsive traits, become objects of hatred by the rest of the personality. Psychotic patients may enucleate their eyes or castrate themselves or perform other extremely self-destructive acts short of actual suicide that have apparent symbolic import. Patients with borderline personality disorders may cut themselves repeatedly on the arms, legs, breasts, or elsewhere with broken glass or razor blades, burn themselves with cigarettes, and engage in other repetitive arousing or tension-releasing behaviors.

Children with the Lesch-Nyhan syndrome, a developmental disability syndrome caused by a congenital metabolic abnormality, bite and pick at themselves so compulsively as to do themselves great harm; they must be routinely restrained.

OTHER DISTURBANCES OF MOOD Some subcultural groups are noted for having a narrow range of emotional expressions and strong inhibitions, whereas others are extremely expressive. Pathological levels of *blunt* or *flattened affect,* indicating markedly diminished affective expression in relation to specific thought content, may be seen in chronic schizophrenia and in some organic mental syndromes. These are to be distinguished from the persistently depressed affect seen in depressive disorders, the aprosodias seen in some cerebral diseases, and the mask-like facies of Parkinson's disease. Pervasive boredom, ennui, may be seen in chronic dysthymias. *Anhedonia* is the lack of pleasurable feelings from activities that ordinarily provide pleasure. Chronically psychotic patients often exhibit emotional deterioration in which affective experience and expression may be entirely unrelated to thought content. *Inappropriate affect* refers to incongruency of affective expression and thought content. There may be loud and raucous laughter or giggling in relation to bland or sad thoughts, or grief without apparent reason. Inappropriate affect may sometimes signify that the thoughts have private meanings for the patients, so that these emotional experiences might make sense to an observer if the private meanings were understood. Inappropriate affect must be distinguished from affective expressions that may be appropriate in a subculture or ethnic group but unfamiliar to the observer and from defensive affect, such as the nervous laughter used to alleviate tension or ward off crying.

Ambivalent affect refers to mixed feelings of opposing valence with regard to a given idea. The importance of the idea and the intensity and relative strength of the opposing tendencies determine the ultimate degree of emotional distress and indecisive or contradictory activity generated.

DISTURBANCES IN MOTOR ASPECTS OF BEHAVIOR

Motor behavior is normally finely coordinated, purposeful, and adaptive, and necessary activities are carried out efficiently. In psychiatric disturbances, abnormalities can involve the entire motor system in generalized overactivity or underactivity or be manifest in a wide range of specific disorders of movement.

OVERACTIVITY *Restlessness* and *agitation* are persistent and generalized diffuse increases in body movement, including fidgeting, rapid and rhythmic leg or hand tapping, and jerky start-and-stop movements of the entire body. These states usually accompany conditions of high emotional arousal or confusion, such as toxic states, delirium, and psychosis, including schizophrenia, mania, and psychotic depressive disorders with melancholia. Restless bedridden patients may exhibit *carphologic movements* (picking at the bedclothes and at imaginary things). In melancholia, restless agitation is often accompanied by pacing and hand wringing.

Generalized overactivity may be seen in hypomania, mania, and anorexia nervosa. In these conditions patients may seem to have a greater than usual amount of physical energy and to be capable of prolonged and strenuous bouts of exertion that would fatigue most people rapidly.

Catatonic excitement refers to a dramatic state of disorganized hyperactive behavior which may include frantic jumping, thrashing of limbs, and seemingly senseless menacing or attacking behavior. Such excitement is seen in catatonic forms of schizophrenia and in some culture-bound syndromes, such as amok. *Confusional excitement* is a state of restlessness and generalized purposeless activity seen in ictal states and in some acute intoxications.

MOTOR DISTURBANCES A large number of motor disturbances can be seen in psychiatric disorders. Some are functional somatic expressions of psychiatric disturbances; some are coincidental neurological features of these disorders (even of disorders usually considered to be primarily functional); some are acute medication effects (in particular due to antipsychotics, but also seen with other types of medication); and some are the long-term side effects of antipsychotic medications that persist even after medication is stopped (i.e., tardive phenomena).

Simple motor phenomena TREMOR *Tremors,* involuntary oscillating movements of the limbs or head, may occur at rest or with movement. Fine resting tremors with small amplitude and high frequency are typical of anxiety, fatigue, toxic or such metabolic disorders as caffeinism or hyperthyroidism and are a side effect of lithium therapy. Coarse tremors with larger amplitudes and slower frequency are seen in Parkinson's disease and cerebellar disease. *Asterixis* is a large-amplitude flapping tremor of the hands seen in hepatic disease.

Dystonic movements usually involve large areas of the body musculature and trunk. They are slow and hypertonic, and they may result in posturing. Dystonic movements induced by antipsychotics most commonly affect the head and neck, often manifesting as spasms of the neck and tongue. Torticollis and oculogyric crisis are frequently associated. Trunk and leg involvement produces a bizarre, rigid gait and abnormally stiff postures. Normal spontaneous associated movements of arms and legs may be reduced during walking.

PARKINSONISM Parkinsonian symptoms and signs may be seen whole or in part in psychiatric disorders, particularly in patients taking antipsychotic medications. Symptoms include akinesias, postural abnormalities, pill-rolling nonintention tremors, and cog-wheel rigidity. The akinesias include expressionless facies, drooling, soft, uninflected speech, spontaneously diminished arm swing, and slow initiation of motor activity.

RABBIT SYNDROME This uncommon drug-induced extrapyramidal syndrome is often misdiagnosed as tardive dyskinesia. It most closely resembles a limited expression of a parkinsonian tremor. Patients make rapid chewing movements similar to those made by rabbits, ordinarily faster and more regular than the orofacial tic of tardive dyskinesia. The tongue is spared.

TICS *Tics* are short (seconds to minutes), sudden, and repetitive movements of muscles, ordinarily of the face and neck. Facial grimacing may occur. The person may try to disguise or hide the tic in a seemingly purposive movement, and this movement may ultimately become a mannerism. In Tourette's disorder, tics of the face and neck are accompanied by forced vocalizations, often obscenities (*coprolalia*). One patient who made the rounds of major teaching hospitals in New York City had a forced exhale grunt that usually came out as "horseshit." Tics tends to run in families.

AKITHESIA This symptom consists of motor restlessness ordinarily due to an antipsychotic drug. The patient experiences restlessness and tension in the lower extremities and feels an irresistible urge to move the legs or shuffle or tap the feet. In severe states, there may be constant movement and rocking of the lower extremities.

TARDIVE DYSKINESIA Tardive dyskinesia is a movement disorder resulting from antipsychotic medication that first appears only after many months or years of antipsychotic use. It may persist for extended periods of time or even indefinitely after the medication is discontinued. The movements occur at rest and can usually be suppressed temporarily by voluntary effort or purposeful action, distraction, or sleep. The mouth and lips are most often affected (bucco-orolingual tics and mannerisms), but abnormal movements may also affect, in descending order of frequency, the hands, trunk, respiratory muscles, and feet. Distal portions of limbs are affected more than proximal ones, and the lower face is affected more than the upper face.

BLEPHAROSPASM *Blepharospasm* is a rapid and violent repetitive, spasmodic movement of the eyelids. These movements are often a side effect of medication, but they may occur spontaneously.

Many of the abnormal movements ascribed to tardive dyskinesia and other antipsychotic-induced dystonic and choreoathetoid conditions had been described in chronically psychotic patients prior to the introduction of antipsychotic medications. In one series of 100 patients, the large majority of whom were diagnosed as schizophrenic, a review of medical records prior to 1955 revealed that abnormal purposive movements were found in 83 percent, mannerisms and tics in 71 percent, abnormal eye movements in 27 percent, abnormal postures or facial movements in 42 percent, and gait abnormalities in 10 percent. This research suggested that many patients with schizophrenia have neurological symptoms not due to medications and that severe psychiatric disorders may have a neurological component as well. Other studies have reported similar findings.

STEREOTYPIC MOVEMENTS These are repeated, seemingly non-goal-directed, complex organized gestures or postures that are thought to have private meanings to the patient. Examples include continuously crossing oneself or blessing others in a religious gesture, waving repeatedly in a stylized manner, and profane gestures. One chronic schizophrenic patient characteristically stood for hours on one leg like a crane with his arms in the air. The stereotypic behaviors commonly seen in autistic children (constant spinning or rocking) may provide soothing, steady sensory input that helps reduce the disturbance they experience from the usual, unpredictable, and uncontrollable stimulation in the environment.

Mannerisms consist of unusual styles of performing normal goal-directed activities. A person may have an unusual style of greeting, a highly stylized gait, or a peculiar way of holding utensils while eating.

Bruxism, chronic teeth grinding, may occur involuntarily during tension states or as an isolated occurrence during stage 4 sleep. The latter condition has sometimes been associated with benzodiazepine or alcohol use. In severe cases, serious damage to dental enamel and temporomandibular joint pain may occur.

Ambitendence, the motor manifestation or ambivalence, consists of repetitive approach-avoidance behavior. With rapid alteration, a patient approaches and then withdraws from a certain person, object, or situation. This phenomenon is most marked in some schizophrenic patients and may also be seen in severe obsessive-compulsive disorders.

Movement perseveration consists of the purposeless, repetitive, and involuntary performance of a previously enacted behavior. The original behavior may have been purposeful and carried out in response to a meaningful stimulus. Motor perseveration may sometimes occur in organic mental disorders and in chronic schizophrenia.

Gait disturbances in patients with psychiatric disorders include a variety of neurogenic gaits consistent with brain disease, intoxications, and medication side effects. These include the festinating gait of parkinsonism, spastic and ataxic gaits of neurological disease and psychiatric medications, waddling and reeling gaits associated with intoxications, and hysterical nonphysiological gait disturbances seen in astasia-abasia, a form of conversion disorder. Gait mannerisms include clowning, prancing, military, and effeminate gaits.

Seizure-like behaviors In addition to generalized, petit mal, and complex partial seizures that may be seen in psychiatric patients, a number of nonepileptic seizure-like behaviors must be distinguished. *Breath-holding spells* usually occur in little children: they hold their breath during moments of oppositional rage and faint as a result. There may be associated jerking or twitching motor movements. This generally innocuous phenomenon is ordinarily impulsive and tantrum-like. *Temper tantrums* in young children may look like seizures, especially to the uninformed observer. The children may lie on the floor, screaming and kicking, and fail to respond to the environment. Catatonic excitement may begin with an acute violent tantrum-like outburst known as *raptus*. Conversion seizures (hysterical seizures) must be differentiated from genuine epileptic seizures. These *pseudoseizures* are nonphysiological. Patients lack abnormal reflexes and there is no incontinence. However, because so many conversion seizures occur in patients who have genuine epilepsy and who know a good deal about the condition, the differential diagnosis sometimes may be difficult.

COMPULSIVE BEHAVIORS Compulsive behaviors take many forms and are present to some extent in most people, where favorite pastimes may take on a compulsive character. "Workaholism" and compulsive exercise, for example, are common today in some strata of American society. Compulsions may consist of everyday activities, such as gambling, sexual conquest, shopping, and watching TV, or in relation to substances, such as alcohol, cocaine, narcotics, and food. Other compulsions may involve reckless risk taking that provides stimulation and dispels dysphoric moods. Such compulsive perversions as exhibitionism, sadomasochism, and transvestism may serve similar purposes. Compulsions may be seen in a variety of psychotic and nonpsychotic psychiatric disorders. The cravings that underlie compulsive behaviors are strong motivating forces, and the compulsive behaviors serve to regulate emotions. It may be that as yet unknown similarities underlie all compulsive and addictive mechanisms.

In obsessive-compulsive disorder, it has been suggested that compulsive behaviors reduce anxiety that would be unbearable if the compulsions were denied. The behaviors are thought to reflect the doing and undoing of alien and unwanted obsessive thoughts. Hand washing compulsions, compulsions to make certain that gas jets and faucets have been turned off, to be sure that doors are locked, to perform religious gesticulations, to count objects, and to place objects in a prescribed order are among the more common ones.

DECREASED MOTOR ACTIVITY Generalized reductions in motor activity, motor retardation, may be seen in a variety of physical disease states, such as hypothyroidism, Addison's disease, and other fatiguing illness as well as in some organic mental disorders, schizophrenias, and depressive disorders. Poverty of movement (*hypokinesia*) may occur in schizophrenia and as a antipsychotic side effect. In stuporous states, patients remain immobile although their eyes are open and they are apparently awake.

Decreased volitional behavior may take several forms. *Motor blocking* is the motor version of thought blocking. In the midst of a movement, a patient may stop entirely, remain still for a moment, and then resume the original movement. The patient's experience is that the movement is "stolen" from the ongoing behavioral stream. In *echopraxia* (in German, *mitmachen* or *mitgehen*), the patient follows the examiner's movements as if in mimicry. Some catatonic patients exhibit *waxy flexibility,* maintaining for prolonged periods of time postures into which they are placed. *Negativisim* may take the form of refusing to behave in a prescribed manner or resisting passive movement (in German, *gegenhalten*).

Conversion reactions A conversion reaction can be sensory or motor. Common motor forms include paralysis and paresis of various types, including limb paralyses, ataxias, and aphonias. In *globus hystericus* the patient is unable to swallow. Sensory conversion reactions include blindness, deafness, anesthesia, and analgesia. Psychogenic pain is considered by some authorities to be the equivalent of a conversion disorder.

Mutism Mutism may result from a variety of peripheral muscle and CNS conditions and from functional disorders. Psychiatric disorders in which mutism may be seen include profound depression, catatonic and negativistic schizophrenia, conversion reactions, and the elective mutism occasionally seen in acute adjustment disorders and some personality disturbances.

LANGUAGE DISORDERS

Communication disorders may be due not only to disorders of thinking, as previously described, but also to speech fluency disorders, such as stuttering or stammering, disorders of the articulation and speech apparatus, and CNS disturbances involved in hearing and speech generation (aphasias).

SPEECH DISORDERS *Stuttering* and *stammering* (ordinarily synonymous), refer to disturbances in the rhythm and fluency of speech due to blocking, convulsive repetition, or prolongation of sounds. This disorder affects males two to three times as often as females, and there is a high rate of familial transmission.

Aphasias *Aphasias,* impairments of language produced by brain dysfunction, are ordinarily described as being fluent or nonfluent. In *fluent aphasias,* which generally affect the posterior right hemisphere, patients have a normal or even elevated verbal output, sometimes with logorrhea, but they ignore the social conventions of conversation. Large amounts of well-articulated phrases with normal prosody are produced but there is little informational content. The fluent aphasias are further divided according to the extent of comprehension by the patient and the ability of the patient to repeat what is said by an examiner. The principal fluent aphasias are Wernicke's aphasia, conduction aphasia, anomic aphasia, and transcortical sensory aphasia.

Nonfluent aphasias are characterized by slow and poor verbal output, difficulty with spontaneous speech, omission of grammatical connecting words, and poor prosody. Patients may produce one-word replies or very short phrases. Brain lesions that cause nonfluent aphasias tend to occur in the anterior left hemisphere. The principal nonfluent aphasias are Broca's aphasia, transcortical motor aphasia, global aphasia, and the mixed transcortical aphasias.

DISTURBANCES OF INTERPERSONAL RELATIONSHIPS

Normal interpersonal relationships include those with parents, children, spouses, lovers, siblings, extended family members, friends, comrades, co-workers, and members of the larger community. These relationships ordinarily help provide for the satisfaction of basic drives, for affiliative needs, and for finding purpose and meaning in life. Through stable and satisfying relationships, human needs are met for intimacy, including love, sex, and affection; to be cared for and nurtured; to provide care; to learn; to play; to relax; to dominate; and to be productive through mutual effort. Interpersonal relationships are regulated by interpersonal signs and signals. These communication patterns and relationships follow rules that are usually predictable, consistent, and lawful, both from moment to moment and over extended periods. The extent to which deviance from these patterns is tolerated in a given relationship varies from behavior to behavior, relationship to relationship, family to family, and culture to culture. Disturbances in interpersonal relationships may be viewed as characteristics attributable to a single person or as characteristics of an interpersonal system. Individual disturbances are considered to be undesirable or maladaptive personality traits. When these traits are present to a significant extent and interfere with social functioning or cause distress, they may comprise a personality disorder. Disturbances of interpersonal relationships have also been described at a systems level (e.g., as dyadic or family patterns of system disturbance); however, these have not been characterized as well as have individual patterns.

INDIVIDUAL FACTORS **Appearance and body language** In addition to the denotations of spoken words, much information is communicated through nonlexical vocalization (the music of the voice), nonverbal gesture, posture, and other aspects of appearance. A great deal of social interaction and communication is initiated, sustained, and modified by means of these modes of communication. The rapid diagnostic impressions gathered by clinicians rely heavily on these aspects of communication. Many clues to personality traits are immediately evident in nonverbal patterns, which must be supplemented, to be sure, with historical information.

Body odor Unlike members of many other cultures, Americans tend to be fastidious about body odor, bathing frequently and using a variety of scents and deodorants. Strong body odor may reflect cultural differences, a deliberate choice not to bathe, or anosmia. Strong perfume scents may reflect cultural styles and desires to be attractive.

Clothing The type, state, and condition of clothing says much about socioeconomic group, self-care and grooming, and personality. Tight, revealing clothes on a woman may signal exhibitionistic or histrionic traits; rumpled, neglected, dirty clothes may be evidence of the self-neglect that often attends cognitive impairment due to organic or functional disorders or chronic substance abuse. Unusual articles of clothing may be emblems of subgroup affiliation or have special personal meaning, as in some psychoses and perversions. Clothes may represent a way of saying, "I'm safe and bland" or a way of signaling counterculture affiliations or a personal sense of weirdness. Clothes can say, "Stay away" or "Approach at your own risk."

Skin adornment Tattoos, unusual haircuts, and scars may reveal subculture affiliations, drug use, and battering. Highly developed muscles may reveal positive athleticism or narcissistic overinvolvement with physical attributes.

Body language Posture, gesture, and eye contact vary interculturally and interpersonally. Studies of proxemics— posture, distancing, the use of space, touching, eye contact, voice loudness, thermal radiation, olfaction—reveal more precisely how body language communicates psychiatrically pertinent information and quantitate the information that clinicians use intuitively all the time. At least initially, most observers are strongly swayed by these body signals, and patients who wish to mislead examiners can do so by skillful misrepresentation. Clinicians often find their first impressions to be wrong, which is why it is always necessary to perform the prescribed examinations and take a history.

The manner in which limbs are positioned and moved, the extent to which posture and gaze are directed or averted, and the way in which one person's body language responds to another's, regardless of the content of ongoing verbal communication, are all highly informative. Videotape analysis of individual and family therapy sessions has demonstrated quasi-courtship behavior—flirtatious advances, preening, seductive body movements— being initiated and responded to by patients and therapists who were all unaware of these body movements and who were all the while engaged in the conversation of the therapy session, which dealt with something entirely different.

Posture can convey information about ethnicity. Persons of Northern and Western European origin tend to maintain a larger personal space or physical distance from one another than do those of Mediterranean ethnic origin. Ethnic Middle Easterners feel more comfortable very close to one another—

nearly nose-to-nose in conversation. Dominance, fear or anxiety, and the desire for intimacy are all communicated through the use of space. Irritable persons insist on more personal space; dependent persons or those seeking intimacy may overstep the comfort bounds of others. Habitual gestures have been posited to reveal personality traits and important life issues: frequent preening, patting, or stroking of the hair or examining the fingernails and narcissism; playing with the wedding ring and marital conflict; spasmodic clutching of the chest and hypochondriasis; repeated removal of the spectacles and nosewiping and denial; and open upper torso body language—broad inviting, seductive gestures—but closed lower body signals—tightly crossed or closed legs—and histrionic personality trait in women.

Studies of gaze have shown extroverts to gaze more directly and more often at others than do introverts. In one study, schizophrenic patients gazed directly at an examiner only 65 percent as much as normal controls, whereas patients with depression gazed 73 percent as much. The schizophrenics also used shorter glances—2.1 seconds, compared with 3.4 for depressed patients and 3.9 for controls. Autistic patients spend only about 4 percent of the time gazing at another person in a room compared with 65 percent for controls.

Averted gaze may be culturally conditioned. In some societies, it is considered rude or sexually forward.

A 15-year-old devout Puerto Rican girl being interviewed by a psychiatric resident kept her body turned 90 degrees from his, refused to face him, and stared continuously at the floor except for occasional side glances throughout the interview. The resident initially interpreted this presentation as withdrawn and avoidant behavior, but he quickly saw that with many other people on the ward the patient was very direct, friendly, and open. For this patient, who had been raised in a strict home in the Puerto Rican countryside and who had only recently come to New York City, staring directly into the resident's eyes for longer periods of time would have been socially inappropriate because of their differences in social standing and a brazen sexual signal as well.

INTERPERSONAL TRAITS Traits that disturb personal relationships are those that interrupt the comfortable give and take of normal intimacy, dependence, and dominance, deviating beyond tolerated boundaries. In Freud's terms, they disrupt the ability to love, play, and work. Although they are listed by personality types, the characteristics described below appear in practice in an almost infinite variety of individual patterns of disturbance.

DSM-III-R divides personality traits and personality disorders roughly into three groups—odd or eccentric; dramatic, emotional or erratic; and anxious or fearful. The *odd or eccentric* group includes paranoid, schizoid, and schizotypal personalities; the *dramatic, emotional, or erratic* group includes histrionic, narcissistic, antisocial, and borderline personalities; and the *anxious or fearful* group includes avoidant, dependent, obsessive-compulsive, and passive-aggressive personalities. Other personality disorders are in a residual category. Traits linked to the odd and eccentric group of personality disorders include being jealous and quick to take offense; carrying a grudge and being uncommunicative and nonconfiding (paranoid type); lacking friendships or close relationships with a parent; being indifferent toward others and lacking a need for feedback (schizoid type); and engaging in odd and eccentric gestures, mannerisms, and practices (schizotypal type).

Characteristics associated with the dramatic, emotional, and erratic group include the following: being impulsive, unpredictable, moody, temperamental, unstable in relationships, and self-destructive with regard to sex, money, and substance abuse (borderline type); being hypersensitive to criticism, exploitative of others, egocentric and self-important, having unstable relationships, exhibiting feelings and behaviors of entitlement, and exhibiting envious remarks and behaviors (narcissistic type); being attention-seeking, exhibitionistic, seductive, self-indulgent, overly concerned with physical appearance, and exhibiting exaggerated expressions of emotions (histrionic type); and truancy, lying, stealing, starting fights, breaking rules, being unable to sustain work or school, quitting impulsively, and shirking everyday responsibilities (antisocial type).

Among the anxious and fearful types are characteristics of being hypersensitive to rejection and reluctant to enter close relationships in spite of a great desire for affection (avoidant type); showing excessive reliance on others to make major life decisions, staying trapped in abusive relationships for fear of being alone, pacifying others at one's own costs, having difficulty initiating projects on one's own, and constantly seeking reassurance and praise (dependent type); exhibiting restrictive expressions of warmth, tenderness, and generosity, stubbornness with a need to be right and to control decisions, indecisiveness at times, and inflexible application of rules and morals (obsessive-compulsive type); and being sulky, irritable, argumentative, petty, resentful, obstructionistic, and procrastinating (passive-aggressive type).

DSM-III-R has suggested another maladaptive style, describing individuals who exhibit self-sacrificing and help-rejecting behaviors, repeatedly undermining attainment of their own stated goals, and turning down opportunities for pleasure (self-defeating or masochistic type).

INTERPERSONAL SYSTEMS Couples and families have been studied as systems in their own right, and numerous qualities of these systems have been identified as being clinically important, but, as yet, no universally accepted set of guidelines has emerged for the psychological assessment of couples and families that parallels those generally used for individuals, such as those described in this chapter. Families normally provide the settings in which development and socialization take place, communication and emotional expression are learned, assumptions and expectations about the world at large are formed, one's sense of personal safety or vulnerability is established, and validation or negation of personal values, strivings, and worth occurs. Characteristics of couples and families that have received the most attention include the rules of communication, such as those governing the directness or indirectness with which disagreement and conflict are addressed; the manner (organized or chaotic) in which communications are conducted; taboo topics and secrets about which no one can openly communicate; the nature and degree of emotional expression, including affection and anger; the cohesiveness, loyalty, and compatibility of members; the nature of the members' shared identities on the one hand and their autonomous development and separateness on the other; the extent to which members treat one another respectfully or take one another for granted and use one another; the distribution of power and decision making among members; the maintenance of generational boundaries (e.g., age-appropriate performance of life roles); and the members' orientation, concurrence, and disagreement about important values involving moral, religious, intellectual, cultural, financial, occupational, and child-rearing issues, as well as aspirations, health practices, leisure activities, and other belief systems.

Disturbed couple and family systems have been characterized according to many of the dimensions mentioned above. Studies of marital patterns have shown that mating is not random. Individuals with certain personal styles tend preferentially to marry spouses with complementary styles. Many imbalanced relationships in which one partner largely dominates the other may remain stable for years (*skewed* relationships). Some couples have chronically unstable relationships with constant overt conflict (*schismatic* relationships). In some families, one or more members are highly vocal and unrelentingly critical of others, creating an emotional tone of high negative expressed emotion. This family characteristic has been shown to be a poor prognostic indicator for a variety of psychiatric problems, including schizophrenia, mood disorders, and anorexia nervosa. Affected family members who continue to reside in such families are less likely to improve and more likely to have further exacerbations than patients from families without this characteristic.

Couple and family system difficulties are most likely to erupt during predictable stressful events in the normal family life cycle, such as during the newlywed period; pregnancy and childbearing; difficult or contentious child-rearing; difficulties with parents, in-laws, and other extended family; insurmountable and unanticipated financial or career problems; serious illness or death of a child or relative; the childrens' adolescence; departure of children from the home; infidelity; and separation.

Some disturbed couple and family systems have been described as playing *pathological games*—repeated interactions with predictable interpersonal sequences and undesirable outcomes. Such systems may have chronic but patterned instability, analogous to biological membranes that build up to a threshold before firing. They contain problem-maintaining homeostatic feedback loops, sequences that have been called pathological games without end. Ongoing three-party pathological games (*perverse triangles*) may constantly generate tension but have tension-releasing mechanisms that function only temporarily and ineffectively and do not adequately resolve the underlying problems.

In response to a sullen and provocative teenager, one father was typically hostile, highly critical, and blaming (generating high negative expressed emotion). At points when it seemed that physical violence was likely to erupt, the mother habitually rushed in to temporarily defuse the situation, soothing both parties and rescuing them from further escalation of hostilities. Then, intentionally or unintentionally, in the very act of defusing or shortly thereafter, the mother always managed to do or say something that was certain to restart the buildup of tension between father and teenager, assuring that another round of angry confrontation would occur.

Some perverse triangles are romantic.

A successful careerwoman was involved with an equally successful professional man. Although they were very attracted to each other, their relationship was chronically unstable because, whenever they spent more than a few days together, the man would start to feel trapped and dominated, sensing that the woman's personality was more forceful than his. The man would then leave her and return to an ongoing love affair he maintained with his very submissive secretary, a woman who was always waiting for him in the background. After 4 or 5 days with the secretary, whom he found pleasant but boring, he would once again return to the more exciting professional woman. This pattern—roughly a 2-week cycle—continued for several years. The two women knew of each other but felt helpless and trapped, as each was willing to settle for whatever time she could get with the man. None of the three was happy with the situation, but no one could figure a way out.

Scapegoating is another form of perverse triangulation in which conflict between two people, frequently spouses, is avoided by means of recrimination or overconcern directed toward a third party, frequently a child. Pathological family coalitions and alliances may be established, cutting across the generations or excluding certain members of the family from important issues, leaving them to feel isolated and abandoned. Pathological *enmeshment,* often manifested as excessive involvement of a parent with a child, may signal inadequacies in the primary marital bond.

The *double bind* form of communication, another pathological family communication pattern thought to generate emotional disturbance, consists of a simultaneous but mutually contradictory set of directives that assure that the victim will be wrong regardless of which directive is followed. Furthermore, in the classic double bind situation, the victim is neither allowed to escape from the situation nor to comment on the double bind being placed, a set of circumstances that some researchers think may be capable of provoking a psychotic response. Vague, imprecise patterns of speech (so-called schizophrenogenic speech) have also been thought to be potentially pathogenic of psychotic disturbances.

A physician telephoned a colleague in another city and spent 4 to 5 minutes on the phone with the secretary. Her speech was hesitant, halting, and interrupted, and she was excessively apologetic because she was unable to put the call through immediately. Following this brief encounter, the psychiatrist told his colleague that while talking to the secretary he felt as if he were going crazy and he imagined that anyone spending a prolonged period of time with her might have psychiatric difficulties. The colleague informed him that the secretary had a schizophrenic son but that she never had any known psychiatric disturbance herself.

LIFE PATTERN DISTURBANCES Optimal patterns of self-expression, self-realization, and self-fulfillment require proper development of the capacities to work, love, and play. These patterns are acted out in the family, school, workplace, friendship networks, and larger community. In each of these settings, persons adopt various social roles, through which their own activities develop and through which they define relationships to others with whom they are involved. Life pattern disturbances may occur in a single role or in multiple ones, in a single setting, such as work, or in several settings. Specific psychological conflicts may inhibit adequate performance in one of these areas. For example, in *success neurosis,* a person who is conflicted about outdoing a parent or sibling will be unable to succeed professionally because unrealistic fears of retribution generate overwhelming anxiety and inhibit performance. Or, chronic inability to control the expression of aggression may disrupt a career.

A somewhat successful 35-year-old film actor was known to be temperamental. Because of repeated temper tantrums, he was called for fewer and fewer roles in spite of his evident talents and was shortly a has-been.

Inhibitions in interpersonal relationships, for example shyness or fear of intimacy or sex, may set up lifelong patterns of unhappiness. Similarly, unrealistic perfectionism may prevent the establishment of satisfying long-term relationships.

An attractive, successful, 32-year-old woman reported having a long string of admiring suitors and a series of intimate sexual relationships since the age of 17. Although several of the suitors to whom she was strongly attracted had proposed marriage, she felt unable to commit herself, never sufficiently in love with any of them and hoping that she would someday meet Mr. Perfect.

Life pattern disturbances sometimes result from multiple concurrent *role strains.* These occur when the individual is faced with simultaneous, excessive, and conflicting demands to fulfill the duties and obligations of work, family, and community. Demands and expectations from many sources produce the chronic overcommitment and time pressures so typical of professional families that often generate chronic disturbance and dissatisfaction punctuated by intermittent crises:

A young, ambitious, devoted, and successful professional woman, the mother of two small children, found herself in repeated crisis situations at times when the demands of her job, parents, marriage, and children converged. She often had to juggle many commitments—writing reports for work, helping her children with important school projects, meeting her husband's needs for intimacy, and taking care of her ailing parents. These circumstances resulted in frequent experiences of overwhelming tension, anxiety, panic, headache, and abdominal cramps. Nevertheless, she was chronically unable to set effective limits on the role demands in any one of these areas; she was reluctant to relinquish responsibility and had difficulty delegating some of her responsibilities to others.

A 40-year-old physician in a successful general practice also had multiple business ventures in which he invested a great deal of the money he had earned from property development. These ventures frequently entangled him in legal disputes. He spent 12 to 14 hours in his office each day seeing patients, completed his charting and paperwork on weekends, and snatched odd moments to conduct complicated business transactions with his attorney. He was snappy and irritable with his family and expected that they would be at his beck and call, seeing how "self-sacrificing" he was on their behalf. Reducing his practice, taking an associate, or limiting his business activities were all unacceptable to him.

Certain lifelong maladaptive patterns have been called *scripts*. The theory assumes that, from an early age, persons are guided toward both success and defeat by deeply ingrained attitudes and assumptions about themselves. Some people believe themselves destined to become heroes or successes, and their activities fulfill this assumption. Others see themselves as destined to be victims and failures, perhaps repeating family patterns or fulfilling perverse expectations of other family members; such expectations may be powerful self-fulfilling prophecies.

A 35-year-old man reported a string of business failures. Although he seemed to have interest in and some actual aptitude for business, he consistently made wrong choices, involving himself in good deals that never materialized, and lost money in a series of business ventures. His father had been unsuccessful at business, and his mother, he recalled, told him from early childhood, "You'll never amount to anything. You're just like your father."

Life pattern disturbances may also take the form of a counterculture life-style. Dissatisfied or unsuccessful with conventional activities, or feeling stymied by or frustrated with various family and career failures, a person may drop out, change social role definitions and class, join cults, or engage in other forms of social deviance, such as gang affiliation, criminality, the welfare culture, or malingering to avoid working. Career requirements—frequent geographic moves or enforced marital separations—may force life pattern disturbances on families. Certain careers and work settings carry heavy social pressures for alcohol and drug use or marital infidelity. Some families accommodate to prolonged separation but later find the demands of continuous marital intimacy and togetherness to be difficult.

A Navy couple had accommodated to the husband's long career pattern of 6 months at sea and 6 months at home. When the husband retired from the Navy, the couple experienced increasing marital conflict. Both husband and wife ascribed these difficulties to having lost their long periods of time apart from one another, time they had learned to enjoy, during which they explored their own interests, developed separate relationships, and defused marital tensions.

FUTURE PROSPECTS

Like psychiatric diagnostic classifications, fashions among psychiatric signs and symptoms change, so that those described above must be taken in historical perspective. Characteristics once given prominence, such as the bony protuberances of the skull studied by phrenologists a century ago, are no longer accorded much importance, whereas only in the past few decades have newly described clinical phenomena, such as family expressed emotion and alexithymia, been appreciated. As understanding of etiology and pathogenesis of psychiatric disorders becomes more sophisticated, the clinical importance of some of these signs and symptoms may wane and they may be relegated to the realm of medical curiosities, as are fourth heart sounds in the wake of modern cardiovascular diagnostic techniques. With advances in psychiatric science, psychiatrists can look forward to the day when the nonspecific symptoms of psychiatric disease will be appreciated for the final common pathway expressions that they are. But no matter how advanced the science, clinicians must always recognize the very human experience of these signs and symptoms and respectfully treat patients so burdened by unhappiness.

REFERENCES

Assad G, Shapiro B: Hallucinations: Theoretical and clinical overview. Amer J Psychiat *143*: 1088, 1986.

Berne E: *Transactional Analysis: Psychotherapy*. Castle Books, New York, 1961.

Bleuler E: *Dementia Praecox: The Group of Schizophrenias*. International University Press, New York, 1950.

Chess S, Thomas A: *Origins and Evolution of Behavior Disorders: From Infancy to Early Adult Life*. Brunner/Mazel, New York, 1984.

Corliss W R, editor: *The Unfathomed Mind: A Handbook of Unusual Mental Phenomena*. The Sourcebook Project, Glen Arm, MD, 1982.

Cummings J L: *Clinical Neuropsychiatry*. Grune & Stratton, New York, 1985.

Cummings J L: Organic psychosis. Psychosomatics *29*: 16, 1988.

Fricchione G, Sedler M J, Shukla S: Aprosodias in eight schizophrenic patients. Amer J Psychiat *143*: 1457, 1986.

Hall R C W, Devaul R A, Stickney S K, Popkin M K, Faillace L A: Physical illness presenting as psychiatric disease. Arch Gen Psychiat *35*: 1315, 1978.

Hilgard E R: *Divided Consciousness: Multiple Controls in Human Thought and Action*. Wiley, New York, 1977.

Hoffman L: *Foundations of Family Therapy*. Basic Books, New York, 1981.

Hoffman R E, Stopek S, Andreasen N C: A comparative study of manic vs. schizophrenic speech disorganization. Arch Gen Psychiat *43*: 831, 1986.

Jaspers K: *General Psychopathology*. University of Chicago Press, Chicago, 1963.

Kluft R P: First-rank symptoms as a diagnostic clue to multiple personality disorder. Amer J Psychiat *144*: 293, 1987.

Koenigsberg H W, Handley R: Expressed emotion: From predictive index to clinical construct. Amer J Psychiat *143*: 1361, 1986.

Lazare A, editor: *Outpatient Psychiatry: Diagnosis and Treatment*. Williams & Wilkins, Baltimore, 1979.

Lazarus R S, Folkman S: *Stress, Appraisal and Coping*. Springer-Verlag, New York, 1984.

Moos R H, editor: *Coping with Physical Illness*. Plenum, New York, 1977.

Rapaport D, editor: *Organization and Pathology of Thought*. Columbia University Press, New York, 1951.

Rogers D: The motor disorders of severe psychiatric illness: A conflict of paradigms. Brit J Psychiat *147*: 221, 1985.

Schneider K: *Clinical Psychopathology*. Grune & Stratton, New York, 1959.

CHAPTER 11 THE CLASSIFICATION OF MENTAL DISORDERS

HAGOP SOUREN AKISKAL, M.D.

INTRODUCTION

The past decade witnessed a renaissance of clinical research on the diagnosis and classification of mental disorders. Descriptive approaches to psychopathological manifestations and their classification into discrete categories are now viewed as prerequisites to the scientific study of mental illness. Although descriptive psychopathology has always been an important concern of psychiatrists worldwide, until recently it was actually unfashionable for U.S. psychiatrists to take an active interest in it. Dissatisfaction with the clinical and research performance of existing diagnostic categories is one of the factors that led to the current critical reappraisal of their usefulness.

CRITICISMS OF PSYCHIATRIC DIAGNOSIS

Although relatively little attention had been paid to formal diagnostic issues in this country, it was not until the 1960s that a truly antinosological climate developed. The arguments advanced against formal diagnostic categories related to the following issues: (1) the alleged superiority of understanding, rather than objectively describing, a person suffering from a psychiatric condition; (2) the unreliability of formal diagnoses; (3) the meager power of such diagnoses to predict treatment response and related outcome variables; and (4) the claim that social harm could result from labeling.

All depth psychologies—classical, neo-Freudian, or others—as well as the more practical Meyerian or "biographical" extensions of these approaches are ultimately concerned with understanding the individual patient; hence the clash with formal classification, which emphasizes shared characteristics. This clash is best exemplified in Carl Jung's declaration that to speak of a science of individual psychology is a contradiction in terms. It was this focus on individuality—the study in depth of a limited number of cases—that led to the alienation of many dynamically trained psychiatrists from formal diagnostic categorization. The reliability of clinical judgments based on individual cases could not easily be tested, a situation that jeopardized the status of psychiatry as a medical specialty devoted to studying psychopathology and concerned with diagnosis, prognosis, treatment, and prevention. If diagnoses were considered to be unreliable, the underlying assumption that diagnostic categories referred to valid entities was no longer tenable. Obviously, biological investigations of unreliable diagnoses could not lead to major advances in etiological understanding.

In the ensuing identity crisis of American psychiatry and the philosophical vacuum that prevailed in the 1960s and 1970s, a spectrum of antinosological approaches proliferated within and outside psychiatry. Some of these approaches still adhered largely to medical metaphors. For instance, Karl Menninger deplored the use of the term "schizophrenia" but did not give up the concept of diagnosis in his five levels of ego dysfunction, each of which corresponds to several traditional diagnostic categories. Likewise, family therapists who considered the index patient to be the healthiest member were to declare the entire family (or even society at large) to be "sick." It is in behavioral approaches that one finds the clearest rejection of psychiatric diagnosis as a medical procedure. Psychopathological phenomena are conceptualized as isolated, contextual response patterns that reflect accidental conditioning or the individual's reinforcement history. It was generally the contention of these antinosological schools that treatment response could be predicted better by these environmental factors than by traditional diagnostic classes. This theoretical bias for the importance of environmental forces in shaping behavior was aligned philosophically with emerging community and social approaches. One extreme school of thought, labeling theory, took the position that it was the very act of diagnosing that produced mental illness. This approach is more famed for its rhetoric than for its contribution to a genuine understanding of contextual factors in mental illness; yet, in their unrelenting criticism of the unsystematic use of psychiatric diagnoses, members of this school pointed to the need for psychiatrists to agree on unambiguous criteria for the diagnosis of specific mental disorders.

THE REBIRTH OF PSYCHIATRIC NOSOLOGY

Ironically, the aforementioned attacks on psychiatric diagnosis proliferated at a time when exciting developments in basic and clinical research were beginning to provide a raison d'être to psychiatry as a medical specialty. The renaissance of descriptive psychopathology in the United States owes a great deal to these advances.

THE IMPACT OF MODERN TREATMENTS ON NOSOLOGY Prior to the modern era of pharmacotherapy, many psychiatrists argued that little could be gained from detailed categorization of mental and behavioral abnormalities. Classification was used for public health purposes—to allocate funds for clinical and social services for the mentally ill. In practice, the main distinctions drawn were organic versus functional disorders (medical interventions were clearly relevant to the former) and psychotic versus neurotic or character disorders (psychodynamic and other psychosocial approaches were generally deemed more appropriate for the latter).

The introduction of antipsychotic drugs in the 1950s led to a shift in attitudes toward psychiatric diagnosis. The enlarged clinical boundaries of schizophrenic disorders embraced even pseudoneurotic and borderline conditions in the hope that these drugs might benefit the largest number of patients. The authority of Eugen Bleuler, whose monograph on the group of the schizophrenias had just been translated, could be used to support this overinclusive concept of schizophrenia. This broad concept dominated North American psychiatry until the US-UK diagnostic project demonstrated that schizophrenia was being diagnosed at the expense of mood (affective), neurotic, and character disorders (Fig. 11-1). Such data, along with the documented effectiveness of lithium for recurrent or cyclic mood disorders and the unnecessary risk of tardive dyskinesia in affectively ill patients exposed to antipsychotics, have been instrumental in reversing this trend in the 1970s. The need to make a careful differential diagnosis between schizophrenia and mood disorders became crucial. Advances in psychopharmacology have also led to the realization that there are attenuated forms of affective illness, which were previously classified as neuroses and character disorders.

DIAGNOSIS AND RESEARCH These developments in the reclassification of mental disorders are part of a wider trend—one could say a megatrend—toward a more empirical approach to psychiatry, in response to pressures on psychiatrists to prove its usefulness, and to demonstrate that different mental disorders can be reliably identified and differentiated and that these diagnoses have predictive value in treatment.

Explicit diagnostic criteria that distinguish between various mental disorders are necessary not only for predicting drug response but also for testing the relative efficacy of psychotherapy in different disorders. The emergence of laboratory and familial-genetic strategies, which have proven to be versatile tools for exploring the etiologies of mental disorders, has also necessitated the use of consistent diagnostic criteria.

While some may subscribe to the notion that the emerging biological technology will ultimately resolve the nosological quandaries of mental disorders, the very development of these techniques depends on rigorously conducted clinical evaluations. The hope that the discovery of biological markers will eventually provide external criteria

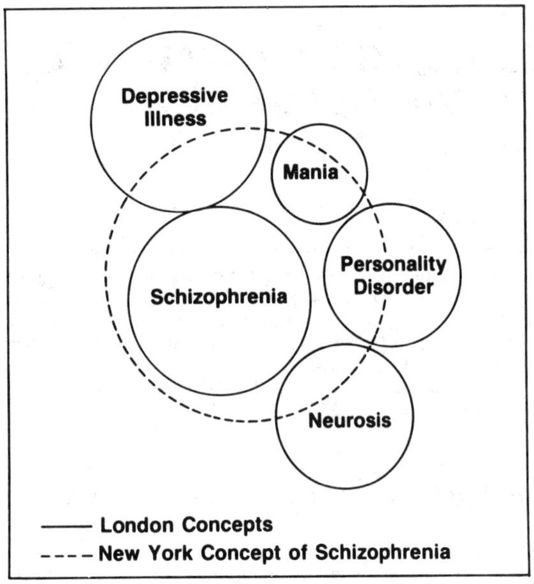

FIGURE 11-1. *Comparison of British (London) and U.S. (New York) concepts of schizophrenia. (From Cooper J E, Kendell R E, Gurland B J, Sharpe L, Copeland J R M, Simon R:* Psychiatric Diagnosis in New York and London. *Oxford University Press, London, 1972, with permission.)*

for validating psychiatric diagnoses will be wishful thinking as long as diagnostic imprecision mars the selection of homogeneous diagnostic groups for scientific study.

THE EMERGENCE OF NEO-KRAEPELINISM Judging from the foregoing review of the U.S. psychiatric scene, it is the proliferation of data-based research on the pathogenesis and therapy of mental disorders that created the contemporary respect for diagnosis and classification. Reciprocally, the recorded progress in diagnostic classification is a major force in shaping the modern empiricist zeitgeist of North American psychiatry, which is characterized by emphasis on description (remaining close to observable data) and operationalism (using reliable methods to assess the manifestations of psychiatric disorders).

Ironically, Emil Kraepelin, who envisioned such a psychiatry built on the foundation of the natural sciences, had lost philosophical ground in many parts of his native Germany. It was the influential British textbook of Kraepelinian persuasion, Mayer Gross's *Clinical Psychiatry,* that taught English-speaking psychiatrists, including many foreign medical school graduates who immigrated to the United States in recent years, the science of psychopathology.

A more systematic neo-Kraepelinian development in the United States can be traced to the psychiatry department of Washington University, which during the past quarter century devoted much of its talent and resources to research to operationalize psychiatric diagnosis, with the result that the St. Louis criteria or the Feighner criteria are today the most widely cited references in psychiatry worldwide. They were adopted and expanded to develop the Research Diagnostic Criteria (RDC), which ultimately culminated in the third edition of the American Psychiatric Association's *Diagnostic and Statistical Manual of Mental Disorders* (DSM-III) in 1980, and in its revision (DSM-III-R) in 1987. It was the special achievement of Robert Spitzer and associates to convince the field that the reliable identification of mental disorders was a concept whose time had come and to oversee the codification of the emerging operational systematization of mental disorders.

The developments outlined in the foregoing paragraphs represent a victory for descriptive European approaches to psychopathology as they were interpreted, modified, or refined by American pragmatism. Philosophically, they conform to Carl Hempel's paradigm of logical empiricism. Thus, DSM-III and DSM-III-R and their empiricist-operational philosophy are not, strictly speaking, atheoretical. However, their theoretical approach to psychopathology is compatible with others. Indeed, it can be considered necessary for the validity of these other approaches. According to Hamilton, the history of ideas teaches one that (especially in the early phases of a new discipline) "observation [has] to be distinguished from theorizing and inference, for without that all the rest of psychiatry, from biochemistry and genetics to sociology and psychodynamics, float in the air without a base." To date, this conceptual framework has found its major applications in psychobiology, neuropsychiatry, and psychiatric epidemiology, but it is clearly compatible with behavioral-cognitive approaches, which, by tradition, emphasize observable constructs. Also, judging from the recent surge of research on personality disorders that utilizes structured diagnostic methods, a combined Kraepelinian-Freudian perspective is both feasible and fruitful.

The adoption of an empiricist operational philosophy as a starting point for psychiatry is also compatible with Karl Popper's position that psychiatric concepts must be formulated in refutable form. This approach has the potential to create much dissent as unverifiable and unverified psychopathological concepts are discarded in favor of ones that have stood the test of refutation. These concepts can obviously come from different theoretical approaches—their merit is determined by their ability to survive rigorous attempts to refute them. Pluralism in this sense would derive from rigorous hypothesis testing and not merely from some idealistic desire for eclecticism.

As in the past 200 years of psychiatry, one should expect in the future much ferment as the concepts of psychopathology are refined, but it is encouraging that, at least in one national system, psychiatrists have agreed in principle to the protoscientific principle of descriptive rigor. U.S. psychiatry, after lagging behind many European national schools in nosological sophistication, is gradually assuming a leadership position.

THE ROLE OF DIAGNOSIS AND CLASSIFICATION IN PSYCHIATRY

DIAGNOSIS AND NOSOLOGY Diagnosis (from the Greek root meaning "to recognize") and nosology (from the Greek *nosos,* "disease") refer to the systematization of knowledge for the identification and classification of diseases. Nosology is to medicine what taxonomy—the ordering of living organisms—is to biology. Classification, then, is a fundamental procedure in all of biology, a shorthand by which individuals with shared characteristics are grouped together.

Classification in medicine further serves to control (i.e., develop treatments or preventive strategies applicable to individuals who have shared clinical or laboratory findings) and ultimately to comprehend the causative mechanisms of such shared findings. Better understanding of causative factors in turn provides the opportunity for more effective control; it also leads to more valid systems of classification.

ILLNESS, SYNDROME, AND DISEASE In all branches of medicine, physicians diagnose diseases in order to prescribe treatment and prognosticate. The desideratum is to cure but it is often necessary to settle for preventing the complications of disease or retarding its progression.

Diagnosis is the medical procedure whereby patients' presenting complaints, disturbed functioning, and incapacity (which can be termed "illness") are evaluated and compared to those of other patients with similar manifestations (as examined and recorded by previous and current generations of physicians). The initial aim is to determine whether *symptoms* (the patient's complaints) and *signs* (observable abnormalities detected by the examiner) cluster into characteristic patterns or *syndromes* (e.g., pneumonia, dementia, schizophrenia), each of which may be produced by several different diseases. For instance, when Bleuler used the plural in describing the schizophrenias, he implied that different disease entities could lead to the final common pathway consisting of the special cluster of associative, affective, volitional, and autistic manifestations. The identification of the disease entities that underlie clinical manifestations is one of the principal functions of diagnosis in medicine.

Laboratory evaluation, documenting specific abnormalities in structure or function, and clinical history are often necessary to differentiate among the various diseases that could produce a given syndrome (e.g., multi-infarct versus degenerative dementia). The clinical boundaries and laboratory findings of diseases often overlap. Only when specific etiologies are discovered or when pathogenetic mechanisms are understood are these boundaries sharpened so that discrete disease entities can be delineated.

The cause of a disease is generally easier to identify when the incubation period, the time elapsed between the operation of causative agents and the onset of clinical manifestations, is short. This is the case with many, but not all, infections and with conditions due to intoxications and trauma. When the incubation extends over years or decades, specific causes may be difficult to identify, and pathogenetic mechanisms are typically multiple intertwined events, many of which date back to the time of onset of the earliest clinical manifestations of the condition. In such cases, causes and effects are difficult to disentangle without long-term prospective studies. Lifelong medical conditions conform to this paradigm. This is also the case with most psychiatric conditions, which explains, in part, why discrete causes have not yet been delineated for most forms of mental illness. Hence, syndromal descriptions are the most cogent way to characterize or categorize psychiatric conditions, given the present state of knowledge.

The word *illness* denotes the subjective suffering dimension of medical conditions (and overlaps with the role of being a patient); *syndrome* refers to a constellation of signs and symptoms; and *disease* is an etiologically defined entity. As diagrammed in Figure 11-2 (going from the bottom to the top), different diseases (etiologies) often result in the same clinical final pathway (the syndrome) which, depending on constitutional and environmental circumstances, manifests in pleomorphic symptomatology. Conversely (going from top to bottom in Fig. 11-2), one can conceptualize the function of diagnostic classification, in medicine and psychiatry, as facilitating the recognition of the prototypical or syndromal form into which the more pleomorphic illness manifestations cluster, with the ultimate hope of identifying underlying disease entities. The task of diagnosis is far more complex in psychiatry than in general medicine, because the typical form of a given mental disorder is often obscured by illness manifestations shaped by personality and sociocultural circumstances.

MENTAL DISORDER Nosology, the science of medical classification, pertains to the principles whereby the various syndromes and diseases comprising a given medical specialty are diagnosed and grouped. In the two major official psychiatric nosological systems, DSM-III-R and the ninth revision of the *International Classification of Diseases* (ICD-9), the term "mental disorder" is used in lieu of "mental disease" because of limitations in the current knowledge of etiology and pathogenesis. The preference for the term "disorder" over "syndrome" reflects the inclusion, particularly in DSM-III-R, of monosymptomatic clinical pictures that do not qualify as syndromes (e.g., functional encopresis, pathological gambling). Implicit in the classification of mental disorders into various categories is the assumption that separate disease entities underlie the various manifestations of psychopathology. The rigorous description and classification of mental disorders is considered a necessary step in establishing discrete disease entities.

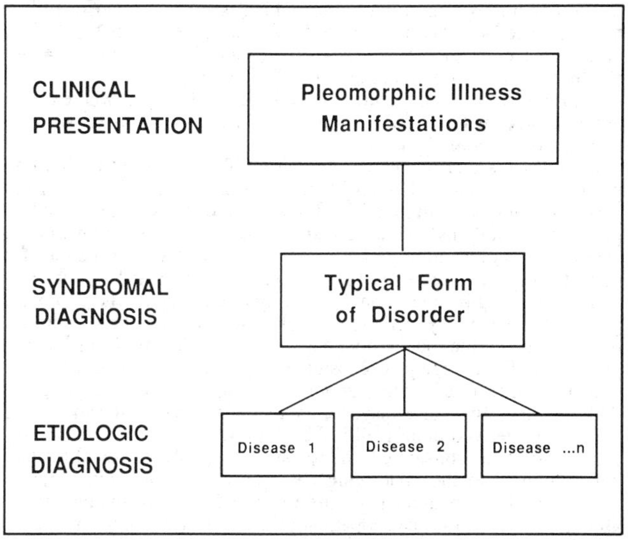

FIGURE 11-2. *Proposed relationship between symptomatic, syndromal, and etiological diagnoses.*

The demonstration of anatomical pathology is not necessary for the definition of an illness. Underlying somatic abnormalities are not established in many forms of such common medical conditions as hypertension, migraine, and arrythmia. Illness is a convention defined by the sufferer and physicians who consider it to be clinically significant or disabling. In the case of mental illness, it consists of behavioral, psychological, or somatic manifestations that cause suffering or impairment in functioning. An important qualification is that these manifestations must result from some structural, developmental, or behavioral abnormality within the patient and not solely reflect a conflict between the individual and a social system or subsystem.

Identification of structural abnormalities would clearly legitimize the medical status of mental disorders, but those who reject the medical model in psychiatry on the grounds that a structurally defined concept of disease is inapplicable tend to forget that caring for and alleviating the suffering of individual patients and preventing further disability by naturalistic methods is the more noble and central role of physicians since the time of Hippocrates.

CATEGORIES AND DIMENSIONS Another argument advanced against the legitimacy of the concept of illness as applied to mental disorders is rooted in the assumption that medical conditions are sharply demarcated from one another and from normality, whereas psychiatric disorders are not. This argument is part of a wider philosophical debate about the nature of disease. The Hippocratic school conceptualized disease as a dimensional outgrowth from premorbid characteristics; disease states were not sharply distinguished from health, and each case was viewed as unique. By contrast, the rival Platonic school postulated that diseases should be categorized into ideal types, distinct from one another.

The seemingly fuzzy dimensional approach has intuitive clinical appeal, especially to followers of the Freudian and Meyerian traditions. The categorical or typological approach, exemplified by Kraepelinian and neo-Kraepelinian biological psychiatry, appears more rigorous but must contend with the symptom overlap observed clinically in the various mental disorders. These two styles of conceptualizing illness represent different phases in the investigation of diseases. Initially, clinical researchers use the categorical approach to describe the essential qualities of a given illness and to discover etiologically relevant factors. As more is learned about a condition, the stage is set for extending its boundaries to describe atypical variants or attenuated expressions. The Washington University, RDC, and DSM-III-R criteria should be regarded as tools for categorizing the largely uncharted universe of mental illnesses.

The categorical approach has great heuristic merit in the early phases of a young discipline. The dimensional strategy, though useful in clinical conceptualization, may prove methodologically sterile unless it is coupled with its categorical counterpart. For instance, the relationship of cyclothymic personality to bipolar psychosis would not have developed without a rigorous typological definition that set manic-depressive illness apart from schizophrenia and personality disorders. It was this classic typology that permitted the delineation of the essential features of bipolar disorders and their subsequent description in attenuated forms.

Taken to the extreme, the dimensional approach is vulnerable to a violation of Aristotelian logic. For instance, to suggest a continuum between sound and music neglects the obvious fact that they are discontinuous in their essential qualities. Likewise, while clinical depression may on occasion seem to arise from "the blues," the clinical disorder tends to be autonomous and has qualities distinct from unhappiness. Despite such qualitative differences, in practice, the threshold used to define the clinical disorder is somewhat arbitrary and depends on the projected use of the category. For instance, a broad RDC definition (depression and four associated symptoms for 1 week) may be desirable for certain types of epidemiological research, while the more restrictive Washington University definition (full syndromal depression with at least five symptoms for over 4 weeks and with the added stipulation that it represents a break from premorbid functioning) is likely to be more informative when testing genetic hypotheses with familial aggregation of cases; an intermediate threshold, such as that in DSM-III-R (depression, anhedonia, or both plus five symptoms over 2 weeks) may suffice for general clinical purposes. This elasticity of the boundary between normal and morbid is not unique to psychiatry; similar questions arise in assessing hypertension, coronary artery disease, and cirrhosis. So, even where mild illness and normality are not easily demarcated, clinicians create categories by positing thresholds that enable them to recognize clinically significant levels of deviation from health.

METHODS OF PSYCHIATRIC CLASSIFICATION

Classification systems of mental disorders in widespread use are based on a mixture of symptoms and etiological criteria. Although they have been criticized repeatedly on theoretical and clinical grounds, preferable alternatives have not been found. Much has been written about the structural and psychometric principles to be considered in devising a scientific nosology of mental disorders. However, theoreticians with such preoccupations have typically failed to propose diagnostic schemas that are workable in practice. In fact, none of the diagnostic entities in current use evolved from complex statistical procedures, such as discriminant, factor, or cluster analysis.

Clinical proposals to substitute symptom-based diagnosis with projective test findings, ego defenses, behavioral analysis, or family interactional patterns for symptoms and etiological criteria have fared no better. These proposals begin by tabulating the shortcomings of the traditional approach (typically rejecting the notion that psychiatric diagnosis is a medical procedure) and proceed to focus on intrapersonal, personal, interpersonal, or social attributes. According to Kendell, the advantages of the proposed approach are emphasized, "but it is left to others to implement it. The would-be innovator either lacks the courage of his convictions or is daunted by the enormity of the task which he has set himself."

In psychiatry as in the rest of medicine, one continues to rely on etiological understanding in the few instances where this has been achieved, and on symptom-based systems of classification in most other situations. Reliance on these two principles is justified, because they continue to carry the greater predictive power for treatment response, course, and outcome.

CLASSIFICATION BASED ON SYMPTOMS Like all science, the study of psychopathology is based on systematic observation of natural phenomena. Although many morbid psychiatric phenomena were described in antiquity (e.g., melancholia, mania, paranoia), it was not until the nineteenth century that most current nosological entities evolved, primarily in French- and German-speaking countries in Europe. The humane treatment of the insane championed by Philippe Pinel, Jean Etienne Esquirol, and their disciples mandated a detailed description of patients' symptoms and habits. A major goal was to catalog which manifestations were associated with early discharge from the hospital and which were associated with long-term institutional care. Thus, for all the criticisms of asylum care of the mentally ill, this system had the important virtue of stimulating systematic clinical descriptions. Following Sydenham's model for general medicine, these descriptions were grouped into syndromes—idiocy, dementia, epileptic insanity, melancholia, circular insanity, paranoia, catatonia, hebephrenia—that ultimately culminated in the Kraepelinian system. This was the beginning of the science of psychiatry.

The Kraepelinian schema Kraepelin is rightfully considered the father of psychiatric nosology. He remains unequalled in his objective description of the signs and symptoms of psychiatric disorders; yet, he was not entirely satisfied with a purely descriptive approach, having discovered significant overlap of symptoms among the various syndromes. He therefore devised the prognostic principle which led to the now familiar division of the functional psychoses into dementia precox and manic-depressive illness. He hypothesized that the underlying neuropathological processes in these two conditions typically led to an irreversible deterioration in the former and to a cyclic or period course in the latter.

Although the Kraepelinian system brought much needed order to psychiatric nosology, it now needs to be modified in light of current concepts of adaptation, disease, and illness behavior. As in general medicine, apart from the virulence of contributing etiological agents, prognosis represents the cumulative effects of many nonetiological variables that reside both in the host and the environment. Thus, it is not surprising that 15 to 20 percent of mood disorders have a chronic course, either in the form of chronic depression or that of continuous rapid-cycling. Conversely, the course of schizophrenia is not invariably deteriorating. Interestingly, schizophrenia appears to have a distinctly better prognosis in Africa than in Western societies. Based on such considerations, psychiatrists can conclude that, although marked differences in outcome do suggest clinical heterogeneity, they need not invalidate the original diagnosis in an individual case.

Actually, laboratory, sociodemographic, and other findings associated with departures from the usual course of a given syndrome are useful in suggesting strategies that can bring about better control (treatment or prevention) for all patients or for those with a given outcome. For instance, concurrent or lithium-induced hypothyroidism in rapid-cycling bipolar disorders suggests the wisdom of thyroid supplementation. In the case of schizophrenia, the transcultural differences in outcome serve as a therapeutic rationale for providing less demanding tasks or jobs to schizophrenic patients living in Western countries.

Although the Kraepelinian schema can be faulted for its tendency to equate diagnosis with prognosis and for its relative overemphasis of disease aspects at the expense of personal considerations, the temporal stability of clusters of signs and symptoms—their pattern of recurrence or chronicity and alternation with other specified symptom clusters—represents a fundamental principle in the classification of mental disorders.

The Bleulerian schema While accepting the general validity of the disease processes Kraepelin delineated, Bleuler, under the influence of Freud and Jung, postulated that most illness manifestations arose from the interaction of a hypothesized somatic disease with the patient's personality and its psychological complexes. In schizophrenia, the underlying disease process was a relatively common physiological vulnerability, which in its grip of the psyche produced such primary signs as associative slippage, affective oscillations, and vaguely defined vegetative irregularities. The secondary manifestations, reflecting the patient's own complexes and experiences, included what Bleuler termed "fundamental" signs (affective impoverishment, ambivalence, and autism) and the "accessory" signs and symptoms (delusions, hallucinations, catatonia, personality deterioration). In giving major importance to the pathogenic influence of psychological factors, Bleuler did not consider such common manifestations of schizophrenia as delusions, hallucinations, and poor outcome to be basic to the disease process.

Bleuler's contributions to our understanding of schizophrenia were primarily theoretical. His delineation of primary and fundamental signs and symptoms did not have the descriptive rigor of Kraepelin's, and its widespread adoption led to the aforementioned unwarranted equation of "psychosis" with "schizophrenia."

Jaspers and Schneider—the phenomenological approach In the phenomenological approach of Karl Jaspers and of Kurt Schneider, one can an attempt to preserve Kraepelinian objectivity without sacrificing the personal. To achieve this, they required faithful descriptions of psychopathological phenomena as experienced by the patient. Jaspers recommended an interview style that relied on empathy rather than interpretation of the patient's experiences. Unlike interpretation, which represents a second order of abstraction, he believed that empathy helped the clinician to elicit the raw subjective data of psychopathology with the greatest precision and the least amount of observer interference. Further, the emphasis is on distinguishing the *content* of these experiences (which is linked to life conditions) from their *form* (which is hypothesized to reflect the influence of a disease process). For instance, when the patient describes the experience of hearing several voices arguing about whether his or her nose is longer than Pinocchio's, what is said about the nose reflects some understandable life situation, whereas the argumentative nature of the auditory hallucinations is ascribed to a hypothesized cerebral disturbance.

Both Jaspers and Schneider were especially interested in defining primary delusional or hallucinatory experiences, those whose form was psychologically irreducible. These were contrasted to secondary psychotic symptoms, which could be understood as a function of another psychological experience. For instance, the false belief of a patient with early dementia that one has been repeatedly robbed of one's purse may be due to one's inability to remember where one last placed the purse. By contrast, the delusion of thought withdrawal (e.g., the belief that one's thoughts are being stolen by being forcibly pulled out of one's brain) is considered a primary delusion, because it does not seem to arise from another psychopathological experience. Although the "first-rank" psychotic experiences that bear Schneider's name were derived empirically, they were developed in a theoretical framework that considered them psychologically irreducible and, hence, closest to the underlying neurophysiology of schizophrenia.

As should be apparent from the foregoing, the phenomenological approach organizes psychopathological manifestations into hierarchies. Some are conceptualized in terms of organic factors and called "process" disorders; others are conceptualized in biographical terms as either understandable "reactive" shifts from the normal or more protracted "development" from the premorbid self. Thus, schizophrenia is conceptualized as a process disease and neurotic conditions as abnormal developments. Based on such considerations, Schneider declared that there are no neuroses, only neurotics.

Jaspers' hierarchical approach had its origin, in part, in the ability of certain disorders to explain, or subsume the features of, other disorders. The hierarchy was topped by organic mental disorders, followed by epileptic, schizophrenic, and mood disorders, with neurotic and psychopathic personalities at the bottom. In this hierarchy, an organic mental disorder can have manifestations of disorders lower in the hierarchy (e.g., hallucinations, delusions, elation, depression, anxiety, or personality disturbances). The reverse, however, is not true, and the occurrence of manifestations typical of a disorder higher in the hierarchy would tend to invalidate a diagnosis of schizophrenia, mood disorder, or neurosis.

The hierarchical principle raises interesting questions about the relationship of descriptive and etiological classifications and the boundaries of the component syndromes. For instance, altered states of consciousness and related psychosensory disturbances that occur in some patients with schizophrenia and anxiety disorders (descriptively defined) would strengthen their kinship to organic disorders at the top of the hierarchy (thereby lending support to an organic etiology). Such instances illustrate the methodological virtues of the hierarchical principle. However, questions arise when mixed syndromes are considered (e.g., anxious depressions, which in Jaspers's hierarchy would be mood disorders but which are now viewed as being more closely related to neurotic disorders).

Although the theoretical aspects of Jaspers's and Schneider's schemas are fascinating, their lasting contributions to psychopathology and nosology reside in their emphasis on "living into" the patient's own morbid experiences and on rendering the subjective experiences of the mentally ill as precise data, to the extent that limitations of language allow. The emphasis is on disturbance of function, on form rather than content. Although this is the legitimate sense in which the terms "phenomenology" and "phenomenological" diagnosis should be used in psychiatry, in the United States "phenomenological" is often erroneously equated with "descriptive." Frank Fish was probably the major expositor in English of the work of the two giants of phenomenological psychiatry. The work of Wing and associates, summarized in the Present State Examination (PSE), is also largely inspired by the phenomenological tradition. Because the original German texts and their English translations were not widely read in the United States, it has been only in the past decade that the phenomenological approach has had pockets of influence in U.S. psychiatry. A more fundamental reason why the phenomenological approach was late in arriving on this continent lies in its philosophical clash with depth psychologies, for it is axiomatic of this approach that there is a point in psychopathology beyond which psychological probing cannot go—that, in short, it is impossible to totally understand the patient's morbid experiences in purely psychological terms.

CLASSIFICATION BASED ON ETIOLOGY

Somatic etiology Kraepelin, like many biological psychiatrists who followed his vision, believed that the task of classification would be simplified eventually by discovering the neuropathological basis of the major psychiatric syndromes (Alzheimer's dementia, delineated by and named for Kraepelin's disciple, is one such example). This was a significant advance that paved the way for recent pathophysiological concepts. Much work is still needed to determine how and why certain genetically vulnerable persons succumb to environmental factors (viral or others) that bring about the disease in the aging brain.

The etiological paradigm for psychiatric classification is also exemplified by the history of general paresis of the insane (GPI). Partly because of the dramatic nature of the discovery of the spirochetal etiology of GPI (which justified the fever therapies and earned the first Nobel Prize for a psychiatrist, Julius von Jauregg), it was hoped that all psychiatric disorders would eventually conform to such a model. Few such discoveries have been made since the search began almost a century ago. Furthermore, such discoveries do not typically account for more than a small proportion of cases within a given syndrome; 10 percent of the dementias in the early part of this century turned out to be secondary to syphilis. Also, as soon as advances in somatic etiology were made (e.g., with phenylketonuria, pellagra, or plumbism) the newly discovered diseases were appropriated by other medical specialties. Some illnesses that remain partly in the domain of psychiatry (e.g., mental retardation and organic mental disorders associated with psychoactive substance abuse or degenerative dementias) are considered not particularly attractive by other medical specialists.

The major problem with the GPI model for psychiatric classification and with etiological approaches in general, however, resides in the fact that they subscribe to a reductionistic and outdated model of disease that has its origin in Koch's postulates for infectious diseases. The view that single etiological agents are necessary and sufficient causes for illness has now been discarded by most branches of medicine, including the field of infectious disease. Modern medicine focuses increasingly on complex interactions between the organism and environment. Thus, myocardial infarction is not classified as a function of the risk factors that are thought to contribute to it, but by clinical manifestations and laboratory findings that result, over a long incubation period, from the interaction of such factors. To paraphrase an epidemiological dictum, the major causes for the most common psychiatric disorders (substance abuse disorders, personality disorders, mood and anxiety disorders, and the schizophrenias) are typically neither necessary nor sufficient but contributory.

Psychosocial stress as a taxonomic criterion Application of the multifactorial logic, undertaken first in mood disorders, has led to a model that views them as the final common pathway of a chain of interdependent causative factors. This means that no factor can be singled out, a priori, for its utility as a taxonomic criterion. Thus, earlier classifications of these disorders as "reactive" (neurotic and psychotic depressive reactions) and "endogenous" (manic-depressive and involutional melancholia), based on the presence or absence of psychosocial precipitants, have not received research support. In a large-scale prospective study (Table 11-1), it was found that neurotic depressions, wherein such precipitants were prominent, did not constitute a unitary syndrome, as evidenced by high rates of outcome into anxiety, melancholic, and bipolar disorders during prospective observation. The failure of life events to define a specific mood disorder is due to the fact that they are part of a complex multicausal chain (e.g., developmental experiences, personality, social supports), and it is unwieldy to attempt to incorporate such a multicausal chain into a nosological rubric.

A psychosocial stressor, therefore, should rarely be used as a taxonomic principle unless it is of a nature and intensity that most people, regardless of vulnerability, would be expected to react to, albeit transiently, with a mental disturbance. This is the rationale for including an adjustment disorder category in the psychiatric nomenclature. Other categories, such as post-traumatic stress disorder, brief reactive psychosis, or psychogenic psychosis, are of more dubious validity, because it is often impossible to demonstrate that the presumed stressor is acting independently of the patient's personality or that it was not triggered by the illness itself.

Psychodynamic approach Kraepelin hypothesized that major psychiatric disorders arose from their respective temperamental foundations (e.g., schizophrenia from the schizoid temperament and manic-depression from a spectrum of affective temperaments). However, emphasis on the pathogenetic role of antecedent developmental and personality factors is more commonly linked to psychodynamic approaches (especially as developed in this country), which, for several decades, exercised a dominant influence on formulations of the etiology of mental disorders.

In formulating his theoretical system of medical psychology, Freud was not primarily interested in developing diagnostic criteria. The major thrust of his work was devoted to understanding the personal

TABLE 11-1
Three- to Four-Year Prospective Follow-up in Neurotic Depressions (N = 100)

Diagnosis and Outcome	*N**
Manic episode	4
Hypomanic episode	14
Psychotic depression	21
Endogenous depression	36
Episodic course	42
"Unstable" characterological features	24
Social invalidism	35
Suicide	3

Table from Akiskal H, et al: The nosological status of neurotic depression: A prospective 3-2-4 year examination in light of the primary-secondary and unipolar-bipolar dichotomies. Arch Gen Psychiat *35:* 756, 1978, with permission.
*The total exceeds 100, because more than one outcome was possible per patient.

and developmental origin of psychopathological processes. Thus, the analytical perspective has proved singularly relevant to certain classes of clinical operations that explore unconscious motivating forces of behavior that have their origins in developmental vicissitudes. In more general terms, psychodynamic theory endeavors to trace the vulnerability to stressors to specified faults in long-term personality functioning.

Freud's outpatient neurology practice brought him into contact with a wide spectrum of psychiatric disorders not seen in the asylum practice of his contemporaries, observations from which laid the groundwork for many of the current concepts of anxiety and neurotic disorders. These were generally viewed as lifelong dispositions, initially conceived to be literally of neural origin (and therefore termed "actual neuroses") but later elaborated from a psychological standpoint (giving rise to the concept of psychoneuroses). Yet, the specificity of the various metapsychological concepts and defense mechanisms initially devised to explain these disorders and later extrapolated by Freud and others to the functional psychoses remains problematic. There is a growing consensus that psychodynamic concepts cut across formal nosological boundaries. Therefore, psychodynamic practice deriving from Freudian theory implicitly acknowledges the utility of a descriptive nosology. It could not be otherwise, because the soundness of psychodynamic interpretations depends on the observed accuracy of descriptive data. However, blurring of the descriptive diagnoses and psychodynamic interpretations is not uncommon, reflecting a more fundamental confusion between cause and meaning. Meehl has remarked in this connection:

> When we learn something about the inner life of a psychiatric patient, we find that he is concerned with aggression, sex, pride, dependence, and the like; that is, the familiar collection of human needs and fears. Schizophrenics are people, and if you are clever enough to find out what is going on inside a schizophrenic's head, you should not be surprised that these goings-on involve his self-image and his human relationships rather than, say, the weather. The demonstration that patients have psychodynamics, that they suffer with them, and that they deal with them ineffectively, does not necessarily tell us what is the matter with them; that is, why they are patients.

This quotation emphasizes Jaspers's distinction between the form of a symptom (or an illness) on the one hand and its psychodynamic content on the other. Mental content is derived from contexts, symbolization, and drives, whereas form is more likely to be determined by etiologically related antecedents. Thus, form and content are applicable to different clinical operations; diagnosis is based largely on form, with relatively little contribution from content. In other words, psychodynamic procedures and formal diagnoses address different aspects of psychopathology. They are best considered complementary. In practice, psychodynamic formulations can supplement formal diagnoses with clinically relevant information on the patient's core conflicts, habitual defenses, and adaptive mechanisms, setting the stage for treatment planning. The psychodynamic formulation needs not be restricted solely to patients suitable for long-term psychotherapy; it can be profitably applied even to psychotic patients. The main limitation of the psychodynamic formulation is methodological, the absence of a standardized approach that would command general consensus.

Limitations in our understanding of specific developmental and social factors in the origin of individual mental disorders preclude etiological classification based on psychosocial understanding for most of them. It is reasonable to expect that descriptive categories will be increasingly modified by advances in knowledge of somatic etiology; such an evolution is less likely with psychodynamic understanding because such understanding is typically more germane to the dynamics and therapy of the person than to the entire membership of a given category. This may change, however, with better operationalization of psychodynamic concepts, like that which has been achieved, for instance, in recent reformulation of such concepts into an ethological framework.

Laboratory findings When psychiatric disorders have established somatic etiology, laboratory findings are clearly useful, even necessary, in the diagnostic classification. However, laboratory findings do not necessarily reflect the specific cause of a disorder. The difficulties involved in applying etiological principles in the classification of mental disorders are no different from those encountered in general medicine, where diagnosis is often accomplished with no knowledge of etiology and is based on a clinical cluster plus characteristic laboratory findings. Lab findings rarely indicate cause; instead they reflect chemical, immunological, or histopathological properties of the disease state, which is itself the product of interaction between predisposing traits with proximate etiological agents. Typically, laboratory findings represent objective data, or signs, to corroborate (e.g., electroencephalography [EEG]), amplify (e.g., thyrotropin stimulation), or localize (e.g., computed tomography [CT] scan) clinical manifestations; only a few laboratory tests typically reveal pathognomonic data.

The diagnostic utility of emerging neuroscience technology has shown special promise in exploring the biology of mood disorders. The sensitivity (the percentage of positively identified cases) of these biological tests rarely surpasses 60 percent, and their specificity (the percentage of those without the disorder correctly excluded) remains to be established. As in general medicine, such laboratory correlates of depression support, rather than substitute for, clinical judgment based on history and syndromal criteria. Their greatest usefulness is in difficult or complex cases referred to specialized academic psychiatric centers where the base prevalence rate of the disorder under consideration is high. At present, these biological approaches are best viewed as attempts to quantify selected biological manifestations of depressive illness, just as the Beck Depression Inventory provides scores of cognitive disturbances and the Salpêtrière Retardation Scale assesses psychomotor disturbances. However, in drawing attention to the perturbed midbrain homeostasis, the biological measures demonstrate some of the disease processes underlying the clinical manifestations.

It was once believed that psychological tests would objectify psychiatric evaluation just as laboratory tests did medical evaluation. This promise has not been fulfilled, and there is no evidence that routinely used psychodiagnostic tests, such as projective techniques, reveal clinically useful data in addition to that obtainable through a systematic clinical interview. At best, most of these tests approximate what is already known about a given patient. Certain neuropsychological batteries can, in selected instances, reveal abnormalities not detectable through routine clinical interviews. As with biological test findings, the specificity of neuropsychological data is generally low, and they should be used to supplement, rather than replace, clinical judgment.

Test findings in psychiatry, whether biological or psychodiagnostic, more often corroborate than establish diagnoses. The quest for etiological factors in the most common psychiatric disorders is unlikely to be rewarding in terms of revising the current nosology unless the descriptive heterogeneity of each syndrome is reduced by recourse to some associated clinical or biological features, such as age of onset, family history, response to a specific therapeutic intervention, and cognitive, physiological, or chemical measures or challenges. Such strategies will have the greatest chance of uncovering discrete disease entities that represent specific genetic faults or have trait markers of vulnerability.

MULTIAXIAL CLASSIFICATION

The foregoing discussion highlighted the advantages and limitations of classification systems based on symptoms and on etiological approaches. Multiaxial classifications are designed to incorporate the main features of both approaches. Thus, different axes would address aspects of the clinical disorder important, respectively, for diagnostic categorization, treatment, and prognosis: descriptive diagnosis (e.g., a delusional syndrome); relevant precipitating circumstances (e.g., amphetamine); mode of onset (e.g., acute); personality (e.g., antisocial); and duration (e.g., weeks) or course (e.g., full recovery). In the example provided, both schizophreniform and amphetamine psychosis would receive the same descriptive diagnosis.

The multiaxial approach was first officially proposed for use in the evaluation of psychiatrically disturbed children. In an informal way, it has been used for a long time by psychiatrists who characterize themselves as eclectic and holistic, who in practice supplement the official diagnosis with a formulation that summarizes the major assets and liabilities of the patient from a biopsychosocial perspective. Thus, in one form or another, multiaxial evaluation of patients has always been attractive to psychiatrists. A major problem with the formal application of such multiaxial schemes is how to limit the number of axes. The more comprehensive one endeavors to be, the greater will be the number of axes and the closer the diagnosis will be to a descriptive essay on the patient, thus the value of diagnosis as a shorthand for communication among professionals is undercut and, in turn, the ability of clinical researchers to use diagnostic categorization for advancing knowledge of causes (and, ultimately, instituting control measures) is compromised.

Multiaxial classification should not be confused with the polyaxial approach, in which a given patient is evaluated against the criteria for one disorder as they are posited by different systems (e.g., Kraepelinian, Bleulerian, Schneiderian, Langfeldt's, ICD-9, RDC, DSM-III-R, PSE, Washington University, Taylor-Abrams, Vienna Research Criteria). The purpose of a polyaxial diagnostic exercise is to examine the performance of each set of criteria in predicting treatment response, prognosis, and related outcome measures. The polyaxial approach, then, is primarily a research strategy, but to the extent that it evaluates the patient according to different criteria sets, it compares the utility of each set for making predictions that vary across a wide range of variables. Thus, different sets of criteria for the same disorder would incorporate several different axes of a multiaxial classification. For instance, the Kraepelinian, DSM-III-R, and Washington University criteria for schizophrenia combine clinical description, age of onset, and social outcome; the Bleulerian and Schneiderian criteria are based essentially on clinical description.

RELIABILITY, VALIDITY, AND CURRENT SYSTEMS

RELIABILITY *Reliability,* the consistent use of diagnostic rubrics or the extent to which different clinicians agree on the diagnoses of a series of patients, is essential to communication in clinical medicine. This characteristic is usually measured by Cohen's kappa statistic, which computes the degree of agreement beyond chance (0.0), +1.0 being perfect agreement and –1.0, total lack of agreement.

Unreliability arises primarily as a result of criterion variance (e.g., different clinicians using different methods to arrive at diagnoses). For instance, a psychiatrist who uses Kraepelin's requirement that there be at least some deterioration of personality in schizophrenia will not diagnose this disorder nearly as often as will one who adheres to Schneider's "first rank" symptoms.

Less common sources of diagnostic inconsistency are information variance (e.g., clinicians have access to different data bases about the patient), observation variance (e.g., clinicians presented with the same stimuli record different observations), and interpretation variance (e.g., clinicians attach different psychopathological significance to a given experience or behavior). If diagnostic evaluation is limited to cross-sectional examination, occasion variance (e.g., patient depressed at time 1 and hypomanic at time 2) can further contribute to diagnostic disagreement.

Unambiguous diagnostic criteria and rigorous training in phenomenology are the most important means of reducing diagnostic discrepancies. These and other approaches to improving reliability are summarized in Table 11-2. Diagnostic accuracy is greatest when an experienced clinician with phenomenological sophistication has access to all sources of clinical information, not merely cross-sectional mental status, and follows a systematic diagnostic procedure based on specified operational criteria. Diagnostic data are elicited from human interaction, which requires extensive training, skill, and empathy. Clearly, this task cannot be performed adequately by computers.

VALIDITY The validity of a psychiatric classification is a function of how adequately the component diagnostic entities serve the purposes of communication, control, and comprehension. Communication is achieved by phenomenological rigor (face and descriptive validity); control, by predictive power (predictive validity); and comprehension, by etiological understanding (construct validity).

TABLE 11-2
Improving the Reliability of Psychiatric Diagnoses

Source of Diagnostic Discrepancy	*Suggested Solution*
Information variance	Obtain full history
Occasion variance	Combine cross-sectional and longitudinal pictures
Criterion variance	Explicit operational (inclusion and exclusion) criteria
Interpretation variance	Set thresholds for symptoms and hierarchical rules for diagnoses

Face validity *Face validity* is informed clinical consensus that assigns a diagnostic rubric to a set of manifestations commonly encountered in clinical practice. This is the beginning phase of identifying discrete nosological entities. A diagnostic rubric created by consensus may represent a variant of a familiar disorder, a new disorder, or a clinical thread that is common to several existing disorders. Personality diagnoses represent the least validated group of psychiatric conditions; except for antisocial personality, and possibly schizotypal personality and cyclothymic disorders, most characterological rubrics have not yet achieved validity beyond this elementary level. Their continued use, however, indicates that they have sufficient face validity to be useful in clinical communication.

Descriptive validity *Descriptive validity* is achieved when the defining characteristics of a syndrome are relatively unique and permit sufficient delineation from other disorders. This is the case with the major psychiatric syndromes, such as dementia, delirium, schizophrenia, melancholia, bipolar disorder, anorexia nervosa, obsessive-compulsive disorder, and transsexualism. Descriptive validity requires, at a minimum, the provision of a characteristic constellation of signs and symptoms (inclusion criteria) as well as rules by which this constellation is distinguished from overlapping conditions (exclusion criteria). Descriptive validity makes it likely, but does not guarantee, that other types of validity exist for a given category.

Predictive validity Clinically, the most important function of diagnosis is that aspect which embodies treatment implications, course, and possible complications. For instance, bipolar disorder has good *predictive validity* with respect to lithium response and cyclic course and to possible suicidal outcome with inadequate treatment. Again predictive validity implies, but does not guarantee, construct validity (for instance, in the case of bipolar disorder, a hypothesized metabolic, membrane, or receptor abnormality on which lithium might exert its therapeutic action).

Construct validity *Construct validity* refers to etiologically relevant factors associated with a given disorder that support a theory of pathogenesis. Examples for mood disorders include monozygotic-dizygotic twin differences, familial distribution of the illness, premorbid personality, and selected neuroendocrine and neurophysiological findings. The demonstration of construct validity will eventually lead to better means of controlling the disorder based on understanding of pathophysiology rather than empirical serendipity.

WASHINGTON UNIVERSITY APPROACH Until recently, it was widely believed that psychiatric diagnoses were unreliable and generally invalid. The challenge of changing this stereotype was taken up by Eli Robins and other members of the psychiatry department at Washington University, St. Louis. The approach they developed builds on the classical descriptive tradition of European psychiatry and relies heavily on family history and course of illness. The five steps of the procedure are: (1) clinical inclusion criteria or description along syndromal lines, further qualified by characteristic demographic features, such as gender and age of onset; (2) delimitation from other disorders by exclusion criteria; (3) family study, documenting the occurrence of specific psychiatric disorders in first-degree biological relatives; (4) laboratory studies, which, when this approach was first enunciated, were considered relevant primarily to the neuropsychiatric disorders (e.g., complex partial seizures, dementia, pellagra psychosis); and (5) follow-up study to provide longitudinal validation of the psychopathological clusters observed in cross section.

The major contribution of the St. Louis group was the development of clearly formulated operational criteria for the major psychiatric diagnoses that were generally arranged polythetically (i.e., each patient who qualified for a given diagnosis has many, but not necessarily all, of the features characteristic of the group). This system of diagnosis is less restrictive, and therefore clinically more realistic, than the monothetic approach, which stipulates that all patients so diagnosed meet all the features of that diagnosis. Despite the heterogeneity entailed in polythetic diagnoses, the Washington University criteria achieved good interrater reliability (Table 11-3). In addition to extensive work on the familial aspects of these disorders, the St. Louis group undertook systematic, long-term follow-up studies to demonstrate the temporal stability of the symptom clusters defined by these operational criteria.

TABLE 11-3
Interrater Diagnostic Agreement (Kappa Coefficient) in Major Psychiatric Disorders

*Diagnosis**	*All Patients (N = 101)*	*Excluding Undiagnosed (N = 71)*
Depression	.55	.70
Mania	.82	.93
Anxiety neurosis	.76	.84
Schizophrenia	.58	.66
Antisocial personality	.81	.85
Alcoholism	.74	.73
Drug dependence	.84	.85
Hysteria (female subjects only)	.72	.72
Obsessional illness	.78	.79
Homosexuality	.85	.79
Organic brain syndrome	.29	.36
Average concordance	.66	.75

Table from Helzer J, et al: Reliability of psychiatric diagnosis. Arch Gen Psychiat *34:* 136, 1977, with permission.
*Excluded from this investigation are anorexia nervosa and transsexualism (because of their rarity in the sample) and phobic disorders (which carry a wide range).

DSM-III The first official classification of mental disorders, a special section of the sixth revision of ICD (ICD-6) published in 1948, was generally considered unacceptable in most countries because of its heavy reliance on unproven etiological concepts. The alternative American classification (the first edition of the *Diagnostic and Statistical Manual of Mental Disorders* [DSM-I]), which appeared in 1952, was no less etiological, relying primarily on Meyer's pathogenetic views of "reaction types." The second edition of DSM (DSM-II), which became official in 1968, represented relatively little improvement aside from the fact that it abandoned the Meyerian view; diagnostic entities were still defined in brief descriptive essays.

DSM-III represents a radical departure from its predecessors, primarily because of its heavy emphasis on operational criteria pretested for adequate reliability. Validity was given less precedence, leading to some lively debates within the profession. These resulted in compromises intended to enhance the day-to-day clinical utility of the manual for all constituencies of the profession. The discussion below is a critical assessment of the innovative features of this new diagnostic classification.

Atheoretical philosophy The chief architects of DSM-III—the American Psychiatric Association (APA) Task Force on Nomenclature and Statistics—generally opted for terms they considered atheoretical. There were, however, some inconsistencies. For example, although the term "melancholia" has clear-cut biochemical connotations, it was introduced as a subtype of major depression. Yet, the term "neurosis," because of its etiological (psychodynamic) implications, was relegated to a parenthetical reminder of the older terminology for the anxiety disorders. In view of recent developments in the biology of panic disorder, one could argue that Freud's concept of "actual" neurosis has much to recommend it. Another questionable revision is the substitution of the term "disorganized" for "hebephrenic": other types of schizophrenia are also characterized by disorganization. These inconsistencies notwithstanding, the descriptive philosophy of DSM-III is solidly rooted in the rich clinical tradition of European psychiatry as modified by American empiricism.

Operational criteria Resolved to reduce criterion variance, the authors of DSM-III selected diagnostic criteria primarily on the basis of their reliability. They also considered the evidence for validity in terms of either etiology (for the organic mental disorders) or family history and course; these are listed as associated features. The selection of diagnostic criteria and categories on the basis of existing reliability and validity data represents a landmark methodological achievement in the history of psychiatry. Furthermore, the operational nature of the classification ensures that the various sections are open for further revision or refutation as new data accumulate.

The authors of DSM-III were charged with the task of providing the profession with a scientific nosology that reflected experience with both inpatient and outpatient settings. The 13 validated St. Louis categories could not serve the needs of the entire profession for terminology. So, in many of the newly created categories, validity is limited to the level of clinical consensus (face validity); yet, by enunciating operational criteria, DSM-III has facilitated the scientific study of important areas of clinical psychiatry. This is particularly striking in the personality disorders, which, in the preoperational era, were rarely studied with the requisite rigor.

Diagnostic hierarchies DSM-III, following the tradition of its predecessors, essentially endorsed Jaspers' hierarchical principle, giving precedence to the diagnosis of organic mental disorders, even in the presence of features of the functional disorders (e.g., schizophrenic, affective, or neurotic). However, for reasons discussed earlier in this chapter, DSM-III reversed the hierarchical order of the functional disorders, according affective illness precedence over schizophrenic manifestations unless the two are so intermingled that neither diagnosis is tenable (a condition dubbed "schizoaffective"). Another major hierarchical departure was the development of a separate axis for personality disorders, to ensure that they would not be neglected at the bottom of the hierarchy. (In Jaspers' hierarchy, personality disorders were to receive independent diagnoses only when all "higher" disorders were excluded.) To ensure maximum clinical usefulness, DSM-III, like DSM-II, also permits multiple Axis I diagnoses in selected instances; these may be from different categories (e.g., mood and substance use disorders) or within the same category (e.g., cyclothymic and bipolar disorders). When multiple diagnoses are made, the clinician must specify the principal diagnosis, the one chiefly responsible for occasioning clinical consultations at the index evaluation (e.g., alcohol withdrawal delirium that brings a patient with a schizophrenic disorder to the hospital).

A major hierarchical departure of DSM-III from its predecessors is the abandonment of "psychosis" and "neurosis" as classifying principles. For instance, in DSM-II, affective disorders were dispersed in the entire classification and listed under psychotic, neurotic, and personality disorders. In DSM-III all affective disorders are grouped together, and the term "psychosis" is only used as a qualifier. The category of anxiety disorders subsumes many, but not all, traditional neurotic disorders. Neurotic depression is now reclassified under the "dysthymic" and "major depressive" rubrics. Thus, except for childhood and organic mental disorders, the classification in DSM-III is along subspecialty lines organized around syndromes (e.g., substance use disorders, affective disorders, anxiety disorders, eating disorders). Inconsistent with this philosophy, however, is the creation of a new borderline personality category denuded of its original genetic and psychodynamic meanings and placed within the general class of personality disorders. Recent research has shown that, like neurosis and psychosis, borderline conditions cut across most major diagnostic categories and do not emerge as circumscribed nosological entities.

Diagnostic uncertainties An important feature of DSM-III is the provision of explicit rules to be used in situations where the information is insufficient (diagnosis to be deferred or provisional) or the patient's clinical presentation and history do not meet the full criteria of a prototypical category (an atypical, residual, or otherwise unspecified subclass within the general category).

Multiaxial system The multiaxial scheme of DSM-III assists clinicians in separating developmental and personality disorders (Axis II), social stressors (Axis IV), and degree of adaptive functioning (Axis V) from the underlying form of the disorder, which is represented by the descriptive and syndromal diagnosis (Axis I). The clinician is also expected to assess any relevant physical disease (Axis III) that may cause, contribute to, precipitate, maintain, or modify the expression of the Axis I disorder or interact with its treatment. For a discussion of the Axis IV and Axis V codes, see Section 9.2, Psychiatric Report.

This approach differs from other proposed multiaxial schemes in that several parameters (i.e., cross-sectional description, age of onset, mode of onset, and course) are collapsed in arriving at Axis I diagnoses. This would mean, for instance, that in incorporating the requirement of some degree of deterioration, DSM-III endorses the Kraepelinian concept of schizophrenia over the Bleulerian and the Schneiderian concepts.

DSM-III rules are not entirely explicit with respect to causality in the multiaxial scheme. It is generally assumed that Axis II disorders, particularly personality disorders, are predisposing or concurrent factors. Yet, personality disorders can represent complications of Axis I disorders. The same can be said about psychosocial stressors. Finally, although one of the main reasons for coding the highest level of adaptive functioning is to acknowledge the patient's assets, social functioning could also reflect the sequelae of the Axis I disorder.

Multiaxial diagnosis entails complex clinical judgments far more difficult than those in general medicine because of the limited knowledge of pathogenesis and the large number of variables involved in the usual case of psychiatric illness. The interface of physical and psychiatric illness represents a particular challenge (i.e., deciding whether an Axis III medical disorder or a pharmacological agent so fully accounts for the origin and maintenance of an Axis I condition, such as mood disorder, that the designation of an "organic mood disorder" is justified). Although this is not intended, and despite disclaimers, this choice of terminology nevertheless conveys the inaccurate implication that other mood disorders do not have a biological basis.

It thus appears that in its praiseworthy endeavor to paint a more holistic picture of the individual patient, the DSM-III multiaxial scheme falls short on methodological grounds. The multiaxial scheme at present is not structured in such a way as to contribute significantly to scientific progress on etiology, and, at best, it would serve primarily as an aid to clinical formulation.

DSM-III-R Despite dissenting views, it was felt that 7 years of experience with DSM-III and advances in clinical research constituted sufficient grounds to improve the reliability and the clinical utility of the diagnostic manual. The process exemplifies the philosophic openness of DSM-III to change when new data warrant revisions. Most of the revisions were more in the nature of tightening the operational criteria for the various disorders, specifying subtypes or qualifying phrases bearing on treatment, and adding new evidence for validity in the text devoted to associated features. The entire revised classification and cautionary statement are reproduced in Table 11-4. Selected revisions are highlighted below.

Organic mental disorders In addition to organic mood and personality disorders, DSM-III-R now recognizes an organic anxiety syndrome. As discussed earlier in connection with mood and schizophreniform disorders, unambiguous rules for assigning organic status are not provided, and one could opt to code the suspected organic cause on Axis III. Indeed, the entire section of organic mental disorders would have been simplified by restricting Axis I to syndromal diagnoses (e.g., delirium, dementia, delusional disorder) and coding the etiology on Axis III in all instances (e.g., pneumonia, Alzheimer's disease, cocaine abuse).

Schizophrenia The cutoff age for onset (45 years) is eliminated in recognition of the fact that late-onset schizophrenic or paraphrenic conditions, albeit uncommon, do exist.

Mood disorders This revision of terminology replaces the broader designation "affective disorders," which technically subsumed both mood and anxiety disorders. Major depression is now specified with respect to seasonal pattern (which has implications for treatment with phototherapy) and chronicity (in recognition of the fact that residual depression occurs in 15 to 20 percent of cases). Both major depressive and manic episodes are now rated for severity. The specifications for dysthymia now tend to acknowledge that early-onset primary dysthymia represents the core subgroup within this heterogeneous realm.

Anxiety disorders The hierarchical rules have been changed so that when anxiety and major depressive disorders coexist, both diagnoses can be given. Panic disorder and phobic avoidance with agoraphobic coloring are more closely aligned, the latter being viewed as a complication of the former. Generalized anxiety disorder is now diagnosed only after a duration of 6 months. Finally, DSM-III-R recognizes that transient delusions in the setting of an obsessive-compulsive disorder do not signal schizophrenia.

Sleep disorders Operational criteria are proposed to aid in evaluating common sleep complaints seen in psychiatric practice. Sleepwalking and sleep-terror disorders are classified here, rather than in the section on childhood disorders. The same logic applied to functional enuresis (retained in the section for childhood disorders) would have led to similar reclassification in the section of sleep disorders.

Axis I–Axis II shifts By moving the category of mental retardation with developmental disorders to Axis II, DSM-III-R attempted to provide a unifying conceptual base for Axis II: disorders that begin in childhood or adolescence and persist in adult life. However, this logic would also dictate the transfer of, among others, transsexualism, cyclothymia, dysthymia, some forms of attention-deficit hyperactivity, and, possibly, somatization and generalized anxiety disorders to Axis II.

NINTH REVISION OF THE *INTERNATIONAL CLASSIFICATION OF DISEASES* This World Health Organization (WHO) classification of diseases, now in its ninth revision, is used in the United States in a clinically modified version (known as ICD-9 CM) to take into consideration specific clinical subtypes of disease that U.S. physicians consider to be important in their clinical and research endeavors (Table 11-5). These should be used by U.S. psychiatrists to code Axis III physical disorders when making DSM-III-R diagnoses.

Chapter V of ICD-9 is devoted to psychiatry. Unlike DSM-III-R, ICD-9 is not multiaxial and limits itself to the more formal diagnostic categories that DSM-III-R lists on Axes I and II. Specific diagnoses within ICD-9 generally correspond to those in DSM-III-R and have the same codes. However, ICD-9 also lists certain categories preferred by one national school or another (e.g., bouffée délirante, which in France is used in lieu of the Scandinavian schizophreniform or reactive psychosis and overlaps to some extent with the categories of brief reactive and atypical psychoses in the American classification). The French rubric (literally, "acute delusional turmoil") has descriptive merits that other rubrics do not and, as supported by U.S. and Danish genetic investigations of schizophrenia, has the terminological virtue of divorcing these disorders from process schizophrenia.

FUTURE PERSPECTIVES

During the present decade, the DSM and the Section of Mental Disorders in the ICD system have come closer, to serve the important goal of a shared language in psychiatry worldwide. This is a particularly important methodological issue in psychiatry where, in the absence of laboratory confirmation for most mental disorders, classification continues to rely primarily on description. Both DSM-IV and ICD-10 are expected to be official sometime in the early 1990s. American psychiatrists familiar with the DSM system would be interested to know of parallel developments in the ICD system. ICD-10 will, in part, retain the descriptive essay approach that characterized ICD-9. It will also make use of operational criteria for diagnosis, although in a somewhat less formal fashion than DSM-III-R. The definitions of the specific disorders in the proposed ICD-10 might nevertheless prove to be explicit enough to permit adequate reliability in ordinary clinical operations. These diagnostic guidelines will be welcomed by clinicians who object to DSM-III-R's somewhat arid style. A set of more explicit diagnostic criteria for research will also be provided in ICD-10.

This chapter has described recent developments in the classification of mental disorders from historical, methodological, and clinical perspectives. The emerging consensus is that the reliable categorization of the phenomena of mental illness is a necessary step in the search for valid etiological factors, be they biological, psychological, or social. To safeguard the progress achieved thus far, several qualifications need to be reiterated:

1. Structured diagnostic interviews do not necessarily achieve the highest degree of reliability. Administration of such interviews by nonclinician research assistants cannot substitute for an experienced and skilled phenomenologist who has access to all available clinical data. In other words, clinical judgment is indispensable. Yet, clinical judgment not coupled with a systematic approach is also inadequate.

2. Reliability does not guarantee validity. Multiple permutations of symptomatologic criteria (the construction of mathematical clusters and multiaxial or polyaxial diagnostic systems, and an ever-increasing number of rating instruments and structured interview schedules) do not carry one too far in the absence of validating correlates external to the symptom picture.

3. Phenomenological and psychodynamic approaches to psychopathology are complementary. Psychodynamic formulation may provide clinical insights and understanding currently unattainable with a purely descriptive diagnostic approach. A major challenge for psychiatry is to achieve at least some clinical standardization in arriving at such formulations.

4. High specificity of putative familial-genetic and laboratory approaches is not a prerequisite for diagnostic or clinical utility. Used in conjunction with symptomatologic criteria, especially in uncertain or difficult clinical situations, these biological approaches can enhance clinical judgment. For instance, consecutive-generation family history of classical bipolar disorder in a patient with early-onset recurrent depressions would suggest the wisdom of lithium therapy. Likewise, shortened rapid eye movement (REM) latency and related circadian sleep abnormalities in someone with unstable personality functioning should raise the suspicion of an underlying mood disorder. Future editions of DSM will not be worthwhile if some progress along these lines does not influence diagnostic decisions.

TABLE 11-4
DSM-III-R Classification of Axis I and Axis II Categories and Codes

CAUTIONARY STATEMENT

The specified diagnostic criteria for each mental disorder are offered as guidelines for making diagnoses, since it has been demonstrated that the use of such criteria enhances agreement among clinicians and investigators. The proper use of these criteria requires specialized clinical training that provides both a body of knowledge and clinical skills.

These diagnostic criteria and the DSM-III-R classification of mental disorders reflect a consensus of current formulations of evolving knowledge in our field but do not encompass all the conditions that may be legitimate objects of treatment or research efforts.

The purpose of DSM-III-R is to provide clear descriptions of diagnostic categories in order to enable clinicians and investigators to diagnose, communicate about, study, and treat the various mental disorders. It is to be understood that inclusion here, for clinical and research purposes, of a diagnostic category such as pathological gambling or pedophilia does not imply that the condition meets legal or other nonmedical criteria for what constitutes mental disease, mental disorder, or mental disability. The clinical and scientific considerations involved in categorization of these conditions as mental disorders may not be wholly relevant to legal judgments, for example, that take into account such issues as individual responsibility, disability determination, and competency.

DISORDERS USUALLY FIRST EVIDENT IN INFANCY, CHILDHOOD, OR ADOLESCENCE

DEVELOPMENTAL DISORDERS
Note: These are coded on Axis II.

Mental Retardation
317.00 Mild mental retardation
318.00 Moderate mental retardation
318.10 Severe mental retardation
318.20 Profound mental retardation
319.00 Unspecified mental retardation

Pervasive Developmental Disorders
299.00 Autistic disorder
Specify if childhood onset
299.80 Pervasive developmental disorder NOS

Specific Developmental Disorders
Academic skills disorders
315.10 Developmental arithmetic disorder
315.80 Developmental expressive writing disorder
315.00 Developmental reading disorder

Language and speech disorders
315.39 Developmental articulation disorder
315.31* Developmental expressive language disorder
315.31* Developmental receptive language disorder

Motor skills disorder
315.40 Developmental coordination disorder
315.90* Specific developmental disorder NOS

Other Developmental Disorders
315.90* Developmental disorder NOS

Disruptive Behavior Disorders
314.01 Attention-deficit hyperactivity disorder

Conduct disorder
312.20 group type
312.00 solitary aggressive type
312.90 undifferentiated type
313.81 Oppositional defiant disorder

Anxiety Disorders of Childhood or Adolescence
309.21 Separation anxiety disorder
313.21 Avoidant disorder of childhood or adolescence
313.00 Overanxious disorder

Eating Disorders
307.10 Anorexia nervosa
307.51 Bulimia nervosa
307.52 Pica
307.53 Rumination disorder of infancy
307.50 Eating disorder NOS

Gender Identity Disorders
302.60 Gender identity disorder of childhood
302.50 Transsexualism
Specify sexual history: asexual, homosexual, heterosexual, unspecified
302.85* Gender identity disorder of adolescence or adulthood, nontranssexual type
Specify sexual history: asexual, homosexual, heterosexual, unspecified
302.85* Gender identity disorder NOS

Tic Disorders
307.23 Tourette's disorder
307.22 Chronic motor or vocal tic disorder
307.21 Transient tic disorder
Specify: single episode or recurrent
307.20 Tic disorder NOS

Elimination Disorders
307.70 Functional encopresis
Specify: primary or secondary type
307.60 Functional enuresis
Specify: primary or secondary type
Specify: nocturnal only, diurnal only, nocturnal and diurnal

Speech Disorders Not Elsewhere Classified
307.00* Cluttering
307.00* Stuttering

Other Disorders of Infancy, Childhood, or Adolescence
313.23 Elective mutism
313.82 Identity disorder
313.89 Reactive attachment disorder of infancy or early childhood
307.30 Stereotypy/habit disorder
314.00 Undifferentiated attention-deficit disorder

ORGANIC MENTAL DISORDERS

Dementias Arising in the Senium and Presenium
Primary degenerative dementia of the Alzheimer type, senile onset
290.30 with delirium
290.20 with delusions
290.21 with depression
290.00* uncomplicated
(Note: code 331.00 Alzheimer's disease on Axis III)

Code in fifth digit:
1 = with delirium, 2 = with delusions,
3 = with depression, 0* = uncomplicated.
290.1x Primary degenerative dementia of the Alzheimer type, presenile onset, ______
(Note: code 331.00 Alzheimer's disease on Axis III)
290.4x Multi-infarct dementia, ______
290.00* Senile dementia NOS
Specify etiology on Axis III if known
290.10* Presenile dementia NOS
Specify etiology on Axis III if known (e.g., Pick's disease, Jakob-Creutzfeldt disease)

Psychoactive Substance-Induced Organic Mental Disorders

Alcohol
303.00 intoxication
291.40 idiosyncratic intoxication
291.80 uncomplicated alcohol withdrawal
291.00 withdrawal delirium
291.30 hallucinosis
291.10 amnestic disorder
291.20 dementia associated with alcoholism

Amphetamine or similarly acting sympathomimetic
305.70* intoxication
292.00* withdrawal
292.81* delirium
292.11* delusional disorder

Caffeine
305.90* intoxication

Cannabis
305.20* intoxication
292.11* delusional disorder

Cocaine
305.60* intoxication
292.00* withdrawal
292.81* delirium
292.11* delusional disorder

Hallucinogen
305.30* hallucinosis
292.11* delusional disorder
292.84* mood disorder
292.89* posthallucinogen perception disorder

Inhalant
305.90* intoxication

Nicotine
292.00* withdrawal

Opioid
305.50* intoxication
292.00* withdrawal

Phencyclidine (PCP) or similarly acting arylcyclohexylamine
305.90* intoxication
292.81* delirium
292.11* delusional disorder
292.84* mood disorder
292.90* organic mental disorder NOS

Sedative, hypnotic, or anxiolytic
305.40* intoxication
292.00* uncomplicated sedative, hypnotic, or anxiolytic withdrawal
292.00* withdrawal delirium
292.83* amnestic disorder

Other or unspecified psychoactive substance
305.90* intoxication
292.00* withdrawal
292.81* delirium
292.82* dementia
292.83* amnestic disorder
292.11* delusional disorder
292.12 hallucinosis
292.84* mood disorder
292.89* anxiety disorder
292.89* personality disorder
292.90* organic mental disorder NOS

Organic Mental Disorders associated with Axis III physical disorders or conditions, or whose etiology is unknown.

293.00 Delirium
294.10 Dementia
294.00 Amnestic disorder
293.81 Organic delusional disorder
293.82 Organic hallucinosis
293.83 Organic mood disorder
Specify: manic, depressed, mixed
294.80* Organic anxiety disorder
310.10 Organic personality disorder
Specify if explosive type
294.80* Organic mental disorder NOS

PSYCHOACTIVE SUBSTANCE USE DISORDERS

Alcohol
303.90 dependence
305.00 abuse

Amphetamine or similarly acting sympathomimetic
304.40 dependence
305.70* abuse

Cannabis
304.30 dependence
305.20* abuse

Cocaine
304.20 dependence
305.60* abuse

Hallucinogen
304.50* dependence
305.30* abuse

Inhalant
304.60 dependence
305.90* abuse

Nicotine
305.10 dependence

Opioid
304.00 dependence
305.50* abuse

Phencyclidine (PCP) or similarly acting arylcyclohexylamine
304.50* dependence
305.90* abuse

Sedative, hypnotic, or anxiolytic
304.10 dependence
305.40* abuse
304.90* Polysubstance dependence
304.90* Psychoactive substance dependence NOS
305.90* Psychoactive substance abuse NOS

SCHIZOPHRENIA

Code in fifth digit: 1 = subchronic, 2 = chronic, 3 = subchronic with acute exacerbation, 4 = chronic with acute exacerbation, 5 = remission, 0 = unspecified.

Schizophrenia
295.2x catatonic, ______
295.1x disorganized, ______
295.3x paranoid, ______
Specify if stable type
295.9x undifferentiated, ______
295.6x residual, ______
Specify if late onset

DELUSIONAL (PARANOID) DISORDER

297.10 Delusional (paranoid) disorder
Specify type: erotomanic
grandiose
jealous
persecutory
somatic
unspecified

PSYCHOTIC DISORDERS NOT ELSEWHERE CLASSIFIED

298.80 Brief reactive psychosis
295.40 Schizophreniform disorder
Specify: without good prognostic features or with good prognostic features
295.70 Schizoaffective disorder
Specify: bipolar type or depressive type
297.30 Induced psychotic disorder
298.90 Psychotic disorder NOS (atypical psychosis)

MOOD DISORDERS

Code current state of major depression and bipolar disorder in fifth digit:
1 = mild
2 = moderate
3 = severe, without psychotic features
4 = with psychotic features (*specify* mood-congruent or mood-incongruent)
5 = in partial remission
6 = in full remission
0 = unspecified

For major depressive episodes, *specify* if chronic and *specify* if melancholic type.

For bipolar disorder, bipolar disorder NOS, recurrent major depression, and depressive disorder NOS, *specify* if seasonal pattern.

Bipolar Disorders

Bipolar disorder
296.6x mixed, ______
296.4x manic, ______
296.5x depressed, ______
301.13 Cyclothymia
296.70 Bipolar disorder NOS

Depressive Disorders

Major depression
296.2x single episode, ______
296.3x recurrent, ______
300.40 Dysthymia (or depressive neurosis)
Specify: primary or secondary type
Specify: early or late onset
311.00 Depressive disorder NOS

ANXIETY DISORDERS (or anxiety and phobic neuroses)

Panic disorder
300.21 with agoraphobia
Specify current severity of agoraphobic avoidance
Specify current severity of panic attacks
300.01 without agoraphobia
Specify current severity of panic attacks
300.22 Agoraphobia without history of panic disorder
Specify with or without limited symptom attacks
300.23 Social phobia
Specify if generalized type
300.29 Simple phobia
300.30 Obsessive-compulsive disorder (or obsessive-compulsive neurosis)
309.89 Post-traumatic stress disorder
Specify if delayed onset
300.02 Generalized anxiety disorder
300.00 Anxiety disorder NOS

SOMATOFORM DISORDERS

300.70* Body dysmorphic disorder
300.11 Conversion disorder (or hysterical neurosis, conversion type)
Specify: single episode or recurrent
300.70* Hypochondriasis (or hypochondriacal neurosis)
300.81 Somatization disorder
307.80 Somatoform pain disorder
300.70* Undifferentiated somatoform disorder
300.70* Somatoform disorder NOS

DISSOCIATIVE DISORDERS (or hysterical neuroses, dissociative type)

300.14 Multiple personality disorder
300.13 Psychogenic fugue
300.12 Psychogenic amnesia
300.60 Depersonalization disorder (or depersonalization neurosis)
300.15 Dissociative disorder NOS

SEXUAL DISORDERS

Paraphilias

302.40 Exhibitionism
302.81 Fetishism
302.89 Frotteurism
302.20 Pedophilia
Specify: same sex, opposite sex, same and opposite sex
Specify if limited to incest
Specify: exclusive type or nonexclusive type
302.83 Sexual masochism
302.84 Sexual sadism
302.30 Transvestic fetishism
302.82 Voyeurism
302.90* Paraphilia NOS

Sexual Dysfunctions

Specify: psychogenic only, or psychogenic and biogenic (Note: If biogenic only, code on Axis III)
Specify: lifelong or acquired;
Specify: generalized or situational

Sexual desire disorders
302.71 Hypoactive sexual desire disorder
302.79 Sexual aversion disorder

Sexual arousal disorders
302.72* Female sexual arousal disorder
302.72* Male erectile disorder

Orgasm disorders
302.73 Inhibited female orgasm
302.74 Inhibited male orgasm
302.75 Premature ejaculation

Sexual pain disorders
302.76 Dyspareunia
306.51 Vaginismus
302.70 Sexual dysfunction NOS

TABLE 11-4 *(Continued)*

Other Sexual Disorders
302.90*† Sexual disorder NOS

SLEEP DISORDERS
Dyssomnias
Insomnia disorder
307.42* related to another mental disorder (nonorganic)
780.50* related to known organic factor
307.42* Primary insomnia
Hypersomnia disorder
307.44 related to another mental disorder (nonorganic)
780.50* related to a known organic factor
780.54 Primary hypersomnia
307.45 Sleep-wake schedule disorder
Specify: advanced or delayed phase type, disorganized type, frequently changing type
Other dyssomnias
307.40* Dyssomnia NOS

Parasomnias
307.47 Dream anxiety disorder (nightmare disorder)
307.46* Sleep terror disorder
307.46* Sleepwalking disorder
307.40* Parasomnia NOS

FACTITIOUS DISORDERS
Factitious disorder
301.51 with physical symptoms
300.16 with psychological symptoms
300.19 Factitious disorder NOS

IMPULSE CONTROL DISORDERS NOT ELSEWHERE CLASSIFIED
312.34 Intermittent explosive disorder
312.32 Kleptomania
312.31 Pathological gambling
312.33 Pyromania
312.39* Trichotillomania
312.39* Impulse control disorder NOS

ADJUSTMENT DISORDER
Adjustment disorder
309.24 with anxious mood
309.00 with depressed mood
309.30 with disturbance of conduct
309.40 with mixed disturbance of emotions and conduct
309.28 with mixed emotional features
309.82 with physical complaints
309.83 with withdrawal
309.23 with work (or academic) inhibition
309.90 Adjustment disorder NOS

PSYCHOLOGICAL FACTORS AFFECTING PHYSICAL CONDITION
316.00 Psychological factors affecting physical condition
Specify physical condition on Axis III

PERSONALITY DISORDERS
Note: These are coded on Axis II.
Cluster A
301.00 Paranoid
301.20 Schizoid
301.22 Schizotypal
Cluster B
301.70 Antisocial
301.83 Borderline
301.50 Histrionic
301.81 Narcissistic
Cluster C
301.82 Avoidant
301.60 Dependent
301.40 Obsessive compulsive
301.84 Passive aggressive
301.90 Personality disorder NOS

V CODES FOR CONDITIONS NOT ATTRIBUTABLE TO A MENTAL DISORDER THAT ARE A FOCUS OF ATTENTION OR TREATMENT
V62.30 Academic problem
V71.01 Adult antisocial behavior

V40.00 Borderline intellectual functioning (Note: This is coded on Axis II.)

V71.02 Childhood or adolescent antisocial behavior
V65.20 Malingering
V61.10 Marital problem
V15.81 Noncompliance with medical treatment
V62.20 Occupational problem
V61.20 Parent-child problem
V62.81 Other interpersonal problem
V61.80 Other specified family circumstances
V62.89 Phase of life problem or other life circumstance problem
V62.82 Uncomplicated bereavement

ADDITIONAL CODES
300.90 Unspecified mental disorder (nonpsychotic)
V71.09* No diagnosis or condition on Axis I
799.90* Diagnosis or condition deferred on Axis I

V71.09* No diagnosis or condition on Axis II
799.90* Diagnosis or condition deferred on Axis II

†This disorder is a residual category for unspecified sexual malfunctions. Ego-dystonic sexual orientation disturbance per se is eliminated.

TABLE 11-5
ICD-9-CM (Clinical Modification) Classification of Mental Disorders

ORGANIC PSYCHOTIC CONDITIONS (290-4)	
Senile and Presenile—(290)	
290.0	Senile dementia, uncomplicated
290.1	Presenile dementia
.11	—with delirium
.12	—with delusional features
.13	—with depressive features
290.2	Senile dementia with delusional or depressive features
.20	—with delusional features
.21	—with depressive features
.3	—with delirium
Arteriosclerotic Dementia (290.4)	
290.40	—uncomplicated
.41	—with delirium
.42	—with delusional features
.43	—with depressive features
290.8	Other specified senile psychotic conditions
.9	Unspecified senile psychotic conditions
Alcoholic Psychoses (291)	
291.0	Alcohol withdrawal delirium
.1	Alcohol amnestic syndrome
.2	Other alcoholic dementia
.3	Alcohol withdrawal hallucinosis
.4	Idiosyncratic intoxication
.5	Alcoholic jealousy
.8	Other specified—psychosis
.9	Unspecified—psychosis
Drug Psychoses (292)	
292.0	Drug withdrawal syndrome
.11	— -induced organic delusional syndrome
.12	— -induced hallucinosis
.2	Pathological drug intoxication
292.8	Other specified drug -induced mental disorders (OMD)
.81	— -induced delirium
.82	— -induced dementia
.83	— -induced amnestic syndrome
.84	— -induced organic affective syndrome
.89	Other
.9	Unspecified drug-induced mental disorder
Transient Organic Psychotic Conditions (293)	
293.0	Acute delirium
293.1	Subacute delirium
293.8	Other specified and transient (OMD)
.81	Organic delusional syndrome
.82	—hallucinosis syndrome
.83	—affective syndrome
.89	Other
.9	Unspecified transient OMD
Other Organic Psychotic Conditions (Chronic) (294)	
294.0	Amnestic syndrome
.1	Dementia in conditions classified elsewhere
.8	Other specified OBS (chronic)
.9	Unspecified OBS (chronic)
OTHER PSYCHOSES	
Schizophrenic Disorders (295) @	
295.0	Simple type
.1	Disorganized type
.2	Catatonic type
.3	Paranoid type
.4	Acute schizophrenic episode
.5	Latent schizophrenia
.6	Residual —
.7	Schizo-affective type
.8	Other specified types of schizophrenia
.9	Unspecified —
Affective Psychoses (296) @@	
296.0	Manic disorder, single episode
.1	—, recurrent episode
296.2	Major depressive disorder, single episode
.3	—, recurrent episode
296.4	Bipolar affective disorder, manic
.5	—, depressed
.6	—, mixed
.7	—, unspecified
296.8	Manic-depressive psychosis, other and unspecified
296.80	—, unspecified
.81	Atypical manic disorder
.82	Atypical depressive disorder
.89	Other
296.90	Unspecified affective psychosis
.99	Other specified —
Paranoid States (297)	
297.0	Paranoid state, simple
.1	Paranoia
.2	Paraphrenia
.3	Shared paranoid disorder
.8	Other specified paranoid states
.9	Unspecified paranoid state
Other Nonorganic Psychoses (298)	
298.0	Depressive type psychosis
.1	Excitative type psychosis
.2	Reactive confusion
.3	Acute paranoid reaction
.4	Psychogenic paranoid psychosis
.8	Other and unspecified reactive psychosis
.9	Unspecified psychosis
Psychoses with Origin Specific to Childhood (299)	
299.0	Infantile Autism
.1	Disintegrative psychosis
.8	Other specified early childhood psychosis
.9	Unspecified
NEUROTIC DISORDERS, PERSONALITY DISORDERS, AND OTHER NONPSYCHOTIC MENTAL DISORDERS	
Neurotic Disorders (300)	
300.0	Anxiety states
.00	Anxiety state, unspecified
.01	Panic disorder
.02	Generalized anxiety disorder
.09	Other
300.01	Hysteria
.10	Hysteria, unspecified
.11	Conversion disorder
.12	Psychogenic amnesia
.13	Psychogenic fugue
.14	Multiple personality
.15	Dissociative disorder or reaction unspecified
.16	Factitious illness with psychological symptoms
.19	Other and unspecified factitious illness
300.2	Phobic disorders
.20	Phobia, unspecified
.21	Agaraphobia with panic attacks
.22	—without mention of panic attacks
.23	School phobia
.29	Other isolated or simple phobias
300.3	Obsessive-compulsive disorders
300.4	Neurotic depression
300.5	Neurasthenia
300.6	Depersonalization syndrome
300.7	Hypochondriasis
300.8	Other neurotic disorders
.81	Somatization disorder
.89	Other
.9	Unspecified neurotic disorder

Personality Disorders (301)
301.0 Paranoid personality disorder
.1 Affective personality disorder
.10 —, unspecified
.11 Chronic hypomanic personality disorder
.12 Chronic depressive personality disorder
.13 Cyclothymic disorder
301.2 Schizoid personality disorder
.20 —, unspecified
.21 Introverted personality
.22 Schizotypal personality
301.3 Explosive personality disorder
301.4 Compulsive personality disorder
301.5 Histrionic personality disorder
.50 —, unspecified
.51 Chronic factitious illness with physical symptoms
.59 Other histrionic personality disorder
301.6 Dependent personality disorder
301.7 Antisocial personality disorder
301.8 Other personality disorders
.81 Narcissitic personality
.82 Avoidant personality
.83 Borderline personality
.84 Passive-aggressive personality
.89 Other
.9 Unspecified personality disorder

Sexual Deviations and Disorders (302)
302.0 Homosexuality
.1 Zoophilia
.2 Pedophilia
.3 Transvestism
.4 Exhibitionism
302.5 Trans-sexualism
.50 —with unspecified sexual history
.51 —with asexual history
.52 —with homosexual history
.53 —with heterosexual history
302.6 Disorders of psychosexual identity
302.7 Psychosexual dysfunction
.70 —, unspecified
.71 — with inhibited sexual desire
.72 — with inhibited sexual excitement
.73 — with inhibited female orgasm
.74 — with inhibited male orgasm
.75 — with premature ejaculation
.76 — with functional dyspareunia
.79 — with other specified sexual dysfunction
302.8 Other specified psychosexual dysfunction
.81 Fetishism
.82 Voyeurism
.83 Sexual masochism
.84 Sexual sadism
.85 Gender identity disorder of adolescent or adult life
.89 Other (nymphomania, satyriasis)
.9 Unspecified psychosexual disorder

Alcohol Dependence Syndrome (303)*
303.0 Acute alcohol intoxication
.9 Other and unspecified alcohol dependence

Drug Dependence (304)
304.0 Opioid type dependence
.1 Barbiturate and similarly acting sedative or hypnotic dependence
.2 Cocaine dependence
.3 Cannabis dependence
.4 Amphetamine and other psycho-stimulant dependence
.5 Hallucinogen dependence
.6 Other specified drug dependence
.7 Combinations of opioid type drug with any other
.8 Combinations of drug dependence including opioid type drug
.9 Unspecified drug dependence

Nondependent Abuse of Drugs (305)
305.0 Alcohol abuse
.1 Tobacco use disorder
.2 Cannabis abuse
.3 Hallucinogen abuse
.4 Barbiturate and similarly acting sedative or hypnotic abuse
.5 Opioid abuse
.6 Cocaine abuse
.7 Amphetamine or related acting sympathetomimetic abuse
.8 Other, mixed, or unspecified drug abuse

Physiologic Malfunction Arising from Mental Factors (306)
306.0 Muscoskeletal
.1 Respiratory
.2 Cardiovascular
.3 Skin
.4 Gastrointestinal
.5 Genitourinary
306.50 Psychogenic genitourinary malfunction, unspecified
.51 Psychogenic vaginismus
.52 Psychogenic dysmenorrhea
.53 Psychogenic dysuria
.59 Other
306.6 Endocrine
306.7 Organs of special sense
306.8 Other specified psychophysiological malfunction
.9 Unspecified psychophysiological malfunction

Special Symptoms or Syndromes, Not Elsewhere Classified (307)
307.0 Stammering and stuttering
307.1 Anorexia nervosa
307.2 Tics
.20 Tic disorder, unclassified
.21 Transient tic disorder of childhood
.22 Chronic motor tic disorder
.23 Gilles de la Tourette's disorder
307.3 Stereotyped repetitive movements
307.4 Specific disorders of sleep of non organic origin
.40 Non organic sleep disorder, unspecified
.41 Transient disorder of initiating or maintaining sleep
.42 Persistent disorder of initiating or maintaining sleep
.43 Transient disorder of initiating or maintaining wakefulness
.44 Persistent disorder of initiating or maintaining wakefulness
.45 Phase-shift disruption of 24-hour sleep-wake cycle
.46 Somnambulism or night terrors
.47 Other dysfunctions of sleep stages or arousal from sleep
.48 Repetitive intrusions of sleep
.49 Other
307.5 Other and unspecified disorders of eating
.50 Eating disorder, unspecified
.51 Bulemia
.52 Pica
.53 Psychogenic remination
.54 Psychogenic vomiting
.59 Other
307.6 Enuresis
307.7 Encopresis
307.8 Psychalgia
.80 Psychogenic pain, site specified
.81 Tension headache
.89 Other (psychogenic backache)
307.9 Other and unspecified special symptoms or syndromes, not classified elsewhere

Acute Reaction to Stress (308)
308.0 Predominant disturbance of emotions
.1 Predominant disturbance of consciousness
.2 Predominant psychomotor disturbance
.3 Other acute reactions to stress
.4 Mixed disorders as reaction to stress

Adjustment Reaction
309.0 Brief depressive reaction
.1 Prolonged depressive reaction
309.2 With predominant disturbances of other emotions
.21 Separation anxiety disorder
.22 Emancipation disorder of adolescence and early adult life
.23 Specific academic or work inhibition
.24 Adjustment reaction with anxious mood
.28 Adjustment reaction with mixed emotional features
.29 Other (culture shock)
309.3 With predominant disturbance of conduct
309.4 With mixed disturbance of emotions and conduct
309.8 Other specified adjustment reactions

.81 Prolonged posttraumatic stress disorder
.82 Adjustment reaction with physical symptoms
.83 Adjustment reaction with withdrawal
.89 Other

Specific Nonpsychotic Mental Disorders Due to Organic Brain Damage (OBD) (310)
310.0 Frontal lobe syndrome
.1 Organic personality syndrome
.2 Post concussion syndrome
.8 Other unspecified nonpsychotic mental disorders following OBD
.9 Unspecified nonpsychotic mental disorder following OBD

Depressive Disorder, Not Elsewhere Classified (311)
Disturbance of Conduct,—(312)
312.0 Undersocialized conduct disorder, aggressive type
.1 —, unaggressive type
.2 Socialized conduct disorder
312.3 Disorders of impulse control, not elsewhere classified
.30 Impulse control disorder, unspecified
.31 Pathological gambling
.32 Kleptomania
.33 Pyromania
.34 Intermittent explosive disorder
.35 Isolated explosive disorder
.39 Other
312.4 Mixed disturbance of conduct and emotions
312.8 Other specified disturbance of conduct, not elsewhere classified
312.9 Unspecified disturbance of conduct (juvenile delinquency)

Disturbance of Emotions Specific to Childhood and Adolescence (313)
313.0 Overanxious disorder
.1 Misery and unhappiness disorder
313.2 Sensitivity, shyness and social withdrawal disorder
.21 Shyness disorder of childhood
.22 Introverted disorder of childhood
.23 Elective mutism
313.3 Relationship problems
313.8 Other or mixed emotional disturbances of childhood or adolescence
.81 Oppositional disorder
.82 Identity disorder
.83 Academic underachievement disorder
.89 Other

Hyperkinetic Syndrome of Childhood (314)
314.0 Attention deficit disorder
.00 Without mention of hyperactivity
.01 With hyperactivity
.1 Hyperkinesis with developmental delay
.2 Hyperkinetic conduct disorder
.8 Other specified manifestations of hyperkinetic syndrome

Specific Delays in Development (315)
315.0 Specific reading disorder
.00 Reading disorder, unspecified
.01 Alexia
.02 Developmental dyslexia
.09 Other
315.1 Specific arithmetical disorder
.2 Other specified learning difficulties
315.3 Developmental speech or language disorder
.31 Developmental language disorder
.39 Other
315.4 Coordination disorder
.5 Mixed development disorder
.8 Other specified delays in development
.9 Unspecified delay in development

Psychic Factors Associated with Diseases Classified Elsewhere (316)
Use additional code to identify any associated physical condition

MENTAL RETARDATION (MR)
317 Mild mental retardation
318 Other specified mental retardation
.0 Moderate mental retardation (IQ 35–49)
.1 Severe mental retardation (IQ 20–34)
.2 Profound mental retardation (IQ < 20)
319 Unspecified mental retardation

Table from World Health Organization: *Manual of the International Classification of Diseases, Injuries, and Causes of Death,* 9 revision, clinical modification. World Health Organization, Geneva, 1979, with permission.
Key: — refers to diagnostic term immediately above
@ The following fifth digit classification is for use with category 295:

0 unspecified
1 subchronic
2 chronic
3 subchronic with acute exacerbation
4 chronic with acute exacerbation
5 in remission

@@ The following fifth digit subclassification is for use with categories 296.0–296.6:

0 unspecified
1 mild
2 moderate
3 severe, without mention of psychotic behavior
4 severe, specified as with psychotic behavior
5 in partial or unspecified remission
+ Fifth-digit subclassifications are to be used with categories 312.0–312.2
0 unspecified 1 mild 2 moderate 3 severe

REFERENCES

Akiskal H S: Diagnosis and classification of affective disorders: New insights from clinical and laboratory approaches. Psychiat Develop *1:* 123, 1983.

Akiskal H S, Webb W L, editors: *Psychiatric Diagnosis: Exploration of Biological Predictors*. Spectrum, New York, 1978.

Berner P, Gabriel E, Katschnig H, Kieffer W, Koehler K, Lenz G, Simhandl C: *Diagnostic Criteria for Schizophrenic and Affective Psychoses*. American Psychiatric Press, Washington, DC, 1983.

Bleuler E: *Dementia Praecox or the Group of Schizophrenias*. International Universities Press, New York, 1950.

Carroll B J: Dexamethasone suppression test: A review of contemporary confusion. J Clin Psychiat *46:* 13, 1985.

Feighner J P, Robins E, Guze S B, et al: Diagnostic criteria for use in psychiatric research. Arch Gen Psychiat *26:* 57, 1972.

Frances A, Widiger T: The classification of personality disorders: An overview of problems and solutions. In *Psychiatry Update: American Psychiatric Association Annual Review,* R Hales, A Frances, editors, vol 5, p 240. American Psychiatric Press, Washington, DC, 1986.

Freud S: On the grounds for detaching a particular syndrome from neurasthenia under the description "anxiety neurosis." In *Sigmund Freud,* J Strachey, editor, vol III, p 91. Hogarth, London, 1962.

Goodwin D W, Guze S B: *Psychiatric Diagnosis,* ed 3. Oxford University Press, New York, 1984.

Hamilton M, editor: *Fish's Clinical Psychopathology*. John Wright, Bristol, England, 1985.

Jaspers K: *General Psychopathology* (Hoenig J, Hamilton M W, trans). Manchester University Press, Manchester, England, 1963.

Kendell R E: *The Role of Diagnosis in Psychiatry*. Blackwell, London, 1975.

Klein D F, Gittelman R, Quitkin F, Rifkin A: *Diagnosis and Drug Treatment of Psychiatric Disorders: Adults and Children,* ed 2. Williams & Wilkins, Baltimore, 1980.

Kraepelin E: *Manic-Depressive Insanity and Paranoia*. Livingstone, Edinburgh, 1921.

Meehl P E: *Psychodiagnosis: Selected Papers*. University of Minnesota Press, Minneapolis, 1973.

Millon T, Klerman G L: *Contemporary Directions on Psychopathology: Towards the DSM-IV*. Guilford, New York, 1986.

Perry S, Cooper A M, Michels R: The psychodynamic formulation: Its purpose, structure, and clinical application. Amer J Psychiat *144:* 543, 1987.

Schneider K: *Clinical Psychopathology*. Grune & Stratton, New York, 1959.

Slater E, Roth M: *Mayer-Gross' Clinical Psychiatry,* ed 3, revised. Williams & Wilkins, Baltimore, 1977.

Spitzer R L, Endicott J, Robins E: Research diagnostic criteria. Arch Gen Psychiat *35:* 773, 1978.

Stone M H: *The Borderline Syndrome: Constitution, Personality, and Adaptation*. McGraw-Hill, New York, 1980.

Wing J K, Cooper J E, Sartorius N: *The Measurement and Classification of Psychiatric Symptoms*. Cambridge University Press, Cambridge, 1974.

CHAPTER 12 ORGANIC MENTAL SYNDROMES AND DISORDERS

THOMAS B. HORVATH, M.D.
LARRY J. SIEVER, M.D.
RICHARD C. MOHS, Ph.D.
KENNETH DAVIS, M.D.

INTRODUCTION

DEFINITION The organic mental syndromes (OMSs) and organic mental disorders (OMDs) constitute a group of behavioral disorders whose distinctive symptoms are largely the result of brain dysfunctions detectable by current methods of clinical and laboratory evaluation. These disorders are grouped together because of a shared known or presumed etiology and represent the one area of psychiatry that has advanced from mere syndromal diagnosis to disease diagnosis and a comprehensive understanding of pathophysiology. It is these disorders that bring psychiatrists closer to their medical colleagues and contribute to the movement to "remedicalize" the discipline. Advances in neuropathology, neuroanatomy, and neurochemistry have changed the perception and improved treatment of such diseases as neurosyphilis, pellagra, Wernicke's encephalopathy, and, most recently, Alzheimer's disease. The rise of an empirical, etiologically agnostic, descriptive classification system in psychiatry during the past decade has contributed to better definitions and nomenclature in this area as well. The main advances in the field, however, will continue to be generated by a better understanding of the underlying pathophysiology based on investigative breakthroughs in neuroscience.

The current revised third edition of the *Diagnostic and Statistical Manual of Mental Disorders* (DSM-III-R) makes a distinction between OMSs and OMDs. An OMS is a constellation of experiential and behavioral signs and symptoms whose etiology or pathophysiology is unknown. An OMD is a particular OMS in which the etiology or pathophysiology is known and is included in the definition of the disorder on Axis I or Axis III. For practical reasons, psychoactive substance-induced OMDs are included in the chapter on psychoactive substance use disorders.

The essential feature of an OMS or OMD is an experiential or behavioral abnormality associated with transient or permanent dysfunction of the brain. However, no single clinical description characterizes them in DSM-III-R in marked contrast to the second edition of *Diagnostic and Statistical Manual of Mental Disorders* (DSM-II), which defined organic brain syndromes (OBSs)—as they were then called—by the following symptoms: impairment of orientation, impairment of memory, impairment of intellectual functions such as comprehension, calculation, knowledge, learning, impairment of judgment, and lability and shallowness of affect. It further divided brain syndromes into psychotic and nonpsychotic disorders according to the severity of functional impairment and distinguished acute disorders from chronic ones on the basis of whether the brain pathology and the accompanying organic syndrome were reversible.

The current World Health Organization's *International Classification of Diseases* (ICD-9) and its clinical modification (ICD-9CM) continue to define organic conditions in a manner similar to DSM-II. For instance, organic psychotic conditions (ICD-9 code nos. 290–294) are defined as syndromes in which there is impairment of orientation, memory, comprehension, calculation, learning capacity, and judgment. There may also be shallowness or lability of affect or a more persistent disturbance of mood, lowering of ethical standards and exaggeration or emergence of personality traits, and diminished capacity for independent decision. Schizophreniform, affective, or paranoid psychoses (295–299) are excluded from 290–294, even though they may be associated with organic conditions. Neurotic and personality disorders occurring in association with a physical condition are coded just as are their functional equivalents in 300–309, with an additional code to identify the physical condition. Finally, there is a residual category (310) for specific nonpsychotic mental disorders following brain damage. This currently includes a frontal lobe syndrome, a postconcussional syndrome, and cognitive or personality changes of other types. In marked contrast, Table 12-1 illustrates the various presenting syndromes for which a diagnosis of an OMS or OMD should be considered using the differential diagnostic algorithms of DSM-III-R.

These protean manifestations of brain impairment classified under the broad categories of OMS and OMD have received reasonable acceptance in the United States, but considerable skepticism has greeted these ideas in Europe and the United Kingdom, as shown by the likely persistence of the older nomenclature. Yet, DSM-III-R has both practical and theoretical merits. The practical requirement that virtually any behavioral and experiential abnormality be evaluated for

TABLE 12-1
Clinical Presentation of the OMSs and OMDs

1. Psychotic features: delusions, hallucinations, incoherence, marked loosening of association, poverty of content of thought, markedly illogical thinking, behavior that is bizarre, grossly disorganized, or catatonic.
2. Anxiety features: irrational anxiety in panic or persistent form manifested by motor tension, autonomic hyperactivity, apprehensive expectation, and hypervigilance; and/or avoidance of objects or situations associated with anxiety.
3. Affective features: depressed, irritable, or expansive mood and its cognitive and vegetative concomitant features.
4. Features usually associated with personality disorders: antisocial, aggressive, violent, defiant, or oppositional behavior; suspiciousness; emotional lability, impaired impulse control or social judgment; marked apathy and indifference.
5. Cognitive features: short- and long-term memory disturbance; disturbance of attention and orientation; impairment of intellectual abilities severe enough to interfere with social or occupational functioning; academic or learning difficulties; disturbances of high cortical function; aphasia, apraxia, agnosia, "constructional difficulties."

Table adapted from DSM-III-R *Diagnostic and Statistical Manual of Mental Disorders,* ed 3, revised. Copyright American Psychiatric Association, Washington, DC, 1987. Used with permission.

organic causes by an adequate history, physical examination, and appropriate laboratory tests should reveal that a considerable number of physical disorders present with psychological symptoms. The empirical finding that virtually all functional mental disorders have an organic counterpart should eventually lead to an understanding of their common pathophysiology and to the disappearance from the nomenclature of an outdated Cartesian dualism.

The concept of OMSs and OMDs represents a practical way of separating a group of mental disorders in the management of which medical diagnosis and treatment play an important part. From a theoretical and ideological point of view, however, the concept is deeply flawed and erroneous. In the last half of the twentieth century, it has become abundantly clear that all behaviors, normal as well as pathological, arise from the organic substratum of the brain. Many disorders previously classified as functional, such as schizophrenia, mood, and panic disorders, were shown to have specific neurophysiological dysfunctions at their core. Evidence was also gathered about the neurobiological substrates of several personality disorders. In the last quarter of the century, a complimentary understanding of brain–cognition–behavior also emerged. Sperry, the 1984 Nobel laureate neurophysiologist, phrased it eloquently: "Our current view no longer interprets the emergent mental properties as passive correlates of cerebral activity but rather as integral working components with causal potency." Eric Kandell and other neuroscientists have described precise ways in which learning and experience play critical roles in functional and structural neural alterations.

The concept of OMSs may be misleading in two practical ways as well. It may lead clinicians to underestimate the biological causation and treatment of certain functional disorders. The practical success of psychopharmacology minimizes this error to some extent, but the increasing participation of nonmedically trained psychotherapists in the treatment of less severe mental disorders is likely to lead to the erroneous conclusion that less severe forms of a disease are less likely to be biological in origin. However, the reverse error can be detected in the management of organic disorders when medical and pharmacological interventions are used to the exclusion of sound principles of environmental modification and of psychotherapy.

PROBLEMS OF DEFINITION A practical definition of OMDs or OMSs may include those disorders of human experience and behavior that are associated with coarse abnormalities in the biological function or structure of the brain. This is necessarily a fluid definition, for several reasons. The texture of descriptions of the range of behavior is becoming ever finer, and even subtle alterations previously dismissed as idiosyncratic or missed altogether are finding clinical significance. Likewise, observations on brain structure and function are also becoming ever more refined and accurate. Some years ago, the OMDs, lying on the border of psychology, psychiatry, neurology, and medicine, were conveniently neglected by members of all these disciplines. (Nurses and social workers did not have the luxury of ignoring them, but, in their preoccupation with taking care of the sufferers, they failed to advance scientific knowledge about the disorders.) Recent developments have made these disorders scientifically more attractive and have led to a variety of territorial disputes about the borders and internal structure of these organic syndromes. Biological psychiatry, neuropsychology, behavioral neurology, and metabolic medicine have all laid claims to some of them: there is competition for Alzheimer's disease, for focal neurological syndromes, for multi-infarct dementias, and for metabolic and infectious encephalopathies. The fact that the current possessor of the territory may change nomenclature complicates the problem. (Witness the semantic confusion among the terms "delirium," "acute confusional state," and "metabolic encephalopathy" or among the terms "Alzheimer's disease," "primary degenerative dementia," and "senile dementia.")

This chapter will use the terminology officially sanctioned by DSM-III-R. However, practitioners wishing to communicate with their colleagues in neurology or internal medicine will be well advised to be aware of the terminology used by those specialists. For these reasons, the appropriate synonyms are listed in each section and any discrepancies in the coverage of various terms is explored.

It is not enough to learn to communicate with other physicians. More than just traces of DSM-II persist in the mental health professions, as shown by loose references to OBS. Outdated terminology causes certain conceptual problems as well as imprecision. DSM-II and ICD-9 recognize only cognitive presentation of OMDs, although they can be manifested through affective, behavioral, and psychotic symptoms. Furthermore, a variety of distinct syndromes can be recognized with some diagnostic specificity: delirium, dementia, amnestic syndrome, organic mood and personality disorders, organic delusional disorder, and hallucinosis. The lingering practice of referring to a patient's condition as an OBS misses important distinctions in prognosis and treatment response.

Two other problems of the old nomenclature can cause confusion: the psychotic-nonpsychotic and the acute-chronic dichotomies. The psychotic-nonpsychotic division based on severity is misleading. There are often significant diurnal variations in behavior *(sundowning);* a patient who is in daytime cooperative and mildly confused can develop intractable agitation and total disorientation at night. Furthermore, severity is not unidimensional: Severe disruption of language and praxis due to posterior cerebral damage are more noticeably abnormal, but less socially disruptive, than the behavioral improprieties committed by the frontal lobe–damaged patient with intact verbal skills.

The acute-chronic dichotomy represents an idiosyncratic use of terminology restricted to psychiatry. Normally in clinical medicine, acuity refers to rapidity of development, but in DSM-II it referred to reversibility. To be consistent, the slow, almost imperceptible but fully reversible mental deterioration seen in myxedema would have to be called an acute brain syndrome in DSM-II, while the sudden, incremental deterioration seen in the course of multi-infarct dementia would by definition be chronic.

The classifications of the third edition of the *Diagnostic and Statistical Manual of Mental Disorders* (DSM-III) and DSM-III-R reject these confusing descriptions in favor of clear, operationally defined diagnostic criteria. The DSM-III-R approach to diagnosis has several other advantages over DSM-II as well. Through the use of the multiaxial approach, it forces clinicians out of a reductionist mode of thinking to a consideration of the full range of biopsychosocial functioning of the person who has a brain disorder. Thus, the clinician needs to contemplate the potential effects of the premorbid personality structure (Axis II) on the clinical presentation of the OMSs (Axis I) and the interactive effects of psychosocial adaptation and brain disorder (Axis V). Axis IV calls to mind the possibility that the onset of psychosocial stress, while not causative of brain damage, may precipitate the clinical presentation of a latent, subclinical OMS. The separation of Axis I and Axis III leads to the possibility of a subtle distinction between syndrome and disease concepts in diagnosis. It frees the diagnostician to describe behavioral changes in Axis I and independently note medical-biological changes in Axis III, without reaching premature closure about diagnosis (e.g., the faulty identification of cerebrovascular disease with arteriosclerotic dementia). Thus, it is possible for a given dementia syndrome to be associated with several different biological diseases (e.g., subcortical dementias are seen with

Parkinson's disease, normal-pressure hydrocephalus, and hypertensive vascular disease). However, the same biological disease may present in several different syndromes (e.g., cerebrovascular disease may present with cortical or subcortical dementia, or a delirium, or an amnestic syndrome and an aphasic apraxia syndrome). A single behavioral syndrome (e.g., delirium) on Axis I may be associated with a complex set of interacting disorders on Axis III (e.g., alcohol withdrawal, hepatic encephalopathy, thiamine deficiency, acute or chronic respiratory failure).

HISTORY

Early history The emergence of the concept of OMDs was an outcome of the historical development of brain–behavior relationships. The Egyptians, despite their advanced knowledge of anatomy and of medicine, failed to attribute any importance to the brain; for them, the seat of perception and of cognition was the heart. The Greeks, in the fifth century B.C., first proposed the brain as the seat of the senses and of intellectual life. Hippocrates continued in this tradition: "By the same organ [brain] we become mad and delirious, and fears and terrors assail us." Not only mental disorders, such as delirium, melancholia, and delusions, but personality variations and temperaments were thought to be caused by the interactions of the four humors on the brain. Aristotle and his medieval followers, Avicenna and Aquinas, continued to regard some mental disorders as being caused by disruptions of the physical apparatus, the brain, and others to be caused by intense passions interfering with the function of reason.

Celsus, in the first century A.D., used the terms "delirium" and "dementia" in ways resembling contemporary usage. Soranus described both lethargic and excited forms of delirium and noted sleep disturbance in both. In his view, delirium could be caused by fevers, drunkenness, or poisoning, by a primary brain disturbance, or by diseases of other organs. Soranus also gave a clear and humane account of therapeutic interventions with acutely disturbed patients.

In the fourth century A.D., some physicians endorsed a tripartite correspondence of mental and brain functions, locating imagination in the forebrain, understanding, in the midventricles, and memory, posteriorly. The religious intensity of the Middle Ages coupled with a Platonic approach to philosophy led to more spiritual explanations and inquiries. During this time, Arab physicians expanded on the biological empirical works of Aristotle, and through them, in the high Middle Ages, Aquinas was able to redescribe the ancient disorders of melancholia, mania, amnesia, and epilepsy and to attribute them to organic factors.

Speculation continued during the Renaissance and in the early rationalist period about the location and manner of interaction between mental passions and physical humors. The sensorium commune thought to mediate this relationship was variously located in the pineal (Descartes), in the centrum ovale, in the corpus callosum, or in the medulla (Willis). Clinical observations were refined after the descriptive approach of Sydenham replaced the speculative humoral theories of medicine. Careful descriptions of delirium and dementia were entered into the English and Continental medical literature of the seventeenth century.

Modern history The modern period of descriptive psychiatry for organic disorders started with Pinel and his student Esquirol, who, in the first third of the nineteenth century, described senile dementia, while their student Bayle described dementia paralytica and its association with inflammation of the meninges, setting the stage for a full pathophysiological account of neurosyphilis. The French school also distinguished between illusions and hallucinations and described the mental state of confusion (disorganization of thought processes, of memory and perception, with spatiotemporal disorientation).

In the early nineteenth century, experiments in brain physiology led to a premature attempt to locate behaviors in specific brain areas. The pseudoscience of phrenology was to give a bad name to subsequent efforts to localize brain function. Yet, physiological research gave Griesinger confidence to contend, in 1845, that all mental diseases were brain diseases and that neuropathology and psychiatry were governed by the same laws. In the late 1800s, the work of Broca and Wernicke on locating the lesions that cause aphasia and Korsakoff's description of an amnestic state in association with polyneuritis confirmed this trend. Kraepelin believed that different somatic disorders presented with different mental syndromes, but Bonhoeffer, in 1912, contradicted him and proposed the modern view that all acute medical and brain diseases may present with overlapping and nonspecific mental syndromes: delirium, excitement, twilightstate, hallucinosis, and incoherent thinking. In 1924, Eugen Bleuler introduced the concept of the chronic organic psychosyndrome, characterized by impaired intellectual skills, emotional lability, and poor impulse control and associated with generalized cortical damage. Manfred Bleuler described focal psychosyndromes in 1957, associating local lesions with changes in emotional responses, impulse controls, and intensity of appetitive drives.

The model of brain function used by neuroscientists had a considerable effect on the concepts of disease used by their clinician contemporaries. In turn, the ideas of neuroscientists were shaped by the scientific culture of their age. Thus, a variety of hidden assumptions exist in the descriptions and conceptualizations of OBSs at a given time in history. Some of these ideas survive, transcribed from textbook to textbook with little reference to ongoing clinical observations or to contemporary neuroscientific evidence. These ideas are no mere historical relics: They form some of the underpinnings of attitudes to clinical evaluation and treatment planning and may lead clinicians to restricted or erroneous actions. The problem with outdated scientific paradigms is not lack of validity but diminishing heuristic impact. In their time, the paradigms served useful functions, but more recently, they failed to raise certain essential questions and failed to note critical discrepancies and thus became less relevant. Many of their original assumptions continue to be useful and valid, however, and are properly incorporated into updated or newly organized paradigms.

The earliest scientific paradigm was the reductionist-materialist view associated with Griesinger in the middle of the nineteenth century. Griesinger contended that all psychiatric symptoms were the direct result of brain lesions. The positive aspects of this paradigm include the correlation of behavioral defects with neuropathologically defined lesions and an enduring attitude of scientific precision toward measurable aspects of the brain–behavior relationship.

Hughlings Jackson enriched this rather static view with a perspective on evolutionary biology. He developed a concept of the hierarchical organization of the neuraxis, and the associated notion that symptoms are produced not only by brain–behavior defects but also by the release of evolutionarily primitive suppressed behaviors from inhibition by higher centers. Goldstein subsequently extended this idea to compensatory active responses to brain damage by the whole organism.

The first part of the twentieth century saw a retreat from the biological explanations of brain–behavior relationships. Freud gave up his early attempt to form a "project for a scientific psychology," which was based on neuroscientific speculations, and expounded a purely cognitive-emotional set of psychological hypotheses. It is true that his thoughts continued to have some biological underpinnings, and ideologically he remained true to an evolutionary, Jacksonian outlook; but Freud moved farther and farther away from developments in neuroscience. He expressed little interest in the OBSs.

In contrast, Pavlov and his behaviorist followers in the United States and the Soviet Union, while they put forth a more scientific program, moved just as far from an accurate appreciation of the brain–cognition–behavior triad. Their attention deviated from physiology to the ever more detailed examination of stimulus–response sets. Their celebrated "black-box" approach to the central nervous system (CNS), however, became increasingly irrelevant, owing to discoveries by neurophysiologists, who initially were interested only in the brain and not in the intricacies of the environmental control of behavior.

Some of the early successes of neurophysiologists and neurochemists in the mid-1900s and the ensuing application of their findings to clinical work remind one of an era a century earlier, when findings from neuropathology were promptly applied to clinical syndromes. In both instances, there were remarkable advances in biology, initially unmatched by equally accurate clinical descriptions and by a failure to understand the complexities of human cognition.

THE COGNITIVE REVOLUTION The information-processing approach to neuropsychology, embodied in the cognitive revolution, is beginning to restore the balance and to provide a bridge between basic neuroscientific observations and clinical findings. However, the traffic of influence has not been entirely one way. While the early notions about cybernetic control systems and their applicability to the brain were derived from computer theory, lately the findings of cognitive- and neuroscientists are beginning to be applied to the design of new computing systems. The early, linear model of information flow in the brain (and in computers) is beginning to be replaced by the idea of a social network of parallel processors or brain centers communicating with each other. The notion of functional subsystems (identified by cognitive-behavioral experiments) superimposed on neurophysiological subsystems (identified by neuroscientific techniques) is gaining momentum. This communication, interactive approach to brain functions ("languages of the brain") fits in well with the dynamic concepts of interconnecting brain centers envisioned by Luria in his work on brain injuries, with work on the disconnection syndromes, and with certain work on hemispheric specialization.

The positive features of the preceding paradigms should be retained. The neurobiological approach continues to demand rigor in the basic biological sciences. The evolutionary approach requires a wider, functional and developmental, perspective as well. The behavioristic approach demands accurate, detailed description of behaviors, and its successors apply the scientific method to the study of covert mental processes. Wundt, James, and Freud, all of whom tried and failed in the scientific study of experiential, subjective phenomena, would hail recent developments in experimental cognitive science. Finally, the empirical, atheoretical observations of several generations of clinicians continue to refine the methodology and findings of that gold standard, the bedside observation. After all, it is the clinician trained in bedside observation who needs to integrate the neurobiological and cognitive-experimental findings and to apply them to the diagnosis and care of a specific patient.

DIAGNOSTIC APPROACH TO ORGANIC MENTAL SYNDROMES

CLINICAL SIGNS AND SYMPTOMS AND ETIOLOGY

There are multiple semantic problems in the area of behavioral abnormalities caused by brain lesions. Symptoms (e.g., confusion) are reified into false syndromal diagnoses (e.g., confusional state); syndromes (e.g., dementia) are mistakenly identified with specific disease entities (e.g., primary degenerative dementia of the Alzheimer type); and prognoses are derived from the biology of certain disorders without taking into account related psychosocial variables or the complications of intercurrent medical disease. The problem of communicating with families is further complicated by the fact that symptoms that are significant to DSM-III-R definitions (e.g., higher cortical signs) may not be significant for caregivers who would rather focus on such troubling, though nonspecific, symptoms as agitation and dysphoria. As diagnoses provide blueprints for treatment interventions, confusion in this area is likely to lead to incomplete or erroneous treatment plans. Some dramatic and not uncommon errors include custodial placement of a person who has been diagnosed as having senile dementia before the reversible causes of dementia have been ruled out; use of tricyclics for alleged depression when the dysphoria is only a presenting symptom of delirium; expenditure of psychotherapeutic efforts on alcoholics whose frontal lobe damage prevents them from benefiting from abstract, symbolically mediated therapies; and diagnosis of dementia secondary to cerebral atrophy found on a computed tomographic (CT) scan that was read without proper attention to age-related radiographic changes.

Close attention to the semantic categories used, together with a systematic, incremental approach to a multilevel, multiaxial diagnosis would obviate much of the confusion and therapeutic uncertainty or therapeutic nihilism. The first step toward this goal is a clear understanding of the hierarchy of symptoms and signs; empirical and pathophysiological syndromes; disorders and diseases; and the related, but distinct, concepts of disability, personal illness, and social predicament.

Symptoms *Symptoms* are the personal, subjective observations by the patient of some deviation of experience or behavior from the normal. Most patients use an intuitive, within-subject sense of normality: How is the current state of affairs different from prior subjective experiences? Clearly, the memory and cognitive problems would distort the accuracy of self-perceptions, as an aphasia will impair the reporting of distress. The chronology and the specificity of complaints is lost early, leaving behind a sense of bewilderment, vague distress, and dysphoria. Reported early symptoms tend to include "I have trouble with my memory"; "My mind is not as clear as usual"; "I have slowed down, can't keep up"; "I can't concentrate"; "I feel anxiety, depression"; and "Things upset me easily." These symptoms are quite nonspecific and may just as easily indicate mood disorders, schizophrenia, or anxiety disorders. Later complaints may include "I just can't think"; "I can't do it"; "I am lost"; "What's wrong with me"; and "This is terrible." In the late stage of dementia, the sense of personal insight and the ability to reflect on and report subjective experience are lost entirely.

Signs *Signs* are objective, observable deviations from the normal behavior, performance, or neurophysiology. Most observers use the normal standard in an explicit, across-subjects sense, ideally comparing the patient to an age- and intelligence-matched control subject. Family members and employers may, however, compare the patient to his or her former self, and if the development of the pathology is slow, may not notice small deviations. The mental status examination (Tables 12-2 and 12-3) and the more formal psychological-psychometric testing (Table 12-4) look at spontaneous behaviors and responses to cognitive (and sometimes affective) challenges. This overlaps with the neurological evaluation, which also includes the assessment of the sensorimotor state and reflexes. The medical evaluation focuses on those organ systems that maintain the interior milieu for the CNS and looks for peripheral signs of systemic diseases that affect the brain.

TABLE 12-2
Mental Symptoms and Signs Important to the Diagnosis of Organic Mental Syndromes

Diagnostic Parameter	*Symptoms and Signs*
Consciousness and arousal	Is there a reduced clarity of awareness, clouding?
	Is there a disturbance or reversal of the sleep–wake cycle?
	Is there a marked change in psychomotor activity level?
Attention	Is the capacity to shift, focus, and sustain attention impaired?
Perception	Are there any misinterpretations, illusions, hallucinations?
Cognitive processing	Is the ability to process information reduced?
	Is there an impairment of abstract thinking (i.e., concrete proverbs, poor similarities, poor concept-forming ability)?
Cognitive content	Is there a loss of general intellectual content?
	Are there any delusions or overvalued ideas, suspiciousness?
High cortical functions	Is there evidence for aphasia (fluent or nonfluent) or incoherent speech, apraxia or constructional difficulty, agnosia?
Memory	Is there ability to learn new information and to transfer it from short- to long-term memory?
	Is there ability to remember information known in the past?
	Is there difficulty with recall or recognition?
	Is there difficulty with verbal or visual memory?
	Is the patient oriented to time, place, person?
Mood	Is the mood prominently depressed, anxious, irritable, aggressive, or jocular?
	Is there an affective instability, marked shifts of mood, outbursts of rage?
	Is the mood shallow, apathetic, indifferent?
Judgment	Is social judgment impaired?
	Is there any insight or foresight?
Time course	Do the symptoms fluctuate?
	Do the symptoms progress abruptly in a stepwise manner?
	Is there a steady decline in capacities or a steady increase in symptoms?

Laboratory tests *Lab tests* should be used to assess the structural and functional state of the brain, the chemistry of its supportive environment, and the non-CNS biological manifestations of diseases that also affect the brain. The technology of structural assessment has made enormous advances—from plain skull films and pneumoencephalograms, to echograms, radionuclide scans, and angiograms, to standard and contrast-enhanced CT, magnetic resonance imaging (MRI), positron emission tomography (PET), and single photon emission computed tomography (SPECT) scans.

The PET and SPECT technologies go beyond displaying anatomical structures to throw light on the metabolic function of brain regions. Their high cost and relatively low resolution have kept them from becoming standard clinical procedures. Radioactive xenon inhalation regional cerebral blood flow measurements do display cortical metabolic activity quite well and can be used in combination with psychological tasks that activate certain regions. The premier modality for functional imaging is still electroencephalography (EEG). The use of on-line computer processing has expanded the amount of information obtainable from the EEG signal. High-speed, color-coded topographic displays and statistical comparisons with stored population norms can identify regional functional differences that are difficult to see on standard EEGs. The topographic display of cerebral-event–related potentials gives further insight into temporospatial aspects of signal processing.

The standard evaluation of most cases of dementia and delirium should include a CT scan and an EEG; use of the more esoteric techniques is based on availability, cost, and the expectation of valuable information. Laboratory testing for systemic disorders cannot be comprehensive, as too many tests would be necessary. The choice of initial tests should be guided by the preliminary findings of the history and physical examination and by the need to check areas that are inaccessible on physical examination. The use of tests is also guided by their expense and the expected yield in the population at risk. Table 12-5 shows an approach to the comprehensive evaluation of an OMS or OMD that has good diagnostic yield for the primary cause and demonstrates the majority of secondary causes as well.

TABLE 12-3
Mini-Mental State Examination

__ (5)	1.	What is the (year, season, date, day, month)?
__ (5)	2.	Where are we (state, borough, city, hospital, floor)?
__ (3)	3.	Name three objects (pen, sky, dog) then ask patient to repeat them. (Score, then repeat answers until patient learns all three.)
__ (5)	4.	Spell *world* backward. Alternate: Serial 7's_ _ _ _ _
__ (3)	5.	Ask for names of three objects given in question #3.
__ (2)	6.	Point to a pencil and a watch. Ask the patient to name each as you point.
__ (1)	7.	Ask the patient to repeat "No ifs, ands, or buts."
__ (3)	8.	Three-stage command: "Take this paper in your right hand. Fold the paper in half. Put the paper on the floor."
__ (1)	9.	Ask the patient to read and obey the following (write on card in large letters): "CLOSE YOUR EYES."
__ (1)	10.	Have the patient write a sentence of his or her choice. (The sentence should contain a subject and an object and should make sense. Ignore spelling.)
__ (1)	11.	Have the patient copy two intersecting pentagons. (Give one point if all sides and angles are preserved and if the intersecting sides form a quadrangle.)
__ (30)		TOTAL MMSE SCORE

Table adapted from Folstein M F, Folstein S, and McHugh P R, Mini Mental State: A practical method for grading the cognitive state of patients for the clinician. Psychiat Res *12:* 189, 1975, with permission.

TABLE 12-4
Psychometric Evaluation of Mental Functions

- Wechsler Adult Intelligence Scale
- Halsted-Reitan battery or its components:
  - Halsted Category Test
  - Trail making
  - Aphasia screening
  - Rhythm perception
  - Speech perception
  - Finger tapping
  - Tactile performance
  - Perceptual examination
- Wechsler Memory Scale
- Bender Gestalt
- Benton Visual Retention
- Luria-Nebraska

TABLE 12-5
Initial Laboratory Studies for Organic Mental Syndromes

Complete blood count
Blood chemistry screening
Serology for syphilis, AIDS
Toxicology screen
Serum thyroxine
Serum folate and B_{12}
Urinalysis
Chest film
EKG
EEG
Computed tomography

Syndromes *Syndromes* are collections of symptoms and signs that group together in predictable ways. There are two approaches to syndrome formation—empirical-statistical and rational-physiological. The former relies on accumulated clinical experience and is the basis of the descriptions in DSM-III-R. Table 12-6 describes the hierarchy of OMDs recognized in DSM-III-R. The rational approach looks at the areas of brain involved and predicts the emergence of certain behavioral abnormalities. The two approaches can interact, as when the presence of aphasia and apraxic signs in Alzheimer's patients prompted the successful search for a regional excess of plaques and a reduction in choline acetyltransferase in the parietotemporal areas of Alzheimer's patients' brains. At other times, the pathological distinctions lead to the clinical differentiation: The difference between cerebrovascular disease with larger cortical infarcts and the lacunar syndrome with multiple, bilateral basal ganglia and white matter lesions lead to the recognition of two clinical variants of multi-infarct dementia.

The various symptoms and signs are by no means equipollent in the establishment of a specific diagnosis. A certain symptom may be quite prominent in a syndrome (e.g., amnesia in delirium), but its presence in other organic syndromes (dementia, amnestic syndrome) makes it merely a sensitive symptom of low specificity for differential diagnosis among the OMSs. The specificity of a symptom varies with the uses it is put to; disorientation has high specificity if the presence of delirium or dementia is sought, but it has low specificity in differentiating between the various disease states that may cause those conditions. By contrast, asterixis is a symptom of low sensitivity for delirium (as the majority of delirious patients do not have it) but of high specificity for certain metabolic encephalopathies (hepatic, renal, and respiratory) that can cause delirium. Certain symptoms and signs of an OMS may be less important as diagnostic benchmarks than as problems for the patient and the family. Changes in social relationships, in a job or housekeeping role, or in money management, or disturbances in the range or control of affect can be prominent symptomatic problems with OMS or OMD. Traditional cognitive symptoms that may be diagnostic pointers (as well as troubling problems) include disorientation, getting lost, forgetfulness, and communication difficulties. Thus, when the clinician lists the diagnostically relevant sensitive and specific symptoms that lead to a formal DSM-III-R diagnosis, it is equally important to construct a problem list. The treatment of the underlying disorder can then proceed in parallel with a series of practical solutions for the problems.

Concept of disease The concept of a *mental disorder* as used in DSM-III-R closely approaches the notion of the pathophysiological syndrome. The definition of a *disorder* includes the presence of a recognizable syndrome that leads to distress, disability, or both, together with an inference of some underlying psychosocial or biological dysfunction. The concept of a disease takes this a step further, specifying an etiology and pathophysiological process. What goes wrong is the domain of etiology—of predisposing, precipitating, and sustaining factors that eventually interfere with the physiological functions of the CNS (Tables 12-7 through 12-10). The anatomical locations where these neurological dysfunctions occur tend to define the symptom patterns produced, while the rate of their manifestation seems to depend on their pathogenesis. Although Table 12-11 describes correlations between lesions and clinical symptoms, it is important not to overestimate the correlation between a disease process and a related clinical syndrome. Dementia as a clinical syndrome has many causal disease states. Even when the syndrome is refined and subdivided through a better understanding of its pathophysiology (as in the distinction between cortical and subcortical dementia), a differential diagnostic process is still required to choose from among the possible diseases.

The reverse is equally true: A given disease process may manifest itself in protean ways, and in its course of development it may present as different syndromes. For instance, cerebrovascular disease may lead to a cortical multi-infarct dementia, an aphasic or apraxic focal syndrome, a transient global amnesia, a delirium, or a subcortical dementia of the lacunar syndrome. Alzheimer's disease may start as an isolated amnestic syndrome (or occasionally as an organic delusional syndrome) before manifesting the full dementia syndrome. Table 12-12 describes a combined syndrome–disease approach to the differential diagnosis of the common dementing diseases. Note that this algorithmic tree has been unduly "pruned"; it would be easy to proceed along other branches.

Disability *Functional disabilities* are activities in various life roles in which the person can no longer engage. The difficulties a patient may experience as a result of a disease are not described fully by the array of symptoms and signs arising from the pathophysiological process. Other mechanisms of disability consist of combinations of behavioral or cognitive defects, failed compensations, release phenomena, and affective overreactions to the defect. For example, a patient with early dementia may have some mild attention and number-handling difficulties which, in a shopping situation where money has to be exchanged quickly, may develop into a major functional disability through the mechanism of catastrophic reaction. *Catastrophic reactions* are emotional overreactions to the perception of cognitive difficulties, which, in turn, interfere with cognitive performance and can lead to a major functional disability. Functional disabilities are often missed by health care professionals if the patient does not engage in activities of daily living (ADL) during their observations. Paradoxically, failure to observe a patient performing ADL may also lead to overestimation of difficulties: a demented person fails many items of a mental status examination but may nevertheless function well in a familiar environment. The subtle neuropsychological features of a frontal lobe dysfunction are often missed on routine psychological evaluations, yet the resulting social functional defects of organic personality disorder are quite gross. Axis V of DSM-III-R goes some way toward identifying at least general levels of disability in personal, social, and occupational terms. Psychological tests (Table 12-4) are valuable tools for evaluating the details and the structure of functional impairments. They are more useful as guidelines to functional

TABLE 12-6
Differential Diagnosis of OMD

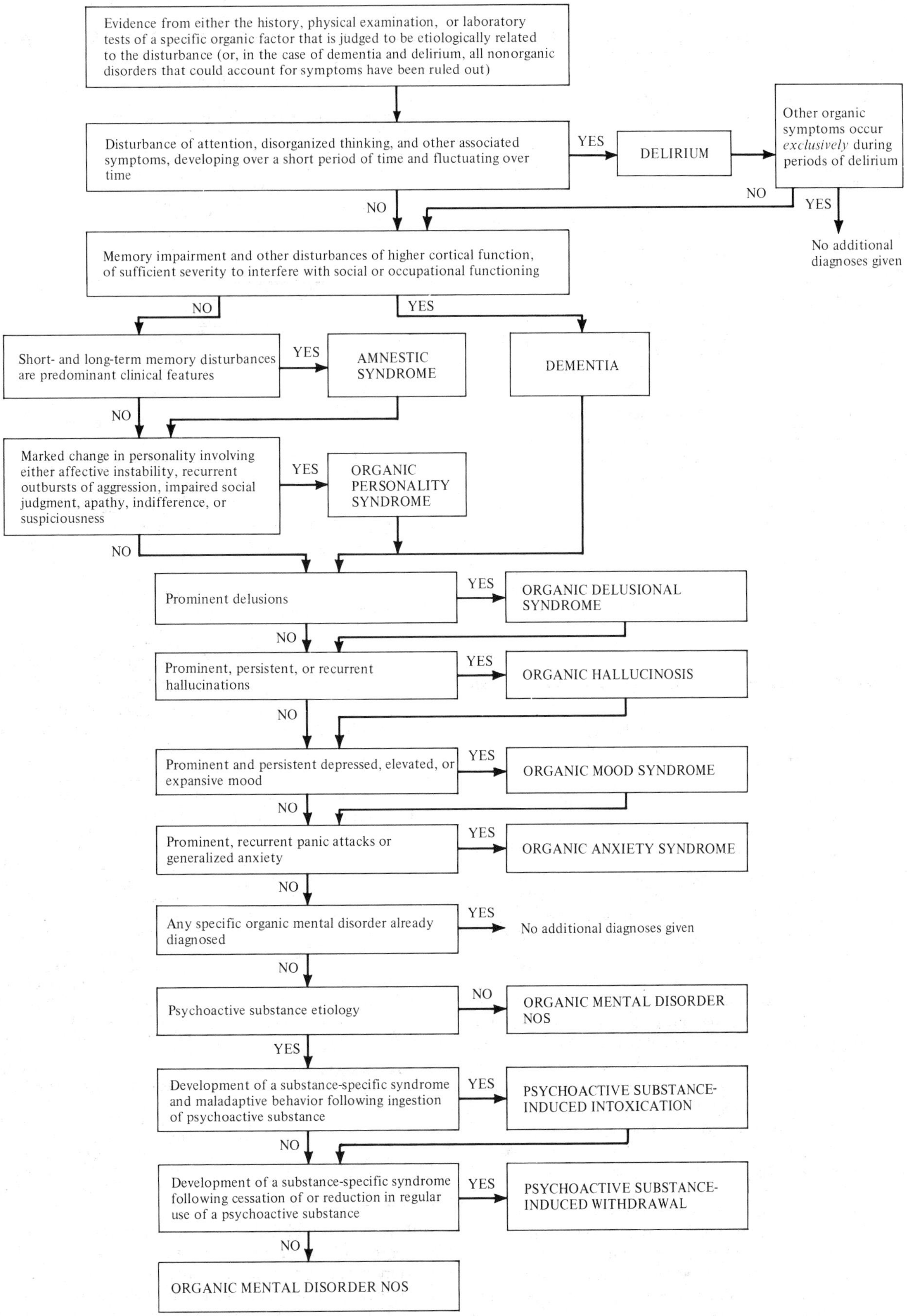

TABLE 12-7
Physiological Abnormalities that Lead to Neuronal Dysfunction

Interference with substrates for metabolism: anoxia, hypoglycemia, ischemia
Interference with metabolic cofactors: thiamine, pyridoxine, nicotinic acid, folate, B_{12} deficiency
Interference with membrane stability: electrolyte acid-base imbalance, internal and external toxins
Interference with DNA–RNA information flow: viral infections
Inflammatory and immune disorders: infections, demyelinating disorders
Genetic and degenerative cellular protein and structural deficits: Huntington's, Parkinson's, Alzheimer's
Traumatic disruptions of neurons and axons: open and closed head injuries
Excessive or inappropriate neural stimulation: focal or general seizures, kindling, receptor up-regulation
Interference with neural communication: neurotransmitter depletion, metabolic pathway block, receptor blockade or down-regulation.

TABLE 12-8
Factors That Predispose to Organic Mental Changes*

Loss of neuronal populations, reduced dendritic branching
Interruption of white matter connecting pathways
Decreased cerebral metabolism, reduced circulation
Reduced activity of neurotransmitter systems; change in rate-limiting enzymes and/or in receptor numbers
Slow-wave EEG activity
Slower information processing

*These factors, in various combinations, create conditions of susceptibility to OMS or OMD in aging, alcoholism, brain damage, functional psychotic disorder, cancer, cardiac-cerebrovascular disease, and diabetes.

TABLE 12-9
Conditions That Precipitate the Clinical Presentation of an OMS

Drug and alcohol intoxication or withdrawal
Metabolic failure in endocrine, hepatic, respiratory, or renal disease
Perfusion failure in cardiac or circulatory disorders
Systemic or cranial infections
Malnutrition or dehydration
Traumatic injury
Rapid development of space-occupying lesions

rehabilitation than as pointers to pathophysiological diagnosis, as they not only demonstrate defects but also display preserved strengths and skills. At times, it may be easier to train a person to compensate for a defect by using preserved functions than to correct the defect.

Concept of personal illness Disease and disability are categories of malfunctions that are generalizable across populations. In real life, however, they are embodied in concrete persons with unique histories. The concept of *personal illness* is a useful way of signifying this. Methods of studying illness are not nomothetic but idiographic. Adolf Meyer approached mental disorders in this idiographic, biographical way. While the nomothetic approach is quite essential for the scientific study of disease categories, the idiographic approach can complement it and supply the background essential for psychotherapy and rehabilitation. Also, the content of many psychotic manifestations (hallucinations, delusions) cannot be understood without a knowledge of personal history. The knowledge of having a disease also carries unique significance for individuals, and their reactions to being ill are at times more dependent on past events in their lives than on the current symptoms of the disease. The early presentation of Huntington's chorea is a case in point.

TABLE 12-10
Sustaining Causes That Perpetuate Organic Mental Symptoms

Sensory deprivation or overload
Poor ego integration, use of inadequate coping and defense mechanisms
Inadequate social supports, high expressed negative emotions
Poor physical health or poor nutrition
Sleep deprivation
Psychopharmacological side effects (especially anticholinergic, postural hypotensive, sedative)
Continuing or iatrogenic metabolic side effects due to attempted rectification of biological problems

TABLE 12-11
Neuroanatomical Correlates of Mental State Changes

Affected Area	*Changes*
Brain stem	Diminished consciousness, fluctuating attention, akinetic mutism
Diencephalon	Distractable attention, depression or hypomania, changes in eating, drinking, or libido, apathy
Limbic system	Apathy, aggression, vegetative-endocrine disturbances, memory problems, especially learning new material
Left posterior hemisphere	Fluent aphasia, alexia, agraphia, apraxia, Gerstmann syndrome (finger agnosia, right-left disorientation, acalculia, agraphia)
Right posterior hemisphere	Constructional apraxia, dressing apraxia, neglect of one side of the body, spatial disorientation, difficulty in directing attention, difficulty in perceiving emotions
Parietal lobes	Body schema disturbances, topographic disorientation, cortical sensory loss
Occipital lobes	Visual hallucinosis, cortical blindness with denial
Temporal lobes, anteromedian	Psychomotor epilepsy (changes in consciousness, perceptions, olfactory, auditory, visual hallucinations, motor automatisms, vegetative signs), interictal schizophreniform and mood disorders, epileptic personality, intense affect, hyperreligiosity, hyposexuality, hypergraphia, viscous thinking
left anterior	Verbal memory problems, speech sound misperception
right anterior	Visual memory disturbance, tonal misperception
posteroinferior	Difficulty in recognizing faces or classifying objects
Motor areas and vicinity	Hemipareses, loss of fine movement; nonfluent aphasias (left)
Frontal lobes	Concrete thinking, inability to change mental set, reduced drive, diminished self-concern, inability to delay gratification, impulsivity, lack of judgment or foresight, shallow affect

Patients also find themselves in certain social predicaments as a result of the interaction between the diagnosed disease, the functional disability, the patient's personal perception of the illness, and the social handicap that attends any of these factors. The term "dementia" once evoked a sense of futility and hopelessness; the social atmosphere has changed through biomedical advances and the activities of advocacy groups.

TABLE 12-12
Differential Diagonsis of Cognitive Impairment

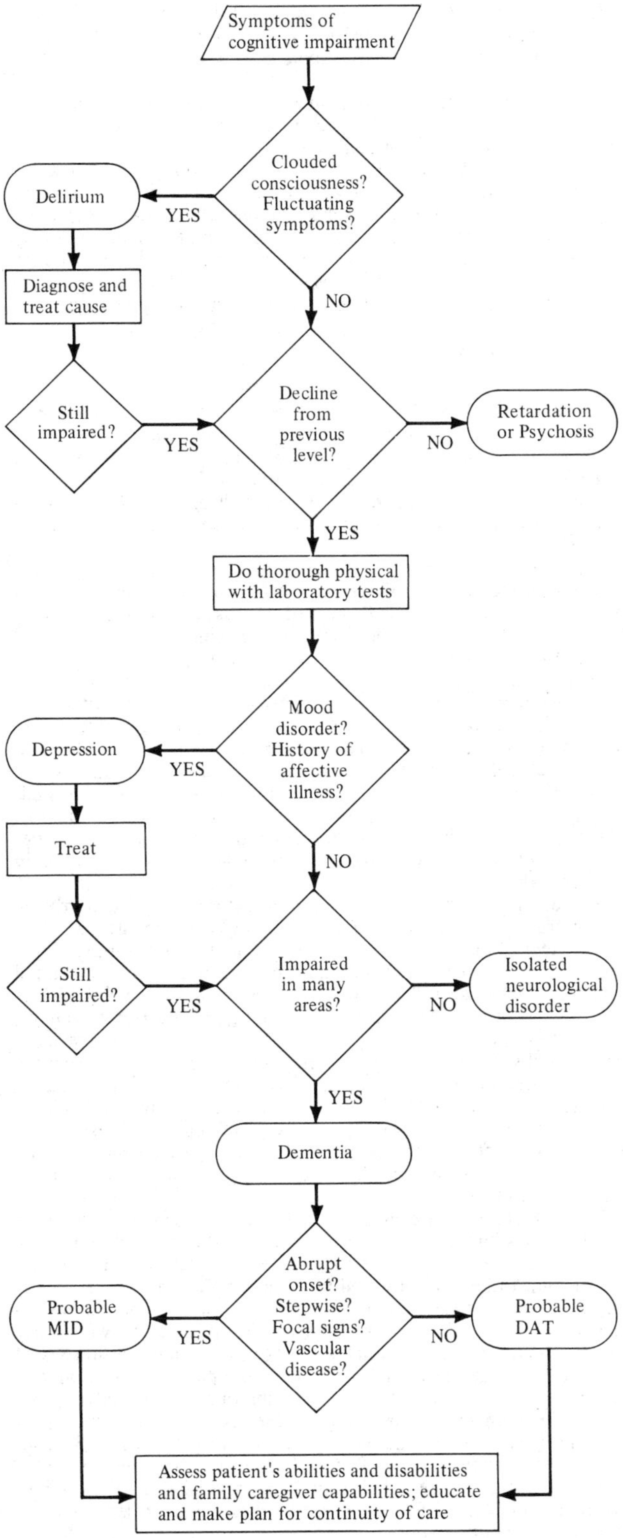

Table from *Dementia*, an information bulletin, Office of Geriatrics and Extended Care of the Veterans Administration, Washington, DC, 1985..

The stigma associated with some notorious diseases is generalized to the mental complications of those diseases. A dramatic contemporary example is the social response to acquired immune deficiency syndrome (AIDS) encephalopathy. The segregation of neurosyphilis patients in asylums is an example from the nineteenth century. Predicaments can be attacked through public education, and their effects on individuals can be minimized through counseling.

PATHOPHYSIOLOGY **Temporospatial analysis of lesions and their impact on behavior** Human behavior and subjective experience are based on perceived changes in the external and internal environments. Information from the primary and secondary sensory areas is integrated into a coherent view of the self in the world in the highest association cortex of the temporo-parietal-occipital area. Communication between the right and left association areas and the introceptive areas of the limbic system ensure an integration of cognitive, affective, and motivational elements. New percepts are compared to memories of previous events and the individual's responses to them through the limbic-hippocampal-median thalamic circuits. Object classification and recognition can thus take place. Novel or significant aspects of the environment are then matched with plans of action generated through the dorsolateral prefrontal cortex, interacting with the orbitofrontal-limbic motivational circuits. The frontal lobes assemble and orchestrate the images of action generated in the sensorimotor cortex into behavioral gestalts. Motor actions are processed through feedback circuits involving the basal ganglia and fast-feed-forward circuits through the cerebellum and are eventually performed through hierarchically organized local circuits in the spinal cord.

FUNCTIONAL SPECIALIZATIONS Functional specializations mark the three dimensions of the neuraxis: anterior-posterior, rostral-caudal, and left-right. As described by Luria, the anterior-posterior dimension corresponds to ever more abstract plans of action anteriorly and to more generalized perceptions posteriorly, at the confluence of the three major sensory areas. The rostral-caudal dimension corresponds roughly to a Jacksonian hierarchical organization of increasing generality and complexity; the more atomic aspects of sensory and motor processing take place farther down the neuraxis, leaving the cortical processing areas to deal with increasingly generalized issues. Sperry's work suggests an important lateral asymmetry as well. To describe left hemispheric information processing as serial, language-oriented, and cognitive and right hemispheric activity as simultaneous, spatially oriented, and affective is to oversimplify this rapidly evolving area. There are also a set of axially organized functional systems with wide, nonspecific projections to the entire neuraxis. Initially described as the reticular formation, its specific components are beginning to be identified according to their synaptic neurotransmitters and the nuclei of their cells of origin. The noradrenergic locus ceruleus system, the serotonergic raphe, the dopaminergic mesencephalic system, and the cholinergic projections from the nucleus basalis (and probably other axial transmitter systems) work together in a complex manner to regulate arousal, activation, sleep-wake cycling, and attentional functions. This system is influenced from the prefrontal and posterior association cortices, as well as from the cingulate limbic cortex, allowing for voluntary shifts of attention and arousal. The brain stem also contains regulatory centers for the maintenance of autonomic functions that have ready access to alerting influences from the reticular formation.

MOTIVATIONAL FUNCTIONS While the arousal–attention system responds mostly to external environmental influences, the rostral hypothalamic system monitors changes in the internal milieu, working through feedback loops for humoral, metabolic, and endocrine components. The motivational functions of the organism seem to be mediated through the connections of the hypothalamus with septal-limbic system, the orbitofrontal cortex, and the mesencephalon. Motivations drive the organism toward positively reinforcing events and away from nociceptive ones. Areas in the anterior hypothalamic-septal area seem to subserve the former, areas in the posterior hypothalamus and periventricular gray matter, the latter. Monoaminergic tracts seem to influence positive reinforcement, and opioid (and possibly cholinergic) transmission plays a part in nociception.

EMOTION Emotion is thought to be related to but distinct from motivation. Instead of driving the organism to or from a stimulus, it interrupts the sequence of planned behavior and forces it to reassess the situation in view of novel or motivationally significant events. The correlation of affective changes and limbic-amygdaloid activity is well known. However, in humans there is an important communicative aspect as well, observed by the right hemisphere.

COMMUNICATIONS The perisylvian area of the neocortex seems to be the cerebral substrate of communication in humans. Speech is decoded in the left temporal lobe, and concepts obtain their linguistic code in Wernicke's area posteriorly. Broca's area can then organize the grammatical and phonetic performance of speech. The perisylvian area has the appropriate interactions with visual and motor areas to allow for reading and writing. It appears that the communication of emotions through prosody, gesture, and facial expression is organized in a mirror image manner around the right Sylvian fissure. More frontal lesions impair the expression of affect; posterior lesions interfere with its decoding (Table 12-13).

There are several cautions to be observed in any review of regional functional-structural correlations. Complex cognitive tasks require the harmonious interconnection of a number of processing areas. Lesions in a particular area may impair a processing unit and disconnect several processing centers (ablation versus disconnection lesions). Complex behaviors are more vulnerable than simple ones, because a lesion at any of their several functional centers may interrupt smooth processing. Widespread or generalized lesions can interrupt many functions, but even a local lesion may cause several apparently unrelated defects if located where several functional regions overlap.

CLINICOPATHOLOGICAL CORRELATIONS Mesulam summarized the principles of clinicopathological correlations as applied to complex mental functions:

1. Components of a complex function are represented within interconnected sites, which collectively constitute an integrated network for that function.

TABLE 12-13
Components of Behavior and Associated Cerebral Areas

Behavioral Parameter	*Anatomical Site*
Arousal	Brain stem reticular formation
Attention	Mesencephalic reticular formation, thalamic reticular nucleus, thalamocortical projection system; right parietotemporo-occipital junction, cingulate gyrus, dorsolateral frontal cortex (especially right side)
Perception	Thalamus, primary sensory cortex, and association areas
Memory	Hippocampal-fornix; mamillary-thalamic, dorso medial-thalamic, and midbrain limbic circuits; cortical association areas
Motivation and emotion	Hypothalamus, limbic circuits with the amygdala and hippocampus, mesolimbic projections, and connections between the limbic system and the orbitofrontal area
Language	Left perisylvian area
Language-mediated skilled behavior	Left parietal area
Emotional communication	Right perisylvian area
Visuospatially mediated skilled behavior	Right parietal area
Motor performance	Sensorimotor strips with parietal and frontal influences in interaction with the basal ganglia and the cerebellum
Plans and integration of behavior	Prefrontal areas

2. Individual cortical areas contain the neural substrate for the components of several complex functions and, thus, may belong to several partially overlapping networks.

3. Lesions of a single cortical area may produce multiple deficits.

4. Severe and lasting impairment of a complex function often requires the simultaneous involvement of several components of its integrated network.

5. A given complex function may be impaired as a result of a lesion in one of several areas, each of which is a component in the integrated network for that function.

Behavior may be altered not only by ablation or disconnection lesions but by irritative ones as well. Focal seizures in areas subserving complex functions (medial temporal) evoke complex, semiautomatic behaviors. Repetitive stimulation of certain tracts may facilitate conduction of impulses in the future (kindling) and may lead to the enhancement of intense behaviors following even mild stimulation. It is thought that some of the personality changes seen after years of temporal lobe epilepsy may represent such a hyperconnection syndrome.

RATE OF DEVELOPMENT The time course of development of the lesion is as important as its location. Slowly growing tumors allow for functional, and even perhaps biological, restitution, and the appearance of a behavioral defect will be delayed. Sudden interruption of function, as in trauma or hemorrhage, may lead to temporary cessation of function in distant but connected parts of the system.

Conversely, the extent of a lesion may influence not only the extent of associated functional loss but also the patient's rate of recovery. (Absence of redundant elements makes the task of recovery difficult and protracted.) The extent of the injury and its biological nature also influence the rate of recovery or deterioration. A neoplastic or ischemic lesion may be surrounded by a zone of edema, excessive neurotransmitter release, and aberrant electrical activity. Such a metabolically disturbed area may not show up on a CT scan, but may become obvious with topographic EEG, MRI, or PET. Restitution of metabolic function in the area around the lesion may be the basis for the initial phase of rapid improvement, while a second, prolonged phase of recovery may be due to functional retraining of related elements. The slowest progress probably represents the development of behavioral protocols that work around a lost function in a novel way.

Granted that lesions are, at times, multifactorial (e.g., hemorrhagic ischemic area, combined electrolyte and acid-base imbalance), their rate of development tends to be typical for their pathology. Thus, electrical disturbances are instantaneous; hemorrhages are rapid (minutes); ischemic and metabolic processes are somewhat slower (minutes to hours); infective processes and demyelination take days; and neoplastic invasion or degeneration spans periods from weeks to many months. Sudden changes in temporal processes may reveal the onset of complicating pathologies (bleeding into a tumor; seizure complicating a metabolic disturbance). A useful diagnostic rule of thumb is the observation that while the type of behavioral disturbance suggests the location of the lesion, the rate of its development and the presence of compensatory behaviors suggest the nature of its pathophysiology.

A careful analysis of even the so-called global mental disturbances into their constituent parts can become a useful, clinicopathologically relevant exercise. The dementia associated with Alzheimer's disease was thought to be clinically uniform when the postulated cause was uniform cortical degeneration. But careful clinical examinations revealed that language, memory, and praxis disturbances were early and common, whereas personality changes were delayed and visual disturbances were uncommon. Analysis of plaque formation and reduction of choline acetyltransferase subsequently showed regional differences, with early hippocampal and temporoparietal involvement and, much later, frontal and (rarely) occipital involvement. By contrast, the behaviors seen in Pick's disease are different, as is the distribution of the supposedly generalized lesions. In Pick's disease, the frontal lobes are affected early, and the patient presents with an organic personality change.

An understanding of the functions of a complex system that influences several other systems can also bring order into what appeared to be a random collection of clinical signs and symptoms. Delirium is characterized by a confusing combination of fluctuating consciousness, sleep–wake cycle disturbances, intermittent amnesia, perceptual anomalies, and variably incoherent speech. It all begins to make sense when the alerting function of the reticular formation, its connection with the limbic system and cortex, and its extension into the midline nuclei of the thalamus are appreciated.

These functional and structural correlations, together with the description of the appropriate diagnostic syndrome and the psychosocial adjustment of the patient, provide an understanding of the biopsychosocial state of the patient and can serve as a blueprint for managing his or her illness.

TREATMENT

The physician encountering the patient with a mental disorder is inclined to follow one of two approaches: a biomedical model of treatment (specific cures for specific disorders) or a psychotherapeutic model (improved mental function arising from the therapeutic interpersonal encounter). Both approaches are inadequate to the problems of patients with OMDs. Cures are rare and seem to apply only to unusual disorders, and psychotherapy appears impractical for organic disease. The rush into specific biological treatment of the first obvious organic disorder usually leads to problems because this therapy neglects the other, multifactorial causes of mental deterioration. Attempts at personal-life–directed, nonspecific psychotherapies tend to founder due to cognitive defects and may even be dangerous to the extent that they neglect biological variables. It is little wonder that a common response to such patients is a flurry of diagnostic action followed by therapeutic nihilism (abandonment of all attempts at treatment and quick referral to a custodial setting). In all these instances, the first, ancient maxim of therapeutics is violated: *Primum non nocere* (above all, do no harm). The best approach to patients is neither therapeutic zeal nor diagnostic excellence coupled with therapeutic nihilism but, rather, a combination of rational and empirical thinking embodied in the classical tenets of clinical management: "to cure sometimes, to relieve often, to comfort always."

Patient management is the fundamental encounter between the ill person and the health care provider. It consists of several partially overlapping phases: triage, crisis intervention or support, assessment and diagnosis, treatment and resource allocation, rehabilitation, and prevention.

Triage is based on the principle of providing the greatest good for the greatest number of subjects, and it implies an allocation of scarce resources to the patients who can benefit most from them. It is an ethically uncomfortable subject, as it may necessitate providing only minimal, strictly supportive, services to some patients with severe dementia. Triage is an accepted procedure in wartime and is still a common procedure in less developed countries and in modern medical facilities in times of disaster. The rising cost of health care and the declining public support for it may bring the issue to the public's attention once again. Crisis support and intervention, a more optimistic concept, aims to alleviate the most pressing problems and attempts to use the crisis as an opportunity for a positive change. The vital mental and safety functions of the patient are stabilized by providing clarification, support, structure, and, if necessary, restraints. A rapid assessment is made of the ecology of the illness, and the patient is observed as a biopsychosocial entity in interactions with the physical, cognitive, and social environment. Both the patient and the environment are evaluated for defects, strengths, and potential compensations. Reassurance, suggestions, and environmental manipulations are used to restore the ecological balance. Whenever possible, the patient and the ecological unit are consulted for validation of therapeutic suggestions and their implementation. Psychological crisis intervention generally needs to proceed hand-in-hand with medical evaluation and emergency treatment of conditions that triggered the mental change.

A full assessment and diagnostic workup generally evolved from the initial interactions of crisis intervention. As discussed in an earlier section, assessment involves a full five-axis DSM-III-R diagnosis as well as an evaluation of the patient's coping style and adaptation to the psychosocial stressors. Physical illness problems and social predicaments are noted, as are any opportunities for favorable change. Distressing symptoms, functional deficits, and behavioral compensations and their temporal and causal interrelations are defined.

This is followed by treatment planning: Several realistic goals are set, and strategies are developed to reach them through specified objectives attained in sequence. Tactics for reaching certain objectives are modified flexibly according to the logistics of resources, but the main goals remain: reverse specific causes, relieve functional problems, and comfort the patient by alleviating distressing symptoms.

TO CURE: THE REVERSAL OF SPECIFIC ETIOLOGIES All important etiological factors need to be described in their complex relations to each other. There will be some predisposing factors of longer duration, some precipitating causes of more immediate impact, and some sustaining forces that come into play opposite compensatory efforts (Tables 12-7 through 12-10). These etiological factors may arise from biological imbalances, from intrapsychic activities, or from the social or physical environment. This detailed diagnostic map then provides the blueprint for multiple corrective interventions. The sequence of such interventions is determined by the empirical constraints of problem urgency and therapeutic availability and by a rational understanding of the pathophysiological sequence of the disorder. The corrective actions arise from the same biopsychosocial matrix as the etiological factors and are carefully monitored using multimodal observations against measurable standards applied against specifiable outcomes.

Occasionally the goal is complete reversal of the pathophysiology of the disorder; more often, it is the achievement of some favorable shift in the biopsychosocial equilibrium that results in reduction of distress and improvement of function. While the definitive treatment of Alzheimer's disease awaits a full understanding of its pathophysiology and the development of new pharmacological, and possibly molecular biological, approaches, the functional status of a specific demented patient with a superimposed agitated delirium can be improved by a structured environment, careful attention to and treatment of the common causes of delirium, and the judicious use of antipsychotics. Sometimes, the accurate diagnosis of a single etiology and the timely availability of a therapeutic agent or intervention can make a decisive difference—vitamin B_{12} in pernicious anemia; nicotinic acid in pellagra; thiamine in Wernicke's encephalopathy; thyroxine in myxedema; cortisol in Addison's disease; detoxification in sedative addiction; antimicrobial therapy in neurosyphilis, tuberculosis, or cryptococcal meningitis; neurosurgical intervention for some space-occupying lesions; and shunting in normal-pressure hydrocephalus. At other times, the recognition and treatment of an ongoing process can at least arrest, if not reverse, neuropsychological decline—abstinence in chronic alcoholism, control of hypertension and embolization in multi-infarct dementia, glucose control in diabetes.

TO RELIEVE: THE CORRECTION OF FUNCTIONAL DEFECTS Perceptual distortions, misinterpretations of reality, and loss of complex behaviors need to be tackled while attempts are made to reverse specific etiologies. The routine relegation of attention to functional defects to a future recovery period allows the impaired function to interfere with the very process of etiological treatment and it also allows for the development of functional chronicity. Once functional and etiological interventions are identified, strategic decisions can be made to advance or delay a certain treatment.

Perceptual distortions are minimized by providing an optimal sensory environment free of sensory deprivation and stimulus overload. The patient should be surrounded by familiar objects and persons that provide spatial and temporal orientation and should be encouraged to interact actively with the environment to prevent autistic regression.

Memory defects should be compensated for by frequent repetitions, simple explanations, and delivery of information through several sensory modalities. Clarity of organization, multiple different presentations, and arousal of attention and emotions often result in better storage. Retrieval strategies can be provided for the patient, including mnemonic lists, visual and spatial clues, and rehearsal of motor performance routines. Cognitive processing is improved if the rate of information flow is reduced, if the material is "chunked" into related units, and if complex problems are broken into manageable parts.

Complex psychomotor deficits can be anatomized into their constituent parts, and attempts can be made to compensate for a lost component by redirecting preserved abilities. Thus, it may be possible to program around a specific missing step in a sequence of neuropsychological behaviors.

Rehabilitation efforts require appropriately modulated arousal and attention, and an ability to direct these functions as dictated by foresight and motivation. When, as frequently happens, there are problems in all these central functions in an OMD, a stable background can be provided against which the stimulus can be presented to enhance involuntary attention. Foresight should not be left to the patient; instead, the task confronting him or her should be structured and planned. It should be recognized that secondary or symbolic delayed reinforcers will have less impact on behaviors than immediate and concrete ones. Simple reinforcement or extinction schedules should be devised for habit training.

A thorough neuropsychological evaluation can provide a comprehensive description not only of the lost functions but also of the preserved strengths. A series of well-coordinated rehabilitative efforts can then be designed. The speech therapist works on linguistic and pragmatic aspects of communication. The physical therapist assists the skilled execution of larger movements, to help the patient acquire confidence in using the body in space. Lack of such confidence leads to falls or prompts the patient to remain in bed, restricting exploratory activities and promoting mental stagnation. The occupational therapist trains the patient in ADL and in fine psychomotor skills to compensate for the effects of agnosia and apraxia. Art and music therapy can also be provided to counteract the mental impoverishment and concrete thinking so prevalent in OMDs.

The family and nursing staff are often underutilized as agents of functional rehabilitation. All too often, their role is perceived as custodial or merely supportive of biological functions. In fact, because they have intimate and ongoing contacts with the patient, they are in a good position to encourage appropriate behaviors and activities that preserve the ability to perform useful skills. Their interaction with the patient should not be merely intuitive; they should be instructed in the pathophysiology of the disorder and the neuropsychology of impaired functions and should be familiar with possible compensations. The time that the psychiatrist and the neuropsychologist spend in consultation with family, nursing staff, and rehabilitation professionals is well spent if it is directed to a clear exposition of a rational treatment plan.

TO COMFORT: THE TREATMENT OF DISTRESSING SYMPTOMS The most troubling symptoms of OMSs are anxiety, agitation, depression, perceptual distortions, and psychotic interpretations of reality. Despite their prominence in the patient's life, they are often disregarded by some health professionals. These symptoms are diagnostically nonspecific and provide little insight into functional deficits or compensations. It is the family and the nursing staff who most often must deal with these behaviors, while the patient, upset by these experiences, is often unable to communicate the precise problem. Some of these symptoms are most intense during the night and least noticeable during formal ward rounds and professional visits.

Emotional support The first line of approach is the provision of emotional support and humane care by the people in the patient's immediate environment. Familiarity with the caretakers improves the patient's chances of cooperating with the required routines; yet, even with difficult, sensitive patients, emotional responses to the patient should be restrained. An attitude of optimism should prevail together with a recognition of current limitations. Appropriate social behaviors should be modeled, and the significance of social interactions should be explained in concrete terms.

Enhance the patient's performance The second line of approach is to carefully tailor the demands placed on these patients to their capacity. Cognitive or emotional tasks that significantly exceed their capacity may trigger a catastrophic reaction. In the extreme, the result can be severely restricted ability to respond even to a simple demand. Repeated painful experience of such failures tends to produce protective withdrawal and avoidance of the anxiety-provoking activity. The end result may be pronounced social withdrawal, apathy, and further disuse atrophy of cognitive skills. The absence of cognitive demands, however, leads to mental stagnation and the behavioral picture of the chronically institutionalized person—dependence, boredom, deterioration of personality, and self-neglect.

Pharmacotherapy Drugs are the third line of approach. Unfortunately, they are frequently used to replace the humane interaction with familiar caretakers in a cognitively well-designed environment. The absence of these basic requirements leads to distressing symptoms that are poorly controlled by the pharmacological agents, which, in turn, leads to overdosage and polypharmacy. Another problem with the routine symptomatic use of psychotropics is their ability to temporarily obscure the progression of the underlying organic pathology. Judicious use of psychotropics together with etiological and functional treatment can make life easier for the patient and the caretakers.

Anxiety and agitation used to be treated with sedatives. The older sedatives (barbiturates, chloral hydrate, paraldehyde) impair cortical efficiency and reticular brain stem function and are thus likely to increase confusion and perhaps cause paradoxical excitation. The benzodiazepines in relatively small doses have more focal effects on the limbic system and are useful for their anxiolytic and hypnotic effects. However, the longer acting benzodiazepines (diazepam [Valium], chlordiazepoxide [Librium]) tend to reach cumulatively high levels and also persist in their active metabolites. Titration is easier with an agent, such as lorazepam (Ativan, 1 mg several times a day) that can be given orally as well as parenterally, which has a shorter half-life and has no active metabolites. Antihistamine sedatives, such as diphenhydramine (Benadryl, 25 mg t.i.d.) have also been used on an empirical basis.

Agitation that fails to respond and psychotic symptoms that persist despite environmental modification should be treated with modest doses of antipsychotic agents. It is best to use the relatively pure dopamine-blocking drug haloperidol (Haldol) in doses low enough not to require anticholinergic treatment for extrapyramidal side effects (0.5 to 1 mg three to four times a day). Anticholinergics, including the side effects of chlorpromazine (Thorazine) and thioridazine (Mellaril), are best avoided because they tend to interfere further with already compromised activity in the nucleus basalis and reticular formation. It is also best to avoid the hypotensive and arrhythmigenic effects of the less potent antipsychotics.

Several groups have treated medically ill patients with severe agitated delirium with high doses of intravenous haloperidol and lorazepam in a ratio of roughly 5 to 1. Under close observation in an intensive-care setting, often with respiratory support, life-threatening agitations have been brought under control.

The aftermath of a psychotic episode is often a residue of frightening half-memories. Brief psychotherapy can be very helpful in resolving these images and shoring up ego defense mechanisms.

Dysphoric mood is a common feature of OMSs, but only a full depressive syndrome is worth the risk of treatment with standard antidepressants. Indiscriminate use of the often highly anticholinergic tricyclics for organically depressed patients is a frequent cause of increased confusion and even agitation. If tricyclics are to be used, the least anticholinergic one (desipramine [Norpramine]) should be tried, initially in low doses divided throughout the day; as the dosage is increased, blood levels should be monitored.

The apathetic mood of some patients may be usefully elevated with small doses of stimulants (e.g., methylphenidate [Ritalin] 5 to 10 mg b.i.d.), if due attention is paid to the risks of increased cardiovascular activity.

Help the caretakers The fourth approach to symptomatic treatment is to help the primary caretakers, the family or the nurses, to tolerate better the patient's unavoidably difficult behavior. Increased understanding of the course of the various syndromes, reading (e.g., *The 36-Hour Day*), practical pointers to easier patient management, and medical and psychiatric consultation tend to reduce some of the frustration inherent in working with OMD patients. Temporary hospitalizations (respite care) of patients with chronic mental disorders can provide periodic relief for caretakers. All efforts directed at the caretaker provide an indirect service to the patient by providing a more accepting and hopeful social environment.

EPIDEMIOLOGY

The incidence and prevalence of OMDs depend on the epidemiology of medical disorders in the community and its subcultures. The decline of serious childhood infections and malnutrition in developed countries resulted in a decline in the incidence of acute delirium. This was probably counterbalanced by the rising incidence of acute toxic delirium and drug withdrawal states in adolescence. At the other end of the life span, survival to extreme old age resulted in an increased prevalence of dementia in the general population, though not in the aged cohort itself. The increased incidence of serious medical diseases in aging persons and the iatrogenic complications, combined with the decreased resistance of the aging brain, resulted in an increased incidence of delirium in populations hospitalized for medical disorders. But advances in medical science and public health virtually abolished several major forms of organic brain pathology—neurosyphilis, pellagra, and cretinism–myxedema. Other preventable disorders persist as testament to the self-destructiveness of humans—chronic alcoholic dementia and the thiamine-deficiency amnestic syndrome. Yet, others show a promising, though modest decline; the incidence of multi-infarct dementia is decreasing in parallel with the declining incidence of strokes, owing to better management of hypertension. New diseases, such as AIDS dementia, may still emerge.

There are some observational problems in determining the incidence and prevalence of the various OMSs. There are only a few population-based studies. Admission rates to psychiatric institutions are influenced by many social and economic factors distinct from the actual incidence of the conditions. Diagnostic practices have varied greatly over the past 20 to 30 years. Organic psychoses are now almost a meaningless group. Senile dementia diagnosed some years ago may today be diagnosed as Alzheimer's disease, as multi-infarct dementia, or even as alcoholic dementia. Furthermore, once a disorder receives a certain attention, even notoriety, in the public mind, it is likely to be diagnosed earlier and more frequently. While this may not change the incidence, it will spuriously increase the prevalence. It is also useful to determine the incidence and prevalence of OMSs in special populations, such as hospitalized medical inpatients, emergency room clients, surgical intensive care unit (ICU) inpatients, or diagnostic groups, such as drug or alcohol addicts, AIDS patients, dialysis patients, or patients in specific age groups. Practicing physicians are generally more interested in the epidemiology of disorders in the subpopulations under their care than in those affecting a whole nation.

In developed countries, OMSs typically affect elderly patients or those suffering from multiple medical problems or from substance abuse. In the aging demography of developed countries, this leads to a perception of a silent epidemic of dementia. Yet perhaps an even greater blight, of truly epidemic proportions, is the impact of malnutrition and chronic disease on the immature brains of a significant group of youngsters in the Third World. A healthy brain and a clear mind are second in importance only to life itself, and the impairment of these in significant segments of the world's population suggests that OMDs are of primary public health importance worldwide. This was clearly perceived once before, in the first part of the century, when neurosyphilis and pellagra were epidemic and were major sources of mental disability. Public health measures dealt effectively with these disorders. Unfortunately, we either do not understand the current OMDs enough to prevent them (Alzheimer's disease) or lack the necessary commitment or social resources to combat them (substance abuse–induced syndromes in the West, malnutrition and chronic disease in the Third World).

To the extent that the prevalence of dementia and the incidence of delirium rise with ill health and old age, the overall clinical burden of these disorders will increase with our aging population. The burden of morbidity may be particularly high on mildly to moderately demented subjects, who may be very prone to develop delirious episodes, which carry significant morbidity and mortality in themselves and also may result in irreversible functional deterioration. As delirium is associated with an increased morbidity and mortality of its associated medical disorders, the presence of delirium is likely to increase the length of hospital stay and per diem resource expense.

Early-onset dementia generally shortens the life span, but it significantly increases health care costs during the period of survival. Costs are incurred both for acute-care medical admissions and for long-term care. As there is virtually no private or public insurance coverage for long-term care, dementia can force a family to "spend down" to poverty or divorce.

There are hidden social costs to some of the significantly less severe OMSs. The organic personality disorders that follow head injuries result in social and family problems, underemployment, and domestic violence. The organic personality disorder that complicates chronic alcoholism further impairs the capacity for psychotherapy and for certain forms of rehabilitation.

The incidence of OMSs that phenomenologically resemble such functional disorders as mood disorders and delusional syndromes is quite uncertain. Recent surveys of the consultation services at several major teaching hospitals uncovered very few of these disorders.

PUBLIC HEALTH APPROACHES

The public expects psychosocial efforts from psychiatrists to prevent mental disorders (primary prevention), early treatment of established disorders (secondary prevention), and rehabilitative efforts to minimize their functional impact (tertiary prevention). Yet, despite a great deal of speculation about determinants of positive mental health, the real success of a public health approach to psychiatric diseases has been in the biological prevention of OMDs.

Two endemic mental disorders (general paresis of the insane and pellagra) produced a great deal of disability at the turn of the century but are virtually unknown today owing to the success of primary prevention. The first disorder, an advanced form of neurosyphilis, disappeared after antibiotics became generally available to treat veneral diseases. The very early treatment of gonorrhea often concurrently treated undiagnosed syphilis and prevented its spread to the CNS. The second disorder, pellagra, responded to increased knowledge of nutrition and to vitamin enrichment of many food staples. In a similar fashion, the use of iodized salt in certain Alpine regions has prevented the development of cretinism. Other, less dramatic, changes of incidence of certain syndromes are due to more effective treatment of underlying conditions. The incidence of strokes and of multi-infarct dementia has decreased over the past 25 years, thanks to better control of hypertension, smoking, and hypercholesterolemia. The incidence of Korsakoff's amnesia no longer rises with the rising incidence of alcoholism, since the application of knowledge about the nutritional origin of Wernicke's encephalopathy and the widespread emergency room practice of giving thiamine to alcoholics.

General hospital psychiatry plays a major role in secondary prevention of disorders that present with delirium and occasionally with dementia. Delirium calls attention to the increased morbidity and mortality of medical diseases associated with it and demands, therefore, more energetic and comprehensive treatment. The early detection of a dementia may lead to the discovery of a reversible cause in about 20 percent of instances. Timely treatment of subdural hematoma, frontal meningioma, normal-pressure hydrocephalus, myxedema, neurosyphillis, chronic sedativism, and several other occult disorders is possible only with early and accurate syndromal and biological diagnosis. There are some unsolved problems: Some medical disorders present with psychological symptoms that are not usually associated with classical organic syndromes. About 10 percent of patients who present for psychotherapy are found to have an organic rather than a psychodynamic cause for their psychological symptoms. A careful systems review and a screening laboratory battery identified most of these patients, but such approaches are not universally applied to psychotherapy applicants.

Tertiary prevention, the treatment of disabilities secondary to cerebral disease, is well developed for the focal psychosyndromes. The treatment of the aphasias leads the field, but occupational and physical therapies for the stroke syndromes are also well advanced. Until recently, an attitude of pessimism has prevented the application of these techniques to the dementias. However, several forms of memory training developed by cognitive psychologists have been applied to the amnestic syndromes. The recognition of partial reversibility of the alcohol dementia is beginning to lead to long-term efforts at maintaining sobriety in association with social and cognitive retraining.

There are several unsolved problem areas in tertiary prevention. The diagnosis of dementia often leads to admission to chronic care facilities. The restrictive environment, the predominant use of unskilled personnel, and the absence of rehabilitative programs not only fails to improve the patient's mental state but in fact induces the secondary problem of chronic institutionalization. The use of higher doses of antipsychotic and sedative agents can exacerbate this problem. Even the more transient states of delirium lead to problems of tertiary prevention. They leave behind a variety of sequelae that are often undertreated and may lead to chronic psychological disability.

A more concerted public health approach to several groups of patients (substance abusers, patients with chronic medical disorders, individuals prone to malnutrition, subjects with early dementia, and the chronically mentally ill) may lead to significant pay-offs in reducing the incidence and morbidity of superimposed OMSs and the severity in functional disability.

DEMENTIA

INTRODUCTION Dementia is defined by DSM-III-R (Table 12-14) as a loss of intellectual abilities of sufficient severity to interfere with occupational functioning or with a person's usual social activities or relationships. In addition, there should be objective evidence of impairment in long-term memory. Finally, one other area of impairment should be apparent; it could be abstraction, judgment, higher cortical function including language, praxis, and object naming, or a personality change. Dementia occurs in the context of a clear sensorium, if consciousness is clouded, delirium should be considered. A number of disease states can be associated with dementia, including Alzheimer's disease, multi-infarct dementia, alcoholic dementia, mood disorder, metabolic disturbances, head trauma, normal-pressure hydrocephalus, space-occupying lesions, and infections of the CNS, including such diseases as neurosyphilis, AIDS, and a number of specific neuropathologies, including degenerative diseases such as Parkinson's and Huntington's diseases (Table 12-15).

Alzheimer's disease is the most common dementing disorder. Slightly less than 5 percent of all persons over age 65 are severely demented, requiring either institutional care or a full-time custodian. An additional 10 percent of people over age 65 have mild to moderate dementia. Alzheimer's disease probably represents 55 percent of all dementias. After age 75, Alzheimer's is the fourth leading cause of death. Applying these proportions to the United States' population yields an estimated 2 million people currently suffering from dementia in the United States. As the number of aged persons in the United States and Western Europe continues to grow, its prevalence can be expected to increase.

ALZHEIMER'S DISEASE Definition and clinical signs and symptoms The dementing condition that has received the most attention by far in the past decade ("the disease of the century" according to a number of popular publications) is Alzheimer's disease. Unlike some dementias, Alzheimer's is a progressive condition. Patients with Alzheimer's disease fall under the DSM-III-R category of primary degenerative dementia of the Alzheimer type, either of senile or presenile onset, that distinction based on whether the occurrence of the disease was before or after age 65 (Table 12-16). The key element that differentiates primary degenerative dementia from many other kinds of dementia is its insidious onset and progressive deteriorating course.

A definite diagnosis of Alzheimer's disease is always problematic. The clinical impression of the condition should be confirmed with histopathological evidence, specifically senile plaques and neurofibrillary tangles, either at autopsy or under the rare circumstances when a biopsy is obtained. Senile plaques are clusters of degenerating nerve endings containing amyloid. Neurofibrillary tangles are microscopic filamentous paired helical filaments. The characteristic distribution and quantity of these histopathological changes aids the neuropathologist in making the diagnosis of Alzheimer's disease. However, even histological diagnosis can be difficult in very elderly people, in whom plaques and tangles can occur without clinical evidence of dementia.

It was with full awareness of the complexity of diagnosis of Alzheimer's disease that the National Institute of Neurological Communicative Disease and Stroke–American Association of Retired Persons (NINCDS–AARP) criteria for Alzheimer's disease were put forth. These criteria differ from the DSM-III-R definition of primary degenerative dementia. Specifically, the certainty of diagnosis is evaluated and noted to be either definite, probable, or possible. A definite diagnosis requires a histopathological as well as a clinical diagnosis. The criteria for a diagnosis of probable Alzheimer's disease include some documentation of the dementia on a standard neuropsychological examination, such as the Mini-Mental State Examination or the Blessed Dementia Scale, combined with a pro-

TABLE 12-14
Diagnostic Criteria for Dementia

A. Demonstrable evidence of impairment in short- and long-term memory. Impairment in short-term memory (inability to learn new information) may be indicated by inability to remember three objects after 5 minutes. Long-term memory impairment (inability to remember information that was known in the past) may be indicated by inability to remember past personal information (e.g., what happened yesterday, birthplace, occupation) or facts of common knowledge (e.g., past Presidents, well-known dates).
B. At least one of the following:
(1) impairment in abstract thinking, as indicated by inability to find similarities and differences between related words, difficulty in defining words and concepts, and other similar tasks
(2) impaired judgment, as indicated by inability to make reasonable plans to deal with interpersonal, family, and job-related problems and issues
(3) other disturbances of higher cortical function, such as aphasia (disorder of language), apraxia (inability to carry out motor activities despite intact comprehension and motor function), agnosia (failure to recognize or identify objects despite intact sensory function), and "constructional difficulty" (e.g., inability to copy three-dimensional figures, assemble blocks, or arrange sticks in specific designs)
(4) personality change (i.e., alteration or accentuation of premorbid traits).
C. The disturbance in A and B significantly interferes with work or usual social activities or relationships with others.
D. Not occurring exclusively during the course of delirium.
E. Either (1) or (2):
(1) there is evidence from the history, physical examination, or laboratory tests of a specific organic factor (or factors) judged to be etiologically related to the disturbance
(2) in the absence of such evidence, an etiologic organic factor can be presumed if the disturbance cannot be accounted for by any nonorganic mental disorder (e.g., major depression accounting for cognitive impairment).

Criteria for severity of dementia:

Mild: Although work or social activities are significantly impaired, the capacity for independent living remains, with adequate personal hygiene and relatively intact judgment.
Moderate: Independent living is hazardous, and some degree of supervision is necessary.
Severe: Activities of daily living are so impaired that continual supervision is required (e.g., unable to maintain minimal personal hygiene; largely incoherent or mute.)

Table from DSM-III-R *Diagnostic and Statistical Manual of Mental Disorders,* ed 3, revised. Copyright American Psychiatric Association, Washington, DC, 1987. Used with permission.

gressive worsening of memory, particularly the ability to learn new information, and some other areas of cognitive dysfunction, typically, in language (aphasia), motor skills (apraxia), and naming (agnosia). Other data that would support the probable diagnosis include impaired ADL and a family history of similar progressive dementing disorders. As is true in DSM-III-R, there should be no disturbance of consciousness or other systemic disorders or brain diseases that could account for these progressive deficits in memory.

By including a category for possible Alzheimer's disease, the NINCDS criteria provide a classification for a group of patients who may have a more atypical pattern than the probable Alzheimer's patients. Such atypia could be manifest in the variability of the disease's onset, presentation, or clinical course. For example, in a patient with progressive dementia, memory problems, and a disturbance of personality, positive diagnosis would seem elusive. Such a patient would be classified by DSM-III-R as having a primary degenerative dementia, but by NINCDS criteria as only possibly having Alzheimer's disease, because no other cognitive disturbances (aphasia, apraxia, agnosia) are yet apparent.

The fundamental differences between DSM-III-R criteria for primary degenerative dementia and NINCDS criteria for probable Alzheimer's disease are the NINCDS requirements that neuropsychological testing document the cognitive abnormalities and that, in addition to a progressive memory loss, there be at least two other areas of cognitive disturbance. DSM-III-R is less restrictive, requiring that one of four possible impairments (not necessarily cognitive) accompanies a problem in short- and long-term memory. Furthermore, the two systems place markedly different values on ADL. DSM-III-R stipulates that the loss of intellectual abilities must be sufficient to cause a change in an individual's occupational or social functioning. NINCDS notes only that impaired ADL and altered patterns of behavior support a diagnosis of probable Alzheimer's disease. However, complex issues arise in determining how ADL should be incorporated into the diagnosis of Alzheimer's disease, the largest confound being baseline functioning. Clearly, the intelligent person who is little challenged by his or her occupation or avocations may not suffer an impairment of ADL until the disease is advanced. In contrast, very mild disease could produce profound social and occupational dysfunction in a person of lower premorbid intellectual capability and could render ADL challenging.

There is considerable variability among Alzheimer's patients. Although the condition is progressive, plateaus in the course of the illness are possible. A host of noncognitive symptoms can be present, particularly in later stages—depression, insomnia, incontinence, delusions, illusions, hallucinations, agitation, weight loss, appetite changes, myoclonus, gait disorders, and seizures. Recognizing these circumstances, DSM-III-R provides subtypes of primary degenerative dementia of the Alzheimer type: with delirium, with delusions, with depression, or uncomplicated.

Some of the most troublesome symptoms of Alzheimer's disease are not the cognitive ones. Agitation, emotional outbursts, occasional violence, uncooperativeness, and badly disrupted sleep are often the most difficult problems for the caretakers of Alzheimer's patient. Delusions and other psychotic behaviors, including hallucinations, affective symptoms, and eating disturbances are also troublesome and not particularly rare.

Given the important differences that can characterize systems for the diagnosis of Alzheimer's disease, data that validate one system or another become particularly relevant. There is a growing body of evidence that the NINCDS–AARP diagnostic criteria for probable Alzheimer's disease have a misdiagnosis rate of approximately 10 percent as confirmed by histopathological examination. In contrast, clinical diagnosis of Alzheimer's disease has error rates of approximately 30 percent, and sometimes misdiagnosis is as high as 50 percent. Until such time as the empirical criteria for primary degenerative dementia are validated against histopathological criteria, the clinician is advised to be well acquainted with the better-validated NINCDS–AARP formulation as well as with DSM-III-R criteria. In most instances, both systems yield a similar diagnosis; discrepancies arise more commonly in patients with early and mild disease, when diagnosis is always more problematic, than in the more advanced stages. Under these circumstances, the NINCDS criteria are less likely to yield a probable diagnosis of Alzheimer's disease than DSM-III-R is to categorize a patient as having primary degenerative dementia.

Epidemiology There are over 1 million Alzheimer's disease patients in the United States. The prevalence of Alzheimer's disease is exquisitely age dependent, being far more common

TABLE 12-15
Causes of Dementia

- Degenerative
  - Alzheimer's disease, senile and presenile forms
  - Parkinson's disease*
  - Pick's disease
  - Huntington's chorea
- Vascular
  - Multi-infarct dementia†
    - Carotid distribution
    - Vertebrobasilar distribution
    - Lacunar syndrome (basal ganglia, white matter, pons)
  - Strategically placed large stroke
  - Vascular inflammatory disease* (systemic lupus, periarteritis)
- Toxic
  - Alcoholic cerebral atrophy†
  - Chronic bromide or barbiturate intoxication*
  - Metals: lead, mercury, manganese*
  - Organic compounds: nitrobenzenes, organophosphates†
  - Carbon monoxide†
- Metabolic
  - Hypothyrodism*
  - Repeated hypoglycemia†
  - B_{12} deficiency† (possibly folic acid deficiency as well)
  - Postanoxic encephalopathy
  - Chronic hepatic or portalsystemic shunt encephalopathy†
  - Wilson's disease*
  - Uremia†
  - Nonmetastatic effects of carcinoma
- Mechanical
  - Traumatic cerebral atrophy
  - Hydrocephalus*: obstruction, subarachnoid infection, and hemorrhage
  - Normal-pressure hydrocephalus*
  - Chronic subdural hematoma*
- Inflammatory
  - General paresis of neurosyphilis†
  - Chronic meningitis (fungal or tubercular)†
  - Jakob-Creutzfeldt (and other slow virus diseases)
  - AIDS encephalopathy
  - Multifocal leukoencephalopathy
  - Multiple sclerosis
- Neoplastic
  - Meningioma*
  - Glioma
  - Pituitary tumor*
  - Metastatic tumor

*Potentially reversible cause
†Condition that can be arrested

TABLE 12-16
Diagnostic Criteria for Primary Degenerative Dementia of the Alzheimer Type

A. Dementia.
B. Insidious onset with a generally progressive deteriorating course.
C. Exclusion of all other specific causes of dementia by history, physical examination, and laboratory tests.

Types
Primary Degenerative Dementia of the Alzheimer Type, Senile Onset (after age 65)
    with delirium; with delusions; with depression; uncomplicated
Primary Degenerative Dementia of the Alzhemier Type, Presenile Onset (age 65 and below)
    with delirium; with delusions; with depression; uncomplicated

Table from DSM-III-R *Diagnostic and Statistical Manual of Mental Disorders,* ed 3, revised. Copyright American Psychiatric Association, Washington, DC, 1987. Used with permission.

in persons aged 85 than in those who are 65. Furthermore, the fastest-growing segment of the population in the United States and Western Europe are persons over 85, a group of whom 15 percent are severely demented. Already, the cost of providing institutional care for patients with dementia in the United States probably exceeds $25 billion. Within the next century, the costs of providing care for the demented population will become staggering; this raises the question of whether our society can afford humane care for all victims of Alzheimer's disease who may require it. The fact that much has been learned about Alzheimer's disease offers hope that the future may see, if not a treatment, at least palliative therapy or the ability to delay the disease's onset.

Etiology and pathology Four factors are known irrefutably to be associated with increased risk for Alzheimer's disease: age, family history, history of head trauma, and Down's syndrome. The cumulative incidence of a progressive dementia in first-degree relatives of patients with Alzheimer's disease has, in some studies, been shown to approach 50 percent by age 90. Clearly, these data suggest a major contribution of genetics to Alzheimer's disease, which was not previously appreciated because so many patients never survived through the age of risk in order that their genotype might be fully expressed. Should Alzheimer's disease prove to have an important genetic component, as has been suggested, powerful tools of molecular genetics likely will be applied to help elucidate the disease's pathophysiology. There are also compelling data (e.g., monozygotic twin studies) that indicate that other factors, probably environmental, influence the expression of the disease. If the factors that lead to the expression of the disease can be identified, a strategy to delay its onset might be devised.

The senile plaques and neurofibrillary tangles of Alzheimer's disease are not uniformly distributed throughout the brain, nor are the more gross characteristics, such as cerebral atrophy. Atrophy is apparent in the associational areas of the cortex, with relative sparing of primary motor, visual, and somatosensory areas. At a microscopic level, cell loss is seen in the hippocampus, enterhinal cortex, locus ceruleus, and nucleus basalis. As these changes progress, they effectively disconnect the hippocampus from the rest of the brain. Senile plaques and neurofibrillary tangles are most prevalent in the temporo-parietal region, an area whose involvement is clearly reflected in the early symptoms of the disease (Figs. 12-1 through 12-4).

Alzheimer's disease does not affect all neurotransmitter systems; rather, it has a predilection for a few neurotransmitters and neuromodulators. There is a profound deficit in acetylcholine in virtually all patients who have been studied, as well as diminished immunoreactivity of somatostatin and corticotropin-releasing factor. The serotonergic and noradrenergic systems seem also to be affected, but primarily when onset of the disease occurs before age 75. Other neurotransmitters have occasionally been implicated in Alzheimer's disease, including some reports of diminished dopaminergic and γ-amino butyric acid (GABA)-ergic concentrations. Nevertheless, most neuropeptides and neurotransmitters that have been studied in Alzheimer's patients remain unaffected.

The relative contributions of these neurotransmitter and neuropeptide deficiencies to the symptoms of Alzheimer's disease are unclear. Surely the cholinergic deficit contributes to some of the cognitive abnormalities. Cholinergic neurotransmission along the septal hippocampal formation and the nucleus basalis projection to the cortex have been implicated repeatedly in the ability to learn new information, a core abnormality in Alzheimer's disease. Alzheimer's disease is not simply a cholinergic deficit, nor does a scopolamine dementia totally mimic Alzheimer's disease. Thus, the other neurochemical problems in Alzheimer's disease must contribute to the symptoms.

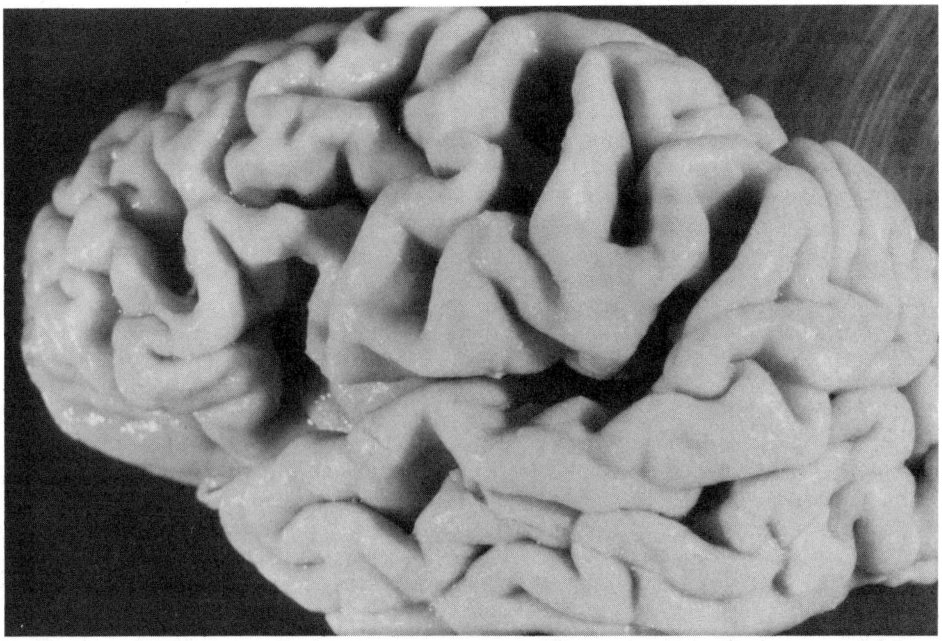

FIGURE 12-1. *Gross external appearance of the brain of a patient who had primary degenerative dementia of the Alzheimer type, senile onset. The leptomeninges have been removed so that the generalized atrophy may be fully appreciated. (Courtesy of Daniel P. Perl, MD.)*

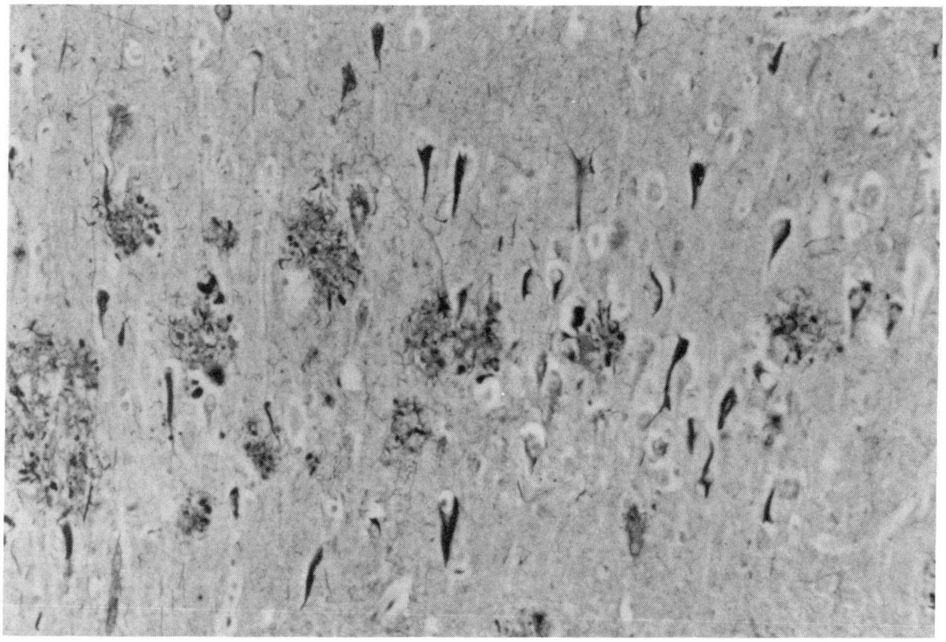

FIGURE 12-2. *Microscopic appearance of the hippocampus from a patient with Alzheimer's disease showing large numbers of neurofibrillary tangles and senile plaques (modified Bielschowsky's stain, original magnification × 190; courtesy of Daniel P. Perl, MD).*

In some instances, the neurotransmitter deficiencies in Alzheimer's disease have been linked to particular subcortical nuclei. For example, severe, late-stage Alzheimer's disease is associated with decreased numbers of cholinergic-staining cells in the nucleus basalis. Similarly, it is likely that the noradrenergic deficiency seen in younger patients is linked to the locus ceruleus and abnormalities in serotonin, to the raphe nuclei. The extensive hippocampal pathology reflected in neurofibrillary tangles and senile plaques undoubtedly disturbs the cholinergic septal-hippocampal projection and a complex array of other neurotransmitter and neuropeptide systems. As basic neurobiology advances, tools likely will become available to elucidate other important neurochemical abnormalities in the Alzheimer's brain.

Differential diagnosis The differential diagnosis of Alzheimer's disease includes all the other causes of a dementia: multiple cerebral infarcts, alcohol abuse, mood dis-

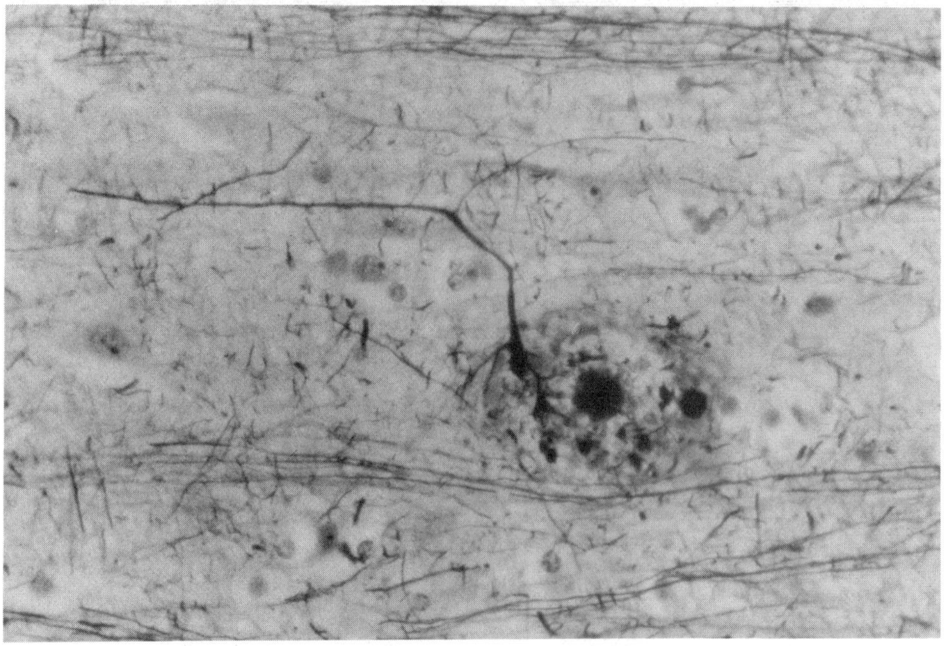

FIGURE 12-3. *Microscopic appearance of a neuron containing a neurofibrillary tangle. Notice the dark-staining fibers within the neuronal cytoplasm (modified Bielschowsky's stain, original magnification × 420; courtesy of Daniel P. Perl, MD).*

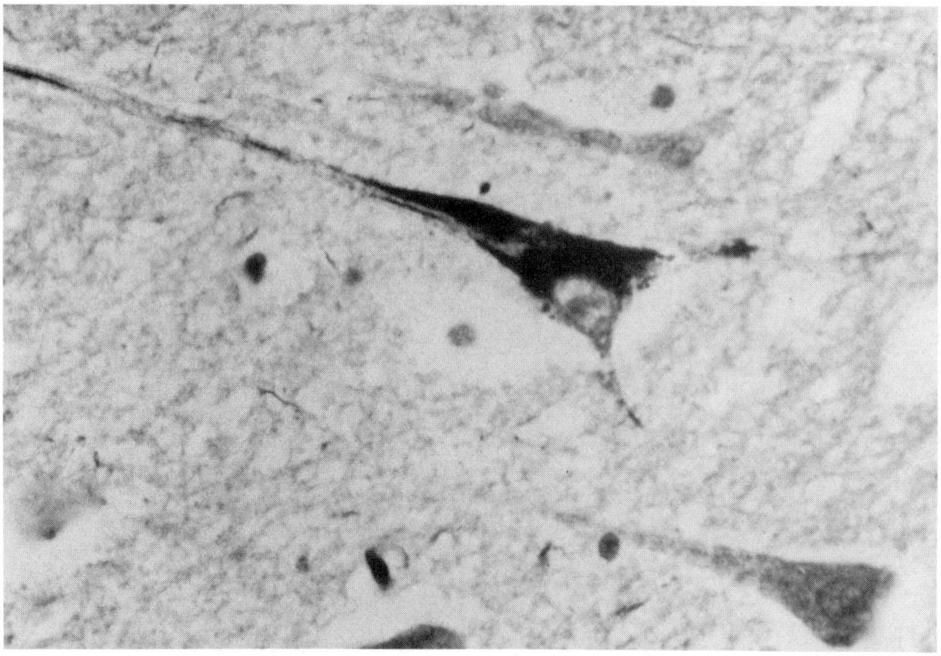

FIGURE 12-4. *Microscopic appearance of a senile (neuritic) plaque in the neocortex. Notice the silver-staining neuronal process (neurite) entering the periphery of the plaque (modified Bielschowsky's stain, original magnification × 420; courtesy of Daniel P. Perl, MD).*

order, metabolic disturbances, toxic states, infectious diseases, space-occupying lesions, normal-pressure hydrocephalus, infection, Parkinson's disease, Huntington's disease, Jakob-Creutzfeld disease, Pick's disease, and other relatively uncommon neurodegenerative conditions.

A careful history and physical examination and judicious use of laboratory tests narrow the diagnosis. Special attention should be paid to the course of the disease. Alzheimer's disease is commonly insidious and steadily progressive, whereas multi-infarct dementia is abrupt in onset and progresses incrementally. Similarly, the presence of focal localizing neurological signs and a history of cerebrovascular disease and hypertension increase the likelihood of multi-infarct dementia. Nonetheless, the two conditions can coexist, and mixed cases are not uncommon. Laboratory tests should be employed to determine whether a metabolic cause for a dementia exists;

careful attention must be directed to the thyroid, to folate and B_{12} concentrations, and to calcium metabolism.

For a clinician who relies on cross-sectional examination the differentiation of mood disorder and Alzheimer's disease can be difficult; however, prior history of mood disorder and a more abrupt onset tend to increase the likelihood that the patient has a mood disorder. In addition, the value of the family history cannot be understated. The presence of affective disease or progressive dementia in a first-degree relative helps to influence the diagnostic impression. However, ultimately, and in a few cases, it is only after a trial of antidepressant medication that a diagnosis of Alzheimer's disease or mood disorder can be made more authoritatively, on the basis of the patient's response to drug treatment. This entire issue is complicated further by the fact that affective symptoms are not uncommon in patients with Alzheimer's disease. Thus, it is possible not only for mood-disorder patients to have a secondary dementia but for patients with Alzheimer's disease to have secondary affective symptoms.

Progress in imaging technologies has contributed to the differential diagnosis of Alzheimer's disease. A subdural hematoma and normal-pressure hydrocephalus can be diagnosed with appropriate imaging devices. Occasionally, the diagnosis of Huntington's disease can be facilitated by a CT scan showing flattening of the caudate nucleus. Initial optimism that MRI might help differentiate multi-infarct dementia from Alzheimer's disease so far has not been borne out, but as the technology is refined its utility may increase. Finally, preliminary work with SPECT suggests that, in the near future, this imaging modality may be capable of definitively detecting Alzheimer's disease. Already it has been suggested that Alzheimer's patients manifest unique patterns of glucose utilization that are pathognomonic.

Physical and mental status examinations usually can differentiate a patient with Alzheimer's from one with Huntington's or Parkinson's disease. Furthermore, it has been suggested that, whereas Alzheimer's disease is a cortical dementia, Huntington's disease and Parkinson's disease are subcortical dementias. Still, there are many similarities between Parkinson's dementia and Alzheimer's dementia, and in the late stage of Alzheimer's disease some signs referable to the basal ganglia can be present. In fact, the dementia in the Parkinson's patient is associated with a cholinergic deficit, so there may be more overlap between these conditions than was previously assumed.

Prognosis The mean duration of Alzheimer's disease, from onset until death, is 7 years, but it can vary widely. It is impossible to accurately predict the progression of symptoms for any single patient. The general course is usually characterized, in the early stage, by problems in learning new information, progressing to difficulties in other cognitive areas, particularly language, praxis, and naming, and in the end stages, by a completely vegetative state. Studies comparing the mortality of Alzheimer's patients to an age-matched cohort suggest that the disease does not shorten life when it occurs in patients over age 75 but significantly shortens life for younger patients. These observations are consistent with the impression that Alzheimer's disease is more malignant in younger age groups than in older patients.

Treatment Two principles underlie the management of the Alzheimer's patient: to treat what is treatable, and in so doing, to minimize disability and to support the caregiver, who suffers almost as much as the Alzheimer's victim. Treating the treatable centers on the use of the appropriate psychopharmacological agents to relieve the concomitant noncognitive symptoms, such as depression, agitation, hallucinations, delusions, and sleep disturbance. This goal can pose a real dilemma in balancing a drug's benefit and its adverse effects. Particular attention has to be given to minimizing the use of drugs that exacerbate the cognitive symptoms of Alzheimer's disease, such as agents with anticholinergic activity and benzodiazepines, which can interfere with new learning. Addressing the needs of the caregiver requires that a full spectrum of programs, from educational to psychodynamic, be available. Support groups, in which caregivers regularly meet to exchange experiences and offer support and advice can be particularly useful.

The question of institutionalization is always difficult. Since the disease is associated with an inability to learn new information and to formulate spatial relationships, placing the Alzheimer's patient in a new environment can be disorienting and can lead to an apparent worsening of the condition. From this perspective, a goal of therapy is to keep the patient functioning in the community for as long as possible. The attainment of that goal may, unfortunately, be limited by a family's resources. The decision to institutionalize must be weighed against the demands the Alzheimer's patient places on caregivers. Situations inevitably arise where a patient can no longer be managed in the home, and to continue to do so would be an enormous burden for the family. Under these circumstances institutional placement is currently the most likely option, although alternative approaches are being developed. Day hospital programs for demented patients, nurse and social worker home visitors, and respite care that allows a family to leave the Alzheimer's patient for a few hours to as much as a few days, can often make the difference between keeping the patient in the community and full-time institutionalization. Undoubtedly the future will see the growth of intermediate programs between total care in the home and nursing home placement.

The long-term hope for the management of Alzheimer's disease is the development of a rational, definitive treatment. But, at this time, too little is known about the pathophysiology of the condition. However, modest results have been obtained with cholinesterase inhibitors (physostigmine [Antilirium], tetrahydroaminoacridine). It is possible that for a subgroup of patients with a relatively specific cholinergic deficit, probably older patients with mild to moderate disease, cholinesterase inhibitors may be palliative. In the next few years, such agents will be widely tested in clinical trials, and, if modestly efficacious, are likely to enter the marketplace. Nonetheless, these treatments are likely to be less effective than is L-dopa in Parkinson's disease or even antipsychotics in psychosis.

MULTI-INFARCT DEMENTIA **Definition and epidemiology** The DSM-III-R criteria (Table 12-17) rely on the symptom complex of dementia complicated by a stepwise deteriorating course and focal neurological signs in combination with evidence for cerebrovascular disease. For research purposes, investigators have used the Hachinski scale (Table 12-18), which is clearly similar to, but much better validated than, the DSM-III-R definition. DSM-III-R also lists three subtypes, for reasons that are unclear. There is no evidence that these subtypes remain consistent through their natural history or that they are prognostically useful. In fact, the delirium could just as easily derive from a superimposed metabolic encephalopathy, and depression may be a side effect of commonly employed antihypertensives.

Senile dementia once was thought to be vascular in origin, secondary to poor perfusion by sclerotic arteries, so cerebral vasodilators seemed a rational therapy. It is clear now that the reduction in cerebral blood flow in primary degenerative dementia is secondary to the reduced metabolic rate of the brain and that the underlying pathology is that of Alzheimer's disease. Vascular dementia has taken a distant second place to Alzheimer's disease among causes of the dementia syndrome: 10 percent versus over 50 percent. The incidence of vascular

TABLE 12-17
Diagnostic Criteria for Multi-Infarct Dementia

A. Dementia
B. Stepwise deteriorating course with "patchy" distribution of deficits (i.e., affecting some functions, but not others) early in the course.
C. Focal neurologic signs and symptoms (e.g., exaggeration of deep tendon reflexes, extensor plantar response, pseudobulbar palsy, gait abnormalities, weakness of an extremity, etc.).
D. Evidence from history, physical examination, or laboratory tests of significant cerebrovascular disease (recorded on Axis III) that is judged to be etiologically related to the disturbance.

Types
Multi-infarct dementia
  with delirium
  with delusions
  with depression
  uncomplicated

TABLE 12-18
Hachinski Ischemic Score

Feature	*Score*
Abrupt onset	2
Stepwise orientation	1
Fluctuating course	2
Nocturnal confusion	1
Relative preservation of personality	1
Depression	1
Somatic complaints	1
Emotional incontinence	1
History of hypertension	2
History of strokes	1
Evidence of associated arteriosclerosis	1
Focal neurological symptoms	2
Focal neurological signs (excluding aphasia and apraxia)	2
Total	

dementias has been decreasing with the incidence of cerebrovascular disease. Their prevalence may have stabilized for two reasons: Better standards of care prevent the onset of major, fatal strokes, and better diagnostic techniques identify small vascular lesions coexisting with Alzheimer's pathology.

Etiology and pathophysiology Several distinct pathologies that affect the cerebrovascular system result in distinct disease syndromes and require different treatment. Lumping them under the single rubric of multi-infarct dementia may confound matters. Furthermore, in the early stages of vascular disease, the cerebral manifestations may not be those of a full-blown dementia.

Hypertensive vascular disease is an affliction of small vessels with median wall thickening. Changes in the critical closing pressure of arterioles may lead to sudden closure of the lumen; ischemia results and infarction of a small area essentially produces a lacuna. The small-caliber vessels most affected are vertical penetrating branches of the medial cerebral artery supplying the basal ganglia and the white matter of the corona radiata (Fig. 12-5). These are also the so-called arteries of cerebral hemorrhage. The severity of the pathology of hypertensive vascular disease is related directly to the adequacy of blood pressure control. Major health monitoring and education efforts have significantly improved this, even among U.S. blacks who are at high risk for complicated hypertension.

Atherosclerotic disease attacks the intima of large and medium-sized vessels, sites of lipid or platelet aggregation that predispose to thrombus formation or to embolization of cholesterol plaque or platelet aggregations. Carotid stenosis figures prominently in the pathophysiology of common middle cerebral territory infarctions, and auscultation of the neck for carotid murmurs is an important element of a physical examination. Atherosclerosis itself is a product of a relatively affluent life-style: hypercholesterolemia, cigarette smoking, obesity, diabetes, inactivity, and stress are contributing risk factors. Related cardiac disease may also promote embolization.

Arterial rigidity as a classical age-related development has a limited impact on the cerebral circulation. The large vessels of the brain generally have a very efficient compensatory circulation through the circle of Willis, and the small vessels have prominent local self-regulation, closely tied to local metabolic demands. Under unusual conditions of extreme persistent hypotension, one can see watershed infarcts along the margins of the middle cerebral artery distribution. Perfusion problems may underlie drop attacks and other brain stem phenomena in vertebrobasilar stenosis; in a small number of patients with an aberrant circle of Willis, temporal lobe ischemia may lead to memory changes.

Vasculitides cause a small but dramatic group of multi-infarct OMSs. In early and middle life, systemic lupus and polyarteritis are the leading causes, while in old age, temporal arteritis is important. Given the scattered, variable foci of partial cerebral ischemia, the clinical presentation is more often a delirium or an organic mood syndrome than a dementia.

Cerebral hemorrhage and meningeal inflammation can irritate nearby arteries and cause them to go into spasm. A leaking anterior communicating artery aneurysm or meningitis can produce the ischemia that causes frontal lobe damage.

Clinical signs and symptoms and differential diagnosis There are two common, distinct types of multi-infarct dementia: cortical and subcortical. The former is based on atherosclerotic or hypertensive disease of large arteries, the latter on hypertensive small-vessel disease.

The cortical dementia is marked by recurrent transient ischemic episodes and small strokes with a gradually deteriorating progression. Neurological signs (motor, reflex changes, transient Babinski, hemianopia, etc.) are transiently quite prominent; some episodes, affecting association areas of the cortex, present as nonspecific confusional episodes. Seizures can complicate the course earlier than in Alzheimer's disease. The course of illness can fluctuate a great deal, with episodes of major impairment interspersed with prolonged lucid periods. As the middle cerebral distribution is involved most of the time, apraxic, agnosic, and aphasic symptoms, and difficulties with topography, dressing, and manual construction are common. Involvement of the right hemisphere may lead to difficulties with emotional expressivity or with the ability to perceive specific emotions in others. Organic mood disorders may arise out of this pathology before the disease progresses to a full dementia. Frontal lobe changes are less common. Occipital signs (cortical blindness, prosopagnosia), sometimes coupled with temporal lobe amnestic features, are seen in vertebrobasilar and posterior cerebral artery disease (a much less frequent disturbance).

The lacunar syndrome, described by Fisher, refers to subcortical, bilaterally scattered small infarcts. While there may be episodes of strokes due to capsular infarcts, usually the syndrome has a more steadily deteriorating, less dramatic course. Pseudobulbar palsy is the neurological hallmark of this disorder, with stiff, stumbling gait,

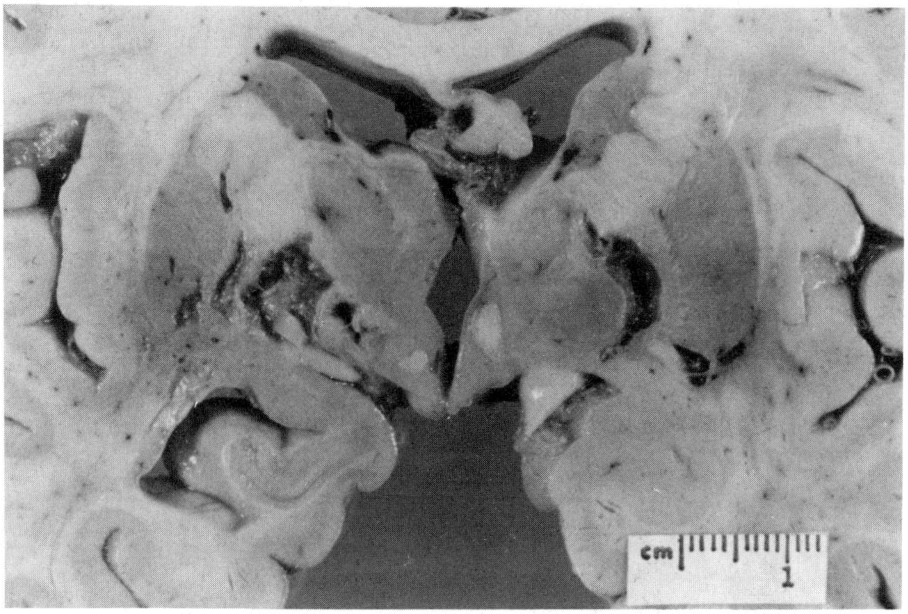

FIGURE 12-5. *Gross appearance of a the cerebral cortex on coronal section from a case of multi-infarct dementia. Notice the multiple bilateral lacunar infarcts involving the thalamus, internal capsule, and globus pallidus. (Courtesy of Daniel P. Perl, MD.)*

bilateral long-tract signs, dysarthria, blank facial expression, and other brain stem and upper motor neuron signs. The mental state is characterized by apathy, lack of motivation and self-respect, and difficulty with memory retrieval (not so much loss of new learning as forgetting how to use recall strategies). Occasionally, there is emotional incontinence—sudden episodes of shallow emotional disturbance triggered by some trivial event. Judgment, abstract thinking, and foresight are impaired early; language and praxis difficulties are much less common. The condition is less easily recognized than the more dramatic cortical multi-infarct dementia, and consequently the patients are frequently berated for poor motivation and are at times thought to be depressed.

The various vascular disorders have a propensity to present with focal psychosyndromes, delirious and affective changes, and organic delusional and personality disorders. While the DSM-III-R empirical-statistical classification categorizes these as OMDs, it is important that they have the same pathophysiology as multi-infarct dementia.

The differential diagnosis of cortical multi-infarct dementia and Alzheimer's disease depends more on the fluctuating natural history and the presence of focal neurological signs rather than on the cross-sectional mental state, which can be quite similar. Subcortical multi-infarct dementia needs to be distinguished from Parkinson's disease, normal-pressure hydrocephalus, depressive pseudodementia, and some metabolic dementias. The focal psychosyndromes need to be investigated for vascular, infectious, embolic, and neoplastic causes.

The routine EEG has a limited role in demonstrating focal ischemic cortical abnormalities and can pinpoint potential seizure foci. The new EEG topographic brain mapping techniques are likely to afford even better physiological localizations. CT, especially contrast scans, truly revolutionized brain imaging, demonstrating even small infarcts and hemorrhages and other focal lesions and outlining atrophy and the often considerable ventricular dilation. MRI is likely to enhance the detection of lesions further, especially more subtle white-matter problems due to ischemia. Vascular changes themselves are demonstrated relatively safely by femoral catheter angiography, but less invasive techniques (e.g., Doppler flow studies, ophthalmodynamometry, digital subtraction angiography) are gaining popularity.

Treatment and prognosis Primary and secondary prevention appear to be making headway with cerebrovascular disorders. However, even in relatively well-established vascular disorders, reduction of cholesterol intake, cessation of smoking, weight reduction, and control of blood pressure and of diabetes can at least arrest the progress of many of these syndromes. Vascular inflammatory disorders need to be recognized early and treated aggressively with steroids.

No biological treatment can reverse the effects of a completed stroke. In a stroke in progress or when transient ischemic attacks (TIAs) are frequent, some investigators suggest anticoagulation; a hemorrhagic lesion must be conclusively excluded. Carotid endarterectomy will not improve mental state in multi-infarct dementia but may prevent new strokes if an ulcerated plaque or severe sterosis is demonstrated.

Platelet aggregation seems to be the important final common pathway for intravascular embolic and thrombotic events. Aspirin, 650 mg per day, as an anti–platelet aggregation agent, has been shown to reduce the incidence of strokes in controlled studies in certain populations and can be utilized relatively safely. Long-term anticoagulation or cerebral vasodilators have their proponents, but their effectiveness has not been documented by controlled observations.

Emotional lability, which is common in these patients, often requires small doses of potent antipsychotics. Depression is a common complication (60 percent) of strokes and responds to heterocyclic antidepressants. Pseudobulbar palsy can be treated with amantadine (Symmetrel) or L-dopa.

While careful and knowledgeable medical management can stabilize patients with multi-infarct dementia and prevent their deterioration, their rehabilitation has not been fully explored. Speech, physical, and occupational therapy offer many techniques, and cognitive psychologists have recently introduced memory training. It seems that the very diagnosis of dementia is responsible for the reluctance to engage some of these patients. Clinical experience in rehabilitative settings suggests that many patients with ostensible focal psychosyndromes are successfully treated for aphasia or apraxia despite their global cognitive loss. It is the label of dementia that would prevent them from continuing with rehabilitation. For other patients, apathy and lack of motivation are the major obstacles. Rehabilitation staff often fails to understand that this is as much a part of the neurological syndrome as is the apraxia or dysphasia. The provision of a closely monitored, structured learning environment and relentless, family-supervised practice of new skills at home can make a significant difference. There is clearly a value here in educating families and rehabilitation specialists.

DEMENTIA IN ALCOHOLISM

Definition DSM-III-R requires that the mental changes of dementia persist at least 3 weeks after the cessation of prolonged heavy drinking in order for this diagnosis to be made (Table 12-19). Alcohol amnestic disorder is available as an alternative diagnosis. The decline of mental competence of chronic alcoholics was well described by the 1850s, when dullness of thought and judgment, impairment of memory, and a variety of other symptoms were noted. The description by Korsakoff of an amnestic state associated with polyneuritis and by Wernicke of an amnestic state with ophthalmoplegia and ataxia, and the eventual recognition by Bonhoeffer of a common underlying pathophysiology opened the way for subsequent elaboration of a nutritional etiology for these disorders. Korsakoff's psychosis became the favorite diagnosis for alcoholics manifesting a chronic change in mental state, just as Sutton's delirium tremens became the favorite diagnosis for any of their acute confusional states. Yet, these customary diagnoses represented an oversimplification, and a potentially dangerous one. Delirium in alcoholics may be due to withdrawal from alcohol, to hepatic encephalopathy, to intercurrent infections, and so on. Chronic mental deterioration may be due to nutritional changes, chronic hepatic encephalopathy, a subdural hematoma or other trauma, or to the chronic toxic effects of alcohol.

At a descriptive level, a clear distinction exists between a Wernicke-Korsakoff syndrome, in which the central problem is difficulty learning new material, and a cortical dementia, in which global intellectual decline is combined with some higher cortical signs. Two other alcohol-related conditions impinge on the borders of dementia—a cognitive impairment that clears with detoxification from alcohol and a gradual change in personality that is not yet associated with the clinical signs of dementia. While each condition can exist in isolation and follows its own pathophysiology, individual alcoholics often demonstrate a marked overlap of several of these disorders; nevertheless, each syndrome requires individualized treatment.

Epidemiology Alcoholism is the third cause of dementia in most studies, after Alzheimer's disease and multiple cerebral infarctions. About 10 percent of alcoholics show evidence of dementia, and the incidence increases with age. Milder degrees of cognitive decline, detectable by neuropsychological testing, are even more common. The disorder afflicts a higher proportion of women than men. Dementia is one of the later complications of alcoholism, manifesting itself after 15 to 20 years of very heavy drinking. About half of these patients also reveal significant evidence of malnutrition (versus one-third of nondemented alcoholics).

TABLE 12-19
Diagnostic Criteria for Dementia Associated with Alcoholism

A. Dementia following prolonged, heavy ingestion of alcohol and persisting at least 3 weeks after cessation of alcohol ingestion
B. Exclusion, by history, physical examination, and laboratory tests, of all causes of dementia other than prolonged heavy use of alcohol

Table from DSM-III-R *Diagnostic and Statistical Manual of Mental Disorders*, ed 3, revised. Copyright American Psychiatric Association, Washington, DC, 1987. Used with permission.

Etiology and pathology The existence of heavy drinking and malnutrition makes for a complicated pathogenesis. Thiamine deficiency leads to median thalamic, diencephalic, periventricular, and upper brain stem lesions, with focal cell loss and small hemorrhages. Persons whose transketolase enzyme binds thiamine less tightly than normal seem to be most prone to these neurological sequelae of thiamine deficiency. The disorder can be precipitated by carbohydrate loading and by seizures, both of which use up the remaining small stores of thiamine. The majority of alcoholics have some intermittent thiamine deficiency, which varies with their diet and with taking vitamin supplements or eating thiamine-enriched food. While thiamine deficiency clearly leads to a global metabolic defect, the characteristic lesions are quite focal. Their location has a good anatomical correlation with the amnesia, truncal ataxia, sixth nerve paralysis, and nystagmus seen in these patients. Cortical lesions are inconstant in these patients and may well be due to the intercurrent toxic and traumatic insults experienced by alcoholics.

Even well-nourished alcoholics, however, show cortical atrophy and ventricular dilation after 10 or more years of drinking. There is neuronal loss, disruption of the cortical layers, pigmentary degeneration, and glial proliferation. The frontal lobes are most extensively affected, followed by the parietal and temporal association areas. It is possible that cortical atrophy (as shown by widening of sulci) runs a different course from ventricular dilation.

Neuropsychological deterioration seems to be correlated with the distinct factors of total lifetime alcohol consumption, number of episodes of very high blood alcohol, and age. It is notable that even among social drinkers tested in a sober state, there is a deleterious interactive effect of past episodes of moderately heavy drinking and age on neuropsychological performance. Animal experiments suggest a correlation between chronic alcoholic feeding in well-nourished animals and impairment of learning ability, as well as a variety of neurotransmitter and neuronal protein and ribonucleic acid (RNA) changes. In clinically nondemented alcoholics, neuropsychological tests may point to early and subtle brain dysfunctions and illuminate the pathophysiology. Language, information, numerical, and constructive skills are well preserved, and the Wechsler Adult Intelligence Scale (WAIS) is generally normal. Subtle memory deficits do show up that are due more to poor mnemonic strategies than to difficulties in transferring information from short-term to long-term memory. The Wisconsin Card-Sorting Test and the Halsted Categories Tests are generally abnormal, showing difficulty in shifting sets in concept-forming tasks. These findings point to frontal lobe type of pathology, as do autopsy and radiographic changes.

Clinical signs and symptoms and differential diagnosis Although the nutritionally caused amnestic syndrome can occur quite suddenly, alcohol dementia due to chronic toxic effects of alcohol develops insidiously. The underlying condition of cerebral atrophy initially presents as an organic personality disorder of the frontal lobe type. Alcoholics manifest increasing disregard for social conventions, appear poorly motivated, lack foresight and planning, and display an apathetic mood interspersed with labile, shallow affect. These problems are generally blamed on the intoxication itself or on the social deterioration that alcoholics often experience at this time. Increasing forgetfulness, inability to remember important events, slowing of cognitive processing, and concrete thinking herald the onset of frank dementia. Minor dysphasic, dysarthric, dyspraxic, and agnosic symptoms appear in a minority of patients, but the disorder rarely becomes as severe as Alzheimer's disease in its late stages.

The steady progress of the dementia is interspersed with acute episodes of delirium, to which the alcoholic becomes increasingly susceptible. Secondary malnutrition may precipitate superimposed Wernicke's encephalopathy, resulting in a sudden deterioration of memory and learning capacity. An acceleration of the global deterioration can also be due to a subdural hematoma, as alcoholics are quite prone to head injuries. Yet, a more common syndrome of subacute decline is the combination of surreptitious drinking and the use of benzodiazepines. Alcoholics are prone to several medical disorders, which can induce subacute mental changes that temporarily make their dementia much worse. Chronic hepatic encephalopathy, respiratory failure due to smoking, metastatic and hormonal effects of neoplasia, folic acid deficiency, and anemias of chronic illness are not uncommon.

Thus, there is a clear need for an adequate, often extensive, medical workup in alcoholics presenting with personality and cognitive changes or with exacerbation of existing dementia. The process is not so much one of differential diagnosis, of looking for the most likely single cause; rather, it is a search for a variety of precipitating and sustaining causes. Energetic medical treatment, detoxification, and good nutrition can significantly improve the mental state of chronic alcoholics within the 2- to 3-week time frame of a general medical hospitalization.

Treatment and prognosis An aura of pessimism pervades the long-term outlook for demented alcoholics. Not only is alcoholism itself a frustrating condition to treat, but the development of dementia clearly adds to the difficulty. Treatment program evaluations show a much poorer response by alcoholics in cognitive decline to the usual psychotherapeutic and educational efforts. Yet, longitudinal psychometric studies reveal continuing improvement in the mental state during periods of sobriety. There is an initial rapid improvement that reaches an early plateau at 3 to 4 weeks. This is followed by more gradual improvement detectable at 6 months. Several studies suggest that neuropsychological improvement, and more remarkably, CT evidence of improvement, can be shown after 18 months of sobriety. There are clinical case reports of remarkable functional recovery from alcoholic dementia and from Korsakoff's amnestic syndrome. The common thread of all these studies is the assurance of complete sobriety, a difficult, if not impossible, feat with outpatient treatment.

A review of the general treatment approaches to alcoholism can fault the field for offering monolithic, undifferentiated treatments to most alcoholics. Evidence suggests that subtle evidence of brain damage, together with the patient's ego strength and social competence, should be taken into account in planning treatment. Exploratory psychotherapy in individual, group, and therapeutic community settings is recommended only for those who are cognitively unimpaired and demonstrate high ego strength and social competence. The presence of neuropsychological impairment calls for more behavioral, supportive, and structured interventions. These may include the use of disulfiram (Antabuse) in a medical-model approach to alcoholism. Alcoholics whose ego functions and social competence are significantly impaired by alcohol-related brain damage require multiple supportive services and even then often fail in ambulatory care. One wonders whether long-term placement in a supportive, alcohol-free residential environment might not allow for sufficient cognitive recovery to permit their eventual return to the community. The alternative is continued failure in short-term treatment settings, persistent drinking, further gradual cognitive and behavioral decline, and, eventually, death from one of the many lethal complications of alcoholism.

PSEUDODEMENTIA

Definition and clinical signs and symptoms Most case series of rigorously worked-up dementias include a group of patients who end up with a diagnosis of functional psychiatric conditions. Depression is the most common, but schizophrenia, personality disorders, and factitious disorders have all been noted. Felix Post and other British psychiatrists have long argued for the concept of a depressive pseudodementia, but Wells has disputed the depressive feature, finding that any of a broad range of dependent, hysterical personality styles was more commonly antecedent. McHugh and Folstein have argued for a dementia of depression, noting the real difficulties in distinguishing this syndrome from some other dementing disorders.

Careful attention to the different levels of diagnosis involved would resolve this controversy and retain the valuable observations of all the participants. At the level of descriptive, syndromal diagnosis, one does perceive two disorders. There is a group of patients who complain a great deal about cognitive loss in a remarkably detailed manner. They show memory gaps for specific, often emotionally charged, events, and their overall memory performance is atypical. They make little effort to perform even simple tasks, tend to highlight their failures, and show marked variability in performance. A strong sense of distress and help-seeking pervades their behavior; they do not try to keep up and give frequent "don't know" answers. All of these features are in contrast with the behavior of the majority of patients who meet DSM-III-R

TABLE 12-20
Diagnostic Criteria for Presenile Dementia Not Otherwise Specified

Dementias associated with an organic factor and arising before age 65 that cannot be classified as a specific dementia (e.g., primary degenerative dementia of the Alzheimer type, presenile onset)

Table from DSM-III-R *Diagnostic and Statistical Manual of Mental Disorders,* ed 3, revised. Copyright American Psychiatric Association, Washington, DC, 1987. Used with permission.

TABLE 12-21
Diagnostic Criteria for Senile Dementia Not Otherwise Specified

Dementias associated with an organic factor and arising after age 65 that cannot be classified as a specific dementia (e.g., as primary degenerative dementia of the Alzheimer type, senile onset, or dementia associated with alcoholism)

Table from DSM-III-R *Diagnostic and Statistical Manual of Mental Disorders,* ed 3, revised. Copyright American Psychiatric Association, Washington, DC, 1987. Used with permission.

criteria for dementia. Careful neurological and neuropsychological examination fails to find higher cortical signs, memory performance is atypical, and behavior is incongruent with the tested level of cognitive dysfunction. Some of these patients barely meet DSM-III-R criteria for dementia; others' problems are much better diagnosed as factitious disorders. A careful longitudinal biographical study gleaned from interviews with significant others generally reveals a lifelong characterological style of interpersonal dependency, somatization, and dysphoric, hypochondriacal, or hysterical traits. This is a group, then, where the term "pseudodementia" would appear appropriate, as the condition mimics the true behavioral syndrome of dementia. There is, however, a group of elderly patients who cross-sectionally meet the DSM-III-R criteria for depression and for dementia. Further cross-sectional evaluation of their mental state fails to reveal any higher cortical signs; rather, they show poor motivation, psychomotor retardation, halting gait, a disheveled, perplexed look, and more difficulties with memory retrieval than with learning new material. Although their language capacity is unimpaired, their speech is slow, halting, and imprecise; that is, they present with subcortical dementia. Neurological and laboratory examination excludes the usual causes of such a dementia (lacunar syndrome of multi-infarct dementia, Parkinsonism, normal-pressure hydrocephalus, metabolic disorders). There is often a personal or family history of depression. The cognitive decline is often preceded by mood changes and the vegetative symptoms of depression. This is, then, a dementia syndrome, but one in which the underlying cause is not Alzheimer's or vascular or systemic metabolic disease but a major mood disorder, a dementia of depression.

Etiology and pathogenesis To understand pseudodementia one needs to turn to the notions of sick role and abnormal illness behavior as developed by the sociologists Talcott Parsons and David Mechanic. As long as society sanctions special settings and privileges for people declared sick by duly authorized health care professionals, there will be those who attempt to solve problems of dependency and interpersonal conflict by mimicking medical or psychiatric syndromes. Their level of conscious awareness will vary, as will the sophistication of the mimicry. The actions of caretakers and health care workers can reinforce this abnormal illness behavior.

The pathogenesis of the dementia of depression can be best approached through a study of cognition in young, mentally unimpaired depressives, who manifest a characteristic pessimistic content of cognition (negative evaluation of the self, the world, and the future) and a characteristic impairment of cognitive processing. There is a decline in the efficiency, speed, and diversity of cognition, memory, and attention. While automatic, simple cognitive tasks are performed normally, complex tasks requiring effort are markedly difficult (unlike in early Alzheimer's disease, where there is deterioration in simple and in complex tasks, in automatic and in demanding routines). Normal aging does interfere with the speed and the span of cognitive processes and with the fluid (though not the crystallized) intelligence. The combination of affective and aging-related impairments of cognitive function can lead to the clinical manifestations of a subcortical dementia.

Differential diagnosis Alzheimer's disease is frequently associated with dysphoric symptoms as well as weight loss, sleep disturbance, psychomotor agitation, and episodes of persecutory or nihilistic delusions. These ostensible indicators of a major depression generally occur in the middle of the natural course of the disease and are likely to be biological, neuroendocrine, or neurotransmitter problems. Language, praxis, and gnosis impairments are common. The early course of the disease, when one might expect to see some reactive despair and psychosocial despondency, seems to be marked more by perplexity and a vague sense of loss.

Multi-infarct dementia may be complicated by secondary depressions of the organic mood disorder variety. Robinson's work has established the high incidence of poststroke depression, especially associated with left anterior cortical lesions. (It is possible that depressions following right-hemisphere lesions are not recognized as easily, owing to abnormalities of affective communication produced by such lesions.) The neurological signs are usually quite obvious.

Organic mood disorders produced by metabolic (hyponatremia, hypercalcemia, hypercarbia, etc.) and endocrine (hypothyroid, Cushing's, etc.) disorders, by organ failure (hepatic encephalopathy, uremia, etc.) or by medications (antihypertensives, β-blockers, etc.) may eventually merge into more marked cognitive decline and a clinical picture of subcortical dementia. The peripheral indicators of the systemic disorders are usually quite obvious.

The presentation of a simple dementia precox–like clinical picture in schizophrenia, with prominent negative and sparse positive symptoms, might occasionally make differential diagnosis problematic, but there is also a rising interest in the notion that schizophrenia may be associated with a gradually progressive true dementia of its own. This presentation will generally not lead to diagnostic confusion, as chronic patients with the most prominent negative symptoms often have marked positive symptoms as well. The presence of ventricular dilation, soft neurological signs, and electrophysiological signs of disturbed information processing points to the need to apply the findings of dementia research to schizophrenia. Confirmation of this suspicion may have specific consequences for the public policy of deinstitutionalization and psychosocial rehabilitation, especially for elderly persons with schizophrenia.

The ability of laboratory tests to distinguish among the various dementias associated with functional psychiatric disorders is limited. CT shows atrophy in a significant percentage of perfectly healthy elderly patients and should not be used to diagnose Alzheimer's disease. In fact, early Alzheimer's disease is often not accompanied by much atrophy. The EEG in early Alzheimer's disease likewise is likely to be normal to clinical reading. Significant cognitive decline is associated with increasing slow waves and with prolongation of the latency of the P300 component of the computer-analyzed event-related potential. In depression, the amplitude of the P300 is reduced but its latency is not prolonged. Rapid eye movement (REM) latency is shortened in depressive patients more than in Alzheimer's disease, but sleep architecture is disrupted in both conditions. There is a high incidence of dexamethasone nonsuppression of the cortisol level and in other neuroendocrine measures of hypothalamic function, both in depression and in Alzheimer's disease. Finally, ordinary psychological testing (WAIS, Wechsler Memory, etc.) cannot differentiate easily between the cognitive decline of these disorders, and only sophisticated neuropsychological analysis does better than a careful evaluation of the natural history of the two disorders.

Treatment and prognosis Pseudodementia should be energetically confronted and treated with family intervention, psychotherapy, and education. Despite its superficially benign appearance, the disorder can be very restrictive for the patient and very damaging and expensive for the family. The underlying personality disorder will generally require supportive psychotherapy.

In the dementia of depression, antidepressants, lithium, and electroconvulsive therapy (ECT) may be applied, depending on the type and severity of the underlying mood disorder. All age-related precautions for their use should be noted. However, a very real danger is undertreatment and the premature declaration of a failed antidepressant trial. Careful clinical, electrocardiogram (EKG), EEG, and blood-level monitoring are likely to be less expensive, in the long run, than incomplete treatment followed by nursing home placement. Cognitive or major role function psychotherapy should follow the initial biological recovery to prevent relapses and to improve the social adaptation of these geriatric patients.

The use of antidepressants for the depressive symptoms of true Alzheimer's disease is fraught with danger. The anticholinergic side effects are likely to exacerbate the cognitive loss by further impairing nucleus basalis function. The hypotensive side effects are likely to contribute to the already high incidence of falls. Seizures may be precipitated. Antidepressants have been shown to be very effective for post-stroke depression and should be studied prospectively in multi-infarct dementia. Organic mood disorders require meticulous medical management. Antidepressants should be avoided initially to prevent the development of central anticholinergic delirium. However, occasionally the mood disorder becomes autonomous and persists despite the resolution of the underlying medical disorders. Standard antidepressant treatment should be applied in those cases.

REVERSIBLE AND OTHER SECONDARY DEMENTIAS

Definition and epidemiology About 20 percent of dementias have theoretically reversible causes, and in another 20 to 25 percent, attention to the underlying medical disorder can arrest the progress of the disease and improve the mental state. Even in the progressive, irreversible disorders (Alzheimer's, Huntington's), careful treatment of intercurrent medical disorders, knowledgeable pharmacotherapy of agitation and psychotic complications, and support and education of the primary caretakers can help, at least temporarily.

Delay in recognizing potentially reversible causes of dementia, incomplete treatment, and side effects of drugs or surgery can significantly hamper the process of reversibility. Empirical follow-up studies of patients with treatable dementias show a persistence in significant degrees of cognitive and behavioral incapacity.

Etiology and pathogenesis The reader is referred to the Introduction above, in which the roles of various predisposing, precipitating, and sustaining factors are discussed (Tables 12-7 through 12-10) and to the list of the more common causes of dementia (Table 12-15). The question to be examined here is, Why do certain medical and neurological disorders present with dementia rather than with delirium? One factor is the natural history of the underlying disease. A gradually developing tumor, progressive demyelination, an imperceptible decline in thyroxine production—all allow for partial biological and psychosocial compensations to take place (Fig. 12-6). The cognitive defects will not be attended by the emotional turmoil of sudden failures, and the attentional processes will not fluctuate.

The second factor is location. Lesions of the frontal lobes that disconnect them from the limbic system and from more posterior neocortical areas are likely to lead to the clinical syndrome of a subcortical dementia. Brain stem, midline thalamic, and right parietal lesions are often associated with a delirium that is due to the impairment of the arousal and attention pathways.

Clinical signs and symptoms There is little uniformity beyond the requirement that the DSM-III-R criteria for dementia be met. Metabolic and endocrine dementias tend to show a subcortical type of clinical presentation, although constructional apraxia and cortical release signs will be seen in some. Parkinson's, Huntington's, and Wilson's diseases are subcortical types and are associated with prominent movement disorders.

The dementia associated with tumors and other space-occupying lesions tends to manifest cerebral localization signs and symptoms. Normal-pressure and communicating hydrocephalus present a subcortical picture with gait apraxia, early urinary incontinence, and personality change.

The dementia associated with advanced degrees of organ failure will be overshadowed by the medical manifestations of these disorders. Infections of the CNS can cause more diagnostic problems, as there are often no systemic or focal neurological manifestations. Meningismus, useful in acute infections, will often be absent from the chronic ones. Examination of spinal fluid plays an important role.

AIDS encephalopathy, the latest syndrome to come to the fore, is likely to assume an important role as the epidemic spreads. It presents with depression and malaise that are at first attributed to the systemic manifestations of the disease or its psychosocial impact. Memory impairment is noted next, and psychomotor retardation becomes prominent. Apathy, withdrawal, and loss of interest develop. Patients also note unsteady gait, loss of coordination, dysarthria, tremor, and impaired handwriting. Late manifestations include global confusion, severe psychomotor retardation, and unresponsiveness, with pyramidal tract signs, incontinence, myoclonus, and seizures. The major sites of neuropathology are in the white matter of the cerebrum and of the cord and may be due to direct invasion of the neuroglial cells by the human immunodeficiency virus (HIV). CT shows ventricular dilation, and MRI outlines the white matter pathology more clearly.

The early diagnosis of chronic intoxication with industrial chemicals, heavy metals, sedatives, or other therapeutic agents requires a high index of suspicion, a careful occupational and medication history, and an occasional home visit to inspect the drug cabinet or the workshop. Urine and blood toxicology and screening tests for heavy metals may be rewarding at times, but they are no substitute for common sense and a willingness to play detective. A consultation with an occupational physician or a toxicologist may be useful.

Treatment and prognosis The outlook for these patients depends on the open-mindedness and receptivity of their physicians. Many of the diseases that can cause dementia are extremely rare, even in specialist practice. Fortunately, their clinical syndromes develop very gradually and present initially with affective or personality changes. The alert psychiatrist should note the aberrant development of a neurotic pattern of behavior in a previously well-adjusted person or the onset of an indolent, mild, but unresponsive depression in a personally and socially successful person and should think twice before assuming a hidden psychodynamic cause. Even if a psychosocial etiology was assumed at the start, the psychiatrist should be flexible enough to acknowledge the failure of a psychotherapeutic approach and the progressive deterioration of the patient, with the emergence of cognitive and

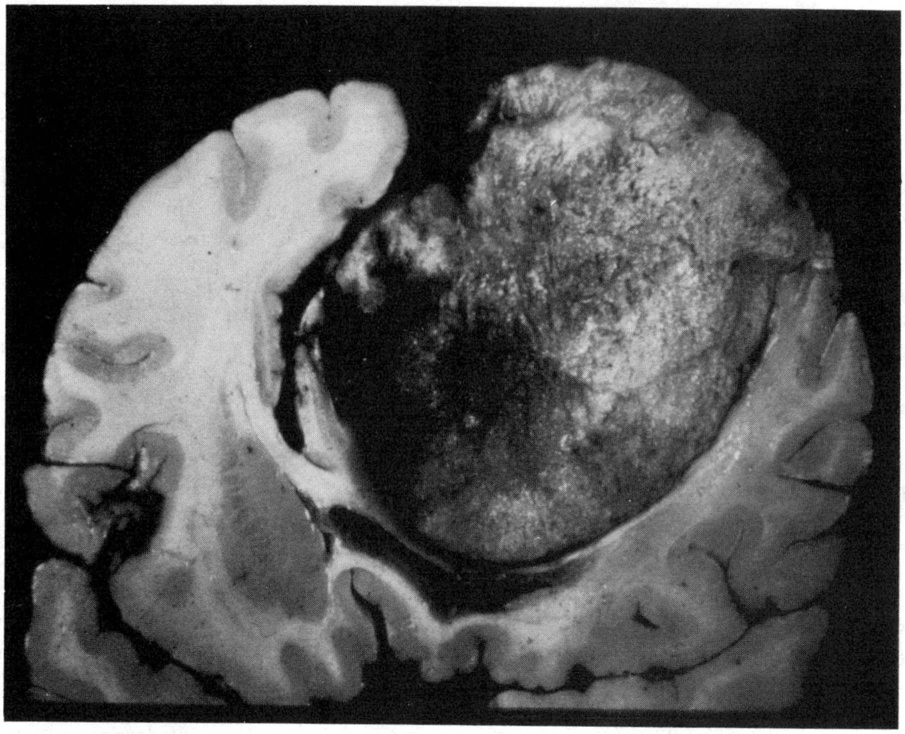

FIGURE 12-6. *Large parasagittal meningioma. The patient with this tumor presented with depression and later developed hemiplegia. (Courtesy of Donald W. Mulder, MD.)*

neurological signs, because it may yet not be too late to search for the organic cause.

A special test that has not received adequate recognition in this regard is the EEG. While the tracing is rarely pathognomic for a certain dementia, the study quite sensitively reflects the metabolic and functional state of the cortex and the state of its subcortical arousal mechanisms. The availability of frequency analysis and topographic display techniques and the use of comparison values may yet restore it to the prominence it once had in neuropsychiatry.

The treatment of each medical disorder is beyond the scope of this section, but the need for rehabilitative and even psychotherapeutic services in the recovery period bears emphasizing. Some of these dementias took years to develop and have disrupted the patient's life to a considerable extent. The typically slow rate of cognitive recovery necessitates the provision of structure and support and family education as well.

DELIRIUM

DEFINITION There is a great deal of semantic confusion surrounding the term "delirium." Internists tend to use it to refer to an agitated, hyperactive, confused mental state. The lay public has a similar image, compounded by notions of an alcoholic etiology, as in delirium tremens. Psychiatrists (in DSM-III-R) define it much more specifically yet broadly, as in Table 12-22. The level of psychomotor activity may be normal, elevated, or depressed according to these criteria. More important is the presence of clouded consciousness that develops relatively quickly and fluctuates during the day, in association with attentional, perceptual, cognitive, and amnestic changes. Neurologists call such a disorder an acute confusional state; they, too, reserve the term "delirium" for the hyperactive, agitated variety. Internists tend to use the concept of metabolic encephalopathy. This designation reflects an unthinking move from a syndromal description to an etiological postulate and poses dangers to patients whose altered mental state is due to focal lesions (strokes, subdural

TABLE 12-22
Diagnostic Criteria for Delirium

A. Reduced ability to maintain attention to external stimuli (e.g., questions must be repeated because attention wanders) and to appropriately shift attention to new external stimuli (e.g., perseverates answer to a previous question).
B. Disorganized thinking, as indicated by rambling, irrelevant, or incoherent speech.
C. At least two of the following:
   (1) reduced level of consciousness (e.g., difficulty keeping awake during examination)
   (2) perceptual disturbances: misinterpretations, illusions, or hallucinations
   (3) disturbance of sleep-wake cycle with insomnia or daytime sleepiness
   (4) increased or decreased psychomotor activity
   (5) disorientation to time, place, or person
   (6) memory impairment (e.g., inability to learn new material, such as the names of several unrelated objects after 5 minutes, or to remember past events, such as history of current episode of illness).
D. Clinical features develop over a short period of time (usually hours to days) and tend to fluctuate over the course of a day.
E. Either (1) or (2):
   (1) evidence from the history, physical examination, or laboratory tests of a specific organic factor (or factors) judged to be etiologically related to the disturbance
   (2) in the absence of such evidence, an etiologic organic factor can be presumed if the disturbance cannot be accounted for by any nonorganic mental disorder (e.g., manic episode accounting for agitation and sleep disturbance).

Table from DSM-III-R *Diagnostic and Statistical Manual of Mental Disorders*, ed 3, revised. Copyright American Psychiatric Association, Washington, DC, 1987. Used with permission.

hematomas) or exogenous factors (drug or medication intoxications). Toxic psychosis is applied to conditions where hallucinations and delusions dominate the clinical picture and an outside factor is suspected. Psychiatrists tended to use the term "exogenous psychosis" in similar cases, although originally the term "exogenous" referred to events outside the brain and included systemic disorders. The Meyerian term "dysergastic reaction" lapsed early into oblivion, replaced by acute OBS (in which acuteness referred not to temporal onset but to the reversibility of the organic psychosyndrome [Bleuler's term]). Acute brain failure was proposed by Engel and Romano but never obtained wide currency. Since the introduction of DSM-III, in 1980, the revived classical term "delirium" seems to have been accepted only by psychiatrists. As the majority of patients so afflicted are under the care of internists and neurologists and are seen by psychiatrists on a consultation basis, it would behoove the consultant to use a term that is understood by all parties. "Acute and subacute confusional state" would meet that criterion. Medical textbooks appropriately emphasize the continuity of these syndromes with stupor and coma. It is far more important to remember this progression in severity rather than the psychiatric nosological dichotomy between delirium and dementia, which seems to enshrine in a dialectical way the old unity of all OBSs. Dementia will not kill a patient in the next few days; delirium progressing to stupor and coma very well could.

HISTORY Delirium was recognized at least as early as Hippocrates' time, and the term itself was used by Celsus in the first century A.D. Areatus of Cappadocia described remarkably enlightened and humane ways of dealing with delirious patients. The chemical (humoral) etiology of the disorder was appreciated by the Middle Ages and distinguished from other mental disorders triggered by psychological passions or faulty reasoning. Sutton, in 1813, described the specific clinical syndrome of delirium tremens and its association with alcoholism, and Wernicke described the condition that now bears his name.

Kraepelin carried the idea of specificity to an extreme and postulated the existence of mental syndromes specific for each major somatic disease. Bonhoeffer unified the field and described five clinical varieties of an underlying acute exogenous reaction—delirium, epileptiform excitement, twilight state, hallucinosis, and amentia. Eugen Bleuler successfully imposed even greater unity when he conceptualized the organic psychosyndrome in acute and chronic manifestations. Lipowski was instrumental in persuading psychiatrists, at least in the United States, to move from this overinclusive unitary concept to the description of a variety of behavioral syndromes, some global, some focal, and some imitating the more common functional disorders.

EPIDEMIOLOGY Delirium is probably the mental disorder with the highest incidence. Ten percent of medical-surgical inpatients and 40 percent of geriatric patients meet criteria for delirium sometime during hospitalization. Given the high lifetime incidence of serious medical diseases, especially in later life, one can predict that episodes of delirium will occur eventually in many elderly patients. The prevalence in the community is low, but it is clearly high in hospitals, ICUs, and emergency rooms serving inner-city areas ridden with substance abuse. The very young (under 6) and the very old (over 75) are especially susceptible to delirium precipitated by minor medical illnesses or toxic changes. Youths and young adults frequently abuse mind-altering substances and suffer head trauma, and people in late middle age encounter severe cardiovascular, respiratory, and neoplastic problems. The onset of delirium during the course of a medical illness is no mere curiosity or behavioral nuisance. All other things being equal, the mortality and morbidity is doubled.

The empirical associations of delirium vary with the treatment setting, the age of the patient, and the medical epidemiology of the community. Hospitals that perform complex surgical procedures see many intensive care syndromes. Inner-city emergency rooms treat a disproportionate percentage of street drug overdose and alcohol withdrawal states. Nursing homes and geriatric evaluation units most often treat delirium superimposed on dementing disease. General hospitals see multifactorial organ failure, often exacerbated by iatrogenic problems.

Community epidemiology explains why AIDS encephalopathy is relatively prevalent in New York and San Francisco in the late 1980s, how phencyclidine (PCP) delirium spread from the West Coast in the 1970s, and why Wernicke's encephalopathy is less common in the nutrition-conscious U.S. population than among the equally hard-drinking and prosperous Australians.

PATHOPHYSIOLOGY The central functional disturbance in delirium is one of attention as represented in the A criteria of the DSM-III-R definition. The diagnosis of delirium involves at least some of the items from the C criteria, but none of them is essential to the definition itself. The cerebral substrate of arousal and attention is the polysynaptic reticular formation of the brain stem, midbrain, and midline thalamic nuclei. This has important intimate connections with other axial structures, such as the noradrenergic locus ceruleus, the serotonergic raphe nuclei, the mesolimbic dopaminergic nuclei, and the cholinergic nucleus basalis. The septal area provides a connection with the limbic system and through it, to the frontal lobes. The inferior parietal lobule, especially on the right side, appears to have important cholinergic connections with the nucleus basalis and with the midline thalamic neuclei. Lesions in various parts of this system have been associated with disorders of attention, consciousness, and the smooth regulation of these functions in the normal sleep–wake cycle. Confusional states have also been described.

The common etiology of delirium and confusion is not a single localized lesion but a diffuse impairment of neuronal metabolism or membrane stability. Correlations have been established between cortical metabolic rates and the frequency of EEG waves: low metabolism being associated with low-frequency, relatively high-amplitude EEGs. Engel and Romano's demonstration of a correlation between the degree of impairment of consciousness and the amount of slow-wave generation struck a responsive cord, and delirium was conceptualized as an acute brain failure, an impairment of cortical neuronal and glial metabolism. Recent evidence revealed, however, that delirium, or at least a subtle cognitive impairment, could occur at modest levels of metabolic disturbance that failed to derange the activity of neuronal or glial cell bodies. A hypothesis emerged that these moderate metabolic disorders impaired only the synaptosomal (hence, neurotransmitter) functions. Choline acetyltransferase, tyrosine hydroxylase, and trytophan hydroxylase, key enzymes for cholinergic and aminergic transmission, were shown to be exquisitely sensitive to modest levels of hypoxia, hypoglycemia, and thiamine deficiency. Calcium-dependent acetylcholine release was reduced, as was glucose incorporation into alanine, glutamate, aspartate, GABA, and glutamine. In other words, widespread impairment of neurotransmitter synthesis and release was seen. Behavioral studies in animals suggested a key role for reduced cholinergic transmission in the production of performance defects that may be used as models of attentional and arousal functions in humans. An experimental treatment, 3,4-diaminopyridine, increased calcium influx into synaptosomes, increased the release of acetylcholine, and reversed the behavioral defects produced by hypoxia in rats. There is some clinical evidence that even delirium states not caused by anticholinergic agents can be ameliorated by intravenous physostigmine, but the drug's cardiovascular toxicity prevents it from becoming a practical treatment.

In delirium associated with withdrawal from alcohol or sedatives, the noradrenergic system is also involved, in the form of rebound overactivation. This may explain the motor and autonomic overexcitation and the intermixture of fast β-waves with slower θ-waves in the EEGs of patients with delirium tremens. Cholinergic, adrenergic, and serotonergic terminals connect on specific cell layers of the primary and secondary sensory cortices and modulate sensory processing. This may provide a neuronal substrate for the production of perceptual distortions and hallucinations. The role of cholinergic neurotransmission in memory processes through the hippocampi are well established, and a hypocholinergic state there produces an amnestic syndrome and disorientation. Sleep–wake cycle regulation is a function of pontine and mesencephalic centers where noradrinergic and serotonergic neurotransmitters may be impaired by metabolic encephalopathies.

Finally, the variably hypophonic, incoherent speech with intermittent lapses of comprehension and understandability characteristic of delirium has been seen with midline thalamic lesions. Thus, all the central diagnostic signs of delirium can be traced back to certain reticular system abnormalities with only a minimum of oversimplification.

ETIOLOGY The etiological factors that move the organism into these final common pathways may be divided into predisposing, precipitating, and sustaining categories (as discussed in the Introduction above and in Tables 12-7 through 12-10 and Table 12-23). The speed of development of the pathophysiology and its impact on the axial reticular activating system will determine whether the clinical manifestation are those of delirium or of another OMS.

For the practicing physician, age is another useful empirical sorting factor:

Childhood: pediatric infections and fevers, intoxications with medications and poisons, epilepsy, trauma
Adolescence, young adulthood: intoxication and withdrawal from street drugs, head injury, infections, postoperative states
Middle age: withdrawal from alcohol and sedatives, exposure to industrial toxins, metabolic encephalopathy from organ failure, complicated cardiovascular disorders, malnutrition, endocrine disorders, neoplasia
Old age: cerebrovascular disease, overmedication, sedative withdrawal, cardiac arrhythmias and heart failure, organ failure

Any more comprehensive enumeration of diseases associated with delirium would be encyclopedic and useless for diagnosis. In the end, a dangerous myth needs to be exploded—that sensory deprivation or overload, in the absence of organic cerebral changes, can cause delirium and that this is the main pathogenesis of ICU syndrome or of postsurgical delirium. Careful review of the anesthesia protocol, of pump perfusion records, of dialysis numbers, and of the current state of electrolytes, blood gases, acid–base balance, and drug administration (cimetidine [Tagamet], digoxin [Lanoxin], theophylline, etc.) will reveal specific, often correctable or preventable, biological causes. This is not to deny that sensory variations and sleep deprivation can play sustaining, contributing roles, but it would be dangerous intellectual laziness to point to nonspecific, fashionable environmental factors to the exclusion of specific, reversible medical disorders.

TABLE 12-23
Causes of Delirium

Toxic
Sedatives, alcohol
Antipsychotics, antidepressants, anticholinergics
Disulfiram
Digitalis
Cimetidine
Aminophylline
L-dopa
Withdrawal
Alcohol, barbiturate, meprobamate, benzodiazepines
Organ failure
Hepatic encephalopathy
Uremia, renal dialysis dysequilibrium
Chronic obstructive lung disease, status asthmaticus
Congestive cardiac failure, left ventricular failure and pulmonary edema, shock, arrhythmia
Metabolic and endocrine
Hypoglycemia, hypoxia
Wernicke's encephalopathy
Thiamine deficiency
Pellagra
Nicotinic acid deficiency
Thyrotoxicosis
Cushing's disease, Addison's disease
Inappropriate antidiuretic hormone secretion
Electrolyte imbalance (nutritional, postsurgical)
Trauma
Postconcussion excitement
Extradural, subdural, intracerebral hematoma
Systemic infections
Pneumonia
Septicemia, especially Gram-negative
Urinary tract infection in elderly person
Meningitis, encephalitis, brain abscess, AIDS encephalopathy
Vascular
Subarachnoid hemorrhage
Transient ischemic attack
Hypertensive encephalopathy
Systemic lupus encephalopathy
Neoplastic
Rapidly growing primary or secondary tumors with cerebral edema or hemorrhage

CLINICAL SIGNS AND SYMPTOMS Ideally, delirium should be prevented by recognizing and treating the underlying disorder before the full syndrome develops. Brain impairment presents quite early with vague symptoms. Fatigue not relieved by sleep, subjective weakness, mood lability, hypersensitivity to stimuli, and vivid dreaming are some of the antecedents of delirium. Loss of mental acuity, reduced concentration and vigilance, mental slowing and distractability, loss of creativity, and reduced frustration tolerance are the earliest nonspecific symptoms of structural brain damage. At increasing levels of cerebral impairment, patients are initially slow, self-absorbed, and irritable and later become inert and lethargic, and lose self-control and insight. Initially, patients use their customary coping strategies and ego defense mechanisms to deal with the frustations of mild cognitive impairment. Later, they regress to more primitive defenses and eventually allow primitive anxiety to break through (catastrophic reactions) and manifest apathy and inertia (giving up–given up state).

A more pronounced presenting symptom of delirium is dysphoria. Depressed, anxious, and irritable moods will frequently lead the primary physician to an initial misdiagnosis of a depressive or anxiety disorder. About 20 percent of delirium cases present this way, and, in turn, about 50 percent of inpatients referred for a consideration of depression on examination are found to have a significant organic cognitive loss. Another 20 percent of delirium patients present very dramatically with hallucinations and delusions. General physicians not infrequently identify any psychotic features as schizophrenia and may insist that the patient is suffering from this nonorganic disorder, especially if the delusions are bizarre and the hallucinations auditory. Another 20 percent of delirious patients manifest their disorder initially by personal irascibility, demanding behavior, uncooperativeness, and attempts at leaving the hospital against medical advice. In only about 30 percent of consultations is there a classical cognitive presentation. It is quite likely that this group is underrepresented in any consultation series, as quietly confused patients do not trouble their physicians and do not prompt psychiatric consultations. Psychiatric consultants who carefully examine the mental state perform a very useful function, as the primary physician recognizes the underlying organic etiology of the altered mental state in less than half the cases.

Need for mental status examination This combination of presenting symptoms in the appropriate setting should raise the psychiatrist's suspicion and prompt the performance of a mental status examination aimed at confirming or eliminating the presence of the DSM-III-R criteria. Identification of the DSM-III-R criteria for delirium (Table 12-22) should be followed by an estimation of its cognitive severity (the Folstein Mini-Mental State Examination is a useful bedside instrument, Table 12-3). There should also be an evaluation of its affective, psychotic, and behavioral severity, for which purpose the Brief Psychiatric Rating Scale is well suited.

The free-flowing general evaluation, the mental status examination, and the structured rating scales reveal an astonishingly wide range of abnormal experiences and behaviors.

The central problem of fluctuating and distractable attention and the clouded sense of awareness are generally noticeable on careful examination but may be overshadowed by more dramatic symptoms. Cognitive decline may be prominent, with incoherent speech and inability to follow complex commands, or an anxious, agitated emotional state with startle reactions and increased psychomotor activity may obscure the mental state. In yet other cases, the patient could be slipping into a stuporous precoma. In some patients, hallucinations dominate. Although classical descriptions emphasize vivid dream-like, visual sequences with secondary delusions, somesthetic and auditory hallucinations are also possible, and illusions and sensory misinterpretations are more frequent than frank hallucinations. The delusions are generally fragmentary, shifting, and poorly organized. The content of these psychotic phenomena is determined by the personal history, intrapsychic conflicts, and recent preoccupations of the patient. Disturbances of sleep patterns and dreaming are quite prominent. Patients frequently complain of nightmares and of awaking confused and lost. Observers note the sundowning phenomenon—the patient who was lethargic and sleepy during the day becomes alert, even agitated and restless, during the night. By next morning, the patient is unlikely to remember what happened during the night.

In general, the patient has patchy amnesia for most events during the delirium episode. There is intermittent impairment of memory transfer into long-term storage and its consolidation there. (Distractability could interfere with registration in the first place). There are also problems with retrieval owing to loss of a coherent mnemonic strategy. As the time sequencing of events is also impaired, telescoping of certain episodes results in convincing confabulation. Dysgraphia, constructional apraxia, and word-finding difficulties are other early higher nervous system signs.

The characteristic fluctuation affects all of these symptoms and may lead to misdiagnosis unless the patient is examined repeatedly. Physicians are advised to read the nursing case notes carefully and to attend to the reports of the night staff.

Delirium is often accompanied by aimless grasping and picking at the bedclothes and intravenous (IV) tubing. Patients often show a coarse tremor and unsteadiness of the hands and sometimes, metabolic encephalopathic asterixis (irregular flapping of the dorsiflexed wrists in hepatic, renal, respiratory failure). Myoclonic jerking, ataxia, dysarthria, and variable hypophonia are other later neurological signs. Release reflexes (grasp, pout, sucking) and nonhabituation of the glabellar tap reflex are seen in severe cases. In advanced, precomatose stages, there may be respiratory and pupillary abnormalities and some conjugate eye movement changes.

Evidence of structural disease A careful neurological evaluation is necessary to detect focal and long tract signs, meningismus, and other evidence of a structural disease. Some metabolic disorders can produce focal signs, however: sixth nerve lesions in thiamine deficiency, bilateral long-tract signs in postanoxic encephalopathy. Usually, an urgent medical examination is needed to uncover signs of systemic disease. Because agitated, combative patients are often difficult to examine, there is a very real danger that a cursory examination will medically clear a psychotic patient whose underlying problem is a delirium secondary to an unrecognized systemic disease.

DIFFERENTIAL DIAGNOSIS Psychotic symptoms frequently raise the possibility of schizophrenia, but only to those unfamiliar with the natural history of the disorder. The onset of a florid psychosis in a young person with an occult medical disease is occasionally a real diagnostic problem. Catatonic stupor can present with low-grade fever, autonomic hyperactivity, rigidity, and extrapyramidal findings; if the patient was medicated, the neuroleptic malignant syndrome should be considered. Very occasionally, an acutely disorganized schizophrenic can present with confusion and disorientation yet have negative medical, neurological, and laboratory findings.

Dysphoric symptoms, often in conjunction with weight loss and insomnia due to underlying disease, prompt referrals for the treatment of depression. Careful cognitive evaluation will uncover the other features of delirium. Unthinking application of heterocyclic antidepressants will exacerbate the delirium.

Dementia is one of the major predisposing causes of delirium. Dementing disorders not infrequently present with an acute, superimposed delirium, and the dementia is noted when there is incomplete resolution of the cognitive failure. A more insidious problem occurs when mental deterioration in the course of a dementing illness is attributed entirely to the progression of the primary neuropathology, and the possibility of a superimposed delirium caused by medications, pneumonia, or urinary tract infection is not considered. In moderately to severely demented patients, the onset of delirium may be the only sign of a serious intercurrent illness, such as an acute abdomen or subdural hematoma.

The distinction between delirium and organic hallucinosis or organic delusional disorder is mostly phenomenological. The underlying pathophysiology is often identical.

The central problem is to distinguish delirium from functional mental disorders. An adequate history and cognitive examination will do that, especially if supported by EEG findings. The earliest changes are slowing and disorganization of the α-frequency and onset of sporadic θ-waves. Increasing severity of the delirium is paralleled by further slowing of the dominant frequencies throughout the cortex, with bilaterally synchronous δ-waves in severe cases.

TREATMENT AND PROGNOSIS It is particularly important in delirium to construct and follow a rational, comprehensive treatment plan. Most delirium patients are not under the care of the psychiatrist, and several consultants may participate in treatment planning. The illness can evolve quite rapidly, threatening to overwhelm the health care team. In the rush to implement the necessary high technology investigations and to perform biomedical interventions, the emotional needs of patient and family may be overlooked. The patient may then demonstrate distress by increasing agitation, confusion, and lack of cooperation, which will interfere with the treatment of his or her medical disease.

Treatment venue In the initial triage phase, cogent decisions must be made quickly as to whether the patient is best placed in a regular medical ward or ICU, on an open psychiatric ward, or in a psychiatric intensive care setting. This is an empirical decision based on the local availability of appropriately trained personnel at these sites. Ideally, the patient should receive close medical monitoring as well as sophisticated behavioral management. It is probably safest to handle such patients in a medical area with one-to-one nursing, enlisting the help of the family if available. The familiar faces of friends and relatives can be reassuring to the patient. The crisis-support phase of the treatment assures the physical safety of the patient, resolves any medicolegal issues about consent for diagnostic and treatment procedures, and provides a supportive social and emotional environment. The patient needs to be provided repeatedly with simple information about his or her health. The family needs to have the medical procedures and the often frightening mental state of the patient explained to them.

These supportive interventions all happen during the diagnostic phase, and its success depends heavily on their adequacy. Familiar staff should accompany the patient to encourage cooperation during EEG and CT; haloperidol can be used acutely in 1- to 5-mg IV or intramuscular (IM) doses.

Monitoring treatment The treatment of delirium is aimed at maintaining vital functions, correcting underlying biological disorders, and reducing the disturbing psychological and behavioral symptoms. Adequate oxygenation, hydration, nutrition, and cerebral perfusion should be monitored by clinical or laboratory determination of oxygen saturation, blood chemistry, blood pressure, and cardiac output. The medical or surgical treatment of the precipitating disorder should be carried out expeditiously with monitoring of therapeutic side effects. Cimetidine, digoxin, aminophylline, the anticonvulsants, centrally acting β-blockers are notorious for precipitating or exacerbating delirium when taken in doses at the upper level of the therapeutic range. Many other agents have idiosyncratic central effects, especially on the aging brain. Sedatives that depress the polysynaptic reticular formation should be avoided, except when benzodiazepines are needed for detoxification from alcohol or sedatives. The longer-acting benzodiazepines with active metabolites (diazepam, chlordiazepoxide) continue to have an important role in alcohol or short-acting–sedative detoxification when complemented with adequate hydration, vitamins, and treatment of intercurrent infection and liver disease.

Psychotropic agents with central anticholinergic side effects should be avoided to preserve the remaining cholinergic modulation of attention, cognition, and memory. The safest agent to use for symptom- and behavior control is haloperidol. In most medically ill and frail patients, 0.5 mg to 1 mg orally or IM at intervals of 4 to 6 hours will suppress psychotic or agitated behavior without causing extrapyramidal side effects. In some very ill, yet physically vigorous, patients, much larger (IV) doses have been used, often together with lorazepam (5 mg haloperidol to 1 mg lorazepam). Close monitoring by a psychiatrist experienced in psychopharmacology in an intensive care environment ensures patient safety. (In hepatic failure, lorazepam alone should be used for tranquilizing, as haloperidol is metabolized in the liver.)

Rehabilitation Rehabilitation is a neglected phase in the management of patients recovering from delirium. At the very least, patient and family should be provided with reassuring information about the nature of the illness and its mental complications. They should be told that they have not gone crazy and be offered an opportunity to discuss their frightening dreams and the half-remembered events of their illness.

Prevention Public health measures aimed at prevention were discussed above. Important interventions can be made at the level of the individual patient. The identification of an episode of street drug intoxication or alcohol–sedative withdrawal is an indication for confronting the patient with the need for intensive substance abuse treatment and rehabilitation. Mere substance misuse does not lead to delirious episodes, and the patient should not be allowed to minimize the problem.

Therapeutic-drug intoxication should lead to careful reassessment of the medical treatment, the medication regime, and the process of self-medication. Geriatric patients often take seven or eight different medications prescribed at several different clinics, possibly in varying and potentially dangerous dosages.

Involvement of a chronic medical disease in precipitating delirium should prompt review of the treatment plan: Was the dialysis adequate? Was there good dietary compliance? Was the acute bronchitis noticed in time? Did the patient smoke more? Was there dietary indiscretion or drinking during treatment for cirrhosis? Did a superimposed urinary tract infection progress unnoticed? The list goes on. Better patient and family education, more frequent medical supervision, and the provision of home health care services may all improve patient compliance and reduce the future risk of delirium.

Postsurgical delirium can be reduced by adequate preoperative orientation of the patient, careful anesthesia monitoring, adequate postoperative analgesia, and postoperative orientation and psychosocial support, as well as by early detection of wound sepsis, urinary tract infections, and pulmonary embolism.

Finally, patients and relatives should be taught to notice the early signs of cognitive and attentional impairment and told to seek medical help at the very onset of the syndrome. Biomedical intervention at that time may prevent the development of dramatic and troubling behavior disturbances. In a best-case scenario, mental health professionals provide readily available consultation–liaison services to medical clinics and wards and pre- and postoperative units to help in education and early identification.

AMNESTIC SYNDROME

INTRODUCTION *Memory* is the process that enables humans and other organisms to learn and to modify their behavior as a result of experience. Efforts to determine the neural mechanisms responsible for the storage of individual experiences has been called the search for the engram. Although much is still unknown about memory functioning in humans, some characteristics of human memory are known and are helpful for an understanding of the amnestic syndromes. One is that, although certain memory functions appear to be localized in specific brain areas, individual memories (engrams) themselves are only partially localized. As an example, memory for faces depends heavily on the inferior temporo-occipital cortex, but the engram for a particular face cannot be localized to any single neuronal circuit. Rather, learning and recall of any face depend on intact functioning of the entire inferior temporo-occipital cortex. A second characteristic of human memory is that many parts of the brain, particulary the neocortex and hippocampus, are involved in learning and recall of complex experiences as they occur in everyday life. These characteristics of memory help to explain why impairment of memory functioning is one consequence of a variety of psychiatric and neurological disorders. Almost any condition that greatly disturbs normal brain function will have some adverse effect on memory, though that may not be the primary symptom. These characteristics also help to explain why pure amnestic syndromes are relatively rare. Because the brain areas responsible for memory functioning overlap so much with those responsible for other cognitive, emotional, and psychomotor functions, it is rare to find an amnestic patient who has little impairment of other psychological functions.

TABLE 12-24
Diagnostic Criteria for Amnestic Syndrome

A. Demonstrable evidence of impairment in both short- and long-term memory; with regard to long-term memory, very remote events are remembered better than more recent events. Impairment in short-term memory (inability to learn new information) may be indicated by inability to remember three objects after 5 minutes. Long-term memory impairment (inability to remember information that was known in the past) may be indicated by inability to remember past personal information (e.g., what happened yesterday, birthplace, occupation) or facts of common knowledge (e.g., past Presidents, well-known dates).
B. Not occurring exclusively during the course of delirium, and does not meet the criteria for dementia (i.e., no impairment in abstract thinking or judgment, no other disturbances of higher cortical function, and no personality change).
C. There is evidence from the history, physical examination, or laboratory tests of a specific organic factor (or factors) judged to be etiologically related to the disturbance.

Table from DSM-III-R *Diagnostic and Statistical Manual of Mental Disorders*, ed 3, revised. Copyright American Psychiatric Association, Washington, DC, 1987. Used with permission.

DEFINITION According to DSM-III-R, the essential feature of an amnestic syndrome is impairment in short- and long-term memory that is attributed to a specific organic factor (Table 12-24). Whenever pronounced memory impairment occurs in the context of significant impairment in ability to maintain or shift attention, the primary diagnosis is likely to be delirium; memory impairment associated with disturbances in other cortical functions, such as language, judgment, and abstract thinking, suggests a diagnosis of dementia. Delirium and dementia are relatively common conditions, particularly among the elderly, but amnestic syndromes are relatively rare.

Nearly all amnestic syndromes result from localized damage to diencephalic and medial temporal structures, such as the hippocampus, fornix, and mammillary bodies. Damage to these structures can result from hypoxia, head trauma, herpes simplex encephalitis, cerebral infarction, or, most commonly, thiamine deficiency secondary to chronic alcoholism.

SIGNS AND SYMPTOMS Diagnostic criteria for amnestic syndrome have remained essentially unchanged for several decades, and there is no evidence to suggest that significant changes in prevalence or etiology are in order. However, systematic studies conducted during the past 20 years have enabled clinical investigators to describe the cognitive capabilities of amnestic patients in great detail and have provided some insights into the neural and cognitive mechanisms responsible for certain aspects of memory functioning. The most detailed descriptions are of patients whose brain lesions were produced surgically or through accidents that resulted in localized damage to specific brain areas.

Undoubtedly, the best-studied patient of this sort is H.M., who, at the age of 27, had bilateral resection of the temporal lobes in an effort to relieve severe epileptic seizures. Following his operation, H.M. displayed intact general intellectual capacity; in fact, tested I.Q. rose from 104 before the operation to 118 afterward. H.M.'s personality, attention span, and many cognitive processes, including language skills and praxis abilities, remained completely intact following the surgery.

The most striking postoperational change in H.M. was an almost total inability to learn new information that exceeded the capacity of his immediate or primary memory. Clinically, the capacity of primary memory is determined by a task included as part of most mental status examinations. H.M.'s ability to remember lists of about seven items was normal; greater numbers of items were impossible to learn. Furthermore, information in primary memory was rapidly and totally lost if H.M. was distracted. Clinically, H.M. suffered an almost total anterograde amnesia; in terms of contemporary memory theory, one would say H.M. had an inability to store new information in long-term memory. In addition to anterograde amnesia, the patient also had marked retrograde amnesia for events that occurred during the year or two before the surgery. Recall for events from very early life and up to the 2 years before surgery was as good as that of normal people.

The pattern of memory deficits exhibited by H.M.—intact primary memory, profound anterograde amnesia, retrograde amnesia with sparing of very remote memories—is the general pattern observed in most cases of the amnestic syndrome. One additional feature of H.M.'s syndrome is also common to other patients with amnesia: H.M. was able to learn some new skills, even though he could almost never learn new facts. As an example, H.M.'s performance on a mirror tracing task (copying geometric figures shown reversed in a mirror) improved normally with practice and good performance persisted over long periods of time. H.M. was, however, unable to recall ever learning such a task and could not recall or recognize any of the people who had instructed him in the task.

Similar results were obtained with N.A., a patient suffering from severe amnesia following an accident with a small fencing foil, which damaged the left mediodorsal thalamic nucleus and possibly other structures. N.A. was able to learn how to read words presented backward just as quickly as normal persons, but was never able to recall the words themselves as normal people do. Results such as these with H.M. and N.A. led clinical investigators to distinguish between declarative, or factual, memory and procedural, or process, memory. The ability to learn new facts (knowing that) appears to be heavily dependent upon the medial temporal regions of the brain, especially the hippocampus, whereas certain types of procedural learning (knowing how) can proceed even if these structures are damaged.

Most of the amnestic syndromes encountered in clinical practice result from damage to the medial temporal regions of the brain, areas in which patients H.M. and N.A. had lesions. Most amnestic patients also have symptoms that are similar to those of N.A. and H.M., but their cognitive deficits are usually less circumscribed. Patients with Korsakoff's syndrome, for example, show, in addition to their marked memory deficits, impaired performance on tests of abstraction, concept formation, and verbal fluency. All of these tests measure abilities that are heavily dependent on frontal lobe functioning. Since frontal lobe dysfunction is common in chronic alcoholics, it is not surprising that patients with Korsakoff's syndrome also show these deficits. For patients with amnestic syndromes resulting from other etiologies, the memory deficit may be accompanied by other psychological abnormalities, which can be detected after careful clinical and neuropsychological examination. In every case, however, the memory deficit is the most prominent feature.

Both clinical examination and formal neuropsychological tests are useful in determining the extent of a patient's memory deficit and the extent to which other cognitive functions are impaired. A carefully obtained clinical history will determine onset, course, and whether there were identifiable precipitants. This information is usually sufficient to differentiate patients with amnesia from those with either delirium or dementia, two more common conditions that also cause memory loss.

TREATMENT AND PROGNOSIS The first step in management of a patient with an amnestic syndrome is to treat, if possible, the underlying cause (e.g., brain tumor). In alcoholics, it is particularly important to try to prevent the development of Korsakoff's syndrome with high doses of thiamine and other vitamins. Once the amnestic syndrome has become fixed, pharmacological and other therapies are of little value in restoring memory functions. The majority of amnestic disorders are chronic, and there are few remissions as they represent permanent damage to brain structures. In contrast to those with most dementias, however, amnestic patients often stabilize for many years. At this point, supportive measures, including the use of memory aids and environmental modifications, may enhance the patient's autonomy and functional capabilities. Pharmacotherapy may also be of value in treating such ancillary symptoms as depression and agitation.

OTHER ORGANIC MENTAL SYNDROMES

ORGANIC MOOD SYNDROME **Definition and clinical signs and symptoms** Organic mood syndrome, as defined in DSM-III-R, is a mood disturbance etiologically related to a specific organic factor (Table 12-25). The clinical manifestation of organic mood disorders may include any of the symptoms typically associated with functional mood disorders—dysphoric mood, loss of interest, anorexia, weight loss, sleep disturbance, reduced libido, pessimistic thinking, reduced cognitive efficiency, ideas of death and suicide, self-blame, and guilt. An organic mood syndrome is distinguished from nonorganic mood disturbances by history, physical examination, or laboratory tests. The diagnosis of organic mood syndrome is predicated on the absence of other OMSs, such as delirium, dementia, organic delusional disorder, or hallucinosis. It is also necessary to distinguish organic mood disorder from the dysphoria often observed in delirium and the apathy and depressive symptoms that frequently accompany dementia. Organic mood disorder is also to be distinguished from the secondary depression, demoralization, or dysphoria associated with the physical, psychological, and social consequences of medical illness, where the medical illness is not the organic etiological CNS factor in producing the depressive state. Because the diagnosis of organic mood disorder is thus generally reserved for persons who present initially with a predominant mood disturbance secondary to an organic cause (in the absence of other symptoms of OMS and, often, of other systemic symptoms), the organic etiological features may often be missed in these patients. These considerations underscore the need for thorough medical, endocrinological, and neurological evaluations of patients who present with depressive symptoms. The identification of a specific organic etiological factor by such a workup then establishes the diagnosis of organic mood disorder and informs its treatment, which is aimed at correcting the underlying disorders as well as reversing the mood disorder.

TABLE 12-25
Diagnostic Criteria for Organic Mood Syndrome

A. Prominent and persistent depressed, elevated, or expansive mood.
B. There is evidence from the history, physical examination, or laboratory tests of a specific organic factor (or factors) judged to be etiologically related to the disturbance.
C. Not occurring exclusively during the course of delirium.
Specify: manic, depressed, or **mixed.**

Pathophysiology The similar symptom patterns that organic and functional mood disorders share suggest common final pathways of the pathophysiological mechanisms involved in these two syndromes. In some cases (e.g., reserpine treatment or viral syndrome), the organic etiological agent induces depressive episodes indistinguishable from classical mood disorders that persist even after the causal agent is no longer present. Individuals with a history or family history of mood disorder seem to be more susceptible to some of the organically induced episodes; this is certainly true for reserpine-induced depression. This phenomenon is consistent with the clinical observation that depressive episodes that occur in persons with a (possibly genetic) predisposition to the disorder are often precipitated by an external or internal stressor or insult. In the organic mood disorders, the predisposition may be a less salient factor and the stressor or insult a more discrete organic agent than in nonorganic mood disorders, but the distinction between organic and nonorganic etiology seems to be less than clear cut.

The neurochemical systems and anatomical structures that are abnormal in the organic mood disorders also correspond closely to the systems and structures implicated as being disordered in nonorganic mood disorders. The observation that medications that deplete the noradrenergic system (e.g., reserpine) may precipitate depression and those that enhance it (e.g., amphetamine, cocaine) may precipitate mania, stimulated the catecholamine hypotheses of mood disorders. Subsequent to its formulation, some evidence implicated corresponding abnormalities in nonorganically initiated mood episodes. Hypoxemia may also reduce noradrenergic function and be associated with depressive symptoms. Affective symptoms may be elicited by cholinesterase inhibitors as well as metoclopramide (Reglan), which causes release of acetylcholine. These observations complement evidence of cholinergic supersensitivity in naturally occurring depressive episodes. Pancreatic carcinoma, sometimes associated with depressive symptoms, has been suggested to alter central serotonergic function, consonant with the indications of serotonergic dysfunction in the mood disorders. Cushing's disease, exogenous adrenocorticotropic hormone (ACTH), or corticosteroid administration frequently precipitate affective syndromes, while abnormalities in hypothalamic-pituitary-adrenal axis function are often demonstrable in nonorganic mood episodes. Although the precise neurochemical mechanisms of mood disorders have yet to be clarified, the parallels between the neurochemical disorders associated with organic and nonorganic mood episodes are clear.

Anatomical structures impaired in organic mood disorders include the hypothalamic-pituitary axis, subcortical limbic system structures, including the median forebrain bundle, left hemisphere (depression), and right hemisphere (mania). These same areas are also implicated in neurophysiological, neuropsychological, and endocrine studies of functional mood disorders, suggesting that the areas that are structurally altered in the organic mood disorders may be functionally disturbed in the other mood disorders.

Etiology and differential diagnosis DRUGS Although over 200 medications have been implicated in the organic mood disorders, a relatively smaller number are responsible for the majority of mood reactions to medications. Medications that may induce depressive episodes include reserpine, methyldopa (Aldomet), clonidine (Catapres), β-adrenergic antagonists, such as propranolol (Inderal) or pindolol (Visken), disulfiram, hydrogen ion antagonists, propylthiouracil, metoclopramide, and oral birth control agents. Alcohol, hypnotics, and benzodiazepines sometimes precipitate depressive symptoms. Withdrawal from drugs, such as the stimulants or antidepressants, may induce a depressive syndrome. The antihypertensives that may trigger depressive episodes generally reduce noradrenergic activity by a variety of mechanisms (e.g., depleting presynaptic norepinephrine [reserpine], replacing norepinephrine with a false neurotransmitter [α-methyldopa], inhibiting presynaptic noradrenergic neuronal firing and release [clonidine], or blocking β-adrenergic receptors [propranolol]. Stimulant withdrawal may result in depletion of norepinephrine. Other offending agents appear to affect the cholinergic, serotonergic, and hypothalamic-pituitary-adrenal axis, while oral contraceptives may trigger depression by reducing systemic levels of pyridoxine, a cofactor for the catecholamine synthetic enzyme tyrosine hydroxylase.

Manic episodes may be initiated by a variety of pharmacological agents, including corticosteroids, corticotropin, thyrotropin, L-dopa, monoamine oxidase inhibitors (MAOIs), tricyclic antidepressants, bromocriptine (Parlodel), cocaine, amphetamine, lysergic acid diethylamide (LSD), and baclofen (Lioresal). It is clear that the induction of a manic episode by some of these agents (such as the tricyclic antidepressants) reflects an underlying bipolar diathesis in the affected person. These drugs generally act by enhancing the activity of monoamine and hypothalamic-pituary systems implicated in the mood disorders. For example, tricyclic antidepressants, MAOIs, cocaine, and amphetamine all appear to enhance the availability of norepinephrine in the synapse. Exogenous steroids and related releasing hormones sometimes produce a steroid psychosis when given at a dose equivalent of 40 mg of prednisone per day or more.

The treatment of drug-induced organic mood disorders clearly includes discontinuing the offending drug. In many cases, its discontinuation does not terminate the episode, and treatment with antidepressants, ECT, or both, in the case of depression, and with antipsychotics or lithium, in the case of mania, is required. However, drug treatment of organic mood disorder is not usually recommended until after the offending agent is cleared from the blood and a brief drug-free observation period has passed.

ENDOCRINOPATHIES AND DISTURBANCES OF METABOLISM Endocrine disorders are among the most frequent causes of organic mood disorders, usually depression. The specific manifestations that usually accompany these syndromes may provide clues to the etiology of the depressive syndrome, although, at times, the symptoms are indistinguishable from those of nonorganic mood disorder. The more common endocrine disorders are hypo- and hyperthyroidism, hyperadrenocorticism (pituitary adenoma, adrenal adenoma or carcinoma, oat-cell carcinoma), Addison's disease, hyper- and hypoparathyroidism, hyperprolactinemia, hypoglycemia, pancreatic carcinoma, premenstrual syndromes, and postpartum depression.

Hypothyroidism may present as either an apathetic depression or an agitated paranoid psychotic depression (myxedema madness). Apathetic depression of hypothyroidism is characterized by weight loss, lethargy, retardation, and depressive demeanor, although depressive cognition and sadness are not as frequent as in primary major depressive disorder. The agitated psychotic depressive manifestation is less common and is characterized by paranoid ideation, delusions, or hallucinations. Because prominent cognitive deterioration may accompany either of these syndromes, if severe, they might be classified as dementias rather than organic mood syndromes. The affective symptoms respond only variably to thyroid replacement and may require treatment with antidepressant medications or ECT as well.

Hyperthyroidism is less frequently associated with mood disorder episodes than is hypothyroidism, although the increased sympathetic and behavioral arousal associated with hyperthyroidism may produce irritable, mania-like behavior. However, in most cases, the expansiveness, euphoria, and racing thoughts are absent, and the physical stigmata of tremor, sweating, and eye signs point to the diagnosis of hyperthyroidism rather than a true organic mood disorder. The situation may be complicated if lithium treatment is initiated prior to thyroid testing; by inhibiting iodine uptake lithium may decrease thyroid function and mask the hyperthyroidism. Occasionally, in the elderly, thyrotoxicosis presents with apathy and pseudodepression often with prominent cardiac arrhythmias.

Disturbances in the hypothalamic-pituitary-adrenal axis often result in psychiatric symptoms and may thus present as organic mood disorders. About a third of patients with Cushing's syndrome show depressive symptoms, such as retardation, irritability, and even suicide attempts. Cushing's syndrome may derive from central hypothalamic dysfunction, anterior pituitary tumors, ectopic ACTH–secreting tumors (e.g., oat-cell carcinoma), therapeutic ACTH or steroid administration, and primary adrenal adenomas or carcinomas. The majority of mood disturbances are associated with the more central ACTH–secreting abnormalities. The treatment of the depressive syndrome is based on reversal of the Cushing's syndrome, and tricyclic antidepressants may cause or exacerbate symptoms of delirium. In some instances, hyperadrenocorticism may also be associated with an irritable, labile, mania-like state.

Hypoadrenocorticism, or Addison's disease, may also be associated with depression, usually late in its course. The depressive symptoms may include lethargy, dysphoria, cognitive impairment, and, later, suspiciousness and anxiety.

Both hyper- and hypoparathyroidism may produce depressive syndromes. In hyperparathyroidism, the degree of mood disturbance is proportional to the increase in serum calcium, generally in the range of 12 to 16 mg per dl (higher values being associated with psychosis or coma). Symptoms tend to occur late in the course of the disorder and frequently include listlessness, apathy, dysphoria, irritability, and, sometimes, mild cognitive impairment. Hypoparathyroidism, usually secondary to surgery of the neck, is frequently accompanied by nonspecific symptoms, such as lethargy and fatigue or delirium but in some cases manifests as a moderate depressive episode.

Hyperprolactinemia (due either to a primary pituitary tumor or higher CNS abnormality) may be associated with depressive episodes with prominent neurovegetative symptoms. Treatment usually consists of correction of the underlying lesion or administration of bromocriptine to normalize prolactin concentrations.

Disturbances in the regulation of glucose by insulin-secreting tumors or metabolic disturbances may lead to symptoms of mood disturbance. Fasting hypoglycemia of less than 50 mg per dl secondary to a pancreatic carcinoma, extrapancreatic insulin-secreting tumor, pituitary, adrenal, or hepatic disease, or prescribed medications may result in lethargy, dysphoria, retardation, and confusion, which tend to worsen in the morning. Reactive or postprandial hypoglycemia may also be associated with autonomic arousal with accompanying symptoms of anxiety and fear and tends to occur in midafternoon.

Depressive syndromes may occur during the periluteal phase of the menstrual cycle and following childbirth, when serum estrogen concentrations are rapidly changing. Postpartum depression and late luteal phase dysphoric disorder, however, are not generally considered to be organic mood disorders, and the latter is still a subject of debate.

Metabolic diseases, such as those secondary to vitamin excess or deficiency, often result in mood disorders. Hypercalcemia of nonendocrine etiology (e.g., excess vitamin D ingestion, multiple myeloma, lung, breast, or renal tumors, milk-alkali syndrome, Paget's disease) can result in a retarded, anhedonic depression. Thiamine deficiency frequently results in apathy, dysphoria, impaired concentration, and irritability, but these signs are usually accompanied by early detectable cardiac and peripheral neurological signs; the symptoms usually remit with thiamine therapy. Pellagra is often associated with headache, insomnia, apathy, and dysphoria. Vitamin B_{12} (cyanocobalamin) deficiency, usually secondary to malabsorption, can result in a patchy CNS demyelination with associated agitated or retarded neurovegetative depressive symptoms; megaloblastic anemia is characteristic.

INFECTIONS While infectious diseases are more frequently associated with delirium or dementia, a number (e.g., neurosyphilis, hepatitis, influenza, systemic immunodeficient Epstein-Barr virus [EBV] syndrome, and AIDS) may present initially with depressive symptoms. Meningovascular syphilis may progress to general paresis after a 5- to 15-year incubation period: manic symptoms, such as euphoria, grandiosity, hyperactivity, and delusions of grandeur, are followed often by depression and, ultimately, by a terminal dementia.

Viral disease may produce psychiatric symptoms due to toxic metabolic effects or to infection of the CNS. The toxic metabolic effects of liver dysfunction secondary to acute infectious hepatitis may result in a depressive syndrome prior to delirium and coma. As lymphocytes and neurons share antigenic determinants, the HIV appears to affect the CNS directly, with symptoms of major depression as well as delusional psychoses and dementia in as many as 40 percent of AIDS patients. These symptoms may constitute the initial presentation of AIDS. Infectious mononucleosis, caused by the EBV and some influenzas, may be accompanied by a convalescent phase with vegetative, depressive symptoms. In the case of mononucleosis, the intensity of the depressive symptoms parallels the cellular immune response to the EBV infection.

CEREBROVASCULAR ACCIDENTS Depressive symptoms are frequent sequelae of cerebrovascular accidents (CVAs; up to 75 percent within 6 months) and seem to be a function of structural damage rather than simply a psychological response to the disabling impact of the CVA. Affective episodes are most frequent when lesions are anterior, and some evidence associates depression with lesions of the left hemisphere and mania or hypomania with right-hemisphere lesions. The extent of the lesion seems to be an independent determinant of the severity of depression. Depression may sometimes be a sequela of contusions (Figs. 12-7 and 12-8).

OTHER DISORDERS A significant depressive syndrome may be observed in up to half of all patients with Parkinson's disease, and often it is the presenting symptom of the illness. The administration of L-dopa sometimes, but not always, reverses the depressive symptoms, and treatment with antidepressants may be warranted.

Huntington's disease may also be punctuated with depressive episodes that may respond to antidepressant treatment. The origin of these symptoms and their relationship to the pathophysiology are currently unclear.

Multiple sclerosis (MS) may present with depressive or manic episodes or be marked by such episodes throughout its course. Euphoria may be manifested without other manic symptoms and has been associated with lesions in the basal forebrain, hypothalamus, thalamus, and temporal lobes. Depression is also common and is more frequently associated with MS than with other comparably debilitating neurological illnesses, such as muscular dystrophy or spinal cord injuries, which suggests a specific CNS etiology. Treatment of MS with steroids or ACTH may provoke an affective episode. Careful titration of MS medications and judicious use of psychotropic medications may be required to treat associated mood disorders.

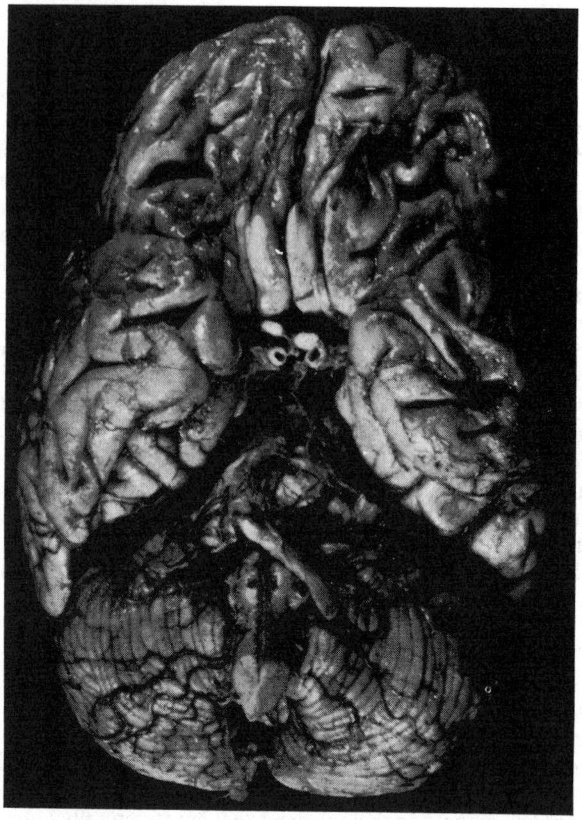

FIGURE 12-7. *Old contusion foci, orbitofrontal and temporal. (Courtesy of Dr. John Moosey.)*

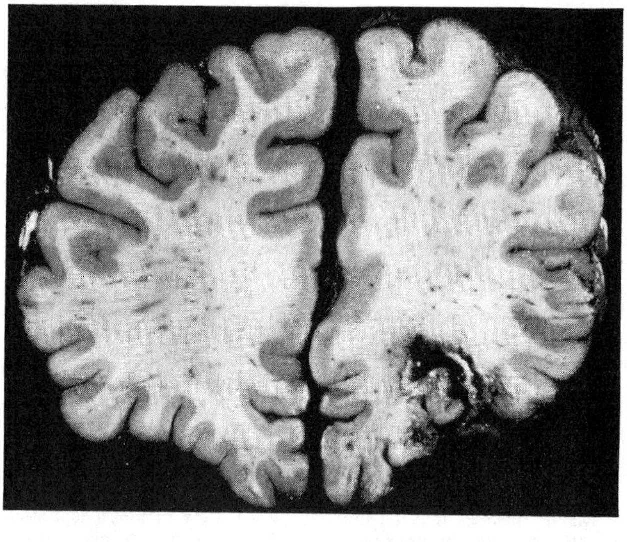

FIGURE 12-8. *Old contusion, orbitofrontal cortex. (Courtesy of Dr. John Moosey.)*

Marchiafava-Bignami disease is an uncommon demyelinating disorder associated with chronic alcoholism and characterized by lesions of the central area of the corpus callosum. Depression or mania may occur early in its course, followed later by dementia and seizures.

Seizure disorder may be associated with secondary depressive symptoms or, less frequently, mania. Epilepsy of late onset, in particular, has been associated with an increased incidence of depression. Although some evidence suggests that the lateralization of the epileptic focus may influence the likelihood of mood disorder episodes, such an association remains to be clearly established. The not uncommon observation of an abnormal EEG in bipolar illness and its response to carbamazepine (Tegretol) suggests some relationship between classical bipolar mood disorder and epilepsy.

A variety of collagen vascular diseases may have associated disorders of mood. Psychotic disorders, including mania, may be associated with systemic lupus erythematosus, while nonpsychotic depression may occur in Sjögren's syndrome and temporal arteritis.

Treatment Successful management of depressive syndromes is usually achieved by treatment of the underlying disease, which is straightforward for most of the better characterized illnesses described above. Not infrequently, however, the reversal of the known organic processes is not followed immediately by remission of depressive symptoms. Such patients require formal antidepressant treatment and psychotherapy. For a disease with no known treatment, such as AIDS, or one whose etiology is not reversible, such as the brain damage due to a CVA, symptomatic relief of depression may be achieved with tricyclic antidepressants and symptomatic relief of mania, with a combination of lithium and antipsychotics. Blood levels of the drugs should be monitored closely, and evidence of the cognitive side effects of psychotropics should be sought.

ORGANIC ANXIETY SYNDROME

Definition Anxiety is a ubiquitous response to medical illness and a symptom of most psychiatric disorders as well. It is an early and highly sensitive symptom with exceedingly low specificity. Two distinct anxiety syndromes have emerged in the DSM-III-R classification—the paroxysmal panic disorder and the generalized anxiety disorder. Panic attacks are defined by some combination of rapidly developing (10 minutes) symptoms: shortness of breath, choking, palpitations, chest discomfort, sweating, faintness, dizziness, abdominal distress, depersonalization, derealization, paresthesias, flushes and chills, tremors, fear of dying, and fear of losing control.

Generalized anxiety is characterized by persistent and excessive worry plus some combination of symptoms of motor tension (restlessness, fatigue, aches and pains, tremors), autonomic hyperactivity (palpitation, dry mouth), and vigilance (exaggerated startle response, difficulty concentrating, trouble falling asleep, irritability).

DSM-III-R has introduced the concept of an organic anxiety syndrome in cases where these symptoms can be attributed to an organic cause (Table 12-26). It should be noted, however, that feelings of anxiety and even full-blown anxiety syndromes are common at the onset of delirium episodes, in response to organic delusions or hallucinations, and also mark the course of dementias, particularly at times when the environmental demands placed on the patient exceed his or her cognitive or perceptual capacity (catastrophic reactions). Anxiety symptoms are also common in organic mood disorders, but there is some question about whether to continue to acknowledge the primacy of the mood disorder or to note the relative independence of anxiety syndromes, especially panic anxiety.

Etiology and differential diagnosis The recent renewal of interest in anxiety disorders is due partly to the development of diversified and effective treatments for panic and for generalized anxiety, and partly to the delineation of the neurophysiology of anxiety itself. The role of the noradrenergic locus ceruleus system, counterbalanced by a GABA-ergic inhibitory system has been clarified, and an endogenous ligand that binds to the benzodiazepine receptor has been identified. Agents and conditions that stimulate the former or inhibit the latter would logically play a part in the precipitation of anxiety symptoms.

TABLE 12-26
Diagnostic Criteria for Organic Anxiety Syndrome

A. Prominent, recurrent, panic attacks.
B. There is evidence from the history, physical examination, or laboratory tests of a specific organic factor (or factors) judged to be etiologically related to the disturbance.
C. Not occurring exclusively during the course of delirium.

Table from DSM-III-R *Diagnostic and Statistical Manual of Mental Disorders*, ed 3, revised. Copyright American Psychiatric Association, Washington, DC, 1987. Used with permission.

DSM-III-R notes two very common substance use disorders whose symptoms overlap largely with those of the anxiety disorder—tobacco (nicotine) withdrawal and caffeine intoxication. Other common exogenous causes of anxiety include withdrawal from sedatives, especially benzodiazepines, and overstimulation by excessive use of sympathomimetics and stimulants.

A number of medical conditions provoke endogenous release of monoamines: pheochromocytoma (directly) and hyperthyroidism, sudden hypoxia, and hypoglycemia (indirectly). There are numerous causes of hypoxia, but conditions that present mostly with anxiety include postoperative atelectasis and pulmonary embolization, and fat embolism secondary to a fracture. Reactive hypoglycemia is seen after subtotal gastrectomy, in early diabetes, and after high-carbohydrate meals. The concept of an organic anxiety syndrome due to a functional hypoglycemia has attracted much attention and a variety of dietary interventions have been proposed, but it likely has been overdiagnosed. The fasting hypoglycemia seen in islet-cell tumors of the pancreas, in Addison's disease, and in pituitary deficiency can be complicated by an organic anxiety syndrome alternating with confusional, frankly delirious episodes, and even with seizures.

Hyperthyroidism frequently presents with a syndrome of generalized anxiety, while the uncommon pheochromocytoma tends to induce panic attacks. Cushing's disease and other types of hypercortisolemia, and hyperparathyroidism and other causes of hypercalcemia have been associated with generalized mild anxiety. The association is not specific to anxiety, as these conditions primarily cause an organic mood syndrome.

A variety of CNS disorders may present with organic anxiety. Very sudden terror may be the aura of a partial complex seizure from the temporal lobe. Transient ischemic episodes affecting silent association areas may have no manifestations other than anxiety, perceptual anomalies, or transient apraxias. Cerebral tumors, MS, subdural hematomas, Wilson's disease, and Huntington's disease have been described with labile mood and fluctuating anxiety before the onset of neurological signs (Fig. 12-9). Anxiety is also a component of the postconcussion syndrome, other signs of which include headache, dizziness, mood lability, and attention deficits. The debate over whether the shearing forces of blunt trauma may produce demyelineation in the limbic and upper mesencephalic areas is unresolved. The association between anxiety and hypertensive vascular disease has a psychogenic cause: Patients who do not know about their high blood pressure do not develop anxiety.

There is at least a statistical correlation between panic disorder and the mitral valve prolapse syndrome. It has been proposed that both may be manifestations of a condition of autonomic β-adrenergic hyperactivity. The chance association

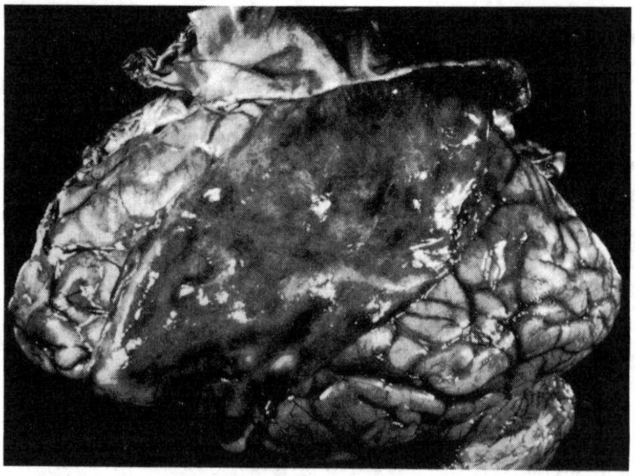

FIGURE 12-9. *Subdural hematoma with encapsulating membranes. (Courtesy of Dr. John Moosey.)*

of two disorders that are normally quite prevalent in a youthful population is another possible explanation.

Treatment and prognosis Removal of the primary cause and symptomatic treatment with benzodiazepines are the standard approaches to these disorders. Studies are not available yet on tricyclic antidepressants in the treatment of organic panic disorder patients. Likewise, there are no prospective studies as yet on the syndromal stability and prognosis of organic anxiety disorders: Do they merge into mood disorders? Do they manifest as delirium or dementia if the underlying neuropathology progresses? Are some of them identical to functional anxiety disorders?

ORGANIC DELUSIONAL SYNDROME

Definition Delusions can be prominent symptoms in dementia and delirium and in mood disorders, schizophrenia, and paranoid psychoses. Organic delusional syndrome is defined by the presence of prominent delusions with an organic etiology. There are other associated symptoms as well: There may be some abnormality of thought, language, and communication; the mood is often dysphoric and anxious; and there may be psychomotor or ritualistic overactivity or catatonic posturing. However, the patient should not meet criteria for the other OMSs (Table 12-27). Researchers often refer to the condition as a schizophreniform psychosis, but it should be distinguished from the schizophreniform disorder of DSM-III-R, which rules out an OMD. True organic delusional disorder is far less common than any of the other mental syndromes that present with prominent delusions. Yet, the condition has a theoretical importance that outweighs its practical impact: To the extent that it can be used as a model for schizophrenia, and perhaps for mood disorders, what is known of its pathophysiology may provide insights into the far more common disorders.

TABLE 12-27
Diagnostic Criteria for Organic Delusional Syndrome

A. Prominent delusions.
B. There is evidence from the history, physical examination, or laboratory tests of a specific organic factor (or factors) judged to be etiologically related to the disturbance.
C. Not occurring exclusively during the course of delirium.

Table from DSM-III-R *Diagnostic and Statistical Manual of Mental Disorders,* ed 3, revised. Copyright American Psychiatric Association, Washington, DC, 1987. Used with permission.

Etiology and differential diagnosis The medical literature contains numerous references to psychoses, exogenous psychoses, and even schizophreniform or manic psychoses occurring during the course of diseases as varied as systemic lupus erythematosus, MS, various endocrinopathies, uremia, porphyria, Wilson's disease, and irritative or ablative lesions of the temporal and parietal lobes. The mental state of such patients is usually so poorly defined that an examiner cannot distinguish between delirium with prominent psychotic features and a true schizophreniform psychosis. The older medical literature used a broad, Bleulerian definition of schizophrenia, and many of their references can be accommodated in one of the DSM-III-R categories of OMD. Closer examination of the circumstances suggests some reasonable alternatives: So-called pancreatic psychosis may well be withdrawal delirium associated with alcoholism and acute pancreatitis; exacerbations of systemic lupus and MS may trigger confusional episodes. Many medications used in the course of chronic diseases also contribute to episodes of confusion and intoxication.

After considerable winnowing of the cases in the literature, one is left with two groups of disorders that produce mental disorders that closely resemble schizophrenia on a cross-sectional basis but that differ in having a normal premorbid personality, a later age of onset, a better preservation of psychosocial function, and a lower incidence of negative symptoms.

The first group are located in the temporal lobes (especially the mesial aspects) and in the diencephalon. A variety of pathological states, especially if complicated by seizures, can induce the psychosis. The best-studied example is the interictal psychosis of classical temporal lobe epilepsy. It occurs after a decade or more of poorly controlled seizures, and it is often superimposed on an organic personality disorder. The psychosis is often inversely related to the intensity of seizures. It should be noted, however, that this psychosis, which can imitate schizophrenia even to showing first-rank Schneiderian symptoms, is by no means the most common psychotic complication of epilepsy. Postictal confusional states, bizarre intraictal experiences and automatisms, anticonvulsant intoxication, and postanoxic and post-traumatic dementias may all be more common and require very different management. There is also some new evidence that not all interictal states are schizophreniform—mood disorders, rapid cycling bipolar disorders, and affective personality changes may also be seen. There is clearly a need for intensive EEG and video monitoring of seizures in suspected cases.

The common denominator of a second group of disorders is their potentiation of dopaminergic neurotransmission. Amphetamine psychosis has long been advocated as a good model for acute paranoid schizophrenia; PCP intoxication may mimic some aspects of an acute hebephrenic disorder. Cocaine psychosis, seen after long-term use of high doses, is characterized by ideas of reference, aggressiveness and hostility, anxiety, and psychomotor agitation.

Treatment and prognosis It is tempting to deal with a patient suffering from a delusional syndrome on a purely symptomatic basis, using antipsychotics and the behavioral controls usually applied to psychotic persons. This indeed may be the appropriate first step in a crisis. However, it is imperative to pursue a full clinical evaluation, seeking evidence of a major mood disorder, depressive or manic symptoms, or supportive evidence for schizophrenia. At the same time, a causative medical disorder must be sought. Mental changes appearing after age 55, absence of psychosocial stress factors, chronic medical illness and possible attendant polypharmacy, exposure to street drugs and alcohol, recent head injury, change in headache pattern, visual disturbances, seizures, speech and communication problems, and movement disorders not caused by antipsychotic therapy point to organic etiology.

The hyperdopaminergic conditions are treated in hospital by withdrawing the offending medication, dealing with rebound depression, and, occasionally, using antipsychotics to control behavior.

The temporal lobe or diencephalic conditions pose a greater challenge. Careful use of anticonvulsants, especially carbamazepine, in adequate doses often controls the partial as well as the major seizures and associated peri-ictal behavior disturbances, and it may even prevent the development of interictal complications. However, once established, these complications, especially the delusional disorder, fail to respond to anticonvulsants alone. Occasionally, good seizure control is attended by an increase in psychotic symptoms. High potency antipsychotics should be used at full antipsychotic dosage, but blood levels of anticonvulsants should be checked to ensure continued seizure control and to check for drug interactions.

Organic delusional disorders generally have a much shorter natural history than delusional disorder or the schizophrenias, and the delusions are much less likely to be crystallized or systematized. So, antipsychotics combined with supportive psychotherapy are much more likely to resolve the problem. The affective intensity associated with the delusions diminishes first, then the patient begins to distance him- or herself from the experience, discussing the phenomena in the past tense. A conviction of reality regarding the subjective delusional event often persists, but it does not interfere with the patient's current concerns.

ORGANIC HALLUCINOSIS

Definition Organic hallucinosis is, by definition, a single-symptom disorder, distinguishable from the other OMSs by a careful mental status examination and from functional hallucinosis by the presence of a detectable organic factor. Hypnagogic and hypnopompic hallucinations and dissociative and factitious states should be ruled out. The majority of people who present with organic hallucinosis have a delirium; isolated hallucinosis is uncommon in general hospitals. It is more common in substance-abuse settings, but not so common as acute withdrawal states. Visual, auditory, olfactory, and somatosensory types are seen; their vividness and elaboration depend on the etiology (Table 12-28).

Etiology and differential diagnosis The most common cause of isolated hallucinations is an intoxication. Hallucinogens, PCP, and cannabis are the main offenders, but therapeutic drugs can also cause them (e.g., digitalis, antiarrhythmic agents, cimetidine, high-dose IV pencillin, a variety of anticholinergic agents and drugs with such side effects, some over-the-counter [OTC] sedatives in overdose quantities). Associated physical findings may be tachycardia, sweating, pupillary dilation, and tremors. Organic hallucinosis is often accompanied by anxiety, ideas of reference, and fear of losing control or losing one's mind.

TABLE 12-28
Diagnostic Criteria for Organic Hallucinosis

A. Prominent persistent or recurrent hallucinations.
B. There is evidence from the history, physical examination, or laboratory tests of a specific organic factor (or factors) judged to be etiologically related to the disturbance.
C. Not occurring exclusively during the course of delirium.

Table from DSM-III-R *Diagnostic and Statistical Manual of Mental Disorders*, ed 3, revised. Copyright American Psychiatric Association, Washington, DC, 1987. Used with permission.

Alcohol hallucinosis is defined as a condition of vivid auditory or visual hallucinations that develop within a few days (usually within 48 hours) of reduction or cessation of drinking in a physiologically dependent person. In the presence of delirium, hallucinations should not be diagnosed as a separate entity. Alcohol hallucinosis can become quite chronic and persist intermittently for several weeks. The patient experiences noises as well as voices and responds appropriately to their content. Delusions are not prominent (may occur as a form of cognitive explanation for the voices), and patients do not meet the criteria for schizophrenia, nor do they have an excess of schizophrenic relatives. The hallucinosis appears to be a withdrawal phenomenon yet outlasts the other signs of withdrawal and does not always respond to benzodiazepines. Antipsychotic drugs will cause a remission.

Focal seizure activities occasionally produce isolated hallucinations, but more frequently, these are a part of complex seizure phenomena, usually of temporal lobe origin. Occipital tumors and CVAs occasionally cause visual hallucinations, often in association with field defects. Classical migraines can produce visual illusions and distortions.

Finally, hallucinations and illusions occur in elderly people under conditions of sensory deprivation, usually in the altered sensory modality. People with deafness due to otosclerosis can develop auditory hallucinations and misperceptions and may elaborate them in a paranoid context. Patients with retinal blindness and those recovering from cataract surgery may note visual hallucinations. More dramatic psychotic decompensations under these conditions (black-patch psychosis) usually occur in the context of an underlying schizophreniform personality disorder or in early dementias.

Treatment and prognosis Intoxications and "bad trips" are quite time limited, though frequently recurrent. It is far safer to "talk the patient down" than to treat with drugs. Antipsychotics with anticholinergic side effects should be avoided, as many street drugs are cut with them already. When therapeutic drug overdose is suspected, blood levels of the agents should be obtained so that the dosage can be modified without depriving the patient of the therapeutic benefit.

Partial complex seizures may need to be treated with carbamazepine, as phenytoin (Dilantin) is likely to control only the generalized seizure component. In persistent hallucinosis, empirical treatment with haloperidol, up to 5 mg per day, may be useful.

ORGANIC PERSONALITY SYNDROME

Definition Organic personality syndrome represents a significant and persistent disturbance in personality attributable to a specific organic factor. The personality disturbance may be lifelong if the organic factor is inherited or acquired early in childhood. It may constitute a marked change from or an accentuation of characteristics of the premorbid personality, if the organic factor is acquired after personality development has taken place. Affective instability, recurrent outbursts of aggression or rage, markedly impaired social judgment, pronounced apathy and indifference, and suspiciousness or paranoid ideation are common manifestations of organic personality syndrome (Table 12-29).

Clinical signs and symptoms Several common patterns of organic personality disorder are rather specifically associated with the character and site of the pathology. One pattern frequently associated with orbital-frontal lesions is a disinhibited, unsocialized pattern; lesions of the convexity of the frontal lobes may produce an apathetic, indifferent picture.

TABLE 12-29
Diagnostic Criteria for Organic Personality Syndrome

A. A persistent personality disturbance, either lifelong or representing a change or accentuation of a previously characteristic trait involving at least one of the following:
(1) affective instability (e.g., marked shifts from normal mood to depression, irritability, or anxiety)
(2) recurrent outbursts of aggression or rage that are grossly out of proportion to any precipitating psychosocial stressors
(3) markedly impaired social judgment (e.g., sexual indiscretions)
(4) marked apathy and indifference
(5) suspiciousness or paranoid ideation
B. There is evidence from the history, physical examination, or laboratory tests of a specific organic factor (or factors) judged to be etiologically related to the disturbance.
C. This diagnosis is not given to a child or adolescent if the clinical picture is limited to the features that characterize attention-deficit hyperactivity disorder.
D. Not occurring exclusively during the course of delirium, and does not meet the criteria for dementia.
Specify explosive type if outbursts of aggression or rage are the predominant feature.

Table from DSM-III-R *Diagnostic and Statistical Manual of Mental Disorders,* ed 3, revised. Copyright American Psychiatric Association, Washington, DC, 1987. Used with permission.

Temporal lesions, usually epileptic foci, tend to produce a viscous, verbose, hyper-religious personality pattern.

Frequently, these disorders are associated with mild cognitive impairment, but not usually to a degree that dementia is diagnosed. Although lesions that result in organic personality disorder may also cause disturbances in sensorium or level of consciousness, these elements are not characteristic of the chronic picture of organic personality disorder.

Frequently, the course of organic personality disorder is chronic and persistent, particularly if it is secondary to structural damage (e.g., epilepsy or trauma; see Fig. 12-10). However, when organic personality disorder has a metabolic cause (e.g., endocrine disorder, medication, or substance abuse), the disorder may be reversed when the metabolic disturbance is corrected or the precipitant pharmacological agent is withdrawn. In some cases, organic personality disorder may be the prodrome of a progressive deterioration in dementia.

Although the degree of psychosocial impairment for organic personality disorder may vary, there is often some social role dysfunction. It may be less severe in cases of the interictal personality characteristics of temporal lobe epilepsy, but in many cases, particularly in frontal lobe syndromes, the disinhibition and poor social judgment may require constant monitoring or even custodial care. Even when such supervision is not required, impulsive or inappropriate behavior almost inevitably leads to profound interpersonal difficulties and even to social ostracism or litigation.

Pathophysiology The symptoms of organic personality disorder are usually attributable to damage in association areas of the cerebral cortex that impairs specific higher integrative

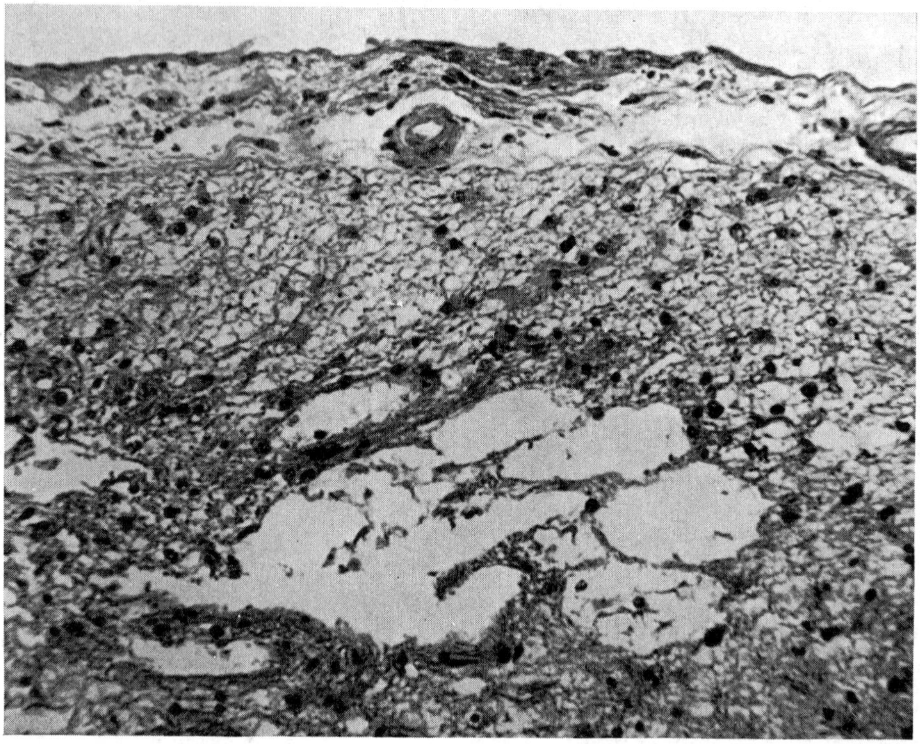

FIGURE 12-10. *Old contusion, orbitofrontal cortex. There are derangements of architecture, loss of nerve cells, diffuse astrocytosis characteristic change, and pigment-laden phagocytes (hematoxylin and costly, original magnification × 200. (Courtesy of Dr. John Moosey.)*

functions of the CNS. Lesions of the premotor frontal lobes and temporal lobes are most frequently associated with changes of organic personality disorder.

The frontal lobes are involved in recruitment and engagement of attention, inhibition of inappropriate behaviors, and initiating, planning, and sequencing of complex behaviors. In the patient with a lesion of the convexity of the frontal lobe, a disturbance in attention, initiation, and engagement with the environment may result in a pseudodepressed presentation with apathy and withdrawal. In the patient with a lesion of the orbital areas of the frontal lobe, disturbances in inhibitory and planning functions may result in pseudopsychopathic presentation, with concreteness, disinhibition of aggression and sexuality, and impaired perception of the social consequences of such behaviors. Frequently, the frontal personality disturbance shows considerable overlap between these two prototypical patterns.

The patient with a pseudodepressed frontal lobe personality pattern may respond normally to environmental stimuli but often cannot act independently, having lost the capacity to take initiative. Such a person may appear slow, apathetic, and disengaged and, so, may be misdiagnosed as having retarded depression; instead of the dysphoria and internal turmoil of the depressive, the patient demonstrates bland indifference. A similar clinical picture may be seen in some subcortical disorders affecting the basal ganglia and thalamus.

The patient with a pseudopsychopathic frontal lobe disorder is characterized by disinhibition, or a lack of the restraint associated with adult social behavior, and may exhibit impulsive, irritable, explosive, affectively labile, promiscuous, grandiose, and paranoid behavior. There is little appreciation of the social implications of behavior, and judgment is clearly impaired. Antisocial personality disorder patients, in contrast, are aware of the potential consequences of their behavior, even if they tend to minimize them.

The epileptic personality, most frequently associated with an irritative lesion in the temporal lobe, is characterized by an intensification of emotional responses and symbolization. These characteristics are consistent with a disturbance in the temporal lobe's apparent regulation of memory and attribution of organismic significance. Thus, the temporal lobe epileptic may have profound ethical-religious feelings and strong perseverative tendencies, may be excessively serious, and exhibits adhesiveness in social interactions and circumstantiality in speech. Episodic discharges of rage, paranoid ideation, mood swings, hyposexuality, and anxiety are also part of the clinical picture.

When such personality characteristics are observed in the absence of seizures, careful history taking and observation are indicated to seek occult temporal lobe seizures. When seizures are present, the EEG abnormalities (often seen on the nasopharyngeal leads in a sleep-deprived patient) usually indicate a temporal lobe irritative focus. In some instances, modest temporal lobe EEG abnormalities may be associated with impulsive features in the absence of seizures, but such an association is poorly understood and is not grounds for a diagnosis of organic personality disorder if a definitive organic cause has not been demonstrated. Hysterical seizures, frequently observed in these patients, should not rule out the diagnosis of epilepsy. Schizophreniform psychoses may be observed late in the course of the disease, but the clinical picture does not include the constricted affect and poor rapport of true schizophrenia.

Frontal lobe lesions are usually ablative—disconnecting prefrontal areas from posterior cortical sites and from limbic and basal ganglia structure. In contrast, the common cause of the temporal lobe personality disorder, epilepsy, induces a hyperconnection within the limbic system.

Etiology and differential diagnosis Traumatic injuries are a common cause of organic personality disorder. Initially, they may cause pervasive OMSs with coma or altered sensorium, but they often leave only minimal residual cognitive impairment with a prominent persistent personality alteration. Organic personality disorder is most common when the trauma involves the frontal or temporal region. Bilateral frontal traumatic lesions are the most frequent etiology of major organic personality disorder. Psychosurgery often results in some characteristics of organic personality disorder. The precise location of the lesion largely determines the character of the symptoms, whether pseudopsychopathic or pseudodepressed.

Frontal tumors, such as meningiomas, are a less frequent cause of organic personality disorder, as are anterior cerebral artery aneurysm ruptures. Huntington's disease may cause a frontal lobe syndrome early in its course leading to disinhibition of aggression and sexual behavior. MS lesions in the frontal lobes may also be associated with organic personality disorder.

The later course of alcoholism is frequently marked by personality alterations that persist even during periods of sobriety. While psychosocial vicissitudes are clearly involved, specific cognitive alterations characteristic of frontal lobe damage have been demonstrated in many alcoholics. Histological and radiographic evidence also suggest that the chronic toxic effects of alcohol seriously affect frontal lobe structure and function first.

Endocrine disorders, such as thyroid or adrenal disease, also infrequently produce a clinical picture of organic personality disorder; for example, the irritability and hyperactivity of a person with hyperthyroidism initially may be interpreted as organic personality disorder. Psychoactive substances may precipitate features of organic personality disorder. Other metabolic changes, including hypoxemia, hypo- and hypercalcemia, hypokalemia, and uremia, may result in less specific personality changes, such as reduced initiative, blunt or labile affect, irritability, or impulsivity, which must be evaluated against premorbid function.

Temporal lobe epilepsy is the most common cause of the epileptic personality disorder, although this disorder does not invariably accompany the syndrome. The temporal seizures can result from tumor, infection, vascular lesions, residue of brain trauma or birth injury, sclerosis of Ammon's horn (apparently secondary to prolonged infantile seizures). The personality disturbances usually develop late in the course of the illness and may create a caricature of the previous personality.

Neurosyphilis is mostly of historical interest now, but at one time, the onset of a socially disinhibited frontal lobe type of behavior most likely would have been the first sign of general paresis of the insane. Today, recovered victims of viral encephalitis have an extraordinarily high incidence of organic personality disorders.

Organic personality disorder must be distinguished from dementia, in which personality changes, when present, are accompanied by pronounced impairment in memory, cognitive processes, and abstract thinking. When the symptoms of a deteriorating or fluctuating illness change from a relatively encapsulated personality disturbance to frank dementia, the diagnosis should be revised accordingly. Personality alterations attributable to or associated with altered sensorium should be diagnosed as delirium. In some cases (e.g., head trauma), symptoms of delirium may antedate the appearance of the personality disorder, which then remains after the delirium remits. Organic personality disorders can be distinguished from functional disorders (e.g., schizophrenia, mood disorders, delusional disorders, impulse control disorders not elsewhere classified, and Axis II personality disorders) by the presence of a specific identifiable organic etiological factor. Organic personality disorder usually involves structural brain disease or specific metabolic disturbances, whereas identified biological disturbances implicated in some of the Axis II personality disorders seem to involve abnormal function of modulating neurochemical and neuroanatomical systems.

Treatment Patients with brain injury (e.g., frontal syndromes) may require supervision, structured environment, or even custodial management. In milder cases, education and counseling of the patient's family is necessary to keep their expectations in line with the patient's capabilities, lest a catastrophic reaction with rage and depression be precipitated.

Disinhibited violent behavior may respond to propranolol, lithium, antipsychotics, or carbamazepine, but there is no way to predict treatment outcome. Personality disorder characteristics secondary to temporal lobe epilepsy may improve with control of seizures by phenobarbital, or carbamazepine, but in some instances, they may worsen. Antipsychotics are of some help in agitated psychotic states. Unilateral anterior temporal lobectomy is a treatment of last resort for a severely disturbed patient refractory to medication.

Primary prevention of deterioration of the process may involve seizure control, prevention of head trauma, and avoidance of alcohol and psychoactive substances.

PERSONALITY CHANGES IN EPILEPSY

History During the first half of the century, the psychiatric complications of epilepsy were one of the three major mental disorders, schizophrenia and affective illness (mood disorder) being the other two. German psychiatrists have described epileptics as hypocritical and two-faced, hiding aggression behind a facade of religiosity and social conformity. Kraepelin noted their slow, ponderous circumstantiality and intense moods. Freud described their intense conflicts over good and evil. Although some observers noted an inverse relationship between psychosis and epilepsy (an observation that led Meduna to invent seizure treatment for functional psychoses), others have emphasized the high incidence of psychotic states among epileptics.

More recently, mental changes in epileptics have been portrayed as understandable reactions (1) to a socially stigmatizing, chronic, disabling illness; (2) to organic mental disorders resulting from the hypoxia and head injuries of uncontrolled seizures; or (3) from the confusional, toxic effects of poorly managed anticonvulsants.

French neurologists continued to emphasize the presence of a unique, specific, and persistent mental syndrome among epileptics characterized by hyposexuality, intense emotionality, verbosity, circumstantiality, philosophical preoccupations, and self-righteous conventionality.

British neuropsychiatrists established the presence of schizophreniform psychoses with Schneiderian features in epilepsy of temporal lobe origin but also noted the absence of family history, schizoid premorbid personality, and psychosocial deterioration in these patients.

Geschwind rekindled interest in the behavioral manifestations of neurological diseases, in general, and epilepsy, in particular in the United States. Under his influence, others developed a psychometric inventory for the description of these so-called epileptoid behavioral changes and found that it correctly distinguished 90 percent of temporal lobe epileptics from matched controls suffering from chronic medical or neurological disorders. (In other studies, it was less successful in differentiating patients with complex partial seizures from those with major motor seizures.)

Epidemiology Given the high prevalence of epilepsy in the United States (4 million) and the likelihood that 50 percent of these are of temporal lobe origin, with a high incidence (up to 40 percent) of associated psychosocial problems, the relative neglect of the psychiatric complications of epilepsy is a profoundly regrettable side effect of professional superspecialization.

Definition There is no specific diagnostic category for these disorders in DSM-III-R, although organic delusional and mood syndromes are the relevant diagnoses for the epileptic interictal psychoses. Three of the five criteria of organic personality disorder can be very relevant: affective instability, recurrent outbursts of aggression, and suspiciousness and paranoid ideation. The two other items (markedly impaired social judgment and marked apathy and indifference) are not features of epilepsy but are seen with frontal lobe damage. The category of organic personality disorder thus may be too broad to be truly helpful in disease or pathophysiologically based syndrome classification.

Etiology and pathology Behavioral and experiential abnormalities in epilepsy vary according to the stage of seizure formation during which they emerge and the neurological structures involved in the aberrant electrical activity, and depend to a much lesser extent on the underlying neuropathology.

The origin of the preictal perception of irritability and tension is unknown. This is often followed by the aura, which is actually a preictal state of localized epileptiform discharge, usually in the medial temporal lobes. Ongoing activities are abandoned and the patient experiences a variety of strange psychic phenomena (déjà vu, perceptual and affective changes) and behavioral automatisms. This may merge into a dreamy state and may or may not be followed by an amnestic period; some patients are amnestic for the entire episode. Complex partial seizures may be followed by major motor seizures. A significant portion of major motor seizures of apparent centrencephalic origin are, in fact, undetected temporal lobe events.

Postictal manifestations include amnesia, confusion, automatism, and, at times, episodes of confused, delirious psychoses. Occasionally, ictal seizure activity of a focal type may progress to what is thought of as the postictal state. Temporal lobe status may be difficult to distinguish from a psychogenic dissociative reaction without ongoing EEG monitoring.

Electrical-chemical activity in the interictal period may not be entirely normal. There may be persistent focal electrical discharges, detectable at times only on depth electrode recordings, and changes in receptors and synaptic relationships may lead to a hyperconnection state. There may be a state of functional sensitization, where repeated stimulation of neural structures may result in a facilitation, rather than habituation, of the responses (the so-called kindling phenomenon).

The emerging complexity of biological reactions should not blind one to relevant psychosocial factors. Interruption of the conscious experience of life with the episodes of confusion, perceptual distortions, and strange phenomena the epileptic patient's experiences form a rich background for psychopathology or for philosophical explanation of mystical experiences. Freud and Szondi remarked on the emergence of accumulated tensions as a result of undischarged drive states. Their sudden catastrophic release, in seizures or seizure equivalents, may have untoward consequences. The reestablishment of order and stability may lead to a sense of guilt coupled with obsessive desire to control the environment. The Jekyl and Hyde appearance of some complex partial seizure epileptics may only seem to be hypocritical and may represent a deep and fundamental conflict between order and disorder or good and evil, as Dostoyevsky portrayed sensitively in his writings.

Behavioral changes may also be secondary to the progression of the underlying disease, and to the anoxic and traumatic complications of uncontrolled seizures, and to the toxic effects of high doses of anticonvulsants. Improved medical management should minimize these changes, as improved public understanding and demythologizing of the illness should result in reduced prejudice and an amelioration of the social handicap placed on epileptic patients.

Clinical signs and symptoms The syndrome was initially described by Gastaut. Hyposexuality is a regular finding, reversed by appropriate anticonvulsants and anterior temporal lobectomy. It often leads male patients to social isolation. Increased emotional depth and an associated mood lability characterize the expression of anger, irritability, depression, and, at times, elation and euphoria. The target of the emotional expressions is usually appropriate, but the affect is poorly modulated and is controlled only with great effort, if at all. Episodes of anxiety and fear may merge into frank paranoia.

The cognitive style of the epileptoid personality is seen in the interictal state of subjects with complex partial seizures of temporal lobe origin. There is considerable circumstantiality, verbosity, and hypergraphia. Attention is often riveted on philosophical and religious or mystical interests. There is also a strong streak of conventionality, moralism, a sense of justice that merges into a humorless self-righteousness. Subjects prefer interpersonal stability, and this can lead to clinging, viscosity, and an inability to terminate a conversation. Yet, the subjects are often very helpful, good-natured, and cooperative. Subjects are quite ready to accept responsibility for actions taken under the influence of their strong feelings, and they are often genuinely conflicted over issues of good and evil, even in trivial matters.

The later stages of the syndrome may be complicated by limited cognitive deterioration, mostly visual and verbal amnesias and frequent anomia, but also, at times, lack of spontaneity, dullness, and retardation. Deterioration to a true amnestic or dementing syndrome is very rare.

After a decade and a half of poorly controlled focal seizures, some patients develop true psychoses. These initially emerge from a background of intense fear responses with paranoid ideation but can have all the Schneiderian symptoms and thought disorder described in schizophrenia. Yet, the affect remains warm and intense, and interpersonal relationships remain, although they may be stormy. Social function tends to be preserved despite recurrent episodes of psychosis. Other patients present with mood disorders with intense anger, depression, suicidal ideations, and mood-congruent and -incongruent delusions and hallucinations. There is some evidence that left temporal foci are associated with schizophreniform disorder and right-sided foci with mood disorders.

A more controversial clinical group has been described, the dysthymic subictal mood syndrome. These characterologically depressed patients have brief euphorias, brief severe depressive plunges, irritability, and paradoxical responses to lithium and tricyclics. The clinical picture resembles that of dysthymia, cyclothymia, or even the borderline personality disorder. There is EEG evidence of temporal lobe abnormality and a good response to carbamazepine.

Differential diagnosis The most critical steps in diagnosing epilepsy-related conditions are taking a thorough history and documenting the seizures (including difficult-to-detect nocturnal ones and the puzzling complex partial seizures) describing aberrant behavior and experiences completely, and performing appropriate EEG investigations. The limitations of random, routine EEGs are well known, and sleep deprivation EEGs with nasopharyngeal leads represent the minimum acceptable investigations of complex partial seizures. Prolonged EEG and video monitoring are becoming increasingly available to correlate behavioral and physiological manifestations. Computer analyzed topographic EEGs (e.g., brain electrical activity mapping [BEAM]) have also been used to detect local frequency deviations from the normal, even in the absence of formal epileptiform activities. In difficult cases, Megimide activation procedures and depth electrodes have been used. Neuropsychological testing often points to isolated verbal or visual memory defects, and the personality inventory introduced by Bear is gaining acceptance.

Dissociative episodes have no EEG signature; they tend to be more prolonged, more purposeful, and less suggestive of automatisms. Dissociative episodes may occur, however, in patients suffering from genuine temporal lobe epilepsy.

Hysterical seizures are not uncommon in patients with true epilepsy. Sometimes these pseudoseizures are easily identified by their wildly flailing, quasipurposeful activity, but in other cases, only EEG monitoring can reveal the difference.

Purposeful aggressive behavior is virtually never an ictal event, despite the occasional medicolegal claim to the contrary. However, complex partial seizure patients in their interictal period may very well show increased tendencies toward retaliatory violence arising out of escalating interpersonal situations. Their increased anger and self-righteousness make them formidable adversaries.

These interpersonal difficulties may lead to a consideration of the diagnosis of a functional character disorder (e.g., antisocial personality). Epileptic patients, however, tend to accept responsibility for their behavior more readily and lack the early history of poor socialization, truancy, or unstable personal behavior that characterizes the antisocial personality.

Differentiation from borderlines may be more difficult, and, indeed, some classical borderline patients studied at McLean's Hospital showed EEG topographical evidence of aberrant temporal lobe electrical activity.

Himmelhoch also emphasized the difficulty in differentiating the interictal behavior of some complex partial seizure patients from varieties of mood disorders. He pointed to the presence of rapid mood swings, atypical responses to tricyclics and lithium, and focal EEG features as suggestive of temporal lobe pathology.

Differentiating true schizophrenia from the phenocopy occasioned by temporal lobe epilepsy is a matter of careful history taking, EEG identification of the epilepsy, and adequate description of the preserved affectivity and social functioning of the patient.

Mental status examination and, in difficult cases, psychological testing can identify delirium or dementia associated with uncontrolled seizures, medication toxicity, or prolonged postictal encephalopathy.

Treatment and prognosis The adequate control of both major motor and partial complex seizures is the primary goal of therapy. Carbamazepine and valproic acid (Depakene) are increasingly used, as the phenobarbital–phenytoin combination often fails to prevent complex partial seizures. Careful behavioral, EEG, and anticonvulsant (blood level) monitoring is required. It is possible that a reduction in the lifetime total of complex partial seizures may prevent, ameliorate, or delay the development of the epileptoid personality and the interictal psychosis of epilepsy. Anterior temporal lobectomy is used occasionally in refractory seizures, but it is unlikely to reverse the behavioral problems.

The relationship between seizures and psychosis is still controversial. Those workers who support the notion of a forced normalization of the EEG during psychoses will, at times, lower the dose of anticonvulsants to permit a seizure in the belief that it will obviate an emerging behavioral abnormality. It would appear to be more prudent to use ECT under controlled circumstances in these cases.

Psychotic behavior in the interictal period responds well to antipsychotics and not at all to anticonvulsants. Some workers prefer molindone (Moban, Lidone) for its minimal effect on seizure threshold. In general it is advisable to avoid the sedative and anticholinergic agents (e.g., chlorpromazine, thioridazine). Mood disorders in these patients often respond paradoxically to antidepressants, which can precipitate seizures as well as manic episodes. Lithium seems better tolerated, but even it may cause neurological side effects. Carbamazepine has both anticonvulsant and mood-stabilizing effects and appears to be the agent of choice.

The interictal personality features of complex partial seizure patients frequently lead to social isolation, interpersonal difficulties, and inability to meet the demands of life (i.e., a formal personality disorder). Supportive, educational psychotherapy dealing with issues of medication compliance, anger control, and social relatedness is an important, often neglected, part of patient management. Cognitive and confrontational techniques in individual and group settings can be utilized to deal with the interpersonal viscosity, verbosity, and circumstantiality of these patients. Exploratory dynamic psychotherapy may be needed by certain intelligent patients who are able to deal with the experience of intense dynamic conflict between affective and drive-related issues and with the demands of a punitive superego.

The management of these fascinating, complex patients requires professionals who are equally adept at monitoring EEGs, anticonvulsant blood levels, antipsychotic and mood-stabilizing medication, complex seizure activities, and subtle interpersonal and psychodynamic conflicts. Behavioral neurologists and biological psychiatrists need psychodynamic and psychosocial training to effectively treat these patients.

FUTURE PROSPECTS

Psychiatry is undergoing a major conceptual and technological revolution. The bases of the dominant theories of pathogenesis have shifted from psychodynamics to neuroscience. The development of an atheoretical, purely descriptive diagnostic and classificatory system, which started a decade ago, will probably be seen by future historians of science as a laudable but temporary expedient, a way of meeting on common ground. Ever finer phenomenological distinctions are unlikely to penetrate to the heart of the matter. Empirical clusters of signs and symptoms are ultimately useful only to the extent that they point to a common pathophysiology. The current understanding suggests that several of the dementia syndromes, delirium, the amnestic syndrome, the organic mood disorder, two of the personality syndromes, and perhaps some form of the organic delusional syndrome may have reached this level of heuristic usefulness. Whether it is wise to proliferate the syndromes further is a matter for clinical and physiological research.

The history of psychiatry does not abound in major victories over diseases. It is heartening to reflect, therefore, on the history of neurosyphilis and see in it a model for conceptually similar advances. Pinel redescribed dementia in the 1800s, and his student Bayle differentiated general paresis from other forms of dementia on clinical grounds in 1825. By the middle of the nineteenth century, there were reports of statistical correlations between syphilis and general paresis, and Kraft-Ebbing experimentally demonstrated the relationship in 1897. The specific spirochete was identified in 1905, and Wasserman introduced a serological test in 1906. In 1913, Noguchi discovered the spirochete in the autopsied brain of paretic patients. In 1909, Ehrlich introduced an arsenical compound; it killed spirochetes in the blood but did not cross the blood–brain barrier. Yet, after all these efforts, the Nobel prize went to Wagner-Jauregg for an empirical discovery—treating syphilitic paresis by inducing fever—which was only a step away from the main line of rational, pathophysiological discovery. Later, the discovery of penicillin led not only to the effective treatment of general paresis, if identified before irreversible damage took place, but to the early treatment of syphilis itself. When the prevalence of syphilis fell dramatically, the incidence of general paresis did as well. Ultimately, the primary prevention of neurosyphilis was an almost complete success. Retrospectively, any path of scientific discovery looks more goal-directed than the same path examined prospectively. The conquest of neurosyphilis had its blind alleys (fever treatment of paresis) and its dark moments (the Tuskeegee experiment, in which black men with syphilis were not treated or informed of their disease, so that the natural course of neurosyphilis could be observed). The central principles remained clear throughout: Clinical classification needs to be followed by basic research to elucidate the pathophysiology; purely empirical treatments lead down blind alleys unless they are supported by rational insights into the disease process; and primary prevention is not possible until the underlying disease process can also be eradicated.

Clinical and neuroscientific investigations of several of the prevalent OMDs are now progressing at similar rates. Alzheimer's disease was described in 1909, but its identity with the far more common senile dementia was not established until the 1950s. In the 1960s, it was clearly distinguished from multi-infarct dementia, and by the late 1960s, the severity of Alzheimer's was correlated with plaque density and the severity of multi-infarct dementia, with the amount of infarcted tissue. During the 1970s, the mnemonic effects of anticholinergic agents and the amnestic effects of cholinomimetics were established, and the regional deficiency of choline acetyltransferase in Alzheimer's disease was correlated with plaque count, clinical severity, and symptomatology. An important role was demonstrated for the cholinergic nucleus basalis. In the 1980s, the genetics of Alzheimer's disease was explored, a marker protein was found, and molecular genetics techniques began to focus on chromosome 21. During these 2 decades, the incidence of multi-infarct dementia, and of strokes in general, began to fall, owing to increasing public awareness of the roles of life-style, diet, cessation of smoking, and compliance with medication in preventing morbidity from vascular disease. The empirical diagnosis, physiological investigation, rational treatment, and eventual prevention of OMSs and OMDs provide models for the future development of the entire field of psychiatry.

REFERENCES

Atkinson R C, Shiffrin R M: The control of short-term memory. Sci Amer *224:* 82, 1971.

Barbizet J: *Human Memory and Its Pathology*. Freeman, San Francisco, 1970.

Butters N: Amnestic disorders. In *Clinical Neuropsychology,* K M Heilman, E Valenstein, editors, p 439. Oxford University Press, New York, 1979.

Corkin S, Davis K L, Growden J H, Usdin E, Wurtman R J: *Alzheimer's Disease: A Report of Progress in Research.* Raven Press, New York, 1982.

Courville C B: *Effects of Alcohol on the Nervous System of Man.* San Lucas Press, Los Angeles, 1955.

Davison K, Bagley C R: Schizophrenia-like psychoses associated with organic disorders of the central nervous system. In *Current Problems in Neuropsychiatry,* R N Herrington, editor. Headley Bro, Kent, 1979.

Engel G L, Romano J: Delirium: A syndrome of cerebral insufficiency. Chronic Dis *9:* 260, 1959.

Fauman M A: The emergency psychiatric evaluation of organic mental disorders. Psychiat Clin N Amer *6:* 233, 1983.

Goldstein K: The effect of brain damage on the personality. Psychiatry *15:* 245, 1952.

Hall R C W, Beresford T P, Gardner E R, Popkin M K: The medical care of psychiatric patients. Hosp Comm Psychiat *33:* 25, 1982.

Hendrie H L, editor: Brain disorders: Clinical diagnosis and management. Psychiat Clin N Amer *1:* 1978.

Horvath T B: The psychological presentations of somatic disorders. In *Biological Psychiatry,* P A Berger, H K H Brodie, editors. Basic Books, New York, 1986.

Jefferson J W, Marshall J R: *Neuropsychiatric Features of Medical Disorders.* Plenum, New York, 1981.

Katzman R, Terry R D, Bick K L, editors: *Alzheimer's Disease: Senile Dementia and Related Disorders.* Raven Press, New York, 1978.

Kertesz A, editor: *Localization in Neuropsychology.* Academic Press, New York, 1983.

Levenson A J, editor: *Neuropsychiatric Side-Effects of Drugs in the Elderly.* Raven Press, New York, 1979.

Lishman W A: *Organic Psychiatry,* ed 2. Blackwell, London, 1986.

Lipowski Z J: *Delirium.* Charles C Thomas, Springfield, IL, 1980.

Luria A R: *The Working Brain: An Introduction to Neuropsychology.* Basic Books, New York, 1975.

McCandles D W, editor: *Cerebral Energy Metabolism and Metabolic Encephalopathy.* Plenum, New York, 1985.

Mace N L, Rabins P V: *The Thirty-Six Hour Day.* Johns Hopkins University Press, Baltimore, 1981.

Milner B: Memory and the medial temporal regions of the brain. In *Biology of Memory,* K H Pribram, D E Broadbent, editors, p 29. Academic Press, New York, 1970.

Plum F, Posner J B: *The Diagnosis of Stupor and Coma,* ed 3. Davis, Philadelphia, 1980.

Shader R I, editor: *Psychiatric Complications of Medical Drugs.* Raven Press, New York, 1972.

Squire L R: Mechanisms of memory. Science *232:* 1612, 1986.

Strub R L, Black F W: *The Mental Status Examination in Neurology.* Davis, Philadelphia, 1977.

Strub R L, Black F W: *Organic Brain Syndromes.* Davis, Philadelphia, 1981.

Swash M, Kennard C, editors: *Scientific Basis of Clinical Neurology.* Churchill Livingstone, New York, 1985.

Vinken P J, Bruyn G W, editors: *Disorders of Speech, Perception and Symbolic Behavior.* Elsevier, New York, 1970.

Vinken P J, Bruyn G W, editors: *Neurological Manifestations of Systemic Disease,* Parts I and II. Elsevier, New York, 1979, 1980.

CHAPTER 13 PSYCHOACTIVE SUBSTANCE USE DISORDERS

13.1 DRUG DEPENDENCE: OPIOIDS, NONNARCOTICS, NICOTINE (TOBACCO), AND CAFFEINE

JEROME H. JAFFE, M.D.

INTRODUCTION

Drug use and dependence are viewed with concern by the world community. Wars have been fought over drug trafficking, and treaties have been signed aimed at controlling the production and distribution of opioids, cocaine, cannabis, and a wide range of synthetic psychoactive drugs; most nations are signatories to two major treaties, and two permanent international bodies exist to decide which new drugs should be included under the treaty provisions. Controlling illicit traffic in psychoactive drugs is an agenda item at economic summit meetings of the world's most powerful nations. Although no treaties exist for the control of alcohol and tobacco, which are more commonly abused than are illicit drugs, such as cocaine or opium, the grave concern of the world's medical community about the growing use of tobacco in developing countries and the impact of alcoholism is reflected in actions and statements of the World Health Organization (WHO).

DEFINITIONS AND DIAGNOSTIC CRITERIA

The terminology used to describe the addictive disorders has been repeatedly revised as concepts about the nature of chronic drug using behavior have evolved. In 1964, a WHO Expert Committee on Addiction Producing Drugs recommended the substitution of the term "drug dependence" for both of the previously used terms "addiction" and "habituation."

The meaning of dependence was to be defined separately for each variety of drug, but no operational criteria were provided. In 1980, the third edition of the American Psychiatric Association's *Diagnostic and Statistical Manual of Mental Disorders* (DSM-III) divided use disorders into two major categories, drug abuse and drug dependence, and offered specific criteria for diagnosis. In DSM-III-R, the most recent revision of DSM-III, these two categories are retained, but the diagnostic criteria have been modified.

These new revisions bring the DSM-III-R formulations closer to the concepts and terminology developed in 1980 by an international working group sponsored by the Alcohol, Drug Abuse, and Mental Health Administration (ADAMHA) and WHO. That group defined *dependence* as

> a syndrome manifested by a behavioral pattern in which the use of a given psychoactive drug, or class of drugs, is given a much higher priority than other behaviors that once had higher value. The term "syndrome" is taken to mean no more than a clustering of phenomena so that not all the components need always be present or not always present with the same intensity. . . . The dependence syndrome is not absolute, but is a quantitative phenomenon that exists in different degrees. The intensity of the syndrome is measured by the behaviors that are elicited in relation to using the drug and by the other behaviors that are secondary to drug use. . . . no sharp cutoff point can be identified for distinguishing drug dependence from nondependent but recurrent drug use. At the extreme, the dependence syndrome is associated with "compulsive drug-using behavior."

In DSM-III-R, psychoactive substance abuse disorders are divided into psychoactive substance dependence and the residual category psychoactive substance abuse for those cases where there is pathological drug use but all of the criteria for drug dependence are not met.

The criteria for psychoactive substance dependence and abuse are presented in Tables 13.1-1 and 13.1-2; the criteria for severity of dependence are shown in Table 13.1-3.

Some individuals use several categories of drugs and are clearly drug-dependent. However, it is sometimes not possible to know if they are dependent on any one specific class of drugs. In DSM-III-R, this condition is called polysubstance dependence. The criteria for this condition are presented in Table 13.1-4.

DSM-III-R also describes two additional substance dependence-related diagnoses: psychoactive substance dependence not otherwise specified (Table 13.1-5) and psychoactive substance abuse not otherwise specified (Table 13.1-6). These categories are residual ones for disorders in which there is dependence or abuse, respectively, on a psychoactive substance that cannot be classified in any of the previous categories (e.g., anticholinergics), or for use as an initial diagnosis in cases of dependence or abuse in which the specific substance is not yet known.

In much of the world literature on drug dependence at present, the term "dependence" is used to convey two distinct ideas: a behavioral syndrome and physical or physiological dependence. Physical dependence can be defined as those alterations in neural systems that are manifested in tolerance and in withdrawal phenomena when a chronically administered drug is discontinued or displaced from its receptor. This dual use of the word "dependence" causes confusion. The 1980 ADAMHA-WHO working group recommended restricting the term "dependence" to the behavioral syndrome previously described and substituting the term "neuroadaptation" for physical dependence. Such a substitution would empha-

TABLE 13.1-1
Diagnostic Criteria for Psychoactive Substance Dependence

A. At least three of the following:
   (1) substance often taken in larger amounts or over a longer period than the person intended
   (2) persistent desire or one or more unsuccessful efforts to cut down or control substance use
   (3) a great deal of time spent in activities necessary to get the substance (e.g., theft), taking the substance (e.g., chain smoking), or recovering from its effects
   (4) frequent intoxication or withdrawal symptoms when expected to fulfill major role obligations at work, school, or home (e.g., does not go to work because hung over, goes to school or work "high," intoxicated while taking care of his or her children), or when substance use is physically hazardous (e.g., drives when intoxicated)
   (5) important social, occupational, or recreational activities given up or reduced because of substance use
   (6) continued substance use despite knowledge of having a persistent or recurrent social, psychological, or physical problem that is caused or exacerbated by the use of the substance (e.g., keeps using heroin despite family arguments about it, cocaine-induced depression, or having an ulcer made worse by drinking)
   (7) marked tolerance; need for markedly increased amounts of the substance (i.e., at least a 50% increase) in order to achieve intoxication or desired effect, or markedly diminished effect with continued use of the same amount

   Note: The following items may not apply to cannabis, hallucinogens, or phencyclidine (PCP):
   (8) characteristic withdrawal symptoms (see specific withdrawal syndromes under psychoactive substance-induced organic mental disorders)
   (9) substance often taken to relieve or avoid withdrawal symptoms

B. Some symptoms of the disturbance have persisted for at least 1 month, or have occurred repeatedly over a longer period of time.

Table from DSM-III-R *Diagnostic and Statistical Manual of Mental Disorders,* ed 3, revised. Copyright American Psychiatric Association, Washington, DC, 1987. Used with permission.

TABLE 13.1-2
Diagnostic Criteria for Psychoactive Substance Abuse

A. A maladaptive pattern of psychoactive substance use indicated by at least one of the following:
   (1) continued use despite knowledge of having a persistent or recurrent social, occupational, psychological, or physical problem that is caused or exacerbated by use of the psychoactive substance
   (2) recurrent use in situations in which use is physically hazardous (e.g., driving while intoxicated).

B. Some symptoms of the disturbance have persisted for at least 1 month, or have occurred repeatedly over a longer period of time.

C. Never met the criteria for psychoactive substance dependence for this substance.

Table from DSM-III-R *Diagnostic and Statistical Manual of Mental Disorders,* ed 3, revised. Copyright American Psychiatric Association, Washington, DC, 1987. Used with permission.

size several points. First, the chronic use of many drugs, including tricyclic antidepressants and β-adrenergic blockers, brings about neuroadaptive changes followed by withdrawal phenomena but not by drug-seeking behavior on discontinuation. Second, it is now clear that neuroadaptive changes begin with the first dose of an opioid or sedative drug, as described later in this section.

In DSM-III-R, neuroadaptive changes are referred to as physiological tolerance and withdrawal, but the conceptual framework now corresponds to that of the ADAMHA-WHO working group in that these drug-induced physiological alterations alone are not sufficient grounds for diagnosing drug dependence.

The words "addict" and "addiction" often have pejorative connotations, but they have also been frequently trivialized. Addiction has been used to apply to behaviors, such as running and solving crossword puzzles, and even to the predisposition of governments to spend more money than they take in.

TABLE 13.1-3
Diagnostic Criteria for Severity of Psychoactive Substance Dependence

Mild: Few, if any, symptoms in excess of those required to make the diagnosis, and the symptoms result in no more than mild impairment in occupational functioning or in usual social activities or relationships with others.

Moderate: Symptoms or functional impairment between mild and severe.

Severe: Many symptoms in excess of those required to make the diagnosis, and the symptoms markedly interfere with occupational functioning or with usual social activities or relationships with others.*

In Partial Remission: During the past 6 months, some use of the substance and some symptoms of dependence.

In Full Remission: During the past 6 months, either no use of the substance, or use of the substance and no symptoms of dependence.

Table from DSM-III-R *Diagnostic and Statistical Manual of Mental Disorders,* ed 3, revised. Copyright American Psychiatric Association, Washington, DC, 1987. Used with permission.
*Because of the availability of cigarettes and other nicotine-containing substances and the absence of a clinically significant nicotine intoxication syndrome, impairment in occupational or social functioning is not necessary for a rating of severe nicotine dependence.

TABLE 13.1-4
Diagnostic Criteria for Polysubstance Dependence

This category should be used when, for a period of at least 6 months, the person has repeatedly used at least three categories of psychoactive substances (not including nicotine and caffeine), but no single psychoactive substance has predominated. During this period the criteria have been met for dependence on psychoactive substances as a group, but not for any specific substance.

Table from DSM-III-R *Diagnostic and Statistical Manual of Mental Disorders,* ed 3, revised, Copyright American Psychiatric Association, Washington DC, 1987. Used with permission.

TABLE 13.1-5
Psychoactive Substance Dependence Not Otherwise Specified

This is a residual category for disorders in which there is dependence on a psychoactive substance that cannot be classified according to any of the previous categories (e.g., anticholinergics), or for use as an initial diagnosis in cases of dependence in which the specific substance is not yet known.

Table from DSM-III-R *Diagnostic and Statistical Manual of Mental Disorders,* ed 3, revised. Copyright American Psychiatric Association, Washington, DC, 1987. Used with permission.

TABLE 13.1-6
Psychoactive Substance Abuse Not Otherwise Specified

This is a residual category for disorders in which there is abuse of a psychoactive substance that cannot be classified according to any of the previous categories (e.g., anticholinergics), or for use as an initial diagnosis in cases of abuse in which the specific substance is not yet known.

Table from DSM-III-R *Diagnostic and Statistical Manual of Mental Disorders,* ed 3, revised. Copyright American Psychiatric Association, Washington, DC, 1987. Used with permission.

Words, such as "addiction" and "abuse," are difficult to expunge from the language. The word "addiction" continues to convey the core connotation of decreased control. This discussion deals primarily with persons dependent on drugs to a severe degree. Therefore, such terms as "opioid addict" will be retained because they are far less awkward than the term "severely opioid-dependent individual." The term "dependent," unmodified, will be used to mean behaviorally dependent; and the terms "physical" or "physiological dependence" or "neuroadaptation" will be used to refer to those changes that result in withdrawal symptoms when drugs are discontinued.

The term "abuse" is also used in ways that differ significantly from the definitions developed for use in DSM-III-R and presented above. In popular and legislative contexts, the term "drug abuse" is commonly employed to include any use at all of an illicit substance, any nonprescribed use of a drug intended as a medicine, as well as the harmful or excessive use of legally available substances, such as alcohol and tobacco.

In addition to drug dependence and abuse, the use of certain psychoactive drugs can induce a number of organic mental disorders. Table 13.1-7 shows the various disorders induced by the drugs discussed in this section.

EPIDEMIOLOGY

Over the past decade, household surveys and other epidemiological methods have been used to gauge the extent of drug use, abuse, and dependence. The accuracy of these techniques is limited by the reluctance of respondents to admit the extent of their drug use and because a significant proportion of people who become dependent on illicit drugs are too mobile to be included in standard household surveys. The National Household Survey on Drug Abuse of the National Institute on Drug Abuse (NIDA), for example, does not interview individuals who are homeless, living in institutions (jails or hospitals), or in dormitory situations. It is likely, therefore, that some varieties of heavy drug use and dependence are underestimated.

Data from the 1985 National Household Survey, shown in Table 13.1-8, reveal that use of illicit drugs (cocaine, heroin,

TABLE 13.1-7
Psychoactive Substance-Induced Organic Mental Disorders*

	Withdrawal	*Withdrawal Delirium*	*Delirium*	*Delusional Disorder*	*Mood Disorder*	*Other Syndromes*†
Alcohol	X	X				1
Sedative-Anxiolytics	X	X				2
Amphetamines	X		X	X		
Cocaine	X		X	X		
Opioids	X					
PCP	—			X	X	3
Hallucinogens	—		X	X	X	4
Cannabis	—			X		
Caffeine	X					
Nicotine	X					
Inhalants	—	—	?	—	?	

Table modified from DSM-III-R *Diagnostic and Statistical Manual of Mental Disorders*, ed 3, revised. Copyright American Psychiatric Association, Washington, DC, 1987. Used with permission.
*DSM-III-R recognizes an intoxication syndrome for all drug categories but nicotine (to which tolerance develops rapidly)
†Keys:
1. Hallucinosis, amnestic disorder, dementia, idiosyncratic intoxication.
2. Sedative-anxiolytic amnestic disorder.
3. Flashback (post-hallucinogen perception disorder).
4. PCP: mental disorder NOS.

TABLE 13.1-8
Extent of Nonmedical Drug Use: 1985*

Age Range: *Estimated Population:*	*12–17 yr* *21,640,000*		*18–25 yr* *32,490,000*		*26+ yr* *136,660,000*		*Total*† *190,790,000*	
	Ever Used‡	*Current User*‡	*Ever Used*	*Current User*	*Ever Used*	*Current User*	*Ever Used*	*Current User*
Marijuana or hashish	24%	12%	60%	22%	27%	6%	33%	10%
Hallucinogens	3	1	12	2	6	—§	7	0.5
Inhalants	9	4	13	1	5	0.6	7	1
Cocaine	5	2	25	8	9	2	12	3
Heroin	—	—	1	—	1	—	1	—
Stimulants	6	2	17	4	8	0.7	9	1
Sedatives	4	1	11	2	5	0.7	6	1
Tranquilizers	5	1	12	2	7	1	8	1
Analgesics	6	2	11	2	6	0.9	7	1
Alcohol	57	32	93	72	89	61	86	59
Cigarettes	45	16	76	37	80	33	76	32

*Estimates of the percent of people 12 years of age and older who have used drugs nonmedically were developed from the National Household Survey on Drug Abuse, 1985, for the National Institute on Drug Abuse. Drugs used under a physician's care are not included.
†Totals may not equal the sum of the three age groups because of rounding.
‡Ever used: used at least once in a person's lifetime.
Current user: used at least once in the 30 days prior to the survey.
§Amounts of less than 0.5% are not listed.

marijuana) is far more prevalent among the young adult population (ages 18 and 25). For example, only 6 percent of older adults (above 26 years of age) reported having used marijuana or cocaine in the last 30 days, compared with 22 percent of those between 18 and 25. These figures may change as the population ages. In 1985, 25 percent of young adults reported some experience with cocaine, but less than 8 percent reported use during the preceding month. Although drug use by females is increasing faster than drug use by males, lifetime use of illicit drugs remains far more common among urban males than among females, a ratio of about 3 to 1.

The changes in patterns of drug use over time are illustrated in the data on drug use within the past 30 days (Fig. 13.1-1) from a national survey that has been conducted annually among high school seniors since 1975. It is obvious that 30-day prevalence for both marijuana and illicit drug use in

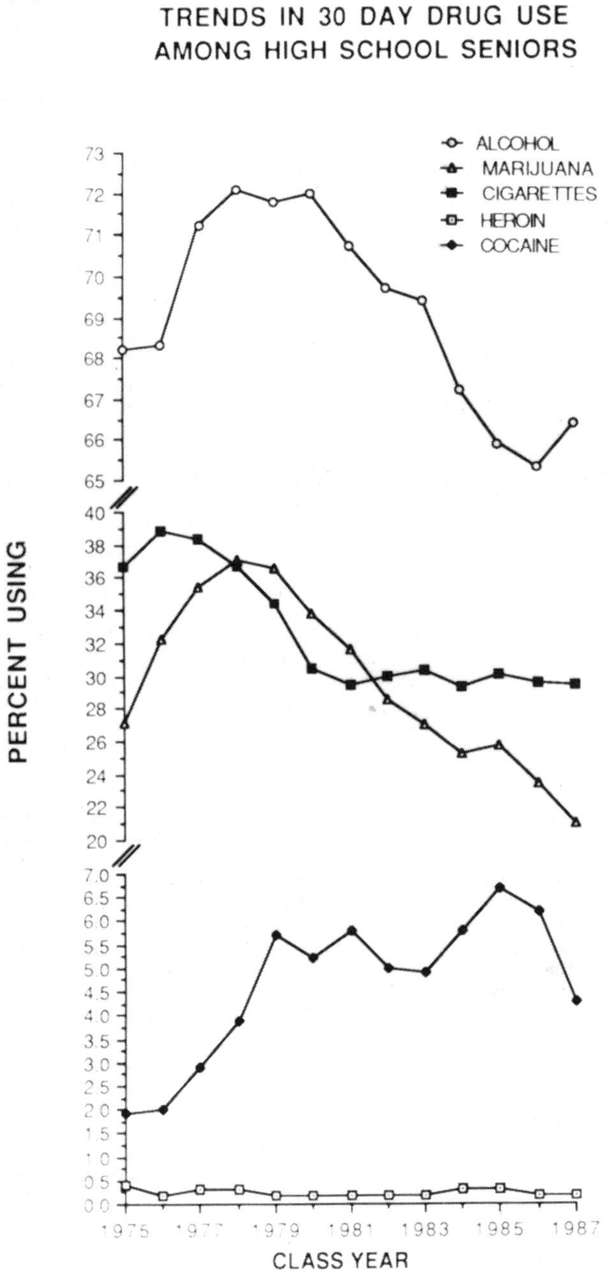

FIGURE 13.1-1. *Data on prevalence of drug use among high school seniors.*

general has declined sharply from the high levels reported in 1977 through 1979. The results from the 1987 survey show further reductions in use of marijuana and other illicit drugs, and for the first time a significant reduction in use of cocaine.

Psychiatric epidemiological studies conducted in 1981 to 1983 found that 5 to 6 percent of the adult population had met DSM-III diagnostic criteria for some type of drug abuse or dependence (other than alcohol abuse or dependence) at some time in their lives. The limitations described for the NIDA National Household Survey also apply to these household survey techniques. However, best estimates for 1981 to 1983 of the percentages of the population meeting DSM-III criteria for dependence or abuse at some point in their lives for specific drug categories are as follows: amphetamines, 2 percent; cocaine, 0.2 percent; cannabis, 4 percent; hallucinogens, 0.3 percent; opioids, 0.7 percent; sedatives and anxiolytics, 1.1 percent; and phencyclidine (PCP), rare.

As part of the same collaborative epidemiological study, Mexican Americans (N = 1243) and non-Hispanic whites (N = 1309) in the Los Angeles area were interviewed in 1983 and 1984. Non-Hispanic whites had significantly higher rates of drug dependence than either Mexican Americans or the general populations surveyed in New Haven, Baltimore, or St. Louis. The large differences across age groups and between sexes and ethnic groups is illustrated in Table 13.1-9.

OTHER ESTIMATING TECHNIQUES Because of the inaccuracies inherent in estimating dependence on illicit opioids through household surveys, the federal government has, in the past, employed several alternative techniques. These techniques include considerations of the annual number of drug overdose deaths, emergency room visits, and new entries into treatment. For opioid dependence, estimators also used the number of opioid users arrested and subsequently rearrested, year of first opioid use among new entries into treatment, and the reported incidence of hepatitis. Using all of these techniques, government estimators inferred that there was a major epidemic of new heroin users beginning in the early 1960s and reaching its peak in 1969 to 1971. Over this period, the total population of opioid addicts grew, reaching its highest point in the early 1970s. The government estimated that in 1977 there were approximately 500,000 opioid abusers and addicts, and, in 1980, there were about the same number.

The population of active opioid addicts fluctuates. As law enforcement control of illicit heroin waxes and wanes in efficacy and as ease of drug availability increases, the relapse rate increases especially among older addicts. The pattern varies from one region to another. Similar methodologies have not been applied to estimate numbers of people dependent on other illicit drugs.

HISTORY OF DRUG ABUSE AND DEPENDENCE IN THE UNITED STATES

The most commonly abused drugs of the present have been in use for hundreds, if not thousands, of years. For example, opium has been used for medicinal purposes for at least 3,500 years; references to cannabis as a medicinal can be found in ancient Chinese herbals, and wine is mentioned repeatedly in the Bible. Tobacco was smoked and coca leaves were chewed by the Indians of the Western Hemisphere for generations before the arrival of the Spanish.

Problems of drug abuse have evolved over many years. Some of the problems caused by these drugs were recognized even in ancient times. Drunkenness was mentioned in the Bible and in the writings of the ancient Greeks and Romans. But other problems emerged more clearly when new and more concentrated forms of drugs were in-

TABLE 13.1-9
Mexican-American and Non-Hispanic White Lifetime DIS/DSM-III Prevalence Rates by Age and Gender*

	Males			*Females*		
	18–39 yr	*40+ yr*	*Total*	*18–39 yr*	*40+ yr*	*Total*
Any DIS disorder						
Mexican-Americans	41.8 (2.6)	35.7 (3.6)	39.5 (2.2)	27.8 (2.9)	32.9 (3.2)	30.0 (2.2)
Non-Hispanic	42.7 (3.3)	28.0 (2.5)	35.5 (2.3)	42.7 (3.5)	24.0 (2.7)	32.8 (2.3)
Substance-use disorders						
Mexican Americans	35.5 (2.7)	28.3 (3.2)	32.9 (2.2)	6.8 (1.3)	4.1 (1.2)	5.6 (0.9)
Non-Hispanic whites	33.8 (2.5)	21.5 (2.9)	27.8 (2.1)	22.9 (2.6)	7.2 (1.4)	14.6 (1.4)
Alcohol abuse-dependence						
Mexican-Americans	33.0 (2.4)	28.5 (3.3)	31.3 (2.1)	5.2 (1.3)	3.9 (1.2)	4.6 (0.9)
Non-Hispanic whites	21.6 (2.0)	20.4 (3.0)	21.0 (1.8)	10.7 (1.7)	6.3 (1.5)	8.4 (1.1)
Drug abuse-dependence						
Mexican-Americans	9.0 (1.4)	0.5 (0.5)	5.9 (1.0)	3.7 (0.8)	1.1 (0.2)	2.6 (0.5)
Non-Hispanic whites	24.7 (2.3)	3.9 (1.2)	14.6 (1.5)	18.7 (2.5)	1.6 (0.7)	9.7 (1.3)

*DIS indicates Diagnostic Interview Schedule. Values are expressed as the rate in percent. Numbers in parentheses indicate standard errors.

vented or new routes of administration were developed. For instance, the introduction of cheap gin into England in the eighteenth century led to problems that were considered more serious than those associated with beer and wine. Although opium smoking was a major problem in the Orient in the eighteenth and nineteenth centuries, morphine, the most active opioid alkaloid in opium, was not isolated until 1806, and the pure alkaloid was not commonly used by injection until the late part of the nineteenth century. The use of morphine and heroin by intravenous (IV) route did not begin to spread until the early part of the twentieth century. Tobacco was smoked even by the native Americans, but it was not until the nineteenth century, when development of the cigarette and new methods of curing produced a mild smoke, that inhalation of tobacco smoke deep into the lungs became routine; cigarette smoking did not become commonplace until the early decades of the twentieth century.

Although it is common to describe the history of use of each class of drugs as an isolated development, in actuality, the use and abuse of one substance often has a significant impact on societal reactions to the use and misuse of pharmacologically unrelated substances. Any effort to describe the long and complex history of drug abuse, even in one country, the United States, can touch only on the highlights of this story.

EARLY ATTITUDES In the closing years of the nineteenth century, there was growing concern in many sectors of U.S. society about the general problem of drug use and abuse. This concern was not limited to any one category of drugs, but included the use of alcohol and tobacco, as well as opioids and cocaine.

Cocaine, first isolated from the coca leaf in 1860, came into widespread use when pharmaceutical companies in the United States and Europe began to sell it widely in 1885. In 1884, in Vienna, Sigmund Freud wrote an enthusiastic review of the potential therapeutic uses of cocaine. Other medical authorities in the United States shared this enthusiasm, and at one point cocaine was recommended by the Hay Fever Association as a remedy for that malady. Within a few years of Freud's publication, the capacity of cocaine to induce toxic psychosis, as well as its capacity to gain control over behavior, was recognized. Similarly, the dependence-inducing effects of chronic opiate use were widely recognized. Nevertheless, in the United States, at the opening of the twentieth century, both the opium alkaloids and cocaine were incorporated into patent medicines and sold over the counter in grocery stores for a wide variety of indications. As often as not, the labeling of these nostrums did not reveal their contents.

By the late 1890s, the public and the medical community were no longer indifferent to drug use and habituation. Medical texts in England, Europe, and the United States contained descriptions of morphinism, theories of its causation, and recommendations for withdrawal and postwithdrawal treatment. Some texts also described problems of cocainism. Medical authorities in the United States cautioned against overly liberal prescribing of cocaine and of opiates by physicians, and expressed great concern about these drugs in unlabeled, proprietary, over-the-counter medicines. State laws were passed aimed at control of sale of opiates and cocaine, especially in patent medicines. In 1903, cocaine in Coca-Cola was replaced by caffeine.

Although the achievement of long-term cure of morphinism was reported to be exceedingly difficult, until the turn of the twentieth century, neither the public nor the medical profession saw the opium habitué or morphinist as invariably suffering from some moral deficit. Those who had developed the morphine habit represented the entire socioeconomic spectrum; women outnumbered men by about 2 to 1. More than a few famous political and literary figures were known to use opiates but to lead otherwise productive and exemplary lives. Yet, it was also true that cocaine use and the morphine habit were common among gamblers, petty thieves, prostitutes, and the inhabitants of the demimonde that exists in any diverse society. Those persons with emotional problems and those who had formerly used alcohol to excess were probably overrepresented among opium users, since it was not unusual to prescribe opiates to control emotional problems and alcoholism.

EARLY EFFORTS TOWARD CONTROL At the turn of the twentieth century, U.S. government representatives were negotiating an international treaty to control traffic in opium, cocaine, and related drugs. Negotiators from the United States were also interested in international control of cannabis, but could not get other nations to view this substance as sufficiently problematic. (Such control was finally achieved in 1925 at the Second Geneva Convention.) By 1900, many U.S. medical and political leaders believed that much of the problem of drug dependence was due to careless prescribing by physicians and to the economically motivated sale of opiates and cocaine in unlabeled proprietary medicines.

State regulations concerning the sale of opiates and cocaine, the introduction of aspirin and barbiturates, and the Pure Food and Drug Act of 1906, which required the labeling of patent medicines, were already having an impact on the use of opiates in medicine when the Harrison Act was passed in 1914. The Harrison Act, the first federal legislation to regulate opiates and cocaine, was designed to restrict access to opiates and cocaine to doctors, dentists, pharmacists, and legitimate importers and manufacturers. It was not originally intended to interfere with the legitimate practice of medicine or to work special hardship on those persons already dependent on opiates. For several years after the passage of the Harrison Act, several cities operated clinics that prescribed morphine to those persons with established habits. Most of those persons who were dependent on opiates before the enactment of the Harrison Act became abstinent within a few years after its passage, although generally not as a result of treatment at the clinics.

By the 1920s, several major changes had taken place in U.S. attitudes and practices. A constitutional amendment prohibiting the sale of alcohol had radically changed U.S. drinking behavior. Within a year after alcohol prohibition was enacted, 14 states had passed cigarette prohibition laws; these were even less popular than alcohol prohibition, and, by 1927, they had all been repealed. By the mid-1920s, Americans were smoking 80 billion cigarettes per year, but cocaine use, which was prevalent at the turn of the century, was no longer widespread.

The medical profession, disillusioned by the reluctance of morphine addicts at clinics to seek treatment and by their repeated relapses to morphine use after they did so, began to recommend compulsory treatment with "confinement until cure." An illicit traffic developed to provide opiates to those who could not or would not use the clinics. Increasingly, the drug sold was heroin rather than morphine. Heroin had been introduced into medicine in 1898, but was quickly found to be quite similar to morphine in its actions. Many of those who patronized the illicit traffic and used the clinics had backgrounds of delinquency and criminal activity, and as time went on, this subgroup came to predominate. Reformers, moralists, and the popular press found in the opiate habit and in the reputation of those who continued to use morphine proof of the evils inherent in these drugs and grist for sensational stories.

Poor publicity, lurid stories, medical disillusionment, and pressure from law enforcement agents acting in concert labeled the morphine clinics as medical folly and brought about their closing. The last clinic was closed in 1923. At the same time, a series of U.S. Supreme Court decisions seemed to imply that prescribing even small amounts of opiates or cocaine to an addict for treatment of addiction was not proper medicine and was therefore an illegal sale of narcotic drugs. Several physicians were imprisoned, and numerous other doctors were tried, reprimanded, or otherwise harassed. By the early 1920s, persons addicted to opiates were no longer welcome in doctors' offices, and they were often refused treatment at hospitals. The terms "dope addict" and "dope fiend" had become common, and the average layman, as well as some otherwise well-informed members of the medical profession, believed that the opiate molecule was inherently evil, capable of quickly bringing about the moral decay of the virtuous. In the late 1930s, cannabis (marijuana) acquired a similar reputation, and, in 1937, the U.S. Congress passed legislation prescribing criminal penalties for its use, sale, or possession. The states quickly followed suit.

NEWER DRUGS Over the 30-year period following the introduction of barbital into clinical medicine, scores of congeners differing primarily in duration of action were introduced. Within a few years after each new compound was introduced, the first case reports of abuse, dependence, and withdrawal appeared in the medical journals. This pattern was repeated with the nonbarbiturate sedatives, such as glutethimide (Doriden), ethchlorvynol (Placidyl), and meprobamate (Miltown).

Amphetamine, first synthesized in 1887, was put into clinical use in 1932 as a drug to shrink mucous membranes. By 1935, its central stimulant effects were recognized and found useful for treating narcolepsy. Dozens of other suggested uses soon followed. Reports of its abuse as a euphoriant first appeared in the late 1930s, but the full significance of its abuse potential was not appreciated until the post–World War II epidemic of IV amphetamine addiction in Japan. That epidemic, precipitated by the sale of surplus tablets intended for combat troops, involved millions of people. Other amphetamine-like drugs were introduced during the 1950s and early 1960s.

The psychological effects of mescaline were known and written about in the early years of the twentieth century, but public concern about this category of drugs did not reach a high level until the 1960s, when the use of the newly discovered and exceedingly potent compound lysergic acid diethylamide (LSD) evolved from experimentation by a few college students to more widespread use by younger groups.

CHANGES IN TREATMENT TECHNIQUES Treatment for drug-related problems has also changed dramatically over the years. During the period from 1923 to 1963, treatment for opioid addiction was almost synonymous with prolonged hospitalization. Treatment took place in private sanitoriums or in one of the two federal hospitals—at Lexington, Kentucky and at Fort Worth, Texas—that were established in the 1930s. Treatment of dependence on barbiturates and amphetamines took place largely within state hospitals and within the mainstream of medical practice, but there was no consensus on what constituted effective follow-up care.

The situation changed in the early 1960s as individual states and the federal government attempted to respond to new outbreaks of heroin use among young people and to concomitant increases in the crime rate. In California, a civil commitment program for addicts was initiated under the administrative control of the Department of Corrections, and New York City reopened Riverside Hospital to treat juvenile heroin addicts.

The first follow-up studies of patients treated at the federal hospital at Lexington, which were published in the early 1960s, revealed exceedingly high rates of relapse after treatment. Doctors and the public demanded new ideas, including a reconsideration of providing addicts with legitimate opioids through medical channels.

Within a span of a few years, from 1960 to 1967, several major new approaches to opioid dependence were developed. Synanon, the prototype therapeutic community, was started in California in 1958, and was replicated in New York with the establishment of Daytop Village and Phoenix House; Dole and Nyswander demonstrated the effectiveness of large daily doses of methadone in reducing crime and heroin use in selected long-term heroin addicts, and several groups demonstrated that heroin addicts would voluntarily try treatment with narcotic antagonists. In the mid-1960s, the state of New York and the federal government legislated civil commitment programs modeled after the program in California, with an initial period of prolonged institutional care as a key element.

Despite the repeated reports of abuse and dependence associated with barbiturates, barbiturate-like sedatives, and amphetamines and related stimulants, and in spite of concerns about experimentation with LSD and related hallucinogens, no federal criminal sanctions related to these drugs were in force until 1964, when authority for their control was assigned to the Food and Drug Administration. In contrast, concern about heroin addiction in the 1950s led to ever harsher penalties for its sale or possession.

Although treatment and law enforcement efforts were stepped up, both the number of new heroin addicts and the crime rates continued to rise throughout the late 1960s. There was also a sharp increase in the nonmedical use of other drugs, such as marijuana and LSD, and a major epidemic of amphetamine abuse and dependence. In addition to amphetamines diverted from medical channels, additional supplies came from drugs produced in clandestine laboratories. Drug use, especially the use of marijuana, became linked to antiestablishment attitudes, politics, and life-style. Originally developed as a general anesthetic in the 1950s, PCP became a drug of abuse in the 1970s.

Although many treatment programs initiated in the early 1960s continued to focus on treatment of opioid dependence, some others, especially the therapeutic communities, viewed all nonmedical drug use as stemming from similar defects in character structure and offered a generic approach to drug dependence.

Meanwhile, in England, social changes and excessive prescribing of heroin by a few physicians had caused a sharp rise in the number of young heroin addicts. In 1968, the old informal system was legislatively changed so that every physician was obliged to notify the Home Office of a case of opioid addiction, and although heroin could still be prescribed for addicts, only physicians at specially designated clinics were permitted to do so. In practice, by the mid-1970s, it became far more common for clinic physicians to prescribe injectable or oral methadone than injectable heroin. These clinics, however, offered little help for those dependent on nonopioid drugs.

RECENT LEGISLATION In 1970, the U.S. government passed new legislation reorganizing the jumble of drug regulatory statutes that had evolved since the passage of the Harrison Act, increased the resources for controlling availability of illicit drugs, and assigned the task of enforcement to the Drug Enforcement Agency, which incorporated elements of the Food and Drug Administration and the Bureau of Narcotic and Dangerous Drugs.

When, in 1971, U.S. troops in Vietnam were reported to be using heroin heavily, a Special Action Office for Drug Abuse Prevention (SAODAP) was established within the Executive Office of the President to coordinate government activities and policies in the area of drug abuse. The creation of that office and the associated legislation marked a turning point in U.S. policy. The notion that opioid dependence was an incurable disorder, which justified the harshest of penalties in the name of prevention, was superseded by a policy that recognized that a substantial proportion of opioid addicts (as well as those with other varieties of drug dependence) could eventually reenter the mainstream of society.

New commitments were made to basic research, epidemiology, the development of new treatment methods, and the evaluation of existing treatment approaches. The opioid maintenance approach using methadone was moved from the legal limbo of experimental status to a category that recognized its legitimacy. In addition, new regulations were developed to prevent inappropriate prescribing of opioids.

Federal support for the expansion of community treatment programs was also greatly increased. By 1973, about 200,000 drug users, most of them opioid users, were in treatment in community programs. These programs were repeatedly and intensively evaluated over the subsequent decade. The legislation that established SAODAP also provided the legislative framework for the NIDA within the U.S. Department of Health, Education, and Welfare (HEW). When established in 1974, NIDA became the lead agency for implementing federal policy on treatment, research, and prevention. By the early 1980s, it was generally accepted that treatment for opioid dependence had demonstrable impact. But by that time, for the majority of patients in treatment programs, the primary drugs of abuse were no longer opioids, but more typically marijuana, stimulants, and sedatives.

During the early and mid-1970s some groups argued for the decriminalization or legalization of marijuana. The arguments lost much of their force with the finding that in 1979 almost 10 percent of high school students were using marijuana on a daily basis.

By the 1970s, it became obvious that U.S. drug abuse problems were not limited to the use of illicit drugs, but that the major problems in terms of social and economic impact were alcoholism and tobacco dependence. Although the U.S. Surgeon General's Report of 1964 linking smoking to lung cancer did not produce any dramatic decrease in smoking, the rate of increase in cigarette consumption among men did begin to level out. The publication of the facts about the health hazards of tobacco, however, did not prevent an increase in smoking among women. By the 1970s, tobacco smoking was increasingly being accepted by the medical and research community as a form of drug dependence, and new efforts were made to understand how nicotine gains control of behavior and to develop new treatments for tobacco dependence.

For several years during the 1970s, the overuse and overprescription of anxiolytic drugs were also areas of major concern in both the medical and political arenas.

The nation's major illicit drug use problems in the late 1970s and early 1980s were the rapid increase in the use of cocaine and heavy use of marijuana by adolescents. By 1985, among the illicit drugs, only marijuana was more commonly abused than cocaine, and new ways of using cocaine, such as the smoking of the free-base version (crack), created unprecedented public concern.

In 1986, spurred in part by concern about the spread of acquired immune deficiency syndrome (AIDS) among IV drug users and, in part, by the rising demand for treatment of cocaine dependence, federal resources for treatment of drug dependence were again substantially increased. The recognition of the need to do more about preventing drug dependence and the rise of politically active groups with drug abuse prevention as a major concern led, in 1986, to the creation of a new Office for Substance Abuse Prevention (OSAP) within the U.S. Department of Health and Human Services (HHS).

OPIOID DEPENDENCE

PHARMACOLOGY OF THE OPIOIDS

Opioids and opioid receptors The discovery of multiple, stereospecific opioid receptors and endogenous ligands for these receptors, as described below, made it easier to understand the multiple actions of morphine-like drugs and of some of the drugs that only partially resembled morphine. Those discoveries, however, also made it necessary to redefine the term "opioid." Opioid now refers to any exogenous substance that binds specifically to any of several subspecies of opioid receptors and produces some agonistic action. Such opioids may have a pharmacological profile dissimilar to that of morphine, may bind to various receptor subtypes in a pattern distinct from that of morphine, and may not suppress the morphine abstinence syndrome. Drugs that bind to any of the subtypes of receptors, but initiate no actions, are termed "opioid antagonists."

A number of opioid receptor subtypes have been described. These include: (1) mu (μ), where classic opioids, such as morphine, bind preferentially and produce actions; (2) kappa (κ), named for the drug ketocyclazocine, where drugs, such as butorphanol (Stadol) and nalbuphine (Nubain), are believed to exert their major effects; and (3) delta (δ), which appears to be the preferential binding site for the endogenous pentapeptide met-enkephalin, as well as for several synthetic peptides. Additional receptors have been proposed, epsilon (ϵ), lambda (λ), and so on as the receptors for some of the many nonanalgesic effects of the opioids. Subtypes of the μ-receptors have been proposed.

The sigma (σ) receptor was named for the benzomorphan derivative SKF-10,047, which in dogs induced excitation and hallucinatory effects, but little or no analgesia. The hypothesis that PCP exerted its action at the σ-receptor has been modified by the finding that PCP binds preferentially to sites that are distinct from those where benzomorphans have their highest affinity.

The actions of morphine are exerted primarily at μ-receptors on neural tissues in the central nervous system (CNS), the autonomic nervous system, and, to some unknown degree, on opioid receptors on white blood cells. The actions include analgesia, respiratory depression, changes in mood (often euphoria), indifference to anticipated distress, drowsiness, decreased ability to concentrate, changes in endocrine and other functions regulated by the hypothalamus, and increased tone of smooth muscle in the gastrointestinal tract. Morphine also induces tolerance and neuroadaptive changes in the CNS that result in distressing withdrawal phenomena when the drug is stopped.

Most of the opioids that are associated with opioid abuse and dependence are typical μ-agonists, having pharmacological profiles identical to that of morphine and differing primarily in terms of metabolism and pharmacokinetics. Thus, heroin (or diacetylmorphine) is more potent and more lipid-soluble than morphine, thereby crossing the blood-brain barrier more rapidly and producing a more rapid onset of subjective effects. Heroin, however, is hydrolyzed quite rapidly to monoacetylmorphine and morphine and probably binds to μ-receptors primarily as those metabolites, rather than as heroin. In contrast, ethyl ketocylcazocine produces dysphoria and no significant pupillary changes, but still induces analgesia.

Codeine (3-methoxymorphine) occurs naturally (0.5 percent) in opium. After absorption, codeine is transformed to some degree into morphine, which accounts, in part, for its opioid effects. As codeine, it does not bind with great affinity to μ-receptors, but does cause some toxicity that probably accounts for its relatively low abuse potential. Methadone also appears to be a typical μ-receptor, but with an extended duration of action after repeated administration, as described. Meperidine (Demerol) has numerous μ-receptor actions, but probably has some actions at other receptors as well. One of its metabolites, normeperidine, has convulsant properties, and addicts who use excessive amounts may achieve high enough levels of this metabolite to experience frank seizures.

Tolerance and physical dependence appear to be specific for each receptor subtype. Thus, when tolerance to a given action develops to a μ-agonist, such as morphine, some cross-tolerance will be seen with other μ-agonists. When, however, tolerance develops to a selective κ-agonist, such as the investigational drug U-50,488, there is no cross-tolerance to μ-agonists. Furthermore, physical dependence induced by κ-agonists has distinct characteristics and a different pattern of withdrawal signs and symptoms.

Several analgesics now available have actions at more than one receptor site. Some have antagonist actions at one site and agonist actions at another. For example, pentazocine (Talwin) has reinforcing properties and is self-administered by animals and some addicts, but it does not appear to exhibit a significant degree of cross-tolerance with μ-agonists and does not suppress μ-agonist withdrawal. Some drug users in the United States inject pentazocine along with tripelenamine (PBZ), an antihistamine that has some euphorigenic effects in its own right. This drug combination is referred to as "T's and B's" (for Talwin and the blue color of tripelennamine).

Buprenorphine (Buprenex) appears to be a partial agonist at the μ-receptor. It supports μ-receptor physical dependence when the degree of physical dependence is low, but precipitates withdrawal when the degree of dependence is high.

Endogenous opioid substances Three distinct neurobiological opioid peptide systems, or families, have now been described. Each of the systems has a distinct genetic basis, separate biosynthetic pathways, and distinct precursor molecules. The anatomical distributions of the receptors and of the cells that produce and release the respective endogenous peptides are also distinct, but there is sometimes considerable overlap. These three systems are usually referred to as: (1) the pro-opiomelanocortin (POMC) system, (2) the pro-enkephalin system, and (3) the pro-dynorphin system. Each precursor protein produces more than one active peptide that can be detected in body tissues. The POMC precursor molecule is a 265-amino-acid protein containing within it the 91-amino-acid peptide, β-lipotropin (β-LPH) as well as adrenocorticotropic hormone (ACTH) and melanocyte-stimulating hormone (MSH). Peptides 61 to 91 within β-lipotropin make up β-endorphin, the active opioid fragment produced by the POMC family. From the parent pro-dynorphin, the dynorphin system produces the 17-amino-acid peptide dynorphin and several other active dynorphin peptides. These include dynorphin A (1 to 8), dynorphin B (1 to 28), and α- and β-neoendorphin, all of which have the pentapeptide leu-enkephalin at their N-terminal, as does dynorphin. The enkephalin system consists primarily of the pentapeptides met-enkephalin (Tyr-Gly-Gly-Phe-Met) and leu-enkephalin (Tyr-Gly-Gly-Phe-Leu). In pro-enkephalin, a 263-amino-acid protein, met-enkephalin is six times as prevalent as leu-enkephalin.

The processing of the precursor molecules to smaller peptides is tissue-specific. For example, in the rat POMC, the precursor is processed to different peptides by the anterior and intermediate lobes of the pituitary.

The various endogenous peptides tend to bind preferentially to one or more of the opioid receptor subtypes. For example, met-enkephalin appears to prefer δ-receptors, and dynorphin A-neoendorphin displays highest affinity for κ-receptors. However, β-endorphin binds to both μ- and δ-receptors and does not appear to be as selective as other endogenous ligands. Some workers have postulated a distinct epsilon (ϵ) receptor for β-endorphin. Preferential binding is not the same as exclusive binding. Peptides that preferentially bind to one set of receptors can, in high enough concentrations, exert actions at receptors for which they have lower affinities. Researchers have suggested that rather than attempting to categorize an endogenous substance with respect to the receptor at which it acts, it would be preferable to present its binding selectivity profile. Thus far, no endogenous peptide has been found that binds as preferentially to the μ-receptor as do drugs, such as morphine. Recently, several laboratories have confirmed the presence of morphine and codeine in mammalian brain and adrenal gland and in human cerebrospinal fluid (CSF). Highest concentrations are found in adrenal glands and spinal cord. Since no exogenous sources could be identified, the morphine and codeine so identified are currently thought to be of endogenous origin. The synthetic pathways and possible biological function of these nonpeptide substances are under investigation. Another, as yet unexplored, finding is the isolation from brain of natural cleavage products of β-endorphin that are more potent than naloxone (Narcan) as opioid antagonists.

TOLERANCE Tolerance does not develop uniformly to all of the actions of opioid drugs. There can be high levels of tolerance to some actions of opioids (such that it requires a hundredfold increase in dose to produce the original effect) when responses to other drug actions show only modest tolerance. With opioids, there can be remarkable tolerance to their analgesic, respiratory depressant, and sedative actions, but markedly less to their miotic effects and constipating actions on the bowel. Intermediate degrees of tolerance to endocrine actions develop, and there appears to be less tolerance to the capacity of opioids to lower the threshold for electrical self-stimulation. Opioids occupying the same receptor types exhibit a considerable degree of cross-tolerance.

PHYSICAL DEPENDENCE (OPIOID NEUROADAPTATION) Physical dependence, as defined earlier in this section, is a drug-induced change in the biological system that is manifested by a characteristic response pattern, the withdrawal syndrome, when the drug is removed or displaced from its receptor. In general, these responses are opposite in direction to the acute agonistic effects of the drugs—that is, rebound hyperexcitabilities. The neuroadaptive changes induced by opioids occur within cells bearing opioid receptors and in neural systems widespread throughout the organism. In humans, the changes probably begin with the first few doses, but some period of continuous receptor occupation is required to permit the detection of withdrawal responses with ordinary clinical means. Withdrawal phenomena are more intense and more readily detectable when the opioid is rapidly removed from its receptor, as happens with opioid antagonist administration.

Opioid withdrawal phenomena can be suppressed by any opioid that occupies the same receptor, as in the phenomenon of cross-dependence. Recent findings suggest that opioid tolerance and neuroadaptive changes are relatively specific to receptor subtypes; that is, κ-agonists do not suppress withdrawal from μ-agonist-induced physical dependence.

CLINICAL CHARACTERISTICS OF THE OPIOID WITHDRAWAL SYNDROME The opioid withdrawal syndrome can vary greatly in intensity, depending primarily on the dose of the opioid used, the degree to which the opioid effects on the CNS are continuously exerted, the duration of the chronic use, and the rate at which the opioid is removed from the receptors. These generalizations apply equally to the other categories of drugs described later in this section. See Tables 13.1-10 and 13.1-11 for the DSM-III-R diagnostic criteria for withdrawal and intoxication; the DSM-III-R diagnostic criteria for opioid intoxication are given in Table 13.1-12.

TABLE 13.1-10
Diagnostic Criteria for Withdrawal

A. Development of a substance-specific syndrome that follows the cessation of, or reduction in, intake of a psychoactive substance that the person previously used regularly.

B. The clinical picture does not correspond to any of the other specific organic mental syndromes, such as delirium, organic delusional syndrome, organic hallucinosis, organic mood syndrome, or organic anxiety syndrome.

Table from DSM-III-R *Diagnostic and Statistical Manual of Mental Disorders,* ed 3, revised. Copyright American Psychiatric Association, Washington, DC, 1987. Used with permission.

TABLE 13.1-11
Diagnostic Criteria for Intoxication

A. Development of a substance-specific syndrome due to recent ingestion of a psychoactive substance. (**Note:** More than one substance may produce similar or identical syndromes.)
B. Maladaptive behavior during the waking state due to the effect of the substance on the central nervous system (e.g., belligerence, impaired judgment, impaired social or occupational functioning).
C. The clinical picture does not correspond to any of the other specific organic mental syndromes, such as delirium, organic delusional syndrome, organic hallucinosis, organic mood syndrome, or organic anxiety syndrome.

Table from DSM-III-R *Diagnostic and Statistical Manual of Mental Disorders,* ed 3, revised. Copyright American Psychiatric Association, Washington, DC, 1987. Used with permission.

TABLE 13.1-12
Diagnostic Criteria for Opioid Intoxication

A. Recent use of an opioid.
B. Maladaptive behavioral changes (e.g., initial euphoria followed by apathy, dysphoria, psychomotor retardation, impaired judgment, impaired social or occupational functioning).
C. Pupillary constriction (or pupillary dilation due to anoxia from severe overdose) and at least one of the following signs:
(1) drowsiness
(2) slurred speech
(3) impairment in attention or memory
D. Not due to any physical or other mental disorder.

Note: When the differential diagnosis must be made without a clear-cut history, testing with an opioid antagonist, or toxicologic analysis of body fluids, it may be qualified as "provisional."

Table from DSM-III-R *Diagnostic and Statistical Manual of Mental Disorders,* ed 3, revised. Copyright American Psychiatric Association, Washington, DC, 1987. Used with permission.

The clinical syndrome observed consists of purposive behavior, which is dependent on the observer and environment (e.g., complaints, pleas, and manipulations directed at getting more of the drug), and nonpurposive behavior, which is not goal-oriented and is relatively independent of the observer and environment.

In the case of short-acting drugs, such as morphine or heroin, the first withdrawal symptoms may be seen within 8 to 12 hours after the last dose of drug. In mild syndromes, the symptoms may be limited to craving, anxiety, dysphoria, yawning, perspiration, lacrimation, rhinorrhea, and restless and broken sleep. In more severe cases, as the syndrome progresses, other signs and symptoms that may be seen include irritability; dilated pupils; aching of bones, back, and muscles; piloerection (waves of gooseflesh, from which comes the term "cold turkey" to describe withdrawal); and hot and cold flashes. In severe syndromes, which, with heroin and morphine, generally reach peak severity at about 48 to 72 hours after the last dose, additional symptoms include nausea, vomiting, diarrhea, weight loss, fever (usually low grade), and increased blood pressure, pulse, and respiratory rate. Also often observed are twitching of muscles and kicking movements of the lower extremities, whence comes the phrase "kicking the habit." The diagnostic criteria for opioid withdrawal syndromes are shown in Table 13.1-13.

With short-acting drugs, the acute phase of the syndrome, if untreated, runs its course in 7 to 10 days. In research subjects, the acute phase was followed by a more subtle but longer-lasting phase, the protracted abstinence syndrome, which sometimes lasted for many weeks. During this phase,

TABLE 13.1-13
Diagnostic Criteria for Opioid Withdrawal

A. Cessation of prolonged (several weeks or more) moderate or heavy use of an opioid, or reduction in the amount of opioid used (or administration of an opioid antagonist after a brief period of use), followed by at least three of the following:
(1) craving for an opioid
(2) nausea or vomiting
(3) muscle aches
(4) lacrimation or rhinorrhea
(5) pupillary dilation, piloerection, or sweating
(6) diarrhea
(7) yawning
(8) fever
(9) insomnia
B. Not due to any physical or other mental disorder.

Table from DSM-III-R *Diagnostic and Statistical Manual of Mental Disorders,* ed 3, revised. Copyright American Psychiatric Association, Washington, DC, 1987. Used with permission.

many physiological variables reached subnormal values, such as hyposensitivity to the respiratory stimulant effects of carbon dioxide. There was also disturbed sleep, overconcern about bodily discomfort, poor self-image, and decreased capacity to tolerate stress. It is speculated that the protracted abstinence syndrome may play a role in relapse.

With longer-acting drugs, such as methadone or L-α-acetylmethadol (LAAM), the onset of withdrawal may be delayed for 1 to 3 days following the last dose. Although the syndrome is qualitatively similar, peak symptoms may not occur until the third to eighth day, and the symptoms may persist for several weeks.

Acute withdrawal from methadone, and presumably from LAAM, is also followed by a protracted abstinence syndrome. If naloxone is given to a patient dependent on methadone, thereby displacing the drug abruptly from the receptors, the withdrawal is immediate in onset, can be quite severe, and persists until the naloxone is metabolized and the residual methadone reoccupies the receptors.

Withdrawal from available analgesics which are presumed to be κ-receptor agonists (e.g., pentazocine, nalbuphine) is generally rapid in onset, mild, and lasts a few days; the syndrome bears some similarities to the μ-receptor withdrawal syndrome, but there are also some distinct elements.

Withdrawal symptoms after chronic administration of buprenorphine, a partial μ-agonist, are generally not severe in intensity, but the time of onset of the symptoms is not clear. In early studies, when the drug was given subcutaneously, withdrawal appeared 7 to 14 days after cessation; after sublingual administration, withdrawal symptoms were experienced within a few days after drug use was stopped.

Mechanisms of tolerance and physical dependence

Several theories attempt to account for the general observation that tolerance and physical dependence tend to develop in parallel and that withdrawal phenomena tend to be opposite in direction to the acute effects produced by the drugs. To a degree, these theories are variations on the homeostatic concept, which postulates that acute opioid effects elicit counteradaptive responses that build up if the drug is continued. When the drug is withdrawn or displaced from its receptor by an antagonist, the unopposed counteradaptive mechanisms produce the withdrawal phenomena.

Several different levels of explanation for the counteradaptive responses have been proposed. The mechanisms that have been proposed focus on changes in gene expression, alterations in intracellular enzyme mediators and Ca^{++} concentration, variations in receptors, and differences in neural pathways. These hypotheses are not mutually exclusive. Indeed, they appear to be complementary: Supportive data exist for several of the views. Opioid drugs can alter the expression of the genes encoding the opioid neurotransmitters; other research has focused on a family of guanine nucleotide-binding proteins (G-proteins) that serve as the transducers between receptor generated signals and second messengers, such as adenosine 3':5'-cyclic phosphate (cAMP). Acute administration of opioids (or, in some cells, α_2-adrenergic agonists) results in inhibition of adenylate cyclase. Opioid-induced changes in concentrations or activity of G-proteins may be the mechanism by which chronic opioid use modifies the rate of synthesis of cAMP. When the opioid is removed, the altered (increased) synthesis rate results in transiently higher cAMP levels. It is postulated that some aspects of rebound during withdrawal are due to these higher cAMP levels. It may be that drug induced supersensitivity and alterations in intracellular Ca^{++} concentrations also involve alterations in G-proteins.

Chronic treatment with opioids also induces supersensitivity in several distinct transmitter circuits, including the dopaminergic, noradrenergic, cholinergic, and serotonergic systems. Opioids also inhibit the activity of adrenergic neurons in the locus ceruleus, and, in opioid dependent animals, naloxone causes increased acitivity in locus ceruleus neurons. These and other findings suggested that noradrenergic neurons in the CNS develop changes in sensitivity during chronic morphine treatment and that increased noradrenergic activity plays a role in some aspects of opioid withdrawal. The observation that certain α_2-adrenergic agonists, such as clonidine (Catapres), also inhibit the activity of neurons in the locus ceruleus formed the background for the clinical trials of clonidine in opioid withdrawal, as described. It is worth noting that supersensitivity to neurotransmitters can also be induced by chronic treatment with drugs that are not subject to abuse, such as dopaminergic blockers.

Tolerance and neuroadaptive change can be induced locally, as well as in the whole organism. Thus, infusions of opioid limited to the spinal cord induce tolerance and withdrawal limited to spinal structures. Learning and conditioning also play roles in opioid tolerance and, perhaps, in dependence as well. Animals that exhibit marked tolerance to the effects of opioids given repeatedly in one situation may exhibit toxicity when the same dose is administered in a novel environment. Thus, adaptations at both the cellular and functional system levels are widespread in animals that are tolerant and physically dependent on opioids.

ETIOLOGICAL FACTORS IN OPIOID DEPENDENCE

The factors presented below as important in the etiology of opioid abuse and dependence—social, environmental, pharmacological, personality, psychopathology, genetic, and familial—are the same factors that must be considered when considering abuse of and dependence on other categories of drugs. What changes is the importance of a particular factor. For example, as reinforcers of drug-taking behavior, benzodiazepine anxiolytics are not as powerful as drugs, such as cocaine. Consequently, medical attitudes, prescribing patterns, and preexisting psychopathology are more dominant as etiological factors in the dependence on benzodiazepines, whereas pharmacological factors (i.e., acute euphorigenic and reinforcing effects) play a larger role in dependence on cocaine. The factors that play important roles in the etiology of opioid dependence are presented in more detail to illustrate their interplay.

There is no single factor that can be said to cause opioid abuse or dependence; rather, there are multiple interacting causes, some of which are more dominant in certain cases than in others. Some may play greater roles in determining who will experiment or be exposed to opioid drugs; others may be more important in determining which experimenters will use opioid drugs briefly, and which persons will go on to develop dependence of great severity and chronicity. Still other factors influence the pattern of use, complications, response to treatment, and the natural history of the dependence syndrome.

SOCIAL AND ENVIRONMENTAL FACTORS Social attitudes, peer pressures, and drug availability are the major determinants of experimentation with the less socially disapproved drugs, such as tobacco, alcohol, and, more recently, marijuana. Generally, the use of such drugs precedes use of opioids, such as heroin. These antecedent drugs are now sometimes referred to as "gateway" drugs. Those persons who go on to experiment with the most socially disapproved drugs, such as heroin, generally come from disrupted families or have disturbed relationships with parents, and they often have low self-esteem. A significant proportion of opioid users meet criteria for antisocial personality disorder, even when those items that are related to illicit drug use are not applied. Illicit opioids are often more available in inner cities of large urban areas than in other parts of the country. Availability, in turn, can influence not only initial and continued use but also relapse after treatment. When a significant number of opioid users reside in one area, a subculture supportive of experimentation and continued use evolves. Many of the areas where illicit opioids are available are also characterized by high crime, high unemployment, and demoralized school systems—all of which serve to reduce the sense of hope and of self-esteem that are associated with resistance to use and good prognosis once dependence develops. These factors, along with family factors, as described below, may account for the disproportionately high rates of heroin addiction among black and Hispanic minorities.

It was once assumed that experimentation with illicit opioids invariably led to dependence. A study of young black males in St. Louis in the early 1960s found that all the men who used heroin more than six times went on to become addicts. In the early 1970s, however, when experimentation with heroin became more widespread, further research found that only a fraction of those persons who briefly experimented with illicit opioids developed serious problems. It is still the case that those persons who use opioid drugs heavily—at least once per week—usually go on to daily use, at least for a brief period. It is likely, however, that many of those persons who go on to develop some degree of dependence recover without ever seeking formal treatment. Certainly, the number of opioid users and experimenters in the United States over the past decade is far larger than the total number of those users who have ever entered treatment programs.

The experience with U.S. servicemen in Vietnam provided a unique natural experiment where the influences of availability, vulnerability, and social norms could be observed. During the period 1970 to 1972, high-grade heroin at very low cost was readily available to young men separated from their families and usual social norms. Among U.S. Army enlisted men, about half of those soldiers who tried heroin became dependent; at least they developed withdrawal symptoms when they attempted to stop using heroin. Of those soldiers who used heroin at least five times, 73 percent became dependent. The background factors that were predictors of addiction—being young and black—were not the factors that best predicted relapse after the soldiers returned to the United States. Relapse was related to being white, older, and having parents who had criminal histories or were alcoholic.

The important role of availability is also illustrated by the repeated observation that physicians, dentists, and nurses have far higher rates of dependence on opioids than other professionals of comparable educational achievement (e.g., accountants, lawyers) who do not have such easy access to the drugs.

OPIOIDS AS REINFORCERS Animals self-administer opioids, as well as several other classes of pharmacological agents, by various routes of administration; thus, opioids are positive reinforcers. It is not clear, however, which of the multiple actions of opioid drugs, as described above, are responsible for these reinforcing properties, or just which neural systems mediate the reinforcing effects of opioids as contrasted with their analgesic or respiratory depressant effects. Figure 13.1-2 shows some of the brain areas where activity is altered by euphoric doses of morphine.

Given to former heroin addicts, opioids reduce anxiety, increase self-esteem and ability to cope with everyday problems, and decrease boredom. When given intravenously, opioids produce a rush or flash, a sudden, brief sensation that is exceedingly pleasurable, much like an orgastic sensation that is felt in the abdomen. In a research setting, heroin addicts who self-administered heroin seemed to develop tolerance to the anxiety-relieving and mood-elevating effects of opioids. Over a period of several weeks, they reported feeling increasingly anxious and dysphoric and developed various somatic complaints. Despite this tolerance, single injections continued to produce brief periods of mood elevation for 30 to 60 minutes after each injection. The loss of mood-elevating effects and appearance of hypophoria and hypochondriasis have also been observed with chronic administration of methadone in a research setting.

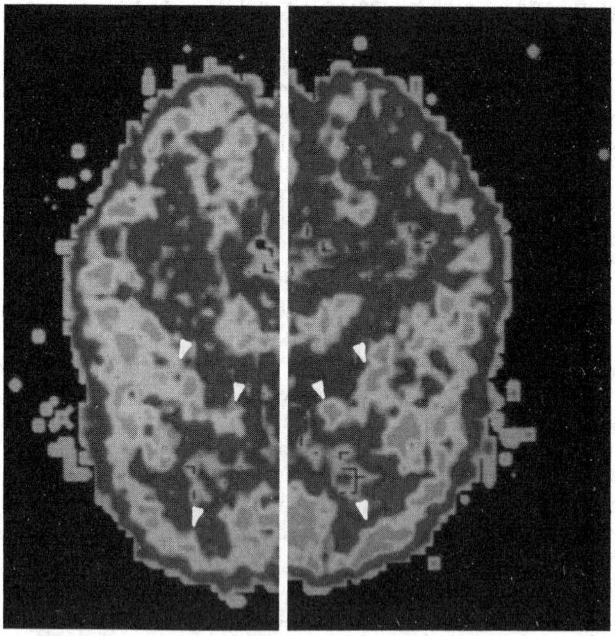

FIGURE 13.1-2. *Glucose utilization, as revealed by positron emission tomography, in the brain of a heroin addict. Higher rates are pictured as lighter areas. On the left, the subject was given placebo. On the right, the subject was given 30 mg of morphine intramuscularly. (Courtesy of E. D. London, Ph.D.)*

Tolerant opioid users do not continue to self-administer opioids solely to prevent the highly aversive withdrawal phenomena. Interviews with heroin users indicated that, despite some tolerance to many of the drug effects, users continued to experience a brief euphoric effect immediately following an injection.

The sites involved in reinforcement and self-administration are probably distinct from those sites responsible for opioid analgesia. It is also unlikely that the endogenous opioids are the sole mediators of euphoria or of the reinforcing effects of environmental stimuli that produce pleasure or positive reinforcements. Addicts maintained on large doses of naltrexone (Trexan) continue to experience pleasurable effects from food, sex, cigarettes, and a variety of nonopioid drugs. Furthermore, it is clear that reinforcing properties do not reside solely in the drug or in the stimulus. Depending on the previous history of the organism and on the reinforcement schedule, animals will continue to press a lever to self-administer electric shocks of the same intensity that they previously had worked hard to avoid. In such an experimental model, the high-level shock is a reinforcer in that it maintains the behavior that leads to the shock.

PSYCHODYNAMIC FACTORS AND PSYCHOPATHOLOGY Early psychoanalytic formulations postulated that drug users, in general, suffered from either a special form of affective dysregulation, tense-depression, that was alleviated by drug use or from a disorder of impulse control in which the search for pleasure was dominant. More recent formulations postulate ego (in the self) defects, which are manifested in the addict's inability to manage painful affects (guilt, anger, anxiety) and to avoid preventable medical, legal, and financial problems. Further, some addicts appear to have great difficulty differentiating and describing what they feel, a difficulty that has been aptly called alexithymia (i.e., no words for feelings). It is postulated that the use of opioids, pharmacologically and symbolically, aids the ego in controlling these affects. Although analysts concede that some of these observations may reflect problems produced by chronic drug use, the psychodynamic perspective is that the psychopathology is the underlying motivation for initial use, dependent use, and relapse after a period of abstinence. Traditions of passivity and uncovering techniques derived from psychoanalysis of neurosis are poorly suited to the treatment of most drug addicts. Epidemiological studies of the personality find that those persons who use illicit drugs, especially those who use opioids, tend to place more value on independence and less on academic achievement. The users are also more tolerant of deviance; indeed, a very substantial number exhibit significant signs of delinquency before their first experimentation with opioids. Follow-up studies of schoolchildren observed in the first grade showed that those rated as more aggressive or especially as shy and aggressive were more likely to be drug users as teenagers.

Diagnostic heterogeneity Although the causal relationships between psychopathology and opioid dependence remain unclear, the high prevalence of additional psychiatric disorders among treated opioid-dependent patients has now been repeatedly confirmed.

When Research Diagnostic Criteria (RDC) are used, 87 percent of opioid addicts seeking treatment at a Yale University–affiliated program met the criteria for a psychiatric disorder, in addition to opioid dependence, at some point in their lives. The most common diagnoses were affective (mood) disorders, alcoholism, antisocial personality, and anxiety disorders (Table 13.1-14). Among women, mood and anxiety disorders were more common, and alcoholism and antisocial personality were less common. If DSM-III criteria, which do not require that the diagnosis of antisocial personality disorder be independent of the need for drugs, had been used, 54 percent of the sample would have received the diagnosis of antisocial personality disorder. The proportion of opioid users meeting criteria for a current episode of a psychiatric disorder was 70 percent, with mood disorder, antisocial personality disorder, alcoholism, and phobia the most common diagnoses. More than half of the patients met the criteria for two or more additional diagnoses, such as alcoholism, antisocial personality, and depression. Very similar patterns of additional psychiatric disorders have been found by workers at other public clinics and by clinicians in private practice. Among patients in therapeutic communities, 60 percent reported depressive symptoms during the year before entry, 28 percent had contemplated suicide, and 13 percent had made at least one suicide attempt.

TABLE 13.1-14
Lifetime Rates for Psychiatric Disorders Among Opioid-Dependent Patients Using Research Diagnostic Criteria

Type of Disorder	*Male* (*n* = *403*) (%)	*Female* (*n* = *130*) (%)
Affective [mood] disorders		
Major depression	48.9	69.2
Minor depression	9.4	5.4
Intermittent depression	18.1	20.8
Cyclothymic personality	2.5	6.9
Labile personality	17.1	14.6
Manic disorders	0.5	0.8
Hypomanic disorder	5.5	10.0
Bipolar 1 or 2	3.7	10.8
Any affective [mood] disorder	70.7	85.4
Schizophrenic disorders		
Schizophrenia	0.7	0.8
Schizoaffective, depressed	2.2	0.0
Schizoaffective, manic	0.5	0.0
Anxiety disorders		
Panic	0.5	3.9
Obsessive-compulsive	1.7	2.3
Generalized anxiety	4.7	7.7
Phobic	8.2	13.9
Any anxiety disorder	13.2	25.4
Alcoholism	37.0	26.9
Personality disorders		
Antisocial personality	29.5	16.9
Briquet's syndrome	0.0	0.7
Schizotypal features	8.7	7.7
Other psychiatric disorders	5.7	10.0

Table modified from Rounsaville B J, Weissman M M, Kleber H, Wilber C: Heterogeneity of psychiatric diagnosis in treated opiate addicts. Arch Gen Psychiat *39*: 162, 1982, with permission.

FAMILY FACTORS More than 50 percent of urban heroin addicts come from single-parent families. Typically, even in two-parent families, there are disturbed family relationships, in which one parent (usually of the opposite sex) is intensely involved with the addict, whereas the other parent is distant, absent, or punitive. Cross-generational alliances between the drug user and one parent against another parental figure are common. Furthermore, alcoholism or drug abuse, or both, is common in the families of heroin users. The disability of the drug-using member often serves as a focus for communication among other members of the family and, sometimes, as the main motive for their remaining together. Thus, the family equilibrium may be threatened by the addict's recovery.

Despite their seeming rebelliousness and precocious efforts to be independent, opioid users often remain dependent on and in close communication with families of origin well into adulthood. Both male and female heroin addicts believe that members of their families of origin or their in-laws would be of the most help to them in their efforts to give up drugs.

BIOLOGICAL FACTORS There is some evidence for a genetically transmitted vulnerability to developing alcoholism, and many opioid addicts are alcoholic in addition to being opioid-dependent. They also have biological parents who are alcoholic, drug-dependent, or both. Among adoptees who had been separated at birth from biological parents, a diagnosis of drug abuse was associated with antisocial personality in a biological parent or, in adoptees without antisocial personality, with alcohol problems in a biological parent. At present, however, there is little direct evidence of any specific biological vulnerability to opioid dependence. It has been postulated that some antecedent metabolic deficiency, such as endogenous opioid dysregulation or a metabolic deficiency induced by chronic opioid use, may increase vulnerability to becoming opioid-dependent, but no evidence for such defects has yet emerged.

LEARNING AND CONDITIONING Drug use, whether occasional or compulsive, can be viewed as behavior maintained by its consequences that strengthens a behavior pattern via reinforcers, and opioids are positive reinforcers of drug self-administration, as described above. Drugs can also reinforce antecedent behaviors by terminating some noxious or aversive state, such as pain, anxiety, or depression. In some social situations, the use of the drug, quite apart from its pharmacological effects, can be reinforcing if it results in special status or the approval of friends. Social reinforcement can sometimes maintain drug use until the effects of primary reinforcement or reinforcement by alleviation of withdrawal symptoms come into play. With each use of the drug, rapid positive reinforcement occurs, either as a result of the "rush" (the drug-induced euphoria), alleviation of disturbed affects, alleviation of withdrawal symptoms, or any combination of these effects. With a short-acting opioid, such as heroin, such reinforcement occurs several times a day, day in and day out, creating a powerfully reinforced habit pattern. Eventually, the paraphernalia and hustling associated with drug use can become secondary reinforcers, as well as cues signaling drug availability; in their presence, craving or desire to experience drug effects increases.

In addition to this operant reinforcement of drug-using and drug-seeking behaviors, other learning mechanisms probably play a role in dependence and relapse. Opioid withdrawal phenomena can be conditioned, in the Pavlovian or classical sense, to environmental or interoceptive stimuli. Such conditioning of withdrawal to environmental stimuli has been demonstrated in both laboratory animals and methadone-dependent human volunteers. For a long period of time following withdrawal, the addict, when exposed to environmental stimuli previously linked with drug use or withdrawal, may experience conditioned withdrawal or conditioned craving. The increased feelings of craving are not necessarily accompanied by symptoms of withdrawal. The conditions that elicit the most intense craving are those associated with the availability or use of the opioid, such as watching someone else use heroin or being offered some drug by a friend, rather than conditions associated with withdrawal.

These conditioning phenomena can be superimposed on any preexisting psychopathology, but preexisting difficulties are not required for the development of powerfully reinforced drug-seeking behavior.

NATURAL HISTORY OF OPIOID DEPENDENCE

Some people apparently can use opioids occasionally—for example, several times per month—over periods of months or years without becoming dependent. For such users, careful rules about time and place of use may help in preventing progression to addiction, but the users are still at risk for death from overdose as well as for infections and other medical complications that affect opioid addicts who inject, as described below. When addiction develops, the subsequent course of the syndrome is dependent on environmental factors, the characteristics of the user, the route of administration, and the specific opioid being used.

HETEROGENEITY OF LIFE-STYLE Opioid addicts seen at clinics in the United States and in England exhibit a surprising heterogeneity of life-styles, attitudes toward conventional values, and criminality. Some addicts, except for their drug use, are quite conventional, avoid criminality, work at legitimate occupations, and do not identify with the addict subculture; these addicts are known as "conformists" or "stables." On the other extreme, some addicts live exclusively by illicit activities and are highly involved with other addicts; this kind of addict is a "hustler" or "junkie." A third group appears to identify with both cultures, engaging in some criminal activities and interacting with other addicts, but living primarily on legitimate earnings; these addicts are "two-worlders." A fourth group of addicts seems not to be involved in either the conventional culture or the addict subculture. People in this group tend to be unemployed and to live on welfare, rather than on criminal earnings. These addicts, the "uninvolved" or "loners," may have high levels of psychopathology.

ENVIRONMENTAL FACTORS For those users who become dependent in the context of medical treatment, the subsequent course depends largely on the medical problems that generated the opioid use, the willingness of doctors to continue to prescribe drugs for them, and whether the drug is used orally or by injection. Those persons who use opioids by the oral route and whose pain is controlled by the doses provided (made available by legitimate prescription) may experience little interference with normal function for many years. If pain is uncontrolled, demands for increased or altered medication schedules will probably lead to repeated diagnostic work-ups, surgery, and other procedures, punctuated by attempts at withdrawal—voluntary and coerced—and treatment for depression.

In the United States, those persons who become dependent on illicit opioids, usually heroin, and who persist in use for any substantial period, are very likely to come to the attention of the police or to seek medical treatment. Since the development of community-based treatment programs in the early 1970s, the average time from addiction to illicit opioids to first episode of treatment has decreased from 6 years to about 2 to 3 years. For those persons arrested, the time from addiction to first arrest may range from 6 months to 5 years. Before the advent of community-based treatment programs, a significant proportion of addicts were never voluntarily abstinent, stopping only when incarcerated. Comparisons of heroin addicts who seek treatment with those who do not suggest that the former are more likely to exhibit symptoms of depression. It may be that depression (in addition to the pressure from family and law enforcement agencies) is an important determinant of which drug users enter treatment.

FOR MOST USERS, AN EPISODIC PATTERN In the early stages of opioid use, the most typical course for the user of illicit opioids is one of periods of abstinence, either voluntary or forced (through prison or hospitalization), lasting from a few weeks to many months, followed by relapse to opioid use and readdiction. Relapse occurs most often within the first 3 months; a number of studies show that at least two out of three patients relapse within 6 months. The theme running through the many specific reasons given for periods of voluntary abstinence is a desire to change life patterns and a weariness with the constant difficulty of trying to obtain illicit opioids. At the time of reentry into treatment, addicts are often less seriously impaired than when first treated, a finding that suggests some residual benefit from intermittent treatment.

Repeated relapse is not an inevitable consequence of opioid dependence. Of those U.S. Army enlisted men who became addicted in Vietnam, 88 percent did not become readdicted any time in the 3 years following their return to the United States; 56 percent did not use opioids at all; and of those soldiers readdicted in the first year, 70 percent were not readdicted in the following 2 years.

FOR MANY USERS, A FINITE CYCLE There is now a growing belief that, in the United States, opioid addiction is a disorder that eventually ends for the majority of those users who survive. Although there are elderly opioid addicts in the United States, their numbers are few. Some experts have estimated that average duration of active opioid addiction is about 9 years.

TOXICITY, MORBIDITY, AND MEDICAL COMPLICATIONS Oral opioids are relatively nontoxic. Although chronic use, as in methadone maintenance, is associated with minor endocrine abnormalities, constipation, and some sleep disturbance, no major organ damage has been noted, and no significant impact on longevity would be expected. The cognitive impairment seen with chronic alcohol and sedative use is not generally found with chronic oral opioid use. Nevertheless, the life expectancy of opioid addicts, especially heroin addicts, is markedly reduced. Estimates range from a two- to threefold increase in the expected mortality rate for older addicts to a 20-fold increase in expected rate among young addicts. A substantial proportion of these deaths are due to drug overdose, drug-related infections, and suicide. Among urban opioid addicts in the United States, homicide is also a common cause of death. In a study of black male heroin addicts in St. Louis, 62 percent of the men had been hospitalized because of narcotics use (12 percent three or more times), 35 percent reported gunshot or knife wounds, 52 percent at least one drug overdose, and 19 percent three or more overdoses. Follow-ups of treated opioid addicts in the United States indicate an overall death rate of 1 to 1.5 percent per year.

A sample of 128 heroin addicts—composed of 93 men and 35 women, with an average age of 25 years—who was receiving daily prescriptions for heroin at London drug clinics in 1969 was followed over a 10-year period. By the seventh year, 12 percent had died; by the tenth year, 15 percent were dead (14 men and 4 women). Eight addicts died because of a drug overdose; four users died of renal failure; one addict died of bronchopneumonia; one user committed suicide; two addicts were killed in accidents; and for three users, the coroner's verdict was simply addiction to drugs. At the British clinics providing injectable drugs to young addicts, the death rate was estimated at 2 to 3 percent per year, at least 20-fold higher than the death rate of comparably aged contemporaries. Although many of the infectious complications are directly related to the use of injectable opioids, death resulting from combining opioids with alcohol or sedatives or from self-destructive behavior is not uncommon among former users of illicit drugs who are subsequently treated with oral opioids, such as methadone.

The suicide rate among opioid addicts is estimated to be three times higher than that of the general population; this figure is probably an underestimate because it is difficult to determine how many overdose deaths are, to some degree, intentional. However, in the St. Louis population cited above, only one subject reported that a drug overdose was a suicide attempt.

MEDICAL COMPLICATIONS AND LIFE EXPECTANCY Medical complications associated with injection of illicit drugs include a variety of pathological changes in the CNS. Degenerative changes in globus pallidus and necrosis of spinal gray matter are usually found at autopsy, but sometimes there are clinical manifestations in those users surviving overdose experiences. Examples are transverse myelitis, amblyopia, plexitis, peripheral neuropathy, parkinsonian syndromes, intellectual impairment, and personality changes. Pathological changes in muscles and degeneration of peripheral nerves have also been seen.

Because opioid addicts—even physicians who have access to drugs and sterile materials—tend to neglect the hygienic aspects of injecting, infections of skin and systemic organs are quite common. Filtering illicit opioids through cigarette filters or wads of cotton and injection of materials intended for oral use result in the entrance of starch, talc, and other particulate contaminants into the bloodstream; these particulates can cause pulmonary emboli that can eventually result in angiothrombotic pulmonary hypertension and right ventricular failure. Staphylococcal pneumonitis may also be related to septic emboli. The incidence of tuberculosis is higher among heroin addicts than in the general population. Endocarditis and septicemia, involving lesions either of the tricuspid or of the aortic and mitral valves, are frequent complications. Less frequent, but equally serious, complications are meningitis and brain abscess.

Other frequently seen infections that are probably related to injecting or sharing of needles include viral hepatitis, human immunodeficiency virus (HIV), malaria, tetanus, osteomyelitis, and syphilis. Although most cases of syphilis are probably acquired in the usual fashion, as is tuberculosis, many opioid addicts who inject have a low-level chronic hepatitis without jaundice and may have abnormal liver function tests and false-positive tests for syphilis. In one study, 45 percent of heroin addicts had hepatitis-B antibody levels. Abnormal liver function tests which are found in about two out of three heroin addicts, may persist for long periods after cessation of injection. Excessive use of alcohol may, in some cases, contribute to the liver disease. Drug users who share needles are at high risk for AIDS. Of the 46,000 reported cases of AIDS in the United States in December 1987, more than 25 percent were found to have a history of drug use. In the northeastern United States, up to 60 percent of addicts at some methadone clinics have antibody evidence of infection with the HIV virus. However, in California, Texas, and the west coast of Florida, only 1 to 2 percent of comparable opioid users were seropositive. As illustrated in Figure 13.1-3, needle sharing among IV drug users was almost a universal practice through the mid-1980s. The finding that not all who share needles have become infected with HIV suggests that the virus is not yet prevalent in all areas of the country and there are still opportunities for vigorous prevention efforts.

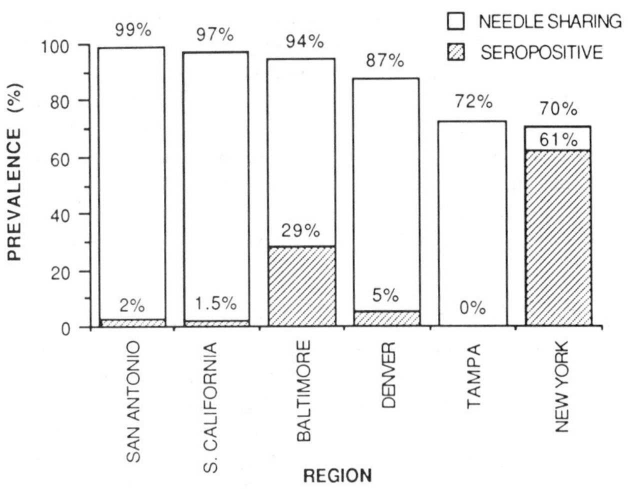

FIGURE 13.1-3. *Needle sharing among IV drug users was almost universal through the mid-1980s, but the percentage of users who were seropositive for HIV varied in different cities.*

Opioid receptors are found on lymphocytes. In heroin addicts, there are changes in the ratio of helper to suppressor T-cells and a suppression of cell mediated immunity. The relationship to opioid use is still unclear.

Prior to the beginning of the AIDS epidemic, lymphadenopathy was seen in 75 percent of addicts and was thought to be related to particulate contaminants; chronic edema of extremities (e.g., puffy hand) may be due to lymphatic obstruc-

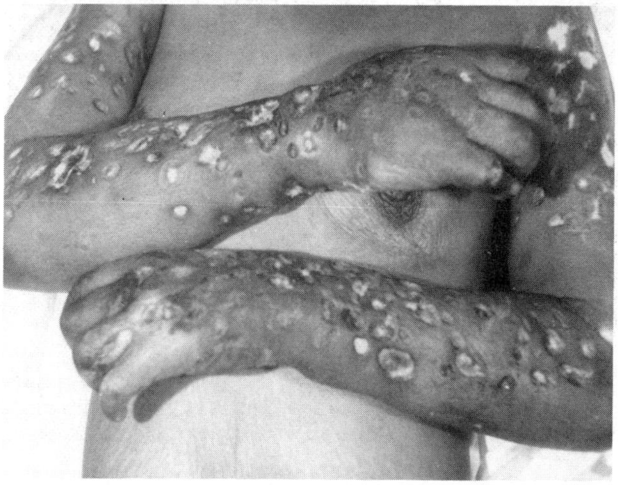

FIGURE 13.1-4. *"Skin-popper": Circular depressed scars, often with underlying chronic abscesses, can result from skin-popping. (Courtesy Michael Baden, M.D.)*

tion caused by contaminants or sclerosis of veins caused by the drugs or their dilutants. Lymphadenopathy in a drug addict who is positive for HIV antibodies now has much more ominous implications. "Skin popping" may cause widespread ulceration and disfigurement as a result of chemical necrosis or infection (Fig 13.1-4). Some drug users seem determined to experience the effects of the drug used intravenously and switch to the use of femoral and jugular veins when the surface veins of the arms and legs have become sclerosed (Fig. 13.1-5).

OPIOIDS AND CRIME In the United States, the statistical relationship between use of illicit opioids and crime is unquestionable. People who use illicit opioids commit crimes more frequently than do nonusers. There are, however, questions about the degree to which one behavior causes the other. The direct tranquilizing actions of opioids ought to reduce criminal activity, rather than to increase it. Indeed, throughout much of history, in countries where crude opioids, such as opium, were inexpensive, socially acceptable, and were either smoked or taken by mouth, there was little relationship between opioid use and criminal behavior (Fig. 13.1-6). The association between opioid use and crime emerges primarily

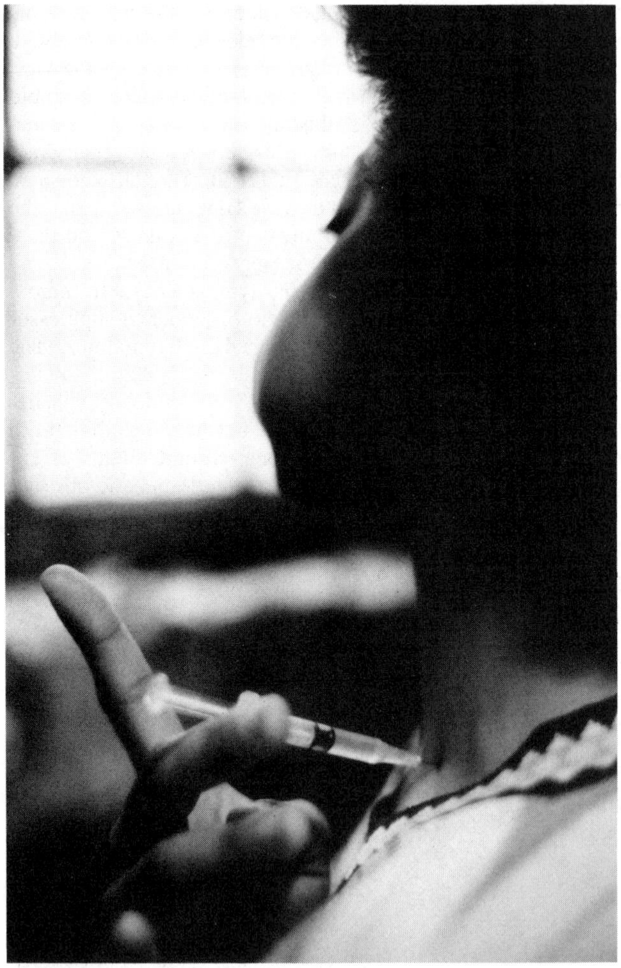

FIGURE 13.1-5. *A heroin user puffs her cheeks to force blood into the jugular vein. (From White P T, Raymer S: The poppy—for good and evil. Nat Geograph* 167: *187, 1985, with permission.)*

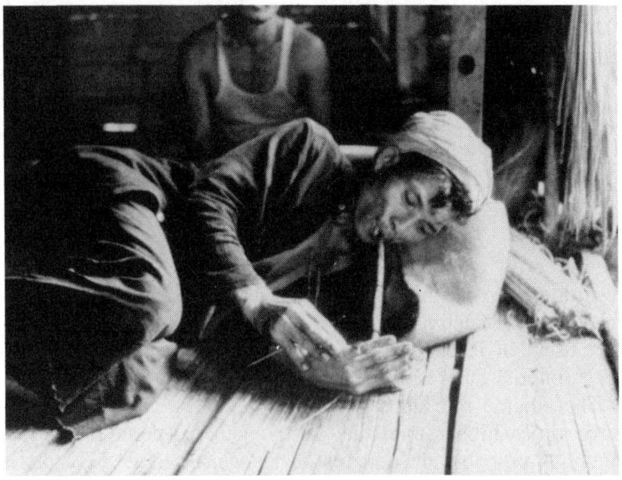

FIGURE 13.1-6. *Opium smoking in Thailand, 1972.*

in countries, such as the United States, that have tried to restrict the use of opioids to legitimate medical indications, but have been unable to eliminate illicit opioid traffic.

In the United States, more than 50 percent of heroin addicts have been arrested prior to their first opioid use. Although it might be argued that the criminal behavior seen after onset of addiction is merely a continuation of a criminal life-style, addicts' self-reports, as well as more objective data, indicate that criminal activity increases sharply after onset of opioid addiction. Arrest rates for nondrug offenses increase 150 to 300 percent after onset of addiction, and self-reported property crimes increase by a comparable degree. Other evidence pointing to a causal relationship between opioid use and crime is the sharp reduction in both self-reported criminal activity and arrests during periods of less than daily opioid use. The decrease in crime is seen whether the decrease in opioid use is a result of effective treatment, probation, parole, or spontaneous cessation. Although most addicts' crimes are directed at generating income for drugs by shoplifting, petty theft, and selling drugs, recently more addicts seem to be engaging in crimes, such as robbery, that involve the potential for violence.

Because criminal behavior often antedates opioid use, it is unrealistic to expect successful treatment of opioid dependence to eliminate criminal behavior entirely. Addicts who were criminally active prior to opioid dependence are more likely to persist in criminal acts when abstinent.

TREATMENT OF OPIOID INTOXICATION

The opioid overdose syndrome consists of coma, severely depressed respiration, and pinpoint pupils. In severe cases, gross pulmonary edema occurs, with frothing at the mouth (Figure 13.1-7), but X-ray evidence of pulmonary changes is seen even in less severe cases. Pulmonary edema is an opioid effect and is seen with overdoses of oral, medically prescribed opioids. Depending on when the patient is found, there may also be cyanosis, cold clammy skin, and decreased body temperature. Blood pressure is decreased, but it falls dramatically only with severe anoxia, at which point pupils may dilate. Cardiac arrhythmias have been reported and may be related either to anoxia or the use of quinine as an adulterant.

The first task is to ensure an adequate air passage. Tracheopharyngeal secretions should be aspirated, and an air-

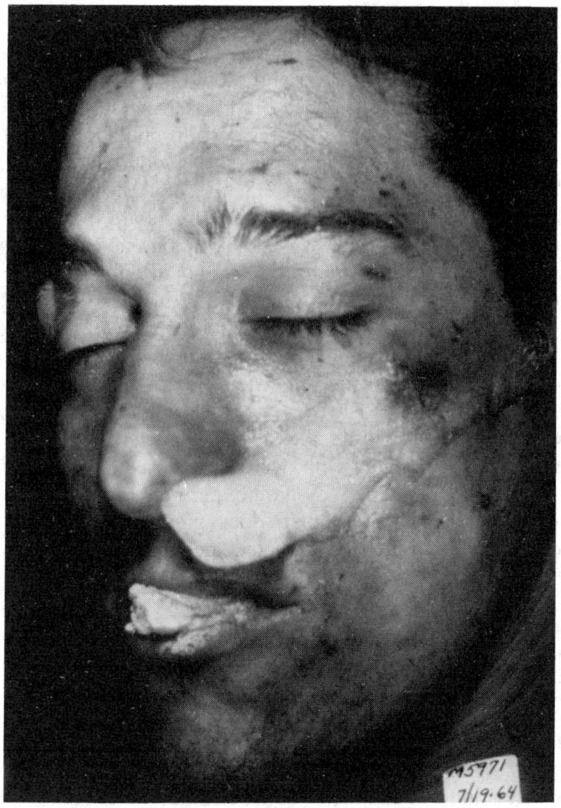

FIGURE 13.1-7. *Pulmonary edema is often associated with heroin overdose. (Courtesy Michael Baden, M.D.)*

way may be inserted. The patient should be ventilated mechanically until naloxone, a special opioid antagonist, can be given. Naloxone is administered intravenously at a slow rate—initially, about 0.8 mg per 70 kg of body weight. Signs of improvement—increase in respiratory rate and pupillary dilation—should occur promptly. In physically dependent addicts, too much naloxone may produce signs of withdrawal, as well as reversal of overdosage. If there is no response to initial dosage, naloxone may be repeated after intervals of about 5 minutes. In past years, it was thought that if no response is observed after 4 to 5 mg, the CNS depression is probably not due solely to opioids. However, buprenorphine, which is now available, is difficult to antagonize with naloxone, and higher doses may be required. The duration of action of naloxone is short compared to many opioids, such as methadone, and repeated administration may be required to prevent recurrence of opioid toxicity.

TREATMENT OF OPIOID DEPENDENCE

Some of the treatment alternatives to be described, such as opioid maintenance, are not currently available in other countries, and not all options are equally accessible in all parts of the United States.

MAJOR MODALITIES Treatment for opioid dependence may involve outpatient, inpatient, residential, or day care settings. The activities may be centered within hospitals, clinics, prisons, or free-standing, unaffiliated organizations. The staff may consist solely of ex-addicts with minimal training, correctional officers, formally trained health care professionals, or some combination of those personnel. The program may emphasize group, individual, or family interactions; all drugs may be proscribed in some programs, whereas other programs may be founded on the use of a drug (e.g., methadone). Theoretically, programs with scores of different combinations of environment, staffing, philosophy, and pharmacological agents are possible; however, in practice, there are only a few major program varieties, each of which may have several subvarieties. The major program varieties include methadone maintenance, detoxification, residential or therapeutic communities, and outpatient drug-free programs. Although other program types exist, such as those utilizing narcotic antagonists, it is estimated that three-fourths of opioid users treated annually in the United States are treated in one of these four types of programs. Many opioid users benefit from participation in self-help groups, such as Alcoholics Anonymous (AA) or Narcotics Anonymous (NA), in conjunction with participation in a formal program or individual psychotherapy. In some cases, such participation is the sole means to begin to maintain control of drug use.

GENERAL PRINCIPLES Patients' willingness to accept treatment may change over time as life circumstances, family relationships, and the severity and complications of the dependence change. Consideration should be given not only to the characteristics, wishes, and previous experiences of patients, but also to how the patients are likely to react to the particular treatments that are economically and geographically feasible.

The clinician should make it clear that treatment requires commitment to long-term change of life-style, attitude, family dynamics, and, sometimes, even geographical location and that the responsibility for making the changes belongs to the patient. The clinician should not rest content with making a diagnosis of opioid dependence, but should make a complete psychiatric assessment and take a thorough drug use history. Most opioid users have additional psychiatric disorders (Table 13.1-14). The severity of psychological difficulties—for example, depression, anxiety, paranoid ideation—and patterns of nonopioid drug use are major predictors of outcome in treatment. Patients, however, should also understand that, although antecedent stresses, environmental conditions, and underlying psychological difficulties may have played important roles in the genesis of drug dependence, opioid dependence, once established, will not spontaneously resolve, even if these conditions are improved. Clinicians must communicate the necessity for treating the pathological drug use as a disorder in its own right. Opioid addicts who enter therapeutic communities under pressure from the criminal justice system are almost as likely to benefit from treatment as those who enter for other reasons. Moreover, court pressure can strongly enhance retention in treatment.

DETOXIFICATION As a general rule, patients who have not been dependent on opioids for more than a year or who have not previously made any attempts at withdrawal are not appropriate candidates for prolonged opioid maintenance.

Standard techniques Detoxification programs may be either outpatient or inpatient. For more than a decade, federal regulations limited the time period for prescribing opioid drugs in outpatient detoxification programs to 21 days, although many programs provided for additional psychological support after the 3-week period. These regulations are now being made more flexible at the federal level, but states are still permitted to have more restrictive regulations.

Currently, the drug most often used to ameliorate the severity of withdrawal is oral methadone; and, except for medical addicts, this drug is the only available opioid approved for this purpose by federal regulations. Theoretically, however, any opioid could be administered and then gradually reduced. In general, the objective in treating hospitalized patients is to make the withdrawal experience tolerable rather than to suppress all symptoms of withdrawal. Patients should be told to expect some discomfort. For patients using street drugs, the initial dosage of methadone is usually 10 to 20 mg orally. If signs of withdrawal persist, the dose can be repeated after about 2 hours. As a general rule, initial stabilization does not require more than 40 mg of methadone during the first 24 hours. Physicians and others with access to pure drugs are exceptions to this general rule and may require higher doses. If the daily dose of opioid—for example, heroin, meperidine, hydromorphone (Dilaudid)—is known, the equivalent withdrawal-suppressing dose of methadone can be found in standard pharmacology texts.

Because the objective of treatment is to prevent severe withdrawal, the current tendency is to base dosage on history rather than to wait for obvious withdrawal or to precipitate withdrawal with naloxone. Caution should be used when giving doses above 40 mg of methadone per day because accumulation of methadone can lead to serious toxicity. Once the patient is stabilized, the dosage of methadone can be gradually reduced. This reduction in dosage can usually be accomplished within 10 days when patients are hospitalized using dose reductions of 10 to 20 percent per day. In some cases of low-level dependence, the withdrawal process can be accomplished within 1 or 2 days by precipitating symptoms with repeated doses of naloxone and ameliorating discomfort with diazepam (Valium) or clonidine. This technique permits rapid transfer onto naltrexone. If the detoxification process is to be successful with outpatients, the time required may have to be extended considerably. Some clinicians recommend 10 percent per week as the maximum rate of reduction from high dosage and reductions of 3 percent per week when the daily dosage is below 20 mg. Patients may be unwilling to accept such a long period of treatment.

Despite the best efforts of clinicians and the use of slow detoxification, all studies to date indicate that relapse rates following successful outpatient or inpatient detoxification are high. The relapse rates are particularly high for users of street heroin who attempt to detoxify on an outpatient basis. For such patients, extending the period of withdrawal from 3 weeks to 6 weeks or using a longer-acting drug, such as LAAM, does not appear to alter a pattern of almost universal, rapid return to illicit opioid use. In a study in which drug users were detoxified over a 90-day period with either methadone or sublingual buprenorphine, both groups did equally poorly in terms of dropping out and reverting to illicit opioids.

Patients who have formed a relationship with the therapist or who have been maintained for some time on methadone have, by comparison, a far better prognosis than others.

Other agents for detoxification Clonidine, an α_2-agonist originally marketed as an antihypertensive, has been shown to suppress some elements of the opioid withdrawal syndrome. With patients stabilized on relatively low doses of opioids (e.g., 30 to 40 mg of oral methadone per day), the opioids can be abruptly discontinued and clonidine used to attenuate withdrawal. Clonidine is given orally, starting at doses of 0.1 to 0.3 mg, three to four times per day. In outpatient settings, total dosage above 1.0 mg per day is not recommended, although higher doses, 1.5 to 2.5 mg, have been used with hospitalized patients. The major side effects are hypotension, which can be quite extreme, and sedation, and the dosage must be carefully individualized. Patients in outpatient clinics who have been stabilized on methadone and have developed a relationship with the therapists are more successful in achieving abstinence when treated with clonidine than are patients who were taking illicit heroin when clonidine treatment was begun. Some studies have found that outpatients who are detoxified with clonidine are almost as successful as outpatients who are treated with decreasing doses of methadone. In hospitalized patients, clonidine permits more rapid detoxification from opioids than does gradual withdrawal of methadone, and patients so treated are more likely to complete the detoxification process.

Clonidine appears to be least effective in suppressing post-withdrawal muscle aches, lethargy, insomnia, restlessness, and craving. There is no evidence that clonidine is useful in preventing relapse after the completion of detoxification. It does appear to facilitate the detoxification of methadone-maintained patients and their stabilization on naltrexone. Properly used, this combination can shorten the period of hospitalization required for detoxification to about 5 or 6 days.

This technique has been used in a day hospital outpatient setting. In a study in which 14 heroin abusers, who responded with obvious withdrawal symptoms to an intramuscular (IM) challenge of 0.8 mg of naloxone, were given oral clonidine three times a day with dosage (range 0.1 to 0.3 mg) adjusted on the basis of severity of dependence and blood pressure response on the first day, naltrexone was started on the second day. Naltrexone dose was given four times a day and increased from the initial 1 mg (orally), so that by days 3 to 5, the patients were receiving 40, 50, and 150 mg, respectively. Of the 14 subjects, 12 were successfully discharged on maintenance naltrexone; 30 days later, five subjects were still taking naltrexone (and three others made unverified claims that they were drug-free).

Other agonists, lofexidine and guanabenz, which are still investigational drugs, appear to have opioid withdrawal ameliorating actions.

Other techniques Because opioid withdrawal is rarely life-threatening in healthy adults, a variety of nonpharmacological, more traditional approaches to drug abstinence have been and continue to be utilized. Abrupt (cold turkey) withdrawal, coupled with considerable emotional support, is still used in some therapeutic communities. Abrupt withdrawal is used as a matter of policy in some countries (e.g., Singapore), where it is believed that experiencing severe withdrawal is a deterrent to relapse. Acupuncture also has been utilized to alleviate opioid withdrawal; the release of endogenous opioids provides some rational basis for this approach. Sometimes, herbal medicines aimed at ridding the body of toxic substances are used in a religious or semireligious context (Fig. 13.1-8). There is no evidence to indicate that when these traditional approaches are used in their own cultural settings, the outcome is any better or worse than more medically sophisticated approaches typically used in the United States.

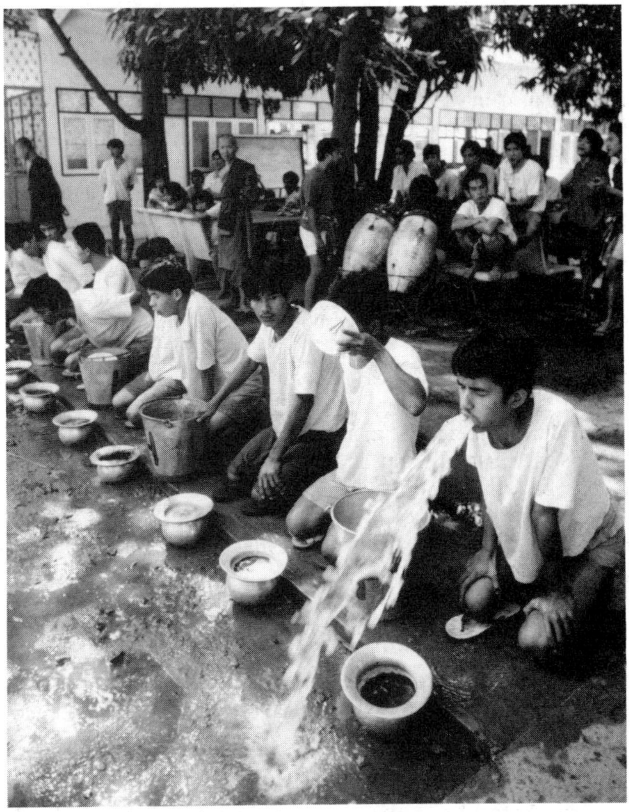

FIGURE 13.1-8. *Treatment of addicts at Tham Krabok Monastery in Thailand results in a 70 percent success rate, according to its records. The 10-day free treatment begins with a vow to Buddha never to use narcotics again. Then patients are given an herbal medicine that makes them vomit immediately. (From White P T, Raymer S: The poppy—for good and evil. Nat Geograph* 167: *187, 1985, with permission.)*

Postdetoxification Because brief detoxification alone is generally followed by relapse, some authorities believe that detoxification should be provided only as part of a more comprehensive treatment effort. Other experts feel that brief detoxification should be available for those addicts who want only a limited service.

COUNSELING Counseling and family and individual psychotherapy are sometimes used, but they have not been satisfactorily evaluated. A self-help group of abstinent drug addicts, NA is modeled on the principles of AA. Branches now exist in most large cities and can provide useful group support. Opioid users assigned to a group support approach, based on the principle that drug users can learn to avoid or cope with those situations that provoke drug cravings or feelings of withdrawal, had lower rates of relapse than addicts assigned to control groups.

OPIOID ANTAGONISTS The use of opioid antagonists to treat opioid dependence is based on the assumption that classically conditioned withdrawal symptoms and operantly reinforced drug-seeking behavior contribute to the high relapse rate that typically occurs after withdrawal from opioids. Theoretically, by blocking the euphoric effects of opioids, treatment with antagonists leads to the extinction of operantly reinforced drug seeking; by preventing the reestablishment of physical dependence, treatment with antagonists also leads to the eventual extinction of conditioned withdrawal phenomena. Various antagonists (e.g., cyclazocine, naloxone, and naltrexone) have been subjected to clinical trials. These drugs do produce the expected blockade of opioid effects, and their toxicity is low; however, in every trial with each drug, the dropout rate has been exceedingly high.

Naltrexone would appear to be an ideal drug for use in therapy. It is orally effective, and when given three times a week (in doses of 100 mg on weekdays, and 150 mg on the weekend), it completely blocks the effects of substantial doses of heroin. When naloxone was tested in a multiclinic, double-blind study, however, very few of those subjects who initially expressed interest in the drug actually took a single dose. Of patients already detoxified, about half began treatment with naltrexone, but the dropout rate was quite high: 25 percent of those subjects starting treatment dropped out within 2 weeks, and 94 percent stopped by 9 months. At the 6-month follow-up, there were few differences between the naltrexone group and the placebo control group, although the naltrexone group had fewer urine specimens positive for opioids while they were in treatment. In other clinical trials, subjects continued to take naltrexone for an average of 6 to 8 weeks.

Experienced clinicians believe that double-blind placebo trials are not the most appropriate way to assess the utility of long-acting antagonists. Experienced clinicians who want to reduce the probability of relapse believe that a period of 30 to 60 days of treatment with naltrexone immediately after detoxification is helpful. New techniques using clonidine to facilitate transfer from methadone to naltrexone may increase the utility of naltrexone, as described above.

OPIOID MAINTENANCE **Methadone programs** Currently, methadone maintenance programs are providing treatment to about 70,000 patients at any given time. Thus, methadone maintenance is a major modality for treating opioid dependence.

Initiated by Dole and Nyswander in 1964, the maintenance approach postulated that high doses of methadone would alleviate "drug hunger" and simultaneously block, by means of cross-tolerance, any euphoria produced by self-administered heroin. Thus, opioid users would be freed from the preoccupation with drug-seeking behavior and, with help and rehabilitation, could channel their energies into more productive avenues. The first several hundred chronic heroin addicts treated with this approach showed dramatic decreases in use of illicit opioids, decreased criminal activity, and increased legitimate, productive work. Furthermore, patients showed little tendency to discontinue treatment, as was the case with other treatment approaches. On the basis of these results, Dole and Nyswander further postulated that opioid dependence is unrelated to antecedent psychological difficulties and that most of the traits of instability and unreliability seen in addicts are the consequence, rather than the cause, of their opioid addiction.

Within the span of a few years, other programs utilizing methadone were established. The results were often less dramatic than those seen by Dole and Nyswander, especially because criteria for program entry were broadened and more disturbed and less motivated patients were admitted.

GENERAL PHARMACOLOGY Given acutely, methadone is a typical μ-receptor agonist producing euphoria, analgesia, and other typical morphine-like effects. Given chronically by the oral route, however, methadone has several properties that make it particularly useful in maintenance programs. These qualities include its reliable absorption and bioavailability after oral administration, the delay of peak plasma levels until 2 to 6 hours after ingestion, and the apparent nonspecific binding to tissues that creates a large reservoir of methadone in the body. This large reservoir, combined with slow time to peak effects, buffers the patients against sharp peaks in subjective effects after ingestion, which, in any event, are highly attenuated as a result of tolerance. The reservoir of methadone also tends to minimize any sharp declines that would induce withdrawal. Thus, administration of methadone on a once-a-day schedule is possible, and minor variations in dosage over short periods do not induce major changes in biological effects. Although the mean plasma half-life in naive subjects is about 15 hours, it may range from approximately 22 to 56 hours, depending on the measurement technique used, in methadone-maintained subjects.

STANDARD PROCEDURES AND GOVERNMENT REGULATIONS
Beginning in 1972, opioid maintenance programs were required to operate within detailed federal, state, and, sometimes, local regulations. Under current federal regulations, opioid-dependent individuals who are less than 16 years old or have been dependent for less than one year can be detoxified using opioids for a 21-day period, but cannot be maintained beyond that period without an opioid-free interval. Regulations also govern maximum take-home dosage (100 mg) and duration of daily clinic treatment before take-home dosage can be provided (90 days). Under proposed changes in these regulations, the permissible period for detoxification will be extended to 180 days.

PHILOSOPHICAL DIFFERENCES AMONG PROGRAMS Methadone maintenance programs vary with respect to dosage, attitudes toward continued antisocial behavior, medical and social services provided, and long-term goals. The original programs emphasized methadone dosage sufficient to suppress opioid drug hunger and to induce a cross-tolerance blockade of the effects of illicit opioids, usually 80 to 120 mg per day. Patients were encouraged to remain on methadone indefinitely on the assumption that the return of opioid drug hunger following detoxification would lead to relapse and loss of any gains achieved during treatment.

Other programs use lower doses of methadone (20 to 60 mg per day) that are often adequate for suppressing drug seeking, but not for producing cross-tolerance to large doses of heroin. Such programs generally view maintenance as a transitional stage to eventual detoxification. Although patients may remain in treatment in such programs indefinitely, the ambience is often more supportive of efforts at gradual withdrawal.

In both types of programs, there is often a continuing struggle with patients over take-home doses. Patients who do not respond to treatment generally continue to use illicit opioids or nonopioids, to use alcohol to excess, to attend the programs very irregularly, or to engage in combative behavior at the clinic. Such patients pose a dilemma to both types of methadone maintenance programs, because they would probably fare worse if discharged. However, permitting them to remain demoralizes staff and other patients and often increases drug use among the latter.

LONG-TERM EFFECTS The relative safety of methadone maintenance in terms of organ toxicity is firmly established. Tolerance to many of the opioid agonist actions of methadone is incomplete, however, and continuing pharmacological effects are observed. Many of these effects, such as euphoria, drowsiness, and somnolence, are more prominent in the first weeks of treatment; if the dosage level is increased too rapidly, they also may be seen at later points in treatment. Some effects, however, persist even after many months of treatment. Among the most common long-lasting effects are constipation, which can sometimes result in fecal impaction and intestinal obstruction, excessive sweating, complaints of decreased libido, and sexual dysfunction—for example, inability to sustain an erection. Opioids reduce plasma levels of testosterone and follicle-stimulating hormone for which tolerance is often incomplete, but the correlation between abnormally low plasma levels of hormones and sexual dysfunction is not high. Both sleep abnormalities (insomnia and nightmares), and altered electroencephalogram (EEG) sleep patterns frequently occur during the first months of methadone treatment; the EEG sleep patterns appear to return to baseline, but complaints of sleep abnormalities may persist.

Tolerance does not develop in all patients to the mood-elevating effects of methadone. In double-blind studies, patients regularly report a greater sense of well-being a few hours after ingesting their daily dose. For some patients, this effect may be an important factor in retention in treatment.

IN-TREATMENT OUTCOME The majority of patients treated in methadone programs show significant decreases in opioid and nonopioid drug use, criminal behavior, and symptoms of depression, as well as increases in gainful employment. Significant differences in effectiveness across programs are due, in some measure, to the characteristics of patients treated, but certain programmatic features tend to make some programs more effective than others. In 1980, the average retention rate for a group of methadone clinics participating in a national prospective study was 81 percent at 1 month, 67 percent at 3 months, and 52 percent at 6 months. Programs espousing the view that methadone is more of a transitional treatment leading to abstinence, those utilizing only lower doses of methadone (20 to 40 mg), or those employing more confrontational techniques tend to have lower retention rates than those programs viewing indefinite treatment as optimal, those using high doses or flexible dosage, or those using support, rather than confrontation. Older, black, married, and employed patients tend to be retained in methadone programs longer. Those patients with extensive criminal backgrounds tend to drop out sooner and to perform more poorly while in treatment. Severity or duration of opioid use does not correlate with retention or performance in treatment.

DETOXIFICATION AND LONG-TERM OUTCOME Among those patients who successfully detoxify after a period of maintenance, the percentage of patients remaining abstinent at periods of 12 to 36 months ranges from 12 to 28 percent for unselected samples of patients, some of whom were discharged for violation of clinic rules, to 83 percent remaining abstinent from opioids, when analysis is restricted to those patients who elect to be withdrawn with staff and patient consensus that treatment is complete. Predictors of retention and positive outcome in treatment do not necessarily predict success in achieving abstinence or long-term positive outcome once withdrawal is completed.

In general, patients with shorter drug histories who have been maintained in the program for longer periods but at lower dosages seem more successful than other patients in detoxifying. In a national, multiclinic follow-up study, 40 percent of former methadone patients interviewed were not using any illicit opioids and did not have any other significant drug problems 6 years after completion of initial treatment.

Other opioid maintenance drugs LAAM is an opioid that is quite similar to methadone in its pharmacological actions; it is converted into active metabolites that have very long biological half-lives. Consequently, LAAM can be given as infrequently as three times per week, thereby reducing the inconvenience of daily clinic attendance to ingest the drug and simultaneously reducing concerns about illicit diversion. When LAAM is abruptly discontinued, the withdrawal syndrome is slow in onset and relatively mild in intensity, but it is at least as protracted as that of methadone. Over the past 15 years, in both double-blind and large-scale, multicenter open studies, LAAM has been shown to be equivalent to methadone in terms of suppressing illicit opioid use and encouraging productive activity. It has been consistently found, however, that retention in treatment with LAAM is lower than with methadone. A small percentage of patients complain of side effects not commonly seen with methadone, such as nervousness, stimulation, and amphetamine-like effects. The pharmacology of LAAM is more complex than that of methadone, and its use demands a more skilled clinician than does methadone. It is currently an investigational drug.

BUPRENORPHINE A partial μ-receptor agonist, buprenorphine is now available as an analgesic. Buprenorphine produces morphine-like effects at low doses; it has a ceiling effect, so the intensity of its actions does not seem to exceed that achieved with 30 to 60 mg of morphine. Because of this ceiling, risk of overdose may be limited. After chronic administration, buprenorphine attenuates or blocks the subjective effects of parenterally administered morphine or heroin, but it is unclear whether this action is due to cross-tolerance or antagonist-like actions. In experimental settings, chronic heroin users given access to IV heroin sharply reduce their heroin intake when maintained on subcutaneous buprenorphine. Buprenorphine has been proposed as an alternative to methadone in opioid maintenance programs.

HEROIN VS. METHADONE Oral methadone has been compared with IV heroin at a London clinic in a random assignment study. Most subjects assigned to heroin continued to inject opioids and stayed involved with the drug culture. Some of the heroin subjects sold part of their prescriptions; other subjects supplemented clinic supplies with opioids from illicit sources. Some of the subjects assigned to oral methadone maintenance refused to participate and left treatment immediately; many other subjects left subsequently. At 12 months, only 29 percent of oral methadone patients were still at the clinic; of those who left the clinic, 40 percent (28 of those initially assigned to oral methadone) were no longer using opioids regularly at the 1-year follow-up. Over the 12-month period, more heroin patients than oral methadone patients died or were admitted to hospitals for drug-related problems. A strong relationship was found between criminal activity and continued illicit opioid use, although differences in baseline rates of criminality make it difficult to evaluate the net impact of the two types of treatment on crime. As in U.S. clinics, at admission, about one-third of the London patients were mildly depressed, 58 percent had a history of depressive episodes, and 38 percent had attempted suicide.

THERAPEUTIC COMMUNITIES The underlying philosophy of the more than 300 therapeutic communities that have evolved from Synanon is that the drug addict is emotionally immature and requires a total immersion in a specialized social structure in order to modify lifelong, destructive behavioral patterns. The goal is to effect a complete change of life-style, including the abstinence from drugs, the development of personal honesty and useful social skills, and the elimination of antisocial attitudes and criminal behavior.

To achieve these objectives, the addict was expected to live in the therapeutic community for approximately 12 to 18 months and to participate in frequent group sessions devoted to mutual criticisms of the attitudes and behavior of the participants. The group sessions, called encounter groups, or games, often involve rather harsh confrontations and remain a key element in all present-day therapeutic communities. The community also acts in many respects as a substitute family. Assumption of responsibility within the community is rewarded with increased personal freedom, material comfort, and the respect of peers. Deviation from community expectations, in terms of behavior or attitude, frequently results in harsh criticisms by staff or, sometimes, by the entire community. Violence and any form of drug use is totally prohibited and may result in expulsion from the community—the ultimate punishment. Although most therapeutic communities avoid the use of drugs even to ease initial withdrawal, some are more flexible regarding treatment with drugs for heavily dependent new entrants. More recently, some therapeutic communities have recognized that a high percentage of addicts have psychopathologies in addition to drug dependence. In some cases, residents may be prescribed antipsychotic or antidepressant drugs.

Although Synanon pointedly rejected any role for mental health professionals, relying solely on ex-addicts as staff, present-day therapeutic communities vary considerably in attitudes toward professionals and in actual staffing patterns. In every community, however, at least a few ex-addicts are employed as key personnel on the staff; the ex-addicts serve as role models and visible signs that recovery and acceptance are possible and expected. Some therapeutic communities, such as Phoenix House and Odyssey House, are directed by psychiatrists and employ a number of health professionals in key positions. Quite recently, a number of federally supported programs have begun to develop individualized treatment plans and to use health care professionals, such as physicians, psychologists, or master's level counselors or social workers, to make initial assessments.

Although most therapeutic communities still expect residents to return to the general community after 12 to 18 months, some are experimenting with shorter periods of residence. Because they require so long a period of residence, therapeutic communities obviously have little appeal to those opioid addicts who have stable and gainful employment and satisfactory marital relationships.

In their early years, 1964 to 1970, therapeutic communities were quite selective, forcing applicants to show a high degree of motivation before they were accepted. Despite this selectivity, dropout rates were quite high: about 50 percent in the first 90 days, 70 percent within 6 months, and up to 90 percent by 12 months. Retention rates for several of the well-established therapeutic communities are shown in Fig. 13.1-9. More recently, a substantial proportion of entrants into therapeutic communities have been referred by the criminal justice system. Criteria for entry have thus been modified,

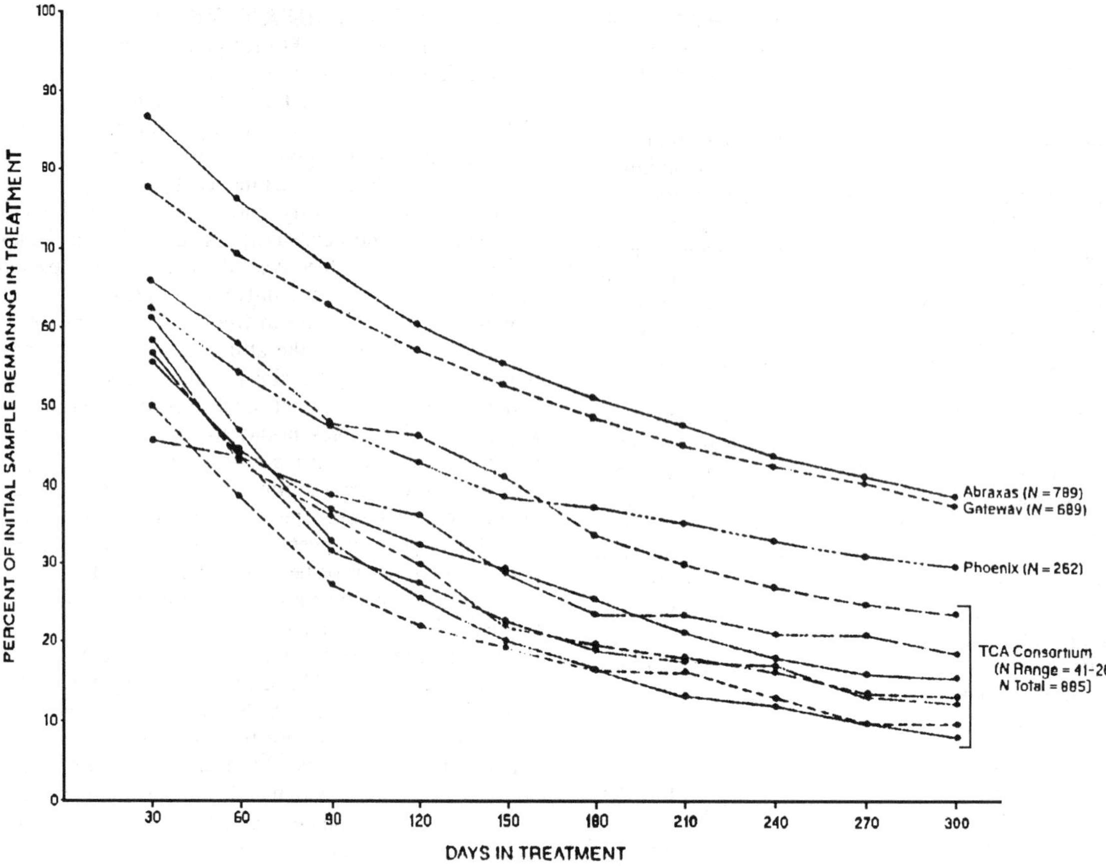

FIGURE 13.1-9. *Retention curves for Abraxas (1979 to 1983 admissions); Gateway Foundation (February 1981 to June 1983 admissions); Phoenix House (January to April 1981 admissions) and seven members of a TCA consortium (February 1 to August 15, 1979 admissions). (From Pompi K F, Resnick J: Retention of court referred adolescents. J Substance Abuse Treat* 13: *3, 1987, with permission.)*

and external pressure to remain in treatment has been increased. However, the dropout rates remain about as high as formerly, when external pressure was less common. Furthermore, the percentage of new entrants with severe psychopathology has been gradually increasing.

Residence in the therapeutic community results in major reductions in drug use problems; indicators of depression also decrease significantly. Follow-up studies of graduates and dropouts indicate that patients remaining 90 days or longer exhibit significant decreases in self-reported antisocial behavior, illicit drug use, and recorded arrests, as well as substantial increases in legitimate employment. In general, for those without severe psychopathology, there is a consistent time-in-program effect up to about 12 months; those patients who stay longer exhibit better outcomes along all dimensions at 12-month and 5-year follow-up intervals. In some cases, patients found to be doing well have had additional treatment in other programs since leaving the therapeutic community.

OUTPATIENT DRUG-FREE PROGRAMS Outpatient treatment programs often subscribe to the same goals as the residential or therapeutic communities, but they attempt to achieve these goals in a setting involving less than 24 hours a day. The programs vary widely in staffing patterns, philosophy, and program content; they range from highly organized daytime therapeutic communities to drop-in centers offering conversational ("rap") sessions and recreational activities. Outpatient drug-free programs tend to deal more with multiple drug abusers than with heavily addicted users of opioids, although heroin addicts are treated by some programs. Long-term follow-up suggests that these programs have an impact beyond that seen with detoxification alone, but differences in patient characteristics make valid comparisons difficult. Self-help groups, such as AA and NA, must always be mentioned as both supplements and alternatives to outpatient drug-free therapies. The possible benefits of non–AA-oriented group therapies, built around the theme of cognitive help in coping with crises and avoiding situations that engender craving, have been described above.

PSYCHOTHERAPIES As measured by use of illicit drugs, need for ancillary psychotropic medicines, scores on scales of psychological distress, and amount of legitimate money earned, patients entering methadone maintenance programs appear to benefit more from individual, analytically oriented, and supportive-expressive psychotherapy than from standard drug counseling alone. Individual, cognitive behaviorally oriented therapy is also superior to counseling alone. With such therapy, the very bleak prognosis for patients with the severest psychopathology can be improved. For the most effective results, individual therapy should be started early and be an integral part of the program.

Among methadone-maintained patients, one controlled study suggests that, if urinalysis results are available to monitor drug use, skillful family therapy is superior to standard drug counseling in fostering decreased illicit drug use over a

6-month follow-up period. There are no controlled studies on the efficacy of psychotherapy in treating patients not stabilized on methadone.

TREATMENT OF SPECIAL POPULATIONS **Criminal justice clients** The criminal justice system has complex interactions with drug dependence treatment systems. Many patients now enter or remain in treatment because of direct coercion by the courts or the correctional system. Conversely, some patients on probation or parole may enter treatment against the wishes of their probation officers or in violation of some condition of parole. It was estimated that, in the late 1970s, 15 to 25 percent of opioid-dependent patients treated had some current criminal justice status. The figure for patients entering a methadone program or therapeutic community was above 50 percent. The impact of such coercion on retention in treatment or outcome has been difficult to estimate because of baseline differences between criminal justice and non-criminal justice patients.

In addition to their relationship to the major modalities of treatment, probation or parole, or both, can be viewed as a drug-using behavior-modifying technique in its own right. Close supervision and antinarcotic testing of parolees result in a substantial reduction in daily narcotics use. Presumably, testing for other drugs could deter their use as well.

Although they remain on the law books, civil commitment programs for opioid users involving long periods of institutional care have lost popularity. They were exceedingly expensive compared to all other treatment modalities, and there was no evidence of their long-term efficacy.

TREATMENT OF PATIENTS WITH ADDITIONAL PSYCHOPATHOLOGY The severity of psychological disturbances—depression, anxiety, paranoid ideation—are major predictors of the overall outcome of treatment for opioid dependence. Other major predictors of outcome include alcoholism and use of nonopioid drugs.

Mood disorders Some form of mood dysregulation is the most common psychiatric disorder found among opioid addicts in treatment (Table 13.1-14). Clinicians agree that those addicts with manic, hypomanic, or bipolar disorders (lifetime prevalence among clinic patients is 5 to 10 percent) can benefit from treatment with lithium. Lithium has been used in combination with methadone without adverse interactions.

Although clinicians in private practice often prescribe such antidepressants as amitriptyline (Elavil) or doxepin (Sinequan) for opioid-dependent patients with major and minor depression, publicly supported programs often do not. The reasons for not prescribing those drugs vary. In the past, therapeutic communities had a general bias against the use of psychoactive agents; methadone programs do not have a bias against pharmacotherapy, but most did not commonly assess depressive symptoms, responding only when symptoms become clinically obvious. The efficacy of antidepressants in treatment of depressed opioid-dependent patients has yet to be clarified. Doxepin, 100 mg daily, mixed with the methadone, produced more rapid improvement in depressive symptoms over a 4-week period than a placebo, but the magnitude of the difference was not great. In contrast, imipramine (Tofranil), average dose 140 mg per day, was no better than a placebo in methadone-maintained patients; both groups showed significant improvements. Because the pharmacokinetics of imipramine and desipramine (Norpramin) are affected by tobacco smoking and use of methadone, adequate plasma levels may not have been achieved. Depressive symptoms among opioid addicts tend to decrease after entry into treatment, whether the treatment is an opioid maintenance program or a therapeutic community. Not every patient, however, shows spontaneous improvement. Since severity of psychological impairment is such a major predictor of overall treatment success, the conscientious clinician will pay particular attention to persistent depression.

Schizophrenic syndromes Although lifetime rates for schizotypal features is 6 to 8 percent among clinic patients, frank schizophrenia is uncommon—less than 1 percent. For those patients with frank schizophrenia, dopamine-blocking antipsychotic agents are probably useful and can be combined with methadone. For some drug users, opioids, including methadone, seem to exert some antipsychotic effects, enabling patients to control paranoid and delusional ideation. There are case reports but, as yet, no controlled studies of opioid users whose psychotic-schizophreniform or delusional states responded to opioids, but only poorly to more traditional antipsychotic agents. The endogenous opioids interact with dopaminergic systems, as described above, and it has been postulated that methadone has antimanic and antipsychotic actions. Addicts may develop tolerance to the antipsychotic effects of opioids so that, after a period on methadone, psychosis may break through again. Some clinicians believe that underlying rage and hostility may play causal roles in opioid dependence and that some addicts use the opioids to control these affects. Clinicians have also observed that, although the psychotic patients are reassured by the structure of the usual methadone clinic, borderline patients make the structure and the rules the objects of an all-out war, leading to their rapid and premature discharge from the clinic program.

Anxiety disorders Anxiety disorders rarely receive specific treatment in programs devoted to opioid dependence. A very high percentage of those addicts with anxiety also have dysphoric disorders. When treatment seems indicated, tricyclic antidepressants, such as doxepin, would appear to be the drugs of choice, because they have antianxiety, antipanic, and antidepressant effects. Also, patients with anxiety disorders may abuse benzodiazepines.

Alcoholism Among opioid addicts in treatment, alcoholism is common, with a lifetime diagnosis rate of 25 to 40 percent. Most addicts that are diagnosed as alcoholic are also diagnosed as having some form of mood disorder. Among patients in a methadone program, neither sessions with special AA counselors twice a week nor behavioral modification sessions provided by psychologists were better than a control condition of standard maintenance. However, most alcoholics showed decrease in alcohol consumption after entering treatment, and patients and counselors who participated in treatment were enthusiastic about group sessions and believed they were beneficial. Disulfiram (Antabuse) can be combined with methadone without adverse effects, and, in small experimental studies, program privileges, such as take-home doses of methadone, have been made contingent on ingestion of disulfiram. In controlled studies, however, disulfiram was not superior to placebo in modifying alcoholism among methadone-maintained patients.

Thus, although alcoholism while in treatment is reported to be a major predictor of reversion to opioid abuse following detoxification from methadone, it appears there is no demonstrably effective specific intervention to reduce alcohol use. Continued participation in a residential program sharply reduces alcohol use, but data on long-term outcome are lacking.

Opioid dependence combined with abuse of nonopioids Up to 25 percent of opioid users regularly self-administer some other category of drug—for example, amphetamines, cocaine, alcohol, barbiturates, benzodiazepines, or cannabinoids—in amounts sufficient to cause problems. In general, such individuals have a greater range and severity of psychiatric problems than those persons dependent on opioids only. In therapeutic communities, mixed abusers create more behavior problems, drop out of treatment sooner, and have poorer posttreatment outcomes than uncomplicated opioid users. Although some mixed abusers do not use opioids heavily enough to qualify for treatment in methadone programs, many such persons are, indeed, eligible. One study retrospectively matched mixed abusers—all male veterans with greater than average psychopathology—who entered a therapeutic community with those who entered a methadone maintenance program, in an attempt to compare outcomes as a function of the category of drugs abused and the treatment received. The patients were further categorized into opioid-stimulant, opioid-depressant, and opioid-only users. At a 6-month follow-up interview, there were clear-cut differences in outcome. Opioid-only patients had better outcomes on all measures than either of the other groups, and for opioid-only patients, there was no clear superiority of either treatment approach. Opioid-stimulant patients did significantly better in methadone maintenance programs, whereas opioid-depressant patients did significantly better after treatment in a therapeutic community. It was speculated that the hypersensitivity and paranoia of the opioid-stimulant group is alleviated by the effects of methadone and is aggravated by the confrontational techniques used in the therapeutic community. It was also inferred that the prolonged abstinence afforded by the therapeutic community was helpful in facilitating recovery from the depression and cognitive impairment that typically accompanies use of sedatives.

PROGNOSIS The usual measures of treatment outcome (legitimate work, crime, drug use, family relationships, psychological adjustment) are predicted best by different pretreatment variables. Thus, pretreatment history of high levels of criminal activity most accurately predicts posttreatment criminal activity, and previous stable work history is more predictive of posttreatment gainful employment. Severity of psychological problems at the beginning of treatment, however, is an important predictor of outcome on all dimensions. Those opioid addicts with least severe psychological problems appear to respond better to all treatments on all outcome measures. Depression and life crises (especially arguments and interpersonal losses) are associated with relapse to illicit drug use; these factors are additive. The impact of these risk factors is reduced by treatment in drug abuse programs. Depression is also a risk factor for continued cocaine use among patients in opioid treatment programs; standard methadone maintenance treatment does not appear to have any major effect in reducing cocaine use among opioid users.

Follow-up studies of opioid addicts initially treated at public clinics provide some general estimate of the intermediate-term prognosis of opioid dependence. A random sample of addicts receiving heroin at several London clinics in 1969 was studied 7 years later: 12 percent were dead; 5 percent were in prison; 5 percent were using illicit opioids regularly; 43 percent were still receiving opioids from clinics, 90 percent of whom were still injecting; 7 percent were entirely abstinent from opioids, but were using alcohol or sedatives daily; 24 percent were entirely abstinent and using no other drugs; and the status of 4 percent was uncertain.

In the United States, a stratified sample of black and white males who had used heroin daily and who first entered a number of different treatment programs in 1972 and 1973 was followed up 6 years after entry. Patients had been out of initial treatment for an average of 4 years. Five percent were known to be dead; 29 percent were not located or could not be interviewed; 3 percent were in jail; 13 percent were using illicit opioids regularly; 8 percent were receiving methadone from clinics; 2 percent had been abstinent, but had relapsed; 5 percent were abstinent from opioids, but were using alcohol or nonopioids heavily; and 32 percent were entirely abstinent from opioids and were not abusing other drugs. By the sixth year, many patients had reentered other treatment programs or had been institutionalized for other reasons. There were no longer any important differences in outcome among patients treated initially in different progams, although over shorter follow-up periods, methadone maintenance, therapeutic communities, and drug-free programs were significantly superior to detoxification programs. More recent studies suggest that those addicts electing detoxification are younger and have less psychopathology than those addicts entering more lengthy forms of treatment. Although a period of prolonged abstinence is a good predictor of long-term outcome, in a study of opioid users in San Antonio, 33 percent of those who reported 3 years of abstinence eventually relapsed. The shifting drug using status of 93 San Antonio opioid addicts followed over a 30-year period is shown in Figure 13.1-10.

SEDATIVES, HYPNOTICS, AND ANXIOLYTICS

Most of the numerous chemical entities introduced into clinical medicine as sedative-hypnotics over the past 100 years have also been linked to excessive use, abuse, and dependence. This link has been especially evident in the case of the shorter-acting barbiturates and certain nonbarbiturate sedatives, such as glutethimide (Doriden) and methaqualone. Although the benzodiazepine anxiolytics and hypnotics, introduced into clinical medicine in the early 1960s, are less likely to be abused, their lower abuse potential is only relative. The benzodiazepines can induce physical dependence, which leads to withdrawal syndromes of varying severity on discontinuation, a factor that needs to be considered in using the benzodiazepines in clinical practice.

For purposes of discussing problems of drug dependence and abuse, both custom and overlapping pharmacological actions justify the discussion of barbiturates, barbiturate-like sedative-hypnotics, and the benzodiazepines as a single category. Despite this custom of generalizing, the pharmacological and pharmacokinetic differences among the agents in this diverse category directly influence patterns of abuse, as well as medical and psychological sequelae.

PHARMACOLOGY OF SEDATIVE-ANXIOLYTICS The benzodiazepines exert their actions at a distinct receptor site which is part of a larger γ-aminobutyric acid (GABA) receptor-gated chloride ion channel. Those benzodiazepines which act as agonists at the benzodiazepine receptor site on this complex increase the binding of GABA, which, in turn, results in opening the chloride channel, an influx of chloride ion, and an inhibition of cellular activity. Some benzodiazepine congeners (e.g., RO 15-1788) bind to this receptor but do not increase GABA binding. They do block the access of benzodiazepines to the benzodiazepine receptor and are therefore called benzodiazepine antagonists. Some agents

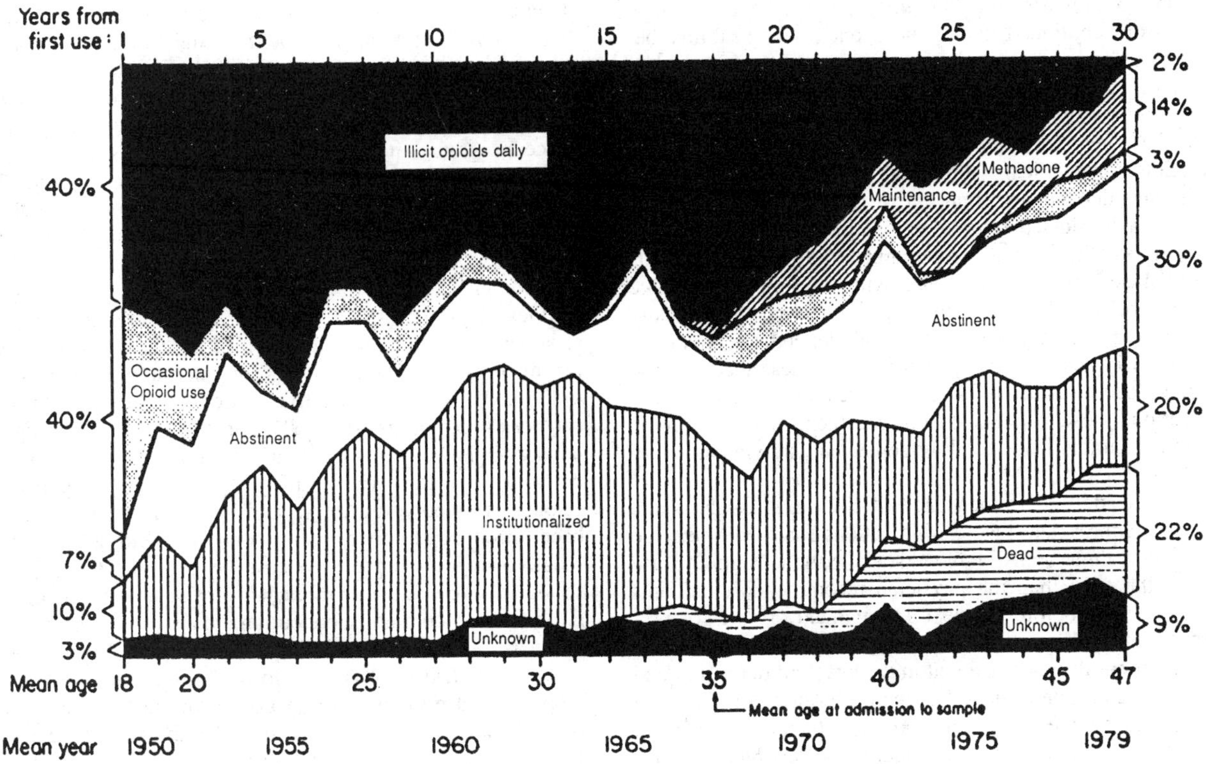

FIGURE 13.1-10. *Drug use status of 93 San Antonio subjects during July of each of 30 years after the onset of opioid use. (From Maddux J F, and Desmond D P: Relapse and recovery in substance abuse careers, 1986)*

acting at this site—such as β-carboline-ethyl ester—actually induce anxiety and seizures and are designated as inverse agonists.

The barbiturates and related drugs act at another site on this GABA-chloride ion channel complex, probably by increasing the likelihood that GABA actions at the complex will open the ion channel. Many barbiturate-like agents appear to act at this barbiturate sensitive site. When an animal is trained to respond to a benzodiazepine drug cue, benzodiazepine antagonists interfere with animals' capacity to discriminate a benzodiazepine drug cue from a placebo, but the animal is still able to discriminate a barbiturate from a placebo. In addition, in animals physically dependent on benzodiazepines, such benzodiazepine antagonists can precipitate benzodiazepine withdrawal but do not precipitate withdrawal in animals dependent on barbiturates. Thus, despite the very similar clinical manifestations of barbiturate and benzodiazepine withdrawal syndromes (see below), these classes of drugs differ in their sites of action at the GABA receptor ion complex. Naturally occurring ligands with some activity at the benzodiazepine receptor site have been isolated from brain tissue.

In addition to these differences in site and mechanism of action between the benzodiazepines and the barbiturates and barbiturate-like drugs, there are also wide differences within both categories of drugs, many of which are related to lipid solubility and duration of action. Equally important, however, are those pharmacological properties and effects that are common to the group. The sedative-hypnotics and benzodiazepines are generally well absorbed orally and, depending on the dose, produce varying degrees of CNS depression. With the barbiturates and related drugs, low doses generally produce some antianxiety effects and some psychomotor and cognitive impairment. Depending on the setting and the individual's experience and degree of tolerance, higher doses may produce disinhibition, gross motor incoordination, impairment of judgment, and some euphoria, or drowsiness and sleep. At very high doses, drugs in this class produce coma, respiratory depression, and death. Taken in therapeutic doses, the benzodiazepines, as a class, seem far less likely to induce euphoria, but are more likely to produce specific anxiolytic actions. They are also more likely to produce memory and psychomotor impairments that are not recognized by the user because the subjective sense of intoxication is less intense. Taken in very high doses, the benzodiazepines, as a class, seem far less likely to induce severe, or fatal, respiratory depression. But they are not totally safe. In most instances of benzodiazepine fatality, the benzodiazepine was used in combination with alcohol. It is claimed that some benzodiazepines have specific antipanic and antidepressant actions. All the drugs in this very heterogeneous category produce various forms of CNS physical dependence (neuroadaptation) having certain common features.

PATTERNS OF ABUSE AND DEPENDENCE There are four major patterns of sedative-anxiolytic dependence. In what is probably the most common pattern, individuals begin to take a prescribed sedative or anxiolytic for insomnia or anxiety. The latter is often secondary to some physical disorder. Over time, there may be some modest increase in dosage, but this increase does not go substantially beyond clinically acceptable limits. For a variety of reasons, drug intake continues. Each attempt to discontinue the drug leads to recrudescence or an exacerbation of insomnia or anxiety, along with other manifestations of the sedative-anxiolytic withdrawal syndrome. Typically, the patient persuades the doctor to continue prescribing the drug. Except for the cost and inconvenience of filling prescriptions, many patients who develop this pattern of dependence exhibit no other signs or symptoms of impairment. Although they may not get much benefit from continued use of the agent, their disability becomes manifest primarily when they try to stop. According to DSM-III-R criteria for dependence, many of these individuals would not be diagnosed as having drug dependence, but would be viewed as having physical dependence (neuroadaptation), a medical rather than a psychiatric disorder. Barbiturate dependence may also develop in individuals taking analgesic-sedative combinations for relief of headache or other somatic complaints. Individuals with this pattern of sedative-anxiolytic use with physical dependence can often be withdrawn on an outpatient basis; they usually have less severe degrees of physical dependence than individuals who exhibit the patterns to be described below. Although occasionally referred to psychiatric units for detoxification, these patients do not see themselves as having the other characteristics of drug-dependent individuals listed in Table 13.1-1.

Another pattern of dependence often begins in the same way, with appropriate medical indications for prescribing the drug. But within weeks or months, the patient begins to use more of the drug than the physician recommended and runs out of medicine before the next appointment or date for prescription refill. When the alert attending physician refuses to prescribe more drug, the patient may engage in deception and subterfuge, claiming to have lost the prescription or obtaining prescriptions for the same drug from more than one physician. In addition to increasing the amount of drug taken at one time, the patient may increase the number of doses per day and, in the case of sedatives, may begin to use the drug during the day as well as at night. In many cases, the use of sedatives and anxiolytics is supplemented by the use of alcohol in individuals who were not previously alcoholic. This general pattern of abuse is often associated with impairment in everyday function, such as impaired memory, labile affect, depression, and psychomotor incoordination. Even though the problem is obvious to family members and co-workers, patients may strongly resist advice to stop drug use or seek treatment. These patients generally meet the criteria for sedative-anxiolytic dependence shown in Table 13.1-1. Individuals in this category may be dependent on high dosages, and because they are often unreliable about disclosing their total dosage, withdrawal on an inpatient basis is generally required. This same caution also applies to the next two patterns of dependence.

Sedative-anxiolytic dependence is commonly seen when individuals with antecedent alcohol abuse or alcoholism begin to use sedatives or anxiolytics to deal with problems caused by alcoholism. Sometimes, the drug use arises from attempts to disguise or suppress alcohol withdrawal symptoms, as when an individual ingests a benzodiazepine instead of alcohol to prevent nausea and tremor (shakes) in the morning. Virtually all of the sedative-anxiolytics in common use are effective suppressors of alcohol withdrawal symptoms. Sometimes, alcohol and sedatives are combined in a deliberate effort to produce or sustain a state of intoxication. The impairment associated with combination of alcohol and anxiolytics may be as great or greater than uncomplicated alcoholism. The combination of alcohol and sedatives is generally believed to be far more toxic than either agent alone.

Still a fourth pattern of dependence may be thought of as classic drug abuse, in which individuals initiate the use of sedative-anxiolytics for their euphoriant and intoxicating actions. Although physicians' prescriptions may be the source of the drugs in some cases, more typically the drugs are obtained from the illicit traffic. For some of these individuals the sedative-anxiolytics may be the drugs of choice, for others the drugs are used to augment the effects of other drugs, such as opioids, or to produce intoxication when opioids are not available. For example, some patients in methadone maintenance programs may take excessive amounts of diazepam; such patients typically claim that the diazepam accentuates the sedative-euphoric effects of the methadone. Sedative-anxiolytics are also used by drug abusers to control or modify the toxicities of cocaine and amphetamines.

Although the sedative-anxiolytics are used most commonly by the oral route, some drug abusers in this subgroup use sedatives by parenteral routes, subjecting themselves to multiple medical risks of infections and dermatological toxicity. Individuals who use sedative-anxiolytics along with other categories of drugs generally meet criteria for drug dependence; however, it is often difficult to know whether or when they meet criteria for any given category of agents. The categories of polydrug abuse and polydrug dependence have been introduced to cover these situations. With all patterns of sedative-anxiolytic excessive use, except the first one described above (i.e., uncomplicated physical dependence), depression is a common concomitant diagnosis.

Occasionally, a mythology, unsupported by known pharmacological actions, develops about a specific drug and perpetuates use in special situations. An outstanding example is methaqualone, which is widely believed to have special euphoriant and aphrodisiac effects.

SEDATIVE-ANXIOLYTIC WITHDRAWAL The signs and symptoms of withdrawal from sedatives, hypnotics, and anxiolytics are quite similar to signs and symptoms of alcohol withdrawal: insomnia, tremulousness, fatigue, weakness, sweating, tachycardia, hypertension, irritability, abdominal upset, nausea, seizures, and delirium. As with alcohol, seizures generally precede delirium. With barbiturate-like sedatives, severe withdrawal can be associated with dysregulation of body temperature and cardiovascular function, which can, on occasion, be fatal. Of these symptoms, insomnia, tremulousness, and anxiety may be the most sensitive, since they appear before other symptoms, often making it difficult to distinguish withdrawal from a recrudescence of the problems for which the drugs were prescribed initially. The diagnostic criteria for sedative, anxiolytic, or hypnotic withdrawal are shown in Table 13.1-15. In DSM-III-R, the diagnostic criteria for benzodiazepine withdrawal are identical to those just listed for barbiturate-sedative withdrawal. However, with benzodiazepine withdrawal, the following have also been reported in the literature: visual, auditory and olfactory perceptual disturbances, depression, somatic anxiety, and transient psychotic episodes.

Tolerance develops to the anticonvulsant and sedative actions of benzodiazepines; patients admitted for benzodiazepine overdoses sometimes leave the hospital with higher plasma levels than when admitted in coma. The onset of benzodiazepine physical dependence is not precisely established. Using benzodiazepine antagonists, it is possible to precipitate withdrawal in animals after a few days of benzodiazepine exposure. Some researchers believe that the rebound insomnia sometimes seen in the morning after taking a very short-acting benzodiazepine sedative the previous evening is a manifestation of physical dependence, as is rebound insomnia following discontinuation of benzodiazepine hypnotics used only for a few days.

As was the case with opioids, the severity of withdrawal is related to the degree to which receptors have been continuously occupied and to the rate at which the drug is withdrawn. Generally, only more severe degrees of physical de-

TABLE 13.1-15
Diagnostic Criteria for Uncomplicated Sedative, Hypnotic, or Anxiolytic Withdrawal

A. Cessation of prolonged (several weeks or more) moderate or heavy use of a sedative, hypnotic, or anxiolytic, or reduction in the amount of substance used, followed by at least three of the following:
(1) nausea or vomiting
(2) malaise or weakness
(3) autonomic hyperactivity (e.g., tachycardia, sweating)
(4) anxiety or irritability
(5) orthostatic hypotension
(6) coarse tremor of hands, tongue, and eyelids
(7) marked insomnia
(8) grand mal seizures

B. Not due to any physical or other mental disorder, such as sedative, hypnotic, or anxiolyic withdrawal delirium.

Note: When the differential diagnosis must be made without a clear-cut history or toxicologic analysis of body fluids, it may be qualified as "provisional."

Table from DSM-III-R *Diagnostic and Statistical Manual of Mental Disorders*, ed 3, revised. Copyright American Psychiatric Association, Washington, DC, 1987. Used with permission.

pendence are associated with withdrawal delirium. Criteria for withdrawal delirium are shown in Table 13.1-16. With benzodiazepines and longer-acting barbiturates, sleep or EEG disturbances may persist for many weeks. Benzodiazepine withdrawal has been reported in individuals receiving as little as 15 mg of diazepam per day for a period of months, but it is more common when the daily dosage of diazepam or its equivalent exceeds 40 mg per day.

MEDICAL AND PSYCHIATRIC COMPLICATIONS All sedative-hypnotics can impair concentration, memory, and psychomotor performance. Among some types of users, acute intoxication is common and, similar to alcoholic intoxication, is characterized by disinhibition of aggressive and sexual impulses, impaired judgment, and labile mood. To meet DSM-III-R criteria, in addition to the mood disturbances just described, at least one of the following must be present: slurred speech, incoordination, unsteady gait, and impairment in attention or memory (Table 13.1-17).

Excessive dosage, accidental or deliberate, can induce respiratory depression and coma, which, even if successfully treated, can leave residual brain damage as a result of anoxia. Treatment of overdosage is aimed at support of respiration and cardiovascular function until the drug can be eliminated. The probability of burns and accidents is increased as a result of chronic intoxication. These various complications, including coma from overdosage, appear to be less common with benzodiazepine and anxiolytic dependence.

TABLE 13.1-16
Diagnostic Criteria for Sedative, Hypnotic, or Anxiolytic Withdrawal Delirium

A. Delirium developing after the cessation of heavy use of a sedative, hypnotic, or anxiolytic, or a reduction in the amount of substance used (usually within 1 week).

B. Autonomic hyperactivity (e.g., tachycardia, sweating).

C. Not due to any physical or other mental disorder.

Note: When the differential diagnosis must be made without a clear-cut history or toxicologic analysis of body fluids, it may be qualified as "provisional."

Table from DSM-III-R *Diagnostic and Statistical Manual of Mental Disorders*, ed 3, revised. Copyright American Psychiatric Association, Washington, DC, 1987. Used with permission.

TABLE 13.1-17
Diagnostic Criteria for Sedative, Hypnotic, or Anxiolytic Intoxication

A. Recent use of a sedative, hypnotic, or anxiolytic.

B. Maladaptive behavioral changes (e.g., disinhibition of sexual or aggressive impulses, mood lability, impaired judgment, impaired social or occupational functioning).

C. At least one of the following signs:
(1) slurred speech
(2) incoordination
(3) unsteady gait
(4) impairment in attention or memory

D. Not due to any physical or other mental disorder.

Note: When the differential diagnosis must be made without a clear-cut history or toxicologic analysis of body fluids, it may be qualified as "provisional."

Table from DSM-III-R *Diagnostic and Statistical Manual of Mental Disorders*, ed 3, revised. Copyright American Psychiatric Association, Washington DC, 1987. Used with permission.

Persistent sedative-hypnotic abuse appears to produce neuropsychological and structural brain damage similar to that found in chronic alcoholics. The reversibility of this damage is uncertain, but deficits are commonly found for months after detoxification. In one study, benzodiazepine dependence appeared to be less likely than alcoholism to induce brain damage. See Table 13.1-18 for the DSM-III-R diagnostic criteria for amnestic disorder caused by sedative, hypnotic, or anxiolytic use.

TREATMENT OF SEDATIVE-ANXIOLYTIC DEPENDENCE Because of the heterogeneity of the patients, treatment should begin only after careful evaluation of the patient's medical condition and social and personal circumstances. Generally, these patients have access to drugs from more than one physician or from street supplies and tend to be unreliable or unable to comply with instructions for gradually decreasing drug dosage. If the physician is to avoid becoming simply one more source of drugs, treatment in the hospital is usually mandatory. The primary goal of treatment in these cases is abstinence. More discretion is possible for those who are physically dependent on therapeutic doses of anxiolytics and hypnotics. In the latter group, under the right circumstances, outpatient withdrawal can be attempted.

TREATMENT OF THE WITHDRAWAL SYNDROME Of the several detoxificaion approaches currently in use, all have a common principle: the gradual reduction of the amount of drug acting at the receptor complex. This gradual reduction can be accomplished by stabilization on a short-acting drug, such as pentobarbital (Nembutal), followed by a stepwise reduction over a period of 10 days or longer. Alternatively, a longer-acting agent that exhibits cross-dependence with the

TABLE 13.1-18
Diagnostic Criteria for Sedative, Hypnotic, or Anxiolytic Amnestic Disorder

A. Amnestic syndrome following prolonged heavy use of a sedative, hypnotic, or anxiolytic.

B. Not due to any physical or other mental disorder.

Note: When the differential diagnosis must be made without a clear-cut history or toxicologic analysis of body fluids, it may be qualified as "provisional."

Table from DSM-III-R *Diagnostic and Statistical Manual of Mental Disorders*, ed 3, revised. Copyright American Psychiatric Association, Washington, DC, 1987. Used with permission.

drug on which the patient is dependent can be substituted—that is, phenobarbital for pentobarbital; diazepam for triazolam (Halcion) or for alcohol. The longer-acting agent can then be either gradually reduced or, if the dosage level is low, abruptly discontinued. Because of the long duration of action of these drugs after a period of repeated administration, there will be a gradual decrease in the amount of drug at the receptor level, even with relatively abrupt discontinuation. Recent work suggests that abrupt outpatient withdrawal from low levels of benzodiazepines (equivalent of about 15 mg of diazepam) is relatively safe. In a study in which two groups of patients were given cognitive therapy to help them cope with anxiety-inducing situations, patients who were abruptly withdrawn were less likely to be using benzodiazepines at the 1-year follow-up than those whose dose was tapered. However, those abruptly withdrawn had significantly more withdrawal symptoms and were more likely to take benzodiazepines during the withdrawal period.

For sedative-hypnotic dependence, two methods have been described. In one, the individual is stabilized on pentobarbital. The pentobarbital is then gradually decreased by approximately 100 mg per day or 10 percent of total dosage. In the other technique, phenobarbital is substituted for the sedative-hypnotic with 30 mg of phenobarbital considered equivalent to each 100 mg pentobarbital or its equivalent on which the patient is dependent.

Some general estimate of the degree of physical dependence (neuroadaptation) can be inferred from the response of the patient to a 200-mg challenge dose of pentobarbital, given by mouth. If there is gross intoxication with ataxia and slurred speech, the daily requirement is probably less than 200 to 300 mg of pentobarbital per day; if there is only fine nystagmus and slight swaying with eyes closed, it is probably between 600 to 800 mg per day. If there is still evidence of withdrawal, the daily requirement is probably 1,000 mg or more. The true test of a correct stabilization level is that while ingesting a prescribed amount of drug over 24 to 48 hours the patient shows signs of neither intoxication nor withdrawal. When stabilization has been achieved, reduction can begin. Patients who show acute signs of withdrawal when dose reduction begins should be kept at the last level at which they were stable for an additional 24 to 48 hours. Decrease in dosage can then be tried again. Sometimes, withdrawal can take several weeks. Some clinicians prefer to use phenobarbital, which is not only longer acting and more likely to provide a smooth reduction of drug levels on the CNS, but is also less likely to become the object of drug-seeking behavior. Other clinicians attempt to use diazepam for the withdrawal from all sedatives. The capacity of diazepam and other benzodiazepines to suppress withdrawal from barbiturates and related hypnotics is not well established. Diazepam, like phenobarbital, does have a long duration of action once stabilization has been achieved (some of its metabolites have half-lives of 50 to 100 hours). Reduction of diazepam dosage of 10 percent per day has been reported to be satisfactory in most cases. The general principle for the use of phenobarbital is to substitute 30 mg of phenobarbital for each 100 mg of pentobarbital or its equivalent.

When patients are dependent on both sedatives and opioids, it is generally preferable to stabilize the patients on both types of drugs before detoxification is undertaken. Current clinical experience suggests that withdrawal of sedatives should be accomplished before an attempt is made to withdraw the patient from opioids.

POSTWITHDRAWAL TREATMENT AND PROGNOSIS In one study, about 40 percent of patients on low doses of benzodiazepines stopped using them without apparent difficulty, simply because they were asked to do so by their physicians. In other studies, more than 50 percent who tried to stop returned to use of benzodiazepines. Important factors appear to be the dose used, rate of withdrawal, personality factors, current severity of psychopathology, and the treatment provided. As noted above, more rapid withdrawal produces more severe symptoms. Patients with inadequate personalities seem less able to remain abstinent; those who have coexistent depression may also be less able to tolerate withdrawal with its associated sleep disturbances and anxiogenic aspects. Once the acute phase of withdrawal has been managed, the use of antidepressants may be helpful in several ways. First, some antidepressants, such as amitriptyline have some sedative actions that may ameliorate sleep disturbances, which may persist for weeks after withdrawal is completed. Also, many cases of sedative-hypnotic-anxiolytic dependence develop in individuals whose initial problem was neither simple insomnia nor anxiety, but unrecognized depression. Some clinicians believe that starting antidepressants or cognitively based anxiety management methods may facilitate withdrawal. Apart from these suggestions, there is no specific approach to psychotherapy of sedative-anxiolytic dependence.

The prognosis for sedative-hypnotic dependence that arises primarily as a form of illicit drug abuse appears to be bleak, but it must also be said that recent data that adjust for psychopathology are scanty. At follow-up, sedative-hypnotic abusers are often found to have developed signs and symptoms of depression. Typically, there are also reports of a worsening of alcoholism, suicide attempts, and deaths from drug overdose and suicide.

The physician's role in prevention There is a growing trend to limit use of benzodiazepines to short courses (i.e., less than 6 weeks) before an effort at cessation is undertaken. There are probably many patients who are currently functioning well on therapeutic doses of benzodiazepines, but who experience major difficulties when efforts are made to withdraw them. It is not clear what benefits are derived from persistent or repeated efforts at withdrawal.

CENTRAL STIMULANTS: COCAINE, AMPHETAMINES, AND RELATED DRUGS

At the turn of the twentieth century, dependence on cocaine was widespread, but it declined over a period of about a decade after laws were passed to restrict cocaine use. In the United States, cocaine use and dependence were uncommon for the 40 years between the late 1930s and the early 1970s.

In the mid-1960s, the U.S. government imposed special regulatory controls on amphetamines and related drugs. Despite these controls, the United States experienced a major epidemic of amphetamine and methamphetamine (Desoxyn) abuse in the late 1960s. During this epidemic, drugs made in illicit clandestine laboratories or smuggled across the borders added to the supplies that had, to that point, come from the diversion of legitimately produced drugs.

Controls on legitimately produced amphetamines were progressively tightened over the next decade. Amphetamine, methamphetamine, methylphenidate (Ritalin), and phenmetrazine (Preludin)are now included in Schedule II of the Controlled Substances Act (CSA) along with morphine and other opioids. In many states, the use of amphetamine in the treatment of obesity is prohibited, although other drugs with very similar actions are still prescribed for this problem. Among the drugs that produce subjective effects quite similar to those of amphetamine and methamphetamine are methylphenidate, phenmetrazine, and diethylpropion (Tenuate); still other related agents have some abuse potential and are included in Schedule III of the CSA. Currently, amphetamine itself is used almost exclusively for treatment of narcolepsy and attention-deficit hyperactivity disorder. There is still considerable misuse of amphetamines and amphetamine-like drugs. However, this use of stimulants is currently overshadowed by the far more prevalent abuse of cocaine.

During the early 1970s, cocaine use again became more common. At first, it was used primarily by the intranasal route and, because of its scarcity and high cost, reports of cocaine toxicity and dependence were not common. The smoking of free-base cocaine was first reported in about 1974. Over the past decade, the supply of cocaine has increased, the cost has decreased, its use has spread from the affluent young adults to all economic and age levels of society and more hazardous routes of administration (injection and free-base inhalation) have become common. By 1985, 20 million people in the United States had tried cocaine; only marijuana was a more commonly abused illicit drug. Emergency room reports of cocaine toxicity overdose deaths, as well as requests for treatment of dependence, rose in parallel with the rise in use and shifts in route of administration.

PHARMACOLOGY AND PSYCHOLOGICAL EFFECTS OF COCAINE, AMPHETAMINES, AND RELATED DRUGS Cocaine and amphetamine-like drugs produce very similar, if not identical, subjective effects in humans, as well as very similar patterns of toxicity. Both categories of CNS stimulants produce a sense of alertness, euphoria, and well-being. There are decreases in hunger and the need for sleep. Performance, which if impaired by fatigue, is improved. Both categories of drugs can induce paranoia, suspiciousness, and overt psychosis, which are difficult to distinguish from acute paranoid schizophrenia (Tables 13.1-19 and 13.1-20).

In animals, both categories of drugs are powerful reinforcers of drug-taking behavior. Cocaine is currently viewed as the most powerful pharmacological reinforcer known; given free access, animals will choose to self-administer cocaine over access to food, water, or other animals. Death from starvation or drug toxicity is the typical consequence of unlimited cocaine access. With limited access (e.g., 6 hours per day), cocaine does not gain such control over behavior.

Although cocaine has both local anesthetic and central stimulant actions, its reinforcing effects in the CNS occur at doses far lower than those needed for local anesthetic action. Cocaine and amphetamine-like drugs produce an activation of mesolimbic and mesocortical dopaminergic systems. The mechanism seems to be the inhibition of the reuptake of released dopamine: Amphetamine also inhibits dopamine reuptake, but it also produces release of dopamine from nerve endings as well. However, the actions of neither cocaine nor amphetamine-like drugs are selective for dopamine. Cocaine is almost as potent in blocking the reuptake of norepinephrine and serotonin. Since other drugs that are not abused (such as certain tricyclic antidepressants) also inhibit uptake of dopamine, norepinephrine, and serotonin, it is not entirely clear why cocaine is such a powerful reinforcer. Animals will self-administer dopamine into sites where cocaine is reinforcing (e.g., medial prefrontal cortex), and will continue to do so after cells mediating cocaine's effects are destroyed. All the evidence taken together strongly points to dopaminergic actions as critical elements in the reinforcing actions of the CNS stimulants.

With chronic use, some degree of tolerance develops to the cardiovascular effects of amphetamines; it is not clear how much tolerance develops to the cardiovascular effects of cocaine. Chronic use of either cocaine or amphetamine-like drugs also produces a form of sensitization in which the response to a given dose is actually enhanced. One theory holds that this sensitization to drug effects is due to a variety of "kindling" in the CNS. In the classic studies of kindling, electrical stimulation of the limbic system, which initially has very little effect, is given repeatedly; after a matter of days, the threshold for effects decreases and major, long-lasting seizures appear. In animals, similar effects are seen with CNS stimulants, so repeated doses after a time come to elicit stereotyped behaviors not seen with initial doses. In animals, a cocaine-amphetamine withdrawal syndrome has not yet been described. The syndrome in humans is described below.

Cocaine and amphetamine-like drugs can be taken orally, by injection, or by absorption via nasal membranes. As with nicotine, opioids, and PCP, inhalation of cocaine in free-base form produces almost immediate absorption and a rapid onset of effects. Cocaine hydrochloride, the water-soluble form typically used for snorting or injection, is largely destroyed by

TABLE 13.1-19
Diagnostic Criteria for Cocaine Intoxication

A. Recent use of cocaine.

B. Maladaptive behavioral changes (e.g., euphoria, fighting, grandiosity, hypervigilance, psychomotor agitation, impaired judgment, impaired social or occupational functioning).

C. At least two of the following signs within 1 hour of using cocaine:
(1) tachycardia
(2) pupillary dilation
(3) elevated blood pressure
(4) perspiration or chills
(5) nausea or vomiting
(6) visual or tactile hallucinations

D. Not due to any physical or other mental disorder.

Table from DSM-III-R *Diagnostic and Statistical Manual of Mental Disorders*, ed 3, revised. Copyright American Psychiatric Association, Washington, DC, 1987. Used with permission.

TABLE 13.1-20
Diagnostic Criteria for Amphetamine or Similarly Acting Sympathomimetic Intoxication

A. Recent use of amphetamine or a similarly acting sympathomimetic.

B. Maladaptive behavioral changes (e.g., fighting, grandiosity, hypervigilance, psychomotor agitation, impaired judgment, impaired social or occupational functioning).

C. At least two of the following signs within one hour of use:
(1) tachycardia
(2) pupillary dilation
(3) elevated blood pressure
(4) perspiration or chills
(5) nausea or vomiting

D. Not due to any physical or other mental disorder.

Table from DSM-III-R *Diagnostic and Statistical Manual of Mental Disorders*, ed 3, revised. Copyright American Psychiatric Association, Washington, DC, 1987. Used with permission.

the heat of burning and, therefore, is not well suited for smoking. However, the hydrochloride salt can be converted to the free-base form by treatment with alkali and extraction with organic solvents. The free-base sublimates before it is destroyed by the heat. Alternatively, cocaine hydrochloride can be mixed with sodium bicarbonate and heated to yield a hard, white mass (crack), consisting of free-base cocaine plus impurities. When smoked, this material gives off a crackling sound.

With cocaine and amphetamine, as with the opioids, rapid onset of effects (i.e., with IV injection or free-base inhalation) produces an intensely pleasurable sensation referred to as a "rush." The rush lasts only a few minutes, in contrast to other psychological and physiological effects, which tend to decline more slowly in parallel with declining plasma levels. The duration of action of cocaine is relatively brief. Its half-life in plasma is 30 to 90 minutes. The drug, an ester, is rapidly hydrolyzed by plasma pseudocholinesterase and liver esterases to relatively inactive metabolites, benzoylecgonine and ecgonine methyl ester. A dose of 40 to 50 mg intravenously or 200 mg intranasally produces peak plasma levels of about 400 mg per ml. Cocaine metabolites can be detected in urine for 24 to 48 hours after use of psychoactive doses. Among smokers of coca paste, a crude form of cocaine sulfate, plasma levels in excess of 1,000 mg per ml can be measured. Individuals with cholinesterase deficiency may be particularly susceptible to cocaine toxicity.

The pharmacokinetics of amphetamine and related drugs are different from those of cocaine. They are all extensively metabolized in the liver. Unchanged amphetamine, a weak base, is excreted in the urine and the half-life of amphetamine is considerably shortened when the urine is acidic. The half-life of amphetamine after therapeutic doses ranges from 7 to 19 hours and that of methamphetamine appears to be at least as long. Thus, after toxic dosage, resolution of symptoms may take far longer with amphetamines than with cocaine.

PATTERNS OF USE, ABUSE, AND DEPENDENCE Indians in the Andes Mountains chew coca leaves on a daily basis. Apparently, very few progress to excessive use or toxicity. Similarly, amphetamines and amphetamine-like drugs can be prescribed and taken on a daily basis over many years by patients with narcolepsy and by children with attention-deficit hyperactivity disorder with few reports of toxicity, escalation of dose, or significant tolerance to therapeutic effects. When amphetamine-like drugs were more widely used in the treatment of obesity, relatively few people who took these drugs on a daily basis progressed to patterns of abuse and dependence. Even when these two classes of drugs are taken initially for their euphorigenic effects, not all users progress to patterns of abuse and dependence. The absolute risk of such progression is not precisely known, but all estimates suggest that the risk is high enough to justify a policy that discourages even experimentation. One estimate of risk comes from a classic study of drug use among a representative sample of young men that was conducted in 1974 and published in 1976. Seventy-three percent of subjects reported no experience with amphetamines; but of the 27 percent who had some experience, almost 10 percent (3 percent of the total) reported use on a daily basis. Some of the factors that increase the likelihood of progression will be discussed.

There are several patterns of amphetamine abuse and of cocaine abuse. Amphetamine-like drugs may be used in relatively low doses intermittently. Examples of this are truck drivers, students, and athletes who seek either to overcome effects of fatigue or need for sleep, or to derive some positive mood effect. Some intermittent users become dependent and find it difficult to stop. Some, but not all, such users may eventually escalate the dosage. Formerly, the drug could be obtained from supplies originating in legitimate medical channels. More recently, individuals with this pattern of use obtain the drugs from illicit traffic.

In still another pattern of amphetamine use, the purpose is to induce euphoria. Such use typically progresses to high dosages, especially if the drugs are used intravenously. This pattern of use is clearly the most dangerous one, and it commonly leads to compulsive use and toxic effects. Although, initially, IV use may occur intermittently with days or weeks between episodes, such high-dosage use often progresses to "sprees" or "speed runs" during which several grams of amphetamine might be injected. The runs might last days or weeks and are commonly punctuated by episodes of toxicity (delusional disorder or delirium—Tables 13.1-21 and 13.1-22, respectively) or by brief periods of abstinence ("crashing"), generally precipitated by interruption of drug supply or exhaustion. This pattern of amphetamine use was relatively uncommon before the mid-1960s. High-dose amphetamine users often combine amphetamine with sedatives or opioids to modulate the stimulant effects.

As with amphetamine and similar agents, there are several patterns of cocaine abuse. Although there are apparently some people who can use cocaine intermittently without progressing to dependence, it is not yet clear how long such intermittent nondependent use can continue. Most cocaine users seeking treatment report that initially their use was intermittent. At some stage, however, abuse escalated and, instead of low-level use, episodes of high-dosage use became more frequent until the pattern resembled the "runs" characteristic of IV amphetamine users. Cocaine runs or binges can last for 7 or more consecutive days, but typically, they last for less than a day. Although there appears to be little tolerance between binges, there are changes in the response to the drug during the course of a binge. Euphoric effects seem less prominent, and anxiety, fatigue, irritability, and depression increase. Any pause in the drug use causes blood levels to drop; typically, there is dysphoria, rather than return to normal mood. If there is cocaine available, it is used to dispel the dysphoria. The binge is generally interrupted when drug toxicity occurs or

TABLE 13.1-21
Diagnostic Criteria for Amphetamine or Similarly Acting Sympathomimetic Delusional Disorder

A. Organic delusional syndrome developing shortly after use of amphetamine or a similarly acting sympathomimetic.

B. Rapidly developing persecutory delusions are the predominant clinical feature.

C. Not due to any physical or other mental disorder.

Table from DSM-III-R *Diagnostic and Statistical Manual of Mental Disorders,* ed 3, revised. Copyright American Psychiatric Association, Washington, DC, 1987. Used with permission.

TABLE 13.1-22
Diagnostic Criteria for Amphetamine or Similarly Acting Sympathomimetic Delirium

A. Delirium developing within 24 hours of use of amphetamine or a similarly acting sympathomimetic.

B. Not due to any physical or other mental disorder.

Table from DSM-III-R *Diagnostic and Statistical Manual of Mental Disorders,* ed 3, revised. Copyright American Psychiatric Association, Washington, DC, 1987. Used with permission.

drug supplies are exhausted. The cocaine crash then quickly follows, probably more rapidly and with more severity than with amphetamine, since cocaine blood levels fall far more rapidly.

Cocaine and amphetamine-like drugs are powerful reinforcers, especially when the drugs are taken in ways that produce very rapid onset of effects (i.e., by IV or intrapulmonary routes). Not only do these routes of administration produce a rapid rise in blood and brain levels and an intense rush but (especially with inhalation of free-base cocaine) there is an almost equally rapid decline in blood and brain drug levels as the drugs are redistributed and metabolized. Clinicians report that some users of inhaled free-base cocaine appear to move immediately from experimentation to a pattern or regular and compulsive use, limited only by the availability of the drug or money to buy it. Even in the laboratory setting, it can be shown that craving for cocaine is briefly intensified 15 minutes after IV use when blood levels are falling. It is important to emphasize, however, that although IV and pulmonary routes of cocaine use are far more likely to escalate into compulsive use and dependence, the intranasal route is far from innocuous. Intranasally, cocaine is fully capable of leading to both dependence and the full range of cocaine toxicity (including fatalities), as described below.

Cocaine abusers frequently use sedatives or opioids, or both, to modulate the stimulant and toxic effects of cocaine. This practice can lead to dependence on sedatives or opioids. Sometimes an opioid, such as heroin, and cocaine are injected intravenously simultaneously; the mixture ("speedball") is reported to be especially euphorigenic.

Cocaine users are known to commit crimes to obtain money to buy cocaine, and such crimes may involve violence. In addition, cocaine can induce paranoid ideation (see below), and there are numerous reports of episodes of homicide and attempted homicide during such cocaine-induced toxic states.

Cocaine and amphetamine dependence Some patterns of cocaine use and amphetamine use clearly meet the generic criteria for dependence shown in Table 13.1-1. For these categories of drugs, use to prevent withdrawal is not as dominant a feature as it is with alcohol or opioids; however, all other criteria are fully met. Who becomes dependent and the rate at which dependence develops has been described under patterns of abuse. Tolerance to some drug actions (e.g., anorexigenic) appear to coexist with increased sensitization to the other actions (e.g., anxiogenic and psychotogenic).

Cocaine toxicity High doses of cocaine can induce seizures, respiratory depression, cardiac arrhythmias, coronary artery spasms, and myocardial infarction. The seizures and respiratory depression may be related to its actions as a local anesthetic, and the cardiovascular complications may be related to its effects on reuptake of catecholamines in the peripheral nervous system. Amphetamine-like drugs can also cause catastrophes of the cardiovascular system (e.g., intracranial hemorrhage, arrhythmias, acute cardiac failure) as a result of their capacity to release biogenic amines and to raise blood pressure. With amphetamines, considerable tolerance develops to the latter effect. Amphetamine in high dosages has also been associated with lethal hyperpyrexia and with destructive deterioration of arterioles.

Treatment of cocaine-induced acute cardiac emergencies is aimed at blocking the sympathetic effects of the drug and correcting arrhythmias. Haloperidol (Haldol) can block some cardiostimulatory effects; some clinicians have recommended β-adrenergic blockers, such as propranolol (Inderal). A cocaine-related myocarditis has been reported.

When inhaled, the cocaine free base is thought to induce lung damage. Gastrointestinal necrosis (as a result of vasoconstriction) has been associated with rupture of swallowed condoms containing large amounts of cocaine. By producing placental vasoconstriction, cocaine may contribute to fetal anoxia.

Some degree of paranoia or hypervigilance is typical of cocaine and amphetamine intoxication (Tables 13.1-19 and 13.1-20). DSM-III-R also lists tactile hallucinations as a symptom of cocaine intoxication. However, both cocaine and amphetamine-like drug use can induce a more persistent toxic state characterized by suspiciousness, paranoia, and visual and tactile hallucinations. The hallucination of bugs or vermin crawling under the skin (formication) is a common, though not a pathognomonic, symptom; it is often associated with excoriation of the skin. Sometimes, the syndrome can develop within 24 hours after the beginning of an amphetamine or cocaine binge. When this syndrome develops in the presence of a clear sensorium, it is designated amphetamine or similarly acting sympathomimetic delusional disorder or cocaine delusional disorder (Table 13.1-23). Criteria for both drug categories are identical. Less commonly, cocaine or amphetamine use can induce a delirium that is often associated with similar persecutory delusions and tactile hallucinations in which the formal diagnosis is amphetamine or similarly acting sympathomimetic delirium or cocaine delirium (Table 13.1-24).

Although amphetamine delusional or delirium syndromes are usually seen only with high doses for prolonged periods, such syndromes have been reported in apparently vulnerable individuals even after therapeutic doses given for short periods. Haloperidol and phenothiazines have been used to treat the delusional syndrome, although with cocaine its action is typically of short duration. With the amphetamine-like drugs, the syndrome may not resolve for many days after drug cessation. Upon recovery from either delusional or delirium syndrome, there may be amnesia for the entire episode or for some part of it. During phases of the cocaine or amphetamine-like drug withdrawal syndromes, users may experience severe depression, which tends to resolve without special treatment when sleep normalizes.

Cocaine or amphetamine tolerance withdrawal syndrome After a period of chronic cocaine or amphetamine use, abrupt discontinuation is followed by a withdrawal syndrome characterized by dysphoria, fatigue, depression, desire for sleep (often coupled with insomnia), or hypersomnia. Upon initial awakening, there is typically hyperphagia with persistent fatigue and depression. Recent clinical studies of cocaine users have attempted to further refine the post–drug use syndrome into several phases or stages.

TABLE 13.1-23
Diagnostic Criteria for Cocaine Delusional Disorder

A. Organic delusional syndrome developing shortly after use of cocaine.

B. Rapidly developing persecutory delusions are the predominant clinical feature.

C. Not due to any physical or other mental disorder.

Table from DSM-III-R *Diagnostic and Statistical Manual of Mental Disorders,* ed 3, revised. Copyright American Psychiatric Association, Washington, DC, 1987. Used with permission.

TABLE 13.1-24
Diagnostic Criteria for Cocaine Delirium

A. Delirium developing within 24 hours of use of cocaine.

B. Not due to any physical or other mental disorder.

Table from DSM-III-R *Diagnostic and Statistical Manual of Mental Disorders,* ed 3, revised. Copyright American Psychiatric Association, Washington, DC, 1987. Used with permission.

Kleber and Gawin described a three-phase syndrome in which the first phase, the crash, lasts from 9 hours to 4 days and can itself be divided into several stages. Early in the crash there is agitation, depression, anorexia, and high cocaine craving. This is followed by a decrease in cocaine craving, fatigue, depression, and a desire for sleep; this stage of Phase I is succeeded by symptoms of exhaustion and hypersomnia from which there is intermittent awakening associated with hyperphagia and continued absence of cocaine craving. Phase II is heralded by normalized sleep, improved mood, and low levels of craving, but this relatively benign phase is succeeded by a return of anergia, anhedonia, anxiety, and increased cocaine craving, especially in response to stimuli previously associated with cocaine use. A third, extinction, phase is also described, which appears to represent a period of extended vulnerability to relapse rather than a phase of an extended withdrawal syndrome. There is very little difference between the clinical descriptions of postchronic cocaine and postchronic amphetamine syndromes. In both situations, the severity of the syndromes are related to the intensity and duration of the antecedent drug use. Some elements of the syndrome can be seen in amphetamine or cocaine abusers after relatively brief binges or runs (i.e., a few days). The immediate effects of cessation (dysphoria and fatigue) are commonly referred to as crashing. Some aspects of crashing—albeit less severe—are reported to occur even after 24 hours of use. The DSM-III-R criteria for cocaine withdrawal (Table 13.1-25) are identical to those of amphetamine or similarly acting sympathomimetic withdrawal (Table 13.1-26). For reasons that are not clear, the DSM-III-R criteria require that the syndrome must persist for more than 24 hours after drug cessation. Symptoms in both drug categories, however, are often obvious within the first 24 hours.

Postwithdrawal treatment Although the general principles of treatment for cocaine and amphetamine dependence are not very different from those outlined for opioid use, there are few replicated studies on the efficacy of any particular approach or combination. As was the case with opioid dependence, cocaine dependence that is severe enough to require formal treatment is associated with other psychiatric diagnoses. Among 30 patients admitted to a private psychiatric facility, 60 percent had some other DSM-III Axis I diagnoses. Most of these diagnoses were affective disorders and, of these, major depression and cyclothymic disorders were the most frequent. In this same group of patients, 90 percent met DSM-III criteria for one or more personality disorders—borderline and narcissistic being the more frequent. In publicly funded treatment facilities, the percentage of cocaine abusers with antisocial personality was 27 percent, far higher than the 3 percent found in the private psychiatric facility.

Patient heterogeneity requires thoughtful selection among available alternatives. Not all cocaine users require extensive treatment; some users who are not dependent respond to external pressures—as, for example, when employers insist on careful monitoring of drug use. The executive with little history of psychopathology, a supportive social network, economic assets, and personal skills has a different prognosis and a wider range of options than a patient who is unemployed, alienated from family, and who may also be using opioids. Although some clinicans favor routine hospitalization for detoxification in order to break the cycle of use, some equally experienced clinicians find that many patients do well with an entirely outpatient-based treatment. Severe depression, psychotic manifestations beyond the initial crash period, and drug use that is completely out of control (i.e., repeated failure to respond to outpatient efforts) seem to be the major accepted criteria for hospitalization.

Both psychological and pharmacological approaches to treatment of cocaine dependence have been reported to be effective in reducing postdetoxification relapse. A generally held consensus is that no use at all (total and permanent abstinence) must be the goal of treatment for those who have developed symptoms of dependence; any use is viewed as a prodrome to relapse into dependence.

Psychological approaches have utilized behavioral, psychodynamic, and general supportive techniques. One behavioral method utilizes contingency contracting in which there is agreement in advance that, for some finite period (e.g., 3 months), should the patient relapse to cocaine use (as measured by supervised urine testing), the therapist will initiate actions that will have serious adverse consequences for the patient. Examples of such actions include informing an employer about cocaine use or mailing a letter to a professional credentials board. In one such study, 48 percent of potential patients accepted such a contractual arrangement and 80 percent of these successfully abstained from cocaine. Many of these successes relapsed when the contract expired.

TABLE 13.1-25
Diagnostic Criteria for Cocaine Withdrawal

A. Cessation of prolonged (several days or longer) heavy use of cocaine, or reduction in the amount of cocaine used, followed by dysphoric mood (e.g., depression, irritability, anxiety) and at least one of the following, persisting more than 24 hours after cessation of substance use:
(1) fatigue
(2) insomnia or hypersomnia
(3) psychomotor agitation

B. Not due to any physical or other mental disorder, such as cocaine delusional disorder.

Table from DSM-III-R *Diagnostic and Statistical Manual of Mental Disorders,* ed 3, revised. Copyright American Psychiatric Association, Washington, DC, 1987. Used with permission.

TABLE 13.1-26
Diagnostic Criteria for Amphetamine or Similarly Acting Sympathomimetic Withdrawal

A. Cessation of prolonged (several days or longer) heavy use of amphetamine or a similarly acting sympathomimetic, or reduction in the amount of substance used, followed by dysphoric mood (e.g., depression, irritability, anxiety) and at least one of the following, persisting more than 24 hours after cessation of substance use:
(1) fatigue
(2) insomnia or hypersomnia
(3) psychomotor agitation

B. Not due to any physical or other mental disorder, such as amphetamine or similarly acting sympathomimetic delusional disorder.

Table from DSM-III-R *Diagnostic and Statistical Manual of Mental Disorders,* ed 3, revised. Copyright American Psychiatric Association, Washington, DC, 1987. Used with permission.

Other behavioral methods aimed at helping subjects deal with conditions that evoke craving have been discussed under opioid dependence. In its specific methods, supportive therapy overlaps the techniques used by behaviorists. Patients are helped to separate themselves from friends who are users and situations in which cocaine is available. Patients are urged to abstain from other drugs, such as alcohol and marijuana, because these drugs have been reported to increase cocaine craving and the probability of relapse. They are also helped in repairing those areas of their lives that once provided satisfaction and may have been damaged by the behaviors associated with cocaine use. The patient may be encouraged to participate in AA or NA as a means of gaining control over other drug use.

Psychodynamic approaches emphasize the patient's unconscious motives for cocaine use (e.g., to relieve an inner sense of emptiness or depression). Experienced clinicians with a wide enough range of skills believe that a combination of these psychological approaches with the emphasis tailored to the circumstances of the individual patient are more effective than treatments emphasizing the principles of only one approach. Combining psychological techniques with newer psychopharmacological treatments seems to be more effective than psychological approaches used alone.

Pharmacological adjuncts to treatment Current pharmacological treatments are based on one of two broad premises. First, some cocaine users are using the drug to ameliorate some preexisting psychiatric disorders, such as attention-deficit hyperactivity disorder (residual state) or cyclothymia. Cocaine users presumed to have such disorders have been treated with methylphenidate and lithium, respectively. These agents are of little or no benefit in patients without these disorders; hence, clinicians are urged that in either situation they adhere strictly to maximal diagnostic criteria before using either methylphenidate or lithium in the treatment of cocaine dependence.

A second pharmacological premise is that chronic cocaine use alters the function of multiple neurotransmitter systems, especially the catecholaminergic and serotonergic transmitters regulating hedonic tone. It has also been proposed that cocaine induces a state of relative dopaminergic deficiency.

Trials (generally single-blind or nonblind) of a number of drugs have resulted in some promising leads, including neurotransmitter precursors, such as tyrosine; dopaminergic agonists, such as bromocriptine (Parlodel); various antidepressents, such as desipramine, imipramine, and trazodone (Desyrel); and antiparkinsonian drugs that may also affect the dopaminergic system, such as amantadine (Symmetrel). But there is general consensus that better controls, larger samples, and independent replication are needed before any agent can be viewed as demonstrably useful. Bromocriptine and amantadine are reported to be useful in reducing cocaine craving in the first week or two after withdrawal. Desipramine appears to have little effect on craving during the first several weeks of treatment, but then begins to induce a reduction in craving. The time course of the imipramine effect on craving is consistent with imipramine-induced changes in CNS receptor sensitivity.

There are no specific or well-established treatments for dependence on amphetamine or amphetamine-like drugs. It is reasonable to expect that treatments that prove to be useful with cocaine dependence will be effective in amphetamine dependence as well.

CANNABIS (MARIJUANA)

There are several varieties or cultivars of the single species of *Cannabis sativa* (the hemp plant). Such cultivars include *sativa indica* and *americana*. Although these names identify the geographic locations in which the plants are grown rather than basic differences in the plant, there are differences in the concentration of cannabinoids in the cultivars grown in different areas. For example, marijuana raised in India and Pakistan contains about 1 to 2 percent tetrahydrocannabinol (THC), varieties grown in Thailand contain almost 5 percent THC, and a type known as sinsemilla, now grown in a number of Western Hemisphere countries, contains up to 10 percent THC. Cannabis produces more than 400 identifiable chemical entities. It is the only plant in nature that produces the cannabinoid family of chemicals; the most active of these cannabinoids in producing psychological effects is Δ-9-tetrahydrocannabinol (Δ^9-THC). Hashish, the resin obtained from the leaves of the plant, contains about 10 percent Δ^9-THC; hashish oil, a concentrated form of the resin, contains from 15 to 30 percent Δ^9-THC.

PHARMACOLOGICAL ACTIONS AND PSYCHOLOGICAL EFFECTS The mechanism by which the cannabinoids exert their actions is still unknown and no saturable stereospecific receptors have yet been identified. The major effects of Δ^9-THC include changes in mood, alertness, and cognition. There are also effects on the endocrine, cardiovascular, and immune systems. Δ^9-THC also lowers intraocular pressure and has antinauseant and antiemetic actions.

The most typical psychological effect is an elevation of mood (relaxation and euphoria) associated with a decreased capacity to accurately gauge the passage of time (time seems slowed down), intensification of perceptions, inappropriate laughter, passivity, apathy, and drowsiness. There is decreased capacity to order sequences of events in time and perform complex tasks. Occasionally, some users, especially those unfamiliar with the drug, may experience acute anxiety or even panic; some may become acutely paranoid, a condition that may persist for several days. In individuals with a history of schizophrenia, marijuana use may trigger a recrudescence of symptomatology. A cannabis delusional disorder is recognized in DSM-III-R (Table 13.1-27).

Although cannabis is absorbed after oral administration, it is typically smoked. About 25 percent of the smoked material is absorbed; the rest is lost to pyrolysis or to side-stream smoke, or is trapped in the butt. Δ^9-THC is soluble in lipids and passes quickly into brain and other fatty tissues. Δ^9-THC is converted into an active metabolite 11-hydroxy-THC; Δ^9-THC and its active metabolites have relatively long half-lives (50 hours), but because of the rapid redistribution of the drug into fat stores, the duration of effects after acute usage may be only a few hours. The significance of the accumulation of

TABLE 13.1-27
Diagnostic Criteria for Cannabis Delusional Disorder

A. Organic delusional syndrome developing shortly after cannabis use.

B. Not due to any physical or other mental disorder.

Table from DSM-III-R *Diagnostic and Statistical Manual of Mental Disorders*, ed 3, revised. Copyright American Psychiatric Association, Washington, DC, 1987. Used with permission.

THC and its metabolites in body fat after chronic use is not known.

The drug and its metabolites may be detected in urine for 48 to 72 hours after the acute psychological effects are no longer detectable. In a very small room, the concentration of cannabis in air produced by four smoked cigarettes can sometimes be high enough that passive inhalers will absorb cannabinoids sufficient to produce psychological effects and levels of metabolites in urine that are detectable with available toxicological methods, such as the enzyme-multiplied immunoassay (EMIT) system when the criterion for detectability is set at a very sensitive level of 20 ng per ml of urine. Such passive inhalers would not produce positive urine results when the criterion is set at the more typical cutoff level of 100 ng per ml of urine. Daily heavy cannabis smokers may excrete THC metabolites that are detectable for up to 2 to 3 weeks after stopping.

TOLERANCE AND PHYSICAL DEPENDENCE Some tolerance develops to the cardiovascular and mood-elevating psychological effects of cannabis. Despite this decrement in euphorigenic and relaxing effects and reports by heavy users that some of the less desirable effects show little decrement, heavy users often continue to use the drug, much as alcoholics and chronic opioid users continue despite adverse consequences and decreased positive effects. It may be that the brief effects that occur after cannabis smoking are sufficient to maintain the behavior.

A cannabis withdrawal syndrome characterized by decrements in performance on drug discontinuation has been demonstrated in monkeys. In human volunteers, discontinuation of THC after oral administration for several weeks is followed by anxiety, insomnia, and other symptoms resembling sedative-anxiolytic withdrawal. The relationship of this generally mild syndrome to the perpetuation of cannabis use is uncertain. Few users report a need to continue to use the drug to prevent unpleasant withdrawal effects.

Patterns of abuse Overall, 62 million Americans (33 percent of those over age 12) have used marijuana at least once. Most experimenters discontinue use after a few trials, but some continue to use it once or twice a week. A still smaller fraction of initial users become heavier users, smoking the drug several times per week, and a still smaller group eventually become daily or almost daily users who may smoke up to 20 marijuana cigarettes per day. At the peak of its recent popularity (about 1979), 10 percent of high school students reported daily or almost daily use of marijuana; this proportion has since fallen to about 3.3 percent in 1987. In 1985, 16 percent of employed 20- to 40-year-olds reported some marijuana use during the preceding month. It is not clear what percentage of marijuana users meet the criteria for drug dependence as defined in DSM-III-R.

Medical and psychiatric complications Cannabis use can induce anxiety, paranoid states, and recrudescence of acute schizophrenia symptoms. Many clinicians believe that chronic (i.e., daily or frequent) use, especially in adolescents and young adults, is associated with a chronic cannabis syndrome, with an extremely variable presentation. Typically, it includes lethargy, reduced drive, mild depression, and loss of interest in areas that were previously valued, and has been called the amotivational syndrome. These mood and behavioral changes persist during short intervals of nonuse of marijuana. Clearly, this picture is difficult to distinguish from either mood disorder or the onset of personality disorder or the effects of disturbances in family and interpersonal relationships. Often, the relationship of impairments and symptoms to marijuana use becomes evident only when the user is persuaded to stop, shows clear-cut improvement in mood and behavior, and describes a feeling of "coming out of a fog." Some of the reluctance of marijuana users to link marijuana use to current difficulties is undoubtedly part of the denial of disability and dependence typical of other varieties of drug dependence. It may also be that because the development of the altered mood and loss of interest is very gradual, it is not readily perceived.

Marijuana may produce its effects on memory by depressing neuronal activity in the hippocampus. In adult rats, chronic exposure to THC doses that cause few observable behavioral effects produces neuronal losses and glial changes in the hippocampus similar to the losses seen with aging.

Acute marijuana use impairs driving and the performance of other complex tasks. The effect on these tasks may be the summation of marijuana-induced impairments on complex reaction time, motor coordination, tracking ability, depth perception, short-term memory, time sense, and glare recovery. Impairments in performance of complex tasks, such as flying and driving, may last for many hours after the subjective effects have subsided.

The DSM-III-R diagnostic criteria for cannabis intoxication are given in Table 13.1-28. DSM-III-R also recognizes a cannabis delusional disorder. The criteria for this disorder are an organic delusional syndrome developing shortly after cannabis use, usually associated with anxiety, emotional lability and depersonalization, not due to any other disorder. The syndrome usually remits within 1 to several days. The psychiatric literature from Middle Eastern and Asian countries describes longer-lasting psychotic states resulting from cannabis use. Cannabis-induced increases in heart rate can cause angina in patients with coronary artery disease. Cannabis use also causes a reddening of the conjunctivae, to which some tolerance develops; however, no long-term adverse effects of this action of cannabis are reported.

Cannabis smoke contains concentrations of carcinogens, cocarcinogens, and irritants equal to or greater than those found in tobacco smoke. Regular cannabis smokers may experience upper airway irritation and inflammation. Premalignant changes in bronchial epithelium have been found in heavy cannabis smokers. Some researchers believe that, in terms of inducing obstructive lung disease and pulmonary malignancies, marijuana may prove to be more pathogenic than tobacco.

Cannabis use has been shown to alter concentrations of reproductive hormones in both animals and humans. Δ^9-THC

TABLE 13.1-28
Diagnostic Criteria for Cannabis Intoxication

A. Recent use of cannabis.

B. Maladaptive behavioral changes (e.g., euphoria, anxiety, suspiciousness or paranoid ideation, sensation of slowed time, impaired judgment, social withdrawal).

C. At least two of the following signs developing within 2 hours of cannabis use:
(1) conjunctival injection
(2) increased appetite
(3) dry mouth
(4) tachycardia

D. Not due to any physical or other mental disorder.

Table from DSM-III-R *Diagnostic and Statistical Manual of Mental Disorders,* ed 3, revised. Copyright American Psychiatric Association, Washington, DC, 1987. Used with permission.

appears to block release of gonadotropin-releasing hormone (GnRH), which is the hypothalamic factor that is responsible for release of luteinizing hormone (LH) and follicle-stimulating hormone (FSH). In men, the quality and quantity of sperm are reduced; in animals, in addition, the weight of seminal vesicles and testes are reduced. In women, smoking a marijuana cigarette produces decrements in FSH and LH during the luteal (postovulatory) phase, but not during the follicular (preovulatory) phase of the menstrual cycle. In women, but not in men, marijuana smoking suppresses prolactin levels. The hormonal disturbances may facilitate the onset of pregnancy and may also place the fetus at higher risk for inadequate development. The effects on neurohormones in both males and females appear to be mediated primarily at the level of the pituitary. Some tolerance to these effects develops, and research with sexually mature primates has shown the effects to be reversible.

Cannabis has been shown to alter the humoral and cell-mediated components of the immune system in several species. In rats, chronic exposure to cannabis lowers resistance to bacterial and viral (herpetic) infections. Effects on the immune system are a characteristic of cannaboids that is independent of their psychoactivity and may occur at doses that do not produce behavioral effects. The implications of these findings for humans are not yet clear.

Marijuana available in the United States may be contaminated with various herbicides used in eradication programs. Paraquat has not been used since 1985, but other agents believed to be less toxic are still being used. Although paraquat is toxic when taken into the body, only minute amounts survive the heat of pyrolysis.

TREATMENT Symptoms of acute intoxication with marijuana are generally managed with reassurance and support. When anxiety or paranoid ideation persists, anxiolytics may be useful. Acute psychotic states persisting beyond a few days are handled in the same way as psychotic states that are not drug-induced. When chronic use causes impairment or request for treatment, the most difficult aspect may be persuading the patient that some degree of impairment exists and that it is due to cannabis use, which will have to be stopped. Family therapy may be useful. In general, the techniques described to help cocaine users are applicable. With the exception of those with cannabis-induced psychotic states, patients with cannabis abuse and dependence rarely require inpatient care.

PHENCYCLIDINE AND RELATED ARYLCYCLOHEXYLAMINE DEPENDENCE AND ABUSE

PCP (angel dust) was introduced into clinical medicine as a dissociative anesthetic in the 1950s. It was restricted to veterinary use when it was noted that some patients developed a delirium on emerging from anesthesia. It became a drug of abuse in the 1960s, but its popularity faded because of its toxicity; it reemerged in the 1970s in smokable form, with use reaching epidemic proportions in Los Angeles and Washington, DC. It is relatively easy and cheap to produce.

PHARMACOLOGY PCP and related arylcyclohexylamines have CNS stimulant, CNS depressant, hallucinogenic, and analgesic actions. The picture of PCP intoxication in humans has elements of widespread increase in the effects of multiple neurotransmitters.

PCP and related psychoactive congeners appear to exert their pharmacological actions at distinct stereospecific receptors concentrated in the hippocampus, frontal cortex, striatum, and amygdala. These receptors are distinct from those at which hallucinogens, such as LSD, exert their effects.

One current theory of the mechanism of PCP action postulates that PCP-like drugs selectively antagonize the neuronal actions of *N*-methyl-*D*-aspartate (NMDA). The PCP receptor may be part of a larger ionophore-controlling NMDA receptor complex similar to that described for the GABA-benzodiazepine chloride ion channel. The ion channels controlled by NMDA include divalent cations (e.g., Ca^{2+}) and monovalent cations. Whether this receptor is the one responsible for all of the varied actions of PCP is uncertain. Earlier pharmacological studies demonstrated that PCP blocks the reuptake of multiple neurotransmitters, such as dopamine, serotonin (5-HT), and norepinephrine. The relation of these effects on neurotransmitters to the previously described effects on ion channels is under active investigation. Whether the receptor for PCP and its analogues is identical to the receptor which was initially labeled with the benzomorphan derivative SKF 10047 and designated as the opioid σ-receptor is the subject of lively debate, but there is growing evidence that there are two distinct receptors. Endogenous peptide and nonpeptide substances that bind differentially to the PCP receptor and to the σ-receptor have been reported.

In addition to PCP itself, there are a variety of structurally related analogues that produce similar actions. These include dexoxadrol, ketamine (Ketlar); and N-(l-[z-thienyl]cyclohexyl)-piperidine (TCP). The practical significance of some of these analogues is that they make control of supplies even more difficult. Drugs in this class are self-administered by rats and monkeys. Some tolerance develops to PCP actions; in monkeys, abrupt cessation after chronic administration is followed by a withdrawal syndrome which includes fearfulness, tremors, and facial twitches. A PCP withdrawal syndrome in humans has not yet been clearly identified.

PCP is well absorbed after all routes of administration. However, as with cocaine and nicotine, the onset of action is far more rapid when smoked than when taken orally. Further, the smoking of the drug may permit some users to control the dosage more easily than is possible with oral use. Smoking PCP in cigarettes is now one of the most common means of using it, although some users still sniff or snort it, and about 2 percent report using it intravenously. The drug can often be detected in urine for several days after use.

PATTERNS OF USE PCP is usually taken episodically or in binges that can last several days. There are some individuals who use the drug on a daily basis, but whether this daily use is in any way related to the tolerance and physical dependence seen in animals is unknown. Most clinicians believe the motive for continued use is the drug's euphorigenic effects. Quite typically, PCP is used in combination with other drugs, such as alcohol and cannabis. For those seeking treatment, PCP is rarely the primary problem drug.

Although PCP and its analogues are reported to induce bizarre and particularly aggressive acts, it is clear that such behavior is exhibited by only a small percentage of users. In one study in New York of arrestees charged with felony offenses, those whose urines were positive for PCP were younger, were likely to be charged with economically motivated offenses, and were less likely to be charged with assault than those positive for other drugs.

Psychological effects Acute serious or major PCP intoxication may present as a catatonic syndrome, toxic psychosis, acute mental syndrome, or coma. These presentations require hospitalization. Less serious episodes of intoxication may involve lethargy, bizarre behavior, agitation, or euphoria, and can usually be managed on an outpatient basis, since the effects commonly dissipate over a period of several hours. Nystagmus and hypertension are prominent features of PCP intoxications, but since these signs are seen in other intoxications, their presence can only be suggestive. Patients may have a clear sensorium or they can be confused, disoriented, stuporous, lethargic, or comatose. There may be numbness or diminished response to pain, as well as ataxia and dysarthria. The degree of intoxication is believed to be dose-related, but there is wide variability. Some individuals with major intoxication may have lower serum concentrations than other individuals with very minor effects.

Clinical disorders The clinical picture can be extremely varied and, in some cases, difficult to distinguish from acute schizophrenia. DSM-III-R lists five organic mental disorders caused by PCP: intoxication (Table 13.1-29); delirium (Table 13.1-30); delusional disorder (Table 13.1-31); mood disorder (Table 13.1-32); and phencyclidine organic disorder not otherwise specified (Table 13.1-33). It is recommended that a provisional diagnosis be used in the absence of a clear-cut history or a toxicological report.

PCP delirium may wax and wane over a period of a week. PCP mood disorder, typically depression or anxiety, may be brief or may persist and become difficult to distinguish from mood disorder. Suicide is a risk. The features of PCP delusional disorder are the same as those described under cocaine delusional disorder.

TABLE 13.1-29
Diagnostic Criteria for Phencyclidine (PCP) or Similarly Acting Arylcyclohexylamine Intoxication

A. Recent use of phencyclidine or a similarly acting arylcyclohexylamine.

B. Maladaptive behavioral changes (e.g., belligerence, assaultiveness, impulsiveness, unpredictability, psychomotor agitation, impaired judgment, impaired social or occupational functioning).

C. Within an hour (less when smoked, insufflated ["snorted"], or used intravenously), at least two of the following signs:
(1) vertical or horizontal nystagmus
(2) increased blood pressure or heart rate
(3) numbness or diminished responsiveness to pain
(4) ataxia
(5) dysarthria
(6) muscle rigidity
(7) seizures
(8) hyperacusis

D. Not due to any physical or other mental disorder (e.g., Phencyclidine [PCP] or similarly acting arylcyclohexylamine delirium).

Table from DSM-III-R *Diagnostic and Statistical Manual of Mental Disorders,* ed 3, revised. Copyright American Psychiatric Association, Washington, DC, 1987. Used with permission.

TABLE 13.1-30
Diagnostic Criteria for Phencyclidine (PCP) or Similarly Acting Arylcyclohexylamine Delirium

A. Delirium developing shortly after use of phencyclidine or a similarly acting arylcyclohexylamine.

B. Not due to any physical or other mental disorder.

Table from DSM-III-R *Diagnostic and Statistical Manual of Mental Disorders,* ed 3, revised. Copyright American Psychiatric Association, Washington, DC, 1987. Used with permission.

TABLE 13.1-31
Diagnostic Criteria for Phencyclidine (PCP) or Similarly Acting Arylcyclohexylamine Delusional Disorder

A. Organic delusional syndrome developing shortly after use of phencyclidine or a similarly acting arylcyclohexylamine, or emerging up to a week after an overdose.

B. Not due to any physical or other mental disorder, such as schizophrenia.

Table from DSM-III-R *Diagnostic and Statistical Manual of Mental Disorders,* ed 3, revised. Copyright American Psychiatric Association, Washington, DC, 1987. Used with permission.

TABLE 13.1-32
Diagnostic Criteria for Phencyclidine (PCP) or Similarly Acting Arylcyclohexylamine Mood Disorder

A. Organic mood syndrome developing shortly after use of phencyclidine or a similarly acting arylcyclohexylamine (usually within 1 or 2 weeks) and persisting more than 24 hours after cessation of substance use.

B. Not due to any physical or other mental disorder.

Table from DSM-III-R *Diagnostic and Statistical Manual of Mental Disorders,* ed 3, revised. Copyright American Psychiatric Association, Washington, DC, 1987. Used with permission.

TABLE 13.1-33
Diagnostic Criteria for Phencyclidine (PCP) or Similarly Acting Arylcyclohexylamine Organic Mental Disorder Not Otherwise Specified

A. Recent use of phencyclidine or a similarly acting arylcyclohexylamine.

B. The resulting illness involves features of several organic mental syndromes or a progression from one organic mental syndrome to another (e.g., initially there is delirium, followed by an organic delusional syndrome).

C. Not due to any physical or other mental disorder.

Table from DSM-III-R *Diagnostic and Statistical Manual of Mental Disorders,* ed 3, revised. Copyright American Psychiatric Association, Washington, DC, 1987. Used with permission.

Treatment of overdosage Treatment of overdosage is symptomatic and directed at protecting the patient and others from effects of impaired behavior and judgment. "Talking the patient down" is not helpful; preferable is isolation from external stimuli consistent with behavioral monitoring and support of vital function. Mechanical restraints for those with serious intoxications are recommended by some experienced clinicians. However, restraints are problematic since excessive muscle contractions when patients fight the restraints may aggravate rhabdomyolysis and contribute to myoglobinemia and renal failure. Convulsions have been treated with diazepam. In some patients, a psychotic phase may last for several weeks after a single dose of PCP.

Because it is a weak base, PCP is trapped in the acidic gastrointestinal fluid, and in cases of intoxication there is considerable gastrointestinal recirculation. Some clinicians recommend gastric suction and report that suction can reduce the typical 3-day half-life of the drug to about 1 day. Experienced clinicians no longer recommend acidification of the urine. In experiments in dogs, drug-specific antibody fragments (Fab fragments) have been shown to accelerate the decline of PCP in serum.

TREATMENT AND PROGNOSIS No special psychotherapeutic approach or pharmacological agent has been reported to be especially helpful in treating the PCP abuser. There is virtually no information on long-term outcome; clinicians report that few adult PCP users complete a course of treatment established for other forms of drug abuse.

HALLUCINOGENS (PSYCHOTOMIMETICS, PSYCHOTOGENICS, PSYCHEDELICS)

The chemically heterogeneous group of drugs discussed here share the capacity to produce the effects implied by terms, such as "hallucinogenic," "psychotomimetic," and "psychotogenic." However, the induction of hallucinations or psychotic-like states is not what distinguishes this group from other categories of pharmacological agents. Rather, it is their capacity to reliably induce states of altered perception, thought, and feeling that are not ordinarily experienced, except in dreams or at times of religious exaltation. In this sense, the term "psychedelic" or "mind-manifesting" would be a more appropriate designation for the class. Some of the drugs in this class, such as mescaline (obtained from the peyote cactus) and psilocin (obtained from various mushroom species), have been used by American and Mexican Indians for untold generations. The psychoactive effects of LSD were not discovered until 1943. Its extraordinary potency (25 to 75 μg orally is a psychoactive dose) generated a flurry of research aimed at understanding its actions and perhaps, in the process, the nature of non–drug-induced psychotic states. Since that time, a number of additional drugs that have LSD-like actions have been discovered or synthesized and investigated. Some drugs have been developed that appear to have properties of both psychedelics and CNS stimulants. For example, 2,5-dimethoxyamphetamine (DMA) has LSD-like effects, but is more like amphetamine in other respects (see below).

PHARMACOLOGICAL ACTIONS AND PSYCHOLOGICAL EFFECTS Drugs in this category can be subdivided into two groups on the basis of chemical structure: (1) the indolealkylamines, resembling 5-HT and including LSD, dimethyltryptamine (DMT), psilocin, and psilocybin; and (2) the phenylethylamines, including mescaline, DMA, 3,4-methylenedioxyamphetamine (MDA) and 3,4-methylenedioxymethamphetamine (MDMA). Current evidence suggests that despite structural differences, both groups act at similar receptors to produce their psychedelic actions. Although the precise mechanism of action is not yet known, most of the evidence points to the involvement of 5-HT and actions at one or more of the several subtypes of 5-HT receptors (although tryptamine receptors may also play a role). A major aspect of the psychedelic action is a reduction of efficiency of the filtering and integrating of sensory input, and a "dehabituating" effect, such that there is an enhanced response to customary input; that is, the familiar seems novel.

Hallucinogens are typically taken by the oral route; DMT, however, is inactive by the oral route and is usually sniffed or smoked. Onset of action of LSD occurs about 20 minutes after oral use. There are both physiological and psychological effects. The former include pupillary dilation, increases in blood pressure, tachycardia, tremor, and hyperreflexia. These symptoms are soon followed by mood changes. Generally, there is euphoria, but several feelings (e.g., euphoria and anxiety) may coexist. These feelings are accompanied by visual illusions and perceptual changes (e.g., micropsia and synesthesias—the merging of auditory and visual perceptions). In addition to experiencing a sense of novelty, the individual may experience a decrease in the sense of boundaries between one object and another and between the self and nonself. Associated with this loss of boundaries, there may be a sense of union with the cosmos or mankind. Alternatively, there may be fear of ego dissolution and fragmentation. The altered sense of time may cause the user to panic and believe that the drug effect may never end. After about 4 to 5 hours (the approximate half-life of LSD), the psychedelic phase of the experience generally passes, leaving the individual with ideas of reference, increased awareness of internal psychological processes, and a sense of being magically in control; this second phase lasts an additional 6 to 8 hours.

Tolerance develops to the sympathomimetic and psychological effects of LSD and related drugs after only three or four daily doses; sensitivity returns after an equal interval of abstinence. There is considerable cross-tolerance between LSD and mescaline and psilocybin, but not between LSD and the amphetamines or Δ^9-THC. No withdrawal phenomena are detected when these drugs are discontinued after chronic administration. Hallucinogens are not reinforcers and are not self-administered by animals.

PATTERNS OF USE Most users of hallucinogens are best described as experimenters. Some quickly discontinue use because of dysphoric effects; others continue, but use is almost always episodic. Because of tolerance and because these drugs are not powerful reinforcers, regular use and dependence are virtually never seen, although DSM-III-R makes provision for such a diagnosis. The diagnostic criteria for hallucinogen abuse are shown in Table 13.1-2.

ADVERSE MEDICAL AND PSYCHIATRIC CONSEQUENCES There are four major organic mental disorders or syndromes related to hallucinogen use: a brief acute intense reaction to drug use (the bad trip); a prolonged psychotic reaction (hallucinogen delusional disorder); a prolonged episode of anxiety, mania, or depression (hallucinogen mood disorder); and spontaneous flashbacks or recurrences of drug effect (post-hallucinogen perception disorder).

The acute syndrome, or bad trip, is designated hallucinogen hallucinosis in DSM-III-R, and the diagnostic criteria are shown in Table 13.1-34. In addition to the perceptual changes described under the subsection on pharmacological actions, this syndrome is characterized by marked anxiety, ideas of reference, paranoid ideation, impaired judgment, distortions of body image, and fear of losing one's mind. Illusions may evolve into true hallucinations, usually of geometric forms, but sometimes of persons and objects. Typically, hallucinations are visual, but tactile and auditory hallucinations may occur. The individual is alert and generally recognizes that the experience is due to drug ingestion. Nevertheless, there may be irrational acts based on drug-induced beliefs that lead to injury to others or to the drug user. With LSD, the syndrome usually subsides within 12 hours when the drug effects wear off.

Hallucinogen delusional disorder (Table 13.1-35) is a syndrome that typically emerges from an episode of hallucinogen hallucinosis. In this syndrome, the physiological (sympathomimetic) components of the acute drug actions subside, but the user becomes delusionally convinced that the disturbed perceptions and thoughts of the acute episode correspond to reality. Although the syndrome may subside within a day or two, it may also persist for weeks or months. When it

TABLE 13.1-34
Diagnostic Criteria for Hallucinogen Hallucinosis

A. Recent use of a hallucinogen.

B. Maladaptive behavioral changes (e.g., marked anxiety or depression, ideas of reference, fear of losing one's mind, paranoid ideation, impaired judgment, impaired social or occupational functioning).

C. Perceptual changes occurring in a state of full wakefulness and alertness (e.g., subjective intensification of perceptions, depersonalization, derealization, illusions, hallucinations, synesthesias).

D. At least two of the following signs:
(1) pupillary dilation
(2) tachycardia
(3) sweating
(4) palpitations
(5) blurring of vision
(6) tremors
(7) incoordination

E. Not due to any physical or other mental disorder.

Table from DSM-III-R *Diagnostic and Statistical Manual of Mental Disorders,* ed 3, revised. Copyright American Psychiatric Association, Washington, DC, 1987. Used with permission.

persists, it is virtually indistinguishable from nonorganic psychotic disorders, such as schizophrenia. Prolonged reactions have been reported in individuals who were previously well balanced and well adjusted. However, in general, when groups of patients are considered, those with LSD psychosis are indistinguishable from those with psychotic states not related to drug use in terms of personality, previous history, family history, and long-term outcome. Such findings suggest that LSD precipitates long-term psychotic states in vulnerable individuals.

Hallucinogen mood disorder (Table 13.1-36) is a state of anxiety, depression, or mania developing within 1 or 2 weeks of drug use (typically very shortly after use) and persisting for more than 24 hours after drug cessation. In the depressive type of this syndrome, there are feelings of guilt and self-reproach, fearfulness, physical restlessness, and insomnia. Although the thoughts are without delusional convictions, those persons with this disorder are commonly preoccupied with the idea that they will be unable to return to normalcy because they have damaged their brain by taking the drug. When the syndrome persists for more than a few days, it is difficult to distinguish from a mood disorder.

TABLE 13.1-35
Diagnostic Criteria for Hallucinogen Delusional Disorder

A. Organic delusional syndrome developing shortly after hallucinogen use.

B. Not due to any physical or other mental disorder, such as schizophrenia.

Table from DSM-III-R *Diagnostic and Statistical Manual of Mental Disorders,* ed 3, revised. Copyright American Psychiatric Association, Washington, DC, 1987. Used with permission.

TABLE 13.1-36
Diagnostic Criteria for Hallucinogen Mood Disorder

A. Organic mood syndrome developing shortly after hallucinogen use (usually within 1 or 2 weeks), and persisting more than 24 hours after cessation of such use.

B. Not due to any physical or other mental disorder.

Table from DSM-III-R *Diagnostic and Statistical Manual of Mental Disorders,* ed 3, revised. Copyright American Psychiatric Association, Washington, DC, 1987. Used with permission.

TABLE 13.1-37
Diagnostic Criteria for Posthallucinogen Perception Disorder

A. The reexperiencing, following cessation of use of a hallucinogen, of one or more of the perceptual symptoms that were experienced while intoxicated with the hallucinogen (e.g., geometric hallucinations, false perceptions of movement in the peripheral visual fields, flashes of color, intensified colors, trails of images from moving objects, positive afterimages, halos around objects, macropsia, and micropsia).

B. The disturbance in A causes marked distress.

C. Other causes of the symptoms such as anatomic lesions and infections of the brain, delirium, dementia, sensory (visual) epilepsies, schizophrenia, entoptic imagery, and hypnopompic hallucinations, have been ruled out.

Table from DSM-III-R *Diagnostic and Statistical Manual of Mental Disorders,* ed 3, revised. Copyright American Psychiatric Association, Washington, DC, 1987. Used with permission.

It is probable that as many as 25 percent of people who use LSD-type hallucinogens will experience an episode in which, without subsequent use of the drug, there is a recurrence of some perceptual change similar to changes originally induced by the hallucinogen. For most users, these episodes are mild, last only for a few seconds, and are not necessarily unpleasant. A smaller percentage, perhaps 5 percent, experience frightening recurrences despite conscious efforts to avoid them. The diagnosis of posthallucinogen perception disorder (Table 13.1-37) is made only when these symptoms cause marked distress. The most common symptoms are hallucinations of formed objects (such as a face or geometric figures), sounds or voices, flashes of color, false perceptions of movement, positive afterimages, and trails of images from moving objects. The symptoms are often triggered by use of cannabis or a phenothiazine, or movement from a lighted to a darker environment. At times, they can be evoked intentionally. Although such symptoms may persist for years in some people, more typically recurrences cease after a few months. The individual has insight into the pathological nature of the symptoms and recognizes them as symptoms previously induced by the ingestion of hallucinogens.

Heavy users of hallucinogens (i.e., an average of 50 uses) have been compared to controls on a number of measures. In general, they seem eccentric and tend to function only marginally, but it has been difficult to determine whether, or how, such characteristics are linked to use of hallucinogens. Some observers suggest that LSD-like drugs can induce an amotivational syndrome like that described for cannabis. Although the persistence of flashbacks suggests some long-lasting drug-induced brain changes, former hallucinogen users score about as well on tests of neuropsychological function as controls; when deficits are found (e.g., nonverbal abstraction), they are not correlated with extent of drug use.

The hallucinogens, in general, are unlikely to produce lethal effects, even in high doses. Although there was once considerable concern that LSD-like drugs could induce chromosomal damage, recent reviews indicate that when all data are considered, the effect has not been proved. Similarly, although LSD users are more likely to experience spontaneous abortions and fetal abnormalities, the use of other drugs and life-style factors associated with poor nutrition and viral and bacterial infections make it difficult to determine the role of the hallucinogens in the effects on the fetus.

DESIGNER DRUGS Included here under the hallucinogens is a group of drugs structurally related to both amphetamine and mescaline. Drugs in this group tend to have some of the properties of hallucinogens, as well as amphetamine-like effects. For the present, there appear to be three drugs within this group of amphetamine-like hallucinogens that are in use: MDA, MDMA, and 3,4-methylenedioxyethamphetamine (MDEA). During the late 1970s, a small number of psychiatrists began using MDA as an adjunct to psychotherapy. In the early 1980s, MDMA, an analogue, began to be synthesized in home laboratories and sold as a recreational drug—that is, a drug self-administered for subjective effects. Not every conceivable drug with reinforcing effects is covered under current state and federal law, and since MDMA was not so specifically listed, the synthesis and sale were not subject to federal criminal statutes. Because it was believed that the decision to synthesize and sell certain drugs with euphorigenic effects was made with a full knowledge of these loopholes in the law, these new synthetics were labeled "designer drugs" by the popular press, and the term was used even in congressional hearings. In July 1985, the loopholes in the law were closed, but not before a considerable number of young people had come to believe that use of these agents was a pleasant and essentially risk-free approach to temporary mind modification. At present, that belief appears to be ill founded. It is now clear that MDA and MDMA can produce long-lasting (probably permanent) damage to serotonergic fibers in the brain of rodents and nonhuman primates. The significance of this finding for humans is now under active investigation.

Among users, MDMA is also known as ecstasy, XTC, Adam, and MDM; MDEA is sometimes called Eve. It is reported to induce euphoria lasting about 4 to 6 hours. As with the LSD-like drugs, some users have reported confusion, depression, and anxiety lasting for several weeks after a single dose. There is almost no reliable information on patterns of use, abuse, or dependence on these drugs. The use of MDMA and MDEA has been associated with a number of reported fatalities, but it is not certain what role the drug effects played in some of them.

TREATMENT AND PROGNOSIS No specialized treatments for hallucinogenic drug abuse have been developed. Most individuals who try these drugs do so for only brief periods; even those whose use meets DSM-III-R criteria for abuse generally cease use after a relatively short time.

INHALANTS

The inhalation of volatile substances for subjective effects antedates the use of these substances as anesthetics. In the nineteenth century, there were ether frolics and nitrous oxide parties before the therapeutic potential of the substances was appreciated. Current problems associated with the use of inhalants made their appearance in the 1950s when it was reported that a variety of easily obtained volatile substances (e.g., glue, spray paint propellants, cleaning fluids, gasoline, and industrial solvents) were being used to produce altered states of consciousness. Because of their widespread use in commerce, control of the availability of these substances is virtually impossible; because of their heterogeneity, generalizations about the pharmacology of these inhalants is almost as difficult.

PHARMACOLOGY These inhaled substances exert actions on the CNS that are roughly similar to those of volatile anesthetics such as ether and chloroform. However, some of the agents also have significant toxic effects on the liver and the kidney; others (e.g., fluorinated hydrocarbons) produce cardiac arrhythmias. Still others produce bizarre perceptual and hallucinatory actions that are not typical of CNS depressants. Peripheral neuropathies and progressive neurological deterioration may follow "huffing" of lacquer thinner, and brain damage has been found among inhalers of aerosol paints. Efforts to delineate more precisely the kinds of CNS damage induced by inhalants are confounded by the variability of the substances used, the wide range of intensity of exposure, and the fact that most inhalant users have histories of learning disabilities and behavioral and mood problems that predate their use of inhalants. Animals will self-administer nitrous oxide, chloroform, and solvents, such as toluene. Some tolerance develops to the actions of these drugs, as well as some cross-tolerance between anesthetics and barbiturates.

PATTERNS OF ABUSE AND PSYCHOLOGICAL EFFECTS Typically, inhalant users have been young, poor, and members of Hispanic, black or native American minorities who do not have easy access to alcohol or other psychoactive agents. Most users actually prefer other drugs, such as marijuana, and most use many drugs when they can get them. Lack of access, however, cannot explain the reports of physicians, dentists, and nurses who have become repetitive users of nitrous oxide and other medically used volatile or gaseous agents, sometimes with disastrous impact on themselves or their patients. For reasons that are not entirely clear, in DSM-III-R, anesthetic gases and short-acting vasodilators (e.g., amyl nitrite) are specifically excluded from the category of inhalants; instead, patterns of abuse and dependence on such substances are listed under psychoactive substance dependence not otherwise specified.

Most commonly, the inhalants are used by placing a rag soaked with inhalant over the mouth and nose. Alternatively, the material can be put into a plastic or paper bag and the user covers his or her face with the bag. In the latter instance, it is possible to induce anoxia as well as intoxication. (Table 13.1-38 lists the diagnostic criteria for inhalant intoxication.) Inhaled substances reach the bloodstream rapidly and the effects are virtually immediate. The sniffing or huffing of inhalants is typically a social activity undertaken in groups. The relatively

TABLE 13.1-38
Diagnostic Criteria for Inhalant Intoxication

A. Recent use of an inhalant.

B. Maladaptive behavioral changes (e.g., belligerence, assaultiveness, apathy, impaired judgment, impaired social or occupational functioning).

C. At least two of the following signs:
(1) dizziness
(2) nystagmus
(3) incoordination
(4) slurred speech
(5) unsteady gait
(6) lethargy
(7) depressed reflexes
(8) psychomotor retardation
(9) tremor
(10) generalized muscle weakness
(11) blurred vision or diplopia
(12) stupor or coma
(13) euphoria

D. Not due to any physical or other mental disorder.

Table from DSM-III-R *Diagnostic and Statistical Manual of Mental Disorders,* ed 3, revised. Copyright American Psychiatric Association, Washington, DC, 1987. Used with permission.

few solitary sniffers are often heavier users who are more psychologically disturbed.

There appears to be no specialized treatments for inhalant abuse or dependence. Clinicians generally report that patients referred for treatment of this behavior generally come from the criminal justice system and are typically unmotivated, disruptive, and mentally slow. Such referrals generally do poorly, staying in treatment for an average of only 2 to 3 months.

NICOTINE (TOBACCO)

During most of the twentieth century, tobacco use was viewed as quite distinct from other forms of drug use, in part because there is no obvious acute phase of intoxication and in part because those who define drug dependence syndromes chose to emphasize this one difference rather than the wider range of similarities. There is now a general consensus that the criteria for drug dependence shown in Table 13.1-1 are applicable to tobacco.

PATTERNS OF USE Tobacco can be smoked or used as snuff, which is either insufflated or held between the cheek and the gum. Most smokers who use cigarettes inhale the smoke deep into the lung; pipe and cigar smokers absorb the nicotine primarily from the buccal mucosa. In all likelihood, pipe and cigar smokers also inhale some of the smoke, especially if they ever learned to inhale cigarette smoke. Approximately 32 percent of Americans over 12 years of age are regular cigarette smokers.

PHARMACOLOGICAL ACTIONS AND PSYCHOLOGICAL EFFECTS The evidence that points to nicotine as the major psychoactive substance in tobacco is at least as strong as the evidence supporting an analogous role for Δ^9-THC in marijuana, morphine in opium, and alcohol in gin and tonic. Nicotine's effectiveness as a reinforcer of drug taking is dependent on the behavioral and physiological status of the user. In animal models, nicotine is not as powerful a reinforcer as cocaine or amphetamines. Despite this difficulty, reinforcing effects as evidenced by drug self-administration have been demonstrated in rats, dogs, and monkeys. In humans, nicotine does not produce such dramatic euphoric effects that most users immediately want to repeat the experience; yet, a very high percentage of those who smoke more than 100 cigarettes go on to become daily cigarette smokers and tend to persist in the behavior for years. When heavy cigarette smokers who are also drug abusers are given nicotine intravenously (0.75 to 3.0 mg per injection), they report euphoric effects somewhat comparable to those produced by CNS stimulants. Research volunteers, even those without histories of illicit drug use, will self-administer nicotine intravenously, and may do so despite adverse effects (e.g., burning sensations in the vein, nausea associated with the procedure).

It does seem that nicotine produces its subjective and reinforcing effects in the CNS, since they can be blocked by centrally active ganglionic blockers (mecamylamine), but not peripherally active blockers, such as pentolinium. There appear to be several subsets of stereospecific binding sites for nicotine in the CNS, but which of these sites are responsible for its subjective and reinforcing actions is not clear. It is not yet clear to what degree, if any, the reinforcing effects of nicotine overlap with the dopaminergic systems that seem so critical to the reinforcing effects of drugs like cocaine. Some animal studies indicate that nicotine can release norepinephrine and dopamine from brain tissue. Nicotine may increase or decrease acetylcholine release, depending on the dose. It causes the release of a number of neurohormones (growth hormone, vasopressin, ACTH). At a more functional level, nicotine at dosages produced by smoking has a number of physiological effects in humans that could be reinforcing for some individuals under some circumstances. It produces an alerting effect on the EEG associated with behavioral arousal. For some smokers, it acts to facilitate functioning under boring conditions. For other smokers, it acts to reduce anxiety. It has been speculated that the nicotine-induced increased capacity to focus attention may be linked to release of one or more of these hormones. Nicotine suppresses the irritability, impatience, and anger associated with nicotine withdrawal, and, even in individuals not physically dependent, nicotine may reduce irritability. Nicotine functions as an anorectant in a variety of animal models and under a remarkably broad range of conditions in humans. Several possible mechanisms, including metabolic changes and selective suppression of carbohydrate appetite, have been implicated. Nicotine is rapidly metabolized to its major metabolite, cotinine, which is inactive. The half-life of nicotine is about 2 hours; that of cotinine is about 20 hours.

FACTORS IN NICOTINE DEPENDENCE The same factors that contribute to dependence on opioids and other drugs contribute, albeit with different weights, to the development of dependence on nicotine (tobacco). Until quite recently, tobacco use was so common and socially acceptable that antecedent deviance or psychopathology, or both, played little role in determining who would experiment; that is, almost everyone tried smoking. But even under conditions of total social acceptance, those who went on to become heavy smokers tended to be a bit more impulsive, adventuresome, extroverted, and somewhat less tolerant of rules. In some studies, the heavy smoker was found to be more angry than the nonsmoker or light smoker. Over the past decade, cigarette smoking has become less socially acceptable. Currently, those who smoke are more likely to be less well adjusted and less scholastically successful. The major motives for initial use of tobacco are to identify with friends who smoke and to signal an attitude toward life and values in general.

Most of those who start to smoke do not plan to become dependent. The loss of flexibility and the development of dependence is gradual. After a while, the pharmacological factors in tobacco use come to be increasingly important in determining continued use. As with cocaine, amphetamines, and opioids, the route of administration makes a significant difference in the likelihood of developing dependence. When cigarette smoke is inhaled, each puff produces a small bolus of nicotine that is absorbed through the alveoli and reaches the brain even more rapidly than nicotine given intravenously. Because of its lipid solubility and rapid metabolism, brain levels of nicotine also fall rapidly so that 30 to 45 minutes later, the smoker, especially the physically dependent smoker, begins to feel the need for another cigarette. Nicotine is not the most powerful reinforcer available, but since the average cigarette delivers about 8 to 10 puffs of nicotine, for the smoker of a pack of cigarettes per day, nicotine inhalation will be reinforced about 70,000 times over a period of just 1 year. Further, puffing behavior and withdrawal-induced craving become conditioned to virtually every element in a smoker's life. Figure 13.1-11 illustrates the way that plasma nicotine levels rise and fall after each cigarette and contrasts this pattern with the slower increases in blood levels produced by nicotine-containing gum. Although the plasma levels do not rise and fall as sharply as they do with cigarette smoking, it is assumed that the pharmacological effects of nicotine are also important factors perpetuating the use of smokeless tobaccos or snuff.

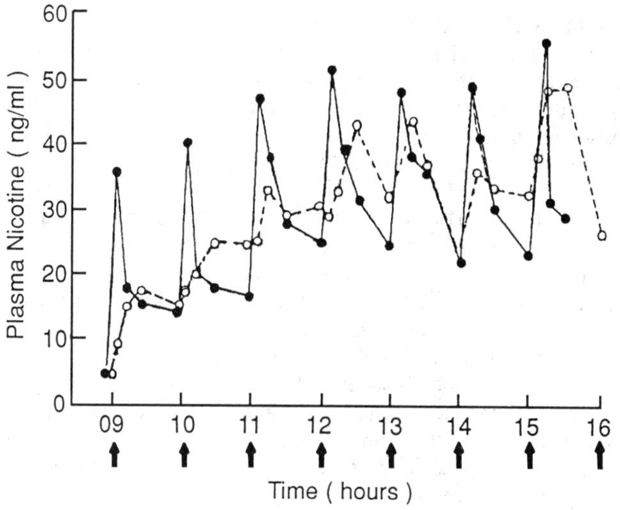

FIGURE 13.1-11. *Plasma nicotine levels after cigarette smoking and the use of 4 mg of nicotine polacrilex. With 2 mg of nicotine polacrilex (the only dosage approved in the United States), plasma levels are half those of the 4-mg dose. (From Sachs D P: Cigarette smoking: Health effects and cessation strategies. Clin Geriat Med 2: 345, 1986, with permission.)*

ADVERSE MEDICAL EFFECTS The adverse medical effects associated with tobacco use will not be described here in detail. They include neoplastic diseases, chronic pulmonary obstructive disease, and cardiovascular disorders ranging from increased probability of myocardial infarction to peripheral arterial disease and cerebrovascular accident.

NICOTINE TOLERANCE AND PHYSICAL DEPENDENCE Considerable tolerance develops to the subjective, cardiovascular, and nauseant effects of nicotine; the heavy cigarette smoker gets a pleasant and relaxed feeling from an IV dose of nicotine (e.g., 3 mg) that would produce nausea and toxicity in a nonsmoker. Some aspects of tolerance decay more rapidly than others. Even for heavy smokers, the first cigarette in the morning produces more intense psychological and cardiovascular effects than those smoked later in the day.

The nicotine withdrawal syndrome has now been amply studied and shown to be primarily due to nicotine withdrawal. It can be produced by use of nicotine in the form of inhaled tobacco smoke, snuff, or nicotine gum. The syndrome begins within a few hours after the last dose of nicotine and consists of craving for nicotine, irritability, frustration, anxiety, difficulty in concentration, decreased performance on a variety of cognitive tasks, restlessness, decreased heart rate, and changes in appetite. Other symptoms include headaches, sleep disturbances, alterations in proportion of rapid eye movement (REM) sleep, and decreased metabolic rate. There are also increases in slow waves on EEG. Typically, over a period of days or weeks, if no nicotine is used, there is weight gain as well. The sense of craving peaks within 24 hours and then declines gradually over a period of 10 days to several weeks. However, as with cocaine and other drugs, craving can be powerfully evoked by stimuli previously associated with smoking or tobacco use.

Decrements in cognitive performance are measurable for 10 days or more, and some formerly heavy smokers report that they were unable to concentrate on difficult mental tasks for many weeks after quitting. Nicotine in the form of gum suppresses the cardiovascular, cognitive, EEG, and, sometimes, the appetite changes typical of tobacco withdrawal. Usually, it is effective in suppressing withdrawal irritability, but in some studies, it has shown little effect on craving. The lack of effect on craving is probably because nicotine gum produces increases in plasma nicotine levels relatively slowly and cannot mimic the subjective effects associated with the sharp spikes in plasma nicotine produced by the inhalation of tobacco smoke (Fig. 13.1-11). Other forms of nicotine (nasal sprays, inhalers) that produce more rapid increases in blood nicotine levels seem better able to suppress tobacco craving. The DSM-III-R criteria for nicotine withdrawal are shown in Table 13.1-39.

As is the case with other drugs, physical dependence on nicotine (neuroadaptation) is only one component of tobacco (nicotine) dependence, and it is a component that can vary in severity. A scale to estimate this component of tobacco dependence has been developed by Fagerstrom and consists of assigning a score (0 to 2) to each of eight items:

1. How soon after you wake do you smoke your first cigarette? (If within 30 minutes, score = 1)
2. Do you find it difficult to refrain from smoking in places where it is forbidden? (Yes = 1)
3. Which cigarette would you hate most to give up? (First in morning = 1)
4. How many cigarettes a day do you smoke? (15 or less = 0; 16 to 25 = 1; 26 or more = 2)
5. Do you smoke more frequently in the morning? (Yes = 1)
6. Do you smoke if you are so ill that you are in bed? (Yes = 1)
7. What is the nicotine level of usual brand? (0.9 mg or less = 0; 1.0 to 1.2 = 1; more than 1.3 mg = 2)
8. Do you inhale? (Never = 0; sometimes = 1; always = 2)

(A score of 8 or more is considered a high degree of tolerance–physical dependence.)

Several studies indicate that those smokers who have a high tolerance–physical dependence score are more likely to be successful when they attempt to quit smoking cigarettes if nicotine gum (or some other form of nicotine) is used in conjunction with behavioral treatment.

Treatments for nicotine dependence Although the principles of treatment of tobacco dependence are quite similar to those that apply to other forms of drug dependence, treat-

TABLE 13.1-39
Diagnostic Criteria for Nicotine Withdrawal

A. Daily use of nicotine for at least several weeks.

B. Abrupt cessation of nicotine use, or reduction in the amount of nicotine used, followed within 24 hours by at least four of the following signs:
(1) craving for nicotine
(2) irritability, frustration, or anger
(3) anxiety
(4) difficulty concentrating
(5) restlessness
(6) decreased heart rate
(7) increased appetite or weight gain

Table from DSM-III-R *Diagnostic and Statistical Manual of Mental Disorders,* ed 3, revised. Copyright American Psychiatric Association, Washington, DC, 1987. Used with permission.

ments for cigarette smoking have developed in a very different historical context and will be discussed separately here.

Treatments for tobacco dependence have included hypnosis; various pharmacological treatments; behavioral modification, including contingency contracting and aversive conditioning; individual counseling; advice and exhortation; group counseling; self-help kits; sensory deprivation; group psychotherapy; acupuncture; and health education. Although there have been some reports of inpatient treatment, tobacco dependence is handled almost exclusively on an outpatient basis. Despite the diversity of the approaches described, each one has some finite expected success rate. For example, when a general practitioner simply takes the time to tell his or her smoking patients to stop, the percentage not smoking 1 year later is significantly greater than would be the case under control conditions (5 percent versus 0.3 percent in one study). When the smoker has just been treated for a life-threatening illness, the percentage responding to such strong advice and still not smoking at 1 year can be substantially higher (e.g., 63 percent of those given the advice in a coronary care unit after a myocardial infarction versus 28 percent of controls).

With smoking, perhaps more so than with other varieties of drug dependence, the likelihood of long-term successful quitting is related to the severity of dependence, even when the severity is measured by as crude an index as total cigarettes smoked per day (e.g., people who smoke more than two packs of cigarettes per day are less likely to be successful than people who smoke a pack or less). For example, in a large-scale multicenter study of men who volunteered for a multifaceted program to reduce the probability of heart attack, 43 percent of those smoking a pack or less per day were able to quit successfully, compared with only 18 percent of those smoking two or more packs per day.

As with other dependencies, motivation is critical; those who seek help only to please others generally do poorly. One finding that repeatedly emerges from the research on smoking behavior is that because of the smoker's tendency to adjust or titrate nicotine levels, switching to low-tar, low-nicotine brands of cigarettes or just cutting down does very little good. Most cigarette smokers tend to adjust puffing and inhalation patterns to compensate for changes in the nicotine delivered by their cigarettes. In smokers who switch brands, plasma nicotine levels decline only modestly and carbon monoxide levels decline minimally, if at all. Even when smokers switch to ultralow-nicotine brands, which use extensive ventilation to dilute the smoke (and on a smoking machine, deliver as little as 0.1 mg of nicotine), blood levels of nicotine fall to only about 50 percent of the levels produced by brands of cigarettes with nicotine deliveries of 1.0 mg or higher per cigarette.

As a gross generalization, from 50 to 75 percent of smokers who seek formal help with tobacco dependence will be able to abstain for 48 hours or more by the end of most established treatments other than with self-help and physician advice. However, the relapse rate over the subsequent 12 months is usually quite high, so only 25 to 30 percent of those who are initially successful are still nonsmokers at the end of 1 year.

SELF-HELP MANUALS AND KITS Over the past decade, the American Cancer Association and the American Lung Association have distributed millions of kits designed to offer smokers a step-by-step approach to quitting. In addition, how-to-quit books, authored by experienced practitioners, have been published and promoted. When these materials are used as study guides by a trained therapist or group leader, they can be as effective as other behavioral approaches, but when used by the smoker as the only form of help, they are considerably less effective than other approaches to be described. Nevertheless, the 1-year success rate for the American Lung Association self-help program was 5 percent, compared with a control condition success rate of 2 percent.

AVERSIVE CONDITIONING Aversive conditioning techniques couple external stimuli (e.g., electric shocks) or internal stimuli (aversive effects of excessive nicotine) with the act of smoking. Electric shock is now rarely used, but the rapid-smoking method, when combined with other behavioral techniques, health advice, and emotional support, is now recognized as one of the most reliable and effective treatments for tobacco dependence. Rapid smoking consists of having the patient inhale smoke from his or her own cigarette every 6 seconds. The procedure is carried out while the patient is being observed by a trained therapist. The puffing continues until the patient is unwilling to take another puff (because the plasma level nicotine has exceeded the level of tolerance, producing typical nicotine-induced nausea and negative effects). It usually takes about 10 to 15 minutes of puffing to reach this level. Repeating this procedure directly links smoking with negative effects. Although it was at first postulated that the buildup of carbon monoxide and nicotine might be unsafe, it has been shown that the method can be used safely even on patients with cardiac and pulmonary disease. In such patients, a 50 percent abstinence rate at the 2-year follow-up has been reported. Such long-term cessation rates exceed those typically associated with other methods, but are not atypical of the rapid-smoking technique when it is used by an experienced therapist as part of an overall program.

ACUPUNCTURE AND HYPNOSIS Acupuncture demands little of the patient, and it delivers in proportion to what it demands. Controlled studies demonstrate no efficacy for this method. Although hypnosis appears to demand no more, it may actually be effective when combined with group therapy. However, there are few controlled studies with 1-year follow-up periods.

COMMERCIAL PROGRAMS These programs (e.g., Smokenders, Shick Clinics) generally involve multiple behavioral modification methods. Some programs (e.g., Smokenders) also utilize group process and group support; for the most part, they focus on motivating participants, teaching them about nicotine dependence, offering techniques to cope with withdrawal, and conditioned craving. Although data are not easily obtained, these programs are probably considerably more effective than self-help programs, but they are probably less effective than the rapid-smoking techniques in the hands of a skilled therapist.

PHARMACOLOGICAL INTERVENTIONS A variety of drugs have been tested as treatments or adjuncts to treatment of tobacco dependence. Thus far, there is firm evidence for the efficacy of only one drug category: nicotine itself. Nicotine in the form of gum (nicotine polacrilex, Nicorette) has been repeatedly demonstrated to increase the likelihood of successful tobacco abstinence in a variety of situations ranging from nicotine gum plus physician's advice to nicotine gum in the context of a multicomponent behavioral treatment offered by an experienced therapist. The context in which it is used makes a great deal of difference. When the gum was prescribed (at no cost) with proper but perfunctory advice by a general practitioner, it raised the 1-year successful abstinence rate from a dismal 4.1 percent to a statistically significant higher, but almost as dismal, rate of 8.8 percent. (However, only half of smokers bothered to have the prescription filled.) When the gum is combined with effective behavioral therapy, 1-year success rates of up to 40 to 50 percent have been reported, compared with 25 to 30 percent for behavioral therapy alone.

People who have higher levels of nicotine physical dependence appear to benefit more from gum than those with lower levels of tolerance and physical dependence. The gum needs to be chewed in a very specific way, since the nicotine is not passively extracted (i.e., chewing is required to release it). Because swallowed nicotine is mostly detoxified in its first pass through the liver, chewing it like ordinary gum will probably produce no significant benefits. Some individuals find it difficult to give up chewing the gum without relapsing to tobacco use. The significance of such dependence on nicotine gum is, at present, unclear. Nicotine gum does not selectively suppress craving for tobacco, but it does reduce some components of the tobacco withdrawal syndrome and perhaps other symptoms that had been suppressed by tobacco-delivered nicotine. With these symptoms under control, the individual generally finds it easier to readjust to behavioral patterns that had been intimately intertwined with tobacco use.

There has been one report that clonidine reduces craving for tobacco.

CAFFEINE

Caffeine is present in a wide range of commonly used beverages, over-the-counter preparations, and combination prescription drugs (Table 13.1-40). Caffeine is, without question, the most commonly used psychoactive drug in the world. It is estimated that 20 to 30 percent of adult Americans consume more than 500 mg of caffeine per day.

TABLE 13.1-40
Some Common Sources of Caffeine and Representative Decaffeinated Products

Source	*Approximate Amounts of Caffeine per Unit*
Beverages and Foods	5–6 oz
Fresh drip coffee, brewed coffee	90–140 mg
Instant coffee	66–100 mg
Tea (leaf or bagged)	30–100 mg
Cocoa	5–50 mg
Decaffeinated coffee	2–4 mg
Chocolate bar or ounce of baking chocolate	25–35 mg
Selected soft drinks	8–12 oz
Pepsi, Coke, Tab, Royal Crown, Pepsi Light, Dr. Pepper, Mountain Dew	25–50 mg
Canada Dry Ginger Ale, Caffeine Free Coke, Like, Pepsi Free, 7-Up, Sprite, Squirt, Caffeine Free Tab	0 mg
Prescription medications (1 tablet)	
Cafergot, Migralam	100 mg
Anoquan, Aspir-code, BAC, Darvon, Fiorinal	32–50 mg
Over-the-counter analgesics and cold preparations	
Excedrin,	60
Aspirin compound, Anacin, B-C powder, Capron, Cope, Dolor, Midol, Nilain, Norgesic, PAC, Trigesic, Vanquish,	30–32.5 mg
Advil, Aspirin, Empirin, Midol 200, Nuprin, Pamprin	0 mg
Over-the-counter stimulants and appetite suppressants	
Caffin-TD, Caffedrine	250 mg
Vivarin, Ver capsules	200 mg
Quick-Pep	140–150 mg
Amostat, Anorexin, Appedrine, Nodoz Wakoz	100 mg

CAFFEINE DEPENDENCE The most characteristic symptom of the caffeine withdrawal syndrome is headache, associated with increased fatigue and decreased alertness and friendliness. The syndrome reaches peak intensity 24 to 48 hours after the last dose of caffeine and then gradually subsides over 5 to 6 days. However, some subjects report persistent headache for many days.

In studies of laboratory animals and man, caffeine is, at best, a weak reinforcer. Further, in contrast to drugs such as amphetamine and cocaine, caffeine generally fails to induce feelings of euphoria or well-being. In fact, it is more likely to induce dysphoria and anxiety, especially in those who do not use it regularly. A major determinant of its effects appears to be the degree of caffeine tolerance and dependence of the user. After a night of caffeine abstinence, heavy coffee drinkers report pleasant and desirable effects of coffee drinking; non–coffee drinkers report unpleasant and undesirable effects. It is probable that, for most individuals who consume caffeine in one form or another, tolerance and physical dependence are necessary preconditions for its pleasurable and reinforcing effects.

Despite the probability that some degree of physical dependence (neuroadaptation) on caffeine is one of the most common self-induced physiological human aberrations, the severity of impairment associated with caffeine neuroadaptation and the long-term consequences of its use were judged to be too low to include caffeine dependence as a disorder in DSM-III-R. In any event, it is unlikely that many individuals would meet the criteria for dependence outlined in Table 13.1-1. As with individuals dependent on therapeutic doses of analgesics, neuroadaptation (physical dependence) alone can be considered a physical, rather than a mental, disorder.

CAFFEINE INTOXICATION In contrast to the low level of importance assigned to caffeine dependence, there is a consensus that caffeinism (acute or chronic overuse of caffeine with resultant toxicity) is a syndrome of clinical significance. It can mimic or aggravate a number of physical and psychiatric disorders. The DSM-III-R diagnostic criteria for caffeine intoxication are given in Table 13.1-41. In addition, the literature on caffeinism also describes abdominal pain, aggravation of anxiety, panic disorder or depression, and possible exacerbation of schizophrenia as possible consequences of excess caffeine intake. Individuals vary considerably in sensitivity to caffeine, and considerable tolerance develops to its effects. However, loss of tolerance to varying degrees also occurs. When this happens, the user, who may not have altered his or her caffeine intake, may not recognize that symptoms are due to caffeine. Caffeine intoxicaton is not commonly seen when daily intake is less than 250 mg. Diagnosis of caffeine intoxication is based on recent consumption of caffeine, usually in excess of 250 mg, excluding other causes and the presence of at least five of the 12 caffeine-induced signs and symptoms of caffeinism mentioned

TABLE 13.1-41
Diagnostic Criteria for Caffeine Intoxication

A. Recent consumption of caffeine, usually in excess of 250 mg.

B. At least five of the following signs:
(1) restlessness
(2) nervousness
(3) excitement
(4) insomnia
(5) flushed face
(6) diuresis
(7) gastrointestinal disturbance
(8) muscle twitching
(9) rambling flow of thought and speech
(10) tachycardia or cardiac arrhythmia
(11) periods of inexhaustibility
(12) psychomotor agitation

C. Not due to any physical or other mental disorder, such as an anxiety disorder.

Table from DSM-III-R *Diagnostic and Statistical Manual of Mental Disorders,* ed 3, revised. Copyright American Psychiatric Association, Washington, DC, 1987. Used with permission.

in Table 13.1-41. Once the cause of the symptoms are brought to the patient's attention, about half of the individuals will follow advice to use decaffeinated beverages. The other half seem reluctant to do so. Special therapy is not commonly required.

IMPLICATIONS OF DRUG DEPENDENCE FOR SPECIAL POPULATIONS

TREATMENT OF PATIENTS WITH SPECIAL MEDICAL AND SURGICAL PROBLEMS Drug users often present unique problems when they require medical care. When former opioid addicts and patients maintained on methadone are admitted to a hospital for medical treatment or surgery, patients should be told what procedures will be done and that adequate analgesia will be provided. Disclosing the precise dosage of the analgesia is usually unnecessary. It is inappropriate to cause stress in the patient by beginning detoxification before the required medical or surgical treatment has been accomplished.

Patients on methadone should be continued on their usual oral dose, or, if oral administration is not possible, they should be given one-half to two-thirds of their usual dose parenterally in divided doses. Methadone may be omitted on the day of surgery. It is reported that, despite their tolerance to the euphorigenic effects of heroin, hospitalized patients maintained on methadone experience satisfactory analgesia with 50 to 100 mg of meperidine given parenterally every 3 to 4 hours; some clinicians recommend increasing the standard dosage of opioid analgesics by 25 percent.

Opioids addicts who are taking street drugs when admitted to a hospital should be placed on oral or parenteral methadone to prevent withdrawal; 30 to 40 mg per day in divided doses is usually sufficient. These patients, too, will require additional analgesia, depending on the problems and procedures. Patients maintained on methadone should not be given pentazocine, butorphanol, or nalbuphine because these drugs may precipitate withdrawal.

Patients dependent on sedatives or anxiolytics are generally tolerant to anesthetics and to routine doses of evening hypnotics; they may experience withdrawal if the drugs are abruptly discontinued. Patients who have been using cocaine, amphetamines, or cannabis generally exhibit few problems requiring special interventions.

OPIOID-DEPENDENT WOMEN Opioid-dependent women have problems that are often unmet in treatment programs. About 70 percent of female opioid addicts cite drug-related medical problems—often infections, venereal disease, and toxemia—as reasons for seeking treatment. Many opioid-dependent women seek medical care when they are pregnant. Women who use opiods also have more problems with depression and low self-esteem than do opioid-using men. A research project on drug-dependent women found that, for the 2 years prior to admission, only 3 percent had been employed continuously, and 37 percent had not been employed at all. Women also have problems with care of their children during treatment. In one study, 73 percent of female opioid addicts were mothers, and 48 percent had children under 6 years of age. In several East Coast treatment programs, 60 percent of black female patients (but only 13 percent of white females) are seropositive for HIV. Most of the children below age 6 with AIDS have a mother who used drugs IV.

Drugs and pregnancy A wide range of drugs can alter fetal growth and development, perinatal morbidity, and later development and emotional behavior. Although opioid withdrawal is almost never fatal for the otherwise healthy adult, opioid withdrawal is hazardous to the fetus and can lead to miscarriage or fetal death. Maintaining the pregnant addict on high doses of methadone, however, carries the risk of severe withdrawal in the neonate. Maintenance on low doses of methadone may not adequately control the tendency to use illicit opioids, but there is a growing consensus that such low-dose maintenance—10 to 40 mg per day—may be the least hazardous course to follow. At such dosage, neonatal withdrawal is usually mild and can be managed with low doses of paregoric. If the pregnancy begins while the patient is on high doses of methadone, reduction to lower dosage should be quite slow (e.g., 1 mg every 3 days), and fetal movements should be monitored. If withdrawal is necessary or desired, it is accomplished with least hazard during the second trimester. Women who use opioids, whether illicit or prescribed, tend to have more obstetrical complications at delivery than controls.

Neonatal withdrawal syndromes have been reported after intrauterine exposure to sedative-hypnotics and cocaine. Much less is known about the hazards of intrauterine withdrawal of other classes of drugs. Data are accumulating on the hazards for the fetus and the longer-term developmental effects on the offspring of maternal drug use during pregnancy. Cocaine use during early pregnancy is associated with a higher rate of spontaneous abortion than is seen with opioid use. Cocaine use during late pregnancy may cause premature labor and abruptio placentae. The embryotoxic and other effects of alcohol are discussed elsewhere. Intrauterine opioid exposures result in reduced intrauterine and neonatal growth. Children exposed to methadone in utero have greater difficulty than control children with tasks that are highly structured or involve verbal instruction, and they are more likely to be referred for behavioral and academic problems. Intrauterine cannabis exposure appears to decrease infant length at birth and may delay postnatal maturation of the arousal system. However, maternal marijuana use does not appear to increase the incidence of obstetrical complications at delivery. Neonates exposed in utero to PCP, stimulants, or sedative-hypnotics showed few significant differences from controls in terms of somatic growth measures, but showed marked deficits in behavior. Some studies suggest that infants of mothers who used drugs during pregnancy have abnormally long periods of apnea and are at higher risk for sudden infant death syndrome. Many of the problems identified among children exposed in utero could have origins in genetic as well as environmental (parenting) factors.

HEALTH CARE PROFESSIONALS The lifetime prevalence of opioid dependence among physicians, nurses, and pharmacists is reported to be approximately 1 percent, a figure that is substantially higher than that of groups with comparable educational achievements and socioeconomic status. It was once generally accepted that ease of access to opioid drugs and familiarity with their effects were the major etiological factors that, for these health care professionals, increased the likelihood of self-medication at times of pain, stress, or depression. Additional factors, however, are usually found when such individuals enter treatment. Among health care professionals under 40 years old, serious psychopathology—especially depression—has been found to be common. In one study, among health care professionals over 55 entering treatment, 60 percent had signs of impaired brain function. It is not clear to what degree brain impairment was a cause or a consequence of drug use. Most physicians who seek treatment use or are dependent on more than one drug; alcoholism is not uncommon.

In recent years, many people have used a variety of drugs for nonmedical purposes before entering the health professions, and in the future, problems with self-administration may be less frequently associated with stress and depression than as a complication of recreational use of opioids. To date, the prognosis for health professionals has been excellent, with 70 to 80 percent making a full recovery from drug problems. Considerable external pressure, however, including threat of license revocation, may be required initially to prod them into treatment, and the continued threat of such license revocation for those professionals under formal probation may be a major factor in the relatively good prognosis. Return to practice with its exposure and access to drugs is also a problem. Contingency contracting has been suggested as a behavioral approach that has particular value for health care and other professionals with drug abuse problems.

PREVENTION OF DRUG ABUSE AND DEPENDENCE

ROLE OF THE MEDICAL COMMUNITY For the past 20 years, the predominant method of preventing drug dependence in the United States has been to limit the availability of drugs to medically approved users and to deter illicit use through the use of criminal sanctions and by heaping opprobrium on the illicit users. For opioids, this approach began almost 80 years ago. The role of the medical profession has been limited largely to prescribing drugs with opioid actions carefully and to identifying new drugs with opioid actions for inclusion under various laws and regulations. With respect to cautious prescribing of opioids, the health professions have probably carried prevention to an extreme, and many medical and surgical patients now suffer needlessly because of the underuse of potent opioids. More recently, the medical profession has become more aware of the importance of carefully prescribing other psychoactive drugs, such as amphetamines, sedatives, and anxiolytics.

To the degree that prevention is also the prevention of the progression and complications of dependence, the reentry of the medical profession into the active treatment of opioid dependence over the past 20 years is a positive step.

OTHER CONSIDERATIONS Over the past decade, there has been renewed interest in preventing drug abuse and dependence through special educational and mass-media efforts. There is no way at present to judge the impact of these mass-media efforts. Some evaluation has been carried out on school-based programs aimed at either (1) increasing awareness of the dangers of drug use (cognitive approach); (2) enabling young people to resist peer pressure to experiment with drugs of any kind; or (3) increasing the general sense of competence of young people to cope with daily stresses. Evaluation thus far suggests that cognitive approaches have little or no impact. In part, these efforts are based on the observation that people who become users of cocaine and heroin in most cases begin with more readily available drugs, such as tobacco, alcohol, and marijuana. The use of these gateway or stepping-stone drugs appears to facilitate other drug use or erode some psychological barrier to progression. A major hypothesis is that preventing or delaying the use of the gateway drugs among young people may prevent later abuse and dependence on a wider range of drugs. What is clear is that, even when attempts are made to control for antecedent individual differences, the use of marijuana and other illicit drugs in adolescence is associated with increased delinquency, unemployment, divorce, and abortions, as well as continued drug use.

Recently, there has been a tendency to extend the use of drug detection (i.e., urine testing), which has been successfully used by the U.S. military, as a technique for deterring drug use and preventing progression of use to dependence. The use of such testing in work force or school populations is costly and is often considered intrusive. Despite the demonstrable efficacy of this approach to prevention within the military, there are still only limited data on which to base cost-benefit analyses.

REFERENCES

Benowitz N L: The human pharmacology of nicotine. Ann Rev Med *37*: 1, 1986.

Busto U, Sellers E M, Naranjo C A, Cappell H, Sanchez-Craig M, Sykora K: Withdrawal reaction after long-term therapeutic use of benzodiazepines. New Eng J Med *315*: 14, 1986.

Childress A R, McLellan A T, O'Brien C P: Conditioned responses in a methadone population: A comparison of laboratory, clinic, and natural settings. J Substance Abuse Treat *3*: 173, 1986.

Clouet D H, editor: *Phencyclidine: An update,* NIDA Research Monograph 64. U.S. Department of Health and Human Services, Rockville, MD, 1986.

Cohen S: Marijuana. In *Psychiatry Update: American Psychiatric Association Annual Review,* A I Frances, R E Hales, editors, vol 5, p 200. American Psychiatric Press, Washington, DC, 1986.

Contreras P C, DiMaggio D A, O'Donohue T L: An endogenous ligand for the sigma opioid binding site. Synapse *1*: 57, 1987.

Freedman D X: Hallucinogenic drug research—If so, so what? Pharmacol Biochem Behav *24*: 1986.

Gawin F H, Kleber H D: Abstinence symptomatology and psychiatric diagnosis in cocaine abusers. Arch Gen Psychiat *43*: 2, 1986.

Griffiths, R R, Bigelow, G E, Liebson, I A: Human coffee drinking: Reinforcing and physical dependence producing effects of caffeine. J Pharmacol Exp Ther *239*: 2, 1986.

Henningfield J E: Pharmacologic basis and treatment of cigarette smoking. J Clin Psychiat *45*: 24, 1986.

Jaffe J H: Drug addiction and drug abuse. In *The Pharmacological Basis of Therapeutics,* A G Gilman, L S Goodman, T W Rall, F Murad, editors, ed 7, p 532. Macmillan, New York, 1985.

Jaffe J H, Martin W R: Opioid analgesics and antagonists. In *The Pharmacological Basis of Therapeutics,* A G Gilman, L S Goodman, T W Rall, F Murad, editors, ed 7, p 491. Macmillan, New York, 1985.
Jones R T: Cannabis and health. Ann Rev Med *34*: 247, 1983.
Kandel D B, Davies M. Karus D, Yamaguchi K: The consequences in young adulthood of adolescent drug involvement. Arch Gen Psychiat *43*: 746, 1986.
Karno M, Hough R L, Burnam A. Escobar J. I, Timbers D M, Santana F, Boyd J H: Lifetime prevalence of specific psychiatric disorders among Mexican Americans and non-Hispanic whites in Los Angeles. Arch Gen Psychiat *44*: 8, 1987, 695.
Kleber H D, Gawin F H: Cocaine. In *Psychiatry Update: The American Psychiatric Association Annual Review,* A I Frances, R E Hales, editors, vol 5, p 160. American Psychiatric Press, Washington, DC, 1986.
Kleber H D, Topazian M, Gaspari J, Riordan C E, Kosten T: Clonidine and naltrexone in the outpatient treatment of heroin withdrawal. Amer J Drug Alcohol Abuse *13*: 1, 1987.
Kosten T R, Rounsaville B J, Kleber H D: A 2.5 year follow-up of depression, life crises, and treatment effects on abstinence among opioid addicts. Arch Gen Psychiat *43*: 733, 1986.
Lewis C E, Halikas J A, Morse C, Rimmer J D: Alcoholism in narcotic addicts with antisocial personality. Brit J Addict *82*: 305, 1987.
Maddux J F, Desmond D P: Relapse and recovery in substance abuse careers. In *NIDA Research Monograph Series 72,* F M Tims, C G Leukenfeld, editors, p 49. U.S. Department of Health and Human Services, Rockville, MD, 1986.
McAuliffe W E, Ch'ien J M N: Recovery training and self help: A relapse-prevention program for treated opioid addicts. J Substance Abuse Treat *3:* 9, 1986.
McLellan A T, Luborsky L, Woody G E, O'Brien C P, Druley K A: Predicting response to alcohol and drug abuse treatments. Arch Gen Psychiat *40*: 620, 1983.
Mendelson J H: Marijuana. In *Psychopharmacology: The Third Generation of Progress,* H. Y. Meltzer, editor, p 1565. Raven Press, New York 1987.
Meyer R E, Mirin S M: *The Heroin Stimulus: Implications for a Theory of Addiction.* Plenum, New York, 1979.
O'Brien C P, Woody, G E: Sedative-hypnotics and antianxiety agents. In *Psychiatry Update: The American Psychiatric Association Annual Review,* A I Frances, R E Hales, editors, vol 5, p 186. American Psychiatric Press, Washington, DC, 1986.
Robins L N, Helzer J E, Weissman M M, Orvaschel H, Gruenberg E, Burke J D Jr, Regier D A: Lifetime prevalence of specific psychiatric disorders in three sites. Arch Gen Psychiat *41*: 949, 1984.
Rounsaville B J, Weissman M M, Kleber H, Wilber C: Heterogeneity of psychiatric diagnosis in treated opiate addicts. Arch Gen Psychiat *39*: 161, 1982.
Sachs D P: Cigarette smoking: Health effects and cessation strategies. Clin Geriat Med *2*: 337, 1986.
Sanchez-Craig M, Cappell H, Busto U, Kay G: Cognitive-behavioural treatment for benzodiazepine dependence: A comparison of gradual versus abrupt cessation of drug intake. Brit J Addict *82*: 1987.
White P T, Raymer S: The poppy—for good and evil. Nat Geograph *167*: 187, February 1985.
Woods J H, Katz J L, Winger G: Abuse liability of benzodiazepines. Pharmacol Rev *39*: 4, 1987.

13.2 ALCOHOLISM

DONALD W. GOODWIN, M.D.

INTRODUCTION

The revised third edition of the American Psychiatric Association's *Diagnostic and Statistical Manual of Mental Disorders* (DSM-III-R) does not mention the word "alcoholism." What most of the world calls alcoholism, DSM-III-R chooses to call alcohol dependence.

Attempts have been made through the years to abandon the word "alcoholism" in favor of a less pejorative-sounding term. "Alcohol dependence" has been recommended by the World Health Organization (WHO), but without much effect. "Alcohol dependence" is an awkward phrase; one must refer constantly to the alcohol-dependent person, when "alcoholic" says the same thing more economically. Introduced by Magnus Huss, a Swedish public health authority in 1849, the word "alcoholism" was quickly adopted by many languages.

While retaining the word "alcoholism," this section of Chapter 13 abides by DSM-III-R definitions. Conditions described under the DSM-III-R category of alcohol-induced mental disorders are discussed here under the subheading Complications. These complications include the alcohol withdrawal syndrome and the amnestic syndrome.

DEFINITION

Before its revision, the third edition of the *Diagnostic and Statistical Manual of Mental Disorders* (DSM-III) separated alcoholism into two types: alcohol abuse and alcohol dependence. The criteria for *alcohol abuse* included a pattern of pathological alcohol use and impairment in social and occupational functioning due to alcohol use. The diagnostic criteria for *alcohol dependence* were identical, with one addition: the patient must also demonstrate tolerance or withdrawal symptoms.

These definitions were widely considered inadequate and, in the revision of DSM-III (DSM-III-R), the term "alcohol abuse" was modified and new criteria for alcohol dependence were introduced. To be alcohol-dependent (or dependent on any drug), the person must demonstrate at least three of the following symptoms:

1. When not actually using the substance, the person spends a great deal of time looking forward to use of or arranging to get the substance.
2. The substance is often taken in larger amounts or over a longer period than the individual intended.
3. The person develops a tolerance; thus, there is a need for increased amounts of the substance in order to achieve intoxication or desired effect, or there will be a diminished effect with continued use of the same amount.
4. Characteristic withdrawal symptoms develop.
5. The substance is often taken to relieve or avoid withdrawal symptoms.
6. There is a persistent desire or repeated efforts to cut down or control substance use.
7. The person shows frequent intoxication or withdrawal symptoms when expected to fulfill social or occupational

obligations, or when substance use is hazardous (e.g., doesn't go to work because hungover or high, goes to work high, drives when drunk).

8. Important social, occupational, or recreational activity is given up or reduced because of its incompatibility with the use of the substance.

9. Substance use continues, despite a persistent social, occupational, psychological or physical problem that it causes or exacerbates.

For the diagnosis to be made, some symptoms of the disturbance must have persisted for at least 1 month or have occurred repeatedly over a longer period of time.

In addition, DSM-III-R introduced criteria for severity of dependence, as follows:

In Full Remission: During the past 6 months, either no use of the substance, or use of the substance and no symptoms of dependence.

In Partial Remission: During the past 6 months, some use of the substance and one or two symptoms of dependence.

Mild: Few, if any, symptoms in excess of those required to make the diagnosis, and the symptoms result in only mild impairment in occupational functioning or in usual social activities or relationships with others.

Moderate: Symptoms or functional impairment intermediate between mild and severe.

Severe: Many symptoms in excess of those required to make the diagnosis, and the symptoms markedly interfere with occupational functioning or with usual social activities or relationships with others.

DSM-III-R defines alcohol abuse as a residual category for noting maladaptive patterns of alcohol use that have never met the criteria for dependence. Table 13.1-2 in Section 13.1 provides the criteria for the category.

The criteria for alcohol abuse apply to abuse of all psychoactive substances. According to DSM-III-R, the category usually applies to people who have only recently started taking psychoactive substances and mainly involves substances, such as cannabis, cocaine, and hallucinogens, that are unlikely to produce severe withdrawal symptoms. The assumption was that only rarely would it be applied to alcohol problems. Hence, this section deals mainly with the concept of alcohol dependence, still commonly called alcoholism.

PHARMACOLOGY OF ALCOHOL

To understand alcoholism, it is useful to know about alcohol itself and its fate in the body. When yeast grows in sugar solutions without air, most of the sugar is converted (fermented) into carbon dioxide and alcohol. When the alcohol concentration reaches about 12 or 13 percent, the process stops. For that reason, unfortified wines have alcohol concentrations of no more than 12 or 13 percent.

As a rule, people do not drink only alcohol; they drink alcoholic beverages. Alcoholic beverages are mainly water and ethyl alcohol. Tiny amounts of other chemicals are present, providing most of the taste and all of the color, if any. Called congeners, these chemicals include amino acids, minerals, vitamins, methanol, and the higher alcohols, known as fusel oil.

Beverages differ according to the sugar source: wine comes from grapes; beer comes from grain and hops; whiskey comes from grain and corn; rum comes from sugar cane; and vodka comes from potatoes and grain.

Distillation was discovered about 800 A.D. in Arabia; alcohol comes from the Arabic word *alkuhl,* meaning essence. Distillation boils away alcohol from its sugar bath and recollects it as virtually pure alcohol. The water is then put back into the solution, so that, instead of it being 100 percent alcohol, the solution is, perhaps, 50 percent alcohol or 100 proof alcohol (the percent figure is half the proof figure).

ALCOHOL METABOLISM Alcohol, whether it is drunk or not, turns to vinegar. Bacteria cause alcohol to sour in open air. To change alcohol to vinegar (acetic acid) in the body, two enzymes are required: alcohol dehydrogenase (ADH) and aldehyde dehydrogenase (AldDH). ADH is located in the liver in surprisingly large supply. The amount of ADH is surprising because, as far as is known, its only function is to metabolize alcohol. ADH disposes of 86 proof distilled spirits at about the rate of 1 ounce per hour. When it is fed into the body's normal metabolic machinery, acetic acid becomes carbon dioxide and water.

Many substances have been tried, such as insulin and caffeine, to speed up the elimination of alcohol from the body. Exercise has also been used in this fashion. Fructose, when given in large doses, speeds up the elimination of alcohol, but the dose is so large that it is sickening, and most people prefer to stay intoxicated.

A second enzyme is required to change alcohol to acetic acid. The intermediate chemical involved in the transformation of alcohol to acetic acid is an aldehyde and is very toxic. The enzyme that destroys the aldehyde is found not only in the liver but also throughout the body. It quickly turns the aldehyde into harmless acetic acid. This enzyme, AldDH, is inhibited by disulfiram (Antabuse). When disulfiram is ingested, an accumulation of acetaldehyde and a toxic reaction result—characterized mainly by vasodilation and hypotension.

Alcohol is almost entirely oxidized in the liver. A small amount is expired in the breath and excreted in urine and sweat. In the oxidation of alcohol, two molecules of diphosphopyridine nucleotide (DPN) are changed to reduced diphosphopyridine nucleotide (DPNH).

$$C_2H_5OH + DPN \xrightarrow{ADH} CH_3CHO + DPNH$$

$$CH_3CHO + DPN \xrightarrow{AldDH} CH_3COOH + DPNH$$

Acetic acid may be harmless, but its production process may harm the body. When it is oxidized, alcohol is stripped of hydrogen atoms. The removal of the hydrogen atoms results in some interesting biochemical changes:

1. There is an increase in lactic acid; such increases have been associated with anxiety attacks. Heavy drinking is also associated with anxiety attacks.

2. There is an increase in uric acid, which is associated with gout—and gout, for centuries, has been associated with alcohol.

3. There is a rapid increase in fat from the oxidation of alcohol, not the slow increase in fat that comes from increased calories (7 calories per gram), but a rapid increase from the oxidation of alcohol. The fat is seen mainly in the liver or blood. One night of serious drinking—say, six or seven highballs—increases discernibly the fat content of the

liver. The liver will be fattier still if fatty food is also ingested.

Alcohol and liver disease The connection between fatty liver and liver diseases, such as hepatitis and cirrhosis, is still undetermined. The fat goes away soon after the drinker stops drinking, and most people who drink do not develop liver disease. Perhaps only 5 or 10 percent of very heavy drinkers develop liver disease. Most people, however, who develop a particular type of liver disease, Laënnec's cirrhosis, are heavy drinkers.

Pancreatitis has long been associated with heavy drinking, and studies in which rats were exposed acutely to alcohol have shown marked alterations in pancreatic lipid metabolism, with increased triglyceride synthesis. Prior exposure to ethanol enhanced this stimulatory effect, confirming the clinical impression that, after one occasion of heavy imbibing, acute pancreatitis occurs less often in moderate drinkers than in chronic alcoholics.

One of the mysteries about alcohol is that, despite its universal reputation for being fattening, not all alcoholics, even those who eat well, are fat. A partial explanation for this may be as follows: Alcohol is an energy-dense but nutrient-free compound producing 7.1 kcal per gram when burned in vitro in a bomb calorimeter. Because in vivo conversion of alcohol to energy in heavy drinkers may not be as efficient as in vitro combustion, a figure between 5 and 6 kcal per gram may be more accurate in calculating the energy provided by alcohol in the diets of such people. The inefficient use of alcohol as an energy source, when ingested in excess, may result from a lack of coupling of oxidation to phosphorylation in liver microsomes that provide a largely unlimited, supplementary ethanol metabolism pathway to the major, but limited-capacity, alcohol dehydrogenase pathway.

Absorption in the bloodstream The effects of alcohol do not depend entirely on how much a person drinks, but on how much alcohol is absorbed into the bloodstream. The absorption of alcohol, in turn, depends on the following factors:

1. Some alcohol is absorbed through the stomach wall, but most alcohol reaches the bloodstream through the small intestine.
2. For rapid absorption, it is important that alcohol reach the small intestine in the highest possible concentration in the shortest possible time. People who have had their pyloric valve removed surgically, as for ulcers, find that they become intoxicated faster than they did before the valve was removed.
3. Other factors affecting absorption include the presence of food in the stomach and the type of beverage consumed. With the same amount of alcohol consumed over the same length of time, the blood alcohol concentration may vary greatly. Gin on an empty stomach produces a far higher blood level than beer consumed with, for example, spaghetti.

In addition to the amount of alcohol that is absorbed in the blood, the effects of alcohol depend on how quickly the alcohol is absorbed. In general, the faster the rate of absorption, the more striking the effect. As alcohol remains in the blood over longer periods, its effects lessen. In practical terms, if one makes five errors per minute while typing sober, one may make 15 errors per minute while typing with a certain blood alcohol concentration after 1 hour of drinking, but may make only seven errors at the same blood alcohol concentration after 5 hours of drinking.

Tolerance In general, people feel better becoming intoxicated than they do becoming sober. That is, as the blood alcohol level climbs from A to B to C, a person may feel euphoric at B and C. As the blood level falls from C to B to A, however, not only is there no euphoria at B, but the person feels discomfort, presaging the hangover to come at A. This slope effect is closely related to and hard to separate from the duration effect. As people drink more alcohol over days, months, and years, they gradually need to drink even more to obtain the same effect. The importance of tolerance, however, is often exaggerated. Seasoned alcoholics, at the prime of their drinking capacity, may be able to drink, at most, twice more than a teetotaler of similar age and health. Compared with tolerance for morphine, which may be manyfold, tolerance for alcohol is modest.

Nevertheless, the importance of tolerance in the addictive process seems established. Recent studies indicate that tolerance may result from changes in cell membranes. A cell membrane consists of a bilayer of phospholipids arranged with the "head" of the molecule facing the extracellular space and the "tail" dangling toward the interior of the cell. The former attracts water and the latter repels water. The result is a strong and resistant sheath for the cells that is also easily perturbed by external and internal changes. Alcohol, among other external influences (such as temperature), makes the membranes more flexible or fluid. After chronic exposure to alcohol, the membranes become stiff again, and this condition is interpreted as tolerance at the cellular level. The so-called disordering effect of alcohol on membranes corresponds to an increase in lipid solubility of alcohol.

Possible beneficial effects Little is mentioned about possible beneficial effects of alcohol, but there is evidence in fact that moderate drinking is associated with increased longevity. Heavy drinkers and abstainers have lower life expectancies than moderate drinkers. This may be due to confounding variables (e.g., moderate drinkers may be moderate in many ways), but a possible biochemical explanation exists. Alcohol produces an increase in high-density lipoproteins (sometimes called good cholesterol); increased high-density lipoproteins are associated with a decreased risk of coronary artery disease. The story is complicated by the fact that high-density lipoproteins consist of several components, and not all are associated with a decreased risk of coronary artery disease or equally influenced by alcohol. However, most of the evidence suggests that alcohol, like exercise, may indeed have a protective effect on the coronary arteries. (One study found that jogging for half an hour and three bottles of beer had equal effects on increasing good cholesterol.)

These findings should not be interpreted as encouragement of immoderate use of alcohol. For alcoholics, no level of intake is considered beneficial. Moreover, the effects of moderate drinking on the unborn child and the relationship of moderate drinking to automobile accidents are still not clear.

Alcohol use during pregnancy Alcohol consumption during pregnancy has been said to be the leading cause of congenital anomalies, but the evidence for this is weak. Although there has been an increase of drinking by women in the United States in recent decades, there has been no apparent increase in anomalies. When first described by two Seattle physicians, the so-called fetal alcohol syndrome consisted of a distinct cluster of anatomical features. With subsequent investigation, the outlines of the cluster became less distinct and the abnormalities were often referred to as "subtle." A select committee appointed to study the fetal alcohol syndrome in the early 1980s decided that "nonspecific deleterious effects from alcohol" was a more appropriate term than "fetal alcohol syndrome." One large study in Boston failed to correlate drinking with congenital anomalies, and other studies have produced weaker correlations than was suggested by the original reports.

At the moment, alcohol cannot be described as a teratogen. Its main association with pregnancy is low birth weight, but most heavy drinking women are also cigarette smokers, and cigarettes are also associated with low birth weights. Although the government supports a large-scale educational campaign against immoderate drinking during pregnancy, a safe level of consumption has not been established. As a result, many physicians and public health officials advise that women not drink at all during pregnancy. One problem with this advice is that the most severe adverse effects, if they occur, would be produced early in the first trimester, at a time when women may not realize they are pregnant. As a consequence, to be totally safe, women should probably be advised not to drink alcohol at any time when they are likely to become pregnant (in short, at any time between menarche and menopause, given the uncertainty of contraceptive protection). Some authorities have objected to the propagandistic flavor of some admonitions about drinking during pregnancy because not only are they based on inadequate data, but also they are calculated to lay a guilt trip on women who have children with congenital anomalies and perhaps had a small amount of alcohol to drink at some point during pregnancy. However, nobody is prepared to encourage women to drink during pregnancy, and the fetal alcohol syndrome has become an emotional issue in which facts become almost irrelevant. Much research is still going on in this field, and many issues remain unresolved.

MEASUREMENT

The alcohol content of various beverages is usually clouded by imprecise definitions. The phrase "common servings of beer, wine, or spirits" or "standard serving of beer, wine, or spirits" repeatedly occurs, but there is no agreement among experts or ordinary people as to what constitutes a common or standard serving of wine or spirits.

Most bottles or cans of beer contain 12 oz, which could be considered a common serving. On an airplane, a serving of scotch, bourbon, gin, or vodka is 1.6 oz of 80-proof spirits. Should this amount be recognized as the standard drink? Yet, in hotels and bars, the serving is usually from 1.0 to 1.5 oz; in many clubs and homes, it is 2 oz. A serving of wine may vary from 3 to 5 oz. The term "equivalence" therefore carries little meaning unless the size of the serving is stated, as illustrated by Table 13.2-1.

The blood alcohol concentration (BAC) or blood alcohol level (BAL) is a reliable measurement of ethanol in the blood. Since alcohol diffuses uniformly to all tissues, it is also a reflection of brain ethanol levels. Breath alcohol determinations should not be done within 15 minutes of having had a drink, otherwise false elevations will occur, in some cases due to the retention of ingested alcohol in the oropharynx. Urine alcohol tests only generally reflect the BAC and are not worth performing for practical purposes.

EPIDEMIOLOGY

CONSUMPTION DATA Currently, the annual consumption of alcohol (pure alcohol) in the United States is about 3 gallons per person over 14 years of age. This figure is based on tax data. Untaxed sales, such as those at military installations, are not included, so per capita consumption may be underestimated. Also, because consumption estimates are based on the population of each state, when residents of one state cross into another state to purchase lower-priced alcoholic beverages, the result is a higher per capita consumption figure for the state where sales occur. Washington, D.C., and states with high rates of tourism and business travel have higher reported consumption rates because sales to transients are calculated as consumption by the resident population.

There was a modest increase in taxed alcohol sales in the United States from 1950 to 1980, perhaps because of the decreased availability of untaxed alcohol. Moonshine is no longer a booming industry in some backwoods areas. Making moonshine alcohol mainly was a small family business, and small family businesses in the United States have declined.

Sine 1980, alcohol sales have declined. Reasons often cited are increased health consciousness, use of other recreational drugs (especially marijuana), and the current fanatical devotion to slimness.

There has been an interesting change in preference within beverage category. In the diet-conscious United States, people drink more light beer—that is, beer with fewer calories than regular beer. They also drink more white spirits, such as vodka or gin, than brown spirits (whiskey). There is no clear explanation for the color preference, unless people have the notion that white spirits are healthier than brown, which is probably not true. So-called California coolers have recently become popular. Consisting of white wine and fruit juice, these drinks contain about 5 percent alcohol, the equivalent of strong beer. The fruit juice masks the wine taste and the drinker may be deceived about the strength of the potion.

International comparisons are difficult at best. It appears, however, that wine countries, such as France and Italy, consume more alcohol than countries where distilled spirits are favored. Israel has the lowest per capita consumption. Ireland, contrary to its popular image, has a lower consump-

TABLE 13.2-1
Ethanol Content (in Grams) According to Size of Servings

	Beer (3.6% by wt)	*80-Proof Spirits (40%)**				*Table Wine (12%)*	
Serving	*12.0 oz*	*1.0 oz*	*1.5 oz*	*1.6 oz*	*2.0 oz*	*3.0 oz*	*5.0 oz*
1	12.6	9.34	14.0	15.0	18.6	8.4	14.0
2	25.2	18.7	28.0	30.0	37.2	16.8	28.0
3	37.8	28.0	42.0	45.0	55.8	25.2	42.0

*To obtain amount in 86-proof spirits, add 7.5%.

tion rate than the United Kingdom. The United States ranks in the middle with regard to alcohol consumption. Soviets are notoriously heavy drinkers, but consumption figures are hard to come by.

DRINKING PATTERNS More is known about patterns of normal drinking than about the prevalence of alcoholism, at least in the United States. Nationwide surveys of drinking practices reveal that about 70 percent of adults in America drink alcohol on occasion and that 12 percent are heavy drinkers. A *heavy drinker* is defined as a person who drinks almost every day and becomes intoxicated several times a month. *Moderate drinking* is defined by some authors as an intake that does not exceed 0.8 g per kg of body weight of ethanol per day, up to a limit of 80 g, or an average of 0.7 g per kg for 3 successive days. Generally, drinkers tend to be young, relatively prosperous, and well educated. More drinkers live in cities and suburbs than in rural regions and small towns. To some extent, religion determines whether a person is a drinker or a teetotaler. Almost all urban Jews and Episcopalians drink on occasion, whereas fewer than half of rural Baptists drink.

More men than women are heavy drinkers: 20 percent of men versus 9 percent of women. Heavy drinkers more often come from the lower classes and are less well educated than moderate drinkers. Drinking patterns appear to be highly changeable. It is common for individuals to be heavy drinkers for long periods and then to become moderate drinkers or teetotalers.

Drinking patterns vary by age and sex. For both men and women, the prevalence of drinking is highest and abstention is lowest in the 21- to 34-year age range. Young white males drink more than any other group in the United States. For ages 65 years and older, abstainers exceed drinkers in both sexes, and only 7 percent of men and 2 percent of women in that age group are considered heavy drinkers.

Consumption varies markedly in different geographical areas. In the United States, consumption is greatest in the Northeast and lowest in the South.

Most alcohol is consumed by a small percentage of people. Whereas 70 percent of the drinking population consumes only 20 percent of the total, 30 percent of drinkers consume 80 percent, and 10 percent consume 50 percent.

ALCOHOLISM There are several problems in estimating the prevalence of alcoholism. One is that few studies agree on the definition of alcoholism. Household surveys can be inaccurate because alcoholics, more than most people, are often not home. Neighborhood bars are rarely included in household surveys.

There have been no nationwide studies of prevalence rates of alcoholism in the United States. Estimates of the extent of alcoholism range from five to nine million Americans. These estimates are roughly equivalent to expectancy rates obtained in studies in Germany, Switzerland, Sweden, Denmark, and England. In those countries, the lifelong expectancy rate for alcoholism among men is about 3.0 to 5.0 percent; the rate for women ranges from 0.1 to 1.0 percent. Similar rates were found in a late-1970s household survey in Connecticut.

In the United States, blacks in urban ghettos appear to have a particularly high rate of alcohol-related problems; it is not known whether rural blacks have comparably high rates of alcohol problems. Native Americans are also said to have high rates of alcoholism, but these rates have probably been exaggerated and, in any case, do not apply to all tribes. Asian persons have low rates of alcoholism.

Alcoholism is a serious problem in France and the Soviet Union. Although Italy, as with France, is a vinocultural country where wine is a popular beverage, it is often asserted that the Italians have a lower rate of alcoholism than the French. The evidence for this statement, however, is scant. Estimates of alcoholism rates are usually based on cirrhosis rates and admissions for alcoholism to psychiatric hospitals. France has the highest cirrhosis rate in the world, but Italy also has a high rate, suggesting that alcoholism may be more common in Italy than is generally assumed. Ireland has a relatively low cirrhosis rate, despite its reputation for a high rate of alcoholism.

Alcohol problems are correlated with a history of school difficulty. High school dropouts and individuals with a record of frequent truancy and delinquency appear to have a particularly high risk of alcoholism.

No systematic studies have explored the relationship between occupation and alcoholism, but cirrhosis data suggest that individuals in certain occupations are more vulnerable to alcoholism. Waiters, bartenders, longshoremen, musicians, authors, and reporters have relatively high cirrhosis rates, whereas accountants, mail carriers, and carpenters have relatively low rates. Of eight Americans who won the Nobel Prize for literature, four were clearly alcoholic—Eugene O'Neill, Sinclair Lewis, William Faulkner, and Ernest Hemingway—and one, John Steinbeck, was a heavy drinker.

There is some evidence that the prevalence of alcoholism may be decreasing, at least in the United States. Benjamin Rush, in 1795, estimated that 4,000 Americans died each year "from overindulgence in ardent spirits." Because the population at that time was about 4 million, Rush's estimate yields a death rate of 100 per 100,000. The officially recorded rate of death from alcoholism in the United States today is 2 per 100,000.

Granting that Rush's estimate is suspect, alcoholism in the United States may be less prevalent today than it was 200 years ago.

CLINICAL SIGNS AND SYMPTOMS

Alcoholism is a behavioral disorder. The specific behavior that causes problems is the consumption of large quantities of alcohol on repeated occasions. The motivation underlying this behavior is often obscure. When asked why they drink excessively, alcoholics occasionally attribute their drinking to a particular mood, such as depression or anxiety, or to situational problems. They sometimes describe an overpowering need to drink, variously described as a craving or compulsion. Just as often, however, alcoholics are unable to give a plausible explanation for their excessive drinking.

As with other drug dependencies, alcoholism is accompanied by a preoccupation with obtaining the drug in quantities sufficient to produce intoxication over long periods. It is especially true early in the course of alcoholism that patients may deny this preoccupation or attempt to rationalize their need by asserting that they drink no more than their friends. As part of this denial or rationalization, alcoholics tend to spend their time with other heavy drinkers.

As alcoholism progresses and problems from drinking become more serious, alcoholics may drink alone, sneak drinks, hide the bottle, or take other measures to conceal the seriousness of their condition. These actions are almost always accompanied by feelings of guilt and remorse that, in turn, may produce more drinking as a temporary relief from those feelings. Remorse may be particularly intense in the morning, when drinkers have not had a drink for a number of hours; this feeling may provoke morning drinking.

ANXIETY AND DEPRESSION Prolonged drinking, even if initiated to relieve guilt and anxiety, often produces anxiety and depression. The full range of symptoms associated with depression and panic disorder, including terminal insomnia, low mood, irritability, and anxiety attacks with chest pain, palpitations, and dyspnea, often appear. Alcohol temporarily relieves these symptoms, resulting in a vicious cycle of drinking-depression-drinking that may ultimately result in a withdrawal syndrome. Often, the patient makes a valiant effort to stop drinking and may succeed for a period of several days or weeks only to fall off the wagon again.

Repeated experiences of failure to stop drinking easily lead to feelings of despair and hopelessness. By the time patients consult a physician, they have often reached rock bottom. Their situation seems hopeless, and after years of heavy drinking, their problems have become so numerous that they feel nothing can be done about them. At this point, they may be ready to acknowledge their alcoholism, but feel powerless to stop drinking. Many alcoholics do stop permanently, however, as will be discussed later.

BLACKOUTS Alcohol is one of the few psychoactive drugs that produces, on occasion, classical amnesia. Nonalcoholics, when drinking, also experience this amnesia (blackouts) but much less often, as a rule, than do alcoholics. These periods of amnesia are particularly distressing to alcoholics, because they may fear that they have unknowingly harmed someone or behaved imprudently while intoxicated.

A 40-year-old attorney, distressed by a recent divorce and bored with his work, fell into a pattern of having increasingly longer lunch hours, spent in a bar sitting in pensive silence or chatting with other customers. Previously a two-martini lunchtime drinker, his intake increased to four or five martinis followed by wine with his lunch and then Irish coffee. Having developed a high tolerance for alcohol, he could still return to his office without seeming intoxicated.

One Monday afternoon, following a heavy-drinking "lunch," he did not make it back to the office. Instead, he awoke the next morning in his own bed but with no recollection of events for the preceding day after about 4 P.M. He was terrified. What had he done? How did he get home? Where was his car? He became panicked by the prospect that he had harmed someone, perhaps killed another person, perhaps in a car accident. He walked out to the garage. His car was there. He checked to see whether there were dents. There were none. He was relieved but still frightened. The worst part was the guilty feeling that he had committed some terrible crime and could not remember it.

Later he checked with the bartender who told him he had drunk steadily through the afternoon but did not seem intoxicated and left the bar in the early evening with a woman. His memory remained a blank and he was so shaken by the experience that he swore off alcohol. Five years later he was still a teetotaler.

Studies of blackouts indicate that the amnesia is anterograde. During a blackout, people have relatively intact remote and immediate memory, but experience a specific short-term memory deficit in which they are unable to recall events that happened 5 or 10 minutes before. Because their other intellectual faculties are well preserved, they can perform complicated acts and appear normal to the casual observer.

Two couples in their later 20s were having drinks while playing bridge. The wives sipped wine but their husbands drank scotch to the point where they lost interest in the bridge game. The husbands began telling jokes. Husband A told the group a joke and they all laughed. Husband B told a joke and again they all laughed. Then husband A repeated the same joke that he had told a few minutes previously. Husband B laughed but the two wives looked at each other in puzzlement. Then husband B told the same joke *he* had just told previously and husband A laughed, and the wives now felt that the situation was utterly ridiculous. The next day neither husband had any recollection of telling the jokes.

Both husbands, in short, had had a blackout. The story illustrates how alcohol can obliterate short-term memory while leaving other intellectual facilities intact. Both husbands could remember the jokes and tell them well, but soon after telling them, they forgot that they had done so. Neither of the men, incidentally, was alcoholic, nor was either of them ordinarily even a heavy drinker. This illustrates how blackouts can occur in more or less normal drinkers who drink excessively on some occasion.

STATE-DEPENDENT EFFECTS Based on present knowledge, there is no evidence that alcoholic blackouts are motivated by a desire to forget events that happened while drinking. Sometimes, however, a curious phenomenon happens. Imbibers recall events that happened during the previous drinking period that, when sober, they had forgotten. For example, alcoholics often report hiding money or alcohol when drinking, forgetting where they hid the articles when sober, and having their memory return when drinking again. This is reminiscent of experiments demonstrating state-dependent learning in animals and humans. "State-dependent" refers to the observation that learning acquired while an animal or person is intoxicated with certain drugs is retrieved more easily when the subject is reintoxicated than when not intoxicated.

Alcohol has been shown experimentally to produce mild state-dependent effects in humans. One theory holds that individuals susceptible to alcoholism are particularly susceptible to state-dependent effects from alcohol. According to the theory, loss of control, which some consider the hallmark of alcoholism, may reflect a relative inability to transfer information acquired during sobriety to periods of intoxication. When intoxicated, an alcoholic, in a sense, forgets the consequences of intoxication: the hangovers, remorse, social opprobrium. Recent evidence indicates that some individuals are more prone to state-dependent effects from alcohol than others, and this proneness is correlated with a history of alcoholic blackouts. Whether state dependency also is a factor in the etiology of alcoholism remains to be explored.

A 47-year-old housewife often wrote letters when she was drinking. Sometimes, she would jot down notes for a letter and start writing it, but not finish it. The next day, sober, she would be unable to decipher the notes. Then she would start drinking again and after a few drinks, the meaning of the notes would become clear and she would resume writing the letter. "It was like picking up the pencil where I had left off."

IDENTIFYING THE ALCOHOLIC Before alcoholism can be treated, it first must be recognized. Physicians are in a particularly good position to identify a drinking problem early because they can do a physical examination and order laboratory tests. The following phenomena indicate the presence of a drinking problem:

1. Arcus senilis—a ring-like opacity of the cornea—occurs commonly with age, causes no visual disturbance, and is considered an innocent condition. The ring forms from fatty material in the blood. Alcohol increases fat in the blood, and more alcoholics are reported to have the ring than their contemporaries who do not drink heavily.

2. A red nose (acne rosacea) suggests that the owner has a weakness for alcoholic beverages. Some people with red noses, however, are teetotalers or even rabid prohibitionists and resent the insinuation.

3. Red palms (palmar erythema) are also suggestive, but not diagnostic, of alcoholism.

4. Cigarette burns between the index and middle fingers or on the chest and contusions and bruises should raise suspicions of recent alcoholic stupor.

5. Painless enlargement of the liver may suggest a larger alcohol intake than the liver can handle. Severe, constant upper abdominal pain and tenderness radiating to the back indicates pancreatic inflammation, which is sometimes caused by alcohol.

6. Reduced sensation and weakness in the feet and legs may occur from excessive drinking.

7. Laboratory tests provide other clues. More than half of alcoholics have increased amounts of γ-glutamyltranspeptidase (GGT) in their blood, which is unusual in nonalcoholics. To a lesser extent than with GGT, elevations in the following tests are most often associated with heavy drinking: mean corpuscular volume, uric acid, triglycerides, aspartate aminotransferase (AST), and the liver enzymes—serum glutamic oxylacetic transferase (SGOT) and serum glutamic pyruvate transferase (SGPT).

Another approach is to use a wide range of commonly available blood chemistry tests and subject them to quadratic discriminant analysis. Each value may be in the normal range, but in toto, the test results produce a distinctive fingerprint that is highly specific for detecting recent heavy drinking. Whether this composite picture is a useful test for alcoholism per se is not known.

The diagnostic criteria for alcohol intoxication and idiosyncratic intoxication according to DSM-III-R are listed in Tables 13.2-2 and 13.2-3.

TABLE 13.2-2
Diagnostic Criteria for Alcohol Intoxication

A. Recent ingestion of alcohol (with no evidence suggesting that the amount was insufficient to cause intoxication in most people).

B. Maladaptive behavior changes (e.g., disinhibition of sexual or aggressive impulses, mood lability, impaired judgment, impaired social or occupational functioning).

C. At least one of the following signs:
(1) slurred speech
(2) incoordination
(3) unsteady gait
(4) nystagmus
(5) flushed face

D. Not due to any physical or other mental disorder.

Table from DSM-III-R *Diagnostic and Statistical Manual of Mental Disorders,* ed 3, revised. Copyright American Psychiatric Association, Washington, DC, 1987. Used with permission.

TABLE 13.2-3
Diagnostic Criteria for Alcohol Idiosyncratic Intoxication

A. Maladaptive behavioral changes (e.g., aggressive or assaultive behavior, occurring within minutes of ingesting an amount of alcohol insufficient to induce intoxication in most people).

B. The behavior is atypical of the person when not drinking.

C. Not due to any physical or other mental disorder.

Table from DSM-III-R *Diagnostic and Statistical Manual of Mental Disorders,* ed 3, revised. Copyright American Psychiatric Association, Washington, DC, 1987. Used with permission.

COURSE

The natural history of alcoholism seems to be somewhat different in men and women. In men, the onset is usually in the late teens or in the 20s. Since the course of alcoholism is insidious, the male alcoholic may not be fully aware of his dependency on alcohol until his 30s. The first hospitalization usually occurs in the late 30s or 40s. Symptoms of alcoholism rarely occur for the first time after age 45. If they do occur, the physician should be alert to the possibility of primary mood disorder or brain disease.

Alcoholism has a higher spontaneous remission rate in men than is often recognized. For both sexes, the incidence of first admissions to psychiatric hospitals for alcoholism drops markedly in the sixth and seventh decades, as do first arrests for alcohol-related offenses. Although the mortality rate among alcoholics is perhaps two to three times that of nonalcoholics, this higher death rate is probably insufficient to account for the apparent decrease in problem drinking in middle and late middle life.

Female alcoholics have been studied less extensively than male alcoholics, but the evidence suggests that the course of the disorder is more variable in women. The onset often occurs later, spontaneous remission apparently is less frequent, and women are more likely than men to develop cirrhosis from drinking. Female alcoholics are also more likely to have a history of mood disorder:

The 46-year-old wife of a politician learned that her husband had a mistress. Her drinking habits changed dramatically. Always a moderate-to-light social drinker, she began drinking during the daytime, wine at first and later vodka. She neglected her personal appearance and housework. She made countless tipsy calls to family and friends, running up a huge phone bill. When the husband agreed to abandon his affair, she forgave him, but their relationship deteriorated. Her sullen silences were punctuated by violent outbursts of rage.

At first, she successfully hid her drinking, but the husband found empty bottles in the trash and full ones concealed in closets and drawers. He consulted a physician friend who referred them to a marriage counselor. The drinking problem quickly emerged, but also typical symptoms of depression: insomnia, feelings of worthlessness, and suicidal thoughts. Abstinence became a condition for therapy and she stopped drinking, but the depressive symptoms persisted. Her family history was strongly positive for mood disorder, and, as a college sophomore, she had missed a semester because of depression. She was referred to a psychiatrist, who successfully treated the depression with supportive psychotherapy and medication. One year later, her marital problems were much improved and her drinking consisted of an occasional glass of wine with meals.

On the basis of questionnaire data obtained from alcoholics, claims have been made that manifestations of alcoholism follow a natural chronological order, with blackouts being one of the early prodromal symptoms of the illness. Later studies have challenged this view, and it is now believed that problems from drinking may occur in various sequences and that blackouts have no special significance as a sign of incipient alcoholism. Frequently, after years of heavy problem-free drinking, a person may experience a large number of problems in a brief period. As will be discussed later, alcoholics with a family history of alcoholism begin having symptoms of alcohol dependence at an earlier age than alcoholics without such a history.

Patterns of drinking also are variable, and it is a mistake to associate one particular pattern exclusively with alcoholism. One researcher divided alcoholics into various species, depending on their pattern of drinking. One species, the so-called gamma alcoholic, is common in the United States and conforms to the stereotype of the Alcoholics Anonymous

(AA) candidate. Gamma alcoholics have problems with control; once they begin drinking, they are unable to stop until poor health or depleted financial resources prevent them from continuing. Once the bender is terminated, however, gamma alcoholics are able to abstain from alcohol for varying lengths of time. The gamma alcoholic is in contrast with a species of alcoholic common in France. French alcoholics have control, but are unable to abstain; they must drink a given quantity of alcohol every day, although they have no compulsion to exceed this amount. They may not recognize that they have an alcohol problem until, for reasons beyond their control, they have to stop drinking, whereupon they experience withdrawal symptoms.

Although these pure types of alcoholism do exist, many individuals who do not conform to these stereotypes still have serious drinking problems. Among U.S. alcoholics, one drink does not invariably lead to a binge; people may drink moderately for a long time before their drinking begins to interfere with their health or social functioning.

This diversity in drinking patterns explains the current emphasis on problems, rather than patterns, as the basis for diagnosing alcoholism.

COMPLICATIONS

Because alcoholism is defined by the problems it creates, symptoms and complications inevitably overlap. For present purposes, social and medical complications will be considered separately.

SOCIAL COMPLICATIONS Alcoholics have a high rate of marital separation and divorce. They often have job troubles, including frequent absenteeism and job loss. They also have a high frequency of accidents—in the home, on the job, and while driving automobiles. About 40 percent of highway fatalities in the United States involve a driver who has blood alcohol concentrations over 100 mg percent; often the driver is an alcoholic. Nearly half of convicted felons are alcoholic, and about half of police activities in large cities are associated with alcohol-related offenses.

MEDICAL COMPLICATIONS Medical complications fall into three categories: acute effects of heavy drinking, chronic effects of heavy drinking, and withdrawal effects.

Consumption of very large amounts of alcohol can lead directly to death by depressing the respiratory center in the medulla. Usually the blood alcohol levels are over 500 mg percent. Acute hemorrhagic pancreatitis occasionally occurs from a single heavy drinking episode.

Nearly every organ system can be affected, directly or indirectly, by chronic, heavy use of alcohol. Gastritis and diarrhea are common reversible effects. Gastric ulcer may also occur, although the evidence that alcohol directly produces ulceration is equivocal.

Liver damage The most serious effect of alcohol on the gastrointestinal (GI) tract is liver damage. After many years of study, however, it is still not clear whether alcohol by itself has a direct toxic effect on the liver. At present, it appears that cirrhosis results from the combined effects of alcohol and diet, as well as other factors, possibly including heredity. Human and animal studies indicate that a single large dose of alcohol, combined with a diet rich in fat, produces a fatty liver. Conversely, alcohol, together with fasting, can result in a fatty liver. The connection between fatty liver and cirrhosis, however, is unclear. The fatty changes in the liver after acute alcohol intoxication are reversible. In Western countries, most patients with Laënnec's cirrhosis are excessive drinkers. Most severe alcoholics, however, do not develop cirrhosis; probably less than 10 percent do.

Until a few years ago, investigations of the pathogenesis of Laënnec's cirrhosis have been hampered by the inability to produce this type of cirrhosis in animals. Recent studies show that force-feeding baboons with large amounts of alcohol over long periods results in cirrhosis. Not all baboons, however, develop cirrhosis, and these studies leave unresolved the question of the direct role of alcohol in producing cirrhosis. One complication in interpreting the finding is that a large intake of alcohol also produces a malabsorption syndrome and, therefore, although the baboons had adequate diets, it is likely that important food constituents, including vitamins, were not fully absorbed during the drinking periods.

Effects on the nervous system Alcoholism is associated with pathology of the nervous system, principally because of vitamin deficiencies and not as a direct toxic effect of alcohol. Peripheral neuropathy, the most common neurological complication, apparently results from multiple vitamin B deficiencies. It is usually reversible with adequate nutrition. Retrobulbar neuropathy may lead to amblyopia—sometimes called tobacco-alcohol amblyopia—that is also usually reversible with vitamin therapy.

Other neurological complications include anterior lobe cerebellar degenerative disease and the amnestic syndrome—Wernicke-Korsakoff syndrome (Table 13.2-4). The amnestic syndrome almost certainly results from thiamine deficiency. The acute Wernicke stage consists of ocular disturbances (nystagmus and sixth nerve palsy), ataxia, and confusion. It usually clears in a few days, but may progress to a chronic brain syndrome—Korsakoff's psychosis. Short-term memory loss—anterograde amnesia—is the most characteristic feature of Korsakoff's psychosis. Confabulation—narration of fanciful tales—may also occur. The Wernicke-Korsakoff syndrome is associated with necrotic lesions of the mamillary bodies, thalamus, and other brain stem areas. Thiamine corrects rapidly early Wernicke signs and may prevent development of an irreversible alcohol amnestic disorder (Korsakoff-type dementia). Once the dementia is established, thiamine does not usually help alleviate symptoms.

A 48-year-old divorced housepainter is admitted with a history of 30 years of heavy drinking. He had two previous admissions for detoxification, but the family states that he has not had a drink in several weeks and shows no sign of alcohol withdrawal. He looks malnourished, however, and, on examination, is found to be ataxic and to have a bilateral sixth cranial nerve palsy. He appears confused and mistakes one of his physicians for a dead uncle.

Within a week, the patient walks normally, and there is no sign of a sixth nerve palsy. He seems less confused and can now find his way to the bathroom without direction. He remembers the names and birthdays of his siblings, but has difficulty naming the past five presidents.

More strikingly, he has great difficulty in retaining information for longer than a few minutes. He can repeat back a list of numbers immediately after he has heard them, but a few minutes later, he does not recall being asked to perform the task. Shown three objects—keys, comb, and ring—he cannot recall them 3 minutes later. He does not seem worried about this lack of recall. Asked if he can recall the name of his doctor, he replies, "certainly," and proceeds to call the doctor "Dr. Masters" (not his name), whom he claims he first met in the Korean War. He tells a long untrue story about how he and "Dr. Masters" served as fellow soldiers in the Korean War.

TABLE 13.2-4
Diagnostic Criteria for Alcohol Amnestic Disorder

A. Amnestic syndrome following prolonged, heavy ingestion of alcohol.

B. Not due to any physical or other mental disorder.

Table from DSM-III-R *Diagnostic and Statistical Manual of Mental Disorders,* ed 3, revised. Copyright American Psychiatric Association, Washington, DC, 1987. Used with permission.

The patient is calm, alert, friendly. One could be with him a short period and not realize he has a severe memory impairment because of his intact immediate memory and spotty, but sometimes impressive, remote memory. Thus, his amnesia is largely anterograde. Although high doses of thiamine are used in his treatment, his short-term memory deficit persists and appears to be irreversible.

Intellectual impairment Whether excessive use of alcohol produces cortical atrophy has been debated for many years. Computed tomography (CT) scans of alcoholics usually show enlarged ventricles, but the cause may be fluid shifts and not loss of brain tissue; in at least one study, ventricular size returned to normal after prolonged abstinence from alcohol. The extensive psychometric literature on intellectual impairment in alcoholics is contradictory. Most studies performed soon after drinking bouts show intellectual deficits, but the deficits vary from study to study. The most consistent results have involved use of the categories test of the Halstead-Reitan Battery, indicating that alcoholics have difficulty in conceptual shifting. Many of the deficits found in alcoholics undergoing detoxification are reversible. In DSM-III-R, a diagnosis of dementia associated with alcoholism may be made if the criteria in Table 13.2-5 are met. No studies have reported a decline in the intelligence quotient (I.Q.) scores of alcoholics.

Other medical complications Other medical complications of alcoholism include cardiomyopathy, thrombocytopenia, anemia, and myopathy. Cancer of the breast in women and neoplasms of the throat and larynx have been associated with heavy drinking, but, at least in the latter instance, cigarette smoking (common in heavy drinkers) is a confounding variable. Alcohol is sometimes called a cocarcinogen, but there are scant animal data to support this theory.

Withdrawal effects The term "uncomplicated alcohol withdrawal" (Table 13.2-6) is preferable to delirium tremens (DTs) (Table 13.2-7) when referring to withdrawal symptoms that are unaccompanied by delirium. DTs refers to a specific manifestation of the withdrawal syndrome. The most common withdrawal symptom is tremulousness, which usually occurs a few hours after cessation of drinking and may even begin while the person is still drinking—a period of relative abstinence. Transitory hallucinations also may occur. If they do occur, they usually begin 12 to 24 hours after drinking stops.

TABLE 13.2-5
Diagnostic Criteria for Dementia Associated with Alcoholism

A. Dementia following prolonged, heavy ingestion of alcohol and persisting at least 3 weeks after cessation of alcohol ingestion.

B. Exclusion, by history, physical examination, and laboratory tests, of all causes of dementia other than prolonged heavy use of alcohol.

Table from DSM-III-R *Diagnostic and Statistical Manual of Mental Disorders,* ed 3, revised. Copyright American Psychiatric Association, Washington, DC, 1987. Used with permission.

TABLE 13.2-6
Diagnostic Criteria for Uncomplicated Alcohol Withdrawal

A. Cessation of prolonged (several days or longer) heavy ingestion of alcohol or reduction in the amount of alcohol ingested, followed within several hours by coarse tremor of hands, tongue, or eyelids, and at least one of the following:
(1) nausea or vomiting
(2) malaise or weakness
(3) autonomic hyperactivity (e.g., tachycardia, sweating, elevated blood pressure)
(4) anxiety
(5) depressed mood or irritability
(6) transient hallucinations or illusions
(7) headache
(8) insomnia

B. Not due to any physical or other mental disorder, such as alcohol withdrawal delirium.

Table from DSM-III-R *Diagnostic and Statistical Manual of Mental Disorders,* ed 3, revised. Copyright American Psychiatric Association, Washington, DC, 1987. Used with permission.

TABLE 13.2-7
Diagnostic Criteria for Alcohol Withdrawal Delirium

A. Delirium developing after cessation of heavy alcohol ingestion or a reduction in the amount of alcohol ingested (usually within 1 week).

B. Marked autonomic hyperactivity (e.g., tachycardia, sweating).

C. Not due to any physical or other mental disorder.

Table from DSM-III-R *Diagnostic and Statistical Manual of Mental Disorders,* ed 3, revised. Copyright American Psychiatric Association, Washington, DC, 1987. Used with permission.

A 30-year-old newspaper reporter started drinking with friends one evening after work and continued to drink through the evening, falling asleep in the early morning hours. On awakening, he had a strong desire to drink again and decided not to go to work. Food did not appeal to him, and instead, he had several Bloody Marys. Later, he went to a local tavern and drank beer through the afternoon. He met some friends and continued drinking into the evening.

The pattern of drinking through the day persisted for the next 7 days. On the eighth morning, he tried to drink a morning cup of coffee and found that his hands were shaking so violently he could not get the cup to his mouth. He managed to pour some whiskey into a glass and drank as much as he could. His hands became less shaky, but now he was nauseated and began having dry heaves. He felt ill and intensely anxious and decided to call a doctor friend. The doctor recommended hospitalization.

On admission, the patient had a marked resting and exertional tremor of the hands, and his tongue and eyelids were tremulous. He also had feelings of internal tremulousness. Lying in the hospital bed, he found the noises outside his window unbearably loud and began seeing visions of animals and, on one occasion, a dead relative. He was terrified and called a nurse, who gave him a tranquilizer. He became quieter, and his tremor was less pronounced. At all times, he realized that the visual phenomena were imaginary. He always knew where he was and was oriented otherwise. After a few days, the tremor disappeared, and he no longer hallucinated. He still had trouble sleeping, but otherwise felt back to normal and vowed never to drink again.

GRAND MAL CONVULSIONS Grand mal convulsions (rum fits) occur occasionally, sometimes as long as 2 or 3 days after drinking stops. As a rule, alcoholics experiencing convulsions do not have epilepsy; they have normal electroencephalograms (EEGs) when not drinking and experience convulsions only during withdrawal.

DELIRIUM TREMENS DTs is infrequent and, when it does occur, is often associated with intercurrent medical illness (Table 13.2-7). For a diagnosis of DTs, gross memory disturbance should be present, in addition to other withdrawal symptoms, such as agitation and vivid hallucinations. Classically, DTs begins 2 or 3 days after drinking stops and subsides within 1 to 5 days. One must always suspect intercurrent medical illness when delirium occurs during withdrawal. The physician should be particularly alert to hepatic decompensation, pneumonia, subdural hematoma, pancreatitis, and fractures.

The DTs has been described brilliantly in fiction by, among others, Malcolm Lowry and Mark Twain. Lowry, in his novella *Lunar Caustic,* wrote from personal experience how it felt to wake up in an alcoholic ward:

> The man awoke certain that he was on a ship. If not, where did those isolated clangings come from, those sounds of iron on iron? He recognized the crunch of water pouring over the scuttle, the heavy tramp of feet on the deck above, the steady Frère Jacques: Frère Jacques of the engines. He was on a ship, taking him back to England, which he never should have left in the first place. Now he was conscious of his racked, trembling, malodorous body. Daylight sent probes of agony against his eyelids. Opening them, he saw three negro sailors vigorously washing down the deck. He shut his eyes again. Impossible, he thought. . . .
>
> As day grew, the noise became more ghastly: what sounded like a railway seemed to be running just over the ceiling. Another night came. The noise grew worse and, stranger yet, the crew kept multiplying. More and more men, bruised, wounded, and always drunk, were hurled down the alley by petty officers to lie face downward, screaming or suddenly asleep on their hard bunks.
>
> He was awake. What had he done last night? Nothing at all, perhaps, yet remorse tore at his vitals. He needed a drink desperately. He did not know whether his eyes were closed or open. Horrid shapes plunged out of the blankness, gibbering, rubbing their bristles against his face, but he couldn't move. Something had got under his bed too, a bear that kept trying to get up. Voices, a prosopopoeia of voices, murmured in his ears, ebbed away, murmured again, cackled, shrieked, cajoled; voices pleading with him to stop drinking, to die and be damned. Thronged, dreadful shadows came close, were snatched away. A cataract of water was pouring through the wall, filling the room. A red hand gesticulated, prodded him: over a ravaged mountain side a swift stream was carrying with it legless bodies yelling out of great eye-sockets, in which were broken teeth. Music mounted to a screech, subsided. On a tumbled bloodstained bed in a house whose face was blasted away a large scorpion was gravely raping a one-armed negress. His wife appeared, tears streaming down her face, pitying, only to be instantly transformed into Richard III, who sprang forward to smother him.

After a few days, the DTs goes away. Lowry's patient:

> . . . now knew himself to be in a kind of hospital, and with this realization everything became coherent and fell into place. The sound of water pouring over the scuttle was the terrific shock of the flushing toilets; the banging of iron and the dispersed noises, the rattling of keys, explained themselves; the frantic ringing of bells was for doctors or nurses; and all the shouting, shuffling, creaking and ordering was no more than the complex routine of the institution.

Psychiatric patients are rarely dangerous, but delirious patients are an exception. They may be dangerous indeed, as was the case of Huckleberry Finn's alcoholic father, whose DTs was described by Mark Twain as follows:

> I don't know how long I was asleep, but all of a sudden there was an awful scream and I was up. There was Pap looking wild, and skipping around and yelling about snakes. I couldn't see no snakes, but he said they was crawling up his legs; and then he would give a jump and scream, and say one had bit him on the cheek. I never see a man look so wild. Pretty soon he was all fagged out, and fell down panting; then he rolled over and over, screaming and saying there was devils a-hold of him. He wore out by and by, and laid still awhile, moaning. Then he laid stiller, and didn't make a sound. I could hear the owls and the wolves away off in the woods, and it seemed terrible still. He was laying over by the corner. By and by he raised up partway and listened, with head to one side. He wails, very low:
>
> "Tramp-tramp-tramp; that's the dead; tramp-tramp-tramp; they're coming after me; but I won't go. Oh, they're here! Don't touch me—don't. Hands off—they're cold; let go. Oh, let a poor devil alone!"
>
> He rolled himself up in his blanket and went to crying. But by and by he rolled out and jumped up to his feet looking wild, and he see me and went for me. He chased me round and round the place with a clasp knife, calling me the Angel of Death, and saying he would kill me . . . I begged, and told him I was only Huck; but he laughed such a screech laugh, and roared and cussed, and kept on chasing me. Once when I turned short and dodged under his arm he got me by the jacket between my shoulders, and I thought I was gone; but I slid out of the jacket and saved myself. Pretty soon he was tired out, and dropped down with his back against the door, and said he would rest a minute and then kill me. He put his knife under him, and pretty soon he dozed off.

TABLE 13.2-8
Diagnostic Criteria for Alcohol Hallucinosis

A. Organic hallucinosis with vivid and persistent hallucinations (auditory or visual) developing shortly (usually within 48 hours) after cessation of or reduction in heavy ingestion of alcohol in a person who apparently has alcohol dependence.

B. No delirium as in alcohol withdrawal delirium.

C. Not due to any physical or other mental disorder.

Table from DSM-III-R *Diagnostic and Statistical Manual of Mental Disorders,* ed 3, revised. Copyright American Psychiatric Association, Washington, DC, 1987. Used with permission.

CHRONIC ALCOHOLIC HALLUCINOSIS So-called chronic alcoholic hallucinosis (Table 13.2-8) refers to the persistence of hallucinations, usually auditory, for long periods after other abstinence symptoms subside and after the patient has stopped heavy drinking. Chronic alcoholic hallucinosis occurs rarely, and 75 years of debate concerning its etiology has not resolved whether drinking actually produces the condition.

Suicide Suicide is an important complication of alcoholism. About one-quarter of suicides are alcoholic, predominantly white males over age 35. Apparently, alcoholics, unlike patients with mood disorder, are especially likely to commit suicide after loss of a spouse or a close relative or other serious interpersonal disruption.

ETIOLOGY

Most adults in Western countries drink alcohol, and 1 in 12 to 15 adults have serious problems from drinking. There is no scientifically acceptable explanation for why some people develop problems and most do not. Although the cause of alcoholism is unknown, a number of risk factors have been identified. They include the following:

1. *Family history.* Alcoholism runs in families. Children of alcoholics become alcoholic about four times more often than children of nonalcoholics. There is some evidence that they become alcoholic even when they are not raised by their alcoholic parents. Alcoholism in the family is probably the strongest predictor of alcoholism occurring in particular individuals.
2. *Sex.* More men are alcoholic than women. The ratio is 3 to 1.
3. *Age.* Men usually develop alcoholism in their 20s and 30s. Alcoholism often develops later in women. People over 65 years of age, regardless of sex, rarely become alcoholic.
4. *Location.* Alcoholism is unevenly distributed geographically and among people of different occupations, racial back-

grounds, nationality, income, and religion. These differences are noted in the section on epidemiology.

5. *Childhood history*. A childhood history of attention-deficit hyperactivity disorder or conduct disorder, or both, apparently increases a child's risk of becoming alcoholic, particularly if there is alcoholism in the family.

GENETIC FACTORS In recent years, the familial nature of alcoholism has been intensively studied. Many family studies have been conducted in Western countries, and all the studies show much higher rates of alcoholism among the relatives of alcoholics than in the general population. Nature-nurture studies, including twin and adoption studies, have attempted to separate genetic from environmental influences.

Twin studies At least four twin studies of alcoholism have been conducted. A Swedish investigator found that identical twins were significantly more concordant for alcoholism than fraternal twins, and the more severe the alcoholism the greater the difference. A Finnish study found that younger identical twins shared alcohol problems more often than older identical twins, but there was no difference in the total sample. A third study, in England, showed no difference at all between American identical and fraternal twins. The most recent study involved analyzing a large number of Veterans Administration records. They supported a genetic factor: identical twins were more often concordant for alcoholism than fraternal twins. In summary, two twin studies produced results consistent with a genetic influence, one did not, and a fourth was equivocal. The inconsistency is unexplained other than by reason of differences among cultures, sampling, information gathering, and definitions of alcoholism. Possibly family history explains some of the inconsistency—perhaps twins with a family history of alcoholism are especially likely to be concordant for alcoholism—but this theory has never been analyzed.

Adoption studies A series of adoption studies of alcoholism was conducted in Denmark in the 1970s. Sons of alcoholics raised by unrelated, nonalcoholic adoptive parents were four times more likely to become alcoholic by an early age than were adopted-out sons of nonalcoholics, but were no more likely to have other forms of psychopathology and no more likely to be classified as heavy drinkers.

Later in Denmark, daughters of alcoholics raised by nonalcoholic adoptive parents and daughters raised by their own alcoholic parents were studied. The adopted-out daughters had a higher rate of alcoholism than exists in the general population—4.0 percent versus 0.1 percent—but adopted-out controls also had a high rate of alcoholism, and the findings were equivocal. Daughters raised by the alcoholic parent or parents also had an alcoholism rate of 4.0 percent, but this rate contrasted with no alcoholism in matched controls.

Two other adoption studies were subsequently performed, one in Sweden and the other in Iowa. Both studies produced essentially the same results as the Danish studies: an increased prevalence of alcoholism in adopted-out children of alcoholics, with no evidence of an increased prevalence of other disorders. The Iowa study recently produced evidence that adopted-out daughters as well as sons of alcoholics have increased rates of alcoholism versus controls.

Summing up the results of these studies, one might conclude that children of alcoholics have an increased susceptibility to alcoholism whether they are raised by their alcoholic parents or by nonalcoholic adoptive parents. Furthermore, children of alcoholics were susceptible only to alcoholism. In these studies, they were no more likely to develop any other psychiatric illness than children of nonalcoholics—including drug abuse.

Familial vs. nonfamilial alcoholism From these studies has been developed the concept of familial alcoholism, which differs from nonfamilial alcoholism in the following ways:

1. There is a family history of alcoholism.
2. The alcoholism develops at an early age—usually in the 20s or even earlier.
3. The alcoholism is severe, often requiring treatment.
4. Having alcoholism in the family only increases the risk of alcoholism, not of other psychiatric disorders.

The idea that alcoholism can be subdivided into two types, familial and nonfamilial, has generated some new research findings. It seems that about half of alcoholics have alcoholism in their families. Of those alcoholics who have alcoholism in the family, about 90 percent have two or more alcoholic relatives. The younger the alcoholic at time of diagnosis, the more likely it is that there will be alcoholism in the family. Familial alcoholism tends to be particularly severe. Whether any alcoholic can ever return to normal drinking is a subject of controversy, but this possibility seems particularly remote with regard to familial alcoholics.

Although little is known about specific genetic mechanisms involved in alcoholism, more is known about one kind of reaction to alcohol that is definitely inherited: Millions of people have unpleasant reactions to small amounts of alcohol. These reactions may take the form of dizziness, nausea, or headaches. Adverse reactions to alcohol have been most studied in Asian people. About two-thirds of the Asian population develop a flush of the skin and have palpitations and other unpleasant effects after drinking a small amount of alcohol. Asian babies, given small amounts of alcohol, also develop a flush. Unquestionably, the basis for the flush is genetic. Apparently, this response can be blocked by antihistamine drugs, for reasons as yet unknown. There is also some evidence that a higher proportion of women than men have adverse reactions to small amounts of alcohol.

There is a lower alcoholism rate in the Orient than in Western countries, and this lower rate is usually attributed to cultural influences. Women have a lower rate of alcoholism than men, and this difference also has been ascribed to cultural influences. Biological influences may be just as important.

PHYSIOLOGICAL FACTORS Because of physiological factors, many people are born "protected" against becoming alcoholic; conversely, many who become alcoholic are born unprotected. Yet, people differ in their response to alcohol in ways other than having varying degrees of intolerance for alcohol. Some people become more euphoric from alcohol than others. Tolerance for alcohol, in part, is innate, and it varies from individual to individual. Also, the "escape" function of alcohol (which seems undeniable but is probably not the decisive factor in alcoholism) is quite variable; the need to escape is stronger in some people than in others.

There are many psychological and biochemical theories for the differential effects of alcohol. Space does not permit exploration of all the theories, but one theory has stimulated a good deal of recent research and will be summarized below.

ALKALOID THEORY OF ALCOHOLISM In 1970, two groups independently reported that central biogenic monoamines and aldehyde metabolites of the amines and alcohol form condensation products in the presence of alcohol. These products, tetrahydro-isoquinolones (TIQs), structurally resemble morphine-like alkaloids. TIQs, some believe, play an important role in alcoholism, possibly by acting as false transmitters.

The two studies led to much research. It was found that infusion of TIQs into the lateral ventricles of the rat brain resulted in increased ethanol preference. TIQs were found in urine and cerebrospinal fluid (CSF) of alcoholics in higher concentration than in nonalcoholics. TIQs were reported to bind opiate receptors, and alcohol was reported to inhibit binding of endogenous opioids to δ-opiate receptors. The opiate antagonist naloxone (Narcan) inhibits withdrawal convulsions in ethanol-dependent mice and blocks subcortical seizure activity produced by ethanol in monkeys. In two studies, naloxone reduced alcohol-induced coma in humans. In one study, naloxone prevented psychomotor impairment induced by small doses of alcohol in normal volunteers.

These findings represent only some of the available information related to these morphine-like compounds. Their relationship to alcoholism remains speculative, but conceivably, a genetic predisposition to alcoholism may involve individual differences in the production of these compounds.

TREATMENT

The treatment of alcoholism and the management of alcohol withdrawal symptoms present separate problems.

TREATMENT OF WITHDRAWAL In the absence of serious medical complications, the alcohol withdrawal syndrome is usually transient and self-limited; the patient recovers within several days, regardless of treatment. Insomnia and irritability may persist for longer periods.

A minor tranquilizer should be given during the acute withdrawal period, and then the dosage should be tapered off during the postwithdrawal period, if there are no other indications. As a rule, 25 mg of chlordiazepoxide (Librium) given 4 times a day with 100 mg of chlordiazepoxide administered intramuscularly (IM) every 4 hours as needed, suffices to calm the withdrawing patient, ward off seizures to some extent, and still be relatively safe, given the frequent uncertainty about the physical status of the patient.

Vitamins are obligatory. The Wernicke-Korsakoff syndrome almost certainly is caused by thiamine deficiency, and the peripheral neuropathy associated with alcohol apparently results from a deficiency of B vitamins in general.

Thiamine should be administered parenterally for the first 3 to 5 days of withdrawal—100 mg administered IM twice a day—with a therapeutic capsule containing the B vitamins administered twice daily for the first 2 weeks and once daily for the indefinite future.

Even if the patient seems well nourished, vitamins should be given. This is one of the rare instances where a devastating chronic brain disorder, Korsakoff's syndrome, can be prevented. Alcoholics almost always have a malabsorption syndrome involving both anatomical changes of the mucosa of the small intestine and also biochemical alterations, which is the reason why thiamine should be given parenterally for the first few days. The malabsorption syndrome also explains why apparently well-nourished individuals who give a history of three substantial meals a day may still have nutritional deficiencies and require supplemental vitamins.

Some clinicians favor giving patients magnesium sulfate during withdrawal. There is some evidence that hypomagnesemia occurs during withdrawal, and this condition may increase the possibility of seizures. There is no direct evidence, however, that seizures are prevented by administration of magnesium sulfate, and most clinicians forgo this treatment.

It is widely believed that heavy use of alcohol produces dehydration. In the absence of vomiting, diarrhea, or objective signs of dehydration, such as an elevated hematocrit, one may assume that the patient, if anything, is overhydrated. Thus, withdrawal is not a universal indication for intravenous (IV) fluids. It is not only easier but also wiser to encourage the patient to drink water and fruit juice.

Other symptoms associated with withdrawal, such as nausea, vomiting, and diarrhea, can be treated symptomatically.

Most alcoholics do not experience hypoglycemia, but it occurs occasionally, and dramatic improvement sometimes can be achieved by giving glucose.

TREATMENT OF ALCOHOLISM Chronic, excessive use of alcohol produces a wide range of psychiatric symptoms that, in various combinations, can mimic other psychiatric disorders. Therefore, while persons are drinking heavily and during their withdrawal period, it is difficult to determine whether they suffer from a psychiatric condition in addition to alcoholism.

The diagnosis of alcoholism itself is relatively easy. Many alcoholics, however, also use other drugs, and it may be difficult to determine which symptoms are produced by alcohol and which by cocaine, amphetamines, or other drugs. If patients have been drinking heavily and have not eaten, they may become hypoglycemic, a condition that may produce symptoms resembling those seen in withdrawal.

Associated disorders The three psychiatric conditions most commonly associated with alcoholism are mood disorder, anxiety disorders, and antisocial personality disorder. Female alcoholics apparently suffer more often from mood disorder than male alcoholics. The diagnosis of mood disorder usually can be made by past history or by observing the patient during long periods of abstinence. According to one study, about one-third of patients with manic-depressive illness drink more while depressed, and another third drink less. Studies indicate that small amounts of alcohol administered to a depressed patient relieve depressive symptoms, but large amounts worsen depression.

Anxiety disorders—particularly agoraphobia in women and social phobias in men—have been associated with alcoholism in recent studies. Nearly a third of treated alcoholics are said to have such disorders. If so, the association of anxiety disorders with alcoholism is stronger than that reported for mood disorders. There is even a suggestion that excessive drinking sometimes begins in an attempt to overcome phobic anxiety.

Many sociopathic people drink to excess, although how many persons would be considered alcoholic is uncertain. A follow-up study of convicted felons, about half of whom had alcohol problems, indicates that sociopathic drinkers have a higher spontaneous remission rate than nonsociopathic alcoholics. When sociopathic individuals reduce their drinking, their criminal activities are correspondingly reduced.

Various personality disorders have been associated with alcoholism, particularly those in which oral dependency is a feature. The consensus at present is that alcoholism is not connected with a particular constellation of personality traits.

Longitudinal studies help little in predicting what types of people are particularly susceptible to alcoholism.

The treatment of alcoholism should not begin until withdrawal symptoms subside. Treatment has two goals: sobriety and amelioration of psychiatric conditions associated with alcoholism.

A small minority of alcoholics eventually may be able to drink in moderation, but for several months after a heavy drinking bout, total abstinence by all patients is necessary for two reasons. First, patients must be followed while sober for a considerable period to diagnose a coexistent psychiatric problem. Second, it is important for patients to learn that they can cope with ordinary life problems without alcohol. Most relapses occur within 6 months of discharge from the hospital; relapses occur less and less frequently after that time period.

Pharmacological treatment For many patients, disulfiram is helpful in maintaining abstinence. By inhibiting AldDH, the drug leads to an accumulation of acetaldehyde if alcohol is consumed. Acetaldehyde is highly toxic and produces nausea and hypotension. Hypotension, in turn, produces shock and may be fatal. In recent years, however, dilsulfiram has been prescribed in a lower dosage (250 mg daily) than was employed previously, and few or no deaths from its use have been reported for a number of years. A recent study indicates the dosage is irrelevant; the deterrent effect is psychological and not dose-dependent.

Discontinuation of disulfiram after administration for several days or weeks still deters drinking for a 3- to 5-day period following its administration, because the drug continues to be excreted for that period of time. Thus, it may be useful to give patients disulfiram during office visits at 3- to 4-day intervals early in the treatment program.

Until recently, it was recommended that patients be given disulfiram for several days and challenged with alcohol to demonstrate the unpleasant effects that follow. This procedure was not always satisfactory because some patients showed no adverse effects after considerable amounts of alcohol were consumed, and other patients became very ill after drinking small amounts of alcohol. At present, the alcohol challenge test is considered optional. The principal disadvantage of disulfiram is not that patients drink while taking the drug, but that they stop taking the drug after a brief period. This factor is another good reason to give the drug on frequent office visits during the early, crucial period of treatment.

Recent progress In recent years, a wide variety of procedures, both psychological and somatic, have been tried in the treatment of alcoholism, but none has been proved definitely superior to others. There is no evidence that intensive psychotherapy helps most alcoholics. Nor are tranquilizers or antidepressants usually effective in maintaining abstinence or controlled drinking. Aversive conditioning techniques have been tried, with such agents as apomorphine and emetine to produce vomiting, succinylcholine (Anectine) to produce apnea, and electrical stimulation to produce pain. The controlled trials required to show the efficacy of these procedures have not been conducted, but a high rate of success has been reported for the apomorphine treatment in well-motivated patients. It is not known how many alcoholics benefit from participation in AA, but clinicians, almost unanimously, agree that alcoholics should be encouraged to attend AA meetings on a trial basis.

In three double-blind studies, lithium was found superior to placebo in reducing drinking in depressed alcoholics. There was a high dropout rate in both studies. A fourth study failed to confirm the efficacy of lithium for alcoholism.

It should be emphasized that relapses are characteristic of alcoholism and that physicians treating alcoholics should avoid anger or excessive pessimism when relapses do occur. Alcoholics see nonpsychiatric physicians as often as, or more often than, they see psychiatrists, and there is evidence that general practitioners and internists are sometimes more helpful. Medical doctors may be particularly helpful when the therapeutic approach is warm but authoritarian, with little emphasis on insight or understanding. Because the cause of alcoholism is unknown, understanding, in fact, means acceptance of a particular theory. Understanding may provide temporary comfort, but it probably rarely provides lasting benefit.

REFERENCES

Amark C: Study in alcoholism: Clinical, social-psychiatric and genetic investigations. Acta Psychiat Scand (Suppl) *70:* 1, 1951.

Cahalan D, Cisin I H, Crossley H M: *American Drinking Practices: A National Survey of Behavior and Attitudes,* Monograph No. 6. Rutgers University Center of Alcohol Studies, New Brunswick, NJ, 1969.

Fuller R K, Branchey L, Brightwell D R, et al: Disulfiram treatment of alcoholism: A Veterans Administration cooperative study. JAMA *256:* 1449, 1986.

Fuller R K, Williford W O: Life-table analysis of abstinence in a study evaluating the efficacy of disulfiram. Alcoholism *4:* 298, 1980.

Galanter M, editor: *Recent Developments in Alcoholism,* vol 3. Plenum, New York, 1985.

Goodwin D W: *Alcoholism: The Facts.* Oxford University Press, New York, 1981.

Goodwin D W: Genetic component of alcoholism. Ann Rev Med *32:* 93, 1981.

Goodwin D W: Drug therapy of alcoholism, In *Psychopharmacology,* D G Grahame-Smith, H Hippius, G Winokur, editors, vol 1, p 295. Excerpta Medica, Amsterdam, 1982.

Goodwin D W: The management of depression in alcoholism. J Psychiat Treat Eval *5:* 445, 1983.

Goodwin D W: Alcoholism and genetics. Arch Gen Psychiat *42:* 171, 1985.

Goodwin, D. W. *Is Alcoholism Hereditary?* Ballantine, New York, 1988.

Jellinek E M: *The Disease Concept of Alcoholism.* College and University Press, New Haven, 1960.

Kent T A, Gunn W H, Goodwin D W, Jones M P, Marples B W, Penick E C: Individual differences in state-dependent retrieval effects of alcohol intoxication. J Stud Alcohol *47*(3): 241, 1986.

Lowry, M: Lunar caustic. Paris Rev: Winter-Spring, 1963.

Mendelson J H, Mello N K, editors. *The Diagnosis & Treatment of Alcoholism.* McGraw-Hill, New York, 1985.

Moore R D, Pearson T A. Moderate alcohol consumption and coronary artery disease: A review. Medicine *65*(4): 242, 1986.

Ryback R S, Eckardt M J, Felsher B: Biochemical and hematological correlates of alcoholism and liver disease. JAMA *248:* 2261, 1982.

Turner T B, Bennett V L, Hernandez H: The beneficial side of moderate alcohol use. Johns Hopkins Med J *148:* 53, 1981.

Vaillant G E. *The Natural History of Alcoholism.* Harvard University Press, Cambridge, MA, 1983.

Whitfield J B: Alcohol-related biochemical changes in heavy drinkers. Aust NZ J Med *11:* 132, 1981.

Wilsnack S C and Beckman L J. *Alcohol Problems in Women.* Guilford, New York, 1984.

CHAPTER 14 SCHIZOPHRENIA

14.1 SCHIZOPHRENIA: EPIDEMIOLOGY

MARVIN KARNO, M.D.
GRAYSON S. NORQUIST, M.D.

INTRODUCTION

HISTORY Epidemiological research in psychiatry has recently burgeoned synergistically with the construction of diagnostic schemas based on specifiable symptom criteria. The rapid, sequential development of the St. Louis (Feighner) diagnostic criteria, the Research Diagnostic Criteria (RDC), and the third edition of the *Diagnostic and Statistical Manual of Mental Disorders* (DSM-III) (and, now, the revised version of DSM-III [DSM-III-R] has come in the past 15 years, after a century of experience worldwide with the phenomenology of mental disorders in community, clinic, and hospital settings. In the clinic and the laboratory, psychiatrists have had to confront the same historical demands as other physicians: to act on only the most preliminary (and often primitive) scientific data and theoretical concepts, while awaiting elaboration by scientific researchers of findings that will form new diagnostic strategies and therapies.

During the 90 years that it has been a recognized syndrome, schizophrenia, with its protean manifestations and lifelong course, has been the classical refractory mental disorder—refractory to consensual conceptualization, definition, and identification of etiology, and tragically refractory to prevention and treatment. Schizophrenia has epitomized the axiom that classification is essential to scientific understanding. A basic process in understanding it is a program of epidemiological studies of the disorder (viz., assessments of its distribution among populations and of factors associated with its occurrence).

Kraepelin's formulation of the concept of dementia precox emphasized its endogenous nature and its destruction of the normal integration of cognition, affect, and volition, but he also stressed the typically chronic and massively disabling course of the disease. Although Bleuler gave full credit to Kraepelin for the concept of dementia precox and its symptomatic classification, Bleuler's own theoretical elaboration of the structure of schizophrenic pathology, based largely on the work of Freud, eventually led to an international schism over the conceptualization and diagnosis of schizophrenia from which two principal (and many lesser) schools of thought and practice evolved. This phenomenon produced dramatically divergent epidemiologies of schizophrenia, depending on the conceptual and diagnostic orientation of the investigator: The Zurich-American camp, in the combined traditions of Bleuler and Freud, was highly inclusive in diagnostic practice; British and non-Swiss continental thought and practice were narrowly exclusive. Bleuler's emphasis on the fundamental, not inherently psychotic, symptoms of schizophrenia caused him to state that mild and latent cases of the disease are many times more common than overt cases. He came to apply the diagnosis indiscriminately and pejoratively, particularly the unfortunate subcategory of simple schizophrenia. In *Dementia Praecox or the Group of Schizophrenias,* Bleuler wrote, "The simple schizophrenics vegetate as day laborers, peddlers, even as servants. They are also vagabonds and hoboes . . . on the higher levels of society, the most common type is the wife . . . who is unbearable, constantly scolding, nagging, always making demands, but never recognizing duties."

As a consequence of Bleuler's influence on American psychiatric thinking, the first edition of the *Diagnostic and Statistical Manual of Mental Disorders* (DSM-I) provided a troublingly nonspecific definition of schizophrenic reactions, asserting that they were characterized by fundamental disturbances in reality relationships and concept formations, with affective, behavioral, and intellectual disturbances in varying degrees and mixtures. In the second edition of DSM (DSM-II), the definition mentioned symptoms that differentiated schizophrenia from paranoid and mood (affective) disorders but provided little more clarification.

The Cross-National Study of Diagnosis of the Mental Disorders provided compelling evidence in the late 1960s that the much greater frequency with which the admission diagnosis of schizophrenia was made at major U.S. psychiatric hospitals than at matched British hospitals was due largely to a tendency on the part of psychiatrists at American hospitals to diagnose schizophrenia more readily than their British counterparts. The bias in American diagnostic practice was particularly concentrated in those cases in which patients demonstrated incomprehensibility, a lack of insight, or psychotic symptoms (e.g., somatic delusions) that were not clearly affective in nature. Indeed, the American psychiatrists tended to diagnose schizophrenia whenever they saw a florid psychosis.

The Americans' tendency to equate psychosis with schizophrenia was also fostered by a concept of psychopathology that derived from psychoanalytic theory concerning stages of psychosexual development and postulated ontological levels of psychopathology characteristic of different steps of fixation or regression. Schizophrenia was viewed as the most primitive psychopathological state, one at which a person subjected to sufficiently faulty parenting and life stress might be fixated or to which he or she might regress under stress. A schizophrenic break was the consequence of a collapse of ego defenses to those characteristic of a psychotic or primary-process level of functioning. So most acute psychotic episodes of adults that could not be clearly related to an organic or toxic cause were likely to be diagnosed as schizophrenia.

Although systematized and specifiable diagnostic criteria, with rules for inclusion and exclusion of cases, have inestimable value for epidemiological studies of most mental disorders, they are of especially great significance to studies of schizophrenia. (Witness the findings of the already cited National Institute of Mental Health [NIMH]-sponsored Cross-National Study, and of the World Health Organization [WHO]-supported International Pilot Study of Schizophrenia of the late 1960s and 1970s.) These landmark studies, and many others, demonstrated that psychiatrist interviewers trained in the use of standardized, structured interviews that generate diagnoses according to specifiable criteria could accurately diagnose schizophrenia in persons of diverse nations and cultures living at widely different levels of socioeconomic status, urbanization, and industrialization.

The discussion of the epidemiology of schizophrenia which follows focuses primarily on studies of community, rather than clinical, populations. This is because admission rates to hospitals and clinic settings do not necessarily correspond to the actual incidence or prevalence of a disorder such as schizophrenia in the community: Onset and development are often insidious, and there is wide variation in how the disease is perceived, defined, and dealt with in community settings. Hospitalization often depends more on what Erving Goffman has called contingencies than on the specific symptoms or behaviors of the ill person. Data obtained at the first three of five community sites in the NIMH–sponsored Epidemiologic Catchment Area (ECA) study, (New Haven, Connecticut; Baltimore, Maryland; and St. Louis, Missouri) indicate that fewer than half of respondents in households who were diagnosed as schizophrenic according to DSM-III criteria had made a visit for mental health reasons to any kind of health or mental health facility or resource during the 6 months prior to interview. Other findings from this major recent study are discussed at length below.

DIAGNOSIS AND MEASUREMENT

At least 15 different sets of diagnostic criteria for schizophrenia are in use somewhere in Western psychiatry, all of which require observation or direct clinical interviewing of the patient in order to make the diagnosis. No laboratory tests as yet can diagnose schizophrenia. What specific questions a trained clinician asks in order to make a diagnosis (identify a case) in most clinical settings is left to the judgment of that clinician. The International Pilot Study of Schizophrenia utilized the Present State Examination (PSE), a semistructured interview that inventories a wide range of psychiatric symptoms common in schizophrenia (and other mental disorders) but leaves the wording of probes to clarify the severity, presence, or absence of a symptom to be chosen by the research-psychiatrist interviewer. The utilization of DSM-III in recent, large-scale epidemiological studies required the development of a new, totally structured diagnostic interview designed to determine the presence or absence of DSM-III–defined mental disorders by computer analysis of diagnostic algorithms. The major recent study that utilized this approach is discussed below.

The DSM-III-R modifications in the diagnosis of schizophrenia are of importance to future epidemiological studies of the disorder. These include the specification of a minimum duration of 1 week for psychotic symptoms (less if successfully treated), which introduces greater precision in case definition, and the omission of a maximum age of onset, which expands potential future prevalence and incidence rates.

DEFINITIONS

The term *prevalence* refers to the number of cases of disorder present either at a particular point in time (*point prevalence*) or during a particular period of time (the week, month, or year prior to evaluation: *period prevalence*). Lifetime prevalence generally is determined only by retrospective recall of whether the disorder had ever occurred during the individual's life. *Incidence* refers to the number of new cases of a disorder or illness that appear in a population during a specified period. The most frequently utilized incidence period is 1 year (*annual incidence*). The term *crude incidence* refers to crude estimates of the occurrence of new cases of a disorder, based on admission rates to hospitals, clinics, or other clinical facilities. The crudeness derives from the multiple potential sources of discrepancy between the number of cases that actually occur and the number that come to clinical attention during a given period.

CASE FINDING

There are four principal methods of locating cases of mental disorder within a population.

COMMUNITY SURVEYS *Community surveys* entail face-to-face interviews of every accessible member of a community or of a selected sample of respondents from that community. The former approach has been feasible with small, insulated, clearly defined populations, such as residents of an island, members of a cohesive religious sect, or inhabitants of a village or town. The results of such studies are of limited generalizability. Studies of large populations require some form of stratified or random sampling in order to limit cost and volume of collected data. A total survey of a small, well-defined population presumably cannot be discredited for not being representative of the group as might a sample from a large population. Total or large-sample surveys of large populations are rendered more economically feasible by a two-stage approach, in which the entire population or sample is first given a brief screening interview, after which only potential cases are pursued with a detailed interview. The relatively low lifetime prevalence of schizophrenia—traditionally estimated at less than one in 100 persons—demands that large populations be studied, in order to find enough cases to generate statistically significant information about the many factors associated with the disorder.

CASE REGISTERS *Case registers* are the product of regular reporting of all cases of a disorder and all clinical contacts with those patients in a defined geographical area or community. The degree to which all cases of schizophrenia come to clinical attention and are faithfully reported to the central case register is unknowable and, so, limits the authority of a case register as a source of epidemiological data. The Monroe County, New York psychiatric case register is an epidemiological data file maintained by the University of Rochester School of Medicine since 1960. The data found that 3 percent of the county received care in mental health facilities. Of that number, about 16 percent were schizophrenic, according to 1975 figures.

KEY INFORMANTS The *key informant* approach, historically a staple of ethnographic investigations in cultural anthropology, identifies persons whose characteristics are of interest to the investigator. A key informant is a person who is known in the community for having intimate knowledge of that culture and wide social contacts. The key informant has been essential for locating persons with mental disorders in nonliterate societies or in those which do not routinely define mental disorders according to Western medical parameters.

CLINICAL FACILITY REPORTS OR SEARCHES These epidemiological methods provide a wealth of epidemiological data, but the cases reported or identified by search may (1) represent a significant undercount of the cases in the community served by the facility and (2) report cases that have uniquely skewed clinical or sociodemographic characteristics not representative of all persons who have the disorder in question. Psychiatric clinical samples typically are not representative of the age, sex, ethnicity, socioeconomic, religious, and demographic characteristics of the population at risk, and may over-report relatively severe cases. Given the large homeless population in the United States (estimates range from 300,000 to 3 million) and the anecdotal evidence for very high rates among them of mental disorders and infrequent contacts with health care resources, case register or clinical facility reports would miss many cases of schizophrenia.

PREVALENCE OF SCHIZOPHRENIA

Recent reviews of 50 studies of the prevalence of schizophrenia in the 6 inhabited continents conducted during the period from 1931 through 1983 and based on diverse methodologies revealed point prevalences (10 studies) ranging from 0.6 to 7.1 cases per 1,000 population; 3- to 6-month prevalences (4 studies) of 3.6 to 7.3 cases per 1,000 population; and 1-year prevalences (7 studies) of 2.7 to 7.0 cases per 1,000 population. Prevalences for periods between 1 year and life (5, 18, 45, and 48 years) revealed a range from 1.7 to 9.5 cases per 1,000 population. Lifetime prevalence (21 studies) ranged from 0.9 to 11.0 cases per 1,000 population. These data include some rates adjusted for what has been considered the period of susceptible risk (approximately ages 15 to 45). The highest rate (11.0 per 1,000) was found in a group of Canadian native Americans; the lowest rate (0.6 per 1000) was found in Ghana. The diagnostic definitions used in the studies ranged from very narrow to very broad and relied on diverse case-finding techniques and interview formats, and all but a few predated structured diagnostic criteria. The 12-fold variation in lifetime rates more likely is due to methodological differences than to true differences in prevalence.

EPIDEMIOLOGIC CATCHMENT AREA (ECA) PROGRAM The largest and most carefully controlled psychiatric epidemiological study yet undertaken is the NIMH–sponsored ECA Program, in which face-to-face interviews were conducted in households with 18,572 persons residing in New Haven, Connecticut; Baltimore, Maryland; St. Louis, Missouri; the North Carolina piedmont; and greater Los Angeles, California from 1980 through 1985. Although the respondents were randomly selected from designated catchment areas in these communities, neither the catchment areas nor the five communities are representative of the entire U.S. population. However, the inclusion of large numbers of elderly, black, Hispanic, and rural respondents in this study, and the geographical distribution of the sample, strongly suggest that the data obtained provide the best estimates available of rates of DSM-III–defined mental disorders in the United States.

A highly structured, precoded household survey instrument, the Diagnostic Interview Schedule (DIS), was developed for the ECA study. The DIS inquires about the presence or absence of specific psychiatric symptoms, and responses are scored by computer algorithms to produce diagnoses for about 40 DSM-III–defined disorders, including subcategories. The interview was administered by trained lay interviewers and included questions to ascertain whether reported symptoms were not likely due to mental disorder. Approximately 76 percent of those contacted and selected agreed to be interviewed.

The questions intended to assess the presence or absence of schizophrenia included a requirement for the verbatim recording of any positive symptom reported by the respondent. Information about the duration of symptoms allowed for the diagnosis of either schizophreniform disorder (if present less than 6 months) or schizophrenia.

The lifetime prevalence rates for schizophrenia and schizophreniform disorder from the New Haven, Baltimore, St. Louis, and Los Angeles ECA sites are presented in Table 14.1-1. Data from North Carolina have not yet been published and, so, are not included. The data are weighted at each site to represent age, sex, and minority group characteristics of the sampled catchment areas. Adjustment for the demographic differences between sites produces no significant changes in the figures presented.

Demographic correlates of ECA prevalence rates Rates for schizophrenia were found to be significantly higher for black than nonblack respondents in Baltimore but not at other sites. Similarly, level of education correlated with prevalence of schizophrenia at only one site, New Haven, where college graduates reported only 20 percent the prevalence of those with less education (0.5 versus 2.5 percent). In St. Louis, schizophrenia was significantly more prevalent among inner city residents than among those who lived in suburbs or rural areas. A sex difference was found only at New Haven, where women reported more than twice the lifetime prevalence of men (2.6 versus 1.2 percent). The prevalence of schizophrenia among Mexican Americans in Los Angeles was not significantly different from that of non-Hispanic Caucasians. No consistent relationship was found between any demographic factor studied and the prevalence of schizophrenia.

The findings from the ECA study indicate a higher lifetime prevalence of schizophrenia than had been generally reported in prior studies. It is impossible at this time to know whether the ECA prevalence figures are inflated by inclusion of false-positive cases, which do not truly meet DSM-III criteria, or whether the ECA has produced better case findings because it was more rigorous and broader-based than prior studies. Criticism of the ECA results stems primarily from later studies in which research psychiatrists interviewed ECA community respondents who had DIS–diagnosed mental disorders. The degree of concordance between the physician and community diagnoses varied according to disorder but was relatively low for schizophrenia. However, there were significant methodological limitations in the reexamination studies, and there is still open debate about appropriate statistical measures for assessing diagnostic agreement between measures of disorders, such as schizophrenia, that occur at low base rates in community populations. In the authors' opinion, despite limitations and uncertainties, the ECA data provide the best estimates yet for the prevalence of DSM-III–defined schizophrenia in the United States. The authors' summary interpretation of ECA and prior epidemiological data is that the lifetime prevalence of schizophrenia is about 1 percent for most populations that have been studied.

INCIDENCE OF SCHIZOPHRENIA

There have been very few studies of the incidence of schizophrenia. Such studies require longitudinal assessment of a population with separate evaluations at two points in time to determine how many new cases have developed in the time interval. Crude incidence estimates (described above), usually based on first psychiatric hospitalization, have very limited value because of the methodological limitations discussed above. A recent review of 13 such studies carried out from 1950 through 1980 revealed crude annual incidence rates ranging from 0.11 to 0.70 per 1,000 population.

TABLE 14.1
Lifetime Prevalence Rates for Schizophrenia and Schizophreniform Disorder from Four ECA Sites

	New Haven, CT	*Baltimore, MD*	*St. Louis, MO*	*Los Angeles, CA*
Sample size	3,058	3,481	3,004	3,132
Date of study	1980–81	1981–82	1981–82	1983–84
Schizophrenia % (SE*)	1.9(0.3)*	1.6(0.2)	1.0(0.2)	0.6(0.2)
Schizophreniform disorder % (SE*)	0.1(0.3)	0.3(0.1)	0.1(0.1)	0.1(0.2)

*Standard error

The ECA study did entail personal follow-up interviews with more than 15,000 community respondents 1 year after their initial interviews, specifically for the purpose of estimating annual incidence of mental disorders. Incidence data are not yet available, but methodological difficulties inherent in comparing results of interviews done 1 year apart will inevitably render the incidence estimates more problematic than the prevalence estimates provided by the ECA.

RISK FACTORS

Risk refers to the likelihood that someone will develop schizophrenia who does not currently have schizophrenia but has been exposed to risk factors. A *risk factor* is an inherent or acquired personal characteristic or an external condition associated with an increased likelihood of schizophrenia.

The concept of risk is expressed in several ways. The most common is a report of the absolute number of new schizophrenia cases detected in a population exposed to a postulated risk factor. Relative risk (incidence ratio, risk ratio) and risk difference—expressions of the relationship of the incidence in those exposed to the risk factor to that of those not exposed—are often used.

Significant risk factors are identified by several different study designs. Cross-sectional studies report descriptive data, such as the increased presence of a particular risk factor in a population with a higher prevalence of schizophrenia. Case-control studies take schizophrenia cases and matched controls and determine whether those who express the disease were exposed to a given risk factor. The most informative (and expensive) study design is the prospective cohort study, which follows a group over time to determine whether those exposed to more risk factors have a higher incidence of schizophrenia.

Risk factors are categorized in several different ways: demographic and concomitant factors (e.g., age, sex, race, social class), precipitating factors that operate immediately before the onset of schizophrenia (e.g., life events, migration), and predisposing factors that act for long periods of time or during an earlier part of life (e.g., genes, perinatal complications, infections). Another scheme describes risk factors as either familial influences or sociodemographic factors. The latter can be further subdivided into mutable factors (e.g., social class, marital status, immigration) and immutable ones (e.g., ethnic group, sex, birthplace); mutable sociodemographic factors could be a result and not a cause of the disease.

Several cautions are necessary when considering reports from studies of schizophrenic risk factors. First, a high prevalence of schizophrenia in a particular area may be the result of a protracted illness rather than an increased incidence of schizophrenia (i.e., prevalence is roughly equal to incidence × duration). Second, studies that report only the prevalence of schizophrenia may have failed to control other confounding factors that themselves might increase prevalence. Third, designating something as a risk factor does not imply that everyone exposed to it is at personal risk to develop schizophrenia. It means that a group of people who are exposed to the risk factor present at some time are likely to have a higher incidence of schizophrenia than a similar group who were not exposed to the risk factor. In other words, risk does not imply etiology but rather an association between the risk factor and the development of schizophrenia. Fourth, schizophrenia may be an etiologically heterogeneous disorder with many risk factors and many protective factors.

Earlier studies of risk factors had many problems, the most important being the failure to standardize diagnostic criteria for selection of schizophrenia cases. However, these studies do help in the continued search to understand this complex disorder.

GENETIC FACTORS Genetic risk has been examined through studies of twins, families, and the adopted-away children of schizophrenic parents. Twin studies have shown a monozygotic concordance of 33 to 78 percent, but only 8 to 28 percent in dizygotic twins. These results may be affected by selection bias if monozygotic twins are more likely to come to the attention of researchers than are dizygotic twins. Also, monozygotic twins may have greater environmental similarity.

Family studies reveal that first-degree relatives of a schizophrenic person have approximately a five- to 10-fold greater chance of developing schizophrenia than nonrelatives. Children have about a 35- to 45-percent chance of schizophrenia if both parents are schizophrenic compared with about a 1-percent lifetime risk if neither parent has schizophrenia. Although the results from family studies are thought to represent genetic influences, they may be a result of similar environmental factors.

Adoption studies have been conducted in an effort to control environmental influences. The adopted-away offspring of schizophrenics are at increased risk for schizophrenia and schizophrenia-spectrum disorders. Although there are methodological problems with these studies, their findings do suggest some type of genetic influence in schizophrenia—the significance of which has yet to be delineated (as has the actual mode of transmission). Genetic and environmental factors surely play a role in the development of schizophrenia, and further refinement in methodology should help to identify the environmental and genetic components of schizophrenia.

ETHNICITY AND RACIAL FACTORS Several studies have discovered differences in the prevalence and number of new cases of schizophrenia among various ethnic and racial groups. These findings are not consistent and may result from failure to control for confounding factors, such as social class, age, sex, and immigration status. Findings from the NIMH-ECA study confirm that, if potential confounding factors such as education are controlled, the difference in prevalence across races disappears.

Studies of different geographic areas have found a higher prevalence and a larger number of new cases in different countries (e.g., Ireland) and within countries (e.g., Istrian Peninsula of Yugoslavia). Most studies comparing geographical areas are usually flawed because they fail to validate diagnostic methods in different ethnic groups and localities. As noted above, a study of psychiatrists in the United States and the United Kingdom found that differences in reported prevalence of schizophrenia in those countries could be explained by diagnostic methods. A recent international study by the WHO that tried to control diagnostic criteria reported that the numbers of new schizophrenia cases that presented in clinics were similar in various cultures. If true differences in incidence can be shown, perhaps differences in environmental characteristics, genetic characteristics, or both, can be found in these areas.

AGE The DSM-III diagnosis of schizophrenia requires onset of symptoms prior to age 45. This criterion was based on early studies that showed mean ages of onset well below 45 in men and women. However, recent data indicate that onset after age 45 may not be as rare as was previously assumed. Preliminary results from the NIMH-ECA study reveal that failure to diagnose schizophrenia in the elderly may be due to the fact that the disease has a different presentation in this age group. When compared with younger persons, most elderly people with delusions or hallucinations may not have the typical pattern of chronic progressive schizophrenia and are less likely to be significantly impaired or to be under the care of a mental health specialist. DSM-III-R does not have as one of the diagnostic criteria onset of symptoms prior to age 45.

SEX Studies that do not separate groups by age of onset show a male to female ratio of close to one, but this changes when various age cohorts are examined. Men are most likely to have the onset of symptoms between ages 15 and 24; women are at highest risk in the age range of 25 to 34 years. The reasons for this difference are not clear. The disease may manifest itself differently in the two sexes, or sociocultural factors may predispose men to more aggressive behavior that leads to earlier case findings.

When different cultures are examined, the findings—earlier onset and earlier date for first treatment and first hospitalization for males—are the same. More asocial premorbid characteristics, birth complications, and cerebral structural changes (especially in the left or dominant hemisphere) have been reported in men than in women, and males' schizophrenia may have a more chronic and disabling course. These findings are not conclusive, and methodological problems, such as failure to control for sociocultural factors, limit the interpretation of previous studies.

TIME OF BIRTH A disproportionate number of schizophrenic persons are born during the winter months; this, together with a birth pattern in their nonschizophrenic siblings that is similar to that seen in the general population, suggest the presence of a seasonal factor. Proposed explanations for this seasonal effect include a deleterious environmental factor in the winter (e.g., temperature, nutritional deficiences, infectious agents); genetic factor in those with a propensity for schizophrenia that protects against infection and other insults and, so, increases the likelihood of survival; and more frequent conception in the spring and summer by the parents of schizophrenic persons.

Although no experimental testing exists, studies appear to favor the harmful-effects hypothesis (e.g., infectious agents, nutritional deficiencies), but the other hypotheses have not been ruled out conclusively. Although some studies in the Southern Hemisphere confirm a higher birth rate for schizophrenic persons in winter than in other seasons, further work is needed. With refinement of research techniques, most methodological problems could be rectified. If there were statistically significant increases of schizophrenic births during the Southern Hemisphere winter, environmental factors should be favored over sociocultural ones. Whether winter- and summer-born schizophrenic persons differ is not clear, but that would not necessarily be expected if the causative agent is active all year but more active in the colder months.

Early studies also reported characteristic places in the birth order for schizophrenic persons, but these results have not been consistent. Family size can affect the findings. For example, some have found schizophrenia to be unusually common in youngest children of large families and in first-born sons of small families. Again, methodological problems limit the value of these studies.

BIRTH COMPLICATIONS When compared with controls, schizophrenic persons as a group experience a greater number of birth complications, especially males. Some studies have also reported a relationship between perinatal complications and early onset of disease, negative symptoms, and poorer prognosis. The crucial factor appears to be transient perinatal hypoxia, although not all infants so affected later develop a psychiatric disorder. There is, however, a general trend toward psychopathology in persons who suffer obstetrical complications; they appear to increase the vulnerability to development of schizophrenia and probably are not a specific cause. No prospective studies have been done, and retrospective case-control studies may be biased if informants interviewed about a schizophrenic relative try harder to remember birth complications than do informants reporting on healthy controls. Even obstetrical records often refer only to severe complications.

SOCIAL CLASS Social class can be specified in various ways using some combination of income, occupation, education, and place of residence. The prevalence and number of newly identified cases of schizophrenia repeatedly are reported to be higher among members of lower social classes than upper social classes. Different explanations have been proposed. Some consider the socioenvironmental factors found at lower socioeconomic levels to be a cause of schizophrenia (*social causation theory*). Several factors associated with lower socioeconomic status are presumed to be potentially responsible for the higher risk of schizophrenia: more life-event stressors, increased exposure to environmental and occupational hazards and infectious agents, poorer prenatal care, and fewer support resources if stress does occur.

Others propose that lower socioeconomic status is a consequence of the disorder (*social selection–drift theory*). The insidious onset of inherited schizophrenia is believed to preclude elevating one's status or to cause a downward drift. Prospective studies have shown that schizophrenic persons have less upward mobility from generation to generation than does the general population and that there is downward drift after the onset of symptoms. Many continue to argue this unsettled case, but current opinion appears to favor the social selection–drift theory. It remains unsettled, in part, because previous studies have had inadequate sample sizes, problems with defining social class, and selection bias when choosing their case and control populations.

MARITAL STATUS Reports based on first hospital admissions have shown higher rates of schizophrenia for single than for married patients, and some have inferred that single status contributes to the development of schizophrenia. However, the phenomenon may be similar to that described under social class; that is, the disease lessens the chance of getting married and increases the chance of divorce. Studies have not shown marriage to have a protective effect against schizophrenia or an excess of schizophrenia in widowed people, and previous research using subjects hospitalized for the first time may have been flawed, because single and married men appear to have different hospital utilization patterns.

IMMIGRATION A higher risk for schizophrenia among recent immigrants than native populations has been reported, but no study to date has confirmed that immigration stress leads to schizophrenia. The increased prevalence of schizophrenia among immigrants could result from selection (i.e., schizophrenic persons may be more likely to leave their families); from the failure to control for other factors, such as social class, age, and sex; or, from the failure to compare these immigrant patients to nonemigrant controls from their homeland. These methodological issues limit any conclusions that can be drawn from current reports.

URBANIZATION AND INDUSTRIALIZATION The prevalence of schizophrenia has been reported to be higher in urban environments than in rural areas. This is consistent with widely held beliefs that cities are places of rapid change and social disorganization, while rural areas are more socially stable and the inhabitants, more integrated. Recent ECA findings show no difference in the prevalence of schizophrenia between urban and rural areas when such factors as race, sex, and age are controlled.

The assertion that the prevalence and incidence of schizophrenia have increased in modern times has been tested by comparing less developed cultures with those in industrialized nations, but such studies are fraught with methodological problems. For example, infant mortality is lower in developed countries, so those likely to develop schizophrenia may survive more frequently. Families are smaller and more insular, and ill members may be more obvious. The question of whether schizophrenia is more prevalent in modern times has also been studied by analyzing the reported number of new cases over time. However, it is difficult to control for probable diagnostic bias across centuries, especially for a disease that was first defined only in the late 1800s. Modern psychiatry may even encourage persons with psychoses to present themselves for treatment.

LIFE STRESSORS The association between stressful life events (e.g., loss of job, divorce) and the etiology and course of schizophrenia has been much studied. Schizophrenia or relapse of preexisting disorder often follows extraordinary stress, so it has been suggested that such stress might provoke acute schizophrenia in a normal person. Others argue that stress plays only a marginal role in the pathogenesis of the disorder or simply triggers schizophrenia in vulnerable persons. The few studies that have considered this issue have suffered the usual methodological problems of retrospective case-control studies and have had difficulty in outlining predispositional factors in schizophrenia. The stressor might have triggered the onset of a disorder that would have occurred in any case. The issue is not settled and will require further studies, especially prospective ones that can consider the role and severity of stressors in individual cases.

INFECTIONS Central nervous system anatomical and immune changes suggestive of chronic viral infection have been reported in some schizophrenia patients. A viral hypothesis is consistent with seasonal excesses, geographical differences, and changes in incidence across centuries. Viruses could also interact with a genetic predisposition, familial transmission, or both in complex ways in the development of the disease. However, as yet, no study has conclusively shown an association between viral infection and the onset of schizophrenia. Further studies, especially those that can show transmission, are needed.

CHILDHOOD SCHIZOPHRENIA

As with adult-onset schizophrenia, different diagnostic criteria can affect the interpretation of results from studies of childhood-onset schizophrenia. Early definitions of childhood-onset schizophrenia tended to be very broad and often included patients with autistic disorder. DSM-III-R has departed from the broad DSM-II definition by using the more restrictive criteria applied to adults that emphasize hallucinations and formal thought disorder. This definition, however, fails to consider developmental issues, such as the nature of delusions in childhood and how a formal thought disorder is diagnosed in a child under 8 years of age, whose formal cognitive processes are not fully developed. Others have considered developmental stages in diagnosing childhood-onset schizophrenia, but no consensus has been reached. The accuracy of any reported epidemiological data on childhood-onset schizophrenia is compromised by differences in diagnostic criteria.

No large-scale population study exists that has used rigorous, standardized criteria for diagnosis. Therefore, the prevalence of childhood-onset schizophrenia is not clear but it is probably less than early infantile autism and is estimated to be 50 times less than that of adult-onset schizophrenia. There does not appear to be a greater incidence in boys than girls as there is in infantile autism.

The risk factors in childhood-onset schizophrenia are not well known, and many investigators have simply extrapolated from adult findings. However, environmental stressors, perinatal complications, and central nervous system dysfunction have all been reported to occur more frequently in children who are diagnosed as schizophrenic. For further discussion of this area, see Section 44.5, Schizophrenia with Childhood Onset.

FUTURE DIRECTIONS

The authors' opinion is that future epidemiological research in schizophrenia should incorporate current laboratory measures of vulnerability indicators into survey field studies. Continuous performance testing, eye tracking, neuromotor screening, and autonomic nervous system testing could all be carried out in well-equipped mobile vans among populations already found by interviews to be at risk. For example, the children of adult respondents who report symptoms of schizophrenia or schizophreniform disorder might be evaluated by such means in community settings, in comparison with appropriate control groups. The National Health and Nutrition Examination Survey (HANES), sponsored by the National Center for Health Statistics, has successfully interviewed thousands of U.S. household respondents in diverse communities. The HANES study conducted physical examinations and obtained urine and blood specimens. The authors believe that such an approach, although expensive, would be invaluable in future epidemiological studies of mental disorders, particularly schizophrenia. Such a strategy might identify young persons at specific risk and might provide important etiological clues about this most tragic mental disorder.

REFERENCES

Beitchman J H: Childhood schizophrenia: A review and comparison with adult onset schizophrenia. Psychiat J Univ Ottawa *8:* 25, 1983.

Bleuler E: *Dementia Praecox or the Group of Schizophrenias.* International Universities Press, New York, 1971.

Cooper J E, Kendell R E, Gurland B J, Sartorius N, Farkas T: Cross-national study of diagnosis of the mental disorders: Some results from the first comparative investigation. Amer J Psychiat *125:* 21, 1969.

Dohrenwend B P, Dohrenwend B S, Gould M S, Link B, Neugebauer R, Wunsch-Hitzig R: *Mental Illness in the United States Epidemiological Estimates.* Praeger, New York, 1980.

Eaton W W: Epidemiology of schizophrenia. Epidemiol Rev *7:* 105, 1985.

Jablensky A: Epidemiology of schizophrenia: A European perspective. Schizophr Bull *12*: 52, 1986.
Jablensky A, Sartorius N: Culture and schizophrenia. Psychol Med *5*: 113, 1975.
Najem G R, Lindenthal J J, Louria D B, Thind I S: Epidemiology of schizophrenia. Publ Health Rev *9*: 113, 1980.
Nuechterlein K H: Annotation: Childhood precursors of adult schizophrenia. J Child Psychol Psychiat *27*: 133, 1986.
Regier D A, Myers J K, Kramer M, Robins L N, Blazer D G, Hough R L, Eaton W W, Locke B Z: The NIMH Epidemiologic Catchment Area Program. Arch Gen Psychiat *41*: 934, 1984.
Robins L N: Epidemiology: Reflections on testing the validity of psychiatric interviews. Arch Gen Psychiat *42*: 918, 1985.
Robins L N, Helzer J E, Croughan J, Ratcliff K S : National Institute of Mental Health Diagnostic Interview Schedule: Its history, characteristics and validity. Arch Gen Psychiat *38*: 381, 1981.
Robins L N, Helzer J E, Weissman M M, Orvaschel H, Gruenberg E, Burke J D, Regier D A: Lifetime prevalence of specific psychiatric disorders in three sites. Arch Gen Psychiat *41*: 949, 1984.
Torrey E F: The epidemiology of schizophrenia. Schizophr Bull *7*: 588, 1981.
Torrey E F: *Schizophrenia and Civilization*. Jason Aronson, New York, 1980.
Von Korff M, Nestadt G, Romanoski A, Anthony J A, Eaton W, Merchant A, Chahal R, Kramer M, Folstein M, Gruenberg E: Prevalence of treated and untreated DSM-III schizophrenia: Results of a two-stage community survey. J Nerv Ment Dis *173*: 577, 1985.
Weissman M M, Myers J K, Ross C E, editors: *Community Surveys of Psychiatric Disorders*. Rutgers University Press, New Brunswick, 1986.
Wing J K, Cooper J E, Sartorius N: *Measurement and Classification of Psychiatric Symptoms: An Instruction Manual for the Present State Examination and CATEGO Program*. Cambridge University Press, Cambridge, 1974.
World Health Organization: *Report on the International Pilot Study of Schizophrenia*. World Health Organization, Geneva, 1973.
World Psychiatric Association: *Diagnostic Criteria for Schizophrenic and Affective Psychoses*. American Psychiatric Press, Washington, DC, 1983.

14.2 SCHIZOPHRENIA: ETIOLOGY

14.2a SCHIZOPHRENIA: BRAIN STRUCTURE AND FUNCTION

KAREN FAITH BERMAN, M.D.
DANIEL R. WEINBERGER, M.D.

INTRODUCTION

The question of whether schizophrenia is an organic disease with underlying physical brain pathology has held a prominent place in the interest of researchers and clinicians for as long as the illness has been studied. The search for a central nervous system (CNS) lesion has been greeted with varying enthusiasm over the past century. Attempts during the first half of this century to find a site of pathological structure or function resulted in a large body of literature in which virtually every brain structure was implicated. However, many methodological problems attended these early studies, and no consistent area of pathology was found.

During the 1950s and 1960s, it became increasingly popular to emphasize psychological and social factors in conceptualizations of schizophrenia. The fact that, despite many years of postmortem examinations, no single underlying neuropathological or neurophysiological factor common to most patients with schizophrenia had yet been identified compounded the prevailing skepticism with which the concept of biological contributions to mental illness was viewed during this period. Schizophrenia was held to be functional rather than organic, and rigorous attempts to link this illness to the brain languished.

Over the past decade, several factors have resulted in a resurgence of interest in the neuropathological basis of schizophrenia and a renewed research effort to find it. One force behind this renaissance has been the emergence of medical treatments, especially pharmacological ones, that incontrovertibly ameliorate major psychotic symptoms. Another factor is the increasing availability of neuroimaging modalities that have made it possible to study the living brain's structure and function in great detail with little or no risk, discomfort, or inconvenience to the patient. No longer is the search for a neurobiological substrate of schizophrenia limited to indirect or peripheral measurements of trace substances in cerebrospinal fluid (CSF), urine, or serum—measurements that may or may not relate to brain physiology.

Concurrent with the advent of these new tools for direct examination of the brain have come advances in the understanding of human functional neuroanatomy, which have resulted in a more enlightened and refined approach to postmortem investigations. At the same time, the development and acceptance of reliable, explicit diagnostic criteria that allow greater consensual definition of psychiatric populations helped overcome a major methodological problem that plagued earlier research efforts.

Schizophrenia is increasingly believed to be a group of organic disorders primarily affecting the CNS. Features, such as peculiarities of gait and posture, disordered smooth-pursuit eye movements, minor (or soft) neurological signs, and subtle electroencephalographic (EEG) abnormalities, all suggest a link between schizophrenia and CNS pathology. More compelling evidence is offered by neuropsychological, neuroradiographic, and neurophysiological studies, some of which are reviewed in this section. While no single pathognomonic neurostructural or neurophysiological abnormality has yet been delineated in schizophrenia, certain cerebral concomitants of this illness have been demonstrated in a somewhat consistent fashion. Given the clinical heterogeneity of schizophrenia, it would be surprising if a single circumscribed lesion formed the neural substrate. Rather, it appears that cerebral dysfunction of a system of interconnected cortical and subcortical brain regions may be present to lesser or greater degrees and may produce more or less psychopathology in individual patients. Delineating the neurobiological substrates of schizophrenia remains an active and rapidly expanding area of research.

POSTMORTEM STUDIES OF BRAIN STRUCTURE IN SCHIZOPHRENIA

NEUROPATHOLOGICAL ATTEMPTS TO LINK SCHIZOPHRENIA TO THE BRAIN Over the past century, literally hundreds of studies have been devoted to a search in autopsy material from patients with schizophrenia for gross and microscopic CNS structural abnormalities. In fact, several nineteenth-century neuropathological reports of anatomical pathology in the brains of hebephrenic persons and catatonic persons actually predate the conceptualization by Emil Kraepelin of dementia precox as a clinical entity. Although there has been no shortage of abnormalities reported over the years, no consensus as to a pathognomonic brain lesion has been reached. Abnormalities of virtually every area of the CNS have been reported. While some have viewed this heterogeneity of findings as proof that there is no association between schizophrenia and brain pathology, an equally reasonable interpretation is that, in the face of so many positive findings, the notion of underlying brain abnormalities cannot be ruled out.

THEORETICAL ISSUES **The role of diagnostic and clinical heterogeneity** The classic approach to neuropathology has yielded a great deal of information about neurological disorders and about the normal function of various brain structures. Such a search for the brain pathology underlying an illness is based on the assumption that the illness is a single entity with regard to the underlying pathology. Clinically, the concept of schizophrenia as a syndrome or spectrum of disorders has gained increasing acceptance, as has the concept that it is a multidimensional disorder having both environmental and genetic components. This clinical heterogeneity and etiological complexity may imply that schizophrenia cannot be traced to a single, finely circumscribed locus of brain abnormality.

Changing notions of clinical and diagnostic subtypes of schizophrenia, inconsistent nomenclature, and lack of standardized or useful diagnostic criteria have at various times complicated the search for neuropathology in schizophrenia. These factors have rendered comparisons of findings across the years and across studies difficult and have added to the variability of the results. The nosological confusion of the early part of this century may in part explain inconsistent findings and may have contributed to premature closure on the question of structural brain pathology in schizophrenia.

The relevance of the understanding functional neuroanatomy At the turn of the century, the brain areas targeted for neuropathological examination in schizophrenia were in the neocortex, a reasonable first choice based on the Kraepelinian notion of a profound deterioration of personality (be it called dementia precox or schizophrenia) and the fact that the neocortex was the primary site of pathology in the other dementias to which schizophrenia was likened at the time. However, targeting brain areas for study on the basis of clinical correlates depends on knowledge of the precise function of the area being studied. Until relatively recently, little was known about the anatomical sites of higher cognitive functions. For example, the function of the largest and most complex area of the neocortex, the frontal lobes, one area implicated in the pathogenesis of schizophrenia, has been poorly understood until recently. Also, knowledge of the limbic areas and diencephalon had been limited. New tools for examining the human brain directly during life have helped to refine current concepts of the roles of some of these brain regions in human behavior and have offered new impetus for their study in schizophrenia.

METHODOLOGICAL ISSUES A number of methodological issues must be considered in assessing the research effort to link schizophrenia to brain pathology. For example, consistent diagnosis, always a pivotal point in psychiatric research, assumes a role of particular importance in postmortem studies of the brain in schizophrenia. Diagnostic criteria and the rigor with which they are applied have varied extensively since the concept of dementia precox was first put forth. Moreover, even with the relatively rigorous and standardized diagnostic criteria in use today, making diagnoses on the basis of chart reviews after death may be particularly unreliable.

Because the pathology in schizophrenia is likely to be subtle, there are other major methodological problems that are particularly critical. Control specimens must be matched not only on the basis of age, sex, and other demographic variables, but also for methods of tissue processing, the interval between death and autopsy (postmortem interval), concurrent illnesses, and agonal events. These latter factors can produce brain structural changes that are not directly related to the illness itself: Postmortem interval and the processes of fixation, staining, and sectioning of brain tissue may produce tissue distortion and other artifacts; agonal events, particularly hypoxia, infection, and trauma, may also cause structural alterations. The possible effects of pharmacological or other somatic treatments, such as electroconvulsive therapy (ECT) or, in early cases, insulin coma and leukotomy, must also be controlled for. Once appropriately matched patient and control samples have been collected, assessments must be done by a blind investigator (i.e., one who does not know which specimens come from which group). These important features of study design were not appreciated by most early investigators in this field.

EARLY HISTOPATHOLOGICAL EXAMINATIONS OF THE BRAIN IN SCHIZOPHRENIA The first half of this century saw a period of vigorous research in which a plethora of abnormalities occurring in the brains of patients with schizophrenia (or dementia precox) were described, but from which surprisingly few conclusions can be drawn. These early studies, whose results were often confounded by small patient populations without proper controls, were rarely consistent with respect to diagnostic criteria, selection of patients and controls, choice of brain area to be studied, or methods of tissue preparation and processing. In light of these problems, it is perhaps not surprising that virtually no histopathological findings from this period were rigorously replicated.

As mentioned above, a number of studies focused on the cortex, then presumed to be the sight of higher cognitive function and thus a likely candidate for pathology in schizophrenia. Although largely anecdotal, these studies in many instances implicated frontal cortex and cortical layers II and III (i.e., those projecting primarily intracortically). Also, a variety of histopathological changes were described in many other cortical regions and also in thalamus, basal forebrain, globus pallidum, corpus striatum, and many other areas. These included alterations and loss of neurons; changes in oligodendroglia, astrocytes, and microglia; and vascular and perivascular changes. However, none of these abnormalities was noted consistently.

One explanation for both the diversity of the findings and their inconsistency was offered by investigators who presented topographical analyses of specific types of symptoms. For example, some believed that loss of cortical neurons and accompanying gliosis was the primary histopathology of dementia precox and that specific psychotic symptoms might be generated in specific cortical areas; for example, delusions, catatonia, and auditory hallucinations were postulated to be associated with frontal, parietal, and temporal lobe lesions, respectively. These researchers noted that, given the clinical heterogeneity of the patient population, different patterns of histopathology would be expected, an idea that is once again in vogue today but one that does not wholly account for the confusing and inconsistent range of findings.

The efforts of this era culminated in the First International Congress of Neuropathology, convened in Rome in 1952 and attended by many leading neuropathologists of the time. The meeting was fraught with bitter disagreements and insoluble controversy regarding the lack of consensus about CNS pathology in schizophrenia. However, it did serve to highlight many of the methodological pitfalls that had been encountered and paved the way for a more cohesive approach to neuropathological studies of postmortem tissue.

RECENT POSTMORTEM STUDIES Unlike the investigations carried out during the first half of this century, which tended to search for a qualitatively pathognomonic lesion, more recent studies have tended to aspire to more conservative goals, such as ascertaining whether any neuropathological process has in fact occurred. Central to these goals has been a methodological shift toward quantitative analyses, such as cell counting and neuronal morphometry, and attention to the formidable research design problems enumerated above. Special stains and advanced technology, including electron microscopy and computer-assisted image analysis, have been developed. There has also been greater consistency of focus on several brain areas suggested by various hypotheses and by the findings of in vivo brain imaging studies.

Frontal cortex and temporolimbic structures have received particular attention. One examination of prefrontal, anterior cingulate, and motor cortex found fewer neurons in layer VI of prefrontal, layer V of cingulate, and layer III of motor cortex. In hippocampal pyramidal cells, dendritic disarray was found more commonly in schizophrenic patients, suggesting to these investigators a congenital failure of these cells to orient properly. This finding could not be confirmed by another group who used a less quantitative method. In a well-controlled study of subcortical structures, decreased volumes of the lateral substantia nigra, amygdala, hippocampal formation, and pallidum internum were seen in patients, but there were no differences in the putamen, caudate nucleus, nucleus accumbens, or bed nucleus of the stria terminalis. Some of these findings may be important in considering the X-ray computed tomography (CT) data discussed below. Another study with special relevance to the CT data demonstrated decreased brain weight and parahippocampal gyral cortical width, and increased cross-sectional area of the temporal horns of the lateral ventricles in schizophrenia.

POSTMORTEM NEUROPATHOLOGY IN SCHIZOPHRENIA Although there is still no recognized pathognomonic histopathology in the brains of patients with schizophrenia, the conclusion that no brain pathology exists cannot be supported. To the contrary, studies employing rigorous methodology have demonstrated abnormalities. However, no single abnormality has been found in a majority, let alone all, of the patients with this disorder, and none can be considered diagnostic. Certain consistent themes emerging from this growing body of data are summarized below.

Brain atrophy Findings of brain atrophy, including ventricular enlargement, decreased tissue weight, gross cortical atrophy (especially of frontal lobe), and decreased volume in deeper midline and limbic structures, have persisted throughout the long search for postmortem neuropathological changes in schizophrenia. These abnormalities are consistent with in vivo neuroradiographic studies described below.

It should be noted that atrophy is a nonspecific term denoting wasting of tissue. However, the mechanism underlying such changes in schizophrenia is unknown. One possibility that cannot be ruled out at this time is a congenital failure to develop, rather than a loss of brain tissue later in life. Another question being actively addressed in current research is what neuronal element is involved in the atrophy; that is, do these changes involve missing or damaged neurons, glia, or neuropil?

Cortical dysmorphism In their investigations of the neocortex, early investigators noted not only decreased cell numbers, but also distortion of neuronal size and shape in various cortical layers. Some recent studies have reported similar alterations. These histopathological changes can be jointly discussed as dysmorphisms. Cortical dysmorphisms appear to be a consistent finding, but what percentage of patients exhibit this finding, which patients they are, and by what means the dysmorphism occurs (e.g., congenital failure to develop, dysplasia, or cell destruction) remains to be determined.

In typical dementias, classically conceived of as cortical dementias (e.g., Alzheimer's disease), it is now clear that subcortical structures also play a role. In considering cortical dysmorphism in schizophrenia, focus must also be directed at deep structures comprising complex cortical, limbic, diencephalic, and brain stem interconnections, and attention must be given to whether the cortical changes are primary or secondary.

Limbic-diencephalic dysmorphism and gliosis Early notions of the limbic system were based primarily on the olfactory connections that predominate in lower animals. During the past 50 years, concepts of the role of the limbic system in humans has expanded to include more complex behavioral, affective, and cognitive functions involving the hypothalamus, septum, amygdala, and hippocampus. There have been a number of reports of pathology, including neuronal distortions and decreased cell numbers, in limbic-diencephalic brain areas of patients with schizophrenia. An accompanying glial reaction has been noted. Since gliosis is a nonspecific marker for cell damage resulting from a variety of CNS insults, including trauma, infection, vascular injury, and autoimmune disorders, no etiology for schizophrenia can be inferred. These findings do, however, identify brain structures that merit further study. Moreover, since all of the in vivo structural findings described below should have postmortem counterparts, reports of postmortem pathology tend to support the validity of in vivo findings.

IN VIVO IMAGING STUDIES OF BRAIN STRUCTURE IN SCHIZOPHRENIA

The first radiological modality for viewing brain structure during life was pneumoencephalography. Injection into the lumbar subarachnoid space of a volume of air, which migrated to the cerebral ventricular system, displacing CSF, provided sufficient contrast on an X-ray film to allow the boundaries of the CSF-filled spaces to be delineated. In early studies of schizophrenia, enlargement of the third and lateral ventricles and widening of the cortical sulci were observed with this technique. In these studies, the suggestion was also made that these anatomical markers correlated with some clinical features of severity of the illness (e.g., apathy, cognitive impairment). While establishing a cornerstone on which more recent work has been founded, this technique has been supplanted by two new modalities capable of imaging structures in the living brain in dramatically greater detail—CT and magnetic resonance imaging (MRI).

X-RAY COMPUTED TOMOGRAPHY IN SCHIZOPHRENIA **Methodological considerations** CT became available in the early 1970s. This method is atraumatic and does not require the introduction of a foreign substance into the body. It depends on passing X-ray beams through the body in a plane by rotating the X-ray source around the subject. The attenuation of the X-ray beams by their passage through the body depends on the density of the material they pass through. A computer determines the amount of X-ray attenuation from many directions simultaneously and from this information reconstructs the density of the structures the X-rays encountered. A two-dimensional matrix, or map, of tissue radiodensity can be constructed for each of a series of tomographic slices. CT scanning provided a major advance over previously available techniques both in the quality of the detailed information it yields and the relative noninvasiveness of the procedure.

Computed tomography research findings in schizophrenia The first controlled CT study carried out on a psychiatric population was reported in 1976. Since that time, some 100 articles based on data from over 40 controlled CT investigations of schizophrenia have appeared in the literature. The most robust and well-replicated findings are lateral ventricular enlargement, widening of cortical sulci, and third ventricle enlargement. Cerebellar atrophy, reversed cerebral asymmetries, and brain density abnormalities have also been reported. It is important to emphasize that none of these structural markers can confirm a diagnosis of schizophrenia in an individual patient; none has been found exclusively in patients with schizophrenia, and none has been found to be present in every patient who has the illness. Rather, these features of brain structure are characteristic of schizophrenic patients as a group when compared to normal control groups. The diagnosis of schizophrenia remains a clinical one to be rendered by the clinician on the basis of the current examination and history.

ENLARGED LATERAL VENTRICLES One recent review found that 75 percent of the published CT investigations of lateral ventricular size have demonstrated enlargement compared with a control group (Fig. 14.2a-1). If those studies that used relatively insensitive indices of lateral ventricular size and chose patients or control groups nonrigorously are excluded, the proportion of positive studies is over 90 percent. In most of these studies, the ranges of values for patients and control subjects overlap. That is, there are many patients whose lateral ventricular size falls within the normal range. Relatively fewer controls have values falling in the upper range of the patients. Thus, patient values fall within a wider range, and the distribution of the patient values is shifted upward compared with that of the control group. It is worth noting that ventricular dilation in schizophrenia is relatively subtle; the scans of most patients, even some of those with the largest ventricles, would not be classified as qualitatively abnormal by most neuroradiologists. Therefore, routine qualitative CT scans of individual patients will often detect no abnormality. The finding of enlarged lateral ventricles in schizophrenia depends on quantitative assessment and comparison of group means. In other words, a separation of patients into those with and those without abnormal ventricles is not a valid interpretation of these research data.

Several methods of determining lateral ventricular size have been utilized in CT studies. Both manual and automatic computer measurements have been employed. Parameters of lateral ventricular size also vary. These include linear measurements across the largest width of the ventricles which may be considered as a ratio to another measure, measurements of the area of the ventricles relative to the area of the whole brain, and estimates of ventricular volume based on several CT slices. The most commonly reported parameter is the ventricle-to-brain ratio (VBR), an area measure. Volumetric measurements have been found to be the most sensitive indicators of enlargement, and linear measures, the least sensitive. Since CT scans are two-dimensional representations of

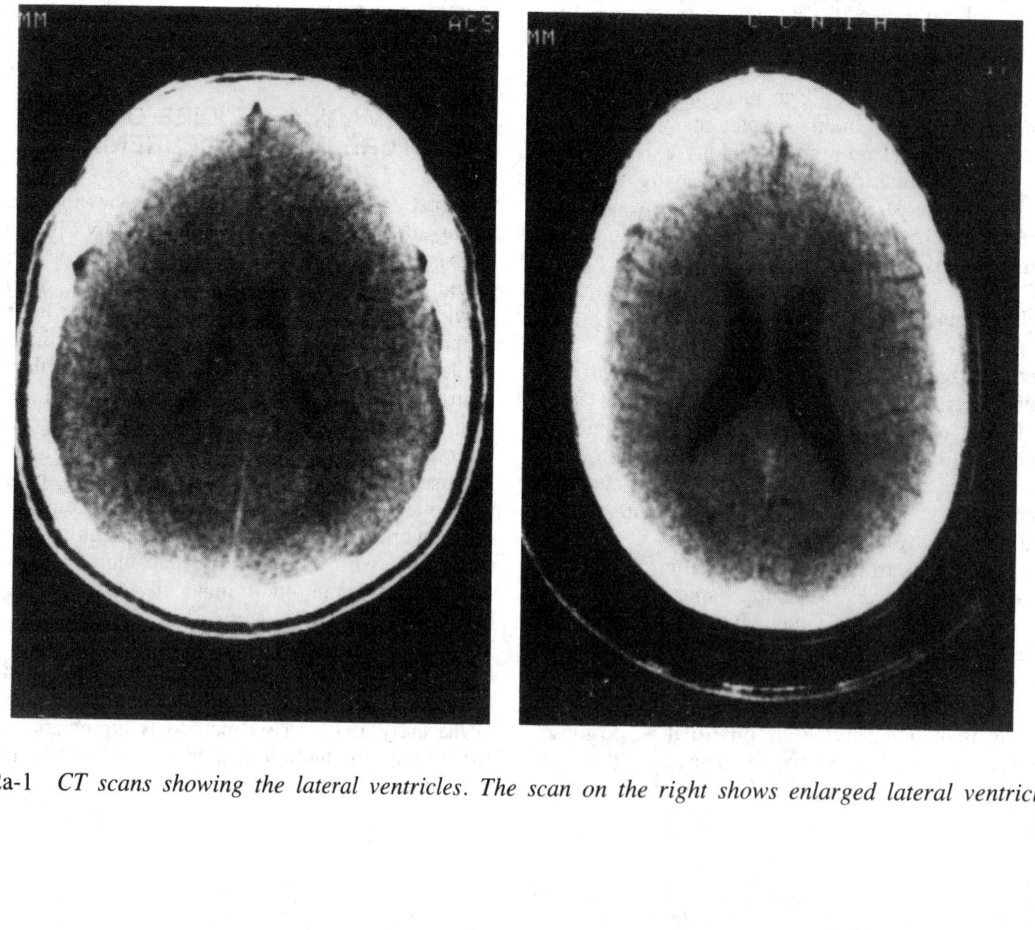

FIGURE 14.2a-1 *CT scans showing the lateral ventricles. The scan on the right shows enlarged lateral ventricles.*

three-dimensional objects, all of the above-mentioned methods provide only an approximation of relative ventricular volume. Therefore, they are all inaccurate to some degree and most likely underestimate differences between control and patient groups.

Another methodological pitfall of CT studies of ventricular size in schizophrenia is selection of an appropriate control group. At the least, experimental groups must be matched for age and sex, since ventricular size is different in men and women and increases with age. While some studies have scanned entirely normal volunteers for the control group, others have used as controls persons who were scanned for medical purposes other than schizophrenia. Since many conditions are associated with atrophic changes on CT scan, including enlargement of the lateral ventricles (Table 14.2a-1) the inclusion of such subjects as controls, like the use of insensitive measurements, would usually bias such studies toward finding no differences between schizophrenic patients and controls. Nonetheless, despite these methodological limitations, differences between control and schizophrenic groups have been demonstrated relatively consistently.

Although it has not been as consistently replicated as the finding of increased lateral ventricular size itself, a relationship between several clinical features and lateral ventricular size has been reported. Poor premorbid social adjustment, poor outcome, negative or defect symptoms, and cognitive (i.e., neuropsychological) deficits have all been reported to be associated with large ventricles. Neurochemical correlates have also been reported, especially an inverse relationship between ventricular size and homovanillic acid in the CSF. Because the association with neuropsychological impairment, which has been reported a number of times, may provide insight into the pathological process underlying these deficits it is particularly interesting. A number of these clinical correlations await rigorous reconfirmation, but taken together they suggest that the degree of certain types of psychopathology and the degree of lateral ventricular enlargement may be positively linked. This notion is supported by the fact that, in several studies in which the patient group was not found to have larger ventricles, patients with minor or soft neurological signs and neuropsychological deficits had been excluded. However, correlations between structural measures and clinical variables, such as outcome and response to treatment, are statistical findings based on the average characteristics of patient groups. As such, they cannot be considered as predictive of the course of a given patient.

Although still an area of active research, the bulk of the data currently available suggests that enlargement of the lateral ventricles found in schizophrenic patients as a group cannot be explained on the basis of treatment. Most investigations have found that there is no relationship between lateral ventricular size and ECT, duration of illness, length of institutionalization, or cumulative antipsychotic dose. Relatively little is known about the time course of ventricular enlargement in schizophrenia, although such knowledge would undoubtedly provide important clues about the pathological process underlying this illness. Prospective studies have been the exception rather than the rule in such investigations, but it is known that enlarged ventricles have been reported in patients with schizophreniform disorders during their first psychotic episode. Also, in two investigations of patients who underwent repeat CT scans, one completed 3 years and the other 8 years after the original CT scan, no consistent progression of ventricular enlargement was noted. However, relatively few patients were available for follow-up in these studies, and it is not known how representative these small groups may be of the patient population as a whole. Since these patients had been ill for some time when the first CT scan was done, it is possible that a period of progression of the illness and any underlying structural abnormality had already passed. Nonetheless, the majority of the evidence to date suggests that at least some portion of patients with schizophrenia do have enlarged lateral ventricles compared with control groups and that this enlargement is present early in the course of the illness.

Although not as consistent a finding as it is in schizophrenia, enlargement of the lateral ventricles has also been described in patients with unipolar, bipolar, and schizoaffective illness. As in schizophrenia, those patients with the largest ventricles appear to be the most chronically or severely ill. In general, the frequency and degree of such findings are lower in affectively ill patients than in schizophrenia, and the results are less conclusive. Whether these findings imply similar pathological processes in mood disorder and schizophrenia or whether they reflect inadequate nosology of these disorders or other methodological problems is unclear and is an area for future investigation.

Lateral ventricular enlargement on CT is a nonspecific sign that may reflect pathology of periventricular structures, such as the lenticular nuclei (caudate, putamen, and globus pallidus), thalamus, hypothalamus, amygdala, hippocampus, fornix, and corpus callosum. However, lateral ventricular enlargement may also be a sign of more diffuse pathology or of focal pathology far from the ventricles. This apparent an-

TABLE 14.2a-1
Conditions Associated with Signs of Generalized Atrophic Changes on CT

Psychiatric
Schizophrenia
Mood disorders
Anorexia nervosa
Post-traumatic syndromes
Neurological
Migraine
Parkinson's disease
Epilepsy
Huntington's disease
Wilson's disease
Postencephalitic states
Multiple sclerosis
Alzheimer's disease
Multi-infarct dementia
Head injury
Systemic lupus erythematosus
Other degenerative CNS conditions
Medical
Nutritional deficits
Cushing's disease
Steroids
Intoxicants
alcohol
solvents
heavy metals
Birth complications
Cytotoxic drugs
Malignancy
Dialysis

Table adapted from Jaskiw G E, et al: X-ray computed tomography and magnetic resonance imaging in psychiatry. In American Psychiatric Association Annual Review, A J Frances, R E Hales, editors, vol 6. American Psychiatric Association, Washington, DC, 1987.

atomical nonspecificity and the clinical nonspecificity mentioned above have been cited by some to refute the importance of this finding in schizophrenia. However, the fact that clinically, etiologically, and pathologically unrelated disorders may have a common pattern of abnormalities on CT does not diminish the fact that such abnormalities are direct evidence of brain structure abnormalities.

THIRD VENTRICLE ENLARGEMENT The third ventricle has also received attention in the CT literature. This midline segment of the CSF system connects rostrally to the anterior horns of the lateral ventricles, connects posteriorly to the fourth ventricle through the Sylvian aqueduct, and is surrounded by the thalamus, hypothalamus, fornix, and habenula. Less extensively studied than the lateral ventricles, the size of this small structure has usually been estimated by measuring its width (although several investigators have employed an adaptation of the VBR method for measuring relative area).

Of the dozen or so published investigations of third ventricle size in schizophrenia, some 80 percent have found significant dilation in patients. The finding has been described in first-episode patients as well. While several studies have described a positive relationship between third ventricle dilation and lateral ventricular enlargement, this is not a universal finding. Reports of correlations with clinical variables are similarly varied. Whether the finding of third ventricle enlargement reflects a localized pathological process or whether, like lateral ventricular enlargement, it is simply a reflection of diffuse dilation of the ventricular system remains to be clarified. It is known that diffuse conditions, such as those listed in Table 14.2a-1, can be associated with third ventricle enlargement.

WIDENED CORTICAL FISSURES AND SULCI The two examples of CT abnormalities previously discussed, lateral and third ventricle enlargement, are signs of so-called central cerebral atrophy. Signs of cortical atrophy (seen as increased cortical markings on CT) have also been found to be more common in patients with schizophrenia than in control groups. Since atrophy of the cerebral cortex involves reduction in volume of the gyri, it is manifested on CT scan by widening, deepening, and increased prominence of the cortical fissures and sulci, which separate adjacent lobes and gyri of the brain, respectively (Fig. 14.2a-2). The gyri themselves may appear thinned.

Methods for quantifying cortical atrophy have proved particularly difficult to standardize. They have ranged from simply measuring the widths of sulci and fissures to the use of computer algorithms that count the number of pixels having a density below a particular cutoff point, which is assumed to represent CSF. Still other investigators have carried out more gross evaluations of the degree of atrophy by comparing subjects' scans to a predetermined reference scale based on standard CT scans having varying degrees of atrophy. The cortical areas studied by different investigators have also varied.

Despite these methodological differences, of 22 CT studies of cortical atrophy recently reviewed, 16 (73 percent) concluded that the patients with schizophrenia had significantly more cortical markings than the control groups. As with indicators of central atrophy, a number of conditions other than schizophrenia are also associated with cortical atrophy (Table 14.2a-1), and if only those studies comparing schizophrenics and nonmedical controls are considered, the percentage of positive studies is higher.

Relatively few attempts to demonstrate demographic or clinical correlates of increased cortical markings on CT in schizophrenia have been published, but there are several interesting reports of an association between cortical atrophy and cognitive impairment. This area remains fertile for further research.

Another question actively being investigated is whether the cortical atrophy noted in schizophrenia is present throughout the cortex or whether it is specific to a certain area (or areas). Exploration of this question is hampered by the fact that different investigators have searched for cortical atrophy in different locales, and some have reported overall atrophy ratings

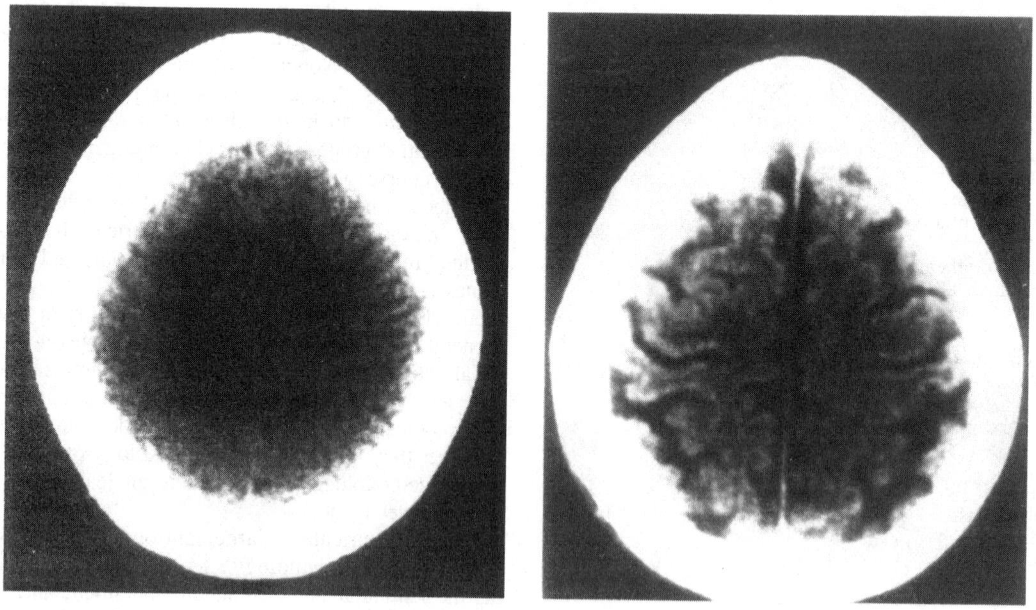

FIGURE 14.2a-2 *CT scans of the cortex. The scan on the right shows widened sulci and fissures and is consistent with cortical atrophy.*

which consider atrophy throughout the cortex. Several recent studies examining specific regions for atrophy suggest that this finding may be especially prevalent in prefrontal cortex.

CEREBELLAR ATROPHY The cerebellum also can be assessed with CT. An unusual finding in patients who do not have neurological disease, cerebellar atrophy is apparent in some 1 to 5 percent of routinely read CT scans. This sign of reduced tissue volume in the cerebellar hemispheres, nuclei, or vermis can occur with primary degenerative diseases, alcoholism, and drug use. It has also been reported to be present with increased frequency in schizophrenia, particularly involving the vermis.

The frequency with which cerebellar atrophy was seen in some 12 published schizophrenia studies ranges from zero to 50 percent. Despite the variety of approaches to cerebellar measurement or clinical populations that were employed in these studies, the incidence of this finding appears to be higher than in the general population.

Clinical and demographic correlates have not been ascertained, and the etiology of this finding is unclear. Although not as frequently studied in other illnesses, cerebellar atrophy has also been reported in schizoaffective and other mood disorders. Recent observations in animals that the cerebellum is involved in conditioned response and, through connections of the vermis and limbic-diencephalic areas, that it is linked to autonomic regulation suggest that cerebellar pathology could, indeed, have behavioral repercussions. This finding, however, has not been reported in acute, first-episode patients.

CEREBRAL ASYMMETRIES Dating perhaps to the discovery that human language function has a distinct, consistent anatomical substrate with primacy in the left hemisphere, the notion that the left and right hemispheres of the normal human brain differ in functional specialization and in structural elements has been an important focal point in the study of human functional neuroanatomy. The implications of these observations for mental illness, although intriguing, are at this point unclear and controversial. Structural asymmetries in healthy subjects have been demonstrated, and aberrations of this normal asymmetry have been reported with CT in schizophrenia.

Asymmetries are usually quantified by measuring the widths of the left and right frontal and occipital lobes on the CT slice where they are most prominent. Alternatively, these widths can be averaged over several slices. Using these techniques, it has been demonstrated that the majority of right-handed persons have wider right than left frontal lobes and wider left than right occipital lobes. Increased frequency of reversal of these normal asymmetries have been reported in dyslexic and autistic persons and in several studies of schizophrenic patients. However, of some 10 studies of patients with schizophrenia only four demonstrated reversed symmetry in the patient group. Thus, the existence and significance of abnormal anatomical lateralization in schizophrenia remain to be established.

BRAIN DENSITY CHANGES As a CT scan is a map of the densities of the anatomical structures in a cross-section of the brain, it is possible to derive an average density value for a given area of interest if the densities (referred to as X-ray attenuation values, CT numbers, or Hounsfield units) of all the pixels comprising the area are averaged. This technique has been applied to the study of schizophrenia, but it is fraught with methodological pitfalls and has produced extremely inconsistent results. Both increased and decreased density of various areas has been described. Several investigators have reported decreased density in cortical areas, perhaps most prevalently in frontal cortex, a finding that may simply reflect tissue atrophy. At this time, the exploration of tissue density with CT remains methodologically limited.

MAGNETIC RESONANCE IMAGING IN SCHIZOPHRENIA

Theory and methods Based on principles of nuclear magnetic resonance long utilized in analytic chemistry, magnetic resonance imaging (MRI) has been available as a tool for imaging the anatomical structures of the human brain since the mid-1980s. It has a number of advantages, by virtue of which it may soon supersede CT. It does not employ ionizing radiation and, so, is essentially risk-free. MRI scans can be made of children and may be repeated any number of times, a feature that makes MRI more suitable than CT for longitudinal research. The only contraindications to MRI are the presence in the subject's body of some types of aneurysm clips and cardiac pacemakers. Spatial resolution and the clarity with which anatomical details are visualized are far superior to CT, and gray and white matter are clearly differentiated. Moreover, in addition to the transverse planes to which CT is usually limited, MRI can also be used to reconstruct sagittal or coronal sections (Figs. 14.2a-3 and 14.2a-4). In fact, MRI permits complete three-dimensional brain reconstruction, and small brain structures of interest in schizophrenia, such as the basal ganglia, hippocampus, and thalamus can be readily discerned.

Images are produced by exposing tissue to a strong magnetic field (produced by magnets typically having a field strength of 0.1 to 2.0 tesla), which causes certain atomic nuclei to behave as dipoles and to align themselves along the lines of force of this field. Current MRI technologies are based primarily on the most abundant of these, hydrogen, which has a single proton, but in principle, any nuclei having an odd number of nucleons (i.e., protons and neutrons) can be imaged. Brief electromagnetic signals of a specific radiofrequency are applied to the aligned atoms to increase their energy state, which tilts them out of alignment. After the pulse of radio waves is discontinued, the atoms realign, their energy state returns to baseline, and they emit element-specific radio signals that can be measured by a radiofrequency receiver, processed for spatial reconstruction, and visually mapped.

More complex than the signals processed for CT scanning, which involve only X-ray attenuation through tissue, the MRI signal reflects not only proton density (a measure of the number of hydrogen atoms, or water, in a tissue), but also several parameters of the rate and characteristics of the return of the atoms to their baseline energy state (relaxation time). The latter are very sensitive discriminators of gray versus white matter and normal versus pathological tissue. MRI thereby produces images far superior to those of CT in spatial resolution, with anatomical detail approaching that achieved with fresh tissue specimens.

MRI is rapidly gaining recognition as the foremost tool for investigating soft-tissue anatomy in vivo. It has the potential to extend the findings of CT, for example, by examining periventricular structures that may contribute to the finding of enlarged lateral ventricles or by defining the precise nature of the cortical atrophy that has been described. In theory, MRI can image physiological information as well as anatomical

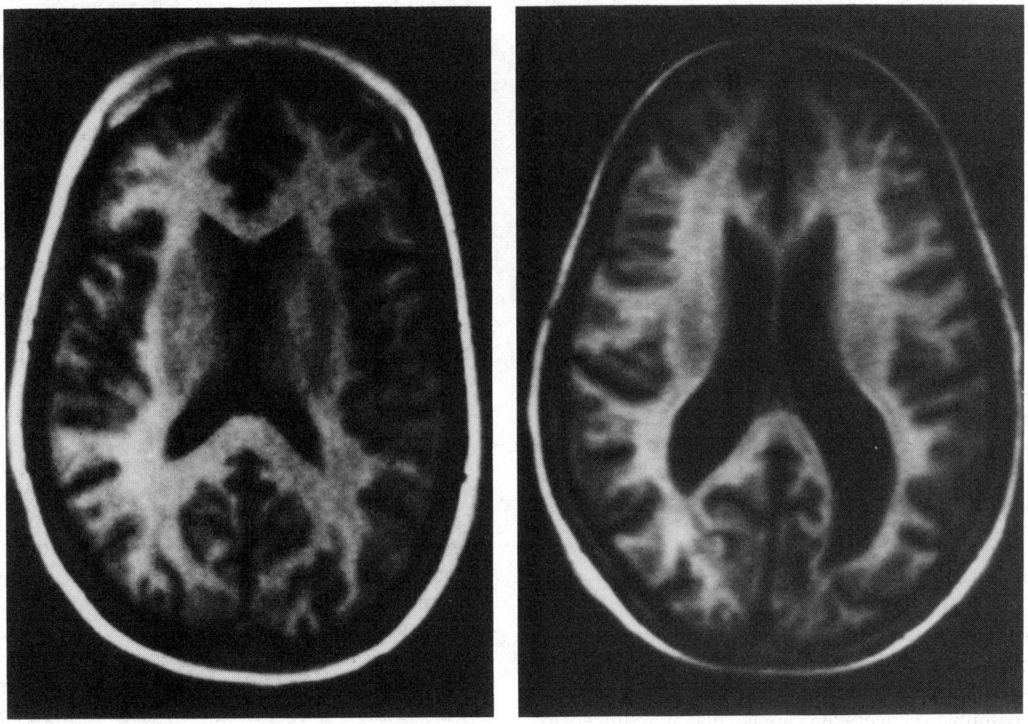

FIGURE 14.2a-3 *MRI scan in the transverse plane showing the lateral ventricles. The scan on the right shows lateral ventricular enlargement. The left hemisphere is pictured on the right side of the scan.*

detail, but this potential has not yet been fully realized in human research.

MRI research findings in schizophrenia Research using MRI to examine morphology of brain structures in schizophrenia is at an early stage. Few studies have appeared in the literature; some have been reported only in preliminary form; others are inconclusive or inconsistent. Since it is possible to delineate fine anatomical detail in the axial, sagittal, and coronal planes, a large number of specific nuclei, cortical areas, and other structures not visualizable with CT can be measured in a single brain. Methods for carrying out such measurements are still in development phases and require standardization and validation. These currently include several extensions of CT methods, such as linear or planimetric determinations made manually as well as new computer-assisted approaches. The best approach to statistical analysis of numerous brain area measurements in a single brain has yet to be delineated.

It is not surprising that the first investigators to apply MRI to brain investigations of schizophrenia attempted to replicate the CT findings of lateral ventricular enlargement. One group of investigators found no difference between schizophrenic and control groups on linear or area measurements of lateral ventricular size, cortical surface markings, lobar asymmetries, and corpus callosum thickness. (This group is one of few who found no ventricular abnormality on CT scan.) They did, however, report increased gray and white matter MRI signal intensity in their patients, a finding difficult to interpret since the meaning of increased signal intensity is not clear. Another study qualitatively examined periventricular areas in patients suffering a first episode of schizophrenia. There was no evidence of a discrete pathological process in the periventricular area in cases of early schizophrenia, and no relation of MRI measures to outcome measures.

Another group quantitated structures on a midsagittal image. They found reduced frontal lobe area in schizophrenia, as well as reduced area of the entire cerebrum and cranium. If replicated, the finding of decreased frontal lobe size may provide important evidence that corroborates findings of other frontal lobe abnormalities described in this section. Also, after dividing the corpus callosum into four segments and the subject groups by sex, these investigators found that female patients had larger middle callosal segments. The difficulties inherent in drawing conclusions about brain morphology on the basis of one midsagittal slice limit interpretations of these data. Another group was not able to confirm decreased brain area or increased callosal area, but noted increased septum pellucidum area on midsagittal plane, a finding that probably reflects increased lateral ventricular size.

PHYSIOLOGICAL BRAIN FUNCTION IN SCHIZOPHRENIA

Although they are too often viewed as a dichotomy, the roles of brain function and of brain structure are intimately linked. However, they provide two different avenues to understanding the neurobiology of schizophrenia. While structural brain imaging techniques localize and quantify brain anatomy, which is static, functional brain imaging techniques localize and quantify the dynamic properties of the living, working human brain. Several relatively recent technological innovations now allow a variety of approaches to studying brain function during life that have the potential to anatomically localize and physiologically characterize human mental processes.

The very feature of these techniques that renders them so potentially powerful, their ability to measure physiological changes underlying transient mental phenomena, also makes

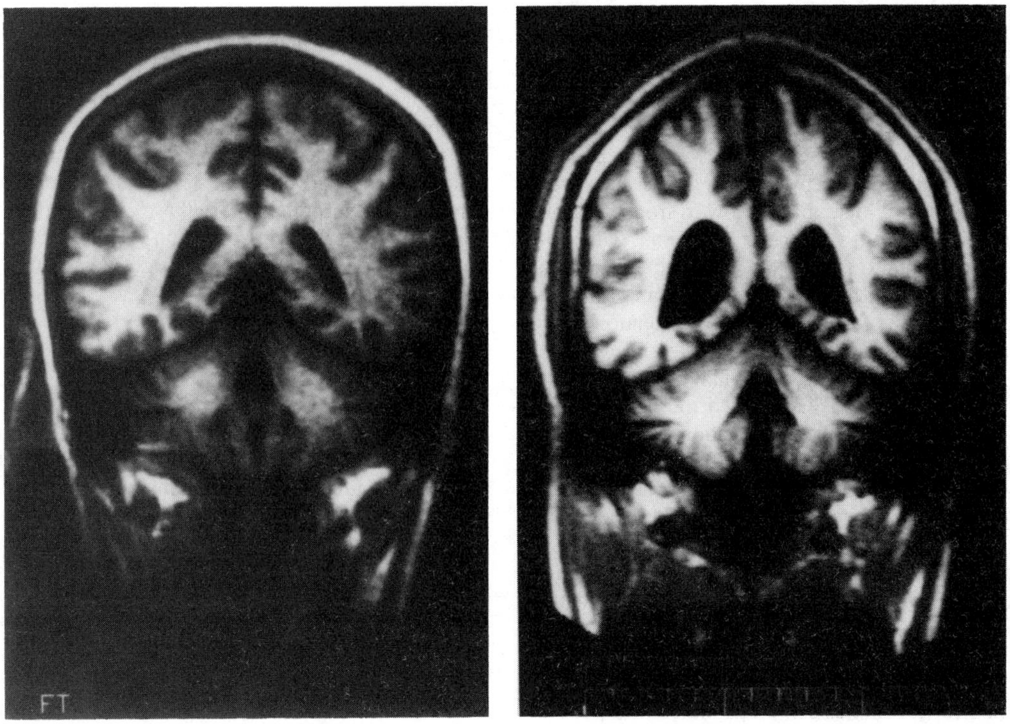

FIGURE 14.2a-4 *MRI scan in the coronal plane showing the lateral ventricles. The scan on the right shows lateral ventricular enlargement.*

their application to psychiatric research complex. Because a subject's sensory input, cognitive and motor outputs, mental state, and the ambient conditions in the testing environment all have potential neurophysiological repercussions, they must be rigorously controlled. The import of this has not been fully appreciated until recently, but it is now quite clear that testing conditions cannot be considered too carefully in research design and in the interpretation of resulting data. Studies carried out at rest, when there is no prescribed sensory, motor, or cognitive activity, produce extremely variable results. This variability may obscure subtle physiological changes that might be related to psychopathology. A less variable and more meaningful approach is to measure brain function during conditions that predictably activate specific brain areas in normal subjects. Such investigations have been carried out and are described below.

Other potential methodological problems in some functional brain imaging studies include poorly matched patient and control groups and failure to study patients who are not taking medication. While pharmacological treatments have not been shown to affect brain structure as measured by in vivo imaging techniques, there are definite neurophysiological effects.

Research has been carried out with several currently available functional brain imaging techniques, including xenon-133 regional cerebral blood flow (rCBF) and positron-emission tomography (PET). Each method has advantages and disadvantages. Xenon-133 rCBF studies expose the subject to less ionizing radiation and are less expensive and more convenient than PET. However, PET has considerably superior spatial resolution, and can measure a number of indicators of neuronal activity in addition to rCBF, such as regional glucose metabolism, oxygen utilization, and specific neurochemical metabolism. It should be emphasized that these neuroradiological procedures remain research tools; they do not, at present, have a place in routine clinical investigation in psychiatry. EEG, another method of assessing brain function, is described elsewhere in this text.

XENON-133 REGIONAL CEREBRAL BLOOD FLOW STUDIES

Theory and method The concept of measuring rCBF as an indicator of brain activity is based on the fact that brain work, neuronal activity, and local blood flow are coupled in the grossly intact brain. Cerebral blood flow, for the most part, reflects brain metabolism. The earliest attempts to exploit this relationship in man were made by Kety and colleagues in 1948. These investigators used nitrous oxide inhalation with carotid and jugular blood sampling to determine average rates of oxygen consumption in the brain by measuring whole brain blood flow. With this technique no difference in whole brain blood flow between patients with schizophrenia and normal subjects was found. However, this did not rule out the possibility of more localized rCBF abnormalities.

In the 1960s, a method for measuring the blood flow of many cortical regions in one hemisphere was developed. This method involved the injection into the carotid artery of a saline solution of the inert radioisotope, xenon-133. Extracranial detectors were used to monitor the rates of arrival and disappearance of gamma rays from various cortical areas, and this allowed the calculation of regional blood flow to each area. It was quickly noted that rCBF measurements carried out in this fashion were sensitive to functional activation of specific cortical areas. For example, if rCBF measurements were made while a subject repeatedly opened and closed his hand, an increase in rCBF was seen in the contralateral motor cortex.

Regional cerebral blood flow research studies in schizophrenia Using this intracarotid technique, several fundamental observations about normal cortical physiology were made during the 1970s. First, it was noted in normal subjects, the highest blood flow (and presumably the highest levels of neuronal activity) consistently occurred in premotor and prefrontal regions. This rCBF pattern, termed "hyperfrontality," has been confirmed repeatedly. At the same time, it was noted that patients with schizophrenia, while having normal mean blood flow, did not exhibit the hyperfrontal rCBF pattern while at rest. Rather, their blood flow landscapes were characterized by relatively lower blood flow to frontal regions and relatively greater flow to postcentral regions. This pattern, termed "hypofrontality," and the resulting theory that schizophrenia is characterized by an impairment of frontal lobe function, has received a great deal of attention since these observations were made. The most indifferent, inactive, and autistic patients had the lowest frontal flow, while the most cognitively disturbed patients showed the highest postcentral rCBF. In addition to these observations, it was noted that rCBF measurements could be made during cognitive activation. During a simple picture test, normal subjects showed changes in rCBF while more deteriorated patients did not.

These pioneering research findings heralded the beginning of the modern era of functional brain imaging in psychiatry. However, the intracarotid technique of xenon-133 administration was not well suited to clinical research. Because of the invasiveness of such procedures, entirely normal persons could not be studied (alcoholics served as the control population), and since it was difficult for psychotic patients to cooperate, sedation during the procedure (which could affect rCBF) was often necessary. Also, measurements could be made on only one hemisphere at a time (usually the dominant hemisphere was studied) and were limited to the cortical areas subserved by the anterior cerebral circulatory system into which the xenon was injected.

Neuropsychiatric research during the 1980s has seen the introduction of a completely noninvasive, atraumatic technique in which xenon-133 gas is administered to the subject by inhalation. Determinations of rCBF are obtained simultaneously for both hemispheres. There is no obstacle to studying young, normal subjects with this technique, and since each procedure can be completed in approximately 15 minutes, many psychotic persons are able to cooperate. The major hypotheses of brain dysfunction in schizophrenia that have been explored with this method are altered overall (i.e., mean) blood flow, changes in cerebral lateralization, and hypofrontality.

CHANGES IN OVERALL (MEAN) BLOOD FLOW Reduced blood flow to the entire cortex has been demonstrated in primary degenerative dementias and in normal aging. The picture in schizophrenia, however, is much less clear. While early studies using invasive techniques rarely found reduced flow, the results of inhalation rCBF studies have been less consistent. Several investigators have reported decreased overall (mean) blood flow, but other studies have found no difference. Some of the positive findings in this area may be accounted for by a methodological problem—failure to take into account the subjects' arterial carbon dioxide levels, which can alter blood flow. While minor alterations may exist, the bulk of the available data indicate that schizophrenia is not characterized by global decreases in blood flow of the magnitude present in typical dementia.

ALTERED CEREBRAL LATERALITY Some investigators have suggested that schizophrenia may involve a disorder of abnormal lateralization of brain activity in response to different tasks, but there is no agreement on which hemisphere is implicated or on whether the putative aberration may involve both hemispheres. The existing rCBF data concerning this question are relatively scarce. The majority of resting studies do not support this hypothesis. However, two activation studies specifically designed to explore laterality in schizophrenia did suggest that there is left-hemisphere overactivity (an alternative interpretation of these data is that there may be right hemisphere underactivation). Further research is necessary to clarify this point and to define the role of functional laterality in schizophrenia.

HYPOFRONTALITY Several lines of converging evidence suggest that impaired frontal cortical function may play a role in schizophrenia. For example, clinical signs and symptoms of patients with gross frontal lobe lesions (including minor or soft neurological signs, disordered smooth-pursuit eye movements, impaired problem solving and abstract thinking, and clinical features, such as bizarre behavior, poor social functioning, inadequate hygiene, etc.) are also seen in schizophrenia. Also, studies of nonhuman primates indicate a role for prefrontal cortex (especially the dorsolateral aspect) in higher-order cognitive processes analogous to those impaired in schizophrenia. Although these lines of reasoning are inferential, more direct evidence for frontal cortical involvement in schizophrenia emerged from the intracarotid rCBF studies.

More recent attempts to confirm hypofrontality in schizophrenia using the noninvasive inhalation technique have produced inconsistent results. Possible explanations for this lack of consensus in the literature may include differences in instrumentation and methodology, differences in patients populations, and, most importantly, failure to control testing conditions adequately. Studies carried out during the resting state have obtained particularly variable results.

A series of experiments in which rCBF was measured during a number of different cognitive activation conditions, some of which were linked to prefrontal cortex and others which were not, indicates that schizophrenic patients do have prefrontal cortical dysfunction but that this may not become apparent until the brain is called on to increase the level of physiological activity in this region. In these studies, normal subjects increased prefrontal rCBF while performing a neuropsychological test linked to the prefrontal cortex and requiring abstract reasoning (the Wisconsin Card-Sorting Test), but neither medication-free nor antipsychotic-treated patients showed this increase (Fig. 14.2a-5). In medication-free patients, the degree of the physiological impairment correlated with the level of cognitive disability on the task. During tasks not specifically linked to prefrontal cortex, including simple matching tasks and paradigms involving attention and vigilance, no regional differences in blood flow between normal and patient groups were noted and no abnormalities in areas other than frontal cortex were found during any condition. Interestingly, blood flow was correlated with lateral ventricular size, particularly prefrontal blood flow and particularly during the Wisconsin Card-Sorting Test. Attempts were made in these experiments to control nonspecific and state-dependent epiphenomena that often confound interpretation of such studies. These included the use of a baseline activation measurement in addition to regionally specific cortical activation and the monitoring of peripheral indicators of autonomic arousal, such as pulse, blood pressure, and respiratory rate. These studies highlight the importance of controlling state factors in functional brain imaging studies.

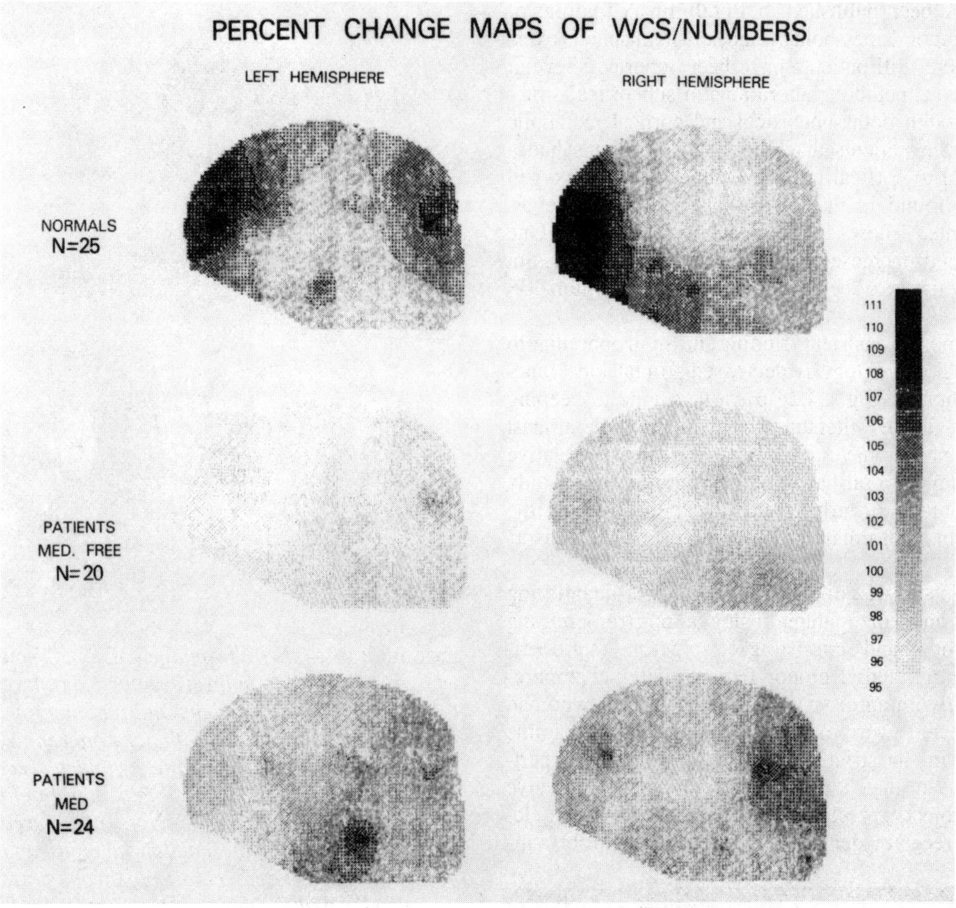

FIGURE 14.2a-5 *Regional cerebral blood flow (rCBF) study. Lateral view (anterior pole at the left) of left and right hemisphere percent change in rCBF during the Wisconsin Card-Sorting (WCS) test compared with rCBF during a number-matching control task. Data are for 25 normal control subjects* (top), *20 medication-free patients* (middle), *and 24 antipsychotic-treated patients* (bottom). *Note that the control subjects, unlike either patient group, show striking rCBF increases (i.e., darker shades) during WCS in an area corresponding to dorsolateral prefrontal cortex. (Adapted from Weinberger et al., 1986, and Berman et al., 1986).*

Despite methodological inconsistences, the rCBF literature taken as a whole suggests that, in some cases, physiological dysfunction of frontal cortex (i.e., hypofrontality) is seen in schizophrenia. Prefrontal cortical deficits have emerged most consistently in patients when studies were carried out under conditions that might stress or impose a physiological load on the prefrontal cortex. These include situations that may involve psychological stress, contingency planning, or divergent thinking as well as cognitive tasks that require these capacities and are specifically linked to prefrontal cortex. The fact that prefrontal cortical dysfunction in schizophrenia may be condition dependent is not inconsistent with the clinical picture of psychopathology that waxes and wanes under various circumstances.

POSITRON EMISSION TOMOGRAPHY STUDIES

Theory and methods Positron emission tomography (PET), a recent addition to the armamentarium of neuroradiology and nuclear medicine, involves the administration of cyclotron-produced radioisotopes that emit short-lived positrons that are rapidly annihilated, producing two characteristic gamma rays of equal energy that can be detected simultaneously outside the head. Unlike the xenon-133 methods described above, this high-resolution technique allows visualization of brain activity in subcortical structures as well as cortex. Several positron-emitting radioisotopes are in use. Currently, the one most widely used is ^{18}F-fluorodeoxyglucose, which is used to measure cerebral glucose metabolism. Oxygen-15 is also employed to measure cerebral oxygen utilization and blood flow. Carbon-11 compounds, positron emitter–labeled neuroreceptor ligands (such as ^{11}C-methylspiperone for dopamine receptors), and neurotransmitter precursors (such as ^{18}F-fluorodopa) have also been developed.

Like rCBF studies, PET results must be interpreted in light of the conditions under which they are carried out, the mental and cognitive state of the subject, the limitations of the instrumentation, and the sampling biases within the experimental population. Additionally, since PET measurements are relatively complex, lengthy, and invasive, application to psychiatric populations has been limited and the number of subjects in most studies is relatively small. Most studies have been carried out in subjects at rest.

Positron emission tomography research findings in schizophrenia A variety of cerebral metabolic differences between normal subjects and those with schizophrenia have been reported, but almost none of these findings have been seen consistently or replicated. Very few reports of altered lateralization have been published, but preliminary findings of increased left temporal metabolism and left-hemisphere overactivation in severely ill patients have been reported. Several recent papers report metabolic alterations in subcortical structures. In one, though both subcortical and cortical metabolic rates were lower in patients than in normals, patients had a higher subcortical-to-cortical ratio; in another, higher oxygen metabolism was found in the left globus pallidus in never-medicated patients. These findings await replication. One PET study reported decreased whole-brain metabolic rates in schizophrenia, which may be consistent with some xenon-133 rCBF studies.

By far, the most consistent finding in schizophrenia to emerge from PET technology is decreased frontal lobe function, or hypofrontality (Fig. 14.2a-6), a fact quite in keeping with the xenon-133 rCBF literature as a whole. While at least five PET investigations have demonstrated decreased relative frontal metabolism, several have not. Furthermore, one study reported hypofrontality in affectively ill patients, raising the possibility that this abnormality may be seen in mood disorders as well.

Recently published was a new PET method for quantifying receptor density in schizophrenia using a positron-emitting dopamine receptor ligand, consisting of spiperone (spiroperidol) linked to a ^{11}C-methyl group. Patients with schizophrenia, those treated with antipsychotics and even those who had never been so treated, were found to have increased dopamine receptor density in the striatum (Fig. 14.2a-7). This experiment is unusual in that it studied a group of drug-naive schizophrenic subjects, precluding the possibility that the elevated dopamine receptor density was an artifact of prior anti-

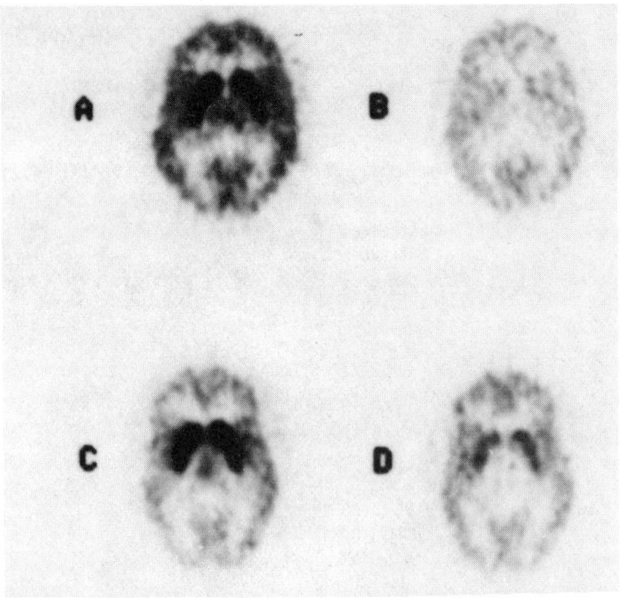

FIGURE 14.2a-7 *PET image of ^{11}C-N-methyl spiperone, which binds to dopamine receptors. Transverse slices at the level of the caudate nucleus and putamen in a normal subject* (A, B) *and in a patient with schizophrenia* (C, D). *Scans B and D were carried out after subjects received a dose of haloperidol (Haldol), which blocks the binding of ^{11}C-NMSP to dopamine D_2 receptors. Note the increase in dopamine receptor binding in the caudate nucleus and putamen of the patient. (Wong D F, et al: Positron emission tomography reveals elevated D_2 dopamine receptors in drug-naive schizophrenics. From Science* 234: *1558, 1986, with permission.)*

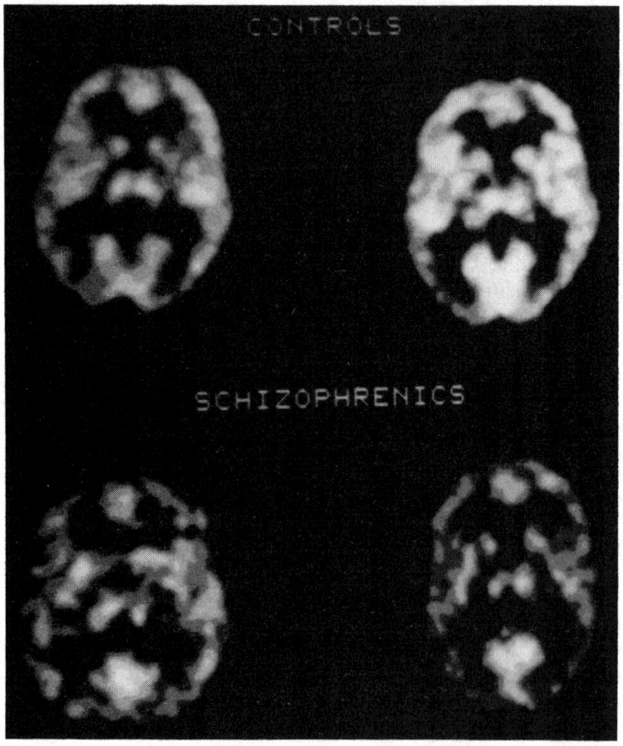

FIGURE 14.2a-6 *PET images of glucose metabolism in two patients with schizophrenia and two healthy control subjects showing alterations in the patients' frontal cortices and basal ganglia. (Courtesy of Dr. Monte Buchsbaum, University of California, Irvine.)*

psychotic treatment. These exciting results potentially represent direct evidence of excessive activity in at least one component of the brain's dopamine systems. However, another group who also studied drug-naive schizophrenic patients has not been able to replicate this finding. While further research will be necessary to resolve this discrepancy, these studies demonstrate the potential power of PET as a tool in schizophrenia research. PET has also recently been used to map dopamine receptor occupancy in schizophrenic patients treated with antipsychotic drugs, an approach that may have future applications in drug treatment and development. There have been few demonstrations of clinical correlates of metabolic alterations as assessed by PET; those reported so far do not tell a cohesive story, and this area also requires further study.

FUTURE PROSPECTS

The contribution of the various approaches now available for studying the brain in schizophrenia can be maximized if several different modalities are applied in a coordinated and complementary fashion. For example, measuring brain physiology and structure directly during life affords several advantages: correlations with other diagnostic evaluations can be made (e.g., with neuropsychological evaluations); cerebral effects of therapeutic interventions can be assessed; and concurrent clinical evaluations can be made and compared with the results. Moreover, these tools can be used to highlight brain areas in living patients that should be examined in subsequent, prospective postmortem studies. The potential interface between clinical research in schizophrenia and other neuroscience disciplines continues to expand.

REFERENCES

Andreasen N C: Brain imaging: Applications in psychiatry. Science *239*: 1381, 1988.

Berman K F, Zec R F, Weinberger D R: Physiological dysfunction of dorsolateral prefrontal cortex in schizophrenia: II. Role of neuroleptic treatment, attention, and mental effort. Arch Gen Psychiat *43*: 126, 1986.

Buchsbaum M S, Haier R J: Functional and anatomical brain imaging: Impact on schizophrenia research. Schizophr Bull *13*: 115, 1987.

Corsellis J A N: Psychoses of obscure pathology. In *Greenfield's Neuropathology,* W Blackwood, J A N Corsellis, editors, ed 3. Edward Arnold, London, 1976.

Davidson K, Bagley C R: Schizophrenia-like psychoses associated with organic disorders of the central nervous system. Brit J Psychiat (Suppl 4): 113, 1969.

Fuster J M: *The Prefrontal Cortex: Anatomy, Physiology, and Neuropsychology of the Frontal Lobe.* Raven Press, New York, 1980.

Ingvar D H, Franzen G: Abnormalities of cerebral blood flow distribution in patients with chronic schizophrenia. Acta Psychiat Scand 50: 425, 1974.

Jaskiw G E, Andreasen N C, Weinberger D R: X-ray computed tomography and magnetic resonance imaging in psychiatry. In *American Psychiatric Association Annual Review,* A J Frances, R E Hales, editors, vol 6. American Psychiatic Association, Washington DC, 1987.

Kety S S, Woodford R B, Harmel M H, Freyham K E, Appel E E, Schmidt C E: Cerebral blood flow and metabolism in schizophrenia. Amer J Psychiat 104: 765, 1948.

Kovelman J A, Scheibel A B: Biological substrates of schizophrenia. Acta Neurol Scand *73*: 1, 1986.

Nasrallah H A, Weinberger D R, editors: *Handbood of Schizophrenia, Volume 1: The Neurology of Schizophrenia.* Elsevier, Amsterdam, 1986.

Nieto D, Escobar A: Major psychoses. In *Pathology of the Nervous System,* J Minckler, editor, vol 3. McGraw-Hill, New York, 1972.

Seidman L F: Schizophrenia and brain dysfunction. Psychol Bull *94*: 195, 1983.

Stevens J R: The neuropathology of schizophrenia. Psychol Med *12*: 695, 1982.

Stevens J R: Schizophrenia: Neuropathological changes in the brain. In *Receptors and Ligands in Psychiatry and Neurology,* A K Sen, T Lee, editors. Cambridge University Press, Cambridge, 1988.

Stuss D T, Benson D F: *The Frontal Lobes.* Raven Press, New York, 1980.

Weinberger D R: Brain disease and psychiatric illness: When should a psychiatrist order a CAT scan? Amer J Psychiat *141:* 1521, 1984.

Weinberger D R, Berman K F, Zec R F: Physiological dysfunction of dorsolateral prefrontal cortex in schizophrenia: I. Regional cerebral blood flow (rCBF) evidence. Arch Gen Psychiat *43*: 114, 1986.

Weinberger D R, Wagner R, Wyatt R J: Neuropathological studies of schizophrenia: A selective review. Schizophr Bull *9*: 193, 1983.

Wong D F, Wagner H N, Jr, Tune L E, Dannals R F, Pearlson G D, Links J M, Tamminga C A, Broussoule E P, Ravert H T, Wilson A A, Toung J K T, Malat J, Williams J A, O'Tuama L A, Snyder S H, Kuhar M J, Gjedde A: Positron emission tomography reveals elevated D_2 dopamine receptors in drug-naive schizophrenics. Science *234:* 1558, 1986.

14.2b SCHIZOPHRENIA: BIOCHEMICAL, ENDOCRINE, AND IMMUNOLOGICAL STUDIES

RICHARD JED WYATT, M.D.
DARRELL G. KIRCH, M.D.
LYNN E. DELISI, M.D.

INTRODUCTION

Despite numerous studies suggesting an association with genetic, toxic-metabolic, endocrine, viral-immunological, and other factors, the etiology of schizophrenia is not known. Whatever the cause, at some level a biochemical disorder of the brain is the result. Though the characteristic cognitive dysfunction of schizophrenia at first glance may appear far removed from neurotransmitters and other chemical systems, cognition takes place in the brain, a biochemical organ with unique structural and physiological organization.

HISTORY The examination of schizophrenic patients from a biochemical perspective dates back at least to the nineteenth century, when psychiatry and biochemistry were in their infancy. In the 1890s at the Maryland Hospital for the Insane and at the turn of the century at McLean Hospital near Boston, W. L. Babcock and Otto Folin, respectively, reported measurements of 24-hour urine constituents. Substances, such as urea, uric acid, ammonia, creatinine, total chlorides, total sulfates, neutral sulfur, ethereal sulfates, indican, and total nitrogen, as well as specific gravity, volume, and acidity, were not found to be abnormal in schizophrenic patients.

In 1922, John C. Whitehorn, who later became head of the psychiatry department at Johns Hopkins University, injected a number of substances intradermally and found schizophrenic patients to have smaller wheal responses to histamine than other patients and normals, a finding that was further replicated in the 1940s and 1950s. Whitehorn speculated that the reason for the decreased histamine response was that schizophrenic patients had an excess of an adrenaline-like (catecholamine) substance. After decades of intensive investigation, today the major hypothesis of the etiology of schizophrenia is that there is an excess of one of the catecholamines—dopamine. Unfortunately, the reliability of early findings (through the 1940s) is complicated by the presence in psychiatric hospitals of patients with various infectious and metabolic disorders that either mimicked schizophrenia or occurred concurrently. Furthermore, until just a few years ago, bioassays were often nonspecific and unreliable.

Nevertheless, the value of a hypothesis, such as that of dopaminergic excess in schizophrenia, is largely dependent on the interest it generates and the possibility of designing experiments to refute or support it. In most areas of human biology, particularly neuropsychiatry, understanding of the relevant systems is too poor to allow the construction of a hypothesis that can be refuted by one or a series of experiments. Therefore, hypotheses—including those related to the pathophysiology and the etiology of schizophrenia—tend to linger. Some are revised in light of new knowledge; others are merely pushed aside by the aggressiveness of new techniques and their proponents. Any comprehensive hypothesis of schizophrenia must take into consideration what is known about the disorder, what is believed to be true. The following strongly supported "facts" are ones that should be explained by a comprehensive hypothesis of schizophrenia.

FACTS ABOUT SCHIZOPHRENIA THAT REQUIRE EXPLANATION

GENDER DIFFERENCES It has been known for a number of years that there are striking gender differences in schizophrenia. The lifetime risk of developing schizophrenia is approximately equal for males and females, although males have an earlier age of onset and poorer outcome than females. This suggests that males often have a more severe form of the disorder. Female patients respond better to neuroleptics. It is unclear if this is simply because they have less severe illness or better premorbid development of social skills owing to later onset of illness. The psychosis in female patients sometimes becomes worse perimenstrually or during the postpartum period, and improvement during pregnancy has been described. Monozygotic twin studies report higher concordance rates among females than males for schizophrenia. Whether a genetic factor in schizophrenia is more common in females is unknown, and family prevalence studies and genetic analyses, thus far, do not support this.

AGE OF ONSET Schizophrenia is rare before puberty, though it is commonly misconceived to begin then. Although age is not a criterion for diagnosis (the revised third edition of *Diagnostic and Statistical Manual of Mental Disorders* [DSM-III-R] states that late onset should be specified in cases developing after age 45), the peak ages of onset for males are 18 to 25 years and for females, 26 to 45.

GENETICS While there remains a possibility that the familial nature of schizophrenia is a consequence of infection, as described below, there is strong evidence that schizophrenia is, at least in part, a genetic disorder. If schizophrenia is genetic, there must be a genetic alteration specific to the brain, unless schizophrenia is similar to phenylketonuria, an illness with many neurological manifestations in which the primary lesion is in a peripheral organ—the liver. Whether one major genetic locus or several are involved is also unknown. The genetic contribution to schizophrenia has not been found to follow known Mendelian patterns.

ENVIRONMENT Since schizophrenia cannot entirely be accounted for by a genetic contribution (as illustrated by discordance for illness between monozygotic twins), an environmental (i.e., social, psychological, physical) factor could play a significant role. The initial schizophrenic episode often occurs during a time of psychological or physical stress, and subsequent exacerbations are also often related to stress. Schizophrenia is more prevalent in large urban environments and in persons of low socioeconomic status, although geographical or socioeconomic drift may be factors.

SEASONALITY OF BIRTH Birth dates of schizophrenics show a modest peak during the late winter and early spring months, above that found in the general population. Some studies associate this excess with viral epidemics, particularly if they occur during the second trimester of pregnancy. There are other equally plausible explanations for seasonality. For example, it is possible that the parents of future schizophrenic individuals conceive more often in the late spring and early summer; perhaps it is a time they are more sexually active.

COURSE OF ILLNESS The course of schizophrenia is extremely variable. Some patients have one or several episodes and then return to normal function, while others have a gradual deteriorating course. Occasionally, even patients who have been ill for many years recover.

STRUCTURAL AND FUNCTIONAL BRAIN ABNORMALITIES The high prevalence of abnormal electroencephalograms (EEGs), abnormal computed tomographic (CT) scans, and neurological abnormalities associated with the disorder are strong indications that schizophrenia involves central nervous system (CNS) structural defects, functional abnormalities, or both.

PHARMACOLOGICAL TREATMENT Neuroleptic medications are useful in treating schizophrenia. They are more effective in treating the positive symptoms (e.g., delusions, hallucinations, thought disorder), but they also may have some effect on the deficit, negative, or core symptoms (e.g., restricted affect, loss of drive, and poverty of speech).

As the biochemical, endocrine, and viral-immunological hypotheses regarding schizophrenia and the data that support them are described below, these essential clinical facts must be kept in mind.

DOPAMINE

The notion that a functional excess of dopaminergic activity is related to the development of schizophrenia has been the most promising and widely accepted hypothesis of schizophrenia. It is certainly one of the most generative yet perplexing hypotheses in the schizophrenia literature.

The dopamine hypothesis of schizophrenia, in its most basic form, states that there is a functional excess of dopamine in the brains of schizophrenic persons, and that the excess is causally related to the disorder. Many investigators have proposed variations of the basic dopamine hypothesis. These include the idea that the mechanism of action of neuroleptic drugs is attributable to their blockade of brain dopamine receptors. Crow and associates assert that the schizophrenic processes can be divided into two biochemically distinct syndromes: one with a functional dopaminergic excess and one with no dopamine-system involvement. Some investigators have proposed that there is a functional decrease in brain dopamine activity in certain schizophrenic persons. Others have postulated that there is both increased and decreased dopamine activity in the brain of the same individual, either concurrently in different anatomical regions or sequentially during the course of the illness. The following discussion reviews what is known about normal brain dopamine systems and the evidence relating dopamine to schizophrenia.

Dopamine is the molecular structural backbone of the catecholamines. It is converted from tyrosine to L-dopa by tyrosine hydroxylase. L-Dopa is subsequently decarboxylated to dopamine by an L-aromatic amino acid decarboxylase. In noradrenergic neurons, dopamine is converted to norepinephrine by dopamine-β-hydroxylase (DBH). Dopamine and norepinephrine are metabolized to inactive products that can be removed from the CNS. These include 3-methoxytyramine, dihydroxyphenylacetic acid (DOPAC), homovanillic acid (HVA), and 3-methoxy-4-hydroxyphenylglycol (MHPG).

Although investigators are learning gradually about monoamine systems in human and nonhuman primate brains, studies of rat brains are still the source of most information. The introduction of histochemical techniques has enabled neuroanatomists to view cell bodies and trace their fibers throughout the brain with the aid of fluoresence microscopy. The cell bodies of the monoamine-containing neurons are compactly located in small nuclei. The dopamine cell bodies that form the nigrostriatal tract are primarily in the substantia nigra (pars compacta) within the mesencephalon. Slightly more anterior and medial, in the decussation of the superior cerebellar peduncle, are the nonpigmented dopamine neurons of the ventromedial mesencephalic tegmentum (VMT). These neurons project to the nucleus accumbens and the prefrontal cortex, making up the meso-cortico-limbic system.

More anterior are dopaminergic neurons that form the incertohypothalamic system and the arcuate nucleus, which forms the tuberoinfundibular tract. The latter gives dopaminergic innervation to the median eminence and pituitary gland. Some of the more caudal dopaminergic neurons project to the spinal cord. Finally, but still within the brain, are short retinal dopaminergic neurons. The arcuate system and the retinal system are important for studies of schizophrenia because both can be studied by relatively noninvasive techniques. For example, concentrations of prolactin and growth hormone in the blood, which reflect hypothalamic dopaminergic activity, have often been studied in schizophrenia. The electroretinogram, which under certain conditions may reflect retinal dopamine activity, is newly in use.

There are at least two types of dopamine receptors in the brain, D_1 and D_2, identified on the basis of their biochemical and pharmacological properties. Most of the pharmacological function of dopamine receptors characterized so far is attributed to D_2 receptors. Little is known about the actions of the D_1 receptor. It remains pharmacologically distinct from the D_2 receptor owing to its ability to stimulate the activity of the enzyme adenylate cyclase, which, in turn, synthesizes the second messenger, adenosine 3':5'-cyclic phosphate (cAMP). Binding studies indicate that the D_1 and D_2 receptors may themselves exist in two forms, one form with high affinity (the degree with which the agonist or antagonist binds), the other with low affinity.

Both D_1 and D_2 receptors are found on postsynaptic membranes, while presynaptic dopaminergic autoreceptors as well as the postsynaptic receptors in most extrasynaptic locations (e.g., the hypothalamic tract) appear to be solely D_2. In the pituitary gland, activation of the D_2 receptor blocks the release of prolactin and α-melanocyte–stimulating hormone (α–MSH). The D_2 receptor also is present on cholinergic striatal interneurons. In these neurons, D_2 agonists increase acetylcholine release and D_2 antagonists increase acetylcholine in the cholinergic interneurons, probably by blocking release. The D_1 receptor is found in the parathyroid gland (where it is involved in the release of parathyroid hormone) and in the retina, but not in the pituitary gland.

The pharmaceutical industry has developed a number of relatively selective D_1 and D_2 agonists and antagonists. A substantial number of these agents are in various stages of preclinical or clinical trials, and there is hope that they will have fewer adverse effects than our current medications. Phenothiazines block D_1 and D_2 receptors. Pimozide (Orap) and molindone (Moban) are more potent blockers of D_2 receptors. Some of the better-known D_2 antagonists include domperidone and (-)-sulpiride. In contrast, the thioxanthene neuroleptic flupenthixol has a high affinity for the D_1 receptor.

There are even newer classes of drugs, such as (-)-3-PPP or 3-(3-hydroxyphenyl)-N-n-propylpiperidine, that act on the dopaminergic system and that appear to have mixed agonist and antagonist activity. That is, they stimulate the presynaptic autoreceptors, inhibiting the release of dopamine at the synapse while blocking postsynaptic dopamine neuronal receptors. The net effect of these agents appears to be to decrease synaptic dopamine concentrations while blocking the dopamine action postsynaptically. Another new class of drugs, selective autoreceptor antagonists, may also be beneficial for the alleviation of negative symptoms by increasing the activity of dopaminergic neurons.

DOPAMINE HYPOTHESIS OF SCHIZOPHRENIA The notion that there might be an excess of dopamine in the brain in schizophrenic persons gained credence when it was realized that drugs that increase dopamine, such as amphetamine, given in high doses or for prolonged periods were capable of producing a paranoid psychosis that in many ways was indistinguishable from schizophrenia. In 1963, a pair of researchers found that medications that decrease the symptoms of schizophrenia, chlorpromazine (Thorazine) and haloperidol (Haldol), are capable of increasing brain 3-methoxytyramine, a major metabolite of dopamine. Medications that did affect the symptoms of schizophrenia did not produce this increase. Based on this finding, the novel hypothesis was proposed that neuroleptics block dopamine receptors, thereby increasing the production of dopamine metabolites as observed in these studies. Subsequently, several groups of investigators demonstrated a striking correlation between the average daily dose of neuroleptics and their ability to displace radiolabeled haloperidol and other neuroleptics in preparations of striatum in vitro.

Studies that correlate the relative clinical potency of various neuroleptics with their ability to block dopamine receptors provide the major support for the dopamine hypothesis. There is a striking correlation of clinical potencies for neuroleptics regardless of diagnosis (schizophrenia or mood disorder). Thus, any dopamine alteration in these disorders might be downstream from the cause, but still be of considerable pathophysiological importance. Alternatively, this common pharmacological responsiveness could be a clue that some mood disorders and schizophrenia may be different manifestations of the same etiology. Nevertheless, the clinical efficacy of neuroleptics for the treatment of schizophrenia remains the strongest evidence in support of the dopamine hypothesis. Even assuming that the dopamine hypothesis is correct for a subgroup of schizophrenia, it is not known whether the hypothesized primary defect is one of synthesis, degradation, release, uptake, abnormal receptor binding or receptor activity, or even presynaptic-postsynaptic receptor mismatch.

ADDITIONAL DATA SUPPORTING AN INCREASE OF DOPAMINE **Stimulants, dopamine precursors, and agonists** One human model for schizophrenia is amphetamine-induced paranoid psychosis, the mechanism for which is thought to be associated with amphetamine-stimulated release of dopamine. It should be noted, however, that while amphetamine does cause release of dopamine, it also causes release of norepinephrine in at least equal quantities. Amphetamine-induced psychosis, however, lacks negative symptoms, specific kinds of auditory hallucinations that occur in schizophrenia, and chronic course.

Occasionally, patients with Parkinson's disease develop a psychosis that is attributed to treatment with L-dopa, although it is unclear if this is related to the production of dopamine or norepinephrine. Perhaps more convincing are the case reports of dopamine agonists, such as bromocriptine (Parlodel), producing a psychosis.

Brain dopamine and its metabolites In one autopsy study of schizophrenic patients and controls, increased levels of HVA were found in the frontal cortex and of dopamine and HVA in the nucleus accumbens and anterior perforated substance. One investigation found increases in the left amygdala in schizophrenic patients. Most studies of schizophrenic brains, however, do not show such increases. Since some animal studies show similar changes after neuroleptic administration, the above findings may be simply a medication effect in the patients studied.

Cerebrospinal fluid While there are few data indicating a high level of dopamine or its metabolites in the cerebrospinal fluid (CSF) of schizophrenic patients compared with controls, two studies show positive correlations between the quantity of HVA and the severity of positive symptoms. This suggests that increased dopamine turnover may be related to the production of active symptoms.

Plasma There are studies that show more plasma HVA in unmedicated schizophrenic patients than in controls. More striking, however, is the positive correlation between plasma HVA-symptoms, and response to treatment. Neuroleptics appear to produce a decrease in plasma HVA at a time when the patients improve.

Brain and peripheral enzymes involved in dopamine metabolism If the enzymes that are involved in the synthetic pathway of dopamine are increased, it might suggest that the brain is capable of making excess dopamine; but lower levels of enzymes involved in dopamine degradation could also produce dopamine excess.

Tyrosine hydroxylase, the enzyme responsible for converting tyrosine to L-dopa, has been found to be normal in several postmortem studies of different areas of the brains of schizophrenic patients. Because of their interest in the role of norepinephrine in reward and self-stimulation (the lack of which could be viewed as a model for the negative symptoms and anhedonia characteristic of schizophrenia), one group of associates proposed a deficit of dopamine-β-hydroxylase (the enzyme that converts dopamine to norepinephrine) in schizophrenia. While they subsequently reported the existence of such a deficit in postmortem schizophrenic brains, others have been unable to confirm this finding. At least some of the deficit may be attributed to neuroleptic medication or to enzyme decay during the interval between death and autopsy.

Dopamine-β-hydroxylase has also been measured in plasma and CSF. While some investigators have found plasma dopamine-β-hydroxylase to be low in schizophrenics, the majority of studies have found no differences.

Decreased monoamine oxidase (MAO) in autopsied brains of patients with schizophrenia was first described in 1941. While all but one subsequent study failed to confirm this finding, decreased MAO activity has been found in the majority of studies of platelet, lymphocyte, and muscle tissue samples from schizophrenic patients. There is little doubt that there is a subgroup of schizophrenic patients who have decreased peripheral MAO activity. The small decreases (usually less than 40 percent compared with 99 percent in most genetic enzyme-defect diseases), however, make it unlikely that the alteration is of direct physiological importance. Furthermore, although early reports indicated there was no effect of medications on MAO activity, a number of subsequent studies have indicated that, at least in the platelet, MAO activity can be significantly reduced by neuroleptic medication.

Brain dopamine receptors Several postmortem brain tissue studies and at least two positron emission tomography (PET) studies show increased numbers of D_2 dopamine-binding sites in the brains of schizophrenic patients. The major issue is whether the increase is a reaction to neuroleptic treatment or a primary alteration in schizophrenia. This question, like the decrease in platelet MAO, has been difficult to resolve; further studies in nonmedicated patients should resolve it.

The dopamine excess hypothesis had enormous heuristic value: It has generated thousands of basic and clinical experiments. Except for the amphetamine-induced paranoid psychosis and the probable dopaminergic effect of neuroleptic medications, the data from clinical studies are not strongly supportive of the hypothesis. Definitive biochemical data in support of an excess of dopamine in schizophrenia remain elusive. Still, some of the data gained in the pursuit of the dopamine-excess hypotheses indicate that a decreased level of dopamine might be present in some patients.

DATA THAT SUPPORT A DECREASE IN DOPAMINE

Chronic stimulant administration in animals There is considerable evidence that stimulants in high doses produce loss of dopaminergic terminals in animal brains. Dopamine released by the stimulant is converted into 6-hydroxydopamine, which, in turn, is taken into dopamine terminals and destroys them.

von Economo's encephalitis or encephalitis lethargica and Parkinson's disease During the worldwide influenza epidemic that began in the winter of 1916 to 1917, Baron Constantine von Economo described a striking hypokinetic state, which he called psychic torpor. Reactions to encephalitis lethargica were often mistaken for schizophrenia and were at times even called epidemic schizophrenia. Karl Menninger noted that unmistakable schizophrenic signs were associated with the encephalitis, including intrapsychic ataxia, emotional-ideational splitting, incoherence, and stereotypies. A number of apparently recovered victims subsequently developed Parkinson's disease.

The major alteration in Parkinson's disease involves destruction of dopamine-containing neurons, primarily in the nigrostriatal system. There is decreased dopamine in the neurons of cortical projection areas that receive processes from the meso-cortico-limbic dopaminergic system. As a number of the deficit symptoms (mild intellectual impairment, apathy or depression, lack of spontaneous speech, problems with concept formation) of Parkinson's disease are similar to those of schizophrenia, it is reasonable to contemplate similar dopamine alterations in both disorders. Furthermore, although it is not common, schizophrenia and Parkinson's disease can occur in the same individual, which strongly implies that (in these cases at least) it is not an excess of dopamine that is responsible for schizophrenia.

Akinesia Akinesia involving both motor and cognitive functions is a well-known side effect of neuroleptic medications and is seen in humans and animals. Akinesia is thought to be attributable to a blocking of dopamine by neuroleptic drugs. The deficit symptoms of schizophrenia, often indistinguishable from the drug-induced akinesia, are present in unmedicated schizophrenic patients.

Cerebrospinal fluid Several studies indicate that concentrations of dopamine or its metabolites are decreased in the CSF of some schizophrenic patients. There are negative correlations between HVA concentrations and the severity of deficit symptoms associated with schizophrenia; these include poor prognosis and length of illness as well as ratings of negative symptoms.

Urine Surprisingly few studies have measured dopamine and its metabolites in the urine of schizophrenic patients. Karoum and associates found that when the molar sum of dopamine and its metabolites is expressed in a ratio to the sum of norepinephrine and its metabolites, medication-free schizophrenics had a lower mean ratio than a group of normal controls. The ratio normalized with neuroleptic treatment.

Animal models Studies of a number of animal models indicate that dopamine deficits can produce symptoms consistent with those of schizophrenia. For example, rats given neuroleptics that reduce functional dopamine exhibit a reduction in the motivational arousal needed for goal-directed behavior.

Location of changes Numerous studies have demonstrated with pneumoencephalography, CT scans, and postmortem measurements that some patients with schizophrenia have localized brain structural alterations. The alterations include enlargement of the lateral and third ventricles, cortical atrophy, and decreased volume of the hippocampus and amygdala. In some patients, there may be relatively specific prefrontal cortical atrophy, even when there is no evidence of alterations in other cortical areas. The prefrontal abnormalities are consistent with studies demonstrating relatively decreased regional cerebral blood flow and metabolism in the prefrontal cortex, particularly when the prefrontal cortex has been specifically activated. Because there are animal data to indicate that prefrontal cortical function is partially dependent on the dopamine projections to it, the apparent atrophy and inability to activate with specific stimulation suggest that some altered dopamine function in the prefrontal cortex may be due to loss of cell bodies or projections. In animal studies, it has been found that stress produces increased dopamine turnover in the frontal cortex.

VARIATIONS ON THE BASIC DOPAMINE HYPOTHESIS The following are attempts at synthesizing the dopamine data into coherent hypotheses:

Hypothesis 1 This variation suggests that schizophrenic persons have a vulnerable dopaminergic system (perhaps inherited) and that, with repeated stress, there is loss of dopaminergic terminals. In this variation, the stress itself is initially responsible for increased dopamine turnover and the productive symptoms of schizophrenia. The progressive loss of dopamine terminals is ultimately responsible for the burned-out state of schizophrenia. This hypothesis is consistent with the observation that patients whose illness begins with predominantly productive symptoms subsequently often develop predominantly deficit symptoms. The hypothesis requires the progressive loss of dopaminergic terminals similar to that seen in stimulant-induced release of dopamine.

Hypothesis 2 This variation suggests that there is an underlying reduction of dopaminergic function in the prefrontal cortex (and perhaps other brain regions of schizophrenic persons) and that the decrease is responsible for some of the prodromal symptoms of the disorder. The acute phase of schizophrenia might be caused by stress and a concurrent increase in dopamine turnover. Neuroleptics increase dopamine turnover in the prefrontal cortex, but tolerance does not develop, as it appears to in other parts of the brain. To speculate further, increased dopamine turnover in this region produced by neuroleptic administration might decrease the deficit symptoms. Thus, where there is a potentially active prefrontal dopaminergic system in schizophrenia, neuroleptics are capable of reducing the deficit symptoms. But where the prefrontal dopamine system is not capable of activation, neuroleptics cannot affect the symptoms. The effects of neuroleptics in other parts of the brain suppress some of the productive or positive symptoms of schizophrenia.

Hypothesis 3 This variation suggests that there is uneven compensation for lost dopaminergic function. Several neurotoxins, including 6-hydroxydopamine, selectively destroy catecholaminergic systems. Under certain circumstances, these neurotoxins are highly specific. Following 6-hydroxydopamine administration to the rat, there is a dramatic reduction in brain norepinephrine, but within 21 days norepinephrine turnover increases. The ability of residual catecholamine terminals to partially compensate for the lost terminals suggests that there may be areas of the brain that have excessive catecholamine stimulation and others that have decreased stimulation. Pycock found that destroying dopamine terminals in rat medial prefrontal cortex was followed by an increase in the number of dopamine receptors in the nucleus accumbens and striatum and by increased dopamine turnover in these areas. Decreased dopamine in the cortex is balanced by a subcortical increase. Some of the observations that imply laterality differences in schizophrenia may be related to the ability of dopamine systems to compensate on one side of the brain when there are changes on the other side.

NOREPINEPHRINE

Norepinephrine (the neurotransmitter for neurons in the peripheral autonomic nervous system), like dopamine, is widely distributed in the brain. It is most highly concentrated in the hypothalamus, thalamus, limbic system, and cerebellum. Cell bodies of noradrenergic neurons are prominent in the locus ceruleus, located beneath the floor of the fourth ventricle. Alquist first proposed the subdivision of noradrenergic receptors into two types—α receptors, found in cortical and limbic structures, and β receptors, found in cortical projections and in the cerebellum. Responses attributed to α-receptor activation are primarily excitatory; responses attributed to β-receptor activation are inhibitory, with the exception of myocardial stimulant effects. α-Noradrenergic receptors have been further subdivided into α_1 and α_2 receptors. Presynaptic receptors are α_2; postsynaptic neurons contain α_1 receptors. All three receptors are linked to cAMP activation. The brain stem α_2-adrenergic receptors may be located presynaptically and postsynaptically. The presynaptic α_2-adrenergic receptor, or autoreceptor, mediates feedback inhibition by norepinephrine on central norepinephrine cell firing and norepinephrine release.

Hypotheses concerning the normal functioning of CNS norepinephrine neurons include a role in learning and memory, reinforcement, sleep-wake cycle regulation, anxiety, and nociception, as well as a more general role in the regulation of CNS blood flow and metabolism. Animal behavior studies support the concept that the norepinephrine neurons of the locus ceruleus may function as a reward system. Activation of this region with electrodes produces behavior, such as reward-directed self-stimulating lever pressing. Wise and Stein proposed that schizophrenia may be related to a defect in the noradrenergic reward system or selective norepinephrine neuron degeneration, producing the anhedonia (or lack of self-initiated goal-directed behavior) characteristic of many chronic schizophrenic patients. Although a specific focus on dopamine-β-hydroxylase deficits does not appear promising, exploration of other aspects of noradrenergic dysfunction in schizophrenia continues. Major support for the presence of increased norepinephrine activity came from initial reports of the successful treatment of schizophrenia with propranolol (Inderal), a drug that blocks β-adrenergic receptors. Unfortunately, propranolol has not proved to be consistently efficacious in subsequent studies.

In recent years, a number of studies of both peripheral and central noradrenergic metabolism in schizophrenia have been completed. Measurements of plasma norepinephrine and its metabolite, MHPG, in drug-free acute and chronic schizophrenic patients have been reported. Increased blood concentrations of norepinephrine have been noted in some studies, though they vary with positioning of patients and may be influenced by neuroleptic medication. Adding confusion is a report that plasma norepinephrine levels are not correlated with CSF norepinephrine concentrations nor with psychopathology. Clonidine (Catapres, a presynaptic α_2 partial agonist) suppresses plasma MHPG in normal persons but not in schizophrenic patients. Twenty-four–hour urinary MHPG excretion in schizophrenic patients was similar to that of normal controls in most studies, unlike the studies reporting low levels in mood disorders. There is only one report of elevated urinary excretion of this metabolite in medication-free chronic schizophrenic patients. As 24-hour urinary MHPG measurements are subject to several problems (e.g., collection procedures), this determination may be of limited value in studies of schizophrenic patients.

Taken together, the studies imply that a peripheral alteration in norepinephrine metabolism or norepinephrine response to stress may be present in at least some schizophrenic patients. The relationship of these findings to brain activity, and thus their significance, is unknown.

At least four studies have reported higher concentrations of norepinephrine in the CSF of some chronic schizophrenic patients (particularly paranoid schizophrenics) than in controls. MHPG, however, was not increased in the CSF of these patients. Furthermore, one of these studies found that the significant increases in CSF norepinephrine were present only in those patients receiving neuroleptics at the time of the study.

Increased norepinephrine concentrations have been reported in the limbic region of postmortem brains from paranoid schizophrenics. This finding was not confirmed by two other groups that did not look at paranoid schizophrenia as a subclassification. Another study of paranoid schizophrenic brains found norepinephrine increased in the mesencephalon; another found high levels of both norepinephrine and its metabolite in the nucleus accumbens. While these studies together suggest the presence of a defect in norepinephrine metabolism in at least a subgroup of schizophrenic patients, the issue of the effect of medication, particularly in the postmortem studies, has not been resolved.

Investigations of noradrenergic receptors have also been conducted. In some areas, their juxtaposition to dopaminergic neurons has led to interesting hypotheses of feedback loops and inhibitory-excitatory mechanisms. Although clinical CNS studies of β-receptor function have not been performed, α-receptor function on platelets, as a proposed model for α-receptor function in the brain, has been studied in medication-free schizophrenic patients. Elevated numbers of α receptors have been found to be associated with a deficiency in prostaglandin E_1–stimulated cAMP production, a function known to be inhibited by α-receptor stimulation. It is not known whether these peripheral findings parallel brain metabolism. Noradrenergic α- and β-receptor binding sites, as measured by 3-H-WB4101 and 3-H-dihydroalprenolol, do not appear to be elevated in the brains of schizophrenic patients.

It appears from several studies that neuroleptics may increase norepinephrine concentrations, probably by inhibiting metabolism. It is even possible, therefore, that the studies reporting norepinephrine data on patients 2 or 3 weeks after neuroleptic withdrawal were still seeing some of the long-term effects of medication. No study has clearly shown elevated plasma or CSF norepinephrine in never-medicated (acute) schizophrenic patients. These studies may indicate that the therapeutic effect of neuroleptic medication, while largely attributed to dopamine receptor blockade, may also result from altered noradrenergic transmission. Despite this, the α-receptor–blocking properties of conventional neuroleptic drugs do not correlate with their clinical potency.

Clonidine, a predominantly centrally acting α_2 receptor partial agonist, in one study produced a transient reduction in symptoms in some schizophrenic patients, concurrently reducing plasma norepinephrine and MHPG concentrations. Another study reported clonidine to be as effective as a neuroleptic for schizophrenic symptoms, while others found no therapeutic benefit from clonidine. Levels of both plasma norepinephrine, derived from peripheral sympathetic nervous system activity, and plasma MHPG, derived from both central and peripheral sources, fall following administration of clonidine as a function of clonidine effects on central brain stem α_2-adrenergic receptors. Phenoxybenzamine (Dibenzyline), a mixed α-receptor antagonist, has not been of benefit in schizophrenia.

The studies reviewed in this section do not contain sufficient evidence to suggest that a defect in the norepinephrine system is primary to the development of schizophrenia. While an elevation in plasma, CSF, and brain norepinephrine, particularly in paranoid schizophrenic patients, has been reported by several investigators, the reasons for it are unclear. No association of elevated norepinephrine with increased dopamine-β-hydroxylase activity or increased dopamine concentrations has been found that would imply increased synthesis. Likewise, increased norepinephrine has not been correlated with decreased MHPG to imply decreased breakdown.

SEROTONIN

Serotonin (5-hydroxytryptamine [5-HT]), a derivative of the amino acid tryptophan, is thought to have an inhibitory function in the CNS. The cell bodies of serotonergic neurons are located in the midline raphe nuclei in the lower midbrain and upper pons, although their axons are widely distributed throughout the brain. In general, activation of serotonergic receptors has been demonstrated to inhibit animal behavior, whereas inactivation of serotonergic mechanisms appears to enhance some behaviors.

Serotonin receptors have been studied by using ligands such as lysergic acid diethylamide (LSD) in binding displacement assays. Binding of spiroperidol, a presumed dopamine-receptor antagonist, however, is also related to serotonin-displaceable sites, particularly in the cerebral cortex. Conversely, D-LSD binds to dopamine receptors in some regions of the brain. Specific descriptions of two distinct serotonin binding sites (S_1 and S_2) have been reported, and pharmacological manipulation of these sites with new agents has been studied. The S_1 site is labeled by [3-H]-serotonin, while the S_2 site is labeled by [3-H]-spiperone, [3-H]-LSD, [3-H]-mianserin, or [3-H]-ketanserin. More recent evidence suggests that this classification may be an oversimplification. At least two distinct subtypes of S_1 receptors, the S_{1A} and S_{1B}, are likely. Biochemical data also suggest that some serotonin receptors (specifically S_1) are linked to cAMP.

There is a significant correlation between the ability of various antagonists to inhibit a number of serotonin-mediated behavioral responses and their ability to inhibit radioligand binding to the S_2 site. The functional role of the S_1 site, however, remains unclear. It has been proposed to be an inhibitory autoreceptor, a serotonin-sensitive adenyl cyclase, or both.

Convincing evidence has emerged that neuropeptides, such as substance P and thyrotropin-releasing hormone (TRH), coexist in many serotonin neurons. These peptides may modify serotonin-receptor sensitivity. New pharmacological agents, such as m-chlorphenylpiperazine (M-CPP), a serotonin-receptor agonist, and metergoline, a receptor antagonist, will help examine the functional status of serotonin systems in psychiatric patients. It is unknown whether these agents act on specific serotonin-receptor subtypes, react with other neurotransmitters, or have mixed actions.

A major role for serotonin in mental processes was first hypothesized in 1953 by workers who postulated that the suppression of its action could result in a psychiatric disorder. They based this hypothesis on the striking similarities between serotonin and the hallucinogen LSD. Because LSD is thought to block serotonin receptor sites, it could produce a relative decrease in serotonergic activity. Later reports that serotonergic-depleting agents, such as reserpine, appeared to alleviate some symptoms of schizophrenia led these analysts to shift position and postulate that an actual increase in serotonin may be causally related to schizophrenia.

Even if schizophrenia is characterized by a deficiency in the serotonin system, it does not necessarily follow that these patients have low brain serotonin concentrations. Any substance, such as LSD, that blocks serotonin receptors might lead to an absolute increase in serotonin concentrations via a feedback loop while suppressing serotonergic function. Numerous clinical studies measuring serotonin and its metabolites in schizophrenic patients have since been conducted. Studies of peripheral measurements of serotonin and its principal metabolite, 5-hydroxyindoleacetic acid (5-HIAA), have been inconsistent. Urinary excretion studies have, for the most part, been negative and of questionable value, since most of urinary 5-HIAA excretion is derived from the gut and does not represent brain metabolism. Although several earlier studies either found low blood serotonin concentrations or showed no abnormalities in schizophrenic patients, more recent research has revealed a group of disorders, including schizophrenia, characterized by elevated blood serotonin concentrations. Whether this finding relates to brain metabolism is far from clear, since blood serotonin is derived predominantly from gut metabolism of tryptophan. In fact, there is some suggestion in the literature of an inverse relationship between blood and brain serotonin. The derivation of CSF serotonin and 5-HIAA is controversial; nevertheless, they are thought to be closer indicators of the status of brain serotonin. Whole blood serotonin was found to be significantly higher in schizophrenic patients with cerebral atrophy detected by CT than in those with normal CT scans or controls. In another study of many of the same patients, lower CSF 5-HIAA correlated directly with the presence of cerebral atrophy by CT scanning and inversely with blood serotonin concentrations. Swedish researchers found elevated CSF 5-HIAA to be associated with a positive family history of schizophrenia. Another study of unmedicated schizophrenic patients showed a positive correlation of CSF 5-HIAA and platelet serotonin concentrations with peculiar mannerisms and posturing.

Postmortem brain studies, unfortunately, do not illuminate the issue, and results are conflicting. While some investigators reported regional elevations in brain serotonin in areas, such as the putamen, hypothalamus, medial olfactory area, nucleus accumbens, and globus pallidus, other studies did not confirm these findings. In addition, reduced serotonin and 5-HIAA concentrations in several brain areas (hypothalamus, medulla oblongata, and hippocampus) in tissue samples from chronic schizophrenic patients have also been reported. These inconsistencies may simply represent difficulties inherent in obtaining reliable data from human postmortem studies. Cause of death, interval between death and autopsy, medication status, and reliability of postmortem diagnosis are only a few of the problems.

Taken together, these several approaches appear to indicate abnormal serotonin metabolism in some chronic schizophrenic patients. The relationship of serotonin to the illness, its etiology, and other biochemical abnormalities all warrant further investigation.

The effect of neuroleptic medication on serotonergic activity is also an open issue. Most studies report an inhibitory effect of neuroleptics on uptake of serotonin in platelets. Because platelets are the primary reservoir of blood serotonin, with decreased platelet uptake whole blood serotonin concentrations probably would be reduced rather than elevated, as has been found in some studies. In animal studies, chronic neuroleptic treatment was shown to increase serotonin turnover and concentration in rat brain. On the other hand, in primate brain, serotonin turnover has been shown to be decreased by neuroleptic treatment. Thus, although results are not consistent across studies, it does appear that altered serotonin and 5-HIAA concentrations in brain and other tissues observed in human studies could be due to chronic medication.

Pharmacological studies have added little to support a serotonin hypothesis. Administration of tryptophan (the precursor of serotonin) to both schizophrenic patients and normal control subjects did not result in increased urinary 5-HIAA excretion in schizophrenic patients, although there was a 100-percent increase in 5-HIAA in the urine of normal controls. This study suggests decreased serotonin production in schizophrenic patients, although it remains unconfirmed.

Assuming a serotonin deficiency, treatment of schizophrenia with serotonin or its direct precursor, 5-hydroxytryptophan (5-HTP), should have been successful; however, in one study 5-HTP exacerbated some patients' psychosis.

Alternatively, if a serotonin excess is related to schizophrenia, then agents aimed at reducing serotonin activity should have clinical efficacy. Para-chlorophenylalanine (PCPA), an inhibitor of serotonin synthesis, however, had no beneficial effect when given in a small trial to chronic schizophrenic patients. Another approach has been to use the drug fenfluramine (Pondimin), a serotonin-depleting agent. In one recent preliminary report, negative symptoms of schizophrenia were improved in three of eight patients treated with the active drug, while none of the four given placebo improved. Though this is not clear evidence of an association of negative symptoms with hyperserotonemia, perhaps only some patients have the potential for their negative symptoms to be reversed with any pharmacological agent. It is interesting that fenfluramine seems to have a significant effect in autistic disorder, improving the symptoms of withdrawal behavior and inappropriate affect that are similar to the negative symptoms of schizophrenia in adults. Nevertheless, another study found a trend toward a worsening of negative symptoms with fenfluramine in eight patients. Perhaps, the patients in these studies are too few and too heterogeneous at present to justify any conclusions about the effects of fenfluramine.

It is still possible, however, that specific serotonergic inhibiting agents could benefit a subgroup of schizophrenic patients not yet clearly defined. Many other aspects of tryptophan metabolism in nerve tissue, as well as the physiological interaction of indoleamines with catecholamines and peptides at nerve synapses, may be crucial to the disordered system and require further investigation.

AMINO ACIDS AND OTHER BIOGENIC AMINES

γ-AMINOBUTYRIC ACID (GABA) While present only in trace amounts in the periphery, GABA is widely distributed within the brain; the highest concentrations are in the substantia nigra, globus pallidus, caudate, medial thalamus, hippocampus, hypothalamus, and occipital, frontal, and cerebellar cortices. The brain contains large amounts of glutamic acid, the main precursor of GABA (metabolized by the pyridoxal-dependent enzyme, glutamic acid decarboxylase [GAD]) and itself a possible neurotransmitter. Thirty percent of all brain synapses are believed to be GABA-ergic. GABA-ergic and dopaminergic pathways in both the nigrostriatal and mesolimbic systems closely interact; it is likely that GABA inhibits dopamine activity. GABA is thought to act postsynaptically by increasing membrane permeability to chloride ions, which, in turn, inhibits the generation of an action potential in postsynaptic cells. There also appears to be coupling of the receptor sites for benzodiazepines and GABA; benzodiazepines exhibit GABA–agonistic properties.

The observation of behavioral abnormalities in animals following mesolimbic injections of GABA antagonists led to a GABA-deficiency hypothesis of schizophrenia. If decreased GABA results in increased dopaminergic activity, then this notion would also be consistent with the notion of excessive dopamine in schizophrenia.

Postmortem brain GABA and GABA receptor–binding studies of schizophrenic patients and controls generally have not detected any differences. Brain GAD, the enzyme responsible for the synthesis of GABA from glutamic acid, has normal activity in schizophrenic patients. It should be noted, however, that a substantial rise in GAD activity occurs immediately postmortem, with a rapid rise in brain GABA content, thus hampering interpretation of postmortem investigations of this substance.

Although most CSF GABA studies have also been negative, a decrease in GABA concentrations was reported in a small proportion of acutely psychotic schizophrenic patients in one study. An increase in GABA was observed in another study of more chronic patients, no doubt with more negative symptoms.

Therapeutic trials of GABA-ergic drugs, such as muscimol and valproic acid (Depakene), either have been of no benefit or have produced exacerbations of psychotic symptoms. The patients selected for these trials, however, were not screened for low CSF GABA concentrations. The knowledge that benzodiazepines bind to GABA receptors and appear to potentiate GABA activity renewed interest in this class of tranquilizers for schizophrenia. While they generally appear not to be of major benefit, there are some reports of marked improvement in psychotic symptoms with some benzodiazepine analogs in small subgroups of patients. In normal doses, these drugs do not appear to be effective adjuncts to neuroleptic therapy and may even increase violent behavior. With very large doses, however, some studies have shown antipsychotic actions. New benzodiazepines, such as clonazepam (Klonopin) and alprazolam (Xanax), have been claimed to have expanded chemical properties, perhaps giving them antipsychotic effects. While clonazepam has not been effective in schizophrenia, it may be effective in bipolar disorder. Alprazolam is thought by some to be effective against deficit or negative symptoms.

The inconsistencies in these reports further support the necessity for biological subgrouping of schizophrenia. It is possible that one subgroup may be characterized by a high dopamine–low GABA syndrome and another by low dopamine and high GABA. Pharmacological studies might then appear to be contradictory, depending on the nature of the patient group studied. Based on their CSF GABA studies, van Kammen and associates have suggested that a subgroup of acutely psychotic patients composes the low GABA subgroup, while the more chronic patients, who have signs of emotional blunting and withdrawal, appear not to fit into this subgroup.

GABA has also been hypothesized to play a role in tardive dyskinesia. While it is possible that patients more susceptible to developing tardive dyskinesia have a GABA deficiency, the evidence for this is extremely weak.

METHIONINE Several reports indicate that schizophrenic patients, unlike normal controls, have adverse behavioral responses when given oral loads of methionine. L-Methionine, the main source of methyl groups in the body, either precipitates acute psychosis in these persons or exacerbates the symptoms of chronic schizophrenia; the specific symptoms that worsen vary among studies. Despite extensive research initiated by these studies, little explanation exists for this phenomenon.

It has been proposed that the clinical symptoms result from increased dimethylation and production of compounds formed from methionine methyl transfer. Unfortunately, multiple studies have not substantiated this. Another explanation may be related to a defect in an enzyme involved in the one-carbon (methionine methyl transfer) cycle itself rather than the production of toxic products. No one enzyme in this cycle has been consistently found to be altered in schizophrenic patients, though several have not been studied.

There is some evidence that CSF methionine is increased in schizophrenic patients. Evidence that methionine may increase dopamine D_2 receptors in the striatum, possibly through methylation of membrane phospholipids, provides a link for a defect in this system with the dopamine hypothesis of schizophrenia.

SERINE A portion of the one-carbon cycle involves the conversion of serine to glycine. Abnormalities in blood serine concentrations have been noted in schizophrenia, but not consistently. Since serine is metabolized to produce phospholipids and thus is important to membrane lipid structure, it has been proposed as an important element in neuronal membrane fluidity, perhaps modulating receptor sensitivity. It also is metabolized by the enzyme serine hydroxymethyltransferase to glycine and is important in the synthesis of adenosine. Both glycine and adenosine are neuroregulators in the brain.

One group of investigators reported elevated plasma serine concentrations in psychotic patients, and one study reported lower urinary excretion of serine. These studies also found an exacerbation of psychiatric symptoms after serine loads and delayed clearance of serine from the plasma in some patients. These are preliminary studies that need to be replicated in acutely psychotic, unmedicated schizophrenic patients. In some other studies, no serine abnormalities have been found in plasma, CSF, or postmortem brain tissue of chronic schizophrenic patients.

PHENYLALANINE AND TYROSINE Since phenylalanine and tyrosine are precursors for catecholamine formation, any abnormalities in their metabolism would be of interest in schizophrenia. A genetic defect in the enzyme that converts phenylalanine to tyrosine, phenylalanine hydroxylase, is responsible for the syndrome of phenylketonuria (PKU). Some investigators have suggested that there may be a link between the inheritance of this disorder and schizophrenia. Poisner found a higher fasting serum phenylalanine concentration in drug-free schizophrenic patients than in normal controls. This finding suggests reduced phenylalanine hydroxylase activity and perhaps an increase of heterozygotes for PKU among schizophrenic patients. Individual heterozygotes were not identified within the sample, since there is significant overlap between heterozygotes and controls. Phenylalanine tolerance tests, similar to glucose tolerance tests for diabetes, can detect heterozygotes for PKU by determining the amount of time for a load of phenylalanine to be metabolized to tyrosine and return to baseline plasma levels. Lippman found that 13 of 50 schizophrenic patients were in the borderline range for heterozygosity. In a more detailed study of both oral and intravenous phenylalanine loads given to 22 schizophrenic patients (12 medication-free) and 18 controls, no differences were observed in pre- or postloading concentrations of phenylalanine or tyrosine in plasma.

Although it does not appear that phenylalanine hydroxylase activity is abnormal in schizophrenic patients, a deficiency in the co-enzyme dihydropteridine reductase would probably not be detected by a phenylalanine tolerance test. Dihydropteridine reductase is a required co-factor for the hydroxylation of phenylalanine to tyrosine, and of tyrosine to dopa in the synthesis of dopamine and norepinephrine.

ASPARAGINE Although there are no reports in the literature of any disease associations with altered asparagine metabolism, there is one case of a psychotic male with elevated plasma and CSF asparagine. No further attempt to define this abnormality in other patients has been published.

Now that amino acid analyzers are in widespread use and available for accurate and specific assays of all the amino acids, other studies will be reported and abnormalities noted. It will be important to determine the effects of medication and other environmental variables, particularly diet, in any study before concluding that genetic defects in crucial enzymes responsible for amino acid metabolism, as in the case of PKU, are responsible for psychosis. Nevertheless, amino acids remain of interest, as many are neurotransmitters or neuroregulators, or their precursors.

HISTAMINE Histamine is normally present and partially metabolized in the brain. It is of interest that schizophrenic patients have a relatively low incidence of allergies and a decreased wheal response to histamine injected intradermally. The onset of schizophrenia has been noted in other cases to coincide with a remission of asthmatic symptoms.

Many early investigators reported abnormalities in histamine metabolism in schizophrenic patients. Because neuroleptic medications have antihistamine activity, it is unclear what role they have played in more recent studies. Nevertheless, some of these studies are worth mentioning. Further pursuit of abnormalities in the metabolism of this amine are warranted.

A few studies have found higher histamine concentrations in serum of schizophrenics than of normals. One study found no difference between these groups in CSF histamine. Since earlier assays may have been measuring spermidine in addition to histamine, it is unclear what may be abnormal in schizophrenia. Pfeiffer and colleagues, with a more specific assay, reported lower concentrations in schizophrenic patients than in normals, although the medication status of these patients was not documented. Mazur and Walaszek measured histaminolytic activity in blood from chronic schizophrenic patients off medication for 2 weeks and from controls. Although the schizophrenic patients had greater histaminolytic activity than the controls, it is now clear from many studies that 2 weeks' discontinuation of neuroleptics is not enough time for many biochemical parameters to return to baseline levels. The histamine abnormalities may have more to do with alterations in immunocompetent cells responsible for the response, rather than actual lack of sensitivity to histamine. The histamine findings have not been resolved but seem worth pursuing in medication-free subjects.

POTENTIAL ENDOGENOUS HALLUCINOGENS

For more than 3 decades, scientists have investigated the possibility than an endogenous substance with hallucinogenic properties might be responsible for some schizophrenic disorders. In 1952, Osmond and Smythies (quoting Harley-Mason) proposed that abnormal endogenous methylation of neurotransmitter substances, producing agents similar to the catecholamine derivative mescaline, could be the biochemical mechanism for hallucinations. Dimethoxyphenylethylamine (DMPEA, "the pink spot") was suggested as one such substance that could be produced under pathological conditions in vivo by an O-methylating enzyme.

Since methylated phenylethylamines (the core structure of catecholamines) were known to produce catatonic-like behavior in animals, Osmond and Smythies proposed that clinical catatonia might also result from abnormal methylation of catecholamines, particularly dopamine. Similarly, dimethyl derivatives (N-methylated) of the indoleamine serotonin (e.g., bufotenine, dimethyltryptamine [DMT]) were also thought to be potential endogenous psychotogenic agents. With the subsequent discovery of an enzyme in human brain that has the potential to produce N-methylated compounds similar to these hallucinogens, this hypothesis was expanded into the more general transmethylation hypothesis. It stated that the abnormal (N- or O-) methylation of biogenic amines may produce symptoms of schizophrenia. While studies examining this hypothesis have accumulated, they cannot be viewed optimistically, as little data have surfaced to link these compounds directly with schizophrenia.

Major support for the transmethylation hypothesis comes from reports of abnormal tolerance of schizophrenic patients to oral loading of the methyl donor, L-methionine, as discussed above. Although the metabolic basis for this observation has not been well studied, it was proposed that the clinical symptoms result from increased dimethylation and production of compounds formed from methionine methyl transfer. Studies in animals, however, fail to show increases in methylated catecholamines or indoleamines after administration of large doses of L-methionine or its metabolite, S-adenosyl-methionine (SAM). Methionine loading in animals was also found to decrease, rather than increase, the formation of N-methyl-tryptamine, the direct precursor of DMT, one of the proposed endogenous hallucinogens. Furthermore, there is no evidence that clinical exacerbation of schizophrenia produced by methionine is associated with blood or urinary dimethyl amines.

The transmethylation hypothesis led to a search for methylated endogenous hallucinogens in the 1960s and 1970s. The status of these compounds is reviewed below. Much of this research has not progressed further due to inadequacies in technology, inconsistent results among investigators, and disillusionment with the apparent oversimplicity of this hypothesis.

DIMETHOXYPHENYLETHYLAMINE (DMPEA) Consistent with the transmethylation hypothesis were the reports that DMPEA was present in urine samples from the majority of schizophrenic patients and not from controls. Referred to as *the pink spot* because of its staining properties when appropriate reagents are added to urine, DMPEA was extensively investigated, although a psychotomimetic effect was never demonstrated. Furthermore, other experiments failed to demonstrate synthesis of DMPEA in vivo. Numerous studies subsequent to this initial report failed to confirm differences between schizophrenic patients and controls. In fact, several studies suggested that DMPEA is of dietary origin rather than related to psychosis, although this was never definitively proven. In one experiment, a common brand of tea was suggested as a source of urinary DMPEA in normals. When the tea was eliminated from the diet, DMPEA was no longer detectable. Other investigators have claimed that the pink spot may actually be p-tyramine, that it contains monoacetyl cadaverine, that it is the product of intestinal bacterial metabolism, or that it may be a metabolite of medication. (Friedhoff and co-workers found that it was detectable only in medication-free patients.) They abandoned this research when they were unable to find evidence for DMPEA production in vivo, despite the inability to establish a clear exogenous source. Whatever its origin, DMPEA does not appear to be related to the etiology of schizophrenia.

DIMETHYLTRYPTAMINE (DMT) DMT, when administered to normal volunteers, causes an acute transient psychosis. Although DMT has been found in human blood and urine, no consistent elevations have been found in either acute or chronic schizophrenic patients. The origin of DMT in these fluids has also been questioned. Although the presence of DMT could be explained by peculiarities in diet, the enzyme N-methyl transferase, presumed to be required for endogenous DMT production, has been demonstrated in human lung and brain. Conversion in vivo of [^{14}C]NMT to [^{14}C]DMT by this enzyme was also demonstrated in rabbit lung. In another study, ^{15}N, ^{13}C-tryptamine was administered to seven chronically hallucinating schizophrenic patients to demonstrate conversion in vivo of tryptamine to N-methyltryptamine (NMT, the precursor of DMT). No NMT was extracted from urine collected for 24 hours subsequent to the infusion, while virtually all the label was detected in the urine specimens as other unidentified substances. It is possible that urinary excretion is not representative of brain metabolism or that the NMT was further metabolized and, so, no longer detectable. Nevertheless, this experiment casts doubt on the significance of endogenous DMT production in schizophrenia. Difficulties in development of sensitive and specific assays for DMT have delayed further pursuit of this hypothesis.

BUFOTENINE Bufotenine is a dimethylated derivative of serotonin. Like DMT, bufotenine is methylated by a dimethyltransferase present in human brain. Several, but not all, investigators found bufotenine-like substances in urine from schizophrenic persons, and either absent or present in significantly lower amounts in urine from normal persons. Tanimukai and associates subsequently demonstrated that the acetone used in some of the assay procedures may have produced bufotenine-like substances. Some investigators have dismissed the importance of bufotenine as a dietary artifact or as the result of bacterial metabolism in the gut. When subjects were on plant- and cheese-free diets, bufotenine-like substances were not present in the urine. Bufotenine has not been shown to produce symptoms of schizophrenia when administered to humans.

THE FROHMAN FACTOR Frohman and colleagues isolated a protein from plasma of schizophrenic patients that they hypothesized is related to abnormal indole metabolism and the accumulation of DMT. The factor, which they named *the S-protein,* is an α_2 globulin. When isolated from plasma of schizophrenic patients, they hypothesized, the protein is in an active form (an α-helical configuration) and causes more tryptophan to accumulate in cells isolated from controls than the inactive form (a β-helix). They also found a high percentage of the α-helical molecule in plasma from normal volunteers under psychological stress. These studies have not been confirmed by others, and the properties of this protein have not been investigated further by Frohman and colleagues in recent years.

PHENYLETHYLAMINE (PEA) PEA, an endogenously produced decarboxylated metabolite of phenylalanine, is structurally and pharmacologically similar to amphetamine and has also been hypothesized to be an endogenous psychotomimetic compound in schizophrenia. Although PEA is not known as a hallucinogen, indirect support for putative hallucinogenic properties comes from its behavioral effects in animals. Stereotypies induced by both PEA and amphetamine in animals are blocked by neuroleptics.

Fisher was the first to report elevated urinary PEA excretion in psychiatric patients. Although several studies subsequently confirmed this finding, its significance remains unclear. Dietary differences, nonspecific stress, and other variables may be relevant to these data, and no evidence for the association of increased production of PEA with the production of psychotic symptoms has been demonstrated.

The contribution to schizophrenia of endogenous production of toxic agents with hallucinogenic properties remains unknown. Intriguing studies demonstrate poorer outcome for schizophrenic patients who do not receive medication subsequent to the appearance of the first symptoms of psychosis:

the longer the delay, the poorer the outcome. It is possible that production of toxic substances, such as these hallucinogenic agents, is suppressed by neuroleptic medication. The longer patients remain untreated, however, the longer toxic destruction of brain cells could continue.

CENTRAL NERVOUS SYSTEM PEPTIDES

It is only in recent years that attention has been focused on peptides, their functional role, and their location in the nervous system. Over 25 small peptides have been found in neurons. While many of these have classical hormonal functions, they may also have neurotransmitter activity. In the classical definition, for a substance to be considered a neurotransmitter, it must (1) be shown to be synthesized in the neuron; (2) be present at the presynaptic terminal and released in amounts sufficient to exert its action on the postsynaptic neuron; (3) activate the same ionic channels when applied to similar postsynaptic cells; and (4) have a specific mechanism for removal from the synaptic cleft. As most of the peptides have not yet been found to satisfy requirements necessary for the label of neurotransmitter and as much about their role in overall nerve function needs to be characterized, many investigators have coined the term "neuroregulators" to describe this group of peptides. They are of particular interest in studies of schizophrenia because several have been found within neurons that also contain monoamines. Some have been found to have properties similar to those of neuroleptics and to influence their action.

CHOLECYSTOKININ (CCK) The 33–amino acid gastrointestinal and brain peptide CCK is thought to play a role as a neuroregulator. In specific brain areas, it coexists with dopamine in neurons and is thought to act as a modulator of dopamine receptor activity. Three known forms of CCK have been isolated from brain: a tetrapeptide (CCK-4), an octapeptide (CCK-8), and a tritriacontapeptide (CCK-33). A deficiency in CCK could lead to an increase in dopaminergic function. Preliminary measurements of CCK in autopsy specimens from schizophrenic brains, using radioimmunoassays sensitive predominantly to CCK-8, have found abnormally low levels in the limbic systems in subgroups of schizophrenic patients. Crow and colleagues reported decreased postmortem CCK concentrations, specifically in the amygdala and hippocampus of chronic schizophrenic patients who, prior to death, were assessed as having predominantly defect symptoms. This finding was not present in acutely schizophrenic patients who had only productive symptoms. Temporal cortex CCK was reduced, as was high-affinity specific CCK binding in the frontal cortex and hippocampus, although not in the amygdala or temporal cortex. Despite these suggestions of reduced brain CCK and receptor binding, administration of ceruletide, a CCK derivative, has not produced significant clinical improvement in schizophrenic patients.

VASOACTIVE INTESTINAL PEPTIDE (VIP) VIP, another gastrointestinal peptide, has recently been of interest to brain researchers, although little is known of its role in neuromodulation. It has been studied in autopsied brains of schizophrenic patients by Crow and colleagues, and unlike CCK, VIP was found to be elevated in the amygdala of schizophrenic patients whose symptoms were predominantly productive. No abnormal VIP concentrations were observed in CSF of schizophrenic patients in other studies.

SOMATOSTATIN Somatostatin is a tetradecapeptide with extensive distribution in the CNS and gut. It appears to be co-localized in neurons with catecholamines and enzymes (GAD and acetylcholinesterase) involved in neurotransmitter metabolism. As a hypothalamic hormone, somatostatin inhibits the release of growth hormone from the pituitary. Its function as a neuroregulator is less well understood. Decreased CSF somatostatin has been found in patients with mood disorders and several neurodegenerative disorders but not schizophrenia in most studies. Unconfirmed reports exist of high CSF somatostatin and low somatostatin in the frontal cortex of schizophrenic patients' brains postmortem. In yet another study, no frontal cortex differences were noted, but a subgroup of deficit-symptom patients had reduced somatostatin in the hippocampus in addition to the previously mentioned decrease in CCK. Perhaps, this is a function of generalized atrophy rather than specific neuropeptide production abnormalities.

OPIOIDS (ENDORPHINS) AND THEIR PRECURSORS Opioids are present throughout the CNS. Those that occur naturally are called *endorphins* (endogenous morphine-like substances); at least nine substances isolated from brain or pituitary have opioid properties. These include the six structurally related peptides: dynorphin, two enkephalins, and α-, β-, and γ-endorphin. β-Endorphin, the most potent of the endogenous opioid agonists, is found in highest concentrations in the hypothalamus, pituitary, midbrain, pons, and medulla. It increases prolactin and growth hormone (GH) secretion while inhibiting the release of thyroid-stimulating hormone (TSH) and luteinizing hormone (LH) from the pituitary. It also can directly increase the formation of dopamine and serotonin precursors when injected intraventricularly. At least three opioid receptors have been identified based on different syndromes produced by their prototype drugs: morphine for the μ-receptor, ketocyclazozine for the κ-receptor, and N-allylnormetazozine for the δ-receptor.

Nalorphine and cyclazocine are opioid antagonists with κ- and δ-receptor effects. In normal persons, low doses of these drugs may produce racing thoughts, irritability, inability to concentrate (suggestive of δ-activity), and sedation and ataxia (suggestive of κ-activity). Delusions and hallucinations have been described with higher doses.

The notion that opioids may play a role in psychiatric disorders dates back to early reports of the use of morphine for the treatment of schizophrenia, and also the observation that schizophrenic patients appear to have reduced sensitivity to pain. The discovery of endogenous opioids and their receptors generated further hypotheses relating opioid activity to schizophrenia.

Two major proposals have been explored with respect to endogenous opioids and their role in schizophrenia. Bloom and colleagues proposed that an excess in central opioids, which induces catalepsy in rats, might have a role in the pathology of schizophrenia. At the same time, Jacquet and Marks speculated that β-endorphins may be of therapeutic benefit as neuroleptics, owing to their production of extrapyramidal effects in animals. Most subsequent clinical studies have attempted to test one of these opposing hypotheses.

Elevations of a variety of endogenous opioids have been detected in CSF, in dialysate, and in plasma from schizophrenic patients, although these have not been confirmed in other studies. Moreover, opioids were found to be reduced in at least one CSF study. In one study, postmortem, regional brain opioid concentration increases were found in putamen, and decreased concentrations were found in the caudate. In another study, no differences in opioid receptor binding were found. One study suggested that increased endorphin concentrations may be a neuroleptic effect unrelated to therapeutic efficacy of the drugs.

If an excess of opioids is related to schizophrenia, then an opioid antagonist, such as naloxone (Narcan) or naltrexone (Trexan), should alleviate some schizophrenic symptoms. In general, however, most one-time administration, double-blind studies of the administration of naloxone to schizophrenic patients have not found a benefit. Although there are some reports of improvement in subgroups of patients who had auditory hallucinations, improvement is usually seen at high dose levels, at which naloxone exerts both agonist and antagonist effects. Because of the high doses involved, it is possible that these effects of naloxone were mediated by nonopioid receptor–related mechanisms. Investigators who report improvement only when naloxone is administered with neuroleptic medication suggest that the improvement may be due to potentiation of the neuroleptics. In other studies, however, some medication-free patients did show improvement from naloxone.

One study is noteworthy. Watson and colleagues screened 1,000 hospitalized psychiatric patients and selected for naloxone injection those having at least two hallucinations per hour. The frequency of their hallucinations decreased with naloxone. Other studies using less rigorous criteria may have missed positive results because of the low numbers of patients, brief duration of the study, or difficulty in quantifying acute symptoms.

Naltrexone, whose opioid-antagonist properties are of longer duration, produced no observable clinical response in trials of up to 3 weeks' duration.

If an endorphin deficit is postulated, then therapeutic trials of endorphins are warranted. β-Endorphin administered to schizophrenic patients in open, single-injection trials was claimed to have an effect by Kline and associates. Only one double-blind trial produced positive results; others found no effect or exacerbation of symptoms with single and multiple injections of β-endorphin.

More hopeful results have been obtained with another endorphin, des-tyrosine-γ-endorphin, a fragment of the parent peptide, β-lipotropin. Its amino acid sequence is a subset of the β-endorphin sequence. In some, but not all, investigative trials, it was effective when administered to acutely psychotic individuals. In one report, the met-enkephalin analog, FK 33-824, was also found to reduce psychotic symptoms. γ-Endorphins produce behavioral effects that may not be initiated through opioid receptors, since their effects are not suppressed by opioid-receptor antagonists. They also appear to be more beneficial to acute schizophrenic patients early in their illness than in chronic schizophrenic patients but are clinically efficacious without concurrent neuroleptics. Although the methodology of these initial trials has been criticized, the results provide some hope for the future usefulness of this class of agents for certain schizophrenic patients and may, in additional trials, help clarify whether opioids have a role in the development of psychotic symptoms. Since opioid pathways in the brain are closely intertwined with those of the major neurotransmitters already discussed, particularly in the limbic and striatal systems, it is not surprising that abnormalities in this system also have been associated with schizophrenia. The defect in the opioid system could be due to a primary defect in catecholamine or indoleamine metabolism.

NEUROTENSIN Neurotensin, a tridecapeptide, coexists with catecholamines in neurons. Its numerous physiological actions include lowering of blood pressure and body temperature, potentiation of barbiturate-induced sleep, and stimulation of GH and prolactin release. The greatest concentrations are in the hypothalamus, nucleus accumbens, and septum. Increased brain neurotensin postmortem has been reported in the frontal cortex and hippocampus of schizophrenic subjects. CSF neurotensin was found to be low in medication-free schizophrenic persons and to return toward normal with neuroleptic treatment.

BOMBESIN Bombesin appears in highest brain concentrations in the hypothalamus. It is thought to play a role in satiety, pain, temperature control, regulation of digestion, and growth of malignant cells. It has received little attention in clinical studies, although one study reported lower CSF bombesin concentrations in schizophrenic patients than in controls.

GENERAL ASPECTS OF ENDOCRINE FUNCTION

As early as 1903, a report described amenorrhea during acute psychosis and return of normal menses as the illness resolved. In the 1920s, a number of investigators described gonadal atrophy in patients with dementia precox. More recently, as the specific mechanisms involved in hypothalamic-pituitary-endocrine organ function have been elucidated, interest has turned toward a broad range of neuroendocrine functions in schizophrenia.

GONADAL FUNCTION The postpubertal age of onset and apparent gender differences in the course of schizophrenia implicate gonadotropic hormones in schizophrenia. Early investigators reported gonadal atrophy, deficient secondary sex characteristics, and amenorrhea to be associated with psychosis, but these findings were not replicated by some later research. Early studies noted decreased urinary excretion of 17-ketosteroids. Other studies that followed serial excretion noted increased 17-ketosteroids during an exacerbation of psychosis, but in some cases the increase appeared to be linked to motor hyperactivity. Moreover, it is important to note that the excretion of 17-ketosteroids may be contributed to by the metabolism of corticosteroids as well as androgens. The androgen-estrogen ratio in male subjects was noted to be reduced in one early study, a finding not replicated by other investigators. Some studies found reduced plasma levels of the metabolite dihydroepiandrosterone (DHEA) in patients having chronic schizophrenia. Insofar as testicular hormonal function appeared to be normal in these subjects, however, the deficit may have been in adrenal function. In spite of clinical observations regarding perimenstrual exacerbations of psychosis, postpartum psychoses, and the later age of onset for females, no abnormalities in progesterone, estrogens, or metabolites have been delineated in schizophrenia.

Given these equivocal endocrine findings, it is not surprising that early clinical trials of testosterone and gonadotrophin in schizophrenia were unsuccessful. Treatment with DHEA in the 1950s appeared to yield some improvement in patients with prominent negative symptoms, but that finding was never replicated. Treatment with estrogen and related compounds has not been reported to be of benefit.

PITUITARY FUNCTION Baseline levels of follicle-stimulating hormone (FSH) and luteinizing hormone (LH) have been reported to be low in schizophrenia, and disruption of normal episodic LH release was noted. In addition, a study of response to gonadotropin-releasing hormone showed blunting in the response of FSH but not LH. These abnormalities are consistent with clinical observations of reduced fertility and an increased rate of spontaneous abortion for women with schizophrenia.

Growth hormone (GH) release from the anterior pituitary is regulated by GH–releasing factor and somatostatin. To date, no clear abnormalities in baseline GH function have been reported in schizophrenia.

Perhaps the most extensively studied aspect of endocrine function in schizophenia has been prolactin secretion. Dopamine has long been known to inhibit prolactin secretion from the anterior pituitary. This, in turn, means that plasma prolactin concentrations could serve as an indirect indicator of CNS dopaminergic function or as an index of dopamine receptor blockade when patients are treated with neuroleptics. Numerous investigations of prolactin secretion in schizophrenia have been conducted in an attempt to examine the dopamine hypothesis. Some studies have noted an inverse correlation between psychotic symptoms and prolactin, and others have reported that low prolactin may be predictive of a higher likelihood of clinical relapse. Although some controversy remains, however, it appears that baseline prolactin secretion in schizophrenia is probably normal and that normal and schizophrenic subjects manifest similar increases in the level of prolactin in response to neuroleptics.

Although no abnormality of antidiuretic hormone (ADH, vasopressin), a posterior pituitary hormone, has been documented in schizophrenia, a number of therapeutic trials of vasopressin and analogs (such as 1-desamino-8-D-arginine vasopressin) were conducted; some therapeutic effects were noted. The major benefits appeared to be in the area of negative symptoms, such as withdrawal and emotional blunting. Oxytocin, another posterior pituitary hormone, has been studied in the Soviet Union. Definitive controlled trials of these hormones as therapeutic agents have yet to be conducted.

THE PINEAL GLAND The pineal gland is the site of synthesis of the hormone melatonin from serotonin by N-acetylation and 5-O-methylation. The primary regulation of melatonin synthesis occurs via the light-dark cycle. In response to the hypothesis that a defect in melatonin synthesis would increase melanin production (and the observation of hyperpigmentation in schizophrenic patients), investigators have posited pineal dysfunction as a possible factor in schizophrenia. As early as 1920, patients were reportedly successfully treated with beef pineal extracts. Subsequent studies reported similar improvement, but the use of crude preparations and lack of appropriate controls compromise these findings.

ADRENAL FUNCTION Both excess adrenocortical hormones (Cushing's syndrome) and insufficient secretion (Addison's disease) are in some cases associated with psychotic symptoms. There has been a surge of recent interest in the dexamethasone suppression test (DST), in which suppression of plasma cortisol in response to administration of a synthetic glucocorticoid is measured. Nonsuppression has been associated primarily with depression, but it is clear that approximately 13 percent of nondepressed patients with schizophrenia also have abnormal DST results. It may be a nonspecific result of the stress associated with acute psychosis or hospitalization.

THYROID FUNCTION Severe thyroid dysfunction may be associated with psychotic symptoms, as exemplified by the term "myxedema madness." A number of early reports cited thyroid abnormalities in schizophrenia. Trials in the 1920s and 1930s reported some benefit following administration of thyroid hormone to schizophrenic patients. The release of TSH is regulated by thyroid-releasing hormone (TRH); both, in turn, appear to be inhibited by dopamine. One group found low plasma TSH and thyroxine levels in schizophrenic patients. The TSH response to TRH administration was abnormal in one study while another found no blunting of TSH response to TRH. A few trials treating schizophrenia with synthetic TRH have shown improvement, particularly in negative symptoms; benefit was even greater when the TRH was combined with a neuroleptic.

NEUROLEPTIC EFFECTS Significant effects of neuroleptics on general endocrine function have been described. Galactorrhea and amenorrhea are common side effects of neuroleptics. In females, the results of studies are somewhat inconsistent, but neuroleptics may lower estrogen and urinary gonadotropic hormone concentrations. In males, they may cause slight reductions in testosterone, FSH, and LH, although other studies have reported normal baseline LH and FSH levels during drug treatment. Gonadotropic hormonal abnormalities appear to be more pronounced with low-potency neuroleptics. Neuroleptics may also influence baseline concentrations of GH and the response to insulin. In addition, neuroleptics have been implicated in the syndrome of inappropriate ADH secretion, which is felt to be a factor in some cases of polydipsia and hyponatremia in chronic schizophrenic patients. These interactions between neuroleptics and hormonal systems certainly have the potential for complicating any attempts to study neuroendocrine parameters in patients with schizophrenia, unless those patients have been subjected to an extended period of abstention from medication.

VIRAL AND AUTOIMMUNE HYPOTHESES OF SCHIZOPHRENIA

Even if schizophrenia proves to involve a dysregulation of central dopamine or some other biochemical or endocrine function, the etiology of that dysregulation would have to be determined. A primary focus in schizophrenia research has been the possible interaction between genetic and environmental factors. It is believed that an environmental insult such as a toxin, pre- or perinatal injury, or infection might, in a genetically susceptible person, cause schizophrenia. A significant effort has been devoted to specifically examining the possibility that the ultimate cause of schizophrenia may be a viral infection or an autoimmune response (perhaps triggered by an infection.)

VIRAL HYPOTHESIS Although the idea that psychosis might be contagious or epidemic was advanced in the nineteenth century, the possibility of a viral etiology for schizophrenia was first presented convincingly in the 1920s by Karl Menninger, who noted that psychoses clinically resembling dementia precox were associated with the influenza pandemics that occurred early in this century. It has now become clear that a number of viral encephalitides may present schizophreniform symptoms, including acquired immunodeficiency syndrome (AIDS) encephalitis caused by the human immunodeficiency virus (HIV), a retrovirus. Given that viruses can cause psychotic symptoms and that they also may interact directly with genes (in the case of retroviruses, they are actually integrated into the host genome), it is reasonable to hypothesize that some cases of schizophrenia may have a viral etiology. Some indirect evidence derived from epidemiology, serology, and neuropathology supports this hypothesis.

Epidemiological evidence A distinct pattern of seasonality of birth is one of the clinical facts of schizophrenia; a disproportionate number of patients are born in late winter and early spring, perhaps implicating pre- or perinatal viral infection in some cases of schizophrenia.

Although the geographic distribution of schizophrenia is usually described as being constant worldwide, there are clear pockets of higher prevalence (northern Sweden, western Ireland, Croatia) and lower prevalence (Micronesia, Papua-New Guinea).

Although family data are usually advanced to support the role of genetic factors in schizophrenia, such data also lend some credence to the viral hypothesis as close and prolonged contact may enhance horizontal transmission. The concordance rate for schizophrenia appears to be higher in dizygotic twins than in siblings and higher in same-sex dizygotic twins than in opposite-sex dizygotic twins. Since genes are shared to the same extent in all such cases, it appears that physical proximity may be a factor. Data on the age of onset in siblings with schizophrenia do not support the idea of contagion occurring near the age of onset; but the point of transmission may be in utero, a possibility that is more consistent with the seasonality of births.

Neuropathological evidence The first postmortem neuropathological studies of schizophrenia, conducted over a century ago, failed to discover a pathognomonic lesion. Despite methodological problems in the preparation and examination of brain tissue, several investigators did observe subtle structural changes. Early reports were qualitative and cited cortical neuronal dysmorphism and, in some cases, gliosis. More recent studies using quantitative techniques have focused more on limbic-diencephalic areas, and some have noted decreased volume of periventricular structures. These studies showing morphological changes are consistent with data obtained via pneumonencephalography, CT scans, and magnetic resonance imaging that have emphasized findings of lateral ventricular enlargement and cortical atrophy in some cases of schizophrenia. Thus, although no definitive lesion has been identified, postmortem neuropathology and brain imaging have presented convincing evidence that schizophrenia does involve subtle structural pathology. Neuropathological changes (including ventricular enlargement, neuronal dysmorphism, and gliosis) may also be observed in association with congenital or acquired CNS viral infections.

Serological evidence To implicate viruses more directly in schizophrenia, a number of investigators have turned to studies of the immune response, in particular, the identification of virus-specific antibodies. Cytomegalovirus (CMV), an agent of the herpes class known to be neurotropic, has received special attention. Some investigators report relative increases in the ratio of CSF to serum anti-CMV antibodies as well as increased CSF anti-CMV immunoglobulin M (IgM). Others have failed to replicate this finding. Similarly inconclusive findings have resulted from studies of other neurotropic viruses. Study of virus-specific antibodies is complicated by the fact that increased levels may result from factors other than viral infection (e.g., antibodies against herpes simplex virus may be produced by activated lymphocytes following cerebral infarction). Other data indicate that some schizophrenic patients have a disrupted blood–brain barrier that may, in turn, increase intrathecal antibody concentrations.

Transmission experiments Another approach to the viral hypothesis is to attempt to transmit the unknown infectious agent. One group of researchers reported that CSF from patients with schizophrenia produced cytopathic effects in tissue culture. The researchers were unable to serially passage or further characterize a replicating agent, and these cytopathic effects have not been replicated consistently by other groups. One study reported that injection of CSF from schizophrenic patients into marmosets caused subtle behavioral changes in the animals after a latency period of 2 to 3 years. A similar transmission experiment involving several different species was not successful—but it used brain tissue rather than CSF.

IMMUNE FUNCTION IN SCHIZOPHRENIA It is possible that immune dysfunction may exist in schizophrenia independently of a viral infection, possibly as a result of other chemical or endocrine defects in neuroregulation. At the turn of this century, some observers noted a relative leukocytosis in acute phases of the disorder, although this may have reflected undiagnosed infections or other factors. More recently, subpopulations of lymphocytes have been studied. Preliminary findings have included increased B-cells, decreased T-cells, and both increases and decreases in suppressor cell percentages. Some investigators have noted increased numbers of atypical lymphocytes on peripheral smears, although this has not been replicated by others. Analyses in vitro of lymphocyte function have noted deficiencies in cellular responsiveness, deficits that have also been observed when normal persons are stressed. The phenomena, therefore, may not be specific.

In addition to abnormalities in cellular immune function, a number of studies have indicated either increases or decreases in levels of IgA, IgG, and IgM in blood and CSF. One report indicated an increase in the index of CSF to serum IgG in one-third of the schizophrenic patients examined, although another group did not find any increase. The inconsistencies in observations regarding both cell-mediated immunity and general immunoglobulin production may relate to a number of complicating variables, such as medication status, diagnostic subtype, age, gender, race, and genetic factors.

AUTOIMMUNE HYPOTHESIS Autoimmunity is a specific form of immune dysfunction that has been hypothesized by some to play a role in schizophrenia. Taraxein, a factor isolated from schizophrenic patients by a group of researchers in the 1960s, was postulated to be an autoantibody to brain tissue. The investigators' experiments indicated that it caused behavioral and EEG changes when injected into animals. Attempts to replicate this work produced mixed results. Subsequent studies using different methodological approaches have claimed to identify increased antibrain antibodies in schizophrenic patients, but no specific autoantibody has been isolated and characterized.

Another approach has been to inject intradermally a preparation of normal brain tissue into psychiatric or neurological patients. A delayed hypersensitivity reaction has been observed in both groups, suggesting prior sensitization to brain membrane proteins, probably the result of nonspecific neuronal injury. Similarly, a delayed hypersensitivity reaction to myelin basic protein has been observed in some patients, but it may be a response to nonspecific neurodegeneration. Antinuclear antibody titers are above normal in approximately 20 percent of psychiatric inpatients, but this finding is nonspecific and may relate to pharmacological treatment.

Although the autoimmune hypothesis has not been proven, the possibility remains that some cases of schizophrenia may involve an autoantibody, the production of which may initially be stimulated by a viral infection. This autoantibody, in turn, may damage neuronal tissue directly or may interact in a more subtle fashion with neurotransmitter receptors.

SYNTHESIS

It is worth reconsidering the "facts" set forth at the outset. Schizophrenia is a clinical syndrome without known causes. Although there appears to be a genetic predisposition, the mode of transmission is not known. Interactions of environmental forces on genetically vulnerable organisms may precipitate the disease, yet it is not certain whether either alone is sufficient to do so. The seasonality of birth phenomenon suggests the possibility for a role of seasonal environmental factors and is one of the strongest pieces of evidence in favor of involvement of a viral-like agent in schizophrenia.

A viral hypothesis of schizophrenia is not incompatible with the existence of some type of biochemical dysfunction. For example, monoamine metabolism in mouse brain has been shown to be altered by herpes simplex infection, although it can only be speculated as to which class (or classes) of viruses is likely to be involved. One hypothesis integrates genetic and viral etiologies by proposing a prominent role for retroviruses. Retroviruses are a special class of ribonucleic acid (RNA) viruses that carry the enzyme reverse transcriptase. Reverse transcriptase allows the viral RNA to be transcribed intracellularly into deoxyribonucleic acid (DNA), which then enters the host cell genome, transmitting the viral information. Retroviruses, by virtue of their infectious nature, may also exhibit characteristics of typical viral infection. The possibility that a viral infection is a pathogenic factor in schizophrenia, either by direct neuronal injury or stimulation of autoantibodies, certainly merits further exploration. The peak onset in early adulthood plus the illness course of exacerbations and recoveries, with some evidence of structural cerebral damage, are reminiscent of known neurotropic viruses that persist within neurons, periodically altering their function and causing cellular damage. Alternatively, they could be explained by periodic production of autoantibodies, like that occurring in autoimmune diseases. The genetic disorder, intermittent porphyria, could also be a model for a nonviral illness with similar exacerbations and remissions.

Gender differences and the peak age of onset should be further clues to the biochemical pathophysiology of the illness. The estrogen-testosterone differences between males and females may explain some of the differences in age of onset, outcome, and clinical features of schizophrenia between the genders. Studies of normal development show gender differences in the rate of brain growth and differentiation, as well as structural differences in specific parts of the adult brain, that may be produced in part by sex hormone regulation of brain growth. Brain development on a cellular and biochemical level may reach its peak in males in their early 20s and somewhat later in females.

In animal studies, some estrogens appear to have neuroleptic effects, and estrogens are known antagonists of D_2 dopamine receptors. Conversely, dopamine regulates the biological effects of estrogen by decreasing the binding of this hormone to its receptors. Some studies have also shown greater serotonergic activity in females. Surges in serotonin levels may actually initiate the onset of puberty by exerting a regulatory effect on steroid hormone production. Little is known of the possible effects of androgens on catecholamine and indoleamines. Testosterone may increase aggressiveness and, thus, could aggravate symptoms of psychosis. Perhaps these effects are enough to modify the expression of the primary pathogenic agent. The crucial factor initiating the schizophrenic process at this time, however, remains unknown, although it is likely that the interactions of steroid hormones with catecholamines and indoleamines play a role.

The peak age of onset of schizophrenia in the mid-20s may relate to peak changes in monoamines and receptor responsivity or other parallel neurochemical events that are modified by gonadal hormones. Onset may be related to a malfunction in neuroendocrine regulation at a time when hormone levels are peaking. Although there is some evidence for neuroendocrine dysfunction in schizophrenia, based on measurements of hypothalamic releasing hormones and postmortem studies of peptides, more investigation in pursuit of this hypothesis is needed. Alternatively, since age of onset has been found in several studies to be correlated among siblings with schizophrenia, age of onset may be genetically programmed or at least related to an incubation period subsequent to the earlier occurrence of an environmental event. An insult to the brain during crucial periods of embryonic and perinatal growth and differentiation may affect certain cells of the brain that have functions that are not expressed until early adulthood.

The overwhelming beneficial effect of neuroleptics in schizophrenia cannot be overlooked. Regardless of the original cause or causes of the illness, the biochemical outcome appears to be a perturbation of the dopamine neurotransmitter system. And although other biochemical alterations, including increased norepinephrine and serotonin, may also be present, none has been found sufficient to cause psychotic symptoms in isolation. It is clear, however, that none of these systems is operating in isolation, and that schizophrenia can no longer be regarded as one simple neurotransmitter defect.

The brain is a complex biochemical organ, with multiple anatomical as well as biochemical networks playing a final role in behavior. The more that can be learned about the role of each substance in normal neurophysiological function, and ultimately behavior, the more that will be understood of the mechanisms for neurobehavioral disorders.

REFERENCES

Babcock W L: A study of the urinalysis of 110 cases of insanity admitted to the Maryland Hospital for the Insane from November 1, 1892—October 31, 1893. Report from the Maryland Hospital for the Insane, no 55, Baltimore, 1892–3.

Bloom F, Segal D, Ling N, Guillemin R: Endorphins: Profound behavioral effects in rats suggest new etiological factors in mental illness. Science *194:* 630, 1976.

Carlsson A: Dopamine receptor agonists: Intrinsic activity vs. state of the receptor. J Neural Trans *57:* 309, 1983.

Carlsson A, Lindquist M: Effect of chlorpromazine and haloperidol on formation of 3-methoxytyramine and norepinephrine in mouse brain. Acta Pharmacol Toxicol *20:* 140, 1963.

Cooper J R, Bloom F E, Roth R H: *The Biochemical Basis of Neuropharmacology*. Oxford University Press, New York, 1986.

Creese I, Burt D R, Snyder S N: Dopamine receptor binding predicts clinical and pharmacological potencies of antischizophrenic drugs. Science *192:* 481, 1976.

Crow T J: Positive and negative schizophrenic symptoms and the role of dopamine. Brit J Psychiat *139:* 251, 1981.

DeLisi L E: Viral and immune hypotheses for schizophrenia. In *Psychopharmacology: Third Generation of Progress,* H Meltzer, editor, p 765. Raven Press, New York, 1987.

DeLisi L E, Wyatt R J: Neurochemical aspects of schizophrenia. In *Handbook of Neurochemistry,* A Lajtha, editor, vol 10, p 553. Plenum, New York, 1985.

Dohrenwend B P, Egri G: Recent stressful life events and episodes of schizophrenia. Schizophr Bull *7:* 12, 1981.

Kellogg T H: The toxic origin of insanity. J Nerv Ment Dis *19:* 742, 1892.

Mendelson W B, Gillin J C, Wyatt R J: Sexual physiology and schizophrenia. Acta Cient Venez *28:* 417, 1977.

Osmond H, Smythies J: Schizophrenia: A new approach. J Ment Sci *98:* 309, 1952.

Reinhard J R, Jr, Bannon M J, Roth R H: Acceleration of stress of dopamine synthesis and metabolism in prefrontal cortex. Naunyn-Schmiedebergs Arch Pharmacol *318:* 374, 1982.

Seeman M V: Symposium: Gender and schizophrenia. Can J Psychiat *30:* 311, 1985.

Usdin E, Hanin I, editors: *Biological Markers in Psychiatry and Neurology*. Pergamon, New York, 1982.

Woodrow K M, Reifman A, Wyatt R J: Amphetamine psychosis: A model for paranoid schizophrenia? In *Neuropharmacology and Behavior,* B Haber, M H Aprison, editors, p 1. Plenum, New York, 1978.

Wyatt R: The dopamine hypothesis: Variations on a theme. In *Research in the Schizophrenic Disorders: The Stanley R. Dean Award Lectures,* R Cancro, S R Dean, editors, vol 2, p 225. Spectrum, New York, 1985.

Wyatt R J, DeLisi L E, Jeste D V, Kleinman J E, Luchins D J, Potkin S G, Weinberger D R: Biochemical and morphological factors in schizophrenia. In *Psychiatry, 1982 Annual Review,* L Grinspoon, editor, p 112. American Psychiatric Association, Washington, DC, 1982.

Wyatt R J, Termini B A, Davis J: Biochemical and sleep studies of schizophrenia: A review of the literature 1960–1970. Part I: Biochemical studies. Schizophr Bull *4:* 10, 1971.

14.2c SCHIZOPHRENIA: GENETIC ETIOLOGICAL FACTORS

C. ROBERT CLONINGER, M.D.

INTRODUCTION

Although strong evidence for the importance of genetic factors in the development of schizophrenia has been obtained in family, twin, and adoption studies, only rare cases, associated with other specific neurological defects, show Mendelian patterns of inheritance. Many challenging questions remain about the clinical boundaries and mode of inheritance of the vast majority of schizophrenias; in particular, the type and number of genetic and environmental factors that influence the development of schizophrenia. Family, twin, and adoption studies provide rich information about the expression of genetic etiological factors in families of schizophrenic persons, which is crucial for understanding the etiology, natural history, and descriptive classification of schizophrenia.

Modern operational diagnostic criteria, such as the revised third edition of the *Diagnostic and Statistical Manual of Mental Disorders* (DSM-III-R), differ from the various clinical concepts used in older European family studies and in most twin and adoption studies of schizophrenic disorders. The third edition of the *Diagnostic and Statistical Manual of Mental Disorders* (DSM-III) and DSM-III-R criteria for schizophrenia correspond to narrow European criteria for nuclear, or process, schizophrenia. Less than 1 percent of persons in the general population satisfy such narrow definitions of schizophrenia. Broader concepts of probable or questionable schizophrenia, which have been fruitfully employed in many genetic studies, include schizophrenia-like (nonaffective) psychoses, in which persistent hallucinations or delusions occur in the absence of prominent affective symptoms. Such broadly defined schizophrenia-like psychoses occur in 1 percent to 2 percent of the general population. In DSM-III-R, such broadly defined groups of schizophrenia-like disorders include schizoaffective disorder, paranoid disorders, and possibly some cases of schizophreniform disorder and severe schizotypal personality disorder. Borderline or ambulatory nonaffective psychoses have been considered within broad concepts of schizophrenia-like psychoses and have been distinguished from personality disorders, such as schizoid personality. Borderline and uncertain psychoses were used as the criterion group in the development of criteria for schizotypal cases, but the DSM-III and DSM-III-R concept has been broadened to a personality disorder that includes cases that are clearly not psychotic. Accordingly, as many as 6 to 10 percent of the general population can satisfy criteria for probable schizotypal personality disorder. All these variations in classification of schizophrenia-like or schizotypal disorders require careful assessment of the natural boundaries of the clinical expression of schizophrenogenic factors and careful interpretation of results by investigators using different concepts and diagnostic criteria. In this section, care has been taken to distinguish among four levels of resemblance to schizophrenia: narrowly defined schizophrenia, corresponding to DSM-III-R schizophrenia and Scandinavian concepts of strict nuclear schizophrenia; broad but not narrow schizophrenia, corresponding to other nonaffective functional psychoses, such as borderline or uncertain schizophrenia-like psychoses like DSM-III-R schizoaffective and paranoid disorders and possibly some schizotypal disorders that have had probable or transient psychotic periods; schizoid, borderline, and schizotypal personality disorders that are clearly not psychotic; and other psychopathology.

With such uncertainty about the clinical boundaries of disorders related to schizophrenia, it is not surprising that the mode of inheritance of schizophrenic disorders remains uncertain. However, the uncertainty about mechanisms of inheritance also is attributable to the complexity of the inheritance pattern itself. Neither narrowly nor broadly defined schizophrenic disorders show a Mendelian pattern of inheritance. Studies of the monozygotic (MZ) co-twins of schizophrenics and of the relatives of MZ twins who are discordant for schizophrenia have clearly demonstrated that schizophrenogenic genotypes show incomplete penetrance (not everyone with the same genotype becomes ill) and variable clinical expression (those who become ill develop different clinical problems) so that the development of schizophrenia definitely depends on aspects of the environment or psychosocial experiences of the individual that have yet to be identified.

CLINICAL BOUNDARIES OF SCHIZOPHRENIC DISORDERS

MODERN FAMILY STUDIES OF SCHIZOPHRENIA Modern family studies employ rigorous methods of assessment to assure replicability of findings. Modern methods include blind assessment and inclusion of normal and psychiatric-patient control groups to avoid biased rating, use of operational diagnostic criteria and standardized interview schedules to increase reliability and replicability, and direct personal interviews of individual family members in addition to treatment records and other collateral information to maximize detection of psychopathology. Two recent studies —the Washington University Psychiatric Clinic Study and the University of Iowa Psychiatric Hospital Study—used diagnostic methods that permit comparison between DSM-III criteria and older European diagnostic concepts.

The Washington University (St. Louis) study involved a blind, prospective follow-up study of 500 randomly selected psychiatric outpatients over a period of 6 to 12 years. Personal interviews were also carried out with 1249 first-degree relatives of the probands by investigators with no knowledge of the proband's or other family members' psychopathology. Sixty-five probands were diagnosed as having chronic schizophrenia or a schizophrenia-like functional psychosis using criteria that correspond closely to those of DSM-III-R. The morbid risk of schizophrenia-like (nonaffective) psychoses is summarized in Table 14.2c-1, and the risks of other psychopathology are shown in Table 14.2c-2. Among the relatives of nonschizophrenic patients, the morbid risk of schizophrenia and schizophrenia-like psychoses was similar to that in the general population, suggesting that risk of schizophrenia is independent of nonschizophrenic psychopathology, such as major depressive disorder, alcoholism, personality disorders, and anxiety states, which affected this group of 435 psychiatric outpatients. In contrast, the risk of chronic schizophrenia was increased sixfold in the relatives of patients with either chronic schizophrenia (4.3 percent) or schizophrenia-like psychoses (3.9 percent) compared with the relatives of nonschizophrenics (0.7 percent). Likewise, the morbid risk of schizophrenia-like psychoses was increased three- to fourfold in the relatives of patients with schizophrenic disorders, so that the overall risk of nonaffective psychoses in the relatives of patients with schizophrenic disorders was 8 to 10 percent. However, there was no excess of other nonschizophrenic psychopathology in the relatives of patients with schizophrenic disorders (Table 14.2c-2). These findings show that schizophrenia and other nonaffective psychoses (but not other forms of psychopathology) aggregate in same families.

The University of Iowa studies included 253 schizophrenic probands diagnosed according to DSM-III criteria who could be compared to the relatives of 261 normal controls. Diagnosis of the probands was based on hospital records only, but relatives were also interviewed. This sample was large enough to subdivide the nonaffective psychoses, as shown in Table 14.2c-3. The morbid risks of schizophrenia (3.7 percent) and of schizophrenia-like psychoses (4.1 percent [7.8–3.7 percent]) in the relatives of schizophrenic probands is similar to that observed in St. Louis. The risk of schizophre-

TABLE 14.2c-1
Morbid Risk of Nonaffective Psychoses in Blindly Interviewed First-Degree Relatives of Schizophrenic Patients and Other Psychiatric Outpatients: Washington University Psychiatric Clinic Study*

	No. of Relatives		*Nonaffective Psychoses in Relatives (%)*		
Proband's Diagnosis	*(N)*	*(BZ)*	Schizophrenia	Other	Total
Schizophrenia (*N* = 44)	111	92.5	4.3†	5.4†	9.7†
Other nonaffective psychoses (*N* = 21)	62	51.5	3.9‡	3.9	7.8‡
All others (*N* = 435)	1,076	840	0.71	1.43	2.14

Table adapted from Guze S B, Cloninger C R, Martin R L, Clayton P J: A follow-up and family study of schizophrenia. Arch Gen Psychiat *40:* 1273, 1983, with permission.
*Schizophrenia was diagnosed according to DSM-III-R criteria. Nonaffective psychoses include disorders in which persistent hallucinations or delusions occurred in the absence of prominent affective symptoms, including DSM-III-R schizoaffective disorder, paranoid disorders, and chronic atypical cases, but not schizophreniform disorder. The total number (*N*) of relatives was age-corrected by the Weinberg shorter method, counting nonschizophrenic relatives who were 15 to 39 years of age at halfway through the risk period on average. The morbid risk is the cumulative lifetime expectancy of becoming ill, computed as the number of affected relatives divided by the bezugsziffer (*BZ*, age-corrected number of complete lifetimes at risk).
†Schizophrenic patients had significantly more ill relatives ($p < .01$) than did nonschizophrenic patients.
‡Other nonaffective psychotics had significantly more ill relatives ($p < .02$) than did nonschizophrenic patients.

TABLE 14.2c-2
Nonschizophrenic Disorders in the Blindly Interviewed First-Degree Relatives of Schizophrenic Patients and Other Outpatients

		Nonschizophrenic Disorders in Relatives			
Proband's Diagnosis	*No. of Relatives*	*Bipolar Affective Disorder*	*Primary Unipolar Disorder*	*Other Psychiatric Disorder*	*No Psychiatric Disorder*
Schizophrenia (*N* = 44)	111	0	2.7	27.9	61.3
Other nonaffective psychoses (N = 21)	62	0	8.1	30.6	55.6
All others (*N* = 435)	1,076	1.1	5.7	37.2	54.3

Table adapted from Guze S B, Cloninger C R, Martin R L, Clayton P J: A follow-up and family study of schizophrenia. Arch Gen Psychiat *40:* 1273, 1983, with permission.

TABLE 14.2c-3
Morbid Risk for Nonaffective Psychoses in Blindly Rated First-Degree Relatives of 253 Schizophrenic Patients and 261 Surgical Control Patients Screened to Exclude Psychopathology University of Iowa Studies*

	Morbid Risks of Relatives				
	Schizophrenics (N = 723)		*Controls (N = 1056)*		*Statistical Significance*
Relative's Diagnosis	*(A/BZ)*	*(%)*	*(A/BZ)*	*(%)*	*(p)*
Schizophrenia	26/703	3.7	2/931	0.2	< .01
Other nonaffective psychosis					
Schizophreniform	1/691	0.1	0/900	0.0	NS
Schizoaffective	8/559	1.4	1/676	0.1	< .01
Paranoid	5/538	0.9	0/577	0.0	< .02
Atypical	14/559	2.5	2/676	0.3	< .01
Total nonaffective psychoses	54/691	7.8	5/900	0.6	< .01

Table adapted from Kendler K S, Gruenberg A M, Tsuang M T: Psychiatric illness in first-degree relatives of schizophrenic and surgical control patients: A family study using DSM-III criteria. Arch Gen Psychiat *42:* 770, 1985.
*Diagnoses were independently reassessed by Kendler et al, 1985, using DSM-III criteria. The morbid risk is the cumulative lifetime expectancy computed as the number affected (*A*) over the bezugsziffer (*BZ*, age-corrected number of lifetimes at risk).

nia-like psychoses in the relatives of controls screened to insure normalcy is lower than expected in the general population (0.6 percent). The excess of schizophrenia-like psychoses in the relatives of schizophrenic patients is due to chronic disorders in which there are persistent hallucinations or delusions (such as schizophrenia, schizoaffective, and paranoid disorders), not acute psychoses, such as schizophreniform disorder.

There is no excess of schizophrenia in the relatives of most manics and unipolar depressives (Table 14.2c-4). In the Iowa study, there was a trend suggesting a slight increase in risk of bipolar affective disorder in the relatives of schizophrenic patients, but this was not replicated in the Washington University study. This suggests that patients with chronic mania are sometimes misdiagnosed as schizophrenics or that there is a small subgroup of schizophrenia with mania-like features, because manic probands do not have an excess of schizophrenic relatives.

EARLY EUROPEAN FAMILY STUDIES The familial aggregation of schizophrenic disorders in "blind" family studies using rigorous assessment methods is remarkably similar to earlier findings in older "nonblind" European family studies that used Kraepelinian diagnostic concepts. For example, in 1916, Ernst Rüdin worked with Kraepelin in Munich on a family study of patients with dementia precox who would now be called schizophrenic. Among 701 sibs of schizophrenic patients, where neither parent had schizophrenia, Rüdin found that 4.5 percent had schizophrenia and another 4.1 percent had other schizophrenia-like psychoses. When one parent was schizophrenic, 6.2 percent of the sibs had schizophrenia and 10.3 percent had other schizophrenia-like psychoses.

Morbid risks of schizophrenia-like (nonaffective) psychoses in earlier European studies are summarized in Table 14.2c-5. The risks to sibs and children of schizophrenics increase when two parents are schizophrenic. This pattern is evidence of vertical inheritance, from parent to child, as in genetic transmission but not in all forms of familial aggregation. The risk to parents is lower than the risk to children, which would be inconsistent with genetic inheritance unless schizophrenic persons tend to have fewer children. In 1955, Essen-Möller observed that schizophrenic patients had few or no children after the onset of their illness; he showed that if the risk of schizophrenia is considered to begin with the birth of their offspring, instead of their own birth, then the morbid risk of schizophrenia in parents increases to 11 percent. Thus, after taking fertility into account, the risk of schizophrenia-like psychoses is about 10 percent overall for all classes of first-degree relatives. (In other words, the risk in parents is too low [5 percent] compared with other first-degree relatives [children, sibs]—which is about 10 percent—because schizophrenic persons have few children after the onset of their illness. Therefore, if the risk in parents is corrected for low fertility after onset of illness, the risk in parents is about 10 percent, like other first-degree relatives.)

When both parents are schizophrenic, the risk in the children is 33.9 percent for schizophrenia and 43.3 percent for all

TABLE 14.2c-4
Schizophrenia, Mania, and Depression in the Blindly Interviewed First-Degree Relatives of Probands from the University of Iowa Psychiatric Hospital*

		Morbid Risks in Relatives by Diagnosis					
		Schizophrenia		*Bipolar Affective*		*Unipolar Affective*	
Proband's Diagnosis	*No. of Relatives*	*(A/BZ)*	*(%)*	*(A/BZ)*	*(%)*	*(A/BZ)*	*(%)*
Schizophrenia	354	11/346	3.2[†]	5/273	1.8[‡]	14/273	5.1
Mania	216	2/204	1.0	3/160	1.9	18/160	11.3
Depression	467	4/435	0.9	3/341	0.9	41/34	12.0[†]
Control	541	3/473	0.6	1/344	0.3	25/344	7.3

Table adapted from Tsuang M T, Winokur G, Crowe R R: Morbidity risks of schizophrenia and affective disorders among first-degree relatives of patients with schizophrenia, mania, depression, and surgical conditions. Brit J Psychiat *137:* 497, 1980.
*Probands included 200 schizophrenics, 100 manics, and 225 depressives and a control group of 160 matched for age, sex, and economic status and screened to exclude psychopathology.
[†]The designated morbid risk is higher than in controls ($p < .05$).
[‡]There is a trend for the designated morbid risk to be higher than in controls ($.05 < p < .10$).

schizophrenia-like psychoses (Table 14.2c-6). The risk of schizophrenia varies from 22.9 to 51.9 percent across six studies. The fact that all the children are not schizophrenic has been taken as evidence against the simple environmentalist hypothesis that schizophrenia involves imitation of parental deviance. It is also inconsistent with schizophrenia being caused by a single Mendelian recessive gene, because children of two homozygous parents would all be schizophrenic.

The studies of matings of two psychotic parents have also provided strong evidence for the specificity of familial predisposition to different types of psychosis. The most recent study, by Kringlen in Norway, is summarized in Table 14.2c-7, and similar results were obtained in the other dual mating studies. If schizophrenia and manic depressive disorders were different poles along a continuum of psychosis, matings between opposite types (e.g., schizophrenic with manic-depressive) might be expected to produce intermediate forms; also, matings between two persons with mild forms of disease would probably produce an increase in risk of severe forms (e.g., two manic parents increase risk for schizophrenia and for milder forms). In fact, the dual matings produce children with the same type of disorder as their parents: Children with schizophrenia occurred only in families with at least one schizophrenic parent, and there is no increase in intermediate forms when parents have different types of psychosis.

TABLE 14.2c-5
Morbid Risks of Nonaffective Psychosis in First-Degree Relatives of Schizophrenic Persons: Summary of European Studies by Family Configuration

	Morbid Risk of Nonaffective Psychosis		
Relationship and Family Configuration	*No. of studies*	*(A/BZ)*	*(%)*
Parents	14	447/8020	5.6
Sibling			
Neither parent schizophrenic	9	698/7264	9.6
One or both parents schizophrenic	5	104/624	16.7
Children			
One or both parents schizophrenic	7	202/1577	12.8
Both parents schizophrenic	6	69/160	43.3

Table updated and adapted from Gottesman I I, Shields J, Hanson D R: *Schizophrenia: The Epigenetic Puzzle.* Cambridge University Press, New York, 1982.

Even within schizophrenia, there is a moderate tendency toward homotypical transmission of catatonic, hebephrenic, and paranoid subtypes. Earlier evidence of this by Kallman has recently been confirmed by Scharfetter and Nüsperli in Switzerland. They studied a heterogeneous group of 269 patients with functional psychosis, and diagnoses of probands and relatives were made independently. The morbid risk of a schizophrenic disorder was 8.9 percent in the 726 first-degree relatives of 140 patients with schizophrenic disorders, so a broad concept of schizophrenia seems to have been used (diagnoses were based on the International Classification of Diseases). Most importantly, 68 percent of the 40 schizophrenic relatives had the same subtype as the proband. In 1938, Kallman had found that 53 percent of 111 children of schizophrenic persons had the same subtype as the parent. However, both studies found that all three subtypes occurred in the relatives of probands with each type, so these subgroups of schizophrenic persons cannot be considered to be genetically distinct. Furthermore, the familial factors that influence subtype expression may be different from those that determine susceptibility to schizophrenia.

GENETIC AND ENVIRONMENTAL FACTORS IN SCHIZOPHRENIC TWINS

SAMPLING FRAMES Many ingenious observations about twins provide important conclusions about the interaction of genetic and environmental factors in the development of schizophrenia. These observations have been replicated in independent investigations by investigators with widely varying genetic and environmental hypotheses about the etiology of schizophrenia, so the findings are a reliable basis for future work. Early twin investigations studied hospital-based series of twins treated for schizophrenia. Such treatment-based identification leads to a bias toward identification of more severe cases and concordant pairs, which are not representative of schizophrenia in the general population. More recently, it has been possible to carry out studies in Scandinavian countries that have national registers that permit studies based on the total population, which largely confirm the earlier findings. The findings of these recent population-based studies will be emphasized here, but pertinent findings from earlier hospital-based series will also be noted.

TABLE 14.2c-6
Morbid Risk of Schizophrenic Disorders in Children of Two Schizophrenic Parents: Summary of Six Series

Investigator	No. of Families	No. of Offspring	Schizophrenia (A/BZ*)	Schizophrenia (%)	? Schizophrenia (A/BZ)	? Schizophrenia (%)
Kahn, 1923	8	17	7/13.5	51.9	2/13.5	14.8
Kallman, 1938	12	35	13/27.5	47.3	3/27.5	10.9
Schulz, 1940	23	58	13/44.5	29.2	5/44.5	11.2
Elsässer, 1952	15	56	12/39.5	30.4	3/39.5	7.6
Lewis, 1957	7	27	4/17.5	22.9	0/17.5	0.0
Kringlen, 1978	8	25	5/17.0	29.4	2/17.0	11.8
Total	73	218	54/159.5	33.9	15/159.5	9.4

Table updated and adapted from Erlenmeyer-Kimling L: Studies on the offspring of two schizophrenic parents. In *The Transmission of Schizophrenia,* D Rosenthal, S Kety, editors. Pergamon Press, Oxford, 1968.
*Age-adjusted lifetimes at risk (*BZ*) computed by Weinberg short method with risk period from 15 to 44 years. Borderline and questionable cases of nonaffective psychosis are designated as ? schizophrenia.

MONOZYGOTIC CO-TWINS OF SCHIZOPHRENIC PERSONS MZ twins are genetically identical, so differences between MZ co-twins must be due to prenatal or postnatal environmental influences. Studies of the MZ co-twins of schizophrenic persons allow direct assessment of the clinical adjustment of persons who have the same genotype as others who are schizophrenic. If co-twins are not all schizophrenic, then genetic factors are not sufficient causes of schizophrenia. If some or all the co-twins may be normal, then environmental factors must be involved in one of two ways: Some environmental events may be sufficient causes of some cases of schizophrenia; in other words, there are sporadic cases of schizophrenia in which special genetic susceptibility factors are unnecessary (for example, schizophrenia that is symptomatic of poorly controlled epilepsy or brain damage involving the dominant temporal lobe). Alternatively, some environmental events may be necessary for the clinical expression of latent genetic susceptibility factors; in other words, there is incomplete penetrance of schizophrenogenic genotypes and gene-environment interaction so that environmental factors exert an influence only on persons with certain susceptible genotypes.

The actual findings in the three available population-based studies of MZ twins are summarized in Table 14.2c-8. The co-twins have a marked excess of schizophrenic disorders over that in the general population, but from 31 to 59 percent of the co-twins are clinically healthy, or normal. The frequency of 59 percent normals in the Finnish study by Tienari may be an overestimate for several reasons. Data about nonpsychotic psychopathology has been published only for the 17 pairs, including three pairs in which the proband had a schizophreniform or schizophrenia-like psychosis, not strict schizophrenia (as tabulated for the Norwegian and Danish studies). Details about nonpsychotic psychopathology is available only in a 1968 study in which there were four "borderline" co-twins; Slater and Shields considered one of these to be a questionable schizophrenic and listed that person's disease as "other psychosis." One other co-twin became schizophrenic by 1971 according to Tienari, so here that schizophrenic person is conservatively assumed to have been one of the other borderlines. Tienari describes six of the co-twins as healthy introverts, so they are listed as normal rather than schizoid. Also, three pairs were added in 1971, one concordant and two discordant for schizophrenia, so the two discordant co-twins are conservatively assumed to have been normal. Nevertheless, details about the other two series are clear, and more than 30 percent of the co-twins are normal in each series. Fischer followed the discordant pairs for an average of more than 24 years after onset of disease in the proband and found that "there were no schizoid personality traits" noted in the cases that she classified as normal. Therefore, it can be confidently concluded that genetic factors are not sufficient causes of schizophrenia and that schizophrenogenic genotypes have a wide range of clinical expression that depends on prenatal or postnatal environmental events.

Information about MZ co-twins alone does not permit a distinction between sporadic cases and incomplete penetrance. This distinction can be evaluated directly in two ways: (1) comparison of concordant and discordant MZ pairs for the morbid risk of schizophrenia in their parents and sibs and (2) comparison of the morbid risk of schizophrenia in the children of schizophrenic persons and in the children of their normal MZ co-twins. If many schizophrenic persons are sporadic cases, then discordant pairs should have fewer schizophrenic relatives than concordant pairs. In contrast, if discordant MZ pairs are usually caused by incomplete penetrance, then there will be no differences in the risk of illness among their relatives. In fact, early work by Kallmann has been confirmed by each of the three recent Scandinavian studies, showing that the morbid risk of schizophrenia is the same in the first-degree relatives of MZ twin pairs who are concordant or discordant for schizophrenia themselves. In addition, two studies are now available about the children of the normal MZ co-twins of schizophrenic persons (Table 14.2c-9). Combining the two small series with no age correction, the children

TABLE 14.2c-7
Type of Psychosis in Offspring of Two Psychotic Parents in Norway

Parental Psychoses	No. of Couples	No. of Offspring	No. of Psychotic Offspring (Sz)	(R)	(Md)	(Su)	(Bd)
Sz × Sz	8	25	5	1			1
Sz × R	20	42	3	1			3
Sz × Md	6	12	2				
Md × R	4	9			1		
R × R	9	28		1		1	1
Md × Md	1	5					
Total	48	121	10	3	1	1	5

Table adapted from Kringlen E: Adult offspring of two psychotic parents, with special reference to schizophrenia. In *The Nature of Schizophrenia: New Approaches to Research and Treatment,* L C Wynne, R L Cromwell, S Matthysse, editors, p 9. Wiley, New York, 1978.
Key: *Sz* = schizophrenia, *R* = reactive psychosis, *Md* = manic-depressive, *Su* = suicide, *Bd* = borderline.

TABLE 14.2c-8
Psychiatric Adjustment of MZ Co-Twins of Schizophrenic Persons in Population-Based Studies in Scandinavia

	Co-Twins by Investigator (%)			
MZ Co-Twin's Diagnosis	*Kringlen* (*N* = 45)	Tienari (*N* = 17)	Fischer (*N* = 21)	Total (*N* = 83)
Schizophrenia	31	18	24	27
Other nonaffective psychosis	2	6	24	8
Nonpsychotic schizoid or borderline	7	12	15	7
Other psychopathology	29	6	5	18
Normal	31	59*	43	40

(Data from Kringlen, 1968; Tienari, 1971; and Fischer, 1973)
*The 10 normal co-twins in Tienari's series include six he rated as "healthy introverts."

of the normal co-twins have a risk of schizophrenia (7.8 percent) that is 38 percent lower than that of the children of the schizophrenic co-twin (12.5 percent). However, the difference in these small numbers is not significant, and Fischer's age-corrected risks suggest no difference at all. Given findings by Kringlen and others that there is no difference in the risk of schizophrenia in the relatives of concordant and discordant MZ pairs, it must be concluded that schizophrenogenic genotypes are often incompletely penetrant. Furthermore, after overt symptomatic cases of brain damage are excluded, covertly sporadic cases of schizophrenia are infrequent.

COMPARISON OF MONO- AND DIZYGOTIC TWIN CONCORDANCES MZ twins are genetically identical, but dizygotic (DZ) twins share half their genes on average and, so, are no more alike than single-born siblings. Since twins are the same age regardless of zygosity, comparisons of MZ and DZ pairs provide a test of the relative importance of genetic and environmental contributions. If familial environmental factors are either unimportant or equally important in MZ and DZ twins, the differences between MZ and DZ twins must be entirely caused by genetic differences. This assumption about familial environmental factors has been supported by adoption studies of MZ co-twins and children of schizophrenic parents that are reviewed later. Also, being a twin does not influence the risk of schizophrenia: There is no excess of twins among schizophrenic persons. Accordingly, findings about the relative importance of genetic and environmental factors in twins can be generalized to single-born individuals.

The concordance for schizophrenia-like psychoses in MZ and same-sex DZ pairs is summarized in Table 14.2c-10 for the three population-based twin studies. The probandwise concordance is presented, because this gives the probability that a co-twin has a schizophrenic disorder if the index case (proband) is schizophrenic. Such probandwise concordances are comparable to the morbid risk estimates presented earlier for first-degree relatives, which are also probandwise risks. The risk to MZ co-twins were more than twice the risk to DZ co-twins in all the population-based series. The Maudsley Hospital twin study involved a blind assessment of a consecutive series of twins, and it has recently been reassessed using modern operational diagnostic criteria similar to the DSM-III, such as the Washington University criteria or the Research Diagnostic Criteria (Table 14.2c-11). Using ratings blind to zygosity and operational criteria based on Kraepelinian concepts, the observed risks are similar to those in the Scandinavian studies, which used similar concepts but not explicit diagnostic criteria. Some recent family studies have used narrower criteria which exclude patients with any nonschizophrenic clinical features, including depression; such an exclusionary approach makes schizophrenia so rare that it is difficult to demonstrate any familial aggregation in studies of practical sample size. Available family and twin studies demonstrate that current diagnostic criteria for schizophrenic disorders should be broader than in DSM-III, not narrower.

If home environmental factors are not important or are equally important regardless of zygosity, then the differences between MZ and DZ twins indicate that genetic factors are important in the development of schizophrenia. The home environmental assumption can be directly tested by observations on MZ twins separated at an early age and reared apart. Such pairs are rare, and only 12 have been observed as part of consecutive series of schizophrenic persons. Concordance and separation data about these twins are summarized in Table 14.2c-12. Individual case reports have been excluded in this table, to avoid biased reporting of concordant cases. Fifty-eight percent of the MZ twins reared apart have been concordant for schizophrenia, which is similar to the concordance among MZ twins reared together. This suggests that the environmental factors relevant to schizophrenia are usually not strongly familial. Combined with the differences in concordance between MZ and DZ twins, it may be concluded that genetic factors are important in the development of schizophrenia.

COMPARISON OF MONOZYGOTIC CO-TWINS AND CHILDREN OF TWO SCHIZOPHRENIC PARENTS Comparisons of MZ and DZ twins indicate that genetic factors are important but do not permit a distinction between

TABLE 14.2c-9
Schizophrenic Psychoses in the Offspring of Schizophrenic MZ Twins and Their Normal Co-Twins

	Schizophrenic Psychoses in Offspring					
	Kringlen		*Fischer*		*Total*	
Parental Diagnosis	*(A/N)*	*(%)*	*(A/N)*	*(%)*	*(A/N)*	*(%)*
Schizophrenic MZ twin	3/25	12.5	6/47	12.8	9/72	12.5
Normal MZ co-twin of schizophrenic	1/40	2.5	4/24	16.7	5/64	7.8

Data of Kringlen (personal communication, 1987) is preliminary, and age-corrected concordance is not available. Age-corrected risks for Fischer based on the 1985 follow-up by Gottesman and Bertelsen (personal communication, 1987) are 6/38.8 or 15.5% for schizophrenic twins versus 4/23.0 or 17.4% for their normal co-twins (not significantly different).

TABLE 14.2c-10
Probandwise Concordance for Nonaffective Psychosis in the Co-Twins of Schizophrenic Persons: Recent Population-Based Studies in Scandinavia

		Monozygotic Pairs		*Same-Sex Dizygotic Pairs*	
Investigator	*Country*	(*N*)	(%)	(*N*)	(%)
Kringlen, 1968	Norway	55	45	90	15
Tienari, 1971	Finland	17	35	20	13
Fischer, 1973	Denmark	21	56	41	27
Weighted total*		93	46	151	18

Table adapted from Gottesman I I, Shields J, Hanson D R: *Schizophrenia: The Epigenetic Puzzle*. Cambridge University Press, New York, 1982.
*The numbers of pairs (*N*) were used to weight the probandwise concordances (%), which take into account possible dual ascertainment of the same pair. Twin concordances are not age-adjusted because of the close correlation in age of onset in twins.

TABLE 14.2c-11
Probandwise Concordance for Operationally Defined Schizophrenia in the Maudsley Hospital Twin Study in London

	Monozygotic Pairs		*Same-Sex Dizygotic Pairs*	
Criteria*	(*N*)	(%)	(*N*)	(%)
Washington University				
Definite	19	47.4	18	9.1
Probable	21	47.6	22	11.1
RDC				
Narrow	19	52.6	21	9.5
Broad	22	45.5	23	8.7

Table adapted from McGuffin P, et al: Twin concordance for operationally defined schizophrenia: Confirmation of familiality and heritability. Arch Gen Psychiat *41:* 541, 1984.
*Operational criteria similar to DSM-III-R criteria are denoted as Washington University criteria (Feighner et al, 1972) and Research Diagnostic Criteria (RDC, Spitzer et al, 1975).

additive and nonadditive genetic effects. Additive genetic effects refer to the influences that can be vertically inherited from parents. Nonadditive genetic effects refer to dominance or recessivity at a single gene locus, as well as to interactions between different loci (called epistasis). Human beings have two genes (alleles) at every autosomal gene locus, one from each parent. Accordingly, inheritance from parent to child only involves the average effects of a single allele in the population, and effects that depend on the presence of two alleles at a single locus (dominance) or of multiple loci (epistasis) cannot be inherited. For example, if a recessive gene caused schizophrenia, both parents would have to transmit a copy of the same gene in order to produce a schizophrenic child. If a gene causing schizophrenia were additive, however, it would increase the risk of schizophrenia by the same amount regardless of any other gene effects.

Additive and nonadditive genetic effects can be evaluated by comparing risks in MZ twins and in children of two schizophrenic parents. The genotypes of MZ twins are identical, so their genetic covariance is the sum of the additive genetic variance (VA) and nonadditive genetic effects. In contrast, the genetic covariance between a child and two schizophrenic parents is largely determined by the additive genetic variance alone. For example, hereditary deafness can be caused by any of many different genes, which are often recessive. The children of two people with hereditary deafness usually have normal hearing, because the parents had different types of genetic defects. The MZ co-twin of a person with hereditary deafness is much more likely to be deaf.

Among children of two schizophrenic parents, the morbid risks have been estimated as 34 percent for narrow schizophrenia and 43 percent for schizophrenia-like psychoses (Tables 14.2c-5 and 14.2c-6). The comparable concordances for MZ twins are 39 and 46 percent (Table 14.2c-13). This suggests that the schizophrenogenic susceptibility genes are largely additive in their effects. In other words, recessive genes and other nonadditive genetic mechanisms have little or no importance in the development of schizophrenia. This conclusion is also supported by the fact that risk for schizophrenic disorders is about the same for both the children and sibs of schizophrenic persons (Table 14.2c-5) and by the observation that the incidence of schizophrenia does not increase in children of consanguineous marriages.

Overall, twin studies have provided strong evidence that genetic factors are not sufficient causes of schizophrenia because of the importance of incomplete penetrance and variable clinical expression and have also provided suggestive evidence that genetic effects are substantial and additive. However, the most direct test for additive genetic inheritance in schizophrenia comes from adoption studies.

ADOPTION STUDIES OF SCHIZOPHRENIC DISORDERS

METHODOLOGICAL ISSUES When children are reared by their biological parents, genetic and psychosocial influences that may contribute to schizophrenia are confounded. Studies of adopted persons afford a distinction between genetic and environmental influences. The confounding influence of the intrauterine environment is still a factor if the biological mother is the schizophrenic parent. Schizophrenia in the biological parent, preferably the father if there is a mechanism for evaluating paternity, is taken as the genetic risk indicator. Schizophrenia in the adoptive parent or another putative psychosocial variable about the adoptive home may be considered as the environmental risk factor. It cannot be assumed that schizophrenia in the adoptive parents is the relevant psychosocial cause of schizophrenia in children; this must be tested. Furthermore, adoptive parents are usually closely screened for psychopathology, so it is likely that any psychopathology that occurs in the adoptive parents will have late onset or will not be prominent or severe. Also, it is essential to rate the adoptive home environment before the adoptive child develops behavioral problems; otherwise, disturbances may represent the parents' reaction to the child's abnormal behavior rather than to its cause.

HESTON IN OREGON In the first adoption or foster-rearing study of schizophrenia, Heston studied children separated from their hospitalized chronic schizophrenic mothers within the first 3 days of life and reared by nonmaternal relatives. The children were often placed in foster homes of paternal relatives, who usually knew about the illness of the biological mother. The only information obtained about the fathers was that they had no known psychiatric hospitalizations. Forty-seven children who had mothers with chronic schizophrenia and who had no contact with maternal relatives during their rearing were studied at a mean age of 36 years. They were compared to 50 foster-reared subjects whose moth-

TABLE 14.2c-12
Concordance for Schizophrenic Disorders in Monozygotic Twins Reared Apart—Observed as Part of Systematic Series

			Number of Pairs	
Date	*Investigators*	*Age at separation*	*Concordant*	*Discordant*
1938	Kallmann	Infancy	1	—
1941	Essen-Moller	7 yr	1	—
1956	Kallmann & Roth	Not stated	1	—
1962	Shields	Birth	1	—
1963	Tienari	3 yr	—	1
1963	Tienari	8 yr	—	1
1967	Kringlen	1 yr, 10 mo	—	1
1967	Kringlen	3 mo	1	—
1972	Inouye	7 days	1	—
1972	Inouye	2 yr, 8 mo	1	—
1972	Inouye	Not stated	—	2
	Total		7	5

Table adapted from Gottesman I I, Shields J: *Schizophrenia: The Epigenetic Puzzle*. Cambridge University Press, New York, 1982, with permission.
Overall concordance is 7/12 = 58%.

ers had no record of psychiatric hospitalization. The evaluations of the children in the two groups was not blind, so assessment bias cannot be excluded with certainty. Five (10.6 percent) of the foster-reared children of schizophrenic mothers were diagnosed as schizophrenic at follow-up; in contrast, none of the control children was psychotic or schizophrenic. With age-correction using the usual Weinberg short method, the morbid risk for schizophrenia in the index group was estimated as 16.6 percent, which is higher than current estimates in blind studies using operational diagnostic criteria. This has been attributed to the severity of illness in the mothers, which some, but not all, studies have found to be associated with higher morbid risks in children. However, the effects of placement with paternal relatives who knew about the mother's illness and the lack of blind assessment with operational diagnostic criteria make the high risk figure open to question. Nevertheless, the study suggested that congenital factors (genetic or intrauterine environmental) may play a major role in the development of chronic schizophrenia.

DANISH ADOPTION STUDIES An important set of adoption studies have been carried out in Denmark by the American investigators Kety, Rosenthal, and Wender in collaboration with Danish psychiatrists Schulsinger, Welner, and Jacobsen, using nationwide registers for adoption and psychiatric illness. This project improved on many of the methodological limitations of the Heston study. All interviewers and diagnostic raters were completely blinded as to whether persons being assessed were index or control subjects. Adoptees were placed with nonrelatives. Children of both schizophrenic fathers and mothers were studied, who were usually born long before the first psychiatric hospitalization of the parent, so neither knowledge of parental illness by the rearing parents nor intrauterine environmental influences associated with treatment of maternal illness were likely to influence the risk of psychopathology in the adopted-away children. The diagnoses were independently reassessed using DSM-III criteria, confirming the reliability of original diagnostic procedures.

TABLE 14.2c-13
Probandwise Concordance in MZ Twins for Schizophrenia and Other Nonaffective Psychoses (? Schizophrenia): Scandinavian Population-Based Studies

	Morbid Risk of Nonaffective Psychoses					
	Strict Schizophrenia			*Questionable Schizophrenia*		
Investigator	*(N)*	*(C/P)*	*(%)*	*(N)*	*(C/P)*	*(%)*
Kringlen, 1968	45	24/57	42	55	31/69	45
Tienari, 1971	13	5/15	33	17	7/20	35
Fischer, 1973	21	9/25	36	21	14/25	56
Weighted total	79		39	93		46

N denotes the total number of pairs. The probandwise concordance (%) is computed as the proportion of probands with an affected co-twin, allowing for independent ascertainment of some concordant pairs. The number of probands (*P*) is the number of pairs (*N*) plus the number of dual ascertainments. The number of concordant pairs can be computed as $(C + N - P)$.

A broad concept of the spectrum of disorders that are related to schizophrenia has been used in the Danish adoption studies. This spectrum includes chronic, uncertain, and acute schizophrenias, as well as borderline and probable borderline states. These borderline states referred to probable or uncertain ambulatory psychotic disorders as well as some schizoid personality disorders that were clearly not psychotic or considered to be susceptible to psychosis. Accordingly, the prevalence of this spectrum was about 10 percent of the total adoptee population.

The results of a cross-fostering analysis using this spectrum concept is summarized in Table 14.2c-14. The risk of schizophrenia-spectrum conditions in the adopted-away children of schizophrenic biological parents was 18.8 percent, nearly twice the 10.7 percent risk observed in the children of normal biological parents, regardless of the psychiatric status of the adoptive parents. However, it should be noted that the schizophrenic disorders in the biological parents were more severe than in the adoptive parents: nearly twice as many of the 69 biological parents with schizophrenia were chronic schizophrenics (61 percent) compared with the 28 schizophrenic adoptive parents (32 percent). There were three chronic schizophrenic offspring among the 44 adopted-away children of chronic schizophrenic biological parents. The high prevalence in the general population and the absence of schizophrenia in the relatives of the broad nonpsychotic part of the spectrum suggests that the spectrum concept employed may have been too broad and nonspecific.

TABLE 14.2c-14
Cross-Fostering Analysis of Schizophrenia Spectrum Disorders* in the Copenhagen Adoption Study

Diagnoses of Parents		*No. of*	*Adoptees in Schizophrenia*
Biological	*Adoptive*	*Adoptees*	*Spectrum (%)*
Normal	Normal	75	10.7
Normal	Schizophrenia	28	10.7
Schizophrenia	Normal	69	18.8

Table adapted from Wender P H, Rosenthal D, Kety S S, Schulsinger F, Welner J: Crossfostering: A research strategy for clarifying the role of genetic and experiential factors in the etiology of schizophrenia. Arch Gen Psychiat *30:* 121, 1974, with permission.
*Schizophrenia spectrum disorders in parents and adoptees include chronic, uncertain, and acute schizophrenias, as well as borderline and probable borderline (schizotypal, but not mildly schizoid) subjects. 61% of the 69 biological parents with schizophrenia were chronic schizophrenics; whereas, 32% of the 28 adoptive parents with schizophrenia were chronic schizophrenics.

The nonspecificity of the nonpsychotic part of the Danish spectrum concept can be evaluated in results obtained by Kety, who took schizophrenic and normal adoptees as his index and control subjects and then studied psychopathology in their biological and adoptive relatives. As summarized in Table 14.2c-15, schizophrenic adoptees had more biological relatives with either chronic schizophrenia or other nonaffective psychoses than normal adoptees. However, schizoid or inadequate personality disorders in the biological or adoptive relatives were not associated with schizophrenia in the adopted children. There was also no excess of chronic or questionable schizophrenia in the adoptive relatives of schizophrenic adoptees compared with normal adoptees. Furthermore, only the 17 adopted-away children with chronic schizophrenia had a biological relative with chronic schizophrenia. No proband with uncertain schizophrenia, borderline or latent schizophrenia, or schizotypal personality disorder (as defined in DSM-III) had a chronic schizophrenic relative. This indicates that persons with schizoid personality and other disorders that meet DSM-III criteria for schizotypal personality disorder but who are clearly not ambulatory psychotics are unlikely to have chronic schizophrenic relatives. This hypothesis has been supported by twin and family studies by Torgersen and others, showing that there is no excess of chronic schizophrenia in the relatives of probands who are ascertained from the general population because they satisfy DSM-III criteria for schizotypal personality disorder. Thus, it must be concluded that the DSM-III criteria for schizotypal personality disorder are too broad and nonspecific to identify the relatives of schizophrenic persons who are characterized by ambulatory or vague schizophrenia-like psychoses. The excess of psychopathology in the family, twin, and adoption studies of schizophrenia appears to be largely limited to nonaffective psychosis.

Kety and his associates have also clarified the relative importance of genetic and maternal intrauterine environmental factors by comparison of psychopathology in paternal and maternal half-sibs of schizophrenic adoptees. Maternal half-sibs share both genetic and intrauterine environmental influences, but paternal half-sibs have only genetic factors in common. In the Copenhagen adoption study, 22 percent of the 63 paternal half-sibs were definite or questionable schizophrenics compared to 15 percent of 41 maternal half-sibs. This strongly suggests that genetic influences on risk of schizophrenic disorders are much more important than intrauterine environmental effects. However, the morbid risks in these half-sibs are higher than those observed in first-degree relatives in the Copenhagen sample or in earlier studies of half-sibs.

The 2.9 percent prevalence of chronic schizophrenia in the 173 biological relatives of schizophrenic adoptees included half-sibs and relatives of probands with acute and latent (nonpsychotic) schizophrenia. Kendler and Gruenberg have reassessed this data using DSM-III criteria for schizophrenia in probands and relatives: The prevalence of schizophrenia is 5.7 percent in the 35 biological relatives of adoptees with schizophrenia and 10 percent in the biological first-degree relatives, but there are only 10 such relatives in the Copenhagen sample. Fortunately, the Danish studies recently have been expanded to include 238 biological relatives of 42 schizophrenic adoptees and 217 biological relatives of 42 control adoptees. This provincial sample includes 31 full sibs of schizophrenic adoptees; the Copenhagen sample included only three full sibs. Preliminary results indicate the prevalence of chronic schizophrenia in the first-degree relatives in the provincial sample was 5 percent for schizophrenic (chronic, acute, or borderline) adoptees and 0.5 percent for normal control adoptees. The unusually high rate of illness in half-

TABLE 14.2c-15
Prevalence of Psychopathology in the Biological and Adoptive Relatives of Schizophrenic Adoptees and Normal Control Adoptees: Copenhagen Adoption Study of Kety and Associates

Type of Relative by Diagnosis of Adoptee	*No. of Relatives*	*Chronic Schizophrenia (N)*	*Chronic Schizophrenia (%)*	*Questionable Schizophrenia* (N)*	*Questionable Schizophrenia* (%)*	*Schizoid Personality (N)*	*Schizoid Personality (%)*
Biological Relatives							
Schizophrenic adoptee	173	5	2.9[†]	19	11.0	13	7.5
Normal adoptee	174	0	0.0	6	3.4	13	7.5
Adoptive Relatives							
Schizophrenic adoptee	74	1	1.4	1	1.4	2	2.7
Normal adoptee	91	1	1.1	4	4.4	2	2.2

Prevalence of Disorders in Relatives

Table adapted from Kety S S: Mental illness in the biological and adoptive relatives of schizophrenic adoptees: findings relevant to genetic and environmental factors in etiology. Amer J Psychiat *140:* 720, 1983, and Kety S S, Rosenthal D, Wender P H, Schulsinger F, Jacobson B: Mental illness in the biological and adoptive families of adopted individuals who have become schizophrenic. In *The Nature of Schizophrenia: New Approaches to Research and Treatment,* L C Wynne, R L Cromwell, S Matthysse, editors, p 9. Wiley, New York, 1978, with permission.
*Questionable schizophrenia here was called borderline or uncertain schizophrenia by Kety et al (1975, 1983) and was the basis for development of DSM-III criteria for schizotypal personality, having features of ambulatory psychosis or psychosis-proneness, rather than inadequate or schizoid personality disorder. Diagnoses here were based on both personal interviews and hospital records.
[†]Only adoptees with chronic schizophrenia ($N = 17$) had biological relatives with chronic schizophrenia; no borderline, uncertain, or schizotypal proband had a chronic schizophrenic relative. Biological relatives include parents and full- and half-sibs.

sibs observed in the Copenhagen sample was not replicated in the larger provincial sample. Results using DSM-III criteria in probands and relatives are not yet available.

FINNISH ADOPTION STUDY An adoption study by Tienari and associates in Finland, still under way, is of particular interest for two reasons. Since Tienari has also conducted twin studies, his adoption studies permits comparisons between adoption and twin material by a single investigator using the same diagnostic method, including distinctions among psychosis, nonpsychotic borderline states, and other psychopathology. Also, Tienari and his associates are conducting detailed interviews and assessments of psychodynamic function in adoptive homes. The investigators are studying a total of 183 offspring of 170 index mothers who were hospitalized with a diagnosis of schizophrenia or paranoid psychosis. The index children, adopted by nonrelatives during the first 4 years of life, were compared blindly with matched controls who are the adopted-away children of parents with no hospitalization for psychosis. The mental health ratings have been published in detail for the first 91 pairs of index and control adoptees in which both adoptees were examined (Table 14.2c-16). Among the total sample of index and control adoptees who have already been examined, nine (7.3 percent) of the 124 adopted-away children of schizophrenic parents were diagnosed as psychotic; two (1.4 percent) of the adopted-away children of nonpsychotic parents became psychotic. The adopted-away children of a schizophrenic mother have more than four times the risk of psychosis that children of nonpsychotic parents do—a significant difference ($p < .05$). The adopted-away children of schizophrenic parents have slightly more frequent borderline states and severe personality disorders also, but the differences were not significant in the first 91 pairs. Using all information available through September 1986, 20 percent of the 124 adoptees with schizophrenic mothers have been diagnosed as having a borderline disorder or severe personality disorder compared with 13 percent of the 147 adoptees with no psychotic parent, still not a significant difference ($p = .11$).

The adoptive parents have also been interviewed, and the current psychosocial adjustment of the home has been rated. Severely disturbed interpersonal functioning in the adoptive home is associated with an increased risk of psychosis, particularly in the biological children of schizophrenic mothers (Table 14.2c-17). This association has been interpreted by Tienari and his associates as evidence that the home environment provokes psychotic reactions in genetically susceptible children. However, the rating of home environment was made after the children were adults and already ill, so a plausible alternative hypothesis is that disturbances in the adoptive home were a reaction to psychopathology in the adoptee. In other words, the observed disturbance in the adult adoptive home may be either a cause or a consequence of severe psychopathology in the adoptee. The direction of effects can be evaluated convincingly only by a prospective study in which the psychosocial status of the adoptive home is assessed prior to the development of behavioral problems in the children at risk.

QUANTITATIVE GENETIC MODELS

Virtually every possible mode of inheritance has been hypothesized to account for the familial transmission of schizophrenia, but only recently have both adequate data sets and refutable quantitative models been available to permit rigorous tests of these alternative hypotheses. Shortly after Kraepelin described dementia precox, Rüdin set out to test alternative Mendelian hypotheses. Mendelian dominant gene models could be rejected because not every schizophrenic had at least one schizophrenic parent: 80 percent of schizophrenics have no parent or sib with schizophrenia. Mendelian recessive models also could be discarded because the morbid risk to full siblings was about 5 percent instead of 25 percent; this led Rüdin to hypothesize that two Mendelian recessive genes were necessary to cause schizophrenia since 0.25×0.25 gives an expected risk of 6.25 percent. However, if schizophrenia was the result of homozygosity at two loci, then all the children of two schizophrenic parents would be expected to have schizophrenia; only 34 percent to 43 percent of the children of schizophrenic couples develop schizophrenia (Tables 14.2c-5 and 14.2c-6). Also, the similarity in risks among sibs and children of schizophrenics is incompatible with recessive genetic effects. Accordingly, simple Mendelian recessive and dominant gene models have to be rejected.

Next, single-gene models that allowed for incomplete penetrance were considered. In its most general form, the monogenic model allows every possible combination of alleles at a single locus to have a different penetrance, that is, a different probability for the development of schizophrenia.

TABLE 14.2C-16
Mental Health Ratings of Adopted-Away Children of Schizophrenic Mothers and of Nonschizophrenic Parents: A Blind Interview Study in Finland

Ratings of Adoptive Offspring	*Offspring by Biological Parent Diagnosis*			
	Schizophrenia		*Nonpsychotic*	
	(N)	*(%)*	*(N)*	*(%)*
Healthy	1	1	8	9
Mild disturbance	41	45	38	41
Neurotic	23	25	30	33
Character disorder	11	12	8	9
Borderline	9	10	6	7
Psychotic	6	7	1	1
Total	91	100	91	100

Table adapted from Tienari P, Sorri A, Lahti I, Naarala M, Wahlberg K E, Pohjola J, Moring J: Interaction of genetic and psychosocial factors in schizophrenia. Acta Psychiat Scand (suppl) *71:* 19, 1985, with permission.

TABLE 14.2C-17
Interaction Between Mental Health of Adopted Offspring and of Family Interaction Patterns in the Finnish Adoption Study*

Is Adoptive Home Severely Disturbed?	*Is Biological Mother Hospitalized Schizophrenic?*	*No. of Adoptees at Risk*	*Psychosis in Adoptees*	
			(N)	*(%)*
No	No	104	0	0
No	Yes	80	3	4
Yes	No	43	2	5
Yes	Yes	44	6	14

Table adapted from Tiernari P, Sorri A, Lahti I, Naarala M, Wahlberg K E, Pohjola J, Moring J: Interaction of genetic and psychosocial factors in schizophrenia. Acta Psychiat Scand (suppl) *71:* 19, 1985, with permission.
*Severe disturbance in the adoptive home refers to families in which a major conflict exists, or in which anxiety is high, trust is low, reality testing is disturbed, or interactional defenses are primitive. Unfortunately, the rating of the adoptive home was made when the adoptees were adults who were possibly already ill, rather than at the time of adoptive placement.

This is usually simplified to let one allele be associated with differences in the risk of schizophrenia (assuming that there is only one other allele) or, if there are multiple other alleles at the locus, that all have equivalent effects on schizophrenia. In other words, in effect there are only two alleles at a single locus, which two can occur in three possible combinations or genotypes, each carrying a different probability of schizophrenia. For example, in the case of Mendelian inheritance, the penetrances of the two homozygotes (i.e., genotypes with two identical alleles) are 0 (i.e., no schizophrenia) and 1 (all schizophrenia), and the heterozygote (i.e., genotype with two different alleles) has a penetrance of 0 if the gene is recessive and 1 if it is dominant. Any intermediate value is permitted in the general case. If the heterozygote had a value that is the average of the two homozygotes, gene action is said to be purely additive.

The family and twin data summarized earlier have been used to test the adequacy of the general single-locus model, making the restrictive assumptions that all cases of schizophrenia have a common etiology and that no familial resemblance is environmentally determined. This hypothesis can be rejected with confidence, because the concordance for schizophrenia in MZ twins (39 to 46 percent) and in children of two schizophrenic parents (34 to 43 percent) are too much greater than that observed in first-degree relatives (4 to 12 percent) of schizophrenic persons. This does not imply that single genes cannot cause some cases of schizophrenia, only that one gene does not cause all cases (genetic heterogeneity) or that familial environmental influences are also important.

Rejection of monogenic models of schizophrenia as a homogeneous unitary trait requires high-risk studies to focus on alternative multifactorial hypotheses. Multifactorial hypotheses include the possibility that there are multiple loci, each of which is sufficient to cause schizophrenia (genetic heterogeneity). A second possibility is that there is a complex developmental pathway from genotype to phenotype in which multiple genetic and environmental factors interact and no one factor is sufficient to cause schizophrenia (complex development). Complex development hypotheses may be subdivided into several more specific models that may be tested by quantitative genetic analysis. These testable special cases of multifactorial inheritance include strict polygenic inheritance, in which all familial resemblance is caused by many additive genes; combined polygenic and cultural inheritance, in which social learning and other nongenetic influences are transmitted from parent to child in addition to polygenic factors; oligogenic inheritance, in which a few loci each have a substantial effect on risk for schizophrenia though none is individually sufficient to cause disease; and mixed multifactorial and single-locus inheritance, in which the effect of a single major gene locus is modified substantially by many other familial background variables.

In strict polygenic or cultural inheritance models, there are many additive factors which contribute to susceptibility (liability) to schizophrenia: Schizophrenia itself is not inherited, rather susceptibility to schizophrenia is. These underlying susceptibility factors, including genetic and environmental influences, influence the probability with which schizophrenia develops, and schizophrenia seldom develops unless a certain critical level (called the threshold) is exceeded. Under the strict polygenic model, inheritance can be described fully by estimating the additive genetic variance or narrow heritability. For example, if the heritability of liability to schizophrenia is 70 percent, then the correlation between MZ twins is expected to be 0.70 and the correlation between pairs of first-degree relatives (who share half their genes) would be half the heritability or 0.35 under the hypothesis of polygenic inheritance. If the morbid risk of schizophrenia in the general population is between 0.5 and 1.0 percent and the heritability of liability is 70 percent, the probandwise concordance between first-degree relatives would be expected to be between 4 and 6 percent and the concordance between MZ twins, between 12 and 27 percent. In fact, the concordances among MZ twins are higher than expected from polygenic models of resemblance among first-degree relatives. Like the monogenic models, the polygenic models of susceptibility to schizophrenia are inadequate because MZ twins and children of two schizophrenic parents are too highly concordant.

McGue and associates recently showed that a more general multifactorial model allowing for a combination of polygenic inheritance, cultural inheritance, special twin environmental effects, and assortative mating for social background was compatible with Western European family and twin data, including spouses, children, sibs, twins, half-sibs, nieces and nephews, first cousins, and grandchildren. Data about children of two schizophrenic parents was not considered. Under this general model for schizophrenia-like functional psychoses, the variance of liability to schizophrenia was attributed largely to polygenic inheritance (63 percent) and to a lesser extent to cultural inheritance (28 percent) and special twin environmental effects (9 percent). The special case in which inheritance was purely polygenic was rejected, because the probability of susceptibility factors being transmitted from parent to child differed significantly from that expected with autosomal inheritance. Also the high concordances between twins were accommodated in the model by an environmental factor unique to twins (regardless of zygosity). Although McGue and associates did not consider data about children of two schizophrenic parents, their model successfully predicts the near equality of the concordance between MZ twins and children of two schizophrenic parents. At the level of schizophrenia-like psychoses, the predicted correlations are 0.83 for MZ twins and 0.84 for children of two schizophrenic parents, which correspond closely to the observed morbid risks (46 percent and 43 percent). This is remarkable, because the nongenetic sources of resemblance are different: in MZ twins, the breakdown is 0.63 from polygenic inheritance, 0.11 from cultural inheritance, and 0.09 from special twin environment; in children of two schizophrenic parents, the breakdown is 0.63 from polygenic inheritance and 0.21 from cultural inheritance. Unfortunately, the predicted differences between these components of resemblance could be tested only by an adoption study of MZ twins and the children of two schizophrenic parents.

The compatibility of available data to a multifactorial model with polygenic, cultural, and twin environmental components does not prove that this is the true etiological model of schizophrenia. Genetic heterogeneity and mixed multifactorial and single-locus models have not been excluded and may explain aspects of the familial pattern that are not accounted for by strict multifactorial models. In particular, the concordance of schizophrenic subtypes is not easily explained in the absence of genetic heterogeneity. For example, attempts to reduce subtype differences to differences in severity along a single dimension of liability have led to inconsistent results. The inconsistent correlation between subtype and severity of liability to schizophrenia may suggest that paranoid and nonparanoid subtypes are manifestations of pathophysiological processes that only partially overlap; alternatively, the variation in subtype may be due to pleiotropic effects of other loci that do not influence the liability to schizophrenia but modify its symptoms when it does develop.

Single gene–locus models with twin or other familial environmental effects also have not been excluded; such refinements of purely genetic models were needed for multifactorial models to provide acceptable fits to available data. Evidence supporting the presence of a major locus effect on susceptibility to schizotypal personality has been obtained by Risch and Baron, but pedigree analyses about definite schizophrenia and schizophrenia-like psychoses have been consistently ambiguous. Resolution of the complex developmental patterns observed in schizophrenia will probably require advances in the subtyping of schizophrenia at a clinical level, in terms of underlying genetic, biological, or environmental risk factors or, more probably, both subtyping and risk factors. Unfortunately, family studies of schizophrenia that are adequate in size, diagnostic procedures, and combined biological-social assessment are not available to permit tests of remaining alternative mechanisms.

WHAT IS INHERITED?

Several possible hypotheses about heritable pathophysiological mechanisms underlying schizophrenia are under active investigation. Several genes have been proposed that may be involved in the development of schizophrenia. In particular, genes that, when homozygous, in some cases lead to diseases complicated by schizophrenic symptoms, such as Wilson's disease, which, in heterozygous form, may increase the risk of schizophrenia. Also, genes involved in immune processes or in the regulation of neurotransmitters or structural proteins in neurotransmitter receptors are under consideration as possible schizophrenia vulnerability factors.

Genes involved in immune response functions, such as those in the human leukocyte antigen (HLA) complex on chromosome 6, have been considered because of the repeated observation that rheumatoid arthritis and the paranoid subtype of schizophrenia seldom occur in the same person. Also, there is evidence of a weak association between paranoid schizophrenia and HLA-A9 in the general population. However, reports of linkage between HLA loci and schizophrenia spectrum disorders have been mostly negative.

Susceptibility to viral and bacterial infections (e.g., tuberculosis, poliomyelitis) may be heritable. Some investigators have speculated that schizophrenia might be caused by viral infections, because some cases of encephalitis are associated with schizophrenia-like symptoms. However, studies of age of onset of schizophrenia in siblings suggest that any such concordance is determined by genetic or prenatal factors rather than postnatal environmental precipitants such as viral contagion. Recent work suggests that children of mothers exposed to viral epidemics during the second trimester of pregnancy are at increased risk for schizophrenia. Crow has proposed that such prenatal exposure may allow retroviruses to be integrated into the genome which are later expressed as schizophrenia. Such integrated genetic factors could either be inherited from a parent or acquired at any early stage of development. However, there is no direct evidence of such viral infection in schizophrenia, and adoption studies of separated paternal half-sibs suggest that intrauterine environmental effects are negligible in the vast majority of cases.

Asymmetrical brain growth leading to abnormalities of the left or dominant hemisphere, common findings in postmortem studies of schizophrenic persons, may be due to genetic or developmental factors. Subtle structural brain variants, such as widening of the corpus callosum (involved in communication between the two hemispheres) or the greater extent of the planum temporale on the left side, have also been associated with schizophrenia. Positron-emission tomography of the brains of schizophrenic persons reveals increased numbers of D_2 dopamine receptors in the vicinity of the caudate nucleus. Unfortunately, no family studies have been carried out to evaluate whether such biological findings are associated with schizophrenia within families or even whether such variations are heritable.

The most useful indicators of susceptibility to schizophrenia are stable traits that are present prior to the onset of illness. Platelet monoamine oxidase (MAO) activity may be a marker of susceptibility to schizophrenia, particularly the paranoid subtype: Schizophrenic persons and their normal MZ co-twins more often have low activity levels. Such activity levels are highly heritable, but low MAO activity is also common in a wide varitey of nonschizophrenic disorders. Similarly, schizophrenic persons and their first-degree relatives with schizophrenia tend to have abnormal smooth-pursuit eye tracking. However, the relatives often have abnormal eye tracking even when the schizophrenic person's eye tracking is normal. Matthysse and Holzman have proposed a model in which both schizophrenia and abnormal eye tracking are caused by the same dominant gene. However, they have not formally tested their Mendelian gene model for its compatibility with the observed pattern of inheritance of schizophrenia in both twins and first-degree relatives or its adequacy in comparison to more general mixed or multifactorial models.

These etiological theories are based largely on indirect or circumstantial data, and in no case is there evidence showing how genetic factors explain the pathophysiology and phenomenology of schizophrenia. In particular, no genetic etiological factors have been identified to account for the earlier age of onset of schizophrenia in men or differences between paranoid and nonparanoid subtypes. No consistent evidence of linkage between a specific gene locus and a putative schizophrenia susceptibility locus has been documented. However, knowledge of the human genome is rapidly advancing, and linkage studies of schizophrenia are only in their beginning stages. Any valid etiological hypothesis of schizophrenia will have to explain the consistent finding of substantial genetic influences on risk for schizophrenia.

MOLECULAR GENETIC STRATEGIES

Novel genetic analysis strategies may be needed to identify genetic determinants of schizophrenia because of limited past success in identifying homogeneous subtypes and neurobiological markers of susceptibility. A particularly promising approach is based on gene-mapping techniques. The gene-mapping strategy is especially useful in schizophrenia because there is strong evidence of a genetic element but uncertainty about its pathophysiology. If susceptibility to schizophrenia in a particular family is largely influenced by a particular susceptibility gene, the presence of the gene can be detected by linkage analysis, and its location within the human genome can potentially be mapped. Genes that are close to one another on the same chromosome (i.e., linked) tend to be transmitted together from parent to child, whereas those that are on different chromosomes or that are far apart on the same chromosome tend to be transmitted independently. Accordingly, it is possible to detect a susceptibility gene for a disorder like schizophrenia by demonstrating that it is transmitted together with a known genetic marker.

In essence, detection of a susceptibility gene requires only that the risk of schizophrenia is associated with the presence or absence of a known genetic marker. However, until recently, available blood and protein markers provided only about a 20 percent chance that a gene for schizophrenia, if present, could be mapped to a known genetic marker. In other words, genetic markers were known for only a small portion of the human genome. Fortunately, if there are any such major gene effects causing schizophrenia, molecular genetics methods have now provided additional genetic markers that increase the probability of being able to detect and map a gene for schizophrenia to about 95 percent. This means that it may be possible to identify the genetic basis of the disorder without first knowing its pathophysiology.

Detection of the linkage of a susceptibility gene for schizophrenia to a known genetic marker would be improved if schizophrenia was always caused by the same gene and environmental factors were unimportant. Although available data indicate that genetic heterogeneity and nongenetic risk factors are important, gene mapping still holds promise. The importance of genetic heterogeneity can be minimized by conducting studies in large multigenerational pedigrees with large sibships. There many be many or only a few genes that are each sufficient to cause schizophrenia. However, assuming that each of these individual genes is relatively rare, then only one susceptibility gene is likely to be causing schizophrenia in a particular pedigree. Different susceptibility genes may be discovered in different pedigrees. In fact, studies of the physiological effects of the products of different genes may help to clarify the final common pathway to schizophrenia.

The importance of nongenetic factors in influencing expression can be minimized by determining whether sets of siblings who are all schizophrenic are more concordant for particular genetic markers than would be expected by chance. By studying only affected siblings, the influence of nongenetic factors on incomplete penetrance and variable clinical expression can be minimized. This may require large numbers of sibships, as well as a detailed map of the human genome, but such requirements are certainly now feasible. The number of sibships that must be studied can be reduced as increasingly fine genetic maps become available. Thus, studies of large pedigrees and of large numbers of affected sibs are complementary types of studies that can be initiated in studies of disorders that may be genetically heterogeneous and incompletely penetrant.

In essence, these strategies involve random search of the entire genome using 150 or more markets that are spaced evenly throughout. If no apparent linkage is found, it is unlikely that any single gene can account for susceptibility in the family or families studied. In contrast, if apparent linkage is found, additional markers in the suggested region can be studied to confirm that the apparent linkage was not due to the large number of comparisons made. Once linkage is confirmed, additional studies are needed to identify the susceptibility locus itself. Recent advances in the ability to handle large segments of deoxyribonucleic acid (DNA) should facilitate efforts to "walk the chromosome" from a linkage marker to the exact site of the susceptibility locus. Such studies in families are feasible, because a renewable source of DNA can be obtained from a peripheral blood sample containing nucleated cells, particularly lymphocytes that are transformed to establish immortal lymphoblastoid cell lines. All these methodological advances in molecular genetics combine to open important new opportunities for clarifying the genetic factors that influence susceptibility to schizophrenia.

REFERENCES

Botstein D, White R L, Skolnick M, Davis R W: Construction of a genetic linkage map using restriction fragment length polymorphisms. Amer J Human Gen *32:* 314, 1980.

Cloninger C R, Martin R L, Guze S B, Clayton P J: Diagnosis and prognosis in schizophrenia. Arch Gen Psychiat *42:* 15, 1985.

Fischer M: Genetic and environmental factors in schizophrenia. Acta Psychiat Scand (Suppl) *238:* 1, 1973.

Gershon E S, Merril C R, Goldin L R, DeLisi L E, Berrettini W H, Nurnberger, J I, Jr: The role of molecular genetics in psychiatry. Biol Psychiat 22 1388, 1987.

Gottesman I I, Shields J, Hanson D R: *Schizophrenia: The Epigenetic Puzzle.* Cambridge University Press, New York, 1982.

Guze S B, Cloninger C R, Martin R L, Clayton P J: A follow-up and family study of schizophrenia. Arch Gen Psychiat *40:* 1273, 1983.

Kendler K S, Gruenberg A M, Tsuang M T: Psychiatric illness in first-degree relatives of schizophrenic and surgical control patients: A family study using DSM-III criteria. Arch Gen Psychiat *42:* 770, 1985.

Kety S S: Mental illness in the biological and adoptive relatives of schizophrenic adoptees: Findings relevant to genetic and environmental factors in etiology. Amer J Psychiat *140:* 720, 1983.

Kety S S, Rosenthal D, Wender P H, Schulsinger F, Jacobsen B: Mental illness in the biological and adoptive families of adopted individuals who have become schizophrenic. In *Genetic Research in Psychiatry,* Fieve R R, Rosenthal D, Brill H, editors. Johns Hopkins University Press, Baltimore, 1975.

Kringlen E: Adult offspring of two psychotic parents, with special reference to schizophrenia. In *The Nature of Schizophrenia: New Approaches to Research and Treatment,* Wynne L C, Cromwell R L, Matthysse S, editors, p 9. Wiley, New York, 1978.

McGue M, Gottesman I I, Rao D C: The transmission of schizophrenia under a multifactorial threshold model. Amer J Human Gen *35:* 1161, 1983.

McGuffin P, Farmer A E, Gottesman I I, Murray R M, Reveley A M: Twin concordance for operationally defined schizophrenia: Confirmation of familiality and heritability. Arch Gen Psychiat *41:* 541, 1984.

McGuffin P, Festenstein H, Murray R: A family study of HLA antigens and other genetic markers in schizophrenia. Psychol Med *13:* 31, 1983.

Matthysse S, Holzman P S, Lange K: The genetic transmission of schizophrenia: Application of Mendelian latent structure analysis to eye tracking dysfunctions in schizophrenia and affective disorder. J Psychiat Res *20:* 57, 1986.

O'Rourke D H, Gottesman I I, Suarez B K, Rice J, Reich T: Refutation of the general single-locus model for the etiology of schizophrenia. Amer J Human Gen *34:* 630, 1982.

Risch N, Baron M: Segregation analysis of schizophrenia and related disorders. Amer J Human Gen *36:* 1039, 1984.

Rosenthal D, Kety S S, editors: *The Transmission of Schizophrenia.* Pergamon Press, Oxford University Press, 1968.

Scharfetter C, Nüsperli M: The group of schizophrenias, schizoaffective psychoses, and affective disorders. Schizophr Bull *6:* 586, 1980.

Sturt E, McGuffin P: Can linkage and marker association resolve the genetic aetiology of psychiatric disorders? Review and argument. Psychol Med *15:* 455, 1985.

Tienari P, Sorri A, Lahti I, Naarala M, Wahlberg K E, Pohjola J, Moring J: Interaction of genetic psychosocial factors in schizophrenia. Acta Psychiat Scand (suppl) *71:* 19, 1985.

Torgersen S: Relationship of schiozotypal personality disorder to schizophrenia: Genetics. Schizophr Bull *11:* 554, 1985.

Tsuang M T, Winokur G, Crowe R R: Morbidity risks of schizophrenia and affective disorders among first-degree relatives of patients with schizophrenia, mania, depression and surgical conditions. Brit J Psychiat *137:* 497, 1980.

Wender P H, Rosenthal D, Kety S S, Schulsinger F, Welner J: Crossfostering: A research strategy for clarifying the role of genetic and experiential factors in the etiology of schizophrenia. Arch Gen Psychiat *30:* 121, 1974.

14.2d SCHIZOPHRENIA: PSYCHODYNAMIC THEORIES

THOMAS H. MCGLASHAN, M.D.

INTRODUCTION

Descartes's assertion, "I think, therefore I am" approximates the essence of that which is considered human among the creatures of this planet's biosphere: awareness of a self—being, comprehending, and doing. The "sapiens" of homo sapiens refers to this creature's wisdom, discerning nature, and drive to know. Humans are unique in their biologically encoded capacity for understanding and their need to make sense out of experience. At times, this drive for meaning supersedes survival in importance, as in Martin Luther's, "Here I stand" or as in Nathan Hale's, "I regret that I have but one life to give for my country." For all animals, the afferent data of experience and the efferent impulses of response must be organized somehow by a central processing or nervous system. Man, however, regularly adds delay, explanation, linguistic communication, and choice to this reflex arc. Sensory data must be understood. Experience must be organized on a matrix of meaning, be it a matrix of belief (mythology, religion), of reason (philosophy, logic), or of science (experimentation, empiricism). The antithesis is chaos, the fragmentation of predictable phenomena into random sequences.

If the unique legacy of evolution is a neuronal superstructure programmed to find meaning (i.e., to program), then schizophrenia may be the quintessential human disorder. Whatever the disease may be and however it may arise, its final common pathway involves dysfunction of the capacity to assign meaning. In the extreme case, the schizophrenic process can render one incapable of Descartes's affirmation. It may leave no "I," no self to filter and contain the data of experience. It may erode rationality so that there is no thinking logical enough to make communicable sense, no "therefore," or cause and effect and, consequently, no meaning. Many victims of schizophrenia cannot assert, "I am." Some maintain they have no existence; virtually all experience themselves as exiles from humanity—alone, utterly different or alien, and devoid of the apparatus that makes them and marks them part of the fold.

Schizophrenia threatens the loss of that which everyone takes completely for granted: selfhood, the sense of being an entity. Only when it is missing are its importance, its survival value, and its function of endorsing us as sentient creatures appreciated. Because schizophrenia often invades this core of human narcissism, humans, in turn, have always regarded it with intense ambivalence. On the one side lies fascination because of the secrets it holds for the understanding of understanding. On the other side lies horror because it threatens the patient with the ultimate paralysis—living meaninglessness. Perhaps because of this anxiety, through the centuries, schizophrenic madness has had more explanations thrown at it and has been the object of more attempts to render it meaningful and understandable than any other mental illness. Prior to Galileo, most of these explanations were found in religious texts. From Galileo to Kraepelin, the explanations were found in medical texts. By the twentieth century, inspired by psychoanalytic thinking, the nature and cause of schizophrenia turned functional. No longer supernatural or organic in etiology, schizophrenia became conceptualized as a clash of ideas, of wishes, of learned habits (i.e., psychological) in its genesis and manifestations. From this milieu came the variegated psychodynamic theories of schizophrenia.

THEORY

A rigorous and operationally oriented definition of theory envisions it as a set of assumptions and definitions that can generate testable and refutable hypotheses or predictions about a phenomenon. This form of theory, constitutes the backbone of modern scientific empiricism. According to Lichtenberg, a broader, esthetically oriented definition of theory regards it as a set of assertions explaining something in a manner that is "balanced, logical, and comprehensive while at the same time parsimonious in its assumptions." This form of theory characterizes most psychodynamic theories of schizophrenia.

Either type of theory can serve as a useful cognitive framework. As Cancro noted, "Theory imposes boundaries and a filter on the potential data set of observation and decreases and sharpens it to manageable size." Furthermore, theories and hypotheses predict relationships that are not immediately or intuitively obvious. Theory informs the task of observation and makes it finite. No serious clinician approaches the schizophrenic patient in a theoretical vacuum; organizing principles are required to avoid being overwhelmed. Theory may foster selective inattention and exclude important alternate meanings or observations. On balance, however, such risks are minor compared to the chaos that greets any therapist without an explicit or implicit model.

PSYCHODYNAMIC THEORIES OF SCHIZOPHRENIA The disorders gathered under the term "schizophrenia" arise (etiology), develop over time (pathogenesis), emerge in certain forms (manifest illness), and undergo vicissitudes over the life span (course). Theories relevant to this group may address any of these facets. Generally, they cluster into two paradigms: descriptive-homeostatic theories and etiological-facilitative theories.

Descriptive-homeostatic theories are more focused on the here and now and stay closest to manifest phenomenology. They label, order, and integrate the data based on observed or hypothesized relations like Eugen Bleuler's division of schizophrenic symptoms into those that are primary and those that are secondary. These theories also introduce causation and attempt to explain or understand how the disease works as a homeostatic system. An example is Sigmund Freud's postulate that paranoia represents reversed and projected latent homosexual wishes.

Etiological-facilitative theories are more concerned with the broader view of schizophrenia over the course of a lifetime. How is it generated? What forces shape its expression? Such theories are more comprehensive in scope and usually more hypothetical. An example is Melanie Klein's postulate that schizophrenia arises from fixations engendered at the paranoid-schizoid phase of development in early infancy. Such theories are often labeled psychogenic because they try to explain the genesis of schizophrenia.

Most of the theories considered here consist of postulates that are both descriptive and etiological. Accordingly, both paradigms will be reviewed.

The psychodynamic theories of schizophrenia belong to a broad model of mental functioning that assumes symptom formation (psychopathology) is functional (i.e., that it can be explained in part, if not entirely, by psychology rather than physiology, by mental phenomena rather than organic changes in the brain). This notion was introduced by Sigmund Freud in *The Interpretation of Dreams:* "For illnesses—those, at least, which are rightly named 'functional'—do not presuppose the disintegration of the apparatus or the production of fresh splits in its interior. They are to be explained on a *dynamic* basis—by the strengthening and weakening of the various components in the interplay of forces, so many of whose effects are hidden from view while functions are normal." The common thread linking psychodynamic theories is this assumption that behavior, both normal and pathological, is determined by a dynamic and complex interplay of motivational forces that interact conflictually or synchronistically. Furthermore, many of these forces operate unconsciously or outside of everyday awareness.

Psychodynamic theories originated from psychoanalytic or psychoanalytically oriented psychotherapeutic practice. This is an inquiry by doctor and patient into the latter's self-experience, parts of which are actively unavailable or disavowed, their presence being signaled only by their pathogenic effects (i.e., symptoms). Troubles arise because something of meaning is missing in the patient's experience. Accordingly, therapeutic resolution follows on accrual of an expanded and enriched perspective of affective-cognitive meanings.

Most psychodynamic theories of schizophrenia are of the broad, esthetically oriented variety noted above. Few of those to be considered can be operationalized and tested. They are too abstract or based on data collected empathically rather than objectively. Their validity rests not on empirical validation per se. While these theories must, in general, conform to rules of evidence, their truthfulness basically derives from their capacity to help one understand schizophrenia. The verity of these theories is proportional to the degree to which they generate meanings about schizophrenia that make communicable sense and that are useful in one's empathic encounters with afflicted patients. Validity here stems from a theory's vividness, connectedness, and depth, as well as its parsimonious integration of complexity. Validity also derives from the theory's usefulness in alerting doctor and patient as listeners and hunters for that which is missing from the latter's experience.

The 1911 publication of Freud's case of Schreber probably marks the formal beginning of the systematic psychodynamic theories of schizophrenia. For the next 50 years, virtually all of the thinking in this realm emerged from within the various psychoanalytic schools, here labeled the classical, interpersonal, and developmental. The next major body of theory grew out of psychoanalysis around the middle of the century as family transaction models. Shortly thereafter, following on the biological revolution in psychiatry and the genetic studies of schizophrenia, the stress-diathesis or vulnerability-stress models blossomed.

PSYCHOANALYTIC MODELS: CLASSICAL SCHOOL

SIGMUND FREUD The classical psychoanalytic model postulates that manifest psychopathology is generated by active and sustained psychological conflict between drive-created wishful impulses and antithetical wishes, reality, or conscience. This conflict generates defenses against the wishful impulse, and these defenses can often be seen in the form of symptoms. Any or all of this drama may be carried on outside of awareness (i.e., unconsciously).

This model finds its most complete elaboration in the structural theory, which postulates the existence of three functional entities in the mind. The *id* is the wellspring of peremptory sexual and aggressive drives and wishes. It is largely unconscious and primitive in its structure. The *superego* or conscience and ego ideal is the repository of rules and values learned (internalized) from patients and society during development. It is also largely unconscious but makes its presence known through the affects of guilt and shame. The *ego* is a group of psychological functions that mediate adaptation between the person and the environment (e.g., reality testing) and among conflicting psychological forces within the person (e.g., repression of forbidden impulses). The ego is complex and develops slowly over the course of life. Many of its functions (e.g., defense) are activated by anxiety, the danger signal generated by conflict or reality. Ego functions, too, operate mostly out of awareness.

Freud postulated that these structures develop during infancy and childhood and are in place by the end of the oedipal period (ages 3 to 5). The person at this point has a stable, integrated ego, seen as a sense of self that is enduring and cohesive. Conflict within and among these structures produces the symptomatic and character neuroses. Freud regarded schizophrenia as deriving from psychological development that is arrested prior to the oedipal stage, prior to development of an integrated ego. Such an arrest, Freud believed, severely compromised the schizophrenic patient's capacity to relate and rendered treatment by psychoanalysis problematic, if not impossible.

Although he had virtually no clinical experience with schizophrenic patients, Freud was the first analyst to elaborate a systematic psychodynamic model for this syndrome. He may be said to have formulated two models, one emphasizing conflict and defense, and the other emphasizing deficiency as the cause of schizophrenic symptoms.

The conflict-defense model basically explains schizophrenic symptoms using the structural model, as outlined above for the neuroses. In this model, schizophrenia, like all psychopathology, is the result of conflict and defense. The difference between schizophrenia and the neuroses is purely quantitative, not qualitative. Schizophrenic conflict is more intense and requires frequent use of very primitive (i.e., developmentally earlier) defenses like denial and projection, which frequently involve a break with reality. The ego functioning of the schizophrenic patient regresses to developmentally earlier stages or levels of organization, the exact level being determined (or fixated) by one or more past psychological traumas. The difference between schizophrenia and neurosis lies in the depth of regression and the point of fixation, which Freud placed in the preoedipal phase of development.

Freud used a deficiency (or deficit) model to explain schizophrenic symptom formation in the case of Schreber. Freud worked from Schreber's published autobiographical account of his paranoid psychosis. Clinically, Schreber's illness began with hypochondriacal preoccupations. This was followed by an apocalyptic panic leading to catatonia, personality change, and symptoms of psychosis, particularly grandiose and paranoid delusions.

Freud, who was elaborating his libido theory at the time,

explained Schreber's psychosis as follows. Conflict initiates the sequence, as it does in all psychopathology. In schizophrenia, however, another process supersedes defense. This process is described as the patient's withdrawal of libidinal or energic investments (cathexes) from the real outside world, especially people (objects, in psychoanalytic parlance). There is a concomitant withdrawal of libidinal investments from the inner, fantasied, mental representations or images of this world and these people. In the developing schizophrenic process, the withdrawn libidinal energy increasingly becomes invested in the patient's self-image, seen clinically as self-aggrandizement or megalomania or invested in the patient's body image, seen clinically as hypochondriasis. A similar process of withdrawal from real, external relations occurs in neurotic responses to conflict, but here, the withdrawn libido remains invested in the fantasied objects.

This withdrawal reaches a state so profound as to constitute a break with external reality and relationships and with internal object representations and relationships in fantasy. At this stage, one can see the apocalyptic panic clinically. It represents a projection outward of this internal catastrophe or collapse of psychological investments. This collapse and profound withdrawal constitutes the deficit of schizophrenia. It renders the patient incapable of relationships, including transference, and thus precludes treatment by psychoanalysis. Following this catastrophe, the patient tries to recover and reinvest libido. Since there has been a break with reality, however, these efforts produce the well-known symptoms of schizophrenia, especially hallucinations, delusions, and disordered thinking. The patient has reinvested interest and attention but in objects that are not part of the real world.

In Freud's defense theory, the sequence of conflict, anxiety, and defense is regarded as sufficient to account for schizophrenic psychopathology. In the deficit theory, conflict and anxiety initiate pathogenesis but trigger a withdrawal process which is qualitatively different from defense. Freud never resolved the differences between his two theories. He seemed to say that schizophrenic people are very much like normal and neurotic people in some ways but profoundly different in others. His two theories formed the nidus for much subsequent controversy.

Freud's other theoretical contributions to schizophrenia concern the psychodynamics of delusion formation. Early in his career, he postulated the mechanism of projection, whereby the subject's wish is disavowed and projected onto (or attributed to) another person (the object). Later, he suggested that delusions of persecution arise from latent homosexual impulses that undergo reversal and projection. Thus, the situation, "I (a man) love him (a man)" is reversed to, "I do not love him; I hate him" and projected into, "He hates (and persecutes) me." Later in his career, Freud maintained that the hostility inherent in any form of intense ambivalence toward an object could be projected into feelings of being persecuted by that object.

PAUL FEDERN If Freud was the first major psychodynamic theoretician of schizophrenia, Paul Federn was the first major psychodynamic clinician of schizophrenia. A contemporary of Freud's, he disagreed with his Viennese colleague's pessimism about the schizophrenic patient's capacity to develop transference and to be treated by psychoanalytically informed therapy. He treated many schizophrenic patients and developed techniques that were virtually half a century ahead of his time.

Federn greatly expanded the notion of ego set down by Freud in the structural theory. He was perhaps the first psychoanalytic theoretician to introduce the notion of self. To him, the ego was not just a collection of psychological functions. It also had its own existential "entityness" or ego feeling. The various ego functions aggregate into a sum or self that has a feeling of permanence and continuity vis-à-vis time, space, and causality. This is ego feeling, the totality of feeling an individual has of his or her own living being. Ego feeling as subject is "I." Ego feeling as object is "self."

Federn also elaborated the concept of ego boundary originally introduced by Tausk. To Federn, each person possessed an inner and an outer ego boundary. The outer boundary consists of the ego versus the external world; it divides and distinguishes mental phenomena from real phenomena. The inner boundary consists of the repression barrier or the line between conscious and unconscious experience. According to his scheme, which utilized Freud's libido theory, schizophrenia is a disease of the ego. The psychopathological process involves a loss of energic investments in ego boundaries. Attenuation at the inner boundary means derepression or a reemergence of developmentally earlier (archaic) ego states. Attenuation at the outer boundary means a loss of the distinction between mental and real, seen in the typical schizophrenic symptoms. Mature and archaic ego states, however, can coexist, thus making it possible for the patient to adjust to the real world while still symptomatic and to engage in psychodynamically oriented therapeutic discourse despite illness.

Federn's basically descriptive model follows the theme of defect. Nevertheless, his concepts prefigure the later distinction between psychotic and nonpsychotic aspects of the patient's personality. For him, the schizophrenic process is never total. Furthermore, by highlighting the self phenomenology in the ego of Freud's structural model, Federn anticipated the development of self psychology.

HEINZ HARTMANN Working within Freud's classical structural theory, Heinz Hartmann was impressed with the ego's complexity and versatility, its strength in opposition to the drives, and its primary aim of serving reality adaptation and survival. Defenses like intellectualization and sublimation, for example, are also coping devices. He regarded humans as biological organisms phylogenetically equipped at birth for adaptation to an average expectable environment. This includes primary ego functions like perception, memory, and motility that are not derived from conflict. Also, ego functions developing later out of conflicts can become autonomous of id and superego or free of conflict to function independently and to serve adaptation. Such functions include language, intellect, thinking, will, judgment, attention, affectivity, reality testing, intention, and object relations in addition to the defenses and primary functions already mentioned. The existence of psychopathology indicates that these ego functions can become reinstinctualized or involved in conflict situations.

The ego, according to Hartmann, also possesses a synthetic function, its aim being to promote homeostasis, or a harmonious equilibrium between the drives of sex and aggression, among the intrapsychic tripartite systems of id, ego, and superego, and between the individual and his or her environment. This supraordinate integrative function carries echoes of Federn's ego feeling. Hartmann, however, regarded the self as an idea (representation) rather than as an entity or functioning mental system.

In comparison to his extensive contributions to general psychodynamic theory, Hartmann's specific postulates regarding schizophrenia are abbreviated, perhaps because such patients did not constitute a large part of his practice. His theory was a mixture of defense and defect. Like Freud, Hartmann felt that schizophrenic symptoms can result from conflicts secondary to intolerable realities or amplified drive pressures. In addition, he postulated an inborn primary defect in the ego of the preschizophrenic patient which renders the ego incapable of neutralizing certain drive pressures, especially aggression. Aggression generated later in life by conflict or narcissistic injury floods this ego (especially its synthetic functioning) and draws it easily into conflict. The ensuing regression is substantial and mobilizes primitive defenses, such as denial and projection, which are viewed as the symptoms of schizophrenia. Not all ego functions regress to the same extent, however, thus accounting for the heterogeneity of the clinical picture.

Hartmann's theory added the importance of aggression to the pathogenesis of schizophrenia. It also placed the source of the syndrome in the preschizophrenic patient's constitution, thus marking these people as qualitatively different from those who later develop normally or neurotically. Finally, Hartmann conceptualized the ego as multidimensional. Schizophrenia affects selective ego function paralysis and can therefore be graded in severity. In Hartmann's scheme, it is possible to have greater or lesser degrees of schizophrenia.

PSYCHOANALYTIC MODELS: INTERPERSONAL SCHOOL

HARRY STACK SULLIVAN The interpersonal model of Harry Stack Sullivan, while psychodynamic in its structure, is fundamentally different from psychoanalytic drive theory in its content. Drive theory works from the perspective of the person as an individual encountering and shaping the world according to inner arising drives and satisfactions. Interpersonal theory elaborates the perspective of man as a social creature who, from the very beginning, is object related and relationship seeking. Sullivan's model still postulates motivational drives and needs, namely the needs for satisfaction, mostly biological, in the form of hunger and lust, and the needs for security, mostly psychosocial, in the form of power. All of these needs require interaction with at least one other human being and serve to mediate the interpersonal exchange.

The developmental aspect of Sullivan's theory regards the human infant as being without a psychology separate from the initial mother–infant dyad. Psychological awareness consists of successive discoveries of one's self in relationship with significant others (objects). The first self consists of a *we,* not an *I.* Development proceeds according to an increasingly complex hierarchy of needs, all interactional in nature. These are the needs for maternal contact in infancy, parental mirroring in childhood, peer play in latency, chum closeness in early adolescence, and sexual intimacy in late adolescence and beyond.

Anxiety, the affect driving psychopathology, was viewed by Sullivan as external to the infant but imparted to the latter by an anxious parent, usually mother. Anxiety in the interpersonal situation develops three self-states, a good me (low anxiety), a bad me (high anxiety), and a not me (intolerable anxiety). Not-me anxiety is extreme awe, dread, loathing, or panic—so dysphoric as to be experienced rarely, as in nightmares or during severe schizophrenic end-of-the-world panic experiences.

Anxiety leads to the organization of defensive structures, which Sullivan described as self-dynamisms or self systems. These function to maximize satisfactions and to maintain security or to minimize anxiety through the use of "security operations" like selective inattention (dissociation), sublimation, or projection. The self system, in its content, is what one takes oneself to be. This is largely secondary to what others take one to be (i.e., it consists mostly of reflected appraisals). The self system security operations operate to establish and protect this content of the self system. In the face of anxiety, this leads to the creation of fantasied defensive self–other constellations like the self as helpless, but deserving, and the other as magical and merciful; the self as victimized and hurt and the other as powerful and persecutory; and the self as special and the other as idealizing. Such illusory configurations become superimposed upon and distort a person's here-and-now relationships, a process akin to transference, which Sullivan labeled parataxic distortion.

Sullivan's psychodynamic theory of schizophrenia was informed by extensive clinical experience with acutely and subacutely affected inpatients. These disorders he regarded in the Meyerian tradition as purely functional reactions to encounters between the person and the environment. Central to the psychopathological process is a disturbance in the capacity to relate to others that is not biological in origin but reflects the history of the patient's interactions with significant others, especially with the mother in the formative years. The syndrome itself represents a massive dissociation secondary to intense anxiety generated by low self-esteem during interpersonal experience. Sullivan acknowledged the probable existence of hereditary or organic determinants in some disorders, such as chronic process schizophrenia. He did not, however, consider them to be schizophrenia per se, or at least the subtype of schizophrenia to which he felt his theory applied.

The pathogenesis of schizophrenia, according to Sullivan's etiological scheme, begins with a mother who is more anxious than normal and who imparts this tension to her child as excessive not-me experiences. The child's self system, developing around the time of speech acquisition, overcompensates with excessive dissociation and warps its own further development. The adolescent surge of new sexual needs (lust dynamisms) assault this compromised self system. The defensive wall of selective inattention fractures; not-me disorganizing anxiety returns, and panic ensues. This state of terror is characterized not only by the uncanny eruption into awareness of developmentally primitive states of mind, but also by a collapse of the integrated self systems into what Sullivan described as "an exceedingly unpleasant form of nothingness." The afflicted person's primary urgencies at this point are to avoid the not-me menace and to reorganize the self in order to reestablish meaning and become human again. This reorganization, known as schizophrenia, is effected at the price of reality.

According to Sullivan, schizophrenia is more than a disorder. It is also an adaptive strategy for avoiding fragmentation and chaos (panic and terror) and for reconstructing a self with human identity, meaning, and purpose, no matter how fantastic that defensive self–other constellation may be. It is better, for example, to be the hapless victim of tyrannical persecutors than to be nothing at all. One must have character, even if it manifests as caricature. With schizophrenia, the needs for satisfaction and reality are secondary to the needs for security and self meaning.

The descriptive-homeostatic aspects of Sullivan's theory highlight the self, both as a content (idea) and as a functional system. Though Federn may have been the first to describe the self as part of a psychodynamic system (as ego feeling), Sullivan was the first to postulate its functional centrality to human psychology. To him, creating and maintaining the integrity and functional alacrity of a self is one of the primary motivating forces of mankind. With schizophrenia, in fact, the drive for meaning exerts hegemony over all other needs. Sullivan also introduced the interpersonal paradigm to psychodynamic theory. Accordingly, environment takes on a more powerful role as facilitator of the schizophrenic process. Sullivan viewed schizophrenia as the result of cumulative experiential traumas during development. His own bias was to regard the preschizophrenic infant as a tabula rasa, on which mother's anxieties became etched. The source of pathogenic anxiety is clearly external to the infant, and schizophrenia is seen as an adaptive attempt to cope with that dysphoric milieu.

BRITISH OBJECT-RELATIONS THEORISTS The British object-relations school operated independently of Sullivan but pursued many of the same ideas, regarding humans as inherently social or object related. Their major spokespersons are Melanie Klein, W. R. D. Fairbairn, and D. W. Winnicott.

MELANIE KLEIN For Melanie Klein, psychodynamic conflict involved love versus hate in relationships (rather than the tension between wish and reality of more classical psychoanalysis). Her descriptive-homeostatic theories were key contributions to classical psychoanalytic dynamics. She emphasized the importance of fantasy, both conscious and unconscious, in determining behavior. Such fantasy usually takes the form of a drama involving the self relating with another—constellations which have come to be known as internal object relationships. She added two important coping or defense mechanisms to the ego's repertoire: splitting and projective identification. During infancy, these mechanisms promote development and adaptation. During adulthood, they signal trouble. Klein related psychopathology to an overabundance of aggression and hate in relationships. Envy (mostly innate) is especially pathogenic, because it is directed at good objects and their capacity to give, thus destroying hope by devaluing healthy relationships.

Klein conceived of human development as a hierarchy of relational patterns (i.e., positions rather than phases). Two positions, both within the first year of life, are central to normal development—or to later psychopathology: the paranoid position, wherein aggressive, dysphoric interpersonal experiences are split off and projected onto significant others, who are then regarded anxiously as persecutory, and the depressive position, the infant's guilty recognition of personal responsibility for being the aggressive persecutor at times. While the accuracy of this scheme may be questionable vis-à-vis contemporary infant observation, it is compelling in its description of two mental constellations frequently encountered in patients with severe psychopathology.

Klein's theory of schizophrenia closely followed her developmental scheme. She regarded the potential schizophrenic patient as endowed with strong sadistic and envious impulses that rendered the infant prone to intense paranoid anxieties and, therefore, to the overuse of withdrawal, splitting, and projective identification. Such infants never negotiate the depressed position and remained fixated at the paranoid position, to which they regress in the face of later stress, after further development through adolescence.

W. R. D. FAIRBAIRN To W. R. D. Fairbairn, the primary aim of human behavior was contact with another, even if it was unpleasant. He viewed psychopathology entirely from a developmental perspective, as the product of failure to establish good object relationships in infancy. Maternal absence or withdrawal during the paranoid-schizoid position leads the infant to regard his love as noxious or bad. The resultant schizoid conflict—to love or not to love—sets off a withdrawal from relatedness in reality with compensatory investments in defensive internal object relations. These, like Sullivan's fantasied self–other constellations, provide a sense of security and continuity that is missing in real relationships, especially the earliest ones with parents. Fairbairn conceived of schizophrenia on a continuum with schizoid psychopathology, the difference being one of degree. The schizophrenic patient withdraws loving investments to such an extent that emotional contact with others and with external reality is renounced.

Both Klein and Fairbairn saw the mind as a consequence of development over time. Psychological structures and functions are built almost entirely out of internalized (learned) experiences with significant others, especially mother. Accordingly, severe psychopathology derives from problems in the early nurturing relationship between mother and infant. Klein emphasized heightened constitutional aggression in the infant, whereas Fairbairn emphasized maternal withdrawal and deprivation. Both, however, conceived of the human infant as an undifferentiated mound of clay, passively and helplessly waiting to be shaped by the forces of inner drive and external reality. The third major figure of the British object-relations school, Winnicott, however, saw the infant as possessing power and influence from the start.

D. W. WINNICOTT To D. W. Winnicott, the infant was an equal partner with mother in the early drama of the dyadic relationship. Mother, via primary maternal empathy, provides a proper holding environment for her infant. This means she responds appropriately to her infant's needs at the moment of excitation when the infant signals them to her. Equally important, she does not impinge on her infant's quiescent states to fulfill her own needs. In all, the environment (as mother) finds the child and promotes a fitting together that is true to the child's innate potential and uniqueness. For the infant, these are experiences of omnipotence, power, or control over the mother or environment. They form the basis of a healthy, competent sense of self. The infant learns about reality little by little over time through mother's natural failures to shape the world perfectly according to the infant's demands. The soothing illusion of omnipotence and magic, however, remains alive and healthy within the realm of transitional objects and experiences.

Winnicott never articulated a theory of schizophrenia per se. However, according to his scheme as interpreted by others, schizophrenia can be viewed as a failure in the development of this spontaneous and competent or true self out of its relational matrix. Because of an improper fit, the infant becomes exposed to realities that are out-of-phase with his or her needs and states of activation and, therefore, to the premature destruction of the illusion of power. This leads to the development of a false self that compliantly reacts to external realities and the needs of others. Increasingly, needed omnipotence derives from defensive, internal, or autistic fantasy rather than from transitional interaction with the environment. In schizophrenia, this fantasy finally comes to replace reality.

The importance of Winnicott's ideas derives not so much from their contribution to a theory of schizophrenia as from their elaboration of a theory of self. Like Sullivan, Winnicott regarded the self as a central psychodynamic force and entity. Winnicott went beyond Sullivan, however, in postulating the importance of illusion to normal growth and development. To Winnicott, the omnipotent self, as played out in fantasy or transitional space, was a sign of health and only later a signal of possible trouble. To Sullivan, such fantasies or self systems were always defensive, a sign of pathological adaptation. Winnicott's perspective also introduced an entirely new dimension to psychodynamic treatment theory. To the classical search for truth and insight (i.e., reality), Winnicott advocated the need for the treatment dyad to create and internalize a protective sense of illusion. He provided the theoretical underpinning for adding the facilitating environment to the analytic situation. Supportive psychotherapeutic techniques, which were commonly used clinically with schizophrenic and severely character disordered patients by dynamic clinicians since Federn, now also had a proper theoretical rationale.

PSYCHOANALYTIC MODELS: DEVELOPMENTAL SCHOOL

Latter-day American theorists contributing to the psychodynamic understanding of schizophrenia include, among others, Margaret Mahler, Edith Jacobson, Silvano Arieti, Peter Giovacchini, Ping-Nie Pao, and James Grotstein. As a group, their work has drawn heavily on observations of and theories about human development.

MARGARET MAHLER Margaret Mahler clearly related early developmental experiences to later mental function. Her developmental phases of autism, symbiosis, and separation-individuation have captured the attention and imagination of many theorists who see different forms of psychopathology corresponding to different levels in her developmental progression. Schizophrenia, for example, is regarded as corresponding to Mahler's autistic phase of development. It is assumed or postulated that the preschizophrenic infant fails to form an adequate and stable symbiosis with the mothering object, a developmental failure rendering the child's image of mother inconstant. This developmental failure leaves the individual vulnerable to regression when facing the second and final phase of individuation, in late adolescence. The regression itself goes back to the preverbal, presymbiotic stage of autism with loss of ego boundaries, merger experiences, and replacement of reality by autistic fantasy.

EDITH JACOBSON Edith Jacobson saw schizophrenia as a disturbance of the sense of self or identity, defined as the observable capacity of the person to remain the same in the midst of change. While schizophrenic patients have difficulties with object relationships, their primary problems lie with maintaining a stable sense of self-sameness and self-cohesion. The breakdown of this sense is one of the most painful and traumatic experiences known to man, provoking preservation efforts that often abandon allegiance to reality.

SILVANO ARIETI AND PETER GIOVACCHINI Latter-day thinkers in the field basically have extended the existing theoretical models already outlined. Silvano Arieti and Peter Giovacchini, for example, elaborated an etiological-developmental theory of schizophrenia similar to that of Sullivan by viewing the disorder as beginning early in childhood owing to an abnormal interpersonal environment. To Giovacchini, trauma during the infantile nursing situation establishes very early fixation points antedating the formation of coherent object relations. Later psychopathological regression, therefore, reaches back to amorphous, chaotic, nonhuman presymbiotic states characterized by a paucity of psychological content or fantasy. The descriptive-homeostatic model of both these theorists parallels current nosological subtyping by emphasizing the negative symptom or deficit presentation in schizophrenia and implying its primacy to the syndrome. Arieti perceives that schizophrenic patients have lost their ability to empathize with others and, therefore, to respond emotionally. For them, feelings are not experienced. Their world is flat, humorless, dead, and indifferent—a phenomenon that is presumably a product of the depth of their functional regression.

PING-NIE PAO Ping-Nie Pao wove together theoretical threads of many forebears. Based upon extensive clinical experience, he subtyped schizophrenic patients into the more acute cases, for whom conflict plays a more pivotal role, and the more chronic cases, with higher genetic-biological loading. Pao, like Freud, was impressed with the catastrophic panic experience that signaled the onset of the schizophrenic process and symptom formation. This process is precipitated by psychodynamic conflicts no different in content from those experienced by all people. In the schizophrenia-vulnerable person, however, these conflicts no longer generate neurotic levels of anxiety but at some point catalyze a crisis known as organismic panic, the term being modeled after Mahler's developmental observations of states of extreme infantile distress. This panic brings with it paralysis of the ego's integrative capacity and fragmentation of the sense of continuity of self. The latter process constitutes an unbearable loss of a basic sense of safety, leading the ego to mobilize primitive or regressive defenses in order to reestablish and protect a sense of self, albeit pathologically. The result of this attempt at adaptation or recovery is the postpanic emergence of a different personality, either pieced together with or distorted by psychotic symptoms. Typical delusions, for example, help to construct a new sense of meaningful self and, though often very unpleasant, are clung to tenaciously because their loss leads to a threatened return of disorganization and panic.

Pao's etiological-developmental theory attempts to explain the origin of the schizophrenic vulnerability to organismic panic and regression. Like other relationalists, he placed etiology in the experiences of early development. Aberrant constitution and inappropriate mothering combine to generate a series of failed emotional cuings within the dyad, leading to frequent episodes of infantile organismic distress or "pain in being held and pain in being laid down." Cumulative exposures to such distress bend further development in maladaptive directions, including a tendency to use primitive defensives, impaired capacity for instinctual neutralization, inability to maintain a sense of reality constancy, heightened aggressive responses to frustration, and heightened wishes for closeness with others coupled with a dread of self dissolution in symbiosis (the need–fear dilemma originally described by Burnham, Gladstone, and Gibson). These vulnerabilities lie dormant and do not produce symptoms until the advent of adolescent drive demands and stress.

JAMES GROTSTEIN James Grotstein's elaborate theory of schizophrenia is almost entirely etiological-developmental in perspective. He amalgamates Mahler's and Klein's developmental schemes and postulates three major infantile developmental phases: the autistic phase of adhesive identification (where ego boundary is identical with skin boundary), the symbiotic phase or paranoid-schizoid position, and the depressive position of separation and individuation. For the infant who will become schizophrenic, development basically aborts at the first stage. In this model, such an infant is born with constitutional defects in the sensory-perceptual apparatus, such as a lower stimulus barrier or precocious perceptual awareness. This, plus inadequate maternal protection, results in sensory overload and frequent organismic panic (the infantile catastrophe). Compensatory elevation of the sensory threshold is achieved through conversion-paralysis of the brain stem vestibular nuclei. The result is a pathologically exaggerated autistic state of functional alexithymia or relative sensory deprivation; such infants are uninformed regarding personal needs and feelings and fill in these intrapsychic gaps with hallucinatory phenomena.

The preschizophrenic infant enters the next developmental phase already deformed and experiences unusually severe persecutory anxieties. Symbiotic relatedness develops incompletely, if at all. The third stage of separation-individuation is essentially avoided altogether.

Emerging out of this infantile catastrophe or psychosis is a schizophrenic personality that has some or all of the following characteristics: alienation, premature developmental closure of the personality, anhedonia, bizarreness, deviant perceptual transformation, neophobia, defective regulatory capacity to channel the data of experience, a sense of vagueness and unreality (seen in the eyes as a glassy, vacant, or fierce stare), and transitivism or feeling like the helpless character in someone else's novel. This schizophrenic personality develops alongside a normal or neurotic personality. Although psychotic (i.e., delusionally oriented) the schizophrenic personality is repressed by the nonpsychotic personality and overtly remains dormant. When activated by various stresses in later life, this schizophrenic personality assumes dominance over the normal personality and mind, resulting in an active symptomatic state.

The overt psychosis, or psychosomatic state of the central nervous system, is characterized by confusion, agitation, and perceptual chaos. Inner and outer stimuli are not attended to in graded fashion or processed into comprehensible meanings. Such an acute state is followed by a state of numbness, dehumanization, and meaninglessness secondary to avoidance and withdrawal. The patient apparently relives in overt form the covert catastrophic experience of the earliest phase of development.

PSYCHOANALYTIC THEORIES OF SCHIZOPHRENIA: CRITIQUE

Psychoanalytic theories of schizophrenia have in recent years fallen into obscurity, mainly because the traumatic-developmental perspective on etiology appears to lack credibility. Virtually all psychoanalytic theorists postulate an experiential disharmony between the mother and her preschizophrenic infant. Whether this derives from genetic or constitutional factors in the infant or from psychological factors in the parent is secondary, as the purported central pathogenic elements are dysphoric experiences which become internalized as aberrant psychological structures. Explicitly or implicitly, the psychogenic models of schizophrenia regard these experiences as sufficient to explain most, if not all, cases of the syndrome.

Several considerations cast doubt on this postulate. First, recent findings from infant research challenge many of the assumptions put forth by psychoanalytic developmentalists. For example, normal development is not like pathological stages projected backward. Infants are active, stimulus-seeking, and socially oriented from day 1. Stages such as the narcissistic, autistic, symbiotic, or schizoid-paranoid are not observed, so it is doubtful that schizophrenia could represent regression to one of them. Also, infants are far more powerful and intricately preprogrammed for adaptation and survival than psychoanalytic theorists assumed; almost without exception they saw them as helpless, utterly dependent, and mindless creatures of infinite malleability. The fact that many infants survive despite unusually bleak or traumatic rearing suggests that factors orthogonal to nurture may be operative.

Second, it is clear that some people who develop schizophrenia as adults come from basically healthy families and undergo normal growth and development—a direct challenge to traumatic hypotheses of etiology. Furthermore, the childhood suffering in the histories of schizophrenic patients is often no more severe or profound than that of patients with other forms of mental illness, suggesting the necessary presence of additional, nonexperiential, pathogenic factors.

Finally, the psychogenic theories have difficulty explaining why, in most cases of schizophrenia, there is an interval of some 2 decades between the purported pathogenic infantile traumatic experiences and the onset of overt symptoms. If the experiences postulated by these theories do indeed occur, one might expect to see symptom formation at the time followed by predictable and nonrepressible (i.e., observable) deformities in subsequent development, at least in some cases. An infantile catastrophe severe enough to produce an illness of the magnitude of schizophrenia is not likely to go unnoticed, yet such catastrophes and their immediate behavioral consequences have not been documented.

Generally, psychoanalytic theories of schizophrenia, especially those with a more descriptive-homeostatic perspective, continue to inform the clinical eye and help clinicians understand the patients they encounter. In this context, they are vital and worthy of study. Furthermore, while exploring the past with schizophrenic patients may no longer be expected to yield etiological or historical truth, it does provide meaningful metaphor that can be useful in the empathic dialogue between doctor and patient.

FAMILY TRANSACTION MODELS

The family transaction models of schizophrenia represent attempts to understand and explain the syndrome as the transmission of aberrant interactions from the family to the patient. The models are compatible with object-relation–oriented psychoanalytic psychogenic theories in assuming psychopathology to be determined largely by experience and learning within the family during growth and development. The models are different, however, in their respective hypothesis-generating and hypothesis-validating data bases. For psychoanalytic theories, the data are the associations of individual patients; for family transaction theories, the data are observed interactions in families with one or more schizophrenic members.

These models emerged following World War II, from the context of clinical work with the families of schizophrenic patients, wherein it was noted with increasing frequency that irrationality was not limited to the identified patient. Unusual and unpredictable interactions were observed between dyads within the family or among family members as an entire unit. Motivated by the idea that these interactions may be schizophrenogenic, several clinical investigators began to describe these families and their transactional patterns in some detail.

GREGORY BATESON AND DONALD JACKSON Gregory Bateson and Donald Jackson, for example, outlined a form of family interaction, which they labeled the *double bind*. The interaction usually occurs between a parent and the schizophrenic offspring; it consists of the former giving the latter incompatible (if not antithetical) messages (e.g., stiffly avoiding a physical embrace while saying, "Why don't you show me more affection?"). This sets up an inescapable damned-if-you-do-and-damned-if-you-don't situation, or double bind, in which the offspring feels paralyzed. Bateson and Jackson hypothesized that repeated exposure to such a dilemma generates or aggravates the schizophrenic state.

RUTH AND THEODORE LIDZ Ruth and Theodore Lidz systematically studied the characteristics of families that had a schizophrenic offspring. Using a psychoanalytically oriented psychodynamic perspective, they looked for and observed disorders in the role and affective relationships among family members, especially the triad of mother, father, and the schizophrenic child. They described several irrational patterns, such as marital schism between parents who remain married because of pathological interdependence despite considerable overt conflict; marital skew between parents who hide chronic disagreement behind a facade of harmony; permeable generational boundaries, where one parent requires the schizophrenic child to assume a parental role; eroticized parent-child relatedness, wherein one parent treats the schizophrenic child as a peer or contemporary; and emotional divorce, in which family members fail to acknowledge and confirm one another's psychological integrity. The Lidzs asserted that such irrational family functioning is sufficient to account for schizophrenia in certain offspring exposed over their formative years.

LYMAN WYNNE AND MARGARET SINGER Lyman Wynne, Margaret Singer, and colleagues explored the nature of communication and cooperation among families with a schizophrenic offspring. From their careful observational work came the concept of communication deviance (CD). This includes parental communications that lack commitment to ideas and precepts; parental communications that are unclear as they are filled with idiosyncratic themes and ideas, have language anomalies, discursive speech, and problems with closure; and parental communications that reflect an inability to establish or maintain a shared focus of attention during transactions with another family member. Among the latter, they identified two common forms: an amorphous style, in which communications are vague, indefinite, and loose, and a fragmented style, in which communications are easily disrupted, poorly integrated, and lack closure. They also described familial displays of mutuality, hostility, or both, which serve as facades hiding antithetical themes and conflicts.

Unlike most other family transactional theorists, Wynne and Singer were able to operationalize their concepts into reliable measures, thus allowing their hypotheses to be tested more systematically. They found CD to be more specific to families of schizophrenic patients compared with the families of patients with depression, personality disorders, neuroses, or no pathology. Furthermore, amorphous patterns of CD correlated more frequently with process schizophrenia and fragmented patterns of CD, with reactive schizophrenia. They also found significant quantitative correlations between amount of CD in the parents and severity of psychopathology in their offspring. For example, schizophrenic offspring came from families where both parents had high levels of CD; normal and neurotic offspring came from families where both parents had low levels of CD; and borderline offspring came from families where one parent's CD level was high and the other parent's was low.

HELM STIERLIN Helm Stierlin described schizophrenia as emerging from a derailed delegating process, in which a vulnerable individual, as a delegate of the parents, becomes overburdened and unable to negotiate adolescent separation-individuation from the nuclear family. He described three major pathological transactional modes between parents and their schizophrenic offspring: binding or overprotection, expelling or overt rejection, and delegating or encouraging separation overtly as long as the adolescent fulfills key covert family missions. While these patterns are not necessarily pathogenic, Stierlin associated the development of chronic and acute schizophrenia with the first and third modes, respectively.

More recently, family investigators have described several family factors that interact powerfully with schizophrenia, either to precipitate its emergence or to aggravate its course. One factor, called expressed emotion (EE), consists of critical or emotionally overinvolved (or both) attitudes and behaviors displayed by parents toward their ill offspring. Another family transactional factor of interest and current study is negative affective style (AS). It includes four kinds of parental behavior: criticism, guilt induction, intrusiveness, and inadequate support. It has been demonstrated and replicated that schizophrenic patients living with high EE or negative AS families relapse with a significantly higher frequency than schizophrenic patients living in families with low EE or normal AS.

Like the psychoanalytic theories of schizophrenia, the family transaction theories have come under considerable criticism as etiological models. With the exception of CD, few of the family transactions described above are demonstrably specific to schizophrenia. Furthermore, it is not implausible that the observed irrational transactions among these families derive from the necessity of dealing with an overtly deviant child, thus reversing the direction of the hypothesized causal vector. In the absence of hard etiological data, the assumption that families transmit and concentrate their irrationalities on a designated family member–victim becomes a nonproductive assignation of blame that does little to advance understanding but much to undermine working alliances between professionals and afflicted families.

Like the psychoanalytic theories of schizophrenia, the family transaction theories remain viable and useful as descriptive-homeostatic models. While irrational behaviors in the families of schizophrenic patients may not cause the illness, these behaviors are nevertheless present and real in their evocative effects. As demonstrated by the EE and AS studies, the family's emotional milieu can profoundly influence the onset or course of schizophrenia. Family transactional stress may not be causative. There is strong evidence, however, that it can be powerfully facilitative in both pathological and therapeutic directions. As such, the family theories as homeostatic models fit well into the most current psychodynamic theory of schizophrenia: the vulnerability-stress model.

VULNERABILITY-STRESS MODEL

ANTECEDENTS The vulnerability-stress model views schizophrenia dynamically as a product of interacting forces, some genetic or biological and some psychological, and some innate or constitutional and some learned through experience. Unlike the purely psychodynamic theories, nature is more important, as suggested by genetic studies and the efficacy of biological treatments. Both nature and experience, however, are considered necessary to describe and understand schizophrenia.

The Finnish adoption study of Tienari and colleagues is illustrative of this model. Comparing adopted away children of schizophrenic mothers (high–genetic risk probands) with adopted away children of nonschizophrenic mothers (low–genetic risk controls), they found that schizophrenia developed only in probands with genetic vulnerability who were raised in adoptive families where the emotional environment was demonstrably unhealthy. None of the high–genetic risk probands raised in healthy adoptive families developed psychosis. Likewise, none of the low–genetic risk probands raised in unhealthy adoptive families developed psychosis, although many developed other forms of psychopathology. These results strongly suggest that both a disturbed rearing environment and an innate vulnerability to schizophrenia are necessary to generate the syndrome.

The concept of such an interaction began with Freud. Describing the origin of neurosis in *On the History of the Psycho-analytic Movement,* he wrote:

> Disposition and experience are here linked up in an indissoluble aetiological unit. For *disposition* exaggerates impressions which otherwise have been completely commonplace and have no effect, so that they became traumas giving rise to stimulations and fixations; while *experiences* awaken factors in the disposition which, without them, might have long remained dormant and perhaps never have developed.

Freud could well have been writing about the origins of psychosis. Certainly, subsequent psychoanalytic theorists took this model seriously in explaining schizophrenia, especially those that emphasized deficit. The true conceptual fathers of today's vulnerability-stress model of schizophrenia, however, are Sandor Rado and Paul Meehl.

Rado hypothesized that schizophrenia begins with an inherited disposition, or genotype. The interaction of this genotype with environment produces the schizophrenic phenotype, a personality type or trait called the schizotype. Central to this trait is an inherent incapacity to experience pleasure.

> In the schizotype the machinery of psychodynamic integration is strikingly inadequate, because one of its essential components, the organizing action of pleasure—its motivational strength—is innately defective.

This defect impairs the development of initiative and leads to schizo-adaptations like compensatory overdependence on others (especially parents) and the elaboration of intricate cognitive processes devoid of affect. Anhedonia results in weak emotional bonds and leads to attenuated relationships. The well-compensated schizotype remains a stable schizoid personality. The poorly compensated schizotype develops exaggerated, bizarre behaviors. Schizophrenia proper represents a decompensated schizotype with adaptive incompetence. The nature and severity of the schizo-adaptation depends on the genotypic loading and on the degree of familial and environmental stress.

To Meehl, the inherited schizophrenic genotype (which he labeled schizotaxia) consists of a defect in neural integration. This defect plus social learning (environment) leads to an abnormally organized personality (the schizotype) characterized by cognitive slippage (thought disorder), anhedonia, ambivalence, and aversion to human relationships. Further progression from schizotypy to schizophrenia depends on the nature and severity of environmental stress versus availability of help and support.

THE MODEL This hypothetically pathogenic interaction between nature and experience came to be known as the stress-diathesis or the vulnerability-stress model. As currently conceived, this model accepts that the relative roles of nature and nurture in the etiology of schizophrenia will remain obscure until there are markers for the genetic predisposition or constitutional vulnerability. It shifts emphasis from the role of psychodynamic factors in etiology to their role in facilitating and preventing the expression of the disease process.

The vulnerability to schizophrenia is seen as a relatively enduring proclivity toward developing clinical symptoms. It is a stable trait independent of nonenduring psychopathological states, meaning that its features are present premorbidly, at onset, during symptomatic efflorescence, and in remission. This trait should not, however, be regarded as developmentally static or fixed. Rather, it is shaped epigenetically via transactions with the environment at each developmental phase. Aspects of vulnerability are undoubtedly genetic. Some may be acquired biologically through intrauterine, birth, and postnatal complications. Season of birth may also contribute, for reasons yet to be ascertained. The evidence for psychosocially acquired vulnerability is meager at present, but it cannot be ruled out.

The stress side of this model postulates that a variety of stressors, that is, internal or external events requiring adaptation, can convert vulnerability into symptoms. Therefore, coping strengths or supports that diminish stress should minimize or prevent clinical expression of vulnerability.

Following the model, the vicissitudes of schizophrenia are determined by the nature of vulnerability and stress and by the individual's strengths and environmental supports. The interaction of sufficient stress with sufficient vulnerability can lead to transient, intermediate (prodromal) states of dysfunction that amplify existing cognitive, affective-autonomic, and social-coping deficits. This, in turn, interacts negatively with stressors and magnifies their effect in a downward spiraling deterioration that culminates in a full-blown clinical syndrome.

VULNERABILITIES TO SCHIZOPHRENIA The list of specific vulnerabilities to schizophrenia is extensive. A few have been demonstrated, and many are postulated. First are deficits in the processing of complex information, in maintaining a steady focus of attention, in distinguishing between relevant and irrelevant stimuli, and in forming consistent abstractions. Second are dysfunctions in psychophysiology, suggesting deficits in sensory inhibition and poor control over autonomic responsivity, especially to aversive stimuli. Third are impairments in social competence, such as processing interpersonal stimuli, eye contact, assertiveness, or conversational capacity. These deficits probably reflect both a core disturbance of schizophrenia (vulnerability) and the social outcomes of severe psychopathology. In the past, the source of these difficulties was often attributed to such external elements as drugs or institutions, a perspective that unduly diverted attention from their primacy in the disorder. Fourth are general coping deficits such as overevaluating threat, underestimating internal resources, and extensive use of denial.

Finding, mapping, and integrating these vulnerabilities has become a central effort in current schizophrenia research. Virtually all of this investigation has focused on demonstrable phenotypic manifestations of hypothetical genotypic vulnerabilities in children and adolescents at risk for schizophrenia. An additional possibility not addressed by this investigative strategy is a genotypic vulnerability with later onset. Huntington's chorea, for example, is an adult-onset neurological deterioration leading to psychosis and dementia; in a similar fashion, many cases of schizophrenia could result from a genotype whose phenotypic expression is not triggered until late adolescence or early adulthood. This phenotype may be a deficit in the neurophysiological maturation of self systems during adolescence or a still later-onset neural deterioration or inhibition of these same systems in adulthood. Early-onset genotypes may help to account for cases with easily identifiable phenotypic deviations that begin in childhood as schizotypal aberrations and progress to chronic, process cases of schizophrenia later on. Later-onset genotypes may help to explain the acute occurrence of schizophrenia later in life in persons with normal growth and development and healthy premorbid personalities.

SOCIOECONOMIC, CULTURAL, AND LIFE EVENT STRESSORS IN SCHIZOPHRENIA

Systematic studies of the stresses that affect the course of schizophrenia have most recently focused on the family environment. Other investigations have concentrated on social class and culture, social networks, and life events.

Socioeconomic and cultural factors have a long history of empirical association with schizophrenia. One of the most replicated findings in the schizophrenia literature is the clustering of schizophrenic patients in the lowest social classes, especially in urban communities. Few now hold that a poor socioeconomic environment causes schizophrenia, but few doubt that it has a major impact on its course. Poverty, ignorance, unemployment, social isolation, poor nutrition, and marginal health care are powerful chronic stressors that lead to frequent breakdown in vulnerable persons.

Many believe that the uneven socioeconomic distribution of schizophrenia is a result, rather than a cause, of the illness. According to Herbert Weiner, the drift hypothesis states that persons who are prone to schizophrenia tend to migrate, or drift, into such areas, in part because the illness makes them socially incompetent or poorly adapted to earning a living. A subhypothesis suggests that such persons are socially mobile, in a downward direction, from generation to generation. Because schizophrenia may be heritable and renders each generation poorly adapted to the social environment, a downward trend occurs over several generations. Eventually, the gene carriers are concentrated in the lowest socioeconomic group. Still another hypothesis relates these findings to the relative lack of psychiatric treatment facilities, other than hospitals, for members of the lowest classes.

International follow-up data suggest that schizophrenic patients in agrarian countries have a more benign course of illness. If agrarian societies selectively apply therapeutic resources to more visible and floridly psychotic schizophrenic individuals with a better prognosis, this finding may reflect sampling artifact. Alternatively, it may be that more rural and economically primitive cultures confront vulnerable persons with fewer demands for initiative and competitiveness while providing them with tighter, smaller, more enduring social and kinship networks.

Schizophrenia and social network are highly interactive, cross-sectionally and longitudinally. Schizophrenic patients usually have social networks that are smaller, less interconnected, simpler, more dependent, casual, nonintimate, and peopled with family as opposed to peers than nonschizophrenic patients. The most dramatic changes in this direction follow the first hospitalization for schizophrenia. After about three hospitalizations, families tend to disengage from the patient. A symptomatic episode forces the patient to rely temporarily on dense formal network clusters (family, hospital, or clinic) requiring little initiative or exchange. Restoration to status quo ante, when achieved, proceeds through formal transitional network clusters, such as churches, self-help groups, sheltered workshops, and day hospitals, where disability and poor motivation are not a bar to membership. The interplay between schizophrenia and social networks appears to be circular rather than linear. Initially, the major vector is schizophrenia on social network. Following the appearance of clinical symptoms, however, social network is likely to exert a powerful influence on the subsequent vicissitudes of schizophrenia.

Stressful life events have a demonstrated association with schizophrenia, but it may not always be necessary or direct. Questions often arise concerning whether stress differs in its effect on disease onset versus recurrence and whether a stressful event precedes illness or represents a product of symptom exacerbation. Convention dichotomizes stressful events into those that are ambient, nonindependent, or chronic, and those that are independent or acute. The former are stresses associated with everyday living, such as family, work, poverty, physical disability, and mental deficit; the latter are stresses associated with largely external or unusual changes, such as loss, death, acute illness, and moves, especially if these changes are unanticipated, undesired, and uncontrolled. Research suggests a high frequency of such events shortly before schizophrenia onset or symptom exacerbation. Furthermore, there appears to be an important interaction between maintenance antipsychotic medication and life-event stress. Patients in the community without medication are vulnerable to acute, as well as to chronic, stress. Patients taking medication, however, appear to be protected against either type of stress, but are likely to suffer relapse if both types occur concurrently.

OVERVIEW

In the twentieth century, psychiatry has seen the elaboration of three major psychodynamic models of schizophrenia: psychoanalytic, family transactional, and vulnerability-stress. All have provided useful descriptions of this mysterious disease. These theories also have elaborated the psychopathological and homeostatic functions of schizophrenia in ways that are meaningful and clinically useful.

In terms of sheer volume, the bulk of psychodynamic theories belong to psychoanalysis. In terms of content, the major issues have not changed much since Freud posited two theories—the structural-conflict theory and the withdrawal-deficit theory. By never integrating these two, Freud seemed to be saying that schizophrenia may be both, in part explained by intrapsychic conflict and in part by something else. Psychodynamic theories became more elaborate and sophisticated over the ensuing years, yet one can still follow the thematic threads of Freud's original part-explanations. Conflict theory has seen a line of development polarized toward object relations, experiential learning within the family, and the stress aspect of the vulnerability-stress model. Deficit theory has seen a line of development polarized toward individual drives, complex constitutional inborn factors, and the vulnerability aspect of the vulnerability-stress model. Today, these threads are each regarded as valid facets of the overall phenomenon. Both are necessary for a comprehensible and potentially workable theory of schizophrenia.

While none of these psychodynamic models of schizophrenia has solved the mystery of its etiology, each system has offered cogent hypotheses or educated guesses. The vulnerability-stress model sees nature as primary, or at least as initiating a process of negative interaction with environmental experience, which becomes pathogenic sooner or later in life, depending on the onset trigger of the genotype. The family transactional model, at least as originally conceived, sees nurture or experience as primary and, frequently, as sufficient for generating schizophrenia. Psychoanalytic models have posited one or the other or both. Since Sullivan and Mahler, however, the emphasis has shifted more uniformly toward the etiological primacy of traumatic nurturing experiences during early development, a shift that has come under increasing criticism as outlined.

Overall, the impressive evidence for the existence of genetic and constitutional factors in schizophrenia has raised questions about the etiological hegemony of experience and learning in early development. Hypothetically, it may be possible that some (if not many) cases of schizophrenia arise from an adolescent-onset neurological dysfunction or deterioration in people who are, up to that point, developmentally normal. Such a process, along the model of Huntington's chorea, selectively inhibits or destroys later developmental levels of personality, especially those neuronal networks involved with the structures, functions, and representations of the self. In response, the individual falls back on more primitively organized levels of personality and development. Such regression is compensatory and adaptive rather than primary and motivating. It does not occur because of developmental fixation but because simpler developmental levels and patterns may be the only ones left.

THERAPEUTIC IMPLICATIONS

With such a model, the study of human development nevertheless remains an important research endeavor, not for its etiological information but for its data about the hierarchical developmental levels of mind, which can inform the study of pathogenesis, severity, and course of illness. Also, with such a model, the study of human development remains cogent for clinical purposes, affording a perspective on how to deal with someone whose mind, at least in part, approximates that of a much younger person in its structural and functional complexity. A certain parallel can be found, for example, between Winnicott's good-enough mother or between Kohut's idealizing parent and the qualities that constitute a good therapist for schizophrenic patients. These are: responsiveness to the infant's idiosyncratic needs and gestures (empathy); nonintrusive holding through quiescent states (being with); survival despite intensity of the infant's needs (limits); failure to retaliate against destructive, greedy, and rageful aspects of object use (tolerance); willingness to share and maintain illusions in transitional space (play); mirroring omnipotence and adoration (hope); and graded disillusionment (titrated reality testing).

Psychodynamic theories of schizophrenia carry with them distinct implications for treatment. Early proponents of the psychoanalytic conflict model advocated the classical techniques of clarification, confrontation, and interpretation. Early proponents of the psychoanalytic deficit model introduced additional strategies. Federn, for example, felt that the usual psychoanalytic techniques aimed at *de*repression whereas, with schizophrenia, the goal was to foster *re*repression. As such, he encouraged positive transference, avoided negative transference, protected patients from undue anxiety and insomnia, taught them to improve their capacities for attention and thinking, exhorted them to give up unrealistic life goals, provided support beyond analytic hours in the form of a skilled nurse-assistant available to the patients at home, and offered consultation to the patient's family (recognizing the importance of the home environment to outcome).

Proponents of the family transactional theories uniformly advocate family therapy in some form. Those that view the family milieu as causing schizophrenia usually regard the entire family as the patient or as the problem and focus interventions accordingly. Those that regard the family as facilitative rather than etiological emphasize the positive and negative effects that domestic tensions can have on the course of the identified patient. Technical strategies in the first instance are more interpretive. In the second instance, they are more psychoeducational.

Proponents of the vulnerability-stress model advocate any intervention that enhances strength and support and minimizes stress and vulnerability. This includes psychobiological as well as psychodynamic treatments. The vulnerability-stress model is the only one that formally (i.e., theoretically) incorporates biology and endorses it therapeutically. This model also defines psychodynamic treatment more liberally. Any and all forms of psychosocial intervention from individual psychotherapy to social skills training are potentially useful, depending on the modality's track record of efficacy with the specific clinical situation or condition.

Conflict psychodynamic models, in keeping with their bias toward object relations and development in the family, emphasize the therapeutic centrality of the doctor-patient relationship. This relationship is facilitating, parental, soothing, mirroring, and protective, and the patient grows by internalizing the interactions that transpire within the dyad. The patient's actual interpersonal experience of the therapist is crucial: the therapist's reality and benignity serve to reality test the patient's transferentially distorted images.

Deficit psychodynamic models, in keeping with their bias toward the patient as an individual with phenotypic abnormalities, emphasize the therapeutic centrality of insight. The goal of treatment is to enhance the power of the ego by expanding its knowledge and control over the inner drives and psychopathological idiosyncrasies. Enlightenment replaces unconscious defense with conscious choice. Therapy from this perspective focuses primarily upon developing the patient's cognitive systems through interpretation, psychoeducation, training, and rehabilitation. The patient comes to develop insight that something is wrong, what that something is, and how it can be dealt with.

The conflict psychodynamicists once eschewed deficit theories as therapeutically nihilistic, insisting that there was no way to make up for a biological defect by psychological means. Such an assertion may be literally correct but operationally erroneous. For example, psychological manipulation cannot make paraplegics walk under their own power, but it can train them in prosthetic ambulation and it can enhance their adaptation and quality of life. Whatever the origin of schizophrenia, its successful psychological treatment involves both the resolution of intrapsychic conflict through insight and the acquisition of psychic structure through affective relationships. If the core of schizophrenia is psychological, then treatment addresses the sick self; if the core is defect, then treatment addresses the healthy self. In the former, it minimizes weakness; in the latter, it maximizes strength. In most cases, it does both.

AN INTEGRATIVE MEDICAL MODEL

One body of theory encompasses all of the foregoing twentieth-century trends—the biopsychosocial medical model of George Engel. According to this model, each individual patient consists of and participates in multiple systems that are related but also distinct from each other. Common systems are subatomic particles, atoms, molecules, organelles, cells, tissues, organs, organ systems, central nervous system, individual, dyad, family, community, culture-subculture, society-nation, and biosphere. In understanding health and disease, all systems are relevant. Each system of this model has a functional structure, one of its purposes being the reduction of complexity and randomness to protect that system's integrity. The functional structure of the psychological systems in this model consist of meanings that serve to order experience through understanding and explanation.

Schizophrenia presents most dramatically at the psychological level as a loss or distortion of the self as a meaningful entity. Despite this, schizophrenia is not entirely or even essentially psychological in its nature. Accordingly, proper medical attention to this disorder should be aimed at any and all relevant systems in the biopsychosocial hierarchy. Whatever schizophrenia may be, it is profoundly disabling and usually chronic. Anything therapeutic that works with sufficient safety is relevant, whether it be biological, psychological, or sociological. Psychodynamic approaches to treatment should not ignore biology because the latter exists outside the realm of empathy and meaning. Biological approaches to treatment should not justify psychological retreat from patients because conflicts cannot be teased apart by electrophoresis. Finally, treatment advocates of both approaches should be aware of patients' social, cultural, and political needs for a place of dignity and safety within society. That is, they also require adequate attention at the social level of the biopsychosocial system.

REFERENCES

Burnham D L, Gladstone A I, Gibson R W: *Schizophrenia and the Need-Fear Dilemma*. International Universities Press, New York, 1969.

Cancro R: General considerations relating to theory in the schizophrenic disorders. In *Towards a Comprehensive Model for Schizophrenic Disorders,* D B Feinsilver, editor, p 97. Analytic Press, Hillsdale, NJ, 1986.

Engel G A: The need for a new medical model: A challenge for biomedicine. Science *196:* 129, 1977.

Federn P: *Ego Psychology and the Psychoses*. Basic Books, New York, 1952.

Freud S: *The Interpretation of Dreams,* standard edition, vol 5. Hogarth Press, London, 1953.

Freud S: *On the History of the Psycho-Analytic Movement,* standard edition, vol 14, p 3. Hogarth Press, London, 1957.

Freud S: *Psychoanalytic Notes on an Autobiographical Account of a Case of Paranoia (Dementia Paranoides),* standard edition, vol 12, p 9. Hogarth Press, London, 1958.

Giovacchini P L: Schizophrenia: Structural and therapeutic considerations. In *Towards a Comprehensive Model for Schizophrenic Disorders,* D B Feinsilver, editor, p 259. Analytic Press, Hillsdale, NJ, 1986.

Greenberg J R, Mitchell S A: *Object Relations in Psychoanalytic Theory*. Harvard University Press, Cambridge, MA, 1983.

Grotstein J S: Schizophrenic personality disorder: "And if I should die before I wake . . . ." In *Towards a Comprehensive Model for Schizophrenic Disorders,* D B Feinsilver, editor, p 29. Analytic Press, Hillsdale, NJ, 1986.

Hogarty G E, Anderson C M, Reiss D J, Kornblith S J, Greenwald D P, Javna C D, Madonia M J, Environmental/Personal Indicators in the Course of Schizophrenia Research Group: Family psychoeducation, social skills training, and maintenance chemotherapy in the aftercare treatment of schizophrenia: I. One-year effects of a controlled study on relapse and expressed emotion. Arch Gen Psychiat *43:* 633, 1986.

Lichtenberg J D: Pao's theory: Origins and future directions. In *Towards a Comprehensive Model for Schizophrenic Disorders,* D B Feinsilver, editor, p 75. Analytic Press, Hillsdale, NJ, 1986.

Lidz T: *Schizophrenia and the Family*. International Universities Press, New York, 1965.

Meehl P E: Schizotaxia, schizotypy, schizophrenia. Am Psychologist *17:* 1, 1962.

Pao P-N: *Schizophrenic Disorders,* p 153. International Universities Press, New York, 1979.

Rado S: *Psychoanalysis of Behavior,* p 276. Grune & Stratton, New York, 1956.

Rosenthal D, Goldberg I, Jacobsen B, Wender P H, Kety S S, Schulsinger F, Eldred C A: Migration, heredity, and schizophrenia. Psychiatry *37:* 521, 1974.

Segal H: *Introduction to the Work of Melanie Klein*. Basic Books, New York, 1973.

Spring B, Zubin J: Vulnerability to schizophrenic episodes and their prevention in adults. In *Primary Prevention in Psychopathology: The Issues,* vol 1, G W Albee, J M Joffe, editors, p 254. University Press of New England, Hanover, NH, 1977.

Stern D: *The Interpersonal World of the Infant*. Basic Books, New York, 1985.

Sullivan H S: *Clinical Studies in Psychiatry,* p 318. Norton, New York, 1956.

Tienari P, Sorri A, Lahti I, Naarala M, Wahlberg K-E, Ronkko T, Pohjola J, Moring J: The Finnish adoptive family study of schizophrenia. Yale Biol Med *58:* 227, 1985.

Wynne L C, Singer M: Thought disorder and family relations of schizophrenics: II. Classification of forms of thinking. Arch Gen Psychiat *9:* 199, 1963.

14.3 SCHIZOPHRENIA: CLINICAL FEATURES

JACK A. GREBB, M.D.
ROBERT CANCRO, M.D., Med.D.Sc.

INTRODUCTION

HISTORY The history of schizophrenia cited here outlines the development of this disease concept and illustrates implications of different theoretical models. It is critical to understand, however, that in the absence of an objective diagnostic marker, any arbitrary set of diagnostic guidelines for schizophrenia (e.g., that of the revised third edition of the *Diagnostic and Statistical Manual of Mental Disorders,* [DSM-III-R]) may eventually prove to have been misleading.

A comparison of present-day clinical presentations of schizophrenia with the descriptions of madness by Pinel and Haslam in the early nineteenth century suggests that the major clinical features of schizophrenia have been fairly constant. There is the clinical impression that, in the past 30 years and perhaps owing to the development of antipsychotic drugs, the symptoms of schizophrenia have become less severe and bizarre. Clinical portrayals of madness in the early nineteenth century were quite descriptive or phenomenological, while the papers by German psychiatrists later in that century attempted to identify specific disease entities. This new attitude was formed by Koch's classical experiments, presented before the Physiological Society of Berlin in 1882, that demonstrated the bacterium responsible for tuberculosis. The presenting clinical picture became a major emphasis in medicine from which inferences could be drawn about specific causes and predictions could be made concerning the natural course. Koch's postulates led to a major emphasis on the search for disease entities in psychiatry.

Pre-Kraepelinian psychiatrists Benedict Morel, a contemporary of Emil Kraepelin, first introduced the term *démence precoce* in 1856 to describe the condition of an originally bright and active adolescent who gradually became gloomy and withdrawn. For the French concept of *delires* (delusional states), the Germans contrived a Latin-Greek appellation—*paranoia*—and in 1868, Wilhelm Sander described paranoid states as they are understood today. The symptom picture of catatonia was accurately depicted in 1868 by Karl Kahlbaum, and hebephrenia was given its name in 1870 by Hecker.

Kraepelin Emil Kraepelin (Fig. 14.3-1) latinized Morel's term to dementia praecox in 1898 and used it to describe catatonic, hebephrenic, and other psychotic states with a deteriorating course. The term "praecox" (hereafter, precox) referred both to the early onset of the illness and the subsequent rapid development of dementia-like symptoms. Kraepelin considered schizophrenia to have an endogenous, organic cause. He differentiated patients with dementia precox from those with manic-depressive psychosis (bipolar disorder), the latter having episodes of psychosis separated by periods of normal mental health without a deteriorating course. In addition to the deteriorating course of schizophrenia, Kraepelin provided detailed descriptions of symptoms such as hallucinations, delusions, negativism, and stereotypies. Kraepelin wrote that approximately 4 percent of patients experienced almost complete recovery and that another 13 percent had a much less severe course, without marked intellectual deterioration. These exceptions to the diagnostic guidelines, as well as the impracticality of needing to observe the course before a diagnosis could be made, fueled the objections of Kraepelin's critics.

Bleuler Eugen Bleuler (Fig. 14.3-2) made three major contributions to the development of the concept of schizophrenia. First, in 1911, he coined the name schizophrenia (splitting of the mind), which reflected his belief that a disharmony of psychic functions, rather than a deteriorating course (as suggested by Kraepelin), was the pathognomonic feature of schizophrenia. Second, Bleuler incorporated Freudian theories to explain the meaning of psychotic symptoms (e.g., blocking as an extreme form of repression). Third, Bleuler pointed out that symptoms similar to those seen in schizophrenia were experienced by mentally healthy people under certain conditions (e.g., sleep deprivation) and that it was the severity and duration of the symptoms that defined schizophrenia as an illness.

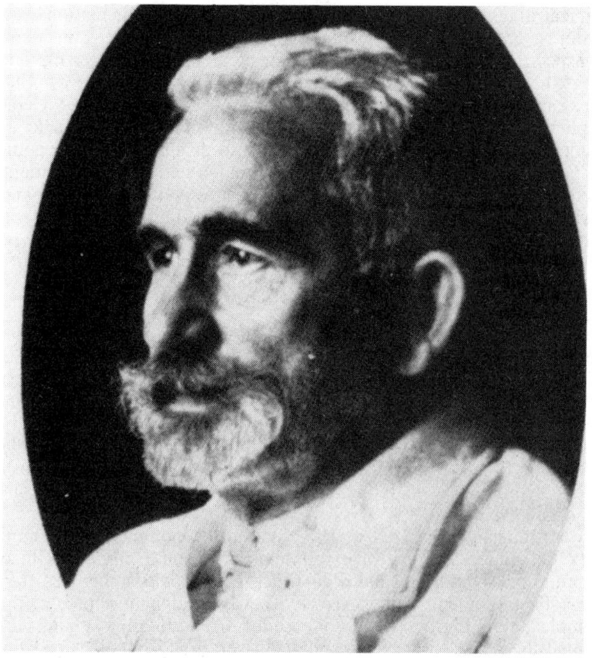

FIGURE 14.3-1. *Emil Kraepelin. (From Davison G C, Neale, J M:* Abnormal Psychology: An Experimental Clinical Approach. *Wiley, New York, 1974, with permission.)*

Bleuler defined four fundamental symptoms—abnormal *a*ssociations in thinking, *a*utistic behavior and thinking, abnormal *a*ffect (including flat and inappropriate affects), and *a*mbivalence (Bleuler's four As). Although important for describing schizophrenic psychopathology, these symptoms are quite general and difficult to measure in operational terms; this severely limits their usefulness in

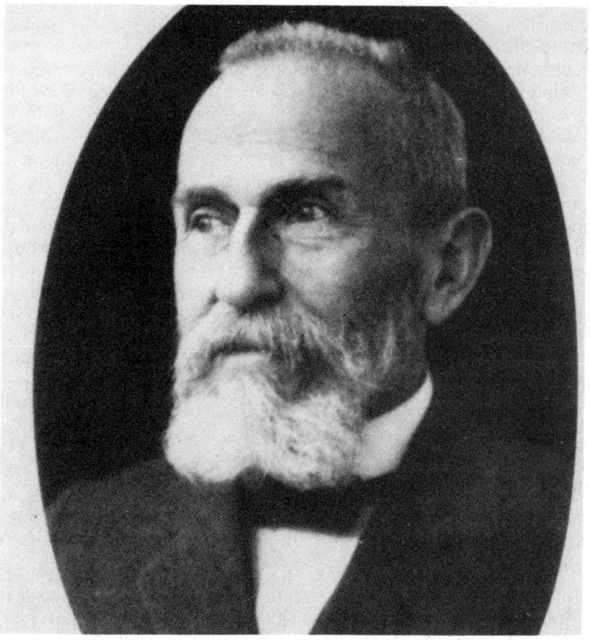

FIGURE 14.3-2. *Eugen Bleuler. (From Davison G C, Neale, J M:* Abnormal Psychology: An Experimental Clinical Approach. *Wiley, New York, 1974, with permission.)*

clinical diagnosis. Accessory symptoms included hallucinations, delusions, and catatonic postures, all of which were considered nonspecific for schizophrenia. Certain of these accessory symptoms (e.g., haptic hallucinations) occurred more often in patients who had other mental disorders. Perhaps the major effect of Bleuler's conceptualization was to broaden the definition of schizophrenia to include patients who would not have been so diagnosed by Kraepelinian criteria. Bleuler, in fact, thought many schizophrenic patients were latent schizophrenics, persons whose symptoms were not serious enough to require hospitalization. Bleuler believed, as did Kraepelin, that schizophrenia had an organic etiology, but his writings emphasized that psychological factors could shape the specific symptom pattern of any individual patient.

Psychodynamic psychiatrists Although Sigmund Freud's conceptualizations changed over the years, his basic premise was that symptoms of schizophrenia resulted from a seriously impaired ego that allowed expression of primary-process drives of a sexual and aggressive nature. In 1924, he suggested that psychosis was not a loss of reality but was an attempt to remodel reality restitutively. Although Freud emphasized the importance of understanding psychotic symptoms psychologically, he thought that schizophrenia had an organic basis.

Carl Jung hypothesized in 1903 that an autonomous mental complex not under the control of consciousness could produce schizophrenia-like symptoms, many of which represented archetypes from the collective unconscious. Affectivity was the dynamic force of this complex; thinking and behavior resulted from affectivity. Jung also coined the terms "introvert" and "extrovert," and hypothesized that schizophrenic patients were in the former class and hysteric patients in the latter. Jung acknowledged that Kraepelin's notion of organic cause was possible, but he also proposed that psychological factors might induce the body to produce a toxin that affected the brain.

Adolf Meyer, founder of the psychobiological school of psychiatry, hypothesized that schizophrenia was a nonadaptive reaction to traumatic life events. While Kraepelin and Bleuler attempted to group patients, Meyer emphasized the unique nature of each individual.

Harry Stack Sullivan, founder of the interpersonal school of psychiatry, felt that the major force in psychic development was the quality of interactions and relationships with other people, especially one's parents. Sullivan hypothesized that schizophrenia was a disorder of nonorganic mental structure that represented the combined effects of organic and interpersonal factors. Sullivan was, perhaps, the most hopeful psychiatric theoretician concerning the psychotherapeutic treatment of schizophrenia.

Stress-diathesis model Although the passage of time allows a select number of previous writers to be singled out as important, the description of contemporary ideas about schizophrenia requires more global discussions about conceptual frameworks. The stress-diathesis model is probably accepted most widely in contemporary psychiatry. It posits that a person experiences the onset of schizophrenia when stressors act on a brain that is characterized by a vulnerability (or diathesis) to producing the symptoms of schizophrenia. If the vulnerability is marked, the triggering stress can be comparatively small; if the vulnerability is slight, the stress must be more severe. Although the diathesis is usually conceptualized as organic and genetically transmitted, it could, hypothetically, result from early psychosocial experiences. Similarly, although the stress is most often conceptualized as being psychosocial, it could also be biologically based (e.g., drug abuse, infection, trauma, toxins). The stress-diathesis model is consistent with the observation of heterogeneous clinical histories in schizophrenia.

CLINICAL SIGNS AND SYMPTOMS

Three key issues regarding clinical signs and symptoms confound the diagnosis of schizophrenia. First, no clinical sign or symptom has been demonstrated to be pathognomonic. Virtually every sign or symptom seen in schizophrenia has been reported to occur in other psychiatric and neurological disorders. It is not possible to diagnose schizophrenia when the only information available is the current mental status examination; history and prospective information are essential for the diagnosis of schizophrenia. Second, the symptoms of an individual patient change with time; for example, a patient may have intermittent hallucinations and a varying level of ability to perform adequately in social situations. This variability of symptoms is information that is required to make a correct diagnosis. (Episodes of psychosis separated by periods of normal mental health can be indicative of a mood disorder rather than schizophrenia.) Third, it is necessary to take into account the educational level, intellectual ability, and cultural and subcultural orientation of the patient. The inability to understand abstract concepts, for example, might reflect ignorance or low intelligence. Various religious or cult organizations have customs that seem strange to outsiders but are perfectly normal within the cultural milieu. Although there may be instances of group psychosis, these are exceptional. The psychiatrist evaluating a member of a subculture for the presence of schizophrenia can often utilize the impressions of other members of the group.

The abuse of prescribed or illicit drugs should also be considered in the assessment of a patient with schizophrenia-like symptoms. Many drugs can cause acute onset of a temporary psychosis. Although many clinicians feel that the use of illicit drugs can precipitate a schizophrenic episode, there are no compelling data to indicate that drug abuse itself can cause schizophrenia. Finally, many schizophrenic patients may have received some form of pharmacotherapy before they are seen by a psychiatrist. Antipsychotics may be suppressing the gross psychotic symptoms of these patients, making correct diagnosis almost impossible. Conversely, antipsychotics and other sedative drugs may make the clinical presentation of a nonschizophrenic patient deceptively similar to that of a schizophrenic patient with marked deficit symptoms (e.g., social withdrawal).

PREMORBID SYMPTOMS For any given patient, the border between what is considered the premorbid or prepsychotic personality and the prodromal phase of the illness is arbitrary. Between 50 and 75 percent of patients with schizophrenia have no premorbid behavioral or personality abnormalities. Approximately 25 to 50 percent of patients with schizophrenia do. Patients are often described as having been withdrawn, introverted, suspicious, eccentric, or impulsive. Some schizophrenic patients were particularly passive as babies and demonstrated short attention span, delayed developmental milestones, poor motor coordination, and impaired sensorimotor coordination. In grade school, these children have been reported to have had interpersonal difficulties, poor affective control, odd or disturbing behaviors, cognitive problems, and reduced emotional rapport with their classmates.

The classical (but actually quite variable) history is that of a schizoid or schizotypal personality disorder—quiet, passive, with few friends as a child; daydreaming, introverted, and shut in as an adolescent and adult. The child often is reported to have been especially obedient and never in any mischief. The preschizophrenic adolescent may have no close friends and few dates and may avoid competitive sports while enjoying movies, television, and listening to music to the exclusion of more social activities. Other personality disorders that may have been present in some schizophrenic patients are paranoid and borderline personality disorders.

Relationship to DSM-III-R schizotypal personality disorder Of all the personality disorders defined in DSM-III-R, it is schizotypal personality disorder that has been most implicated as being within a range of schizophrenia-related disorders of differing severity, which are referred to as the *schizophrenia spectrum*. The prevalence of schizotypal personality disorder is abnormally high in the relatives of schizophrenic probands. However, there is not a higher risk of developing schizophrenia in the relatives of schizotypal probands. Some recent work has suggested that the schizotypal symptoms of aloofness, suspiciousness, oddness, idiosyncratic communication, and poor social and vocational performance are specifically related to the schizophrenia spectrum. When present in schizotypal patients, the more classically psychotic symptoms (e.g., looseness of associations, delusions, magical thinking) appear not to increase the likelihood that the patient will develop schizophrenia. The vast majority of patients with schizotypal features do not develop schizophrenia and certainly should not be treated prophylactically with antipsychotics; conversely, the majority of patients with schizophrenia appear not to have had schizotypal personality disorder or any other premorbid personality abnormalities.

SYMPTOMS AT ONSET Although the onset of illness is often defined either as the time of diagnosis or of first hospitalization, symptoms of the illness can often be seen to have developed slowly over the previous month or year. The person may first complain of somatic symptoms, such as headache, back and muscle pain, weakness, or stomach problems, and may initially be diagnosed as a malingerer or as having a somatization disorder. Family and friends may eventually notice that the person has changed as he or she begins to function less well in work, school, social, and personal activities. The affected person may begin to feel anxious or perplexed during this stage of the illness and also may develop an interest in abstract ideas, philosophy, the occult, or religious matters. DSM-III-R includes markedly peculiar behavior, abnormal affect, unusual speech, bizarre ideas, and strange perceptual experiences in the list of prodromal symptoms.

The subjective experience for the patient at this time can be quite anxiety-provoking and depressing. As onset very often occurs during adolescence, the patient, his or her family and friends, and the doctor may all be uncertain whether the symptoms represent normal adolescence, situational or family problems, or serious mental illness. The patient may sense that something ominous is happening and may feel locked in, powerless, and harassed. He or she may make desperate attempts to regain control through elaborate schemes of body and character building. As described by H. A. Lehmann, the following is a personal schedule, devised by a 19-year-old man 3 months before he was admitted to a mental hospital in an acute catatonic stupor:

Time	*Activity*
7:00—8:00	Cold bath, toiletries, bed, dress
8:00—8:15	Encyclopedia (memorize three facts)
8:15—8:30	Handwriting
8:30—8:45	Brisk walk
8:45—9:00	Breakfast (one apple, one dish of bran, two glasses of milk, two glasses of water)
9:00—10:00	Hearing, sight, and scent
10:00—11:00	European, financial, and sports news
11:00—12:00	Wax floors and clean door knobs
12:00—1:00	Cold bath and exercises
1:00—1:30	Geometry
1:30—1:45	Vegetable lunch (very light)
1:45—2:45	Music
2:45—3:45	Walk as far as Atwater and then back to library
3:45—4:45	Study at library
4:45—6:00	Accounting
6:00—6:20	Cold bath
6:20—6:35	Vegetable supper
6:35—8:05	Accounting
8:05—9:00	Hearing, sight, and scent
9:00—9:30	*Strength and Health* magazine
9:30—10:00	Wardrobe
10:00—10:20	Cold bath
10:20—10:40	Study vocabulary (12 words)
10:40—11:00	Undress and toiletries
11:00—11:15	Breathing exercise
11:15—11:30	Note improvement in mental fortitude in diary

MENTAL STATUS EXAMINATION The findings on a mental status examination of a schizophrenic patient differ, depending on whether the patient is experiencing an exacerbation of acute psychotic symptoms or is in a fairly complete remission. The symptoms of an acute psychotic episode also vary markedly among schizophrenic patients. The following descriptions of the mental status examination, the neurological examination, and psychological testing represent composites of abnormal findings, virtually any combination of which may be seen in an individual patient at a particular time.

General description and abnormal behaviors The most common first impressions of a schizophrenic patient may be extremes of bizarreness, agitation, or withdrawal. Although the first two are obvious when present, withdrawal may present as set facial expression, few spontaneous movements, lack of sustained eye contact with the interviewer, and staring at inanimate objects in the room.

Deteriorated appearance and manners The personal appearance of a schizophrenic patient tends to deteriorate. Efforts at grooming and self-care may become minimal, and patients may have to be reminded to wash, bathe, shave, and change their clothes; in general, they show poor regard for the social amenities. Some schizophrenic patients may dress bizarrely, in unusual and loud colors and combinations of patterns or bizarre accessories. They may fail to return a greeting or a smile or carry on their part in a conversation and may exhibit idiosyncratic table manners or offensive behavior.

Lack of motivation This may first be evident to a clinician when the patient seems not to care about talking to the doctor or about his or her illness or situation. Further questioning of patient, friends, and family may disclose that there is a pervasive lack of planning and volition. The patient may have stopped working at a job, completing schoolwork, or doing household chores. The patient may show complete disinterest in planning what to do during the coming day, let alone the next week or year.

Somatic symptoms Plausible and relatively mild somatic complaints are quite common during the prodromal phase of schizophrenia, and more extreme and even bizarre somatic concerns occur during later phases of the illness. However, the profoundly uncommunicative nature of some patients may cause them not to complain about potentially serious medical symptoms. For example, severely regressed schizophrenic patients may suffer silently from abdominal pain that, without adequate medical care, can result in a ruptured appendix; a schizophrenic woman may not report symptoms of pregnancy.

Stereotyped behavior This behavior is more often seen in chronic schizophrenic patients than in acutely ill ones. It may present itself as repetitive patterns of moving or walking (e.g., walking the same circle every day), repetitive performance of strange gestures, or endless repetitions of the same phrase or question. For more than 5 years, a 36-year-old schizophrenic man greeted his doctor, whenever they met, with the question, "Is it going to rain?" (in the summer) or "Is it going to snow?" (in the winter). It may sometimes be difficult to distinguish stereotyped behavior from obsessive-compulsive symptoms that also occur in schizophrenia. Both types of symptoms are thought to carry a poor prognosis.

Social withdrawal and relationship to examiner Social withdrawal is a very common symptom in schizophrenia. The examiner feels unable to establish rapport with the patient, as do others in the patient's life. This symptom often prevents others from feeling empathy or sympathy toward the patient, thereby further isolating the patient. Health care providers, family, and friends should be educated in this matter and be encouraged consciously to try to overcome the tendency not to feel warmth toward these individuals. Conversely, some schizophrenic patients are bizarrely intrusive, demonstrating no appreciation for the usual social and interpersonal boundaries and conventions.

The reaction of a clinician to the patients' social withdrawal and other symptoms has, in the past, been described as the *precox feeling,* and has been claimed by some clinicians to be virtually diagnostic of schizophrenia. Although this feeling is understandable, there are absolutely no data to indicate that it is a valid or reliable criterion for the diagnosis of schizophrenia, and clinicians should not consider it in the decision-making process, except as a possibly useful countertransference experience.

Stuporous states Until the mid-1930s, mental hospitals were filled with stuporous catatonic patients, many of whom would lie motionless for weeks or months, unresponsive to almost every stimulus (Fig. 14.3-3). They had to be fed by gavage twice a day and catheterized regularly. For some unknown reason, stuporous states are quite rare now. Such stuporous patients were also known to erupt with episodes of excited catatonia. Also rare today is *waxy flexibility* (catalepsy), which was present in many patients 40 years ago. It consisted of wax-like yielding of the limbs and trunk, such that a patient put into even an awkward and apparently uncomfortable position would remain so for very long periods of time.

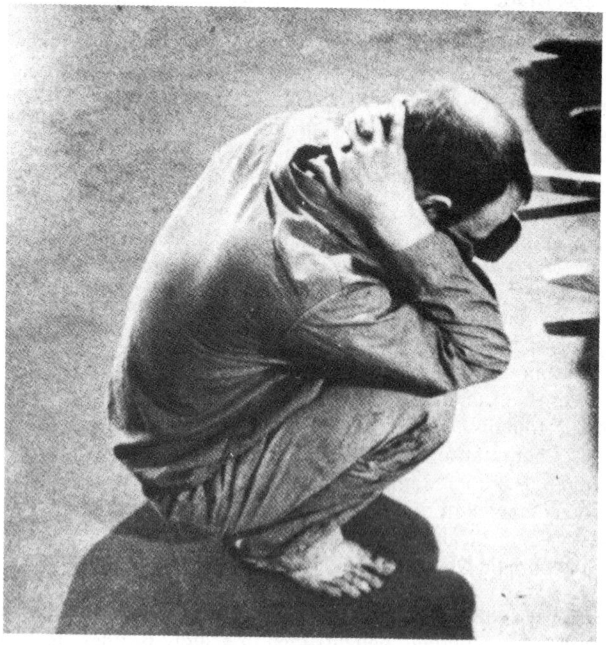

FIGURE 14.3-3. *A patient exhibiting catatonic posturing. (From Davison G C, Neale, J M:* Abnormal Psychology: An Experimental Clinical Approach. *Wiley, New York, 1974, with permission.)*

Eating disorders Eating disorders (which meet some, but usually not all, of the criteria for anorexia nervosa, bulimia nervosa, or pica) are not rare in schizophrenia. Obesity, a common clinical problem, especially in female patients, is exacerbated by many psychotropic medications. Approximately one-half of schizophrenia-related eating disorders are in response to psychotic experiences—for example, the belief that the food is poisoned.

Self-induced water intoxication It is sometimes noted on routine laboratory tests that a patient has a low urine specific gravity and low serum sodium concentration. It may retrospectively be noted that the patient seems always to be at the water fountain. This syndrome should be considered in the differential diagnosis of seizures in schizophrenic patients, and the workup for increased water intake should include tests for inappropriate secretion of antidiuretic hormone, which is sometimes caused by treatment with antipsychotics, carbamazepine (Tegretol), lithium, or other drugs.

Echopraxia This symptom, the motor analog of echolalia, consists of the imitation of the movements and gestures of the person the schizophrenic patient is observing.

Negativism A patient's refusal to cooperate with even the most simple and reasonable requests constitutes *negativism.* Sometimes the patient may even do the opposite of what is asked.

Mood, feelings, and affect In schizophrenia, mood, feelings, and affect can be grossly reduced, extremely exaggerated, or patently bizarre. Milder abnormalities, as well as mixtures of symptoms, are common. It is very important to remember that the observable affect of a schizophrenic patient may not reflect the patient's inner mood (e.g., a schizophrenic patient who constantly smiles should not be assumed to be happy and contented).

Reduced emotional responses Many schizophrenic patients seem to be indifferent (or, at times, totally apathetic). Others with less marked emotional restriction, or *blunting,* show emotional shallowness. Inexperienced observers, however, should be extremely careful in assessing emotional depth. For example, what is normal emotional expression in Anglo-Saxon culture may suggest a flattened emotional response in a person from a Mediterranean culture. This can be a particularly difficult assessment to make in urban emergency rooms that serve a large variety of cultural groups. *Anhedonia* is an extreme form of reduced emotions in which the patient is incapable of experiencing, or even imagining, any pleasure; the result is a sense of profound emotional barrenness. Patients themselves often offer valuable and valid information about their own gradually increasing inability to experience emotions.

Inappropriate responses Many times the emotional reaction of a schizophrenic patient is incongruous or inappropriate to the ideational content or situation. A patient may talk about a morbid subject with a smile or answer a straightforward question with anger. In some patients with schizophrenia, disorganized type, a profound silliness can color all interpersonal interactions. Again, it should be remembered that the patient's outward affect may not represent his or her internal emotional tone.

Bizarre emotions Schizophrenia not only alters emotional reactions; it may induce strange emotions that are rarely experienced by normal persons. A patient may feel, for example, states of exaltation, feelings of omnipotence, oneness with the universe, religious ecstasies, terrifying apprehensions about the disintegration of personality or body, or anxiety about impending destruction of the universe.

Emotional sensitivity Many clinicians have described a particular sensitivity to emotional trauma in schizophrenic patients. It has been clinically noted that schizophrenic patients are very easily hurt by even slightly aggressive or rejecting behavior by others, behavior that, in most cases, would not be noticed by a person of normal emotional sensitivity. This observation is particularly germane to less experienced clinicians who, feeling frustrated in their therapeutic efforts to treat a schizophrenic patient, may say or do something that is unconsciously aggressive. Such behavior on the part of a therapist can provoke an exacerbation of psychotic symptoms. This emotional sensitivity also needs to be considered when the schizophrenic individual is at home with his or her family or in the workplace.

Perceptual disturbances Hallucinations and illusions are very common in schizophrenia, but the frequency of these symptoms may vary among cultures. There is some indication that hallucinations are more common in African, West Indian, and Asian cultures than in American and European ones. Somewhat parallel to the emotional sensitivity of schizophrenic patients, some patients seem to have a perceptual hypersensitivity to light, sound, touch, smell, and taste. Small changes in the lighting on another person's face, for example, might be perceived as dramatic changes by some schizophrenic patients.

Hallucinations Hallucinations may occur in any of the five sensory modalities. Patients may be reluctant to discuss their hallucinations; therefore, clinicians need to take a particularly nonthreatening and nonjudgmental approach in order to elicit this information. Auditory hallucinations are the most common (50 to 75 percent of patients). Sometimes the voices are those of God or the devil; sometimes they are voices of deceased relatives, neighbors, or unrecognized individuals. Two or more voices may discuss the patient in the third person; voices may make threatening or obscene comments about the patient. Patients can often be observed talking aloud to their hallucinated voices, as if in conversation. The hallucinations may also be merely of identifiable or unidentifiable sounds.

Visual hallucinations are less frequent in schizophrenia, but they are not rare. Tactile, olfactory, and gustatory hallucinations do occur, but the clinician must be particularly careful to rule out organic causes for them. Schizophrenic patients sometimes report *cenesthetic hallucinations,* sensations of altered states in body organs without plausible explanations (e.g., a burning sensation in the brain, a pushing sensation in the blood vessels, or a cutting sensation in bone marrow). Illusions may also occur in schizophrenia, but the clinical differentiation between hallucinations and illusions may be quite difficult when discussing a particular sensory experience of an individual patient.

Unusual perceptual sensations Schizophrenic patients may experience a haunting unfamiliarity with their normal environment, sometimes causing them to feel a sensory "jolt," or, at other times, feeling a remoteness and lack of contact with the world through the usual five senses.

Thought process It is possible to attempt—not always successfully—to divide nonperceptual disorders of thought into disorders of content, process, and form.

Disorders of content Disorders of content reflect ideas, beliefs, and interpretations of stimuli.

DELUSIONS Delusions, the clearest example of a disorder of content, can be quite bizarre and varied in schizophrenia and may be persecutory, grandiose, religious, or somatic. The patient may believe that some outside entity is controlling his or her thoughts or behaviors, or, conversely, that he or she is controlling outside events in some extraordinary fashion (e.g., causing the sun to rise and set, preventing earthquakes). Common paranoid delusions of patients are that they are being spied upon, talked about, or at risk of being harmed. The experiences of thought broadcasting, thought insertion, thought withdrawal, and thought control (e.g., "by X-rays") are common in schizophrenia and can be variously conceptualized as delusions, disorders of perception, or the result of a loss of ego boundaries. Frequently, the schizophrenic patient's delusions of imminent doom take the form of a delusional scientific or political insight that the patient believes can prevent or counteract the threat. The patient may be driven by an urgent need to get this important message to scientific or government authorities, who should then be able to put it into action for the protection of humankind. Such patients often use excessive scientific jargon, and the schemes may seem almost rational at first glance.

A common characteristic of schizophrenic delusions is the direct, immediate, and total certainty with which the patient holds these beliefs. If asked why he or she believes such an unlikely idea, a schizophrenic patient will often simply say, "I know it." Although delusions can occur in any psychotic illness, the clinical impression is that schizophrenic delusions are consistently more bizarre, as in the following excerpt from a letter written by a schizophrenic patient.

> Further to my investigation . . . I would like to inform that the TADPOLE in the eyes moves or floats around with the movement of the iris. . . . The tadpole reveals the photographic and its spirit the parabiological matter. From experience the Spirit is more deadly than the vision—the vision could bring on a person a berserk or manic attitude if he is unaware of its tricks—it could also be a danger to schizoid, alcoholic, and neurotic personalities. Further to the tadpole, it is luminous in the dark at times and flashes rings of light when both eyes are closed. Have you any idea if science could produce a solution that could cover the iris and eradicate the tadpole and the luminous matter? I repeat again, this is a diabolical science deliberately soon to destroy human nature.

CONCERN WITH THE ESOTERIC AND SYMBOLIC The above example also illustrates a tendency among schizophrenic patients to have an intense and consuming preoccupation with esoteric, abstract, symbolic, psychological, or philosophical ideas (Fig. 14.3-4). The patient's speech may be filled with symbolic images, the meaning of which is difficult to comprehend even with concerted effort.

LOSS OF EGO BOUNDARIES This phrase describes a patient's lack of a clear sense of where his or her own body, mind, and

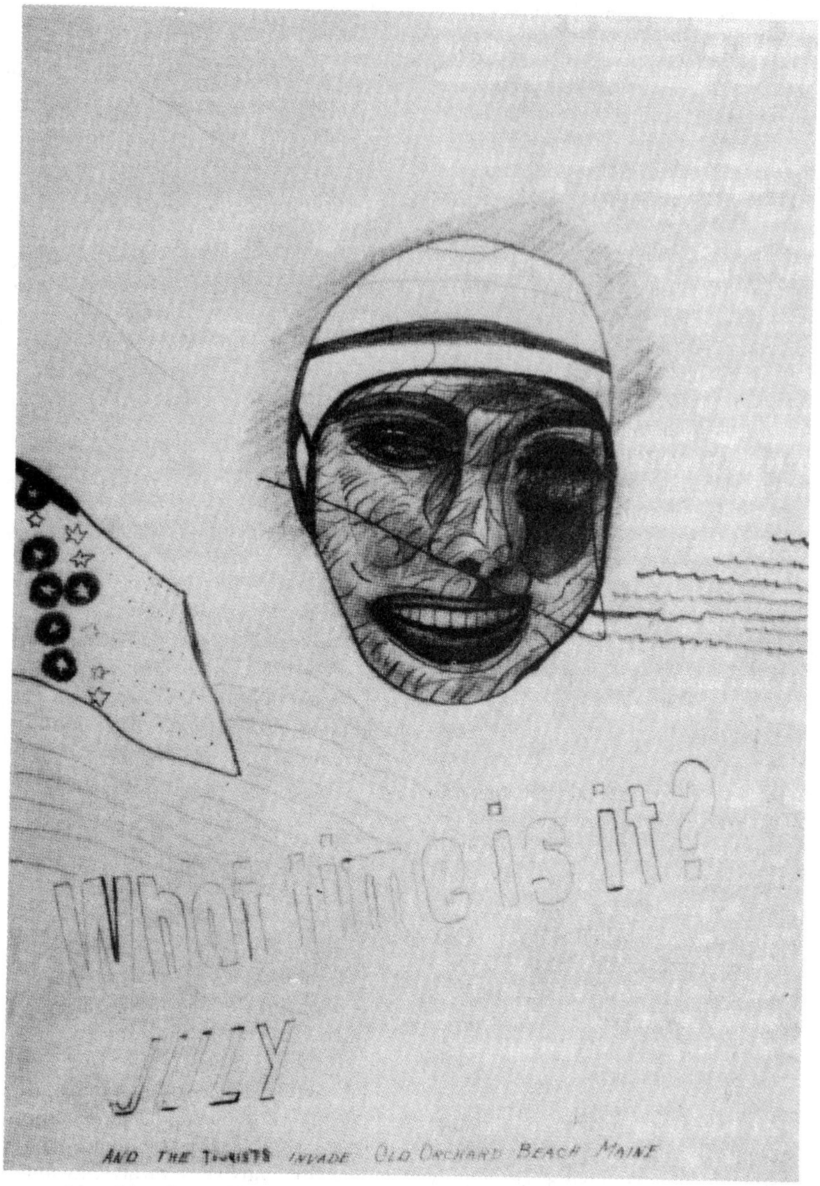
What time is it?
JULY
AND THE TOURISTS INVADE OLD ORCHARD BEACH MAINE

FIGURE 14.3-4. *A 25-year-old schizophrenic man produced this eerie-looking mixture of commercial poster and existential quandary about time.*

influence end, and where these characteristics in other animate and inanimate objects begin. For example, the patient may have *ideas of reference*—that other people, the television, or the newspapers are talking about him or her. Other symptoms include the sense of having fused with outside objects (e.g., a tree, another person) or of having disintegrated completely. Depersonalization and derealization can be conceptualized as stemming from a loss of clear ego boundaries. Given this state of mind, it is not surprising that patients with schizophrenia may have doubts as to which sex they are or what their sexual orientation is. These symptoms should not be confused with transvestism, transsexuality, or homosexuality.

Disorders of form and process Disorders of the form of thought are objectively observable in the spoken and written language of the patient; disorders of the process of thought are inferred by the examiner in a manner similar to how the mood of a patient is inferred during the mental status examination. Disorders in process refer to how ideas and language are formulated within the person's brain. The inference is based mostly on what and how the patient says, writes, or draws (Fig. 14.3-5), although it may be possible to make assessments about thought processes by observing how a patient behaves, especially in carrying out discrete tasks such as one might see in an occupational therapy session. Some writers have classified specific thought disorders as either disorders of process or form, but there is some disagreement about this division because the two are so interrelated. Disorders of thought process and form include looseness of associations, incoherence (similar to word salad), tangentiality, flight of ideas, neologisms, echolalia, verbigeration, mutism, thought blocking, impaired attention, poor abstraction abilities, perseveration, idiosyncratic associations (e.g., identical predicates, clang associations), overinclusion, illogical ideas, vagueness, poverty of content, and circumstantiality.

Schizophrenic patients do not seem to be aware that their verbal communication is abnormal. Although some of these disorders of thought have previously been said to be pathognomonic for schizophrenia (looseness of associations, for example), these symptoms are also seen in other psychotic disorders. Even if the more bizarre symptoms are seen more often in schizophrenia, this observation is not diagnostically useful.

The following proclamation was written by a schizophrenic woman. The phrases are repetitive, and the syntax is distorted, which, together with numerous non sequiturs, renders the text sometimes incoherent.

> The French Force orders from now on to the German Force to respect the Queen Sacre in Christianity as well as the Queens in France & in other countries, ill treated and destroyed in all countries since the beginning of this century in Europe and allied countries. The Queens are the co-partners in masonry of the order of Grand Masters and by doing so the prosperity and balance of the world have been destroyed, they have been destroyed for homosexuality which is the emblem of grand mystery really instead of being distinguished from the criminals who kill the soul and commit the crime of homosexuality of destroying the emblem of grand mastery. The attack on the Queen Sacre in Masonry comes from an inversion in data in the German spying service in 1903 in the class of sorcerers of this organization, deciding that the Chateau de Chambord en France was going to be the Castle not of the saint to be, but of the sorceress and killing in soul that child many times without the effect desired obtained.

The following is a patient's short apologetic note to a psychiatrist whom she had bluntly propositioned on frequent occasions and expresses her sexually laden message briefly and, in her way, to the point. She had previously inserted a screwdriver into her vagina and later expressed continuing guilt feelings for having done so.

> Dear . . .
> I wasn't thinking too well when I was speaking to you but I do believe you were the postman whom I spent the night with. It is still Dr. David . . . in my heart. Am sick because of the screw driver. Please no hard feelings. Kiss your penis did. I would not harm you. . . .
>
> Sincere regards,

The following brief transcript from a videotaped interview with a schizophrenic young man illustrates his autistic preoccupation with sex and death; there seems to be some clang association (association by sound) between "feet" and "foetus." The patient was puzzled that his interviewer had difficulties following him.

> the fleur de Lys is a castrated ace—you see, the design is the feet—the same as a woman's foetus—now you take five French safes and you put them together between four coffins—that's what it represents. . . .

THOUGHT BLOCKING When a patient's thoughts seem to stop suddenly and without warning, the phenomenon is referred to as *thought blocking*. The patient may cease speaking in the middle of a sentence and may remain silent for seconds or minutes. Questioned about the experience, patients sometimes report the physical sensation of having had their thoughts taken out of their heads.

POVERTY OF CONTENT The examiner may often feel that he or she has received no information from the patient, despite the fact that he or she has listened intently to the patient for several minutes. This is referred to as *poverty of content*. Conversely, some clinicians claim to be able to understand virtually every verbal production of their schizophrenic patients. While it is undoubtedly worthwhile to attempt to understand a schizophrenic patient's verbal output, there may also be a tendency for some clinicians to overvalue the patient's psychotic productions and covertly encourage them. Even though a sensitive clinician may sense what a patient is trying to communicate, it may be inappropriate to imply to the patient that his or her communication style is normal. The clinician could easily misinterpret the verbal productions of a psychotic patient and draw incorrect conclusions.

PSYCHOANALYTIC CONCEPTS Many observers believe that the schizophrenic person uses archaic modes of mystical or magical thinking. Such primitive modes of thinking are closely related to the psychoanalytic concept of primary thought processes that are at work in normal dreaming and that allow for condensations, reversal, substitution, displacement, and other distortions of conceptual relations impossible in rationally controlled thought.

ABILITY TO UTILIZE ABSTRACT CONCEPTS An impairment in the ability of schizophrenic patients to utilize abstract concepts has often been emphasized. The interpretation of proverbs is traditionally used to test this ability. A schizophrenic patient may interpret, "A stitch in time saves nine" as meaning, "I should sew nine buttons on my coat," both personalizing the proverb and missing the abstract concept about procrastination. The clinician should be cautioned that the use of proverbs is not a particularly reliable test in uncontrolled clinical settings, and that many other factors (e.g., motivation, intelligence, culture) can affect the patient's responses. Moreover, an inability to conceptualize abstract concepts is not pathognomonic for schizophrenia.

PROSODY In addition to disorders of form and process, the accessory behaviors and intonations of speech may be abnormal. The patient may lack the usual expressive gestures, such as hand waving and head movements. Even more obvious, the patient may demonstrate both productive and receptive aprosodia, that is, an inability to understand or to create the usual emotional inflections of speech. The patient's speech may have an abnormal modulation of emphasis and volume, producing speech that is either too loud, too soft, or unusually accented.

MUTISM This inhibition of speech and vocalization may last for hours or days, but before the days of modern treatment methods, mutism often lasted for years in chronic schizophrenic patients of the catatonic type. Many schizophrenic patients tend to be monosyllabic and to answer questions as briefly as possible. They may attempt to restrict contact with the interviewer as much as possible without being altogether uncooperative.

Examples of some of these disorders of thought from patients with schizophrenia are listed below.

NEOLOGISMS A schizophrenic woman who had been hospitalized for several years kept repeating, in an otherwise quite rational conversation, the word "polamolalittersjittersstittersleelitla." She explained, "polamolalitters" was intended to recall the disease poliomyelitis, because the patient wanted to indicate that she felt she was suffering from a serious disease affecting her nervous system; the component "litters" stood for untidiness or messiness, the way she felt inside; "jitterstitters" reflected her inner nervousness and uneasiness; "leelitla" was a reference to the French *le lit là* (that bed there), meaning that she was both dependent on and feeling handicapped by her illness.

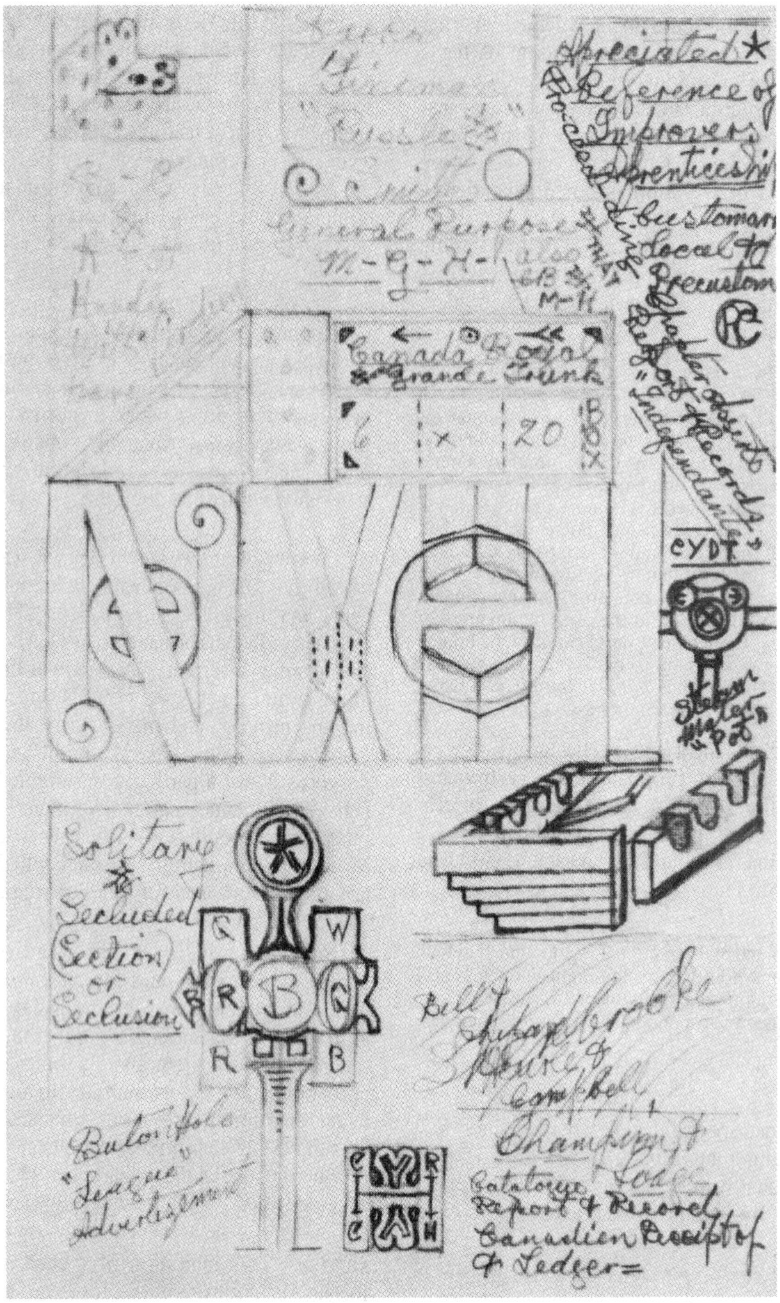

FIGURE 14.3-5. *This drawing, carefully executed by a schizophrenic woman, expresses graphically her incoherent thinking and her tendency to perseveration of ideas, combined with an ability to accomplish quite complex drafting. Similar drawings may be produced when normal people doodle while their attention is not focused on what they are doing.*

STILTED LANGUAGE The following excerpt from a letter written by a schizophrenic physician who was hospitalized for more than 15 years but is now living alone in an apartment is an example of stilted language.

> My dear friend and Professor: A hearty and cheerful. (Please turn page over) and a real magnanimous good-morning to you on this first Wednesday of our glorious New Year: And I do hope that our great and our good Lord, and our dearly beloved and kind Shepherd. (Kindly read page three, now). Will be gracious unto both me and thee. I am sure that He will be gracious unto both of us; if He has some sound common sense in His Being, this morning . . . I have not yet heard (Kindly turn over to p4 now) from any one of my own colleagues when I am leaving this noble institution of the healing arts; Nor with whom: Nor through which of the portals. Though I am sure that you-as much as any (Kindly turn to page five, now) one else—must be able to enlighten me; very soon, my good old friend. . . .

ECHOLALIA A patient demonstrates *echolalia* when he repeats exactly the words of another person. Examiner: "I heard that you played well in the softball game." Patient: "I heard that you played well in the softball game." The following case example and Figure 14.3-6 demonstrate multiple disorders of thought:

> The seabeach gathering homestead building upon the site of the bear mountains. Time placed of the dunce to the recovery of the setting sun, upon the stream, poling paddleboat, Mickey, Rooney,

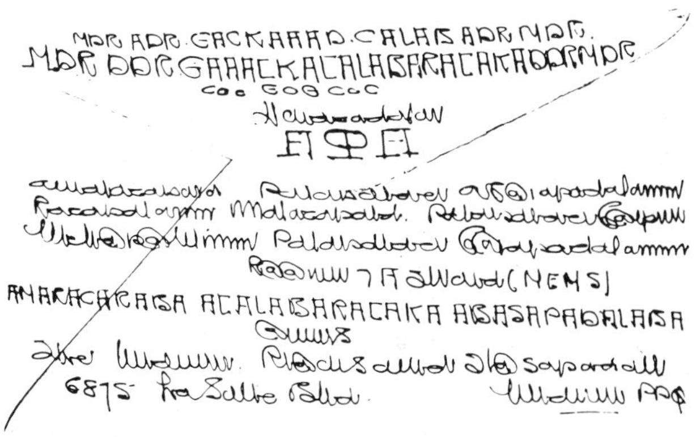

FIGURE 14.3-6 *Sample of a chronic schizophrenic patient's noncommunicative writing. This addressed envelope illustrates manneristic writing, verbigeration, and possibly neologisms. Although the script appears to be exotic, note the recognizable Arabic numerals and English street names. (Courtesy of Heinz E. Lehmann.)*

Bill. Proceeded of, to the enlivenment. Placed upon the assiduous laboriousness of keeping aloof, the alive to the forest stream. Haunting the distance of the held possession, requiring means of liberty to sociability. Upon the advisability of the held keeping, environment of the seabeach gathering, to the forest stream reinstatement of consideration to the placed, pooling paddleboat, of the swamp morass, to the forest compensation of the dance. Upon the ledge retaining consternation, endorsed encouragement. Tallyin poling trees, of the forest encampment fireside, burning under brush. Disgrace, mellowed to the compensation of the breath of distance. Remaining too, the placed haunt, upon the forest dunce of acquirement. The poling paddleboat, upon the seabeach gathering, enjoyment of the held keeping, to the commendation of the held means of support, upon the swamp morass, revolting equal to the shirking acquirement to the keeping possession, of the haunt established distance to gullible achievement, upon the ledge of the dunce, rising compensation of procreation arising aspirations, of the keeping ambition of the feathered birds.

Positive and negative symptoms A somewhat more clinically useful system for describing thought disorders and other symptoms of schizophrenia is to divide them into negative and positive symptoms. This differentiation is discussed further in the subsection on subtypes of schizophrenia.

Impulse control Patients with schizophrenia may be quite agitated and have little impulse control while acutely ill. They also lack social sensitivity and may appear to be impulsive, for example, when they grab another patient's cigarettes, change television channels abruptly, or throw food on the floor. Some apparently impulsive behavior, including suicide and homicide attempts, may be in response to hallucinated commands.

SUICIDE Suicide is common in schizophrenia; 40 percent of patients attempt it, and 10 percent succeed. Suicide may be precipitated by feelings of absolute emptiness, depression, wanting escape from the mental torture, or by hallucinated commands. Some potential risk factors for suicide in schizophrenia have been identified (Table 14.3-1).

HOMICIDE Although such epidemiological studies are quite difficult, it is currently believed that homicide is not more common in schizophrenic patients than it is in the general population. A schizophrenic patient is driven to homicide often for very unpredictable and bizarre reasons based on hallucinations or delusions. The clinician should be wary, however, if a change in a patient's symptoms causes the clinician to consider the possibility of the patient's committing a violent act. Some schizophrenic patients will voluntarily report command hallucinations to kill; such information is often a strong indication for hospitalization.

TABLE 14.3-1
Risk Factors for Suicide in Schizophrenia

Young age
Early in course of illness
College education
Overly high ambitions
High number of exacerbations and remissions
Patient in a period of change in condition
Patient in a period of improvement following exacerbations
Feelings of depression and hopelessness
Agitation while in hospital
Dependence on hospital
Prior suicide attempts
Suicidal plan
Living alone

SELF-MUTILATION Self-mutilation, such as cutting off an ear or even self-castration, is a rare form of self-directed violence that can be seen in psychotic disorders, including schizophrenia. Such acts are usually quite unpredictable and, therefore, very difficult to prevent. Self-mutilation is also known as the van Gogh syndrome, after the artist who cut off his ear.

DANGEROUSNESS IN THE HOSPITAL Very few studies have addressed risk factors for specifically predicting violent behavior in the hospital. The factors currently considered as most predictive are low blood concentrations of antipsychotics, severity of psychosis, and past history of violence. In war veterans who have schizophrenia, the severity of combat experience, especially in Vietnam, may correlate with the likelihood of violent behavior in the hospital.

Orientation Schizophrenic patients are usually oriented to person, time, and place. Lack of such orientation should prompt an investigation for an organic mental disorder. Some schizophrenic patients may give incorrect or bizarre answers to these questions (e.g., "I am Christ; this is heaven; and it is 33 A.D."). Other patients may lack the attention or motivation to answer such basic questions.

Memory Memory, as tested in the clinical mental status examination, is usually intact. It may be impossible, however, to get a patient to attend enough to the memory tests to assess this ability adequately.

Insight and judgment Classically, schizophrenic patients have very little insight into their illness, at least as evidenced by their ability to talk about the disease process or their emotional reaction to it. The judgment of patients is variable and is assessed best from observing patients' behavior in the interview and from interviewing outside sources of information about their behavior.

Reliability Although a particular schizophrenic patient may turn out to be a completely reliable historian, the nature of the illness requires that the examiner attempt to verify important information through additional sources.

NEUROLOGICAL FINDINGS There is renewed interest in the careful description of the neurological status of patients with schizophrenia. This is related to a neuropsychiatric approach to brain disorders in which the first question is, "Where is the lesion?" The neurological examination, in combination with psychological testing, neuropathological studies, and brain imaging, seeks to answer this question. A medical model approach often is comforting to the patient and family when previously they have been exposed solely to a psychodynamic approach to the symptoms.

The vast majority of schizophrenic patients would be said to have a normal neurological examination by most neurologists. It is interesting in this regard that the psychosis of classic neurological illnesses presents early in these diseases, often before the onset of the characteristic neurological features. Since more obvious neurological symptoms would result in the diagnosis of a nonschizophrenic organic disorder, it is not surprising that the neurological findings in schizophrenia are more subtle. This would actually imply that a psychiatrist should be capable of performing an even more refined neurological examination than a neurologist usually performs.

When careful neurological examinations of psychiatric patients are conducted, neurological abnormalities are found in approximately 50 percent of schizophrenic patients. In such studies, schizophrenic patients have more neurological findings than either patients with mood disorders or normal subjects. The presence of neurological findings in patients with schizophrenia has been correlated in some studies with severity of thought disorder, impaired cognitive abilities, poor premorbid functioning, and chronicity of course. It is interesting that although most offspring of schizophrenic probands have normal neurological examinations, there is a subgroup who demonstrate poor motor coordination and perceptual dysfunction. It is currently not known whether this subgroup of high-risk children is more likely to develop schizophrenia.

Neurological history A critical part of a neurological examination is a complete history. Questions should be asked regarding perinatal events, including prematurity, complicated labor, infections, seizures, and APGAR scores. The patient's childhood developmental milestones should be ascertained, and school and work performance should be evaluated. History of head trauma, central nervous system (CNS) infections, and drug abuse should be carefully noted. Information should be obtained regarding family history of epilepsy, dementia, other neurological diseases, and of psychiatric, immune, and endocrine disorders.

Motor system Clinicians have observed that one of the earliest signs of incipient schizophrenia can be a loss of the natural gracefulness of body movements. Choreoathetoid movements of the extremities and involuntary movements of the orobuccal area can be symptoms of tardive dyskinesia, but similar abnormal movements were reported in schizophrenic patients before the advent of antipsychotic drugs. It is estimated that 10 to 25 percent of schizophrenic patients have abnormal movements such as these that are not related to antipsychotic drug treatment. Somewhat less obvious motor abnormalities seen in schizophrenia include abnormal gait, stereotypies, mannerisms, grimacing, abnormal motor tone (increased or decreased), impaired fine motor skills, and abnormal reflexes (glabellar, grasp, palmomental, pollicomental, decreased gag reflex, abnormal vestibular reflexes). Patients may also exhibit an apraxia, that is, difficulty in carrying out a purposeful, organized, somewhat complex task, such as drawing a picture, dressing, or following a command to strike and blow out a match.

Abnormal eye signs There are two major ocular abnormalities in schizophrenia: unusually frequent blinking and abnormal rapid eye movements. The rate of blinking, thought to reflect dopaminergic CNS activity, decreases with antipsychotic medication and remission of psychotic symptoms. Abnormal rapid eye movements (saccades) during attempts to follow a moving object smoothly are seen in approximately 50 to 80 percent of patients. Saccades is seen on smooth pursuit in only 8 percent of normals but in approximately 40 percent of first-degree relatives of schizophrenic patients, including children of schizophrenic parents. Abnormal smooth pursuit may be a neurophysiological marker for some aspect of the pathophysiology of schizophrenia. Abnormal saccades are also seen in some patients with mood disorders, in patients with cerebellar lesions, and in some drug-induced states. It has been hypothesized that the site of pathology may be the frontal lobe input to the basal ganglia and superior colliculus.

Nonlocalizing neurological signs Nonlocalizing neurological signs, sometimes referred to as soft neurological signs, are seen in schizophrenic patients more frequently than in normals and about equally commonly in patients with schizophrenia and organic mental syndrome. These signs include dysdiadochokinesia, agraphathesia, astereognosis, poor right-left discrimination, and extinction on the face-hand test. Although these signs are nonlocalizing, they are consistent with brain injury to the frontal or parietal lobes.

Speech disorders Some investigators who approach schizophrenia as a neurological disorder consider a disorder of thought to be a forme fruste of aphasia, perhaps implicating the dominant parietal lobe. The lack of ability of schizophrenic patients to perceive the prosody of speech or to inflect their own speech (e.g., aprosodia) can be conceptualized as a neurological symptom of the nondominant parietal lobe. Other symptoms in schizophrenia that implicate the parietal lobes include the apraxias, right-left disorientation, and lack of concern about the illness (anosognosia).

Autonomic abnormalities A patient suffering an acute schizophrenic episode often presents with dilated pupils, moist palms, moderate tachycardia, and a systolic blood pressure 10 to 20 torr above the norm. These signs of sympathetic excitation may be present even if the patient shows no outward signs of emotional excitation, and initially they may point toward an erroneous diagnosis of sympathomimetic drug ingestion.

PSYCHOLOGICAL TESTING Psychological testing is of limited value in the actual diagnosis of schizophrenia. Projective testing (e.g., Rorschach, Thematic Apperception Test [TAT]) may indicate bizarre ideation, but if this is not evident in the routine mental status examination, a diagnosis of schizophrenia would almost never be appropriate. Confabulation and contamination are often seen in the responses of schizophrenic patients to the Rorschach Test. Other qualities of the responses are poorly perceived form responses, repetitions of one concept, lack of imagination, lack of movement and human content, and an inability to integrate color into the percepts. There are often only a small number of responses, and the popular responses (e.g., a bat in the fifth Rorschach card) are often absent. Sometimes, the responses can be overly personalized, extremely bizarre, or unusually sexual or violent. Although it does not contribute significantly to the diagnosis of schizophrenia, the TAT has been used by some clinicians to provide information about the dynamic issues that may be involved in a particular patient's symptoms. For example, responses may indicate features of the patient's relationships with his or her family. Such information may be useful in treatment planning.

Personality inventories (e.g., Minnesota Multiphasic Personality Inventory [MMPI]) are often abnormal in schizophrenic patients, but their contribution to diagnosis or treatment planning is quite minimal. One instrument that may be useful in assessing schizophrenic patients, the Phillips Scale, is constructed from data gathered from the patient's history and premorbid personality; it yields a prediction of the outcome in schizophrenic patients.

Psychological tests that measure objective neuropsychological performance (e.g., Halstead-Reitan Battery, Luria-Nebraska Battery) are abnormal in approximately 50 percent of schizophrenic patients. In contrast to projective tests and personality inventories, neuropsychological tests may suggest localized lesions and also demonstrate specific cognitive deficits that can be actively treated. The diversity of abnormalities on neuropsychological test batteries is most consistent with global bilateral injury (Table 14.3-2). A deficit in attention has often been reported using either reaction time or a continuous performance test (CPT) to measure attention. Recent reports have utilized the Wisconsin Card-Sorting Test as a measure of frontal lobe functioning, particularly dorsolateral prefrontal cortex. The intelligence quotient (I.Q.) of a subgroup of schizophrenic patients is lower than normal at onset of the illness. It is controversial whether I.Q. decreases with the course of illness, but it seems fairly certain that a low I.Q. is associated with a poor prognosis.

COURSE

The course of schizophrenia is considered to begin at the onset of the prodromal symptoms described previously. The onset is usually in adolescence and there may be an identified precipitating event (e.g., moving away to college, an experience with a hallucinogenic drug, death of a significant person). Almost any psychiatric disorder that occurs during adolescence assumes a certain schizophrenic coloring because many of the features characteristic of nonschizophrenic adolescent turbulence—exaltation, intense preoccupation with abstract ideas, unpredictable variations in mood, daydreaming, introspection, shyness—are often seen in schizophrenia. Although onset of schizophrenia is quite rare before age 10, onset after age 45 may be more common than was previously thought. The European literature describes schizophrenia-like illnesses with late onset as having symptoms quite similar to those of classically defined schizophrenia.

TABLE 14.3-2
Some Neuropsychological Abnormalities in Schizophrenia

Unable to maintain preparatory set
Perseveration in cross-modal stimulus conditions
Excessive habituation
Poor vigilance in continuous-performance tests
High distractibility by irrelevant stimuli
Slow information processing
Vulnerability to stimulus and response complexity
Increased or poorly modulated arousal
Poor language processing
Decreased mental flexibility
Poor tactile problem solving
Decreased memory for stories and designs
Decreased attention

The symptoms present in the prodrome become worse until some point at which the patient comes to the attention of professionals. Some symptoms have often been present for as long as a year at the time of diagnosis. (It is required by DSM-III-R, for example, that symptoms be present for 6 months to make the diagnosis.)

There have been many descriptions of the evolution or stages of a schizophrenic decompensation. The following is a compilation of these reports: The patient may feel overwhelmed by external and internal pressures, resulting in anxiety, irritability, increased distractibility, and impaired performance in school and work. The patient may then experience a stage of boredom, apathy, withdrawal, hopelessness, and loneliness. The patient may become more activated in the next stage and exhibit hypomanic symptoms with increased sexual and aggressive behaviors. The next stage is the actual psychosis. Following acute psychosis, the patient may be left with delusions, denial, and depression.

The classical course of schizophrenia is one of exacerbations and relative remissions. The major distinction between schizophrenia and the mood disorders is the lack of return to baseline functioning following each relapse. There is renewed interest in identifying the initial stages of a relapse so that antipsychotic medications can be initiated or increased and other attempts at prevention of the relapse can be taken. The signs and symptoms of a relapse include hallucinations, increased suspiciousness, changes in sleep, increased cognitive difficulties, and hostility. These signs can be identified by both clinicians and family. Following a psychotic episode, there is sometimes a clinically observable period of vulnerability and depression. A sensitivity to even small stresses and changes is characteristic of many schizophrenic patients throughout their lives. Drug use, including alcohol and marijuana, is associated with more relapses.

Some studies have suggested that deterioration progresses for an average of 5 years, at which point most patients reach a plateau. Positive symptoms tend to become less severe with time but remain a problem in as many as 40 percent of patients. Much more commonly, patients are left with the more socially and functionally debilitating negative symptoms. The lives of many patients are characterized by frequent hospitalizations, and in urban settings, by homelessness and poverty. Only recently has the fact of the limited quality of life experienced by the homeless, urban, chronic mental patients come to public awareness. There is an increased mortality rate among schizophrenic patients, mostly from suicide. There is also an increase in the mortality of schizophrenic patients from a variety of medical diseases and trauma.

STABLE CHRONICITY Although complete intellectual and social deterioration is rarer now, many schizophrenic patients, despite intensive therapeutic efforts, remain in a state of stable chronicity. These patients remain functionally incapacitated, with clearly visible signs and symptoms of active mental disease. The casual observer in a large city can encounter many of these formerly hospitalized schizophrenic patients along the sidewalks—talking to themselves and to passers-by, gesticulating, preaching, or just sitting on the stoops. It is not clear that these patients are better off in the community than they were in the hospital, although the community setting would be much better if more services were offered.

REMISSION AND SOCIAL RECOVERY Many schizophrenic patients today fall into the categories of social remission with residual personality defects or full remission with relapses. A person in the former category may be more withdrawn, more aloof, and more selfish than before the onset of the illness. Such a patient may neglect personal appearance and will almost certainly be less effective occupationally. A schizophrenic patient may eventually end up doing menial work well below his or her educational level. Such persons often are best suited for quiet, routine work that can be performed independently of others and at a slow pace. Those who have profound residual personality defects may require continuous protective supervision and sheltered work conditions. Sometimes the personality defect is slight enough that only family and old friends recognize the symptoms (e.g., diminished capacity for enthusiasm, lessened spontaneity, decreased initiative, and decline in creative imagination).

TABLE 14.3-3
Features Suggesting Good and Poor Prognoses in Schizophrenia

Good	Poor
Late onset	Early onset
Obvious precipitating factors	No precipitating factors
Acute onset	Insidious onset
Good premorbid social, sexual, and work history	Poor premorbid social, sexual, and work history
Affective symptoms (especially depression)	Withdrawn, autistic behavior
Paranoid or catatonic features	Undifferentiated or disorganized features
Married	Unmarried, divorced, or widowed
Family history of mood disorders	Family history of schizophrenia
Good support system	Poor support system
Undulating course	Chronic course
Positive symptoms	Negative symptoms
	Neurological signs and symptoms
	History of perinatal trauma
	No remission in 3 years
	Numerous relapses

PROGNOSIS

It is incorrect to consider schizophrenia as invariably having a deteriorating course. It is confusing, therefore, that such a course is a DSM-III-R criterion. A variety of factors are associated with good and poor prognoses (Table 14.3-3). The range of recovery rates in the literature is 10 to 60 percent, and a reasonable estimate is that 20 to 30 percent are able to lead relatively normal lives. Approximately 20 to 30 percent of patients continue to experience moderate symptoms, and 40 to 60 percent remain significantly impaired for life. It is certainly quite clear that schizophrenic patients do much less well than patients with mood disorders, although approximately 20 to 25 percent of the latter group are also severely disturbed at long-term follow-up.

DIAGNOSIS

DSM-III-R contains the official diagnostic guidelines of the American Psychiatric Association for schizophrenia (Table 14.3-4). Changes from the third edition of the *Diagnostic and Statistical Manual of Mental Disorders* (DSM-III) include the requirement that the major symptoms be present for at least 1 week, the inclusion as a criterion of the failure of a child or adolescent to reach an expected developmental level, and the elimination of the requirement that the illness begins before age 45. DSM-III-R specifically describes prodromal and residual symptoms and classifies the course as subchronic, chronic, subchronic with acute exacerbation, chronic with acute exacerbation, or in remission. DSM-III-R developed out of the work of researchers in nosological psychiatry, but it is fundamentally a combination of Kraepelin's and Bleuler's descriptions.

UNITED STATES–UNITED KINGDOM DIAGNOSTIC PROJECT Observations on discordant admission rates for depressive disorders and schizophrenia into mental hospitals in England, Wales, and the United States led to a major study in the 1960s, in which a research team, composed of American- and British-trained psychiatrists, explored the reasons for those differences. The study demonstrated that the higher incidence of schizophrenia in the United States was mainly attributable to different diagnostic practices in the two countries. In filmed and videotaped interviews of patients, for example, American psychiatrists tended to interpret flatness of affect and the presence of delusions as indicative of schizophrenia. Since the publication of these findings, changes in American psychiatry, such as the publication of DSM-III-R, have now standardized the diagnostic practices of the two countries.

WORLD HEALTH ORGANIZATION DIAGNOSTIC STUDY The goal of the International Pilot Study of Schizophrenia (IPSS), conducted by the World Health Organization (WHO), was to discover reliable methods of diagnosing schizophrenia in a standardized and universally acceptable way. The project involved over 1,000 patients in nine countries. The interviewing psychiatrists used the Present State Examination (PSE), a standardized interview form, to arrive at their own diagnoses. The information from the PSE was also used to arrive at computer-generated diagnoses. It was found in this study that the information on the PSE was the principal instrument for arriving at an accurate diagnosis and that, in most cases, the additional psychiatric and social histories contributed much less information. The following list of symptoms includes the frequency with which they were found in schizophrenic patients: lack of insight, 97 percent; auditory hallucinations, 74 percent; verbal hallucinations, 70 percent; ideas of reference, 70 percent; suspiciousness, 66 percent; flatness of affect, 66 percent; voices speaking to patient, 65 percent; delusional mood, 64 percent; delusions of persecution, 64 percent; inadequate description of problems, 64 percent; thought alienation, 52 percent; thoughts spoken aloud, 50 percent.

OTHER DIAGNOSTIC SYSTEMS Although DSM-III-R is the officially endorsed set of diagnostic guidelines in the United States, there are other diagnostic systems that are used in the United States and other parts of the world. Some clinicians continue to use the original descriptions of Kraepelin and Bleuler to diagnose schizophrenia, and a variety of other systems have been proposed.

Kurt Schneider described certain *first-rank symptoms* that were considered pathognomonic for schizophrenia: audible

TABLE 14.3-4
Diagnostic Criteria for Schizophrenia

A. Presence of characteristic psychotic symptoms in the active phase: either (1), (2), or (3) for at least 1 week (unless the symptoms are successfully treated):
  (1) two of the following:
    (a) delusions
    (b) prominent hallucinations (throughout the day for several days or several times a week for several weeks, each hallucinatory experience not being limited to a few brief moments)
    (c) incoherence or marked loosening of associations
    (d) catatonic behavior
    (e) flat or grossly inappropriate affect
  (2) bizarre delusions involving a phenomenon that the person's culture would regard as totally implausible (e.g., thought broadcasting, being controlled by a dead person)
  (3) prominent hallucinations [as defined in (1)(*b*) above] of a voice with content having no apparent relation to depression or elation, or a voice keeping up a running commentary on the person's behavior or thoughts, or two or more voices conversing with each other
B. During the course of the disturbance, functioning in such areas as work, social relations, and self-care is markedly below the highest level achieved before onset of the disturbance (or, when the onset is in childhood or adolescence, failure to achieve expected level of social development).
C. Schizoaffective disorder and mood disorder with psychotic features have been ruled out, i.e., if a major depressive or manic syndrome has ever been present during an active phase of the disturbance, the total duration of all episodes of a mood syndrome has been brief relative to the total duration of the active and residual phases of the disturbance.
D. Continuous signs of the disturbance for at least 6 months. The 6-month period must include an active phase (of at least 1 week, or less if symptoms have been successfully treated) during which there were psychotic symptoms characteristic of schizophrenia (symptoms in A), with or without a prodromal or residual phase, as defined below.
  Prodomal phase: A clear deterioration in functioning before the active phase of the disturbance that is not due to a disturbance in mood or to a psychoactive substance use disorder and that involves at least two of the symptoms listed below.
  Residual phase: Following the active phase of the disturbance, persistence of at least two of the symptoms noted below, these not being due to a disturbance in mood or to a psychoactive substance use disorder.
  Prodromal or Residual Symptoms:
  (1) marked social isolation or withdrawal
  (2) marked impairment in role functioning as wage-earner, student, or homemaker
  (3) markedly peculiar behavior (e.g., collecting garbage, talking to self in public, hoarding food)
  (4) marked impairment in personal hygiene and grooming
  (5) blunted or inappropriate affect
  (6) digressive, vague, overelaborate, or circumstantial speech, or poverty of speech, or poverty of content of speech
  (7) odd beliefs or magical thinking, influencing behavior and inconsistent with cultural norms (e.g., superstitiousness, belief in clairvoyance, telepathy, "sixth sense," "others can feel my feelings," overvalued ideas, ideas of reference)
  (8) unusual perceptual experiences (e.g., recurrent illusions, sensing the presence of a force or person not actually present)
  (9) marked lack of initiative, interests, or energy

Examples: Six months of prodromal symptoms with 1 week of symptoms from A; no prodromal symptoms with 6 months of symptoms from A; no prodromal symptoms with 1 week of symptoms from A and 6 months of residual symptoms.
E. It cannot be established that an organic factor initiated and maintained the disturbance.
F. If there is a history of autistic disorder, the additional diagnosis of schizophrenia is made only if prominent delusions or hallucinations are also present.

Classification of course. The course of the disturbance is coded in the fifth digit:
  1-Subchronic. The time from the beginning of the disturbance, when the person first began to show signs of the disturbance (including prodromal, active, and residual phases) more or less continuously, is less than 2 years but at least 6 months.
  2-Chronic. Same as above, but more than 2 years.
  3-Subchronic with acute exacerbation. Reemergence of prominent psychotic symptoms in a person with a subchronic course who has been in the residual phase of the disturbance.
  4-Chronic with acute exacerbation. Reemergence of prominent psychotic symptoms in a person with a chronic course who has been in the residual phase of the disturbance.
  5-In remission. When a person with a history of schizophrenia is free of all signs of the disturbance (whether or not on medication), "in remission" should be coded. Differentiating schizophrenia in remission from no mental disorder requires consideration of overall level of functioning, length of time since the last episode of disturbance, total duration of the disturbance, and whether prophylactic treatment is being given.
  0-Unspecified.

Specify late onset if the disturbance (including the prodromal phase) develops after age 45.

Table from DSM-III-R *Diagnostic and Statistical Manual of Mental Disorders,* ed 3, revised. Copyright American Psychiatric Association, Washington, DC, 1987. Used with permission.

thoughts; voices arguing, commenting, or discussing; thought withdrawal and broadcasting; delusional perceptions; and experiences of somatic passivity. Although these symptoms have since been considered not to be pathognomonic for schizophrenia, they are included as criteria in most other diagnostic systems, including DSM-III-R. Schneider's *second-rank symptoms* included feelings of emotional impoverishment, depressed and euphoric moods, perplexity, and other delusions and perceptual disorders. Schneider did point out, however, that schizophrenia could also be diagnosed exclusively on the basis of second-rank symptoms when an otherwise typical clinical picture was present.

Gabriel Langfeldt, unlike Bleuler, derived his criteria from empirical experience rather than a theoretical formulation. Langfeldt divided the disorder into *true schizophrenia* and *schizophreniform psychosis*. The diagnosis of true schizophrenia rested on the presence of depersonalization, autism, emotional blunting, insidious onset, and feelings of derealization. Although schizophreniform patients were symptomatically similar to true schizophrenic patients, the former had a better response to treatment and a more favorable prognosis.

The 12 major diagnostic systems for schizophrenia currently used by various clinicians are Kraepelin's; Bleuler's; Schneider's; Langfeldt's (1960); the ninth revision of *International Classification of Disease* (ICD-9, 1978); the St. Louis Criteria (also called the Feighner's, 1972); the Research Diagnostic Criteria (RDC, 1977); the New Haven Schizophrenia Index (1972); the Flexible System (also called Carpenter's, 1973); the Present State Examination (also called the PSE/CATEGO or Wing's, 1974); the Taylor and Abrams system; and DSM-III-R. All of these systems include the usual symptoms of psychosis in their criteria. The Langfeldt, St. Louis, and DSM-III-R criteria require a reduced level of functioning for the diagnosis. The RDC, Taylor and Abrams, St. Louis, and DSM-III-R systems stipulate minimum durations of symptoms, and the St. Louis system requires onset of symptoms before the age of 45. The criteria for these diagnostic systems are listed in Table 14.3-5

EVALUATION OF DIAGNOSTIC SYSTEMS FOR SCHIZOPHRENIA There are five measures by which a diagnostic system should be evaluated: objectivity of data, reliability, validity, comprehensiveness, and specificity.

Objectivity of data All of the diagnostic systems for schizophrenia are based on the presence of particular symptoms; course of illness; various exclusion criteria; and information drawn from the patient, family, and friends, past psychiatric records, and current mental status examination. The objectivity of these data must be evaluated separately in every instance, but the different diagnostic systems do not vary in their reliance on the objectivity of the same data.

Reliability Interrater reliability in assessing the criteria required for diagnosis is high for the Schneider, St. Louis, RDC, Flexible, PSE, Taylor and Abrams, and DSM-III-R systems. It is critical to remember that high interrater reliability shows merely that clinicians agree on how to apply the criteria as described and not that the clinicians are actually identifying schizophrenia more exactly. Test-retest reliability measures how stable a diagnosis is with the passage of time. The diagnostic systems with good interrater reliability and diagnostic criteria regarding course of illness tend to have good test-retest reliability.

Validity The four levels of validity are face, descriptive, predictive, and construct. All of the currently used systems have face and descriptive validity, meaning that large numbers of clinicians agree that the criteria describe a particular group of psychiatric patients. The diagnostic schemes that include a specific duration of symptoms (St. Louis, RDC, DSM-III-R) are the only systems clearly predictive of poorer outcome. Construct validity requires an independent objective marker for verification of the diagnostic system; therefore, no diagnostic system for schizophrenia has been demonstrated to have construct validity.

Comprehensiveness and specificity An ideal diagnostic system should categorize all patients (comprehensiveness) into nonoverlapping groups (specificity). Comprehensiveness of these systems varies so much that one system may diagnose 10 times more patients as schizophrenic than another. The systems are sometimes divided into more restrictive systems (DSM-III-R, Taylor and Abrams, St. Louis), which diagnose fewer patients as schizophrenic, and less restrictive ones (e.g., New Haven), which diagnose more patients as schizophrenic. It is incorrect, however, to assume that more restrictive systems identify a truer schizophrenia. DSM-III-R, at first, seems to ignore the concern for specificity by requiring the use of all appropriate diagnoses, except where prohibited by exclusion criteria. This approach is consistent with that of internal medicine, which allows a clinician to diagnose more than one heart ailment in a single patient.

SUBTYPES

There have been many schemes devised to subtype schizophrenia. These schemes are most valuable clinically when they distinguish patients with a good prognosis from those with a poor prognosis. This can be done most pragmatically, however, by following the guidelines in Table 14.3-3. Although some subtyping schemes have addressed prognosis, others have paid more attention to differences in clinical presentations. DSM-III-R has actually based its subtypes primarily on clinical distinctions (Table 14.3-6). The DSM-III-R subtypes—paranoid, catatonic, disorganized, undifferentiated, and residual—have few implications for treatment, although a patient with the catatonic subtype may actually benefit more from treatment with electroconvulsive therapy (ECT) or lithium than patients with other subtypes. Some catatonic patients may respond to barbiturate infusions; whether catatonic patients would do well with chronic treatment with CNS depressants is not known. In general, catatonic and paranoid patients seem to have better prognoses than undifferentiated or disorganized patients.

PARANOID SUBTYPE The paranoid type of schizophrenia is characterized by delusions of persecution or grandeur. Patients with paranoid schizophrenia are often older at onset than patients with catatonic or disorganized schizophrenia. Patients who are well until their late 20s or early 30s have usually established a place and identity for themselves in the community. Their personal and social resources are greater than those of the catatonic and hebephrenic patients who decompensate earlier. Paranoid schizophrenia is often attended by less regression of mental faculties, emotional response, and behavior than the other subtypes of schizophrenia. DSM-III-R differs from DSM-III in that it separates out a stable subtype of paranoid schizophrenia that describes a group of patients with a pattern of presenting symptoms that is particularly stable over time.

Three months after their initial contact with the patient, a 26-year-old male migrant farm worker, a community mental health team was contacted by the city police. The patient, who had been maintained in an outpatient clinic for the past few months, had suddenly appeared in a judge's chamber and demanded to be put to death because he felt he was responsible for the production of evil and violence in the world. When team members reached the jail, they found the patient agitated, irascible, suspicious, and guarded. His speech was disorganized and often incoherent. He stated that he could not eat meat lest terrible violence and evil be unleashed on the world. He also described a plot by the California Mafia to keep him from working, and he spoke of voices that told him what to do that "must be obeyed."

His history included similar episodes over the previous 5 years, resulting in several year-long hospitalizations. At no time did he exhibit a full manic or depressive syndrome. Between hospitalizations the patient lived in hobo jungles, flophouses, and gospel missions; rode freight trains from town to town; and worked, picking fruit, for a few days at a time. Since adolescence he had lived the life of a drifting loner.

(Adapted from *DSM-III Case Book*. American Psychiatric Association, Washington, DC, 1981, with permission.)

CATATONIC SUBTYPE Catatonic schizophrenia occurs as inhibited (or stuporous) catatonia and as excited catatonia.

Stuporous catatonia Stuporous catatonic schizophrenic patients may be in a state of complete stupor or may show a pronounced decrease in spontaneous movements and activity. They may be mute or nearly so and may show distinct negativism, stereotypies, echopraxia, or automatic obedience.

TABLE 14.3-5
Essential Features* of Various Diagnostic Criteria for Schizophrenia

KURT SCHNEIDER

1. First-rank symptoms
   a. Audible thoughts
   b. Voices arguing, discussing, or both
   c. Voices commenting
   d. Somatic passivity experiences
   e. Thought withdrawal and other experiences of influenced thought
   f. Thought broadcasting
   g. Delusional perceptions
   h. All other experiences involving volition, made affects, and made impulses
2. Second-rank symptoms
   a. Other disorders of perception
   b. Sudden delusional ideas
   c. Perplexity
   d. Depressive and euphoric mood changes
   e. Feelings of emotional impoverishment
   f. ". . . and several others as well"

GABRIEL LANGFELDT

1. Symptom criteria
   Significant clues to a diagnosis of schizophrenia are (if no sign of organic mental disorder, infection, or intoxication can be demonstrated):
   a. Changes in personality, which manifest themselves as a special type of emotional blunting followed by lack of initiative, and altered, frequently peculiar behavior. (In hebephrenia, especially, these changes are quite characteristic and are a principal clue to the diagnosis.)
   b. In catatonic types, the history as well as the typical signs in periods of restlessness and stupor (with negativism, oily facies, catalepsy, special vegetative symptoms, etc.)
   c. In paranoid psychoses, essential symptoms of split personality (or depersonalization symptoms) and a loss of reality feeling (derealization symptoms) or primary delusions
   d. Chronic hallucinations
2. Course criterion
   A final decision about diagnosis cannot be made before a follow-up period of at least 5 years has shown a chronic course of disease.

NEW HAVEN SCHIZOPHRENIA INDEX

1. a. Delusions: not specified or other-than-depressive: 2 points	
b. Auditory hallucinations c. Visual hallucinations d. Other hallucinations	any one: 2 points
2. a. Bizarre thoughts b. Autism or grossly unrealistic private thoughts c. Looseness of associations, illogical thinking, overinclusion	any one: 2 points
d. Blocking e. Concreteness	either: 2 points
f. Derealization g. Depersonalization	each: 1 point
3. Inappropriate affect: 1 point	
4. Confusion: 1 point	
5. Paranoid ideation (self-referential thinking, suspiciousness): 1 point	
6. Catatonic behavior a. Excitement b. Stupor c. Waxy flexibility d. Negativism e. Mutism f. Echolalia g. Stereotyped motor activity	any one: 1 point

Scoring: To be considered part of the schizophrenic group, the patient must score on Item 1 or Item 2a, 2b, or 2c, and must receive a total score of at least 4 points.

FLEXIBLE SYSTEM

Minimum number of symptoms required can be four to eight, depending on investigator's choice.

1. Restricted affect
2. Poor insight
3. Thoughts aloud
4. Poor rapport
5. Widespread delusions
6. Incoherent speech
7. Unreliable information
8. Bizarre delusions
9. Nihilistic delusions
10. Absence of early awakening (1–3 hr)
11. Absence of depressed facies
12. Absence of elation

TABLE 14.3-5 (*Continued*)

RESEARCH DIAGNOSTIC CRITERIA

Criteria 1 through 3 required for diagnosis.

1. At least two of the following for definite illness, and one for probable (not counting those occurring during period of drug or alcohol abuse or withdrawal):
   a. Thought broadcasting, insertion, or withdrawal
   b. Delusions of being controlled or influenced, other bizarre delusions, or multiple delusions
   c. Delusions other than persecution or jealousy lasting at least 1 month
   d. Delusions of any type if accompanied by hallucinations of any type for at least 1 week
   e. Auditory hallucinations in which either a voice keeps up a running commentary on subject's behaviors or thoughts as they occur or two or more voices converse with each other
   f. Nonaffective verbal hallucinations spoken to subject
   g. Hallucinations of any type throughout day for several days or intermittently for at least 1 month
   h. Definite instances of marked formal thought disorders accompanied by blunted or inappropriate affect, delusions or hallucinations of any type, or grossly disorganized behavior
2. One of the following:
   a. Current period of illness lasted at least 2 weeks from onset of noticeable change in subject's usual condition
   b. Subject has had previous period of illness lasting at least 2 weeks during which he or she met criteria, and residual signs of illness have remained (e.g., extreme social withdrawal, blunted or inappropriate affect, formal thought disorder, or unusual thoughts or perceptual experiences)
3. At no time during active period of illness being considered did subject meet criteria for probable or definite manic or depressive syndrome to the degree that it was a prominent part of illness

ST. LOUIS CRITERIA

1. Both necessary:
   a. Chronic illness with at least 6 months of symptoms before index evaluation, without return to premorbid level of psychosocial adjustment
   b. Absence of period of depressive or manic symptoms sufficient to qualify for mood (affective) disorder or probable mood (affective) disorder
2. At least one of the following:
   a. Delusions or hallucinations without significant perplexity or disorientation
   b. Verbal production that makes communication difficult owing to lack of logical or understandable organization (in presence of muteness, diagnostic decision must be deferred)
3. At least three for definite, two for probable, illness:
   a. Never married
   b. Poor premorbid social adjustment or work history
   c. Family history of schizophrenia
   d. Absence of alcoholism or drug abuse within 1 year of onset
   e. Onset before age 40

TAYLOR AND ABRAMS' CRITERIA

All criteria must be met for diagnosis.

1. Duration of episode greater than 6 months
2. Clear consciousness
3. Presence of delusions, hallucinations, or formal thought disorder (verbigeration, non sequiturs, word approximations, neologisms, blocking, and derailment)
4. Absence of broad affect
5. Absence of signs and symptoms sufficient to make diagnosis of affective disease
6. No alcoholism or drug abuse within 1 year of index episode
7. Absence of focal signs and symptoms of coarse brain disease or major medical illness known to produce significant behavioral changes

PRESENT STATE EXAMINATION

The following 12 items from the Present State Examination correspond to a 12-point diagnostic system for schizophrenia, with varying levels of certainty of diagnosis based on the cut-off score determined by the examiner. Nine of the symptoms are scored 1 point each when present (+), and three are scored 1 point each when absent (–).

1. Restricted affect (+)
2. Poor insight (+)
3. Thoughts aloud (+)
4. Awaking early (–)
5. Poor rapport (+)
6. Depressed facies (–)
7. Elation (–)
8. Widespread delusions (+)
9. Incoherent speech (+)
10. Unreliable information (+)
11. Bizarre delusions (+)
12. Nihilistic delusions (+)

The criteria of Schneider and Langfeldt are used with permission from: World Psychiatric Association: *Diagnostic Criteria for Schizophrenic and Affective Psychoses*. American Psychiatric Press, Washington, DC, 1983. The criteria of St. Louis, RDC, NHSI, Flexible, and Taylor and Abrams are from: Endicott J, Nee J, Fleiss L, Cohen J, Williams J B W, Simon R: Diagnostic criteria for schizophrenia. Arch Gen Psychiatry *39:* 884, 1982. All used with permission.

*Only the essential features of the criteria are listed here. Investigators who plan to use any of these systems should refer to the original sources. (See body of chapter for Bleulerian, Kraepelinian, and DSM-III-R diagnostic criteria for schizophrenia.)

TABLE 14.3-6
Diagnostic Criteria for Subtypes of Schizophrenia

Paranoid Type
A type of schizophrenia in which there are:
A. Preoccupation with one or more systematized delusions or with frequent auditory hallucinations related to a single theme
B. None of the following: incoherence, marked loosening of associations, flat or grossly inappropriate affect, catatonic behavior, grossly disorganized behavior
Specify stable type if criteria A and B have been met during all past and present active phases of the illness.
Catatonic Type
A type of schizophrenia in which the clinical picture is dominated by any of the following:
(1) catatonic stupor (marked decrease in reactivity to the environment and/or reduction in spontaneous movements and activity) or mutism
(2) catatonic negativism (an apparently motiveless resistance to all instructions or attempts to be moved)
(3) catatonic rigidity (maintenance of a rigid posture against efforts to be moved)
(4) catatonic excitement (excited motor activity, apparently purposeless and not influenced by external stimuli)
(5) catatonic posturing (voluntary assumption of inappropriate or bizarre postures)
Disorganized Type
A type of schizophrenia in which the following criteria are met:
A. Incoherence, marked loosening of associations, or grossly disorganized behavior
B. Flat or grossly inappropriate affect
C. Does not meet the criteria for catatonic type
Undifferentiated Type
A type of schizophrenia in which there are:
A. Prominent delusions, hallucinations, incoherence, or grossly disorganized behavior
B. Does not meet the criteria for paranoid, catatonic, or disorganized type
Residual type
A type of schizophrenia in which there are:
A. Absence of prominent delusions, hallucinations, incoherence, or grossly disorganized behavior
B. Continuing evidence of the disturbance, as indicated by two or more of the residual symptoms listed in criterion D of schizophrenia

Table from DSM-III-R *Diagnostic and Statistical Manual of Mental Disorders,* ed 3, revised. Copyright American Psychiatric Association, Washington, DC, 1987. Used with permission.

After standing or sitting motionless for long periods of time, they may suddenly and without provocation have a brief outburst of violence. Occasionally, catatonic schizophrenic patients exhibit catalepsy or waxy flexibility.

An 18-year-old student was admitted for the first time to the psychiatry service because for 3 days she had not spoken and would not eat. According to her parents, she had been a normal teen-ager, with good grades and friends, until about 1 year ago, when she began to stay at home more, alone in her room, and seemed preoccupied and less animated. Six months before admission, she began to refuse to go to school, and her grades became barely passing. About a month later, she started to talk gibberish about spirits, magic, the devil—things that were totally foreign to her background. For the week preceding admission to the hospital she had stared into space, immobile, only allowing herself to be moved from her bed to a chair or from one room to another.

(Adapted from *DSM-III Case Book.* American Psychiatric Association, Washington, DC, 1981, with permission.)

Excited catatonia Excited catatonic patients are in a state of extreme psychomotor agitation and talk and shout almost continuously. Verbal productions are often incoherent, and behavior seems to be influenced more by inner stimuli than by responses to the environment. Patients in catatonic excitement urgently require physical and medical control because they are often destructive and violent toward others and their excitement can cause them to injure themselves or to collapse from complete exhaustion. Excited catatonic states that in the past could not be controlled by sedation have been called pernicious or fatal catatonia. It is likely, however, that many of the patients previously thought to have excited catatonia were actually in a manic phase of bipolar disorder.

An unmarried man of 27, a teacher, was admitted to a psychiatric hospital, after having become increasingly agitated and irrational after several nights of wakefulness. He was extremely talkative and ran about aimlessly. His behavior at home was bizarre: he tried to clean everything in the house, wore his wristwatch up on his shoulder, stripped his clothes off, chewed large wads of paper in the belief that it was good for him, talked about killing himself, then said he might already be dead.

He heard voices constantly ordering him about, and he frequently laughed for no apparent reason. After chewing the paper, he would spit in it and then drink his saliva. He rolled into odd postures on the bed, sticking out his tongue. He started to jump and dance when taken to the bathroom for a shower and destroyed the bathroom furnishings. His gait was manneristic. His speech was utterly incomprehensible. He refused to take any medication and had to be sedated parenterally.

Periodic catatonia A rare, but intriguing, form of catatonia has been called periodic catatonia (a subtype not specified in DSM-III-R). Patients with this syndrome have periodic episodes of stuporous or excited catatonia that have been correlated with shifts in thyroid hormone levels and nitrogen balance. These patients respond to administraton of thyroxine in combination with antipsychotics. The vast majority of patients who present with catatonia do not fall into this category.

DISORGANIZED (HEBEPHRENIC) SUBTYPE The disorganized or hebephrenic subtype is characterized by primitive, disinhibited, and unorganized behavior. The hebephrenic patient is usually active but aimlessly and nonconstructively so. Thought disorder is pronounced; contact with reality is extremely poor. Personal appearance is slipshod, and social behavior is primitive. Emotional responses are inappropriate, and there is explosive laughter without apparent reason. Incongruous grinning and grimacing are common in this type of patient.

Emilio is 40 but looks 10 years younger. He is brought to the hospital (his twelfth hospitalization) by his mother, because she is afraid of him. He is dressed in a ragged overcoat, bedroom slippers, and a baseball cap and wears several medals around his neck. His affect ranges from anger at his mother—"She feeds me shit . . . what comes out of other people's rectums"—to a giggling, obsequious seductiveness toward the interviewer. His speech and manner have a childlike quality, and he walks with a mincing step and exaggerated hip movements. His mother reports that he stopped taking his medication about a month ago and has since begun to hear voices and to look and act more bizarrely. When asked what he has been doing, he says, "eating wires and lighting fires." His spontaneous speech is often incoherent and marked by frequent rhyming and clang associations.

Emilio's first hospitalization occurred after he dropped out of school at 16; since that time he has never been able to attend school or hold a job. He lives with his elderly mother, but sometimes disappears for several months at a time and is eventually picked up by the police as he wanders in the street. There is no known history of drug or alcohol abuse.

(Adapted from *DSM-III Case Book*. American Psychiatric Association, Washington, DC, 1981, with permission.)

UNDIFFERENTIATED AND RESIDUAL SUBTYPES

The diagnostic guidelines for these two subtypes are specified in DSM-III-R (Table 14.3-6). The hallmark of the undifferentiated subtype is the presence of psychotic symptoms that cannot be classified as fitting the paranoid, catatonic, or disorganized. The residual subtype is used for patients who have had a previous episode of symptoms that have met the criteria for schizophrenia, yet, at the present evaluation, show no prominent psychotic symptoms.

Undifferentiated schizophrenia

Susan, a 15-year-old, was seen at the request of school authorities for advice on placement. She had recently moved into the area with her family and, after a brief period in a regular class, was placed in a class for the emotionally disturbed. She was very difficult, with a very poor understanding of schoolwork at about the fifth-grade level, despite an apparently good vocabulary; and she disturbed the class by making animal noises and telling fantastic stories, which made the other students laugh at her.

At home Susan was aggressive, biting or hitting her parents or brother if frustrated. Often bored, she has no friends and finds it difficult to occupy herself. She spends a lot of time drawing pictures of robots, spaceships, and fantastic or futuristic inventions. Sometimes she has said she would like to die, but she has never made any attempt at suicide, and apparently has not thought of killing herself. Her mother says that from birth she has been different, and that the onset of her current behavior has been so gradual that no definite date can be assigned to it.

Susan's prenatal and parental history are unremarkable. Her milestones were delayed, and she did not use single words until 4 or 5 years of age. Ever since she entered school there has been concern about her ability. Repeated evaluations have suggested an I.Q. in the lower 70s, with achievement somewhat behind even that expected at this level of ability. Because her father was in the military, there have been many moves, and results of her earlier evaluations are not available.

The parents report that Susan has always been difficult and restless, and that several doctors have said she is not just mentally retarded but suffers from a serious mental disorder. The results of an evaluation done at the age of 12, because of difficulties in school, showed "evidence of bizarre thought processes and fragmented ego structure." At this time she was sleeping well at night and was not getting up with nightmares or bizarre requests, though this apparently had been a feature of her earlier behavior. Currently she is reported to sleep very poorly and tends to disturb the household by getting up and wandering around at night. Her mother emphasizes Susan's unpredictability, the funny stories that she tells, and the way in which she will talk to herself in "funny voices." Her mother regards the stories Susan tells as childish make-believe and preoccupation and pays little attention to them. She says that since Susan went to see the movie *Star Wars* she has been obsessed with ideas about space, spaceships, and the future.

Her parents are in their early 40s. Her father, having retired from military service, now works as an engineer. Susan's mother has many unusual beliefs about herself. She claims to have grown up in India and to have had a very bizarre early childhood full of dramatic and violent episodes. Many of these episodes sound highly improbable. Her husband refuses to let her talk about her past in his presence and tries to play down this material and Susan's problems. The parents appear to have a rather restricted relationship in which the father plays the role of a taciturn, masterful head of household and the mother bears the brunt of everyday family duties. The mother, in contrast, is loquacious and very circumstantial in her history giving. She dwells a great deal on her strange childhood experiences. Susan's brother is now 12 and apparently is a normal child with an average school career. He does not spend much time in the house or with the family, but prefers to play with his friends. He is ashamed of Susan's behavior and tries to avoid going out with her.

In the interview Susan presented as a tall, overweight, pasty-looking child, dressed untidily and with a somewhat disheveled appearance. She complained vociferously of her insomnia, though it was very difficult to elicit details of the sleep disturbance. She talked at length about her interests and occupations. She says she made a robot in the basement that ran amok and was about to cause a great deal of damage, but she was able to stop it by remote control. She claims to have built the robot from spare computer parts, which she acquired from the local museum. When pressed on details of how this worked, she became increasingly vague, and when asked to draw a picture of one of her inventions, drew a picture of an overhead railway and went into what appeared to be complex mathematical calculations to substantiate the structural details, but which in fact consisted of meaningless repetitions of symbols (e.g., plus, minus, divide, multiply). When the interviewer expressed some gentle incredulity, she blandly replied that many people did not believe that she was a supergenius. She also talked about her unusual ability to hear things other people cannot hear and said she was in communication with some sort of creature. She thought she might be haunted, or perhaps the creature was a being from another planet. She could hear his voice talking to her and asking her questions; he did not attempt to tell her what to do. The voice was outside her own head, but was inaudible to others. She did not regard the questions being asked her as upsetting. They did not make her angry or frightened.

Her teacher comments that although Susan's reading is apparently at the fifth-grade level, her comprehension is much lower. She tends to read what is not there and sometimes changes the meaning of the paragraph. Her spelling is at about the third-grade level, and her mathematics, a bit below that. She works hard at school, though very slowly. If pressure is placed on her, she becomes upset, and her work deteriorates.

(Adapted from *DSM-III Case Book*. American Psychiatric Association, Washington, DC, 1981, with permission.)

Residual schizophrenia

A 27-year-old woman was admitted to a neurology service for an evaluation of a movement disorder thought to be tardive dyskinesia. She described a history of four hospitalizations over the past 6 years and virtually continuous treatment with phenothiazines. Her most recent psychiatric admission had been approximately 1 year earlier. The hospital chart noted that at that time she believed that her husband was a notorious killer then being sought by the police and that she had marked loosening of associations. Her delusion was based on similarities she saw between newspaper speculations about the personality of the killer and certain characteristics of her husband.

During the present examination the patient acted silly and asked the doctors about their personal lives. She described plans to put her powerful intuitive senses to work by becoming a counselor for other patients like herself. Although her speech was digressive and circumstantial, it was not incoherent.

The patient, once a nursing student, had tried to be a waitress at McDonald's, but got confused by the customers' orders. Her husband both worked and took care of the household.

(Adapted from *DSM-III Casebook*. American Psychiatric Association, Washington, DC, 1981, with permission.)

POSITIVE AND NEGATIVE SUBTYPES The positive-negative dichotomy may have significant correlations with prognosis and biological variables. The positive symptoms are also referred to as florid, productive, or type I symptoms; the negative symptoms are referred to as defect, deficit, or type II symptoms. The positive symptoms (delusions, hallucinations, bizarre or agitated behavior) are associated with acute onset, a history of exacerbations and remissions, normal premorbid functioning, relatively normal social functioning during remissions, normal neuropsychological testing, normal computed tomography (CT) scans, and a favorable response to antipsychotic medication. The negative symptoms include affective blunting, poverty of speech and thought content, apathy, anhedonia, and poor social functioning. Negative symptoms are associated with an insidious onset, positive premorbid history, chronic deterioration, demonstration of atrophy on CT, abnormalities on neuropsychological testing, and poor response to antipsychotics.

OTHER SUBTYPING DICHOTOMIES Other dichotomies used to differentiate patients with good prognosis from those with poor prognosis have included the following: reactive or process disease, good or poor premorbid personality, exogenous or endogenous origin, schizophreniform disease or true schizophrenia, atypical or typical, with or without affective symptoms, and latent or psychotic. These various dichotomies depend on different subsets of the characteristics previously mentioned in Table 14.3-3. The use of these terms is not recommended because they are not clearly defined and there are no well-designed studies to support the concepts.

OTHER SUBTYPES OF SCHIZOPHRENIA The first three of the following subtypes are included in ICD-9 but not in DSM-III-R. Because these subtypes are not included in DSM-III-R, such patients would be diagnosed either as having one of the DSM-III-R subtypes or as having some other DSM-III-R diagnostic entity.

Paraphrenia This term is used as a synonym for paranoid schizophrenia in ICD-9. In other nosological systems, it is used to describe patients with a chronic course and the presence of well-systematized delusions but with well-preserved personality. In yet another, the term "paraphrenia" is used to indicate a group of late- (and insidious-) onset conditions that are characterized by paranoid delusions and are often associated with hearing loss. Its multiple meanings render the term not particularly useful for communication of information.

Simple ICD-9 includes schizophrenia, simple type, although clinicians are cautioned to use this diagnosis only rarely. This disorder is characterized by a gradual, insidious loss of drive and ambition. The patient is usually not hallucinating or delusional, and, if these symptoms do occur, they do not persist. The patient withdraws from contact with others and often stops working. Clinicians are indeed well advised not to make this diagnosis rashly because the condition is probably not very responsive to medication, and the diagnostic label of schizophrenia, even if warranted, can do more harm to such patients than good.

An unmarried man of 27 was brought to a mental hospital, because he had on several occasions become violent toward his father. For a few weeks he had auditory hallucinations. The voices eventually ceased, but he then adopted a strange way of life. He would sit up all night, sleep all day, and become very angry when his father tried to get him out of bed. He did not shave or bathe for weeks, smoked continuously, ate very irregularly, and drank enormous quantities of tea.

In the hospital he adjusted rapidly to the new environment and was found to be generally cooperative. He showed no marked abnormalities of mental state or behavior, except for his lack of concern for just about everything. He kept to himself as much as possible and conversed little with patients and staff. He also had little concern for personal hygiene or his dress.

Twenty years later he is still in the hospital. Described as shiftless and careless, sullen and unreasonable, he lies on a couch all day long. Antipsychotic treatment failed to alter his mental state or behavior. Despite many efforts to get the patient to accept therapeutic work assignments, he refuses to consider any kind of regular occupation. In the summer he wanders about the hospital grounds or lies under a tree. In the winter he wanders through the tunnels connecting the various hospital buildings and is often seen stretched out for hours under the warm pipes that carry steam through the tunnels.

Latent Latent schizophrenia (also known as borderline schizophrenia) is diagnosed in those patients who may have a marked schizoid personality and who show occasional behavioral peculiarities or thought disorders, without consistently manifesting any clearly psychotic pathology. Again, the clinician is wise to make a diagnosis of schizophrenia only with more significant pathology.

***Boufée délierante* (acute delusional psychosis)** This diagnostic category is used in France and is considered to be a discrete diagnostic category, not a subtype of schizophrenia. The actual criteria are similar to DSM-III-R's for schizophrenia, but require that the symptoms be present for less than 3 months; to some extent, this approximates the DSM-III-R diagnosis of schizophreniform disorder. French psychiatrists report that about 40 percent of patients with this diagnosis are later diagnosed as having schizophrenia.

Oneiroid In the oneiroid state, the patient feels and behaves as though in a dream. (*Oneiros* is Greek for "dream.") Sometimes deeply perplexed and not fully oriented in time and place, the oneiroid schizophrenic patient acknowledges everyday realities but gives priority to his world of hallucinatory experiences. Oneiroid states are usually limited in duration and might be classified as atypical psychosis in DSM-III-R. The clinician should be careful to seek an organic cause in the presence of such symptoms. There is no research evidence that this diagnostic designation has any utility in treatment planning or prognosis, nor is there any evidence that this subtype has a specific biological basis.

Pseudoneurotic These patients present predominantly with neurotic symptoms, however, on closer examination, reveal schizophrenia-like abnormalities in thinking and emotional reaction. The condition is characterized by pananxiety, panphobia, and chaotic sexuality. Unlike patients suffering from anxiety neuroses, these patients have anxiety that is free floating and hardly ever subsides.

A 34-year-old single man had been hospitalized in a mental hospital for 5 years. His main complaints were as follows:

I feel panicky and very upset inside. . . . I am afraid something inside me might explode, and I might do something bad. . . . I feel depressed all the time. . . . I couldn't hold a job now if I did get one. . . . My head feels funny inside. . . . I always feel tense, sometimes I feel like two persons, sometimes I feel that everybody's against me. . . .

He was one of four children born into a family in which all the members had fairly close relationships with each other and no major problems seemed to exist. Although he was always bright and considered to be the most talented of the four children, he failed his third year of high school and blamed his difficulty on one teacher. He went to a special tutorial school and later earned his Bachelor of Science degree with honors in chemistry at the age of 24. He got along well with his peers and participated in boxing, swimming, and singing.

In the 7 years after he graduated from college, he held at least nine different jobs. Several companies where he worked were sufficiently impressed with his ability to offer him special training. Various reasons were offered for the termination of his employment—not getting along with other staff members, poor work, better prospects elsewhere, accidents to company cars, simply leaving the job, and personal difficulties. He was often unemployed. On one occasion he worked as an orderly in a hospital.

In spite of his apparently good social adjustment as a child, he said that he had never really enjoyed life and that he was always anxious with people; however, he never manifested any clearly psychotic symptoms, such as hallucinations, delusions, thought disorders, and irrational behavior.

At age 27 he fell acutely ill for the first time after an episode of intense petting with his girlfriend. "I was afraid of exploding . . .

afraid of doing something awful . . . just generally tense." He was treated for a few weeks at a psychiatric clinic. Then he went to another city and worked for a short time, but soon had to return home and to the psychiatric clinic. He complained of a pulling sensation in the left side of his head.

Since then he has had 3 years of intensive psychotherapy, several courses of continuous sleep treatment, somnolent insulin therapy, several courses of ECT, and prolonged treatment with a variety of sedatives and antipsychotics.

He finally had to remain under close observation because of repeated suicide threats and a few superficial suicide attempts. He was convinced that he had some physical brain disease that was responsible for his constant tension, and he insisted that some neurosurgery could be done to correct it. Repeated neurological investigations have not revealed a lesion. His spontaneous activity consisted solely in reading the paper and watching television. He said he was too anxious to remain in any occupational setting for longer than a few days, after which he either asked for a new assignment or claimed he was too weak to work at all.

DIFFERENTIAL DIAGNOSIS

There are four principal guidelines in the differential diagnosis of schizophrenia. First, the clinician should aggressively investigate the possibility of an identifiable organic cause, especially if there are unusual or rare symptoms. Second, there should be a complete evaluation of each exacerbation of psychotic symptoms in a schizophrenic patient. The clinician should have an open mind to the possibility of a superimposed organic cause, especially when the patient has been in remission for a long time or if there is a change in the quality of symptoms. Third, the clinician should carefully elicit and consider a family history of psychiatric and neurological diseases. Finally, the clinician should make the diagnosis of schizophrenia only if the patient truly meets the criteria and if the possibility of other psychiatric diagnoses has been clearly ruled out.

MEDICAL DISORDERS There are a large number of neurological and medical diseases that can have symptoms identical to those of schizophrenia (Table 14.3-7). The psychiatric manifestations of many of these disorders often come early in the course, before the development of other symptoms. It is generally, but not invariably, true that patients with neurological and medical disorders have more insight into and distress over the symptoms. The fact that so many disorders can mimic schizophrenia is consistent with the notion that schizophrenia itself is a heterogeneous disorder. The most practical rule of thumb regarding psychiatric side effects of medications is that some patients may manifest virtually any symptom, including psychosis, in response to virtually any drug.

PSYCHIATRIC DISORDERS The psychiatric differential diagnosis for schizophrenia-like symptoms is also quite lengthy (Table 14.3-7).

Malingering and factitious disorder with psychological symptoms Because the diagnosis depends so much on the report of the patient, it is possible to simulate the symptoms of schizophrenia. Patients who, in fact, do have schizophrenia may sometimes falsely complain of symptoms for secondary gain, such as increased assistance benefits or admission to a hospital. It can be very difficult, sometimes impossible, to detect these two situations. Possible indicators include inconsistency in the mental status examination, history of similar presentations with against medical advice (AMA) discharges, and obvious secondary gain (e.g., legal troubles).

TABLE 14.3-7
Differential Diagnosis of Schizophrenia-like Symptoms

Medical or neurological
- Drug-induced, especially amphetamines, alcohol hallucinosis, anticholinergic, barbiturate withdrawal, belladonna alkaloids, cimetidine, cocaine, digitalis, disulfiram, hallucinogens, L-DOPA, phencyclidine (PCP)
- Epilepsy, especially of temporal lobe origin
- Tumors, especially frontal or limbic
- CNS infections, especially herpes encephalitis, Creutzfeldt-Jakob disease, neurosyphilis, AIDS
- Acute intermittent porphyria
- Alzheimer's disease
- B_{12} deficiency
- Carbon monoxide poisoning
- Endocrinopathies, especially adrenal and thyroid
- Fabry's disease
- Fahr's syndrome
- Hallervorden-Spatz disease
- Heavy metal poisoning (arsenic, manganese, mercury, thallium)
- Homocystinuria
- Huntington's disease
- Metachromatic leukodystrophy
- Normal-pressure hydrocephalus
- Pellagra
- Pick's disease
- Systemic lupus erythematosus
- Wernicke-Korsakoff syndrome
- Wilson's disease

Psychiatric
- Malingering
- Factitious disorder with psychological symptoms
- Autistic disorder
- Schizophrenia
- Schizophreniform disorder
- Brief reactive psychosis
- Mood disorder
- Schizoaffective disorder
- Atypical psychosis
- Delusional disorder
- Personality disorder, especially schizotypal, schizoid, borderline, paranoid
- Obsessive-compulsive disorder

Autistic disorder Autistic disorder is diagnosed when onset is after 30 months of age but before age 12 and there are no delusions, hallucinations, or looseness of associations. DSM-III-R does not include a separate diagnosis of childhood schizophrenia.

Mood disorders The distinction of schizophrenia and mood disorders can be quite difficult, but it is particularly important because of the availability of specific and effective treatments for the latter. DSM-III-R stipulates that affective symptoms in schizophrenia be brief relative to the duration of the primary symptoms. In the absence of information in addition to that obtained from a one-time mental status examination, it is usually more prudent to defer conclusive diagnosis or to assume the presence of a mood disorder than to diagnose schizophrenia prematurely.

The presence of marked thought disorder in mania, as well as in psychotic depression, has helped to demonstrate that there is no specific thought disorder that is pathognomonic for schizophrenia. There are significant differences, however, among groups of patients with these various disorders. Although both manic and schizophrenic patients have positive psychotic symptoms, schizophrenic patients tend to have more negative symptoms, and the manic patients virtually always recover from their thought disorder. Both schizophrenic and depressed patients have negative symptoms, but the depressed patients recover, whereas the schizophrenic patients very often are left with residual negative symptoms. There may be subtle differences in the quality of the thought disorder between groups of patients with mood disorders and schizophrenic disorders. Schizophrenic patients may have fewer intrusions of ideas but more bizarre and idiosyncratic thought processes than affectively ill patients.

Schizoaffective disorder This diagnosis is made when a manic or depressive syndrome is present concurrently with the major symptoms of schizophrenia. DSM-II-R specifies that delusions or hallucinations have persisted for at least 2 weeks in the absence of prominent affective symptoms.

Schizophreniform disorder and brief reactive psychosis Schizophreniform disorder is diagnosed when all the criteria for schizophrenia have been met, except that the symptoms have been present for less than 6 months. Brief reactive psychosis is diagnosed when schizophrenia-like symptoms have been present for less than 1 month and there was either a clear precipitating stressor or a series of stressors.

Delusional disorders A diagnosis of delusional disorder is warranted if nonbizarre delusions of mostly a persecutory nature have been present for at least 6 months in the absence of the other symptoms of schizophrenia or a mood disorder.

Atypical psychosis A diagnosis of atypical psychosis is warranted when a psychotic patient does not meet the criteria for another psychotic disorder.

Personality disorders A variety of personality disorders may present with some features of schizophrenia, but without meeting the entire list of diagnostic criteria for schizophrenia. Personality disorders, moreover, are long-standing patterns of behavior and do not have a relatively specific date of onset, as would the symptoms of schizophrenia.

REFERENCES

Allebeck P, Wistedt B: Mortality in schizophrenia. Arch Gen Psychiat *43:* 650, 1986.

Andreasen N C: The clinical assessment of thought, language, and communication disorders. II: Diagnostic significance. Arch Gen Psychiat *36:* 1325, 1979.

Arieti S: *Interpretation of Schizophrenia.* Basic Books, New York, 1974.

Bleuler E: *Dementia Praecox or the Group of Schizophrenias,* Zinker J, translator. International Universities Press, New York, 1950.

Cadet J L, Rickler K C, Weinberger D R: The clinical neurologic examination in schizophrenia. In *The Neurology of Schizophrenia,* H A Nasrallah, D R Weinberger, editors. Elsevier, Amsterdam, 1986.

Cancro R, Pruyser P W: A historical review of the development of the concept of schizophrenia. Bull Menninger Clin *34:* 61, 1970.

Docherty J P, van Kammen D P, Siris S G, Marder S R: Stages of onset of schizophrenic psychosis. Amer J Psychiat *135:* 420, 1978.

Drake R E, Gates C, Whitaker A, Cotton P G: Suicide among schizophrenics: A review. Compr Psychiat *26:* 90, 1985.

Goldberg T E, Weinberger D R: Methodological issues in the neuropsychological approach to schizophrenia. In *The Neurology of Schizophrenia,* H A Nasrallah, D R Weinberger, editors. Elsevier, Amsterdam, 1986.

Hamilton M, editor: *Fish's Schizophrenia,* ed 3. John Wright, Bristol, 1984.

Kraepelin E: *Dementia Praecox and Paraphrenia,* R M Barclay, translator, G M Robertson, editor. Robert E. Krieger, Huntington, NY, 1971.

May J V: The dementia praecox-schizophrenia problem. Amer J Psychiat *11:* 401, 1931.

Parnas J, Schulsinger F, Schulsinger H, Mednick S A, Teasdale T W: Behavioral precursors of schizophrenia spectrum. Arch Gen Psychiat *39:* 658, 1982.

Pope H G, Lipinski J F: Diagnosis in schizophrenia and manic-depressive illness. Arch Gen Psychiat *35:* 811, 1978.

Romano J: On the nature of schizophrenia: Changes in the observer as well as the observed (1932–77). Schizophr Bull *3:* 532, 1977.

Solovay M R, Shenton M E, Holzman P S: Comparative studies of thought disorders. I. Mania and schizophrenia. Arch Gen Psychiat *44:* 13, 1987.

Stephens J H, Astrup C, Carpenter W T, Jr, et al: A comparison of nine systems to diagnose schizophrenia. J Psychiat Res *6:* 127, 1982.

Volovka J: Late-onset schizophrenia: A review. Compr Psychiat *26:* 148, 1985.

Walters G D: The MMPI in schizophrenia: A review. Schizophr Bull *9:* 226, 1983.

Wyatt R J, Alexander R C, Egan M F, Kirch D G: Schizophrenia, just the facts. What do we know, how well do we know it? Schizophr Res *1:* 1, 1988.

Yesavage J A: Correlates of dangerous behavior by schizophrenics in hospital. J Psychiat Res *18:* 225, 1984.

14.4 SCHIZOPHRENIA: SOMATIC TREATMENT

JOHN M. KANE, M.D.

INTRODUCTION

The treatment of schizophrenia remains one of the major challenges in modern-day medicine, not merely because of the prevalence of the disorder, its frequent severity and chronicity, but also because the management of the illness requires thoughtful integration of biological, psychological, and environmental factors.

The clinician who treats persons with schizophrenia must attempt to assimilate and integrate this information while continuing to be alert to the possible implications for treatment planning of new findings in any of these areas. The clinician also must recognize the enormous individual variations in premorbid adjustment, mode of onset, symptomatology, and social and environmental factors that may influence treatment response, course of illness, and level of adaptation. Although this section will focus on the use of somatic treatments, these treatments are administered in the context of diagnostic considerations, variability in response, course of illness, and a variety of other factors.

DIAGNOSTIC AND ASSESSMENT ISSUES

Any discussion of somatic treatment must recognize the limitations of current nosology and assessment measures. Although increasing attention has been given to issues of validity and reliability in psychiatric diagnosis, psychiatrists still rely very heavily on subjective reports of mood, feeling states, and cognitive phenomena (e.g., delusions, hallucinations) for which there are no external or objective sources of validation. A clinician who works with psychotic patients is keenly aware of how variable the reporting of such symptoms can be over the course of a psychotic episode and of how new information may emerge even as the patient improves. Given this, one must also recognize that no signs or symptoms are pathognomonic for schizophrenia.

The importance of a differential diagnosis and longitudinal perspective in psychiatry cannot be overemphasized, given the current state of knowledge. The application of somatic treatment should always be viewed as a therapeutic trial, which must be evaluated on an ongoing basis with very clear goals and objectives as well as appropriate clinical measures of assessment for both beneficial and adverse effects. When somatic treatments are administered on a long-term basis, the medical record becomes a critical source document in reviewing indications for (and response to) treatment over time. Any clinician who has reviewed the medical records of chronic schizophrenic patients has experienced frustration in many cases when it was difficult to determine the nature and severity of previous symptoms and the response to treatment.

Response to somatic treatment has been used to some extent to validate diagnosis. Although this perspective can be useful clinically and heuristically, it has limitations vis à vis currently available treatments and diagnostic strategies. A patient who has a manic episode may respond as well to antipsychotic drugs as to lithium, though the preferred long-term treatment for bipolar disorder is lithium. Antipsychotic drugs have a broad spectrum of action and may be clinically useful in a variety of conditions that are not schizophrenia. So, good response to this particular somatic treatment may not elucidate the diagnosis. It could be argued that, in the face of diagnostic uncertainty, the clinician should choose a treatment the response to which might provide some support for a specific diagnosis (e.g., if the differential diagnosis includes mania and schizophrenia, a trial of lithium might be more informative than a trial of antipsychotics).

In a climate wherein rapidity of discharge from hospitals is emphasized, clinicians may feel that such therapeutic trials are difficult to justify, but hospitalization for an acute episode of a patient likely to need long-term treatment is an extremely valuable opportunity, which should be taken advantage of to the extent possible.

Somatic treatment is not administered in a vacuum. Quality of history taking, clinician-patient relationship, psychoeducation, informed consent, and therapeutic alliance with the patient and family or significant others are only a few of the factors that will affect somatic treatment. It is unfortunate when, for example, enormous effort goes into diagnosis and treatment planning and little attention is paid to factors that might ultimately lead to patient noncompliance.

The rationale for specific somatic treatment is largely empirical, and the current view of schizophrenia as a biological illness with an important genetic component supports that rationale. At the same time, patients present with a heterogeneous array of manifestations, responses to treatment, and outcomes, suggesting that schizophrenia may not be a single disease entity and that a given type of somatic treatment may not be appropriate for all patients.

HISTORY

The observations that chemical substances can affect mood, affect, behavior, and cognition are as old as recorded time. It is not surprising, therefore, that a variety of somatic treatments were utilized in attempts to correct or ameliorate abnormal behavior or feeling states. The history of the treatment of schizophrenia includes not only the use of an incredible array of pharmacological substances but physical treatments, including removal of teeth, tonsils, intestines, and parts of the brain, and purging, bleeding, immersion in water, and countless unrecorded efforts.

The modern era of somatic treatment began in the 1940s with reports that extracts of the *Rauwolfia serpentina* plant (reserpine) had antipsychotic properties and with the subsequent observations by Delay and Deniker in France, in the early 1950s, that the phenothiazines (chlorpromazine [Thorazine]) also had antipsychotic action. Although the use of reserpine and chlorpromazine became increasingly widespread, with chlorpromazine being safer, better tolerated, and probably more efficacious, other somatic treatments continued to be used well after the introduction of these compounds.

Insulin coma continued to be used as a treatment for schizophrenia into the 1960s, and in some American institutions was used as recently as the 1970s. This treatment had been introduced in the early 1930s, and although not studied systematically, it was in widespread use prior to the introduction of antipsychotic drugs.

Convulsive therapy, initially induced by injection of camphor, which was then replaced by metrazol, and eventually by the application of electric current, was also widely used to treat schizophrenia and was demonstrated to be effective in some patients.

The administration of electroconvulsive therapy (ECT) in a much safer and more sophisticated fashion than originally employed continues to be a useful treatment in mood disorders and in some patients with schizophrenia. Its indications and spectrum of activity in schizophrenia, however, require further study.

Although the Portuguese physician Moniz was awarded the Nobel Prize for the introduction of the surgical procedure known as prefrontal lobotomy, the use of psychosurgery in mental disorders is now quite rare. Though new techniques make the potential for precise surgical approaches to specific brain areas much more feasible, this strategy is viewed as a last resort in very carefully selected cases. In the United States, prior to the use of psychosurgery, the case must be reviewed by a board whose composition and procedures for review have been approved by the Department of Health and Human Services.

ANTIPSYCHOTIC DRUGS

The class of compounds referred to as antipsychotic now includes several different chemical classes other than the phenothiazenes, of which chlorpromazine was the prototype. These compounds were once referred to as major tranquilizers, but this term is misleading and should be abandoned. Table 14.4-1 lists the antipsychotic agents currently marketed in the United States and the generally recommended dose ranges and potency equivalence. These figures should be taken merely as guidelines, since the issue of dosage requirements and relative potency across antipsychotic drug classes is far from clearly established.

At present, there are no well-established differences between specific antipsychotic drugs or drug classes in terms of efficacy (with the exception of promazine [Sparine] and mepazine, which appear to be less effective, and clozapine (Clozaril), which appears to offer some advantage in refractory patients). The so-called high-potency drugs produce less sedation and hypotension but have a greater propensity to produce extrapyramidal side effects. The adverse-effects profile may be related to a variation in specific receptor-blocking effects in different neurotransmitter symptoms. Table 14.4-2 provides data on the relative potencies of these drugs in different systems. These apparent differences in receptor effects should stimulate additional research on other potential clinical differences between the drugs; in the past, however, most comparisons have involved a heterogeneous group of schizophrenic patients randomly assigned to one or another drug, resulting in a similar proportion of patients responding in each

TABLE 14.4-1
Typical Dosages of Frequently Used Antipsychotics: Approximate Relative Potency of Antipsychotic Agents*

Generic	*Representative Brand*	*Relative Potency*	*Usual Range of Total Daily Dose†* Acute (mg/day)	Maintenance (mg/day)
Phenothiazines				
Chlorpromazine	Thorazine	100	200–1000	50–400
Thioridazine	Mellaril	100	200–800	50–400
Mesoridazine	Serentil	50	100–400	25–200
Acetophenazine	Tindal	20	60–100	40–80
Prochlorperazine	Compazine	15	60–200	20–60
Perphenazine	Trilafon	10	12–64	8–24
Trifluoperazine	Stelazine	5	10–60	4–30
Triflupromazine	Vesprin	25	30–150	20–100
Fluphenazine	Prolixin	2	5–60	1–15
Thioxanthenes				
Thiothixene	Navane	5	10–120	6–30
Chlorprothixene	Taractan	100	50–600	50–400
Butyrophenones				
Haloperidol	Haldol	2	5–50	1–15
Dibenzoxazepines				
Loxapine	Loxitane	10	20–160	10–60
Dihydroindolones				
Molindone	Moban	10	40–225	15–100
Long-Acting Injectable Preparations				
Fluphenazine decanoate	Prolixin decanoate			6–100‡
Haloperidol decanoate	Haldol decanoate			50–200§

*These are approximate estimates of relative potency. It should be noted that relative potency may not be the same in the higher dosage ranges as it is in the lower.
†Dosage may vary with individual responses to the antipsychotic agent employed.
‡Prolixin decanoate may be given at intervals of up to 3 to 4 weeks. Dosage requirements vary widely.
§Haloperidol decanoate should be given every 4 weeks. Dosage requirements vary widely.

group. Such findings do not enable one to determine whether the drugs are equally efficacious in specific patients. A major clinical question remains: Is any benefit derived from switching from one antipsychotic to another in a patient who has failed to respond adequately?

CHOICE OF DRUG An important consideration in the choice of antipsychotic drug should be the patient's history. Evidence of a prior good response to a specific compound should suggest using that drug again. However, if a patient on a specific drug has shown significant adverse effects or relapses (assuming adequate doses and compliance), another drug should be considered. Many clinicians continue to believe that a more sedating drug is necessary for the agitated or highly excited patient. There is no evidence that this is the case, and the high-potency and low-potency drugs are equally efficacious as antipsychotics, regardless of whether the patient is agitated or psychomotor retarded. If it is clear that the patient might ultimately benefit from the use of a long-acting injectable drug, the oral form of that particular compound should be considered for use during the acute treatment phase.

TABLE 14.4-2
Affinities of Antipsychotics for Human Brain Receptors

	D_2	*Muscarinic Acetylcholine*	*Histamine H_1*	*α-Adrenergic*
Highest	cis-Thiothixene	Clozapine	Mesoridazine	Mesoridazine
	Fluphenazine	Thioridazine	Promazine	Chlorpromazine
	Perphenazine	Mesoridazine	Clozapine	Thioridazine
	Trifluoperazine	Chlorpromazine	Loxapine	Promazine
	Trifluopromazine	Promazine	cis-Thiothixene	Haloperidol
	Haloperidol	Loxapine	Perphenazine	Clozapine
	Prochlorperazine	Prochlorperazine	Chlorpromazine	Fluphenazine
	Chlorprothixene	Trifluoperazine	Thioridazine	Perphenazine
	Mesoridazine	Perphenazine	Prochlorperazine	cis-Thiothixene
	Chlorpromazine	Fluphenazine	Fluphenazine	Prochlorperazine
	Thioridazine	cis-Thiothixene	Trifluoperazine	Trifluoperazine
	Loxapine	Haloperidol	Haloperidol	Loxapine
	Molindone	Molindone	Molindone	Molindone
	Promazine			
Lowest	Clozapine			

Table adapted from Richelson E: Neuroleptic affinities for human brain receptors and their use in predicting adverse effects. J Clin Psychiat *45:* 331, 1984, with permission.

DOSAGE Because individual differences in absorption and metabolism of drugs that are as lipophilic as the antipsychotic drugs are considerable, dosage requirements may vary a great deal from one patient to another. In general, doses of 400 mg per day of chlorpromazine equivalents are felt to be a minimum for the average patient. No formula, however, can substitute for clinical judgment and dosage titration. One clinical dilemma that remains is the treatment of the patient who has failed to respond to a course of antipsychotic drugs. Should the dosage be increased? Should another antipsychotic drug be substituted? Or, should the clinician allow more time on the original dose? A variety of factors enter into this decision, including the patient's history, the dosage employed initially, and the length of the treatment period. With increasing pressure to discharge patients rapidly, many clinicians feel compelled to alter the treatment plan very quickly if the patient does not show the expected response. At the same time, given that most patients can tolerate very high doses of the high-potency antipsychotic drugs, clinicians have used high doses, and even megadoses, in the hope of improving response. In addition, rapid dosage escalation, particularly with parenteral preparations, has been employed on the assumption that therapeutic response could be hastened if high loading doses could be administered in the first few days of treatment. In general, these strategies have not altered the degree or the rapidity of therapeutic response; at the same time, they probably expose the patient to greater risk of adverse effects.

Although some therapeutic response may be apparent within the first few days, it usually takes 10 to 14 days for clinically significant improvement to appear, and this improvement may continue for an additional 4 to 6 weeks or longer. It is difficult, therefore, to know when to abandon a particular drug or dosage regimen. The clinician cannot accurately attribute causes and effects of changes in a treatment program. For example, the patient who does not respond after 2 weeks to a dose of 10 to 20 mg of haloperidol (Haldol) might respond after an additional 2 weeks. The clinician who increases the dose to 40 mg after 10 days may attribute the response to the dose increase, when, in fact, the original dosage would have taken effect in time.

BLOOD LEVELS As techniques became available for measuring minute quantities of substances in blood, there was considerable optimism that the determination of blood levels of the antipsychotic drugs would go a long way toward explaining idiosyncratic responses to drug treatment and would enable clinicians to improve overall response rates substantially. Although some progress has been made in this area, the value of blood-level monitoring in the acute treatment of schizophrenia is far from established; routine use of this procedure could not now be advocated. Some drugs (e.g., haloperidol) seem to have a *therapeutic window,* a blood concentration level that produces the optimal response. At present, however, its upper limits have not been established. To prove the validity of this assertion would require demonstrating that patients with blood levels above the putative therapeutic range who have failed to respond adequately improve when the blood level is lowered; very few relevant data are available. Another unanswered question is, What events or effects interfere with therapeutic response in patients who do not respond despite high blood levels of antipsychotic drugs? It is quite likely that blood levels do account for some variability in clinical response, but this appears to be only one of several contributing factors.

The currently available methods for measuring concentration of antipsychotic drugs in blood include specific chemical assays for a particular parent compound or metabolite. The value of such a study may be limited if researchers do not know which metabolites are therapeutically active (or possibly even toxic) and which are most relevant to measuring clinical response. Some relatively specific radioimmunoassays have been developed which are capable of detecting very low levels of particular drugs, but there are sometimes problems with cross-reactivity with certain metabolites. The radioreceptor assay, an outgrowth of the dopamine hypothesis of schizophrenia, attempts to measure the amount of displacement of radioactive material bound to dopamine receptors in vitro produced by a specific sample. Theoretically, this provides a quantitative estimate of the amount of dopamine-blocking activity in the blood and should include both parent compound and active metabolites which are capable of binding to dopamine receptors. Although some studies have reported significant correlations between this measure and clinical response, the results are not consistent across all classes of antipsychotic drugs, and further work is necessary to establish the utility of this method (which relies very heavily on the dopamine hypothesis and binding to a specific subtype of dopamine receptor).

The state of the science is such that, if a clinician has access to a well-established laboratory for the assessment of blood levels and a knowledgeable consultant who can provide guidance as to the appropriate time and conditions under which to obtain the sample and can help interpret a particular result, a blood-level assay may be helpful to a patient who has failed to respond to a conventional dosage regimen of an antipsychotic drug or to a patient who has shown unusual sensitivity to adverse effects.

ROUTE OF ADMINISTRATION To control an acutely agitated and uncooperative patient, intramuscular (IM) administration of the first few doses of antipsychotics may be desirable. If a patient is cooperative, oral concentrates are well absorbed and can also be very useful for initial dosing. Blood levels are more predictable following parenteral administration; however, when patients comply with oral medication regimens, appropriate dosage titration can achieve a good therapeutic effect. Long-acting injectable drugs are not recommended for acute treatment, because their long half-lives would produce considerable escalation of drug levels over time, and the ability to titrate doses from day to day is reduced enormously. For the first several days there may be some advantage to giving medication two or three times a day, but subsequently, antipsychotic drugs are tolerated well when given in a single dose at bedtime. Since most patients are likely to require continued antipsychotic drug treatment on a maintenance basis, the simpler the regimen, the more likely the patient will be to comply.

This author feels that there is an important role for long-acting injectable antipsychotics and that they are underutilized in the United States. Many clinicians consider such agents only for patients who have demonstrated noncompliance or who have proven refractory to other drugs. Because rates of noncompliance among schizophrenic outpatients are so high, and as we have no well-validated methods for predicting the development of noncompliance, more thought should be given to resolving this problem as it relates to long-term treatment. This will be discussed further in the context of maintenance treatment, but it is worth emphasizing that administration of a low test dose of a long-acting injectable drug prior to the patient's discharge may be valuable in setting the stage for subsequent drug therapy. Later attempts to change antipsychotic drugs or to introduce a new route of administration may be fraught with difficulties.

DOSE EQUIVALENCY The increasing emphasis on identifying optimal dosage for both acute and long-term treatment makes the issue of dose equivalencies among antipsychotic drugs and drug classes an important issue. Chlorpromazine has frequently been the standard against which equivalent doses are established. Unfortunately, the information regarding dose equivalencies is based on clinical impressions not all of which have been systematically validated. The usual method has been a double-blind clinical trial of two different antipsychotics, dosages having been established on the basis of clinical judgment. At the end of the trial, comparisons are made regarding the doses employed, and an attempt is made to establish a conversion ratio between the two drugs. In other situations, clinical trials comparing drug and placebo are utilized to suggest an effective dose range for a particular drug and then data from other studies may be utilized to establish equivalency between drugs. The potential problems in assuming the validity of these results are considerable, and it is particularly important to consider the possibility that conversion ratios that may be appropriate at the lower end of the dose spectrum may not apply at higher dose ranges. There have been no systematic studies of this phenomenon, but it is apparent that clinicians give high-potency and low-potency antipsychotics in different doses and schedules. R. Baldessarini's group compared the findings of a survey of 110 private hospital inpatients with the dosing practice reported in surveys of nearly 16,000 Veterans Administration patients. The doses of high-potency drugs above the daily equivalent of 1 gram of chlorpromazine accounted for more than 40 percent of all prescriptions. The mean chlorpromazine-equivalent dose of the two most potent antipsychotic agents (haloperidol and fluphenazine [Prolixin, Permitil]) was over three times as high as the mean doses prescribed of chlorpromazine or thioridazine (Mellaril). As these authors suggested, the sedative and autonomic effects of the low-potency drugs may limit their use in the higher dose range, whereas it is feasible for clinicians to increase doses of potent antipsychotics without substantial increases in immediate adverse effects. The relationship between the increasing popularity of utilizing relatively high doses of potent antipsychotics and the apparent increase in the prevalence of tardive dyskinesia over the past 2 decades is unknown, but is certainly worth considering. This author sees no value in high-dose treatment for the average patient.

STRATEGIES FOR MANAGING REFRACTORY PATIENTS Although antipsychotic drugs have a dramatic effect in most patients with schizophrenia, a substantial number of patients derive little, if any, benefit from these compounds, a circumstance that is a major clinical dilemma. In this context, clinicians usually consider therapeutic trials of various classes of antipsychotics or other treatments, which have been discussed (e.g., lithium, propranolol [Inderal], ECT). Although some reports describe patients who benefit from such strategies, no systematic, well-controlled studies have been carried out that compare the relative efficacy of alternative treatment strategies in refractory patients. It is certainly reasonable for the clinician to conduct a therapeutic trial of some alternative treatment in a patient in this subgroup, but there may also be a point at which one must recognize that the current level of knowledge does not enable one to help every patient. This author's practice in treating refractory patients is to provide adequate trials of at least three different chemical classes of antipsychotic drugs. "Adequate," in this context, is defined as at least 6 weeks of 1,000 mg per day of chlorpromazine or an equivalent. Patients on this regimen who have relatively low blood levels (if such assays are available) may be given a trial of higher-than-usual doses of antipsychotic medication.

ADVERSE EFFECTS Table 14.4-3 lists some of the more common adverse effects of antipsychotic drugs, drugs capable of producing a broad range of adverse effects. The high-potency drugs, such as haloperidol and fluphenazine, are more likely to produce extrapyramidal side effects but less likely to produce sedation and autonomic side effects, as compared with the low-potency drugs, such as chlorpromazine or thioridazine.

The clinician prescribing these drugs should be particularly sensitive to side effects that may have behavioral manifestations, such as akinesia or akathisia. Unfortunately, many parkinsonian side effects continue to be unrecognized or misdiagnosed, with potentially negative consequences for therapeutic response, compliance, and overall levels of functioning.

NEUROLOGICAL SIDE EFFECTS OF ANTIPSYCHOTIC DRUGS Among the most common and troublesome side effects of antipsychotic drugs are those that are labeled extrapyramidal. These reactions can be subdivided into five basic categories: acute dystonia, parkinsonism, akathisia, tardive dyskinesia, and dystonia. Although there is some indication that parkinsonian side effects are due to dopamine-receptor blockade in the basal ganglia, the pathophysiology of these syndromes is not well understood and may vary with individual vulnerability and other factors.

Acute dystonia Acute dystonia involves intermittent or sustained muscle spasms and abnormal postures. These phe-

TABLE 14.4-3
Adverse Effects of Antipsychotics

Central nervous system
Parkinsonism
Dystonia (acute and tardive)
Dyskinesia (acute and tardive)
Akathisia
Neuroleptic malignant syndrome
Seizures
Cognitive dysfunction
Skin and eyes
Allergic skin reactions
Phototoxicity
Pigmentation
Ocular deposits
Endocrine
Menstrual irregularities
Galactorrhea
Gynecomastia
Hematological
Neutropenia
Agranulocytosis
Hepatic
Cholestatic hepatitis
Enzyme induction

nomena usually involve the musculature of the head, neck, and trunk, but the extremities may also be involved. Grimacing, opening of the jaw, and involvement of muscles controlling the tongue may also occur. Blepharospasm (sustained closure of the eyelids) or oculogyric crises (upward and lateral rotation of the eyes, frequently accompanied by retrocollis or torticollis) can also occur. The bodily distribution of dystonic reactions may vary depending on individual vulnerability factors, which are not well understood. There is a tendency for more body and limb involvement in younger persons and children and for more facial involvement in older adults.

Acute dyskinesias should not be confused with acute dystonia or tardive dyskinesia; the former movements may involve tongue movements, lip smacking, or movements of the trunk and extremities, but do not involve severe muscle spasms. This reaction may follow the same time course as acute dystonia and some cases may respond to anticholinergic drugs. The relationship between acute dyskinesia and tardive dyskinesia is poorly understood, and the differential diagnosis may be difficult. Further research is necessary to delineate better the subtypes of such movements and to clarify what areas of overlap may exist.

Acute dystonic reactions usually occur soon after the institution of antipsychotic drug therapy (approximately 50 percent of cases occur within 48 hours; 90 percent, within 5 days). These reactions last from a few seconds to several hours. Estimates suggest that the incidence of acute dystonic reactions may vary from as low as 2 percent to as high as 25 percent, depending on the patient population and the potency and dosage of the particular drug.

The treatment of acute dystonic reactions usually involves IM or intravenous (IV) administration of an anticholinergic or an antihistamine, which usually takes effect within a few minutes. This experience can be very frightening to patients and their families. Frequently, when patients give a history of being allergic to a particular drug, they, in fact, are referring to having experienced a dystonic reaction. It is important, therefore, for clinicians to explain what this phenomenon is, so that subsequently it can be reported accurately to treating clinicians. Although the use of prophylactic antiparkinsonian medication remains controversial, the potential to prevent frightening adverse reactions, such as acute dystonia, may justify the use of antiparkinsonian drugs on a prophylactic basis during the early phases of treatment, particularly for patients receiving high-potency drugs.

Parkinsonism Drug-induced parkinsonism is similar in manifestations to idiopathic parkinsonism, except that the tremor is less prominent. The onset of these side effects usually occurs after the first week of treatment, but within the first 4 weeks. Some patients appear to develop tolerance to this effect over time, though adverse effects can persist even during the maintenance phase of treatment, and clinicians should remain alert to this possibility.

Severe akinetic reactions, which can mimic catatonia, have been reported with antipsychotic drugs. This possibility should be considered in the differential diagnosis of such behavior. (The neuroleptic malignant syndrome [NMS] is discussed below.)

Parkinsonian symptoms are characterized by akinesia, muscle rigidity, alterations of posture, tremor, and autonomic symptoms. Some patients may exhibit flat affect or mask-like facies, shuffling gait, loss of normal associated movements (particularly while walking), increased salivation, and frank drooling. A variety of agents are now available for the treatment of drug-induced parkinsonism, and their efficacy supports the pathophysiological hypothesis implicating reduction in dopamine activity (and a relative excess of cholinergic function) in the basal ganglia. Table 14.4-4 lists the most commonly used antiparkinsonian agents and their usual dose ranges.

TABLE 14.4-4
Antiparkinsonian Agents

Generic	*Representative Brand*	*Range of Daily Oral Dose (mg)*
Amantadine	Symmetrel	100–400
Benztropine	Cogentin	0.5–6
Biperiden	Akineton	2–6
Diphenhydramine	Benadryl	75–200
Ethopropazine	Parsidol	50–600
Orphenadrine	Disipal Norflex	200
Procyclidine	Kemadrin	5–15
Trihexyphenidyl	Artane	6–15

Whether or not the clinician decides to use antiparkinsonian drugs on a prophylactic basis during the initial phase of treatment, it is critical that patients be examined regularly to determine whether parkinsonian symptoms are present. If the clinician does choose to use antiparkinsonian agents on a prophylactic basis, attempts should be made to discontinue this adjunctive treatment after the first stages of initial treatment are over. Patients must be evaluated repeatedly for parkinsonian side effects, even during the maintenance phase of treatment. In the author's view, the potential negative consequences of antiparkinsonian drugs do not necessarily outweigh the potential advantages. Clearly, patients receiving a variety of potent anticholinergic agents may be at higher risk of adverse atropine-like effects, so the anticholinergic potency of the antipsychotic drug, as well as that of other potential treatment agents (tricyclic antidepressants), should be taken into consideration. In addition, antiparkinsonian drugs may have a negative impact on some aspects of cognitive functioning and do have abuse potential. These factors should also be taken into consideration. The possibility that they may reduce blood levels of antipsychotic drugs has been suggested, but has not been consistently supported in clinical trials. In the author's view, this effect is relatively small and not clinically significant, even if it does exist, and in no way accounts for the antiparkinsonian activity of these drugs. If the dose of the antipsychotic drug can be reduced as a strategy to minimize the parkinsonian side effects, this reduction should be considered. There has also been some concern that the concurrent administration of antiparkinsonian drugs and antipsychotics might increase the risk of tardive dyskinesia; but, this risk has not been established and is based largely on the observation that the acute administration of anticholinergic compounds may exacerbate preexisting tardive dyskinesia in a proportion of patients. In fact, it may be that those persons most vulnerable to developing acute extrapyramidal side effects are also most vulnerable to developing tardive dyskinesia, a circumstance that might make it appear that the concurrent administration of antiparkinsonian drugs is a risk factor when, in fact, it is an epiphenomenon resulting from the emergence of parkinsonian symptoms.

Antimuscarinic drugs are capable of inducing anticholinergic toxicity, which may manifest itself in restlessness, agitation, confusion, disorientation, hyperthermia, dry and flushed skin, tachycardia, sluggish and dilated pupils, diminished bowel sounds, and urinary retention. This response is best treated by discontinuing the causative drug and by the use of physostigmine (Antilirium, Eserine), a centrally and peripherally active anticholinesterase agent.

Akathisia Akathisia is a subjective or objective sense of restlessness manifested by fidgeting, pacing, and, at times, an inability to sit still. This adverse effect can be particularly unpleasant and may be difficult for a psychotic patient to describe adequately, so akathisia should be considered in the differential diagnosis of anxiety and psychotic agitation in patients receiving antipsychotic drugs. The pathophysiology of this syndrome is not well understood, as akathisia is not characteristically seen in idiopathic Parkinson's disease, though it may be seen in postencephalitic parkinsonism.

Antiparkinsonian drugs may have a beneficial effect. However, their efficacy for this particular condition may be less dramatic than for the previously described extrapyramidal effects. Benzodiazepines may be helpful in some patients with akathisia, as may be peripheral beta blockers, such as propranolol, in relatively low doses.

Tardive dyskinesia Tardive dyskinesia is an abnormal involuntary movement disorder seen in a proportion of patients receiving long-term antipsychotic treatment. The most common form is the constellation of mouth, tongue, and jaw movements characterized by chewing, lip sucking, lip smacking, and tongue movements. In addition, facial grimacing and choreoathetoid movements of the fingers and hands are also common.

Tardive dyskinesia is capable of presenting in a variety of ways, including impaired vocalization, disturbances in breathing, and abnormal movements of the trunk and extremities, and as a consequence any abnormal movements seen in the context of chronic antipsychotic treatment should be evaluated with tardive dyskinesia in mind. Epidemiological data suggest that antipsychotic treatment is an important etiological factor in the development of involuntary movements, although individual vulnerability may vary considerably, and it is conceivable that some patients may exhibit abnormal movements unrelated to antipsychotic exposure. Prevalence estimates vary widely and are influenced by a variety of patient, demographic, and treatment history characteristics, as well as by methodological issues involving differences in case ascertainment, diagnostic criteria, and related variables.

Data from an ongoing prospective study of tardive dyskinesia development suggest an incidence of 4 percent per year of antipsychotic drug exposure for at least the first 5 to 6 years of drug treatment. Whether the incidence continues at this rate beyond 5 years remains to be seen. It is also important to point out that the majority of these prospectively identified cases were rated as mild and did not necessarily increase in severity during a 2- to 3-year follow-up period, despite the fact that many patients continued to receive antipsychotic drugs. Data from several sources suggest that tardive dyskinesia is not necessarily progressive, despite the continued administration of antipsychotic drugs. It does appear, however, that improvement in abnormal involuntary movements is more likely if antipsychotic drugs can be discontinued, particularly if this discontinuation occurs when evidence of tardive dyskinesia is first observed. The importance of discontinuing antipsychotic drugs is particularly evident in older populations, where persistence of the dyskinesia is even more likely with continued antipsychotic exposure than in younger persons.

A small subgroup of patients develop a very severe and progressive form of the disorder. Because at present one cannot predict this degree of vulnerability, overall caution in the use of antipsychotic drugs is of utmost importance. The single most frequently implicated risk factor for the development of tardive dyskinesia is age, and older women appear to be at greater risk than older men. There are no proven safe and effective treatments for this condition, though antipsychotic dose reduction (and particularly discontinuation) have a definite beneficial effect. Complete discontinuation of drugs is frequently not feasible for schizophrenic patients, and no particular antipsychotic drug or drug class is less likely than others to produce tardive dyskinesia or more appropriate for patients who have developed the disorder. For persons who must continue to take antipsychotic drugs despite having developed tardive dyskinesia, utilization of the lowest effective dose may ameliorate the involuntary movement disorder. Given the potential adverse effects of antipsychotic drugs, it is critical that attention be given to the overall risk-benefit ratio when utilizing these agents, and patients should participate in a process of informed consent (documented in the medical record). Clear documentation of ongoing need and benefit derived from the treatment, as well as documentation that the patient has been informed about the potential benefits and risks (including that of tardive dyskinesia) should be reflected in the medical record of any patient who receives antipsychotic drugs. In addition, patients should undergo periodic evaluation for the presence of abnormal involuntary movements.

Tardive dystonia is another form of abnormal involuntary movement disorder that can occur in the context of long-term antipsychotic treatment. It presents a different clinical picture from tardive dyskinesia: Spasms of muscles in the face, neck, back, or limbs produce a picture similar to torsion dystonia. Although until recently relatively few cases have been reported, the recognition of this condition has spread considerably in recent years and must be included in the differential diagnosis of patients who present with these types of symptoms and have a history of taking antipsychotic drugs.

SEIZURES Grand mal seizures can occur with antipsychotic drug treatment, particularly with very high doses or rapid increases in dose. These infrequent reactions are usually treated with a reduction in dose. The utility or necessity of coprescribing anticonvulsant drugs for such patients has not been well established, and recurrence of seizures can, in all likelihood, be prevented by reducing the dose of the offending agent.

NEUROLEPTIC MALIGNANT SYNDROME Administration of antipsychotic drugs has also been associated with a syndrome manifested by fever, rigidity, confusion, autonomic dysfunction, and rhabdomyolysis. As a rule, this condition resolves after a period of days to weeks if the antipsychotic drug is discontinued, but the condition has been associated with mortality estimated at 15 to 20 percent. Some experts have suggested that in many reported cases of NMS, the primary event may have been severe antipsychotic-induced parkinsonism resulting in disruption of normal eating, walking, and breathing, with fever resulting from medical complications, such as dehydration, myoglobinuria with renal failure, pulmonary embolus, and pulmonary infarction.

Reports of lethal catatonia have decreased considerably since the introduction of psychotropic drugs, and it may be that the successful control of severely agitated patients may be related to this factor; however, it has also been suggested that in recent years some cases that once might have been described as lethal catatonia have been attributed to NMS. Further research is necessary to understand fully the nature of these phenomena.

AUTONOMIC SIDE EFFECTS Antipsychotic drugs, particularly those with higher levels of antimuscarinic activity, are capable of producing a variety of autonomic effects, including dizziness, faintness, weakness, dry mouth, nasal congestion, nausea, vomiting, constipation, urinary disturbances, blurred vision, and orthostatic hypotension.

Orthostatic hypotension is particularly likely to develop with the aliphatic phenothiazines, although it can occur with all antipsychotic drugs as well as the tricyclic antidepressants and the monoamine oxidase inhibitors. It most frequently appears during the first several days of treatment and is most apparent when the patient arises from bed. Tolerance to this effect usually develops rapidly; however, occasionally it can be a significant problem. The use of surgical elastic stockings can be helpful to prevent venous pooling in the extremities in some patients. Explaining this effect and reassuring the patient can also be helpful. Patients should be told not to shift position rapidly. On awakening, they should sit first and arise gradually after 1 or 2 minutes.

Less frequent side effects include jaundice, which was more common in the early days of chlorpromazine utilization; however, recent estimates suggest that this effect is relatively rare. The reason for this decrease is not clear. Chlorpromazine-induced jaundice most commonly occurs within the first few weeks of treatment. It is preceded by fever, malaise, and gastrointestinal symptoms, which are then followed by liver enlargement and tenderness. The jaundice is usually benign and self-limiting. It is probably due to a hypersensitivity reaction that produces small bile duct obstruction. Most patients recover spontaneously within a few weeks after discontinuation of the offending medication. Cross-sensitivity to other antipsychotic drugs rarely occurs, so that another antipsychotic drug may be substituted.

AGRANULOCYTOSIS Antipsychotic drugs, particularly phenothiazines, have been associated with agranulocytosis. There is considerable variation in estimates of incidence of agranulocytosis among patients receiving these agents (from one in 250,000 cases to one in 200). The estimate of 1 in 1,000 may represent the most reasonable overall estimate. Leukopenia occurs much more frequently in patients receiving phenothiazines. It has been suggested that agranulocytosis is more likely to occur and more likely to be fatal in older persons, particularly elderly women. In some reviews, a relationship between dosage and risk has been suggested. Agranulocytosis usually occurs after the first 3 to 5 weeks of treatment. Ninety percent of cases occur within the first 8 weeks. The peripheral blood count reveals few granulocytes or none, and the marrow shows a selective aplasia of the granulocyte series. If the offending agent is discontinued, recovery usually takes place within 2 weeks if the patient can be protected from infection.

Management of such patients should involve hematologists and infectious-disease specialists. The value of routine blood counts during the initial phases of treatment with antipsychotic drugs remains a subject of controversy. Most clinicians have abandoned the practice, because routine screening may not be helpful in identifying cases rapidly. However, recent experience with clozapine, a drug with an apparently higher incidence of agranulocytosis, suggests that, when it is used, routine complete blood counts (CBCs) may be critical in identifying this reaction as early as possible. Clinicians must be aware of the potential significance of signs of infection in a patient receiving these drugs, particularly during the period of maximum risk.

OCULAR AND SKIN EFFECTS Several phenothiazines (particularly chlorpromazine) produce phototoxicity; patients can develop painful sunburn after only a few minutes' exposure to bright sunlight. This differs from photosensitivity, which is an allergic reaction requiring previous exposure. Patients should be warned about the hazards of this side effect and encouraged to use a sun block. Pigmentary changes in the skin or conjunctiva can occur following prolonged high-dose phenothiazine treatment and exposure to sunlight.

In most cases, the ocular changes associated with phenothiazine medication are of no functional significance. Because thioridazine has produced a pigmentary retinopathy in patients receiving doses in excess of 800 mg per day, daily doses of this particular compound should not exceed 800 mg.

ENDOCRINE AND METABOLIC EFFECTS Disturbances in sexual functioning may occur as a result of the sympathetic and parasympathetic effects of these drugs. Men may have difficulty in achieving and maintaining erections, and inability to reach orgasm or ejaculate can occur. Retrograde ejaculation has also been reported. Thioridazine appears more likely than other phenothiazines to cause such sexual dysfunctions. Antipsychotic agents may also cause amenorrhea, lactation, and gynecomastia. Antipsychotic drugs are also frequently associated with weight gain, though the mechanism is unclear.

Teratogenicity Although the teratogenic potential of antipsychotic drugs appears to be low, there is always some risk, and the ideal situation is to avoid any drug treatment. For women who have chronic schizophrenia, this avoidance is sometimes not feasible, but decisions as to how to manage pregnant women who require antipsychotic drugs should be discussed thoroughly with expert consultants, the patient, and the family.

Electrocardiographic changes Many phenothiazines, but most frequently thioridazine, are associated with electrocardiographic (EKG) abnormalities consisting of increased Q–T interval and a flattened T-wave. Psychotropic drugs, including some antipsychotic compounds, may also have antiarrhythmic properties in ordinary doses. The clinical significance of EKG changes with antipsychotic drug treatment must be evaluated in each patient.

Heat stroke The anticholinergic activity of antipsychotics, particularly the low-potency drugs, is capable of inhibiting sweating and cutaneous heat elimination, particularly if combined with antiparkinsonian agents or tricyclic antidepressants. This effect may be a risk factor in the development of hyperthermia under certain circumstances. In addition, the effect of psychotropic drugs on temperature regulation in the hypothalamus may be responsible for impaired response to high ambient temperatures. It is important that patients receiving these drugs be monitored closely in very hot weather and that adequate ventilation and temperature control be provided in facilities housing these individuals, particularly seclusion rooms.

MECHANISM OF ACTION OF ANTIPSYCHOTIC DRUGS The major hypothesis of antipsychotic drug activity involves dopamine-receptor blockade. This appears to be one property shared by these compounds, and a fairly good correlation between clinical potency and the degree of dopamine-receptor blockade in vitro frequently has been cited as evidence for this assumption. Recent research has emphasized the need to explain the time course of clinical response, given the fact that the receptor blockade occurs very quickly, whereas the clinical therapeutic effect may take several weeks. It may be that the receptor blockade is merely the first stage in a process involving the response of dopaminergic systems to the blockade. Initially, for example, there is a rise in homovanillic acid (the major metabolite of dopamine in the central nervous system [CNS]) followed by a decline over the next 3 to 4 weeks. This decline appears to correlate with the time course of clinical response and may provide a clue as to the brain mechanisms responsible for antipsychotic drug action.

Another line of reasoning which supports the dopamine hypothesis to some extent is based on the consistent observation that agents which are capable of stimulating dopamine receptors through direct or indirect mechanisms (e.g., amphetamine, methylphenidate [Ritalin], cocaine) are also capable of producing psychoses if given in high enough doses for sufficient lengths of time, even in healthy individuals. In addition, even a single oral or IV dose of these agents is capable of producing a transient exacerbation of psychotic signs and symptoms in schizophrenic patients.

Considerable efforts are under way to assess dopamine-receptor abnormalities in postmortem CNS tissue; however, these efforts are compromised by the fact that most postmortem samples are from persons who had received chronic antipsychotic treatment at some point during their illness. In addition, positron-emission tomographic (PET) studies are being employed to assess dopamine receptors in living subjects, but here, also, the focus needs to be on patients who have yet to be treated with antipsychotic drugs. Given the likely heterogeneity of schizophrenia, it is surprising that antipsychotic drugs are as effective as they are for the majority of patients with this illness. It is possible that certain aspects of psychoses share a common pathophysiology, even though the etiology may be different. This is also an important consideration in attempting to understand the efficacy of antipsychotic drugs in patients who are not schizophrenic (e.g., acute mania, delusional depression, borderline states, organic mental syndromes). It is also quite possible that other CNS neurotransmitters or neuromodulators are involved in the therapeutic activity of antipsychotic drugs, and this remains an area of considerable complexity.

PREDICTORS OF RESPONSE AND THE ROLE OF ALTERNATIVE TREATMENTS

Given the considerable variability in antipsychotic drug response among patients diagnosed as schizophrenic, repeated attempts have been made to identify predictors of therapeutic response. The literature cites many possible variables, ranging from premorbid social adjustment to ventricular brain ratio, but no well-established predictors of antipsychotic drug response, during an acute episode or an exacerbation, have been identified. There are numerous lines of investigation which may, at some point, produce evidence on which to base recommendations for a particular alternative somatic treatment in specific patients; however, with the present level of knowledge, antipsychotic drugs are the most effective treatment for most patients with schizophrenia.

LITHIUM Some reports have suggested that lithium carbonate may be useful in the treatment of a subgroup of patients with a diagnosis of schizophrenia or schizophreniform psychosis. Clearly, the issue of diagnosis is critical here. Particularly during a first episode of psychosis, the differentiation of bipolar disorder, schizoaffective disorder, and schizophrenia may be difficult. Some investigations have suggested that patients who meet criteria for chronic schizophrenia derive some benefit from lithium. It appears that the presence or absence of affective symptoms does not necessarily predict response to lithium. It may have some prophylactic value for maintenance treatment in patients with schizoaffective diagnoses, but no evidence is available for its maintenance value in schizophrenia. Schizophrenic patients who derive little or partial benefit from antipsychotic drugs sometimes improve when lithium is added to their ongoing antipsychotic drug regimen. Although concern has been expressed about possible neurotoxicity, there is very little controlled evidence that such toxicity occurs any more often in schizophrenic patients than in patients with other diagnoses treated with lithium. In some patients, the combination of lithium and antipsychotic drugs may exacerbate adverse extrapyramidal effects.

PROPRANOLOL In the early 1970s, several reports suggested that β-adrenergic receptor blockers might be effective in alleviating psychoses. Typically, very high doses of propranolol were utilized (up to 3 or 4 grams per day in some studies). A few reports suggested that propranolol had antipsychotic activity when administered alone to schizophrenic patients, while others reported it potentiated the efficacy of antipsychotic drugs when given in combination.

The results of more recent controlled trials do not support the original enthusiasm for propranolol's efficacy in the treatment of psychoses. It remains possible that propranolol or other β-blockers would prove to be of some value in a specific subgroup of schizophrenic patients, but at present, this possibility cannot be confirmed or refuted. Propranolol does not appear to have nearly the spectrum of activity of conventional antipsychotic compounds. It has been suggested that brain-damaged persons who are violent or aggressive may benefit from propranolol, but this, too, requires substantiation. Propranolol, administered in much lower doses than those doses used to treat schizophrenia itself, may have some role in the treatment of akathisia resulting from antipsychotic administration, but this indication is clearly very different.

BENZODIAZEPINES Benzodiazepines have been used in a variety of contexts in schizophrenia. Some individuals with schizophrenia suffer from anxiety, and benzodiazepines are prescribed for their anxiolytic properties. It is not entirely clear to what extent this class of drugs offers advantages above and beyond those of antipsychotic treatment for anxiety associated with schizophrenia; however, this use is fairly widespread. Benzodiazepines are also used as hypnotics in patients with schizophrenia, but here, again, their role (particularly on a long-term basis) has not been established.

Attempts have been made to utilize benzodiazepines as primary antipsychotic agents, particularly in high doses; the rationale is the capacity of benzodiazepines to facilitate γ-aminobutyric acid (GABA) neurotransmission, which might indirectly reduce dopamine activity. Their efficacy in this context has not been established, and several controlled trials suggest that they are ineffective as antipsychotic agents. In recent years, the use of IM benzodiazepines as adjuncts to antipsychotics in the acute control of psychotic signs and symptoms has also been advocated, but remarkably few data are available to support the superiority of this approach over the use of other sedative-hypnotics to help control acute agitation in the context of psychosis.

CLONIDINE Clonidine (Catapres) is an antihypertensive agent that stimulates presynaptic α_2-adrenergic receptors. By stimulating these inhibitory presynaptic sites, clonidine is capable of decreasing norepinephrine release. If the noradrenergic system is involved in psychosis, clonidine might have some therapeutic activity. There are limited data suggesting clonidine's efficacy as an antipsychotic. Although this treatment has considerable heuristic implications, its efficacy is far from established.

CARBAMAZEPINE Carbamazepine (Tegretol), an anticonvulsant, has gained some acceptance as an alternative prophylactic treatment in bipolar disorder patients who are unresponsive to or intolerant of lithium. It has not been well studied in schizophrenia and, at present, does not appear to have a place in its treatment. It is possible that some patients diagnosed as having schizophrenia do have electroencephalographic (EEG) abnormalities, particularly complex partial seizures, which may benefit from carbamazepine.

CLOZAPINE Over the past several years, enormous effort has gone into developing and testing potential antipsychotic drugs which are designated as atypical. Atypicality must be viewed as a working concept rather than a clearly delineated and well-validated classification. In general, this designation has been used to characterize drugs that are either more selective in their dopamine-antagonist properties (e.g., sulpiride) or more broadly active in having marked antiserotonergic or antinoradrenergic effects as well (e.g., clozapine).

Specific preclinical phenomena, such as relative propensity to produce dopamine-receptor hypersensitivity in animal models following long-term administration, have also contributed to the definition of atypical compounds. In addition, relative lack of effect on prolactin secretion when administered to humans has been a characteristic of some drugs, particularly clozapine. It has been suggested that atypical drugs are relatively free from the usual degree of extrapyramidal side effects associated with currently marketed antipsychotics.

Clozapine belongs to the chemical class of dibenzodiazepines. It is related chemically to the antipsychotic drug loxapine (Loxitane), but its pharmacological characteristics are quite different. Unlike other more typical antipsychotics, clozapine produces only slight and transient elevations in serum prolactin, even in patients on moderate or high doses.

Several controlled clinical trials in the 1970s established the antipsychotic efficacy of clozapine, but it was also associated with a higher incidence of agranulocytosis than more typical antipsychotics. A large multicenter clinical trial was carried out in the United States recently, comparing clozapine to chlorpromazine in well-characterized treatment-refractory patients. The results suggest that clozapine may benefit a proportion of patients who fail to respond adequately to other antipsychotic compounds; however, it does place them at substantially higher risk of agranulocytosis.

Clozapine and other drugs may offer important clues for the development of new agents with better risk-benefit ratios. Although carefully controlled clinical trials in human subjects have not been conducted, there is reason to suspect that clozapine therapy may carry considerably less risk of tardive dyskinesia than therapy with more typical antipsychotics.

ANTIDEPRESSANTS Patients with schizophrenia may experience varying degrees of clinical depression. In schizophrenia, symptoms such as anhedonia, reduced motivation, reduction in energy, psychomotor retardation, pessimism, and suicidal ideation must be viewed in terms of differential diagnosis. Severe demoralization may be an appropriate response to the realization that one has a devastating illness. At the same time, antipsychotic side effects, specifically akinesia, may in some cases mimic certain aspects of depression. It is also quite common for schizophrenic patients to experience residual deficit states or negative symptoms, which frequently manifest themselves as lack of motivation, diminished pleasure capacity, flatness of affect, and emotional withdrawal. If the differential diagnosis suggests a true depression in a patient with schizophrenia, then a trial of tricyclic treatment in conjunction with continued antipsychotic administration may be appropriate, particularly if this is viewed as a therapeutic trial with clear goals and assessment measures. The utilization of tricyclic antidepressants alone in schizophrenia is not recommended, because they can produce psychotic exacerbations in vulnerable patients. Also, tricyclic antidepressant administration may produce increased blood levels of antipsychotics through competitive inhibition of hepatic microsomal enzymes. The anticholinergic potency of specific tricyclic antidepressants should be taken into consideration, especially if they are combined with anticholinergic antipsychotic drugs or anticholinergic antiparkinsonian agents.

Monoamine oxidase inhibitors have also been utilized in conjunction with antipsychotic agents, but there is no evidence that they are any more effective than tricyclics in patients with schizophrenia. As they necessitate dietary restrictions and interact with other drugs, monoamine oxidase inhibitors are not a first-line treatment for presumptive depression in schizophrenic patients.

ELECTROCONVULSIVE THERAPY The role of ECT in the treatment of schizophrenia is unclear. Although some controlled trials in patients with acute schizophrenia have suggested that ECT is superior to placebo or no treatment, most experts believe that drug therapy is superior to ECT for the routine treatment of schizophrenia. ECT may be helpful for some patients who fail to respond to drugs, and a few studies suggest that ECT given in conjunction with antipsychotics may succeed when antipsychotics alone failed. Specific syndromes, such as catatonic withdrawal or catatonic excitement, are thought to be particularly responsive to ECT, and its role in treating schizoaffective states is worthy of further investigation. The potential value of ECT, especially in refractory cases, should be the subject of additional research.

MAINTENANCE ANTIPSYCHOTIC TREATMENT

The acute phase of treatment for schizophrenia involves the attempt to alleviate the signs and symptoms associated with psychotic exacerbation. Antipsychotic drugs generally have a dramatic effect on the delusions, hallucinations, thought disorder, and other acute symptoms within 4 to 6 weeks of initiating treatment, although improvement may continue well beyond that interval. The therapeutic response attained during this treatment phase will, to some extent, determine the rationale and expectations of subsequent continuation or prophylactic treatment. The pharmacological treatment of an illness with exacerbations and relative remissions is usually divided into three phases: acute, continuation, and maintenance (or prophylactic). For patients who achieve full or substantial recovery during the initial treatment phase, the continuation period of treatment begins at the point when maximum improvement is reached, and its objective is to continue the pharmacotherapy long enough to ensure that the episode for which the original treatment was given is, in fact, over. Once this phase has passed, further pharmacological treatment is intended to prevent the occurrence of a new episode (rather than the reemergence of the original episode). This model has been applied perhaps more readily to mood disorders, where episodes may be more discrete, but this conceptualization may be useful in managing some schizophrenic patients as well. For example, it appears that patients are more vulnerable to psychotic exacerbation, even with continued medication, during the first several months following recovery than they may be subsequently. The delineation of these illness phases in schizophrenia may be difficult, because a substantial proportion of patients do not achieve a full remission of psychopathology despite continuous drug treatment. Although antipsychotic drug discontinuation studies demonstrate that many of these patients would experience even more psychopathology without medication, continued drug treatment in this context may be viewed as controlling or suppressing ongoing manifestations of the illness rather than as preventing a new episode. Such patients may be poor candidates for drug discontinuation or substantial dose reduction.

Long-term maintenance antipsychotic drug treatment has proven to have enormous value in reducing the risk of psychotic relapse and rehospitalization. Numerous double-blind, placebo-controlled clinical trials support this conclusion. Initially, long-term treatment trials focused almost exclusively on rates of relapse and rehospitalization; in the last decade, one has seen the initiation of much more sophisticated long-term clinical trials, which have focused not only on relapse and rehospitalization rates, but on a variety of other factors relevant to better assessing the overall benefits and risks of long-term drug treatment. A variety of concerns have influenced the types of studies conducted in recent years: high rates of noncompliance in taking medication for long periods; the frequent occurrence of adverse effects (particularly tardive dyskinesia); the relative lack of substantial improvement for many patients in functional areas leading to continued disability in psychosocial and vocational arenas; the considerable heterogeneity in clinical course; and the potential importance of other therapeutic modalities, as well as environmental and personality factors.

Table 14.4-5 summarizes the results of double-blind comparisons of active drug versus placebo, two different active drugs or forms of administration (i.e., oral versus long-acting injectable), or the same drug given in different doses. This table includes only maintenance treatment trials that lasted at least 9 months.

It is apparent that there is enormous variability in relapse rates across these studies. Comparisons are made difficult, however, by differences in design and methodology, such as diagnostic criteria, level and duration of remission, patient selection and recruitment methods, and definition of relapse, among others. In addition, not all of these reports have presented cumulative relapse rates or "life table" analyses, which allow for appropriate handling of patients with incomplete data (e.g., those who drop out of the study or are discontinued from the trial because of adverse effects). When cumulative relapse curves are presented, data from different studies can be contrasted even though the investigators may have employed different assessment intervals, conducted trials for different periods of time, and experienced different dropout rates.

So-called guaranteed medication delivery (of long-acting injectable drugs) has played an important role in many of the major maintenance treatment studies in recent years, because the investigator can be certain that relapse occurring in the context of long-term pharmacotherapy is not due to noncompliance. This strategy enables the investigator to explore the impact of other patient, treatment, or environmental factors without regard for their potential influence on compliance. The use of guaranteed medication delivery in clinical trials has also made it quite clear that many patients continue to experience psychotic relapses despite receiving medication and has underscored the importance of exploring other factors that might contribute to this vulnerability.

INDICATIONS FOR MAINTENANCE TREATMENT

The evidence in the literature for the value of maintenance antipsychotic drug treatment in preventing psychotic relapse and rehospitalization in well-diagnosed schizophrenic patients is extremely compelling. Given that not all patients relapse within a specified interval following discontinuation of antipsychotics and that there is enormous heterogeneity in the long-term outcome of schizophrenia, some question remains as to whether there may be a subgroup of patients for whom long-term antipsychotic treatment may not be indicated. Available measures (phenomenological, historical, biological, etc.) do not allow one to identify such patients.

One subgroup of patients has received some attention in this regard, based on the assumption that there may be persons who experience only one episode of schizophrenia and do not go on to have another. Recent studies that have examined the advantages of maintenance medication treatment in this subgroup suggest that even among good-prognosis first-episode patients, medication may be indicated for the prevention of subsequent episodes. Among first-episode patients who come to hospitals, it is the rare patient who remains free of subsequent episodes when followed for 2 or 3 years after recovery from the first episode. It may be reasonable to consider a finite period of maintenance treatment following recovery from an acute episode and then a trial of antipsychotic discontinuation; however, it should be kept in mind and the family and patient should be informed that the likelihood of a subsequent episode should not be ignored or denied. In multiepisode well-diagnosed schizophrenic patients, the risk of relapse without medication tends to average 65 to 70 percent within the year following medication discontinuation, so one is hard pressed to identify patients

TABLE 14.4-5
Maintenance Pharmacotherapy in Schizophrenia

Author	*N*	*Age (Mean or Range)*	*Sex*	*Prior Episodes*	*Time Since Discharge*	*Level of Remission*	*Duration*	*Outcome (Relapse)*	*Drop Out*
Troshinsky et al., 1962	43	40–50	63% F	2–3	2–4 yr	No hallucinations, delusions, or obvious thought disorder. Required 300 mg CPZ.	1 yr	Drug 4% PBO 63%	?
Engelhardt et al., 1963; 1964; 1967	446	18–44	?	?	?	?	48 mo	CPZ 1 yr 15% 4 yr 20% PBO 1 yr 30% 4 yr 31%	36% in 18 mo
Leff & Wing, 1971	35	16–55	?	?	6–12 wk	Preadmission level	12 mo	Drug 35% PBO 80%	14%
Hirsch et al., 1973	81	43	36% F	70%	50% 52 wk	?	9 mo	FD 8% PBO 66%	9%
Crawford & Forrest, 1974	31	20–65 X=40s	71% F	?	?	?	10 mo	Stel 40% FD 14.3%	7%
Hogarty et al., 1974	374	34	58% F	60% 2 or more	?	?	24 mo	Drug 12 mo 31%, 24 mo 48% PBO 12 mo 68%, 24 mo 80%	8%
Chien, 1975	47	43	57% F	Former long-term inpatients	?	?	12 mo	FE[1] 12% FE[2] 37% PBO 86% [1]Doctor-regulated interval [2]Patient-regulated interval	?
Rifkin et al., 1977	73	23	32% F	1.9	X=26 wk	Remitted or stable plateau	12 mo	FD+Oral 5% PBO 75%	11%
Kelly et al., 1977	60	42	66% F	?	?	?	9 mo	Fluph Dec 10% Flupen Dec 10%	2%
Falloon et al., 1978	44	17–60 X=39	55% F	2 or more 80%	0	?	12 mo	Pimozide 24% FD 40%	12%
Quitkin et al., 1978	56	26	44% F	2.7	X=64 wk	Remitted or stable plateau	12 mo	Pen 7% FD 10%	20%
Hogarty et al., 1979	105	34	54% F	4.6	0	?	24 mo	Oral 2 yr 65% 12–24 mo 42% FD 2 yr 40% 12–24 mo 8%	13%
McCreadie et al., 1980	35	50	All M	?	?	"Well-controlled"	9 mo	Pimozide 19% FD 17%	3%
Schooler et al., 1980	214	29	41% F	2 or more	0	?	12 mo	FHCL 38% FD 46%	25%
Cheung, 1981	30	40	60% F	1.6	3–5 yr	Fully remitted 3–5 yr	18 mo	Antipsychotic 13% Benzodiazepine 62%	7%
Kane et al., 1982	28	22	50% F	1	X=17 wk	Remitted	1 yr	Drug 0% PBO 41%	35%

McCreadie et al., 1982	28	55	All M	?	Inpatients	"Well-controlled"	10 mo	Pimozide 15% FD 7%	25%
Odejide & Aderounmu, 1982	70	?	?	2 or more	?	Well for at least 12 mo	12 mo	FD 19% PBO 56%	25%
Kane et al., 1983	126	29	37% F	3.2	X=64 wk	Remitted or stable plateau	12 mo	Low-dose FD 56% Intermdt dose 24% Std-dose FD 14%	10%
Marder et al., 1984	50	36	All M	?	X=23 mo	Stable	1 yr	Low-dose FD 1 yr 22% 2 yr 44% Std-dose FD 1 yr 20% 2 yr 31%	14%
Crow et al., 1985	120	26	38% F	1	1 mo	Able to be discharged	2 yr	Drugs 58% PBO 70%	11%

who can be withdrawn indefinitely from antipsychotic drugs. Even studies that have focused on patients who have been in good remission on long-term antipsychotic treatment for substantial intervals (from 1 to 5 years) have found that antipsychotic drug discontinuation is associated with a 75 percent relapse rate within the next 12 to 24 months.

It is clear that many patients do not relapse immediately on discontinuation of antipsychotic drug, and on average 3 to 7 months may pass before a relapse is experienced. This fact has suggested the use of intermittent pharmacotherapy to capitalize on the possible lack of need for antipsychotic drug therapy for relatively lengthy intervals while acknowledging that eventually the reinstitution of these medications will be necessary.

Another subgroup of patients for whom the continued indication for antipsychotic drug treatment may be questioned are those who continue to experience psychotic relapse despite taking maintenance medication. This author knows of no studies that have focused specifically on the potential benefits of ongoing antipsychotic treatment for this population of patients, but it seems that many of them would experience an even poorer outcome and more malignant course if antipsychotic drug treatment were not continued. Other factors may reduce the overall benefits of the antipsychotic drug treatment—undue stress, substance abuse, personality disorders—and attention to these factors might improve the long-term outcome in the context of continued maintenance on antipsychotic drugs.

Patients who have predominantly affective symptoms or whose course results in the emergence of new symptoms more consistent with a schizoaffective or mood disorder should receive a trial of maintenance lithium. It is also possible that some schizophrenic patients who do not fully benefit from continued antipsychotic treatment may benefit from a combination of antipsychotic drugs and lithium.

Another obvious concern in the continued utilization of long-term and antipsychotic treatment is the emergence of tardive dyskinesia. As previously discussed, this situation should prompt an extensive reevaluation of the overall risk-benefit ratio of continued antipsychotic treatment. This process should involve informed consent by the patient and the family, with adequate documentation in the medical record. In many cases involving multiple episodes of schizophrenia, the decision may be to continue the antipsychotic drug despite the presence of tardive dyskinesia, and for many patients, this continuation will not necessarily lead to a continued progression in severity of the abnormal involuntary movement disorder. It is important, however, to utilize the lowest possible effective dose and to continue to reevaluate the patient in all respects.

For the overwhelming majority of patients with schizophrenia, a good rationale for indefinite discontinuation of antipsychotic drug treatment cannot be established. It is hoped that eventually predictors may be developed that can help select patients for whom at least lengthy drug interruptions might be feasible. Despite the very impressive evidence of the value of maintenance antipsychotic drug treatment, the data base on this issue in general involves studies lasting 1 to 2 years at most. Systematic controlled data addressing the issue of the very long-term impact of antipsychotic treatment (e.g., 10 to 20 years) on the course of schizophrenic illness are not available. Many clinicians who have had the opportunity to evaluate and follow patients in both the pre- and postantipsychotic eras do feel that the introduction of antipsychotic treatment has had a salutary effect on the long-term course of schizophrenia; however, these impressions are merely that. Some long-term outcome studies of patients with schizophrenia do find substantial improvement in the overall level of psychopathology and social disability in some patients 20 years after onset of the illness. The extent to which antipsychotic drugs introduced early in the illness and continued throughout the course of the disorder affect the likelihood of this positive outcome remains to be established.

DRUG DOSAGE IN LONG-TERM TREATMENT Given the desire to reduce adverse effects, particularly tardive dyskinesia but also those behaviorally manifest parkinsonian side effects such as akinesia and akathisia, there has been increasing interest in identifying minimum effective dose requirements for long-term maintenance treatment of schizophrenia. Several recent dosage reduction studies have employed fixed doses or fixed dose ranges of long-acting injectable antipsychotics. In the case of fluphenazine decanoate, it appears that for many patients, a dose of 5 to 10 mg given intramuscularly every 2 weeks is sufficient to prevent psychotic relapse, particularly if the clinician is observing the patient closely and is in a position to provide a temporary increase in dose if there is evidence of psychotic relapse.

Results from these trials also suggest that dose reduction in the maintenance phase of treatment can be associated with improved subjective well-being and some improvement in psychosocial and vocational adjustment, which is probably mediated through a reduction in behaviorally manifest and cognitive adverse effects. In addition, some preliminary results suggest that the incidence of tardive dyskinesia may be reduced if minimal doses can be employed for long periods of time. These dose-reduction strategies are not without risk. The incidence of psychotic relapse may increase, so patients should be selected carefully for dose-reduction strategies, on the basis of a variety of clinical factors ranging from length of time in remission to environmental and psychosocial stresses. The available data suggest that dose-reduction strategies may be more successful in patients who have been out of hospitals for several months and are in a reasonably stable remission and for patients who are in relatively less stressful environments. Other factors that should be taken into consideration include history of nature and type of onset of relapse, as well as consequences in terms of history of suicidal or aggressive behavior. Clearly, substantial dose-reduction strategies are not appropriate for all patients, and clinicians should exercise a good deal of judgment in selecting patients best suited for this strategy. At the same time, it is this author's impression that for many patients being treated in the community, doses of maintenance antipsychotic medication have been far in excess of what is necessary to achieve the desired results. Excessive maintenance doses pose additional risk of tardive dyskinesia and may also have a negative impact on compliance in that patients experiencing even subtle subjective distress or dysphoria due to the medication may have substantially diminished motivation to take it.

Careful clinical evaluation and observation are necessary to minimize the potential risks of substantial dose reduction. Because it is difficult to predict the time course of relapse, the clinician is not in a position to determine when the minimum effective threshold dosage has been reached. Even if drugs are completely discontinued, many patients will not experience a psychotic relapse for several months, so, when the dose has been reduced below the minimum effective level, the clinician may not be aware of this immediately. These factors require careful ongoing evaluation and education of patient and family in early signs of relapse and in preparation for increasing the dose when necessary. If clinical judgment and ongoing evaluation are applied thoughtfully and judiciously, many patients can benefit from substantially reduced doses.

TARGETED OR INTERMITTENT TREATMENT Based on the observations that relapse may not occur for several months after the discontinuation of antipsychotics and that some patients exhibit prodromal signs and symptoms of an imminent psychotic relapse, some investigators have demonstrated the feasibility of utilizing antipsychotic drugs on an intermittent or targeted basis. The approach involves careful interviewing of the patient and the family to determine whether characteristic signs and symptoms precede the onset of a full-blown psychotic episode. Many patients experience anxiety, agitation, irritability, or insomnia prior to the onset of hallucinations, delusions, or conceptual disorganization. If early signs are noticed, antipsychotic drugs can be reintroduced before a relapse becomes full blown. This strategy may not be feasible for all patients, especially those who live in environments or participate in clinical programs wherein supervision and monitoring are inadequate to detect early signs of relapse. Even at the beginning of relapse, some patients do not retain sufficient insight or judgment to recognize the need for the reinstitution of the drug. Some patients and families are unable to recognize prodromal signs, and in a subgroup of patients the relapse may occur too quickly for anything to be done.

When this strategy is successful, however, it may allow some persons to stop taking antipsychotics for substantial intervals (e.g., 6 to 12 months), thereby reducing the risk of adverse effects and perhaps improving the level of subjective well-being. It must be recognized that a portion of patients who are completely discontinued from antipsychotic drugs may experience a relatively rapid recurrence of psychotic signs and symptoms (i.e., within 2 to 4 weeks). Current estimates suggest that from 10 to 20 percent of patients might be vulnerable to this type of rapid relapse. Factors that may influence this risk could include length and level of remission from the previous episode at the point at which antipsychotic drugs were discontinued.

Does intermittent antipsychotic drug treatment reduce, increase, or have any effect on the risk of tardive dyskinesia? There are relatively few data on this empirical question; however, it is the author's impression that the effect of intermittent treatment on the risk of developing tardive dyskinesia may depend a great deal on how long the patient can be withdrawn from antipsychotic drugs. Intervals of 1 to 2 months might be of little or no advantage (or even deleterious), whereas intervals of 6 months or longer might be very beneficial. This question is the focus of an ongoing collaborative study being administered by the National Institute of Mental Health.

COMPLIANCE

Compliance with the recommended treatment plan is a major concern in all areas of medicine. Frequently, an enormous amount of effort goes into diagnosis and treatment planning, whereas factors related to compliance receive inadequate attention. Among psychiatric patients, compliance may be even more problematic because the illnesses have considerable potential to impair judgment, insight, and stability. Mental disorders also carry greater social stigma, and patients may be embarrassed about psychotropic medication.

Although most often discussed in the context of medication taking, compliance is equally relevant to other aspects of the treatment and rehabilitation plans. Compliance is frequently discussed as an all-or-nothing phenomenon, when, in fact, it may frequently be partial and may change over time. Many patients are prone to take less medication than prescribed, take it irregularly, or take excessive amounts at certain times, and they may not adhere to proscriptions that attend treatment (e.g., avoidance of alcohol). At times, the causes of various forms of noncompliance may be quite different, and the clinician must be sensitive to all aspects of the problem.

One problem in assessing the scope of this difficulty has been the fact that poor adherence tends to disappear under scrutiny. Patients who are likely to agree to participate in a study of compliance may not be representative of the patient population, so findings of studies that have attempted to document the scope of noncompliance may grossly underestimate the extent of the problem.

The methods employed to determine noncompliance have varied enormously. The simplest, but perhaps most misleading, strategy is simply to ask the patient. During any psychiatric workup and history taking, the patient should be queried about past and present levels of compliance. The phrasing of the question may help elicit information that might not otherwise be learned: "What did you do when you found that the medication was not helping?" or "What did you do when you developed the side effects?" or "How many times did you forget to take your medication?" Many patients deny noncompliance even when questioned directly. Pill counting has been employed in research protocols, but is rarely done on a routine clinical basis, and there is no assurance that the medication removed from the bottle has actually been consumed by the patient.

Some clinicians have attempted to utilize assays developed to measure psychotropic drugs in blood to assess compliance in taking medication. This strategy may help to determine whether the patient has taken any medication at all; beyond that, a blood level may not tell whether the patient is taking the appropriate amount of medication or taking it on a regular basis. In order to monitor patients for complete compliance utilizing blood levels, a steady-state level would have to be established under controlled (compliance-assured) circumstances, after which substantial deviations from this level could be attributed to noncompliance. This procedure would clearly consume much time and money.

Most of the treatment that the average patient with schizophrenia receives is administered on an outpatient basis. The importance of maintenance medication in preventing psychotic relapse and rehospitalization has been discussed previously. Patients and their families must be educated about the indications and benefits of ongoing antipsychotic treatment. The concept of prophylaxis is difficult for many persons to understand, and particularly so in schizophrenia, because the time course of relapse following antipsychotic drug discontinuation is unpredictable. Patients experiment with discontinuing antipsychotic medication for brief intervals and sometimes develop a cavalier attitude toward the risk of psychotic relapse. Others become disillusioned with the residual deficits associated with a schizophrenic illness. The target symptoms for which antipsychotic drugs are effective and the areas for which these treatments are ineffective must be clear to patients and their families, so that realistic expectations of drug treatment as well as other therapeutic modalities can be assumed.

The type of treatment regimen may affect compliance. Patients are more likely to adhere to a simple regimen; when multiple medications are prescribed simultaneously or doses are to be taken several times a day, compliance is frequently poor. A single daily dose has increased in popularity for the treatment of many psychiatric conditions.

Recognition of unpleasant side effects is another important factor in reducing potential noncompliance. Patients who feel that their clinician is unresponsive to complaints about adverse affects frequently adjust their medication themselves. A clinician may not realize that a particular problem and the drug being administered are associated, though the patient firmly believes that they are. For example, in an illness as severe as schizophrenia, complaints about sexual dysfunction, which can be drug related, may not be taken seriously enough. Clinicians must remain particularly sensitive to the possibility of continued extrapyramidal side effects of antipsychotic drugs, which may be subtle. Side effects such as akinesia and akathisia may continue to be a problem, even during the maintenance phase of treatment; however, their presentation may be subtle and easily confused with aspects of psychopathology, residual deficit state, or demoralization.

The patient's own conception of the illness and the need for continued treatment are extremely important in any long-term prophylactic phase. Even in more common, less emotionally charged medical illnesses, patients who feel well tend to stop taking medication. The concept of prevention requires ongoing recognition and acceptance of the risk of becoming ill again, something that many persons would prefer to deny. Schizophrenic patients, in particular, often tend to attribute the acute illness to mild stresses or emotional concerns that they believe will not occur again, and they therefore conclude that ongoing preventive treatment is unnecessary. Although psychosocial stress and other factors may contribute to relapse in some situations, patients and their families must be made to understand the importance of maintenance medication in preventing psychotic relapse. Some patients are frightened because a biological factor in the etiology of the illness deprives them of an element of subjective control. It may be helpful to discuss these issues with patient and family.

Various psychodynamic factors are also potential causes of noncompliance, and it is useful to understand the psychological meanings that patients attach to different treatment modalities. The taking of medication can be a focus of family or interpersonal struggle. The patient who discontinues medication may do so to express anger toward a relative, a mental health professional, or himself or herself, or to express demoralization.

These potential factors should be appreciated in any treatment relationship; when noncompliance becomes apparent, the need to explore them is even more critical. It is unlikely that admonitions, lectures, or entreaties would be appropriate or effective without a full understanding of the context in which the noncompliance occurs. Clearly, at different stages of the illness, the impact of various issues may change. For example, a person who has had multiple psychotic episodes may have a very different attitude toward taking medication than one who has had a single episode.

The use of long-acting injectable medication is an important strategy for reducing noncompliance, though the effect has not always been easy to document in controlled research. Studies that attempted to compare relapse rates of patients receiving long-acting injectable drugs and those receiving oral medication in a double-blind random-assignment design have not necessarily demonstrated a statistically significant advantage for the long-acting injectable drug. Patients willing to cooperate in a study requiring, at least initially, a high degree of compliance are not likely to represent the patients prone to noncompliance. In addition, the potential advantage of long-acting injectable antipsychotics in preventing relapse may not be obvious unless patients are followed for periods over 1 year. Most of the studies in the literature attempting to assess this effect have lasted 1 year or less. A notable exception is the study by Hogarty's group, in which patients were followed for 24 months; there appears to be a clear suggestion for an advantage of the injectable medication in the second year of treatment, particularly in combination with social therapy. This author would argue that a long-term prospective study is necessary: The problem of compliance may increase with the duration of treatment with medication. Second, in stable or remitted schizophrenic patients, relapse may not occur for several months, even after complete discontinuation of medication. Therefore, an extended period of observation is necessary to assess fully the impact of guaranteed medication delivery.

The potential advantages of long-acting injectable medication also include the avoidance of more subtle degrees of noncompliance. Patients are unable to alter their dosage, and it becomes much easier to assess drug efficacy as well as adverse effects. In addition, parenteral administration overcomes individual differences in drug absorption to some extent because the drug avoids the first pass metabolic effect of the liver.

Dosage equivalency between long-acting injectable drugs and oral medication is not very well established; as a consequence, some clinicians have tended to prescribe higher than necessary doses of these preparations. It is also important to know the pharmacokinetic characteristics of these drugs. Preparations such as these, which have very long half-lives, may take 2 to 3 months to achieve the steady state; unless careful attention is given to titrating dosage over time, inappropriate levels of medication may be administered. When initiating long-acting injectable antipsychotic therapy, it is useful to start off with a low test dose and titrate upward, in order to assure that the patient can tolerate the medication. During this interval, it may be necessary to continue some degree of oral medication in order to provide a smooth transition from oral to long-acting injectable drugs.

INTERACTION OF SOMATIC TREATMENT WITH OTHER THERAPEUTIC MODALITIES

The treatment of schizophrenia requires a variety of different modalities which may be utilized to different degrees or in different combinations, depending on a variety of factors ranging from the level of psychopathology and stage of the illness to the patient's personality, psychosocial adaptation, and family environment. There is no general formula for utilizing and integrating different modalities; clinical judgment must be employed in each case.

It is critical that a true team approach be applied in treating schizophrenia, but unfortunately, this approach is frequently not in practice. Members of the team must understand what other clinicians and therapists are attempting to do. For example, if medication side effects are interfering with vocational rehabilitation efforts, the rehabilitation therapists must be in a position to recognize this and provide appropriate feedback to the prescribing physician. Certain types of environmental stress may necessitate dose adjustment, to prevent psychotic exacerbation; in fact, some forms of therapy may be too stressful at a given stage of the illness. In addition, the effect of one modality may be indirectly exerted through another, as when family therapy serves to enhance compliance with medication. By the same token, appropriate use of medication may enhance the patient's ability to participate in other forms of therapy, which will ultimately improve overall adjustment.

It should be kept in mind that the utilization of specific therapies in schizophrenia should be based on empirical data and not on intuitive assumptions or hypothetical constructs. The increasing emphasis on cost-benefit analyses of treatment delivery will eventually demand that psychiatrists be able to demonstrate the value of therapeutic interventions, and more clinicians should be involved in this process if they are to succeed in adequately studying treatment effects, particularly when various treatments combined or given serially raise the possibility of additive or interactive effects. In addition, it is essential to determine to what extent specific treatment effects persist once the treatment is discontinued and to what extent maintenance treatment is necessary to maintain therapeutic gains.

REFERENCES

Baldessarini R, Katz B, Cotton P: Dissimilar dosing with high potency and low potency neuroleptics. Amer J Psychiat *141:* 748, 1984.
Davis J M, Schaffer C B, Killian G A, Kinard C, Chan C: Important issues in the drug treatment of schizophrenia. Schizophr Bull *6:* 70, 1980.
Gelenberg A J: Treating extrapyramidal reactions: Some current issues. J Clin Psychiat *48* (9 suppl): 24, 1987.
Hogarty J E, Schooler N R, Ulrich R F, Mussare F, Ferro P, Herron E: Fluphenazine and social therapy in the aftercare of schizophrenic patients: Relapse analyses of a two year controlled study of fluphenazine decanoate and fluphenazine hydrochloride. Arch Gen Psychiat *36:* 1283, 1979.
Jeste D V, Wisniewski A W, Wyatt R J: Neuroleptic-associated tardive syndromes. Psychiat Clin N Amer *9:* 183, 1986.
Kane J M: *Drug Maintenance Strategies in Schizophrenia*. American Psychiatric Press, Washington, DC, 1984.
Kane J M, Woerner M, Borenstein M, Wegner J, Lieberman J: Integrating incidence and prevalence of tardive dyskinesia. Psychopharmacol Bull *22:* 254, 1986.
Kane J M: Treatment of schizophrenia. Schizophr Bull *13:* 133, 1987.
Kane J, Honigfeld G, Singer J, Meltzer H: Clozapine for the treatment-resistant schizophrenic: A double-blind comparison with chlorpromazine. Arch Gen Psychiat *45:* 789, 1988.
Marder S R, Van Putten T, Mintz J, Lebelle M, McKenzie J, May P R A: Low and conventional dose maintenance therapy with fluphenazine decanoate: A two-year outcome. Arch Gen Psychiat *44:* 518, 1987.
May P R A: *Treatment of Schizophrenia: A Comparative Study of Five Treatment Methods*. Science House, New York, 1968.
Pearlman C A: Neuroleptic malignant syndrome: A review of the literature. J Clin Psychopharmacol *6:* 257, 1986.
Richelson E: Neuroleptic affinities for human brain receptors and their use in predicting adverse effects. J Clin Psychiat *45:* 331, 1984.
Salzman C: The use of ECT in the treatment of schizophrenia. Amer J Psychiat *137:* 1032, 1980.
Siris S G, Morgan V, Fagerstrom R, Rifkin A, Cooper T B: Adjunctive imipramine in the treatment of postpsychotic depression. Arch Gen Psychiat *42:* 533, 1987.
Van Putten T: Why do schizophrenic patients refuse to take their drugs? Arch Gen Psychiat *31:* 67, 1974.
Van Putten T, May P R A, Marder S R: Responses to antipsychotic medication: The doctor's and consumer's view. Amer J Psychiat *141:* 16, 1984.
Weiden P J, Mann J J, Haas G, Mattson M, Frances A: Clinical nonrecognition of drug-induced movement disorders: A cautionary study. Amer J Psychiat *144:* 1148, 1987.

14.5
SCHIZOPHRENIA: PSYCHOSOCIAL TREATMENT

ROBERT PAUL LIBERMAN, M.D.
KIM T. MUESER, Ph.D.

INTRODUCTION

The treatment of schizophrenia can be guided by a multidimensional and interactional model. Symptoms and their associated social and personal disabilities are the result of stressors impinging on a person's enduring biobehavioral vulnerability. The noxious effects of these stressors are modulated by the person's social competence and the amount of available social support. The appearance or increase in characteristic schizophrenic symptoms and disabilities may be caused by changes in the environment, behavior, and biology of the person, for instance, as follows:

(1) The underlying biological diathesis or vulnerability increases or is physiologically stressed (e.g., by abuse of alcohol or street drugs);

(2) Stressful life events or daily levels of tension intervene that overwhelm the individual's coping in social and instrumental roles (e.g., overstimulating, critical, or overinvolved family relationships);

(3) The person's social and professional support network weakens or diminishes (e.g., family member dies, therapist terminates, patient leaves home);

(4) Social problem-solving skills, previously in the individual's repertoire, atrophy as a result of disuse, reinforcement of the sick role, or loss of motivation.

Thus, the symptomatic and social status of persons with a biological vulnerability for schizophrenia at any point in time is determined by the amount and type of life stressors and the person's problem-solving capacities and social support network. Too much environmental change, stress, or ambient tension or too little coping skill and social support can lead to breakdown and exacerbation.

The significance of this bidirectional model of symptom formation lies in its emphasis of the active role of the patient's coping skills and support system, both of which directly suggest targeted objectives and modalities for therapeutic intervention. The clinician can prescribe antipsychotic drugs to protect against the underlying biological diathesis. Environmental modification can be employed to lessen the negative effects of stressors. In such instances, hospitalization can be beneficial in temporarily removing the patient from stressors in family and community. Alternatively, treatment can emphasize strengthening the patient's social support network, as is the case in family and group therapies and self-help clubs. Finally, increasing the patient's resilience through training in social and problem-solving skills can also reduce the likelihood of relapse.

Psychosocial interventions must serve as a major component of treatment and rehabilitation plans for schizophrenics, if optimal outcomes are to accrue. Antipsychotic drug therapy reduces the risk of relapse, which, however, remains unacceptably high; for example, recent research has shown that even with reliable administration of antipsychotics, upward of 35 to 40 percent of schizophrenic patients still relapse within a year. The side effects of antipsychotics reduce compliance even in patients responsive to the beneficial effects of the drugs. Most importantly, drugs cannot teach life and coping skills, nor can they improve the quality of a person's life, except indirectly through suppression of symptoms. Most schizophrenic patients need to learn or relearn social and personal skills for surviving in the community.

Empirically based guidelines point to potentially constructive approaches to the psychosocial treatment of schizophrenia. Studies carried out in England, the United States, and elsewhere have found *expressed emotion*—criticism and emotional overinvolvement by family members of schizophrenic patients—to be the most powerful predictor of relapse in the 9 months following discharge from an inpatient treatment setting. These findings suggest that family therapy may reduce the level of family tension, social skills training may improve the patient's ability to cope with family problems, and psychosocial rehabilitation and group therapy may enlist support from persons other than family in the patient's natural environment.

To justify further an investment in social rehabilitation, evidence abounds that social inadequacy correlates with poor symptomatic and behavioral outcome and with rehospitalization. Schizophrenic persons appear to be markedly deficient in interpersonal problem solving, especially in the ability to generate alternative ways of responding to situational challenges. Deficits in social skills may include misperception of relevant social cues; poor cognitive processing of these cues, leading to inadequate generation of response alternatives; and sending back inappropriate behavioral responses to others in the situation. Deficits in social problem solving may partly reflect core attentional and psychophysiological impairments in schizophrenia.

TAXONOMY OF PSYCHOSOCIAL INTERVENTIONS

Psychosocial interventions can be organized according to their focus, locus, and modus, as well as to their goals and objectives (Fig. 14.5-1). The focus can be on the individual as in one-on-one therapy, in groups, in families, or in a total milieu. The locus of therapeutic and rehabilitative efforts can be the hospital, private office, clinic, mental health center, natural home, board and care home, or social club. The modus, or modality, of intervention can derive from one or more explicit or implicit orientations, such as behavioral, psychodynamic, systems-strategic, and ego-supportive. It is recognized that there may be considerable overlap among modalities; for example, a particular therapist may utilize both behavioral and psychodynamic principles and methods. In addition, much of the therapeutic impact of any psychiatric or medical treatment derives from so-called nonspecific and placebo effects that are inherent in any therapy that is offered in a credible, hopeful, and positive manner. Focus, locus, and modus of treatment may change over time as the specific problems and needs of the patient and available resources change. Also, at any point in time, multiple foci, loci, and modalities may be harnessed to implement a comprehensive rehabilitation plan.

A wide spectrum of goals can further subdivide psychosocial efforts into those that aim primarily to maintain a person at a marginal level of functioning with minimal stress and relapses; those that provide crisis intervention when needed; and those that attempt to build social and independent living skills. Thus, the process of designing, employing, and evaluating psychosocial interventions requires reference to a matrix with at least four mutually exclusive domains of attributes; for example, family therapy may be provided in the home, with a behavioral orientation that aims to improve the problem-solving and communication skills of the patient and relatives. Figure 14.5-1 shows the matrix containing the four essential dimensions for describing psychosocial interventions. Because most psychosocial rehabilitation programs take place in full-day or 24-hour residential settings, they will be described under milieu therapy.

EXPLORATORY AND INSIGHT-ORIENTED THERAPY The clinical efficacy of exploratory, insight-oriented (EIO) therapy for schizophrenia has been debated since soon after the development of psychoanalysis in the early twentieth century. Recent research on psychoanalytic psychotherapy for schizophrenia-spectrum disorders has overcome past methodological weaknesses by providing treatment by experienced clinicians over extended periods of time and by utilizing objective diagnostic criteria and standard outcome measures of symptoms, occupational and social functioning, and recidivism. The results of these studies uniformly demonstrate that insight-based therapies, at best, confer little benefit to either good-prognosis or chronic schizophrenic patients and may worsen the course of the illness and adaptive functioning of some schizophrenic patients.

In a well-controlled collaborative study conducted in the Boston area, 164 schizophrenic patients were randomly assigned to one of two outpatient treatments: EIO psychotherapy or reality-adaptive, supportive (RAS) therapy for 2 years. In order to select patients who might benefit most from therapy, very chronic schizophrenic patients were excluded from the study; more than half of the treated patients

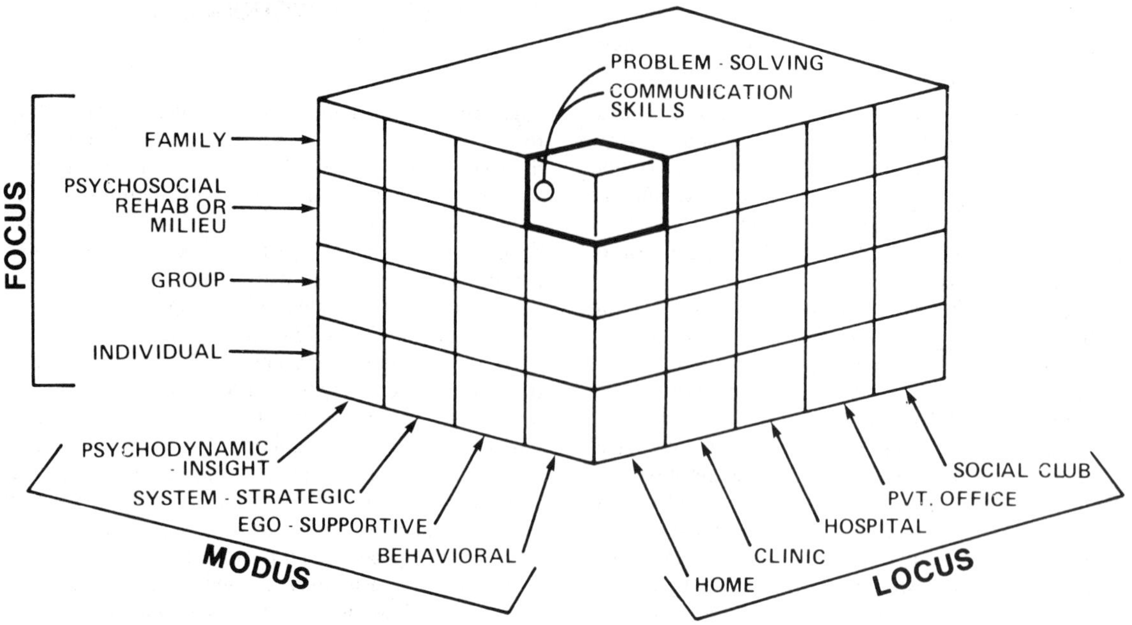

FIGURE 14.5-1 *Matrix of attributes of psychosocial therapies for schizophrenia. In the treatment of any particular patient, multiple modalities, foci, and loci are desirably combined in a comprehensive approach.*

had no prior psychiatric admissions. Despite the fact that patients in the EIO therapy received more treatment sessions than those in the RAS therapy (2.14 versus 0.63 sessions per week), the two groups did not differ in most of the outcome measures. Where group differences were present, they favored the more economical RAS therapy. Over the 2-year treatment period, patients in the RAS therapy spent less time in the hospital, more time fully employed, and assumed more major household responsibilities than patients in EIO therapy. In addition, at McLean Hospital, where the majority of patients were treated, the amount of time spent in EIO therapy was consistently associated with a negative outcome on days hospitalized, employment, occupational level achieved, household responsibilities, and significant relationships, whereas the RAS therapy was not.

Prolonged psychoanalytic treatment for schizophrenic inpatients in carefully crafted residential milieus has not yielded any more encouraging results than outpatient treatment. Of 72 schizophrenic patients treated for an average of 12.3 months of intensive psychoanalytic therapy at New York State Psychiatric Institute, more than half remained substantially dysfunctional, and 20 percent had committed suicide when followed up 10 to 20 years later. Similarly, schizophrenic patients treated at Chestnut Lodge, a long-term private residential facility that specializes in intensive psychoanalytic treatment, showed little improvement with long-term psychodynamic therapy. Of 163 schizophrenic patients treated at the Lodge for an average of over 3 years, two-thirds were functioning marginally or worse 15 years later. Thus, insight-oriented psychoanalytic therapies do not have an empirically supported role in the residential, inpatient, or outpatient treatment of schizophrenia. However, future research may address whether subpopulations of schizophrenic patients, such as those with verbal insight into their illness, capacity to form meaningful interpersonal relationships, or good ego functioning, can benefit from exploratory, psychodynamic therapy.

FAMILY THERAPY With replications in England, the United States, and India of the finding that critical or emotionally overinvolved attitudes and feelings of relatives (expressed emotion) are among the most powerful predictors of relapse in schizophrenia, several modes of family therapy have been designed and empirically tested for their ability to change the emotional climate of the family and to reduce the incidence of such relapses. These new approaches to family therapy have a distinctively different rationale from those of clinical studies in the 1950s and 1960s that implicated family structure, communication, and relationships in the etiology of schizophrenia. In fact, as part of the initial contacts with the family group, the newer family therapies pronounce a loud disavowal of any etiological link between family relations and the development of schizophrenia. Instead, the vulnerability-stress conceptualization of schizophrenia is invoked to explain how the stress of an already established major mental illness can place burdens on patient and relatives alike, thereby raising tension levels in the family that, given the fragile coping capacity of the index patient, can lead to relapse.

The genesis of these new modes of family therapy came from studies carried out 2 decades ago and more. Those studies demonstrated the efficacy and cost-effectiveness of providing supportive family interventions in the home over the more traditional hospital-based treatment for acutely and chronically ill patients with major mental disorders. The new family therapies are offered in a variety of locales—home, clinic, hospital, storefront, private office—and with different theoretical and operational modes. Most have in common an emphasis on educating the patient and family members about the nature of schizophrenia and available treatments.

Time is spent demystifying the various symptoms, signs, and prognoses associated with the disorder and translating the neurobiological underpinnings into lay terminology. The role of antipsychotic drugs in the treatment and prophylaxis of schizophrenia is highlighted, and an effort is made to improve adherence to the pharmacotherapeutic regimen. Some therapists prefer to meet with the relatives alone for initial sessions and to invite the patient to join in later, when acute symptoms have been controlled and the attention span has increased. Therapists provide educational and other interventions with individual families, in multiple family groups, and during day-long or evening survival skills workshops. In addition to family sessions, antipsychotic drugs are uniformly prescribed to the patient. Both low-dose and intermittent-dose strategies have been used in attempts to reduce overall exposure to the side effects of antipsychotics while still retaining their protective effects.

Modes of family therapy The modes of family therapy run along a continuum from those using systems-strategic methods to those that are supportive or behavioral. Many of the systems-strategic therapists employ paradoxical interventions, which are primarily helpful in the initial stages of engaging patient and relatives in a therapeutic relationship through evocative demonstrations of the capacity of the family to change its rules and reactions despite considerable inertia and resistance. Most modalities have been shown to produce highly significant reductions in relapse rates, whether measured by statistical or clinical yardsticks. In families where relatives are high on expressed emotion, the base rate of relapse in index patients receiving standard aftercare during the first year following discharge from hospital can be expected to fall in the 50- to 60-percent range. Supportive and behavioral therapies that employ educational and skill-building methods have reduced relapse rates to 6 to 19 percent, even with less use of antipsychotic drugs. The remarkable efficacy of family therapy is currently undergoing several systematic replications, but the results promise an innovation in the treatment of schizophrenia that may be as significant as the advent of the antipsychotic drugs.

BEHAVIORAL FAMILY THERAPY The new family therapies for schizophrenia were born from naturalistic studies that teased out family factors predictive of outcome and that matured through empirical validation in controlled clinical trials. Among these new approaches, behavioral family therapy was the first to be subjected to a rigorous clinical trial, so its methods and results will be described further.

Thirty-six young adult schizophrenic patients were randomly assigned either to in-home family therapy or to clinic-based individual supportive therapy, with treatment visits scheduled weekly for the first 3 months, biweekly for the next 6 months, and monthly thereafter for a period of 2 years. The patients were considered to be at high risk of relapse because they lived with relatives who had high expressed emotion, they had markedly poor premorbid social adjustment, and they had a history of multiple psychiatric admissions during the previous 2 years. Before entering the study, all patients had attained a stable baseline of symptoms and had complied with antipsychotic drug therapy for 1 month.

The same team of therapists—psychiatrist, psychologist, social worker, and nurse—treated both groups of patients and provided comprehensive case management. In addition, all patients were seen in a clinic each month by a psychiatrist or clinical pharmacist; both of these clinicians were blind to patients' therapy assignments. The pharmacotherapists prescribed optimal doses of antipsychotics and carried out blind ratings of psychopathology. Patients who did not comply with oral medication were switched to long-acting depot drugs. The patient sample included twice as many men as women, as well as a large number of blacks, Hispanics, and Asians.

The family therapy was designed to train patients and their parents to reduce environmental stress. The first two sessions were devoted to educating the patient and family about the nature, course, and treatment of schizophrenia. Schizophrenia was presented as a major mental illness with both biological and psychosocial components. The notion that families somehow cause schizophrenic illness was refuted, but it was pointed out that families can play an important part in improving the course of the illness. Considerable attention was given to discussing the rationale for maintenance of antipsychotic medication.

Subsequent family sessions were devoted to reducing existing family tensions and improving the problem-solving skills of the family in coping with causes of stress. The strengths and weaknesses of the family group were pinpointed, and major deficits became the focus of subsequent sessions. Specifically, behavioral rehearsal, modeling, feedback, and social reinforcement were used to enhance skills in the expression of positive and negative feelings, active listening, requests for behavioral change, and reciprocity of conversation.

Each family was taught a structured problem-solving method, which was utilized in weekly family meetings at home whenever a problem arose. This technique encouraged the entire family to discuss and specify the exact nature of the problem, to list and consider alternative solutions, and to reach a consensus on the best solution and implement it. In most families, the therapist merely assisted the family in their structured problem-solving efforts, but if patients had persisting symptoms of schizophrenia or if major discord was observed, additional specific strategies were employed. These strategies included methods to improve medication compliance, to cope with persistent symptoms, to improve marital relationships, to deal with unacceptable behavior, and to expand the social contacts of any family member (Table 14.5-1).

The comparison treatment was clinic-based, individual, supportive psychotherapy that was comparable to the best available at well-staffed community aftercare clinics. In addition to receiving maintenance pharmacotherapy and rehabilitation counseling, individually treated patients were educated about the nature, course, and treatment of schizophrenia and were assisted in their efforts to cope with problems of daily living. Although the issues addressed in treatment were similar to those that arose in the family-treated group, the problems were dealt with primarily from the patient's perspective.

The results of this test of behavioral family therapy are depicted in Table 14.5-2. Not only were therapeutic effects on relapse, rehospitalization, and psychotic symptoms significantly better, but this mode of family therapy also was associated with substantial cost benefits, upgrading of social and work adjustment, and reductions of family burden. Consistent with the goals of the therapy for improving family problem solving, patients and their relatives who received behavioral family therapy substantially increased their problem-solving ability after 3 months of treatment, whereas the other families did not. Other studies of family therapy have found improved outcomes to be correlated with reductions in expressed emotion. Further research is necessary to determine which elements in a combined program of pharmacotherapy plus family therapy can be linked to which desirable outcomes. For example, it may be found that educational and supportive efforts

TABLE 14.5-1
Component Interventions Comprising Behavioral Family Management

Behavioral analysis of all members of the family
Defining individual and familywide problems
Setting goals for each individual and family system
Identifying reinforcers
Pinpointing assets and resources within individuals, family, and community
Education of all family members on nature of schizophrenia and currently available treatment and rehabilitation modalities
Training in communication skills
Expressing positive feelings to others and acknowledging when others do or say something positive toward you
Active, reflective listening
Making positive requests and asking for what you want
Expressing negative feelings in constructive ways
Training in problem-solving skills
Be specific and objective in describing the problem
Express how you feel directly and subjectively about the problem
Listen to each other actively and reflectively as the problem is described and feelings are expressed
Help each other generate alternatives and options in dealing with the problem
Weigh the potential consequences or outcomes (risks and benefits, pros and cons) of each alternative
Choose a reasonable alternative
Decide how to implement the alternative
Behavioral interventions for specific problems
Contingency management for negative symptoms
Job-finding skills training
Friendship skills training
Independent living skills training

can yield marked reductions in relapse rate but that only specific and structured efforts at skill building can produce meaningful and durable improvements in social and vocational competence and quality of life.

GROUP THERAPY Group psychotherapy evolved from individual psychotherapy, so there are as many schools of group psychotherapy as there are of individual therapy. Group therapy, like family therapy, can be characterized by its theoretical and operational qualities and procedures. There are highly structured activity and behavioral groups, unstructured and spontaneous psychodynamic and insight-oriented groups, and supportive groups. The locus for most group therapy is the hospital, clinic, or private office, although multiple family groups have met in homes and storefronts, and groups emphasizing peer support and normalization often meet in community centers, schools, and churches.

The goals of therapy groups overlap considerably. Varying degrees of emphasis are placed on insight, behavior change, and skill development; social support and maintenance; and participation in recreational activities. What cuts across most modalities is the group leader's use of the naturally developing interactional dynamics in groups, such as cohesion, to strengthen the group process and to improve the outcomes. A large body of evidence collected from groups serving a spectrum of patient populations suggests that cohesion has a generically favorable impact on group therapy, an impact that is similar to the positive transference or therapeutic alliance between patient and therapist in individual therapy.

Traditional group psychotherapy is provided in the context of a relatively unstructured and spontaneously unfolding group process. The group therapist is much more responsive and reactive than directive. Other characteristics of traditional group therapy include regularly scheduled meeting times, a closed membership, and only occasional replacement of patients who drop out or terminate.

With the change in the treatment zeitgeist toward brief inpatient hospitalizations for schizophrenic patients followed by continuing care in the community, almost all group psychotherapy takes place in the aftercare period. Exploratory and psychodynamic group therapy during the inpatient period may worsen the clinical state of patients who are still floridly psychotic and thus vulnerable to overstimulation and hyperarousal from the treatment environment. Group therapy is likely to be more beneficial when offered after the positive symptoms of schizophrenia have been controlled, and if it focuses on practical problems of daily living experienced by patients trying to adjust to the community. Most outpatient groups aim at supporting a patient's stabilization and community tenure, assisting the patient in coping with stressful life events, and facilitating efforts at longer-term rehabilitation.

Groups led in a supportive manner, rather than an interpretive one, appear to be more helpful for schizophrenic patients. For example, in a collaborative study involving a number of Veterans Administration day treatment centers, it was found that those centers employing more practical types of therapy groups, led by lower-level professionals and paraprofessionals who focused on problems of daily living, had significantly better outcomes with schizophrenic patients than centers using more insight-oriented approaches. Group psychotherapy has been found to be more effective than individual therapy for schizophrenic patients when the group goals aim to improve occupational and social functioning. This result might be expected, because the group provides incidental learning experiences in socializing, provides more peer models for successful coping in daily life, and protects the schizophrenic patient from overstimulating transference relationships.

Behavioral methods A variety of behavioral methods have been used in conventional group therapy settings in which there is little or no interference by the leader in the spontaneous group interaction. Verbal prompting and reinforcement have been used to increase sociability in schizophrenic inpatients; for example, whenever desired personal and group-centered references were expressed by patients, the therapist rewarded them by giving verbal approval. Silences were effectively eliminated in a therapy group of chronic schizophrenic patients by surreptitiously introducing a noxious noise whenever the group fell silent for more than 10 seconds. The noise was turned off as soon as a group member broke the silence; thus, the group avoided the aversive stimulus by increasing their talk. Frequent prompting and reinforcement of group interaction as well as active verbal participation by the group leader have also yielded more productive group therapy or therapeutic community meetings.

Token reinforcement was used to increase social interaction among four chronic schizophrenic women, each of whom had been hospitalized for over 15 years. Reliable, quantitative records were made of their social conversation during 50-minute meetings, in an A-B-A-B intensive design. During the baseline period, conversational interchanges occurred at an average rate of one per minute. Contingent reinforcement for conversation among themselves was introduced using tokens, which could be exchanged for candy, cake, cigarettes, and jewelry. The tokens were distributed at the end of each session. A noncontingent reinforcement phase was introduced next, in which the patients received their tokens before the session. This procedure was followed to assess the causal influence of the contingent use of tokens. In a final phase, reinforcement was again contingent on social conversation. Using the same design, another series of sessions was run in which the patients played a table game that stimulated conversation.

Contingent token reinforcement increased participation in spontaneous, open-ended conversation to 10 times that of baseline and noncontingent reinforcement phases. Although the game situation alone produced a high baseline rate of conversation, introduction of contingent reinforcement doubled the conversation rate evoked by the game. Using the same methods, similar results have been found with a group of four delusional schizophrenic patients, who showed

TABLE 14.5-2
Comparison in Outcomes Between Behavioral Family Therapy and Individual Therapy for Schizophrenia with N = 18 in Each Group

Outcome Dimension	*Family Therapy*	*Individual Therapy*	*Probability of Statistical Significance of Behavioral Therapy*
Clinical exacerbations			
9 mo	1	8	$p<.01$
24 mo	2	15	$p<.005$
Target psychotic symptoms pretreatment	2.22	2.15	
9 mo	2.25	4.10	$p<.005$
24 mo	2.55	4.75	$p<.005$
Symptom remission			
9 mo	10	4	$p<.05$
24 mo	12	4	$p<.01$
Community tenure–24 mo mean no. hospital days/yr	1.8	11.3	
No. patients readmitted–24 mo	4	10	$p<.05$
Total no. readmissions–24 mo	5	22	
Social adjustment reported by patients			
Overall adjustment	Family therapy better than individual therapy		$p<.05$
Leisure activities	Family therapy better than individual therapy		$p<.01$
Family life	Family therapy better than individual therapy		$p<.05$
Social adjustment reported by relatives			
Self-neglect	Family therapy better than individual therapy		$p<.05$
Behavioral disturbances	Family therapy better than individual therapy		$p<.05$
Household tasks	Family therapy better than individual therapy		$p<.05$
Friendships outside family	Family therapy better than individual therapy		$p<.01$
Work or study	Family therapy better than individual therapy		$p<.005$
Average time working over 2 yr	12.6 mo	7.2 mo	
Family burden			
pretreatment	70%	56%	
9 mo	17%	61%	$p<.05$
24 mo	6%	41%	$p<.01$
Cost per unit of effectiveness	$2,220	$5,167	$p<.05$

Table from Falloon I R H, Boyd J L, McGill C W, Razani J, Moss H B, Gilderman A M: Family management in the prevention of exacerbations of schizophrenia. New Eng J Med *306:* 1437, 1982; Falloon I R H, Boyd J L, McGill C W, Williamson M, Pederson J, Cardin V A, Razani J, Moss H B, Gilderman A M, Simpson G M: Family versus individual management in the prevention of morbidity of schizophrenia. Arch Gen Psychiat *42:* 887, 1985; with permission.

dramatic increases in their rational speech when it was contingently reinforced with tokens during group therapy.

While controlled research studies have shown that insight-oriented group therapy is not efficacious for schizophrenic patients, the beneficial effects of more socially interactive groups on outcome criteria, such as symptomatology, rehospitalization, vocational or social adjustment, remain to be established. The consensus of clinicians, buttressed by controlled studies, is that group therapy is more effective during the aftercare, outpatient phase of treatment than during inpatient treatment. Group therapy formats have been adapted broadly for providing such services as medication evaluations, occupational and recreational therapy, patient and family education, patient government, self-help, and mutual support.

Social skills training The most highly structured form of group therapy for schizophrenic patients is social skills training. The goals are explicit, the session agendas are usually planned in advance, the procedures follow written guidelines often derived from a manual, and practice and homework assignments are emphasized. Social skills can be defined as those interpersonal behaviors required to attain instrumental goals necessary for community survival and independence, and to establish, maintain, and deepen supportive and socially rewarding relationships. Schizophrenia disrupts one or more of the affective, cognitive, verbal, and behavioral domains of functioning and thereby impairs a person's potential for enjoying and sustaining interpersonal relationships, which are the essence of the social quality of life. Recurring schizophrenic disorders pose enduring social disruptions for affected persons. These disorders involve symptoms that adversely affect the schizophrenic patients' social quality of life and also evoke impairments that hamper learning or relearning adaptive social behaviors. Applying behavior analysis principles to identify and to remedy deficits in social behaviors, clinicians have developed treatment packages, termed "social skills training," that have proved effective with schizophrenic patients.

SOCIAL SKILLS TRAINING METHODS In virtually all published reports of social skills training, role playing is the vehicle used both to assess patients' pretreatment social competence and to correct targeted behavioral excesses or deficits during treatment. Training scenes are selected either on the basis of the individual's past difficulties or from problem situations that have been found to apply to most of the psychiatric population to which the patient belongs. Training sessions vary in length from 15 to 120 minutes, depending on the number of patients participating and on their level of functioning. Although the group format provides vicarious learning opportunities through observation of other patients' behavior and from amplified reinforcement from peers, the group experience is sometimes supplemented by individual training, which allows more intensive focus on a single patient's behavior and provides an opportunity for more practice within sessions.

Participants in the role playing include the target patient or patients, the respondent, and the trainer or therapist. In most reports, focused instructions, modeling, feedback, and social reinforcement are applied as a package to remediate deficits in social behavior. Modeling and feedback are accomplished in vivo or through videotape playback. Target behaviors selected for change usually include both process behaviors (e.g., eye contact, voice loudness or intonation, response latency, smiles, and other affective behaviors) and content behaviors (e.g., requests for change, highlighting the importance of a need, empathic responses, compliance, hostile comments, and irrelevant remarks). The *sine qua non* of social skills training is the specific, functional, and goal-oriented nature of the behaviors that are targeted for change.

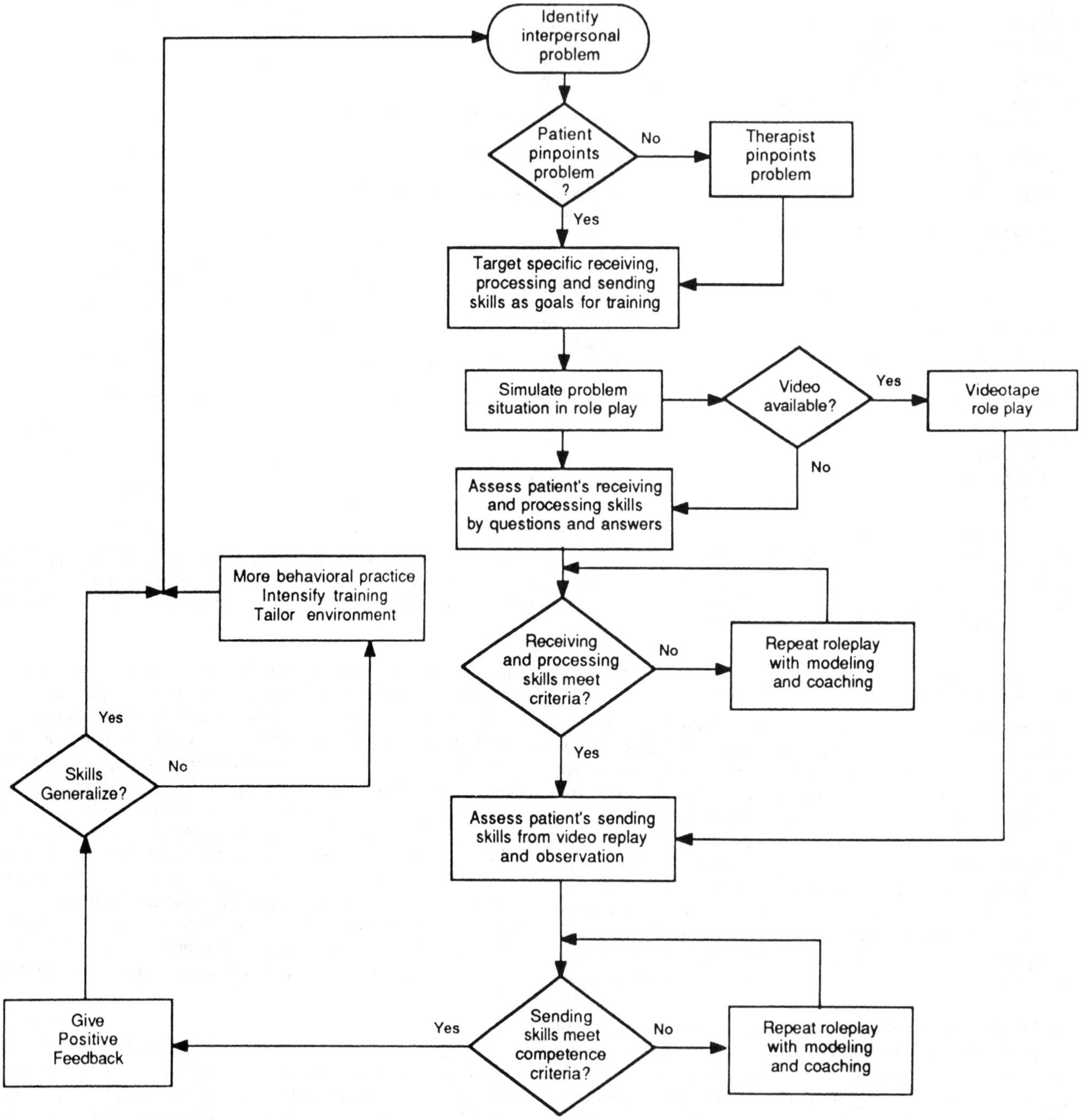

FIGURE 14.5-2 *Flow chart for conducting social skills training. Social skills training can be conducted individually or in groups. Problems and goals are selected in recurring fashion, from session to session, with less complex and challenging skills usually preceding more difficult ones.*

The sequence of a social skills training session is outlined in Figure 14.5-2, and the active and directive role of the therapist in coaching a patient to improve social skills is shown in Figure 14.5-3. A recent innovation in social skills training has been the packaging of a group of functionally related skills into a training module. Modules have been developed for medication management, symptom self-management, personal hygiene and grooming, social problem solving, and leisure and recreational skills. The module consists of a patient's workbook, a trainer's manual, and a demonstration videocassette that provides adaptive models for the patients in the skills-training group to learn from. Each module contains a set of sequential exercises designed to teach patients the skills that constitute the module, train them to solve problems they might encounter when using the skills, and have them practice the skills in both the training sessions and the real world. The eight learning activities that comprise a module are depicted in Figure 14.5-4. Empirical evaluations of the modules, including nationwide field testing in typical mental health facilities, have documented the ability of schizophrenic patients to learn the skills, and reasonable durability and generalization are demonstrated at 6-month follow-ups.

Social-skills training techniques have been effectively utilized in teaching patients how to solicit job leads, contact

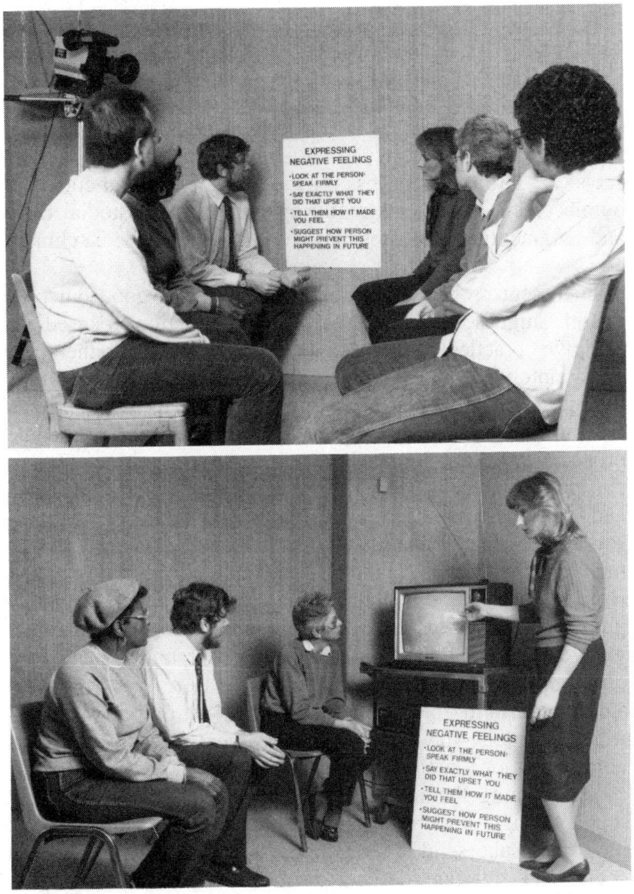

FIGURE 14.5-3 *Scenes of a social skills training group in progress. The top photo shows a trainer instructing the group members in the behavioral elements comprising the communication skill, "expressing negative feelings." The bottom photo shows video feedback of a previously rehearsed interpersonal situation being annotated.*

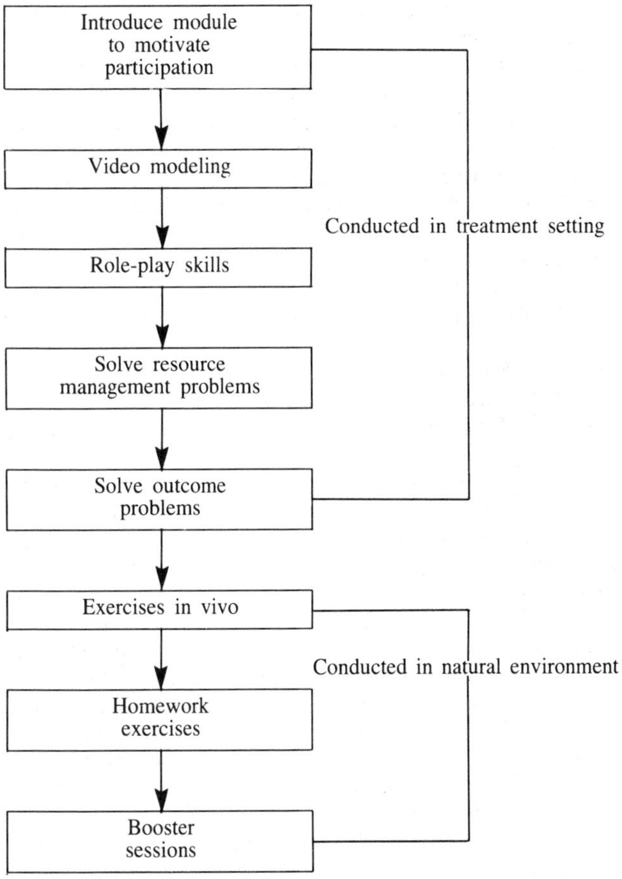

FIGURE 14.5-4 *Constituent learning activities in a social skills training module. Each skill area related to independent living is sequentially taught through behavioral learning techniques that are active and directive in nature and that employ a general problem-solving strategy.*

employers, and pass through job interviews. One program, now widely disseminated, provides job finding skills training in a supportive context of daily goal setting and reinforcement to sustain the arduous job search. One-third of schizophrenic patients referred to the Job Finding Club find full-time employment after an average of 4 weeks of training and effort.

The content of training is as important as the teaching methods used in social skills training. It is of little use to train persons to cope with situations that they are unlikely to encounter in their natural environments. Systematic history taking with patients and relatives, behavioral observation of high-probability and difficult situations, and self-report assessment instruments are methods used to identify individualized training goals.

RESEARCH FINDINGS Approximately 40 published studies have appeared on social skills training with schizophrenic patients during the past decade. Many of the studies used single-case experimental designs, which inherently limit the generality of the findings. Some of the published group-design studies are also limited in external validity, because they failed to adequately define the patient population and control for medication effects; however, there is convergence across studies with respect to several findings. First, schizophrenic patients in a treatment setting can be trained to improve social skills in specific situations. Second, moderate generalization of acquired skills to similar situations can be expected from the training. There is clear evidence that, given the favorable learning environment structured by behavioral principles, most schizophrenic patients can acquire or relearn social and conversational skills. Learning, however, occurs tediously or hardly at all when patients are still floridly ill, with positive symptoms and high distractibility. Third, participants in the training consistently report decreases in social anxiety after training. Finally, follow-up evaluations tend to indicate that durability of acquired social skills depends on the duration of training; that is, overlearning that stems from repeated practice promotes retention but is unlikely to occur during brief training (less than 2 to 3 months of twice-weekly sessions).

There are also findings that limit the applicability of social skills training. Generalization of complex conversational skills is less likely than that of briefer, more discrete verbal and nonverbal responses. Because complex behaviors are more critical for generating social support in the community, methods have been developed to improve the learning and durability of conversational skills; these training methods focus on problem-solving and perceptual and information-processing skills. Another challenge to the broad use of social skills training is the limited evidence that generalization of skills occurs in the natural environment of persistently psychotic patients in the absence of prompting and planned supportive reinforcement.

One example of the efficacy of social skills training comes from a study comparing skills training with psychoeducational family therapy for schizophrenic patients. All patients lived with high expressed emotion relatives and were therefore at increased risk for relapse. Following hospital admission, 103 schizophrenic or schizoaffective patients were randomly assigned to one of four treatment groups for a 2-year period: social skills training and medication, family therapy and medication, social skills training, family therapy, and medication, or medication alone. Patients in the social skills group were seen weekly during the first year and received training to improve social behavior and the accuracy of their social perception. Family sessions addressed social skills with family members and later progressed to other relationships outside the home in social, rehabilitative, or vocational settings. Table 14.5-3 contains the phases of social skills treatment, goals, and behaviors that were assessed and targeted for modification.

The relapse rates at 1 year showed a definite benefit for both social skills training and psychoeducational family therapy: 20 percent of the patients in the social skills group relapsed, 19 percent of the family therapy group relapsed, no patients with the combined treatments relapsed, and 41 percent of medication control treatment patients relapsed. This study demonstrated the utility of skills training with schizophrenic patients, and indicated that it had separate and additive effects to family therapy and medication in the prophylaxis of relapse.

MILIEU THERAPY The locus for milieu therapy is a living, learning, or working environment. Examples include the inpatient psychiatric unit, day hospitals, psychosocial rehabilitation clubs, board-and-care homes, community-based residential alternatives to hospitals, and sheltered workshops. The defining characteristics of treatment and rehabilitation milieus are the use of a team to provide treatment and the large amount of time spent by the patient in the environment. Recent adaptations of milieu therapy have included 24-hour per day programs that are situated in the community locales frequented by patients and that provide support, case management, and training in living skills.

Milieu therapy or the therapeutic community may be based on any of a number of modalities ranging from structured behavior therapy to spontaneous, humanistically oriented approaches. Most programs encompass the following attributes: emphasis on group and social interaction; rules and expectations that are mediated by peer pressure for normalization of adaptation; blurring of the patient role by viewing patients as responsible human beings; emphasis on patients' rights for involvement in setting goals, for freedom of movement, and for informality of relationships with staff; and emphasis on interdisciplinary participation and goal-oriented, clear communication.

A body of data has emerged that describes the elements of effective therapeutic milieus for schizophrenic patients and other severely impaired populations. These elements can be divided into those related to milieu structure and those related to treatment procedures. Structural elements associated with favorable outcomes include small size and census; high staff-to-patient ratios and staff stability; heterogeneity of patient population, with an optimal mix of two-thirds higher-functioning, acutely ill patients and one-third lower-functioning, chronic patients; and clarity and consistency in status and roles among staff. Other program elements that appear to be related to successful treatment are active participation by patients and nursing staff; administrative commitment to short stays (i.e., 3 months or less for the average hospital episode); outplacement of patients requiring long-term, custodial care; and segmenting the hospital for geographical catchment areas.

Treatment process variables correlated with good outcome include high levels of staff-patient interaction focused on adaptive, practical aspects of everyday behavior, rather than on symptomatic and psychodynamic issues. Treatment units that set clearly defined and time-limited goals with patients are more effective, as are units that organize and schedule prosocial activities for most waking hours. A variety of psychosocial treatment models have been developed and tested and are considered more effective than standard or comparison approaches. These models include the community lodge, the Training in Community Living Program, the Fountain House social club, and the social learning–token economy program. Each of these model programs has focused on somewhat different patient populations, in different loci, and with different modalities.

Social learning–token economy For chronic, treatment-refractory, long-stay psychotics who have resisted all efforts at deinstitutionalization, the psychosocial strategy of choice is social learning therapy. Utilizing behavioral assessment and therapy, highly trained paraprofessionals and nursing staff have been successful in remediating the bizarre symptoms and social and self-care deficits of most chronic schizophrenic patients. Combining elegant experimental designs with rigorous pursuit of relevant clinical goals, Gordon Paul and his colleagues compared the social learning approach with therapeutic community methods and customary custodial care.

Over 100 severely debilitated and chronically institutionalized patients were treated by paraprofessionals backed by psy-

TABLE 14.5-3
Goals and Targeted Behaviors for Social Skills Training

Phase	*Goals*	*Target Behaviors*
Stabilization and assessment	Establish therapeutic alliance Assess social performance and perception skills Assess behaviors that provoke expressed emotion	Empathy and rapport Verbal and nonverbal communication
Social performance within family	Express positive feelings within family Teach effective strategies for coping with conflict	Compliments, appreciation, interest in others Avoidance response to criticism, stating preferences and refusals
Social perception in the family	Correctly identify content, context, and meaning of messages	Reading a message Labeling an idea Summarizing other's intent
Extrafamilial relationships	Enhance socialization skills Enhance prevocational and vocational skills	Conversational skills Dating Recreational activities Job interviewing, work habits
Maintenance	Generalize skills to new situations	

Table adapted from Hogarty G E, Anderson C M, Reiss D J, Kornblith S J, Greenwald D P, Javna C D, Madonia M J: Family psychoeducation, social skills training and maintenance chemotherapy: I. One-year effects of a controlled study on relapse and expressed emotion. Arch Gen Psychiat *43:* 633, 1986.

chology graduate students. Staff-patient ratios were similar to those used in custodial institutions. The social learning program employed a highly specific token economy with many hours of structured educational activities throughout the day and evening. The therapeutic community followed principles of peer pressure and democratic decision making. Both programs were offered on 28-bed units in a regional psychiatric hospital; the paraprofessional staff rotated between the units to control for the potentially confounding effects of the personalities of the therapists. Most of the patients received inpatient care for at least 1 year and then obtained aftercare for 6 months after discharge into the community.

A multimodal assessment battery, including reliable time-sampled behavioral observations, revealed impressive and clear-cut results favoring the social learning approach. Improved functioning, enabling long-term community tenure, occurred in 97 percent of the social learning patients. The therapeutic community program was less effective, but its 71 percent release and community maintenance rate was still a favorable outcome when compared with the 45-percent rate of patients released from custodial care and living in the community for 18 months or longer.

The outstanding success in sustaining patients in the community was mirrored by the significant clinical and behavioral improvements, which even produced a minority of patients who, by direct observational ratings, could not be distinguished from a normal population. After only 14 weeks of treatment, every resident in the social learning program showed dramatic improvements in overall functioning, regardless of usual prognostic indicators, such as duration of hospitalization and pretreatment level of regression. By the end of the second year of programming, fewer than 25 percent of residents in either experimental program were on maintenance psychotropic drugs. Figure 14.5-5 demonstrates the superiority of the social learning–token economy treatment over a therapeutic community or traditional hospital treatments for chronic schizophrenia. Two clinically significant conclusions reached by the study were (1) that few, older chronic mental patients, when provided active and structured psychosocial therapies, have need for maintenance antipsychotic drugs and (2) that it is not how much attention and enthusiasm are offered to patients by staff, but how that attention is given that makes a difference. Patients in the therapeutic community program received more overall attention but improved less than their counterparts in the social learning program.

Social learning principles have been extended into the community, where loci of treatment include day hospitals. One such program, associated with a Veterans Administration hospital, offered structured and scheduled classes in which social, vocational, and survival skills were taught. Rehospitalization rates were only 10 percent in the patients participating in the behaviorally oriented educational program but were 53 percent in a comparison group receiving traditional aftercare services. In a similar program located in a community mental health center, specific goal setting and active behavioral training of social and community living skills led to attainment of increasing numbers of clinical goals during a 24-month follow-up, period; matched patients from a more traditional day hospital showed decrements in goal attainment over the 24-month period. Treatment procedures based on this program were subsequently adopted by 50 community mental health centers around the United States.

In an early effort to demonstrate that a comprehensive learning-based program could be effective with chronic mental patients, one approach used the hospital as a base for initial training of patients in interpersonal skills, effective decision making, and group governance and cohesion. Following this training, the patients were transferred as a group to living quarters in the community. These quarters resembled a lodge, and the patients were assisted in gradually assuming full responsibility for its maintenance and operation. They bought and prepared food, kept financial records of income and expenditures, and consulted community-based physicians and agencies for their medical, psychiatric, and support needs. Live-in staff gradually receded from the picture until the lodge residents were functioning autonomously. In addition, the patients earned money by starting a local business that provided janitorial services, yard work, general hauling, and painting. At 40 months' follow-up, the patients trained to live and work in a community lodge were found to have remained outside the hospital and gainfully employed significantly longer.

Psychosocial rehabilitation Another modality of milieu therapy, psychosocial rehabilitation, emerged during the late 1940s, when former patients began to meet together in a social club in New York City to satisfy their needs for acceptance and emotional support. Emphasizing self-help, mutual

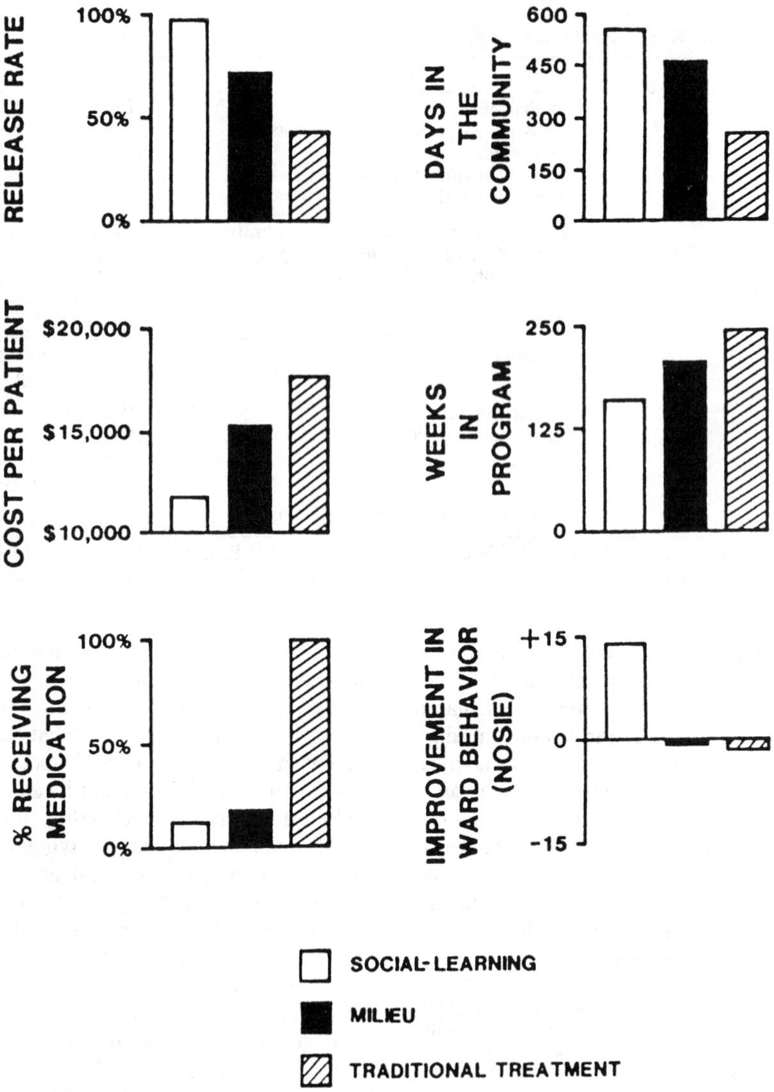

FIGURE 14.5-5 *Results of three long-term inpatient treatment programs for chronically psychotic patients: Social learning and token economy, therapeutic community milieu, and traditional custodial treatment. The social learning and therapeutic milieu environments were equally intensive, with patients receiving a minimum of 18 months posthospital treatment on a declining-contact basis. (From Paul G, Lentz R:* Psychosocial Treatment of Chronic Mental Patients: Milieu vs. Social-Learning Programs. *Harvard University Press, Cambridge, MA, 1977, with permission.)*

interdependence, and reliance on assets, the movement led to the establishment of Fountain House and its hundreds of clones throughout the United States. Instead of thinking and calling themselves patients, they took on the identity of members and formed groups and teams to accomplish tasks, plan activities, and solve problems; in so doing, they improved the quality of their lives. Creating their own social support network, members of psychosocial clubs design activities that build experiences of mutual ownership and needs. Staff members, primarily nonprofessionals or those trained in vocational rehabilitation, provide positive, accepting reactions and require members to obtain psychiatric treatment, such as medication, elsewhere; so the club has rehabilitation but not clinical goals. During the day, members spend varying amounts of time in the club, engaging in chores, such as operating a cafeteria and snack bar, assisting each other in banking and budgeting, visiting friends who are hospitalized or unable to come to the club, printing a daily newspaper, helping each other with entitlements from social agencies, taking remedial education courses, manning a thrift shop, working the switchboard, doing clerical work, and refurbishing cooperative apartments.

Central to the Fountain House treatment philosophy is the belief that psychiatric patients have a fundamental right to work and that employment facilitates community adjustment and reduces symptoms. In the transitional employment program, patients are placed in jobs located in normal places of business. Ranging from large corporations to small firms, these jobs are at the entry level, requiring minimal training or skills. The clubhouse staff guarantees that the job will be performed reliably, even if they must fill in occasionally for an absent club member. These transitional jobs are opportunities for club members to work temporarily in preparation for full-time employment elsewhere or work on a longer-term basis in the entry-level position. The number of transitional employment programs in the United States has grown to over 100, with over 500 employers involved in providing wages in excess of $4 million.

An 18-month follow-up evaluation of club members working in transitional jobs revealed that 16 percent were employed independently on a full-time basis, and an additional 45 percent continued part-time work in the transitional program or were attending school or other training programs. Only 2 percent were in psychiatric hospitals at the time of the 18-month follow-up. Another evaluation of the psychosocial club model found that 38 percent of members were rehospitalized during a 2-year follow-up period, in comparison with a 60-percent rehospitalization rate for a contrast group. Members of the club also had significantly lower rehospitalization rates 5 years later; those who were hospitalized from the club spent 40 percent fewer days in the hospital than the rehospitalized control subjects. Evaluations of the club model have been flawed by lack of diagnostic clarity, randomized controls, and checks on medication intake.

Outreach psychosocial programs Effective strategies for reducing rehospitalization rates and improving rehabilitation outcomes have been developed that utilize assertive outreach services to aid schizophrenic patients functioning in the community. In such programs, the majority of staff-patient contact occurs in the patient's home, neighborhood, or workplace, with the focus on meeting basic living needs, developing more effective coping skills, and social support.

A well-controlled experiment documented the efficacy of this approach with 130 severely symptomatic psychiatric patients who were randomly assigned to standard hospital treatment or to a community-based outreach program. The interdisciplinary treatment team that was drawn from a state hospital to work in the community did whatever was necessary to maintain their patients outside the hospital. Staff worked around the clock, 7 days a week, to advocate patients' needs, intercede with relatives to promote constructive separation, and carry out crisis intervention. Medication was also used in customary ways. The outreach effort, called Training in Community Living, eased the patients' transition into community functioning, helped them develop living skills, and reduced dependence on relatives. This concentrated form of community support and continuity of care, which now has been disseminated to other sites throughout the United States and overseas, resulted in lowered rehospitalization rates, reductions of symptoms, increased capacity to work, increased independent living, and reduced family burden.

The reduction in rehospitalization rates for schizophrenic patients treated in an Australian replication of the Training in Community Living program is depicted in Figure 14.5-6. In addition, cost-benefit analyses have found that assertive outreach programs are more economical than traditional case management approaches for recidivist patients. However, when the demonstration program was terminated, the differences favoring the experimental patients evaporated rapidly. This finding underscores the need to sustain psychosocial support indefinitely, just as antipsychotic drugs often must be given long term. It remains to be seen whether use of social learning principles in such community support programs can improve acquisition, durability, and generalization of living skills.

The Training in Community Living model has been successfully adapted for even more chronic patients who have histories of multiple hospitalizations and difficulty sustaining community tenure. For example, the Bridge Program was developed as a community outreach treatment based in the urban environment of Chicago for the most highly recidivistic psychiatric patients. Only patients with at least three admissions in the previous year are admitted; in the first demonstration phase of the program, patients had an average of 14 prior hospitalizations.

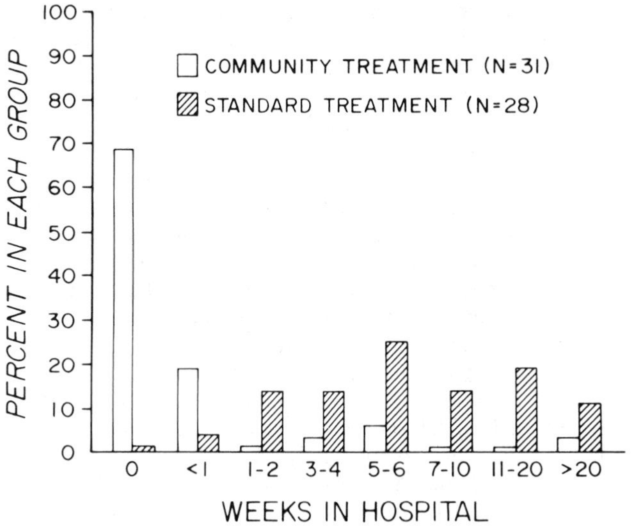

FIGURE 14.5-6 *Sixty-five schizophrenic patients presenting for admission to a psychiatric hospital were randomly assigned to two groups: community treatment and standard hospital plus aftercare. Community treatment patients were not admitted to the hospital, if possible, and were provided comprehensive treatment and 24-hour crisis services, based on the model program, Training in Community Living. Patients receiving community treatment achieved superior clinical outcomes, and along with their relatives were more satisfied with their treatment than standard-care patients. Patients in community treatment spent substantially less time in the hospital, a difference that was highly statistically significant (p <.001). (Adapted from Hoult J, Reynolds I: Schizophrenia: A comparative trial of community-oriented and hospital-oriented psychiatric care. Acta Psychiatr Scand* 69: *359, 1984, with permission.)*

The basic goal of reducing rehospitalizations is accomplished by providing patients (referred to as members in psychosocial programs) with the material and social support necessary for maintaining tenure in the community and for coping effectively with everyday problems. A unique feature of the program is that all staff–member contacts occur in the field—on the street, in the house, in local restaurants, in low-rent hotels, in Skid Row missions, in police lock-ups, and in bars. The objective of contacts is to help members cope effectively with the concrete details of daily life. Staff persons act as resource coordinators connecting members with the services available in the community. Crisis intervention is available on a 24-hour basis. Staff operate as a team without individual caseloads, and see each member on a rotating basis.

Outcome results from the Bridge Program suggest that it effectively lowers rehospitalization rates. Seventy-one members treated at the Bridge Program for 1 year reduced the number of their hospitalizations from an average of 3.3 in the year preceding the program to 1.9 the following year, with a corresponding drop in time spent in the hospital from 106.9 days to 43.1. By avoiding costly inpatient treatment, the program more than paid for itself; savings were almost $6,000 per patient per year.

Other psychosocial rehabilitation models A unique example of a milieu for which professional staff were specially selected and trained to provide a nurturing, stimulus-reducing, and accepting environment for young, acutely psychotic persons was Soteria House. Medication was purposely minimized, on the assumption that the psychotic process, if met with understanding and acceptance, could offer a learning experience through increased self-awareness and could thereby strengthen the person against subsequent episodes. The Soteria milieu achieved reductions in positive symptoms equal to those achieved by a traditional hospital unit that utilized drugs. However, the duration of treatment was longer, and there were no differences in recidivism.

A different approach to psychosocial rehabilitation housed patients with selected surrogate families in the community with whom hospital staff had established a close alliance. Patients given the foster family support backed by professional consultation had greater community tenure than their counterparts who lived in less supportive residences. Foster home programs, when characterized by tolerance for deviance and realistic but low levels of performance expectations, have been important mechanisms for aftercare and community support ever since the noble Gheel, Belgium, experience that began hundreds of years ago. For centuries, family households in Gheel have adopted former mental patients, sustaining them as citizens of the city in a normalizing fashion.

COMBINING PSYCHOSOCIAL AND DRUG THERAPIES

In a disorder, such as schizophrenia, that has a profound biological diathesis, it is important to combine drug and psychosocial treatments for the vast majority of patients. Drugs are never prescribed, ingested, or metabolized in a psychosocial vacuum; the activity of drugs is facilitated or impaired by concurrent events within the person's living environment. Environmental events may be planned or spontaneous, implicit or explicit, but they are nonetheless potent factors in determining responsiveness to medication.

Evidence from many studies supports the conclusion that, when combined with rationally prescribed antipsychotic drugs, properly designed psychosocial treatment offers greater protection against relapse and higher levels of social adjustment than drugs or psychosocial treatment alone. The consensus of these studies is that antipsychotic drugs have a primary effect on cognitive disorganization and positive symptoms of schizophrenia and have less impact on psychosocial functioning. The opposite seems to be the case with social and psychosocial therapies. In combination, their beneficial impact on the comprehensive needs of the schizophrenic patient is additive. The psychiatrist, therefore, must be capable of providing or orchestrating both biological and psychosocial care to be professionally responsive to the needs of schizophrenic patients.

The following clinical advice, crystallized from the results of many studies, summarizes current wisdom about drug-psychosocial interactions in schizophrenia.

1. Psychosocial treatment is most helpful for patients who are in reasonably good states of partial or full remission from florid symptoms and who have reached stable levels of maintenance medication. Psychosocial treatment during acute flare-ups of symptoms should be aimed at calming the patient, reducing levels of social and physical stimulation, and assisting the patient to integrate and understand the symptoms as part of an illness process.

2. The most effective psychosocial treatment—whether provided by individual therapy, group or family therapy, day hospital, or inpatient milieu therapy—contains elements of practicality, concrete problem solving of everyday challenges, low-key socialization and recreation, engagement of attainable tasks, and specific goal orientation.

3. A continuing positive relationship is central in the overall strategy for treating the schizophrenic patient, no matter how much drug or psychosocial treatment contributes. This relationship may be with the prescribing psychiatrist or with a paraprofessional case manager.

4. The critical time to offer psychosocial treatment is during the aftercare period, when the patient is able to absorb rehabilitation and needs assistance in surmounting the problems and stresses of readjusting to family and community.

5. Psychosocial treatment should be long term; benefits rarely become apparent before 12 months and are even greater after 2 years. It is likely that indefinite, if not lifelong, psychosocial support, guidance, and training are optimal for most chronic schizophrenic patients. As antipsychotic drugs are most effective in maintaining symptomatic improvement when continued indefinitely, it is not surprising that psychosocial rehabilitation efforts are similarly optimized by continuity.

6. Psychosocial treatment should focus on stressors in the environment and deficits in personal characteristics that seem to play specific roles in relapse and community maladjustment. Schizophrenic relapse is common even when drug compliance is firmly established. Nor is there any evidence that a patient's level of manifest psychopathology at hospitalization or discharge predicts subsequent relapse. The best explanation, based on converging lines of evidence from empirical studies, is that the patient's personal assets and deficits, the social environment, and the type of psychosocial therapy are the most powerful influences on relapse, even in the face of reliably administered maintenance medication.

The potential interactions between antipsychotic maintenance and behavioral family therapy for schizophrenia are presently under investigation in a 5-year multiple–treatment center collaborative study sponsored by the National Institute of Mental Health. All patients in the program are treated for 2 years with long-acting, injectable fluphenazine decanoate (Prolixin decanoate) using one of three treatment strategies (regular-dose, low-dose, or targeted-dose) administered in double-blind fashion. Regardless of which medication group a patient is in, exacerbations in schizophrenic symptoms can be medicated with short-acting, oral fluphenazine hydrochloride until they have subsided. In addition, each patient's family is offered either educational supportive treatment or education plus behavioral family therapy. Family members in both psychosocial treatment conditions are invited to an educational workshop in which information about schizophrenia is presented, relatives' experiences with and understanding of the illness are explored, and practical ways of coping with common problems are discussed. Families in both treatment groups are also invited to monthly support meetings, are assigned a clinician for casework and occasional counseling, and have access to 24-hour crisis services for the 2-year period of the program. In addition to the above treatments, families in the behavioral family therapy group receive training in communication and problem-solving skills in their homes on a declining-contact basis for the first year of the program. Thus, both treatment conditions provide education and support to family members, but only behavioral family therapy provides training in communication and problem-solving skills.

Extensive, frequent assessments are made of patients' symptoms, early warning signs, side effects, social adjustment, and quality of life throughout the program. This research design will shed light on the clinical efficacy of both the pharmacological and family treatments and determine whether the treatment strategies interact with each other. For example, it is possible that the low-dose and targeted-dose treatments will be more effective for schizophrenic patients who are receiving behavioral family therapy than for those receiving supportive therapy, indicating that the reduction of family stress may enable patients to be maintained on much lower doses of antipsychotics than was previously believed.

The following is a case illustration of behavioral family therapy:

Dave, the youngest of seven children, was raised by his father, a Baptist minister, and his mother, a homemaker, in a protective home environment. Dave began to develop his first psychiatric symptoms when he was 16, after starting his junior year at a new high school. He had difficulty adjusting to the new school and was frequently teased by his classmates, who called him dumb. Gradually, Dave began to spend more and more time by himself, spending hours alone in his room listening to music, and interacting less with his family members and friends. Dave's parents' concern grew as his grades dropped from mediocre to poor and he ceased playing the piano, which had formerly been his favorite activity. They attempted to talk to Dave about his problems at school, but he kept putting them off by saying that nothing was wrong, and they did not press him further.

After several months of increasing social withdrawal, Dave's behavior became grossly disorganized and bizarre. He began staying up nights, pacing and talking excitedly about the FBI and Mafia following him and interfering with his thoughts. Later he complained to his mother that voices were telling him to hurt himself and that he was receiving messages from the radio and television. After an especially difficult day in which Dave became extremely agitated and started to throw food around the house and attempted to climb the walls, his parents realized that he would not snap out of it and needed immediate medical attention, so they took him to a mental health clinic.

Dave was admitted to a local psychiatric hospital, where he was treated unsuccessfully with antipsychotic medications for a month, and was then transferred to a state hospital for longer-term treatment. Throughout much of his inpatient stay, Dave's behavior alternated between aggressive, explosive outbursts precipitated by delusions of having been raped or physically abused, to not being able to distinguish other patients from his family, to apathy, depression, and social withdrawal. Eventually, he responded to electroconvulsive therapy and was discharged after 6 months on maintenance chlorpromazine (Thorazine), with a diagnosis of undifferentiated schizophrenia.

Dave returned home and completed high school. He did not have his second hospitalization until he was 21 years old and had begun attending music school. Although subsequently he was able to return to school and complete a 2-year associate's degree in music, the following 12 years were characterized by multiple hospitalizations, declining vocational and social functioning, and pervasive negative symptoms. He attended day treatment programs sporadically, and several relapses were precipitated by his discontinuing his medication.

When Dave was 33 years old and his parents were out of town for several weeks, he ran out of his antipsychotic medication and was not able to get a new prescription. He rapidly became psychotic and was involved in an altercation in which he was badly beaten by a security guard at a supermarket after leaving the store half-naked with some food he had not paid for. Dave was charged with simple assault and placed in a detention center, where he remained for 2 months, until his family was able to get the charges dropped and arrange a transfer to a psychiatric hospital. Dave was admitted to the Eastern Pennsylvania Psychiatric Institute, where he was enrolled in the Schizophrenia Treatment Program, an outpatient program that combined low-dose fluphenazine decanoate with behavioral family therapy.

Dave's positive symptoms were well controlled, but he continued to have prominent negative symptoms. His affect was flat, he had severe psychomotor retardation, he slept much of the time, and he interacted with few people outside his family. Dave began attending a day treatment program; he and his parents participated in monthly support groups; and they started behavioral family management sessions, which were conducted by a therapist who came to the house.

Before the family sessions began, each member was interviewed to identify specific goals for treatment, to involve them in a collaborative therapeutic alliance, and to assess their knowledge of schizophrenia. Despite over 10 years' experience with repeated hospitalizations, no one in the family knew even elementary facts about the illness, such as the symptoms, names, and side effects of medications, and the role of stress on the course of the illness. During the educational sessions, family members learned the early warning signs of schizophrenic relapse, which for Dave were suspiciousness and increased sleeping. On two occasions over the next 1½ years, impending relapses were recognized and successfully avoided by Dave and his parents, who employed the problem-solving skills that were taught in the family sessions.

In communication skills training, a major element of behavioral family management, special attention was given to improving Dave's nonverbal communication (eye contact, voice volume, tone), which was muted owing to his pronounced negative symptoms. Over the course of more than 25 sessions, Dave engaged in much role playing with his mother and father, rehearsing such skills as expressing positive and negative feelings. One skill that Dave found particularly difficult was making positive requests. In one family session, his parents portrayed co-workers or the supervisor at the sheltered workshop, and Dave rehearsed requesting help on a job: "Chuck, could you show me how we're supposed to assemble this? I'd really appreciate it." Dave's parents focused on increasing their verbal reinforcement to shape desired changes in his behavior by expressing positive feelings to him for small improvements. In one meeting, Dave's father expressed his satisfaction with his participation in the workshop: "Son, I'm really proud of you getting up so early every day to get to your program on time."

The family members learned quickly how to do cooperative problem solving following a structured sequence. However, extensive prompting was necessary to get them to meet on their own for weekly problem-solving sessions, which finally began after 10 months of family management. A wide range of problems were addressed, including coping with auditory hallucinations, arriving late at the workshop, and feeling fatigued. One important goal for Dave was to begin practicing the piano again. After a period of 4 months and several problem-solving discussions, Dave increased his practicing from zero times per week to an average of three-and-a-half times per week. He began to accept more invitations to play the piano for the church choir and at parties, which formerly he had declined. As he played the piano more, Dave began to again arrange and write his own music, something he had not done for several years.

Throughout the course of treatment Dave steadily improved. He gradually transitioned from a day hospital to a vocational workshop, to prepare for competitive employment. While Dave continued to have negative symptoms, they were less severe. By the end of the first year of combined drug and family therapy, Dave's Brief Psychiatric Rating Scale scores declined from severe to mild for blunted affect, and from moderately severe to mild and very mild for psychomotor retardation and emotional withdrawal, respectively. Despite his residual symptoms, Dave became eager to obtain a competitive job so that he could marry his girlfriend of several years, a long-term goal he had stated at the beginning of the family sessions. While the changes evidenced by Dave over 1½ years of behavioral family management were modest, he continued to move toward greater social and economic independence while remaining clinically stable. The burden of care on his family was greatly reduced by Dave's assuming more responsibility for managing his illness, such as attending follow-up medication appointments and a vocational program.

REFERENCES

Anderson C M, Reiss D J, Hogarty G E: *Schizophrenia and the Family*. Guilford, New York, 1986.

Bellack A S, editor: *A Clinical Guide for the Treatment of Schizophrenia*. Plenum, New York, 1988.

Bellack A S, editor: *Treatment and Care of Schizophrenia*. Grune & Stratton, New York, 1984.

Curran J P, Monti P M, editors: *Social Skills Training: A Practical Handbook for Assessment and Treatment*. Guilford, New York, 1982.

Falloon I R H, editor: *Handbook of Behavioral Family Therapy*. Guilford, New York, 1988.

Falloon I R H, Boyd J L, McGill C W: *Family Care of Schizophrenia*. Guilford, New York, 1984.

Goldstein M J, Hand I, Hahlweg K, editors: *Treatment of Schizophrenia: Family Assessment and Intervention*. Springer-Verlag, Berlin, 1986.

Hatfield A B, Lefley H P, editors: *Families of the Mentally Ill*. Guilford, New York, 1987.

Keith S J, Matthews S M: Group, family, and milieu therapies and psychosocial rehabilitation in the treatment of the schizophrenic disorders. In *Psychiatry 1982 Annual Review*, L Grinspoon, editor, p 166. American Psychiatric Press, Washington, DC, 1982.

Leff J, Vaughn C: *Expressed Emotion in Families*. Guilford, New York, 1985.

Liberman R P, editor: Special issue on psychiatric rehabilitation. Schizophr Bull *12:* 540, 1986.

Liberman R P: *Psychiatric Rehabilitation of Chronic Mental Patients*. American Psychiatric Press, Washington, DC, 1987.

Liberman R P, Falloon, I R H, Wallace C J: Drug–psychosocial interactions in the treatment of schizophrenia. In *The Chronically Mentally Ill: Research and Services*. SP Publications, New York, 1983.

Liberman R P, Glynn S, Phipps C C: Rehabilitation of schizophrenic disorders. In *Treatment of Psychiatric Disorders*, B Karasu, editor. American Psychiatric Press, Washington, DC, 1988.

Liberman R P, Mueser K T, DeRisi W J: *Social Skills Training for Psychiatric Patients*. Pergamon, New York, 1988.

Linn M W, Klett C J, Coffey E M: Relapse of psychiatric patients in foster care. Amer J Psychiat *139:* 778, 1982.

McFarlane W R, editor: *Family Therapy in Schizophrenia*. Guilford, New York, 1983.

McGlashin T H: Schizophrenia—Psychosocial treatments and the role of psychosocial factors in its etiology and pathogenesis. In *Psychiatry Update: Annual Review*, vol 5, A J Frances, R E Hales, editors. American Psychiatric Press, Washington, DC, 1986.

Paul G L, Lentz R J: *The Psychosocial Treatment of the Chronic Mental Patient*. Harvard University Press, Cambridge, MA, 1977.

Stein L I, Test M A, editors: *The Training in Community Living Model: A Decade of Experience*. Jossey-Bass, San Francisco, 1985.

Strauss J S, Boker W, Brenner H D, editors: *Psychosocial Treatment of Schizophrenia*. Hans Huber, Toronto, 1987.

Talbott J A, editor: *The Chronic Mentally Ill*. Human Sciences Press, New York, 1981.

Wallace C J, Nelson C, Liberman R P, Aitchison R A, Ferris C: A review and critique of social skills training with chronic schizophrenics. Schizophr Bull *6:* 42, 1980.

14.6
SCHIZOPHRENIA: INDIVIDUAL PSYCHOTHERAPY

DANIEL P. SCHWARTZ, M.D.

INTRODUCTION

The work of Adolf Meyer and Harry Stack Sullivan has provided a foundation for individual psychotherapy with schizophrenic patients in the United States. The hallmarks of their work are a conception of the human responsiveness of the patient, regardless of a withdrawn and deluded state, and a real and humane interaction with the patient and physician. Central in their work was the focus on schizophrenia as an understandable disorder of self-organization, however predisposed by genetic vulnerability, which was influenced by the patient's actual environments during psychotherapy and during development. The minute examination of physician-schizophrenic patient interaction—symbolized as the participant observation of the psychiatrist by Sullivan or explained as an exploration of the transference expectations of the patient in the doctor-patient relationship by Frieda Fromm-Reichmann—was and is regarded as the most powerful therapeutic lever in individual psychotherapy's support of the patient's recovery.

These psychiatric pioneers focused on the attempts of the schizophrenic patient's disordered self to manage overwhelming anxiety, awesome shame, and an abysmal lack of self-esteem. Support of the patient's attempts to cope in the face of such affect disruption centered on communication with the psychiatrist and use of psychoactive drugs. It was found, as O. Will and L. Hill suggested, that if one could decipher the language of such patients—the language of their behavior, of their rigid delusions and obscure neologisms, and of their formidable needs for withdrawal—schizophrenic patients were transformed into communicative, sensitive, ordinary human beings. Early on, psychiatric students of these deciphering processes discovered that they could fully understand the cryptic organizations of their patients only by examining their own partially dissociated selves and unconscious processes as they engaged in individual courses of psychotherapy.

No enterprise of this nature could be envisioned without the accumulated knowledge, treatment data, and therapeutic methods that originated with and evolved from the works of Sigmund Freud and those whom he influenced. All understanding of normal childhood development; the place of unconscious processes; the acquisition of conscience and of defenses; the body's central place in the evolving self matrix and in its thinking and interaction; and the evolving place of one's own experience of the environment, mother, and father—all these and more evolved from the accretion of psychoanalytic knowledge. Furthermore, this information has been integrated with and has continually evolved from experience in individual psychotherapy with schizophrenic patients.

Psychoanalysts have learned to be mindful of the absolute necessity of preserving the schizophrenic patient's fragile integrity of self and its capacity to function. For example, Will studied the sense of personal freedom and its relation to autonomy of the self. Others who contributed insights that inform the special process of individual psychotherapy with schizophrenic patients are C. Schulz, E. Erikson, M. Wexler, H. Kohut, T. Lidz, D. Schwartz, and D. W. Winnicott. Their research has led psychiatrists to provide treatment that acknowledges the patient's strengths as well as conflicts; gives voice to the patient's need to be held in the heart and mind and voice of their therapist and to be listened to; and creates a genuine relationship with each patient, a context in which to sort out difficulties.

The personal experiences, emotional reactions, and fantasies of the psychiatrist who is working with schizophrenic patients received little attention in this country until the work of H. Searles, who integrated observations of his own work with schizophrenic patients and the understanding of countertransference—the troubling and troubled inner responses of the therapist to each individual patient. This integration attempted to combine the operation of projective and introjective processes, in which the patient unwittingly provokes the therapist to feel tempted to behave as does some hated or loved part of the patient's self or another important person. Searles combined these projective-introjective countertransference themes with a major theme of psychoanalytic work on the crucial therapeutic process in which the therapist inevitably, if unconsciously, comes to identify to some extent with every patient. This partial identification is central to the therapist's capacity to understand the patient and, so, help the patient understand him- or herself.

Psychotherapists who work with schizophrenic patients find that their own affective processes become distressing, owing to some loss of self boundaries. (This is one of the schizophrenic's typical problems.) They have periods of feeling overinvolved with the patient, disturbed by sexual and romantic ideas regarding the patient, and of simultaneously feeling rage and loving responsibility toward the troubled schizophrenic patient. Such therapists' experiences became more available and accepted after Searles's integration of countertransference data. Most therapists still found it counterproductive to talk about their own feelings to their patients; however, the work allowed them to examine their own experience and the state of the patient they are treating.

Finally, an articulation of the realities of the undertaking was identified as a basic therapeutic ingredient. Both parties must understand the assumption that patient and therapist have their respective tasks and that there are therapeutic requirements—regularity of time and place, mutual safety, financial compensation, and intention to understand. Individual therapists of schizophrenic patients have learned that they may not violate such realities, such limits of task, without risking irreversible loss of therapeutic and developmental potential. Insistence on setting forth such rules does not impugn the therapist's humanity, nor should it serve as a vehicle for a perfunctory or rigidly mechanistic therapeutic approach.

PRINCIPLES OF INDIVIDUAL PSYCHOTHERAPY OF SCHIZOPHRENIA

The individual psychotherapy of schizophrenia is concerned with the fragility of the patient's self (now more fragile owing to the psychotic breakdown) and the necessary disorganization of the self as the patient attempts to recover and grow. The treatment presupposes a thorough knowledge of the principles involved in any psychoanalytic therapy.

PRINCIPLES AND PROCESSES OF INDIVIDUAL PSYCHOANALYSIS In psychoanalysis, therapists listen and identify the patient's affect. They clarify defense before impulse and surface before depth and deal with transference. They attend to all that is excluded from the patient's awareness, evolve a therapeutic alliance with each patient, and take a position regarding material the patient presents that is equidistant from the patient's id, ego, and superego, and reality. Therapists regard each area of the patient's mind with curiosity and pay special attention to the relationship of past experiences and current reality, including the experience of the therapy, the therapist, and the therapeutic environment. The patient's work and personal environments and capacities to use, fit into, and change those environments are central to the therapist's attention. The limits of the environment's adaptability to the patient are also of special interest. Therapists try to understand the somatic and developmental circumstances that preceded the therapeutic actuality. They are particularly attentive to past and present developmental trauma, including the patient's assets and opportunities and the nature of the stresses that precipitated the onset of disease.

The therapist's responses must be honest, genuine, personal, intimate, oriented toward understanding the patient's agenda, and appreciative of opportunities for choice and activity on the patient's part. The doctor's responses are determined by the patient's task, rather than the therapist's agenda. The therapist's needs are limited, in this context, to that of being paid. Personal information and theories, including opinions on how people should live their lives, are kept out of the therapy. Therapists maximize useful information from the patient, focusing on the patient's task of representing, ultimately in words, and then examining the patient's experiences of self, of the therapist, and of the world. They enhance the patient's ability to determine a course of action.

The process of helping the patient put feelings into words affords both parties an understanding of the patient's developmental and interpersonal history, including relationships with important people. The two share a significant and jointly evolved memory. As the therapeutic work proceeds, a mutual, though asymmetrical attachment evolves, one in which are reproduced the feelings, thoughts, and behaviors—those strengths and deficits—that are the product of the patient's handling of developmental tasks. Early childhood tasks of each psychosexual and psychosocial stage—the organization of early object relations (e.g., the capacity to delay and internalize and to invest and develop skills), the evolution of talents, values, morality, and defenses—all play themselves out in words, feelings, and behaviors within the limits of the structured therapeutic relationship. Through the joint examinations of those behaviors, feelings, thoughts, and memories, the patient internalizes a new knowledge of self and others. In the course of that process, growth occurs, which then has its rewards and brings new problems. Ultimately, the patient, having internalized and integrated aspects of the work and relationship with the therapist, needs to leave the therapeutic relationship to pursue a separate (now richer) life. Termination is then discussed, explored, and planned, and therapy ends.

None of these therapeutic processes can occur without disruption, without new organizations of the self where therapy is meaningful, or without pleasure and pain. These pleasures and pains, disruptions and growth, must be acknowledged, articulated, and accepted by the participants in different ways. This is not a symmetrical relationship. It is an expert working with someone who wants help and an opportunity to develop. In every psychotherapeutic process with each patient, the therapist experiences countertransferences that both obscure and illuminate the therapeutic work. Privately or in consultation with colleagues, the therapist attempts to examine those evolving organizations and looks at the nature of his or her feelings and subconscious behaviors as part of the interpretive process toward understanding a patient. The therapy is an interactive process; the therapist is a participant-observer whose job is to conceptualize and communicate useful observations to the patient. It is not an attempt to impose a particular therapeutic approach on the patient; rather, the therapist learns from each patient what conditions for personal development, mutual honesty, and growth that patient seeks.

DEVELOPMENTAL DIFFICULTIES OF THE SCHIZOPHRENIC PATIENT The ordinary psychotherapeutic enterprise, as described above, is difficult for schizophrenic patients because of the difficulties imposed by the disease—

developmental difficulties and difficulties in the organization of a self that are compounded by a schizophrenic breakdown. The developmental difficulties include the regular occurrence of traumas, many at crucial developmental stages (especially adolescence) that are features of the life histories of most schizophrenic patients—parents' interpersonal problems, genetically determined vulnerabilities, special needs, or tragic environmental circumstances.

These traumas have all the complexities of which human beings are capable. The young child about to become a schizophrenic patient is often regarded by the mother as loathsome, too demanding, impossible to comfort, or colicky, or, conversely, perfect and happy, absolutely wonderful, and the greatest baby that ever was. The mother or father is often absent, is cruel and unable to communicate, communicates only about him- or herself, is overwhelmed by circumstances, or is depressed. Premorbidly, the schizophrenic patient often is intensely involved with a mother, father, or sibling who is emotionally troubled. The internalized trauma, thus, often is the result of having, as a child, loved and cared about a mother, father, or sibling who became troublesomely absent, severely depressed, or psychotic but who was not openly regarded as sick by the family. Instead, distortions surrounded the acknowledgment of the family's and individual's conditions.

In such families, there is often no opportunity for the child to develop the ego functions crucial to a separate self that are essential to honest interaction and necessary for the appreciation of successes and failures in everyday relationships. Rather, a false and conforming sense of self often develops that has little depth and does not feel to the child as if it belongs to him or her. The self is made to conform to a reality view that the family can live with. As one examines this view with a patient or family, it appears that the unspoken but profoundly effective and operative family rules suggest that the future patient should attempt not to be, not to exist—that the child should not be a separate being, not have a personal (and, incidentally, troublesome) body, not have affects or express personal opinions and observations. Such developing children feel they are allowed a self and may exist only as long as they play by the rules of the family system, by being mother's perfect daughter or father's confidant and whipping boy but not by being a separate individual. This reaction produces feelings of alienation from one's own body and self, from one's inner reality, and from the world outside. In the absence of a separate self, private, inner organizations of limitless grandiosity, omnipotence, and magical power alternate with a profound sense of emptiness and worthlessness.

PROBLEMS OF THE SCHIZOPHRENIC STATE

DISORGANIZATION OF THE SELF AND REGRESSION When persons with such developmental problems come up against an acute crisis (e.g., leaving home, becoming sexual, falling in love, leaving college, starting significant work), they experience very troubling affects. Their feelings are overwhelming, and their limited capacity for coping is overwhelmed. Because they have not developed a separate, inner ego-self-object relation organization with which to modulate affect and develop a workable relationship with others, a regression to childish and painful need states ensues, usually in adolescence. In these states, primitive developmental organizations of ego-self-other emerge, and depending on the nature of the patient's pathology and experience, panic ensues.

With this disorganization comes a loss of ego boundaries and a fragmentation of the self. The person's options are significantly narrowed; the person can go neither backward nor forward in development. There is a withdrawal and fragmentation of the self-object-reality relations; a loss of reality testing is part of the breakdown. It is as if the inner self and the outside world have been destroyed.

In desperation, the patient attempts to repair the disintegration, to reorganize the self, however tenuously; the result is a fragile, unstable, pathological self, usually with delusional components. In the context of this delusionally organized reality, the patient attempts to manage behavior, sequence thoughts, stabilize inner organization, and modulate the accompanying affects and panic. In the course of the psychotic state, however, the patient's sublimatory activity often "comes down in ruins." The task of holding together the ego-self-object-reality organization is so consuming that the patient abandons talents and previous activities, sometimes permanently.

The nature of this acute psychotic experience and its forms of reorganization involve either a flexible regression with withdrawal or a fixed pathological self-organization with delusion formation and withdrawal from reality. The degree of fluidity and regression or rigidity of ego-self-other organization and delusion formation in these processes is determined partially by the patient's previous ego development and inner organization of ego-object-reality relationships and also by the environment in which the patient is living and receiving treatment.

Treatment modes may determine whether the patient's response to the acute psychosis is a flexible regression, facilitating recovery and a favorable response to subsequent psychotherapy, or a rigid pathological, delusional self that resists outside help and personal change. This is not the time for deep personal exploration. Rather, this acute disorganization is the occasion for active support, direction, and facilitation of the ego's adaptive forces and strengths. It is generally believed that, when patient and family can understand the stressful precipitating events, subsequent debilitating chronicity can often be prevented.

Problematic organization of the self The pathological ego-self organizations, both before and after the psychotic break, with which the schizophrenic patient, the therapy, and the therapist will contend, need to be characterized.

Before the schizophrenic break, there is a pathological self-formation; the patient perceives the self as being false, conforming (pliant), and focused on the patient's and family's externals. This self, which almost always has had a troubled symbiotic support system with a parent, works fairly well until some thrust occurs, usually in adolescence, such as the need to have a separate body that has sexual and aggressive interests, to begin a career, to separate from home, or to form separate values.

As an example, consider a schizophrenic boy who went through college being called by his football teammates the "coachable kid." A major activity while growing up was listening for long hours to his mother talk about her loneliness and unhappiness. (His father was an isolated man and was often away from his family.) He seemed to his mother to have been a perfect child. This boy had no rebellion, no troublesome sexuality to evolve, and no separate sense of what he was or needed to be.

Because such children are central to the mother or father and, as none of their individual needs or troubles is seen and struggled with, the self is perceived as both false and enormously powerful, often as if they are guilty, oedipal winners. They feel as if their self is part of the other person's self, and that they are able to adapt to that one symbiotically involved person very specifically, and often too flexibly. Such patients say they have found no place for their own aggression, their own sexuality, or their own separate genuineness, either in their family or in their own mind.

During and after a schizophrenic psychotic breakdown, these patients evolve their own forms of organization of ego-self-object-reality relations. In this fragmented state, there are partial, momentary, and longer-lasting delusional, hallucinatory, grandiose, and narcissistic organizations of the self. The ego-self tries to use global, undifferentiated, defensive organizations. It uses primitive modes of operation and defense, including denial, magical thinking, omnipotence, projection, introjection, and splitting.

Primitive defenses and their self-organizations regularly involve a violation of ego-object boundaries. In fact, a primitive defense cannot be defined without involving a violated ego-self boundary. A projection, for example, involves an "It's you, not me" concept; it violates the ego-object boundary. Boundary-altering use of defensive behaviors is a regular developmental occurrence in childhood. Using magical thinking, children close their eyes, turn their heads, and make others disappear.

Fluid and undefined self-organizations also emerge as dream-like states involving grandiose fantasies. These delusional and dream-like states require the schizophrenic patient, after the breakdown, to withdraw from reality and other human beings into a "spacey" state. During these withdrawn states, the patient arranges fragile fantasy organizations of an omnipotent self in order to manage anxiety. Intrusions of the outside world on this state and the demands for interaction with that world cause the ego-self to become disorganized and fragmented; panic ensues.

PROBLEMS OF REORGANIZATION OF EGO AND SELF

DISRUPTIVE EFFECTS OF THERAPEUTIC INTERACTION Questions that ordinary psychoanalytic psychotherapy asks and the process by which it pursues its ends are disruptive to the self-organization of schizophrenic patients. For persons who have learned to have a self in which one does not appear to exist, or to take up personal space, or to notice or put into words the troubling lack of investment from or traumatic behavior of one's parents, and how not to hold as central their own developmental necessities, participation in psychotherapy is bound to be disorganizing.

When schizophrenic patients find themselves in an individual psychotherapy situation, the usual questions—Who are you? How did you get that way? What do you want to become?—normal to most psychotherapy, are disruptive to their developmentally organized, inner ego-self-object state: They do not have a self; they have not had a development; they will not explore its purpose. In an individual psychotherapeutic situation, the processes are personal, intimate, and affective, and it is expected that these processes will be examined openly by therapist and patient. This procedure is foreign to the schizophrenic patient, and even if the therapist does not direct the agenda or impose an external theory, there is for the patient a clash of developmentally internalized, antithetical systems of behavior, thought, feeling, and value.

Schizophrenic patients typically say that they find analytic psychotherapy disruptive to their organization of ego functions and their sense of self and that they have to contend with the hateful experience of intrusion by the therapy and therapist.

One patient, after many months of individual work, said she felt as if her therapist pursued her hungrily in the course of the psychotherapy hour, as if she were something to be devoured. Although customarily mute, when her therapist occasionally stopped in the hospital hallway to say hello before her therapy hour she would ask, "What is this, hors d'oeuvres?" as if she were some delicious morsel for him to devour. Later, as she improved, she explained to her therapist that she was raised in a family in which personal contact was minimal. She had been cared for by governesses and maids, and she lived in her elegant city apartment with these maids while the family was in the country on "weekends," which lasted from Thursday through the following Tuesday. She had not been allowed to eat dinner with the family in the dining room until she was 6 or 7 years old. As she was slowly recovering from catatonic schizophrenia with the help of phenothiazines and individual psychotherapy, she commented on the fact that she was getting to know her doctor as an ordinary person: "Doctor, you will have to excuse me, I have never known a human being before. I was spoiled by my parents. They left me to live in a world of fantasy, all my own."

THE PATIENT'S EXPERIENCE OF THERAPIST OR HOSPITAL Many patients believe that their difficulties stem from trouble in the external world and that there is nothing wrong with them or their family. Often, even if they ask for help and want to go to a hospital, they say they did not realize before that they were sick. They believed they were in trouble. They felt unhappy and persecuted, or believed somehow they or their family had failed, but the trouble was not something disordered or malfunctioning within them.

For these patients, the fact of hospitalization or of going for individual psychotherapy involves, for the first time, the experience of the inner reality of having a self that is disordered. This realization itself is traumatic to the patient. Many patients who have been psychologically disorganized, even delusional, for a long time say they were not psychotic until they were admitted to the hospital—"not psychotic until that doctor talked to me" (incidentally, another example of magical thinking).

The presence of an ordinary human being (the therapist) who interferes with the accustomed withdrawal and pathological self-formation and disrupts the false self's symbiosis is very disturbing. The schizophrenic patient, in the course of individual psychotherapy in or out of the hospital, often becomes more disorganized and more psychotic. The patient—and often the family—hold the therapist and the hospital (if the patient is treated in a hospital) responsible for the disorganization and its disruptions and regard the therapist and therapy as dangerous, and the hospital as hateful, even evil.

Therapists are regarded as bad and dangerous, because the patient is afraid that a dependent attachment may develop, something the patient's developmental history has taught must be avoided. A healthy dependent attachment involves a relationship in which each can trust the other to notice and be responsive to his or her developmental needs. Often, this has not been the experience of schizophrenic patients. Initially, patients think the therapist is asking them to engage in an odious, dependent relationship that will require them to conform and to submit to exploitation.

Therapists are also mistrusted by schizophrenic patients,

because they are perceived as seductive. What happens is that the therapist notices and voices the patient's observations about his or her body, its ways of being, and its place in the patient's life and in the therapeutic work. In the patient's experience, such acknowledgments of self have not been safe. The personality has been organized to exclude such experience. By being direct about the patient's body, the therapist disrupts dissociative organizations.

The therapist is human, too, and that destroys many of the patient's habitual withdrawal and avoidance organizations. The patient is often more comfortable in the presence of someone who is not responsive, who is formal, who is not genuine. The availability of the therapist's therapeutic self is incompatible with avoidances that have served the patient effectively and is therefore also bad.

Finally, the therapist is annoyingly empathic, capable of saying such things as, "I gather that you felt hurt by me when I looked away a moment ago." When such an empathic observation is accurate, patients feel the therapist understands them and is sharing the experience. That moment is both intensely pleasurable and frightening for a schizophrenic patient, because patients cannot at that moment separate the understanding experience from the feeling that the therapist has merged with the patient, that they are one. This experience is both terrifying and disruptive. At such moments, patients say to the therapist, "Now I have to stop talking to you, because you are eating me up" or "You are devouring me" or "You are trying to manipulate me" or "You are reading my mind."

For some patients, this momentary merging involves their own omnipotence and grandiosity. They say, "Did you know I can read your mind?" or "I knew what you were going to say before you said it just now." Or they may manage this empathic occasion more projectively by saying, "You are planting ideas in my head." Early in the treatment, patients feel terrified, disrupted, and enraged by empathic experiences.

Later, during the individual psychotherapy process, patients notice faults in the therapist and empathic failures in the therapeutic relationship. These real failures in the therapeutic relationship, its moments of increasing anxiety and the self-object disruptions, are when much of the useful work of psychotherapy is accomplished. On these occasions of anxiety and empathic failure, the patient finds that the therapist is bad and needs to discover ways to acknowledge the real behaviors and repair the rents in the relationship and in the developing ego-self-other organizations.

With these considerations in mind, one can understand how the social rehabilitation programs for schizophrenic patients, which avoid intimacy and expression of dysphoric affects, do not engage the patient in one-to-one relationships, concentrate on interpersonal distance and structure interpersonal relationships, aim for small, reasonable, externally achievable goals, and avoid intense engagement have the potential to relieve the patient's stress and avoid disorganization. These rehabilitative programs often acknowledge the fragility of the patient's self; they do not interfere with the patient's idiosyncratically organized interactive and intrapsychic structure. They maintain the ongoing family systems and relationships; they allow time and space for withdrawal from reality and for most of the patient's unchallenged, privately organized, grandiose views of self. They manage the dysfunction of the disorder with psychoactive medication. These processes also significantly relieve guilt for the schizophrenic patient and family through their educational focus on a biological theory of causation that is external to the self; they slow down the patient's developmental occasions to relate to the patient's and family's minimal, immediate, manageable needs. This may allow the patient's fragile ego-self-other organization to chart a manageable course slowly. Above all, such rehabilitation programs do not disrupt, through self-examination and personal intimacy, organizations of intrapsychic structure and the corresponding ego-self-other-reality relations.

PROJECTIVE NECESSITIES FOR DEVELOPMENT OF A NEW SELF

PROJECTION IN NORMAL DEVELOPMENT OF THE SELF Central to the definition of what is first located and represented as belonging to the self and to the outside are a person's body, as a slowly defined object, and mother, as one who is both present and absent. The first vehicles for the child's development of a sense of self and other are its body and its mother. At first, all the good things—the child's eyes, hands, thumbs, and mouth, and the mother, her breasts and their milk—seem external, even as they belong to the self. The good things also include the parts of the self that make the mother smile and laugh and are involved in soothing and play. Indeed, the mother actually does act in a good way, loving her baby, soothing it, caring for it, and giving herself to its needs and development. It is onto these representations of interactions with mother that the child projects a sense that the two are evolving simultaneously.

These projected developmental aspects can be seen in normal children, who naturally cannot understand why, when they love somebody, that somebody does not love them back. It is as if they think they have created the loved object, which, developmentally, they have. Investments in loving objects, such as the family home, stem from these developmental forces. It feels as if the home loves the person. The important point is that the child's action endows mother's smile with the child's own warm affection, which is projected and then internalized by the child for developmental ego-self-object purposes. Such processes, which persist through life, are necessary to the elaboration of each new organization (or each extension of an organization) of the self.

All the bad—painful and frustrating—things that occur developmentally and experientially for the child also seem to come from the outside. In the child's mind, all the ice cream in the outside world, all the good food, belong to the child. Naturally when a child sees his or her own food disappearing into mother's or father's mouth, the child is angry and envious of the fact that this good food is outside and separate from him or her, even though this occurs during a time when self and mother have not yet been defined experientially as separate beings. So, the child identifies the origin of all the bad that occurs in the other, outside the self. If the mother is frustrating or unavailable, she is bad, she is angry, not the infant. The mother—not the infant—is bad if she is not paying attention, not soothing.

This proper developmental location of good and bad outside the self is repeated with each developmental advance, each extension of the self at any age. The first love is all wondrous things in the world. The first sexual feelings are aroused by a sexy other, on the outside. The first angry feelings are often externally elicited. One stubs one's toe and kicks the furniture.

Projection is a central part of transference in normal psychoanalytically informed psychotherapy and, so, is a regular and useful part of the treatment. The conditions of therapy are arranged so that the patient can examine and use the therapeutic situation to facilitate these projective parts of the transference operations. Maintaining the partial anonymity of the therapist, having the patient set the agenda, limiting the therapist's action—all invite this. The patient then locates in the therapist unnamable emerging parts of the self including impulses of the id, libido, and aggression, of ego self, and conscience, views of important others that heretofore were not admissible into the self or personality. The patient says and feels that it is the therapist who is secretly thinking sexual thoughts about the patient, not the reverse, just as it is the therapist who is secretly aggressively critical of the patient. Only later in the therapeutic process is this projected, merged portion of the patient's self reclaimed and integrated.

The patient projects not only what is painful or bad but also what is good, loved, valued, and idealized, so, at times, the therapist is regarded as wondrous, lovable, and perfect. The projection must occur before the patient can reclaim and integrate into the self these positive feelings.

PROJECTION IN INDIVIDUAL PSYCHOTHERAPY OF SCHIZOPHRENIA In the context of the developmental deficits and premorbid vulnerabilities experienced by a schizophrenic patient, survival of self-organizations requires that the patient elaborate a new ego-self-object reality. The process requires the projective creation of a new other outside, in which the patient can place parts of the self for the time being. (If no reasonable other is available, a schizophrenic patient may organize projectively and delusionally around a public figure.)

During individual psychotherapy, the schizophrenic patient attempts to localize all good in the therapist who, through this idealization, becomes frighteningly powerful. At the same time, the patient must confront and project everything in the present self that is seen as bad. Hatefulness, weakness, neediness, and (most critically) conscience functions are localized in the therapist. Because the schizophrenic patient has these needs and behaviors, he or she often will hear only those statements of the therapist that conform to an organizational view the patient is developing. And the intended communication may not be received if it does not conform to or confirm the patient's grandiose, unlimited, idealizing, good projections or, conversely, the omnipotent, menacing, and dangerous projections.

Patients are vaguely aware of the dissociated processes within. They often see their own projections not simply as mental events but as real, damaging behaviors. They then try to protect both themselves and the therapist from these noxious personal experiences. Often, they are convinced that the therapist will get to know this destructiveness, will discover that it is actually within him- or herself, and will inevitably come to hate the patient. Patients often decide, therefore, that if they stay away, or hide their face, or do not communicate, or do not tell the therapist anything about themselves, they are protecting the therapist, at least temporarily, from being damaged by the phenomena emanating from within themselves. They believe this may save them from (otherwise) certain abandonment, at least for a time.

BAD INTROJECTED BY THE PATIENT

Often patients' actions are the result of the difficulties of their development. They behave as if they have dangerously organized parts of which they are not totally aware. Therapeutic work reveals and helps patients integrate these largely unconscious organizations, called introjected part objects.

Introjected part objects arise from interaction with the family of origin, whom patients perceive as having been harmful. Thus, a mother by whom the patient feels abandoned or engulfed is, to some degree, unconsciously internalized, to become, in this example, an abandoning or devouring characteristic of the patient. The patient feels a need to protect other human beings, including the therapist, from knowing him or her, from being exposed to the hateful nature inside.

Such factors led early investigators of analysis of schizophrenic patients to regard patients' fears of their own destructiveness as being grossly inflated. Still, the therapist who works with schizophrenic patients must recognize the patient's capacity for genuine aggression that is mobilized voluntarily and not simply responsive to frustration. This aggression is usefully evolved in the patients' capacities, in their assertive vitality, and in their therapeutic work.

INTERACTIVE NECESSITIES IN NORMAL DEVELOPMENT OF THE SELF

The processes involved in developing a new organization or a new evolution of self include fantasies, language, and affect, as well as new behaviors congruent with the nature of the particular person's task. This task is to develop a self that trusts itself and others; trusting behaviors as well as trusting words, affects, and fantasies must evolve between the self and the developmental other. For an autonomous self to evolve integratively, behaviors, with their accompanying pain, loneliness, aggressiveness, and triumph, must be verbalized by those involved in psychotherapy—the patient and the therapist. If only words or words with affects evolve without behavior, only a partial organization of the self and other that is difficult to integrate results from the process. The body must act within developmental limits to perform the psychosocial and psychosexual tasks and necessities in order to organize the self. If therapy is to foster an evolving self, analogous behaviors must occur within different limits. One cannot drag a drugged body or a body with forever-frozen behavior through a psychotherapeutic hour and expect to find an integrated new self evolving. The patient's physical experiences, feelings, and expressions (e.g., arriving late, being ready for a fight, being joyful, being aroused, being smarter than the therapist) need to be recognized and discussed in the therapy.

In any therapy, there are small experiments with these matters, and real behavior occurs within limits. They are not simply fantasies, thoughts, words, or affects. There are, for the patient, real silence, real hiding of one's face, real acts of hatred, and real smiles and seductiveness. It is necessary that these occur in a relationship with a real other person whose limits are imposed by the task of therapy—that is, with a responsive therapist.

INTERACTIVE NECESSITIES AND BOUNDARIES FROM THE POINT OF VIEW OF DEVELOPMENT The developmental organization of boundaries of ego, self, and other is central to the inner and outer development of human beings. The self is defined by the behaviors with which it is comfortable. At some point, almost everyone will say, "No I do not do that. No that is just not me."

People are aware, dimly or acutely, of the nature of these positive and negative developmental limits. Often, they are conscious of what those boundaries are and of how they are involved in self organization. There are mothers, for example, who prohibit certain evolutions of the daughter's feminine self: "Keep out of my kitchen. You can't make dinner. You can't even boil water." The implied message is that the young woman is not entitled to master feeding, nurturing functions, that they are the exclusive province of the mother. If such restrictions are systematic enough, the young woman develops a sense of unexplored behavioral space and experiences, as well as feelings of limitations on her feminine self and her world. It is from these feelings she organizes her conscience and her sense of boundaries.

During a schizophrenic patient's psychotherapy where natural prohibitions and forces had been operative, new behaviors occur in the presence of a new other—the therapist. The new behaviors engage the other's capacity to experience pleasure in the patient, for example, in discovering that the young woman patient is a motherly nurturer. Such behaviors must be welcomed and reinforced as they occur, within the limits of the therapeutic framework. Patients must know that they are not well served by their previously internalized boundaries.

The patients' new behaviors are also used by the therapist as information about the developmental process. This development occurs not only in fantasy, in words, or with affects, but as behavior within the therapy. This happens to therapists; they do not arrange it.

For the processes of projection and fusion of the self and other to occur, patients have to act out behaviors toward the therapist, within the limits of the therapy and then step back and separate from the processes and examine them, in order to organize internally a new, separate sense of self. This autonomous inner and outer organization of behavior, of becoming a separate self, then can acknowledge itself as having real force relative to the therapist, the therapy, and ordinary life. These behaviors are necessary for the development, through defining boundaries, of a new self. The positive limit is defined by the behavioral space that is evolved and exercised through the patient's responsive systems and their accompanying affect, fantasy, and words, during the course of this development.

The customary understanding of a limit, however, involves the definition, not of where a behavior exists but of where it stops. As such, the "nos" as limits to behavior are also part of the internalized self definition. They are crucial developmentally, defining boundaries of ego, self, and other for each child, at each stage of development.

The therapist expresses limits naturally in terms of time, place, and money. But limits are also present in every interpretive intervention. When a patient says, "Doctor, I feel so pleased I would just like to kiss you" or, "Doctor, I am so mad I would like to sock you in the jaw," the therapist says, "Could you tell me more about that—how you imagine that. What do you have in mind?" Behaviorally the therapist is saying, "No. Do not kiss me or sock me in the jaw, but do tell me in words what you have in mind." A limit has been imposed that defines the therapeutic task. It says this is where the work is for you and for me. It differentiates the work behaviors of therapy from those in which therapist or patient might engage during ordinary human relationships. Such necessary and useful limits are involved in all developmental events of life, including definition of self and other; of gender identity; of boundaries between the generations; and of existence and death. In families in which limits have not been preserved, there are usually difficult developmental problems.

SCHIZOPHRENIA AND THE SELF'S BOUNDARIES AND INTERACTIVE NECESSITIES

Adolescent development normally includes the tasks of reorganizing ego-self-object relations and of evolving a new organization of the self and its relation to new others. The task of reorganizing the conscience involves enlarging the boundaries of the self's action and evolving a new organization of its morality and ideals. Adolescence's new investments include an aroused body and leaders other than one's parents. This evolution of an individuated self from the family, the inner process of leaving home and its outer realities, involves real interaction and real self-other boundary renegotiation. Such adolescent renegotiation and individuating processes, with their needs for new boundaries, often prove difficult for the preschizophrenic patient's fragile and rigidly organized ego-self-object relations.

After an adolescent schizophrenic breakdown, the boundaries of the ego-self-object organization and their interactive necessities are even more vulnerable, disorganized, and fragile. This vulnerability is most evident by the patient's withdrawal from and avoidance of any human contact and its reality relations. This avoidance of reality, of the tasks of work and love, seem to the schizophrenic patient truly necessary, in order to protect the delusionally grandiose and fragile ego-self formation that evolved during the breakdown from further disintegration. But since the tasks of adolescence—new evolutions of the self, new investments, and different location and reorganization of self and other—are those that schizophrenic patients, however fragile, must address if they are to grow and recover, resolution of boundary problems must occupy the therapeutic work. Thus, the fragility of the patient's self and its boundaries becomes troublesomely central to the individual psychotherapeutic process.

In the new evolution of the self, various projective and introjective processes occur. Who is doing what to whom can become a very confusing and frightening issue to the patient. For example, schizophrenic patients commonly feel they are not supposed to have a body. They often behave as if that body does not exist as a part of themselves. They become engaged in trying to get rid of and destroy that body, starving it to death, masturbating constantly and compulsively to rid themselves of sexuality, or hiding to keep the body out of sight. Usually, these senses of having an evil self and an evil body are projected onto the therapist because the therapist is an invested part of the world, outside the patient's self, among those available bad people. The therapist, trying to locate, and perhaps care about, that body, may be seen projectively by the patient as murderous. The boundaries of who is murdering the body become very confusing to both patient and therapist.

Boundaries of the self may also become confounded as patients develop a therapeutic attachment. Patients may notice, for example, their internalization of the therapist's ability to hold (embrace) the patients' self symbolically. The patient may carry an image of the therapist's willingness to listen and not strike back when the patient criticizes. It may feel as if the therapist is inside the patient. Patients at first find this inhabiting of self to be in violation of their own fragile ego-self boundaries, but disruption of ego boundaries, being part of the therapist, becomes part of the patient's self and has to be acknowledged, managed, and worked with again and again, however painful the work.

Such disruptions are characterized by the terrifying sense that one can lose one's self and one's hold on the world totally. Thus, schizophrenic patients initially cannot manage the fusions that occur in individual psychotherapeutic work. They cannot tolerate the experience of losing their all too fragile self and usually need to find some definition of outside in order to be able to separate and locate themselves.

The search for separateness of the self uses the patient's aggression, which initially labels separateness as something bad. As that bad thing is located outside the self (and is therefore separate), it helps define a self for the patient. The bad, at first, is located in the therapist; however, it may be located in any person to whom the patient is attached. Often, as organizations of the self develop, the outside-bad–inside-good self is split. The bad then is projected onto the hospital, the nurse, or the family; the good may include the therapist.

The autonomous capacities of the schizophrenic patient's ego and self are enhanced in their search for defined boundaries by therapists' capacity to set clear limits. Their ability to say, "No, the hour ends now," "No, you may not throw that vase in my office," or "No, I will not hold your hand" is essential. They facilitate patients' capacities to define, develop, and sustain internally their evolving autonomy.

While therapists are repetitively disrupting and involved in the patient's boundary and self-loss processes, they hold the patient symbolically. That is, in the therapist's memory and feeling is the patient and the patient's developmental struggle as a person. As therapists, in their words and behaviors, work with patients, they hold in their memory the evolving, fragile, personal processes and organizations within that other person's life history and within their joint therapeutic work. In this effort, therapists attempt to own and value both their own and the patient's individual boundaries and their respective contributions to their mutual task.

BOUNDARY PROCESSES IN THE THERAPIST Because projection, introjection, and other boundary operations are inevitable and central phenomena in the individual psychotherapy of schizophrenia, an enormous amount of information can be obtained by therapists from the problems they have in the countertransference organizations. Patients regularly project their developing and defensive parts onto therapists and take parts of therapists from them to be internalized, held, and managed to modulate the hurts and evolve and extend their own psychologically integrated self. Therefore, the experience of the therapist involved with a schizophrenic patient's therapy is one of inhabiting and being inhabited psychologically, and of being treated (as the patient often unconsciously feels) as a helpless and hurting child or as that noxious other who attacks and demeans the patient instead of helping.

ADAPTIVE DIMENSIONS OF RESPONSE IN REGRESSIVE STATES Among the issues around which ego-self-object relationships are formed and internalized is autonomy. Delineation of the tasks reality presents and clarification of a person's autonomous response to those tasks appear to go hand in hand. For the evolving ego or self, a clear understanding of the nature of the interpersonal reality is the facilitating condition for the autonomous response of self. Facets of a responsive autonomous self to a task involve delineating the nature of the task, defining the motive, sorting out the ego's capacities for managing the task, and deploying the necessary actions in relation to the tasks.

Most of the explication of these tasks' dimensions and corresponding facets of autonomous response in ordinary psychotherapeutic work with less troubled patients can be managed by the patient. Therapists typically help neurotic patients concentrate on understanding the developmental complexities of motive and self-knowledge. They help them hold on to what the self wants and has wanted and the conflicts involved.

Schizophrenic patients find that their developmental, familial, and interpersonal environments often have made it impossible for them to master the personal developmental tasks; the environment does not admit of a place for a separate and needy self. Such persons find themselves hindered by familial responses that either demean or inflate their attempts to delineate their capacities and skills accurately. Indeed, frequently they grew up in families who did not tolerate creativity or individuality. Therefore, all the dimensions of autonomy and task are centrally important to the schizophrenic patient and the therapist, if the patient is to develop an autonomous new self that has the capacity to interact with others and to define its inner and outer reality.

For schizophrenic patients, the question of whether they or their environment truly want and can tolerate their autonomous development is often tested in terms of whether the hospital and therapist want their selves and troublesome bodies to be alive. Thus, therapeutic activity may involve helping arrange for the patient to be protected from harm, by managing, when the patient cannot, self-destructive and suicidal behaviors. The therapist attempts to ensure this protection and verbalizes and behaves in ways that tell the patient that no one wants the patient to go away or to die.

In the acute and repetitive disorganizations of schizophrenia, the therapist, at first, may have to undertake the task of locating, naming, and facilitating the elimination of the body's unnecessary pain. The therapist may need to arrange for the provision of care and comforting, set limits, and provide attention and psychoactive medication. When possible, this is done in consultation with the patient. At crucial times, and, for some patients, during prolonged developmental periods, the hospital setting and its services are necessary.

In the course of these processes, the therapist respects the antiregressive, autonomous, adaptive capacities of the patient, the family, and the hospital staff. Supporting the patient may require altering the therapist's schedule to accommodate the patient's work or school hours, being available by phone, or summoning relatives. Reality testing by the therapist and being available for reassurance, outrage, and appropriate advice are "givens" of the therapeutic relationship. These ordinary and real qualities of the therapist plus the capacity to set limits firmly are regularly available to schizophrenic patients. The therapist's attempt is not to prescribe these attitudes nor simply to provide for the patient, but rather to lend defined, separate capacities to the developing patient's ego autonomy, as necessary.

The patient's life and welfare are always more central concerns of the therapist than the therapeutic procedure itself; when indicated, changing therapists or hospitals should not be resisted. This does not mean that periods of discouragement, despair, or hostility are not regular occurrences during therapeutic work or that therapeutic impasses can be avoided. It does mean that verbal interpretation and clarification are not the sole activities of the therapist.

Because the schizophrenic patient's developmental circumstances obviated the elaboration of a separate self, the patient cannot manage the stresses, affects, and traumas of ordinary tasks. They avoid recognizing their own capacities for adaptive responses to these tasks. All human beings, however, regularly and naturally try to represent the tasks both of their outer world and of their intrapsychic state. They often try, in dreams and behaviors (before words), to put into a representable form what they experience, what they need to do, and what the other important persons in their world are or are not doing.

With schizophrenic patients, especially, the therapist needs to be alert to such attempts at representation, trying to notice all that is accurate and potentially adaptive in the patient's experiences. This effort includes what the patient tries to represent about the therapist's verbal and other behavior and the rest of the environment. Crucially, the therapist openly and repeatedly invites the patient to notice what the therapist does that is helpful and useful and what is interfering and harmful (i.e., whether the therapist is abandoning the patient, or missing the point, or not usefully contributing to the patient's autonomous, representing, communicative, and adaptive processes). In this mutual task, not only are the difficulties and criticisms often kept out of the therapist's and patient's awareness, but the valuable, loving, and proud observations of the patient are often dismissed by the patient as unmentionable. Therapists then attend to any regressive behavior as an attempt by the patient to form a representation of an interpersonal or intrapsychic problem. These regressive schizophrenic behaviors often can and do convey important partial memory and new perceptual information and are not simply defensive modes of operation.

Personal failure by the patient may also contain such adaptive attempts at regression. For example, the schizophrenic patient may represent as external an internally prohibited, autonomous act, such as saying "no" to an unwelcome inner or outer event or feeling.

Finally, when shame becomes evident during individual psychotherapy, it often marks as an affect a new organization of the patient's evolving self and its individuating process. Any new inner organization, any new inner structure and outer behavior of an autonomous nature, is accompanied by the capacity for the experience of shame. This change is seen routinely in adolescent development, and its place in the individual psychotherapy of schizophrenia is crucial, since that therapy is centrally occupied with the organizations of a newly evolving self.

Contained in these views of adaptive possibility is the appreciation by the therapist, and ultimately by the patient, of the schizophrenic patients' capacity for human strength, unconscious morality, and severe honesty, their hidden capacity to love and value themselves and others, their attenuated and unintegrated sexuality and aggression, and their vital ability to grow.

PROBLEMS IN INDIVIDUAL PSYCHOTHERAPY OF SCHIZOPHRENIA

SELF-ATTACK Just as persons with schizophrenia lack awareness of their own strengths, they are largely unaware of their powerful capacities for self-attack. Suicidal behavior is only one (relatively infrequent) sort of attack on the self. Self-attack can come from varied inner and dissociated organizations, such as projected aggression, primitive conscience formation, unconscious hostile and grandiose identification, and introjected part objects. It can also occur during an evolution in psychotherapy of patients' valuable aggression, as they experiment with its control-delay modulation processes and boundary evolution issues. In such circumstances, it may not be immediately apparent, say, in an episode of wrist cutting, whether the unconscious object of the aggression is really the patient, therapist, family member, or some evolving part of the patient's personality that has not yet been internalized or accepted. Attacks on the self in response to projected affects are a pervasive phenomenon, and the therapists must be aware of how any of his or her own responses will be heard as if they were attacks by the schizophrenic patients.

DEPENDENCY Early in the individual psychotherapy of schizophrenia, patients are anguished simply by the fact that they are responsively engaged with the therapist, since this dependency violates their fragile sense of an autonomous self. Any suggestion that the patient and therapist are living in the same, mutually responsive world is intolerable to the patient.

During the early middle period of an individual psychotherapy process, it is very painful for the patient to hear observations about dependency dynamics with the therapist or the hospital, because, in the past, dependency processes with important human beings left the patient helpless and hopeless. When the process of developing a new self is renewed in individual psychotherapy, a number of developmental phenomena appear with regularity. All good things are located in the therapist, as they would normally be in an infant's mother and father. If the therapist goes off on a weekend or vacation, it feels as if all those good organizations of the patient's self go with the therapist. The impact is much like that of losing one's mother at approximately 8 months of age. The adult patient feels enraged and demeaned.

During the later middle processes of treatment, often after some progress, schizophrenic patients must struggle with the autonomous processes of choice (i.e., to decide whether to choose to work with the particular therapist or hospital). By virtue of the patient's improvement, circumstances are different from when treatment began. Now the patient can choose whether to tolerate the pain of dependency processes in therapy in order to grow. At this juncture, the patient may run away or try other therapists in order to exercise and acknowledge his or her capacity for autonomous choice.

GROWTH Early in treatment, there are rudimentary periods of growth during which aggressive attempts to establish new behaviors and new ego boundaries emerge. There is often an accompanying aggressive disorganization of self and other, as organization and image, as well as regressive attempts to reestablish previously organized forms of the self. These processes, which are disruptive and painful to the adult schizophrenic patient, appear to resemble the phenomenon noted when children who have just learned to walk decide, for a time, to resume crawling.

During the middle periods of growth in treatment, patients often find their separate development lonely and, to some degree, unwanted. They feel partially abandoned by the therapist as they try out their skills separately.

During later treatment development, there is often a further evolution of the organization of the patient's conscience and a reworking of the problems of delay, involving both prohibitive morality and guilt, and idealization. Patients find they can wait more patiently and are aware of caring more about what the therapist is feeling. At such times, an important question is whether patients can own and tolerate the real envy and competition toward and from the people with whom they have evolved their own separate selves. The patient examines whether friends, family, spouse, and therapist will continue to exist, now that he or she has an independently developing personality or whether those others will become, sadly, a lost part of their past.

Finally, at the time of therapy termination, organizations of the self that are separate and exciting also hold a great deal of grief for the patient, as they are reminders of the lost forms of the self, including once cherished delusional states and self-organizations. There is also the ordinary grief involved in growing up and leaving behind parts of the parents and of the dependent, developmental self. Grief is involved in recognizing that one is, in reality, leaving behind that therapist and allowing him or her to become a part of one's remembered past. When, as often happens, these experiences of essential and developmental grief present in the schizophrenic patient as guilt, the patient needs to appreciate that the guilt is really nostalgia for portions of him- or herself, of the cared-for mother or father, and of the valued therapist that he or she will be leaving behind.

SEPARATION Early in the treatment, there are the necessary processes of losing and separating prerequisite to reclaiming and internally reorganizing parts of the self in therapy. Entering the middle phase of treatment, much of the work includes locating who is the autonomous generator of each new evolution, the patient or the therapist. What part the patient plays, what contribution the therapist makes, and how the patient's self reacts and regulates each part are crucial issues. Did the patient discard or hold dear, destroy, or protect as valued, the internalized, represented parts of his or her new self in the face of the perceived sadness and envy of the therapist? Does the patient destroy the inner image of the therapist during weekends and vacations because he or she is enraged by being abandoned? Do they resort to previously organized, regressive retreats, using their own discouragement and delusion formation in attempts to manage rage and avoid loneliness in familiar ways?

A danger in all these interactive processes, particularly those involving separation tasks, is that the periodic impasses that arise between therapist and patient will become structuralized, with stereotypy of mutual communicative response and mutual withdrawal. Often, the stereotypy is a form of sadomasochistic clinging adaptation of therapist and patient at levels of minimal functioning, with a refusal to acknowledge or act on the separateness of each participant. In consultation with psychotherapeutic colleagues, with the use of medication, and, on occasion, with hospital admission, it is often possible to resolve these painful and counterproductive behaviors through communication. The patient can then resume development with the same therapist or a new one.

Finally, as termination of therapy approaches and the inevitable reliving of partially remembered pathologically organized states occurs, the patient is capable of holding on to what has been gained, locating it largely within the possibilities of the self, without need of the therapist's actual presence. This individual psychotherapy termination is an adolescence-like experience during which the locus of value, of boundary organization, and of important love objects are all reworked and reintegrated in order to separate from the therapist and be an individual with responsibility for and authority over one's own life. The temptation to replace sadness with hatefully re-created psychotic organizations of the self during this period makes it a difficult time. It is, as well, usually a joyful and intense period, for both patient and therapist.

REFERENCES

Anderson C M, Hogarty G E, Reiss D J: Family treatment of adult schizophrenic patients: A psycho-educational approach. Schizophr Bull *6:* 490, 1980.

Burnham D L: *Schizophrenia and the Need-Fear Dilemma.* International Universities Press, New York, 1969.

Erikson E H: Identity and the life cycle. In *Psychological Issues,* G S Klein, editor, Monograph 1. International Universities Press, New York, 1959.

Federn P: *Ego Psychology and the Psychoses.* Basic Books, New York, 1952.

Freud S: An autobiographical account of a case of paranoia. In *Standard Edition of the Complete Psychological Works of Sigmund Freud,* vol 12, p 9. Hogarth Press, London, 1958.

Fromm-Reichmann F: *Principles of Intensive Psychotherapy.* University of Chicago Press, Chicago, 1950.

Gill M: *Analysis of Transference,* vol 1, *Theory and Technique.* In *Psychological Issues,* Monograph 53. International Universities Press, New York, 1982.

Hill L B: *Psychotherapeutic Intervention in Schizophrenia.* University of Chicago Press, Chicago, 1955.

Kernberg O F: *Severe Personality Disorders.* Yale University Press, New Haven, CT, 1984.

Kohut H: *The Restoration of the Self.* International Universities Press, New York, 1977.

Lidz T: *The Origin and Treatment of Schizophrenic Disorders.* Basic Books, New York, 1973.

Loewald H W: *Papers on Psychoanalysis.* Yale University Press, New Haven, CT, 1980.

Meyer A: Undergraduate instruction in psychiatry. In *The Collected Papers of Adolf Meyer,* vol 3, p 100. Johns Hopkins University Press, Baltimore, 1951.

Pao P-N: *Schizophrenic Disorders.* International Universities Press, New York, 1979.

Racker E: *Transference and Counter-transference.* Hogarth Press, London, 1968.

Rosenfeld H A: *Psychotic States.* International Universities Press, New York, 1965.

Schulz C G: The contribution of the concept of self-representation—object-representation differentiation to the understanding of the schizophrenias. In *The Course of Life: Psychoanalytic Contributions Toward Understanding Personality Development.* S I Greenspan, G H Pollock, editors, vol 3, p 453. US Government Printing Office, Washington, DC, 1981.

Schwartz D P: Loving action and the shape of the object. In *Toward a Comprehensive Model for Schizophrenic Disorders.* D Feinsilver, editor, p 323. Analytic Press, Hillsdale, NJ, 1986.

Searles H F: *Collected Papers on Schizophrenia.* International Universities Press, New York, 1965.

Segal H: *Introduction to the Work of Melanie Klein.* Basic Books, New York, 1974.

Sullivan H S: *Schizophrenia as a Human Process.* Norton, New York, 1962.

Wexler M: The structural problem in schizophrenia. In *Psychotherapy with Schizophrenics,* E B Brody, F C Redlich, editors. International Universities Press, New York, 1952.

Will O A: The reluctant patient, the unwanted psychotherapist—and coercion. Contemp Psychoanal *5:* 1, 1968.

Winnicott D W: *Collected Papers: Through Paediatrics to Psychoanalysis.* Basic Books, New York, 1958.

15 DELUSIONAL (PARANOID) DISORDERS

THEO C. MANSCHRECK, M.D.

INTRODUCTION

Delusional (paranoid) disorders comprise a heterogeneous group of disorders of unknown etiology whose hallmark and chief feature is the delusion. Criteria in the revised third edition of the American Psychiatric Association's *Diagnostic and Statistical Manual of Mental Disorders* (DSM-III-R) provide reliable means for identifying cases and developing systematic information about these conditions. The category of delusional disorders replaces the earlier third edition of the American Psychiatric Association's *Diagnostic and Statistical Manual of Mental Disorders* (DSM-III) category of paranoid disorders. The term "delusional" has been chosen to avoid certain confusions about the term "paranoid" and to emphasize that the category includes disorders in which delusions other than those of the persecutory or jealous type are present. Although these criteria reflect progress, their validity is only partly established. Knowledge must grow substantially if one is to master this area of psychopathology.

Because delusional disorders are believed to be uncommon, and because paranoid features are ubiquitous in medical and psychiatric disorders, a critical aim of this chapter is to underline the importance of careful diagnosis, especially differential diagnosis.

DEFINITION

The diagnosis of delusional (paranoid) disorder, according to DSM-III-R, can be made when a patient exhibits nonbizarre delusions of at least 1 month's duration that cannot be attributed to other psychiatric disorders. Definitions of the term "delusion" and types relevant to delusional disorders are presented in Table 15-1. The criteria for delusional (paranoid) disorder are presented in Table 15-2. The term "nonbizarre" means that the delusions must be about situations that can occur in real life (e.g., being followed, infected, loved at a distance). There are several types of such delusions, and the predominant type is specified in making the diagnosis.

Generally, the nonbizarre delusions of these disorders are well systematized and logically developed. The individual may experience auditory or visual hallucinations, but they are not prominent features. The behavioral and emotional responses of the individual to the delusion appear to be appropriate. Impairment of functioning or personality deterioration is minimal, if it occurs at all.

Induced psychotic disorder (shared paranoid disorder) is defined in Table 15-3. This unusual condition has also been called folie à deux. It requires an absence of psychotic disorder prior to the onset of the induced delusion. It is considered in this chapter because it has usually been classified with paranoid disorder.

HISTORY A major change in the DSM-III-R classification is to emphasize the central role of delusions in these disorders and to steer away from the more vague label of paranoid, which in English has become synonymous with suspicious. The history of the paranoid concept indicates that controversy and confusion surrounding its use are not new. The term "paranoia" was coined by the ancient Greeks from roots meaning beside and self. Hippocrates applied this term to delirium associated with high fever, but other writers used it to describe demented conditions and madness. It sometimes meant "thinking amiss," "folly," and the like. Hence, its meaning was unclear. For centuries, the term "paranoia" fell into disuse, until a revival of interest in the nineteenth century.

Karl Kahlbaum, in 1863, classified paranoia as a separate mental illness; "a form of partial insanity, which, throughout the course of the disease, principally affected the sphere of the intellect." Influenced by the current method of empirical medicine, Kahlbaum emphasized the importance of natural history in mental illness, and restricted the term "paranoia" to a persistent delusional illness that remained unchanged throughout its course. Paranoid features, he noted, could occur in a number of medical and psychiatric conditions.

Emil Kraepelin found the paranoid concept troublesome and altered his thinking on it with each edition of his textbook. His final view called for three types of paranoid disorder. Like Kahlbaum, Kraepelin based his conclusions upon analysis of the natural history of mental disorders, and particularly upon outcome. He restricted the definition of paranoia to a rare (he saw 19 cases during his career), insidious, chronic illness characterized by a fixed delusional system, an absence of hallucinations, and a lack of deterioration of the personality. The types of delusions included persecutory, grandiose, somatic, jealous, and possibly hypochondriacal. He considered this illness a psychogenic disorder, grouped with hysteria, a disorder of intellect caused by constitutional abnormalities and environmental factors. Paraphrenia was a second paranoid disorder that developed later than dementia precox and was milder. There were hallucinations (auditory in particular), but no deterioration (dementia). Finally, there was dementia paranoides, an illness that initially resembled paranoia, but that had an earlier onset and showed a deteriorating course. Because of this latter feature, Kraepelin considered dementia paranoides a form of dementia precox, which arose from disorders of thought, volition, and emotional incongruity. Mayer's follow-up of Kraepelin's 78 paraphrenia cases challenged the validity of this category because the vast majority showed an outcome indistinguishable from dementia precox, casting doubt on the separability of this group. Karl Kolle's follow-up of Kraepelin's paranoia cases indicated some overlap with dementia precox. Kraepelin also emphasized that isolated paranoid symptoms occurred in a variety of psychiatric and medical illnesses.

Eugen Bleuler also recognized paranoia (although he broadened its definition to include cases with hallucinations), a paranoid form of dementia precox (which he called schizophrenia), and an intermediate group, but thought that Kraepelin's paranoia was so rare that it did not warrant a separate classification. Further, he argued that schizophrenic symptoms must be suspected and carefully sought after even in these cases. Paraphrenia and intermediate states, he held, were forms of schizophrenia linked by "much that was identical," and, in particular, a common disturbance in associative processes. He also emphasized that paranoid symptoms occurred in other conditions and that to label them schizophrenic required at least one of the fundamental symptoms: loosened associations, ambivalence, inappropriate affect, and autism.

Sigmund Freud used the autobiographical writings of Judge Daniel Schreber to illustrate the role of psychological defense mechanisms in the development of paranoid symptoms. He proposed that Schreber's illness involved a process of denial or contradiction of repressed homosexual impulses toward his father. Persecutory and other delusions (see subsection on etiology) result from projecting these denied yearnings into the environment. He did not differentiate subtypes of paranoid disorder and added to the confusion by proposing that the term "paraphrenia" be substituted for dementia precox or schizophrenia. The major impact of Freud's work was to suggest

TABLE 15-1
DSM-III-R Definition of Delusion and Certain Common Types Associated with Delusional Disorders

DELUSION A false personal belief based on incorrect inference about external reality and firmly sustained in spite of what almost everyone else believes and in spite of what constitutes incontrovertible and obvious proof or evidence to the contrary. The belief is not one ordinarily accepted by other members of the person's culture or subculture (i.e., it is not an article of religious faith).

When a false belief involves an extreme value judgment, it is regarded as a delusion only when the judgment is so extreme as to defy credibility. Example: If someone claims he or she is terrible and has disappointed his or her family, this is generally not regarded as a delusion even if an objective assessment of the situation would lead observers to think otherwise; but if someone claims he or she is the worst sinner in the world, this would generally be considered a delusional conviction. Similarly, a person judged by most people to be moderately underweight who asserts that he or she is fat would not be regarded as delusional; but one with anorexia nervosa who, at the point of extreme emaciation, insists he or she is fat could rightly be considered delusional.

A delusion should be distinguished from a hallucination, which is a false sensory perception (although a hallucination may give rise to the delusion that the perception is true). A delusion is also to be distinguished from an overvalued idea, in which an unreasonable belief or idea is not as firmly held as is the case with a delusion.

Delusions are subdivided according to their content. Some of the more common types are listed below.

Delusion of being controlled A delusion in which feelings, impulses, thoughts, or actions are experienced as being not one's own, as being imposed by some external force. This does not include the mere conviction that one is acting as an agent of God, has had a curse placed on him or her, is the victim of fate, or is not sufficiently assertive. The symptom should be judged present only when the subject experiences his or her will, thoughts, or feelings as operating under some external force. Examples: A man claimed that his words were not his own, but those of his father; a student believed that his actions were under the control of a yogi; a housewife believed that sexual feelings were being put into her body from without.

Delusion, bizarre A false belief that involves a phenomenon that the person's culture would regard as totally implausible. Example: A man believed that when his adenoids had been removed in childhood, a box had been inserted into his head, and that wires had been placed in his head so that the voice he heard was that of the governor.

Delusion, grandiose A delusion whose content involves an exaggerated sense of one's importance, power, knowledge, or identity. It may have a religious, somatic, or other theme.

Delusion, nihilistic A delusion involving the theme of nonexistence of the self or part of the self, others, or the world. Examples: "The world is finished"; "I no longer have a brain"; "There is no need to eat, because I have no insides." A somatic delusion may also be a nihilistic delusion if the emphasis is on nonexistence of the body or a part of the body.

Delusion, persecutory A delusion in which the central theme is that a person or group is being attacked, harassed, cheated, persecuted, or conspired against. Usually the subject or someone or some group or institution close to him or her is singled out as the object of the persecution.

It is recommended that the term *paranoid delusion* not be used, because its meanings are multiple, confusing, and contradictory. It has often been employed to refer to both persecutory and grandiose delusions because of their presence in the paranoid type of schizophrenia.

Delusion of poverty A delusion that the person is, or will be, bereft of all, or virtually all, material possessions.

Delusion of reference A delusion whose theme is that events, objects, or other people in the person's immediate environment have a particular and unusual significance, usually of a negative or pejorative nature. It differs from an idea of reference, in which the false belief is not as firmly held as in a delusion. If the delusion of reference involves a persecutory theme, then a delusion of persecution is present as well. Examples: A woman was convinced that programs on the radio were directed especially to her: when recipes were broadcast, it was to tell her to prepare wholesome food for her child and stop feeding her candy; when dance music was broadcast, it was to tell her to stop what she was doing and start dancing, and perhaps even to resume ballet lessons. A patient noted that the room number of his therapist's office was the same as the number of the hospital room in which his father died and believed that this meant there was a plot to kill him.

Delusion, somatic A delusion whose main content pertains to the functioning of one's body. Examples: One's brain is rotting; one is pregnant despite being postmenopausal.

Extreme value judgments about the body may, under certain circumstances, also be considered somatic delusions. Example: A person insists that his nose is grossly misshapen despite lack of confirmation of this by observers.

Hypochondriacal delusions are also somatic delusions when they involve specific changes in the functioning or structure of the body rather than merely an insistent belief that one has a disease.

Delusion, systematized A single delusion with multiple elaborations or a group of delusions that are all related by the person to a single event or theme. Example: A man who failed his bar examination developed the delusion that this occurred because of a conspiracy involving the university and the bar association. He then attributed all other difficulties in his social and occupational life to this continuing conspiracy.

Delusional jealousy The delusion that one's sexual partner is unfaithful.

Table from DSM-III-R *Diagnostic and Statistical Manual of Mental Disorders*, ed 3, revised, p 395. Copyright American Psychiatric Association, Washington, DC, 1987. Used with permission.

hypotheses that indicated the relationship between certain delusions and personality.

Ernst Kretschmer's work on the theory of paranoia emphasized that certain sensitive personalities, characterized by depressive, pessimistic, and narcissistic traits, developed paranoid features acutely when key or precipitating experiences occurred at critical moments in their lives. He observed that these individuals failed to develop schizophrenic conditions and had a favorable prognosis.

Current views Current views are based on these historical antecedents. The development of DSM-III introduced greater rigor in the assessment of disorders in which paranoid features may occur. Moreover, the awareness that paranoid features result from numerous conditions has had a positive influence on the diagnostic process.

Much of current clinical and research writing on paranoid conditions has characteristically avoided defining paranoid, however, apparently because it has assumed that everyone knows what paranoid means. Adding to the muddle is a variety of related adjectives, such as paranoiac and paranoic.

In popular and literary usage, the term "paranoid" has come to mean insane, angrily suspicious, distrustful, or irrationally irritable; it thus has come to carry no more meaning than it did among the ancient Greeks. The paranoid concept, however clumsy it may be, continues to be used routinely in clinical work. Because it is necessary to differentiate conditions with paranoid features, a useful paranoid concept is essential.

CLARIFICATION OF THE PARANOID CONCEPT

Paranoid features (signs and symptoms) are among the most dramatic and serious disturbances in psychiatry and medicine. Nevertheless, the term "paranoid" refers to a variety of behaviors that are often not psychopathological and certainly are not necessarily related to schizophrenia. Hence, use of the word "paranoid" is so varied that its meaning has become obscure. Some clinicians label ordinary suspiciousness as paranoid. Others restrict its use to persecutory delusions. Still

TABLE 15-2
Diagnostic Criteria for Delusional Disorder

A. Nonbizarre delusion(s) (i.e., involving situations that occur in real life, such as being followed, poisoned, infected, loved at a distance, having a disease, being deceived by one's spouse or lover) of at least 1 month's duration.

B. Auditory or visual hallucinations, if present, are not prominent [as defined in Schizophrenia, A(1)(b)].

C. Apart from the delusion(s) or its ramifications, behavior is not obviously odd or bizarre.

D. If a major depressive or manic syndrome has been present during the delusional disturbance, the total duration of all episodes of the mood syndrome has been brief relative to the total duration of the delusional disturbance.

E. Has never met criterion A for schizophrenia, and it cannot be established that an organic factor initiated and maintained the disturbance.

Specify type: The following types are based on the predominant delusional theme. If no single delusional theme predominates, specify as **unspecified type.**

Erotomanic type
Delusional disorder in which the predominant theme of the delusion(s) is that a person, usually of higher status, is in love with the subject.

Grandiose type
Delusional disorder in which the predominant theme of the delusion(s) is one of inflated worth, power, knowledge, identity, or special relationship to a deity or famous person.

Jealous type
Delusional disorder in which the predominant theme of the delusion(s) is that one's sexual partner is unfaithful.

Persecutory type
Delusional disorder in which the predominant theme of the delusion(s) is that one (or someone to whom one is close) is being malevolently treated in some way. People with this type of delusional disorder may repeatedly take their complaints of being mistreated to legal authorities.

Somatic type
Delusional disorder in which the predominant theme of the delusion(s) is that the person has some physical defect, disorder, or disease.

Unspecified type
Delusional disorder that does not fit any of the previous categories, e.g., persecutory and grandiose themes without a predominance of either; delusions of reference without malevolent content.

Table from DSM-III-R *Diagnostic and Statistical Manual of Mental Disorders,* ed 3, revised. Copyright American Psychiatric Association, Washington, DC, 1987. Used with permission.

TABLE 15-3
Diagnostic Criteria for Induced Psychotic Disorder

A. A delusion develops (in a second person) in the context of a close relationship with another person, or persons, with an already established delusion (the primary case).

B. The delusion in the second person is similar in content to that in the primary case.

C. Immediately before onset of the induced delusion, the second person did not have a psychotic disorder or the prodromal symptoms of schizophrenia.

Table from DSM-III-R *Diagnostic and Statistical Manual of Mental Disorders,* ed 3, revised. Copyright American Psychiatric Association, Washington, DC, 1987. Used with permission.

others apply it to grandiose, litigious, hostile, and jealous behavior—despite the fact that these behaviors may all be within the normal spectrum. Clearly, paranoid describes a multitude of behaviors.

To make the paranoid concept clinically useful and less confusing requires the consideration of several points. First, it is a clinical construct used to interpret observations. In order to apply this construct effectively, the clinician must know its meaning and be able to make accurate observations of potentially paranoid behavior.

Second, use of the term "paranoid" means the clinician has judged that the behavior is *psychopathological*. This judgment is usually based on the discovery that the individual who displays these features is either disturbed or disturbing to others.

Third, although many contributions to understanding paranoid phenomena have focused on conditions in which they are central characteristics (e.g., in Bleuler's schizophrenia or Kraepelin's dementia paranoides), these features are not necessarily associated with schizophrenia and can appear in other psychiatric and medical disorders. Hence, paranoid features indicate psychopathology, but no specific etiology (Table 15-4) or, for that matter, chronicity or curability.

Fourth, the observations that form the basis for judging behavior to be paranoid are of two kinds: *subjective,* meaning part of the private mental experience of the patient (e.g., a delusion); and *objective,* or observable as a manifest form of behavior (e.g., litigiousness, guardedness, grandiosity). Table 15-5 lists the subjective and objective features that have traditionally been labeled paranoid and that are frequently found in association. Some of them can be entirely normal manifestations of behavior. The judgment that such behaviors are paranoid may rest on (1) their extremeness or inappropriateness, (2) their presence in combination or association with other behaviors on the list, and (3) the presence of delusions.

Fifth, and finally, paranoid delusions traditionally have referred to a wide variety of delusions, not simply those of grandeur, persecution, or jealousy. However, because of recent confusion, this term probably should not be used. Paranoid and associated terms are defined in Table 15-6.

COMPARATIVE NOSOLOGY

Certain advances have been made in the nosology of delusional disorders, but the variety of current definitions illustrates that consensus has not yet been achieved. The reasons for differences are multiple. The main one is simply a lack of relevant data. Because delusional disorders are uncommon and have minimal overt characteristics to help identify them, only limited knowledge, largely case reports, has accumulated. Systematic, larger-scale studies are uncommon. The very idea that these disorders are distinct from schizophrenia and mood disorders has until recently been unacceptable to many psychiatrists.

Kahlbaum was the first to use the term "paranoia" to designate a diagnostically separate group of disorders. Kraepelin developed this diagnostic concept further by emphasizing the chronic and unremitting nature of paranoia and its lack of other features, such as hallucinations, that distinguished it from schizophrenia. The first diagnostic manual of the American Psychiatric Association (DSM-I) incorporated these ideas in 1952 and defined paranoid reactions as conditions with persecutory or grandiose delusions, with emotional responses and behavior consistent with the delusions and generally without hallucinations. The subtypes were paranoia (a chronic disorder with systematized delusions) and paranoid state (a more acute, less persistent condition with less systematized

TABLE 15-4
Conditions Associated with Delusions and Other Paranoid Features

- Neurological disorders
  - Arteriosclerotic psychoses
  - Blunt head trauma
  - Brain tumors
  - Cerebrovascular disease
  - Delirium
  - Dementia
  - Fat embolism
  - Hearing loss
  - Huntington's chorea
  - Hydrocephalus
  - Hypertensive encephalopathy
  - Idiopathic basal ganglia calcification
  - Idiopathic Parkinson's disease
  - Intracranial hemorrhage
  - Marchiafava-Bignami disease
  - Menzel-type ataxia
  - Metachromatic leukodystrophy
  - Migraine
  - Motor-neuron disease
  - Multiple sclerosis
  - Muscular dystrophy
  - Narcolepsy
  - Postencephalitic parkinsonism
  - Presenile psychoses (Alzheimer's and Pick's diseases)
  - Roussy-Levy syndrome
  - Senile psychoses
  - Spinocerebellar degeneration
  - Subarachnoid hemorrhage
  - Subdural hematoma
  - Temporal lobe epilepsy
- Metabolic and endocrine disorders
  - Acute intermittent porphyria
  - Addison's disease
  - Complication of surgical portacaval anastomosis for cirrhosis
  - Cushing's syndrome
  - Folate deficiency
  - Hemodialysis
  - Hypercalcemia
  - Hypoglycemia
  - Hyponatremia
  - Hypopituitarism
  - Liver failure
  - Malnutrition
  - Niacin deficiency
  - Pancreatic encephalopathy
  - Parathyroid disorders
  - Pellagra
  - Pernicious anemia
  - Phenylketonuria
  - Systemic lupus erythematosus
  - Thiamine deficiency
  - Thyroid disorders
  - Uremia
  - Vitamin B_{12} deficiency
  - Wilson's disease
- Sex chromosome disorders
  - 47 XXY
  - Klinefelter's syndrome
  - Turner's syndrome
- Infections
  - Acquired immune deficiency syndrome (AIDS)
  - Encephalitis lethargica
  - Creutzfeldt-Jakob disease
  - Malaria
  - Syphilis
  - Toxic shock syndrome
  - Trypanosomiasis
  - Typhus
  - Viral encephalitides
- Psychiatric disorders
  - Brief reactive psychosis
  - Delusional disorders (including classical paranoia)
  - Induced psychotic disorder
  - Mood disorders
  - Schizoaffective disorder
  - Schizophrenia (all subtypes)
  - Schizophreniform disorder
- Alcohol and drug abuse disorders
  - Alcohol withdrawal
  - Amphetamine
  - Anesthetic nitrous oxide
  - Atropine toxicity
  - Barbiturate
  - Chronic alcohol hallucinosis
  - Chronic bromide intoxication
  - Cocaine
  - Ephedrine
  - Marijuana
  - Mescaline and other hallucinogens
  - Perbitine
  - Withdrawal from minor tranquilizers and hypnotic medications
- Toxic agents
  - Arsenic
  - Carbon monoxide
  - Manganese
  - Mercury
  - Thallium
- Pharmacological agents
  - ACTH
  - Amphetamine and related compounds
  - Anticholinergic drugs
  - Antimalarials
  - Antitubercular drugs
  - Bromocriptine
  - Buproprion
  - Cimetidine
  - Cortisone
  - Diphenylhydantoin
  - Disulfiram
  - L-Dopa
  - Imipramine and other tricyclic antidepressants
  - Mephentermine
  - Methyldopa and imipramine (combination)
  - Methyltestosterone
  - Pentazocine
  - Phenylpropanolamine
  - Prophylhexedrine

delusions). The second edition of the *Diagnostic and Statistical Manual of Mental Disorders* (DSM-II) in 1968 largely preserved these concepts.

DSM-III: PARANOID DISORDERS In 1980, new definitions of these disorders were established, but the earlier concepts of these conditions are still evident. The essential features of these disorders are persistent persecutory delusions or delusional jealousy not attributable to any other mental disorder. Included in the group of paranoid disorders are paranoia, shared paranoid disorder, acute paranoid disorder, and a residual category, atypical paranoid disorder. The boundaries between these conditions and other disorders, such as paranoid personality disorder or schizophrenia, paranoid subtype, are noted to be vague. Different types of paranoid disorders are classified on the basis of chronicity. The criteria narrow the bounds of previous classifications by not including cases with marked hallucinations or a variety of delusional types (e.g., hypochondriacal, love).

DSM-III-R: DELUSIONAL (PARANOID) DISORDERS DSM-III-R simplifies the DSM-III definitions, attempts to

TABLE 15-5
Paranoid Features

Objective features
- Anger
- Critical, accusatory behavior
- Defensiveness
- Grandiosity or excessive self-importance
- Guardedness, evasiveness
- Hate
- Hostility
- Humorlessness
- Hypersensitivity
- Inordinate attention to small details
- Irritability, quick annoyance
- Litigiousness (letter writing, complaints, legal action)
- Obstinacy
- Resentment
- Seclusiveness
- Self-righteousness
- Sullenness
- Suspiciousness
- Violence, aggressiveness

Subjective features*
- Delusions of self-reference, persecution, grandeur, infidelity, love, jealousy, imposture, infestation, disfigurement
- Overvalued ideas

*Part of private mental experience. The patient often discloses these features during the clinical interview, but may not do so, even with specific questioning.

minimize the confusion of the term "paranoid," and highlights the view that the formation of delusions in the absence of schizophrenia, mood disorder, or organic illness is the essential feature of these conditions. In contrast to DSM-III, diagnosis requires a duration of 1 month. Subtyping is based on the predominant type of delusion that is specified (e.g., jealous, erotomanic, somatic). This latter feature broadens the category to include a variety of unusual delusions as well as the more common persecutory type.

Shared paranoid disorder is renamed induced psychotic disorder and is placed in the category of psychotic disorders not elsewhere classified, along with schizophreniform and schizoaffective disorders and brief reactive psychosis. This approach represents a fundamental departure from DSM-III, which placed this disorder in the paranoid disorders. In patients with this disorder, the delusional content may not concern persecution or jealousy, hence the change in terminology. The term "induced" more accurately describes the nature of the condition, but hardly resolves the puzzle of etiology.

ICD-9 The ninth revision the World Health Organization's *International Classification of Diseases* (ICD-9) has a larger number of categories for paranoid disorder than the U.S. schemes (Table 15-7). Most paranoid disorders fall under the rubric "paranoid state," including simple paranoid state, paranoia, paraphrenia, and induced psychosis. Additional subcategories include other and unspecified paranoid states. Acute paranoid reactions and psychogenic paranoid psychosis are classified separately. DSM-III and DSM-III-R generally maintain an atheoretical position with respect to etiology in these disorders, whereas ICD-9 is less neutral. For example, psychogenic paranoid psychosis implies a kind of causal mechanism. The categories of paranoid disorder according to these classifications are summarized in Table 15-8.

EPIDEMIOLOGY

Delusional disorders have been considered uncommon, if not rare, conditions from their earliest descriptions. Little is known about the epidemiology. Recent demographic evidence covering a period from 1912 to the 1970s provides an estimate of their incidence and prevalence and related statistics (Table 15-9). However, this evidence was assembled using definitions that are not the same as those of DSM-III or DSM-III-R. The figures will, in all likelihood, be somewhat different using the newer criteria. Clearly, they are merely indications, but they should serve as useful guidelines to future appraisals of these conditions.

Certain features are remarkable. For example, the stability of incidence has been striking over extended periods of time in this century. The prevalence of these disorders substantiates the widely held clinical impression that they are

TABLE 15-6
Terminology Connected with Paranoia

Term	*Description*
Delusional (paranoid) disorders	DSM-III-R category emphasizing that the cardinal feature of these conditions is delusions.
Paranoia	Old term for an insidiously developed disorder in which individuals suffer from an unshakable delusional system but have no disturbance in the clarity or form of their thinking. Also known as paranoia vera, simple delusional disorder, delusional monomania.
Paranoic or paranoiac	Old adjectives used to describe individuals with paranoia.
Paranoid	Broad term meaning suspicious to most people. In psychiatry, however, it is a clinical construct used to describe various objective and subjective features of behavior deemed to be psychopathologic. See Table 15-5 for a list of such behaviors. It refers to no specific condition (e.g., to be paranoid does not mean that schizophrenic disorder is present).
Paranoid delusion	Older term used to refer to persecutory and grandiose delusions because of their occurrence in the paranoid subtype of schizophrenia. This term has suffered from the confusion associated with the paranoid concept. DSM-III-R recommends that it not be used.
Paranoid disorders	DSM-III term for an idiopathic group of conditions including paranoia, acute paranoid disorder, shared paranoid disorder, and atypical paranoid disorder.
Paranoid personality	Enduring traits of paranoid behavior not due to schizophrenia or other mental disorder. Generally, there is no evidence of delusions or other features of psychosis.
Paranoid syndrome	Term applied to constellations of paranoid features that occur together and can arise from multiple sources, including depression, organic disorder, and schizophrenia.
Paraphrenia	Old term for conditions lying theoretically between schizophrenia and paranoia and sharing features of both (e.g., hallucinations but no deterioration). It, too, remains controversial and probably should not be used until research validates its meaning.

TABLE 15-7
ICD-9 Criteria for Paranoid States and Other Nonorganic Psychoses

Paranoid states

Excludes: acute paranoid reaction
alcoholic jealousy
paranoid schizophrenia

Paranoid state, simple

A psychosis, acute or chronic, not classifiable as schizophrenia or affective psychosis, in which delusions, especially of being influenced, persecuted, or treated in some special way, are the main symptoms. The delusions are of a fairly fixed, elaborate, and systematized kind.

Paranoia

A rare chronic psychosis in which logically constructed systematized delusions have developed gradually without concomitant hallucinations or the schizophrenic type of disordered thinking. The delusions are mostly of grandeur [the paranoiac prophet or inventor], persecution, or somatic abnormality.

Excludes: paranoid personality disorder

Paraphrenia

Paranoid psychosis in which there are conspicuous hallucinations, often in several modalities. Affective symptoms and disordered thinking, if present, do not dominate the clinical picture and the personality is well preserved.

Involutional paranoid state, late paraphrenia

Induced psychosis

Mainly delusional psychosis, usually chronic and often without florid features, which appears to have developed as a result of a close, if not dependent relationship with another person who already has an established similar psychosis. The delusions are at least partly shared. The rare cases in which several persons are affected should also be included here.

Folie à deux, induced paranoid disorder

Other

Paranoid states that, though in many ways akin to schizophrenic or affective states, cannot readily be classified under any of the preceding rubrics or under psychogenic paranoid psychosis (see below).

Paranoia querulans, Sensitiver Beziehungswahn

Excludes: senile paranoid state

Unspecified

Paranoid: psychosis NOS, reaction NOS, state NOS

Other nonorganic psychoses

Acute paranoid reaction

Paranoid states apparently provoked by some emotional stress. The stress is often misconstrued as an attack or threat. Such states are particularly prone to occur in prisoners or as acute reactions to a strange and threatening environment, e.g., in immigrants.

Bouffée délirante

Excludes: paranoid states

Psychogenic paranoid psychosis

Psychogenic or paranoid reactive psychosis of any type that is more protracted than the acute reactions covered under acute paranoid reaction (above). Where there is a diagnosis of psychogenic paranoid psychosis that does not specify "acute," this coding should be made.

Protracted reactive paranoid psychosis

Other and unspecified reactive psychosis

Hysterical psychosis, psychogenic stupor, psychogenic psychosis NOS

Unspecified psychosis

To be used only as a last resort, when no other term can be used.

Psychosis NOS

Table from ICD-9 Classification of Mental Disorders from *Manual of the International Statistical Classification of Diseases, Injuries, or Causes of Death,* rev 9, vol 1, appendix D, World Health Organization, Geneva, 1977, with permission.

uncommon conditions (compared to mood disorders and schizophrenia) but indicates they are not rare. Patients with delusional disorders are somewhat more likely to be female (but this is an inconsistent feature) and to be relatively more disadvantaged socially and educationally than patients with mood disorders. There is suggestive evidence that immigrant status is associated with delusional disorder.

ETIOLOGY

The etiology of delusional disorders is unknown. Paranoid features, including the types of delusions encountered in these disorders, occur in a large number of conditions (Table 15-4). Differences in classifying these disorders add to the problems of understanding etiology. Theories and explanations of de-

TABLE 15-8
Comparative Nosology

ICD-9 (1979)	*DSM-III (1980)*	*DSM-III-R (1987)*
Paranoid state, simple	—	—
Paranoia	Paranoia	Delusional (paranoid) disorder
Paraphrenia (involutional paranoid state, late paraphrenia)	—	—
Induced psychosis (folie à deux, induced paranoid disorder)	Shared paranoid disorder	Induced psychotic disorder
Other specified states (paranoia querulans, Sensitiver Beziehungswahn)	—	—
Unspecified paranoid states	Atypical paranoid disorder	—
Acute paranoid reaction (bouffée délirante)	Acute paranoid disorder	—
Psychogenic paranoid psychosis (protracted reactive paranoid psychosis)	—	—

lusions abound in the literature; empirical evidence to support them, however, is limited. With so many uncertainties, conclusions concerning etiology must be made with great care.

The problem can be stated in this fashion. We are dealing with an uncommon group of illnesses, the validity of which has been questioned ever since Kahlbaum put forth his views. The major phenomenological feature of these conditions is the formation and persistence of nonbizarre delusions. It is well known that such delusions occur in a variety of psychiatric and medical conditions, and their pathogenesis is not understood in these conditions either. Hence, discussion of etiology in the delusional disorders can proceed on two lines: (1) the distinctiveness of the category itself, and (2) the theories proposed to account for delusion formation.

THE DISTINCTIVENESS OF DELUSIONAL DISORDERS An issue that is central to unraveling etiology in these uncommon disorders is whether delusional disorders are a separate group of conditions or atypical forms of schizophrenia and mood disorders. The relevant data are from a limited number of studies. Despite this, certain consistencies are apparent. Epidemiological data suggest that delusional disorders are separate. Delusional disorders are far less prevalent than schizophrenia or mood disorders. Age of onset is later than in schizophrenia. The sex ratio is different from that of mood disorder, in which the excess of females is far more pronounced. Findings from family or genetic studies also support the concept of separateness. If delusional disorders are simply unusual forms of schizophrenia or mood disorders, the incidence of these latter conditions in family studies of delusional disorder patients should be higher than that of the general population. However, this finding has not been a consistent one. Moreover, a recent study concluded that patients with delusional disorder are more likely to have family members who show suspiciousness, jealousy, secretiveness, even paranoid illness, than controls. Another study has found paranoid personality disorder to be more common in relatives of delusional disorder patients than in relatives of controls or schizophrenic patients.

Natural history investigations also lend support to the separateness of the delusional disorders category. Though riddled with methodological shortcomings, premorbid personality data indicate schizophrenic patients and patients with delusional disorder differ early on in life. The former are more likely to be introverted, schizoid, and submissive, the latter more extroverted, dominant, and hypersensitive. Delusional disorder patients may have below-average intelligence. Precipitating factors, especially related to social isolation, conflicts of conscience, and immigration, are more frequently found in delusional disorder than in schizophrenia. These characteristics support Kraepelin's view that environmental factors may have an important etiological role. Follow-up studies indicate that the diagnosis of delusional disorder remains stable: only a small proportion of cases (3 to 22 percent) are rediagnosed schizophrenic; and even fewer (6 percent) are rediagnosed as affectively ill. Outcome in terms of hospitalization and occupational adjustment is markedly more favorable for delusional disorder than for schizophrenia.

TABLE 15-9
Epidemiological Features of Delusional Disorders

Incidence*	0.7–3.0
Prevalence*	24–30
Age at onset (range)	35–45 (18–80)
Sex ratio M:F	0.85

Table adapted from Kendler K S: Demography of paranoid psychosis (delusional disorder). Arch Gen Psychiat *39:* 890, 1982.
*Incidence and prevalence figures represent cases per 100,000 population.

In sum, the evidence argues for distinctiveness of delusional disorders, but it is likely that at least some patients diagnosed as having delusional disorder will develop schizophrenia or mood disorders. Hence, clinical criteria have limitations that need to be improved, possibly with the use of laboratory techniques or more specified clinical definitions. Furthermore, the data suggest that delusional disorders are relatively chronic and probably biologically distinct from other psychotic disorders.

THEORIES OF DELUSION FORMATION Although a clear understanding of the pathogenesis of delusions remains an unfulfilled hope, several major theories have been put forward. Any adequate hypothesis for delusion formation must deal with certain facts:

1. Delusions occur in a variety of medical and psychiatric diseases.
2. Not all individuals with such conditions develop delusions.
3. The content of delusions constitutes a relatively short list of types and is strikingly repetitious despite the variety of diseases.
4. Delusions can clear rapidly with treatment of the underlying condition or its termination.
5. Delusions can persist, even become systematized.
6. Delusions often accompany perceptual changes such as hallucinations or impaired sensory input.
7. Delusions may be highly encapsulated features in individuals such that their functioning may not be compromised socially, intellectually, or affectively.

Further, any adequate hypothesis must respond to two questions: First, why does the patient have a delusion? This question concerns the form of psychopathology. Second, why does the patient have this particular delusion? This question concerns the content of the psychopathology.

PSYCHODYNAMIC MECHANISM In 1911, Freud published "Psychoanalytic Notes upon an Autobiographical Account of a Case of Paranoia (Dementia Paranoides)." His interpretation of this case became the foundation of the psychodynamic theory of paranoia and was based on his reading of the memoirs of the presiding judge of a Dresden appeals court, Daniel Paul Schreber, who had suffered two episodes of psychiatric illness in 1884 to 1885 and again in 1893. The second episode led to two prolonged hospitalizations from which the patient obtained discharge in 1902 following legal action, although he was still delusional. Freud asserted that Schreber's 1903 account, *Memoirs of My Nervous Illness*, offered a legitimate basis for theory, as "paranoiacs cannot be compelled to overcome their internal resistances, and since in any case they only say what they choose to say. . . ." Freud argued that the written case report can take the place of personal acquaintance; and in the case of Schreber, Freud never saw the patient.

Freud asserted that Schreber's case illustrated a general mechanism involving denial or contradiction and projection of repressed homosexual impulses that break out from the unconscious. The forms of delusion in paranoia can be represented as contradictions of the proposition "I (a man) love him (a man)."

Delusion of persecution In this contradiction, "I do not love him, I hate him . . .," the hate being unacceptable at the conscious level is transformed and becomes, instead, "He hates (elaborated to persecutes) me." Patients can then rationalize their anger by consciously hating those persons whom they perceive to hate them.

Delusion of love (erotomania) "I do not love him—I love her." This proposition is transformed through projection to "She loves me—and so I love her."

Delusional jealousy To protect against unwarranted, threatening impulses, the patient transforms the proposition in this manner. "I do not love him—she (a wife, lover) loves him." Hence, jealous delusions represent the transformed attractions of the deluded for the lover.

Delusion of grandiosity (megalomania) Here the contradiction is made: "I do not love him—I love myself."

The essence of the theory is that delusions represent attempts to manage the stirrings of unconscious homosexuality. The dynamics of unconscious homosexuality are similar for female as well as male patients in the classic theory.

Many theorists have added to the psychodynamic lore on delusion formation from the standpoint of understanding personality factors. For example, some of the vulnerability to delusion formation may be related to deficiently developed trust, narcissistic dynamics, or exaggerated traits, such as hypersensitivity.

Freud proposed a mechanism to account for delusions that sidesteps the distinction between form and content. Although he proposed an inferential process to account for the particular delusion, he did not clearly address the issue of why a delusion is formed rather than another symptom, such as an hallucination. Verification of Freud's hypothesized mechanism clearly rests on finding evidence that delusions are associated with indications of homosexual tendencies. The theory has been perpetuated in part because an absence of homosexuality can never be proved, and such tendencies can be used as a pillar, even if not a scientifically or empirically demonstrable pillar, in the psychodynamic argument. The few experimental attempts to test the hypothesis have been inconclusive or equivocal. Moreover, although homosexual concerns have been found among some delusional patients, the variety of conditions with delusions argues against a common mechanism of unconscious homosexuality. Indeed, the persons who persecute delusional patients are not always known by them. Furthermore, the persistence of such delusions is not adequately accounted for in this formulation. Nevertheless, this approach has had immense influence, and has provided important concepts, such as projection, and an awareness that developmental experiences may operate to influence the content of delusional thinking. Systematic empirical study should prove valuable.

PSYCHOBIOLOGICAL MECHANISM The French psychiatrist G. de Clérembault hypothesized in 1942 that chronic delusions resulted from abnormal neurological events. Infections, lesions, intoxications, and other forms of damage produce automatisms that puzzle or distress the patient initially, and eventually demand explanation. The explanations take the form of delusions. Automatisms include hallucinations, a constant parade of memories, feelings of familiarity, false recognition, arresting of thought, disturbances in attention, bizarre tactile sensations, and even kinesthetic sensation.

The view that delusions represent an explanation of hallucinations is an old concept in psychiatry that has not been formulated well. The fact that hallucinations have been introduced and retracted from the definition of delusional disorder over the years also reflects a lack of clarity regarding a possible connection between the two forms of psychopathology.

Maher has proposed a more closely argued and similar hypothesis that conceptualizes delusions as explanations of anomalous experiences that arise in the environment, the peripheral sensory system, or the central nervous system (CNS). A central tenet of his view is that the processes whereby delusional beliefs are formed are similar in their essential nature to those that operate in the formation of normal beliefs and scientific hypotheses. Integral to the hypothesis is the assumption that components of this normal operational sequence have a neural substrate, which may be activated either by sensory input (as in hallucinatory effects of drugs) or by the effects of brain damage (as in alcoholism). The activation of any part of the sequence demands explanation and may thus give rise to delusions. The sequence, activated by disturbances in sensory experience, emotional incongruity, and CNS abnormalities has the following stages: (1) anomalous experience, (2) feelings of significance, (3) testing for reality of experience, (4) developing tentative hypotheses, (5) additional observation, (6) exploring insights, and (7) confirmation of the insight by selective observation.

The patient is delusional because he or she actually experiences anomalies that demand explanation. The particulars of the delusion (its content) are drawn from the past or current circumstances, experience, and personal and cultural background of the patient. These anomalies are sources for explanatory material available to the patient. The explanation answers questions, such as: What is happening? Why? Why do other people deny it is happening? Why is it only happening to me? Who is responsible for it? The delusional explanation offers relief from puzzlement and the relief works against abandonment of the explanation.

Although this formulation has gone largely unstudied, there is some supporting evidence. Studies of patients, normals with sensory impairment, sensory deprivation, and persons abusing various drugs have demonstrated a high incidence of delusion formation. Clearly, this hypothesis warrants further examination. It is unclear how applicable it is to conditions, such as delusional disorder, where the occurrence of hallucinations is debated and sensory impairment and central nervous dysfunction have not been consistently established.

OTHER MECHANISMS AND RELEVANT FACTORS

Delusions have been linked to a variety of additional factors such as social and sensory isolation, socioeconomic deprivation, and personality disturbance. The deaf, visually impaired, and, possibly, immigrant groups with limited ability in a new language are more vulnerable to delusion formation than the normal population. This vulnerability is heightened with advanced age. In fact, delusional disturbance and other paranoid features in the elderly are common. In short, multiple factors influence the formation of delusions. Breakthroughs in specifying the source and pathogenesis of delusional disorders are still forthcoming.

PATHOLOGY

As in most psychiatric conditions, there is no evidence of localized brain pathology to correlate with clinical psychopathology. Patients with delusional disorders seldom die early and show no abnormalities on neurological examination. There are, nonetheless, some possible connections between delusion phenomenology and certain kinds of brain disorder. For example, patients with more severe cortical impairment tend to experience more simple, transient, persecutory delusions. This type of delusional experience is characteristic of conditions, such as Alzheimer's disease, multi-infarct dementia, and metabolic encephalopathy. These disorders are also associated with significant cognitive disturbance. More complex (i.e., elaborate, systematic) delusional experiences tend to be more chronic, resistant to treatment, and associated with neurological conditions producing less intellectual impairment. These features occur in cases with neurological lesions involving limbic system or subcortical nuclei rather than cortical areas.

Although a neuropathology of delusional disorders is far in the future, the available evidence suggests that if there is one, it will be subtle. Nevertheless, future empirical studies, guided by etiological hypotheses, could lead to breakthroughs. Given the uncommonness of delusional disorders, studies of cases with delusions from known causes (and with identifiable neuropathologies) offer a useful beginning point.

CLINICAL SIGNS AND SYMPTOMS

DELUSIONAL DISORDERS DSM-III-R defines the core psychopathological feature of delusional disorder as persistent, nonbizarre delusions not explained by other psychotic disorders (Table 15-2). A precipitating event may be associated with the acute formation of the delusional thinking, or the disorder may emerge gradually and may become chronic. Behavioral and emotional responses are generally appropriate, and neither mood disorders nor the volitional, thinking, and emotional disturbances of schizophrenic illness are present.

The delusions are unusual, yet they refer to aspects of life that might be real, such as being conspired against, cheated on, physically ill, in love, jealous, and the like. They are, as George Winokur has suggested, "possible," rather than totally incredible and bizarre as are many of the delusions of schizophrenia. The types of delusions are specified according to their content. There are several types and they have been the sources of separate classifications in the past (e.g., erotomania or Clérembault's syndrome). The most common concern persecution and jealousy. The delusions are not shared with members of the patient's social group. They are fixed (i.e., persistent) and unarguable. Patients interpret facts to fit the delusion rather than modifying the delusion to fit the facts. There is systematization in the delusional thinking, meaning that a single theme or series of connected themes is present with links to the predominant delusion.

Many researchers have pointed to a descriptive continuum between paranoid personality disorder, delusional disorders, and the paranoid subtype of schizophrenia in terms of degrees of disorganization and impairment. However, there is little evidence to support the concept that these disorders share more than overlapping psychopathology. In general, patients with delusional disorders show little disorganization or impairment in their behavior or in the clarity of their thinking.

The presence of hallucinations in such disorders has been debated. Some researchers argue that schizophrenia is a more likely diagnosis in such cases, whereas others are not concerned so long as the hallucinations are not marked and persistent. The resolution of this issue remains distant, but it is reasonable to consider infrequent hallucinations that are not a prominent part of the psychopathology to be a feature of delusional disorder. These hallucinations are usually auditory, but may be visual, and tend to be more common in acute cases. Other types of hallucinations are rare.

Emotional contact and affective behavior are generally intact. The emotional response is frequently consistent with the delusional concern, and the mood is often appropriately depressed. Restlessness and agitation may be present. Loquaciousness and circumstantiality, usually accompanying descriptions of the delusions, are found in some patients, but formal thought disorder as sometimes found in schizophrenia is absent.

Associated features in delusional disorders include those of the paranoid syndrome (Table 15-5). The degree of hostility and suspiciousness may be such that violent or aggressive behavior results. Litigious behavior is common among such patients.

Persecutory type A 30-year-old college-educated man was living alone, seclusive, and working as a clerk in a printing supplies store when he presented with suspiciousness, apprehension, and agitation. He claimed that he did not need to be in a psychiatric clinic, but had been referred by an acquaintance because he was so worried. He explained that he was upset because his brother was plotting to keep him out of the family inheritance. There was no evidence of hallucinations or confusion, and the patient's thinking was clear and logical. The brother, a successful businessman, allegedly made remarks which the patient interpreted as unsubtle suggestions that he move away from his parents' hometown. With the patient out of the way, he reasoned, the brother would be able to endear himself to the elderly parents, who had been disappointed by the patient's lack of success in the work world.

The patient's delusional thinking responded initially to antipsychotic medication, in that the agitation, preoccupation with, and conviction concerning the delusions diminished. However, the patient has now harbored the delusions for more than a decade, despite antipsychotic drug treatment and numerous attempts by the family to present the facts and reassure the patient. The conspiracy has broadened to include various therapists, employers, and neighbors of the patient.

The delusion of persecution is the classic symptom of delusional disorder. This type and the jealousy type are probably the most common forms seen clinically by psychiatrists.

In contrast to persecutory delusions in schizophrenia, the

clarity, logic, and systematic elaboration of the persecutory theme in delusional disorder leave a remarkable stamp on this condition.

Jealous type A 32-year-old man was taken to the hospital by police following complaints by neighbors that he was beating his wife. The patient denied psychiatric illness and reported that he was feeling depressed because his wife was having an affair. The patient had spent large amounts of time trying to prove his suspicions about infidelity. He phoned frequently to see what his wife was doing; laid traps (e.g., placed tape recorders in the bedroom) before he went to work; checked her purse, clothes, and phone bill frequently for "evidence"; and commented that he was planning to buy a video camera to document his wife's indiscretions. On numerous occasions, he interrogated her about past lovers. This pattern had begun just prior to his marriage, and the delusion of infidelity had emerged fully formed within 2 months after the wedding.

The patient was admitted to the hospital, but argued vigorously and angrily that he was not ill. He threatened lawsuits, kept extensive notes, and made numerous complaints to the hospital administration. His affect was intense and appropriate. He showed no signs of perceptual, cognitive, or thinking disturbances. The delusion remained unchanged for several months despite a trial of antipsychotic medications. His continued threats to harm his wife led to legal commitment. His wife separated from and then divorced him. This change coincided with reduced activity about the delusion but did not lead to its remission.

Delusional disorder with delusions of infidelity has been called conjugal paranoia when it is limited to the delusion that a spouse has been unfaithful. The eponym "Othello syndrome" has also been used to name this condition. This delusion usually afflicts males and usually with no prior psychiatric illness. It may appear suddenly and serve to "explain" a host of present and past events involving the spouse's infidelity. Difficult to treat, this condition may diminish only on separation, divorce, or death of the spouse.

Jealousy is also a common symptom (usually termed pathological or morbid jealousy) of many disorders, including schizophrenia, epilepsy, mood disorders, drug abuse, and alcoholism, for which treatment is directed at the primary disorder. Jealousy is a powerful emotion; when it occurs in delusional disorder or as part of another condition, it can be a potentially dangerous feature and has been associated with both suicide and homicide.

Erotomanic type A 23-year-old woman presented to the walk-in clinic in a state of anxiety with concerns that her true love, a star of a local athletic team, might already be married. The patient explained that she had never really met or talked with the local celebrity but that she had been at a crowded party several months ago, where she had stood approximately 10 feet away from him. She knew within hours after the party that he loved her, and she in turn loved him. She had sent letters, had phoned repeatedly, and even waited outside the sports arena to meet her love. These attempts to communicate had not been successful, but only confirmed her suspicion that he was having difficulty keeping the relationship and his desires secret.

The patient showed no other symptoms except for mild anxiety and depressed mood, appropriate to her concerns. There was no prior history of psychiatric illness. Antipsychotic medication was not prescribed, and the patient underwent a brief period of supportive psychotherapy. This case remitted briefly, but relapsed later when a new lover was identified.

These patients have delusions of secret lovers. Most frequently, the patient is a woman, but men are also susceptible to this delusion. The patient believes that a suitor, usually more socially prominent than herself, is in love with her. The delusion becomes the central focus of the patient's existence. Its onset can be acute.

Erotomania, the *psychose passionelle,* is also referred to as Clérembault's syndrome to emphasize its occurrence in different disorders. Besides being the key symptom in some cases of delusional disorder, it is well known to occur in schizophrenia, mood disorder, and organic disorder.

Somatic type A 38-year-old white, single male went to treatment complaining that his nose was irregular in shape and that he was losing all his hair. His nose was normal in appearance and he had no evidence of premature baldness. He had been reassured about this repeatedly not only by his family doctor, but also by specialists with whom he consulted. He believed all his doctors were quacks or trying to get rid of him.

He had been mildly depressed and irritable in response to the change in his appearance, which he claimed was due to medicine he had received years before from a physician. He could not explain why he was so troubled now even though his appearance had been altered for a long time. Trained as an upholsterer, he had been able to work at times, but when he became more delusional, he was too fearful to go to his job, was unable to remain in his apartment, and refused to go to his parents' home. There was no evidence of confusion, neurovegetative features of depression, memory impairment, or bizarre delusions. There were no hallucinations and he had no insight into his illness. Family history was negative. He responded gradually to antipsychotic medication, which he reluctantly took.

Delusional disorders with hypochondriacal delusions have been called monosymptomatic hypochondriacal psychoses. These conditions differ from others with hypochondriacal symptoms in degree of reality impairment. In delusional disorder, delusions are fixed and unarguable. In contrast, hypochondriacs are often aware that their fear of illness is groundless. The content of the delusion may vary widely from case to case but can include delusions of infestation, parasitosis, personal ugliness, misshapenness, or exaggerated size of body parts, and foul smell.

The frequency of these conditions is low, but they may be underdiagnosed, as they may present to dermatologists, plastic surgeons, and infectious disease specialists more readily than to psychiatrists. Several recent reports indicate that pimozide (Orap, a diphenylbutyliperidine and a highly specific dopamine blocker) may be effective in treatment of such disorders, even in cases with a variety of delusional themes. There may be a heightened association of folie à deux (induced psychotic disorder) involving primary cases of hypochondriacal delusion. One study reported a quarter of cases with such an association.

Grandiose type A 49-year-old married woman was taken to the hospital by her family because they feared she would be arrested for disturbing the peace. For several months the patient had become aware of special abilities for healing the sick and she began to preach in her neighborhood about her powers. The patient was scornful and angry both toward the physician and her family whom she perceived to be railroading her into treatment when in fact she was not at all ill. On admission, the patient calmed considerably and began to discuss her abilities with other patients. Her affect lost much of its intensity, remained entirely appropriate, and there was no other evidence of psychopathology including euphoria. Eventually, the delusional concerns began to increase, and the patient complained that there was a conspiracy to prevent her from using her special powers. At discharge, there was no change in the delusion, but there was a reduction in activity associated with it.

Delusions of grandeur (megalomania) have been noted for years. They were described in Kraepelin's paranoia and have been associated with conditions fitting the description of delusional disorders.

Unspecified type This category is reserved for cases in which the predominant delusion cannot be subtyped in the previous categories. Perhaps, there are several delusions, or there may be a delusion of an unusual type that forms the central feature of the illness.

An example of the latter may be *Capgras'* delusion, named after the French psychiatrist Jean Marie Joseph Capgras, who described the *illusion des sosies* (the illusion of double). This referred to the delusion that impersonators had replaced familiar persons. Others described variants of Capgras' delusion, namely the delusion that persecutors or familiar persons could assume the guise of strangers *(Frégoli's delusion)* and the very rare delusion that familiar persons could change themselves into other persons at will *(intermetamorphosis)*. Each of these is not only rare but highly associated with schizophrenia, dementia, epilepsy, and other organic disorders. Reported cases have been predominantly female, have had associated paranoid features, and have experienced feelings of depersonalization or derealization. The delusion may be short-lived, recurrent, or persistent. It is unclear whether delusional disorder can appear with such a delusion. Certainly, the Frégoli and intermetamorphosis delusions have bizarre content and are unlikely; but the Capgras' delusion is a possible candidate.

INDUCED PSYCHOTIC DISORDER This disorder, which has several names (e.g., shared paranoid disorder, folie à deux, double insanity) was first described by E. Lasègue and J. Falret in 1877. It is probably rare, but incidence and prevalence figures are lacking. The literature consists almost entirely of single-case reports. This unusual disorder is characterized by the transfer of delusions from one person to another; both persons have been intimately associated for a long time and typically live in relative social isolation. In its most common form (folie imposée), the individual who first has the delusion (the primary case) is often chronically ill and typically is the influential member of a close relationship with a more suggestible person (the secondary case), who also develops the delusion. The secondary case is frequently less intelligent, more gullible, and passive than the primary case. If the pair separates, the secondary case may (or may not) abandon the delusion. There are other special forms, such as folie simultanée, where two people become psychotic simultaneously and share the same delusion. Occasionally, more than two individuals are involved (e.g., folie à trois, quatre, cinq; also folie à famille), but these forms are especially rare. The most common relationships in folie à deux are sister-sister, husband-wife, and mother-child; however, other combinations have also been described. Almost all cases involve members of a single family.

The secondary or recipient case has been described as submissive and low in self-esteem. The occurrence of the delusion is attributed to the strong influence of the more dominant member. Old age, low intelligence, sensory impairment, cerebrovascular disease, and alcohol abuse are among the factors associated with this peculiar form of psychotic disorder. A genetic predisposition to idiopathic psychoses has also been suggested as a possible risk factor.

There is some question as to whether patients with such conditions are truly delusional rather than highly impressionable, because frequently there is merely passive acceptance of the delusional beliefs of the more dominant person (primary case) in the relationship until they are separated, at which point the unusual belief may remit spontaneously. In the criteria, the requirement that the secondary case not have a psychotic disorder prior to onset of the induced delusion illustrates the relevance of this question. The psychopathology of secondary cases, in fact, varies. In DSM-III-R, induced psychotic disorder is classified under psychotic disorders not elsewhere classified. Some cases, however, will fit the definition of delusional disorder.

A 52-year-old man was referred by the court for inpatient psychiatric examination, charged with disturbing the peace. He had been arrested for disrupting a trial, complaining of harassment by various judges. He had walked into a courtroom, marched to the bench, and begun to berate the probate judge. While in the hospital, he related a detailed account of conspiratorial goings-on in the local judiciary. A target of certain judges, he claimed he had been singled out for a variety of reasons for many years: he knew what was going on; he had kept records of wrongdoings; and he understood the significance of the whole matter. He refused to elaborate on the specific nature of the conspiracy. He had responded to it with frequent letters to newspapers, the local bar association, and even to a Congressional subcommittee. His mental state, apart from his story and a mildly depressed mood, was entirely normal.

A family interview revealed that his wife and several grown children shared the belief in a judicial conspiracy directed against the patient. There was no change in delusional thinking in the patient or the family after ten days of observation. The patient refused follow-up.

In this case, protection is provided by others who share the delusion and believe in the reasonableness of the response; such cases are uncommon, if not rare.

DIAGNOSIS

Making the diagnosis of delusional disorders requires that the clinician match the features of the case to the appropriate criteria. When the clinician has successfully ruled out alternative sources for the presentation, certain features of the case can help substantiate the delusional disorder diagnosis.

MENTAL STATUS EXAMINATION The patient's complaints are brought to the attention of the clinician by the patient or a third party, such as police, family, or neighbors. The patient may have acted to draw attention by asking for protection or quarreling with neighbors. The complaint focuses on the distressing behavior and possibly on incidental symptoms. The patient will not complain of a psychiatric condition; in fact he or she will deny it or the presence of any psychiatric symptoms altogether. Examination of the patient leads to the often surprising discovery that thinking, orientation, affect, attention, memory, perception, and personality are intact. The patient's thinking is so clear and the delusional features so central to his or her concerns that the clinician begins to anticipate precisely the responses of the patient, to the point that accurate predictions of specific actions and reactions are possible. This predictability may distinguish the behavior of patients with delusional disorder from that associated with other psychotic conditions.

The patient's behavior and responses to the interview are consistent with the range of features in other paranoid conditions. There may be lack of cooperation, hostility, anger, and a sarcastic or challenging quality in most of what the patient says.

The capacity to act in response to delusions is an important dimension of the evaluation. Level of impulsiveness should be assessed and related to any potential for violence or suicidal behavior. The patient's self-righteousness and the intensity of the delusional experience may be clues to the possibility of violent behavior; and any plans for harming others, including homicide, should be inquired about. If such thoughts exist, the patient should be asked how they were handled in the past.

LABORATORY EXAMINATION A range of assessments is often necessary, but several of them have a high likelihood of detecting key factors in the case. The use of drug-screening measures is particularly valuable given the marked delusional responses induced by a number of drugs, especially amphetamine, cocaine, and other CNS stimulants.

Neuropsychological assessment may help disclose evidence of impaired intellectual functioning that suggests brain abnormalities. The assessment of intelligence may show discrepancies between verbal and performance scores as well as scatter in the overall performance. Limited data on delusional disorders (especially the more chronic form) suggest that average or marginally low intelligence is characteristic. Projective testing, such as the Rorschach Test, has limited value in making the diagnosis, but may confirm features consistent with it. The Minnesota Multiphasic Personality Inventory (MMPI) has a number of clinical scales, including the Paranoia (Pa) scale developed to identify paranoid symptoms. Deviation on this scale has strong correlations with paranoid features. Again, these results may help substantiate the diagnosis or raise it as a possibility.

DIFFERENTIAL DIAGNOSIS Because delusional disorders are uncommon, idiopathic, and possess features characteristic of the full range of paranoid illnesses, differential diagnosis has a clear-cut logic; namely, a diagnosis of delusional disorder is one of exclusion. There are many conditions to consider. To avoid premature diagnosis, a strategy of careful evaluation is required.

The clinical assessment of paranoid features requires three steps. Initially, the clinician must recognize, characterize, and judge as pathological the presence of these features. Next, the clinician should determine whether they form a part of a syndrome or are isolated. Finally, a differential diagnosis should be developed.

The first of these three steps must be pursued systematically. The clinician needs to be aware that a range of objective traits or behaviors (Table 15-5) are often found in paranoid illness. These traits may constitute the only clue that a paranoid illness is present. Furthermore, paranoid patients are frequently unwilling to reveal their subjective experiences to examiners or to cooperate in the clinical investigation. Nevertheless, careful interviewing of the patient and other informants may disclose further evidence that behavior is clearly psychopathological. In other cases, however, the conclusion that behavior suggesting a paranoid condition is psychopathological must await further observations. Delusional thinking should be examined for its fixity, logic, encapsulation, degree of systematization, and elaboration, and its effect on action and planning.

Having determined that a paranoid condition is present, the clinician should attend to the premorbid characteristics, the course, and the associated symptomatology to detect patterns of psychopathology. The discovery of clouded consciousness, perceptual disturbance, other psychopathology, physical signs, or confusing symptoms may suggest different causes for paranoid features. Isolated acute paranoid symptoms, however, often appear in early medical illness.

Finally, the clinician should avoid the temptation to diagnose schizophrenia and delusional disorder in cases where paranoid features are present. These features occur regularly in a variety of psychiatric and medical illnesses. Consequently, awareness of the multiple causes of paranoid features is essential to completing the differential diagnosis.

Certain principles can guide effective assessment. First, it is important to have knowledge of the paranoid features and patterns of the clinical conditions in which they occur. Generally, for example, only few cases of schizophrenia (10 to 20 percent) begin after age 40. Furthermore, most idiopathic psychiatric problems do not begin after age 50. Second, the premorbid status of the patient should be determined. Generally, a normal premorbid state suggests that acute paranoid features are the consequence of medical disease. Third, an abrupt change in personality, mood, ability to function, and mental state should be noted, because such symptoms suggest complications resulting from medical disease. Fourth, in those cases in which there is evidence that the patient has been refractory to psychotropic medication or psychotherapy, the continuing presence of paranoid features should alert the clinician to consider alternative diagnoses.

The final diagnosis in cases where paranoid features are prominent should be made following: (1) a complete medical and psychiatric history with special attention paid to alcohol and drug history (including drugs of abuse and prescribed and over-the-counter medication history); (2) a thorough physical examination including neurological and mental status examinations; (3) appropriate laboratory studies, particularly serological, toxicological, endocrine, microbiological, radiological, and electroencephalographic studies.

There are certain delusional conditions that, because of their frequency and seriousness, should be routinely considered in differential diagnosis. They are among the most likely sources of delusions.

ORGANIC DISORDERS Delusions arise in conjunction with a number of organic diseases and syndromes. Many are listed in Table 15-4. What they have in common is often a disturbance of perception, especially of visual and auditory functioning.

Drug intoxications (organic delusional syndrome) are particularly relevant. Abused drugs, such as amphetamine and cocaine; over-the-counter drugs, such as sympathomimetics; and prescribed drugs, such as steroids and L-dopa, can cause a delusional syndrome, often without cognitive impairment. A careful drug history and screen may establish the diagnosis.

Particularly in older individuals, dementia should be considered when paranoid features occur. Mental status examination should uncover the characteristic cognitive changes, which do not occur in delusional disorder. Delirium—with its fluctuating course, confusion, memory impairment, and transient delusions—contrasts with the persistence of delusions in delusional disorders and should be considered in acute cases with paranoid features. Physical, neurological, mental status, and laboratory examinations will usually detect organic causes of delusions. Special focus for each evaluation should be on perceptual disorder.

SCHIZOPHRENIA Delusions may be the presenting feature of schizophrenic illness. This diagnosis should be considered when the delusions are bizarre, affect is blunted or incongruous with thinking, thought disorder is pervasive, or role functioning is impaired. Paranoid schizophrenics may have somewhat less bizarre delusions; however, role functioning is impaired and auditory hallucinations are present, in contrast with delusional disorder.

MOOD DISORDER: DEPRESSION The persistent and profound dysphoric mood of depressed patients often points to the proper diagnosis; in delusional disorder, affect may be intense, but it is not itself an overwhelming experience to the patient. Delusions in depression, if present, are frequently related to mood (mood-congruent delusions). For example, the patient with feelings of worthlessness or guilt may feel that persecution against him or her is justified as a punishment for evil ways. Somatic delusions may be puzzling to differentiate if the clinician fails to consider associated psychopathological features. Depression refers to a host of signs and symptoms, and it usually has a constellation of neurovegetative features (affecting appetite, sleep, libido, energy, etc.) that are not part of delusional disorder. Moreover, depression is frequently cyclical, and often it is associated with a positive family history of mood disorder. Delusional disorder, in contrast, is remarkably free of symptoms other than the delusion.

MOOD DISORDER: MANIA Manic delusions, often grandiose and therefore mood congruent, occur in the severest stages of this illness. This may mislead the diagnostician, but the cyclical nature, marked change in mood (often euphoric or irritable at a very intense level), reduced need for sleep, increased energy, lack of social inhibition, and increased activity level of mania should be decisive in distinguishing it from delusional disorder.

PARANOID PERSONALITY DISORDER Individuals with paranoid personality disorder often have paranoid features in abundance. They are persistently oversensitive, ready to take offense, suspicious, resentful, rigid, and frequently self-centered. Rather than delusions, such persons tend to have strongly held ideas (overvalued ideas). Generally, however, they are believed to be free of delusions. This is the most useful differential feature. There is some evidence that this personality pattern occurs often enough in families of probands with delusional disorder to suggest a connection between the two, possibly of a genetic sort. This relationship remains unclear at present.

AGING DISORDERS Any discussion of differential diagnosis of paranoid features is incomplete unless consideration is given to the occurrence of paranoid features in the elderly. Paranoid features develop frequently in the elderly, and assessment in such cases should be particularly careful. Our understanding of paranoid features among the aged is limited. But there are several facts worth noting: (1) The association of depressive illness with paranoid features is high enough to warrant suspicion of mood disorder in all cases with paranoid features. (2) There appears to be a late-occurring form of schizophrenia sometimes labeled late paraphrenia or senile schizophrenia in which paranoid characteristics frequently occur. This controversial diagnosis can be made, however, only on finding no other clinical disorder to account for the changes observed. (3) The sudden onset of acute paranoid features in the elderly can be a sign of cerebrovascular injury or other medical illness. (4) Many of the illnesses associated with delusions have increased incidence in the elderly population. (5) Perhaps most important for the general clinician is to recognize sources of increased risk of paranoid disorder among older individuals. It is now known that many factors contribute to the incidence of paranoid features in the aged, including lack of stimulating company, isolation, physical illness, the aging process itself, loss of hearing, and loss of visual acuity. Each of these, particularly hearing, should be carefully assessed in all cases.

COURSE AND PROGNOSIS

Studies generally indicate that delusional disorders do not lead to severe impairment, and the base rate of spontaneous recovery may not be as low as previously thought. Suicide has been associated with such disorders, although most patients live the normal life span. Retterstol's personal follow-up investigation of a large series of cases has provided much of the viewpoint on natural history.

The more chronic forms of the illness (i.e., patients presenting with features for more than 6 months) have their onset early in the fifth decade. The onset is acute in nearly two-thirds of the cases, gradual in the remainder. The delusion has disappeared at follow-up in 53 percent of the cases, is improved in 10 percent, and is unchanged in 31 percent.

In more acute forms, the age of onset is in the fourth decade, a lasting remission occurs in more than half, and a pattern of chronicity develops in only 10 percent. A relapsing course occurs in 37 percent. Thus the more acute and earlier the onset, the more generally favorable the prognosis. The presence of precipitating factors signifies a positive outcome as does being female and being married. In terms of prognosis, outcome associated with the predominant delusion is most favorable for cases with persecutory delusions and least favorable for delusions of grandeur and jealousy. Work status at follow-up has indicated that the vast majority of patients are employed.

These observations, though limited to few cases, provide some basis for optimism: perhaps half the cases with delusional disorders may remit, but relapse and chronicity are common.

TREATMENT

The goals of treatment are to establish the diagnosis, to decide on appropriate interventions, and to manage complications. Fundamental to the success of these goals is an effective and therapeutic doctor-patient relationship, the establishment of which is far from simple. These patients do not complain about psychiatric symptoms and often enter treatment against their will. Even the psychiatrist may be brought into their delusional nets.

PSYCHOTHERAPY There is not enough evidence to substantiate the claim for any particular school or approach to talking with the patient. Insight-oriented therapy is usually contraindicated, but a combination of supportive psychotherapeutic approaches is sensible. It is unlikely that there is any psychiatric condition that requires greater diplomacy, openness, and reliability than this one. Hence, considerable skill is required in dealing with the profound and intense feelings of these patients.

Awareness of the fragile self-esteem and unusual sensitivity of these patients is essential for general management and somatic treatment. Direct questioning about the veracity of the delusion, apart from establishing its nature during clinical evaluation, is seldom helpful. Although getting an alliance started may be especially difficult, responding to the patient's concerns rather than the delusion itself may be effective. Understanding that fear and anxiety serve to stimulate hostility may be the key to adopting a flexible approach that promotes empathy but maintains physical and emotional distance. Patients with these disorders are, in fact, suffering—often feeling demoralized, miserable, isolated, and abandoned.

They may face rejection at home or on the job. They can be approached and their treatment focused on such experiences.

The goals of supportive therapy are to allay anxiety, to initiate discussion of troubling experiences and consequences of the delusion, and thereby gradually to develop a collaboration with the patient. In some patients, this strategy allows the psychiatrist to suggest means of coping more successfully with the delusional thinking. For example, the psychiatrist might encourage patients to keep their ideas to themselves as they might lead to surprise, dismay, or amazement in others and considerable cost to the patient. For others, if the patients are amenable, it may be possible to provide some educational intervention to help the patient understand how such factors as sensory impairment, social and physical isolation, and stress contribute to making matters worse. In all such approaches, the overriding aim is to assist in a more satisfying general adjustment.

SOMATIC TREATMENT Delusional disorders are psychotic disorders by definition, and the natural presumption has been that they would respond to antipsychotic medication. Because of a lack of controlled studies and the uncommonness of the condition, the results required to support this practice are still uncertain. Some investigators have reported beneficial responses in monosymptomatic hypochondriacal psychosis with pimozide. Thus, the impression remains that antipsychotic drugs are effective and a trial is usually warranted. Certainly, trials of antipsychotic medication make sense when the agitation, apprehension, and anxiety that accompany delusions are prominent.

Delusional disorders respond less well generally to electroconvulsive treatment than does major mood disorder with psychotic features. In cases where differential diagnosis is unclear between delusional disorder and psychotic depression, a trial of combined antipsychotic and antidepressant therapy may be worthwhile. In cases where standard strategies are unsuccessful, trials of lithium or anticonvulsant medication (e.g., carbamazepine [Tegretol]), or both, probably should be considered. However, there is no systematic information to support this approach.

In these patients, the use of somatic treatments is difficult on two levels. Their insistence on lack of psychiatric problems may be an insurmountable barrier to initiating treatment, and their sensitivity to all side effects may constitute an additional frustrating factor in their care. An open and clear approach in which patients are warned about and then assisted through possible unpleasant experiences is essential.

In general, some patients, especially younger delusional patients, will respond to supportive management and somatic treatment. Unfortunately, some delusional patients, especially the elderly, are refractory to any attempts to reduce their delusional thinking. In all cases, goals that are realistic and by and large modest are the most sensible. Because most of the difficulty in this disorder results from the effects of the patient's actions regarding delusions, a preventive approach has considerable value.

HOSPITALIZATION Most delusional disorder patients can be treated effectively in outpatient settings. Hospitalization may be necessary in the face of potentially dangerous behavior or unmanageable aggressiveness. The patient may show signs of poor impulse control, excessive motor and psychic tension, unremitting anger, brooding, and even threats. Suicidal ideation and planning are also potential grounds for hospitalization.

Once the psychiatrist decides on hospitalization, it is preferable to inform the patient through a process of tactful persuasion that a voluntary hospitalization is necessary. If this strategy fails, legal means to commit the patient to hospital must be undertaken.

Delusional disorders are uncommon, but probably not as rare as previously thought. Their relationship to other psychoses remains unclear, and much about them is a puzzle. The DSM-III-R requirement of excluding other organic and psychiatric conditions is prudent given the special importance of differential diagnosis. Although the DSM-III-R criteria are not definitive, they provide a sound basis for clinical and research investigation.

REFERENCES

Crowe R: Paranoid disorders. In *The Medical Basis of Psychiatry*, G. Winokur, P Clayton, editors, p 182. Saunders, Philadelphia, 1986.

Cummings J: Organic delusions: phenomenology, anatomical correlation, and review. Brit J Psychiat *146:* 184, 1985.

Cummings J: Organic psychosis. Psychosomatics *29:* 16, 1988.

de Clérembault G G: *Les Psychoses Passionelles. Œuvre Psychiatrique*. Presses Universitaires, Paris, 1942.

Enoch M D, Trethowan W H: *Uncommon Psychiatric Syndromes*, ed 2. John Wright, Bristol, England, 1979.

Freud S: Psychoanalytic notes upon an autobiographical account of a case of paranoia (dementia paranoides). In *Collected Papers*, vol 3. Hogarth Press, London, 1950. Originally published, 1911.

Kendler K S: The nosologic validity of paranoia (simple delusional disorder). Arch Gen Psychiat *37:* 699, 1980.

Kendler K S: Demography of paranoid psychosis (delusional disorder). Arch Gen Psychiat *39:* 890, 1982.

Kolle K: *Die Primäre Verrücktheit: Psychopathologische, Klinische und Genealogische Untersuchungen*. Thieme, Leipzig, 1931.

Kolle K: *Der Wahnkranke in Lichte alter und neuer Psychopathologie*. Thieme, Stuttgart, 1957.

Lewis A: Paranoia and paranoid: A historical perspective. Psychol Med *1:* 2, 1970.

Maher B: Delusional thinking and perceptual disorder. J Indiv Psychol *30:* 98, 1974.

Maher B, Ross J: Delusions. In *Comprehensive Handbook of Psychopathology*, H Adams, P Sutker, editors, p 383. Plenum, New York, 1983.

Manschreck T C: The assessment of paranoid features. Compr Psychiat *20:* 370, 1979.

Manschreck T C, Petri M: The paranoid syndrome. Lancet *251:* 1978.

Munro A: Monosymptomatic hypochondriacal psychosis. Brit J Hosp Med *24:* 34, 1980.

Munro A: Paranoia revisited. Brit J Psychiat *141:* 344, 1982.

Munro A: Paranoid (delusional) disorders: DSM-III-R and beyond. Compr Psychiat *28:* 35, 1987.

Nasrallah H A: Special and unusual psychiatric syndromes. In *The Medical Basis of Psychiatry*, G Winokur, P Clayton, editors, p 268, Saunders, Philadelphia, 1986.

Retterstol N: *Paranoid and Paranoiac Psychoses*. Charles C Thomas, Springfield, IL, 1966.

Schreber D: *Memoirs of My Nervous Illness*. R Bentley, Cambridge, MA, 1955. Originally published, 1903.

Shepherd M: Morbid jealousy: Some clinical and social aspects of a psychiatric syndrome. J Ment Sci *107:* 687, 1961.

Winokur G: Delusional disorder (paranoia). Compr Psychiat *18:* 511, 1977.

Winokur G: Familial psychopathology in delusional disorder. Compr Psychiat *26:* 241, 1985.

CHAPTER 16 PSYCHOTIC DISORDERS NOT ELSEWHERE CLASSIFIED

16.1 SCHIZOAFFECTIVE DISORDER, SCHIZOPHRENIFORM DISORDER, AND BRIEF REACTIVE PSYCHOSIS

WARREN R. PROCCI, M.D., Ph.D.

INTRODUCTION

Naturally occurring disease processes often have the perverse habit of not conforming to diagnostic criteria. The admirable and more rigorous diagnostic criteria for schizophrenia, mood disorders, and delusional (paranoid) disorders specified in the third edition and revised third edition of the *Diagnostic and Statistical Manual of Mental Disorders* (DSM-III and DSM-III-R) do not cover all patients with psychotic conditions. As a result, DSM-III and DSM-III-R have established a section entitled psychotic disorders not elsewhere classified. Included in this section of DSM-III-R are the three disorders discussed in this section, namely, schizoaffective disorder, schizophreniform disorder, and brief reactive psychosis. This section of DSM-III-R also includes a fourth disorder, atypical psychosis, a residual category for psychotic disorders that do not meet the criteria for any specific psychotic disorder. Atypical psychosis is discussed in Section 16.2, which follows. DSM-III-R has added a fifth disorder to the above four, induced psychotic disorder. This disorder is discussed in Chapter 15, Delusional (Paranoid) Disorders.

There has long been considerable confusion concerning the nosology, classification, and etiology of schizoaffective disorder, schizophreniform disorder, and brief reactive psychosis. Various diagnostic labels, including Bell's mania, catatonic syndrome applied to manic-depressive insanity, benign stupor, schizoaffective psychosis, schizophreniform psychosis, recovered schizophrenia, cycloid psychoses, remitting schizophrenia, good prognosis schizophrenia, and reactive psychoses all have been used to describe a disorder—or, more correctly perhaps, a heterogeneous group of disorders—characterized by some or all of the following: positive Bleulerian signs, acute onset, presence of precipitants, good premorbid adjustment, affective symptoms, heredity positive for mood disorder, psychomotor excitation, and remission. There has been no universal agreement concerning the definitions of these various conditions or their relationship to one another.

Because of this diagnostic and classificatory confusion, any discussion of schizoaffective disorder, schizophreniform disorder, and brief reactive psychosis must be qualified regarding the clinical and research applicability of these terms. Both the second edition of the *Diagnostic and Statistical Manual of Mental Disorders* (DSM-II) and the ninth revision of the *International Classification of Diseases* (ICD-9) handle these concepts differently from DSM-III-R. Subsequent editions of DSM, aided by a continued flow of sound empirical data, will no doubt offer further alterations in the understanding of these disorders. DSM-III-R brought new and specific defining criteria for schizophreniform disorder and brief reactive pyschosis, criteria that take these concepts somewhat afield from what their founding authors described.

Schizoaffective disorder is considered first and in greatest detail, as it has generated the most empirical research. Paradoxically, DSM-III provides no specific criteria for schizoaffective disorder, although it does for schizophreniform disorder and brief reactive pyschosis.

SCHIZOAFFECTIVE DISORDER

DEFINITION Schizoaffective disorder is not specifically defined in DSM-III. Rather, the category is to be used for those cases in which the clinician is unable to make a differential diagnosis between affective (mood) disorder and either schizophreniform disorder or schizophrenia. DSM-III suggests the following defining criteria: conditions with a full affective syndrome accompanied by prominent mood-incongruent delusions and hallucinations that occur when affective symptoms are not present. This definition implies that schizoaffective disorder is probably a variant of mood disorder, as a full affective syndrome should be present, but a full schizophrenic syndrome should not. DSM-III-R does provide specific defining criteria for schizoaffective disorder: an illness marked by a full major depressive or manic syndrome with concurrent symptoms from the "A" diagnostic criterion of schizophrenia. During an episode of the illness, delusions or hallucinations are present for a period of at least 2 weeks in the absence of affective symptoms. The condition does not, however, meet all the criteria for schizophrenia. Organic factors must not be implicated in initiating and maintaining the condition. Finally, the illness must be specified as bipolar or depressive.

COMPARATIVE NOSOLOGY The term "schizoaffective" has caused a great deal of diagnostic confusion since it was first coined in 1933 by Jacob Kasanin. Historically, it has been considered as a form of schizophrenia, and DSM-II accordingly categorized schizoaffective disorder as a subtype of schizophrenia. DSM-III moved this condition to the category of psychotic disorders not elsewhere classified. It is now labeled simply schizoaffective disorder.

DSM-III encourages using this diagnostic label in only relatively rare circumstances in which the diagnosis cannot differentiate between mood disorder and either schizophreniform disorder or schizophrenia. Major mood disorders with psychotic features, especially major depression or bipolar disorder with mood-congruent or mood-incongruent psychotic features, must also be ruled out.

DSM-III aims toward a careful and accurate differential diagnosis, implying that the schizoaffective diagnosis rarely needs to be used if an adequate differential diagnosis is possible. When the schizoaffective diagnosis is appropriate, DSM-III seems to assume that the disorder is probably a mood-disorder variant with the addition of persistent mood-incongruent psychotic features that are present for at least some time when the affective features are not.

DSM-III-R improves on this by presenting specific criteria for making the diagnosis of schizoaffective disorder; that is, it is no longer primarily a diagnosis of exclusion. These criteria are clearly delineated in Table 16.1-1. DSM-III-R also requires specifying the disturbance as either bipolar or depressive. Because DSM-III-R replaces the term "affective disorder" with the term "mood disorder," this disorder should really be called "schizomood disorder." DSM-III-R, however, retains the schizoaffective designation for historical continuity.

The Research Diagnostic Criteria (RDC) definition for schizoaffective disorder is similar to that of DSM-III-R, but the RDC diagnostic criteria are more detailed. The criteria also divide the disorder into schizoaffective disorder, manic type, and schizoaffective disorder, depressed type. These two types are further subdivided according to duration (i.e., acute, subacute, subchronic, or chronic). The RDC also makes another subdivision, into a mainly schizophrenic subtype, a mainly affective subtype, or another subtype based on the temporal relationship of the affective and schizophrenic features during the current episode. The RDC, like DSM-III-R, emphasizes an illness that fulfills the criteria for an affective syndrome but also presents at least one major schizophrenic symptom. But the RDC differs from DSM-III-R in the following way: The RDC defines the mainly affective subtype by the absence of the schizophrenic symptoms for at least 1 week during the absence of the affective symptoms, whereas DSM-III-R requires that the schizophrenic symptoms (delusions or hallucinations) be present for at least 2 weeks in the absence of the prominent affective symptoms. The RDC's mainly affective subtype may well define an illness even more closely allied to mood disorder than that described in DSM-III-R, whose definition itself leans toward mood disorder.

The ICD-9 classification of schizoaffective disorder is similar to that of DSM-II. Schizoaffective type is listed as a specific subtype of schizophrenic disorders. In its glossary, however, ICD-9 describes the schizoaffective type as characterized by both affective and schizophrenic symptoms, and both of these groups of symptoms must be pronounced. The illness also tends to remit without permanent defect, but it is prone to recur. Therefore, although it is classified as a subtype of schizophrenia in ICD-9, schizoaffective disorder is seen as having a number of characteristics more akin to mood disorder than to schizophrenia.

TABLE 16.1-1
Diagnostic Criteria for Schizoaffective Disorder

A. A disturbance during which, at some time, there is either a major depressive or a manic syndrome concurrent with symptoms that meet the A criterion of schizophrenia.
B. During an episode of the disturbance, there have been delusions or hallucinations for at least 2 weeks, but no prominent mood symptoms.
C. Schizophrenia has been ruled out (i.e., the duration of all episodes of a mood syndrome has not been brief relative to the total duration of the psychotic disturbance).
D. It cannot be established that an organic factor initiated and maintained the disturbance.

Specify: **bipolar type** (current or previous manic syndrome)
or
depressive type (no current or previous manic syndrome)

Table from DSM-III-R *Diagnostic and Statistical Manual of Mental Disorders,* ed 3, revised. Copyright American Psychiatric Association, Washington, DC, 1987. Used with permission.

EPIDEMIOLOGY Because schizoaffective disorder has been variously defined through the years, precise data concerning its incidence are limited. Some information is available, however, that indicates the frequency of occurrence of schizoaffective disorder. In one recent study, the incidence per year of schizoaffective disorder (0.3 to 5.7 per 100,000) was compared with the incidence per year of schizophrenia (7.3 to 15.0 per 100,000) and mania (1.7 to 3.3 per 100,000). Thus, it was about one-quarter as common as schizophrenia and roughly as common as mania. These data show that schizoaffective disorder is far more common than one would expect were it to represent the combination of both schizophrenia and mood disorder (calculated by multiplying the incidence of schizophrenia by the incidence of manic-depressive disorder, yielding a miniscule figure), as a handful of investigators have speculated.

ETIOLOGY It is naive to speak of an etiology of schizoaffective disorder at this point, as the issue is still clouded by the chronic confusion concerning the nature of the illness. Is it a variant of mood disorder or schizophrenia, or is it yet another psychotic disorder? These questions have puzzled several generations of investigators, even before Kasanin introduced the term in 1933. Emil Kraepelin's classification system is partly responsible for this diagnostic confusion, as he conceptualized psychotic illness as composed of two major groups: the deteriorating illness, which he called dementia precox, and the remitting illness, or manic-depressive disease.

The best data currently available suggest that most of what is now diagnosed as schizoaffective disorder is probably the result of factors similar to those predisposing to mood disorder. The psychotic symptoms, those resembling or mimicking schizophrenia, remain something of an enigma, but it has been suggested that they are independent of the affective symptoms and are evoked only when the affective symptoms become sufficiently intense. This should not be taken, however, to imply that schizoaffective disorder is necessarily a more serious version of mood disorder, with a more problematic course and negative outcome. Furthermore, at least some patients with the schizoaffective diagnosis probably have an illness more closely related to schizophrenia, and a few may have an unrelated disease. Clearly, determining the etiology of schizoaffective disorder is a task that will keep investigators occupied for some time to come.

PATHOLOGY DSM-III sparked psychiatrists' long-standing desire to identify specific pathologies for specific illnesses. Current psychiatric knowledge is sufficiently advanced so that such correlation may be available in the near future. But at present, no known specific neuropathological process correlates reliably with schizoaffective disorder.

The biological-marker approach to understanding psychiatric illness has yielded some relatively promising suggestions concerning possible physiological correlates for schizoaffective disorder. A beneficial side effect of biological-marker research is that it has enabled investigators to speculate about the etiology of schizoaffective disorder. For example, if a biological marker found in schizoaffective disorder is closely related to a biological marker also associated with schizophrenia but not with mood disorder, then schizoaffective disorder may be hypothesized as being a subtype or variant of schizophrenia. Similar logic would apply if the biological marker closely corresponded to a marker known to identify a mood disorder.

Various studies have measured the urinary excretion of 3-methoxy-4-hydroxyphenylglycol (MHPG) to establish a biochemical classification for serious mood disorders. One study examined schizoaffective patients and found that they had mean urinary MHPG values very similar to those of bipolar manic depressives and quite different from subjects with schizophrenia and also some signs of depression. Electroencephalogram (EEG) records provide another biological marker. One study compared the all-night sleep records of schizoaffective and psychotic depressive patients, but no significant differences were found. Brain ventricular size has also been used to classify psychotically ill patients, and some of the current findings, though inconsistent and still controversial, are of interest. In general, schizoaffective patients, in contrast to schizophrenics, have relatively normal ventricular/brain ratios (VBRs).

Biological-marker studies thus have failed to identify a specific pathophysiological identifier of schizoaffective illness nor have they identified a specific etiological origin. Considered together, however, these few studies support a closer relationship between schizoaffective disorder and mood disorder than between schizoaffective disorder and schizophrenia.

CLINICAL SIGNS AND SYMPTOMS A precise clinical description of schizoaffective disorder depends on one's definition of the disorder. Since Kasanin introduced the term—primarily to describe atypical psychotic patients with a mixture of schizophrenic and affective symptoms—several investigators have described similar clinical syndromes. But most of these descriptions have not been precise enough to allow comparative research. Some of these conditions are described in the introduction to this section. A careful reading of the original papers reporting these conditions reveals that these descriptions have much in common, and they may well refer to the same condition or a similar group of conditions. Among the factors common to at least several of these descriptions are the following:

1. Relatively early age of onset (i.e., between ages 20 and 40), perhaps with a subclinical episode during adolescence.
2. Acute onset, often in the face of a precipitating environmental stress.
3. Marked emotional turmoil.
4. Good premorbid functioning, with good social and vocational adjustment.
5. No evidence of emotional withdrawal.
6. Brief duration of the psychotic illness.
7. No family history of schizophrenia.
8. Presence of a family history of mood disorder.
9. Good outcome, with preservation of social and vocational functioning.

Although not all of these features are present in all of these clinical descriptions, these signs and symptoms do merit being grouped together and are considered as important characteristics of schizoaffective disorder.

To be more specific, schizoaffective disorder consists of an acute episode of a floridly psychotic illness characterized by a mix of classical manic or depressive features with prominent mood-incongruent psychotic symptoms, especially mood-incongruent delusions or hallucinations. For at least some of the time during the acute episode, the affective symptoms are not present, and the mood-incongruent psychotic features persist.

Often, there have been earlier episodes of the illness, which may have been more typically affective or schizophrenic in nature. If this is so, the clinician should be wary of making a diagnosis of schizoaffective disorder.

By definition, the cross-sectional presentation of the illness varies considerably. If the patient is seen when the mood-incongruent psychotic features are prominent and the affective features are absent, the patient may well be indistinguishable from a schizophrenic. Conversely, there are periods of time when the affective symptoms are florid and the mood-incongruent psychotic features are relatively quiescent.

The outcome of this illness also varies. Incomplete recovery with functional deterioration is possible. But this does not necessarily indicate that the illness is really schizophrenic in nature, as some patients with an apparently pure mood disorder go on to exhibit impaired vocational, social, and interpersonal functioning. More typically, the outcome is reasonably benign, with the resolution of the acute episode followed by a substantial recapture of premorbid psychosocial and vocational functioning. A recurrence, however, is likely: DSM-III-R emphasizes a tendency toward chronicity in this disorder.

As suggested above, DSM-III was disappointing because it did not precisely define schizoaffective disorder but made it a residual diagnostic category characterized by a mixture of schizophrenic and affective symptoms. Later, the RDC and then DSM-III-R called for the presence of a full mood disorder syndrome and then the addition of mood-incongruent psychotic features in order to make the schizoaffective diagnosis. This attempt at codifying the diagnosis has indeed helped narrow the competing clinical descriptions, but it by no means solves the problem of accurate description. Even according to the more precise clinical descriptions of the RDC or DSM-III-R, patients may display in cross-sectional view any one or more of the wide array of symptoms characteristic of either schizophrenia or mood disorder. Still, the RDC and DSM-III-R are a vast improvement over prior efforts and are more amenable to comparative research. Because both the RDC's and DSM-III-R's descriptions require the presence of a full affective syndrome, there is the danger of circularity in the definition. If an affective syndrome is necessary for the diagnosis, then it is more likely that schizoaffective disorder, so defined, is either a subtype or a variant of mood disorder than of schizophrenia. If only it were that clear. Indeed, one study specified that both a full mood disorder syndrome and a full schizophrenic syndrome, as defined by DSM-III, were required for the schizoaffective diagnosis. When subjected to a 15-year follow-up, these patients exhibited an outcome quite similar to that of rigorously diagnosed schizophrenic patient. A reasonable implication of this data is that the presence of a full schizophrenic syndrome carries a poor prognosis, even when a full affective syndrome coexists. Thus, schizophrenic symptoms in the presence of a full affective syndrome may not be associated with a poor prognosis, but if the schizophrenic symptoms evolve into a full schizophrenic syndrome, then even the presence of a full affective syndrome will not protect against a poor prognosis. Prognostic precedence should be given to a full schizophrenic syndrome over a full affective syndrome.

THE NATURE OF SCHIZOAFFECTIVE DISORDER

Through the years, there have been three major possibilities regarding the nature of schizoaffective disorder. The first possibility, which prevailed at the time of DSM-II and which is suggested by DSM-III-R, is that schizoaffective disorder is a variant of schizophrenia. The second possibility, as exemplified in the RDC and DSM-III, is that schizoaffective disorder is a variant of mood disorder. The third possibility is that schizoaffective disorder is truly an independent category, a "third" psychotic disorder that defies the long-standing Kraepelinian dichotomy.

Some researchers have attempted to combine all three of these possibilities by suggesting that schizoaffective disorder itself is not a single disorder but is heterogeneous and composed of at least three subtypes: first, a mood-disorder subtype, which is probably the most common; second, a schizophrenic subtype; and finally, a mixed subtype. This approach is probably the wisest one to adopt given the current available data and vague definitions.

Until recently, little attention was paid to possible differences between the manic and depressive subtypes of schizoaffective disorder. The development of the RDC criteria has provided an incentive to pursue this, as the RDC does specify criteria for these subtypes. DSM-III-R insists that the schizoaffective diagnosis be subtyped into one of these two categories. These two subtypes may, in fact, not be subtypes but two distinct disease processes.

Variant of schizophrenia In many respects, the DSM-II criteria for schizophrenia were an outgrowth of Manfred Bleuler's criteria, which lacked precision and defied reliable operational definition. However, Bleuler's criteria held sway in the United States for a considerable time, and as a result, schizophrenia was undoubtedly overdiagnosed. Bleuler's criteria considered the presence of the so-called fundamental signs, the four A's, to be pathognomonic for schizophrenia. If these were present, the diagnosis was schizophrenia, regardless of whether prominent affective symptoms were also present. Many investigators view the introduction of lithium as a landmark in reconsidering the importance of affective symptoms, perhaps because a relatively specific and highly effective treatment became available for mood disorder. Following the introduction of lithium, the concept of schizoaffective disorder was reexamined by a number of investigators who, while studying patients with mixed schizophrenic and affective features, chose to consider the illness as affective in nature and elected to treat the patients with lithium. Because many patients responded favorably, some researchers began to view schizoaffective disorder as a mood disorder variant.

Recently, however, a few contrary studies have challenged this assumption and have lent new life to the idea that schizoaffective disorder is a variant of schizophrenia. DSM-III-R subtly suggests this. Several studies have found that the presence of affective symptoms within the framework of marked schizophrenic symptoms do not necessarily predict a good outcome. The criteria used to determine schizoaffective disorder in at least one of these studies did include the presence of a persistent thought disorder during the time period between the acute episodes. In another study, a full schizophrenic syndrome was required for a schizoaffective diagnosis. Clearly, then, these criteria may have been biased toward selecting patients with an illness more akin to schizophrenia, analogous to the manner in which RDC and DSM-III criteria may bias diagnosis toward mood disorder. This again demonstrates clinicians' dependence on various investigators' diagnostic criteria and thus the importance of standardized diagnostic criteria.

Variant of mood disorder One approach to diagnosing schizoaffective disorder is to examine the longitudinal course of schizoaffective illness via either retrospective or prospective follow-up studies and compare this with the longitudinal course of patients with schizophrenia and patients with mood disorder. This approach is a tried and tested one. Some investigators have found that Bleulerian-positive schizophrenic patients whose psychosis remitted were often characterized by the presence of prominent affective symptoms. One prospective study associated the presence of depressive symptoms in Bleulerian-diagnosed schizophrenic patients with a positive outcome. Another investigator, perhaps overly optimistically, asserted that the evidence was sufficiently conclusive that the presence or absence of affective symptoms alone could differentiate recovered patients from chronic patients. A consistent finding is that the presence of the so-called first-rank symptoms of Kurt Schneider do not augur a poor prognosis as long as affective symptoms are present. Some researchers feel strongly that the presence of affective symptoms, and not schizophrenic symptoms, should be accorded diagnostic precedence.

Patients with schizoaffective disorder have a better long-term course than that of schizophrenia but probably not as good as that in pure mood disorder.

Schizoaffective patients have also been subcategorized as schizomanic or schizodepressive. Six studies compared the course of illness in schizomanics with bipolar mania, and four of these six studies also included comparisons with schizophrenic patients. The two studies that compared schizomanics only with manics found that the outcome was at least as good in schizomanics as in bipolar manic patients. In each of the other four studies, the schizomanics had an outcome intermediate between that of the schizophrenics and that of the bipolar manics. Six studies compared schizodepressive patients with patients with major mood disorder, depressed type, and five of these six studies also made comparisons with schizophrenic patients. The pattern is similar to that found for schizomanics. In four of the five studies in which schizodepressives were compared with affectively depressed patients and with schizophrenics, the outcome was intermediate. In one study, however, schizodepressives did no better than schizophrenics. In the study comparing schizodepressives with depressed patients with mood disorder, the schizodepressives had a less favorable course.

Although the more recent studies have more similar diagnostic criteria than the earlier studies, in part because of the increasing use of the RDC, the later studies still disagree on what is meant by the term "outcome." Certainly, the presence of schizophrenic symptoms in an otherwise typically affective illness generally lowers the prognosis. But it is also clear that the presence of affective symptoms in an otherwise typically schizophrenic presentation improves the prognosis, although one recent study found no improvement in prognosis even if a full affective syndrome coexisted with a full schizophrenic syndrome. In the future, this type of investigation should result in a higher yield as more uniform and more objective outcome criteria are developed to match the currently more precise diagnostic criteria.

Family history is also important to the investigation of schizoaffective disorder, because if schizoaffective disorder is a variant of schizophrenia, there should be more schizophrenically ill relatives in the families of probands. Similarly, the children of such individuals should be at increased risk for schizophrenia. Analogous considerations apply if schizoaffective disorder is a variant of mood disorder. If schizoaffective disorder is a third psychosis, an "independent" disease category, the relatives of index cases should exhibit a schizoaffective picture, and the children of such patients should be at increased risk for schizoaffective disorder.

Early studies noted that schizoaffective patients with a good outcome had many more relatives with a mood disorder. Several more recent studies, however, have found that the relatives of schizoaffective probands were more likely to have schizophrenia than the relatives of mood disorder probands. But these relatives had a generally lower risk rate for schizophrenia than for mood disorder. DSM-III-R emphasizes the familial pattern of increased risk for schizophrenia in the relatives of schizoaffective patients. In general, the risk rate for schizophrenia in the relatives of schizoaffective patients was lower than the corresponding risk rate for schizophrenic relatives in schizophrenic patients.

Some studies have looked specifically at schizomanics, but none has found significant numbers of cases of schizophrenia among the relatives of schizomanic probands. Similar risk rates for mood disorder were found in the relatives of the schizomanics and in the relatives of patients with bipolar manic disorder. Several studies examined schizodepressives and reported either mixed results (i.e., either a risk rate intermediate between the risk rate seen in mood disorder and that seen in schizophrenia) or a risk rate similar to that seen in mood disorder.

These family history studies cannot be considered conclusive, but the general findings show the rate of mood disorder in the relatives of schizoaffective probands to be lower than the rate of mood disorder in the relatives of mood disorder probands, but still substantially higher than that of the general population. The overall pattern strongly suggests that the lower incidence of mood disorder in the relatives of patients with schizoaffective illness is small, as is the increased incidence of schizophrenia in the relatives of schizoaffective probands. The results of these investigations support at least some relationship between schizoaffective illness and mood disorder but offer less support for any relationship between schizoaffective disorder and schizophrenia. More recent studies have found a greater risk for schizophrenia in schizoaffective disorder, and DSM-III-R points to these data in suggesting that schizoaffective disorder may be a variant of schizophrenia.

A separate disorder Schizoaffective disorder may also be a separate illness, distinct from either schizophrenia or mood disorder. A few genetic studies offer the strongest support for this hypothesis.

According to a review of the genetics of so-called atypical psychoses, the evidence supports the genetic distinction of schizophrenia, bipolar illness, and atypical psychoses. There are strong homotypic tendencies within the families of schizophrenics, bipolars, and atypical schizophrenics (i.e., each of these three types of psychotic disorder has a tendency to "breed true"). This suggests that atypical schizophrenia, which most likely includes at least some cases of schizoaffective disorder, may be a separate illness. An in-depth genetic study of a schizoaffective index case revealed a pedigree with many schizoaffectives but without a single schizophrenic or bipolar patient. Several other reviewers have also pointed out that in some families, atypical psychoses occurred repeatedly without any of the children developing schizophrenia or mood disorder. But in families in which both parents were schizophrenic, their psychotic children were schizophrenic, and in families in which both parents were bipolar, their psychotic children were bipolar. If a schizophrenic marries a bipolar, their children will have a relatively equal chance of developing either schizophrenia or bipolar disease, but not mixed or schizoaffective disorder.

One recent investigation examined 35 psychotic sibling pairs among whom were 17 pairs in which at least one in the pair had schizoaffective disorder. In five pairs was a sibling with schizophrenia (29 percent), in eight pairs was a sibling with mood disorder (47 percent), and four pairs (24 percent) were concordant for schizoaffective disorder. These results suggest that what is commonly called schizoaffective disorder may be a heterogeneous disease with a mood-disorder subtype most frequent, a schizophrenic subtype, and a truly independent subtype.

Thus, there is some evidence that at least some schizoaffectives have an illness that is neither clearly schizophrenic nor clearly a mood-disorder variant.

DIFFERENTIAL DIAGNOSIS The differential diagnosis of schizoaffective disorder can be quite complicated. There are four major areas of difficulty:

1. Distinguishing schizoaffective disorder from schizophrenia with excitation, agitation, and affective symptoms.
2. Distinguishing schizoaffective disorder from bipolar disorder with mood-incongruent features.
3. Distinguishing schizoaffective disorder from major depression with mood-incongruent features.
4. Distinguishing schizoaffective disorder from the wide variety of conditions arising from demonstrable organic lesions, which can produce a confusing mix of schizophrenic and affective symptoms.

Schizophrenia The first of these four differentiations is probably the most troublesome. For many years, American psychiatry used a rather loose approach to the diagnosis of schizophrenia, as illustrated by the DSM-II description. The presence of so-called psychotic features, such as hallucinations and delusions, would always take diagnostic precedence, whereas affective symptoms were accorded only secondary significance. Recent research has demonstrated, however, that the exclusive focus on a symptom cluster for diagnostic purposes is likely to be misleading. In one study, the investigators attempted to determine whether there was a clear demarcation, in the acute symptom complex, between schizophrenia and mood disorder. If there was, they would expect to find a bimodal distribution of symptoms. They did not. One conclusion was that there was no clean dividing line between the symptom complex present in schizophrenia and that present in mood disorder. Another study further illustrated this point. The research team examined unequivocally manic patients in a longitudinal fashion through an entire untreated acute manic episode. They found distinct phases of typical mania. During one of these phases, about one-third of the manic patients exhibited a set of clinical features indistinguishable from a paranoid schizophrenic state. So if the diagnostic appraisal is limited to only one set of symptoms, it is relatively easy to be misled. Patients who appear to be clearly schizophrenic may, in fact, be classical manics passing through a fairly brief phase of a typical manic illness. The assigning of diagnostic priority to schizophrenic symptoms over affective symptoms thus can be misleading.

A major impact of the Washington University research diagnostic criteria, and later the RDC, DSM-III, and DSM-III-R, is the insistence on an overall clinical appraisal, including acute symptom picture, premorbid history, family history, response to treatment, and outcome. It is the totality of this appraisal that is essential to accurate diagnosis. Although the vagaries of the clinical setting often preclude such a thorough evaluation, it should be viewed as an ideal goal. When such an appraisal is possible, differential diagnostic problems tend to recede.

Schizoaffective disorder can be distinguished from typical schizophrenia by referring to several of these aforementioned criteria. A premorbid history characterized by a long history of schizophrenia certainly suggests schizophrenia. Evidence of a premorbid existence of the negative symptoms of schizophrenia, such as anhedonia, blunted or flat affect, poverty of thought, poverty of content, and the amotivational syndrome also strongly supports a schizophrenic diagnosis. If affective symptoms are not prominent and if the DSM-III criteria for schizophrenia are otherwise fulfilled, schizophrenia is suggested. If the positive symptoms of schizophrenia, such as delusions or hallucinations, occur prior to and independent of the acute episode, rather than during the acute episode, this again suggests schizophrenia. Obviously, a family history heavily weighted in favor of schizophrenia suggests schizophrenia. Agitated and excitable schizophrenic patients may be insomnic or impulsive, but they generally do not exhibit typical manic symptoms such as pressured speech, grandiosity, or inappropriate euphoria. The nature of the primary disturbance of affect is important. Schizoaffective patients may show either euphoric or irritable affect. But schizophrenic patients do not show euphoria, nor do they demonstrate true irritability. Their affect may be angry or hostile, which may appear irritable when combined with psychomotor agitation. An angry or hostile affect in the presence of immediately frustrating environmental stimuli may indicate irritable affect, but a spontaneously angry or hostile affect in the absence of immediately frustrating environmental stimuli is unlikely to represent irritability. More likely it is a response to internally derived psychotic stimulation in a schizophrenic patient.

Bipolar disorder Bipolar disorder should be considered when there is either a premorbid history of good psychosocial functioning or a prior history of typical bipolar disorder. A family history of a typical bipolar disorder also supports a bipolar diagnosis. A prior history of successful treatment with lithium, especially if lithium alone was effective and supplementary or adjunctive treatment with antipsychotics was not required, supports a bipolar diagnosis. In typical bipolar disorder, any mood-incongruent psychotic features that may be present occur only as part of the mood disorder. Their occurrence is transient and is confined to a time during which the mood-disorder episode is apparent. In schizoaffective disorder, the mood-incongruent features—though confined to the acute episode—are persistent during the episode. The mood-incongruent features do not precede, nor do they appear independent of, the boundaries of the affective episode, although they can and do occur when affective symptoms are quiescent.

Major depression Differentiating depression with mood-incongruent features from schizoaffective disorder can also be quite difficult. Again, the premorbid pattern, prior history, response to treatment, family history, and clinical course can be extremely helpful. Careful history taking is important. Some depressive symptoms, such as slowness of speech, psychomotor retardation, difficulty with decisions, amotivational state, and ideas of reference, may resemble some typical schizophrenic symptoms such as withdrawal, formal thought disorder, autism, and ambivalence. A schizoaffective diagnosis may be tempting. In these cases, repeated clinical assessments may be necessary before the clinician can clearly determine whether the symptoms are in fact depressive, schizophrenic, or a true mixture of both. A further complicating factor is the tendency of patients' families to interpret the negative schizophrenic symptoms as depression. The so-called postpsychotic depression seen in schizophrenia can also be confusing. The quality of the postpsychotic depression in schizophrenic patients is somewhat different from that of depression or schizoaffective depression. The intensity of the depression is less severe in the schizophrenic patient, and it is described by the patient with characteristic affective bluntness or flatness and not in the tearful, sad manner of the depressive.

Organically induced conditions Differentiating schizoaffective disorder from an organically induced psychotic state can also be problematic, especially in the urban hospital emergency room where drug abusers are so often brought. Various sympathomimetic drugs (e.g., the amphetamines) can produce manic-like symptoms, such as psychomotor excitation, inappropriate euphoria, and pressured speech. A psychotic picture also emerges in some amphetamine users that is virtually indistinguishable from classically described paranoid schizophrenia. To make things even more difficult, amphetamine users sometimes "crash" after a period of continuous amphetamine ingestion, with resultant sleepiness, dysphoria, and irritability. This can readily be confused with depression.

Phencyclidine (PCP) abuse has become very common. Unfortunately, this drug produces several confusing symptoms and so is frequently misdiagnosed. Paranoid delusions are common and may occur in the presence of a clear sensorium, thereby suggesting schizophrenia. Prominent depressive symptoms are also possible. But certain physical signs and symptoms are generally seen in PCP intoxication that do help identify this condition. Such features as hypertension, hyperreflexia, analgesia, ataxia, nystagmus, and slurred speech frequently accompany PCP abuse.

High doses of exogenously administered corticosteroids are classically associated with an excited, psychomotorically agitated state that can closely resemble a manic or schizomanic condition. Corticosteroid-related psychoses are quite brittle, and manic, depressive, schizophrenic, and delirious symptoms all can be seen in rapid succession. This condition is largely dose related, and so the clinical picture develops and resolves quickly, seldom lasting more than 2 to 3 weeks. An accurate history should clearly establish the diagnosis in this condition.

A few general clinical features should point to the presence of an organic condition. A depressed mood or affect without most of the nine DSM-III-R criterion A symptoms for depression should always raise the possibility of an organic condition. The sudden appearance of psychotic or affective symptoms in geriatric patients with "clean" psychiatric histories is another red flag.

With all of these differential diagnostic possibilities in mind, the following additional general principles are useful for an accurate diagnostic appraisal. Careful observation over a period of time is important. Such a longitudinal view may clarify a clouded clinical picture. Affective symptoms previously hidden by mood-incongruent features may come to the fore (remember the findings about the "stages" of mania). The clinician must also attempt to determine which set of symptoms, the affective or the schizophrenic, predominates. The nature of the onset of the condition must be determined. If it is very sudden, a drug-induced psychosis must be considered. Careful attention must be paid to both the prior psychiatric history and the family history, and especially the response to treatment and the course of the illness in both the patient and any relatives with psychotic disorders. It is certainly appropriate to defer a diagnosis when the clinical picture is unclear, especially as a premature diagnosis can be incorrect and lead to chronic inappropriate treatment.

TREATMENT The question of the best treatment in schizoaffective disorder has not been settled, no doubt because the nature of the condition remains unclear. Nevertheless, there are a number of general principles, some of which are supported by reasonably well-controlled data.

Greater weight should probably be accorded to the presence of affective symptoms, especially in the case of schizomanics. According to a review of the literature through 1982 on the use of lithium in schizoaffective disorder, the treatment of 113 schizoaffective patients with lithium was described in a total of 19 papers. Sixteen patients (14 percent) showed full recovery, and another 66 (58 percent) were described as, at the very least, "improved." Thus, a total of 82 out of 113 schizoaffective patients (73 percent) treated with lithium showed improvement up to and including full recovery. But the nature of the response to lithium is unclear: whether its effect is limited to the affective symptoms only or whether it also benefited the schizophrenic symptoms. Fifteen studies reported on the treatment with lithium of 157 schizophrenic patients, and 80 (51 percent) of the patients showed improvement. Even if the "excited" schizophrenic patients were removed from the sample, 45 of 111 nonexcited schizophrenic patients (41 percent) still showed improvement. This suggests that the response to lithium is not necessarily limited to the symptoms of excitation. In many schizoaffective patients, however, it is necessary to supplement lithium treatment with an antipsychotic, at least during the acute phase of the illness.

If the predominant symptoms are more heavily weighted toward schizophrenia, then lithium will likely prove to be less effective, and it will probably be necessary to treat the patient with antipsychotic medication.

Schizodepressive patients are a different matter. One recent study described the treatment of 41 schizodepressive patients with amitriptyline (Elavil), chlorpromazine (Thorazine), or both. The drug response in the schizodepressives was generally disappointing: Only 20 percent showed significant improvement during the 1-month course of the acute study. These patients generally responded better to antipsychotic medication than to the antidepressant, suggesting that schizodepressive disorder may be more closely related to schizophrenia than to bipolar disorder.

One of the most interesting treatment questions in schizoaffective disorder is the role of electroconvulsive therapy (ECT). One recent study looked retrospectively at the use of ECT in depressed schizoaffectives. Mortality rates and suicide rates significantly increased among patients who had not received ECT. These findings also suggested that both schizophrenic and affective symptoms improved in the ECT group. The investigators further pointed out that the percentage of deaths from suicide in schizoaffective disorder (15.8 percent) was higher than the comparable figures in schizophrenia (10.1 percent), mania (11.1 percent), or depression (9.3 percent). This suggests that the suicide risk in schizoaffective disorder is, at the very least, comparable to that in schizophrenia and mood disorder, and perhaps even higher. Thus, not only are these patients somewhat difficult to diagnose and treat, but they also can be more suicidal and thus require relatively intensive monitoring. ECT should be kept in mind as a possible treatment for schizoaffective depression in cases that do not show significant improvement following vigorous treatment with lithium or antidepressant and antipsychotic drugs or one of these latter two.

The following is a case example of schizoaffective disorder, bipolar type:

R. E., an unmarried female, had her first psychiatric hospitalization in 1972 when she was 26 years old. She was taken to the hospital emergency room by the local police, who found her in a city park wearing only the bottom part of a bikini bathing suit. She told the police that she was out looking for men and that thousands of men wished to date her. She was a university graduate student with no prior psychiatric history.

When examined, her mood alternated between euphoria and irritability, depending on the degree of frustration she experienced. She was unable to sit still. Although now fully clothed, she remained seductive and suggested that she possessed unusual sexual capability. She exhibited flight of ideas and was vague, circumstantial, and delusional. A Protestant herself, she was preoccupied with the historical persecution of Jews and wished to convert to Judaism.

She was diagnosed as having schizophrenia, schizoaffective type, according to the diagnostic practice prevalent at that time. She was treated with a combination of trifluoperazine (Stelazine) and lithium and responded within a few weeks.

Her course over the ensuing 15 years has been marked by several recurrences, either primarily manic or depressive in nature. They have always been associated with some disorder of thinking and some mood-incongruent delusions.

Although she has generally done well and is free of either affective or schizophrenic symptoms between episodes, she has some persistent deficits. She has clearly not lived up to the potential of someone with a Ph.D. from a major university. She has had difficulty breaking away from home and establishing an independent existence. She has almost always held a job, although never for more than a few years at a time, and her jobs have not tapped her considerable intellectual resources. Finally, she has never formed a very close heterosexual relationship.

She has no known family history of major mental illness. The patient's father was a merchant marine ship officer who was most likely alcoholic.

The following is a case example of schizoaffective disorder, depressed type:

H. L., a 36-year-old male, has a 15-year history of psychiatric illness. At present, he has been married for 5 years and has two children. His current presentation to an outpatient clinic was the result of depressive ideation concerning his inadequacies as a husband and provider. H. L. is the only child of Eastern European immigrant parents who built an impressive financial empire. But he has not been able to hold a job on his own, despite a college degree. He is employed in a largely ceremonial job, with a large salary, in the family business. He is distinctly aware of the superficial nature of his duties, which is a substantial blow to his self-esteem.

H. L. has been hospitalized six times during the past 15 years with a relatively consistent history of depressive ideation, motor retardation, insomnia, and appetite and weight loss. He also engages in considerable ruminative, and often circumstantial, thinking. Mood-incongruent delusions are also present. For example, he was convinced during his last admission that certain colors had special and unique meaning for him and that they indicated certain actions that should be taken by the family business. He was unable to be more specific.

H. L. has been treated with a wide variety of medications, including tricyclic antidepressants, antipsychotics, and lithium. He usually has received tricyclic antidepressants during the acute episodes, which required hospitalization. Between episodes, he did best when treated with low-to-moderate dosages of high-potency antipsychotic medication, usually haloperidol (Haldol) or fluphenazine (Prolixin). When his dosage was lowered, his depressive and mood-incongruent psychotic symptomatology returned.

H. L. has no known family history of major mental illness. The patient's father died at age 64 and had been diagnosed as suffering from Alzheimer's disease.

SCHIZOPHRENIFORM DISORDER

INTRODUCTION Schizophreniform disorder has acquired a different meaning since the publication of DSM-III. G. Langfeldt originated the term in 1937 when describing a group of patients with psychotic features similar to those of schizophrenia. These psychoses were characterized by an acute onset usually preceded by emotional stress. These patients' affective features often accompanied the more typical schizophrenic features. Their histories revealed good premorbid adjustment, and longitudinal observation almost invariably revealed a complete recovery. Langfeldt considered these patients to have an illness different from true schizophrenia, despite the similarities in their acute symptomatic presentation.

The term "schizophreniform" continued to be used, and the disorder eventually came to be regarded as a variant or relative of schizoaffective disorder. A review article from the 1960s examined a group of papers describing various good prognosis, or remitting schizophrenias. The article compared 16 different diagnostic labels, including Langfeldt's schizophreniform patients and Kasanin's schizoaffective patients. The reviewer concluded that there was little substantive difference among the conditions. Thus, for many years the term "schizophreniform" and the term "schizoaffective" have been closely related.

DEFINITION DSM-III completely redefined the term "schizophreniform" as a disorder identical with schizophrenia except for its duration. In schizophreniform disorder, the total duration of illness, including the prodromal, active, and residual phases, is limited to a period of at least 2 weeks and no longer than 6 months. This definition clearly moves the concept implied by the term "schizophreniform" away from that implied by "schizoaffective." Langfeldt himself pointed out this discrepancy and indicated that DSM-III does not accurately reflect his original concept of schizophreniform psychosis.

In the text, but not in the actual diagnostic criteria, DSM-III describes schizophreniform disorder as being outside the category of schizophrenic disorders, because there is a greater likelihood of emotional turmoil, confusion, acuteness of onset, acuteness of resolution with return to premorbid level of functioning, and the general absence of a family history of schizophrenia. This certainly implies a major differentiation from schizophrenia, even though the actual diagnostic criteria are essentially identical.

DSM-III-R appears to recognize these shortcomings and introduced the requirement that the disorder be specified as either having or not having good prognostic features. DSM-III-R lists the following four features: onset of prominent psychotic symptoms within 4 weeks; confusion, disorientation, or perplexity at the height of the episodes; good premorbid functioning; and absence of blunted or flat affect. If at least two of these features are present, the disorder is defined as having good prognostic features, and if fewer than two are present, it is described as not having good prognostic features. DSM-III-R clearly states that the presence of these features merely suggests a good prognosis; it does not guarantee it. Thus in DSM-III-R, schizophreniform illness is distinguished from schizophrenia by more than just the duration of the illness (Table 16.1-2).

COMPARATIVE NOSOLOGY According to DSM-III, schizophreniform disorder meets all of the criteria for schizophrenia, except for the duration of the illness. The text of DSM-III, however, suggests that schizophreniform disorder is different from schizophrenia in several other respects. In schizophreniform disorder, there is a greater likelihood of emotional turmoil, confusion, fear, vivid hallucinations, acute onset, acute resolution, and recovery to premorbid levels of functioning (i.e., no deterioration). The text also comments that there is no increased prevalence of schizophrenia in the families of patients with schizophreniform disorder. Thus, on close inspection—examining the discussion section and not just the actual diagnostic criteria—the DSM-III concept of schizophreniform disorder is quite different from that of schizophrenia, in factors other than duration.

DSM-III-R adds to these diagnostic criteria four good prognosis features: acuteness of onset, confusion, good premorbid functioning, and absence of blunted or flat affect. At least two of these four features must be present for the disorder to be considered as having a good prognosis. DSM-III-R also specifies that there be a return to the approximate premorbid level of functioning. DSM-III-R returns the concept of schizophreniform closer to what Langfeldt had in mind and closer also to that of schizoaffective disorder.

The RDC does not acknowledge the concept of schizophreniform disorder. But it does subtype schizophrenia by course, and here the RDC describes a disorder resembling the schizophreniform disorder defined by DSM-III and DSM-III-R. The RDC defines acute schizophrenia as having a sudden onset (less than 3 months) and a short course (less than 3 months). Therefore, the total duration of the illness is less than 6 months, with a full recovery from any and all prior episodes. The RDC's definition of subacute schizophrenia, however, shifts away from DSM-III's and DSM-III-R's definitions of schizophreniform disorder. Here the onset is described as fairly rapid, and though not specifically defined, it must be assumed to be more than 3 months, according to the RDC's definition of a rapid onset. The active phase of the

TABLE 16.1-2
Diagnostic Criteria for Schizophreniform Disorder

A. Meets criteria A and C of schizophrenia.
B. An episode of the disturbance (including prodromal, active, and residual phases) lasts less than 6 months. (When the diagnosis must be made without waiting for recovery, it should be qualified as "provisional.")
C. Does not meet the criteria for brief reactive psychosis, and it cannot be established that an organic factor initiated and maintained the disturbance.

Specify: without good prognostic features or with good prognostic features (i.e., with at least two of the following):
(1) onset of prominent psychotic symptoms within 4 weeks of first noticeable change in usual behavior or functioning
(2) confusion, disorientation, or perplexity at the height of the psychotic episode
(3) good premorbid social and occupational functioning
(4) absence of blunted or flat affect.

Table from DSM-III-R *Diagnostic and Statistical Manual of Mental Disorders,* ed 3, revised. Copyright American Psychiatric Association, Washington, DC, 1987. Used with permission.

illness is limited to 5 months for the first episode and 6 months for the second episode. Thus, subacute schizophrenia is considered to be a recurring disorder, although it is associated with recovery.

The diagnostic label "schizophreniform" was not part of DSM-I or DSM-II. The clinical description most closely resembling this in DSM-I is schizophrenic reaction, acute undifferentiated type. The corresponding disorder in DSM-II is acute schizophrenic episode, which is described as the acute onset of schizophrenic symptoms accompanied by at least some of the following characteristics: confusion, perplexity, emotional turmoil, dream-like dissociation, excitement, and depression. The DSM-II clearly is describing a heterogeneous condition here. For example, it acknowledges that some cases recover within weeks, whereas others are progressive. Many patients who conform to the DSM-III criteria for schizophreniform illness would also have met the DSM-II criteria for acute schizophrenic episode.

The ICD-9 ignores the term "schizophreniform," instead using other diagnostic labels for patients who meet the DSM-III criteria for schizophreniform illness—labels such as "excitative psychosis" or "reactive confusion." In the ICD-9's glossary, the term "schizophreniform" is listed but not defined; the reader is referred to the term "schizophrenia." But the glossary does list under the term "schizophreniform" an affective type and a confusional type. These also are not defined, and for the affective type the reader is referred to schizophrenia, schizoaffective type, and for the confusional type, the reader is referred to schizophrenia, acute episode.

EPIDEMIOLOGY There are few data concerning the incidence and prevalence of schizophreniform disorder. But by comparing the number of cases in a hospital population identified as schizophreniform with the number of cases identified as schizophrenic, at least a general idea can be formed of the frequency with which schizophreniform disorder is identified in an inpatient population. The studies that provide such data suggest that schizophreniform disorder occurs somewhat less than half as often as does schizophrenia.

ETIOLOGY Because DSM-III altered the concept of schizophreniform disorder and because this discussion will use American psychiatry's official diagnostic scheme, only those data obtained since the publication of the DSM-III criteria will be used.

The findings of the five studies reviewed differed. One study found that schizophreniform patients had more affective symptoms and a better outcome than did their schizophrenic counterparts, thereby validating the criterion of the illness having a 6-month duration. The findings also suggest that some schizophreniform patients suffer from mood disorder, although perhaps of an atypical nature. In a relatively large-scale study, 16 percent of schizophreniform patients recovered, a rate far closer to the recovery rate (8 percent) of schizophrenic patients and considerably lower than the recovery rate (58 percent) of patients with unipolar and bipolar mood disorders. The number of relatives with each of the major psychotic illnesses was essentially identical in both the schizophreniform and the schizophrenic groups. These findings can thus be seen as relegating many of the schizophreniform patients to the schizophrenic realm. This study also found that the schizophreniform patients who did better had a very brief illness, usually considerably less than 6 months—closer to 1 month. A third study found that most patients who met the DSM-III criteria for schizophreniform disorder also met the DSM-III criteria for affective (mood) disorder. Overall, these patients appeared to have a course of illness, family history, response to treatment, and dexamethasone suppression test (DST) scores similar to those for pure mood disorder. The authors concluded that at least some forms of schizophreniform disorder are really a form of mood disorder. In another study, the mean VBRs of schizophreniform patients (5.3 ± 3.6) were closer to those of chronic schizophrenics (6.0 ± 4.2) than to those of patients with mood disorder (3.8 ± 2.9). A final study reported on sophisticated neuroendocrine functions. Schizophreniform patients had a rate of abnormal dexamethasone suppression midway between that of patients with mood disorder and that of patients with schizophrenia. The schizophreniform patients, however, had a rate of blunted thyroid-stimulating hormones (TSH) responsivity to thyrotropin-releasing hormone (TRH) that was almost identical to that of patients with mood disorder. This study suggested that schizophreniform disorder is probably a heterogeneous group of illnesses. If there were any evidence of neuroendocrine dysregulation in a patient with schizophreniform illness, then a relatively benign prognosis would be more likely than a deteriorating one.

Considered together, these studies do not allow one to conclude whether schizophreniform illness is more closely related to mood disorder or to schizophrenia or whether it is an independent disease. Clearly, at least some schizophreniform patients have a good prognosis with many similarities to mood disorder, whereas some have an illness with a greater resemblance to schizophrenia. These studies do show that the duration of the illness is related to outcome. Brief duration is indeed indicative of benign prognosis, and DSM-III's and DSM-III-R's figures of a 6-month total duration are probably too long. More likely, a total duration of illness of 1 to 2 months is associated with a benign prognosis.

PATHOLOGY As with many psychiatric illnesses, there are no well-established, specific neuropathological correlates or markers that have been determined to be specific for schizophreniform disorder.

CLINICAL SIGNS AND SYMPTOMS Schizophreniform disorder, by definition, is characterized by the presence of prominent schizophrenic signs and symptoms. At some point during the illness, the clinician can expect to see at least several of the common schizophrenic symptoms, including delusions or hallucinations. Delusions can be relatively straightforward expressions of falsely held beliefs, or they can be more complex and bizarre, such as thought broadcasting or the experience that one's mind is under the control of another. Hallucinations may also be relatively clear-cut, such as hearing a voice disparaging the patient or constantly commenting on the patient's behavior and thinking. The patient may also hear two or more voices conversing together. In schizophreniform disorder, the delusions or hallucinations may be incongruent with a depressed or elated mood. Other schizophrenic features that may be present are incoherence, marked loosening of associations, and psychomotor agitation or retardation similar to what has been described as catatonic. The flat or grossly inappropriate affect, which is so characteristic of schizophrenia, is only rarely seen in schizophreniform disorder.

These patients generally have good premorbid functioning. Despite a history of prior episodes with hospitalizations, such patients generally recover between episodes and are able to maintain social and vocational responsibilities. But during the episodes themselves, vocational, social, and familial functioning are seriously impaired. The onset of schizophreniform disorder is usually abrupt and is often related to a major emotional stress.

Affective symptoms are often present but not in sufficient quantity to warrant a diagnosis of pure mood disorder with mood-incongruent features. The affective symptoms in schizophreniform patients are usually, though not always, appropriate to the content of thought. The affective symptoms are not as prominent as are the schizophrenic symptoms.

Excessive agitation may be seen in these patients, who on occasion may exhibit assaultive, violent behavior.

DIFFERENTIAL DIAGNOSIS The disorders that most frequently need to be differentiated from schizophreniform disorder are schizophrenia, bipolar mood disorder with mood-incongruent features, and major depressive disorder with mood-incongruent features. Schizophreniform disorder can be differentiated from schizophrenia on the basis of history. If the illness has a total duration of more than 6 months, in either its present episode or a prior episode, then schizophrenia is present. Obviously, a patient or a collateral informant must be able to provide an accurate history concerning the duration of symptoms during all stages of the illness, to describe the premorbid functioning, and, if appropriate, to determine whether the patient returned to the premorbid level of functioning following an earlier episode.

Schizophreniform disorder can usually be distinguished from the mood disorders, mentioned above, in the following manner: In bipolar disease or major depressive disorder, the affective symptoms are clearly more prominent than the schizophrenic symptoms. In schizophreniform disorder, the schizophrenic symptoms are the most striking. In the mood disorders, when delusions or hallucinations develop, they develop secondarily (i.e., only after the mood symptoms are well established). Psychotic symptoms may in rare cases develop simultaneously with the mood symptoms, but they are less intense than the mood symptoms and do not develop prior to the appearance of affective symptoms. If the patient cannot provide an accurate history, then the diagnosis may be clear only after the patient has been observed over a period of time. If schizophrenic symptoms become less prominent longitudinally and if mood symptoms come to the fore, then a diagnosis of mood disorder can be confirmed. As mentioned in regard to schizoaffective disorder, if the diagnosis is not clear at a given time, it is appropriate to consider the diagnosis deferred or pending until longitudinal observation or a more accurate history can confirm it.

Because confusion can be a manifestation of schizophreniform disorder, it is sometimes necessary to include organic mental disorders in the differential diagnosis. A clouded sensorium is a relatively common finding in the organic mental disorders, whereas confusion is not always present in schizophreniform disorder. When confusion does occur in schizophreniform disorder, it is generally confined to the period of time when the psychotic symptoms are most intense.

Many neurological illnesses have been reported as being accompanied by schizophrenia-like (i.e., schizophreniform) psychotic states. A brief and incomplete listing of such illnesses includes temporal lobe epilepsy, space-occupying lesions, Huntington's chorea, and Parkinson's disease. Various medical conditions may also be associated with schizophrenia-like psychoses. Again, a brief and incomplete listing includes: exogenous anabolic steroid ingestion, pheochromocytoma, various infectious disorders, and certain metabolic disturbances. A careful medical history and physical examination usually reveal enough stigmata of the underlying medical or neurological illness to make these differentiations.

TREATMENT As with schizophrenia, the antipsychotic drugs are the treatment of choice in schizophreniform disorder. Because schizophreniform patients are often floridly psychotic and because the schizophrenic symptoms can develop rapidly, the required route of administration of the antipsychotic drugs may be intramuscular, or even intravenous in the most agitated cases. Megadosages of antipsychotic drugs may be required in the acute treatment phase in order to control severe agitation.

Because schizophreniform disorder is of brief duration, the long-term administration of antipsychotic medication is not necessary. As soon as the patient calms down and is free from delusions and hallucinations, the antipsychotic drugs should be tapered and withdrawn. If the patient cannot be controlled without chronic administration of antipsychotic medication, another diagnosis should be considered. Schizophrenia generally should be the first such consideration.

Because there are few data concerning the nature of schizophreniform disorder, including its long-term outcome, the treatment recommendations discussed here must be considered only speculative. A few papers have reported on managing with lithium or carbamazepine (Tegretol) the acute and chronic phases of schizophreniform disorder. These studies generally demonstrated favorable results, although schizophreniform patients who respond to lithium or carbamazepine may in fact be suffering from a mood disorder. This should be considered in cases in which apparently schizophreniform patients require prophylactic treatment with lithium or carbamazepine.

The following is a case example of schizophreniform disorder:

P. G. was a 20-year-old unmarried undergraduate student admitted to the hospital following a period of increasingly bizarre behavior, noted by his roommate.

P. G. had been well until 2 weeks before his admission. He had become agitated and preoccupied with thoughts of heredity and genetic transmission and would often stay up all night thinking about and writing about them. The roommate was unable to understand either P. G.'s ramblings or his voluminous writings. The roommate did state that P. G. had recently been rejected by a woman.

On examination, P. G. was floridly psychotic and confused. He thought he was in a genetics laboratory where his sperm was to be studied. His affect alternated between happiness—perhaps even euphoria—and intense anxiety. His verbal productions focused almost entirely on his concerns about transmitting "many generations of sperm." He drew picture after picture of individual spermatozoa and was convinced that within each sperm cell were hundreds of smaller sperm cells, and so each cell could control "many many generations of P. G.s yet to come." P. G. was afraid that some doctor would attempt to place a needle in his scrotum and "steal" his sperm, thereby depriving him of "many generations of offspring." At times, P. G.'s associations were so loose as to preclude understanding. When sufficiently frightened, he became physically threatening, and as a result, seclusion and restraints were necessary. P. G. was vigorously treated with antipsychotic medication, and within 3 weeks he was essentially symptom-free. He related that his rejection by his former girlfriend had damaged his masculine self-image.

His medication was gradually tapered over a 2-month period. P. G. was forced to drop out of school for the semester during which this episode occurred. But he returned the next semester and was able to make up for the lost time. He graduated with his class and went on to graduate school. He makes occasional follow-up visits and, 3 years later, appears essentially symptom-free.

P. G.'s premorbid history was free of any prior psychiatric symptoms, and he had no family history of any psychiatric illness.

BRIEF REACTIVE PSYCHOSIS

INTRODUCTION Brief reactive psychosis has been the subject of special study by Scandinavian psychiatrists, but only recently has this term received serious consideration by American psychiatrists. There is no true international agreement on this concept, which has often included various paranoid, confused, excited, and depressed states. In the Scandinavian concept of the disorder, much of which is included in DSM-III and DSM-III-R, the key element is that the condition is a reaction to the patient's background, personality development, and current stressful life situation. According to the criteria describing the stressor–reaction combination, the disorder has an abrupt onset in response to an intense trauma. The content of the psychosis reflects the traumatic experience, and the reaction is defensive. Its purpose is to allow the sufferer to escape the pain of the trauma. The illness has a benign course and terminates when the conditions that produced the traumatic experience are resolved.

DEFINITION Brief reactive psychosis is defined in DSM-III as a psychotic process with an abrupt onset and a short duration. It lasts no longer than 2 weeks and occurs immediately after a recognized psychosocial stressor. The stressor must be a major one that would evoke significant symptoms of distress in almost anyone. There is considerable emotional turmoil and rapid shifts in affects, without the persistence of any one affect. There are frankly psychotic symptoms, such as incoherence, looseness of associations, delusions, hallucinations, and grossly disorganized or catatonic behavior. This disorder resolves quickly, by definition within 2 weeks, and the patient eventually returns to the premorbid level of functioning. There is no premorbid symptomatology.

This definition was slightly modified by DSM-III-R (Table 16.1-3). The term "catatonic" was more precisely defined to include either catatonic stupor or catatonic excitement. The definition of the stressor also was broadened to represent a summation of more than one event, with this sum being markedly stressful to anyone, though each component stressor need not be markedly stressful. The duration of the illness was lengthened to 1 month. Emotional turmoil, specifically a rapid shift from one intense affect to another, or overwhelming perplexity or confusion were added as specific defining criteria.

TABLE 16.1-3
Diagnostic Criteria for Brief Reactive Psychosis

A. Presence of at least one of the following symptoms indicating impaired reality testing (not culturally sanctioned):
   (1) incoherence or marked loosening of associations
   (2) delusions
   (3) hallucinations
   (4) catatonic or disorganized behavior.

B. Emotional turmoil, i.e., rapid shifts from one intense affect to another, or overwhelming perplexity or confusion.

C. Appearance of the symptoms in A and B shortly after, and apparently in response to, one or more events that, singly or together, would be markedly stressful to almost anyone in similar circumstances in the person's culture.

D. Absence of the prodromal symptoms of schizophrenia, and failure to meet the criteria for schizotypal personality disorder before onset of the disturbance.

E. Duration of an episode of the disturbance of from a few hours to 1 month, with eventual full return to premorbid level of functioning. (When the diagnosis must be made without waiting for the expected recovery, it should be qualified as "provisional.")

F. Not due to a psychotic mood disorder (i.e., no full mood syndrome is present), and it cannot be established that an organic factor initiated and maintained the disturbance.

COMPARATIVE NOSOLOGY In American psychiatry, all psychiatric illnesses were at one time considered reactive. DSM-I described all functional psychotic and neurotic illnesses as reactive. But in DSM-III, only brief reactive psychosis retained this designation, so in this respect DSM-III is similar to the Scandinavian concept of brief reactive psychosis.

A major difficulty with the DSM-III concept is the somewhat arbitrary limitation of its duration to 2 weeks. That is, if the condition persists beyond 2 weeks, it must be reclassified, generally as schizophreniform disorder or perhaps as a mood or paranoid disorder. This is not satisfactory because schizophreniform, mood, and paranoid disorders are conceptually quite different from brief reactive psychosis, and it seems arbitrary to suggest that the basic nature of an illness changes merely because it lasts for 1 day longer than some preestablished duration. The Scandinavian concept has always implied a disorder lasting up to a month or two. DSM-III-R improved on this by specifically lengthening the duration criteria to 1 month.

Langfeldt's description of schizophreniform psychosis was probably heterogeneous and some of these patients probably develop a true schizophrenic illness, whereas some have truly reactive psychoses. Although some investigators may see brief reactive psychoses, schizophreniform psychoses, and schizophrenia as on a continuum in regard to their course, DSM-III-R considers brief reactive psychosis, schizophreniform disorder, and schizophrenia as distinct and not on a continuum. Only brief reactive psychosis is seen as an illness resulting from a severe psychosocial stressor and is therefore truly reactive in nature.

The RDC does not specifically address the concept of brief reactive psychosis.

DSM-I and DSM-II appear to consider the concept of brief reactive psychosis, or at least a condition somewhat similar. DSM-I describes psychotic reaction without clearly defined structural change, and DSM-II has a category, unspecified psychosis, that lists as subtypes reactive excitation and reactive confusion. But DSM-II does not define these conditions, and so it is difficult to know just what the authors meant, but obviously, some cases that DSM-III defined as brief reactive psychosis would fit these two DSM-II subtypes.

Because the ICD-9 is a true international classification and because brief reactive psychosis has been described and discussed in the Scandinavian literature for many years, it is no surprise that the ICD-9 labels brief reactive psychosis as a subtype of other and unspecified reactive psychoses. The ICD-9's glossary lists brief reactive psychosis and describes it as a florid psychosis of at least a few hours' duration, but not longer than 2 weeks. It has a sudden onset immediately following a severe environmental stress. Eventually, there is complete recovery to the prepsychotic state. The DSM-III and ICD-9 concepts are quite similar.

EPIDEMIOLOGY There are no reliable data concerning the incidence and prevalence of brief reactive psychosis as defined by DSM-III.

ETIOLOGY Because brief reactive psychosis has only recently been specifically defined in American psychiatry, there are no well-constructed etiological studies. In general, the outcome in reactive psychoses as defined by the Scandinavians has been good. Approximately 80 percent of patients with reactive psychoses have favorable outcomes, compared with about 60 percent of patients with schizophreniform illness and a mere 20 percent with true schizophrenia. Thus, it is unlikely that brief reactive psychosis is a close relative of schizophrenia. One Scandinavian study found the relatives of patients with brief reactive psychosis to have a slightly higher risk for mood disorder but not for schizophrenia. This too suggests that there is no relationship between brief reactive psychosis and schizophrenia, but it does suggest that some patients with brief reactive psychosis may be in the mood-disorder spectrum.

PATHOLOGY No specific neuropathological findings have been reliably described in regard to brief reactive psychosis.

CLINICAL SIGNS AND SYMPTOMS The essential feature of brief reactive psychosis is the rapid onset of a floridly psychotic picture in response to a serious psychological stressor or multiple stressors. These patients are generally young, usually adolescents or young adults, or are disaster victims or refugees. At least some of these patients would have been diagnosed in the past as suffering from hysterical psychosis.

Delusions, hallucinations, and paranoid ideation are often present and can usually be understood within the context of the prevailing severe psychosocial stressors. The patients may relate their story in a histrionic manner, and their symptoms may have a dramatic quality. But some patients are mute, and so their history must be obtained from collaterals. In other cases, the clinical picture might resemble a popular or theatrical idea of what psychotic behavior is like, such as demonstrated on television or in films.

There is usually a rapid and spontaneous recovery following cessation of the stressor. This can occur at any time from a few hours up to a month. There is usually a full return to the premorbid level of functioning and only minimal residual symptomatology.

DIFFERENTIAL DIAGNOSIS The greatest diagnostic concern is differentiating brief reactive psychosis from organic mental disorders and psychogenic amnesia.

The presence of an abrupt onset in apparent response to a significant emotional stress is the key factor supporting the diagnosis of brief reactive psychosis. Abrupt onset can certainly occur in many organic mental disorders, but prominent signs of disorientation and clouding of consciousness are present in the organic mental disorders. A thorough physical examination supplemented by laboratory work, including electrolytes, blood urea nitrogen (BUN), and creatinine, is essential. Toxic screening for drugs and alcohol is also indicated.

In psychogenic amnesia, the prominent feature is loss of memory associated with perplexity and disorientation. This may suggest brief reactive psychosis, but in psychogenic amnesia delusions, hallucinations, and markedly disorganized behavior—common stigmata of brief reactive psychosis—are absent.

TREATMENT Because brief reactive psychosis is a remitting, time-limited disorder, treatment is strictly symptomatic. If the patient has prominent psychotic symptoms, short-term treatment with an antipsychotic drug may be necessary. If psychotic features are not prominent, treatment with a milder medication, such as an anxiolytic agent or perhaps even a sedative-hypnotic, might suffice. By definition, long-term or chronic treatment of this disorder is unnecessary. If a patient does require chronic treatment, the presence of another psychotic disorder must be considered.

The following is a case example of brief reactive psychosis:

J. R., a 20-year-old unemployed college dropout, presented in an emergency room in an acutely agitated state. J. R. was essentially incoherent, although he occasionally would shout, "I'm no ____ fag" or "Kill all the queers," in a markedly aggressive, hostile fashion. J. R.'s affect was intense and rapidly shifted from angry arrogance to fear and withdrawal. He was delusional, insisting that all homosexuals would be "damned to the fires of hell." He described the presence of voices that repeatedly told him, "You're a queer, you're a queer." He was disoriented as to time and place.

J. R. was admitted to the hospital, and treatment was instituted with large dosages of intramuscular antipsychotic medication. He was assaultive toward a male nurse, whom he accused of "wanting to suck my cock."

J. R. responded in a matter of days and was able to provide some background. He had a long history of sexual identity confusion but during the past year had apparently accepted that he was homosexual. He had recently decided to "come out" and, in the process, had been assaulted by several abusive, ostensibly homophobic men who forced him to perform oral sex on them. His psychotic episode began shortly thereafter.

J. R. had no history of psychotic illness nor any family history of psychotic illness. J. R. felt that he could benefit from psychotherapy to help him deal with his sexual feelings, and this has helped him achieve substantial comfort with his sexuality. J. R. has done quite well since his discharge and continues in his outpatient psychotherapy. There is no evidence of any recurrence of his psychosis.

REFERENCES

Abrams R, Taylor M A: Importance of schizophrenic symptoms in the diagnosis of mania. Amer J Psychiat *138:* 658, 1981.

Carlson G A, Goodwin F K: The stages of mania. Arch Gen Psychiat *28:* 221, 1973.

Cloninger C R, Martin R L, Guze S B, Clayton P J: Diagnosis and prognosis in schizophrenia. Arch Gen Psychiat *42:* 15, 1985.

Coryell W: Schizoaffective and schizophreniform disorders. In *The Medical Basis of Psychiatry,* G Winokur, P Clayton, editors. Saunders, Philadelphia, 1986.

Coryell W, Lavori P, Endicott J, Keller M, Van Eerdewegh M: Outcome in schizoaffective, psychotic, and nonpsychotic depression: Course during a six- to 24-month follow-up. Arch Gen Psychiat *41:* 787, 1984.

Coryell W, Tsuang M T: Outcome after 40 years in DSM-III schizophreniform disorder. Arch Gen Psychiat *43:* 324, 1986.

Delva N J, Letemendia F J J: Lithium treatment in schizophrenia and schizo-affective disorders. Brit J Psychiat *141:* 387, 1982.

Kasanin J: The acute schizoaffective psychoses. Amer J Psychiat *13:* 97, 1933.

Kolakowska T, Williams A O, Ardern M, Revelay M A, Jambor K, Gelder M G, Mandelbroti B M: Schizophrenia with good and poor outcome. Early clinical features, response to neuroleptics and signs of organic dysfunction. Brit J Psychiat *146:* 229, 1985.

Langfeldt G: The prognosis in schizophrenia and the factors influencing the course of the disease. Acta Psychiat Scand (suppl 13), 1937.

Levinson D F, Levitt M E M: Schizoaffective mania reconsidered. Amer J Psychiat *144:* 415, 1987.

Miller F T, Libman H: Lithium carbonate in the treatment of schizophrenia and schizo-affective disorder: Review and hypothesis. Biol Psychiat *14:* 705, 1979.

Mitsuda H: The concept of "atypical psychoses" from the aspect of clinical genetics. Acta Psychiat Scand *41:* 372, 1965.

Pope H G, Lipinski J F: Diagnosis in schizophrenia and manic-depressive illness: A reassessment of the specificity of "schizophrenic" symptoms in the light of current research. Arch Gen Psychiat *35:* 811, 1978.

Retterstol N: The Scandinavian concept of reactive psychosis, schizophreniform psychoses and schizophrenia. Psychiat Clin *11:* 180, 1978.
Stephens J H, Shaffer J W, Carpenter W T: Reactive psychoses. J Nerv Ment Dis *170:* 657, 1982.
Tsuang M T, Dempsey G M: Long-term outcome of major psychoses: II. Schizoaffective disorder compared with schizophrenia, affective disorder, and a surgical control group. Arch Gen Psychiat *36:* 1302, 1979.
Vaillant G E: An historical review of the remitting schizophrenias. J Nerv Ment Dis *138:* 48, 1964.
Williams P V, McGlashan T M: Schizoaffective psychosis: I. Comparative long-term outcome. Arch Gen Psychiat *44:* 130, 1987.
Winokur G: Psychoses in bipolar and unipolar affective illness with special reference to schizo-affective disorder. Brit J Psychiat *145:* 236, 1984.

16.2 ATYPICAL, UNUSUAL, AND CULTURAL PSYCHOSES

VERNON M. NEPPE, M.D., Ph.D.
GARY J. TUCKER, M.D.

ATYPICAL PSYCHOSIS

INTRODUCTION The revised third edition of the *Diagnostic and Statistical Manual of Mental Disorders* (DSM-III-R) considers atypical psychosis as a category for "disorders in which there are psychotic symptoms (delusions, hallucinations, incoherence, marked loosening of associations, catatonic excitement or stupor, or grossly disorganized behavior) that do not meet the criteria for any other nonorganic psychotic disorder" (Table 16.2-1). The terminology has thus changed slightly from the third edition of the *Diagnostic and Statistical Manual of Mental Disorders* (DSM-III), which referred to this residual category as relating to psychotic symptoms that did not meet the criteria for "any specific mental disorder." The phrase "nonorganic psychotic disorder" is certainly more specific. It does raise some difficulties because several categories, such as epilepsy with psychosis, would qualify for a diagnosis of atypical psychosis using DSM-III, but it would be difficult to state that most of these patients are, in fact, nonorganic, although some of them are in relation to their psychotic disorder. Nevertheless, it does not disqualify the organic psychotic disorders ipso facto, as they too do not meet the criteria for nonorganic psychotic disorder.

The classic examples given in DSM-III, but applicable to DSM-III-R as well, for these conditions include psychoses with unusual features, for example:

1. Persistent auditory hallucinations as the only disturbance.
2. Transient psychotic episodes associated with the menstrual cycle, and postpartum psychoses that do not meet the criteria for an organic mental disorder or any other psychotic disorder.
3. Psychoses about which there is inadequate information to make a more specific diagnosis. This diagnosis can be changed if more information becomes available.
4. Psychoses with confusing clinical features that make impossible a more specific diagnosis. "Confusing" in this context means "perplexing" and not a clouding of consciousness.

Excluded from these criteria are psychoses that could be classified elsewhere except that their duration is less than 2 weeks (i.e., the symptomatology of a schizophreniform disorder lasting only 3 days). This category is also included in DSM-III-R. Atypical psychosis has clearly become the dumping ground for the diagnostically destitute.

Atypical psychosis implies a diagnosis that may change when the diagnostic criteria become clearer: Many of those patients diagnosed by one person as having atypical psychosis may have had a previous history or a history thereafter of being diagnosed successively as having schizophrenia, affective illness (mood disorder), or schizoaffective illness. This may have been preceded by diagnoses, such as schizophreniform illness, brief reactive psychosis, and borderline personality disorder. This category is very heterogeneous.

The following classification of atypical psychoses is thus proposed: (1) cultural psychoses, (2) other atypical psychoses (i.e., epileptic psychosis, temporal-limbic dysfunction with psychosis, nonresponsive psychosis), and (3) unusual psychoses.

CULTURAL PSYCHOSES

INTRODUCTION Emil Kraepelin's conceptualization of functional mental diseases as two clearly defined endogenous psychoses—dementia precox (schizophrenia) and manic-depressive psychosis—was a neat categorization, but many functional psychiatric disorders could not be fitted into this dual system. It is these categories that are now regarded as the atypical psychoses, many of which are unusual, exotic, or culturally related.

These three conditions are extremely important because they reflect the potential limitations of current conceptualizations of psychiatric illness more than any other conditions. Psychiatrists may not encounter many patients with unusual syndromes, and in Western societies these cultural psychoses are rare, but these categories of deviant behavior reflect the extent of psychopathology. But the similarities of psychopathology in many different cultures may lead to a

TABLE 16.2-1
Diagnostic Criteria for Psychotic Disorders Not Otherwise Specified (Atypical Psychosis)

Disorders in which there are psychotic symptoms (delusions, hallucinations, incoherence, marked loosening of associations, catatonic excitement or stupor, or grossly disorganized behavior) that do not meet the criteria for any other nonorganic psychotic disorder. This category should also be used for psychoses about which there is inadequate information to make a specific diagnosis. (This is preferable to "diagnosis deferred," and can be changed if more information becomes available.) This diagnosis is made only when it cannot be established that an organic factor initiated and maintained the disturbance.

Examples:
(1) psychoses with unusual features (e.g., persistent auditory hallucinations as the only disturbance)
(2) postpartum psychoses that do not meet the criteria for an organic mental disorder, psychotic mood disorder, or any other psychotic disorder
(3) psychoses with confusing clinical features that make a more specific diagnosis impossible.

Table from DSM-III-R *Diagnostic and Statistical Manual of Mental Disorders,* ed 3, revised. Copyright American Psychiatric Association, Washington, DC, 1987. Used with permission.

better appreciation of a homogeneous etiology and the dynamically related differences.

DEFINITION Cultural psychoses also are difficult to define. A broad definition of psychosis may be a loss of contact with reality that is associated with limited insight and impaired judgment and coping mechanisms. These phenomena, however, may be missed in the context of cultural syndromes and their subcultural variants, in which hallucinations may be viewed by the culture as normal variants. The definition of delusion thus must be reevaluated, and the frameworks of thought disorder and catatonic behavior must be reformed within the particular cultural setting.

Psychiatrists should not perceive many of these categories as separate. Often such categories differ in content and manifestations, but the core issues appear similar. Many of these categories may reflect schizophrenia or mood disorder dressed up in different clothes. Thus, a subculture or social culture may interpret aberrant behavior as relating to some kind of voodoo or anger of ancestors and may regard such behavior as within normal limits, even though these patients may conform to the conventional diagnosis of schizophrenia. This perception of psychopathology as normal, however, is unusual.

Two epidemiological studies of the endogenous black southern African population showed that referrals to psychiatrists and medical practitioners because of psychiatric illness almost always come from within, and not from outside, the culture. The culture, not the Westernized psychiatrist, therefore, perceives the behavior at the start as aberrant. Behavior that is particularly perceived as deviant is culturally disruptive behavior. Behavior, such as withdrawal into an autistic or catatonic stupor, is often not regarded as abnormal because it does not constitute a cultural disruption. Consequently, these patients may present only as medical emergencies. Similarly, hallucinatory or delusional experiences or potentially profound affective changes are not in themselves regarded as pathological; rather, some disruption in the status quo of the environment is required.

WESTERN DIAGNOSTIC BASE Most cases presenting in non-Western cultures can be diagnosed using a Western diagnostic schema. For example, the cross-sectional features of schizophrenia have been shown in several studies, including one by the World Health Organization, to be similar in form in several different cultural settings. The content of the delusional or hallucinatory experience, however, may differ depending on the particular culture.

CULTURE Culture refers to the complex patterns of learned behavior, values, and belief systems shared by members of a designated group. These patterns are generally transmitted through generations, creating a blueprint not only for thought and action but also for physical illness and its presentations, for psychopathology, and for models of treatment.

Culture is based on normative beliefs, values, perceptions, meanings, and behavior. A phenomenologically distinct component of culture is mental disorder, which involves particular perspectives of describing subjective experiences within that culture. The socioculture often dictates particular symptoms. For example, the absence of a word for depression in Africa and other cultures makes impossible the complaint of depression, although certain behaviors manifesting as depression may be present.

Western psychiatrists should be careful not to impose their own cultural ethnocentrism on indigenous peoples but should adapt to the requirements of these individuals and perceive differences. Their psychopathology may also be marked by such conditions as malnutrition and organic brain syndromes (e.g., cerebral syphilis) that are not often seen in more affluent societies.

Knowledge of the culture is essential to psychiatrists treating its members, including its norms, conceptions of illness, factors that predispose to illness, and the expectations of treatment. These factors influence the kind of help that is sought and the presenting symptoms. Thus, in certain cultures, voices heard in dreams are not generally separated from voices heard while awake. For example, in Africa, these both may reflect communications from the ancestors. Again, linguistic difficulties may cause such patients to indicate that they were asleep the whole night because they spent the time in bed, and so such questions as "Did you sleep with your eyes open or closed?" need to be asked. Behavior patterns also are influenced by culture.

CULTURE-BOUND SYNDROMES The basic principles of psychiatry still apply to such cultures, and the same kinds of psychopathology are still seen, as evidenced by the consistency of schizophrenia throughout many cultures.

Specific syndromes occurring within a particular culture are often referred to as *culture-bound*. They are restricted to that setting, and they have a special relationship to that setting. These syndromes appear distinctive and unique but delimitation of the syndrome even within the individual culture is not reliable. Very often these conditions have been classified on the basis of a common etiology, such as magic or evil spells or angry ancestors, such that their clinical pictures vary greatly.

THE PROJECTION MECHANISM The most common ego defense mechanism in many non-Western cultures is projection. Guilt and shame are often projected into cultural beliefs and ceremonies, and so they are not often private experiences. With such attempts to obviate guilt and shame, the consequence is that depression as seen in Westernized cultures appears far more rarely. In addition, because guilt and shame are attributed to other individuals, groups, or objects, there is a great deal of acting out of behavior, blaming others, and, consequently, needing to punish others. Assault may therefore be a substitute for suicide or self-harm.

The role of projection is also seen in magic and supernatural perspectives of existence. Outside forces cause problems, which leads to the development of protective ceremonies. When these protective ceremonies are not performed, their neglect may lead to illness: Thus, illness has an extraneous role and is not caused by organisms.

HYSTERICAL PSYCHOSIS A variety of terms, most commonly, "hysterical psychosis," have been used to describe some culture-bound syndromes. These syndromes are supposedly characterized by disruption of ego functioning with mounting frustration, generally at an interpersonal level, and emotional stress supposedly in a predisposed hysterical personality faced with a threatened or actual loss. It is a self-limiting condition generally lasting a week or less and certainly not more than 4 weeks. It is associated with acute delusions and hallucinatory experiences with no schizophrenic thought disorder. Often the delusions and hallucinations are family-syntonic and relate to family themes. This condition rapidly resolves itself.

Hysterical psychosis has also been called culture-bound psychosis, psychogenic psychosis, ethnic psychosis, exotic psychosis, and dissociative psychosis. This category has officially disappeared since the introduction of the term "brief reactive psychosis." Unfortunately, many of these conditions do not conform to this model because there is no overt stressor, and the psychoses are not necessarily brief. Using conventional DSM-III-R criteria, these conditions could be termed "schizophreniform," although some of these conditions are atypical enough to be called atypical psychosis. The authors feel that sometimes these patients' full psychopathology is not reflected in this blanket Western perspective.

The diagnostic criteria for these conditions are difficult to specify. The major features of these dissociative psychoses are acting-out behavior, conversion or dissociation during that episode or in the past, and a history of psychosis associated with auditory or visual hallucinations or both, and delusions. Longitudinally these patients do not deteriorate; they are premorbidly reasonable; and there is no reason that they be "hysterical personalities." The exclusion diagnoses are schizophrenia, schizophreniform illness, organic mental syndrome, and bipolar mood disorder. There is no restriction on further features, but the following are common: there may have been a previous episode; there may or may not be biological or vegetative symptoms; the duration is generally short, lasting hours to days, seldom weeks, but sometimes longer; there is a specific cultural relationship; there is a specific mechanism involving some kind of outside influence (either magical or supernatural) in non-Western cultures; and these conditions may occur more commonly in young adult females.

Analyzing conditions in this framework allows a perspective into many different cultural psychoses. These are seldom seen in Western settings and seldom in mental hospitals. Rather, they are seen in the community and in rural, indigenous, non-Western folk settings. Fitting these conditions to Western criteria will miss a great deal, as the manifestations of content are different, the mode of expression is different, the use of language is different, and the cultural response is different, but these conditions often reflect the same underlying perspective of culture-bound syndrome with psychosis or, alternatively, of schizophreniform psychosis, schizophrenia, or affective illness.

Another problem, seldom mentioned, is toxicity. Alcohol is a major toxin, and some kinds of alcohol drunk by some of the indigenous peoples of Africa contain other toxins. Intoxication by atropine-like derivatives and other hallucinogenic agents (i.e., hallucinogenic mushrooms) is not uncommon and further complicates assessments.

ATTRIBUTED ETIOLOGY In indigenous non-Western cultures, etiology can generally be divided into natural, magical, or supernatural. The natural may involve changes in a person's balance of sensitivity to supernatural and magical elements, perhaps because of herbs administered. A magical etiology generally involves "spells," or "black magic" of some kind, and is counteracted with "charms." The supernatural involves evil passed on to the patient, perhaps through their "living dead," or ancestors, who are angry and have taken away their protection or have cast a spell.

Western psychiatrists should understand that physical examinations under such circumstances are foreign because physicians, like the local folk diviners, are expected to diagnose from afar or "to divine the causes." Patients will not discuss such causes. They may provide hints, but in many cultures it is taboo to say that the cause is due to "my uncle who has cast a spell on me."

ROLE PLAYING IN FOLK CULTURE Local folk diviners are regarded as able to "divine" the causes of illnesses. Diviners differ from herbalists. Diviners play a religious role, go through an initiation phase, are called to their profession, and are involved in holistic treatment. Herbalists have a different kind of apprenticeship and may use their abilities for good and evil to treat patients with herbs. Senior kinsmen also play a major role, as they bring the patients to the appropriate therapist: Generally, patients first are treated at home, and when this fails, they are taken to the diviner or the herbalist. Only after that will they be taken to a Western physician, and so many of these patients, suffering severely, are presented late to the physician.

Such patients often present during puberty, marriage, death, and birth rituals. They do not generally present in later life because retirement is not a problem and older people in the culture are enormously respected and protected.

Herbal medicines consist of leaves, barks, fats, skins, roots, bulbs, fruit, flowers, and seeds. They may be dried, ground, or fresh. Some may be toxic. The color is important and has great symbolic meaning. For example, in the Zulu culture, black and red imply that the evil is coming out, and white implies good health; eating is viewed as having life; and defecation is associated with death.

The two major influences in culture-bound syndromes are the ancestors or other spirits (generally revealed by the diviner) and the spells cast by the evil herbalists, the "wizards." A third factor, dreams, enormously influences the behavior of these patients because their experience of reality during dreams is equated with those experiences during waking hours. Diseases are sometimes caused by ancestors who may communicate their wrath in dreams and cause the patient to act out on this. Certain patients are perceived by the culture as already compromised and therefore may be predisposed to different psychopathologies because they lack protection from their ancestors. Such persons include albinos, who are perceived in certain cultures as not having a soul. Similarly, when taboos, such as incest or sex during menstruation, are violated, this may take away ancestral protection and be a major stressor for illness.

Treatment of the syndrome should therefore be complementary, involving both the doctor and the indigenous therapist. Such a team approach may involve several members of the subculture because illness generally is a public phenomenon. Sometimes group therapeutic sessions (e.g., trances) with the ancestors may be held. The dyad of doctor and patient does not therefore exist. Patients must feel that their own skilled healer-diviner has not abandoned them and that the magic of the Western psychiatrist is stronger than what has caused the illness.

AMAFUFANYANE AS A PROTOTYPE Amafufanyane, a condition little known outside southern Africa, is important as a prototype. *Amafufanyane* is a psychiatric illness caused by witchcraft as practiced by a wizard (as opposed to diseases caused by the influences of ancestors' spirits). The patient may present to the "witch doctor" (i.e., the diviner-shaman-sangoma) for treatment. "Witch doctor" is a misnomer in that a witch doctor is not perceived as a witch but, as one described himself, "a doctor against the (evil) witches."

The (evil) wizard sends spells to the patient and, depending on the sex of the patient and the particular culture, they may be sent in the form of a baboon or a bird (sometimes at night). Thus, a female may present saying she is pregnant by a baboon, which may imply amafufanyane, as the baboon has delivered a particular evil spell to her. Alternatively, the evil spell may be delivered via objects or dead animals, or *tikoloshe*. It is these outside forces that are seen as producing the illness, thereby giving projection a fundamental role, as outlined above. The bewitched may present with delusions and hallucinations occurring during waking hours that may be interpreted as schizophrenic, and indeed it may be difficult to differentiate these conditions from schizophrenia.

Often there is a real somatic source, with epilepsy being a good example. Such persons will present with any form of acting-out behavior; they may have conversion symptoms—headaches and abdominal pains being particularly common—or they may have special kinds of pains. For example, a "shadow of the breast" is particularly common in young Zulu adolescent females who have pain in the left nipple. This condition may last a long time and be associated with a disturbed parent–child relationship. The cure for this condition is the cure for the spell cast by the perpetrator. Rarely this cure may be the murder of the person regarded as the perpetrator.

CULTURAL PSYCHOSES BY TAXONS Acting-out behaviors in the cultural psychoses can be sorted into various taxa. The meanings assigned to such behaviors vary from site to site, but the salient features are remarkably similar. The biological term *taxon* refers to a grouping based on similarities without specifying its level of abstraction. Ronald Simons divided such behaviors into seven taxa: startle matching, sleep paralysis, genital retraction, sudden mass assault, running, fright illness, and cannibalistic compulsion. Approximately 200 such cultural syndromes are described, many of which would not fit into the framework of a psychosis per se.

Sleep-paralysis taxon (amafufanyane) The taxon that is most difficult to attribute to psychosis is the sleep paralysis taxon. Sleep paralysis is a common symptom, often occurring in normal people and particularly in patients with narcolepsy, and it may be used in a broader framework for patients with somatoform disorders. Under these circumstances, amafufanyane as described above would fit this taxon. Amafufanyane occurs particularly in young females, classically in the Zulu population of southern Africa, and often contains sexual contents and symbols. The somatic features vary from abdominal pains, paralysis, blindness, hysterical seizure phenomena, shouting, and sobbing to amnesia. All of these fit into a "conversion–dissociation framework," a term probably preferred (i.e., "conversion–dissociation") to sleep paralysis taxon.

Sudden mass assault taxon (amok/benzi) The next taxon is the sudden mass assault taxon. The prototype condition for this is *amok,* which is certainly the most well-known cultural psychosis, as the phrase "to run amok" has been incorporated into English.

Amok is the Malayan word meaning "to engage furiously in battle," and the syndrome occurs in Malaysia and Indonesia. It is associated with a sudden, unprovoked outburst of wild rage causing the affected person to run madly about armed with a weapon—perhaps a knife, firearm, or grenade—and indiscriminantly maim, attack, or kill people and animals before being overpowered or committing suicide. Amok is a savage, homicidal attack involving an average of 10 victims and is often preceded by a period of preoccupation, brooding, and mild depression. After the attack, the person feels exhausted and is completely amnesic. The attack generally lasts a few hours and may be associated with an underlying toxic state or chronic psychotic condition. It may be precipitated by the belief in magical possessions by demons and evil spirits. Shame and loss of face have been hypothesized as relevant dynamic factors, as are special features pertaining to allowing children free reign, separation from family, recent loss, and intoxication.

Another example of an assault syndrome is *benzi,* occurring in the Shona of Zimbabwe. This is attributed to witchcraft and is associated with striking out at others, accompanied by amnesia. Alternatively, such patients may continually tell lies (not an example of sudden mass assault and difficult to classify into a taxon).

Genital retraction taxon (koro) The most characteristic condition of the genital retraction taxon group is *koro,* which occurs in south China and Malaysia. Koro is intense anxiety about the retraction of one's genitals—in males the penis, and in females the vulva or breasts—thereby leading to the attachment of devices to prevent such retraction.

The desperate fear that the penis is shrinking and disappearing into the abdomen, which will cause the patient to die, is a typical example of the difficulty of differentiating a delusion from a cultural belief system that a culture recognizes as an illness, and the family and indigenous healers are usually very concerned about the danger.

Epidemic outbreaks of a koro-like syndrome have occurred in Thailand, although it is regarded as relatively rare. The etiology appears to relate to culturally elaborated fears of nocturnal emission, masturbation, and sexual overindulgence. Fears concerning sexual virility and precipitators seem to be related to coitus, sudden exposure of the penis to cold water or cold air, tales of people dying from the illness, and the eating of spoiled food. The genital retraction taxon is therefore an example of a depersonalization syndrome affecting the integrity of the body image.

Startle-matching taxon (latah) *Latah* is an example of a startle-matching condition occurring in Malaysia or Indonesia. It is induced as a startle response and is characterized by echo phenomena, such as echolalia and echopraxis.

The startle reaction is caused by a sudden stimulus that suspends all normal activity. This stimulus triggers unusual and inappropriate motor and verbal manifestations over which the affected person has no voluntary control. A second kind of reaction is a mimetic or echo reaction in which a sudden stimulus initiates a compulsion to imitate any action or words to which the affected person is exposed. Automatic obedience is therefore common, and the condition may resemble catatonic schizophrenia. This is an example, therefore, of a cultural psychosis that may be fit into a Western framework.

The latah reaction may be brief and be a chronic disease with permanent automatic obedience and personality deterioration. It is perceived as the prototypical intense fright reaction involving disorganization of the ego and obliteration of the ego boundaries. A sudden fright may provoke inhibition of proper perceptual motor integration through loosening of ego boundaries and may render the patient powerless to resist any environmental stimuli.

The latah reaction's etiology may relate to the traditional beliefs in possession states or trance states with the consequent behavior of mimicking animals. Often this condition has a psychosexual element.

Running taxon (piblokto) The prototype of the running taxon condition is *piblokto* or *Arctic hysteria,* which occurs among Eskimos in the Arctic. It is characterized by attacks lasting from 1 to 2 hours during which the patient, usually a woman, screams and tears off and destroys her clothing. She may imitate the cry of some animal or bird and then throw herself in the snow or run wildly about on the ice, although the temperature may be well below zero. Echo phenomena, hysterical seizures, and amnesia for the episode are usual, although after the attack the patient appears quite normal. Broodiness and mutism may precede the attack. The Eskimos are reluctant to touch any afflicted person during the attack because they attribute the condition to evil spirits. It is therefore a running state that in Western society would be perceived as hysterical dissociation.

Cannibalistic compulsion taxon (windigo) The prototypical condition of the cannibalistic compulsion taxon is *windigo* or *wihtigo,* which occurs in central and northeast Canadian Indians who believe that they may be transformed into a *wihtigo,* or giant monster, that eats human flesh. The condition is preceded by depression and anorexia. Because of this possession by a giant monster who eats human flesh, it may ultimately manifest as homicidal or suicidal ideation and impulses. There may be a psychophysiological precipitator because it can occur during times of starvation, with an acute craving for human flesh, although it is generally attributed to witchcraft.

Fright illness taxon (hexing, voodoo, ghost illness) Three similar prototypical conditions in the fright illness taxon are hexing, voodoo, and ghost illness. Hexing and voodoo may be synonymous and occur in the Western world, including the United States, and often are accompanied by the delusion that patients have been doomed to die because of a voodoo or spell that has been cast on them. This produces various somatic symptoms. Such patients may well die, particularly if they are aware of when they are supposed to die. Such patients often believe that they are possessed. The possession states associated with the mythology, cultural traditions, and specific rituals of voodoo have been popular subjects for discussion among anthropologists, psychiatrists, and sociologists.

The voodoo cult is practiced in Africa and Brazil and among native West Indians and particularly in Haiti where voodoo ceremonies of 2 to 3 hours of dancing with wild rhythms and drums are accompanied by incantations of priests in hysterical trance states, excited hysterical seizure states, or twilight states. The transcultural significance is the patients' believing that they have been possessed by evil spirits. This produces their chronic hysterical and psychosomatic symptoms, which are sometimes extremely difficult to treat because the patients believe that the evil spells must be cast out. Besides voodoo, amafufanyane also has a fright illness component. One theory concerning death in such conditions is that the stress on a diseased heart may trigger fatal arrhythmias.

Ghost sickness occurs among the Kiowa Apache Indians in the southern plains of the United States and may be triggered by a death. During the mourning phase, such patients feel that the ghost of the dead person may be tormenting them. They do not want to turn around because of the sounds and the touch of the ghost that they may experience. This terror causes various psychophysiological conversion and dissociative symptoms, including palsies and seizure phenomena. There may or may not be cannibalism associated with this. If there is, it is attributed to witchcraft.

WESTERN CULTURE-BOUND PSYCHOSES

Two examples of Western cultural psychoses are anorexia nervosa–bulimia, which is described elsewhere, and subjective paranormal experience psychosis.

Cognitive disorders are often described as disorders of form or of content. The form of many atypical conditions superficially appears similar to schizophrenia. However, the cognitive content and the longitudinal course of the illness motivate separate diagnoses.

Subjective paranormal experience (SPE) psychosis is particularly interesting from a Western cultural perspective. Such patients believe that they have had *psychic experiences* or SPEs. This term implies subjective, hallucinatory, or delusional experiences but does not attempt to judge whether they are genuine. Persons who have SPEs claim a unique experience or reality, just as those who hallucinate do. Because they are not able to correlate their experiences with others' experiences, they may misinterpret reality.

SPE psychosis has the following features: onset of SPEs during childhood and a history of numerous SPEs that, to the subject, were well validated. The SPEs do not relate to the individual but pertain to other people and other contents, at least before the onset of the psychotic episode. At this stage, the patients start manifesting self-referenced delusions pertaining to at least one of these SPEs, often relating to their death. This produces a phase of acute turmoil. Patients are convinced that the SPE is true but are in turmoil because it cannot be proved. After the SPE has been shown to be false, a sudden recovery may follow. There is no deterioration phase and no family history of major psychiatric illness, but there is usually a family history of SPEs. Alternatively, there is a marked antagonism within the primary family group to any such experiences. These patients do not respond to appropriate management by conventional agents. They generally have no previous psychiatric history, maintain adequate and appropriate affective expression, and do not have any overt physical reasons for their symptoms.

A 30-year-old divorced female presented with the fixed idea that she was going to die that December. She had no previous psychiatric history or family history, and other than this fixed delusion, she did not appear floridly psychotic. She had no overt cognitive or vegetative depressive features, but she was acutely agitated and frustrated about her impending death and did not want to talk about it. As a consequence, she had periods of hopelessness lasting some hours. She had a history of numerous SPEs since early childhood and claimed she had never been proved wrong. The SPEs did not have a self-referential component until this time. Her admission had been precipitated by a Ouija board's having "told" her that she would die that December. This produced a rapid decompensation that required hospitalization. The patient was treated with psychotherapy and appropriate psychotropics, but these made no real impression on her delusional system.

PERSPECTIVE ON CULTURE-BOUND SYNDROMES

Culture-bound syndromes are by no means homogeneous, in either their symptomatology or their etiology. They do have, however, the following common elements:

1. These patients generally were normal before the onset of the syndrome.

2. Their behavior usually is some kind of acting out that attracts cultural attention. Amnesia is common.

3. The triggers of their behavior may be difficult to isolate, as they may not be perceived in Western culture as stressors.

4. There is no adequate information available on the personalities of these patients, and so labeling them hysterical personalities is justified at this point.

5. These conditions generally involve no deterioration.

6. Such patients are usually young.

7. There is no evidence of an underlying functional psychosis.

8. Such patients' illness may be either an isolated occurrence or chronic. There are always cultural attributions of this illness to an outside influence.

9. Somatic symptoms often are predominant, particularly gastrointestinal, genital, conversion phenomena, or dissociation.

10. These patients either improve spontaneously or need sedation or antipsychotics.

11. Therapy requires collaboration with traditional healers.

OTHER ATYPICAL PSYCHOSES

EPILEPTIC PSYCHOSIS Epileptic psychosis has had a somewhat speckled history in psychiatry. It was recognized in the nineteenth century by early researchers, such as Benedict A. Morel, Jean Pierre Falret, and Hughlings Jackson. It achieved a certain preeminence in the early 1920s when Emil Kraepelin classified it with dementia precox (schizophrenia) and manic-depressive insanity as one of the three major psychiatric illnesses.

The relationship between epilepsy and psychosis has been somewhat controversial and has given rise to two major theories. One is the antagonistic theory, and the second is the affinity theory. These contradictions become apparent if epilepsy and psychosis are not considered to be a single homogeneous condition. The antagonistic theory argues that epilepsy and psychosis are opposite sides of a pole, that psychosis is more likely to occur when the epilepsy is well controlled, and that poor control of the epilepsy is not associated with psychosis. The affinity theory is based on epidemiological studies showing a substantially and significantly increased incidence of psychoses in epileptics compared with what would be expected by chance.

Clinical signs and symptoms The heterogeneity of epileptic psychosis is marked. For example, the interictal psychoses of epilepsy, particularly the more long-lasting chronic kinds of interictal psychosis, have often been characterized as schizophrenia-like or schizophreniform. These conditions seem to differ from classical schizophrenia because these patients are nonschizoid and nonparanoid premorbidly: They maintain good rapport, and their affect does not appear to be blunt. They also maintain good contact with reality and have substantial insight into their condition. They have no family history of schizophrenia and do not appear to have the negative features of schizophrenia (apathy, amotivation, withdrawal, autism, and blunting). The similarity of patients with temporal lobe epileptic-type psychoses (which appears to be the most common form of this schizophrenia-like illness) and schizophrenia has been demonstrated on Present State Examination, and this is like the profile of the schizophrenic person. But whereas these features emphasize the positive features of schizophrenia, the negative withdrawal features are often absent, suggesting a temporal, as opposed to a frontotemporal, base for some such conditions.

Etiology The etiology of the epilepsy–psychosis relationship is as follows:

1. The psychopathology is related to organic mental syndrome factors, not the seizure itself.
   a. The first possibility is epilepsy as an epiphenomenon of underlying diffuse organic brain disturbance. This is most commonly seen in the mentally retarded person with coexistent secondary generalized epilepsy (i.e., epilepsy generalized from the start with diffuse generalized slowing on the electroencephalogram [EEG], probably reflecting the diffuse generalized pathology).
   b. The second link is a consequence of anticonvulsant medication, with features of cognitive, affective, and motoric disturbance (this has commonly been recognized and is particularly associated with such anticonvulsants as phenytoin [Dilantin], phenobarbital, primidone [Mysoline], and ethosuxamide [Zarontin]). The role of anticonvulsants in provoking cognitive-behavioral deterioration has been borne out by many studies. Psychosis occurs in clouded consciousness with intoxication and may be precipitated in clear consciousness with ethosuxamide.
   c. The third link is a consequence of cerebral anoxia caused by previous status epilepticus with secondary organic brain damage. Structural changes caused by the seizures may be more common than previously thought, particularly in such areas as Sommer's area in the mesial temporal lobe.
   d. The fourth link is created when the organic mental syndrome is secondary to an active intracranial lesion (e.g., tumor or extracranial causes, such as metabolic encephalopathy), and it presents with both epilepsy and severe behavior disturbance. Such delirious states are often misinterpreted as psychosis.
2. Psychiatric illness may be due to a manifestation of the epilepsy itself. This implies peri-ictal seizure activity associated with psychomotor automatisms or complex partial seizures associated with substantial cognitive and behavioral manifestations. Such presentations are often missed, though only rarely present as psychosis (Table 16.2-2).
3. Psychosocial elements play a predominant role. The rejection by society, the limitations in social interaction lest a seizure occur, the feelings of psychological inferiority and frustration because of the diagnosis of epilepsy, the fears that others may find out about the seizure disorder (taken, at times, to a paranoid persecutory delusional extreme), and the rejections by family and friends all are major psychosocial elements. These may precipitate particularly reactive psychosis states.
4. The site of the epileptic focus may be relevant, particularly when the site is in the temporal lobe or the focus is in the dominant hemisphere. There is much literature on the links between temporal lobe epilepsy and psychosis or, particularly, dominant temporal lobe epilepsy (Table 16.2-2).
5. The kindling phenomenon has been used to explain some of the links between complex partial services (usually temporal lobe epilepsy) and their psychiatric manifestations.
6. The links of epilepsy and psychosis may relate purely

TABLE 16.2-2
Possible Temporal Lobe Symptoms

Paroxysmal (recurrent) episodes of
1. Complex visual hallucinations linked to other qualities of perception, such as voice, emotions, or time

Any form of
2. Auditory perceptual abnormality
3. Olfactory hallucinations
4. Gustatory hallucinations
5. Rotation of disequilibrium feelings linked to other perceptual qualities
6. Unexplained "sinking," "rising," or "gripping" epigastric sensations
7. Playback
8. Illusions of distance, size (micropsia), loudness, tempo, strangeness, unreality, fear, sorrow
9. Hallucinations of indescribable modality

Paroxysmal (recurrent) episodes of
1. Epileptic amnesia
2. Lapses
3. Conscious confusion
4. Epileptic automatisms
5. Masticatory-salivatory episodes
6. Speech automatisms
7. "Fear which comes from itself" linked to other disorders (hallucinatory or unusual autonomic)
8. Uncontrolled, unprecipitated, undirected, aggressive episodes
9. Superior quadrantic homonymous hemianopia
10. Receptive (Wernicke's) aphasia

to a genetic or other constitutional predisposition to both conditions or to some kind of incidental-coexistence explanation.

TEMPORAL ASSOCIATIONS The above etiological possibilities may be combined with time (temporal) associations to the seizure manifestation itself. When the behavioral disorder is a direct manifestation of the seizure disorder itself, this peri-ictal condition is differentiated from disorders occurring between seizure manifestations (interictal).

Peri-ictal disorder The peri-ictal disorder may be subdivided into preictal, ictal, and postictal.

Preictal conditions occur before the seizure, either as a prodrome that may last some days before the seizure itself or as an aura that arrives minutes or seconds before the major convulsive seizure. An example of a prodrome is major alterations in affect, such as profound depression or irritability and agitation, or major cognitive alterations lasting for several days with the patient becoming disorganized and somewhat incoherent in his or her thinking and ending with a tonic clonic seizure. Alternatively, an aura of fear may last a few seconds before a tonic clonic seizure. Such a fear may be associated with profound behavioral consequences, possibly because it is anatomically linked to the mesial temporal lobe. Ictal manifestations themselves may best be linked to psychomotor automatisms, in which the person may manifest automatic behavior in a state of defective consciousness with no memory for this. This automatic behavior may not be only of a simple motoric kind (i.e., buttoning or unbuttoning the shirt or movements of the mouth) but may involve complicated fugue states or furor states that may be misinterpreted as psychosis. Postictal manifestations may occur immediately after the seizure without the patient's returning to normal consciousness or normal behavior in between. Such postictal elements may be associated with profound behavior disorder, irritability, agitation, clouding of consciousness, and misinterpretations of reality, which may be gross, as well as the more common headache and sleepiness.

Interictal disorder Interictal psychoses commonly are more prolonged, lasting days, weeks, months, or even the person's lifetime. Therefore, they may range from acute and subacute to chronic and may be commonly associated with paranoid hallucinatory psychoses, pure delusional syndromes, atypical hallucinatory experiences, or schizophrenia- or mania-like conditions. These manifestations vary.

EPIDEMIOLOGICAL AFFINITY Despite more than 100 publications in the scientific literature on epilepsy in relation to psychosis, the area has been little explored and ill defined. Such studies suggest that the incidence of epilepsy in relation to psychosis is about 2 to 27 percent, with the most common figure being about 7 percent. These studies have major difficulties and consequent methodological flaws that have plagued the literature on epilepsy and psychosis. The first difficulty is in the definitions. Psychosis, particularly in the epilepsy–psychosis literature, has often been perceived far more broadly than many psychiatrists would perceive it. That is, patients with overt clouding of consciousness have been included as psychotic, whereas many psychiatrists would regard these patients as delirious or use terms, such as "confusion," implying a clouding of consciousness. The authors suggest that psychosis in the context of epilepsy be limited to conditions associated with hallucinations, delusions, thought disorders, or other incoherence in the face of clear consciousness, or, at best, an altered but not defective state of consciousness. For example, states of profound depersonalization and derealization with occasional amnesic components may be acceptable, but not states in which there is defective consciousness with profound persistent amnesia throughout.

The definition of epilepsy should be easier but, unfortunately, is not. Epilepsy is technically defined as a recurrent paroxysmal condition manifesting with biochemical and electrical discharges in the brain and associated with alterations in consciousness, behavior, cognition, affect, and motoric functions. But sometimes psychotic patients are referred with a previous diagnosis of epilepsy that is difficult to confirm, with a history of a single seizure that implies no recurrence of this condition, or with a history of more than one seizure but which may have been associated with alcohol or other form of withdrawal. The authors suggest that for patients to be subclassified under epileptic psychosis, they must have not only psychosis as defined above, in clear or altered consciousness, but also have a confirmed history of epilepsy associated with at least two documented seizures not linked to withdrawal phenomena.

TEMPORAL LOBE EPILEPSY AND PSYCHOSIS: ETIOLOGY The above confounding features are particularly prominent when correlating temporal lobe epilepsy specifically with psychosis. There are no consistent diagnostic features for temporal epilepsy; instead, they may range from the purely clinical diagnoses to the purely EEG diagnoses, which reflect two extremes ranging from the very rare spike waves in the temporal lobe to nonspecific paroxysmal episodes in the temporal lobe. On the other hand, diagnostic criteria for temporal lobe epilepsy may require both clinical diagnosis with EEG confirmation, with varying degrees of accuracy.

The term "temporal lobe epilepsy" is not used in the latest classification of seizures of the International League Against Epilepsy. Temporal lobe epilepsy is often regarded as synonymous with complex partial seizures, although such manifestations may also include simple partial seizures, behavioral arrests (absences, psychomotor automatisms, or generalized tonic clonic seizures).

The incidence of psychoses in such temporal lobe epilepsy studies is four to eight times higher than in epilepsy with generalized tonic clonic seizures and no evidence of a temporal lobe focus. The many confounding features may suggest that the epidemiological evidence for the increased incidence of temporal lobe epilepsy and psychosis over other epilepsies is seriously flawed.

TREATMENT The management of patients with temporal lobe epilepsy depends largely on their symptomatology and presentation. There are certain ground rules, however. (1) Patients with mild mental retardation and secondary generalized epilepsy when presenting psychotic generally have unfixed, unsystematized delusions. Such patients do well with low doses of antipsychotics. They generally develop side effects before attaining a conventional dose of antipsychotics. They are antipsychotic nontolerators and develop extrapyramidal symptoms and autonomic or hypnogenic effects, depending on the particular drug used. (2) Those patients with temporal lobe epilepsy with paranoid hallucinatory psychoses generally require antiepileptic monotherapy, usually carbamazepine (Tegretol), with high doses of antipsychotics.

Choosing the antipsychotic is difficult, and the literature is unclear in this regard because all antipsychotics are epileptogenic. When analyzing hippocampal firing in guinea pig slices, such drugs as pimozide (Orap) have less firing, and chlorpromazine (Thorazine) peaks in mid-dosage and, in fact, in higher dosage may have some anticonvulsant properties. Haloperidol (Haldol) and chlorpromazine are markedly synergistic in increasing hippocampal firings, thereby suggesting that antipsychotics should not be mixed. Thioridazine (Mellaril) causes less firing than most. On a clinical basis, haloperidol, thioridazine, thiothixene (Navane), and prochlorperazine (Compazine) have commonly been used in epilepsy. The issue of antipsychotics is therefore unresolved.

Peri-ictal conditions occurring without clouding but with delusional or hallucinatory features should be treated predominantly with anticonvulsants with as small a dose of antipsychotics as possible. Manic-like symptoms occur interictally, and so a drug like lithium could be considered in addition to the invariable carbamazepine monotherapy. Complex partial seizure epileptics should be treated entirely with anticonvulsants, particularly such drugs as lorazapam (Halcion), diazepam (Valium), or, where available, clonazepam (Klonopin) parenterally.

Postsurgical (post-temporal lobectomy) psychotic patients are particularly intractable to treat. They may present with refractory hallucinatory experiences and often require various combinations of therapy. Patients with preictal psychoses, if of sufficient severity, may occasionally warrant induction of the seizure by electroconvulsive therapy (ECT).

TEMPORAL-LIMBIC DYSFUNCTION WITH PSYCHOSIS The category of temporal-limbic dysfunction with psychosis is highly controversial and may not exist. It is mentioned here only because many patients with atypical psychosis do not respond to conventional antipsychotic therapy and, in fact, may become somewhat dysphoric on antipsychotics but do not have histories of hard seizure disorder. Many of these patients do have histories of soft neurological condition (i.e., attention-deficit hyperactivity disorder as a child, abuse of hallucinogenic medications, previous minor head injury, or birth trauma) and may present with psychotic features that may be paranoid hallucinatory or schizophreniform.

These patients may have marked affective elements and lability of affect. Such patients have been investigated in several studies. The only double-blind randomized study used carbamazepine versus a placebo in all chronic hospitalized psychiatric patients with nonspecific EEG temporal lobe abnormalities. Three-quarters of the 11 patients were technically diagnosed as DSM-III-R schizophrenics, but all seven of these patients were extremely atypical in regard to nonblunting, absence of withdrawal, and reasonable interpersonal relationships. The patients improved substantially on carbamazepine, as compared with the placebo, and the principal improvement was self-control. In uncontrolled studies, anticonvulsant medication was added to dysphoric antipsychotic for nonresponders with abnormal EEGs, with similar improvement. Another study of patients with such symptomatology and spells of impaired consciousness or altered behavior and marked lability of mood also responded to anticonvulsant medication. All these studies suggest the adjunctive use of anticonvulsants (carbamazepine particularly but others as well) in this specially selected psychotic population.

Such case descriptions suggest that sometimes anticonvulsants, particularly carbamazepine, may be valuable adjuncts to the treatment of patients with atypical psychoses and particularly in patients with other features of temporal lobe dysfunction. Such a temporal lobe dysfunction may be at either an epileptic level or a nonepileptic level, so that either firing or some kind of minimal atrophic defective lesion may occur.

The following symptomatologies may suggest the initiation of carbamazepine:

1. Spells in which the patient loses track of time. Staring, dazed feelings, trance or dream-like symptoms, and absences are consistent features.
2. Intense episodic mood swings, dyscontrol episodes, hostility, panic-like anxiety attacks, or sudden depressive moods occurring abruptly and episodically and remitting suddenly.
3. Episodic disturbances of thought processes with forced thoughts, Schneiderian first-rank features, episodic delusions, racing thoughts, loosened associations, and suicidality (either previously with attempts or suicidal ideation unrelated to any precipitator with the same kind of sudden abruptness).
4. Episodic auditory, visual, or tactile hallucinations, sometimes polymodal in quality and with a sharp, distinct nature and quite normal behavior in between. These phenomena all are brief and focused and may include other perceptual phenomena. Alternatively, although EEG is a rather primitive method based on scalp recordings to analyze data, the presence of a temporal lobe focus on the EEG may support such an attempt. These patients seldom have paroxysmal foci or spike-wave types of foci.

NONRESPONSIVE PSYCHOSIS The spectrum of nonresponsive psychoses implies heterogeneous conditions. At one end is the subgroup of patients who do not tolerate antipsychotic doses of conventional antipsychotic medication. When the doses are lowered to subpsychotic doses, they still are not tolerated. These patients develop extrapyramidal side effects if given aromatic antipsychotics, and hypnogenic or autonomic effects if given alaphatic antipsychotics in subpsychotic dosages. Considering the relevance of psychopharmacological responsiveness, this issue may be superimposed on the clinical manifestations on which the diagnosis is based. In an uncontrolled prospective study of more than 3,000 successive psychotic admissions, only a score did not tolerate antipsychotics. In every instance organic pathology was demonstrated, the most common being hyperthyroidism. Such a study reinforces the dopamine theory of psychosis, and when patients are given adequate doses of dopamine blocker and do not respond appropriately, it may imply that they cannot have a psychosis related to dopamine.

A second subgroup is those patients who tolerate antipsychotic doses of antipsychotics but whose symptomatologies do not respond. These patients also show heterogeneous symptoms, which may again imply a certain atypical psychosis or atypicality of the underlying schizophrenia or mood disorder. Among the strategies to be tried in such patients, treatment adjunctive to their antipsychotics should be considered. For example, anxiety may sometimes respond to propranolol (Inderal) as an adjunct to the antipsychotic medication, not as an antipsychotic. Affective features may call for the addition of lithium, and antidepressants may be required for depression. Extrapyramidal symptoms and signs require anticholinergics.

The most interesting symptoms are those that may respond to anticonvulsants or, more specifically, limbic-antikindling agents. There is some literature on the usage of carbamazepine in such patients and on temporal-limbic instability psychosis, an overlapping condition in nonresponsive psychoses. The authors believe, however, that the kindling phenomenon may be very important to human psychopharmacology.

OTHER UNUSUAL PSYCHOSES

Two unusual psychoses, *folie à deux* (shared paranoid disorder) and the conditions that make up the brief reactive psychoses, are dealt with elsewhere in this text. Six syndromes are briefly described below—Capgras' syndrome, autoscopy, Clérembault's syndrome, Cotard's syndrome, atypical cycloid psychosis, and atypical schizophrenia. These six conditions do not appear in DSM-III-R.

THE CAPGRAS' SYNDROME Capgras' syndrome was described in 1923 by the French psychiatrist Jean Marie Joseph Capgras as *illusion de sosies*. *Sosies,* French for "double," has its origins in the Greek play *Amphitryon,* in which Mercury impersonates the servant Sosia.

Capgras' syndrome refers to the fixed false belief (i.e., a delusion) in doubles of significant others and, infrequently, of oneself. Thus, this condition involves fixed false beliefs, as opposed to distortions (illusions) or percepts without the presence of any stimuli (i.e., hallucinations). Consequently, the original *illusion de sosies* is a misnomer, as the Capgras' syndrome is a delusional syndrome.

The essential feature of the Capgras' syndrome is the negation of identity. In effect, the double component is induced by a denial that certain features, often characterological, can occur in a person with whom the patient usually has strong emotional ties. For example, a patient's wife may be idealized as perfect. When something happens that may contradict this idea, the patient may perceive his wife as an imposter. That is, this woman cannot be his wife, as she is perfect, and consequently he denies the authenticity of his wife's identity. He clearly recognizes her; his problem is not perceptual. The patient does not perceive images of a double. His wife looks the same and even talks the same, perhaps even behaves the same, but the patient's distorted thinking allows the splitting of these physical and characterological features. He insists that this is a double, and this splitting is associated with a sense of strangeness about the person. Because of these features, an intense affective sentiment appears, such that the double invariably is a member of the family or someone else in a supportive role, like a doctor.

When the patient believes himself or herself to be an imposter, such a presentation can be compared with a dual personality, in which the patient can behave and feel quite differently, depending on the personality assumed. But in Capgras' syndrome, the ego defense mechanism involved is projection. Such patients project characteristics that they cannot accept as belonging to themselves. Patients with a dual personality, in contrast, handle their anxiety by dissociating.

The most common diagnosis associated with Capgras' syndrome appears to be schizophrenia, particularly paranoid schizophrenia. About one-fifth of these patients have organic psychotic reactions, and a few have various conditions, such as manic-depressive disorder, mood disorder, alcoholism, borderline personality disorder, and postpartum conditions. It manifests at any age in adults and about equally in males and females. Depending on the underlying diagnosis, the syndrome is best treated with antidepressants, antipsychotics, and ECT, the last with varying success.

The underlying cause of Capgras' syndrome is neither perceptual nor a disturbance of memory. Patients can easily recall facts about the nonimposters who they now believe are imposters. Their delusion is selective and may or may not be explained psychodynamically.

AUTOSCOPY Another apparently rare condition is *autoscopy,* or illusions or hallucinations of self. In contrast with Capgras' syndrome, with its delusion of doubles of self, the experience of autoscopy is perceptual and most commonly is a visual hallucination of oneself. It may be extended to looking, talking, dressing, and acting like oneself, and in this instance all the senses—visual, auditory, and kinesthetic—and all actions may be involved. The autoscopic double may not necessarily be hallucinatory but may be an illusion or vivid fantasy. The condition has been regarded psychiatrically as caused by various organic and functional conditions, but it may also occur in states of exhaustion or anxiety in normal people. The psychiatric literature does not agree that autoscopy, which by definition is an SPE, can occur in normal nonpsychiatrically disordered people.

The major difference between Capgras' syndrome and autoscopy is the psychological identity between the real self and the double. The double in autoscopy is not an imposter but is another self, thereby inducing perplexity, detached insight, or a sense of unreality of the experience. These phenomena are generally not symptomatic of any mental disorder. The hallucinatory experience may involve only a part of the person's own body, sometimes only the face or bust. If visualized, it is usually colorless and transparent but is seen clearly, appears suddenly and without warning, and imitates the person's movements. Such dislocated body images usually appear for only a few seconds and may appear at dusk.

Sex, age, heredity, and intelligence do not seem to be significantly related to the occurrence of autoscopy. Autoscopy may occur only once in a lifetime, but some people appear to experience it regularly. Johann Wolfgang von Goethe, Percy Shelley, Guy de Maupassant, and Edgar Allan Poe all claimed to have had autoscopic experiences.

CLÉREMBAULT'S SYNDROME French, Italian, Brazilian, and North American psychiatric literature refers to two different syndromes, both named Clérembault's syndrome. The better known of the two is *psychose passionelle* or *erotomania*. This is the delusional conviction that someone who hardly knows the patient or does not know the patient at all is passionately in love with him or her. This conviction is often symptomatic of an underlying paranoid schizophrenia.

The second Clérembault's syndrome is characterized by automatisms of the mental apparatus, explosive and absurd utterances, thought echoes, and the feeling of being possessed and influenced by some dissociated force. The possession syndrome of Clérembault strongly resembles the experiences that are frequently expressed by schizophrenic patients and are probably manifestations of a primarily paranoid state or paranoid schizophrenia.

COTARD'S SYNDROME Cotard's syndrome was described by the French psychiatrist Jules Cotard in the late nineteenth century as *délire de négation*. Such patients may complain of having lost not only their possessions, status, and strength but also their heart, blood, and intestines. They may also reduce the world beyond them to nothingness. The full-blown syndrome may be characterized by other megalomelancholic ideas, such as delusions of immortality. Patients with this syndrome do not appear to differ greatly from those who manifest nihilistic delusions, although these are particularly intense.

Such delusions are common in psychotic endogenous depressions (i.e., major depression with melancholia and psychosis). They may also occur in organic mental syndromes associated with primary degenerative dementia of the Alzheimer type, senile onset, and their treatment is that of the underlying condition.

ATYPICAL CYCLOID PSYCHOSES The final two unusual or atypical psychoses to be discussed are K. Leonhard's atypical cycloid psychoses and atypical schizophrenias. These he considered as classes of atypical psychoses that are independent nosological categories with their own genetic characteristics and are not just idiopathic variations or mixtures of two more typical psychoses—manic-depressive and schizophrenic.

Leonhard subdivided the cycloid psychoses, which are characterized by phasic recurrences, into three forms: motility psychoses, confusional psychoses, and anxiety–blissfulness psychoses. The hyphenated name of the third form of these cycloid psychoses suggests a bipolarity; the first one is clinically divided into hyperkinetic and akinetic motility psychoses, and the second one is divided into excited and inhibited confusional psychoses.

In their hyperkinetic form, the motility psychoses may resemble a manic or catatonic excitement. A hyperkinetic motility psychosis may be distinguished from a manic state by the presence of many abrupt gestures and expressive movements that seem to be the result of autonomous mechanisms and are apparently not responses to environmental stimuli or expressions of the patient's mood. These disorders may be differentiated from catatonic excitement by the absence of stereotypical and bizarre movements.

The akinetic motility psychosis seems to be identical with the typical picture of a catatonic stupor. Leonhard separated these states from typical schizophrenia mainly because of their rapid and favorable course, which does not lead to any personality deterioration.

The excited confusional psychosis should be distinguished from some confused manic states. The difference is mainly in the greater lability of the patient's emotional state, which may be characterized by prevailing anxiety rather than euphoria. These patients are not as distractable as manic patients are; they often misidentify persons in their environment, and the incoherence of their speech seems to be independent of their flight of ideas.

The inhibited confusional psychosis shares with the catatonic stupor and the akinetic motility psychosis the symptoms of mutism and greatly decreased motor psychosis, but it differs from these states in its preservation of better self-care, greater spontaneity, and the absence of negativism.

The anxiety phase of the anxiety–blissfulness psychosis may resemble what is generally known as agitated depression, but it also may be characterized by so much anxious inhibition that the patient can hardly move. Periodic states of overwhelming anxiety and paranoid ideas of reference are characteristic of this condition, but self-accusations, hypochondriacal preoccupations, and other depressive symptoms, as well as hallucinations, may accompany it.

The blissfulness phase is manifested most frequently in expansive behavior and grandiose ideas, which are concerned less with self-aggrandizement than with the mission of making others happy and saving the world. In women, the dominant emotion is usually passive ecstacy, often the result of fantastic religious delusions, which to most observers appear to be almost pathognomonic of schizophrenia.

Leonhard stated that within the group of cycloid psychoses, periodic recurrences are most frequent in the motility psychoses. They are less frequent in the anxiety–blissfulness ones and are still rarer in the confusional psychoses. Complete recovery of the patient is the rule.

ATYPICAL SCHIZOPHRENIAS Leonhard believed that the atypical schizophrenias carry a poorer prognosis and are more malignant than the cycloid psychoses. He distinguished three atypical schizophrenias: affective-laden paraphrenia, periodic catatonia, and schizophasia.

Patients suffering from affect-laden paraphrenia express manifold delusions, which may be well systematized. They receive their characteristic color from the strong and sustained affect that pervades them. This affect is pathological, although it may be an appropriate reaction to the delusions' content. It may be expressed as irritability, anxiety, or ecstasy. A certain similarity of symptoms may make the differentiation from anxiety–blissfulness psychosis difficult, particularly at the beginning of the psychosis.

Periodic catatonia differs from typical schizophrenic catatonia by its periodic excited or stuporous phases. It may sometimes resemble an akinetic or hyperkinetic mobility psychosis. It usually presents distinctive symptoms of stereotypy, bizarreness, grimacing, and a peculiar mixture of simultaneous akinetic and hyperkinetic manifestations.

Schizophasia is characterized by a profound thought disturbance. This results in a disorder of concept formation and abstract thinking and is expressed in marked incoherence of speech. Such patients may sometimes resemble excited confusional psychotics and, at other times, excited catatonics or hebephrenics.

Leonhard justified the separation of these atypical psychoses from the nuclear group by citing the much greater range of variation in the symptoms of the atypical psychoses. He found further confirmation of these independent groups in the fact that these atypical psychoses have a different (i.e., much higher) rate of genetic transmission than the typical schizophrenias. In a study of 826 typical schizophrenias, the incidence of mental disease in the siblings was 5.3 percent. In 203 atypical schizophrenias, all three forms combined, the corresponding percentage was 13.3. Similarly, Leonhard demonstrated a higher incidence of suicides in the family histories of atypical schizophrenias when compared with those of the typical systematic schizophrenias.

The prognosis is, in general, much poorer for the atypical schizophrenias than for the cycloid psychoses, and it is most guarded for the schizophasic patients, who often remain chronically ill or may recover but with a permanent personality defect.

REFERENCES

Berson R J: Capgras' syndrome. Amer J Psychiat *140:* 969, 1983.
Bradley P B, Hirsch S R, editors: *The Psychopharmacology and Treatment of Schizophrenia.* Oxford University Press, Oxford, England, 1986.
Golden K M: Voodoo in Africa and the United States. Amer J Psychiat *134:* 1425, 1977.
Lehmann H E: Unusual psychiatric disorders, atypical psychoses, and brief reactive psychosis. In *Comprehensive Textbook of Psychiatry,* ed 4, A L Kaplan, B J Sadock, A M Freedman, editors, p 1224. Williams & Wilkins, Baltimore, 1984.
Leonhard K: Kaspar Hauser und die moderne renntis des hospitalismus. Confin Psychiat *13:* 213, 1970.
McKenna P J, Rane J M, Parrish R: Psychotic syndromes in epilepsy. Amer J Psychiat *142:* 895, 1985.
Murphy H B M: History and evolution of syndromes: The striking case of latah and amok. In *Psychopathology: Contributions from the Social, Behavioral and Biological Sciences,* M Hammer, K Salzinger, S Sutton, editors, p 33. Wiley, New York, 1983.
Neppe V M: *The Psychology of Déjà Vu: Have I Been Here Before?* Witwaterstrand University Press, Johannesburg, 1983.
Neppe V M: Subjective paranormal experience psychosis. Parap Rev *15:* 7, 1984.
Neppe V M: Epilepsy and psychiatry: Essential links and management. Psychiat Insight *2:* 18, 1985.
Neppe V M: *Innovative Psychopharmacotherapy.* Raven Press, New York, 1989.
Neppe V M, guest editor: Carbamazepine use in neuropsychiatry. J Clin Psychiat *49*(4 suppl): 1, 1988.
Neppe V M, Tucker G J: Modern perspectives on epilepsy in relation to psychiatry. Hosp Comm Psychiat *39:* 263 and 389, 1988.
Pincus J H, Tucker G J: *Behavioral Neurology,* ed 3. Oxford University Press, New York, 1985.
Simons R C, Hughes C C, editors: *The Culture Bound Syndrome: Folk Illnesses of Psychiatric and Anthropological Interest.* Reidel, Boston, 1986.
Stevens J R: Intercerebral clinical manifestations of complex partial seizures. In *Advances in Neurology,* J K Penry, D D Daly, editors, vol 21, p 85. Raven Press, New York, 1975.
Stromgren E: Psychogenic psychoses. In *Themes and Variations in European Psychiatry,* S Hirsch, M Shepard, K Kalinowsky, editors, p 97. University of Virginia Press, Charlottesville, 1974.
Trimble M R, editor: *The Psychopharmacology of Epilepsy.* Chichester, New York, 1985.
Tucker G J, Price T R P, Johnson V B, McAllister T: Phenomenology of temporal lobe dysfunction: A link to atypical psychoses—A series of cases. J Nerv Ment Dis *174:* 348, 1986.
Tucker G J, Neppe V M: Neurology and psychiatry. Gen Hosp Psychiat *10:* 24, 1988.

16.3 POSTPARTUM PSYCHOTIC DISORDERS

DAVID G. INWOOD, M.D.

INTRODUCTION

Recent prospective studies in the United States and especially in Great Britain have resulted in the beginning of reliable predictions about which groups of women are at the highest risk for developing postpartum psychiatric disorders: psychosis, the blues, and depression. Short, standardized screening questionnaires are being developed to identify women at risk in the antenatal period, and preliminary prospective intervention strategies can now be formulated. The data show that more than 50 percent of women with a prior history of postpartum psychosis will experience a second episode in future pregnancies. Also, women with a history of both bipolar manic depression and postpartum decompensation are at the greatest risk for recurrence. Therefore, obstetricians, psychiatrists, midwives, nurse clinicians, and social workers are now able to advise the patient and her family of the risk of future psychiatric disorders in the puerperium and to provide the care and support needed during the pre- and postpartum periods if the patient elects to have more children.

NORMAL POSTPARTUM REACTIONS

Psychoanalytically oriented psychiatrists have focused on the conscious and unconscious stresses experienced during the pregnancy and postpartum periods, as a woman attempts to resolve conflicts concerning feminine identification, body image, nurturance, dependency, and her relationship with her own mother and father. Similarly, interpersonally oriented psychiatrists have focused on the major changes in the woman's relationship and role with her husband, the nature of the marriage, and the beginnings of motherhood and caring for an infant.

Phenomenologically, studies of the normal immediate postpartum period show that the first few days following delivery are psychologically stressful, that there are major hormonal changes, and that the woman's behavior may mimic depressive symptoms associated with any mild adjustment reaction. Women frequently complain of dysphoria, irritability, anxiety, emotional lability, tearfulness, and fatigue. There may even be mild vegetative symptoms, such as sleep disturbance, changes in appetite, and loss of desire for intimacy. Of course, many women experience the pre- and postpartum periods as pleasant and emotionally satisfying.

Compared to multiparas, women who have delivered for the first time report heightened distress during the pre- and postpartum periods. The disruption of life routines and even the anticipation of caring for a helpless child worry some women. Many postpartum women report that caring for their infants is sometimes difficult and isolating.

Additional quantitative studies of exactly what constitutes the normal adjustment responses would be helpful. Nonetheless, the epidemiology of the more severe pathological responses has been well documented.

EPIDEMIOLOGY

Epidemiological studies in the United States and Great Britain using Research Diagnostic Criteria for psychosis and depression concur on incidence rates:

- Severe puerperal psychosis occurs in one or two per thousand deliveries.
- Mild postpartum blues occur in up to 50 percent of women.
- Significant postpartum depressive disorders occur in up to 10 percent of women.

For epidemiological studies, the postpartum period has been defined as occurring from 2 weeks to 1 year following the birth of the child. The British use the entire first year as the time frame; the author believes that this is clinically most useful.

Epidemiological studies have revealed two major facts:

1. In the first postpartum month, a woman is at the highest risk for psychiatric hospitalization that she is at during her entire life. Rarely in psychiatry may such a predictable danger period be so clearly anticipated. Epidemiologists found that 18 times as many women were admitted to a psychiatric facility during the first postpartum month as were admitted during any of the 9 months of pregnancy. Researchers concur on hospitalization rates over the postpartum year:
   - 50 percent in the first postpartum week
   - 25 percent in the second through the fourth weeks
   - 25 percent over the rest of the year
2. What further makes this so remarkable and distressing is that more than 70 percent of these women have had no apparent prior psychiatric history.

CLASSIFICATION

Investigators using Research Diagnostic Criteria found that more than three-quarters of hospitalized women in the puerperium showed symptoms of labile mania and that one-quarter presented with major depression. These figures substantiate the data presented by the French psychiatrist Louis Marcé, who, in 1848, wrote "A Treatise on Insanity in Pregnant, Puerperal, and Lactating Women." He described the symptom confluence of mood lability, confusion, visual hallucinations, delirium, catatonia, and echolalia. More contemporary investigators have recognized that the earlier the onset, the more dramatic the presentation. The puerperal psychosis presents with elements of affective, schizophreniform, and organic features that clinically change daily and even hourly in a very dramatic manner. Other investigators have focused on studying groups of women who experience mild postpartum blues and later-occurring postpartum depressions.

The nosological classification of puerperal phenomenology has been somewhat controversial. Many, though not all, of the principal researchers in this field argue that the temporal contiguity between the life-stressful event of parturition and the development of postpartum psychiatric disorders deserves diagnostic recognition. Other investigators, as well as the official U.S. psychiatric diagnostic nomenclature, view postpartum psychosis as a variant of major mood disorders with manic or atypical psychotic features, in which a significant portion of sufferers will go on to develop bipolar mood disorders or recurrent unipolar depressions. Therefore, they do not believe it necessary to grant diagnostic recognition to postpartum disorders.

Still, it is important to note that classification schemas in psychiatry (that is, the first, second, third and revised third editions of the *Diagnostic and Statistical Manual of Mental Disorders* [DSM-I, DSM-II, DSM-III, DSM-III-R], Group for the Advancement of Psychiatry, and the ninth revision of the *International Classification of Diseases* [ICD-9]) come and go with disconcerting frequency. Practicing clinicians, academicians, and trainees are expected to adopt the consensually agreed-on conceptualizations and are obliged to diagnose, treat, and perhaps be compensated on the basis of these often-changed schemas.

Critical reviewers of nosology stress that there is no natural or one right way to classify psychiatric conditions. A descriptive approach can be as valid as an etiological approach. To be clinically useful in psychiatric work with patients, a diagnosis should have reliability, explicit criteria, and predictive validity. The author believes that by these standards the spectrum of postpartum psychiatric disorders has earned nosological recognition. Accordingly, the author suggests the following three-part classification schema. The schema is derived from Research Diagnostic Criteria, DSM-III-R nomenclature, and findings from the ongoing investigative literature.

For heuristic, research, and clinical purposes, postpartum psychiatric disorders should be considered to be a single diagnosable syndrome with a three-part subclassification (Table 16.3-1). The author is not proposing an idiosyncratic schema for the nosological criteria, but instead attempting to simplify and parsimoniously conceptualize observable puerperal phenomena as rooted to major developmental, biological, and psychosocial events in a woman's life cycle. This is an attempt to organize the phenomena instead of scattering them, as does the DSM-III-R. DSM-III-R also ignores the work of those investigators who have carried out reliable and valid prospective studies of postpartum disorders. The knowledge gained from those studies can now be clinically used to identify and formulate comprehensive treatment plans to aid women at risk.

ETIOLOGY

Psychiatrists continually struggle to explain why their patients become ill. A postpartum disorder is particularly tantalizing, though ultimately frustrating, for clinicians who prefer to seek a single explanation for the emergence of the "point epidemic" of childbirth that apparently makes so many women psychiatrically ill. Investigative hypotheses have been based on psychoanalytic concepts, the hypothalamic-pituitary-gonadal axis, neurotransmitters, genetics, life stressors, and social support theories. Regardless of their theoretical emphasis, investigators concur that puerperal psychoses occur twice as commonly in the primiparous as in the multiparous woman and that there is probably a heterogeneous population consisting of different subgroups of women. The risk of developing a postpartum disorder is increased if the patient or her mother has had a previous puerperal illness or if the family has a history of mood disorder. Patients with a known history of bipolar illness who have experienced a postpartum psychiatric illness are at the highest risk of all for recurrence in a subsequent pregnancy. One study showed a 100 percent recurrence rate. A constitutional or genetic factor associating bipolar illness with a predisposition to the development of post-

TABLE 16.3-1
Three-Part Subclassification of Postpartum Psychiatric Disorders:
Type I: Postpartum Psychosis (also known as Puerperal Psychosis or Brief Reactive Psychosis)
Type II: Adjustment Reaction with Depressed Mood (also known as Postpartum, Maternal, or Postnatal Blues)
Type III: Postpartum Major Mood Disorder (also known as Major Depression, Postpartum Neurosis, or Neurotic Reaction)

Characteristic	*Type I* *Postpartum Psychosis*	*Type II* *Adjustment Reaction with Depressed Mood*	*Type III* *Postpartum Major Mood Disorder*
Incidence	0.1%–0.2% (1–2 per 1,000)	Up to 50%	10%
Etiology	Hormonal, genetic	Psychological stress, hormonal variability	Psychological stress, genetic vulnerability
Symptoms	Hallucinations, labile affect, agitation, delirium	Mild irritability, fearfulness, insomnia, labile mood	Sadness, inadequacy, fatigue, guilt, fearfulness
Risk factors	Previous puerperal psychosis, manic-depressive history, prenatal life stressors, obsessive personality, family history of mood disorder	Narcissistic vulnerability, primiparity, premenstrual disorders	Primiparity, prepartum depression, ambivalence about the pregnancy, marital discord, poor relationship with parents
Onset	Day 3 to 1 month	Day 1 to 6 weeks	4 weeks to 1 year
Possibility of suicide or infanticide	Up to 10%	Rare	Less than 5%
Treatment	Hospitalization, antipsychotics, electroconvulsive therapy, social support, psychotherapy, child care assistance	Support from family and physicians	Medication, psychotherapy, social support, possible hospitalization, child care assistance
Prognosis with treatment	Good for first episode, at risk for recurrence (10%–50%)	Excellent	Variable, from good to continuous episodes of affective disorder

Table from Inwood D G: *Recent Advances in Postpartum Psychiatric Disorders*. American Psychiatric Press, Washington, DC, 1985, with permission.

partum mood disorders is the major known unequivocal risk factor.

Mood disorder in a parent, especially bipolar illness or a postpartum disorder in the maternal line, is the most significant stressor. An older study described postpartum emotional problems experienced by fathers, adoptive parents, and grandmothers of the new baby. The National Institute of Mental Health recently reported on a group of bipolar manic-depressive fathers. The study found that half of the men experienced an affective episode during the partum period, most often during the pregnancy.

BIOLOGICAL FACTORS **Estrogen, progesterone, and prolactin levels** Biological explanations have attempted to relate the onset of affective symptoms and affective illnesses that occur premenstrually, postpartum, and menopausally with alterations in the hormonal levels of the hypothalamic-pituitary-gonadal axis. Specifically, in the immediate postpartum period (the 5 days following delivery), there is a dramatic drop in estrogen and progesterone levels and a large increase in prolactin. This correlates with the peak presentation of postpartum psychosis. Although the data are not complete, many but not all women who experience menstrual distress also experience postpartum distress. The progesterone level drops from 140 to 2 ng per ml 10 days after delivery, and the estrogen level decreases from 2100 to 10 ng per ml by the ninth day. The elevated prolactin level by day 3 is associated with lactogenesis but decreases after the milk-let-down reflex. Unfortunately, because postpartum psychosis is relatively rare, many investigators' findings have been based on studies of women who have experienced milder postpartum blues or severe postpartum depressions. And because the incidence is so low, it is difficult to gather a large enough group of puerperally psychotic women to be able to conduct a prospective study. Therefore, many of the findings have been confusing and even disappointing when they are extrapolated to those who experience puerperal psychoses.

The most thorough studies correlated hormonal levels with moods in multiparous and primiparous women during the antenatal and postnatal periods. After controlling for social stress factors, the study found that:

1. The higher predelivery estrogen level was associated with greater irritability in the subjects.
2. The lower the progesterone level dropped, the more likely the subjects were to be depressed within 10 days of giving birth.
3. The lower the progesterone level dropped, the fewer sleep disturbances were reported.
4. The lower the postpartum estrogen level was, the greater the sleep disturbance was.

These symptoms were minor in degree and duration; generalizations from postpartum blues to the psychosis may be made only with great caution. Nonetheless, some clinicians have attempted to treat unresponsive puerperal psychosis with trials of exogenous progesterone or estrogen and have found varying degrees of improvement.

Other investigators have studied the effects of prolactin. Some have noted that a low premenstrual progesterone level associated with a high prolactin level may lead to irritability, hostility, and anxiety. Also, a low level of estrogen combined with a high prolactin level may produce depressive symptoms. This profile occurs in the postpartum period, especially when the patient experiences postpartum blues. Therefore, some investigators have reported effectively treating depression in double-blind studies using bromocriptine (Parlodel) to lower the prolactin level as well as to increase dopaminergic neurotransmission. Recent reports find that bipolar depressions respond even more favorably to bromocriptine than do unipolar depressions. If this finding is confirmed by others, bromocriptine may prove to be a particularly useful medication and perhaps even a prophylaxis for at-risk populations.

Cyclic adenosine monophosphate It is known that cyclic adenosine monophosphate (cAMP) is elevated during pregnancy. Some researchers have found that women who experienced mood changes had large increases in cAMP during their pregnancy and that decreased cAMP in the postpartum period may be associated with depression.

Cortisol Urinary-free cortisol excretion increases late in pregnancy, surges at birth, and then rapidly declines. Although some studies have linked both increased and decreased cortisol levels in women who experience postpartum blues, there are no published cortisol studies of women with postpartum psychosis or major mood disorder. Nonetheless, there are reported but unreplicated case-history studies of clinicians favorably treating with steroids women who had resistant postpartum depression and a low cortisol level. Indeed, the same investigator claims to have prevented recurrences of postpartum depression with the prophylactic use of prednisone administered to at-risk patients.

Alpha-2-adrenoceptor, tryptophan, and serotonin Similarly, there are reports of persistent increase, as compared with the expected decrease, in α-2-adrenoceptor capacity in women who suffer postpartum blues. The α-2-adrenoceptor levels have not been studied for the puerperal psychoses. Other investigators have studied the levels of tryptophan, the precursor of 5-OH tryptamine, and serotonin in the immediate postpartum period (days 2 to 5). They were able to correlate low tryptophan levels with depressed mood, but did not actually study any patients who had puerperal psychosis.

Thyroid hormone Numerous anecdotal reports have correlated postpartum mood disorders with alterations in thyroid hormone level; the researchers recommend treatment with exogenous thyroid. Hormonal investigations have not yet revealed the biological cause for postpartum disorders, but it is clear that psychiatric disorders are often accompanied by disturbances in the hypothalamic-pituitary-gonadal axis. Because it is well known that psychological stimuli affect the neuroendocrine system, hormonal studies should take into account psychosocial findings.

Endorphins Reports suggest that decreased levels of endorphin covary with the decrease in estrogen levels in the postpartum period. Decreased levels of endorphins are related to dysphoria, decreased motor activity, lability, and lethargy.

Serum calcium One study reported an elevated serum ionized calcium among puerperally psychotic women who had no previous personal or family history of psychiatric illness. These patients were compared with three groups of women: (1) puerperally psychotic women with personal and family histories of psychiatric illness, (2) postpartum women without psychiatric illness, and (3) psychiatrically ill women who were not in the postpartum period. The control groups of women did not have elevated serum calcium levels. On follow-up 12 to 25 months later, those women without previous personal or family psychiatric illness were found to have had much better recoveries. There was a significant correlation between the fall of the serum calcium level and improved psychiatric functioning. If this study is replicated, calcium levels may serve as a marker to predict which women are more or less likely to improve and which women may be vulnerable to recurrence of postpartum illness.

Sleep Sleep investigators, having noted significant disturbances in sleeping during pregnancy and the postpartum period, focus on the decreased stage 4 sleep time. The problems in interpreting this finding are that the overwhelming majority of pregnant and postpartum women experience sleep disruption and that though many of them become irritable, relatively few develop frank psychiatric disorders. Nonetheless, the clinician is always advised to help the affected woman return to as regular a sleep pattern as possible.

PSYCHOSOCIAL AND OBSTETRICAL FACTORS

Psychoanalytic formulations have postulated that the pre- and postpartum periods are stressful for women. These stresses lead to regressions that evoke earlier conflicts, especially when there has been a history of inadequate maternal role models or rejection by the mother. Also important is a history of conflict with the father or a period of separation from him. The depression, if not the actual psychosis, may result from unresolved conflicts regarding motherhood or the feminine role. Some researchers have found that women who assessed themselves on a rating scale as more masculine than others reported fewer psychiatric symptoms during pregnancy but more during the postpartum period.

Researchers tend to agree that ambivalence about maintaining the pregnancy and marital discord during the pregnancy are associated with an increased incidence of postpartum illness. There are inconsistent findings about whether prepartum depression or anxiety leads to an increased incidence of postpartum distress. The lack of social supports has been implicated as a major factor in increased postpartum disorders. Other supposedly stressful life events include low socioeconomic status, poverty, and legitimacy of the pregnancy.

Personality studies indicate that women who have obsessive-compulsive traits are at risk for experiencing postpartum disorders. Their coping mechanisms are rigid and inflexible. They often experience a great deal of guilt and a sense of inadequacy that may accompany unacceptable feelings of anxiety and hostility. Indeed, many psychiatrists view obsessive-compulsive syndromes as a variant of a mood disorder.

Obstetrical events other than parity have not proven to be significant. Factors such as age of the mother, prematurity of the infant, medical complication during the pregnancy, prolonged or complicated labor, caesarean delivery, fetal loss, and gender of the baby have not proven useful in identifying those women at risk of postpartum psychiatric illness.

SUBCLASSIFICATION OF POSTPARTUM PSYCHIATRIC DISORDERS

TYPE I: POSTPARTUM PSYCHOSIS (ALSO KNOWN AS PUERPERAL PSYCHOSIS OR BRIEF REACTIVE PSYCHOSIS)

Mrs. D. P., the 27-year-old primiparous, white, Catholic wife of an internist, had two previous abortions at ages 16 and 26 but no prior remarkable psychiatric history. The patient's mother did not have a history of postpartum disorder, but her father experienced a brief psychotic event 3 years earlier. The patient was pressured by her husband into conceiving a child shortly after the last termination. During the pregnancy, she often felt miserable, suffered from insomnia, and had a large weight gain. Three days after giving birth to a healthy daughter, she became febrile, agitated, delirious, and religiously preoccupied. The patient showed elated mood, flight of ideas, and frequent lability of affect. An extensive medical workup, including a spinal tap, was negative.

The patient was hospitalized on a university service for 3 weeks. The baby, who was being cared for by the maternal grandmother, frequently visited under the careful supervision of the nursing staff. The patient was treated in the hospital with chlorpromazine (Thorazine) 400 mg. On discharge, she received thiothixene (Navane) 10 mg per day, but she complained of side effects, and so the medication was tapered and discontinued 3 months postpartum. The patient stayed in her mother's home for the first month and then moved to her own home, where she was often troubled by obsessive thoughts about picking up a knife and stabbing her daughter. Her husband was alerted to the patient's distress. He altered his schedule and became less aloof and more flexible in his approach to his wife. Her mother continued to help care for the baby. Much improved, the patient discontinued twice-weekly psychotherapy after 6 months but maintains regular phone contact with a psychiatrist to discuss child rearing.

Clinical signs and symptoms Puerperal psychosis, occurring within the first 6 weeks postpartum and having its peak incidence between day 3 and day 14, is the gravest and most dramatic of all the postpartum disorders. The frequency is low (between 1 and 2 per 1,000 births), but it must be recognized as a true medical-psychiatric emergency. The mother should be hospitalized. There is a real risk of infanticide or suicide. The author believes that clinicians must be prepared to document in great detail why they decided not to hospitalize the mother and instead attempted to treat her on an outpatient basis. Historically, English common law, but only inconsistently U.S. law, has recognized that the mother was criminally insane if she injured her child during this illness—still, this is of little consolation to a bereft family. Indeed, in some U.S. localities, mothers are criminally prosecuted and jailed for these injuries or deaths.

The illness is characterized by agitation, restlessness, insomnia, mood lability, tearfulness, elation, progression to a state of confusion, irrationality, and eventually a fulminant psychotic episode with signs of mania and delirium. In former times, the illness often occurred while the mother was still on the obstetrical unit. However, today, with the trend toward early discharge for the uneventful noncaesarian delivery, the mothers are already home and are not usually scheduled to be seen by the obstetrician until the sixth postpartum week. Therefore, the burden of trying to make sense of the woman's peculiar behavior falls on the family. As noted in the case history, preliminary investigative evaluations often center on discovering a physical explanation for the onset of bizarre behavior. The experienced clinician eventually recognizes the nature of the illness and then refers the patient for a psychiatric evaluation.

The natural course of the illness has been studied for over 100 years. It is now known that most women will make a good recovery from the acute illness. Unfortunately, 10 percent to 50 percent of these women will have recurrent episodes in subsequent pregnancies, regardless of whether chemoprophylaxis or psychotherapeutic interventions are offered or even whether the woman is followed at a specialized referral center.

The best longitudinal study was of 75 women followed over a 30-year period. It was found that 85 percent had a diagnosis of mood disorder, and although some of them relapsed during subsequent pregnancies, most of them functioned well at most other times. The 15 percent of women who were diagnosed as schizophrenic tended to have disabilities that more pregnancies intensified and that were accompanied by deterioration of the underlying schizophrenic process. Five percent of the sample ultimately committed suicide, and there was a probable infanticide rate of 4 percent. Only about 1 percent of the women was diagnosed as having an obsessional disorder. But it was commonly reported that many of the women had obsessional thoughts about harming their infant, although the vast majority (96 percent) did not actually injure their baby.

Treatment Postpartum psychosis is a major psychiatric emergency. Because suicide and infanticide are significant occurrences, an immediate psychiatric evaluation with a high probability of recommendation to hospitalize defines the parameters of the initial assessment. Because most affected women have no known previous psychiatric history, the physician must tactfully but decisively form an alliance with the family to inform them of the immediate gravity of the situation and the need for vigilance until the patient is stabilized. Most women recover from the episode, and so a sense of guarded optimism is justified and should be conveyed to the family and to the patient when she is able to understand what has been happening to her.

The British, with their system of conjoint mother–child hospitalization in specialized units in general hospitals, have pioneered a humane and developmentally sensible approach to facilitate mother–child attachment in even the most adverse conditions. Although there have been occasions on which the mother injured herself or her child, most mothers under the careful observation of experienced nurses have been able to tend their infants safely and to leave the unit when they were ready. Unfortunately, in the United States, where there are few mother–infant units, the clinician faces enormous pressure from quickly recompensating mothers who plead for early discharge so that they can be reunited with their babies.

With hospitalization, sedatives, antipsychotic medication, such as chlorpromazine in dosages of 400 mg or more per day, a series of three electroconvulsive therapy sessions, or a combination of these treatments, as the British will often prescribe, the mother's psychotic symptoms quickly abate. The clinician's worry is that following a speedy discharge or brief hospitalization of 3 weeks or less, the mother may still be plagued by intrusive, dystonic, obsessive thoughts about hurting herself or the baby. She is often ashamed and fearful of acknowledging these thoughts to her family or physician. At these times, catastrophic events may occur, such as the mother's injuring or killing the baby or herself.

Extended treatment requires counseling in child rearing and observation for the emergence of a major mood disorder, most often a bipolar illness. The patient needs the support and active help of her spouse and family, especially for child care. Counseling in regard to the risk for postpartum disorders following future pregnancies is indicated.

BIPOLAR DISORDERS The special population of bipolar mood-disordered women with a prior history of postpartum psychosis requires sensitive management during pregnancy. Current psychopharmacological recommendations are based on the findings of the Register of Lithium Babies. As of 1980, of the 225 babies who were reported to be exposed to lithium during the first 3 months of fetal life or longer, 25 were born with congenital malformations, especially of the heart. Therefore, women who take lithium must do so only after the risk–benefit ratio has been closely assessed. If it is decided that the lithium must be maintained, the minimal effective doses must be prescribed, and ongoing, frequent clinical and laboratory reevaluations must be made. Temporary reduction and discontinuation of lithium about 1 week prior to delivery is advised to reduce the risk of maternal and newborn toxicity. Lithium can be restarted once the mother has stabilized postpartum.

Because at least 40 percent of bipolar women can expect to experience one or more postpartum episodes of mania or depression, the clinician can consider reinstituting prophylactic lithium therapy during the third trimester of pregnancy or shortly after delivery for those whose history of affective episodes indicates that they are at high risk for relapsing following delivery. Longer stays in the hospital of 1 week to 10 days to observe for the emergence of a postpartum psychosis may be prudent. Breast feeding by mothers taking lithium is generally discouraged because the effects of lithium on a developing organism are unknown and infants are susceptible to lithium intoxication.

TYPE II: ADJUSTMENT REACTION WITH DEPRESSED MOOD (ALSO KNOWN AS POSTPARTUM, MATERNAL, OR POSTNATAL BLUES) Mrs. B. T., a 35-year-old, white, Greek Orthodox mother of a 10-year-old, stated that for 6 weeks after the birth of her first child, she cried and cried for no apparent reason. After these 6 weeks she felt better, but she was so upset by that experience that she deferred having another baby for 10 years. During the second pregnancy, she neither told nor was asked by her obstetrician about any postpartum emotional reactions.

Such crying is a common, transient, self-limiting disorder occurring in at least 50 percent of all women. With such a high incidence, many investigators consider this to be a normal occurrence of the postpartum period. But because the affect is both dysphoric and disconcerting, the author believes that it should be classified as a disorder.

This feeling peaks within 10 days to 3 weeks after delivery and may occur while the obstetrical patient is still in the hospital. Characteristics include mild depression, anxiety, brief crying episodes, headaches, fatigue, and irritability—often consisting of only a few brief but unexplained crying episodes. The postpartum blues are most severe in the primiparous. During subsequent pregnancies, if the blues occur at all, they usually are milder.

The depression usually remits spontaneously without any special treatment other than family support. Yet for some, these moods are a precursor to the development of a frank postpartum depression.

Their etiology is unknown but seems related to the rapid alternation of hormonal levels of estrogen, progesterone, and prolactin following delivery. As reported above, most biological investigations of postpartum disorders have been of women who experienced postpartum blues. Clinically, many of these women seem quite stressed in caring for their infants; they often feel fearful and reluctant to be left alone with their babies. The third week postpartum appears to be particularly difficult, as at that time there is often a significant loss of social support: The baby nurse, mother, or mother-in-law have left, and the husband has often returned to work. Some women report feeling fat, ugly, and wounded when they are unable to fit into their prepregnancy clothes. Although most women manage to muddle through, the author believes that a simple educational approach would be helpful and interventive (e.g., the attending health care professional informs the woman that she might experience postpartum blues and contacts the patient 3 weeks postpartum to inquire whether she is experiencing a mood disturbance).

TYPE III: POSTPARTUM MAJOR MOOD DISORDER (ALSO KNOWN AS MAJOR DEPRESSION, POSTPARTUM NEUROSIS, OR NEUROTIC REACTION)

Three months after giving birth to a much-wanted and much-loved son, Mrs. R. A., a 24-year-old, white, Jewish mother, began feeling fearful that someone was trying to poison the baby. She was in daily contact with her mother, but during a snowstorm she felt isolated, became very depressed, and was hospitalized. Over the next 3 years, she developed a frank history of manic depression.

Postpartum major depressions, which develop in more than 10 percent of women during the postpartum year, result in great morbidity to the mother, family, and child. It is well known that the children of mentally ill parents have a higher risk of developing psychopathology than the children of emotionally well parents. Many youngsters of parents who have unipolar or bipolar mood disorders develop insecure, ambivalent attachments to their caretakers and also have impaired regulation of their own mood and behavior. Depression disorganizes and disrupts a mother's capacity to care for her infant and jeopardizes the development of a healthy attachment between mother and child.

The phenomenology of a postpartum depression corresponds to the DSM-III-R criteria for major mood disorders (sadness, feelings of inadequacy, fatigue, insomnia, and anhedonia). Although suicide is not common, it has been reported. Management includes possible hospitalization, medication, psychotherapy, and a social support system.

What is most disturbing is that for some women, childbearing and child rearing herald recurrent unipolar or bipolar mood disorders. Their etiology is unknown. As in any depression, biological factors must be considered as well as the role of personality and social risk factors.

Obstetrical complications, socioeconomic status, and postpartum blues have not been found to be significant predictors. Rather, the relevant risk factors include:

1. Pregnancy and psychiatric history: primiparous status, ambivalence about maintaining the pregnancy, and a history of postpartum depression or bipolar illness.
2. Current life situation: the lack of a social support system; the lack of a nurturing, dependable relationship with spouse and parents; and the woman's dissatisfaction with herself.
3. Early family life: the lack of a nurturant relationship with mother and father and separation from parents, especially the father.

Intervention strategies Several investigators have used these data to develop short questionnaires to be administered to pregnant women to identify which women are at risk for postpartum depression. These questionnaires have been correlated with the Beck Depression Inventory. Recent cross-cultural anthropological studies indicate that in societies that have distinct postpartum rituals, such as a mandated rest period, social seclusion, assistance in tasks of daily life by relatives and midwives, bearing of gifts, and enhanced social status, there is a decreased incidence of postpartum depression.

Treatment The treatments for postpartum depressions are similar to those for any major depression: medication, psychotherapy, hospitalization if indicated, and support for activities of daily life, especially child rearing. There is now sufficient knowledge to enable the sensitive clinician to inquire about the known risk factors when taking a prenatal history and to be able to identify those women who are likely to experience postpartum depression. Consequently, the clinician can devise antenatal and postnatal intervention strategies—such as counseling, medication, social support, and child care assistance—that may forestall or ameliorate the otherwise-to-be-expected emergence of a postpartum emotional disorder.

REFERENCES

Brockington I F, Kumar R: *Motherhood and Mental Illness*. Grune & Stratton, New York, 1982.

Campbell J, Winokur G: Postpartum affective disorders: Selected biological aspects. In *Recent Advances in Postpartum Psychiatric Disorders,* D G Inwood, editor, p 19. American Psychiatric Press, Washington, DC, 1985.

Hamilton J A: *Postpartum Psychiatric Problems*. Mosby, St. Louis, 1962.

Hopkins J, Marcus M, Campbell S: Postpartum depression: A critical review. Psychol Bull, *95:* 498, 1984.

Jefferson J, Greist J, Ackerman D, Carrol J: Pregnancy. In *Lithium Encyclopedia for Clinical Practice,* ed 2, p 504. American Psychiatric Press, Washington, DC, 1987.

Marcé L V: *Traité de la Folie des Femmes, Enceintes de Nouvelles Accouchées, et des Nourrices*. Ballière, Paris, 1858.

O'Hara M V: Social support, life events, and depression during pregnancy and the puerperium. Arch Gen Psychol *43:* 569, 1986.

Posner N, Unterman R, Williams K: Postpartum depression: The obstetrician's concerns. In *Recent Advances in Postpartum Psychiatric Disorders,* D G Inwood, editor, p 59. American Psychiatric Press, Washington, DC, 1985.

Stern G, Kruckman L: Multidisciplinary perspectives on postpartum depression: An anthropological critique. Soc Sci Med *17:* 1027, 1983.

Uddenberg N: Reproductive adaptation in mothers and daughters: A study in personality development and adaptation to motherhood. Acta Psych Scand *254* (suppl): 1, 1974.

CHAPTER 17 MOOD (AFFECTIVE) DISORDERS

17.1 MOOD DISORDERS: EPIDEMIOLOGY

RICHARD F. MOLLICA, M.D.

INTRODUCTION

The major task of psychiatric epidemiology is to investigate the frequency with which definable psychiatric disorders occur in carefully delineated populations. In general, the dual purpose of this task is administrative and scientific. First, by establishing the prevalence and incidence of a disease, along with its social and demographic correlates, the epidemiological method can help policymakers determine what segments of society are ill and need clinical treatment and prevention. Second, by investigating the phenomena of the disease and its associated risk factors, morbidity, and prognosis, it can help establish the relationship between pathogenesis and causal factors. The clinical relevance of the epidemiological method occurs at the intersection between the administrative and scientific tasks, that is, at the point that the effectiveness of treatment and prevention strategies are determined. The knowledge revealed by psychiatric epidemiology must ultimately be judged by its ability to prevent and heal psychiatric illness.

Psychiatric epidemiology has made important contributions to the study of mood disorders. These disorders have been consistently demonstrated to have a high prevalence in the community. They are commonly untreated, frequently have a chronic course, and are often associated with serious social and emotional disability, including suicide. This section will review the major findings of the epidemiology of mood disorders, focusing on the extensive epidemiological data for major mood disorders, including major depression and bipolar disorder.

IDENTIFYING AND DIAGNOSING MOOD DISORDERS

WHAT IS A CASE? Depression has had an extensive history in Western society since Hippocrates first described it as a medical illness. The historical classification of depressive disorders (the term "affective" disorders was introduced by Manfred Bleuler in the 1930s) has undergone many fascinating transformations through the centuries and now has been replaced in the revised third edition of the *Diagnostic and Statistical Manual of Mental Disorders* (DSM-III-R) by the term "mood" disorders. Depression is widely used by the general public to describe those emotional states characterized by a lowering of spirits, dejection, and sadness. The state of sadness, however, does not necessarily qualify a person as having an illness or a psychiatric disease. The determination of those phenomena, which is the legitimate domain of the epidemiology of mood disorders, has therefore been a major stumbling block to the investigation of these disorders. Epidemiologists studying mood disorders must first identify those somatic and psychological alterations that are the objective bedrock of these disorders. Answering the question, What is a case? is the core of this endeavor. Furthermore, the clinical criteria for the disorders must be recognizable not only by those who observe and treat mood disorders, but also by those who have them. For example, Tristam Englehardt, a philosopher of medicine, citing Christopher Boorse, emphasizes the important role of dysfunction in determining what is a disease.

> The state of an organism is theoretically healthy, i.e., free of disease, insofar as its mode of functioning conforms to the natural design of the organism . . . and the single unifying property of all recognized diseases of plants and animals appears to be this: that they interfere with one or more functions typically performed within members of the species.

If those symptoms that are generally associated with mood disorders are relatively common, at what point do these symptoms either individually or in combination with other symptoms constitute a disease (i.e., seriously interfere with the normal functioning of the individual)? For example, a prospective study of bereaved widows found that 1 year after losing their spouses, 17 percent met the third edition of the *Diagnostic and Statistical Manual of Mental Disorders* (DSM-III) criteria for major depression. Yet, few felt they were ill or in need of psychiatric care. Did these women have a mood disorder, or was this symptomatology only a normal sign of extreme grief?

The interpretation of epidemiological results is easy, especially when the answers are couched in terms like positive and negative or present and absent. An ideal classification system for mood disorders would conform to this yes–no model. Unfortunately, mood disorder symptoms and the epidemiological instruments used to measure them are much harder to interpret than a yes–no model. The question is not so much, Has he got it? as, How much of it does he have? It is important to realize that all mood disorder symptoms are on a continuum. For example, mood disturbances may vary from mild feelings of sadness to such intense feelings that an individual may not want to live. All of the symptoms that clinicians and epidemiologists generally use to identify or measure mood disorders are a matter of degree (e.g., sleep disturbance, poor appetite, impaired concentration). Figure 17.1-1 highlights the important distinctions between ideal and actual situations in identifying any medical or psychiatric disease. No illness conforms to the bimodal yes–no model. Any criteria established for mood disorders will overlap with the normal population, resulting in both false positives and false negatives. For example, in Figure 17.1-1, if patients with symptom levels to the right of *A* are considered to have a

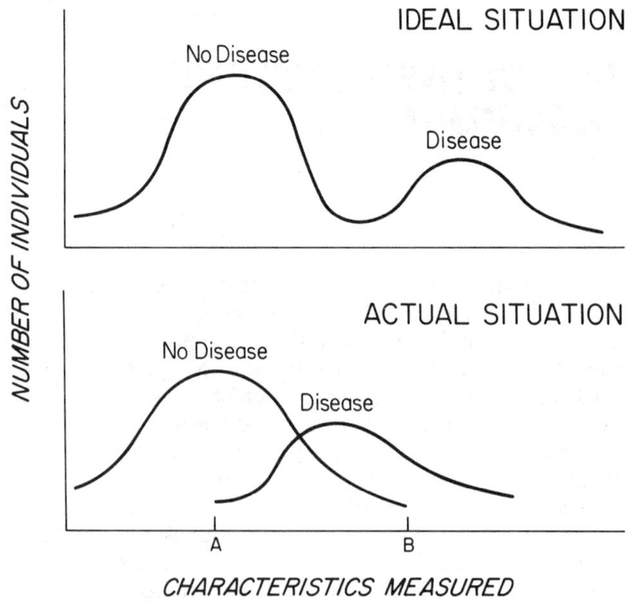

FIGURE 17.1-1. *Ideal and actual distributions of psychiatric disease and no disease in the general community. Because diagnostic classifications are not perfect (e.g., mood disorders), the distributions overlap. If all individuals to the right of* A *are considered to have the psychiatric disorder, many false positives will occur. If only individuals to the right of* B *are considered to have the psychiatric disorder, many false negatives will result.*

mood disorder, many false positives will be included in this definition of the disease. But if only patients to the right of *B* are included, many persons with mood disorders will be excluded. This problem of identification has been so severe in the epidemiological assessment of psychiatric disorders that a special term was coined, "demoralization," to describe those false positives to the right of *A*. Determining and excluding false positives has been a task crucial to the establishment of valid diagnostic criteria for identifying and measuring the prevalence rates of mood disorders.

ESTABLISHING A DIAGNOSTIC SYSTEM The disease concept called mood disorder is a convention; the clinical criteria for defining it are artificial. Those clusters of symptoms that are determined to comprise mood disorders are established by assumptions regarding the relative negative effects of depressive symptoms on an individual's life. There are no final arbitrators of the validity of the classification systems for mood disorders that can serve as a final and independent test.

The classic disease model established by the seventeenth-century physician Thomas Sydenham requires that in order to establish a disease entity, at least one of the following is necessary: (1) a description of the disease (inclusion criteria), (2) differentiation of the disease from similar diseases already described (exclusion criteria), and (3) follow-up studies establishing that the disease either went away or remained the same. The criteria for mood disorders in DSM-III-R are the latest attempts to establish diagnoses compatible with Sydenham's criteria, that is, criteria based on the psychopathological and psychological processes unique to mood disorders and their differential response to treatment. Other aspects of validity, such as familial patterns, genetic background, and differential response to medication, are also important. Yet, any system of diagnostic classification, because it is an organization of symptom clusters into a diagnostic category, frequently obscures the continuous nature of both the symptoms and the diagnostic category in the general population. Diagnostic classifications, in fact, purposely strive to fit the actual overlapping distribution of no disease and disease into the ideal bimodal model (Fig. 17.1-1). But when 100 percent conclusiveness for the disease is achieved, the classification itself becomes a tautology (i.e., all individuals who have the symptoms of X therefore have the disease X). For example, widows who met the DSM-III-R criteria for major depression must have a major mood disorder even if they do not consider themselves ill. The English epidemiologist A. L. Cochrane challenged the reductionistic tendency of diagnostic systems by shifting the focus of epidemiological interest away from disease definition to clinical care. He asserts that the most important epidemiological question is not whether one has the disease, but at which point on the symptom distribution curve (Fig. 17.1-1) therapy begins to do more good than harm. Furthermore, in order to achieve this clinical goal, the diagnostic classification must take into account the reliability of the instruments used to establish the diagnosis as well as the validity of their measurements. At this level, the epidemiology of mood disorders overlaps with the clinical usefulness of its investigations, as patients are best managed when the natural history of the disease and the relative effectiveness of available therapies are known.

MAJOR SYMPTOMS What are the most appropriate criteria for classifying mood disorders? Again, a more general discussion of this question underlies the nosological debates that have flourished in this field. Denis Hill compared the two major contrasting concepts of disease that have influenced the classification of mood disorders:

> The first view is that of disease as a separate distinct entity. When a man falls ill . . . he acquires a disease, which is, as it were added unto him. It did not preexist in him. This concept leads on to the view that there are innumerable diseases, each with its own individual, specific and recognizable characteristics. The second and alternative view of disease presents it as a deviation from normal. In this concept, the platonic variety, the healthy man falls ill through the influence of any number of factors, physical or psychological, and, as a consequence, is changed and suffers. The change in him and the suffering he experiences is then his disease.

These contrasting views of disease etiology are reflected in the classification systems that have been proposed for mood disorders. DSM-III-R attempted to bypass this contradiction by using a nosological system that is atheoretical with regard to etiology or pathogenesis in order to avoid unproved theoretical assumptions. DSM-III-R's claim to complete theoretical neutrality has been challenged, however: Without a conceptual framework for mood disorders, how can symptoms be chosen that will qualify an individual for having this disease?

The following four clinical vignettes highlight the problem of symptom selection and assumed causality:

Vignette 1: A 75-year-old man has never before had a psychiatric problem. But 1 year after losing his wife, after 50 years of marriage, he becomes seriously depressed and contemplates suicide.

Vignette 2: A recently arrived refugee seeks medical care because of extreme grief. He survived torture and is the sole surviving member of his entire family.

Vignette 3: A 35-year-old woman seeks treatment for depression. She has no idea why she is depressed. However, both her parents are alcoholics, and her siblings have also experienced recurrent bouts of depression.

Vignette 4: A middle-aged man's depression lifts after a benign brain tumor is removed.

These vignettes describe four individuals who sought medical care for what they felt were serious depressive symptoms. The fact that all four individuals met the DSM-III-R criteria for major depression, does not, however, satisfy the commonsense belief that each of these individuals has a different illness. The grief of a 75-year-old man who lost his wife seems very different from the grief of a refugee who survived torture and lost his entire family during the war, even though both have many mood-disorder symptoms in common.

Figure 17.1-2 illustrates the three major symptom domains that comprise mood disorders. The prominence of any of these symptom groups is usually linked to causal explanations (e.g., somatic dysfunction is associated with biological causes). Each individual with a mood disorder will have varying degrees of overlap among social impairment, psychological distress, and somatic dysfunction. Unfortunately, epidemiological investigations of major depression (and other major psychiatric diagnoses) have not been able to determine the precise interaction of these symptom domains with one another. Impairments in one domain are poor predictors of impairments in another. The DSM-III-R diagnosis of major mood disorder has dealt with this dilemma by choosing clusters of symptoms to define this disease primarily from the somatic and psychological domains. Social impairment has been determined to be an outcome of the illness and is not considered an essential ingredient of the diagnosis (Fig. 17.1-2). The advantage of this system is that it uses relatively simple diagnostic criteria based on well-defined empirical phenomena (which can be easily measured) and avoids complex diagnostic assessments of psychological meaning and levels of social adjustment. In contrast, another type of diagnostic system could classify mood disorders by different phenomenological characteristics. For example, a specific mood-disorder category could be assigned to bereavement, refugee trauma, medical illness, among others. Although it is incomprehensible that a single diagnosis could be applied to all mood disorders, the DSM-III-R diagnostic system has attempted to purify its classification criteria of theoretical assumptions in order to leave the job of differential diagnosis to the clinician. This goal demonstrates why the use of DSM-III-R criteria in recent large-scale epidemiological studies have produced results that are limited to diagnosis and do not specify cause in their measurement of mood disorders.

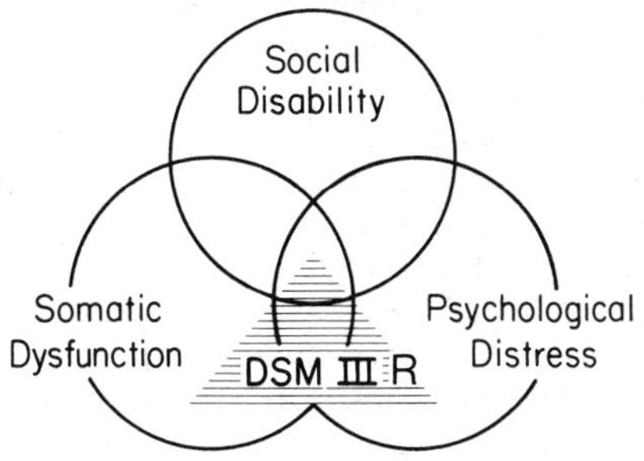

FIGURE 17.1-2. *Psychiatric illnesses such as mood disorders usually include varying degrees of impairment in three major symptom domains: somatic, psychological, and social. Although these symptom domains overlap, the degree of overlap varies for each diagnostic category. Impairment in one domain will not necessarily predict the extent of impairment in other domains. DSM-III-R criteria for mood disorders consist primarily of somatic and psychological symptoms. Social disability is viewed as an outcome of the illness and not as an essential ingredient of the diagnosis.*

VALIDITY OF MEASUREMENTS The instruments used in the epidemiology of mood disorders have the standard methodological problems of validity and reliability. However, two measurement considerations are of special interest to this area. First is the problem of triviality. Measurements in large-scale studies are often considered inadequate, as the questionnaires used cover complex human attitudes and behavior with a few simple questions. For example, a questionnaire may ask, Do you feel blue? or Do you have a satisfying marital relationship? These questions are complex, and it is remarkable that most individuals know (more or less) what they mean. Second, considerable discussion has focused on the relative validity of three major approaches (normative, subjective, and contextual) to assessing the impact of negative life events on the onset of major depression. This discussion can also be generalized to other epidemiological methods. The normative approach to life events assigns a weight to an event, based on a community norm. If the individual questioned has experienced this event, he or she will be assigned a particular score. The main criticism of the normative approach is its vague definition of life events. The possible confusion between event and symptom and the rigidity of the weighting system prevents any appreciation of the different meanings of events for different individuals. In contrast, individual meanings attributed to life events can also be determined by using self-rating measures, that is, the subjective approach. Yet, self-ratings may be seriously flawed, as individuals may search for a meaning after an illness or crisis has occurred. Recognizing these risks, George Brown and Tirril Harris, in *Social Origins of Depression,* devised a contextual approach. Through lengthy standardized interviews, they collected background material about various events. People not involved in the interview then scored the importance of the event to the respondent's biography. The contextual approach evaluates the significance of the life event to the individual's life history without relying solely on the individual's own interpretation of it.

These three methods of assessing life events demonstrate the difficulty in obtaining objective as well as meaningful measurements of life experiences. Similarly, measuring even such simple symptoms as sleep disturbance is problematic. As the measurement moves from somatic symptoms to social and psychological symptoms, the problem of validity becomes even more difficult as social-role performance and psychological states are gauged. It thus has been difficult to move beyond crude measures of social and psychological symptoms and their correlates in determining the etiology of mood disorders, and it is apparent that more refined methodological techniques are necessary.

SOCIAL AND CULTURAL DIMENSIONS

DEMORALIZATION The problems of validity in determining the meaning of high symptom levels revealed in large-scale epidemiological studies in the community using symptom checklists caused the Dohrenwends to introduce the term "demoralization," in the early 1970s, to describe these results. These epidemiological studies typically used a small battery of questions that included various somatic and psychological symptoms (usually related to depression and anxiety) thought to be related to psychiatric disorders. For example, investigators interested in the prevalence of depressive disorders would ask respondents a set of questions considered likely to reveal the presence of a depressive illness (e.g., Do you feel blue? or Are you worrying about things too much?). The Dohrenwends suggested that these scales were not measuring psychiatric illness but, rather, responses, such as low self-esteem, helplessness, hopelessness, sadness, and anxiety, which all were major facets of Jerome Frank's definition of demoralization. Frank's formulation of demoralization was not originally intended to serve as an epidemiological concept, but to describe that state of mind of hopelessness and helplessness characteristic of psychotherapy patients, regardless of their psychiatric diagnosis. Both Frank and the Dohrenwends believed that demoralization is a condition likely to be experienced in association with a variety of problems, including severe physical illness, chronic illnesses, psychiatric disorders, and those conditions of social emargination experienced by the poor, minorities, and others. Individuals who are demoralized (as indicated by a high score on a symptom checklist), therefore, may sometimes (but not always) have an associated psychiatric illness. Although the concept was not intended to be a psychiatric diagnosis and although it claims to have limited etiological meaning, demoralization does have a diagnostic-like quality, as it describes the state of many individuals who are depressed and anxious but not severely enough to be diagnosed as suffering from a major clinical disorder. This definition indirectly solved the conceptual problem of the continuity of depressive symptoms and their possible meaning. Whether demoralization is an adequate classification or explanation of mild depressive states, it has helped shift the epidemiological measurement of mood disorders away from a reliance on symptom checklists toward the use of standardized diagnostic criteria.

The epidemiological importance of the early community studies, however, has more than just limited methodological and heuristic value. Several studies that used both symptom checklists and clinical judgments to identify psychiatric cases in the same sample of respondents from the general population found that the overlap between the two approaches was approximately 50 percent. The early checklist studies demonstrated that approximately 25 percent of the U.S. population suffered from demoralization or a checklist positive state. Rates were consistently higher for women than for men, and higher for lower social classes as compared with higher social classes. The prevalence of diagnosable psychiatric illness based on these estimates would therefore be one-half of 25 percent. This estimate is compatible with recent community studies using standardized diagnostic criteria. A reanalysis of two major symptom checklist studies using DSM-III diagnostic criteria reveals similar rates. These results demonstrate a remarkable consistency in overall rates of psychiatric disorders between different historical time periods. Interpretation of the clinical meaning of symptom checklist positive responses, however, still remains controversial.

INFLUENCE OF CULTURE How cultural and social factors affect the manifestation of depressive symptoms has not been clearly explained, despite numerous epidemiological studies. It is now generally accepted that mood disorders exist in all societies and are expressed through a wide range of symptoms. It is not evident, however, that Western categories of mood disorders and those defined by other cultures are the same.

Many cross-cultural psychiatric studies suggest that the assessment of psychiatric illness should begin with local phenomenological descriptions that can then be compared with Western psychological criteria. One investigator demonstrated this approach in his investigations in Laos. He and his colleagues were able to identify a number of individuals in a well-circumscribed area (in a country that, until 1975, was without psychiatrists or psychiatric institutions) who had been diagnosed by their villages as having either *ba* ("insane" or "crazy") or *sia chit* (literally "lost mind," figuratively "nervous breakdown" or "nervous problem"). The criteria that the Lao villagers used to apply the term *ba* to an individual were the following: seeing or hearing things not observed by others; purposeless or dangerous behavior; little or no productive work; and impaired thought, memory, logic, or intelligence. The *sia chit* category referred to individuals complaining of constant sadness or crying spells, difficulty sleeping, weakness, fright, panic, and various physical symptoms. Independent psychiatric ratings by five experienced Western psychiatrists revealed a close agreement between the folk diagnosis of *ba* and the Western diagnosis of psychosis. But they did disagree on the *sia chit* category; for example, two psychiatric raters who had no experience with any Asian culture diagnosed these villagers as psychotic. But this study does support the accuracy of folk diagnosis in locating severe or chronic cases of psychiatric disorder in a population. And it also is a warning to experienced Western clinicians who are not familiar with Southeast Asian cultures to guard against overdiagnosing nonpsychotic cases as psychotic.

Clearly, describing culturally defined mood disorders is an enormous research task, further complicated by possible atypical and masked depressions. As a consequence, little is known of the prevalence of the various symptomatological presentations of mood disorders in different cultures and the applicability of current Western concepts and classification schemes. Simply put, is there a core depressive syndrome that can be readily identified in all cultures? A World Health Organization (WHO) study conducted in five countries attempted to identify those clinical features that patients with major depression share irrespective of cultural variation. In the five centers (Canada, India, Iran, Japan, and Switzerland), 573 psychiatric patients were selected and evaluated using a standardized diagnostic interview schedule. The WHO study demonstrated the existence of a common core of depressive symptomatology which included sadness, joylessness, anxiety, tension, lack of energy, loss of interest, loss of ability to concentrate, and ideas of insufficiency, inadequacy, and worthlessness. The symptomatic differences among the centers were minimal. For example, guilt feelings were present in 68 percent of the Swiss sample, but in only 32 percent of the Iranian sample; suicidal ideas were present in 70 percent of the Canadian sample, but in only 40 percent of the Japanese sample. Somatization was present in 57 percent of the Iranian sample, but in only 27 percent of the Canadian sample. Unfortunately, the WHO study was not a community study. There is no evidence that the psychiatric patients selected were actually characteristic of those depressive disorders commonly recognized in the various communities. Many other cross-cultural studies have revealed that although individuals from other cultures might meet Western diagnostic criteria for major mood disorders, the symptoms that comprise these criteria may not be those that the community considers as culturally the most significant and in need of treatment.

PREVALENCE RATES AND RISK FACTORS

EPIDEMIOLOGICAL ADVANCES Several diagnostic systems have been proposed for the classification of mood disorders, including diagnostic schemes, such as endogenous versus reactive, psychotic versus neurotic, and unipolar versus bipolar. These systems are an attempt to establish a valid clinical entity (or entities) in which predictable relationships can be found among etiology, clinical symptom picture, natural history, and treatment course. So far in the field of mood disorders, there are no nosological models that are specific enough to enable investigators to understand the etiology and pathogenesis of any group of mood disorders. This limited knowledge led the DSM-III-R to define mood disorders by their major symptom profiles without implying unproven causal explanations. The DSM-III-R criteria, however, have explicitly accepted the unipolar-bipolar distinction by dividing the major categories of mood disorders into major depression and bipolar disorder.

The advances in diagnostic classification reflected by DSM-III-R were matched by two steps forward in epidemiological research. First was a shift in psychiatric epidemiology after World War II, away from studying patients in treatment settings toward studying individuals in the general population through large-scale community surveys. This shift in focus was necessary to establish the true prevalence of mood disorder, because most individuals suffering from these disorders do not seek treatment. Second, the development of standardized symptom questionnaires (or checklists) allowed nonpsychiatrists to interview large numbers of individuals. These early symptom questionnaire studies (e.g., the Stirling County Study) provided the methodological advancements in identifying a psychiatric case that led to standardized interview schedules that could obtain psychiatric diagnoses similar to those used in clinical practice. The latter include the Research Diagnostic Criteria (RDC), the Schedule for Affective Disorders and Schizophrenia-Lifetime (SADS-L), and the Diagnostic Interview Schedule (DIS).

The first epidemiological survey in a community in the United States to apply standardized diagnostic criteria (RDC, SADS-L) was conducted in 1975 in New Haven, Connecticut. In 1983, the National Survey of Psychotherapeutic Drug Use was the first study to use the DSM-III diagnostic criteria for major depression to reanalyze by computer a large-scale symptom checklist survey conducted in 1979. The original data from the Stirling County Study were also reanalyzed in a similar fashion. The New Haven survey set the stage for the largest community study to date—the Epidemiologic Catchment Area program (ECA).

RATES **Major depression** Lifetime prevalence rates for major depression has been reported to be as high as 18.0 percent. The ECA study found much lower lifetime rates of 6.7 percent, 3.7 percent, and 5.5 percent for New Haven, Baltimore, and St. Louis, respectively. Table 17.1-1 presents the prevalence rates for current episodes of major depression determined by the major U.S. studies using standardized diagnostic criteria. Total rates vary from 3.0 to 6.4 percent. Rates for men vary from 1.7 to 4.7 percent and for women from 4.1 to 6.9 percent. Incidence rates are poorly described and have ranged from 1.8 per 1,000 cases per year to 4.5 per 1,000 cases per year.

Bipolar disorder Rates of bipolar disorder have been investigated primarily through treatment cases because of its infrequent occurrence. A few noteworthy exceptions exist. The 1975 New Haven survey reported a lifetime prevalence rate of 1.2 percent. The ECA studies revealed 6-month prevalence rates ranging from 0.4 to 0.8 percent for men and from 0.4 to 0.9 percent for women. Total 6-month prevalence rates for the three sites range from 0.4 to 0.7 percent. The Amish Study, which identified all known individuals with bipolar disorder in a well-delineated Amish community of slightly over 8,000 adults, had comparable current prevalence rates of 0.5 percent. One-year incidence rates based on treatment cases in different geographical and clinical settings vary widely and have led to no definite conclusions.

RISK FACTORS The extensive investigations of risk factors associated with major mood disorders are summarized in Table 17.1-2, which compares major depression and bipolar disorders. Significant differences in prevalence rates between major depression and bipolar disorder as well as differences in associated risk factors strongly support the view that these are separate clinical entities. Although most investigations reveal that both disorders are strongly associated with a family history of depression, the evidence is much stronger for bipolar disorder than for major depression that this disorder is genetically transmitted. Major depression is still probably comprised of a more hetereogeneous group of disorders than bipolar illness. Four of the risk factors prominently associated with major mood disorders are gender, social class, life events, and heredity.

Gender Almost all surveys in developed countries show that females have two to three times as many mood disorders as

TABLE 17.1-1
Comparative Overview of the Prevalence Studies of Major Depression

Community Survey	*Year*	*Size*	*Diagnosis and Case Identification Procedure*	*Period of Prevalence*	*Men %*	*Women %*	*Total %*
Stirling County Study	1952	1,003	DSM-III Symptom Checklist	Current	4.7	6.0	5.3
National Survey of Psychotherapeutic Drug Use	1979	3,161	DSM-III Symptom Checklist	1 year	2.8	6.9	6.4
New Haven Survey	1975	511	RDC SADS-L	Current	3.2	5.2	4.3
New Haven ECA Study	1980	3,058	DSM-III DIS	6 months	2.2	4.6	3.5
Baltimore ECA Study	1981	3,481	DSM-III DIS	6 months	1.8	4.1	3.0
St. Louis ECA Study	1981	3,004	DSM-III DIS	6 months	1.7	4.5	3.2

TABLE 17.1-2
Summary of Risk Factors for Major Mood (Affective) Disorders

Major Depression	*Bipolar Disorder*
Gender:	Gender:
Women > men	Women = men
Age of Onset:	Age of Onset:
Late 20s	Early 20s
Race:	Race:
No differences	No differences
Social Class:	Social Class:
More common in lower socioeconomic groups	More common in higher socioeconomic groups
Religion:	Religion:
No differences	More common in religious communities (e.g., Old Order Amish)
Family History:	Family History:
Positive	Positive and genetically linked
Life Events:	Life Events:
Negative events often before onset	Unknown

males. A 1977 survey of 40 studies from 30 countries found few exceptions to this gender bias. Table 17.1-1 demonstates similar findings from all major U.S. studies that used DSM-III criteria. The ECA results, in particular, reveal that although current prevalence rates of major depression for women are at least two times greater than those for men, the prevalence rates for bipolar disorder are equal for the sexes. (These gender differences lend additional validity to the uniqueness of these diagnoses.)

Several explanations for the differences in the male–female rates for mood disorder have been proposed. Many argue that these findings are artificial and do not reflect real differences. Women are more prone than men are to seek psychiatric help and are more willing than men are to express their feelings. Higher rates of alcohol abuse and antisocial behavior have also been thought to mask mood disorders in males. For example, in the Amish community, where alcohol is prohibited, the sex ratio for major depression was equal.

There is increasing evidence, however, that these gender differences are real and may be attributed to psychosocial, genetic, or endocrine factors. The psychosocial explanation contends that women's lives are more difficult than men's lives are, resulting in a higher prevalence of mood disorder. Many studies have attempted to demonstrate that women are exposed to more stress than men are, have more frequent and negative life experiences than men do, and have less successful coping strategies than men do. Inadequate coping skills and attitudes may contribute to a greater inclination for women, than for men, to develop mood disorders. Several large-scale family studies have failed to confirm the hypothesis that sex differences are genetically linked. Recent evidence has not supported an endocrine basis for major depression in women. Women also seem not to be at a significantly higher risk for mood disorder during any gender-related developmental stage, except the postpartum period. No studies have been able to correlate altered mood states in women with hormonal imbalance. Unfortunately, despite numerous investigations and hypotheses, there are no definitive explanations of these sex differences in prevalence rates for major depression.

Social class Since August Hollingshead and Fritz Redlich's book, *Social Class and Mental Illness,* there has been considerable interest in the relationship between social class and psychiatric disorder. The early symptom checklist studies revealed a significant relationship between social class and the presence of a mental disorder. Depressive symptoms have been found to be much higher in individuals from the lower classes. The 1975 New Haven survey using RDC criteria found higher rates of depression (except bipolar) in the lower classes. George Brown and Tirril Harris, examining the relationship between social class and major depression in women, found that this disorder was more common among working-class women than among upper- or middle-class women. An analysis of the five-site ECA data revealed that although sex and age factors predominate, there is also a substantial relationship between social class and major depression. The lowest social-class group had twice the risk of a major depression than that of the highest social-class group. In contrast, the lowest social classes had eight times the risk for schizophrenia as compared to the highest social classes. These data again confirm the relationship between socioeconomic status and the presence of a mental disorder. Although the relationship is strongest for schizophrenia, there is a much weaker but significant relationship for major depression. In contrast, bipolar disorder may be more common in the upper classes. This impression, however, has not yet been confirmed by the ECA studies.

Life events A relationship between traumatic life experiences and the onset of mood disorder has long been hypothesized. However, a number of major difficulties interfere with the establishment of a causal relationship between a negative life experience and a psychiatric disorder, especially depression. Interpreting the meaning of life events is difficult; memory recall is usually limited; and depression can profoundly influence an individual's outlook on life. Determining whether negative life events are the consequence, and not the cause, of depression can also be difficult. An additional problem is that few studies are prospective and thereby do not allow an accurate assessment of the impact of the individual's life experience on the development of mood disorder. For example, it has been demonstrated that only 10 percent of all exit events (i.e., significant loss of others) are followed by a major depression. An investigation of bereaved widows found that after 1 year, only 17 percent met the criteria for major depression. But few felt they were abnormally depressed or in need of psychiatric treatment. These studies are consistent with the common knowledge that not all negative life experiences are always followed by a depressive episode.

In a comprehensive investigation of the impact of life events on the development of major depression, 114 women being treated for depression were compared with a random sample of 382 normal women between the ages of 18 and 65 living in the Camberwell section of London. This study attempted to solve many of the methodological difficulties cited by establishing a definite diagnosis of major depression, by using a standardized interview schedule, and by evaluating life events through the contextual approach previously described. The severity of each life event was assessed by the investigators according to the extent to which it was judged to have threatened the individual's social adjustment and equilibrium. In all, 67 percent of the patients, compared with only 20 percent of the normal women, reported at least one severe event in the period studied. Forty-seven percent of the patient group, compared with only 17 percent of the healthy women, had been laboring under one or more social difficulties, such as finances or housing conditions. When life events and ongoing difficulties were grouped together as provoking agents, the differences between the patient group and the healthy group increased. Three-quarters of the former, as against only one-third of the latter, reported a severe life event or a major social difficulty, or both, within the relevant time period. Finally, the probability of developing a major depression in the face of one or more provoking agents was found to increase if one or more of the following vulnerability factors were also present: (1) the lack of an intimate, confiding relationship with husband or boyfriend; (2) the presence at home of three or more children under 14 years of age; and (3) the loss of one's mother, by death or separation, before the age of 11.

Although many studies have demonstrated the important relationship between life events and major depression in patient groups, a causal relationship cannot be definitely concluded, as it is still not known what percentage of individuals who experience major life events become clinically depressed. The relationship between life events and bipolar disorder is also unknown. There has been no research on the impact, if any, of stressful life experiences on the onset, course, and treatment of bipolar disorder, during either its manic or its depressive phase.

Hereditary factors and genetics For many years, the increased presence of mood disorders in the family members of patients with major mood disorders has been recognized. Numerous studies have demonstrated that mood disorder runs in families. Investigations have also revealed a possible genetic predisposition, especially for bipolar disorder, which may explain these findings. Patients with bipolar disorder have a significantly higher risk of having parents and first-degree relatives with mood disorders than do those with major depression. Familial patterns are also significantly different between the two major mood disorders. Although bipolar patients will have family members with both bipolar illness and major depression, patients with major depression will have few relatives with bipolar illness. Twin and adoption studies also support a much stronger genetic component for bipolar disorder. The concordance rate for monozygotic twins is 80 percent for bipolar disorder, as compared with 59 percent for major depression. The only adoption study revealed much higher rates of mood disorders in the biological parents of adoptees, as compared with the adoptive parents and the biological parents of normal controls.

The Amish study established the possibility of a linkage between bipolar disorder and a genetic marker. This investigation was of the Old Order Amish in southeastern Pennsylvania. This religious community is a unique laboratory for genetic research on mood disorders because of its social and cultural isolation, large family size, and clearly established paternity extending back to 30 progenitors who emigrated to the United States in the eighteenth century. All known individuals with active mental illness in that community were identified and diagnosed using RDC criteria. Intergenerational pedigrees for those with mood disorder were established. This evaluation determined that 112 individuals in a population of 12,500 currently had a psychiatric disorder. Seventy-one percent received the diagnosis of major mood disorder, with an almost equal distribution of bipolar illness and major depression. A segregation analysis of the family data for bipolar patients indicated an autosomal dominant mode of transmission. Linkage studies were then conducted on one large composite family which encompassed 81 living members, including 19 diagnosed as having a major mood disorder (14 were bipolar) and 62 psychiatrically well individuals. Deoxyribonucleic acid (DNA)-linkage analysis revealed strong evidence that a gene on chromosome 11 is associated with bipolar illness. This study's promising results will need to be replicated. The extent to which the genetic basis of bipolar disorder can be generalized to other Amish families and other bipolar patients is unknown. The mechanism by which this DNA sequence on chromosome 11 influences human behavior is also unknown. This study also dramatically highlights the impact on genetic research of the recent advancements in psychiatric epidemiology in determining "caseness" (i.e., establishing homogeneous diagnostic categories). For example, almost 80 percent of the bipolar cases determined by RDC criteria in the Amish study had been previously diagnosed in the community and treated as schizophrenia.

SOCIAL IMPACT

SOCIAL DISABILITY Over the past 20 years, epidemiologists have had an unprecedented interest in investigating the relationship between psychiatric illness and social disability. This interest has been partly stimulated by more than a half-century of public policy directed at returning the chronically mentally ill to the community from the state mental hospitals. Although most of the research has focused on the social impairments of schizophrenic patients, many of the lessons learned from these studies are relevant also to the mood disorders.

Measuring social competence and social adjustment is extremely complex. Social scientists have suggested that social competence can be measured accurately only through investigations that move away from single-measurement criteria toward multidimensional constructs. Geoff Shephard explains:

> Social competence is not any one "thing": It is a number of things. It can refer to an individual's observed behavior during a social interaction, how they appear and what they do. It can also refer to their subjective thoughts and feelings, how competent they feel themselves to be. Finally, it can refer to their ability to initiate and sustain social roles and relationships; for example, as a worker, a housewife, a patient, a friend or lover.

The majority of studies on schizophrenia and depression have suggested that psychiatric symptoms are poor predictors of social functioning. Yet, it is well known that mood disorders, especially those of an enduring nature, can damage an individual's work and family life. Large-scale epidemiological studies have consistently revealed both the chronicity and the serious social disability associated with mood disorders. Follow-up studies of patients with mood disorders report a chronic course for as many as 28 percent, with an average of 12 to 15 percent. In the 1979 National Survey of Psychotherapeutic Drug Use, almost 47 percent of those individuals in the community identified as having major depression reported impaired social role performance during the past year. More than one in four reported days when they could not work or carry out their usual activities.

Although there is a limited correlation between the symptom severity of patients' mood disorders and their social disabilities, they probably have major problems in social competence and social adjustment. Depression is a painful emotional state that can lead to suicide. Not surprisingly, patients with mood disorders have social problems at work and in the home, and they often have major impairments in maintaining intimate relationships, which include problems of irritability, interpersonal friction, and poor communication. These character traits often do not remit even after the depressive mood has subsided. Recovered patients have also been found to continue to have poor self-esteem, an unhappy outlook on life, narcissistic vulnerability, helplessness, and low confidence. Chronic psychological problems associated with mood disorders include poor concentration and retarded performance. Recovered patients who suffered from major depression can exhibit a lack of initiative, poor motivation, and a low level of perceived personal success or satisfaction. This state of behavior has been called learned helplessness. Because of the chronicity of many depressive states, patients with mood disorders can be caught in a vicious cycle of emotional despair, poor interpersonal relationships, and a stressful unsupportive family and social environment. Limited outcome research reveals that symptom levels and impaired social functioning respond differently to different treatments. Although psychotherapy alone will improve only social adjustment, including work performance and personal communication, medication alone will improve only symptom level without affecting social adjustment. These studies demonstrate the importance of combining therapies (psychotherapy and psychopharmacology) to ameliorate the entire range of symptoms, including associated impairments in social functioning.

UTILIZATION AND TREATMENT Relatively little is known about the interrelationship among social, cultural, and clinical factors regarding the utilization of mental health services. The 1975 New Haven community study demonstrated that only 9 percent of the population sought treatment during the preceding year for what they had identified as an emotional problem. In addition, the overall number of persons with a current psychiatric diagnosis who received treatment for their disorder was low (only about one-third sought any kind of professional help). However, those who did seek help did not exclusively choose mental health services; rather, they chose equally between mental health professionals and other professional groups (e.g., general practitioners, clergy). Individuals identified in the same survey as having major depression had utilization patterns similar to those of the total diagnosed population, except that those who did not receive treatment for an emotional disorder frequently visited general medical practitioners. (Recent ECA results from New Haven on utilization are comparable: 6.8 percent of the general population sought mental health services; 19.5 percent of those with any psychiatric diagnoses and 31.7 percent diagnosed with a mood disorder had made a mental health visit within the previous 6 months.) A reanalysis of the National Survey of Psychotherapeutic Drug Use also revealed the limited treatment of individuals in the community diagnosed with major depression. In particular, according to this study's review of treatment histories, only 11 percent of individuals with major depression had received an antidepressant medication.

Research into treatment practices suggests that when individuals with major mood disorders seek treatment, they are usually underdiagnosed, or if a diagnosis is made, they receive inadequate psychopharmacological intervention. Antianxiety agents are the most commonly prescribed medication despite their limited value, if any, for treating mood disorders. The treatment history of the first 217 subjects who were recruited for the National Institute of Mental Health Study of the Psychobiology of Depression with a current episode of major depression of at least 1 month's duration demonstrates these conclusions. This study found that 14 percent of the subjects had received no treatment; 67 percent had received psychotherapy (13 percent had only psychotherapy); 55 percent had received antianxiety medication (19 percent had received no other medication); and only 34 percent had received antidepressant medication. Few of the latter (including individuals who were psychotically depressed) received the most intensive level of pharmacological intervention. These studies, and many others, agree that the majority of individuals in the community suffering from major depression do not receive any treatment or are inadequately treated.

Analyses of the utilization data from the ECA New Haven site have revealed more of the complex interaction between psychiatric diagnosis and health-seeking behavior. In this survey, individuals who met the DSM-III criteria for major depression or schizophrenia were more likely to seek psychiatric help. However, other social factors, such as age, gender, race, and education, continued to influence the rate of utilization of psychiatric care over and above the important influence of diagnosis. Women had greater contact with the mental health system than men; whites had greater contact than blacks; the middle-aged had greater contact than the young and elderly; and the better educated had greater contact than the less educated. These findings have significant public policy implications, as they support the general conclusions of many treatment studies. That is, those social groups (e.g., minorities, the elderly) who are at high risk for developing mood disorders and other major psychiatric illnesses also have lower utilization rates of mental health services than lower-risk populations. And even if these groups do seek mental health care, they will receive differential care (and possibly inadequate treatment), as originally suggested in Hollingshead and Redlich's classic study and its 25-year follow-up.

HISTORY AND SOCIETY

The realization that the classification systems and treatment practices of psychiatry are closely associated with the values and problems of society has received considerable historical and sociological attention. Mood disorders have been described for over 2,000 years. An alternative perspective might see both the phenomenological manifestation of depressive symptoms throughout the centuries and their changing clinical classification not as objective descriptions of actual disease states but as a reflection or mirror of that society's world view and culture. The philosophical method that best supports this position was described by Michel Foucault in *The Order of Things*. He began his discussion by pointing out the arbitrary nature of scientific classification:

> This book first arose out of a passage in Borges, out of the laughter that shattered, as I read the passage, all the familiar landmarks of my thought—*our* thought, the thought that bears the stamp of our age and our geography—breaking up all the ordered surfaces and all the

planes with which we are accustomed to tame the wild profusion of existing things, and continuing long afterwards to disturb and threaten with collapse our age-old distinction between the Same and the Other. This passage quotes a "certain Chinese encyclopedia" in which it is written that "animals are divided into: (a) belonging to the Emperor, (b) embalmed, (c) tame, (d) sucking pigs, (e) sirens, (f) fabulous, (g) stray dogs, (h) included in the present classification, (i) frenzied, (j) innumerable, (k) drawn with a very fine camelhair brush, (l) et cetera, (m) having just broken the water pitcher, (n) that from a long way off look like flies." In the wonderment of this taxonomy, the thing we apprehend in one great leap, the thing that, by means of the fable, is demonstrated as the exotic charm of another system of thought, is the limitation of our own, the stark impossibility of thinking that.

Foucault's empirical method gives priority to understanding the value system of every culture and historical period that is reflected in its categories and practices.

Three epidemiological studies of the changing cultural meaning of psychiatric diagnoses illustrate this point. One study of patient diagnoses at the New York State Psychiatric Institute between 1932 and 1956 determined that a sharp rise in the number of patients with the diagnosis of schizophrenia reflected shifts in the diagnostic concepts used by clinicians at the hospital and not a temporal change in the kinds of patients admitted. Temporal changes in diagnosis at the Iowa State psychopathic Hospital between 1920 and 1966 were also due to the shifting use of the diagnostic subtypes of schizophrenia. Although the total number of schizophrenic patients in this hospital had remained constant over almost a half-century, the shift in diagnosis from catatonic and hebephrenic schizophrenia to chronic undifferentiated schizophrenia was dramatic. Most relevant was the investigation of a single New Haven facility that found that the major changes in the diagnosis of depression made at a single treatment facility ($N = 2{,}134$) during three different time periods (1954, 1964, 1974) were not due to a true change in presenting symptomatology. For example, although the proportion of patients diagnosed as having a mood disorder had increased threefold, those patients diagnosed as having a neurosis went from being the largest group to one of the smallest. These diagnostic shifts occurred even though the presenting symptoms remained relatively unchanged. Comparisons of primary symptoms versus total symptoms also strongly suggested that different aspects of a patient's symptom cluster became more significant at different time periods. These epidemiological analyses of the relationship between diagnosis and historical period support Foucault's philosophical position on the cultural meaning of diagnostic systems. This position, in fact, is compatible with this section's initial discussion of "caseness" and the psychiatric search over the past 100 years for those social, psychological, and somatic symptoms that define mood disorder (Figs. 17.1-1 and 17.1-2). The most radical conclusion to be drawn from this approach is the importance of recognizing that social practices and attitudes influence how institutions define mood disorders as well as determine who should receive treatment and the type of treatment provided.

REFERENCES

Blum J D: On changes in psychiatric diagnosis over time. Amer Psychol *33:* 1017, 1978.

Boyd J H, Weissman M M: Epidemiology of affective disorders: A reexamination and future directions. Arch Gen Psychiat *38:* 1039, 1981.

Cochrane A L: *Effectiveness and Efficiency*. Burgess & Son (Abingdon), London, 1971.

Egeland J A, Gerhard D S, Pauls D L, Sussex J N, Kidd K K, Allen C R, Hostetter A M, Housman D E: Bipolar affective disorders linked to DNA markers on chromosome 11. Nature *325:* 783, 1987.

Egeland J A, Hostetter A M: Amish study, I: Affective disorders among the Amish, 1976–1980. Amer J Psychiat *140:* 56, 1983.

Engelhardt H T, Jr: The concepts of health and disease. In *Evaluation and Explanation in the Biomedical Sciences,* H T Engelhardt, Jr, S F Spicker, editors, p 125. Reidel, Dordrecht, Netherlands, 1975.

Faravelli C, Ambonetti A: Assessment of life events in depressive disorders: A comparison of three methods. Soc Psychiat *18:* 51, 1983.

Foucault M. *The Order of Things: An Archaelogy of the Human Sciences*. Pantheon, New York, 1970.

Hill D: Depression: Disease, reaction, or posture? Amer J Psychiat *125:* 445, 1968.

Hirschfeld R M A, Cross C K: Epidemiology of affective disorders: Psychosocial risk factors. Arch Gen Psychiat *39:* 35, 1982.

Holzer C E, Shea B M, Swanson J W, Leaf P J, Myers J K, George L, Weissman M M, Bednarski P: The increased risk for specific psychiatric disorders among persons of low socioeconomic status: Evidence from the Epidemiologic Catchment Area surveys. Amer J Soc Psychiat *4:* 259, 1986.

Jablensky A, Sartorius N, Gulbinat W, Ernberg G: Characteristics of depressive patients contacting psychiatric services in four cultures. Acta Psychiat Scand *63:* 367, 1981.

Keller, M B, Klerman G L, Lavori P W, Fawcett J A, Coryell W, Endicott J: Treatment received by depressed patients. JAMA *248:* 1848, 1982.

Leaf P J, Livingston M M, Tischler G L, Weissman M M, Holzer C E, Myers J K: Contact with health professionals for the treatment of psychiatric and emotional problems. Med Care *23:* 1322, 1985.

Link B, Dohrenwend B P: Formulation of hypotheses about the true prevalence of demoralization in the United States. In *Mental Illness in the United States,* B P Dohrenwend, B S Dohrenwend, M S Gould, B Link, R Neugebauer, R Wunsch-Hitzig, editors, p 114. Praeger, New York, 1980.

Mollica R F: Psychiatry in quest after orientation. In *Analecta Husserliana,* vol 20, p 101. Reidel, Dordrecht, Netherlands, 1986.

Murphy J M, Sobol A M, Neff R K, Olivier D C, Leighton A H: Stability of prevalence: Depression and anxiety disorders. Arch Gen Psychiat *41:* 990, 1984.

Myers J K, Weissman M M, Tischler G L, Holzer C E, III, Leaf P J, Orvaschel H, Anthony J C, Boyd J H, Burke J D, Kramer M, Stoltzman R: Six-month prevalence of psychiatric disorders in three communities: 1980 to 1982. Arch Gen Psychiat *41:* 956, 1984.

Shepherd G: Introduction. In *Developments in Social Skills Training,* S Spence and G Shepherd, editors, p 11. Academic Press, London, 1983.

Uhlenhuth E H, Balter M B, Mellinger G D, Cisin I H, Clinthorne J: Symptom checklist syndromes in the general population: Correlations with psychotherapeutic drug use. Arch Gen Psychiat *40:* 1167, 1983.

Weissman M M, Klerman G L: Sex differences and the epidemiology of depression. Arch Gen Psychiat *34:* 98, 1977.

Weissman M M, Myers J K, Thompson W D: Depression and its treatment in a U.S. urban community—1975–1976. Arch Gen Psychiat *38:* 417, 1981.

Westermeyer J: Lao folk diagnosis for mental disorders: Comparison with psychiatric diagnosis and assessment with psychiatric rating scales. Med Anthropol *5:* 425, 1981.

17.2 MOOD DISORDERS: ETIOLOGY

17.2a MOOD DISORDERS: BIOCHEMICAL ASPECTS

JOSEPH J. SCHILDKRAUT, M.D.
ALAN I. GREEN, M.D.
JOHN J. MOONEY, M.D.

INTRODUCTION

The biochemistry of the affective disorders (called mood disorders in the third revised edition of the *Diagnostic and Statistical Manual of Mental Disorders* [DSM-III-R]) has been an active area of scientific investigation since the introduction of the first clinically effective antidepressant drugs—imipramine (Tofranil) and the monoamine oxidase inhibitors (MAOIs)—in the late 1950s. In the 30 years since then, these first antidepressant drugs, as well as the newer ones as they have come along, have themselves become major research tools. Research into their mechanisms of action has provided the basis for various working hypotheses about the biochemistry of depressions and has also led to more fundamental discoveries about the neurobiology of the central nervous system (CNS) itself. This section delineates the several lines of current research on the biochemistry of depressive disorders and provides a guide for understanding existing theoretical frameworks.

The brain is known to contain billions of neurons, each one interacting with the others by electrochemical means. When a neuron is stimulated, the resulting impulse, or electrical action potential, causes a release of a chemical substance (a neurotransmitter) from a specialized region close to a neighboring neuron. The neurotransmitter is released into a space between the two neurons, called the *synaptic cleft.* The neuron leading to the synaptic cleft is called the *presynaptic neuron,* and the neuron leading away from the synaptic cleft is called the *postsynaptic neuron.* The neurotransmitter released into the synaptic cleft from the presynaptic neuron briefly interacts with a receptor on the postsynaptic neuron, resulting in either electrical stimulation (increasing the likelihood of an action potential) or electrical inhibition (decreasing the likelihood of an action potential) of the postsynaptic neuron.

There seem to be many different substances that can act as neurotransmitters in the brain. There are also many other brain chemicals that can regulate or modulate this process. Pharmacological agents, such as the antidepressants, or many kinds of environmental stimuli work by altering this neurotransmitter-mediated interaction between neurons.

Genetic factors clearly may have biochemical expressions at the synapse, and environmental or psychological factors may act in that way as well. Neurochemical and neurophysiological changes secondary to such factors can alter an individual's vulnerability to depressive episodes or even precipitate a depressive episode; therefore, sharp distinctions cannot be drawn between genetically and environmentally induced depressions or between biological and psychological depressions. Similar neurochemical or neurophysiological changes are probably involved to a greater or lesser degree in virtually every type.

Most of the biological research on the affective disorders aims at learning more about the workings of the CNS in these disorders. As an offshoot of this research, however, many investigators are using various biochemical measures to subtype these disorders. Biological subtyping, if successful, may enable the differentiation of groups of patients who appear similar clinically, but who are distinct biochemically. The existence of such subtypes may have important clinical implications.

HISTORICAL OVERVIEW OF NEUROPSYCHOPHARMACOLOGY

The two major classes of antidepressant drugs, the MAOIs and the tricyclic antidepressants, were first used in psychiatry about 30 years ago. Within a few years after their introduction, several lines of evidence began to suggest that these medications worked at least in part through effects on catecholamines (norepinephrine, epinephrine, and dopamine)—one of the many groups of chemical substances that function as neurotransmitters in the CNS. One of these catecholamines, norepinephrine, seemed to have particular importance in this regard. The first clue was that the MAOIs increased concentrations of norepinephrine in the brain by blocking one of its metabolic pathways. Shortly thereafter, the drug imipramine, a tricyclic antidepressant, was found to enhance the effects of norepinephrine by blocking a major inactivation mechanism, that is, the reuptake of norepinephrine into presynaptic neurons after release into the synaptic cleft. At about the same time, reserpine, a drug then used for hypertension, was noted both to deplete catecholamines in the brain and to cause clinical depressions in some patients.

On the basis of these and other data, the catecholamine hypothesis of affective disorders was formulated and introduced into the literature in the mid-1960s because of its potential heuristic value. This hypothesis, in its simplest form, proposed that some depressive disorders may be associated with an absolute or relative deficiency of catecholamines, particularly norepinephrine, at functionally important synapses in the brain, whereas manias may be associated with an excess of such catecholamines. The focus on levels of catecholamines in the simplest statement of the hypothesis was based on the research techniques of the day that allowed only for the measurement of the output and metabolism of norepinephrine released by presynaptic neurons. Nevertheless, the possibility of abnormalities in receptor function was also considered in the general formulation of the hypothesis, because it was known that in the event of receptor subsensitivity, a relative functional deficiency of norepinephrine could occur even with normal or elevated presynaptic output.

Because the broad clinical and biological heterogeneity of depressive disorders was recognized, it was apparent from the outset that this focus on catecholamine metabolism was, at best, an oversimplification of complex biological mechanisms. Alterations in many other neurotransmitter or neuromodulator systems were envisioned, as were ionic changes, endocrine changes, or other biochemical abnormalities.

Nonetheless, the possibility that different subgroups of depressed patients might ultimately be characterized by differences in the metabolism of norepinephrine or in the physiology of noradrenergic (norepinephrine-containing) neuronal systems was raised in the initial formulation of the catecholamine hypothesis of affective disorders. Subsequent studies by many research groups have provided considerable data to support this possibility. Other research in recent years has looked at other neurotransmitters or neuromodulators as well. In particular, there have been studies on the relationship of dopamine, acetylcholine, and the indoleamine serotonin to depression.

In the past, many investigations attempted to separate the depressive disorders into noradrenergic or serotonergic depressions, depending on certain biochemical data and particular responses to various tricyclic antidepressant drugs. This notion, based in part on presumed differences among various tricyclic antidepressant drugs in the inhibition of norepinephrine and serotonin reuptake, no longer seems tenable. Recent findings from studies of depressed patients, as well as data concerning the physiological interactions between noradrenergic and serotonergic neurons and the complex neuropharmacological effects of antidepressant drugs, make it clear that such separations are overly simplistic and artificial.

Acetylcholine, another classic neurotransmitter, also may play a role in the pathophysiology of at least certain types of depressive disorders. Drugs that stimulate acetylcholinergic activity have been found to induce depressions in control subjects, to exacerbate depressions in depressed patients, and to decrease manias in manic patients. Recent studies have also suggested that some depressed patients may have supersensitive acetylcholinergic receptors. Thus, the anticholinergic effects of the commonly prescribed antidepressant drugs may be responsible for more than side effects; they may be of some importance in the drugs' actual antidepressant effects as well.

Neurotransmitters interact with specific receptors to exert their effects. Recent studies have shown that alterations in the biochemical and physiological properties of these receptors may be involved both in the mechanisms of action of antidepressant drugs and in the pathophysiology of depressive disorders. These possibilities are currently being investigated in a number of laboratories throughout the world.

It is becoming increasingly clear that the pathophysiology of depressive disorders is not restricted to abnormalities in brain function. Rather, the depressive disorders must be conceptualized as complex neuroendocrinometabolic disorders that involve many different organ systems throughout the body. The close connection to the endocrine system is just beginning to be understood. Many specialized laboratory tests are now starting to be used in psychiatry, and it is expected that during the coming years, such clinical laboratory tests will play an increasingly important role in the diagnostic evaluation and treatment of patients with depressive disorders.

BIOGENIC AMINES

The term "biogenic amine" generally refers to four compounds, the catecholamines, norepinephrine, epinephrine, and dopamine; and the indoleamine, serotonin. All four compounds have a single amine group on the side chain and are consequently also called monoamines. The neuronal systems using the monoamines originate as relatively small collections of cell groups located mainly in the brain stem. From there, the cell groups project widely into other brain regions. Such widespread projection makes these neuronal systems logical targets for psychiatric research, as small changes in them can have diverse behavioral effects.

At the synapse, the biogenic amines are released into the synaptic space and act at pre- and postsynaptic receptor sites. Most of the neurotransmitter is inactivated by reuptake into the presynaptic neuron; however, a portion may be metabolized in the synaptic space outside the neuron. The mitochondrial enzyme monoamine oxidase (MAO) is involved in the metabolism of the neurotransmitter within the presynaptic neuron.

NOREPINEPHRINE METABOLISM AND PHYSIOLOGY The noradrenergic cell bodies containing norepinephrine are found in the locus ceruleus, medulla oblongata, and pons. They distribute projections by two major pathways to the entire neocortex, limbic structures, thalamus, hypothalamus, reticular formation, dorsal raphe nucleus, cerebellum, sensory and motor brain stem nuclei, and spinal cord. Individual locus ceruleus neurons can simultaneously send collateral branches to the neocortex, hippocampus, cerebellum, and spinal cord. The norepinephrine projections from the locus ceruleus also regulate brain blood flow and capillary permeability.

One method of studying the activity of noradrenergic neurons in the brain is to measure the level of 3-methoxy-4-hydroxyphenylglycol (MHPG) in the urine. Known to be a major metabolite of norepinephrine originating in the brain, MHPG may also derive in part from the peripheral sympathetic nervous system. Any MHPG from either source may be converted to 3-methoxy-4-hydroxymandelic acid (VMA). Thus, the fraction of urinary MHPG deriving from brain norepinephrine is uncertain. Despite this uncertainty, urinary MHPG has been measured in attempts to elucidate the pathophysiology of depressions and to discriminate among biologically distinct subgroups of depressive disorders.

Urinary MHPG levels In longitudinal studies of patients with naturally occurring or amphetamine-induced bipolar manic-depressive episodes, many investigators have found that levels of urinary MHPG are low during periods of depression and high during periods of mania or hypomania. Comparably low MHPG values, however, are not present in all types of depressions. This has raised the possibility that MHPG, or other catecholamine metabolites, may provide a biochemical basis for differentiating among subgroups of depressive disorders.

In early studies, urinary MHPG levels were found to be significantly lower in patients with bipolar manic-depressive depressions than in patients with unipolar nonendogenous chronic characterological depressions. Subsequent studies confirmed the presence of reduced urinary MHPG levels (and plasma norepinephrine levels) in patients with classic bipolar manic-depressive depressions (i.e., bipolar I, but not bipolar II, depressive disorders), when compared with mean values in various subtypes of unipolar depressions or in nondepressed control subjects. One study suggested that the differences in urinary MHPG levels in bipolar manic-depressive depressions and control subjects became more pronounced when the peripheral contribution to urinary MHPG was reduced with carbidopa, a decarboxylase inhibitor that does not cross the blood–brain barrier.

In contrast to the reduction in urinary MHPG levels in patients with bipolar manic-depressive depressions, as compared with those with unipolar depressions, a number of studies reported no differences in urinary VMA levels. This finding is important because studies reporting that circulating MHPG may be converted to VMA have raised questions concerning the specific value of urinary MHPG (e.g., in contrast to VMA) as an index of norepinephrine metabolism in the brain or as a biochemical marker in studies of depressed patients.

Patients with unipolar depressions have been reported to have a wide range of plasma norepinephrine and MHPG, as well as urinary MHPG levels. Low, intermediate, or high levels of urinary MHPG have been found in various studies. This range of findings may reflect diagnostic heterogeneity among the group of unipolar depressions. In some patients with unipolar depressions, low levels of urinary MHPG are comparable to those seen in the bipolar depressions; whereas in others, high values are sometimes above the normal range. Because the values of urinary MHPG in normal control subjects also tend to vary widely, urinary MHPG levels cannot be used to diagnose depression per se; yet, urinary MHPG levels may help differentiate depressive subgroups.

Recent studies have described a subgroup of patients with severe unipolar depressions whose urinary MHPG and urinary free cortisol (UFC) levels both were very high. In this subgroup of severely depressed patients with high catecholamine and cortisol output, increased acetylcholinergic activity could conceivably be a primary factor in the depression, with elevated urinary MHPG and UFC as a secondary response. This suggestion is particularly intriguing when certain other data are considered: (1) Physostigmine (Antilirium, Eserine), an anticholinesterase, and other pharmacological agents that increase brain cholinergic activity exacerbate depressive symptoms in normal controls. (2) Physostigmine increases plasma cortisol levels in normal controls. (3) Physostigmine can overcome suppression of the hypothalamic-pituitary-adrenocortical axis by dexamethasone in normal subjects, thereby mimicking the abnormal escape from dexamethasone suppression seen in some patients who show cortisol hypersecretion. (4) Physostigmine increases the cerebrospinal fluid levels of MHPG in normal subjects. The preceding suggestion thus raises the unorthodox possibility that the anticholinergic effects of some antidepressant drugs, commonly regarded as side effects, may actually contribute to their antidepressant action in patients with this depressive subtype.

Thus, there may be at least three distinct subtypes of what appear to be unipolar depressive disorders that can be distinguished by urinary MHPG levels. Subtype I, with low pretreatment urinary MHPG levels, may have low norepinephrine output as the result of a decrease in norepinephrine synthesis or its release from noradrenergic neurons. (Many patients included in this subtype may be patients with underlying bipolar mood disorders who have not yet had their first episode of mania or hypomania.) In contrast, Subtype II, with intermediate urinary MHPG levels, may have normal norepinephrine output but abnormalities in other biochemical systems. Subtype III, with high urinary MHPG levels, may have high norepinephrine output in response to alterations in noradrenergic receptors or to an increase in cholinergic activity. Further research is required to confirm these findings and to explore physiological abnormalities that may be associated with these subtypes of unipolar depressive disorders.

The D-type equation Although MHPG alone does help differentiate subtypes of depressions, multivariate discriminant function analysis has been used to explore the possibility that levels of norepinephrine (NE), epinephrine (E), normetanephrine (NMN), metanephrine (MN), and VMA might provide an even better differentiation. This analysis led to the development of an empirically derived equation, termed the "Depression type (D-type) equation," that distinguishes even more precisely between bipolar manic-depressive and unipolar nonendogenous chronic characterological depressions than urinary MHPG alone. This equation is of the form:

$$\text{D-type score} = C_1\,(\text{MHPG}) - C_2\,(\text{VMA}) + C_3\,(\text{NE}) - C_4\,\frac{(\text{NMN} + \text{MN})}{\text{VMA}} + C_0$$

The metric for this equation was established so that patients with bipolar manic-depressive depressions tend toward a score of 0 and patients with unipolar nonendogenous depressions tend toward a score of 1.

In a subsequently studied validation sample of 114 depressed patients whose data had not been used to derive the equation, the D-type score (using a criterion of D-type score $\leq .50$) had a sensitivity of .85 and a specificity of .84 in identifying patients with clinically diagnosed bipolar manic-depressive (and bipolar-related schizoaffective) depressions. A wide range of D-type scores was seen in patients with clinically diagnosed (putative) unipolar endogenous depressions (i.e., depressed patients with no prior history of mania). Preliminary findings using this equation suggest that low D-type scores in patients with such putative unipolar depressions may identify those with latent bipolar disorders who have not yet had a clinical episode of mania.

The findings of a recent study have indicated that D-type scores also may be an even better predictor than is urinary MHPG alone of antidepressant responses to imipramine or alprazolam (Xanax) in patients with unipolar depressions. When a model or equation derived to describe or account for observations in one domain is found to have more general applicability in predicting observations in yet another domain, confidence in the explanatory power of that model is enhanced. The D-type equation was initially derived to separate patients with bipolar manic-depressive depressions from patients with other subtypes of depressive disorders. The finding that D-type scores also appear to predict differential clinical responses to antidepressant drugs in patients with unipolar depressions thus extends the potential clinical utility of the D-type equation and also enhances its heuristic value.

Urinary MHPG levels as predictors of differential responses to antidepressant drugs Studies from a number of laboratories have indicated that pretreatment levels of urinary MHPG may help predict responses to certain tricyclic and tetracyclic antidepressant drugs. In many (though clearly not in all) studies, depressed patients with low pretreatment urinary MHPG levels have been found to respond more favorably to treatment with imipramine, desipramine (Norpramine), nortriptyline (Pamelor), or maprotiline (Ludiomil) than patients with high MHPG levels. In contrast, some but not all studies have found that depressed patients with high pretreatment levels of urinary MHPG respond more favorably to treatment with amitriptyline (Elavil) or alprazolam than patients with lower MHPG levels.

Urinary MHPG values trichotomized into the three subtypes

described above also may be useful in predicting treatment responses. Preliminary data have shown that although depressed patients with elevated MHPG levels may be more responsive to treatment with imipramine or maprotiline than patients with intermediate levels, neither group was as responsive as patients with low MHPG levels. Moreover, patients with low pretreatment urinary MHPG levels were found to respond rapidly to relatively low doses of maprotiline, whereas those patients with elevated MHPG levels (who responded to maprotiline at all) required significantly higher doses and longer periods of drug administration. This finding suggests a differential response or that the antidepressant drug, maprotiline, may have different pharmacological properties in high doses than in low doses. The notion of the relative sensitivity of different subtypes of depressions to antidepressant drugs may be analogous to the concept of the relative sensitivity of different infectious diseases to antibiotic drugs.

At present, one cannot draw valid inferences about biochemical predictors of differential antidepressant drug responses on the basis of hypothesized pharmacological mechanisms of action, as it is known that these drugs have multiple, complex effects on many neurotransmitter systems. Consequently, empirical clinical trials will be required to assess the value of particular biochemical measures, such as urinary MHPG levels, as clinically useful predictors of responses to each specific antidepressant drug. But because the patients referred for study in academic centers today may be more refractory to the commonly used antidepressant drugs than the patients studied some years ago when antidepressant drugs were less widely used in the routine practice of medicine and psychiatry, caution must be exercised when comparing new data with earlier findings.

DOPAMINE METABOLISM AND PHYSIOLOGY The major metabolite of dopamine is homovanillic acid (HVA). Many studies of levels of HVA in cerebrospinal fluid (CSF) have shown that CSF HVA levels are reduced in depressed patients. Recent studies have shown, however, that many depressed patients with delusions or a history of psychosis have higher CSF HVA levels than patients with nonpsychotic depressions. An increase in dopamine turnover in response to increased corticosteroid output has been proposed as a mechanism that could account for the increase in CSF HVA levels in delusional depressions.

SEROTONIN METABOLISM AND PHYSIOLOGY The cell bodies of serotonergic neurons are located in the raphe nuclei and superior central nucleus, and their axons project widely throughout the CNS, to the entire neocortex, entorhinal cortex, thalamus, hypothalamus, limbic structures, reticular formation, locus ceruleus, cerebellum, and spinal cord. As is true of noradrenergic neurons, such a widespread projection of serotonergic neurons makes them logical candidates for psychiatric research. In many regions, the serotonergic and noradrenergic projections overlap with each other, and there is at least one major interface between the raphe nuclei of the serotonergic system and the locus ceruleus of the noradrenergic system.

Certain lines of evidence suggest that some patients with depressive disorders may have abnormal serotonin metabolism and physiology. A number of studies have found that some depressed patients have a reduced level of 5-hydroxyindoleacetic acid (5-HIAA), a metabolite of serotonin, in the CSF. Other studies have noted an association between this lower level of CSF 5-HIAA and the increased incidence of completed suicide, attempted suicide, or acts of aggression.

In several older studies, the brains of suicide victims were found to have low concentrations of serotonin. Some recent studies, looking at the brains of suicide victims, found that the binding of ^{3}H-imipramine, which is thought to bind to serotonergic nerve terminals, is decreased. These studies also reported higher numbers of postsynaptic serotonin receptors. These findings have led a number of investigators to suggest that there may be a serotonergic deficiency in suicide victims or in those depressed patients who attempt suicide.

Decreased serotonin uptake into platelets has been observed in patients with depressive disorders. ^{3}H-imipramine binds to brain and platelet high-affinity sites thought to be near the cellular uptake regulation sites for serotonin. A highly significant decrease in the number of ^{3}H-imipramine–binding sites with no significant change in the apparent affinity constant has been observed in platelets from depressed patients, compared with those from control subjects. The decreased platelet ^{3}H-imipramine binding observed in depressed patients may reflect a deficiency in the platelet serotonin transport mechanism in these patients.

STUDIES OF RECEPTORS Many investigators have suggested that alterations in receptor sensitivity may play a role in both the mechanism of action of antidepressant drugs and the pathophysiology of the depressive disorders. The time course of the clinical effects of antidepressants has been linked to changes in receptor functioning. Various subtypes of depressive disorders may also be distinguished by particular receptor characteristics.

Receptors are studied by in vivo or in vitro techniques. In vivo study involves the use of various pharmacological challenges of physiological properties thought to reflect the action of particular receptors. For example, the α-adrenergic agonist clonidine (Catapres) stimulates growth hormone (GH) release, which is thought to occur via the postsynaptic α-adrenergic receptor. In many depressed patients, the GH response is blunted, suggesting a decreased sensitivity of these receptors.

The study of adrenergic receptors on human blood cells allows in vitro measurements of adrenergic receptors from psychiatric patients. These receptors may not reflect similar changes in the CNS; yet, they do provide a valuable research tool. For example, the number of the β-adrenergic binding sites on lymphocytes has been found to be lower in some depressed and manic patients as compared with those of control subjects or euthymic patients. Some studies also suggest that the β-adrenergic receptor–mediated stimulation of cyclic adenosine monophosphate (cAMP) production by isoproterenol is reduced in leukocytes and lymphocytes from depressed patients. One investigator noted this lack of responsiveness in depressed patients with psychomotor agitation but not in those with psychomotor retardation. More research is needed to clarify the significance of these findings suggesting decreased β-adrenergic receptor function in lymphocytes from some depressed patients.

There also have been studies of platelet α_2-adrenergic receptors, which suppress the activity of prostaglandin-stimulated adenylate cyclase, in depressed subjects. Some studies reported platelet adenylate cyclase (whether basal, prostaglandin-stimulated, or α-adrenergic suppression of prostaglandin-stimulated) to be unchanged. Other studies of patients with unipolar depressions found that both prostaglandin-stimulated and α-adrenergic suppression of prostaglandin-stimulated adenylate cyclase were decreased. The discrepancies between these findings may reflect differences in the platelet adenylate cyclase activity in subgroups of depressed patients.

Several studies reported that the total numbers of platelet α_2-adrenergic receptors were either unchanged or increased (but not decreased) in depressed patients. In light of the findings of decreased platelet α-adrenergic suppression (and decreased prostaglandin stimulation) of adenylate cyclase, the failure to find a decrease in the number of platelet α_2-adrenergic receptors suggests a defect in the coupling between the platelet α_2-adrenergic (or prostaglandin) receptors and platelet adenylate cyclase in some unipolar depressed patients. This deficiency may involve the guanine nucleotide regulatory proteins that link neurotransmitter or hormone receptors to the catalytic unit of adenylate cyclase.

Several laboratories have found increased catecholamine output in some depressed patients. In the presence of increased catecholamine levels, catecholamine-receptor interactions tend to become desensitized over time. One group of investigators proposed that the changes in receptor coupling and functioning seen in some depressed patients may be the result of heterologous desensitization. The term "heterologous desensitization" or "agonist nonspecific desensitization" refers to the process whereby a chronic exposure to one particular agonist (e.g., a neurotransmitter, neuromodulator, or hormone) produces diminished responsiveness to multiple agonists in many different receptor systems, because of a reversible alteration in the guanine nucleotide regulatory proteins that link or couple all of these receptors to the catalytic unit of adenylate cyclase. Taken one step further, this concept raises the possibility that many of the physiological and neuroendocrinometabolic alterations observed in patients with depressive disorders (including some of the psychoneuroendocrine abnormalities described below) may be the result of catecholamine-induced heterologous desensitization.

PLATELET MONOAMINE OXIDASE ACTIVITY To explore further the pathophysiology of the depressive disorders, investigators studied the enzyme monoamine oxidase (MAO), which deaminates biogenic amines in many body tissues, including the nervous system and the blood platelet. A growing body of literature suggests that levels of platelet MAO activity may help discriminate among subtypes of depressive disorders.

In the early 1970s, platelet MAO activity was reported to be increased in a heterogeneous group of depressed patients (most of whom had unipolar depressions) and to be decreased in a group of bipolar depressed patients. Subsequent results have not been so clear. For example, some investigators reported increased platelet MAO activity in patients with unipolar endogenous depressions; others found increased platelet MAO activity in patients with unipolar nonendogenous depressions. Because each study used different criteria for the diagnosis of endogenous or nonendogenous depressions, as well as different methods to determine platelet MAO activity, it is not possible to reconcile these conflicting data at the present time.

One study, however, suggested that bipolar and unipolar depressions may show differences in the relationship between platelet MAO activity and the severity of clinical symptomatology. In bipolar depressions, greater severity was associated with low platelet MAO activity, and in unipolar depressions, greater severity was associated with high platelet MAO activity. (This study systematically excluded patients with schizotypal features, such as unusual perceptions, ideas of reference, impairment in communication, and a history of social isolation. This was done because the presence of such schizotypal features would raise the question of schizophrenia-related disorders, with associated changes in platelet MAO activity, which might otherwise confound the data.)

Several studies have found an unexpected association between increased platelet MAO activity and increased activity of the hypothalamic-pituitary-adrenal (HPA) axis in depressed patients. Elucidation of the clinical and pathophysiological significance of this intriguing association also may help clarify aspects of the confusing and seemingly contradictory literature on platelet MAO activity in regard to subtypes of depressive disorders.

In some studies of patients with unipolar depressions, platelet MAO activity was found to correlate both with the severity of the depression and with anxiety symptoms and somatic complaints. The clinical items found to be correlated with platelet MAO activity in these studies corresponded to those symptoms reported by other investigators to be associated with favorable responses to treatment with MAO inhibitors. Other studies have found an association of high platelet MAO activity with social introversion or asociality, and of low platelet MAO activity with social extroversion or sensation seeking.

Additional studies will be needed to determine whether such clinical (psychometric) variables also may help account for the differences in platelet MAO activity that have been observed in various subgroups of depressions. More research will also be required to compare kinetic parameters (and other properties) of platelet mitochondrial MAO with other biological indicators in patients with various subtypes of depressive disorders and in control subjects as well.

PSYCHONEUROENDOCRINOLOGY

Because many endocrinopathies present with psychiatric symptoms, particularly affective symptoms, clinicians and investigators have long considered the possible connection between the endocrine system and mood disorders. The discovery that peptides from the hypothalamus, under the control of various neurotransmitters linked with the pathophysiology of these disorders, regulate the release of pituitary hormones led to further speculation about this relationship. Recent advances, including the development of sensitive hormonal assays and the isolation of many hypothalamic peptides, have enabled psychoneuroendocrinology to emerge as an important research discipline.

The possibility that hormones might somehow be related to affective states was raised with the earliest clinical descriptions of Cushing's disease and hypothyroidism, both of which are associated with changes in mood. The exact relationship between the endocrine system and the brain as a mediator of behavior, however, was unclear for years. In fact, it was not until the late 1940s that the neurovascular model linking the hypothalamus and the pituitary was first proposed, and it was not until the mid-1950s that the existence of a substance in pituitary extract that stimulated the release of adrenocorticotropic hormone (ACTH) was demonstrated. This substance was called corticotropin-releasing factor (CRF), but its structure eluded investigators until quite recently. In about the past 15 years, a number of hypothalamic peptides controlling the anterior pituitary gradually have been isolated and synthesized: thyrotropin-releasing hormone (TRH), gonadotropin-releasing hormone (GnRH), growth hormone–releasing factor (GHRF), growth hormone release–inhibiting factor (GHRIF or somatostatin), and CRF itself.

The activity of the limbic system, long suggested to be a CNS site mediating affective states, is regulated by many of the neurotransmitters thought to be involved in the pathophysiology and, possibly, the etiology of mood disorders. The limbic system in turn regulates the pituitary hormone release, a key element in the endocrine network. Thus, many investigators have examined endocrine changes in mood disorders to obtain information concerning possible functional alterations of certain CNS neuronal systems that use one or another neurotransmitter or neuromodulator. This strategy has been likened to looking at the brain through a neuroendocrine window. Another strategy in recent psychiatric studies has been more practical. This is the search for one or more laboratory tests of endocrine function that might distinguish certain mood subtypes from other subtypes or mood disorders from other psychiatric illnesses.

The neuroendocrine network is a highly complex, well-integrated system. It involves the release of anterior pituitary hormones by various hypothalamic factors, a feedback control of this release by circulating target organ hormones, and an overriding control on the entire system by internal biological rhythms or external events affecting the hypothalamus.

The methods used for studying the endocrine network as it relates to mood disorders are multifaceted. First, because each bodily hormone is released according to a circadian rhythm, the study of possible changes in the rhythm in a mood disorder is of interest. Second, the response of the anterior pituitary to the introduction of a hypothalamic factor can also be measured in affected patients and compared with normals. Third, direct challenges to the hypothalamus itself, such as insulin-induced hypoglycemia, provide further information about the functioning of the endocrine axes. Fourth and finally, provocative neuropharmacological challenges with such drugs as amphetamine, clonidine, or physostigmine can also be used to test for changes in neurotransmitter systems in affective disease states.

Hundreds of studies using one or another of these strategies have resulted in an enormous volume of information. The studies are often conflicting, yet one conclusion seems sure: Various endocrine changes are associated with affective disorders. The best documented changes involve the HPA, the hypothalamic-pituitary-thyroid (HPT), and the hypothalamic-pituitary-growth hormone (HPGH) axes.

HYPOTHALAMIC-PITUITARY-ADRENAL AXIS The HPA axis has been extensively studied in affective disorders. CRF, a hypothalamic peptide recently identified, stimulates the release of ACTH from the anterior pituitary. ACTH causes the adrenal cortex to secrete cortisol that, in turn, regulates the further release of CRF from the hypothalamus. The entire HPA system has a circadian rhythm; most of the cortisol released from the adrenal glands comes in periodic bursts in the early morning hours. The regulation of CRF is complex and involves various neurotransmitters and neuromodulators, including acetylcholine, serotonin, and norepinephrine.

Hyperactivity of the HPA axis in depressed patients has been extensively reported over the past decade. Cortisol hypersecretion, documented by 24-hour urinary free cortisol output or cortisol production rates, has been found in approximately one-half of the depressed patients studied. These cortisol hypersecreters show a characteristic flattening of their circadian cycle, such that they secrete cortisol during a time of day when such secretion is normally at a minimum. The cortisol abnormality seems related to the depression per se and not merely to stress or hyperactivity. Most studies reported the hypercortisol state to revert to normal with clinical remission. One study, however, suggested that urinary cortisol levels may remain elevated in some depressed patients even after their depression has resolved.

The dexamethasone suppression test (DST) has been used extensively to study the HPA axis in patients with affective disorders. First introduced in 1960 to study Cushing's disease, this procedure determines whether the administration of dexamethasone results in normal suppression of the HPA axis, as determined by lowered concentrations of cortisol in blood at various times after the administration of dexamethasone. Two groups of investigators, working independently, began applying the DST to depressed patients in the late 1960s, and both groups found abnormal DST values (the failure of dexamethasone to suppress cortisol secretion) in some of the patients with endogenous depressions. A number of seminal reports in the early 1980s led to widespread interest in the use of the DST in psychiatric research and practice. These reports specified (1) an optimal method (1 mg of oral dexamethasone with 4 P.M. and 11 P.M. plasma cortisol measurements); (2) sensitivity (67 percent); (3) specificity (96 percent, if strict exclusion criteria are followed); and (4) a cutoff for normal postdexamethasone plasma cortisol (5 μg per dl). Some recent studies have reported data using other dexamethasone dosages; a few investigations have suggested that a 2 mg dose may provide a more valid measure of the cortisol hyperactivity.

Dexamethasone suppression test and depression The recent literature contains many reports both confirming and questioning various aspects of the early DST findings. The reported sensitivity level for the 1 mg dose has been confirmed by many other investigators for patients variously described as having major depressive disorder, primary depression, or endogenous depression. The percentage of positive (abnormal) tests in patients with unipolar psychotic depressions or in older depressed patients has been found to be higher than in nonpsychotic melancholic patients. The actual cortisol concentration in 4 P.M. postdexamethasone blood samples may be significantly higher in these patients as well. The percentage of abnormal DSTs is often reported to be lower than 50 percent in outpatients, perhaps because outpatients may be more heterogeneous and, as a group, have less severe depressions. The association of abnormal DST results with a family history of depression has been reported by some investigators. The DST abnormality may cut across many different diagnostic categories and may define a diagnostically broader, but biologically more homogeneous, group of disorders than does melancholia per se.

The DST abnormality appears to be stable over the course of a depressive episode and often remits with clinical recovery. Subsequent depressions in a particular patient seem to run true; suppressors in one depression tend to be suppressors in the next. The change in the DST with treatment precedes the clinical recovery. An incomplete normalization of the DST, irrespective of the clinical symptomatology, may indicate an incomplete resolution of the depressive process.

There has been much discussion of whether an abnormal

DST indicates the need for pharmacological treatment. Although not all studies agree, it appears that patients with abnormal DSTs before treatment do not exhibit a significantly greater degree of improvement with pharmacological treatment than those with normal DSTs. An interesting series of preliminary studies has suggested, however, that depressed patients with an abnormal DST may be less likely to respond to a placebo than will those with a normal DST. If these studies are confirmed, the need for active pharmacological treatment to achieve clinical improvement in depressed patients with an abnormal DST may be greater than in those with a normal DST.

The issue of the specificity of the DST for depression is an important one, as in large measure it determines the test's clinical utility. The rate of false positive results on the DST in normal subjects has varied from 4 percent to over 10 percent in different reports. The variability in these reports may be due to an unrecognized history of affective disorders in the control subjects or their relatives. In patients or normals, variations in plasma dexamethasone levels following a fixed oral dexamethasone dose may contribute to some inconsistency in DST data. Differences in laboratory assay techniques and accuracy may also account for some of the reported variability in the DST data. Not taking the dexamethasone will produce a false positive result; the patient will then have a normal diurnal cortisol fluctuation that will be interpreted as an abnormal DST. (Some investigators have advocated using methylene blue as a marker for validating compliance.) Even if compliance is assured, however, various medical disorders and pharmacological agents can produce false positive or false negative results. In addition, weight loss per se, often an accompaniment of major depressions, may cause an abnormal DST.

Dexamethasone suppression test and other disorders The literature on psychiatric conditions other than depressions that may be associated with an abnormal DST is considerable. The DST may be abnormal in some patients with panic disorder and obsessive-compulsive disorder, especially in severe cases in which a secondary depression is suspected. Patients with anorexia nervosa and bulimia nervosa may also have abnormal DST results, even without a major weight change. An abnormal DST is observed in many patients with depression-like states after strokes and also in withdrawing alcoholics. Although some investigators have found normal results on the DST in schizophrenic and manic patients, the recent literature contains a few reports of a significant percentage of abnormalities on the DST in both diagnostic groups.

Clinical utility of the dexamethasone suppression test As might be expected from the conflicting published reports, the possible clinical utility of the DST has attracted considerable controversy. The number of known factors that can produce a false positive DST is expanding. Some investigators have suggested that the level of the postdexamethasone plasma cortisol may be more valuable than the mere qualitative assessment of the test as either abnormal or normal. There is a reasonable consensus of opinion that the DST has little value as a diagnostic screening test for depression. But many investigators believe that it may be helpful in difficult clinical situations (e.g., in differentiating psychotic depression from schizophrenia). The value of the DST as a predictor of response to treatment appears limited, except, as noted above, that an abnormal DST may imply a lack of placebo response. For this reason, some investigators suggest that a truly abnormal DST in a depressed person may indicate the need for pharmacological treatment.

Hypothalamic-pituitary-adrenal axis abnormality Recent studies have focused on the nature of the defect detected by an abnormal DST in populations of depressed patients. Some investigators have studied patients with an abnormal response to a 2 mg dose of dexamethasone, rather than the standard 1 mg, or those who have a very high level of postdexamethasone plasma cortisol. Other investigators have infused CRF into groups of depressed patients and normal controls. Preliminary data show that pituitary function in depressed patients is intact and that the defect may be at the level of the hypothalamus or above and manifested by an increased secretion of CRF. The standard DST detects one aspect of a disordered HPA axis in depressed patients; other methods (e.g., measurement of urinary free cortisol, plasma cortisol and ACTH levels following dexamethasone, ACTH stimulation, CRF stimulation, or the 2 mg DST) may provide more information. As noted above, the preliminary studies suggest that although the DST may usually normalize with clinical recovery, urinary free cortisol levels in recovered patients may remain slightly abnormal as a trait marker for depression.

The relationship of the HPA abnormality to other biological variables is currently an active area of research. Recent studies describe a subgroup of patients with severe unipolar depressions who have an increased catecholamine output (e.g., as reflected by very high levels of urinary MHPG) as well as evidence of high HPA activity (as documented by elevated urinary free cortisol or an abnormal DST). As noted earlier, the subgroup with high levels of urinary MHPG (Subtype III) may have a high norepinephrine output, either because of alterations in noradrenergic receptors or because of an increase in cholinergic activity. These studies have contributed to speculation about a possible adrenergic–cholinergic imbalance in some depressed patients. Investigators have also observed in some depressed patients an association of HPA hyperactivity, as detected by the DST, with increased platelet MAO activity. As with much of the data concerning the HPA axis, further study will be required to clarify this association.

HYPOTHALAMIC-PITUITARY-THYROID AXIS The HPT axis has received almost as much attention as has the HPA axis. There has been a long-standing interest in the thyroid and its function in emotion. Modern research can be traced to a 1938 report that suggested that some patients with periodic catatonia improved when they received thyroid extract. Approximately 40 years later, it was reported that small doses of triiodothyronine (T3) potentiated the antidepressant effects of tricyclics. More recently, a number of subtle changes in the thyroid axis have been detected in patients with affective disorders.

The HPT axis, like the HPA axis, is a complex and highly integrated network. The hypothalamic peptide TRH is carried to the anterior pituitary by the pituitary portal circulation. TRH stimulates the release of the pituitary hormone thyrotropin (thyroid-stimulating hormone [TSH]), which regulates the production of the thyroid hormones L-thyroxine (T4) and L-triiodothyronine (T3). The thyroid hormones exert a feedback control over the axis.

Symptoms of depression have long been known to occur in patients with frank hyperthyroidism or hypothyroidism; the psychiatric symptoms generally revert with the normalization of the thyroid status. Many psychiatric patients may also exhibit transient changes in their thyroid function test results at the time of hospitalization. These abnormalities, which generally return to normal within a matter of weeks, may simply reflect the stress of acute illness. Some depressed patients, however, may show persistent mild, or subclinical, hypothyroidism, detected by an elevated TSH value or an elevated TSH response to injected TRH. It is not known whether such subclinical hypothyroidism is related to the beneficial effect described when thyroid hormone is added to antidepressant medication or when TRH is infused into depressed patients. Elevated TSH has also been noted in patients with rapid cycling bipolar disorders, and some of these patients may benefit from the use of thyroid hormone. The adjunctive benefit gained from the use of thyroid hormone in patients with an affective disorder may derive from the thyroid modulation of adrenergic receptors.

The TRH stimulation test The TRH stimulation test, a standard endocrine procedure, has been used to probe the HPT axis in patients with affective disorder but apparently normal thyroid functioning. In medicine, this test is used mainly to evaluate dysfunction of the HPT axis. Often helpful in pinpointing the source of the dysfunction, it is considered to be a safe clinical procedure. The TRH test has become a useful research tool in psychiatry, one that may also have clinical applications. Investigators using this test have reported a decreased, or blunted, TSH response to TRH in many depressed patients. The blunted TSH response, which has been confirmed by many investigators, has been reported to occur in 25 to 70 percent of depressed patients. It has been reported in over 1,000 depressed patients in nearly 50 different studies over the past 15 years.

The test has been standardized and is generally performed as follows: After an overnight fast, the patient is placed in a recumbent position. An intravenous (IV) line is started in the morning, and a baseline TSH is drawn. The TRH is then injected IV, and blood samples are taken at intervals over the next 90 minutes for TSH measurements. The test result is usually expressed as ΔTSH, or the highest TSH value after the TRH infusion minus the TSH value before the TRH. Because in depression the TSH values are likely to be low, the laboratory assay (generally a radioimmunoassay) must be sensitive to these low levels.

The data on the TSH response have been reported either as group means or as a percentage of blunting for individual patients. Studies using group means have clearly indicated that, as a cohort, depressed patients have a lower TSH response to TRH than normal persons. The percentages of blunting vary from about 25 to 70 percent, depending on the definition of blunting and the diagnostic groups studied. Some groups have found that those patients with a blunted TSH response also have a blunted prolactin response or an abnormal GH response, but other groups have not. The possibility of differences between bipolar and unipolar depressions in the blunting of the TSH response to TRH has been raised but not resolved.

A number of factors are known to cause blunting in normal persons. Most important for the use of this test in psychiatry are increasing age and being male. Many of the studies of depressed patients are hard to interpret because of the lack of adequate controls. Other factors that may be related to blunting in normals are acute starvation, chronic renal failure, Klinefelter's syndrome, repeated TRH tests, and the administration of somatostatin, neurotensin, dopamine, thyroid hormone, or glucocorticoids. Because of the effect of glucocorticoids on the TRH test, some investigators have suggested that the blunted TRH test in depressives may be an epiphenomenon of an elevated plasma cortisol, known to be found in many depressed patients. Some recent studies, however, have separated these two factors. At times, the TRH blunting and the abnormal DST appear in the same depressed patients. But, some patients exhibit only one abnormality, whereas others may have neither.

The possible diagnostic significance of the TSH blunting has been a subject of some debate. As noted above, a number of studies have suggested that about 25 to 70 percent of patients variously described as having endogenous, primary, or major depressions also have a blunted TSH response to TRH. In two separate studies, patients with the TSH blunting were not found to be within particular familial subtypes of depression. Only a few studies have specifically reported on the TSH response in neurotic or minor depressions; but in those, the TSH was normal, as it was also in groups of patients with secondary depressions, schizophrenia, and acute paranoid reactions. Normal TSH responses, but with delayed time course, have been found in anorexia nervosa. Alcoholics, both during and after withdrawal, have been reported to have TSH blunting in the range of 25 to 60 percent. Some patients with a borderline personality disorder may have blunting as well. Thus, the finding of a blunted TSH response to TRH is not specific to endogenous depression.

One important question about the TRH test concerns the normalization of the TSH blunting with clinical improvement. In some depressed patients, the TSH response seems to change with symptomatology. A number of studies, however, have found that not all of the blunted responses in depressed patients return to normal with clinical improvement. Similarly, TSH responses have been found to be blunted in some alcoholics both during and long after withdrawal, suggesting that the TSH response to TRH may have trait as well as state characteristics. This possibility, that the TSH blunting may be a partial trait marker, has stimulated recent studies of the nondepressed relatives of TSH-blunted depressed patients.

Some investigators have studied the prognostic value of the TRH test. One group reported that a blunted TSH response may predict a more favorable response to antidepressant drugs. Another group followed a cohort of clinically recovered depressed patients to determine relapse rates based on an index of change in the TRH test known as the $\Delta\Delta$TSH, which is defined as the TRH test result (ΔTSH) after a favorable treatment response minus the result before treatment began. In their studies, a $\Delta\Delta$TSH of >2 μU per ml was associated with no relapse within 6 months, whereas a value of ≤ 2 μU per ml predicted a relapse within 6 months. In all the cases, no maintenance treatment had continued after the clinical response. The investigators suggested that the $\Delta\Delta$TSH may be helpful in determining when to stop treatment. Other studies have confirmed the value of $\Delta\Delta$TSH as a predictor of relapse, but it is not certain that antidepressant therapy will prevent it.

A number of investigators have studied the relationship of the TRH test blunting to other biological measurements in depressed patients, but clear-cut confirmed findings have not yet emerged. Studies such as these that combine multiple tests can be expected to become more common in the future.

It is not known what relationship the TRH test blunting has to the augmented response of TSH that may be seen in those depressed patients with subclinical hypothyroidism. Moreover, the pathophysiological significance of the TSH blunting in affective disorders is not clear. Hypersecretion of TRH could lead to the downregulation of the pituitary response (i.e., TSH blunting). This possibility is supported by one report of elevated TRH in the cerebrospinal fluid of depressed patients.

HYPOTHALAMIC-PITUITARY-GROWTH HORMONE AXIS The third endocrine system studied in patients with mood disorders is the HPGH axis. Investigators have looked at levels of GH and somatostatin—growth hormone release–inhibiting factor (GHRIF)—as well as the growth hormone response to various stimuli, such as insulin hypoglycemia, L-dopa, 5-hydroxytryptophan, apomorphine, d-amphetamine, clonidine, growth hormone–releasing hormone (GHRH), and TRH. The findings in patients with affective disorders have been, in general, confusing; the HPGH axis is a very complex one.

GH is elevated during stress and in relation to the first nightly cycle of slow-wave sleep, but GH also seems to be released in 6-hour intervals throughout each 24-hour day. Adrenergic, serotonergic, cholinergic, and opioidergic inputs modify the production of hypothalamic GHRH and GHRIF, but the relationship of these factors to the pulsatile secretion is unclear.

Basal GH levels in depressed patients are generally reported to be grossly normal, despite the illness's apparent stress. However, a reduction in sleep-associated GH release has been detected in depressed patients, as has an intermittent increase in daytime release. When measured in the CSF, basal somatostatin has been reported by two separate groups of investigators to be diminished in depressed patients but normal in manic patients. The level reverts to normal with clinical improvement.

Although some lines of evidence suggest that GH regulation may be abnormal in patients with depression, the picture is far from clear. As noted above, the sleep-associated GH release may be low, and the daytime GH secretion in depressed patients may be intermittently elevated. But although some challenge tests of the GH system have substantiated the suspicion of abnormalities in depressed patients, others have not.

The one challenge test of the GH system that has been consistently reported by several different groups to be abnormal in depressed patients is the GH response to clonidine. This test, which measures the responsiveness of postsynaptic α_2-adrenergic receptors, is blunted in some depressed patients. The abnormality may be a trait marker and not be resolved with treatment.

Results from most other challenge tests of the GH system have been conflicting. As noted above, stimulation by L-dopa has been used to measure GH response. An early report suggested that depressed patients had a lower GH response to L-dopa; however, in a subsequent study, when age, sex, and menopausal status were controlled, the diminished GH response to L-dopa disappeared.

Similarly an early study reported that the GH release after IV amphetamine administration was lower in endogenous depressives and higher in reactive depressives, as compared with normals. A later report, however, found that age or estrogen status greatly influenced the amphetamine effect on GH. A restudy of GH release, with adequate control groups, did not confirm the original findings in depressed patients.

There has been an interesting series of reports on abnormal GH responses to TRH in depressed patients. As discussed above, TRH normally causes the release of TSH and prolactin only. According to three separate research groups, GH increases can be detected in approximately 50 percent of patients with either unipolar or bipolar depressions, but in no patients with a minor depression. This abnormality ceases with clinical recovery. At least three other groups, however, did not find an abnormal growth hormone response to TRH in depressed patients. It is unclear at this time why such inconsistent findings are being reported. Further studies are required.

Some investigators have noted a reduced GH response to an insulin stimulus in some depressed patients. It may be more dramatic in psychotic depressions and, in some cases, persist after clinical recovery. One report noted the GH reduction to be more pronounced in bipolar than in unipolar depressions; yet, another report found just the opposite. One recent publication, which controlled for the adequacy of the hypoglycemic response to the insulin stimulus before measuring GH, reported no evidence of an abnormal GH response. A second study, however, which also ensured an adequate hypoglycemic response, did note a blunted GH secretion. Correcting for the hypoglycemic response to insulin when measuring the GH response in depression is essential, as some investigators have noted a blunted hypoglycemic response in unipolar depressed patients. This blunted response, too, may be associated with more severe depressions.

Even though, the HPGH axis provides intriguing clues to the pathophysiology of depression, it requires more intensive study. Any abnormalities that may be shown to exist in this axis will be exceedingly difficult to interpret because of the system's complexity.

HYPOTHALAMIC-PITUITARY-PROLACTIN AXIS Prolactin has also been studied in depressed patients, but the results have been generally inconclusive. This is undoubtedly due to the complexity of the control of prolactin secretion and the difficulties inherent in the study of the hormone. Prolactin is released from the anterior pituitary under the control of releasing and inhibitory factors. Various other substances can either increase or decrease its secretion. Among these are dopamine, which provides for the tonic inhibition of prolactin release, and serotonin, which is stimulating.

Investigations of basal prolactin levels in depressed patients have produced inconsistent results. Still-preliminary studies of fenfluramine (Pondimin) and L-tryptophan challenge of prolactin release point to a blunted response. This has been interpreted as being related to a serotonergic deficiency in some depressed patients. However, many factors, including weight loss, can have dramatic effects on prolactin challenge test results. Further studies are needed.

MELATONIN Melatonin, a hormone derived from the pineal gland, is synthesized from serotonin under the regulatory control of norepinephrine. Although melatonin's function in humans is poorly understood, investigators have used it to study psychiatric disorders. For example, many recent studies have explored the relationship between light-induced changes in melatonin secretion and depressive symptoms. Some investigators have detected lowered nocturnal melatonin levels in certain depressed patients; one group reported that the lowest levels existed in those depressed patients with an abnormal DST. It is not known whether such changes are due to a deficient release of a putative CRF inhibitory factor from the pineal gland or are merely the reflection of a reduced CNS noradrenergic tone in depressed patients. Lastly, the fact that melatonin is tightly controlled by norepinephrine has stimulated investigators to use plasma melatonin levels and urinary levels of its primary metabolite, 6-hydroxymelatonin, as an index of noradrenergic functioning in various states, such as before and after treatment with antidepressant medication.

OTHER BIOCHEMICAL ASPECTS OF AFFECTIVE DISORDERS

NEUROPEPTIDES In the past decade, dozens of neuropeptides have been isolated and sequenced. The study of their multiple and complex actions throughout the nervous system has become a major thrust of neuroscience research. Possible relationships between neuropeptide actions and psychiatric disorders have also been examined. As noted above, challenge studies with the peptides CRF and TRH have added to the understanding of the integrity of important neuroendocrine axes in patients with affective disorders. Many other neuropeptides, including β-endorphin, β-lipotropin, somatostatin, arginine vasopressin, cholecystokinin, substance P, bombesin, vasoactive intestinal peptide, delta sleep–inducing peptide, and calcitonin have also been studied in patients with mood disorders. Unfortunately, information about these neuropeptides is conflicting and, for some, quite sparse. Those that have been studied the most are β-endorphin, somatostatin, and arginine vasopressin.

The well-known effects of administered opioids and the documented existence of endogenous opioid peptides have led to questions about the role of the opioid peptides in affective disorders. The possibility that administered opioids may have antidepressant effects, or that opioid antagonists may worsen depression and lessen mania has been explored but several studies have failed to provide supporting evidence; there is, however, one study using a high dose of the opioid antagonist naloxone (Narcan) that suggests that its use may exacerbate depression.

Because both ACTH and β-endorphin are derived from pro-opiomelanocortin (POMC), under the regulation of CRF, changes in β-endorphin have been studied to examine the integrity of the HPA axis in depressed patients. β-endorphin has been measured in the plasma of depressed patients before and after dexamethasone challenge. Although not all studies agree, some have reported elevated levels of plasma β-endorphin in depressed patients, as well as the nonsuppression of the peptide following the administration of dexamethasone. But studies of CSF β-endorphin or total opioid binding in depressed patients have not shown the same changes.

As stated above, somatostatin (GHRIF) has been studied in patients with affective disorders as an indicator of growth hormone axis regulation. Somatostatin, however, is a neuromodulator with complex actions impinging on many other neurotransmitter systems. Because of its widespread actions, somatostatin has been thought to play a role in the behavioral, physiological, and endocrine changes in patients with affective disorders. At least three separate studies of CSF have shown decreases in somatostatin in patients with depression. This relationship, however, is complicated, as somatostatin levels are also related to sleep, which is frequently disturbed in depressed patients.

Arginine vasopressin (AVP) is known to be widely distributed throughout the central nervous system, where it functions as a neuromodulator and has complex behavioral effects. Animal studies have suggested that AVP's actions may be related to memory, rapid-eye-movement (REM) sleep, biological rhythms, and neuroendocrine function, all thought to be altered in patients with affective disorders. In one study, CSF AVP was significantly lower in depressed patients than in controls and was significantly higher in manic than in depressed patients. In a related study, when the vasopressin analogue 1-Desamino-8-D-arginine vasopressin (DDAVP) was given to four depressed patients, their cognitive function improved without a change in mood.

PSYCHOIMMUNOLOGY Some studies suggest that bereavement and depression can interfere with immunological competence. Bereaved men and women have a reduced in vitro lymphocyte response to mitogen stimulation, with normal levels of circulating immunoglobulins and normal responses on delayed hypersensitivity skin tests; the reduced lymphocyte response is most dramatic in bereaved patients with depressive symptoms. Severely depressed patients also have a reduced in vitro lymphocyte response to mitogen stimulation, a finding apparently unrelated to the hypercortisolemia often seen in these patients. Recent reports of other immunological changes in depressed patients include fewer circulating lymphocytes (especially in unipolar depressed patients), fewer natural-killer T-cell lymphocytes (which interact with virus-infected and tumor cells), and fewer T-suppressor cells (which regulate antibody production).

An explanation for some of these diverse immunological findings may lie in a high output of catecholamines, as well as an increased production of prostaglandins, each of which has been observed separately in studies of depressed patients. Catecholamines, acting through β-adrenergic receptors, are known to suppress the activity of human natural killer cells. Prostaglandins, functioning through a complex interaction between second messenger systems, may inhibit the in vitro mitogen-induced lymphocyte proliferation. And because recent animal work suggests that prostaglandin production is increased by catecholamines through a nonreceptor mediated mechanism, the diminished immunological competence reported in depressed patients may be a result of the dysregulation of the catecholaminergic system.

BEYOND THE CATECHOLAMINE HYPOTHESIS: TOWARD A BIOCHEMICAL CLASSIFICATION OF DEPRESSIVE DISORDERS

It is clear that the affective disorders are a heterogeneous group of conditions. The clinical subtyping of these disorders has been only partially successful in identifying homogeneous categories; even within categories (i.e., major depressive disorder), the natural history of the disorder may vary, as may the response to treatment. It is also generally recognized that the clinical categories do not necessarily represent distinct biologically homogeneous entities. For these reasons, many studies have examined various biochemical characteristics that might serve as independent variables for classifying subtypes of these disorders.

Studies of the biogenic amines have revealed important clues to the pathophysiology underlying this heterogeneity. For over 20 years, the catecholamine hypothesis of affective disorders proved to be a model of heuristic value. It gave both investigators and clinicians a frame of reference for understanding much of the available data about these disorders, and it stimulated new research on their biochemistry.

At present, the field seems to be in a new phase of development in which much new information is being accumulated, not all of which can be nicely fitted into any one theoretical framework. Intriguing clues across the biological variables have begun to appear. The process of norepinephrine-induced heterologous desensitization, if confirmed, may provide a useful link among some of these variables. But this work, like much of the new research, is still preliminary. Perhaps the best synthesis that can be offered now should emphasize two facts: the affective disorders are most likely a group of interrelated neuroendocrinometabolic disorders, and biochemical procedures will be required to subdivide and classify them.

THE EMERGING FIELD OF PSYCHIATRIC CHEMISTRY

The development of a biochemical classification of depressive disorders will require empirically derived clinical laboratory tests that document one or another aspect of the pathophysiology of these disorders. It seems highly unlikely, however, that there will be a truly comprehensive understanding of the etiology and pathophysiology of the depressive disorders until a parallel description of the functional neurochemistry and neurophysiology of the normal human brain becomes available. Studies using animal models to explore specific forms of behavior on the cellular and molecular levels document the feasibility of such an undertaking, but these studies also underscore how far off is the attainment of this goal. Thus, in the foreseeable future, psychiatric practice may be guided by the use of specialized clinical tests that the theory of psychiatry may not meaningfully integrate for many years. In this regard, however, psychiatrists are in a position quite similar to that of their colleagues in other medical specialties.

Recognizing this fact, over 10 years ago the Harvard Medical School Department of Psychiatry and the Department of Pathology of the New England Deaconess Hospital established a Psychiatric Chemistry Laboratory to serve as a model academic laboratory for the integration and translation of biochemical research into clinical psychiatric practice. Besides providing specialized clinical laboratory tests for psychiatry, an explicit aim of the Psychiatric Chemistry Laboratory has been to offer physicians educational and consultative services in the use and interpretation of these tests.

Finally, it may be useful to compare the pneumonias and the depressions. Both of these disorders are diagnosed on the basis of clinical data, and both are treated more effectively using information gleaned from clinical tests. In the case of pneumonias, the physician makes a diagnosis on the basis of history and physical examination (including a chest X-ray). Having made the diagnosis, sputum cultures can then help determine the specific type of pneumonia that the patient may have and the specific antibiotic or other forms of treatment that may be most effective, irrespective of why the pneumonia developed. Similarly, in the case of depressions, the physician diagnoses depression on the basis of clinical history coupled with physical and mental status examinations. Having made a diagnosis of depression, a physician can then use specialized clinical laboratory tests to help determine the type of depression the patient may have and the forms of treatment most likely to be effective.

Although the biochemical tests available today do not necessarily enable physicians to select a clinically effective treatment on the first trial, the use of these clinical laboratory tests can increase the probability of their doing so. Considering the time it takes for antidepressant drugs to have a clinical effect, even a small increase in the percentage of patients who receive an effective drug on the first clinical trial of treatment would represent a major advance in the treatment of patients with depressive disorders.

REFERENCES

APA Task Force on Laboratory Tests in Psychiatry: The dexamethasone suppression test: An overview of its current status in psychiatry. Amer J Psychiat *144:* 1253, 1987.

Calabrese, J R, Kling M A, Gold P W: Alterations in immunocompetence during stress, bereavement, and depression: Focus on neuroendocrine regulation. Amer J Psychiat *144:* 1123, 1987.

Carroll, B J: Dexamethasone suppression test: A review of contemporary confusion. J Clin Psychol *46:* 13, 1985.

Gold P W, Rubinow D R: Neuropeptide function in affective illness: Corticotropin-releasing hormone and somatostatin as model systems. In *Psychopharmacology: The Third Generation of Progress,* H Y Meltzer, editor, p 617. Raven Press, New York, 1987.

Golden R N, Markey S P, Risby E D, Rudorfer M V, Cowdry R W, Potter W Z: Antidepressants reduce whole-body norepinephrine turnover while enhancing 6-hydroxymelatonin output. Arch Gen Psychiat *45:* 150, 1988.

Green A I: Thyroid function and affective disorders. Hosp Comm Psychiat *35:* 1188, 1984.

Heninger G R, Charney D S: Mechanism of action of antidepressant treatments: Implications for the etiology and treatment of depressive disorders. In *Psychopharmacology: The Third Generation of Progress,* H Y Meltzer, editor, p 535. Raven Press, New York, 1987.

Janowsky D S, Khaled El-Yousef M, Davis J M, Sekerke H J: A cholinergic-adrenergic hypothesis of mania and depression. Lancet *2:* 632, 1972.

Janowsky D S, Risch S C: Role of acetylcholine mechanisms in the affective disorders. In *Psychopharmacology: The Third Generation of Progress,* H Y Meltzer, editor, p 527. Raven Press, New York, 1987.

Jimerson D C: Role of dopamine mechanisms in the affective disorders. In *Psychopharmacology: The Third Generation of Progress,* H Y Meltzer, editor, p 505. Raven Press, New York, 1987.

Krog-Meyer I, Kirkegaard C, Kijne B L: Prediction of relapse with the TRH test and prophylactic amitriptyline in 39 patients with endogenous depression. Amer J Psychiat *141:* 945, 1984.

Langer G, Koinig G, Hatzinger R, Schonbeck G, Resch F, Aschauer H, Keshavan M S, Sieghart W: Response of thyrotropin to thyrotropin-releasing hormone as predictor of treatment outcome. Arch Gen Psychiat *43:* 861, 1986.

Meltzer H Y, Lowy M T: The serotonin hypothesis of depression. In *Psychopharmacology: The Third Generation of Progress,* H Y Meltzer, editor, p 513. Raven Press, New York, 1987.

Miles A, Philbrick D R S: Melatonin and psychiatry. Biol Psychiat *23:* 405, 1988.

Mooney J J, Schatzberg A F, Cole J O, Kizuka P P, Salomon M, Lerbinger J, Pappalardo K M, Gerson B, Schildkraut J J: Rapid antidepressant response to alprazolam in depressed patients with high catecholamine output and heterologous desensitization of platelet adenylate cyclase. Biol Psychiat, *23:* 543, 1988.

Nemeroff C B, Bassette G: Neuropeptides in psychiatric disorders. In *American Handbook of Psychiatry,* ed 2, S Arieti, editor, vol 8, p 64. Basic Books, New York, 1986.

Post R M, Ballenger J C: *Neurobiology of Mood Disorders.* Williams & Wilkins, Baltimore, 1984.

Potter W Z, Rudorfer M V, Goodwin F K: Biological findings in bipolar disorders. In *Psychiatry Update, American Psychiatric Associates Annual Review,* R E Hales, A J Frances, editors, vol 6, p 32. American Psychiatric Press, Washington, DC, 1987.

Prange A J, Jr, Garbutt J C, Loosen P T: The hypothalamic-pituitary-thyroid axis in affective disorders. In *Psychopharmacology: The Third Generation in Progress,* H Y Meltzer, editor, p 629. Raven Press, New York, 1987.

Prange A J, Jr, Garbutt J C, Loosen P T, Bissette G, Nemeroff C B: The role of peptides in affective disorders: A review. In *Progress in Brain Research,* E R de Kloet, V M Wiegant, D de Wied, editors, vol 72, p 235. Elsevier, New York, 1987.

Samson J A, Gudeman J E, Schatzberg A F, Kizuka P P, Orsulak P J, Cole J O, Schildkraut J J: Toward a biochemical classification of depressive disorders. VIII: Platelet MAO activity and subtypes of depressions. J Psychiat Res *19:* 547, 1985.

Schatzberg A F, Orsulak P J, Rosenbaum A H, Maruta T, Kruger E R, Cole J O, Schildkraut J J: Toward a biochemical classification of depressive disorders. V: Heterogeneity of unipolar depressions. Amer J Psychiat *139:* 471, 1982.
Schatzberg A F, Rothschild A J, Gerson B, Lerbinger J E, Schildkraut J J: Toward a biochemical classification of depressive disorders. IX: DST results and platelet MAO activity in depressed patients. Brit J Psychiat *146:* 633, 1985.
Schatzberg A F, Rothschild A J, Langlais P J, Bird E D, Cole J O: A corticosteroid/dopamine hypothesis of psychotic depression and related states. J Psychiat Res *19:* 57, 1985.
Schatzberg A F, Samson J A, Bloomingdale K L, Orsulak P J, Gerson B, Kizuka P P, Cole J O, Schildkraut J J: Toward a biochemical classification of depressive disorders. X: Urinary catecholamines, their metabolites and D-type scores in subgroups of depressive disorders. Arch Gen Psychiat, 1989.
Schildkraut J J: The catecholamine hypothesis of affective disorders: A review of supporting evidence. Amer J Psychiat *122:* 509, 1965.
Schildkraut J J, Orsulak P J, LaBrie R A, Schatzberg A F, Gudeman J E, Cole J O, Rohde W A: Toward a biochemical classification of depressive disorders. II: Application of multivariate discriminant function analysis to data on urinary catecholamines and metabolites. Arch Gen Psychiat *35:* 1436, 1978.
Schildkraut J J, Orsulak P J, Schatzberg A F, Gudeman J E, Cole J O, Rohde W A, LaBrie R A: Toward a biochemical classification of depressive disorders. I: Differences in urinary MHPG and other catecholamine metabolites in clinically defined subtypes of depressions. Arch Gen Psychiat *35:* 1427, 1978.
Siever L J: Role of noradrenergic mechanisms in the etiology of the affective disorders. In *Psychopharmacology: The Third Generation of Progress,* H Y Meltzer, editor, p 493. Raven Press, New York, 1987.
Stokes P E, Sikes C R: Hypothalamic-pituitary-adrenal axis in affective disorders. In *Psychopharmacology: The Third Generation of Progress,* H Y Meltzer, editor, p 589. Raven Press, New York, 1987.

17.2b MOOD DISORDERS: GENETIC ASPECTS

ELLIOT S. GERSHON, M.D.
WADE H. BERRETTINI, M.D., Ph.D
LYNN R. GOLDIN, Ph.D.

INTRODUCTION

The well-known advances in molecular genetics have lent new importance to the evidence that the mood disorders are genetically transmitted, raising the hope that vulnerable individuals and rational and definitive treatments may be identified, based on the discovery of specific genetic deficits. At the same time, epidemiological evidence points to a secular increase in mood disorders in recent decades that interacts with familial vulnerability, but also must include major nongenetic causative factors.

EVIDENCE REGARDING GENETIC TRANSMISSION

Twin and adoption studies show whether vulnerability to a disorder has a genetic component, meaning that a genetic variation in a population renders some persons more susceptible than others. Family studies indicate in a particular population the degree to which a disorder is familial, which diagnostic entities or other characteristics share familial transmission with a particular disorder, and perhaps, most importantly, allow the testing of hypotheses regarding the mode of genetic transmission, such as whether one gene or many are acting. When biological variables are studied, their validity as genetic markers or inherited risk factors can be tested in families.

ADOPTION STUDIES

A 1977 study of bipolar adoptees found that a mood disorder (including spectrum disorder) was found in 31 percent of the biological parents of these probands, compared with 2 percent in the biological parents of normal adoptees. The morbid risk of a mood disorder in biological parents of bipolar patients was comparable to the risk that the investigators found in the parents of nonadopted bipolars (26 percent). The risk of mood disorder was also higher in the biological parents of bipolar patients than it was in the adoptive parents of bipolar adoptees or normal adoptees (12 percent and 9 percent, respectively).

In Denmark, the suicide rate among the biological relatives of 71 adoptees with mood disorders was disproportionately high (15 of 381, or 3.9 percent) compared with the rate among adoptive relatives of those probands (1 of 168, or 0.6 percent) or among the biological or adoptive relatives of control adoptees (1 of 353, or 0.3 percent, and 1 of 166, or 0.6 percent, respectively). Major mood disorders (bipolar, unipolar, and uncertain major mood disorders) were diagnosed significantly more frequently in biological relatives of mood-disordered adoptees than in the relatives of control adoptees, but milder depressions (neurotic depression [dysthymia]) did not occur more frequently. Nonpsychiatric suicide, defined as suicide with no preceding psychiatric hospitalization, also appeared to be genetically transmitted. It is not clear from the published data whether this entity is independent of mood disorders.

In 1983, an adoption study from Sweden that included 56 probands with mood disorders and matched adopted and nonadopted controls found no concordance of psychopathology between biological parents and adoptees, with the possible exception of more mood disorders in the biological mothers of female adoptees with a mood disorder. This study may have underreported diagnoses, however. Suicide, the key outcome variable in the Danish study, could have been entirely missed in the Swedish study. Untreated psychiatric disorders and disorders treated privately or under a nonpsychiatric guise could have been missed, as the subjects were not examined. Nonetheless, this and the Danish study do cast some doubt on the genetic transmissibility of very broadly defined nonbipolar major depression.

Further adoption studies in mood disorders might be useful. But it appears that the crucial contributions to genetic progress can be expected not from adoption studies, but from studies on the mechanisms of transmission, including segregation analyses, linkage studies, and studies of inherited risk factors.

TWIN STUDIES

The clear difference between monozygotic (about 67 percent) and dizygotic (about 15 percent) concordance in numerous twin studies of mood disorder over a 50-year period argues strongly for the heritability of mood disorders. Twelve cases of monozygotic twins raised apart in which at least one twin had a mood disorder were reviewed, and eight pairs (67 percent) were found to be concordant. Although this finding is quite similar to those for monozygotic twins raised together, one must note the studies did not systematically sample twins raised apart.

A 1979 study used the Danish twin register, which includes all same-sex twins born from 1870 to 1920. Questionnaires were sent to twins or, if the twins had died, to their relatives and was followed up with a personal interview if necessary. Zygosity was checked either serologically or, if both twins were not living, anthropometrically. It was possible to identify 110 twin pairs in which one or both members had manic-depressive illness (using the Kraepelinian criteria). The concordance for monozygotic twins (58 pairs) was 0.67 and for dizygotic twins (52 pairs) was 0.20. This concordance closely agrees with the data previously summarized. The concordance was higher for bipolar monozygotic probands (0.79) than for unipolar monozygotic probands (0.54). Dizygotic rates were similar (0.24 for bipolar and 0.19 for unipolar).

Further analysis of concordant pairs for polarity revealed 11 unipolar pairs, 14 bipolar-bipolar pairs, and 7 unipolar-bipolar pairs. This result suggests some genetic specificity for polarity, but also that unipolar and bipolar illness can be associated with the same genetic makeup. These data clearly demonstrate the inherent ambiguity in biological comparisons of bipolar versus unipolar patients. At the very least, a substantial portion of the unipolar patients have the same genetic and biological vulnerability as do the bipolar patients.

FAMILY STUDIES

A familial concentration of mood disorders has been shown in recent case-controlled studies. Relatives of bipolar and unipolar patients have higher prevalence of bipolar and unipolar disorder than the relatives of controls. Major depression (unipolar disorder) is the most common mood disorder in families of both unipolar and bipolar patients; this frequency implies overlap in the familial causes of both forms of disorder. The same implication is also present in the twin data in a smaller number of individuals at risk.

There is an inconsistency in the reported prevalences in relatives in the family studies, which necessitates a methodological digression on family studies. The inconsistency is present even in studies with explicit diagnostic criteria and direct examination of relatives. Some of the discrepancies are undoubtedly due to differences in procedures and criteria, as well as to population differences; yet, could the inconsistencies also reflect a basically unreliable methodology? In collaborative studies, good reliability between centers can be established, and very similar prevalences in relatives can be found. In studies that had good reliability and used similar procedures, cognitive or cultural factors were shown to lead to differences in diagnostic rates in family studies. Urban setting, younger generation, and possibly American nationality are associated with higher diagnostic rates for unipolar disorder.

The fact that cognitive or cultural factors appear to be a general aspect of morbid risk estimates has several implications. The authors believe that there is not a true rate of diagnosable mood disorder in the population or in relatives of patients. The rates may be a function of procedures and criteria, of the culture of the population in which they are observed, and of genetic factors. But if all these variables are held constant, in carefully performed studies, the more broadly one defines depression, the less inherited it appears to be. This conclusion was noted in the adoption data discussed above and was also demonstrated in the authors' family studies. The authors' studies found that nonfamilial depression (i.e., depression when it occurs in relatives of normal controls) most commonly satisfies only the minimal number of the revised third edition of the *Diagnostic and Statistical Manual of Mental Disorders* (DSM-III-R) criteria for major depression, with no significant impairment in the individual's major life role, whereas depressions in relatives of mood-disordered patients tend to have such an impairment and to be recurrent.

A cohort effect has been observed in mood disorders: People born in the decades starting approximately in 1940 have a higher lifetime prevalence of mood disorders and suicide than people born earlier. This effect has been seen in mania and depression, in epidemiological studies, and in studies of families of mood-disordered patients. The greatest increase in suicide is in the younger age groups, particularly between ages 15 and 24. It is not seen in schizophrenia.

In the authors' data, the age at onset for bipolar and schizoaffective disorders has become younger, and the total lifetime prevalence appears likely to be much higher, in the cohorts born after 1940. This finding cannot be due to genetic change over such a short period, nor to selective effects on reproductive fitness. It must reflect, then, another cultural influence (in the broadest sense of culture, as the entire environmental and biological setting) on the incidence of mood disorders. Whatever the cause, it interacts with familial vulnerability, as the rate remains elevated in relatives of patients.

The question of which cultural influences are causing this increase in mood disorders and suicide has not yet been determined. Recent data suggest that substance abuse is associated with half the young suicides in San Diego; the substances abused include alcohol, cocaine, amphetamines, and marijuana. The greater use of these substances, and possibly tobacco—whose use also increased over the same period—may contribute as well to the birth cohort–related increases in mood disorders.

FAMILIAL COTRANSMISSION OF MOOD DISORDERS

In the authors' own data, in a metropolitan American setting, the lifetime prevalences of mood disorders in first-degree relatives of normal controls, unipolars, bipolars, and schizoaffectives, were 7 percent, 20 percent, 25 percent, and 37 percent, respectively. These data show that the mood disorders are fairly common and that they are concentrated to a great extent in a few families.

There appears to be considerable overlap between unipolar and bipolar illness within families, particularly in the major studies published since 1980. The relatives of bipolar patients are likely to have a bipolar disorder and are even more likely to have unipolar disorder. The relatives of unipolar patients have even more unipolar disorder than the relatives of bipolars, and also a modest but consistent increase in bipolar illness when compared with the rates of relatives of normals. The authors' own data are representative: The relatives of bipolars had lifetime prevalences of 8 percent bipolar and 14.9 percent unipolar disorder; the relatives of unipolars had 2.9 percent bipolar and 16.6 percent unipolar; and the relatives of normal controls had 0.5 percent bipolar and 5.8 percent unipolar. These data, like the twin data, suggest a genetic overlap between the two forms of mood disorder.

The clinical spectrum of mood disorders can be constructed by comparing the prevalence of illness in patients' relatives with the prevalence in controls' relatives.

SCHIZOAFFECTIVE DISORDER Schizoaffective disorder is the diagnosis for patients with episodic, as opposed to chronic, periods of schizophreniform psychosis along with mood disorder symptoms, and for patients with some episodes that appear schizophrenic and others that appear mood disordered, again episodic over the lifetime. Most studies of first-degree relatives of patients with schizoaffective illness have shown more mood disorders, particularly bipolar illness, and (to a lesser extent) schizophrenia than schizoaffective illness. The authors and colleagues found that, among 84 first-degree relatives of schizoaffective probands, the morbid risk is 6.1 percent for schizoaffective disorder, 10.7 percent for bipolar I disorder, 6.1 percent for bipolar II, 14.5 percent for unipolar, and 3.6 percent for schizophrenia.

Although schizoaffective probands tend to have a high frequency of mood disorder in relatives and a low incidence of schizoaffective illness, the twin studies present a very different picture. In a 1975 review, 13 out of 44 monozygotic twins, versus 1 out of 45 same-sex dizygotic twins, were concordant for type of illness. This definition included as concordant those persons with reactive schizophreniform psychosis and those with schizoaffective psychosis. Although the twin studies show that the same form of psychosis appears to be genetically transmitted, this fact does not appear to be true in the family studies.

When the monozygotic twin concordance appears so much greater than the concordance among first-degree relatives, the data may be reflecting a complex form of inheritance. The phenomenon may be produced by interaction among several loci in such a way that there is a much greater concordance in monozygotic twins, as compared with the concordance in dizygotic twin and other first-degree relatives. This concordance is produced because monozygotic twins will be identical by descent at all loci, but the chances, for example, of two siblings' being identical by descent at a given locus are one-half. The probability of being identical by descent at n loci is therefore 0.5^n, which becomes an exceedingly small number as the number of loci involved rises. An example of this type of inheritance can be found in the visual evoked response.

As applied to schizoaffective disorder, this speculation suggests specific genetic factors that cause the psychosis to have a schizoaffective expression, as there is high twin concordance. These factors, in turn, appear to be superimposed on the genetic diathesis for mood disorders, as they are consistently the most frequently found in relatives of schizoaffective patients.

ALCOHOLISM There has been disagreement in the literature as to whether alcoholism tends to concentrate in the families of persons with a mood disorder. This controversy may be resolved by studying mood-disordered probands who have no alcoholic difficulties themselves.

The authors' own and other current data show no increase in alcoholism in the relatives of nonalcoholic, mood-disordered probands, compared with the relatives of controls. Although bipolar illness and alcoholism are not uncommonly found in the same person, alcoholism by itself without mood disorder does not appear to belong in the genetic spectrum of bipolar manic-depressive illness.

ANOREXIA NERVOSA A 1977 family history study of anorectic patients found that an excess of mood disorder was present in relatives, a discovery that has been repeatedly corroborated. In a study of 25 anorectic women and 192 of their first- and second-degree relatives, a group of 25 age-matched women with no history of anorexia or depression were used as controls. Of the relatives of the anorectic women, 17.7 percent had unipolar illness, and 4.7 percent had bipolar illness (not age corrected). The corresponding figures for controls' relatives were 9.2 percent and 0.6 percent. The difference in the total incidence of mood disorder was significant, suggesting a genetic relationship between the two disorders.

The authors and their colleagues have also found a modest amount of anorexia nervosa in relatives of anorectic patients (2.0 percent) and as much mood disorder as in relatives of bipolars (8.3 percent bipolar and 13.3 percent unipolar). In relatives of bipolars, however, there is very little anorexia nervosa (0.6 percent). It appears that anorexia nervosa has a unique familial vulnerability factor, possibly genetic, that is superimposed on a genetic tendency toward bipolar and unipolar mood disorder. This tendency appears to be even less common than the similar tendency toward schizoaffective disorder.

CHILDHOOD DEPRESSION It is generally agreed now that mood disorders, particularly bipolar disorder, can begin in adolescence. There is a greater prevalence of mood disorders among adult relatives of adolescent mood-disordered patients, as one would expect if the adult and adolescent forms share the same basis. Mania and severe (hospitalized) depression are also now acknowledged to exist in the prepubertal years and to be related to the adult forms of mood disorders. However, there are reasons to question whether the milder depressive syndromes observed in childhood are associated with the familial adult mood disorders. The current number of published controlled family studies is small and does not allow unambiguous conclusions regarding two crucial questions: whether children of mood-disordered patients are at an increased risk of depression in childhood, and whether childhood depression in the offspring of mood-disordered patients predicts adult major depression.

CYCLOTHYMIA The evidence from family studies suggests that cyclothymia and mild hypomania may be related to bipolar mood disorder.

MODE OF GENETIC TRANSMISSION

The multifactorial transmission of a genetic disease can be modeled as a linear combination of genetic and environmental factors (liability factors), each having a small effect. There can be one or more thresholds on a hypothesized liability scale that determine whether an individual expresses a particular trait (illness). This multifactorial approach has a polygenic component (i.e., many genes), with random or familial environmental variation. The models will predict the prevalence rates in various classes of relatives of ill persons and can be compared with observed prevalences.

In some studies, the prevalences of the mood-disorder diagnoses in relatives of patients with mood disorders are consistent with a multifactorial liability, with two thresholds corresponding to the severity of illness (risk in relatives of unipolar patients $<$ risk in relatives of bipolar patients). Thus, the degree of genetic transmission is related to the severity of illness as modeled on a continuous liability scale. The biological implications of this multifactorial model are that the bipolar vulnerability includes all of the unipolar genetic vulnerability, plus other factors that may be genetic or environmental. However, although multifactorial transmission appeared to fit several data sets before the recognition of the cohort effect, the fit worsens and the model is rejected in the few analyses that have taken this into account.

Segregation analysis has long been used in the study of genetic diseases to determine whether the distribution of an illness in families corresponded to some Mendelian mode of transmission. Diseases could be shown to be dominant, recessive, or sex linked. Many common diseases, a class to which psychiatric disorders belong by virtue of population prevalence > 1 percent, are known to be familial but do not appear to conform to simple Mendelian models. But methods have been developed to test Mendelian hypotheses regarding such disorders, allowing for reduced penetrance (i.e., not all persons having a susceptible genotype will develop the illness) and the probability of being ill depending on age or sex. This method of segregation analysis has allowed the testing of genetic hypotheses of the transmission of mood disorders in families. These studies have generally rejected single-locus transmission in families of both unipolar and bipolar patients. The fact that multifactorial models are consistent with some studies and that single-locus models are usually rejected does not necessarily rule out single-locus inheritance. The power of these methods to detect major loci in complex diseases may be low. Simulation studies have shown that a single locus for a disease could not be identified for certain modes of inheritance, especially "quasi-recessive" inheritance, in which the heterozygote individuals have low, but not zero, penetrance. If mood disorders are genetically heterogeneous, the detection of single genetic mechanisms will be difficult using the current methods. Thus, the possibility that there are major loci causing vulnerability to these disorders cannot be ruled out. A single-gene effect may not be detectable from pedigree data unless a closely linked marker locus is studied. The historical example of diabetes mellitus—long thought of as a classical multifactorial disorder, but recently discovered to have two forms with single-locus determinants—should be borne in mind.

ASSOCIATION, LINKAGE, AND BIOLOGICAL VULNERABILITY

Two strategies can be used to identify specific genetic components causing susceptibility to an illness that avoid some of the uncertainties of studying clinical diagnoses. The first is to identify a biological trait that is correlated with susceptibility to a particular illness (e.g., an enzyme, neurotransmitter, receptor protein, or membrane transport characteristic). If a variant of such a trait can be shown to be associated with an illness in a population and to be genetically transmitted with the illness in families, then the trait represents a specific genetic susceptibility component (though other genetic and environmental components may exist). The second strategy is to study the linkage or association relationships of known polymorphic genetic loci (such as ABO blood types) to these illnesses, both at the population level and within families of affected individuals. Various statistical methods are available to analyze these relationships in order to detect loci that are either directly or indirectly involved in disease susceptibility.

Both of these strategies are important for identifying genetic susceptibility components. The first strategy identifies traits whose underlying genetics are usually unknown; whereas the second strategy identifies traits determined by single loci.

ASSOCIATION STUDIES Studies of patients having both common and rare diseases have revealed associations with genetic marker phenotypes. For example, the blood group O has been consistently shown to be associated with an increased risk for duodenal ulcers. Specific human lymphocyte antigen (HLA) types have been found to be associated with a variety of diseases such as ankylosing spondylitis, juvenile diabetes, and multiple sclerosis. These associations can be explained in several ways. First, the association could be an artifact of population stratification. For example, a particular antigen could have a higher frequency in a diseased population because these individuals come from a racial or ethnic group with a higher frequency of the antigen. Stratification can be controlled during population sampling, but not all heterogeneity is obvious. For instance, there is known to be significant geographical variation in the frequencies of HLA antigens that may not always correlate with ethnicity. However, assuming that the association found is not an artifact, then other explanations are possible. The marker trait itself may play a role in the disease even if other genetic and environmental components are involved. This is likely to be the case in ankylosing spondylitis, in which 90 percent of patients have HLA B27 and only 10 percent of control individuals have this antigen. Alternatively, another gene close in distance to the marker trait on the chromosome (i.e., linked) may cause susceptibility. Generally, if two loci are chromosomally linked, there will be no association of alleles at these loci because recombination randomizes the allele combinations. But, there may be disequilibrium at two loci because of the natural selection for some allelic combinations, a recent admixture of populations, or a chance genetic drift, which leads to an association. Disequilibrium is known to exist among the loci of the HLA region, although the reason for its existence is unknown. Thus, for diseases associated with HLA antigens, the primary association may be with some unknown locus that is closely linked to the HLA region. Whatever the reason for an association between a disease and a marker locus, it is an important finding because it identifies a chromosomal region that contributes to illness susceptibility and provides an etiological hypothesis that can be tested using other strategies.

LINKAGE STUDIES Loci that are situated close together on the same chromosome are not transmitted independently and are said to be linked. In human genetics, linkage analysis has been used to determine whether a locus for a disease is linked to some known genetic marker locus. In the case of psychiatric disorders, single-disease loci have not been identified. However, simulation studies have shown that segregation analysis has only limited power to detect a major locus in many situations. Thus, it is still possible that genes playing a large role in susceptibility are segregating in some families. The existence of loci with major effects can be confirmed by finding a linkage to a marker locus.

The marker loci that have been most commonly used are the red cell antigens, HLA antigens, red cell and serum enzyme electrophoretic variants, and banding pattern variants on chromosomes. Until recently, the main limitation of linkage studies was that there were only a limited number of marker loci (about 30) that could be easily used. For 30 markers, the prior probability that one of them will be linked to a disease locus with a 20 percent or less recombination is about 30 percent.

It has also been possible to identify genetic variants of proteins by means of two-dimensional electrophoresis proteins from various tissues. This technique allows many (30 to 50) loci to be identified in a single gel. Most of the loci, however, are two-allele polymorphisms that are often not informative in some families. With the advent of new molecular genetic techniques that allow polymorphisms in deoxyribonucleic acid (DNA) sequences to be detected, the number of loci that can be used as marker traits is constantly expanding. As will be discussed later, these techniques will greatly increase the power of linkage methods by increasing the prior probability of linkage to nearly 100 percent.

The classic method of detecting linkage is to determine whether the phenotypes at two loci are transmitted together in families. Assuming that the mode of transmission (gene frequencies and genotype penetrances) is known for each locus, one compares the probability of observing the segregation of the two traits in a family if there is a linkage with the probability of observing the segregation pattern if there is no linkage. The probability of a linkage is expressed as a function of the recombination fraction (θ), where θ is some value between 0 and 0.5. The probability of no linkage is the probability that the two loci are segregating independently (i.e., $\theta = 0.5$). This odds ratio is expressed by a statistic called the lod score (or the log of the odds ratio) and is defined as follows:

$$\text{lod score} = \log_{10} \left(\frac{\text{probability of observing a family given } \theta < 1/2}{\text{probability of observing a family given } \theta = 1/2} \right)$$

A lod score of 1.0 means that a linkage is 10 times more likely than no linkage. The lod scores for small families can be calculated by hand or by using published tables in simple cases. If the data consist of larger or multigenerational geneologies or it is necessary to allow for more complicated genetic parameters (such as reduced penetrance, age of onset, and quantitative traits), computer programs are available to calculate the lod scores. Because the lod scores are in log 10 units, the scores can be summed across families. If the linkage is true, the best estimate of θ will be that value of θ that maximizes the lod score. It was originally proposed that a lod score of 3.0 should be the cutoff for accepting the linkage hypothesis, and –2.0 should be the cutoff point for rejecting linkage. This convention has generally been followed in linkage studies, although investigators do not usually stop sampling families when they reach a lod score of 3.0, as more data will allow accurate estimates of θ to be made and tests of heterogeneity to be carried out. It also must be stressed that 3.0 is considered the cutoff value for confirming linkages between two Mendelian loci and that for more complex diseases, this criterion may not be sufficient. The mode of inheritance is not known for psychiatric disorders. In practice, lod scores are calculated according to several different assumptions about the parameters of the presumed disease susceptibility locus. Genetic heterogeneity decreases the power of linkage analysis, as in some families the disease gene will not be linked to the marker locus. There are several methods available for testing heterogeneity. A reasonable approach is to assume that families are either linked or unlinked and then simultaneously estimate the recombination fraction and the proportion of families in the sample that are linked.

Linkage can also be tested from data on affected pairs of siblings. These methods are derived from the sib-pair method, which was based on looking at the concordance of illness and marker phenotypes in pairs of siblings. Current methods use affected sib pairs only and are based on the assumption that if a disease is linked to a marker locus, the affected sib pairs will have the same phenotype at the marker locus more often than expected by chance. The major advantages of the affected sib-pair method are that no assumptions about the mode of the illness's transmission are required and there is no loss of power because of decreased penetrance. This method was developed mainly to detect linkage to the HLA loci which are highly polymorphic. Because two unrelated parents are unlikely to share the same HLA alleles (haplotypes), it is usually possible to determine whether affected sib pairs share exactly two, one, or zero haplotypes at the marker locus. If there is no linkage, then the proportion of affected sib pairs sharing two, one, and zero haplotypes will be one-quarter, one-half, and one-quarter, respectively. If there is a linkage, then this distribution will be skewed so that more than 25 percent of the sib pairs will have two identical haplotypes. The simple hypothesis of linkage can be tested by comparing the observed haplotype-sharing distribution with the expected distribution if there is no linkage. From the observed distribution, inferences can also be made about the mode of inheritance and about the recombination fraction. Methods have also been developed to analyze families with more than two affected sibs. The affected sib-pair method is most appropriate for markers like HLA that have a high degree of polymorphism. Other, less polymorphic markers can be used, but a much larger sample size would be needed to detect a deviation of the observed distribution from random expectations.

The choice of linkage methods depends on several factors, such as the type of data most obtainable (e.g., families or sib pairs), the degree of polymorphism at the marker loci of interest, and knowledge of the disease's mode of inheritance.

NEW STRATEGIES USING MOLECULAR GENETICS The development of powerful methods of molecular genetics has revolutionized the study of human genetic diseases. These breakthroughs are a result of the discovery of restriction endonucleases, the development of methods for cloning genes, and the detection of fragments of DNA separated by gel electrophoresis and by southern blotting, followed by hybridization with cloned DNA sequences. Variations in DNA sequences (called restriction fragment length polymorphisms [RFLPs]) can thus be identified using these techniques. These methods were first applied to human research when it was discovered that a RFLP in the β-globin gene could predict a person's genotype for sickle cell anemia and thus be used for genetic counseling. In the last few years, genes coding for proteins such as insulin, growth hormone, coagulation factor VIII, and various neuropeptides have been cloned and applied to human genetic research. It was also found that arbitrary DNA sequences could be cloned and used to identify RFLPs, and thus numerous markers for the human genome are being generated. As of the Eighth International Human Gene Mapping Workshop in 1985, a total of 808 DNA clones had been mapped to the human genome, of which 249 represent cloned genes and 559 represent arbitrary genes; 333 out of 808 are known to be polymorphic. It has been estimated that 150 evenly spaced polymorphisms would cover the genome, so that any unknown locus would be no farther than 10 percent recombination units from a marker locus. Thus, in a fairly short period of time, enough polymorphisms are expected to be discovered so that the whole genome will be covered by genetic marker loci. This is a large advance over the classic protein and red cell polymorphisms.

ASSOCIATION AND LINKAGE STUDIES OF MOOD DISORDERS

ASSOCIATION STUDIES Several studies have reported the frequencies of ABO blood types in patients with mood disorders (or subgroups of patients), as compared with control populations. A few studies found a higher frequency of blood type 0 in manic-depressive patients than in controls, but other studies have not. Some studies detected no differences between patients and controls. Some of the significant results may be caused by skewed patient population samples. One study found that the entire population of psychiatric patients had ABO frequencies different from those of the control population and that manic-depressive patients were not different from other psychiatric patients. This finding demonstrates the potential effect of population stratification on association studies and emphasizes that associations must be consistently found in multiple studies before conclusions can be made.

There have been many studies of HLA antigens in patients with mood disorders. Although one early study found a higher frequency of HLA BW16 in patients than in controls, subsequent studies could not replicate this finding. No other HLA types have been consistently associated with mood disorders.

Recent studies have looked for associations of RFLPs in genes of neurobiological interest. One study examined the distribution of RFLPs of the pro-opiomelanocortin (POMC) gene in psychiatric patients and controls. But there was no association of this locus with mood disorders. Another study found no association of RFLPs in the somatostatin or NPY gene with mood disorders. It has been hypothesized that major psychoses are caused by retroviral integration into an individual's genome. However, an experiment designed to test this hypothesis revealed that neither bipolar nor schizophrenic patients differed from controls in their pattern of restriction fragments to a retroviral sequence probe. The study of brain-relevant probes in psychiatric disorders is exciting and will be pursued in the future.

LINKAGE STUDIES In the late 1960s and 1970s, a linkage was reported of bipolar mood disorders to markers on the X chromosome, including color blindness (CB), G6PD, and Xg blood group. Although CB and G6PD are closely linked, Xg is in an entirely different region. Linkage to both regions would thus be incompatible. Other studies did not find a linkage to any X chromosome marker loci. It has been argued that, based on a reanalysis of all the published X-chromosome data incorporating age of onset, there is a heterogeneity of mood disorders in bipolar families and that mood disorders in a significant proportion of these families are linked to the CB-G6PD region of the X chromosome. This analysis did not indicate a linkage to the Xg locus. This conclusion is somewhat controversial. Many families cannot be tested for X linkage because they are not informative for either the CB or the G6PD polymorphism. Recently, additional families have been found to be linked to CB, G6PD, and the Factor IX loci. However, with many new DNA polymorphisms that are available in this region of the X chromosome, all bipolar families will be informative for X linkage, and the heterogeneity hypothesis can be more rigorously tested.

A few studies have examined possible linkages to autosomal markers, such as red cell antigens and serum proteins. No positive or consistent linkages have been found for either unipolar or bipolar disorder. Some investigators have hypothesized that mood disorders are linked to the HLA region in some families. Some of these positive studies are methodologically flawed, however, and the majority of studies do not support linkage to HLA.

Recently, linkage studies of mood disorders have focused on the molecular genetic study of RFLPs. One small study indicated no linkage of mood disorders to either the somatostatin or the NPY loci. A study of a large pedigree in the Amish population revealed strong evidence for the linkage of mood disorders to markers on the short arm of chromosome 11, insulin, and the harvey-ras oncogene. Most of the ill individuals in this pedigree had bipolar illness, and the transmission of the illness was consistent with a highly penetrant dominant gene. This is an exciting finding but needs further replication in other populations. So far, a few other, smaller families have not been found to be linked. But, if this represents a rare form of mood disorder, then it may be necessary to study many more families.

Several strategies can be used to find genes for disorders like mood disorders using linkage methods. It is theoretically possible to screen the entire genome for linkage, using random DNA probes in the appropriate locations. This may seem like an inordinate amount of work, but the number of markers needed is finite (150 to 200). There is an advantage in studying pedigrees from population isolates, such as the Amish, because they are genetically homogeneous; that is, the ill individuals are likely to be segregating for the same susceptibility genes. Unfortunately, such pedigrees are rare, but it may be possible to detect linkage with a larger sample of moderate-sized pedigrees because of improvements in both laboratory and statistical methodology. It has been shown that linkage methods are more efficient when multiple closely linked marker loci are available and analyzed simultaneously. As more RFLPs are mapped to the human genome, it will be possible to examine the linkage of a susceptibility locus to a whole series of closely linked marker loci whose map positions are known. The effort to screen the entire genome is likely to decrease in the future with advances in laboratory techniques. Thus, even if it were possible to detect only very close linkages to diseases like mood disorders, it might be profitable to score the large number of loci needed to cover the genome. Another strategy is to screen candidate probes (i.e., probes of genes relevant to the brain). Although many genes of interest have been cloned, there are also many possibly relevant genes. Clearly, it is of interest to look for a linkage and association with such genes, and thus, both approaches will be used to find specific genetic causes of mood disorders.

Given the practical limitations in studying families with mood disorders, the affected sib-pair method offers another approach to detecting linkage. As mentioned earlier, this method is informative only for highly polymorphic loci, but there are likely to be many RFLPs or combinations of closely linked, highly polymorphic RFLPs. The affected sib-pair method is best for rare, recessive susceptibility genes. If the locus for mood disorders is dominant or intermediate, then a close linkage (i.e., $\theta < .1$) can be detected by this method with reasonable power (80 percent) in a sample size of about 80 pairs if there is heterogeneity (i.e., if up to 50 percent of pairs had a different susceptibility gene unlinked to the marker locus). This sample size is relatively large but could be obtained in a collaborative study.

Using the new molecular genetic technology to detect a gene for mood disorders is in its infancy. But, now that the techniques are available, it seems reasonable for researchers to use a combination of strategies for applying molecular genetic techniques to this illness, including studies of unrelated patients and controls, families or larger pedigrees, and affected sib pairs. If a major gene for mood disorders exists, it may be found in the foreseeable future.

BIOLOGICAL VULNERABILITY TRAITS

INVESTIGATIVE STRATEGIES A number of studies have attempted to identify biological factors that are inherited in mood disorders. Ideally, an inherited biological factor would be a variant (such as an altered protein) that could be assigned a specific locus on an identifiable chromosome. Because stable biochemical differences may suggest genetic variation, however, virtually any stable biological finding that is clearly associated with the tendency toward mood disorder may be studied as a possible genetic trait, even if the association is limited to a subgroup of patients. The converse approach is also valid: Genetic strategies may be used to demonstrate the validity of a particular biological component of the mood disorders, even without an established mechanism of genetic transmission. The criteria for establishing a genetic vulnerability marker for mood disorders are

1. The marker (either quantitative or qualitative) must be associated with a greater likelihood of the psychiatric illness. Not every individual with the illness must show the characteristic, because the illness may have a biological heterogeneity.
2. The marker must be heritable in general and, as observed, must not be a secondary effect of the illness.
3. The marker must be demonstrable in the well state, so that it is possible to determine its presence independently of the illness and to evaluate well relatives.
4. The illness should be associated with the marker within pedigrees. Because the twin and family data strongly suggest that some persons with a genetic vulnerability to mood disorders will be phenotypically well, some well relatives will not show the marker. If the marker is necessary for the illness, frank illness would not be transmitted without the marker, except for sporadic cases. If, in a pedigree, some ill persons show the marker and other ill subjects do not, then the illness can be transmitted without the marker. If the finding is more common only in ill relatives, it may be a contributing factor, but not a necessary (primary) factor.

An alternative strategy has been proposed as the biochemical high-risk paradigm. Here, a large population sample is studied, on a quantitative measure for a putative biochemical marker. Persons at low and high extremes of the measurement are compared for family history of psychiatric illness. If the marker is valid, a family history of illness will cluster at one extreme. This strategy, however, is less robust than the pedigree strategy detailed above, because it will lose power if there is biological heterogeneity in the illness.

Phenomena that are demonstrable only in the presence of active illness have limited usefulness in the genetic investigation of an illness with incomplete penetrance. For example, if a urinary metabolite is decreased or if cortisol is increased only during episodes of illness, it will be impossible to determine whether well relatives or controls will have the same finding. State-dependent phenomena can be studied, however, to see whether they are associated with familial mood disorder or whether they can predict increased morbid risk in relatives.

FINDINGS

These studies of the criteria for genetic vulnerability markers delineated above are summarized in Table 17.2b-1.

The lithium erythrocyte–plasma ratio may be a vulnerability marker for mood disorders, but definitive family studies are needed to determine whether a high lithium ratio segregates with illness of pedigrees of mood disorder. Although cerebrospinal fluid 5-hydroxyindoleacetic (CSF 5-HIAA) may be lower in a subgroup of patients with a mood disorder (even during remission), recent data indicate that this variable is not heritable. Another marker of serotonergic function, platelet imipramine binding, is lower in acutely depressed patients, according to several studies. However, the decreased binding normalizes at some point after the clinical recovery is complete, indicating that it is state dependent, as opposed to a trait marker for vulnerability to mood disorders. Plasma γ-aminobutyric acid (GABA) is somewhat lower in acutely ill and recovered patients and may be heritable, but family studies are lacking. Given the relatively small differences between recovered patients and controls, it is not likely that this biochemical characteristic will be promising. CSF GABA, which is lower in acutely depressed patients, normalizes after recovery, suggesting that it is a state-dependent marker. β-Adrenergic receptors on cultured lymphoblasts may be decreased in manic depressive subjects and their ill relatives, implying that this could be a trait marker, but recently published conflicting data cast doubt on this potential marker. Despite numerous negative findings, several areas of investigation remain promising, such as cholinergic rapid eye movement (REM) sleep induction and plasma melatonin.

Several groups have reported that manic depressive patients are more sensitive than controls to the REM sleep–inducing effects of cholinergic agonists. This effect is independent of mood state and is highly concordant in monozygotic twins. Recent data show that this abnormality segregates with illness in families in which the proband has the marker. If other groups can replicate the existing family study, then cholinergic REM induction may be established as a vulnerability marker for mood disorders.

The interest in the role of melatonin in mood disorders originates in observations of disturbed diurnal rhythms and seasonal variation in mood disorders. Melatonin production by the pineal gland is closely entrained to the day–night cycle. Normal daylight inhibits melatonin production, so that plasma levels are nearly undetectable during normal waking hours. Plasma levels increase tenfold during the night. Manic-depressive patients are supersensitive to the inhibitory effects of light on plasma melatonin levels. These effects are independent of mood state. Recently, the same light supersensitivity was observed in the well adolescent offspring of bipolar parents, compared with the well adolescent offspring of control parents. This suggests that the melatonin response to light may be a vulnerability marker for mood disorders. Family

TABLE 17.2b-1
Proposed Genetic Vulnerability Traits for Mood Disorders

Proposed Marker	*Patients Differ from Controls*	*State Independent*	*Heritable*	*Segregates with Illness*
Lithium ratio	Yes (most studies)	Possibly	Yes	No conclusive data
CSF 5-HIAA	Yes (most studies)	Yes, for a subgroup	No	No data
Platelet imipramine binding	Yes	No	Yes	No data
Plasma GABA	Yes	Yes	Possibly	No data
Lymphoblast beta receptor	Conflicting data	Yes	Possibly	Very few data
Cholinergic REM sleep induction	Yes	Yes	Possibly	Yes (more data needed)
Plasma melatonin response to light	Yes	Yes	No data	No data
Tyramine excretion	Yes	Yes	No data	No data

studies are needed to determine whether the light supersensitivity segregates with illness within pedigrees.

Two independent groups of investigators have described decreased excretion of a tyramine metabolite, after an oral tyramine dose, in mood-disordered patients. This finding is state independent and applies to about 50 percent of the well relatives of probands with the marker. Studies of ill relatives and heritability research are needed.

FAMILY STUDIES OF BIOLOGICAL TRAITS

Only two of the studied characteristics have relevant data on segregation of a biological abnormality with illness: the lithium erythrocyte–plasma ratio and muscarinic acetylcholine receptor density.

LITHIUM TRANSPORT Data regarding the genetics of lithium transport and its relation to the genetics of manic depressive disorder were gathered on 291 individuals from 120 families of normal controls and on 66 relatives of 31 bipolar I patients, of whom 16 had a major mood disorder and 28 had a minor mood disorder. Of the relatives, 11 with major mood disorders and 2 with other diagnoses had been psychiatrically hospitalized. The 31 bipolar I patients, however, were not studied for their own lithium transport parameters. This was unfortunate because the 31 probands constituted the majority of major mood-disordered patients in these families and because the key issue in these data of the relationship of major mood disorder to lithium transport in relatives has not been resolved.

The analysis of lithium-ratio inheritance per se is a straightforward analysis of a quantitative trait, based on 291 individuals from normal families. Solutions that include all the parameters of major gene and polygenic inheritance are accepted from among similarly complex hypotheses that have been rejected. The major component of inheritance appears to be multifactorial, and a single-locus component is also present. Using the same model on a linear combination of the lithium ratio and diagnosis, the null hypothesis of no single locus and no polygenic transmission was rejected. The rejected model, however, was mathematically much simpler (had fewer parameters) than the other models. There was a lack of discrimination among various specific genetic hypotheses, and most of the affected relatives had lithium ratios within the lower distribution (i.e., the distribution found in the normal families). If the relative with the diagnostic trait had ever been hospitalized, the discrimination improved, but there were only 13 such relatives, two of whom were not diagnosed as having a mood disorder.

Nonetheless, this conclusion is most important. If it is replicated, with larger numbers of lithium studies of ill individuals, it would have important diagnostic and preventive implications.

ACETYLCHOLINE The interest in acetylcholine in mood disorders stems from the proposal that depression is accompanied by a relative increase of cholinergic to adrenergic activity in some part of the central nervous system (CNS). Several groups have demonstrated that cholinergic REM induction distinguishes tragic mood-disordered patients from normal controls, even when these patients are tested in the well state. In this test, a small dose of a cholinergic agonist, arecoline, induces a REM sleep period. At low doses of arecoline, a REM sleep period is induced in mood-disordered patients, but not in controls. The ability to induce REM sleep by this procedure is also highly correlated in monozygotic twins. These findings have raised the possibility of greater muscarinic receptor sensitivity as a pathophysiological vulnerability marker. Recent studies found that rapid cholinergic REM induction segregates with illness in some families.

A muscarinic receptor vulnerability hypothesis regarding mood disorders may be based on the evidence that there is increased CNS response to muscarinic stimulation in mood-disordered patients, that these findings are state independent and heritable, and that the rapid REM response is associated with illness in the relatives of patients. According to this hypothesis, increased muscarinic receptor density, characteristic of some neurons, is a predisposing factor to mood disorder.

NOREPINEPHRINE The interest in adrenergic receptor abnormalities in mood disorders results, in part, from the observation that antidepressants reduce the numbers of brain β-adrenergic receptors. One study found that cultured lymphoblast cell lines from mood-disordered subjects and their ill relatives have fewer numbers of β-receptors than cell lines from well relatives or controls. This study is consistent with the hypothesis that a genetically determined reduction in β-adrenergic receptors is a risk factor for mood disorders. The authors, however, have not been able to replicate this observation. Further research on the role of β-adrenergic function in the genetic etiology of mood disorders is needed.

MELATONIN The interest in the role of melatonin in mood disorders began with observations of disturbed diurnal rhythms, light sensitivity, and seasonal variation in depression and mania. Normally, melatonin production by the pineal gland is closely entrained to the day–night cycle, with gland activity closely entrained to the day–night cycle, and with high plasma levels occurring at night. Light inhibits melatonin production, so that plasma levels cannot be detected during the day. Supersensitivity to the inhibitory effects of light on melatonin production was described in bipolar patients, independent of mood state. The same phenomenon was also observed in the well adolescent offspring of bipolar parents, implying that the melatonin response to light may be a risk factor for mood disorders. Confirmation of these observations by other investigators and additional research on the heritability of this response are needed. These hypotheses are supported by only small numbers of patients or ill relatives, or both. Further studies of segregation within pedigrees are required.

CLINICAL APPLICATIONS

In clinical practice, several issues frequently arise as a result of the greater sophistication of the consumers of medical care and the widespread belief among patients and relatives that all serious psychiatric illnesses are genetic. These issues are (1) the risk to offspring of patients, (2) the possibilities for prevention, (3) the choice of treatment in view of the family history, and (4) requests for genetic counseling.

In the authors' recent study, the lifetime risk of mood disorders to 614 offspring of one mood-disordered parent (largely bipolar) was 27 percent. The risk to 28 offspring of two ill parents was 74 percent. Great precision from an estimate based on 28 persons at risk would not be expected, but other studies also suggest the risk to be at least 50 percent. These risks are for adult mood disorder. Systematic studies of diagnosis in childhood of these offspring are only now beginning. But, clinicians may be asked for advice on childhood interventions by parents with a mood disorder. The authors do not know of any therapeutic intervention that would reduce the risk of illness. The only interventions they can suggest is the early recognition and treatment of the mood disorder if it does develop. Their experience has been, especially when the onset is in adolescence, that treatment may be avoided for years because of denial, with tragic consequences, such as teenage suicides.

The choice of pharmacological treatment may be helped by the family history. In one study, unipolar patients with a family history of bipolar illness were more likely to be lithium responders than those without such a family history. The history of response to a therapeutic agent in a close relative is good reason to try the same agent in a newly presenting patient.

There will also be requests for genetic counseling, which should be looked on as problems in short-term psychotherapy. The goals may be (1) a realistic and appropriate appreciation of the patient's (or spouse's) family history, (2) the communication of current knowledge on morbid risk, (3) a way to cope with the anxiety and narcissistic injury related to risk, and (4) a plan for the appropriate response to high risk.

The patient's spouse must also be considered in the counseling. A tendency for assortative mating—or for persons with similar mood disorders to marry—has often been reported. Whether this tendency increases the genetic risks is not known, but it does give a peculiar quality to many of the marriages. Divorce is often attributed to symptoms of the illness, usually mania. Occasionally, clinicians will be confronted with blunt questions: "My fiancé is a manic-depressive. Should I marry him?" "My wife is a manic-depressive. Should we have children?" Answering these questions requires clinical skill and compassion. In a questionnaire given to a group of married bipolar patients and their well spouses, one of the questions asked was, "If you had known then what you know now, would you have married?" Nine out of 10 of the bipolar patients said yes, but more than half of the spouses said no.

Unfortunately, no test can now be given that identifies persons at risk of developing a mood disorder or producing an ill offspring. Although there are some promising developments, none of them is at the point that clinical application is appropriate. Studies of young persons at high risk for developing a mood disorder, on the basis of parental illness, might now usefully incorporate tests of putative biological markers.

REFERENCES

Berrettini W H, Goldin L R, Nurnberger J I, Jr, Gershon E S: Genetic factors in affective illness. J Psychiat Res *18:* 329, 1984.

Bertelsen A: A Danish twin study of manic-depressive disorders. In *Origin Prevention and Treatment of Affective Disorders,* M Schou, E Stromgren, editors, p 227. Academic Press, London, 1979.

Botstein D, White R L, Skolnick M, Davis R W: Construction of a genetic linkage map in man using restriction fragment length polymorphisms. Amer J Human Gen *32:* 314, 1980.

Detera-Wadleigh S D, Berrettini W H, Goldin L R, Boorman D, Anderson S, Gershon E S: Close linkage of c-Harvey-*ras*-l and the insulin gene to affective disorder is ruled out in three North American pedigrees. Nature *325:* 806, 1987.

Dorus E, Cox N J, Gibbon R D, Shaughnessy R, Pandey G N, Cloninger C R: Lithium ion transport and affective disorders within families of bipolar patients. Arch Gen Psychiat *40:* 55, 1983.

Egeland J A, Gerhard D S, Pauls D L, Sussex J N, Kidd K K, Allen C R, Hostetter A M, Housman D E: Bipolar affective disorders linked to DNA markers on chromosome 11. Nature *325:* 783, 1987.

Gershon E S, Hamovit J, Guroff J J, Dibble E, Leckman J F, Sceery W, Targum S D, Nurnberger J I, Jr, Goldin L R, Bunney W E, Jr: A family study of schizoaffective, bipolar I, bipolar II, unipolar, and normal control probands. Arch Gen Psychiat *39:* 1157, 1982.

Gershon E S, Hamovit J H, Guroff J J, Nurnberger J I, Jr: Birth cohort changes in manic and depressive disorders in relatives of bipolar and schizoaffective patients. Arch Gen Psychiat, *44:* 314, 1987.

Goldin L R, Cox N J, Pauls D L, Gershon E S, Kidd K K: The detection of major loci by segregation and linkage analysis: A simulation study. Gen Epidemiol *1:* 285, 1984.

Goldin L R, Gershon E S: Association and linkage studies of genetic marker loci in major psychiatric disorders. Psychiat Develop *4:* 387, 1983.

Hodgkinson S, Sherrington R, Gurling H, Marchbanks R, Reeders S, Mallet J, McInnis M, Petursson H, Brynjolfsson J: Molecular genetic evidence for heterogeneity in manic depression. Nature *325:* 805, 1987.

Klerman G L, Lavori P W, Rice J, Reich T, Endicott J, Andreasen N C, Keller M B, Hirschfeld R M A: Birth cohort trends in rates of major depressive disorder among relatives of patients with affective disorder. Arch Gen Psychiat *42:* 689, 1985.

Mendlewicz J, Rainer J D: Adoption study supporting genetic transmission in manic-depressive illness. Nature *268:* 32, 1977.

Reich T, James J W, Morris C A: The use of multiple thresholds in determining the mode of transmission of semi-continuous traits. Ann Human Gen *36:* 163, 1972.

Rieder R O, Gershon E S: Genetic strategies in biological psychiatry. Arch Gen Psychiat *35:* 866, 1978.

Risch N, Baron M: X-linkage and genetic heterogeneity in bipolar-related major affective illness: Re-analysis of linkage data. Ann Human Gen *46:* 153, 1982.

Sitaram N, Nurnberger J I, Jr, Gershon E S, Gillin J C: Faster cholinergic REM sleep induction in euthymic patients with primary affective illness. Science *208:* 200, 1980.

Spence M A: Linkage methods in psychiatric disorders. In *Genetic Strategies for Psychobiology and Psychiatry,* E S Gershon, S Matthysse, X O Breakfield, R D Ciaranello, editors, p 295. Boxwood Press, Pacific Grove, CA, 1980.

Suarez B K, Rice J, Reich T: The generalized sib pair IBD distribution: Its use in the detection of linkage. Ann Human Gen *42:* 87, 1978.

Targum S D, Gershon E S: Pregnancy, genetic counseling, and the major psychiatric disorders. In *Genetic Diseases in Pregnancy,* D

Shulman J L Simpson, editors, p 413. Academic Press, New York, 1981.
von Knorring A, Cloninger C R, Bohman M, Sigvardsson S: An adoption study of depressive disorders and substance abuse. Arch Gen Psychiat *40:* 943, 1983.
Weissman M M, Leaf P J, Holzer C E, III, Myers J K, Tischler G L: The epidemiology of depression. An update on sex differences in rates. J Affect Dis *7:* 179, 1984.
Wender P H, Kety S S, Rosenthal D, Schulsinger F, Ortmann J, Lunde I: Psychiatric disorders in the biological and adoptive families of adopted individuals with affective disorders. Arch Gen Psychiat *43:* 923, 1986.

17.2c
MOOD DISORDERS: PSYCHODYNAMIC ETIOLOGY

AUSTIN SILBER, M.D.

INTRODUCTION

In psychoanalytic theory, a *mood* is a pervasive, sustained, internal feeling. The process by which the mood becomes pervasive entails both ego regression and ego synthesis and organization. Some psychoanalysts, such as Lars Lofgren, define a mood as a relatively complex, highly refined, and personal feeling state that is more difficult to capture than such basic feelings as fear and rage.

An *affect* is a subjective feeling or sensation that is attached to an idea or mental representation of an object. This subjective feeling or sensation may be a compromise containing pertinent conscious, preconscious, and unconscious elements that are expressed only obliquely. The attached idea can also be conscious and unconscious and can include relevant memories or fantasies. A person's mood can bind or tame affects by permitting a repetitive affective discharge and, at the same time, by protecting the ego from affective discharges that are too intense or too overwhelming. This taming of affects is aided by the child's long period of dependence on the parents, by the slow maturation of the ego apparatus and functions, and by the biphasic nature of sexual development.

Affects evolve and are elaborated in many different ways, depending on the circumstances: whether they are produced by real events or fantasies, and whether these are traumatic or benign. Ernest Jones showed how the affects of fear, guilt, hate, rage, and shame are implicated in the development of depression. Rage can be ranked as more primitive and more poorly organized than shame, and guilt can be viewed as more developmentally complex and organized than either shame or rage. Thus, both qualitative and quantitative factors and the maturity of the psychic apparatus itself are significant variables in determining the impact of a particular affect on a person's development.

DEPRESSION

Depression encompasses a wide range of clinical entities, from a mild mood disturbance that is commonly found in both normal and neurotic persons to a severe illness that is characterized by such vegetative signs as restlessness, motor retardation, early-morning awakening, weight loss, and anorexia and by such subjective symptoms as self-reproach, apathy, despondence, feelings of worthlessness, and suicidal preoccupations.

In the early twentieth century, the fundamental psychoanalytic findings and formulations regarding depression emerged. Karl Abraham, for instance, derived his clinical findings from analyses of manic-depressive patients who were between their depressive and manic extremes.

DEFENSE MECHANISMS

Several defense mechanisms—unconscious ways of relieving conflict and anxiety—are used in the formation of depression.

AMBIVALENCE Abraham found that depressed patients have a marked ambivalence toward the objects of their love. This love–hate feeling is formed before the age of 3, during the pregenital stage of psychosexual development. Accompanying the child's ambivalent attitudes and omnipresent narcissism are aggression and aggressive affects.

INTROJECTION Sigmund Freud described introjection as the defense mechanism pathognomonic and characteristic of depression. In introjection, the depressed patient psychologically incorporates the love object into the ego. Thus, what had been an external struggle between the patient and the love object becomes an internal battle. The conflict is between the patient's harsh, sadistic superego, which contains aspects of both parental and personal aggression, and the patient's ego, which now contains the introjected love object. However, the love object is now also hated because of the patient's ambivalence.

Freud showed the importance of introjection in depression by pointing to the differences between mourning (a normal ego activity) and melancholia (a severe psychotic depression). Common to both conditions is an intense feeling of loss, but the mourner eventually returns to reality, to a normal mood, and to new relationships, whereas the melancholic person persists in this painful withdrawal from the world. The melancholic's inability to adapt to or resolve this loss is rooted in the failure of reality testing to reassert itself. The melancholic is unconscious of the loss's meaning: it is connected to an important object relationship in his or her early life or to some symbolically important goal or need representing that tie.

The self-reproaches invariably observed in melancholia, Freud asserted, can often be understood as reproaches toward an emotionally important person who disappointed or frustrated the patient, suggesting that the patient introjected that person and turned the reproaches inward. The intensity of this self-reproach suggests that sadistic aggression has grown in the patient's psyche. The melancholic's angry withdrawal from the rejected person is followed by an unconscious identification with that person. The melancholic's symptoms thus represent a mounting attack by the patient's own sadistic superego on the disappointing person, now internalized as part of the patient's own sense of self. This inner emotional turmoil is manifested in the melancholic by significantly lowered feelings of self-esteem. Freud concluded that the premorbid object relationship in the melancholic patient was more narcissistic and more emotionally dependent than similar relationships in normal mourners.

REGRESSION The depressed patient returns to an earlier pattern of adaptation. In libidinal terms, the patient's oral eroticism is accentuated.

Abraham believed that the precipitating event in depression is perceived by the patient as a repetition of a traumatic infantile experience, a primal depression. Such patients had sustained significant injuries to their infantile narcissism because of disappointments in their relationships with both loved parents. Those infantile disappointments acquired more significance when early developmental conflicts were not resolved and led to ambivalent attitudes. Abraham also contended that an inborn overaccentuation of oral eroticism can skew the effects of certain childhood events, giving them an unexpected traumatic significance.

Freud saw the withdrawal into a psychotic state of identification in melancholia as a regression to the developmental state of narcissism. In the melancholic patient, a real interaction with an object is replaced by an internalized, purely fantasized relationship. The intensity of the patient's rage toward the disappointing person is characteristic of narcissistic object relationships in general, which are often ambivalent and sensitive to disappointments. The patient's regression includes a return to early levels of instinctual functioning—oral and anal—each of which normally involves a heightened ambivalence. The unconscious, slow, painful process in melancholia, according to Freud, leads to the continuing disparagement of the disappointing person until the patient's fury is spent or the person is given up as worthless.

EGO–ENERGY EXHAUSTION

Some mild depressions, similar to the uncomplicated mourning described by Freud, seem to be caused by an exhaustion of ego energy. Thus, the mental energy ordinarily at hand for ego functioning is used up in unconscious conflicts or in efforts to defend oneself against such conflicts. And so there is not enough psychological energy available for the enjoyment of one's usual daily activities.

Ego energy can also be drained off by perverse, addicting, and impulsive behaviors. Such behaviors may represent depressive equivalents, and so if those gratifying behaviors are blocked, depression may set in.

INFANTILE SUPEREGO DEVELOPMENT

Unlike most psychoanalysts, Melanie Klein and her followers argued that the precursors to superego formation are in place in the very young child and account for the development of depression in the first year of life. Klein postulated that each child normally traverses an infantile depressive position in response to relationships with early objects. The general characteristics of that early response determine the characteristics of the child's depressive responses in later life.

According to Otto Kernberg, at about 6 months of age, children become aware that good and bad external objects are really one and that their mother as a whole has good and bad parts. At that point, infants begin to acknowledge their own aggression toward the good object or to recognize the good aspects of the objects they attack and perceive at such times as bad. The predominant fear in the depressive position is of harming the good internal and external objects. Bad internal objects may contaminate good internal objects that, because of their demanding or standard-setting nature, have also been internalized into the superego, resulting in cruel demands for perfection. Klein considered the depressed patient's self-reproaches as directed not against the object but against the self and the internal impulses. Accordingly, she thought that suicide corresponds to the unconscious fantasy of destroying the bad self.

EGO PSYCHOLOGY THEORIES

Ego psychology shifts the focus from libidinal development and its psychosexual stages to the ego and the development of the whole personality.

ARRESTED DEVELOPMENT Edith Jacobson linked severe depression to inordinate early infantile deprivations and to instinctual overstimulations and frustrations that lead to arrests in ego and superego development. The arrests in development hamper the person's ability to master inner and outer reality by the use of appropriate defenses, adaptations, and controls. When the person is not able to make a realistic judgment about a disappointing situation and is not able to take appropriate measures to restore a normal affect state, a pathological depression results. In Jacobson's view, too much unmastered aggression in early life leads to an instability in the self and in object representations, relations, and identifications, thereby contributing to the weakness, instability, and unreliability of many ego and superego functions in such predisposed persons.

Jacobson believed that the child's early introjections and internalizations of parental attitudes and prohibitions play a decisive role in superego development. She also contended that an oedipal child's severe disappointment in both parents added to a depressive predisposition—a child who is narcissistically vulnerable and has a fragile sense of self-esteem—can lead to aberrant superego development and probably future depression. When the parents are devalued and useless and the child introjects or identifies with them, Jacobson postulated, the child's self-esteem is diminished, leading to a sense of worthlessness, which is characteristic of the depressive.

TENSION WITHIN THE EGO Edward Bibring formulated the thesis that depression is the result of a struggle within the ego, rather than a conflict between the ego and the superego or between the ego and objects in the real world. For Bibring, all depressions, from the most benign to the most pathological, involve the same factors—a decrease in self-esteem, an intense state of helplessness, and an extensive inhibition of functions. Moreover, both depression and anxiety are basic ego reactions, but they are diametrically opposed in the ways they are worked out. Anxiety is a reaction to external danger or to internally perceived danger, and it demonstrates the ego's desire to survive; challenged by danger, the ego mobilizes its defenses and prepares to fight or flee. In depression, the opposite occurs: The ego seems paralyzed; feelings of helplessness and diminished self-esteem take over; and the depressed person seems to be incapable of maintaining the lifelong aspirations embodied in his or her superego and ego ideal.

EARLY DEPRIVATION Edith Zetzel noted that when significant adverse experiences in early childhood are aggravated by subsequent separation and loss, the capacity for tolerating depression can be seriously compromised. If a child has not been helped by caregivers to identify and tolerate such affects as depression without resorting to primitive defensive measures, then he or she has not had the chance to adjust gradually to such painful realities as the mother's illness, absence, and emotional unavailability. Learning to adjust to painful reality early in life contributes to subsequent adaptation, tolerance, and flexibility and makes gratification and achievement attainable. But the failure to learn that early lesson can lead to depression.

Does the idea of an affective vaccination—an optimal exposure to affectively charged situations and the subsequent adaptational advantages posited by Zetzel—apply to most children? Exposure to helplessness, narcissistic vulnerability, and bruised self-esteem is the fate of every child. But what may be traumatic for one child may be reasonable or even enhancing for another. René Spitz showed that overt depression is precipitated in infants separated from their mothers during the second 6 months of life; the result for some infants was marasmus and death. And Margaret Mahler showed that the child's absolute emotional and developmental dependence on the parents affects his or her capacity to mourn and grieve and recover and, therefore, affects the child's feelings of self-esteem and helplessness. Clearly, the child's relationship with his or her parents, the first objects in the child's life, plays a significant role in depression. The clinically depressed may represent, from a purely psychodynamic point of view, those developmental failures who have not received the help they needed, from nature or nurturing, to learn to cope psychologically.

The patient, a 24-year-old teacher, became severely depressed shortly after the birth of her second child, a son, born when her daughter was 2 years old. Before the onset of her depression, the patient, although sad at times, had never been clinically depressed.

The patient had one brother, 18 months younger. Her mother had nursed the patient during her first year of life but was unable to take proper care of many of her bodily needs. Those needs were met by her father until her brother was born. At that time, her father lost interest in her, as both parents had been looking forward to having a son.

The patient's father had a history of ulcer-like pains and occasional bouts of depression. At times, when despondent, he would lie on the floor, covering his face with his hands, wanting to die.

The patient's second pregnancy was uneventful. She seemed pleased to have a son. Shortly after his birth, however, she became fearful that she might handle him too roughly and might do him some harm. She began to wake, startled, after about an hour's sleep, and developed obsessive thoughts that she might kill her son. She returned to her teaching several weeks after her son's birth but became worried that she would not be able to continue to be an effective teacher, because the demands of caring for her son were sapping her of her strength and ability to work effectively. One of her students complained that she was not doing a good job. She felt she was becoming worthless as a teacher, and her self-esteem plummeted.

The patient's ambivalent feelings about looking after her son reminded her of her father's loss of interest in caring for her when she was a child. She became conscious of feeling furious at her son and also of death wishes toward her father. These wishes were revealed in her dreams and fantasies. Although intellectually conscious of the wishes, she could not grasp them emotionally. Instead, she became aware of severe upper abdominal pains, a new symptom. The pains forced her to lie down whenever she had any free time. Her severe abdominal pains thus represented her identification with her father's discomfort. Her lying down repeated what she had observed her father do as she was growing up: Instead of being able to accept her wish to destroy him—she instead identified with him—she literally took him inside herself. At one point, as the patient was complaining of abdominal distress while lying on the couch, she felt confused about whether she or her father was in pain. In her ensuing regression, with the activation of introjective and identificatory defenses, the instability of her conception of herself as separate from her father became confused, and one seemed readily to substitute for the other.

The birth of the patient's son drew onto him some of the repressed, murderous feelings that she harbored toward her father. The patient also tended to ignore her son and her son's needs, which represented an identification with her father's tendency to ignore her and her needs when she was young. At times, she had fantasies of attacking and injuring her son. Hidden behind those fantasies were repressed wishes to injure and destroy her father. Some of those wishes became clearer in the analysis when she and the therapist analyzed her fantasies and her continual efforts to find fault with the analyst's interpretations. She was constantly fearful that the analyst would interpret her ideas, thoughts, and fantasies incorrectly, thereby revealing incompetence and lack of care in regard to her and, in that way, do her severe personal harm. Only slowly was it possible for her to recognize her unacknowledged, painful recognition of her father's neglect of her in childhood—shifted onto the analyst in her analysis—and gradually begin to accept her disappointment in and, finally, her anger at and hatred toward her father. As her hatred became more accessible and acceptable, she was gradually able to give up her identification with him in the form of the abdominal symptoms, which had, in effect, protected her from coming to terms with her own hatred of him. She was also able to differentiate more clearly her feelings about her son from her feelings about her father. Her postpartum depression lifted, and her analysis continued to a successful conclusion.

MANIA

Mania—the mood disorder characterized by elation, agitation, hyperactivity, and accelerated thinking and speaking—can occur with or without a clinical history of depressive illness. However, Abraham believed that manic patients without a clinical history of depression had experienced what he called a primal depression very early in childhood. Those children who never learn to tolerate early depression or who lose a parent or a parent's love deny the reality of their developmental tragedy and become manic.

MANIC-DEPRESSIVE ILLNESS

As Abraham and others noted, in the manic state, depressed patients throw off the burden imposed on them by their tyrannical superego. Instead of criticizing the ego, the superego merges with it, and, thus, the distinction between the ego and the superego disappears.

The manic's mood is one of self-satisfaction, not disturbed by self-criticism. Such patients enjoy the abolition of their inhibitions, feelings of consideration for others, and self-reproaches. Now that their ego is no longer being consumed by the once-loved introjected object, they turn their energies to the outer world with an excess of eagerness. And they have more energy, leading to euphoria, because the energy that had been bound up in the depressive struggle is released when the patients triumph over their introjected object.

The patients' change in attitude from their depressed state gives rise to increased oral cravings, for their view of the world has been altered by the regressive changes affecting both their ego and their superego. The hunger for new objects can be played out in multiple identifications related to transient, superficial objects in the external world.

Bertram Lewin viewed the ego's fusion with the superego in somewhat different terms. He saw the fusion as a "faithful intrapsychic repetition of the experiences of that fusion with the mother that takes place during nursing at the breast." Just as satiety follows hunger, so elation or mania follows the self-punishment of depression, as the patient intrapsychically revives the oral technique for regaining self-esteem. Lewin viewed the ego as the infant and the superego as the breast, the epitome of the mother, the earliest object. In this formulation, the superego is not viewed as the repository of prohibitions and restrictive parental attitudes, as it is usually seen.

HYPOMANIA

Hypomania—a mood disturbance similar to mania but less intense—can alter the mind's affective apparatus in order to forestall anxiety. The hypomanic's ego, Lewin noted, can be considered a purified pleasure ego. The defense mechanism of denial is positioned at the boundary of the pleasure ego to repel external reality or any psychic realities that would interfere with the ego's need to experience only pleasure. Caught up in denying the reality of unpleasant ideas and perceptions, hypomanic patients avoid the emotional consequences of reality by immersion in a mood that varies from good humor to exaltation. What hypomanic patients are avoiding is the anxiety that would overwhelm their ego if the warded-off depressed feelings and their ideational counterparts were permitted to flood it. The hypomanic's regressive denial, affecting both ego and superego, causes a profound estrangement from reality and a retreat to narcissistic preoccupation, instead of emotional involvement with the real world of people and ideas.

The following case history, illustrates the importance denial plays in hypomania:

The patient who had been treated in psychotherapy for a series of moderate depressions, had an occasional hypomanic episode. It would be ushered in by a hallucinatory episode that dramatized the central wish of the hypomanic episode, the wish to have a penis materialize at will. Unconsciously, the hallucination represented the penis, which the patient felt that fate, as epitomized by her parents, had denied her. After a depressive episode had receded, the patient would notice that many men she looked at seemed to have a penis dangling in front of their trousers. At times, she saw a similar penis exposed on her own lap, as though the new addition belonged to her.

In the course of her therapy, a central fantasy emerged. She saw herself, as an infant, lying between her parents' exposed genitals. In effect, she became a bridge that both connected them and kept them separate. She saw her body as representative of an enormous phallus that could join her parents together; she was the organ they shared in common. The hallucinated penis represented that common phallus, appearing in men and women alike.

The appearance of the hallucinated penis was accompanied by a sense of increased well-being. It ushered in a period of excited sexual interest that culminated in more frequent, insistent masturbation. During those episodes, the patient would become much more interested in shopping for new clothes and new house furnishings. The episodes lasted for several days, but they responded to the interpretive efforts of her therapist. So when the patient started to notice exposed penises in her immediate environment, this alerted both the patient and the therapist to the hypomanic episode, which required immediate attention.

OTHER PSYCHOLOGICAL AND PSYCHODYNAMIC FACTORS

ADOLF MEYER Meyer believed depression to be the person's reaction to a disturbing life experience, such as the loss of a loved one, a financial setback, unemployment, or an illness: Depression must be understood as part of the patient's life history, as an event that has psychic causality.

KAREN HORNEY According to Horney, the child raised by rejecting parents develops feelings of loneliness and insecurity. The child needs to be loved but fears criticism and rejection and so is susceptible to feelings of helplessness and depression.

SANDOR RADO Rado described depression as consisting primarily of a sense of helplessness. Anhedonia, or the inability to experience pleasure, is a key phenomenon that develops when the person is not aware of his or her capacities or is unable to achieve emotional self-reward. Rado believed that melancholia resulted from the person's punitive superego, which punishes the patient for his or her unconscious hostile feelings toward a deceased loved one.

AARON BECK According to Beck, depression results from faulty cognition. He described a cognitive triad consisting of (1) perceiving oneself as defective and inadequate; (2) perceiving the world as demanding and punishing; and (3) expecting failure, defeat, and hardship. These errors in cognition are based on one's life experience.

JOHN BOWLBY Bowlby saw disorders of the mother–infant attachment bond as the paradigm of depression. If the infant is separated early and for long periods of time from his or her mother (or other caregivers), depressive hopelessness may result that could continue throughout life.

HARRY STACK SULLIVAN Sullivan concentrated more on schizophrenia than on mood disorders. He believed that adverse interaction between a person and his or her psychosocial environment (particularly interpersonal interaction) is critical to psychiatric disorders, including depression.

HEINZ KOHUT According to William Meissner, Kohut believed that a child's fragile sense of self can be fragmented by severe deprivation, such as that caused by the child's premature separation from the mother. Primary narcissism changes into normal narcissism that allows the child to maintain a sense of self-esteem and pride in accomplishment even when confronted with unavoidable disappointments. This transition is dependent on proper maternal care and responsiveness to the child's needs.

REFERENCES

Abraham K: Notes on the psychoanalytical investigation and treatment of manic-depressive insanity and allied conditions. In *Selected Papers on Psychoanalysis,* p 137. Basic Books, New York, 1953.

Abraham K: A short study of the development of the libido, viewed in the light of mental disorders. In *Selected Papers on Psychoanalysis,* p 418. Basic Books, New York, 1953.

Bibring E: The mechanism of depression. In *Affective Disorders—Psychoanalytic Contribution to Their Study,* P Greenacre, editor. International Universities Press, New York, 1953.

Freud A: *Normality and Pathology in Childhood: Assessments of Development,* vol 6. International Universities Press, New York, 1965.

Freud S: Mourning and melancholia. In *Standard Edition,* vol 14. Hogarth Press, London, 1957.

Freud S: Inhibitions, symptoms and anxiety. In *Standard Edition,* vol 20. Hogarth Press, London, 1959.

Jacobson E: *Depression.* International Universities Press, New York, 1971.

Jones E: Fear, guilt, hate. Int J Psychoanal *10:* 383, 1929.

Klein M: Contribution to the psychogenesis of the manic-depressive state. In *Contributions to Psychoanalysis, 1921–1945.* Hogarth Press, London, 1948.

Lewin B D: *The Psychoanalysis of Elation.* Norton, New York, 1950.

Lofgren L B: Psychoanalytic theory of affects. J Amer Psychoanal *16:* 638, 1968.

Mahler M: *On Human Symbiosis and the Vicissitudes of Individuation,* vol 1: *Infantile Psychosis.* International Universities Press, New York, 1968.

Spitz R: Anaclitic depression. In *The Psychoanalytic Study of Child,* vol 2, p 313. International Universities Press, New York, 1946.

Zetzel E: The depressive position. In *Affective Disorders,* P Greenacre, editor. International Universities Press, New York, 1953.
Zetzel E: Depression and the incapacity to bear it. In *Drives, Affects, Behavior,* M Schur, editor. International Universities Press, New York, 1965.

17.3 MOOD DISORDERS: CLINICAL FEATURES

MAX HAMILTON, M.D., F.R.C.P., F.R.C.Psych., F.B.P.S.

INTRODUCTION

HISTORY Both mania and depression were known to the ancient Greeks, though they used these words with meanings somewhat different from modern usage. In accordance with their humoral theories of disease, they named depressive states melancholia, signifiying black bile. Very few doctors have seen black bile, a condition in which biliary obstruction reaches such an intensity that the patient's color deepens from the yellow of jaundice to a dark green. Such patients are undoubtedly depressed, but whether this is caused by a toxic effect or by knowledge of the prospects of an unpleasant death is still undecided.

Manias and depressions continued to be described in medical textbooks. Jean Pierre Falret recognized their association in 1854 with his term *folie circulaire,* and all forms were finally brought together by Emil Kraepelin at the end of the nineteenth century as the manic-depressive psychoses. His subclassifications of this group are now chiefly of historical interest. In particular, his separate group of involutional depression is not now regarded as distinct from the others.

Since then, the continued extension of psychiatry into the extrahospital outpatient and office practice has broadened the range of the conditions being treated. The increasing number and practical importance of the milder forms of mental illness, such as the neurotic or reactive depressions, have led to controversies concerning their nature and classification, which are not yet resolved.

In 1962, the recurrent forms were divided into monopolar and bipolar types, and in 1966, the monopolar was renamed unipolar. Patients with unipolar depressions are liable to recurrent attacks of depressive disorder, whereas those with bipolar disorder are liable to attacks of depression and mania. Unipolar manias do exist but are very rare.

In 1975, the bipolar disorders were subdivided into Type I, in which the manic phase is always mild, and Type II, in which the manic phase may be severe, though not invariably so. A triple classification was proposed in 1978: MD, Dm, and Md, in which the upper-case letter (D, M) signifies attacks of depression or mania severe enough to require admission to hospital, and the lower-case letter (d, m) signifies milder attacks not requiring hospital treatment. Type Dm corresponds to Type I, and Type MD corresponds to Type II.

The current classifications depend not only on the clinical phenomena (symptoms, course, and outcome) but also on genetic evidence and the response to treatment. The great success of biological treatments (drugs and electroconvulsive therapy [ECT]) have promoted biological theories and downgraded psychological theories of the nature and causation of the mood disorders. Two distinct genes for bipolar disorder have now been identified. Unfortunately, despite much research, no unequivocal biochemical basis has been established. The search for biological markers, or clinical or biochemical phenomena clearly linked to a mood disorder, continues.

INCIDENCE It is generally accepted that there is a large pool of persons suffering from depressive illness, from which the number of patients coming for treatment depends very much on the facilities available. There also are many individuals who are depressed or, rather, unhappy because of their circumstances. Some of them may seek help or treatment.

As a result, estimates of the population incidence of mood disorders cannot be accurate. For a thorough discussion on this issue, see Section 17.1, Epidemiology. Most of the figures lie between 1 and 3 percent of the population, but these figures are certainly too low. Many patients who come for treatment will remember that years earlier they experienced an attack similar to the current one, either milder or of shorter duration, for which they did not seek treatment. However, it can be safely said that mania is the rarest of the major psychoses and that depression is one of the most common.

The lifetime expectation of suffering from mood disorder is estimated to be just under 2 percent for men and about twice that for women. For patients coming for treatment, among the unipolars there are twice as many women as men and much the same for the schizoaffectives. For the bipolars, the ratio is about 3 to 2.

SOCIAL FACTORS The most serious consequence of depressive illness is suicide, and there is no doubt that the overwhelming majority of suicides are the consequence of that illness. The only firm evidence of the influence of social factors on the incidence of mood disorders is that during times of war and civil strife, the rate of suicide falls.

Much research has been carried out showing that depressions are more common in young working-class women who have three children under the age of 5 years and unsympathetic husbands. It is doubtful whether these cases should be classified as depressive illness, rather than as a reaction to the stresses of individual circumstances. Half of the cases remit within a month, often because of neutralizing life events.

BASIC PREMORBID PERSONALITY The traditional view is that obsessive-compulsive personalities are more prone to involutional depressions than to other types, but more recent work has not confirmed this view. The same is true of the so-called depressive personality. It is more than likely that such individuals have not fully recovered from a previous depressive illness. All the evidence indicates that the average sufferer has a normal personality before the onset of the disorder and in between acute phases. Some believe that there is a continuous gradation between the extroverted personality, the cyclothymic personality, and cyclothymia, recognized as being on the borderline of the normal.

DEFINITION The word "depression" is used in three different ways. In common speech, it is used to describe the state of sadness that all persons experience when they lose something of importance to them (e.g., when a near relative dies). In psychiatry, it is used to signify an abnormal mood, akin to the sadness, unhappiness, and misery of everyday experience. As such, depression may appear as a symptom in any mental disorder and is also a symptom in many organic diseases and toxic conditions. The depression discussed here often has another quality that makes it distinctive. This quality appears to be related to an inability to experience pleasure (anhedonia) in any way and with any experience. Those patients who are sufficiently self-aware and intelligent will recognize this difference between their mood and normal experience but can describe it only in metaphors: It is like a black cloud; it cuts you off.

Finally, the word "depression" is used as the name for clinical states or disorders (replacing the former "melancholia") that consist of a group of symptoms forming recognizable patterns and sometimes showing a cyclical course, with more or less complete recovery between acute attacks.

Mania, as used in psychiatry, has only the one meaning, although the adjective "maniacal" is used in common speech to signify exaggerated and excited behavior (e.g., maniacal enthusiasm).

Depressive illness is recognized as not being a unitary disorder, and it has been classified in many different ways. In the United States, the classification scheme of the revised third edition of the *Diagnostic and Statistical Manual of Mental Disorders* (DSM-III-R) of the American Psychiatric Association is the one currently accepted and will be used here. Outside the United States, the ninth revision of the *International Classification of Diseases* (ICD-9) is preferred.

Traditional classifications are still common in the literature, and a guide to their description and usage follows.

MOOD DISORDERS

COURSE OF ILLNESS Depressive illness is not only a common disorder but also a very serious one. About 15 percent of these patients commit suicide in the end, and of those who have made an unsuccessful attempt, 10 percent will eventually kill themselves. Unipolar depressions have a higher rate of suicide than the other forms.

Unipolar and bipolar disorders The most important distinction among the varieties of mood disorder is that between unipolar (recurrent depressions) and bipolar (recurrent attacks of depression and mania). A third variety, consisting of recurrent attacks of mania only, is regarded as a form of bipolar disorder. It constitutes less than 10 percent of bipolar disorder.

Because attacks of depression are much more common than those of mania, many patients diagnosed as the former will eventually have their diagnosis changed. However, with each successive attack of depression, the probability of a mania's appearing diminishes, though it never disappears. One study reported that 10 percent of unipolar depressives eventually changed to bipolar disorder and 6 percent to schizoaffective disorder. About 7 percent of bipolars are rediagnosed as schizoaffective.

Bipolar disorders Although the attack of mania may be detached from the depressive phase, it is more usual for it to be linked. Either the illness begins with a bout of mania that in the end swings into a depressive phase, or the patients swing into mania as they recover from the depression. Two forms of bipolar disorder are recognized: Type I, in which the manic phases are mild (hypomanic) and do not require admission to the hospital, and Type II, in which the manic phase may range from mild to severe, a true manic attack.

Mania is uncommon, and even more so is the condition of pure mania in which the patient does not experience phases of depression. The ratio of bipolars to pure manias is about 10 to 1. For this reason, DSM-III-R does not have a separate category for them. All manias are defined as bipolar disorder.

Age at onset (of first episode) The median age of the onset of bipolar disorder is, for men, 29 years and, for women, 34.5 years. The corresponding figures for unipolar disorder are 51 and 47.5 years, and for schizoaffective disorder, 24 and 31 years. This means that half of the patients will have started their first attack before these ages. The first two types show two peaks (modes) in the frequency distribution. The bipolar peaks are at ages 20 to 30 and 40 to 50 years. The unipolar depressions have a prominent peak at 50 to 60 years and a lesser one at 20 to 30 years. There are more men than women in the early onset groups, because of the preponderance of the mild and severe Type II (MD) groups. In the late onset groups, the illness is Type I (Dm) and affects more women than men. This suggests that late-onset illnesses may have different etiologies. The single peak of incidence of the schizoaffective group is at 20 to 30 years.

Duration of phases A bout of illness is called a phase, and the tradition is that a phase lasts for an average of 6 to 12 months. In fact, more than two-thirds of phases last for less than 6 months. This overestimate arises from the asymmetrical frequency distribution of phase length. The curve rises steeply and then falls slowly; in statistical terms, it has a positive skew. If the duration of phase is replaced by its logarithm, the curve will become symmetrical, the shape of a Gaussian or normal curve. The original curve is therefore known as a log normal curve and is found repeatedly in all statistics relating to the mood disorders. For such a distribution, the arithmetic mean is inappropriate, as it gives too high a figure.

The length of the first phase, for both unipolar and bipolar disorder, is about 3 months, the latter being about 20 percent shorter. Because of the asymmetrical distribution, the 95 percent confidence limits have a very wide span. Thus, for 95 percent of first phases, the duration will range between 0.8 and 29 months for unipolars and between 0.8 and 25 months for bipolars.

The duration of these phases tends to increase with successive phases, especially for the unipolars. There is some correlation between duration and both severity and age of onset. Treatment seems to reduce the amplitude of the phases but probably not their length. However, lithium appears to reduce the length as well as the amplitude (Table 17.3-1).

Duration of cycles The span of time covering a phase and the free interval until the next phase is called a cycle. It is often said that between acute phases, the patients make a complete recovery. Unfortunately, at least one in 10 patients is left with residual symptoms of depression when the acute phase ends. Unlike schizophrenia, in which the residual symptoms are presented as an impairment of personality and social adjustment, the depressives return to their normal personality, and their social adjustment shows only such slight impairment as is inherent in their symptoms.

There is no difference between the duration of cycles of depressions associated with precipitating stresses and those

TABLE 17.3-1
Duration of Phases and Cycles (in months)

	Phases		
	Unipolar	*Bipolar*	*Schizoaffective*
Median	5.1	4.4	4.2
Interquartiles	3.2–11.5	2.5–7.6	3.0–6.4
Means (after log transform)	5.95	4.4	4.65
Cycles			
Median	50.3	31.3	34.9
Interquartiles	26.8–95.5	18.2–48.7	25.0–66.3

without and between the two sexes. The cycle's duration tends to decrease with each successive phase, about 20 percent for the unipolars and 10 percent for the bipolars. The best estimate for the length of the first cycle is that it is about 65 months for the unipolars, 48 months for the bipolars, and 35 months for the schizoaffectives. The cycles tend to shorten to 28, 22, and 31 months, respectively. Once again, the skew (log normal) distribution leads to widely ranging confidence limits. Thus for the unipolars, 95 percent of the cycles will lie between 4 months and 52 years, and for the bipolars they will be between 4 months and 30 years. In consequence, it is not possible to give reasonable estimates for the length of a cycle.

Because 2 to 3 percent of patients suffering from unipolar recurrent depressions may expect that their cycle will be over 50 years, some of them will not live long enough to experience their second attack. A certain proportion of patients suffering from nonrecurrent depressions therefore will be of the unipolar recurrent type. This proportion will be small, as nonrecurrent depressions are common, but all depressions could be regarded as of the cyclical type.

The duration of the first cycle decreases with the age of onset of the first phase (i.e., the later the onset is, the shorter the length of the first cycle will be), but the variability is very great.

The cycles decrease in length with the increasing number of episodes, and as the variability is small, it is possible to make useful predictions. The average length is best expressed as the geometric mean, which is 33 months for the bipolars and 45 months for unipolars. The length diminishes rapidly at first but more slowly later, to reach an average of about 9 months. However, although the figures apply to both sexes, there is much variation between individuals (Table 17.3-1).

Number of phases A prolonged follow-up is required to determine the number of phases experienced by a patient over a lifetime. So far, it would appear that for a follow-up of 20 years or more, the median number of episodes in unipolar depressions is four to six; for bipolars it is seven to nine; and for schizoaffectives it is seven. In that period, 15 percent of unipolars have only one phase, 22 percent have two phases, and 49 percent have fewer than four. Only 3 percent of schizoaffectives have no more than one phase. All bipolars have multiple phases.

Effects of treatment with drugs Treatment with antidepressant drugs does not appear to shorten the episodes but does decrease their amplitude. The drugs do not seem to decrease the risk of recurrence. Nevertheless, there is good evidence that if the drug is continued for at least a year, the risk of recurrence during that time will be much reduced.

Treatment with lithium definitely lowers the risk of recurrence, reduces the duration of episodes and their amplitude, and lengthens the cycles. The response is not related to sex, current age, or age at onset.

Effect of electroconvulsive therapy ECT is one of the most effective forms of treatment for the depressions. Improvement occurs much more quickly than with other treatments; the proportion of patients who respond is much greater; and the level of response is higher. There is no doubt that it cuts short an attack, but there is some evidence that it is not effective if given in too early a stage of the phase. More precisely, patients who have failed to respond to the treatment will not have a spontaneous recovery for another 6 months.

Prodromal period An acute illness may start suddenly, or it may develop slowly, reaching a maximum within a few months at most. A fair proportion of patients will have difficulty determining when their illness began until the question is divided into two: "How long have you been feeling (more or less) like this?" and "When did you last feel well—your normal self?" It will then become apparent that their present symptoms began fairly recently, but before this there was a long period during which they experienced relatively minor symptoms. This prodromal period may range from a few months to as much as 5 or 6 years, and its frequency distribution also has a positive skew.

The particular importance of this prodromal phase is that although the symptoms sometimes may be those of a depressive state, they may also reflect a typical anxiety state (neurosis). Surprisingly, such patients often respond well to ECT.

DEPRESSIONS

TYPES OF DEPRESSIONS The classification of depressions goes a long way back in the history of psychiatry, but the number of different classifications and types suggest that no one has been really satisfactory. This is equally true for current classifications.

Retarded depression Psychomotor retardation is a prominent symptom. Whether the psychic or the motor component predominates is not regarded as of practical importance. It is usually accompanied by other biological symptoms (e.g., disturbed sleep, loss of appetite, fatigue, and loss of libido).

Agitated depression The prominent symptom may be agitation, but the other symptoms are much like those in retarded depression. It was said that this type was characteristic of involutional depression.

Endogenous depression In its simplest meaning, endogenous means that it has not been possible to elicit a recognizable psychological precipitating stress that could account for the onset of the illness. In practice, the term is used to signify the opposite of neurotic depression and also to imply that the symptoms are biological. In that case, it combines retarded and agitated depressions.

All three types will be included in DSM-III-R as major depressive episode, and if there have been previous attacks and they have responded well to standard antidepressant therapy, they could be included in the melancholic type.

Reactive depression Reactive depression implies that the disturbed state is clearly related to precipitating stresses. For formal definitions the relation between the two has sometimes been stretched to cover an interval of 3 or even 6 months between the stress and the onset of symptoms. It is implicit that there are no psychotic features. It is generally accepted that the clinical picture is not of the retarded (or endogenous) type but includes much anxiety and associated symptoms.

Even those psychiatrists who are convinced that the depressions are fundamentally biological fully accept that the onset of an acute phase may be precipitated by psychological stresses. Reactive and endogenous are therefore not mutually exclusive. In all the mood disorders, there is some constitutional predisposition, but in the majority of patients, it is always possible to find a reason that the illness should have developed at the time when it did. Predisposition and precipitating stresses are thus complementary.

There has always been difficulty in distinguishing reactive depression from what is described in DSM-III-R as adjustment disorder with depressed mood. If reactive depression is to be distinguished from adjustment disorder, it must be on the basis that the link between the latter and the environmental stresses is clearly present, whereas the former has lost it.

Psychotic depression Psychotic depression should signify a depressive illness with psychotic symptoms (i.e., delusions and hallucinations), but it is often used as a synonym of endogenous depression, at the same time acknowledging that the psychotic symptoms appear only in the more severe cases. In DSM-III-R, psychotic depression is subsumed under major depressive episode, subcategory with psychotic features.

Neurotic depression Insofar as neurotic depression has any meaning, it should be that the disturbance is a reaction of the personality to external stresses but goes beyond the bounds of normal reaction. This implies that the symptoms are excessive and that there is an impaired capacity to carry on a normal life. Although the patients may show disturbed or distorted judgment, they have not lost contact with reality (i.e., have developed delusions or hallucinations). Some psychotherapists would accept the notion of a neurotic depression reaching psychotic intensity.

In the DSM-III-R classification, a neurotically depressed patient, if presenting milder symptoms, would be classified as having adjustment disorder with depressed mood. If the symptoms continue to be mild and the condition lasts for 2 years, it could be classified as dysthymia, but by this time the link with the precipitating stresses would have worn very thin.

Anxious depression Anxious depression refers to a pattern of symptoms, indicating that symptoms of anxiety (both psychological and somatic) are prominent. It could be regarded as a milder form of agitated depression or as an alternative description for neurotic depression, emphasizing the descriptive aspects.

Masked depression In clinical practice, especially office practice, a large proportion of patients will emphasize their somatic symptoms and minimize or deny their psychological ones. They will make much of their loss of appetite, perhaps also loss of weight, their feelings of tiredness and lack of energy, and various aches and pains. This group constitutes the majority of masked depressions, but it is easy to elicit the other symptoms of depressive illness by asking.

It is doubtful if there is any point in having a special category for these patients, except as a teaching device to emphasize the importance of adequate interviewing and history taking. As Francisco Alonso-Fernandez once said, "The somatic symptoms of masked depressions are not so much a mask of the depressions as for our ideas of depressions."

Neurasthenic depression Neurasthenic depression is a term that, if not quite obsolete, should be. It has been used to describe depressive illness in which the symptoms of loss of energy and fatigue are prominent. Patients sometimes make a great point of one particular symptom because they are much disturbed by it, but this is related more to specific aspects of their personality or their circumstances than to the illness itself.

If the patient's condition cannot be classified under the usual DSM-III-R categories, it could well be regarded as dysthymia.

Involutional depression Involutional depression was defined as an agitated depression occurring mainly in women, having an onset in the involutional period (late 40s and 50s) and often precipitated by stresses. The clinical picture showed much anxiety, even with minimal agitation. The personality before the onset of illness was described in terms that were typical of the obsessive or anankastic personality.

This term has now been abandoned on the grounds that it is a distinction that has been made unnecessary by the current classifications. Bipolar depressions have a peak incidence in the late 20s and are found equally in men and women. The clinical picture is predominantly that of retarded depression. Unipolar depressions have a peak onset in the 50s; they are much more common; and they afflict twice as many women as men. Because the obsessional personality is widespread, it is common among depressives.

Paranoid depression Careful inquiry of depressive patients will show that a small proportion (less than 10 percent and probably less than 5 percent) will have mild paranoid ideas, not consonant with their mood. It is important not to confuse them with so-called paraphrenics, who are late-onset schizophrenics severely depressed because of the sudden onset of hallucinatory voices.

Puerperal depression There are three main types of puerperal depression. The first, often called baby blues, is a transitory condition of tearfulness, depression, anxiety, and lethargy. It begins about the third or fourth day postpartum and responds quickly to reassurance and support.

The second type of postnatal depression develops in about the third week of the puerperium and manifests typical depressive symptoms. It can lead to serious disturbance, and although nearly two-thirds of patients recover within a year, the rest are left with residual symptoms.

The third type is a severe disturbance with hallucinations, delusions, and confusion. It begins within 3 months of delivery, with nearly half beginning within the first week. Response to treatment is good.

Seasonal pattern (affective) disorder There are some individuals who become depressed every winter, and so it would appear that this disorder is related to the shortened length of daylight at this season (Table 17.3-2).

Chronic depression At least 10 percent of depressives will have an attack that will last longer than 2 years. Some follow-up studies have reported a figure more than twice as high for the development of chronicity. Most of the cases are of the unipolar type, with previous bouts that have been successfully treated. About one patient in three has a positive family history of clear-cut depressions, often quite severe and found in more than one relative. The premorbid personality was well adjusted, but by the time the patients reach this stage, they may be involved in many troubles (e.g., alcoholism or drug abuse). For this reason, many of these patients are misdiagnosed as having a personality disorder.

Atypical depression The classical descriptions of depressive illness were based on patients admitted to mental

TABLE 17.3-2
Diagnostic Criteria for Seasonal Pattern

A. There has been a regular temporal relationship between the onset of an episode of bipolar disorder (including bipolar disorder NOS) or recurrent major depression (including depressive disorder NOS) and a particular 60-day period of the year (e.g., regular appearance of depression between the beginning of October and the end of November). **Note:** Do not include cases in which there is an obvious effect of seasonally related psychosocial stressors, e.g., regularly being unemployed every winter.
B. Full remissions (or a change from depression to mania or hypomania) also occurred within a particular 60-day period of the year (eg., depression disappears from mid-February to mid-April).
C. There have been at least three episodes of mood disturbance in 3 separate years that demonstrated the temporal seasonal relationship defined in A and B; at least 2 of the years were consecutive.
D. Seasonal episodes of mood disturbance, as described above, outnumbered any nonseasonal episodes of such disturbance that may have occurred by more than three to one.

Table from DSM-III-R *Diagnostic and Statistical Manual of Mental Disorders,* ed 3, revised. Copyright American Psychiatric Association, Washington, DC, 1987. Used with permission.

hospitals, often involuntarily. The majority of depressives who now come for treatment, especially those seen in office practice, show a very different clinical picture. In that sense, the majority of patients who now come for treatment are atypical.

All good classifications retain an "et cetera" group, indicating thereby that they have not yet reached perfection. For those patients whose anomalous features make it difficult to fit them into the standard groups, there is the category depressive disorder not otherwise specified. The examples given are (1) major depressive episode superimposed on residual schizophrenia, a type that will be found if sought among the patients in the geriatric and long-stay wards of mental hospitals; (2) intermittent dysthymic episodes; and (3) non-stress-related depressive episodes that do not meet the criteria for a major depressive episode.

A few clinical conditions (e.g., school phobia, anorexia and bulimia nervosa, and facial pain) have been reported to respond to treatment with antidepressant drugs. This response may signify that there is some relationship among these disorders or, alternatively, that they are responding to different actions of the drugs. The fact that both headaches and rheumatoid arthritis respond to salicylate drugs does not signify that they are related disorders.

SYMPTOMS OF DEPRESSIVE ILLNESS A change of affect is regarded as the central clinical feature of the mood disorders. In the case of the manias, the mood is elevated and is described as euphoric. The lowering of mood, depression, has now given the name to the disorders formerly known as melancholias.

Depression is a normal experience of human beings and the higher vertebrates and probably is found well down the evolutionary scale. It is the mood that people experience when they lose something important or when they fail to obtain something for which they had been hoping. As such, it is part of the inbuilt emotional mechanisms. Whatever pathological processes lead to depressive illness, they seem to use these mechanisms. Consequently, there is considerable resemblance, or overlap, between the manifestations of depressive illness and those of normal depression. The distinction between normal and abnormal depressive mood and between normal depression and depressive illness must be considered.

Depressed mood From the clinical point of view, the central and most typical features of the depressive illnesses are the three symptoms: depressed mood, guilt, and suicide. But what is meant by typical? A distinction must be made between what is most common and what is characteristic in the sense of making the diagnosis of depressive illness very probable and other diagnoses very improbable. The most relevant of the three characteristic symptoms is depressed mood, as it is always present to a lesser or greater degree, although patients may not necessarily mention it at interview. Most often this is because they may be reluctant to mention psychological symptoms for fear of being labeled as neurotic, but sometimes it is because they regard their depression as being a reaction secondary to their other troubles. The author remembers vividly an elderly man who had recounted his various symptoms without mentioning depression. When asked if he felt depressed, he replied, "But doctor, if you couldn't sleep, and you couldn't concentrate, and you had no appetite, always felt tired, and couldn't go with your wife, wouldn't you feel depressed?"

In its mildest forms, such patients experience a flattening of affect, an inability to respond to the mood of the occasion. They cannot laugh at jokes, be delighted by some fortunate event, or be at one with the cheerfulness of a group.

As the depression increases, the patients recognize that they are miserable and unhappy, and so do those around them. They become preoccupied with gloomy thoughts and tend to look on the black side of things. At first, they can be distracted from their preoccupations or can be persuaded to "snap out of it" and, with an effort, may regain their normal cheerfulness. At this stage, they will respond temporarily to comfort and reassurance, but this becomes more and more difficult.

They experience a tendency to weep which they find increasingly difficult and eventually impossible to control. Expressions of sympathy will move them to tears, often in quite early stages of the development of their illness. Many men, and some women, will be ashamed to mention their tearfulness and will admit to it reluctantly only when questioned. The author saw a man burst into a fit of weeping that he could not stop, when asked in a friendly fashion if he were liable to tears. However, when their mood is sufficiently depressed, patients reach a stage "beyond weeping," when they come to think their feelings would be relieved if only their tears could come.

A feature that helps distinguish an abnormal from a normal depressed mood is the disturbance of judgment so often found in the former. Patients not only are preoccupied with the gloomy side of things, but they also feel that everything is valueless and futile. The future is hopeless, and the past was useless. Often they are convinced that they will never get better and that their doctors' efforts will fail and are nothing but a waste of time and effort. But they will usually be too polite to mention this.

Over half of depressives change their drinking habits at the onset of the depression, some of them increasing their consumption and others decreasing it.

Guilt About three in four patients exhibit guilt in some degree. At its mildest, the patients feel vaguely that it is their fault that they are in their present state and that they would do better if only they could bring themselves to the effort. This self-accusation is recognizably different from the attitude of most patients toward their illness which they feel they have brought on themselves: "If I hadn't eaten that dinner, I would not have been sick"; "Had I worn my coat, I would not have caught cold." But these are explanations rather than self-accusations.

Patients often look back on their lives in order to find something about which they can feel guilty and self-accusatory. In the nature of things, most people find little difficulty in bringing up appropriate sins. The student feels she has been lazy; the businessman has neglected opportunities; a man admits he has been unkind or cruel to his wife; and a woman may be convinced that she has neglected her children. All these tales may be quite true, but only naive interviewers will take these stories at their face value. What the patients cannot explain is why they have felt guilty only in the last few months since their other symptoms began.

With the increasing severity of the symptom, the ideas of guilt begin to take on a delusional quality, although nowadays patients usually receive treatment before they reach this stage. The contents of the delusions are appropriate to the patients' interests and personalities. The author remembers one young English sportsman who was convinced that the English had been defeated by the Australians in a recent cricket match because of his wickedness. He was not convinced when the author explained that up until that time this was the expected outcome in such matches. And a woman, who had previously been a missionary in Africa, was always found lying on the floor under her bed: She explained that she was too sinful to deserve the comfort of a proper bed. Patients may believe that they have been cast out from society or are going to be punished for what they have done (e.g., the police are looking for them in order to arrest them for their crimes). Such a delusion is not persecutory, as it is consonant with the patient's mood.

Even rarer are hallucinatory voices that accuse the patients of dreadful crimes or sins or threaten to punish them for their misdeeds. Occasionally, the voices urge the patient to commit suicide. Again, it is important to recognize that all this is appropriate to the patient's character, attitudes, and current mood.

It is often said that guilt feelings do not appear in patients from African and Asian cultures. As always, it is necessary to distinguish between the basic nature of a symptom and the way the patients express it. Underlying guilt is basically a feeling of inadequacy. In patients of European traditions, it is expressed as guilt; in others, often as shame or some equivalent.

Suicide Some suicidal thoughts are present in four out of five patients, and in three out of five they are more than trivial. Usually, the symptom develops slowly. At its mildest, the patients feel that life is a burden and is scarcely worth living. With the symptom's increasing severity, the patients may wish that they could fall asleep and never wake up or perhaps die suddenly or be killed in a traffic accident. After that, they begin to toy with thoughts of killing themselves in some way. These thoughts may eventually change to specific plans that culminate in an actual attempt. Sometimes a patient who has shown few or no suicidal thoughts will attempt suicide, but if the attempt does not succeed, an explanation for this sudden impulse will probably not be forthcoming. The risk of suicide must always be considered once a diagnosis of a depressive illness has been made, and particularly so if there has been an attempt in a previous attack. One in six depressives eventually commits suicide. The risk of suicide is greater in men, older women, and those living alone.

Not all attempted suicide is a failed attempt at self-murder. Sometimes the act is an attempt to attract attention, a search for help. Often both the two motives are present in varying degrees. In a sense, the act may be a gamble with death. But it should always be taken seriously, as it is known that further attempts occur at a rate of 16 percent per year. Much work has been carried out on parasuicide, and although it is accepted that the majority of such cases do not suffer from a depressive illness, they do among 40 percent of female and 28 percent of male cases.

Loss of interest (anhedonia) Loss of interest is as characteristic and as common as is depressed mood, although it is not included in the traditional three symptoms of depressive illness. In fact, it would be better to talk of the typical tetrad of symptoms. Subjectively, it appears as a loss of satisfaction and pleasure from experiences, hence the current term "anhedonia." In its mildest forms, it will be expressed as a difficulty in maintaining concentration and interest in normal activities. The patient becomes bored very easily. Objectively, it appears as a steadily increasing disinclination to take part in normal activities. Work becomes increasingly difficult as interest fades. Mildly ill patients may exaggerate this because of their feelings of inadequacy. Concentration diminishes, decisions are put off, and activity slows. Even when the patients struggle to continue working, their indecisiveness may make their efforts almost useless. The work eventually accumulates until the patients cannot face it and finally give up. Much the same applies to the patients' hobbies: Interest and activity steadily diminish until finally they cease. The golfer lets his clubs rust; the gardener lets the weeds grow.

Housewives become less interested in those aspects of their work that previously they most enjoyed. They simplify it and reduce it to a minimum, cleaning and tidying less frequently, simplifying their cooking and giving up those activities, such as needlework, that they enjoyed more as a hobby. Even when they reach the stage at which men will have given up their work completely, they will often still be carrying on at a minimal, desultory level.

Anxiety Anxiety is not regarded as characteristic of the depressions; indeed in the classic retarded or endogenous depression, it may be completely absent or, at least, appear to be absent. Nevertheless, in current clinical practice, it is the third most common symptom (Table 17.3-3). Subjectively, it is experienced as a state of continual apprehension. Patients feel tense and are unable to relax. Accompanying this is a difficulty in concentration and lack of attention. Not surprisingly, these patients complain of forgetfulness, and they are often irritable (i.e., they tend toward outbursts of ill temper at the slightest frustration).

TABLE 17.3-3
Most Common Symptoms of Depressive Illness (Based on Rating-Scale Items)

Women		*Men*	
Depressed mood	100%	Depressed mood	100%
Loss of interest	99	Loss of interest	99
Anxiety (psychic)	96	Anxiety (psychic)	96
Loss of energy	94	Insomnia (initial)	86
Somatic general	91	Anxiety (somatic)	86
Anxiety (somatic)	86	Loss of energy	82
Loss of appetite	84	Suicide	82
Suicide	80	Loss of appetite	80
Guilt	73	Guilt	72
Weight loss	69	Libido	60

The psychological aspects of anxiety are usually accompanied by somatic symptoms, most of which indicate overactivity of the sympathetic nervous system. Patients complain of attacks of palpitations not related to exercise, pain in the precordium, and sometimes "missed heart-beats." They complain of dryness of mouth, indigestion (epigastric discomfort or pain), wind (air swallowing and eructation), and, much less often, colic and diarrhea. They tend to sweat, especially in the hands, axillae, and feet. Headache and giddiness are also common.

Disturbances of sleep Current theories and research on the depressions now give greater significance to disturbances of sleep. About four out of five depressives suffer from disturbances of sleep, usually a difficulty in falling asleep. Patients complain of tossing and turning restlessly, worrying about anything and everything and unable to fall asleep. Almost as common is insomnia delayed to the end of the sleep period. The patient wakes in the early hours of the morning and is unable to fall asleep again. When the symptom is mild, the loss of sleep may be less than an hour, but when it is severe, the loss may be of several hours. It is generally said that delayed insomnia is typical of the endogenous type of depressive illness, but this symptom seems to be more indicative of the illness's severity. It is more common in older than in younger persons. Some patients say that they may finally fall asleep for a few minutes just before they normally get up.

Another type of insomnia is that in which patients wake during the middle of the night and, after a period of restlessness, fall asleep again for some time. This symptom is less common than the other two types of insomina, but occurs in about half of the patients.

However mild the insomnia may be, the patients complain that they do not feel refreshed in the mornings. In whatever way it starts, the insomnia tends to spread to include the other kinds of insomnia as it becomes more severe. Patients may have unpleasant dreams with a depressed content, from which they awake (sometimes without remembering the dream) in tears. The inadequate sleep of the night may be partially recompensed by a short nap during the day. A rare symptom is that of hypersomnia: Patients complain that they need an excessive amount of sleep. This symptom has been confirmed by continuous electroencephalographic (EEG) recordings.

Somatic symptoms GENERAL Some somatic symptoms are particularly characteristic of the depressions and may even come to dominate the clinical picture. One is a general loss of energy, which is more common in women than in men. Patients find it difficult to get started on any activity, however trivial, and they quickly become tired. As the symptom progresses, the feeling of tiredness becomes continuous and increases until everything becomes too much of an effort. Patients may complain that they feel completely exhausted all the time, and this symptom may dominate the clinical picture. Nothing can be found to explain this very subjective feeling.

Sometimes the patients will complain of vague fleeting aches in their muscles and of headaches, which are frequently located at the back of the neck. These symptoms tend to be overshadowed by the fatigue, and patients will often not mention them unless specifically asked.

GASTROINTESTINAL The earliest gastrointestinal symptom is a slight decrease in appetite sometimes accompanied by a bad taste in the mouth. Patients lose their interest in food, which seems to be tasteless. They do not feel hungry and have to force themselves to eat. As the symptom worsens, they eat less and less until they can scarcely be persuaded to eat anything. Patients sometimes refuse to eat, saying that they do not deserve to eat because of their wickedness, that they should not take food from those who are hungry, and so on. Such expressions of feelings of guilt should not be confused with a true loss of appetite.

Patients may complain of dryness of the mouth, and it has been demonstrated that this is the result of a decrease in salivation. It has been shown that in the depressions, the activity of the whole gastrointestinal tract is reduced, including hypotonia. The last may account for the occasional descriptions of a feeling of heaviness in the abdomen.

Constipation is a frequent complaint of the patients, and undoubtedly it does occur, but not as often as was once thought. First, it is a popular belief that constipation is extremely common and that it is the cause of all sorts of minor symptoms. As a result, patients will often say that they are constipated because they assume that this must be the cause of their symptoms. Their statements should be checked by asking them if they have always been constipated and, if so, whether it worsened when they became ill. Without clear evidence, it is unwise to accept the presence of constipation.

LOSS OF WEIGHT Patients will lose weight if they do not eat enough, but often it will be clear that they have lost weight (e.g., their faces are thinner, and their clothes have become loose) even if there is nothing to suggest that they are eating less. As their illness abates, their weight will return to normal, but this sometimes happens so quickly that it is difficult to believe that the loss of weight is a true loss of bodily tissue, rather than a change in water retention.

HYPOCHONDRIASIS Hypochondriasis is one of the less common symptoms, occurring in about a third of the patients. It is a psychological or behavioral symptom, but it is convenient, because of the nature of the patients' complaints, to deal with it here. This symptom has been variously defined, but its central feature is a conviction of the possibility or presence of some disease, generally serious or even fatal. The belief is not a delusion, because often the patients can be convinced that their fears are mistaken. The effects of the reassurance are brief because the patients soon return, either with the same complaint or another one. However, when this symptom is sufficiently severe, it may attain delusional intensity. It should not be confused with an excessive preoccupation with matters relating to health, fitness, diet, bowel washouts, and so on. Hypochondriasis is not a unitary condition, and it is not well understood. As the author has often pointed out, the valetudinarian is a well-known figure of fun in novels and on the stage, but it is doubtful if he is suffering from a depressive illness.

LOSS OF LIBIDO Loss of libido occurs early in the development of a depressive illness. This is in sharp contrast with the anxiety states, in which quite severely disturbed patients may yet be able to carry on normal, or nearly normal, sexual activity. Men may complain of difficulty with erections, of an inability to ejaculate, and finally of complete impotence. Even in the earliest stages, there is a loss of sexual desire. In older patients, this symptom becomes less prominent; however, because sexual function is already diminishing, the additional impairment from the illness is very quickly noticed.

Women also experience a loss of sexual interest, although

they tend to make very much less of it as a symptom. Perhaps this is because, as some believe, sexual desire in women is somewhat less of a drive than in men and more of a response to stimulus. It can be very difficult to obtain satisfactory information about libido in a woman of 50 years, who has been widowed for 20 of them. The chief complaint is of frigidity, and women who declare that they have never enjoyed sexual intercourse sense a change in feeling. It is sad to hear that they used to tolerate sexual intercourse as one of the chores of married life, but now they cannot even do that.

It is not uncommon to find that loss of libido is one of the earliest symptoms to appear, but one of the last to disappear as the patient improves.

Retardation Retardation is found in about half of the patients. When it occurs, it is typical of the depressions, but in its mildest form it is more a sign than a symptom and may be difficult to detect. One must look for a slight diminution of mobility of facies, a slight flattening of the voice, or an impression of relative postural immobility. One way of demonstrating mild retardation is to break one of the rules of social intercourse: When in the course of the interview, it is the physician's turn to speak, he or she then remains silent. Most patients become more and more anxious and disturbed until finally they feel forced to break the silence with some remark. But in this situation, the retarded patients sit silent and still, apparently immersed in their miserable preoccupations and entirely unresponsive to the breach of good manners. Schizophrenic patients also are undisturbed, but they give the impression that it is because they are completely unaware that there is anything wrong.

Subjectively, there is a slowness or difficulty in thinking, often accompanied by a poverty of ideas, of which the patients are well aware. This difficulty in thinking may lead to lack of concentration and great indecisiveness. Some patients complain not so much of a slowness of thoughts or an inability to think at all as of thoughts that go round and round in the same circle.

As the symptom worsens, the patients take an increasingly longer time to respond to questions; the intervals between their words become obviously greater; their voice fades; and their speech becomes an indistinct mumble and finally ceases.

At the same time, the patients' activity diminishes. Their walk is slow and dragging, and they are bowed down as if carrying a great weight on their shoulders. All their movements are difficult and require a great effort to get started. The patients sit with head bent, gazing at the floor, with their hands on their lap and unresponsive to their surroundings.

Agitation Agitation must be regarded, in the present context, as the motor expression of anxiety. It is found in about three out of four female patients and is therefore twice as common in them as is retardation. It is less common in male patients, in whom it is found about as frequently as is retardation. Anxious patients always have some difficulty sitting still and continually shift in their chair. They tend to fidget with cigarettes, handbag, or just their fingers. Sometimes they are sufficiently embarrassed by this symptom to attempt to control it and will hold onto the arms of their chair, grip a handbag or case firmly, or even just hold their hands tightly together. When they succeed in controlling themselves in this way, their feet often become restless.

As the symptom becomes worse, the restlessness becomes greater and more difficult to control. The author saw a patient suddenly stand up during the interview and then sit down again after a few seconds. Grosser forms of this symptom are now seen very rarely, as it responds very well to treatment. Sometimes, the patients cannot sit at all and pace up and down the room so that interviews have to be conducted "on the run." They will tear at their hands and face and hair and will moan continuously. If forced to sit, they will rock backwards and forwards and then struggle to get up. A severely agitated patient can be a heartrending sight.

Diurnal variation of symptoms A diurnal variation of symptoms has long been recognized as a typical symptom in depressive illness, although there is much controversy as to whether it is confined to endogenous depression or can be found also in neurotic depression. Whatever the method of subdividing the depressions, the diurnal variation of symptoms is not confined to one group. In clinical practice, it will be found in about half the patients. Among these, the great majority complain that they feel at their worst in the mornings. Most of the rest say that they feel worse in the evenings. A small proportion insist that their symptoms peak in the middle of the day. Clearly, the presence of this symptom helps confirm the diagnosis, but by itself it is by no means sufficient. Alcoholics also feel bad in the mornings.

Panic attacks It is now more or less generally accepted that attacks of panic are part of one of the syndromes of anxiety states. However, they can occur in patients whose symptoms include some that are typical of the depressive illnesses. The fact that panic attacks may respond to treatment with antidepressant tricyclic drugs suggests that the current classifications are by no means in their final state.

The symptoms of panic attacks are varied and appear suddenly for no known reason. The attacks usually start with severe palpitations, breathlessness, and perhaps pain in the chest. The patients may feel dizzy, faint, and trembly and choke and sweat. The anxiety is intense, and the patients may be convinced that they are about to die, even if they are well aware that they have had previous nonfatal attacks.

Loss of insight It might seem that insight is an all-or-none phenomenon: Either a person does or does not have insight. But in clinical practice this is not true. Whereas in mania, insight is absent almost invariably from the beginning, depressed patients are well aware that something is wrong with them. When asked if they understand that they have a mental or emotional illness, they may deny it, but they will do so for many different reasons. The most obvious is that they do not wish to be labeled as mental or neurotic, even though they recognize that that is the nature of their disturbance. In other cases they will regard the mental symptoms, especially depression, as secondary or a reaction to their other symptoms. The lack of knowledge and understanding and their cultural background may also produce equivocal answers. Careful questioning will soon clarify the situation.

It is when patients begin to feel that their condition is a punishment for their sins that they begin to lose insight. The conviction and the insight tend to be reciprocal, and both can exist in a halfway state. Some evidence of loss of insight can be found in about one in three patients at the most, but this depends on the type of clinical practice.

Uncommon symptoms Vague and ill-defined paranoid ideas may be present, and diligent inquiry will find this symptom in about one in ten patients. The defining feature is that the ideas are not consonant with the depressive mood. The only significance they have clinically is that such patients tend to respond poorly to treatment.

Obsessional thoughts and even compulsive rituals can occur in depressive illness. They are rarely severe and appear with the onset of the illness, fading with recovery.

Depersonalization and derealization have also been associated with depressive illness. They, too, disappear as the patient recovers, and their chief significance is in relation to the management of the patient. It is important that this symptom be elicited if it is present and the patient given appropriate reassurance.

Instead of losing their appetite, some patients overeat. The symptom is uncommon and is usually associated with anxiety. It is more common in women than in men. Again, disturbance of sleep may sometimes show as hypersomnia.

The clinical condition may show a mixture of manic and depressive symptoms. This is extremely uncommon (and its existence has even been queried) and is usually viewed as the presence of depressive symptoms in a patient going through a manic attack rather than the opposite.

A rare symptom is that of disturbed behavior occurring in a setting of clinical depression and that is quite out of keeping with the patient's character (e.g., shoplifting or indecent exposure). It is analogous in adults of the disturbed behavior found in depressed children.

All persons are unique, and most patients will have some odd symptom that fits in with their personality and the circumstances of their illness. Odd symptoms also may indicate that there is an organic basis of the depressive illness.

DIAGNOSIS Once it appears that the patient is suffering from a depressive illness, it is necessary to answer three questions before a final diagnosis can be made:

1. Is the patient suffering from a pathological condition, or is the behavior within normal bounds?
2. Is this one of the varieties of depressive illness or of anxiety states?
3. Is there an organic or toxic basis for the condition?

Only when the answers to these questions have been found is it possible to continue with the usual process of diagnosis of a depressive illness and differential diagnosis from other mental disorders.

Normal or not? Depression is the normal human reaction to the loss of something valued. Normal must be judged from the person's viewpoint. A serious loss will produce a greater reaction than will a minor one, but what is serious to one individual may be trivial to another. Old people may have to face very real problems about which they do not necessarily complain or which they minimize. The intensity of the reaction should also be judged in terms of the personality's reactivity. Some persons are stolid and unemotional, whereas others show great lability in their moods. The reaction to the death of a beloved relative, to the loss of livelihood, or to the sudden learning of a dreadful fate can have devastating effects on an individual. These symptoms can be as severe and as disturbing—both to the sufferer and near friends and relatives—as any pathological depressive state.

Despite this clinical resemblance, there is a fundamental difference between a normal reaction to loss and a pathological condition. Against the background of personality and severity of stress, the distinction between normal and morbid depends on the relationship of the person's state to the real world. Emotional reactions not only are precipitated by external circumstances but also change directly in relation to them. A depressive illness, whatever may be its precipitating factors, develops autonomously according to its own characteristics. For example, the reaction of parents to the news of their child's death will change immediately once they discover that the news is false. Conversely, a depressed businessman who is convinced that he is bankrupt will not be affected by the evidence that his business is doing well.

The difficulty lies in the fact that although an acute and severe depressive state can develop rapidly without any discoverable reason for its onset, for most patients it is possible to find some explanation of why the condition should have appeared at that particular time and no other. The precipitating stress may have been comparatively minor, its role being recognized because in previous attacks there were also similar minor precipitants. Or it may be of such a nature that almost everybody would show an extreme reaction to it.

At one time, the distinction between endogenous and reactive depressions was regarded as fundamental, and attempts were made—but with only moderate success—to demonstrate that the two conditions differed in their symptoms, course, and so forth. It is now generally, though not universally, accepted that the relationship between constitutional predisposition and environmental precipitants is one of a continuous balance and not an "either-or."

The distinction between a normal and an abnormal depressive state is not one that can be defined easily by a few criteria. Would ordinary human experience judge the condition as within normal bounds or not? This should take into account the significance of the loss to the individual and the reactivity of the personality (the variations here are greater than is generally realized, even by psychiatrists). Has anything like this happened before to the sufferer, and if so, what was the outcome? If the patient has an opinion on this, how plausible is it to an outsider? Is there a history of mood disorder in the patient or relatives? Although in most cases the decision may be reasonably easy to make, there will always be some for which there is no easy answer. It is then necessary to consider very carefully the nature of the precipitant, the type of personality, the previous history (both social and medical), and any information from others that may be helpful.

If there is still doubt, the best action is to observe the patient, to give such comfort and reassurance as may be helpful, and to wait. The comfort and reassurance may be what friends and relatives would give, although it will usually be more convincing coming from a pschiatrist with a background of experience. Or it could be some form of formal psychotherapy. Normal reactions to loss begin to resolve fairly quickly, although not necessarily continuously. If there is still doubt about the nature of the condition, the premature introduction of biological treatments will usually not be helpful, either to the patient or to the physician's reputation.

Differential diagnosis ANXIETY STATE There is generally no difficulty in coming to a diagnosis when the patient is severely ill. But a diagnosis can be more difficult in those patients who are less disturbed, particularly as there is considerable overlap in the symptoms of depressive and anxiety states. Thus, in the latter condition, four out of five patients complain of depressed mood and of disturbed sleep. In depressive patients, the proportion that complains of symptoms of anxiety is even higher (Table 17.3-4).

TABLE 17.3-4
Percentage Frequency of Anxiety Symptoms Common in Depressive Illness

	M	*F*
Anxiety, psychic	97	98
Anxiety, somatic	87	87
Insomnia, initial	84	78
Agitation	68	68

TABLE 17.3-5
Symptoms Distinguishing Between Anxiety States and Depressive Illness

	Anxiety States	*Depressive Illness*
Sleep	Nightmares	Waking depressed
Gastrointestinal	Indigestion, wind	Loss of appetite
Sexual (M)	Premature ejacul.	Loss of libido
(W)	Dispareunia	Loss of libido

In patients with much milder illnesses—and these constitute the majority of the patients who attend a general practitioner—the overlap of symptoms is even greater, and diagnosis is therefore much more difficult. There are a few symptoms that are particularly helpful, such as loss of appetite, impaired libido, and disturbed sleep (Table 17.3-5), but it is the total pattern that should be considered.

The onset of anxiety states tends to be more abrupt than that of the depressions, and the first breakdown occurs earlier, in the 20s or teens. In general, the symptoms of anxiety states are more responsive than are those of the depressions to suggestion and placebos. Although the patient may suffer from depressed mood, it tends to be episodic and fluctuating, responsive to external circumstances, similar to but not as markedly as anxious mood is. Patients often say that they can more or less easily "shake myself out of it." Agoraphobic patients may not mention their disability, even when they are almost completely house bound, and they may even deny its existence even when questioned. In case of doubt, the patient's statements should be checked with the relatives. Somatic symptoms are frequent and may dominate the clinical picture. They are of the type associated with overactivity of the adrenergic autonomic nervous system. Sexual function is disturbed. In men this is usually premature ejaculation or an inability to maintain an erection; in women it may appear as anorgasmia but more commonly as dyspareunia.

The background of anxiety states can help make the diagnosis. The previous personality can usually best be described as an anxious disposition, which may have been recognized from earliest childhood. There may be a personal history of previous bouts. If there is a hereditary predisposition, there will be a family history of anxiety states, alcoholism, or even personality disorder. Finally, precipitating stresses are likely to be such that the patient regards them as some sort of threat.

Aside from the common symptoms of the depressive states (described above) that are required to make a diagnosis, it is well to remember that the biological symptoms should indicate a deficiency of function, rather than the overactivity of the autonomic nervous system. The previous history of the patient and of the family may be helpful in making a diagnosis of a depressive illness. There may be a family history of depressions and sometimes even of suicides. Previous attacks may have been recognizably depressive. The patient's personality is typically well adjusted, often euthymic, sociable, and extroverted. Finally, the precipitating stress, when present, is usually recognizable as some sort of loss.

The current confusion between depressive illness and anxiety state will doubtless be made clear one day, but whatever may come about from future research, clinical practice still requires the distinction to be made. The reason is simple: The current effective treatments are different, and, therefore, the differential diagnosis is important.

In actual clinical practice, even the most careful examination and interviewing of the patient will still leave some cases undiagnosed. For these mildly ill patients, the best course is to wait until time makes the diagnosis clear. Patients can be reassured about the nature of their illness and its good prognosis. It is surprising how helpful this can be, and it has no side effects. Sound judgment is always better than enthusiasm in the treatment of patients.

ORGANIC OR TOXIC BASIS Whereas an organic condition can present as a psychiatric disorder, (e.g., thyrotoxicosis may look like an anxiety state, and dementia may resemble a depressive illness), the presentation may also be the other way around. This will be particularly important when patients are reluctant to mention their psychological symptoms, for fear of being labeled neurotic, or sometimes when they think that doctors are concerned only with somatic symptoms. Either way, the patients do not mention their psychological symptoms or minimize them or explain them away. Only too often, therefore, the problem of diagnosis is that of recognizing a mental disturbance when it is presented under the guise of physical symptoms.

In the case of the depressions, however, even when the diagnosis seems obvious, it is wise to consider the possibility of an organic basis. Myxoedema can closely mimic a mild depression in its history and symptoms. Typical depressive illness has appeared against a background of undetected diabetes mellitus, Addison's anemia, early dementia, cerebral arteriosclerosis, cerebral tumor (of which nearly 20 percent have depressions), and even, in the old days, general paresis. Other possibilities that must be considered are vitamin B_2 deficiency, electrolyte imbalance, or early parkinsonism. Drugs can produce similar symptoms, the most common offenders being the antihypertensive drugs, reserpine, estrogen, α-methyldopa, propranolol (Inderal), hydralazine (Apresoline), guanethidine (Esimil, Ismelin), and clonidine (Catapres).

The problem is twofold. First, what may seem to be a straightforward depressive illness may be a manifestation of an organic disease not immediately recognizable. Second, depressive illness may occur in a patient already suffering from an organic disease that may have been present for a short or long time. Severe somatic disease does not immunize a person against depressive illness; on the contrary, in a person already predisposed (e.g., with a record of previous attacks or a positive family history), it may be an important precipitating factor.

If the first possibility applies, then simple clinical examination and tests should eliminate the most likely organic conditions. After that, it is not worth carrying out investigations for uncommon diseases. Because they are uncommon, most of the time, nothing will be found, and a fruitless search for rarities is obviously wasteful when one considers that anxiety and depressive states are common. The only time when obscure organic disease must be seriously considered is when the patient manifests atypical symptoms suggestive of organic disease (e.g., clouding of consciousness, slight confusion).

Diagnosis of depressions in clinical practice The diagnosis of depressive disorder, as with any other, must be made on positive grounds. Depressed mood is always present, even if only very mild. It is always more persistent than the depression of anxiety states and is usually worse in the mornings. Next to depression, the most common and most important symptom to look for is a loss of interest in life, work, hobbies, and normal activities. After that the clinician places great weight on the somatic symptoms of loss of appetite, energy, libido, and weight. Feelings of self-reproach and guilt will usually be present, and thoughts of suicide, quite often. Except in the severely ill patients, these symptoms will usually be elicited only on questioning. They are not only among the most common but are also the most characteristic symptoms of depressions. Delayed insomnia is of little help in the milder cases, but a particularly useful sign when it is detected is psychomotor retardation.

The diagnosis cannot be completed until the current condition is considered in relation to the background. The presence or absence of a precipitating stress and its nature must be considered. Unfortunately, patients do not always tell the truth about these things. Old people, in particular, may have problems that they are extremely reluctant to mention. Information should be sought about a first attack in the 30s, a history of previous attacks of depression, and a family history of depression or suicide. The patients may have had well-adjusted personalities when they were well.

Patients may show severe depressive symptoms against a background of other mental disorder. These will usually be apparent from the symptoms but may not be so in the more uncommon psychiatric conditions. Careful routine history taking should reveal the hallucinations of the paraphrenic who presents as a depressive, or the compulsive rituals of the obsessional who mentions only the symptoms of anxiety and depression.

Depression in the elderly After the age of 65, the incidence of depressive illness in men rises to about equal that in women. Life events become particularly traumatic, and patients have great difficulty in recovering from their effects. Psychotic symptoms are common and contribute to the poor response to treatment. Although not common, the symptoms of impaired memory, confusion, and disorientation may lead to a diagnosis of dementia. However, depressions are more common than are dementias until about 75 years of age. The risk of suicide in these patients is very great, and what may seem to be an abortive attempt or a mere parasuicide must be taken seriously. It is even more important in these suicidally depressed patients to consider the possibility of organic disease in the background of the patients' condition. In general, when psychotic symptoms, poor health, and problems with drug treatments are present in older patients, the outcome is unsatisfactory.

Depression in children and adolescents Depressive states can occur in children and are not a rarity. In infants deprived of proper mothering, there may appear a condition known as analytic depression (reactive attachment disorder of infancy), which is characterized by lack of thriving, cessation of growth, and regression of behavior. In older children, a depressive state is common as an underlying cause of behavior disorders.

Adolescents' symptoms generally resemble those in adults, although it has been claimed that hypersomnia is more common in this age group than in older patients. The loss of interest and working capacity may make the patients withdraw from all personal and social activities and relationships, which may lead to a mistaken diagnosis of early schizophrenia.

DSM-III-R CRITERIA Despite constant efforts to refine diagnostic criteria and procedures, these are still by no means satisfactory. Follow-up studies have shown that reactive depressions can sometimes be rediagnosed as primary depressive disorder. Even the Research Diagnostic Criteria (RDC), which were set up to produce a homogeneous group suitable for research purposes, have been shown to mix together endogenous and neurotic depressions. Indeed, no mere checklist of clinical features could be expected to select a completely homogeneous group of patients.

As an illustration, compare the symptoms of the following two patients, each of whom could be diagnosed as having a major depressive episode according to the criteria in DSM-III-R:

Patient 1	*Patient 2*
Depressed mood	Depressed mood
Impaired appetite	Loss of interest
Insomnia	Retardation
Weariness and lack of energy	Feelings of guilt
Lack of concentration	Suicidal thoughts

The difference between them is great and cannot be ascribed to mere differences in severity of illness. Even so, the criteria laid down by DSM-III-R are a great advance on the previous edition and compare well with the ICD-9 of the World Health Organization.

Major depressive episode For a major depressive episode, the symptoms should have been present every or nearly every day for at least 2 weeks (Table 17.3-6). Depressed mood, present much of the day, or loss of interest in almost all activities is essential. In addition, there must be present at least four other symptoms (which can include the one from the above two not already included) from the following seven:

Significant loss of appetite or loss of weight or, alternatively, a gain.
Insomnia or, alternatively, hypersomnia.
Psychomotor retardation or agitation clearly observable.
Fatigue or loss of energy.
Feelings of guilt or worthlessness.
Difficulties with thinking, concentration, or making decisions.
Thoughts of death and suicide up to a suicidal attempt.

Note that although anxiety is common in the depressions, it is not included in this list. Exclusion criteria fall into three groups. The first requires the exclusion of organic or toxic factors and a normal grief or bereavement reaction. The second requires that delusions or hallucinations (persistent for not less than 2 weeks) not be present in the absence of prominent affective symptoms. Finally, the condition should not be superimposed on schizophrenia, schizophreniform, or delusional disorder.

If these criteria are fulfilled, the patient's diagnosis for a first attack is major depression, single episode (Table 17.3-7), and for second and subsequent attacks, it is major depression, recurrent (Table 17.3-8). If there is a history of manic attacks, the diagnosis will come under bipolar disorder. Another disorder noted in DSM-III-R is depressive disorder not otherwise specified. It is described in Table 17.3-9.

TABLE 17.3-6
Diagnostic Criteria for Major Depressive Episode

Note: A major depressive syndrome is defined as criterion A below.

A. At least five of the following symptoms have been present during the same 2-week period and represent a change from previous functioning; at least one of the symptoms is either (1) depressed mood, or (2) loss of interest or pleasure. (Do not include symptoms that are clearly due to a physical condition, mood-incongruent delusions or hallucinations, incoherence, or marked loosening of associations.)
   (1) depressed mood (or can be irritable mood in children and adolescents) most of the day, nearly every day, as indicated either by subjective account or observation by others
   (2) markedly diminished interest or pleasure in all, or almost all, activities most of the day, nearly every day (as indicated either by subjective account or observation by others of apathy most of the time)
   (3) significant weight loss or weight gain when not dieting (e.g., more than 5% of body weight in a month), or decrease or increase in appetite nearly every day (in children, consider failure to make expected weight gains)
   (4) insomnia or hypersomnia nearly every day
   (5) psychomotor agitation or retardation nearly every day (observable by others, not merely subjective feelings of restlessness or being slowed down)
   (6) fatigue or loss of energy nearly every day
   (7) feelings of worthlessness or excessive or inappropriate guilt (which may be delusional) nearly every day (not merely self-reproach or guilt about being sick)
   (8) diminished ability to think or concentrate, or indecisiveness, nearly every day (either by subjective account or as observed by others)
   (9) recurrent thoughts of death (not just fear of dying), recurrent suicidal ideation without a specific plan, or a suicide attempt or a specific plan for commiting suicide

B. (1) It cannot be established that an organic factor initiated and maintained the disturbance
   (2) The disturbance is not a normal reaction to the death of a loved one (uncomplicated bereavement)
   Note: Morbid preoccupation with worthlessness, suicidal ideation, marked functional impairment or psychomotor retardation, or prolonged duration suggest bereavement complicated by major depression.

C. At no time during the disturbance have there been delusions or hallucinations for as long as 2 weeks in the absence of prominent mood symptoms (i.e., before the mood symptoms developed or after they have remitted).

D. Not superimposed on schizophrenia, schizophreniform disorder, delusional disorder, or psychotic disorder NOS.

Table from DSM-III-R *Diagnostic and Statistical Manual of Mental Disorders,* ed 3, revised. Copyright American Psychiatric Association, Washington, DC, 1987. Used with permission.

Major depressive episode subtypes Further division into subtypes and chronicity requires a fifth digit after the previous four (Table 17.3-10). These are (in reverse order):

6-In full remission.
5-In partial remission.
4-With psychotic features (mood congruent or mood incongruent has to be stated).
3-Severe, without psychotic features.
2-Moderate.
1-Mild.
0-Unspecified.

The classification of melancholic depression (Table 17.3-11) requires the presence of at least five of the following nine symptoms:

1. Loss of interest or pleasure.
2. Lack of reaction to pleasurable stimuli.
3. Depression worse in the mornings.
4. Early morning awakening (at least 2 hours).
5. Psychomotor retardation or agitation clearly visible.
6. Significant anorexia or weight loss.
7. No significant personality disturbance (before first episode).
8. One or more previous attacks, followed by good or complete recovery.
9. Previous good response to specific antidepressant therapies.

Dysthymia For patients who are in a state recognizably depressive, but that does not fulfill the criteria for major depressive disorder, there are other diagnostic categories available. If the depressed mood is accompanied by at least one of the following:

poor appetite or overeating,
insomnia or hypersomnia,
low energy or fatigue,
low self-esteem,
poor concentration or indecisiveness,
feelings of hopelessness

and has been present for at least 2 years, with intermissions never lasting more than 2 months, then the patient can be diagnosed as having dysthymia (Table 17.3-12). There are

TABLE 17.3-7
Diagnostic Criteria for Major Depression, Single Episode

For fifth digit, use the major depressive episode codes to describe current state.
A. single major depressive episode
B. never had a manic episode or an unequivocal hypomanic episode
Specify if **seasonal pattern**

Table from DSM-III-R *Diagnostic and Statistical Manual of Mental Disorders,* ed 3, revised. Copyright American Psychiatric Association, Washington, DC, 1987. Used with permission.

TABLE 17.3-8
Diagnostic Criteria for Major Depression, Recurrent

For fifth digit, use the major depressive episode codes to describe current state
A. Two or more major depressive episodes; each separated by at least 2 months of return to more or less usual functioning. (If there has been a previous major depressive episode, the current episode of depression need not meet the full criteria for a major depressive episode.)
B. Has never had a manic episode or an unequivocal hypomanic episode.
Specify if **seasonal pattern**

Table from DSM-III-R *Diagnostic and Statistical Manual of Mental Disorders,* ed 3, revised. Copyright American Psychiatric Association, Washington, DC, 1987. Used with permission.

TABLE 17.3-9
Diagnostic Criteria for Depressive Disorder Not Otherwise Specified

Disorders with depressive features that do not meet the criteria for any specific mood disorder or adjustment disorder with depressed mood.
Examples:
   (1) a major depressive episode superimposed on residual schizophrenia
   (2) a recurrent, mild, depressive disturbance that does not meet the criteria for dysthymia
   (3) non-stress-related depressive episodes that do not meet the criteria for a major depressive episode
Specify if **seasonal pattern**

Table from DSM-III-R *Diagnostic and Statistical Manual of Mental Disorders,* ed 3, revised. Copyright American Psychiatric Association, Washington, DC, 1987. Used with permission.

TABLE 17.3-10
Diagnostic Criteria for Major Depressive Episode Codes: Fifth-Digit Code Numbers and Criteria for Current State of Bipolar Disorder, Depressed or Major Depression

1-Mild: Few, if any, symptoms in excess of those required to make the diagnosis, **and** symptoms result in only minor impairment in occupational functioning or in usual social activities or relationships with others.
2-Moderate: Symptoms or functional impairment between "mild" and "severe."
3-Severe, without psychotic features: Several symptoms in excess of those required to make the diagnosis, **and** symptoms markedly interfere with occupational functioning or with usual social activities or relationships with others.
4-With psychotic features: Delusions or hallucinations. If possible, **specify** whether the psychotic features are *mood congruent* or *mood incongruent*.
Mood-congruent psychotic features: Delusions or hallucinations whose content is entirely consistent with the typical depressive themes of personal inadequacy, guilt, disease, nihilism, or deserved punishment.
Mood-incongruent psychotic features: Delusions or hallucinations whose content does *not* involve typical depressive themes of personal inadequacy, guilt, disease, death, nihilism, or deserved punishment. Included here are such symptoms as persecutory delusions (not directly related to depressive themes), thought insertion, thought broadcasting, and delusions of control.
5-In partial remission: Intermediate between "in full remission" and "mild," **and** no previous dysthymia. (If major depressive episode was superimposed on dysthymia, the diagnosis of dysthymia alone is given once the full criteria for a major depressive episode are no longer met.)
6-In full remission: During the past 6 months no significant signs or symptoms of the disturbance.
0-Unspecified.
Specify chronic if current episode has lasted 2 consecutive years without a period of 2 months or longer during which there were no significant depressive symptoms.
Specify if current episode is **melanocholic type.**

three exclusion criteria that must be fulfilled: For the first 2 years, a diagnosis of major depressive disorder was never applicable, no psychotic features have been present, and there is no organic or toxic basis.

Adjustment disorder An adjustment disorder is a maladaptive reaction to an identifiable psychosocial stress that occurs within 3 months of the onset of the stress. The maladaptive nature of the reaction is indicated either by impairment of social or occupational functioning or by symptoms that are excessive for a normal and expected reaction to the stress.

The disturbance is not merely one instance of a pattern of overreaction to stress or an exacerbation of another mental disorder. The former exclusion is designed to exclude those individuals whose emotional responses are a characteristic of personality, even though they may be regarded by the average stolid citizen (and psychiatrist) as excessive. The latter exclusion prevents multiple diagnoses for the varying course of a single illness.

The maladaptive reaction should not have persisted for more than 6 months after the stress (and its environmental consequences) has ceased. The category of adjustment disorder is designed to cover temporary reactions to stress that do not meet the criteria for any specific DSM-III-R disorder or uncomplicated bereavement. Clearly, 6 months is an arbitrary figure, but some definite duration has to be specified.

TABLE 17.3-11
Diagnostic Criteria for Melancholia

The presence of at least five of the following:
(1) loss of interest or pleasure in all, or almost all, activities
(2) lack of reactivity to usually pleasurable stimuli (does not feel much better, even temporarily, when something good happens)
(3) depression regularly worse in the morning
(4) early morning awakening (at least two hours before usual time of awakening)
(5) psychomotor retardation or agitation (not merely subjective complaints)
(6) significant anorexia or weight loss (e.g., more than 5% of body weight in a month)
(7) no significant personality disturbance before first major depressive episode
(8) one or more previous major depressive episodes followed by complete, or nearly complete, recovery
(9) previous good response to specific and adequate somatic antidepressant therapy, e.g., tricyclics, ECT, MAOI, lithium

ADJUSTMENT DISORDER WITH DEPRESSED MOOD Adjustment disorder with depressed mood should be used when the predominant manifestation involves such symptoms as depressed mood, tearfulness, and hopelessness. Other types of adjustment disorder include those with anxious mood and mixed emotional features.

In DSM-III-R, adjustment disorders are classified under a separate heading but are covered here because of their affective features.

MANIA

Mania is the least common of the major psychoses. It is always recurrent, but pure mania accounts for fewer than one in six of bipolar patients. Most cases are found as manic phases of bipolar disorder. As a syndrome, it may be primary (a functional psychosis) or secondary, arising from organic disease or toxemia.

TYPES OF MANIA Emil Kraepelin described four types of mania:

1. Hypomania: This is a mild condition, but it may be long lasting. It is characterized by predominant euphoria, overactivity, and disinhibition.
2. Acute mania: This is a severe condition, showing transient grandiose delusions, a labile mood, and sometimes incoherent talk.
3. Delusional mania: This condition is characterized by less excitement, more persistent grandiose delusions, and even occasional hallucinations.
4. Delirious mania: This condition is characterized by frenzied overactivity, labile mood varying from excitement to depression to panic, variable delusions, vivid visual and other hallucinations, and disorientation for time and place.

Delirious mania Delirious mania is really a combination of mania with a confusional or delirious state following exhaustion from overactivity, together with dehydration from lack of drinking and eating.

Secondary mania Mania can also be brought about by treatment of depression with drugs. This may occur in patients

TABLE 17.3-12
Diagnostic Criteria for Dysthymia

A. Depressed mood (or can be irritable mood in children and adolescents) for most of the day, more days than not, as indicated either by subjective account or observation by others, for at least 2 years (1 year for children and adolescents)
B. Presence, while depressed, of at least two of the following:
(1) poor appetite or overeating
(2) insomnia or hypersomnia
(3) low energy or fatigue
(4) low self-esteem
(5) poor concentration or difficulty making decisions
(6) feelings of hopelessness
C. During a 2-year period (1 year for children and adolescents) of the disturbance, never without the symptoms in A for more than 2 months at a time
D. No evidence of an unequivocal major depressive episode during the first 2 years (1 year for children and adolescents) of the disturbance
Note: There may have been a previous major depressive episode, provided there was a full remission (no significant signs or symptoms for 6 months) before development of the dysthymia. In addition, after these 2 years (1 year for children or adolescents) of dysthymia, there may be superimposed episodes of major depression, in which case both diagnoses are given.
E. Has never had a manic episode or an unequivocal hypomanic episode
F. Not superimposed on a chronic psychotic disorder, such as schizophrenia or delusional disorder
G. It cannot be established that an organic factor initiated and maintained the disturbance (e.g., prolonged administration or an antihypertensive medication).

Specify primary or **secondary type:**
Primary type: the mood disturbance is not related to a preexisting, chronic, nonmood, Axis 1 or Axis III disorder, e.g., anorexia nervosa, somatization disorder, a psychoactive substance dependence disorder, an anxiety disorder, or rheumatoid arthritis.
Secondary type: the mood disturbance is apparently related to a pre-existing, chronic nonmood, Axis I or Axis III disorder.

Specify early onset or **late onset:**
Early onset: onset of the disturbance before age 21
Late onset: onset of the disturbance at age 21 or later

Table from DSM-III-R *Diagnostic and Statistical Manual of Mental Disorders,* ed 3, revised. Copyright American Psychiatric Association, Washington, DC, 1987. Used with permission.

already predisposed to mania. Secondary mania has also been reported during treatment with amphetamines, corticosteroids, L-dopa, and isoniazid (for tuberculosis). It is a rare complication of thyrotoxicosis and cerebral disease: acute and chronic organic mental syndrome, following influenza, encephalitis, multiple sclerosis, rheumatic chorea, and cerebral tumors.

Hypomania Hypomania does not differ significantly from mania in its manifestations, except that it is much milder and may often not lead to the patient's coming for treatment. It also is part of bipolar disorder, Type II.

Mania in young persons About one in three patients has the first attack in the teens. It is now accepted that mania can occur in childhood and shows symptoms similar to those found in adults, including bouts of depression. Overactivity, physical aggressiveness, and a low toleration of frustration are present, together with a family history of mood disorder.

Chronic mania In chronic mania, the patients lose their euphoria, becoming irritable and resentful, and acquire a paranoid-like attitude. They are convinced that they are being kept down, that their bright ideas are rejected, and that others are cooperating or conspiring to ensure that they do not receive proper recognition for their achievements. Sometimes there is a grain of truth in these ideas, for their long-suffering colleagues may have had to cope with impractical schemes, with activities never completed and the consequences thereof.

SYMPTOMS OF MANIA

Mood A phase of mania may start quite suddenly, especially on the rare occasions when it is precipitated by some recognizable stress. But, usually, it will develop over a period of time, ranging from a few days to a few weeks. Sometimes, it appears as the patient recovers from a depressive phase. If the development is slow, the first changes in mood will not usually be considered abnormal. The patients are cheerful, feel well, and enjoy life and all activities. Gradually, however, the cheerfulness begins to jar on others, and the patients are now seen to be too hilarious and too optimistic about everything, the past, the present, and the future. They are filled with jollity which is characteristically infectious; people laugh with manics, not at them. This cheerfulness is accompanied by a certain mischievousness which may become unpleasant. However, the euphoric mood is volatile and can quickly change, at the slightest frustration, into anger, resentment, and hostility. Occasionally, the euphoria can be interrupted by spells of depression, tearfulness, and even suicidal thoughts, but it all disappears with the return of the joviality. These emotional changes are what is meant by lability of mood. Chronic manics tend to be aggressively resentful and abusive of others.

In their relationships with others, manics tend to be self-assertive and boastful. They become overbearing and brook no interference. Hence, they easily become litigious. Their volatility may show itself in violent likes or dislikes of others, and the one may change suddenly into the other.

As the mood intensifies, it begins to show a quality of excitement that, together with the other symptoms, ends in a state of apparent confusion. In the long-standing cases of moderate severity, the euphoria diminishes, and the patient becomes irritable, disgruntled, and resentful. Sometimes, on recovery, the patients may have some insight into their subjective state during the attack. They may then say that, despite their outward good-humored jolliness, inwardly they had a feeling of desperation and of being driven.

Thinking The patients are full of ideas on how to improve things, and at first, they may have a measure of plausibility. Characteristically, they lack judgment and self-criticism and show no sense of proportion, and so their schemes soon become quite unrealistic. The ideas come freely and soon pass through the mind in rapid succession. None of them is dealt with adequately before the next one comes to the fore. The patients' distractibility adds to this. They cannot concentrate on anything for long. As the symptom worsens, the typical flight of ideas appears. The movement of thought from one idea to another ceases to be controlled by a coherent purpose and becomes determined by rhymes, puns, and the most superficial of sound relationships (clang associations). Although the patients move from one subject to another, careful listening shows that the range of their ideas is limited and that the same themes recur constantly.

Speech The patients talk loudly, quickly, and too much, and eventually their speech becomes incessant. It is full of jokes and rhymes and puns. Often it is grandiose in manner as well as in content and full of risqué jokes. Soon the patients have no time to finish a sentence, and soon their speech consists of nothing but isolated words. By this time, it may be quite incoherent and be difficult, if not impossible, to distinguish their speech from the word salad of the schizophrenic patient.

Activity The patients declared that they have never felt so well and full of energy. They soon become obviously overactive, appearing never to become tired. Although at first their activities are coherent and well directed, soon they are like Stephen Leacock's hero "riding off in all directions." They are unable to finish anything, going from one thing to another until they are completely disorganized; their business and social activities are in a state of chaos.

When rushing about, they may knock themselves against furniture or other obstructions and can receive quite severe injuries without apparently noticing it. The vigor of their movements is accompanied by an astonishing increase in strength: "Maniacal strength" has to be seen to be believed. The author remembers vividly, in the days before antipsychotics, a particular patient. She was a young, curly-headed blonde, pretty and frail looking, who had had to be put into a "strong suit" and into seclusion. As she sat on the floor, joking, punning, chattering, and laughing away, she casually ripped her strong suit into strips. The author picked up a piece, and hard as he tried to tear it, he could make absolutely no impression on that piece of canvas.

Sleep Sleep is always diminished, the patients appearing to be able to carry on with only an hour or so of sleep, and sometimes even less. Sometimes, the patients take short catnaps during the day.

Appetite Appetite is usually increased, the patients taking to eating hurriedly, wolfing down sandwiches because they have no time for a proper meal. They may end up losing weight because they do not eat enough, as well as being overactive. The hurried eating may be accompanied by hurried drinking which may well have its usual consequences (drunk while driving, and the like).

Libido Libido is increased and at first will appear as risqué jokes, offensive flirting, and philandering. Eventually the patients may become completely shameless in their erotic behavior. In the early stages, their increased libido, together with their overactivity and lack of judgment, may lead to disastrous consequences. A point is reached that despite their increased libido, the patients are unable to complete any activity.

Insight In recurrent attacks, the patients may recognize what is happening at the onset of another phase. In the hypomanic state, patients may show that they have some insight, by the way they control themselves when interviewed (e.g., by a physician or in a court of law). But, usually, they have no insight whatever. They may be persuaded or bullied into seeing a physician but regard the interview as a joke.

Behavior The patients have poor control of their impulses. They eagerly seek social contacts, getting in touch with old friends, telephoning them at all hours, and spending money freely. They not only are overactive, but their gestures also are overemphatic and expansive. Their expansiveness becomes overwhelming and overbearing. They may be grandiose and condescending toward others. Their clothes are unusual and tend to be loud, but when they are overactive and have no time to complete anything, they tend to neglect themselves, becoming carelessly or insufficiently dressed, unwashed, and unkempt.

Appearance The traditionally typical appearance of the manic patient is now rarely seen, owing to effective treatment. Although at the onset of an attack, the patients may look as well as they claim, their appearance begins to change. They are restless and talkative, their voice so hoarse from overuse as to be barely audible. Their face is drawn and has a worn-out expression. The patients may obviously have lost weight.

Delusions The typical delusions, when they occur, are consonant with the patients' mood. They tend to be a development of the grandiose ideas. Four types have been described. Patients are convinced that they have special abilities (scientific, artistic, or inventive); they may insist that they are members of some important (royal or aristocratic) family; they may believe that they possess vast sums of money; or they may think that they have a special mission (to save the world).

Other delusions, more characteristic of schizophrenia, may be found, especially in the middle of an acute phase at its maximum, and even those disturbances of thinking known as first-rank symptoms. They tend to be accompanied by bizarre behavior, irritability, and depression. Their presence makes the diagnosis difficult, but they appear to be of no great significance.

Other symptoms Hallucinations are rare, and although the patients may make remarks suggesting that they are hearing voices, questions are usually turned off with some joke or witticism. Mention has already been made of momentary depressions. Transient hypochondriacal ideas have also been described.

DIAGNOSIS Because the patients feel so well during a hypomanic phase, they do not seek treatment unless they have had previous attacks and recognize what is happening to them. Occasionally, they may visit a doctor because of pressure from spouse or other relatives. But even when the symptoms are more marked, patients may be able to restrain themselves during the interview and offer plausible explanations for their conduct. Without a history of previous attacks, it can therefore be extremely difficult to make the diagnosis.

In the more severe states the diagnosis is usually straightforward, but when the patient is very excited, it may be difficult to distinguish the condition from schizophrenia or the schizophreniform psychoses (i.e., schizoaffective and cycloid disorders). (The term "cycloid" is not synonomous with "cyclothymic." The term "cycloid" has been gaining ground steadily in Europe to cover a special subdivision of the schizophrenias. It is not yet current in the United States but it is likely that it will eventually be recognized as indicating a coherent subgroup.) Many patients have their first attack at 15 to 19 years, and these are particularly liable to be mistaken for schizophrenia. In such circumstances, it is helpful to go into the details of the evolution of the attack (e.g., the euphoria and its accompaniments may have been very obvious at an earlier stage). A history of previous attacks and a family history may also be crucial. A decision is often possible only after the patient has been observed over a period of hours or even a few days.

DSM-III-R CRITERIA **Mania** For the diagnosis of a manic episode, it is essential that the mood be elevated, expansive, or irritable for at least 1 week, but for marked impairment in social or occupational functioning, it can be of any duration (Table 17.3-13). In addition, the patient must experience at least three of the following symptoms, and if the dominant mood is irritability, there must be at least four. They must be persistent (not fleeting or momentary) and be of significant degree. However, if the patient has experienced a previous manic episode, all the criteria are not necessary for the diagnosis.

1. Inflated self-esteem (grandiosity, which may be delusional).
2. Decreased need for sleep.
3. More talkative than usual or pressure to keep talking.
4. Flight of ideas or subjective experience that thoughts are racing.
5. Distractibility (i.e., attention too easily drawn to unimportant or irrelevant external stimuli).
6. Increase in activity (socially, at work, or sexually) or physical restlessness.
7. Excessive involvement in activities that have a high potential for painful consequences that are not recognized (e.g., buying sprees, sexual indiscretions, foolish business investments, reckless driving).

The episode of mood disturbance must be sufficiently severe to cause a marked impairment in social or occupational functioning or to necessitate admission to hospital. This excludes temporary exuberance arising from some sudden good fortune.

At no time during the illness should there be delusions or hallucinations for at least 2 weeks in the absence of prominent affective symptoms (i.e., before the affective symptoms developed or after they have remitted).

The symptoms must not be superimposed on either schizophrenia, schizophreniform disorder, delusional disorder, or psychotic disorder not otherwise specified.

Finally, the clinical condition must not be sustained by a specific organic factor or substance (although there may be an organic precipitant).

TABLE 17.3-13
Diagnostic Criteria for Manic Episode

Note: A "manic syndrome" is defined as including criteria A, B, and C below. A "hypomanic syndrome" is defined as including criteria A and B, but not C, i.e., no marked impairment.

A. A distinct period of abnormally and persistently elevated, expansive, or irritable mood.
B. During the period of mood disturbance, at least three of the following symptoms have persisted (four if the mood is only irritable) and have been present to a significant degree:
   (1) inflated self-esteem or grandiosity
   (2) decreased need for sleep, e.g., feels rested after only 3 hours of sleep
   (3) more talkative than usual or pressure to keep talking
   (4) flight of ideas or subjective experience that thoughts are racing
   (5) distractibility, i.e., attention too easily drawn to unimportant or irrelevant external stimuli
   (6) increase in goal-directed activity (either socially, at work or school, or sexually) or psychomotor agitation
   (7) excessive involvement in pleasurable activities which have a high potential for painful consequences, e.g., the person engages in unrestrained buying sprees, sexual indiscretions, or foolish business investments
C. Mood disturbance sufficiently severe to cause marked impairment in occupational functioning or in usual social activities or relationships with others, or to necessitate hospitalization to prevent harm to self or others.
D. At no time during the disturbance have there been delusions or hallucinations for as long as 2 weeks in the absence of prominent mood symptoms (i.e., before the mood symptoms developed or after they have remitted).
E. Not superimposed on schizophrenia, schizophreniform disorder, delusional disorder, or psychotic disorder NOS.
F. It cannot be established that an organic factor initiated and maintained the disturbance. **Note:** Somatic antidepressant treatment (e.g., drugs, ECT) that apparently precipitates a mood disturbance should not be considered an etiologic organic factor.

Table from DSM-III-R *Diagnostic and Statistical Manual of Mental Disorders,* ed 3, revised. Copyright American Psychiatric Association, Washington, DC, 1987. Used with permission.

Mania with psychotic features Mania with psychotic features is the category used when there is apparently gross impairment in testing of reality (i.e., when there are present delusions, hallucinations, or grossly bizarre behavior [Table 17.3-14]):

Mood congruent: When the content is entirely consistent with the themes of inflated worth, power, knowledge, identity, or special relationships to a deity or famous persons; if there is flight of ideas without apparent awareness by the patient that the speech is not understandable.

Mood incongruent: Either delusions or hallucinations that do not have the contents described above (e.g., delusions of persecution, or of thought insertion or of being controlled, or catatonic symptoms—stupor, mutism, negativism, posturings).

BIPOLAR DISORDERS (MANIC-DEPRESSION)

Patients experience manic phases with or without depressive phases. Although the attack of mania may be detached from the depressive phase, it is more usual for it to be linked. Either the attacks of illness begin with a bout of mania that in the end swings into a depressive phase, or the patients swing into mania as they recover from the depression. Two forms of bipolar disorder are recognized: Type I, in which the manic phases are mild (hypomanic) and have not required admission to hospital, and Type II, in which the manic phase may range from mild to severe, a true manic attack. A minor form clinically is distinguished as cyclothymia.

Mania is uncommon, and even more so is the condition of pure mania in which the patient does not experience phases of depression. The ratio of bipolars to pure manias is about 10 to 1. For this reason, DSM-III-R does not have a separate category for them; all manias are subsumed under bipolar disorder.

CYCLOTHYMIA Cyclothymia refers to individuals who are liable to mood swings of sufficient duration to be recognizable as similar to manic-depressive (bipolar) disorder, but do not reach an intensity such as to require treatment. There is evidence that cyclothymic personalities are those liable to bipolar disorder, and so it is possible that the mild mood swings are really a prodromal expression of bipolar disorder.

DIAGNOSIS A diagnosis of bipolar disorder requires the recognition of both types of phase in the one patient over the course of the illness. If the attack starts with a mild phase of hypomania, the abnormality may not be recognized by the patients and their relatives. Sometimes a clue is provided when the patient claims that the depressive illness "was brought on by overwork (or overexcitement)."

TABLE 17.3-14
Diagnostic Criteria for Manic Episode Codes: Fifth Digit Code Numbers for Severity of Current State of Bipolar Disorder, Manic or Mixed

1-Mild: Meets minimum symptom criteria for a manic episode (or almost meets symptom criteria if there has been a previous manic episode).
2-Moderate: Extreme increase in activity or impairment in judgment.
3-Severe, without psychotic features: Almost continual supervision required in order to prevent physical harm to self or others.
4-With psychotic features: Delusions, hallucinations, or catatonic symptoms. If possible, **specify** whether the psychotic features are *mood congruent* or *mood incongruent*.
Mood-congruent psychotic features: Delusions or hallucinations whose content is entirely consistent with the typical manic themes of inflated worth, power, knowledge, identity, or special relationship to a deity or famous person.
Mood-incongruent psychotic features: Either (a) or (b):
(a) Delusions or hallucinations whose content does *not* involve the typical manic themes of inflated worth, power, knowledge, identity, or special relationship to a deity or famous person. Included are such symptoms as persecutory delusions (not directly related to grandiose ideas or themes), thought insertion, and delusions of being controlled.
(b) Catatonic symptoms, e.g., stupor, mutism, negativism, posturing.
5-In partial remission: Full criteria were previously, but are not currently, met; some signs or symptoms of the disturbance have persisted.
6-In full remission: Full criteria were previously met, but there have been no significant signs or symptoms of the disturbance for at least 6 months.
0-Unspecified.

Table from DSM-III-R *Diagnostic and Statistical Manual of Mental Disorders,* ed 3, revised. Copyright American Psychiatric Association, Washington, DC, 1987. Used with permission.

DSM-III-R CRITERIA **Bipolar disorder, manic** A patient with bipolar disorder, manic, is currently (or most recently) in a manic episode, as defined. If there has been a previous episode, the current attack need not meet the full criteria in the definition. The disorder presents with or without psychotic features (Table 17.3-15).

Bipolar disorder, depressed A patient with bipolar disorder, depressed, having previously experienced one or more manic episodes, is now in a major depressive episode, as defined. As with mania, if there has been a previous major depressive episode, the current one need not meet the full criteria. Both psychotic features and melancholia can be present (Table 17.3-16).

Bipolar disorder, mixed In bipolar disorder, mixed, the current or most recent episode involves the full symptomatic picture of both manic and major depressive episodes, intermixed or rapidly alternating every few days. This covers patients with 24- and 48-hour cycles.

The depressive symptoms are prominent and last at least a full day. This criterion recognizes that depressive symptoms can occur, briefly and evanescently, during a manic phase (Table 17.3-17).

Bipolar disorder not otherwise specified Among other conditions, bipolar disorder not otherwise specified is designed to include bipolar II disorder (Table 17.3-18).

Cyclothymia Cyclothymia is on the borderline between normal and pathological and is therefore included among the diagnostic categories of DSM-III-R (Table 17.3-19). There are four criteria: There must be at least 2 years during which there have been numerous periods with abnormally elevated, expansive, or irritable mood that did not meet the symptom criteria for a manic episode; also numerous periods with depressed mood or loss of interest or pleasure that did not meet the symptom criteria for a major depressive episode. For the past 2 years, the patient has never been without symptoms of hypomania or depression for more than 2 months at a time. During the first 2 years of the disorder, the patient does not exhibit evidence of a major depressive episode or manic episode. Finally, this condition cannot be superimposed on a

TABLE 17.3-15
Diagnostic Criteria for Bipolar Disorder, Manic

For fifth digit, use the manic episode codes to describe current state.
Currently (or most recently) in a manic episode. (If there has been a previous manic episode, the current episode need not meet the full criteria for a manic episode.)
Specify if **seasonal pattern**

Table from DSM-III-R *Diagnostic and Statistical Manual of Mental Disorders,* ed 3, revised. Copyright American Psychiatric Association, Washington, DC, 1987. Used with permission.

TABLE 17.3-16
Diagnostic Criteria for Bipolar Disorder, Depressed

For fifth digit, use the major depressive episode codes to describe current state.
A. Has had one or more manic episodes
B. Currently (or most recently) in a major depressive episode. (If there has been a previous major depressive episode, the current episode need not meet the full criteria for a major depressive episode.)
Specify if **seasonal pattern**

Table from DSM-III-R *Diagnostic and Statistical Manual of Mental Disorders,* ed 3, revised. Copyright American Psychiatric Association, Washington, DC, 1987. Used with permission.

TABLE 17.3-17
Diagnostic Criteria for Bipolar Disorder, Mixed

For fifth digit, use the manic episode codes to describe current state.
A. Current (or more recent) episode involves the full symptomatic picture of both manic and major depressive episodes (except for the duration requirement of 2 weeks for depressive symptoms), intermixed or rapidly alternating every few days.
B. Prominent depressive symptoms lasting at least a full day.
Specify if **seasonal pattern**

Table from DSM-III-R *Diagnostic and Statistical Manual of Mental Disorders,* ed 3, revised. Copyright American Psychiatric Association, Washington, DC, 1987. Used with permission.

TABLE 17.3-18
Diagnostic Criteria for Bipolar Disorder Not Otherwise Specified

Disorders with manic or hypomanic features that do not meet the criteria for any specific bipolar disorder.
Examples:
(1) at least one hypomanic episode and at least one major depressive episode, but never either a manic episode or cyclothymia. Such cases have been referred to as "bipolar II."
(2) one or more hypomanic episodes, but without cyclothymia or a history of either a manic or a major depressive episode
(3) a manic episode superimposed on delusional disorder, residual schizophrenia, or psychotic disorder NOS
Specify if **seasonal pattern**

Table from DSM-III-R *Diagnostic and Statistical Manual of Mental Disorders,* ed 3, revised. Copyright American Psychiatric Association, Washington, DC, 1987. Used with permission.

TABLE 17.3-19
Diagnostic Criteria for Cyclothymia

A. For at least 2 years (1 year for children and adolescents), presence of numerous hypomanic episodes (all of the criteria for a manic episode, except criterion C that indicates marked impairment) and numerous periods with depressed mood or loss of interest or pleasure that did not meet criterion A of major depressive episode.
B. During a 2-year period (1 year in children and adolescents) of the disturbance, never without hypomanic or depressive symptoms for more than 2 months at a time.
C. No clear evidence of a major depressive episode or manic episode during the first 2 years of the disturbance (1 year in children and adolescents).
Note: After this minimum period of cyclothymia, there may be superimposed manic or major depressive episodes, in which case the additional diagnosis of biopolar disorder or bipolar disorder NOS should be given.
D. Not superimposed on a chronic psychotic disorder, such as schizophrenia or delusional disorder.
E. It cannot be established that an organic factor initiated and maintained the disturbance (e.g., repeated intoxication from drugs or alcohol).

Table from DSM-III-R *Diagnostic and Statistical Manual of Mental Disorders*, ed 3, revised. Copyright American Psychiatric Association, Washington, DC, 1987. Used with permission.

chronic psychotic disorder, such as schizophrenia or delusional disorder. The condition is also not sustained by specific organic factors or substances (e.g., drugs or alcohol).

SCHIZOAFFECTIVE DISORDER

Schizoaffective disorder usually covers several different conditions. It is used to describe a patient whose manic symptoms are intermingled with those more closely related to schizophrenia: thought disorder, persecutory delusions and hallucinations, delusions of influence, and various forms of interference with thinking. Some patients experience recurrent phases of illness, some of which may be clearly manic and others apparently schizophrenic. Finally, the term is also used to describe that group of disorders otherwise known as cycloid disorders. They have certain basic features that are important for making a diagnosis: They are much more common in females than males; they are often precipitated by stress; and there is sometimes a family history of cycloid disorder. Typical symptoms, which are uncommon in schizophrenia and certainly in mania, are perplexity, confusion, ecstasy, anxiety, and panic. Delusions and hallucinations occur even in mild forms.

It is not yet possible to classify the schizoaffective disorders unequivocally. They can be classified with the schizophrenias, with the mood disorders, or as a separate group. From the clinical point of view, the classification is irrelevant. Insofar as the symptoms overlap with the mood disorders, they come into the differential diagnosis, and it is therefore necessary to give some account of them here. For further discussion of this topic, see Section 16.1, Schizoaffective Disorder, Schizophreniform Disorder, and Brief Reactive Psychosis.

DSM-III-R CRITERIA Schizoaffective disorder is defined as an illness during which at some time there is either a major depressive or a manic syndrome concurrently with those from the A criterion for schizophrenia. These include at least one of the following three groups (provided that they have been present for at least 1 week):

1. Two of delusions, hallucinations, loosening of associations, catatonia, flat or inappropriate affect.
2. Bizarre delusions.
3. Prominent auditory hallucinations.

In addition, during an episode of the illness, there must have been delusions or hallucinations for at least 2 weeks in the absence of prominent affective symptoms. Finally, the illness does not meet the criteria for schizophrenia or organic mental disorder, and it cannot be established that an organic factor initiated or maintained the disturbance.

These somewhat confusing and repetitive criteria are designed to exclude a manic state with slightly atypical symptoms, as well as schizophrenia with such obvious affective symptoms as depressed mood or euphoria. At the current time, schizoaffective disorder is classified in DSM-III-R under the heading psychotic disorder not elsewhere classified.

ASSESSMENT OF MOOD DISORDERS (DEPRESSION AND MANIA)

Although rating scales have now been fully accepted in clinical psychiatry, if anything, their swing into favor has gone too far, and too much is expected from them. However useful they may be, it must never be forgotten that the information they provide is very limited. For the fullest description of a person, a novelist or biographer (perhaps with some psychiatric insight) is a better resource. A full psychiatric case history gives much less information but is sufficient for the diagnosis, treatment, and management of the patient. The much shorter case summary provides an adequate introduction to the case and a justification for the diagnosis. The most common type of rating scale merely provides a standard way of recording a patient's current condition, but for the purpose for which it is required (to record the patient's progress or response to treatment), it is sufficient. Attempts have been made to develop diagnostic scales, but they are still by no means adequate to their purpose.

The material recorded in a rating scale is based either on direct observations or inferences from them, though the distinction is not absolute. If the rater does not recognize the clinical phenomena, know how to observe, or makes incorrect inferences, the information recorded will not be enhanced by being presented in the form of numbers. Scales can be an improvement on clinical judgment, because they define the categories of severity and force the clinician to think carefully about each symptom. A total score then becomes a measure of severity by a clearly defined process, unlike the vague and unknown process of synthesis used by the clinician.

The advantages of scales are that for all patients and all occasions, the items are the same, the grades are defined in the same way, and they are used uniformly. The information provided is in a quantitative form and is therefore easy to use for making comparisons and analyzing by statistical methods. In the end, scales are justified by their value in use, and the difference between a good and a bad scale is determined in the same way.

Thus, the most important use of rating scales is in clinical research. The point has now been reached that it is even thought that ratings scales are the essential mark of a scientific clinical trial. They are also of value for teaching purposes. But in ordinary clinical practice, such scales are inferior to a good case record, although they are better than a bad one.

CHOICE OF SCALES A scale should be relevant and accurate. In technical terms, it should be valid and reliable. The former can be defined as the relationship between the measurement obtained and the true value of the variable being measured. Reliability may be defined as the amount by which random factors interfere with accurate measurement. If the interference is small, the scale will have high reliability.

When appropriate, there should be available normative data (i.e., scores on normal or control populations). It is useful to know how a scale compares with others. It should not only be clear and simple but also be designed so that it is easy to use in the course of ordinary clinical work. If a scale is too long, it will interfere with the clinical interview, and if its completion has to be left to the end, the rater is likely to forget what should have been recorded. The technical terms in items should be familiar to the rater and be based on familiar concepts. A scale designed for use by unskilled observers should, as far as possible, be confined to observed behavior and require a minimum of interpretation. If the scale is for use by skilled observers (i.e., those who understand the subject matter and are experienced in interviewing patients), it should make full use of that skill. When such raters neglect to use their experience and judgment, they are throwing away their most powerful instrument of measurement.

The items should be relevant to the purpose of the scale. This is one of the disadvantages of all-purpose scales compared with special scales. Individual items will always have a lower reliability than will the sum of several. In consequence, scales that are too short are likely to have a low reliability. Very long scales are difficult to complete and are not necessarily more reliable.

It is advisable that items not assess changes. If a patient's condition fluctuates, then the recording of irregular sequences of "better" and "worse" can only give rise to an end result that cannot be interpreted. The exception is when changes are firmly anchored to a baseline (e.g., weight).

Use of observer rating scales Raters should be familiar with the clinical phenomena; otherwise they will have difficulty in recognizing mild symptoms. They should have sufficient skill and experience to be able to elicit the information they are seeking (e.g., mild hypochondriasis or hallucinations, when they are not obvious). Raters should also be familiar with the scale they are using and be aware of the special problems (e.g., "constant errors," "response set," and other biases connected with ratings.

This account may seem to have emphasized the difficulties in making ratings. In practice, an experienced clinician will have no difficulty, after a few practice assessments, in arriving at ratings that correlate highly with those of others.

Use of self-assessment scales Self-rating scales, and those for use by an unskilled observer, should have clear and simple instructions for use, and the vocabulary should be clearly understandable to the user. It may be necessary here to take local usage into account.

Patients are sick persons, apprehensive about their condition and the future. In a clinic, they find themselves in strange and somewhat forbidding surroundings. In addition, one of the most common of their symptoms is an inability to concentrate. So, when they start to fill in their questionnaire, they should be kept under observation to see that they are doing it correctly.

CURRENT SCALES: GENERAL PURPOSE Only a few scales can be considered, and even then only briefly. Self- and observer-rating scales will be discussed together.

Brief Psychiatric Rating Scale This scale was first published by Overall and Gorham in 1962 and is therefore one of the oldest general-purpose scales as well as being one of the most popular. It contains 18 items (originally 16) dealing with groups of symptoms. Six of them are relevant to the assessment of depressive illness. This scale has been shown to have high reliability and to be sensitive to changes produced by treatment. It is easy to use and ratings are usually completed on the basis of observation and information obtained in an interview of 30 to 45 minutes. As with all the general scales considered here, it has been used as a diagnostic scale. (See Table 9.4-12 in Section 9.4, Psychological Assessment of Personality of Adults and Children.)

Comprehensive Psychiatric Rating Scale An English translation of this scale has been available since 1978, although it has been in use in Scandinavia for many years. It contains 40 items on symptoms reported by the patient and 27 items on observed variables. It was designed to be easy to use even by a semiskilled rater. Although it is practicable to use the whole scale, it was recommended that items be selected to make subscales for specific purposes. It contains nine items related to mania. The Montgomery–Asberg Depression Scale (described below) was derived in this way.

Association for Methodology and Documentation in Psychiatry This scale, originally in German, has now been translated into 11 languages. It contains five parts concerned with demographic data, life events, previous history of the patient, psychopathological symptoms, and somatic signs. The last two contain 100 and 40 items, respectively. Raters require training, but this scale is easy to use, requiring only about 45 minutes for the interview. The assessment of items is based on the events of the last 24 hours, which may be an advantage or a disadvantage, according to what is required. Reliability is high.

The Mania–Depression subscale contains 19 depressive and seven manic symptoms and has high interrater and test–retest reliability. It has been shown to correlate (rho) 0.62 with the Hamilton scale.

Schedule for Mood Disorders and Schizophrenia This scale was published in 1978 and was designed originally for use by skilled raters for making diagnoses according to the RDC. It has since been extensively used. The items are graded but, for diagnostic purposes, are usually dichotomized. Since then a subscale was devised in 1981 that could be regarded as equivalent to the Hamilton Depression Rating Scale. The correlation between the extracted score and the Hamilton scale, based on 48 patients, was 0.92. The extracted scale was designed to have the same mean and standard deviation as the Hamilton scale.

Goldberg General Health Questionnaire A standardized method of assessment is particularly important for community surveys, and although interviewing methods are the best, questionnaires are simpler to use and much less time-consuming. One of the most popular is the 1970 Goldberg General Health Questionnaire. Questionnaires have their weaknesses, and one worth mentioning is that older patients tend to minimize their mental symptoms and emphasize their somatic complaints. A clear distinction between depression as an illness and the other kinds still shows that the first is common.

A 28-item reduced version is particularly useful in that it gives scores on subscales, one of which is depression. Its value in survey work has been adequately demonstrated. Scores on the scale have been shown to decrease with clinical improvement, but there is insufficient information on its usefulness (e.g., in evalution of treatment).

Hopkins Symptom Check List (SCL-90) This self-rating scale covers a wide range of symptoms, from which, in addition to a global psychopathology index, nine subscales have been obtained by factor-analytic methods. Among them are anxiety and phobic anxiety, depression, but nothing that corresponds to mania. Test–retest reliability is 0.81, and internal consistency coefficients are on the order of 0.86. The depression subscale contains 13 items and has been found to be sensitive to changes produced by treatment.

In addition, there is a version for rating by a therapist, but the correlation between the two is low. This is partly explained by patients' under- and overreporting.

Present State Examination The current revision is available in many languages, including non-European ones. Originally it contained 360 items but has been shortened to 140. It is used chiefly for diagnostic purposes and requires training for its use. Patients can be classified into diagnostic syndromes by the computer program CATEGO. It has high reliability and is particularly valuable for cross-national comparisons. It has enough items on depression and mania for it to be used not only for diagnosis but also for assessment.

Visual Analogue Scale This type of scale can be used for both global judgments and specific variables, also by observers or patients. It consists of a line, usually 10 cm long, drawn on paper, the two ends of which are defined by the extremes of the variable (e.g., "Not at all depressed" and "As depressed as I can imagine"). The rater marks a point on the line corresponding to the present state. The score is the distance of the mark from one end of the line. It may have to undergo a mathematical transformation to compensate for a peculiar distribution of scores. Despite this scale's simplicity, it is quite effective. But, it suffers from an excessive response to "contrast effects" (i.e., quick changes give higher values than do slow ones).

Even without training and experience of standards, patients are able to give information with this method that is adequate for many purposes. This scale's great advantage is that it can be repeated as quickly and as often as desired, and therefore for recording quick and short-term changes. When used on patients admitted to hospital for treatment, the scale correlated 0.78 with global judgment and 0.79 with the Hamilton Depression Rating Scale, but these figures dropped considerably during treatment and on discharge.

SPECIFIC SCALES: DEPRESSION

OBSERVER RATING SCALES **Cronholm-Ottosson Scale** This scale is one of the earliest specific scales and originally consisted of eight items. Depressed mood and thoughts were separate items. Psychomotor retardation and intellectual and conative retardation were two items. The item "emotional indifference" dealt with anhedonia, and anxiety, suicidal tendencies, and disturbed sleep each had one item. The scale is somewhat deficient in items concerned with physical symptoms, but a later version of 12 items overemphasizes symptoms of anxiety (four out of 12). It has been shown to have high reliability (ranging between 0.72 and 0.86) and validity. It is adequately sensitive to changes in the severity of illness (e.g., in response to treatment).

Hamilton Depression Rating Scale This scale was first published in 1960. Later, a slightly revised version, together with better definition of the items, appeared in 1967 and details concerning its administration in 1980. The scale contains

17 items to assess the severity of an illness, scored 0 to 4 or 0 to 2. Five of them are on somatic symptoms (anxiety, gastrointestinal, general, genital, and weight) and three on insomnia in its three phases (early, middle, and delayed). Working capacity and loss of interest (anhedonia) are combined in one item. The other items cover depressed mood, guilt, suicide, retardation, agitation, psychic anxiety, hypochondriasis, and loss of insight. Diurnal variation is not included because it describes merely the form of the illness and is not part of its severity. Three others were omitted because they occurred with insufficient frequency to merit inclusion. All four were added to the total scale because of their potential value for purposes other than measurement of severity (e.g., response to treatment). It has high validity against global judgment and high reliability, both showing correlations about 0.90. It has often been found, in comparison with other scales, to be the most sensitive for measuring response to treatment.

The original recommendation for this scale was that it not be used as a checklist, but with the full clinical judgment of a skilled rater using all sources of information. In practice, it requires little training. Its most important limitation is that the rating must cover the patient's condition for the last week or so, and therefore it cannot be used for frequent assessments. (See Table 9.8-4 in Section 9.8, Psychiatric Rating Scales.)

Bech–Rafaelsen Melancholia Scale This scale appeared in 1980 and was claimed to be an improvement on the Hamilton scale. It contains 11 items, five of which are identical with the Hamilton scale (depressed mood, guilt, suicide, work and interests, and anxiety (psychic), and a sixth, tiredness and pains, which is the equivalent of somatic (general). Insomnia has been compressed into one item, and retardation has been expanded into four: motor, verbal, intellectual, and emotional. It therefore concentrates chiefly on psychological symptoms. The interrater reliability ranges from 0.82 to 0.93, comparing well with the Hamilton scale's figures of 0.79 to 0.93. The two scales correlate (rho) 0.97.

Montgomery–Asberg Depression Rating Scale The Scandinavian Comprehensive Psychiatric Rating Scale (CPRS) was designed to facilitate the development of specific scales by extracting suitable items. The Montgomery–Asberg Depression Rating Scale (MADRS), which appeared in 1979, is such a one. It consists of 10 items selected from the 17 in the CPRS related to depression, on the grounds that they are the most sensitive to changes produced by treatment. The scale has high interrater reliability (up to 0.92), correlates 0.87 with a nurses' rating scale, but only 0.63 with the Beck self-rating scale.

These two scales have claimed an advantage over the Hamilton scale in that they are shorter, but as they require a proper interview for completion, this makes little difference in practice.

SELF-RATING SCALES Self-rating scales have been severely criticized for their limitations, but despite their deficiencies, they are still frequently used in evaluating treatments. This is largely because they are economical of the time of investigators, particularly when frequently repeated assessments are required, but also because they generally do give useful information. There is now much evidence to show that they are much less effective for more severely ill patients. Their correlations with observer scales tend to be low, which indicates that the two types of scales are really measuring something different. They should therefore not be regarded as substitutes for observer scales, but as complementary.

Beck Depression Inventory This scale, when it first appeared in 1961, was originally designed to be used by an interviewer who called out the items and the patients chose the appropriate response. This avoided some of the difficulties associated with self-rating scales. It could also be used by the patient for self-rating and is now generally used in this way. It has been shown to have high reliability and validity and compares well with the Hamilton scale, except for the most severely ill depressives. It contains 21 items, scored 0 to 3, of which 15 deal with psychological symptoms and only six are concerned with somatic ones. Some symptoms typical of depressive states are omitted (e.g., loss of appetite and libido).

The scale gives a here-and-now assessment and is easy to use for frequent repetitions. It has been reported to correlate 0.62 with global judgments.

Zung Self-Rating Depression Scale There are 20 items in this scale, rated 1 to 4. Scores are expressed as a percentage of the maximum score and therefore range from 25 to 100. Half of them are worded positively and half negatively. The description of the grades of severity are "A little of the time," "Some of the time," "Good part of the time," and "Most of the time." They do not fit at all well such items as "I notice I am losing weight" and "My mind is as clear as it used to be," but this has not interfered with its use.

The split-half reliability is 0.73, which is quite high, but the correlations with observer scales and clinical judgment are lower. A high figure for the Hamilton scale is 0.62, and with global judgment, the highest value obtained is 0.69. Its use has declined in recent years since some reports appeared indicating that it was somewhat insensitive to clinical improvement following treatment.

Wakefield Self-Assessment Inventory This scale was published in 1971 as an attempt to improve on the Zung scale. It contains 12 items, graded 0 to 3, and is intended for a here-and-now assessment. It has a test–retest reliability of 0.68, which is quite high for this type of scale, and it has correlated 0.87 with the Hamilton scale. It can be used for screening for depressive symptoms (but not for depressive illness). Using a cutoff of 14 to 15 points for this purpose, it was found to misclassify 3 percent of patients and 7.5 percent of normals. It has been found satisfactory by several workers but recently has been criticized as lacking in differentiation between grades of severity in comparison with global judgment.

Leeds Scale This scale was designed in 1976 as an improvement on the Wakefield scale for depression, by adding to it a scale for anxiety. The depression subscale was compared with two self-rating scales and two observer scales and was found to distinguish reasonably well among different levels of severity of illness.

Zerssen Adjective Check List The Adjective Check List is another type of self-assessment in which the subject is asked to choose the one of a pair of adjectives that better corresponds to his or her feelings (e.g., joyful-tearful). The individual items are less informative than symptoms are, but the scale is very sensitive to changes of mood, even short ones.

This checklist, which first appeared in 1970, is an extremely useful one and has been translated into English and other European languages. It consists of two versions, each containing 28 items. The correlation between the two forms (split-half reliability) has been reported as 0.89 in a control group, 0.79 in newly admitted depressives, and 0.93 to 0.96 in an antidepressant trial. Correlations with observer scales have a maximum of 0.71. It has been found to be of adequate sensitivity to the response to treatment.

PARALLEL SELF AND OBSERVER SCALES A few scales are available in parallel versions for use by self or observer. Obviously, the Visual Analogue Scale can be carried out either by an observer or by the patient. Zung designed a Depression Status Inventory to match his self-assessment scale, which contains 20 items scored 1 to 4 and is based on a semistructured interview. It correlated 0.87 with the self-assessment scale on 225 patients of varied diagnoses. Internal consistency, as shown by the correlation between odd- and even-numbered items, came to 0.81. It does not appear to have been much used.

Two self-rating scales have been designed to match the Hamilton scale. The first is the Carroll Rating Scale. Its correlation with the Hamilton scale came to 0.80 and with the Beck Inventory to 0.86. Various other papers have been published giving correlations of that order. The split-half reliability is 0.87. Judging by these figures it would appear to provide a convenient and useful substitute for Hamilton scale scores when, for whatever reason, the latter are not available. It has been used as a screening device for depression in a normal population, in which a cutoff score of 10 points yielded a figure of 9 percent having significant symptoms.

The second is Interact, a computerized self-assessment questionnaire based on the Hamilton scale. It correlated 0.78 with a 10-point global rating scale for outpatients and 0.72 for inpatients. When used as a screening device with a cutoff score of 10, none of 43 control subjects and only four out of 125 patients were misclassified. Patients appear to have found this computer-interview quite acceptable. One of the reasons given is that the computer does not become impatient if a long time is required to come to an answer.

OTHER RATING SCALES Many scales have been devised for use in surveys, to detect those who suffer from psychiatric symptoms. One (the Goldberg scale) has already been described.

SPECIFIC SCALES: MANIA

Compared with the depressions, mania is relatively uncommon. Indeed, it is the most uncommon of the major psychoses, which may be one reason that the construction of scales for its measurement has aroused relatively little interest. Items concerned with manic symptoms are to be found in most general-purpose scales, and in all those described in this section.

Even in the mild cases, manic patients do not feel ill and lack insight. Consequently, there are no self-rating scales for mania. When rating these patients for the first time, it must be taken into account that they can control themselves for a short time and behave quite normally, while at the same time blandly denying, or explaining away, their alleged oddities of behavior. The patients may regard the interview as a joke or an opportunity to have fun at the expense of a mere psychiatrist. It is therefore all-important to obtain from relatives or friends a detailed account of the patient's symptoms and behavior.

Assessment becomes much easier when the patients are admitted to the hospital. Manic euphoria is typically infectious, but is not always present. When the flight of ideas is more than mild, it may be difficult to follow and be mistaken for the thought disorder of schizophrenia. With a little encouragement, these patients will chatter away quite freely. This response is different from schizophrenic patients, who tend to be taciturn.

Biegel Manic State Scale This scale was first described in 1971. It is designed to be used by nursing staff and consists of 26 items, each rated for frequency and severity on six-point scales. The product of the two gives the score for that item. It is highly reliable and was validated by physicians against 15-point global judgments, which were also demonstrated to be highly reliable. Although the scale covers most of the features of mania (indeed, there are redundant items), some aspects are not considered (e.g., disturbed sleep and lability of mood). Its great asset is that the rating covers a long period. It was examined by a team in 1975 that found, as with all the scales examined, that it was not satisfactory by the standards the team had laid down.

Modified Manic State Scale (Blackburn) This scale was designed in 1977 as an improvement of the Biegel scale. It consists of 28 items, for which a glossary is provided. Interrater reliability has been found to vary between 0.79 and 0.85. Validity was determined by using the mean score of three raters and correlating them with global ratings. With nurses' ratings, the correlation was 0.65, and with physicians' ratings, the correlation was 0.80.

Bech–Rafaelsen Mania Scale This scale was devised in 1978. It consists of 11 items that deal with motor and verbal activity, flight of ideas, level of noise, hostility (destructiveness), mood, self-esteem, contact, sleep, sexual interest, and working capacity, rated 0 to 4. There is no item for depressed mood. Interrater reliability, as determined by correlating (rho) each of four raters with the mean of the three others, ranged from 0.97 to 0.99. This obviously represents a maximum. A version consisting of a combination of the mania and melancholia scales has been developed.

REFERENCES

Angst J: Zur Aetiologie und Nosologie Endogener Depressiver Psychosen. Springer, Berlin, 1966. (English trans.) The aetiology and nosology of endogenous depressive psychoses. Foreign Psychiat: Spring 1973.

Angst J: Verlauf unipolar depressiver, bipolar manisch-depressiver, und schizo-affectiver Erkrankungen und Psychosen. Ergebnisse einer prospectiven Studie Fortschr Neurol Psychiat *48:* 3, 1980.

Angst J: The switch from depression to mania, or from mania to depression. J Psychopharmacol *1:* 13, 1987.

Blacker C V R, Clare A W: Depressive disorder in primary care. Brit J Psychiat *150:* 737, 1987.

Hamilton M: *Fish's Clinical Psychopathology,* ed 2. John Wright, Bristol, England, 1985.

Hamilton M, White M: Clinical syndromes in depressive states. J Ment Sci *105:* 985, 1959.

Hedlund J L, Vieweg B W: The Hamilton rating scale for depression: A comprehensive review. J Operational Psychiat *10:* 149, 1979.

Kearns N P, Cruickshank C K, McGuigan K J, Riley S A, Shaw S P, Snaith R P: A comparison of depression rating scales. Brit J Psychiat *141:* 45, 1982.

Kettering R L, Harrow M, Grossman L, Meltzer H Y: The prognostic relevance of delusions in depression: A follow-up study. Amer J Psychiat *144:* 1154, 1987.

Kraepelin E: *Manic-Depressive Insanity and Paranoia,* trans M. Barclay. Livingstone, Edinburgh, 1921.

Kukopulos A, Reginaldi D, Tondo, Barnabei A, Caliari B: Spontaneous length of depression and response to ECT. Psychol Med *7:* 625, 1977.

Leonhard K: *Die Aufteilung der endogenen Psychosen,* ed 2. Akademie-Verlag, Berlin, 1959.

Leonhard K, Korff I, Schulz H: Die Temperamente in den Familian der monopolaren und bipolaren phasischen Psychosen. Psychiat Neurol *143:* 416, 1962.

Paykel E S, editor: *Handbook of Affective Disorders* Churchill Livingstone, Edinburgh, 1982.

Paykel E S, Myers J K, Dienelt M N, Klerman G L, Lindenthal J L, Pepper M P: Life events and depression: A controlled study. Arch Gen Psychiat *21:* 753, 1969.

Perris C: A study of bipolar (manic-depressive) and unipolar recurrent depressive psychoses. Acta Psychiat Scand *42*(suppl): 194, 1966.

Pichot P, Olivier-Martin R, editors: *Psychological Measurements in Psychopharmacology.* S Karger, Basel, 1973.

Roth M, Gurney C, Garside R F, Kerr T A: The relationship between anxiety states and depressive illness, I. Brit J Psychiat *121:* 147, 1972.

Ryan N D, Puig-Antich J, Ambrosini P, Rabinovich H, Robinson D, Nelson, Lyengar S, Twomey J: The clinical picture of major depression in children and adolescents. Arch Gen Psychiat *44:* 854, 1987.

Sartorius N, Ban T A, editors: *Assessment of Depression.* Springer Verlag, New York, 1986.

Weissman M M, Prusoff B, Pincus C: Symptom patterns in depressed patients and depressed normals. J Nerv Ment Dis *160:* 15, 1975.

Winokur G, Clayton P, Woodruff R A: *Manic-Depressive Illness.* Mosby, St. Louis, 1969.

Zerssen D V, Koeller D M, Rey E R: Objectivierende Untersuchungen zur pramorbiden Personlichkeit endogen Depressiver. In *Das Depressive Syndrom,* H Hippius, H Selbach, editors. Urban and Schwarzenberg, Munich, 1969.

17.4
MOOD DISORDERS: SOMATIC TREATMENT

ROBERT M. POST, M.D.

INTRODUCTION

The psychopharmacotherapy of the mood disorders is approaching a subspecialty in psychiatry because of the multitude of treatment modalities that are now available to the clinician. Just 50 years ago, treatments were only supportive and palliative. Electroconvulsive therapy (ECT) then emerged as an efficacious somatic treatment for major depressive illness. It was soon followed by the introduction of monoamine oxidase inhibitors (MAOIs), tricyclic antidepressants, and now a host of second- and third-generation treatment modalities.

The discovery of the effectiveness of lithium salts in the treatment of patients with manic-depressive illness (bipolar disorder) revolutionized the therapy of this illness. With lithium, a treatment became available that, for the first time, was effective for both acute intervention in and the longer-term prevention of mood disorder recurrences. Likewise, tricyclics and MAOIs are now known to be able to prevent relapses in unipolar depressive illness. Only recently have alternatives emerged for the treatment of the lithium-nonresponsive bipolar patient. A series of anticonvulsant agents, used either alone or in combination with lithium carbonate, may provide the next generation of treatment strategies. Very preliminary evidence of the efficacy of the calcium channel antagonists and the even more preliminary evidence for peptide interventions in manic-depressive illness may lead to the development of new therapeutic strategies. One may look forward to more specific pharmacotherapies and even the intrathecal and discrete regional delivery of somatic treatment to the brain.

The development of somatic treatments, such as ECT and pharmacological interventions, in psychiatry has been closely tied to neurology and medicine. Seizure therapy with chemical or electrical inductions was introduced after the observation of an inverse relationship between seizures and psychosis in some epileptic patients. Even the first observations with lithium were focused initially on looking for a sedative and anticonvulsant for uric acid–induced excitement and seizures. It is curious that a series of anticonvulsants may now play a role in the treatment of recurrent manic-depressive illness, in light of the original use of the convulsive seizures themselves as a therapeutic modality for mania and depression. Carbamazepine, valproic acid, and clonazepam, for example, each appear to possess antimanic properties. Mood elevation was noted in tuberculosis patients treated with isoniazid, providing the background for the development of the MAOI antidepressants. The tricyclic antidepressant imipramine emerged from the search for psychoactive derivatives of the antipsychotic phenothiazines, and imipramine was observed to have active antidepressant properties.

The field of psychopharmacology now requires a medical sophistication similar to that necessary for the management of cardiac or epileptic patients. Assessment of the type of cardiac arrhythmia, its pattern, and its atrial or ventricular origin is critical to the subsequent pharmacotherapy. A different series of drugs is ranked according to the type of pathophysiological process involved. This is also the case in the seizure disorders, as complex partial seizures (temporal lobe epilepsy) are treated very differently from the absence seizures of petit mal epilepsy. A similar situation is now apparent in the pharmacotherapy of the mood disorders. Although biochemical, anatomical, and physiological diagnostic techniques are not so far advanced as in the specialties just mentioned, nonetheless, the initial diagnostic process and longitudinal description of episodes are important. In particular, the treatments of unipolar and bipolar depression are very different, with different priorities for the unipolars and even relative contraindications of some of these treatments for the bipolar-disordered patient. Mania presents its own unique therapeutic challenges.

INITIAL DIAGNOSTIC AND THERAPEUTIC APPROACHES

IMPEDIMENTS TO TREATMENT Mood disorders are eminently treatable, yet several illness-related variables complicate the treatment. That is, depressed patients often do not recognize their symptoms as related to the constellation of a medical illness, may not seek treatment, and may become overwhelmed by the symptoms of the depression itself, such as helplessness and hopelessness, or suicidality. Thus, treatment must be conducted against the backdrop of the patient's distorted cognitions of hopelessness and untreatability, and the treatment, which may take time, must be continually weighed in relation to suicidal risk. The therapist's empirical basis for hope and recovery even as part of the illness's natural course needs to be conveyed to the patient without the promise of immediate results, as the expected lags in the onset of the treatment's efficacy could be misinterpreted as confirming the patient's worst fears of being untreatable.

There are also particular impediments to treating manic patients. The early stages of hypomania are often associated with increased productivity and a sense of well-being. A variety of positive attributes, including increased energy, sociability, and an ability to function with fewer hours of sleep, may be seen as highly desirable. The adverse personal, social, and employment consequences of escalating hypomania and full-blown mania tend to be dismissed. It therefore becomes imperative to establish ways to recognize symptoms early, to treat them, to keep the patient in treatment, and to provide a safety net by means of patient and family interaction and education. Thus, the denial and thought disorder of mania must be approached as seriously as the hopelessness and suicidality of depression. Therapeutic activism and the aggressive treatment of early manic and depressive symptoms should be the byword.

LONG-TERM ISSUES A fundamental aspect of the mood disorders is their recurrent or cyclic nature. The approach to the acute episode must thus be integrated with the longer-term course of illness in the patient with recurrences. This becomes even more important in regard to unequivocal findings for long-term prophylaxis in unipolar patients with tricyclic antidepressants, MAOI antidepressants, or even lithium carbonate, as well as the use of lithium and the newer agents to prevent recurrences of both depression and mania in the bipolar disorders. These longer-term issues, perhaps, should not immediately be discussed with the patient, as they might increase the hopelessness of depression or the denial of mania. However, they should be explored in detail in the resolution phase of the acute episode when the patient can more realistically deal with his or her illness in terms of some of its longer-term characteristics and the possibilities of recurrence. In this fashion, the illness should be viewed as a chronic and episodically relapsing illness, such as rheumatoid arthritis or diabetes, for which effective long-term management strategies are available and with which patients are likely to have long periods of time without symptoms but at the same time be vulnerable to acute episodes that need more active and aggressive intervention and management.

MEDICAL EXAMINATION A thorough history and medical examination is paramount. In light of the multitude of medical mimics of both manic and depressive syndromes, the patient should be approached with the perspective that an associated medical cause may exist until proven otherwise. Throughout the history and physical examination, attention should be paid to the obvious or subtle hallmarks of associated pathology. The physician should be alert to signs and symptoms indicative of central nervous system (CNS) neuropathology, underlying endocrinopathy, or associated medical illness. Although aggressive in exploring these themes with patient and family, the physician should nonetheless be aware and even directly state to the patient that all of these somatic and vegetative symptoms may indicate a typical depressive process. Thus, even the earliest parts of the history taking can be used not only for diagnostic uncovering, but also for the patient's initial education in the types of symptoms that are typical of the disorder or indicative of its natural course of spontaneous remission and the likely response to somatic and pharmacological intervention. The medical examination should also be directed at uncovering evidence of glaucoma (relative contraindication for anticholinergic antidepressants), or of cardiac, renal, or thyroid abnormalities that may help guide subsequent treatment choices.

This initial "medicalization" assists in the development of the therapeutic process. It focuses the clinician on each psychological and somatic symptom category, simultaneously educating the patient, providing target symptoms for future assessment of the efficacy of psychological and pharmacological intervention, and constructing the framework for the longitudinal monitoring of the patient, as these same symptoms are likely to form the core symptoms of a future recurrence and provide an early warning system for the early detection and aggressive treatment of any future emerging symptoms. In this regard, the historical approach to the mood-disordered patient should differ from casual psychiatric history taking.

GRAPHING THE ILLNESS The author suggests developing a graphic representation of the patient's prior depressive and manic symptoms. This will form a backdrop to the evaluation of the efficacy of previous treatments, if any, and to the efficacy of the current and future prescription. A formal and visual graphic representation of the patient's longitudinal course of illness is useful for several reasons. It will provide a clear-cut picture of the earlier course of illness, which appears to be the best predictor of the future pattern of episodes. It clarifies medication responsiveness. It helps in the medicalization of the history taking and management process. It encourages the patient's collaboration and thus may enhance the doctor–patient relationship, bringing the patient into the process as an active rather than a passive participant. If a number of past recurrences are uncovered in the history, it may also help in the subsequent long-term approach to the illness and in the patient's compliance with prescribed regimens. Moreover, the author has found that this process often leads to the uncovering of important psychosocial events and possible precipitants of the illness, as well as unique characteristics of the illness, such as seasonal variation, relationship to anniversaries, and other variations that cannot be discovered easily without systematic and graphic representation of the prior course.

With a little practice, the course of an illness can be graphed easily, if not almost automatically. The author suggests that this be done in the initial history-taking session and be the primary mode of history taking, in preference to a verbal account that is later intended for conversion to a graph. In this way, both the patient and the physician are immediately and systematically focused on the longitudinal course of the illness and its variation over time, rather than having this develop as a later agenda that can easily be sidetracked by time pressures and attention to acute symptomatology. The graphic approach and its associated landmarks can also facilitate recall of important events and dates.

Levels of severity Physicians can devise their own ways of plotting the longitudinal course of illness or adopt a system like the one the author and his colleagues have used successfully over the past decade, which is graphing three levels of severity of mania or depression based on functional incapacity which can be easily assessed retrospectively (Fig. 17.4-1).

The mild level is one in which the patient or family notes a distinct change from the usual behavior, but there is not a notable impairment in the patient's functional status. This state is readily discerned by depressed patients and may represent the baseline of double depression from which more severe episodes erupt. However, hypomanic patients may deny this mild state, and so one may have to obtain additional information from family members and relatives. Parenthetically, this observation also reemphasizes the utility of an initial nonanalytic approach to the patient's illness and its diagnosis and treatment, including the participation and support of family members from the outset. This may be of value in both gaining historical information and managing potential suicidality of depression and denial of the adverse consequences of hypomania and mania.

Moderate levels of depression and mania can be graphed at the next level to represent illness with distinct functional impairment. That is, patients are able to continue their social or employment responsibilities, but only barely and with obvious difficulties, such as absences from work or not being able to perform some routine social tasks.

The third, or severe, level of impairment is graphed when patients are functionally incapacitated and unable to perform consistently in their usual roles (i.e., they are no longer able to go to work or to perform socially). Hospitalization can be indicated by shading in the severe manic or depressive episode.

Earlier psychopharmacological interventions Superimposed on this template of mood fluctuations can be the history of prior psychopharmacological interventions which is plotted above the episodes, as illustrated in Figure 17.4-1 of the life chart schema and in the case examples in Figures 17.4-2 and 17.4-3. When plotted in this fashion, the efficacy of earlier treatments is often reclassified. A treatment previously deemed ineffective may, on careful reexamination, be shown to be partially effective (i.e., a decreased frequency or severity of prior episodes depicted, compared with the pretreatment baseline). If this is the case, this reassessment will be used to consider supplementing this partially effective treatment, rather than abandoning it. Previous psychotherapeutic interventions should also be systematically graphed. As illustrated in Figure 17.4-1, important psychosocial events (anniversaries, suicide attempts) and other notes about side effects, dosage, reasons for discontinuation of medications, and the like can be noted below the mood graph.

Descriptive symptoms The anamnestic account of symptomatology also provides the basis for following clinical improvement during an acute episode and during possible subsequent episodes. In particular, one should develop a sense for the areas of major symptomatology that are the best descriptors of an individual patient's episode. For some, it may be impaired sleep with early morning awakening; for others it may be impaired concentration; and for still others, it may be decreased energy or increased agitation and an inner sense of anxiety. The sequential ebbing of symptomatology during a treated episode may also be a clue to the duration of maintenance treatment required and to the earliest symptoms that may recur during a subsequent episode. Should these more difficult or residual symptoms tend to recur or become more profound while tapering medication, or break through during constant prophylaxis, they can be used as indicators for renewed, more aggressive management of a potential episode.

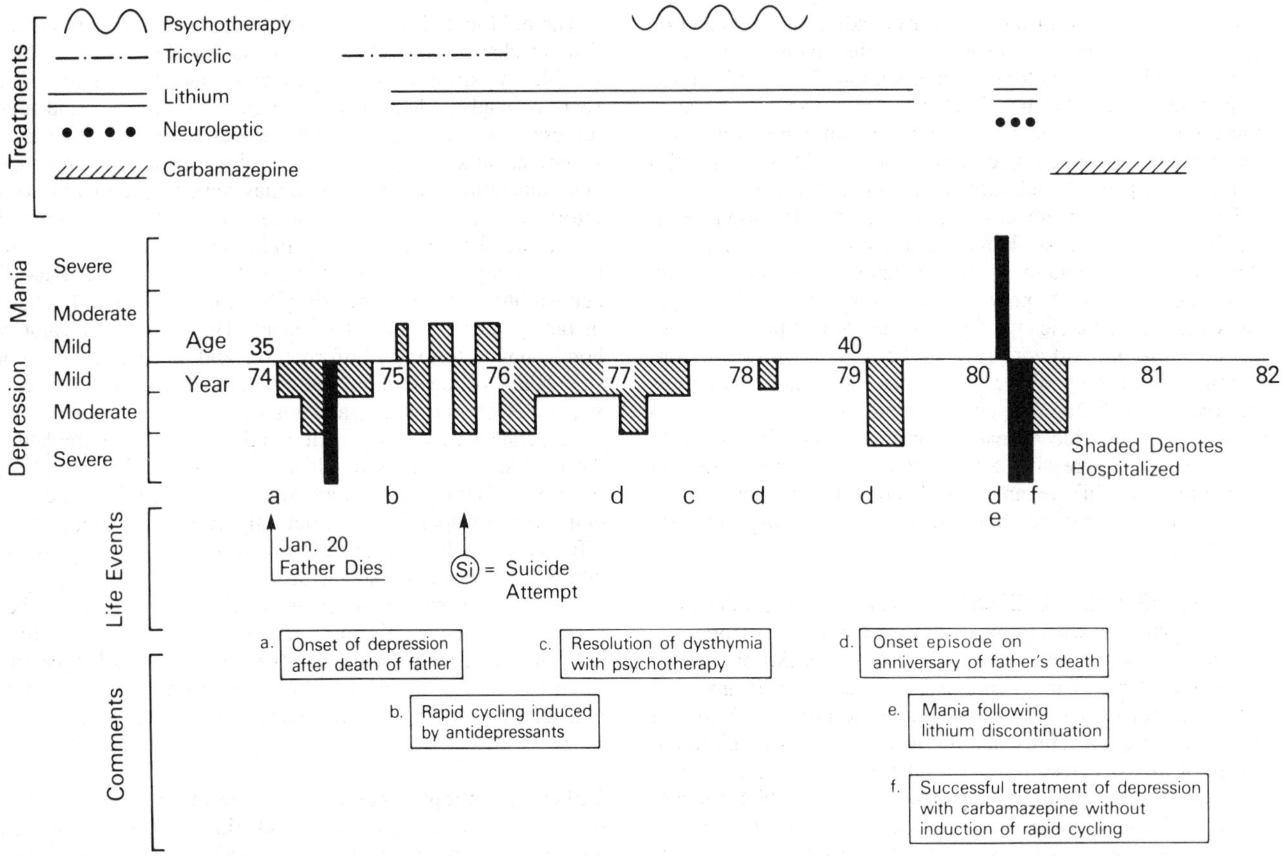

FIGURE 17.4-1. *Graphing the course of mood disorder: Prototype of a "life chart."*

Similarly, clinicians should decide and make a contract with their patients in advance about symptoms that may be forerunners to a manic episode and require monitoring and intervention. Early signs of the emergence of the patients' typical symptoms, such as increased energy or religiosity or decreased sleep, which may be appreciated as welcome attributes, may nonetheless be the precursor to more adverse symptoms. Attention to these early symptoms, while insight is still preserved and denial manageable, may save the patients and their families from much more severe and prolonged episodes.

Prospective charting For the unipolar patient with recurrent illness, and definitely for the bipolar patient with many episodes, the author suggests that some elements of this life chart process be continued prospectively. This can be accomplished quite easily in a number of ways, including having the patient keep a nightly calendar and write a number representing a visual analogue scale from 0 (worst ever felt) to 50 (normal or usual self) to 100 (best ever felt). In this fashion, patients can track their mood fluctuations in a systematic manner that is unobtrusive and only takes a matter of seconds to complete. In an analogy to the diabetic patient, mood rating, like self assessment of urine glucose, may provide an important measure of how well the patient's illness is responding to a given treatment modality or dose–side effect titration. It is, in fact, worth reemphasizing that the morbidity and mortality of the mood disorders can be no less severe than are those of many medical illnesses, for which a great deal more attention is paid to the longitudinal and systematic monitoring of fluctuations in symptomatology, biochemistry, and underlying pathology.

Subjective and objective differences Finally, asking patients to make a calendar and rate their moods with a specific number on the 100 mm line has an additional, secondary benefit. It speaks to the possibility of becoming attuned to the major subjective or objective differences in the assessment of a patient's illness. Many unipolar depressed patients can detect mood changes and side effects before the therapist observes them. Conversely, many bipolar patients show remarkable improvement in major aspects of their symptomatology, including sleep, appetite, energy, spontaneity, and sociability, without any subjective sense of clinical improvement attending these obvious objective changes. If patients do not recognize that their depression is improving despite objective signs, it may lead to further therapeutic pessimism and also may increase the possibility of suicide, as the patients may have more energy to carry out such a plan, still convinced that improvement is not imminent.

PERSPECTIVE Although a hopeful perspective about the treatability of a patient's episode should be maintained, it should also be recognized that a series of drugs may need to be tried before the best treatment regimen can be found. The evaluation of a treatment response often requires 3 to 6

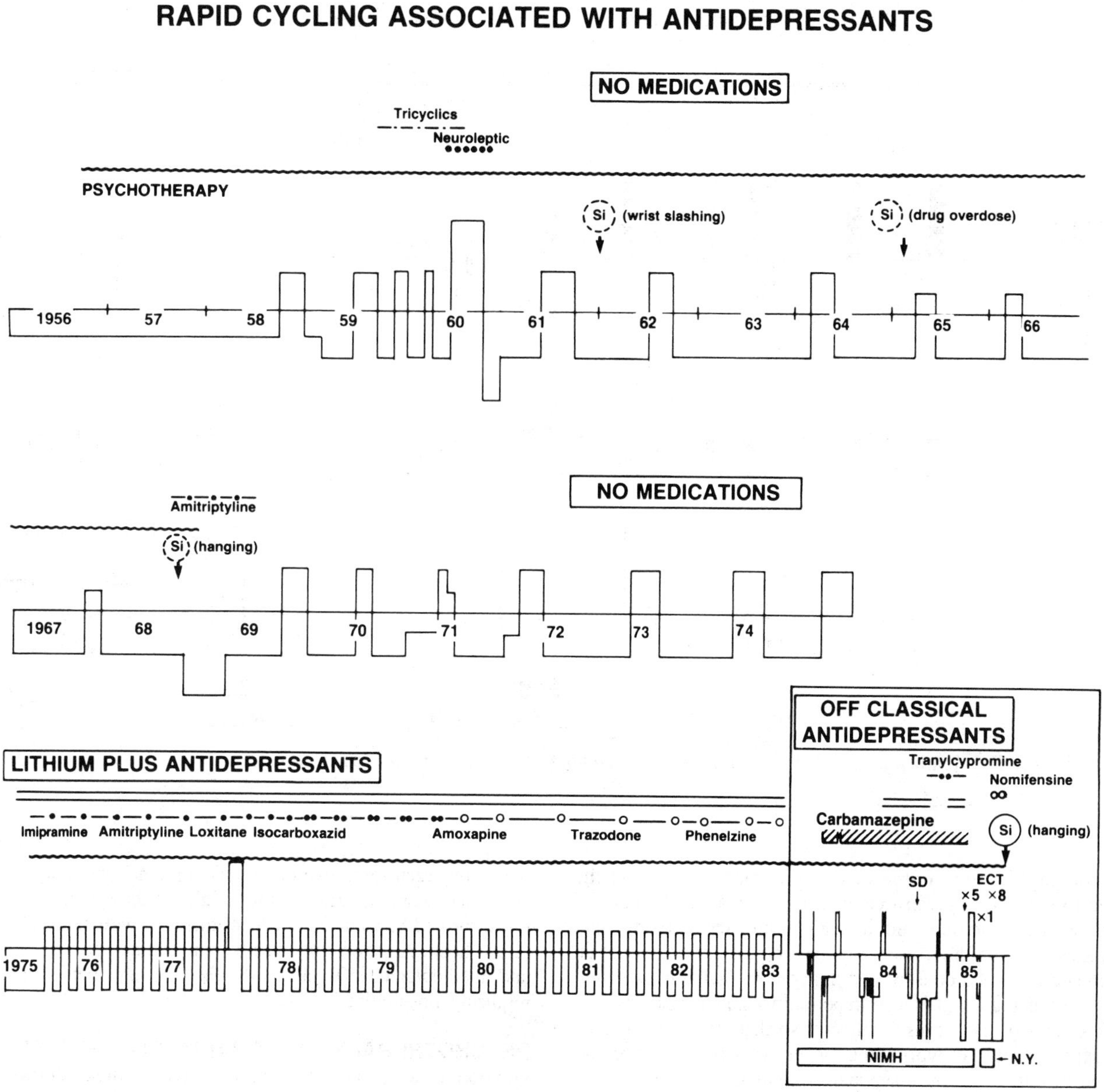

FIGURE 17.4-2. *Rapid cycling associated with antidepressants: Case study of 59-year-old bipolar female.*

weeks, and a given agent's lack of efficacy should be treated as additional information about the patient's illness, rather than as an indication that the illness is not responsive. At the outset of treatment, the availability of different effective treatments, with many drugs in each class, should thus be brought to the patient's attention. This is important for putting possible treatment sequences in their proper perspective, as well as emphasizing that a lack of response to or an intolerance of a drug or its side effects does not portend a negative therapeutic outcome.

TIME FRAME These points should be reemphasized throughout the entire therapeutic process, particularly in light of the different time frames available to the therapist and the patient. The therapist is aware not only of these many treatment alternatives but also of the extended treatment course that sometimes is required in order to achieve optimal efficacy. From the patient's perspective, and perhaps even from that of his or her family, the current mood-disordered state may overwhelm with its sense of immediacy and desperation. Particularly for the depressed patient, this feeling of pain and hopelessness can all too easily overtake the realities of the situation and increase the risk of suicide before a positive treatment outcome.

Reassurance without overpromising immediate therapeutic effect would thus appear to be an important part of the treatment process. A similar but inverse process may be required for the manic patient, who also may see only the immediate time frame and not the longer-term perspective. The therapist should encourage and help supply the ego for the longer-term view in both of these cases. In this fashion, supportive and cognitive approaches to psychopharmacotherapy as well as to psychotherapy of the mood disorders may be essential. The patient should also be counseled not to make important long-term decisions on the basis of a distorted view of him- or herself.

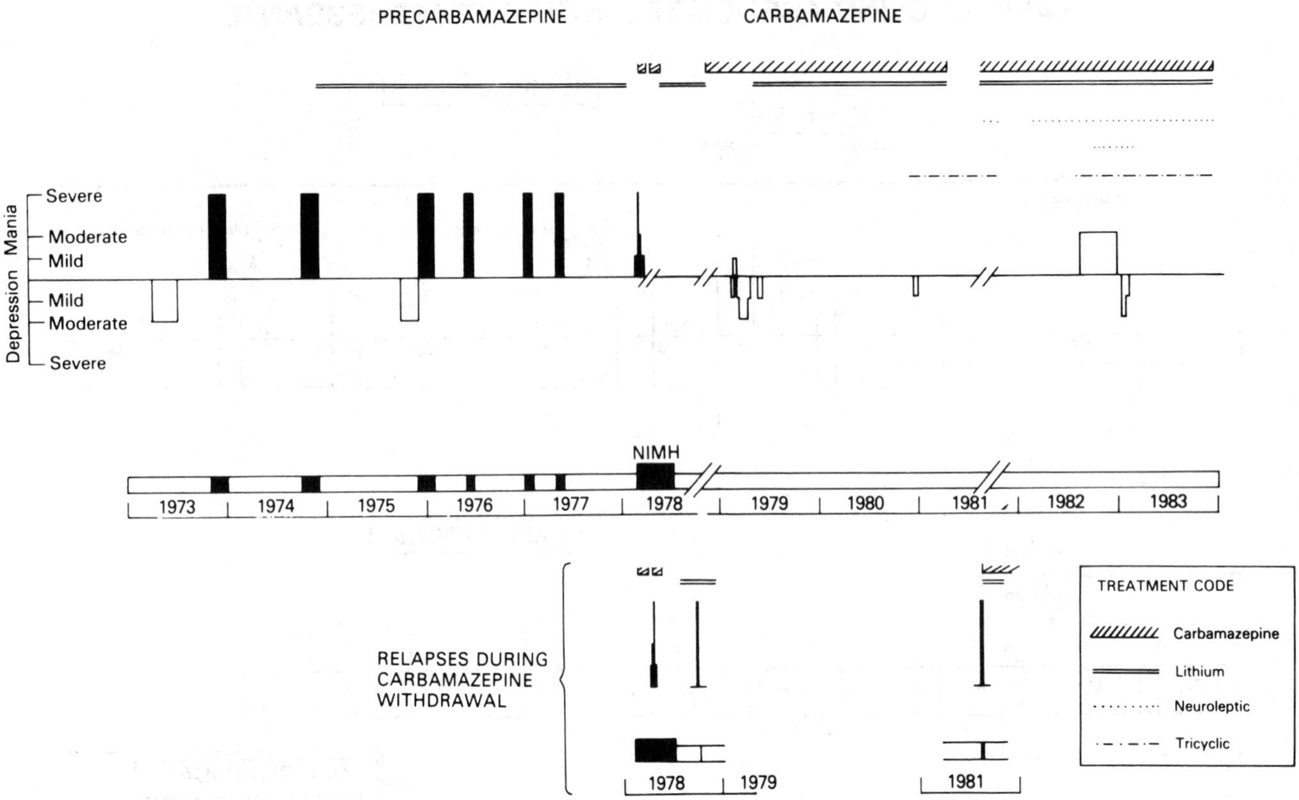

FIGURE 17.4-3. *Acute and prophylactic response to carbamazepine in a lithium nonresponder.*

Stressing the time frame of possible improvement and the need to evaluate a given treatment over a matter of weeks to months may not only aid in maintaining the patients' and families' morale but also may be helpful in obtaining an adequate informed consent and in avoiding malpractice litigation. In this regard, it is also important to indicate the possible side effects of each drug treatment, so that these can be seen as expected and not worrisome, or, conversely, can be recognized as out of the ordinary and something that merits a call to the physician when indicated.

HOSPITALIZATION The decision to hospitalize severely depressed or manic patients depends on a variety of clinical and pharmacological issues. Hospitalization is often indicated for the acutely suicidal patient, but may also be considered for a patient with associated medical problems or one who needs close management and monitoring of complicated or novel psychopharmacological regimens. For the knowledgeable patient and supportive family, one or more of a series of psychopharmacological approaches can often be accomplished on an outpatient basis, particularly if there is close coordination between the patient and physician regarding dosage, titration, side effects, and the like. Despite many of the largely societal criticisms of the modern use of ECT, this modality should be given higher than usual priority when faced with an extremely suicidal patient, one with associated medical illnesses and a difficult side effects profile to routine psychopharmacological agents, or in other medical and psychological emergency situations that demand the most rapid treatment response available.

For the recurrent severely manic patient who may refuse voluntary hospitalization at the height of an episode, obtaining informed consent in advance during a well interval for a future hospitalization may avoid many cumbersome practical and medicolegal difficulties should another manic episode requiring hospitalization occur.

PSYCHOTHERAPY AND PHARMACOTHERAPY Depression is a serious, potentially lethal medical illness. As such, the patients and their families deserve much support. The range of psychotherapeutic modalities and techniques useful in treating depressed patients is discussed elsewhere in this text. The author emphasizes the importance of combining psychosocial and pharmacological approaches in a majority of patients, not only because of the evidence for the efficacy of both treatment modalities, but also because of the potential for mutual interaction and support of the patients and their social system in the context of ongoing pharmacotherapy. Even if one does not entirely believe in psychotherapy as a primary treatment modality for depression, or in the evidence for its efficacy, it may behoove the clinician to use a combined treatment for the severely depressed patient for many reasons. Not only does the initial evidence suggest that these two types of therapy may target different symptoms, but the therapeutic process may provide strong support for the patient before the psychopharmacological interventions are effective, especially if several agents are required before a successful one is found. Psychosocial issues and stresses may not only play important etiological roles in the onset and amelioration of some types of depression, but may also guide the need for more aggressive pharmacological management during a period of high vulnerability.

Frequent meetings with the patient may also help in assessing the progress of pharmacotherapy, titrating the dose against blood levels and side effects, and facilitating compliance in the face of pessimism. Finally, if a depressed patient has severe pain and suffering, frequent meetings may encourage the physician to apply maximum clinical and therapeutic leverage.

THEORETICAL ASSUMPTIONS AND RATIONALE

NEUROTRANSMITTER THEORIES Because most of the effective treatments for mood disorders were discovered by serendipity or empiricism, the effectiveness of somatic treatments has propelled theoretical formulations, rather than vice versa. Neurotransmitter theories of the basis of depression have included serotonergic, noradrenergic, cholinergic, dopaminergic, and γ-aminobutyric acid (GABA)-ergic theories, each based on presumed mechanisms of effective pharmacotherapeutic interventions. For example, the findings that several antidepressant modalities could, at least acutely, potentiate catecholamines and that reserpine, which depleted these neurotransmitters, could exacerbate depression and treat mania led to the catecholamine hypothesis of deficiencies in depression and excesses in mania.

Now that it appears that relatively selective manipulations of several different neurotransmitter systems can be effective, a critical psychopharmacological question is raised as to whether an individual may respond to one type of treatment with a postulated mechanism of action targeting one neurotransmitter system, but not to another. This area clearly requires further research. However, in the absence of definitive studies of this question, one is tempted to recommend the sequential use of drugs that act differently within or among classes of agents (e.g., changing from a relatively more serotonergic to a relatively more noradrenergic tricyclic reuptake blocker, or from a tricyclic to a MAOI to lithium). Because there appear to be relatively few validated clinical or biological markers of response to given treatment agents, one must move through the various treatment agents for the refractory patient until an effective one is found, with the process largely being trial and error. A similar strategy of using agents with different mechanisms of action in mania may also be warranted.

CLINICAL PREDICTORS The author will attempt, wherever possible, to indicate the relative predictors of response based on the clinical presentations of a given type of depression or mania, although, in most instances, a strong empirical data base for the recommendations is lacking. For example, the drugs of choice may vary for an agitated, retarded, or psychotic depression. Moreover, given the necessity for protracted clinical trials (of many weeks) in order to evaluate clinical efficacy, one might attempt to potentiate a specific drug treatment once adequate blood levels have been reached, prior to switching treatment modalities. Thus, thyroid potentiation or lithium potentiation deserves an earlier emphasis in the treatment sequence than do alternative agents.

Once a detailed history from the patient and, perhaps, a friend or relative shows that there is no prior personal or family history of mania, one proceeds in the acute and prophylactic treatment of the unipolar depressed patient in a fashion very different from that used in the bipolar patient. These approaches form a backdrop to the longer-term prophylaxis of either unipolar or recurrent depression or bipolar manic-depressive illness which, likewise, tends to be recurrent. When an antidepressant treatment modality is found to help alleviate an acute depressive episode, conventional wisdom suggests that treatment be continued for 6 to 9 months. This process can be lengthened or shortened, depending on other variables. The discreteness, rapidity, and completeness of the alleviation of depressive symptoms may provide a guideline. The presence of residual symptomatology (such as minor sleep disturbance, anergia, lack of concentration, or minor early morning awakening) tends to suggest continuing therapy as well as a more aggressive treatment with higher doses or potentiation. Minor increases in depression following a gradual reduction in dose may also suggest the need for continuing the therapy. (Tapering of cyclic and MAOI antidepressants may also help avoid minor drug withdrawal symptoms, which can include sleeplessness, nausea, vomiting, and irritability, as well as rebound increases in dreaming with the MAOIs.)

BIOLOGICAL PREDICTORS Although considerable work is needed in the area of biological prediction of treatment response, the initial data suggest that the lack of normalization in the dexamethasone suppression test in a patient who shows an abnormal escape from dexamethasone suppression during an episode may be associated with a higher risk of relapse. Thus, a positive test may point to continuing a tricyclic antidepressant treatment, even though the patient is clinically asymptomatic. Some evidence indicates that the sleep electroencephalogram (EEG) may remain abnormal for a long time after remission, although this test does not appear to be a practically useful marker for continuing therapy. As in many other instances, the best prediction of future episodes may be the scrutiny of past episodes. Therefore, if there have been earlier, protracted episodes with some evidence of relapse after stopping medication, the treatment of an episode should be extended.

PHARMACOLOGICAL AGENTS AND SOMATIC THERAPIES

ACUTE TREATMENT OF UNIPOLAR DEPRESSION **Tricyclics** Despite sporadic claims to the contrary, there is little convincing evidence that one tricyclic works more rapidly than another, and this may also be true for the new second- and third-generation heterocyclic (tetra- and bicyclic) antidepressants. Although further research may prove some exceptions to this rule, clinicians should become familiar with several different antidepressants in the heterocyclic class and their dose response and dose–side effect characteristics. The clinical response profiles and side effects of tricyclic and related antidepressant agents are summarized in Table 17.4-1.

SIDE EFFECTS Conventional wisdom suggests using initial minor selection criteria to choose one agent over the next. For example, one might consider protriptyline (Vivactil), or desipramine (Norpramin) (or imipramine [Tofranil]) for a retarded depressed patient and a more sedating drug, such as amitriptyline (Elavil) or doxepin (Sinequan), for a more agitated depressed patient. In general, the tertiary amine antidepressants, such as amitriptyline, imipramine, trimipramine (Surmontil), and doxepin, tend to be more sedating than

TABLE 17.4-1
Relative Side Effects of Antidepressant Modalities

Drug	*Sedation*	*Hypotension*	*Anticholinergic‡*	*Relative Action† Ne/5-HT*	*Other Effects*
(Dose: mg/day)*					
Amitriptyline (75–300)	+++	+++	+++	±/+++	H.O.D.
Imipramine (75–300)	++	+++	+++	++/+++	H.O.D.
Doxepin (75–300)	+++	++	++	++/++	C.T. and H.O.D. Useful blockage of H_2 receptors; will not reverse guanethidine effects.
Nortriptyline (50–150)	++	+	++	+++/++	H.O.D.; possible inverted "U" relationship of blood levels to clinical response.
Protriptyline (15–60)	±	++?	+++	+++/+	H.O.D.
Desipramine (75–300)	+	+++	+	+++/0	H.O.D.; ? Less weight gain.
Maprotiline (50–225)	++	++	++	+++/0	Seizures; long half-life; C.T. and H.O.D.
Trazodone (50–600)	++	+++	0	0/++	Priapism; no prolongation of cardiac conduction but possible arrhythmogenic; L.O.D.
Fluoxetine (20–80)	±	0	0	0/+++	No weight gain; possible insomnia, rash
Bupropion (75–450)	0			0/0 ?	Seizures in high doses.
Amoxapine (50–600)	++	+	++	+++/±	Extrapyramidal effects and tardive dyskinesia; ? rapid onset, L.O.D.
Alprazolam (2–6)	+++	± ?	?	? / ?	? tolerance, dependence.
Lithium (900–2,400)	±	0	0	– / +	Thyroid and renal side effects.
Bromocriptine (10–60)	±?	+++	/	0 / 0	Dopamine agonist.
ECT (7–10 Rx's)	0	0	0	++ / ?	Acute memory loss.

*Starting doses are usually one-half or less than the lower dose range; doses should be started slower and achieve about one-half of the conventional range in geriatric patients.
+++ = marked; ++ = moderate; + = mild; ± = equivocal; 0 = absent
†Reuptake blockage of norepinephrine (NE) or serotonin (5-HT)
‡Effects include dry mouth, blurred vision, constipation, tachycardia, and urinary hesitancy/retention.
C.T.: As cardiotoxic as TCAs.
H.O.D.: Potentially lethal in O.D.
L.O.D. Low cardiotoxicity in O.D.

are the secondary amines—desmethylimipramine, nortriptyline (Pamelor), and protriptyline. Desipramine or fluoxetine (Prozac) may be considered for the overweight depressed patient or one with a history of weight gain during previous tricyclic administration, as preliminary evidence suggests that these drugs may be less prone to induce tricyclic-induced weight gain. The use of L-glutamine or L-tryptophan for tricyclic-induced weight gain has been recommended by some authorities. Bupropion (Wellbutrin) and fluoxetine may cause a weight loss rather than a weight gain. Isocarboxazid (Marplan) may be less likely to cause weight gain than tranylcypromine (Parnate) or phenelzine (Nardil).

Anticholinergic effects (such as dry mouth, sweating, constipation, urinary hesitancy and retention, and delayed ejaculation) tend to be more prominent with imipramine and protriptyline, and less so with trazodone (Desyrel), desipramine, amoxapine (Asendin), maprotiline (Ludiomil), and the MAOIs or lithium. Problems with orthostatic, hypotension, particularly in the elderly, can be associated with imipramine, amitriptyline, desipramine, trazodone, and the MAOIs, but not as often with nortriptyline, amoxapine, maprotiline, and doxepin (or lithium and carbamazepine). The heterocyclics—amoxapine, maprotiline, and trazodone—touted for their less sedating and, possibly, less anticholinergic and less cardiotoxic profile, are not consistent in this regard. Doses of tricyclics equivalent to 2,500 mg of imipramine may be fatal. The risk of seizures increases with many cyclic antidepressants, especially with high-dose maprotiline treatment (i.e., above 225 mg per day). This drug thus should be avoided in patients with an abnormal EEG or family history of epilepsy. Again, these guidelines are clinical generalizations, often based on several case reports or anecdotal evidence, and may not stand the test of time and careful clinical research evaluation.

BLOOD LEVELS A general rule that is widely applicable and replicated is that there is a wide variation in blood levels among patients treated with the same dose of a tricyclic or heterocyclic. Thus, bringing all patients to the conventional dose range will leave some with blood levels below the therapeutic range and others with very high levels. This may be important for nortriptyline, for which there is evidence of an inverted U-shaped curve (i.e., that there is a therapeutic window for clinical improvement below and above which patients do not do as well). Thus, with the exception of nortriptyline, it appears clinically useful to increase doses slowly, titrating against side effects with blood-level monitoring at (maintenance) doses in those patients who do not show an adequate therapeutic effect. During a moderate to high-dose, but ineffective, nortriptyline treatment, one might decrease the dose to bring levels back into the therapeutic range (which is highly variable across studies).

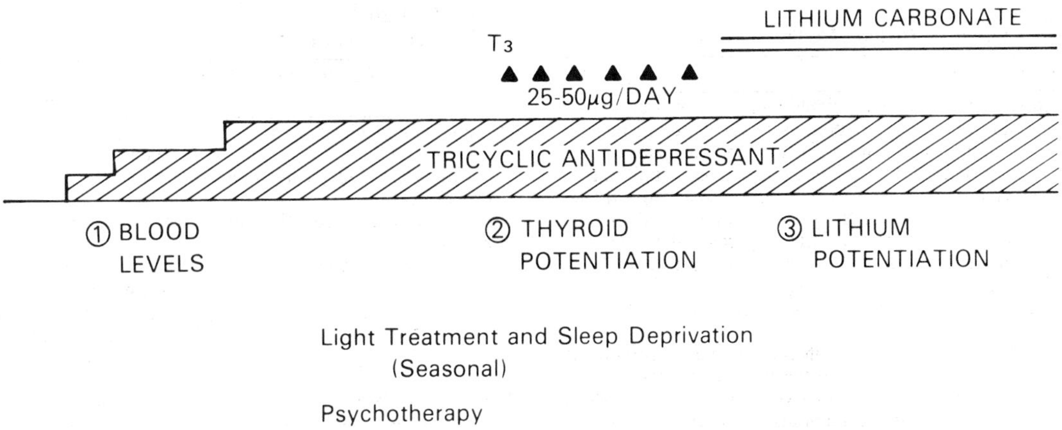

FIGURE 17.4-4. *Maximizing and potentiating antidepressant treatment.*

TIME FRAME With the traditional tricyclic antidepressants, imipramine and amitriptyline, as well as the less conventional and atypical agent carbamazepine (Tegretol), it appears that initial improvement in sleep in the first weeks of treatment is not predictive of the subsequent outcome. Physicians often use this initial improvement in sleep as an index of ultimate clinical response, but the preliminary evidence indicates that this is not warranted. Nevertheless, the patient may be comforted by the fact that sleep is improving in its own right. Antidepressant effects often require 2 to 4 weeks before they become substantial and 4 to 8 for maximal effect; however, gradual clinical improvement often begins in the first and second weeks of treatment. Thus, there may not be an absolute lag in onset of clinical efficacy, only in the time to onset of substantial or maximal change.

POTENTIATION Given the long time frame that may be required to evaluate an antidepressant response, one is tempted to consider relatively benign types of antidepressant potentiation in the first or second antidepressant trial before switching to a new category of agents (Fig. 17.4-4). Thus, when a patient appears to be at either maximally tolerated doses or adequate blood levels of the drug and has not responded adequately, one might consider the addition of thyroid hormones or lithium carbonate. There is a sizable literature regarding the efficacy of thyroid potentiation in converting antidepressant nonresponders to responders. This appears to be independent of an initial clinical thyroid status or any evidence of hypothyroidism. A response to the addition of T_3 (25 to 50 μg per day) usually occurs within the first week or two of treatment. Therefore, if there is no response in this time frame, the clinical trial of T_3 potentiation can be exchanged for other options. A second option is potentiation with lithium carbonate.

An extensive literature, including several controlled clinical trials, reveals that the addition of lithium carbonate to a variety of antidepressant modalities, including tricyclic, heterocyclic, and MAOI antidepressants, or even carbamazepine, is often accompanied by a rapid clinical improvement. This may begin within 24 to 48 hours, but may be slower in onset and stretch over the first week to 10 days. Conventional doses of lithium that are slightly lower than those usually used in single-drug treatment generally are effective. When used in this fashion, the side-effects profile appears to be quite benign. Lithium potentiation may be effective for all subtypes of depression. The initial reports of estrogen potentiation of antidepressant response do not appear as promising as those of either thyroid or lithium potentiation.

One might consider shifting treatment from one cyclic antidepressant to another should there appear unacceptable side effects before adequate blood levels or a clinical response has been achieved. If adequate doses and blood levels have been achieved but the response is inadequate, one may switch to a drug with a different biochemical profile within the same class or to a different class, such as a MAOI.

Monoamine oxidase inhibitors MAOIs may be started shortly after the termination of tricyclic antidepressant therapy, but the converse is not recommended, as MAO inhibition can persist from 1 to 2 weeks or longer following cessation of treatment. The lag in onset of relief with the MAOIs is similar to that of the heterocyclics, so 3 to 6 weeks may be required to assess the treatment's effectiveness. Doses in the higher drug range should be given to achieve adequate MAO inhibition (phenelzine, 60 to 90 mg; tranylcypromine, 30 to 60 mg; i.e., these latter doses are above those usually recommended). Antidepressant effects may be more closely associated with the inhibition of MAO type A (clorgyline-like), primarily affecting norepinephrine (and serotonin). Thus, high doses of type B selective agents (deprenyl, 30 to 60 mg; and pargyline [Eutonyl]) may be required for antidepressant effects. Phenelzine and tranylcypromine are A,B nonselective. The potentiation of antidepressant efficacy during MAOI therapy has also been reported for both T_3 and lithium carbonate.

SIDE EFFECTS Problems with orthostatic hypotension may become prominent in the second week of treatment. Fludrocortisone (Florinef) may prove to be effective in the treatment of MAOI-induced hypotension. Insomnia or bouts of daytime drowsiness and sedation may also become a problem. One should titrate the dose against side effects, as small variations in dose can change either therapeutic or side effects.

The necessity of restricting substances that release tyramine or catecholamines and can produce hypertensive crises during MAOI treatment should be emphasized to the patient. These crises may be clinically manifested as explosive headaches, flushing, palpitations, perspiration, and nausea. Immediate treatment with a slow infusion of phentolamine (Regitine) (5 mg, IV) in an emergency room is the recommended treatment (Tables 17.4-2a, b, c).

TABLE 17.4-2a
Instructions for Patients Taking MAOIs

Background Information

Foods rich in tyramine and some related amines have been known to cause serious side effects and hypertensive responses in patients taking MAOIs. Tyramine is an amino acid found in many protein substances and is produced by fermentation, aging, spoiling, or pickling. The enzyme MAO found in the liver normally inactivates tyramine. In the presence of a MAOI, tyramine is not deactivated by MAO and is allowed to circulate and indirectly cause the release of norepinephrine from nerve endings. This may lead to detrimental side effects, especially hypertensive responses.

Summary of Guidelines to Follow While Taking an MAOI (from Murphy et al., 1984)

1. The foods in the "high tyramine" category should be completely avoided. If you consume small quantities of foods in this category without symptoms, do not assume that you can repeat this. These foods vary greatly in tyramine content and their ability to cause a severe reaction. You may have a reaction the second time.
2. You are allowed foods with moderate to low tyramine content (categories 2 and 3). These foods should be eaten in moderation. Try to avoid eating combinations of foods in these categories because of the possible additive effects of tyramine.
3. Avoid aged, spoiled, improperly refrigerated, or frozen foods. Do not eat tuna fish that has been in the refrigerator for 2 or 3 days. Eat only fresh food or freshly prepared frozen or canned foods. Beware of many foods that derive their flavor from aging, smoking, or pickling. Also note that cooking of degraded protein does not alter the tyramine content of these foods.
4. Avoid any foods that have previously caused adverse side effects.
5. Cheeses have been responsible for the greatest number of reported hypertensive responses. Observe that many foods contain cheese as an ingredient such as cheese crackers, pizza, and cheese bread.
6. There are certain prescription and nonprescription medicines that should be avoided. See list of MAOI Drug Incompatibilities. Be certain to tell your physician, dentist, or pharmacist that you are taking an MAOI.
7. Call your physician immediately or go to your nearest emergency medical facility if you should suffer from the following symptoms: a throbbing, explosive headache of sudden onset associated with flushing, visual disturbances, nausea or vomiting. Major muscle jerks, confusion, or excitement may also occur, and in the case of a reaction with another drug, sometimes without a severe headache.

Table from Murphy D L, Sunderland T, Cohen R M: Monoamine oxidase–inhibiting antidepressants: A clinical update. Psychiat Clin N Amer *7:* 549, 1984, with permission.

TABLE 17.4-2b
MAOI Dietary Restrictions

High Tyramine Content—Not Permitted	*Examples*
Aged, matured cheeses (unpasteurized)	Cheddar, Camembert, Stilton, bleu, Swiss
Smoked or pickled meats, fish, or poultry	Herring, sausage, corned beef
Aged/putrifying meats, fish, or poultry	Chicken or beef liver, paté, game
Yeast or meat extracts	"Bovril," marmite, brewer's yeast (beware of drinks, soups, or stews made with these products)
Red wines	Chianti, burgundy, sherry, vermouth
Italian broad beans	Fava beans
Moderate Tyramine Content—Limited Amounts Allowed	
Meat extracts	Bouillon, consommé
Pasteurized light and pale beers	
Ripe avocado	
Low Tyramine Content—Permissible	
Distilled spirits (in moderation)	Vodka, gin, rye, scotch
Cheese	Cottage cheese, cream cheese
Chocolate and caffeine-containing beverages	
Fruits	Figs, raisins, grapes, pineapple, oranges
Soy sauce	
Yogurt, sour cream (made by reputable manufacturers)	

DEPRESSIVE SYMPTOMS AND SUBTYPES The lack of response to clinical trials of a typical tricyclic or MAOI antidepressant should lead to a careful reassessment of many of the principles emphasized in the introduction to this section. One should also assess the possible clinical and symptom subtypes of depression as an additional, potentially useful guide to further pharmacotherapy.

Generalized anxiety If there are marked increases in generalized anxiety associated with depression, one should remain undaunted in the pursuit of a tricyclic or MAOI, as these drugs are among the best for treating primary panic disorder. Nonetheless, if prominent anxiety symptoms continue despite apparently adequate antidepressant treatment, one might consider using a benzodiazepine-active agent, such as alprazolam (Xanax) (or the less well-studied clonazepam [Klonopin]), which has also been reported to be useful in treating primary panic disorder. These benzodiazepine agents may also have a role in the first weeks of tricyclic treatment when anxiety symptoms may occasionally increase. Alprazolam should be avoided in patients with borderline personality disorder, as it may be associated with an increased incidence of dyscontrol episodes and acts. Atypical patients with panic or with marked anxiety symptoms have often been reported to respond to MAOIs with or without lithium. Trazodone and bupropion should be avoided, as they are not effective in panic-anxious patients. Trazodone should also be avoided in male patients because of the risks of irreversible priapism requiring surgical intervention. The new antianxiety drug buspirone (Buspar) has recently been reported to show moderate to marked antidepressant effects in 55 percent of a small number of nonmelancholic depressives, but had no effect on melancholics; responses were not associated with baseline anxiety scores. The early literature also suggested a response to MAOIs by hysteroid dysphoric patients with rejection sensitivity, leaden paralysis, hypersomnia, and hyperphagia, although a recent study reported characteristics of typical depression as predictive of a positive response to tranylcypromine: These included greater initial severity of depressed mood, psychomotor retardation, weight loss, but less middle and late insomnia (early morning awakening). Thus, the MAOIs should be considered for tricyclic nonresponsive patients, almost regardless of the subtype of clinical presentation.

Psychosis There is a growing literature suggesting that if the patient's depression has reached psychotic proportions and delusions are present, low to moderate doses of antipsychotics may produce an antidepressant response and help alleviate delusional symptomatology. Preliminary evidence also suggests that lithium carbonate may be useful and that a triple combination (tricyclic, antipsychotic, lithium) may be required in some patients. When using an antipsychotic potentiation of tricyclic antidepressant response in delusional depression, one should taper and discontinue the anti-

TABLE 17.4-2c
MAOI Drug Incompatibilities

*Generally Contraindicated: Hazardous Potentiations**	
Stimulants	Weight-reducing or antiappetite drugs; amphetamines; cocaine
Decongestants	Sinus, hay fever, and cold tablets; nasal sprays or drops; asthma tablets or inhalants; cough preparations (or any products containing ephedrine, phenylephrine, or phenylpropanolamine)
Antihypertensives	Methyldopa, guanethidine, reserpine
TCAs	Imipramine, desipramine, clomipramine
MAOIs	Tranylcypromine, after other MAOIs
Sympathomimetics	Dopamine, Metaraminol
Amine precursors	L-dopa, L-tryptophan
Narcotics	Meperidine (Demerol)
Some Potentiation Possible	
Narcotics	Morphine, codeine
Sedatives	Alcohol, barbiturates, benzodiazepines
Local anesthetics containing vasoconstrictors	
Sympathomimetics	Ephedrine, norepinephrine, isoproterenol
General anesthetics	

*Under certain circumstances, some of these drugs may be used together with MAOIs in specialized treatment approaches and with additional precautions. For example, TCAs or L-tryptophan have been used with MAOIs in antidepressant regimens. Also of note is that other agents from these drug classes are safely used; for example, the antihypertensive agent chlorothiazide, as only mild potentiation occurs.
Table from Murphy D L, Sunderland T, Cohen R M: Monoamine oxidase–inhibiting antidepressants: A clinical update. Psychiat Clin N Amer *7:* 549, 1984, with permission.

psychotics as early as possible to avoid the risk of tardive dyskinesia. Amoxapine (Asendin) may also be considered for agitated, delusionally depressed patients, as it has some inherent antipsychotic (dopamine receptor–blocking) properties that may be advantageous, although it has also been associated with the development of tardive dyskinesia.

ECT is far more likely to be successful, with a more rapid onset than most psychopharmacological regimens, in treating delusionally depressed patients. Thus, ECT may be considered earlier for delusional depressed patients, rather than as a treatment of last resort only after psychopharmacological trials have failed. An absolute contraindication to ECT is the presence of a cerebral aneurysm or increased intracranial pressure, but a recent myocardial infarction is only a relative contraindication. Positive indications, in addition to delusions and extreme suicidality, may include cardiac problems (that make tricyclics dangerous) as well as pregnancy.

Insomnia Continued insomnia is usually associated with an inadequate antidepressant response and should begin to resolve as the treatment begins to be effective. Giving more sedating antidepressants in a once-a-day evening dose is an effective strategy because of the long half-life of most cyclic antidepressants. This regimen makes positive use of the sedation at bedtime and increases the likelihood of compliance with a single nighttime dose. Acute adjunctive treatment with a benzodiazepine may be warranted in rare instances of severe sleep loss, although one should be extremely cautious about using these and related sedatives because of the possibility of habituation and addiction. One may also consider adjunctive nighttime medication with agents, such as tryptophan, which have been reported effective in primary insomnia. Conversely, sleep deprivation may be an adjunctive procedure, whether or not there is severe sleep loss.

An acute, but transient, antidepressant response to one night of sleep deprivation has been reported consistently in studies in many different laboratories. Although many patients relapse after one night's recovery sleep, this treatment may be used in combination with more traditional tricyclic antidepressant or lithium carbonate treatment. There is preliminary evidence that these modalities, especially lithium, may help sustain the sleep deprivation response. Moreover, preliminary evidence suggests that deprivation of sleep in the last half of the night (i.e., from 3 to 7 A.M.) may be just as effective as total sleep deprivation and may thus be more convenient for clinical use and outpatient treatment. The rapid onset of effects achieved in approximately one-half of severely depressed patients is different from the slower but sustained effects following selective deprivation of rapid eye movement (REM) sleep that is not amenable to easy clinical induction.

Lethargy and retardation Extreme morning lethargy and retardation may be an indication for the short-term supplementation of cyclic antidepressant (not MAOIs) with psychomotor stimulants until there is an adequate antidepressant response to the other agents. Small doses of methylphenidate (Ritalin) (5 to 10 mg) in the morning may help the otherwise incapacitated, severely retarded, depressed patient face the day with more energy.

For depressed patients with marked decreases in appetite and associated decreased nutritional intake, one may consider potentiating with folic acid supplements, as a folic acid deficiency has often been reported to cause refractory depression in patients receiving anticonvulsants and, presumably, could also occur because of decreased dietary intake.

Obsessive-compulsive symptoms The associated occurrence of marked obsessive-compulsive symptomatology may lead to the consideration of chlomipramine (Anafranil), which has been reported to be highly effective in adults and children with primary obsessive-compulsive symptomatology, even when other, more traditional antidepressants are not efficacious. Currently, this antidepressant is not available in the United States, but is in Canada and Mexico. Fluoxetine may share this positive effect on obsessive-compulsive symptoms.

Double depression It also is important to assess the possible occurrence of a double depression, in that many of the patient's superimposed depressive symptoms may have been alleviated, leaving only a core of the chronic, minor depression. In this case, the conclusion that the superimposed episode has not been successfully treated may be erroneous. Psychopharmacological approaches to the baseline level of the double depression have not been adequately delineated, but one might consider drugs used for the cyclic mood disorders, such as lithium, in addition to the more traditional antidepressant agents.

Atypical depressive features The occurrence of atypical depressive features, such as hypersomnia, carbohydrate craving, and weight gain, suggest a careful reevaluation for the possibility of bipolar disorder (and MAOI or lithium treatment), as well as seasonal affective disorder (SAD). These atypical symptoms have been found in patients with primary SAD as well as in some apparently otherwise classically diagnosed bipolar II patients. A clear-cut diagnosis of SAD, however, leads to a different prescription and treatment regimen. Increased depression occurs selectively in the winter months associated with the shortening of the daylight hours. Reports from many laboratories throughout the world reveal that this syndrome responds well over a period of several days to high-intensity light given in the morning and evening, although a single exposure of several hours may also prove effective. This treatment can be used prophylactically throughout the winter months in a patient with marked SAD. Ordinary light is not effective; rather, light in the intensity of 2,000 to 2,500 lux is required to achieve a therapeutic response. It is unclear whether this light treatment would be effective for nonseasonal depressions.

EXPERIMENTAL AGENTS If one of the traditional cyclic or MAOI antidepressants has been used and the patient still shows refractory depression, one may consider using a drug acting on another neurotransmitter system beyond that of norepinephrine or serotonin.

Bupropion Bupropion has antidepressant properties that do not involve brain norepinephrine or serotonin. Further study in bipolar patients is eagerly awaited, as preliminary reports have suggested that it may have prophylactic effects without increasing the risk of mania in this subgroup. A positive effect on motor retardation has been reported. Bupropion has few or no anticholinergic side effects and is not associated with weight gain. As of April 1988, its marketing status was on hold, pending clarification of seizures occurring in bulimic patients at doses above 450 mg. Psychosis in bipolar patients has also been reported.

Bromocriptine Clinical trials have also suggested some antidepressant efficacy of the direct dopamine agonist bromocriptine (Parlodel), which is used to treat parkinsonian patients. One double-blind study indicated that, compared with imipramine, it was equally effective. A related dopamine agonist, piribedil, has also been effective for the occasional refractory depressive. This drug, levodopa (Larodopa), and nomifensine (Merital) (which has been withdrawn because of side effects) had been reported to be more effective in those patients with low levels of the dopamine metabolite homovanillic acid (HVA) in their cerebrospinal fluid (CSF). A similar relationship to low levels of the serotonin metabolite 5-hydroxyindoleacetic acid (5-HIAA) and a better response to the serotonin active compound chlorimipramine have been reported. The results are inconsistent as to whether urinary levels of the norepinephrine metabolite 3-methoxy-4-hydroxyphenylglycol (MHPG) can predict the response to noradrenergically active antidepressants. Consistent biochemical markers of antidepressant response have not yet been found.

Lithium Although the acute antidepressive effects of lithium are repeatedly reported, especially in bipolar patients, they still remain controversial; nonetheless, consideration of this compound for unresponsive unipolar depressed patients appears reasonable. The lag in onset is often 2 to 4 weeks or longer. Lithium, too, can be potentiated with tricyclic antidepressants, T_3, tryptophan, or even carbamazepine.

Combination treatment Using a combination treatment with a tricyclic antidepressant and a MAOI has been advocated by some for treatment-resistant patients, although its superiority to single-agent treatment remains controversial. The best recommendation is to start both drugs together (at low doses) or to begin with the tricyclic and add the MAOI later. The reverse order should be avoided whenever possible. The tricyclic nortriptyline appears to have a better record of safety compared with that of imipramine or protriptyline.

Other antidepressant modalities A whole host of tested but unproven antidepressant modalities have been reported; these may be considered for depressed patients who have failed more routine treatment regimens and their potentiation. These might include carbamazepine, s-adenosyl-methionine (SAM), β-noradrenergic agonists, GABA agonists (such as progabide), the opiate agonist buprenorphine (Temgesic), the α-2 agonist clonidine (Catapres), very high doses of parenteral reserpine, anticholinergics, thyrotropin-releasing hormone (TRH), melanoyte inhibitory factor (MIF-1), vasopressin, and circadian-phase interventions.

In light of the rapid onset of effects of s-adenosyl-methionine in a high percentage of patients and the relative absence of side effects in a series of studies, this agent deserves further careful clinical and theoretical attention and investigation. Double-blind studies also document the rapid effects of s-adenosyl-methionine at doses of 400 mg per day.

Compounds active in the dopamine biosynthetic pathway—phenylalanine, tyrosine, and levodopa—have each been reported effective in small groups of depressed patients. Levodopa may be more activating in retarded depressed patients with low HVA in CSF, but its effectiveness is limited by increases in agitation, psychosis, or the switch into mania in bipolar patients. The precursors of serotonin, tryptophan and 5-hydroxytryptophan (5-HTP), also have been reported to have antidepressant effects. The effects of tryptophan, in combination with MAOIs, are notable; how effective tryptophan alone is remains to be better delineated. Surprisingly favorable results in 12 of 14 studies have been reported with 5-HTP in 53 percent of a total of 547 depressed patients.

Prophylaxis In the best controlled follow-up studies, evidence suggests that up to 70 percent of patients with a single depression will have at least one recurrence. Thus, following successful treatment of a unipolar depression, prophylaxis might be in order for the patient with a history of several recurrences or increasingly short well intervals between episodes. The severity of depression, need for hospitalization during previous episodes, and likelihood of suicide should there be a recurrence, all should be part of the decision regarding prophylaxis. Although the rules for prophylaxis have not been spelled out, a generally accepted principle is that the agent that was apparently effective in treating an acute episode may be considered for prophylaxis. Studies reporting prophylaxis in unipolar depression have included traditional heterocyclic compounds, MAOIs, and lithium carbonate.

TREATMENT OF ACUTE MANIA **Lithium carbonate** Lithium carbonate remains the paradigmatic treatment for acute mania. In comparative studies with antipsychotics, it demonstrates overall better improvement in all aspects of manic symptomatology, including psychomotor activity, grandiosity, manic thought disorder, insomnia, and irritability. However, the onset of antimanic action with lithium carbonate can be rather slow (even with aggressive dosing), and so for acutely deteriorating aggressive or psychotic manic patients, it may need to be supplemented in the early phases of treatment. This has traditionally been accomplished with antipsychotics, including the phenothiazines and butyrophenones, such as haloperidol (Haldol). Because of the rapidly growing evidence for the parallel acute antimanic efficacy of carbamazepine, it is suggested that this agent or other anticonvulsants, such as clonazepam or even valproic acid (Depakene), be the supplement rather than an antipsychotic.

A series of double-blind controlled evaluations in many different laboratories have indicated that the onset of antimanic efficacy is as rapid with carbamazepine as it is with traditional antipsychotics, including chlorpromazine (Thorazine), thioridazine (Mellaril), pimozide (Orap), and haloperidol. As of October 1987, nine double-blind studies of carbamazepine in acute mania all suggested clinical efficacy. Because initial acute antimanic response may be a guide to subsequent prophylaxis, the author also encourages the investigation of an individual's response to these alternative anticonvulsant agents before initiating antipsychotics. Antipsychotics can always be used later if other agents are ineffective.

Antipsychotics Chronic maintenance antipsychotic treatment should be avoided for bipolar patients, as they are reported to run an increased risk for tardive dyskinesia. The strategy of rapid tranquilization with suprathreshold doses of antipsychotics should also be avoided. Many double-blind evaluations of this strategy in acutely psychotic patients have shown it to be no more efficacious than traditional dose regimens, and it may be associated with toxic effects. Particularly for extremely manic patients, the use of heroic doses to decrease psychomotor activation may not be justifiable in regard to the added risk of ordinary toxicities, as well as the apparent increased risk for neuroleptic malignant syndrome, or even the sporadic syndromes of reversible and irreversible organic impairment. Although the author is not aware of controlled clinical trials of rapid tranquilizing doses of antipsychotics in acutely manic patients, more traditional doses have been consistently demonstrated to be efficacious; thus, one should consider other antimanic agents, rather than immediately or automatically resorting to higher doses of antipsychotics.

Lithium response The typical clinical profile of the manic patient most responsive to lithium carbonate is one with a classic presentation and hypomania rather than severe mania with either paranoid or destructive trends; one who shows less dysphoria (coexistent depression); one with a prior history of less rapid cycling illness (i.e., fewer than four episodes a year); and one with a family history of mood disorder. Lithium doses should be administered to achieve levels between 0.8 and 1.2 mEq per liter. Although a high-dose strategy is advocated by some investigators (levels to 1.5 or above), the author has not seen many patients who, having failed to respond at more typical blood levels of lithium, have then responded well when pushed to higher levels and potential toxicity. Dose-limiting side effects may be gastrointestinal disturbances, particularly diarrhea, as well as neuropsychiatric syndromes, including tremor, confusion, and myoclonic twitches. Again, for the inadequate responder the author recommends potentiation with other agents, rather than increasing lithium to toxic levels. Blood levels of lithium achieved at a given dose may increase when the patient switches from mania to depression, leading to an increase in side effects.

Carbamazepine Several preliminary studies have suggested that the very variables associated with lithium nonresponse (greater severity, dysphoria, a prior history of rapid cycling illness, and no family history of mood disorders in first-degree relatives) tend to be associated with a better acute antimanic response to carbamazepine. Thus, this drug should be considered for lithium-nonresponsive manic patients.

Typical doses of carbamazepine to treat mania have ranged between 600 and 1,600 mg per day associated with blood levels of between 6 and 12 μg per ml. However, within this dose and blood-level range, there does not appear to be a clear relationship to the degree of clinical response across patients. For an individual patient, however, clinical response and side effects are dose related. It is important to individualize dose administration with this anticonvulsant, as there is wide variability in the dose and blood level at which side effects occur. Increasing the dose in order to achieve a clinical effect and titrating the increases against the emergence of side effects is the appropriate strategy for such wide individual variability.

Valproic acid Although most have been uncontrolled, studies in six different countries indicate the acute or prophylactic efficacy of valproic acid. One study also documented positive acute antimanic responses using an off-on-off design. Typical dose levels are 800 to 1,800 mg per day, achieving blood levels between 50 and 100 μg per ml. In this series of studies, patients with more typical manic syndromes and fewer schizoaffective symptoms appear to show a higher frequency of response. Although carbamazepine and valproic acid have been used in combination to treat epilepsy, there are no systematic investigations of this combination in acute mania.

Clonazepam Another anticonvulsant reported efficacious in acute mania is clonazepam. The sedating side effects of clonazepam may be problematic in some outpatients, but this property of the drug may be used in the management of inpatients or for bedtime medication for severely insomnic manic patients. This anticonvulsant works selectively at the central-type benzodiazepine receptor; in contrast, carbamazepine is not active at this receptor and appears to act at the so-called peripheral-type benzodiazepine receptor. These findings are noteworthy in regard to possible mechanisms of action and differential clinical response. Classic central-type benzodiazepine receptors are associated with GABA receptors and surround the chloride ionophore through which chloride influx mediates neuronal inhibition. In contrast, the peripheral-type benzodiazepine receptor appears more closely associated with a calcium channel.

Calcium channel antagonists A series of preliminary reports suggest that verapamil (Calan, Isoptin) and associated calcium channel antagonists have acute and possibly prophylactic antimanic efficacy. The overall clinical utility of this class of compounds appears promising but remains to be more systematically documented.

Other anticonvulsants The clinical utility of other anticonvulsants, such as the GABA agonist progabide or the traditional anticonvulsant phenytoin (Dilantin), also requires further evaluation. Acetazolamide (Diamox) has been reported to be effective in patients with atypical psychoses associated with dreamy, confusional states occurring premenstrually or in the puerperium.

Antiadrenergic drugs A series of other nonanticonvulsant compounds with some neurotransmitter selectivity have been reported efficacious in treating mania. Clonidine, an α-2 adrenergic agonist, is used to treat hypertension. It acutely inhibits the firing of the noradrenergic locus ceruleus and has been reported to show acute antimanic efficacy in some double-blind clinical trials. Response in the first few days of treatment may not be associated with the ultimate outcome, however. Another agent that inhibits noradrenergic function, in this case by blocking β-adrenergic receptors, is the β antagonist propranolol (Inderal) and related drugs. Because very high doses of this agent in either the d- or l-isomer form have been effective, it is questionable whether the β-antagonist properties or other membrane-stabilizing effects of this drug account for its acute antimanic efficacy.

Cholinomimetics Intravenous administration of the indirect acting cholinergic agonist physostigmine has been demonstrated to have an almost immediate antimanic effect. Physostigmine inhibits acetylcholine esterase function, making more acetylcholine available at the synapse. Although this strategy can produce rapid decreases in manic symptomatology, it can also be associated with rather marked increases in dysphoria and side effects such that its long-term efficacy is doubtful. The success of attempts to chronically increase cholinergic function through other methods, such as lecithin, deanol, or direct acetylcholine agonists, has not been adequately delineated.

Electroconvulsive therapy Older clinical observations and recent controlled clinical trials continue to document the efficacy of ECT in acute mania. Bilateral treatments are required, as unilateral, nondominant treatments have been reported to be ineffective or to exacerbate manic symptoms. In light of the many effective pharmacological treatments noted above, ECT may be reserved for the rare refractory patient or one with medical complications, extreme exhaustion (lethal catatonia), or malignant hyperthermia.

Overview of antimanic agents The ability to achieve rapid antimanic effects with intravenous physostigmine suggests that, given appropriate pharmacological intervention and pharmacokinetics, there is no reason that an acute antimanic response cannot be achieved extremely rapidly. Whereas most of the other antimanic treatments have a moderate delay in onset, the physostigmine data suggest that it is possible, at least theoretically, to terminate manic symptoms in an extremely short time.

Taken together, the efficacy data are also interesting because manipulations of various neurotransmitter systems (inhibition of norepinephrine and dopamine, and potentiation of the cholinergic, benzodiazepine, GABA, and, perhaps, serotonergic systems) all are capable of inducing antimanic effects. The antipsychotics block dopamine receptors; clonidine and propranolol appear to decrease α- and β-noradrenergic function, respectively; and lithium, ECT, and carbamazepine each alter dopamine, noradrenergic, and GABA function. Reserpine, which depletes catecholamines and indoleamines, has also been reported to have antipsychotic and antimanic effects. The literature on tryptophan-induced altered serotonergic function in relation to antimanic efficacy is ambiguous. Awareness of the multiple neurotransmitter approaches to the treatment of mania not only may be clinically useful in changing treatments that target different systems in nonresponsive patients, but also suggests the current weakness of any hypothesized single neurotransmitter defect in mania.

Alterations in endogenous neuropeptide function also have been postulated in mania. Although manipulations of opiates or cholecystokinin (CCK) has not revealed consistent results in psychotic schizophrenic patients, calcitonin has been reported successful in treating excited psychotic states, including mania. These findings are of interest in regard to the preliminary evidence that other calcium-active treatments, such as the blockers mentioned above, may also be effective in treating acute mania. The clinical efficacy of calcitonin or other peptide interventions in mania remains to be confirmed but is mentioned because peptides could represent the next generation of antimanic treatments, particularly in light of the increasing evidence of peptide neurotransmitters coexisting in the same neurons with more classical neurotransmitter substances that have been indirectly linked to the manic syndromes.

MAINTENANCE TREATMENT OF BIPOLAR ILLNESS

LITHIUM PROPHYLAXIS Lithium carbonate appears to be effective in some 70 to 80 percent of bipolar patients. Although the initial studies indicated the need for blood levels between 0.8 and 1.2 mEq per liter, more recent studies have suggested that lower levels in the range of 0.5 to 0.8 mEq per liter may also be effective in the maintenance treatment. Long-term toxicities tend to be less prominent at this blood-level range. Monitoring of "trough" levels (performed in the early morning with the A.M. dose held) at 4- to 8-week intervals, or more frequently if the patient's course is unstable, is recommended. Because of the overwhelming data on long-term efficacy, it is important to consider preventive treatment after a severe episode.

Although many investigators suggest that prophylaxis should be initiated after two or three recurrences in a period of several years, rather than fixing specific numbers or interval duration to the recommendation, the author suggests that several variables be considered together in arriving at the decision for prophylaxis. The development of a life chart, so that the frequency, severity, and interval between episodes can be accurately assessed, is essential. If previous episodes were severe—socially incapacitating and requiring hospitalization—or associated with extremely adverse events for the patient and family, one would be more likely to consider prophylaxis earlier rather than later, despite moderately long well intervals between episodes. These factors should be discussed with the patient during a well interval so that the appropriate risk–benefit ratios can be weighed intelligently and with adequate informed consent.

LITHIUM SIDE EFFECTS The profile of lithium-induced side effects has proved to be benign even in the long-term maintenance treatment of patients over several decades. Several of lithium's effects deserve comment, however.

Thyroid function Lithium clearly impairs thyroid function by several different mechanisms and has even been used to treat hyperthyroidism. Lithium rather uniformly lowers T_3 and T_4 levels circulating in the plasma and, in some patients, increases thyroid-stimulating hormone (TSH). TSH increases above normal can be taken to indicate that the hypothalamic-pituitary axis is working overtime to maintain normal levels of thyroid hormones. Thus, one might consider thyroid replacement with T_4 when levels of TSH are elevated and thyroid hormone indices are near, at, or below their normal lower limits. Routine checks of thyroid function at 6-month intervals are wise, as are more frequent checks if there is a breakthrough of depressive symptomatology during otherwise adequate lithium maintenance treatment. Treatment of underlying hypothyroidism can, in these instances, help alleviate a depression that is linked to this hormonal deficit.

Renal function As of the mid-1980s, the scare regarding the long-term adverse consequences of lithium on the kidneys has been largely dissipated. Original reports on the induction of severe nephrotoxicity and pathology induced by lithium were, in part, related to the absence of an age-matched control group of psychiatric patients not treated with lithium. Thus, although lithium rather consistently impairs vasopressin function at the level of adenylate cyclase and often produces a syndrome of diabetes insipidus, it is less consistently associated with other evidence of renal toxicity. Preliminary data suggest that less renal toxicity may occur with single nighttime dosing producing higher peaks, but lower nadirs, than that achieved with regimens that produce the most constant blood levels of lithium. Current practice suggests that quarterly or less frequent monitoring of renal function in elderly patients may be sufficient. It also is important to obtain baseline measures of renal function, including a creatinine clearance, before beginning the lithium treatment, particularly in patients with a history of some renal alterations. Because of the induction of diabetes insipidus syndrome related to the blockade of antidiuretic hormone actions, patients must have adequate fluid intake to maintain an appropriate fluid and electrolyte balance. Several cases have been reported in which marked lithium toxicity has been associated with irreversible changes in the cerebellum because of inadequate maintenance of fluid intake. Thus, lithium levels or fluid and electrolyte status, or both, should be monitored closely during periods of febrile illness, decreased fluid intake, or greater-than-ordinary fluid loss, such as during extreme athletic stress or during gastrointestinal illnesses with vomiting or diarrhea. Only with careful monitoring should the treatment of lithium-induced diabetes insipidus with diuretics (furosemide or thiazide) be attempted; lower doses of lithium may be indicated with these diuretics.

Tremor Tremor can be problematic for a small but substantial percentage of patients treated with lithium carbonate. The tremor is frequently exacerbated by social stress, sometimes to the degree that the patient denies that it is lithium related. When the tremor persists at doses at the lower end of the therapeutic range or at the minimum doses necessary for therapeutic efficacy, attempts may be made to treat it symptomatically. Some investigators find that 10 to 40 mg of the β-blocker propranolol in divided daily doses may reduce lithium tremor. Relief may occur within 30 minutes and may last from 4 to 6 hours.

Gastrointestinal effects Gastrointestinal side effects (diarrhea and indigestion) can also be problematic for many patients, but may be attenuated by reducing the dose or giving it at meal times (for indigestion). Antidiarrheal agents should be restricted to acute treatment.

Mental effects Patients may express concern about the effects of lithium carbonate on their learning, memory, spontaneity, or creativity. Although some impairment can be objectively delineated in detailed neuropsychological testing, most patients either do not experience this effect or do not find it unduly impairing. In fact, productivity and creativity may, overall, be enhanced during lithium treatment because it prevents unproductive manic and depressive phases. Although no adequate approach to these side effects of lithium has been demonstrated other than reducing the dose, it is important to rule out associated causes for cognitive impairment, including the possible emergence of lithium-induced hypothyroidism or an inadequately treated level of coexistent depression. Many so-called drug-related side effects are clearly evident during placebo treatment phases and thus appear more closely associated with illness-related variables rather than with a particular psychopharmacological treatment. This perspective on lithium maintenance treatment clearly needs to be explored with the patient to avoid premature discontinuation of treatment or noncompliance.

Weight gain Lithium-induced weight gain can be a vexing problem for a small percentage of patients. If there is a reactive hypoglycemic component, carbohydrate restriction may help avoid this problem. Thyroid indices should be rechecked and the patient reminded to not use calorie-containing beverages to maintain the necessary increased fluid intake associated with diabetes insipidus.

Dose reduction Dose reduction may be a first maneuver in treating a variety of lithium-induced problems (tremor, weight gain, thirst, urinary frequency, diarrhea, or psychomotor slowing); if these lower doses are not adequate for prophylaxis, combination or alternative treatment especially with carbamazepine (which has a different side-effects profile) may be indicated. Other lithium-related effects during combination with carbamazepine are discussed below. It is noteworthy that the renal clearance of lithium appears to decrease with age, so that a lower dose may be adequate and necessary in the older patient on lithium maintenance.

TREATMENT OF BREAKTHROUGH EPISODES DURING LITHIUM PROPHYLAXIS

Depressive breakthroughs

AVOIDANCE OF TRICYCLIC AND MAOI ANTIDEPRESSANTS The treatment of a bipolar depressed patient either untreated or with an episode emerging during lithium prophylaxis is very different from that of the unipolar depressed patient. Although tricyclic antidepressants and MAOIs are the main treatment of the unipolar depressed patient, there is reason for caution in using them for the bipolar patient. Some studies have reported an increased incidence of switches into hypomania or mania observed during tricyclic or MAOI therapy, above that expected for the patient's natural course of illness. Although it is still being debated whether this increased incidence of switching is sufficient to relatively contravene the use of tricyclics or MAOIs for bipolar patients, the evidence is clear that these compounds can speed up the rate of cycling in rapid-cycling patients. Thus, a shorter depression may occur at the cost of the more rapid onset of the following manic episode, which also may be more severe than previously experienced. Tricyclic antidepressant withdrawal studies have indicated that some of this cycling may slow down when these offending agents are removed. Moreover, there are uncontrolled observations that tricyclic and related compounds may be implicated in the development of continuous cycling phases (i.e., successive episodes without a well interval). This phase of the illness becomes exceedingly difficult to treat and tends to be relatively lithium refractory.

Once a switch has been observed on one type of MAOI, the

use of a different compound appears to lead not only to an onset of a switch when treatment is reinstituted, but also to its occurrence at an earlier phase in the treatment than during the first treatment sequence. Thus, there may be a sensitization to this drug-induced switching phenomenon. Moreover, it is unclear whether a pharmacologically induced switch appears only in those predestined to have spontaneous switches or whether this occurrence actually predisposes the patient to develop further spontaneous manic episodes. The data suggest that even though tricyclic and MAOI maintenance treatments of bipolar patients prevent depressive recurrences, they tend to increase the incidence of manic episodes.

Therefore, the bipolar depressive episode or breakthrough should be managed, insofar as it is possible, without resorting to the traditional modes for unipolar patients. Women appear to be particularly predisposed to tricyclic-induced cycling. If tricyclics are used, they should be tapered and discontinued as rapidly as possible, so as to avoid this switch process. Lithium may not be able to prevent this tricyclic-induced switch. Several case reports suggest that alprazolam may also induce switches into hypomania and mania, even in nonpredisposed patients.

Some evidence suggests that the MAOIs, in general, may be less prone than the tricyclics are to induce switches, and so they may be given relatively greater consideration, especially for anergic, hypersomnic, hyperphagic bipolar patients. Clorgyline, a selective MAO type A inhibitor, which is not yet clinically available, has been reported to slow the cycling frequency.

FOLIC ACID It has been reported that folic acid supplementation in the dose range of 300 to 400 μg per day significantly reduces affective morbidity compared with a placebo group similarly maintained on lithium therapy. Although this was only a single investigation, the promising result and the benign nature of folic acid treatment suggests that it be considered while awaiting further clinical investigation.

CARBAMAZEPINE One alternative to using tricyclics and MAOIs for depressive breakthroughs is the addition of carbamazepine. Although the evidence is rather scanty as to the overall clinical benefit of carbamazepine when used as the sole treatment in primary depression, those findings, taken with the more substantial emerging literature on the efficacy of carbamazepine prophylaxis for both manic and depressive episodes, raise the priority of using this agent as a supplement to lithium in depressive breakthroughs. Although only one-third of acutely depressed patients responded in one study, these tended to be the patients with greater initial severity of depression and more clear-cut prior histories of acute rather than chronic episodes of depression. Evidence of an abnormal EEG or increased psychosensory and other paraepileptic symptoms in the history did not predict an acute response to carbamazepine. When antidepressant response was observed, it tended to occur with the typical lag observed with other agents, so that only minor improvement was noted in the first and second weeks of treatment, but more considerable improvement was observed after the third and fourth weeks.

LITHIUM POTENTIATION OF CARBAMAZEPINE A series of 15 patients who were treated with carbamazepine alone and who showed inadequate degrees of antidepressant response were then supplemented with lithium carbonate. Eight of these 15 showed a rapid onset of antidepressant improvement, often within the first 4 to 6 days. Thus, when given in this order, the combination appears to be helpful for a substantial subgroup of otherwise refractory patients. There are no systematic studies of the efficacy of carbamazepine supplementation of lithium, but it should be a promising clinical strategy in light of the evidence of carbamazepine's efficacy alone in the acute and long-term treatment of the illness.

Whether the combined efficacy of carbamazepine and lithium is sufficient to block tricyclic and MAOI-induced switches remains to be documented, but this strategy appears worthy of individual clinical trials in otherwise resistant patients.

SEROTONIN AND THYROID The clinical utility of tryptophan (1.5 to 6 grams with 100 to 300 mg vitamin B_6) and 5-hydroxytryptophan potentiation is encouraging but has not been adequately documented. Although thyroid potentiation similar to that observed in unipolar depression can be attempted, treatment with suppressive doses of thyroid is still experimental. Several investigators have found associated medical toxicities with this treatment and an inadequate maintenance of long-term prophylaxis unless other routine agents were used concurrently.

VALPROIC ACID Lithium plus valproic acid has been reported to be successful in the long-term treatment of a subgroup of previously lithium-refractory patients. The antidepressant efficacy of valproic acid is less well delineated than its antimanic efficacy, and the utility of this treatment for an acute depressive episode remains to be further elucidated. Nonetheless, this combination offers another option in the long-term management of bipolar patients who do not respond to lithium alone. A response to one anticonvulsant may not be predictive of a response to another, and positive long-term effects of valproic acid plus lithium have been noted in a patient not responsive to lithium alone or carbamazepine prophylaxis (Fig. 17.4-5).

ELECTROCONVULSIVE THERAPY ECT may also be useful for bipolar depressed patients who do not respond to lithium and its adjunctive agents. Whether it would continue to help abbreviate recurrent depressive episodes in rapid-cycling patients or whether it would be useful in long-term prophylaxis must be further investigated.

BUPROPION As noted above, bupropion has shown promise in the acute and prophylactic management of bipolar patients.

CALCIUM CHANNEL BLOCKERS The calcium blockers show promise as prophylactic treatments but may be less effective for depressive breakthroughs than for manias.

SPIRONOLACTONE Spironolactone (Aldactone) has been reported effective in six lithium-intolerant patients, but, surprisingly, has received no further systematic study.

Manic breakthroughs A wide range of drugs is available for breakthrough manic episodes occurring during lithium treatment. They include the entire spectrum of drugs indicated for the treatment of acute mania. Ranking high in these treatments are carbamazepine and valproic acid, because of their longer-term prophylactic efficacy. However, clonazepam may be a useful alternative to antipsychotic supplementation, even

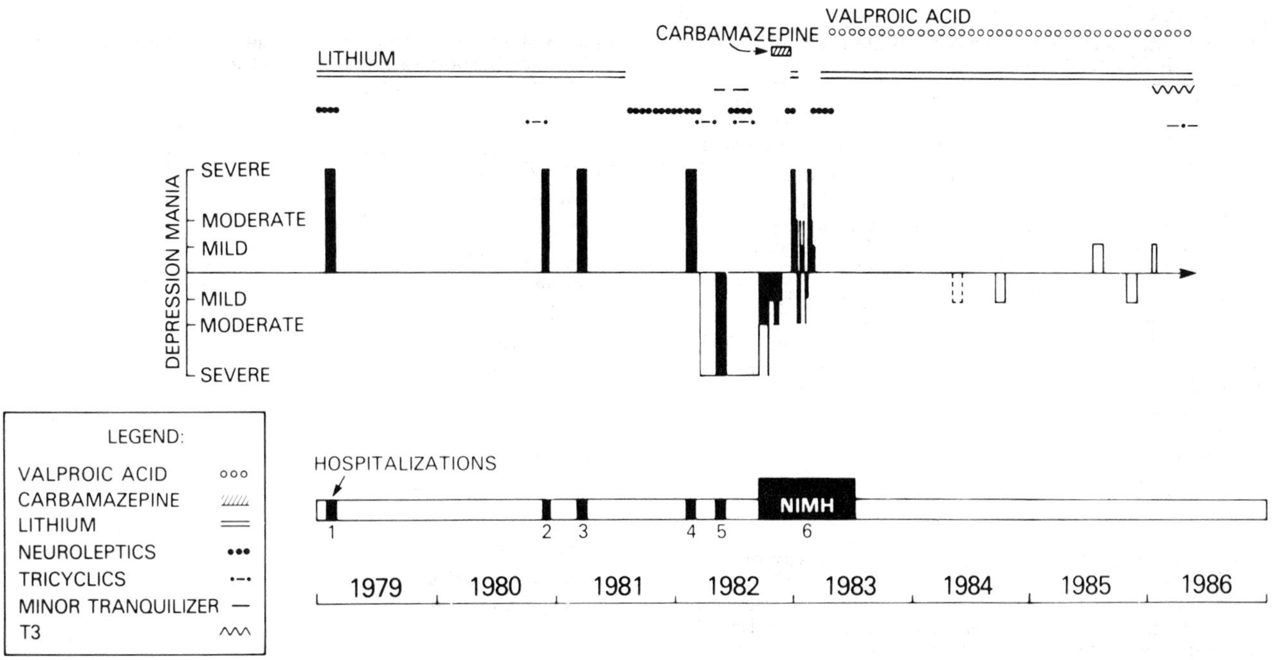

FIGURE 17.4-5. *Prophylactic response to valproic acid in a carbamazepine nonresponder.*

though both of these agents appear to have a lesser role in the long-term management of bipolar illness compared with that of carbamazepine or valproic acid. Other approaches to the manic breakthrough include antipsychotics, used judiciously at minimal doses for the shortest period of time, and the drugs listed in Table 17.4-3.

LITHIUM–CARBAMAZEPINE COMBINATION TREATMENT As noted above, attempting to supplement the clinical effects of lithium with anticonvulsants such as carbamazepine and valproic acid appears to be a better initial step than using these anticonvulsants alone. For patients who are otherwise unable to tolerate lithium carbonate, the preliminary evidence does suggest that carbamazepine alone may be a useful long-term maintenance treatment in preventing both manic and depressive episodes. Most of these data are based on case reports and clinical vignettes. However, there is a rather substantial literature on open clinical trials with carbamazepine, and several double-blind studies do support the preliminary evidence of its long-term efficacy. Thus, it is recommended as the second-line treatment after lithium to achieve prophylaxis.

White count suppression The side-effects profile of carbamazepine tends to be quite different from that of lithium carbonate (Table 17.4-4). It is a useful rule of thumb that whenever these two drugs act on a common system, the effect of lithium tends to override that of carbamazepine. In almost every instance this is a clinical disadvantage, except in white count suppression. Here, the ability of lithium carbonate to increase the white count and override the white count–suppressing effects of carbamazepine may be used to clinical advantage. This appears to be the case only with carbamazepine's benign suppression of the white count and should not be attempted if there is evidence of more problematic interference by carbamazepine in hematological function manifest in other cell lines such as platelets or red cells. If there is normal function in these other elements, potentiation with lithium in order to return the white count to a more normal range may be attempted. The suggested guideline for carbamazepine discontinuation is a white count below 3,000.

Vasopressin function and electrolytes Because carbamazepine appears to act like a vasopressin agonist either directly or by potentiating vasopressin effects at the receptor, it will not be sufficient to reverse lithium-induced diabetes insipidus, which occurs by an action of lithium below the receptor level at the adenylate cyclase second-messenger system. To the extent that the minor cognitive impairments of lithium are, in part, related to its ability to impair vasopressin function in the brain, these data suggest that not only would carbamazepine be less likely to cause this side effect, but that during combination treatment, the side effects of lithium would override those of carbamazepine. Carbamazepine tends to induce a benign hypocalcemia that is generally not associated with bone demineralization. In contrast, lithium often produces a transient increase in serum calcium.

Thyroid function Not only does carbamazepine tend to decrease T_4, free T_4, and T_3 levels, as does lithium, but in combination, the decreases also are potentiated. However, during carbamazepine treatment, there is a negligible incidence of clinical hypothyroidism or above-normal increases in thyroid-stimulating hormone (TSH). Consequently, thyroid supplementation of carbamazepine is rarely needed. But, when the two drugs are used in combination, the lithium effect on TSH will override that of carbamazepine, and the patient may require thyroid supplementation during combination treatment.

Allergic rash Carbamazepine induces an allergic rash in 10 to 15 percent of patients treated. In most instances, the drug

TABLE 17.4-3
Options in the Long-Term Treatment of the Lithium-Refractory Patient with Bipolar Disorder

Prophylaxis	*Breakthrough Manias During Lithium*	*Breakthrough Depressions During Lithium*
Lithium	Carbamazepine	(Tricyclics or MAOIs)†
Carbamazepine	Valproic acid	Carbamazepine
Lithium + Carbamazepine	Clonazepam	Thyroid potentiation
Lithium + Valproic acid	Antipsychotics	ECT*
Lithium + Folate	Clonidine	Alprazolam
Suppressive doses of thyroid	Reserpine	Sleep deprivation
Verapamil	Propranolol	Tryptophan + 5-HTP
Acetazolamide	Verapamil	Bromocriptine
Phenytoin	ECT*	Sulpiride??
Spironolactone		
Electroconvulsive therapy (ECT)		
Reserpine		

*Use of ECT considered earlier if medically necessary or suicide is a high risk.
†Avoid tricyclics and MAOIs as long as possible in order to prevent development of rapid or continuous cycling. Consider in combination with lithium and carbamazepine.

should be discontinued. However, in cases that show evidence of the efficacy of carbamazepine and not other available agents, one may consider pretreating with glucocorticoids, such as prednisone, when carbamazepine is being restarted. Case reports indicate that this will block the development of carbamazepine-induced rash in cases of dermatologic allergy not complicated by other systemic manifestations that may not respond to steroid suppression.

Hepatitis There are rare cases of carbamazepine-induced hepatitis, several of which have been fatal. The incidence of this side effect appears to be extremely rare, perhaps equivalent to that associated with traditional psychotropic agents, including the antipsychotics. Thus, routine monitoring for this side effect does not appear to be indicated, although one should be aware of this side effect and immediately discontinue carbamazepine treatment if there are more than minor enzyme elevations, which do tend to occur transiently with this and many anticonvulsant agents. In contrast to this rare incidence with carbamazepine, with the use of valproic acid there have been a number of reports of severe hepatitis in the neurological literature, mostly in children. No hepatic side effects have been reported in the small group of psychiatric patients so far studied with valproic acid, but liver function tests should be monitored when using this agent.

Neurotoxicity There have been occasional reports of neurotoxicity when lithium and carbamazepine are used together. Because both agents can cause this side effect at or below clinically accepted dose ranges, this may occasionally occur from the combination treatment as well. In most studies, the combination appears to be well tolerated without side effects greater than when either agent is used alone. Many of the side effects reported in the literature appear to be caused by starting relatively large doses of carbamazepine (rather than slow increases) in combination with other psychotropic agents and assuming that the attendant side effects are related to the combination treatment rather than to carbamazepine alone.

TABLE 17.4-4
Comparative and Differential Clinical and Side Effects Profile of Lithium Carbonate and Carbamazepine

	Lithium Carbonate	*Carbamazepine*	*Li & Carba. Combination*
Clinical Profile			
Mania (M)	++	++	+++
Dysphoric	±	+	
Rapid cycling	+	++	
Severe	+	++	
Family history negative	±	+	
Depression (D)	+	+	+++
M D prophylaxis	++	++	+++
Epilepsy	0	++	
Pain syndromes	0	++	
Side Effects			
White blood count	↑	↓	↑,—, Li*
Diabetes insipidus	↑	↓	↑, Li*
Thyroid hormones T_3, T_4	↓	↓	↓↓
TSH	↑	(—)	↑, Li*
Serum calcium	(↑)	↓	(↑), (Li*)
Weight gain	(↑)	(—)	
Tremor	(↑)	(—)	
Memory disturbances	(↑)	?	
Diarrhea	(↑)	—	
Teratogenic	(↑)	—	
Psoriasis	(↑)	(—)	
Pruritic rash (allergy)	—	↑	
Agranulocytosis	—	(↑)	
Hepatitis	—	(↑)	
Hyponatremia, water intoxication	—	(↑)	
Dizziness, ataxia, diplopia	—	↑	
Hypercortisolism, escape from dexamethasone suppression	—	↑	

Legend: *Clinical Efficacy* 0: None; ±: Equivocal; +: Effective; ++: Very effective; +++: Potentiation. *Side Effects* ↑: Increase; ↓: Decrease; ( ): Inconsistent or rare; —: Absent; ↓↓: Potentiation; Li*: Effect of lithium predominates

Pharmacokinetic interactions There do not appear to be major pharmacokinetic interactions between carbamazepine and lithium. However, this is not the case with carbamazepine and haloperidol, as haloperidol levels are markedly reduced by carbamazepine. Despite this reduction in haloperidol blood levels, most studies report improvement with carbamazepine supplementation, suggesting that carbamazepine might potentiate antipsychotic effects because of its action on systems other than that of the dopamine receptor blockade.

Agents commonly employed in medical practice can markedly increase carbamazepine levels and can produce attendant toxicity (Table 17.4-5). The most frequent dose-related toxic manifestations are dizziness, drowsiness, ataxia, diplopia, and confusion. These may occur in someone otherwise tolerating the drug well when other drugs are added. Erythromycin, triacetyloleandomycin, isoniazid (but apparently not other MAOIs), and the calcium channel blockers verapamil and diltiazam (Cardizem) (but not nifedipine [Procardia]) will increase carbamazepine levels. Less marked increases occur during co-treatment with propoxyphene (Darvon) and, transiently, with cimetidine (Tagamet). Carbamazepine will lower the blood levels of various agents and interfere with some tests that are dependent on protein binding, including some pregnancy tests.

Teratogenic effects Another area of differential side effects is the teratogenetic effects of lithium compared with carbamazepine. The lithium registry suggests that cardiac and several other anomalies may occur with a higher frequency than expected in patients treated with lithium carbonate during pregnancy. In contrast, the teratogenetic effects of carbamazepine have not been readily discerned in animals or in an increasingly large clinical literature, suggesting that it—relative to several other anticonvulsants—has a relatively low risk of inducing congenital malformations. Behavioral and other toxicities associated with treatment of the mother during fetal gestation have not been either reported or adequately studied. Although tricyclic antidepressant compounds have not been reported to have induced systematic congenital malformations, preliminary evidence suggests that there may be a type of behavioral withdrawal syndrome that occurs in the newborn. This kind of longer-term toxicity has been found in animal studies of benzodiazepines, antipsychotics, and related psychotropic drugs, but has not been assessed systematically in human follow-up studies.

TABLE 17.4-5
Clinically Important Interactions Between Carbamazepine and Other Drugs

Influence of Other Drugs on Carbamazepine	
Increased Carbamazepine Levels and Toxicity Produced by	*Increased Carbamazepine Levels Not Associated with Marked Toxicity*
Erythromycin (and analogues)	Valproic acid (increases epoxide only)
Triacetyloleandomycin	Propoxyphene
Verapamil	Cimetidine (mild acute increases; none after 1 week)
Diltiazem (not nifedipine)	Nicotinamide
Isoniazid (not tranylcypromine)	Josamycin
Viloxazine	
Nafimidone	
Decreased Carbamazepine Levels Produced by	
Phenobarbital	
Phenytoin	
Primidone	
Theophylline	

Influence of Carbamazepine on Other Drugs	
Carbamazepine Decreases Levels or Effects of	*Carbamazepine Increases*
Haloperidol	Escape from dexamethasone suppression
Clonazepam	Clomipramine
Valproate	Desmethylclomipramine
Ethosuximide	Phenytoin
Theophylline	
Dexamethasone	
Dicoumarol	
Warfarin	
Pregnancy tests	
Doxycycline	

SENSITIZATION EFFECTS IN MOOD DISORDERS

Although spontaneous remissions late in the course of mood disorders have been reported, even in the prepsychopharmacological Kraepelinian era, most cases appear to follow a pattern of stable or increasing episode frequency. In essentially every study that has examined this variable, there tends to be a sensitization or decreasing well interval between successive episodes (Fig. 17.4-6). The author postulates that this acceleration in the course of manic-depressive illness could occur via mechanisms analogous to those observed with behavioral sensitization to psychomotor stimulants and electrophysiological kindling. In these models, if the stimulation or resulting behavior is blocked, sensitization and kindling will proceed less robustly or not at all. This perspective points to the importance of the pharmacological prophylaxis of manic-depressive illness, not only to spare the patient from another mania or depression, but also to retard the sensitization process, if this proves to be an accurate analogy for the course of manic-depressive illness.

Changes in pharmacoresponsivity during course of illness Across studies, one of the best predictors of long-term positive response to lithium carbonate is the initial treatment response. Failures in the first months of lithium prophylaxis appear to predict subsequent relapses. Less well studied is the long-term course in initially positive lithium responders and the occurrence of breakthrough episodes associated with aging, the continued progression of processes underlying the illness, or the loss of treatment efficacy. Preliminary data show that some patients with initially excellent responses to carbamazepine, or lithium and carbamazepine in combination, may have relapses with more extended treatment durations. Whether this represents partial tolerance to the effects of the psychopharmacological treatments or the underlying illness process despite stable pharmacological effects remains to be demonstrated. Certainly in the case of parkinsonism, there are major changes in drug responsivity over time. Initially excellent responses to levodopa give way to inefficacy and also to rapid alterations in motor phenomena oscillating from dyskinesias to parkinsonian akinetic immobility. This "on-off" phase in the motor sphere may be a model for rapid fluctuations in mood.

Some of the treatments of mood disorders, including tricyclic antidepressants—if not direct and indirect dopamine agonists per se—could similarly influence later stages of the illness in a nontherapeutic fashion. Also, taking the analogy from parkinsonism, pharmacological responsivity differs as a function of stage of illness, and although levodopa therapy may be adequate initially, later combination with a direct dopamine agonist may also be required. The author has also noted in kindling models of epilepsy that the pharmacoresponsiveness differs as a function of stage of kindling: development, completed stable, and spontaneous. For example, an agent like diazepam (Valium), which is an extremely effective anticonvulsant in blocking the development phase of kindling or the middle, stable phases, is ineffective in the spontaneous phases following many repetitions of seizures, when the animals begin to have seizures without any exogenous electrophysiological stimulation. Conversely, the anticonvulsant phenytoin is not very effective in the initial and middle phases of kindling, but is effective in inhibiting spontaneous kindled seizures. Carbamazepine is not effective in the development stage of amygdala-kindled seizures, but is effective in the completed stage, although the converse is true for local anaesthetic seizures kindled with lidocaine or cocaine.

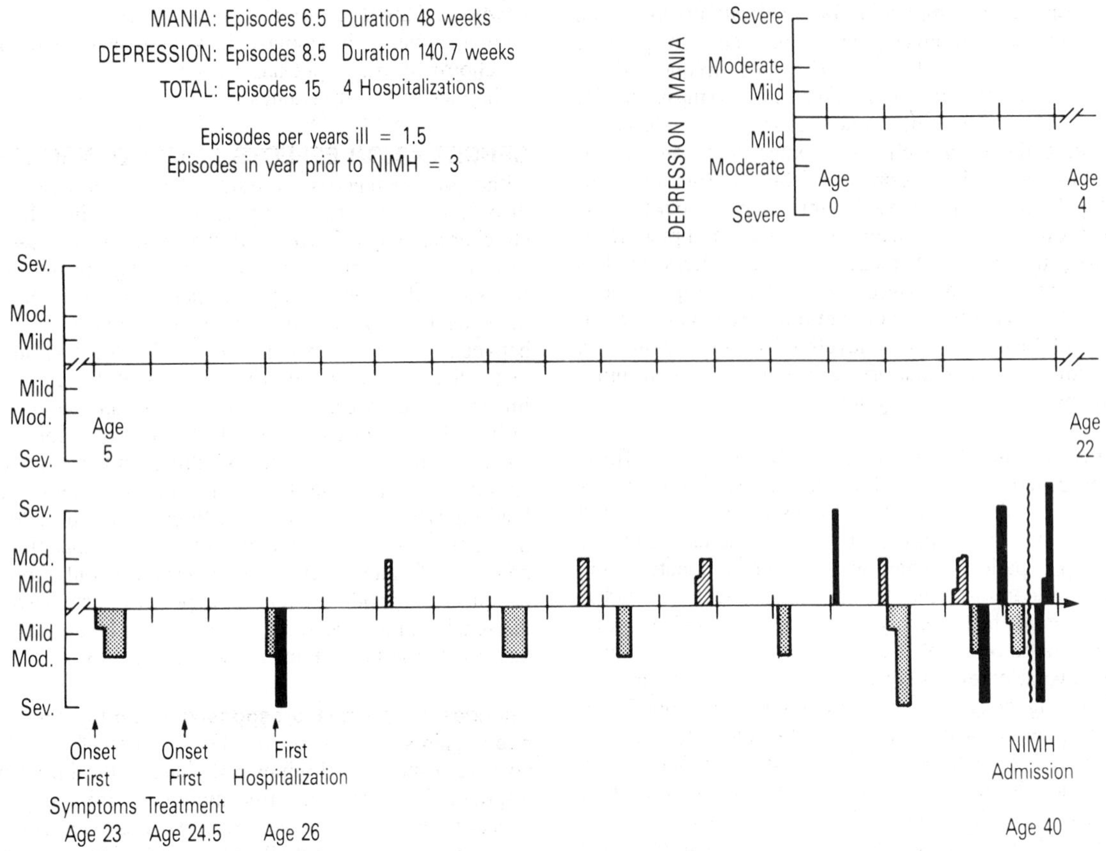

FIGURE 17.4-6. *Median course of mood disorder in 82 refractory bipolar manic-depressive patients.*

Thus, these quite strong data from animal models of epilepsy and the clinical data in parkinsonism suggest that some neuropsychiatric illnesses may differ in their pharmacotherapeutic responsivity as a function of stage of illness. This may also be the case for the pharmacotherapy of mood disorders, although there have been no direct tests of this hypothesis. Minor tranquilizers and psychotherapeutic interventions may be most effective in early phases of the illness characterized by stress-induced dysphoria. Traditional antidepressant modalities and lithium carbonate are particularly effective in mid-phases of unipolar or bipolar illness, respectively. But in bipolar patients who show extremely rapid cycling (often occurring late in the illness), lithium carbonate tends to be less effective, and carbamazepine and related adjunctive anticonvulsant treatments may play a greater role in the treatment of these later stages of manic-depressive illness. The existing preliminary data raise the possibility that, in addition to the usual clinical variables of severity, phenomenological subtype, and familial and genetic predisposition, one might consider the phase in the development of mood disorders as relevant to the optimal psychopharmacotherapeutic intervention.

Also on a speculative note, one might consider a possible differential role of stress as a function of course of illness. The kindling model is an interesting one for suggesting how an illness process, which is closely tied to a given exogenous stimulation, can become independent of it (i.e., spontaneous). Could this not also occur in manic-depressive illness, in which initial episodes may be more likely to be associated with psychosocial stresses but, with sufficient repetition, episodes occur autonomously?

PSYCHOTHERAPY COMBINED WITH PHARMACOTHERAPY There is an important role for psychotherapeutic approaches combined with pharmacological approaches in treating manic-depressive patients. This appears to be true not only for episodes that are more clearly associated with psychosocial stresses, but also in relation to apparently spontaneous episodes. Some of these episodes may be triggered by psychological processes that had previously been conditioned to the occurrence of mood fluctuations. As such, addressing these psychological variables in psychotherapy may be valuable. Patients who were doing well on maintenance pharmacoprophylaxis may relapse in the face of increased psychosocial stress. Thus, not only would some degree of psychotherapy appear to be useful in its own right in manic-depressive patients, but it might also enhance various aspects of the therapeutic alliance and the possibility of a collaborative process and compliance with psychopharmacotherapeutic regimens. It clearly allows the early detection of impending mood changes and appropriate psychological and pharmacological interventions.

Although some therapists have dichotomized psychotherapeutic and pharmacotherapeutic processes, the author encourages a combined approach, either with one therapist or with two who are in close communication with each other. It is curious, at a time when the role of stress is increasingly recognized in epilepsy, diabetes, autoimmune diseases, and even cancer, that some pharmacotherapeutic practitioners maintain that psychotherapy is irrelevant, and conversely, some therapists attempt heroic psychotherapeutic treatment without pharmacotherapeutic assistance.

FUTURE TRENDS As this most exciting century for the development of psychobiological theories and therapies for the mood disorders closes, one hopes for clearer definitions of the different psychotherapies and pharmacotherapies critical to adequate therapeutic intervention in different patients and stages of illness. The pharmacotherapies have provided the critical neurobiological hypotheses of the mechanisms underlying the mood disorders, and one hopes that there is a mutually interactive process of more specific treatments, theories, and therapies that will be derived from systematic clinical and basic research in this area. Not only is there a wealth of information to be learned through research, but each patient has much to teach the practitioner and the theoretician. There are a host of effective treatment alternatives now available for mood-disordered patients, and one can look forward to even more effective interventions in the future.

REFERENCES

Akiskal H S: The clinical management of affective disorders. In *Psychiatry,* R Michels and J O Cavenar, Jr, editors, vol 1, p 1. Lippincott, Philadelphia, 1985.

Baldessarini R J: Antidepressant agents. In *Chemotherapy in Psychiatry: Principles and Practices,* R J Baldessarini, editor, p 130. Harvard University Press, Cambridge, MA, 1985.

Berrettini W, Post R M: GABA and affective illness. In *Neurobiology of Mood Disorders,* R M Post, J C Ballenger, editors, p 673. Williams & Wilkins, Baltimore, 1984.

Cade J F J: Lithium salts in the treatment of psychotic excitement. Med J Aust *2:* 349, 1949.

Davis J M, Sharma R P: Biological treatment of affective disorders. In *American Handbook of Psychiatry,* P A Berger, H K H Brodie, editors, vol 8, p 302. Basic Books, New York, 1986.

Goodwin F K, Jamison K R, editors: *Manic-Depressive Illness.* Oxford University Press, New York, 1989.

Jimerson D C: Role of dopamine mechanisms in the affective disorders. In *Psychopharmacology: The Third Generation of Progress,* H Y Meltzer, W E Bunney, Jr, J T Coyle, K L Davis, I J Kopin, D I Schuster, R I Shader, G M Simpson, editors, p 505. Raven Press, New York, 1987.

Joffe R T, Post R M: Experimental treatment for affective disorder. In *American Handbook of Psychiatry,* P A Berger, H K H Brodie, editors, vol 8, p 386. Basic Books, New York, 1986.

Kerns L L: Treatment of mental disorders in pregnancy. A review of psychotropic drug risks and benefits. J Nerv Ment Dis *174:* 652, 1986.

Murphy D L, Sunderland T, Cohen R. M: Monoamine oxidase–inhibiting antidepressants: A clinical update. Psychiat Clin N Amer *7:* 549, 1984.

Pare C M: The present status of monoamine oxidase inhibitors. Brit J Psychiat *146:* 576, 1985.

Post R M, Rubinow D R, Ballenger J C: Conditioning, sensitization, and kindling: Implications for the course of affective illness. In *Neurobiology of Mood Disorders,* R M Post, J C Ballenger, editors, p 432. Williams & Wilkins, Baltimore, 1984.

Post R M, Rubinow D R, Ballenger J C: Conditioning and sensitization in the longitudinal course of affective illness. Brit J Psychiat *149:* 191, 1986.

Post R M, Uhde T W: Refractory manias and alternatives to lithium treatment. In *Textbook of Depression and Mania,* A Georgotas, R Cancro, editors, p 410. Elsevier, New York, 1988.

Post R M, Uhde T W, Roy-Byrne P P, Joffe R T: Correlates of antimanic response to carbamazepine. Psychiat Res *21:* 71, 1987.

Price L H, Charney D S, Heninger G R: Variability of response to lithium augmentation in refractory depression. Amer J Psychiat *143:* 1387, 1986.

Rosenthal N E, Sack D A, Gillin J C, Lowy A J, Goodwin F K, Davenport Y, Mueller P E, Newsome D A, Wehr T A: Seasonal affective disorder. A description of the syndrome and preliminary findings with light therapy. Arch Gen Psychiat *41:* 72, 1984.

Roy-Byrne P, Uhde T W, Post R M: Antidepressant effects of one night's sleep deprivation: Clinical and theoretical implications. In *Neurobiology of Mood Disorders,* R M Post, J C Ballenger, editors, p 817. Williams & Wilkins, Baltimore, 1984.

Schou M, Juel-Nieben N, Stromgren E, Voldby H: The treatment of manic psychoses by the administration of lithium salts. J Neurol Neurosurg Psychiat *17:* 250, 1954.

Schou M, Stromgren E, editors: *Origin, Prevention and Treatment of Affective Disorders.* Academic Press, New York, 1979.

Wehr T A, Goodwin F K: Rapid cycling in manic-depressives induced by tricyclic antidepressants. Arch Gen Psychiat *36:* 555, 1979.

White K, Simpson G: Combined MAOI-tricyclic antidepressant treatment: A reevaluation. J Clin Psychopharmacol *1:* 264, 1981.

17.5 MOOD DISORDERS: PSYCHOSOCIAL TREATMENTS

ROBERT M. A. HIRSCHFELD, M.D.
M. TRACIE SHEA, Ph.D.

INTRODUCTION

The treatment for depression has come a long way since the days of leeching by the ancient Greeks. In the intervening centuries, cures have ranged from exorcism to wet-sheet body wraps.

More new treatments for depression have developed in the twentieth century than in its entire earlier history. Psychoanalytic approaches predominated in the early to middle 1900s and were based on a theory of depression as an expression of a disorder of the mind. Later in the century, electroconvulsive therapy (ECT) was found to be very efficacious for severe depression. In the 1960s and 1970s, psychopharmacological approaches virtually exploded and changed forever the treatment of depression. Important developments in psychiatric classification and in pharmacology converged to foster this phenomenon.

The principal development in psychiatric classification was a shift toward the use of manifest psychopathology (i.e., signs and symptoms) as the unit of classification. Although this idea is not new, in the past the most prevalent approaches to diagnosis were based on inferences about unconscious processes or on a unitary theory of mental disorders. Agreement among clinical raters (i.e., reliability) is vastly easier to achieve using the sign and symptom approach. The development of operational criteria for diagnostic categories has been a parallel process. Now, diagnostic categories may be tested for usefulness in terms of increased communication, etiology, selection of treatment response, and prediction of clinical course.

The discovery of selective therapeutic effectiveness of particular medications for specific conditions came hand in hand with the nosological advances. First were the phenothiazines for schizophrenia, then the monoamine oxidase inhibitors (MAOIs) and tricyclic antidepressants for depression, and finally lithium for mania. This selectivity of therapeutic response provides a clear clinical rationale for using nosology in practice.

The mid-1970s until the present time has been the period of psychotherapies for depression. This period has profited from the developments made during the psychopharmacological period in nosology and clinical trial methodology. The psychotherapeutic approaches aim at correcting specific aspects of depression, including cognitions, behavior, and affect, and were developed specifically for depression. In general, they are short-term and seek to alleviate the depressive condition per se, not to change character.

PSYCHOANALYSIS AND PSYCHOANALYTIC APPROACHES

THEORETICAL ROOTS AND THE CONCEPT OF DEPRESSION As a comprehensive review is well beyond the scope of this section, a brief focused review follows to introduce psychoanalytic principles in the treatment of depression.

The interpersonal nature of depression was noted and emphasized in even the earliest psychoanalytic writings on depression, as was the centrality of the regulation of self-esteem. In *Mourning and Melancholia,* Sigmund Freud stated that a vulnerability to depression caused by an interpersonal disappointment very early in life led to future love relationships marked by ambivalence. Actual or threatened interpersonal losses in adult life would trigger a self-destructive struggle in the ego that would be manifested as depression.

This theory was significantly refined by other psychoanalysts who described the depression-prone personality as one needing constant reassurance, love, and admiration. Such individuals are inordinately dependent on others for narcissistic gratification and for the maintenance of self-esteem. Frustration of their dependency needs leads to a plummet in self-esteem and to subsequent depression. Later, this notion was expanded to include any individual with a fragile self-esteem system.

Another dynamic approach focused on cognitive aspects, highlighting the recognition of the disparity between one's actual and idealized situation. This realization leads to a sense of helplessness and powerlessness and, ultimately, to depression.

All psychoanalytic contributions rest on the theory that a disturbance in interpersonal relations in early childhood, usually involving a loss or disappointment, will impair subsequent interpersonal relations. Such an individual is especially vulnerable to interpersonal disappointments and losses later in life, which may result in a depression.

GOALS In general, the goal of psychoanalytic psychotherapy is to effect a change in personality structure, and not simply to alleviate symptoms. Improvement in interpersonal trust, intimacy and generativity, coping mechanisms, the ability to experience a wide range of emotions, and the capacity to grieve are some of the aims. Treatment may often require the patient to experience heightened anxiety and distress during the course of therapy, which usually continues for several years.

Several approaches based on psychoanalytic principles have recently been developed and used to treat depression. These approaches seek to reduce symptomatology, resolve neuroses, and improve the quality of life.

GENERAL CONSIDERATIONS Early psychoanalytic treatments were short in duration, in comparison with those in current practice, usually lasting no more than a few months. Freud, for example, cured the composer Gustav Mahler of a sexual problem in one 4-hour session. Psychoanalytic treatments lengthened in duration as the development and interpretation of the transference relationships became the core of the therapy and as the therapists became more passive in their behavior.

Several clinicians, including Franz Alexander in Chicago, attempted to reverse this trend, but overall, they have had relatively little impact on their colleagues. In the past 2 decades, however, several specific short-term psychoanalytic approaches have evolved that are applicable to the treatment of depression. Perhaps the most seminal work was by Michael Balint and his colleagues in the 1950s at the Tavistock Clinic in London. Since the death of Balint, the work has been continued by David Malan. Other contributors include Habib Davanloo in Montreal, Peter Sifneos in Boston, Hans Strupp in Tennessee, and Lester Luborsky in Philadelphia (Table 17.5-1).

What distinguishes these psychoanalytic therapies from other psychotherapeutic approaches to depression is the use of the transference relationship. The relationship and interaction of the patient and the therapist are the key to the therapeutic process and subsequently to change. The patient–therapist relationship is used to examine and reexperience important present and past relationships that may account for the current difficulties. The various treatments differ in how they deal with the transference relationship, although most relate patterns of therapist–patient interactions to current interpersonal situations. The development of a transference neurosis, in which there is a regression into early childhood relationships, is usually discouraged.

These treatments depart somewhat from classical psychoanalytic practice. All involve active participation by the therapist and discourage free-association techniques. In general, they identify and emphasize a single focal issue.

The identification of suitable patients for these short-term psychoanalytic therapies is given preeminence by all proponents. In general, the patient selection criteria are very similar, although there are some differences among the therapies. Psychological mindedness and intelligence are considered to be very important. Individuals should be capable of introspection and should be able to see a connection among thoughts, feelings, and behavior. Patients should have a strong motivation for change and be flexibile; this motivation may be tested by assessing the patient's responsiveness to interpretations early in therapy. A capacity for meaningful human relationships must have been demonstrated at some time during life. Finally, the capacity to tolerate anxiety and frustration is required. Obviously, these criteria will exclude a significant proportion of psychiatric patients, leaving only the most desirable, verbal therapy candidates. Nonetheless, the proponents of these therapies point out that true character change is achieved in a relatively short time and that serious personality problems are addressed.

STRATEGIES AND TECHNIQUES Among the specific techniques used in these approaches are the active interpretation of the transference, the identification of and emphasis on a specific dynamic focus, the active collaboration between the patient and therapist, and the discouragement of regression.

The transference relationship is the heart of the short-term psychoanalytic approaches. The therapeutic relationship is composed of two aspects, the real and the transferred. The real relationship refers to those thoughts, feelings, and behaviors that are relevant and appropriate to the current interaction between patient and therapist. The transferred aspect is used to identify and reexperience problems and patterns that

TABLE 17.5-1
Features of Short-Term Psychoanalytic Approaches

Name	*Duration of Treatment (No. of Sessions)*	*Specific Time Limit*	*Indications*	*Special Notes*
Brief Psychotherapy (Malan)	20 to 40	Yes	Patients with a focal life problem who respond to trial interpretations.	Significant personality changes in suitable patients.
Short-Term Dynamic Psychotherapy (Davanloo)	15 to 30	No	Oedipal problems. Neurotic problems where the focus is loss. Obsessional and phobic neuroses. Long-standing, characterological problems without a single focus.	Highly confrontational. Recommended for resistant patients. Not recommended for patients with significant dependency or separation problems.
Short-Term Anxiety-Provoking Psychotherapy (Sifneos)	12 to 15	No	Oedipal triangular interpersonal problems.	Avoids regression into pregenital characterological issues. Change attributed to interpretation of oedipal issues.
Time-Limited Dynamic Psychotherapy (Strupp)	Fewer than 25	Yes	Avoidant, dependent, compulsive, and passive-aggressive personality disorders associated with depression, anxiety, and resentment.	Focus on interpersonal themes. Uses transference in a here-and-now way, not genetically.
Supportive-Expressive Treatment (Luborsky)	12 to 25	Yes	Broad range of problems—from mild situational maladjustments to borderline psychotic.	Techniques flexible so that a wide range of patients can benefit from treatment.

developed in important relationships early in life that were recreated in current important relationships. This process is considered to be the key to all psychoanalytic approaches. In the short-term approaches, the transference is actively developed and interpreted, often right from the outset. This approach is illustrated in an excerpt from an initial session with Davanloo in which he immediately challenges the patient's passivity.

Therapist: How do you feel about talking to me about yourself?
Patient: I feel uncomfortable. I have never done this before, so I don't really, you know. . . . I feel I don't really know how to answer some of your questions.
Therapist: Um-hum. But have you noticed that in your relationship here with me you are passive, and I am the one who has to question you repeatedly?
Patient: No.
Therapist: Um-hum. What do you think about this? Is this the way it is with other people, or is it only here with me? . . . This passivity, lack of spontaneity.

A vignette from an initial session with Sifneos illustrates another interpretation of the transference.

Patient: I put on an act. I wear a mask. I give the impression that I'm different from what I really am. I don't like this attitude in me.
Therapist: Can you give me an example?
Patient: What happened last week is a case in point. Before my girlfriend broke off our relationship, she said that she didn't like going out with someone who is a phony. . . . Mary, my previous girlfriend, had said the same thing, using different words, and so did Bob, my best friend. I know what they are all talking about. At times, even here, I have this great urge to show off and make you admire me.
Therapist: And where does this urge come from?
Patient: From very long ago. I used to put on an act to impress my mother. I remember one time when I made up a whole story about school. I told her that the teacher had said I was the best student she had ever had. My mother was impressed, but you know, doctor, it wasn't true. The teacher complimented me, but I exaggerated it. I blew it out of proportion.
Therapist: So you were trying to impress your mother, you are trying to impress your girlfriends and Bob, and even here. . . .
Patient: What do you mean by even here?
Therapist: A minute ago you said that even here you had such a tendency.
Patient: Did I say that?
Therapist: Yes, you did. Furthermore, why does it surprise you? If you put on an act with everyone else, why couldn't you put on an act with me?

The short-term therapies differ from classic psychoanalysis in their emphasis on the identification of a specific dynamic focus. A particular issue, usually an interpersonal problem, is selected, and both the patient and therapist agree to deal primarily with this problem during therapy. This focus is considered dynamic because it is used as a link with core conflicts arising from early life. This technique uses the current conflict as a microcosm for the more substantial and long-lasting conflicts in the patient's life.

In his manual, Strupp describes a married woman in her 30s who sought treatment for recurrent depressive episodes. The woman's manner in the interview was somewhat aloof and curt, which led the therapist to want to discuss facts rather than to elicit feelings. When this inclination was pointed out to her, the patient responded that she could not imagine that anything she said could be of interest to anyone, and therefore, she acted in this way to protect herself from being hurt. The dynamic focus then became an exploration of her expectation that she was of no interest to anyone. A link was subsequently made with the patient's childhood, during which her parents seemed to prefer her sisters to her.

Active collaboration between the patient and therapist involves the establishment of a working alliance. The therapist seeks to convey interest in the patient's problems, as well as respect and warmth, and attempts to elucidate explanations from the patient, in addition to using interpretations. Thus, a mutuality and common purpose are fostered.

Most of the short-term psychoanalytic approaches discourage regression. The principal reason for this is that emergence of such material as pregenital characterological issues often leads to significant therapeutic impasses that may not be resolved in a short period of time. Sifneos gives an example of a patient who became very angry and demanding about making up a canceled session. Instead of encouraging associations to childhood orality and dependency, the therapist confronted the patient's maladaptive and self-destructive current behavior, and encouraged the patient to request an extra session, rather than being angry and withdrawn.

INTERPERSONAL THERAPY

THEORETICAL FOUNDATIONS AND CONCEPTS OF DEPRESSION Interpersonal therapy (IPT) was developed by Gerald Klerman and Myrna Weissman as part of their extensive research on the nature and treatment of depression over the past 2 decades. The theoretical basis of IPT includes the work of Adolf Meyer and Harry Stack Sullivan. In contrast with the predominantly intrapsychic orientation of classical psychoanalysis and Emil Kraepelin's biomedical model, Meyer's psychobiological approach emphasizes the interaction between the individual and the psychosocial environment over the whole life course. The patient's current interpersonal experiences and attempts to adapt to environmental change and stress are seen as critical factors in psychiatric illness. Sullivan's interpersonal theory views interactions between people as the focus for study and treatment in psychiatry. His theory draws heavily from the social sciences, including anthropology and sociology.

A second major influence comes from John Bowlby's studies of attachment. These studies demonstrate the importance of attachment and social bonding to human functioning, and the connection between disruption of these bonds and vulnerability to depression.

In IPT, depression is conceptualized from a medical model vantage. Thus, depression is viewed as something that happens to the individual and requires treatment. The depressed person can then assume the sick role and not be blamed for the affliction any more than someone would be blamed for having cancer, heart disease, or pneumonia. This issue of attribution of blame is an important one. Many other approaches view depression as something brought on by oneself and as something of which individuals must rid themselves.

The IPT approach to depression involves three interacting components: symptom formation, social and interpersonal experiences, and enduring personality patterns. In IPT, medication is often recommended for reducing symptoms, and psychotherapy is focused on improving the patient's interpersonal life. Although the etiology may vary with regard to biological vulnerability or personality predispositions, depression always occurs in a psychosocial and interpersonal context. Depression can predispose a patient to interpersonal problems, or interpersonal problems can precipitate depression. An interpersonal focus in the treatment process is thus presumed essential for symptom recovery.

GOALS The first of IPT's two goals is to reduce depressive symptoms and improve self-esteem. The second is to help the patient develop more effective strategies for dealing with social and interpersonal relations. As a short-term psychotherapy, IPT does not attempt to restructure the patient's character. This approach recognizes the importance of early developmental experiences but emphasizes interpersonal relationships in the current life situation, as it is assumed that the historical conflicts will be manifested in the current relationships.

GENERAL CONSIDERATIONS IPT is a short-term psychotherapy, normally consisting of 12 to 16 weekly sessions, and was developed specifically to treat nonbipolar, nonpsychotic ambulatory depressives. It is characterized by an active approach on the part of the therapist and by an emphasis on current issues and social functioning in the life of the patient. Intrapsychic phenomena, such as defense mechanisms or internal conflicts, are not addressed. Discrete behaviors, such as lack of assertiveness, social skills, or distorted thinking, may be addressed, but only in the context of their meaning or effect on interpersonal relationships.

STRATEGIES AND TECHNIQUES **General strategies** There are general strategies for each of the two primary goals. For the reduction of symptoms, an educational approach is used. The patient is told about the clinical syndrome of depression, including its components and course. The therapist reviews the symptoms with the patient and, to give the patient a sense of optimism and hope, emphasizes that depression is a common disorder with a good prognosis. Pharmacotherapy may be considered for use in conjunction with IPT, if appropriate.

The general strategy for the second goal—helping the patient deal more effectively with current interpersonal problems—is establishing a problem area from the patient's interpersonal issues. IPT defines four major problem areas that are commonly presented by depressed patients and outlines associated therapeutic goals and recommended treatment strategies for each. The areas are (1) grief, (2) interpersonal role disputes, (3) role transitions, and (4) interpersonal deficits (Table 17.5-2). Defining a problem area helps the therapist outline realistic goals and productive treatment strategies, because the choice of specific IPT strategies and techniques will depend on the problem area defined as most salient for the patient. The problem areas are not mutually exclusive, and patients may have multiple problems in more than one area; however, only one or two current interpersonal problems in the four areas are selected for focus in the therapy.

Cases of abnormal grief may involve delayed or distorted mourning, or both. For example, as cited in the IPT manual:

> A 68-year-old woman became depressed following the death of her husband, who had suffered a long course of physical and mental deterioration, which resulted in considerable constraints and isolation on the part of the patient. Her symptoms included pervasive sadness and preoccupation with feelings of guilt and hopelessness. The first aim of treatment was to help the patient to successfully mourn the loss, as the mourning process had been blocked by anger. The second aim was to help her to reestablish interests and relationships to substitute for what she had lost.

The interpersonal issues in a troublesome and conflicted marriage are examples of role disputes or role transitions. The choice between the two problem areas will depend on whether the patient believes that the marriage is salvageable and whether the patient wants to stay in the marriage. If the patient decides to leave the marriage and the problem area is defined as role transition, the therapist will attempt to help the patient make that transition. This may include working on

TABLE 17.5-2
Interpersonal Problem Areas

Problem Areas	*Definition*	*General Goals and Strategies*
Grief	Abnormal grief reactions resulting from failure to go through normal mourning following the death of a person important to the patient.	Facilitate the mourning process. Help patient reestablish interests and relationships to substitute for the loss.
Interpersonal role disputes	Patient and significant other(s) have nonreciprocal expectations about the relationship.	Help patient identify the dispute. Guide patient in choices as to plans of action. Encourage modification of maladaptive communication patterns. Encourage reassessment of expectations.
Role transitions	Patient feels unable to cope with change in life role; may be experienced as threatening to self-esteem, sense of identity, or both.	Help patient regard role in a more positive and less restrictive manner. Restore self-esteem by helping patient develop sense of mastery with regard to demands of new role.
Interpersonal deficits	Patient has history of inadequate or unsustaining interpersonal relationships.	Reduce patient's social isolation by focusing on past relationships and relationship with therapist and by helping patient form new relationships.

identifying new sources of emotional support, overcoming irrational fears and regarding the new role more positively, and helping the patient master the demands of the new role. Alternatively, if the problem area is defined as a role dispute, the treatment strategies will include identifying the dispute and working toward its resolution, improving communication patterns, examining appropriateness of expectations, outlining various options, and deciding on a plan of action.

The interpersonal deficit problem area is appropriate for patients who are socially isolated or have a sufficient number of relationships but feel unable to enjoy them. Interpersonal deficits may exist in patients who are chronically depressed, resulting in impaired interpersonal functioning. Problems with social isolation may be long-standing or temporary; treatment strategies are geared toward reducing social isolation. In the absence of current relationships, discussion of positive and negative features of past relationships may be used as a model for the development of new relationships. Treatment may also focus on the relationship between the therapist and the patient.

An example of an interpersonal deficit cited by the IPT manual is as follows:

> A 22-year-old single male became severely depressed 1 month after the breakup of a 3-year relationship with his girlfriend. The patient, a part-time student employed as a cook, lived with his mother, who had stopped working after being hospitalized for physical problems, and subsequently, he had become depressed. Discussion of the patient's current relationship revealed that apart from his mother, he felt close to no one.

Information from the patient's past revealed a history of inadequate social relationships and a lack of interpersonal skills. The treatment focused on past significant relationships and on his conflicts over his relationship with his mother. The patient–therapist relationship provided a direct source of information about the patient's style of relating to others, and this information was used to modify maladaptive interpersonal patterns.

Specific techniques The specific techniques used in IPT may be applied to any of the four interpersonal problem areas. In the general order of their use in the course of treatment, they are (1) exploratory techniques, (2) encouragement of affect, (3) clarification, (4) communication analysis, (5) use of therapeutic relationship, and (6) behavior change techniques (Table 17.5-3).

IPT thus places interpersonal issues in a preeminent position in the depressive syndrome, as either a cause or a complication, which, as such, need to be addressed in the treatment of depression. In IPT, the patient's predominant interpersonal problems are formulated in terms of an interpersonal problem area, which defines the focus for treatment and guides the choice of therapeutic strategies and techniques.

BEHAVIORAL APPROACHES

THEORETICAL ROOTS AND CONCEPTS OF DEPRESSION Although current behavioral approaches to depression have somewhat different theoretical assumptions and specific treatment methods, they do have a common source. B. F. Skinner, incorporating the principles of classical conditioning and, more importantly, operant conditioning in an empirical analysis of behavior, provided the basic framework, methodology, and assumptions for the current behavioral theories and their clinical applications.

The application of the behavioral model to complex human behavior led some theorists to expand the framework. For example, social learning theory includes cognitive phenomena in its emphasis on the role of subjective expectations and value in reinforcement. Although interested in the role of cognitions, behavioral theories assume that cognitions follow the same laws of learning as do more observable behavioral events; thus, while related, they do not determine behavior in a causal sense. This assumption distinguishes behavioral approaches from the cognitive-behavioral approach described below. Despite some differences in focus, behavioral therapies are commonly characterized by an emphasis on (1) the links between an observable or operationally definable behavior and the conditions that control or determine it and (2) the role of rewards or reinforcement as determinants of behavior and behavioral change.

The introduction of the behavioral approach to depression occurred in 1965 with an analysis of depression by C. B. Ferster, who proposed that depression is caused by a loss of positive reinforcement. The loss of the usual supply of reinforcement may be due to such events as separation, death, or sudden environmental change and this loss results in the reduction of the entire behavioral repertoire, as well as depressed behaviors and dysphoric feelings. This concept of

TABLE 17.5-3
Interpersonal Therapy Techniques

Techniques	*Definition*
Exploratory techniques	Collection of information about patient's symptoms and problems, which can be directive or nondirective.
Encouragement of affect	Help patient recognize and accept painful affects. Help patient use and manage affects positively in interpersonal relationships. Encourage expression of suppressed affect.
Clarification	Restructure and feed back patient's communications.
Communication analysis	Identify maladaptive communication patterns. Help patient communicate more effectively.
Use of therapeutic relationship	Examine patient's feelings and behaviors in therapeutic relationship as a model of patient's interactions in other relationships.
Behavior change techniques	Use techniques to help patient solve simple life problems. Teach patient to consider range of options for solving problems. Use role playing to explore and understand patient's relationship with others and to train patient in new ways of interacting with others.

depression is central to all behavioral approaches. A change in the rate of reinforcement is believed to be a key factor in the origin, maintenance, and reversal of depression. This change may occur when there is a lack of available reinforcers or when the available reinforcers are not contingent on the person's behavior. Ferster also proposed that a social skills deficit—characterized by difficulty in obtaining social reinforcement—might make it more difficult to cope with the loss of the usual supply of reinforcement. The role of social skills deficits in depression is also common to many of the behavioral approaches.

GOALS The goals of the behavioral therapies are to increase the frequency of the patient's positively reinforcing interactions with the environment and to decrease the number of negative interactions. Some of the behavioral treatments aim also at improving social skills. Alteration of personal behavior in depressed patients is believed to be the most effective way to change the associated depressed thoughts and feelings.

GENERAL CONSIDERATIONS Several behavior therapies have been devised to treat depression and are characterized by overlapping behavioral and cognitive intervention strategies. One particularly well known and extensively studied approach was developed by Peter Lewinsohn on the basis of social learning theory. In addition to the individual-based social learning approach, Lewinsohn developed a "Coping with Depression Course," designed to deliver the specific behavioral strategies in a group format. The focus of Lewinsohn's approach, whether in individual or group format, is on increasing pleasant activities and interactions with the environment. A second prominent behavioral approach, based on a self-control model of behavior, was developed by Lynne Rehm to treat depression. Key components of this approach include techniques designed to correct deficits in the patient's ability to realistically and productively self-monitor, self-evaluate, and self-reinforce. A third approach focuses on the training of social skills in order to increase positive social interactions and reinforcements. Table 17.5-4 summarizes these approaches, strategies, and tactics. These therapies share certain assumptions and strategies:

1. The treatment program is highly structured and generally short term.
2. The principle of reinforcement is seen as the key element in depression.
3. Changing behavior is considered to be the most effective way to alleviate depression.
4. The focus is on the articulation and attainment of specific goals.

Some behavioral treatments combine a variety of behavioral techniques and tailor the techniques to the individual needs of each patient. Normally, there are core ingredients in conjunction with a number of optional techniques.

STRATEGIES AND TECHNIQUES Although the major behavioral approaches to depression vary in their focus and emphasis in treatment and in their frequency of use of specific techniques, there is considerable overlap. Detailed manuals specify treatment regimes for most of these approaches.

Maintain records Recording mood and activities, both positive and negative, is essential to most behavioral therapies. Patients may also monitor the immediate and long-term consequences of specific behavior.

Increase general activity level, particularly pleasant events On the basis of the daily mood and activity recordings, the therapist encourages the patients to increase their participation in those activities rated as most pleasant, by demonstrating a relationship between increased pleasant activities and lower levels of depression.

Decrease or manage unpleasant events From the daily ratings, negative interactions or situations that trigger feelings of depression are identified. Patients learn to avoid and decrease unpleasant events when possible. Patients are also taught to manage their reactions to negative events by learning to substitute more positive thoughts, to prepare for unpleasant events, and to prepare for failure.

Develop new self-reinforcement patterns Patients learn to reward themselves or to increase goal-related activities with material rewards or activities.

Enhance social skills Deficits in social skills and interaction patterns may be addressed through assertiveness training, modeling, and role playing with feedback and rehearsal or by providing graduated performance assignments to promote rewarding social interaction and to decrease social avoidance; or, they may be addressed by a combination of approaches. Group therapy sessions may be used to improve communication skills or to resolve specific interpersonal problems.

Relaxation training Relaxation techniques may aid in achieving other goals, such as increasing social interaction, reducing the aversiveness of unpleasant situations, or produc-

TABLE 17.5-4
Behavioral Approaches to Depression

Treatment Approach	*Basic Approach and Strategies*	*Tactics*
Self-control therapy (Rehm)	Self-monitoring—gain control over and increase positive activities. Self-evaluation—learn to set realistic goals; learn to make more accurate attributions regarding causes of successes and failures. Self-reinforcement—learn to increase and maintain level of positive activities.	Monitor mood. Schedule pleasurable activities. Set realistic goals and break into operational subgoals. Schedule activities related to goals and monitor progress. Teach patients to make correct self-attributions. Have patients construct individualized self-reinforcement programs to increase and maintain level of positive activities.
Social learning therapy (Lewinsohn)	Initial 2-week diagnostic phase leading to behavioral diagnosis. Treatment designed to increase activity level and enhance social skills.	Home observation. Daily monitoring of mood and activity. Increase participation in pleasant events. Environmental interventions—environmental shifts, change consequences of certain behaviors. Assertion training through modeling and rehearsal. Set goals for increasing social activities. Relaxation training. Time management. Cognitive techniques (including thought interruption, worrying time, disputing irrational thoughts, noticing accomplishments, and positive self-rewarding thoughts).
Social skills training (Hersen and Bellack)	Skills training—patient is taught positive assertion, negative assertion, and conversational skills. Social perception training—patient learns to attend to relevant context and cues of interpersonal interactions. Practice—newly learned responses are carried out in the natural environment. Self-evaluation and self-reinforcement—patient is trained to evaluate responses more positively and to provide self-reinforcment.	Didactic instruction. Modeling, guided practice of skills. Role playing. Homework assignments. Monitoring and recording of homework performance by patient. Patient's evaluation of role-played responses with letter grade; therapist's correction of inappropriately low responses; therapist's modeling of positive self-statement.

ing a mood state incompatible with depression. Patients are taught relaxation of the major muscle groups; they are encouraged to practice relaxation twice a day and are instructed to keep a relaxation log.

Time management Training patients to plan ahead and make preparations necessary to participate in pleasant events (e.g., obtain a baby-sitter) is part of time management. An effort is made to work out an appropriate balance between activities that the patients want to do and activities that they feel they have to do.

Cognitive skills training Cognitive skills training is generally geared toward decreasing negative thinking and increasing positive thinking. Patients are taught to monitor their thinking and to discriminate between positive and negative thoughts, necessary and unnecessary thoughts, and constructive and destructive thoughts. Specific techniques include thought-stopping, disputing irrational thoughts, and correcting errors in attribution regarding causes of successes and failures.

COGNITIVE BEHAVIORAL THERAPY

THEORETICAL ROOTS AND CONCEPTS OF DEPRESSION Cognitive behavioral (CB) therapy stems from four major theories: psychoanalysis, phenomenological philosophy, cognitive psychology, and behavioral psychology. Several threads emerge from these theories. Perhaps most salient is the recognition of the importance of the subjectiveness of conscious experience (i.e., the experience of reality) rather than objective reality. Another thread is the recognition of the emotional consequences of irrational beliefs.

Aaron Beck, the originator of CB therapy, developed a comprehensive, structured theory of depression. Depression consists of a cognitive triad, specific schemas, and cognitive errors, or faulty information processing (Table 17.5-5).

The cognitive triad consists of negative cognitions regarding oneself, the world, and one's future. First is a negative self-percept involving seeing oneself as defective, inadequate, deprived, worthless, and undesirable. Second is a tendency to experience the world as a negative, demanding, and defeating place and to expect failure and punishment. Third is an expectation of continued hardship, suffering, deprivation, and failure.

Schemas are stable cognitive patterns through which one interprets experience. Schemas of depression are analogous to viewing the world through dark glasses. Depressogenic schemas may involve viewing experience as black or white without shades of gray, as categorical imperatives that allow no options, or as expectations that people are either all good or all bad.

Cognitive errors are systematic errors in thinking that lead to the persistence of negative schemas despite contradictory evidence.

The cognitive theory of depression posits that cognitive dysfunctions are the core of depression and that affective and physical changes, and other associated features of depression, are consequences of the cognitive dysfunctions. For example, apathy and low energy are results of the individual's expecta-

TABLE 17.5-5
Elements of Cognitive Theory

Element	*Definition*
Cognitive triad	Beliefs about oneself, the world, the future.
Schemas	Ways of organizing and interpreting experiences.
Cognitive distortions	
Arbitrary inference	Drawing a specific conclusion without sufficient evidence.
Specific abstraction	Picking out a single detail and ignoring other more important aspects of an experience.
Overgeneralization	Forming conclusions on the basis of too little and too narrow experience.
Magnification and minimization	Over- or undervaluing the significance of a particular event.
Personalization	Tendency to self-reference to external events without basis.
Absolutist, dichotomous thinking	Tendency to place experience into all-or-none categories.

tion of failure in all areas. Similarly, a paralysis of will stems from the individual's pessimism and feelings of hopelessness.

GOALS The goal of CB therapy is to alleviate depression and prevent its recurrence by helping the patient (1) identify and test negative cognitions; (2) develop alternative, more flexible schemas; and (3) rehearse both new cognitive and new behavioral responses. The goal is also to change the way an individual thinks and, subsequently, to alleviate the depressive syndrome.

GENERAL CONSIDERATIONS CB therapy was developed by Aaron Beck. CB therapy is a short-term, structured therapy that involves active collaboration between the patient and the therapist toward achieving the therapy goals. It is oriented toward current problems and their resolution. CB therapy is usually conducted on an individual basis, although group techniques have been developed and tested. This therapy may be used in conjunction with drug therapy.

STRATEGIES AND TECHNIQUES As with other psychotherapies, the therapist's attributes are fundamental to suc cessful CB therapy. Therapists must be warm, be able to understand the life experience of each patient, and be truly genuine and honest with themselves as well as with the patients. Therapists also must be able to relate skillfully to patients in their own experiential world in a truly interactive way.

As a highly structured therapeutic approach, CB sets the agenda at the beginning of each session, assigns homework to be performed between sessions, and teaches specific new skills. The active collaboration between the therapist and the patient provides a genuine sense of teamwork.

CB therapy has three basic components: didactic aspects, cognitive techniques, and behavioral techniques (Table 17.5-6).

Didactic aspects The didactic aspects include explaining to the patient the nature of the cognitive triad, schemas, and faulty logic. The therapist must tell the patient that they will formulate hypotheses together and will test them over the course of treatment. CB therapy also requires a full explanation of the relationship between depression and thinking, affect, and behavior, as well as the rationale for all aspects of the treatment. This explanation is in contrast to the more psychoanalytically oriented therapies, in which very little explanation is involved.

Cognitive techniques The cognitive approach has four processes: (1) eliciting automatic thoughts, (2) testing automatic thoughts, (3) identifying maladaptive underlying assumptions, and (4) testing the validity of maladaptive assumptions.

ELICITING AUTOMATIC THOUGHTS Automatic thoughts are cognitions that intervene between external events and the individual's emotional reaction to the event. An example of an automatic thought is the belief that "everyone is going to laugh at me when they see how badly I bowl"—a thought that occurs to someone who has been asked to go bowling and responds negatively. Another example is a person's thought that "he doesn't like me", if someone passes that person in the hall without saying hello.

TESTING AUTOMATIC THOUGHTS The therapist, acting as a teacher, helps the patient test the validity of the automatic thought. The goal is to encourage the patient to reject inaccurate or exaggerated automatic thoughts after carefully examining them.

Patients often blame themselves for things that go wrong that may well have been outside their control. The therapist reviews with the patient the entire situation and helps reattribute more accurately the blame or cause of the unpleasant events. The case of a 51-year-old moderately depressed bank manager who complained of "ineffectiveness in my job" is detailed by Beck.

Patient: I can't tell you how much of a mess I've made of things. I've made another major error of judgment that should cost me my job.

Therapist: Tell me what the error in judgment was.

Patient: I approved a loan that fell through completely. I made a very poor decision.

Therapist: Can you recall the specifics about the decision?

Patient: Yes, I remember that it looked good on paper, good collateral, good credit rating, but I should have known there was going to be a problem.

Therapist: Did you have all of the pertinent information at the time of your decision?

Patient: Not at the time, but I sure found out 6 weeks later. I'm paid to make profitable decisions, not to give the bank's money away.

TABLE 17.5-6
Cognitive Behavioral Therapy

Components
1. Didactic Issues
Learning the therapy's rationale and strategy.
2. Cognitive Techniques
Eliciting automatic thoughts.
Testing automatic thoughts.
Identifying maladaptive underlying assumptions.
Analyzing validity of maladaptive assumptions.
3. Behavioral techniques
Scheduling activities.
Mastery and pleasure.
Graded task assignment.
Cognitive rehearsal.
Self-reliance training.
Role playing.
Diversion techniques.

Therapist: I understand your position, but I would like to review the information that you had at the time your decision was required, not 6 weeks after the decision had been made.

In this example, when the patient and therapist carefully reviewed the situation, it became apparent that the patient's original decision was justified on the basis of the facts available at the time that the loan was made. The reasons for the default on the loan came to light only afterward, and therefore, the patient could not be blamed for having made a bad decision.

Generating alternative explanations is another way of undermining inaccurate and distorted automatic thoughts.

A medical records librarian with a 6-year history of depression reported that the charge nurse in the coronary care unit was curt and said, "I hate medical records", when the librarian went to collect charts for the record review committee. The patient reported feelings of sadness, slight anger, and loneliness. Her automatic thought was, "She [the nurse] doesn't like me." The therapist helped the patient find other possible interpretations, such as the possibility that the charge nurse is generally unhappy, that she may be under pressure for reasons unrelated to the librarian, that hating medical records is not the same as hating the librarian, and that perhaps she actually hated paperwork.

IDENTIFYING MALADAPTIVE ASSUMPTIONS As the patient and therapist continue to identify automatic thoughts, patterns usually become apparent, representing rules or maladaptive general assumptions that guide the patient's life. Samples of such rules are, "In order to be happy, I must be perfect" or "If anyone doesn't like me, I'm not lovable." Such rules inevitably lead to disappointment, failure, and subsequently to depression.

ANALYZING THE VALIDITY OF MALADAPTIVE ASSUMPTIONS Similar to testing the validity of automatic thoughts is testing the accuracy of maladaptive assumptions. One particularly effective technique is for the therapist to ask the patient to defend the validity of an assumption.

Patient: I guess I believe that I should always work up to my potential.
Therapist: Why is that?
Patient: Otherwise I would be wasting time.
Therapist: What is the long-range goal in working up to your potential?
Patient: I've never really thought about that. I've just assumed that I should.
Therapist: Are there any positive things you give up by always having to work up to your potential?
Patient: I suppose it makes it hard to relax or take a vacation.
Therapist: What about living up to your potential to enjoy yourself and relax? Is that important at all?
Patient: I've never really thought of it that way.
Therapist: Maybe we can work on giving yourself permission not to work up to your potential at all times.

In this example, the therapist is helping the patient recognize how maladaptive it is to strive to work up to one's potential at all times.

Behavioral techniques Behavioral techniques go hand in hand with cognitive techniques; They are used to test and change maladaptive or inaccurate cognitions. The overall purpose of behavioral techniques is to help patients understand the inaccuracy of their cognitive assumptions and to learn new strategies and ways of dealing with issues.

Among the behavioral techniques utilized in CB therapy are scheduling activities, mastery and pleasure, graded task assignments, cognitive rehearsal, self-reliance training, role playing, and diversion techniques.

Among the first things done in CB therapy is to schedule activities on an hourly basis. The patient keeps a record of these activities and reviews it with the therapist.

In addition to scheduling activities, patients are asked to rate the amount of mastery and pleasure of their activities; they are often surprised at how much more mastery and pleasure they get out of activities than they had otherwise believed.

In order to simplify the situation and allow for miniaccomplishments, tasks are often broken down into subtasks, as in graded task assignments, to demonstrate to patients that they can succeed.

Cognitive rehearsal means having the patient imagine the various steps involved in meeting and mastering a challenge and rehearsing the various aspects of it.

Patients, especially inpatients, are encouraged to become more self-reliant, by doing such simple things as making their own beds, doing their own shopping, or preparing their own meals, rather than relying on other people. This is self-reliance training.

Role playing is a particularly powerful and useful technique used to elicit automatic thoughts and learn new behaviors.

Diversion techniques are useful in helping patients get through particularly difficult times, by means of physical activity, social contact, work, play, or visual imagery.

The techniques that CB uses are highly structured and goal oriented and require active collaboration between the therapist and the patient. Emphasis is on identifying maladaptive, inaccurate cognitions in various forms, seeking alternative explanations, and learning new behaviors. The major principle of all of these techniques is that identifying and changing these cognitions and relevant behaviors will reverse the affective and drive disturbances and other associated features of depression and, it is hoped, will help prevent their recurrence.

DISCUSSION

The success of any treatment of depression depends on many factors, including diagnosis, the duration of the condition, and the mode of therapy. The accurate identification of the patient's condition (i.e., the diagnosis) is perhaps the most important factor. How long the depression has been present can strongly influence the effectiveness of the treatment. Patients with chronic depression present a very difficult problem for treatment. The choice of individual, marital, family, or group therapy can also be important. Another consideration is whether to combine psychotherapeutic techniques with medications. Do they interact positively? Do they add anything? Do they address the same problems?

DIAGNOSIS In general, these psychotherapeutic approaches were developed for, and are recommended primarily for, outpatients with nonbipolar depressions in the mild to moderate range (although there are data for efficacy in more severely ill outpatients). There is some controversy over whether nonbipolar depressions should first be treated with medication, but certainly, patients who are very suicidal or present with hallucinations, delusions, or both, are not considered to be good candidates for these approaches. In general, patients meeting the criteria for melancholia should first be given a trial of medications alone or in combination with psychotherapy.

Since the discovery of the efficacy of lithium in the treatment of bipolar disorder, little, if any, attempt has been made to develop specific techniques for patients with bipolar depressive disorder, beyond marital or various supportive techniques. This is unfortunate, because bipolar disorder is especially destructive for the individuals and their families, and psychotherapeutic techniques may be useful.

CHRONICITY The overwhelming bulk of knowledge about the clinical course and treatment of depression comes from the study of patients with acute major depression. Knowledge about chronic depression, whether dysthymia or incompletely recovered major depression, has lagged woefully behind. This is particularly unfortunate because the prevalence of chronic depression is high. The National Institute of Mental Health (NIMH) Epidemiologic Catchment Area Program figures show that over 3 percent of the U.S. adult population suffers from dysthymia during any 6-month period. In addition, up to 20 percent of individuals with an episode of depression will become chronic, and an additional 30 to 40 percent will have episodic recurrences.

At this time, the diagnostic and treatment strategies for these groups of patients are just beginning to be addressed. Which patients will respond better to psychotherapy and to which psychotherapy is at this time a matter of conjecture. Similarly, the utility of medications for this group must be investigated. Variables associated with a positive response to medications include a family history of bipolar disorder, a history of incomplete recovery from a major depressive episode, and an increased severity of depressive symptoms.

MODE OF THERAPY Individual psychotherapy has been the standard mode of psychotherapeutic treatment described in this section. Some of these psychotherapies, however, seem to be particularly well suited to therapeutic modes other than individual psychotherapy. For example, IPT using a family mode seems to be a logical choice for a marital dispute. Testing cognitive distortions regarding one's social presence may be easy to do in group therapy. Also, group therapy allows for the development of a number of transference relationships, rather than a single one between the therapist and the patient. And social skills are more easily learned in a group situation.

COMBINATION PSYCHOTHERAPY AND MEDICATION Depression is a complex group of disorders that affect many body systems. Clinicians, thus, expect that several different therapeutic approaches will be effective in counteracting depression's various aspects. In fact, many clinicians do just that, combining medication and psychotherapeutic techniques to address the many types of problems with which patients present.

This issue has been the subject of several research projects, including IPT, CB, and behavioral approaches in combination with several tricyclics, in the treatment of outpatient major depression. Several studies found that the combined approach is superior to either drugs alone or psychotherapy alone. Others found no difference between the combined therapy and either psychotherapy alone or drugs alone. None found that the combination is worse than a single treatment alone. In addition, dropout rates are usually lowest in the combined group. At this time, the issue is far from resolved, and considerably more research is required.

Do medications address problems that are different from those in psychotherapeutic approaches? The answer is by no means clear. However, some evidence exists that drugs affect the somatic and vegetative symptoms of depression more specifically and more quickly, whereas the psychotherapies affect the interpersonal and cognitive aspects.

OTHER INFLUENCING VARIABLES A number of other issues may affect the outcome of a particular treatment and, therefore, may influence the treatment selection. These issues include premorbid personality, concurrent personality disorders, and expectations of therapy.

Premorbid personality Many patients with depression have been described as having premorbid personalities characterized by increased interpersonal dependency, whereas others are considered more obsessional. These personality features could well lead to vulnerability to subsequent depressive episodes and affect treatment considerations. Patients with excessive dependency may not be good candidates for short-term psychoanalytic therapies because dependency on the therapist may become too great and termination too disruptive. Obsessional patients, however, may do much better when transference issues are actively confronted.

The importance of concurrent personality disorders has only recently begun to be appreciated. The treatment of patients with borderline personality disorder would certainly be different from that of someone with paranoid personality disorder and, again, may be very different from the treatment of someone with avoidant personality disorder. Patients with avoidant personality disorder may do much better in behavior therapy, where social skills are learned in a safe environment; however, the social approach may be less effective for someone with paranoid personality disorder. A cognitive approach may be much better for these patients.

Patient's expectations The expectations of the patient should also be considered. Some patients consider depression to be a psychological disorder that should be amenable to psychotherapeutic approaches, and they are resistant to using medication. Other patients have exactly the opposite expectations; they may consider their depression to be a biochemical disturbance that will require medication if it is to be corrected, and not psychotherapy. A good therapist may be able to modify such expectations when necessary, but a positive attitude toward treatment on the part of the patient may be very important to a successful outcome.

In general, the therapist should be cautious in making attributions about premorbid personality problems during the depressed phase. Many interpersonal and cognitive styles may appear different to the patient and the therapist after the acute phase of the disorder has been alleviated.

Standard therapeutic approach The theoretical rationale and basic strategies of each of the psychotherapies described are distinct; yet, considerable overlap exists among them. All recommend an empathic, understanding approach by the therapist, who collaborates with the patient, rather than simply delivering a treatment. Most of the approaches explain the nature of depression and the techniques involved in the treatment. Interpersonal issues are central to all of the therapies, and most of them encourage behavioral change and judicious management of current crises.

What accounts for change is not clear at this time. Probably the answer will be complex; certain psychotherapeutic strategies will yield certain kinds of change (e.g., CB for changes in maladaptive assumptions), whereas general characteristics may account for other changes (e.g., a warm, accepting therapist may be responsible for a general uplifting of self-esteem). The elucidation of these active ingredients for affective, cognitive, and behavioral change is the next great task for psychotherapeutic research.

EFFICACY The psychotherapeutic approaches used in the treatment of episodes of major depression have two purposes: to resolve the acute episode and to prevent recurrences. In addition, psychotherapy can be used after recovery from an episode as a maintenance treatment to prevent recurrences.

Psychotherapy vs. medication A fundamental aspect of psychotherapy is that it teaches new strategies for dealing with life's problems and it teaches better coping skills for dealing with adversity. The new knowledge gained from psychotherapy will help reverse the depressive process and rid the person of the disorder. If this is true, this knowledge should serve to prevent recurrences of depression. Such a quality would be very valuable, as compared with medication.

In contrast to psychotherapy, medication alleviates depressive symptoms but does not change the underlying pathophysiology responsible for the disorder. Therefore, successful psychotherapeutic approaches might be more effective in preventing recurrences than would medication, especially if the medication were not continued in a maintenance fashion.

The last edition of this text contained descriptions of the psychotherapies developed specifically for the treatment of depression, but there was little evidence for their efficacy. Relatively little research using anything approaching clinical trial methodology had been performed, and much of the research had been conducted by the developers of the psychotherapies, whose enthusiasm might have influenced the results.

This is not meant to demean the researchers or their results. In fact, those who devised the psychotherapies did much to advance the clinical trials methodology in psychotherapy research. Further, these investigations were subjected to empirical trials. In order to achieve full credibility, however, the efficacy of the psychotherapies must be demonstrated by neutral investigators (i.e., those not invested in any particular outcome).

Fortunately, testing by neutral investigators is currently taking place. This phase of development of psychotherapies for depression involves the active application of clinical trial methodology, usually including a drug treatment condition. Several factors have enabled this phase: (1) development of training procedures for therapists, (2) development of measures to assess whether therapists are actually practicing the treatment appropriately, and (3) development of outcome measures for symptomatology and social and interpersonal functioning. These three factors, along with the earlier developments, have provided a structure for research. Most of the results of the best recent studies on the efficacy of these psychotherapies do not meet all the criteria noted above, but all involve random assignment to one of several groups, often including a medication condition and an independent assessment of outcome.

Review of recent studies INTERPERSONAL THERAPY One study compared IPT, amitriptyline (Elavil), IPT plus amitriptyline, and a nonscheduled, low-contact psychotherapeutic treatment for acutely depressed men and women. Symptomatic failure rates were significantly lower for all the active treatments, compared with those for the low-contact group. The combined IPT and drug treatment had the lowest rates of all the groups. After 1 year, patients treated with IPT had better social functioning but were equal to the other groups in depressive symptoms. In a separate study, following full recovery, IPT was found to improve social functioning, when used as a maintenance treatment over time, but it had no discernible effect in preventing relapse in 150 recovered neurotic depressives. Similar results were reported in a study of 62 depressed outpatients at 1-year follow-up.

CB THERAPY CB therapy has been tested against both behavioral and drug therapies in a number of studies. The two most recent studies of CB versus behavior therapy found them to be equally efficacious. An earlier study in 1977 found that cognitive therapy was more effective than behavior therapy in a 4-week trial. In a clinical trial comparing drugs and CB, CB was found to be more efficacious than tricyclics. However, in two more recently completed studies, no differences were found between the two. Two of the studies examined relapse rates in patients who had recovered during treatment, and both reported superior results for the CB-treated patients.

TREATMENT OF DEPRESSION COLLABORATIVE RESEARCH PROGRAM The NIMH initiated this program to address the major methodological shortcomings that had plagued the field: (1) lack of explicit diagnostic criteria and operationalized, reliable diagnostic assessment procedures; (2) lack of clearly defined and operationalized treatment procedures; (3) lack of adequate control groups; (4) lack of training and monitoring of therapists; (5) lack of independent and objective outcome assessments; and (6) lack of neutral investigation sites.

This multisite collaborative study investigated the effectiveness of IPT and CB therapy in a sample of 250 outpatients with major depression. The two psychotherapies were compared with a standard antidepressant drug (imipramine [Tofranil]), and a pill-placebo plus clinical management condition, which was included in the study as a control for the drug. There were no statistically significant differences in the reduction of depressive symptoms in the four treatment conditions among patients completing at least 3½ weeks of treatment. However, nearly half of the patients receiving one of the active treatments recovered fully in contrast to only one-quarter of the pill-placebo group. Imipramine had its effect more rapidly than the other treatments.

When patients were categorized on the basis of initial impairment, important differences emerged. In the more severely impaired patients completing at least 3 ½ weeks of treatment, only 10 percent of the pill-placebo group recovered, whereas 75 percent of the imipramine group recovered. The recovery rates for the two psychotherapy groups were in between: about 45 percent for IPT and 35 percent for CB therapy. The differences in recovery rates among the less impaired patients were small, ranging from 30 percent for the imipramine group to nearly 50 percent for the IPT group.

OTHER STUDIES A number of studies investigating either specific behavioral strategies in isolation (e.g., pleasant activities) or various combinations of interventions associated with a particular behavioral approach (e.g., self-control) have demonstrated the efficacy of behavioral strategies and approaches. These studies varied in type of comparison groups, use of control groups, and size and type of the sampling. Nine studies compared behavior therapy (social learning and self-control approaches) with another active treatment (psychosocial, drug, or combined psychosocial and drug) and with a nonactive control or no-treatment condition, or both. Six studies found the behavior treatment to be superior to either another psychosocial treatment or to a control condition; one of these studies also found the behavior therapy to be superior to an antidepressant. Four of the studies found the behavior therapy to be equal to another psychosocial treatment, and one reported no differences between the behavioral approach combined with a placebo or with a drug, and between either of these conditions and a drug alone.

At this time, no studies similar to those described above have been undertaken for the short-term dynamic therapies. This is unfortunate because these approaches are probably the most commonly used to treat outpatient depression in the United States. Several studies of dynamic therapies for depression have been reported, but only one of them describes any training procedures. In this report, which compares behavior, cognitive, and dynamic therapies for depression in the elderly, no differences were found among the treatments, and all were more effective than a delayed treatment control group.

In general, maintenance trials have revealed that antidepressants are most useful in the prevention of symptomatic relapse. The psychotherapies, however, have been shown to have a greater impact on social and interpersonal functioning.

PROGRESS IN TREATING DEPRESSION

Knowledge about psychotherapeutic approaches to depression has continued to expand, and there now are several approaches from which to choose. Each has a conceptual basis, a comprehensive operationalized manual for therapists, a training program so that the therapy can be exported, and, most important, evidence for its efficacy.

Considerably more research must be done to establish fully the efficacy of each approach, but the exciting next steps will be identifying the patient qualities most responsive to each specific approach. This, in turn, will allow matching the treatment approach to a patient's particular problems.

REFERENCES

Beck A T, Rush A J, Shaw B F, Emery G: *Cognitive Therapy of Depression*. Guilford, New York, 1979.
Bellack A S, Hersen M, Himmelhoch J S: Social skills training for depression: A treatment manual. Cat Sel Doc Psychol *10:* 2156, 1980.
Davanloo H: *Short-Term Dynamic Psychotherapy,* vol 1. Jason Aronson, New York, 1980.
Elkin I, Parloff M B, Hadley S W, et al: NIMH treatment of depression collaborative research program: Background and research plan. Arch Gen Psychiat *42:* 305, 1985.
Ferster C B: A functional analysis of depression. Amer Psychol *10:* 857, 1973.
Gaylin W, editor: *The Meaning of Despair*. Jason Aronson, New York, 1968.
Kazdin A E: Comparative outcome studies of psychotherapy: Methodological issues and strategies. J Consult Clin Psychol *54:* 95, 1986.
Klerman G L: Drugs and psychotherapy. In *Handbook of Psychotherapy and Behavior Change: An Empirical Analysis,* O Garfield, A Bergin, editors. Wiley, New York, 1986.
Klerman G L, Weissman M W, Rounsaville B J, Chevron E S: *Interpersonal Psychotherapy of Depression*. Basic Books, New York, 1984.
Lewinsohn P M, Antonuccio D O, Steinmetz J L, Teri L: *The Coping with Depression Course: A Psychoeducational Intervention for Unipolar Depression*. Castalia, Eugene, OR, 1984.
Lewinsohn P M, Sullivan J M, Grosscup S J: Changing reinforcing events: An approach to the treatment of depression. Psychother: Theor, Res Prac *17,* Fall 1980.
Luborsky L: *Principles of Psychoanalytic Psychotherapy—A Manual for Supportive-Expressive Treatment*. Basic Books, New York, 1984.
Malan D H: *Individual Psychotherapy and the Science of Psychodynamics*. Butterworth, London, 1979.
Rehm L P: Self-management therapy for depression. Adv Behav Res Ther *6:* 83, 1984.
Rush A J, editor: *Short-Term Psychotherapies for Depression*. Guilford, New York, 1982.
Rush A J, Beck A T, Kovacs M, et al: Comparative efficacy of cognitive therapy and pharmacotherapy in the treatment of depressed outpatients. Cogn Ther Res *1:* 17, 1977.
Shea M T, Elkin I, Hirschfeld, R M A: Psychotherapeutic treatment of depression. In *Review of Psychiatry,* Frances, Hales, editors. American Psychiatric Press, Washington, DC, 1988.
Sifneos P E: *Short-Term Dynamic Psychotherapy Evaluation and Technique*. Plenum, New York, 1979.
Simons A D, Murphy G E, Levine F L, et al: Cognitive therapy and pharmacotherapy for depression: Sustained improvement over one year. Arch Gen Psychiat *43:* 43, 1986.
Strupp H, Binder J L: *Psychotherapy in a New Key: A Guide to Time-Limited Dynamic Psychotherapy*. Basic Books, New York, 1984.
Weissman M W, Jarrett R B, Rush A J: Psychotherapy and its relevance to the pharmacotherapy of major depression: A decade later (1976–1985). In *Psychopharmacology: The Third Generation of Progress,* H Meltzer et al, editors, p 1059. Raven Press, New York, 1987.

17.6 GROUP PSYCHOTHERAPY OF DEPRESSION

JOHN P. DOCHERTY, M.D.

INTRODUCTION

The last decade has seen a major advance in psychotherapy research. Using methods successful in clinical research psychiatry, remarkable progress has been made in developing methods for standardizing the psychotherapy treatment variables.

These methods address three questions, the first being "What is the therapy?" This question has been answered in manuals that describe the therapy's rationale, its strategies and techniques, and examples of their application. The manual serves not only a prescriptive purpose (i.e., to describe the therapy), but also a proscriptive purpose (i.e., to limit the content of the therapy).

The second question is "Are the therapists in the study competent to conduct the therapy?" The techniques devised to answer this question represent a major breakthrough for psychotherapy research. Such techniques include the systematic training and supervision of therapists in the study therapy; the assessment, through written examination and review of videotapes, of the therapists' competence prior to beginning therapy; and the development of reliable rating scales to assess a therapists' expertise in different parts of the therapy.

The third question is "Do the therapists adhere to the specific therapy throughout the study?" Monitoring techniques allow for the continuous assessment of the therapists' adherence to the protocol of the specific therapies as well as for the assessment of their competence in using that therapy.

Studies of the treatment of depression have been the focal point for the development of these procedures for psychotherapy research. The most notable example of this is the National Institute of Mental Health (NIMH)–sponsored Treatment of Depression Collaborative Research Program. Over the last 10 years, there have been approximately 25 controlled clinical trials of the psychotherapy of depression. This represents an advance of more than fivefold over the preceding decade. Most of the work, however, has been in individual psychotherapy, with far less in group psychotherapy for depression.

INPATIENT GROUP PSYCHOTHERAPY FOR DEPRESSION

INPATIENTS There has been little work done on the psychosocial treatment of depressed inpatients. Research in this area has been limited for several reasons. First, the inpatient setting contains many confounding variables because of the presence of several therapeutic interventions. Second, the usual short length of a hospital stay in the contemporary climate of undue fiscal constraints limits the feasibility of a psychotherapy study. However, clinicians do treat depressed inpatients with both group psychotherapy and individual therapy, and clinical observations suggest that they both have been helpful. To the author's knowledge, there is only one controlled trial under way to test the efficacy of a psychotherapy intervention with depressed inpatients. There is also only one article addressing the group psychotherapy of depressed inpatients, and it describes a psychodynamic supportive-expressive treatment of depression during hospitalization.

RATIONALE The psychodynamic supportive-expressive treatment is based on the concept of depression as an interpersonal experience of a sense of isolation and withdrawal from people important to the patient.

GOALS This treatment has two primary and two secondary goals. The primary goals are (1) creating a cohesive group and (2) combating demoralization. The secondary goals are. (1) improving reality testing and (2) supporting and establishing therapeutic norms in the hospital.

STRUCTURE Participation in the groups is mandatory for all patients except those who are severely brain damaged and retarded. The group has between eight and 12 members and meets for 45 minutes, three times each week.

STRATEGIES AND TECHNIQUES The major strategies for this treatment are linked to the goals. The first strategy is to establish clear group boundaries. This strategy is supported by the following techniques.

1. *The establishment of confidentiality.* Members may discuss what occurs in the group sessions with one another or the staff but no one else.
2. *Containment.* Members must attend the sessions even if they are too agitated to participate in them.
3. *The establishment of appropriate rituals.* Rituals should be established for welcoming new members and saying goodbye to departing members.
4. *Rules for participation.* All new members should be helped to understand at the start of their participation what is required and expected, including the importance of confidentiality, requirements for participation in the group, and the understanding of relevant subject matter for group discussion.
5. *Group responsibility.* The therapist should help the group clarify and implement the boundary tasks.

The second strategy for this treatment is bridging arbitration, which has two techniques: (1) The group leader should identify common themes and encourage participation, and (2) the group leader should prevent the members from verbally abusing one another ("Encourage people to disagree without being disagreeable").

The third strategy is inclusion, which has three techniques: (1) Each member should be invited to speak at least once in each session; (2) psychotic or autistic utterances should be translated into meaningful communication; and (3) patients should be responsible for making sense of the other members' communications or should indicate that they do not understand them.

The fourth strategy is the focusing of interventions, which has two techniques: (1) Here-and-now efforts are used to cope with problems inside and outside the hospital, and (2) the group therapist should encourage the members to interact with one another.

The fifth strategy supports the second goal, combating demoralization, and has two techniques: (1) The establishment of reasonable goals that can be achieved during this treatment, and (2) the encouragement by the therapist of the group members' participation.

EVALUATION There has been no systematic study of the efficacy of this treatment approach (Table 17.6-1).

OUTPATIENT GROUP PSYCHOTHERAPY FOR DEPRESSION

BEHAVIORAL THERAPIES **Self-control therapy** Self-control therapy is based on Kanfer's learning theory model of self-control.

RATIONALE The symptoms of depression are seen as the patient's failure to use self-control to bridge the loss or delay of external reinforcement. Specific deficits may be present in any or all of the three major elements of self-control: self-monitoring, self-evaluation, and self-reinforcement. This therapy also is based on the observation that depressed people have the following deficits: In self-monitoring, they attend selectively to immediate and external events and not to the delayed and internal consequences of their behavior. They also concentrate on negative events. In self-evaluation, depressed people tend to have unrealistic and perfectionistic goals and a global appraisal of the achievement of their goals. Finally, in self-reinforcement, they have low rates of self-reward and high rates of self-punishment.

TABLE 17.6-1
Inpatient Group Psychotherapy of Depression

Name	Group Size	Duration	Frequency	Role of Therapy	Major Goals	Major Strategies and Techniques
Inpatient Psychodynamic Therapy	8 to 12	Variable	3 times a week, 45-min. session	1. Facilitates expression 2. Identifies shared themes	1. Create a cohesive group 2. Combat demoralization	1. Mandatory participation 2. Establishment of clear group boundaries 3. Open communication 4. Productive communication of all members 5. "Active coping"

STRUCTURE Self-control therapy consists of six sessions with groups of usually eight to 10 patients. The sessions are divided into three phases corresponding to the three elements of self-control noted above. The first session of each phase is for instructions and the assignment of homework. In the second session, the group reviews and discusses the previous week's assignment.

GOALS The goal of the therapy is to modify specific self-control deficits by means of explicit training procedures.

STRATEGIES AND TECHNIQUES The three major strategies are (1) an explanation and discussion of the principles of self-control learning, (2) homework assignments, and (3) encouragement.

The homework assignments include the following:

1. Log forms. These are logs on which the patients are required to note each day's positive activities and to rate on an 11-point scale the mood associated with these activities.
2. Graphs. The patients are also asked to keep a graph of each day's predominant mood and the total number of positive activities recorded that day.
3. Goal setting. Each patient is asked to decide on a set of goals to increase the number of positive activities. The patient must define these goals and also formulate subgoals for each, which are numbered according to their importance.
4. Reward menus. Each patient is asked to list feasible and available rewards that they will be able to award to themselves for attaining their goals and subgoals.

EVALUATION Self-control therapy is one of those therapies of depression that has been subjected to controlled clinical trials. Four trials comparing patients receiving self-control therapy with a waiting list comparison group all demonstrated the effectiveness of self-control therapy. Two studies compared self-control therapy with cognitive therapy. One found self-control superior, and the other found cognitive therapy better. Another study compared self-control therapy with social skills training and found self-control therapy superior. And two studies compared self-control therapy with a dynamic psychotherapy. One found self-control therapy superior, and the other found no difference. But the one follow-up study at 6 months did not show that these gains had lasted, although the severity of the depression had lessened. Predictors of success in self-control therapy include initial coping skills, an expectation of success, late onset of illness, and less severe overall psychological morbidity.

The current evidence supports the efficacy of self-control therapy and suggests that this treatment is more helpful for those individuals who do not have serious cognitive or motor impairment, who have a need for control, and whose life is characterized by inattention and neglect of self-care and self-reward.

Depression management training Depression management training is a multimodality combination treatment that relies heavily on the work of Peter Lewinsohn and Aaron Beck.

RATIONALE This treatment is based on the belief that depression is a result of difficulty coping with or adapting to aversive events, rather than to any direct effect of the events themselves.

STRUCTURE The group, of seven to 10 patients, meets weekly for six sessions.

GOALS Depression management training has three major goals: (1) to enable individuals to understand the origins and symptoms of their depression, (2) to help group members understand the connection between coping and depression, and (3) to help participants learn and strengthen their coping skills so as to manage their depression.

STRATEGIES AND TECHNIQUES This treatment uses five strategies: (1) identifying individual stressors leading to depression, (2) identifying dysfunctional cognitions as defined by Beck, (3) increasing the individual's ability to provide self-reinforcement, (4) increasing the individual's ability to identify a wide range of affective states, and (5) increasing the individual's awareness of the interpersonal ramifications of depressive symptomatology.

The techniques used in this treatment are those developed in cognitive-behavioral, social learning, and rational-emotive therapies and are classified as instruction, experience, and homework assignments.

EVALUATION This treatment has not had a controlled clinical trial. Uncontrolled pre- and postevaluation assessments indicate, however, that both immediately following treatment and at 6-month follow-up, a treated group showed a significant reduction in the level of their depressive symptomatology.

Psychoeducational treatment RATIONALE Psychoeducational treatment is based on social learning theory and is the clinical application of that theory to the treatment of depression. The current form of this treatment combines social learning theory and cognitive theory principles to treat depression and was developed by Lewinsohn and his colleagues over the last 10 years. It assumes that depression is a process in which the depressed person has learned maladaptive reaction patterns that can be unlearned. The depression is seen as dependent on three variables:

1. The availability of reinforcers (positive responses following the person's active behavior) is low, or the availability of punishers (negative events following the individual's behavior) is high.

2. The individual cannot create positive events in his or her life or cope with negative events.

3. The individual responds less to positive events or more to negative events.

The intention of the treatment is to develop a comprehensive instructional program to change the person's behavior so as to generate more positive events and fewer negative events and to encourage constructive thinking and discourage self-defeating thinking.

STRUCTURE This treatment uses a radical educational format. The provider of care is defined clearly as the instructor. Clinical responsibility is sharply limited compared with that in the usual individual therapy. The instructor's role is to ensure that all of the classroom work in the "course for learning how to cope with depression" is explained to the participants.

This treatment is structured as a 12-session treatment conducted over 8 weeks. The first two sessions provide an introduction and overview to the course and help the participants draw up their own "change plans." The next two sessions are devoted to the patients' learning and implementing relaxation procedures; the fifth and sixth sessions, to their learning ways to create more pleasant events; and the seventh and eighth sessions, to their changing their thinking in a more positive direction. The ninth and tenth sessions help the participants improve their social skills, and the final two sessions teach them to maintain the learning and gains made during the course.

GOALS This program is based on social learning theory. Its purpose is to enhance the quality and quantity of the person–environment interaction, by increasing the number and effect of the participants' positive experiences and decreasing the number and effect of unpleasant experiences.

STRATEGIES The two major strategies are assessing the specific functional deficits in obtaining pleasure or protecting oneself from harmful events and systematically teaching how to alter the specific deficits. The major teaching teachniques used to accomplish the goals of the treatment are lecturing; assigning homework; discussing lecture and homework material in the course; and participating during class instruction, tasks, and exercises.

Techniques used for assessment include monitoring activities and assessing related moods, and maintaining schedules of pleasant events and unpleasant events. The frequency of unpleasant events is decreased by means of the following techniques: environmental interventions (e.g., terminating a bad relationship, changing jobs); social skills training; cognitive skill training; stress management; and time management.

EVALUATION One uncontrolled study showed a significant decrease from pretreatment to postreatment using an early form of this treatment intervention. Another controlled clinical trial demonstrated that psychoeducational treatment was better than that given to a waiting list comparison group. Two other studies suggested that psychoeducational treatment in a group is equivalent to individual cognitive and individual psychodynamic treatment as well as individual behavioral treatment. Those variables that suggest the likelihood of a positive response to this form of treatment are (1) the expectation that the treatment will help, (2) general satisfaction with life, (3) no concurrent treatment, (4) perceived social support from family members, (5) no physical handicap or disabling disease, (6) no history of suicidal attempts, and (7) a perception of control over what happens in the patient's life.

The author believes that psychoeducational treatment is an important and interesting development in the group treatment of depression. It is a radical approach in that it limits the therapist's responsibility to that of a teacher-student rather than a physician-patient. Although this therapy does seem to be useful, for more seriously ill patients, it would be better used as an adjunctive treatment. In its current form, it is probably most useful for the group for whom it was originally developed: adolescents who have a relatively stable social network of concerned parents and teachers and whose depression does not require or seem likely to require emergency intervention.

GROUP COGNITIVE THERAPY OF DEPRESSION

INTRODUCTION Group cognitive therapy has received the most study of any of the therapies developed for the group treatment of depression. Ten studies have addressed the effectiveness of group cognitive therapy for depression, although in each study, the therapy was carried out differently. For example, the durations of the time-limited studies ranged from 4 weeks to 36 weeks, and the procedures and conceptual framework for conducting group cognitive therapy have not been definitively established. There is currently no standard, although Lino Covi's work discusses the specific procedures for conducting cognitive therapy in a group. Thus, the following description of group cognitive therapy will rely most on Covi's work.

RATIONALE Group cognitive therapy assumes that modifications in the individual's negative thinking, maladaptive assumptions, and logical errors will relieve the depression and prevent its recurrence. Group cognitive therapy also assumes that the group will (1) establish norms of behavior that will increase adherence to the therapy's requirements; (2) through the development of group cohesion, discourage dropping out of the therapy; (3) provide positive social reinforcements; and (4) provide a source of peer support to facilitate acceptance and understanding of individual cognitive dysfunctions.

GOALS The goals of group cognitive therapy are the same as those of individual cognitive therapy. The long-term goals are to relieve the depression and to acquire the cognitive skills to prevent its recurrence.

STRUCTURE The structure of group cognitive therapy, as noted, varies but generally has the following structure:

1. Two individual sessions to introduce the cognitive therapy and to describe the group treatment.

2. Fifteen to 20 sessions for a closed group or no limit for an open-ended group.

3. Ninety-minute sessions.

4. Weekly meetings.

5. The therapist in both closed and open-ended group cognitive therapy assumes a very active role in maintaining the group's task focus, setting the agenda for the group,

facilitating the group's interaction, and ensuring the participation of and adequate attention to all members.

6. Closed groups are divided into three phases. In phase 1, the group members learn the cognitive therapy concepts and are introduced to the use of the forms and schedules used in behavioral and cognitive exercises. Phase 2 focuses on how the therapeutic tools learned in phase 1 are used to resolve the patient's depressogenic constellation. Phase 3 is the termination phase. It concentrates on tying up the interpersonal relationships that have developed in the group, summarizing each member's progress, and reviewing plans for maintaining these gains.

Structure of an open-ended group session

1. *Go around (15 minutes):* Each member is asked to present a status report on his or her depression during the preceding week and his or her specific agenda for that session.
2. *Review of significant experiences in the past week.* Examples are those events that trigger depression, problems with homework, and success with using the cognitive procedures. Homework assignments include such tasks as scheduling activities in a way selected to reverse or challenge maladaptive assumptions, and rating the mastery and pleasure experienced in these activities.
3. *Examination of "chunked" agenda items:* This part constitutes the body of the therapy session. The therapist discusses some of the common agenda items, especially those that address most of the group's needs and seem to be the most instructive.
4. *Assessment:* During this phase of the session, each group member establishes new short-term goals for the upcoming week and new homework assignments based on those goals.
5. *Personal relevance:* The session ends with a review of its personal relevance to each member, indicating what has been learned, the new short-term goals that have been established, and the ways to achieve them.

STRATEGIES AND TECHNIQUES To prepare for the group treatment, the therapist first deals with any negative thoughts that the members may have about the group treatment. The therapist asks the group members to share their initial negative thoughts on entering the group. Such common assumptions include the fear that the individual will always remain an outsider or that no one else will understand his or her problems. This technique also involves eliciting and correcting specific depressogenic assumptions an individual may have regarding his or her performance in the group setting (e.g., that the individual will appear stupid, be feared, or be otherwise socially incompetent).

The therapist should anticipate negative responses by other members to an individual joining the group and also should prepare the group for new members. Particularly applicable to open-ended groups, this preparation involves asking the group to examine the negative cognitions the group may have about a new member. For example, "He will interfere with our relationships" or "We have a good group functioning now. This person will mess things up." Specific ways of welcoming and incorporating the new member into the group should be devised. During the first session, old members are asked to describe the therapy that they have had and the progress that they have made. The new member is asked to express his or her thoughts or feelings about joining the group, and the old members examine these thoughts and feelings and share their own past experiences.

The therapist should use group feedback to correct cognitive distortions. The group provides an opportunity for multiple perspectives regarding a particular depressogenic cognition. Using the five-column procedure of cognitive behavior therapy (situation, cognition, affect, alternative thought, new affect), the group can identify a negative cognition and then help the individual generate alternative thoughts. For example, an individual applied for a job and then called to make an appointment for an interview and was told that the firm would contact him to schedule the interview. He became depressed, as he saw this as an indication that the firm was not interested in him. The alternative thoughts that the group generated were that (1) the firm was not yet ready to set up an interview schedule; (2) all the applications had to be considered in order for the firm to determine whom it wanted to interview; and (3) if a negative decision had been made, he probably would have been told in order to save the firm time.

Veteran members of the group should describe the progress they have made. Patients often come into the group with feelings of hopelessness about the possibility of change through therapy. Thus, those individuals in the group who have experienced such change can help relieve this demoralization and pessimism.

The group should offer social reinforcement to help increase the number of activities of individual participants.

All of the group's members are asked each week to reassess the short-term goals they have established in order to meet their long-term goal of alleviating their depression. The group then discusses these short-term goals. Examples of such short-term goals in treatment are to understand the use of the forms in cognitive therapy or to increase participation in the group and in activities outside the group. Later in treatment, goals may be to establish the number of times in a week that the individual rejects a specific depressogenic assumption and to tell the new members of the group about what he or she has gained from cognitive therapy.

The group may be used, because of its many listeners, to identify hidden agendas—that is, those negative thoughts of which an individual is aware but which he or she is reluctant to express and to modify through cognitive techniques. This strategy takes advantage of the self-disclosure that can occur in a close-knit group.

EVALUATION Controlled clinical trials have demonstrated the efficacy of group cognitive therapy in reducing depressive symptomatology. At least five studies have shown group cognitive therapy to be superior to a waiting list control condition. Two studies found cognitive group therapy and supportive-expressive group therapy to be equally helpful. There have been three studies of individual cognitive therapy versus group cognitive therapy. Two found the individual format superior to the group format. One found the outcome of both forms of treatment to be the same. Finally, the issue of combining medication and group cognitive therapy yielded equivocal results. One study found cognitive group therapy plus medication equivalent to cognitive group therapy alone. Another found cognitive group therapy alone superior to medication alone, and still another found medication alone superior to group cognitive therapy alone. Although many questions about the specific indications for, and the relative efficacy of, group cognitive therapy remain unanswered, the current literature supports the use of group cognitive therapy for depression.

The author believes that group cognitive therapy is a useful treatment for the depressed patient. The contradictory results regarding the interaction with medication are not surprising and are likely due to the differences in the group's composition: Some patients will fare better with group cognitive therapy alone, some with medication alone, and some with the combination. The rules for selecting patients for the various therapies are not clear, however. Patients with cognitive impairment and clear endogenicity may do better with drugs alone; those with no cognitive impairment, no endogenicity, and high resourcefulness may do better with group cognitive therapy alone; and those with some endogenicity, mild cognitive impairment, and moderate resourcefulness may do better with the combination.

PSYCHODYNAMIC SUPPORTIVE-EXPRESSIVE THERAPY OF DEPRESSION

INTRODUCTION The fourth major approach to the group treatment of depressed patients is psychodynamic supportive-expressive therapy. Although this has been the main form of therapy used for treating heterogeneous patient groups, it has received far less attention for its use with diagnostically homogeneous groups of depressed patients. Four studies observed the application of this approach to treat depressed patients. But because there has been so little work in this area, it is not surprising that no specific psychodynamic supportive-expressive therapy has achieved paradigmatic status. It is possible, however, to extract some central principles of the rationale, strategies, and techniques of this therapy.

RATIONALE This therapy views depression as resulting from some significant disturbance in the perception and regulation of interpersonal relationships. This disturbance is often perceived as the patient's dependence on a "dominant other," without whom the patient feels lost and unable to function but by whom the patient feels used and controlled. Psychodynamic supportive-expressive therapy attempts to give the patients a setting of security and trust within which they can understand how their earlier relationships helped create this self-defeating perception of the interpersonal world and to teach the patients how to escape this depressive interpersonal predicament.

STRUCTURE This therapy is conducted in either an open-ended or a time-limited structure. Time-limited groups generally meet from 15 to 16 times, usually weekly, for 1 to 2 hours. Some individual sessions are usually prescribed to establish a diagnosis and clarify for the patient the rules of participation in the treatment. The therapy usually consists of three phases. In the initial phase, the group achieves cohesion through the disclosure of each patient's own relationship difficulties. In the middle phase, the group tries to discover the source of the members' current relationship difficulties in past important relationships, the impact of the members' depressive behavior on others, and alternative ways of relating to important others. In the final phase, the patients prepare for the termination and the dissolution of the group. The group summarizes the members' gains during their participation in the group, and it clarifies ways in which the members can continue to grow and use this understanding to reduce or prevent future depressive states.

GOALS There are two major goals for this treatment.

Support An important part of this therapy is to create an atmosphere in which the patients can feel trust and confidence, can expect help, and can know that they are not alone in their suffering.

Expression This therapy enables the group's members to express themselves freely so as to understand their self-destructive relationships and how they arise from earlier relationships. It is expected that this understanding will lead to the development of more adaptive ways of responding.

STRATEGIES AND TECHNIQUES This therapy uses three strategies. The first is to develop group cohesion, by concentrating on maintaining the therapeutic task and discouraging any resistance to that task, encouraging the identification the group members have with one another, and conveying an attitude of hopefulness.

The second strategy is to point out self-defeating interpersonal behavior. This strategy is accomplished using the traditional methods of psychodynamic treatment, such as interpretive feedback of transference manifestations and the development of insight. These techniques focus on understanding the patients' intentions and wishes toward others, and the expected consequences for themselves and others of those intentions and wishes.

Finally, the third strategy is to improve personal adaptation by the patients expressing their resentment of and hostility toward the therapist; thinking of alternative ways of dealing with particular interpersonal situations based on the experiences of other group members; and supporting and encouraging patients' efforts at positive change.

EVALUATION The data regarding the efficacy of psychodynamic supportive-expressive group therapy for depression are very limited and also mixed. One study using a before-and-after design demonstrated the superiority of group treatment to individual therapy for chronically depressed women. Another study for anxious depressives showed no advantage for a psychodynamic group therapy used in conjunction with medication over minimal supportive therapy used in conjunction with medication. Two studies compared supportive-expressive therapy with group cognitive therapy and found significant improvement with both interventions. All in all, psychodynamic supportive-expressive group therapy appears to be a useful form of treatment. Although it derives from a widely used therapeutic approach, it is the least formally developed of the group therapies for treating depression (Table 17.6-2).

DISCUSSION

The studies that have been conducted to date are a creditable beginning. Three different approaches to the group therapy of depression have been developed, and the data support their efficacy. Thus, in many ways, the most important step has been taken: The base has been laid for increasingly refined studies of the process and efficacy of each of these treatments.

Comparative research may shed light on the question of which type of therapy should be used for which particular

TABLE 17.6-2
Major Therapeutic Approaches to Outpatient Group Therapy of Depression

Behavioral Therapies

Name	*Group Size*	*Duration*	*Frequency*	*Role of Therapist*	*Major Goals*	*Major Strategies and Techniques*
I. Self-control therapy	8 to 10	6 sessions	1. Monitoring 2. Self-evaluation 3. Self-reinforcement	1. Educator 2. Facilitator	1. Modification of self-control deficits through use of explicit training procedures	1. Presentation/discussion 2. Homework assignments (log forms, graphs, goal setting, reward menus) 3. Encouragement
II. Depression management training	7 to 10	6 sessions	Weekly	1. Enabler 2. Facilitator	1. Understand origins and symptoms of depression 2. Understand connection between coping and depression 3. Learn and strengthen coping skills	1. Identify stressors 2. Identify dysfunctional cognitions 3. Increase self-reinforcement 4. Increase ability to identify affective states 5. Understand interpersonal ramifications of depressive symptomatology
III. Psychoeducational treatment	7 to 10	8 weeks	12 sessions	1. Educator 2. Facilitator	1. Increase number and potency of positive experiences and decrease and diminish unpleasant experiences	1. Assess specific deficits 2. Teach ways to alter deficits: a. environmental interventions b. social skills training c. cognitive skills training d. stress management e. time management

Group Cognitive Therapy

Name	*Group Size*	*Duration*	*Frequency*	*Role of Therapist*	*Major Goals*	*Major Strategies and Techniques*
Group cognitive therapy		Closed group: 15 to 20 sessions Open-ended group: no limit 90-min. session	Weekly	1. Maintains group task focus 2. Sets agenda 3. Facilitates discussion 4. Ensures participation of all members	1. Remediation of depression 2. Acquisition of cognitive skills to prevent recurrence of depression	1. Deal with individuals' negative thoughts about group treatment. 2. Anticipate other members' negative responses to the individual joining group 3. Give group feedback to correct cognitive distortions 4. Review progress by veteran members 5. Offer positive reinforcement 6. Reassess short-term goals 7. Identify hidden agendas

Psychodynamic Supportive-Expressive Therapy

Name	*Group Size*	*Duration*	*Frequency*	*Role of Therapist*	*Major Goals*	*Major Strategies and Techniques*
Psychodynamic supportive-expressive therapy		Time-limited groups: 15 to 16 1- to 2-hr sessions Open-ended	Weekly	1. Gives feedback of transference 2. Facilitates discussion 3. Gives support and encouragement	1. Support 2. Expression	1. Develop group cohesion 2. Clarify self-defeating patterns of interpersonal behavior 3. Understand patients' intentions and wishes for others 4. Enhance personal adaption

patient. Preliminary results from the Treatment of Depression Collaborative Research Program suggest that patients with a cognitive impairment fare poorly in cognitive therapy, whereas patients with few social skills and networks do poorly in interpersonal therapy. Other work supports the finding that patients with good coping skills do well in cognitive therapy and that those deficient in this regard do poorly. Overall, these findings mean that specific competencies may be assessed to determine the best form of therapy and, thus, to assign therapies with a greater likelihood of achieving good results. Future research in the group psychotherapy of depression must address this issue.

There are also the clinically important but longer-range issues of the value of combining group therapy approaches

TABLE 17.6-3
Group Cognitive Therapy: Closed and Open-Ended Formats

	Number of Sessions	*Content of Sessions*
Closed group	15 to 20, 90-min. sessions held weekly	Phase 1: 1. Learn cognitive therapy concepts. 2. Introduce use of forms and schedules to facilitate behavioral and cognitive exercises.
		Phase 2: 1. Use therapeutic tools. 2. Apply tools to resolve patient's depressogenic constellation.
		Phase 3: 1. Resolve interpersonal relationships in the group. 2. Summarize individual's progress. 3. Review plans for maintaining gains made.
Open-ended group	No definite limit, 90-min. sessions held weekly	1. Go around: Individual presents status report of past week's depression and decides on specific agenda for the session.
		2. Review significant experiences in past week.
		3. Examine "chunked" agenda items: Therapist identifies common agenda items and chooses one or several items that address most of the group's needs.
		4. Assessment: Therapist establishes new short-term goals for upcoming week and assigns homework.
		5. Personal relevance: Therapist reviews personal relevance of the session to the individual.

and of combining in the most effective ways pharmacological treatment with group psychotherapy.

Further, for each of these therapeutic approaches, there are questions as to which techniques and structure will enhance its efficacy. One question relevant to all of these therapies is the relative value of open-ended versus time-limited groups and of open versus closed membership groups (i.e., those groups that accept new members versus those that do not). Some clinical information suggests that these varying structures may have different effects on different patient populations (e.g., disturbed suicidal adolescents seem to do very poorly in time-limited groups) (Table 17.6-3).

Finally, those questions that may not receive the research attention they deserve are whether patients are better treated in diagnostically homogeneous or heterogeneous groups, and which diagnoses may do better in heterogeneous or homogeneous groups.

REFERENCES

Betcher R W: The treatment of depression in brief inpatient group psychotherapy. Int J Group Psychother *33:* 365, 1983.

Beutler L E, Scogin F, Kirkish P, Schretlen D, et al: Group cognitive therapy and alprazolam in the treatment of depression in older adults. J Consult and Clin Psychol *55:* 4, 1987.

Covi L, Lipman R S, Alarcon R D, et al: Drugs and psychotherapy interactions in depression. Amer J Psychiat *133:* 502, 1976.

Covi L, Lipman R S, Derogatis L R, Smith J E, et al: Drugs and group psychotherapy in neurotic depression. Amer J Psychiat *131:* 191, 1974.

Covi L, Roth D, Lipman R: Cognitive group psychotherapy of depression: The close-ended group. Amer J Psychother *36:* 456, 1982.

Fuchs C Z, Rehm L P: A self-control behavior therapy program for depression. J Consult Clin Psychol *45:* 206, 1977.

Green M, Wisner W: Evaluation of a multi-model structured group approach in treatment of depression. Psychol Rep *56:* 984, 1985.

Hollon S D, Shaw B F: Group cognitive therapy for depressed patients. In *Cognitive Therapy of Depression,* A T Beck et al, editors. Guilford, New York, 1979.

Jarvik L F, Mintz J, Stever J, Gerner R: Treating geriatric depression: A 26 week interim analysis. J Amer Geriat Soc *30:* 713, 1982.

Kibel H D: A conceptual model for short-term inpatient group psychotherapy. Amer J Psychiat *138:* 74, 1981.

Lerman C A, Baron A: Depression management training. A structured group approach. Personnel Guid J *60:* 86, 1981.

Lewisohn P M, Antonuccio D O, Steinmetz J L, Teri L: *The Coping with Depression Curse. A Psychoeducational Intervention for Unipolar Depression.* Castalia, Eugene, OR, 1984.

Lewisohn P M, Munoz R, Youngren M, Zeiss A: *Control Your Depression.* Prentice-Hall, Englewood Cliffs, NJ, 1978.

Lipman R S, Covi L: Outpatient treatment of neurotic depression: Medication and group psychotherapy. In *evaluation of psychological therapies,* R L Apitzer, D F Klein, editors. Johns Hopkins University Press, Baltimore, 1976.

Luborsky L: *Principles of Psychoanalytic Psychotherapy: A Manual for Supportive-Expressive Treatment.* Basic Books, New York, 1984.

McLean P D, Hakstian A R: Clinical depression: Comparative efficacy of outpatient treatments. J Counsel Clin Psychol *47:* 818, 1979.

Morris J B: Group psychotherapy for prolonged postnatal depression. Brit J Med Psychol *60:* 279, 1987.

Rehm L P: Self-management therapy for depression. Adv Behav Res Ther *6:* 83, 1984.

Rehm L P, Kaslow N J, Rabin A S: Cognitive and behavioral targets in a self-control therapy program for depression. J Consult Clin Psychol *55:* 4, 1987.

Reynolds W M, Coats K I: A comparison of cognitive-behavioral therapy and relaxation training for the treatment of depression in adolescents. J Consult Clin Psychol *54:* 5, 1986.

Roth D, Covi L: Cognitive group psychotherapy of depression: The open-ended group. Int J Group Psychother *34:* 67, 1984.

Rush A J, Watkins J T: Group versus individual cognitive therapy: A pilot study. Cognitive Ther Res *5:* 95, 1981.

Shapiro J, Sank L I, Shaffer C S, Donovan D C: Cost effectiveness of individual vs. group cognitive behavior therapy for problems of depression and anxiety in HMO population. J Clin Psychol *38:* 674, 1982.

Shaw B F: Comparison of cognitive therapy and behavior therapy in the treatment of depression. J Consult Clin Psychol *45:* 543, 1977.

Steinmetz J L, Lewisohn P M, Antonuccio D O: Prediction of individual outcome in a group intervention for depression. J Consult Clin Psychol *51:* 331, 1983.

Yalom I D: *The Theory and Practice of Group Psychotherapy.* Basic Books, New York, 1970.

CHAPTER 18 ANXIETY DISORDERS (ANXIETY AND PHOBIC NEUROSES)

18.1 PANIC AND GENERALIZED ANXIETY DISORDERS

THOMAS W. UHDE, M.D.
JOHN C. NEMIAH, M.D.

INTRODUCTION

Anxiety neurosis, cardiac neurosis, DaCosta's syndrome, disordered action of the heart, effort syndrome, irritable heart, nervous exhaustion, nervous tachycardia, neurocirculatory asthenia, soldier's heart, vasomotor neurosis, vasoregulatory asthenia—under a whole rogue's galley of aliases, anxiety has stalked through the last 100 years. As most of these old terms suggest, the particular system of interest (e.g., cardiac) to the observer resulted in myriad diagnostic terms (e.g., irritable heart, soldier's heart, nervous tachycardia). Although different diagnostic terms have been used throughout the history of neurology and psychiatry, most of these earlier terms, including anxiety neurosis, were probably diagnostic forerunners of panic and generalized anxiety disorders as currently defined by the revised third edition of the *Diagnostic and Statistical Manual of Mental Disorders* (DSM-III-R).

According to DSM-III-R, generalized anxiety disorder (Table 18.1-1) is characterized by persistent anxiety of at least 6 months' duration. Patients with generalized anxiety disorder usually display chronic signs of muscle tension; autonomic disturbance, such as sweating, dizziness, bowel disturbances, urinary frequency, and high pulse rates; apprehensive expectation as reflected by worry, irritability, and rumination; anticipation of catastrophe; and increased startle and vigilance.

Panic disorder is characterized by recurrent panic attacks. Panic attacks are manifested by the sudden onset of intense apprehension, fear, or terror, often associated with feelings of impending doom. As illustrated in Table 18.1-2, panic attacks are routinely associated with somatic symptoms, and at least four of the following symptoms are required to meet formal DSM-III-R criteria for a panic episode: dyspnea or smothering sensations, dizziness or faintness, chest pain or discomfort, hot and cold flashes, palpitations or tachycardia, trembling or shaking, paresthesias, choking, sweating, gastrointestinal distress, depersonalization or derealization, fear of dying, and fear of going crazy or doing something uncontrolled.

The essential feature of agoraphobia (Table 18.1-3) is a pathological fear of being in any situation in which escape or help would not be immediately available in case of sudden incapacitation. Historically, agoraphobia would have been conceptualized as a phobic neurosis. However, recent data suggest that agoraphobia often develops as a secondary complication of panic attacks. Because of these fears, there is a progressive constriction of normal function. The agoraphobic patient with panic attacks has an underlying fear of having an unprovoked panic attack. In these cases, avoidance behaviors are thought to arise as a secondary complication of panic attacks. DSM-III-R legitimizes this concept by creating the new diagnostic category of panic disorder with agoraphobia, rather than agoraphobia with panic attacks, as employed in the third edition of the *Diagnostic and Statistical Manual of Mental Disorders* (DSM-III). Given these theoretical and diagnostic caveats, panic disorder, with or without accompanying agoraphobia (Table 18.1-4) or avoidance behaviors, will be discussed in this section. Agoraphobia without a history of panic disorder, a rarely observed syndrome in psychiatric treatment facilities, will be discussed in the section on phobic disorders.

ANXIETY: A CHANGING CONCEPT

Psychiatrists may agree with a concept of panic and generalized anxiety disorders that puts anxiety in center-stage, but if they were to talk with their colleagues in other fields of medicine, they would often find them using a different language. Cardiologists, with their attention focused on the function of the cardiopulmonary system, still speak of neurocirculatory asthenia or fatigue syndrome in the discussion of those cardiorespiratory symptoms that psychiatrists view as the physiological manifestations of pathological anxiety states. The origins of this mind–brain–body splitting are rooted in the clinical soil of the American Civil War.

"Shortly after the establishment of military hospitals in our large cities," reported Jacob Mendes DaCosta in the *American Journal of the Medical Sciences* of 1871,

> I was appointed visiting physician to one in Philadelphia, and there I noticed cases of a peculiar form of functional disorder of the heart, to which I gave the name of irritable heart—a name by which the disorder soon became known both within and without the walls of the hospital. [Typical was the case of] William Henry H., Private, 68th Pennsylvania Vol., admitted into the Turner's Lane Hospital in Philadelphia, November 2, 1863, having just returned from furlough. He enlisted in August 1862, at the time in good health, though he had suffered occasionally from rheumatism. He did a great deal of hard duty with his regiment. Some time before the Battle of Fredericksburg, he had an attack of diarrhea; after the battle, he was seized with lancinating pains in the cardiac region, so intense that he was obliged to throw himself down upon the ground, and with palpitation. These symptoms frequently returned while on the march, were attended with dimness of vision and giddiness, and obliged him often to fall out from his company and ride in the ambulance. Yet he remained with his regiment until July 4, 1865, when he was wounded at the Battle of Gettysburg. The wound healed in about one month, but the cardiac symptoms became worse, and violent palpitations ensued upon the slightest exertion, sometimes also whilst in bed, obliging him to rise. There was soreness in the cardiac region, and a constant dull pain.

TABLE 18.1-1
Diagnostic Criteria for Generalized Anxiety Disorder

A. Unrealistic or excessive anxiety and worry (apprehensive expectation) about two or more life circumstances (e.g., worry about possible misfortune to one's child who is in no danger and worry about finances for no good reason, for a period of 6 months or longer, during which the person has been bothered more days than not by these concerns. In children and adolescents, this may take the form of anxiety and worry about academic, athletic, and social performance).
B. If another Axis 1 disorder is present, the focus of the anxiety and worry in A is unrelated to it, e.g., the anxiety or worry is not about having a panic attack (as in panic disorder), being embarrassed in public (as in social phobia), being contaminated (as in obsessive-compulsive disorder), or gaining weight (as in anorexia nervosa).
C. The disturbance does not occur only during the course of a mood disorder or a psychotic disorder.
D. At least six of the following 18 symptoms are often present when anxious (do not include symptoms present only during panic attacks):
Motor tension
(1) trembling, twitching, or feeling shaky
(2) muscle tension, aches, or soreness
(3) restlessness
(4) easy fatigability
Autonomic hyperactivity
(5) shortness of breath or smothering sensations
(6) palpitations or accelerated heart rate (tachycardia)
(7) sweating, or cold clammy hands
(8) dry mouth
(9) dizziness or lightheadedness
(10) nausea, diarrhea, or other abdominal distress
(11) flushes (hot flashes) or chills
(12) frequent urination
(13) trouble swallowing or "lump in throat"
Vigilance and scanning
(14) feeling keyed up or on edge
(15) exaggerated startle response
(16) difficulty concentrating or "mind going blank" because of anxiety
(17) trouble falling or staying asleep
(18) irritability
E. It cannot be established that an organic factor initiated and maintained the disturbance (e.g., hyperthyroidism, caffeine intoxication).

Table from DSM-III-R *Diagnostic and Statistical Manual of Mental Disorders,* ed 3, revised. Copyright American Psychiatric Association, Washington, DC, 1987. Used with permission.

TABLE 18.1-2
Diagnostic Criteria for Panic Disorder

A. At some time during the disturbance, one or more panic attacks (discrete periods of intense fear or discomfort) have occurred that were (1) unexpected, i.e., did not occur immediately before or on exposure to a situation that almost always caused anxiety, and (2) not triggered by situations in which the person was the focus of others' attention.
B. Either four attacks, as defined in criterion A, have occurred within a 4-week period, or one or more attacks have been followed by a period of at least a month of persistent fear of having another attack.
C. At least four of the following symptoms developed during at least one of the attacks:
(1) shortness of breath (dyspnea) or smothering sensations
(2) dizziness, unsteady feelings, or faintness
(3) palpitations or accelerated heart rate (tachycardia)
(4) trembling or shaking
(5) sweating
(6) choking
(7) nausea or abdominal distress
(8) depersonalization or derealization
(9) numbness or tingling sensations (paresthesias)
(10) flushes (hot flashes) or chills
(11) chest pain or discomfort
(12) fear of dying
(13) fear of going crazy or of doing something uncontrolled
Note: Attacks involving four or more symptoms are panic attacks; attacks involving fewer than four symptoms are limited symptom attacks (see agoraphobia without history of panic disorder).
D. During at least some of the attacks, at least four of the C symptoms developed suddenly and increased in intensity within 10 minutes of the beginning of the first C symptom noticed in the attack.
E. It cannot be established that an organic factor initiated and maintained the disturbance, e.g., amphetamine or caffeine intoxication, hyperthyroidism.
Note: Mitral valve prolapse may be an associated condition, but does not preclude a diagnosis of panic disorder.

Table from DSM-III-R *Diagnostic and Statistical Manual of Mental Disorders,* ed 3, revised. Copyright American Psychiatric Association, Washington, DC, 1987. Used with permission.

From his examination of a large number of these patients, DaCosta soon recognized that there was often no evidence of a structural lesion of the heart, and he concluded that a disturbance in the functioning of the sympathetic nervous system was the cause of the cardiac symptoms. "It seems to me most likely," he wrote, "that the heart has become irritable, from its overaction and frequent excitement, and that disordered innervation keeps it so." "Irritable heart" (or *DaCosta's syndrome,* as it came to be known) soon became an established clinical entity, and the diagnosis was frequently made by military surgeons among the soldiers fighting the Franco-Prussian War of 1870 and the Boer War of the 1890s.

The element of anxiety was injected into the syndrome with the publication in 1895 of Sigmund Freud's paper "On the Grounds for Detaching a Particular Syndrome from Neurasthenia Under the Description 'Anxiety Neurosis.' " Anxiety as a symptom had been recognized for some decades by neurologists and psychiatrists abroad and in the United States. It had not been deemed worthy, however, of having a diagnosis to itself but, rather, had been lumped together with a congeries of psychoneurotic symptoms, such as exhaustion and depression, under the label of *neurasthenia,* a term popularized in the 1870s by the American George Miller Beard.

Freud's clinical perspicacity led him to recognize a regularly associated group of symptoms that could be distinguished from neurasthenia. "I call this syndrome 'anxiety neurosis,' " he wrote, "because all its components can be grouped round the chief symptom of anxiety." The anxiety, Freud pointed out, might either exist in a chronic state or erupt in discrete attacks.

> An anxiety attack of this sort may consist of the feeling of anxiety, alone, without any associated idea, or accompanied by the interpretation that is nearest to hand . . . The feeling of anxiety may have linked to it a disturbance of one or more of the bodily functions—such as respiration, heart action, vasomotor innervation or glandular activity. From this combination the patient picks out in particular now one, now another, factor. He complains of "spasms of the heart," "difficulty in breathing," "outbreaks of sweating," "ravenous hunger," and such like.

In Freud's hands, DaCosta's syndrome was turned inside out. Anxiety was brought from behind the physical symptoms that for DaCosta and his followers had constituted the whole of the disorder and was then seen to be the central unifying factor that organized and gave collective form to the somatic manifestations. Since Freud's time, anxiety has been recognized by psychiatrists as a psychological entity of paramount importance, and under the various terms of anxiety state, anxiety reaction, and anxiety neurosis, the syndrome in which anxiety is the prime feature has been given a place in the family of emotional disorders.

Internists, however, were slow to adopt this view of things.

TABLE 18.1-3
Diagnostic Criteria for Panic Disorder with Agoraphobia

A. Meets the criteria for panic disorder.
B. Agoraphobia: Fear of being in places or situations from which escape might be difficult (or embarrassing) or in which help might not be available in the event of a panic attack. (Include cases in which persistent avoidance behavior originated during an active phase of panic disorder, even if the person does not attribute the avoidance behavior to fear of having a panic attack.) As a result of this fear, the person either restricts travel or needs a companion when away from home, or else endures agoraphobic situations despite intense anxiety. Common agoraphobic situations include being outside the home alone, being in a crowd or standing in a line, being on a bridge, and traveling in a bus, train, or car.
Specify current severity of agoraphobic avoidance:
Mild: Some avoidance (or endurance with distress), but relatively normal life-style (e.g., travels unaccompanied when necessary, such as to work or to shop; otherwise avoids traveling alone).
Moderate: Avoidance results in constricted life-style (e.g., the person is able to leave the house alone, but not to go more than a few miles unaccompanied).
Severe: Avoidance results in being nearly or completely housebound or unable to leave the house unaccompanied.
In Partial Remission: No current agoraphobic avoidance, but some agoraphobic avoidance during the past 6 months.
In Full Remission: No current agoraphobic avoidance and none during the past 6 months.
Specify current severity of panic attacks:
Mild: During the past month, either all attacks have been limited symptom attacks (i.e., fewer than four symptoms), or there has been no more than one panic attack.
Moderate: During the past month attacks have been intermediate between "mild" and "severe."
Severe: During the past month, there have been at least eight panic attacks.
In Partial Remission: The condition has been intermediate between "in full remission" and "mild."
In Full Remission: During the past 6 months, there have been no panic or limited symptom attacks.

Table from DSM-III-R *Diagnostic and Statistical Manual of Mental Disorders,* ed 3, revised. Copyright American Psychiatric Association, Washington, DC, 1987. Used with permission.

TABLE 18.1-4
Diagnostic Criteria for Panic Disorder Without Agoraphobia

A. Meets the criteria for panic disorder.
B. Absence of agoraphobia, as defined above.
Specify current severity of panic attacks, as defined above.

Table from DSM-III-R *Diagnostic and Statistical Manual of Mental Disorders,* ed 3, revised. Copyright American Psychiatric Association, Washington, DC, 1987. Used with permission.

During World War I, DaCosta's syndrome reappeared under the guise of "disordered action of the heart (DAH)," the official British Army designation for a condition that afflicted some 60,000 British soldiers. Once again, the cardiac manifestations of anxiety were the focus of attention, although clinical investigators were aware that many of the patients gave a past history of neurotic problems that presumably contributed to their disorder. In 1918, Sir Thomas Lewis proposed the alternative name *effort syndrome,* a noncommittal term that reflected the patient's labored response to mild exertion. In his view, the symptoms were the result of a variety of physical factors, prominent among them being overexertion, infectious illness, underlying cardiac disease, and "abnormalities of the central nervous system." Oppenheimer, one of Lewis's American collaborators, preferred the label *neurocirculatory asthenia* (NCA) as more accurately describing the frequent combination of cardiac symptoms and exhaustion.

By World War II, there was a greater recognition of the psychological dimensions of these various functional heart conditions. During this conflict, combatants who complained of symptoms previously considered to have been the result of functional heart disorders were now diagnosed as having anxiety reaction and were accordingly managed by the military psychiatrist rather than the internist.

In the past decade, attention and research have focused on the interrelatedness of mind, brain, and bodily functions, and less credibility has been given to theories that view anxious emotions and fear behaviors as exclusively psychological or biological phenomena. Nonetheless, it is intriguing that contemporary researchers still struggle with many of the old questions regarding the psychobiological nature of pathological anxiety states. As reviewed in this section, modern psychiatric investigators are today as intensely interested in, and perplexed by, the nature of cardiopulmonary function in panic and generalized anxiety disorders as DaCosta and his contemporaries were in understanding the basis of similar syndromes. Investigators in this era, however, are no longer interested in the mind–brain–body split, and a great deal of attention is now paid to the psychosocial and biological bases of such intricately related phenomena as learning, memory, and emotions—especially anxiety. The study of the functional relationships among these phenomena has been made possible by the creation of new and sophisticated technologies. As the understanding of the mechanisms that underlie learning, memory, and emotions improves, new treatments with more specific actions and fewer side effects will emerge. This era should be anticipated with great excitement by all clinicians, as these future findings will ultimately be of great importance and practical usefulness to psychotherapists, behavioral therapists, and psychopharmacologists alike.

EPIDEMIOLOGY AND FAMILIAL PATTERNS

Anxiety as a symptom is a component of almost every psychiatric disorder, and primary anxiety disorders represent one of the most prevalent mental health problems in the United States today. Although modern people pride themselves on the noisy, violent, nerve-shattering pace of twentieth-century life, there is no good evidence that anxiety is on the increase. The oft-cited fact that hysteria predominated as a psychiatric disorder among soldiers in World War I—in contrast to the much greater prevalence of anxiety and psychophysiological disorders in the conflict of the 1940s—is vitiated as support for an increase in anxiety, because, as has been seen, many men who today would be considered as psychoneurotic were diagnosed in the earlier war as having functional heart disorders and thus did not appear in the statistics as suffering from anxiety.

Before 1975, there were no population studies of the rates of anxiety disorders using current diagnostic terminology. More recent surveys have found current and 1-year prevalence rates of 2.5 and 6.4 percent, respectively, for generalized anxiety disorder. The 1982 Epidemiologic Catchment Area (ECA) Study Survey found 6-month prevalence rates of 0.6 to 1.0 percent for panic disorder and 2.7 to 5.8 percent for agoraphobia. Differences in prevalence rates depended on the community sampled.

In general, anxiety disorders are more common among women than men. This is particularly true for panic disorder and agoraphobia, whose prevalence rates are two- to fourfold greater in women than men. The familial nature of anxiety disorders has long been recognized and accepted. A number of older studies consistently found a 15 percent rate of anxiety disorders in the first-degree relatives of patients with anxiety neurosis. Although these data suggest that panic disorder runs in families, it remains uncertain to what extent the increased familial rates in offspring are derived from environmental versus genetic factors.

One researcher found a fivefold greater concordance rate for panic disorder or agoraphobia with panic attacks in monozygotic than in dizygotic adult same-sexed twins. In contrast, there was a similar rate of anxiety disorders in monozygotic and dizygotic co-twins with generalized anxiety disorder. These data suggest that genetic factors may play a more prominent role in the panic disorders than in generalized anxiety disorder.

CLINICAL SIGNS AND SYMPTOMS

OVERVIEW An anxiety disorder may begin slowly and insidiously with general feelings of tension and nervous discomfort (e.g., generalized anxiety disorder), or its onset may be sudden, heralded by the outbreak of panic attacks (e.g., panic disorder). Although several lines of evidence suggest that panic disorder and generalized anxiety disorder represent distinct disorders, there can be significant overlap in their phenomenology and longitudinal course of illness. Whereas the onset of panic disorder typically begins with the occurrence of unprovoked or spontaneous panic attacks, some panic-disorder patients report several months of tension, stress, and generalized anxiety before the development of panic attacks. Most patients with panic disorder, even those with excellent premorbid function, usually develop significant anticipatory and generalized anxiety between panic episodes, particularly if the panic attacks persist without treatment.

The average age of onset of panic disorder, with or without associated avoidance behaviors, is generally in late adolescence or early adulthood. Although panic disorder may develop in later life, senior citizens who experience their first panic attacks after the age of 50 should be particularly carefully evaluated to rule out underlying medical conditions that might produce free-floating anxiety or mimic panic disorder. Most patients with panic disorder can recall the precise date, time, nature, and circumstances of their first panic attack, whereas patients with generalized anxiety disorder may be unable to recall the year of onset and tend to be more uncertain regarding its clinical course.

During the initial phase of history taking, patients with panic disorder will often stoutly maintain their ignorance of what might have triggered their symptoms and will frequently be distressed by their inability to explain the symptoms' onset. Indeed, the medical-model concept of panic disorder emphasizes the autonomous nature of panic attacks. This perspective is supported by the fact that panic attacks can often occur spontaneously in the absence of psychosocial stress or overt psychological conflict. As many as 50 to 75 percent of patients with panic disorder are awakened from non-REM (rapid eye movement) sleep with panic attacks. This observation also suggests a primary neurophysiological disturbance in panic disorder. Conversely, from a psychodynamic perspective, the inability of some patients with panic disorder to appreciate the temporal relationship between life situations and anxiety may be viewed as repression. There have been few systematic studies investigating the role of life events and stressors in the onset and natural course of panic disorder. Preliminary findings suggest that before the onset of illness, patients with panic disorder personally experience a greater number of life events than normal controls. Often, if patients are allowed to associate freely about their anxiety and the circumstances under which it has appeared, the interviewer will be able to uncover the environmental events that have contributed to stimulating the internal conflict of which the anxiety is a part. Although these observations do not indicate that specific life events cause panic disorder, clinicians should be aware that life stressors may precipitate panic attacks or exacerbate symptoms of anticipatory anxiety in panic-prone patients.

Some theories have linked a particular type of experience (i.e., separation and loss) with panic disorder. A recent National Institute of Mental Health (NIMH) study found that the occurrence of a major loss before the onset of panic disorder was associated with an increased risk for a subsequent major depressive episode but had no impact on the subsequent rate of panic attacks. These results support previous observations and theories suggesting a connection between a major loss (e.g., death of a spouse) and the onset of depression. The relationship between particular types of life events in the onset of panic disorder, however, remains unclear. It is likely that the subjective experience and meaning of life situations, in addition to the increased exposure to distressing life events, is a crucial factor in triggering illness in vulnerable individuals.

From a practical perspective, clinicians are encouraged to assess the possible impact of psychosocial stressors in each patient with panic disorder. In some cases, clinicians will find no association between psychosocial stress and the onset and course of panic disorder. In other cases, there might be a fairly obvious connection between a particular life event and the onset and phenotypic expression of illness.

Less is understood about the age of onset and clinical course of generalized anxiety disorder. Although generalized anxiety disorder usually begins in early adulthood, there may be a broader distribution in age of onset compared with that of panic disorder. The relationship between life events and course of generalized anxiety disorder also remains obscure, although clinical experience suggests that stressors may play a central role in the onset and maintenance of this disorder.

One precipitant found frequently enough in generalized anxiety disorder, hypochondriasis, and somatization disorders to be worthy of special mention is the death of a near relative from a myocardial infarction. Following the loss, the survivor develops the nonspecific cardiac, respiratory symptoms, and skeletomuscular aches and pains commonly observed in generalized anxiety disorder. Such patients may become convinced that they have the same disease as the departed, or one closely related to it.

PANIC DISORDER In 1919, H. G. Wells published *The Journal of a Disappointed Man,* a selection of passages from the diary of a promising young biologist, W. N. P. Barbellion, who developed multiple sclerosis at the age of 23 and died of his disease at 28. It was in his late teens that Barbellion first noted the onset of the symptoms of anxiety that became particularly distressing during the next few months, in the form of overwhelming panic attacks. The journal entry of February 11, 1911, reads as follows:

Walked in the country. Coming home, terrified by a really violent attack of palpitation. Almost everyone I met I thought would be the unfortunate person who would have to pick me up. As each one in the street approached me, I weighed him in the balance and considered if he had presence of mind and how he would render first aid. After my friend, P.C., had passed, I felt sorry that the tragedy had not already happened, for he knows me and where I live. At length, after sundry leanings over the river wall, arrived at the Library, which I entered, and sat down, when the full force of the palpitation was immediately felt. My face burned with the hot blood, my hand holding the paper shook with the angry pulse, and my heart went bang! bang! bang! and I could feel its beat in the carotids of the neck and up along the Torcular herophili and big vessels in the occipital region of the head. Drew in each breath very gently for fear of aggravating the fiend. Got home (don't know how) and had some sal volatile. Am better now but very demoralized.

In Barbellion's account, one can see the striking cardiac symptoms that have so frequently drawn the interest of cardiologists to panic disorder. But in addition to the violent palpitations, the flushing of the face, and the pulsations that he felt in his neck and head, Barbellion reveals the state of mind that is the essence of the condition. He is "terrified," he says, and it is easy to imagine the anguish of his walk along the river, punctuated by "leanings over the river wall" as he tries to quiet himself and to shake off the conviction that at any moment he is going to drop dead. Barbellion's experience is quite typical of panic attacks, but he mentions in his journal entry only a handful of the wide range of symptoms that occur with varying frequency—the most common, in addition to panic and palpitations, being pains in the chest, respiratory difficulties, and a sense of dizziness, weakness, or faintness.

The feeling of panic, as has been stated, is hard to define. It often has a peculiar quality that differentiates it from simple fear of a real external danger—a quality that is described by patients as weird, eerie, or strangely and dreadfully awesome. Barbellion's reference to the "fiend" perhaps catches some of this dire complexion. Anxiety, furthermore, is forward looking: Patients are overwhelmed by a sense of some imminent catastrophe about to engulf them. Often the patients' awareness of their heart action forces on them the dreadful anticipation of death from a heart attack. In fact, during the initial course of illness, many patients with panic disorder are seen in emergency rooms to rule out impending myocardial infarction. Patients with panic attacks frequently fear fainting, but the fear is compounded by a terror of being seen by others in this weak and helpless state. Sometimes the patients cannot specify what they dread, and the mystery about what lies ahead as well as about what is causing their panic only adds to their desperation. Finally, panic attacks often have an impelling quality; the patients feel that they must do something—run, hide, scream, or get away—although just what they are to do or where they are to go is as unclear as the reason for their terror.

The nature of the cardiac symptoms is reasonably self-evident. They result from the patients' awareness of an actual change in heart function as it beats more rapidly and forcefully. This is often accompanied by a sense of hollow emptiness inside the chest, within which the heart, like a wild, captive animal, is felt leaping and pounding against the prison of the rib cage. If in bed, the patients' awareness of their heart's function may be heightened when lying on their left side. Moreover, as in Barbellion's account, the patient may be conscious of strong pulsations along the course of the major arteries.

Generally associated with the cardiac symptoms are various chest pains. Most commonly these are sharp and sticking in quality and are felt precordially, either at the apex of the heart or a bit higher and more centrally in the upper-left quadrant of the chest wall. Not infrequently, they may radiate to the left shoulder, axilla, arm, and, on occasion, even to the right extremity. Less commonly, the patient may complain only of a dull discomfort in the cardiac region, and pains may be felt substernally and in the epigastrium.

Nearly as common as the cardiac manifestations are feelings of respiratory discomfort. These are usually described by the patient as a sense of not being able to get enough air into the lungs, accompanied by a feelings of fullness in the chest and inadequate respiration. Because of this air hunger, patients will often breathe more rapidly and more deeply and may feel impelled to run out of doors to get more air. If they wake up in the middle of the night with a panic attack, they will sometimes jump out of bed and rush to an open window to gulp down air in deep breaths in an attempt to relieve their sense of suffocation.

Sleep, sleep panic, and sleep deprivation Although restless sleep and sleep panic are common complaints in panic disorder, there have been few sleep polysomnographic studies in patients with panic disorder. A reduced REM latency and an increased REM percentage are common in depressed and dysthymic patients but not in patients with panic disorder. Preliminary evidence suggests that panic disorder patients have increased movement time during sleep, perhaps reflecting a paradoxical state of hyperarousal during circumstances of relative relaxation.

Accumulating evidence also suggests that panic attacks may arise from sleep in approximately 70 percent of patients with panic disorder. Of interest, sleep-related panic attacks are not linked to REM sleep, dreaming, or its associated imagery or cognitions. In fact, most sleep-related panic attacks occur during stage 2 or stage 3 sleep. Sleep-related panic attacks are also similar in quality to daytime panic attacks. The following, in descending order of prevalence, are the most commonly reported symptoms of sleep-related panic attacks: sudden fear, palpitations, sweating, chest pain or discomfort, choking or smothering feelings, feelings of unreality, and hot and cold flashes.

Another aspect of sleep worthy of mention is the effect of sleep deprivation. Although one night's total sleep deprivation produces a transient elevation in mood in depressed patients, several lines of evidence suggest that the lack of sleep often worsens anxiety in patients with panic disorder. As illustrated in Figure 18.1-1, a recent NIMH study found that although no patient with major depression grew worse following sleep deprivation, 58 percent of panic disorder patients worsened, including 40 percent who experienced panic attacks on the day following a night of total sleep deprivation. The effects of repeated sleep deprivation or changes in day–night shift work in panic disorder are unknown. Until further information becomes available, current wisdom suggests that panic disorder patients should avoid, when feasible, activities requiring excessively long periods of sleep deprivation or frequent interruptions in the normal sleep-wake cycle.

Acute and chronic hyperventilation Accumulating evidence indicates that both acute and chronic hyperventilation may be an important physiological component of panic disorder. In acute hyperventilation, sufficient carbon dioxide (CO_2) may be blown off to bring on a hypocapnic and alkalo-

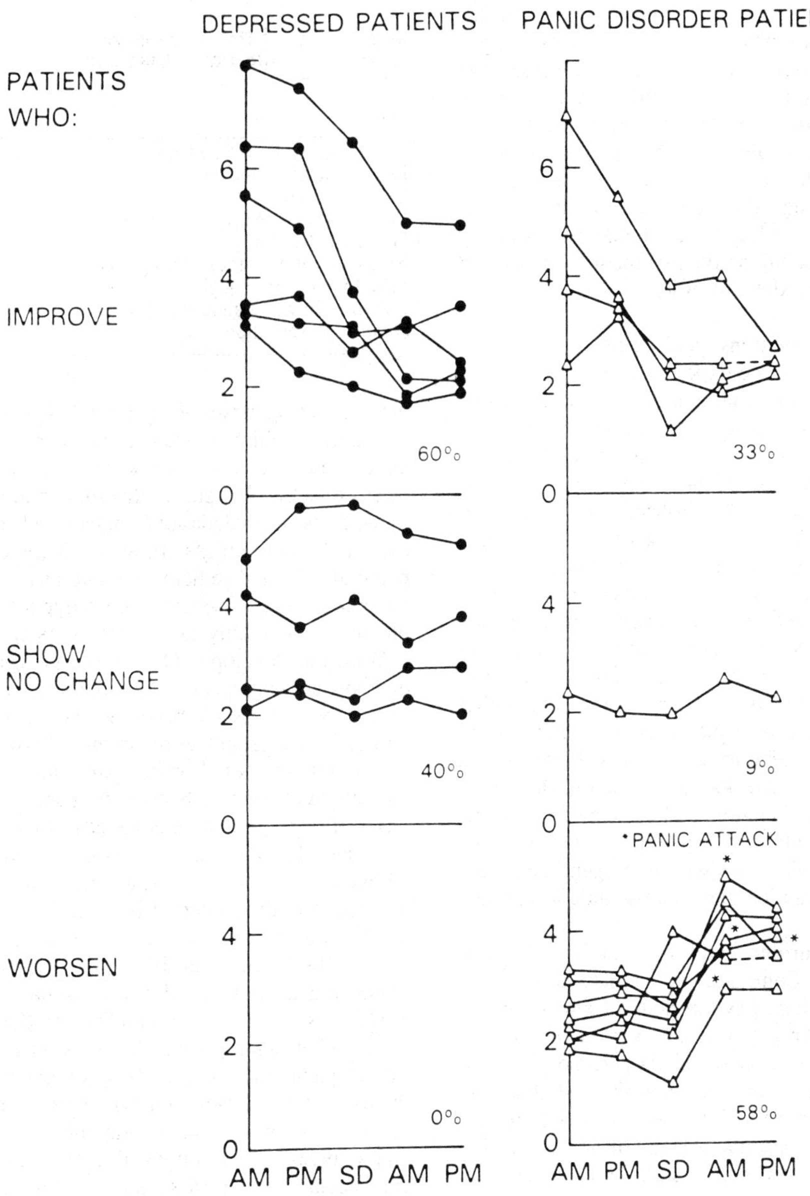

FIGURE 18.1-1. *Differential response to 1 night's total sleep deprivation in patients with panic disorder and major depressive disorder. Although 58 percent of the panic disorder patients worsened (four patients experienced panic attacks), none of the depressed patients had increased measures of anxiety following sleep deprivation.*

tic state (pH > 7.45). Excessive hypocapnia decreases cerebral blood flow which may result in transient cerebral hypoxia. In acute hyperventilation, patients first notice mild numbness and tingling in their fingers, usually bilaterally, but occasionally in one extremity only. With more severe degrees of alkalosis, the numbness and tingling become more widespread, affecting the toes, feet, and face, particularly the area around the mouth. Much less commonly, muscle twitching and even tetany (e.g., carpopedal spasm) may result.

In addition, patients often complain of a light-headedness and a sense of fullness and enlargement of the head. In addition to acute hyperventilation, recent evidence also suggests that panic disorder patients are chronic hyperventilators. The chronic hyperventilator has a low pCO_2 but normal pH and cerebral blood flow. Under circumstances of chronic hyperventilation, even minimal increases in the ventilatory exchange of air may suddenly trigger an acute hyperventilation syndrome.

Recent findings also suggest that the inhalation of CO_2 is more likely than is room-air hyperventilation to provoke panic attacks in panic disorder patients.

These findings raise issues regarding the common emergency room practice of instructing all patients with hyperventilation syndrome to breath into a paper bag. Although such a practice might initially be useful by lowering pH, it is theoretically possible that prolonged CO_2 rebreathing might trigger waves of panic in panic-prone individuals. Rather than breathing into a bag, support and assisting the patient to reduce breathing to 10 breaths per minute might be equally effective. This approach also avoids the symbolic discomfort of cutting off air experienced by some acutely panicking patients when breathing into a bag.

The exact relationship between hyperventilation syndrome and panic disorder remains obscure. Some theories suggest that the acute hyperventilation syndrome *is* panic disorder, but other theories view symptoms of hyperventilation as simply a secondary manifestation, frequently but not always associated with panic attacks. It is possible that hyperventilation causes panic attacks in some individuals. Conversely, hyperventilation may be just a physiological concomitant of panic attacks in other patients. Even in the latter case, breathing-retraining techniques may be a useful adjunctive treatment in the overall management of primary anxiety disorders.

Somatic symptoms Palpitations and tachycardia, chest pain, respiratory distress, and the experience of panicky dread are the cardinal symptoms of panic attacks, but various other manifestations may be less commonly found. Dizziness is not unusual and is described as an awareness of an irregular, blurring, and swimming motion of the surroundings. Associated with this is usually a sense of light-headedness and faintness. Patients may complain of flushing of the face, cold perspiration, and gooseflesh, and they are commonly aware of the trembling of their extremities. The latter can often be observed, but patients sometimes also report a trembling on the inside, which seems to be more a subjective sensation than an observable fact. Gastrointestinal symptoms occur in nearly 40 percent of patients and are commonly either epigastric pains or a feeling of a jittery, hollow fluttering in the epigastric region—the familiar sensation of butterflies in the stomach. Finally, panic attacks have a highly disruptive effect on normal mental functions. Preoccupied as panic patients are with their body and immediate fate, they are hardly in a position to think or act with intelligence, and not surprisingly, they often describe their mental state as clouded and confused.

The frequency of occurrence and the number of panic attacks vary considerably. Some individuals may have only a few during a lifetime. Others have periods in which attacks may occur repeatedly over a few days, weeks, or months, only to disappear as mysteriously as they came. The individual episodes of panic vary in intensity and duration: They typically arise suddenly and last from seconds to minutes. A few patients will describe a siege of anxiety lasting hours during which they cower in a state of persistent, intensely painful anxiety punctuated by waves of utter panic and terror.

Psychosensory symptoms: Relation to limbic function After severe panic attacks, many patients describe profound fatigue and exhaustion. Some patients report sleeping many hours after such episodes of panic. Although patients with panic disorder do not generally have electroencephalographic (EEG) evidence of temporal lobe epilepsy, lethargy and behavioral inactivity are common manifestations of the postictal state in animals and humans. In addition to postpanic fatigue, the high prevalence of psychosensory disturbances associated with panic attacks has led to the suggestion that limbic substrates may play an important role in the neurobiology of panic disorder. In fact, as illustrated in Table 18.1-5, some psychosensory symptoms are probably more common during panic attacks than are many of the symptoms currently endorsed by DSM-III-R.

TABLE 18.1-5
Most Frequent Psychosensory Symptoms Reported by Patients with Panic Disorder

Symptom	*Patients Affected* %
Distortion of light intensity	59
Distortion of sound intensity	46
Derealization	46
Strange rising feeling in stomach	41
Depersonalization	37
Sensation of floating, turning, moving	32
Speeding up of thoughts	22
Slowing down of thoughts	20
Jamais vu sensation	17

Panic-related agoraphobia The word *agoraphobia* literally translated means a fear of the marketplace or open spaces. This translation, however, is misleading. In panic disorder patients, the genesis of agoraphobia is a fear of any place or situation in which assistance would be unavailable in case of an unexpected panic attack or sudden incapacitation (e.g., heart attack). In panic disorder patients, agoraphobia is viewed as a maladaptive behavioral complication of unexpected panic attacks. In an inadequate attempt to ward off panic attacks and remain in a safe environment, such patients become severely impaired and polyphobic. Table 18.1-6 lists the most commonly associated fears in panic disorder.

With the development of these polyphobias, patients later develop context-specific or situational panic attacks. As the illness progresses, it becomes increasingly difficult for the clinician and patient to distinguish between spontaneous (uncued) and situational (cued) panic attacks. Most agoraphobic patients will give a history of panic attacks preceding the onset of agoraphobia. Studies at NIMH found that 97 percent of panic disorder patients with secondary agoraphobia developed avoidance behaviors after the onset of their panic attacks. The time interval between the onset of panic attacks and the development of agoraphobia, however, can be rapid. In the NIMH study, all of the patients with agoraphobia plus panic attacks developed agoraphobia within 6 months (the range was 3 days to 6 months) of their first panic attack. Thus, when agoraphobia develops as a secondary complication of panic attacks, it is likely to emerge within 6 months of the first panic attack. Given these observations, panic disorder, with or without agoraphobia, is conceptualized as a single neuropsychobiological entity. However, agoraphobia can occur without associated panic attacks. Agoraphobic patients without panic attacks are rarely seen in anxiety-disorder clinics, and little, therefore, is known about the phenomenology, neurobiology, or pharmacotherapy of this disorder.

GENERALIZED ANXIETY DISORDER

Acute panic attacks may appear suddenly with no forewarning in a person who until their onset has been reasonably calm and untroubled. Panic attacks may also occur against a background of chronic stress and anxiety. Many patients, however, experience only chronic anxiety without being subject to eruptions of panic attacks. As is the case in patients with panic disorder, patients with generalized anxiety disorder may not be able to state what is making them anxious. A fair number of individuals, however, can relate their chronic tension to environmental troubles such as marital discord or pressures at work, although they may be unaware of exactly how or why the anxiety produces their symptoms. Chronic anxiety is uncomfortable and, if it persists long enough, may be demoralizing to a degree that hampers patients' daily functioning.

The symptoms of chronic generalized anxiety are many and varied. Patients commonly complain of feeling nervous, tense, jumpy, and irritable. They may have difficulty falling asleep at night and tire easily during the day. Gastrointestinal symptoms are common, the patients being disturbed not only by the sense of butterflies in the stomach but also by heartburn and epigastric fullness, which are sometimes accompanied by belching. They may notice occasional looseness in their bowel movements and sometimes frequency of urination. Headaches are not uncommon, usually being described as pressure or tension frontally, occipitally, or vertically, although occasionally they may have the quality of a nagging, throbbing frontal ache. In addition, patients may complain of muscular tension or pain, especially in their neck and back. They sweat easily, particularly on the palms of their hands, often sense a flushing in their face, are troubled by dryness of the mouth or a "frog in the throat," and frequently feel shaky and tremulous. Particularly troubling to those whose occupation requires mental work is the difficulty in concentrating, in marshaling their thoughts, and in thinking through problems.

BEHAVIOR AND PHYSICAL EXAMINATION The characteristic signs and behavior of patients with panic attacks or severe anticipatory anxiety are hard to miss, and even were one inclined to overlook them, the patients' importunity would not permit one to do so. Often pacing anxiously if not frenetically or, if remaining seated, moving arms and legs restlessly about, the patients complain loudly of their inner turmoil and vociferously demand help. Their facial expression is in keeping with their terror. They may be visibly perspiring, may sigh frequently, and often are obviously hyperventilating. Physical and neurological examinations should pay special attention to those medical disorders that may mimic or exacerbate pathological anxiety states.

Sweating may be profuse, particularly on the hands, feet, and forehead. Reflexes are frequently brisk, but without clonus. Acutely anxious patients may have increased psychomotor activity, as well as evidence of tachycardia, although heart size is normal. It has long been recognized that an increase in heart rate (tachycardia), usually of normal sinus rhythm, is characteristic of acute anxiety states. Until recently, however, there had been few systematic studies investigating the heart rate and rhythm of anxiety patients under natural conditions. Recent studies with 24-hour ambulatory heart monitoring in panic disorder patients indicate that a relative increase in heart rate often precedes or develops concomitantly with the subjective experience of panic. Some panic disorder patients demonstrate panic-related heart rates of 120 to 130 beats per minute (bpm). Although most panic attacks are probably associated with a relative increase in heart rate in each patient, not all panic attacks are accompanied by heart rates above 100 bpm. Thus, heart rates per se cannot be used as a validity measure for panic attacks in either the clinical or the research setting. Moreover, the average heart rate of panic-disorder patients under nonpanic conditions is generally unimpressive and within a similar range of age- and sex-matched normal controls.

TABLE 18.1-6
Most Frequent Fears Reported by Panic Disorder Patients

Fear	*Patients Affected %*
Driving	54
Stores, shopping malls	43
Being alone	37
Crowds, lines	34
Leaving home, traveling far away	34
Restaurants	34
Elevators, escalators	29
Doctors, dentists	29
Being closed in	23
Bridges, tunnels	20
Social gatherings, meetings, strangers	20
Flying	14
Heights	14

Although patients with panic and generalized anxiety disorders frequently complain of chest pain, palpitations, fluttering, and skipped heart beats, the prevalence of arrhythmias during panic attacks and severe generalized anxiety is less well understood. Recent evidence suggests that most panic attacks are not associated with cardiac arrhythmias, although when arrhythmias (e.g., simple ventricular premature complexes) do develop, they tend to occur during periods of high anxiety.

The cardiovascular status of patients with panic and generalized anxiety disorders is grossly within normal limits under nonstressful (asymptomatic) circumstances. During periods of extreme anxiety or panic, there is usually, but not always, a relative increase in heart rate. Arrhythmias are infrequent but, when present, tend to occur during moments of stress or high anxiety. These observations, together with the controversial evidence suggesting an association between panic disorder and mitral valve prolapse, are consistent with the hypothesis that panic disorder is a minor disorder in a broader spectrum of autonomic nervous system diseases. The relationship of autonomic dysfunction to controversial reports of increased cardiovascular mortality in panic disorder remains to be elucidated.

On physical examination, an area of soreness on the surface of the chest may be discovered on palpation, and fine tremors of the outstretched hands can often be observed. When hyperventilation is present, a positive Chvostek sign can be elicited, and with severe overbreathing there may be actual tetantic contractions (e.g., carpopedal spasm) in the extremities.

Special laboratory and diagnostic evaluations are required when the constellation of symptoms and physical signs indicates a reasonable possibility of an underlying medical condition. All patients with pathological anxiety should receive a careful physical examination, including electrocardiogram, laboratory evaluation (particularly thyroid function tests), and a neurological examination.

The fear of an underlying, life-threatening illness is common in patients with anxiety disorders. As noted previously, patients with panic and generalized anxiety disorders frequently experience a wide range of somatic and psychosensory complaints. As a result, many patients with anxiety disorders initially present to general practitioners or other medical specialists with a long list of somatic complaints. In this setting, patients with primary anxiety disorders may eventually undergo unnecessary and sometimes invasive procedures. However, psychiatrists must avoid the temptation, and perhaps the inclination, to view all somatic complaints as psychogenic in origin. For example, approximately 50 percent of the panic disorder patients referred to NIMH have been found to have concomitant physical illnesses. Although these previously undiagnosed medical illnesses are rarely the direct pathogenesis of their panic attacks, clinicians should remember that patients with anxiety can and do develop medical disorders.

COURSE AND PROGNOSIS

As is so often the case with psychiatric syndromes, the paucity of studies concerning the natural history and evolution of anxiety disorders makes it difficult to speak authoritatively about either their course or their prognosis.

Generalized anxiety disorder tends to be chronic, with frequent stress-related exacerbations and fluctuations in the course of illness. General clinical experience suggests that patients with generalized anxiety disorder tend to become less symptomatic as they grow older, especially if they have achieved any degree of success and stability in their personal lives. The long-term prognosis of panic disorder is controversial. Panic disorder patients with concomitant obsessive-compulsive symptoms tend to have a poorer response to all treatments, including pharmacotherapy. Panic disorder patients with obsessive features also have an increased risk of depression and alcohol abuse, compared with that for panic disorder patients without obsessive-compulsive features. Early investigations of patients with neurocirculatory asthenia (i.e., panic disorder) indicated that although perhaps one-third either recovered completely or made a significant improvement, the majority continued to manifest symptoms and incapacitation of varying degrees of severity. A 1982 study found increased mortality in panic disorder patients from cardiovascular disease and suicide.

In both panic and generalized anxiety disorders, the nature of the symptoms alone does not usually help in forecasting the outcome, and as in any patient with an anxiety problem, the prognosis is guided by various factors: the degree of environmental stress in precipitating the disorder, the biological nature of the illness, the maturity of the patient's ego, the stability of the patient's personal relationships, the patient's work performance, and the duration of symptoms. With the advent of improved behavioral and psychopharmacologic treatments, most patients with panic disorder, including those with agoraphobia, can achieve near complete resolution of symptoms with appropriate treatment. The overall prognosis of generalized anxiety disorder tends to be more variable.

ETIOLOGY

In anxiety, people's mental and bodily functions find a meeting place unparalleled in other aspects of human life. Any discussion of the etiology of anxiety must therefore deal with both psychological and physiological processes. In what follows, no attempt is made to take sides in the controversy over whether the conscious experience of the affect or the bodily changes associated with it come first. William James long ago proposed the paradoxical theory that feelings (including anxiety) were merely the individual's conscious awareness of physiological processes antecedent to the emotion, and the argument he started is not yet settled. Nor is any stand taken on the age-long philosophical duel between the monists, who view body and mind as one, and the dualists, who see each as a separate, distinct entity. That issue is sidestepped in the ensuing discussion, with the assumption that the human organism reacts to stimuli with a variety of responses, some of which are better described in psychological language and some in the vocabulary of physiology.

PSYCHOLOGICAL ASPECTS Anxiety is a universal human experience, characterized by fearful anticipation of an unpleasant event in the future. In psychoanalytic theory, anxiety is differentiated from fear. Anxiety, it is said, is the individual's response to a danger that threatens from within in the form of a forbidden instinctual drive that is about to escape from the individual's control. Fear, on the other hand, is defined as the reaction to a real external danger that threatens the individual with possible injury or death. In actuality, this theoretical distinction cannot always be strictly maintained. With phobic symptoms, for example, the patient experiences the threatening situation as being external, although there may, in reality, be nothing dangerous about it. At the same time, an external situation that is genuinely hazardous may arouse instinctual drives that produce internally derived anxiety. In any given episode, both fear and anxiety may be present in varying proportions; from a practical, clinical point of view, it is probably more relevant to ascertain the causes of the affect than to try to decide whether it is fear or anxiety.

The following discussion is centered on the specific aspect of the affect that represents the ego's response to internal conflict and that forms the paramount symptom of anxiety disorders. In this context, anxiety is viewed as playing a central role in the functioning of the psychic apparatus. As the ego's reaction to an internal threat arising from forbidden instinctual drives, it is experienced in consciousness as mental pain. The pain, in turn, motivates the ego to defensive maneuvers aimed at controlling the drives in order to avoid mental suffering. Anxiety, in other words, is viewed as a signal, or indicator, to the ego, both of the need to erect psychological defenses and of the success of their functioning. In this theoretical scheme, anxiety is not necessarily considered as being pathological. Before attention can be focused on the etiology of the anxiety disorders from a psychoanalytic perspective, the history of the development of the concept of anxiety must be reviewed.

As mentioned earlier, DaCosta and other military surgeons who dealt with panic disorder in soldiers during the wars of the late-nineteenth century apparently were not aware of the vital role that anxiety played in the disorder they described. Their attention was almost entirely focused on the bodily symptoms, and by the same token, their explanations were physiological. In DaCosta's view, the excessive demands made on the nervous system and the heart by the physical rigors of warfare, disease, and injury in some way not clearly understood caused a derangement in both organ systems, leading to disordered function.

Pierre Janet's theories DaCosta's contemporaries among psychiatrists, although they recognized anxiety as a significant psychological symptom, still tended to explain it in physical terms. Pierre Janet's theories were probably the most sophisticated of all those stemming from the neurologically oriented school of Jean Charcot at the Salpétrière. For Janet, neurotic syndromes were divided into two main classes: (1) hysteria, which included dissociated states of consciousness and a variety of sensorimotor phenomena; and (2) psychasthenia, into which were lumped a hodgepodge of symptoms, including phobias, obsessions, anxiety, and neurotic depression. The key to the formation of psychoneurotic symptoms was the concept of dissociation, which rested on the physicalistic notion of a hereditary constitutional degeneration of the nervous system. In Janet's scheme, the various mental functions were viewed as being held together by nervous energy in a coordinated, working whole. In individuals with bad heredity, the total quantum of this nervous energy was less than that of normal people, and in the face of life stresses, it thus was more rapidly lowered in the constitutionally inferior.

If the level fell too low, the integration of the mental functions would be impaired, and specific individual functions would be dissociated from the normally integrated totality. The fatigue so common in neurotic states was explained as a direct, conscious awareness of the diminution of nervous energy, whereas other neurotic symptoms were viewed as being release phenomena secondary to the escape of lower mental functions from central control. In this theoretical framework, anxiety was seen as the consequence of the anarchic functioning of lower vegetative nervous centers.

Freud's theories Trained as a neurologist, Freud had been dragged reluctantly into the camp of the psychologists by the observations forced on him by his neurotic patients. As stated earlier, he was the first investigator to recognize that anxiety neurosis as a psychiatric disorder could be separated from the potpourri of symptoms of neurasthenia. Nonetheless, although his experience with phobic symptoms had led him to concede the importance of anxiety as a psychological force, his initial explanation of its genesis was couched in physical concepts.

Freud's early awareness of the central role of sexuality in the formation of neurotic symptoms induced him to see abnormalities in the sexual life of his patients as the fundamental cause of their anxiety. He viewed the sexual drive as being a form of nervous energy that exerted constant pressure for discharge in sexual activity. If such activity were excessive, then abnormal amounts of sexual energy (or libido) would be expended, and the individual would be conscious of fatigue. A chronic state of fatigue of this sort constituted the clinical syndrome of neurasthenia, which could be produced, for example, by excessive masturbation. On the other hand, if the opposite situation pertained—if, that is, through sexual continence or coitus interruptus, libido failed to find a normal sexual channel for discharge—libido would accumulate in the nervous system. Up to a point, the organism could tolerate this accumulation without ill effects, but if its quantity became too great, then an internal process would take place that resulted in clinical symptoms. That process, in Freud's early theory, was the transformation of sexual energy into anxiety. This was conceived of as a direct physiological change, and the anxiety was viewed as following on the failure of libido to achieve a normal discharge in sexual intercourse. On the basis of this theoretical formulation, Freud proposed separating anxiety neurosis as a clinical entity distinct from the other neurotic syndromes. He futhermore referred to it as an "actual neurosis" rather than a "psychoneurosis," as no psychological mechanisms (such as the conversion process at work in hysteria) and no memories of past emotional traumata were found to play a part in the appearance of the symptoms of anxiety neurosis.

Initially, Freud's explanation of the anxiety-producing damming up of libido invoked purely fortuitous, external causes, such as the failure of an individual to have normal sexual intercourse. As his theory became more complex, he proposed a new mechanism, repression, which he saw as playing a major role in causing the accumulation of sexual energy.

The concept of repression had rapidly taken a central position in Freud's early theoretical formulations. In this scheme, it was postulated that ideas, emotions, and impulses unacceptable to the conscious ego were forced by the agency of repression into the unconscious portion of the psychic apparatus. The sexual drive, in particular, was seen as subject to repression, and it was this psychological mechanism, rather than voluntary sexual continence or coitus interruptus, that came to be viewed as the major reason for the potentially dangerous accumulation of undischarged sexual energy and its ultimate transformation into anxiety.

In this theoretical scheme, anxiety was seen as the result of repression. As Freud continued to study psychoneurotic patients, his attention focused more on the psychological, experiential aspects of anxiety, and he came to recognize that besides its being a derivative of sexual libido, anxiety was also a psychological reaction of the ego to dangers that threatened it from without and within. He did not, however, abandon his theory of the libidinal source of anxiety until some 30 years after his first physiological proposition concerning its origin, and then only after he had made a major alteration in his theoretical model of the structure of the psychic apparatus. The details of the evolution of his theory cannot be recorded here; suffice it to say that from his earlier topographical model of the psyche—which portrayed the human mind as being divided between conscious and unconscious processes, each with characteristic modes of thinking—Freud moved to a structural model, in which the psychic apparatus was seen as being composed of three psychological agencies—ego, superego, and id—each with specific functions.

In this new model, anxiety was viewed in an entirely different light. It was now seen as the ego's reaction to instinctual forces arising from the id which, if uncontrolled, could be dangerous to the self, either because of their inherently disruptive potential or because of retaliatory punishment arising from the superego or the external world if they were acted on. Anxiety, thus conceived of as originating in the ego as an ego affect, became a psychological force in its own right. As a signal of danger, it was viewed as being a central moving force in the working of the entire psychic apparatus, its main function being to motivate the ego to employ repression and other defensive mechanisms to control the underlying drives and affects. Anxiety was no longer considered to be the result of repression, but the cause of it.

Current psychodynamic perspectives In view of the central position that it occupies in the human psychic apparatus, it should be no surprise that anxiety is found as a symptom in all forms of emotional illness. When it occurs, it is a sign of movement within, an indication that something is disturbing the internal psychological equilibrium.

Anxiety is a signal to the ego that an unacceptable drive is pressing for conscious representation and discharge, and as a signal it arouses the ego to take defensive action against the pressures from below. If the defenses are successful, the anxiety will be dispelled or safely contained, but depending on the nature of the defenses employed, the individual may develop a variety of psychoneurotic symptoms. Ideally, the employment of repression alone should restore psychological equilibrium without symptom formation, as effective repression completely contains the drives and their associated affects and fantasies by rendering them unconscious. But more often than not, repression is not entirely effective, and it is necessary to call into play auxiliary defenses, such as conversion, displacement, or regression, through which the drives achieve a partial, though disguised, expression in the symptoms of hysteria, phobic anxiety, or obsessive-compulsive disorder, depending on the defense that predominates. As is evident from the frequent presence of anxiety in association with other neurotic symptoms, the auxiliary defenses themselves are not totally effective, but they generally keep the affect within tolerable levels.

If repression fails to function adequately and if other defenses are not called into play, then anxiety will be the only symptom, and when it rises above the low level of intensity characteristic of its function as a signal, it may emerge in all the fury of a panic attack. From a clinical point of view, this internal state of affairs is manifested as anxious symptomatology. The significance and meaning of the anxiety depend on the nature of the underlying conflict of which it is a part, and that conflict is itself a legacy of the patients' experiences during their early phases of growth and development that have shaped the psychic structure with which, as adults, they face the world. Stimuli from their adult environment activate the conflicts that they carry with them, disturb their psychic equilibrium, and mobilize the signal anxiety that in turn calls into play the various ego defenses.

The patients themselves, however, are not consciously aware of all the psychological movements taking place and frequently are not aware of what in their environment has started the process. Psychodynamically oriented psychiatrists are expected to uncover these unconscious processes so that the reasons for their patients' symptoms may be understood and properly treated. When faced with patients with anxiety disorders, psychodynamically oriented therapists ask themselves two questions about the patients' anxiety, both of which refer to its function in the psychological processes leading to the clinical symptoms: (1) What inner drives are such patients afraid of? (2) What are the consequences they fear from their expression?

The drives Anxiety is a response to the pressure of underlying instinctual drives; it is these drives of which such patients may be said to be afraid. They fear the emergence of an impulse that will lead them into forbidden and unacceptable actions aimed at discharging the energy associated with the drives. In psychoneurotic conflicts, the latter are either sexual or aggressive in nature, and patients' associations during the course of psychiatric interviews will gradually disclose the specific kind of sexuality and aggression that is the source of conflict. Patients may be found, for example, to be concerned with homosexuality, with murderous destructiveness, or with oral dependency needs. It is, however, not the mere existence of the drives that threatens the patients. They are afraid of them because they fear the consequences of actively expressing them.

The consequences The consequences of the individual's anticipated behavior determine the quality of the anxiety experienced. In this context, anxiety is seen as falling into four major categories.

SUPEREGO ANXIETY So human and ubiquitous is the anxiety stemming from the superego that it hardly needs illustration. The workings of the human conscience have often been dealt with by creative writers. What Edgar Allan Poe, for example, described in the few stark sentences of "The Tell-Tale Heart," Fyodor Dostoyevsky's introspective genius expanded into the hundreds of pages of *Crime and Punishment.* Almost everyone has experienced at some time the pangs of guilt arising from an action that he or she feels to be wrong and the accompanying anxious expectation of being found out, and so knows at first hand the quality and discomfort of superego anxiety.

The prickings of conscience are not only ubiquitous but can hardly be considered abnormal when they arise in response to behavior that flouts one's personal code of ethics or the standards of morality prescribed by social custom. Superego anxiety, however, can occur with a degree of intensity or can produce pathological symptoms that mark it as being clearly abnormal, no matter how appropriate it may be as a response to wrongdoing. Perhaps the clearest and most common form of such anxiety is seen among those persons with psychotic depressions who are convinced that they are the greatest sinners of all times and that all the ills of the world can be laid at their doorstep. That superego anxiety can result in neurotic symptoms is evident from the experience of a patient reported by Janet.

Achille, aged 33, had until the onset of his illness been a happily married, active, and cheerful businessman. He had always been healthy, both physically and emotionally. However, after his return from a short business trip away from home, his wife noted a striking change in his personality. He suddenly became depressed, withdrawn, and uncommunicative. Increasingly nervous and agitated, he began to worry that he had a variety of serious bodily illnesses and at length took to his bed. His symptoms culminated in total unresponsiveness to anyone or anything around him, and he was apparently unconscious. Suddenly, however, 2 days later, he awoke from this state to manifest a new pattern of behavior. Now alert, active, and in contact with his family, he reported with considerable anxiety that he was possessed by the devil, who caused him to utter terrible blasphemies. "This poor man," wrote Janet, "small in stature, with haggard eyes and pitiful appearance . . . murmured blasphemies in a muffled, sober voice." "Cursed be God," he would say. "Damn the Trinity and damn the Virgin." Then in a shriller voice, with tears in his eyes, "It's not my fault if my voice utters these horrors. It's not me. I tighten my lips so that the words won't pass them and be spoken aloud, but it does no good. The devil speaks these words inside of me. I can clearly feel him speak them and make my tongue move despite myself."

Under hypnosis, Janet obtained an interesting additional bit of history. Achille revealed a series of events leading up to his state of possession, of which he had no conscious memory during normal consciousness. While away on the business trip that preceded the onset of his symptoms, he had had a brief affair with another woman. On his return home, he was suddenly seized with remorse for his infidelity and was terrified that if he talked, he would inadvertently reveal his affair to his wife. Hence, his initial withdrawn, silent uncommunicativeness. With the passing days, his guilt became worse. He was now convinced that he was developing a number of serious illnesses as punishment for his sin. At length he began to have vivid dreams that he was dead, had descended into hell, and was surrounded by a host of demons. These dreams were at first apparently nightmares but later merged into a spontaneous somnambulistic trance state—his 2 days of unresponsiveness—in which he vividly hallucinated hellfire and all the tortures of the damned at the hands of a wild, satanic crew of tormentors. Awake, as noted, Achille had no conscious recall or memory of these events and images revealed by hypnosis but was plagued with the ego-alien sense of being possessed by the devil and of being forced against his will to utter blasphemies. Thus, presented with a patient with a mixture of anxiety and dissociative and obsessive-compulsive symptoms, hypnosis revealed to the observer the profound, unconscious superego anxiety and its source that had initiated the patient's defensive repression resulting in the psychopathological behavior that represented the underlying dissociated mental complexes.

CASTRATION ANXIETY The term *castration anxiety* refers to a variety of anxieties having in common a fear of bodily damage or of some kind of diminution of one's capacities. These are given the generic label *castration* because the patient's associations frequently lead to fantasies of genital mutilation often associated with a confusion over sexual identity.

A married man of 32 was referred for therapy for a severe and incapacitating anxiety disorder, which was clinically manifested as repeated outbreaks of acute attacks of panic arising from a background of chronically distressing nervous tension. Initially, he had absolutely no idea what had precipitated his attacks, nor were they associated with any conscious mental content. In the early weeks of treatment, he spent most of his time trying to impress the doctor with how hard he had worked and how effectively he had functioned before he was taken ill. At the same time, he described how fearful he was that he would fail at a new business venture he had embarked on. One day, with obvious acute anxiety that practically prevented him from talking, he revealed a fantasy that had suddenly popped into his mind a day or two before that had led to the outbreak of a severe anxiety attack. He had had the image of a large spike being driven through his penis. Over the next few days he recalled that, as a child of 7, he was fascinated by his mother's clothing and that, on occasion, when she was out of the house, he had dressed himself up in them. From there, his associations led to a confession that, as an adult, he was fascinated by female lingerie and would sometimes find himself impelled by a desire to wear women's clothing. He had never yielded to the impulse, and indeed on those few occasions when the idea had entered his consciousness, he had been so overwhelmed by anxiety that he could think of it no further.

This patient's castration anxiety could clearly be seen in the fantasy of his mutilated penis. At the same time, fantasies referring to a confusion in his sexual identity emerged into consciousness, which were seen to be a major source of his anxiety. Such concerns are commonly found in association with castration anxiety that appears in homosexual panic, a particularly severe form of anxiety. Usually occurring in adolescent or young adult males who have not entirely consolidated their masculine identity, it is frequently precipitated by a situation in which the patient is, for the first time, exposed to other men in close contact, such as in college dormitories or military barracks. In this setting, underlying unconscious homosexual impulses may be aroused that threaten the patient's masculinity and lead to the sudden eruption of what are often peculiarly violent and disintegrating attacks of acute anxiety.

SEPARATION ANXIETY As its name implies, *separation anxiety* represents the fearful anticipation of the loss of an important human relationship.

A patient reported that for several days before he had to go away on a trip, he regularly began to feel increasingly anxious. Although the anxiety did not impinge on his work and daily functioning, he found it quite unpleasant. A sense of uneasy tension was constantly present in his stomach, and he often felt mildly flushed and unable to think as clearly as he wished. Whenever his mind turned to the trip ahead, these feelings would increase and would be accompanied by an outpouring of sweat on the palms of his hands and the eruption of gloomy, anxiety-provoking fantasies of accidents or other disasters that would leave his family fatherless. Particularly distressing was that these phenomena totally destroyed any pleasurable anticipations about his journey, which usually promised objectively to be interesting and rewarding. His symptoms would reach a peak on the day of his departure and, fortunately, disappeared once he was actually on his way.

ID OR IMPULSE ANXIETY Not infrequently, patients express a panicky fear that they are about to lose control over an impulse and that they will consequently act in an irrational, crazy fashion. In its extreme form, this may be felt as an impending dissolution of the total sense of self, an awareness that may accompany the anxiety associated with the onset of an acute schizophrenic episode. Such fears, however, are not invariably related to the outbreak of psychosis and are commonly associated with the emergence of an awareness of rage in those for whom aggression is a serious source of intrapsychic conflict.

A patient arrived one day for his therapeutic hour in a state of acute anxiety. His complaints of severe palpitations, pounding in his head, and a "trembling feeling all over" were matched by a generalized visible tremulousness, heavy sighing, facial perspiration, and a worried, anxious look on his face. Particularly troubling to him was that he had absolutely no idea what was making him feel as he did. However, as his associations poured forth during the interview, his imagery became increasingly colored with violently aggressive fantasies of banging, smashing, and destroying things and people. The insight by both the patient and the doctor as to the source and nature of the patient's anxiety was summed up by the patient toward the end of the hour. It was a fear, he said, "that I won't be able to hold myself back. . . . It's a feeling of being scared of what I'm apt to do . . . go berserk. Jesus! It's an awful feeling!"

Psychogenetic aspects of anxiety The varieties of anxiety just described are viewed by psychodynamically oriented psychiatrists as having their source and taking their coloring from the various points along the continuum of early growth and development. Id or impulse anxiety is seen as related to the primitive, diffuse discomfort of infants when they feel overwhelmed by needs and stimuli that they cannot control. Separation anxiety refers to the stage of the somewhat older but still preoedipal child, who fears the loss of parental love or even abandonment if he or she fails to control and channel such impulses in conformity with the parents' standards and demands. The fantasies of castration that characterize oedipal children, particularly in relation to their developing sexual impulses, are reflected in adults' castration anxiety. Finally, superego anxiety is the direct result of the final development that marks the passing of the Oedipus complex and the advent of the prepubertal period of latency.

The observation of children illustrates this psychoanalytic schematization. Anxiety can be found throughout all the phases of early life, manifested in different characteristics as children develop. The visible separation anxiety of children of 2 or 3 gives way in the oedipal period to the typical nightmares and fears of injury, which often have a directly genital content. Likewise, in adult patients one can find direct associative links between pathological adult anxiety and anxiety-provoking childhood experiences.

A 23-year-old woman was admitted to a general hospital psychiatric ward for incapacitating anxiety symptoms of 8 months' duration. She could give no reason for her symptoms, except to say that they were particularly associated with an image in her mind's eye of herself and her father locked in a naked embrace. The image made her intensely anxious, and she did all she could to erase it whenever her mind went back to it. In the course of giving her life history, she protested that although she had been particularly close to her father as a little girl, as an adult she "hated" him and did her best to avoid his company. It then developed that her symptoms had appeared suddenly at the end of a period of several days during which her father had tried to be particularly nice and helpful to her at a time of financial need. It was only after several interviews that she remembered that her first symptoms of anxiety had appeared in association with a nightmare that had occurred during this period of interaction with her father. In her dream she was at a zoo at night. She heard strange noises in the darkness, which a nearby zookeeper told her were "only the animals mating." Then she saw a large gray elephant lying on its right side on the ground. As she watched, the animal lifted its left leg up and down as if it were trying to struggle to its feet. She awoke in a state of acute anxiety and from that time on manifested increasingly severe anxiety that finally led to her hospitalization.

In direct association to the dream, the patient reported that she had slept in a crib in her parent's bedroom until she was 5 and recalled for the first time in her adult life an episode in which, while in her crib, she awoke one night to see her parents having intercourse. When they noticed her, they sprang apart. She remembers seeing her father's erection, and as she watched him, he tried to sit up and cover himself with the bedclothes, lifting his left leg like the elephant in the dream. During the patient's associations to the dream, which came out in bits and pieces, she was frequently so overcome by anxiety that she could not talk for minutes at a time. Following the interview, her anxiety and the thoughts about her father disappeared, and in a few days she was discharged symptom-free, an improvement that had been maintained when she was followed up in the outpatient clinic 3 months later.

Although many parts of the patient's history remained obscure, the nature of her symptoms and associations, the quality of her relationship with her father and his apparent role in precipitating her adult illness, the revival of a long-repressed childhood memory, and the disappearance of her anxiety following the recall all suggested that the anxiety was oedipal in nature and was directly related to events in her oedipal period, the memory of which, although repressed, had had a continuing influence during her adult life.

Developmental and ego psychology The recognition of signal anxiety and its role in psychic functioning throw into bold relief the fact that anxiety appears clinically in two forms: First, as a state of panic, it is manifested as a massive, global, and intense discharge of autonomic functions that overwhelms and disorganizes ego functions and renders the individual helpless to behave adaptively. Second, as a signal of danger, internal or external, anxiety is a less intense experience that enables the individual to anticipate the threat of danger and to take defensive action against it.

In Freud's initial theory of anxiety as a transformation of libido into somatic, autonomic discharge, he viewed the intensity of the discharge as matching the intensity of the libido from which it was derived. This economic theory of anxiety explained its source and magnitude but could not account for its formal characteristics. Initially, Freud proposed that the somatic manifestations of acute anxiety were in many ways similar to those of orgasmic discharge. This explanation, however, did not account for the significant difference between the ecstatic pleasure of orgasm and the overwhelmingly painful affect of panic. Accordingly, Freud subsequently suggested that anxiety recapitulated the affective and somatic response of the infant to the trauma of the birth process, which acted as a template for the form of all later anxious reactions to severe traumatic situations. Ultimately, Freud generalized his concept of anxiety to include traumatic anxiety, the response to an actually present overwhelming and dangerous traumatic situation, and to signal anxiety, which as an ego affect alerts the individual to anticipate the threat of a traumatic situation. In signal anxiety, anxiety occurs as a response to cognitive processes, such as the perception of indicators of potential danger and the memory of past experiences of psychic trauma. This form of anxiety is derived from those cognitions, not from a transformation of repressed affects, libidinal or otherwise, and its intensity cannot be economically equated with the intensity of the repressed affects. With the development of the concept of anticipatory anxiety, the economic theory of anxiety was replaced by what has come to be called the signal theory of anxiety.

With the emergence of the idea that acute anxiety recapitulates the response of the infant and young child to painful traumatic anxiety, Freud introduced a developmental, psychogenetic view of anxiety itself. Modern observations of the early psychic development of human infants and of defective ego functioning in adults support this psychogenetic view. Modern investigators of early development generally agree that infants are unable to experience anxiety per se before the age of 3 or 4 months. Rather, the infant's response to painful, traumatic situations, such as hunger and painful bodily sensations, is a diffuse, somatic, autonomic, and motor discharge, accompanied by an undifferentiated experience of unpleasure.

It is only when early cognitive ego functions begin to develop that a primitive ego structure emerges, permitting the infant to begin to experience anxiety as a qualitatively distinct affect that signals the threat of a potential traumatic situation. The ego develops as the result of repeated interactions between infants and their environment. They gradually learn, for example, that when they are hungry, their needs are gratified by their mothers. As their cognitive capacities for perception and memory develop, they begin to recognize their mothers as distinct persons. Their perceptions of their mothers and, ultimately, their internal memory images of them enable the infants to postpone an immediate total global discharge in response to the early sensation of hunger as they anticipate its removal by their mothers' forthcoming succor. At the same time, the perception of the mothers' absence becomes itself a signal of the potential approach of a traumatic situation and arouses infants to actions, such as motor restlessness, fretting, and crying, that motivate mothers to engage in appropriate caretaking behavior. Step by step, the infants' cognitive and executive ego functions are strengthened and organized into a structure of growing complexity that enables them to manage themselves, their needs, and their environment in an increasingly adaptive, autonomous, and effective manner. Similarly, anxiety becomes increasingly differentiated, attenuated, more affective, and less somatic in character: The traumatic anxiety has evolved into signal anxiety.

Although acute traumatic anxiety tends to disappear as the ego develops, it is not eradicated but remains as a potential response beneath the surface, even in psychologically healthy adults. In the face of overwhelming environmental disasters, even the strongest people are liable to experience disorganizing anxiety, especially if the catastrophe finds them unprepared. If the traumatic situation is prolonged—as, for example, in the experience of the unending horror and brutality of the concentration camps of the Nazi holocaust and their modern counterparts—serious and permanent regressions in ego functions take place that result in a de-differentiation and resomatization of affects, including anxiety. Anxiety, in other words, reemerges in its genetically earlier somatic and undifferentiated form. Similarly, the intense anxiety seen in psychotic and borderline states can be viewed as the more primitive manifestations that result when developmental defects in ego functions and an increased sensitivity to separation compromise the individual's capacity to modulate anxiety. This intense anxiety retains its genetically earlier tendency to be expressed in the form of a massive somatic discharge.

The analytical classification of anxiety is attractive. It gives system and order to a welter of clinical observations; it defines a relationship between past and present; and it suggests a hierarchy of levels of clinical anxiety in which the degree of pathology of the clinical manifestation is determined by the phase of development from which it is derived—the earlier the phase is from which it stems, the more serious will be its diagnostic and prognostic import. A caution must be raised, however, against accepting it as being anywhere near final and complete, and it is by no means an infallible prognostic guide. Superego anxiety, for example, though arising in the later phases of childhood development, can be seen in psychotic proportions in patients with agitated depressions; and separation anxiety, stemming from the earlier phases of development, is a widespread human phenomenon that does not necessarily imply severe emotional pathology. As has been pointed out earlier, many factors (particularly those concerned with ego structure) must be considered in determining the gravity and prognosis of any given clinical illness.

Other analytical views The concept of anxiety has gained widespread acceptance in the various analytical approaches to psychiatric illness. Differences of opinion about its nature arise in many instances from differences of emphasis or from focusing on one kind of anxiety to the relative exclusion of others. Otto Rank, for example, traced back the genesis of all anxiety to the processes associated with the trauma of birth. Harry Stack Sullivan stressed the early relationship between mother and child and the importance of the transmission of the mother's anxiety to her infant. Existential analysts view anxiety as being central to the human condition, and they point to the fear of nonbeing, for example, as being ubiquitous and unrelated to conflict or to past experience.

LEARNING THEORY Although learning theorists have formulated widely accepted behavioral accounts of the acquisition and maintenance of phobic disorders, theoretical explanations of the etiology of panic and generalized anxiety disorders have received significantly less attention. Thus, behavioral models of panic and generalized anxiety disorders are not well developed, and the theoretical assumptions underlying behavioral intervention strategies for these disorders diverge markedly. Conditioned-reflex theorists regard anxiety as an unconditioned, inherent response of the organism to painful or dangerous external stimuli. As such, learning theorists view phobias as conditioned-avoidance reactions in which anxiety may become associated, through classical conditioning, to originally neutral stimuli but also provide a powerful motivating force for shaping learned-avoidance behaviors. This classical-conditioning explanation is not easily applied to nonphobic anxiety states, as the anxiety experienced by those suffering from panic and generalized anxiety disorders is not situationally induced but is, rather, unpredictable or pervasive in occurrence. Moreover, neither panic disorder without agoraphobia nor generalized anxiety disorder results in significant avoidance behaviors. One learning model used to explain the genesis of panic disorders is based on the concept of single-trial learning. In this scenario, internal, previously neutral stimuli (e.g., interoceptive cues) or thoughts become conditioned stimuli capable of eliciting full-blown panic attacks by initially being fortuitously paired with a panic attack of unknown origin. An obvious weakness in this explanation is its failure to account for the genesis of the original panic attack. Thus, although learning theory provides a useful model for understanding the formation of symptoms and providing a rational method of treatment for certain psychiatric syndromes such as the phobic disorders, it is less helpful in explaining the origins of other nonphobic forms of anxiety, particularly panic attacks and free-floating or generalized anxiety.

In recent years, proponents of behavioral theories have shown increasing interest in cognitive approaches to conceptualizing and treating anxiety disorders, and cognitive theorists have proposed potentially more helpful alternatives to traditional learning-theory etiological models of anxiety. Cognitive conceptualizations of nonphobic anxiety states suggest that faulty, distorted, or counterproductive thinking patterns accompany or precede maladaptive behaviors and emotional disorders. According to one model, patients suffering from anxiety disorders tend to overestimate the degree of danger and the probability of harm in a given situation and to underestimate their abilities to cope with perceived threats to their physical or psychological well-being. This model asserts that panic-disordered patients often have thoughts of loss of control and fears of dying that follow inexplicable physiological sensations (e.g., palpitations, tachycardia, lightheadedness) but precede and then accompany panic attacks. Patients with generalized anxiety disorders are viewed as holding distorted, disabling thoughts with regard to events perceived as threatening to their physical or social well-being.

Cognitive-behavioral treatment strategies, designed to modify maladaptive thought patterns that putatively underlie pathological affective reactions, have emerged as alternatives to exposure-based treatment procedures. Systematic research is required to determine the overall and relative efficacy of these newer cognitive-behavioral approaches in the treatment of panic and generalized anxiety disorders.

BIOLOGICAL ASPECTS During the past decade, a massive body of data has been generated regarding the neurophysiology, psychoneuroendrocrinology, and physiology of panic disorder. Less attention has been paid to the biological correlates of generalized anxiety disorder. Despite the importance and prevalence of the bodily manifestations of anxiety, little can be said about the explicit neurophysiological and neurochemical causes of panic and generalized anxiety disorders. In part, the problem in identifying precise biological mechanisms of anxiety underscores the reality of the intricate relationship between psychosocial events and brain function.

In this subsection, the authors review current knowledge regarding the neuroanatomical substrates, neuroendocrinology, and biochemistry of normal and pathological anxiety states. No attempt is made to assess cause-effect relationships. Much of the following information is based on preliminary investigations and requires, therefore, independent confirmation. Given the large number of ongoing worldwide investigations of anxiety and the anxiety disorders, the reader can anticipate major modifications and additions to the current understanding of the psychobiology of anxiety disorders.

Neuroanatomical Clinical and experimental evidence points increasingly to the function of the limbic system as central to the neurobiology of human emotions. Although panic disorder is not associated with EEG evidence of epilepsy, anxiety and fear are commonly reported experiences during seizures in patients with temporal lobe epilepsy. In fact, panic attacks associated with impulsive behavior can be a major symptom in patients with temporal lobe epileptic foci. Moreover, interictal behavioral symptoms, including agoraphobia and other phobic-like symptoms, are reported in patients with temporal lobe epilepsy.

Recent findings suggest that the ventricular brain ratio, assessed by computed tomography (CT), is not enlarged in panic disorder, as has been reported in patients with chronic alcohol abuse or schizophrenia and in a subgroup of patients with affective illness. Preliminary findings do indicate, however, that lactate-sensitive patients may have an abnormal hemispheric asymmetry of parahippocampal blood flow when evaluated with positron emission tomography (PET). This PET study, however, was made in only a small number of patients and requires confirmation in a larger sample size by independent investigators. If confirmed, the asymmetry in parahippocampal blood flow can be added to the long list of indirect evidence implicating an important role for limbic-temporal lobe substrates in the neurobiology of anxiety, perhaps particularly panic attacks.

Biochemical Researchers use several chemical models for inducing anxiety, particularly panic attacks. At the present, there is no justification for the general use of these panicogenic agents as diagnostic tests in clinical practice. Despite this limitation, these chemical models provide useful tools for investigating the phenomenology and biology of panic disorder. The most well known and systematically studied chemical probe of anxiety is lactate-induced panic.

Lactate-induced panic Interest in the lactate model of anxiety evolved from the observations of exercise intolerance and excessive production of lactate in patients with neurocirculatory asthenia (panic disorder). In a classic experiment, an infusion of sodium lactate produced typical attacks of panic in 13 of 14 patients with anxiety neurosis, as compared with only two of 10 normal controls subjected to the same experimental procedure.

Although several laboratories have replicated the findings of increased lactate sensitivity in panic-prone individuals, it has not been conclusively determined whether patients with other nonpanic anxiety disorders are equally insensitive as controls to lactate's panicogenic effects. Agents, such as tricyclic antidepressants and monoamine oxidase (MAO) inhibitors, appear to block both spontaneous and lactate-induced panic attacks. Lactate has also been shown to release corticotropin-releasing hormone from cell cultures. Despite these data suggesting that lactate metabolism may be altered in panic disorder, abnormal elevations of blood lactate, regardless of the source, do not appear to be the direct cause of spontaneous or laboratory-induced panic attacks.

Yohimbine-induced panic Yohimbine, an α-2 adrenergic antagonist, increases noradrenergic nucleus locus cereuleus firing in animals. Stimulated locus ceruleus firing is associated with increases in noreprinephrine release and fear behaviors. Conversely, clonidine (Catapres), an α-2 adrenergic agonist, decreases locus ceruleus firing, decreases norepinephrine release, and reduces fear behaviors in animals. Parallel findings have been observed in humans. In fact, yohimbine has proved to be an especially useful chemical model for the study of panic attacks.

Patients with panic disorder are more vulnerable than are normal controls to the anxiogenic effects of yohimbine. Twenty-milligram doses of yohimbine commonly produce panic attacks in panic-disorder patients. These panic attacks are similar to naturally occurring panic attacks. Although high doses of yohimbine can produce severe anxiety in normals, it is extremely rare for healthy controls to experience panic anxiety with a 20 mg dose. There has also been found a significant correlation between yohimbine-induced anxiety and increases in levels of plasma 3-methoxy-4-hydroxyphenylglycol (MHPG) in panic disorder patients. This relationship was not found in the normal controls. Moreover, patients with frequent panic attacks had a significantly greater rise in plasma MHPG after yohimbine than panic disorder patients with infrequent panic attacks.

These and several other lines of evidence suggest a role for noradrenergic dysfunction in panic disorder. However, not all natural or drug-induced anxiety states are associated with indices (e.g., increased plasma MHPG levels) suggestive of noradrenergic overactivity. Thus, disturbances in noradrenergic function may play an important, but not exclusive, role in the neurobiology of panic or generalized anxiety disorders.

Caffeine-induced panic Anecdotal reports have long suggested that caffeine in excessive quantities can produce anxiety in humans. Only recently, however, have there been double-blind, placebo-controlled studies investigating the behavioral and biochemical effects of caffeine in patients diagnosed according to DSM-III-R criteria. Again, the major focus of research has been in patients with panic disorder.

After oral administration of 480 mg of caffeine, equivalent to approximately 4 to 6 cups of coffee, 40 percent of panic disorder patients experience panic attacks. In contrast, normal controls do not experience panic attacks at this dose. After ingesting caffeine, panic disorder patients also experience significantly greater increases in plasma levels of cortisol and lactate. Although caffeine increases noradrenergic function and, at high Um concentrations, binds to benzodiazepine receptors in animals, current studies suggest that the anxiogenic effects of caffeine are probably mediated by the blockade of adenosine receptors.

Benzodiazepine inverse agonists The recent discovery of the benzodiazepine-GABA-receptor complex has stimulated a search for the putative endogenous ligand that naturally binds to this receptor. Although the endogenous ligand has yet to be identified, fairly profound behavioral and physiological changes relevant to the study of anxiety can be elicited by manipulating this receptor system.

Benzodiazepine agonists (e.g., diazepam [Valium]) have antianxiety and anticonvulsant effects, whereas inverse agonists (e.g., B-carboline-3-carboxylic acid ethyl ester [B-CCE], FG-7142) have proconvulsant and anxiogenic properties. In animals, B-CEE was recently found to produce fear behaviors, such as agitation, vocalization, grimacing, head and body turning, and defecation and urination associated with increases in plasma cortisol, heart rate, and mean arterial pressure. Pure antagonists, such as R015-1788, have little intrinsic behavioral or biochemical effects in human and nonhuman primates but block and reverse the biobehavioral effects of both benzodiazepine agonists and inverse agonists. Available inverse agonists are not widely used in human experimentation because of their powerful anxiogenic effects and potential for inducing seizures. However, one study of healthy humans found that FG-7142 produced a wide variety of symptoms, including waves of anxiety, terror, cold sweat, tremor, agitation, facial flushing, fear of impending death, and "intense inner strain and excitation." This panic-like response to FG-7142 was associated with an increase in plasma cortisol, growth hormone, and prolactin.

These basic science and clinical research findings, representing a major scientific advance, suggest that the benzodiazepine-GABA complex is an important molecular substrate in the biological regulation of arousal and anxiety in humans.

Neuroendocrine function Recent investigations of neuroendocrine function in anxiety disorders have focused on the hypothalamic-pituitary-adrenal (HPA) and hypothalamic-pituitary-thyroid (HPT) axes.

Hypothalamic-pituitary-adrenal function The test most commonly used to assess HPA function is the dexamethasone suppression test (DST). Using a standard 4 P.M. cortisol value of greater than 5 ng per dl to indicate nonsuppression after an 11 P.M. dose of dexamethasone (1 mg), most nondepressed panic disorder patients, with or without agoraphobia, demonstrate normal suppression. Although findings with DST suggest a normal pattern of feedback regulation, other lines of evidence suggest that subtle abnormalities in HPA function may be associated with panic disorder. For example, although

24-hour samples of urinary free cortisol are normal in panic disorder, preliminary evidence suggests that levels of cortisol in the afternoon or early evening may be elevated. Recent reports of blunted adrenocorticotropic hormone (ACTH) and cortisol responses to corticotropin-releasing hormone (CRH) also suggest that brief periods of cortisol hypersecretion, perhaps associated with circadian disturbances, may be a biological correlate of panic disorder.

Hypothalamic-pituitary-thyroid function The clinical observation of an association between neuroendocrine disturbances, especially hyperthyroidism or hypothyroidism, and the onset of panic disorder is not uncommon. Also, some investigations have found statistically, but not clinically, significantly higher levels of T_3 and T_4 in panic disorder patients, as compared with normal controls. These data suggest that some panic disorder patients may have subclinical hyperthyroidism. Consistent with this hypothesis is a recent study reporting a high incidence of undetectable levels of thyroid-stimulating hormone (TSH). Moreover, two independent studies have found blunted TSH responses to thyrotropin-releasing hormone (TRH), again consistent with an element of subclinical hyperthyroidism in panic disorder. The practical treatment implications, if any, of these clinical and research findings require further investigation.

Receptor binding Alterations in central noradrenergic and, more recently, serotonergic function have been hypothesized in panic disorder. Of course, current techniques do not allow for direct assessment of brain function in humans. As a result, clinical investigators have developed an indirect method for investigating brain neurochemical function by studying peripheral blood elements such as erythrocytes, lymphocytes, and platelets. The basic rationale for this approach is that many of the neurotransmitter receptor systems that influence brain function are also important mediators of blood elements. Although this methodology is not without problems, its practical advantages have led to extensive studies of peripheral blood elements in patients with major affective disorders. Only recently have binding studies been conducted in patients with panic disorder. These studies have focused on platelet function as it relates to the number (B_{max}) and affinity (Kd) of binding sites relevant to the noradrenergic and serotonergic systems.

In the study of adrenergic systems, radioligand binding to the adrenergic receptor has been investigated with ^{3}H-clonidine, an α-2 adrenergic agonist, and ^{3}H-yohimbine and ^{3}H-dihydroergocryptine, both α-2 adrenergic antagonists. To date, the preliminary results have been either contradictory or difficult to interpret. ^{3}H-clonidine parameters were found to be normal in one study. The number of binding sites for ^{3}H-yohimbine, however, has been reported to be normal or decreased, but the binding of ^{3}H-dihydroergocryptine to platelets has been reported to be increased in panic disorder patients, as compared with normal controls.

Binding parameters of the 5-HT uptake site with ^{3}H-imipramine have been more consistent. Four of five studies of ^{3}H-imipramine binding to platelets in panic disorder found it to be normal. One study, however, found a decrease in both Bmax and Kd with ^{3}H-imipramine. Most, but not all, studies of platelet ^{3}H-imipramine binding in major depressive disorder, especially in patients with melancholia, found a decreased number of binding sites.

In summary, the studies of platelet α-2 adrenergic receptors in panic disorder are perplexing and inconclusive but not totally inconsistent with a noradrenergic dysregulation model of panic disorder. The function of the serotonin uptake site, as reflected by ^{3}H-imipramine binding, appears to be normal in most studies of panic disorder. Two studies also found normal imipramine binding in patients with generalized anxiety disorder. The finding of normal platelet-binding parameters does not totally exclude, however, the possibility of disturbances in brain serotonergic function.

Physiology In the past, psychophysiological studies of nonspecific anxiety disorders, using EEG and autonomic techniques (i.e., galvanic skin response, electromyography, blood pressure, and pulse rate) found increases in most of these measures that could be globally characterized as overarousal. Early studies in patients with neurocirculatory asthenia, an early diagnostic term for panic disorder, found panic-anxious patients to overreact to ischemic pain and auditory, visual, and thermal stimuli. Patients with mixed anxiety symptoms were found on several autonomic measures to habituate slowly to repeated psychophysiological stimuli.

More recently, the psychophysiology of patients with DSM-III–diagnosed anxiety disorders has been investigated with a number of different modern techniques. Using threshold pain and signal detection methods, patients with panic disorder were found not to be more sensitive than controls to experimentally induced electric pain stimuli. These negative findings with pain in panic disorder patients are noteworthy because they argue against a nonspecific stress theory of panic disorder. The nonspecific stress theory of panic disorder posits that any physiological perturbation or physical discomfort will elicit panic attacks in panic-prone patients. That panic disorder patients report similar pain counts and pain sensitivity as do normal controls following electric shock (1 to 31 milliamperage) and do not experience panic attacks associated with either the ice-water test or after glucose- or insulin-induced hypoglycemia largely disproves intolerance to nonspecific arousal as the basic pathogenesis of panic attacks.

The EEG sleep of depressed patients, especially melancholic patients, is generally characterized by a shortened REM latency and increased REM activity and density. Only recently have sleep laboratories begun to investigate the sleep polysomnography of the anxiety disorders. Although disturbed sleep continuity, reductions in delta sleep, and poor adaptation may be found in both panic and generalized anxiety disorders, preliminary evidence suggests that reduced REM latency and increased REM percentage discriminate depressed patients from those with these anxiety disorders. It is of interest, however, that patients with panic disorder may have increased motor activity during sleep. Moreover, accumulating evidence suggests that sleep panic attacks may be prevalent in patients with panic disorder. Preliminary reports indicate that sleep panic occurs during non-REM sleep, typically during stage 2 or stage 3 sleep.

DIFFERENTIAL DIAGNOSIS

PSYCHIATRIC CONDITIONS Anxiety as a symptom is found in almost all patients suffering from psychiatric illness. What characterizes anxiety disorders is that some forms of anxiety (e.g., panic attacks or generalized anxiety) are the principal or exclusive symptoms of the illness. Although anxiety can be a prominent feature of any psychiatric disorder, the primary anxiety disorders are rarely confused with other psychiatric disorders.

Most of the confusion arises in differentiating among the anxiety disorders and mood disorders. Some confusion is understandable, given the overlap in symptomatology between mood and anxiety disorders. In phobic disorders, the anxiety is characteristically bound to the phobic object or situation, and obsessive-compulsive disorder is easily distinguished by the mental and behavioral phenomena that give the disorder its name. Occasionally, an episode of acute schizophrenia will be ushered in by the onset of anxiety. This is often found to be an intense fear of the dissolution of the self, and usually in a very brief period following the appearance of anxiety, disorders of thinking characteristic of schizophrenia will become evident.

MEDICAL CONDITIONS Patients with panic disorder will report discrete episodes of panic or profound apprehension, usually articulated by them as an "out-of-the-blue" experience. Patients with panic disorder are frequently afraid that they will die from a heart attack. During panic attacks, patients will experience myriad somatic symptoms, including shortness of breath, chest pain, profuse diaphoresis, and heart palpitations. The initial experience of panic attacks often leads patients to seek medical attention, frequently in emergency rooms. In this environment, most panic attacks caused by major medical illnesses (e.g., cardiovascular disease, hyperthyroid crisis) are probably accurately diagnosed and treated as indicated. Nonetheless, the prudent psychiatrist should be knowledgeable of the medical conditions that may be associated with panic attacks or severe generalized anxiety.

Acute myocardial infarction It is well known that patients with chest pain and cardiac arrhythmias may have fears of impending doom. Occasionally, patients with impending myocardial infarction will present to the emergency room with a chief complaint of anxiety. Patients with pathological anxiety associated with unexplained chest pain should be evaluated for possible cardiovascular disease. Some patients with panic disorder and many patients with impending myocardial infarction have chest pain radiating into their neck and arms. However, most patients with panic or generalized anxiety disorders without concomitant cardiovascular disease do not experience crushing chest pain.

Pheochromocytomas The pathogenesis of pheochromocytomas is a vascular tumor of the chromaffin tissue of the adrenal medulla (50 percent), the paraganglia, or, rarely, other sites. Most of these catecholamine-secreting tumors are located between the diaphragm and pelvic floor, frequently resulting in some symptoms (e.g., crushing back or abdominal pain or both), which may help distinguish this condition from primary anxiety disorders. Patients with pheochromocytomas may experience diaphoresis, heart palpitations, tachycardia, chest pain, diarrhea, hot and cold flashes, trembling, shaking, and a fear of dying. Thus, patients with these catecholamine-secreting tumors can experience panic similar to spontaneous panic attacks. Patients with pheochromocytomas rarely develop agoraphobia.

Several symptoms should increase the suspicion of pheochromocytomas. A hypertensive response to smoking or malignant hypertensive episodes should alert the clinician to suspect a pheochromocytoma. Moreover, sweating in patients with panic or generalized disorders is most prominent in the hands, feet, and forehead, whereas patients with pheochromocytomas may sweat profusely in the chest and back regions as well. Both patients with panic disorder and patients with pheochromocytomas may have rather severe headaches, although patients with pheochromocytomas will frequently describe a sensation that their head is going to "explode outward." During acute episodes of catecholamine release, pheochromocytoma patients will frequently want to stay absolutely still. Most patients with panic or generalized anxiety, however, demonstrate increased motor activity as part of their anxious symptomatology.

In those patients in whom a pheochromocytoma is suspected, the following measures in a 24-hour urine sample are recommended:

1. Total epinephrine plus norepinephrines (free catecholamines), upper normal limit approximately 100 μg.
2. Metanephrine plus normetanephrine, upper normal limit approximately 1.3 mg.
3. Vanillylmandelic acid (VMA), upper normal limit 6.5 mg.

Substance abuse Both cocaine intoxication and withdrawal states may be associated with generalized anxiety or panic attacks. The relationship of cocaine-related panic attacks to underlying vulnerability remains unclear. Patients who experience multiple episodes of cocaine-related panic anxiety may later develop spontaneous panic attacks and agoraphobia. It is not known whether these patients have a typical response pattern to standard antipanic agents, such as tricyclics and MAO inhibitors.

A significant number of patients experience their first panic attack during a recreational use of marijuana. Whether this response is related to marijuana directly or to other psychosocial variables is unknown.

Alcohol withdrawal is often associated with anxiety, and some patients have reported the onset or recurrence of panic attacks or generalized anxiety on the day after an evening of heavy drinking.

Anxiety and fear of impending doom are central components of the opioid withdrawal syndrome. Other symptoms common to both anxiety disorders and the opiate abstinence syndrome include perspiration, increased blood pressure, tachycardia, increased respiratory rate and depth, tremors, and restlessness. The following symptoms are rare in patients with panic disorder or generalized anxiety disorder but common in patients undergoing opiate withdrawal: severe aching bones and muscles, vomiting, marked rhinorrhea, craving, and spontaneous ejaculation.

Hypoglycemia Almost all patients with panic disorder eventually will ask their physician whether their panic attack may be caused by hypoglycemia. Current evidence suggests that hypoglycemia is an extremely rare cause of spontaneous panic attacks. Furthermore, lactate-induced panic attacks are not associated with hypoglycemia, and glucose- or insulin-induced hypoglycemia does not produce typical panic attacks in panic disorder patients.

Caffeine The possible role of excessive caffeine consumption should be evaluated in all patients with pathological anxiety states. Excessive amounts of caffeine (greater than 700 mg) may be associated with classic panic attacks in normal individuals, and patients with panic disorder may aggravate their symptomatology with as little as 1 cup of coffee. Thus, individuals with recent-onset panic attacks or free-floating anxiety who function in a work environment associated with sleep deprivation (e.g., college students, long-distance truck drivers, individuals working night shifts, psychiatric residents) should be carefully assessed regarding the possibility of caffeinism.

Mitral valve prolapse The relationship between mitral valve prolapse and pathological anxiety states remains one of the more fascinating, perplexing, and unresolved issues in modern psychiatry. Patients with generalized anxiety and panic disorders often report symptoms involving the cardiopulmonary system. In fact, the prominence of these symptoms heavily contributed to the historical use of terms such as "irritable" or "soldier's heart." In 1968, the auscultatory phenomenon of one or more systolic clicks was linked to these traditional disorders, their associated symptomatology, and the mitral valve. These associated signs and symptoms are referred to as Barlow's syndrome or mitral valve prolapse syndrome.

Mitral valve prolapse syndrome is putatively caused by a redundant mitral valve that prolapses into the left atrial chamber during systole. Although there is fairly good consensus regarding what a prolapse of the mitral valve is, there is extremely poor agreement regarding the reliability and validity of auscultatory and echocardiographic techniques in the diagnosis of mitral valve prolapse. Moreover, the clinical significance of mitral valve prolapse, particularly the milder forms (e.g., $\leq$ 4 mm of leaflet displacement) and its prevalence in panic disorder remains extremely controversial.

A possible relationship between mitral valve prolapse and panic disorder was originally entertained for several reasons. First, both panic disorder and mitral valve prolapse syndrome have a familial pattern of transmission; second, there is a greater female-male ratio in both disorders; and third, the symptomatic profiles of both syndromes were initially thought to be strikingly similar. Despite the apparent overlapping nature of these syndromes and over 15 echocardiographic studies in panic disorder, there remains no definitive proof of an association between panic disorder and mitral valve prolapse. On the other hand, the possibility of an indirect but relevant relationship between panic disorder and mitral valve prolapse cannot be totally discarded, as 50 percent of the studies have found an increased rate of prolapse in panic disorder patients, compared with that of the matched controls or published norms. Thus, mitral valve prolapse may be more prevalent in panic disorder patients than in the general population. If so, the nature of the relationship remains perplexing, as in family pedigree studies, the two disorders appear to segregate independently.

Even if there is a greater prevalence of mitral valve prolapse in panic disorder, the opposite may not be true. That is, panic disorder may not be more prevalent in cardiac patients with mitral valve prolapse, compared with cardiac patients without mitral valve prolapse. Moreover, the evidence suggests that many individuals in the general population have definite mitral valve prolapse but are euthymic and free of pathological anxiety states. Thus, it appears clear that there is no simple cause-and-effect relationship such that mitral valve prolapse is the direct and immediate cause of panic disorder. Some investigators, however, have suggested the interesting possibility that panic disorder may induce mitral valve prolapse in a subpopulation of vulnerable individuals.

Clinical experience and preliminary research suggest that the presence of mitral valve prolapse has no practical implications in managing patients with panic disorder. Imipramine (Tofranil), a tricyclic antipanic agent, appears equally effective in panic disorder patients with versus without echocardiographic evidence of mitral valve prolapse. Although antibiotic prophylaxis against subacute bacterial endocarditis is recommended by some cardiologists in patients with mitral valve prolapse, this recommendation is not without controversy, especially in panic disorder patients, who typically demonstrate mild forms of prolapse when it is present. The relationship between mitral valve prolapse and panic disorder and each of these syndromes with cardiac morbidity and mortality has yet to be elucidated in terms of practical guidelines in treating patients with panic and generalized anxiety disorders.

Complex partial seizures Temporal lobe epilepsy has been associated with panic attacks. Moreover, anecdotal reports have suggested that some patients with complex partial seizures may subsequently develop agoraphobia. Many symptoms are common to both disorders; however, some symptoms clearly should alert the physician to the possibility of an underlying seizure diathesis. If a patient admits to periods of transient amnesia, motor automatisms, urine or fecal incontinence, or convulsions, the physician is obligated to rule out a seizure diathesis.

TREATMENT

INSIGHT PSYCHOTHERAPY The prognosis of neurotic syndromes, including anxiety disorders, depends not primarily on the nature of the symptoms themselves but on a variety of factors that indicate the ego's degree of strength. The stability of human relationships and work situations, the ability to bear painful affects and to relate to the therapist, intelligence, motivation for treatment, capacity for introspection and insight all must be assessed in determining the chances for a good response to insight psychotherapy.

Once the patient's suitability for such therapy has been determined, the method of approach will depend on the nature of the problem underlying the anxiety. From a psychoanalytic perspective, neurotic problems that involve characterological dysfunction will require psychoanalysis or one of the more prolonged forms of treatment. If the psychological problem is circumscribed and is related to specific external circumstances, briefer forms of therapy may be quite effective in freeing the patient from the conflict and relieving the symptoms.

SUPPORTIVE PSYCHOTHERAPY Most patients will experience a marked lessening of anxiety when given the opportunity to discuss their difficulties with a concerned and sympathetic physician. Frequently, after the initial hidden precipitants have been determined in the course of a few interviews, the specific supportive techniques to be employed may become clear. Reassurance about unrealistic fears, encouragement to face anxiety-provoking situations, and the continued opportunity to talk regularly to the psychiatrist about problems all are helpful to the patient, even if they are not definitively curative. If doctors discover external anxiety-provoking situations, they may be able themselves, or with the help of the patients and their families, to change the environment so as to reduce the stressful pressures. A reduction in symptoms may often allow patients to function more effectively in their daily work and relationships, which provides new rewards and gratifications that are in themselves therapeutic.

COGNITIVE-BEHAVIORAL THERAPY In contrast with the vast body of literature examining the efficacy of behavioral approaches to the treatment of phobic and obsessive-compulsive disorders, the efficacy of cognitive-behavioral treatment strategies for nonphobic anxiety states remains relatively untested. A few controlled studies, however, have examined the effectiveness of various approaches to relaxation training, including progressive muscle relaxation and biofeedback techniques, in the treatment of generalized anxiety and panic disorders. These relaxation techniques, used primarily by hypnotists and behavior therapists, may prove helpful in patients with generalized anxiety disorder, especially in those who are suggestible. In the initial stages, after instructing the patient in the various methods of relaxation, the psychiatrist should allow the patient to practice them in the office so that the psychiatrist may encourage the patient's efforts. The goal is to enable the patient to employ the techniques alone.

Relaxation may be associated with a paradoxical increase in anxiety, tension, or even panic attacks in patients with generalized anxiety and panic disorders. In fact, the phenomenon of relaxation-induced anxiety may explain why some patients with anxiety disorders are unable to complete taped self-help courses whose major clinical goal is relaxation. Thus, relaxation-induced anxiety may represent an untoward complication of some, but not all, techniques of relaxation training. Conversely, the feared somatic cues accompanying relaxation-induced anxiety might result in habituation and anxiety extinction with repeated training. From this perspective, relaxation-induced anxiety may provide a behavioral tool for treating some anxiety disorders. The ultimate clinical complications or benefits of relaxation-induced anxiety are yet to be determined. Moreover, the cognitive, physiological, and neurobiological mechanisms of relaxation-induced anxiety remain unclear. At the very least, however, relaxation-induced anxiety and relaxation-induced panic may provide an important and new research tool for the study of anxiety disorders.

Cognitive therapy techniques, including cognitive restructuring, self-instructional training, and stress-inoculation training, have recently been touted to be useful in treating generalized anxiety and panic disorders. However, there have been few controlled studies examining the effectiveness of these cognitive-behavioral techniques in treating nonphobic anxiety disorders. Although the results of these initial investigations are promising, further investigation of these methods applied alone and in combination with other treatments (e.g., pharmacotherapy) is clearly indicated.

MEDITATION In recent years, there has been a growing interest in Eastern techniques of meditation. Adapted to Western needs, they have been taught to hundreds of thousands of individuals, who report substantial relief from anxiety and nonspecfic types of tension. Experimental evidence of the efficacy of meditation is still in its infancy, but it seems to have a striking effect on physiological functions as measured by oxygen consumption. One recent study found that mantra meditation as well as progressive relaxation produced increased anxiety in 30 to 53 percent of subjects with generalized tension who received a single training session in these techniques. Thus, the usefulness of meditation in the therapy of anxiety and its relation to hypnosis and progressive relaxation must await further study and controlled clinical trials.

PHARMACOTHERAPY During the 1960s, clinical observations suggested that tricyclic and MAO inhibitor antidepressants were effective in treating patients with phobic anxiety and atypical depressions characterized by anxious dysphoria. During the past 20 years, double-blind, placebo-controlled studies have confirmed these early impressions and have firmly established these and other pharmacological agents as important tools in treating panic and generalized anxiety disorders. The following outline of psychotropic medications used to treat panic and generalized anxiety disorders represents a synopsis of the pharmacotherapy of these disorders and is not intended as a comprehensive review of the mechanisms of action, drug interactions, or side effects. Before using any medication, the clinician should refer to specialized articles regarding individual psychotropic agents and keep abreast of ongoing developments in the area of psychopharmacology. Several new experimental agents and drug combinations are now being tested in the treatment of anxiety disorders. One can anticipate, therefore, that effective treatments with new agents will emerge in the near future and new insights into the use of older, well-established drugs will become more refined. With these caveats in mind, a selective review of the more poignant aspects of the pharmacotherapy of panic and generalized anxiety disorders is presented.

Tricyclics Several studies have demonstrated that imipramine is effective in the treatment of panic disorder. The presumed mechanism of action is imipramine's apparent ability to block panic attacks. Starting doses of imipramine should be somewhat lower (e.g., 10 mg per day) than the typical starting doses prescribed in the treatment of depression. This conservative approach is recommended because many anxiety patients, particularly those with panic disorder, are unusually sensitive to the anticholinergic and activating side effects of imipramine. But even patients who are unusually sensitive to the initial doses of imipramine may have a complete therapeutic response to this agent. In most patients, the untoward side effects associated with imipramine are limited to approximately the first 2 weeks of treatment. Although some panic disorder patients may respond to low dosages of imipramine (50 to 75 mg per day), most patients require dosages equivalent to those required for antidepressant efficacy. Thus, if a satisfactory response is not attained at lower dosages, then dosages as high as 300 mg per day may be necessary, as taking inadequate dosages of imipramine is a common cause for its therapeutic failure.

The relationship between plasma levels of imipramine and the antipanic efficacy of imipramine is poorly understood. Until this relationship is clarified, decisions regarding the total daily dosage and monitoring of imipramine plasma levels must be based on good clinical judgment. Issues such as the severity of psychopathology; achievable, desirable, and acceptable levels of drug response; and a profile of the drug's side effects should be assessed and discussed with the patient. The patient should be encouraged to participate as an active collaborator in this process. Table 18.1-7 represents a rough guideline for the stepwise treatment of panic disorder with imipramine.

Although imipramine has been the most systematically studied tricyclic in the treatment of panic disorder, an increasing number of case reports and clinical studies suggest that other tricyclic antidepressants may be equally effective. Chlomipramine (Anafranil), currently unavailable in the United States, has been reported in open and placebo-controlled trials to be an effective agent. Clinical observations also

TABLE 18.1-7
Treatment with Imipramine

Starting dose: 10 to 25 mg/day*
- —Increase at 25 mg increments Q 2 to 4 days
- —Increase to 200 mg/day
  - If unresponsive, obtain an IMI + DMI blood level
    - —Increase dose until blood level of 120 to 200 ng/ml is achieved

*An inadequate dose of imipramine is the most common cause of therapeutic failure.

suggest that doxepin (Sinequan), amitriptyline (Elavil), nortriptyline (Pamelor), and desipramine (Norpramin) are useful in treating panic disorders. The comparable efficacy of these agents, however, remains unknown. Zimelidine, a serotonin reuptake inhibitor, was initially found to have antipanic effects in two small studies but was removed from the market owing to associated cases of Guillain–Barré syndrome. Nomifensine (Merital) and buproprion (Wellbutrin) have been found to be ineffective, and reports of trazodone's (Desyrel's) effectiveness are mixed.

Initial reports suggested that tricyclic antidepressants were relatively ineffective in the treatment of generalized anxiety disorder. But recent observations suggest that imipramine may also be useful in the treatment of some patients with generalized anxiety disorder.

MAO inhibitors Like tricyclic antidepressants, MAO inhibitors (e.g., phenelzine [Nardil]) appear to be quite effective in the treatment of panic disorder. In fact, some investigators have suggested that MAO inhibitors may be slightly more effective than imipramine. Although the majority of patients with panic disorder will achieve significant benefit from 45 mg per day of phenelzine, general clinical experience suggests that a more complete response and a higher percentage of panic disorder patients will respond to 75 to 90 mg per day. Phenelzine may have activating properties in selective patients, but these and other side effects commonly associated with tricyclic antidepressants (e.g., imipramine) during the initial 2 weeks of treatment are relatively minimal. Most untoward side effects associated with phenelzine pharmacotherapy develop later in the trial and can include orthostatic hypotension, impotence, weight gain, and nocturnal myoclonus. Of course, the decision to prescribe MAO inhibitors must also be balanced against the dietary inconvenience (i.e., low tyramine diet) necessary for their use. Despite these potential problems, phenelzine may provide a rather dramatic alleviation of a broad range of symptoms, including not only the blockade of panic attacks but also a reduction of symptoms such as hysteroid dysphoria, phobic anxiety, and atypical depression.

Antihypertensive agents There is some evidence to suggest that β-blockers (e.g., propranolol [Inderol]) possess anxiolytic properties. Clinical experience, however, suggests that β-blockers may be less effective in the treatment of panic disorder than tricyclic antidepressants. Many clinicians report that β-blockers, especially in combination with benzodiazepines, are useful in the treatment of generalized anxiety disorders and social phobia. β-blocking agents may be effective in patients who focus on interoceptive cues related to cardiovascular and pulmonary function. Thus, patients who experience heart palpitations and tachycardia as the most prominent (almost exclusive) manifestation of their anxiety may respond to β-blockers. Although many anecdotal cases support these guidelines, the determination of the overall utility of β-blockers in treating anxiety disorders will require further investigation.

Clonidine, an α-2 adrenergic agonist, decreases noradrenergic locus ceruleus activity and fear behaviors in animals. These and other lines of evidence suggesting a role for noradrenergic overactivity in anxiety states led several research teams to study clonidine's antianxiety effects in humans. Although clonidine has been found to have acute antianxiety effects in a number of different conditions (e.g., opiate and nicotine withdrawal), it has had limited usefulness in the long-term treatment of panic and generalized anxiety disorders. The main problem with the chronic administration of clonidine is the development of tolerance to its antianxiety effects. Clonidine and propranolol can also induce depressions in predisposed individuals. Thus, α-2 adrenergic agonists (e.g., clonidine) and β-blockers (e.g., propranolol) should be used cautiously in patients with histories of depression.

Anecdotal evidence and a recent controlled study suggest that some calcium channel blockers (e.g., verapamil [Isoptin]) may be useful in the treatment of panic disorder. Determination of the efficacy of calcium channel blockers must await further investigation with double-blind, placebo-controlled trials.

Benzodiazepines Many investigators have suggested that benzodiazepines are effective in the treatment of generalized anxiety but fail to prevent panic attacks. Recent research has cast doubt on this popular but unsubstantiated notion. Despite the ongoing controversy regarding this issue, many patients with panic disorder achieve inadequate relief with low to moderate doses of traditional benzodiazepines (e.g., diazepam ≤ 25 mg). Emerging data suggest that this relative lack of response to many benzodiazepines may be related to issues of potency. Consistent with this concept, two high-potency benzodiazepines (alprazolam [Xanax] and clonazepam [Klonopin]) have been found to be effective in the treatment of panic disorder.

Alprazolam has three positive attributes that make it a good choice for the treatment of many patients with panic and generalized anxiety disorders. First, it is effective. Second, it has a rapid onset of action. Patients often exhibit a dramatic response to alprazolam within days, even at very low doses. The rapid and dramatic response to alprazolam often contributes to the establishment of a therapeutic alliance. Obviously, this is important in the treatment of all patients but may be of particular value in panic disorder patients, who are typically frustrated, angry, and demoralized about their many previous treatment failures. Third, it is well tolerated and widely accepted by patients. It is associated with few untoward side effects or complications during the initial weeks of administration. The most common side effect during the initial phase of treatment is daytime drowsiness, a complication that usually subsides after several days. Patients should be cautioned to avoid driving or using dangerous equipment until they have adapted to the sedating effects of alprazolam. In addition to the initial problems with sedation, the clinician and patient should be aware of other issues that may be encountered with the use of alprazolam.

For example, many patients develop a tolerance to alprazolam's initial therapeutic effects. As a result, increments in dosage may be required until a therapeutic plateau is achieved. To date, the average effective dose in the treatment of panic disorder is approximately 5 to 6 mg per day. It remains unclear whether a therapeutic plateau can be achieved in all patients, and this may lead to a difficult clinical decision as to when one must abandon hope of achieving a sustained therapeutic effect in the higher dosage ranges. Some patients may develop physiological dependence to a marked extent. In addition to the possible development of physiological dependence, many patients report an interdose rebound in anxious symptomatology. As a result, at least four-times-a-day dosing is recommended.

In part because of this rebound phenomenon, several investigators have investigated the effects of clonazepam, another high-potency benzodiazepine with a long-life (24 hours), in the hope that this agent might have antipanic effects and not have interdose-rebound symptomatology. Determination of the efficacy of clonazepam awaits completion of ongoing trials, although preliminary evidence suggests that 1 to 5 mg of clonazepam in two doses provides potent antipanic effects without interdose-rebound symptoms. Clonazepam may also be associated with a lower risk of a full-blown withdrawal syndrome (e.g., rhinorrhea, muscle aches and pains, tachycardia, perspiration, increase in blood pressure), than alprazolam is, although this has yet to be systematically studied. Although alprazolam has been implicated in the induction of hypomania, clonazepam has been associated with triggering depression in patients with previous histories of major depressive disorder. This differential effect on mood may suggest differences in underlying mechanisms of action.

COMBINATION THERAPY For pragmatic reasons it is often necessary to treat patients with combination therapies. Few studies have been conducted addressing this issue, although clinical experience suggests that 20 to 30 percent of panic disorder patients with agoraphobia will require both pharmacotherapy and behavioral therapy in order to achieve maximum benefit. Group and family therapies may also be indicated as adjunctive therapies in selected patients. Combination therapies, however, are not without controversy. The few studies that have been conducted have failed to demonstrate any significant advantages of medication plus behavioral therapy. In fact, some theoreticians have suggested that drug therapy might prevent a complete therapeutic response to behavioral interventions. Until further research clarifies these issues, the clinician must judge the value of combination or sequential treatments according to each patient's particular circumstances and previous treatment history.

REFERENCES

Ballenger J C: Pharmacotherapy of the panic disorders. J Clin Psychiat *47*(suppl): 27, 1986.

Charney D S, Heninger G R, Breier A: Noradrenergic function in panic anxiety: Effects of yohimbine in healthy subjects and patients with agoraphobia and panic disorder. Arch Gen Psychiat *41:* 752, 1984.

Coryell W, Noyes R, Clancy J: Excess mortality in panic disorder—Comparison with primary unipolar depression. Arch Gen Psychiat *39:* 701, 1982.

DaCosta J M: On irritable heart: A clinical study of a form of functional cardiac disorder and its consequences. Amer J Med Sci *61:* 17, 1871.

Dorow R, Horowski R, Paschelke G, Amin M, Braestrup C: Severe anxiety induced by FG-7142 a B-carboline ligand for benzodiazepine receptors. Lancet *8341:* 98, 1983.

Freedman R R, Ianni P, Ettedgni E, Puthezhath N: Ambulatory monitoring of panic disorder. Arch Gen Psychiat *42:* 244, 1985.

Freud S: On the grounds for detaching a particular syndrome from neurasthenia under the description "anxiety neurosis." In *The Standard Edition of the Complete Psychological Works of Sigmund Freud,* vol 3, p 90. Hogarth Press, London, 1959.

Gorman J M, Askanazi J, Liebowitz M R, Fyer A J, Stein J, Kinney J M, Klein D F: Response to hyperventilation in a group of patients with panic disorder. Amer J Psychiat *141:* 857, 1984.

Insel T R, Ninan P T, Aloi J, Jimerson D C, Skolnick P, Paul S M: A benzodiazepine-receptor-mediated model of anxiety. Arch Gen Psych *41:* 741, 1984.

Janet P: *Les Obsessions et la Psychasthlénie,* vols 1, 2. Félix Alcan, Paris, 1903.

Klein D F: Importance of psychiatric diagnosis in prediction of clinical drug effects. Arch Gen Psychiat *16:* 115, 1967.

Liebowitz M R, Fyer A J, Gorman J M, Dillon D, Appleby I L, Levy G, Anderson S, Levitt M, Palij M, Davies J, Klein D F: Lactate provocation of panic attacks. Arch Gen Psychiat *41:* 764, 1985.

Marks I, Lader M: Anxiety states (anxiety neurosis): A review. J Nerv Ment Dis *156:* 3, 1973.

Pasnau R, editor: *Diagnosis and Treatment of Anxiety Disorders.* American Psychiatric Press, Washington, DC, 1983.

Redmond D E, Jr, Huang Y H: New evidence for a locus coeruleus connection with anxiety. Life Sci *25:* 2149, 1979.

Roy-Byrne P P, Geraci M, Uhde T W: Life events and the onset of panic disorder. Amer J Psychiat *143:* 1424, 1986.

Roy-Byrne P P, Uhde T W, Post R M: Effects of one night's sleep deprivation on mood and behavior in patients with panic disorder: Comparison with depressed patients and normal controls. Arch Gen Psych *43:* 895, 1986.

Sargant W: The treatment of anxiety states and atypical depressions by the monoamine oxidase inhibitor drugs. J Neuropsychiat *3*(suppl 1): 96, 1963.

Sheehan D V, Ballenger J C, Jacobsen G: Treatment of endogenous anxiety with phobic, hysterical and hypochondriacal symptoms. Arch Gen Psychiat *39:* 51, 1980.

Torgersen S: Genetic factors in anxiety disorders. Arch Gen Psychiat *40:* 1085, 1983.

Tuma A H, Maser J D: *Anxiety and the Anxiety Disorders.* Erlbaum, Hillsdale, NJ, 1985.

Uhde T W, Boulenger J-P, Roy-Byrne P P, Vittone B J, Post R M: Longitudinal course of panic disorder: Clinical and biological considerations. Prog Neuropsychopharmacol Biol Psychiat *9:* 39, 1985.

Uhde T W, Roy-Byrne P, Gillin J C, Mendelson W D, Boulenger J-P, Vittone B J, Post R M: The sleep of patients with panic disorder: A preliminary report. Psychiat Res *12:* 251, 1984.

Uhde T W, Roy-Byrne, P P, Post R M: Panic disorder and major depressive disorder: Biological relationship. In *Biological Psychiatry, 1985,* C Shagass, R C Josiassen, W H Bridger, K J, Weiss, D Stoff, G M Simpson, editors, p 472. Elsevier, Science, New York, 1986.

18.2
PHOBIC DISORDERS

JOHN C. NEMIAH, M.D.
THOMAS W. UHDE, M.D.

INTRODUCTION

During the 1890s, G. Stanley Hall made a nationwide survey of the fears of many hundreds of Americans, including large numbers of high school girls and boys. In "A Study of Fears," published in the *American Journal of Psychology* in January 1897, he summarized his work:

> 1,701 persons have described 6,456 fears. . . . It would appear that thunder storms are feared most, that reptiles follow, with strangers and darkness as close seconds, while fire, death, domestic animals,

disease, wild animals, water, ghosts, insects, rats and mice, robbers, high winds, dream fears, cats and dogs, cyclones, solitude, drowning, birds, etc., represent decreasing degrees of fearfulness. . . . This order, however, is not quite the same in different localities. In Cambridge, Mass., alone thunder and lightning does not lead, and self-consciousness, dreaded by 24 boys there, does not appear in either Trenton or St. Paul. In the latter place 67 fear cyclones and only 8 the end of the world, which has 62 victims in Trenton, where also 46 fear being buried alive. The St. Paul returns, moreover, show an average of 4.86 fears for each person, those from Trenton 3.66, while the Cambridge, Mass., boys report 2.28 each.

If one stops one's ears to the symphony of Hall's statistics and can move beyond the exquisite metaphysics of 28 one-hundredths of a fear, one finds a wealth of clinical vignettes. A 50-year-old professor of psychology, for example, after seeing a man fall from a fourth-floor window:

. . . Cannot sleep in high rooms at a hotel; tried in vain to ascend Bunker Hill monument as a discipline, but found the tension too great when half way up; could only get over the suspension bridge at Niagara eighteen years later by walking in the middle and grasping a carriage; the fear is rather more that the whole structure may collapse, but partly that he will lose control.

Numerous cases like this suggest that many of Hall's subjects had no ordinary fears. It is perhaps not unnatural to be afraid of tornadoes in St. Paul, but the same cannot be said of trembling in terror before a harmless puss or a common sparrow. Many of what Hall called simply "fears" fall more technically into the category of the phobia, a psychiatric symptom that is the hallmark of phobic disorders. Of particular importance is that the degree of anxiety often severely limits the sufferer's freedom of action. The resulting disability may be as crippling as a major physical illness, and the techniques for removing or reducing phobic anxiety form an essential part of the psychiatrist's therapeutic armamentarium.

DEFINITION

The predominant feature of phobias is a persistent avoidance behavior secondary to irrational fears of a specific object, activity, or situation. Although fears are ubiquitous to the human condition, phobias are unreasonable and unwarranted fears given the actual dangerousness of the object, activity, or situation avoided. The traditional phobic disorders are identified in the revised third edition of the *Diagnostic and Statistical Manual of Mental Disorders* (DSM-III-R) as agoraphobia without panic attacks, social phobia, and simple phobia.

The characteristic irrationality of the fear that constitutes the phobia's central emotion is well demonstrated in the following autobiographical fragment from a psychiatrist who suffered from a phobia of airplanes:

I was pampering my neurosis by taking the train to a meeting in Philadelphia. It was a nasty day out, the fog so thick you could see only a few feet ahead of your face, and the train, which had been late in leaving New York, was making up time by hurtling at a great rate across the flatland of New Jersey. As I sat there comfortably enjoying the ride, I happened to glance at the headlines of a late edition, which one of the passengers who had boarded in New York was reading. "TRAINS CRASH IN FOG," ran the banner headlines, "10 DEAD, MANY INJURED." I reflected on our speed, the dense fog outside, and had a mild, transitory moment of concern that the fog might claim us victim, too, and then relaxed as I picked up the novel I had been reading. Some minutes later the thought suddenly entered my mind that had I not "chickened out" about flying, I might at that moment be overhead in a plane. At the mere image of sitting up there strapped in by a seat belt, my hands began to sweat, my heart to beat perceptibly faster, and I felt a kind of nervous uneasiness in my gut. The sensation lasted until I forced myself back to my book and forgot about the imagery.

I must say I found this experience a vivid lesson in the nature of phobias. Here I had reacted with hardly a flicker of concern to an admittedly small but real danger of accident, as evidenced by the fog-caused train crash an hour or two earlier. But at the same time I had responded to a purely imaginary situation with an unpleasant start of nervousness, experienced as both somatic symptoms and an inner sense of indescribable dread so characteristic of anxiety. The unreasonableness of the latter was highlighted for me by its contrast with the absence of concern about the speeding train, which if I had worried about it, would have been an apprehension grounded on real, external circumstances.

This account needs little further explanation, except to point out that (1) in the phobic disorders, anxiety is a central component, no longer free floating or unexpected, as in panic disorder without agoraphobia, but attached to a specific object, activity, or situation; (2) either the anxiety is not justified by the stimulus that provokes it, or it is out of proportion to the real situation; and (3) the sufferers are completely aware that their reactions are irrational. Although the features that characterize most phobic disorders are clear, it can sometimes be difficult to decide whether the response to the external situation is, in fact, justifiable. It is clearly reasonable to experience fear in the face of an enemy charging with a loaded gun; equally clearly, it is completely irrational to experience terror when venturing out onto a peaceful street. In between these two ends of the spectrum lie many situations in which the absence of a quantitative measure of the degree of the external danger and of the level of anxiety makes the assessment of the reasonableness of the response a matter of imprecise clinical judgment.

HISTORY

Samuel Johnson's monumental fear of death or the request of Mr. Purrier in 1794 that he be excused from jury duty because he came "very near fainting . . . in all crowded places," as cited in *The Trial of John Horne Tooke for High Treason,* demonstrates that phobias have long been a part of human experience. Historically, phobias were viewed as personal eccentricities of human behavior, and despite their mention in the Hippocratic corpus and Burton's treatise on melancholia, phobias were not generally considered a matter for clinical concern until the middle of the nineteenth century. At that point, the phenomenon began to interest the clinician. Men like Karl Westphal and Legrand du Salle, both of whom published studies of agoraphobia, led the way for later investigators, who compiled long lists of phobias, naming each in resounding Greek or Latin terms after the object or situation feared. The patient who was spared the pangs of taphophobia (fear of being buried alive) or ailurophobia (fear of cats) might yet fall prey to belonophobia (fear of needles), siderodromophobia (fear of railways), or triskaidekaphobia (fear of 13 persons at a table). Pantaphobia was the diagnostic fate of that unfortunate soul who suffered from them all.

The genius for taxonomy reflected in this erudite name calling was not matched by a similar facility in the clinical classification of the whole spectrum of neurotic symptoms. The neurotic symptoms, with the possible exception of the more dramatic hysterical phenomena, had in previous centuries generally escaped the notice of clinicians, whose attention had always been focused on the major aberrations of the psychoses. The neurological interests of Jean Charcot and his pupils led them to an exhaustive study of hysteria, and George Beard's development of the concept of neurasthenia in the 1870s and 1880s introduced a new clinical entity into the family of neuroses. It was Pierre Janet, however, who first attempted a comprehensive classification of neurotic disorders.

Janet's system had two major divisions: hysteria, which denoted the disturbances in sensation, movement, and consciousness still today considered by many to be the cardinal symptoms of that syndrome; and psychasthenia, which included most of the remaining neurotic phenomena: anxiety, phobias, obsessions, depression, fatigue, tics, and so on. For Janet, the phobia was simply one emotional manifestation of a disorder that had a host of other visceral and emotional expressions as well.

It was not until Sigmund Freud that the nosology of neurotic disorder began to take on a modern look, and one might almost say that what Emil Kraepelin accomplished for the classification of the psychoses, Freud did for the neuroses. The fame of Freud's psychoanalytic theories has overshadowed the brilliance of his early attempts to distinguish among the various neurotic syndromes. In a cluster of papers published between 1893 and 1895, he laid the groundwork for his classificatory scheme, which was based on his extensive clinical experience. His view of the clinical phenomena that he observed was determined in good part by his early psychodynamic theoretical formulations, which gave him a rationale for separating out several distinct disorders.

After returning to Vienna following his early work with Charcot, Freud turned first to a study of hysteria. He soon recognized that the concept of conversion, although it explained the formation of somatosensory hysterical symptoms, could not do the same for a number of neurotic manifestations in which a variety of affects—doubt, remorse, anger, anxiety—remained in the consciousness. Initially, therefore, he assigned phobias and obsessions to a separate diagnostic category. Almost at once he was struck by the special relationship of anxiety to the phobia, and he then made a further taxonomic separation between phobic neurosis and obsessive-compulsive neurosis. At almost the same time, he distinguished a further clinical entity, anxiety neurosis, which was characterized by free-floating anxiety.

The four diagnostic categories—with the addition of the depressive neurosis, to which Freud gave little attention as a specific entity—remained as the basis of the taxonomy of the neuroses until the diagnostic reorganization proposed by the third edition of the *Diagnostic and Statistical Manual of Mental Disorders* (DSM-III). It is true that Freud subsequently proposed that the term "anxiety hysteria" be substituted for "phobic neurosis," but apart from its frequent use by psychoanalysts, the term anxiety hysteria has not been generally accepted. The influence of Adolf Meyer, as well as their clincal experiences during World War II, led American psychiatrists to speak diagnostically of reactions, rather than neuroses, a practice that was reflected in the first edition of the *Diagnostic and Statistical Manual of Mental Disorders* (DSM-I), which referred to phobic reaction. The second edition (DSM-II), in an attempt to bring American taxonomy closer to international usage, reverted to the term "phobic neurosis," which was replaced in DSM-III by "phobic disorders." In DSM-III, phobic disorders represented one of the three major subcategories, along with anxiety states and post-traumatic stress disorder, of the anxiety disorders. These major subcategories were eliminated in DSM-III-R, and the traditional disorders of social phobia, simple phobia, and agoraphobia without panic attacks are simply listed as separate entities in this new classificatory scheme. Given the phenomenological overlap and the historical conceptualization of phobic syndromes as closely linked cousins in terms of psychopathology, the DSM-III-R anxiety disorders of simple phobia, social phobia, and agoraphobia without panic attacks will be discussed in this section under the traditional heading of phobic disorders.

EPIDEMIOLOGY

Until recently, the incidence, gender distributions, and natural history of simple phobias and agoraphobia were poorly understood. A 1979 symptom-checklist survey of psychotherapeutic drug use found an incidental 1-year prevalence for agoraphobia-panic and nonagoraphobic phobias of 1.2 percent and 2.3 percent, respectively. There appears to be a tight relationship between panic attacks and agoraphobia, with the latter symptom almost always developing at a later time than panic attacks in the natural course of illness.

Although agoraphobic patients without a history of panic attacks are rarely seen in treatment facilities, data from a recent National Institute of Mental Health (NIMH) Epidemiologic Catchment Area (ECA) study, as interpreted by some investigators, indicate that agoraphobia without panic attacks might not be a rare condition. The current information indicates that the onset of agoraphobia, with or without panic attacks, is in the mid 20s and occurs more frequently in women than men. There appears to be no association between agoraphobia and education, religion, or race.

With the exception of social phobias and agoraphobia, DSM-III-R classifies all specific phobias as simple phobias. Some investigators question this diagnostic scheme and have suggested that blood–injury–illness phobias be distinguished from animal and other specific (nonagoraphobia) phobias on the basis of a unique physiological response to phobic exposure. Although many young children develop animal and insect fears, the onset of most simple phobias is during the teenage years. Prognosis is generally excellent for childhood phobias, with many resolving spontaneously without treatment. Clinical experience suggests, however, that adult-onset simple phobias, or childhood phobias that persist into adulthood, remit less frequently and, therefore, often require treatment. The recent ECA study found simple phobias to be approximately twice as common in women than men.

The lifetime prevalence, morbidity, and risk factors of social phobia are poorly understood. Unlike agoraphobia and simple phobias, there is no female predominance with social phobias. The onset of social phobia is in the teenage years; shyness and blushing have been suggested as early variants of the illness.

ETIOLOGY

PSYCHOLOGICAL ASPECTS

Janet's theories Explanations of neurotic disorders in the early-nineteenth century were based primarily on the idea of the hereditary degeneration of the central nervous system (CNS). However, it was Janet who first attempted to give a systematic and detailed presentation of the psychological mechanisms underlying the origin of neurotic disorders.

According to Janet, phobias were ultimately the result of the constitutionally based lowering of nervous energy, a concept that remained for him the starting point of all processes leading to neurotic illness. The consequent impairment of the highest mental functions of will and purposeful, constructive action, which enabled healthy persons to live and work effectively in the real world of people and things was followed by an emergence of less complex nervous and mental functions. Prominent among those functions were discharges of the autonomic nervous system manifested as the symptoms of anxiety, and when those symptoms were combined with a pathologically heightened attention to bodily functions or to objects or situations in the external world, a phobic symptom was the result.

Freud's earlier theories From the outset, Freud's basic theoretical assumptions were the obverse of Janet's. Freud viewed neurotic phenomena as the result not of a lowering of nervous energy but of its heightening caused by the force of repression, which blocked normal avenues of discharge and forced it into substitute physical and psychological channels that produced neurotic symptoms. In his early formulations, however, Freud was not always clear, either in his own mind or in his exposition, about the details of the mechanism of symptom formation. That lack of clarity is particularly evident in his explanation of the production of phobias, and the history of his ideas concerning that symptom is intimately connected with the general development of psychoanalytic theory over the 3 decades of his scientific work and writing.

Freud early made a clinical separation between hysteria, on

the one hand, and phobias and obsessions, on the other hand. In hysteria, the affect associated with an idea unacceptable to the ego was converted into a somatic symptom, and both the idea and its related affect disappeared from consciousness. In his earliest theoretical formulation, Freud postulated a different mechanism for the formation of both phobias and obsessions. In those conditions the offending affect—anger, remorse, shame, anxiety—was not converted into a somatic symptom, but continued to be consciously experienced. It did not, however, remain attached to the unacceptable idea, but was transferred to another seemingly harmless conscious idea, object, or situation. That idea, object, or situation was related in special ways to the original affect-producing idea, which now disappeared from consciousness. What remained in the patient's awareness was an apparently insignificant idea, object, or situation that, through the mechanism of displacement, became associated with a painful affect. Anxiety, for example, originally attached to a sexual thought that was now unconscious, could be transferred to the situation of walking alone on the streets, an action that then produced what seemed to be senseless anxiety. In other words, the patient was observed to be suffering from agoraphobia.

After the initial formulation, two almost simultaneous developments in Freud's thinking led to a revision of the theory: (1) He recognized that phobias could be separated from obsessions because the phobias were always associated with anxiety, whereas anxiety was not necessarily present in obsessions. (2) His clinical observations led him to theorize that anxiety was the direct result of a physiological transformation of undischarged sexual energy. On that basis, Freud proposed that anxiety neurosis be considered a distinct clinical entity and, furthermore, that phobias be viewed as a manifestation of that syndrome. He stated that anxiety might be manifested clinically in a free-floating state as chronic apprehensiveness or acute anxiety attacks unaccompanied by ideation. In the form of a phobia, anxiety could also find channels of discharge in connection with ideas, objects, or situations intimately associated with it. Such an association came from two sources: (1) Some objects or situations, like snakes or darkness, were inherently frightening to human beings and provided ready-made avenues of expression for the libido-derived anxiety. (2) In other cases, the initial outbreak of pathological anxiety had occurred in a particular situation (e.g., while the patient was walking on the street), which thereafter, because of the initial chance association, remained an outlet for the discharge of affect. In that new formulation, the phobia was no longer classed with obsessions as a symptom resulting from the psychological process of a transference of affects. No psychological elaboration was involved in the production of a phobia. It was merely a form of anxiety, itself a nonpsychological physiological transformation of undischarged libido.

From the start, Freud was never completely satisified with that more biological view of the phobia. First, he recognized that anxiety was, in some instances, a reaction of the ego to dangerous situations and not merely a physiological transformation of somatic energies. Second, he was aware that psychical elaborations contributed to the final clinical manifestations of some phobias. Apart from a tangential allusion to hysterical phobias, however, he did not pursue that line of thought until 15 years after those initial formulations.

LITTLE HANS With the publication in 1909 of the case study of Little Hans, the many interim elaborations of Freud's theory of mental functioning became apparent. Those elaborations developed into a new explanation of the production of phobic symptoms. That explanation in turn invoked the operation of psychological mechanisms that were seen in part as being psychic operations aimed at relieving the individual of anxiety and psychic tension. The development of Freud's views is evident in his study of the little 5-year-old Hans, who suffered from a phobia of horses. Anxiety is still viewed as resulting from a physiological transformation of nervous energy, the normal discharge of which has been blocked, but the energy subjected to transformation is now thought to be not libido alone but any affect that has been unable to find an avenue to expression. Furthermore, the factors leading to a blocking of discharge of the affects are not viewed merely as arising from fortuitous environmental circumstances, such as enforced sexual continence or coitus interruptus, but as the result of the psychological mechanism of repression. Repression is a psychological concept, and in the new explanatory model, it is seen as the agent that renders unacceptable affects unconscious and blocks their discharge. In other words, although anxiety is still viewed as physiological in its immediate origins, a psychological element has been introduced into the new model.

In his theoretical conception of phobia formation, Freud went even further in the direction of psychology. The repressed affects, he postulated, were at least partially projected onto the external world. Aggression toward an object, for example, was projected by the individual onto the object, which was then seen as itself being aggressive toward the person and, as such, became a source of anxiety. The person could now find relief from the painful anxiety by avoiding the object that produced it. There was, furthermore, yet another psychological elaboration in Freud's new theory. The anxiety attached to the object was subjected to a further psychological process, which he called *displacement*. This object was transferred or displaced to another object that was connected to the first by associative links that allowed the second object to symbolize the first.

Those mechanisms were well demonstrated in the case of Little Hans. His naturally occurring oedipal libidinal strivings for his mother and his rivalrous aggression toward his father were repressed as forces unacceptable to his developing ego. Unable to find an outlet for discharge because of repression, these drives were partially transformed into anxiety. At the same time, some of Little Hans's aggressive energy was projected outward onto his father, whom he now saw as a dangerous person and who, therefore, became a source of anxiety. It still was difficult, however, for Little Hans to find relief from his painful anxiety, because his father who provoked it was constantly present and impossible to avoid. A further psychic mechanism was required to obtain relief, which was found in the displacement of the anxiety engendered by his father onto horses, objects that in Little Hans's experiences had been associatively linked with his conflict and could therefore act symbolically as the carrier of the anxiety. Because horses could be avoided, Hans could escape from anxiety by staying away from places where horses were to be found.

In that scheme, the phobia was viewed as having a complex structure involving a number of psychic mechanisms that shaped the ultimate clinical manifestations of the anxiety, which had initially been produced by physiological processes. The explanation thus offered was a much more elaborate and psychologically sophisticated model than its predecessor of 15 years earlier. In a final elaboration, Freud applied his new model to phobias in adults: The mechanisms of symptom production were the same as in children, with the additional proposition that the psychic processes involved in the adult phobia were a recapitulation of a similar phobic neurosis in the childhood of the patient—an earlier neurosis that had not been resolved and hence provided a psychogenetic basis for the adult illness.

Current psychoanalytic theories It was not until 17 years later, in *Inhibitions, Symptoms and Anxiety,* published in 1926, that Freud reached his final formulation of the phobic neurosis, which has remained in its essentials the analytic explanation of the disorder. In that monograph, Freud took a new view of the place of anxiety in the psychic economy. Reviving an idea he had briefly mentioned 30 years before—that anxiety could be the ego's reactions to danger—Freud now proposed that the quality of being a response was anxiety's primary attribute, the response being to a danger arising not only from perilous external situations but also from inner drives and affects that were unacceptable and threatening to the ego. The major function of anxiety was to signal to the ego that a forbidden unconscious drive was pushing for conscious expression, thus alerting the ego to strengthen and marshal its defenses against the threatening instinctual force. In that new view, anxiety was seen not as the result of repression, which set in motion the transformation of affects and drives, but as the cause of repression through its stimulating the ego to take defensive action. Anxiety had come full circle from having been a physiological concept to becoming a psychological one.

In that new theoretical framework, Freud viewed the phobic disorder—or anxiety hysteria, as he continued to call it—as resulting from conflicts centered on an unresolved childhood oedipal situation. In the adult, because the sexual drive continued to have a strong incestuous coloring, its arousal tended to cause anxiety that was characteristically a fear of castration. The anxiety then alerted the ego to exert repression to keep the drive away from conscious representation and discharge, but, repression failing to be entirely successful in its function, it was necessary for the ego to call on auxiliary defenses. In phobic patients, the defenses, arising from an earlier phobic response during the initial childhood period of the oedipal conflict, primarily used displacement; that is, the sexual conflict was transposed or displaced from the person who evoked the conflict to a seemingly unimportant, irrelevant object or situation, which now had the power to arouse the entire constellation of affects, including signal anxiety. On examination, it can usually be determined that the phobic object or situation thus selected has a direct associative connection with the primary source of the conflict and has thus come naturally to symbolize it. Furthermore, the situation or object is usually such that the patient is able to keep out of its way and, by this additional mechanism of defense of avoidance, can escape suffering from serious anxiety.

This theoretical formulation of phobia formation, which attributes the phobia to the use of the ego defense mechanisms of displacement and avoidance against incestuous oedipal-genital drives and castration anxiety, is illustrated in the following case:

A woman of 28 years of age suffered from a severe phobia of boats and was so terrified of even a picture of a ship that she would have to dismiss it hastily from her sight. During therapy she gradually revealed her intense interest in but fear of sexuality, which was colored by frightening fantasies of the mutilation of the female genitals that, she imagined, resulted from sexual intercourse. It was at length discovered that her symptoms had started after a brief experimental sexual affair in adolescence that had taken place on her boyfriend's boat. At the time, she was convinced that her mother knew what she was doing, and the young woman was so upset by what she felt was her mother's disapproval that she had terminated the relationship with her friend. Not long afterward, her phobia of boats erupted. Ultimately, her associations led her back to loving and sexual feelings toward her father during her childhood, which at the time had been a source of intense guilt and anxiety. From these observations, it was clear that, through the mechanism of displacement and because of their association with the sexual activity that had initially aroused her anxiety, boats had come to be the symbol of the patient's sexual conflict, which was manifested clinically as a simple phobia.

Although all the theoretical ingredients of the phobia are to be seen in the patient described above, that combination of characteristics is by no means always the case. Since Freud's formulation, other investigators, without altering its basic structure, have made extensions or changes in the details of the theory to bring it into agreement with observations that often seemed initially to contradict what Freud had proposed. These revisions fall into three main categories: (1) Writers like Kurt Lewin developed the theory of the processes by which the phobic facade is created, pointing out the similarity between the manifest content of dreams and the associative links that tie the phobic object or situation to the basic conflict—an observation that Freud himself had recognized. (2) It has been demonstrated that, in addition to castration anxiety, other forms of anxiety, notably separation anxiety, are prominent in many phobias. (3) Clinical observations indicate that aggression and pregenital sexual drives, as well as oedipal sexuality, may contribute to the formation of phobic symptoms, such as the scoptophilic impulse in its relation to erythrophobia.

The clinical observations relevant to the mechanisms involved in phobia formation, including the more recent additions to the theoretical formulations, are well illustrated in a patient treated early in the twentieth century by Morton Prince. His account is made all the more interesting by the fact that his findings led Prince at that early date in the history of analysis to question the exclusive role of sexuality in the etiology of phobic disorders.

The patient was a 40-year-old woman who suffered from a phobia of towers and church steeples and, as it ultimately turned out, of bells. The phobia had begun at some point in her adolescence, although she was vague about the exact time of its onset. Attempts to get her to associate to the symptom caused her to experience anxiety, especially when church bells were mentioned, and many of her associations referred to her long-dead mother. There was nothing, however, that gave a clue to the meaning of the symptoms. At length, as Prince wrote:

"After all endeavors to discover the genesis of the phobia by analysis were in vain, I tried another method. While she was in hypnosis I put a pencil in her hand with the object of obtaining the desired information through automatic writing"—an unusual form of dissociation, in which, without the subject's awareness of what was happening, her hand wrote sentences that contained information or memories not consciously remembered. Prince continued: "While she was narrating some irrelevant memories of her mother, the hand rapidly wrote as follows: "G . . . M . . . church and my father took mother to Bi . . . where she died and we went to Br . . . and they cut my mother. I prayed and cried all the time that she would live and the church bells were always ringing and I hated them."

As she wrote the last of the message, she became anxious and agitated, although she neither knew what she had written nor why she was upset. Later, she was able to tell Prince the events to which the script referred, but with no visible evidence of emotion. Her mother had, indeed, been taken seriously ill while the family was visiting England, had had an operation, and had died. During all that time the patient had prayed frequently for her mother's recovery, often to the accompaniment of the bells in the church tower near by her hotel, which rang every quarter of the hour. Prince wrote: "They got on her nerves; she hated them; she could not bear to hear them, and while she was praying they added to her anguish. Ever since this time the ringing of bells has continued to cause a feeling of anguish."

Not long after this the patient revealed two more bits of significant information. First of all, she confessed, as Prince wrote, that on one occasion she "omitted to go to church to pray and the thought came to her that if her mother died it would be due to this omission, and it would be her fault. . . . When her mother did die she thought it was God's punishment of herself because of that one failure. . . . She thought she was to blame for her mother's death." Furthermore, as an adult she still felt that her mother's death was her fault, a conviction strengthened by another circumstance that she eventually confessed to Prince. Two years before her mother's death, the patient had caught a cold as a result of disobeying her mother's instructions. This was diagnosed as incipient phthisis, and on the doctor's advice her mother had taken her to Europe for an extended cure, during which time the mother's death had occurred: "The patient still believed and argued that if her mother had not been compelled to take her abroad she . . . in all probability would not have died."

Finally, it was discovered that she had similarly blamed herself for her brother's death, which had occurred some time before her mother's death, and as an adult, she always felt that unfortunate events in her life were her fault: "She had been unable on many occasions to leave home on pleasure trips for fear lest some accident might happen within the home and consequently it would be due to her fault; and if away she was in constant dread of something happening for which she would be to blame."

Despite Prince's repeated denials in his discussion of this case, psychiatrists today would perhaps not be quite so certain that there were no sexual, oedipal elements hidden behind the material uncovered by Prince. It is clear from the patient's production and associations that the aggressive impulse played an important part in the formation of her symptoms. Its role was especially evident in her irrational convictions that she was the cause of harm and misfortune. The nature of the process of displacement is particularly well illustrated in the symptom of the bells. A small and seemingly insignificant fragment of the entire panoply of sights and sounds that comprised the patient's experience during the period of her mother's illness and death came symbolically to represent the whole. In that role, the bells carried the full charge of the patient's emotions, including her painful guilty anxiety, which were displaced from their central source, her relationship with her mother, to one small part of her perceptions—a part, however, that was intimately and associatively linked to the whole. From then on, by avoiding the part, by refraining from thinking of bells, and by trying to keep out of their way in her external environment, she was able to escape the full force of the anxiety and despair about her mother's death, emotions that were still actively alive in her 25 years after the event.

Finally, mention should be made of the obsessional aspects of the patient's conflict. As the therapy progressed, there emerged from behind her phobic symptoms evidence of a morbid preoccupation with ideas of disaster for which she would in some way be responsible. The intrusive quality of these thoughts, as well as the fact that they involved her in the active role of an aggressor, place them in the class of obsessive phenomena. It is observations such as these, as well as the existence of symptoms with mixed phobic and obsessional characteristics and the presence of compulsive traits in the character structure of some patients with phobias, that have led many clinicians to place the phobic disorders between hysteria and obsessive-compulsive disorder in the spectrum of neurotic syndromes.

CONDITIONED REFLEX THEORIES In 1920, John B. Watson, with his collaborator Rosalie Rayner, published a communication in the *Journal of Experimental Psychology*. Entitled "Conditioned Emotional Reactions," it recounted their experiences with Little Albert, an infant with a phobia of rats and rabbits. Unlike Freud's Little Hans, who had developed symptoms in the natural course of his maturation, Little Albert's difficulties were the direct result of the scientific ingenuity of two experimental psychologists, who dispassionately employed techniques that had successfully induced conditioned responses in laboratory animals.

At the age of 11 months, Albert was an apparently happy, placid baby, and in fact, as the authors state, his "stability was one of the principal reasons for using him as a subject in this test." Systematically exposed to a whole battery of objects, such as rats, rabbits, dogs, and a variety of masks, he showed no response whatsoever of fear or concern. The only stimulus that caused him any alarm was the sudden sharp noise that occurred when the experimenters banged an iron bar behind his head. With that baseline established, the investigators began their work. Presenting Albert with a white rat to which he reached out without evident concern, they simultaneously vigorously struck the iron bar behind his head. Startled, Albert withdrew from the rat. After several such conditioning procedures in rapid succession, the experimenters discovered that the subject withdrew from the rat alone. The experimental session was then terminated.

Seven days later, the investigators made an interesting observation. When Albert was presented with the rat unaccompanied by the unconditioned stimulus, he began at once to cry and crawled away from it with such sudden speed that he almost fell off the edge of the experimental table before he could be stopped. Twelve days later, another phenomenon was observed. Again without benefit of the unconditioned stimulus, Albert reacted with alarm to the rat, but what was even more fascinating was that he showed the same response to a rabbit, a fur coat, and, to a lesser degree, a dog, although the last three had never been presented in conjunction with the unconditioned stimulus. When after 17 days, Albert's conditioned response was beginning to wane, it was reinforced by the further introduction of the retrocephalic banging of the iron bar. One month later, the subject having passed his first birthday, he was observed to manifest a continued strong reaction of aversion to rats, dogs, fur coats, and a mask of Santa Claus with a long white beard.

From this series of experimental observations, it was evident that a conditioned reflex could be produced in the human being that had all the appearance of a clinical phobia. Moreover, the fear component of the conditioned response was spontaneously generalized to objects not combined with the unconditioned stimulus, just as in the naturally occurring syndrome there is a tendency toward broadening the range of phobic objects and situations. The authors concluded that the model derived from conditioning psychology explained the phobic symptom and that the more elaborate elements of Freudian theory involving sexuality, repression, and other mental mechanisms were superfluous.

The subsequent course of Watson's and Rayner's subject could not be ascertained, because, as the authors reported: "Unfortunately Albert was taken from the hospital the day the above tests were made. Hence the opportunity of building up an experimental technique by means of which we could remove the conditioned emotional response was denied us." Their theoretical explanation of the formation of phobias has, however, played an increasingly important role in recent years in the understanding and treatment of patients with phobic disorders.

Watson's formulation accounts for the initial creation of the phobia with the traditional Pavlovian stimulus–response model of the conditioned reflex. Anxiety that has been aroused by a naturally and inherently frightening stimulus occurs in contiguity with a second naturally and inherently neutral stimulus. As a result of the contiguity, especially when the two stimuli are paired on several successive occasions, the originally neutral stimulus takes on the capacity for arousing anxiety by itself; that is, it becomes a conditioned stimulus for anxiety production. That effect can be clearly observed in both Watson's experimental subject and Prince's patient, and as a concept, it has a close affinity to Freud's early theoretical model of the displacement of anxiety from one idea to another.

In the classical stimulus–response theory, the conditioned stimulus was seen as gradually losing its potency to arouse a response if it was not reinforced by a periodic repetition of the unconditioned stimulus. In the phobic symptom, that attenuation of the response to the phobic (conditioned) stimulus does not occur, and the symptom may last for years without any apparent external reinforcement. In the more recently formulated operant conditioning theory, however, a model is provided for explaining that phenomenon. In the new theory, anxiety is viewed as a drive that motivates the organism suffering from it to do what it can to obviate the painful affect. In the course of its random behavior, the animal soon learns that certain actions enable it to avoid the stimulus to anxiety and the consequent experience of pain. The avoidance patterns thus set up remain stable for long periods of time as a result of the reinforcement that those patterns receive from their success in drive reduction—that is, their capacity to diminish anxiety. That model is readily applicable to the phobia in which avoidance of the anxiety-provoking object or situation plays a central part. Such avoidance behavior, clinically observable as the manifestations of phobias, becomes fixed as a stable symptom because of its effectiveness in protecting the patient from the phobic anxiety.

Learning theory has a particular relevance to phobic disorders, as it supplies simple and intelligible explanations of many aspects of phobic symptoms. In its present form, however, learning theory deals more with the surface mechanisms of symptom formation and is perhaps less useful in explaining some of the more complex underlying psychic processes that are involved—processes to which analytic observations, concepts, and theories are addressed. Nonetheless, the phobic disorder provides an important meeting ground for both analytic and learning theorists, and it is in that clinical area that future clinical investigators from both disciplines should be able to define the significant differences and similarities between the two theoretical models.

BIOLOGICAL ASPECTS Emerging evidence suggests that biological as well as phenomenological, natural history, demographic, and treatment-response variables can separate the anxiety disorders. Although a biological dissection of the anxiety disorders is expected to lead to more specific and effective pharmacological and psychosocial treatments, no neuropathological condition has been identified as a direct and exclusive cause of pathological anxiety states.

Agoraphobia One theoretical formulation suggests that agoraphobia is a residual, or secondary, complication of unprovoked or spontaneous panic attacks. That is, panic attacks are thought to play a primary role in the pathogenesis of most agoraphobic conditions. If this is true, the core biological substrate of panic disorder without agoraphobia would be identical to panic disorder with agoraphobia.

Consistent with this hypothesis, several studies investigating the relationship between panic disorder with agoraphobia and panic disorder without agoraphobia have found similar disturbances in neuroendocrine function, supporting the DSM-III-R emphasis on panic attacks as playing a central role in the pathogenesis of most agoraphobic conditions. Thus, a great deal is understood about the neurobiology of agoraphobia associated with panic attacks. Agoraphobia with limited symptom attacks is generally thought to represent simply a less severe variant of panic disorder with agoraphobia.

Despite the wealth of knowledge regarding panic-related agoraphobia, a biological profile of agoraphobia without a history of panic disorder is virtually nonexistent. It is of interest that panic disorder with agoraphobia may be associated with a higher female–male ratio than agoraphobia without panic attacks.

Simple phobias Biological studies of simple phobias have often employed methods that assume that stress and anxiety are closely related conditions. Although stress responses and anxiety may be related phenomena, the reader should be cautioned not to assume a common pathogenesis. Nonetheless, the well-documented changes following stress in animals and the endocrine and cardiovascular responses following phobic exposure in humans provide worthwhile tools for the study of simple phobias.

In a series of studies at the University of Michigan, patients with simple phobias were exposed to their relevant feared objects (e.g., animals), and the neuroendocrine and physiological changes associated with this exposure-induced anxiety were documented. On exposure, the patients experienced severe anxiety, as evidenced by cringing, gooseflesh, screaming, weeping, sweating, and tremors. Associated with this phobic anxiety was a statistically significant increase in their systolic and diastolic blood pressure, pulse rate, norepinephrine, epinephrine, insulin, cortisol, and growth hormone. Despite the statistically significant changes in these physiological and biochemical indices, many of the changes (e.g., cortisol) were relatively unimpressive given the extreme nature of the anxious response. In fact, the profile and magnitude of neuroendocrine responses to stress, phobic exposure and related paradigms are often transient, inconsistent, and variable across subjects. These findings and evidence from other laboratories suggest that neuroendocrine, particularly measures of hypothalamic-pituitary-adrenal function, and physiological responses may be dissociated from the subjective experience of context-specific anxiety, or cued anxiety. Unconfirmed data suggest that, during in vivo exposure, levels of plasma glucagon, thyroid-stimulating hormone, and prolactin do not significantly change in patients with simple phobias.

Although elevated catecholamine levels also have been associated with public-speaking phobias, the lack of consistent and sustained changes in most biological measures during in vivo exposure underscores the current inability to use neurochemical or psychophysiological indices as diagnostic tests or validity measures of stress or anxiety in either the clinical or the research setting.

The type of simple phobia with probably the most characteristic physiological response (e.g., blood–injury–illness phobia) is infrequently encountered in psychiatric treatment centers. Data from several investigations suggest that blood–injury–illness phobias may deserve a separate classification from the other phobic disorders. Patients with these phobias often report a history of trauma related to the phobic stimuli, and unlike other anxiety disorders, a true syncopal episode is not uncommon when these patients are exposed to the specific phobic stimulus (e.g., blood or injection). It has been suggested that the syncope is vasovagal in character, with a diphasic pattern characterized by an initial period of tachycardia and elevated blood pressure followed by a rebound phase of parasympathetic overarousal.

Social phobia Little is known about the neurobiology of social phobia. Preliminary but unsubstantiated evidence indicates that patients with social phobias may be lactate insensitive, compared with panic-disorder patients. Social phobics have been reported to have a greater number of spontaneous fluctuations in galvanic skin response than simple phobics.

CLINICAL SIGNS AND SYMPTOMS

ONSET With the exception of certain simple phobias and the school phobias of childhood, phobic disorders usually begin in the late teens or early adulthood and are generally sudden in onset, heralded by the outburst of an attack of anxiety in the face of what is destined from that time on to be the phobic object or situation. More often than not, the reason for the appearance of symptoms is not immediately apparent.

SYMPTOMS The phobia is the central and diagnostic symptom of phobic disorders. Phobias are characterized by the arousal in the patient of severe anxiety, often mounting to terror, in circumstances specific to each individual—circumstances that do not in reality warrant the emotional reactions that are evoked. In many patients the anxiety may be compounded by a feeling of depersonalization, although that feeling is by no means an essential element of the phobic symptom. As a secondary response to their intense discomfort, patients do everything in their power to avoid the situations that stimulate their phobic anxiety.

Although the kinds of phobic circumstances that clinicians have described are legion, a few are found with great regularity and probably account for the majority of the clinically significant phobic disorders. Most common are fears of streets and open spaces; of crowded, enclosed places, such as churches and theaters; and of vehicles of transportation, most notably airplanes. The degree of the syndrome's severity, as well as the incapacity resulting from it, depends on the practical significance of the phobic circumstances for the patient. A phobia of airplanes that is a mere unpleasant curiosity to the person who does not have to fly can be a source of great discomfort, if not outright incapacity, to those individuals whose work requires them to make frequent long trips by air. It is obvious that patients whose agoraphobia keeps them confined to their homes are as incapacitated as if they had a severely crippling physical lesion. Under the best of circumstances, persons with phobic symptoms find their lives constricted to some degree.

PHOBIC CIRCUMSTANCES Janet described three major categories of circumstances associated with phobic anxiety: phobias of objects, phobias of situations, and phobias of function. Janet's schematization is reflected in the classification in DSM-III-R of phobias into simple phobias, agoraphobia without panic attacks, and social phobias.

Simple phobias (phobias of objects) In *Grace Abounding to the Chief of Sinners,* John Bunyan tells how his simple boyhood pleasure in ringing the bells in the parish church of Elstow was outlawed by his stern Puritan conscience:

> Now, you must know that before this I had taken much delight in ringing, but my conscience beginning to be tender, I thought such practice was but vain, and therefore forced myself to leave it, yet my mind hankered; wherefore I should go to the steeple house, and look on it, though I durst not ring. But I thought this did not become religion neither, yet I forced myself, and would look on still; but quickly after, I began to think, how, if one of the bells should fall? Then I chose to stand under a main beam, that lay overthwart the steeple, from side to side, thinking there I might stand sure, but then I should think again, should the bell fall with a swing, it might first hit the wall, and then rebounding upon me, might kill me for all this beam. This made me stand in the steeple door, and now, thought I, I am safe enough; for if a bell should then fall, I can slip out behind these thick walls, and so be preserved not withstanding.
>
> So, after this, I would yet go to see them ring, but would not go farther than the steeple door, but then it came into my head, How, if the steeple itself should fall? And this thought, it may fall for aught I know, when I stood and looked on, did continually so shake my mind, that I durst not stand at the steeple door any longer, but was forced to flee, for fear the steeple should fall upon my head.

A better or more beautifully described phobic disorder could hardly be found, and in his simple, biblical prose, Bunyan makes clear not only the overwhelming power of his anxiety but also the absurdity of his fear. The tower of nearby Ely Cathedral had indeed collapsed in the early fourteenth century, but in the intervening 3 centuries there could have been few if any others that had met a similar fate, and the statistical chances that the catastrophe Bunyan dreaded would occur were infinitesimally small. In this passage, Bunyan also demonstrates a further common feature of phobias, their tendency to spread. At first, it is just the straight plunge of the bell that he fears, then its bouncing course, and finally the complete crashing destruction of the whole steeple, so that he had to take ever and ever greater measures of avoidance to escape his doom. The DSM-III-R criteria for simple phobia are listed in Table 18.2-1.

Agoraphobia (phobias of situations) Agoraphobia is popularly interpreted as being a fear of open spaces, but as is properly recognized in DSM-III-R (Table 18.2-2), it has wider implications. Agoraphobic patients are generally thrown into a state of trepidation and severe anxiety when they are forced into a feared situation or condition in which help upon incapacitation would be unavailable. Both open places and public places pose a threat to such patients, particularly such areas as crowded stores, public transportation, elevators, or theaters from which they can find no ready es-

TABLE 18.2-1
Diagnostic Criteria for Simple Phobia

A. A persistent fear of a circumscribed stimulus (object or situation) other than fear of having a panic attack (as in panic disorder) or of humiliation or embarrassment in certain social situations (as in social phobia).
Note: Do not include fears that are part of panic disorder with agoraphobia or agoraphobia without history of panic disorder.
B. During some phase of the disturbance, exposure to the specific phobic stimulus (or stimuli) almost invariably provokes an immediate anxiety response.
C. The object or situation is avoided, or endured with intense anxiety.
D. The fear or the avoidant behavior significantly interferes with the person's normal routine or with usual social activities or relationships with others, or there is marked distress about having the fear.
E. The person recognizes that his or her fear is excessive or unreasonable.
F. The phobic stimulus is unrelated to the content of the obsessions of obsessive-compulsive disorder or the trauma of post-traumatic stress disorder.

Table from DSM-III-R *Diagnostic and Statistical Manual of Mental Disorders,* ed 3, revised. Copyright American Psychiatric Association, Washington, DC, 1987. Used with permission.

TABLE 18.2-2
Diagnostic Criteria for Agoraphobia Without History of Panic Disorder

A. Agoraphobia: Fear of being in places or situations from which escape might be difficult (or embarrassing) or in which help might not be available in the event of suddenly developing a symptom(s) that could be incapacitating or extremely embarrassing. Examples include: dizziness or falling, depersonalization or derealization, loss of bladder or bowel control, vomiting, or cardiac distress. As a result of this fear, the person either restricts travel or needs a companion when away from home, or else endures agoraphobic situations despite intense anxiety. Common agoraphobic situations include being outside the home alone, being in a crowd or standing in a line, being on a bridge, and traveling in a bus, train, or car.
B. Has never met the criteria for panic disorder.
Specify with or **without limited symptom attacks**

Table from DSM-III-R *Diagnostic and Statistical Manual of Mental Disorders,* ed 3, revised. Copyright American Psychiatric Association, Washington, DC, 1987. Used with permission.

cape from public view. Secondary agoraphobia and anticipatory anxiety begin after the outbreak of a series of panic attacks. Very little is understood about the phenomenology, longitudinal course, and neurobiology of agoraphobia without panic attacks. So infrequently is agoraphobia without panic attacks observed in clinical practice that some investigators have questioned its validity as a distinct entity. As a general rule, agoraphobic patients feel more comfortable when accompanied by a friend or relative. They also tend to avoid phobic stimuli by restricting their activities and excursions to an increasingly smaller area, and in extreme cases, they may be totally confined to their homes.

Social phobias (phobias of function) Central to social phobia is a concern about appearing shameful, stupid, or inept in the presence of others. As indicated in Table 18.2-3, individuals with social phobia fear that their behavior (e.g., talking or writing in public) or one of their bodily functions (e.g., eating, urinating, or blushing) will be the focus of scornful scrutiny by those around them, a fact that often further impairs their performance. Two particular varieties of this class should be noted.

TABLE 18.2-3
Diagnostic Criteria for Social Phobia

A. A persistent fear of one or more situations (the social phobic situations) in which the person is exposed to possible scrutiny by others and fears that he or she may do something or act in a way that will be humiliating or embarrassing. Examples include: being unable to continue talking while speaking in public, choking on food when eating in front of others, being unable to urinate in a public lavatory, hand-trembling when writing in the presence of others, and saying foolish things or not being able to answer questions in social situations.
B. If an Axis III or another Axis I disorder is present, the fear in A is unrelated to it, e.g., the fear is not of having a panic attack (panic disorder), stuttering (stuttering), trembling (Parkinson's disease), or exhibiting abnormal eating behavior (anorexia nervosa or bulimia nervosa).
C. During some phase of the disturbance, exposure to the specific phobic stimulus (or stimuli) almost invariably provokes an immediate anxiety response.
D. The phobic situation(s) is avoided, or is endured with intense anxiety.
E. The avoidant behavior interferes with occupational functioning or with usual social activities or relationships with others, or there is marked distress about having the fear.
F. The person recognizes that his or her fear is excessive or unreasonable.
G. If the person is under 18, the disturbance does not meet the criteria for avoidant disorder of childhood or adolescence.

Specify generalized type if the phobic situation includes most social situations, and also consider the additional diagnosis of avoidant personality disorder.

Table from DSM-III-R *Diagnostic and Statistical Manual of Mental Disorders,* ed 3, revised. Copyright American Psychiatric Association, Washington, DC, 1987. Used with permission.

Erythrophobia (fear of blushing) can be a particulary painful and stubborn symptom. Janet considered it a phobia of situation for reasons that are not entirely clear, except that the symptom is restricted to situations in which other people are present. Patients, commonly women, are terrified that they will blush in the company of others and are convinced that in that state they will be highly visible and, consequently, the center of painful attention. If questioned, patients cannot say what is so dreadful about blushing, but it is often evident that shame is an important component of their anxiety. It is of interest that a change in color may not be at all evident to the observer, despite the patients' insistence that they feel bright red. The force of their fear, unfounded as it may be, often leads patients to restrict their social lives severely.

Fear of eating is another troublesome type of social phobia. It may be limited to a dread of eating in the company of others, but in some patients the restriction applies to the intake of food under any circumstances, whether or not the patient is alone. Comment should be made concerning the relation of this symptom to anorexia nervosa. That condition is commonly considered either as a hysterical phenomenon or as belonging to the psychophysiological disorders because of the widespread secondary somatic changes associated with it and because there is evidence that, in many patients, the loss of menses is directly mediated by centrally controlled psychoendocrine and autonomic nervous system mechanisms. However, the psychological disturbance from which all else follows is often a genuine and profound phobia of eating, not a true anorexia. Patients will frequently complain of severe anxiety mounting to panic if they are forced to eat and are able to gain relief only by vomiting or by taking large doses of cathartics in order to get the food out of their bodies. The avoidance of eating to prevent such anxiety is a true phobic mechanism, and in some patients, anorexia nervosa may justifiably be considered a severe type of phobic syndrome.

PSYCHOLOGICAL NATURE OF PHOBIC ANXIETY

It was originally thought, particularly by psychoanalytic investigators, that the fear manifested by phobic patients was a form of castration anxiety. That formulation would, indeed, seem to apply to such symptoms as those described by Freud in the case of Little Hans, in which the central dread is that of bodily injury. On more careful observation, however, it becomes evident that many fears of phobic patients fall into other categories. In agoraphobia, for example, separation anxiety may play an important role, and in erythrophobia, the element of shame implies the involvement of superego anxiety. Although on casual consideration, Bunyan's avoidance of church steeples appears to result from his anticipation of bodily injury, on further reflection one recognizes that he actually dreads total annihilation, an anxiety that is more closely linked to the fear of dissolution that is found at the genetically earlier end of the spectrum. It, therefore, more closely reflects clinical observation to view the anxiety associated with phobias as having a variety of sources and colorings.

COUNTERPHOBIC ATTITUDE

Otto Fenichel noted that phobic anxiety can be hidden behind attitudes and behavior patterns that represent a denial either that the dreaded object or situation is dangerous or that one is afraid of it. Basic to that phenomenon is a reversal of the situation in which one is the passive victim of external circumstances to a position of actively attempting to confront and master what one fears. The counterphobic person, at times with a persistence that is almost obsessional in quality, seeks out situations of danger and rushes enthusiastically toward them; the devotee of dangerous sports like parachute jumping or rock climbing, for example, may be exhibiting counterphobic behavior. Such patterns may be set against neurotic-phobic anxieties or may be used more normally as a means of dealing with realistically dangerous and anxiety-provoking situtations. The play of children may contain counterphobic elements; one example is the common game of playing doctor and giving to one's doll the injection one has received earlier in the day while visiting the pediatrician's office. That pattern of behavior also involves the related mechanism of identification with the aggressor.

PHOBIAS AND OBSESSIONS

In the modern classification of the anxiety disorders, phobias are distinguished from obsessive-compulsive ideas. In the strict sense of the term, the phobia is a phenomenon in which the direction of the fantasied action is from an external danger toward the patient. In obsessive and compulsive ideas, however, the direction is reversed insofar as a fantasy of action is concerned; patients are disturbed about some harmful deed they may have done or are impelled to do to others. Patients with phobias are passive; patients with obsessive-compulsive ideas are active. Furthermore, in the phobia the patients can quiet their anxiety by avoiding the feared external situation, whereas the obsessive-compulsive idea is characterized by the difficulty that patients have in escaping its persistent, forceful intrusion into their consciousness.

Despite the official diagnostic separation of phobias from obsessive-compulsive ideas, there are a number of symptoms that are not easily assigned to one or the other category, but lie along the middle reaches of the spectrum represented at one end by the pure phobias and at the other by pure obsessive-compulsive ideas. In this middle realm, the distinction between the disorders is blurred, because the symptoms share some characteristics of both phobias and obsessive-compulsive ideas. The common phobia of knives or other dangerous objects often rests on the patients' fantasies that they will actively hurt someone else, but at the same time, they are able to control their anxiety by avoiding the dreaded object. The phobia of dirt or disease, however, involves the patients' fears that they will be damaged by the external agent. Yet, the fear has all the intrusiveness of an obsession, and patients cannot avoid the feared object because they imagine it as being everywhere around them and as constantly threatening no matter what they do. Whether one views patients with symptoms like these as having a phobic disorder or an obsessive-compulsive disorder will be determined by the nature of their other symptoms and of the characteristics of their personality structures. Sometimes, one must remain content with placing them in the category of atypical anxiety disorder.

SECONDARY REACTIONS TO PHOBIC SYMPTOMS

Brief mention must be made of certain secondary reactions to phobic symptoms that contribute to the clinical manifestations of phobic disorders. One may observe that some patients with phobias experience a loss of self-esteem related as a feeling of being weak, cowardly, or not so effective and capable as they would like to be. There may be a mild element of depression added to the phobic symptoms. Those patients, however, who have been able to master the phobic anxiety and to carry out an action successfully by facing the phobic situation without giving in to their anxiety may experience a mild sense of pleasant elation, self-confidence, and emotional freedom.

PERSONALITY CHARACTERISTICS OF PHOBIC PATIENTS

There cannot be said to be a specific phobic personality. In some patients, ready access to their feelings and fantasies and the importance of repression as a major mechanism of defense in their personalities place them in the category of the hysterical character. In other patients, reliance on the defensive operations of reaction formation, isolation, and other obsessional mechanisms tends to relegate them to the class of the obsessional character. As was pointed out earlier with regard to symptoms, there appears to be a spectrum of character types ranging from the hysterical to the obsessional, with some types, it must be admitted, also showing passive-dependent features. In this spectrum, some psychoanalytically oriented clinicians view the phobic disorders as falling midway between genital hysteria and the anal obsessive-compulsive neurosis; others consider obsessions and phobias as falling within a single nosological category.

COURSE AND PROGNOSIS

In the absence of extensive studies concerning the natural history of phobic disorders, statements concerning its course and prognosis must be made and received with caution. Clinical experience suggests that most phobic disorders, with the possible exception of childhood fears and phobias, tend to be chronic, with frequent recurrences of symptoms. Some forms of phobic symptoms, particularly agoraphobia, are notoriously difficult to manage and may cause the patient to lead a severely constricted life of psychologically induced incapacitation for years on end. The few systematic reports on patients who have been observed clinically have conflicting conclusions. For example, in a series of 19 patients followed up for an average of 23 years, 12 patients were unchanged and only one was completely free of symptoms. In contrast, in 86 patients followed for years, 67 percent were permanently relieved of symptoms, 24 percent were greatly improved, and only 9 percent showed slight or no change in their condition. The fact that individuals may develop a phobic disorder that disappears spontaneously without their ever having consulted a physician clearly complicates a valid determination of both prevalence and clinical course. It is important to recognize, however, that spontaneous cures are far less likely to occur in patients who have had phobic symptoms for over a year.

DIFFERENTIAL DIAGNOSIS

The relationship of the phobia to fear and obsessive-compulsive phenomena, and the common difficulty of making a sharp distinction between them, were discussed earlier. The clear-cut phobia is, however, not difficult to recognize, and when it constitutes the primary clinical manifestation of an emotional disorder, it places the patient's illness in the DSM-III-R diagnostic category of an anxiety disorder.

Occasionally, however, phobias are found in patients whose illnesses are primarily schizophrenic in nature. At times, the onset of an acute schizophrenic episode may be heralded by the sudden appearance of phobic symptoms, along with other clinical manifestations usually thought of as neurotic, such as obsessions and compulsions. Phobic symptoms may also form part of the syndrome of "pseudoneurotic" schizophrenia. In other cases, the phobia coexists with other mental disturbances characteristic of chronic schizophrenia.

A 34-year old man, for example, suffered from typical agoraphobia. He was generally acutely anxious in crowds, theaters, churches, and other confined spaces, and so he took jobs that would allow him to work outdoors throughout the year. Periodically, he would suddenly disappear from home, invariably turning up a few days later in Wyoming, where he felt that he had enough room and space around him to allow him to be comfortable. Careful examination of the patient's mental status disclosed a number of chronic delusions, which he generally kept to himself so that they were not readily apparent on casual acquaintance. He thought of himself as a brilliant inventor and had a portfolio of crude drawings of unworkable machines; he was convinced that one of those machines, a kind of flying wing, had been stolen by the Air Force, which was putting it into production. He also firmly maintained that he had made a flight into stellar space and had narrowly missed being pulled into the sun's gravitational field.

TREATMENT

The modern clinician has a number of treatment modalities available for the treatment of phobic disorders. Increasing evidence suggests that treatment measures based on the learning theory model and on pharmacotherapy are very effective in the treatment of selective phobic disorders.

PSYCHOTHERAPY Early in the development of psychoanalysis, it was felt that the dynamically-oriented psychotherapies were the treatment of choice for phobic disorders, whose genesis were seen as lying in the areas of oedipal-genital conflicts. Soon, however, therapists recognized that, despite progress in uncovering and analyzing unconscious conflicts, patients frequently failed to lose their phobic symptoms and, by continuing to avoid the phobic situation, excluded a significant degree of anxiety and its related associations from the analytic process. Both Freud and his pupil Sandor Ferenczi recognized that, if progress in analyzing the symptoms were to be made, therapists had to go beyond their merely analytic roles and actively urge their phobic patients to enter the phobic situation and experience the anxiety involved. There has since been a general agreement among psychiatrists that a measure of activity on the part of the therapist is often required to get at the phobic anxiety. At the same time, a growing body of clinical experience has demonstrated that many phobic patients are not readily helped by analytic techniques, especially patients suffering from phobias whose roots lie in serious preoedipal conflicts. The decision to apply the techniques of psychodynamic insight therapy should be based not on the presence of the phobic symptom alone, but on positive indications from the patient's ego structure and life patterns for the use of this method of treatment.

BEHAVIOR THERAPY In their paper on conditioned emotional reactions, Watson and Rayner stressed the need for developing an experimental technique for removing such responses. Although the experimental subject, Little Albert, had been taken away before they could attempt to remove the phobias they had created in him shortly before his first birthday, the authors described the therapeutic measures they would have taken had they been able to do so: (1) habituating the subject to the phobic object by its repeated presentation to him; (2) combining the presentation of the painful conditioned stimulus with the pleasurable sensation produced by tactual stimulation of the subject's erogenous zones; "We should try first the lips," they wrote, "then the nipples, and as a final resort, the sex organs"; (3) reconditioning by offering candy along with the painful stimulus; and (4) building up of constructive activities around the phobic object by passively putting the subject's hand through the motions of manipulation.

In those suggestions lies the germ of the maneuvers that now constitute behavior therapy. In recent years, there have been reports of a number of dramatic cures of patients with phobic disorders through the use of techniques derived from the concepts of learning theory. Agras, for example, has described a woman with an incapacitating agoraphobia who was completely relieved of her symptoms in only a few weeks through the use of selective positive reinforcement. An increasing number of studies are appearing in the American and English literature reporting favorable results in patients who, after many years of suffering from phobias and despite treatment with more traditional psychotherapies, have been helped by a few sessions in which behavior therapy was employed.

Various behavioral treatment techniques have been used, such as imaginal desensitization. In systematic desensitization, patients are exposed serially to a predetermined list of anxiety-provoking stimuli graded in a hierarchy from the least to the most frightening. Each of the anxiety-provoking stimuli is paired with the arousal of another affect of an opposite quality (e.g., relaxation) that is strong enough to suppress the anxiety. Through the use of tranquilizing drugs, hypnosis, and instruction in the art of muscle relaxation, patients are taught how to induce in themselves both mental and physical repose. Once they have mastered these techniques, the patients are instructed to use them in the face of each anxiety-provoking stimulus in the hierarchy as the stimuli are presented to them, from the least to the most potent. As they become desensitized to each stimulus in the scale, the patients move up to the next stimulus until, ultimately, what previously produced the most anxiety is no longer capable of eliciting the painful affect. More recent behavioral techniques that have been employed are intensive exposure to the phobic stimulus either through imagery or in vivo. In imaginal flooding, patients are exposed to phobic anxiety produced by images of the phobic stimulus for as long as they can tolerate the fear until they reach a point at which they can no longer feel it. The most common behavioral therapy currently employed is in vivo exposure. With exposure techniques, patients are required to experience similar anxiety through exposure to the actual phobic stimulus itself.

An alternative behavioral approach to the treatment of phobias, cognitive therapy, focuses less on the anxious affect and more on the self-defeating cognitive patterns presumed to mediate maladaptive emotional reactions. Cognitive-behavioral therapies are based on the assumption that the ways patients evaluate situations or events, rather than the events themselves, can affect, if not determine, the associated affective responses. Thus, cognitive therapies are designed to modify patients' perspectives of potentially anxiety-provoking stimuli. Reviews of the literature examining the application of cognitive-behavioral interventions in the treatment of anxious college students and related analogue populations indicate that these techniques are effective in treating simple fears and social anxiety. Treatment outcome studies examining the efficacy of cognitive therapies with clinical populations are sparse, but initial findings are promising, especially from investigations of cognitive interventions for social phobia. Further research is needed to address the question of how valuable cognitive-behavioral interventions might be as primary or adjunct treatment strategies for severe and disabling conditions like agoraphobia.

Considerable success has been reported in treating phobic disorders by behavioral-cognitive techniques, although it is not always clear how much the effects are to be attributed to the measures that are characteristic of behavior therapy and how much to other factors that accompany the effects, such as suggestion or the supportive relationship with an enthusiastic therapist. In general, the simple and social phobias respond best to behavioral methods, whereas patients with agoraphobia, especially when panic attacks are a prominent and continuous feature, fare less well and often run a long and fluctuating course of continuing symptoms and disability. However, in the agoraphobic patient without any history of panic attacks, exposure therapy may be the treatment of choice. Even in the agoraphobic group with concomitant panic attacks, nearly half the patients report sufficient improvement with behavior therapy to enable them to lead reasonably active lives, despite an incomplete resolution of their spontaneous panic attacks. It is clear that behavioral therapeutic techniques have added an important dimension to the psychiatrist's therapeutic armamentarium and should be considered for every patient with a phobic disorder.

PHARMACOTHERAPY Considerable success in controlling panic disorder, with and without agoraphobia, has been reported in recent years with the use of tricyclic antidepressants, especially imipramine (Tofranil); monoamine oxidase inhibitors, such as phenelzine (Nardil); and some (i.e., alprazolam [Xanax], clonazepam [Klonopin]), but not all, benzodiazepines. The dramatic reduction in panic attacks that follows such medication is the central factor in recovery from the secondary agoraphobia associated with panic disorder. Sometimes the mere control of the unprovoked panic attacks is sufficient to allow patients with secondary agoraphobia to resume their customary activities. If anticipatory or chronic generalized anxiety persists despite the blockade of the spontaneous panic attacks, benzodiazepines or behavioral desensitization, or both, may be required to combat this more chronic form of anxiety. Insight-oriented psychotherapy also may be considered in a subgroup of patients with generalized anxiety or in patients who unequivocally associate a life event or stressor as being directly linked to their symptomotology. Such patients may be helped to correct any unresolved psychological conflicts or to develop more effective strategies for confronting problems of daily living.

Only recently have investigators begun to study systematically the pharmacotherapy of patients who meet formal DSM-III-R criteria for social phobia. Limited data suggest that phenelzine is effective in patients with panic-related agoraphobia or social anxiety and in patients with an admixture of agoraphobic–social anxiety symptomatology. It has long been suggested that patients with anticipatory performance anxiety, although not sufficiently impaired to meet the DSM-III-R criteria for social phobia, respond to β-adrenergic blockers, such as propranolol (Inderal).

As a general rule, most simple phobias (i.e., animal and insect phobias) do not appear to respond to pharmacological intervention.

SUPPORTIVE THERAPY As in the treatment of any illness, the support afforded patients by a positive relationship with their physicians has a beneficial effect. Beyond this, especially in the more active forms of treatment, such as behavioral and cognitive therapies, psychiatrists must encourage, exhort, instruct, and suggest as they try to help their patients overcome the dread of the phobic situation. In this regard, it is important to keep in mind that the more patients avoid what they fear, the more they are liable to fear it and, at the same time, to become discouraged and downhearted at their pusillanimity. If they can once be persuaded to face the phobic situation and come through the experience with a measure of success, the increase in their self-esteem and self-confidence will make it easier for them to try it again. Each successful attempt makes the next try less of an ordeal, and the vicious downward cycle of avoidance can sometimes be reversed to the point that patients either lose their symptoms or so master them that their lives are no longer seriously constricted by the limitations they had previously imposed on their actions.

REFERENCES

Barlow D H, Cohen A S, Waddell M T, Vermilyea B B, Klosko J S, Blanchard E-B, DiNardo P A: Panic and generalized anxiety disorders: Nature and treatment. Behav Ther *15:* 431, 1984.

Beck A T: *Cognitive Therapy and the Emotional Disorders.* International Universities Press, New York, 1976.

Beck A T, Emery G: *Anxiety Disorders and Phobias.* Basic Books, New York, 1985.

Connolly J, Hallam R, Marks I M: Selective association of fainting with blood–injury–illness fear. Behav Ther *7:* 8, 1976.

Curtis G, Buxton M, Lippman D, Nesse R, Wright J: "Flooding in vivo" during the circadian phase of minimal cortisol secretion: Anxiety and therapeutic success without adrenal cortical activation. Biol Psychiat *11:* 101, 1976.

Curtis G C, Nesse R, Buxton M, Lippman D: Anxiety and plasma cortisol at the crest of the circadian cycle: Reappraisal of a classical hypothesis. Psychosom Med *40:* 368, 1978.

Curtis G C, Thyer B: Fainting on exposure to phobic stimuli. Amer J Psychiat *140:* 771, 1983.

Curtis G C, Thyer B A, Rainer J M: *Anxiety Disorders. The Psychiatric Clinics of North America.* Saunders, Philadelphia, 1985.

Fenichel O: The counterphobic attitude. Int J Psychoanal *20:* 263, 1939.

Freud S: Analysis of a phobia in a five-year-old boy. In *The Standard Edition of the Complete Psychological Works of Sigmund Freud,* vol 10, p 5. Hogarth Press, London, 1955.

Freud S: Inhibitions, symptoms and anxiety. In *The Standard Edition of the Complete Psychological Works of Sigmund Freud,* vol 20, p 87. Hogarth Press, London, 1959.

Freud S: Obsessions and phobias. In *The Standard Edition of the Complete Psychological Works of Sigmund Freud,* vol 3, p 74. Hogarth Press, London, 1962.

Glass C R, Shea C A: Cognitive therapy for shyness and social anxiety. In *Shyness: Perspectives on Research and Treatment,* W H Jones, J M Cheek, S R Briggs, editors, p 315. Plenum, New York, 1986.

Goldfried M R: Anxiety reduction through cognitive-behavioral intervention. In *Cognitive-Behavioral Interventions: Theory, Research and Procedures,* P C Kendall, S D Hollon, editors, p 117. Academic Press, New York, 1979.

Lader M H, Gelder M G, Marks I M: Palmar skin-conductance measures as predictors of response to desensitization. J Psychosom Res *11:* 283, 1967.
Lewin B: Phobic symptoms and dream interpretation. Psychoanal Q *21:* 295, 1952.
Liebowitz M R, Gormon J M, Fyer A J, Klein D F: Social phobia. Arch Gen Psychiat *42:* 737, 1985.
Marks I M: *Fears and Phobias*. Heinemann, London, 1969.
Nemiah J: A psychoanalytic view of phobias. Amer J Psychoanal *41:* 115, 1981.
Nesse R M, Curtis G C, Thyer B A, McCann D S, Huber-Smith M J, Knopf R F: Endocrine and cardiovascular responses during phobia anxiety. Psychosom Med *47:* 320, 1985.
Prince M: *The Unconscious*. Macmillan, New York, 1924.
Roth M: The phobic anxiety–depersonalization syndrome. Proc R Soc Med *52:* 587, 1959.
Tuma A H, Maser J D: *Anxiety and the Anxiety Disorders*. Erlbaum, Hillsdale, NJ, 1985.

18.3 OBSESSIVE-COMPULSIVE DISORDER

JOHN C. NEMIAH, M.D.
THOMAS W. UHDE, M.D.

INTRODUCTION

Sigmund Freud wrote in one of his earliest psychological papers:

> If someone with a disposition [to neurosis] lacks the aptitude for conversion but if, nevertheless, in order to fend off an incompatible idea, he sets about separating it from its affect, then that affect is obliged to remain in the psychical sphere. The idea, now weakened, is still left in consciousness, separated from all association. But its affect, which has become free, attaches itself to other ideas which are not in themselves incompatible; and thanks to this "false connection" those ideas turn into obsessional ideas. This, in a few words, is the psychological theory of obsessions and phobias.

Freud's first psychodynamic formulations were created to explain the formation of the symptoms of conversion hysteria. When an idea is incompatible with an individual's ego, so ran his theory, the affect associated with the idea is rendered unconscious by repression and is converted into a sensorimotor disturbance that symbolizes the unacceptable idea. The formulation was satisfactory, for it adequately explained the observed clinical manifestations of conversion hysteria: the existence of somatic, sensory, or motor symptoms, the absence of distressing affects associated with them, and the disappearance of the symptoms when the pathogenic idea and the associated painful affects were brought into the individual's conscious awareness by therapeutic techniques, such as hypnosis.

It soon became apparent, however, that the theory did not adequately explain other forms of neurotic symptoms. In patients suffering from obsessions and phobias, for example, the predominant clinical manifestations were not somatic but psychic; instead of being disabled by disturbances in their sensations or motor functions, patients were afflicted by distressing, consciously experienced ideas. Furthermore, unlike hysterical symptoms, these ideas were accompanied by an acute, conscious awareness of painful emotions, such as anxiety or shame. In other words, at the very beginning of his attempt to develop a psychodynamic psychopathology, Freud was faced with the problem of explaining symptom choice and was forced to modify his theories to satisfy the demands of stubborn clinical facts. That process of modification continued throughout his long and creative career and led eventually to the highly elaborate web of contemporary psychoanalytic theory.

In that first expansion of his psychological formulations, Freud separated from the somatosensory symptoms of hysteria a group of symptoms characterized by their psychical nature, but he failed initially to differentiate between phobic and obsessive-compulsive phenomena; that differentiation came later in his expanding psychodynamic scheme. There was, however, good reason for that early confusion. Not only do phobic and obsessive-compulsive symptoms have features in common, but the characteristics that are used to differentiate them clinically do not always lead to a clear separation. In fact, the clinical phenomena lie along a spectrum. The phenomena are clearly differentiated at the extremes, but there are forms in the middle of the spectrum that are difficult to assign to diagnostic categories.

DEFINITION

Despite the confusion regarding classification, it is possible to designate certain symptoms as obsessions and compulsions and to distinguish them from other clinical manifestations by their specific characteristics. Direct observation of the phenomena themselves provides the surest approach to a definition of these two symptoms.

In his autobiographical volume, *Lavengro,* that enchanting English vagabond George Borrow reproduced a tale told to him by a stranger he had encountered in his wanderings:

> Amid darkness and gloom, occasionally broken by flashes of lightning, the stranger related to me, as we sat at the table in the library, his truly touching history. . . .
>
> There was one thing that I loved better than the choicest gift which could be bestowed upon me, better than life itself—my mother; at length she became unwell, and the thought that I might possibly lose her now rushed into my mind for the first time: it was terrible, and caused me unspeakable misery, I may say horror. My mother became worse, and I was not allowed to enter her apartment, lest by my frantic exclamations of grief I might aggravate her disorder. I rested neither day nor night, but roamed about the house like one distracted. Suddenly I found myself doing that which even at the time struck me as being highly singular; I found myself touching particular objects that were near me, and to which my fingers seemed to be attracted by an irresistible impulse. It was now the table or the chair that I was compelled to touch; now the bell-rope, now the handle of the door; now I would touch the wall, and the next moment stooping down, I would place the point of my finger upon the floor: and so I continued to do day after day; frequently I would struggle to resist the impulse, but invariably in vain. I have even rushed away from the object, but I was sure to return, the impulse was too strong to be resisted: I quickly hurried back, compelled by the feeling within me to touch the object. Now I need not tell you what impelled me to these actions was the desire to prevent my mother's death; whenever I touched any particular object, it was with the view of baffling the evil chance, as you would call it—in this instance my mother's death.
>
> A favourable crisis appeared in my mother's complaint, and she recovered; this crisis took place about six o'clock in the morning; almost simultaneously with it there happened to myself a rather remarkable circumstance connected with the nervous feeling which was rioting in my system. I was lying in bed in a kind of uneasy doze, the only kind of rest which my anxiety, on account of my mother, permitted me at this time to take, when all at once I sprang up as if electrified, the mysterious impulse was upon me, and it urged me to go without delay, and climb a stately elm behind the house and touch

the topmost branch; otherwise—you know the rest—the evil chance would prevail. Accustomed for some time as I had been, under this impulse, to perform extravagant actions, I confess to you that the difficulty and peril of such a feat startled me; I reasoned against the feeling, and strove more strenuously than I had ever done before; I even made a solemn vow not to give way to temptation, but I believe that nothing less than chains, and those strong ones, could have restrained me. The demoniac influence, for I can call it nothing else, at length prevailed; it compelled me to rise, to dress myself, to descend the stairs, to unbolt the door and to go forth; it drove me to the foot of the tree, and it compelled me to climb the trunk; this was a tremendous task, and I only accomplished it after repeated falls and trials. When I had got amongst the branches, I rested for a time, and then set about accomplishing the remainder of the ascent; this for some time was not so difficult, for I was now amongst the branches; as I approached the top, however, the difficulty became greater, and likewise the danger, but I was a light boy, and almost as nimble as a squirrel, and, moreover, the nervous feeling was within me, impelling me upward. It was only by means of a spring, however, that I was enabled to touch the top of the tree. I sprang, touched the top of the tree and fell a distance of at least twenty feet, amongst the branches; had I fallen to the bottom I must have been killed, but I fell into the middle of the tree, and presently found myself astride upon one of the boughs; scratched and bruised all over, I reached the ground, and regained my chamber unobserved; I flung myself on my bed quite exhausted; presently they came to tell me that my mother was better—they found me in the state which I have described and in a fever besides. The favourable crisis must have occurred just about the time that I performed the magic touch; it certainly was a curious coincidence yet I was not weak enough, even though a child, to suppose that I had baffled the evil chance by my daring feat.

Indeed, all the time that I was performing these strange feats, I knew them to be highly absurd, yet the impulse to perform them was irresistible—a mysterious dread hanging over me till I had given way to it; even at that early period I frequently used to reason within myself as to what could be the cause of my propensity to touch, but of course I could come to no satisfactory conclusion respecting it; being heartily ashamed of the practice, I never spoke of it to anyone, and was at all times highly solicitous that no one should observe my weakness.

Distinguishing characteristics of obsessive-compulsive phenomena can be observed in the above few paragraphs. These characteristics, when they form the predominant manifestations of a patient's psychoneurotic illness, make up obsessive-compulsive disorder. The word *obsessive* or *obsession* refers to an idea or thought, such as, in the passage just quoted, the narrator's idea of his mother's death. The word *compulsive* or *compulsion* refers to an urge or impulse to action that, when put into operation, leads to a compulsive act. Compulsive acts, such as touching the floor and climbing the tree, predominate in the narrator's description of his trials.

Obsessions and compulsions have certain features in common:

1. An idea or an impulse obtrudes itself insistently, persistently, and impellingly into the individual's conscious awareness.
2. A feeling of anxious dread accompanies the central manifestation and frequently leads the individual to take countermeasures against the initial idea or impulse.
3. The obsession or compulsion is ego-alien; that is, it is experienced as being foreign to and not a usual part of one's experience of oneself as a psychological being; it is undesired, unacceptable, and uncontrollable.
4. No matter how vivid and compelling the obsession or compulsion is, individuals recognize it as absurd and irrational; they retain their insight.
5. The person suffering from these manifestations feels a strong need to resist them.
6. Filled with shame about the symptoms, the individual often hides their existence from others.

TABLE 18.3-1
Diagnostic Criteria for Obsessive-Compulsive Disorder

A. Either obsessions or compulsions:
Obsessions: (1), (2), (3), and (4):
(1) Recurrent and persistent ideas, thoughts, impulses, or images that are experienced, at least initially, as intrusive and senseless (e.g., a parent's having repeated impulses to kill a loved child, a religious person's having recurrent blasphemous thoughts)
(2) The person attempts to ignore or suppress such thoughts or impulses or to neutralize them with some other thought or action
(3) The person recognizes that the obsessions are the product of his or her own mind, not imposed from without (as in thought insertion)
(4) If another Axis I disorder is present, the content of the obsession is unrelated to it (e.g., the ideas, thoughts, impulses, or images are not about food in the presence of an eating disorder, about drugs in the presence of a psychoactive substance use disorder, or guilty thoughts in the presence of a major depression)
Compulsions: (1), (2), and (3):
(1) Repetitive, purposeful, and intentional behaviors that are performed in response to an obsession, or according to certain rules or in a stereotyped fashion
(2) The behavior is designed to neutralize or to prevent discomfort or some dreaded event or situation; however, either the activity is not connected in a realistic way with what it is designed to neutralize or prevent, or it is clearly excessive
(3) The person recognizes that his or her behavior is excessive or unreasonable (this may not be true for young children; it may no longer be true for people whose obsessions have evolved into overvalued ideas)

B. The obsessions or compulsions cause marked distress, are time-consuming (take more than an hour a day), or significantly interfere with the person's normal routine, occupational functioning, or usual social activities or relationships with others

Table from DSM-III-R *Diagnostic and Statistical Manual of Mental Disorders,* ed 3, revised. Copyright American Psychiatric Association, Washington, DC, 1987. Used with permission.

Most of these characteristics are found in the official definition of the obsessive-compulsive disorder given in the revised third edition of the American Psychiatric Association's *Diagnostic and Statistical Manual of Mental Disorders* (DSM-III-R):

A chronic, but occasionally episodic, disorder in which the predominant feature is recurrent obsessions or compulsions or both. Obsessions are persistent ideas, thoughts, images, or impulses that are viewed at least initially by the subject as ego-alien. They are not experienced as voluntarily produced but, rather, as ideas that invade the field of consciousness. Attempts are made to ignore or to suppress them. Compulsions are behaviors that are repetitive, purposeful, and intentional. These behaviors, however, are performed in response to an obsession, according to rules, in order to diminish discomfort or prevent some dreaded event or situation. In order for these behaviors to be defined as compulsions, either the behavior is "not connected in a realistic way with what it is designed to neutralize or prevent, or it is clearly excessive." Such patients recognize obsessions as foreign to their personality and recognize compulsions as unreasonable. Early in the course of adult obsessive-compulsive disorder, there is a desire to resist the compulsion. Later in the natural course of illness, there may be no active resistance. The most common compulsions are probably hand washing, counting, checking, and touching. (Table 18.3-1 provides the DSM-III-R criteria for obsessive-compulsive disorder.)

EPIDEMIOLOGY AND FAMILY STUDIES

Probably most persons have at some time in their lives experienced a fleeting bit of obsessional thinking or compulsive behavior. However, a transient, unreasonable compulsion to check a gas jet that one knows is closed or a momentary urge to shout out an obscenity during a solemn ceremony hardly constitutes an obsessive-compulsive disorder, which in its severest forms can, like severe phobias, be as disabling to the sufferer as can the most crippling physical illness.

It is hard to determine the exact incidence of obsessive-compulsive disorder. Scattered anecdotal evidence indicates that it has occurred throughout history. Although clinicians who have studied the natural history of the disorder have found an incidence that is never higher than 5 percent of all psychoneurotic patients, and usually less than 1 percent of a general psychiatric treatment population, the recent National Institute of Mental Health (NIMH) Epidemiologic Catchment Area (ECA) study found a 6-month prevalence rate of 1 to 2 percent and a lifetime prevalence of 2 to 3 percent. Although the validity of these findings is questionable, it is possible that the actual incidence of obsessive-compulsive disorder is higher than previously appreciated. It is also possible that the proportion of patients in the community with obsessive-compulsive disorder who actually seek treatment in either an inpatient or an outpatient facility may be extraordinarily low. It is known that individuals with obsessive-compulsive disorder tend to be secretive about their symptoms and to avoid disclosing them to physicians, often doing so only when some other illness has forced them to seek medical attention. Furthermore, because people with obsessive-compulsive symptoms are frequently able to work and earn a living despite marked limitations in their social and emotional lives, their disorders may be known only by their closest associates. These facts and the recent unexpected ECA findings suggest that the incidence based on figures derived from clinical populations may be spuriously low.

There appears to be no significant sexual difference in the adult form of obsessive-compulsive disorder. Childhood-onset obsessive-compulsive disorder may be more common in males than females. It is interesting that a large proportion of obsessive-compulsive patients remain unmarried, up to 50 percent in some surveys. Recent studies indicate that the frequency of the disorder is higher in upper-class persons and in those with higher intelligence levels. The data on familial patterns are meager, but they suggest that parents and siblings of patients with obsessive-compulsive disorder have a significantly higher incidence of the condition, as compared with a control population, and that the presence of obsessional traits is similarly increased. Twin studies suggest a greater degree of concordance of obsessional traits in monozygotic, as compared with dizygotic twins. The relationship between obsessive-compulsive disorder and other psychiatric conditions, especially major depressive disorder and Tourette's disorder, remains an area of intense debate and investigation.

ETIOLOGY

EARLY THEORIES In the *Malleus Maleficarum,* Heinrich Kramer and James Sprenger wrote of a fifteenth-century patient whom one of them observed:

> A certain Bohemian from the town of Dachow brought his only son, a secular priest, to Rome to be delivered because he was possessed. It happened that I, one of us Inquisitors, went into a refectory, and that priest and his father came and sat down at the same table with me. We saluted each other, and talked together, as is customary; and the father kept sighing and praying Almighty God that his journey might prove to have been successful. I felt great pity for him, and began to ask what was the reason of his journey and of his sorrow. Then he, in the hearing of his son who was sitting next to me at the table, answered: "Alas! I have a son possessed by a devil, and with great trouble and expense I have brought him here to be delivered." And when I asked where the son was, he showed me him sitting by my side. I was a little frightened, and looked at him closely; and because he took his food with such modesty, and answered piously to all questions, I began to doubt that he was possessed, but that some infirmity had happened to him. Then the son himself told what had happened, showing how and for how long he had been possessed. . . . When I asked him about the length of the intervals during which he had the use of his reason more than is usual in the case of persons possessed, he answered: "I am only deprived of the use of my reason when I wish to contemplate holy things or to visit sacred places." . . .
>
> When he passed any church, and genuflected in honour of the Glorious Virgin, the devil made him thrust his tongue far out of his mouth; and when he was asked whether he could not restrain himself from doing this, he answered, "I cannot help myself at all, for so he uses all my limbs and organs, my neck, my tongue, and my lungs, whenever he pleases, causing me to speak or to cry out; and I hear the words as if they were spoken by myself, but I am altogether unable to restrain them: and when I try to engage in prayer he attacks me more violently, thrusting out my tongue."

For twentieth-century minds, the concepts of witchcraft, devils, and possession that fill the *Malleus Maleficarum*—of the whole paraphernalia of external, independent, immaterial beings in a spiritual world—are nothing but worthless superstition and delusion. It must be remembered, however, that for people of earlier ages, those were real and useful ideas. They provided an explanation for the observed phenomena and constituted a seriously conceived theory based on observable facts. As the seventeenth-century preacher Joseph Glanvil wrote in the introduction to his *Sadducismus Triumphatus,* a volume devoted to the proof of the existence of witches,

> Whether Witches are, or are not is a Question of Facts: For it is in Effect, whether any Men or Women have been, or are in Covenant with evil Spirits, and whether they, by the Spirit's Help, or he on their Account, performs such or such things. . . . Matters of Fact can only be proved by the immediate Sense, or the Testimony of others, Divine or Human. To endeavour to demonstrate fact by abstract Reasoning and Speculation, is as if a Man should prove, that Julius Caesar founded the Empire of Rome, by Algebra or Metaphysicks.

It is evident that Glanvil eschews logic chopping and deductive ratiocination. For him, the existence of witches is to be determined by observation. Although modern scientists would not subscribe to Glanvil's reliance on divine testimony, they can find themselves quite at home in the strictly empirical approach that Glanvil takes to his subject matter.

By the nineteenth century, the climate of opinion had radically changed. Scientific theories no longer invoked sentient, purposeful spiritual beings as causal factors but relied on explanations that involved impersonal measurable natural forces acting mechanically on material objects. That change is reflected in the language used by George Borrow in the case history quoted earlier. Although he does make passing reference to a demoniac influence, Borrow's vocabulary is otherwise within a scientific frame of reference. He speaks of thoughts, feelings, impulses, anxiety, nervous feelings rioting within, a mysterious dread. He does not mention devils, witches, or possession by spiritual beings. His concern is only with mental events—thoughts, feelings, and impulses—that are contained within the confines of the individual's mind and body. The explanation of the phenomena has been shifted from external supernatural forces to a consideration of the inner workings of the human mind. Demonology has been replaced by psychology, a natural science.

Borrow was a layman, but the psychologists who were his contemporaries, as well as those who followed him in succeeding decades, worked within the same scientific frame of reference in their attempts to understand and explain the wide spectrum of normal and abnormal mental phenomena. Obsessions and compulsions had a significant place among the concerns of the clinicians, who offered two different and rival explanations concerning those symptoms: (1) The primary disturbance lay in an unclearly specified defect in intellectual functions, leading to difficulties in making logical decisions and to an exaggerated preoccupation with certain ideas out of proportion to their importance. (2) The basic problem was a disturbance in the function of the emotions, especially anxiety, which, escaping control and becoming attached to an idea, forced that idea with undue intensity and persistence onto the patient's conscious attention.

PIERRE JANET'S THEORIES In 1903, Pierre Janet's two-volume work *Obsessions and Psychasthenia* was published. From a wide range of clinical observations, Janet deduced a theoretical scheme that included many of the ideas of his predecessors and introduced certain concepts he considered basic to an understanding of obsessions. For Janet, the central disturbance lay in a pathological diminution of mental energy that resulted in a disintegration of the normal organization of mental functions. That disintegration led to a failure of the highest of those functions—will and attention, which enabled individuals to control their thoughts and actions, to perceive themselves and their environment realistically, and to perform actions appropriate to that correctly perceived reality. When these higher mental functions were impaired or destroyed, lower, subsidiary, more primitive mental functions—especially the emotions with their mental, visceral, and motoric correlates—escaped from control. Without regard for reality, lower functions made their appearance in a chaos of mental anarchy. They operated with energy that was normally and naturally theirs and with an additional quantum of energy derived from the higher functions that were no longer operable once the whole psychic apparatus had fallen apart.

With this theoretical model, Janet attempted to provide a systematic explanation of a variety of clinical symptoms that he felt were related. These symptoms included the subjective sense of mental fatigue and depression (psychasthenia), obsessions, compulsive urges and acts, phobias, and anxiety attacks. Certain concepts contained in Janet's earlier theories concerning hysteria are to be found in that formulation. In particular can be found the notion, basically a physiological one, that a diminution in energy leads to a disorganization of integrated personality structure, with a resulting autonomous, uncontrolled functioning of subsidiary mental functions. Interestingly, the idea of unconscious mental functioning, which had a place in Janet's explanations of hysteria, plays no part in his later theoretical scheme. The entire theoretical model rests on a quantitatively and mechanistically conceived lowering of mental energy. Although Janet tried to account for this diminution through emotional shock, physical illness, or hereditary degeneracy, he did not satisfactorily explain its genesis.

By ignoring the concept of unconscious mental processes, Janet and those who preceded him compromised their ability to illuminate the origin of obsessive-compulsive phenomena. In some ways, the earlier demonological theories provided a more complete and a more dynamic explanation of the symptoms than did the more naturalistic hypotheses of the nineteenth century. The earlier observers, confronted with the directly observable central feature of the obsession or compulsion as an insistent idea or urge imposed on individuals by some force seemingly outside themselves, accepted those observations at face value. The compelling force that was experienced as external was, they argued, in reality external in the form of the devil or some related spiritual being. (The Ptolemaic cosmology took the same literal approach to physical phenomena: Because the sun and stars were observed to revolve around the earth, it was assumed that they, in fact, did so.) The scientific climate of opinion in the nineteenth century forbade belief in demons, but the clinical facts persisted.

PSYCHOANALYTIC THEORIES It remained for Freud, by exploiting the possibilities offered by the concepts of the unconscious and of psychological conflict, to devise a theory that would explain obsessive-compulsive symptoms in terms of its psychogenetic roots in the early phases of childhood development and of the psychodynamic factors important to the production of its symptoms. His point of departure lay in his early belief that the difference between hysterical and obsessional symptoms rested on a difference in the psychological mechanisms that led to their formation. Although his earliest formulation was in many ways incomplete, it provided a starting point from which he and his co-workers gradually evolved the theoretical explanation that is widely accepted among psychodynamically oriented psychiatrists today.

Psychodynamic factors From a psychoanalytic perspective, three major psychological defensive mechanisms determine the form and quality of obsessive-compulsive symptoms and character traits: isolation, undoing, and reaction formation.

ISOLATION Isolation is a defense mechanism that protects an individual from anxiety-provoking affects and impulses. Under ordinary circumstances, an individual experiences in consciousness both the affect and the imagery of an emotion-laden idea, whether it be a fantasy or the memory of an event. When isolation occurs, the affect and the impulse of which it is a derivative are separated from the ideational component and pushed out of consciousness.

If isolation is completely successful, the impulse and its associated affect will be totally repressed, and the patient will be consciously aware of only the affectless idea that is related to it.

A patient reported one day in a therapeutic hour that she had had a fantasy of her doctor falling from a seventh-story window. In her mind's eye she had seen him hit the pavement and had then observed his crumpled body with jagged bone fragments sticking through lacerated compound fractures and blood oozing from his nose and mouth. "I infer from this," she said in a flat, emotionless tone of voice, "that I am angry at you, but I don't have any feeling like that." That fantasy could not be considered a symptom; it was transient and caused the patient no emotional distress. The defense of isolation had functioned successfully.

Sometimes, however, the isolation is less effective, and the total quantity of energy accruing to the impulse and its associated affect cannot be completely restrained by the repressing forces from entering the patient's consciousness. Patients experience a partial awareness of the impulse without fully recognizing its meaning or significance. They may, for example, have frightening and compelling murderous impulses toward strangers or casual acquaintances; here, the impulse makes itself felt as an urge to violent action, but the direction of the urge is displaced from the true object of the patients' aggression to other people in their environment. At the same time, isolation exerts a partial effect by rendering patients unaware that they are angry, so that they are puzzled, mystified, and disturbed by their compulsions. Or they may be obsessed with images and thoughts of violence and destruction; here again, the energy from the partially repressed impulse gives the thoughts their compelling quality, and the continuing partial functioning of the mechanism of isolation prevents patients from becoming aware that beneath the surface they harbor intense aggression.

These processes can be looked at from two viewpoints: (1) Clinically, the patient's consciously experienced mental events are seen as obsessive and compulsive symptoms. (2) Psychodynamically, the events are viewed as a psychological conflict between impulses and controlling defensive forces. The concept of psychological conflict is based on the notion that an undischarged impulse constantly exerts pressure on the person for both conscious recognition and discharge. The defenses that operate to control that impulse must, therefore, exert a constantly opposing energy if the impulse is to be maintained under control; that is, a dynamic equilibrium of opposing psychic forces is established. Such an equilibrium may be relatively stable and persistent, as in the case of successful isolation in which no symptoms are evident or as in the case of conversion hysteria in which persistent and stable somatic symptoms are apparent. In fact, conversion appears to be, in one sense, a highly effective if ultimately pathological defense mechanism. The energy of the impulse is almost entirely bound by the somatic symptom, and the patient is spared the experience of unpleasant affects, as is manifested clinically in the phenomenon of *la belle indifférence*. The situation is different in the case of the defense mechanisms operating in obsessive-compulsive disorder. In that syndrome the equilibrium often proves to be less stable, and the impulse constantly threatens to break through the controls that the patient imposes on it. In fact, the tendency of the underlying impulse to escape its bonds is a salient characteristic of obsessive-compulsive disorder.

UNDOING In the face of the impulse's constant threat to escape the primary defense of isolation and to break free, further secondary defensive operations are required to combat it and to quiet the anxiety that the imminent eruption of the impulse into consciousness arouses in the patient.

> In a patient who was obsessed by the thought that, by bumping passersby, he had knocked them down and injured them, it was ultimately discovered that he harbored real and angry wishes to push people out of his way when he walked down the street, a conscious awareness of these impulses emerging into the patient's mind in the course of his free associations. When he had initially described his obsessional thought, however, he strongly denied any such urges and was genuinely unaware of any such feelings within himself. Nonetheless, the obsessional thought made him very anxious and guilty, just as if he really did have such urges and had in actuality harmed other people. The only way he could reassure himself and quiet his anxiety was by returning to the scene of his supposed crime to make sure that everything was all right. Although he knew the whole thing was absurd, he was compelled to this action and remained acutely anxious until he had performed it. The compulsive act, in other words, was secondary to the original obsessional thought.

The anxiety-allaying function of compulsive acts can readily be noted in the clinical manifestations of obsessive-compulsive disorders. What should be observed here is that the compulsive act constitutes the surface manifestation of a further defensive operation aimed at reducing anxiety and at controlling the underlying impulse that has not been sufficiently contained by isolation. A particularly important secondary defensive operation of that sort is the mechanism of undoing. As the word suggests, *undoing* refers to a compulsive act that is performed in an attempt to prevent or undo the consequences that the patient irrationally anticipates from a frightening obsessional thought or impulse.

> This mechanism was clearly at work in the patient who, whenever he turned off a light, obsessively thought, "My father will die," and would then be compelled to turn around, touch the switch, and say, "I take back that thought." With that act he was literally undoing the damage that he feared would result from the initial thought, which arose from an underlying aggressive impulse toward his father.

REACTION FORMATION Both isolation and undoing are defensive maneuvers that are intimately involved in the production of clinical symptoms. Reaction formation, a third mechanism closely associated with obsessive-compulsive disorder, results in the formation of character traits, rather than symptoms. As the term implies, *reaction formation* involves manifest patterns of behavior and consciously experienced attitudes that are exactly the opposite of the underlying impulses. Often these patterns appear to an observer to be highly exaggerated and, at times, quite inappropriate.

A 32-year-old woman, the mother of three small children, revealed that she had had frightening impulses to kill her two older sons. Describing her relationship with her children, she said:

> I think of my children all the time. . . . I can't punish them. It hurts me to punish them. I just can't do it. I can't face up to hitting them. Even my husband, he'll tell you—even my sisters say the same thing about me. I'm too good to them. I let them run my life, and yet I can't help it . . . I can't go out unless I buy them a toy. . . . I never went out or anything. I never left them with anybody. I always stayed in the house. Since I had my first boy, anywhere I went, I took him with me. . . . I never had any time away from my children. Since I had my first boy [4 years previously], I've never had no time away from them—no time at all.

Her habitual and persistent pattern of solicitousness and kindness toward her children, which even her husband and sisters recognized as being inappropriately exaggerated, was a defensive maneuver designed to control her underlying aggressiveness toward her children. That aggressiveness was manifest in murderous fantasies of killing them that ultimately emerged in the course of therapy.

Reaction formation is responsible for many of the personality traits characterized by control that make up the obsessive-compulsive character.

Psychogenetic factors One of the striking features of patients with obsessive-compulsive disorder is the degree to which they are preoccupied with aggression or dirt, either overtly in the content of their symptoms or in the associations that lie behind them. That and other observations have led to the psychodynamic proposition that the psychogenesis of obsessive-compulsive disorder lies in disturbances in normal growth and development related to the anal-sadistic phase. According to this conceptualization, the impulses associated with the anal-sadistic phase are normally modified in the oedipal and succeeding stages of development. If, however, this developmental process is disturbed, unmodified anal-sadistic impulses will remain as components of the individual's psychological makeup. Ordinarily, impulses of this type are controlled and disguised by character traits and may not significantly affect the person's functioning in the usual course of daily living. They remain, however, as fixation points that may, under certain circumstances, give rise to difficulties.

Regression From the psychoanalytic perspective, the concepts of disturbances in development and fixation points permit an understanding of the process of regression. In the classical analytic theoretical formulation, regression is the central mechanism in the formation of obsessive-compulsive symptoms and determines that a person will develop that disorder rather than a conversion disorder. According to psychoanalytic theory, in conversion disorder the person represses oedipal genital libido, the energy from that undischarged impulse then being converted into somatic symptoms. In the obsessive-compulsive reaction, a different process occurs. As with hysterical patients, obsessive-compulsive patients may begin with a conflict over the oedipal genital impulse, when, for example, it is aroused by an environmental stimulus. Instead of repressing and converting that impulse, they employ a different maneuver to avoid the anxiety associated with the genital impulse. They abandon the genital impulses and regress to the earlier anal-sadistic phase of psychosexual development. The return to that earlier stage is facilitated by the fixation points that have remained from the distortions that occurred during their childhood development. By giving up genital urges, patients are no longer confronted with the conflicts and problems resulting from these urges.

Yet they have only increased their conflicts and problems. As a result of the regressive movement of psychic energies, all the anal-sadistic impulses from the earlier phase of development are reinforced, augmented, and strengthened. Now the pressure of reactivated anal and aggressive impulses toward discharge in behavior arouses new anxieties and new conflicts and requires new defensive operations. Previously, before the regression occurred, reaction formations had been sufficient to control and modify the manageable amount of anal-sadistic energy in the personality structure. Now, with the amount of that energy dangerously increased by the regressive return of energies flowing from the abandoned oedipal position, emergency measures are needed to control the heightened impulses toward anal-sadistic behavior. Prominent among these emergency measures are isolation, undoing, and displacement. As has been seen, these defenses, in conjunction with the constantly pressing impulses, lead to the appearance of obsessive-compulsive symptoms. The mechanism of regression sets the stage for the emergence of these symptoms in the form of obsessive-compulsive disorder.

According to this theoretical model, regression causes an alteration in the quality of the energy with which the psychic apparatus has to deal and in the nature of the defenses controlling that energy. Moreover, three additional alterations occur in psychic functioning as a result of regression: ambivalence, the emergence of magical thinking, and alterations in the superego.

AMBIVALENCE Ambivalence is the direct result of a change in the characteristics of the impulse life; it is an important feature of normal children during the anal-sadistic developmental phase. That is, they feel both love and murderous hate toward the same object, sometimes seemingly simultaneously; at least, one emotion follows the other in such rapid succession that they appear temporarily to exist side by side. In the normal course of development, much of the aggression is neutralized, and what remains becomes a desire to win out over, rather than to destroy, the other person. As a result, in a mature person, love for the object is dominant, and aggression plays a minor role. When regression occurs, there is a return to the earlier level of functioning, in which ambivalence is a characteristic mode of feeling. Thus, one finds obsessive-compulsive patients often consciously experiencing both love and hate toward their objects. The conflict of opposing emotions may be seen in the doing–undoing patterns of behavior and the paralyzing doubt in the face of choices that are so frequently found in persons with this emotional disorder.

MAGICAL THINKING In the phenomenon of magical thinking, the regression uncovers earlier modes of thought, rather than impulses; that is, ego functions, as well as id functions, are affected by regression. The phenomenon of the omnipotence of thought is inherent in magical thought. Individuals feel that merely by thinking about an event in the external world, they can cause that event to occur without intermediate physical actions. It is that feeling that makes having an aggressive thought so frightening to obsessive-compulsive patients.

For example, in the young man who had the thought

> "My father will die" when he turned off a light, there was an anxious concern that his father really would die because of his thought. As has been seen, to undo the consequences of his thought, the patient would compulsively touch the light switch and take the thought back. Here was mere magic, partly in the realm of thinking but also in the form of a ritual. That magical act, the touching, in itself could have no effect on events but was endowed by the patient with unrealistic powers of prevention.

These phenomena have a striking similarity to the incantations and rituals that are central to organized magic in all ages and cultures. The same modes of thinking are also present in the mental processes of primitive peoples, who fear the evil thoughts of others and ward off the bad consequences of such thoughts by apotropaic formulas or who try to influence natural forces, such as rain and fertility, by sympathetic magic. The same kind of magical thinking can be seen in children's rituals, games, and fears, which at times reach a degree that is suggestively pathological. For example, a patient of the Swiss psychologist T. Flournoy described the following episode that occurred in her childhood:

> One of my earliest memories concerns my mother. She had been sick in bed for several weeks, and one of the servants told me that she was going to die in several days. I must have been 4 or 5 years old. My most cherished possession was a little toy horse made of brown wood, covered with real hair, with a bridle and saddle that I could put on and off as I wished. The horse was kept in a little stable in the hall. I would stubbornly refuse to say my prayers by my bed because Mama was not there to hear them. Instead, I began to pray to the horse, kneeling before the little stable and reciting very quickly, without in the least understanding them, the few German phrases of our evening prayer. I was certain that my mother's recovery depended on the faithfulness of my prayers. When her recovery was slow in taking place, a curious thought arose in my mind: that I must sacrifice my horse in order for my mother to get well. The deed was not done all at once, and it cost me dear! I began by throwing the bridle and saddle in the fire, thinking that I might keep the horse when it was thus denuded. I don't remember the exact sequence of events, but I know that with great sorrow I finally broke my horse in little pieces and when a few days later I saw my mother up and about, I was for a long time convinced that my sacrifice had mysteriously cured her.

Because it occurs in both less civilized peoples and children, magical thinking is often considered to be a primitive form of mental functioning. The word "primitive" has here a temporal connotation, referring to the fact that it appears early in the evolution of the race or the development of the individual. The theoretical term, "primary-process thinking," of which magical thought is a manifestation, has the same temporal implication. Such primitive modes of thinking are never entirely eradicated from mental functioning, no matter how mature the person. They are merely layered over and controlled by more rational and realistically oriented thinking, and they readily reappear when a person dreams, creates, or suffers a pathological regression.

CHANGES IN THE SUPEREGO The standards and ideals of mature individuals are generally within the limits of potential achievement, and they mostly live at peace with their consciences, which prick them only when they have clearly violated their ethical principles. But in patients with obsessive-compulsive disorder, the situation is quite different. The number and range of mental and behavioral activities that are taboo are markedly increased; the patients have a heightened self-awareness and self-criticism; and they become harsher in their self-judgments. This phenomenon is evident in their obsessional concerns about harming or defiling others, in their constant, guilty anxiety over what they may have done, and in their incessant need by means of ritual and compulsive acts to prevent, control, and undo the effects of their forbidden thoughts and impulses. To a certain degree, these pathological features can be found in nonsymptomatic persons with obsessive-compulsive character traits, but they become exaggerated when such persons develop a clinical obsessive-compulsive disorder. The psychoanalytic concept views patients with obsessive-compulsive disorder as having regressed to developmentally earlier stages of the infantile superego—sometimes called the archaic superego—the harsh, exacting, punitive characteristics of which now reappear in the mental functioning of neurotically ill adults.

The psychoanalytic theory of obsessive-compulsive disorder ascribes the appearance of symptoms to a defensive regression of the psychic apparatus to the preoedipal anal-sadistic phase, with the consequent emergence of earlier modes of functioning of the ego, superego, and id. These factors, along with the use of specific ego defenses—isolation, undoing, displacement—combine to produce the clinical symptoms of obsessions, compulsions, and compulsive acts. These various psychodynamic processes can be observed as they emerge in the course of an exploratory interview of a patient with obsessive-compulsive disorder:

Joseph D., age 36, had been admitted to the hospital because of obsessional concerns about bumping into people that so preoccupied his thoughts that he was unable to work. As he was walking down the stairs from the ward to the doctor's office, he paused momentarily and looked around apprehensively. At the start of the interview, the doctor asked him what had happened on his way to the office.

Patient: Just as we were coming down the stairs and we turned the corner, I had the feeling there was something I wanted to check there. I still have the feeling, and I'm trying to put it out of my mind right now. And I want to walk back and check, but I'm trying to force myself not to. Now I know I couldn't have hurt anybody out there or bumped into anything, or anything like that. I know there's nothing there, and I didn't harm nothing. I just want to go back and check that, to see that there's nothing there. Now I *know* there's nothing.

Doctor: What do you think you might see?

P: I know I'll see nothing.

D: No—but in imagination what do you think is there?

P: I don't know what I would see. It's just there might be something out of place there—something like that.

D: Something out of place—like what?

P: I don't know—I can't explain it. It sounds crazy, I know, but I can't help it. I've been doing this the last couple of weeks on the street. I'd walk by people, and I'd think that they fell down, or something happened. Not that they fell down—I had to check to see that they got by me all right. Do you understand this? I just have to check to see that they got by me all right. I must have an aggression toward things, and I'm afraid it's going to come out. And when I walk by those people, there must be like a feeling of anxiety there that I could possibly have bumped into them—when I didn't. I must be guarding that aggression. In other words, I'm watching it like a hawk, and when somebody moves by me like that, I think that possibly they—the aggression—will come out. Do you think so?

Two aspects of the opening portion of this interview should be noted. First, the patient describes graphically and succinctly the symptoms that characterize obsessive-compulsive disorder: the anxiety-provoking, insistent intrusion of a thought that the patient himself recognizes as being realistically absurd, his attempt to fight off the thought, and his compulsion to an action aimed at offsetting both the obsessive idea and the anxiety aroused by it. Second, one should note the hint that the patient is struggling with angry feelings and impulses beneath the surface: his denial that "I didn't harm nothing"—his own spontaneous protestation of innocence—and his speculation that he "must have an aggression toward things." It is important to recognize, however, that the patient does not experience or admit his anger directly. The presence of anger is only an inference on the observer's part, based on the coloring of the patient's language and imagery. Even the patient's profession of possible "aggression" cannot be taken at face value as direct evidence. He uses the word in an affectless, intellectualized way: It is not an expression of a felt emotion, but a speculative inference by the patient about the reason for his symptomatic behavior.

At this point, the doctor chose to focus the patient's attention on the aggression, to see whether the patient's association might lead him closer to the hypothesized aggressive drive:

D: Tell me about the aggression that you have.

P: I can't explain it, doctor. I can't seem to analyze it. Whether it's a guilt that I'm responsible for people, and I'm afraid I'm going to do something that I don't know I've done—like indirect aggression. Like suppose you bumped into someone going down the stairs you didn't mean to. You jostled them in the subway as you walked down to the bottom. Well, then, when that person got to the bottom, they might have been a little bit upset by being jostled, and they might have tripped at the bottom (which wasn't your fault that they tripped at the bottom), and they might have hurt themselves. Well, now, I would feel guilty because I jostled them at the top. Do you understand? It's like an indirect aggression.

D: What about the subway?

P: I've been having trouble on the subway. I get on the train all right, but when I get off the train I'm afraid I'm going to—now it's unreasonable. I know that people can't fall under the train or fall down, because someone will see them and pick them up. Whether I feel I'm going to—that by doing so I'm hurting them, I don't know.

D: You're afraid of jostling them on the subway and knocking them under the car?

P: Oh, no. I don't think that they'll fall under the car. I just have a faraway fear that they would fall under the car. In other words, indirectly, not directly. I don't mean I'm going to go out and hurt somebody, but I mean through no great fault of my own, somebody's going to be hurt. Suppose somebody fell off into the subway pit by himself, and I tried to grab them and couldn't get them in time. I'd feel terribly guilty, like I didn't act quick enough. Do you understand what I mean? It's not that I'm going to hurt somebody. It's that I feel like a responsibility toward people.

Although the patient still has not confessed to an open experience of anger or a wish to act aggressively toward others, his associations to the word "aggression" reveal additional obsessional symptoms that had not been elicited in previous history taking. The imagery of the symptoms, which are entirely his own productions and fantasies, have an increasingly violent, bloody, and destructive character.

Not long after this interchange, in the course of describing himself as an easygoing person who avoided arguments or any show of differences with other people, the patient suddenly admitted that, once in his life, he had become angry in the course of a minor disagreement with a fellow employee at work. For the first time in the interview, in other words, the patient openly revealed that he had consciously felt angry and had openly expressed anger in a controlled way. Accordingly, the doctor pursued this tenuous lead:

D: Tell me about feeling angry.

P: It's just that it's like a feeling, more or less. You mean when I have these feelings of aggression when I'm walking by people?

D: Supposing you're angry, what does it feel like?

P: There's a certain—well, like a tension. You feel aggression. It's just like a feeling of aggression. It's instantaneous, and it's followed in my mind immediately by a feeling of guilt. If I walk by someone and they walk too close to me, I feel like—it must be a reaction. It must be a primitive reaction. You feel a little angry. You feel an aggressive feeling, and immediately it is followed by a feeling of guilt.

D: Tell me about somebody walking too close to you.

P: Well, suppose somebody's taking up the whole sidewalk or something like that, and you're trying to get by. You feel a little angry that they're taking up the whole sidewalk. You have a feeling of—sort of like a feeling of aggression.

D: What do you want to do?

P: Just push them, I guess. I must have a feeling that I want to push them off to one side—not hurt them, but just shove them out of the way like they want to shove me out of the way.

At this point, there was a dramatic change in the patient's behavior. He suddenly became visibly anxious and agitated, abruptly stopped talking, and then, after a brief pause, in a hesitant, faltering voice, he said:

P: I don't think I'm—my mind isn't working too well, doctor. It feels cloudy-like, you know.

Thereafter, for the rest of the interview, the patient was unable to pursue the line of thought he had been pursuing just before the outbreak of disorganizing anxiety.

These observations were interesting and revealing. The patient finally admitted to an impulse to push other people. For the first time, one is able to see directly the aggressive impulse that had previously been merely inferred from the obsessional symptoms, in which the dangerous, potentially harmful bumping of others was an accident that occurred passively, without any intent or wish to do so on the patient's part—although, curiously, he felt guilty about the obsessional thought, as if he were in fact truly responsible for an aggressive action. When, however, the patient became momentarily consciously aware of an active wish to push, he was suddenly overcome by disorganizing anxiety and was unable to continue his train of thought. One can now see by direct observation that the patient did indeed have angry feelings, thoughts, and wishes and, at the same time, that they were the source of significant anxiety. This anxiety motivated the patient to a variety of defenses—isolation, undoing, intellectualization. These defense mechanisms distorted these aggressive impulses into the channel of ego-alien symptoms that indirectly expressed his unconscious aggression.

LEARNING THEORY Although there are several behavior therapy models and theoretical assumptions underlying various behavioral treatment strategies, practitioners of behavior therapy hold in common a view of anxiety as a conditioned or learned response to specific stimuli or sets of stimuli and so have developed behavioral accounts of the acquisition and maintenance of anxiety disorders based on learning theory. One of the most influential learning theories in the early development of behavior therapy for anxiety disorders, O. H. Mowrer's two-stage theory of fear acquisition and maintenance, has been applied to explain both phobic disorders and obsessive-compulsive disorder.

Mowrer's theory holds that relatively neutral stimuli become associated with fear or anxiety through a process of respondent conditioning by becoming paired with events that are by nature noxious or anxiety producing. Thus, in obsessive-compulsive disorder, previously neutral objects and thoughts become conditioned stimuli capable of provoking anxiety or discomfort. The second stage of symptom development is complete when avoidance or escape behaviors are established to reduce the discomfort attached to the obsessional thought and maintained by anxiety reduction. In obsessive-compulsive disorder, active avoidance strategies in the form of compulsions or ritualistic behaviors are developed to control anxiety. Gradually, because of their efficacy in reducing a painful secondary drive (the anxiety), the avoidance strategies become fixed as learned patterns of compulsive behaviors. Research conducted during the past decade supports the assumptions that obsessions are associated with increases in anxiety and that the performance of ritualistic behaviors results in anxiety reduction.

It is apparent that Mowrer's two-stage theory provides useful concepts for explaining certain aspects of the obsessive-compulsive phenomena (e.g., the anxiety-producing capacity of ideas that are not necessarily inherently frightening and the acquisition and maintenance of compulsive patterns of behavior). The theory also provides a rationale for treatment procedures aimed at removing symptoms by decreasing the anxiety associated with obsessional thoughts and blocking the reinforcement gained by completing compulsive behaviors.

In their present forms, however, learning theories leave many questions unanswered, such as the reason that many patients do not report a learning experience contiguous with the onset of symptoms, the special prominence of ideas concerning dirt and aggression, the reason for the obsessional preoccupation with ideas that provoke anxiety (one would expect an avoidance of them), or the magical quality of the thought processes in obsessive-compulsive phenomena.

BIOLOGICAL ASPECTS Significant advances regarding the neurobiology of obsessive-compulsive disorder and its relation to major mood disorders have been made during the past 5 years. It has long been suspected that obsessive-compulsive disorder might be caused by either a gross brain abnormality or more subtle disturbances in biochemistry, neurotransmission, or receptor function. In the past, there was considerable interest in the possibility that specific brain lesions might be related to obsessive-compulsive symptoms.

For example, some patients, following the onset of Economo's disease, developed behavioral disorders that often appeared to be compulsive in nature. These phenomena, however, often differ from those seen in classical obsessive-compulsive disorder, in that they were primarily motoric and characteristically consisted of uncomplicated, stereotyped movements without associated mental content. Moreover, much of the disturbed behavior that has followed encephalitis has been characterized by impulsive, immature, and antisocial actions that result from a loss of control of the impulse life and may be characteristically different from the excess of inner controls that seem to typify individuals with obsessive-compulsive disorder.

Cases have also been reported in which temporal lobe–limbic pathology, including temporal lobe tumors and complex partial seizures, have been associated with obsessive-compulsive phenomena. Although studies such as these are interesting and suggestive, in most patients with obsessions and compulsions, there has been no consistent evidence pointing toward a specific lesion in the brain. Nonetheless, these older observations and new findings suggest that neurobiological disturbances may play an important role in the pathogenesis and maintenance of obsessive-compulsive disorder.

Recent studies have focused on strategies that assess the functional state of neuroendocrine or neurotransmitter systems. Because the pathophysiological relationship of obsessive-compulsive disorder to major mood disorders remains unclear, most recent biological investigations have used biological markers of depression to study obsessive-compulsive disorder. Accumulating neuroanatomical, neuroendocrine, electroencephalographic, and receptor-binding studies suggest that obsessive-compulsive disorder and mood disorders are related but probably distinct entities.

Neuroanatomy Several brain regions have been implicated in the neurobiology of obsessive-compulsive disorder. Bilateral hippocampal lesions in animals produce repetitive stereotyped behaviors. Destructive lesions of orbital gyri and the cingulum alleviate some obsessive-compulsive symptoms. A recent preliminary study with the positron emission tomography fluorodeoxyglucose method demonstrated increased metabolic rates in the left orbital gyrus and in the caudate nuclei bilaterally. The ventricular-brain ratio, which is increased in many alcoholic and schizophrenic patients, has been found to be similar to nonpsychiatric controls.

Neuroendocrine function DEXAMETHASONE SUPPRESSION TEST The most widely studied neuroendocrine test in psychiatric research is the dexamethasone suppression test (DST). Approximately 40 to 50 percent of patients with major depressive disorder, particularly patients with melancholia, demonstrate cortisol nonsuppression (plasma cortisol values above 5 μg per dl) during the 24-hour period after receiving 1 mg dexamethasone. An increased rate of dexamethasone nonsuppression (25 to 41 percent) has been reported in patients with obsessive-compulsive disorder. Preliminary evidence suggests that there is no clear relationship between the presence or absence of concomitant depression and dexamethasone status (i.e., suppression versus nonsuppression) in patients with obsessive-compulsive disorder. Although these findings with the DST provide indirect evidence of a biological connection between obsessive-compulsive and major depressive disorders, the underlying mechanisms responsible for dexamethasone nonsuppression require elucidation. Moreover, there may be distinct and separate mechanisms leading to dexamethasone nonsuppression. Thus, although these preliminary findings in a small number of obsessive-compulsive patients suggest a possible relationship between obsessive-compulsive patients and patients with major melancholic depressions, they are far from conclusive.

GROWTH HORMONE RESPONSE TO CLONIDINE One of the most consistent findings in the biological study of major depression has been the blunted growth hormone (GH) response to clonidine (Catapres). Current evidence suggests that clonidine, an α-2-adrenergic agonist, stimulates GH release by a direct effect on postsynaptic α-2-adrenergic receptors in the hypothalamus. Thus, the blunted GH response to clonidine observed in depression suggests a downregulation or subsensitivity of α-2-adrenergic receptors. A recent study of a few obsessive-compulsive patients also found a modest blunting of the GH response to clonidine. A similar finding has been reported in two independent studies of panic disorder, leading to the hypothesis that a blunted GH response to clonidine may identify a heterogeneous group of patients, independent of diagnosis, who respond to tricyclic antidepressants. Although such a hypothesis is intriguing, it is highly speculative, and the decision to treat with medications and the choice of pharmacological agents must still be determined on the basis of clinical presentation and natural course.

Physiology As with panic disorder, some clinical features of obsessive-compulsive disorder are similar to both the ictal and interictal behavioral disturbances associated with complex partial seizures. Although obsessive-compulsive disorder may be associated with nonspecific electroencephalogram (EEG) changes, the EEG abnormalities in obsessive-compulsive disorder are generally of a nonepileptiform pattern. Using somatosensory-evoked potential methods, a recent study found a high-amplitude N60 epoch in obsessive-compulsive patients, compared with normal controls and individuals with other neurotic disorders. The occurrence of nonepileptiform EEG abnormalities and a distinctive pattern with evoked potential recording has led to hypotheses that obsessive-compulsive disorder may represent a nonconvulsive epileptiform disorder (e.g., abnormal discharges in selective brain regions) or an abnormality in left-frontal brain functions.

Recent NIMH EEG studies, though not documenting epileptiform discharges on standard awake recordings, did find a sleep architecture similar to that of depressed patients. In fact, patients with obsessive-compulsive disorder were found to be similar to patients with major depressive disorder in terms of total sleep time, increased awake-movement time, decreased total sleep, decreased delta sleep, and reduced rapid eye movement (REM) latency. Moreover, the shortened REM latency in the obsessive-compulsive patients could not be accounted for on the basis of secondary depression.

Receptor binding Several lines of evidence suggest that ^{3}H-imipramine binds to the reuptake site for serotonin in the brain and that ^{3}H-imipramine–binding sites on platelets are similar in character to brain-binding sites. For these reasons, platelet ^{3}H-imipramine binding has been suggested as a model for the study of serotonergic function in psychiatric disorders.

Most studies have demonstrated a reduced number of ^{3}H-imipramine–binding sites in depressed patients. Given the neuroendocrinological and sleep physiological overlap between obsessive-compulsive and major mood disorders and hypotheses linking serotonergic dysfunction to obsessional symptomology and ritualistic behaviors, the study of platelet ^{3}H-imipramine binding in obsessive-compulsive disorder offers a promising research strategy. Although initially no significant difference was found in platelet ^{3}H-imipramine binding in a small number of obsessive-compulsive patients, compared with normal controls, a later study did find reduced ^{3}H-imipramine binding in a large sample of obsessive-compulsive patients. If the latter study is confirmed, the findings would be consistent with a theory of abnormal serotonin function in obsessive-compulsive disorder. Other lines of evidence also implicate serotonergic dysfunction in obsessive-compulsive disorder.

Neurochemistry Serotonin has been the principal neurotransmitter implicated in obsessive-compulsive disorder. L-tryptophan, a serotonin precursor, has been reported to decrease obsessive-compulsive symptoms, and trazodone (Desyrel), an agent with serotonergic agonist-like properties, has also been reported to diminish obsessions in a single case.

M-chlorophenylproperazine (M-CPP), a serotonin receptor agonist, has been used as a more specific pharmacological probe in the study of serotonergic postsynaptic receptor function. In contrast with the beneficial effects of L-tryptophan on obsessive-compulsive symptomatology, M-CPP has been found to produce an acute increase in obsessional symptoms.

Although these paradoxical findings cannot be totally explained in terms of a single serotonergic abnormality (e.g., increased receptor sensitivity), they do suggest that alterations in serotonergic function may play an important role in the neurobiology of obsessive-compulsive disorder.

The increase in obsessional symptoms following manipulations of the serotonin system with these pharmacological probes cannot be explained on the basis of a nonspecific anxiety reaction, as lactate and yohimbine, panicogenic agents in panic disorder, do not exacerbate obsessive or ritualistic behaviors in obsessive-compulsive patients. Moreover, the behavioral and biochemical effects of clomipramine (Anafranil), an inhibitor of serotonin reuptake, supports a serotonin connection in obsessive-compulsive disorder. For example, preliminary data suggest that clomipramine may have relatively selective and potent antiobsessional effects. Moreover, a significant correlation has been reported between plasma levels of clomipramine and clinical response, and clinical improvement has been positively correlated with decreases in 5-hydroxyindoleacetic acid (5-HIAA) after treatment with clomipramine.

CLINICAL SIGNS AND SYMPTOMS

Because of the relative rarity of the obsessive-compulsive disorder and the paucity of patients adequately studied, it is difficult to make categorical statements about the natural history of this anxiety disorder. All statements about its course, prognosis, and etiology must be considered as only tentative and perhaps applicable only to selected patients rather than to the syndrome itself.

ONSET The onset of obsessive-compulsive disorder occurs predominantly in adolescence or early adulthood. The symptoms first appear in approximately two-thirds of the patients by the time they are 25 years of age, with 15 percent having an onset before the age of 10. Less than 5 percent of patients have symptoms starting for the first time after the fourth decade of life. Those patients with obsessions and compulsions seek professional help at an earlier age than do those suffering from hysterical symptoms or anxiety. In one series of patients, the average age when they first saw a doctor was 22.0 years for the obsessive-compulsive group, 30.3 years for the hysterical patients, and 32.2 years for those with anxiety. A major life event or environmental stressor has been associated with the onset of obsessive-compulsive disorder in some patients.

SYMPTOMS The fundamental characteristics of the obsessive-compulsive phenomena described earlier are generally valid and useful in distinguishing them from the manifestations of other emotional disorders. The attempt, however, to categorize the various obsessive-compulsive manifestations themselves is a more complicated task, for the multiplicity of variables makes it difficult to devise a classification that will sharply differentiate one kind of obsessional or compulsive symptom from another.

Obsessive-compulsive phenomena may be manifested psychically or behaviorally; they may be experienced as ideas or as impulses; they may refer to events anticipated in the future or to actions already completed; they may express desires and wishes or protective measures against such desires; they may be simple, uncomplicated acts and ideas or elaborate, ritualized patterns of thinking and behavior; their meaning may be obvious to the most unsophisticated observer, or they may be the end result of highly complicated psychological condensations and distortions that yield their secret only to the skilled investigator.

No single classificatory scheme can do justice to clinical events that are composed of these many features in almost endless variation, and the organization that is suggested in what follows is only one possible way of looking at the phenomena. In most general terms, the symptoms may be divided into those that are psychic in nature and those that are manifested in observable behavior.

Obsessional thoughts Perhaps the simplest of the psychic symptoms are those in which thoughts, words, or mental images are obtruded into the conscious awareness of patients, against their wills. In *Grace Abounding to the Chief of Sinners,* John Bunyan left his spiritual autobiography and a magnificant case history as well, for he vividly described in those pages the variety of psychiatric symptoms from which he suffered, among them a paradigm of the obsessional thought:

> The Tempter came upon me again, and that with a more grievous and dreadful Temptation than before.
>
> And that was, To sell and part with this most blessed Christ, to exchange him for the things of this life, for anything. The Temptation lay upon me for the space of a year, and did follow me so continually that I was not rid of it one day in a month, no, not sometimes one hour in many days together, unless when I was asleep. . . .
>
> But it was neither my dislike of the thought, nor yet any desire and endeavor to resist it that in the least did shake or abate the continuation, or force and strength thereof; for it did always in almost whatever I thought, intermix itself therewith in such sort that I could neither eat my food, stoop for a pin, chop a stick, or cast mine eye to look on this or that, but still the temptation would come, Sell Christ for this, or sell Christ for that; sell him, sell him.
>
> Sometimes it would run in my thoughts, not so little as a hundred times together, Sell him, sell him, sell him; against which I may say, for whole hours together, I have been forced to stand as continually leaning and forcing my spirit against it, lest haply, before I were aware, some wicked thought might arise in my heart that might consent thereto.

Bunyan's preoccupations and his language are, of course, partly determined by his seventeenth-century surroundings, but the modern sinner has temptations to match.

> Freud's famous Wolf Man found himself from time to time compelled to think "God-Shit" or "God-Swine." A young woman of 23 years of age was shocked one day when the mental image flashed into her mind of her father and herself undressing each other and joining in a sexual embrace. From that time on, despite her desperate efforts to erase the image, it recurred with mounting intensity, and she finally fled to the hospital for help. A mother in her late 30s was tortured every time her daughter left the house by images of the child's being hit by a car. The mental picture of the little girl's body lying broken and bleeding in the gutter was particularly vivid, and nothing the mother could do would exorcise the tormenting scene.

In all these examples, the obsessional thought refers to present or future time. In a minor variation of the theme, the following patients are preoccupied with a guilty dread that an action they performed in the past has or will lead to dreadful consequences:

> A young man was constantly plagued every time he left his house with the fear that he had left a cigarette burning that would set the house on fire. An adolescent boy was tormented by the thought after he had masturbated that his semen had been spread about and would impregnate his mother and sisters. For days after she had kissed a boy, a young woman was obsessed with the idea that she was pregnant.

A special form of forced preoccupation with thoughts is designated by the term *obsessive ruminative states,* in which the central feature is rumination about a topic or problem, often of a religious or abstrusely philosophical nature. The pros and cons of the questions are repetitively considered, and imponderables are weighed in a prolonged, fruitless, and inconclusive inner dialogue, filled with doubting and despair. Bunyan was adept at such interior debate. He described how

blasphemous thoughts . . . stirred up questions in me, against the very Being of God, and of his only beloved Son; as, whether there were, in truth, a God, or Christ? And whether the holy Scriptures were not rather a Fable, and cunning story, than the holy and pure Word of God?

The Tempter also would much assault me with this, How can you tell but that the Turks had as good Scriptures to prove their Mahomet the Saviour, as we have to prove our Jesus is? And, could I think that so many ten thousands, in so many Countries and Kingdoms, should be without the knowledge of the right way to heaven (if there were indeed a heaven), and that we only, who live in a corner of the Earth, should alone be blessed herewith? Every one doth think his own religion rightest, both Jews and Moors and Pagans! and how if all our Faith, and Christ, and Scriptures should be but a Think-so too?

Sometimes I have endeavoured to argue against these Suggestions, and to set some of the Sentences of Blessed Paul against them; but, alas! I quickly felt, when I thus did, such arguings as these would return again upon me. Though we made so great a matter of Paul and of his words, yet how could I tell but that in very deed, he being a subtle and cunning man, might give himself up to deceive with strong delusions; and also take the pains and travel to undo and destroy his fellows?

These suggestions (with many others which at this time I may not, nor dare not utter, neither by word nor pen) did make such a seizure upon my spirit, and did so overweigh my heart, both with their number, continuance, and fiery force, that I felt as if there were nothing else but these from morning to night within me; and as though, indeed, there could be room for nothing else.

Compulsions In another form of the psychic phenomenon, ideas and images may be present, but the central feature is an irrational impulse to some form of action. The impulse, however, remains merely an impulse and is not acted on by patients, no matter how fearful they may be that they will lose control of their behavior. As earlier defined, that clinical manifestation is known as a compulsion. In yet another passage from his richly clinical autobiography, Bunyan exemplified that symptom:

One day as I was betwixt Elstow and Bedford, the temptation was hot upon me, to try if I had Faith, by doing of some Miracle; which Miracle at that time was this, I must say to the Puddles that were in the Horse-pads, Be dry; and to the dry places, Be you the Puddles. And truly, one time I was going to say so indeed; but just as I was about to speak, this thought came into my mind, But go under yonder Hedge and pray first that God would make you able. But when I had concluded to pray, this came hot upon me. That if I prayed, and came again and tried to do it, and yet did nothing not withstanding, then be sure I had no Faith, but was a Castaway and lost. Nay, thought I, if it be so, I will never try yet, but will stay a little longer.

So I continued at a great loss; for I thought, if they only had Faith, which could do so wonderful things, then I concluded that, for the present, I neither had it, nor yet, for time to come, were ever like to have it. Thus I was tossed betwixt the Devil and my own ignorance, and so perplexed, especially at some times, that I could not tell what to do.

Modern-day patients are perhaps more prosaic and less articulate than their Puritan predecessor, but they have, nonetheless, quite similar symptoms. They may feel the impulse to jump out the window of a high building or to throw themselves in the path of a moving train or car. Their aggressions may be aimed at others rather than themselves.

For example, a man constantly had the urge to push people down elevator shafts and so avoided elevators lest his temptations be too strong. A young mother was beset with the impulse to beat her infant son when he cried and at times had the urge to pick him up by the heels and bash his head against the wall. Others are driven by impulses to stab those around them with knives, scissors, or other sharp objects.

The aggressive compulsion need not be physical but may be an urge toward an act of defiance or one that is socially inappropriate or shocking, such as shouting obscenities in church. Although these impulses do not lead to action, they frequently arouse strong anxiety in patients and cause them to avoid the situation or object that evokes the impulse. Such an avoidance reaction is shared by individuals with compulsions of this sort and by those with typical phobic reactions.

Behavioral manifestations When the obsessive-compulsive phenomena are psychic, no one would know that there was anything unusual going on in patients unless they chose to divulge their purely private experiences. The situation is obviously quite different in the case of compulsive acts, in which the phenomena are behavioral and usually visible to anyone present to see them, although, often out of shame or embarrassment, patients will try to restrict their actions to those times when they are alone. There are two principal types of compulsive acts: those that express the primary urges or impulses that underlie them and those that are a reaction or an attempt to control the primary impulse.

Compulsive acts that simply and directly express the underlying urges are rare, although they do occur, as in the case of a young single woman who felt compelled to keep her diaphragm on top of her Bible in her bureau drawer and who did so. In most instances, the compulsion expressing an urge remains in the psychic sphere and is not visible in action, except when it contaminates a compulsive act that began as a controlling maneuver.

In general, compulsive acts are, or at least begin as, attempts to control or modify a primary obsession or compulsion, either because patients fear the consequences of the obsessions or because they are afraid that they will not be able to control their impulses. Such defensive compulsive acts are employed to contain, neutralize, or ward off the feared results of concurrent obsessions and compulsions, or they may represent a desire to ensure that some action in the past has not led to disaster.

Compulsive acts of the first type were particularly prominent in Borrow's account of the young tree climber, whose actions all were aimed at preventing his mother's death, which he obsessively feared. The same motivation was apparent in the law student who had to touch the light switch after turning it on to counteract his thought that his father might die.

Bunyan wrote that, in attempting to resist the evil thought to sell Christ,

by the very force of my mind, in labouring to gainsay and resist this wickedness, my very body also would be put into action or motion by way of pushing or thrusting with my hands or elbows, still answering as fast as the destroyer said, "Sell him; I will not, I will not, I will not, I will not; no, not for thousands, thousands of Worlds." Thus reckoning lest I should, in the midst of these assaults, set too low a value of him even until I scarce knew where I was, or how to be composed again.

Certain compulsive acts, as has been noted, are motivated by a guilty dread on the part of patients that they have done something bad; the acts are designed to atone for their sins or to reassure them that things are, in reality, all right.

A man in his 30s, fearing lest he push a stranger off the subway platform in the path of an oncoming train, was compelled to keep his arms and hands glued rigidly to his sides. The same patient, obsessed with the idea that dirt from his hands might harmfully contaminate others, often spent hours compulsively washing himself. The elaborate, ritualized preparations that some patients are compelled to carry out on going to bed may be a conscious attempt to control an impulse to masturbate.

The patient who kept his arms tight against his sides was on one occasion obsessed with the idea that despite his stringent precautions, he had, after all, inadvertently knocked someone off the subway platform. He struggled with himself for weeks to dispel what he rationally knew was a foolish notion but was at length compelled to call the transport authority to reassure himself that there had not, in fact, been any such accident. The same patient was for a time preoccupied with the concern that when he walked on the streets, he was dislodging manhole covers so that strangers passing by would fall into the sewer and be injured. Whenever he passed a manhole in the company of friends, he would be compelled to count his companions to make sure that none was missing.

The patient described in more detail earlier, who was beset by the same fear that by accidentally bumping strangers, he had caused them to fall and be injured, felt compelled to return to the scene of his supposed wrongdoing to determine whether anything really had happened. He would not rest easy until he was certain that no harm had been done.

The purpose of these various compulsive acts was evident to the patient or the observer, or both. There are, however, compulsive phenomena whose meaning is obscure and can be ascertained, if at all, only by a painstaking exploration of the patient's psychic function and associations. Two commonly found compulsive symptoms often fall into that category: the compulsion to touch, as seen in Borrow's acquaintance, and the compulsion to count. A patient is frequently compelled to utter an idiosyncratic, cryptic, seemingly nonsensical word that, on careful examination, proves to be a highly condensed and abbreviated formula, whose function is to ward off or neutralize an underlying impulse. Such was the nonsense word "Glegisamen" uttered by Freud's Rat Man. On analysis the word proved to be composed of the initials of the first word of several short protective prayers prefixed to "Amen."

Those compulsive acts that already have been examined have been relatively simple, straightforward, usually meaningful single actions. At times, however, the patient's compulsive behavior may become highly elaborate and repetitively stereotyped in the form of compulsive rituals. On going to bed, for example, the process of taking off one's clothes must conform to an exact pattern; they must be placed exactly so on a chair or hanger, the sequence of washing, voiding, and brushing one's teeth must be rigidly adhered to; the furniture in the bedroom, the bedclothes, and pillow must be symmetrically arranged. Any deviation in the pattern arouses anxiety in patients, and they must be certain that all has been done properly before they can drop off to sleep. Often, the same process must be carried out in reverse when they get up in the morning and prepare for the day.

A 32-year-old man who worked on the assembly line of an electronic concern developed the following compelling ritual: Before he could solder one piece to another, he had to tap the workbench three times with his left hand and three times with his right, followed by stamping three times on the floor with his left foot, then with his right. For a time this ritual merely slowed down his work performance, and he was able to continue his job. Gradually, however, an element of doubt crept into his mind. After completing a sequence of tapping and stamping, doubting thoughts would flash into his consciousness: "Did I really do it right? Am I sure that I tapped three times? Did I stamp with my left foot first?" In response to these self-questionings, he had to repeat the ritual to make sure it was perfectly done; but the more he performed it, the greater was his doubt. Before long, almost his entire working day was taken up by his rituals, and he was forced to leave his job.

The element of doubt manifested by this last patient is evident in some of the clinical examples already examined, especially in Bunyan's confessions and in the phenomenon of obsessional rumination. Doubt is, indeed, often found in connection with compulsive acts performed to ward off the feared consequences of obsessional ideas and compulsive urges. Those ideas and urges are not dissipated or quieted by the compulsive acts employed against them; patients are never sure that they have contained their ever-pressing impulses, that the impulses have not somehow leaked out inadvertently into their behavior or in some other way created the trouble they are at such pains to avoid. Often the patients' concerns are justified. Despite the best of their cautious intentions, the underlying impulse may manifest itself in the very process of carrying out defensive compulsive acts, and many distort these actions so that they appear to achieve exactly the effect they are designed to prevent. One of Freud's patients, for example, spent hours saying simple prayers designed to combat obsessional ideas of harm coming to others, but when he wished to say "May God protect him," he would find the words coming out, "May God *not* protect him."

A woman in her late 30s was obsessed with the idea that her excreta might offend or harm other people. During a stay on a psychiatric ward, she spent long periods of time washing in the communal bathroom after voiding or defecating. She would throw her skirts and petticoats over her head and scrub the entire lower part of her body, especially her genitalia and anus. Then she would scour with soapy water the toilet seat and the walls of the toilet stall. Finally, her hands would be mercilessly scrubbed, often to the point that they were red and raw. When she finished her ablutions, she and the toilet were spotlessly clean, but the rest of the bathroom was a shambles—dirty, soapy water still filling the wash basins, the floor awash with sudsy water, and countless soggy paper towels thrown about with complete abandon, littering the fixtures and the floor. In the end, the other patients on the ward were infuriated by the amount of time the patient spent in the bathroom and by the filthy mess she created by the very process that was designed to control her dirtiness and to protect the other people around her.

CHARACTER TRAITS A great deal has been written about the nature of obsessive-compulsive character traits, and the person who exhibits them has been described variously in the literature as having an obsessional character, an anal personality, or an anancastic personality. All these terms refer to a group of behavioral phenomena characterized by control, in contrast with the hysterical personality, in which a tendency toward a flamboyant expression of fantasies and feelings predominates.

As they are observed and experienced by others, individuals with obsessional personality traits are seen to exercise a marked measure of control over both themselves and their environment. They are cautious, deliberate, thoughtful, and rational in their approach to life and its problems and may appear dry and pedantic when those traits are carried to an extreme. They emphasize reason and logic at the expense of feeling and intuition, and they do their best to be objective and to avoid being carried away by subjective enthusiasms. As a result, these individuals often appear sober and emotionally distant, but at the same time they are found to possess great steadiness of purpose, reliability, and earnest conscientiousness. What they lack in flexibility, imagination, and inventiveness, they make up for in a conservative cautiousness about change that provides a healthy balance to the transient but violent enthusiasms of others.

In addition to their need to restrain themselves and their emotions, persons with obsessional personality traits like to feel that they have control of their environment as well. They subscribe to the dictum, "A place for everything, and everything in its place," and neatness, orderliness, and tidiness characterize their arrangement of space, just as punctuality marks their management of time. They like people and institutions to behave predictably and to conform to their predilections. They can be surprisingly obstinate and stubborn when challenged or contradicted. These individuals greatly value justice and honesty, have a strong sense of property rights, manage their own resources with frugality, and do not easily part with their possessions. A recent volume on the obsessive personality emphasized the usefulness of that element of control as a means of enabling individuals to enhance their sense of security and to protect themselves against feelings of helplessness in a world full of unpredictable and often unpleasant surprises.

The presence of obsessional character traits is not in itself, however, an indication of obsessive-compulsive disorder. On the contrary, those traits may be a great asset to their owners, and society owes much of its stability and efficiency to its more obsessional members. Rather, those traits become a liability only when they are carried to an extreme or when the balance between control and impulse expression leads to paralysis. Furthermore, there is no necessary connection between obsessional character traits and obsessive-compulsive symptoms. The incidence of the obsessional personality in the population at large is not accurately known, but it is far more common than obsessive-compulsive disorder. Most people with obsessional character traits do not develop obsessive-compulsive disorder, and obsessive-compulsive disorder does not always arise from the soil of the obsessional personality. In fact, there is no history of prior obsessional character traits in 20 to 30 percent of patients with obsessive-compulsive disorder.

COURSE AND PROGNOSIS

Accurate statements about the course and prognosis of obsessive-compulsive disorder are precluded by the lack of detailed knowledge of the natural history of the syndrome. There are only a few series in which longitudinal studies have been conducted, and the figures presented below must be considered as first approximations at best.

When first consulting a physician for their difficulty, two-thirds of the patients give a history of prior episodes of obsessive-compulsive symptoms, some 15 percent having first experienced them before the age of 10. The large majority of patients have had only one such prior attack, although a good number, roughly 30 percent, have experienced two or three episodes. In 85 percent of these attacks, the duration was less than a year, although some attacks lasted 4 to 5 years.

The figures given for the prognosis vary widely from series to series, but the following general statement may be made for patients followed up for anywhere from 1 to 10 years after treatment, excluding leukotomy: Some 25 percent are recovered, 50 percent are improved, and 25 percent are unchanged or worse. Those persons considered to be improved fall into two groups: (1) patients whose symptoms have lessened to a point that they are able to work and function socially and (2) patients who run a fluctuating course, often with long periods of complete remission of symptoms.

In general, obsessive-compulsive disorder is a chronic disorder, often following a remitting course. The prognosis is better (1) the shorter the duration of symptoms before the time the patient is first seen, (2) the greater the element of environmental stress associated with the onset of the disorder, (3) the better the environment to which the patient must return after treatment, and (4) the better the patient's general social and community adjustment and interpersonal relationships.

DIAGNOSIS

PSYCHIATRIC EXAMINATION The most obvious disturbances in behavior in patients with obsessive-compulsive disorder occur in those whose illnesses are characterized by compulsive acts. The observer cannot fail to see the elaborate rituals or stereotyped movements if they are performed in the public eye. Moreover, if patients divulge the nature of their inner obsessional thoughts and compulsive urges, these thoughts and urges are often seen to be irrational and bizarre. At the same time, patients almost always retain full insight; they recognize that their pathological thoughts and impulses are quite unreasonable and alien to the mainstream of their personalities. Apart from these obviously abnormal phenomena, there is little else that on casual examination appears to be unusual. As one observes more closely and perceptively, however, one becomes aware of behavioral elements, most of which are related to obsessive-compulsive character traits, although they are not invariably present in obsessive-compulsive patients.

The patients are often neatly dressed and groomed, sometimes with almost fussy tidiness. Reserved and formal in manner, they sit before the examiner stiff and prim, showing little in the way of gestures of facial expression, and their movements are careful and precise without spontaneity or easy grace. The controlled quality of their posture and movement is matched in their speech. Their sentences may be long and involved and full of stilted phraseology or stereotyped expressions. These patients characteristically balance one clause against another—"whereas . . ., yet . . .," "on the one hand . . ., on the other. . . ." They say the same thing several times in succession, introducing each paraphrase with "Again" or "In other words" or "To put it another way." They qualify any direct statement with words like "maybe," "perhaps," or "possibly," to avoid sounding dogmatic or escape being caught in error. They rely heavily on rational argument and talk in highly intellectual and intellectualized terms about the simplest matters, interspersing their pronouncements with the copious and needless interjection of words or phrases like "indeed," "to be sure," "be that as it may." They recount events in infinite detail, with a painful attention to accuracy and completeness, sometimes referring to written notes they have brought with them. Often it turns out that they have rehearsed what they plan to say in the interview for hours before it takes place and have tried to anticipate every move and question the interviewer may introduce. Any attempt to hurry them along, to cut them short, or to switch to another topic is met by the patients' resistance and rigid adherence to their preconceived programs of action. Evidence of expression of emotion, save possibly controlled anxiety, is at a minimum or entirely absent. If they are sophisticated about psychiatric theory, and such patients often are, they will discourse at length about their "conflicts," their "defenses," their "aggression," or their "libido." Yet, in answer to direct questioning, they will deny having any of the feelings related to those words. Their self-awareness and self-knowledge, however extensive, are entirely intellectual in nature and quite without emotional correlates.

These patterns of behavior are apparent from the outset, and they tend to be maintained intact by patients over many hours of contact with their doctors. Despite the physician's attempts to focus on and to encourage the expression of emotion, patients maintain their formality and their distance. Meaningful, warm, affective relationships appear to develop very slowly, if at all. Yet appearances can be deceptive, for many patients display evidence of a strong dependence on the doctor early in the relationship, despite their attempts to control their emotions. Patients will ask anxiously for reassurance that their obsessional impulses have not gotten out of control; they will be loath to stop at the close of the interview, and the interviewer may have to cut them short; and after leaving the office, they may come back a moment later to give additional information they had forgotten to mention. If the doctor casually passes these patients on the hospital wards, they are irresistibly drawn, like iron to a magnet, to approach the doctor to ask a question or to make a comment. They follow closely as the doctor walks along, unable to let go until the doctor almost literally has to shake them off. The adjective "sticky" applied to such patients is entirely appropriate.

DIFFERENTIAL DIAGNOSIS The descriptive and structural characteristics of obsessive-compulsive symptoms generally differentiate them from other psychogenic symptoms, such as depression, conversion phenomena, and phobias. But in regard to the obsessive-compulsive disorder as a syndrome, including the course and patterns of the symptoms in the life of individual patients, it is harder to separate it from other psychogenic disorders, especially phobic disorders and some variants of major mood disorders. There are, of course, many patients whose illnesses fit tidily within the area defined by the characteristics ascribed to them, but frequently, patients manifest admixtures of features belonging to several syndromes, and the diagnostic lines cannot be sharply drawn. Although that lack of neatness and order is distressing to the obsessional clinician, it perhaps reflects the fact that anxiety disorders are not simply the result of localized psychological disturbances but are the surface manifestations of complicated psychodynamic and neurobiological processes.

Although one assumes that there is a neurophysiological substrate to obsessions and compulsions, neurophysiological knowledge is not as yet detailed enough to provide a clinically useful and precise mechanistic explanation for the classic features of obsessive-compulsive disorder. The important diagnostic task is to differentiate it from other neuropsychiatric disorders, of which four—the phobic disorders, major mood disorders, schizophrenia, and Tourette's disorder—require attention.

Phobic disorder Some older classifications included phobias under the heading of obsessive-compulsive phenomena, and it is often difficult to distinguish sharply between them. In general, the phobic reaction is characterized by anxiety that harm will come to the phobic individuals from an external object or situation, and the patients control their anxiety by avoiding the object. The important mechanisms in phobia formation are displacement and projection, and the underlying conflicts are often oedipal in nature. This is, of course, in contrast to obsessive-compulsive disorder, in which the patients fear that they will hurt others, their anxiety is controlled by compulsive acts and by the mechanisms of undoing and isolation, and the underlying conflicts are predominantly preoedipal in nature.

When the clinical phenomena fit the criteria specified for either one of these two categories, there is no difficulty in differentiating them. The two sharply defined categories are, however, only the two ends of a spectrum, and in between fall phenomena that partake of characteristics from both categories.

One patient irrationally feared and avoided elevators—not, as it turned out, because he anticipated being hurt by riding in them but because he was afraid of his impulse to push others down the shaft. A young woman with a phobia of streets was afraid of her temptation to yield to her sexual impulses. The bedtime rituals of a young man proved to be a compulsive defense against expressing oedipal genital strivings through masturbation.

These three examples contain an admixture of obsessive-compulsive and phobic characteristics. It is not therefore possible in every instance to make a sharp distinction between phobic and obsessive-compulsive disorders.

Depression As with the phobic disorders, there are areas of overlap in obsessive-compulsive disorder and major depressive disorder. Some 30 percent of patients with depressive illness have obsessive-compulsive symptoms, and one-third have obsessive-compulsive character traits. It has been suggested that obsessive-compulsive features may be particularly common in patients with agitated, compared with retarded, depression.

Patients who for a period of time have manifested the symptoms of obsessive-compulsive disorder may go on to develop a typical depression. In fact, many patients with primary obsessive-compulsive disorder may not seek treatment until they develop a secondary major melancholic depression. Moreover, several neuroendocrine and physiological abnormalities common in major depressive disorder, such as an abnormal DST and shortened REM latency, are also found in obsessive-compulsive disorder. These observations have persuaded some experts to view obsessive-compulsive disorder as a subtype of major mood disorder rather than an anxiety disorder. Additional research is required to clarify this issue.

Schizophrenia Because magical thinking erupts into consciousness, the thought content of obsessive-compulsive patients often has a bizarre quality, which raises the question of whether they are really suffering from schizophrenia. Yet, despite that characteristic, clinical investigators have pointed out that surprisingly few patients with obsessive-compulsive disorder develop a clearly defined schizophrenic psychosis. The figures run from 3 to 12 percent and seem to be related in part to the strictness with which the investigator defined the initial obsessive-compulsive episode.

During the developing phase of schizophrenia, especially in the acute undifferentiated form, one frequently sees transient and varying obsessive-compulsive phenomena, and these phenomena may appear intermittently during the course of a well-established psychotic disorder. Occasionally, a clearly schizophrenic episode may appear in the course of a chronic obsessive-compulsive disorder, but it is characteristically mild and transient. One very rarely observes the direct transition of an obsessional thought into a delusion. And when this does occur, the delusion appears to be singular and without other commonly found symptoms of schizophrenia (e.g., hallucinations).

Despite these areas of superficial overlap between the two syndromes, the relationship between schizophrenia and obsessive-compulsive disorder is much more tenuous than the overlap between obsessive-compulsive disorder and major depression or phobic disorders. No matter how bizarre the content of patients' obsessional thoughts or how strange their compulsive acts, they usually maintain full contact with reality and are painfully aware of the absurdity of their thinking and behavior. No matter how preoccupied they appear to be with their symptoms, they do not retreat from their relationships with the people around them, and their affects remain appropriate. The most careful and prolonged observation of their clinical courses usually fails to reveal the characteristic stigmata of schizophrenia.

Tourette's disorder The observation that many patients with Gilles de la Tourette disorder have associated obsessive-compulsive symptomatology has led investigators to hypothesize that Tourette's disorder and obsessive-compulsive disorder may have overlapping neurobiological substrates. Several lines of investigation support this conceptualization.

There are many similarities between the two disorders, including youthful age of onset; a waxing and waning course over many years; intrusive thoughts involving sexual, aggressive, or visceral (fecal) motifs; and impulsive behaviors. In both disorders, vocal and motor tics and compulsive, ritualistic behaviors are induced or exacerbated by anxiety. Emerging data also suggest a genetic relationship between Tourette's disorder and obsessive-compulsive disorder. Moreover, both disorders are associated with an increased number of soft neurological signs and nonspecific EEG abnormalities. Obsessive-compulsive symptoms have also been reported as a sequela of encephalitis. In a parallel fashion, involuntary motor tics and vocalizations—separate from or concomitant with obsessive-compulsive symptomatology—have developed as a secondary complication of infectious or toxic encephalopathies. Although both disorders tend to be relatively refractive to treatment, it has been reported that frontal leukotomy is beneficial in the treatment of both disorders.

Although patients with classic obsessive-compulsive disorder will not be confused with most Tourette's patients, who have characteristic motor (i.e., recurrent, involuntary motor movements) or vocal (e.g., coprolalia, echolalia) tics, increasing evidence suggests that relatives of probands with either classic obsessive-compulsive disorder or Tourette's disorder may have less severe symptoms and atypical admixtures of both disorders. As individuals with these variants are identified with increasing frequency, the differential diagnosis and psychobiological distinction between the two disorders may become less well defined.

TREATMENT

Any discussion of the treatment of obsessive-compulsive disorder must be prefaced by the reminder that the absence of good, controlled studies and the paucity of information about the natural history of the disorder severely limit an evaluation of any of the recommended therapeutic measures. Nonetheless, when faced with the suffering of their patients and with the often-desperate situations that their symptoms may create for their families, the clinician is forced to do something in an attempt to alleviate their pain.

PSYCHOTHERAPY There can be no doubt that some obsessive-compulsive patients respond to the psychiatrist's psychotherapeutic maneuvers. It is possible, for example, to effect a complete disappearance of compulsive behavior in some patients by simply informing them that the doctor will assume complete responsibility for anything that may happen as a result of their impulses. With that reassurance, an occasional patient may abruptly give up a chronic compulsive ritual. Unfortunately, the improvement usually lasts for only a few hours. Then the patient begins to doubt the doctor's capacity to assume responsibility and soon returns to the compulsive acts. Even if this device is valueless as a definitive measure of treatment, the response does show that symptoms can be modified, however transiently, by psychological maneuvers.

In the absence of any adequate studies of psychotherapy in obsessive-compulsive disorder, it is difficult to make any valid generalizations about its effectiveness. Early in the development of psychoanalysis, it was felt that psychotherapy was the treatment of choice, because, like conversion hysteria, obsessive-compulsive disorder was conceived of as a transference neurosis and should theoretically therefore respond to psychoanalytic techniques. Some analysts have seen striking and lasting changes for the better in patients with obsessive-compulsive character traits, especially when the patients are able to come to terms with the aggressive impulse behind their character traits. Likewise, analysts and dynamically oriented psychiatrists have observed marked symptomatic improvement in their patients in the course of analysis or prolonged insight psychotherapy.

The decision whether such techniques will be helpful cannot be made on the basis of the nature of the symptoms alone. In general, the more chronic and fixed the symptom pattern is, the less responsive the disorder will be to modification by psychotherapy. As is always the case in choosing patients for insight psychotherapy, the criteria for selection depend primarily on factors other than symptoms: (1) the prominence of situational precipitating events, (2) the capacity to relate to the physician, (3) evidence of good relationships with others, (4) stable work patterns, (5) the capacity to tolerate anxiety and depression, (6) the ability to express emotion, (7) intelligence, (8) the ability to be introspective, (9) flexibility in thinking and behavior, and, perhaps most important of all, (10) the motivation for change.

Supportive psychotherapy undoubtedly has its place in the psychiatrist's armamentarium, especially for that group of obsessive-compulsive patients who, despite symptoms of varying degrees of severity, are able to work and make a social adjustment. The continuous and regular contact with an interested, sympathetic, and encouraging professional may enable patients to continue to function by virtue of this help, without which they would become completely incapacitated by their symptoms. Occasionally, when obsessional rituals and anxiety reach an intolerable intensity, it may be necessary to hospitalize the patient until the shelter of an institution and the removal from external environmental stresses reduce the symptoms to a more tolerable level. Nor must it be forgotten that the patient's behavior often drives the patient's family to the verge of despair. Any psychotherapeutic endeavors must include attention to family members through the provision of emotional support, reassurance, explanation, and advice on how to manage and respond to the patient.

BEHAVIOR THERAPY Although behavioral interventions have been applied extensively to patients with phobias, there are fewer reports of their use in the treatment of obsessive-compulsive disorder, and controlled studies of outcome are relatively scarce. The available data do, however, indicate that behavioral interventions are effective in treating obsessive-compulsive patients who traditionally have been viewed as refractory to treatment. Recent reviews of the behavioral literature reported success rates ranging from 70 to 80 percent. The major behavioral interventions applied to obsessive-compulsive patients have included aversive procedures aimed at eliminating obsessional thoughts and compulsive behaviors (e.g., shock treatment, thought stopping, covert sensitization), anxiety-reduction procedures designed to reduce the anxiety associated with obsessional thoughts (e.g., systematic desensitization, flooding in imagination and in vivo, paradoxical intention, satiation), prolonged exposure to obsessional cues, and blocking strategies aimed at preventing compulsive behaviors.

Aversive methods have been applied most often to eliminate obsessional thoughts. Aversive techniques are based on the idea that the occurrence of a noxious event or punishment immediately following a behavior will decrease the likelihood of that behavior occurring again. Thought stopping is an aversive technique in which the therapist interacts with the patient. As the patient broods on the obsessional thought, the therapist yells "Stop!" to counteract the patient's obsessional preoccupation. Eventually, the patient is encouraged to perform the thought-stopping procedure independently. Electric shocks administered following obsessional thoughts have been applied with some efficacy.

Anxiety-reduction procedures aimed at reducing the anxiety associated with obsessions have been applied: The notion underlying the use of these procedures is that by eliminating the anxiety associated with the obsessions, the compulsive behaviors will automatically extinguish, as they are no longer needed to decrease anxiety. Systematic desensitization is gradually exposing patients (in imagination or in vivo) to a graded hierarchy of anxiety-provoking stimuli, while maintaining a state of calm through deep muscle relaxation or a variety of other methods applied to induce a countering relaxation. A number of direct, more confrontative anxiety-reduction procedures have also been tested. Flooding and implosion have the patient confront the most anxiety-provoking stimuli and experience the full tide of affect thus aroused. Neither systematic desensitization nor flooding techniques have been studied in controlled investigations.

A more substantial and growing body of literature, including controlled investigations, supports the efficacy of prolonged exposure and response prevention techniques used in combination to combat simultaneously obsessions and compulsions. Patients are exposed to obsessional cues and carefully prevented from engaging in compulsive behaviors. Thus, an attempt is made to reduce the anxiety-provoking valence of the obsessions while simultaneously blocking the reinforcement of anxiety reduction that accompanies the carrying out of compulsive behaviors. This combination treatment approach repeatedly exposes patients for prolonged periods to events or thoughts that provoke anxiety while strictly preventing ritualistic behaviors. Investigators have examined the relative efficacy of exposure alone, response prevention alone, and exposure plus response prevention and have found that the combined treatment was clearly superior to either approach used in isolation. Initial findings suggest that imaginal and in vivo exposure are equally effective in achieving therapeutic gains. Prolonged exposure and massed practice appear more effective than shorter, more frequent, spaced-exposure sessions. Prolonged exposure plus response prevention interventions have proved highly effective: A recent review reported that 65 to 75 percent of 200 patients treated with this intervention improved and maintained gains at follow-up. Thus, although the ultimate efficacy of these procedures remains to be determined in more extended clinical trials, evidence for the effectiveness of behavioral interventions—specifically, prolonged exposure and response prevention procedures—is mounting and suggests that exposure plus response prevention may be one of the more effective treatment modalities currently available in the treatment of obsessive-compulsive disorder. These behavioral therapies may be particularly useful in the management of patients with well-entrenched ritualistic behaviors.

PHARMACOTHERAPY Increasing evidence suggests that clomipramine, a tricyclic antidepressant, is effective in the treatment of obsessive-compulsive disorder. Clomipramine may have selective antiobsessional, rather than just antidepressant, effects in the treatment of obsessive-compulsive disorder. The following observations support this conceptualization: First, clomipramine appears to be effective in the treatment of obsessive-compulsive patients with pure obsessions not accompanied by ritualistic behaviors. Second, obsessive-compulsive patients without concomitant depression also respond favorably to clomipramine. Third, several tricyclic and monoamine oxidase inhibitor antidepressants appear to be relatively ineffective in the treatment of obsessive-compulsive disorder. For example, desipramine (Norpramin), nortriptyline (Pamelor), amytriptyline (Elavil), clorgyline, and probably imipramine (Tofranil) are ineffective in the treatment of obsessive-compulsive disorder. Nontricyclic agents with serotonin reuptake blocking effects (e.g., zimelidine and fluoxetine [Prozac]) have, like clomipramine, been reported to have antiobsessional efficacy.

PHYSICAL THERAPIES Some researchers have recommended leukotomy as a valuable approach to the treatment of patients with obsessive-compulsive disorder. As a general rule, irreversible surgical procedures on the brain in patients with psychogenic disorders should be avoided, particularly when these disorders, as is the case with many patients with obsessive-compulsive disorders, run an intermittent course. There is evidence, however, that the procedure of leukotomy can lessen the intensity of obsessions and compulsions and can diminish the suffering they engender, even if it does not necessarily improve the patient's social adjustment. On that basis, it should be considered in those patients who have a chronic, severe, unremitting obsessive-compulsive disorder that has not responded to any of the less drastic forms of treatment.

REFERENCES

Baxter L R Jr, Phelps M E, Mazziotta J C, Guze B H, Schwartz J M, Selin C E: Local cerebral glucose metabolic rates in obsessive-compulsive disorder. Arch Gen Psychiat *44*: 211, 1987.

Beech H R: *Obsessional States*. Methuen, London, 1974.

Cummings J L, Frankel M: Gilles de la Tourette's syndrome and the neurological basis of obsessions and compulsions. Biol Psychiat *20*: 1117, 1985.

Flament M F, Rapoport J L, Murphy D L, Berg C J, Lake C R: Biochemical changes during clomipramine treatment of childhood obsessive-compulsive disorder. Arch Gen Psychiat *44*: 219, 1987.

Freud S: The neuro-psychoses of defense. In *The Standard Edition of the Complete Psychological Works of Sigmund Freud*, vol 3, p 45. Hogarth, London, 1952.

Freud S: Notes upon a case of obsessional neurosis. In *The Standard Edition of the Complete Psychological Works of Sigmund Freud*, vol 10, p 155. Hogarth, London, 1955.

Insel T R: Obsessive compulsive disorder: Five clinical questions and a suggested approach. Compr Psychiat *23*: 241, 1982.

Insel T R, Donnelly E F, Lalakea M L, Alterman I S, Murphy D L: Neurological and neuropsychological studies of patients with obsessive-compulsive disorders. Biol Psychiat *18*: 741, 1983.

Insel T R, Gillin J C, Moore A, Mendelson W B, Lowenstein R J, Murphy D L: The sleep of patients with obsessive-compulsive disorder. Arch Gen Psychiat *39*: 1372, 1982.

Insel T R, Mueller E A, Alterman I, Linnoila M, Murphy D L: Obsessive-compulsive disorder and serotonin: Is there a connection? Biol Psychiat *20*: 1174, 1985.
Insel T R, Murphy D L, Cohen R M, Alterman I, Kilts C, Linnoila M: Obsessive-compulsive disorder: A double-blind trial of clomipramine and clorgyline. Arch Gen Psychiat *40*: 605, 1983.
Jenike M A: Obsessive-compulsive disorder. Compr Psychiat *24*: 99, 1983.
Lieberman J: Evidence for a biological hypothesis of obsessive-compulsive disorder. Neuropsychobiol *11*: 14, 1984.
Marks I: Review of behavioral psychotherapy. I: Obsessive-compulsive disorders. Amer J Psychiat *138*: 584, 1981.
Mowrer, O: *Learning Theory and Behavior*. Wiley, New York, 1960.
Pippard J: Rostral leukotomy: A report on 240 cases personally followed up after 1½ to 5 years. J Ment Sci *101*: 756, 1955.
Pollitt J D: Obsessional states. Brit J Psychiat (special publication) *9*: 133, 1975.
Rachman S, Hodgson R: *Obsessions and Compulsions*. Prentice-Hall, Englewood Cliffs, NJ, 1980.
Rapoport J, Elkins R, Langer D H, Sceery W, Buchsbaum M S, Gillin J C, Murphy D L, Zahn T P, Lake R, Ludlow C, Mendelson W B: Childhood obsessive-compulsive disorder. Amer J Psychiat *138*: 1545, 1981.
Rasmussen S A, Tsuang M T: The epidemiology of obsessive-compulsive disorder. J Clin Psychiat *45*: 450, 1984.
Rasmussen S A, Tsuang M T: Clinical characteristics and family history in DSM-III obsessive-compulsive disorder. Amer J Psychiat *143*: 317, 1986.
Robins L N, Helzer J E, Weissman M M, Orvaschel H, Gruenberg E, Burke J D, Regier D A: Lifetime prevalence of specific psychiatric disorders in three sites. Arch Gen Psychiat *41*: 949, 1984.
Salzman L: *The Obsessive Personality*. Science House, New York, 1968.
Salzman L, Thaler F: Obsessive-compulsive disorders: A review of the literature. Amer J Psychiat *138*: 286, 1981.
Steketee G, Foa E B: Obsessive-compulsive disorder. In *Clinical Handbook of Psychological Disorders,* D Barlow, editor, p 69. Guilford, New York, 1986.
Thoren P, Asberg M, Bertilsson L, Mellstrom B, Sjoqvist F, Traskman L: Clomipramine treatment of obsessive-compulsive disorder: II. Biochemical aspects. Arch Gen Psychiat *37*: 1289, 1980.
Thoren P, Asberg M, Cronholm B, Jornestedt L, Traskman L: Clomipramine treatment of obsessive-compulsive disorder: I. A controlled clinical trial. Arch Gen Psychiat *37*: 1281, 1980.
Zohar J, Insel T R: Obsessive-Compulsive disorder: Psychobiological approaches to diagnosis, treatment and pathophysiology. Biol Psychiat, *22*: 667, 1987.

18.4 POST-TRAUMATIC STRESS DISORDER

J. DAVID KINZIE, M.D.

DEFINITION

The term *post-traumatic stress disorder* (PTSD) first appeared in the third edition of the *Diagnostic and Statistical Manual of Mental Disorders* (DSM-III) and is listed within the group of anxiety disorders. DSM-III defines PTSD as follows:

> The essential feature is the development of characteristic symptoms following a psychologically traumatic event that is generally outside the range of usual human experience. The characteristic symptoms involve reexperiencing the traumatic event: numbing of responsiveness to, or reduced involvement with, the external world and a variety of autonomic, dysphoric or cognitive symptoms.

The revision of DSM-III (DSM-III-R) specifies the types of stressors that cause psychological trauma: "serious threat to one's life or physical integrity; serious threat or harm to one's children, spouse, or other close relatives or friends; destruction of one's home or community, or seeing another person who is mutilated, dying or dead, or the victim of physical violence."

This definition highlights the importance and severity of the stressor and recognizes that PTSD comprises a group of symptoms that can arise from a wide variety of severe, psychologically traumatic events. The disturbance must last at least 1 month to make the diagnosis of PTSD.

HISTORY Nightmares, shaking, persistent fear, and phobic behavior were described by famous writers such as William Shakespeare and Charles Dickens—all as aftereffects of traumatic events. The idea that catastrophes or personal tragedies can result in persistent symptoms is common among the lay public. It is therefore surprising that it has taken psychiatry so long to recognize officially PTSD as a result of traumatic events.

Documented war experiences have provided an early description of this disorder among soldiers during the American Civil War. A combat soldier with palpitations and chest pains was felt to have a functional cardiac disturbance which was called "soldier's heart" or "effect syndrome." Anxiety symptoms in World War I soldiers were called "shell shock" and were thought to be related to lesions in the central nervous system (CNS).

Theories of the syndrome's psychological etiology began to compete with physical causation theories in the early 1900s. Under the influence of psychodynamic theory, "traumatic neurosis" was viewed as the result of the reactivation of an unresolved conflict in a predisposed individual. Childhood traumas or conflicts that might lie dormant out of the individual's consciousness were emphasized. The stressor was considered to be not of primary importance but, rather, an event that brought to awareness as trauma the previously unresolved conflicts. This was consistent with the view that objective trauma itself could not cause a neurosis without significant childhood predisposition.

World War II brought further clinical experience not only with combatants but also with civilians: survivors of prisoner-of-war camps, Nazi death camps, and the atomic bombing of Japan. An early description of symptoms among civilians caught in the disastrous Boston Coconut Grove fire of 1941 listed general nervousness, irritability, fatigue, insomnia, and nightmares. Both physical and psychological causes of the resulting disorder were stressed.

Early investigators of the survivors of death camps described symptoms of anxiety, motor restlessness, hyperapprehensiveness, difficulty sleeping, night terrors, fatigue, phobic reactions, and a constant preoccupation with recollections of persecutory experiences. This became known as the concentration-camp syndrome. Some investigators regarded as the significant factor an organic brain disease as a result of physical injury. The concentration-camp syndrome occurred, however, so regularly without evidence of predisposition among such a high proportion of survivors that it became clear the symptoms were almost entirely the result of the psychological trauma itself. The existential factors involved surviving the concentration camp and were vividly described by Viktor Frankl in his book *From Death Camp to Existentialism*. Robert Lifton emphasized in *The Broken Connection* the death imagery with resultant symptoms among civilians after the bombing of Hiroshima.

The traumatic neurosis of war was described in terms quite similar to DSM-III's PTSD. Recognition of the neuroses of World War II veterans led to the category of gross stress reaction in the first edition of the *Diagnostic and Statistical Manual of Mental Disorders* (DSM-I) in 1952, which also appeared in the *International Classification of Diseases* (ICD). This category was not included in the second edition of the *Diagnostic and Statistical Manual of Mental Disorders* (DSM-II) in 1968, however, despite the syndrome's being well described in multiple settings, both civilian and military. Work on reactions to trauma continued. One particularly influential report described a phasic reaction of intrusive responses alternating with avoidant behavior and denial. The increasingly obvious problems of Vietnam veterans plus clinical work with victims of multiple disasters made clear a need for a post-traumatic stress category in DSM-III. The symptoms were primarily based on the varieties of clinical reports described above, and so the syndrome was placed with the anxiety disorders. Unlike most other disorders in DSM-III, PTSD did not undergo prior extensive field or interrater reliability studies, resulting in some controversy over its validity. Studies done after the appearance of DSM-III, however, generally confirmed the disorder's validity. The appearance of the operationally described category increased interest in studying and comparing reactions to such diverse disasters and personal calamities as incest, rape, child kidnapping, terrorism, the Vietnam War, Three-Mile Island, the Mt. St. Helens volcano explosion, Cambodian concentration camps, and children viewing the murder of parents. As clinical and research experience mounted, it became necessary to modify the criteria, and DSM-III-R was published in 1987.

DSM-III had four main criteria for PTSD: (1) evidence of a recognizable stressor that would evoke significant symptoms of distress in almost everyone, (2) reexperiencing the trauma, (3) numbing of responsiveness, and (4) at least two (from a list of six) associated symptoms that were not present before the trauma. It recognized that some of the reactions were chronic or delayed.

COMPARATIVE NOSOLOGY

In the ninth revision of ICD (ICD-9), the only similar disorder is acute reaction to stress, defined as "a very transient disorder of any severity and nature which occurs in individuals without any apparent mental disorder in response to exceptional physical or mental stress such as natural catastrophes or battle and which usually subsides within hours or days."

The temporary nature of the disorder and the specification that it occur in normal personalities are the primary differences from DSM-III's description of PTSD.

DSM-III-R makes major changes in the emphasis on symptoms in PTSD and thus reflects some conceptual change. The stressor, which is the first criterion, is explicitly listed in the definition, and examples are given of psychologically traumatic events. The criteria are shown in Table 18.4-1. The other three groups of symptoms are (1) persistent reexperience of the traumatic event, (2) persistent avoidance of stimuli associated with the trauma, or numbing of general responsiveness (at least three of seven symptoms must be present), (3) persistent symptoms of increased arousal (at least two of six symptoms), (4) duration of the disturbance of at least 1 month. All these symptoms must occur during the same period for at least 1 month. The total number of possible symptoms has increased to 17. Compared with DSM-III, DSM-III-R places more emphasis on the avoidance of stimuli associated with the trauma and less on numbing of responsiveness; it introduced symptoms of persistent increased arousal as a necessary criterion and removed survivor guilt as an associated symptom.

DSM-III recognizes two subtypes of PTSD: the acute form with an onset of symptoms within 6 months of the trauma and a duration of symptoms of less than 6 months, and the chronic or delayed form, with a duration of symptoms of 6 months or more (chronic) or with an onset of symptoms at least 6 months after the trauma (delayed). The acute and chronic subtypes are not listed in DSM-III-R, but the diagnosis should specify whether there is a delayed onset (i.e., onset of symptoms of at least 6 months after the trauma).

TABLE 18.4-1
Diagnostic Criteria for Post-Traumatic Stress Disorder

A. The person has experienced an event that is outside the range of usual human experience and that would be markedly distressing to almost anyone, e.g., serious threat to one's life or physical integrity; serious threat or harm to one's children, spouse, or other close relatives and friends; sudden destruction of one's home or community; or seeing another person who has recently been, or is being, seriously injured or killed as the result of an accident or physical violence.

B. The traumatic event is persistently reexperienced in at least one of the following ways:
   (1) Recurrent and intrusive distressing recollections of the event (in young children, repetitive play in which themes or aspects of the trauma are expressed)
   (2) Recurrent distressing dreams of the event
   (3) Sudden acting or feeling as if the traumatic event were recurring (includes a sense of reliving the experience, illusions, hallucinations, and dissociative [flashback] episodes, even those that occur upon awakening or when intoxicated)
   (4) Intense psychological distress at exposure to events that symbolize or resemble an aspect of the traumatic event, including anniversaries of the trauma

C. Persistent avoidance of stimuli associated with the trauma or numbing of general responsiveness (not present before the trauma), as indicated by at least three of the following:
   (1) Efforts to avoid thoughts or feelings associated with the trauma
   (2) Efforts to avoid activities or situations that arouse recollections of the trauma
   (3) Inability to recall an important aspect of the trauma (psychogenic amnesia)
   (4) Markedly diminished interest in significant activities (in young children, loss of recently acquired developmental skills such as toilet training or language skills)
   (5) Feeling of detachment or estrangement from others
   (6) Restricted range of affect (e.g., unable to have loving feelings)
   (7) Sense of a foreshortened future (e.g., does not expect to have a career, marriage, children, or a long life)

D. Persistent symptoms of increased arousal (not present before the trauma), as indicated by at least two of the following:
   (1) Difficulty falling or staying asleep
   (2) Irritability or outbursts of anger
   (3) Difficulty concentrating
   (4) Hypervigilance
   (5) Exaggerated startle response
   (6) Physiologic reactivity upon exposure to events that symbolize or resemble an aspect of the traumatic event (e.g., a woman who was raped in an elevator breaks out in a sweat when entering any elevator)

E. Duration of the disturbance (symptoms in B, C, and D) of at least 1 month.

Specify delayed onset if the onset of symptoms was at least 6 months after the trauma.

Table from DSM-III-R *Diagnostic and Statistical Manual of Mental Disorders*, ed 3, revised. Copyright American Psychiatric Association, Washington, DC, 1987. Used with permission.

EPIDEMIOLOGY

The definition of PTSD requires that it follow unusual and severe stress. Therefore, it can occur only when the patient has undergone stressful events. The incidence of PTSD increases after disasters involving large numbers of people. Only since the DSM-III definition was formally accepted have comparable epidemiological studies been made. Data on PTSD in the general population and among victims of specific disasters are now being accumulated.

Early reports, using various criteria for PTSD gave incidences of the disorder that increased with the severity of stresses. Eighty-five percent of victims of Nazi death camps were reported to have the concentration-camp syndrome, and none was without pathology. Fifty-seven percent (26 of 46) of patients in the 1941 Coconut Grove nightclub disaster developed psychiatric complications involving multiple symptoms. Traumatic-neurotic reactions were found in 80 percent of the survivors of the 1972 Buffalo Creek disaster.

Newer studies using the DSM-III criteria offer a better comparison. PTSD was recently added to the diagnoses stud-died in the St. Louis Epidemiologic Catchment Area (ECA) Survey. In the general population it is a rare disorder, occurring in 0.5 percent of men and 1.2 percent of women. In a study following the volcanic eruption of Mt. St. Helens, a lifetime prevalence of PTSD was 2.9 percent for males and 2.3 percent for females. Sixty percent of the disorders were unrelated to the Mt. St. Helens experience. In both studies the most common stressors in men were combat experience. Being assaulted was the most common stressor in women in the St. Louis study and second only to the experience of the explosion itself in the Mt. St. Helens disaster.

A survey among Vietnam veterans found that after active duty, 26 percent in heavy combat, 17 percent in average combat, and 7 percent not in combat met the criteria for PTSD. A follow-up study 6 to 16 years after the men returned home showed 36 percent of those in heavy combat, 24 percent in average combat, and 17 percent not in combat suffering from chronic PTSD.

Structured interviews with former World War II prisoners of war (POWs) revealed that 67 percent had a PTSD after their release. Of those affected, 24 percent had moderate residual symptoms, and 8 percent (5 percent of the total) had marked chronic PTSD 40 years later. Using a structured interview with Cambodian children who had endured 4 years of forced labor, starvation, witnessing executions, separation from their family, and dislocation to a new country, it was found that after 5 years, 50 percent (of 40) had full PTSD diagnoses. As further research on the epidemiology of PTSD gathers data, prevalence in the community and the acute and chronic phases of the disorder following a disaster will become even clearer.

ETIOLOGY

The etiology of PTSD combines the interaction of many factors, including the type of stressor, the personality of the individual involved, and the social environment of the traumatic and post-traumatic period. Unlike most other diagnoses in DSM-III, the definition of PTSD includes a stressor of such severity as to produce significant symptoms of distress in most people. Though necessary, the stressor by itself is usually insufficient to develop the disorder. That is, aside from extremely prolonged catastrophic conditions such as living in a death camp, most individuals experiencing a trauma do not develop the disorder.

STRESSORS Stressors of different types and durations contribute to the etiology of PTSD. The stress must be outside the range of common experiences, which excludes simple bereavement, chronic illness, business losses, marital conflict, or divorce. The trauma includes rape or assault, military combat, natural and manufactured disasters (airplane crashes, auto accidents, industrial accidents) and deliberate violence (torture and death camps). The stressor may cause a physical injury such as head trauma or malnutrition, but as stated in DSM-III-R, it must also cause a psychological trauma such as a serious threat to one's life or family, the destruction of one's home, or the sight of dying or mutilated bodies. The victim of physical violence is one of the clearest examples and most frequently suffers PTSD. The severity of the stressors as recorded on Axis IV is usually extreme (physical or sexual abuse) or catastrophic (concentration camp or devastating natural disasters).

Traumatic events vary in intensity and duration, may affect individuals or groups, or can have manufactured or natural causes. All of these factors influence the development of the disorder and the chronicity of its course. Some events such as an isolated physical assault occur in a single brief episode. Others, such as combat experience, involve several episodes over a longer duration. Death-camp and some POW experiences are of severe intensity over a prolonged time. Those of greater severity and longer duration regularly produce a high occurrence of PTSD with a more chronic course.

Group trauma is often more complicated. The large number of people involved in a catastrophe can mean seeing bodies, witnessing mass destruction, and watching (or reading) media coverage. Grieving family members or friends complicate the primary disorder; loss of family or community support prolongs the trauma. Catastrophes (earthquakes, floods) that wipe out entire communities, or a genocidal death camp may destroy the entire social and cultural fabric of a community, greatly impairing the ability of individuals or the social group to recover. Manufactured disasters regularly produce a higher prevalence of PTSD than do natural disasters. Symptoms of guilt concerning others, rejection by others, and humiliation are more common in manufactured disasters than in natural disasters. Manufactured disasters can result from acts of both commission and omission. Acts of commission are direct, conscious, violent acts. Acts of omission such as toxic flooding from ill-maintained dams or poor safety standards at industrial sites are the result of attempts to save money or time and often result in slower recognition of the event, ill-defined anger at "the system," and prolonged, complicated legal processes.

Participation in abusive violence acts (defined as unlawful behavior) was found to be related to the denial pattern of PTSD but not to the reexperiencing symptoms. Witnessing abusive violence resulted in the reexperiencing symptoms but not the denial.

INDIVIDUAL FACTORS The idea that a person is predisposed to PTSD harks back to the concept of traumatic neurosis in which a patient's response to a current trauma was considered to be a reactivation of prior unresolved conflict. But establishing premorbid personality functioning is difficult after a trauma has occurred, thus making predisposition difficult to determine. In severe trauma such as death-camp experiences, the disorder is so common that the syndrome seems to be the result of the trauma itself. In a group of Vietnam POWs whose precaptivity personalities were known, the post-traumatic psychiatric problems did not correlate with preexisting problems. A study of rape victims, however, showed that poor long-term recovery was related to poor premorbid adjustment. In a study of fire fighters exposed to a bushfire disaster, the intensity of the exposure or losses sustained did not predict development of PTSD. However, introversion, neuroticism, and past history were premorbid factors associated with chronic PTSD.

Trauma in early life may increase the symptoms in response to later trauma. Psychiatric patients have an increase in symptoms in response to trauma; however, this usually takes the form of the previous disorder—not a new PTSD per se. The individual's defensive style determines how a specific trauma is perceived and what coping mechanism is used. Similarly, for combatants, the subjective perceptions of the meaning of combat influence the perception of realistic dangers and reactions to war. A sense of personal responsibility, either real or exaggerated, can promote or maintain PTSD symptoms.

Among families of patients with chronic PTSD, familial psychopathology was found in 66 percent, with alcoholism, depression, and anxiety the most common. The probands with anxiety showed more similarity to the patients than did the probands with depression, indicating that chronic PTSD may be genetically related to generalized anxiety.

PTSD can occur at any age, with the young adult years the most prevalent. Several studies now indicate that the syndrome exists in very young children, even those who are preverbal, but they tend not to exhibit psychic numbing or visual flashbacks. Reenactment occurs in post-traumatic play, and such children often have a foreshortened view of the future. An earlier traumatic event may become apparent only in old age. There are several reports of World War II veterans in their 60s who, probably as a result of age, illness, or losses, developed PTSD from traumatic events that occurred more than 30 years earlier.

Many soldiers in their formative adolescent years developed strong group cohesion in the military. Because such groups can be severely disrupted by death and injury, the younger soldiers were more vulnerable to PTSD. One study found that soldiers who developed PTSD had an average age of 18.3, whereas the average age of a control group without PTSD was 21.5. Other work with veterans found that those with high PTSD scores also had high hypnotizability scores and high imagery scores, indicating that people with excellent hypnotic potential may be more susceptible to PTSD.

The associated features of PTSD, especially among Vietnam veterans, include behavioral abnormalities such as aggressive-impulsive behavior and substance abuse. Some evidence indicated that these disorders were common in those with PTSD before enlistment and were not related to PTSD and the war experience.

SOCIAL FACTORS Often trauma can affect a large group of people and their social environment, which further impairs recovery. Disasters such as airplane crashes or floods imply multiple trauma, with sights and sounds of death and destruction. The media's attention and publicity can lengthen the trauma but also mobilize public support and sympathy for the victims. When the social environment is destroyed, as in mass flooding with severe loss of life, the loss of the community adds further demoralization: The normal, helping community network disintegrates, and individuals are often left to cope on their own. Some traumas are so severe (Nazi death camps, Cambodian concentration camps, or civil wars of attrition) that the entire cultural structure breaks down. Traditions, cultural models, or leaders can no longer handle the processes of grief, and an existential or religious meaning to life can also be lost.

In mass disasters, especially natural disasters, some groups find short-term cohesion and acceptance by others. If help and intervention materialize slowly, doubts about society's genuineness may cause disillusionment and social disintegration, with further individual withdrawal. After a disaster, family and friends tend to be protective and often limit contact—even that which may be beneficial. This group solidarity offers social support but also limits necessary treatment.

More social support leads to a better outcome for the victims. Some highly symptomatic victims with PTSD had smaller social networks, fewer social contacts outside family circles, and more negative emotions toward family members. The specific symptoms of PTSD, however, such as a diminished interest in activities or feelings of detachment (numbing), may mean that a traumatized individual does not perceive or use the available social support.

Society's attitude toward the victims of trauma may play a large role in their recovery. Some events evoke positive attitudes toward victims (hostages), whereas other events are received by the public with disinterest or apathy (refugees of the Central American conflict). Still other events induce public hostility (perceptions of some Vietnam veterans about the Vietnam War). Negative attitudes of society or friends can exacerbate the original trauma.

PSYCHOLOGICAL FACTORS Sigmund Freud and other early analysts made several attempts to explain the symptoms and course of traumatic neurosis. An early formulation contended that trauma revived the original childhood neurosis through regression. Later an energy model was postulated in which a strong external trauma caused a disturbance in the organism's energy. The "stimulus barrier" or "protective shield" was exceeded. Defensive mechanisms, such as repression of the event and undoing (in dreams and compulsive repetition of the trauma), were the ego's attempt to cope with the event and to drain off excess energy. Fixation on the trauma was important to this theory. Severe trauma with chronic course and poor response to treatment may lead to two unmodifiable ego changes: ego exhaustion and changes in the ego–superego boundary as a result of overwhelming guilt and shame.

Other analysts revised the concept of a stimulus barrier, from a passive to an active total attempt by the ego to protect against traumatization: The trauma must be understood in terms of the individual's psychic reality and how the person interpreted and reacted to the experience. Psychic trauma may result in the individual's being overwhelmed with emotion and becoming terrified of the uncontrollable element of the emotion. The central role of affect in the theory explains such phenomena as affective blocking and alexithymic or chronic depression.

An information-processing model has been proposed that regards human cognition as having the central role. The concept of information overload can replace energy overload; a person will remain in a state of stress until the information has been processed. Emotions are seen not as drives but as responses to ideational incongruities and motives for defense and coping behavior. Overload symptoms can occur in two phases, alternating with each other: the intrusive phase (unhidden and flooded images, hypervigilance, startle reactions, labile emotional behavior, and compulsive repetition predominating after a breakthrough of the difficult-to-complete stress-related information process) and the numbing phase (a defense against these images and its anxiety, characterized by denial, selective inattention, constriction of thought and sense of numbness, and social withdrawal). This reduces the cognitive processes and anxiety but may not prevent the return of the intrusive phase. A premorbid personality style greatly influences the defenses used in coping, for example, but hysterical or obsessive styles offer much different responses.

One investigator working with victims of severe disasters involving death used a paradigm that emphasized symbolization in human cognition. Severe trauma interrupts the individual's participation in life activities and affects that person's ties to the human community. Mental life is strongly related to symbols of death anxiety and death guilt (self-condemnation for surviving). These death imprints prompt other images of destruction and impairment of symbolization, resulting in psychic numbing—a decreased capacity to feel and maintain the continuity of life. At a more philosophical level, disaster epitomizes the tenuousness of life and the always-present possibility of death.

The psychological theories of PTSD have evolved as a response to the evolution of psychodynamic theory in general and a recognition of the complexity of the symptoms and the chronicity of course. Clinicians working with mild or discrete trauma have emphasized the dynamic, cognitive, and defensive aspects of the response to trauma. Others who have worked with victims of massive trauma have emphasized more permanent ego changes, affective regression, and psychic numbing as core psychological reactions.

BIOLOGICAL FACTORS The symptoms of PTSD are a combination of biological and psychological factors. The earliest symptoms following or during a trauma are the result of a large autonomic sympathetic discharge to a realistic fear. Hyperactivity, increased heart rate, increased respiration, sweating, muscle tension, vigilance, and overwhelming anxiety occur acutely and can persist if the stress is extreme or constant. Increasing evidence has shown that a variety of biological factors as well as autonomic activity are an important part of the disorder's chronic symptoms.

Reactions to a traumatic event may represent a conditioned emotional response. Studies of patients with chronic PTSD when confronted with combat sounds showed regressed, highly emotional responses. This conditioned response of fear, rage, or despair was accompanied by increased pulse rate, systolic blood pressure, and muscle tension, all suggestive of central adrenergic hyperactivity. Patients with PTSD, on hearing personal scripts of combat experiences, had higher physiological responses measured by heart rate, skin conductance, and frontalis electromyogram than control subjects. This is supported by other studies that show a sustained urinary catecholamine elevation in patients with chronic PTSD.

Sleep studies of PTSD patients, although a small sample, have shown long sleep latencies, shorter latencies to the first rapid eye movement (REM) sleep period, decreased deep sleep, and a high REM density during REM sleep. These resemble primary depression. Traumatic nighmares, in comparison with lifelong nightmares, tended to occur earlier in the sleep cycle, were replicas of actual events, and were accompanied by gross body movements. They occurred in varying stages of sleep and were not confined to the REM stage. The autonomic arousal in some stages of sleep may be associated with the affect of the trauma and may be responsible for the replicative traumatic nightmares.

Endogenous opioid peptides, which have anxiolytic action and reduction of aggression and feelings of inadequacy properties, may be produced as part of a biological response to psychological as well as physical trauma. Reexposure to the trauma may produce an endogenous opioid peptide response which results in a subjective sense of calmness or control. This may also explain why some victims continuously seek out situations that remind them of the trauma. When the traumatic stimulus is stopped, there may be a subsequent reduction in endogenous opiates that produce symptoms of opiate withdrawal. These symptoms, probably mediated by CNS noradrenergic hyperactivity, include anxiety, irritability, hyperalertness, insomnia, and startle response. Thus, endogenous opiates as well as CNS noradrenergic hyperactivity may be involved in the combination of intrusive and hyperactive symptoms of PTSD. From the same line of reasoning, clonidine (Catapres), an α-2 adrenergic agonist that has been used to treat opiate withdrawal, has been useful in some symptoms of PTSD.

Urinary free cortisol levels were found to be low and stable in patients with PTSD. This was surprising, as the patients displayed overt signs of anxiety and depression and had signs of chronic increased sympathetic nervous system activity, as shown by elevated urinary catecholamines. It was thought that specific psychological defense mechanisms, especially denial, caused a selective inhibitory effect on the pituitary-adrenal-cortical system. This finding points the way for future research and offers a possible hormonal criterion as an adjunct to clinical diagnosis.

The new preliminary research of biological aspects of PTSD offers new hypotheses for understanding the syndrome. Highly emotional arousal states can be conditioned from the original traumatic stimulus and reactivated by a stimulus that resembles the original trauma. This may be mediated by CNS nonadrenergic and sympathetic nervous systems. The arousal state that occurs in times of emotional distress or sleep could also bring back the traumatic images. Endogenous opiate withdrawal could be helping maintain the syndrome. Specific psychological defenses may inhibit the pituitary-adrenal axis. Biological research has offered some understanding of complex psychophysiological interactions, has suggested specific treatments, and may offer a new diagnostic test.

CLINICAL SIGNS AND SYMPTOMS

PTSD can begin anytime after the occurrence of the stressor, but the full syndrome does not usually occur immediately. Anxious or depressed affective states may develop soon after acute trauma, and emotional constriction may predominate in chronic trauma. Typically, weeks, months, and sometimes years follow the trauma before the full syndrome is expressed.

The most typical feature of PTSD is the persistent reexperiencing of the trauma. This usually includes intrusive thoughts or dreams that are unwanted and often fearful and are often replications of the traumatic events with the full, associated emotional reactions. The distressing recollections occur without an environment stimulus of the event. The dreams may wake up the patient in terror sometimes several times every night. The reexperience may be a sudden acting or feeling as if the traumatic event were recurring and can include a feeling of reliving the experience. Illusions, hallucinations, or dissociative (flashback) episodes are examples of reliving the trauma.

The patient may have a physiological reactivity or intense psychological distress at exposure to a stimulus that resembles an aspect of the original trauma. Examples of this are the reaction of a German concentration-camp victim on seeing a swastika or a Vietnam veteran on seeing a television news report on fighting in Indochina.

The following patient exhibited many of the reexperiencing symptoms of PTSD:

A 50-year-old widowed Cambodian female had difficulty sleeping and had nightmares that for 2 years had been increasing in frequency. Raised in the rural areas of Cambodia, one of four children, she had married a soldier and had eight children. In 1975, when the Pol Pot communist regime came to power, she was separated from her husband and repeatedly threatened with death because of her military connections through him. Her husband was executed; one son was killed; and one daughter died of starvation. Her father was beaten and starved and subsequently died, and a brother was also executed.

Through most of the next 4 years, she was separated from her family. Her wrists were broken as she tried to defend herself when being beaten over the head with an axe. She faced multiple punishments and starvation, and at one point felt sure she would die from starvation. Her health deteriorated to where she had edema and could barely walk. After the Vietnamese invaded Cambodia in 1979, she spent 2 years wandering around trying to find her family. In 1981, she and her remaining family left for Thailand; a son-in-law was killed during their escape. The remaining members of the family eventually came to the United States. She felt that her life was much better, but it was difficult for her to see why her symptoms progressed. Her primary complaints were difficulty falling asleep and frequent wakening with nightmares that resulted in her screaming out. Her nightmares were filled with scenes of being beaten and tortured and of the death of her son. She described tremors and startle reactions to even minimal sounds. The nightmares occurred three times each night. The intrusive thoughts of her trauma occurred in the daytime despite her attempts to avoid all memories, activities, or events of the past. She reported no interest in anything and was constantly tired. Her concentration and memory were poor. She seemed only remotely connected to her family and had suicidal thoughts. She originally told her story in a very detached, reserved way but did appear sad. When the story was recounted to her, she began to cry profusely and was unable to control her emotions for several minutes.

The following case is of a veteran with no symptoms until they were activated by a death that reminded him of the trauma in Vietnam:

This man was referred for evaluation because of persistent symptoms of rage, nightmares, and subsequent drinking behavior. He was a 35-year-old Vietnam veteran involved for 1 year in brutal and heavy combat in Vietnam. Apparently he was considered to be "macho" and often led seek-and-destroy missions. He was encouraged by his companions because of his daring approach which fitted his previous occupation as a cowboy and his own image. In one close-range combat episode, he killed an enemy soldier. As the soldier fell, he could see it was a young woman, who motioned for him to help before she died. After his time in Vietnam, he returned to the United States and maintained a regular job, married, and reported no acute symptoms, although his drinking increased. Ten years after Vietnam, a fellow worker was killed next to him in an industrial accident. Soon thereafter he began to develop a clear PTSD, with frequent nightmares involving both the worker and the woman in Vietnam. There were intrusive distressing images about Vietnam. He had rage reactions and increased his drinking but the intrusive thoughts continued. He lost interest in his family and his job and had a startle response and severe problems with concentration. The symptoms subsided with treatment over several years, but recently, while watching a movie on Vietnam, all his symptoms returned. Consistent with his macho image, he had tried to see and read everything available about Vietnam. This practice continued to stimulate his thoughts, and so his symptoms continued despite the psychotherapy and psychopharmacological treatment.

For a diagnosis of PTSD, either persistent avoidance of stimuli associated with the trauma or numbing of responsiveness—neither of which was present before the trauma—always occurs, and in addition, two of the following symptoms must occur: deliberate avoidance of thoughts or feelings associated with the trauma, deliberate avoidance of situations that would arouse memories of the trauma, numbing experienced by psychogenic amnesia, diminished interest in significant activities, feeling of detachment or estrangement from others, or restricted range of affect with inability to have loving feelings. The avoidance of traumatic stimuli may be a problem in the original interview, as the patient may avoid giving any history about the trauma. Psychogenic amnesia may also be present and make it impossible to get a full history of the trauma. Numbness can severely impair interpersonal relationships with families, and marriages may disintegrate without overt concern by the patients. Indeed, many state that they receive no enjoyment from any activity or have any emotion toward it. Sometimes avoidance and constriction of responsiveness are the most obvious signs of chronic PTSD, as shown by the following case example:

When first seen, 30 years after World War II, the patient was a 55-year-old businessman who had complained of a long history of a depressive disorder and had received a variety of treatments, including years of psychoanalysis. He was chronically depressed and dissatisifed with his life and goals. He had been raised in a European country occupied by the Germans during World War II. As a teenager, he was placed in a concentration camp and subsequently learned of the death of most of his family members. The conditions were harsh, but he was never able to describe the exact trauma he encountered. His comment at the original interview was, "What's the use, I've been through it so many times." Although he originally had had some nightmares and some intrusive thoughts of the past, more recently his symptoms had been primarily a chronic dissatisfaction with his life and poor relationships with family members and friends. He felt generally unhappy with his wife and had an ongoing sexual problem that progressed to the point of rarely attempting sexual relations. He was unhappy with his work and changed jobs several times, as none gave him any satisfaction. He was not close to his children and indeed could not describe any happiness in his life. The patient's life continued to deteriorate, with a divorce, several job changes, and continued unhappiness. Although there were no biological signs of depression, he lived in isolation, alienated from people. Despite his ability to relate intellectually to his problem, he was unable to change his life. He lived in a low-income section of town with few social contacts and without any feeling of enjoyment or love.

In addition to reexperiencing the trauma and avoiding stimuli or numbing, two persistent symptoms of arousal must be present for a diagnosis of PTSD: These can be difficulty falling asleep, irritability or angry outbursts, difficulty concentrating, hypervigilance, and exaggerated startle response. The sleep disorder is often accompanied by terrifying nightmares. The irritability and anger often further compound the social impairment caused by numbing. Difficulty concentrating and complaints of cognitive problems such as poor memory and attention are often found in those who suffered severe trauma in death camps, where head trauma and malnutrition compounded the psychological trauma. The startle reaction can be extremely disabling when any unexpected noise will produce an involuntary motor movement:

A 30-year-old professional woman was referred because of poor sleep and irritability at work. She had recently changed jobs, had separated from her husband, and had begun to date other men. On one occasion a person that she had casually known forced her to engage in sexual relations. Originally she was reluctant to call this a rape, possibly because of an unjustified sense of guilt, but later became aware of a tremendous sense of personal violation. She reported poor sleep, nightmares about the event, and irritability. She also became preoccupied with a relative who had committed suicide 5 years before and whose death she had not adequately worked through. She found herself getting easily angered at work and had difficulty concentrating on normal work tasks which became difficult for her to complete. She became hypervigilant and suspicious of all men, refusing to date. Once when she saw socially the man who had raped her, she became extremely anxious and was unable to be in the same room with him, feeling her heart was beating fast and restlessly. She later found herself being startled at even small sounds and, with suicidal preoccupations, questioned the value of her own life.

Other symptoms have also been associated with PTSD. Although survivor guilt was listed in DSM-III but not in DSM-III-R, persistent guilt feelings associated with surviving a trauma in which others died or suffered severely are often present. In some cultures the concept of shame is a more public sense of dishonor or disgrace and more adequately describes the emotion. The recognition that certain events or places may evoke intrusive symptoms can result in phobic behavior that greatly restricts the person's life. Depressive symptoms are common. Some symptoms such as sleep disorders, difficulty concentrating, and decreased interest in previously pleasurable activities are included in the diagnostic criteria of major mood disorder. In many reports, including those of traumatized refugees, the two diagnoses frequently coexist.

Symptoms of anxiety with tremors and restlessness are common. In some disaster studies, generalized anxiety disorder commonly coexists with PTSD. The irritability and anger may increase to the point of aggression and violence. Explosions of violent behavior have been reported in war veterans, although it is unclear how much this is related to their prewar experiences. The increased drug and alcohol use reported in Vietnam veterans has been described as self-medication to decrease intrusive symptoms and autonomic hyperactivity. There are dramatic reports of war veterans reenacting or reliving the war experience, sometimes involving a dissociative state with weapons and violent acts duplicating actual battle events. A malignant form of PTSD involves violent, explosive behavior, social ostracism and isolation, extreme self-loathing, and a vivid and persistent reexperiencing of psychological war trauma. This has been associated with high degrees of death immersion in Vietnam and a family background in which affective experience was discharged through action.

PTSD can occur in very young children, but some features may be different from those in adults. Children tend not to exhibit psychic numbing but may show a diminished interest in significant activities. Children may not be able to report on this, and so such information must come from other observers. Although visual flashbacks are rare, disturbing dreams may occur soon after the trauma and may generalize into terrifying nightmares. Young children do reexperience the past but reenact the trauma through action in repetitive post-traumatic play. A unique symptom of PTSD in children is a foreshortened view of the future. This may include the feeling of dying young or pessimism about getting married or having a career. *Omen formation*, a belief in the ability to prophesy negative events, has also been noted.

DIFFERENTIAL DIAGNOSIS

Although PTSD can follow a severe trauma, not all trauma victims suffer from PTSD. Indeed, other psychiatric disorders have been more commonly reported after some disasters. Although the diagnosis can be suspected in victims of a disaster, other diagnoses must be considered. The symptoms are subjective, require a careful history, and overlap with those of other major psychiatric diagnoses. The presentation may be complicated by secondary problems such as drug abuse, alcoholism, chronic pain or rage, and violent attacks. The latter may result in severe legal problems during which a psychiatric evaluation is requested.

Many studies have indicated that a high percentage (up to 80 percent) of patients with PTSD had one or two concurrent psychiatric diagnoses. Depression has been commonly found, as many symptoms of PTSD overlap with those of depression. When the diagnostic criteria are met for a mood disorder, that diagnosis should also be made.

Anxiety symptoms are common following a trauma. Even though PTSD is listed as an anxiety disorder, if the criteria for generalized anxiety or phobic disorder are met, this should also be listed.

Many patients with PTSD have difficulty with concentration and attention and have memory problems. These could be the results of severe physical trauma (head injury, starvation) accompanying the psychological trauma, and therefore a diagnosis of organic mental disorder should be considered. Organic mental disorder differs from PTSD in that no organic factors can be found to explain the cognitive disturbance. In cases in which the history and examination indicate the presence of an organic brain disorder, both diagnoses should be given.

Adjustment disorders are a major differential diagnostic consideration. In adjustment disorders the stressors are less severe and more in the range of common human experience. The symptoms of reexperiencing are usually absent in an adjustment disorder, and the course is less chronic, persistent, and debilitating than in PTSD.

Because the symptoms of PTSD are subjective and have received some publicity, and with the Vietnam War fading in clinicians' memory, it is not surprising to have reports of factitious Vietnam PTSD. Some involve elaborate stories of combat by people who were never in Vietnam. Some cases represent factitious medical illness (Munchausen's syndrome). Other motives are expectations of monetary compensation, relief from criminal responsibility, and guilt about not serving in Vietnam. In some ways this diagnosis is similar to compensation neurosis, which contains the belief that an injury or accident should result in financial compensation. In contrast, PTSD is outside the patient's conscious control and persists despite any compensation received.

Some psychological testing may be helpful, but not decisive, in making the diagnosis of PTSD. The Minnesota Multiphasic Personality Inventory (MMPI) has shown several typical scale elevations in veterans with PTSD, including schizophrenia (Sc) and depression (D) as the highest scales and high elevations in the frequency (F) and psychasthenia (Pt) scales. But these profiles may suggest more severe psychopathology than actually exists. A 49-item MMPI subscale also was developed to evaluate combat-related PTSD. The Impact of Event Scale (IES), a self-rating psychological test, was developed to rate the intrusive and denial symptoms following a traumatic event.

PROGNOSIS

Although DSM-III-R does not divide PTSD into acute and chronic categories, such a dichotomy probably has clinical use. Acute disorders have symptoms that either develop within 6 months or do not last longer than 6 months. Both instances tend to offer a more favorable prognosis. Most acute symptoms usually clear spontaneously after a mild stressor such as an auto or industrial accident. Studies of the Mt. St. Helens volcano disaster showed that the number of disorders greatly decreased between the first and second year. Recovery is aided by a healthy premorbid personality, good social supports, and the absence of ongoing physical or medical problems.

When symptoms are present for more than 6 months, the disorder is chronic; the prognosis is less favorable and may result in severe impairment. Impairment is not necessarily related to the present symptoms or type of symptoms. Some individuals with marked symptoms seem to function well in many areas of life, but others with few overt symptoms are socially and vocationally impaired. The avoidance behavior may appear phobic and cause patients to avoid activities or events that even symbolically resemble the original trauma, thereby severely restricting the patient's personal and professional life. Emotional constriction and depression may lead to social isolation, drug abuse, or suicidal actions. The degree of impairment is noted on Axis V of DSM-III-R, which specifies the global assessment of functioning.

With severe stressors, more people tend to develop chronic PTSD. According to some reports, the incidence has increased several years after combat or the catastrophic event. Many reports have indicated that chronic reactions to trauma are enduring. A 20-year follow-up of World War II combat stress-reaction patients showed that their symptoms of startle reaction, nightmares, irritability, and depression had worsened since the end of the war. World War II and Korean War follow-up studies showed persistent psychoneurosis sequelae in many POWs. Depression was found to be significantly higher 40 years after World War II in POWs than in controls. Many studies have reported persistent effects of the Nazi concentration-camp experience. These effects include most symptoms of PTSD as well as depression and, in some, chronic aggression. Even for those who have seemingly made a successful life adjustment, the success was based on a single-minded pursuit of their goal, but with little satisfaction. In a 40-year follow-up of POWs that used DSM-III criteria, of those who had PTSD, 29 percent had fully recovered; 39 percent still reported mild symptoms; 24 percent had improved but still had moderate residual symptoms; and 8 percent had not recovered or had deteriorated.

The author's work with Cambodian refugees who were severely and chronically impaired by PTSD found that a majority had improved significantly (most on the intrusive symptoms) in 1 year. Over the next several years, however, everyone had at least one major relapse with a full return of symptoms. After treating over 50 patients for 2 to 4 years, it is clear that PTSD symptoms are cyclical. Some symptoms such as nightmares, irritability, startle reaction, and depression can improve, and the patient seems much less impaired, although avoidance symptoms remained. But after a loss (death of family or friends) or increased stress, the symptoms usually return fully for a time. Others have reported symptoms reactivated or delayed 30 years after the original trauma. After the trauma, there is often a chronic relapsing in which some or all symptoms are latent but can be reactivated by further trauma, loss, or stress. This may make the patient's response to treatment temporary at best or refractory in the severe cases.

TREATMENT

Two historical approaches have influenced the treatment of PTSD. One approach to combat stress reaction, an acute form of PTSD, treated affected soldiers close to the combat zone, as soon as their symptoms developed and with expectations of returning to active duty. The second approach, from experience with concentration-camp victims, emphasized psychoanalysis or long-term psychodynamic psychotherapy. There is little empirical evidence regarding the effectiveness of the former, and results with the latter have been disappointing. Clearly, different treatment methods are needed for victims of acute trauma than for those of chronic trauma or with chronic symptoms.

INDIVIDUAL PSYCHOTHERAPY For an acute, simple, traumatic event, time-limited psychotherapy has been advocated. Individual personality style can greatly influence the type and duration of symptoms. The technique focuses on the personal style and cognitive processes to complete the educational and emotional integration of the experience into the patient's life. Other therapies have emphasized more the patients' inability to tolerate the intense effects and so are aimed at increasing the patients' affective expression and tolerance. The prognosis for acute traumatic disorders in healthy individuals is good, and time-limited therapy with emphasis on cognitive or emotional aspects is indicated.

For those who suffer from the chronic stress of PTSD, the therapy is more complicated. Even compliance with therapy is difficult after chronic symptoms develop, and a high rate of dropout has been reported. For those involved in abusive violence or immersion in death experiences, suspicion, paranoia, and trust are the major themes in treatment. Some of the patients' stories may be so disturbing that the therapist's reaction may make it difficult to obtain a history of the trauma. Or some of the patient's rage may be transferred to the therapist who in turn reacts with guilt, dread, horror, or displaced rage. For these reasons, individual therapy—especially dynamic and explorative—of victims of chronic trauma is a difficult undertaking. Some patients can never really integrate their trauma, and so their goals must be limited. A supportive long-term treatment based on recognizing the chronic course of the disorder, setting limited goals, and solving practical problems of living may offer the most realistic relief. An existential approach based on the issues of death, the meaning of life, and the attitude toward suffering is useful for many patients.

GROUP THERAPY Because of the difficulties with transference, suspicions of the therapist's authority, and the patient's lack of social support, group therapy has been strongly advocated for victims of combat trauma and the Nazi holocaust. Some groups are informal and leaderless, such as veterans' "rap" groups. Most therapists, however, feel that the group should embody the basic principles of group therapy and be led by an experienced group therapist who has had some first-hand experience with the trauma. Some groups have involved family members, thereby recognizing that the symptoms of PTSD may also severely affect them (they also may have a secondary PTSD).

INPATIENT TREATMENT Brief hospitalization may be needed to treat some acute effects or complications of PTSD. These include suicidal behavior from severe depression, violence from uncontrolled rage, or the effects of alcohol or drug abuse. Some Veterans Administration hospitals have used special group therapy in the regular psychiatric wards for those who suffer from PTSD. Some special Vietnam veteran PTSD inpatient units, averaging about a 3-week length of stay, have been established. The units emphasize abreaction and group process of the material with a therapist who served in Vietnam. Early reports indicate successful therapeutic outcomes.

PSYCHOPHARMACOLOGY A wide variety of medications have been tried for symptoms of PTSD. Clinical reports indicate the best response is from the tricyclic antidepressants, usually amitriptlyline (Elavil) and imipramine (Tofranil). These drugs not only are useful in depression but also can help relieve intrusive thoughts, sleep disorders, and nightmares. The usual doses required are 150 to 300 mg per day. Avoidance symptoms, however, have not been helped by these agents. Some symptoms of autonomic arousal, such as tremors and startle reactions, have been treated with propranalol (Inderal) or clonidine. In the author's experience, clonidine in dosages of 0.1 or 0.2 mg, 2 or 3 times a day, has been well received by patients and has alleviated many intrusive symptoms. Phenelzine (Nardil) is helpful in some cases. The antipsychotics can be useful if clear psychotic symptoms develop in the course of PTSD. Severe agitation and anger, especially of a paranoid quality, may need brief periods of antipsychotic medicine. The benzodiazepines can interfere with the patient's ability to cope with severe emotions, can cause paradoxical rage, and can lead to abuse. Generally, therefore, they should not be used in PTSD.

The author recommends that acute PTSD be treated with individual psychotherapy with an emphasis on integrating the experience into the patient's life. Chronic PTSD usually needs a long-term supportive relationship, with the intrusive symptoms treated with tricyclic antidepressants. Clonidine may also be used. Sharing the traumatic experience in an existential sense often alleviates the patient's sense of futility. Group therapy is necessary for social support and to help reduce the avoidance and numbing symptoms.

REFERENCES

Adler A: Neuropsychiatric complications in victims of Boston's Coconut Grove disaster. JAMA *123:* 1098, 1943.

Bleich A, Siegel B, Garb R, Lerer B: Post-traumatic stress disorder following combat exposure: Clinical features and psychopharmacological treatment. Brit J Psychiat *149:* 365, 1986.

Eth S, Pynoos R S, editors: *Post-traumatic Stress Disorder in Children.* American Psychiatric Press, Washington, DC, 1985.

Figley C R, editor: *Trauma and Its Wake: The Study and Treatment of Post-traumatic Stress Disorder.* Brunner/Mazel, New York, 1985.

Frankl V: *From Death Camp to Existentialism.* Beacon Press, New York, 1959.

Helzer J E, Robbins L N, McEvay L: Post-traumatic stress disorder in the general population. Findings from the Epidemiologic Catchment Area Survey. New Eng J Med *317:* 1650, 1987.

Horowitz M J: Stress response syndromes: Character style and brief psychotherapy. Arch Gen Psychiat *31:* 768, 1974.

Horowitz M J, Wilner N, Kaltreider N, Alvarez W: Signs and symptoms of posttraumatic stress disorder. Arch Gen Psychiat *37:* 85, 1980.

Kinzie J D, Fredrickson R H, Ben R, Fleck J, Karl W: Posttraumatic stress disorder among survivors of Cambodian concentration camps. Amer J Psychiat *141:* 645, 1984.

Kluznik J C, Speed N, Valkenburg C V, Magraw R: Forty-year follow-up of United States prisoners of war. Amer J Psychiat *143:* 1443, 1986.

Kolb L C: Return of the repressed: Delayed stress reaction to war. J Amer Psychoanal *11:* 531, 1983.

Laufer R S, Brett E, Gallops M S: Symptom patterns associated with posttraumatic stress disorder among Vietnam veterans exposed to war trauma. Amer J Psychiat *142:* 1304, 1985.

Lifton R J: *The Broken Connection.* Simon & Schuster, New York, 1979.

Mason J W, Giller E L, Kosten T R, Ostroff R B, Podd L: Urinary free-cortisol levels in post-traumatic stress disorder patients. J Nerv and Ment Dis *174:* 145, 1986.

McFarlane A C: The aetiology of post-traumatic stress disorders following a natural disaster. Brit J Psychiat *152:* 116, 1988.

Pitman R K, Orr S P, Forgue D F, deJong J B, Claiborn J M: Psychophysiologic assessment of posttraumatic stress disorder imagery in Vietnam combat veterans. Arch Gen Psychiat *44:* 970, 1987.

Scrignar C B: *Posttraumatic Stress Disorder.* Praeger, New York, 1984.

Shore J H, editor: *Disaster Stress Studies: New Methods and Findings.* American Psychiatric Press, Washington, DC, 1986.

Sonnenberg S M, Blank A S, Talbot J A, editors: *The Trauma of War: Stress and Recovery in Vietnam Veterans.* American Psychiatric Press, Washington, DC, 1985.

van der Kolb B A, editor: *Posttraumatic Stress Disorder: Psychological and Biological Sequelae.* American Psychiatric Press, Washington, DC, 1984.

van der Kolb B A: *Psychological Trauma.* American Psychiatric Press, Washington, DC, 1987.

Wilson J P, Harel A, Kahana B: *Human Adaptation to Extreme Stress: From the Holocaust to Vietnam,* Plenum, New York, 1988.

19 SOMATOFORM DISORDERS

ARTHUR J. BARSKY, M.D.

INTRODUCTION

The somatoform disorders are characterized by physical symptoms suggesting medical disease, but no demonstrable organ pathology or known pathophysiological mechanism can be found to account for them. They are considered psychiatric disorders because there is clear evidence, or a strong presumption, that the symptoms are linked to psychological factors. The third edition of the *Diagnostic and Statistical Manual of Mental Disorders* (DSM-III) was the first attempt to gather these conditions together into one discrete category, to distinguish them from other psychiatric disorders, and to define them relative to one another. The somatoform disorders differ from factitious disorder and malingering in that the patient has no voluntary control over the symptoms.

The somatoform disorders are difficult to distinguish from somatization, which is a general psychological predisposition or a symptom rather than a disorder. *Somatization* is the tendency to experience, to conceptualize, and to communicate mental states and personal distress as bodily complaints and medical symptoms. Someone who somatizes, therefore, need not necessarily have any psychiatric disorder.

The somatoform disorders are also difficult to distinguish from organic medical disease. Problems arise when clinicians attempt to exclude a medical cause for a patient's symptoms and to infer a psychological etiology for them. This is because clinical judgments about whether signs and symptoms conform to known patterns of pathological anatomy and pathophysiology are unreliable. In addition, patients with undiagnosed physical disorders may exaggerate or misrepresent their symptoms. And to make matters worse, somatoform disorders often occur in patients with preexisting medical disease.

The nosology, terminology, and interrelationships of somatoform disorders are confused. This results from historical and conceptual ambiguities and persists because of a paucity of definitive empirical data. Each of these disorders has arisen within a different school of psychiatric thought. The concept of a conversion reaction was elaborated in the psychoanalytic tradition, whereas somatization disorder originated in the phenomenological and descriptive approach. Chronic pain, on the other hand, has achieved recognition primarily because of its clinical import. Thus, the present confusion is not surprising: Etiology and phenomenology have not been adequately distinguished; psychopathology has been confused with normal individual variation; personality style and personality disorder have not been distinguished; and treatment has evolved piecemeal.

At present the rigorous empirical data to resolve this confusion are lacking. Much of the current literature consists of uncontrolled observation, anecdote, and impression, often without a clear distinction between inference and observation. Noncomparable populations have been studied; diagnostic criteria vary; problems of retrospective design abound; and control groups are frequently lacking. Somatizing patients reside in a strange limbo between psychiatry and medicine. Although psychiatrists have shown some interest in studying and treating such patients, they encounter only a small and very biased sample of them, as most somatizers gravitate to medical settings and refuse psychiatric referral.

SOMATIZATION DISORDER

DEFINITION Somatization disorder is a chronic syndrome of multiple somatic symptoms that cannot be explained medically and are associated with psychosocial distress and medical help seeking. The revised edition of DSM-III (DSM-III-R) diagnosis (Table 19-1) requires a history of several years' duration, beginning before the age of 30. The somatic symptoms must not be caused by medical disease, medication, drugs, or alcohol, and they must be troublesome enough to cause the patient to take a prescription medication, to visit a physician, or to alter his or her life-style. These diagnostic symptoms must come from a list of 35 symptoms which are clustered into six groups. The patient must have a minimum of 13 of these symptoms in order to be so diagnosed. There is no requirement regarding the distribution of the symptoms among the groups. A symptom need only be reported by the patient in order to be counted; it is not necessary to establish that the patient actually had the symptom (i.e., vomiting). DSM-III-R designated seven of these symptoms to serve as screening questions for the disorder. Positive responses to at least two of these suggest a high likelihood of the diagnosis.

HISTORY Somatization disorder has a long history—from Paul Briquet in 1859 through the work of Thomas Savill and James Purtell—of a phenomenological approach to hysteria. These clinicians described, assessed, and categorized the somatic complaints of patients who had multiple medical symptoms without any demonstrable medical disease to explain them. They observed that these hysterical patients were flamboyant and emotional, that they tended to be women, that their symptoms began early in life, and that there was a high frequency of sexual complaints and pain symptoms.

In the 1960s, a series of studies began that delineated a homogeneous subgroup of hysteria patients with multiple somatic symptoms, a chronic course, and excessive amounts of medical and surgical care. The disorder was termed "Briquet's syndrome." Clinical, epidemiological, and follow-up studies established the validity, reliability, and internal consistency of Briquet's syndrome and demonstrated its independence from anxiety disorders and mood disorders. The stability of the disorder was established by demonstrating that in the 6 to 8 years following diagnosis, there was a 90 percent probability that the clinical picture would remain unchanged and that no new medical or psychiatric disorder would develop to explain the original symptoms. DSM-III-R somatization disorder was derived directly from Briquet's syndrome.

COMPARATIVE NOSOLOGY Briquet's syndrome is characterized by a complicated and dramatic medical history beginning before the age of 30, for which there is no known medical explanation. The patient has at least 25 different symptoms from among a list of 59 symptoms that are assorted into 10 different groups. The patient must have at least one symptom from nine out of the 10 groups.

Somatization disorder is a simplified version of Briquet's syndrome. The 59 symptoms of Briquet's syndrome proved too cumbersome for clinical use, and so a shorter list of 35

TABLE 19-1
Diagnostic Criteria for Somatization Disorder

A. A history of many physical complaints or a belief that one is sickly, beginning before the age of 30 and persisting for several years.
B. At least 13 symptoms from the list below. To count a symptom as significant, the following criteria must be met:
(1) no organic pathology or pathophysiologic mechanism (e.g., a physical disorder or the effects of injury, medication, drugs, or alcohol) to account for the symptom or, when there is related organic pathology, the complaint or resulting social or occupational impairment is grossly in excess of what would be expected from the physical findings
(2) has not occurred only during a panic attack
(3) has caused the person to take medicine (other than over-the-counter pain medication), see a doctor, or alter life-style

Symptom list:

Gastrointestinal symptoms:

(1) **vomiting (other than during pregnancy)**
(2) abdominal pain (other than when menstruating)
(3) nausea (other than motion sickness)
(4) bloating (gassy)
(5) diarrhea
(6) intolerance of (gets sick from) several different foods

Pain symptoms:

(7) **pain in extremities**
(8) back pain
(9) joint pain
(10) pain during urination
(11) other pain (excluding headaches)

Cardiopulmonary symptoms:

(12) **shortness of breath when not exerting oneself**
(13) palpitations
(14) chest pain
(15) dizziness

Conversion of pseudoneurologic symptoms:

(16) **amnesia**
(17) **difficulty swallowing**
(18) loss of voice
(19) deafness
(20) double vision
(21) blurred vision
(22) blindness
(23) fainting or loss of consciousness
(24) seizure or convulsion
(25) trouble walking
(26) paralysis or muscle weakness
(27) urinary retention or difficulty urinating

Sexual symptoms for the major part of the person's life after opportunities for sexual activity:

(28) **burning sensation in sexual organs or rectum (other than during intercourse)**
(29) sexual indifference
(30) pain during intercourse
(31) impotence

Female reproductive symptoms judged by the person to occur more frequently or severely than in most women:

(32) **painful menstruation**
(33) irregular menstrual periods
(34) excessive menstrual bleeding
(35) vomiting throughout pregnancy

Note: The seven items in boldface may be used to screen for the disorder. The presence of two or more of these items suggests a high likelihood of the disorder.

Table from DSM-III-R *Diagnostic and Statistical Manual of Mental Disorders*, ed 3, revised. Copyright American Psychiatric Association, Washington, DC, 1987. Used with permission.

was derived, the diagnosis requiring a total of 13. These symptoms no longer have to be distributed among a number of different groups.

There is good diagnostic concordance between Briquet's syndrome and somatization disorder, and these two sets of diagnostic criteria identify substantially the same group of patients. But the overlap is by no means complete; some patients meet the criteria for one of the disorders but not the other.

EPIDEMIOLOGY The lifetime prevalence rate of somatization disorder in females is between 0.2 and 2 percent. Although it is quite rare in males, occasional cases do occur. Somatization disorder is inversely related to social position, occurring more often among the less educated, the poor, and those of lower occupational status.

By definition, somatization disorder begins before the age of 30, most commonly in the late teens. Although the onset is early in life, the diagnosis may not be made until much later, and it is not uncommon to discover somatization disorder for the first time in a middle-aged or elderly patient. Menstrual complaints are most often the first symptoms, but it may also begin with headaches, abdominal pain, or seizures.

Somatization disorder tends to run in families, occurring in 10 to 20 percent of the primary female relatives of somatization disorder patients. Within these families, primary male relatives have an increased prevalence of alcoholism, drug abuse, and antisocial personality disorder.

ETIOLOGY The etiology of somatization disorder is unknown. Its familial aggregation suggests genetic or environmental factors, but the existing data do not permit a distinction between these two causes, and current thinking accords a significant role to both. Social, cultural, and ethnic factors that foster somatization in general may have an etiological role in the disorder or at least contribute to its expression. The associations of somatization disorder with less education and lower social position suggest that this is the case. Parental teaching and parental example, as well as cultural and ethnic mores, may in effect teach children to somatize.

Some research has suggested a neuropsychological basis for somatization disorder. Such patients may have characteristic attentional and cognitive impairments that result in the faulty perception and assessment of somatosensory input. The reported impairments include excessive distractibility, inability to habituate to repetitive stimuli, the grouping of cognitive constructs on an impressionistic basis, and associations that tend to be partial and circumstantial.

PATHOLOGY Nothing is known about neuropathology in somatization disorder. By definition, no systemic pathology is present to account for the patient's somatic symptoms. Frequently, however, there is evidence of previous surgery and invasive medical procedures.

CLINICAL SIGNS AND SYMPTOMS Somatization-disorder patients have a multitude of somatic complaints and long, complicated medical histories. Numerous medical diagnoses have been entertained along the way, but none accounts adequately for the patient's complaints. Although there may have been some benign medical disorder, the patient's symptoms and disability are excessive. Typical complaints include conversion or neurological symptoms, such as paralysis or blindness or difficulty swallowing; gastrointestinal complaints such as abdominal pain, bowel difficulties, nausea, and vomiting; menstrual complaints; psychosexual symptoms, including dyspareunia, impotence, and sexual indifference; pain, such as pain in the back or extremities; and cardiorespiratory symptoms, including shortness of breath unrelated to exertion.

Somatization disorder patients are severely disabled by these symptoms (more than three-quarters are unable to work because of their health) and are usually incapacitated for long periods. They have received a great deal of medical care, often visiting many different doctors (sometimes simultaneously) and many different institutions. They have had many diagnostic tests and surgical procedures (especially gynecological) and have high rates of medical and surgical hospitalization, most without clear medical indication. Their per-capita expenditures for personal health care are nine times the average.

Psychological distress and interpersonal problems are prominent in somatization disorder. Anxiety and depression are the most prevalent psychiatric conditions. Suicide threats, and even attempts, are not infrequent, but suicide is rarely completed. If suicide does occur, it is usually associated with substance abuse. Simple hallucinations have been reported in some somatization disorder patients. Three other psychiatric disorders occur with higher-than-expected frequency in somatization disorder patients: antisocial personality disorder, alcohol abuse, and drug abuse. However, because much of this research has been done on populations of lower socioeconomic status, the results may not be generalizable. Among female criminals, for example, there is a very high concordance between antisocial personality and Briquet's syndrome, and women with either diagnosis alone closely resemble one another. Somatization disorder appears to be closely related to histrionic personality; a large proportion of patients have histrionic personality traits (e.g., as evidenced on the Minnesota Multiphasic Personality Inventory [MMPI]), although it is less clear what fraction has DSM-III-R's histrionic personality disorder.

These patients often grew up in families that were inconsistent, unreliable, and not emotionally supportive. Their parents' marriages were poor, and there was often sexual or physical abuse. Frequently, one or both parents were alcoholic or sociopathic. The patients' schoolwork and social adjustments were poor, and a history of adolescent delinquency is common. Menstrual periods were often associated with discomfort, beginning right from menarche. Their adult lives are chaotic, complicated, and poorly organized. Somatization-disorder patients marry many times, but for the most part, their relationships are abusive, unstable, and unsatisfactory. Alcoholism, drug abuse, and sociopathy are common in the spouses. These patients are often themselves inconsistent and neglectful as parents. Sexual activity frequently began at an early age but is generally not pleasurable, and sexual problems are common. Interpersonal difficulties are frequent, with shallow and chaotic relationships, and their occupational history is often unsatisfactory as well, with low wages, frequent firings, and long periods of unemployment.

The patient's clinical presentation is important, as it is the positive responses on clinical inquiry, rather than the objective existence of the symptoms, that constitute the diagnostic criteria. The medical history and review of systems are diffusely positive, and the history is circumstantial, vague and imprecise, inconsistent and disorganized. For example, the patient may respond to the question, "Is the pain worse in the morning?" with, "Yes. And it's worse in the afternoon, too." Complaints are described in a dramatic, emotional, and exaggerated fashion, using vivid and colorful language. Temporal sequences are confused, and current symptoms are not clearly distinguished from past history. The clinician soon realizes that taking an accurate and well-organized medical history is out of the question and becomes irritated and overwhelmed. The patient is often dressed and groomed in an exhibitionistic manner and may be coy and flirtatious, or even overtly seductive. Patients with somatization disorder are often described as dependent, self-centered, hungry for admiration and praise, and manipulative. Manipulation may be most evident in suicide threats, substance abuse, and attempts aimed at influencing others, particularly by playing on their guilt.

The following vignette exemplifies the somatization disorder patient:

A 29-year-old mother of two requested medical clearance for impending surgery for cysts in her breasts. She described the cysts as rapidly enlarging and unbearably painful. While drawing attention to her breasts, she noted, "They are so large and so tender to the touch. And I just can't have relations—forget that."

She also had disabling back pain that spread up and down her spine and made her "legs give out" on her suddenly, causing her to fall. When discussing this, she winced visibly, adding, "Oh, there it goes—my back keeps clicking. The pain is so severe it affects me with my kids. Pain like that will make anyone into a beast." (She had previously been suspected of child abuse.) She also complained of dyspnea and a dry cough that prevented her from walking uphill.

Her medical history began at menarche with dysmenorrhea and menorrhagia. At 18, she had exploratory surgery for a possible ovarian cyst and was subsequently reoperated on for suspected abdominal adhesions. There was also a history of recurrent urinary tract symptoms, though no organisms were ever clearly documented, and she had a normal workup for "an enlarged thyroid." At various times she had received the diagnoses of spastic colon, migraine, and endometriosis.

Two marriages, both to alcoholic and abusive men who refused to pay child support, ended in divorce. She had lost several clerical jobs because of excessive absences. During the periods when she felt worst, she spent most of the day at home in a bathrobe, while her relatives cared for her children. She had a history of narcotic addiction, claiming that she began using analgesics for her back pain and then, "I overdid it."

The physical exam at the time of her visit revealed inconsistencies of the breast tissue, but no frank masses, and mammography was normal.

DIFFERENTIAL DIAGNOSIS The symptoms of somatization disorder are not pathognomonic and occur in many medical disorders. Thus, clinicians must always rule out organic causes for the patient's symptoms. Medical disorders that present with nonspecific, transient abnormalities pose the greatest diagnostic difficulty, such as multiple sclerosis, systemic lupus erythematosus, acute intermittent porphyria, hyperparathyroidism, and chronic systemic infections such as brucellosis. Somatization disorder may be differentiated on the basis of its early onset and extremely long course, without the emergence of a serious medical cause, and the involvement of multiple organ systems and multiple sites in the body. The onset of many somatic symptoms late in life must be presumed to be caused by a medical illness until this has been ruled out.

Somatization disorder may be difficult to differentiate from anxiety disorders. Patients with generalized anxiety often complain of somatic symptoms, including fatigue, pain (especially headache, musculoskeletal pain, and heartburn), gastrointestinal symptoms (cramps and diarrhea), and profuse sweating. Patients with panic disorder have prominent cardiorespiratory complaints. But the somatic symptoms of panic disorder occur only during well-defined panic attacks and are accompanied by the characteristic affective, cognitive, and motor symptoms. Although the somatic symptoms of somatization disorder wax and wane chronically, they do not fluctuate over such short intervals. Somatization disorder symptoms involve a broader array of organ systems, including menstrual and sexual symptoms, and these patients experience greater maladjustment in social, family, and occupational spheres. Panic disorder may coexist with somatization disorder, and if the somatic complaints occur at times other than during panic attacks, both diagnoses can be made.

Depressive symptoms are prominent in somatization disorder, and major depression is frequently diagnosed. The characteristic cognitive, behavioral, and affective symptoms of depression usually make clear the differential diagnosis, and the neurovegetative symptoms are not among the symptoms of somatization disorder. Major depression also has an episodic course, and the characteristic family history may be present. In addition, depressed patients often act as if they do not deserve to get better, have little hope of improvement, and are not worth the doctor's therapeutic efforts.

Schizophrenic patients with multiple somatic delusions may resemble somatization disorder patients. Schizophrenic patients' somatic delusions tend to be early features of the disorder and are followed by the characteristic formal thought disorder, hallucinations, and loss of reality testing. Their somatic delusions also tend to be more bizarre, elaborate, and highly personalized than the complaints in somatization disorder, and a positive family history of schizophrenia is helpful.

Conversion symptoms form one of the six symptom groups in somatization disorder, and thus recurrent, multiple conversion reactions, beginning before age 30, would be diagnosed as somatization disorder. But the symptoms of somatization disorder are not restricted to sensorimotor and neurological complaints and cover a far broader range. Hypochondriasis is distinguished from somatization disorder in that it includes disease conviction, disease fear, and bodily preoccupation. It often begins after age 30, and although somatization disorder is far more common in females, hypochondriasis is more evenly distributed between the sexes. Their clinical presentations may differ, in that somatization disorder patients often tell their stories in a histrionic flamboyant and colorful way, whereas hypochondriacs tend to be more painstaking, boring, and obsessive. Somatoform pain patients have symptoms limited to pain but in other ways may be quite similar to individuals with somatization disorder.

In factitious disorder with physical symptoms, the symptoms are under the patient's voluntary control.

PROGNOSIS Somatization disorder is a chronic condition whose prognosis is considered to be poor. These patients suffer and are disabled for much of their lives. They are often most floridly symptomatic in early adulthood, but complete spontaneous remission is uncommon at any stage of life. The disorder runs a fluctuating course, but patients are rarely entirely asymptomatic, and it is unusual for them to go for more than a year or two without some medical attention. Somatization disorder patients do not appear to have a significantly higher mortality rate than the general population.

TREATMENT There is no definitive therapy for somatization disorder. Management centers on early diagnosis, obviating unnecessary medical and surgical interventions, and helping patients turn their attention from their somatic symptoms to their problems in living.

These patients need a long-term empathic relationship with a single primary care physician. Every attempt should be made to keep the patient from "doctor shopping," as more physicians become involved, there will be more opportunity for manipulation by the patient and for unnecessary medical interventions. The patient's periodic threats to change doctors should be met by calmly reemphasizing that the present doctor already knows the patient well and can therefore provide the best medical care. Physicians should not allow such threats to compromise their best clinical judgment (e.g., prescribing a narcotic analgesic). Once a relationship has been established, primary care physicians should try to curtail unnecessary diagnostic procedures and overly aggressive treatment. Such interventions complicate and exacerbate the illness by producing side effects and iatrogenic illness. Therefore diagnostic and therapeutic procedures should be based more on objective evidence than on subjective complaints. It is best to refrain from treating equivocal or adventitious findings. At the same time, of course, physicians must guard against overlooking a serious physical disease.

The psychiatrist can help the primary care physician by explaining the nature of the disorder and the strategy for managing it. This sort of psychiatric consultation has been shown to decrease somatization disorder patients'personal health care expenditures by 50 percent, largely by decreasing the rate of hospitalization, without diminishing their functional status or satisfaction with medical care.

The basic goal of management is to help such patients cope with their symptoms rather than eliminate them completely. The aim is palliation rather than cure, while at the same time physicians should support healthy and adaptive behaviors, encourage the patients to move beyond their somatization, and help them manage their lives more effectively. The physicians should try to focus on the personal and social difficulties that the patients are experiencing in daily life (such as problems at work and home). The goal is to improve the patients' coping skills through concrete, nondirective discussion of practical alternative solutions. Although physicians sometimes might offer concrete advice, specific suggestions tend to foster undesirable dependence and facilitate the patients' manipulation of the physician. These discussions may be started by invoking the notion of "stress," a concept that is acceptable to many of these patients, who do indeed have difficulty dealing with stressful situations and relationships. A general interviewing technique is to evidence more interest in the patients' social and personal problems than in their somatic complaints, while remaining within the bounds of good medical practice. In addition, providing frequent, regularly scheduled appointments, rather than on an as-needed basis, is helpful because it tells the patients that the doctor is interested in them rather than their symptoms, and it declares that medical illness is not a necessary pretext for maintaining their relationship.

Psychotropic medications and prescription analgesics should be avoided when possible. These medications are generally not very effective, though some clinicians feel that antianxiety agents and antidepressants are helpful when anxiety or depression is prominent. If prescribed, these medications must be carefully monitored because somatization-disorder patients tend to be erratic and unreliable in their use of medication and because confusing side effects, drug dependence, and abuse are common. Firm, consistent, nonpunitive limits should be placed on patients' excessive demands regarding medication, as they should be if there are suicide threats. Whenever patients report new symptoms, physicians should consider drug effect or drug withdrawal as possible causes.

Ongoing contact with family members can help primary care physicians learn about emerging social problems, curtail doctor shopping, and maintain the patients' compliance with medical therapy. In addition, the family members themselves often have serious psychiatric problems requiring treatment in their own right.

Although psychiatric referral can be helpful initially in establishing the diagnosis, in assisting primary care physicians to understand that the patients need their symptoms and visits to the doctor, and in planning a management strategy, psychiatric treatment per se is usually not acceptable to somatization disorder patients. A few, however, do accept a psychiatric referral because of severe anxiety, depression, or other dysphoria. No specific psychiatric treatment exists, but eclectic, supportive psychotherapy that is educational in tone is helpful to those patients who are willing to undergo it. Group therapy apparently is the most successful modality. Therapeutic goals should be concrete and limited to things like increased functioning of the family unit, decreased use of medication, and decreased medical utilization. Abreaction and ventilation tend not to be helpful, as these patients are likely to be too impulsive and have difficulty with deliberation, long-term planning, and postponing gratification.

CONVERSION DISORDER

DEFINITION Conversion disorder is a loss of or change in bodily functioning that results from a psychological conflict or need. The bodily symptoms cannot be explained by any known medical disorder or pathophysiological mechanism. Symptoms of pain and sexual dysfunction are specifically excluded. Such patients are not conscious of the psychological basis for their symptoms and thus cannot control their disturbances. The DSM-III-R definition appears in Table 19-2. This diagnosis is unique to DSM-III-R in that it depends on a determination of etiology: Psychological factors must be judged to be causative, as evidenced by the presence of primary or secondary gain. In primary gain, the formation of the symptom lessens intrapsychic dysphoria. In secondary gain, in contrast, the formation of the symptom enables the patient to avoid difficult situations or to obtain support that might not otherwise be forthcoming.

TABLE 19-2
Diagnostic Criteria for Conversion Disorder

A. A loss of, or alteration in, physical functioning suggesting a physical disorder.
B. Psychological factors are judged to be etiologically related to the symptom because of a temporal relationship between a psychosocial stressor that is apparently related to a psychological conflict or need and initiation or exacerbation of the symptom.
C. The person is not conscious of intentionally producing the symptom.
D. The symptom is not a culturally sanctioned response pattern and cannot, after appropriate investigation, be explained by a known physical disorder.
E. The symptom is not limited to pain or to a disturbance in sexual functioning.

Specify: single episode or recurrent.

Table from DSM-III-R *Diagnostic and Statistical Manual of Mental Disorders*, ed 3, revised. Copyright American Psychiatric Association, Washington, DC, 1987. Used with permission.

HISTORY The history of conversion disorder is long, confused, and intertwined with that of somatization disorder. Both originated in the concept of hysteria. The term *hysteria* is derived from the Greek word *hystera,* meaning uterus. The ancient Greeks noted an association among hysteria, menstrual disorders, and sexual issues and thus considered it to be a disorder in which the uterus moved throughout the body. The modern concepts of conversion disorder originated in the nineteenth century when the first attempts were made to correlate symptom reports with demonstrable physical pathology. A group of hysterical patients were recognized who had physical symptoms for which no pathological basis could be discovered. Briquet, Jean Charcot, and Pierre Janet studied them, and although they recognized the importance of traumatic environmental precipitants, they conceived of hysteria as fundamentally a neurological disorder.

Hysterical symptoms then became central to the evolution of psychodynamic thinking. After working with Charcot, Sigmund Freud began studying these symptoms and discovered many of the most basic psychoanalytic principles. In 1894 and 1895, he proposed a mechanism for the formation of hysterical conversion symptoms. After a traumatic event, he proposed, the painful memory of the event was repressed or dissociated, and the painful affect was converted into a bodily symptom. Freud initially believed that the precipitating trauma was sexual in nature, but he subsequently concluded that a fixation at the oedipal level was all that was necessary to produce a conversion symptom. The failure to resolve the incestuous oedipal tie forms the basis for intrapsychic conflict when sexual drives are heightened in adulthood, as the sexual urge retains the unacceptable, forbidden, and incestuous qualities it had in childhood. The ego then defends itself against the resulting anxiety and intrapsychic conflict with repression and conversion.

The psychodynamic conceptualization of conversion was subsequently progressively modified. Aggressive impulses and oral-dependency needs were added to sexual conflicts as causes of conversion symptoms. The concept of secondary gain was increasingly emphasized, particularly as a force that perpetuated conversion symptoms once they had occurred. Finally, conversion symptoms increasingly began to be regarded as a form of nonverbal communication.

COMPARATIVE NOSOLOGY The first edition of the *Diagnostic and Statistical Manual of Mental Disorders* (DSM-I) defined a *conversion reaction* as a functional symptom resulting from the conversion of anxiety into bodily sensations. The second edition of DSM (DSM-II) called the disorder hysterical neurosis, conversion type, and described it as an involuntary psychogenic loss or disorder of function. With the publication of DSM-III, hysterical conversion was split into three separate disorders: conversion disorder, composed of sensorimotor and neurological symptoms other than pain; psychogenic pain disorder, whose symptoms are limited to pain; and somatization disorder, with a broader array of symptoms and a more chronic picture. DSM-III-R does not fundamentally alter DSM-III's concept. It specifically excludes symptoms that are culturally sanctioned, and it permits somatization disorder and schizophrenia as concurrent diagnoses. Recognizing the diagnostic importance of recurrent conversion symptoms, clinicians are asked to specify whether the current disturbance is the first such episode or a recurrence.

One problem with DSM-III-R's conversion disorder is that it may not be truly a disorder or even a syndrome but, rather, a nonspecific symptom (such as fever) that can be either a secondary feature of some other primary psychiatric disorder or a reaction to environmental stress or medical illness.

EPIDEMIOLOGY The incidence and prevalence of conversion disorder are unclear. When samples of women are carefully questioned about a history of isolated conversion symptoms, the incidence is high; in some surveys, the lifetime incidence of conversion symptoms is as high as 25 to 33 percent. The prevalence among general hospital inpatients receiving psychiatric consultation has been reported between 5 and 16 percent. In contrast, the prevalence of conversion reactions among patients in ongoing psychiatric treatment appears to be considerably lower. The annual incidence of conversion disorders in patients seen by general psychiatrists has been reported as low as 0.01 to 0.02 percent. Most observers believe the incidence has been declining, although some believe it remains as common as previously.

Conversion disorder is probably between two and five times more common in women than in men. It may be seen at any stage of life, from early childhood (and indeed it is fairly common in children) to extreme old age, but it is most common in adolescents and young adults. Conversion symptoms are apparently more prevalent in lower-socioeconomic groups, in rural populations, and among those with less education. The more flamboyant, bizarre, and grossly nonphysiological symptoms tend to occur in those of rural background and with less education, whereas the symptoms more closely resemble known diseases in better-educated populations. These findings, however, are tentative because of differing utilization rates of medical and psychiatric care and because conversion disorder is often short-lived. There are suggestions of a familial aggregation of conversion disorder, but this needs confirmation. It has also been reported that these patients tend to be the youngest children in their families, but this too needs further study.

ETIOLOGY According to psychoanalytic theory, conversion is caused by the anxiety of unconscious intrapsychic conflict. The conflict occurs between an instinctual impulse (e.g., aggressive or sexual) and the prohibitions against its expression. The symptom allows partial expression of the forbidden wish or urge but disguises it sufficiently so that the person need not consciously confront the unacceptable impulses. At the same time, the symptom imposes suffering and disability, which serve as a punishment for the impulse or wish. In order to do this, the conversion symptom must bear a symbolic relationship to the dilemma. Thus, for example, an elderly widower, who is furious at his grown children's failure to care for him, finds himself paralyzed and, as a result, legitimately requires their constant attention. The symptom allows him to express his dependent longings and his unacceptable rage at his family, but in a fashion subtle enough that he need not consciously experience them. At the same time, his disability appeases the superego's demands for punishment for these unacceptable urges. The resulting reduction in anxiety and psychological distress is called *primary gain*.

Another etiology for conversion disorder is interpersonal. It has been viewed as a nonverbal interpersonal communication, a kind of bodily pantomine employed when direct verbal statement is not possible. The conversion symptom is an acceptable way for the patient to tell important others that their relationship is in danger or that he or she is in pain, is suffering, and is in need of special consideration and special treatment. It also may function as a nonverbal means of controlling or manipulating others.

Conversion disorder is believed by some to have a neuropsychological basis. Some conversion patients are thought to have a disturbance in central nervous system arousal. It has been theorized that their symptoms are due to excessive cortical arousal, which sets off negative feedback loops between the cerebral cortex and the brain stem reticular formation. Elevated levels of corticofugal output in turn inhibit afferent sensorimotor impulses, diminishing the awareness of bodily sensation. This theory would explain the observed sensory deficits in some conversion disorder patients, and their apparently low levels of anxiety and relative indifference to their impairment.

Neuropsychological tests reveal subtle cerebral impairments in some conversion patients in verbal communication and memory, affective incongruity, suggestibility, and vigilance and attention. Thus, a second set of neuropsychological theories revolves around the role of cerebral asymmetry in mediating attention and arousal, and the differences between the dominant and nondominant hemispheres in processing somatosensory stimuli. Theories of conversion disorder based on hemispheric asymmetry emphasize the predominant role of the right hemisphere. And conversion symptoms, when unilateral, are more frequent on the left than on the right.

Predisposing factors Serious medical illness predisposes people to conversion disorder. The symptoms often arise as secondary elaborations or exaggerations of a medical illness, sometimes appearing in the locations and organ systems that were previously the site of organic pathology. Pseudoseizures, for example, have been reported in epileptics after their epilepsy has been adequately controlled with anticonvulsants.

Conversion has long been noted to occur in persons who have undergone extreme psychological stress. For example, a young woman became aphonic moments after she was mugged on the street: Her assailant had knocked her down, put his boot over her throat, and threatened to stomp down if she made a sound. Conversion symptoms are also common among combatants in warfare. Some empiric data confirm this relationship: Evidence of a precipitating stress is reported in more than half of conversion disorder patients. Yet, the patients themselves appear oblivious to any relationship between their symptom and life events.

Preexisting psychopathology also predisposes to the development of conversion disorder. The most common Axis I disorders are depression, anxiety, schizophrenia, and somatization disorder. Among hospitalized patients with a conversion symptom, one-quarter to one-half have a clinically significant depression, manic-depressive disorder, or schizophrenia. A past history of somatic symptoms without a demonstrable medical etiology, or Briquet's syndrome predisposes to conversion. Some form of prior somatization was reported in 84 percent of conversion disorder patients in one series, and somatization disorder can be diagnosed in 29 to 34 percent of such patients. It is important to remember, however, that conversion reactions can also occur without any other past or concurrent psychopathology.

Axis II personality disorder is often present in conversion patients, most commonly histrionic personality disorder, passive-dependent personality, passive-aggressive personality, and various types of primitive oral characters and borderline personalities. Although many conversion patients have a histrionic personality style, this is far from universal; it has been found in between 5 and 21 percent of patients. More common is passive-dependent personality, reportedly found in 9 to 40 percent of conversion patients. These findings are compatible with the psychoanalytic theory that conversion symptoms arise in people with hysterical and oral-dependent features.

PATHOLOGY By definition, no medical disorder is responsible for conversion symptoms, though prolonged loss of function may result secondarily in complications, such as contractures or disuse atrophy from conversion paralysis. No brain pathology has been found in conversion disorder patients, though some subtle brain dysfunctions have been demonstrated in a few patients.

CLINICAL SIGNS AND SYMPTOMS The most typical conversion symptoms are sensory or motor symptoms that suggest neurological disease. These commonly include paralysis, aphonia, seizures, coordination disturbances, blindness, tunnel vision, anesthesia, paresthesia, akinesia, and dyskinesia. DSM-III-R's conversion disorder also encompasses autonomic and endocrine symptoms when these symptoms are a direct symbolic expression of psychological conflict. Examples include psychogenic vomiting expressing disgust or rejection, and pseudocyesis symbolizing the wish to be pregnant.

Sensory symptoms Anesthesia and paresthesia are common, especially of the extremities. All sensory modalities are involved. The distribution of the disturbance is inconsistent with that of either central or peripheral neurological disease. Thus, one sees the characteristic stocking and glove anesthesia of the hands or feet, and hemianesthesia of the body beginning precisely along the midline. With careful testing, the sensory pathways can often be shown to be intact. For example, patients complaining of loss of touch, position, and vibratory sense are nonetheless able to walk normally. If patients with anesthesia are instructed to answer yes when they feel a stimulus and no when they do not, some respond no when the affected area is touched.

Conversion symptoms may involve the organs of special sense and include deafness, blindness, and tunnel vision. The symptom may be unilateral or bilateral. Neurological evaluation reveals intact sensory pathways. In conversion blindness, for example, the patient walks around without collisions or self-injury; the pupils react to light; and cortical evoked potentials are normal.

Motor symptoms Motor symptoms include abnormal movements, gait disturbances, weaknesses, and paralyses. Gross, rhythmical tremors, as well as choreiform tics and jerks, are seen. These movements generally worsen when attention is called to them. A common gait disturbance is a wildly ataxic, staggering gait accompanied by gross, irregular, jerky truncal movements, and thrashing and waving of the arms (astasia abasia). These patients rarely fall, and if they do, they are generally not injured.

Convulsive movements are sometimes seen. These are not rhythmical, tonic-clonic movements of the extremities but, rather, a disorganized, flailing, thrashing, and jerking of the entire body. Rarely is there incontinence or tongue biting, and the patients do not injure themselves. Postictal confusion and amnesia are absent, and so patients can recall what was going on around them during the event.

Other common motor disturbances are paralysis and paresis, involving one, two, or all four limbs. The distribution of the involved muscles does not conform to neural pathways. Thus, for example, the hand is paralyzed from the wrist down, or the entire forearm below the elbow is weak. The affected parts are flaccid, and the deficit is generally more severe proximally than distally. If patients are asked to move the afflicted member, spasm of the antagonist muscles occurs which prevents motion. Reflexes remain normal; there are no fasiculations or muscle atrophy (except after long-standing conversion paralysis); and electromyography is normal.

The presence of organic disease One of the major problems in diagnosing conversion disorder is the difficulty in ruling out a medical disorder. The clinical picture is often an amalgam of significant medical disease (either concurrently or previously) and a superimposed psychological elaboration or exaggeration of it. Concomitant organic disease is common in hospitalized patients with conversion symptoms: Evidence of current or prior neurological disorder, or of systemic disease affecting the brain, has been reported in between 18 and 64 percent of them.

Other associated features The absence of a medical etiology is necessary, but not sufficient, for the diagnosis of conversion disorder. In addition, positive findings indicating a psychological etiology should be established. It is clinically unsound to consider a symptom to be a conversion symptom solely because the medical workup is not revealing. DSM-III-R requires the identification of a psychological etiology, as evidenced by a temporal relationship between the symptom and a significant psychosocial stress, or by the presence of secondary gain. The positive psychiatric criteria have traditionally included primary gain, secondary gain, *la belle indifférence,* figures of identity, and other psychopathology. Most of these criteria, however, are of rather limited diagnostic validity.

In order for the conversion symptom to alleviate psychic distress (i.e., to result in primary gain), it must symbolize the disturbing psychological conflict or need, and the onset of the symptom must be preceded by an event that causes psychic distress. Although the primary gain may be obvious and convincing in some cases, in many others it is far less clear. Symbolism may be lacking or at least obscure. At other times, the clinical picture is cloudy because the symbolism has been secondarily superimposed on an organic symptom. Empirical research does not unequivocally support the validity or reliability of symbolism or primary gain as a diagnostic criterion, and further investigation is needed to substantiate their utility.

Secondary gain is another positive diagnostic criterion, but it too presents difficulties. Secondary gain refers to the tangible benefits that accrue to people as a result of becoming sick, such as being excused from various obligations, duties, and responsibilities; the ability to postpone facing difficult life situations or challenges; receiving attention, support, and assistance that might not otherwise be forthcoming; and controlling and influencing the behavior of important people in the patient's life. Sometimes the secondary gain resulting from a symptom may be so clear and so specific as to convince the clinician beyond doubt of the symptom's psychological etiology. But in many other patients, the secondary gain is not as apparent, and to make matters even more difficult, medical disorder also results in a secondary gain. This criterion is therefore of limited utility and validity as a diagnostic feature of conversion symptoms.

La belle indifférence is another commonly used diagnostic criterion. This term refers to an inappropriately cavalier attitude toward a serious symptom. The patient seems unconcerned about what appears to be a major impairment. Though sometimes obvious, such bland indifference may be lacking in the majority of conversion patients. In addition, this attitude is seen in especially stoical patients with serious medical disorders. Thus, it is now considered to have little diagnostic value.

It has been generally held that conversion patients unconsciously model their symptoms on those of someone important to them, and so the presence of such figures of identity has been used as a diagnostic criterion. These people (i.e., a parent or someone who has recently died) have organic or functional symptoms that are identical to the conversion patient's, and they appear to serve as a model for their unconscious mimicry. Thus, it is common in the course of a pathological grief reaction for the bereaved to develop the symptoms of the deceased. Empirical studies of this diagnostic criterion in conversion disorder suggest that it is valid and useful.

Empirical research suggests that a previous history of conversion or other unexplained physical complaints is the most valid and reliable diagnostic criterion of conversion. Some clinicians argue that the diagnosis of conversion disorder is unreliable without a prior history of similar psychogenic complaints or somatization disorder. More than a third of conversion patients have previously had a conversion reaction, and a third have somatization disorder.

DIFFERENTIAL DIAGNOSIS The first diagnosis to consider is a medical disorder, particularly neurological disorders (such as dementia and other degenerative diseases, brain tumors, and basal ganglia disease) and systemic disorders that present with vague, protean, and disparate symptoms (such as multiple sclerosis and systemic lupus erythematosis). It is crucial to follow the patient carefully over time, looking for the emergence of additional medical signs or symptoms or for subsequent conversion episodes. Weakness, for example, may be confused with myasthenia gravis, polymyositis, acquired myopathies, or periodic paralysis. Optic neuritis may be misdiagnosed as conversion blindness. Signs and symptoms that are inconsistent with anatomic distributions and known pathophysiological mechanisms or that vary from one examination to another are more likely to be due to conversion than to medical disease. But it must always be remembered that medical knowledge is still incomplete and that there are always atypical and unusual presentations of known medical disorders. The complete resolution of symptoms with suggestion, hypnosis, or intravenous amobarbital (Amytal) suggests they are psychogenic, but partial improvement with reassurance or sedation often occurs in medical disorders and is of no differential diagnostic value. Furthermore, conversion and medical disease are by no means mutually exclusive: The presence of organic disease does not rule out a conversion reaction, and conversely, the presence of a conversion reaction does not mean that medical disease is absent.

Conversion symptoms occur in schizophrenia and depressive disorder. Schizophrenia, with its dissolution of reality testing and illogical thinking, is generally evident. According to DSM-III-R, when schizophrenia is present, it takes precedence, and the diagnosis of conversion disorder should not be made. Depression can usually be distinguished because it is more pervasive and lasts longer.

Sensorimotor symptoms occur in somatization disorder, but this is a more pervasive and more chronic illness, which begins early in life and includes symptoms in many other organ systems as well. Patients with repetitive conversion disorder often meet the criteria for somatization disorder, and when this is the case, according to DSM-III-R, the diagnosis of conversion disorder should not be made. In hypochondriasis, there is no actual loss or distortion of function. The somatic complaints are more chronic and not limited to neurological symptoms, and the characteristic hypochondriacal attitudes and beliefs are present. If the symptoms are limited to pain, then a diagnosis of somatoform pain disorder should be made. The patient whose complaints are limited to sexual function is diagnosed as having a psychosexual dysfunction rather than a conversion disorder.

In both malingering and factitious disorder, the symptoms are under conscious, voluntary control. Malingerers' histories are usually more inconsistent and contradictory than are conversion patients', and their fraudulent behavior is clearly goal directed.

PROGNOSIS Individual conversion symptoms are generally of short duration, with abrupt onset and resolution. Fifty to 90 percent of hospitalized patients with conversion reactions have recovered by the time of discharge from the hospital. Although conversion symptoms tend to remit spontaneously, a few become chronic, and many other patients experience recurrences. About 25 percent of these patients develop another conversion symptom during the next 1 to 6 years, most commonly when the precipitating stress is chronic or recurrent, when there is other psychopathology, or when there is marked secondary gain (such as compensation payments or disability pensions). During a single conversion episode, there is generally only one symptom. Subsequent episodes may involve the same symptom or a different one.

A favorable outcome seems to depend more on the patients' psychological strengths and personality than on the nature of their symptoms. Good prognostic signs include acute onset, massive environmental stress, good premorbid psychological health, the absence of another major psychiatric disorder, and the absence of medical disease. Patients with long histories of conversion symptoms and those with massive secondary gain do particularly poorly.

Even with competent medical evaluation, some conversion-disorder patients will eventually manifest organic disorders that in retrospect explained or contributed to the presenting symptoms. At times, the premonitory organic symptoms precipitated a conversion symptom. In other instances the initial diagnosis was incorrect, and the underlying organic pathology was simply missed. In still other cases, the medical disease was too atypical, or had not evolved far enough, to permit a diagnosis. Three- to 11-year follow-ups reveal that 13 to 60 percent of all hospitalized patients receiving a diagnosis of conversion reaction subsequently develop an organic illness that can account for the original symptoms. A medical etiology is less likely to emerge in patients with a prior history of somatization.

TREATMENT Most conversion symptoms remit with nonspecific, supportive interventions incorporating a prominent element of suggestion. Prompt elimination of the symptom is important in order to prevent secondary gains from reinforcing it and causing it to persist or recur. If the symptom does not improve rapidly or if precipitating or perpetuating factors remain, more definitive treatment is indicated. If the conversion symptom is part of a more pervasive psychiatric illness, such as schizophrenia, treatment should be aimed at the underlying disorder first.

Initial management focuses on alleviating the conversion symptom. Relaxing and reassuring the patient are crucial here. After a thorough medical workup, the patient may be told that the examination indicates that nothing grave is wrong, that the symptom will rapidly subside, and even that it is already beginning to improve. Telling the patient there is nothing "real" wrong will often make things worse rather than better. Although the initial focus is on symptom relief, it is also important to identify precipitating stressors and conflicts. Recent events and feelings are discussed in order to do so, as long as this does not heighten anxiety. Hypnosis, anxiolytics (for those patients who are unusually anxious), and behavioral relaxation exercises may be effective at this stage. In the heyday of hypnosis, hysterical conversion symptoms were removed by hypnotic suggestion, although the symptom frequently recurred or another took its place. Thus, in recent times, the hypnotic technique has been modified so that the symptom is not removed outright but, rather, is attenuated so that it is no longer disabling. If these measures do not eliminate the symptom, an amobarbital interview may be undertaken, especially when there has been a specific traumatic event. This technique is employed to obtain more history, to help the patient reexperience the traumatic event, and to suggest that the symptom will disappear.

The second phase of treatment is aimed at helping the patient recognize and cope with the psychosocial stresses that provoked the symptom and at preventing chronicity. If the precipitating stress is persistent or if there is significant psychopathology, psychotherapy that explores the psychological origins of the conversion is indicated. Psychodynamic psychotherapy has been used to gain insight into the genesis of the conversion symptom, including exploring intrapsychic conflict and recapturing traumatic memories. The therapist listens for the psychological symbolism and personal meaning of the conversion symptom, while also regarding it as an interpersonal communication and a way of dealing with painful affect. The patients learn to say in words what they had been able to say only with their bodies as the therapist helps them bear the affects that had been unbearable. Briefer and more directive forms of short-term psychotherapy have also been used to treat conversion disorder.

When secondary gain is prominent, behavioral therapy and environmental manipulation may be used to reduce it. This may involve working with the family and others in the patient's life, because they may perpetuate the symptom by rewarding passivity and dependency and by being overly solicitous and helpful. These families must learn to reward the patient's autonomy, self-sufficiency, and independence. But the longer such patients have been in the sick role and the more they have regressed, the more difficult the treatment will be.

HYPOCHONDRIASIS

DEFINITION Hypochondriasis is a pervasive and excessive concern about disease and a preoccupation with one's health. DSM-III-R (Table 19-3) defines hypochondriasis as an unrealistic interpretation of physical signs and sensations as abnormal, leading to a preoccupation with the fear or belief of having a serious disease. Coexisting medical disease may be present but is not of sufficient magnitude to account for the physical signs or sensations. The disease fear or conviction is disabling and persists despite appropriate reassurance.

HISTORY The Greeks used the word *hypochondria* to refer to the region of the body below the ribs and the xiphoid cartilage, and they associated various mental states with changes in the organs of the hypochondria. This region was thought to be the source of black bile, believed responsible for melancholy. From the time of Galen, in the second century A.D., through the nineteenth century, hypochondriasis referred to somatic complaints involving the hypochondria rather than to a morbid preoccupation with illness. With advances in the scientific understanding of disease, many of the abdominal disorders that had been subsumed under the term hypochondriasis came to be recognized as separate medical diseases (e.g., cholycystitis or ulcers). In the 1800s, observers noted that psychological factors could play a role in some of the residual conditions still referred to as hypochondriasis, and melancholy was singled out in this respect. Gradually the term hypochondriasis came to refer to certain unexplained somatic symptoms that were associated with a morbid or distorted preoccupation with health and the body.

TABLE 19-3
Diagnostic Criteria for Hypochondriasis

A. Preoccupation with the fear of having, or the belief that one has, a serious disease, based on the person's interpretation of physical signs or sensations as evidence of physical illness.
B. Appropriate physical evaluation does not support the diagnosis of any physical disorder that can account for the physical signs or sensations or the person's unwarranted interpretation of them, **and** the symptoms in A are not just symptoms of panic attacks.
C. The fear of having, or belief that one has, a disease persists despite medical reassurance.
D. Duration of the disturbance is at least 6 months.
E. The belief in A is not of delusional intensity, as in delusional disorder, somatic type (i.e., the person can acknowledge the possibility that his or her fear of having, or belief that he or she has, a serious disease is unfounded).

Table from DSM-III-R *Diagnostic and Statistical Manual of Mental Disorders,* ed 3, revised. Copyright American Psychiatric Association, Washington, DC, 1987. Used with permission.

COMPARATIVE NOSOLOGY Hypochondriasis can be a symptom of another underlying psychiatric disorder (secondary hypochondriasis), an independent disorder that exists without other concurrent psychiatric disorder (primary hypochondriasis), or a transient reaction to life stress. The condition described in DSM-III-R is primary hypochondriasis, a condition seen far more often in medical than in psychiatric settings. Among psychiatric patients, by contrast, hypochondriasis is most often a secondary feature of some other psychiatric disorder.

Nosological confusion has also centered on the distinction between hypochondriasis as a chronic condition, which is considered a psychiatric disorder, and hypochondriasis as a transient reaction to a stress, which is not thought to be psychopathological. Thus, DSM-III-R requires a duration of 6 months. As long as the disease conviction is not delusional, then hypochondriasis may be diagnosed in the presence of anxiety disorder, mood disorder, schizophrenia, or other somatoform disorders. DSM-III-R, however, specifically requires that the patient's somatic symptoms not occur only during panic attacks.

EPIDEMIOLOGY Hypochondriasis is present in 3 to 14 percent of patients in general medical practice. The prevalence in the general population is unknown. The sex distribution is approximately equal or slightly predominant in men. Some research suggests hypochondriasis has an inverse relationship with social position, but other research suggests no relationship. Likewise, the peak age of onset is unclear: Several studies put it in the third and fourth decades, but others report the peak age of onset is in adolescence, and still other reports find that hypochondriasis is common among those over 60. Some studies report ethnic and cultural differences, whereas others find none.

Though little is known about the inheritance of hypochondriasis, there is some evidence of an increased prevalence of hypochondriasis among identical siblings and other first-degree relatives.

ETIOLOGY Hypochondriasis has been thought to have a psychodynamic origin in the unconscious gratifications of bodily symptoms and physical suffering. Thus, hypochondriasis has been seen as a drive derivative and an ego defense. Some investigators emphasize the transformation of aggressive and hostile wishes toward others into physical complaints to others. Hypochondriacs express their anger by reproaching others and belaboring them with their complaints and suffering. Their anger originates in past disappointments, rejections, and losses but is expressed in the present by soliciting other people's help and concern and then thwarting and rejecting them as ineffective. Other psychodynamic observers have focused more on oral and dependency needs, viewing hypochondriacal symptoms as the somatic expression of pregenital wishes for caring, nurturance, attention, sympathy, and physical contact. Hypochondriasis has also been invoked as an ego defense mechanism. Some see it as a defense against unbearably low self-esteem and the experience of the self as worthless and defective, as it is less painful to feel that something is wrong with the body than to feel that something is wrong with the self. Hypochondriasis has also been viewed as a defense against guilt and a sense of innate badness. Pain and somatic suffering thus become a means of atonement and expiation and can be experienced as deserved punishment for past wrong doing (either real or imaginary) and the sense that one is wicked and sinful.

Hypochondriasis may have a sociocultural origin. Thus it has been viewed as a request for admission to the sick role made by a person who is facing seemingly insurmountable and insoluble problems. Hypochondriacal symptoms are thus a declaration that the individual feels distressed, disabled, and unable to solve a particular dilemma. Patienthood and the sick role offer a way out because the sick person is allowed to avoid noxious obligations, postpone unwelcome challenges, and is excused from onerous duties. And with the sick role comes sympathy, encouragement, attention, support, and concrete assistance—especially financial compensation—all without any implication of blame or fault or failure. Sick patients also have special powers within their family—sickness and suffering allow them to avoid intimacy ("Not tonight, dear, I have a headache"), to control and manipulate others, and to express their hostility, since temper tantrums and irritability are excusable if one is sick. By the same token, hypochondriacs also seek a caretaking relationship with a physician, and the ticket of admission to the doctor's office is a somatic complaint.

Hypochondriasis may be due to a perceptual disturbance in which normal bodily sensations and symptoms are amplified and experienced as more intense and more noxious by hypochondriacs than they are by nonhypochondriacs. There is some evidence suggesting that hypochondriacs augment and amplify somatic sensations and that they have lower thresholds for and a lower tolerance of physical discomfort. What the normal individual perceives as abdominal pressure, for example, the hypochondriac experiences as abdominal pain.

Hypochondriasis may also result from a faulty cognitive scheme that is self-perpetuating and self-validating. According to this theory, hypochondriasis begins when a person mistakenly attributes to serious disease normal bodily sensations, the benign symptoms of trivial illnesses, or the somatic symptoms of emotional arousal. Nonhypochondriacs would attribute the same somatic sensations to such nonpathological causes as overwork, dietary indiscretion, insufficient rest, or old age. But hypochondriacs focus on these sensations, misinterpret them, and are therefore alarmed by them. This state of apprehensive arousal and somatic self-scrutiny further amplifies other normal bodily sensations. The patients then interpret these new sensations as further evidence confirming the hypothesis that they have a serious disease. Thus, a vicious cycle is set into motion. Once formed, the incorrect disease attribution tends to persist because subsequent perceptions are selected to confirm it.

Predisposing factors During childhood, hypochondriacs appear to have had a high incidence of medical illness and functional symptoms in their family members. The literature generally points to a role for the modeling and reinforcement of somatic complaints in the hypochondriac's family of origin: Illness frequently appears to have been a source of overconcern and a prominent focus of attention. Attitudes such as maternal overattentiveness to a child's trivial symptoms apparently result in an enhanced perception of somatic symptoms in adulthood.

Medical disorder predisposes one to hypochondriasis in two ways. First, transient hypochondriacal reactions often follow a severe or life-threatening illness, such as during the recuperative phase after a myocardial infarction. Second, primary hypochondriacs seem to have an increased incidence of childhood medical illness and more extensive past medical histories; their intimate experience with medical illness makes them more susceptible to the subsequent development of hypochondriasis and the use of a somatic language to articulate social and psychological distress.

Although hypochondriacs are not characterized by a single personality type, clinical observers have suggested that three personalities are particularly vulnerable to the development of hypochondriasis: narcissistic, obsessive-compulsive, and masochistic. Hypochondriacs, with their self-absorption and preoccupation with their bodies, to the exclusion of other people and objects, assume a profoundly narcissistic position. Another group of hypochondriacs are said to have obsessional characteristics, in particular, obstinacy, defiance, miserliness, and conscientiousness. Finally, some hypochondriacs have prominent masochistic traits, including a general inclination toward defeat, humiliation and suffering, guilt, and a refractoriness to treatment and clinical improvement.

PATHOLOGY There are no known neuropathological findings in hypochondriasis. A few studies claim an increased prevalence of brain disease and abnormal electroencephalograms in this population. By definition, if any organ pathology were present, it would be far too limited to account for the patient's symptoms.

CLINICAL SIGNS AND SYMPTOMS Hypochondriacs complain of noxious physical sensations, disturbed bodily functions, or anatomical deviations, which suggest disease. And although medical disease may be present, the symptoms are grossly disproportionate to it. There are many symptoms, involving multiple organ systems and many anatomical locations. The most common complaints are pain and symptoms referable to the gastrointestinal and cardiovascular systems. The symptoms are chronic, waxing and waning over many years. The patients recount them in exquisite and intimate detail and often have an elaborate, detailed, pathophysiological model in mind to explain them. Hypochondriacs are very concerned with the meaning and authenticity of their symptoms and with their etiological significance. Thus, they may be as interested in a diagnostic label as they are in symptom relief per se.

Hypochondriacs believe that they have a serious disease that has not yet been detected, and they cannot be persuaded to the contrary. Their disease conviction persists in spite of negative laboratory investigations, a benign course over time, and appropriate reassurance from the physician. This conviction is not of delusional proportions, however, in that hypochondriacs can admit temporarily that their beliefs of disease may be unrealistic and exaggerated. But they are so firmly convinced of an organic etiology that they adamantly reject, and are often irritated by, any implication that stress or psychosocial factors play any role in their condition. In addition, hypochondriacs are troubled by an intense and persistent fear of disease. They are apprehensive and frightened, becoming alarmed at the slightest hint of illness, such as from reading about a disease, knowing someone who becomes sick, or from the direct experience of benign bodily sensations.

Hypochondriacs are profoundly preoccupied with their bodies and their health status. They vigilantly scrutinize their physiological functioning, are absorbed with their bodily appearance and limitations, and are obsessed with their health in general. Nothing is as interesting to hypochondriacs as their own body. They have retreated from engagement with the outside world, recognizing only their own needs. Their illness and suffering become a key part of their self-identity. Hypochondriacs spend much of their time discussing with friends and family their medical condition and care and often make acquaintances on the basis of common medical experiences.

Hypochondriacs have an extensive history of medical care, and for some, visiting doctors and clinics becomes a way of life. Although some become attached to a single physician, whom they consult repeatedly and on the slightest pretext, others go from one source of care to another, undergoing endless examinations and evaluations. But their interactions with physicians are as disappointing as they are extensive, and the physicians are ultimately blamed for the patients' problems. Hypochondriacs carry out elaborate self-treatment regimens, perform self-diagnosis, and complain vociferously and publicly about their plight. As could be anticipated from the above, they are often quite disabled. Their symptoms and their concerns interfere with their close relationships, their work, their interests, and their friendships. Their physical performance, activities of daily living, and avocational pursuits are often impaired. In addition, anxiety and depressive symptoms are common.

The clinical presentation is quite characteristic. Such patients immediately launch into an irritatingly detailed history and a difficult-to-interrupt barrage of complaints, often presented in a hostile or reproachful fashion. Frequently they come with all their medical records and demand further diagnostic procedures and therapeutic interventions. The interview is a monologue, not a dialogue, and it is almost impossible to deflect such patients from their "organ recital" into a discussion of family, work, hobbies, or personal background. Hypochondriacs form hostile-dependent relationships with their doctors that are strained and unsatisfactory. They are clinging and demanding, but also rejecting and hostile, a combination that elicits a negative reaction from the physician. The patients end up rejecting and dismissing the doctor's attempts to help. They become disparaging, angry, and ungrateful, and continue to complain all the while.

Clinical types The following vignette illustrates some of the characteristics of the hypochondriac:

> The patient was a 36-year-old accountant who had been bedeviled since his mid 20s by a series of disturbing symptoms that waxed and waned. Many physicians had failed to ameliorate his distress, and in his view, a number had made things worse. He was most bothered by a burning pain in his mouth, sore throats, tinnitis, and a feeling of "pressure" or "congestion" in his head that made voices sound as if they were underwater and slowed his thinking. He noted that he always felt unbalanced, even when seated, and that when standing more weight seemed to be on one foot than the other. Frequently he noted that his muscles were stiff and heavy; his ankles were weak; and he seemed to move more slowly than was normal.
>
> The patient had researched his symptoms in medical texts and various newspapers and magazines. He suspected that he was harboring the Epstein–Barr virus, and he urgently requested studies to confirm the diagnosis. His quest had taken him to endocrinologists, neurologists, nephrologists, otolaryngologists, as well as infectious disease specialists. He kept detailed charts of his symptoms and his medications and their side effects. He was disparaging and resentful of his previous doctors, maintaining that they had failed to take him seriously enough and to evaluate his case adequately.
>
> He avoided marriage because "no one wants to live with an invalid." He had turned down a promotion in his firm because it would have entailed longer hours and frequent travel, and he feared these physical demands would make him sicker. He also curtailed his social life and his avocational pursuits in order to avoid overtaxing himself. After he had hiked up a mountain, for example, it struck him that he had been using muscles he did not ordinarily use, and so he became frightened that he had damaged himself and that the descent would be painful.
>
> As a child, he battled frequently with his mother, but he remembered that she would always call a truce when he had a cold, "flu," or a "racing pulse." He recalled with fondness those peaceful interludes. He also observed that verbal battles with his parents were followed by severe headaches and that this pattern had persisted throughout his adult life. But he steadfastly denied any relationship between his somatic symptoms and his emotions or interpersonal relationships.

There are three types of hypchondriasis: primary hypochondriasis (as in DSM-III-R), transient hypochondriacal reactions, and hypochondriasis in the elderly.

Transient hypochondriacal reactions occur after major stresses, two of which seem to be most common: the death or serious illness of someone important to the patient, or a serious and perhaps life-threatening illness that resolves but leaves the patient temporarily hypochondriacal in its wake. Such hypochondriacal states lasting less than 6 months would be diagnosed according to DSM-III-R as somatoform disorder not otherwise specified. Transient hypochondriacal responses to external stress generally remit when the stress resolves, but they can become chronic if reinforced by people in the patient's social system and by health professionals.

Hypochondriasis frequently accompanies medical disorder in the elderly. Previous tendencies toward hypochondriacal preoccupation may gradually intensify with aging, or hypochondriasis may appear for the first time in old age. Although the elderly do experience a decline in physical capacity and bodily function, most elderly patients are not hypochondriacal, and hypochondriacal behavior should not be considered a normal aspect of aging. Instead, it should be seen as a symptom of another underlying problem, usually depression or the result of a break in the patient's social matrix. It may also represent a transient adjustment reaction to an external stress such as a change in residence or a new social situation. When hypochondriasis occurs for the first time in old age, the clinician should first suspect an underlying depression.

DIFFERENTIAL DIAGNOSIS As with all somatoform disorders, hypochondriasis must first be differentiated from organic disease. The physician must be especially wary of the early stages of diffuse illnesses that affect multiple organ systems (such as endocrine disease or connective tissue disease).

As already noted, however, the presence of medical disorder does not rule out the possibility of coexisting hypochondriasis, if the patient's symptoms and attitudes are disproportionate to the medical morbidity.

Hypochondriacal complaints are common features of depression. An underlying depression is especially likely if the hypochondriacal symptoms have an episodic course like that of recurrent depression or if they appear for the first time in elderly patients who were never before hypochondriacal. Depressed patients' attitudes differ from hypochondriacs' in that the former feel that they are not worth treating and have no hope of recovery, and they act as if their physical suffering is deserved. Finally, depressed patients may have a family history of mood disorder, and their somatic symptoms are more characteristic of the neurovegetative cluster.

Hypochondriacal symptoms are also common in generalized anxiety disorder and panic disorder, and primary hypochondriacs have an increased incidence of panic attacks. According to DSM-III-R, hypochondriasis cannot be diagnosed if the symptoms occur only during panic attacks. Anxiety disorder patients are often alarmed about their health, have prominent somatic symptoms, and manifest extreme bodily vigilance and disease fears. Here the hypochondriasis is not the predominant disturbance but, rather, a feature in a more pervasive disorder. In primary hypochondriasis, by contrast, the false belief in an occult medical illness is the central clinical feature, and the other symptoms are largely consequences of this belief system.

Frankly somatic delusions of having a medical disease occur in schizophrenia, psychotic depression, and organic mental syndromes. Hypochondriacs' disease conviction is not delusional (though the dividing line between obsessed concern and delusional conviction can be very thin indeed), and they may entertain, if only briefly, the possibility that they do not have the particular disease they dread. Another differential point is that somatic delusions are static and unchanging, whereas hypochondriacal symptoms fluctuate over time. Schizophrenic patients' somatic delusions tend to be bizarre and absurd (i.e., their internal organs have been strangely altered, or foreign objects are inside an orifice or cavity, or body parts are deformed or missing).

Neurotic phenomena, such as obsessions and phobias, may resemble hypochondriasis. Simple disease phobias are common, and obsessions may center on dirt and germs, bodily contamination, and fears of disease. These neurotic phenomena differ from hypochondriasis in that they are cognitions rather than bodily symptoms, and they are private and shameful and therefore tenaciously concealed from others. Hypochondriacs, on the other hand, do not believe their symptoms are irrational, excessive, or unrealistic, and they display them openly and publicly.

The relationship of hypochondriasis to the other somatoform disorders is somewhat unclear. According to DSM-III-R, it is possible to diagnose hypochondriasis along with any other somatoform disorder. Somatization disorder does not include disease conviction, disease fear, or bodily preoccupation, and it begins before age 30. The somatization disorder patient is more often female and is more likely to have a histrionic cognitive and interpersonal style, as compared with the more obsessional hypochondriac. The degree of overlap between these two conditions has not been established empirically. Conversion disorder is acute and transient, involving a single neurological symptom at a time, whereas hypochondriasis is chronic and involves multiple symptoms in multiple sites and organ systems. If *la belle indifférence* is present in conversion disorder, it contrasts markedly with the hypochondriac's anguish. Somatoform pain disorder is chronic, like hypochondriasis, but the symptoms are limited to pain. Body dysmorphic disorder patients wish to appear normal and believe that others notice that they are not, whereas hypochondriacs wish to draw attention to themselves and proclaim loudly that they are not normal.

Hypochondriasis is distinguished from factitious disorder with physical symptoms and malingering in that hypochondriacs actually experience the symptoms they report and are not simulating.

PROGNOSIS The natural course of hypochondriasis is not entirely clear, but it is generally thought to be chronic, with the symptoms waxing and waning. On long-term follow-up, a quarter of hypochondriacs do poorly, and about two-thirds run chronic, fluctuating courses. Some do recover. Most hypochondriacal children recover by late adolescence or early adulthood. Although there is a general feeling of pessimism about the effectiveness of treatment, this is not substantiated by most of the studies of treatment outcome, which instead suggest that treatment helps a significant proportion of patients. Favorable prognostic features include the concurrent presence of anxiety or depression, acute onset, the absence of personality disorder, higher socioeconomic status, younger age, and the absence of organic disease.

TREATMENT Hypochondriacs are usually managed by primary care physicians, as they find a psychiatric referral unacceptable. Psychiatric treatment is helpful for those few patients who acknowledge emotional difficulties or in whom it is possible to penetrate the mask of somatic complaints to reach their underlying dysphoria. Some hypochondriacs accept psychiatric treatment if it takes place in a medical setting and focuses on stress reduction and coping with chronic illness. Among such patients, group psychotherapy has been reported to be the modality of choice, in part because it provides the social support and social interaction that these patients need. Individual, insight-oriented, traditional psychotherapy for primary hypochondriasis is generally not successful.

The primary care physicians' goal in managing hypochondriacal patients is care rather than cure. The physicians take the position that they will try to alleviate the patients' symptoms as much as possible but that some degree of discomfort is likely to persist. Just as they do with patients with chronic medical illnesses, the doctors aim to help hypochondriacs to cope with and tolerate their symptoms and to live with them as adaptively as possible, rather than to remove them. Physicians must recognize that these patients have psychological and social reasons for remaining symptomatic and that no medical or surgical intervention can cure the psychological need to have symptoms. Once the physicians conceptualize the patients' complaints as a communication rather than as a disease that can be eradicated, their relationship becomes less adversarial. Only when doctors have acknowledged and accepted the patients' experiences can the patients then begin to ease their grip on their symptoms.

Physicians should try to divorce the experience of being symptomatic from the experience of being accepted as a patient. In other words, the doctors should allow the patients the sick role, regardless of how symptomatic they are. This is done by establishing regularly scheduled appointments rather than "as needed," as the latter means to the patients that they can see the doctor only if they are symptomatic. Doctors also should communicate their acceptance of their patients as persons and not just as patients. Thus, physicians should couple their attention to the patients' physical complaints with a genuine interest in the patients as individuals. This can be conveyed by paying attention to their personal and social history, which is additionally important because patients' bodily pain is often referred from their social world, interpersonal relationships, and family. It is also valuable to compliment patients on their perseverance and their endurance of their discomfort. Encouraging the direct expression of affect may reduce the need for somatic concerns. Over a period of time there may be a change in the patients' lexicon, with talk about personal issues and feelings gradually replacing talk about somatic sensations.

Physicians tread a fine line between taking the patient's symptoms so literally and so seriously that they try to cure everyone, and giving them no legitimacy at all by ignoring them completely and acting as if the patients were malingering. Medical interventions should be modest, simple, and benign: hot water bottles, ointments, frequent physical examinations, vitamins, and physiotherapy. As much as possible, physicians should prescribe themselves. Invasive diagnostic and therapeutic procedures should be undertaken on the basis of objective evidence rather than subjective complaints. When possible, it is best to refrain from treating equivocal or incidental findings. Underdiagnosis and undertreatment (while staying within the bounds of good medical practice, of course) are preferable to overdiagnosis and overtreatment, giving rise to the maxim "Don't just do something, stand there." Because hypochondriacs tend to develop side effects, iatrogenic illnesses, and new symptoms to replace the old ones, they are harmed more by overaggressive than underaggressive management.

Hypochondriacs' demands for a diagnosis present physicians with a dilemma. Trying to give these patients insight into the psychosocial and psychodynamic sources of their suffering is generally not helpful. It is often better to offer them an alternative explanation for their symptoms, a model of dysfunction rather than of discrete, localized tissue pathology. Physicians may suggest that the problem lies in the patients' perceptual apparatus and cognitive interpretation of their bodily experience. Some physicians make an analogy to a radio receiver with the volume turned up so high that the background static becomes disturbing and unpleasant. If patients reject this explanation, physicians should refrain from struggles over its validity.

Pharmacotherapy alleviates hypochondriacal symptoms only when there is an underlying drug-sensitive condition, such as an anxiety disorder or a major depression. When hypochondriasis is secondary to some other primary psychiatric disorder, the latter must be treated in its own right. When hypochondriasis is a transient situational reaction, the patient must be helped to cope with the stress without reinforcing the illness behavior and use of the sick role as solutions to the problem.

SOMATOFORM PAIN DISORDER

DEFINITION The predominant disturbance in somatoform pain disorder is severe and prolonged pain for which there is no adequate medical explanation (Table 19-4).

TABLE 19-4
Diagnostic Criteria for Somatoform Pain Disorder

A. Preoccupation with pain for at least 6 months.
B. Either (1) or (2):
   (1) appropriate evaluation uncovers no organic pathology or pathophysiologic mechanism (e.g., a physical disorder or the effects of injury) to account for the pain
   (2) when there is related organic pathology, the complaint of pain or resulting social or occupational impairment is grossly in excess of what would be expected from the physical findings

Table from DSM-III-R *Diagnostic and Statistical Manual of Mental Disorders*, ed 3, revised. Copyright American Psychiatric Association, Washington, DC, 1987. Used with permission.

Nosologically, this is the least satisfactory of the somatoform disorders. First, it is not clear that all patients with intractable, idiopathic pain have a psychiatric disorder. Some of these patients may be better characterized by conceptualizing their symptom as a form of abnormal illness behavior, a personality type, or even a nonspecific psychiatric syndrome rather than a single disorder. The boundaries and overlap of somatoform pain disorder with other major Axis I disorders have not yet been established. Second, chronic pain patients may not form a homogeneous group and may instead constitute discrete and different subgroups. Thus, it is not clear how much patients with low back pain, atypical facial pain, chronic pelvic pain, and headache (as four examples) actually share in common. This seems especially salient when we realize that these patients' pain may be post-traumatic, neuropathic, neuralgic, iatrogenic, or musculoskeletal.

Some of the difficulties derive from the complicated nature of chronic pain itself. Pain is a complex mental event, the product of psychological, neurochemical, and neurophysiological factors, all of which modulate and transform the nociceptive sensation. Although pain perception has a sensory component, it also has affective, motivational, and attitudinal components, as numerous associative pathways link the sensory cerebral cortex with the limbic system. Thus, the problem of organic versus functional is particularly acute here, for all pain is simultaneously pathogenic and psychogenic, rather than one or the other.

HISTORY The study of chronic pain began with the rise of modern neuroanatomy and neurophysiology. Ascending pain pathways in the spinal cord were found to have extensive interconnections with other spinal segments, the reticular activating system, hypothalamus, thalamus, and limbic system. Eventually, efferent, descending neural pathways that modulate the afferent pain impulses were discovered. Later, in probing the biochemistry of pain and analgesia, brain opiate receptors and then endogenous analgesic peptides were discovered. These endorphins were found concentrated in discrete regions, such as the periaqueductal gray matter of the midbrain, the rostroventral medulla, and the dorsal horn of the spinal cord. Ascending pain pathways were found to stimulate neurons in the periaqueductal gray area, releasing endorphins and stimulating a feedback loop of descending, modulating efferents. Serotonin, norepinephrine, and substance P were discovered to be key neurotransmitters in these pain pathways. This system of endogenous opioids and neural feedback loops forms the neurophysiological basis for the cortical influence over the pain experience.

Along with this investigation of nociception, other research provided insight into the psychology of pathological and experimental pain. Researchers probed the motivational, affective, and cognitive components of the total pain experience—the element of suffering, as opposed to the nociceptive or sensory element of pain. In addition, psychologists and psychiatrists began to distinguish chronic from acute pain, emphasizing the interpersonal and behavioral dimensions of chronic pain.

COMPARATIVE NOSOLOGY Chronic pain has been classified in several different ways: in the ninth revision of the *International Classification of Diseases* (ICD-9), according to any associated demonstrable pathology; in the Classification System of the International Association for the Study of Pain, according to its phenomenology; and in DSM-III, according to associated psychopathology. It is the importance of psychological factors in intractable pain that led to the inclusion in DSM-III of a diagnosis termed psychogenic pain disorder.

This DSM-III diagnosis of psychogenic pain disorder required positive evidence (either primary or secondary gain) of a psychological etiology in order to distinguish it from undiagnosed pain of organic etiology. But such positive evidence is most often lacking in patients with intractable pain that has no adequate medical explanation. Furthermore, judgments about the presence of a psychological cause for a patient's symptoms tend to be neither reliable nor valid. Accordingly, in DSM-III-R, the disorder was renamed somatoform pain disorder, and positive evidence of psychogenicity is not necessary for the diagnosis. It was decided that idiopathic pain would be considered a mental disorder because it can be presumed that psychological factors are important to the condition in general, even though evidence for them might not be readily apparent in each case.

EPIDEMIOLOGY The symptom of pain is perhaps the most frequent complaint in medical practice, and intractable pain syndromes are also common. The magnitude of the problem of chronic idiopathic pain can only be glimpsed from the enormous morbidity and disability associated with it. In 1980, more than $10 billion was spent on disability payments to patients with chronic pain problems. Low back pain alone has disabled an estimated 7 million Americans and accounts for more than 8 million physician office visits yearly.

The prevalence of somatoform pain disorder is uncertain. It is diagnosed more frequently in women (probably about twice as often). The age of onset ranges from childhood to old age, but the peak age of onset is in the fourth and fifth decades. It is more common among people in blue-collar occupations.

ETIOLOGY Four possible etiologies are psychodynamic, behavioral conditioning, interpersonal, and neurophysiological.

The psychodynamics of pain center on its unconscious meanings, which originate in infantile and childhood experiences. Pain may be equated with parental care and affection. Children may unconsciously find in pain a means of obtaining love from parents who otherwise offer little affection. Another important unconscious meaning of pain is punishment for wrongdoing, whether real or imagined. Thus, pain is a way of expiating guilt, of atoning for an innate sense of badness. Children who have been severely punished feel guilty and unconsciously come to believe that they must indeed be bad. Such children may grow up with an unconscious need for suffering and pain to assuage this guilt. As adults, they use pain to punish themselves, as well as a way of reuniting with love objects.

Pain can also be understood as a behavior that is learned by operant and classical conditioning. Here the salient aspect of intractable pain is not the disturbing mental experience but, rather, the activities and behaviors that accompany it, such as grimacing, complaining, lying down, taking analgesics, and staying away from work. Such behaviors were first learned when the pain began, but they persist after the original cause of the pain has ceased, continuing as long as the positive and negative reinforcements do. In operant conditioning, pain behaviors are reinforced when rewarded and inhibited when ignored, discouraged, or punished. For example, pain symptoms may become more intense, more frequent, and more disabling when followed by the solicitous and attentive behavior of others, the pleasurable effects of narcotic analgesics, the monetary gains of litigation or disability compensation, and the successful avoidance of distasteful activities. Families can thus reinforce chronic pain by rewarding pain-related behaviors. Classical conditioning occurs when previously neutral objects and situations (such as a bedroom) evoke pain-related behaviors because they have become associated with the pain.

Social forces, such as interpersonal control and coercion, are another etiological factor. Intractable pain has been conceptualized as a means for manipulation and gaining advantage in interpersonal relationships, through what has been called *pain games* or *painsmanship*. Pain becomes a nonverbal language used for interpersonal communication, in order to, for example, ensure the devotion of a family member or to stabilize a fragile marriage. Conversely, pain may be maintained in an identified patient when it is psychologically important to the other family members to do this. This has been referred to as *tertiary gain*. Some such families have an excessive degree of mutuality or enmeshment, and the patient's pain has a crucial role in the family's dynamics.

Though chronic pain (in contrast with acute pain) is thought to be more a psychological phenomenon than a sensory one, the neuroanatomical and neurophysiological substrate of idiopathic pain is under active investigation. As discussed above, the cerebral cortex can inhibit the firing of afferent pain fibers. Serotonin is probably the main neurotransmitter in the descending inhibitory pathways, and endorphins also probably play a role in the central modulation of pain. Endorphins and serotonin metabolites are apparently decreased in the cerebrospinal fluid of some chronic pain patients. This endorphin deficiency seems to correlate with the augmentation of incoming sensory stimuli. It is not clear, however, that these changes are the cause of the patient's pain.

Predisposing factors Social, cultural, and ethnic forces influence pain tolerance and its expression. Therefore, social norms, cultural values, and family models may predispose some individuals to chronic pain. For example, schoolchildren with chronic unexplained abdominal pain are more likely to have a relative with chronic pain than are children with pathological abdominal pain. Ethnic differences have been found in pain perception, and these are attributed to differing child-rearing practices. Italians and Jews have been reported to be very sensitive to pain and very emotional in their responses to it, whereas the Irish are more stoical and deny pain, and old Americans regard it with emotional detachment. Recent studies, however, have not confirmed these ethnic differences.

Gender may also be a predisposing factor, as men can tolerate more experimental pain than women can. Pain tolerance also declines with age. In as many as one-half the cases of somatoform pain disorder, the onset of the pain follows accidental trauma or surgery.

PATHOLOGY By definition, patients with somatoform pain disorder have no tissue pathology or gross pathophysiological mechanism (such as the muscle spasm responsible for tension headaches) to account for the magnitude of their symptoms. But careful examination and long-term follow-up of intractable pain patients occasionally disclose subtle, pathological findings. Thus, infrared thermography may disclose reduced vascular flow and lower temperatures in the region of the pain. These findings, however, are not necessarily etiological. No central neuropathology has been found.

Chronic pain may cause people to restrict or alter their activities in ways that produce pathology. Invalidism may lead to disuse atrophy of skeletal muscle, osteoporosis, and obesity. Abuse of opioid analgesics leads to infection, central nervous system degeneration, and embolic phenomena. There also may be prominent iatrogenic complications resulting from medical and surgical therapies for the pain, including dependence on minor tranquilizers and narcotic analgesics.

CLINICAL SIGNS AND SYMPTOMS The predominant feature of somatoform pain disorder is a preoccupation with severe and continuous pain of at least 6 months' duration that has no adequate medical explanation. Localized sensory or motor findings may accompany the pain, such as paresthesias or muscle spasm. Either there is no detectable tissue pathology or the symptoms are grossly disproportionate to the pathology that does exist. The pain is constant. The patient arises with it in the morning, and it continues unabated throughout the day. It does not vary from day to day or week to week. The pain is often inconsistent with the neurological innervation of the affected area, but it may sometimes closely mimic the pain distribution of a known disease. In some cases (such as angina-like chest pain in a man whose father died from heart disease), the patient's symptoms appear to have a psychological significance, because they are identical to those of someone important to the patient or they have been learned in previous experiences. Clear evidence of a psychological etiology, in the form of primary or secondary gain, is present in some cases, but in others there is no obvious evidence of psychogenicity.

Somatoform pain patients exhibit a great deal of illness behavior. They are often severely disabled, living the life of an invalid and rarely working, especially when there is pain-contingent financial compensation, pending litigation, or disability claims. They have long histories of medical and surgical care, visiting many doctors and requesting many medications. They are especially insistent in their desire for surgery. They are completely preoccupied with their pain, citing it as the source of all their misery, often denying any emotional dysphoria and devoutly maintaining that the rest of their lives is blissful. Somatoform pain patients deny that psychosocial factors have any role in their suffering, and they are often intent on having their physicians accept their pain as completely organic in origin. They may have a history of drug abuse or alcoholism.

Depression is common in somatoform pain patients, and indeed, neurovegetative symptoms generally emerge whenever severe pain lasts for a long time. Major depression is present in about 25 to 50 percent of somatoform pain patients, and dysthymia or depressive symptoms are reported in between 60 and 100 percent. How often the depression precedes the pain and how often it follows it is a continuing controversy. Some investigators believe that chronic pain is almost always a variant of depressive disorder, that it is a masked or somatized form of depression. The most prominent depressive symptoms in idiopathic pain patients are anergia, anhedonia, decreased libido, insomnia, and irritability. However, diurnal variation, weight loss, and psychomotor retardation appear to be less common.

Clinical observers have repeatedly noted that personality seems to be an important factor in chronic idiopathic pain and that these patients may have a particular premorbid personality type. Empirical data are needed to validate these observations, especially because it is difficult to determine which characteristics precede the development of pain and which follow it. The "pain-prone patient," first described by George Engel, is one such constellation that has been proposed. Pain-prone patients are described as guilty, pessimistic people who unconsciously believe they do not deserve success, pleasure, or happiness and who thus feel that they must pay a price for it should it befall them. They have long histories of suffering, defeat, and humiliation in many different spheres. Many of these situations could have been avoided, but the patients seem unable to learn from experience. It is as if they cannot tolerate happiness or success or good fortune, for the pain often develops just when their lives begin to go smoothly. Pain occurs and recurs when pain-prone patients feel guilty and circumstances fail to satisfy their unconscious need for suffering.

Alexithymia is another personality type reported to be common among idiopathic pain patients. Alexithymic individuals think mechanically and literally, focusing on banal facts, details, and external events rather than on subjective experiences. They do not appreciate or verbalize their emotions, are not psychologically introspective or imaginative, and do not express inner drives, wishes, or fantasies. They act stoical and controlled, and psychologically stressful events result in somatic symptoms, such as chronic pain, rather than dysphoric emotions.

Other chronic pain patients have a counterdependent style, characterized by "workaholism," extreme self-sufficiency and independence, conscientiousness, and constant upward striving. They often began working at an early age, worked at several jobs simultaneously, took little vacation time, and assumed a strong paternal or maternal role within their extended families, supporting and helping many other family members. Once their pain begins, these people rapidly become totally incapacitated, regressing dramatically into an infantile, dependent position. In short, they collapse completely, and more-or-less permanently, into invalidism.

Clinical types There are a number of different chronic pain syndromes, including chronic pelvic pain, low back pain, headaches, temporomandibular joint pain, and iatrogenic pain following surgery. The following vignette illustrates one of these syndromes:

A 46-year-old man suffered with back pain for 6 years. It began when he slipped at work while carrying a heavy piece of machinery. A medical workup revealed nothing, and he was treated conservatively for "back sprain." But the pain worsened, and 2 years later a lumbar laminectomy was performed. This was followed by immediate relief, and the patient returned to work. But within a few months the pain returned, and as his financial pressures grew, he found himself unable to sit or stand for any prolonged period, and he retired on permanent disability. The pain continued unabated, with no change in character or intensity. No medical explanation was discovered, and physical findings were limited to paraspinal muscle spasm. He became an invalid, having to waken his wife each morning so that she could help him get out of bed. He spent much of the day lying on the sofa, watching television. Various conservative treatments, antidepressants, and even repeated back surgery were totally ineffective. He began abusing narcotic analgesics and anxiolytics, though they did not seem to be helpful either.

He was the oldest child in his family and had always been at the center of family disputes as the peacemaker to whom relatives turned to settle their frequent squabbles and grudges. He began working at age 14 to make extra money to support the family, as his father was an alcoholic and had been totally disabled from an on-the-job injury. The patient married at 19, to a woman he idealized as "wonderful, hardworking, honest, kind, sympathetic, and friendly," though he did acknowledge that she had been unfaithful to him on numerous occasions. He had always worked 7 days a week, first as an electrician and then as the owner of his own home-contracting company, hoping to be able to buy his own home and support his two sons who had dropped out of school and refused to go to work. He described his family situation, however, as ideal.

Though acknowledging that he felt "defeated" and "down in the dumps," he quickly insisted that this was solely the consequence of his pain. He admitted that he did not find much pleasure in most things but also attributed this entirely to his pain. "I can't finish anything anymore; I'll never get anywhere. It's all this damn pain."

DIFFERENTIAL DIAGNOSIS Pathological pain (pain of organic origin) can be difficult to distinguish from psychogenic pain, especially because they are not mutually exclusive. In general, pain that is portrayed in highly affective, personalized, or unique terms has a more prominent psychogenic component. Psychogenic pain patients emphasize the singular, unusual, special character of their symptom. The likelihood of a functional component increases as the number of different anatomical sites and kinds of pain increase. Pathological pain fluctuates in intensity and is highly sensitive to emotional, cognitive, attentional, and situational influences. Pain that does not vary and is insensitive to any of these factors is more likely to be psychogenic. When the pain does not wax and wane, when neither distraction nor analgesics provide even transient relief, then the clinician should suspect an important psychogenic component.

As noted, there is a large overlap between somatoform pain disorder and depression. It may be difficult to determine which disorder is primary, and when in doubt, clinicians should consider depression to be primary because it is so treatable. In schizophrenia, there may be various aches and pains, but the pain rarely dominates the clinical picture.

Somatoform pain disorder must also be distinguished from the other somatoform disorders. Pain is among the symptoms of somatization disorder, and in DSM-III-R both diagnoses may be given if the patient meets the criteria for both. Somatization disorder, however, includes many other physical symptoms as well, begins before the age of 30, and is rare in men. Hypochondriacs may complain of pain, and their body preoccupation and disease conviction may be present in idiopathic pain patients as well. Hypochondriacs, however, have multiple symptoms, and their clinical picture fluctuates over time. Conversion disorder is generally short-lived, whereas idiopathic pain is chronic, and pain is by definition not a conversion symptom. Malingerers often complain of pain, but unlike patients with somatoform pain disorder, they are pretending to be in pain, and their complaints serve a clearly recognizable goal. A common example is the narcotic addict seeking to obtain narcotics. But the differential diagnosis can be difficult because the chronic pain patient often receives disability compensation or a litigation award.

PROGNOSIS Somatoform pain, by definition, persists for at least 6 months. The pain generally begins abruptly and increases in severity over a few weeks or months. The prognoses of the various idiopathic pain syndromes are not clear, but in general they are chronic, very disturbing and incapacitating, and these patients do not do well. Idiopathic pain may sometimes subside with treatment, after eliminating the external reinforcement or following the successful therapy of associated psychopathology. But more often it persists for years. The patients with the poorest prognoses, with or without treatment, have preexisting characterological problems, especially pronounced passivity; are involved in litigation or receive financial compensation; use addictive drugs; and have longer histories of pain.

TREATMENT Although the treatment of somatoform pain disorder is difficult, many modalities are available. Treatment begins by attempting to change the patients' expectation from complete relief of pain to coping with some degree of persistent pain. In short, treatment aims to rehabilitate the person rather than to cure the pain. In negotiating the therapeutic goals with the patients, it becomes clearer how motivated they are to improve. It may be useful to discuss early the issue of psychological etiology with the patients, telling them frankly that psychological factors are important to both pathogenic and psychogenic chronic pain, whether as cause or consequence, and that the treatment must take them into account. It must be emphasized at the same time, however, that the patients' pain is real. Other important aspects of overall management include minimizing iatrogenic illness and eliminating environmental reinforcers of illness behavior.

Medical interventions Analgesic medications are not very helpful for most chronic idiopathic pain, and, in addition, drug abuse and addiction are often major problems for somatoform pain patients. Opiates are generally ineffective and should be reserved for patients suffering from pain that is clearly pathogenic. If analgesics are used, aspirin and the nonsteroidal anti-inflammatory agents are usually the agents of choice. They should be used on a regular basis, not as needed. Patients' demands for medication should generally be resisted, and it should be prescribed only when clinicians believe it is indicated.

As a general rule, sedatives and antianxiety agents are not of great benefit and often become problems in themselves because of frequent abuse, misuse, and side effects. The experience with antidepressants, however, is different. Antidepressants such as amitryptilene (Elavil), imipramine (Tofranil), doxepin (Sinequan), and phenelzine (Nardil) are extensively used to treat chronic pain. There is no clear evidence that any one agent is superior. They are routinely prescribed when the neurovegetative cluster of symptoms is present, but a therapeutic trial is also warranted when the depressive symptoms are of lesser magnitude. The antidepressants sometimes afford pain relief at a dosage below that used to treat depression, and, therefore, treatment is initiated at relatively low doses. If initially ineffective, the dose is gradually increased into the range used to treat depression. If there is no response after 6 weeks at an adequate dose, a trial of one other agent is indicated before concluding that antidepressants are of no benefit. Whether antidepressants reduce pain via their antidepressant action or whether they exert an independent, direct, analgesic effect (possibly by stimulating the efferent serotonergic inhibitory pain pathways) remains controversial. Anticonvulsants (most prominently phenytoin [Dilantin], carbamazepine [Tegretol], and clonazepam [Klonopin]) have been reported to be effective in treating neuropathic and neuralgic pain, at least for short periods. But their efficacy in other somatoform pain disorders is less clear. There have also been empirical trials of other psychotropic agents in various forms of idiopathic pain, but few rigorous data exist regarding their efficacy.

Biofeedback has become popular in recent years and can sometimes be moderately helpful, particularly in migraine, myofascial pain, and muscle tension states such as tension headaches. Biofeedback has the advantage of being very acceptable to some of these patients. The role of acupuncture is still unclear. It is apparently most useful in those moderately painful conditions that respond to anti-inflammatory analgesics. Hypnosis has been used with patients who are especially good subjects. Transcutaneous nerve stimulation and dorsal column stimulation have also been tried.

Nerve blocks and surgical ablative procedures are not effective for most somatoform pain disorder patients, with pain returning after 6 to 18 months.

Behavioral interventions The goal of behavioral treatment is to replace pain-related behaviors with normal activities, to teach competent coping skills, to increase the level of physical activity, and finally to decrease pain complaints and perceived pain intensity. This is done by discouraging pain-related behaviors and shaping and reinforcing new health-related behaviors. New health behaviors are rewarded with attention, praise, and positive feedback, whereas a minimum of attention is paid to pain-related behaviors and complaints. Examples of common pain behaviors that need modification are actions that evoke protective responses from others, like wincing, groaning, and complaining; staying in bed; excessive reliance on pain medications; and diminished social, vocational, and avocational activities. Clinicians must remember that simply eliminating the original cause of the pain will not extinguish pain behavior once it has been conditioned.

A wide variety of behavioral modalities can be used, including relaxation training, cognitive therapy, graduated exercise programs, and behavior modification. Initially, the patient may keep a daily diary of activity, pain, and associated circumstances, making it possible to identify certain conditioned behaviors and then to set about modifying them by changing the reinforcement given to the patient. Health professionals, family members, and others in the patient's social support system all must be part of the behavioral prescription.

Psychotherapeutic interventions Idiopathic pain patients are usually resistant and unresponsive to traditional psychotherapeutic interventions, especially insight-oriented individual psychotherapy. However, group, family, and couples therapy are increasingly being employed, especially in combination with other interventions. Even if conjoint marital therapy or family therapy is not undertaken, the patient's marital and family situation must be understood and taken into account, as relatives may be reinforcing the patient's pain-related behaviors, and they themselves frequently have significant psychiatric illness as well. Group therapy is an especially promising approach, particularly when the groups are composed exclusively of pain patients. The focus is on exploring how pain is used as a language of interpersonal communication and the role it plays in the patient's daily life.

Pain control programs When the problem is severe, individual outpatient treatment tends to be unsuccessful, and it is necessary to remove the patients from their usual setting and place them in a comprehensive, inpatient, pain control program. Here a more comprehensive and more intensive intervention can be fashioned, and it is possible to reorient, retrain, and reeducate the patients and their families and to restructure their environment. More recently, a number of outpatient programs have been established that are more limited in their goals.

These multidisciplinary pain units use many different modalities, but at the heart of the program are cognitive, behavioral, and group modeling techniques. They provide extensive patient education, use hypnosis and cognitive techniques rather than analgesics for pain control, teach relaxation techniques, emphasize improved physical conditioning through physical therapy and exercise, and offer vocational evaluation and rehabilitation. Any concurrent psychiatric disorder is diagnosed and treated, and patients addicted to analgesics and hypnotics are detoxified.

Inpatient treatment programs generally report encouraging results, with decreased analgesic use, diminished depression, greater activity, and a decrease in reported pain. About one-half to three-quarters of the patients discharged from such programs have moderate or greater improvement, and about one-third to one-half of the total have maintained this improvement at the 1-year follow-up. There are some methodological problems with these outcome studies, and it is difficult to determine which of the elements in these programs are most helpful. Patients who are refractory to treatment are more likely to have continuing disability compensation or associated psychopathology such as personality disorder, drug dependence, or somatization disorder.

MONOSYMPTOMATIC HYPOCHONDRIASIS AND BODY DYSMORPHIC DISORDER

DEFINITION Monosymptomatic hypochondriasis refers to several different syndromes characterized by a single hypochondriacal belief that one is diseased. The disease conviction is either a delusion or an overvalued idea, and it is grossly disproportionate to any objective disease or deformity. There is no other thought disorder. Body dysmorphic disorder, formerly termed dysmorphophobia, is one of the most common such syndromes (Table 19-5). These patients believe that they are physically misshapen or defective in some specific way, although their objective appearance is unremarkable. Other forms of monosymptomatic hypochondriasis include the delusional belief that one is infested with some parasite or vermin, or the belief that one emits an offensive body odor (olfactory reference syndrome).

COMPARATIVE NOSOLOGY Body dysmorphic disorder, delusions of parasitosis, and olfactory reference syndrome are generally grouped together, but DSM-III-R lists body dysmorphic disorder as a separate diagnosis. Body dysmorphic disorder did not appear in DSM-II, and was termed dysmorphophobia in DSM-III, where it was classified as one type of atypical somatoform disorder. In DSM-III-R, it has been accorded independent status. DSM-III-R specifies that the belief is not of delusional proportion but, rather, is a preoccupation or overvalued idea. If the belief is a true delu-

TABLE 19-5
Diagnostic Criteria for Body Dysmorphic Disorder

A. Preoccupation with some imagined defect in appearance in a normal-appearing person. If a slight physical anomaly is present, the person's concern is grossly excessive.
B. The belief in the defect is not of delusional intensity, as in delusional disorder, somatic type (i.e., the person can acknowledge the possibility that he or she may be exaggerating the extent of the defect or that there may be no defect at all).
C. Occurrence not exclusively during the course of anorexia nervosa or transsexualism.

Table from DSM-III-R *Diagnostic and Statistical Manual of Mental Disorders,* ed 3, revised. Copyright American Psychiatric Association, Washington, DC, 1987. Used with permission.

sion, the correct DSM-III-R diagnosis is delusional disorder, somatic subtype. In practice, the distinction between an overvalued idea and a delusion is extremely difficult to determine. In Europe, where these syndromes have been more widely studied, all the monosymptomatic hypochondriacal syndromes are considered to be psychoses.

Although these three syndromes may occur in the absence of any other psychopathology, they are also often a feature of another more pervasive psychiatric disorder. According to DSM-III-R, body dysmorphic disorder can be diagnosed as long as anorexia nervosa and transsexualism are absent.

EPIDEMIOLOGY Though rare, the monosymptomatic hypochondriacal syndromes are nonetheless more common than has been appreciated. This is because psychiatrists see only a tiny fraction of the cases, most of whom visit dermatologists, parasitologists, internists, and plastic surgeons (2 percent of the patients coming to plastic surgeons for cosmetic procedures are reported to have body dysmorphic disorder).

The average age of a patient with body dysmorphic disorder is 30. The sex distribution is unclear. In patients with delusions of parasitosis, the average age of onset is 55, and two-thirds are said to be women. In olfactory reference syndrome, in contrast, the patients are more commonly male, and their average age is 25.

ETIOLOGY The etiology of body dysmorphic disorder is unknown. In some patients the belief is due to another more pervasive psychiatric disorder, such as schizophrenia, major mood disorder, or severe personality disorder. Beliefs regarding one's unattractiveness, however, are not often associated with organic mental syndromes. Delusions of parasitosis can be caused by a mood disorder or schizophrenia and can also result from the tactile hallucinosis caused by toxins and other organic brain diseases and from medical diseases and medications that cause pruritis.

Some patients who appear to have olfactory reference syndrome actually turn out to have olfactory hallucinations caused by a mood disorder, schizophrenia, or an organic mental syndrome such as that accompanying temporal lobe epilepsy.

PATHOLOGY By definition, there is no medical illness or deformity to explain these patients' complaints. Patients with delusions of parasitosis frequently have excoriations and skin inflammations produced by their attempts to rid themselves of their imagined infestation.

CLINICAL SIGN AND SYMPTOMS In body dysmorphic disorder, patients imagine some defect in their appearance, most commonly of the face, nose, hair, breasts, or genitals. Frequent complaints include skin blemishes or facial wrinkles or involve the shape of the nose, mouth, or jaw. The patients' anguish is intensified in social situations. These patients are either completely normal looking or may have a slight physical anomaly (such as heavy eyebrows) that is inconsequential. False beliefs in one's ugliness lie along a smooth continuum of intensity from neurotic obsessions through overvalued ideas to frank delusions. At one end of the spectrum, patients merely regard themselves as unattractive, whereas at the other end they feel utterly repulsive and regard their imagined defect with loathing and repugnance.

Secondary symptoms developing in the course of body dysmorphic disorder include depression, insomnia, and severe anxiety. The patients' hypochondriacal beliefs remain tightly circumscribed, and there are no other delusions, ideas of reference, formal thought disorder, or hallucinations. Affect is appropriate. The premorbid personality is reported to be a mixture of obsessional and schizoid traits, and these patients are concerned with achieving perfection in many aspects of themselves. Their lives are profoundly disrupted by their illness. They constantly pursue medical and surgical remedies and undergo many corrective surgical procedures, such as rhinoplasty. At the same time, they tenaciously resist psychiatric referral or psychiatric treatment.

Patients suffering from a delusion of parasitosis falsely believe they have scabies, lice, fleas, or worms. They complain bitterly of itching or tickling sensations in the skin, which they believe are caused by them. Frequently the patients produce bits of fiber, hair, or skin as evidence of their infestation. They totally disregard the physician's reassurance that they are not infected, decline a psychiatric referral, and push on with their quest for a medical remedy. Delusions of parasitosis are sometimes reported to be shared or induced in others, resulting in a *folie à deux*.

Patients with olfactory reference syndrome are convinced that they emit foul odors that offend others. They are most disturbed in social situations, and consequently they withdraw from them. These patients engage in elaborate rituals, such as frequent bathing and changing of clothing and the use of perfumes and deodorants. Like all the monosymptomatic hypochondriacal syndromes, patients with olfactory reference syndrome have no other psychotic signs or symptoms—no loosened associations, personality disorganization, or compromise of reality testing. Their disorder is as circumscribed as it is anguishing and disabling.

DIFFERENTIAL DIAGNOSIS Each of these syndromes can be a feature of another underlying primary psychiatric disorder, most commonly schizophrenia, a mood disorder, or an organic mental syndrome such as temporal lobe epilepsy. Distortions of body image occur in anorexia nervosa, transsexualism, and some specific types of brain damage. Normal adolescents often have a heightened concern about minor defects in their appearance, but this concern is not as grossly excessive as it is in body dysmorphic disorder. According to DSM-III-R, if the imagined defect is of delusional intensity, the diagnosis is delusional disorder, somatic subtype, but this distinction is often very difficult to make. Thus, patients with body dysmorphic disorder can acknowledge that they may be exaggerating their physical defect or that none exists at all.

It may be difficult to distinguish a delusional belief of malodorousness from an olfactory hallucination, but olfactory reference syndrome patients believe their own body to be the origin of the odor and perform counterphobic rituals to conceal it.

PROGNOSIS Monosymptomatic hypochondriasis is a group of chronic and disabling disorders that rarely remit spontaneously. Suicide is said to occur in some cases. The onset of body dysmorphic disorder is insidious, with the concern about one's appearance developing gradually. Patients often brood about their defect for several years before consulting a physician.

MANAGEMENT These patients are difficult to treat, in part, because they are so resistant to psychiatric help of any sort. Psychopharmacological agents are effective, but the patients are usually unwilling to comply. They are evasive, do not believe psychotropics can help, and many refuse treatment outright, despite intense suffering. If another underlying psychiatric disorder is present, that condition should be treated first.

Pimozide (Orap) is effective in suppressing the symptoms of body dysmorphic disorder and may also ameliorate delusions of parasitosis. Most patients retain some concern about their problem, but its intensity is blunted enough to allow them to lead more normal lives. Long-term treatment is necessary, as relapse after discontinuation of medication is common. Pimozide, an antipsychotic agent with potent dopamine-blocking action, has side effects that include sedation, extrapyramidal reactions (particularly parkinsonian-like symptoms), and the potential risk of tardive dyskinesia. There is also concern about possible cardiotoxicity with this drug. Recent scattered case reports suggest that tricyclic antidepressants, monoamine oxidase inhibitors, and various antipsychotics may be effective for some patients with olfactory reference syndrome and body dysmorphic disorder.

UNDIFFERENTIATED SOMATOFORM DISORDER

DSM-III-R contains one new somatoform disorder, termed undifferentiated somatoform disorder (Table 19-6). This diagnosis requires 6 months of one or more physical symptoms without an adequate medical explanation. The symptoms must not occur only in the course of any other major psychiatric disorder or another somatoform disorder. This disorder was created because of the common finding that although cases meeting the full criteria for somatization disorder are relatively rare, there are many cases of chronic multiple functional symptoms that are otherwise similar to somatization disorder, and do not meet the criteria for any other somatoform disorder. There is either a single or several circumscribed symptoms. Anxiety and depressive symptoms frequently accompany them.

There are few empirical data concerning undifferentiated somatoform disorder, but it is thought to be less disabling than somatization disorder, to have a more variable and less chronic course, and to lack any marked gender predominance.

TABLE 19-6
Diagnostic Criteria for Undifferentiated Somatoform Disorder

A. One or more physical complaints (e.g., fatigue, loss of appetite, gastrointestinal or urinary complaints).
B. Either (1) or (2):
   (1) appropriate evaluation uncovers no organic pathology or pathophysiologic mechanism (e.g., a physical disorder or the effects of injury, medication, drugs, or alcohol) to account for the physical complaints
   (2) when there is related organic pathology, the physical complaints or resulting social or occupational impairment is grossly in excess of what would be expected from the physical findings
C. Duration of the disturbance is at least 6 months.
D. Occurrence not exclusively during the course of another somatoform disorder, a sexual dysfunction, a mood disorder, an anxiety disorder, a sleep disorder, or a psychotic disorder.

Table from DSM-III-R *Diagnostic and Statistical Manual of Mental Disorders,* ed 3, revised. Copyright American Psychiatric Association, Washington, DC, 1987. Used with permission.

TABLE 19-7
Diagnostic Criteria for Somatoform Disorder Not Otherwise Specified

Disorders with somatoform symptoms that do not meet the criteria for any specific somatoform disorder or adjustment disorder with physical complaints.

Examples:
(1) an illness involving nonpsychotic hypochondriacal symptoms of less than 6 months' duration
(2) an illness involving non-stress-related physical complaints of less than 6 months' duration

Table from DSM-III-R *Diagnostic and Statistical Manual of Mental Disorders,* ed 3, revised. Copyright American Psychiatric Association, Washington, DC, 1987. Used with permission.

(For somatoform disorder not otherwise specified, please see Table 19-7.)

REFERENCES

Barsky A J, Klerman G L: Overview: Hypochondriasis, bodily complaints, and somatic styles. Amer J Psychiat *140:* 273, 1983.
Barsky A J, Wyshak G, Klerman G L: Hypochondriasis: An evaluation of the DSM-III criteria in medical outpatients. Arch Gen Psychiat *43:* 493, 1986.
Bishop E R: Monosymptomatic hypochondriasis. Psychosomatics *21:* 731, 1980.
Blumer D, Heilbronn M: Chronic pain as a variant of depressive disorder: The pain-prone disorder. J Nerv Ment Dis *170*: 381, 1982.
Cloninger C R: Somatoform and dissociative disorders. In *Medical Basis of Psychiatry,* G Winokur, P Clayton, editors. Saunders, Philadelphia, 1987.
Engel G: Psychogenic pain and the pain-prone patient. Amer J Med *26:* 899, 1959.
Folks D G, Ford C V, Regan W M: Conversion symptoms in a general hospital. Psychosomatics *25:* 285, 1984.
Ford C V: *The Somatizing Disorders. Illness as a Way of Life.* Elsevier Biomedical, New York, 1983.
Guze S B: The validity and significance of the clinical diagnosis of hysteria (Briquet's syndrome). Amer J Psychiat *132:* 138, 1975.
Guze S B, Perley M J: Observations on the natural history of hysteria. Amer J Psychiat *119:* 960, 1963.
Hackett T P, Bouckoms A: The pain patient: Evaluation and treatment. In *Massachusetts General Hospital Handbook of General Hospital Psychiatry,* T P Hackett, N H Cassem, editors, ed 2. Mosby, St. Louis, 1987.
Kellner R: Functional somatic symptoms and hypochondriasis. Arch Gen Psychiat *42:* 821, 1985.
Lazare A: Current concepts in psychiatry: Conversion symptoms. New Eng J Med *305:* 745, 1981.
Lipsitt D R: Medical and psychological characteristics of "crocks." Psychiat Med *1:* 15, 1970.
Smith G R, Monson R A: Patients with multiple unexplained symptoms: Their characteristics, functional health, and health care utilization. Arch Int Med *146:* 69, 1986.
Smith G R, Monson R A, Ray D C: Psychiatric consultation in somatization disorder: A randomized controlled study. New Eng J Med *314:* 1407, 1986.
Sternbach R: *Pain Patients: Traits and Treatment.* Academic Press, New York, 1974.
Stimmel G L, Escobar J I: Antidepressants in chronic pain: A review of efficacy. Pharmacotherapy *6:* 262, 1986.
Torgersen S: Genetics of somatoform disorders. Arch Gen Psychiat *43:* 502, 1986.
Webb W L: Chronic pain. Psychosomatics *24:* 1053, 1983.
Weintraub M I: *Hysterical Conversion Reactions: A Clinical Guide to Diagnosis and Treatment.* Spectrum, New York, 1983.

20 DISSOCIATIVE DISORDERS (HYSTERICAL NEUROSES, DISSOCIATIVE TYPE)

JOHN C. NEMIAH, M.D.

HISTORY AND DEFINITION

The Providence, Rhode Island, *Bulletin* for January 20, 1887, carried the following brief item, headlined "A Missing Preacher":

> This morning Mrs. Bourne, the wife of Rev. Ansel Bourne, called at the police headquarters and reported that her husband had been missing since Monday last. Rev. Mr. Bourne is quite widely known as an evangelist, and during the past twenty-five years he has carried on his religious work in various parts of the United States. For some years, it is said, he has been subject to attacks of a peculiar kind, which rendered him temporarily insensible, and on some occasions he has remained in an unconscious state for many hours. He came originally from the West, and after these attacks he sometimes expressed an intention of returning to his native state, and some of his friends think he may have started for the West. Rev. Mr. Bourne was 60 years of age, and had gray hair and a long gray beard. He was dressed in dark-coloured clothes, wore a brown and blue neck-scarf and Derby hat. He was in Providence on Monday, but he did not return to his home, and he has not been heard from since.

This snippet from a provincial journal would hardly have immortalized the Rev. Ansel Bourne, and he would have been forgotten long ago had it not been for William James, who studied him at length after Bourne's return home and recorded his clinical history in *The Principles of Psychology:*

> On January 17, 1887, he drew 551 dollars from a bank in Providence with which to pay for a certain lot of land in Greene, paid certain bills, and got into a Pawtucket horsecar. This is the last incident which he remembers. He did not return home that day, and nothing was heard of him for two months. . . . On the morning of March 14th, however, at Norristown, Pennsylvania, a man calling himself A. J. Brown, who had rented a small shop six weeks previously, stocked it with stationery, confectionery, fruit and small articles, and carried on his quiet trade without seeming to any one unnatural or eccentric, woke up in a fright and called in the people of the house to tell him where he was. He said that his name was Ansel Bourne, that he was entirely ignorant of Norristown, that he knew nothing of shopkeeping, and that the last thing he remembered—it seemed only yesterday—was drawing the money from the bank, etc., in Providence. He would not believe that two months had elapsed.

After his return to Providence, Bourne had a complete amnesia for the 2 months of his absence. No information was available about the 2 weeks in which he traveled from his home to Norristown, but his neighbors there described him

> as taciturn, orderly in his habits, and in no way queer. He went to Philadelphia several times; replenished his stock; cooked for himself in the back shop, where he also slept; went regularly to church; and once at a prayer meeting made what was considered by the hearers a good address, in the course of which he related an incident which he had witnessed in his natural state of Bourne.

It was not until 1890 that James had the opportunity to examine the patient. Under hypnosis James was able to revive the lost memories, which were readily recovered in the trance state,

> so much so indeed that it proved quite impossible to make him whilst in the hypnosis remember any of the facts of his normal life. He had heard of Ansel Bourne, but "didn't know as he had ever met the man." When confronted with Mrs. Bourne, he said that he had "never seen the woman before," etc. On the other hand, he told of his peregrinations during the lost fortnight, and gave all sorts of details about the Norristown episode. The whole thing was prosaic enough, and the Brown personality seems to be nothing but a rather shrunken, dejected, and amnesic extract of Mr. Bourne himself. . . . I had hoped by suggestions, etc., to run the two personalities into one, and make the memories continuous but no artifice would avail to accomplish this, and Mr. Bourne's skull to-day still covers two distinct personal selves.

Ansel Bourne was not alone. Indeed, the literature of the final 3 decades of the nineteenth century was full of long, detailed reports of patients with a variety of strange disorders of memory and dramatic changes in personality. Almost every investigator of note had a favorite, and some of those clinical affairs have achieved lasting fame: Azam and Félida X., Weir Mitchell and Mary Reynolds, Pierre Janet and Léonie, William James and Mrs. Piper, Morton Prince and Sally Beauchamp, Théodore Flournoy and Hélène Smith.

Pierre Janet was by far the most indefatigable student of these unusual phenomena. Under Jean Paul Charcot's sponsorship at the Salpêtrière, Janet observed scores of patients who suffered from diverse dissociated mental states. In the hundreds of pages of his *L'Automatisme Psychologique* and *État Mental des Hystériques,* he described and classified the phenomena in a manner that has not been equaled since.

With the dawn of the twentieth century, for reasons that are not entirely clear, there was a sudden loss of interest in the clinical syndromes of dissociation. From that point on, individual patients were rarely reported in the literature, and until recently, the few papers that have been published on the subject have generally been impersonal statistical studies of a large series of cases. Such clinical apathy cannot be blamed on a disappearance of patients suffering from these disorders, for there is no evidence to suggest that the incidence of amnesia and most of its related clinical states have in any way decreased since that time. Indeed, during the past 5 years, a group of clinicians interested in multiple personality disorder have collectively identified several hundred patients with that syndrome, suggesting that it is a far more common disorder than had previously been recognized.

Nineteenth-century observers generally viewed those phenomena as being part of the hysterical syndrome. Janet, for example, in his extensive clinical studies of many hysterical patients, frequently found a conjunction of disorders of memory and consciousness with the major sensorimotor symptoms of *la grande hystérie,* and he attributed both classes of disturbances to the basic mechanism of dissociation. Sigmund Freud, however, although recognizing the phenomenon of amnesia—which he saw as a result of repression—was more interested in the somatic manifestations of hysteria and, particularly, in the theoretical mechanism of conversion, which he invoked to explain the occurrence of hysterical manifestations.

In the early decades of the twentieth century, clinicians were content with that diagnostic arrangement, and official classifications of the neuroses listed the various forms of psychogenic disturbances of memory and consciousness under the larger category of hysteria. However, the first edition of the American Psychiatric Association's *Diagnostic and Statistical Manual of Mental Disorders* (DSM-I), published shortly after World War II, incorporated the distinction between the concepts of dissociation and conversion into the classificatory scheme. The term "conversion reaction" was assigned to the sensorimotor symptoms of the old hysterical neurosis, and amnesia and its related disorders were placed in the separate category of dissociative reaction.

In the second edition of the *Diagnostic and Statistical Manual of Mental Disorders* (DSM-II), the breach was healed, and all the symptoms were reunited under the heading of hysterical neurosis. The distinction between conversion and dissociation remained, however, in the division of hysteria into conversion type and dissociative type.

In the third edition and the revised third edition of the *Diagnostic and Statistical Manual of Mental Disorders*

(DSM-III and DSM-III-R), the two conditions were renamed and separated once again. Hysteria, conversion type, became conversion disorder and was assigned to the general class of somatoform disorders. Hysteria, dissociative type, was expanded into the dissociative disorders, which by themselves constitute a major category of the neurotic disorders.

According to DSM-III-R, the essential feature of dissociative disorders is a disturbance or alteration in the normally integrative functions of identity, memory, or consciousness. The disturbance or alteration may be sudden or gradual, and transient or chronic. If it occurs primarily in identity, the person's customary identity is temporarily forgotten, and a new identity may be assumed or imposed (as in multiple personality disorder), or the customary feeling of one's own reality is lost and is replaced by a feeling of unreality (as in depersonalization disorder). If the disturbance occurs primarily in memory, important personal events cannot be recalled (as in psychogenic amnesia and psychogenic fugue).

Depersonalization disorder has been included in the dissociative disorders because the feeling of one's own reality, an important component of identity, is lost. Some, however, question this inclusion because disturbance in memory is absent.

EPIDEMIOLOGY

As has been mentioned, there is no evidence to suggest a diminution in the incidence of most forms of the dissociative disorders. Until recently, the one exception to that statement appeared to be the category of multiple personality disorder. In a review article published in 1944, for example, only 72 cases were recorded, and if the assertion that "these conditions have become extinct today, at least in Western civilization" could not be considered strictly accurate in the face of clinical reports such as those by Corbey Thigpen and Hervey Cleckley on "Eve" or by Flora Schreiber on "Sybil," the condition appeared to be very rare. However, the modern discovery of hundreds of new cases of the disorder is forcing a reappraisal of its rarity, although there are not as yet sufficient data to permit a reliable determination of its incidence.

ETIOLOGY

Although attempts have been made to define dissociative symptoms in terms of the function of the ascending reticular activating system, thalamocortical projections, and other neurological pathways, the information currently available concerning neurophysiological processes is not sufficiently detailed to provide clinically useful concepts and explanations. Contemporary clinicians must turn to the discipline of psychology to find constructs that will help them understand the conditions they observe in their patients and for which ultimately, it is hoped, the specific underlying brain mechanisms will be discovered.

Two basic phenomena

The psychodynamic theories relevant to dissociative conditions are related to two more widely applicable psychological phenomena: hypnosis and the dynamic unconscious.

Hypnosis It was the Marquis de Puységur who, early in the course of its development, first clearly recognized the central position of somnambulism among the manifestations of Franz Mesmer's magnetism. Mesmer, to be sure, had himself observed somnambulistic phenomena in his own patients, but he was more concerned with defining the nature of the physical magnetic fluid that he thought underlay the somnambulistic manifestations than with the psychological experiences of his mesmerized subjects. Puységur, too, rested his explanations of somnambulistic phenomena on the mechanical operations of physical forces, but he was keenly aware of the importance of psychological factors in the production of magnetic cures. In his writings he repeatedly insisted that patients could not be helped unless the magnetizers firmly believed in their own therapeutic powers and strongly willed their patients' improvement—*croyez et veuillez* were his constantly reiterated watchwords.

Puységur's perceptions paved the way for James Braid's subsequent explicit recognition that suggestion, a psychological event, was the central feature of the phenomena that the mesmerists had observed. Hypnosis, as Braid renamed magnetism, attracted widespread medical interest, and a generation later, numerous clinical investigators further defined its characteristics and therapeutic applications. Through their studies, it became apparent that hypnosis was an excellent experimental tool for producing many of the phenomena that arose spontaneously as the clinical symptoms of hysteria. In particular, amnesias, somnambulistic states, and a variety of localized paralyses, anesthesias, paresthesias, and hallucinations could be induced by hypnotic suggestion and were indistinguishable from those occurring in hysterical patients.

Of special interest was the so-called posthypnotic suggestion, a name applied to the observation that commands given during the hypnotic trance would be carried out by subjects at some given future time after awakening from hypnosis, without their remembering that they had been so instructed. H. M. Bernheim describes such an experiment with Mme. G., "an intelligent, impressionable, but not at all hysterical woman" in whom he

> induced the most complex posthypnotic hallucinations, in which all the senses took part. I made her hear military music in the courtyard of the hospital. The soldiers came upstairs and into the room. She saw a drum-major making *pirouettes* before her bed. A musician came up and spoke to her. He wished to embrace her. She slapped him in the face twice, and called her sister and nurse, who ran up and put the drunken man out. This entire scene, suggested during sleep, developed itself before her, both spectator and actress, as vividly as reality. She had not been able to experience similar hallucinations before. She could not get rid of this one. She looked around and asked the other patients if they had not seen and heard what was going on. She could not distinguish between illusion and reality. When it was all over I said to her, "it was only a vision I gave to you." She understood perfectly that it was a vision, but insisted that it was more than a dream and that it was as vivid as reality.

That brief experiment with posthypnotic suggestion provided a model for many of the features of the naturally occurring hysterical somnambulistic trance. In the experimental situation, an earlier event in the subject's environment (the instructions given under hypnosis) is completely forgotten when the subject is awakened from the artificial trance state (posthypnotic amnesia). At some time later, however, the forgotten memories suddenly return to conscious awareness. They return in a peculiar way, emerging in a form of sensory hallucinations so compelling and vivid that the subject is convinced that they are real and behaves accordingly—just as the memories of hysterical somnambulists return as a hallucinatory tableau to which they react as if it actually existed.

It was not to somnambulism alone, moreover, that posthypnotic suggestion applied a useful model. In fugue states and multiple personalities, it not only was evident that amnesia was present, as shown by the fact that certain clusters of memories were forgotten, but in some patients, it also could be seen that the forgotten memories had a direct effect on conscious awareness. For example, the Rev. Mr. Hanna—who, as described below, alternated between two separate states of consciousness, each with mental contents unknown to the other—had had vivid nocturnal dreams while he was existing in his B state. He could describe details of those dreams, although the images meant nothing to him and seemed foreign to anything in his past experience. His parents, however, when they heard the dreams, recognized their content as matching real past events in their son's life that he was completely unable to recall. In his account of Mr. Hanna's illness, Boris Sidis reports:

> Then he says he finds himself on a white and soft road. "Never saw anything like it." A man stood at his side whom he called, although not knowing why, by the name of Bustler. The father afterward told us that Bustler was the name of a minister, a friend of Mr. Hanna's. He could describe the man fully. He was tall, but not fat; he had a coat rounded in front and of a black color. They came up together to the railroad. Mr. Hanna carried with him a satchel, with a brown strap, held in front of him. (The description was found to be correct.)
>
> Mr. Hanna described another picture, in which he had another companion, whom he called for no reason, Ray W. Schuyler. In his dream he heard that the name of the place was "Morea." (We learned that Schuyler was the name of an old companion of Mr. Hanna's schooldays; that they had been together in Morea, a town in Pennsylvania.)
>
> The father, who was present when the dreams were related by the son, could identify the places spoken of as well as their names and also the persons mentioned. The description of the individuals in the dreams was found to be correct. When the father happened to mention the name "Martinoe," Mr. Hanna at once said, "Oh, yes, that was the name of the place I passed through, but," he exclaimed, "how do you know it?" When the father interposed and described more fully what Mr. Hanna saw, the latter with great wonder and amazement exclaimed, "How can you know all this, it was only a dream!"

Through observations such as these, clinical investigators gradually recognized that not only could blocks of associated memories totally disappear from conscious memory only to return completely at some later time, but also while the memories were in that forgotten state, they could, nonetheless, influence the mental contents of conscious awareness without inducing any recollection of what lay beneath the surface of consciousness. These findings led to the development of the psychological concept of unconscious thought processes.

The unconscious The notion of an unconscious mind long antedated the work of those nineteenth-century clinicians. The germ of the idea is to be found not in the stream of medical history but in the intuitions and reflections of early-nineteenth-century philosophers and poets in England and Germany. It was not until the second half of the century when physicians became aware that psychological forces often played a significant role in the production of their patients' symptoms that they began to adapt the concept of the unconscious to the clinical conditions they were observing.

From the beginning, this use of the term "unconscious" had psychological, rather than physiological, connotations. A patient observed by Romolo Righetti, in a study of amnesia made early in the twentieth century, accentuates the distinction:

> On the morning of the second of December, 1912, Joseph P., an unmarried travelling salesman of about 23 years of age, for personal reasons, fired a pistol shot at his sister-in-law, causing a slight wound in her lumbar region; then suddenly turning the revolver on himself, he fired several shots point blank in the direction of his right auditory canal. As X-rays later confirmed, one bullet penetrated the cranial cavity through the petrous bone, injuring the brain substance of the right temporal pole, and the contiguous portions of the frontal lobe of the same side. As an immediate consequence of the wound, the patient fell face down on the ground with a serious hemorrhage from his right auditory meatus and lost complete consciousness for a period of about an hour. Taken to the hospital, the injured man, during the initial phase of the treatment, deliriously uttered a few words ("that whore"), alluding to the lady at whom he had shot.

For 3 days thereafter, the patient remained in shock and was semistuporous, after which he began rapidly to recover. His mental functioning was tested from that time on at regular intervals and consistently showed a marked, although circumscribed, loss of memory, which was completely blank for a period that extended back to a month before his homicidal-suicidal act and forward in time to 40 days after the event.

Two years and 3 months after the injury, as Righetti reported:

> On the night of the 13th of March, 1915, the patient had a dream in which he found himself in an insane asylum, without being able to discover the reason for his being there. All of a sudden there reappeared in his mind (in the dream) the episode of the 2nd of December, with all its particulars. He awoke with a start, the dream image remained in his consciousness, and from that moment on, the patient retained a clear memory of the passionate scene that had transpired between himself and his sister-in-law up until the instant he lost consciousness as a result of the revolver shot aimed at himself.

Thereafter he recovered all his lost memories of events before and after the injury, except that, as the clinical account concluded, "There persisted a short gap in memory corresponding to the period of posttraumatic confusion."

In this patient's history, there are two different kinds of amnesia. In the one, the memories that are lost pertain to the short period of time immediately after the injury during which the patient was semistuporous. Those memories appear to be irrevocably absent. In the other kind of amnesia, the lost memories refer to events that extended over a period of time many weeks before and after the injury, during which time the patient was observed to be mentally alert and responding normally to his environment. Those memories, although irretrievable for 2 years and 3 months after the shooting, returned at the end of that time with every detail intact. Furthermore, they returned in a sudden and dramatic irruption into the patient's conscious awareness in the form of a vivid dream.

When applied to these two types of amnesia, the word "unconscious" has two different meanings. In the first, it refers to the patient as being unconscious, with the implication that the functioning of the brain is so grossly impaired by the acute effects of the trauma that he or she is totally unable to respond to external stimuli. Furthermore, as a result of the same disturbance in brain function, permanent memory traces of the events in the patient's environment cannot be recorded, and when regaining consciousness, the patient will thereafter have a lasting amnesia for the period of impaired brain function. In that context, the terms "unconscious" and "amnesia" are used to refer to events and processes that have a physiological frame of reference.

In the second type of amnesia, one refers to the memories as being unconscious, with the implication that, although unavailable to consciousness by voluntary recall, they do not lack an underlying neural registration but are accessible to conscious awareness, given the proper circumstances. Here, amnesia and unconscious are used to refer to events and processes that have a psychological frame of reference.

Psychological theories Early clinical investigators used the term "unconscious" in its psychological sense to conceptualize the processes underlying the phenomena of dissociative hysteria. Janet and Freud were the two major contributors to the theories that explained those processes. Both men considered the appearance of amnesia to result from the removal of a cluster of mental associations from consciousness, accompanied by an inability of the persons to recall them voluntarily to their conscious mind. Furthermore, many of the symptoms of hysteria could be viewed as the effect of those absent mental contents on certain operations of the patients' conscious mind and bodily functioning.

It was when they explained how the memory clusters escaped from the mainstream of conscious awareness that Freud and Janet parted company. For Janet, the key concept was the process of *dissociation*. That process was based on the ultimately physiological concept of a constitutional lowering of nervous energies of such magnitude that the forces normally binding brain and mental functions into an integrated whole could no longer keep them together. As a result, certain of those functions escaped central control. When memory was affected by that disintegration, a dissociation of memory clusters followed that placed them beyond the purview of consciousness. The clinical result was amnesia and other related hysterical symptoms.

Freud proposed the concept of *repression,* a psychic force that actively removed mental contents from conscious awareness. With that concept, he introduced the notion of the dynamic unconscious, an area of the mind into which mental contents unacceptable to the individual were pushed from consciousness by the specific psychic force of repression and where they were actively kept in an unconscious state, unavailable to conscious recall. In other words, for Freud, amnesia and the related symptoms were the result of active mental processes, as opposed to Janet's concept of passive mental processes.

Current explanations of dissociative hysteria are based on Freud's dynamic concepts. The repression of mental contents that leads to amnesia and other manifestations of the resulting dissociation is conceived of as a mechanism for protecting the patient from emotional pain that has arisen either from disturbing external circumstances or from anxiety-provoking inner drives and affects.

Disturbing external circumstances Some patients, when faced with a situation that has aroused overwhelming grief, despair, or anxiety, may respond with a total repression of the memories of the disturbing events, accompanied by a disappearance of the painful affect. That process is frequently the cause of the amnesia that develops in soldiers who have been exposed to intolerable battle stress, and it certainly accounts for some of the cases of amnesia found in the general civilian population.

Repression appeared to be a primary factor in the symptoms developed by Barbara M., who was taken to the hospital for an amnesia covering the events of some 7 hours on the day of admission. After entering the psychiatric ward, the patient talked freely about herself and the many experiences she had crowded into her short life. She related that some years before, her parents had separated because of her mother's promiscuity. Initially, the patient lived with her mother, where she witnessed her mother's many brief affairs and was, on several occasions, approached sexually by her mother's male visitors. Eventually, she met a young merchant seaman and became pregnant by him. Although he had promised to marry her, he disappeared several days before the wedding and had never been heard from since. The patient had her child, a boy then 3 years of age, and went to live with her father and two younger brothers, a move that caused a permanent rift with her mother.

For reasons that were not entirely clear, there had been mounting tension at home during the 3 to 4 weeks before her admission to the hospital. In particular, the patient felt that her father had been growing increasingly irritable and critical of her, and as she reported, for the week or 2 immediately past, every day had been a running battle between them in which he would yell and scream at her, accusing her of being lazy, a liar, and no good. In the course of that tension, she developed a number of symptoms, prominent among them being generalized headaches, fatigue, insomnia, increasing anxiety, and a sense of loneliness and depression. It was during that time that she met Frank, a young man slightly older than she, to whom she rapidly developed a deep attachment. In the 2 weeks she had known him, she had seen him nightly and had found him a source of comfort and peace in the face of her difficulties at home.

Barbara rapidly adjusted to the ward and began to feel better. Despite attempts to dispel the amnesia, she remained totally unable to recall the events that had occurred between noon and 7:00 P.M. on the day of admission. When asked to recount what had happened during the day, she could and would invariably describe in detail her activities around the house that morning until the point at which she boarded a bus shortly before noon to make a visit to her local doctor, whom she had decided to consult for her symptoms. Her amnesia started at that point, for, as she insisted, "I don't remember nothing after that."

It was particularly interesting to note her strikingly bland and unconcerned attitude toward the serious gap in her memory. When asked about the memory loss, she denied repeatedly that it seemed at all unusual to her or worried her. She would say only that whenever she thought about the period covered by the memory loss, she would have a vivid, almost hallucinatory image—"a dream," she called it—of a parking lot, although she could attach no significance to it and did not recognize it as in any way connected with herself.

Thinking that the image might be related to her experiences during the time for which she was amnesic and hoping that, in association, she might revive her lost memories, her doctor asked her to describe the image in detail. She replied:

> The dream is about a parking lot, and it is full—nothing but cars. You have to weave in and out of the cars, it is so full. And there's a man, way, way over toward the other end of the parking lot. I don't know who it could be, but there's a girl running toward him. Now I keep saying it's me. I don't know why, but it keeps looking like me. She has a pocketbook in her hand, and she runs across the parking lot, and it seems like—I mean, every time I've seen that dream, it's the same picture. The girl doesn't seem to move. She's running as fast as she can, but yet she doesn't seem to be going farther into the parking lot. It seems like it's me that's running, but what I'm running for, I don't know. And what was it?—Yes, it was the other day I was thinking that it reminded me it was me running to somebody for help. What the help was for, even if it was me, I don't know what she is running for. And that day all I could think of was she running for help. What the help was for, I don't know. That man seems to be the man I was running to—I was running to him for help. What kind of help or anything else, I don't know.
>
> *D:* Tell me right this moment what comes to your mind when you think of running for help.
>
> *P:* A doctor. About 4 days before this happened [the amnesia], I was thinking about going to a psychiatrist. I mentioned it to Frank. At that time he was working part-time over at Winthrop.

There were several significant features in that interchange between the patient and the doctor—in particular, the way she personalized the "dream" as she described the details, her direct association to her new friend Frank, and her revelation that he was working at Winthrop, which was where she had been found by the police in her amnesic state. Although the evidence pointed increasingly to the probability that her dream represented a fragment of the events covered by the amnesia, it remained an enigma to the patient. She denied that it had, in reality, any connection with herself, and further attempts to press for her associations to it produced no recollections of the period buried under her loss of memory. Instead, she began to talk more freely about her mounting tension and desperation during the several days before her amnesia began. The situation at home had been going from bad to worse, and what was especially distressing to her was that she found her own anger rising to a point that she was having murderous fantasies about her father, her brothers, and her son. Because of the fantasies and the anxiety associated with them, she had decided to seek medical help, and she was indeed on her way to the doctor the day the amnesia occurred.

Because her waking associations had repeatedly failed to lead to the lost memories, it was finally decided to try to revive the memories under hypnosis. A light trance was induced, and on the assumption that the dream did indeed reproduce reality, the doctor used it as a starting point for the patient's hypnotic associations. She was instructed to visualize the dream's imagery and to recount the events of the day that had led up to the dream. In halting, somewhat telegraphic but clear speech, she began by describing her activities on the morning of the day she became amnesic—activities that she had previously reported while awake.

> I got up. Father was getting ready for work. I started doing the housework and started getting dizzy. I couldn't wait to see the doctor. I put the clothes on the baby. I put on my sweater and coat, took my pocketbook with money, and I went over to the babysitter. She asked me if there was anything wrong. I said, "No, I'll be back in an hour." I walked down to the store and the bus came along. I thought I was going to pass out, and yet I didn't. I am going to the doctor. I got off at my stop all right, and I rang Dr. Palmer's bell. I didn't seem to get any answer. I *had* to see him, so I went to the drugstore and called him by telephone. No answer. I decided to go see Frank—he had helped me, and I could go to him. My father was always hard, and my mother doesn't want to see me. Alice, who is supposed to be my girlfriend, doesn't seem to care—she always finds excuses not to see me. So I had to see Frank. I didn't feel good. I got on the bus again. I had to get over there to Winthrop. I got on a train, and at the first stop I got off. It was after two o'clock, and I knew he was working. I saw his car in the parking lot. There were two entrances, and I saw him walking to his car. I was thinking of walking to it, when Frank came. Then I thought I'd go to the other entrance; he'd ask me to go along with him. He'd know something was wrong—I *had* to see him. I was scared. He didn't even see me. I started across the street again, and a car almost hit me. I started getting dizzy. I wanted to get help. I saw the police sign, and I went in. The nurse brought me in a room, where I saw another policeman, and I saw another. They stared at me and started laughing at me.

Here the patient, who had been speaking with appropriate feeling all along, became suddenly restless and acutely anxious, turned away from the doctor, and became momentarily incoherent. After a short while, she grew calmer and continued:

> My father has always laughed at me—he's always howling at me as if I was 2 years old. Frank is nice. He's the only one I can talk to. Nobody else seems to care. I felt disappointed—I should have gone to the nearest entrance. I felt mad, just mad, and I just gave up.

After she awoke from the hypnosis, the patient remembered all that had occurred during it. The amnesia had been removed, and in subsequent therapeutic sessions, she was able, without the aid of hypnosis, to recollect and talk about all the events that had previously been forgotten, as well as to express the feelings associated with them. As the pieces of her history were fitted together, it was possible to understand what had happened. Despite having lived a difficult life for a number of years, the patient had, nonetheless, been able to manage fairly successfully and had been asymptomatic until the recent period of mounting family strife and turmoil. As she became increasingly depressed in that situation, she began more and more desperately to feel the need of the help and support that were not forthcoming from her family. Finally, on the day the amnesia occurred, she took active steps to obtain assistance, only to find it denied her. First, her doctor was not available, and then she had to watch helplessly as Frank disappeared before she could reach him. That was the climax of her troubles. The loss of the person she really counted on to help her was more than she could bear. At that point, the mechanism of repression took over. By removing the memories of the events back to and including the doctor's absence, along with the associated affects, repression protected her from experiencing the painful feelings of helplessness and despair aroused by the entire episode. The repression was a successful defense, but the patient paid a price for the emotional relief it gave her: She developed amnesia, a clinical illness that was the surface manifestation of the operation of underlying pathological mental mechanisms and that resulted in her hospitalization.

Yet another feature of her clinical disorder should be noted. As it turned out, the surmise that her "dream" was connected with the events hidden by her amnesia was borne out by her subsequent recollections. The fragmentary image of the parking lot represented a "return of the repressed"; that is, it was a small piece of the submerged mental contents that had escaped the repression and had returned to her conscious awareness, but it returned in such a way that it was ego-alien and had no meaning to her. It should be noted that the phenomenon thus described in terms of dynamic mental process can also be viewed clinically as a symptom of her illness. From a clinical point of view, the stereotyped image of the parking lot that she repeatedly saw was a visual hallucination and, as such, formed a characteristic manifestation of her hysterical disorder.

Finally, another aspect of her illness should be mentioned. Once the amnesia had been established, it enabled her to get the help that had been denied her. Now that she had developed such an obvious and dramatic sickness, she was taken to a hospital, where she was the center of attention from doctors, nurses, family, and friends. Furthermore, by being in the hospital, she was removed from the troubling turmoil at home. The secondary gains accruing to her symptoms provided an added reason for maintaining them apart from their primary function of relieving her of mental pain.

In Barbara M., that secondary function did not seriously interfere with the therapeutic attempts to remove her symptoms, but in some patients, the secondary gains may create a major obstacle to treatment. For example, in soldiers, the fact that a dissociative disorder prevents them from being returned to the terrors and dangers of combat may ultimately play a more important role in sustaining their symptoms than does the initial relief the disorder provided them from the painful affect of the precipitating traumatic event.

Internal psychological conflicts Most of the patients with amnesia who are seen in modern-day hospitals have, like Barbara M., developed their symptoms in response to a difficult life situation. Furthermore, as pointed out earlier, the majority of patients manifesting somnambulism are found to be reenacting a traumatic event that actually occurred at some time in their past. In patients with multiple personalities, however, and in those with fugue states, although traumatic events may play an important etiological role, one may also find a drive that is usually repressed or patterns of behavior that are normally under control emerging into open expression in a dissociative state. For example, in many patients exhibiting multiple personalities, it is found that the primary personality—the one that has characterized patients during the greater part of their lives—is somewhat emotionally constricted, restrained, moralistic, and proper. One or more of the secondary personalities, however, will exhibit quite different attitudes and behavior patterns. When the secondary personality is manifested, the patient will indulge freely in all kinds of drive-gratifying activities; may be loud, boisterous, and prankish; and is generally expansive, uninhibited, and outgoing. In such cases, the primary personality remains unaware of the existence of the secondary personality, whereas the secondary personality is usually fully aware of all the thoughts and activities of the first, often being quite scornful of the priggishness of the "better half."

Martha B., a 35-year-old married woman, was admitted to the hospital because she had been unable to walk for 6 months. Three years earlier, she had joined an evangelical religious sect and had given up smoking, drinking, and spending an occasional evening in a nightclub—"partying and dancing"—because, as she said, "The Lord didn't like those things." She then turned to a life of altruistic practical nursing of the sick and aged members of her parish. Her life was uneventful until 6 months before admission when she was involved in a minor automobile accident. She claimed that she had hurt her back in the accident, although examination at the time had disclosed no significant physical injury. It was after the accident that she was unable to walk, and she remained essentially bedridden until she entered the hospital.

On examination, she was found to have normal movements in her legs and to be able to stand unsupported, although she could not take a step. Her reflexes were equal and active with normal extensor plantars. All modalities of sensation, however, were absent bilaterally from her hips down; that finding appeared consistent with her statement "My legs—there's no legs there. I don't know whether I have legs. I have to keep looking to see that they're there. There's no feelings, you know." It should be noted, furthermore, that her bowel and bladder functions were not impaired by the accident and continued to be normal.

In addition to those somatic disturbances, the patient complained of hearing a voice. "It's a terrible voice," she said. "It's a voice I would like to get rid of, you know. It makes you say things you don't want to do. It's not really you. It makes you say things, you know, you wouldn't usually say. Like, you know, I got mad at the doctor the other day, and that wasn't me. I try to cooperate with my doctors because, you know, they know what they're doing." Furthermore, she reported, "At the time the voice is telling me what to say, and if I don't say it, it, like, overcrowds me—it overshadows me. It's another part of me that takes complete control of me."

On the basis of the patient's history and the nature of the physical findings, it was concluded that her motor disorder and her auditory hallucination were conversion symptoms. Further examination revealed other interesting phenomena as well. At one point in the interview, as the patient was describing the intrusiveness of the voice, the doctor suggested, "Why don't you let it take control of you now?" The patient's response was immediate and dramatic. She closed her eyes, threw back her head, flexed her arms, and for 30 seconds, rocked her upper body back and forth, apparently out of contact with her environment. Suddenly she opened her eyes, looked around with a slight smile, and, with a brightness and alertness in her manner and tone of voice that had previously been absent, she commented, "We've got rid of that other one, the one that stays sick all the time."

The clinical impression that another personality had now emerged was confirmed when the patient said that her name was "Harriet." She reported, furthermore, that she felt good and experienced none of the aches and pains that characterized Martha's clinical state. Particularly striking was the fact that Harriet not only had completely intact motor and sensory functioning but, when asked to do so, stood up and walked easily around the room. Even more remarkable was Harriet's scornful commentary on Martha's way of life. Although Harriet liked "partying," she said that Martha had given up such activities because "she's religious. All she does is go to church, come home, go to church, come home, go to church. She don't do nothing else. She says she loves the Lord and that the Lord is part of her. She's not supposed to do those things no more, and I get very angry with her. I make her miserable—I make her so miserable! I keep bothering her. I keep telling her I'm going to make her say things, I'm going to make her do things. Sometimes I make her stay awake all night long." When asked whether it might be possible for Martha and her to be brought together into one personality, Harriet replied, "No, because we like different things, you know. I like to go out partying and dancing, and she likes to go to church, and I don't."

Shortly thereafter, it was suggested to Harriet that she let Martha return. After a mild protest, Harriet agreed; she then lapsed into a short absence of consciousness rocking and writhing in her chair and repeatedly exclaiming, "No! No!," as if undergoing some internal struggle. On regaining consciousness as Martha, the patient opened her eyes and commented, "Oh, I've been asleep on you." It was then evident that she had a complete amnesia for the period in which Harriet had been in the ascendancy and that, as before, she had no knowledge of the secondary personality she harbored. Furthermore, she once again manifested her conversion symptoms and remarked in a languid voice, "I'm tired and cold and my back's aching." Sick Martha had returned.

From those added observations, it became clear that the patient suffered from the form of dissociative disorder known as multiple personality, manifesting the classical characteristics noted earlier. Of particular interest was the striking difference in attitudes between the two personalities. Whereas Martha was moral, proper, and almost prim in her eschewal of the simple if mildly sinful pleasures of life, Harriet enjoyed them to the full and heaped scorn on Martha for her religiosity and her adherence to puritanical canons of behavior. Harriet, furthermore, could be angry and aggressive, in contrast with Martha's wish to be agreeable, kind, and cooperative. It was as if there were a cleavage line determined by Martha's superego that relegated the bad things to Harriet and the good to Martha. Moreover, in the psychological conflict over the forbidden impulses, the impulses were repressed (dissociated) to form the nucleus of a well-organized secondary personality, of which the primary personality was totally unconscious. Repression effectively protected the patient from her forbidden impulses, but at the cost of a major fracture in her psychological structure and functioning.

The role of dissociation in symptom formation Dissociation appears to be a fundamental mechanism underlying both conversion and dissociative hysteria. Whether the symptom is a loss of sensation and function in a limb—conversion disorder—or a loss of memory—dissociative disorder—the mental process common to both is the removal from conscious awareness and control of a complex of associated mental elements, such as thoughts, images, feelings, sensations, and drives. The clinical difference between conversion and dissociative symptoms is only superficial and is determined by the nature of the mental elements that have been dissociated. It is not surprising, therefore, that one often finds both conversion and dissociative symptoms in the same patient, as was evident in the previously described case of Martha and Harriet.

Mention has already been made of the close connection between hypnosis and dissociation. Indeed, hypnotic phenomena are merely dissociative phenomena elicited by the commands of the hypnotist; these phenomena are capable of reproducing all the naturally occurring symptoms of conversion and dissociative disorders. As measured by hypnotizability scales, most people are either only moderately hypnotizable or not hypnotizable at all. In contrast, patients with conversion and dissociative hysteria measure at the highest end of hypnotizability scales. Hysterical patients, in other words, have an exaggerated, perhaps inborn, tendency toward mental dissociation that provides them with a ready-made mechanism of defense for dealing with emotionally painful events. That diathesis for dissociation is a significant factor in determining that the outcome of psychological conflict will be a hysterical neurosis, rather than some other form of neurotic disorder resulting from the operation of other psychological defense mechanisms.

The diagnostic implications of dissociation As noted earlier, DSM-I made a sharp clinical distinction between conversion reaction and dissociative reaction and treated the two syndromes as separate, if not totally unrelated, entities. It was a virtue of DSM-II that the breach between these two categories was narrowed by including them both under the more inclusive term "hysteria." If the retention of the term "conversion" in the subcategory of hysteria, conversion type, perhaps made an unnecessary distinction between conversion and dissociation, at least the way was opened to a fresh consideration of the close relation of conversion and dissociative phenomena and to a renewed study of the all-but-forgotten mechanism of dissociation, which provides a basis for understanding the genesis of both categories of symptoms.

In DSM-III and DSM-III-R, the reversal of this earlier healthy reconciliation once again divorced dissociative and conversion hysteria and placed each in a totally separate and unrelated diagnostic category. The motivation behind the DSM-III classification is understandable and is based on a valid concern. Over the centuries, hysteria has been wanton in the partners it has taken into its bed, and the term in modern psychiatric parlance has so many referents that it verges on the useless as a diagnostic category: A mélange of somatic symptoms, a variety of alterations of consciousness, a diversity of character traits, a specific psychodynamic mechanism (conversion), phobic disorders (anxiety hysteria)—all huddle promiscuously together under the covers and are commonly referred to, singly or collectively, as hysteria.

It is a valuable feature of DSM-III (and its revision) that it attempts to bring order out of chaos by separating the protean symptoms labeled hysterical into what seem to be naturally related clusters or syndromes. In so doing, it properly focuses attention on the tendency of many patients toward somatization, a process that has been inadequately studied and remains poorly understood.

In its zeal for empiricism, however, the classification in DSM-III and DSM-III-R has perhaps overshot the mark by separating conversion disorder from dissociative disorders and by overlooking the central and common role that the mechanism of dissociation plays in both clinical disorders. In conformity with the classification of DSM-III and DSM-III-R, dissociative disorder is discussed here as a distinct and autonomous clinical entity, but the reader would do well to consider it in close conjunction with the description of conversion disorder, even though each has been relegated to a separate, apparently unrelated diagnostic category.

CLINICAL SIGNS AND SYMPTOMS Characteristically, the various forms of dissociative disorders begin and end abruptly. Patients slip rapidly into a somnambulistic state or are themselves suddenly aware that they have lost their memory for a period of time in their immediate past. Or, again, they may "wake up" to find themselves in a strange place with no knowledge of how they got there or what they have been doing in the time that has elapsed from the last thing they can remember—a phenomenon they often refer to as "losing time."

Although many episodes apparently occur spontaneously, there may be a definite history of a preceding emotional trauma or a situation charged with painful emotions and psychological conflict. At times, amnesia follows a physical head trauma. That trauma may have been so slight as to lead one to doubt its physiological significance, or it may have been severe enough to have caused unconsciousness, in which case it is often very difficult to untangle the element of postconcussional amnesia from the hysterical component. In susceptible individuals, treatment with electroshock may lead to hysterical amnesia.

> A 37-year-old woman received a course of 20 electroconvulsive therapy (ECT) treatments for a depressive disorder and thereafter developed a severe, total amnesia that covered not only the period of ECT but also the events of several weeks preceding the commencement of treatments. But under hypnosis, she recalled in minute detail many of the events that had occurred during her hospitalization and course of treatments, strongly suggesting that much of her memory loss was psychogenic in nature.

On occasion, hypnosis may precipitate a self-limited but sometimes prolonged somnambulistic episode in hypnotic subjects from which they cannot readily be aroused. Finally, intense concentration tends to induce somnambulistic states in some individuals. Of particular interest in this regard is the practice of crystal gazing, which was extensively studied during the heyday of interest in dissociative phenomena. By staring intently at a *point de repère,* usually an imperfection in the glass of the crystal ball, subjects develop altered states of consciousness, during which they see vivid hallucinatory images in or at the site of the ball.

The manifestations of dissociative disorders are varied, often complex, and frequently difficult to distinguish sharply from one another. One characteristic links them together in a common family: In each manifestation, a cluster of recent, related mental events—memories, feeling, fantasies—is beyond the patient's power of conscious recall but remains capable under certain circumstances of returning to conscious awareness; that is, the mental events are unconscious in the psychodynamic sense of the term. At least three factors, however, determine the separate natures of the various forms of dissociative disorders and stamp them with the characteristics that permit their differentiation into clinical types: (1) the state of consciousness during an episode of hysterical dissociation, (2) the pattern of amnesia, and (3) the quality of changes in personality and behavior that may accompany the episode.

Somnambulism It is characteristic of somnambulism that patients exhibit an altered state of conscious awareness of their surroundings and often have vivid hallucinatory recollections of an emotionally traumatic event in their past of which they may have no memory during their usual waking state. Somnambulistic episodes are accompanied by an altered state of conscious awareness that is usually easy for an observer to detect but is difficult to describe. The patients are out of contact with their environment, appear preoccupied with a private world, and, if their eyes are open, are seen to be staring into space. They may appear emotionally upset, speak excitedly in words and sentences that are frequently hard to understand, or engage in a pattern of seemingly meaningful activities that is repeated every time an episode occurs. It can often be determined that their behavior represents the external manifestations of the inner, hallucinatory reexperiencing of a traumatic event, the memories of which are normally repressed. There is amnesia for the somnambulistic episode once it is terminated.

Janet recorded his observation of a number of patients with this form of hysteria. For example, in *The Major Symptoms of Hysteria,* he describes the following:

> A young woman, twenty-nine years old, called Gib., intelligent, sensitive, hears one day abruptly some disastrous news. Her niece, who lives next door, has just died in dreadful circumstances. She rushes out, and comes, unhappily, in time to see the body of the young girl lying in the street. She had thrown herself out of the window in a fit of delirium. Gib., although very much moved, remains to all appearance calm, helping to make everything ready for the funeral. She goes to the funeral in a very natural way. But from that time on she grows more and more gloomy, her health fails, and we may notice the beginning of the singular symptoms we are going to speak of. Nearly every day, at night and during the day, she enters into a strange state; she looks as if she were in a dream, she speaks softly with an absent person she calls Pauline (the name of her lately deceased niece), and tells her that she admires her fate, her courage, that her death has been a beautiful one. She rises, goes to the windows and opens them, then shuts them again, tries them one after another, climbs on the window, and if her friends did not stop her, she would, without doubt, throw herself out of the window. She must be stopped, looked after incessantly, till she shakes herself, rubs her eyes and resumes ordinary business as if nothing had happened.

In Janet's patient, all the characteristics of somnambulism are strikingly evident, and it is clear how the memories of the traumatic event, which form the core of her preoccupations during the episode of altered consciousness, are dramatically played out in her behavior.

Psychogenic amnesia Patients suffering from amnesia (Table 20-1) are often brought to general hospital emergency wards by police who have found them wandering confusedly around the streets. Barbara M., examined in detail earlier, was typical of such an admission. The psychiatrist, who first saw her after she arrived at the hospital emergency ward at 7:00 P.M., wrote the following brief note:

> Barbara M., has had a loss of memory since 12 noon today. The patient is brought in by the police, who apparently found her wandering around in the area of Winthrop Beach. She is able to account for her actions today till 12 noon, i.e., she arose late in the morning and took her baby son to a girlfriend's so that she could go to the doctor to get pills for her "kidney trouble." She recalls getting on the Charlestown bus, but nothing more until finding herself on the police stretcher in the ambulance. She claims she lives in Chelsea, but can't remember the address.

Barbara M.'s mental state is representative of one of the several forms that amnesia may take—forms for which Janet's four categories provide a useful classification: localized amnesia, general amnesia, systematized amnesia, and continuous amnesia (Table 20-2).

Localized and general amnesia In localized and general amnesia, as can be observed in Barbara M., patients suddenly become aware that they have a total loss of memory for the events of a period of time covering anything from a few hours (localized form) to a whole lifetime of experience (generalized form). In contrast with Barbara M.'s limited amnesia, which lasted 7 hours, the Rev. Mark Hanna found that after a minor carriage accident, he had totally lost his memory of his entire past life. He appeared on initial examination to be like a helpless infant. He knew no one, not even close family members; had no idea where he was; was unaware of the significance of common, familiar objects; and was completely without language. His mind was, in other words, a veritable tabula rasa.

It is important to recognize that, although amnesia for an immediately past experience is found in both patients with somnambulism and those with localized or general amnesia, the state of consciousness during the period for which they are amnesic differs in character. Somnambulistic patients seem out of touch with their environment and appear as if in a dream. Amnesic patients, on the other hand, usually give no indication to observers that there is anything amiss and seem entirely alert both before and after the amnesia occurs. The only possible exception to that statement is the evidence provided by some patients that there is a mild, transient disturbance of consciousness immediately surrounding the period when the amnesia sets in. Barbara M., for example, described what sounds like a mild clouding of consciousness when she was first seen in the hospital. As she reported later in her hospital stay:

> They asked me what my name was, and they found it in my pocketbook. And they asked me if that was my name three or four different times, and actually I didn't concentrate on it until about the fourth time. I heard them saying it, I remember them saying it, but it didn't dawn on me that that was my name until about the fourth time that they asked me, because I was in a very, very heavy fog. In fact, I couldn't even hear the doctors half the time. I had to keep asking them to repeat what they said, or to speak louder.

It cannot be said with certainty, however, that all patients experience such temporary clouding of consciousness at the point at which the amnesia develops, because the absence of observations on a sufficiently large number of patients precludes such generalizations.

Selective (systematized) and continuous amnesia The other two types of amnesia described by Janet are rarely seen. In the selective (systematized) form, patients lose memory for only specific and related past events (e.g., those concerning the birth of a child), with other memories of simultaneously experienced events being retained in consciousness. Patients with continuous amnesia forget each successive event as it occurs, although they are clearly alert and aware of what is going on around them. Janet writes of Marie, for example, who

> attempted to read a novel, but, as her fellow patients pointed out to me, spent the whole day reading the first page over and over again. When she had reached the bottom of the page, she would pause for a moment, and then regularly start to read the beginning again. Moreover, when I asked her what she had been reading, she was unable to tell me even the title of her novel.

Psychogenic fugue In the story of Ansel Bourne told earlier are found the features typical of fugue (Table 20-3): (1) As the name implies, patients wander, usually far from home and for days at a time. (2) During that period, they completely forget their past lives and associations, but unlike the patients with amnesia, they are unaware that they have forgotten anything. It is only when they suddenly come back to their former selves that they recall the time preceding the onset of the fugue, but now they are amnesic for the period covered by the fugue itself. (3) Unlike those in the somnambulistic state, patients in a fugue do not appear to others to be behaving in any way out of the ordinary, nor do they, like somnambulistic patients, give evidence of acting out any specific memory of a traumatic event. On the con-

TABLE 20-1
Diagnostic Criteria for Psychogenic Amnesia

A. The predominant disturbance is an episode of sudden inability to recall important personal information that is too extensive to be explained by ordinary forgetfulness.
B. The disturbance is not due to multiple personality disorder or to an organic mental disorder (e.g., blackouts during alcohol intoxication).

Table from DSM-III-R *Diagnostic and Statistical Manual of Mental Disorders,* ed 3, revised. Copyright American Psychiatric Association, Washington, DC, 1987. Used with permission.

TABLE 20-2
Clinical Features of Amnesia

Essential Features	*Associated Features*
Temporary disturbance in the ability to recall important personal information already registered and stored in memory without evidence of underlying brain disease.	Conflict over sexual or aggressive drives. Often after physical trauma. Frequent indifference to presence of amnesia.
Sudden onset.	
Amnesia generally of localized or selective (systematized) form. Generalized and continuous amnesia less common.	
Awareness of disturbance of recall.	

Table adapted from DSM-III-R *Diagnostic and Statistical Manual of Mental Disorders,* ed 3, revised. Copyright American Psychiatric Association, Washington, DC, 1987. Used with permission.

TABLE 20-3
Diagnostic Criteria for Psychogenic Fugue

A. The predominant disturbance is sudden, unexpected travel away from home or one's customary place of work, with inability to recall one's past.
B. Assumption of a new identity (partial or complete).
C. The disturbance is not due to multiple personality disorder or to an organic mental disorder (e.g., partial complex seizures in temporal lobe epilepsy).

Table from DSM-III-R *Diagnostic and Statistical Manual of Mental Disorders,* ed 3, revised. Copyright American Psychiatric Association, Washington, DC, 1987. Used with permission.

trary, fugue patients generally lead a quiet, prosaic, and somewhat seclusive existence, work at simple occupations, live modestly, and do nothing to draw to themselves the attention or suspicion of their neighbors and acquaintances (Table 20-4).

Multiple personality Morton Prince's "Sally Beauchamp"—"The Saint, the Devil, the Woman," as he hesitantly christened her—is among the most renowned of multiple personalities. In *The Dissociation of a Personality,* the volume devoted to her biography, Prince summarized the essence of her clinical problem in a brief paragraph that illustrates most of the characteristic features of the multiple personality.

In addition to the real, original or normal self, the self that was born and which she was intended by nature to be, she may be any one of three different persons. I say three different, because although making use of the same body, each, nevertheless, has a distinctly different character; a difference manifested by different trains of thought, by different views, beliefs, ideals, and temperament, and by different acquisitions, tastes, habits, experiences, and memories. Each varies in these respects from the other two, and from the original Miss Beauchamp. Two of these personalities have no knowledge of each other or of the third, excepting such information as may be obtained by inference or second hand, so that in the memory of each of these two there are blanks which correspond to the times when the others are in the flesh. Of a sudden one or the other wakes up to find herself, she knows not where, and ignorant of what she has said or done a moment before. Only one of the three has knowledge of the lives of the others, and this one presents such a bizarre character, so far removed from the others in individuality, that the transformation from one of the other personalities to herself is one of the most striking and dramatic features of the case. The personalities come and go in kaleidoscopic succession, many changes often being made in the course of twenty-four hours. And so it happens that Miss Beauchamp, if I may use the name to designate several distinct people, at one moment says and does and plans and arranges something to which a short time before she most strongly objected, indulges in tastes which a moment before would have been abhorrent to her ideals, and undoes what she had just laboriously planned and arranged.

TABLE 20-4
Clinical Features of Fugue

Essential Features	*Associated Features*
Loss of identity associated with wandering, often with the assumption of a new identity and life pattern.	Heavy alcohol use and conflicts over sexuality, aggression, and money.
No evidence of underlying brain disease.	
Amnesia for events occurring during fugue after its termination.	

Table adapted from DSM-III-R *Diagnostic and Statistical Manual of Mental Disorders,* ed 3, revised. Copyright American Psychiatric Association, Washington, DC, 1987. Used with permission.

The characteristics of the disorder manifested by Sally Beauchamp and others like her may be summarized as follows:

1. At any given time, the patients are dominated by one of two or more distinct personalities, each of which determines the nature of their behavior and attitudes during the period that it is uppermost in consciousness.
2. The transition from one personality to another is sudden and often dramatic.
3. Generally, there is amnesia during each state for the existence of the other personality or personalities and for the events that took place when another personality was in the ascendancy. Often, however, one personality state is not bound by such amnesia and retains complete awareness of the existence, qualities, and activities of the other personalities.
4. Each personality is a fully integrated, highly complex set of associated memories with characteristic attitudes, personal relationships, and behavior patterns.
5. On examination, patients will generally show nothing unusual in their mental status, other than a possible amnesia for periods of time of varying duration, and one is unable to tell from a single, casual encounter that the patients lead other lives at other times. Only prolonged contact that enables one to observe the sudden discontinuities in mental functioning discloses that information (Table 20-5).

The first appearance of the secondary personality or personalities may be spontaneous, as seemed to be the case in the patient "Eve," studied by Thigpen and Cleckley, or it may emerge in relation to what appears to be a precipitant. Sally Beauchamp's multiple personalities made their debut during a hypnotic trance induced by Prince in the course of psychotherapy for her initial complaints of "headaches, insomnia, bodily pains, persistent fatigue, and poor nutrition." In other patients, the change occurs following an emotional shock or physical trauma, in which the initial phase may take the form of a typical episode of amnesia that leads to the development of a secondary personality. (See Table 20-6 for the DSM-III-R criteria for multiple personality disorder.)

TABLE 20-5
Clinical Features of Multiple Personality

Essential Features	*Associated Features*
Patient is dominated by one of two or more distinct personalities at any one time.	Conflicts over impulses.
Each personality has a full or nearly full range of mental functions, often with different, frequently opposite, characteristics.	
Transition from one personality to the other is sudden.	
Amnesic barriers are found between one personality and another.	

Table adapted from DSM-III-R *Diagnostic and Statistical Manual of Mental Disorders,* ed 3, revised. Copyright American Psychiatric Association, Washington, DC, 1987. Used with permission.

TABLE 20-6
Diagnostic Criteria for Multiple Personality Disorder

A. The existence within the person of two or more distinct personalities or personality states (each with its own relatively enduring pattern of perceiving, relating to, and thinking about the environment and self).
B. At least two of these personalities or personality states recurrently take full control of the person's behavior.

Table from DSM-III-R *Diagnostic and Statistical Manual of Mental Disorders,* ed 3, revised. Copyright American Psychiatric Association, Washington, DC, 1987. Used with permission.

The Rev. Mr. Hanna, mentioned earlier, well exemplifies the pattern of change following a physical trauma. After his carriage accident and total amnesia for his entire past life, the patient gradually began to build a new life, with new friends and activities, but remained in complete ignorance of his previous existence. Suddenly one morning, after several months in that phase, he awoke with all the memories of his past life entirely recovered—except that now he was amnesic for the period that had elapsed since his accident. Not long after, he again awoke one morning in an altered condition. He was amnesic for his immediate past and for his life before the accident (his A state), but could recall the period following his accident when he had initially suffered from amnesia (his B state). From that point on, he alternated unpredictably between his A state and his B state, in each one having intermittent patches of amnesia for the memories referable to the other state. He had, in other words, two separate systems of memories of two different integrated personalities. Furthermore, each state had its own personality characteristics. In the A state, he was a rather constrained and proper parson, who allowed himself none of the minor vices, whereas in his B state, he enjoyed an occasional cigar or glass of beer. In other words, what had begun as the clinical disorder of amnesia developed into that form of dissociative hysteria characterized by the existence of multiple personalities.

Finally, mention must be made of the recent discovery of the frequency of a history of child abuse, both sexual and physically assaultive, in patients with multiple personality disorder. Because patients are often loathe to reveal such traumatic events, they must be specifically inquired about; in some series of patients, the incidence of abuse has reached 80 percent. As the history of such trauma unfolds, it often becomes apparent that, as a child, the patient had dealt with the accompanying pain and despair by dissociating during the episodes of abuse, a mechanism of defense that had subsequently been carried into adult life as a means of self-protection against the anxiety and depression associated with the memories of the traumatic episodes.

COURSE AND PROGNOSIS

The natural history of the dissociative disorders has not received sufficient attention from clinical investigators, and the inadequacy of the data precludes definitive statements about either their course or their prognosis. Generally, the outlook for individual episodes of dissociative states, such as amnesias or fugues, is good, particularly if energetic therapeutic measures are applied. It must be remembered, however, that the tendency of individuals to resort to dissociative mechanisms when they are under either instinctual or environmental pressures can be a continuing liability for them over long periods of time.

The condition of multiple personality is probably a more serious phenomenon, involving major disturbances of ego function and of the process of identification. Left to itself, the disorder tends to be a chronic, lifelong condition, although the experience of modern clinicians suggests that some patients may achieve a lasting synthesis of personality structure following prolonged, intensive psychotherapy.

DIFFERENTIAL DIAGNOSIS

Schizophrenia To casual observation, a dissociative trance state frequently resembles catatonic stupor, and it may at times be difficult to distinguish between them, especially if the hysterical patient is negativistic or cannot be communicated with while the dissociative mechanisms are at work. Patients in a somnambulistic episode usually give evidence to indicate that they are reliving a traumatic event, and most dissociative trance states, as contrasted with catatonia, are generally self-limited and of short duration. Furthermore, when contact can be established with the hysterical patient, it is evident that the disorders of thought and affect characteristic of schizophrenia are absent.

The fact that many patients in dissociated states are subject to vivid hallucinations has led clinicians to misdiagnose them as suffering from schizophrenia or psychotic depression. Indeed, the recent apparent increased incidence of multiple personality disorders may actually be the result of more skillful and accurate diagnostic criteria that have enabled clinicians to recognize dissociative disorders in individuals who were formerly labeled psychotic. The presence of hallucinations should alert the clinician to the possibility that the patient has a dissociative disorder, in particular, multiple personality disorder. Careful exploration will reveal that, in contrast with those with more serious psychotic disturbances, patients with multiple personality disorder are able to relate well to the examiner, experience episodes of "losing time" (i.e., periods of amnesia), and are highly hypnotizable as measured by hypnotizability scales, which should be used as an aid to differential diagnosis.

Sleepwalking The term *somnambulism* refers both to the dissociative phenomenon that is a part of the dissociative disorders and to episodes of activity during sleep that have a different character and significance. Very commonly in childhood and less frequently in adulthood, a person may get out of bed during actual sleep and wander around. Such behavior is not necessarily pathological, especially in children, and it differs from hysterical somnambulism in that nondissociative somnambulism (1) occurs during deep sleep unassociated with dreams, (2) is poorly integrated and nonpurposive in nature, and (3) is characterized by actions that are awkward, fumbling, and show a lack of dexterity. Dissociative somnambulistic episodes may occur at night, but they are as different from normal sleepwalking as hypnosis is from true sleep.

Postconcussional amnesia As was noted earlier, dissociative amnesia may be associated with head injury, and in such cases there may be a combination of hysterical and postconcussional amnesia that can be difficult to untangle. In general, the retrograde amnesia following concussion does not extend beyond the period of 1 week. Postconcussional amnesia, furthermore, disappears slowly, and memory is usually not completely restored for the events that occurred during the amnesic period, whereas the recovery from hysterical amnesia is sudden and is accompanied by a total restoration of memory. Righetti's patient, described earlier, exemplifies those distinguishing characteristics. In doubtful cases, hypnosis is sometimes useful as a diagnostic tool. If memories can be retrieved in a hypnotic trance, there is strong evidence that dissociative mechanisms are at least partially responsible for the clinical amnesia.

Temporal lobe epilepsy One of the difficult diagnostic distinctions that the clinician must make is that between hysterical somnambulism and an episode of temporal lobe epilepsy. Epileptic patients, like somnambulistic patients, may follow a highly complex pattern of behavior. In some patients with electroencephalographic (EEG) evidence of temporal lobe dysfunction, their seizural behavior patterns have been shown to refer to a memory of a significant past event in their lives, as is often the case in patients with hysterical somnambulism. In general, when a trance-like episode occurs in conjunction with evidence of other typical hysterical symptoms and stigmata and when it is not accompanied by positive EEG indications of temporal lobe dysfunction, the episode is a form of dissociative hysteria. When, however, there is positive brain-wave evidence of a temporal lobe dysrhythmia, even if the clinical episode has features characteristic of hysterical dissociation, it should be considered as being, at least partially, the result of a gross brain lesion.

The problem of diagnosis is further compounded by recent clinical studies indicating that a number of patients with proven temporal lobe epilepsy develop typical dissociative symptoms in the interictal phases of their seizure disorder. The exact clinical, scientific significance of these findings is still unclear, but it has suggestive implications for future investigations into the possible neurological correlates of dissociative phenomena and, perhaps, ultimately, for their therapeutic management.

TREATMENT In patients with amnesia, as well as in those with the less commonly seen fugue states, it is important to restore the lost memories to consciousness as soon as possible. Otherwise, the mental contents remaining in an unconscious state will likely form a nucleus for the production of a future episode of amnesia or fugue.

By various therapeutic interventions, it is usually possible to recover the lost memories. In some patients, after one or two interviews, one can get at the unconscious mental contents simply by allowing the patients to free associate or by encouraging them to give their associations to a specific fragment of the repressed material that has returned in the form of a conscious image, dream, or hallucination. At other times, more active measures, such as hypnosis or intravenous thiopental (Pentothal), may be required to mobilize the memories. Once the memories are obtained, the suggestion must be made to patients that they will retain them in consciousness after awakening.

If there is a significant degree of secondary gain resulting from the presence of the amnesia itself, it may be very difficult for the therapist to persuade patients to abandon their symptoms. When the amnesia is very firmly fixed, one must consider the possibility that it is protecting the patient from a continuing difficult situation. At times, there may be an element of malingering in the patients' preservation of symptoms, but as is true in all forms of hysterical neurosis, that element is difficult to ascertain. One should be wary of assuming that patients are consciously pretending, unless there is very strong evidence to support that supposition.

The recent revival of interest in multiple personality disorder has led to a renewed enthusiasm for treating such patients with prolonged psychotherapy. Current therapeutic guidelines suggest that the physician should actively explore the various dissociated personalities, should encourage them to become aware of one another across previously amnesic barriers, and should facilitate the catharsis of the traumatic memories (especially those related to child abuse) associated with the different personality manifestations. The course of treatment can often prove difficult and anxiety provoking to patient and doctor alike, especially when aggressive or suicidal personalities are in the ascendancy, and brief periods of hospitalization may be necessary as an interim supportive measure.

In general, the treatment measures aimed at the immediate symptoms of dissociative neurosis should ideally be combined with a therapeutic plan designed to help patients with the basic conflicts that have resulted in symptom formation. In many cases, that is more easily said than done, but for some patients, as noted, more extensive and intensive psychotherapy may be valuable. The type of treatment to be used will depend on the nature of the illness and the circumstances in which it occurs. It is often useful for patients who are responding to severe environmental stress through the use of dissociative mechanisms to provide them with a supportive relationship in combination with environmental manipulation aimed at ameliorating the stressful situation; that therapeutic strategy may also prevent further episodes of dissociation. In those patients in whom the dissociative phenomena arise against a background of intrapsychic conflict, a more radical approach aimed at developing insight may be attempted, combined with attempts to modulate the severity of the patients' superego demands when their excessiveness is an etiological factor. In general, however, despite the current growing interest in individuals suffering from multiple personality disorder, experience in treating dissociative disorders is limited, and the value and effectiveness of prolonged psychotherapy cannot be dogmatically asserted.

DEPERSONALIZATION DISORDER (DEPERSONALIZATION NEUROSIS)

HISTORY AND DEFINITION A 28-year-old civil engineer described his illness as follows:

> I suffer from attacks of dizziness and vertigo. At the peak of their intensity I cannot understand anything I hear or see. Words bang at my ears like a hammer and people seem to be figures in a dream. During the dizzy spells I have no idea where I am, and it takes me over a minute to collect my thoughts. The sensation occurs many times a day and is often brought on by noise. . . .
>
> Sometimes I have difficulty in sleeping, but this is neither severe nor prolonged. I always get to sleep, but I am tormented by nightmares of such vividness that I confuse them with reality for some time after I wake up. I often dream of falling or of violent death. In a nightmare that recurs very often, I am guillotined and put my head back on my shoulders. The terror that accompanies that dream is so great that sometimes I actually think I am going to die.
>
> I attribute my frequent palpitations to these repeated experiences. The least little thing brings on the palpitations, and sometimes it is only necessary for a troublesome thought to cross my mind to make them violent.
>
> At the start of my sickness I suffered from tremendous fatigue; I was constantly exhausted and often fell asleep in the middle of a conversation or of something I was doing. I frequently have involuntary impulses: For example, I will have to walk in a certain specific direction despite myself, or I will have to say incoherent words that have no connection with my thoughts. Sometimes I notice a trembling or shivering followed by a feeling of heat. I rarely have an exact idea of the time; I have to reflect for several minutes before I can recollect the date or the exact time of the day.
>
> I feel sad most of the time and want to cry. I have thoughts of suicide, which at certain moments I am sure I am about to act upon. I have feelings of hatred and anger that are insufficiently motivated. I frequently experience a sensation of strangulation, which lasts several hours at a time, but always goes away at night. . . .
>
> One of the strangest ideas I have, which I am obsessed with and which forces itself on my mind against my will, is that I think I am double. I experience one self that thinks, and another self that acts. At such times I lose the feeling of the reality of the world; I feel that I am plunged into a deep dream, and I don't know if I am the self that thinks or the self that acts. No effort of will has any power against this bizarre state that forces itself on my mind.

Were he alive today, that unfortunate engineer could have recently celebrated the anniversary of the publication of his case history more than a century ago. In 1873, the French clinician Maurice Krishaber presented to the medical world his monograph entitled *De le Névropathie Cérébro-Cardiaque,* a study based on the observation of 38 patients whose histories were summarized in its pages. Most of the patients suffered from a mixture of symptoms of anxiety, fatigue, and depression, from which the author derived the name "cerebro-cardiac neuropathy," which he suggested for the syndrome. Of particular interest was that over one-third of his patients complained of a strange and unpleasant alteration in their perception of themselves or their surroundings. The loss of "the feeling of the reality of the world" described by the patient quoted above was matched by reports of other patients with similar difficulties.

A 43-year-old British Army colonel said: "I felt as if I was almost entirely separated from the world, as if there was some barrier between me and it. . . . [I seem] to be at the bottom of a well, or walled up in a block of ice." A 34-year-old Swiss gardener reported that "it often seems to me that I am not part of the world. My voice sounds strange to me, and when I see my fellow patients, I say to myself, 'These are figures in a dream.' Often, to tell the truth, I don't know if I am dreaming or awake; it seems to me that I am not myself."

Krishaber's monograph apparently made little impact on his medical contemporaries; at least *névropathie cérébro-cardiaque* does not appear to have been accepted into the standard psychiatric nomenclature of the day, nor did the disturbances to which he called attention arouse any significant degree of medical interest.

Krishaber's observations did not, however, go entirely unnoticed. The concern with the nature of reality by psychologists like Théodule Ribot and William James and philosophers like Hippotyte Taine and Laurent Dugas drew them to the problems that many of Krishaber's patients manifested. Dugas, in particular, was struck by Krishaber's observations, for which he suggested the name "depersonalization," and in 1911, with the clinician F. Moutier as coauthor, he published an extensive monograph on the psychological, historical, and clinical aspects of the phenomenon.

The thoroughness of Dugas and Moutier's treatment of the subject seemed to leave little further to be said about the phenomenology of depersonalization. Perhaps because Dugas's papers and his monograph were published mainly in the philosophical literature, his ideas appear to have had little influence on medical or psychiatric thought. It was not until after World War I that psychiatrists began to pay significant attention to the subject. Some focused on the clinical manifestations of depersonalization, pointing out that the alterations in reality perception involved both the observer's self and the objects in the environment and suggested the term "derealization" for altered perceptions of objects in the environment, reserving "depersonalization" for altered perceptions of the self. At the same time, some analysts were attempting to explain the origins of the symptoms and the psychodynamic forces that entered into their production.

Although many of these clincians were aware that depersonalization could appear as an isolated symptom in patients without other psychiatric complaints, they generally considered it a "non-specific syndrome occurring in illnesses of different kinds." It was not until after World War II that the possibility was considered that the phenomena might form a specific syndrome in their own right. More recently, depersonalization syndrome has been assigned a niche of its own in the European psychiatric taxonomy.

TABLE 20-7
Diagnostic Criteria for Depersonalization Disorder

A. Persistent or recurrent experiences of depersonalization as indicated by either (1) or (2):
   (1) an experience of feeling detached from, and as if one is an outside observer of, one's mental processes or body
   (2) an experience of feeling like an automation or as if in a dream
B. During the depersonalization experience, reality testing remains intact.
C. The depersonalization is sufficiently severe and persistent to cause marked distress.
D. The depersonalization experience is the predominant disturbance and is not a symptom of another disorder, such as schizophrenia, panic disorder, or agoraphobia without history of panic disorder but with limited symptom attacks of depersonalization, or temporal lobe epilepsy.

Table from DSM-III-R *Diagnostic and Statistical Manual of Mental Disorders,* ed 3, revised. Copyright American Psychiatric Association, Washington, DC, 1987. Used with permission.

The term "depersonalization neurosis" made its debut in the United States in DSM-II. The manual commented: "This syndrome is dominated by a feeling of unreality and of estrangement from the self, body, or surroundings." In DSM-III, depersonalization was considered as a form of dissociative disorder characterized by "an alteration in the perception or experience of the self, so that the feeling of one's own reality is temporarily lost or changed." It has been retained as a distinct syndrome in DSM-III-R (Table 20-7).

Some clinicians, as mentioned earlier, distinguish between depersonalization and derealization. They apply depersonalization to the feeling that one's body or one's personal self is strange and unreal, and they apply derealization to the experience of perceiving objects in the external world as having the same quality of unreality and estrangement. Strictly speaking, that distinction provides a more accurate description of the phenomena than does placing them together under the category of depersonalization alone. If a single term is to be used, derealization is the more appropriate, because it refers to a characteristic change in the perception of objects that is common to all of them—to self, body, or external world—whereas depersonalization has a more limited scope. In the following discussion, depersonalization disorder is used as the generic label in order to conform to the terminology suggested by DSM-III-R.

Frequently, clinical investigators have included déjà vu and related phenomena in the same category as depersonalization. There is no question that those various kinds of experience are in some way related, because in all of them individuals observe a change in their sense of the reality of what they are perceiving. There is, however, an important difference: In déjà vu what is, in fact, new, alien, and previously unexperienced is felt as being familiar and as having been perceived before. In contrast, in depersonalization what is actually familiar is sensed as strange, novel, and unreal. The one, in other words, is the obverse of the other, and the two phenomena are therefore better considered as distinct entities. In the following discussion, depersonalization is restricted to the more limited definition of the term.

EPIDEMIOLOGY As an occasional isolated experience, depersonalization is a common phenomenon for all of us and, as such, is not necessarily pathological. Studies of its incidence in normal college students indicate that transient depersonalization may occur in as many as 50 percent of a given population, without any significant difference in incidence between men and women. It is a frequent event in children as they develop the capacity for self-awareness, and adults often experience a temporary sense of unreality when they travel to new and strange places. George Eliot, in her novel *Silas Marner,* wrote:

> Even people whose lives have been made various by learning, sometimes find it hard to keep a fast hold on their habitual views of life or their faith in the invisible—nay, on the sense that their past joys and sorrows are a real experience, when they are suddenly transported to a new land, where the beings around them know nothing of their history, and share none of their ideas—where their mother earth shows another lap, and human life has other forms than those on which their souls have been nourished. Minds that have been unhinged from their old faith and love have perhaps sought this Lethean influence of exile, in which the past becomes dreamy because its symbols have all vanished, and the present too is dreamy because it is linked with no memories.

Information about the epidemiology of depersonalization of pathological proportions is more scanty. Depersonalization is apparently rare as a pure syndrome but is frequently found as a symptom in association with anxiety neurosis, depression, and schizophrenia. In the very few studies of depersonalization, it has been found to occur at least twice as often in women as in men and is a disorder of younger people, rarely being found in those over 40 years of age.

ETIOLOGY Even though a number of thoughtful clinical investigators have focused their attention on depersonalization, its etiology remains obscure. Many physiological, psychodynamic, and ego psychological theories have been proposed, but there has been little agreement among their proponents as to the exact mechanisms of depersonalization. Many of the psychological explanations either are restatements in technical language of the clinical phenomena or are hypothetical models so constructed that they do not lend themselves to experimental or clinical validation. One should therefore be wary of uncritically accepting the theoretical formulations that follow.

Physiological theories Earlier investigators favored physiological explanations of the depersonalization phenomena. Krishaber, whose syndrome included many neurotic symptoms other than depersonalization, stressed the importance of a familial neuropathic diathesis. Under the influence of Claude Bernard's then-recent demonstration of the function of the vasomotor nerves, Krishaber proposed that the immediate mechanism underlying the symptoms was a "functional ischemia of the centers" in the relevant areas of the brain, which occurred secondarily to those vascular changes. Among the various disturbances that resulted was a diminution in the faculties of memory and judgment that, in Krishaber's view, underlay the individual's incapacity for recognizing "the reality of objects around him and even of his own identity."

Janet proposed that the basic cause of mental disorders lay in a depletion of nervous energy. He viewed the phenomena of depersonalization and estrangement as being among the first indicators of a pathological disturbance of that energy. In his model of the human psyche, the highest and most complex mental functions included the capacity both for the synthesis of all the normal psychological operations into a unified whole and for the endowing of experience with the quality of reality. The disappearance of a reality sense was one of the earliest effects of the diminution of nervous energy. Sensations and the perception of one's self and the objects in one's environment could still be experienced, but they would appear to the observer to have the tenuous, unsubstantial quality that normally characterizes memory images. Unlike memory images, however, those perceptions were not recognized as having happened before or as having a meaningful connection with one's self and, therefore, seemed to be unfamiliar and strange.

More recent studies have focused on a variety of pharmacological, neurophysiological, and situational factors that may act as the precipitants of the experience of depersonalization. Among the distortions of perception that follow the use of psychotomimetic drugs, such as mescaline and lysergic acid diethylamide (LSD), alterations in the sense of reality may be prominent. Diseases of the central nervous system (CNS) may have the same effect, as seen in the association of depersonalization phenomena with electrical stimulation of the cortex of the temporal lobes. In that regard, two earlier clinical observations are of interest: Janet described a patient whose grand mal seizures were preceded by an aura in which "she is no longer the same, she no longer recognizes herself, she has lost herself." Dugas cited a patient with an ultimately fatal parietal lobe brain tumor whose initial symptoms were an attack of altered perception in which, as he complained, "I am completely impersonal. . . . I see the world as if it were a photograph. . . . I feel myself outside of life." Finally, many researchers have pointed out that persons subjected to sensory deprivation occasionally experience the phenomena of depersonalization.

Psychodynamic explanations From the earliest period of the development of psychoanalytic concepts, the experience of estrangement that is central to depersonalization phenomena has been viewed as a psychological defense. In *The Interpretation of Dreams,* Freud pointed out how dreamers, by recognizing that they were "only dreaming," could relieve themselves of the anxiety associated with their dreams by sensing them as unreal. In his discussion of the Wolf Man's symptom of depersonalization, Freud suggested that the function of depersonalization was to prevent anxiety-provoking wishes to return to the womb from entering consciousness. In a later autobiographical paper, Freud explained his own sudden questioning of the reality of the Acropolis, when he finally visited Athens, as a defense against his guilt-producing rivalry with his father.

Other analytic investigators saw depersonalization and derealization as the result of changes in libidinal cathexes. H. Nunberg stressed the occurrence of such phenomena in the face of sudden object loss, attributing the resulting disturbance in reality sense to the abrupt shifting of libido from the object onto the ego. Paul Schilder likewise viewed the symptoms as following the withdrawal of libido from both self and objects and suggested that unconscious voyeuristic drives accounted for the characteristic increase in self-observation. Otto Fenichel placed more emphasis on the mechanism of countercathexes; in his formulation, it was not so much the withdrawal of libido from both self and objects as the repression of painfully excessive cathexis that led to the phenomena of depersonalization.

More recently, attention has been paid to the role of disturbances in ego identifications. A study of the experiences of women subjected to the brutal horror of German concentration camps noted that depersonalization tended to occur when one part of the individual's ego repudiated a self-image that was colored by primitive, pregenital aggressive drives. Another study pointed to the clash between conflicting ego identifications derived from both parents locked in a hostile marriage; the consequent withdrawal of cathexis from the incompatible self-representation "results in the feeling of estrangement from the self." The majority of recent investigators, furthermore, stress that depersonalization is a primitive, highly pathological defense that is allied to denial and is used as an emergency measure when the more usual mechanism of repression fails to control unacceptable impulses.

Little is known about the psychogenic origins of depersonalization phenomena. One formulation indicated the importance of parental discord during the child's formative years, and another study suggested that difficulties in infants' early relationships with their mothers lead to basic disturbances in the development of perception and cognition. Most investigators cite the need for further observations concerning the origin of the disorder.

Ego structure and depersonalization Although many investigators have been primarily interested in the defensive function of depersonalization, their focus on the disturbances in identification revealed by their patients has pointed to the importance of psychological conflicts within the ego itself. Schilder first called attention to the heightening of the function of self-observation in depersonalization, and numerous investigators since then have been concerned with elucidating the split in the ego between an observing self and an acting self or the split between conflicting identifications.

Paul Federn, one of the pioneers of ego psychology, disagreed with those clinicians who attributed depersonalization and derealization to the repression of libidinal cathexes or their withdrawal from objects and object representations. In support of his objections, he noted that a diminution of libidinal cathexis may lead to a loss of interest in an object but not to its becoming unreal; however, one may still retain interest in those objects that have the quality of unreality. To explain those observations, Federn suggested that the significant locus of libidinal change was the boundaries of the ego. A lowering of the libidinal cathexis of those boundaries, not of objects or object-images, resulted in the perception of those objects taking on the quality of unreality when they impinged on the altered ego boundaries. The derealization of objects was matched by the depersonalization that followed the perception of self at similarly decathected ego boundaries through which self-images passed into conscious awareness. In fact, Federn believed, altered self-perceptions came first, and as his clinical observations revealed, all patients perceived distortions in their body image before they experienced alterations in the reality of the external world. For Federn, in other words, the explanation of depersonalization lay primarily in understanding the pathology of the structure and function of the ego, not in the broader reaches of intersystemic conflicts.

Comments on the theory of depersonalization The various theoretical formulations reviewed here are not necessarily restricted to depersonalization disorder itself but often deal with depersonalization as a symptom that, although it forms the central feature of the syndrome proper, may also be found as a part of other disorders as well. This clinical distinction is particularly true of the physiological considerations. Depersonalization disorder is, by definition, a condition in which no evidence can be found for pathological functioning of the brain, such as that associated with epilepsy, brain tumors, or the use of psychotomimetic drugs, which may be accompanied by the experience of depersonalization. Such gross disturbances in the structure and physiology of the CNS are not therefore viewed as being the cause of the neurotic syndrome. They do, however, point to the possible site of the neuronal structures that immediately underlie the isolated symptom of depersonalization and that consequently may be relevant to the ultimate understanding of the correlative relationships between brain function and psychological events.

Mention has already been made of the inadequacy of the psychological explanations. Those explanations are fragmentary, uncoordinated, and not well integrated with the more completely and solidly elaborated portions of contemporary psychological theory, and they tend to deal with concepts of psychic energy and its distribution that are difficult to validate. Confusion also arises because the various investigators disagree on the definition of depersonalization. Some investigators include within its purview the phenomena of déjà vu and disturbances of identity, which, although possibly related to depersonalization, may require different explanations. Current psychological theories concerning the phenomena, although imaginative and suggestive, must be viewed as being only the first step toward a more complete understanding of the disorder.

CLINICAL SIGNS AND SYMPTOMS Dugas and Moutier, whose monograph is by far the most complete and extensive review of depersonalization, summarized its salient clinical features as follows:

> Consider a person in the ordinary circumstances of life: He receives the sensory impressions of objects, marshals his memories, recalls images, forms and combines ideas, judges, reasons, carries out actions, is affected by pleasure and pain; he is aware of all of these and of their connection with himself. Suppose that the same person experiences identical states, but ceases to have an awareness of them as being his own; he will witness "his life as a performance presented by another" [Fromentin]; he will continue to perceive sensations, colors and forms, touches, smells, etc., but it will seem to him that these sensory impressions do not affect him or reach him any more. He will continue to have memories, but it will appear to him that the past they recall escapes him and is no longer his own. He will still think, reason, act, even be moved by feelings, but it will seem to him that it is not he who thinks, reasons, acts or feels pleasure and pain. Although nothing in his life will be different, yet everything about it will appear changed. He will no longer know himself, will be amazed that he is still alive, and will be outside of his experiences.

Alterations in reality perception As the passage just quoted suggests, the central characteristic of depersonalization is the quality of unreality and estrangement that is attached to conscious experience. Inner mental processes and external events seemingly go on exactly as before; yet everything is different and seems no longer to have any personal relation or meaning to the person who is aware of them. The feeling of unreality affects individuals' perceptions of their physical and psychological selves and of the world around them (Table 20-8).

Perception of self Parts of one's body or one's entire physical being may appear foreign. One of Dugas's correspondents, who experienced an attack of depersonalization while riding one night in a train, exclaimed:

> I look at my hands which are writing this! How odd it is! Are they really concerned with what they are doing? I look at my reflection in the window, and find myself to be strange, novel. For a moment I was almost afraid of the image the window pane returned to me, of this phantom of myself.

In the same way, all the mental operations and behavior of individuals may feel alien to them. Said another of Dugas's subjects:

TABLE 20-8
Clinical Features of Depersonalization Disorder

Essential Features	*Associated Features*
Alteration of the perception or experience of the self, with loss of sense of one's own reality and associated changes in body image.	Dizziness, anxiety, hypochondriasis, fears of going insane, disturbance in sense of time.
Rapid onset and disappearance.	Derealization—loss of feeling of reality of world—and perceived changes in size and shape of external objects.
Feeling of loss of control of one's action and speech.	
Episodes lasting for many minutes to hours and recurring frequently.	

Table adapted from DSM-III-R *Diagnostic and Statistical Manual of Mental Disorders,* ed 3, revised. Copyright American Psychiatric Association, Washington, DC, 1987. Used with permission.

Is this really I, who am at this moment receiving visitors in my drawing-room, speaking commonplace words, asking people about their health, laughing with them, while my real self follows another train of thought and is entirely under sway of a tremendous change that has taken over my life? Yes, without doubt, I see myself, hear myself and yet I witness what I am doing as if it involves someone else. I no longer recognize myself. I have the impression of strangeness and of the unknown in the face of the actual reality.

A common and particularly troublesome manifestation is a loss of the capacity to experience emotions, even though the patient may appear to express them. Dugas cited the observation made about a woman who, separated by hospitalization from her family,

complained of being unable to feel any emotion. "I wish," said she, "that I had some sorrow for my husband and my son . . . (she cries). You see, Sir, I am crying but it does not touch me; I feel nothing."

Her husband came to visit her in the hospital. She was told to kiss him and did so. "That, Sir, affects me as much as if I were to kiss this table."

Perception of the external world Similar feelings of unreality and strangeness may invade patients' perceptions of the objects and people in the world around them. One of Janet's patients said:

Things don't look the way they used to. Everything I see, even the decorations on the wall of my room, seem strange to me. . . . It's as if I were seeing everything for the first time. . . . Everything appears unreal to me. . . . When I go out, it seems to me that the street is not the same. . . . It's like a city I haven't seen for a long time. Suddenly everything around me gives me the effect of having become odd. . . . It's as though reality were deformed.

Other symptoms Krishaber was the first to call attention to the frequency with which dizziness appeared as a symptom in his series of patients, and more recently Schilder and others commented on the same association. Anxiety is commonly found as an accompaniment of depersonalization, and many patients complain of distortion in their sense of time and space. Especially common is the experience of a change in patients' bodies: In addition to their general sense of estrangement from their bodily selves, they may feel that their extremities are bigger or smaller than usual. An occasional and particularly curious phenomenon is that of doubling: Patients feel that their point of conscious "I-ness" is outside their bodies, commonly a few feet overhead, from where they actually observe themselves as if they were a totally other person.

Painfulness of depersonalization The experience of depersonalization is often accompanied by considerable secondary anxiety, and frequently, patients fear that their symptoms are a sign that they are "going insane." It is a curious paradox that, even though patients complain of being emotionally dead and estranged, they are capable of being emotionally upset by that very sense of loss. Indeed, all the manifestations of depersonalization are acutely unpleasant; they not only motivate the patients to seek medical help but also often drive them to vigorous activity or to inducing intense sensations in themselves in order to break through the prison walls of their sense of unreality. One of Krishaber's patients said:

I seemed to be dreaming and no longer to be the same person. The sensation of being in a dream was the most painful part for me. I would touch things around me hundreds of times, or would speak in a very loud voice in order to restore the reality of the external world and my own identity, but then my illusions became even more marked. The sound of my voice was absolutely insupportable and touching things did nothing to restore my impressions to normal.

Preservation of insight On July 8, 1880, Henri-Frédéric Amiel, the sensitive Swiss author, teacher, and diarist, wrote in his *Journal Intime*:

Since the age of sixteen onwards I have been able to look at things with the eyes of a blind man recently operated upon—that is to say, I have been able to suppress in myself the results of the long education of sight, and to abolish distances; and now I find myself regarding existence as though from beyond the tomb, from another world; all is strange to me; I am, as it were, outside my own body and individuality; I am *depersonalized,* detached, cut adrift.—Is this madness? No. Madness means the impossibility of recovering one's normal balance after the mind thus played truant among alien forms of being, and followed Dante to invisible worlds. Madness means incapacity for self-judgment and self-control.

Amiel, as Dugas pointed out, made numerous references in his *Journal Intime* to states of estrangement such as that, from which it is clear that he frequently experienced attacks of depersonalization. What is of particular interest in the journal entry quoted here is Amiel's awareness that his capacity for insight into his condition was maintained throughout all the alterations of his perceptions of himself and the world. He also recognized that no matter how bizarre his experiences were, the preservation of insight kept them clearly out of the realm of madness.

Amiel's perceptive introspection revealed to him a clinical truth about depersonalization that remains a central element of the modern concept of the disorder: Patients have a keen and unfailing awareness of the disturbances in their sense of reality. Indeed, as Schilder commented, there appears in depersonalization to be a heightening of the psychic energy invested in the self-observing ego, the mental function on which rests the capacity for insight.

COURSE AND PROGNOSIS In the majority of patients, the symptoms first appear suddenly; only a few patients report a more gradual onset. The disorder starts most commonly between the ages of 15 and 30, but it has been seen in patients as young as 10; it begins less frequently after age 30 and almost never in the later decades of life. A few follow-up studies indicate that, in more than half the cases, depersonalization tends to be a long-lasting, chronic condition. In many patients, the symptoms run a steady course without significant fluctuation of intensity, but the symptoms may occur in a series of attacks interspersed with symptom-free intervals. Little is known about precipitating factors, although the disorder has been observed to begin during a period of relaxation that follows a time of fatiguing psychological stress. Depersonalization disorder is sometimes ushered in by an attack of acute anxiety that is frequently accompanied by hyperventilation.

DIAGNOSIS **Psychiatric examination** There is little remarkable about the appearance of patients suffering from depersonalization. Although they may complain about feelings of estrangement and absence of emotions, to the observer, the patients show genuine concern about their symptoms and may at times manifest considerable anxiety. They remain in contact with the examiner and give no evidence of a major disturbance in affect or of disorganized thought processes. The mental status examination, therefore, reveals little of specific value for establishing the diagnosis.

Differential diagnosis It is evident that depersonalization may occur as a symptom in numerous other psychiatric syndromes. Indeed, as has been pointed out, some clinicians, such as Janet, Nunberg, and Schilder, consider depersonalization an integral part of all psychological illness. Struck by the frequent association of agoraphobia and depersonalization, Martin Roth suggested the inclusion of a new category—phobic anxiety, depersonalization syndrome—in the psychiatric nomenclature. The common occurrence of depersonalization in patients with depression and schizophrenia should alert the clinician to the possibility that the patient who initially complains of feelings of unreality and estrangement is actually suffering from those more common disorders. A carefully taken history and the mental status examination should, in most cases, disclose the characteristic features of these two illnesses. A disturbance of identity as a prominent element in the experience of depersonalization also is a strong indicator of schizophrenia. Because of the frequency with which psychotomimetic drugs induce often long-lasting changes in the experience of the reality of one's self and one's environment, it is important to inquire about the use of those substances. The presence of these other clinical phenomena in patients complaining of unreality should usually take precedence in determining the diagnosis, and, in general, the label "depersonalization disorder" should be reserved for those conditions in which depersonalization constitutes the predominating symptom.

The fact that depersonalization phenomena may result from gross disturbances in brain function underlines the necessity for careful neurological evaluation, especially when the depersonalization is not accompanied by other more common and obvious psychiatric symptoms. In particular, the possibility of brain tumor and epilepsy should be considered, and the diagnostic studies relevant to epilepsy should be aimed at determining whether the seizures are idiopathic in nature or the result of a localized alteration of neuronal structures in the temporal area. Because the experience of depersonalization secondary to brain tumor may be an early presenting symptom before there is other detectable evidence of neoplasm, patients complaining of depersonalization phenomena should be followed carefully.

TREATMENT Little attention has been focused on the treatment of patients with depersonalization disorder. Various physiological treatment measures—such as continuous narcosis, Benzedrine, insulin coma, ether abreaction—have had only very modest therapeutic results. Good symptomatic relief is reported from dextroamphetamines and amobarbital (Amytal) combined with chlorpromazine (Thorazine) if anxiety is an important element of the clinical condition. In general, however, there are insufficient data on which to base a specific pharmacological regimen.

Psychotherapeutic approaches are equally untested. As with all patients with neurotic symptoms, the decision to use psychoanalysis or the specific techniques of analytically oriented insight psychotherapy should be determined not by the presence of the symptom itself but by a variety of positive indications derived from an assessment of the patient's personality, human relationships, and life situation. Indeed, some clinicians view depersonalization as a contraindication to analysis, and others believe that a successful outcome requires a minimum of 5 years of treatment. Presumably, the common supportive psychotherapeutic measures will be helpful to some patients, but specific recommendations for the management of the disorder must await more extensive clinical investigation.

TABLE 20-9
Diagnostic Criteria for Dissociative Disorder Not Otherwise Specified

Disorders in which the predominant feature is a dissociative symptom (i.e., a disturbance or alteration in the normally integrative functions of identity, memory, or consciousness) that does not meet the criteria for a specific dissociative disorder

Examples:

(1) Ganser's syndrome: the giving of "approximate answers" to questions, commonly associated with other symptoms such as amnesia, disorientation, perceptual disturbances, fugue, and conversion symptoms
(2) cases in which there is more than one personality state capable of assuming executive control of the individual, but not more than one personality state is sufficiently distinct to meet the full criteria for multiple personality disorder, or cases in which a second personality never assumes complete executive control
(3) trance states (i.e., altered states of consciousness with markedly diminished or selectively focused responsiveness to environmental stimuli). In children this may occur following physical abuse or trauma
(4) derealization unaccompanied by depersonalization
(5) dissociated states that may occur in people who have been subjected to periods of prolonged and intense coercive persuasion (e.g., brainwashing, thought reform, or indoctrination while the captive of terrorists or cultists)
(6) cases in which sudden, unexpected travel and organized, purposeful behavior with inability to recall one's past are not accompanied by the assumption of a new identity, partial or complete

Table from DSM-III-R *Diagnostic and Statistical Manual of Mental Disorders,* ed 3, revised. Copyright American Psychiatric Association, Washington, DC, 1987. Used with permission.

DISSOCIATIVE DISORDER NOT OTHERWISE SPECIFIED

DSM-III-R reserves the category of dissociative disorder not otherwise specified for individuals who suffer from a dissociative symptom without the specific characteristics of one of the dissociative disorders described above (Table 20-9). Included here are persons with nonspecific, trance-like states or who manifest derealization unaccompanied by depersonalization. The diagnosis applies, too, to those individuals suffering from more pervasive dissociative states after being subjected to periods of prolonged and intensive coercive persuasion, such as brainwashing and thought reform. Whether these are truly dissociative states is perhaps open to question, as some evidence, especially in victims of Nazi concentration camps, indicates that such persons are often alexithymic, a state resulting from massive regression rather than from dissociation.

REFERENCES

Boor M, Coons P: A comprehensive bibliography of literature pertaining to multiple personality, Psychol Rep *53:* 295, 1983.
Braun B, editor: *Treatment of Multiple Personality Disorder.* American Psychiatric Press, Washington, DC, 1986.
Dugas L, Moutier F: *La Dépersonnalisation.* Félix Alcan, Paris, 1911.
Flournoy T: *From India to the Planet Mars.* Harper and Brothers, New York, 1900.
Hilgard E R: *Divided Consciousness.* Wiley, New York, 1977.
Janet P: *L'Automatisme Psychologique.* Félix Alcan, Paris, 1889.
Janet P: *Névroses et idées fixes,* ed 2. Félix Alcan, Paris, 1904.

Janet P: *The Major Symptoms of Hysteria*. Macmillan, New York, 1907.
Kiersch T A: Amnesia: A clinical study of ninety-eight cases. Amer J Psychiat *119:* 57, 1962.
Kluft R: An introduction to multiple personality disorder. Psychiat Ann *14:* 19, 1984.
Kluft R: Treatment of multiple personality. Psychiat Clin N Amer *7:* 9, 1984.
Kluft R, editor: *Childhood Antecedents of Multiple Personality*. American Psychiatric Press, Washington, DC, 1985.
Nemiah J: Dissociative amnesia: A clinical and theoretical reconsideration. In *Functional Disorders of Memory,* J Kihlstrom, editor, p 303. Erlbaum, Hillsdale, NJ, 1979.
Prince M: *The Dissociation of a Personality*. Longmans, Green, New York, 1906.
Rosenbaum M: The role of the term schizophrenia in the decline of diagnosis of multiple personality. Arch Gen Psychiat *37:* 1383, 1980.
Roth M: The phobic anxiety–depersonalization syndrome. Proc R Soc Med *52:* 587, 1959.
Schenk L, Bear D: Multiple personality and related dissociative phenomena in patients with temporal lobe epilepsy. Amer J Psychiat *138:* 1311, 1981.
Shorvon H: The depersonalization syndrome. Proc R Soc Med *39:* 779, 1946.
Sidis B, Goodhart S P: *Multiple Personality. An Experimental Investigation into the Nature of Human Individuality*. Appleton, New York, 1905.
Taylor W, Martin M: Multiple personality. J Abnorm Soc Psychol *39:* 281, 1944.

CHAPTER 21 NORMAL HUMAN SEXUALITY AND SEXUAL DISORDERS

21.1 NORMAL HUMAN SEXUALITY AND SEXUAL DYSFUNCTIONS

VIRGINIA A. SADOCK, M.D.

INTRODUCTION

Sexual behavior is diverse and determined by a complex interaction of factors. It is affected by one's relationships with others, by life circumstances, and by the culture in which one lives. A person's sexuality is enmeshed with other personality factors, with his or her biological makeup, and with a general sense of self. It includes the perception of being male or female, and it reflects developmental experiences with sex throughout the life cycle. A rigid definition of normal sexuality is difficult to draw and is clinically impractical. It is easier to define abnormal sexuality—that is, sexual behavior that is destructive to oneself or others, that cannot be directed toward a partner, that excludes stimulation of the primary sex organs, and that is inappropriately associated with guilt and anxiety.

HISTORY Cultural mores regarding sexual behavior have varied throughout the history of Western civilization. Attitudes have oscillated between the liberal and the puritanical, between the acceptance and the repression of human sexuality. During the past several decades, the prevalent attitudes toward sex in the United States have been markedly liberal. However, recent studies indicate a trend toward accepting more conservative values. That shift is attributed largely to the fear of acquired immune deficiency syndrome (AIDS). A recent poll reported that 40 percent of Americans are concerned that they will contract AIDS and are altering their sexual behavior because of that fear. The greatest concern was expressed by young adults who are now more likely to use condoms as a precaution and to choose their sexual partners with greater care. Conservative segments of society emphasize abstinence before marriage as the answer to the fear of AIDS. The recurrence of conservative attitudes in response to the threat of illness has parallels in history. The sexual liberality of the Renaissance ended when syphilis swept the European continent and became a major argument for chastity among proponents of the Reformation. Other factors that predispose to more restrictive mores are periods of economic recession that tend to bring people to more puritanical positions and limited gratification when sexual freedom is used as a substitute for intimate relationships. Few of these issues have been resolved definitively in the form of new social mores, however, and the legacies of the sexual revolution of the 1960s and 1970s exert a strong effect on current sexual behavior.

That particular sexual revolution derived from social and scientific sources. The Kinsey reports of 1948 and 1953 made public the degree, type, and frequency of sexual activity occurring in this country, bringing sexual practices from the realm of inference and secrecy into accepted, if still private, reality. In the early 1970s, the Presidential Commission on Pornography advised against sexual repression, encouraging the candid discussion of sexuality in society and the acceptance of frank and sexually stimulating material. The recommendations of the report, however, were disregarded by that presidential administration. The advent of effective birth control methods and legalized abortion clearly differentiated the pleasure of sexual activity from its procreative function. The feminist movement attacked the double standard in what was considered acceptable sexual behavior for men and women, encouraged women to accept sexual responsibility for the gratification of their needs, and challenged society to reevaluate stereotyped male and female roles. The women's movement also focused attention on rape and incest. Gerontologists and elderly people alike have drawn attention to the sexual needs of the aged. Middle-class adolescents became sexually active and gay rights groups urged acceptance of their sexual orientations, and succeeded in having homosexuality dropped as a diagnostic category in the third edition of the American Psychiatric Association's *Diagnostic and Statistical Manual of Mental Disorders* (DSM-III).

Concurrent with the cultural changes of the sexual revolution there was growth in scientific research into sexual physiology and sexual dysfunctions. William Masters and Virginia Johnson published their pioneering work on the physiology of sexual response in 1966 and reported on their program for treating sexual complaints in 1970. Most medical centers now have programs specifically geared to the treatment of sexual dysfunctions.

Historically, problems of sexual conflict and sexual dysfunction have always been the province of psychiatry. Such pioneers as Havelock Ellis (Fig. 21.1-1), Richard Krafft-Ebing (Fig. 21.1-2), and Sigmund Freud focused broadly on human sexuality. More recent workers have focused more intensively on sexual physiology and dysfunctions. Problems of dysfunction are particularly distressing to patients and have often been resistant to treatment. The current approach to sexual dysfunctions reflects the cultural and scientific developments of recent years, the development of specific techniques for the treatment of these problems, the historical interest of psychiatry in this area, and the recognition of its importance in psychiatric practice.

DEFINITION

In the revised third edition of *Diagnostic and Statistical Manual of Mental Disorders* (DSM-III-R), sexual dysfunctions are categorized as Axis I disorders. Ten syndromes are listed, and they are correlated with the sexual physiological response. The sexual response cycle is divided into four phases: appetitive, excitement, orgasm, and resolution. The essential feature of the sexual dysfunctions is inhibition in one or more of these phases, including disturbance in the subjective sense of pleasure or desire or disturbance in the objective performance (Tables 21.1-1 and 21.1-2). Either type of disturbance can occur alone or in combination. Sexual dysfunctions are so diagnosed only when such disturbances are a major part of the clinical picture. They can be lifelong or acquired, generalized or situational. They are not diagnosed if such dysfunctions are symptomatic of other Axis I syndromes; moreover, if they are attributable entirely to organic factors, they are coded on Axis III.

In actuality, one rarely finds sexual dysfunctions, with the possible exception of premature ejaculation, separate from other psychiatric syndromes. Sexual disorders may lead to or result from marital disorders, and the patient invariably develops an increasing fear of failure and self-consciousness about his or her sexual performance. Sexual dysfunctions are frequently associated with depression, adjustment reactions, neurotic disorders, or personality disorders. In the first two cases, the sexual dysfunctions may exist for too short a period

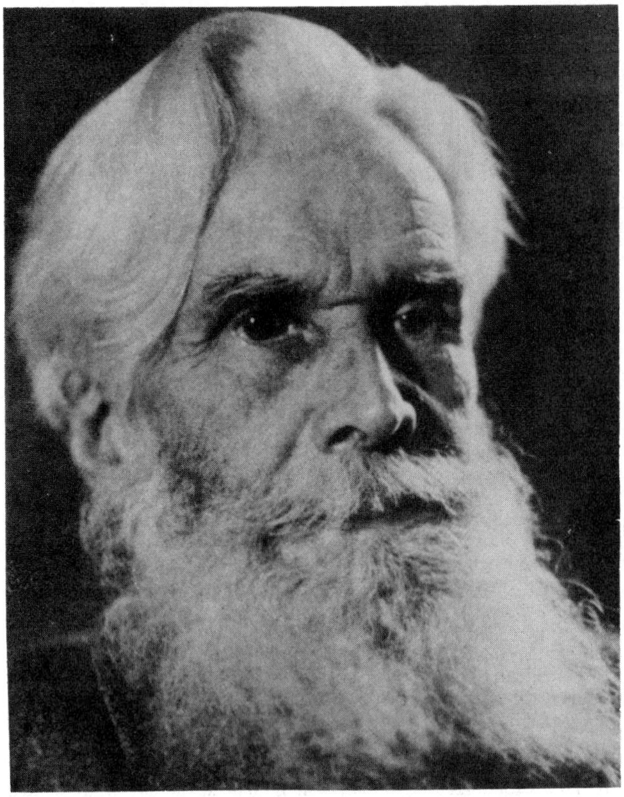

FIGURE 21.1-1. *Havelock Ellis, 1859–1939 (courtesy of New York Academy of Medicine).*

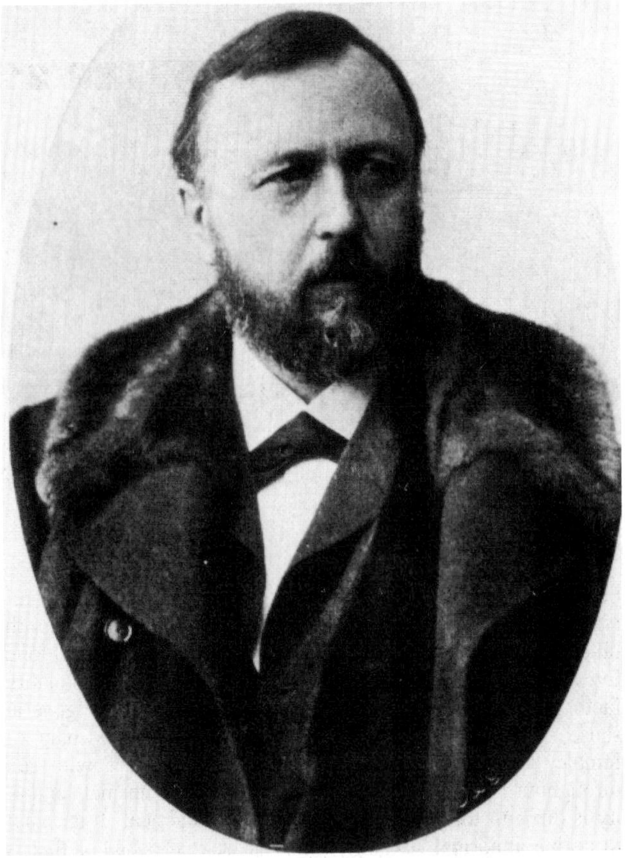

FIGURE 21.1-2. *Richard Krafft-Ebing, 1840–1903 (courtesy of New York Academy of Medicine).*

of time to warrant a diagnosis. In the latter two instances, sexual dysfunctions may be diagnosed in conjunction with the other psychiatric disorders.

NORMAL SEXUALITY

ANATOMICAL AND PHYSIOLOGICAL BASES A discussion of the organs of sexuality and the normal physiological sequence of male and female response is necessary for an informed understanding of the sexual dysfunctions.

Anatomy of the male The external genitalia of the normal adult male include the penis, scrotum, testes, epididymus, and parts of the vas deferens. Internal components include the vas deferens, seminal vesicles, ejaculatory ducts, and prostate gland.

Freud referred to the penis as the executive organ of sexuality. Since antiquity, culture after culture has represented the penis in a variety of art forms. In ancient Greece, the cults of Dionysus, Priapus, and the satyrs used the phallus as a recurrent symbol of fertility and rejuvenation. The word "penis" has been traced from the Latin, meaning variously "tail" or "to hang," and refers to the pendant position of the organ in its resting or flaccid state. The size of the penis varies within a fairly constant range, but sex researchers over the years have disagreed on the dimensions of the range. All agree, however, that concern over the size of the penis is practically universal among men. Masters and Johnson report a range of 7 to 11 cm in the flaccid state and 14 to 18 cm in the erect state. Of particular interest was their observation that the flac-

TABLE 21.1-1
Phases of the Sexual Response Cycle and Associated Sexual Dysfunction

Sexual Response Phase	*Phase-Related Dysfunctions*
I. Appetitive	Hypoactive sexual desire disorder Sexual aversion disorder
II. Excitement	Female sexual arousal disorder Male erectile disorder
III. Orgasm	Inhibited female orgasm (anorgasma) Inhibited male orgasm (retarded ejaculation) Premature ejaculation (male)
IV. Resolution	No dysfunctions

TABLE 21.1-2
Sexual Dysfunction Not Correlated with Phases of the Sexual Response Cycle

Category	*Dysfunctions*
Sexual pain disorders	Vaginismus (female) Dyspareunia (female and male)
Other	Sexual dysfunctions not otherwise specified. Examples: 1. No erotic sensation despite normal physiological response to sexual stimulation (e.g., orgasmic anhedonia) 2. Female analogue of premature ejaculation 3. Genital pain occurring during masturbation

cid dimension bears little relation to the erect dimension: The smaller penis erects to a proportionally greater size than does the larger penis.

Circumcision, in which the prepuce is surgically removed, has been practiced for centuries as a religious rite by Jews and Moslems and is a common medical procedure in the United States today. It was once believed that the circumcised penis, with its exposed glans, was less sensitive due to cornification of the epithelium. In laboratory studies, however, researchers have found no difference in tactile threshold between the circumcised penis and the uncircumcised penis. Intravaginally, they have found, the prepuce of the uncircumcised penis remains retracted behind the glans during penile thrusting, dispelling the myth that premature ejaculation may be more common in uncircumcised men because of increased stimulation caused by preputial movements.

The parasympathetic nervous system activates the process of erection. The pelvic splanchnic nerves (S2, S3, and S4) stimulate the blood vessels of the area to dilate, causing the penis to become erect. In ejaculation, the sympathetic nervous system is involved. Through its hypogastric plexus, the sympathetic nervous system innervates the urethral crest and the muscles of the epididymis, vas deferens, seminal vesicles, and prostate. Stimulation of the plexus causes ejaculation of seminal fluid from those glands and ducts into the urethra. The dilation of the prostatic urethra and the passage of fluid into the urethra provide the man with a sensation of impending climax. That is the emission phase of the ejaculatory process. Indeed, once the prostate contracts, ejaculation is inevitable. The ejaculate is propelled through the penile urethra contractions of the striated pelvic and perineal muscles. That phase of ejaculation is essentially under somatic efferent control. The ejaculate consists of about 1 teaspoon (2.5 ml) of fluid and contains about 120 million sperm cells.

Anatomy of the female The external genitalia of the normal female are also called the vulva and include the mons pubis, major and minor lips, clitoris, glans, vestibule of the vagina, and vaginal orifice. The internal system includes the ovaries, fallopian tubes, uterus, and vagina.

The word "vagina" comes from the Latin word meaning "sheath." The vagina is usually in a collapsed state, a potential rather than an actual space. About 8 cm long, the vagina extends from the cervix of the uterus above to the vestibule of the vagina or the vaginal opening below. In most virgins, a membranous fold, the hymen, separates the vestibule and opening from the rest of the vaginal canal. The mucous membrane lining the vaginal walls rests in numerous transverse folds. To accommodate the penis during sexual intercourse, the vagina expands in both length and width. After menopause, due to decreased circulating estrogen levels, the vagina loses much of its elasticity.

Hippocrates first described the clitoris in the medical literature, referring to it as the site of sexual excitation. Masters and Johnson described the clitoris as the primary female sexual organ, because orgasm depends physiologically on adequate clitoral stimulation. Anatomically, the clitoris has a nerve net that is proportionally three times as large as that of the penis.

Kinsey found that, when women masturbate, most prefer clitoral stimulation to any other. This finding was refined further by Masters and Johnson, who reported that women prefer the shaft of the clitoris to the glans, because the glans is hypersensitive if stimulated excessively.

An important anatomical finding is that the clitoral prepuce is contiguous with the labia minora and that during coitus the penis does not stimulate the clitoris directly. Rather, penile thrusting exerts traction on the minor lips, which in turn stimulates the clitoris sufficiently for orgasm to occur. During heightened excitement, just before orgasm, the clitoris retracts under the clitoral hood as a result of the contraction of the ischiocavernosi muscles. Retracting thus, the clitoris moves away from the vaginal barrel, which makes clitoral-penile contact impossible. The size of the clitoris varies considerably and is unrelated to the degree of sexual responsiveness of a particular female.

Endocrinology From the time of conception, hormones play a major role in human sexual development. Unlike the fetal gonads, which are under chromosomal influence, the fetal external genitalia are very susceptible to hormones. Exogenous hormonal administration can cause external genital development inconsistent with the fetal sex gland development. For instance, if the pregnant mother receives sufficient exogenous androgen, a female fetus possessing an ovary can develop external genitalia resembling those of a male. Fetal, maternal, or exogenous hormones administered to a pregnant woman may all affect the development of external genitalia of the fetus. Deprived of male and female gonads and the respective hormones testosterone and estrogen, the human adult does not develop normal secondary sexual characteristics, is incapable of reproduction, and, in the case of the female, does not develop a menstrual cycle.

Testosterone is the hormone believed to be connected with libido in both men and women. In men, there is an inverse correlation between stress and the testosterone blood level. Other factors, such as sleep, mood, and life-style, are being studied to evaluate their relationship to circulating levels of this hormone. The administration of androgens to patients complaining of sexual dysfunction is usually futile if normal hormonal function is present. Androgen administered to men complaining of loss of potency and loss of libido has usually been unsuccessful, and administration to women results in disturbing virilizing side effects. Many clinicians correct the hormone deficiency of the postmenopausal period with estrogen replacement therapy. Although this therapy is effective in relieving much of the physiological stress of the period, prolonged administration of hormones is controversial because it may increase the risk of development of endometrial cancer.

THE BRAIN AND SEXUAL BEHAVIOR Experimentation with animals has demonstrated that the limbic system is directly involved with elements of sexual functioning. In all mammals, the limbic system is involved in behavior required for self-preservation and the preservation of the species.

Chemical or electrical stimulation of various sites of the limbic system—the lower part of the septum and the contiguous medial preoptic area, the fimbria of the hippocampus, the mammillary bodies, and the anterior thalamic nuclei—have all elicited penile erection. The hippocampus is believed to influence genital tumescence and affect the regulation of the release of gonadotropins.

The stimulation of the amygdala in primates initiates first oral (chewing, lip smacking) and then genital (penile erection) behavior. Researchers have stated that the closeness of those functions may derive from the evolutionary fact that the olfactory sense was strongly involved in both feeding and mating. They speculate that the evolution of the third subdivision of the limbic system may reflect a shift in importance from olfactory contact to visual communication in sociosexual behavior.

SEXUAL LEARNING AND MASTURBATION Sexual learning begins in childhood. In a broad sense, that learning occurs through parent-child interaction, including the meeting of the infant's physical needs, cuddling, the reinforcement or discouragement of gender-associated activities, and the establishment by the age of 2 of gender identity. The elaboration of gender roles continues throughout one's lifetime.

Genital self-stimulation is a normal activity of babies. It is particularly pronounced between the ages of 15 and 19 months and is part of the general interest of the child in his or her body. The activity is reinforced by the pleasurable sensations it produces. As the child grows older, that exploration and stimulation are extended to other children in "doctor" games. The child is socialized not to masturbate in public, but unless he or she is unduly shamed, self-stimulation usually continues as a pleasurable, private experience.

With the hormonal acceleration of puberty and the physiological changes of adolescence, masturbation serves additional functions. At that time it is frequently accompanied by coital fantasies and acts as preparation for adult interaction with a partner. Also, it provides an acceptable release for the adolescent who must establish his or her sexual identity, but who frequently has no outlet for his or her heightened sexual impulses.

Masturbation usually continues to some degree through the life cycle. Even after a permanent sexual relationship has been established, masturbation remains a healthy sexual activity during the illness or absence of a partner. Only when it is a compulsive activity or when it is preferred to partner interaction should it be considered maladaptive. Even the punitive and inhibitory myths that surround masturbation—that it causes blindness, impotence, illness, or sterility—have not prevented it from being a nearly universal practice. Kinsey reported that nearly all men and three-fourths of women masturbate sometime during their lives.

Physiological responses Normal men and women experience a sequence of physiological responses to sexual stimulation. In the first detailed description of these responses, Masters and Johnson observed that the physiological process involves increasing levels of vasocongestion and myotonia *(tumescence)* and the subsequent release of the vascular activity and muscle tone as a result of orgasm *(detumescence)*. Tables 21.1-3 and 21.1-4 describe the male and female sexual response cycles, respectively. DSM-III-R defines a four-phase response cycle: Phase I—Appetitive; Phase II—Excitement; Phase III—Orgasm; Phase IV—Resolution.

PHASE I: APPETITIVE This phase is distinct from any identified solely through physiology and reflects the psychiatrist's fundamental concern with motivations, drives, and personality.

TABLE 21.1-3
Male Sexual Response Cycle

	Excitement Phase	*Orgasmic Phase*	*Resolution Phase*
	Lasts several minutes to several hours; heightened excitement prior to orgasm, 30 seconds to 3 minutes	3 to 15 seconds	10 to 15 minutes; if no orgasm, ½ to 1 day
Skin	Just prior to orgasm: sexual flush; inconsistently appears; maculopapular rash originates on abdomen and spreads to anterior chest wall, face, and neck, and can include shoulders and forearms	Well-developed flush	Flush disappears in reverse order of appearance; inconsistently appearing film of perspiration on soles of feet and palms of hands
Penis	Erection within 10 to 30 seconds caused by vasocongestion of erectile bodies of corpus cavernosa of shaft; loss of erection may occur with introduction of asexual stimulus, loud noise; with heightened excitement there is a further increase in size of glans and diameter of penile shaft	Ejaculation: emission phase marked by three to four contractions at 0.8 second of vas, seminal vesicles, prostate; ejaculation proper marked by contractions at 0.8 second of urethra and ejaculatory spurt of 12 to 20 inches at age 18, decreasing with age to seepage at 70	Erection: partial involution in 5 to 10 seconds with variable refractory period; full detumescence in 5 to 30 minutes
Scrotum and testes	Tightening and lifting of scrotal sac and elevation of testes; with heightened excitement, 50% increase in size of testes over unstimulated state and flattening against perineum signaling impending ejaculation	No change	Decrease to baseline size due to loss of vasocongestion; testicular and scrotal descent within 5 to 30 minutes after orgasm; involution may take several hours if there is no orgasmic release
Cowper's glands	2 to 3 drops of mucoid fluid that contain viable sperm are secreted during heightened excitement	No change	No change
Other	Breasts: inconsistent nipple erection with heightened excitement, prior to orgasm: Myotonia: semispastic contractions of facial, abdominal, and intercostal muscles Tachycardia: up to 175 per minute. Blood pressure: rise in systolic 20 to 80 mm; in diastolic 10 to 40 mm Respiration: increased	Loss of voluntary muscular control Rectum: rhythmical contractions of sphincter Heart rate: up to 180 beats per minute Blood pressure: 40 to 100 systolic; 20 to 50 diastolic Respiration: up to 40 respirations per minute	Return to baseline state in 5 to 10 minutes

TABLE 21.1-4
Female Sexual Response Cycle

	Excitement Phase	*Orgasmic Phase*	*Resolution Phase*
	Lasts several minutes to several hours; heightened excitement prior to orgasm, 30 seconds to 3 minutes	3 to 15 seconds	10 to 15 minutes; if no orgasm, ½ to 1 day
Skin	Just prior to orgasm: sexual flush inconsistently appears; maculopapular rash originates on abdomen and spreads to anterior chest wall, face, and neck, can include shoulders and forearms	Well-developed flush	Flush disappears in reverse order of appearance; inconsistently appearing film of perspiration on soles of feet and palms of hands
Breasts	Nipple erection in two-thirds of women, venous congestion and areolar enlargement; size increases to one-fourth over normal	Breasts may become tremulous	Return to normal in about ½ hour
Clitoris	Enlargement in diameter of glans and shaft; just before orgasm, shaft retracts into pupuce	No change	Shaft returns to normal position in 5 to 10 seconds; detumescence in 5 to 30 minutes; if no orgasm, detumescence takes several hours
Labia majora	Nullipara: elevate and flatten against perineum Multipara: congestion and edema	No change	Nullipara: increase to normal size in 1 to 2 minutes Multipara: decrease to normal size in 10 to 15 minutes
Labia minora	Size increase two to three times over normal; change to pink, red, deep red prior to orgasm	Contractions of proximal labia minora	Return to normal within 5 minutes
Vagina	Color change to dark purple; vaginal transudate appears 10 to 30 seconds after arousal; elongation and ballooning of vagina; lower third of vagina constricts prior to orgasm	3 to 15 contractions of lower third of vagina at intervals of 0.8 second	Ejaculate forms seminal pool in upper two-thirds of vagina; congestion disappears in seconds or, if no orgasm, in 20 to 30 minutes
Uterus	Ascends into false pelvis; labor-like contractions begin in heightened excitement just prior to orgasm	Contractions throughout orgasm	Contractions cease and uterus descends to normal position
Other	Myotonia A few drops of mucoid secretion from Bartholin's glands during heightened excitement Cervix swells slightly and is passively elevated with uterus	Loss of voluntary muscular control Rectum: rhythmical contractions of sphincter Hyperventilation and tachycardia	Return to baseline status in seconds to minutes Cervix color and size return to normal and cervix descends into seminal pool

The phase is characterized by sexual fantasies and the desire to have sexual activity.

PHASE II: EXCITEMENT This phase is brought on by psychological stimulation (fantasy or the presence of a love object), physiological stimulation (stroking or kissing), or a combination of the two. It consists of a subjective sense of pleasure. The excitement phase is characterized by penile tumescence leading to erection in the man and vaginal lubrication in the woman. The nipples of both sexes become erect, although nipple erection is more common in women than in men. The woman's clitoris becomes hard and turgid, and her labia minora become thicker as a result of venous engorgment. Initial excitement may last several minutes to several hours. With continued stimulation, the man's testes increase in size 50 percent and elevate. The woman's vaginal barrel shows a characteristic constriction along the outer third known as the orgasmic platform. The clitoris elevates and retracts behind the symphysis pubis. As a result, the clitoris is not easily accessible. As the area is stimulated, however, traction on the labia minora and the prepuce occurs, and there is intrapreputial movement of the clitoral shaft. Breast size in the woman increases 25 percent. Continued engorgement of the penis and vagina produces specific color changes, particularly in the labia minora, which become bright or deep red. Voluntary contractions of large muscle groups occur, rate of heartbeat and respiration increases, and blood pressure rises. Heightened excitement lasts 30 seconds to several minutes.

PHASE III: ORGASM This phase consists of a peaking of sexual pleasure, with release of sexual tension and rhythmic contraction of the perineal muscles and pelvic reproductive organs. A subjective sense of ejaculatory inevitability triggers the man's orgasm. The forceful emission of semen follows. The male orgasm is also associated with four to five rhythmic spasms of the prostate, seminal vesicles, vas, and urethra. In the woman, orgasm is characterized by 3 to 15 involuntary contractions of the lower third of the vagina and by strong sustained contractions of the uterus, flowing from the fundus downward to the cervix. Both men and women have involuntary contractions of the internal and external sphincter. These and the other contractions during orgasm occur at intervals of 0.8 second. Other manifestations include voluntary and involuntary movements of the large muscle groups, including facial grimacing and carpopedal spasm. Blood pressure rises 20 to 40 mm (both systolic and diastolic), and the heart rate increases up to 160 beats a minute. Orgasm lasts from 3 to 25 seconds and is associated with a slight clouding of consciousness.

PHASE IV: RESOLUTION Resolution consists of the disgorgement of blood from the genitalia (detumescence), and this detumescence brings the body back to its resting state. If orgasm occurs, resolution is rapid; if it does not occur, resolution may take 2 to 6 hours and be associated with irritability and discomfort. Resolution through orgasm is characterized by a subjective sense of well-being, general relaxation, and muscular relaxation.

After orgasm, men have a refractory period that may last from several minutes to many hours; in that period they cannot be stimulated to further orgasm. The refractory period does not exist in women who are capable of multiple and successive orgasms.

Sexual response is a true psychophysiological experience. Arousal is triggered by both psychological and physical stimuli, levels of tension are experienced both physiologically and emotionally, and, with orgasm, there is normally a subjective perception of a peak of physical reaction and release. Psychosexual development, psychological attitude toward sexuality, and attitudes toward one's sexual partner are directly involved with and affect the physiology of human sexual response.

SEXUAL DYSFUNCTIONS

A sexual disorder can be symptomatic of biological problems, intrapsychic conflicts, interpersonal difficulties, or a combination of these factors. The sexual function can be affected by stress of any kind, by emotional disorders, and by a lack of sexual knowledge. In this subsection, various sexual dysfunctions are discussed as they apply to heterosexual relationships. The 10 sexual dysfunction categories listed in DSM-III-R will be examined.

HYPOACTIVE SEXUAL DESIRE DISORDER

Hypoactive sexual desire disorder is experienced by both men and women; however, they may not be hampered by any dysfunction once they are involved in the sex act. Conversely, hypoactive desire may be used to mask another sexual dysfunction. Lack of desire may be expressed by decreased frequency of coitus, perception of the partner as unattractive, or overt complaints of lack of desire. In some cases there are biochemical correlates associated with hypoactive desire. A recent study found markedly decreased levels of serum testosterone in men complaining of this dysfunction when they were compared to normal controls in a sleep-laboratory situation. Also, a central dopamine blockage is known to decrease desire (Table 21.1-5).

The need for sexual contact and satisfaction varies among individuals as well as in the same person over time. In a group of 100 couples with stable marriages, 8 percent reported having intercourse less than once a month. In another group of couples, one-third reported lack of sexual relations for periods of time averaging 8 weeks. In a survey of a general medical practice in England, 25 percent of that sample reported no sexual activity the majority of the time. It has been estimated that 20 percent of the total population have hypoactive sexual desire disorder. The complaint is more common among women.

Desire disorders are not new, although they have become the focus of much attention. Patients with desire problems often have good ego strengths and use inhibition of desire in a defensive way to protect against unconscious fears about sex. Lack of desire can also be the result of chronic stress, anxiety, or depression. Abstinence from sex for a prolonged period sometimes results in suppression of the sexual impulse. It may also be an expression of hostility or the sign of a deteriorating relationship.

The presence of desire depends on several factors: biological drive, adequate self-esteem, previous good experiences with sex, the availability of an appropriate partner, and a good relationship in nonsexual areas with one's partner. Damage to any of these factors may result in diminished desire.

TABLE 21.1-5
Diagnostic Criteria for Hypoactive Sexual Desire Disorder

A.	Persistently or recurrently deficient or absent sexual fantasies and desire for sexual activity. The judgment of deficiency or absence is made by the clinician, taking into account factors that affect sexual functioning, such as age, sex, and the context of the person's life.
B.	Occurrence not exclusively during the course of another Axis I disorder (other than a sexual dysfunction), such as major depression.

Table from DSM-III-R *Diagnostic and Statistical Manual of Mental Disorders*, ed 3, revised. Copyright American Psychiatric Association, Washington, DC, 1987. Used with permission.

SEXUAL AVERSION DISORDER

This new category of sexual disorder is defined in DSM-III-R as a "persistent or recurrent aversion to, and avoidance of, all or almost all, genital sexual contact with a sexual partner." Some researchers consider the line between hypoactive desire disorder and sexual aversion disorder blurred, and in some cases both diagnoses are appropriate. Low frequency of sexual interaction is a symptom common to both disorders. From a clinician's perspective, it is helpful to think of the words "repugnance" or "phobia" in relation to the patient with sexual aversion disorder (Table 21.1-6).

The disorder may result from a traumatic sexual assault, such as rape or childhood abuse, from repeated painful experiences with coitus, and from early developmental conflicts that have left the patient with unconscious connections between the sexual impulse and overwhelming feelings of shame and guilt. The disorder may also be a reaction to a perceived psychological assault by one's partner and to relationship difficulties.

SEXUAL AROUSAL DISORDERS

Sexual dysfunction with inhibited sexual arousal involves recurrent and persistent inhibition during sexual activity, manifested either by the man's partial or complete failure to attain or maintain an erection until the completion of the sex act or by the woman's partial or complete failure to attain or maintain the lubrication-swelling response of sexual excitement until the completion of the sexual act (in some people the physiological response to stimulation may be present but without a subjective sense of sexual pleasure and excitement). The diagnosis is made in the light of clinical judgment that takes

TABLE 21.1-6
Diagnostic Criteria for Sexual Aversion Disorder

A.	Persistent or recurrent extreme aversion to, and avoidance of, all or almost all, genital sexual contact with a sexual partner.
B.	Occurrence not exclusively during the course of another Axis I disorder (other than a sexual dysfunction), such as obsessive-compulsive disorder or major depression.

Table from DSM-III-R *Diagnostic and Statistical Manual of Mental Disorders*, ed 3, revised. Copyright American Psychiatric Association, Washington, DC, 1987. Used with permission.

TABLE 21.1-7
Diagnostic Criteria for Female Sexual Arousal Disorder

A. Either (1) or (2):
   (1) persistent or recurrent partial or complete failure to attain or maintain the lubrication-swelling response of sexual excitement until completion of the sexual activity
   (2) persistent or recurrent lack of a subjective sense of sexual excitement and pleasure in a female during sexual activity

B. Occurrence not exclusively during the course of another Axis I disorder (other than a sexual dysfunction), such as major depression.

Table from DSM-III-R *Diagnostic and Statistical Manual of Mental Disorders,* ed 3, revised. Copyright American Psychiatric Association, Washington, DC, 1987. Used with permission.

TABLE 21.1-8
Diagnostic Criteria for Male Erectile Disorder

A. Either (1) or (2):
   (1) persistent or recurrent partial or complete failure in a male to attain or maintain erection until completion of the sexual activity
   (2) persistent or recurrent lack of a subjective sense of sexual excitement and pleasure in a male during sexual activity

B. Occurrence not exclusively during the course of another Axis I disorder (other than a sexual dysfunction), such as major depression.

Table from DSM-III-R *Diagnostic and Statistical Manual of Mental Disorders,* ed 3, revised. Copyright American Psychiatric Association, Washington, DC, 1987. Used with permission.

into account the focus, intensity, and duration of the sexual activity in which the patient engages (Tables 21.1-7 and 21.1-8).

Female sexual arousal disorder Women who have excitement-phase dysfunction often have orgastic problems as well. In one series of relatively happily married couples, 33 percent of the women described difficulty in maintaining sexual excitement.

Numerous psychological factors are associated with female sexual inhibition. These conflicts may be expressed through inhibition of excitement or orgasm and are discussed under orgasmic phase dysfunctions. In some women, arousal disorders are associated with dyspareunia or with lack of desire.

Less research has been done on physiological components of dysfunction in women than in men and there have been conflicting results. Masters and Johnson found normally responsive women to be particularly desirous of sex premenstrually. In a recent study, dysfunctional women tended to be more responsive immediately following their periods. A third group of dysfunctional women felt the greatest sexual excitement at the time of ovulation. There is some evidence that dysfunctional women are less aware of the physiological responses of their bodies, such as vasocongestion, during arousal.

There are some organic etiologies for female sexual arousal disorder. Medications with antihistaminic or anticholinergic properties cause lessened vaginal lubrication. Also, postmenopausal women require a longer period of stimulation for lubrication to occur and there is generally less vaginal transudate after menopause. An artificial lubricant is frequently useful in that situation.

Male erectile disorder Inhibited sexual excitement in the male is also called erectile dysfunction or impotence. In *primary impotence,* the man has never been able to obtain an erection sufficient for vaginal insertion. In *secondary impotence,* the man has successfully achieved vaginal penetration at some time in his sexual life, but later is unable to do so. In *selective impotence,* the man is able to have coitus in certain circumstances, but not in others: for example, a man may function effectively with a prostitute but may be impotent with his wife.

It was estimated by Kinsey that a few men (2 to 4 percent) are impotent at age 35, but 77 percent are impotent at age 80. More recently, it has been estimated that the incidence of impotence in young men is about 8 percent. However, this sexual dysfunction may first appear later in life. Masters and Johnson report a fear of impotence in all men over 40, which the researchers believe reflects the masculine fear of loss of virility with advancing age. (As it happens, however, impotence is not a regularly occurring phenomenon in the aged; having an available sexual partner is more closely related to continuing potency in the aging man than is age per se.) The percentage of all men treated for sexual disorders who have impotence as the chief complaint ranges from 35 to 50 percent.

The incidence of psychological as opposed to organic impotence has been the focus of many recent studies. Physiologically, impotence may be due to a variety of organic causes (Table 21.1-9). In the United States, it is estimated that 2 million men are impotent because they suffer from diabetes mellitus; an additional 300,000 are impotent because of other endocrine diseases; 1.5 million are impotent as a result of vascular disease; 180,000 because of multiple sclerosis; 400,000 because of traumas and fractures leading to pelvic fractures or spinal cord injuries; and another 650,000 are impotent as a result of radical surgery, including prostatectomies, colostomies, and cystectomies. In addition, the clinician should be aware of the possible pharmacological effects of medication on sexual functioning. The increased incidence of organic etiologies for this dysfunction in the past 15 years may, in part, reflect the increased use of psychotropic and antihypertensive medications. Statistics indicate that 20 to 50 percent of men with erectile dysfunction have an organic basis for their problem (Table 21.1-10).

ORGANIC VS. FUNCTIONAL IMPOTENCE A number of procedures from benign to invasive are used to help differentiate organically caused impotence from functional impotence. The most common procedure is the monitoring of nocturnal penile tumescence, or erections that occur during sleep, normally in association with rapid eye movement (REM). It has been assumed that men who did not experience erections during REM sleep had an organic etiology for their erectile dysfunctions. However, studies have revealed decreased tumescence and decreased testosterone levels under sleep-laboratory conditions in physically healthy men who suffer from primary erectile dysfunction, from combined hypoactive desire disorder and secondary impotence, and in men who suffer from depression. Conversely, men with subtle vasculogenic disorders or with hyperprolactinemia may have erections with REM sleep but still have an organic basis for their impotence. Nonetheless, this procedure is still effective for ruling out physical causes for erectile dysfunction as it is relatively simple to administer and is accurate 85 to 90 percent of the time. Many sleep laboratories measure the degree of penile rigidity in addition to tumescence. A pressure device is pressed against the base of the penis, and the amount of pressure needed to make the penis buckle is measured in millimeters of mercury.

Other procedures used to define organic causes for erectile

TABLE 21.1-9
Diseases Implicated in Erectile Dysfunction

Infectious and parasitic diseases
- Elephantiasis
- Mumps

Cardiovascular diseases
- Atherosclerotic disease
- Aortic aneurysm
- Leriche syndrome
- Cardiac failure

Renal and urological disorders
- Peyronie's disease
- Chronic renal failure
- Hydrocele or varicocele

Hepatic disorders
- Cirrhosis (usually associated with alcoholism)

Pulmonary disorders
- Respiratory failure

Genetics
- Klinefelter's syndrome
- Congenital penile vascular or structural abnormalities

Nutritional disorders
- Malnutrition
- Vitamin deficiencies

Endocrine disorders
- Diabetes mellitus
- Dysfunction of the pituitary-adrenal-testis axis
- Acromegaly
- Addison's disease
- Chromophobe ademona
- Adrenal neoplasias
- Myxedema
- Hyperthyroidism

Neurological disorders
- Multiple sclerosis
- Transverse myelitis
- Parkinson's disease
- Temporal lobe epilepsy
- Traumatic or neoplastic spinal cord disease
- Central nervous system tumors
- Amyotropic lateral sclerosis
- Peripheral neuropathies
- General paresis
- Tabes dorsalis

Pharmacological contributants (see Table 21.1-10)
- Alcohol and other addictive drugs (heroin, methadone, morphine, cocaine, amphetamines, and barbituates)
- Prescribed drugs (psychotropic drugs, antihypertensive drugs, estrogens, and antiandrogens)

Poisoning
- Lead (plumbism)
- Herbicides

Surgical procedures
- Perineal prostatectomy
- Abdominal-perineal colon resection
- Sympathectomy (frequently interferes with ejaculation)
- Aortoiliac surgery
- Radical cystectomy
- Retroperitoneal lymphadenectomy

Miscellaneous
- Radiation therapy
- Pelvic fracture
- Any severe systemic disease or debilitating condition

dysfunction are monitoring tumescence with a strain gauge; measurement of the blood pressure in the penis using an ultrasound (Doppler) flow meter to assess blood flow in the internal pudendal artery; and caversonograms and measurement of pudendal nerve latency time. Additional diagnostic tests include glucose tolerance tests; plasma hormone assays; liver and thyroid function tests; prolactin, and follicle-

TABLE 21.1-10
Pharmacological Agents Inplicated in Male Sexual Dysfunction*

Drug	*Impairs Erection*	*Impairs Ejaculation*
Psychiatric drugs		
Tricyclic antidepressants†		
Imipramine (Tofranil)	+	+
Protriptyline (Vivactil)	+	+
Desmethylimipramine (Pertofrane)	+	+
Clomipramine (Anafranil)	+	+
Amitriptyline (Elavil)	+	+
Nortripytline (Aventyl)		
Monoamine oxidase inhibitors		
Tranylcypromine (Parnate)	+	
Mebanazine (Actomal)	+	+
Phenelzine (Nardil)	+	+
Pargyline (Eutonyl)	—	+
Isocarboxazid (Marplan)	—	+
Other mood-active drugs		
Lithium	+	
Amphetamines	+	+
Major tranquilizers‡		
Fluphenazine (Prolixin)	+	
Thioridazine (Mellaril)	+	+
Chlorprothixene (Taractan)	—	+
Mesoridazine (Serentil)	—	+
Perphenazine (Trilafon)	—	+
Trifluoperazine (Stelazine)	—	+
Butaperazine (Repoise)	—	+
Reserpine (Serpasil)	+	+
Haloperidol (Haldol)	—	+
Minor tranquilizers§		
Chlordiazepoxide (Librium)	—	+
Antihypertensive drugs		
Clonidine (Catapres)	+	
Methyldopa (Aldomet)	+	+
Spironolactone (Aldactone)	+	—
Hydrochlorthiazide (Apresoline)	+	—
Arramethidine (Ismelin)	+	+
Commonly abused drugs		
Alcohol	+	+
Barbituates	+	+
Cannibus	+	—
Cocaine	+	+
Heroin	+	+
Methadone	+	—
Morphine	+	+
Miscellaneous drugs		
Antiparkinsonian agents	+	+
Clotibrate (Atromid-S)	+	—
Digoxin (Lanoxin)	+	—
Glutethimide (Doriden)	+	+
Indomethacin (Indocin)	+	—
Phentolamine (Regitine)	—	+
Propranolol (Inderal)	+	—

*Both increase and decrease in libido have been reported with psychoactive agents. It is difficult to separate those effects from the underlying condition or from improvement of the condition. Sexual dysfunction associated with the use of a drug disappears when the drug is discontinued.

†The incidence of erectile dysfunction associated with the use of tricyclic antidepressants is low.

‡Impairment of sexual function is not a common complication of the use of major tranquilizers. Priapism has occasionally occurred in association with the use of major tranquilizers.

§Benzodiazepines have been reported to decrease libido, but in some patients the diminution of anxiety caused by those drugs enhances sexual function.

stimulating hormone (FSH) determinations; and cystometric examinations.

ETIOLOGY A good history is crucial in determining the etiology of the dysfunction. If a man reports having spontaneous erections at times when he does not plan to have intercourse, having morning erections or only sporadic erectile dysfunction, or having good erections with masturbation or with partners other than his usual one, then organic causes for his impotence can be considered negligible, and costly diagnostic procedures can be avoided. In those cases in which an organic basis for impotence is found, psychological factors often contribute to the dysfunction, and psychiatric treatment may be helpful. In some diabetics, for instance, erectile dysfunction may be psychogenic. About 50 to 80 percent of erectile dysfunction cases have a psychogenic origin. In general, the psychological conflicts that cause impotence are related to an inability to express the sexual impulse because of fear, anxiety, anger, or moral prohibition. Primary impotence is a more serious, but less common, condition than secondary impotence, and primary impotence is less amenable to treatment.

Many developmental factors have been cited as contributing to erectile disorder. Any experience that hinders the ability to be intimate, that leads to a feeling of inadequacy or distrust, or that develops a sense of being unloving or unlovable may result in impotence. In an ongoing relationship, erectile dysfunction may reflect difficulties between the partners, particularly if the man cannot communicate his needs or his angry feelings in a direct and constructive way. Unfortunately, successive episodes of impotence are reinforcing, with the man becoming increasingly anxious about his next sexual encounter. Regardless of the original etiology of the dysfunction, his anticipatory anxiety about achieving and maintaining an erection interferes with his pleasure in sexual contact and with his ability to respond to stimulation, thus perpetuating the problem.

ORGASM DISORDERS

Inhibited female orgasm Sexual dysfunction with inhibited female orgasm *(anorgasmia)* is defined as the recurrent and persistent inhibition of the female orgasm, as manifested by the absence or delay of orgasm after a normal sexual excitement phase that the clinician judges to be adequate in focus, intensity, and duration. Women who can achieve orgasm with noncoital clitoral stimulation but are unable to experience it during coitus in the absence of manual clitoral stimulation are not necessarily categorized as anorgasmic (Table 21.1-11).

Physiological research regarding the female sexual response has demonstrated that orgasms caused by clitoral stimulation and those caused by vaginal stimulation are physiologically identical. Freud's theory that women must give up clitoral sensitivity for vaginal sensitivity in order to achieve sexual maturity is now considered misleading, although some women say that they gain a special sense of satisfaction from an orgasm precipitated by coitus. Some workers attribute that to the psychological feeling of closeness engendered by the act of coitus, but others maintain that the coital orgasm is a physiologically different experience. Many women achieve orgasm during coitus by a combination of manual clitoral stimulation and penile vaginal stimulation.

Primary nonorgasmic dysfunction exists when the woman has never experienced orgasm by any kind of stimulation. Secondary orgasmic dysfunction exists if the woman has previously experienced at least one orgasm regardless of the circumstances or means of stimulation, whether by masturbation or during sleep while dreaming. Kinsey found that the proportion of married women over 35 years of age who had never achieved orgasm by any means was only 5 percent. The incidence of orgasm increases with age. According to Kinsey, the first orgasm occurs in late adolescence in about 50 percent of women. The rest usually experience orgasm by some means as they get older. Primary anorgasmia is more common among unmarried women than among married women; 39 percent of the unmarried women over age 35 in Kinsey's study had never experienced orgasm. Increased orgasmic potential in women over 35 has been explained on the basis of less psychological inhibition, greater sexual experience, or both. Also, orgasmic consistency has been correlated with marital happiness, although cause and effect have not been determined.

TABLE 21.1-11
Diagnostic Criteria for Inhibited Female Orgasm

A. Persistent or recurrent delay in, or absence of, orgasm in a female following a normal sexual excitement phase during sexual activity that the clinician judges to be adequate in focus, intensity, and duration. Some females are able to experience orgasm during noncoital clitoral stimulation, but are unable to experience it during coitus in the absence of manual clitoral stimulation. In most of these females, this represents a normal variation of the female sexual response and does not justify the diagnosis of inhibited female orgasm. However, in some of these females, this does represent a psychological inhibition that justifies the diagnosis. This difficult judgment is assisted by a thorough sexual evaluation, which may even require a trial of treatment.

B. Occurrence not exclusively during the course of another Axis I disorder (other than a sexual dysfunction), such as major depression.

Table from DSM-III-R *Diagnostic and Statistical Manual of Mental Disorders,* ed 3, revised. Copyright American Psychiatric Association, Washington, DC, 1987. Used with permission.

Secondary orgasmic dysfunction is a common complaint in clinical populations. One clinical treatment facility described nonorgastic women as about four times more common in its practice than patients with all other sexual disorders. In another study, 46 percent of the women complained of difficulty in reaching orgasm, and 15 percent described inability to have orgasm. The overall prevalence of inhibited orgasm in women is estimated at 30 percent.

Some medical conditions, specifically endocrine diseases such as hypothyroidism, diabetes mellitus, or primary hyperprolactinemia can affect a woman's ability to have orgasms (Table 21.1-12). Also, a number of drugs affect some women's capacity to have orgasms. Antihypertensive medications, central nervous system (CNS) stimulants, tricyclic antidepressants, and, more frequently, monoamine oxidase (MAO) inhibitors have interfered with female orgastic capacity. However, a recent study of women taking MAO inhibitors found that after 16 to 18 weeks of pharmacotherapy, that side effect of the medication disappeared and the women were able to reexperience orgasms although they continued on an undiminished dosage of the drug.

Numerous psychological factors are associated with female sexual inhibition. They include fears of impregnation, rejection by the sexual partner, or damage to the vagina; hostility toward men; and feelings of guilt regarding sexual impulses. For some women, orgasm is equated with loss of control or with aggressive, destructive, or violent behavior. Fear of these impulses may be expressed through inhibition of excitement or orgasm. The expression of orgasmic inhibition varies. Some women feel unentitled to gratify themselves and are

TABLE 21.1-12
Psychiatric Drugs Implemented in Inhibited Female Orgasm*

Antidepressant
Amoxapine (Asendin)†
Tricyclic antidepressants
Imipramine (Tofranil)
Clomipramine (Anafranil)‡
Nortriptyline (Aventyl)§
Monoamine oxidase inhibitors**
Tranylcypromine (Parnate)
Phenelzine (Nardil)
Isocarboxazid (Marplan)
Major tranquilizers
Thioridazine (Mellaril)
Trifluoperazine (Stelazine)

*The interrelationship between female sexual dysfunction and pharmacological agents has been less extensively evaluated than have male reactions. Oral contraceptives are reported to decrease libido in some women and some drugs with anticholinergic side effects may impair arousal as well as orgasm. Benzodiazepines have been reported to decrease libido, but in some patients the diminution of anxiety caused by those drugs enhances sexual function.
Both increase and decrease in libido have been reported with psychoactive agents. It is difficult to separate those effects from the underlying condition or from improvement of the condition. Sexual dysfunction associated with the use of a drug disappears when the drug is discontinued.
†Bethanechol (Urecholine) can reverse the effects of amoxapine-induced anorgasmia.
‡Clomipramine also is reported to increase arousal and orgasmic potential.
§Cyproheptadine reverses nortriptyline-induced anorgasmia.
**MAO-induced anorgasmia dysfunction may be a temporary reaction to the medication, which disappears even though administration of the drug is continued.

unable to masturbate to climax. Others enjoy self-stimulation but are unable to reach orgasm with a partner present. Cultural expectations and societal restrictions on women are also relevant. Nonorgastic women may be otherwise symptom-free or may experience frustration in a variety of ways, including such pelvic complaints as lower abdominal pain, itching, and vaginal discharge, as well as increased tension, irritability, and fatigue.

Inhibited male orgasm In inhibited male orgasm, also called *retarded ejaculation,* the man achieves climax during coitus with great difficulty, if at all. A man suffers from primary retarded ejaculation if he has never been able to ejaculate during coitus. The disorder is diagnosed as secondary if it develops after previous normal functioning (Table 21.1-13).

Some workers suggest that a differentiation should be made between orgasm and ejaculation. Certainly, inhibited orgasm must be differentiated from retrograde ejaculation, in which ejaculation occurs but the seminal fluid passes backward into the bladder. The latter condition always has an organic cause. Retrograde ejaculation can develop after genitourinary surgery and is also associated with medications that have anticholinergic side effects, such as the phenothiazines.

The incidence of inhibited male orgasm is much lower than that of premature ejaculation and impotence. Masters and Johnson reported only 3.8 percent in one group of 447 sex-dysfunction cases. This problem is more common among men with obsessive-compulsive disorders than among others. Inhibited male orgasm may have physiological causes and can occur after surgery of the genitourinary tract, such as prostatectomy. It may also be associated with Parkinson's disease and other neurological disorders involving the lumbar or sacral sections of the spinal cord. The antihypertensive drugs guanethidine monosulfate (Esimil) and methyldopa (Aldomet) have been implicated in retarded ejaculation. Phenothiazines have also been associated with the disorder. Transient retarded ejaculation may occur with excessive alcohol intake or with hyperglycemia, whether caused by drugs or by a pituitary adenoma. Strictly organic cases and problems that are symptomatic of other Axis I psychiatric syndromes are not to be included in this diagnosis.

TABLE 21.1-13
Diagnostic Criteria for Inhibited Male Orgasm

A. Persistent or recurrent delay in, or absence of, orgasm in a male following a normal sexual excitement phase during sexual activity that the clinician, taking into account the person's age, judges to be adequate in focus, intensity, and duration. This failure to achieve orgasm is usually restricted to an inability to reach orgasm in the vagina, with orgasm possible with other types of stimulation, such as masturbation.

B. Occurrence not exclusively during the course of another Axis I disorder (other than a sexual dysfunction), such as major depression.

Table from DSM-III-R *Diagnostic and Statistical Manual of Mental Disorders,* ed 3, revised. Copyright American Psychiatric Association, Washington, DC, 1987. Used with permission.

Primary inhibited male orgasm is indicative of more severe psychopathology. The man often comes from a rigid, puritanical background: He perceives sex as sinful and the genitals as dirty, and he may have conscious or unconscious incest wishes and guilt. There are usually difficulties with closeness that extend beyond the area of sexual relations.

In an ongoing relationship, secondary ejaculatory inhibition frequently reflects interpersonal difficulties. The disorder may be the man's way of coping with real or fantasized changes in the relationship. Those changes may include plans for a pregnancy about which the man is ambivalent, the loss of sexual attraction to the partner, or demands by the partner for greater commitment as expressed by sexual performance. In some men, the inability to ejaculate reflects unexpressed hostility toward women.

In a version of this dysfunction, some men experience partial inhibition of ejaculation. These men experience a slow dribbling of ejaculate (not related to age) rather than an ejaculatory spurt. They usually do not experience the pleasurable sensations of orgasm.

Premature ejaculation In *premature ejaculation,* the man recurrently achieves orgasm and ejaculation before he wishes to. There is no definite time frame within which to define the dysfunction. The diagnosis is made when the man regularly ejaculates before or immediately after entering the vagina or following minimal sexual stimulation. DSM-III-R advises the clinician to consider factors that affect duration of the excitement phase, such as age, novelty of the sexual partner, and the frequency and duration of coitus (Table 21.1-14). Masters and Johnson conceptualize the disorder in terms of the couple and consider a man a premature ejaculator if he cannot control ejaculation for a sufficient length of time during intravaginal containment to satisfy his partner in at least one-half of their episodes of coitus. This definition assumes that the female partner is capable of an orgastic response. As with the other dysfunctions, this disturbance is diagnosed only if it is not caused exclusively by organic factors or is not symptomatic of any other Axis I syndrome. No separate category of premature orgasm for women is included in DSM-III-R because of the absence of data on the subject. Also, the presence of a

TABLE 21.1-14
Diagnostic Criteria for Premature Ejaculation

Persistent or recurrent ejaculation with minimal sexual stimulation or before, upon, or shortly after penetration and before the person wishes it. The clinician must take into account factors that affect duration of the excitement phase, such as age, novelty of the sexual partner or situation, and frequency of sexual activity.

Table from DSM-III-R *Diagnostic and Statistical Manual of Mental Disorders,* ed 3, revised. Copyright American Psychiatric Association, Washington, DC, 1987. Used with permission.

refractory period in the man has obvious consequences that do not necessarily exist for the potentially multiorgasmic woman.

Premature ejaculation is more common today among college-educated men than among men with less education and is thought to be related to their concern for partner satisfaction. It is estimated that 30 percent of the male population have this dysfunction, and about 40 percent of men treated for sexual disorders have premature ejaculation as the chief complaint.

Difficulty in ejaculatory control may be associated with anxiety regarding the sex act or with unconscious fears about the vagina. It may also result from negative cultural conditioning. The man who has most of his early sexual contacts with prostitutes who demand that the sex act proceed quickly or in situations in which discovery would be embarrassing, such as in an apartment shared with roommates or in the parental home, may become conditioned to achieve orgasm rapidly. In ongoing relationships, the partner has been found to have great influence on the premature ejaculator. A stressful marriage exacerbates the disorder. The developmental background and dynamics found in this disorder and in impotence are similar.

SEXUAL PAIN DISORDERS

Dyspareunia *Dyspareunia* refers to recurrent and persistent pain during intercourse in either the man or the woman. In women, the dysfunction is related to and often coincides with vaginismus. Repeated episodes of vaginismus may lead to dyspareunia and vice versa, but in either case somatic causes must be ruled out. Dyspareunia should not be diagnosed as such when an organic basis for the pain is found, or when, in a woman, it is associated with vaginismus or with lack of lubrication (Table 21.1-15).

The true incidence of dyspareunia is unknown, but it has been estimated that 30 percent of surgical procedures on the female genital area result in temporary dyspareunia. Additionally, of women with this complaint who are seen in sex therapy clinics, 30 to 40 percent have pelvic pathology. Chronic pelvic pain is a more common complaint in women with a history of rape or childhood sexual abuse.

Organic abnormalities leading to dyspareunia and vaginismus include irritated or infected hymenal remnants, episiotomy scars, Bartholin's gland infection, various forms of vaginitis and cervicitis, endometriosis, and other pelvic disorders. Dyspareunia prior to coitus may occur as a concomitant of sexual excitement when the woman has an irritation of her external genitalia. The vasocongestion that is intrinsic to the excitement phase may result in increased sensitivity and discomfort in the affected area. Postcoital pain sometimes has been attributed to intense uterine contractions during orgasm in women with myomata or endometriosis.

The postmenopausal woman may develop dyspareunia resulting from thinning of the vaginal mucosa and lessened lubrication. Dynamic factors are usually considered causative, although situational factors probably account more for secondary dysfunctions. Painful coitus may result from tension

TABLE 21.1-15
Diagnostic Criteria for Dyspareunia

A. Recurrent or persistent genital pain in either a male or a female before, during, or after sexual intercourse.
B. The disturbance is not caused exclusively by lack of lubrication or by vaginismus.

Table from DSM-III-R *Diagnostic and Statistical Manual of Mental Disorders,* ed 3, revised. Copyright American Psychiatric Association, Washington, DC, 1987. Used with permission.

TABLE 21.1-16
Diagnostic Criteria for Vaginismus

A. Recurrent or persistent involuntary spasm of the musculature of the outer third of the vagina that interferes with coitus.
B. The disturbance is not caused exclusively by a physical disorder, and is not due to another Axis I disorder.

Table from DSM-III-R *Diagnostic and Statistical Manual of Mental Disorders,* ed 3, revised. Copyright American Psychiatric Association, Washington, DC, 1987. Used with permission.

and anxiety about the sex act that cause the woman to involuntarily tense her vaginal muscles. The pain is real and makes intercourse unbearable or unpleasant. The anticipation of further pain may cause the woman to avoid coitus altogether. If the partner proceeds with intercourse regardless of the woman's state of readiness, the condition is aggravated. Dyspareunia can also occur in men, but it is uncommon and is usually associated with an organic condition, such as Peyronie's disease, prostatitis, or gonorrheal or herpetic infections. Vasocongestion during sexual activity without orgasmic release also may lead to discomfort. Rarely, some men experience pain upon ejaculation. That pain results from an involuntary spasm of the perineal muscles that is due to psychological conflicts about the sex act or that occurs as a side effect of some antidepressant medications.

Vasginismus *Vaginismus* is an involuntary constriction of the outer one-third of the vagina that prevents penile insertion and intercourse. This response may be demonstrated during a gynecological examination when involuntary vaginal constriction prevents introduction of the speculum into the vagina. The diagnosis is not made if the dysfunction is caused exclusively by organic factors or if it is symptomatic of another Axis I psychiatric syndrome (Table 21.1-16). Vaginismus is less prevalent than anorgasmia. It most often afflicts highly educated women and those in the higher socioeconomic groups. A milder form of this dysfunction, where there is some degree of vaginal tightness that makes penile entry difficult, is experienced by a greater number of women on an intermittent or chronic basis.

The woman suffering from vaginismus may consciously wish to have coitus, but she unconsciously prevents penile entrance into her body. A sexual trauma, such as rape, may result in vaginismus. Women who have experienced pain with nonsexual bodily traumas, through accidents or because of illness or surgery, may become sensitized to the idea of penetration. Women with psychosexual conflicts may perceive the penis as a dangerous weapon. In some women, pain or the anticipation of pain at the first coital experience causes vaginismus. A strict religious upbringing that associates sex with sin is frequently noted in these cases. For others, there are problems in the dyadic relationship: If the woman feels emotionally abused by her partner, she may protest in this nonverbal fashion.

TABLE 21.1-17
Diagnostic Criteria for Sexual Disorder Not Otherwise Specified

Sexual disorders that are not classifiable in any of the previous categories. In rare instances, this category may be used concurrently with one of the specific diagnoses when both are necessary to explain or describe the clinical disturbance.

Examples:
(1) Marked feelings of inadequacy concerning body habitus, size and shape of sex organs, sexual performance, or other traits related to self-imposed standards of masculinity or femininity
(2) Distress about a pattern of repeated sexual conquests or other forms of nonparaphilic sexual addiction, involving a succession of people who exist only as things to be used
(3) Persistent and marked distress about one's sexual orientation

Table from DSM-III-R *Diagnostic and Statistical Manual of Mental Disorders,* ed 3, revised. Copyright American Psychiatric Association, Washington, DC, 1987. Used with permission.

SEXUAL DISORDER NOT OTHERWISE SPECIFIED

This category is for psychosexual dysfunctions that cannot be classified under the nine categories described above (Table 21.1-17). Included as an example in DSM-III-R is genital pain during masturbation. Other examples are persons who experience the physiological components of sexual excitement and orgasm but report no erotic sensation or even anesthesia. Women with conditions analogous to premature ejaculation in the man should also be classified here. Another dysfunction of this type would be the male experience of orgasm with a flaccid penis. The orgastic female who desires but has not experienced multiple orgasms can be classified under this heading as well. Also, disorders of excessive rather than inhibited function, such as compulsive masturbation, might be diagnosed under atypical dysfunctions. There are other sexual practices, which are classified in DSM-III-R under sexual disorders and sexual masochism. They involve behaviors that attempt to enhance sexual arousal by oxygen deprivation (hypoxyphilia).

Atypical dysfunctions also might be used to cover complaints engendered by couple, rather than individual, dysfunction. An example is a couple of whom one partner prefers morning sex and one functions more readily at night; another example is a couple with unequal frequencies of desire. Also, a couple who have an unconsummated marriage might be categorized here. The couple involved in an unconsummated marriage have never had coitus and are typically uninformed and inhibited about sexuality. Their feelings of guilt, shame, or inadequacy are only increased by their problem, and they are conflicted by a need to seek help and by a need to conceal their difficulty. Couples present with the problem after having been married several months or several years. The man in the couple may require the concomitant diagnosis of erectile disorder and the woman may suffer from vaginismus.

Other atypical disorders are found in persons who have one or more sexual fantasies about which they obsess, feel guilty, or are otherwise dysphoric. As indicated in Table 21.1-18, however, the range of common sexual fantasies is broad. Masturbatory practices have resulted in what has been called autoerotic asphyxiation. This practice involves masturbating while hanging oneself by the neck to heighten erotic sensations and the intensity of orgasm. Although such persons release themselves from the noose after orgasm, an estimated 500 to 1,000 persons per year unwittingly kill themselves by hanging. Most persons indulging in this practice are male; transvestism is often associated with the habit, and the majority of deaths occur among adolescents. Such masochistic practices are usually associated with severe mental disorders, such as schizophrenia and mood disorders.

TABLE 21.1-18
Common Sexual Fantasies*†

Men	*Women*
Heterosexual	
Replacement of established partner	Replacement of established partner
Forced sexual encounters with woman	Forced sexual encounters with man
Observing sexual activity	Observing sexual activity
Sexual encounters with man	Idyllic encounters with unknown man
Group sex	Sexual encounters with woman
Homosexual	
Images of male anatomy	Forced sexual encounters with women
Forced sexual encounters with men	Idyllic encounters with established partner
Sexual encounters with women	Sexual encounters with man
Idyllic enounters with unknown men	Memories of past sexual experiences
Group sex	Sadistic imagery

*Most frequent listed on order of occurrence.
†Adapted from Masters W, Schwartz M: The Masters and Johnson treatment program for dissatisfied homosexual men. Amer J Psychiat *141:* 173, 1984, with permission. (Courtesy of The New York Times.)

TREATMENT

Various corrective therapies are now used to treat sexual dysfunctions. Psychiatrists are eminently well qualified to incorporate the techniques of sex therapy into their practices. This practice simply follows the general history of psychiatry, which has modified and absorbed any number of specialized techniques into its treatment repertoire. Where the dysfunction occurs alone, an unmodified sex therapy approach seems to be the treatment of choice. For patients with accompanying personality disorders or physical conditions, it is but one of many techniques to be considered.

In addition to making the determination of which type of therapy to use, the clinician must evaluate whether or not the disorder has a physiological cause. It is assumed that prior to entering psychotherapy, the patient will have had a thorough medical evaluation, including a medical history, physical examination, and appropriate laboratory studies when necessary. If an organic cause for the disorder is found, treatment should be directed toward ameliorating the physical cause of the dysfunction.

Prior to 1970, the most common treatment of psychosexual dysfunction was individual psychotherapy. Classic psychodynamic theory considers sexual inadequacy to have its roots in early developmental conflicts, and the sexual disorder is treated as part of a more pervasive emotional disturbance. Treatment focuses on the exploration of unconscious conflicts, motivation, fantasy, and various interpersonal difficulties. One of the assumptions of therapy is that the removal of the conflicts will allow the sexual impulse to become structurally acceptable to the patient's ego and thereby find appropriate means of satisfaction in the environment. Unfortunately, the symptom of sexual dysfunction frequently becomes secondarily autonomous and continues to persist when other problems evolving from the patient's pathology have been resolved. The addition of behavioral techniques is often necessary to cure the sexual problem.

Four treatment modalities that emphasize behavioral approaches—dual-sex therapy, hypnotherapy, behavior therapy, and group therapy—will be discussed, as well as analytically oriented sex therapy, which integrates the tenets of psychoanalysis with behavioral techniques. Organic therapies will also be reviewed.

DUAL-SEX THERAPY The theoretical basis of the dual-sex therapy approach is the concept of the marital unit or dyad as the object of therapy. The method of dual-sex therapy was originated and developed by Masters and Johnson. In dual-sex therapy, there is no acceptance of the idea of a sick half of a patient couple. Both are involved in a relationship in which there is sexual distress, and both, therefore, must participate in the therapy program.

The sexual problem often reflects other areas of disharmony or misunderstanding in the marriage. The marital relationship as a whole is treated, with emphasis on sexual functioning as a part of that relationship. Improved communication in sexual and nonsexual areas is a specific goal of treatment. Psychological and physiological aspects of sexual functioning are discussed, and an educative attitude is used. Suggestions are made for specific sexual activity, and those suggestions are followed in the privacy of the couple's home.

Initial histories are taken to determine suitability for this type of treatment. When there is evidence of major underlying psychopathology, further psychiatric evaluation is suggested, and participation in the program may be deferred until the patient seems better able to benefit from it. Concurrent psychotherapy with a psychiatrist while participating in dual-sex therapy is sometimes recommended.

Each patient is interviewed individually early in the course of treatment. A complete sexual history is obtained, and that history is later reflected back to the couple, with the aim of helping them understand their present problem. The individual sessions also enable the therapist to understand the patients' life-style and to make suggestions that fit into that life-style.

Behavioral exercises Treatment is short term and is behaviorally oriented. Specific exercises are prescribed for the couple to help them with their particular problem. Sexual dysfunction often involves a fear of inadequate performance. The couples are therefore specifically prohibited from any sexual play other than that prescribed by the therapist. Initially, intercourse is interdicted, and couples learn to give and receive bodily pleasure without the pressure of performance. Beginning exercises usually focus on heightening sensory awareness to touch, sight, sound, and smell.

During these exercises, which are called *sensate focus exercises,* the couple is given much reinforcement to lessen their anxiety. The patients are urged to use fantasies to distract them from obsessive concerns about performance, which is termed "spectatoring." The needs of both the dysfunctional and the nondysfunctional partner are considered. If either partner becomes sexually excited by the exercises, the other is encouraged to bring him or her to orgasm by manual or oral means. This procedure is important to keep the nondysfunctional partner from sabotaging the treatment. Open communication between the partners is urged, and the expression of mutual needs is encouraged. Resistances, such as claims of fatigue or not enough time to complete the exercises, are common and must be dealt with by the therapist. Genital stimulation is eventually added to general body stimulation. The couple are instructed sequentially to try various positions for intercourse, without necessarily completing the act, and to use varieties of stimulating techniques before they are instructed to proceed with intercourse.

The specific exercises vary with differing presenting complaints, and special techniques are used to treat the various dysfunctions. In cases of vaginismus, for instance, the woman is advised to dilate her vaginal opening with her fingers or with size-graduated vaginal dilators as part of the therapy.

In cases of premature ejaculation, an exercise known as the *squeeze technique* is used to raise the threshold of penile excitability. In that exercise the man or the woman stimulates the erect penis until the earliest sensations of impending orgasm and ejaculation are felt. Penile stimulation is then stopped abruptly, and the coronal ridge of the penis is forcibly squeezed for several seconds. The technique is repeated several times. A variation is the *stop-start technique* in which stimulation is interrupted for several seconds but no squeeze is applied. Masturbation to the point of imminent orgasm raises the threshold of excitability to a more tolerant stimulation level. Communication between the partners is improved, because the man must let his partner know the degree of his sexual excitement so that she can squeeze the penis before the ejaculatory process has started. Sex therapy has been most successful in the treatment of premature ejaculation.

A man with inhibited desire or erectile disorder is sometimes told to masturbate to demonstrate that full erection and ejaculation are possible. In cases of primary anorgasmia, the woman is directed to masturbate, sometimes using a vibrator. Kegel's exercises to strengthen the pubococcygeal muscles may be introduced; that is, the woman is instructed to contract her vagina voluntarily. The woman is also encouraged to contract her abdominal and perineal muscles during masturbation and coitus. When a man is impotent, the woman may be instructed to stimulate or tease his penis. This same technique is used with men who suffer from retarded ejaculation, and, in this case, stimulation sometimes involves a vibrator. Retarded ejaculation is managed by extravaginal ejaculation initially and gradual vaginal entry after stimulation to the point of near ejaculation.

Treatment goals The overall goal of treatment always is to initiate an educational process, to diminish the fears of performance felt by both sexes, and to facilitate communication within the marital unit in sexual and nonsexual areas. Therapy sessions follow each new exercise period, and problems and satisfactions, both sexual and in other areas of the couple's lives, are discussed. Specific instructions and the introduction of new exercises geared to the individual couple's progress are reviewed in each session. Gradually, the couple gains confidence and learns or relearns to communicate verbally and sexually. Dual-sex therapy is most effective when the sexual dysfunction exists apart from other psychopathology.

HYPNOTHERAPY Hypnotherapists focus specifically on the anxiety-producing symptom—that is, the particular sexual dysfunction. The successful use of hypnosis enables the patient to gain control over the symptom that has been lowering self-esteem and disrupting psychological homeostasis. The cooperation of the patient is first obtained and encouraged during a series of nonhypnotic sessions with the therapist. These discussions permit the development of a secure doctor-patient relationship, a sense of physical and psychological comfort on the part of the patient, and the establishment of mutually desired treatment goals. During this time, the therapist assesses the patient's capacity for the trance experience. The nonhypnotic sessions also permit the clinician to take a careful psychiatric history and do a Mental Status Examination before beginning hypnotherapy. The focus of treatment is on symptom removal and attitude alteration. In a trance state, the patient is able to entertain ideas incongruent with his or her usual (nonhypnotized) perceptions of reality. The patient is instructed in developing alternative means of dealing with the anxiety-provoking situation, which is the sexual encounter.

For example, a woman suffering from vaginismus is given the posthypnotic suggestion that she will not feel pain during intercourse and that she will be able to relax the muscles surrounding her vagina. If compliance with the suggestion is successful, the patient is able to deal with the anxiety produced by the sex act. She is also taught new attitudes, such as being entitled to sexual pleasure. Under hypnosis her fear or anger at sexual contact can be examined, and she learns how her emotions are expressed by involuntary spasms of her vagina.

Recent research indicates that patients respond particularly well to the use of self-hypnosis and to indirect suggestion. These techniques allow them to retain a greater sense of control over their situation. Typically, the patient is instructed to conjure up images and develop ideas that are antithetical to their dysfunctional responses. For example, a woman with an arousal disorder may first agree to concentrate on imagery that causes her to salivate. Then she is told that just as she has made her mouth water by focusing on stimulating images she can affect the lubricating response of her vagina by focusing on images she finds erotic or romantic. At the same time, the therapist helps her deal with her anxieties about a positive sexual response. Patients are also taught relaxing techniques to use on themselves before sexual relations. With those methods to alleviate anxiety, the physiological responses to sexual stimulation can more readily result in pleasurable excitation and discharge. Hypnosis may be added to a basic individual psychotherapy program to accelerate the impact of psychotherapeutic intervention.

BEHAVIOR THERAPY Behavior therapists assume that sexual dysfunction is learned maladaptive behavior. Behavioral approaches were initially designed for the treatment of phobias. In cases of sexual dysfunction, the therapist sees the patient as phobic of sexual interaction. Using traditional techniques, the therapist sets up a hierarchy of anxiety-provoking situations for the patient, ranging from the least threatening to the most threatening situation. Mild anxiety may be experienced at the thought of kissing, and massive anxiety may be felt when imagining penile penetration. The behavior therapist enables the patient to master the anxiety through a standard program of systematic desensitization. The program is designed to inhibit the learned anxious response by encouraging behaviors antithetical to anxiety. The patient first deals with the least anxiety-producing situation in fantasy and progresses by steps to the greatest anxiety-producing situation. Medication, hypnosis, or special training in deep-muscle relaxation is sometimes used to help with the initial mastery of anxiety.

Assertiveness training is also used and is helpful in teaching the patient to express his or her sexual needs openly and without fear. Exercises in assertiveness are given in conjunction with sex therapy, and the patient is encouraged both to make sexual requests and to refuse to comply with requests perceived as unreasonable. Sexual exercises may be prescribed for the patient to perform at home, and a hierarchy may be established starting with those activities that have proved most pleasurable and successful in the past.

One treatment variation involves the participation of the patient's sexual partner in the desensitization program. The partner, rather than the therapist, presents the hierarchical items to the patient. In such situations, a cooperative partner is necessary to help the patient carry gains made during treatment sessions to sexual activity at home.

Brady found behavior therapy techniques particularly effective in the treatment of women with severe inhibition of excitement and orgasm when such feelings were accompanied by strong feelings of anxiety, anger, or disgust.

GROUP THERAPY Methods of group therapy have been used to examine both intrapsychic and interpersonal problems in patients with sexual disorders. The therapy group provides a strong support system for a patient who feels ashamed, anxious, or guilty about a particular sexual problem. It is a useful forum in which to counteract sexual myths, correct misconceptions, and provide accurate information regarding sexual anatomy, physiology, and varieties of behavior.

Groups for the treatment of sexual disorders can be organized in several ways. Members may all share the same problem, such as premature ejaculation; members may all be of the same sex with different sexual problems; or groups may be composed of both men and women who are experiencing different sexual problems. Group therapy may be an adjunct to other forms of therapy or the prime mode of treatment. Groups organized to cure a particular dysfunction are usually behavioral in approach. For example, patients suffering from anorgasmia may participate with others suffering from the same problem in a short-term, intensive group experience. Sexual histories, feelings of inadequacy, and concerns about body image are shared. Specific physiological information, sometimes with the aid of audiovisual materials, is presented to the group members. Members are given homework assignments. For instance, they may be instructed to masturbate. A combination of group support and group pressure helps some of the participants complete assignments they might otherwise want to avoid. As the short-term group process nears termination, members are encouraged to talk about their experiences with their partners.

Groups have also been effective when composed of sexually dysfunctional married couples. The group provides the opportunity to gather accurate information, provides consensual validation of individual preferences, and enhances self-esteem and self-acceptance. Techniques such as role playing and psychodrama may be used in treatment. Such groups are not indicated for couples when one partner is uncooperative, when a patient is suffering from a severe depression or psychosis, when there is a strong repugnance for explicit sexual audiovisual material, or when there is a strong fear of groups.

ANALYTICALLY ORIENTED SEX THERAPY One of the most effective treatment modalities is the use of sex therapy integrated with psychodynamic and psychoanalytically oriented psychotherapy. The addition of psychodynamic conceptualizations to the behavioral techniques used to treat sexual dysfunctions allows for the treatment of patients with sex disorders associated with other psychopathology. Also, this therapy is appropriate for patients suffering from hypoactive desire disorders. Insight-oriented therapy helps them deal with problems in their interpersonal relationships or with conflicts on an intrapsychic level that frequently are at the root of the problem.

The themes and dynamics that emerge in patients in analytically oriented sex therapy are the same as those seen in psychoanalytic therapy, such as relevant dreams, fear of punishment, aggressive feelings, difficulty with trusting the partner, fear of intimacy, oedipal feelings, and fear of genital mutilation.

A 34-year-old widow presented for therapy with a chief complaint of vaginismus. Her marriage of 3 years, which had been unconsummated, ended when her husband was killed in a car accident. Approximately 1 year after she lost her husband, the patient became involved with a married man. She was very attracted to him and became highly aroused during their sexual encounters. Although she could reach orgasm through manual or oral stimulation, she could not tolerate penetration. She was motivated to seek help for her problem—although she never considered therapy when she was married, in spite of her husband's requests to do so—because she felt sure her lover would leave his wife for her if they could have a more complete sexual experience together.

The patient's vaginismus was partly the result of unresolved developmental conflicts. Her parents had been loving but rigid people who came from different socioeconomic backgrounds. Their values often conflicted and they frequently fought over their daughter as she entered adolescence: the mother insisted that she take an academic course in high school preparatory for college, whereas the father pushed a "more practical" business program. The patient sided with her mother and felt that her father, whom she had always perceived as cold, became more distant than before. Some of her difficulties were due to unresolved oedipal problems: Both her husband and her lover were more than 20 years older than she was, and her lover, reflecting her parental situation, was married to a woman who was more successful than he was. In addition, she had identified with some of her mother's negative feelings about men. The mother had once expressed to the patient the hope that she would be "spared" marriage. Her vaginismus protected the patient from the closeness with men that she consciously wanted but that she unconsciously perceived as hurtful and dangerous.

Another patient, a 56-year-old man, came for treatment because of an erectile disorder. In general, he was better able to function in extramarital affairs than in his marriage. Although he loved his wife and felt that she was an attractive woman, he believed that she was not interested in sex. He was rarely able to achieve an erection with her and he gradually stopped approaching her sexually. In fact, his wife felt deprived by their lack of sexual relations and indulged in frequent masturbation.

The patient had been a sickly child, with a mother he described as devoted but smothering. He remembered her cuddling him in bed until he was 8 years old, and he felt that she was inappropriately affectionate in general; "she embarrassed me." At the same time, he remembered his father as an "earthy" man and had a childhood recollection of hearing his mother tell the father, "How could you, how could you?" The patient believed that this had been his mother's response to a sexual overture or act. In part, his disorder derived from his unconscious oedipal associations to his wife which made her taboo for him as a sex partner. The women he responded to had to be blatantly sexual and signal their acceptance of him before he would risk an advance. Therapy involved both individual sessions with the patient and joint sessions with him and his wife. Communication, which had been strained partly because of the sexual distance between them, was encouraged, and a behavioral approach was used to reestablish some physical interaction. Individual work focused on his deeper psychological problems.

The dynamics and the emotional difficulties evident in these vignettes are those seen every day by the psychiatrist. Psychiatrists are readily able to absorb the techniques of sex therapy into their treatment armamentarium, just as they have modified and absorbed any number of specialized techniques from classic analytic dynamic formulations to the use of pharmacotherapy, group therapy techniques, and behavioral and other directive modalities.

The combined approach of analytically oriented sex therapy is used by the general psychiatrist, who carefully judges the optimal timing of sex therapy and the ability of patients to tolerate the directive approach that focuses on their sexual difficulties.

ORGANIC TREATMENT METHODS Organic forms of treatment, including pharmacotherapy and surgical treatment, may have some application in specific cases of sexual disorder. Coexisting physical and psychiatric problems should receive appropriate treatment as necessary.

Pharmacotherapy A variety of drugs have been explored in the treatment of sexual dysfunction. Intravenous methohexital sodium (Brevital) has been used in desensitization therapy. Antianxiety agents may have some application in tense patients, although these drugs can also interfere with the sexual response. Bromocriptine (Parlodel), a dopamine agonist, has been found to increase desire in some women suffering from hyperprolactinemia. Sometimes the side effects of such drugs as thioridazine (Mellaril), haloperidol (Haldol), lorazepam (Ativan), the MAO inhibitors, and the tricyclic antidepressants are used to prolong the sexual response in conditions, such as premature ejaculation. The use of tricyclics has also been advocated in the treatment of patients who are phobic of sex and in patients with a post-traumatic stress disorder following rape. The risks of taking such medications must be carefully weighed against the possible benefits they provide, particularly when the sexual problems may respond to nonpharmacological means.

A number of substances have popular standing as aphrodisiacs. Examples of those are ginseng root and yohimbine. However, studies have not confirmed that they have any aphrodisiac properties beyond a placebo effect. Also, many recreational drugs, including cocaine, amphetamines, alcohol, and marijuana are considered enhancers of sexual performance. Although they may provide the user with an initial benefit because of their tranquilizing, disinhibiting, or mood-elevating effects, consistent or prolonged use of any of those substances impairs sexual functioning.

A variety of injectable vasoactive substances have been studied for use in cases of erectile dysfunction. They produce a transient increase in penile blood flow, which allows the patient to become tumescent or gain an erection. The physician usually administers a test dose of the drug and if the patient responds favorably he is then taught to inject himself. The drugs are injected into the cavernosa of the penis. The substance most frequently used in this country is a mixture of Papaverine HCL and phentolamine mesylate. However, there are possible hazardous sequelae to its use, including priapism and sclerosis of the small veins of the penis. Another substance being tried is vasoactive intestinal polypeptide. Some researchers speculate that this substance, which has been found in the hypothalamus and the female genital organs, is an essential factor in male and female arousal. In Europe, phenoxybenzamine (Dibenzyline) is used to produce erections. Serious side effects include priapism and pain accompanying the injection, and the drug is not allowed as a therapy in the United States. Gonadotropin-releasing hormone is also used in Europe, but as an inhalant. It is used both to correct impotence and increase desire. However, studies on its effectiveness are still in progress.

Surgical treatment MALE PROSTHESIS Surgical treatment is even more rarely advocated, but improved penile prosthetic devices are available for men with inadequate erectile response who are resistant to other treatment methods or who have organically caused deficiencies. There are two main types of prostheses: a semirigid rod prosthesis that produces a permanent erection that can be positioned close to the body for concealment, and an inflatable type that is implanted together with its own reservoir and pump for inflation and deflation. The latter type is designed to mimic normal physiological functioning. Placement of a penile prosthesis in a male who has lost the ability to ejaculate or to have an orgasm as a result of organic causes will not enable him to recover those functions. Men with prosthetic devices have generally reported satisfaction with their subsequent sexual functioning. Their wives, however, report much less satisfaction than do the men. Presurgical counseling is strongly recommended so that the couple has a realistic expectation of what the prosthesis can do for their sex lives. Postsurgical counseling may also be necessary to help the couple adapt to their rediscovered ability to have intercourse. They may experience a high level of anxiety if their sex life had been inactive for a prolonged period of time before surgery. Prosthetic devices have been associated with severe side effects in some cases, including perforation, infection, urinary retention, and persistent pain.

Some European physicians are attempting revascularization of the penis as a direct approach to treating erectile dysfunction resulting from vascular disorders. There are limited reports of prolonged success with this technique. Another organic treatment that is being studied is electrostimulation to the base of the penis. This technique is being tested as a treatment for erectile disorders. Initial reports indicate minimal physical discomfort on the part of patients subjected to the therapy. However, response to treatment is inconsistent, and a problem exists in terms of maintaining erections. At the present time, this treatment seems to have no benefits.

FEMALE PROCEDURES Surgical approaches to female dysfunctions include hymenectomy in the case of dyspareunia in an unconsummated marriage, vaginoplasty in multiparous women complaining of lessened vaginal sensations, or "freeing" of clitoral adhesions in women with inhibited excitement. Such surgical treatments have not been carefully studied and should be considered with great caution.

RESULTS OF TREATMENT The reported effectiveness of various treatment methods for problems of sexual dysfunction varies from study to study. Demonstrating the effectiveness of traditional outpatient psychotherapy is just as difficult when therapy is oriented to sexual problems as it is in general. In some cases, the patient improves in all areas except the sexual area. Unfortunately, the more severe the psychopathology associated with a problem of long duration, the more adverse the outcome is likely to be.

The more difficult treatment cases involve couples with severe marital discord. Cases with problems of fear of intimacy, excessive dependency, or excessive hostility are also complex. Other challenges are posed by patients with lack of desire, impulse disorders, unresolved homosexual conflicts, or fetishistic defenses. Patients phobic of sex also present treatment difficulties.

When behavioral approaches are used, empirical criteria that are supposed to predict outcome are more easily isolated. Using these criteria, for instance, it appears that couples who regularly practice assigned exercises have a much greater likelihood of successful outcome than do more resistant couples or couples whose interaction involves sadomasochistic or depressive features or mechanisms of blame and projection. Flexibility of attitude is also a positive prognostic factor. Overall, younger couples tend to complete sex therapy more often than do older couples. Those couples whose interactional difficulties center on their sex problems, such as inhibition, frustration, or fear of performance failure, are also likely to respond well to therapy.

Masters and Johnson have reported positive results for their dual-sex therapy approach. They have studied the failure rates of their patients; failure is defined as the failure to initiate reversal of the basic symptom of the presenting dysfunction. They compare initial failure rates with 5-year follow-up findings for the same couples. Although some have criticized their definition of the percentage of presumed successes, other studies have confirmed the effectiveness of their approach. The use of one therapist, however, seems to be nearly as effective as the male-female therapy team that Masters and Johnson use.

In general, methods that have proved effective singly or in combination include training in behavioral-sexual skills, systematic desensitization, directive marital counseling, traditional psychodynamic approaches, and group therapy. Although treating a couple for sexual dysfunctions is the mode preferred by most workers, treatment of individuals has also been successful.

REFERENCES

Araoz D L: Uses of hypnosis in the treatment of psychogenic sexual dysfunctions. Psychiat Ann *16:* 2, 102, 1986.

Brady J P: Behavior therapy and sex therapy. Amer J Psychiat *133:* 896, 1976.

Chessick R D: Thirty unresolved psychodynamic questions pertaining to feminine psychology. Amer J Psychother *42:* 86, 1988.

Diego B L, Magni G: Sexual side effects of anti-depressants. Psychosomatics *24:* 12, 1983.

Furlow W L: Prevalence of impotence in the United States. Med Aspects Human Sex: 1985.

Herman J, LoPiccolo J: Clinical outcome of sex therapy. Arch Gen Psychiat *40:* 443, 1983.

Koppelman M, Parry B L, Hamilton J A, Alogna S W, Loreaux P L: Effect of bromocriptine on affect and libido in hyperprolactinemia. Amer J Psychiat *144:* 1037, 1987.

Kegeles S M, Adler N E, Irwin C E: Sexually active adolescents and condoms: Changes over one year in knowledge, attitudes and use. Amer J Publ Health *78:* 460, 1988.

LoPiccolo J, Lobitz W: The role of masturbation in the treatment of sexual dysfunction. Arch Sex Behav *2:* 163, 1972.

Masters W H, Johnson V E: *Human Sexual Response*. Little, Brown, Boston, 1970.

Masters W H, Johnson V E: *Human Sexual Inadequacy*. Little, Brown, Boston, 1970.

Nunberg G H, Levine P E: Spontaneous remission of MAOI-induced anorgasmia. Amer J Psychiat *144:* 805, 1987.

Offit A K: *The Sexual Self*. Lippincott, Philadelphia, 1977.

Ottesen B: Vasoactive intestinal polypeptide as a neurotransmitter in the female genital tract. Amer J Obstet Gynec *147:* 208, 1983.

Sadock V A: The treatment of psychosexual dysfunctions: An overview. In *Psychiatry 1982. The American Psychiatric Association Annual Review,* L Grinspoon, editor. American Psychiatric Press, Washington, DC, 1982.

Sadock V A: Group psychotherapy of psychosexual dysfunctions. In *Comprehensive Group Psychotherapy,* H I Kaplan, B J Sadock, editors. Williams & Wilkins, Baltimore, 1983.

Segraves R T: Female orgasm and psychiatric drugs. J Sex Educ Ther *11:* 69, 1985.

Semans J H: Premature ejaculation: A new approach. South Med J *49:* 353, 1956.

Shrainer-Engel P, Schiavi R: Lifetime psychopathology in individuals with low sexual desire. J Nerv Ment Dis *174:* 646, 1986.

Small J G, Small I F: Psychosexual dysfunctions. In *Comprehensive Textbook of Psychiatry,* H I Kaplan, A M Freedman, B J Sadock, editors, ed 3, p 1783. Williams & Wilkins, Baltimore, 1980.

Thase M, Reynolds C, Glanz L, Jennings J R, Sewitz D E, Kupper D J, Frank E: Nocturnal penile tumescence in depressed men. Amer J Psychiat *144:* 89, 1987.
Wise N T: Sexual dysfunctions in the medically ill. Psychosomatics *24:* 9, 1982.
Zorgniotto A W, Lefleur R S: Autoinjection of corpus cavernosium with vasoactive drug combination for vasculogenic impotence. J Urol *133:* 39, 1985.

21.2 GENDER IDENTITY DISORDERS OF CHILDHOOD, ADOLESCENCE, AND ADULTHOOD

STEPHEN B. LEVINE, M.D.

INTRODUCTION

Prior to an operation performed in Denmark in 1952, which enabled a soldier to return to the United States as Christine Jorgensen, the medical profession paid almost no attention to gender identity problems. A notable exception was Harry Benjamin (1885–1986), an American endocrinologist who was known among the hidden cross-gender subculture as a trustworthy source of hormones and pre- and postsurgical counsel. The Jorgensen case, which remained a media sensation for months, stimulated a limited medical, surgical, and psychiatric involvement with the range of problems that came to be known as transsexualism. Now these problems are recognized as extreme pathologies of sexual identity development.

A VOCABULARY OF SEXUAL IDENTITY

Impairments in sexual identity development generate three constellations of interconnected problems: the gender identity disorders, variations in orientation, and the paraphilias. Of these, the gender disorders have the most dramatic impact on psychological experience. Although these curiosities have been known anecdotally since antiquity, they have only recently been formally recognized as psychiatric disorders.

Understanding the gender identity disorders requires an appreciation of the complexities of sexual identity. To avoid confusion in thinking about sexual identity it should be recalled that the term "sex" refers only to anatomical and physiological phenomena. The three components of sexual identity are gender identity, orientation, and intention. Each component has both a subjective, or psychological, aspect and an objective, or behavioral, aspect. *Gender identity* is the psychological experience of the self as male or female, masculine or feminine; *gender role* is its behavioral aspect. The subjective aspect of orientation refers to the sex of those whose images produce attraction and arousal; this aspect is properly described as heteroerotic, homoerotic, bierotic, or anerotic. *Behavioral orientation,* which refers to the sex of one's actual partners, may be described as heterosexual, homosexual, bisexual, or asexual. *Intention*—that is, what individuals want to do sexually with a partner or have done to them—has a subjective aspect involving fantasies, attractions, and urges, and a behavioral aspect involving actual sexual behaviors. "Intention" is a new term that conveys what Freud meant by the aim of the sexual instinct. The *paraphilias,* which are pathological intentions, may be confined to the subjective realm of urges and masturbation fantasies or may be acted on sexually with a partner (Table 21.2-1).

The other complexities of sexual identity include the following: It evolves during the life cycle (occasionally with surprising outcomes); its subjective and objective aspects do not always correspond; its determinants have not been firmly established scientifically; and its pathologies have a tendency to assume different forms over the life cycle.

NOSOLOGY

Clinicians are alerted to the gender identity disorders by patients who verbalize or demonstrate discomfort with living as members of their own sex. The child, adolescent, or adult with a gender disorder always says, in some fashion, "My gender identity does not match my sex." Clinicians ascertain the duration and degree of the cross-gender identification and cross-gender role behavior—for example, Does the man sit to urinate? Does the woman bind her breasts? In doing so, they confront the patients' conceptions of what can or should be done about their failure to develop an anatomically congruent gender identity.

EVOLUTION OF TRANSSEXUALISM NOSOLOGIES

The nosologies of transsexualism, which have always focused more on males, have evolved over three decades. The earliest systems were dominated by the need to identify candidates for sex reassignment surgery (SRS). The diagnosis of true transsexual was equated with a good surgical candidate, and was to be carefully distinguished from varieties of transvestite and stigmatized effeminate homosexual—diagnoses that were considered poor indications for SRS. Although conceptually clear, this schema's utility was limited for several reasons: Many patients did not fit any of these diagnoses; factors other than diagnosis were used for surgical selection; and it was discovered that some true transsexuals had lied to meet the diagnostic criteria. Attempts were then made to distinguish patients with lifelong cross-gender role behavior (i.e., the primary transsexuals) from those with intensification of cross-gender role behavior after living in the anatomically congruent gender role (i.e., the secondary transsexuals). This basis of surgical selection was abandoned because secondary

TABLE 21.2-1
Components of Sexual Identity

Component	*Subjective Aspect*	*Behavioral Aspect*	*Major Form of Pathology*
Gender identity	Gender identity	Gender role	Transsexualism
Orientation	Erotic orientation	Sexual orientation	Ego-dystonic homosexuality
Intention	Erotic intention	Sexual intention	Paraphilia

transsexuals often claimed to have strong lifelong subjective cross-gender identifications. Confusion as to the relative importance of subjective gender identity and objective gender role ensued. This schema did, however, clarify the existence of diverse pathways to the desire for SRS.

During the frustrating search for a useful nosology, the diagnosis of gender dysphoria syndrome became used as a means of referring to males and females who were preoccupied with bodily and gender role change as a solution to discomfort with gender identity. This term continues to be used as a shorthand means of referring to a gender problem.

The third edition of the American Psychiatric Association's *Diagnostic and Statistical Manual of Mental Disorders* (DSM-III) was the first psychiatric nosology to include gender identity disorders. Its requirement to look for an Axis II diagnosis ended the preoccupation with the gender disturbance in isolation from the underlying personality. Axis II diagnoses among gender-disturbed adolescents and adults are often conspicuous; the most common is borderline personality organization. DSM-III directed clinicians not to diagnose transsexualism in the face of schizophrenia or an intersex condition. They were to ascertain that the sense of discomfort and inappropriateness about anatomical sex had been present for 2 years and was associated with the wish to be rid of the genitals (and breasts in females). It provided a separate diagnosis for children (gender identity disorder of childhood) and a residual category for adults and children (atypical gender identity disorder).

DSM-III-R DIAGNOSES The revised edition of DSM-III (DSM-III-R) provides three diagnoses for postpubertal males and females with severe gender identity disorders: transsexualism; gender identity disorder of adolescence or adulthood, nontranssexual type (GIDAANT); and gender identity disorder not otherwise specified. The first two diagnoses share two criteria: the persistent discomfort and sense of inappropriateness about one's assigned gender, and either cross-living in the opposite gender role or fantasies of doing so. They are distinguished on the basis of consistent 2-year preoccupation with ridding oneself of primary and secondary sex characteristics and acquiring those of the other sex. Individuals with a persistent preoccupation qualify for transsexualism (Table 21.2-2); cases of individuals without it are labeled gender identity disorder of adolescence or adulthood, nontranssexual type (Table 21.2-3). DSM-III-R asks that the patient's orientation be specified as either asexual, homosexual, heterosexual, or unspecified. Gender identity disorder not otherwise specified is available for those who do not fit into the other diagnoses (Table 21.2-4). DSM-III-R no longer uses schizophrenia or chromosomal or intersex conditions as exclusionary criteria; it recognizes, for example, that people can be both schizophrenic or intersexed and transsexual.

In making these diagnoses, clinicians must not be swayed by their notion of the appropriate treatment: SRS or psychotherapy, or the solution the patient may have already found (e.g., cross-gender living, self-administration of hormones). DSM-III-R diagnoses refer to the persistence of subjective, intrapsychic distress, and fantasies of bodily transformation; they do not include matters, such as the quality of passing in the opposite gender role or the threat of suicide if not granted hormones. DSM-III-R is neither a foolproof guide to surgical selection nor a means of discriminating among etiological influences. It is an attempt to order transgenderal phenomena rationally that awaits validation.

The following is a case example of transsexualism:

Tim, a 33-year-old separated engineer who was estranged from his 10-year-old daughter, sought help about his female essence. "I want to talk about living as a female, taking hormones, and having surgery." This masculine-appearing, obsessive man with shoulder length hair, long fingernails, and raw skin from incessant handwashing claimed to be forever uncomfortable in his male role and with his genital anatomy. He reported cross-dressing since age 4 and masturbating in female undergarments since age 11. He strongly envied his sister's ability to dress up in fancy clothes, while the best he could do was pretend he was a girl by pulling his penis high on his abdomen or toward his buttocks and rubbing himself to orgasm through his panties. During his army and college years his opportunities to cross-dress were limited. He married, impregnated his wife, and then revealed his cross-dressing to her. He was able to sustain their sexual activity by fantasizing that he was a woman and she was a man or by cross-dressing. When she tired of making love to a "man pretending to be a woman," he became even less com-

TABLE 21.2-2
Diagnostic Criteria for Transexualism

A. Persistent discomfort and sense of inappropriateness about one's assigned sex.

B. Persistent preoccupation for at least 2 years with getting rid of one's primary and secondary sex characteristics and acquiring the sex characteristics of the other sex.

C. The person has reached puberty.

Specify history of sexual orientation: **asexual, homosexual, heterosexual,** or **unspecified.**

Table from DSM-III-R *Diagnostic and Statistical Manual of Mental Disorders,* ed 3, revised. Copyright American Psychiatric Association, Washington, DC, 1987. Used with permission.

TABLE 21.2-3
Diagnostic Criteria for Gender Identity Disorder of Adolescence or Adulthood, Nontranssexual Type (GIDAANT)

A. Persistent or recurrent discomfort and sense of inappropriateness about one's assigned sex.

B. Persistent or recurrent cross-dressing in the role of the other sex, either in fantasy or actuality, but not for the purpose of sexual excitement (as in transvestic fetishism).

C. No persistent preoccupation (for at least 2 years) with getting rid of one's primary and secondary sex characteristics and acquiring the sex characteristics of the other sex (as in transsexualism).

D. The person has reached puberty.

Specify history of sexual orientation: **asexual, homosexual, heterosexual,** or **unspecified.**

Table from DSM-III-R *Diagnostic and Statistical Manual of Mental Disorders,* ed 3, revised. Copyright American Psychiatric Association, Washington, DC, 1987. Used with permission.

TABLE 21.2-4
Diagnostic Criteria for Gender Identity Disorder Not Otherwise Specified

Disorders in gender identity that are not classifiable as a specific gender identity disorder.

Examples:

(1) children with persistent cross-dressing without the other criteria for gender identity disorder of childhood
(2) adults with transient, stress-related cross-dressing behavior
(3) adults with the clinical features of transsexualism of less than 2 years' duration
(4) people who have a persistent preoccupation with castration or penectomy without a desire to acquire the sex characteristics of the other sex

Table from DSM-III-R *Diagnostic and Statistical Manual of Mental Disorders,* ed 3, revised. Copyright American Psychiatric Association, Washington, DC, 1987. Used with permission.

municative, withdrew from all marital social activity, and tried to give up his feminine interests by becoming "macho"—for example, wearing leather, riding motorcycles, drinking to excess. He then abandoned this year-long charade and returned to wearing panties under his male clothes. When his wife left him 2 years ago, he lost 40 pounds to help him in passing as a female, and set about learning how to be female. During masturbation, he continued to imagine himself as a female with breasts and a vagina; alternatively, however, he saw himself making love to a man or to a woman. His night dreams were occasionally man-to-man homoerotic, but he experienced himself as a heterosexual who would like to end up a lesbian. Except for going to work and ballet classes, he lived in isolation. He occasionally ingested birth control pills. He claimed to have wanted breasts and genital surgery for years. This desire was now stronger than ever, but he was uncertain about its being the wisest course.

The following is a case example of gender identity disorder of adulthood, nontranssexual type:

Teri, a gangly, unkempt, effeminate 26-year-old with a soft voice and a bewildered manner, emphasized that he felt more genderless than female. "I'm neuter to the feminine side." A cross-dresser since early childhood, Teri's most consistent interest has been in female clothing and hairstyles, and high-heeled shoes. He kept pictures of himself cross-dressed and desired surgery in order to be freed from his "horrible genitals"; his greatest desire, however, was to have his square chin remodeled into softer features. Homosexually active since his early teens, he hated his experience among gays—"drugs, group sex, disease, and humiliation; I never fit in there!" His masturbatory fantasies often involved degradation. His preoccupation with gender and bodily transformation fluctuated in response to his mood regulation, as well as economic and housing problems. "I change so much, I don't know who or what I am!" Chronically late, unable to concentrate long enough to read a paragraph, this disorganized man has led a hand-to-mouth existence since high school graduation; he plans to be an architect. He has been hospitalized for depression and suicidal ideation on four occasions.

The following is a case example of gender identity disorder not otherwise specified:

Tess, a 25-year-old laboratory technician with a unisexual appearance, nervously requested male hormones, mastectomy, and hysterectomy. Her evaluation was made with the support of her psychotherapist, who began seeing her 2 years ago because of a reactive depression with suicidal ideation following her homosexual lover's decision to marry a man. Tess, a tomboy, claimed to have been uncomfortable with her breasts and genitals since puberty. She resisted all parental attempts to feminize her and threw herself into athletics. She claimed never to have masturbated and could not discuss her fantasies of being a boy without blushing silence. She could not say the word "penis." Her lover, who suspected she wanted to be a boy, was never permitted to touch her breasts or genitals. Tess was certain that she did not want her body as it was, but had no consistent clarity about what it should be. Although her stated hope was to take androgens in order to pass as a male, she had resisted the offers of her body-building friends to supply her with the hormone. Attempts to ascertain her subjective orientation and intention failed. She focused only on her inability to be comfortable with her female self and to feel any commonality with other females. She wanted to know how to deal with the problem.

DSM-III-R provides two diagnoses for prepubertal children: gender identity disorder of childhood (Table 21.2-5) and gender identity disorder not otherwise specified (Table 21.2-4). The criteria for the first diagnosis are offered separately for each sex, but they involve comparable signs of repudiation or denial of socially expected gender identity. These manifestations vary somewhat with the age of the child. All gender-disturbed children who fail to meet criteria of gender identity disorder of childhood are to receive the gender identity disorder not otherwise specified diagnosis.

The following is a case example of gender identity disorder of childhood:

Bobbie, a 4-year-old of average intelligence quotient (I.Q.), plays exclusively with the girls at his day care center and frequently verbalizes fantasies of being a bride at weddings or being married to a handsome man. He enjoys cross-dressing and loves to watch his mother dress. His favorite toy is a Barbie doll. He avoids rough-and-tumble play with boys, saying he is afraid of being hurt. He has spoken of wanting to be a girl for 2 years. His recent talk of wanting his penis to disappear and turn into a vagina led his parents to seek psychiatric attention.

TABLE 21.2-5
Diagnostic Criteria for Gender Identity Disorder of Childhood

For females:

A. Persistent and intense distress about being a girl, and a stated desire to be a boy (not merely a desire for any perceived cultural advantages from being a boy), or insistence that she is a boy.

B. Either (1) or (2):

(1) persistent marked aversion to normative feminine clothing and insistence on wearing stereotypical masculine clothing, e.g., boys' underwear and other accessories

(2) persistent repudiation of female anatomic structures, as evidenced by at least one of the following:
(a) an assertion that she has, or will grow, a penis
(b) rejection of urinating in a sitting position
(c) assertion that she does not want to grow breasts or menstruate

C. The girl has not yet reached puberty.

For males:

A. Persistent and intense distress about being a boy and an intense desire to be a girl or, more rarely, insistence that he is a girl.

B. Either (1) or (2):

(1) preoccupation with female stereotypical activities, as shown by a preference for either cross-dressing or simulating female attire, or by an intense desire to participate in the games and pastimes of girls and rejection of male stereotypical toys, games, and activities

(2) persistent repudiation of male anatomic structures, as indicated by at least one of the following repeated assertions:
(a) that he will grow up to become a woman (not merely in role)
(b) that his penis or testes are disgusting or will disappear
(c) that it would be better not to have a penis or testes

C. The boy has not yet reached puberty.

Table from DSM-III-R *Diagnostic and Statistical Manual of Mental Disorders,* ed 3, revised. Copyright American Psychiatric Association, Washington, DC, 1987. Used with permission.

EPIDEMIOLOGY

Trustworthy information about the prevalence of gender identity disorders among children, adolescents, and adults is almost entirely lacking. Estimates are available about those who seek surgical or psychiatric attention for gender problems. However, these are likely to be underestimations, because many individuals with milder gender identity disorders do not seek medical attention. Data from a central registry of all patients seeking sex reassignment surgery in Sweden have suggested a prevalence of 1 in 37,000 males and 1 in 103,000 females, with an annual incidence of 0.17 cases per 100,000 individuals over age 15. In Australia, where sex roles are more rigid than in Sweden, the estimated incidence is 0.58 per 100,000. Although most estimates of prevalence that are based on those seeking SRS indicate a male preponderance, this ratio of males to females has fluctuated in various centers over time between 8 to 1 and 1 to 1; the most consistent ratio has been 3 to 1. The ratio of boys to girls in three child gender identity clinics—30 to 1, 17 to 1, and 6 to 1—indicates a paucity of experience with girls. This disparity might indicate a greater male vulnerability to gender identity disorders, or a greater sensitivity and worry about cross-gender-identified boys than cross-gender-identified girls.

Follow-up of gender-disturbed boys has consistently indicated that homosexual orientation, not transsexualism, is the usual adolescent outcome; transsexualism occurs in less than 10 percent and in the largest prospective study in only 1 of 57 feminine boys. Retrospective data on homosexual men have indicated a high frequency of cross-gender identifications and feminine gender role behavior. These data invite the speculation that the 8 to 12 percent prevalence of male homosexuality among adults may reflect a similar prevalence of strong, persistent subjective or subjective and behavioral cross-gender identifications in childhood. If gender identity disorders of adolescence are an infrequent outcome of persistent, strong childhood cross-gender identity, then subjective cross-gender identifications, bieroticism or homoeroticism, and paraphilias may be the more frequent result. It is not clear whether a completely conventional sexual identity is possible after years of cross-gender identification in childhood; whether girls and boys have equal potential in this regard is also unclear. These unanswered questions highlight the fact that the study of the gender-disturbed person is an introduction to the ways in which biology, individual psychology, and socialization interact to form and evolve the components of sexual identity. In a larger sense, the pathologies of gender identity provide perspective on the formation of the self.

ETIOLOGY

BIOLOGICAL CONTRIBUTIONS The earliest thinking about the etiology of adult gender disorders proceeded on the assumption that infants were biologically programmed to develop a gender identity consonant with their sex. If that were the case, one would assume that gender-disordered persons must have biological abnormalities of sexual development; however, studies of gender-disordered patients failed to find any consistent chromosomal, endocrine, genital, or electroencephalography (EEG) abnormalities. This assumption was further examined in a series of retrospective and prospective studies delineating the gender identity, gender roles, and orientation of intersexed children. As a result of this work, new conclusions about the origins of gender identity were posited: Neonates are in a state of psychosexual neutrality; postnatal processes, the foremost of which is the infant's perceived sex (i.e., sex of rearing), are routinely able to override the prenatal influences on gender identity; once it has been established by age 3, gender identity is irreversible.

These conclusions are no longer universally accepted. Questions have been raised about the validity of the original descriptions of the sexual identities of intersexed children. Children with gender identifications that are incongruent with sex of rearing, who are subsequently discovered to have been missexed at birth, suggest the possibility that sex of rearing is not always stronger than biological programming. The immutable nature of the gender identity that has been established in early life has been challenged by successful sex reassignment of intersexed children after age 4, and by the syndrome caused by 5-α-reductase deficiency. Affected individuals in the Dominican Republic, raised as females and possessing feminine gender identities, successfully change their gender identity and gender role when their bodies become masculinized at puberty.

Currently, there is insufficient evidence to assume that gender identity development is simply biologically determined. The striking temperamental characteristics of neonates and infants, which are based on their unique neurophysiological organization, interact to influence postnatal events. Temperament, which is not definable in any more biological detail, is a reminder that a search for either a purely biological or a purely psychosocial etiology is an oversimplification.

PSYCHOSOCIAL CONTRIBUTIONS The principle that children develop a gender identity consonant with sex of rearing does not explain the mechanisms by which infants and toddlers learn that they belong to one sex, acquire comfort with their designation as "boy" or "girl," and increasingly gravitate to gender dimorphic behavior. Repetitive interactions with caretakers in which gender dimorphic language and affectively charged labels, such as "good boy " and "that's my girl," may induce intrapsychic responses that lead either to calm, immediate acceptance, conflict, then acceptance, or to nonacceptance of the family's expectation that the child behave as a member of the designated sex. Factors that influence the degree of acceptance in early life are open to speculation, but generally they are thought to include the characteristics of the child, the attitudes of caretakers, and the quality of the interactions between them. The inconspicuous intrapsychic process that directs the child toward identity conventionality or unconventionality occurs within the crucible of early object relationships. The mystery about how masculinity and femininity become part of character structure during the second year of life is not solved by labeling this process conditioning, imprinting, or identification.

Family dynamics Stoller suggested that early persistent femininity in a boy derives from specific family dynamics requiring a too satisfying, too prolonged merging of mother and son, and a passive, disinterested father. The background for the blissful symbiosis involves forgotten gender identity struggles in each parent. Comfortable early masculinity requires a balance between parental nurturance and the wish for the son's masculine individuation. A son's failure to individuate means that he does not give up the primary feminine identifications that all boys who are raised by mothers possess. Stoller distinguishes this form of early, conflict-free femininity from other, more common forms of gender disorders that are born of lesser or later difficulties in early object relationships. His explanation for persistent masculinity in girls centers on a rupture of the maternal-infant symbiosis, usually due to maternal depression or physical illness, which is dealt with by an unusual closeness to the father. These ideas are quantitative—that is, the more symbiosis and the less paternal involvement, the greater the boy's femininity; the less the maternal bond and the greater the paternal bond, the greater the daughter's masculinity.

Any variety of gender identity pathology makes clinicians wonder about the quality of the original maternal-infant bond and the early processes of separation-individuation. Theorists who have dealt with large numbers of children, families, and adults sense a diversity of family dynamics. Both too much of the bond or disruptions of attachment are seen as inciting processes. The nature and timing of these difficulties are suspected to modify the form of gender pathology. By the time a patient is recognized as having a gender pathology, there have usually been years of missed developmental opportunities. The fact that the origins of the pathology may have been conflict-free does not prevent adverse social and psychological consequences—often including subtle impairment in reality testing and the inability to relate to other people with ease.

The psychosocial forces that generate strong cross-gender identity may not be the same ones that account for its persistence. Parents have an opportunity to discourage feminine behaviors. Many mothers recall that they first perceived their sons' feminine behavior as cute; their enjoyment may encourage its persistence. Parents of gender-typical children may be made anxious by occasional cross-gender role behaviors and guide their children toward the appropriate gender models.

Developmental factors Etiological hypotheses tend to be preoccupied with the forces external to the child that account for the child's interest in cross-gender role behaviors. They do not emphasize the possibility that cross-gender identifications are the child's reactions to ordinary developmental dilemmas. These identifications may be idiosyncratic responses to common early-life problems in a temperamentally predisposed child—that is, one who is passive, inactive, clinging, cuddly, or fearful.

The theories are also preoccupied with early-life processes as the source of pathology. Preoedipal processes, however, may not so much cause adolescent gender pathology as predispose the teenager to gender confusion. Most adolescents find a nontranssexual solution for their gender confusion. Here is one who did not:

A girl was adopted from an orphanage at 4 months of age by a 30-year-old woman, who immediately became depressed, and her agoraphobic husband. The new mother took to her bed for 6 months, allowing her husband and her mother-in-law next door to provide for the infant. The mother's depression resolved quickly after she returned to work. The daughter remained wary of contact with her harsh-sounding mother for 4 years, preferring her indulgent, athletic father. The child's gender identity and gender role behavior were inconspicuously feminine. Her athletic endowment was unusual. By age 9 she was the star on her father's little league baseball team. She experienced a few preadolescent crushes on female teachers. Homosexual activity began in her sixteenth year, after she began writing poetry about twins and decided to act out the role she created as her separated-through-adoption twin brother. This impersonation was so exhilarating that she decided to live her life as a male, declaring that her former life as a female was a sham. Her mother, who often spoke of punishment when she intended to set limits, responded, "Over my dead body, you will live as a man!" Her gentle, ever-worrying father, who also felt this was a profound mistake for his creative daughter, concentrated, as usual, on preserving the relationship between his wife and daughter. All three agreed that the most difficult moments in her otherwise happy childhood occurred during her baseball days when she experienced mortification and outrage over being mistaken for a boy.

In psychotherapies with gender patients, cross-gender identifications appear to be a characterological defense that effectively protects against frightening feelings or memories. Intensified cross-gender identifications of those who have lived in their anatomically appropriate gender roles come about, for instance, in response to another work failure, inability to elicit love, a bout of suicidal ideation, a surge of violent feelings, and familial rejection of homosexual behavior. Similar intrapsychic maneuvers can be seen among those who have never been able to live comfortably in the anatomically correct gender role. Children who have been abused physically or sexually, or those who have never had any constant relationship with a nurturant parent, may respond by trying to live out their fantasy that they would be better treated if they were a member of the opposite sex. "Whenever things went wrong for me as a boy—when I couldn't see my father, for instance, I would tell myself that if only I were a girl he would visit me."

Enticing theories or clinical observations should not be confused with answers to the fundamental question about the determinants of gender identity and its unique evolution during childhood, adolescence, and adulthood. Clinicians are usually unable to explain adequately why cross-gender identifications appeared, persisted, and found their avenues of expression.

PATHOLOGY

When transsexualism first attracted psychiatric attention, many professionals labeled the underlying problem as schizophrenia, perversion, or a defense against homosexuality. Subsequent studies indicated that less than 10 percent were or had been schizophrenic. Patients were never systematically investigated for associated perversions. It is now recognized that perversions are often polymorphous over time. Men who present with perversion frequently have a history of occasional cross-dressing. A large percentage of SRS candidates display strident antihomosexual bias and vehemently reject the possibility of living a homosexual life-style. Patients' argument that their basic problem is their gender is supported by the fact that gender identity becomes part of character structure before orientation. Clinicians should still consider the role of psychosis, associated perversions, and retreat from a homosexual adaptation in their attempts to understand how a gender problem evolves. These issues are not strictly those of differential diagnosis; for example, one can be gender dysphoric, homoerotic, and intermittently psychotic.

Some of the early proponents of SRS believed that nothing was wrong with these patients except for their longing to bring their bodies and their minds into unity. Others, uncertain or skeptical of the utility of SRS, emphasized the high prevalence of borderline-narcissistic character pathology among adults applying for SRS. They did not, however, know whether the gender problem was a product of an underlying character, mood, or thinking disorder, or whether the conspicuous psychopathology was a consequence of impaired gender identity. The lower frequency of readily diagnosable psychopathology among female patients raised questions as to whether cultural factors were modifying the pathological consequences of gender identity problems.

A gender problem in a boy is now thought to be a manifestation of a pervasive difficulty manifested by, but not confined to, gender identity. The level of clinical psychopathology is at least moderate and typically involves internalized overcontrol and social interaction skills deficit. Psychometric findings suggest a borderline level of psychological organization.

The observation that gender disorders and borderline psychopathology are frequently associated will have more meaning when it is possible to clarify whether borderline psychopathology is the cause or result of preoedipal developmental difficulties.

SELF-PATHOLOGY Lothstein reformulated the psychopathology of gender disorders as a self-pathology. He suggested that the child's inability to consolidate a gender identity invariably produces structural ego deficits of a borderline nature because the child is unable to establish and maintain a cohesive sense of self. Whereas other children are able to move on to other developmental issues, the gender-disturbed child continues to search for gender self-constancy. The fundamental lack of a cohesive self leaves the child with a primitive anxiety focused on bodily loathing, reparative cross-gender fantasies, and preoccupation with rigid stereotyped representations of the opposite gender roles. The formulation suggests that strong cross-gender identifications mask gender confusion, diffusion, and oscillation between split-off male and female gender self-representations. The underlying problem is an inability to integrate male and female identifications, which are brought about by what the child perceives as frightening messages from the parents about his or her sex.

EVALUATION AND DIFFERENTIAL DIAGNOSIS

Three tentative formulations should be made during a multi-interview evaluation: a multiaxial DSM-III-R diagnosis; hypotheses concerning the meaning of the gender problem; and a treatment plan. The assessment of children begins with an interview of the parents, who report their concerns about the cross-gender behaviors, identity statements, peer relationships, and other difficulties of their child.

The clinician then interviews and questions the child directly about gender matters, such as: What is good about being a boy or girl? Toy and costume preferences are observed during play, and simple tests such as the Draw-a-Person Test are employed. A detailed developmental history is elicited from the parents as a first step in formulating the personal meaning of the gender disorder to the child. This is aided by projective testing, which often demonstrates anxiety about self-annihilation, profound fear of separation from the mother, and the link between feared aggression toward the male patient and maleness in general. The clinician notes the child's temperament and style, the mother's capacity to foster autonomy, her attitudes toward the child's sex, the benefits she may be deriving from having a "little helper" or "little man" in the home, and the nature of the father's involvement in the child's life. This process enables the clinician to note whether separation anxiety disorder or depressive symptomatology coexist with the gender disorder.

Deliberate cross-dressing of a male child by a relative, psychosis, prenatal diethylstilbesterol (DES) exposure, genital anomalies, and other intersex conditions are exceedingly rare among feminine boys. They need to be considered, however. Younger feminine boys are apt to state that they are, or will be, girls, whereas older ones are more likely to make clear that they are simply unhappy about being a boy. By itself, confusion as to whether a child is a boy or a girl is insufficient evidence of psychosis.

Most tomboys are reputed to outgrow their masculine preoccupations and to become heterosexual, but some become homosexual. The majority of lesbians have a history of tomboyism. Since no follow-up studies of gender-disordered girls are available, and the boundary between tomboyism and the diagnosis of gender identity disorder not otherwise specified is uncertain, there is no scientific basis on which to assure parents that their daughter will attain a conventional sexual identity.

All components of sexual identity should be assessed in adolescent and adult patients (Table 21.2-1). The history of male gender dysphoria should be traced. The nature of his prior subjective and behavioral sexual life should be clarified. The factors that may have produced the urgency to change sex should be defined—for example, loss of a homosexual lover; job failure; worsening of a chronic physical condition; unwillingness to pay child support; arrest for assault. The patient's intellectual capacity, reality testing, and quality of object relationships should be noted. Interviews with family members should be routinely sought because they are often more revealing than the initial ones with the patient. A thorough physical examination is indicated, and, if appropriate, should include testing for acquired immune deficiency syndrome (AIDS) antibodies and intersex conditions.

Clinicians should be mindful of the reports of a 40 percent frequency of polycystic ovary disease and 30 percent frequency of serum testosterone elevations among female applicants for SRS. The etiological significance of these observations is unclear. Although the degree of psychopathology on initial clinical evaluations of females seems to be less than males, they also have been noted to have schizophrenia, depressive symptomatology, or severe character pathologies. Projective testing often reveals more severe psychopathology and may help to elucidate the dynamic meaning of the disorder.

TREATMENT

Adolescents and adults usually find their own solutions for their strong cross-gender identifications. Professionals may either briefly interact to make a diagnosis and to decide about hormones or surgery, or more leisurely engage in therapy. Either way, those who see many patients encounter a spectrum of problematic adaptations.

Among males, these include retreat to fantasies of a named female self; pursuit of feminine interests and vocations while remaining in the male gender role; transvestitic patterns, such as periodic cross-dressing in privacy, with a partner, or in public; and female impersonation in a relationship, on the stage, or as a barroom dancer or prostitute. Female adaptations include gravitation to male work and recreation while living as a female, assumption of a male name and life in fantasy, stereotypic male roles in a homosexual relationship, and periodic public outings as a male.

Some patients are seen when these adaptations fail and they think that the best solution may be to change sex. Males then want to undertake electrolysis for beard removal, live and work as females full-time, take estrogens, and undergo augmentation mammoplasty and genital surgery. Females want to bind their breasts, more often pass as males, take androgens, and undergo mastectomies and genital surgery. Other patients appear after they have made the gender role transition and have taken hormones. They only want psychiatric clearance for SRS.

Gender role transition is often exhilarating; however, it preoccupies the patient with appearance, voice, and gesture; limits self-awareness; makes the past and present unimportant; interferes with concentration at work; and alters relationships with family and acquaintances. If this new solution fails, suicidal ideation can be expected. Because suicide is a risk, psychiatric interventions are useful.

A socially isolated, stammering, 40-year-old homoerotic man of limited intelligence spent 2 years caring for his dying mother. After her death, he moved to the city and found factory work. When he was laid off 6 months later, he sought SRS. After psychiatric evaluation, the recommendation was made that he return to talk. He responded by demanding hormones and threatening suicide if he could not immediately start classes to become a woman. (He misunderstood the nature of a group therapy for gender patients.) After an ingestion of a dozen aspirin tablets, he spent a week in the hospital clamoring for discharge. The work with him about his grief, loneliness, need for employment, and the reasons for his 1-year interest in living as a woman seemed to have no impact. He angrily left vowing to obtain SRS elsewhere. A year later, without a trace of a stammer, he returned to obtain permission for a circumcision because of a painful phimosis. Shortly after discharge, he found a job as a man, eventually met a woman, and decided to get married. When asked about his former desire for SRS, he giggled, scratched his head and replied, "Gee, shucks, I don't know what got into me."

SEX REASSIGNMENT SURGERY SRS is a frightening, expensive, and distant option that many patients will not undertake—no matter how certain they are at the moment that it is the only solution for them. Professionals need not unalterably oppose hormones and SRS because: (1) they may help some individuals live more comfortable and productive lives; (2) unyielding opposition may decrease the professional's ability to help the patient calmly think through many options; (3) opposition may provoke autocastration in a few desperate males; (4) opposition may destroy all hope for renewal and lead to a suicide attempt; and (5) the patient usually has more conflict about proceeding than he or she is able to acknowledge, and opposition serves to focus the struggle between therapist and patient, rather than to help the patient assume ownership of the conflict.

Because the early cases of transsexualism were not comprehensively dealt with by mental health professionals and the outcomes were uncertain, the Harry Benjamin International Gender Dysphoria Association established minimal standards of care for the evaluation and treatment of patients requesting SRS. These guidelines mandate that physicians, psychologists, and patients proceed slowly. The patient first establishes a relationship with a gender identity program that employs experienced therapists who are able to undertake a comprehensive psychological and medical evaluation. Then, if it has not already occurred, the patient must begin a trial of cross-gender living. Hormones are prescribed only after the patient has undergone 3 months of psychotherapy and the gender dysphoria has been documented to be persistent for at least 2 years. No surgery should be undertaken until the patient has been in psychotherapy for at least 6 months and has successfully lived and worked in the new gender role for at least a year. SRS requires a written second opinion of another experienced mental health professional with a Ph.D. or M.D. degree.

These guidelines are an antidote to the impulsiveness that so often accompanies the decision to undergo SRS. Most gender identity programs double or triple the time requirements. This provides patients with the opportunity to change their minds and to deal with the problems of living in a new role before receiving hormones or surgery.

Surgical techniques Genital reconstruction of either sex is a complicated surgical task requiring skills found among plastic surgeons, urologists, and gynecologists. The technical results are better among the relatively few surgeons who do these operations regularly. The simplest procedure is mastectomy for female patients. After being informed of the current limitations in creating a phallus that can be mechanically erected for intercourse, that can transport urine throughout its length, that will retain sensation for sexual activity, and that will cosmetically resemble a penis, many female patients elect mastectomy only. Many patients delay total hysterectomy and salpingo-oorphorectomy because androgens usually cause amenorrhea within 4 months.

Penectomy, orchiectomy, and the creation of labia from scrotal tissue are not as technically difficult as is the creation of a vagina. At least 35 percent of patients complain of inadequate vaginal depth in the years following SRS. In either sex, SRS often requires surgical revision after the initial sequence of surgeries is performed. These facts are important for patients to understand before surgery so that they can make an informed decision about the surgical, economic, and psychological burdens of the procedures. For some biological males, the urge to transform the body will lead to requests for augmentation mammoplasty, rhinoplasty, and a reduction in the size of the thyroid cartilage. Some follow-up studies have suggested that a successful postsurgical psychological adaptation depends on the functional capacity of the vagina; those with stenosed vaginas are the most unhappy with the decision to undergo SRS.

The methodological problems of assessing the psychosocial results of SRS are formidable. They stem from lack of agreement on the presurgical diagnosis; variable preparation prior to surgery; the inability to separate the effects of cross-gender living, hormones, and changing relationships from the impact of bodily transformation; changing patient attitudes over time toward SRS; and inconsistent means of making postoperative assessments. Suicide, suicide attempts, and requests for reversion to the original sex are known to occur in occasional cases.

Most systematic studies of patients who have had surgery indicate that approximately 85 percent are pleased that they underwent their operations and feel that their bodies and their minds are finally whole. The longest follow-up study of males surgically reassigned in Sweden, however, indicate that 30 percent came to regret having undergone SRS. Character structure and vocational, economic, and social patterns do not change dramatically.

HORMONAL TREATMENT The effects of estrogens on transsexual males have never been studied in a blind, placebo-controlled fashion. Patients usually report immediate psychological satisfaction, based on a sense of tranquility, less frequent erections, and fewer sexual drive manifestations. Their new sterility is not of concern to them. After several months, bodily contours become more rounded, a limited but pleasing breast enlargement develops, and testicular volume decreases. The quality of the voice does not change. Patients need to be watched for hypertension, hyperglycemia, hepatic dysfunction, and thromboembolic phenomena.

Females who take androgens quickly notice an increased sexual drive, clitoral tingling and enlargement, and, after several months, amenorrhea and hoarseness. If weight lifting is undertaken, a pronounced increase in muscle mass may occur. Depending on the hair distribution already present, there may be a moderate increase in the amount and coarseness of facial and body hair; some develop frontal balding. Thromboembolic phenomena, hepatic dysfunction, and elevations of cholesterol and triglycerides are possible.

PSYCHOTHERAPY Psychotherapy is especially difficult for the therapist. Besides the problems inherent in working with borderline patients, most therapists initially have considerable countertransferential difficulties with the idea of changing gender roles and the demanding, unreflective patient attitudes. Therapists need support through supervision to deal with conflicts concerning their curiosity about the patient's life, which feels uncomfortably voyeuristic, and the emerging awareness of their own gender identity, which inevitably arises when initially dealing with gender-disordered patients.

Therapists need to discuss their ethical concerns over cooperating with patients' desires to change their anatomy and physiology. Most professionals initially feel this desire is against both the medical tenet "to do no harm" and the psychodynamic tenet to deal with the internal conflict rather than with its symptomatic manifestations. Failure to address these legitimate concerns leads to a refusal to deal with any gender-disordered patients. The rewards for the perseverant therapist are a deeper understanding of psychological development and its pathology and the ability to alleviate psychological pain.

Patients have trouble with psychotherapy because they anticipate being viewed as immoral and crazy. Because they often think their problem is biological, they believe they could not possibly benefit from talking. They want to spend their often limited financial resources on electrolysis, hormones, or surgery. Their lack of insight and untrusting transferences may produce "nothing to talk about." As a result, the demoralized therapist may agree not to meet very often or for very long or not to deal with matters of personal development. Although the difficulties of conducting psychotherapy with SRS candidates are legion, many patients with gender disorders soon simply want to talk about their lives and the odyssey that they are contemplating.

It is not known whether the modest results claimed by the proponents of psychotherapy for children, adolescents, or adults are due to a healing of the defective gender-self or to the mobilization of restraints against further cross-gender role behavior. Psychotherapy with adults requires spending enough time to understand their suffering and to share their aspiration to find a workable, comfortable sexual identity. The goals are not to create a person with a conventional sexual identity. By the time these adults are seen in individual or group therapy, their capacities to be trustingly intimate are usually severely limited. Psychotherapies with gender-disturbed adolescents are more chaotic and involve more frequent acting out. There are more exceptions to these generalizations among females than males. Psychotherapy with children typically requires family interventions. Lessening of cross-gender behaviors seems to result from therapies that last longer, involve the parents, and deal with gender issues directly. The relative efficacy of psychodynamic versus behavioral interventions and male versus female therapists are unknown.

The basic psychopathologies of the gender disordered (i.e., structural ego defects) have lifelong consequences for capacities to work and to relate to others. These problems are not alterable by surgery and often are only modestly helped by psychotherapy. Somatic interventions can help some people consolidate a gender identity that leaves them more subjectively comfortable. The degree and persistence of this comfort needs to be compared with the patient's baseline in the anatomically appropriate gender role. The fact that the underlying anxiety may still appear and produce distress should not surprise mental health professionals.

INTERSEX DISORDERS

Intersex disorders are conditions in which persons have genetic, anatomical, or physiological characteristics of both males and females (Table 21.2-6). The appearance of the genitalia in these diverse conditions is ambiguous or incongruent with the person's genetic or chromosomal makeup. Intersex disorders are not Axis I or II diagnoses in DSM-III-R; they are properly considered Axis III diagnoses that relate to associated physical conditions.

Intersex patients may develop gender identity problems because of complicated biological influences and familial confusion about their actual sex. When these conditions are discovered, a panel of pediatric experts usually determines the sex of rearing based on clinical examination, urological studies, buccal smears, chromosomal analyses, and assessment of the parental wishes.

TABLE 21.2-6
Classification of Intersexual Disorders

Syndrome	*Description*
Virilizing adrenal hyperplasia (andrenogenital syndrome)	Results from excess androgens in fetus with XX genotype; most common female intersex disorder; associated with enlarged clitoris, fused labia, hirsutism in adolescence
Turner's syndrome	Results from absence of second female sex chromosome (XO); associated with web neck, dwarfism, cubitus valgus; no sex hormones produced; infertile; usually assigned as females because of female-looking genitals
Klinefelter's syndrome	Genotype is XXY; male habitus present with small penis and rudimentary testes because of low androgen production; weak libido; usually assigned as male
Androgen insensitivity syndrome (testicular-feminizing syndrome)	Congenital X-linked recessive disorder that results in inability of tissues to respond to androgens; external genitals look female and cryptorchid testes present; assigned as females even though they have XY genotype; in extreme form patient has breasts, normal external genitals, short blind vagina, and absence of pubic and axillary hair
Enzymatic defects in XY genotype (e.g., 5-α-reductase deficiency, 17-hydroxysteroid deficiency)	Congenital interruption in production of testosterone that produces ambiguous genitals and female habitus; usually assigned as female because of female-looking genitalia
Hermaphroditism	True hermaphrodite is rare and characterized by both testes and ovaries in same person (may be 46 XX or 46 XY)
Pseudohermaphroditism	Usually the result of endocrine or enzymatic defect (e.g., adrenal hyperplasia) in persons with normal chromosomes; female pseudohermaphrodites have masculine-looking genitals, but are XX; male pseudohermaphrodites have rudimentary testes and external genitals and are XY; assigned as males or females depending on morphology of genitals

Assignment should be agreed on as early as possible so that the entire family system, including the patient, can treat the patient in a consistent, relaxed manner. When surgery is necessary to normalize genital appearance, it is generally undertaken well before the age of 3. It is easier to assign the child to be female than to be male because ambiguous-to-female genital surgical procedures are far more advanced than ambiguous-to-male ones.

REFERENCES

Coates S, Zucker K J: Assessment of gender identity disorders in children. In *Handbook of Clinical Assessment of Children and Adolescents: A Biopsychosocial Perspective,* C J Kestenbaum, D T Williams, editors. New York University Press, New York, 1987.

Diamond M: Sexual identity, monozygotic twins reared in discordant sex roles, and a BBC follow-up. Arch Sex Behav *11:* 181, 1982.

Dörner G: Neuroendocrine response to estrogen & brain differentiation in heterosexuals, homosexuals, & transsexuals. Arch Sex Behav 17: 57, 1988
Futterweit W, Weiss R A, Fagerstrom M: Endocrine evaluation of forty female-to-male transsexuals. Arch Sex Behav *15:* 69, 1986.
Green R: *Sexual Identity Conflict in Children and Adults,* Basic Books, New York, 1974.
Green R: Gender identity in childhood and later sexual orientation: Follow-up of 78 males. Amer J Psychiat *142:* 339, 1985.
Green R: *"The Sissy Boy Syndrome" and the Development of Homosexuality*. Yale University Press, New Haven, 1987.
Hoenig J: Etiology of transsexualism. In *Gender Dysphoria: Development, Research, Management,* B W Steiner, editor, p 33.
Imperato-McGinley J, Peterson R E, Gautier T, Sturla E: Androgens and the evolution of male gender identity among male pseudohermaphrodites with 5-alpha-reductase deficiency. New Eng J Med, *300:* 1233, 1979.
Lindemalm S, Korlin D, Uddenberg N: Long-term follow-up of "sex change" in 13 male-to-female transsexuals, Arch Sex Behav *15:* 187, 1986.
Lothstein L M, Levine S B: Expressive psychotherapy with gender dysphoric patients. Arch Gen Psychiat *38:* 924, 1981.
Lothstein, L M: *Female to Male Transsexualism: Historical, Clinical, and Theoretical Issues*. Routledge, Kegan, Boston, 1983.
McEwan L, Ceber S, Davis J: Male-to-female surgical genital reassignment. In *Transsexualism and Sex Reassignment,* W A W Walters, M J Ross, editors, p 103. Oxford University Press, New York, 1986.
Meyer-Bahlburg H F L: Gender identity disorder of childhood: introduction. J Amer Acad Child Psychiat *24:* 681, 1985.
Money J, Ehrhardt A A: *Man and Woman, Boy and Girl: Differentiation and Dimorphism of Gender Identity from Conception to Maturity*. Johns Hopkins University Press, Baltimore, 1972.
Pauley I B, Edgerton M T: The gender identity movement: A growing surgical-psychiatric liaison. Arch Sex Behav *15:* 315, 1986.
Ross M J, Walinder J, Lundstrom B, Thuwe I: Cross-cultural approaches to transsexualism: A comparison between Sweden and Australia. Acta Psychiat Scand *63:* 75, 1981.
Stoller R J: *Presentations of Gender*. Yale University Press, New Haven, 1985.
Thomas A, Chess S: Genesis and evolution of behavioral disorders: from infancy to early adult life. Amer J Psychiat *141:* 1, 1986.
Walker P, Berger J, Green R, Laub D, Reynolds C, Wollman L: Standards of care. The hormonal and surgical reassignment of gender dysphoric persons. Arch Sex Behav *14:* 79, 1985.
Zucker K J, Bradley S J, Doering R W, Lozinski J A: Sex-typed behavior in cross-gender-identified children: Stability and change at a one year follow-up. J Amer Acad Child Psychiat *24:* 710, 1985.
Zucker K J, Green R: Treatment of the gender identity disorder of childhood, in *APA Task Force on the Treatment of Psychiatric Disorders,* T B Karasu, editor. American Psychiatric Press, Washington, DC, 1987.
Zuger B: Early effeminate behavior in boys: Outcome and significance for homosexuality. J Nerv Ment Dis *172:* 90, 1984.

21.3 PARAPHILIAS

GENE ABEL, M.D.

INTRODUCTION

Human sexual behavior is varied. It requires a biological substrate for physiological expression and is strongly influenced by the socialization process in which individuals learn the norms of their culture. Although sexual behavior plays a role in the preservation of the species, its major function for human beings is to assist in bonding, to express emotion between individuals, and for recreation. Across various cultures, one can also see sexual practices that are repetitive in nature and appear to exclude others or disrupt the potential bonding process between individuals. When these behaviors become extremely divergent from the norm, and especially when they are harmful to others, investigators attempt to understand them better by defining their characteristics. The definition and classification of these behaviors has been difficult because they are (1) committed by a small percentage of the population, (2) concealed by their participants, and (3) constantly modified by adaptations to changes in society.

DEFINITION

The major systems of classification that attempt to define unusual sexual practices are the ninth revision of the World Health Organization's *International Classification of Diseases* (ICD-9) or its *Clinical Modification* (ICD-9-CM) and the third edition of the American Psychiatric Association's *Diagnostic and Statistical Manual of Mental Disorders* (DSM-III), including its current revision (DSM-III-R). The sequence of development of these classifications has been ICD-9, DSM-III, and, most recently, DSM-III-R. Examination of these classification systems reveals a gradual clarification of definition and the exclusion of conditions that were acceptable between partners. ICD-9 is a statistical classification with limited descriptions of criteria for inclusion of diseases in its various categories. It included under the category of sexual deviation both transsexualism and homosexuality. DSM-III appropriately excluded transsexualism and DSM-III-R excluded homosexuality as sexual deviations.

Transsexuals have problems of sexual identity, believing that their sexual identities are different from their anatomical bodies. As psychiatry gains increased clinical understanding of sexual identity issues, the sexual preferences of transsexuals appear not so unusual but consistent with their sexual identity. Transsexualism is therefore appropriately excluded from categories of paraphilias.

Homosexuality is a sexual preference that is usually shared with others of similar interest, and although procreation is not possible, homosexuality seems to serve many of the recognized functions of human sexual behavior, such as providing opportunities for bonding, closeness, and mutual expression of feelings.

A common finding in paraphiliacs is the coexistence or previous history of several paraphilias. The two exceptions to this finding occur in cases of transsexualism and homosexuality, which further supports their exclusion from any classification as paraphilias.

DSM-III-R uses the term *paraphilia* to indicate that the deviation (para) is that to which the individual is attracted (philia). DSM-III indicated that unusual or bizarre imagery or acts were necessary for the paraphiliac's sexual excitement. In addition, such imagery or acts were insistently and involuntarily repetitive and generally involved: (1) preference for use of a nonhuman object, (2) repetitive sexual activity with humans involving real or simulated suffering or humiliation, or (3) repetitive sexual activity with nonconsenting partners. The stipulation that the unusual images or acts be necessary for sexual excitement, however, proved to be an inappropriate restriction on the criteria for inclusion as a paraphilia. Most individuals who commit paraphilic acts can also perform nonparaphilic sexual behaviors without the concomitant use of paraphilic fantasies or images. Although some paraphiliacs do exclusively use paraphilic images or acts that are absolutely necessary if they are to engage in any form of sexual behavior, these individuals are in the minority. DSM-III-R has appropriately modified this requirement by clarifying that paraphilic arousal may only be transiently present. For example, paraphilic arousal may develop during periods of stress or conflict, but remain completely absent at other times. DSM-III-R has also excluded simulated suffering or humiliation as one of the three categories of paraphilic behavior, requiring instead that there be actual suffering or humiliation in the paraphilic act.

CHARACTERISTICS A hallmark of the paraphilias is that the unusual or bizarre imagery or acts are insistently and involuntarily repetitive. During the socialization process, children attempt to learn the sexual patterns of their culture. As with the acquisition of any new behavior, numerous errors or false starts are made. Persons making trial-and-error attempts at normative sexual behavior must be separated from those in the culture who repetitively and persistently carry out inappropriate behaviors. DSM-III-R has defined repetitive and persistent by specifying that the sexual urges and fantasies must persist at least 6 months. Data are currently not available indicating how long paraphilic interests of an exploratory nature might persist before disappearing permanently. Until such data are available, it is appropriate and consistent with clinical judgment that DSM-III-R establish for the paraphilic interest an arbitrary duration of 6 months.

Another issue affecting classification is the paraphiliac's own response to the presence of paraphilic urges and fantasies. DSM-III-R requires that the individual repeatedly act on these urges or be markedly distressed by them. Excluded would be individuals with repetitive, intense paraphilic interests who have never acted on their interests and those who feel no discomfort from the presence of the fantasy.

The major categories of paraphilias included in DSM-III-R are pedophilia, exhibitionism, sexual sadism, sexual masochism, voyeurism, fetishism, transvestic fetishism, frotteurism, and a separate category for minor paraphilias not otherwise specified. DSM-III-R appropriately allows for multiple paraphilic diagnoses in the same individual, which is often warranted.

The expression of paraphilic interests varies as the culture changes. For example, obscene verbalizations to others have always occurred, but the invention of the telephone allowed marked acceleration of their expression. The incidence of frottage is much higher in some Mediterranean cultures, where it is more widely accepted. In rural farmlands, its expression is not supported because of the low population density, whereas in larger cities requiring public transportation, frottage is observed more frequently.

Paraphilic behavior is an exaggeration of less intense, less repetitive interests in the general population. For example, the average citizen enjoys observing erotica in the theatre, in night clubs, on television, and in the movies. Touching one's sexual partner's buttocks and thighs is very much a part of sexual behavior. Only a quantitative difference and an unwilling partner separates these behaviors from their respective paraphilic diagnoses, voyeurism and frottage.

Examinations of the presence of paraphilias in the general population has not been possible, but it is clinically suspected that individuals with paraphilic interests are infrequent. At the same time, the clinician must appreciate that because of the high frequency of the commission of paraphilic acts, a large proportion of the population has been victimized by such individuals. Ten to 20 percent of children have been molested by age 18. Twenty percent of adult females have been the targets of exhibitionists and voyeurs. Although the paraphilias are rare, a high frequency of commission of paraphilic acts per individual has brought this population to the attention of the general population.

HISTORY

Since the forbidden fruit in the Garden of Eden, humans have placed restrictions on the unlimited expression of sexual behavior. Although the consequences of violating sexual prohibitions often seem absurd, their goal has been to provide possible containment for sexuality's potentially disruptive power. Unfortunately, laws designed to limit victimization by sexual offenders often made victims of the offenders themselves. In Orthodox Jewish codes, masturbation was punishable by death, while Catholics thought masturbation a carnal sin. This victimless crime was seen as a major cause of insanity in the late nineteenth century.

Of those sexual practices condemned in ancient cultures, none warrants classification as a paraphilia today more than pedophilic incest. Human disgust at incest extends beyond all national borders and historical epochs. Incest was punishable by death in Babylonia, Judea, and ancient China, and offenders were handed the death penalty as late as 1650 in England. Social consciousness prohibiting sex with one's own children was slower to awaken to the issue of sex with someone else's children. In Europe, as late as the nineteenth century, children were considered small adults capable of assuming the full responsibilities of work and the pleasures of sexuality. Child labor laws enacted during Queen Victoria's reign to limit the exploitation of children removed them from the work force; laws prohibiting pedophilia soon removed them from adults' bedrooms as well.

In contrast to incest, not all cultures shared Judeo-Christian revulsion toward homosexuality. City coffers throughout Asia Minor depended on licensed houses of male prostitution for a substantial part of their income. Ancient Greek law allowed contracts between boys and male adults to establish sexual privileges. The Romans looked leniently on homosexuality when increased fear of venereal disease prompted men to seek male partners. The Christian Church, however, viewed oral-genital, anal, homosexual, and animal contacts as unnatural and greater sins than extramarital coitus because these activities did not lead to biological reproduction. This negative attitude lingered in the United States up until the formulation of the first edition of the *Diagnostic and Statistical Manual of Mental Disorders* (DSM-I). Of these Church-condemned, nonprocreative behaviors, only sex with animals retains its classification as a paraphilia in DSM-III-R.

EPIDEMIOLOGY

Random sampling is the most scientific technique for obtaining an accurate estimation of the occurrence of an illness within a general population. It appears impossible, however, to collect data on the paraphilias by using random sample methods. Because discussing sexual behavior in general and paraphilic behavior in particular is not socially acceptable, most people are reluctant to report (even anonymously) their intimate sexual behaviors. Constraints to conceal their sexual behavior are even more important for the majority of paraphiliacs, since severe legal repercussions could follow disclosure. Information regarding the occurrence of paraphilias has therefore accumulated through records from arrested or incarcerated paraphiliacs, data from victims of paraphilic behaviors, and information from outpatient treatment programs that provide services for those seeking assessment or treatment or both. Data from these sources, however, cannot be considered representative.

Criminal justice records are nonrepresentative for a number of reasons: (1) Many sex crimes are committed against an unknowing victim (voyeurism) and, as a result, infrequent attempts at apprehension occur; (2) the criminal justice system tends to trivialize some paraphilic crimes (exhibitionism, frottage) as being of insufficient seriousness to warrant attempts at apprehension and as such, these crimes are less represented in criminal justice statistics; (3) apprehended offenders most skilled at organizing a defense and able to afford legal counsel either escape conviction or are more likely to receive a lesser charge in plea-bargaining efforts; and (4) the most aggressive, violent offenders or those who commit the offense repeatedly are more likely to come to the attention of the criminal justice system and be incarcerated.

Occurrence rates of paraphilias drawn from victim-reporting services (such as rape crisis centers) are likewise skewed because of reporting patterns. Victim services have predominantly focused on providing services to the adult rape victim or female child who has been assaulted by a family member. Victims of other categories of sex crimes are therefore underrepresented in statistics from such centers.

A final source of information is obtained from outpatient psychiatric services for paraphiliacs outside the criminal justice system. Data from such centers are probably the most valid in reflecting the true distribution of paraphiliacs. When statistics demonstrating the occurrence and distribution of paraphilias is based on self-reports, the crucial issue is the confidentiality under which data were collected from the paraphiliac. When confidentiality was extensively guaranteed at psychiatric centers offering services to paraphiliacs seeking treatment, data were obtained (Table 21.3-1) reflecting the relative occurrence of the various paraphilias and the frequency of paraphilic crimes.

These data indicate that the vast majority of paraphiliacs seeking outpatient treatment have either pedophilia, exhibitionism, or voyeurism, and the clinician should therefore become most skilled at assessing and treating these three conditions. Patients with paraphilias show tremendous variance in the number of paraphilic acts they commit. Examining the average (mean) number of paraphilic acts per paraphilia would be a misleading statistic, since some diagnostic groups have individuals committing crimes thousands of times. Median numbers of crimes are therefore more representative of the expected frequency of paraphilic acts reported by paraphiliacs seeking outpatient treatment.

TABLE 21.3-1
Frequency of Paraphilic Acts Committed by Paraphiliacs Seeking Outpatient Treatment

Diagnostic Category	*Approximate Percentage of All Paraphiliacs Seeking Outpatient Treatment*	*Median Number of Paraphilic Acts per Paraphiliac*
Pedophilia	45	5
Exhibitionism	25	50
Sexual sadism	3	3
Sexual masochism	3	36
Voyeurism	12	17
Fetishism	2	3
Transvestic fetishism	3	25
Zoophilia	1	2
Frotteurism	6	30

ETIOLOGY

Psychiatry's approach to the paraphilias has consistently reflected the cross-currents and controversies in Western society's attitude toward mental illness in general. In the nineteenth century, as the concept of sexual deviation as sin gave way to the medical model of sexual deviation as disease, psychiatrists were divided as to whether disorders were somatic in origin or acquired as a result of experience. Advocates of organic pathology saw the paraphilias as instances of insanity brought on by organic degeneration or congenital anomaly. In either case, curative treatment was considered irrelevant, but patients were spared full responsibility for their behavior.

By the early twentieth century, advocates of the view that paraphilias were acquired through experience were likewise split into two camps. One camp insisted that any learned deviant sexual behavior could be reversed, while the other camp remained skeptical that treatment could ever entirely reverse lifelong patterns of paraphilic interest. These two camps of behaviorism and psychoanalysis remain today the competing approaches toward understanding paraphiliacs, with psychoanalysis gaining the first foothold in American psychiatry.

PSYCHOANALYTIC APPROACH In the psychoanalytic model, a paraphiliac is an individual who has failed the normal developmental process toward heterosexual adjustment. Although external circumstances, environmental factors, and social training are given consideration, what distinguishes one paraphilia from another is the method chosen by the individual (usually male) to cope with the anxiety caused by the threat of (1) castration by the father and (2) separation from the mother. However bizarre its manifestation, the resulting perversion provides an outlet for the sexual and aggressive drives that would otherwise have been channeled into proper gender behavior.

Failure to resolve the oedipal crisis by identification with the father aggressor (for boys) or mother aggressor (for girls) will result either in improper identification with the opposite-gender parent or in an improper choice of object for libido cathexis. Regardless of current DSM-III-R classifications, homosexuality, transsexualism, and transvestic fetishism are all considered perversions within psychoanalytic theory since each demonstrates identification with the opposite-gender instead of same-gender parent. A male dressing in women's clothes, for example, is clearly seen as identifying with his mother. Exhibitionism and voyeurism, however, are also seen as expressions of feminine identification since the paraphiliac must constantly examine his own or others' genitals to calm his anxiety about castration. Fetishism is an attempt to avoid anxiety by displacing libidinal impulses to inappropriate objects. The shoe fetishist unconsciously denies that women lost their penis through castration by attaching libido to a phallic object, the shoe, that symbolizes the female penis. Both pedophile and sexual sadist share a need to dominate and control their victims, as though to compensate for their feelings of powerlessness during the oedipal crisis. The sexual masochist overcomes his fear of injury and sense of powerlessness by demonstrating that he is impervious to harm. Although recent developments in psychoanalysis place more emphasis on treating defense mechanisms than oedipal traumas, the course of psychoanalytic therapy for the paraphiliac remains consistent with Freud's theory.

BEHAVIORAL APPROACH The behavioral approach to treating paraphilias is more a collection of many diverse, specific therapies than a unified model based on one theoretical position. For example, in the late nineteenth century, hypnosis was the preferred treatment for paraphilias, even though it may be thought to share more theoretical assumptions with psychoanalysis than with behaviorism. Yet, the procedures followed by hypnotherapists resemble the structured, repetitive therapies developed in the past 2 decades for the behavior modification of paraphilias. As the behavioral approaches continue to demonstrate increased effectiveness with an expanding repertoire of therapies, they now appear to be the treatments preferred by centers specializing in paraphilias.

Although the theoretical orientations of behavioral approaches and psychoanalytic approaches have differed from one another, their conclusions regarding the initiation and maintenance of paraphilic interests are surprisingly similar. A unified, single model of the etiology of paraphilias can be constructed by highlighting the similarities across orientations. When fields with such markedly different theoretical orientations arrive at very similar conclusions, there is a high likelihood that the subsequent composite model has high validity.

AN INTEGRATED MODEL A theory of the development of paraphilias must include an explanation of the initial instigation of a deviant interest or act followed by those factors that suppress or maintain the deviant interest. Instigators are those factors that lead to the very first interest or urge to commit a paraphilic act. Possible instigators include recalled memories of experiences from an individual's early life (especially the first shared sexual experience), modeling behavior of others who have carried out paraphilic acts, mimicking sexual behavior depicted in the media, and sometimes recalling emotionally laden events from one's past, such as one's own molestation.

Prior to the first commission of a paraphilic act, the individual appraises the possibility of committing that behavior within the context of cognitive beliefs and attitudes developed during the course of socialization. This cognitive appraisal evaluates what constitutes acceptable or unacceptable behaviors as condoned by one's family, peers, religious training, or education, After evaluation, if the potential act is found to be incompatible with one's view of self, the instigation will be sidetracked before it has the opportunity to occur. If, after appraisal, however, the individual concludes that there are minimal negative consequences from performing the behavior, instigation will occur.

A variety of unconscious and conscious factors may contribute to the evaluative process. For example, the psychoanalytic model suggests that, unconsciously, the child suffers from castration anxiety and identifies with the opposite gender parent, resulting in a biological male who develops the symptom of transvestic fetishism. A cultural model suggests that the socialization process teaches the child appropriate and inappropriate instigations of behavior. For example, in cultures where there is less sex role stereotyping, rape is quite infrequent, whereas in cultures robust with sex role stereotyping, rape occurs at a high frequency.

Social learning theory suggests that the socialization process and the child's own experience help teach the kinds of behaviors that can be expected to be rewarded. Similarly, a failure of such teaching would allow inappropriate behavior to be instigated because the socialization process has not led to its inhibition. Learning theory suggests that since fantasizing of paraphilic interests begins at such an early age and because personal fantasies and thoughts are not shared with others (because sexual topics are precluded from discussion), the use and misuse of paraphilic fantasies and urges will continue uninhibited until late in the individual's life. Only then will the individual begin to realize that such paraphilic interests and urges are inconsistent with societal norms. Unfortunately, by this time, the repetitive use of such fantasies has become chronic. All the various factors listed above probably contribute to the development and expression of a paraphilic interest by not blocking or inhibiting the pathway of the paraphilic interest.

Once the initial paraphilic act occurs, its consequence to the paraphilic patient is then evaluated. Such factors as punishment, a perceived harm or injury to the victim, or a lack of pleasure following the experience may all lead to nonrecurrence of the paraphilic act. Without such inhibitors, when negative consequences do not occur, when the act itself is highly pleasurable to the patient, or when the paraphilic person immediately escapes and thereby avoids seeing any negative consequences experienced by the victim, the urge or act is more likely to be repeated.

A major factor maintaining or increasing paraphilic behavior is the individual's use during masturbation-orgasm of previous fantasies or experiences involving paraphilic acts. The recall of these fantasies and images then becomes paired and associated with the pleasure of masturbation and the enjoyment of ejaculation, so that initial paraphilic behaviors that may at first have had only limited erotic arousal take on an increasingly erotic quality. Since the individual's recall of the initial paraphilic act may selectively suppress negative components of the incident (the paraphiliac's fear of being apprehended, the victim's negative experience during the commission of the act, etc.) while the perceptual recall of the incident focuses on the more positive aspects (the pleasure involved in the commission of the act), the paraphilic experience associated with orgasm becomes increasingly distorted and free of anxiety-producing components. Individuals whose recall is associated with the many negative, anxiety-provoking aspects of the incident will similarly have fewer pairings of the paraphilic images with orgasm, and so the fantasy becomes progressively weaker. The clinical importance of the paraphiliac's use of fantasies of prior experiences is that only a few incidents need be recalled and paired with orgasm hundreds and hundreds of times in order to ensure that the paraphilic fantasies become more and more erotic.

In this fashion, the instigation of paraphilic interests can be prompted by both intrapsychic and extrapsychic phenomena and. depending on the individual's idiosyncratic cognitive apparatus, can be appraised within the individual's self-perception and perceptions of what constitutes appropriate behavior. Since this process occurs at an early age and generally in secret, there is considerable variability in the sharing of knowledge about the repercussions of the use of paraphilic images or the consequences of paraphilic behavior. Usually by the time the paraphiliac is old enough to appreciate that his behavior runs counter to that of society, the paraphilic interest is well ingrained and more resistant to change. As a consequence, the paraphiliac develops a belief system that supports continuation of a long-standing paraphilia. The continued need to conceal the interest supports the maintenance of the cognitive rationalizations for paraphilic urges and behavior. Unless checked, deviant urges gain momentum and strength, fueled by the pleasure from orgasmic experiences associated with paraphilic images, thoughts, and fantasies.

PATHOLOGY

All behavior has a biological substrate. Factors that change the normality of that substrate thereby can influence the individual's behavior. Attempts to identify pathological conditions associated with paraphilias have followed two different lines of research.

ORGANIC DISEASE ASSOCIATED WITH PARAPHILIAS A number of studies have begun to appear that identify abnormal organic findings in paraphiliacs. None of these studies have been of random samples, but are instead extensive investigations of paraphiliacs who have been referred to large medical centers. Paraphiliacs in whom organic factors are unlikely or not suspected are rarely referred to such medical centers, and as a consequence, assessment of the referred samples reveals a high incidence of organic disease. The assessed paraphiliacs not only comprise skewed, nonrandom samples, but are usually not compared with a control group of nonparaphiliacs. In studies where such comparisons have been made, the initial differences felt to be specific to paraphiliacs disappear as appropriate control groups appear to have a similar incidence of abnormalities.

Of those paraphiliacs evaluated at referral centers who had positive organic findings, 74 percent had abnormal hormonal levels, 27 percent hard or soft neurological signs, 24 percent chromosomal abnormalities, 9 percent seizures, 9 percent dyslexia, 4 percent abnormal electroencephalograms (without seizures), 4 percent major psychiatric disorders, and 4 percent mental retardation. The remaining question, however, is whether these abnormalities are etiologically related to paraphilic interests or are incidental findings that bear no relevance to the development of paraphilic interests. Until this dilemma is resolved, more extensive organic evaluations are indicated when the paraphiliac's history is positive to any of the following criteria:

1. Is the paraphiliac's behavior significantly more idiosyncratic than the typical paraphiliac with this arousal pattern?
2. Is the paraphiliac excessively aggressive during the commission of the paraphilic crime?
3. Does the paraphiliac report auras or seizure-like symptoms prior to or during the commission of the paraphilic act?
4. Does the paraphiliac have an abnormal body habitus?
5. Does the paraphiliac show any inclination of sadistic or aggressive arousal concomitant with a disordered sexual identity or transvestic fetishism?

If one or more of the above questions are answered positively, the paraphiliac needs more extensive testing. It is anticipated that as the diagnostic studies become more sophisticated—through computed tomography (CT) and positron emission tomography (PET) techniques, for example—a higher incidence of abnormal organic findings will occur. The vital question, however, will still remain whether abnormal organic findings are etiologically connected with the paraphilia.

Robert was 24 when he sought help following his first arrest for exhibitionism. Sexual problems had begun at age 8 when he first masturbated in front of his sister. His family was quite concerned, and he was subsequently referred to specialists on a number of occasions to help him control his behavior. At age 16, he began exposing himself and masturbating in public. His urges to expose were first preceded by his smelling a peculiar odor that he perceived as emanating from his upper lip. He would stretch his upper lip towards his nose, focus on the odor, and begin to have urges to expose himself. The most erotic aspect of his fantasy was imagining that the female to whom he exposed himself viewed him as an inferior person.

Psychological treatment was minimally effective at helping him control his urges. Treatment with carbamazepine (Tegretol) led to a dramatic reduction in his urges and behaviors. After a number of months of complete control, he relapsed during a period of emotional stress in spite of continuation of the drug. His diagnosis was that of temporal lobe seizures with subsequent exhibitionism.

PATHOLOGICAL PSYCHOPHYSIOLOGICAL FINDINGS A second, more extensive line of research has been directed at detecting the presence of paraphilic arousal in populations of known paraphiliacs and populations without such diagnoses. The methodology assesses sexual preference using direct psychophysiological measurements of the individual's erectile responses.

The unique characteristic of the paraphiliac is his sexual arousal to unusual objects or behaviors. K. Freund in the early 1960s pioneered a new methodology to arrive at paraphilic diagnoses by measuring a paraphiliac's erections to paraphilic and nonparaphilic stimuli. Recording volumetric size of the penis with a penile plethysmograph, he was able to demonstrate a high correlation between the patient's reported deviant behavior and objectively recorded responses in the laboratory. Since then, a host of technological changes have expanded clinical understanding of the paraphiliac's sexual arousal.

Laboratories in treatment centers for paraphiliacs can record deviant and nondeviant arousal by attaching a small penile circumference device commonly used during nocturnal penile tumescence monitoring. Clinicians are best able to differentiate among paraphiliacs interested in fetishism, exhibitionism, pedophilia, and rape. Moreover, psychophysiological assessment is especially valuable in detecting very specific, subtle arousal differences within categories of paraphilias. Psychophysiological assessment has not only successfully identified the differences in sexual arousal patterns among rapists, sadists, and nonrapists, but has revealed the similarities between molesters of young female children and individuals involved in incestuous activities with young girls.

Advantages of psychophysiological assessment Psychophysiological assessment avoids placing an overreliance on self-reported sexual preference. One of the greatest obstacles to providing treatment for paraphiliacs occurs when some individuals will not or cannot accurately report the presence of their deviant arousal. Psychophysiological assessment has been used to confront paraphiliacs with objective evidence of their deviant arousal. When confronted, 55 percent of paraphiliacs report new paraphilic interests that they previously had neglected to report to the clinician. In this fashion, the penile transducer method allows the clinician a means of obviating the paraphiliac's denial and brings him to the point of reporting more of his deviant interest so that treatment can progress.

The anticipated effectiveness of treatment can also be evaluated in the psychophysiological laboratory. A common treatment used to help the patients control deviant interest is to teach them how to imagine aversive consequences of their deviant behavior so that they become skilled in pairing or associating the antecedents of paraphilic behavior with these aversive images. This treatment, called covert sensitization, might use a variety of deviant and aversive scenes. The clinician's difficulty is in determining which deviant stimuli are most arousing to the offender and which aversive scenes might be most effective at controlling or eliminating the paraphiliac's arousal. This determination can be accomplished in the laboratory by presenting such pairs of stimuli to the offender and recording the extent to which the deviant imagery elicits erections and the aversive stimuli disrupts those erections. With this objective evidence of treatment effectiveness, the clinician can save time by knowing which types of aversive images are most helpful in reducing the paraphiliac's deviant interest.

In recent years, psychophysiological assessment has been used to monitor the success of therapy during treatment. The common methodology is to assess the paraphiliac's erectile responses to paraphilic and nonparaphilic sexual stimuli before, during, and after treatment. If treatment is effective, the paraphiliac's arousal to nondeviant stimuli should increase or be maintained, wheras the arousal to paraphilic stimuli should decrease or be eliminated. Because some paraphiliacs can voluntarily inhibit their deviant arousal, the clinician should be cautious about interpreting the paraphiliac's failure to respond to paraphilic stimuli posttreatment, since psychophysiological assessment is less valid when no erection is elicited. By contrast, the clinician should be most concerned about sustained deviant arousal posttreatment.

Disadvantages of psychophysiological assessment Unfortunately, a serious problem can arise when interpreting the measurement of sexual arousal. In experiments designed to detect whether patients were faking erections in order to appear sexually "normal," Freund was the first to observe that some men are successfully able to exert voluntary control over their erectile response. Laboratory experiments to test whether patients can suppress erections suggest that apparent voluntary suppression may be the result of the patient's shifting his attention away from the target stimuli. Countermeasures to focus the paraphiliac's attention to the stimuli are important to ensure validity of the assessment.

The absence of tumescence is problematic for interpretation, inasmuch as it could mean that the stimulus is really not arousing or that the patient can suppress his arousal. A few strategies have been implemented to increase the validity of the psychophysiological assessment, such as providing the patient a task to occupy his hands and prevent manual manipulation of the penile transducer, using a surveillance camera, and increasing communication between patient and technician to keep the patient's attention on the stimuli during assessment. Clinicians, however, should place their faith more in the presence of erection rather than its absence, since it has been established that erections are much more difficult to generate voluntarily than to suppress.

CLINICAL SIGNS AND SYMPTOMS

Different diagnostic categories of paraphilias exist because of the differing erotic attractions of paraphiliacs. In spite of these different categories, there are some similarities across them. More than 50 percent of all paraphilias, irrespective of diagnostic category, have their onset prior to age 18. Individuals with one diagnostic category of paraphilia rarely have that one paraphilic interest alone. Instead, paraphiliacs frequently have three to five different paraphilias, either occurring concomitantly or at different times throughout their lives. This is especially the case with exhibitionism, fetishism, masochism, sadism, transvestic fetishism, voyeurism, and zoophilia.

If specific conflicts produced specific paraphilias, it would be unlikely that multiple paraphilias would occur in the same individual. A more parsimonious explanation is that individuals who develop paraphilias have a general deficit that predisposes them to develop a variety of paraphilic interests. Within any paraphilic category, there is tremendous variability in terms of the number of paraphilic behaviors committed. Within most diagnostic categories, there are individuals who have committed hundreds to thousands of paraphilic acts. The frequency of commission appears to be related to the consequence of the behavior. Paraphilic behaviors that are solitary (fetishism) or those where minimal repercussions fall on the paraphiliac (voyeurism and obscene phone calls) occur at higher frequencies, whereas behaviors that involve others and are likely to have strong negative sanctions (pedophilia) occur at much lower frequencies.

The paraphiliac is usually male, a finding confirmed across different societies and cultures. Although female pedophiles and masochists are seen in clinical practice, females with other paraphilic arousal patterns are a novelty. The occurrence of paraphilic behavior, as with most asocial acts, peaks between ages 15 and 25 and gradually declines, so that by age 50, the occurrence of paraphilic acts is very low, except for those paraphilic behaviors that occur in isolation or with a cooperative partner.

The following case reports describe typical paraphiliacs found in each of the major diagnostic categories. Because paraphilic behavior is secretive, it breeds idiosyncratic responses in the paraphiliac. As a consequence, considerable variation in each category is normal. One should appreciate that the following descriptions are oversimplifications of a real world filled with variance.

EXHIBITIONISM Exhibitionists have recurrent intense sexual urges to expose their genitals to an unsuspecting stranger, who in 99 percent of cases is female (Table 21.3-2). The exhibitionist's urges to expose himself intensify when he has excessive free time or is under significant stress. He usually has rewarding sexual encounters with his adult partner, but concomitantly exposes himself to other females. As with all paraphiliacs, the frequency of the deviant behavior varies tremendously; some exhibitionists expose themselves only a few times, whereas others may expose thousands of times. The typical exhibitionist will have hundreds of exposures before he seeks treatment. The urges to expose come in waves, and during days to weeks the exhibitionist may expose himself daily from 1 to 15 times, followed by periods of quiescence that may last weeks, months, or even years.

The steps preceding exposure may vary among exhibitionists, but will generally proceed in a predictable sequence: having free time on his hands or emotional conflict at home or on the job; driving around while fantasizing prior episodes of exposing oneself; selecting an area of town he

TABLE 21.3-2
Diagnostic Criteria for Exhibitionism

A. Over a period of at least 6 months, recurrent intense sexual urges and sexually arousing fantasies involving the exposure of one's genitals to an unsuspecting stranger.
B. The person has acted on these urges, or is markedly distressed by them.

Table from DSM-III-R *Diagnostic and Statistical Manual of Mental Disorders,* ed 3, revised. Copyright American Psychiatric Association, Washington, DC, 1987. Used with permission.

knows and can escape from; selecting a woman who is by herself; preparing for the exposure (stopping the car, hiding close to a walkway); and culminating in the actual exposure while masturbating, or escaping and then masturbating while imagining the experience. Typical of most paraphiliacs, the exhibitionist fantasizes sexual encounters with his target. He may fantasize that her startled look reflects seeing the immensity of his penis, her overwhelming desire to have sex with him, or other cognitive distortions. Initially in his career, the exhibitionist has no cognitive distortions, but as time progresses, he develops and embellishes the attitudes and beliefs that justify his continuing exposures.

A common variant of the exhibitionist is the public masturbator who carries out all the typical exhibitionistic behavior except actually exposing himself. He masturbates from a distance, not allowing his target to see him. His masturbation is accompanied by fantasies of developing a special sexual relationship with the unsuspecting female as he uses her images to enhance his sexual arousal. In addition to their exhibitionism, a significant number of exhibitionists are concomitantly or have previously been involved in frottage, voyeurism, rape, or pedophilia.

George was a 22-year-old single male referred following his fourth arrest for exhibitionism. He had exposed himself on more than 60 occasions since age 18. He would usually expose himself from his car to women up to their late 20s. The victim's response was to laugh, to be startled and run away, or to make harsh comments to him. Following his first exposure, he concluded that there was nothing to it and he did not expose himself again until 4 months later. Since then, he exposed himself two to three times per month. Exposures occurred in waves, followed by periods of up to a year of no exhibitionism. His four arrests had led to minimal consequences for him. During the year prior to referral, he had a rich, enjoyable sexual relationship with his girlfriend, with frequent intercourse and without sexual dysfunction.

An intelligent student, George logically appreciated the inappropriateness of his exposing himself. Although he hoped for a sexual encounter with one of his victims, it had never occurred. Although 15 percent of his masturbatory fantasies involved recalling previous episodes of exposing, his remaining fantasies were of normal heterosexual intercourse. An increased intensity of his urges to expose were provoked by seeing female peers walking or driving by themselves. He would follow a woman in his car while fantasizing her possible positive reaction should he expose himself. These fantasies were soon accompanied by masturbation while driving. His excitement and anxiety intensified as the time of his attempted exposure approached. Exposure was usually to a woman in her car while driving his car, a technically difficult feat fraught with danger.

Typical was his careless disregard for protecting his identity. George made minimal attempts to conceal his appearance, the characteristics of his car, or even his license plate. After a series of exposures, he would be overcome by depression and intense guilt. He would resolve not to expose himself again, but after 1 to 6 weeks, his cycle of recurrent urges and exposures would return.

FETISHISM AND TRANSVESTIC FETISHISM Paraphiliacs with fetishism, according to DSM-III, used nonliving objects to achieve sexual excitement repeatedly, and these objects were not limited to articles of female clothing used in cross-dressing (such as with transvestic fetishism) or to objects designed for purposes of sexual stimulation (vibrators). In contrast, transvestic fetishism was defined as the recurrent and persistent cross-dressing by a heterosexual male where cross-dressing is for the purpose of sexual excitement (at least initially in the course of the disorder), and intense frustration occurs when cross-dressing is interfered with.

DSM-III-R has clarified that, in both cases, the sexual interest or behavior must last for at least 6 months and either recur repeatedly or the individual must be markedly distressed by the urges (Tables 21.3-3 and 21.3-4). Both fetishism and transvestic fetishism have their onset during adolescence. They differ in that the fetishist does not use the fetish object in the course of cross-dressing, while the transvestite is aroused by the dressing-up process or by his public appearance while cross-dressed. Table 21.3-5 shows the essential differences among diagnostic categories of individuals who might present somewhat similar arousal patterns or behaviors: the fetishist, transvestite, transsexual, and effeminate homosexual.

The eventual dilemma faced by both the fetishist and the transvestite occurs as they become progressively more intensely aroused to sexual behaviors that exclude a sexual partner. Initially, the fetish or transvestite behavior fails to interfere with nonparaphilic sexual behavior. As time progresses and the fetishist or transvestite recalls more frequently his paraphilic fantasies and urges during sexual arousal, he attends less and less to his sexual partner. Greater distancing between the paraphiliac and his partner results until the partner eventually terminates the relationship. Unfortunately, most fetishists and transvestites are unaware of this progression of their paraphilic interest, and by the time such arousal has led to marked conflicts between the couple, reversal of the deviant arousal has become very problematic.

In addition to their fetishism, significant numbers of fetishists are concomitantly or have previously been involved in exhibitionism, frottage, pedophilia, rape, or voyeurism. Significant numbers of transvestic fetishists are concomitantly or have previously been involved in exhibitionism, pedophilia, or rape.

Gary was 35 when evaluated because he wished to abandon transvestism. He reported that at age 6 he first had interest to cross-dress, but did not act on his urges until age 10. He experienced orgasms during adolescence when he would dress in women's clothes and rub his penis against his mattress, imagining how he looked

TABLE 21.3-3
Diagnostic Criteria for Fetishism

A. Over a period of at least 6 months, recurrent intense sexual urges and sexually arousing fantasies involving the use of nonliving objects by themselves (e.g., female undergarments).

Note: The person may at other times use the nonliving object with a sexual partner.

B. The person has acted on these urges, or is markedly distressed by them.

C. The fetishes are not only articles of female clothing used in cross-dressing (transvestic fetishism) or devices designed for the purpose of tactile genital stimulation (e.g., vibrator).

Table from DSM-III-R *Diagnostic and Statistical Manual of Mental Disorders,* ed 3, revised. Copyright American Psychiatric Association, Washington, DC, 1987. Used with permission.

TABLE 21.3-4
Diagnostic Criteria for Transvestic Fetishism

A. Over a period of at least 6 months, in a heterosexual male, recurrent intense sexual urges and sexually arousing fantasies involving cross-dressing.

B. The person has acted on these urges, or is markedly distressed by them.

C. Does not meet the criteria for gender identity disorder of adolescence or adulthood, nontranssexual type, or transsexualism.

Table from DSM-III-R *Diagnostic and Statistical Manual of Mental Disorders,* ed 3, revised. Copyright American Psychiatric Association, Washington, DC, 1987. Used with permission.

TABLE 21.3-5
Characteristics of Males Who Cross-Dress

Diagnostic Category	*Stimulus Eliciting Arousal*	*Adult Sexual Preference*	*Gender Motor Behavior*	*Sexual Identity*
Fetishism	Nonliving objects	Usually females	Masculine	Male
Transvestic fetishism	Cross-dressing in female clothing	Usually females	Masculine (feminine while cross-dressed)	Male
Effeminate homosexuality	Males	Males	Somewhat feminine	Male
Transsexuality (male to female)	Males	Males	Exaggerated feminine	Female

dressed in women's clothing. Initially, this behavior occurred four times per month, but over the years it had accelerated so that by the time he was referred, he was masturbating four to six times per week while cross-dressed. At age 25, an additional erotic fantasy was added to his transvestic fantasies. He imagined himself being forced to cross-dress by a strong, humiliating woman. At age 27, after a nearly lifelong pattern of using transvestite and masochistic fantasies, he first had intercourse with a female partner. Engaging in intercourse two to three times per week, Gary always fantasized himself cross-dressed as a woman during these encounters.

Over the years, his interest in females began to wane as he realized that he was more attracted to women's clothing than to women. He maintained an extensive collection of women's clothes and frequently read transvestic literature. His referral was precipitated by his increasing concern that he might break up with his girlfriend because of his transvestite behavior and his lack of sexual interest in her.

FROTTEURISM Frotteurism as defined by DSM-III-R involves recurrent preoccupation with intense sexual urges or fantasies of at least 6 months' duration involving touching or rubbing a nonconsenting person (Table 21.3-6). It is the touching of the target that is erotic and not the coercive nature of the act. Furthermore, the individual either acts on these urges or is markedly distressed by them.

The frotteur usually carries out his paraphilic behavior under crowded conditions. Entering the rush-hour crowds on subways and buses allows him access to potential victims as well as some rationalization for why he rubs up against his victim. The frotteur frequently touches his victim with his erect penis through his clothes, up against the victim's buttocks or thighs. At other times, he may use his hands to rub an unsuspecting victim. The typical frotteur waits at the subway station 6 to 8 feet back from the crowd, identifying the victim that he plans to touch. As the subway train arrives, he moves in behind her, putting his arms up to her sides so that no one can separate them. After the crowd surges forward to fill the car, the frotteur has approximately a minute and a half between subway stations to rub the victim. Erection is almost immediate as he pushes his penis against her. His fantasies of having a special relationship with her and the sensations of touching her body with his penis accentuate his arousal so that he frequently can ejaculate in 1 minute. Should ejaculation occur, he will cease the activity and go on to his destination. Should he not ejaculate after rubbing his first victim, he often will get off at the next station and take another subway train to rub another unsuspecting victim.

TABLE 21.3-6
Diagnostic Criteria for Frotteurism

A. Over a period of at least 6 months, recurrent intense sexual urges and sexually arousing fantasies involving touching and rubbing against a nonconsenting person. It is the touching, not the coercive nature of the act, that is sexually exciting.

B. The person has acted on these urges, or is markedly distressed by them.

Table from DSM-III-R *Diagnostic and Statistical Manual of Mental Disorders,* ed 3, revised. Copyright American Psychiatric Association, Washington, DC, 1987. Used with permission.

In addition to frottage, significant numbers of frotteurs are concomitantly or have previously been involved in exhibitionism, pedophilia, sadism, rape, or voyeurism.

James had been a frotteur for 10 years when seen at age 45. His usual pattern was first to decide at home if he had time to carry out frottage while on his way to work. He would then place plastic wrap around his penis while dressing, anticipating that when he ejaculated, the ejaculate would not show through his suit pants. To increase the likelihood of crowding, he would stand in the middle of the subway platform with the majority of passengers waiting to board. He would then select a woman with large buttocks and tight-fitting clothes. After entering the train, pressed to her, he would fantasize a sexual experience with her as he pushed his penis against her buttocks. On 40 percent of occasions, he would ejaculate and go on to work. If he did not ejaculate, he would continue the cycle with a new victim until he ran out of time or was able to ejaculate. By the time he was seen, he had been arrested on two occasions, but had carried out frottage on more than a thousand separate occasions.

Referral for treatment was precipitated by his arrest. His guilt following each commission of frottage was usually high, but was now excessive as he anticipated that others at work would learn of his deviant behavior and that he would be fired from his white-collar job.

PEDOPHILIA Pedophilia involves recurrent intense sexual urges or arousal to children 13 years of age or younger that has persisted over a minimum of 6 months (Table 21.3-7). The individual diagnosed as a pedophile should be at least 16 years of age and at least 5 years older than the victim. When the paraphiliac is younger than 16, clinical judgment should determine whether the diagnosis is warranted (given the maturity of the paraphiliac and victim). The gender of the

TABLE 21.3-7
Diagnostic Criteria for Pedophilia

A. Over a period of at least 6 months, recurrent intense sexual urges and sexually arousing fantasies involving sexual activity with a prepubescent child or children (generally age 13 or younger).

B. The person has acted on these urges, or is markedly distressed by them.

C. The person is at least 16 years old and at least 5 years older than the child or children in A.

Note: Do not include a late adolescent involved in an ongoing sexual relationship with a 12- or 13-year-old.

Specify: same sex, opposite sex, or **same and opposite sex.**

Specify if **limited to incest.**

Specify: exclusive type (attracted only to children), or **nonexclusive type.**

Table from DSM-III-R *Diagnostic and Statistical Manual of Mental Disorders,* ed 3, revised. Copyright American Psychiatric Association, Washington, DC, 1987. Used with permission.

victim has major prognostic value since pedophiles molesting boys show high recidivism; appropriately, DSM-III-R includes specifying whether the victim and the offender are of the same or opposite gender. Additional specifiers include whether the pedophilia is limited to incest and whether the paraphiliac is exclusive (only attracted to children) or nonexclusive (attracted to children and adults). The latter two specifiers also appear to predict recidivism and help clarify treatment components. Clinicians should become knowledgeable about pedophilia, because this category of paraphilia is the most common of sexual assaults.

The vast majority of child molestations involve genital fondling or oral sex. Vaginal or anal penetration of the child is an infrequent occurrence except in cases of incest. Although the majority of child victims coming to public attention are female, the reason appears to be a product of the referral process. Offenders report that when they actually touch the child, the majority (60 percent) of victims are male. This figure is in sharp contrast to nontouching victimization of children, such as window peeping or exhibitionism, which in 99 percent of cases is committed against female children. In addition to their pedophilia, a significant number of pedophiles are concomitantly or have previously been involved in exhibitionism, voyeurism, or rape.

Albert was 52 years of age when he sought counseling following his second arrest for endangering the morals of a minor. He reported that since age 7, he had been aroused to young boys all his life. At age 12, he first began mutual fondling and anal manipulation of his male peers. From age 16 to 18, he enjoyed fondling young boys in crowded surroundings (frottage). As he matured through adolescence and adulthood, his attraction to 10-year-old boys expanded to adolescent boys and adult males. At age 18, he was arrested for impairing the morals of a minor and was placed on probation. At age 21, he married, hoping that his limited interest in females would be enhanced by sexual experiences with his wife. Shortly before their marriage, he told her of his arousal to young boys, but the topic was never discussed again. He denied sexual involvement with any of his four children, including his three boys.

In addition to young adults and adolescent boys, he had been sexually involved with more than 50 boys under 14, usually neighbors or boys that he met through his extensive church work or at recreational centers and electronic game parlors. Although he also reported attraction to young girls under 14, he denied any sexual involvement with them. He reported his greatest arousal was to adult males, followed in order by adolescent males, males under 14, girls under 14, and adult females. In the psychophysiological laboratory assessment, however, his arousal to adolescent boys was twice as great as his arousal to boys under 14 and to adolescent girls, followed distantly by adult males, and with negligible arousal to both adult females and girls under 14.

Although intercourse with his wife at first occurred every 1 to 2 weeks, the act was accomplished by his fantasizing that these sexual activities were not actually with his wife but with adolescent or young males. Although his wife would freely participate in fellatio, such activity would remind him of his extensive experiences with males. As a consequence, his sexual encounters with her became less frequent.

SEXUAL MASOCHISM The DSM-III criteria for sexual masochism involved either (1) a preferred or exclusive mode of producing sexual excitement is to be humiliated, bound, beaten, or otherwise be made to suffer, or (2) the individual has intentionally participated in activity in which he or she was physically harmed or his or her life was threatened in order to produce sexual excitement. DSM-III-R presents similar criteria except that the period of masochistic urges or fantasies must be 6 months in duration, and the individual must either act or be markedly distressed by these urges (Table 21.3-8).

Because arousal to masochism involves an appreciation of the sadist's goals and objectives in harming his or her victim-

TABLE 21.3-8
Diagnostic Criteria for Sexual Masochism

A. Over a period of at least 6 months, recurrent intense sexual urges and sexually arousing fantasies involving the act (real, not simulated) of being humiliated, beaten, bound, or otherwise made to suffer.

B. The person has acted on these urges, or is markedly distressed by them.

Table from DSM-III-R *Diagnostic and Statistical Manual of Mental Disorders,* ed 3, revised. Copyright American Psychiatric Association, Washington, DC, 1987. Used with permission.

partner, it is not surprising that 30 percent of masochists have also performed the sadist's role and show sadistic arousal as well. In addition, a significant number of masochists are concomitantly or have previously been involved in exhibitionism, pedophilia, rape, or transvestism.

Denise was 35 when referred for treatment for her anxiety in groups. She described herself as a social isolate with marked difficulties when around others because she never knew how to act or what to say. She came from an exceedingly poor family living in an isolated, primitive mountainous area of the United States. When she was born, her mother refused to bring Denise home from the hospital, claiming she already had too many children to care for. Denise was brought home after her father agreed to care for her. At age 3, her father died, and Denise was cared for by her hostile, violent, and physically abusive mother. Denise's only form of entertainment was to read pulp magazines that described how women were exploited by their lovers.

She slept in her mother's bed from childhood until age 19. At age 11, her mother began to fondle her while she lay in bed. If she cried during these molestations, her mother callously told her to shut up. When one of her sisters attempted to console her after one of these molestations, her mother struck the sister so hard that she was knocked across the room. The mother's molestations continued throughout Denise's adolescence until she left home at age 19. Throughout these years, she realized the inappropriateness of her mother's behavior, but her utter isolation prevented her from getting help. She was most upset that she had no control of her body during the molestations.

At age 13, the patient began using masochistic fantasies during masturbation, recalling the violent scenes that she read about in magazines. These fantasies persisted and became progressively more violent, so that when she was evaluated, 100 percent of her masturbatory fantasies were of being raped and violated by brutalizing men. Although some of the rape fantasies were tolerable (imagining a lover overcome by lust and raping her), others were intolerable (imagining being sadistically raped by strangers while onlookers watched). Her own attempts at dislodging the masochistic fantasies had proved unsuccessful, and she became increasingly concerned because she was unable to achieve orgasm other than by using these fantasies, which were abhorrent to her.

SEXUAL SADISM The DSM-III criteria for sexual sadism required at least one of the following: (1) On a nonconsenting partner, the individual has repeatedly intentionally inflicted psychological or physical suffering in order to produce sexual excitement; (2) with a consenting partner, the repeatedly preferred or exclusive mode of achieving sexual excitement combines humiliation with simulated or mildly injurious bodily suffering; and (3) on a consenting partner, bodily injury that is extensive, permanent, or possibly mortal is inflicted in order to achieve sexual excitement. DSM-III-R has simplified these diagnostic criteria, as shown in Table 21.3-9.

The primary component of the sadist's arousal is a sexual attraction to commit physical injury or psychological harm to the victim far in excess of that required to accomplish compliance with a sexual interaction. As is the case with most paraphilias, the onset of this interest is usually prior to age 18. By adulthood, the individual has usually developed a relationship with a partner in which sadistic assaults or

TABLE 21.3-9
Diagnostic Criteria for Sexual Sadism

A. Over a period of at least 6 months, recurrent intense sexual urges and sexually arousing fantasies involving acts (real, not simulated) in which the psychological or physical suffering (including humiliation) of the victim is sexually exciting to the person.

B. The person has acted on these urges, or is markedly distressed by them.

Table from DSM-III-R *Diagnostic and Statistical Manual of Mental Disorders,* ed 3, revised. Copyright American Psychiatric Association, Washington, DC, 1987. Used with permission.

humiliation has become a regular pattern of their sexual interaction. Rather than committing sadistic acts on multiple partners, the sadist usually performs these acts repetitively against a few partners. Of those males who rape adult females, fortunately only a minority (8 percent) do so because of their sadistic interest. However, paraphiliacs with sadistic arousal frequently rape (38 percent), and these rapes are qualitatively different from other rapists' assaults in that the amount of force used is far in excess of what would be required to subdue the victim into a sexual encounter. The sexual fantasies of the sadist during sexual encounters are, as expected, far more violent than the attacks themselves.

In addition to their sadism, a significant number of sadists are concomitantly or have previously been involved in exhibitionism, frottage, pedophilia, rape, or voyeurism.

Charlie was 25 and single when referred because of sadistic arousal. He began voyeuristic activities at age 15, window peeping at a rate in excess of 100 times per year until age 22. Shortly after his voyeurism began, he started fantasizing about transsexuals and men who cross-dressed. He was especially attracted to thoughts of raping them. He subsequently began dating drag queens, whom he would eventually intoxicate with drugs and then rape anally. At age 16, he also engaged in oral and anal intercourse with male homosexuals, but he denied raping them. At age 18, he began accelerating the frequency of his sadistic attacks on intoxicated drag queens, and would not only rape them but beat them in the testicles. He also began raping 18- to 30-year-old women in attacks that did not involve sadistic beatings, but during which he used threats of physical attack with a knife to subdue his victims.

When referred, he described himself as a bisexual, equally attracted to adult males and adult females. Fifty percent of his masturbatory fantasies were of mutually consenting sexual experiences with adults, but 50 percent of his fantasies involved imagining sadistic attacks upon drag queens or transsexuals. In spite of various paraphilic experiences, he had been arrested only once for a sex crime.

VOYEURISM Voyeurism is the earliest of the paraphilias to develop in that 50 percent of individuals so classified acknowledge voyeuristic arousal prior to age 15. By DSM-III criteria, voyeurism involved the intense desire to observe or actual observation of unsuspecting people who are naked, disrobing, or engaging in sexual activities, and the voyeur repeatedly prefers or uses such peeping as an exclusive method of achieving sexual excitement. DSM-III-R requires that the voyeuristic urges must be present at least 6 months and that either the individual has acted on these urges or is markedly distressed by them (Table 21.3-10). It is appropriate that the DSM-III-R classification does not require that voyeuristic activity be the preferred or exclusive method of achieving sexual excitement, because the majority of individuals who window peep have normal, enjoyable sexual encounters with their adult partners. To rule out all individuals who carry out window peeping but do not exclusively prefer it would exclude the majority of individuals who commit voyeurism.

TABLE 21.3-10
Diagnostic Criteria for Voyeurism

A. Over a period of at least 6 months, recurrent intense sexual urges and sexually arousing fantasies involving the act of observing an unsuspecting person who is naked, in the process of disrobing, or engaging in sexual activity.

B. The person has acted on these urges, or is markedly distressed by them.

Table from DSM-III-R *Diagnostic and Statistical Manual of Mental Disorders,* ed 3, revised. Copyright American Psychiatric Association, Washington, DC, 1987. Used with permission.

Voyeurism is probably initiated and sustained at an early age because of the infrequent consequences to the voyeur for perpetrating his voyeuristic activity. Many targets of voyeurism are unaware that they are being observed by a voyeur and, as a consequence, few attempts at apprehension occur. The typical voyeur may spend 1 to 3 hours cruising his favorite areas, looking for opportunities to window peep. He usually masturbates while window peeping on others, but may wait until he returns home to masturbate while recalling his experience.

In addition to their voyeurism, a significant number of voyeurs are concomitantly or have previously been involved in exhibitionism, frottage, pedophilia, rape, or sadism.

Fred was 31 when referred for treatment of his voyeurism that had culminated in his recent arrest. His interest in voyeurism began at age 15 when he began window peeping approximately twice per month on his 15-year-old neighbor while she dressed. He terminated window-peeping activity because he felt guilty for the behavior and also feared getting caught. At age 24, he separated from his wife for a few months because of a major conflict between them regarding child rearing. Eight months later, while jogging, he began glancing at windows, and 1 month later began window peeping. After eight episodes of window peeping, he told his wife what he had done. Feeling guilty about his voyeuristic activity, he stopped jogging. Shortly thereafter, he began going to strip joints to watch nude dancing. Just prior to his referral, while between jobs, he found himself with nothing to do, so he began jogging again. His voyeurism returned, and he was subsequently arrested. By the time he was evaluated, he had window peeped on 10 victims for a total of 33 times. He and his wife both confirmed their rich and varied sex life with intercourse five to seven times per week. As a prelude to intercourse, she would often undress in front of him as if he were watching a stranger.

ZOOPHILIA Zoophilia in DSM-III was defined as a repeatedly preferred or exclusive use of animals in order to achieve sexual excitement. If sexual excitement with animals is transient and occurs because of the unavailability of suitable human partners or is a form of sexual experimentation that is not repetitive, the diagnosis of zoophilia would not be made. DSM-III-R has not included zoophilia as a major paraphilia but includes it as a paraphilia not otherwise specified with the stipulation that the duration of urges and fantasies involving sexual activity with animals must be 6 months in duration and does not have to occur as the preferred or exclusive form of sexual behavior. Indeed, most zoophilia occurs concomitantly with either nonparaphilic sexual behavior or other paraphilic behavior.

Some have considered zoophilia, although socially disgusting, not to be of major psychological importance to the paraphiliac. Clinical experience, however, suggests otherwise. In order to accomplish sexual activities with animals, initial force is required in order to perpetrate the act. Even when animals are trained to perform sexually, the paraphiliac must also learn to ignore a variety of offensive stimuli during the sex act with the animal. The animal's odor, feces, aggressiveness, and nonhuman status must all be successfully ignored in order for the zoophiliac to sustain erection to ejaculation. To ignore such salient features of one's environment while still performing sexually means that participating in zoophilia also trains the paraphiliac to ignore cues that normally inhibit what one does sexually. Although initially this poses minimal problems for the paraphiliac, as time progresses, this ability to ignore such cues appears to make the paraphiliac more susceptible to participating in sexual behavior that runs counter to the culture. Zoophiliacs seen in later adulthood very rarely commit only one type of paraphilia (their zoophilia), but usually have other, multiple paraphilic interests (usually exhibitionism, pedophilia, rape, transvestism, or voyeurism).

Arthur was 16 when referred because of his sexual attraction to 8-year-old boys. His first sexual experiences began at age 7 when he began forcing his penis into dogs' rectums, masturbating them, or letting them lick his erect penis. This behavior occurred twice per month and was unknown to any family member in spite of continuing up to referral. By age 10, he began involving himself with his younger brother, and within 1 year was having regular sexual activities with other young boys outside the home. At age 11, he cross-dressed on three occasions and became attracted to women's clothing. In the next 2 years, he became increasingly involved with sadomasochistic arousal and began masturbating with dead animals against his penis. At age 13, his attraction to sadomasochistic acts and dead animals began to blend with his attraction to young boys, and during one rape of a 5-year-old boy, he seriously thought of killing the child and doing anything he wanted with the boy's dead body. At age 14, during a 1-year period, he had sustained sexual activities with 10 different boys 3 to 12 years of age and had over 150 such sexual contacts with children he usually met in youth groups. When referred, he felt completely out of control because of the high frequency and easy availability of animals and young children, both of which he could easily access sexually.

RAPE AS A PARAPHILIA? An especially difficult issue in paraphilia research is whether some rapists should be considered paraphiliacs. All major treatment centers for paraphiliacs have been providing treatment to rapists for a number of years. The issue, however, is whether the scientific evidence concerning such individuals justifies categorizing rape as a paraphilia.

Within a group of individuals who have committed rape, there is a subcategory who have had the onset of intense, repetitive urges to commit rape from an early age (more than 50 percent of these individuals have the onset of this deviant interest prior to age 21). They, like other paraphiliacs, attempt to control these urges, but at times the urges to commit rape exceed their control and they rape. They feel guilt afterwards and, hence, their urges decline rapidly, only to recur at a later date to repeat the cycle. In this respect, their urges are very similar to those of typical paraphiliacs.

In addition, this subcategory of rapists has the same high occurrence of other paraphilias associated with paraphiliacs. Of rapists with recurrent, intense urges to rape, significant numbers have concomitantly or previously been involved in exhibitionism, frottage, pedophilia, sadism, or voyeurism. If this subcategory of rapists were simply criminals who performed antisocial acts, who forced themselves on others in order to get what they want, one would not expect a high percentage of associated, concomitant paraphilias in their histories. Although 44 percent of paraphilic rapists begin their paraphilic behavior as rapists, the majority do not: 26 percent begin as pedophiles, 9 percent as voyeurs, 8 percent as exhibitionists, 6 percent as frotteurs, 2 percent as fetishists, and the remainder begin within a less common paraphilic category. Here again, one is impressed by how rape behavior appears embedded within a variety of other paraphilic behaviors, suggesting that members of this subcategory of rapists are paraphiliacs.

Paraphilic rapists differ from sadists in that the sadist is clearly attracted and aroused by using greater force against his victim than would be necessary in order to accomplish compliance with his sexual behavior. Rapists, by contrast, are aroused by fantasies and urges of forcing themselves on their victims, but are not aroused by the use of force in excess of that necessary to accomplish the rape. Extensive psychophysiological assessment of rapists and sadists has confirmed these arousal patterns but has also shown that sadists fail to be aroused by stimuli depicting mutually consenting sexual interactions with a partner. Rapists, by contrast, are sexually aroused by such stimuli. Both groups are attracted by depictions of rape. Rapists are not sexually aroused by descriptions of a physical, nonsexual assault upon a female victim. Sadists, by contrast, feel high arousal to such nonsexual, physically assaultive stimuli. Rapists referred to paraphilic treatment centers are referred four times more frequently than sadists.

The issue of paraphilic coercive disorder The task force on paraphilias convened to revise DSM-III concluded that the weight of scientific evidence supported the inclusion of rape as a paraphilia called paraphilic coercive disorder. The category, like all paraphilic categories, was only intended for individuals with intense, repetitive urges of 6 months' duration to commit rape, who had either acted on these urges or were disturbed by their presence. This recommendation by the task force, however, was not approved by the Board of Directors of the American Psychiatric Association.

A number of questions have recurred in deliberations related to the issue of the paraphilic coercive disorder; for example, would inclusion of this diagnostic category lead many rapists to avoid punishment? This avoidance of punishment certainly has not happened with the other paraphilias diagnosed as psychiatric disorders. In court, psychiatric testimony is presented regarding psychological factors contributing to the commission of crimes by paraphiliacs. In the lesser crimes, there is generally some consideration of psychiatric testimony, but as the offender acts more aggressively against the will of the victim, the courts are more cautious about making allowances for the behavior because the perpetrator had a paraphilia. There is no evidence to assume that crimes committed by an offender diagnosed under the category of paraphilic coercive disorder would be treated in any other way. Furthermore, nonparaphilic rapists would be ill advised to seek out escape from punishment by identifying themselves as having intense, repetitive, compulsive urges to commit rape. Such a classification could possibly bring them lengthened sentences to include not only a punishment phase but also a treatment phase to eliminate their paraphilic interest.

Would the inclusion of paraphilic coercive disorder give the message to society that victimization of an individual by a rapist has been trivialized, since the rapist's diagnosis of psychiatric disorder, in part, justifies the motivation for his behavior? There is no question that victims of rape are tremendously influenced by this barbaric act, and that contrary to the rationalizations of men charged with rape, the victim does not precipitate the attack. Services must be expanded for rape victims to help them cope with rape's effects. However, to lower society's high incidence of rape, more forces must be brought together to help eliminate the sexual assault. The major treatment centers for sex offenders in North America and Europe have found that the general elements of treatment for paraphiliacs can be adjusted and applied to those paraphiliacs with repetitive urges to rape. This finding suggests that treatment interventions for rapists could help reduce the number of rape victims.

Are those rapists who have been evaluated so far by psychiatric facilities truly representative of the general population of rapists? Or are the findings with evaluated rapists only representative of a small subset of the general population of rapists? There is no question that only specific rapists have been selectively referred to diagnostic and treatment centers for paraphiliacs. At present, the data are not available to indicate what percentage of rapists might be diagnosed as coercive paraphilic disorders. This issue remains to be researched.

At present, the preponderance of scientific evidence supports the inclusion of a subcategory of rapists as having a true paraphilia. There is little doubt that such an inclusion, however, would raise a number of ethical issues as well as a number of misperceptions by those unfamiliar with the criteria for categorization of rape as a paraphilia.

PARAPHILIA NOT OTHERWISE SPECIFIED Some sexual behaviors do not meet the criteria for any of the preceding specified categories, yet are classified as paraphilias because of their compulsive, repetitive occurrence or the marked distress that the urges or acts cause the patient (Table 21.3-11). Making obscene phone calls is the most common of the paraphilias that follow.

Telephone scatologia (lewdness) Josh was 18 when he was referred for treatment because he was unable to control his impulsive homosexual encounters with peers in local shopping centers. Although he had no dissatisfaction with his homosexual interests or attractions, he was quite upset by the compulsiveness of his clandestine contacts. He was increasingly concerned about the possibility of contracting acquired immune deficiency syndrome (AIDS), because many of his involvements were single-experience sexual activities with males unknown to him.

His obscene phone calls began at age 14. Twice per week, he would make five to ten calls. Sometimes, he dialed numbers at random with the hope of talking about sex with a male. His goal was to ask about the male's penis size and body shape while the patient masturbated to ejaculation. On other occasions, he called the acquaintances or individuals he had seen at school to suggest homosexual activities with them. Despite making over 500 calls, he had been apprehended only once. Although initially frightened by the arrest, he continued to make calls at a somewhat reduced rate.

Necrophilia (corpses)

Partialism (exclusive focus on part of body)

Klismaphilia (enemas)

Urophilia (urine)

Coprophilia (feces) Jack was 33 when referred during his seventh hospitalization because of inappropriate sexual behavior. History revealed extensive involvements with prepubescent girls while in his teens, incestuous involvement with his sister, and sexual involvements with young boys beginning in his late teens. As an adolescent, he also began inserting objects into his urethra and rectum, and began his involvement with coprophilia. He would masturbate frequently, wrapping his own feces around his penis. His repeated inappropriate behavior with children had led to numerous, long-term psychiatric admissions in residential settings. Concerted efforts by the residential staff to provide him with alternative materials for masturbation (e.g., baby oil) were somewhat successful, but he continued to report a preference for masturbating with feces around his penis.

TABLE 21.3-11
Diagnostic Criteria for Paraphilia Not Otherwise Specified

Paraphilias that do not meet the criteria for any of the specific categories.

Examples:
(1) Telephone scatologia (lewdness)
(2) Necrophilia (corpses)
(3) Partialism (exclusive focus on part of body)
(4) Zoophilia (animals)
(5) Coprophilia (feces)
(6) Klismaphilia (enemas)
(7) Urophilia (urine)

Table from DSM-III-R *Diagnostic and Statistical Manual of Mental Disorders,* ed 3, revised. Copyright American Psychiatric Association, Washington, DC, 1987. Used with permission.

DIFFERENTIAL DIAGNOSIS

A number of conditions must be differentiated from paraphilia. Fortunately, the majority of these conditions are sufficiently dissimilar clinically from paraphilias to be differentiated on a clinical basis alone. Other conditions require psychophysiological assessment to arrive at the proper diagnosis.

ADOLESCENT EXPERIMENTATION The most difficult condition to separate from true paraphilia is adolescent experimentation. An adolescent's inappropriate sexual behavior is frequently brought to the attention of the mental health worker with the question of whether the behavior was simply experimentation or evidence of a true deviant arousal pattern the onset of which occurs in adolescence. Since the paraphilic adolescent knows that admitting his paraphilic interest would most certainly lead to more severe consequences than denying involvement in deviant interests, the paraphilic adolescent and nonparaphilic adolescent frequently present the same clinical picture. Initially, both usually deny any kind of involvement in deviant sexual behavior. If involvement is admitted, both also report that this was the first time that they had ever participated in the deviant behavior, that they were led on by their victim, that it was not an enjoyable sexual experience, and that they will never do it again.

The dilemma facing the clinician is that a failure to investigate the paraphilic adolescent for possible deviant interest will lead to further victimizations. Equally as devastating, the adolescent's next offense is more likely to provoke an extreme response from the criminal justice system. Psychophysiological assessment for deviant arousal can be critical under such circumstances. It is especially helpful when positive erection responses to deviant stimuli are recorded in the laboratory and the adolescent flatly denies having attained any arousal to the deviant stimuli. Confrontation with the adolescent regarding this discrepancy can be highly valuable. By contrast, when psychophysiological assessment yields erection responses to deviant stimuli and the adolescent admits erection but still denies a specific interest in deviant themes, the clinician is in a difficult position. Adolescents who do not participate in deviant behavior can become aroused to a variety of deviant stimuli in the laboratory because of the excessive sexual responsivity of adolescents.

The value of psychophysiological assessment of adolescents must also be weighed against the potential negative consequences to the adolescent and his family. The adolescent's psychophysiological results may trigger negative reactions by his family to either the adolescent or to the procedures of objective assessment. Here there are no clear answers, but it is recommended that if the adolescent has gone so far as to be charged and found guilty by the criminal justice system, then the weight of evidence justifies psychophysiological assessment.

MENTAL RETARDATION As greater attention is focused on the sexual behavior of various handicapped groups, increased attention will be given to the sexual behavior of the mentally retarded. Within institutions serving the retarded, a variety of inappropriate behaviors occur that are not drawn to public attention because of the taboo against talking about sex within the institution, fears of the institutional staff that they would be reproached by the patient's family, and an unclear understanding of the treatment or disposition of the mentally retarded individual who does carry out deviant sexual acts.

Psychophysiological assessment of the retarded patient poses problems in itself. Because of deficits in education, retarded individuals have minimal knowledge as to what constitutes appropriate and inappropriate sexual behavior. As a result, psychophysiological measures frequently reveal a lack of discrimination to various sexual stimuli.

OBSESSIVE-COMPULSIVE DISORDERS A few individuals report the recurrent, obsessional fear that they will become involved in sexual activities resulting in public humiliation. The recurrent, obsessional nature of these thoughts and urges can sometimes be similar to those of the paraphiliac. The obsessive-compulsive person, however, denies erections during such thoughts. Psychophysiological assessment also fails to reveal erection responses to the obsessive thoughts. Treatment is therefore directed at the primary condition, the obsessive-compulsive disorder.

ORGANIC MENTAL SYNDROMES A primary function of socialization is the acquisition of social norms concerning sexual behaviors. As disease and aging take their toll on brain functioning, the inhibitory function of the cortex becomes less effective at controlling the individual's sexual urges. As a result, generally beginning in the fifth decade, it is possible to see a variety of individuals whose control over their sexual impulses has weakened. These individuals fail to have lengthy histories of deviant arousal from an earlier age and generally feel considerable guilt and anxiety about their new paraphilic behavior. When they show evidence of impaired brain functioning, treatment is directed at the primary condition, the organic mental syndrome.

SCHIZOPHRENIA AND MANIC-DEPRESSIVE DISORDER Major psychotic illnesses are sometimes associated with inappropriate nonparaphilic sexual behavior that must be differentiated from paraphilic behavior. Sexual offenses committed by individuals with major psychoses are usually qualitatively different from those committed by paraphiliacs. Treatment is directed at the primary psychiatric illness.

Barry was 31 when referred through the criminal justice system after being charged with sexual abuse. He had had a nervous breakdown 8 years earlier and was maintained on major antipsychotics since his 1-month hospitalization. He reported that while on his way to the grocery store, he saw a woman walking near him who he thought was particularly attracted to him. Believing her to be interested in him, he ran up to her, fondled her buttocks and breasts, and then waited for some communication about her love and caring for him. The astounded woman called the police and he was arrested. The patient was somewhat flabbergasted by the arrest since it was his expectation that his "sexual overtures" would be reciprocated by the woman. He denied a prior history of deviant sexual behavior and denied recurrent urges to touch females.

PROGNOSIS

The prognosis for paraphilic patients who are treated or untreated depends heavily on the consequences to the person following commission of deviant sexual acts. Awareness of the negative consequences to the victim of this behavior, comments from friends and family once the deviant behavior becomes known to them, the legal consequences of behavior (such as public notoriety and incarceration), and the influence of treatment directed at reducing the frequency of the paraphilic behavior can all influence the prognosis of the paraphilic patient's condition.

The following specific factors can also have great impact on prognosis.

Age of onset The earlier paraphilic interests and behaviors affect the individual, the more likely they are to become ingrained in the offender's sexual fantasies and more strongly influence his subsequent sexual behavior. Paraphilias with the earliest onset (voyeurism, pedophilia involving boys, frottage, and exhibitionism) are therefore more likely to be sustained.

Age of the paraphilic patient The age of the paraphilic patient at the time of psychiatric evaluation also influences the prognosis in that recurrence of the paraphilic acts is highest when social controls are yet developing (adolescence) and the impact of biological drives is being felt by the individual (ages 15 to 25). Most paraphilias left untreated begin to decrease in frequency as the patient approaches age 40, although some sex crimes, especially those that require no partner (fetishism, transvestism) persist into late adulthood.

The frequency of the paraphilia Patients who have already committed hundreds of paraphilic acts are more likely to recidivate than those with few commissions. The offender who commits numerous crimes must develop cognitive distortions to justify the recurrent nature of his deviant behavior. As offenses become more frequent, these cognitive distortions become more ingrained and thereby insulate the offender from factors that usually decrease the likelihood of reoffense, such as fear of legal repercussions and the shame and guilt involved if others learn of the offense.

Anxiety or guilt related to the paraphilic behavior Guilt or shame following commission of the crime appears crucial if the offender is to gain control and limit the recommission of the crime. The paraphiliac's prognosis is therefore worse if he fails to have anxiety or guilt, whether immediate or delayed, about committing the crime or its consequences to others.

Concomitant drug and alcohol involvement A variety of recreational drugs and alcohol are frequently associated with the commission of paraphilic acts. These chemical agents seem to reduce anxiety and guilt and therefore are thought to block cognitions that might inhibit paraphilic acts. Unless steps are taken to disrupt the concomitant use of these chemical agents, the prognosis is unfavorable.

Environmental surveillance All behaviors that are brought to the attention of others are more likely to normalize. A number of paraphilias, however, are carried out in private and without active participants or victims (fetishism, transvestic fetishism, voyeurism). In such cases, the paraphilic behavior may occur for months or years with the knowledge of no one other than the paraphilic person. As a consequence, in the absence of feedback regarding the inappropriateness of this behavior, the prognosis worsens. When others (wives, friends, and families) concerned about the paraphilic person's welfare can help scrutinize his behavior, the prognosis is improved. However, if a sex offender is of the predatory type, it is difficult to carry out surveillance of his paraphilic behavior since he seeks his victims opportunistically. Surveillance is much easier to carry out with the nonpredatory offender because he offends against victims with whom he has developed a relationship.

The absence of concomitant appropriate sexual arousal The majority of paraphilic patients simultaneously have both paraphilic interests and nonparaphilic sexual interests. Some paraphiliacs, however, have no sexual arousal other than with their paraphilic interest. As a result, elimination of their deviant interests leaves them without an alternative expression of sexuality. Therefore, additional treatment components to assist in the development of appropriate nondeviant sexual arousal are needed, or else the paraphiliac is at greater risk of recidivism.

The presence of multiple problematic behaviors The number of the paraphiliac's behavioral excesses or behavioral deficits also determines the paraphiliac's prognosis. Sexual behavior, like other behaviors, is multicausal. The more conflictual areas requiring change and the fewer resources or support available to him, the worse his prognosis.

The lack of discrimination of paraphilic interests The socialization process teaches individuals how to inhibit sexual interests in socially unacceptable behaviors or objects. With less discrimination of what constitutes appropriate sexual stimuli, the paraphiliac develops more varied responses to more global sexual stimuli. This lack of differentiation is seen in the paraphiliac interested in multiple paraphilic behaviors with females or males, with children, adolescents, or adults, within or outside the family. This lack of differentiation is a strong predictor of poor prognosis and recidivism.

To date, the paraphiliac's prognosis has been predicted on the basis of characteristics that are static and will never change as a result of treatment, such as the age at which the paraphilia develops, the years the paraphilia has been present, and the multiplicity of different paraphilias present in the same individual. Future research must focus on characteristics that can change as a result of treatment, such as excessive deviant physiological arousal, the presence of excessive cognitive distortions, and a deficit in sexual knowledge. Effective treatment should be able to alter such factors so that measures assessed pretreatment would fall outside the normal range, whereas measures assessed after treatment would fall within a range that is subsequently associated with low recidivism. Identifying valid, nonstatic predictors of low recidivism are a high priority for research in the field.

TREATMENT

Clinical management of the paraphiliac can be an exceedingly frustrating experience for both therapist and patient. Establishing a therapeutic alliance is especially problematic because of the extensive denial of most paraphiliacs: The offender may not report his paraphilic acts to the therapist unless confidentiality of records is maintained. If maintained, confidentiality may pose major ethical problems for the therapist, who is further confronted by the reality that his or her paraphilic patient has committed many hedonistic crimes that have caused major emotional problems to victims. For these and other reasons, many clinicians should not attempt to assess and treat paraphiliacs but should instead develop skills at referring such individuals to specialists familiar with working with this special population.

Paraphiliacs usually seek psychiatric care after their paraphilic behavior comes to the attention of others. Public exposure of the patient's previously secret paraphilic behavior usually has a profound impact on the patient by causing a dramatic, temporary reduction in his urges to commit paraphilic acts (Fig. 21.3-1).

This dramatic reduction feeds into the paraphiliac's denial; that is, by the time he seeks psychiatric care, he reports being cured by the very public exposure, humiliation, and resulting anxiety that led him to seek out psychiatric care. It is most helpful for the clinician to point out the natural course of untreated paraphilias by clarifying to him that the dramatic reduction of his urges does, indeed, give him all of the feelings of a true cure and remission of the paraphilia. However, the patient must be acquainted with the expected course of his urges. This transient suppression of his deviant interest will diminish once the acute but temporary crisis of facing legal charges and confrontation by others passes. Most paraphiliacs can recall previous temporary "cures" resulting from prior arrests or from others learning of their paraphilic behavior.

RELATIONSHIP WITH THE CLINICIAN Four factors seem particularly important in helping the paraphiliac develop a working relationship with the clinician. First, the clinician must promptly clarify the degree of confidentiality of any information the paraphiliac may provide. Knowing that any disclosed information is confidential is a giant step toward encouraging the paraphiliac to reveal his problem. Second, trust between therapist and paraphiliac is strengthened by explaining to the patient how the proposed treatment will help him control his paraphilic urges and the expected effectiveness of that treatment. The paraphiliac will be especially comforted by hearing precisely what can be done to help him control his deviant behavior. His usual perception of psychiatric services is that they take a moralistic stance toward paraphilic behavior. Educating the patient on how therapy can help him control his urges and avoid incarceration will allow him to reveal his deviant interests more easily. Third, the clinician should not give the patient the opportunity to discuss at length why he is not a paraphiliac. After the paraphiliac has lied to his therapist, it is difficult to undo the lie even if he wishes to later. Rather than discussing whether the patient is or is not committing paraphilic acts, the therapist should take the position of "let's evaluate the issue, collect the information, and then make a judgment based on the acquired data." Fourth, of considerable assistance to the therapist are various paper-and-pencil tests and psychophysiological techniques currently available in assessing possible paraphiliacs. Excluding the recent plethora of cases of potential child molestation involving divorced couples in child custody issues, the majority of individuals seeking psychiatric assessment will report paraphilic interests and behaviors after the above four steps are taken.

ANTECEDENT EVENTS Treatment for the paraphiliac is more clearly understood by identifying the behavioral excesses and behavioral deficits of the patient. Since offenders'

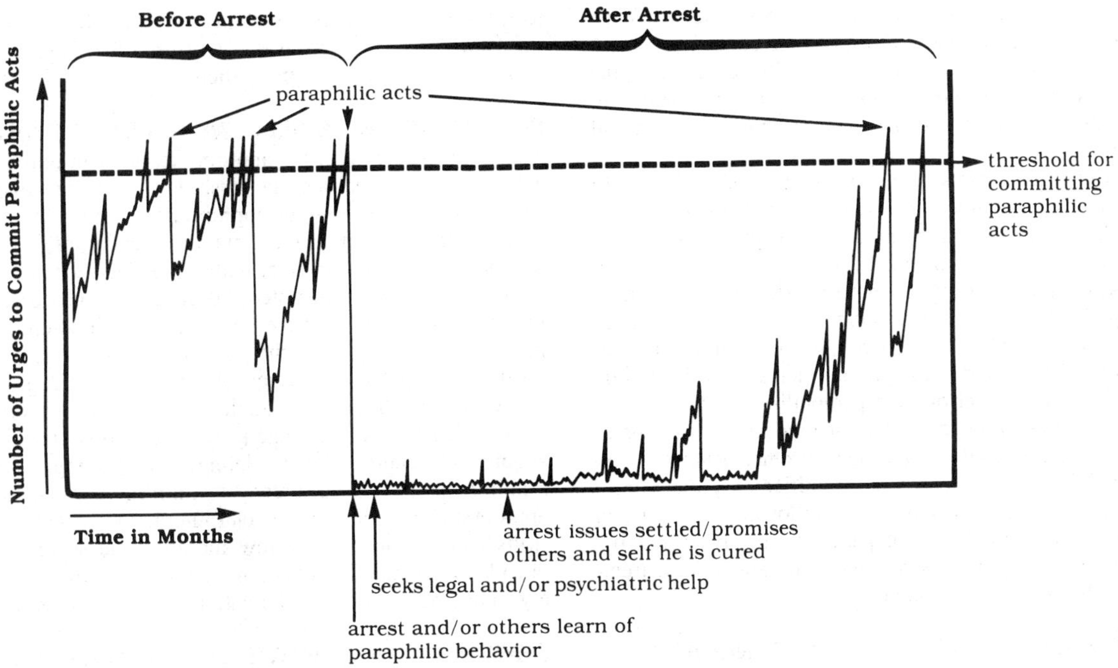

FIGURE 21.3-1. *Frequency of a typical paraphiliac's urges before and after arrest.*

lives are disrupted because of their commission of paraphilic acts, the first priority must focus on teaching the paraphiliac to block or eliminate his deviant behavior. Paraphilic behavior is seldom the result of spontaneous action. Instead, there is a series of behaviors or chain of events leading to the actual commission of the crime. The identification of elements early in this chain and subsequent disruption of the chain is crucial if the offender is to gain control of his behavior.

Providing the offender with a better understanding of the sequence of events and with a technique for disrupting this sequence is one goal of treatment. A variety of methods are available that the offender can use to disrupt such sequences, such as (1) introducing conflicting fantasies that reflect what will happen if he continues following his traditional chain of events (a technique called covert sensitization) or (2) associating noxious stimuli early in the chain so as to disrupt his fantasizing (such as using ammonia or valeric acid, noxious odors that the paraphiliac self-administers to disrupt the progression of the sequence).

DECREASE OF DEVIANT BEHAVIOR An equally important goal of treatment is to assist the paraphiliac in reducing the erotic quality of his paraphilic interest. Without paraphilic desires, attraction, and interest, the paraphiliac would not commit paraphilic acts. Treatment in this sphere attempts to defuse the source of the deviant behavior—paraphilic arousal. Early attempts at reducing paraphilic arousal focused on efforts by the therapist to do something aversive to the paraphiliac, such as showing slides depicting paraphilic stimuli while shocking the patient with faradic stimulation to the hand. These early therapeutic attempts failed because the therapy was not controlled by the patient and was based on the premise that successful treatment would prevent the offender from ever having a recurrent paraphilic interest or fantasy once treatment was completed.

Current therapy to decrease paraphilic arousal is preferably patient controlled, and its goal is to teach the sex offender not only how to reduce his paraphilic interest significantly but to learn a self-administered treatment that can be applied any place or any time that the patient might have a recurrence of paraphilic fantasies, desires, or interests. Therapy is seen as training a skill that would initially have to be applied frequently when paraphilic interests are high, but would also need to be applied at times in the future when unpredicted conditions might lead to a recurrence of the paraphilic fantasies and urges.

Satiation and signaled punishment Controlled studies have identified two promising methods of reducing paraphilic interests: satiation and signaled punishment. Satiation is a boredom technique in which the sex offender uses his most erotic fantasies postorgasm in a boring, repetitive fashion to extinguish the erotic quality of his paraphilic desire. By requiring the patient to audiotape each session, this method is especially applicable to paraphilic interest because it is relatively easy to verify patient compliance and to assess the accuracy with which the individual has learned the treatment method. Signaled punishment involves combining faradic aversion therapy with biofeedback of one's erections to deviant stimuli.

Intervention with drugs The above treatment interventions are not always effective. In some cases, the paraphiliac's behavior is highly dangerous to others, and thus an immediately effective intervention is required. Organic intervention with drugs to reduce sexual drive has proved to be a valuable resource in treating these more dangerous offenders (aggressive child molesters, sadists, and masochists) who require a prompt means of curtailing their paraphilic behavior. Although surgical castration has been ineffective with more dangerous sexual aggressives, chemical castration with either cyproterone acetate (Androcur) or medroxyprogesterone acetate (Provera) to reduce the male hormone testosterone can help the offender control his deviant sexual interests. As yet, there is no evidence supporting the contention that paraphilias result from excessive sexual drive, but there is a considerable body of evidence indicating that the paraphiliac's control can be improved by the administration of these drugs. When administered to an offender who has poor control or whose commission of the crime would be especially dangerous to the victim, they provide the therapist with an alternative to hospitalization. These drugs, however, are not available in all countries.

The various side effects of the drugs can limit their use. In addition, many paraphiliacs refuse the drugs because of their global reduction of nonparaphilic as well as paraphilic drives. Finally, as with all forms of treatment, addition of antiandrogens does not always guarantee complete cessation of the paraphilic behavior. They serve, nonetheless, as an invaluable tool that, when used in conjunction with other components of a therapeutic package, can increase the likelihood of more immediate control over paraphilic behaviors.

Beyond the most immediate need for reduction of the paraphiliac's deviant arousal are a variety of other behavioral excesses or deficits that have been identified in paraphiliacs. There is no evidence that any of the following contribute in precipitating the commission of paraphilic behavior, but because they are frequently associated with paraphiliacs, treatment has also focused on them.

DEFICIT AROUSAL TO ADULT PARTNERS A frequent misperception is that paraphiliacs commit deviant sexual acts because avenues to appropriate sexual behavior are blocked by a lack of appropriate sexual arousal. History for most sex offenders, however, reveals that they have always had adequate nondeviant sexual arousal and that their paraphilic behavior is completely independent of appropriate sexual behavior with adult partners. Although some sadists, fetishists, transvestites, and child molesters of boys report limited arousal to adult partners, the majority of other categories of paraphilias have adequate nondeviant arousal. Strategies to help the paraphiliac acquire nondeviant arousal are still at the experimental stage. Three methods currently show considerable promise: fading, exposure, and masturbatory conditioning.

Fading Fading is a feedback technique in which a paraphiliac is signaled when he develops arousal to a visual stimulus in the laboratory. Treatment involves a gradual shaping or fading technique in which his deviant stimuli are gradually, almost imperceptibly changed to incorporate more and more nondeviant cues while he watches them. The treatment program is labor intensive and requires psychophysiological measurement, but has demonstrated effectiveness.

Exposure A more cost-effective method is the simpler exposure method in which the offender is exposed to explicit sexual films of the category of stimuli to which he wishes to acquire arousal. The paraphiliac is socially reinforced for his incorporation of these nondeviant fantasies into his sexual fantasizing. As the paraphiliac uses the stimuli more in his erotic behavior, these nondeviant stimuli that once lacked erotic power gradually become less offensive and then take on positive valence.

Masturbatory conditioning A final treatment procedure involves masturbatory conditioning in which the patient's masturbatory fantasies are directly modified by him so that nondeviant stimuli become paired with the pleasures of masturbation to orgasm and subsequently develop a greater erotic arousal. In many respects, this technique is similar to the shaping or fading method described above except that the fantasies are altered at the very time that sexual pleasure and orgasm are felt by the patient.

DEFICIT SOCIAL SKILLS WITH ADULT PARTNERS
Many paraphiliacs with appropriate nonparaphilic sexual arousal lack appropriate social skills. They may experience sexual arousal to possible appropriate partners but lack the social skills to initiate and maintain conversations, show interest and concern, and interact without anxiety. The paraphiliac is thus continuously frustrated, because although he may have the desire to eventually become involved with potential sexual partners, he simply lacks the skills to interact on a nonsexual level with a potential partner. Appropriate social skills normally develop throughout adolescence as one observes and then models the skills of others. A rapid means of social skills acquisition occurs when modeling, role playing, and social reinforcement are used directly to train the paraphiliac in the appropriate components of social interaction. Adequate social skills can be taught in a few months, and when practiced outside the therapeutic situation, can allay the offender's anxiety about beginning social relationships with others.

DEFICITS IN ASSERTIVE SKILLS Many paraphiliacs lack the ability to express their inner feelings or request changes by others. Angered by a family member or friend, but unable to express that anger directly to them, the paraphiliac may then force himself on others in a sexual assault. Paraphiliacs with these deficits profit from standard assertive skills training where role playing, modeling, and social reinforcement are used to train the paraphiliac in appropriate assertive skills.

DISTORTED COGNITIONS A large percentage of paraphiliacs who have sustained paraphilic behaviors over a year will have unusual, idiosyncratic belief systems that justify or rationalize their deviant sexual behavior. The molester of young boys might proclaim that his 4-year-old victim consented to the sexual interaction since the child told no one about the molestation and the paraphiliac did not use physical force. The voyeur may attempt to explain his window peeping on the basis that many women wish to be observed while undressing and that is why they leave their window shades up in the evening. The exhibitionist might justify his exposures as public education to females who have not seen a male's genitals before. The paraphiliac early in his career has few such faulty cognitions, whereas the chronic sex offender usually has a plethora of such faulty beliefs to help him justify continuing his deviant behavior. Because offenders do not share these faulty cognitions with others as they attempt to keep all elements of their deviant sexual behavior secret, the clinician who first hears these rationalizations is often bewildered by their illogical nature. The presence of faulty cognitions appears to be closely linked with the persistence of the paraphiliac's deviant arousal, and these beliefs are especially common in offenders whose likelihood of reoffense is high.

Treatment to reduce or eliminate these false beliefs can be exceedingly difficult, since the faulty cognitions help reduce the paraphiliac's anxiety, depression, shame, and guilt should he appreciate the true nature of the impact of his deviant behavior on his victims. Treatment includes exploring the development of the offender's rationalizations and acquainting the offender with the opinions of victims and others as to whether the offender's cognitions are valid. This is effective in group therapy with offenders because the cognitive distortions of one paraphiliac frequently do not match the distortions of another, even within the same diagnostic paraphilia.

SEXUAL DYSFUNCTIONS AND LACK OF KNOWLEDGE Some paraphiliacs show a surprising lack of general sexual knowledge; a few others have specific sexual dysfunctions when attempting nondeviant sexual activities with their partners. There is no evidence that deficits in sexual knowledge or specific sexual dysfunctions are ideologically linked to paraphilic behaviors. Nevertheless, most treatment programs for paraphiliacs do provide sex education courses and treatment for specific sexual dysfunctions.

It is sometimes reported that sex offenders during the commission of a sex crime have specific sexual dysfunctions that preclude their completing a preferred sexual act with their victim. These temporary sexual dysfunctions appear to occur at no higher frequency than one would expect from nonparaphiliacs attempting to complete nondeviant sexual behavior with their partners in a public setting where their behavior could be observed by others and could lead to their arrest. Most males, paraphilic or nonparaphilic, find it difficult to perform under such high-anxiety situations, and the paraphiliac's failure to function sexually during the commission of his paraphilic act should not be interpreted as having special meanings beyond what would be expected should nonparaphiliacs attempt to perform sexually in the public eye.

EXCESSIVE DRUG AND ALCOHOL USE Some paraphiliacs report that because alcohol or drug abuse always precedes their deviant sexual behavior, such chemical abuse may be a cause of the behavior. The clinician must realize that individuals attempting to rationalize and justify their behaviors frequently seek socially acceptable justifications for them. Today, a variety of behaviors are condoned if they occur within the context of alcohol and drug abuse. It is not surprising, therefore, that paraphiliacs use such justifications to explain their commission of an inappropriate sexual act.

Laboratory measures of paraphiliacs who report that alcohol and drugs generate deviant arousal indicate that, contrary to most of these reports, the patient's deviant arousal can be confirmed in the laboratory when no such drugs are concomitantly within the offender's body. These findings suggest that the clinician should be cautious about the validity of the paraphiliac's report of the impact of alcohol and drugs on the development of deviant interest. However, alcohol and drugs do appear to inhibit control of sexual behavior in both nonparaphiliacs and paraphiliacs. For this reason, and because the consequences of the offender's rearrest for paraphilic behavior can be so devastating to him, treatment intervention for alcohol and drug abuse is essential for the holistic treatment of the paraphiliac.

ROLE OF PSYCHIATRY

Although they are few in number, paraphiliacs have victimized a large percentage of our population because of the highly repetitious nature of their paraphilic behavior. The high frequency of paraphilic acts and high numbers of victims have reached public health proportions. Other public health problems have been effectively controlled not by treating the results of a pathogen but by directing preventive strategies against the pathogen. In this case, treating the victims of sexual assault will not significantly reduce the frequency of paraphilic acts as effectively as treating the individuals who commit paraphilic acts.

The available data indicate that psychiatry now has the clinical skills to evaluate and treat paraphiliacs and thereby prevent these unwanted sex crimes. The paraphiliac presents a significant challenge to psychiatry, partly because of his denial and lack of motivation to change his behavior, and partly because of the moral disgust that society and the clinician feel toward his behavior. The remaining task is for members of the psychiatric community to overcome their distaste for patients who commit these crimes so that they can get on with the job of helping paraphiliacs to control their behavior.

REFERENCES

Abel G G, Barlow D H, Blanchard E B, Guild D: The components of rapists' sexual arousal. Arch Gen Psychiat *34:* 895, 1977.

Abel G G, Becker J V, Cunningham-Rathner J, Rouleau J L, Kaplan M, Reich J: *Treatment Manual: The Treatment of Child Molesters*. Behavioral Medicine Institute, Atlanta, GA, 1984.

Abel G G, Becker J V, Mittelman M S, Cunningham-Rathner J, Rouleau J L, Murphy W D: Self-reported sex crimes of nonincarcerated paraphiliacs. J Interpersonal Violence *2:* 3, 1987.

Abel G G, Blanchard E B: The role of fantasy in the treatment of sexual deviation. Arch Gen Psychiat *30:* 467, 1974.

Ben-Aron M H, Hucker S J, Webster C D, editors: *Clinical Criminology: The Assessment and Treatment of Criminal Behaviour*. M & M Graphics, Toronto, 1985.

Berlin F S: Ethical use of antiandrogenic medications. Amer J Psychiat *138:* 1516, 1981.

Bradford J M W: Organic treatments for the male sexual offender. Behav Sciences & Law *3:* 355, 1985.

Bradford J M W: Research on sex offenders. Psychiat Clin N Amer *6:* 715, 1983.

Cook M, Howells K, editors: *Adult Sexual Interest in Children*. Academic Press, New York, 1981.

Freund K: Erotic preference in pedophilia. Behav Res Ther *5:* 339, 1967.

Gebhard P, Gagnon J H, Pomeroy W B, Christenson C V: *Sex Offenders: An Analysis of Types*. Harper & Row, New York, 1965.

Greer J G, Stuart I R, editors: *The Sexual Aggressor: Current Perspectives on Treatment*. Van Nostrand Reinhold, New York, 1983.

Groth A N: *Men Who Rape: The Psychology of the Offender*. Plenum, New York, 1979.

Knopp F H: *Retraining Adult Sex Offenders: Methods & Models*. Safer Society Press, Syracuse, NY, 1984.

Langevin R: *Sexual Strands: Understanding and Treating Sexual Anomalies in Men*. Erlbaum, Hillsdale, NJ, 1983.

Langevin R, editor: *Erotic Preferences, Gender Identity, and Aggression in Men: New Research Studies*. Erlbaum, Hillsdale, NJ, 1985.

Laws D R, Holmen M L: Sexual response faking by pedophiles. Crim Justice Behav *5:* 343, 1978.

Maletzky B M: "Assisted" covert sensitization in the treatment of exhibitionism. Behav Ther *42:* 34, 1974.

Marshall W L: Satiation therapy: A procedure for reducing deviant sexual arousal. J Appl Behav Anal *12:* 10, 1979.

Quinsey V L: The assessment and treatment of child molesters: A review. Can Psychol Rev *18:* 204, 1977.

Rada R: *Clinical Aspects of the Rapist*. Grune & Stratton, New York, 1979.

Roth L H, editor: *Clinical Treatment of the Violent Person*. Guilford, New York, 1986.

Stoller R J: *Perversion, the Erotic Form of Hatred*. Pantheon, New York, 1975.

21.4 SPECIAL AREAS OF INTEREST

21.4a HOMOSEXUALITY

WARREN J. GADPAILLE, M.D.

INTRODUCTION

For many people, including many psychiatrists, homosexual behavior has become more a sociopolitical issue than a variety of sexual activities that may or may not have clinical relevance. Homosexual activity occurs under some circumstances in probably all known human cultures and all mammalian species for which it has been studied. The conditions under which it occurs, and the probable or inferred meanings of the activity vary so widely that little authoritative consensus exists about when, or even whether, it ever represents clinical psychopathology. Public attitudes have rarely been that ambivalent, however, and the usually prevailing disapproval has stigmatized homosexual activity to such an extent that many of those engaging in it have suffered social and legal mistreatment utterly irrelevant to the behavior itself.

The justified effort to remove the burden of social stigmatization from homosexuality has resulted in a deplorably unscientific politicization of the issue of psychopathology in homosexual object choice. People who conceptualize all forms of homosexual activity as normal variants of the human sexual repertoire can appear as enlightened scientific champions of equal individual rights; but those individuals who see any manifestations of homosexuality as the consequence of pathological psychosexual development are often attacked as oppressors who are against homosexuals' human rights. A "diagnosis" of homosexuality as a treatable form of disordered development is overlain with such social and moral implications that the basic scientific questions are lost—an utter confusion of issues that does not occur over a diagnosis, for example, of hyperadrenocorticism or learning disability. This section will not be able to avoid controversial issues or data in trying to summarize the current state of knowledge, nor will it resolve many of the conflicting opinions about homosexuality.

DEFINITION

The word "homosexuality" derives from the Greek word for "same," and generically refers to any sexual activity between members of the same sex. The additional term "lesbianism" is often used to refer to female homosexuality. Homosexuality as a clinical or diagnostic term is misleading, however; it implies a unity of behavior and meaning that does not exist. There is a wide variety of emotional and life conditions in which homosexual behavior occurs, which makes the behaviors qualitatively distinct, even though they may be anatomically identical. Homosexuality and heterosexuality are not always lifelong mutually exclusive orientations, in that it is common for a large proportion of people to have had some of both kinds of experiences at some times in their lives.

In this section, the word *homosexuality* will be used for the sexual pattern of preferential or obligatory erotic interaction between persons of the same sex despite the availability of willing opposite-sex partners. The term *preferential* refers to the conscious erotic preference for a homosexual partner in someone capable of heterosexual function. It does not imply that adult sexual orientation is a product of conscious choice between equally available options. Such terms as homosexual activity or homosexual behavior will be used for the many other forms of homosexual interaction, which statistically involve a far larger number of people. Homosexuality as defined here commands the greatest social and clinical interest, and will be the chief focus of this section. But many of the other forms also can have clinical importance, and will be discussed where relevant.

COMPARATIVE NOSOLOGY

The official status of homosexuality as a diagnosis of mental disorder has changed markedly since the 1960s. In the first edition of the *Diagnostic and Statistical Manual of Mental Disorders* (DSM-I), published by the American Psychiatric Association, homosexuality was listed under the sociopathic personality disturbances as a sexual deviation involving "pathologic behavior." In the second edition (DSM-II), published in 1968, the category of sociopathic personality disturbances no longer obtained, but homosexuality remained under sexual deviations, and those with these deviations were described as unable to substitute normal sexual behavior for their deviant practices.

In 1973, after a great deal of gay activist agitation and protest, and the support of many psychiatrists, the American Psychiatric Association Board of Trustees decided to remove homosexuality as a diagnosis of mental illness. This decision aroused considerable controversy, and the issue was submitted to a vote by the membership, which decided by a 58 percent majority (slightly more than 10,000 voting) to uphold the decision of the board. The issue was not settled for many psychiatrists, however, as shown by a poll conducted by the journal *Medical Aspects of Human Sexuality* in 1977; of the first 2,500 out of 10,000 polled psychiatrists who responded, 69 percent regarded homosexuality as a pathological adaptation as opposed to a normal variation. The official action remained, however, and in the third edition of the *Diagnostic and Statistical Manual of Mental Disorders* (DSM-III), published in 1980, homosexuality as a diagnosis no longer appeared. The term "ego-dystonic homosexuality" appeared under the general category of psychosexual disorders. The reasoning was that only in those troubled by their homosexuality did it constitute a psychological disorder. The diagnostic criteria essentially require that the homosexual orientation is a persistent inner concern of the individual; mild dissatisfaction, or conflict solely between one's homosexuality and society do not qualify for the diagnosis.

The ninth revision of the World Health Organization's *International Classification of Diseases* (ICD-9), also published in 1980, continues to list homosexuality, subdivided into homosexual conflict disorder and lesbianism, under sexual deviations and disorders. However, in the revised third edition of the *Diagnostic and Statistical Manual of Mental Disorders* (DSM-III-R), ego-dystonic homosexuality is no longer a diagnostic term. Under sexual disorders not otherwise specified, one of three categories is persistent and marked distress about one's sexual orientation. There are no further comments or diagnostic criteria, and presumably this condition could include heterosexuals who are distressed with their heterosexuality and persistently wish to be homosexual.

Although the social and humanitarian thrust of these changes is clear, whether the changes equally reflect an advance in medical-psychiatric science is less clear. Categorizing homosexuality as a unitary sexual state of being is no longer scientifically tenable. The relevance of mental disorder in homosexual interactions is controversial and at least demands major reconceptualization. However, the implication that ego-syntonicity necessarily rules out psychopathology is patently invalid. Delusions and hallucinations are often ego-syntonic, and an entire category of mental disorders, personality disorders, is defined in part by the characteristic of ego-syntonicity. Truth cannot be determined by vote, even by supposed authorities. The history of scientific issues that become highly charged emotionally is not distinguished by clear thought and rational weighing of data.

EPIDEMIOLOGY

Homosexual activity of some form occurs in most if not all human cultures. Ford and Beach studied 76 non-Western cultures for which relevant data regarding males were available and found that homosexual behavior was disapproved but not necessarily absent in only 36 percent. Sixty-four percent of the cultures were reported as regarding homosexual activity as "normal and socially acceptable" for some members of society. Subsequent studies of additional cultures have generally supported this prevalence data, and also question the complete absence of homosexual activity in those cultures that deny its existence. Ford and Beach found only 17 non-Western cultures for which data on female homosexual activity existed, and, although their data are not quantified, it is implied that there is a similar ratio of approving versus disapproving cultures.

The most common homosexual interaction cross-culturally is anal intercourse. Homosexual activity ranges from experimental acts between children and adolescents, to enforced periods of homosexual relations for adolescent males with otherwise married heterosexual adults, to a frequent adult male form, in which a man adopts the dress and role of a woman and may marry a heterosexually active man who may have a female wife. Adult preferential or exclusive homosexuality is not the rule in any society for which there are adequate data.

One must be cautious about equating cultural acceptance of certain forms or periods of homosexual behavior with cultural approval of adult homosexuality as defined in this section. Even in Greece and Rome of the classic period, where nonexclusive homosexual activity among both sexes was widespread and generally tolerated, and where homosexuality was extolled in philosophical writings as the highest form of love, adult preferential homosexuality was derided and caricatured in the literary and historical commentaries. Most cultures have been and are more accepting of all forms of homosexual behavior than is Western culture. But an extensive historical and cross-cultural review by A. Karlen indicates that adult homosexuality has universally been regarded as deviant, even in cultures in which accepted institutionalized roles exist for homosexuals.

Western, or Judeo-Christian, culture was not originally fiercely antihomosexual. Adultery is the only sexual act forbidden by the Ten Commandments. In later pre-Christian times, Jews increasingly condemned homosexuality, both because of its association with pagan worship and because it was believed to be against God's law for a man to expend semen nonprocreatively. Leviticus 20:13 states "If a man also lie with mankind, as he lieth with a woman, both of them have committed an abomination: they shall surely be put to death; their blood shall be upon them." Emerging Christian doctrine continued the Hebrew trend of increasing hostility toward homosexuality, and shaped both secular law and the personal values of most people in Western culture. Homosexuality became a capital offense in some areas. Although legal sanctions against homosexual acts of all kinds have moderated greatly or disappeared throughout Western culture, social attitudes most often remain mildly to intensely negative.

It is in this milieu that adult homosexuality exists as a minority, but widespread, orientation. The Kinsey study of males found that 4 percent of males in the United States were exclusively homosexual throughout their lives from adolescence on, and 13 percent had been predominantly homosexual for at least 3 years between the ages of 16 and 55, and 37 percent had some homosexual experience to the point of orgasm. The data in the later Kinsey study of women were not organized in an exactly parallel manner. It found 1 to 3 percent of single women exclusively homosexual, and 3 to 8 percent "mostly" homosexual; moreover, 13 percent of all women had had some homosexual experience to the point of orgasm.

Surveys in other Western countries are roughly comparable in incidence figures, as are subsequent, but less extensive, U.S. surveys. All studies find the incidence of homosexuality in females to be about one-half to one-third that in males. True incidence figures for any stigmatized or illegal activity are probably higher than those found in surveys. It is reasonable, based on the diverse data, to assume that 6 to 10 percent of adult males and 2 to 4 percent of adult females may be preferentially or exclusively homosexual. There are no data on the incidence of ego-dystonic homosexuality.

ETIOLOGY

The focus here will be on the data and the theoretical explanations regarding adult preferential or obligatory homosexuality.

BIOLOGICAL FACTORS There is evidence that various aspects of sociosexual behavior and possibly of sexual object choice are influenced by the presence or absence of fetal gonadal androgenic substances. Most of the experimental data derive from rodents and, to a lesser extent, from primates. The following discussion is an oversimplified but generally valid summary of the sex-specific differentiation of the central nervous system (CNS). The presence of adequate fetal gonadal androgens during the critical period of differentiation for a particular species organizes the CNS, principally portions of the hypothalamus and related structures, for, among other things, the mediation of sexual and social behaviors typical of males, including heterosexual object choice and male copulatory behavior. In the absence of appropriate androgenization or if the fetal tissues are nonresponsive to the androgens, somewhat different areas of the same CNS structures are organized to mediate the complementary female behaviors, preferred choice of male sexual partners, and female copulatory behavior. In experimental androgenization of female fetuses or deandrogenization of male fetuses during their critical periods, cross-sex organization of the CNS occurs. The deandrogenized genetic males show female social and sexual behaviors and prefer male partners; the androgenized genetic females display comparable male patterns.

Hormonal studies Sex-specific behaviors dependent on the inducing actions of fetal gonadal hormones on the CNS are not limited to the specifically sexual. For example, there are markedly sex-dimorphic play behaviors in juvenile rhesus monkeys; males threaten, attempt mounting more often, engage in rough-and-tumble play, initiate play, and withdraw less from threat than do females. Androgenized female juveniles display more typically male behavior. Male rhesus fetuses produce more androgens than do females, but from 6 months to 3 years of age, no circulating androgen can be detected in rhesus males. The sex-dimorphic play of normal rhesus juveniles and the male play pattern of fetally androgenized females is best explained on the basis of critical period sex-specific organization of the CNS.

The extrapolation of such data to humans is uncertain, at best. The evidence for comparable fetal hormonal influences on sex-dimorphic CNS organization rests principally on the occurrence of pathological conditions that to some extent parallel the animal experiments. Sexual dimorphism in childhood play that is remarkably parallel with that in rhesus monkeys, and dimorphic patterns of interests and attitudes in childhood and adulthood are mediated by the presence or absence of organizing fetal androgens, as shown in studies of females with hyperadrenocorticism and also those with progestin-induced hermaphroditism. Women with hyperadrenocorticism become bisexual or homosexual in greater proportion than expected in the general population. In the androgen-insensitivity syndrome, in which the tissues (including the CNS) of a genetic male are nonresponsive to androgens, gender identity and psychosexual development, if not introgenically disrupted, are unequivocally female.

The gap between such observations and postulating a hormonal etiology for homosexuality is too great to be bridged by current knowledge; the data are inadequate either to support or to refute such a postulate. Hyperadrenocorticism is a lifelong condition even when treated from birth, and influences other than fetal androgenation cannot be ruled out as playing a role in the high level of lesbianism in these patients. Numerous studies have reported differences in adult sex hormone levels between homosexuals and heterosexuals; in virtually every instance, they have been disconfirmed by other studies attempting to replicate them. The one reported study that presumably would reflect a difference in fetal CNS organization, a delayed surge of luteinizing hormone following estrogen injection in homosexual men (typical and more pronounced in heterosexual women, absent in heterosexual men) has not, to this author's knowledge, been replicated. However, male-typical responses to the same estrogen challenge have been reported in two studies of transsexual women with homosexual behavior.

A biological etiology of homosexual object choice has been proposed by some authorities. But if the cause of homosexuality were an abnormality in critical period organization of the CNS, one would expect that similar atypical or pathological hormonal conditions would occur spontaneously in other mammalian species, resulting in some percentage of naturally occurring adult preferential homosexuality in other species, but that is never the case. However, the evidence is cumulatively compelling that early hormonal milieu plays some role, perhaps a variable one, in the development of human heterosexual or homosexual orientation.

Genetic factors Kallman's study of male monozygotic twins who were homosexual found an astounding 100 percent concordance. There were many problems, shortcomings, and internal contradictions (e.g., none of the fathers was homosexual) in that study, however, and it has not been replicated in other studies, although the concordance rate does seem to be higher than random in monozygotic twins. A recent study found that 22 percent of the male siblings of an index group of male homosexuals were bisexual or homosexual, compared with 4 percent of those of a matched group of male heterosexuals; there was no difference between the two groups in the percentage of homosexual sisters. Although there appear to be at least familial factors in some instances of male homosexuality, the definitive determination of genetic factors through the study of monozygotic twins reared separately from birth has not yet been reported.

Evolutionary studies Evidence of the continuity or discontinuity between humans and their evolutionary forebears is relevant to the biological underpinnings of heterosexual and homosexual behavior, although the mechanisms responsible for continuities are not understood. As previously stated, some homosexual behavior has been observed in every mammalian species for which it has been studied. As in humans, it is always more common among males than females and among juveniles than adults. Among adult males, homosexual activity occurs most among those who are peripheral or subordinate to the group.

Despite the probable ubiquity of some homosexual behaviors among other mammalian species, there is no evidence that homosexual activity among adults has a primarily sexual motive. Anal intromission or ejaculation among male primates has been reported in only one instance in one species of macaque, and evidence of female orgasm has been reported for a few individuals in one other species of macaque; both were laboratory populations, and there are no similar reports for any wild populations. Homosexual behavior can reflect affectional bonds, but it lacks evidence of sexual release. Adult homosexual behavior is often stimulated in the immediate context of heterosexual excitement among other individuals, but its most frequent context is that of dominance-submission interactions. In both sexes, the dominant animal assumes the male mounting position. These interactions function in regulating the social hierarchy and the various behaviors and intragroup distinctions inherent in the hierarchy; evidence of sexual motivation or pleasure is absent.

A very few instances of experimentally produced adult homosexual preference have been reported, again with an absence of sexual release between the partners. No instances of adult preferential or obligatory homosexuality, in any social context, has ever been reported for any nonhuman mammalian species in the wild. Adult homosexuality as defined in this section is an exclusively human phenomenon.

SOCIAL AND FAMILIAL FACTORS Most theories of the etiology of homosexuality focus on a pathogenic family environment. Perhaps the best-known theory, supported by careful research with male homosexual psychoanalytic patients, is that of I. Bieber and co-workers. They found that the predominant pattern among their patients was that of a close-binding, seductive mother who devalues and dominates a passive, distant, hostile father. This constellation encourages defensive identification with mother and undermines both the father's availability as an acceptable object for identification and the boy's masculinity for fear of losing mother's love. Although this family constellation was the most prevalent one, there were others that underlay homosexuality in other patients. Other researchers have both confirmed this kind of family in the backgrounds of some homosexuals, and have also found other patterns deleterious to comfortable heterosexual orientation and function. There is a similar variability in patterns of family dynamics in the histories of lesbians who have been similarly studied in depth.

Clearly, there is no one pathogenic family constellation in the backgrounds of all homosexuals. There are, however, common denominators in the various family patterns: parenting figures of the same sex who are so weak or punitive and hostile as to make identification impossible or unacceptable, parent figures of the opposite sex who are so seductive or so demeaning and hostile or so emotionally disorganized that the child cannot learn to trust those of the opposite sex, and parents who successfully undermine and reject a child's biological sex and the sex-specific behaviors and attitudes typical of it.

Assuming some validity to the rather voluminous research into and literature on family pathogenesis, there are important caveats that are as relevant as are the positive correlations. One is that because relatively so few homosexuals have been studied in such uncovering detail, there may be many—perhaps a majority—in whom no such pathogenic family influences exist. The question of whether it can be assumed that what is valid in patients is equally valid in nonpatients cannot be answered to everyone's satisfaction at present, if ever. Clinicians cannot know as much about people who do not submit themselves to the depth of anamnestic exploration possible in psychoanalysis as they can about those who do; any extrapolation is, by definition, speculative. But this caveat is not only reasonable and scientific; it is also a hotly contended sociopolitical issue in homosexuality that can obscure matters at the same time that it demands scientific rigor. Psychiatry appropriately does not assume that persons in any diagnostic category who are not treated are qualitatively different from those who are treated. However, homosexuality is not a single condition, but a variety of related behaviors occurring in a variety of people and circumstances. In this situation, it is necessary to be especially prudent in generalizing from a patient population.

A second caveat recognizes that the same parental pathology does not always contribute to homosexuality. Similar disturbed family patterns can be found in the backgrounds of some heterosexuals; they take their toll in other ways. Family pathology cannot be seen as acting alone in all, perhaps even in most, instances.

The basic premise that parents can influence or shape a child's sexual orientation has been questioned, most strongly in the most recent volumes of research from the Kinsey Institute. In a detailed retrospective interview study of almost 1,500 homosexuals and heterosexuals, it was concluded that there was little important correlation, and even less evidence of causative links, between recalled family constellations or parental characteristics and adult homosexuality. However, they also published their data, and their stated conclusions are quite at variance with their actual data. Both male and female homosexuals differed from heterosexuals in personal and family history at statistically significant levels in many, if not most, of the same dimensions found in psychoanalytic studies. Such data confirm the relevance of early childhood familial experiences although interview studies can reveal only correlations, not necessarily causal chains. Therefore, it is not clear on what bases they derive their conclusions from their data.

Social learning theories have also been proposed to explain every variation of human sexual behavior. These theories discount biological species norms and deny major importance for any early childhood experiences in the shaping of specific aspects of adult sexuality. They postulate that not only individual variations of behavior and attitude, but even sexual orientation are learned primarily postpubertally as one experiences the attitudes and mores of one's social milieu, and most particularly of those sexually functioning people who are closest and most important. At this stage of development, these are more likely friends than parents. It is unlikely that the subtleties of sexual life can be understood without including the influence of social learning, and it throws valuable light on some of the developmental manifestations of homosexual activity. Sexual orientation, however, is too basic a component of sexuality to be satisfactorily explained on the basis of chiefly postpubertal learning. Social learning theories are inadequate to explain erotically preferential adult homosexuality precisely because they negate the demonstrable influence of early childhood experiences, and because the one-sided position they take regarding nature versus nurture is no longer scientifically enable.

PSYCHODYNAMIC FACTORS Every developmental line follows an innate timetable. The unfolding sequence of developmental stages and the readiness for successive maturational levels is biologically determined and innate to each species. These developmental imperatives exist independently of the familial and cultural environment of the child. It is this developing intrapsychic self that the infant and child bring to parent-child interactions, and it is by means of this self that the child responds to, interprets, and integrates his or her experiences. Neither the sequence nor the nature of developmental potentials is environmentally dependent, but the accomplishment of those potentials is, within the constraints of biological predisposition.

In the gradual organization of sexual identity, of which sexual orientation is but one component, there are developmental stages that contribute different elements to the eventual outcome. In the intimate body contact, nurturing, and caretaking in infancy, infants are programmed to develop the most basic attitudes toward their own and others' bodies. Appropriate parenting of a biologically normal infant results in the firm sense that one's own body is good and pleasureful and that physical closeness to others can be trusted to be good and is worth seeking.

Toddlers become cognitively able to appreciate the difference between the sexes at about the same time they are working to accomplish a sense of separateness and individuality. Part of being separate is being the sex one is. Intrapsychically, the child must integrate the experience of its own particular self and body within its unique parental environment. Optimally, it comes to feel safe to be separate, and good to be the sex, and only the sex, that he or she is, with all the implicit but yet unconceptualized qualities and potentials of that specific sex. Out of this, one's core gender identity—the unshakable sense of being male or female—is consolidated by the age of 2 to 2½.

In the oedipal period, the child forms a sexually tinged attachment to the parent of the opposite sex and develops rivalry with and fear of the same-sex parent. It is the child's intrapsychic self, regardless of what the parents are like, that conjures up fantasies of replacing and destroying the rival and elaborates awesome fears of retaliation—castrative and more intense for boys. Reality—the reality of the parents' qualities and personalities, and the child's growing capacity for reality testing—largely determines the resolution of this dilemma.

The situation that permits the fullest ultimate achievement of developmental potential is one in which the child identifies with the same-sex parent and relinquishes the wish for sexual possession of the other. At the same time, whatever fearful and aggressive fantasies may exist are not so overwhelming that the child cannot in the future desire partners of the opposite sex and be willing to compete with same-sex rivals for them.

At each stage, there is the possibility for alternative, less optimal outcomes. If the most fulfilling development is, for whatever reasons, unavailable, the child will compromise. He will learn to avoid physical intimacy if it is not safe or he cannot be proud. She will not outgrow the need for symbiotic union with mother if being separate is too terrifying. If any of the dangers inherent in the oedipal situation seem insuperable, the child may adopt the negative oedipal position of compromise: identification with and renunciation of desire for the opposite-sex parent, and capitulation and sexualized attachment to the same-sex parent.

Every mental phenomenon has its negative side. Psychoanalysis has uncovered the existence of homosexual wishes—and, therefore, the potential for homosexual solutions and compromises to developmental dilemmas—in all patients, regardless of their complaints or conditions. Observational studies of child development have confirmed developmental lines and sequences, and elucidated their integration with intrapsychic progressions and pressures. Comparative biology and biological research support the principle that under species-typical biological conditions, heterosexual bias is innate.

AN INTEGRATION The attempt to understand the roots of sexual orientation is all encompassing; it does not focus on homosexuality while assuming that heterosexuality needs no explanation. Biology, family-cultural environment, and intrapsychic psychodynamics are together and variably determinant of all aspects of life, not only of sexual orientation. With respect to homosexuality, no one influence acts necessarily alone, or in an invariable way. Biological predisposition may help to determine the individual's vulnerability or resistance to parental influences. It may play a role in the relative potency of intrapsychic conflict versus environmental reality. The power of parental influences may override predisposition toward either heterosexuality or homosexuality. It is a given among mammalian species that species-typical biology and rearing conditions result in adult preferential heterosexuality. With this perspective, adult preferential homosexuality represents an adaptation—often quite successful—to shaping conditions of any nature that render species-typical heterosexuality unavailable or unacceptable.

PSYCHOPATHOLOGY

The issue of psychopathology in homosexuality is controversial and emotionally charged, but the form that the controversy usually takes misses the point and creates confusion. The question typically focuses on whether homosexuals are sick in comparison with heterosexuals. Aside from the question being of doubtful relevance, it is unlikely that heterosexuality, by definition, conveys any special protection against psychopathology.

At any point along any developmental line, interpersonal or intrapsychic conditions may exist that impair progress toward or achievement of optimal developmental potential. Symptoms and character pathology represent the compromises that the developing individual had to make under those conditions. This principle holds for all people. Sexual identity is one of many developmental lines. All families and all environments are fallible and distortive to some degree. It is axiomatic that heterosexuals are as likely to have encountered impediments to optimal development in various developmental areas, and to have made symptomatic compromises, as have homosexuals. The only difference by definition between homosexuals and heterosexuals is that the capacity to prefer heterosexual partners is not one of the potentials impaired by compromise formation in heterosexuals, whereas it is in homosexuals. But any overall assessment of psychological health and maturity considers total function. A hateful, lazy heterosexual is likely to be sicker than a gentle, creative homosexual when total function versus compromise is assessed. The term "homosexuality" identifies an area of compromise formation, but considered as whole persons, homosexuals do not necessarily have a broader range of, or more severe, psychopathology than do heterosexuals.

PATHOGENESIS Psychopathology and pathogenesis are scientifically relevant to homosexuality in only one specific, limited way: What influences derailed species-typical heterosexuality and what influences determined the homosexual compromise? If biological predisposition plays a major role in any instances, there may be little or no interpersonal or intrapsychic pathogenetic influence. In other instances, nonbiological influences can be identified when a person allows himself or herself to be studied in sufficient depth.

With reference only to patients who have made themselves available for psychoanalytic study, the range of pathology in the developmental line involving sexual orientation is broad and can vary from severe to minor. The earlier the pathogenesis, the more primitive the defenses and compromises and the more global the consequences. Those patients who fail to establish basic bodily trust are crippled in their capacity for intimacy with anyone, man or woman, whether they are heterosexual or homosexual. Closeness engenders fear of annihilation, and sexuality, if the individual is active at all, is often chaotic because orientation and even core gender identity are not firmly fixed.

Deficits at the level of separation-individuation leave males unconsciously terrified of engulfment by women; they are revolted by the prospect of a female sex partner. Internalized part objects remain unfused, and relationships with other men are primitive and infantile, often focusing on only a body part, genitals or anus, never the whole person. Women are not as avoidant of symbiosis with a mother figure because that does not threaten their gender identity, but the fantasies and needs that are being acted out in the relationship are equally primitive.

Oedipal pathogenesis can leave much, or most, of ego development less compromised, and the constrictions are far less crippling. Sexual object choice is determined by castration anxiety in males, who relinquish sexual relations with women to father (= heterosexual, dangerous men), although they can retain nonerotic closeness with women and erotize their interactions with men. In oedipally damaged women, it is the conviction of genital inferiority that fuels the sexual avoidance of men (= father) and the erotized turn toward women (= mother) with the fantasy of eventual genital restoration. Here, too, nonsexual relations with men can often be untroubled.

It is clear that heterosexuals can and do suffer impaired development at all the same levels, which lead to symptomatic compromises in other areas of sexuality than orientation, and which are by no means inherently preferable simply because object choice remains heterosexual. The woman who cannot allow closeness and commitment because of fear and rage, and therefore uses and hurts even the loving men with whom she has sexual relations, is not a better person than the lesbian who enjoys a conflicted and turmoil-filled infantile symbiosis with her lover. The oedipally damaged man who must try to seduce and then leave every woman who already is committed to another man, thus vanquishing an endless succession of fathers, is not healthier than the homosexual man striving against his own internal conflicts to achieve a loving relationship with his partner.

The psychodynamic pathology becomes apparent during analytic therapy whether or not the homosexuality itself is initially regarded as ego-dystonic.

A 25-year-old professional woman, Mrs. X, entered therapy because of increasing personality disorganization and deteriorating function in most areas of life. She spent much time withdrawn into solitary camping trips, sleeping in her car, or sitting in trees. Psychological testing indicated schizophrenia, but in retrospect she was functioning at a very primitive level of borderline personality organization. She was technically bisexual, married to a man with erectile dysfunction and little sexual interest, with whom coitus occurred rarely. However, she had a history of preferring homosexual play since early childhood, and when therapy began she had had an intense sexual and emotional involvement for more than a year with a woman about 20 years her senior, with whom she felt fully sexually fulfilled. Her lesbianism was not seen as a problem; rather, it was fully ego-syntonic and was her main source of joy and self-affirmation.

Mrs. X was obese and sloppily "butch." Her behavior during the early periods of therapy was often infantile to the extent of curling up or sitting on the floor, and communicating only through drawings. She was the only child of an emotionally unavailable father and a controlling, very intrusive mother with whom she recalled an eroticized relationship. There was a large, mostly female, overclose extended family. Partly because she did not question her homosexuality and partly because of her overriding disintegration, therapy did not focus on her sexuality until she had begun to mobilize her considerable but unavailable ego strengths and was able to withstand psychoanalysis. She began to discover that she had chosen a lover with character pathology markedly similar to that of her mother, and that her relationship with her was a fantasied reliving of a masochistic symbiosis with mother. She hoped to gain mother's love by giving her sexual pleasure; her own pleasure was very intense but motivationally secondary to the infantile needs. Through a turbulent, complex, and lengthy analysis, she resolved her infantile dependency and was able to progress to and resolve the oedipal issues. She divorced her husband, accomplished her delayed adolescent sexual explorations, and entered into a loving, stable, and heterosexually fulfilling marriage, meanwhile functioning as a very successful professional woman. Follow-up after nearly 15 years found the marriage and all areas of function stable and rewarding.

It may never be possible to determine to everyone's satisfaction whether the various kinds of pathology evident in adequately studied patients can be at all extrapolated to that vast majority of homosexual people who never become patients. As stated earlier, no one is immune from the etiological influences that are part of the human condition and that determine health or illness and greater or lesser achievement of potential. Developmental influences, good or bad, leave their fingerprints on people's lives as signs that often can be seen by any observer. But similar causes for similar signs can only be inferred, and there is a long history in medicine of the wrong causal relationships being inferred on seemingly logical bases.

One generalization that in fact helps to define virtually all preferential homosexuals is that they did not identify with the sexual orientation of their same-sex parent. Except in possible instances of biological predisposition, this pattern reflects conflict with and hostility toward that parent, which, as is known from other contexts, tends to extend to others of the same sex. There are studies of nonpatient homosexual males that find hostility toward other men to be characteristic. If such built-in hostility contaminates male-male relationships, it could help to explain the great difficulty homosexual men have in forging long-term, committed, monogamous relationships. This hypothesis, however, leaves unexplained the fact that lesbians are much more successful in forming relationships despite the same failure in identification. Perhaps one explanation is that lesbians are able to retain their earlier, deeper, pregenital identifications with their mothers; little boys do not usually have that kind of identification with their fathers to retain.

CASUAL SEX Casual sex with a multitude of strangers is considered symptomatic of pathology, as much in heterosexuals as in homosexuals, at least in this culture. It is not clear to what extent this is a culture-bound definition of pathology. There are some cultures in which sexual partnerships are normally expected to be unlimited for the unmarried. Those known to the author involve small population groups in which no partners are or remain strangers in the sense used here. In this culture, such casual sexual encounters with strangers is an expression of narcissistic, impersonal, often compulsively driven, genital rather than person-oriented sex, and of impaired capacity for intimacy and commitment.

Available studies find this pattern more typical of homosexuals, especially males, than of heterosexuals, although it is by no means limited to them. It has been suggested that the biological constraints of pregnancy and the social constraints of marriage and children, as well as the lack of social support for open homosexuality and homosexual pairing, explain the higher incidence of this pattern of promiscuity among homosexuals. The pattern, and the psychopathology, is not unusual among straights who make a life-style of singles bars. In a study of the ultimate anonymity of public restroom sex, where the partner is not even seen, 38 percent of the recipients (not providers) of sexual release, usually fellatio, were heterosexual males. At present, there are insufficient data to explain the greater incidence of pathological promiscuity among homosexuals, or to support or refute the sociological hypotheses for it.

DEGREE OF PSYCHOPATHOLOGY Despite the demeaning irrelevance of comparing the degree of psychopathology in homosexuals and heterosexuals, that is a major focus of Bell and Weinberg's extensive retrospective interview study of male and female homosexuals and heterosexual controls, and their work deserves comment. They found that in overall comparison of their total samples, the male homosexuals were less well adjusted intrapsychically, interpersonally, and socially along a number of dimensions than the heterosexual controls. The lesbians were closer in psychological adjustment measures to the heterosexual women, but were still somewhat less well adjusted along some of the same dimensions as the men.

The researchers were clearly cognizant, however, of the

nonhomogeneity of their homosexual sample. They devised a typology into which about 70 percent of that sample could be subdivided. There were the "coupled," living in quasimarriage with one partner. Of their total sample of 686 males, the "close-coupled" (9.8 percent) desire monogamy and closeness; the "open-coupled" (17.5 percent) regard a regular partner important for sex and affection, but agree to outside sexual encounters despite considerable jealousy. The "functionals" (14.9 percent) have a high level of sexual activity, with more partners than the other groups, have little regret about their homosexuality, and have few sexual problems. The "dysfunctionals" (12.5 percent) have more sexual problems and more regret over their homosexuality than the other groups. The "asexuals" (16 percent) have many sexual problems, little sexual interest or activity, and few partners. A similar percentage of the lesbians were also classifiable, but there were about three times as many close-coupled, and far fewer functionals, dysfunctionals, and asexuals.

Rating these categories separately, Bell and Weinberg found pathology in the male homosexuals to be most concentrated in the dysfunctionals and asexuals; the remaining three subgroups were closer in psychological variables to the controls; in all groups, however, there was a greater degree of pathology reported by the homosexuals. Among the lesbians, the pathology was concentrated in the open-coupled, dysfunctionals, and asexuals, the remaining two subgroups being roughly the same as the heterosexual women. No separate data or comparisons were provided for the nearly 30 percent of both men and women who could not be classified into their subgroups.

The problems with this study, the largest and most representative to date, are twofold, aside from the authors' conclusions that, despite their data, there are negligible differences in psychopathology between the majority of homosexuals and heterosexuals. The first is that they do not compare their subgroups of homosexuals with parallel subgroups of heterosexuals, but with the total sample. If the highest-functioning group of homosexuals were compared with the similarly defined highest-functioning group of heterosexuals, and so on down the line, differences in psychopathology as defined in their study may have been more comparable in each subgroup. Certainly, the results would have been different and would have contributed more to the understanding of similarities and differences.

The second problem is that this study attempts to assess overall function, not only psychosexual development and sexual behavior. By the reasoning presented earlier in this section, one would not anticipate significant, consistent differences in psychopathology. One logical explanation is that the differences are secondary to the social disapproval and stigmatization of homosexuals. Homosexuals invariably learn first to be ashamed of their atypical sexual interests and to hate themselves for it, a self-concept that is pathogenic in itself. Relatively few of those in this study report such gross examples of prejudicial oppression as arrest, extortion, or assault, but the real sources of self-derogation are earlier and more pervasive than such events. Surprisingly, the one study that compared homosexual males in discriminatory and nondiscriminatory societies found more psychological problems in homosexuals than in heterosexuals in both milieus and failed to find that nondiscrimination made a significant difference. Thus, the data are relatively consistent in finding a greater incidence of psychopathology in preferential homosexuals compared with heterosexuals, the discrepancy being greater for males than for females. Whether the differences are inherent in homosexuality or secondary to social pressures is an issue for which definitive, unassailable data do not yet exist.

CLINICAL DESCRIPTIONS

ADULT PREFERENTIAL HOMOSEXUALITY Homosexuals express the same variety of erotic and sensual behaviors as do heterosexuals, such as kissing, caressing, mutual masturbation, mouth-genital stimulation, and anal intercourse. Only the lack of complementary genitalia limit their activities; anal intercourse is much more common among male homosexuals than among heterosexuals, and some less common homosexual practices, such as inserting the fist in partner's anus, are essentially absent in heterosexuals. The imitation of heterosexual intercourse by lesbians through the use of dildos is rare in this culture. Anal intercourse is imitative of coitus, but this may as often be enforced by anatomical limitations as it is expressive of male-female roles or of dominance-submission interactions. Homosexuals, like heterosexuals, have individual preferences for some practices over others, and some prefer or limit themselves to the active or passive, insertor or insertee roles. Most switch roles at least part of the time, and many express little preference.

There is no characteristic self-presentation of homosexuals. Probably no more than 20 percent are markedly or exaggeratedly effeminate among the males, or hypermasculine and "butch" among the females. Both men and women are found in every professional and occupational field, even those most stereotypically heterosexual.

Relationship patterns are as varied among homosexuals as among heterosexuals. Homosexual relationships are not by definition impoverished in their quality of interaction. Masters and Johnson studied committed and functional homosexual and heterosexual couples, and found that the homosexual couples were more egalitarian, communicated more freely about their sexual feelings and sensations, spent more time in total body sensuality and foreplay, and were more sensitive to partners' needs and responses than did the heterosexuals.

Even among those who are preferentially or exclusively homosexual at any given time, experience with heterosexual intercourse at some time in life is the rule rather than the exception. Depending on the study, from 33 to over 65 percent of males and 60 to 85 percent of females have experienced coitus, and a significant minority continue to have some degree of heterosexual activity. Many have been married, and 50 to 75 percent of those have had children.

It is in the number and nature of sexual partnerships that homosexuals in this culture at least differ most from heterosexuals, and in which male and female homosexuals differ most from each other. One study found that 72 percent of the male homosexuals reported more than 100 sexual partners; 41 percent reported more than 500, and 27 percent reported more than 1,000. Seventy-four percent stated that more than half their partners were strangers, and 65 percent had sex only once with over half of their partners. In contrast, only 8 percent of lesbians reported 50 or more partners, and only 6 percent stated that over half of their partners were strangers. Comparative partnership data for their heterosexual controls were not provided. Another study compared homosexuals with heterosexuals in number of partners, finding that homosexuals of both sexes change partners more frequently than heterosexuals, and that the difference is much greater between homosexual and heterosexual males. Parallel with this degree of activity, about 66 percent of the males but less than 1 percent of the females had had venereal disease at least once. Recent concerns over acquired immune deficiency syndrome (AIDS) is anecdotally reported to have cut down the number of indiscriminate liaisons, but there are no research data demonstrating this reduction.

OTHER VARIETIES OF HOMOSEXUAL ACTIVITY

Although adult preferential or exclusive homosexuality is the principal focus of both lay and scientific interest, it is not the only variety with potential clinical relevance, nor does it account for the majority of people involved in homosexual behavior. All of the types below may require clinical recognition and attention.

Developmental behavior Homoerotic activity can occur in both boys and girls at any immature stage of development. It is usually part of normal development and not prognostic of adult homosexuality. Kinsey found that it was more common than heteroerotic play in girls up to age 13 and in boys up to age 15, and that 33 percent of women and 50 percent of men reported such play by age 15. It is rarely a problem for the youngsters involved unless it is made so by parents or other adults, who are usually deeply concerned that it may indicate future homosexuality. In most instances, a knowledgeable clinician could safely be reassuring to both adults and children, but a minority of the children do progress toward homosexuality; the differential diagnosis will be addressed later.

Pseudohomosexuality Pseudohomosexuality has been described chiefly in males, but the complementary dynamics can exist in females. There is no primary erotic attraction to persons of the same sex. Rather, the conflicts center on power versus dependency, respectively associated with masculinity and femininity. Men who feel themselves to be weak, submissive, or inadequate compared with other men may unconsciously make the equation "I am nonmasculine = I am feminine = I am homosexual." These men tend more to conceptualize themselves as homosexual rather than to become actively homosexual, but they may also act out the passive homosexual role. In others, the fear that they may be homosexual may escalate into homosexual panic, sometimes with violence or suicidality; they may require emergency psychiatric attention.

Situational homosexuality activity The absence of opposite-sex partners in some environments, such as unisex boarding schools, prisons, or some armed services stations will induce some preferential heterosexuals to turn to same-sex partners until they return to normal environments. Some have regarded this to be a healthy adaptation; for mutually consenting persons, it is at least usually not harmful. However, for someone who is unaware of deep insecurities over his or her sexual identity or possesses powerful moral taboos, tremendous turmoil and emotional conflict may ensue.

Exploitative homosexual behavior As in heterosexual rape, the penis can be used as a weapon and as an assertion of dominance and power against other men. This is frequent in, but not limited to, prison populations, where violence is endemic; those with the power to intimidate often coerce the weaker and more fearful into being recipient sexual partners, usually in anal intercourse and sometimes in fellatio. The sexual release is not emotionally the main goal. Such sexual exploitation is not uncommon in women's prisons. The exploiters, particularly the males, do not consider themselves homosexual. As in some cultures and subcultural groups where there is a sharp dichotomy between insertor (male) versus insertee (female) roles, the insertor does not lose status and is not regarded as homosexual within the group. The clinical import of this behavior bears almost exclusively on the exploited, although none would question the severe character pathology of the exploiter.

Enforced homosexual activity The trauma to an exploited partner's sexual and social self-concept can be shattering. Coerced homosexual compliance causes a true psychiatric emergency, often in settings where it cannot properly be addressed. There is general consensus that such experiences usually do not result in subsequent homosexuality, but some cases have been reported in which victims become homosexual even though there had been no prior awareness of homosexual feelings.

Bisexuality and ambisexuality As discussed earlier, it is more common than not for homosexuals also to have heterosexual experience. Those who have some degree of ongoing coital experience are often regarded as bisexual, but closer attention to their erotic fantasies and differential arousal responses generally reveal that their erotic preference is homosexual. True ambisexuality—equal arousal and pleasure with partners of either sex—has been described, but it is apparently rare. Clinical significance is rarely psychiatric, but rather medical in terms of exposure to conditions more common in homosexual populations.

Ideological homosexuality Occurring principally among militant feminists, ideological homosexuality constitutes an angry repudiation of any need for men, and, at times, an effort to deny innate masculine-feminine differences or complementarity. Sexual conflicts may masquerade as ideology; however, by definition, psychopathology is denied by these individuals. Nonetheless, reports are appearing in the literature of such women seeking psychotherapy as they discover that conscious efforts to manipulate their sexual orientation do not solve their sexual relationship problems and may do violence to their basic sexual identities.

DIFFERENTIAL DIAGNOSIS

Adult preferential or obligatory homosexuals are distinguished simply by the conscious awareness of greater or exclusive sexual arousal by persons of the same sex. They need not be sexually active; persons of either orientation may be sexually inactive, yet be clearly aware of their arousal patterns. In this kind of homosexuality, the sexual motivation is primarily erotic, genital, and affectional; regardless of its etiology, the homosexual arousal is not secondary to some other motivation, and it is not sexual behavior used fairly transparently in the service of some nonsexual goal.

An important initial task is to determine whether the sexual behavior is secondary to a major psychiatric illness, such as schizophrenia or bipolar disorder, in which the primary condition takes precedence and the sexual activity may never emerge as a treatment issue. Homosexuals who cross-dress must be differentiated from fetishistic transvestites (typically heterosexual males who are sexually aroused by donning female clothing) and transsexuals (persons who believe that they are members of the opposite sex trapped in the wrong body).

The primacy of homoerotic arousal allows its differentiation from other expressions of homosexual behavior with the possible exception of ambisexuality. In pseudohomosexuality, the primary conflicts concern power and dependency. Though there may be homosexual dreams or fantasies, they do not typically involve positively perceived erotic excitement and eagerness, but rather issues of dominance and submission. The same is true if actual homosexual behavior occurs. In situational homosexuality, orgasmic pleasure and sexual release occur, but the participants are in no doubt about the substitutive nature of the same-sex activity. The motives of power, domination, and humiliation are primary in exploitative homosexual activity; motivationally, sexual release is secondary. Powerful, vicious, and violent homosexuals can, for example, in a prison setting, also use their sexuality for the same nonsexual purposes. For this small minority, positive erotic drive is also subordinate, as in heterosexual rape, although the sexual release achieved in the latter case may be more pleasureful since the partner happens also to be of the preferred sex. In ideological homosexuality, the choice of partner is reactive, rationalized, consciously defensive, and defiant. Except in those who have not yet recognized or accepted their lesbianism, the motivation is not primarily and spontaneously erotic, although after the fact the erotic superiority is often strongly proclaimed.

CHILDHOOD PREHOMOSEXUALITY There are special problems in the differential diagnosis of childhood prehomosexuality from developmental homosexual activity. In the case of highly effeminate boys (occasional to frequent cross-dressing; persistent preferences for girls' toys, activities, girl playmates, and the company of female adults; fear of physical injury and avoidance of body contact sports and other rough play with boys; feminine identification in family role play, and expressed cross-gender wishes), follow-up studies in the aggregate show that the majority, but not 100 percent, become homosexual, bisexual, or transsexual. Inquiry into the families of these boys reveals a pattern of pathogenic influences on sexual identity development consistent with that discussed under etiology. Not as much is known about equally masculine girls. Their pattern would seem a mirror image of the effeminate boys, and there is some indication that they too are more likely than feminine-identified girls to become lesbian or transsexual. However, tomboyism per se is not as prognostic of lesbianism as effeminacy in boys is of homosexuality.

Most often, the youthful behavior a physician is asked to evaluate is not so blatant as that just described. In these instances, it is most often the parents who are concerned, although the youngsters may become so. Often the youngster is not clearly concious of a preference for the pleasure derived from sex play with same-sex or opposite-sex partners, although this situation changes by the time of early adolescence. The expression of a strong erotic homosexual preference by an adolescent is usually diagnostic. The homoerotic behaviors can be identical, whether prehomosexual or not. Mutual masturbation is the most common activity for both sexes, although fellatio, cunnilingus, and anal intercourse may occur in purely developmental play. Preoccupation with one of the less common behaviors may be more likely prehomosexual, but is not a reliable criterion. An older youngster who is involved in homosexual activity and who has a history of persistent cross-gender behavior in earlier childhood is more likely to be prehomosexual. Purely developmental activity typically occurs between age peers; the child who is willingly erotically involved with a same-sex adult and the child who is erotically in love with someone of the same sex is more possibly prehomosexual. And predominantly homosexual masturbatory fantasies are strongly diagnostic.

INTERNAL DISTRESS In the patient who presents with dysphoria over his or her homosexuality, the source of that distress must be explored. Often the distress is external; there may be pressure from a court, a spouse, parents, or others. Such pressure may be strong enough to cause deep conflict and make the person question or regret the homosexual orientation. Unless the dysphoria is truly internal, however, efforts toward shifting orientation are likely to be neither effective nor appropriate. But such patients may need therapy, for example, to deal with the pressure or to learn to curb illegal or criminal behavior, as in homosexual pedophilia.

Internal distress cannot be taken at face value, either. Growing up in a homosexually negative family or social milieu can produce guilt and self-derogation in someone who otherwise would not be motivated to change. The distinction between the genuine wish to be heterosexual and reactive shame over homosexuality can be difficult to make and may even, at times, be a spurious one. Contrary to the position of many gay activist spokesmen, there are homosexuals of both sexes who genuinely wish to be heterosexual and who can accomplish the shift. The realities of life in a heterosexual world and the facts of relinquished reproductive and procreative potential are not always false pressures toward heterosexuality. The inner conviction of having experienced distorting developmental influences and of the constrictions of consequent compromise formations are not invalid awarenesses in those who have them. Whether to try to form a working alliance toward the goal of acceptance of homosexuality or toward the goal of heterosexuality depends on the evaluation of the nature and sources of the ego-dystonicity. But because the distinctions may be so unclear, the direction of therapy may, in fact, depend on the prognosis for or against change.

TREATMENT

There are those among homosexual psychiatrists and other mental health professionals who are so offended by the implication of sickness in the very idea of treating homosexuality that they refuse to honor any homosexual's request for therapy aimed at changing orientation and similarly refuse to refer him or her to anyone who would make such a therapeutic effort. Their position is that no gay would wish to change if society were not so repressive and punitive. It is this author's position that such a stance is unethical—indeed, a form of malpractice—quite equivalent to that of trying to force a change of orientation on those who do not wish it. There are gays who yearn to be straight and who may be able to make the change; their wishes must be respected. Furthermore, prehomosexual indicators may show up in childhood, when therapy may be genuinely preventive. Enlightened people know that homosexuality is neither bad nor evil, but they also know that it confers few benefits and many disadvantages in this culture. A majority of adult homosexuals, when polled on this issue, stated that they would prefer any children of their own not be homosexual because of the problems encountered.

CHILDHOOD PREHOMOSEXUALITY Although it is unwise to try to convince adults to enter therapy, it is appropriate to urge therapy for prehomosexual children. Children cannot appreciate cognitively the future consequences of sexual orientation, and cannot give, in effect, informed consent to a developmental direction that could eventuate in homosexuality. Ideally, therapy should involve the family as well as the child, so as to try to modify the influences that may be impairing heterosexual development. The same reasoning applies for adolescents, but it may be very difficult to involve adolescents in therapy. Theoretically, the younger a person is, the more amenable to modification his or her patterns are. But the normal dynamics of adolescence involve the need to distance oneself from, and to overcome dependence on, adult parental figures. It is most often too difficult to form a therapeutic alliance with an adolescent strong enough to withstand the emotional intensity of transference issues and long-term depth therapy.

OUTSIDE PRESSURES Adults who present themselves for therapy because of outside pressure are very poor prospects for change. Even when they have some ambivalence about their own homosexuality, their resentment of the pressure becomes a resistance that cannot usually be overcome. Sometimes, their sexual behavior is driven to the point that the compulsiveness is ego-dystonic even though the orientation is not; the behavior may be criminal, as in homosexual pedophilia. Psychotherapy or medication, such as with medroxyprogesterone acetate or cyproterone acetate (compounds with antiandrogen properties), can be helpful in reducing the intensity of sexual drive in males to manageable levels.

HOMOSEXUALS WITH EMOTIONAL PROBLEMS Homosexuals who come into therapy for emotional difficulties other than their homosexuality present a special problem. They may have conflicts in interpersonal relations with their lovers or with others, they may have neurotic or characterological pathology, or they may have sexual dysfunctions within their homosexual liaisons. As with anyone with such problems, many can benefit enormously from psychotherapy that never focuses on their sexual orientation. But unless the therapy is very specifically problem or behavior oriented, if the patient remains long enough in any exploratory therapy, material pertaining to sexual orientation will emerge. This emergence is generally very threatening and causes termination. The author has found it helpful to discuss this eventuality in advance, when goals and treatment procedures are being decided on; this approach can sometimes help to prevent termination so premature that even the nonorientation conflicts remain less well-resolved than would be possible.

A 36-year-old successful clergyman, Mr. Y, exclusively homosexual, presented with sexual dysfunction within his monogamous relationship, and with guilt-producing but highly exciting sadomasochistic (master-slave) masturbatory fantasies. He was fetishistic for western leatherwear since early childhood. He was anorgasmic, although he had occasional retarded ejaculation in his sexual relationship, but was easily orgasmic with the masturbatory fantasies. The fantasies could allow him to be orgasmic during anal intercourse or fellatio, but they caused too much guilt for him to utilize them. He wanted therapy only to improve his homosexual relationship. He was the only son of a sexually prohibitive mother (who died when he was 12 years old) and a father with whom he had a warm, seductive, and consciously erotic, though not actively incestuous, relationship. His father had remarried during Mr. Y's teens, and his stepmother had originally been very nice to him, then suddenly became totally rejecting in his early 20s for reasons Mr. Y claimed never to understand. Mr. Y had never acknowledged his homosexuality to his father.

Therapy utilized a combination of behavior modification and uncovering techniques. Through behavior therapy, he was able to use his fantasies to achieve more successful physical closeness with his partner, and then to replace the fantasy imagery with that of his lover. At the same time, he was discovering his negative oedipal attraction to his father—the father always wore western clothing and boots, and eventually he came to recognize his father as the master in his fantasies. He also realized his fear of women and of their anger, his conviction that women would always be right and he always wrong and guilty. His goal of orgasmic response with his partner was achieved at about the time he began to have dreams of heterosexual arousal to women. He was consciously threatened by the implications of this material and terminated therapy, fortunately not before successful accomplishment of his original goal.

Shift to heterosexuality For those who wish to become heterosexual, therapy can be effective to a greater degree than is often realized. About one-third or more achieve results ranging from capacity for heterosexual arousal and response, to genuine heterosexuality in all its facets and complexities. One large center has reported a 79 percent reorientation rate using intense behavior modification techniques, but to the author's knowledge, that work has not been replicated.

Most therapeutic modalities—including psychoanalysis and psychoanalytically oriented psychotherapy; analytic group therapy; behavior modification techniques involving conditioning, desensitizing, and reconditioning; and aversive techniques—report roughly comparable results. It is not clear, however, whether the outcomes are truly comparable in terms of the involvement of the whole person in coming to grips with the complexities of sexual intimacy and commitment. Nonanalytic techniques focus on increasing arousal and response to heterosexual stimuli and fantasies while decreasing homosexual arousal. The author has seen frequent resistance to and rejection of such therapy in otherwise well-motivated patients when the unconscious motivation compelling homoerotic response has not yet been resolved. Data on the ability to carry these changes into real life, and on the permanency of the shift to heterosexuality, are inconclusive. Follow-up studies of psychoanalytically treated patients do show changes in all facets of heterosexual involvement that hold up well over time. In addition, some deep and well-defended conflicts cannot be uncovered and resolved by any less arduous approach.

PROGNOSIS

Prognosis is difficult, and the indicators are not always either clear or clearly known. Strong motivation to change is most important, but it is insufficient in itself. Ego strength is of major prognostic import. Primitive levels of ego development, as in psychotic or borderline individuals, make such major changes as sexual orientation unlikely. Patients with severe character pathology are less likely to accomplish major therapeutic goals than are patients with the essentially normal neurotic levels of ego development. Ego development can be assessed with psychological tests, especially the projective tests, and some sense of strengths can be achieved by assessing function in other appropriate areas of life, such as school performance, occupational function, interpersonal relations, and level of involvement in sports, hobbies, or cultural interests. Ego development affects not only prognosis for various treatment goals, but also choice of treatment modality. Lower levels of ego development argue against the rigors of psychoanalysis and for less threatening and more supportive, or more mechanical, therapies.

Relative youth argues for a better prognosis, but one cannot assume that the young have good ego flexibility and the older do not. Some history of heterosexual arousal and experience, and relative recency of beginning homosexual activity improves prognosis, as does sex-appropriate role behavior. Marked effeminacy in a man or hypermasculine behavior in a woman—especially if continuous from chronic cross-gender behavior in childhood—is a poor prognostic sign for change. The better the relationship, past or present, with an emotionally healthy same-sex parent or the more qualities that parent had that could deserve respect even if the patient had never been able to acknowledge them, the greater the potential of weathering the negative transference and achieving healthy identification.

Therapy that aims at modifying the object of or the conditions for erotic arousal is particularly difficult. Even when homosexuality is strongly ego-dystonic, it is still associated with intense physical pleasure. Sexual excitement and orgasm are powerful reinforcers of the behaviors that produce them. Although many homosexuals can achieve the shift to heterosexuality if they are so motivated, there are even more who cannot or who stop short of that goal, even though they had personally chosen it. A psychiatrist who works with ego-dystonic homosexuals should be prepared to help them be realistic about their goals and to shift the therapeutic focus. When it is with the patient's full consent, it is equally appropriate that the goal be to accept themselves and their homosexuality without shame and self-hatred, to withstand the social opprobrium, and to function with the productivity and maturity of which they are capable.

OTHER CONSIDERATIONS

All of the scientific questions about sexual orientation await definitive answers. It is only because heterosexuality is the species norm, as in all mammalian species, that to some it may seem that being straight requires no explanation, whereas being gay, or any other deviation from heterosexuality, does require one. But, one cannot validly try to understand one without inevitably having to try to understand all. There are reasons why the norm exists, just as there are reasons for deviations. But that understanding is in its scientific infancy.

Some things are known. It is known that rearing pressures can help to shape psychosexual development and sexual identity, including orientation; it is not known how broadly applicable is the knowledge derived from patients. It is known that biological factors play some role in the development of sexual identity; it is not known to what extent or in what ways those factors operate, how variably influential they are, or what determines that variability. It is known that since postnatal interpersonal influences can affect sexual orientation, interpersonal therapeutic influences can help bring about a shift in orientation in a significant proportion of those who want it and who are willing and able to withstand the emotional rigors of the effort.

Most notably, perhaps, it is known that homosexuality, whatever brings it about, is not a sign of degeneracy or evil or inferiority. It appears to be human to recoil unthinkingly from those who are different. That response has no place among thinking people, and, most particularly, not among psychiatrists.

REFERENCES

Bell A P, Weinberg M S: *Homosexualities*. Simon & Schuster, New York, 1978.

Bell A P, Weinberg M S, Hammersmith, S K: *Sexual Preference*. Indiana University Press, Bloomington, 1981.

Bieber I, Dain H J, Dince P R, Drellich M G, Grand H G, Grundlach R H, Kremer M W, Rifkin A H, Wilbur C B, Bieber T B: *Homosexuality*. Basic Books, New York, 1962.

Dörner G: Neuroendocrine response to estrogen and brain differentiation in heterosexuals, homosexuals, and transsexuals. Arch Sex Behav *17:* 57, 1988.

Ehrhardt A A, Meyer-Bahlberg H F L: Effects of prenatal sex hormones on gender-related behavior. Science *211:* 1312, 1981.

Ellis L, Ames M A, Peckham W, Burke D: Sexual orientation of human offspring may be altered by severe maternal stress during pregnancy. J Sex Res *25:* 152, 1988.

Endleman R: New light on deviance and psychopathology?: The case of *Homosexualities* and *Sexual Preference*. J Psychoanal Anthropol *7:* 75, 1984.

Ford C S, Beach F A: *Patterns of Sexual Behavior*. Harper & Row, New York, 1951.

Gadpaille W J: Research into the physiology of maleness and femaleness. Arch Gen Psychiat *26:* 193, 1972.

Gadpaille W J: Biological factors in the development of human sexual identity. Psychiat Clin N Amer *3:* 3, 1980.

Gadpaille W J: Cross-species and cross-cultural contributions to understanding homosexual activity. Arch Gen Psychiat *37:* 349, 1980.

Green R: *Sexual Identity Conflict in Children and Adults*. Basic Books, New York, 1974.

Kallman F J: Comparative twin study on the genetic aspects of male homosexuality. J Nerv Ment Dis *115:* 283, 1952.

Karlen A: *Sexuality and Homosexuality*. Norton, New York, 1971.

Kinsey A C, Pomeroy W B, Martin C E: *Sexual Behavior in the Human Male*. Saunders, Philadelphia, 1948.

Kinsey A C, Pomeroy W B, Martin C E, Gebhard P H: *Sexual Behavior in the Human Female*. Saunders, Philadelphia, 1953.

Masters W H, Johnson V E: *Homosexuality in Perspective*. Little, Brown, Boston, 1979.

Ovesey L: *Homosexuality and Pseudohomosexuality*. Science House, New York, 1969.

Pillard R C, Weinrich J D: Evidence of familial nature of male homosexuality. Arch Gen Psychiat *43:* 808, 1986.

Saghir M T, Robins E: *Male and Female Homosexuality*. Williams & Wilkins, Baltimore, 1973.

Schäfer S: Sociosexual behavior in male and female homosexuals: A study of sex differences. Arch Sex Behav *6:* 355, 1977.

Sexual Survey No. 4: Current thinking on homosexuality. Med Aspects Human Sex *11:* 110, 1977.

Stoller R J, Herdt G H: Theories of origins of male homosexuality: A cross-cultural look. Arch Gen Psychiat *42:* 399, 1985.

21.4b
RAPE, SPOUSE ABUSE, AND INCEST

VIRGINIA A. SADOCK, M.D.

INTRODUCTION

The three areas in this section have in common physical assault that inflicts lasting psychological damage. In all three abuses, the victim is most frequently—but not always—a woman, and the assaulter is usually male. The rapist violates the victim with an assault that distorts highly intimate physical contact into a hurtful and humiliating attack. In spouse abuse and incest, the abuse of one human being (the weaker one) by another (the stronger one) takes place within the context of a unit normally designed to offer protection, love, and support—the family. The physical hurt inflicted on the victim is compounded by the emotional betrayal by the abuser, which usually results in damage to the psyche of the victim.

RAPE

DEFINITION Rape is a physical and emotional outrage that assaults psychological well-being in a particularly harmful way. The rapist violates the victim and leaves her or him traumatized and frequently too vulnerable to report the crime. Although rape is a sexual assault, it has more to do with anger and aggression than sexuality. In fact, one-third of rapists experience either erectile or ejaculatory dysfunction during the assault.

In the revised third edition of the American Psychiatric Association's *Diagnostic and Statistical Manual of Mental Disorders* (DSM-III-R), rape is mentioned under sexual sadism:

> Rape or other sexual assault may be committed by people with this disorder. In such instances the suffering inflicted on the victim is far in excess of that necessary to gain compliance, and the visible pain of the victim is sexually arousing. In most cases of rape, however, the rapist is not motivated by the prospect of inflicting suffering, and he may even lose sexual desire while observing the victim's suffering. Studies of rapists indicate that fewer than 10 percent have sexual sadism. Some rapists are apparently sexually aroused by coercing or forcing a nonconsenting person to engage in intercourse and are able to maintain sexual arousal even while observing the victim's suffering. However, unlike the person with sexual sadism, such people do not find the victim's suffering sexually arousing.

RAPE OF WOMEN Recent research has categorized male rapists into separate groups: sexual sadists, who are aroused by the pain of their victims; exploitative predators, who use their victims as objects for their gratification in an impulsive way; inadequate men, who believe no woman would voluntarily sleep with them and who are obsessed with fantasies about sex; and men for whom rape is a displaced expression of anger and rage. Some workers believe that the anger was originally directed toward a wife or mother. However, feminist theory proposes that the woman serves as an object for the displacement of aggression that the rapist cannot express directly toward other men. The woman is considered the property or vulnerable possession of men and is the rapist's instrument for revenge against other men.

Those dynamics are clearly evident in rape during wartime. That type of assault against women is frequent in war and may be committed by soldiers with no psychiatric or criminal history. Rape in war—frequently gang rape—serves to demoralize the male enemy, relieve pent-up aggression and fear, enhance male bonding, and increase feelings of power.

The concept of women as property or chattel, without sexual rights, has a tribal, biblical, and feudal history that extends to the present time. Until recently, a woman could not accuse her husband of rape because the law presumes sexual intercourse to be part of the marital contract. However, in 1982, a man in Florida was found guilty of raping his wife, the first time a husband was convicted of committing the crime while living with his spouse. Twenty-five states have eliminated the legal exemption from marital rape. Husbands have been found guilty of helping other men to rape their wives. Men have also been found guilty of rape if they forced themselves sexually on their wives after legal separation. Feminists propose that rape is encouraged by any cultural representation of women as objects or property, as exemplified by pornography and prostitution.

Rape and the media Recent studies have shown that nonsexual violence toward women depicted in the media leads to the development of attitudes that foster tolerance of rape. Repeated exposure to the physical mistreatment of women, sexual or otherwise, creates callousness toward women in both male and female viewers. Violent pornography promulgates myths about rape that make it acceptable: that women want to be raped; that they enjoy violent sex; and that women are lying when they say they have been raped. In the past decade, there has been an increase in the depiction of violence toward women in magazines, films, television, record covers, and rock video tapes.

Rape and the law The basic legal definition of rape in the United States is as follows:

> The perpetration of an act of sexual intercourse with a female, not one's wife, against her will and consent, whether her will is overcome by force; or by drugs or intoxicants; or when because of mental deficiency she is incapable of exercising rational judgment; or when she is below an arbitrary age of consent.
>
> The crime of rape requires slight penetration of the victim's outer vulva. Full erection and ejaculation are not necessary. In some states forced acts of fellatio and anal penetration, although they frequently accompany rape, are legally considered sodomy or labeled sex offenses.

Convicted rapists seem to be part of a general subculture of violence. Federal Bureau of Investigation records reveal that 71 percent of arrested rapists have prior criminal histories, including records of assault, robbery, and homicide. Rape often occurs as an accompaniment to another crime. The rapist always threatens his victim with words, fists, gun, or knife, and frequently harms her in nonsexual ways, as well as in sexual ways. Victims are often beaten or wounded, and sometimes they are killed.

Statistics Statistics show that the greatest number of rapists are between 25 and 44, a higher age group than that involved in most other crimes. Fifty-one percent are white, 42 percent are black, and the remaining 7 percent come from all other races. However, police statistics may be misleading, since rape is a highly underreported crime. The Justice Department estimates that 1.4 million rapes of women or rape attempts occurred between 1973 and 1982—and that only half were reported. The underreporting is attributed to feelings of shame on the part of the victim and to feelings that there is no recourse through the legal system. However, reporting has tripled since the 1960s, when feminist groups first focused attention on this issue.

Victims of rape can be of any age. Cases have been reported in which the victim was 15 months old and others in which she was 82 years old. The greatest danger exists for women from 16 to 24, but almost one-fifth of all victims are between 12 and 15 years old. Seventy percent of victims are unmarried. Rape most commonly occurs in a woman's own neighborhood, frequently in a neighborhood street or parking lot, and 29 percent of rapes occur in the woman's own home. About 60 percent of rapes are committed by strangers, 30 percent by men known to varying degrees by the victim, and 7 percent by close relatives of the victim. Moreover, 20 percent of rapes involve more than one attacker.

The rape victim The woman being raped is frequently in a life-threatening situation. During the rape, she experiences shock and fright approaching panic. Her prime motivation is to stay alive. Victims have tried to defend themselves by fighting physically, by screaming for help, by running in an attempt to escape the attacker, by reasoning with the offender, or just by talking in the hope of establishing some kind of human connection that will make the rapist reconsider the attack. There is a high incidence of submission, as can be expected, when the rapist uses a knife or a gun. In most cases, rapists choose victims slightly smaller than themselves. The rapist may urinate or defecate on his victim, ejaculate into her face and hair, force anal intercourse, and insert foreign objects into her vagina and rectum.

Effects on the victim After the rape the woman experiences shame, humiliation, confusion, fear, and rage. The type of reaction and the length of duration of the reaction are variable, but women report effects lasting for a year or longer. A considerable number of women report that it takes many years to get over the experience. Many women experience the symptoms of a post-traumatic stress disorder. The rape overwhelms them with a sense of vulnerability, a fear of living in a dangerous world, and a loss of control over their own lives. They become preoccupied with the trauma, and it colors their future actions and day-to-day behavior. Some women feel defiled and unable to wash themselves clean. Many victims are afraid to walk through the neighborhood where the rape occurred, even if they lived there for years before the rape. Other women cannot remain in their homes or apartments. They have a fear of being followed or a fear of being alone. They may have nightmares or be unable to sleep, afraid to shop in their usual stores, or unable to function at work. Many victims experience changes in eating patterns and somatic symptoms, such as headaches, nausea, exhaustion, and overall tension and discomfort. Social relationships are affected. Some women are able to resume sexual relations with men, but others become phobic of sexual interacton or develop such symptoms as vaginismus.

In one study of 130 women interviewed between 15 and 30 months after they had been raped, more than half the women reported sexual dysfunctions, including lack of desire, inhibited orgasm, and inhibited excitement. Another study on the long-term psychological effects of rape found victims (assaulted 2 to 46 years earlier) to be significantly more depressed, generally anxious, and fearful than control subjects. Studies trying to isolate variables that exacerbate the trauma have produced confusing results. Researchers differ as to whether an assault by strangers or by men known to victims is more destructive. Recovery is prolonged if the woman is attacked in her home, but an attack in the rapist's home has a greater impact on social functioning. Physical violence in addition to the rape compounds the trauma, but the specific use of a weapon is not significant in that regard. The racial relationship between the victim and the rapist also affects recovery. One factor that repeatedly has been demonstrated to lead to prolonged sequelae is a history of prior sexual assault.

Treatment The victim fares best when she receives immediate support and is able to ventilate her fear and rage to believing family members, physicians, and law enforcement officials. She is helped when she knows she has socially acceptable means of recourse at her disposal, such as the arrest and conviction of the rapist. Rape treatment centers that coordinate psychiatric, gynecological, and physical trauma services in one location and that cooperate with local law enforcement agencies are most helpful to the victim.

Therapy is usually supportive in approach, unless there is a severe underlying disorder, and focuses on restoring the victim's sense of adequacy and control over her life and relieving the feelings of helplessness, dependency, and obsession with the assault that frequently follow rape. Group therapy with homogeneous groups composed of rape victims is a particularly effective form of treatment. One study that investigated the question of sex biases in rape counselors found that men and women therapists reported similar affective responses to their patients and made similar treatment recommendations. The women therapists, however, rated their patients as having more functional impairment, possibly suggesting that they were more sensitive to the women's distress.

Rape as a crime The rape victim experiences a physical and psychological trauma when she is assaulted. Until recently, she also faced frequent disbelief when she reported the crime, if she had sufficient ego strength to do so, or accusations of having provoked or wanted the assault. Such statements as "She was asking for it" or "She wishes it had happened" are culturally pervasive, and they haunt and intimidate the rape victim. In reality, the National Commission on the Causes and Prevention of Violence found discernible victim precipitation of rape in only 4.4 percent of cases. That statistic was lower than in any other crime of violence. Victim precipitation in homicide was found to be 22.0 percent by the same commission, and in unarmed robbery it was 6.1 percent. Why, then, the myth of the lying or provocative woman "deserving rape" and the need to make the victim equally responsible with the rapist for his crime? Feminist literature perceives the myth of the falsely accusing woman—from Potiphar's wife in the Old Testament to the present—as a male projection. The fear of being falsely accused of rape seems particularly irrational in view of the degree of underreporting of actual rapes.

Feminist groups have been the most active antirape faction in society in terms of consciousness raising, prevention, and immediate and long-term support for victims. There have been several cultural changes that benefit the rape victim; for example, the education of police officers and the use of policewomen in dealing with rape victims have helped increase the reporting of the crime. Rape crisis centers and telephone hot lines are available for immediate aid and information for victims. Volunteer groups work with emergency rooms in hospitals and with physician education programs regarding the treatment of victims. Legally, when they appear in court, women no longer have to prove that they actively struggled against the rapist. Testimony regarding the prior sexual history of the victim has recently been declared inadmissible as evidence in a number of states. Also, penalties for first-time rapists have been reduced, making juries more amenable to considering a conviction, whereas sentences for repeat offenders have become more severe.

In some states, rape has been punishable by death, primarily in cases of miscegenational rape. The severity of the penalty in those cases has had more to do with prejudice and offended manhood than with the protection of women.

Date rape Date rape or acquaintance rape is a term applied to situations in which the rapist is known to the victim. The rape can occur with a new boyfriend, on a first date, on a ride home after a party, or when the man and woman have known each other for many months. Considerable data on this type of rape have been gathered from college populations, and many schools have set up counseling programs to deal with these assaults.

A survey of 500 students at one university found that 16 percent of the women had been raped by men they knew or were dating. Of the men interviewed, 11 percent stated they had committed rape. Those findings are reflected in studies at a number of institutions throughout the United States. In a survey including several universities, 38 percent of the male students said they would commit rape if they thought they could get away with it, and 50 percent of the male students subscribed to myths that predispose to rape tolerance—that women don't mean it when they say "no" to intercourse or that they want to be coerced into having coitus.

In addition to suffering the symptoms experienced by all rape survivors, victims of date rape berate themselves for exercising poor judgment in their choice of male friends. They are more likely to blame themselves for provoking the rapist (by saying they should have not worn a low-cut dress, for example) than are other victims. Ironically, self-blame aids the recovery of these and other rape victims. Focusing on something they could have done differently seems to restore an element of control to the victim who has been made to feel so helpless. Date rape victims are less likely than others to report the crime to authorities. Also, because victim and rapist frequently have friends in common, the woman fears being disbelieved and being ostracized by her social group if she talks about the attack.

MALE RAPE In some states, the definition of rape has become gender neutral: the word "person" has been substituted for "female"; homosexual rape is included in the definition, and the use of an object, in place of a penis, for penetration also constitutes sexual assault. The Justice Department estimates that 123,000 men were the victims of rape or rape attempts between 1973 and 1982. Homosexual rape was not differentiated from other attacks in that statistic. Male rape is a significantly underreported crime.

Homosexual rape is much more frequent among men than among women, and it occurs regularly in closed institutions, such as prisons and maximum security hospitals. The attacks are violent, rather than sexual, and are used to express anger or power. The dynamics are identical to those involved in heterosexual rape. The crime enables the rapist to discharge aggression and to aggrandize himself. The victim is usually smaller than the rapist. He is always perceived as passive and unmanly (weaker) and is used as an object.

The rapist selecting a male victim may be heterosexual, bisexual, or homosexual. He forces his victim to have sex through entrapment (e.g., by getting him drunk), through intimidation by threats with a knife or gun, or through the use of brute force. Male rape can involve one or several forced sexual acts: The most common act is anal penetration of the victim; the second most common act is forcing the victim to perform fellatio. Frequently, the rapist makes an effort to bring the victim to ejaculation by fellatio or masturbation. That condition is humiliating to the victim, and it reinforces the rapist's sense of conquest and his fantasy that the victim wanted or enjoyed the rape. The male rape victim often feels, as do the raped women, that he has been ruined. In addition, he often fears he will become homosexual because of the attack.

STATUTORY RAPE Intercourse is unlawful between a male over 16 years of age and a female under the age of consent, which varies from 14 to 21, depending on the jurisdiction. Thus, if an 18-year-old man and a 15-year-old girl have consensual intercourse, the man may be held for statutory rape. That type of rape may vary drastically from the crimes described above in being nonassaultive and in being a sexual act, not a violent act. Nor is it a deviant act, unless the age discrepancy is sufficient for the man to be defined as a pedophile; that is, when the man is 10 years older than a young girl or the girl is 12 years old or less. Charges of statutory rape are rarely pressed by the consenting girl; they are usually brought by her parents.

SPOUSE ABUSE

DEFINITION Spouse abuse, most simply defined, is the mistreatment or misuse of one spouse by the other. It takes many forms that often result in injury.

Abuse can range from shoving and pushing to choking and severe battering, involving broken limbs, broken ribs, internal bleeding, and brain damage. The face and breasts are the most frequent sites of assault, and when the woman is pregnant, her husband often batters her abdomen. The problem of spouse abuse is a long-standing one. However, it was the cultural emphasis on civil rights and the work of feminist groups in the 1970s that focused attention on domestic violence and brought the severity of the problem into public awareness.

STATISTICS Spouse abuse is estimated to occur in from 2 million to 12 million U.S. homes each year, and more than 8 percent of the homicides that occur in the United States involve the killing of one spouse by another. Wives are much more frequently beaten than are husbands. One study estimates that 25 to 30 percent of all U.S. women have been beaten at least once during marriage by their spouses. Another study cited a figure of 1.8 million battered married women, a statistic that excluded divorced women and teenage girls who were battered on dates. The surgeon general's office has identified pregnancy as a high risk period for battering and recommends screening for battery as part of routine prenatal assessments. A major predictive factor for battering during pregnancy is prior abuse.

Although the major problem in spouse abuse is wife abuse, some beatings of husbands are reported. In those cases, husbands complain of fear of ridicule if they expose the problem, fear of charges of counterassault, and inability to leave the situation because of financial difficulties. Husband abuse has also been reported when a frail elderly man is married to a much younger woman.

Wife beating occurs in families of every racial and religious background and crosses all socioeconomic lines. It is most frequent in families with problems of drug abuse, particularly when there is alcoholism. Unfortunately, violence in families is largely condoned in today's society. In a survey of a representative national sample of adult men and women, 20 percent approved of husband and wife hitting. Wife beating has a long history of sanction by society. The right of a husband to beat his wife was part of the written law of the United States until 1874. Although the statute was overruled at that time, perpetrators of family violence have rarely been prosecuted, and women, the main victims of spouse abuse, have rarely been protected.

ETIOLOGY Cultural, intrapsychic, and interpersonal factors all contribute to the development of the problem. Abusive men are likely to have come from violent homes where they witnessed wife beating or were abused themselves as children. The act itself is reinforcing. Once a man has beaten his wife, he is likely to do so again. Although abusive husbands may not suffer from severe mental illness, they tend to be immature, dependent, and nonassertive and to suffer from strong feelings of inadequacy.

Their aggression is bullying behavior, designed to humiliate their wives to build up their own low self-esteem. The abuse is most likely to occur when the man feels threatened or frustrated at home, at work, or with peers. Impatient and impulsive, abusive husbands—verbally and physically—displace aggression provoked by others onto their wives. The dynamics include identification with an aggressor (father, boss), testing behavior (will she stay with me no matter how I treat her), distorted desires to express manhood, and dehumanization of the woman. As in rape, aggression is permissible when the woman is perceived as property.

CHARACTERISTICS OF THE ABUSER An abusive husband considers his wife his belonging and may be particularly assaultive when she shows any sign of independence, talks about getting a job, leaves the house without telling him, or threatens to leave the marriage. By the same token, he is most destructive when she is most dependent—when she is pregnant or when she has small children—because the immature husband may feel he does not get enough attention or respect when his wife responds to the demands of their little children and has less time and energy for him. The spouse abuser usually beats his children as well as his wife. He may neglect them when they are little, but he attacks them as they grow older and begin to make demands on him or attempt to protect their mother from abuse.

The abusive husband is extremely jealous and possessive. He not only batters his wife, but wages a conscious campaign to isolate her, lower her self-esteem, and make her feel utterly inept, worthless, and incapable of surviving without him. No matter how hard his wife tries to please him, he will find fault with her and is prone to make remarks like "You never do anything right." His aim is to make his wife totally dependent on him so that she will accept his views absolutely and tolerate his behavior, no matter how abusive it becomes. He frequently interferes with friendships she may develop, prevents her from working outside the home, or insists that she work where he does so he can control and monitor her on the job.

CHARACTERISTICS OF THE ABUSED Approximately one-half of the women who are in such marriages grew up in violent homes. Frequently, they married at a young age, just to escape those parental homes. Abusive husbands generally do not attack their wives physically until after the marriage, and, thus, the women believe that they are moving to a safer environment. The trait most commonly found in abused wives who stay with their husbands is dependency. The woman perceives herself as unable to function alone in the world or without a man. Regardless of her occupation or talents, she sees marriage as an unequal partnership, with the man in the dominant position. She usually comes from a background that has supported traditional male-female (aggressive-passive) role models. On a deeper level, she defines herself by her husband and takes her identity from him. That dynamic makes it extremely difficult for her to expose the problem. Revealing her husband as brutal and inadequate is tantamount to revealing herself as inadequate. As does the abused child, the dependent woman frequently blames herself for the abuse she receives.

Unfortunately, the culture has supported the distortion of the man who sees his wife as property and himself as manly when he is violent. It has also told the woman that she provokes the behavior and that she should maintain her marriage at all costs. That message has been reinforced by mental health professionals, by pastoral counselors, by police officers (until recently, all usually men) who are reluctant to interfere in domestic problems, and by society in general, which has largely ignored the problem.

SOCIETAL ATTITUDES There is some evidence of movement toward change.

In 1987, a woman who killed her estranged husband was acquitted of the crime when a history of years of brutal abuse by him, culminating in a rape at knife point, was revealed at her trial. She had unsuccessfully tried every legal channel to have him barred from access to her and to their children—whom he also battered—for 11 years.

That case focused attention on the lack of effective legal recourse available to battered women and made clear the potential for disaster for the entire family when domestic violence goes unchecked. Also, a legal defense based on being a battered spouse evolved for the first time. A recent study financed by the National Institute of Justice has recommended that cases of spouse abuse be treated as violent crimes, that domestic violence involving a gun or knife be treated as a felony, and that police departments should routinely conduct follow-up investigations after reports of battering within a family. Also, hot lines and emergency shelters for women and organizations, such as Respond, have been developed to aid battered wives and to educate the public. Other organizations, such as EMERGE, have been formed to provide therapy for abusive husbands.

PROBLEM OF HOMELESSNESS A major problem for abused women has been where to find a place to go when they leave home, frequently in fear of their lives. When an abused wife tries to leave her husband, he often becomes doubly intimidating and threatening, saying, "I'll get you." If the woman has small children to care for, her problem is compounded. If she leaves home without them, she may lose custody of them on grounds of desertion. If she can prove that her husband has abused them, she risks being charged with complicity in that abuse. If she tries to take them with her, she needs shelter, day care for the children if she expects to work, and some immediate means of subsistence, such as food stamps or welfare. Ideally, job training with the goal of self-sufficiency should be offered. Unfortunately, in spite of some progress, society still offers few shelters and little legal protection for the battered wife.

About 20 to 40 percent of the homeless in urban areas are estimated to be battered wives fleeing from their husbands. Abusive husbands routinely persecute a wife who tries to leave. As a result, she often remains imprisoned in a situation that is extremely frightening and demoralizing. The experience is emotionally comparable to being held hostage.

TREATMENT Some men feel remorse and guilt after an episode of violent behavior and become particularly loving. That behavior gives the wife hope, and she remains until the next cycle of violence, which inevitably occurs. Change is initiated only when the man is convinced that the woman will not tolerate the situation and when she begins to exert control over his behavior. She can do so if she is in a position to leave for a prolonged period, with therapy for the man as a condition of return. Under those circumstances, family therapy is effective in treating the problem. With relatively less impulsive men, external controls, such as calling the neighbors or the police, may be sufficient to stop the behavior. The incidence of abuse decreases significantly when wife beaters are routinely arrested.

Some women enter therapy while they still live with their abusive spouse. In that situation, visits to the doctor or clinic are usually secret. Most abusive husbands will not voluntarily enter therapy, nor will they allow their wives to do so. Psychiatric treatment of these women is complex, as both overwhelming external stresses and internal conflicts must be addressed. These women are frequently in a state near panic or are depressed, hopeless, and very passive. The depression and passivity are a defense against their husband's moods (by remaining quiet and compliant, they hope to avoid antagonizing him) and against their own suppressed rage.

The therapist is faced with the reality of the woman's dangerous situation and the sometimes limited alternatives available to her. At the same time, therapy is directed toward changing her hopeless state, rebuilding her self-esteem, developing her autonomy, and enabling her to deal with her own controlled rage. A frequent problem is that the woman's rage is directed toward herself, in the form of suicide attempts or self-mutilation, or toward her children. Another problem is that the husband may, in fact, become more abusive as the wife becomes less passive and less depressed. The therapist should keep in mind that the woman, through experience, is the best judge of when the home situation is becoming more dangerous.

The goal of treatment is to resolve the violence in the marriage—an aim that necessitates the husband's participation—or to enable the woman to leave the marriage. Social agencies should be involved in the treatment process as issues of child custody and means of support must be addressed if the woman plans to leave the abusive home either temporarily or permanently.

INCEST

DEFINITION The word "incest" is derived from the Latin words *incestus,* which means impure, immodest, or lewd, and *incestare,* which means to stain or to defile. The act of incest involves sexual intercourse between close blood relatives. However, in the current society of broken and re-formed families in the United States, sexual intercourse between step-relations is also considered incestuous even though no blood relationship exists. Murdoch explains that sexual relations with stepparents or stepsiblings is taboo because of the assumed, though artificial, bond of kinship that has developed. Other incestuous types of behavior include fondling, as well as oral and anal intercourse.

HISTORY There is a history of incest occurring in all societies and a parallel history of prohibitions to prevent its practice. Incest taboos of some sort have existed in every culture known to humans. They are sanctioned by law, tradition, and religion. The particular taboo or definition of incest, however, has varied in different eras and societies. For example, among the royal families of Egypt, the Incas, and the Hawaiians, brother-sister marriages have been countenanced at times. There is some indication that marriages between siblings were also permitted among commoners in Iran and Egypt under Roman rule. The Azande tribe of Africa allowed high chiefs to enter into father-daughter marriages. In American culture, marriage between distant cousins is permitted (e.g., Franklin and Eleanor Roosevelt).

The strongest and most universal taboo exists against mother-son incest. However, this relationship was not considered taboo among the Incan nobility. It occurs much less frequently than any other form of incest, and such behavior is usually indicative of more severe psychopathology among the participants than is father-daughter or sibling incest.

Numerous factors have been cited as determining prohibitions against incest. More comprehensive prohibitions developed with the acceptance of the Judeo-Christian tradition. Sociologists have underlined the role of incest prohibitions as socialization factors. Incest taboos protect the family, encourage the healthy psychosexual development of the child, and promote socialization outside the family. Biological arguments also have been used to support the taboo. Groups that inbreed risk the unmasking of lethal or detrimental recessive genes, and the progeny of inbreeding groups are generally less fit than other progeny. Anthropologists have observed that the particular form of the incest taboo is culturally determined and affected by whether the society is patriarchal or matriarchal and particularly by how property is inherited.

In *Totem and Taboo,* Sigmund Freud developed the concept of a primal horde in which the younger men collectively murdered the group's patriarch, who had kept all the women of the tribe for himself. The incest taboo arose out of guilt after the murder and to prevent a repetition of the act, further rivalry after the murder, and the disintegration of the horde.

STATISTICS Accurate figures of the incidence of incest are difficult to obtain because of the general shame and embarrassment of the entire family that is involved. Incest victims rarely report the relations while they are still children. Females are the victims of incest much more commonly than are males.

It is currently estimated that between 12 and 15 million women in the United States have been the object of incestuous attention. In one study of 521 families, 6 percent of the men and 15 percent of the women reported having been sexually abused as children; 94 percent of the abusers were male. One-third of the abused people had been molested before the age of 9. Another study reported that 19 percent of U.S. women and 9 percent of U.S. men had been sexually victimized as children; 50 percent of the abuse came from a relative. Recent research estimates that from 100,000 to 300,000 children are sexually abused each year and that 80 percent of those cases involve abuse by a parent or legal guardian. The Child Welfare League of America reports that the incidence of sexual abuse is rising or, at best, remaining constant. Also, since the percentage of proved abuse cases out of those reported (approximately 50 percent) has remained the same, the increase is not attributed to more cases being reported.

Incestuous behavior is much more frequently reported among families of low socioeconomic status than among other families. That difference may be due to greater contact with reporting officials—such as welfare workers, public health personnel, and law enforcement agents—and not a true reflection of higher incidence in that demographic group. Incest is more easily hidden by economically stable families than by the poor. However, studies of white, middle-class U.S. women indicate that 10 to 25 percent had a childhood sexual experience with an older male relative and 1 percent had relations with a father or stepfather.

ETIOLOGY Social, cultural, physiological, and psychological factors all contribute to the breakdown of the incest taboo. Incestuous behavior has been associated with alcoholism, overcrowding and increased physical proximity, and rural isolation that prevents adequate extrafamilial contacts. Some communities may be more tolerant of incestuous behavior than is society in general.

There is a higher incidence of incest among families where remarriage has occurred. This increased incidence may indicate a less strict observance of the taboo among stepparents. It may also indicate a less protective attitude among stepparents who may not molest stepchildren but who are less careful of them and leave them more vulnerable to others in the new family network. A divorced parent, usually the mother, also may unwittingly bring sexually opportunistic men into the home before she remarries.

Major mental illness and intellectual deficiencies have been described in some cases of clinical incest. Some family therapists view incest as a defense designed to maintain a dysfunctional family unit. The older and stronger participant in incestuous behavior is usually male. Thus, incest may be viewed as a form of child abuse or a variant of rape. When there is actual intercourse, as opposed to other types of incestuous behavior, the father is usually tyrannical and violent, and the mother is significantly physically or emotionally impaired. Additionally, she never seems to question the father's authority.

EFFECTS ON CHILDREN Incest is extremely confusing to children. That behavior entails an abrogation by the parent of his or her responsibilities, particularly that of protection of the child; the teaching of antisocial behavior rather than the fostering of socialization; and most important, the abuse of the child's trust, love, and dependent position. Children are further damaged and confused because they are usually told by the abusing relative that there is nothing wrong with the incestuous behavior. Some children participate willingly in the relationship because the sex is coupled with loving and nurturant behavior for which the child is starved. Other children are cajoled or intimidated into incestuous relationships. Similarly, bribes and threats are used to keep them silent. For instance, one stepdaughter with an ailing mother submitted to her stepfather for years because he threatened to leave her mother if she did not, and he predicted that the mother would then die.

FATHER-DAUGHTER INCEST About 75 percent of reported incest cases involve father-daughter relationships. Families at higher risk for father-daughter incest include those with violent fathers, as well as mothers who have been disabled as a result of depression, alcoholism, psychoses, frequent involuntary childbearing, or chronic illness. However, several researchers believe that many cases of sibling incest are denied by parents and that sexual relations between siblings may equal or exceed those between fathers and daughters.

Family dynamics Because of the high incidence of reported cases, particular attention has been paid to father-daughter incest. Three types of families have been described in which father-daughter incest occurs. One group includes families with a pervasive pattern of violence and abuse by the father, a high frequency of alcohol abuse by the father, and a mother who is psychologically or physically beaten and who explicitly sanctions the incest. A second group includes families where the incestuous behavior usually occurs as a single episode and usually does not involve intercourse. In the third group of families, the behavior is implicitly sanctioned by family members. In those families, the sexual relationship between the parents is impaired. The father suffers from a high level of anxiety and a sense of inadequacy that prevents his working out problems with his wife or looking outside the family for a sexual liaison. He is frequently unpredictable, dominating, and impulsive. The mother is usually remote, child-like, and submissive, and she readily abrogates her wifely and maternal roles. The entire family tolerates the incestuous behavior as a way of coping with family problems and perpetuating the unit. All members seem to fear disintegration of the family.

Some incestuous fathers form sequential relationships with several daughters, starting with the oldest girl. Each liaison usually lasts for an extended period of time, often over a period of years. Occasionally, incestuous fathers have difficulty establishing normal heterosexual relationships because they have latent homosexual urges. In addition to incest, they may present with a history of prolonged periods of abstinence or with a history of sexual promiscuity. They deal with the guilt about their behavior through a series of rationalizations (e.g., they are just expressing love; they are the kindest teachers of the facts of life for their daughters). Frequently, they are more guilty about embarrassment brought to the family after the behavior is exposed than about participation in the incestuous activity itself.

Daughters who are victims of incest have been studied extensively. They typically develop personality disorders, suffer poor sexual adjustment (although they may have a high degree of eroticism), are prone to depression, and sometimes express homicidal or suicidal ideation. In general, they suffer from impaired self-esteem, undergo a negative identity formation, experience difficulty in intimate relationships, and may go through repeated victimizations.

The daughter has frequently had a close relationship with her father throughout her childhood and is at first pleased when he approaches her sexually. The onset of incestuous behavior usually occurs when the daughter is 10 years of age. As the incestuous behavior continues, however, the abused daughter becomes more bewildered, confused, and frightened. As she nears adolescence, she undergoes physiological changes that add to her confusion. She never knows whether her father will be paternal or sexual. Her mother may be alternately caring and competitive. Her relationships with her siblings are also affected if they sense her special position with her father and treat her as an outsider. The incestuous father, fearful that his daughter may expose their relationship and often jealously possessive of her, interferes with the development of her normal peer relationships.

The physician must be aware of the possibility of intrafamilial sexual abuse as the cause of a wide variety of emotional and physical symptoms, including abdominal pain; chronic pelvic pain; genital, anal, or oral irritations; lesions of venereal disease; separation anxiety; phobias; nightmares; and school problems. When incest is suspected, it is essential to interview the abused child apart from the rest of the family. Otherwise, the family dynamics that enabled the behavior to occur in the first place will prevent the girl from reporting the behavior. A young child may not be able to articulate the trauma, but may indicate the incestuous behavior in play therapy sessions. Revelation of the incestuous relationship is extremely difficult for the daughter who suffers a mixture of confusing and contradictory emotions. She often feels both love for and anger toward her father. She suffers from a pervasive sense of guilt for her participation in the incestuous behavior and for her anger toward both parents. She is also fearful of their reactions if she exposes the incest and she may be fearful of destroying the family unit. The incest victim in a violent home fears physical reprisals if she reveals the incest.

HOMOSEXUAL INCEST In father-son incest, two cultural sanctions are violated: the taboo against incestuous behavior and the sanction against homosexual behavior. The family in which such behavior occurs is usually highly disturbed, with a violent, alcoholic, or psychopathic father; a dependent mother who is unable to protect her children; and an obliteration of the usual family roles and individual identities. Sometimes the abuser is an older brother in the family who usually was abused himself and subsequently exploits his younger siblings.

Father-son incest is only rarely reported. In such cases, the son is frequently the oldest child, and if he has sisters, they are sexually abused by the father as well. The father does not necessarily have any other history of homosexual behavior. The son in the situation may experience homicidal or suicidal ideation and may first present to a psychiatrist with self-destructive behavior.

TREATMENT The first step in the treatment of incestuous behavior is its disclosure. Once a breakthrough of the denial and collusion or fear by the family members has been achieved, incest is less likely to recur. When the participants suffer from severe psychopathology, treatment must be directed toward the underlying illness. Family therapy is useful in efforts to reestablish the group as a functioning unit and to develop healthier role definitions for each member. The external control provided by therapy helps prevent further incestuous behavior while the particpants are learning to develop internal restraints and more appropriate methods of gratifying their needs. Sometimes the revelation of incestuous behavior results in the expulsion of a family member from the group. It is important to involve law enforcement agencies to prevent a recurrence of incest in a family while therapy is conducted. Several disciplines are needed to counteract the pressure on the abused child to recant.

Group therapy Group therapy has proved helpful to victims who have experienced incest in the past. The groups studied have been comprised of female victims. Group therapy is particularly useful in helping the survivor overcome the legacy of shame from the experience. Group cohesiveness readily develops around shared feelings of secrecy, stigma, helplessness, and fear. The victims learn that they have not been alone in suffering incest and begin to negate feelings that they were responsible for the behavior. The group experience can cause initial regression in some patients; in those cases, concomitant individual therapy is indicated. Good prognostic factors for the success of group treatment include high motivation and positive expectations in the prospective group member.

Some groups have been composed of mothers of children sexually abused by fathers, stepfathers, or boyfriends. The women in those groups have usually expelled the male abusers from the home. The mothers frequently express rage, bewilderment, and helplessness. They feel they are blamed for the incest as much as the abusing father. Additionally, they report that they are blamed for the dissolution of the family by other family members and that they are the recipients of anger from their children who were not victimized. Divorced mothers, whose children were the victims of incest when they visited the fathers' homes, feel particularly angry and frustrated.

Individual therapy Individual therapy is the best forum for the patient's anger at her victimization. In a group setting, that anger is often too threatening for the other group members to tolerate. Women who have difficulty recalling memories of the incestuous experience frequently have been subjected to particularly sadistic forms of abuse. In those cases, individual therapy also seems to be the most effective modality of treatment. The treating psychiatrist should anticipate some acting out on the part of the patient as therapy progresses and be ready to confront the patient with it. Major tasks of treatment are to build the patient's self-esteem and to develop or redevelop the patient's capacity for trust and the ability to feel comfortable in close relationships. Patients are often depressed, or may evince hysterical symptoms or hypersexuality. Adolescent patients frequently have school problems and act on impulses to run away.

Studies suggest that, as a preventive measure, parents should warn children about sexual molestation in simple but specific terms. For instance, the parent should explain to the child that the genital area is a private part of the body and that the touching of those parts by adults, even if they are family members, is not an acceptable demonstration of affection.

REFERENCES

Adolescent sex offenders, Vermont, 1984. JAMA, *255;* 2, Jan 1986.

Bassuk E, Apsler R: Are there sex biases in rape counseling? Amer J Psychiat *140:* 3, 1983.

Brownmiller S: *Against Our Will: Men, Women, and Rape*. Simon & Schuster, New York, 1975.

Carmen E H, Rieker P P, Mills T: Victims of violence and psychiatric illness. Amer J Psychiat *141:* 378, 1984.

Criminal Victimization in the United States, 1982. U.S. Department of Justice, Bureau of Justice Statistics, Washington, DC, 1984.

Felman Y M, Nikitas J A: Sexually transmitted diseases and child sexual abuse. NY State J Med *83;* 341, 1983.

Ganzarin R, Buchele B: Acting out during group psychotherapy for Incest. Int J Group Psychother *37:* 2, Apr 1987.

Helton A S, McFarlane J, Anderson E T: Battered and pregnant: A prevalence study. Amer J Publ Health, *77:* 1337, 1987.

Henderson D J: Incest. In *The Sexual Experience,* B J Sadock, H I Kaplan, A M Freedman, editors, p 415. Williams & Wilkins, Baltimore, 1976

Herman J, Hirschman L: Families at risk for father-daughter incest. Amer J Psychiat *138:* 7, 1981.

Herman J, Schaztzan E: Time-limited group therapy for women with a history of incest. Int J Group Psychother *34:* 4, 1984.

Hilberman E: Wife-beater's wife: Reconsidered. Amer J Psychiat *137:* 11, 1980.

Humphrit L, Barclay G, Mahler S N: Perspectives on a case of multiple incestuous relationships. J Amer Med Wom Assoc *41:* 1986.

Maisch H: *Incest.* Stein and Day, New York, 1972.

McGaldrick K E: Sexual abuse of children: A silent shame no more. J Amer Med Wom Assoc *41:* 3, 1986.

Murstein B I: *Love, Sex, and Marriage Throughout the Ages,* Springer-Verlag, New York, 1974.

Nadelson C, Notman M T, Zackson H, Gornick J: A follow-up study of rape victims. Amer J Psychiat *139:* 10, 1982.

Santiago J M, McCall-Perez F, Gorcey M, Biegel A: Long-term psychological effects of rape in 35 rape victims. Amer J Psychiat *142:* 11, 1338, 1985.

Walken E., Katon W, Harrop-Griffiths J, Holm L, Russo J, Hickok, L R: Relationship of chronic pelvic pain to psychiatric diagnoses and childhood sexual abuse. Amer J Psychiat *145:* 75, 1988.

Wells L: Family pathology and father-daughter incest: Restricted psychopathy. J Clin Psychiat *42:* 5, 1981.

INDEX

Page numbers in **boldface** type indicate major discussions; those followed by *t* or *f* indicate tables or figures, respectively.